OTHER PMIC TITLES OF INTEREST

CODING AND REIMBURSEMENT TITLES
Collections Made Easy!
CPT & HCPCS Coding Made Easy!
CPT Coding Guides by Medical Specialty
CPT Plus! Coders Choice®
DRG Plus!
E/M Coding Made Easy!
Getting Paid for What You Do
HCPCS Coders Choice®,
Health Insurance Carrier Directory
HIPAA Compliance Manual
ICD-9-CM, Coders Choice®,
ICD-9-CM Coding for Physicians' Offices
ICD-9-CM Coding Made Easy!
ICD-9-CM, Home Health Edition
Medical Fees in the United States
Medicare Compliance Manual
Medicare Rules & Regulations
Physicians Fee Guide
Reimbursement Manual for the Medical Office

PRACTICE MANAGEMENT TITLES
Accounts Receivable Management for the Medical Practice
Achieving Profitability With a Medical Office System
Encyclopedia of Practice and Financial Management
Managed Care Organizations
Managing Medical Office Personnel
Marketing Strategies for Physicians
Medical Marketing Handbook
Medical Office Policy Manual
Medical Practice Forms
Medical Practice Handbook
Medical Staff Privileges
Negotiating Managed Care Contracts
Patient Satisfaction
Performance Standards for the Laboratory
Professional and Practice Development
Promoting Your Medical Practice
Starting in Medical Practice
Working With Insurance and Managed Care Plans

OTHER PMIC TITLES OF INTEREST

RISK MANAGEMENT TITLES
Malpractice Depositions
Medical Risk Management
Preparing for Your Deposition
Preventing Emergency Malpractice
Testifying in Court

FINANCIAL MANAGEMENT TITLES
A Physician's Guide to Financial Independence
Business Ventures for Physicians
Financial Valuation of Your Practice
Personal Money Management for Physicians
Personal Pension Plan Strategies for Physicians
Securing Your Assets

DICTIONARIES AND OTHER REFERENCE TITLES
Dictionary of Coding & Billing Terminology
Drugs of Abuse
Health and Medicine on the Internet
Medical Acronyms and Abbreviations
Medical Phrase Index
Medical Word Building
Medico Mnemonica
Medico-Legal Glossary
Spanish/English Handbook for Medical Professionals

MEDICAL REFERENCE AND CLINICAL TITLES
Advance Medical Directives
Clinical Research Opportunities
Gastroenterology: Problems in Primary Care
Manual of IV Therapy
Medical Care of the Adolescent Athlete
Medical Procedures for Referral
Neurology: Problems in Primary Care
Orthopaedics: Problems in Primary Care
Patient Care Emergency Handbook
Patient Care Flowchart Manual
Patient Care Procedures for Your Practice
Physician's Office Laboratory
Pulmonary Medicine: Problems in Primary Care
Questions and Answers on AIDS

ICD·9·CM

International Classification of Diseases
9th Revision

Clinical Modification
Sixth Edition

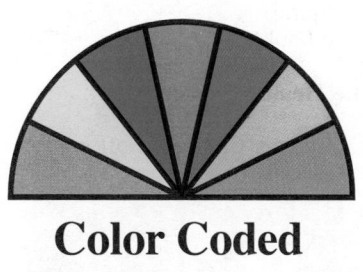

Color Coded
2013

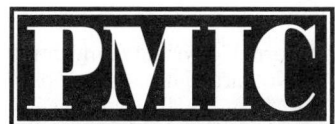

Volumes 1 & 2 : Office Edition

ISBN 978-1-936977-18-5 (Coder's Choice® Soft cover)
ISBN 978-1-936977-19-2 (Spiral)
ISBN 978-1-936977-23-9 (e-book)

Volumes 1, 2, & 3 : Hospital Edition

ISBN 978-1-936977-20-8 (Coder's Choice® Soft cover)
ISBN 978-1-936977-21-5 (Spiral)
ISBN 978-1-936977-24-6 (e-book)

Volumes 1, 2, & 3 : Home Health Edition

ISBN 978-1-936977-22-2 (Coder's Choice® Soft cover)
ISBN 978-1-936977-25-3 (e-book)

Practice Management Information Corporation [PMIC]
4727 Wilshire Boulevard, Suite 300
Los Angeles, California 90010
1-800-MED-SHOP
http://www.pmiconline.com

Printed in China

Preface

Health care professionals have long used coding systems to describe procedures, services, and supplies. However, most described the reason for the procedure, service or supply with a diagnostic statement. Of those health care professionals who do code the diagnosis, either due to a requirement for a computer billing system and/or electronic claims filing, many do not code completely or accurately. With the passage of the Medicare Catastrophic Coverage Act of 1988, diagnostic coding using *ICD-9-CM* became mandatory for Medicare claims. In the area of health care reimbursement rules and regulations, the typical progression is that changes required for Medicare are followed shortly by similar changes for Medicaid and private insurance carriers.

To some professionals, the requirement to use diagnostic coding may have seemed like a burden or simply another excuse for Medicare intermediaries to delay or deny payment. However, it is important to understand that the proper use of coding systems for both procedures and diagnoses gives the professional absolute control over his or her billing and reimbursement. Accurate diagnosis coding is not easy. It requires a good working knowledge of medical terminology and a fundamental understanding of *ICD-9-CM*. In addition, the coder must know the rules and regulations required to comply with Medicare requirements for coding.

This edition of the *International Classification of Diseases, 9th Revision, Clinical Modification (ICD-9-CM)* is published by Practice Management Information Corporation in recognition of its responsibility to promulgate this classification throughout the United States for morbidity coding and billing purposes. *The International Classification of Diseases, 9th Revision*, originally published by the World Health Organization (WHO) is the foundation of the *ICD-9-CM* and continues to be the classification employed in cause-of-death coding in the United States.

The *ICD-9-CM* is recommended for use in all clinical settings, but is required for reporting diagnoses and diseases to all U.S. Public Health Service and Department of Health and Human Services programs, such as Medicare and Medicaid. This version faithfully follows and contains the same information found in the official U.S. government version of the *ICD-9-CM*.

All official authorized addenda effective October 1, 2012, have been included in this edition. A new revision will be available approximately September 15th of each year. Revised editions may be purchased from:

Practice Management Information Corporation
4727 Wilshire Boulevard, Suite 300
Los Angeles, California 90010
1-800-MED-SHOP

Or by contacting our web site at http://www.pmiconline.com.

Disclaimer

This publication includes all official ICD-9-CM codes, descriptions, annotations and guidelines as maintained by the U.S. Department of Health and Human Services with the exception that this publication includes special symbols to indicate additions and revisions from the previous edition and special symbols to facilitate identification of diagnostic codes that require 4th or 5th digit specificity, the use of color coding to alert the user to special coding considerations, and thumb indexing to make locating codes easier. This publication is revised annually so that we may present the most current information possible. Though all of the information is carefully researched and checked for accuracy and completeness, the publisher accepts no responsibility with regard to errors, omissions, misuse or misinterpretation.

Table of Contents

TABLE OF CONTENTS

TABLE OF CONTENTS

[1] These listings appear only in the three volume edition

Introduction to ICD-9-CM

ICD-9-CM is an acronym for *International Classification of Diseases, 9th Revision, Clinical Modification*, published under different names since 1900. *ICD-9-CM* is a statistical classification system that arranges diseases and injuries into groups according to established criteria. Most *ICD-9-CM* codes are numeric and consist of three, four or five numbers and a description. The codes are revised approximately every 10 years by the World Health Organization and annual updates are published by Center for Medicare and Medicaid Services (CMS).

HISTORICAL PERSPECTIVE

The *International Classification of Diseases, 9th Revision, Clinical Modification (ICD-9-CM)* is based on the official version of the *World Health Organization's (WHO) 9th Revision, International Classification of Diseases (ICD-9)*. *ICD-9* is designed for the classification of morbidity and mortality information for statistical purposes, and for the indexing of medical records by disease and operations, and for data storage and retrieval. *ICD-9-CM* replaced the Eighth Revision International Classification of Diseases, Adapted for Use in the United States commonly referred to as *ICDA*.

The concept of extending the International Classification of Diseases for use in hospital indexing was originally developed in response to a need for a more efficient basis for storage and retrieval of diagnostic data. In 1950, the U.S. Public Health Service and the Veterans Administration began independent tests of the International Classification of Diseases for hospital indexing purposes. In the following year, the Columbia Presbyterian Medical Center in New York City adopted the International Classification of Diseases, 6th Revision for use in its medical record department. A few years later, the Commission on Professional and Hospital Activities adopted the International Classification of Diseases for use in hospitals participating in the Professional Activity Study (PAS).

In view of the growing interest in the use of the International Classification of Diseases for hospital indexing, a study was undertaken in 1956 by the American Medical Association and the American Medical Record Association of the relative efficiencies of coding systems for diagnostic indexing. Following this study, the major uses of the International Classification of Diseases for hospital indexing purposes consolidated their experiences and an adaptation was published in December 1959. A revision containing the first "Classification of Operations and Treatments" was published in 1962.

In 1968, following a study by the American Hospital Association, the United States Public Health Service published the Eighth Revision International Classification of Diseases, Adapted for Use in the United States. This publication became commonly known as ICDA, and served as the basis for coding diagnostic data for official morbidity and mortality statistics in the United States.

ICD-9-CM Background

In February 1977, a committee was convened by the National Center for Health Statistics to provide advice and counsel for the development of clinical modification of the ICD-9. The organizations represented on the committee included:

American Association of Health Data Systems
American Hospital Association
American Medical Record Association
Association for Health Records
Commission on Professional and Hospital Activities
Council on Clinical Classifications, sponsored by:

American Academy of Pediatrics
American College of Obstetricians and Gynecologists
American College of Physicians
American College of Surgeons
American Psychiatric Association

Health Care Financing Administration
WHO Center for Classification of Diseases

The resulting *ICD-9-CM* is a clinical modification of the *World Health Organization's International Classification of Diseases, 9th Revision (ICD-9)*. The term "clinical" is used to emphasize the modifications intent; namely, to serve as a useful tool in the area of classification of morbidity data for indexing of medical records, medical care review, ambulatory and other medical care programs, as well as for basic health statistics.

In use since January 1979, *ICD-9-CM* provides a diagnostic coding system that is more precise than those needed only for statistical groupings and trend analysis. Official addenda (updates) to *ICD-9-CM* are issued in October each year by the National Center for Health Statistics (NCHS), part of the Centers for Disease Control (CDC).

Use of ICD-9-CM Codes for Professional Billing

Until passage of the Medicare Catastrophic Coverage Act of 1988, health care professionals were not required to report *ICD-9-CM* codes when billing government or private insurance carriers for reimbursement. The exception to this requirement was for those health care professionals who filed insurance claims electronically and those who used "code driven" computer billing services or computer systems.

Most health care professionals simply included the text or description of the injury, illness, sign or symptom that was the reason for the encounter. Insurance carriers who used *ICD-9-CM* coding had to code the diagnostic statements prior to input into their computer systems for reimbursement processing.

A specific requirement of the Medicare Catastrophic Coverage Act of 1988 required health care professionals to include *ICD-9-CM* codes on their Medicare claim forms effective April 1, 1989. After a two-month grace period, the requirement was officially implemented on June 1, 1989. The Medicare Catastrophic Coverage Act was repealed in November, 1989; however the ICD-9-CM coding requirement was continued.

TERMINOLOGY

There are terms used throughout this publication that are important for a proper understanding of *ICD-9-CM*. The following terms are defined specifically as they are used for *ICD-9-CM* with the knowledge that some terms may have other definitions and meanings.

acute   refers to the condition that is the primary reason for the current encounter.

addenda   official updates to ICD-9-CM published continuously since 1986, that become effective on October 1st of each year.

adverse   any response to a drug that is noxious and unintended and occurs with proper dosage.

aftercare   an encounter for something planned in advance, for example, cast removal.

AHFS   American Hospital Formulary Service.

alphabetic index   the portion of ICD-9-CM that lists definitions and codes in alphabetic order. Also called Volume 2.

category   refers to diagnoses codes listed within a specific three-digit category, for example category 250, Diabetes Mellitus.

cause   that which brings about any condition or produces any effect.

chronic   continuing over a long period of time or recurring frequently.

coding   the process of transferring written or verbal descriptions of diseases, injuries and procedures into numerical designations.

combination   a code that combines a diagnosis with an associated secondary process or complication.

complication   the occurrence of two or more diseases in the same patient at the same time.

concurrent   when a patient is being treated by more than one provider for different care conditions at the same time.

conventions   refers to the use of certain abbreviations, punctuation, symbols, type faces, and other instructions that must be clearly understood in order to use ICD-9-CM.

CPT   Current Procedural Terminology. Listing of codes and descriptions for procedures, services and supplies published by the American Medical Association. Used to bill insurance carriers.

diagnosis   a written description of the reason(s) for the procedure, service, supply or encounter.

down coding   the process where insurance carriers reduce the value of a procedure, and the resulting reimbursement, due to either 1) a mismatch of CPT code and description or 2) ICD-9-CM code does not justify the procedure or level of service.

E codes   specific ICD-9-CM codes used to identify the cause of injury, poisoning and other adverse effects.

eponyms   medical procedures or conditions named after a person or a place.

etiology   the cause(s) or origin of a disease.

HCFA1500	Uniform health insurance claim form used for billing services to Medicare and other insurance carriers.
hierarchy	a system that ranks items one above another.
ICD-9-CM	International Classification of Diseases, 9th Revision, Clinical Modification.
ICD-10	International Classification of Diseases, 10th Revision
late effect	a residual effect (condition produced) after the acute phase of an illness or injury has ended.
main term	refers to listings in the Alphabetic Index appearing **BOLDFACE** type.
manifestation	characteristic signs or symptoms of an illness.
multiple	refers to the need to use more than one ICD-9-CM code to fully identify coding a condition.
primary code	the ICD-9-CM code that defines the main reason for the current encounter.
residual	the long-term condition(s) resulting from a previous acute illness or injury.
rule out	refers to a method used to indicate that a condition is probable, suspected, or questionable but unconfirmed. ICD-9-CM has no provisions for the use of this term.
secondary	code(s) listed after the primary code that further indicate the cause(s) code for the current encounter or define the need for higher levels of care.
sections	refers to portions of the Tabular List that are organized in groups of three-digit code numbers. For example, Malignant Neoplasm of Lip, Oral Cavity and Pharynx (140-149).
sequencing	the process of listing ICD-9-CM codes in the proper order.
specificity	refers to the requirement to code to the highest number of digits possible, 3, 4 or 5, when choosing an ICD-9-CM code.
sub term	refers to listings appearing in the Alphabetic Index under MAIN TERMS and always indented two spaces to the right.
subcategories	refers to groupings of four-digit codes listed under three-digit categories.
Tabular List	the portion of ICD-9-CM that lists codes and definitions in numeric order. Also referred to as Volume 1.
V codes	specific ICD-9-CM codes used to identify encounters for reasons other than illness or injury, for example, immunization.
Volume 1	see TABULAR LIST
Volume 2	see ALPHABETIC INDEX
Volume 3	procedure codes used only for hospital coding. Volume 3 contains both a numeric listing and an alphabetic index.

FORMAT OF ICD-9-CM

The *International Classification of Diseases, 9th Revision, Clinical Modification* was originally published as a three volume set (2nd edition). Newer versions of *ICD-9-CM* are available as two separate books containing Volume 1 and Volume 2 in one book and Volumes 1, 2 and 3 in the other. It is also now available on CD-ROM from the U.S. Government.

This edition of *ICD-9-CM* includes all official addenda from October 1986 through October 2012.

The Tabular List (Volume 1)

The Tabular List (Volume 1) is a *numeric* listing of diagnosis codes and descriptions consisting of 17 chapters that classify diseases and injuries, two sections containing supplementary codes (V codes and E codes) and four appendices.

Classification of Diseases and Injuries

The Classification of Diseases and Injuries includes the following 17 chapters:

Chapter 1   Infectious and Parasitic Diseases (001-139)

Chapter 2   Neoplasms (140-239)

Chapter 3   Endocrine, Nutritional and Metabolic Diseases, and Immunity Disorders (240-279)

Chapter 4   Diseases of the Blood and Blood-Forming Organs (280-289)

Chapter 5   Mental, Behavioral and Neurodevelopmental Disorders (290-319)

Chapter 6   Diseases of the Nervous System and Sense Organs (320-389)

Chapter 7   Diseases of the Circulatory System (390-459)

Chapter 8   Diseases of the Respiratory System (460-519)

Chapter 9   Diseases of the Digestive System (520-579)

Chapter 10   Diseases of the Genitourinary System (580-629)

Chapter 11   Complications of Pregnancy, Childbirth, and the Puerperium (630-677)

Chapter 12   Diseases of the Skin and Subcutaneous Tissue (680-709)

Chapter 13   Diseases of the Musculoskeletal System and Connective Tissue (710-739)

Chapter 14   Congenital Anomalies (740-759)

Chapter 15   Certain Conditions Originating in the Perinatal Period (760-779)

Chapter 16   Symptoms, Signs and Ill-defined Conditions (780-799)

Chapter 17   Injury and Poisoning (800-999)

Each chapter of the Tabular List (Volume 1) is structured into four components, namely:

Sections: groups of three-digit code numbers

Categories: three-digit code numbers

Subcategories: four-digit code numbers

Fifth-Digit Subclassifications: five-digit code numbers

Supplementary Classifications

There are two supplementary classifications included in the Tabular List (Volume 1). These are:

V Codes   Supplementary Classification of Factors Influencing Health Status and Contact with Health Services (V01-V91)

E Codes   Supplementary Classification of External Causes of Injury and Poisoning (E000-E999)

Appendices

The Tabular List (Volume 1) includes four appendices. These are:

Appendix A Morphology of Neoplasms

Appendix C Classification of Drugs by American Hospital Formulary Service List Number and Their ICD-9-CM Equivalents

Appendix D Classification of Industrial Accidents According to Agency

Appendix E List of Three-Digit Categories

Appendix F List of Three-Digit Categories Mapped to ICD-10

Specifications for the Tabular List

1.   Three-digit rubrics and their contents are unchanged from *ICD-9*.

2.   The sequence of three-digit rubrics is unchanged from *ICD-9*.

3.   Three-digit rubrics are not added to the main body of the classification.

4.   Unsubdivided three-digit rubrics are subdivided where necessary to:

   a) Add clinical detail

   b) Isolate terms for clinical accuracy

5.   The modification in *ICD-9-CM* is accomplished by the addition of a fifth digit to existing *ICD-9* rubrics, except as noted under number 7 below.

6.   Four-digit rubrics are added to subdivided three-digit codes only when there is no other means of achieving desired detail. These codes, unique to *ICD-9-CM* (28 three-digit categories) are marked with the symbol in the Tabular List.

7.   The optional dual classification in *ICD-9* is modified.

   a) Duplicate rubrics are deleted:

      1) Four-digit manifestation categories duplicating etiology entries.

      2) Manifestation inclusion terms duplicating etiology entries.

   b) Manifestations of diseases are identified, to the extent possible, by creating five digit codes in the etiology rubrics.

   c) When the manifestation of a disease cannot be included in the etiology rubrics, provision for its identification is made by retaining the *ICD-9* rubrics used for classifying manifestations of disease.

8.   The format of *ICD-9-CM* is revised from that used in *ICD-9*.

   a) American spelling of medical terms is used.

   b) Inclusion terms are indented beneath the titles of codes.

   c) Codes not to be used for primary tabulation of disease are printed in italics with the notation, "code also underlying disease."

The Alphabetic Index (Volume 2)

The Alphabetic Index (Volume 2) of *ICD-9-CM* consists of an alphabetic list of terms and codes, two supplementary Sections following the alphabetic listing, plus two special tables found within the alphabetic listing. The Alphabetic Index (Volume 2) is structured as follows:

MAIN TERMS: appear in **BOLDFACE** type

SUBTERMS: are always indented two spaces to the right under main terms

CARRY-OVER
LINES: are always indented more than two spaces from the level of the preceding line

Supplementary Sections

The supplementary sections following the Alphabetic Index are:

TABLE OF DRUGS AND CHEMICALS

This table contains a classification of drugs and other chemical substances to identify poisoning states and external causes of adverse effects.

INDEX TO EXTERNAL CAUSES OF INJURIES & POISONINGS (E-CODES)

This section contains the index to the codes that classify environmental events, circumstances, and other conditions as the cause of injury and other adverse effects.

Special Tables

The two special tables, located within the Alphabetic Index, and found under the main terms as underlined below, are:

HYPERTENSION TABLE

NEOPLASM TABLE

Specifications for the Alphabetic Index

1. Format of the Alphabetic Index follows the format of the ICD-9.

2. Main terms in the Alphabetic Index are printed in bold face type.

3. When two codes are required to indicate etiology and manifestation, the manifestation code appears in brackets, e.g., diabetic cataract 250.5 *[366.41]*.

Procedures: Tabular List and Alphabetic Index (Volume 3)

Volume 3 consists of two sections, a Tabular List of codes and an alphabetic index. These codes define procedures instead of diagnoses. Frequently used incorrectly by health care professionals, codes from Volume 3 are intended only for use by hospitals.

The ICD-9-CM Procedure Classification is a modification of WHO's *Fascicle V, Surgical Procedures*, and is published as Volume 3 of ICD-9-CM. It contains both a Tabular List and an Alphabetic Index. Greater detail has been added to the ICD-9-CM Procedure Classification necessitating expansion of the codes from three to four digits. Approximately 90% of the rubrics refer to surgical procedures with the remaining 10% accounting for other investigative and therapeutic procedures.

Tabular List of Procedures

The Tabular List includes 16 chapters containing codes and descriptions for surgical procedures and miscellaneous diagnostic and therapeutic procedures.

Alphabetic Index to Procedures

The Alphabetic Index provides an alphabetic index to the Tabular List of Volume 3

Specifications for the Procedure Classification

1.   The ICD-9-CM Procedure Classification is published in its own volume containing both a Tabular List and an Alphabetic Index.

2.   The classification is a modification of *Fascicle V Surgical Procedures* of the ICD-9 Classification of Procedures in Medicine, working from the draft dated Geneva, 30 September-6 October 1975, and labeled WHO/ICD-9/Rev. Conf. 75.4.

3.   All three-digit rubrics in the range 01-86 are maintained as they appear in *Fascicle V,* whenever feasible.

4.   Nonsurgical procedures are segregated from the surgical procedures and confined to the rubrics 87-99, whenever feasible.

5.   Selected detail contained in the remaining fascicles of the *ICD-9 Classification of Procedures in Medicine* is accommodated where possible.

6.   The structure of the classification is based on anatomy rather than surgical specialty.

7.   The *ICD-9-CM* Procedure Classification is numeric only, i.e., no alphabetic characters are used.

8.   The classification is based on a two-digit structure with two decimal digits where necessary.

9.   Compatibility with the *ICD-9 Classification of Procedures in Medicine* was not maintained when a different axis was deemed more clinically appropriate.

CONVENTIONS USED IN THE TABULAR LIST

The *ICD-9-CM* Tabular List (Volume 1) makes use of certain abbreviations, punctuation, symbols, and other conventions that must be clearly understood. The purpose of these conventions is to first, provide special coding instructions, and second, to conserve space.

Abbreviations

NOS   Not Otherwise Specified. Equivalent to Unspecified. This abbreviation refers to a lack of sufficient detail in the statement of diagnosis to be able to assign it to a more specific sub division within the classification.

NEC   Not Elsewhere Classified. Used with ill-defined terms to alert the coder that a specified form of the condition is classified differently. The category number for the term including NEC is to be used only when the coder lacks the information necessary to code the term to a more specific category.

Punctuation

( )   PARENTHESES are used to enclose supplementary words that may be present or absent in a statement of disease without affecting the code assignment.

[ ]   SQUARE BRACKETS are used to enclose synonyms, alternate wordings or explanatory phrases.

:   COLONS are used after an incomplete phrase or term that requires one or more of the modifiers indented under it to make it assignable to a given category. EXCEPTION to this rule pertains to the abbreviation NOS.

Symbols

●   A filled BLACK CIRCLE preceding a code indicates that the code is new to this revision of ICD-9-CM. A symbol key appears on all left-hand pages of the Tabular List, Volume 1 and Volume 3.

▲   A filled BLACK TRIANGLE preceding a code indicates that there is a revision to the text of an existing code. A symbol key appears on all left-hand pages of the Tabular List, Volume 1 and Volume 3.

④ ⑤   A circle containing the number 4 or the number 5 preceding a code indicates that a fourth or fifth digit is required for coding to the highest level of specificity. Valid digits are in [brackets] under each code if the fourth- and fifth-digit codes themselves are not listed. Definitions of valid fifth digits are found under the major category.

Other conventions

Type Face:

    BOLD: Bold type face is used for all codes and titles in the Tabular List.

    Italics: Italicized type face is used for all exclusion notes and to identify those rubrics that are not to be used for primary tabulations of disease.

Format: ICD-9-CM uses an indented format for ease in reference.

ALERT!   References alternate codes for personal history/late effects or other coding alerts.

DEFINITION   Definition of a common word or phrase.

Instructional Notations

Instructional terms define what is, or what is not, included in a given subdivision. This is accomplished by using both inclusion and exclusion terms.

INCLUDES: Indicates separate terms, such as, modifying adjectives, sites and conditions, entered under a subdivision, such as a category, to further define or give examples of, the content of the category.

Excludes: Exclusion terms are enclosed in a box and are printed in italics to draw attention to their presence. The importance of this instructional term is its use as a guideline to direct the coder to the proper code assignment. In other words, all terms following the word EXCLUDES: are to be coded elsewhere as indicated in each instance.

NOTES   These are used to define terms and give coding instructions. Often used to list the fifth-digit subclassifications for certain categories.

SEE   The "see" instruction following a main term in the index indicates that another term should be referenced. It is necessary to go to the main term referenced with the "see" note to locate the correct code.

SEE CATEGORY   A variation of the instructional term SEE. This refers the coder to a specific category. You must *always* follow this instructional term.

SEE ALSO   A "see also" instruction following a main term in the index instructs that there is another main term that may also be referenced that may provide additional index entries that may be useful. It is not necessary to follow the "see also" note when the original main term provides the necessary code.

CODE FIRST   This instructional note is used for those codes not intended to be used as a principal diagnosis, or not to be sequenced before the underlying disease. The note requires that the underlying disease (etiology) be coded first with the code the note is applied to being coded second. This note appears only in the Tabular List (Vol. 1).

USE ADDITIONAL CODE   This instruction is placed in the Tabular List in those categories where the coder may wish to add further information, by using an additional code, to give a more complete picture of the diagnosis or procedure.

Related terms

AND   The word "and" should be interpreted to mean either "and" or "or" when it appears in a title.

WITH   The word "with" in the alphabetic index is sequenced immediately following the main term, not in alphabetical order.

COLOR CODING

A PMIC versions of ICD-9-CM include color-coding to alert the user to special coding situations or conditions that require additional attention. The use of color-coding is found in the Tabular List of Volume 1 and the Tabular List of Volume 3. The color is applied as solid rectangular bars over the codes only so that the descriptions remain clear and legible. The color codes and definitions are printed at the bottom of all right-sided pages of Volume 1 and Volume 3.

Volume 1

Three digit codes. Coding to fourth or fifth digit specificity is required.

Unspecified code. Descriptions include the term "unspecified." Use only if a more specific diagnosis is not known or available.

Nonspecific code. Descriptions include the term "nonspecific, unspecified, other specified or other." A report *may* be required by insurance carriers.

Manifestation codes. Used only to code the manifestation of an underlying disease. Code the underlying disease first.

Medicare secondary payer (MSP) alert. Diagnoses that may trigger a post-payment review by Medicare. Medicare is usually the secondary payer for these diagnoses.

Secondary diagnosis only. V codes that may only be used as additional codes, not as first-listed codes.

Primary diagnosis only. V codes which are only acceptable as first listed codes.

Volume 3*

Noncovered operating room procedure. An operating room procedure that is not covered by Medicare.

Non-operating room procedure. A procedure that is not performed in the operating room that affects DRG assignment.

Bilateral procedure.

Valid operating room procedure. Prompts a change in DRG assignment.

Nonspecific operating room procedure. Choose a more precise code if possible.

---

*These colors appear only in the three-volume edition

ICD-9-CM OFFICIAL GUIDELINES FOR CODING AND REPORTING

Guidelines effective as of publication date. For updates, visit http://pmiconline.com
The guidelines include the updated V Code Table

The Centers for Medicare and Medicaid Services (CMS) and the National Center for Health Statistics (NCHS), two departments within the U.S. Federal Government's Department of Health and Human Services (DHHS) provide the following guidelines for coding and reporting using the International Classification of Diseases, 9th Revision, Clinical Modification (ICD-9-CM). These guidelines should be used as a companion document to the official version of the ICD-9-CM as published on CD-ROM by the U.S. Government Printing Office (GPO).

These guidelines have been approved by the four organizations that make up the Cooperating Parties for the ICD-9-CM: the American Hospital Association (AHA), the American Health Information Management Association (AHIMA), CMS, and NCHS. These guidelines are included on the official government version of the ICD-9-CM, and also appear in "Coding Clinic for ICD-9-CM" published by the AHA.

These guidelines are a set of rules that have been developed to accompany and complement the official conventions and instructions provided within the ICD-9-CM itself. The instructions and conventions of the classification take precedence over guidelines. These guidelines are based on the coding and sequencing instructions in Volumes I, II and III of ICD-9-CM, but provide additional instruction. Adherence to these guidelines when assigning ICD-9-CM diagnosis and procedure codes is required under the Health Insurance Portability and Accountability Act (HIPAA). The diagnosis codes (Volumes 1-2) have been adopted under HIPAA for all healthcare settings. Volume 3 procedure codes have been adopted for inpatient procedures reported by hospitals. A joint effort between the healthcare provider and the coder is essential to achieve complete and accurate documentation, code assignment, and reporting of diagnoses and procedures. These guidelines have been developed to assist both the healthcare provider and the coder in identifying those diagnoses and procedures that are to be reported. The importance of consistent, complete documentation in the medical record cannot be overemphasized. Without such documentation accurate coding cannot be achieved. The entire record should be reviewed to determine the specific reason for the encounter and the conditions treated.

The term encounter is used for all settings, including hospital admissions. In the context of these guidelines, the term provider is used throughout the guidelines to mean physician or any qualified health care practitioner who is legally accountable for establishing the patient's diagnosis. Only this set of guidelines, approved by the Cooperating Parties, is official.

The guidelines are organized into sections. Section I includes the structure and conventions of the classification and general guidelines that apply to the entire classification, and chapter-specific guidelines that correspond to the chapters as they are arranged in the classification. Section II includes guidelines for selection of principal diagnosis for non-outpatient settings. Section III includes guidelines for reporting additional diagnoses in non-outpatient settings. Section IV is for outpatient coding and reporting.

SECTION I. CONVENTIONS, GENERAL CODING GUIDELINES AND CHAPTER SPECIFIC GUIDELINES

The conventions, general guidelines and chapter-specific guidelines are applicable to all health care settings unless otherwise indicated. The conventions and instructions of the classification take precedence over guidelines.

A. Conventions for the ICD-9-CM

The conventions for the ICD-9-CM are the general rules for use of the classification independent of the guidelines. These conventions are incorporated within the index and tabular of the ICD-9-CM as instructional notes. The conventions are as follows:

1. Format:

The ICD-9-CM uses an indented format for ease in reference

2. Abbreviations

a. Index abbreviations
NEC   "Not elsewhere classifiable"
This abbreviation in the index represents "other specified." When a specific code is not available for a condition the index directs the coder to the "other specified" code in the tabular.

b. Tabular abbreviations
NEC   "Not elsewhere classifiable"
This abbreviation in the tabular represents "other specified". When a specific code is not available for a condition the tabular includes an NEC entry under a code to identify the code as the "other specified" code.
(See Section I.A.5.a. "Other" codes").

NOS   "Not otherwise specified"
This abbreviation is the equivalent of unspecified.
(See Section I.A.5.b., "Unspecified" codes)

3. Punctuation

[ ]   Brackets are used in the tabular list to enclose synonyms, alternative wording or explanatory phrases. Brackets are used in the index to identify manifestation codes.
(See Section I.A.6. "Etiology/manifestations")

( )   Parentheses are used in both the index and tabular to enclose supplementary words that may be present or absent in the statement of a disease or procedure without affecting the code number to which it is assigned. The terms within the parentheses are referred to as nonessential modifiers.

:   Colons are used in the Tabular list after an incomplete term which needs one or more of the modifiers following the colon to make it assignable to a given category.

4. Includes and Excludes Notes and Inclusion terms

Includes: This note appears immediately under a three-digit code title to further define, or give examples of, the content of the category.

Excludes: An excludes note under a code indicates that the terms excluded from the code are to be coded elsewhere. In some cases the codes for the excluded terms should not be used in conjunction with the code from which it is excluded. An example of this is a congenital condition excluded from an acquired form of the same condition. The congenital and acquired codes should not be used together. In other cases, the excluded terms may be used together with an excluded code. An example of this is when fractures of different bones are coded to different codes. Both codes may be used together if both types of fractures are present.

Inclusion terms: List of terms is included under certain four and five digit codes. These terms are the conditions for which that code number is to be used. The terms may be synonyms of the code title, or, in the case of "other specified" codes, the terms are a list of the various conditions assigned to that code. The inclusion terms are not necessarily exhaustive. Additional terms found only in the index may also be assigned to a code.

5. Other and Unspecified codes

a. "Other" codes

Codes titled "other" or "other specified" (usually a code with a 4th digit 8 or fifth-digit 9 for diagnosis codes) are for use when the information in the medical record provides detail for which a specific code does not exist. Index entries with NEC in the line designate "other" codes in the tabular. These index entries represent specific disease entities for which no specific code exists so the term is included within an "other" code.

b. "Unspecified" codes

Codes (usually a code with a 4th digit 9 or 5th digit 0 for diagnosis codes) titled "unspecified" are for use when the information in the medical record is insufficient to assign a more specific code.

6. Etiology/manifestation convention ("code first", "use additional code" and "in diseases classified elsewhere" notes)

Certain conditions have both an underlying etiology and multiple body system manifestations due to the underlying etiology. For such conditions, the ICD-9-CM has a coding convention that requires the underlying condition be sequenced first followed by the manifestation. Wherever such a combination exists, there is a "use additional code" note at the etiology code, and a "code first" note at the manifestation code. These instructional notes indicate the proper sequencing order of the codes, etiology followed by manifestation. In most cases the manifestation codes will have in the code title, "in diseases classified elsewhere." Codes with this title are a component of the etiology/manifestation convention. The code title indicates that it is a manifestation code. "In diseases classified elsewhere" codes are never permitted to be used as first listed or principal diagnosis codes. They must be used in conjunction with an underlying condition code and they must be listed following the underlying condition.

There are manifestation codes that do not have "in diseases classified elsewhere" in the title. For such codes a "use additional code" note will still be present and the rules for sequencing apply.

In addition to the notes in the tabular, these conditions also have a specific index entry structure. In the index both conditions are listed together with the etiology code first followed by the manifestation codes in brackets. The code in brackets is always to be sequenced second.

The most commonly used etiology/manifestation combinations are the codes for Diabetes mellitus, category 250. For each code under category 250 there is a use additional code note for the manifestation that is specific for that particular diabetic manifestation. Should a patient have more than one manifestation of diabetes, more than one code from category 250 may be used with as many manifestation codes as are needed to fully describe the patient's complete diabetic condition. The category 250 diabetes codes should be sequenced first, followed by the manifestation codes.

"Code first" and "Use additional code" notes are also used as sequencing rules in the classification for certain codes that are not part of an etiology/manifestation combination.

See - Section I.B.9. "Multiple coding for a single condition".

7. "And"

The word "and" should be interpreted to mean either "and" or "or" when it appears in a title.

8. "With"

The word "with" should be interpreted to mean "associated with" or "due to" when it appears in a code title, the Alphabetic Index, or an instructional note in the Tabular List. The word "with" in the alphabetic index is sequenced immediately following the main term, not in alphabetical order.

9. "See" and "See Also"

The "see" instruction following a main term in the index indicates that another term should be referenced. It is necessary to go to the main term referenced with the "see" note to locate the correct code.

A "see also" instruction following a main term in the index instructs that there is another main term that may also be referenced that may provide additional index entries that may be useful. It is not necessary to follow the "see also" note when the original main term provides the necessary code.

B. General Coding Guidelines

1. Use of Both Alphabetic Index and Tabular List

Use both the Alphabetic Index and the Tabular List when locating and assigning a code. Reliance on only the Alphabetic Index or the Tabular List leads to errors in code assignments and less specificity in code selection.

2. Locate each term in the Alphabetic Index

Locate each term in the Alphabetic Index and verify the code selected in the Tabular List. Read and be guided by instructional notations that appear in both the Alphabetic Index and the Tabular List.

3. Level of Detail in Coding

Diagnosis and procedure codes are to be used at their highest number of digits available. ICD-9-CM diagnosis codes are composed of codes with 3, 4, or 5 digits. Codes with three digits are included in ICD-9-CM as the heading of a category of codes that may be further subdivided by the use of fourth and/or fifth digits, which provide greater detail.

A three-digit code is to be used only if it is not further subdivided. Where fourth-digit subcategories and/or fifth-digit subclassifications are provided, they must be assigned. A code is invalid if it has not been coded to the full number of digits required for that code. For example, Acute myocardial infarction, code 410, has fourth digits that describe the location of the infarction (e.g., 410.2, Of inferolateral wall), and fifth digits that identify the episode of care. It would be incorrect to report a code in category 410 without a fourth and fifth digit.

ICD-9-CM Volume 3 procedure codes are composed of codes with either 3 or 4 digits. Codes with two digits are included in ICD-9-CM as the heading of a category of codes that may be further subdivided by the use of third and/or fourth digits, which provide greater detail.

4. Code or codes from 001.0 through V91.99

The appropriate code or codes from 001.0 through V91.99 must be used to identify diagnoses, symptoms, conditions, problems, complaints or other reason(s) for the encounter/visit.

5. Selection of codes 001.0 through 999.9

The selection of codes 001.0 through 999.9 will frequently be used to describe the reason for the admission/encounter. These codes are from the section of ICD-9-CM for the classification of diseases and injuries (e.g., infectious and parasitic diseases; neoplasms; symptoms, signs, and ill-defined conditions, etc.).

6. Signs and symptoms

Codes that describe symptoms and signs, as opposed to diagnoses, are acceptable for reporting purposes when a related definitive diagnosis has not been established (confirmed) by the provider. Chapter 16 of ICD-9-CM, Symptoms, Signs, and Ill-defined conditions (codes 780.0 - 799.9) contain many, but not all codes for symptoms.

7. Conditions that are an integral part of a disease process

Signs and symptoms that are associated routinely with a disease process should not be assigned as additional codes, unless otherwise instructed by the classification.

8. **Conditions that are not an integral part of a disease process**

Additional signs and symptoms that may not be associated routinely with a disease process should be coded when present.

9. **Multiple coding for a single condition**

In addition to the etiology/manifestation convention that requires two codes to fully describe a single condition that affects multiple body systems, there are other single conditions that also require more than one code. "Use additional code" notes are found in the tabular at codes that are not part of an etiology/manifestation pair where a secondary code is useful to fully describe a condition. The sequencing rule is the same as the etiology/manifestation pair - , "use additional code" indicates that a secondary code should be added.

For example, for infections that are not included in chapter 1, a secondary code from category 041, Bacterial infection in conditions classified elsewhere and of unspecified site, may be required to identify the bacterial organism causing the infection. A "use additional code" note will normally be found at the infectious disease code, indicating a need for the organism code to be added as a secondary code.

"Code first" notes are also under certain codes that are not specifically manifestation codes but may be due to an underlying cause. When a "code first" note is present and an underlying condition is present the underlying condition should be sequenced first.

"Code, if applicable, any causal condition first", notes indicate that this code may be assigned as a principal diagnosis when the causal condition is unknown or not applicable. If a causal condition is known, then the code for that condition should be sequenced as the principal or first-listed diagnosis.

Multiple codes may be needed for late effects, complication codes and obstetric codes to more fully describe a condition. See the specific guidelines for these conditions for further instruction.

10. **Acute and Chronic Conditions**

If the same condition is described as both acute (subacute) and chronic, and separate subentries exist in the Alphabetic Index at the same indentation level, code both and sequence the acute (subacute) code first.

11. **Combination Code**

A combination code is a single code used to classify:

— Two diagnoses, or
— A diagnosis with an associated secondary process (manifestation), or
— A diagnosis with an associated complication

Combination codes are identified by referring to subterm entries in the Alphabetic Index and by reading the inclusion and exclusion notes in the Tabular List.

Assign only the combination code when that code fully identifies the diagnostic conditions involved or when the Alphabetic Index so directs. Multiple coding should not be used when the classification provides a combination code that clearly identifies all of the elements documented in the diagnosis. When the combination code lacks necessary specificity in describing the manifestation or complication, an additional code should be used as a secondary code.

12. Late Effects

A late effect is the residual effect (condition produced) after the acute phase of an illness or injury has terminated. There is no time limit on when a late effect code can be used. The residual may be apparent early, such as in cerebrovascular accident cases, or it may occur months or years later, such as that due to a previous injury. Coding of late effects generally requires two codes sequenced in the following order: The condition or nature of the late effect is sequenced first. The late effect code is sequenced second.

Exceptions to the above guidelines are those instances where the late effect code has been expanded (at the fourth and fifth-digit levels) to include the manifestation(s), or the classification instructs otherwise. The code for the acute phase of an illness or injury that led to the late effect is never used with a code for the late effect.

13. Impending or Threatened Condition

Code any condition described at the time of discharge as "impending" or "threatened" as follows:

If it did occur, code as confirmed diagnosis.

If it did not occur, reference the Alphabetic Index to determine if the condition has a subentry term for "impending" or "threatened" and also reference main term entries for "Impending" and for "Threatened."

If the subterms are listed, assign the given code.

If the subterms are not listed, code the existing underlying condition(s) and not the condition described as impending or threatened.

14. Reporting Same Diagnosis Code More Than Once

Each unique ICD-9-CM diagnosis code may be reported only once for an encounter. This applies to bilateral conditions or two different conditions classified to the same ICD-9-CM diagnosis code.

15. Admissions/Encounters for Rehabilitation

When the purpose for the admission/encounter is rehabilitation, sequence the appropriate V code from category V57, Care involving use of rehabilitation procedures, as the principal/first-listed diagnosis. The code for the condition for which the service is being performed should be reported as an additional diagnosis.

Only one code from category V57 is required. Code V57.89, Other specified rehabilitation procedures, should be assigned if more than one type of rehabilitation is performed during a single encounter. A procedure code should be reported to identify each type of rehabilitation therapy actually performed.

16. Documentation of BMI and Pressure Ulcer Stages

For the Body Mass Index (BMI) and pressure ulcer stage codes, code assignment may be based on medical record documentation from clinicians who are not the patient's provider (i.e., physician or other qualified healthcare practitioner legally accountable for establishing the patient's diagnosis), since this information is typically documented by other clinicians involved in the care of the patient (e.g., a dietitian often documents the BMI and nurses often document the pressure ulcer stages). However, the associated diagnosis (such as overweight, obesity, or pressure ulcer) must be documented by the patient's provider. If there is conflicting medical record documentation, either from the same clinician or different clinicians, the patient's attending provider should be queried for clarification.

The BMI and pressure ulcer stage codes should only be reported as secondary diagnoses. As with all other secondary diagnosis codes, the BMI and pressure ulcer stage codes should only be assigned when they meet the definition of a reportable additional diagnosis (see Section III, Reporting Additional Diagnoses).

17. Syndromes

Follow the Alphabetic Index guidance when coding syndromes. In the absence of index guidance, assign codes for the documented manifestations of the syndrome.

18. Documentation of Complications of care

Code assignment is based on the provider's documentation of the relationship between the condition and the care or procedure. The guideline extends to any complications of care, regardless of the chapter the code is located in. It is important to note that not all conditions that occur during or following medical care or surgery are classified as complications. There must be a cause-and-effect relationship between the care provided and the condition, and an indication in the documentation that it is a complication. Query the provider for clarification, if the complication is not clearly documented.

C. Chapter-Specific Coding Guidelines

In addition to general coding guidelines, there are guidelines for specific diagnoses and/or conditions in the classification. Unless otherwise indicated, these guidelines apply to all health care settings. Please refer to Section II for guidelines on the selection of principal diagnosis.

1. Chapter 1: Infectious and Parasitic Diseases (001-139)

a. Human Immunodeficiency Virus (HIV) Infections

1) Code only confirmed cases

Code only confirmed cases of HIV infection/illness. This is an exception to the hospital inpatient guideline Section II, H. In this context, "confirmation" does not require documentation of positive serology or culture for HIV; the provider's diagnostic statement that the patient is HIV positive, or has an HIV-related illness is sufficient.

2) Selection and sequencing of HIV codes

(a) Patient admitted for HIV-related condition

If a patient is admitted for an HIV-related condition, the principal diagnosis should be 042, followed by additional diagnosis codes for all reported HIV-related conditions.

(b) Patient with HIV disease admitted for unrelated condition

If a patient with HIV disease is admitted for an unrelated condition (such as a traumatic injury), the code for the unrelated condition (e.g., the nature of injury code) should be the principal diagnosis. Other diagnoses would be 042 followed by additional diagnosis codes for all reported HIV-related conditions.

(c) Whether the patient is newly diagnosed

Whether the patient is newly diagnosed or has had previous admissions/encounters for HIV conditions is irrelevant to the sequencing decision.

(d) Asymptomatic human immunodeficiency virus V08

V08 Asymptomatic human immunodeficiency virus [HIV] infection, is to be applied when the patient without any documentation of symptoms is listed as being "HIV positive," "known HIV," "HIV test positive," or similar terminology. Do not use this code if the term "AIDS" is used or if the patient is treated for any HIV-related illness or is described as having any condition(s) resulting from his/her HIV positive status; use 042 in these cases.

(e) Patients with inconclusive HIV serology

Patients with inconclusive HIV serology, but no definitive diagnosis or manifestations of the illness, may be assigned code 795.71, Inconclusive serologic test for Human Immuno deficiency Virus [HIV].

(f) Previously diagnosed HIV-related illness

Patients with any known prior diagnosis of an HIV-related illness should be coded to 042. Once a patient has developed an HIV-related illness, the patient should always be assigned code 042 on every subsequent admission/encounter. Patients previously diagnosed with any HIV illness (042) should never be assigned to 795.71 or V08.

(g) HIV Infection in Pregnancy, Childbirth and the Puerperium

During pregnancy, childbirth or the puerperium, a patient admitted (or presenting for a health care encounter) because of an HIV-related illness should receive a principal diagnosis code of 647.6X, Other specified infectious and parasitic diseases in the mother classifiable elsewhere, but complicating the pregnancy, childbirth or the puerperium, followed by 042 and the code(s) for the HIV-related illness(es). Codes from Chapter 15 always take sequencing priority.

Patients with asymptomatic HIV infection status admitted (or presenting for a health care encounter) during pregnancy, childbirth, or the puerperium should receive codes of 647.6X and V08.

(h) **Encounters for testing for HIV**

If a patient is being seen to determine his/her HIV status, use code V73.89, Screening for other specified viral disease. Use code V69.8, Other problems related to lifestyle, as a secondary code if an asymptomatic patient is in a known high risk group for HIV. Should a patient with signs or symptoms or illness, or a confirmed HIV related diagnosis be tested for HIV, code the signs and symptoms or the diagnosis. An additional counseling code V65.44 may be used if counseling is provided during the encounter for the test.

When a patient returns to be informed of his/her HIV test results use code V65.44, HIV counseling, if the results of the test are negative.

If the results are positive but the patient is asymptomatic use code V08, Asymptomatic HIV infection. If the results are positive and the patient is symptomatic use code 042, HIV infection, with codes for the HIV related symptoms or diagnosis. The HIV counseling code may also be used if counseling is provided for patients with positive test results.

b. **Septicemia, Systemic Inflammatory Response Syndrome (SIRS), Sepsis, Severe Sepsis, and Septic Shock**

1) **SIRS, Septicemia, and Sepsis**

(a) The terms septicemia and sepsis are often used interchangeably by providers, however they are not considered synonymous terms. The following descriptions are provided for reference but do not preclude querying the provider for clarification about terms used in the documentation:

(i) Septicemia generally refers to a systemic disease associated with the presence of pathological microorganisms or toxins in the blood, which can include bacteria, viruses, fungi or other organisms.

(ii) Systemic inflammatory response syndrome (SIRS) generally refers to the systemic response to infection, trauma/burns, or other insult (such as cancer) with symptoms including fever, tachycardia, tachypnea, and leukocytosis.

(iii) Sepsis generally refers to SIRS due to infection.

(iv) Severe sepsis generally refers to sepsis with associated acute organ dysfunction.

(b) The coding of SIRS, sepsis and severe sepsis requires a minimum of 2 codes: a code for the underlying cause (such as infection or trauma) and a code from subcategory 995.9 Systemic inflammatory response syndrome (SIRS)..

(i) The code for the underlying cause (such as infection or trauma) must be sequenced before the code from subcategory 995.9 Systemic inflammatory response syndrome (SIRS).

(ii) Sepsis and severe sepsis require a code for the systemic infection (038.xx, 112.5, etc.) and either code 995.91, Sepsis, or 995.92, Severe sepsis. If the causal organism is not documented, assign code 038.9, Unspecified septicemia.

(iii) Severe sepsis requires additional code(s) for the associated acute organ dysfunction(s).

(iv) If a patient has sepsis with multiple organ dysfunctions, follow the instructions for coding severe sepsis.

(v) Either the term sepsis or SIRS must be documented to assign a code from subcategory 995.9.

(vi) See Section I.C.17.g), Injury and poisoning, for information regarding systemic inflammatory response syndrome (SIRS) due to trauma/burns and other non-infectious processes.

(c) Due to the complex nature of sepsis and severe sepsis, some cases may require querying the provider prior to assignment of the codes.

2) Sequencing sepsis and severe sepsis

(a) Sepsis and severe sepsis as principal diagnosis

If sepsis or severe sepsis is present on admission, and meets the definition of principal diagnosis, the systemic infection code (e.g., 038.xx, 112.5, etc) should be assigned as the principal diagnosis, followed by code 995.91, Sepsis, or 995.92, Severe sepsis, as required by the sequencing rules in the Tabular List. Codes from subcategory 995.9 can never be assigned as a principal diagnosis. A code should also be assigned for any localized infection, if present.

If the sepsis or severe sepsis is due to a postprocedural infection, see Section I.C.1.b.10 for guidelines related to sepsis due to postprocedural infection.

(b) Sepsis and severe sepsis as secondary diagnoses

When sepsis or severe sepsis develops during the encounter (it was not present on admission), the systemic infection code and code 995.91 or 995.92 should be assigned as secondary diagnoses.

(c) Documentation unclear as to whether sepsis or severe sepsis is present on admission

Sepsis or severe sepsis may be present on admission but the diagnosis may not be confirmed until sometime after admission. If the documentation is not clear whether the sepsis or severe sepsis was present on admission, the provider should be queried.

3) Sepsis/SIRS with Localized Infection

If the reason for admission is both sepsis, severe sepsis, or SIRS and a localized infection, such as pneumonia or cellulitis, a code for the systemic infection (038.xx, 112.5, etc) should be assigned first, then code 995.91 or 995.92, followed by the code for the localized infection. If the patient is admitted with a localized infection, such as pneumonia, and sepsis/SIRS doesn't develop until after admission, see guideline I.C.1.b.2.b).

If the localized infection is postprocedural, see Section *I.C.1.b.10* for guidelines related to sepsis due to postprocedural infection.

Note: The term urosepsis is a nonspecific term. If that is the only term documented then only code 599.0 should be assigned based on the default for the term in the ICD-9-CM index, in addition to the code for the causal organism if known.

4) Bacterial Sepsis and Septicemia

In most cases, it will be a code from category 038, Septicemia, that will be used in conjunction with a code from subcategory 995.9 such as the following:

(a) Streptococcal sepsis

If the documentation in the record states streptococcal sepsis, codes 038.0, Streptococcal septicemia, and code 995.91 should be used, in that sequence.

(b) Streptococcal septicemia

If the documentation states streptococcal septicemia, only code 038.0 should be assigned, however, the provider should be queried whether the patient has sepsis, an infection with SIRS.

5) Acute organ dysfunction that is not clearly associated with the sepsis

If a patient has sepsis and an acute organ dysfunction, but the medical record documentation indicates that the acute organ dysfunction is related to a medical condition other than the sepsis, do not assign code 995.92, Severe sepsis. An acute organ dysfunction must be associated with the sepsis in order to assign the severe sepsis code. If the documentation is not clear as to whether an acute organ dysfunction is related to the sepsis or another medical condition, query the provider.

6) Septic shock

(a) Sequencing of septic shock and postprocedural septic shock

Septic shock generally refers to circulatory failure associated with severe sepsis, and, therefore, it represents a type of acute organ dysfunction.

For cases of septic shock, the code for the systemic infection should be sequenced first, followed by codes 995.92, Severe sepsis and 785.52, Septic shock or 998.02, Postoperative septic shock. Any additional codes for other acute organ dysfunctions should also be assigned. As noted in the sequencing instructions in the Tabular List, the code for septic shock cannot be assigned as a principal diagnosis.

(b) Septic shock and postprocedural septic shock without documentation of severe sepsis

Since septic shock indicates the presence of severe sepsis, code 995.92, Severe sepsis, can be assigned with code 785.52, Septic shock, or code 998.02 Postoperative shock, septic, even if the term severe sepsis is not documented in the record.

7) Sepsis and septic shock complicating abortion and pregnancy

Sepsis and septic shock complicating abortion, ectopic pregnancy, and molar pregnancy are classified to category codes in Chapter 11 (630-639). See section I.C.11.i.7. for information on the coding of puerperal sepsis.

8) Negative or inconclusive blood cultures

Negative or inconclusive blood cultures do not preclude a diagnosis of septicemia or sepsis in patients with clinical evidence of the condition, however, the provider should be queried.

9) Newborn sepsis

See Section I.C.15.j for information on the coding of newborn sepsis.

10) Sepsis due to a Postprocedural Infection

(a) Documentation of causal relationship

As with all postprocedural complications, code assignment is based on the provider's documentation of the relationship between the infection and the procedure.

(b) Sepsis due to postprocedural infection

In cases of postprocedural sepsis, the complication code, such as code 998.59, Other postoperative infection, or 674.3x, Other complications of obstetrical surgical wounds should be coded first followed by the appropriate sepsis codes (systemic infection code and either code 995.91or 995.92). An additional code(s) for any acute organ dysfunction should also be assigned for cases of severe sepsis. See Section see Section I.C.1.b.6 if the sepsis or severe sepsis results in postprocedural septic shock.

(c) Postprocedural infection and postprocedural septic shock

In cases where a postprocedural infection has occurred and has resulted in severe sepsis and postprocedural septic shock, the code for the precipitating complication such as code 998.59, Other postoperative infection, or 674.3x, Other complications of obstetrical surgical wounds should be coded first followed by the appropriate sepsis codes (systemic infection code and code 995.92). Code 998.02, Postoperative septic shock, should be assigned as an additional code. In cases of severe sepsis, an additional code(s) for any acute organ dysfunction should also be assigned.

11) External cause of injury codes with SIRS

Refer to Section I.C.19.a.7 for instruction on the use of external cause of injury codes with codes for SIRS resulting from trauma.

12) Sepsis and Severe Sepsis Associated with Noninfectious Process

In some cases, a non-infectious process, such as trauma, may lead to an infection which can result in sepsis or severe sepsis. If sepsis or severe sepsis is documented as associated with a non-infectious condition, such as a burn or serious injury, and this condition meets the definition for principal diagnosis, the code for the noninfectious condition should be sequenced first, followed by the code for the systemic infection and either code 995.91, Sepsis, or 995.92, Severe sepsis. Additional codes for any associated acute organ dysfunction(s) should also be assigned for cases of severe sepsis. If the sepsis or severe sepsis meets the definition of principal diagnosis, the systemic infection and sepsis codes should be sequenced before the non-infectious condition. When both the associated non-infectious condition and the sepsis or severe sepsis meet the definition of principal diagnosis, either may be assigned as principal diagnosis. *See Section I.C.1.b.2.a for guidelines pertaining to sepsis or severe sepsis as the principal diagnosis.*

Only one code from subcategory 995.9 should be assigned. Therefore, when a non-infectious condition leads to an infection resulting in sepsis or severe sepsis, assign either code 995.91 or 995.92. Do not additionally assign code 995.93, Systemic inflammatory response syndrome due to non-infectious process without acute organ dysfunction, or 995.94, Systemic inflammatory response syndrome with acute organ dysfunction. *See Section I.C.17.g for information on the coding of SIRS due to trauma/burns or other non-infectious disease processes.*

c. **Methicillin Resistant** *Staphylococcus aureus* **(MRSA) Conditions**

1) **Selection and sequencing of MRSA codes**

(a) Combination codes for MRSA infection

When a patient is diagnosed with an infection that is due to methicillin resistant *Staphylococcus aureus* (MRSA), and that infection has a combination code that includes the causal organism (e.g., septicemia, pneumonia) assign the appropriate code for the condition (e.g., code 038.12, Methicillin resistant Staphylococcus aureus septicemia or code 482.42, Methicillin resistant pneumonia due to Staphylococcus aureus). Do not assign code 041.12, Methicillin resistant Staphylococcus aureus, as an additional code because the code includes the type of infection and the MRSA organism. Do not assign a code from subcategory V09.0, Infection with microorganisms resistant to penicillins, as an additional diagnosis.

See Section C.1.b.1 for instructions on coding and sequencing of septicemia.

(b) Other codes for MRSA infection

When there is documentation of a current infection (e.g., wound infection, stitch abscess, urinary tract infection) due to MRSA, and that infection does not have a combination code that includes the causal organism, select the appropriate code to identify the condition along with code 041.12, Methicillin resistant Staphylococcus aureus, for the MRSA infection. Do not assign a code from subcategory V09.0, Infection with microorganisms resistant to penicillins.

(c) Methicillin susceptible *Staphylococcus aureus* (MSSA) and MRSA colonization

The condition or state of being colonized or carrying MSSA or MRSA is called colonization or carriage, while an individual person is described as being colonized or being a carrier. Colonization means that MSSA or MSRA is present on or in the body without necessarily causing illness. A positive MRSA colonization test might be documented by the provider as "MRSA screen positive" or "MRSA nasal swab positive".

Assign code V02.54, Carrier or suspected carrier, Methicillin resistant Staphylococcus aureus, for patients documented as having MRSA colonization. Assign code V02.53, Carrier or suspected carrier, Methicillin susceptible Staphylococcus aureus, for patient documented as having MSSA colonization. Colonization is not necessarily indicative of a disease process or as the cause of a specific condition the patient may have unless documented as such by the provider.

Code V02.59, Other specified bacterial diseases, should be assigned for other types of staphylococcal colonization (e.g., *S. epidermidis*, *S. saprophyticus*). Code V02.59 should not be assigned for colonization with any type of *Staphylococcus aureus* (MRSA, MSSA).

(d) MRSA colonization and infection

If a patient is documented as having both MRSA colonization and infection during a hospital admission, code V02.54, Carrier or suspected carrier, Methicillin resistant Staphylococcus aureus, and a code for the MRSA infection may both be assigned.

2. Chapter 2: Neoplasms (140-239)

General guidelines

Chapter 2 of the ICD-9-CM contains the codes for most benign and all malignant neoplasms. Certain benign neoplasms, such as prostatic adenomas, may be found in the specific body system chapters. To properly code a neoplasm it is necessary to determine from the record if the neoplasm is benign, in-situ, malignant, or of uncertain histologic behavior. If malignant, any secondary (metastatic) sites should also be determined.

The neoplasm table in the Alphabetic Index should be referenced first. However, if the histological term is documented, that term should be referenced first, rather than going immediately to the Neoplasm Table, in order to determine which column in the Neoplasm Table is appropriate. For example, if the documentation indicates "adenoma," refer to the term in the Alphabetic Index to review the entries under this term and the instructional note to "see also neoplasm, by site, benign." The table provides the proper code based on the type of neoplasm and the site. It is important to select the proper column in the table that corresponds to the type of neoplasm. The tabular should then be referenced to verify that the correct code has been selected from the table and that a more specific site code does not exist.

See Section I. C. 18.d.4. for information regarding V codes for genetic susceptibility to cancer.

a. Treatment directed at the malignancy

If the treatment is directed at the malignancy, designate the malignancy as the principal diagnosis. The only exception to this guideline is if a patient admission/encounter is solely for the administration of chemotherapy, immunotherapy or radiation therapy, assign the appropriate V58.x code as the first-listed or principal diagnosis, and the diagnosis or problem for which the service is being performed as a secondary diagnosis.

b. Treatment of secondary site

When a patient is admitted because of a primary neoplasm with metastasis and treatment is directed toward the secondary site only, the secondary neoplasm is designated as the principal diagnosis even though the primary malignancy is still present.

c. Coding and sequencing of complications

Coding and sequencing of complications associated with the malignancies or with the therapy thereof are subject to the following guidelines:

1) Anemia associated with malignancy

When admission/encounter is for management of an anemia associated with the malignancy, and the treatment is only for anemia, the appropriate anemia code (such as code 285.22, Anemia in neoplastic disease) is designated as the principal diagnosis and is followed by the appropriate code(s) for the malignancy. Code 285.22 may also be used as a secondary code if the patient suffers from anemia and is being treated for the malignancy. If anemia in neoplastic disease and anemia due to antineoplastic chemotherapy are both documented, assign codes for both conditions.

2) Anemia associated with chemotherapy, immunotherapy and radiation therapy

When the admission/encounter is for management of an anemia associated with chemotherapy, immunotherapy or radiotherapy and the only treatment is for the anemia, the anemia is sequenced first. The appropriate neoplasm code should be assigned as an additional code.

3) Management of dehydration due to the malignancy

When the admission/encounter is for management of dehydration due to the malignancy or the therapy, or a combination of both, and only the dehydration is being treated (intravenous rehydration), the dehydration is sequenced first, followed by the code(s) for the malignancy.

4) Treatment of a complication resulting from a surgical procedure

When the admission/encounter is for treatment of a complication resulting from a surgical procedure, designate the complication as the principal or first-listed diagnosis if treatment is directed at resolving the complication.

d. Primary malignancy previously excised

When a primary malignancy has been previously excised or eradicated from its site and there is no further treatment directed to that site and there is no evidence of any existing primary malignancy, a code from category V10, Personal history of malignant neoplasm, should be used to indicate the former site of the malignancy. Any mention of extension, invasion, or metastasis to another site is coded as a secondary malignant neoplasm to that site. The secondary site may be the principal or first-listed with the V10 code used as a secondary code.

e. Admissions/Encounters involving chemotherapy, immunotherapy and radiation therapy

1) Episode of care involves surgical removal of neoplasm

When an episode of care involves the surgical removal of a neoplasm, primary or secondary site, followed by adjunct chemotherapy or radiation treatment during the same episode of care, the neoplasm code should be assigned as principal or first-listed diagnosis, using codes in the 140-198 series or where appropriate in the 200-203 series.

2) **Patient admission/encounter solely for administration of chemotherapy, immunotherapy and radiation therapy**

If a patient admission/encounter is solely for the administration of chemotherapy, immunotherapy or radiation therapy assign code V58.0, Encounter for radiation therapy, or V58.11, Encounter for antineoplastic chemotherapy, or V58.12, Encounter for anti-neoplastic immunotherapy as the first-listed or principal diagnosis. If a patient receives more than one of these therapies during the same admission more than one of these codes may be assigned, in any sequence. The malignancy for which the therapy is being administered should be assigned as a secondary diagnosis.

3) **Patient admitted for radiotherapy/chemotherapy and immunotherapy and develops complications**

When a patient is admitted for the purpose of radiotherapy, immunotherapy or chemotherapy and develops complications such as uncontrolled nausea and vomiting or dehydration, the principal or first-listed diagnosis is V58.0, Encounter for radiotherapy, or V58.11, Encounter for antineoplastic chemotherapy, or V58.12, Encounter for antineoplastic immunotherapy followed by any codes for the complications.

f. **Admission/encounter to determine extent of malignancy**

When the reason for admission/encounter is to determine the extent of the malignancy, or for a procedure such as paracentesis or thoracentesis, the primary malignancy or appropriate metastatic site is designated as the principal or first-listed diagnosis, even though chemotherapy or radiotherapy is administered.

g. **Symptoms, signs, and ill-defined conditions listed in Chapter 16 associated with neoplasms**

Symptoms, signs, and ill-defined conditions listed in Chapter 16 characteristic of, or associated with, an existing primary or secondary site malignancy cannot be used to replace the malignancy as principal or first-listed diagnosis, regardless of the number of admissions or encounters for treatment and care of the neoplasm.

h. **Admission/encounter for pain control/management**

See Section I.C.6.a.5 for information on coding admission / encounter for pain control/management.

i. **Malignant neoplasm associated with transplanted organ**

A malignant neoplasm of a transplanted organ should be coded as a transplant complication. Assign first the appropriate code from subcategory 996.8, Complications of transplanted organ, followed by code 199.2, Malignant neoplasm associated with transplanted organ. Use an additional code for the specific malignancy.

3. **Chapter 3: Endocrine, Nutritional, and Metabolic Diseases and Immunity Disorders (240-279)**

   a. **Diabetes mellitus**

   Codes under category 250, Diabetes mellitus, identify complications/ manifestations associated with diabetes mellitus. A fifth-digit is required for all category 250 codes to identify the type of diabetes mellitus and whether the diabetes is controlled or uncontrolled.
   See I.C.3.a.7 for secondary diabetes

   1) **Fifth-digits for category 250:**

   The following are the fifth-digits for the codes under category 250:

   0 type II or unspecified type, not stated as uncontrolled
   1 type I, [juvenile type], not stated as uncontrolled
   2 type II or unspecified type, uncontrolled
   3 type I, [juvenile type], uncontrolled

   The age of a patient is not the sole determining factor, though most type I diabetics develop the condition before reaching puberty. For this reason type I diabetes mellitus is also referred to as juvenile diabetes.

   2) **Type of diabetes mellitus not documented**

   If the type of diabetes mellitus is not documented in the medical record the default is type II.

   3) **Diabetes mellitus and the use of insulin**

   All type I diabetics must use insulin to replace what their bodies do not produce. However, the use of insulin does not mean that a patient is a type I diabetic. Some patients with type II diabetes mellitus are unable to control their blood sugar through diet and oral medication alone and do require insulin. If the documentation in a medical record does not indicate the type of diabetes but does indicate that the patient uses insulin, the appropriate fifth-digit for type II must be used. For type II patients who routinely use insulin, code V58.67, Long-term (current) use of insulin, should also be assigned to indicate that the patient uses insulin. Code V58.67 should not be assigned if insulin is given temporarily to bring a type II patient's blood sugar under control during an encounter.

   4) **Assigning and sequencing diabetes codes and associated conditions**

   When assigning codes for diabetes and its associated conditions, the code(s) from category 250 must be sequenced before the codes for the associated conditions. The diabetes codes and the secondary codes that correspond to them are paired codes that follow the etiology/manifestation convention of the classification (See SectionI.A.6., Etiology/manifestation convention). Assign as many codes from category 250 as needed to identify all of the associated conditions that the patient has. The corresponding secondary codes are listed under each of the diabetes codes.

(a) Diabetic retinopathy/diabetic macular edema

Diabetic macular edema, code 362.07, is only present with diabetic retinopathy. Another code from subcategory 362.0, Diabetic retinopathy, must be used with code 362.07. Codes under subcategory 362.0 are diabetes manifestation codes, so they must be used following the appropriate diabetes code.

5) **Diabetes mellitus in pregnancy and gestational diabetes**

(a) For diabetes mellitus complicating pregnancy, see Section I.C.11.f., Diabetes mellitus in pregnancy.

(b) For gestational diabetes, see Section I.C.11, g., Gestational diabetes.

6) **Insulin pump malfunction**

(a) Underdose of insulin due to insulin pump failure

An underdose of insulin due to an insulin pump failure should be assigned 996.57, Mechanical complication due to insulin pump, as the principal or first listed code, followed by the appropriate diabetes mellitus code based on documentation.

(b) Overdose of insulin due to insulin pump failure

The principal or first listed code for an encounter due to an insulin pump malfunction resulting in an overdose of insulin, should also be 996.57, Mechanical complication due to insulin pump, followed by code 962.3, Poisoning by insulins and antidiabetic agents, and the appropriate diabetes mellitus code based on documentation.

7) **Secondary Diabetes Mellitus**

Codes under category 249, Secondary diabetes mellitus, identify complications/manifestations associated with secondary diabetes mellitus. Secondary diabetes is always caused by another condition or event (e.g., cystic fibrosis, malignant neoplasm of pancreas, pancreatectomy, adverse effect of drug, or poisoning).

(a) Fifth-digits for category 249:

A fifth-digit is required for all category 249 codes to identify whether the diabetes is controlled or uncontrolled.

(b) Secondary diabetes mellitus and the use of insulin

For patients who routinely use insulin, code V58.67, Long-term (current) use of insulin, should also be assigned. Code V58.67 should not be assigned if insulin is given temporarily to bring a patient's blood sugar under control during an encounter.

(c) Assigning and sequencing secondary diabetes codes and associated conditions

When assigning codes for secondary diabetes and its associated conditions (e.g. renal manifestations), the code(s) from category 249 must be sequenced before the codes for the associated conditions. The secondary diabetes codes and the diabetic manifestation codes that correspond to them are paired codes that follow the etiology/manifestation convention of the classification. Assign as many codes from category 249 as needed to identify all of the associated conditions that the patient has. The corresponding codes for the associated conditions are listed under each of the secondary diabetes codes. For example, secondary diabetes with diabetic nephrosis is assigned to code 249.40, followed by 581.81.

(d)   Assigning and sequencing secondary diabetes codes and its causes

The sequencing of the secondary diabetes codes in relationship to codes for the cause of the diabetes is based on the reason for the encounter, applicable ICD-9-CM sequencing conventions, and chapter-specific guidelines.

If a patient is seen for treatment of the secondary diabetes or one of its associated conditions, a code from category 249 is sequenced as the principal or first-listed diagnosis, with the cause of the secondary diabetes (e.g. cystic fibrosis) sequenced as an additional diagnosis.

If, however, the patient is seen for the treatment of the condition causing the secondary diabetes (e.g., malignant neoplasm of pancreas), the code for the cause of the secondary diabetes should be sequenced as the principal or first-listed diagnosis followed by a code from category 249.

(i)   Secondary diabetes mellitus due to pancreatectomy

For postpancreatectomy diabetes mellitus (lack of insulin due to the surgical removal of all or part of the pancreas), assign code 251.3, Postsurgical hypoinsulinemia. Assign a code from subcategory 249, Secondary diabetes mellitus and a code from subcategory V88.1, Acquired absence of pancreas as additional codes. Code also any diabetic manifestations (e.g. diabetic nephrosis 581.81).

(ii)   Secondary diabetes due to drugs

Secondary diabetes may be caused by an adverse effect of correctly administered medications, poisoning or late effect of poisoning. *See section I.C.17.e for coding of adverse effects and poisoning, and section I.C.19 for E code reporting.*

4. Chapter 4: Diseases of Blood and Blood Forming Organs (280-289)

a. Anemia of chronic disease

Subcategory 285.2, Anemia in chronic illness, has codes for anemia in chronic kidney disease, code 285.21; anemia in neoplastic disease, code 285.22; and anemia in other chronic illness, code 285.29. These codes can be used as the principal/first listed code if the reason for the encounter is to treat the anemia. They may also be used as secondary codes if treatment of the anemia is a component of an encounter, but not the primary reason for the encounter. When using a code from subcategory 285 it is also necessary to use the code for the chronic condition causing the anemia.

1) Anemia in chronic kidney disease

When assigning code 285.21, Anemia in chronic kidney disease, it is also necessary to assign a code from category 585, Chronic kidney disease, to indicate the stage of chronic kidney disease.
See I.C.10.a. Chronic kidney disease (CKD).

2) Anemia in neoplastic disease

When assigning code 285.22, Anemia in neoplastic disease, it is also necessary to assign the neoplasm code that is responsible for the anemia. Code 285.22 is for use for anemia that is due to the malignancy, not for anemia due to antineoplastic chemotherapy drugs. Assign the appropriate code for anemia due to antineoplastic chemotherapy. *See I.C.2.c.1 Anemia associated with malignancy. See I.C.2.c.2 Anemia associated with chemotherapy ,immunotherapy and radiation therapy.*

5. Chapter 5: Mental Disorders (290-319)

Reserved for future guideline expansion

6. Chapter 6: Diseases of Nervous System and Sense Organs (320-389)

a. Pain - Category 338

1) General coding information

Codes in category 338 may be used in conjunction with codes from other categories and chapters to provide more detail about acute or chronic pain and neoplasm-related pain, unless otherwise indicated below.

If the pain is not specified as acute or chronic, do not assign codes from category 338, except for post-thoracotomy pain, postoperative pain, neoplasm related pain, or central pain syndrome. A code from subcategories 338.1 and 338.2 should not be assigned if the underlying (definitive) diagnosis is known, unless the reason for the encounter is pain control/management and not management of the underlying condition.

(a) Category 338 Codes as Principal or First-Listed Diagnosis

Category 338 codes are acceptable as principal diagnosis or the first-listed code:

■ When pain control or pain management is the reason for the admission/encounter (e.g., a patient with displaced intervertebral disc, nerve impingement and severe back pain presents for injection of steroid into the spinal canal). The underlying cause of the pain should be reported as an additional diagnosis, if known.

■ When an admission or encounter is for a procedure aimed at treating the underlying condition (e.g., spinal fusion, kyphoplasty), a code for the underlying condition (e.g., vertebral fracture, spinal stenosis) should be assigned as the principal diagnosis. No code from category 338 should be assigned.

■ When a patient is admitted for the insertion of a neurostimulator for pain control, assign the appropriate pain code as the principal or first listed diagnosis. When an admission or encounter is for a procedure aimed at treating the underlying condition and a neurostimulator is inserted for pain control during the same admission/encounter, a code for the underlying condition should be assigned as the principal diagnosis and the appropriate pain code should be assigned as a secondary diagnosis.

(b) Use of Category 338 Codes in Conjunction with Site-Specific Pain Codes

(i) Assigning Category 338 Codes and Site Specific Pain Codes

Codes from category 338 may be used in conjunction with codes that identify the site of pain (including codes from chapter 16) if the category 338 code provides additional information. For example, if the code describes the site of the pain, but does not fully describe whether the pain is acute or chronic, then both codes should be assigned.

(ii) Sequencing of Category 338 Codes with Site Specific Pain Codes

The sequencing of category 338 codes with site-specific pain codes (including chapter 16 codes), is dependent on the circumstances of the encounter/ admission as follows:

■ If the encounter is for pain control or pain management, assign the code from category 338 followed by the code identifying the specific site of pain (e.g., encounter for pain management for acute neck pain from trauma is assigned code 338.11, Acute pain due to trauma, followed by code 723.1, Cervicalgia, to identify the site of pain).

■ If the encounter is for any other reason except pain control or pain management, and a related definitive diagnosis has not been established (confirmed) by the provider, assign the code for the specific site of pain first, followed by the appropriate code from category 338.

2) Pain due to devices, implants and grafts

Pain associated with devices, implants or grafts left in a surgical site (for example painful hip prosthesis) is assigned to the appropriate code(s) found in Chapter 17, Injury and Poisoning. Use additional code(s) from category 338 to identify acute or chronic pain due to presence of the device, implant or graft (338.18-338.19 or 338.28-338.29).

3) Postoperative Pain

Post-thoracotomy pain and other postoperative pain are classified to subcategories 338.1 and 338.2, depending on whether the pain is acute or chronic. The default for post-thoracotomy and other postoperative pain not specified as acute or chronic is the code for the acute form.

Routine or expected postoperative pain immediately after surgery should not be coded.

(a) Postoperative pain not associated with specific postoperative complication

Postoperative pain not associated with a specific postoperative complication is assigned to the appropriate postoperative pain code in category 338.

(b) Postoperative pain associated with specific postoperative complication

Postoperative pain associated with a specific postoperative complication (such as painful wire sutures) is assigned to the appropriate code(s) found in Chapter 17, Injury and Poisoning. If appropriate, use additional code(s) from category 338 to identify acute or chronic pain (338.18 or 338.28). If pain control/management is the reason for the encounter, a code from category 338 should be assigned as the principal or first-listed diagnosis in accordance with Section I.C.6.a.I.a above.

(c) Postoperative pain as principal or first-listed diagnosis

Postoperative pain may be reported as the principal or first-listed diagnosis when the stated reason for the admission/encounter is documented as postoperative pain control/management.

(d) Postoperative pain as secondary diagnosis

Postoperative pain may be reported as a secondary diagnosis code when a patient presents for outpatient surgery and develops an unusual or inordinate amount of postoperative pain.

The provider's documentation should be used to guide the coding of postoperative pain, as well as *Section III. Reporting Additional Diagnoses* and *Section IV. Diagnostic Coding and Reporting in the Outpatient Setting.*

See Section II.I.2 for information on sequencing of diagnoses for patients admitted to hospital inpatient care following post-operative observation.

See Section II.J for information on sequencing of diagnoses for patients admitted to hospital inpatient care from outpatient surgery.

See Section IV.A.2 for information on sequencing of diagnoses for patients admitted for observation.

4) Chronic pain

Chronic pain is classified to subcategory 338.2. There is no time frame defining when pain becomes chronic pain. The provider's documentation should be used to guide use of these codes.

5) Neoplasm Related Pain

Code 338.3 is assigned to pain documented as being related, associated or due to cancer, primary or secondary malignancy, or tumor. This code is assigned regardless of whether the pain is acute or chronic.

This code may be assigned as the principal or first-listed code when the stated reason for the admission/encounter is documented as pain control/pain management. The underlying neoplasm should be reported as an additional diagnosis.

When the reason for the admission/encounter is management of the neoplasm and the pain associated with the neoplasm is also documented, code 338.3 may be assigned as an additional diagnosis. *See Section I.C.2 for instructions on the sequencing of neoplasms for all other stated reasons for the admission/encounter (except for pain control/pain management).*

6) Chronic pain syndrome

This condition is different than the term "chronic pain," and therefore this code should only be used when the provider has specifically documented this condition.

b. Glaucoma

1) Glaucoma

For types of glaucoma classified to subcategories 365.1-365.6, an additional code should be assigned from subcategory 365.7, Glaucoma stage, to identify the glaucoma stage. Codes from 365.7, Glaucoma stage, may not be assigned as a principal or first-listed diagnosis.

2) Bilateral glaucoma with same stage

When a patient has bilateral glaucoma and both are documented as being the same type and stage, report only the code for the type of glaucoma and one code for the stage.

3) Bilateral glaucoma stage with different stages

When a patient has bilateral glaucoma and each eye is documented as having a different stage, assign one code for the type of glaucoma and one code for the highest glaucoma stage.

4) Bilateral glaucoma with different types and different stages

When a patient has bilateral glaucoma and each eye is documented as having a different type and a different stage, assign one code for each type of glaucoma and one code for the highest glaucoma stage.

5) Patient admitted with glaucoma and stage evolves during the admission

If a patient is admitted with glaucoma and the stage progresses during the admission, assign the code for highest stage documented.

6) Indeterminate stage glaucoma

Assignment of code 365.74, Indeterminate stage glaucoma, should be based on the clinical documentation. Code 365.74 is used for glaucomas whose stage cannot be clinically determined. This code should not be confused with code 365.70, Glaucoma stage, unspecified. Code 365.70 should be assigned when there is no documentation regarding the stage of the glaucoma

7. Chapter 7: Diseases of Circulatory System (390-459)

a. Hypertension

Hypertension Table

The Hypertension Table, found under the main term, "Hypertension", in the Alphabetic Index, contains a complete listing of all conditions due to or associated with hypertension and classifies them according to malignant, benign, and unspecified.

1) Hypertension, Essential, or NOS

Assign hypertension (arterial) (essential) (primary) (systemic) (NOS) to category code 401 with the appropriate fourth digit to indicate malignant (.0), benign (.1), or unspecified (.9). Do not use either .0 malignant or .1 benign unless medical record documentation supports such a designation.

2) Hypertension with Heart Disease

Heart conditions (425.8, 429.0-429.3, 429.8, and 429.9) are assigned to a code from category 402 when a causal relationship is stated (due to hypertension) or implied (hypertensive). Use an additional code from category 428 to identify the type of heart failure in those patients with heart failure. More than one code from category 428 may be assigned if the patient has systolic or diastolic failure and congestive heart failure.

The same heart conditions (425.8, 429.0-429.3, 429.8, and 429.9) with hypertension, but without a stated causal relationship, are coded separately. Sequence according to the circumstances of the admission/encounter.

3) Hypertensive Chronic Kidney Disease

Assign codes from category 403, Hypertensive chronic kidney disease, when conditions classified to category 585 or code 587 are present with hypertension. Unlike hypertension with heart disease, ICD-9-CM presumes a cause-and-effect relationship and classifies chronic kidney disease (CKD) with hypertension as hypertensive chronic kidney disease.

Fifth digits for category 403 should be assigned as follows:

0 with CKD stage I through stage IV, or unspecified.

1 with CKD stage V or end stage renal disease.

The appropriate code from category 585, Chronic kidney disease, should be used as a secondary code with a code from category 403 to identify the stage of chronic kidney disease.

See Section I.C.10.a for information on the coding of chronic kidney disease.

4) Hypertensive Heart and Chronic Kidney Disease

Assign codes from combination category 404, Hypertensive heart and chronic kidney disease, when both hypertensive kidney disease and hypertensive heart disease are stated in the diagnosis. Assume a relationship between the hypertension and the chronic kidney disease, whether or not the condition is so designated. Assign an additional code from category 428, to identify the type of heart failure. More than one code from category 428 may be assigned if the patient has systolic or diastolic failure and congestive heart failure.

Fifth digits for category 404 should be assigned as follows:

0 without heart failure and with chronic kidney disease (CKD) stage I through stage IV, or unspecified

1 with heart failure and with CKD stage I through stage IV, or unspecified

2 without heart failure and with CKD stage V or end stage renal disease

3 with heart failure and with CKD stage V or end stage renal disease

The appropriate code from category 585, Chronic kidney disease, should be used as a secondary code with a code from category 404 to identify the stage of kidney disease. *See Section I.C.10.a for information on the coding of chronic kidney disease.*

5) Hypertensive Cerebrovascular Disease

First assign codes from 430-438, Cerebrovascular disease, then the appropriate hypertension code from categories 401-405.

6) Hypertensive Retinopathy

Two codes are necessary to identify the condition. First assign the code from subcategory 362.11, Hypertensive retinopathy, then the appropriate code from categories 401-405 to indicate the type of hypertension.

7) Hypertension, Secondary

Two codes are required: one to identify the underlying etiology and one from category 405 to identify the hypertension.Sequencing of codes is determined by the reason for admission/encounter.

8) Hypertension, Transient

Assign code 796.2, Elevated blood pressure reading without diagnosis of hypertension, unless patient has an established diagnosis of hypertension. Assign code 642.3x for transient hypertension of pregnancy.

9) Hypertension, Controlled

Assign appropriate code from categories 401-405. This diagnostic statement usually refers to an existing state of hypertension under control by therapy.

10) Hypertension, Uncontrolled

Uncontrolled hypertension may refer to untreated hypertension or hypertension not responding to current therapeutic regimen. In either case, assign the appropriate code from categories 401-405 to designate the stage and type of hypertension. Code to the type of hypertension.

11) Elevated Blood Pressure

For a statement of elevated blood pressure without further specificity, assign code 796.2, Elevated blood pressure reading without diagnosis of hypertension, rather than a code from category 401.

b. Cerebral infarction/stroke/cerebrovascular accident (CVA)

The terms stroke and CVA are often used interchangeably to refer to a cerebral infarction. The terms stroke, CVA, and cerebral infarction NOS are all indexed to the default code 434.91, Cerebral artery occlusion, unspecified, with infarction.

Additional code(s) should be assigned for any neurologic deficits associated with the acute CVA, regardless of whether or not the neurologic deficit resolves prior to discharge.

See Section I.C.I8.d.3 for information on coding status post administration of tPA in a different facility within the last 24 hours.

c. **Postoperative cerebrovascular accident**

A cerebrovascular hemorrhage or infarction that occurs as a result of medical intervention is coded to 997.02, Iatrogenic cerebrovascular infarction or hemorrhage. Medical record documentation should clearly specify the cause- and-effect relationship between the medical intervention and the cerebrovascular accident in order to assign this code. A secondary code from the code range 430-432 or from a code from subcategories 433 or 434 with a fifth digit of "1" should also be used to identify the type of hemorrhage or infarct.

This guideline conforms to the use additional code note instruction at category 997. Code 436, Acute, but ill-defined, cerebrovascular disease, should not be used as a secondary code with code 997.02.

d. **Late Effects of Cerebrovascular Disease**

1) **Category 438, Late Effects of Cerebrovascular disease**

Category 438 is used to indicate conditions classifiable to categories 430-437 as the causes of late effects (neurologic deficits), themselves classified elsewhere. These "late effects" include neurologic deficits that persist after initial onset of conditions classifiable to 430-437. The neurologic deficits caused by cerebrovascular disease may be present from the onset or may arise at any time after the onset of the condition classifiable to 430-437.

Codes in category 438 are only for use for late effects of cerebrovascular disease, not for neurologic deficits associated with an acute CVA.

2) **Codes from category 438 with codes from 430-437**

Codes from category 438 may be assigned on a health care record with codes from 430-437, if the patient has a current cerebrovascular accident (CVA) and deficits from an old CVA.

3) **Code V12.54**

Assign code V12.54, Transient ischemic attack (TIA), and cerebral infarction without residual deficits (and not a code from category 438) as an additional code for history of cerebrovascular disease when no neurologic deficits are present.

e. **Acute myocardial infarction (AMI)**

1) **ST elevation myocardial infarction (STEMI) and non ST elevation myocardial infarction (NSTEMI)**

The ICD-9-CM codes for acute myocardial infarction (AMI) identify the site, such as anterolateral wall or true posterior wall. Subcategories 410.0-410.6 and 410.8 are used for ST elevation myocardial infarction (STEMI). Subcategory 410.7, Subendocardial infarction, is used for non ST elevation myocardial infarction (NSTEMI) and nontransmural MIs.

2) **Acute myocardial infarction, unspecified**

Subcategory 410.9 is the default for the unspecified term acute myocardial infarction. If only STEMI or transmural MI without the site is documented, query the provider as to the site, or assign a code from subcategory 410.9.

3) **AMI documented as nontransmural or subendocardial but site provided**

If an AMI is documented as nontransmural or subendocardial, but the site is provided, it is still coded as a subendocardial AMI. If NSTEMI evolves to STEMI, assign the STEMI code. If STEMI converts to NSTEMI due to thrombolytic therapy, it is still coded as STEMI.

See Section I.C.18.d.3 for information on coding status post administration of tPA in a different facility within the last 24 hours.

8. **Chapter 8: Diseases of Respiratory System (460-519)**

See I.C.17.f. for ventilator-associated pneumonia.

a. **Chronic Obstructive Pulmonary Disease [COPD] and Asthma**

1) **Conditions that comprise COPD and Asthma**
The conditions that comprise COPD are obstructive chronic bronchitis, subcategory 491.2, and emphysema, category 492. All asthma codes are under category 493, Asthma. Code 496, Chronic airway obstruction, not elsewhere classified, is a nonspecific code that should only be used when the documentation in a medical record does not specify the type of COPD being treated.

2) **Acute exacerbation of chronic obstructive bronchitis and asthma**

The codes for chronic obstructive bronchitis and asthma distinguish between uncomplicated cases and those in acute exacerbation. An acute exacerbation is a worsening or a decompensation of a chronic condition. An acute exacerbation is not equivalent to an infection superimposed on a chronic condition, though an exacerbation may be triggered by an infection.

3) **Overlapping nature of the conditions that comprise COPD and asthma**

Due to the overlapping nature of the conditions that make up COPD and asthma, there are many variations in the way these conditions are documented. Code selection must be based on the terms as documented. When selecting the correct code for the documented type of COPD and asthma, it is essential to first review the index, and then verify the code in the tabular list. There are many instructional notes under the different COPD subcategories and codes. It is important that all such notes be reviewed to assure correct code assignment.

4) Acute exacerbation of asthma and status asthmaticus

An acute exacerbation of asthma is an increased severity of the asthma symptoms, such as wheezing and shortness of breath. Status asthmaticus refers to a patient's failure to respond to therapy administered during an asthmatic episode and is a life threatening complication that requires emergency care. If status asthmaticus is documented by the provider with any type of COPD or with acute bronchitis, the status asthmaticus should be sequenced first. It supersedes any type of COPD including that with acute exacerbation or acute bronchitis. It is inappropriate to assign an asthma code with 5th digit 2, with acute exacerbation, together with an asthma code with 5th digit 1, with status asthmatics. Only the 5th digit 1 should be assigned.

b. Chronic Obstructive Pulmonary Disease [COPD] and Bronchitis

1) Acute bronchitis with COPD

Acute bronchitis, code 466.0, is due to an infectious organism. When acute bronchitis is documented with COPD, code 491.22, Obstructive chronic bronchitis with acute bronchitis, should be assigned. It is not necessary to also assign code 466.0. If a medical record documents acute bronchitis with COPD with acute exacerbation, only code 491.22 should be assigned. The acute bronchitis included in code 491.22 supersedes the acute exacerbation. If a medical record documents COPD with acute exacerbation without mention of acute bronchitis, only code 491.21 should be assigned.

c. Acute Respiratory Failure

1) Acute respiratory failure as principal diagnosis

Code 518.81, Acute respiratory failure, may be assigned as a principal diagnosis when it is the condition established after study to be chiefly responsible for occasioning the admission to the hospital, and the selection is supported by the Alphabetic Index and Tabular List. However, chapter-specific coding guidelines (such as obstetrics, poisoning, HIV, newborn) that provide sequencing direction take precedence.

2) Acute respiratory failure as secondary diagnosis

Respiratory failure may be listed as a secondary diagnosis if it occurs after admission, or if it is present on admission, but does not meet the definition of principal diagnosis.

3) Sequencing of acute respiratory failure and another acute condition

When a patient is admitted with respiratory failure and another acute condition, (e.g., myocardial infarction, cerebrovascular accident, aspiration pneumonia), the principal diagnosis will not be the same in every situation. This applies whether the other acute condition is a respiratory or nonrespiratory condition. Selection of the principal diagnosis will be dependent on the circumstances of admission. If both the respiratory failure and the other acute condition are equally responsible for occasioning the admission to the hospital, and there are no chapter-specific sequencing rules, the guideline regarding two or more diagnoses that equally meet the definition for principal diagnosis (Section II, C.) may be applied in these situations.

If the documentation is not clear as to whether acute respiratory failure and another condition are equally responsible for occasioning the admission, query the provider for clarification.

d. Influenza due to certain identified viruses

Code only confirmed cases of avian influenza (codes 488.01-488.02, 488.09, Influenza due to identified avian influenza virus), 2009 H1N1 influenza virus (codes 488.11-488.12, 488.19), or novel influenza A (codes 488.81-488.82, 488.89, Influenza due to identified novel influenza A virus). This is an exception to the hospital inpatient guideline Section II, H. (Uncertain Diagnosis).

In this context, "confirmation" does not require documentation of positive laboratory testing specific for avian, 2009 H1N1 or novel influenza A virus. However, coding should be based on the provider's diagnostic statement that the patient has avian influenza, 2009 H1N1 influenza, or novel influenza A.

If the provider records "suspected" or "possible" or "probable" avian, 2009 H1N1, or novel influenza A, the appropriate influenza code from category 487, Influenza should be assigned. A code from category 488, Influenza due to certain identified influenza viruses, should not be assigned.

9. Chapter 9: Diseases of Digestive System (520-579)

Reserved for future guideline expansion

10. Chapter 10: Diseases of Genitourinary System (580-629)

a. Chronic kidney disease

1) Stages of chronic kidney disease (CKD)

The ICD-9-CM classifies CKD based on severity. The severity of CKD is designated by stages I-V. Stage II, code 585.2, equates to mild CKD; stage III, code 585.3, equates to moderate CKD; and stage IV, code 585.4, equates to severe CKD. Code 585.6, End stage renal disease (ESRD), is assigned when the provider has documented end-stage-renal disease (ESRD).

If both a stage of CKD and ESRD are documented, assign code 585.6 only.

2) Chronic kidney disease and kidney transplant status

Patients who have undergone kidney transplant may still have some form of CKD, because the kidney transplant may not fully restore kidney function. Therefore, the presence of CKD alone does not constitute a transplant complication. Assign the appropriate 585 code for the patient's stage of CKD and code V42.0. If a transplant complication such as failure or rejection is documented, see section I.C.17.f.2.b for information on coding complications of a kidney transplant. If the documentation is unclear as to whether the patient has a complication of the transplant, query the provider.

3) Chronic kidney disease with other conditions

Patients with CKD may also suffer from other serious conditions, most commonly diabetes mellitus and hypertension. The sequencing of the CKD code in relationship to codes for other contributing conditions is based on the conventions in the tabular list.

See I.C.3.a.4 for sequencing instructions for diabetes. See I.C.4.a.I for anemia in CKD. See I.C.7.a.3 for hypertensive chronic kidney disease. See I.C.I7.f.2.b, Kidney transplant complications, for instructions on coding of documented rejection or failure.

11. Chapter 11: Complications of Pregnancy, Childbirth, and the Puerperium (630-679)

a. General Rules for Obstetric Cases

1) Codes from chapter 11 and sequencing priority

Obstetric cases require codes from chapter 11, codes in the range 630-679, Complications of Pregnancy, Childbirth, and the Puerperium. Chapter 11 codes have sequencing priority over codes from other chapters. Additional codes from other chapters may be used in conjunction with chapter 11 codes to further specify conditions. Should the provider document that the pregnancy is incidental to the encounter, then code V22.2 should be used in place of any chapter 11 codes. It is the provider's responsibility to state that the condition being treated is not affecting the pregnancy.

2) Chapter 11 codes used only on the maternal record

Chapter 11 codes are to be used only on the maternal record, never on the record of the newborn.

3) Chapter 11 fifth-digits

Categories 640-649, 651-676 have required fifth-digits, which indicate whether the encounter is antepartum, postpartum and whether a delivery has also occurred.

4) Fifth-digits, appropriate for each code

The fifth-digits, which are appropriate for each code number, are listed in brackets under each code. The fifth-digits on each code should all be consistent with each other. That is, should a delivery occur all of the fifth-digits should indicate the delivery.

b. Selection of OB Principal or First-listed Diagnosis

1) Routine outpatient prenatal visits

For routine outpatient prenatal visits when no complications are present codes V22.0, Supervision of normal first pregnancy, and V22.1, Supervision of other normal pregnancy, should be used as the first-listed diagnoses. These codes should not be used in conjunction with chapter 11 codes.

2) Prenatal outpatient visits for high-risk patients

For routine prenatal outpatient visits for patients with high-risk pregnancies, a code from category V23, Supervision of high-risk pregnancy, should be used as the first-listed diagnosis. Secondary chapter 11 codes may be used in conjunction with these codes if appropriate.

3) Episodes when no delivery occurs

In episodes when no delivery occurs, the principal diagnosis should correspond to the principal complication of the pregnancy, which necessitated the encounter. Should more than one complication exist, all of which are treated or monitored, any of the complications codes may be sequenced first.

4) When a delivery occurs

When a delivery occurs, the principal diagnosis should correspond to the main circumstances or complication of the delivery. In cases of cesarean delivery, the selection of the principal diagnosis should be the condition established after study that was responsible for the patient's admission. If the patient was admitted with a condition that resulted in the performance of a cesarean procedure, that condition should be selected as the principal diagnosis. If the reason for the admission/encounter was unrelated to the condition resulting in the cesarean delivery, the condition related to the reason for the admission/encounter should be selected as the principal diagnosis, even if a cesarean was performed.

5) Outcome of delivery

An outcome of delivery code, V27.0-V27.9, should be included on every maternal record when a delivery has occurred. These codes are not to be used on subsequent records or on the newborn record.

c. Fetal Conditions Affecting the Management of the Mother

1) Codes from category 655 and 656

Codes from categories 655, Known or suspected fetal abnormality affecting management of the mother, and 656, Other known or suspected fetal and placental problems affecting the management of the mother, are assigned only when the fetal condition is actually responsible for modifying the management of the mother, i.e., by requiring diagnostic studies, additional observation, special care, or termination of pregnancy. The fact that the fetal condition exists does not justify assigning a code from this series to the mother's record. *See I.C.18.d. for suspected maternal and fetal conditions not found*

2) In utero surgery

In cases when surgery is performed on the fetus, a diagnosis code from category 655, Known or suspected fetal abnormalities affecting management of the mother, should be assigned identifying the fetal condition. Procedure code 75.36, Correction of fetal defect, should be assigned on the hospital inpatient record.

No code from Chapter 15, the perinatal codes, should be used on the mother's record to identify fetal conditions. Surgery performed in utero on a fetus is still to be coded as an obstetric encounter.

d. HIV Infection in Pregnancy, Childbirth and the Puerperium

During pregnancy, childbirth or the puerperium, a patient admitted because of an HIV-related illness should receive a principal diagnosis of 647.6X, Other specified infectious and parasitic diseases in the mother classifiable elsewhere, but complicating the pregnancy, childbirth or the puerperium, followed by 042 and the code(s) for the HIV-related illness(es).

Patients with asymptomatic HIV infection status admitted during pregnancy, childbirth, or the puerperium should receive codes of 647.6X and V08.

e. Current Conditions Complicating Pregnancy

Assign a code from subcategory 648.x for patients that have current conditions when the condition affects the management of the pregnancy, childbirth, or the puerperium. Use additional secondary codes from other chapters to identify the conditions, as appropriate.

f. Diabetes mellitus in pregnancy

Diabetes mellitus is a significant complicating factor in pregnancy. Pregnant women who are diabetic should be assigned code 648.0x, Diabetes mellitus complicating pregnancy, and a secondary code from category 250, Diabetes mellitus, or category 249, Secondary diabetes to identify the type of diabetes.

Code V58.67, Long-term (current) use of insulin, should also be assigned if the diabetes mellitus is being treated with insulin.

g. Gestational diabetes

Gestational diabetes can occur during the second and third trimester of pregnancy in women who were not diabetic prior to pregnancy. Gestational diabetes can cause complications in the pregnancy similar to those of pre-existing diabetes mellitus. It also puts the woman at greater risk of developing diabetes after the pregnancy. Gestational diabetes is coded to 648.8x, Abnormal glucose tolerance. Codes 648.0x and 648.8x should never be used together on the same record.

Code V58.67, Long-term (current) use of insulin, should also be assigned if the gestational diabetes is being treated with insulin.

h. Normal Delivery, Code 650

1) Normal delivery

Code 650 is for use in cases when a woman is admitted for a full-term normal delivery and delivers a single, healthy infant without any complications antepartum, during the delivery, or postpartum during the delivery episode. Code 650 is always a principal diagnosis. It is not to be used if any other code from chapter 11 is needed to describe a current complication of the antenatal, delivery, or perinatal period. Additional codes from other chapters may be used with code 650 if they are not related to or are in any way complicating the pregnancy.

2) Normal delivery with resolved antepartum complication

Code 650 may be used if the patient had a complication at some point during her pregnancy, but the complication is not present at the time of the admission for delivery.

3) V27.0, Single liveborn, outcome of delivery

V27.0, Single liveborn, is the only outcome of delivery code appropriate for use with 650.

i. The Postpartum and Peripartum Periods

1) Postpartum and peripartum periods

The postpartum period begins immediately after delivery and continues for six weeks following delivery. The peripartum period is defined as the last month of pregnancy to five months postpartum.

2) Postpartum complication

A postpartum complication is any complication occurring within the six-week period.

3) Pregnancy-related complications after 6 week period

Chapter 11 codes may also be used to describe pregnancy-related complications after the six-week period should the provider document that a condition is pregnancy related.

4) Postpartum complications occurring during the same admission as delivery

Postpartum complications that occur during the same admission as the delivery are identified with a fifth digit of "2." Subsequent admissions/encounters for postpartum complications should be identified with a fifth digit of "4."

5) Admission for routine postpartum care following delivery outside hospital

When the mother delivers outside the hospital prior to admission and is admitted for routine postpartum care and no complications are noted, code V24.0, Postpartum care and examination immediately after delivery, should be assigned as the principal diagnosis.

6) **Admission following delivery outside hospital with postpartum conditions**

A delivery diagnosis code should not be used for a woman who has delivered prior to admission to the hospital. Any postpartum conditions and/or postpartum procedures should be coded.

7) **Puerperal sepsis**

Code 670.2x, Puerperal sepsis, should be assigned with a secondary code to identify the causal organism (e.g., for a bacterial infection, assign a code from category 041, Bacterial infections in conditions classified elsewhere and of unspecified site). A code from category 038, Septicemia, should not be used for puerperal sepsis. Do not assign code 995.91, Sepsis, as code 670.2x describes the sepsis. If applicable, use additional codes to identify severe sepsis (995.92) and any associated acute organ dysfunction.

j. **Code 677, Late effect of complication of pregnancy**

1) **Code 677**

Code 677, Late effect of complication of pregnancy, childbirth, and the puerperium is for use in those cases when an initial complication of a pregnancy develops a sequelae requiring care or treatment at a future date.

2) **After the initial postpartum period**

This code may be used at any time after the initial postpartum period.

3) **Sequencing of Code 677**

This code, like all late effect codes, is to be sequenced following the code describing the sequelae of the complication.

k. **Abortions**

1) **Fifth-digits required for abortion categories**

Fifth-digits are required for abortion categories 634-637. Fifth digit assignment is based on the status of the patient at the beginning (or start) of the encounter. Fifth-digit 1, incomplete, indicates that all of the products of conception have not been expelled from the uterus. Fifth-digit 2, complete, indicates that all products of conception have been expelled from the uterus.

2) **Code from categories 640-649 and 651-659**

A code from categories 640-649 and 651-659 may be used as additional codes with an abortion code to indicate the complication leading to the abortion.

Fifth digit 3 is assigned with codes from these categories when used with an abortion code because the other fifth digits will not apply. Codes from the 660-669 series are not to be used for complications of abortion.

3) Code 639 for complications

Code 639 is to be used for all complications following abortion. Code 639 cannot be assigned with codes from categories 634-638.

4) Abortion with Liveborn Fetus

When an attempted termination of pregnancy results in a liveborn fetus assign code 644.21, Early onset of delivery, with an appropriate code from category V27, Outcome of Delivery. The procedure code for the attempted termination of pregnancy should also be assigned.

5) Retained Products of Conception following an abortion

Subsequent admissions for retained products of conception following a spontaneous or legally induced abortion are assigned the appropriate code from category 634, Spontaneous abortion, or 635 Legally induced abortion, with a fifth digit of "1" (incomplete). This advice is appropriate even when the patient was discharged previously with a discharge diagnosis of complete abortion.

12. Chapter 12: Diseases Skin and Subcutaneous Tissue (680-709)

a. Pressure ulcer stage codes

1) Pressure ulcer stages

Two codes are needed to completely describe a pressure ulcer: A code from subcategory 707.0, Pressure ulcer, to identify the site of the pressure ulcer and a code from subcategory 707.2, Pressure ulcer stages.

The codes in subcategory 707.2, Pressure ulcer stages, are to be used as an additional diagnosis with a code(s) from subcategory 707.0, Pressure Ulcer. Codes from 707.2, Pressure ulcer stages, may not be assigned as a principal or first-listed diagnosis. The pressure ulcer stage codes should only be used with pressure ulcers and not with other types of ulcers (e.g., stasis ulcer).

The ICD-9-CM classifies pressure ulcer stages based on severity, which is designated by stages I-IV and unstageable.

2) Unstageable pressure ulcers

Assignment of code 707.25, Pressure ulcer, unstageable, should be based on the clinical documentation. Code 707.25 is used for pressure ulcers whose stage cannot be clinically determined (e.g., the ulcer is covered by eschar or has been treated with a skin or muscle graft) and pressure ulcers that are documented as deep tissue injury but not documented as due to trauma. This code should not be confused with code 707.20, Pressure ulcer, stage unspecified. Code 707.20 should be assigned when there is no documentation regarding the stage of the pressure ulcer.

3) Documented pressure ulcer stage

Assignment of the pressure ulcer stage code should be guided by clinical documentation of the stage or documentation of the terms found in the index. For clinical terms describing the stage that are not found in the index, and there is no documentation of the stage, the provider should be queried.

4) Bilateral pressure ulcers with same stage

When a patient has bilateral pressure ulcers (e.g., both buttocks) and both pressure ulcers are documented as being the same stage, only the code for the site and one code for the stage should be reported.

5) Bilateral pressure ulcers with different stages

When a patient has bilateral pressure ulcers at the same site (e.g., both buttocks) and each pressure ulcer is documented as being at a different stage, assign one code for the site and the appropriate codes for the pressure ulcer stage.

6) Multiple pressure ulcers of different sites and stages

When a patient has multiple pressure ulcers at different sites (e.g., buttock, heel, shoulder) and each pressure ulcer is documented as being at different stages (e.g., stage 3 and stage 4), assign the appropriate codes for each different site and a code for each different pressure ulcer stage.

7) Patients admitted with pressure ulcers documented as healed

No code is assigned if the documentation states that the pressure ulcer is completely healed.

8) Patients admitted with pressure ulcers documented as healing

Pressure ulcers described as healing should be assigned the appropriate pressure ulcer stage code based on the documentation in the medical record. If the documentation does not provide information about the stage of the healing pressure ulcer, assign code 707.20, Pressure ulcer stage, unspecified.

If the documentation is unclear as to whether the patient has a current (new) pressure ulcer or if the patient is being treated for a healing pressure ulcer, query the provider.

9) Patient admitted with pressure ulcer evolving into another stage during the admission

If a patient is admitted with a pressure ulcer at one stage and it progresses to a higher stage, assign the code for highest stage reported for that site.

13. **Chapter 13: Diseases of Musculoskeletal and Connective Tissue (710-739)**

a. **Coding of Pathologic Fractures**

1) **Acute Fractures vs. Aftercare**

Pathologic fractures are reported using subcategory 733.1, when the fracture is newly diagnosed. Subcategory 733.1 may be used while the patient is receiving active treatment for the fracture. Examples of active treatment are: surgical treatment, emergency department encounter, evaluation and treatment by a new physician.

Fractures are coded using the aftercare codes (subcategories V54.0, V54.2, V54.8 or V54.9) for encounters after the patient has completed active treatment of the fracture and is receiving routine care for the fracture during the healing or recovery phase. Examples of fracture aftercare are: cast change or removal, removal of external or internal fixation device, medication adjustment, and follow up visits following fracture treatment.

Care for complications of surgical treatment for fracture repairs during the healing or recovery phase should be coded with the appropriate complication codes.

Care of complications of fractures, such as malunion and nonunion, should be reported with the appropriate codes. *See Section I. C. 17.b for information on the coding of traumatic fractures.*

14. **Chapter 14: Congenital Anomalies (740-759)**

a. **Codes in categories 740-759, Congenital Anomalies**

Assign an appropriate code(s) from categories 740-759, Congenital Anomalies, when an anomaly is documented. A congenital anomaly may be the principal/first listed diagnosis on a record or a secondary diagnosis.

When a congenital anomaly does not have a unique code assignment, assign additional code(s) for any manifestations that may be present.

When the code assignment specifically identifies the congenital anomaly, manifestations that are an inherent component of the anomaly should not be coded separately. Additional codes should be assigned for manifestations that are not an inherent component.

Codes from Chapter 14 may be used throughout the life of the patient. If a congenital anomaly has been corrected, a personal history code should be used to identify the history of the anomaly. Although present at birth, a congenital anomaly may not be identified until later in life. Whenever the condition is diagnosed by the physician, it is appropriate to assign a code from codes 740-759.

For the birth admission, the appropriate code from category V30, Liveborn infants, according to type of birth should be sequenced as the principal diagnosis, followed by any congenital anomaly codes, 740-759.

15. Chapter 15: Newborn (Perinatal) Guidelines (760-779)

For coding and reporting purposes the perinatal period is defined as before birth through the 28th day following birth. The following guidelines are provided for reporting purposes. Hospitals may record other diagnoses as needed for internal data use.

a. General Perinatal Rules

1) Chapter 15 Codes

They are never for use on the maternal record. Codes from Chapter 11, the obstetric chapter, are never permitted on the newborn record. Chapter 15 code may be used throughout the life of the patient if the condition is still present.

2) Sequencing of perinatal codes

Generally, codes from Chapter 15 should be sequenced as the principal/first-listed diagnosis on the newborn record, with the exception of the appropriate V30 code for the birth episode, followed by codes from any other chapter that provide additional detail. The "use additional code" note at the beginning of the chapter supports this guideline. If the index does not provide a specific code for a perinatal condition, assign code 779.89, Other specified conditions originating in the perinatal period, followed by the code from another chapter that specifies the condition. Codes for signs and symptoms may be assigned when a definitive diagnosis has not been established.

3) Birth process or community acquired conditions

If a newborn has a condition that may be either due to the birth process or community acquired and the documentation does not indicate which it is, the default is due to the birth process and the code from Chapter 15 should be used. If the condition is community-acquired, a code from Chapter 15 should not be assigned.

4) Code all clinically significant conditions

All clinically significant conditions noted on routine newborn examination should be coded. A condition is clinically significant if it requires:

- clinical evaluation; or
- therapeutic treatment; or
- diagnostic procedures; or
- extended length of hospital stay; or
- increased nursing care and/or monitoring; or
- has implications for future health care needs

Note: The perinatal guidelines listed above are the same as the general coding guidelines for "additional diagnoses", except for the final point regarding implications for future health care needs. Codes should be assigned for conditions that have been specified by the provider as having implications for future health care needs. Codes from the perinatal chapter should not be assigned unless the provider has established a definitive diagnosis.

b. Use of codes V30-V39

When coding the birth of an infant, assign a code from categories V30-V39, according to the type of birth. A code from this series is assigned as a principal diagnosis, and assigned only once to a newborn at the time of birth.

c. Newborn transfers

If the newborn is transferred to another institution, the V30 series is not used at the receiving hospital.

d. Use of category V29

1) Assigning a code from category V29

Assign a code from category V29, Observation and evaluation of newborns and infants for suspected conditions not found, to identify those instances when a healthy newborn is evaluated for a suspected condition that is determined after study not to be present. Do not use a code from category V29 when the patient has identified signs or symptoms of a suspected problem; in such cases, code the sign or symptom.

A code from category V29 may also be assigned as a principal code for readmissions or encounters when the V30 code no longer applies. Codes from category V29 are for use only for healthy newborns and infants for which no condition after study is found to be present.

2) V29 code on a birth record

A V29 code is to be used as a secondary code after the V30, Outcome of delivery, code.

e. Use of other V codes on perinatal records

V codes other than V30 and V29 may be assigned on a perinatal or newborn record code. The codes may be used as a principal or first-listed diagnosis for specific types of encounters or for readmissions or encounters when the V30 code no longer applies.

See Section I.C.18 for information regarding the assignment of V codes.

f. Maternal Causes of Perinatal Morbidity

Codes from categories 760-763, Maternal causes of perinatal morbidity and mortality, are assigned only when the maternal condition has actually affected the fetus or newborn. The fact that the mother has an associated medical condition or experiences some complication of pregnancy, labor or delivery does not justify the routine assignment of codes from these categories to the newborn record.

g. **Congenital Anomalies in Newborns**

For the birth admission, the appropriate code from category V30, Liveborn infants according to type of birth, should be used, followed by any congenital anomaly codes, categories 740-759. Use additional secondary codes from other chapters to specify conditions associated with the anomaly, if applicable.

Also, see Section I.C.14 for information on the coding of congenital anomalies.

h. **Coding Additional Perinatal Diagnoses**

1) **Assigning codes for conditions that require treatment**

Assign codes for conditions that require treatment or further investigation, prolong the length of stay, or require resource utilization.

2) **Codes for conditions specified as having implications for future health care needs**

Assign codes for conditions that have been specified by the provider as having implications for future health care needs.

Note: This guideline should not be used for adult patients.

3) **Codes for newborn conditions originating in the perinatal period**

Assign a code for newborn conditions originating in the perinatal period (categories 760-779), as well as complications arising during the current episode of care classified in other chapters, only if the diagnoses have been documented by the responsible provider at the time of transfer or discharge as having affected the fetus or newborn.

i. **Prematurity and Fetal Growth Retardation**

Providers utilize different criteria in determining prematurity. A code for prematurity should not be assigned unless it is documented. The 5th digit assignment for codes from category 764 and subcategories 765.0 and 765.1 should be based on the recorded birth weight and estimated gestational age.

A code from subcategory 765.2, Weeks of gestation, should be assigned as an additional code with category 764 and codes from 765.0 and 765.1 to specify weeks of gestation as documented by the provider in the record.

j. **Newborn sepsis**

Code 771.81, Septicemia [sepsis] of newborn, should be assigned with a secondary code from category 041, Bacterial infections in conditions classified elsewhere and of unspecified site, to identify the organism. A code from category 038, Septicemia, should not be used on a newborn record. Do not assign code 995.91, Sepsis, as code 771.81 describes the sepsis. If applicable, use additional codes to identify severe sepsis (995.92) and any associated acute organ dysfunction.

16. Chapter 16: Signs, Symptoms and Ill-Defined Conditions (780-799)

Reserved for future guideline expansion

17. Chapter 17: Injury and Poisoning (800-999)

a. Coding of Injuries

When coding injuries, assign separate codes for each injury unless a combination code is provided, in which case the combination code is assigned. Multiple injury codes are provided in ICD-9-CM, but should not be assigned unless information for a more specific code is not available. These traumatic injury codes are not to be used for normal, healing surgical wounds or to identify complications of surgical wounds.

The code for the most serious injury, as determined by the provider and the focus of treatment, is sequenced first.

1) Superficial injuries

Superficial injuries such as abrasions or contusions are not coded when associated with more severe injuries of the same site.

2) Primary injury with damage to nerves/blood vessels

When a primary injury results in minor damage to peripheral nerves or blood vessels, the primary injury is sequenced first with additional code(s) from categories 950-957, Injury to nerves and spinal cord, and/or 900-904, Injury to blood vessels. When the primary injury is to the blood vessels or nerves, that injury should be sequenced first.

b. Coding of Traumatic Fractures

The principles of multiple coding of injuries should be followed in coding fractures. Fractures of specified sites are coded individually by site in accordance with both the provisions within categories 800-829 and the level of detail furnished by medical record content.

Combination categories for multiple fractures are provided for use when there is insufficient detail in the medical record (such as trauma cases transferred to another hospital), when the reporting form limits the number of codes that can be used in reporting pertinent clinical data, or when there is insufficient specificity at the fourth-digit or fifth-digit level. More specific guidelines are as follows:

1) Acute Fractures vs. Aftercare

Traumatic fractures are coded using the acute fracture codes (800-829) while the patient is receiving active treatment for the fracture. Examples of active treatment are: surgical treatment, emergency department encounter, and evaluation and treatment by a new physician.

Fractures are coded using the aftercare codes (subcategories V54.0, V54.1, V54.8, or V54.9) for encounters after the patient has completed active treatment of the fracture and is receiving routine care for the fracture during the healing or recovery phase. Examples of fracture aftercare are: cast change or removal, removal of external or internal fixation device, medication adjustment, and follow up visits following fracture treatment.

Care for complications of surgical treatment for fracture repairs during the healing or recovery phase should be coded with the appropriate complication codes.

Care of complications of fractures, such as malunion and nonunion, should be reported with the appropriate codes.

Pathologic fractures are not coded in the 800-829 range, but instead are assigned to subcategory 733.1. *See Section I.C.13.a for additional information.*

2) **Multiple fractures of same limb**

Multiple fractures of same limb classifiable to the same three-digit or four-digit category are coded to that category.

3) **Multiple unilateral or bilateral fractures of same bone**

Multiple unilateral or bilateral fractures of same bone(s) but classified to different fourth-digit subdivisions (bone part) within the same three-digit category are coded individually by site.

4) **Multiple fracture categories 819 and 828**

Multiple fracture categories 819 and 828 classify bilateral fractures of both upper limbs (819) and both lower limbs (828), but without any detail at the fourth-digit level other than open and closed type of fractures.

5) **Multiple fractures sequencing**

Multiple fractures are sequenced in accordance with the severity of the fracture. The provider should be asked to list the fracture diagnoses in the order of severity.

c. **Coding of Burns**

Current burns (940-948) are classified by depth, extent and by agent (E code). Burns are classified by depth as first degree (erythema), second degree (blistering), and third degree (full-thickness involvement).

1) **Sequencing of burn and related condition codes**

Sequence first the code that reflects the highest degree of burn when more than one burn is present.

(a.) When the reason for the admission or encounter is for treatment of external multiple burns, sequence first the code that reflects the burn of the highest degree.

(b.) When a patient has both internal and external burns, the circumstances of admission govern the selection of the principal diagnosis or first-listed diagnosis.

(c.) When a patient is admitted for burn injuries and other related conditions such as smoke inhalation and/or respiratory failure, the circumstances of admission govern the selection of the principal or first-listed diagnosis.

2) Burns of the same local site

Classify burns of the same local site (three-digit category level, 940-947) but of different degrees to the subcategory identifying the highest degree recorded in the diagnosis.

3) Non-healing burns

Non-healing burns are coded as acute burns. Necrosis of burned skin should be coded as a non-healed burn.

4) Code 958.3, Posttraumatic wound infection

Assign code 958.3, Posttraumatic wound infection, not elsewhere classified, as an additional code for any documented infected burn site.

5) Assign separate codes for each burn site

When coding burns, assign separate codes for each burn site. Category 946 Burns of Multiple specified sites, should only be used if the location of the burns are not documented. Category 949, Burn, unspecified, is extremely vague and should rarely be used.

6) Assign codes from category 948, Burns

Burns classified according to extent of body surface involved, when the site of the burn is not specified or when there is a need for additional data. It is advisable to use category 948 as additional coding when needed to provide data for evaluating burn mortality, such as that needed by burn units. It is also advisable to use category 948 as an additional code for reporting purposes when there is mention of a third-degree burn involving 20 percent or more of the body surface.

In assigning a code from category 948:

- Fourth-digit codes are used to identify the percentage of total body surface involved in a burn (all degree).

- Fifth-digits are assigned to identify the percentage of body surface involved in third-degree burn.

- Fifth-digit zero (0) is assigned when less than 10 percent or when no body surface is involved in a third-degree burn.

Category 948 is based on the classic "rule of nines" in estimating body surface involved: head and neck are assigned nine percent, each arm nine percent, each leg 18 percent, the anterior trunk 18 percent, posterior trunk 18 percent, and genitalia one percent. Providers may change these percentage assignments where necessary to accommodate infants and children who have proportionately larger heads than adults and patients who have large buttocks, thighs, or abdomen that involve burns.

7) Encounters for treatment of late effects of burns

Encounters for the treatment of the late effects of burns (i.e., scars or joint contractures) should be coded to the residual condition (sequelae) followed by the appropriate late effect code (906.5-906.9). A late effect E code may also be used, if desired.

8) Sequelae with a late effect code and current burn

When appropriate, both a sequelae with a late effect code, and a current burn code may be assigned on the same record (when both a current burn and sequelae of an old burn exist).

d. Coding of Debridement of Wound, Infection, or Burn

Excisional debridement involves surgical removal or cutting away, as opposed to a mechanical (brushing, scrubbing, washing) debridement. For coding purposes, excisional debridement is assigned to code 86.22. Nonexcisional debridement is assigned to code 86.28

e. Adverse Effects, Poisoning and Toxic Effects

The properties of certain drugs, medicinal and biological substances or combinations of such substances, may cause toxic reactions. The occurrence of drug toxicity is classified in ICD-9-CM as follows:

1) Adverse Effect

When the drug was correctly prescribed and properly administered, code the reaction plus the appropriate code from the E930-E949 series. Codes from the E930-E949 series must be used to identify the causative substance for an adverse effect of drug, medicinal and biological substances, correctly prescribed and properly administered. The effect, such as tachycardia, delirium, gastrointestinal hemorrhaging, vomiting, hypokalemia, hepatitis, renal failure, or respiratory failure, is coded and followed by the appropriate code from the E930-E949 series.

Adverse effects of therapeutic substances correctly prescribed and properly administered (toxicity, synergistic reaction, side effect, and idiosyncratic reaction) may be due to (1) differences among patients, such as age, sex, disease, and genetic factors, and (2) drug-related factors, such as type of drug, route of administration, duration of therapy, dosage, and bioavailability.

2) Poisoning

(a) Error was made in drug prescription

Errors made in drug prescription or in the administration of the drug by provider, nurse, patient, or other person, use the appropriate poisoning code from the 960-979 series.

(b) Overdose of a drug intentionally taken

If an overdose of a drug was intentionally taken or administered and resulted in drug toxicity, it would be coded as a poisoning (960-979 series).

(c) Nonprescribed drug taken with correctly prescribed and properly administered drug

If a nonprescribed drug or medicinal agent was taken in combination with a correctly prescribed and properly administered drug, any drug toxicity or other reaction resulting from the interaction of the two drugs would be classified as a poisoning.

(d) Interaction of drug(s) and alcohol

When a reaction results from the interaction of a drug(s) and alcohol, this would be classified as poisoning.

(e) Sequencing of poisoning

When coding a poisoning or reaction to the improper use of a medication (e.g., wrong dose, wrong substance, wrong route of administration) the poisoning code is sequenced first, followed by a code for the manifestation. If there is also a diagnosis of drug abuse or dependence to the substance, the abuse or dependence is coded as an additional code. *See Section I.C.3.a.6.b. if poisoning is the result of insulin pump malfunctions and Section I.C.19 for general use of E-codes.*

3) Toxic Effects

(a) Toxic effect codes

When a harmful substance is ingested or comes in contact with a person, this is classified as a toxic effect. The toxic effect codes are in categories 980-989.

(b) Sequencing toxic effect codes

A toxic effect code should be sequenced first, followed by the code(s) that identify the result of the toxic effect.

(c) External cause codes for toxic effects

An external cause code from categories E860-E869 for accidental exposure, codes E950.6 or E950.7 for intentional self-harm, category E962 for assault, or categories E980-E982, for undetermined, should also be assigned to indicate intent.

f. Complications of care

1) General Guidelines for Complications of Care

(a) Documentation of complications of care

See Section I.B.18. for information on documentation of complications of care.

(b) Use additional code to identify nature of complication

An additional code identifying the complication should be assigned with codes in categories 996-999, Complications of Surgical and Medical Care NEC, when the additional code provides greater specificity as to the nature of the condition. If the complication code fully describes the condition, no additional code is necessary.

2) Transplant complications

(a) Transplant complications other than kidney

Codes under subcategory 996.8, Complications of transplanted organ, are for use for both complications and rejection of transplanted organs. A transplant complication code is only assigned if the complication affects the function of the transplanted organ. Two codes are required to fully describe a transplant complication, the appropriate code from subcategory 996.8 and a secondary code that identifies the complication.

Pre-existing conditions or conditions that develop after the transplant are not coded as complications unless they affect the function of the transplanted organs. *See I.C.18.d.3) for transplant organ removal status. See I.C.2.i for malignant neoplasm associated with transplanted organ.*

(b) Kidney transplant complications

Patients who have undergone kidney transplant may still have some form of chronic kidney disease (CKD) because the kidney transplant may not fully restore kidney function. Code 996.81 should be assigned for documented complications of a kidney transplant, such as transplant failure or rejection or other transplant complication. Code 996.81 should not be assigned for post kidney transplant patients who have chronic kidney (CKD) unless a transplant complication such as transplant failure or rejection is documented. If the documentation is unclear as to whether the patient has a complication of the transplant, query the provider.

Conditions that affect the function of the transplanted kidney, other than CKD, should be assigned code 996.81, Complications of transplanted organ, Kidney, and a secondary code that identifies the complication.

For patients with CKD following a kidney transplant, but who do not have a complication such as failure or rejection, see section I.C.10.a.2, Chronic kidney disease and kidney transplant status.

3) Ventilator associated pneumonia

(a) Documentation of Ventilator associated pneumonia

As with all procedural or postprocedural complications, code assignment is based on the provider's documentation of the relationship between the condition and the procedure.

Code 997.31, Ventilator associated pneumonia, should be assigned only when the provider has documented ventilator associated pneumonia (VAP). An additional code to identify the organism (e.g., Pseudomonas aeruginosa, code 041.7) should also be assigned. Do not assign an additional code from categories 480-484 to identify the type of pneumonia.

Code 997.31 should not be assigned for cases where the patient has pneumonia and is on a mechanical ventilator but the provider has not specifically stated that the pneumonia is ventilator-associated pneumonia. If the documentation is unclear as to whether the patient has a pneumonia that is a complication attributable to the mechanical ventilator, query the provider.

(b) Patient admitted with pneumonia and develops VAP

A patient may be admitted with one type of pneumonia (e.g., code 481, Pneumococcal pneumonia) and subsequently develop VAP. In this instance, the principal diagnosis would be the appropriate code from categories 480-484 for the pneumonia diagnosed at the time of admission. Code 997.31, Ventilator associated neumonia, would be assigned as an additional diagnosis when the provider has also documented the presence of ventilator associated pneumonia.

g. SIRS due to Non-infectious Process

The systemic inflammatory response syndrome (SIRS) can develop as a result of certain non-infectious disease processes, such as trauma, malignant neoplasm, or pancreatitis. When SIRS is documented with a noninfectious condition, and no subsequent infection is documented, the code for the underlying condition, such as an injury, should be assigned, followed by code 995.93, Systemic inflammatory response syndrome due to noninfectious process without acute organ dysfunction, or 995.94, Systemic inflammatory response syndrome due to non-infectious process with acute organ dysfunction. If an acute organ dysfunction is documented, the appropriate code(s) for the associated acute organ dysfunction(s) should be assigned in addition to code 995.94. If acute organ dysfunction is documented, but it cannot be determined if the acute organ dysfunction is associated with SIRS or due to another condition (e.g., directly due to the trauma), the provider should be queried.

When the non-infectious condition has led to an infection that results in SIRS, *see Section I.C.Lb.12 for the guideline for sepsis and severe sepsis associated with a non-infectious process.*

18. Classification of Factors Influencing Health Status and Contact with Health Service (Supplemental V01-V91)

Note: The chapter specific guidelines provide additional information about the use of V codes for specified encounters.

a. Introduction

ICD-9-CM provides codes to deal with encounters for circumstances other than a disease or injury. The Supplementary Classification of Factors Influencing Health Status and Contact with Health Services

(V01.0 - V91.99) is provided to deal with occasions when circumstances other than a disease or injury (codes 001-999) are recorded as a diagnosis or problem.

There are four primary circumstances for the use of V codes:

1) A person who is not currently sick encounters the health services for some specific reason, such as to act as an organ donor, to receive prophylactic care, such as inoculations or health screenings, or to receive counseling on health related issues.

2) A person with a resolving disease or injury, or a chronic, long term condition requiring continuous care, encounters the health care system for specific aftercare of that disease or injury (e.g., dialysis for renal disease; chemotherapy for malignancy; cast change). A diagnosis/symptom code should be used whenever a current, acute, diagnosis is being treated or a sign or symptom is being studied.

3) Circumstances or problems influence a person's health status but are not in themselves a current illness or injury.

4) Newborns, to indicate birth status

b. V codes use in any healthcare setting

V codes are for use in any healthcare setting. V codes may be used as either a first listed (principal diagnosis code in the inpatient setting) or secondary code, depending on the circumstances of the encounter. Certain V codes may only be used as first listed, others only as secondary codes. *See Section I.C.18.e, V Codes That May Only be Principal/ First-Listed Diagnosis.*

c. V Codes indicate a reason for an encounter

They are not procedure codes. A corresponding procedure code must accompany a V code to describe the procedure performed.

d. Categories of V Codes

1) Contact/Exposure

Category V01 indicates contact with or exposure to communicable diseases. These codes are for patients who do not show any sign or symptom of a disease but have been exposed to it by close personal contact with an infected individual or are in an area where a disease is epidemic. These codes may be used as a first listed code to explain an encounter for testing, or, more commonly, as a secondary code to identify a potential risk.

Codes V15.84 – V15.86 describe contact with or (suspected) exposure to asbestos, potentially hazardous body fluids, and lead.

Subcategories V87.0 – V87.3 describe contact with or (suspected) exposure to hazardous metals, aromatic compounds, other potentially hazardous chemicals, and other potentially hazardous substances.

2) Inoculations and vaccinations

Categories V03-V06 are for encounters for inoculations and vaccinations. They indicate that a patient is being seen to receive a prophylactic inoculation against a disease. The injection itself must be represented by the appropriate procedure code. A code from V03-V06 may be used as a secondary code if the inoculation is given as a routine part of preventive health care, such as a well-baby visit.

3) Status

Status codes indicate that a patient is a carrier of a disease, has the sequelae or residual of a past disease or condition, or has another factor influencing a person's health status. This includes such things as the presence of prosthetic or mechanical devices resulting from past treatment. A status code is informative, because the status may affect the course of treatment and its outcome. A status code is distinct from a history code. The history code indicates that the patient no longer has the condition.

A status code should not be used with a diagnosis code from one of the body system chapters, if the diagnosis code includes the information provided by the status code. For example, code V42.1, Heart transplant status, should not be used with code 996.83, Complications of transplanted heart. The status code does not provide additional information. The complication code indicates that the patient is a heart transplant patient.

The status V codes/categories are:

V02   Carrier or suspected carrier of infectious diseases

Carrier status indicates that a person harbors the specific organisms of a disease without manifest symptoms and is capable of transmitting the infection

V07.5x Use of agents affecting estrogen receptors and estrogen level

This code indicates when a patient is receiving a drug that affects estrogen receptors and estrogen levels for prevention of cancer.

V08   Asymptomatic HIV infection status

This code indicates that a patient has tested positive for HIV but has manifested no signs or symptoms of the disease.

V09   Infection with drug-resistant microorganisms

This category indicates that a patient has an infection that is resistant to drug treatment. Sequence the infection code first.

V21   Constitutional states in development

V22.2   Pregnant state, incidental

This code is a secondary code only for use when the pregnancy is in no way complicating the reason for visit. Otherwise, a code from the obstetric chapter is required.

V26.5x Sterilization status

V42 Organ or tissue replaced by transplant

V43 Organ or tissue replaced by other means

V44 Artificial opening status

V45 Other postsurgical states

Assign code V45.87, Transplant organ removal status, to indicate that a transplanted organ has been previously removed. This code should not be assigned for the encounter in which the transplanted organ is removed. The complication necessitating removal of the transplant organ should be assigned for that encounter.

See section I.C17.f.2. for information on the coding of organ transplant complications.

Assign code V45.88, Status post administration of tPA (rtPA) in a different facility within the last 24 hours prior to admission to the current facility, as a secondary diagnosis when a patient is received by transfer into a facility and documentation indicates they were administered tissue plasminogen activator (tPA) within the last 24 hours prior to admission to the current facility.

This guideline applies even if the patient is still receiving the tPA at the time they are received into the current facility.

The appropriate code for the condition for which the tPA was administered (such as cerebrovascular disease or myocardial infarction) should be assigned first.

Code V45.88 is only applicable to the receiving facility record and not to the transferring facility record..

V46 Other dependence on machines

V49.6 Upper limb amputation status

V49.7 Lower limb amputation status

Note: Categories V42-V46, and subcategories V49.6, V49.7 are for use only if there are no complications or malfunctions of the organ or tissue replaced, the amputation site or the equipment on which the patient is dependent.

V49.81 Asymptomatic postmenopausal status (age-related) (natural)

V49.82 Dental sealant status

V49.83 Awaiting organ transplant status

V49.86 Do not resuscitate status

This code may be used when it is documented by the provider that a patient is on do not resuscitate status at any time during the stay.

V49.87 Physical restraint status

This code may be used when it is documented by the provider that a patient has been put in restraints during the current encounter. Please note that this code should not be reported when it is documented by the provider that a patient is temporarily restrained during a procedure.

V58.6x Long-term (current) drug use

Codes from this subcategory indicate a patient's continuous use of a prescribed drug (including such things as aspirin therapy) for the long-term treatment of a condition or for prophylactic use. It is not for use for patients who have addictions to drugs. This subcategory is not for use of medications for detoxification or maintenance programs to prevent withdrawal symptoms in patients with drug dependence (e.g., methadone maintenance for opiate dependence). Assign the appropriate code for the drug dependence instead.

Assign a code from subcategory V58.6, Long-term (current) drug use, if the patient is receiving a medication for an extended period as a prophylactic measure (such as for the prevention of deep vein thrombosis) or as treatment of a chronic condition (such as arthritis) or a disease requiring a lengthy course of treatment (such as cancer). Do not assign a code from subcategory V58.6 for medication being administered for a brief period of time to treat an acute illness or injury (such as a course of antibiotics to treat acute bronchitis).

V83 Genetic carrier status

Genetic carrier status indicates that a person carries a gene, associated with a particular disease, which may be passed to offspring who may develop that disease. The person does not have the disease and is not at risk of developing the disease.

V84 Genetic susceptibility status

Genetic susceptibility indicates that a person has a gene that increases the risk of that person developing the disease.

Codes from category V84, Genetic susceptibility to disease, should not be used as principal or first-listed codes. If the patient has the condition to which he/she is susceptible, and that condition is the reason for the encounter, the code for the current condition should be sequenced first. If the patient is being seen for follow-up after completed treatment for this condition, and the condition no longer exists, a follow-up code should be sequenced first, followed by the appropriate personal history and genetic susceptibility codes. If the purpose of the encounter is genetic counseling associated with procreative management, a code from subcategory V26.3, Genetic counseling and testing, should be assigned as the first-listed code, followed by a code from category V84. Additional codes should be assigned for any applicable family or personal history.

See Section I.C. 18.d.14 for information on prophylactic organ removal due to a genetic susceptibility.

V85   Body Mass Index (BMI)

V86   Estrogen receptor status

V88   Acquired absence of other organs and tissue

V90   Retained foreign body

4) History (of)

There are two types of history V codes, personal and family. Personal history codes explain a patient's past medical condition that no longer exists and is not receiving any treatment, but that has the potential for recurrence, and therefore may require continued monitoring. The exceptions to this general rule are category V14, Personal history of allergy to medicinal agents, and subcategory V15.0, Allergy, other than to medicinal agents. A person who has had an allergic episode to a substance or food in the past should always be considered allergic to the substance.

Family history codes are for use when a patient has a family member(s) who has had a particular disease that causes the patient to be at higher risk of also contracting the disease.

Personal history codes may be used in conjunction with follow-up codes and family history codes may be used in conjunction with screening codes to explain the need for a test or procedure. History codes are also acceptable on any medical record regardless of the reason for visit. A history of an illness, even if no longer present, is important information that may alter the type of treatment ordered.

The history V code categories are:

V10   Personal history of malignant neoplasm

V12   Personal history of certain other diseases

V13   Personal history of other diseases

> Except: V13.4, Personal history of arthritis, and subcategory V13.6, Personal history of congenital (corrected) malformations. These conditions are life-long so are not true history codes.

V14   Personal history of allergy to medicinal agents

V15   Other personal history presenting hazards to health

Except: Codes V15.7, Personal history of contraception; V15.84, Contact with and (suspected) exposure to asbestos; V15.85, Contact with and (suspected) exposure to potentially hazardous body fluids; and V15.86, Contact with and (suspected) exposure to lead.

V16   Family history of malignant neoplasm

V17   Family history of certain chronic disabling diseases

V18   Family history of certain other specific diseases

V19   Family history of other conditions

V87   Other specified personal exposures and history presenting hazards to health

Except: Subcategories V87.0, Contact with and (suspected) exposure to hazardous metals; V87.1, Contact with and (suspected) exposure to hazardous aromatic compounds; V87.2, Contact with and (suspected) exposure to other potentially hazardous chemicals; and V87.3, Contact with and (suspected) exposure to other potentially hazardous substances

5) Screening

Screening is the testing for disease or disease precursors in seemingly well individuals so that early detection and treatment can be provided for those who test positive for the disease. Screenings that are recommended for many subgroups in a population include: routine mammograms for women over 40, a fecal occult blood test for everyone over 50, an amniocentesis to rule out a fetal anomaly for pregnant women over 35, because the incidence of breast cancer and colon cancer in these subgroups is higher than in the general population, as is the incidence of Down's syndrome in older mothers.

The testing of a person to rule out or confirm a suspected diagnosis because the patient has some sign or symptom is a diagnostic examination, not a screening. In these cases, the sign or symptom is used to explain the reason for the test. A screening code may be a first listed code if the reason for the visit is specifically the screening exam. It may also be used as an additional code if the screening is done during an office visit for other health problems. A screening code is not necessary if the screening is inherent to a routine examination, such as a pap smear done during a routine pelvic examination.

Should a condition be discovered during the screening then the code for the condition may be assigned as an additional diagnosis.

The V code indicates that a screening exam is planned. A procedure code is required to confirm that the screening was performed.

The screening V code categories:

V28   Antenatal screening

V73-V82 Special screening examinations

6) Observation

There are three observation V code categories. They are for use in very limited circumstances when a person is being observed for a suspected condition that is ruled out. The observation codes are not for use if an injury or illness or any signs or symptoms related to the suspected condition are present. In such cases the diagnosis/symptom code is used with the corresponding E code to identify any external cause.

The observation codes are to be used as principal diagnosis only. The only exception to this is when the principal diagnosis is required to be a code from the V30, Live born infant, category. Then the V29 observation code is sequenced after the V30 code. Additional codes may be used in addition to the observation code but only if they are unrelated to the suspected condition being observed.

Codes from subcategory V89.0, Suspected maternal and fetal conditions not found, may either be used as a first listed or as an additional code assignment depending on the case. They are for use in very limited circumstances on a maternal record when an encounter is for a suspected maternal or fetal condition that is ruled out during that encounter (for example, a maternal or fetal condition may be suspected due to an abnormal test result). These codes should not be used when the condition is confirmed. In those cases, the confirmed condition should be coded. In addition, these codes are not for use if an illness or any signs or symptoms related to the suspected condition or problem are present. In such cases the diagnosis/symptom code is used.
Additional codes may be used in addition to the code from subcategory V89.0, but only if they are unrelated to the suspected condition being evaluated.

Codes from subcategory V89.0 may not be used for encounters for antenatal screening of mother. See Section I.C.18.d., Screening).

For encounters for suspected fetal condition that are inconclusive following testing and evaluation, assign the appropriate code from category 655, 656, 657 or 658.

The observation V code categories:

V29   Observation and evaluation of newborns for suspected condition not found

           For the birth encounter, a code from category V30 should be sequenced before the V29 code.

V71   Observation and evaluation for suspected condition not found

V89   Suspected maternal and fetal conditions not found

7) **Aftercare**

Aftercare visit codes cover situations when the initial treatment of a disease or injury has been performed and the patient requires continued care during the healing or recovery phase, or for the long-term consequences of the disease. The aftercare V code should not be used if treatment is directed at a current, acute disease or injury. The diagnosis code is to be used in these cases. Exceptions to this rule are codes V58.0, Radiotherapy, and codes from subcategory V58.1, Encounter for chemotherapy and immunotherapy for neoplastic conditions. These codes are to be first listed, followed by the diagnosis code when a patient's encounter is solely to receive radiation therapy or chemotherapy for the treatment of a neoplasm. Should a patient receive both chemotherapy and radiation therapy during the same encounter code V58.0 and V58.1 may be used together on a record with either one being sequenced first.

The aftercare codes are generally first listed to explain the specific reason for the encounter. An aftercare code may be used as an additional code when some type of aftercare is provided in addition to the reason for admission and no diagnosis code is applicable. An example of this would be the closure of a colostomy during an encounter for treatment of another condition.

Aftercare codes should be used in conjunction with any other aftercare codes or other diagnosis codes to provide better detail on the specifics of an aftercare encounter visit, unless otherwise directed by the classification. The sequencing of multiple aftercare codes is discretionary.

Certain aftercare V code categories need a secondary diagnosis code to describe the resolving condition or sequelae, for others, the condition is inherent in the code title.

Additional V code aftercare category terms include fitting and adjustment, and attention to artificial openings.

Status V codes may be used with aftercare V codes to indicate the nature of the aftercare. For example code V45.81, Aortocoronary bypass status, may be used with code V58.73, Aftercare following surgery of the circulatory system, NEC, to indicate the surgery for which the aftercare is being performed. Also, a transplant status code may be used following code V58.44, Aftercare following organ transplant, to identify the organ transplanted. A status code should not be used when the aftercare code indicates the type of status, such as using V55.0, Attention to tracheostomy with V44.0, Tracheostomy status.*See Section I. B.16 Admissions/Encounter for Rehabilitation*

The aftercare V category/codes:

V51.0   Encounter for breast reconstruction following mastectomy

V52   Fitting and adjustment of prosthetic device and implant

V53   Fitting and adjustment of other device

V54   Other orthopedic aftercare

V55   Attention to artificial openings

V56   Encounter for dialysis and dialysis catheter care

V57   Care involving the use of rehabilitation procedures

V58.0   Radiotherapy

V58.11 Encounter for antineoplastic chemotherapy

V58.12 Encounter for antineoplastic immunotherapy

V58.3x Attention to dressings and sutures

V58.41 Encounter for planned post-operative wound closure

V58.42 Aftercare, surgery, neoplasm

V58.43 Aftercare, surgery, trauma

V58.44 Aftercare involving organ transplant

V58.49 Other specified aftercare following surgery

V58.7x Aftercare following surgery

V58.81 Fitting and adjustment of vascular catheter

V58.82 Fitting and adjustment of non-vascular catheter

V58.83 Monitoring therapeutic drug

V58.89 Other specified aftercare

8) Follow-up

The follow-up codes are used to explain continuing surveillance following completed treatment of a disease, condition, or injury. They imply that the condition has been fully treated and no longer exists. They should not be confused with aftercare codes that explain current treatment for a healing condition or its sequelae. Follow-up codes may be used in conjunction with history codes to provide the full picture of the healed condition and its treatment. The follow-up code is sequenced first, followed by the history code.

A follow-up code may be used to explain repeated visits. Should a condition be found to have recurred on the follow-up visit, then the diagnosis code should be used in place of the follow-up code. The follow-up V code categories:

V24   Postpartum care and evaluation

V67   Follow-up examination

9) Donor

Category V59 is the donor codes. They are used for living individuals who are donating blood or other body tissue. These codes are only for individuals donating for others, not for self donations. They are not for use to identify cadaveric donations.

10) Counseling

Counseling V codes are used when a patient or family member receives assistance in the aftermath of an illness or injury, or when support is required in coping with family or social problems. They are not necessary for use in conjunction with a diagnosis code when the counseling component of care is considered integral to standard treatment.

The counseling V categories/codes:

V25.0   General counseling and advice for contraceptive management

V26.3   Genetic counseling

V26.4   General counseling and advice for procreative management

V61.x   Other family circumstances

V65.1   Person consulted on behalf of another person

V65.3   Dietary surveillance and counseling

V65.4   Other counseling, not elsewhere classified

11) Obstetrics and related conditions

See Section I.C.11., the Obstetrics guidelines for further instruction on the use of these codes.

V codes for pregnancy are for use in those circumstances when none of the problems or complications included in the codes from the Obstetrics chapter exist (a routine prenatal visit or postpartum care). Codes V22.0, Supervision of normal first pregnancy, and V22.1, Supervision of other normal pregnancy, are always first listed and are not to be used with any other code from the OB chapter.

The outcome of delivery, category V27, should be included on all maternal delivery records. It is always a secondary code.

V codes for family planning (contraceptive) or procreative management and counseling should be included on an obstetric record either during the pregnancy or the postpartum stage, if applicable.

Obstetrics and related conditions V code categories:

V22   Normal pregnancy

V23   Supervision of high-risk pregnancy

Except: V23.2, Pregnancy with history of abortion. Code 646.3, Recurrent pregnancy loss, from the OB chapter is required to indicate a history of abortion during a pregnancy.

V24   Postpartum care and evaluation

V25   Encounter for contraceptive management

Except V25.0x
(See Section I.C.18.d.11, Counseling)

V26   Procreative management

Except V26.5x, Sterilization status, V26.3 and V26.4
(See Section I.C.18.d.11., Counseling)

V27   Outcome of delivery

V28   Antenatal screening
(See Section I.C.18.d.6., Screening)

V91   Multiple gestation placenta status

12) Newborn, infant and child

See Section I.C.15, the Newborn guidelines for further instruction on the use of these codes.

Newborn V code categories:

V20   Health supervision of infant or child

V29   Observation and evaluation of newborns for suspected condition not found

(See Section I.C.18.d.7, Observation)

V30-V39 Liveborn infant according to type of birth

13) Routine and administrative examinations

The V codes allow for the description of encounters for routine examinations, such as, a general check-up, or examinations for administrative purposes, such as a pre-employment physical. The codes are not to be used if the examination is for diagnosis of a suspected condition or for treatment purposes. In such cases the diagnosis code is used. During a routine exam, should a diagnosis or condition be discovered, it should be coded as an additional code. Pre-existing and chronic conditions and history codes may also be included as additional codes as long as the examination is for administrative purposes and not focused on any particular condition.

Pre-operative examination and pre-procedural laboratory examination V codes are for use only in those situations when a patient is being cleared for a procedure or surgery and no treatment is given.

The V codes categories/code for routine and administrative examinations:

V20.2   Routine infant or child health check

Any injections given should have a corresponding procedure code.

V70   General medical examination

V72   Special investigations and examinations

Codes V72.5 and V72.62 may be used if the reason for the patient encounter is for routine laboratory/radiology testing in the absence of any signs, symptoms, or associated diagnosis. If routine testing is performed during the same encounter as a test to evaluate a sign, symptom, or diagnosis, it is appropriate to assign both the V code and the code describing the reason for the non-routine test.

14) Miscellaneous V codes

The miscellaneous V codes capture a number of other health care encounters that do not fall into one of the other categories. Certain of these codes identify the reason for the encounter, others are for use as additional codes that provide useful information on circumstances that may affect a patient's care and treatment.

Prophylactic Organ Removal

For encounters specifically for prophylactic removal of breasts, ovaries, or another organ due to a genetic susceptibility to cancer or a family history of cancer, the principal or first listed code should be a code from subcategory V50.4, Prophylactic organ removal, followed by the appropriate genetic susceptibility code and the appropriate family history code.

If the patient has a malignancy of one site and is having prophylactic removal at another site to prevent either a new primary malignancy or metastatic disease, a code for the malignancy should also be assigned in addition to a code from subcategory V50.4. A V50.4 code should not be assigned if the patient is having organ removal for treatment of a malignancy, such as the removal of the testes for the treatment of prostate cancer.

Miscellaneous V code categories/codes:

V07   Need for isolation and other prophylactic or treatment measures

Except V07.5X, Use of agents affecting estrogen receptors and estrogen levels

V40.31   Wandering in diseases classified elsewhere

V50   Elective surgery for purposes other than remedying health states

V58.5 Orthodontics

V60   Housing, household, and economic circumstances

V62   Other psychosocial circumstances

V63   Unavailability of other medical facilities for care

V64   Persons encountering health services for specific procedures, not carried out

V66   Convalescence and Palliative Care

V68   Encounters for administrative purposes

V69   Problems related to lifestyle

15) Nonspecific V codes

Certain V codes are so non-specific, or potentially redundant with other codes in the classification, that there can be little justification for their use in the inpatient setting. Their use in the outpatient setting should be limited to those instances when there is no further documentation to permit more precise coding. Otherwise, any sign or symptom or any other reason for visit that is captured in another code should be used.

Nonspecific V code categories/codes:

V11   Personal history of mental disorder

       A code from the mental disorders chapter, with an in remission fifth-digit, should be used.

V13.4 Personal history of arthritis

V13.6 Personal history of congenital malformations

V15.7 Personal history of contraception

V23.2 Pregnancy with history of abortion

V40   Mental and behavioral problems
       Exception: V40.31 Wandering in diseases classified elsewhereMental and behavioral problems

V41   Problems with special senses and other special functions

V47   Other problems with internal organs

V48   Problems with head, neck, and trunk

V49   Problems with limbs and other problems
       Exceptions:

       V49.6   Upper limb amputation status

       V49.7   Lower limb amputation status

> V49.81 Asymptomatic postmenopausal status (age-related) (natural)
>
> V49.82 Dental sealant status
>
> V49.83 Awaiting organ transplant status
>
> V49.86 Do not resuscitate status
>
> V49.87 Physical restraints status
>
> V51.8 Other aftercare involving the use of plastic surgery
>
> V58.2 Blood transfusion, without reported diagnosis
>
> V58.9 Unspecified aftercare
>
> *See Section IV.K. and Section IV.L. of the Outpatient guidelines.*

e. V Codes That May Only be Principal/First-Listed Diagnosis

The list of V codes/categories below may only be reported as the principal/first-listed diagnosis, except when there are multiple encounters on the same day and the medical records for the encounters are combined or when there is more than one V code that meets the definition of principal diagnosis (e.g., a patient is admitted to home healthcare for both aftercare and rehabilitation and they equally meet the definition of principal diagnosis). These codes should not be reported if they do not meet the definition of principal or first-listed diagnosis.

See Section II and Section IV. A for information on selection of principal and first-listed diagnosis.

See Section II. C for information on two or more diagnoses that equally meet the definition for principal diagnosis.

V20.X Health supervision of infant or child

V22.0 Supervision of normal first pregnancy

V22.1 Supervision of other normal pregnancy

V24.X Postpartum care and examination

V26.81 Encounter for assisted reproductive fertility procedure cycle

V26.82 Encounter for fertility preservation procedure

V30.X Single liveborn

V31.X Twin, mate liveborn

V32.X Twin, mate stillborn

V33.X Twin, unspecified

V34.X Other multiple, mates all liveborn

V35.X Other multiple, mates all stillborn

V36.X Other multiple, mates live- and stillborn

V37.X Other multiple, unspecified

V39.X Unspecified

V46.12 Encounter for respirator dependence during power failure

V46.13 Encounter for weaning from respirator [ventilator]

V51.0 Encounter for breast reconstruction following mastectomy

V56.0 Extracorporeal dialysis

V57.X Care involving use of rehabilitation procedures

V58.0 Radiotherapy

V58.11 Encounter for antineoplastic chemotherapy

V58.12 Encounter for antineoplastic immunotherapy

V59.X Donors

V66.0 Convalescence and palliative care following surgery

V66.1 Convalescence and palliative care following radiotherapy

V66.2 Convalescence and palliative care following chemotherapy

V66.3 Convalescence and palliative care following psychotherapy and other treatment for mental disorder

V66.4 Convalescence and palliative care following treatment of fracture

V66.5 Convalescence and palliative care following other treatment

V66.6 Convalescence and palliative care following combined treatment

V66.9 Unspecified convalescence

V68.X Encounters for administrative purposes

V70.0 Routine general medical examination at a health care facility

V70.1 General psychiatric examination, requested by the authority

V70.2 General psychiatric examination, other and unspecified

V70.3 Other medical examination for administrative purposes

V70.4 Examination for medicolegal reasons

V70.5 Health examination of defined subpopulations

V70.6   Health examination in population surveys

V70.8   Other specified general medical examinations

V70.9   Unspecified general medical examination

V71.X   Observation and evaluation for suspected conditions not found

19. Supplemental Classification of External Causes of Injury and Poisoning (E-codes, E800-E999)

Introduction

These guidelines are provided for those who are currently collecting E codes in order that there will be standardization in the process. If your institution plans to begin collecting E codes, these guidelines are to be applied. The use of E codes is supplemental to the application of ICD-9-CM diagnosis codes.

External causes of injury and poisoning codes (categories E000 and E800-E999) are intended to provide data for injury research and evaluation of injury prevention strategies. Activity codes (categories E001-E030) are intended to be used to describe the activity of a person seeking care for injuries as well as other health conditions, when the injury or other health condition resulted from an activity or the activity contributed to a condition. E codes capture how the injury, poisoning, or adverse effect happened (cause), the intent (unintentional or accidental; or intentional, such as suicide or assault), the person's status (e.g. civilian, military), the associated activity and the place where the event occurred.

Some major categories of E codes include:

> transport accidents
> poisoning and adverse effects of drugs, medicinal substances and biologicals
> accidental falls
> accidents caused by fire and flames
> accidents due to natural and environmental factors
> late effects of accidents, assaults or self injury
> assaults or purposely inflicted injury
> suicide or self inflicted injury

These guidelines apply for the coding and collection of E codes from records in hospitals, outpatient clinics, emergency departments, other ambulatory care settings and provider offices, and nonacute care settings, except when other specific guidelines apply.

a.   General E Code Coding Guidelines

1)   Used with any code in the range of 001-V91

An E code from categories E800-E999 may be used with any code in the range of 001-V91, which indicates an injury, poisoning, or adverse effect due to an external cause.

An activity E code (categories E001-E030) may be used with any code in the range of 001-V91 that indicates an injury, or other health condition that resulted from an activity, or the activity contributed to a condition.

2) Assign the appropriate E code for all initial treatment

Assign the appropriate E code for the initial encounter of an injury, poisoning, or adverse effect of drugs, not for subsequent treatment.

External cause of injury codes (E-codes) may be assigned while the acute fracture codes are still applicable.

See Section I.C.17.b.1 for coding of acute fractures.

3) Use the full range of E codes

Use the full range of E codes (E800 - E999) to completely describe the cause, the intent and the place of occurrence, if applicable, for all injuries, poisonings, and adverse effects of drugs.

See a.1.), j.), and k.) in this section for information on the use of status and activity E codes.

4) Assign as many E codes as necessary

Assign as many E codes as necessary to fully explain each cause.

5) The selection of the appropriate E code

The selection of the appropriate E code is guided by the Index to External Causes, which is located after the alphabetical index to diseases and by Inclusion and Exclusion notes in the Tabular List.

6) E code can never be a principal diagnosis

An E code can never be a principal (first listed) diagnosis.

7) External cause code(s) with systemic inflammatory response syndrome (SIRS)

An external cause code is not appropriate with a code from subcategory 995.9, unless the patient also has another condition for which an E code would be appropriate (such as an injury, poisoning, or adverse effect of drugs.

8) Multiple Cause E Code Coding Guidelines

More than one E-code is required to fully describe the external cause of an illness, injury or poisoning. The assignment of E-codes should be sequenced in the following priority:

If two or more events cause separate injuries, an E code should be assigned for each cause. The first listed E code will be selected in the following order:

E codes for child and adult abuse take priority over all other E codes.

See Section I.C.19.e., Child and Adult abuse guidelines.

E codes for terrorism events take priority over all other E codes except child and adult abuse.

E codes for cataclysmic events take priority over all other E codes except child and adult abuse and terrorism.

E codes for transport accidents take priority over all other E codes except cataclysmic events, child and adult abuse and terrorism. Activity and external cause status codes are assigned following all causal (intent) E codes.

The first-listed E code should correspond to the cause of the most serious diagnosis due to an assault, accident, or self-harm, following the order of hierarchy listed above.

9) If the reporting format limits the number of E codes

If the reporting format limits the number of E codes that can be used in reporting clinical data, report the code for the cause/intent most related to the principal diagnosis. If the format permits capture of additional E codes, the cause/intent, including medical misadventures, of the additional events should be reported rather than the codes for place, activity or external status.

b. Place of Occurrence Guideline

Use an additional code from category E849 to indicate the Place of Occurrence. The Place of Occurrence describes the place where the event occurred and not the patient's activity at the time of the event. Do not use E849.9 if the place of occurrence is not stated.

c. Adverse Effects of Drugs, Medicinal and Biological Substances Guidelines

1) Do not code directly from the Table of Drugs

Do not code directly from the Table of Drugs and Chemicals. Always refer back to the Tabular List.

2) Use as many codes as necessary to describe

Use as many codes as necessary to describe completely all drugs, medicinal or biological substances.

If the reporting format limits the number of E codes, and there are different fourth digit codes in the same three digit category, use the code for "Other specified" of that category of drugs, medicinal or biological substances. If there is no "Other specified" code in that category, use the appropriate "Unspecified" code in that category.

If the reporting format limits the number of E codes, and the codes are in different three digit categories, assign the appropriate E code for other multiple drugs and medicinal substances.

3) If the same E code would describe the causative agent

If the same E code would describe the causative agent for more than one adverse reaction, assign the code only once.

4) If two or more drugs, medicinal or biological substances

If two or more drugs, medicinal or biological substances are reported, code each individually unless the combination code is listed in the Table of Drugs and Chemicals. In that case, assign the E code for the combination.

5) When a reaction results from the interaction of a drug(s)

When a reaction results from the interaction of a drug(s) and alcohol, use poisoning codes and E codes for both.

6) Codes from the E930-E949 series

Codes from the E930-E949 series must be used to identify the causative substance for an adverse effect of drug, medicinal and biological substances, correctly prescribed and properly administered. The effect, such as tachycardia, delirium, gastrointestinal hemorrhaging, vomiting, hypokalemia, hepatitis, renal failure, or respiratory failure, is coded and followed by the appropriate code from the E930-E949 series.

d. Child and Adult Abuse Guideline

1) Intentional injury

When the cause of an injury or neglect is intentional child or adult abuse, the first listed E code should be assigned from categories E960-E968, Homicide and injury purposely inflicted by other persons, (except category E967). An E code from category E967, Child and adult battering and other maltreatment, should be added as an additional code to identify the perpetrator, if known.

2) Accidental intent

In cases of neglect when the intent is determined to be accidental E code E904.0, Abandonment or neglect of infant and helpless person, should be the first listed E code.

e. Unknown or Suspected Intent Guideline

1) If the intent (accident, self-harm, assault) of the cause of an injury or poisoning is unknown

If the intent (accident, self-harm, assault) of the cause of an injury or poisoning is unknown or unspecified, code the intent as undetermined E980-E989.

2) If the intent (accident, self-harm, assault) of the cause of an injury or poisoning is questionable

If the intent (accident, self-harm, assault) of the cause of an injury or poisoning is questionable, probable or suspected, code the intent as undetermined E980-E989.

f. Undetermined Cause

When the intent of an injury or poisoning is known, but the cause is unknown, use codes: E928.9, Unspecified accident, E958.9, Suicide and self-inflicted injury by unspecified means, and E968.9, Assault by unspecified means.

These E codes should rarely be used, as the documentation in the medical record, in both the inpatient outpatient and other settings, should normally provide sufficient detail to determine the cause of the injury.

g. Late Effects of External Cause Guidelines

1) Late effect E codes

Late effect E codes exist for injuries and poisonings but not for adverse effects of drugs, misadventures and surgical complications.

2) Late effect E codes (E929, E959, E969, E977, E989, or E999.1)

A late effect E code (E929, E959, E969, E977, E989, or E999.1) should be used with any report of a late effect or sequela resulting from a previous injury or poisoning (905-909).

3) Late effect E code with a related current injury

A late effect E code should never be used with a related current nature of injury code.

4) Use of late effect E codes for subsequent visits

Use a late effect E code for subsequent visits when a late effect of the initial injury or poisoning is being treated. There is no late effect E code for adverse effects of drugs.

Do not use a late effect E code for subsequent visits for follow-up care (e.g., to assess healing, to receive rehabilitative therapy) of the injury or poisoning when no late effect of the injury has been documented.

h. Misadventures and Complications of Care Guidelines

1) Code range E870-E876

Assign a code in the range of E870-E876 if misadventures are stated by the provider. When applying the E code guidelines pertaining to sequencing, these E codes are considered causal codes.

2) Code range E878-E879

Assign a code in the range of E878-E879 if the provider attributes an abnormal reaction or later complication to a surgical or medical procedure, but does not mention misadventure at the time of the procedure as the cause of the reaction.

i. Terrorism Guidelines

1) Cause of injury identified by the Federal Government (FBI) as terrorism

When the cause of an injury is identified by the Federal Government (FBI) as terrorism, the first-listed E-code should be a code from category E979, Terrorism. The definition of terrorism employed by the FBI is found at the inclusion note at E979. The terrorism E-code is the only E-code that should be assigned. Additional E codes from the assault categories should not be assigned.

2) Cause of an injury is suspected to be the result of terrorism

When the cause of an injury is suspected to be the result of terrorism a code from category E979 should not be assigned. Assign a code in the range of E codes based circumstances on the documentation of intent and mechanism.

3) Code E979.9, Terrorism, secondary effects

Assign code E979.9, Terrorism, secondary effects, for conditions occurring subsequent to the terrorist event. This code should not be assigned for conditions that are due to the initial terrorist act.

4) Statistical tabulation of terrorism codes

For statistical purposes these codes will be tabulated within the category for assault, expanding the current category from E960-E969 to include E979 and E999.1.

j. Activity Code Guidelines

Assign a code from category E001-E030 to describe the activity that caused or contributed to the injury or other health condition.

Unlike other E codes, activity E codes may be assigned to indicate a health condition (not just injuries) resulted from an activity, or the activity contributed to the condition. The activity codes are not applicable to poisonings, adverse effects, misadventures or late effects.

Do not assign E030, Unspecified activity, if the activity is not stated.

k. External cause status

A code from category E000, External cause status, should be assigned whenever any other E code is assigned for an encounter, including an Activity E code, except for the events noted below. Assign a code from category E000, External cause status, to indicate the work status of the person at the time the event occurred. The status code indicates whether the event occurred during military activity, whether a non-military person was at work, whether an individual including a student or volunteer was involved in a non-work activity at the time of the causal event.

A code from E000, External cause status, should be assigned, when applicable, with other external cause codes, such as transport accidents and falls. The external cause status codes are not applicable to poisonings, adverse effects, misadventures or late effects.

Do not assign a code from category E000 if no other E codes (cause, activity) are applicable for the encounter.

Do not assign code E000.9, Unspecified external cause status, if the status is not stated.

SECTION II. SELECTION OF PRINCIPAL DIAGNOSIS

The circumstances of inpatient admission always govern the selection of principal diagnosis. The principal diagnosis is defined in the Uniform Hospital Discharge Data Set (UHDDS) as "that condition established after study to be chiefly responsible for occasioning the admission of the patient to the hospital for care."

The UHDDS definitions are used by hospitals to report inpatient data elements in a standardized manner. These data elements and their definitions can be found in the July 31, 1985, Federal Register (Vol. 50, No, 147), pp. 31038-40.

Since that time the application of the UHDDS definitions has been expanded to include all non-outpatient settings (acute care, short term, long term care and psychiatric hospitals; home health agencies; rehab facilities; nursing homes, etc).

In determining principal diagnosis the coding conventions in the ICD-9-CM, Volumes I and II take precedence over these official coding guidelines. (See Section I. A., Conventions for the ICD-9-CM)

The importance of consistent, complete documentation in the medical record cannot be overemphasized. Without such documentation the application of all coding guidelines is a difficult, if not impossible, task.

A. Codes for symptoms, signs, and ill-defined conditions

Codes for symptoms, signs, and ill-defined conditions from Chapter 16 are not to be used as principal diagnosis when a related definitive diagnosis has been established.

B. Two or more interrelated conditions, each potentially meeting the definition for principal diagnosis.

When there are two or more interrelated conditions (such as diseases in the same ICD-9-CM chapter or manifestations characteristically associated with a certain disease) potentially meeting the definition of principal diagnosis, either condition may be sequenced first, unless the circumstances of the admission, the therapy provided, the Tabular List, or the Alphabetic Index indicate otherwise.

C. Two or more diagnoses that equally meet the definition for principal diagnosis

In the unusual instance when two or more diagnoses equally meet the criteria for principal diagnosis as determined by the circumstances of admission, diagnostic workup and/or therapy provided, and the Alphabetic Index, Tabular List, or another coding guidelines does not provide sequencing direction, any one of the diagnoses may be sequenced first.

D. Two or more comparative or contrasting conditions.

In those rare instances when two or more contrasting or comparative diagnoses are documented as "either/or" (or similar terminology), they are coded as if the diagnoses were confirmed and the diagnoses are sequenced according to the circumstances of the admission. If no further determination can be made as to which diagnosis should be principal, either diagnosis may be sequenced first.

E. A symptom(s) followed by contrasting/comparative diagnoses

When a symptom(s) is followed by contrasting/comparative diagnoses, the symptom code is sequenced first. All the contrasting/comparative diagnoses should be coded as additional diagnoses.

F. Original treatment plan not carried out

Sequence as the principal diagnosis the condition, which after study occasioned the admission to the hospital, even though treatment may not have been carried out due to unforeseen circumstances.

G. Complications of surgery and other medical care

When the admission is for treatment of a complication resulting from surgery or other medical care, the complication code is sequenced as the principal diagnosis. If the complication is classified to the 996-999 series and the code lacks the necessary specificity in describing the complication, an additional code for the specific complication should be assigned.

H. Uncertain Diagnosis

If the diagnosis documented at the time of discharge is qualified as "probable", "suspected", "likely", "questionable", "possible", or "still to be ruled out", or other similar terms indicating uncertainty, code the condition as if it existed or was established. The bases for these guidelines are the diagnostic workup, arrangements for further workup or observation, and initial therapeutic approach that correspond most closely with the established diagnosis.

Note: This guideline is applicable only to inpatient admissions to short-term, acute, long-term care and psychiatric hospitals.

I. Admission from Observation Unit

1. Admission Following Medical Observation

When a patient is admitted to an observation unit for a medical condition, which either worsens or does not improve, and is subsequently admitted as an inpatient of the same hospital for this same medical condition, the principal diagnosis would be the medical condition which led to the hospital admission.

2. Admission Following Post-Operative Observation

When a patient is admitted to an observation unit to monitor a condition (or complication) that develops following outpatient surgery, and then is subsequently admitted as an inpatient of the same hospital, hospitals should apply the Uniform Hospital Discharge Data Set (UHDDS) definition of principal diagnosis as "that condition established after study to be chiefly responsible for occasioning the admission of the patient to the hospital for care."

J. Admission from Outpatient Surgery

When a patient receives surgery in the hospital's outpatient surgery department and is subsequently admitted for continuing inpatient care at the same hospital, the following guidelines should be followed in selecting the principal diagnosis for the inpatient admission:

- If the reason for the inpatient admission is a complication, assign the complication as the principal diagnosis.

- If no complication, or other condition, is documented as the reason for the inpatient admission, assign the reason for the outpatient surgery as the principal diagnosis.

- If the reason for the inpatient admission is another condition unrelated to the surgery, assign the unrelated condition as the principal diagnosis.

SECTION III. REPORTING ADDITIONAL DIAGNOSES

General Rules For Other (Additional) Diagnoses

For reporting purposes the definition for "other diagnoses" is interpreted as additional conditions that affect patient care in terms of requiring:

clinical evaluation; or
therapeutic treatment; or
diagnostic procedures; or
extended length of hospital stay; or
increased nursing care and/or monitoring.

The UHDDS item #11-b defines Other Diagnoses as "all conditions that coexist at the time of admission, that develop subsequently, or that affect the treatment received and/or the length of stay. Diagnoses that relate to an earlier episode which have no bearing on the current hospital stay are to be excluded." UHDDS definitions apply to inpatients in acute care, short-term, long term care and psychiatric hospital setting. The UHDDS definitions are used by acute care short- term hospitals to report inpatient data elements in a standardized manner. These data elements and their definitions can be found in the July 31, 1985, Federal Register (Vol. 50, No, 147), pp. 31038-40.

Since that time the application of the UHDDS definitions has been expanded to include all non-outpatient settings (acute care, short term, long term care and psychiatric hospitals; home health agencies; rehab facilities; nursing homes, etc).

The following guidelines are to be applied in designating "other diagnoses" when neither the Alphabetic Index nor the Tabular List in ICD-9-CM provide direction. The listing of the diagnoses in the patient record is the responsibility of the attending provider.

A. Previous conditions

If the provider has included a diagnosis in the final diagnostic statement, such as the discharge summary or the face sheet, it should ordinarily be coded. Some providers include in the diagnostic statement resolved conditions or diagnoses and status-post procedures from previous admission that have no bearing on the current stay. Such conditions are not to be reported and are coded only if required by hospital policy.

However, history codes (V10-V19) may be used as secondary codes if the historical condition or family history has an impact on current care or influences treatment.

B. Abnormal findings

Abnormal findings (laboratory, x-ray, pathologic, and other diagnostic results) are not coded and reported unless the provider indicates their clinical significance. If the findings are outside the normal range and the attending provider has ordered other tests to evaluate the condition or prescribed treatment, it is appropriate to ask the provider whether the abnormal finding should be added.

Please note: This differs from the coding practices in the outpatient setting for coding encounters for diagnostic tests that have been interpreted by a provider.

C. Uncertain Diagnosis

If the diagnosis documented at the time of discharge is qualified as "probable", "suspected", "likely", "questionable", "possible", or "still to be ruled out" or other similar terms indicating uncertainty, code the condition as if it existed or was established. The bases for these guidelines are the diagnostic workup, arrangements for further workup or observation, and initial therapeutic approach that correspond most closely with the established diagnosis.

Note: This guideline is applicable only to inpatient admissions to short-term, acute, long-term care and psychiatric hospitals.

SECTION IV. DIAGNOSTIC CODING AND REPORTING GUIDELINES FOR OUTPATIENT SERVICES

These coding guidelines for outpatient diagnoses have been approved for use by hospitals/providers in coding and reporting hospital-based outpatient services and provider-based office visits.

Information about the use of certain abbreviations, punctuation, symbols, and other conventions used in the ICD-9-CM Tabular List (code numbers and titles), can be found in Section IA of these guidelines, under "Conventions Used in the Tabular List." Information about the correct sequence to use in finding a code is also described in Section I.

The terms encounter and visit are often used interchangeably in describing outpatient service contacts and, therefore, appear together in these guidelines without distinguishing one from the other.

Though the conventions and general guidelines apply to all settings, coding guidelines for outpatient and provider reporting of diagnoses will vary in a number of instances from those for inpatient diagnoses, recognizing that:

> The Uniform Hospital Discharge Data Set (UHDDS) definition of principal diagnosis applies only to inpatients in acute, short-term, long-term care and psychiatric hospitals.

> Coding guidelines for inconclusive diagnoses (probable, suspected, rule out, etc.) were developed for inpatient reporting and do not apply to outpatients.

A. Selection of first-listed condition

In the outpatient setting, the term first-listed diagnosis is used in lieu of principal diagnosis.

In determining the first-listed diagnosis the coding conventions of ICD-9-CM, as well as the general and disease specific guidelines take precedence over the outpatient guidelines.

Diagnoses often are not established at the time of the initial encounter/visit. It may take two or more visits before the diagnosis is confirmed.

The most critical rule involves beginning the search for the correct code assignment through the Alphabetic Index. Never begin searching initially in the Tabular List as this will lead to coding errors.

1. Outpatient Surgery

When a patient presents for outpatient surgery, code the reason for the surgery as the first-listed diagnosis (reason for the encounter), even if the surgery is not performed due to a contraindication.

2. Observation Stay

When a patient is admitted for observation for a medical condition, assign a code for the medical condition as the first-listed diagnosis.

When a patient presents for outpatient surgery and develops complications requiring admission to observation, code the reason for the surgery as the first reported diagnosis (reason for the encounter), followed by codes for the complications as secondary diagnoses.

B. Codes from 001.0 through V91.99

The appropriate code or codes from 001.0 through V91.99 must be used to identify diagnoses, symptoms, conditions, problems, complaints, or other reason(s) for the encounter/visit.

C. Accurate reporting of ICD-9-CM diagnosis codes

For accurate reporting of ICD-9-CM diagnosis codes, the documentation should describe the patient's condition, using terminology which includes specific diagnoses as well as symptoms, problems, or reasons for the encounter. There are ICD-9-CM codes to describe all of these.

D. Selection of codes 001.0 through 999.9

The selection of codes 001.0 through 999.9 will frequently be used to describe the reason for the encounter. These codes are from the section of ICD-9-CM for the classification of diseases and injuries (e.g. infectious and parasitic diseases; neoplasms; symptoms, signs, and ill-defined conditions, etc.).

E. Codes that describe symptoms and signs

Codes that describe symptoms and signs, as opposed to diagnoses, are acceptable for reporting purposes when a diagnosis has not been established (confirmed) by the provider. Chapter 16 of ICD-9-CM, Symptoms, Signs, and Ill-defined conditions (codes 780.0-799.9) contain many, but not all codes for symptoms.

F. Encounters for circumstances other than a disease or injury

ICD-9-CM provides codes to deal with encounters for circumstances other than a disease or injury. The Supplementary Classification of factors Influencing Health Status and Contact with Health Services (V01.0-V91.99) is provided to deal with occasions when circumstances other than a disease or injury are recorded as diagnosis or problems. See Section I.C. 18for information on V-codes.

G. Level of Detail in Coding

1. ICD-9-CM codes with 3, 4, or 5 digits

ICD-9-CM is composed of codes with either 3, 4, or 5 digits. Codes with three digits are included in ICD-9-CM as the heading of a category of codes that may be further subdivided by the use of fourth and/or fifth digits, which provide greater specificity.

2. Use of full number of digits required for a code

A three-digit code is to be used only if it is not further subdivided. Where fourth-digit subcategories and/or fifth-digit subclassifications are provided, they must be assigned. A code is invalid if it has not been coded to the full number of digits required for that code.

See also discussion under Section I.b.3., General Coding Guidelines, Level of Detail in Coding.

H. ICD-9-CM code for the diagnosis, condition, problem, or other reason for encounter/visit

List first the ICD-9-CM code for the diagnosis, condition, problem, or other reason for encounter/visit shown in the medical record to be chiefly responsible for the services provided. List additional codes that describe any coexisting conditions. In some cases the first-listed diagnosis may be a symptom when a diagnosis has not been established (confirmed) by the physician.

I. Uncertain diagnosis

Do not code diagnoses documented as "probable", "suspected," "questionable," "rule out," or "working diagnosis" or other similar terms indicating uncertainty. Rather, code the condition(s) to the highest degree of certainty for that encounter/visit, such as symptoms, signs, abnormal test results, or other reason for the visit.

Please note: This differs from the coding practices used by short-term, acute care, long-term care and psychiatric hospitals.

J. Chronic diseases

Chronic diseases treated on an ongoing basis may be coded and reported as many times as the patient receives treatment and care for the condition(s)

K. Code all documented conditions that coexist

Code all documented conditions that coexist at the time of the encounter/visit, and require or affect patient care treatment or management. Do not code conditions that were previously treated and no longer exist. However, history codes (V10-V19) may be used as secondary codes if the historical condition or family history has an impact on current care or influences treatment.

L. Patients receiving diagnostic services only

For patients receiving diagnostic services only during an encounter/visit, sequence first the diagnosis, condition, problem, or other reason for encounter/visit shown in the medical record to be chiefly responsible for the outpatient services provided during the encounter/visit. Codes for other diagnoses (e.g., chronic conditions) may be sequenced as additional diagnoses.

For encounters for routine laboratory/radiology testing in the absence of any signs, symptoms, or associated diagnosis, assign V72.5 and a code from subcategory V72.6. If routine testing is performed during the same encounter as a test to evaluate a sign, symptom, or diagnosis, it is appropriate to assign both the V code and the code describing the reason for the non-routine test.

For outpatient encounters for diagnostic tests that have been interpreted by a physician, and the final report is available at the time of coding, code any confirmed or definitive diagnosis(es) documented in the interpretation. Do not code related signs and symptoms as additional diagnoses.

Please note: This differs from the coding practice in the hospital inpatient setting regarding abnormal findings on test results.

M. Patients receiving therapeutic services only

For patients receiving therapeutic services only during an encounter/visit, sequence first the diagnosis, condition, problem, or other reason for encounter/visit shown in the medical record to be chiefly responsible for the outpatient services provided during the encounter/visit. Codes for other diagnoses (e.g., chronic conditions) may be sequenced as additional diagnoses.

The only exception to this rule is that when the primary reason for the admission/encounter is chemotherapy, radiation therapy, or rehabilitation, the appropriate V code for the service is listed first, and the diagnosis or problem for which the service is being performed listed second.

N. Patients receiving preoperative evaluations only

For patients receiving preoperative evaluations only, sequence first a code from category V72.8, Other specified examinations, to describe the pre-op consultations. Assign a code for the condition to describe the reason for the surgery as an additional diagnosis. Code also any findings related to the pre-op evaluation.

O. Ambulatory surgery

For ambulatory surgery, code the diagnosis for which the surgery was performed. If the postoperative diagnosis is known to be different from the preoperative diagnosis at the time the diagnosis is confirmed, select the postoperative diagnosis for coding, since it is the most definitive.

P. Routine outpatient prenatal visits

For routine outpatient prenatal visits when no complications are present, codes V22.0, Supervision of normal first pregnancy, or V22.1, Supervision of other normal pregnancy, should be used as the principal diagnosis. These codes should not be used in conjunction with chapter 11 codes.

APPENDIX I : Present On Admission (POA) Reporting Guidelines

Introduction

These guidelines are to be used as a supplement to the ICD-9-CM Official Guidelines for Coding and Reporting to facilitate the assignment of the Present on Admission (POA) indicator for each diagnosis and external cause of injury code reported on claim forms (UB-04 and 837 Institutional).

These guidelines are not intended to replace any guidelines in the main body of the ICD-9-CM Official Guidelines for Coding and Reporting. The POA guidelines are not intended to provide guidance on when a condition should be coded, but rather, how to apply the POA indicator to the final set of diagnosis codes that have been assigned in accordance with Sections I, II, and III of the official coding guidelines. Subsequent to the assignment of the ICD-9-CM codes, the POA indicator should then be assigned to those conditions that have been coded.

As stated in the Introduction to the ICD-9-CM Official Guidelines for Coding and Reporting, a joint effort between the healthcare provider and the coder is essential to achieve complete and accurate documentation, code assignment, and reporting of diagnoses and procedures. The importance of consistent, complete documentation in the medical record cannot be overemphasized. Medical record documentation from any provider involved in the care and treatment of the patient may be used to support the determination of whether a condition was present on admission or not. In the context of the official coding guidelines, the term "provider" means a physician or any qualified healthcare practitioner who is legally accountable for establishing the patient's diagnosis.

These guidelines are not a substitute for the provider's clinical judgment as to the determination of whether a condition was/was not present on admission. The provider should be queried regarding issues related to the linking of signs/symptoms, timing of test results, and the timing of findings.

General Reporting Requirements

All claims involving inpatient admissions to general acute care hospitals or other facilities that are subject to a law or regulation mandating collection of present on admission information. Present on admission is defined as present at the time the order for inpatient admission occurs -- conditions that develop during an outpatient encounter, including emergency department, observation, or outpatient surgery, are considered as present on admission. POA indicator is assigned to principal and secondary diagnoses (as defined in Section II of the Official Guidelines for Coding and Reporting) and the external cause of injury codes. Issues related to inconsistent, missing, conflicting or unclear documentation must still be resolved by the provider. If a condition would not be coded and reported based on UHDDS definitions and current official coding guidelines, then the POA indicator would not be reported.

Reporting Options
Y   -   Yes
N   -   No
U   -   Unknown
W   -   Clinically undetermined
Unreported/Not used (or "1" for Medicare usage) - (Exempt from POA reporting)

Reporting Definitions
Y   =   present at the time of inpatient admission
N   =   not present at the time of inpatient admission
U   =   documentation is insufficient to determine if condition is present on admission
W   =   provider is unable to clinically determine whether condition was present on admission or not

Timeframe for POA Identification and Documentation
There is no required timeframe as to when a provider (per the definition of "provider" used in these guidelines) must identify or document a condition to be present on admission. In some clinical situations, it may not be possible for a provider to make a definitive diagnosis (or a condition may not be recognized or reported by the patient) for a period of time after admission. In some cases it may be several days before the provider arrives at a definitive diagnosis. This does not mean that the condition was not present on admission. Determination of whether the condition was present on admission or not will be based on the applicable POA guideline as identified in this document, or on the provider's best clinical judgment.

If at the time of code assignment the documentation is unclear as to whether a condition was present on admission or not, it is appropriate to query the provider for clarification.

Assigning The POA Indicator

Condition is on the "Exempt from Reporting" list

Leave the "present on admission" field blank if the condition is on the list of ICD-9-CM codes for which this field is not applicable. This is the only circumstance in which the field may be left blank.

POA Explicitly Documented

Assign Y for any condition the provider explicitly documents as being present on admission.

Assign N for any condition the provider explicitly documents as not present at the time of admission.

Conditions diagnosed prior to inpatient admission

Assign "Y" for conditions that were diagnosed prior to admission (example: hypertension, diabetes mellitus, asthma)

Conditions diagnosed during the admission but clearly present before admission

Assign "Y" for conditions diagnosed during the admission that were clearly present but not diagnosed until after admission occurred.

Diagnoses subsequently confirmed after admission are considered present on admission if at the time of admission they are documented as suspected, possible, rule out, differential diagnosis, or constitute an underlying cause of a symptom that is present at the time of admission.

Condition develops during outpatient encounter prior to inpatient admission

Assign Y for any condition that develops during an outpatient encounter prior to a written order for inpatient admission.

Documentation does not indicate whether condition was present on admission

Assign "U" when the medical record documentation is unclear as to whether the condition was present on admission. "U" should not be routinely assigned and used only in very limited circumstances. Coders are encouraged to query the providers when the documentation is unclear.

Documentation states that it cannot be determined whether the condition was or was not present on admission

Assign "W" when the medical record documentation indicates that it cannot be clinically determined whether or not the condition was present on admission.

Chronic condition with acute exacerbation during the admission

If the code is a combination code that identifies both the chronic condition and the acute exacerbation, see POA guidelines pertaining to combination codes.

If the combination code only identifies the chronic condition and not the acute exacerbation (e.g., acute exacerbation of CHF), assign "Y."

Conditions documented as possible, probable, suspected, or rule out at the time of discharge

If the final diagnosis contains a possible, probable, suspected, or rule out diagnosis, and this diagnosis was based on signs, symptoms or clinical findings suspected at the time of inpatient admission, assign "Y."

If the final diagnosis contains a possible, probable, suspected, or rule out diagnosis, and this diagnosis was based on signs, symptoms or clinical findings that were not present on admission, assign "N".

Conditions documented as impending or threatened at the time of discharge

If the final diagnosis contains an impending or threatened diagnosis, and this diagnosis is based on symptoms or clinical findings that were present on admission, assign "Y".

If the final diagnosis contains an impending or threatened diagnosis, and this diagnosis is based on symptoms or clinical findings that were not present on admission, assign "N".

Acute and Chronic Conditions

Assign "Y" for acute conditions that are present at time of admission and N for acute conditions that are not present at time of admission.

Assign "Y" for chronic conditions, even though the condition may not be diagnosed until after admission.

If a single code identifies both an acute and chronic condition, see the POA guidelines for combination codes.

Combination Codes

Assign "N" if any part of the combination code was not present on admission (e.g., obstructive chronic bronchitis with acute exacerbation and the exacerbation was not present on admission; gastric ulcer that does not start bleeding until after admission; asthma patient develops status asthmaticus after admission)

Assign "Y" if all parts of the combination code were present on admission (e.g., patient with diabetic nephropathy is admitted with uncontrolled diabetes)

If the final diagnosis includes comparative or contrasting diagnoses, and both were present, or suspected, at the time of admission, assign "Y".

For infection codes that include the causal organism, assign "Y" if the infection (or signs of the infection) was present on admission, even though the culture results may not be known until after admission (e.g., patient is admitted with pneumonia and the provider documents pseudomonas as the causal organism a few days later).

Same Diagnosis Code for Two or More Conditions

When the same ICD-9-CM diagnosis code applies to two or more conditions during the same encounter (e.g. bilateral condition, or two separate conditions classified to the same ICD-9-CM diagnosis code):

Assign "Y" if all conditions represented by the single ICD-9-CM code were present on admission (e.g. bilateral fracture of the same bone, same site, and both fractures were present on admission)

Assign "N" if any of the conditions represented by the single ICD-9-CM code was not present on admission (e.g. dehydration with hyponatremia is assigned to code 276.1, but only one of these conditions was present on admission).

Obstetrical conditions
Whether or not the patient delivers during the current hospitalization does not affect assignment of the POA indicator. The determining factor for POA assignment is whether the pregnancy complication or obstetrical condition described by the code was present at the time of admission or not.

If the pregnancy complication or obstetrical condition was present on admission (e.g., patient admitted in preterm labor), assign "Y".

If the pregnancy complication or obstetrical condition was not present on admission (e.g., 2nd degree laceration during delivery, postpartum hemorrhage that occurred during current hospitalization, fetal distress develops after admission), assign "N".

If the obstetrical code includes more than one diagnosis and any of the diagnoses identified by the code were not present on admission assign "N". (e.g., Code 642.7, Pre-eclampsia or eclampsia superimposed on pre-existing hypertension).

If the obstetrical code includes information that is not a diagnosis, do not consider that information in the POA determination. (e.g. Code 652.1x, Breech or other malpresentation successfully converted to cephalic presentation should be reported as present on admission if the fetus was breech on admission but was converted to cephalic presentation after admission (since the conversion to cephalic presentation does not represent a diagnosis, the fact that the conversion occurred after admission has no bearing on the POA determination).

Perinatal conditions
Newborns are not considered to be admitted until after birth. Therefore, any condition present at birth or that developed in utero is considered present at admission and should be assigned "Y". This includes conditions that occur during delivery (e.g., injury during delivery, meconium aspiration, exposure to streptococcus B in the vaginal canal).

Congenital conditions and anomalies
Assign "Y" for congenital conditions and anomalies, except for categories 740-759, Congenital anomalies, which are on the exempt list. Congenital conditions are always considered present on admission.

External cause of injury codes
Assign "Y" for any E code representing an external cause of injury or poisoning that occurred prior to inpatient admission (e.g., patient fell out of bed at home, patient fell out of bed in emergency room prior to admission)

Assign "N" for any E code representing an external cause of injury or poisoning that occurred during inpatient hospitalization (e.g., patient fell out of hospital bed during hospital stay, patient experienced an adverse reaction to a medication administered after inpatient admission)

Categories and Codes Exempt from Diagnosis Present on Admission Requirement

Note: "Diagnosis present on admission" for these code categories are exempt because they represent circumstances regarding the healthcare encounter or factors influencing health status that do not represent a current disease or injury or are always present on admission

Categories or subcategories listed are inclusive of all codes within those categories or subcategories, unless otherwise indicated. In order to streamline the POA exempt list and make it easier to read, where all of the codes in a code range are POA exempt, only the code range is shown, rather than listing each of the individual codes in the range.

137-139	Late effects of infectious and parasitic diseases
268.1	Rickets, late effect
326	Late effects of intracranial abscess or pyogenic infection
412	Old myocardial infarction
438	Late effects of cerebrovascular disease
650	Normal delivery
660.7	Failed forceps or vacuum extractor, unspecified
677	Late effect of complication of pregnancy, childbirth, and the puerperium
740-759	Congenital anomalies
905-909	Late effects of injuries, poisonings, toxic effects, and other external causes
V02	Carrier or suspected carrier of infectious diseases
V03	Need for prophylactic vaccination and inoculation against bacterial diseases
V04	Need for prophylactic vaccination and inoculation against certain viral diseases
V05	Need for other prophylactic vaccination and inoculation against single diseases
V06	Need for prophylactic vaccination and inoculation against combinations of diseases
V07	Need for isolation and other prophylactic or treatment measures
V10	Personal history of malignant neoplasm
V11	Personal history of mental disorder
V12	Personal history of certain other diseases
V13	Personal history of other diseases
V14	Personal history of allergy to medicinal agents
V15	Other personal history presenting hazards to health
V16	Family history of malignant neoplasm
V17	Family history of certain chronic disabling diseases
V18	Family history of certain other specific conditions
V19	Family history of other conditions
V20	Health supervision of infant or child
V21	Constitutional states in development
V22	Normal pregnancy
V23	Supervision of high-risk pregnancy
V24	Postpartum care and examination
V25	Encounter for contraceptive management

V26	Procreative management
V27	Outcome of delivery
V28	Antenatal screening
V29	Observation and evaluation of newborns for suspected condition not found
V30-V39	Liveborn infants according to type of birth
V42	Organ or tissue replaced by transplant
V43	Organ or tissue replaced by other means
V44	Artificial opening status
V45	Other postprocedural states
V46	Other dependence on machines and devices
V49.60-V49.77	Upper and lower limb amputation status
V49.81-V49.85	Other specified conditions influencing health status
V50	Elective surgery for purposes other than remedying health states
V51	Aftercare involving the use of plastic surgery
V52	Fitting and adjustment of prosthetic device and implant
V53	Fitting and adjustment of other device
V54	Other orthopedic aftercare
V55	Attention to artificial openings
V56	Encounter for dialysis and dialysis catheter care
V57	Care involving use of rehabilitation procedures
V58	Encounter for other and unspecified procedures and aftercare
V59	Donors
V60	Housing, household, and economic circumstances
V61	Other family circumstances
V62	Other psychosocial circumstances
V64	Persons encountering health services for specific procedures, not carried out
V65	Other persons seeking consultation
V66	Convalescence and palliative care
V67	Follow-up examination
V68	Encounters for administrative purposes
V69	Problems related to lifestyle
V70	General medical examination
V71	Observation and evaluation for suspected condition not found
V72	Special investigations and examinations
V73	Special screening examination for viral and chlamydial diseases
V74	Special screening examination for bacterial and spirochetal diseases
V75	Special screening examination for other infectious diseases
V76	Special screening for malignant neoplasms
V77	Special screening for endocrine, nutritional, metabolic, and immunity disorders
V78	Special screening for disorders of blood and blood-forming organs
V79	Special screening for mental disorders and developmental handicaps
V80	Special screening for neurological, eye, and ear diseases
V81	Special screening for cardiovascular, respiratory, and genitourinary diseases
V82	Special screening for other conditions
V83	Genetic carrier status

V84	Genetic susceptibility to disease
V85	Body Mass Index
V86	Estrogen receptor status
V87.32	Contact with and (suspected) exposure to algae bloom
V87.4	Personal history of drug therapy
V88	Acquired absence of other organs and tissue
V89	Suspected maternal and fetal conditions not found
V90	Retained foreign body
V91	Multiple gestation placenta status
E000	External cause status
E001-E030	Activity
E800-E807	Railway accidents
E810-E819	Motor vehicle traffic accidents
E820-E825	Motor vehicle nontraffic accidents
E826-E829	Other road vehicle accidents
E830-E838	Water transport accidents
E840-E845	Air and space transport accidents
E846-E848	Vehicle accidents not elsewhere classifiable
E849	Place of occurrence (except E849.7)
E883.1	Accidental fall into well
E883.2	Accidental fall into storm drain or manhole
E884.0	Fall from playground equipment
E884.1	Fall from cliff
E885.0	Fall from (nonmotorized) scooter
E885.1	Fall from roller skates
E885.2	Fall from skateboard
E885.3	Fall from skis
E885.4	Fall from snowboard
E886.0	Fall on same level from collision, pushing, or shoving, by or with other person, In sports
E890.0-E890.9	Conflagration in private dwelling
E893.0	Accident caused by ignition of clothing, from controlled fire in private dwelling
E893.2	Accident caused by ignition of clothing, from controlled fire not in building or structure
E894	Ignition of highly inflammable material
E895	Accident caused by controlled fire in private dwelling
E897	Accident caused by controlled fire not in building or structure
E917.0	Striking against or struck accidentally by objects or persons, in sports without subsequent fall
E917.1	Striking against or struck accidentally by objects or persons, caused by a crowd, by collective fear or panic without subsequent fall
E917.2	Striking against or struck accidentally by objects or persons, in running water without subsequent fall
E917.5	Striking against or struck accidentally by objects or persons, object in sports with subsequent fall
E917.6	Striking against or struck accidentally by objects or persons, caused by a crowd, by collective fear or panic with subsequent fall
E919	Accidents caused by machinery (except E919.2)
E921	Accident caused by explosion of pressure vessel

E922	Accident caused by firearm and air gun missile
E926.2	Visible and ultraviolet light sources
E928.0-E928.8	Other and unspecified environmental and accidental causes
E929.0-E929.9	Late effects of accidental injury
E959	Late effects of self-inflicted injury
E970-E978	Legal intervention
E979	Terrorism
E981	Poisoning by gases in domestic use, undetermined whether accidentally or purposely inflicted
E982	Poisoning by other gases, undetermined whether accidentally or purposely inflicted
E985	Injury by firearms, air guns and explosives, undetermined whether accidentally or purposely inflicted
E987.0	Falling from high place, undetermined whether accidentally or purposely inflicted, residential premises
E987.2	Falling from high place, undetermined whether accidentally or purposely inflicted, natural sites
E989	Late effects of injury, undetermined whether accidentally or purposely inflicted
E990-E999	Injury resulting from operations of war

POA Examples

The POA examples have been removed from the guidelines.

ICD-10

Subject to possible legislative delays, ICD-10-CM codes must be used on all HIPAA transactions, including outpatient claims with dates of service, and inpatient claims with dates of discharge on and after October 1, 2013. In addition, ICD-10-PCS will replace the current ICD-9-CM Volume 3 procedures list. This change does not affect CPT coding for outpatient procedures and there will continue to be ICD-9-CM updates until ICD-10-CM is implemented.

Differences Between ICD-10-CM and ICD-9-CM

ICD-10-CM uses 3-7 alpha and numeric digits and full code titles, but the format is very much the same as ICD-9-CM. Primarily, changes in ICD-10-CM are in its organization and structure, code composition, and level of detail.

Format of ICD-10-CM

■ 3-7 digits

■ Digit 1 is alpha; Digit 2 is numeric

■ Digits 3-7 are alpha or numeric (alpha characters are not case sensitive)

■ Decimal is used after third character.

Examples of ICD-10-CM Codes

A78   Q fever

A69.21   Meningitis due to Lyme disease

S52.131A Displaced fracture of neck of right radius, initial encounter for closed fracture.

Due to the additional digits, there will be over 85,000 potential codes in ICD-10-CM versus about 16,000 codes in ICD-9-CM.

WHERE TO GET ANSWERS TO QUESTIONS ABOUT ICD-9-CM

Questions regarding the use and interpretation of the *International Classification of Diseases, 9th Revision, Clinical Modification* should be directed in writing to any of the organizations listed below.

Coding Advice/Central Office on ICD-9-CM
American Hospital Association
One North Franklin
Chicago, Illinois 60606
Vols. 1 and 2: kayala@aha.org

World Health Organization Collaborating Center
    for Classification of Diseases in North America
National Center for Health Statistics
Department of Health and Human Services
6525 Belcrest Road
Hyattsville, Maryland 20782

Morbidity Classification Branch
National Center for Health Statistics
Department of Health and Human Services
6525 Belcrest Road, Room 1100
Hyattsville, Maryland 20782

Center for Medicare and Medicaid Services (CMS)
Division of Prospective Payment
Mail Stop C5-06-27
7500 Security Blvd.
Baltimore, MD 21244-1850
Vol. 3: pbrooks@cms.hhs.gov

Comments, questions or suggestions regarding the PMIC version of ICD-9-CM should be directed in writing to:

Managing Editor
Practice Management Information Corporation
4727 Wilshire Boulevard, Suite 300
Los Angeles, California 90010
http://www.pmiconline.com

Anatomical Illustrations

A fundamental knowledge and understanding of basic human anatomy and physiology is a prerequisite for accurate diagnosis coding. While a comprehensive treatment of anatomy and physiology is beyond the scope of this text, the large scale, full color anatomical illustrations on the following pages are designed to facilitate the diagnosis coding process for both beginning and experienced coders.

The illustrations provide an anatomical perspective of diagnosis coding by providing a side-by-side view of the major systems of the human body and a corresponding list of the most common diagnoses categories used to support medical, surgical and diagnostic services performed on the illustrated system.

The diagnostic categories listed on the left facing page of each anatomical illustration are three-digit categories and may not be used for coding. These categories are provided as "pointers" to the appropriate section of the ICD-9-CM Volume 1 where the complete listings, including 4th and 5th digits if appropriate, may be found.

PLATE 1. SKIN AND SUBCUTANEOUS TISSUE — MALE

Viral diseases accompanied by exanthem	050-057

Neoplasms

Malignant melanoma of skin	172
Other malignant neoplasm of skin	173
Malignant neoplasm of male breast	175
Kaposi's sarcoma	176
Benign neoplasm of skin	216
Carcinoma in situ of skin	232

Infections of skin and subcutaneous tissue

Carbuncle and furuncle	680
Cellulitis and abscess of finger and toe	681
Other cellulitis and abscess	682
Acute lymphadenitis	683
Impetigo	684
Pilonidal cyst	685
Other local infections of skin and subcutaneous tissue	686

Other inflammatory conditions of skin and subcutaneous tissue

Erythematosquamous dermatosis	690
Atopic dermatitis and related conditions	691
Contact dermatitis and other eczema	692
Dermatitis due to substances taken internally	693
Bullous dermatoses	694
Erythematous conditions	695
Psoriasis and similar disorders	696
Lichen	697
Pruritus and related conditions	698

Other diseases of skin and subcutaneous tissue

Corns and callosities	700
Other hypertrophic and atrophic conditions of skin	701
Diseases of nail	703
Diseases of hair and hair follicles	704
Disorders of sweat glands	705
Diseases of sebaceous glands	706
Chronic ulcer of skin	707
Urticaria	708
Other disorders of skin and subcutaneous tissue	709
Symptoms involving skin and other integumentary tissue	782

Symptoms, signs and ill-defined conditions	780-799

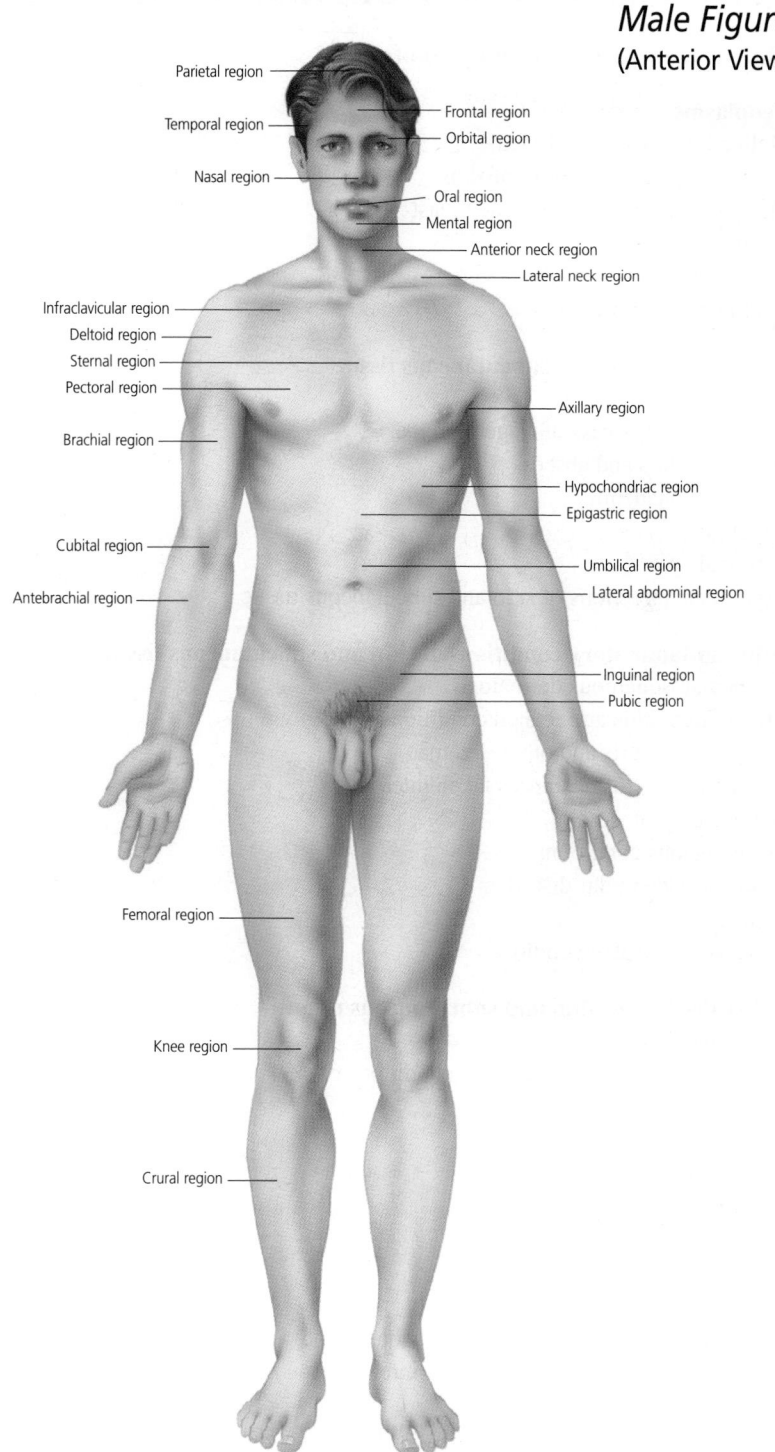

Male Figure
(Anterior View)

Parietal region

Frontal region
Orbital region

Temporal region

Nasal region

Oral region
Mental region

Anterior neck region
Lateral neck region

Infraclavicular region

Deltoid region
Sternal region
Pectoral region

Axillary region

Brachial region

Hypochondriac region
Epigastric region

Cubital region

Umbilical region

Antebrachial region

Lateral abdominal region

Inguinal region
Pubic region

Femoral region

Knee region

Crural region

PLATE 2. SKIN AND SUBCUTANEOUS TISSUE — FEMALE

Viral diseases accompanied by exanthem   050-057

Neoplasms
Malignant melanoma of skin	172
Other malignant neoplasm of skin	173
Malignant neoplasm of female breast	174
Kaposi's sarcoma	176
Benign neoplasm of skin	216
Carcinoma in situ of skin	232

Infections of skin and subcutaneous tissue
Carbuncle and furuncle	680
Cellulitis and abscess of finger and toe	681
Other cellulitis and abscess	682
Acute lymphadenitis	683
Impetigo	684
Pilonidal cyst	685
Other local infections of skin and subcutaneous tissue	686

Other inflammatory conditions of skin and subcutaneous tissue
Erythematosquamous dermatosis	690
Atopic dermatitis and related conditions	691
Contact dermatitis and other eczema	692
Dermatitis due to substances taken internally	693
Bullous dermatoses	694
Erythematous conditions	695
Psoriasis and similar disorders	696
Lichen	697
Pruritus and related conditions	698

Other diseases of skin and subcutaneous tissue
Corns and callosities	700
Other hypertrophic and atrophic conditions of skin	701
Other dermatoses	702
Diseases of nail	703
Diseases of hair and hair follicles	704
Disorders of sweat glands	705
Diseases of sebaceous glands	706
Chronic ulcer of skin	707
Urticaria	708
Other disorders of skin and subcutaneous tissue	709
Symptoms involving skin and other integumentary tissue	782

Symptoms, signs and ill-defined conditions   780-799

Female Figure
(Anterior View)

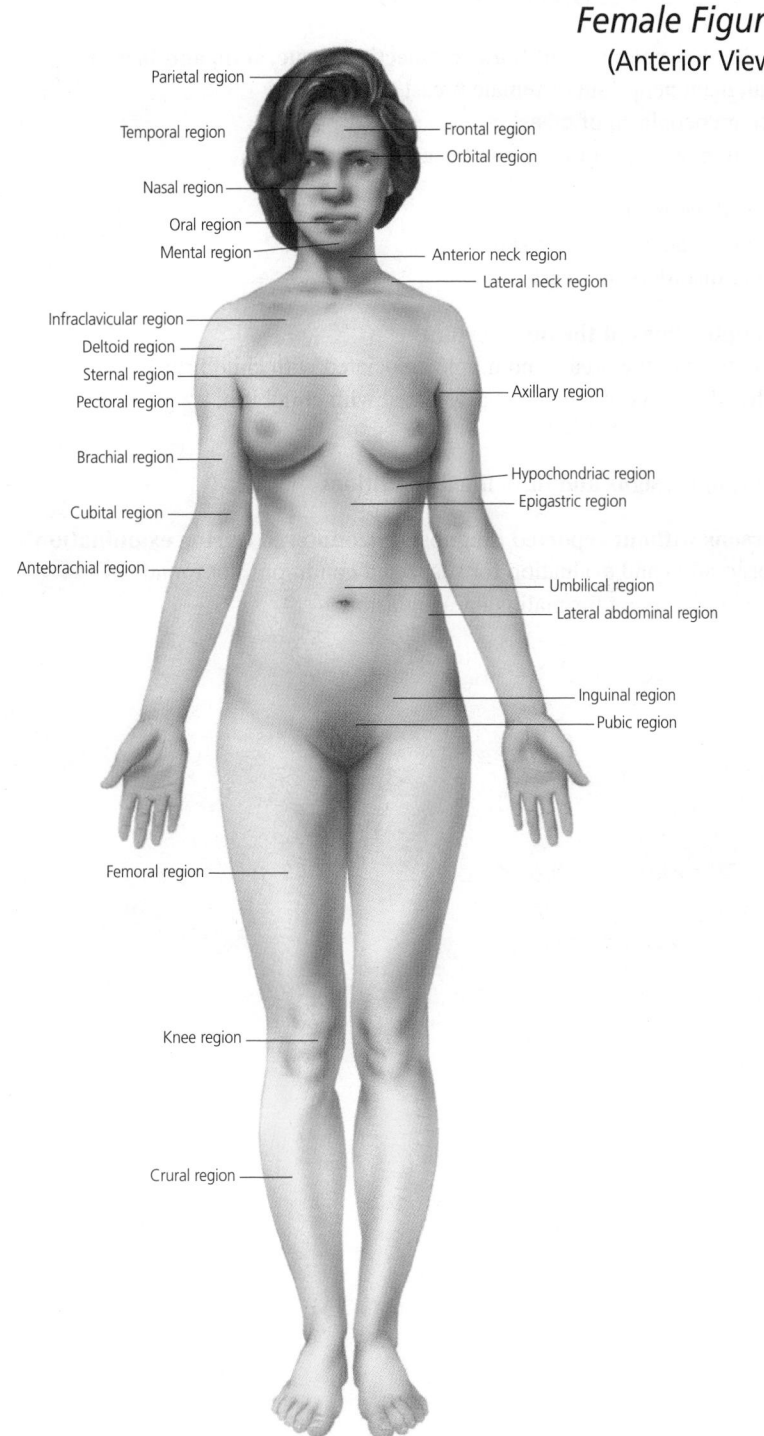

Parietal region

Temporal region

Nasal region

Oral region

Mental region

Frontal region

Orbital region

Anterior neck region

Lateral neck region

Infraclavicular region

Deltoid region

Sternal region

Pectoral region

Axillary region

Brachial region

Cubital region

Hypochondriac region

Epigastric region

Antebrachial region

Umbilical region

Lateral abdominal region

Inguinal region

Pubic region

Femoral region

Knee region

Crural region

PLATE 3. FEMALE BREAST

Female Breast

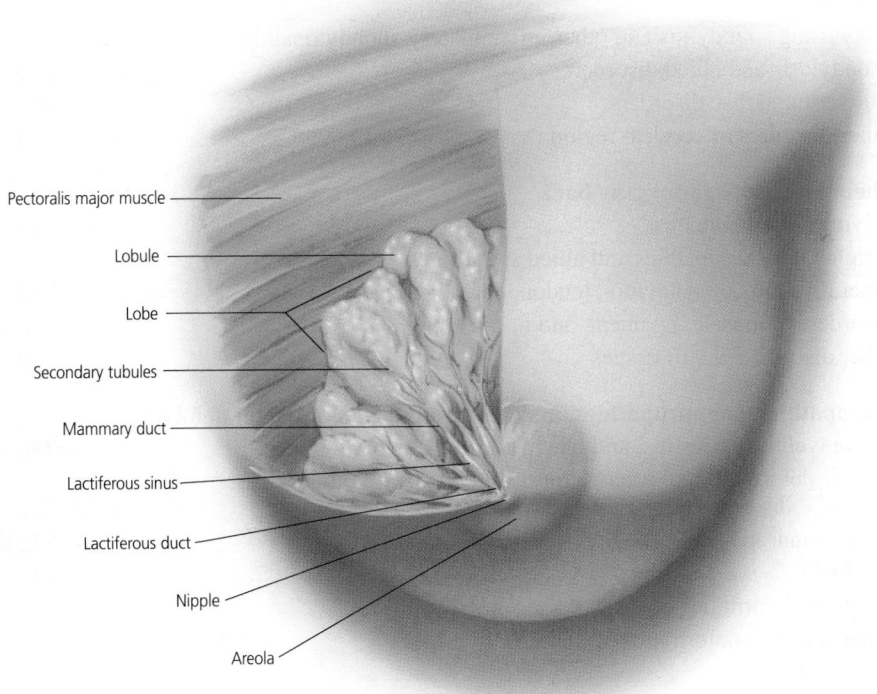

Pectoralis major muscle

Lobule

Lobe

Secondary tubules

Mammary duct

Lactiferous sinus

Lactiferous duct

Nipple

Areola

PLATE 4. MUSCULAR SYSTEM AND CONNECTIVE TISSUE — ANTERIOR VIEW

Muscular System
(Anterior View)

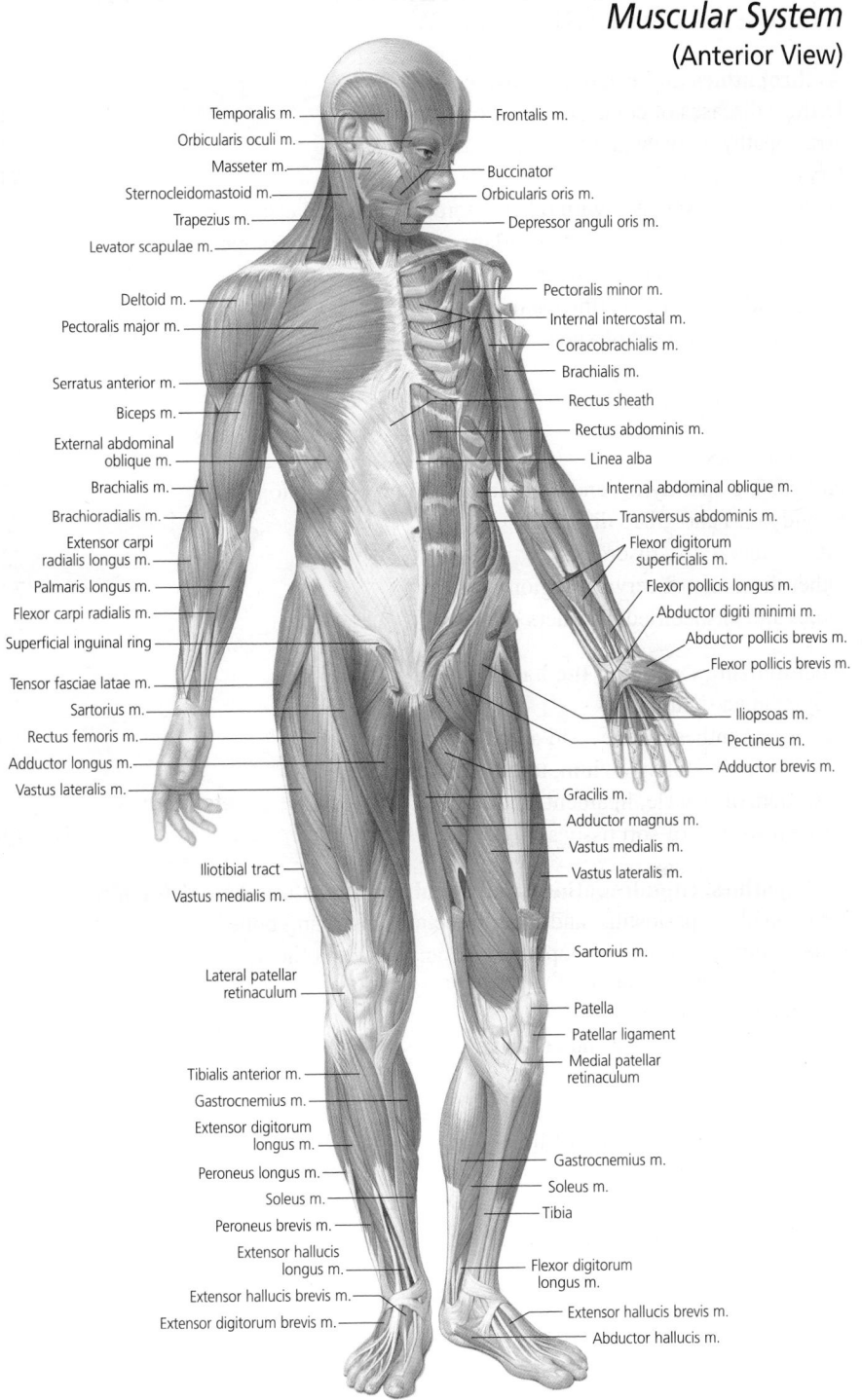

Temporalis m.
Orbicularis oculi m.
Masseter m.
Sternocleidomastoid m.
Trapezius m.
Levator scapulae m.

Frontalis m.
Buccinator
Orbicularis oris m.
Depressor anguli oris m.

Deltoid m.
Pectoralis major m.

Pectoralis minor m.
Internal intercostal m.
Coracobrachialis m.
Brachialis m.
Rectus sheath
Rectus abdominis m.
Linea alba
Internal abdominal oblique m.
Transversus abdominis m.
Flexor digitorum superficialis m.
Flexor pollicis longus m.
Abductor digiti minimi m.
Abductor pollicis brevis m.
Flexor pollicis brevis m.
Iliopsoas m.
Pectineus m.
Adductor brevis m.

Serratus anterior m.
Biceps m.
External abdominal oblique m.
Brachialis m.
Brachioradialis m.
Extensor carpi radialis longus m.
Palmaris longus m.
Flexor carpi radialis m.
Superficial inguinal ring
Tensor fasciae latae m.
Sartorius m.
Rectus femoris m.
Adductor longus m.
Vastus lateralis m.

Gracilis m.
Adductor magnus m.
Vastus medialis m.
Vastus lateralis m.
Sartorius m.

Iliotibial tract
Vastus medialis m.

Lateral patellar retinaculum

Patella
Patellar ligament
Medial patellar retinaculum

Tibialis anterior m.
Gastrocnemius m.
Extensor digitorum longus m.
Peroneus longus m.
Soleus m.
Peroneus brevis m.
Extensor hallucis longus m.
Extensor hallucis brevis m.
Extensor digitorum brevis m.

Gastrocnemius m.
Soleus m.
Tibia
Flexor digitorum longus m.
Extensor hallucis brevis m.
Abductor hallucis m.

©Scientific Publishing Ltd., Rolling Meadows, IL

PLATE 5. MUSCULAR SYSTEM AND CONNECTIVE TISSUE — POSTERIOR VIEW

Muscular System
(Posterior View)

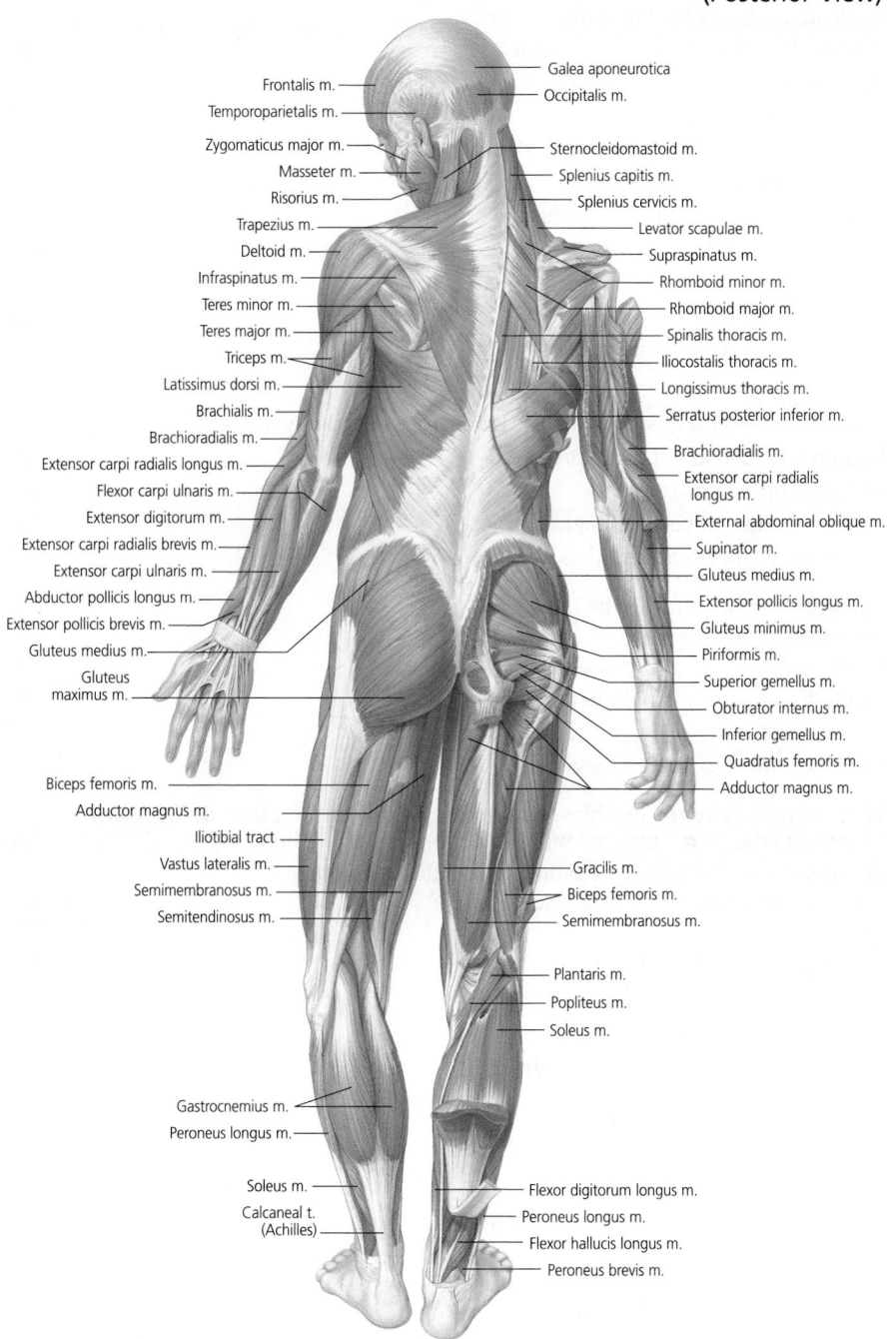

Frontalis m.
Temporoparietalis m.
Zygomaticus major m.
Masseter m.
Risorius m.
Trapezius m.
Deltoid m.
Infraspinatus m.
Teres minor m.
Teres major m.
Triceps m.
Latissimus dorsi m.
Brachialis m.
Brachioradialis m.
Extensor carpi radialis longus m.
Flexor carpi ulnaris m.
Extensor digitorum m.
Extensor carpi radialis brevis m.
Extensor carpi ulnaris m.
Abductor pollicis longus m.
Extensor pollicis brevis m.
Gluteus medius m.
Gluteus maximus m.
Biceps femoris m.
Adductor magnus m.
Iliotibial tract
Vastus lateralis m.
Semimembranosus m.
Semitendinosus m.
Gastrocnemius m.
Peroneus longus m.
Soleus m.
Calcaneal t. (Achilles)

Galea aponeurotica
Occipitalis m.
Sternocleidomastoid m.
Splenius capitis m.
Splenius cervicis m.
Levator scapulae m.
Supraspinatus m.
Rhomboid minor m.
Rhomboid major m.
Spinalis thoracis m.
Iliocostalis thoracis m.
Longissimus thoracis m.
Serratus posterior inferior m.
Brachioradialis m.
Extensor carpi radialis longus m.
External abdominal oblique m.
Supinator m.
Gluteus medius m.
Extensor pollicis longus m.
Gluteus minimus m.
Piriformis m.
Superior gemellus m.
Obturator internus m.
Inferior gemellus m.
Quadratus femoris m.
Adductor magnus m.
Gracilis m.
Biceps femoris m.
Semimembranosus m.
Plantaris m.
Popliteus m.
Soleus m.
Flexor digitorum longus m.
Peroneus longus m.
Flexor hallucis longus m.
Peroneus brevis m.

PLATE 6. MUSCULAR SYSTEM — SHOULDER AND ELBOW

Shoulder and Elbow
(Anterior View)

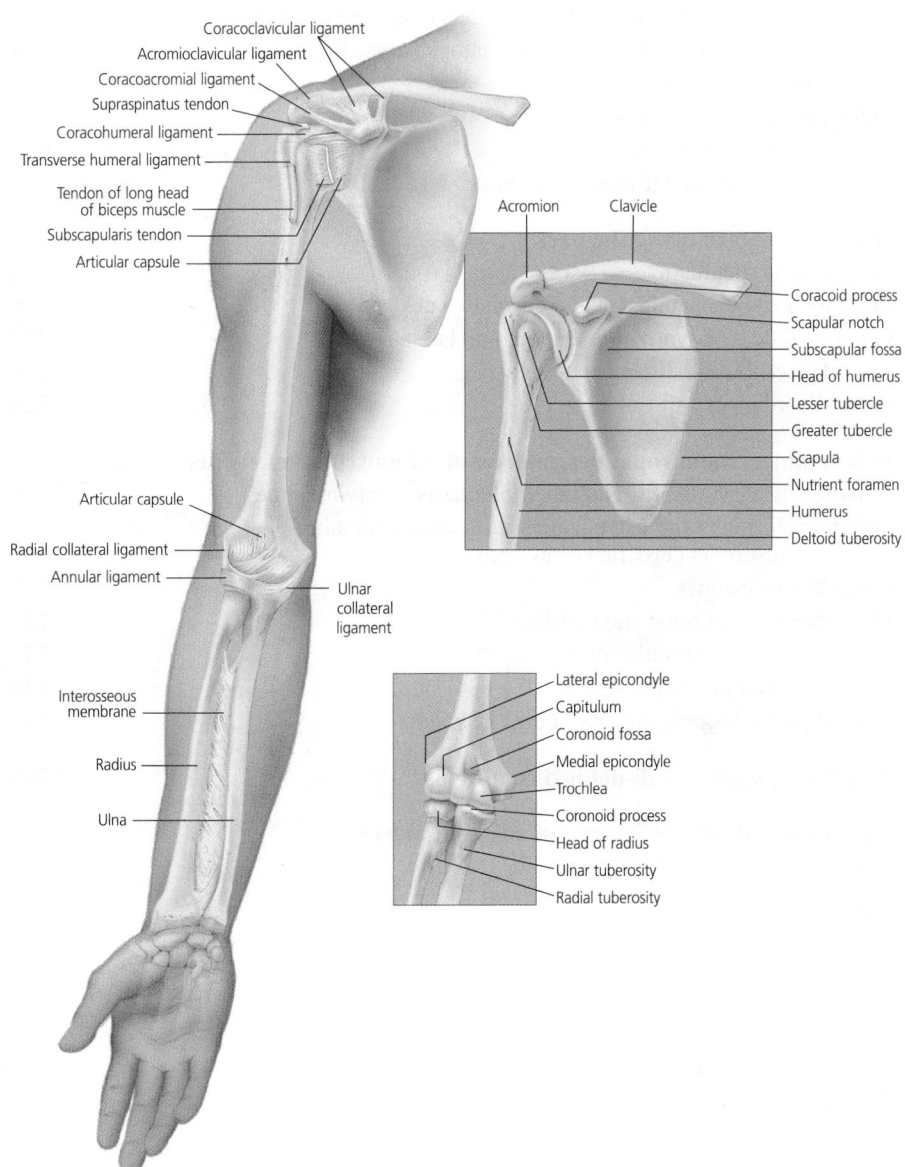

Coracoclavicular ligament
Acromioclavicular ligament
Coracoacromial ligament
Supraspinatus tendon
Coracohumeral ligament
Transverse humeral ligament
Tendon of long head of biceps muscle
Subscapularis tendon
Articular capsule

Acromion   Clavicle

Coracoid process
Scapular notch
Subscapular fossa
Head of humerus
Lesser tubercle
Greater tubercle
Scapula
Nutrient foramen
Humerus
Deltoid tuberosity

Articular capsule
Radial collateral ligament
Annular ligament

Ulnar collateral ligament

Interosseous membrane
Radius
Ulna

Lateral epicondyle
Capitulum
Coronoid fossa
Medial epicondyle
Trochlea
Coronoid process
Head of radius
Ulnar tuberosity
Radial tuberosity

PLATE 7. MUSCULAR SYSTEM — HAND AND WRIST

Hand and Wrist

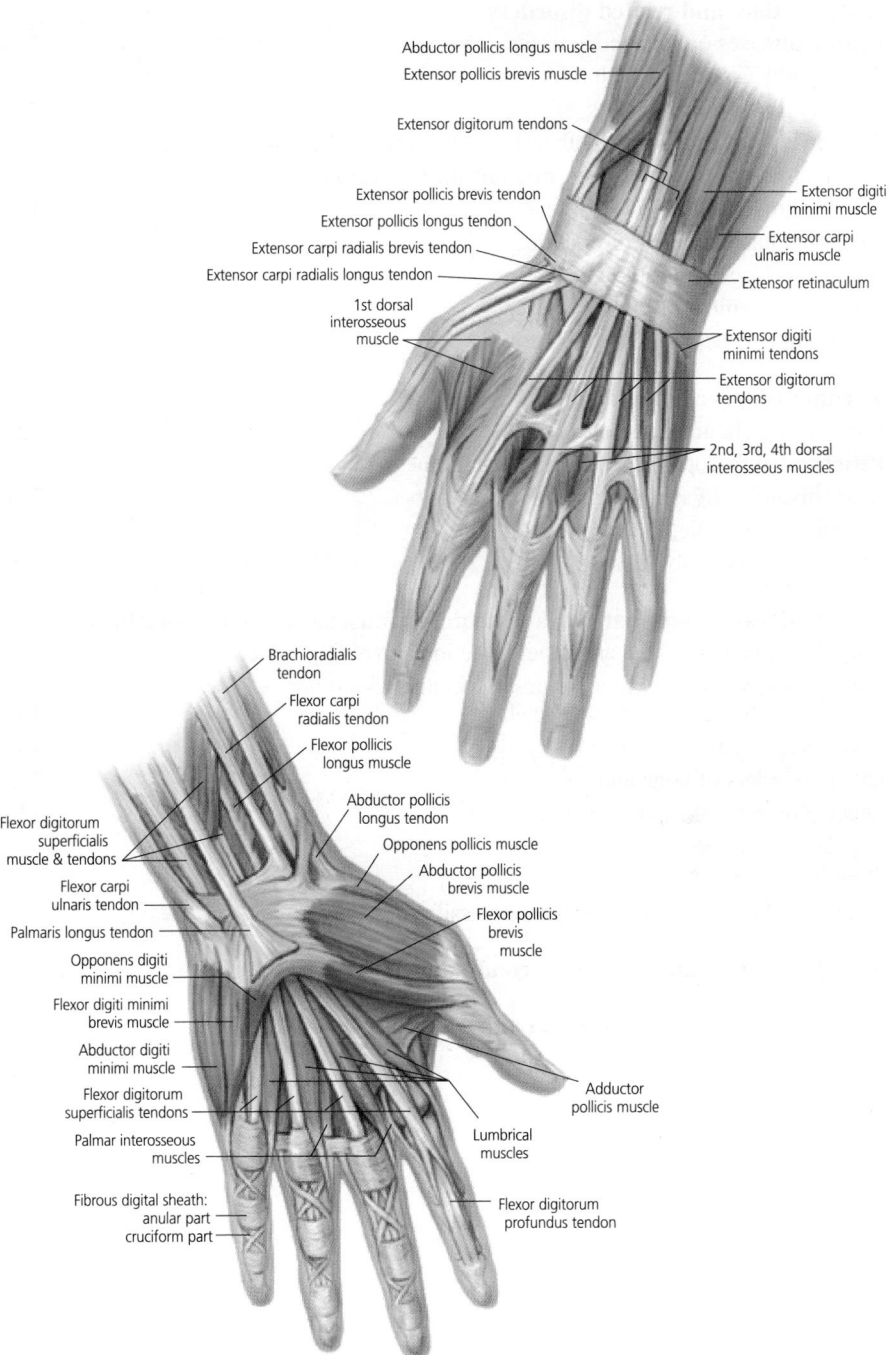

Abductor pollicis longus muscle

Extensor pollicis brevis muscle

Extensor digitorum tendons

Extensor pollicis brevis tendon

Extensor pollicis longus tendon

Extensor carpi radialis brevis tendon

Extensor carpi radialis longus tendon

1st dorsal interosseous muscle

Extensor digiti minimi muscle

Extensor carpi ulnaris muscle

Extensor retinaculum

Extensor digiti minimi tendons

Extensor digitorum tendons

2nd, 3rd, 4th dorsal interosseous muscles

Brachioradialis tendon

Flexor carpi radialis tendon

Flexor pollicis longus muscle

Abductor pollicis longus tendon

Flexor digitorum superficialis muscle & tendons

Opponens pollicis muscle

Abductor pollicis brevis muscle

Flexor carpi ulnaris tendon

Palmaris longus tendon

Opponens digiti minimi muscle

Flexor digiti minimi brevis muscle

Abductor digiti minimi muscle

Flexor digitorum superficialis tendons

Palmar interosseous muscles

Fibrous digital sheath:
anular part
cruciform part

Flexor pollicis brevis muscle

Adductor pollicis muscle

Lumbrical muscles

Flexor digitorum profundus tendon

PLATE 8. MUSCULOSKELETAL SYSTEM — HIP AND KNEE

Hip and Knee
(Anterior View)

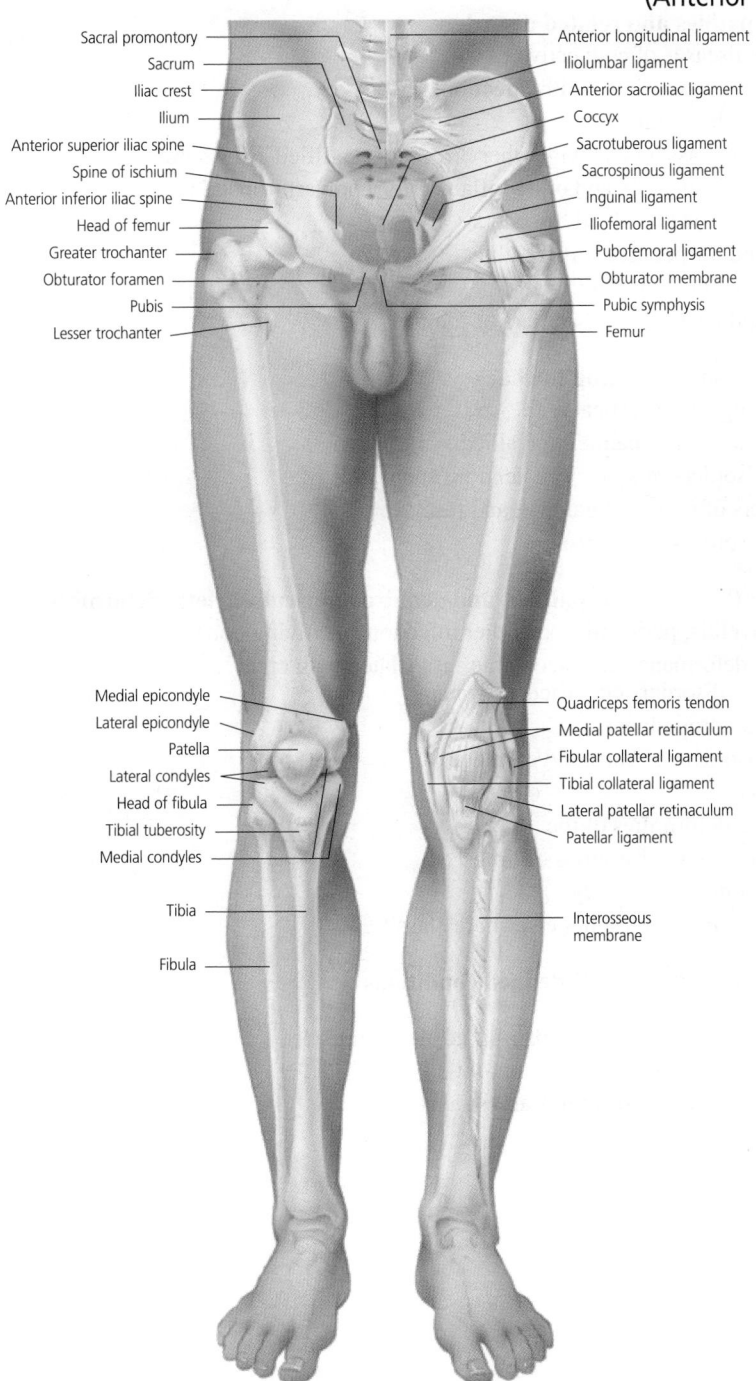

Sacral promontory

Sacrum

Iliac crest

Ilium

Anterior superior iliac spine

Spine of ischium

Anterior inferior iliac spine

Head of femur

Greater trochanter

Obturator foramen

Pubis

Lesser trochanter

Anterior longitudinal ligament

Iliolumbar ligament

Anterior sacroiliac ligament

Coccyx

Sacrotuberous ligament

Sacrospinous ligament

Inguinal ligament

Iliofemoral ligament

Pubofemoral ligament

Obturator membrane

Pubic symphysis

Femur

Medial epicondyle

Lateral epicondyle

Patella

Lateral condyles

Head of fibula

Tibial tuberosity

Medial condyles

Tibia

Fibula

Quadriceps femoris tendon

Medial patellar retinaculum

Fibular collateral ligament

Tibial collateral ligament

Lateral patellar retinaculum

Patellar ligament

Interosseous membrane

PLATE 9. MUSCULOSKELETAL SYSTEM — FOOT AND ANKLE

Foot and Ankle

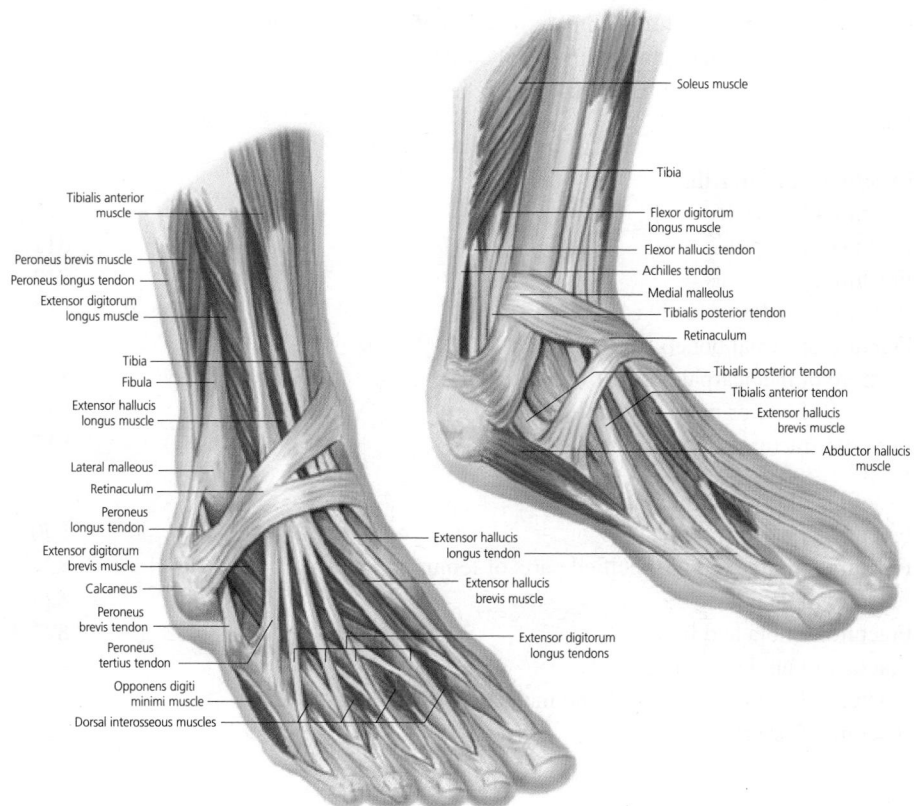

Tibialis anterior muscle

Peroneus brevis muscle
Peroneus longus tendon
Extensor digitorum longus muscle

Tibia
Fibula
Extensor hallucis longus muscle

Lateral malleous
Retinaculum
Peroneus longus tendon
Extensor digitorum brevis muscle
Calcaneus
Peroneus brevis tendon
Peroneus tertius tendon
Opponens digiti minimi muscle
Dorsal interosseous muscles

Soleus muscle

Tibia

Flexor digitorum longus muscle
Flexor hallucis tendon
Achilles tendon
Medial malleolus
Tibialis posterior tendon
Retinaculum

Tibialis posterior tendon
Tibialis anterior tendon
Extensor hallucis brevis muscle
Abductor hallucis muscle

Extensor hallucis longus tendon
Extensor hallucis brevis muscle
Extensor digitorum longus tendons

PLATE 10. SKELETAL SYSTEM — ANTERIOR VIEW

Symptoms, signs and ill-defined conditions   780-799

Fracture of skull

Fracture of vault of skull	800
Fracture of base of skull	801
Fracture of face bones	802
Multiple fractures involving skull or face with other bones	804

Fracture of neck and trunk

Fracture of vertebral column without mention of spinal cord injury	805
Fracture of vertebral column with spinal cord injury	806
Fracture of rib(s), sternum, larynx and trachea	807
Fracture of pelvis	808

Fracture of upper limb

Fracture of clavicle	810
Fracture of scapula	811
Fracture of humerus	812
Fracture of radius and ulna	813
Fracture of carpal bone(s)	814
Fracture of metacarpal bone(s)	815
Fracture of one or more phalanges of hand	816
Multiple fractures of hand bones	817

Fracture of lower limb

Fracture of neck of femur	820
Fracture of other and unspecified parts of femur	821
Fracture of patella	822
Fracture of tibia and fibula	823
Fracture of ankle	824
Fracture of one or more tarsal and metatarsal bones	825
Fracture of one or more phalanges of foot	826

Dislocation

Dislocation of jaw	830
Dislocation of shoulder	831
Dislocation of elbow	832
Dislocation of wrist	833
Dislocation of finger	834
Dislocation of hip	835
Dislocation of knee	836
Dislocation of ankle	837
Dislocation of foot	838

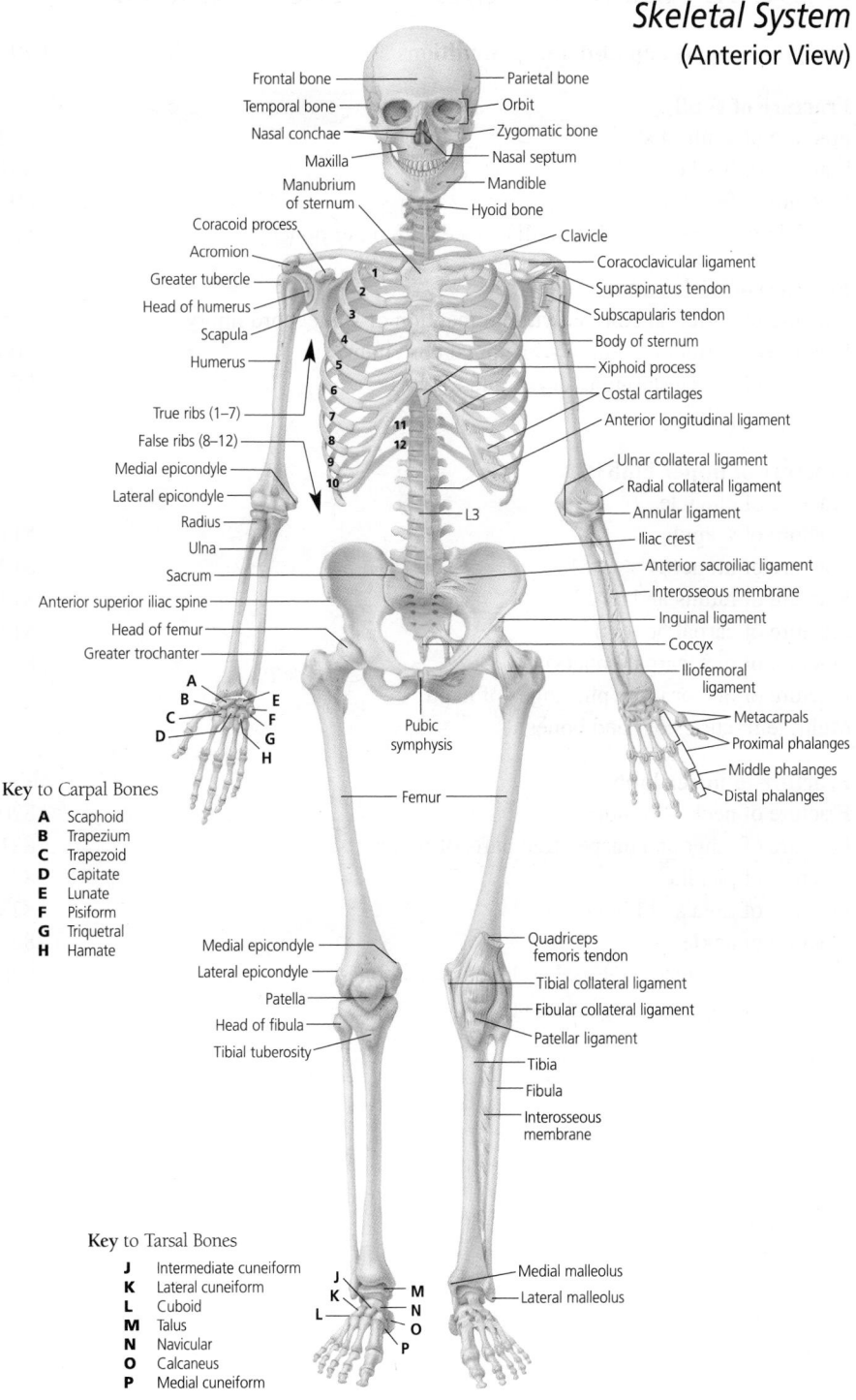

Skeletal System
(Anterior View)

Frontal bone — Parietal bone
Temporal bone — Orbit
Nasal conchae — Zygomatic bone
Maxilla — Nasal septum
Manubrium of sternum — Mandible
— Hyoid bone
Coracoid process — Clavicle
Acromion — Coracoclavicular ligament
Greater tubercle — Supraspinatus tendon
Head of humerus — Subscapularis tendon
Scapula — Body of sternum
Humerus — Xiphoid process
— Costal cartilages
True ribs (1–7) — Anterior longitudinal ligament
False ribs (8–12) — Ulnar collateral ligament
Medial epicondyle — Radial collateral ligament
Lateral epicondyle — Annular ligament
Radius — Iliac crest
Ulna — Anterior sacroiliac ligament
Sacrum — Interosseous membrane
Anterior superior iliac spine — Inguinal ligament
Head of femur — Coccyx
Greater trochanter — Iliofemoral ligament
Metacarpals
Proximal phalanges
Pubic symphysis — Middle phalanges
— Distal phalanges
Femur

Key to Carpal Bones
A Scaphoid
B Trapezium
C Trapezoid
D Capitate
E Lunate
F Pisiform
G Triquetral
H Hamate

Medial epicondyle — Quadriceps femoris tendon
Lateral epicondyle — Tibial collateral ligament
Patella — Fibular collateral ligament
Head of fibula — Patellar ligament
Tibial tuberosity — Tibia
— Fibula
— Interosseous membrane

Key to Tarsal Bones
J Intermediate cuneiform
K Lateral cuneiform
L Cuboid
M Talus
N Navicular
O Calcaneus
P Medial cuneiform

Medial malleolus
Lateral malleolus

PLATE 11. SKELETAL SYSTEM — POSTERIOR VIEW

Skeletal System
(Posterior View)

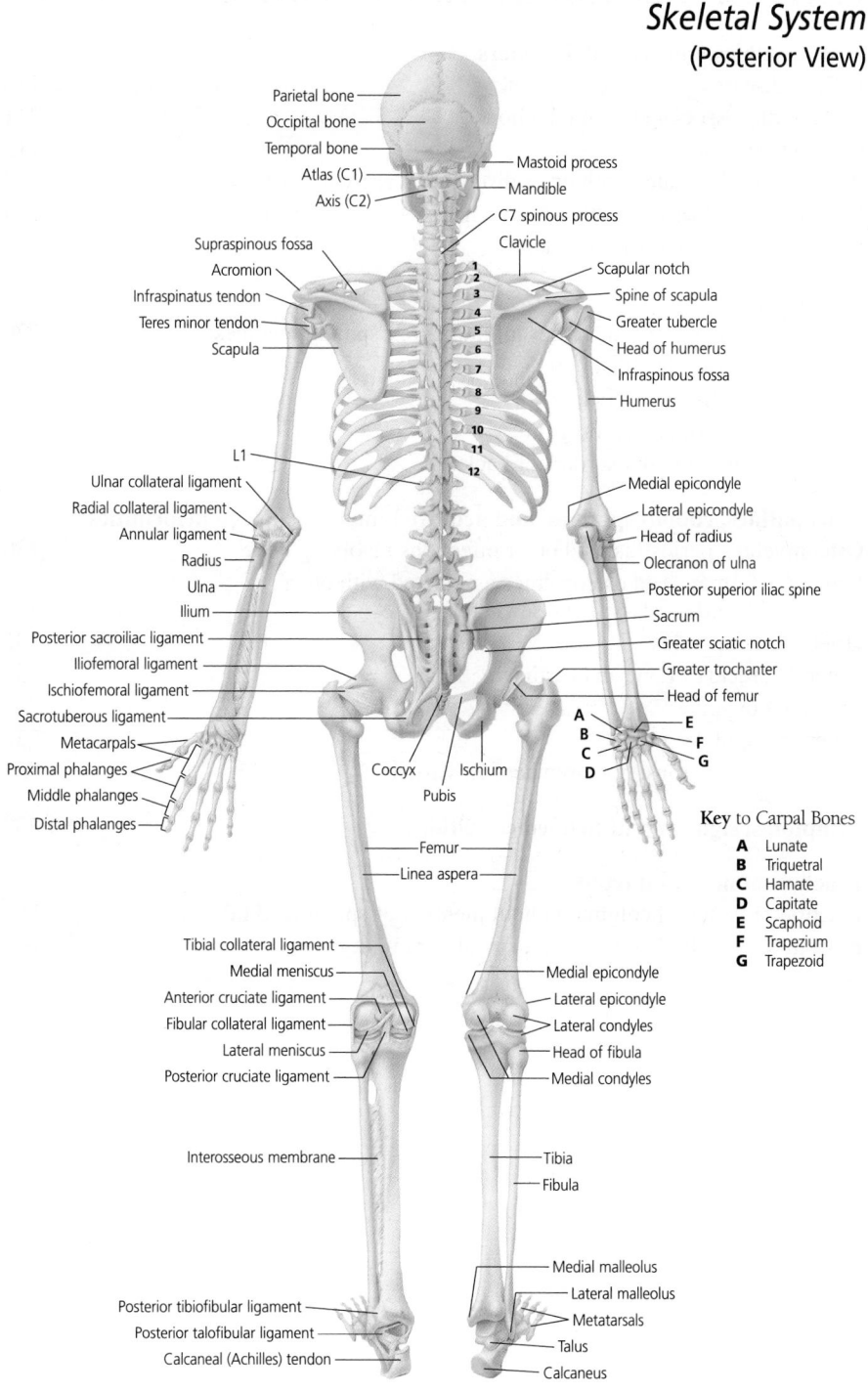

Parietal bone
Occipital bone
Temporal bone
Atlas (C1)
Axis (C2)
Mastoid process
Mandible
C7 spinous process
Clavicle
Supraspinous fossa
Acromion
Infraspinatus tendon
Teres minor tendon
Scapula
Scapular notch
Spine of scapula
Greater tubercle
Head of humerus
Infraspinous fossa
Humerus
L1
Ulnar collateral ligament
Radial collateral ligament
Annular ligament
Radius
Ulna
Ilium
Medial epicondyle
Lateral epicondyle
Head of radius
Olecranon of ulna
Posterior superior iliac spine
Sacrum
Posterior sacroiliac ligament
Iliofemoral ligament
Ischiofemoral ligament
Sacrotuberous ligament
Greater sciatic notch
Greater trochanter
Head of femur
Metacarpals
Proximal phalanges
Middle phalanges
Distal phalanges
Coccyx   Ischium
Pubis
A
B
C
D
E
F
G

Key to Carpal Bones
A Lunate
B Triquetral
C Hamate
D Capitate
E Scaphoid
F Trapezium
G Trapezoid

Femur
Linea aspera
Tibial collateral ligament
Medial meniscus
Anterior cruciate ligament
Fibular collateral ligament
Lateral meniscus
Posterior cruciate ligament
Medial epicondyle
Lateral epicondyle
Lateral condyles
Head of fibula
Medial condyles
Interosseous membrane
Tibia
Fibula
Medial malleolus
Lateral malleolus
Metatarsals
Posterior tibiofibular ligament
Posterior talofibular ligament
Calcaneal (Achilles) tendon
Talus
Calcaneus

©Scientific Publishing Ltd., Rolling Meadows, IL

PLATE 12. SKELETAL SYSTEM — VERTEBRAL COLUMN

Vertebral Column
(Lateral View)

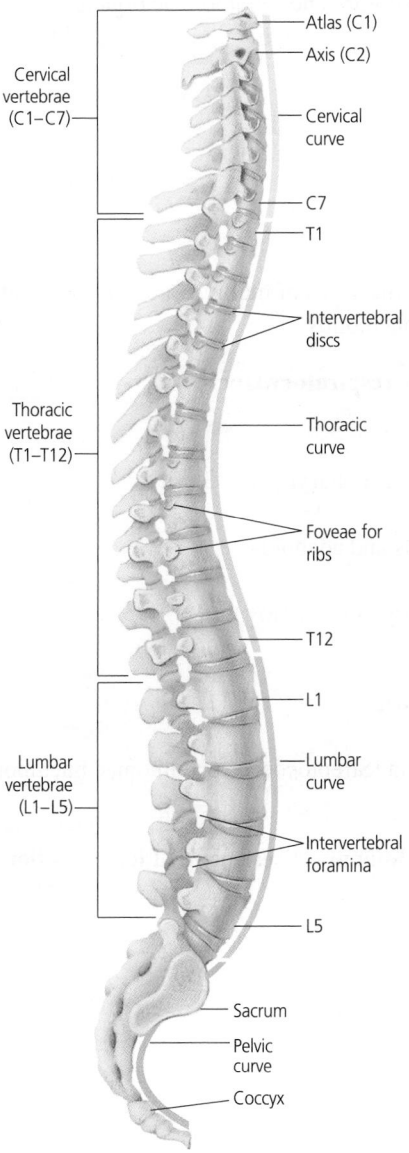

Cervical
vertebrae
(C1–C7)

Thoracic
vertebrae
(T1–T12)

Lumbar
vertebrae
(L1–L5)

Atlas (C1)

Axis (C2)

Cervical
curve

C7

T1

Intervertebral
discs

Thoracic
curve

Foveae for
ribs

T12

L1

Lumbar
curve

Intervertebral
foramina

L5

Sacrum

Pelvic
curve

Coccyx

PLATE 13. RESPIRATORY SYSTEM

Respiratory System

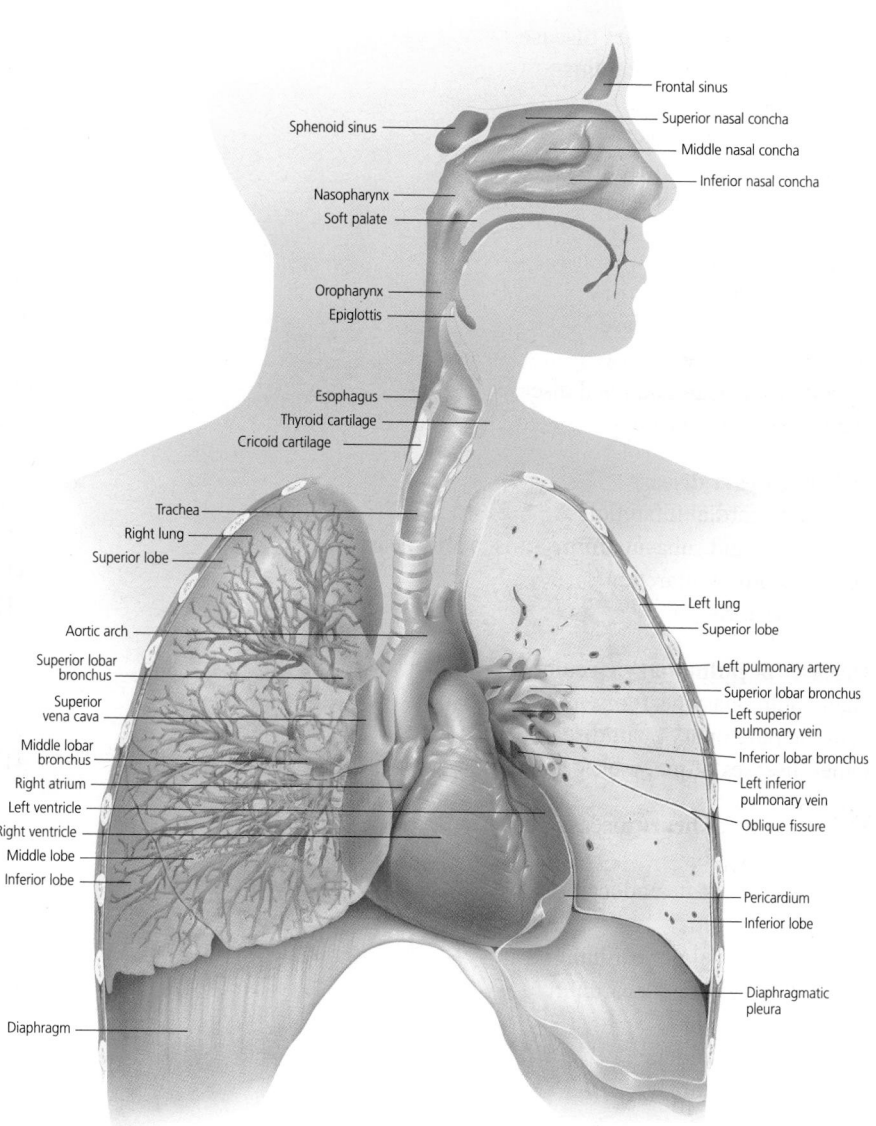

Frontal sinus
Sphenoid sinus
Superior nasal concha
Middle nasal concha
Inferior nasal concha
Nasopharynx
Soft palate
Oropharynx
Epiglottis
Esophagus
Thyroid cartilage
Cricoid cartilage
Trachea
Right lung
Superior lobe
Left lung
Superior lobe
Aortic arch
Superior lobar bronchus
Left pulmonary artery
Superior lobar bronchus
Superior vena cava
Left superior pulmonary vein
Middle lobar bronchus
Inferior lobar bronchus
Right atrium
Left inferior pulmonary vein
Left ventricle
Right ventricle
Oblique fissure
Middle lobe
Inferior lobe
Pericardium
Inferior lobe
Diaphragmatic pleura
Diaphragm

PLATE 14. HEART AND PERICARDIUM

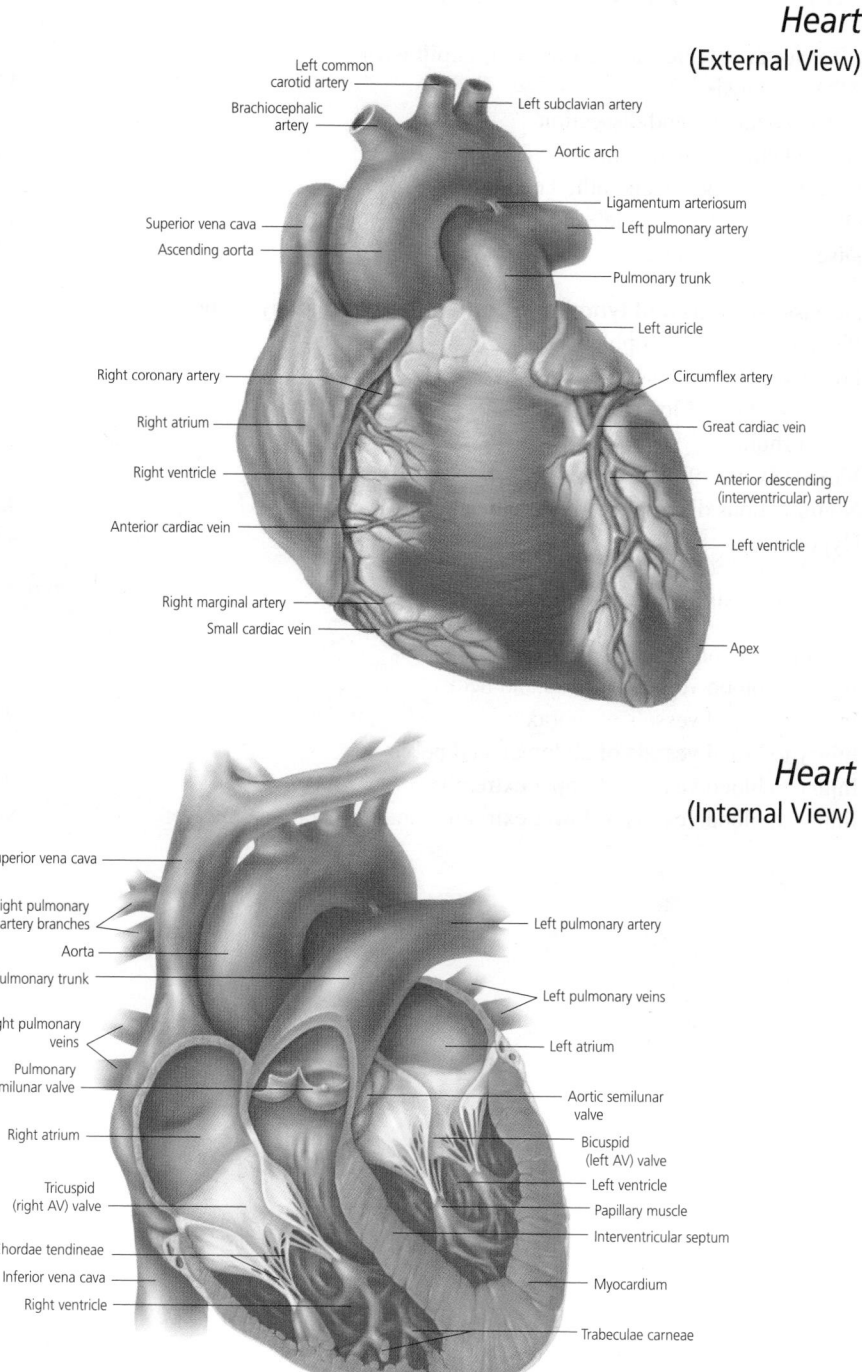

Heart
(External View)

Left common carotid artery

Brachiocephalic artery

Left subclavian artery

Aortic arch

Ligamentum arteriosum

Superior vena cava

Left pulmonary artery

Ascending aorta

Pulmonary trunk

Left auricle

Right coronary artery

Circumflex artery

Right atrium

Great cardiac vein

Right ventricle

Anterior descending (interventricular) artery

Anterior cardiac vein

Left ventricle

Right marginal artery

Small cardiac vein

Apex

Heart
(Internal View)

Superior vena cava

Right pulmonary artery branches

Left pulmonary artery

Aorta

Pulmonary trunk

Left pulmonary veins

Right pulmonary veins

Left atrium

Pulmonary semilunar valve

Aortic semilunar valve

Right atrium

Bicuspid (left AV) valve

Tricuspid (right AV) valve

Left ventricle

Papillary muscle

Chordae tendineae

Interventricular septum

Inferior vena cava

Myocardium

Right ventricle

Trabeculae carneae

PLATE 15. CIRCULATORY SYSTEM

Vascular System

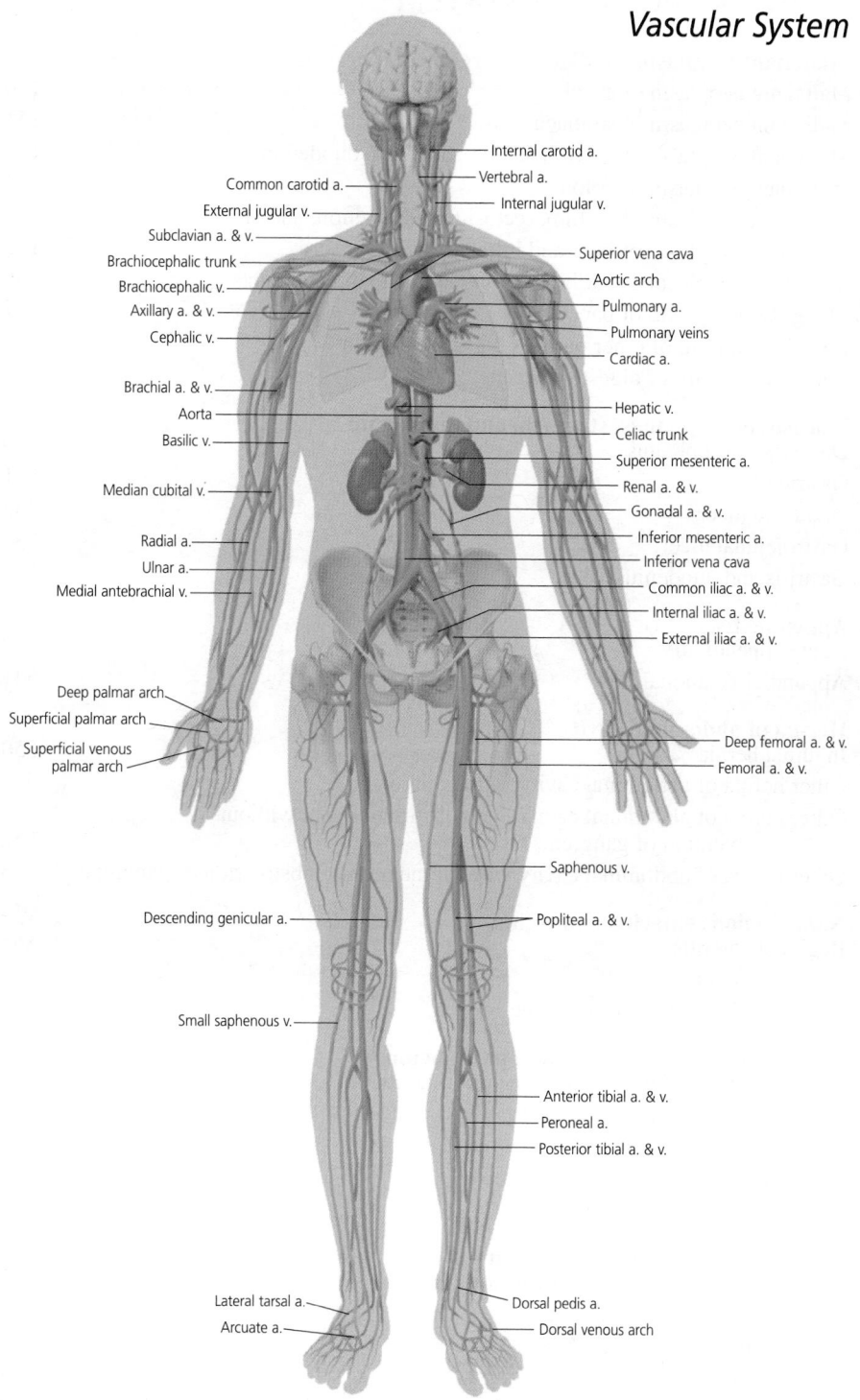

Internal carotid a.
Common carotid a.
Vertebral a.
External jugular v.
Internal jugular v.
Subclavian a. & v.
Superior vena cava
Brachiocephalic trunk
Aortic arch
Brachiocephalic v.
Pulmonary a.
Axillary a. & v.
Pulmonary veins
Cephalic v.
Cardiac a.
Brachial a. & v.
Hepatic v.
Aorta
Celiac trunk
Basilic v.
Superior mesenteric a.
Renal a. & v.
Median cubital v.
Gonadal a. & v.
Radial a.
Inferior mesenteric a.
Ulnar a.
Inferior vena cava
Medial antebrachial v.
Common iliac a. & v.
Internal iliac a. & v.
External iliac a. & v.
Deep palmar arch
Superficial palmar arch
Superficial venous palmar arch
Deep femoral a. & v.
Femoral a. & v.
Saphenous v.
Descending genicular a.
Popliteal a. & v.
Small saphenous v.
Anterior tibial a. & v.
Peroneal a.
Posterior tibial a. & v.
Lateral tarsal a.
Dorsal pedis a.
Arcuate a.
Dorsal venous arch

PLATE 16. DIGESTIVE SYSTEM

Digestive System

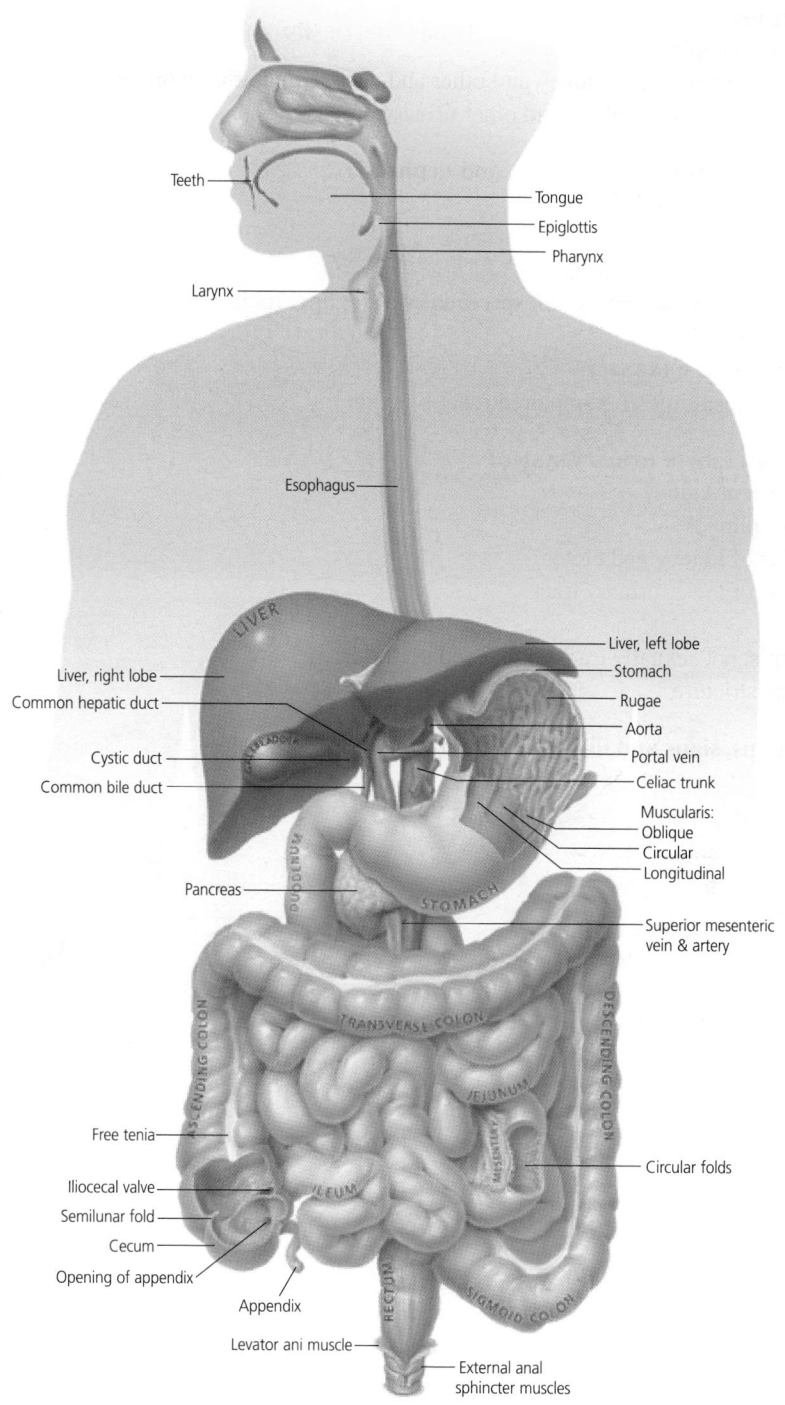

Teeth

Tongue
Epiglottis
Pharynx

Larynx

Esophagus

Liver, right lobe
Common hepatic duct

Liver, left lobe
Stomach
Rugae
Aorta
Portal vein
Celiac trunk

Cystic duct
Common bile duct

Muscularis:
Oblique
Circular
Longitudinal

Pancreas

Superior mesenteric
vein & artery

Free tenia

Circular folds

Iliocecal valve
Semilunar fold
Cecum
Opening of appendix

Appendix

Levator ani muscle

External anal
sphincter muscles

PLATE 17. GENITOURINARY SYSTEM

Neoplasms

Nephritis, nephrotic syndrome, and nephrosis

Other diseases of urinary system

Urinary System

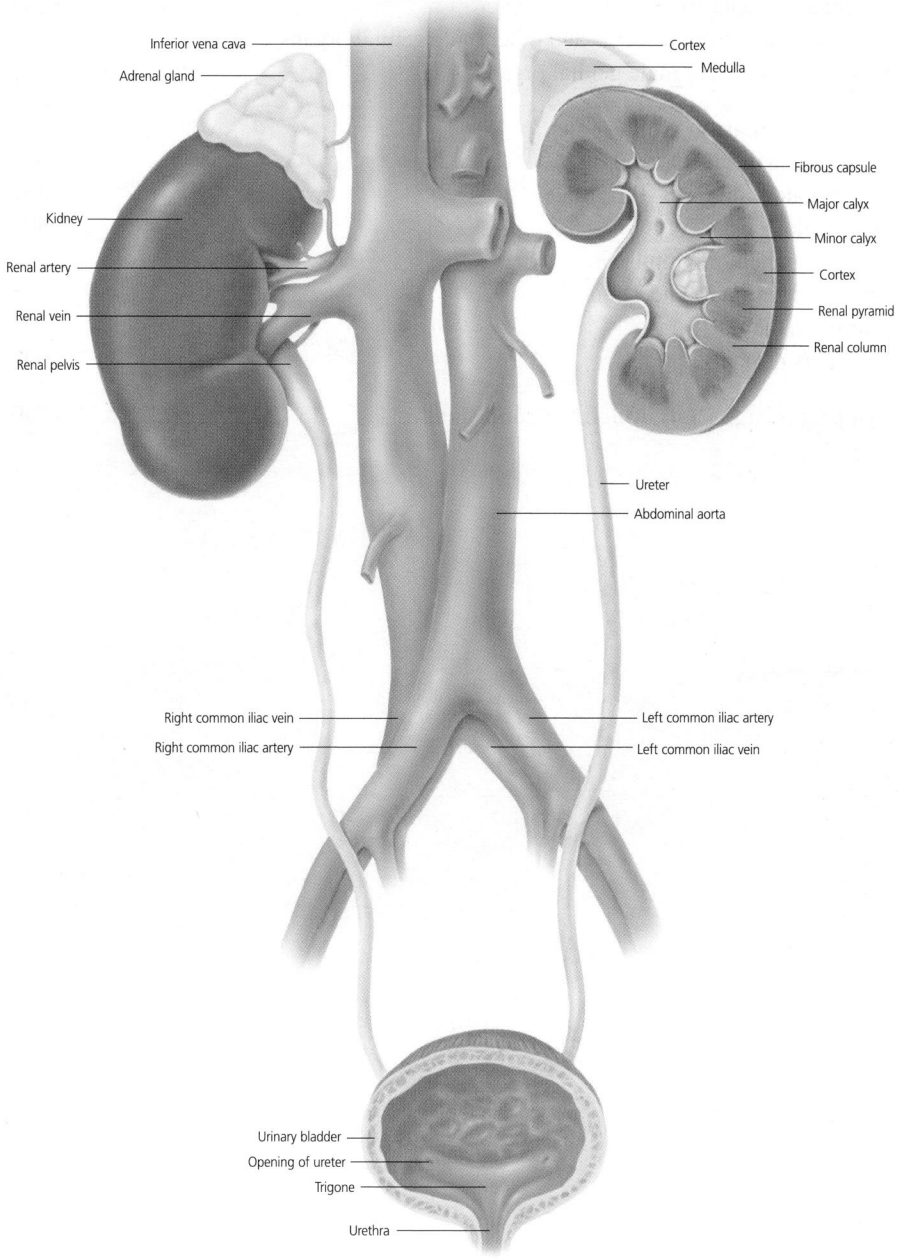

Inferior vena cava

Adrenal gland

Cortex

Medulla

Fibrous capsule

Major calyx

Kidney

Minor calyx

Renal artery

Cortex

Renal vein

Renal pyramid

Renal pelvis

Renal column

Ureter

Abdominal aorta

Right common iliac vein

Left common iliac artery

Right common iliac artery

Left common iliac vein

Urinary bladder

Opening of ureter

Trigone

Urethra

PLATE 18. MALE REPRODUCTIVE SYSTEM

Male Reproductive System

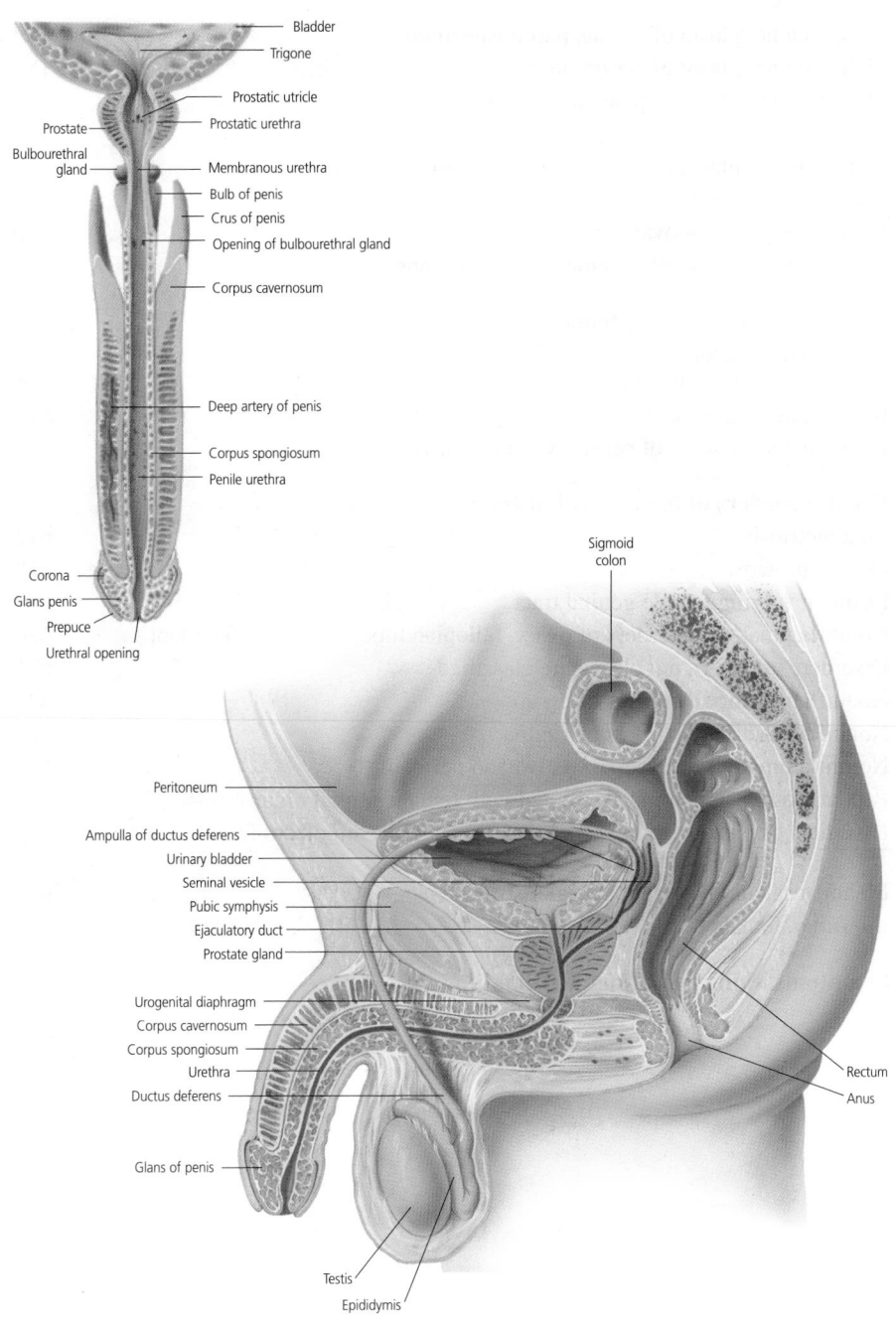

PLATE 19. FEMALE REPRODUCTIVE SYSTEM

Female Reproductive System

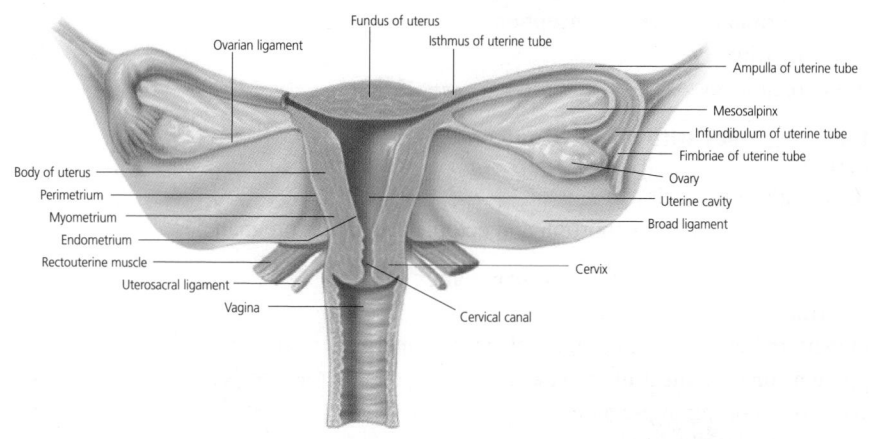

Fundus of uterus
Ovarian ligament
Isthmus of uterine tube
Ampulla of uterine tube
Mesosalpinx
Infundibulum of uterine tube
Fimbriae of uterine tube
Ovary
Uterine cavity
Broad ligament
Body of uterus
Perimetrium
Myometrium
Endometrium
Rectouterine muscle
Uterosacral ligament
Vagina
Cervix
Cervical canal

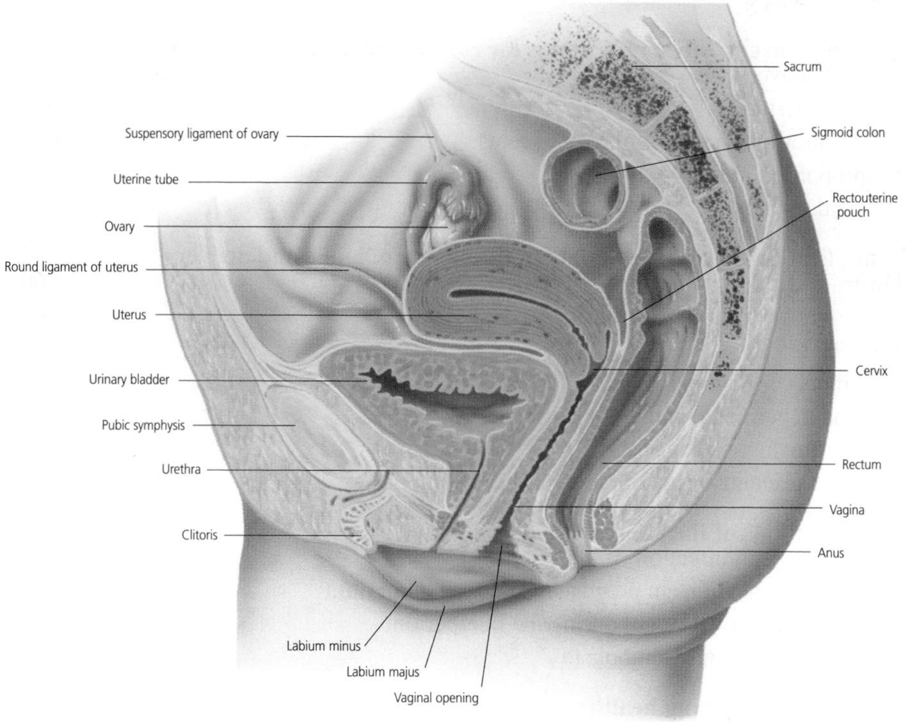

Suspensory ligament of ovary
Uterine tube
Ovary
Round ligament of uterus
Uterus
Urinary bladder
Pubic symphysis
Urethra
Clitoris
Labium minus
Labium majus
Vaginal opening
Sacrum
Sigmoid colon
Rectouterine pouch
Cervix
Rectum
Vagina
Anus

PLATE 20. PREGNANCY, CHILDBIRTH AND THE PUERPERIUM

Female Reproductive System: Pregnancy
(Lateral View)

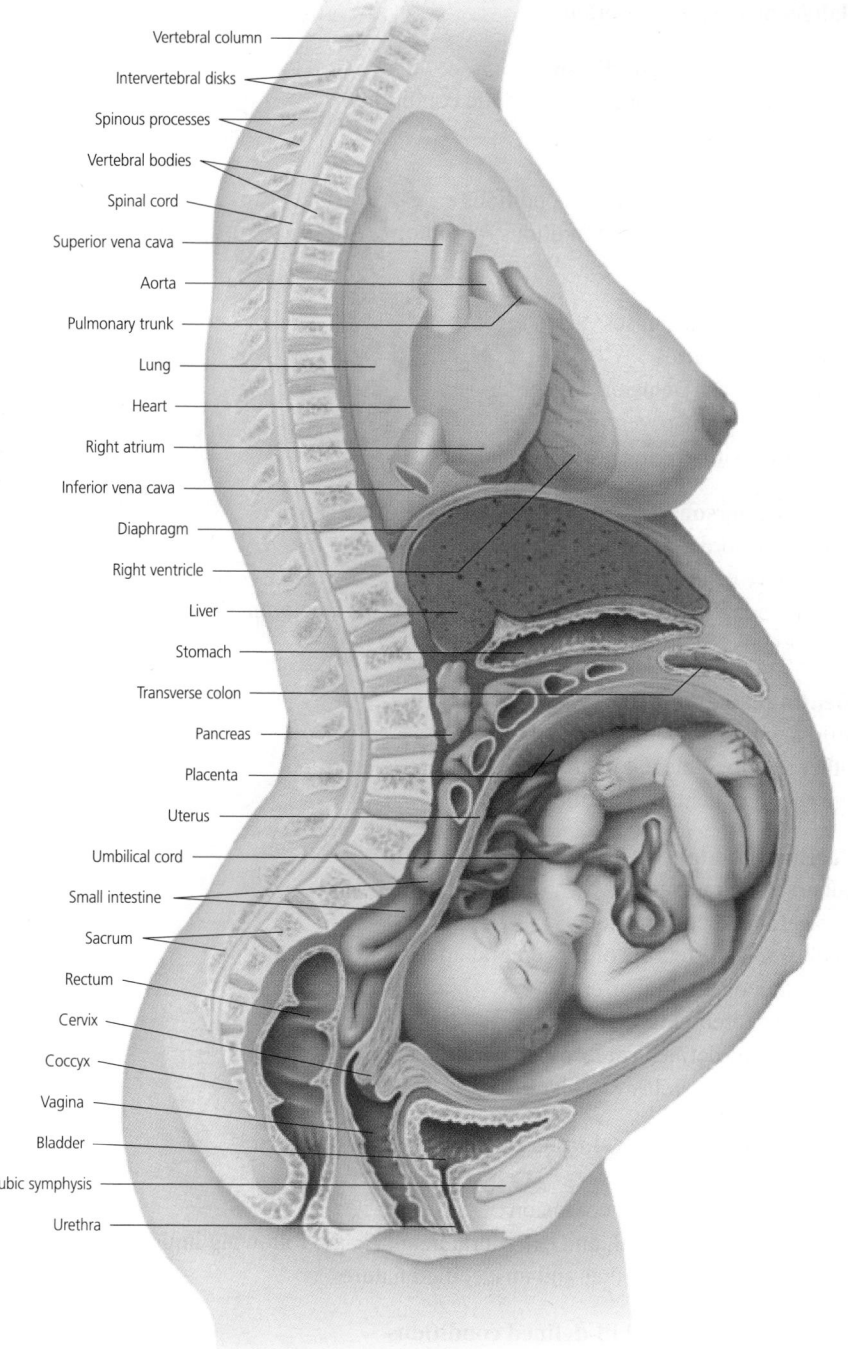

Vertebral column
Intervertebral disks
Spinous processes
Vertebral bodies
Spinal cord
Superior vena cava
Aorta
Pulmonary trunk
Lung
Heart
Right atrium
Inferior vena cava
Diaphragm
Right ventricle
Liver
Stomach
Transverse colon
Pancreas
Placenta
Uterus
Umbilical cord
Small intestine
Sacrum
Rectum
Cervix
Coccyx
Vagina
Bladder
Pubic symphysis
Urethra

PLATE 21. NERVOUS SYSTEM — BRAIN

Brain
(Base View)

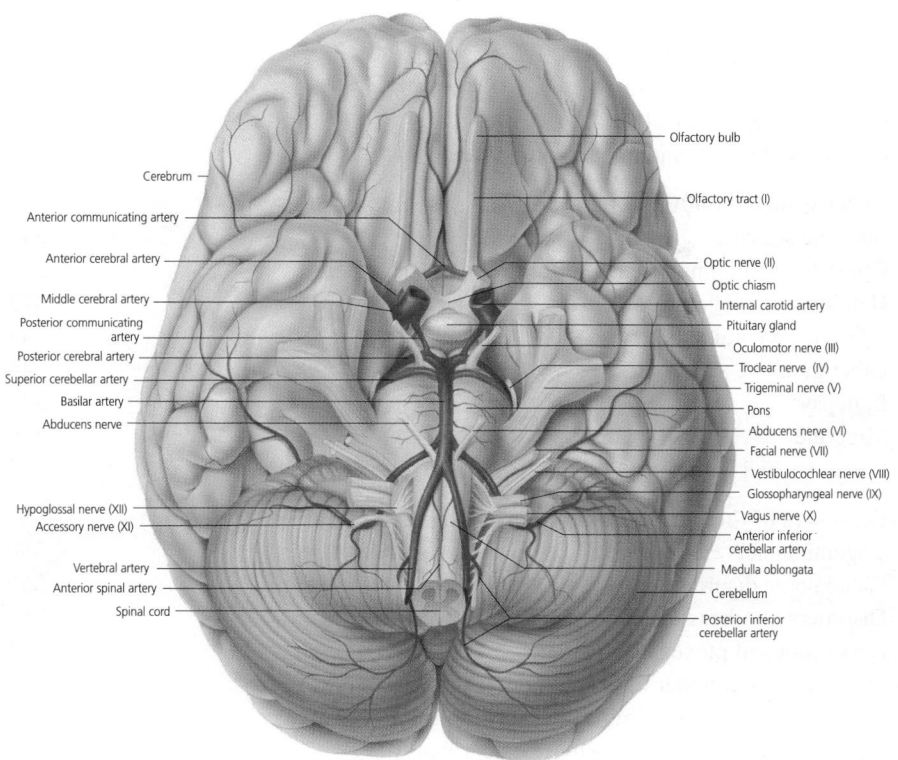

Olfactory bulb

Cerebrum

Anterior communicating artery

Anterior cerebral artery

Middle cerebral artery

Posterior communicating artery

Posterior cerebral artery

Superior cerebellar artery

Basilar artery

Abducens nerve

Hypoglossal nerve (XII)

Accessory nerve (XI)

Vertebral artery

Anterior spinal artery

Spinal cord

Olfactory tract (I)

Optic nerve (II)

Optic chiasm

Internal carotid artery

Pituitary gland

Oculomotor nerve (III)

Troclear nerve (IV)

Trigeminal nerve (V)

Pons

Abducens nerve (VI)

Facial nerve (VII)

Vestibulocochlear nerve (VIII)

Glossopharyngeal nerve (IX)

Vagus nerve (X)

Anterior inferior cerebellar artery

Medulla oblongata

Cerebellum

Posterior inferior cerebellar artery

PLATE 22. NERVOUS SYSTEM

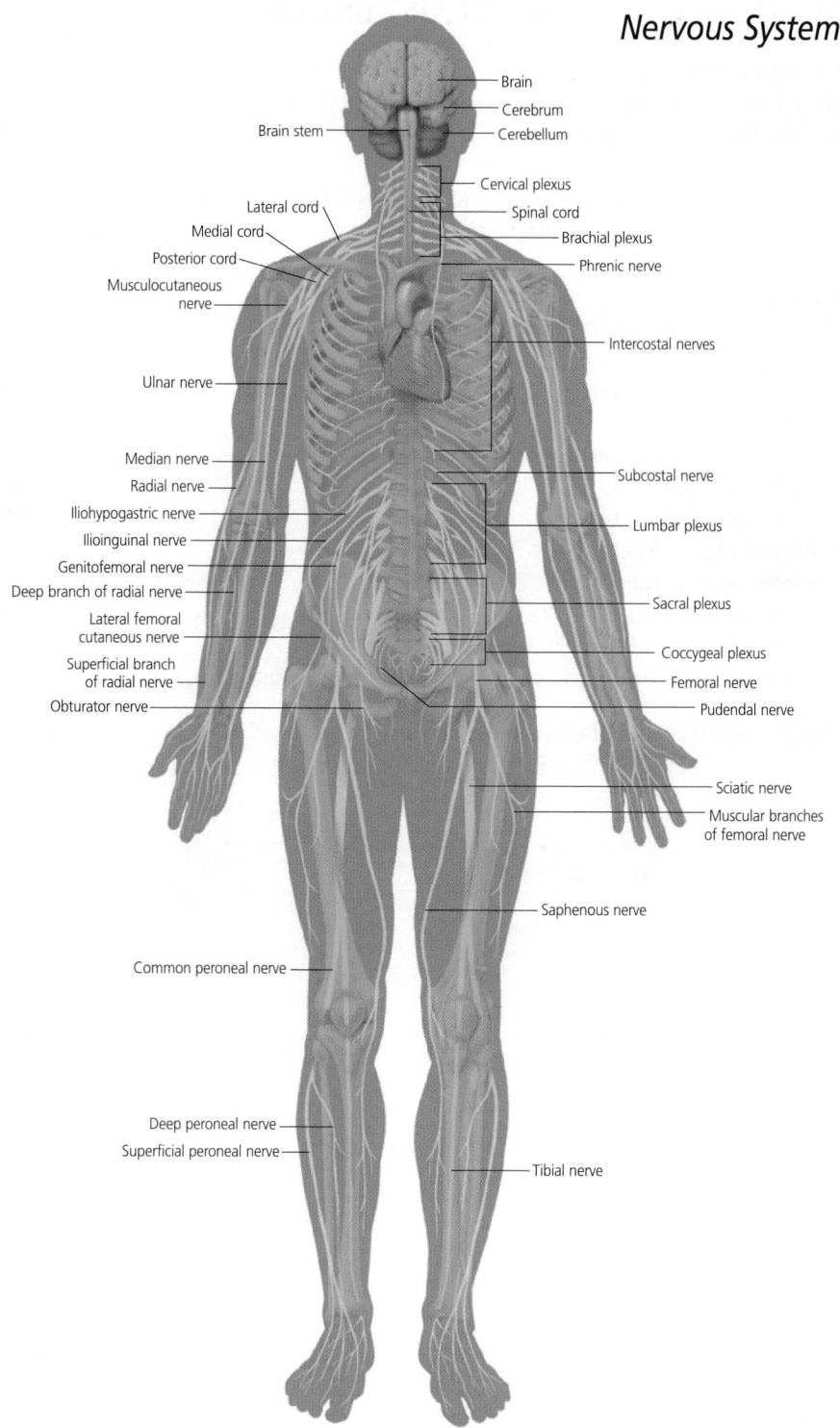

Nervous System

Brain
Cerebrum
Cerebellum
Brain stem
Cervical plexus
Lateral cord
Spinal cord
Medial cord
Brachial plexus
Posterior cord
Phrenic nerve
Musculocutaneous nerve
Intercostal nerves
Ulnar nerve
Median nerve
Subcostal nerve
Radial nerve
Iliohypogastric nerve
Lumbar plexus
Ilioinguinal nerve
Genitofemoral nerve
Deep branch of radial nerve
Sacral plexus
Lateral femoral cutaneous nerve
Superficial branch of radial nerve
Coccygeal plexus
Obturator nerve
Femoral nerve
Pudendal nerve
Sciatic nerve
Muscular branches of femoral nerve
Saphenous nerve
Common peroneal nerve
Deep peroneal nerve
Superficial peroneal nerve
Tibial nerve

PLATE 23. EYE AND OCULAR ADNEXA

Right Eye
(Horizontal Section)

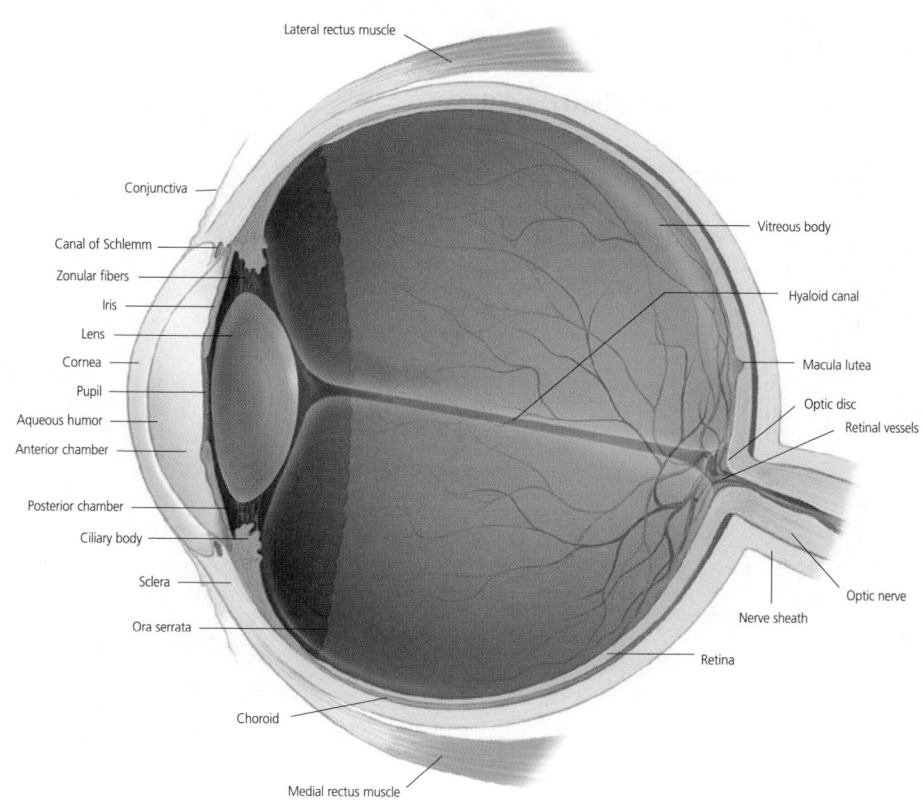

PLATE 24. AUDITORY SYSTEM

The Ear

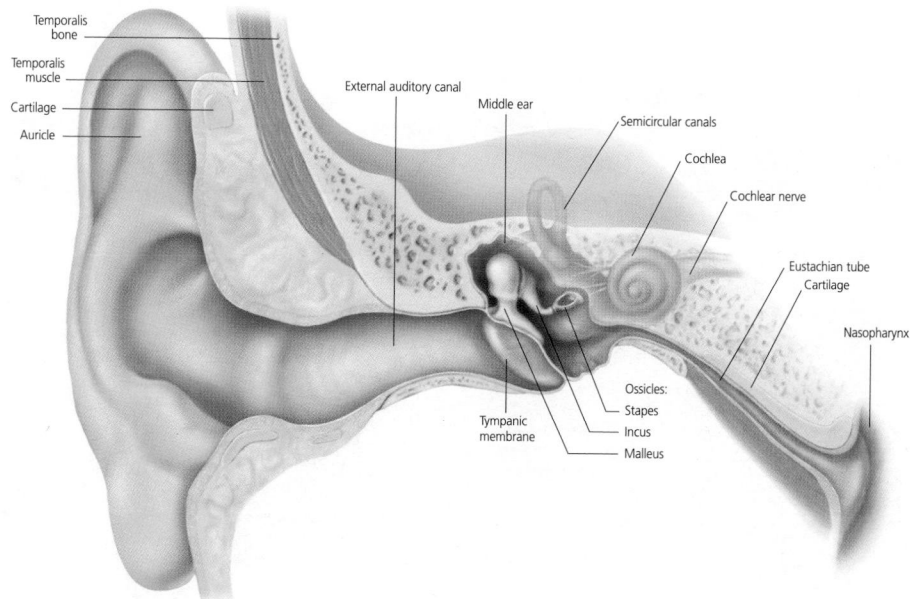

Temporalis bone

Temporalis muscle

Cartilage

Auricle

External auditory canal

Middle ear

Semicircular canals

Cochlea

Cochlear nerve

Eustachian tube

Cartilage

Nasopharynx

Ossicles:

Stapes

Incus

Malleus

Tympanic membrane

This page intentionally left blank.

DISEASES: TABULAR LIST

VOLUME 1

This page intentionally left blank.

Chapter 1: Infectious and Parasitic Diseases (001-139)

DEFINITIONS AND CODING ALERTS

This chapter includes definitions of selected key words, terms and phrases and coding alerts for adding points to the clinical domain, references to coding late effects where appropriate, and references to personal history V-codes in situations where the acute or chronic condition is no longer active. An example from this chapter is as follows:

049 **Other non-arthropod borne viral diseases of central nervous system**

> **DEFINITION** Non-arthropod-borne viral diseases refers to diseases caused by a virus that is not carried by insects, spiders, crustaceans, centipedes or millipedes
> **ALERT!** For coding late effects of viral encephalitis see 139.0.
> **ALERT!** For personal history of other specified infectious and parasitic disease see V12.09.

MULTIPLE CODING FOR A SINGLE CONDITION

In addition to the etiology or manifestation convention that requires two codes to fully describe a single condition that affects multiple body systems, there are other single conditions that also require more than one code. "Use additional code" notes are found in the tabular at codes that are not part of an etiology or manifestation pair where a secondary code is useful to fully describe a condition. The sequencing rule is the same as the etiology or manifestation pair - , "use additional code" indicates that a secondary code should be added. For example, for infections that are not included in chapter 1, a secondary code from category 041, Bacterial infection in conditions classified elsewhere and of unspecified site, may be required to identify the bacterial organism causing the infection. A "use additional code" note will normally be found at the infectious disease code, indicating a need for the organism code to be added as a secondary code.

"Code first" notes are also under certain codes that are not specifically manifestation codes but may be due to an underlying cause. When a "code first" note is present and an underlying condition is present the underlying condition should be sequenced first.

"Code, if applicable, any causal condition first", notes indicate that this code may be assigned as a principal diagnosis when the causal condition is unknown or not applicable. If a causal condition is known, then the code for that condition should be sequenced as the principal or first-listed diagnosis. Multiple codes may be needed for late effects, complication codes and obstetric codes to more fully describe a condition. See the specific guidelines for these conditions for further instruction.

COMBINATION CODE

A combination code is a single code used to classify: two diagnoses, or a diagnosis with an associated secondary process (manifestation) A diagnosis with an associated complication Combination codes are identified by referring to subterm entries in the Alphabetic Index and by reading the inclusion and exclusion notes in the Tabular List.

Assign only the combination code when that code fully identifies the diagnostic conditions involved or when the Alphabetic Index so directs. Multiple coding should not be used when the classification provides a combination code that clearly identifies all of the elements documented in the diagnosis. When the combination code lacks necessary specificity in describing the manifestation or complication, an additional code should be used as a secondary code.

CODING LATE EFFECTS

A late effect is the residual effect (condition produced) after the acute phase of an illness or injury has terminated. There is no time limit on when a late effect code can be used. The residual may be apparent early, such as in cerebrovascular accident cases, or it may occur months or years later, such as that due to a previous injury. Coding of late effects generally requires two codes sequenced in the following order: The condition or nature of the late effect is sequenced first. The late effect code is sequenced second.

An exception to the above guidelines are those instances where the code for late effect is followed by a manifestation code identified in the Tabular List and title, or the late effect code has been expanded (at the fourth and fifth-digit levels) to include the manifestation(s). The code for the acute phase of an illness or injury that led to the late effect is never used with a code for the late effect.

	Add 4th or 5th digit		Nonspecific code		Unspecified code		Manifestation code

HUMAN IMMUNODEFICIENCY VIRUS (HIV) INFECTIONS

Code only confirmed cases

Code only confirmed cases of HIV infection or illness. This is an exception to the hospital inpatient guideline Official Guidelines, Section II, H. In this context, "confirmation" does not require documentation of positive serology or culture for HIV; the provider's diagnostic statement that the patient is HIV positive, or has an HIV-related illness is sufficient.

Selection and sequencing of HIV codes

A. Patient admitted for HIV-related condition

If a patient is admitted for an HIV-related condition, the principal diagnosis should be 042, followed by additional diagnosis codes for all reported HIV-related conditions.

B. Patient with HIV disease admitted for unrelated condition

If a patient with HIV disease is admitted for an unrelated condition (such as a traumatic injury), the code for the unrelated condition (e.g., the nature of injury code) should be the principal diagnosis. Other diagnoses would be 042 followed by additional diagnosis codes for all reported HIV-related conditions.

C. Whether the patient is newly diagnosed

Whether the patient is newly diagnosed or has had previous admissions or encounters for HIV conditions is irrelevant to the sequencing decision.

D. Asymptomatic human immunodeficiency virus V08

Asymptomatic human immunodeficiency virus [HIV] infection, is to be applied when the patient without any documentation of symptoms is listed as being "HIV positive," "known HIV," "HIV test positive," or similar terminology. Do not use this code if the term "AIDS" is used or if the patient is treated for any HIV-related illness or is described as having any condition(s) resulting from his or her HIV positive status; use 042 in these cases.

E. Patients with inconclusive HIV serology

Patients with inconclusive HIV serology, but no definitive diagnosis or manifestations of the illness, may be assigned code 795.71, Inconclusive serologic test for Human Immunodeficiency Virus [HIV].

F. Previously diagnosed HIV-related illness

Patients with any known prior diagnosis of an HIV-related illness should be coded to 042. Once a patient has developed an HIV-related illness, the patient should always be assigned code 042 on every subsequent admission or encounter. Patients previously diagnosed with any HIV illness 042 should never be assigned to 795.71 or V08.

G. HIV Infection in Pregnancy, Childbirth and the Puerperium

During pregnancy, childbirth or the puerperium, a patient admitted (or presenting for a health care encounter) because of an HIV-related illness should receive a principal diagnosis code of 647.6X, Other specified infectious and parasitic diseases in the mother classifiable elsewhere, but complicating the pregnancy, childbirth or the puerperium, followed by 042 and the code(s) for the HIV-related illness(es). Codes from Chapter 15 always take sequencing priority.

Patients with asymptomatic HIV infection status admitted (or presenting for a health care encounter) during pregnancy, childbirth, or the puerperium should receive codes of 647.6X and V08.

H. Encounters for testing for HIV

If a patient is being seen to determine his or her HIV status, use code V73.89, Screening for other specified viral disease. Use code V69.8, Other problems related to lifestyle, as a secondary code if an asymptomatic patient is in a known high risk group for HIV. Should a patient with signs or symptoms or illness, or a confirmed HIV related diagnosis be tested for HIV, code the signs and symptoms or the diagnosis. An additional counseling code V65.44 may be used if counseling is provided during the encounter for the test.

When a patient returns to be informed of his or her HIV test results use code V65.44, HIV counseling, if the results of the test are negative.

● Code new
to 2012 edition
▲ Revision of
existing code
④ ⑤ Fourth or fifth
digit required

If the results are positive but the patient is asymptomatic use code V08, Asymptomatic HIV infection. If the results are positive and the patient is symptomatic use code 042, HIV infection, with codes for the HIV related symptoms or diagnosis. The HIV counseling code may also be used if counseling is provided for patients with positive test results.

SEPTICEMIA, SYSTEMIC INFLAMMATORY RESPONSE SYNDROME (SIRS), SEPSIS, SEVERE SEPSIS, AND SEPTIC SHOCK

SIRS, Septicemia, and Sepsis

A. The terms septicemia and sepsis are often used interchangeably by providers, however they are not considered synonymous terms. The following descriptions are provided for reference but do not preclude querying the provider for clarification about terms used in the documentation:

1) Septicemia generally refers to a systemic disease associated with the presence of pathological microorganisms or toxins in the blood, which can include bacteria, viruses, fungi or other organisms.

2) Systemic inflammatory response syndrome (SIRS) generally refers to the systemic response to infection, trauma or burns, or other insult (such as cancer) with symptoms including fever, tachycardia, tachypnea, and leukocytosis.

3) Sepsis generally refers to SIRS due to infection.

4) Severe sepsis generally refers to sepsis with associated acute organ dysfunction.

B. The Coding of SIRS, sepsis and severe sepsis requires a minimum of 2 codes: a code for the underlying cause (such as infection or trauma) and a code from subcategory 995.9 Systemic inflammatory response syndrome (SIRS).

1) The code for the underlying cause (such as infection or trauma) must be sequenced before the code from subcategory 995.9 Systemic inflammatory response syndrome (SIRS).

2) Sepsis and severe sepsis require a code for the systemic infection (038.xx, 112.5, etc.) and either code 995.91, Sepsis, or 995.92, Severe sepsis. If the causal organism is not documented, assign code 038.9, Unspecified septicemia.

3) Severe sepsis requires additional code(s) for the associated acute organ dysfunction(s).

4) If a patient has sepsis with multiple organ dysfunctions, follow the instructions for coding severe sepsis.

5) Either the term sepsis or SIRS must be documented to assign a code from subcategory 995.9.

6) See Official Guidelines, Section I.C.17 g, Injury And Poisoning, Due To Non-Infectious Process, for information regarding systemic inflammatory response syndrome (SIRS) due to trauma or burns and other non-infectious processes.

C. Due to the complex nature of sepsis and severe sepsis, some cases may requirequerying the provider prior to assignment of the codes.

Sequencing sepsis and severe sepsis

A. Sepsis and severe sepsis as principal diagnosis

If sepsis or severe sepsis is present on admission, and meets the definition of principal diagnosis, the systemic infection code (e.g., 038.xx, 112.5, etc) should be assigned as the principal diagnosis, followed by code 995.91, Sepsis, or 995.92, Severe sepsis, as required by the sequencing rules in the Tabular List. Codes from subcategory 995.9 can never be assigned as a principal diagnosis. A code should also be assigned for any localized infection, if present.

If the sepsis or severe sepsis is due to a postprocedural infection, see Official Guidelines, Section I.C.10 for guidelines related to sepsis due to postprocedural infection.

B. Sepsis and severe sepsis as secondary diagnoses

When sepsis or severe sepsis develops during the encounter (it was not present on admission), the systemic infection code and code 995.91 or 995.92 should be assigned as secondary diagnoses.

	Add 4th or 5th digit		Nonspecific code		Unspecified code		Manifestation code

C. Documentation unclear as to whether sepsis or severe sepsis is present on admission

Sepsis or severe sepsis may be present on admission but the diagnosis may not be confirmed until sometime after admission. If the documentation is not clear whether the sepsis or severe sepsis was present on admission, the provider should be queried.

Sepsis or SIRS with Localized Infection

If the reason for admission is both sepsis, severe sepsis, or SIRS and a localized infection, such as pneumonia or cellulitis, a code for the systemic infection (038.xx, 112.5, etc) should be assigned first, then code 995.91 or 995.92, followed by the code for the localized infection. If the patient is admitted with a localized infection, such as pneumonia, and sepsis or SIRS doesn't develop until after admission, see Official Guidelines, Section I.c.1.b.2.b).

If the localized infection is postprocedural, see Official Guidelines, Section I.c.10 for guidelines related to sepsis due to postprocedural infection.

Note: The term urosepsis is a nonspecific term. If that is the only term documented then only code 599.0 should be assigned based on the default for the term in the ICD-9-CM index, in addition to the code for the causal organism if known.

Bacterial Sepsis and Septicemia

In most cases, it will be a code from category 038, Septicemia, that will be used in conjunction with a code from subcategory 995.9 such as the following:

A. Streptococcal sepsis

If the documentation in the record states streptococcal sepsis, codes 038.0, Streptococcal septicemia, and code 995.91 should be used, in that sequence.

B. Streptococcal septicemia

If the documentation states streptococcal septicemia, only code 038.0 should be assigned, however, the provider should be queried whether the patient has sepsis, an infection with SIRS.

Acute organ dysfunction that is not clearly associated with the sepsis

If a patient has sepsis and an acute organ dysfunction, but the medical record documentation indicates that the acute organ dysfunction is related to a medical condition other than the sepsis, do not assign code 995.92, Severe sepsis. An acute organ dysfunction must be associated with the sepsis in order to assign the severe sepsis code. If the documentation is not clear as to whether an acute organ dysfunction is related to the sepsis or another medical condition, query the provider.

Septic shock

A. Sequencing of septic shock

Septic shock generally refers to circulatory failure associated with severe sepsis, and, therefore, it represents a type of acute organ dysfunction.

For all cases of septic shock, the code for the systemic infection should be sequenced first, followed by codes 995.92 and 785.52. Any additional codes for other acute organ dysfunctions should also be assigned. As noted in the sequencing instructions in the Tabular List, the code for septic shock cannot be assigned as a principal diagnosis.

B. Septic Shock without documentation of severe sepsis

Septic shock indicates the presence of severe sepsis.

Code 995.92, Severe sepsis, must be assigned with code 785.52, Septic shock, even if the term severe sepsis is not documented in the record. The "use additional code" note and the "code first" note in the tabular support this guideline.

● Code new
to 2012 edition

▲ Revision of
existing code

④ ⑤ Fourth or fifth
digit required

Sepsis and septic shock complicating abortion and pregnancy

Sepsis and septic shock complicating abortion, ectopic pregnancy, and molar pregnancy are classified to category codes in Chapter 11 (630-639).

Negative or inconclusive blood cultures

Negative or inconclusive blood cultures do not preclude a diagnosis of septicemia or sepsis in patients with clinical evidence of the condition, however, the provider should be queried.

Newborn sepsis

Code 771.81, Septicemia [sepsis] of newborn, should be assigned with a secondary code from category 041, Bacterial infections in conditions classified elsewhere and of unspecified site, to identify the organism.

Sepsis due to a Postprocedural Infection

A. Documentation of causal relationship

As with all postprocedural complications, code assignment is based on the provider's documentation of the relationship between the infection and the procedure.

B. Sepsis due to postprocedural infection

In cases of postprocedural sepsis, the complication code, such as code 998.59, Other postoperative infection, or 674.3x, Other complications of obstetrical surgical wounds should be coded first followed by the appropriate sepsis codes (systemic infection code and either code 995.91or 995.92. An additional code(s) for any acute organ dysfunction should also be assigned for cases of severe sepsis.

External cause of injury codes with SIRS

An external cause code with systemic inflammatory response syndrome (SIRS) is not appropriate with a code from subcategory 995.9, unless the patient also has an injury, poisoning, or adverse effect of drugs.

Sepsis and Severe Sepsis Associated with Noninfectious Process

In some cases, a non-infectious process, such as trauma, may lead to an infection which can result in sepsis or severe sepsis. If sepsis or severe sepsis is documented as associated with a non-infectious condition, such as a burn or serious injury, and this condition meets the definition for principal diagnosis, the code for the noninfectious condition should be sequenced first, followed by the code for the systemic infection and either code 995.91, Sepsis, or 995.92, Severe sepsis. Additional codes for any associated acute organ dysfunction(s) should also be assigned for cases of severe sepsis. If the sepsis or severe sepsis meets the definition of principal diagnosis, the systemic infection and sepsis codes should be sequenced before the non-infectious condition. When both the associated non-infectious condition and the sepsis or severe sepsis meet the definition of principal diagnosis, either may be assigned as principal diagnosis.

See Official Guidelines, Section I.C.1.b.2.a for guidelines pertaining to sepsis or severe sepsis as the principal diagnosis.

Only one code from subcategory 995.9 should be assigned. Therefore, when a non-infectious condition leads to an infection resulting in sepsis or severe sepsis, assign either code 995.91 or 995.92. Do not additionally assign code 995.93, Systemic inflammatory response syndrome due to non-infectious process without acute organ dysfunction, or 995.94, Systemic inflammatory response syndrome with acute organ dysfunction.

SIRS Due To Trauma Or Burns Or Other Non-Infectious Disease Processes

The systemic inflammatory response syndrome (SIRS) can develop as a result of certain non-infectious disease processes, such as trauma, malignant neoplasm, or pancreatitis. When SIRS is documented with a noninfectious condition, and no subsequent infection is documented, the code for the underlying condition, such as an injury, should be assigned, followed by code 995.93, Systemic inflammatory response syndrome due to noninfectious process without acute organ dysfunction, or 995.94, Systemic inflammatory response syndrome due to non-infectious process with acute organ dysfunction. If an acute organ dysfunction is documented, the appropriate code(s) for the associated acute organ dysfunction(s) should be assigned in addition to code 995.94. If acute organ dysfunction is documented, but it cannot be determined if the acute organ dysfunction is associated with SIRS or due to another condition (e.g., directly due to the trauma), the provider should be queried.

| | Add 4th or 5th digit | | Nonspecific code | | Unspecified code | | Manifestation code |

METHICILLIN RESISTANT STAPHYLOCOCCUS AUREUS (MRSA) CONDITIONS

Selection and sequencing of MRSA codes

A. Combination codes for MRSA infection

When a patient is diagnosed with an infection that is due to methicillin resistant Staphylococcus aureus (MRSA), and that infection has a combination code that includes the causal organism (e.g., septicemia, pneumonia) assign the appropriate code for the condition (e.g., code 038.12, Methicillin resistant Staphylococcus aureus septicemia or code 482.42, Methicillin resistant pneumonia due to Staphylococcus aureus). Do not assign code 041.12, Methicillin resistant Staphylococcus aureus, as an additional code because the code includes the type of infection and the MRSA organism. Do not assign a code from subcategory V09.0, Infection with microorganisms resistant to penicillins, as an additional diagnosis.

See Section C.1.b.1 for instructions on coding and sequencing of septicemia.

B. Other codes for MRSA infection

When there is documentation of a current infection (e.g., wound infection, stitch abscess, urinary tract infection) due to MRSA, and that infection does not have a combination code that includes the causal organism, select the appropriate code to identify the condition along with code 041.12, Methicillin resistant Staphylococcus aureus, for the MRSA infection. Do not assign a code from subcategory V09.0, Infection with microorganisms resistant to penicillins.

C. Methicillin susceptible Staphylococcus aureus (MSSA) and MRSA colonization

The condition or state of being colonized or carrying MSSA or MRSA is called colonization or carriage, while an individual person is described as being colonized or being a carrier. Colonization means that MSSA or MSRA is present on or in the body without necessarily causing illness. A positive MRSA colonization test might be documented by the provider as "MRSA screen positive" or "MRSA nasal swab positive".

Assign code V02.54, Carrier or suspected carrier, Methicillin resistant Staphylococcus aureus, for patients documented as having MRSA colonization. Assign code V02.53, Carrier or suspected carrier, Methicillin susceptible Staphylococcus aureus, for patient documented as having MSSA colonization. Colonization is not necessarily indicative of a disease process or as the cause of a specific condition the patient may have unless documented as such by the provider.

Code V02.59, Other specified bacterial diseases, should be assigned for other types of staphylococcal colonization (e.g., S. epidermidis, S. saprophyticus).

Code V02.59 should not be assigned for colonization with any type of Staphylococcus aureus (MRSA, MSSA).

D. MRSA colonization and infection

If a patient is documented as having both MRSA colonization and infection during a hospital admission, code V02.54, Carrier or suspected carrier, Methicillin resistant Staphylococcus aureus, and a code for the MRSA infection may both be assigned.

● Code new
to 2012 edition ▲ Revision of
existing code ④ ⑤ Fourth or fifth
digit required

1. INFECTIOUS AND PARASITIC DISEASES (001-139)

[ALERT!] For personal history of infectious and parasitic disease see V12.0

Note: Categories for "late effects" of infectious and parasitic diseases are to be found at 137-139.

Includes: diseases generally recognized as communicable or transmissible as well as a few diseases of unknown but possibly infectious origin

[*Excludes:*] *acute respiratory infections (460-466)*
carrier or suspected carrier of infectious organism (V02.0-V02.9)
certain localized infections
influenza (487.0-487.8, 488.01-488.19)

INTESTINAL INFECTIOUS DISEASES (001-009)

[*Excludes:*] *helminthiases (120.0-129)*

001 Cholera

[DEFINITION] Cholera, aka asiatic or epidemic cholera, is an infectious gastroenteritis caused by enterotoxin-producing strains of the bacterium vibrio cholerae.

001.0 Due to Vibrio cholerae

001.1 Due to Vibrio cholerae el tor

001.9 Cholera, unspecified

002 Typhoid and paratyphoid fevers

[DEFINITION] Typhoid fever, aka enteric fever, salmonella typhi is an illness caused by the bacterium salmonella enterica serovar typhi.

002.0 Typhoid fever
Typhoid (fever) (infection) [any site]

002.1 Paratyphoid fever A

002.2 Paratyphoid fever B

002.3 Paratyphoid fever C

002.9 Paratyphoid fever, unspecified

003 Other salmonella infections
Includes: infection or food poisoning by Salmonella [any serotype]

[DEFINITION] Salmonellosis is an infection with salmonella bacteria. Most persons infected with salmonella develop diarrhea, fever, vomiting, and abdominal cramps.

003.0 Salmonella gastroenteritis
Salmonellosis

003.1 Salmonella septicemia

[5] **003.2 Localized salmonella infections**

003.20 Localized salmonella infection, unspecified

003.21 Salmonella meningitis

003.22 Salmonella pneumonia

003.23 Salmonella arthritis

003.24 Salmonella osteomyelitis

003.29 Other

003.8 Other specified salmonella infections

003.9 Salmonella infection, unspecified

004 Shigellosis
Includes: bacillary dysentery

[DEFINITION] Shigellosis, aka bacillary dysentery, is a food borne illness caused by infection by bacteria of the genus shigella.

004.0 Shigella dysenteriae
Infection by group A Shigella (Schmitz) (Shiga)

004.1 Shigella flexneri
Infection by group B Shigella

004.2 Shigella boydii
Infection by group C Shigella

004.3 Shigella sonnei
Infection by group D Shigella

004.8 Other specified shigella infections

004.9 Shigellosis, unspecified

005 **Other food poisoning (bacterial)**

> *Excludes:* salmonella infections (003.0-003.9)
> > *toxic effect of:*
> > *food contaminants (989.7)*
> > *noxious foodstuffs (988.0-988.9)*

DEFINITION Food poisoning (bacterial) is any illness resulting from the consumption of contaminated food.

005.0 **Staphylococcal food poisoning**
Staphylococcal toxemia specified as due to food

005.1 **Botulism food poisoning**
Botulism NOS
Food poisoning due to Clostridium botulinum

> *Excludes:* infant botulism (040.41)
> > wound botulism (040.42)

DEFINITION Botulism is food poisoning resulting from the toxin produced by botulinus bacteria, sometimes found in foods improperly canned or preserved; often fatal.

005.2 **Food poisoning due to Clostridium perfringens [C. welchii]**
Enteritis necroticans

005.3 **Food poisoning due to other Clostridia**

005.4 **Food poisoning due to Vibrio parahaemolyticus**

⑤ **005.8** **Other bacterial food poisoning**

> *Excludes:* salmonella food poisoning (003.0-003.9)

005.81 **Food poisoning due to Vibrio vulnificus**

005.89 **Other bacterial food poisoning**
Food poisoning due to Bacillus cereus

005.9 **Food poisoning, unspecified**

006 **Amebiasis**
Includes: infection due to Entamoeba histolytica

> *Excludes:* amebiasis due to organisms other than Entamoeba histolytica (007.8)

DEFINITION Amebiasis is an inflammation of the intestines caused by infection with entamoeba histolytica characterized by frequent, loose stools flecked with blood and mucus.
DEFINITION Amebic dysentery is an inflammation of the intestines caused by endamoeba histolytica; usually acquired by ingesting food or water contaminated with feces; characterized by severe diarrhea.

006.0 **Acute amebic dysentery without mention of abscess**
Acute amebiasis

006.1 **Chronic intestinal amebiasis without mention of abscess**
Chronic:
amebiasis
amebic dysentery

006.2 **Amebic nondysenteric colitis**

006.3 **Amebic liver abscess**
Hepatic amebiasis

006.4 **Amebic lung abscess**
Amebic abscess of lung (and liver)

006.5 **Amebic brain abscess**
Amebic abscess of brain (and liver) (and lung)

006.6 **Amebic skin ulceration**
Cutaneous amebiasis

006.8 **Amebic infection of other sites**
Amebic: Ameboma
appendicitis
balanitis

> *Excludes:* specific infections by free-living amebae (136.21-136.29)

006.9 **Amebiasis, unspecified**
Amebiasis NOS

● Code new
  to 2012 edition
▲ Revision of
  existing code
④ ⑤ Fourth or fifth
  digit required

007 **Other protozoal intestinal diseases**
Includes: protozoal:
colitis
diarrhea
dysentery

DEFINITION Protozoal intestinal diseases refers to diseases of the intestinal system caused by protozoa, which are single-cell organisms that can only divide within a host organism. Malaria ,giardia and toxoplasmosis are examples of diseases caused by protozoa.

ALERT! For personal history of other specified infectious and parasitic disease see V12.09.

007.0 Balantidiasis
Infection by Balantidium coli

007.1 Giardiasis
Infection by Giardia lamblia
Lambliasis

007.2 Coccidiosis
Infection by Isospora belli and Isospora hominis
Isosporiasis

007.3 Intestinal trichomoniasis

007.4 Cryptosporidiosis

007.5 Cyclosporiasis

007.8 Other specified protozoal intestinal diseases
Amebiasis due to organisms other than Entamoeba histolytica

007.9 Unspecified protozoal intestinal disease
Flagellate diarrhea   Protozoal dysentery NOS

008 **Intestinal infections due to other organisms**
Includes: any condition classifiable to 009.0-009.3 with mention of the responsible
organisms

Excludes: *food poisoning by these organisms (005.0-005.9)*

⑤ **008.0 Escherichia coli [E. coli]**

008.00   E. coli, unspecified
E. coli enteritis NOS

008.01   Enteropathogenic E. coli

008.02   Enterotoxigenic E. coli

008.03   Enteroinvasive E. coli

008.04   Enterohemorrhagic E. coli

008.09   Other intestinal E. coli infections

008.1 Arizona group of paracolon bacilli

008.2 Aerobacter aerogenes
Enterobacter aerogenes

008.3 Proteus (mirabilis) (morganii)

⑤ **008.4 Other specified bacteria**

008.41   Staphylococcus
Staphylococcal enterocolitis

008.42   Pseudomonas

008.43   Campylobacter

008.44   Yersinia enterocolitica

008.45   Clostridium difficile
Pseudomembranous colitis

008.46   Other anaerobes
Anaerobic enteritis NOS
Bacteroides (fragilis)
Gram-negative anaerobes

008.47   Other Gram-negative bacteria
Gram-negative enteritis NOS

Excludes: *Gram-negative anaerobes (008.46)*

008.49   Other

008.5 Bacterial enteritis, unspecified

⑤ **008.6 Enteritis due to specified virus**

008.61   Rotavirus

	Add 4th or 5th digit		Nonspecific code		Unspecified code		Manifestation code

008.62 Adenovirus

008.63 Norwalk virus
Norovirus
Norwalk-like agent

008.64 Other small round viruses [SRV's]
Small round virus NOS

008.65 Calicivirus

008.66 Astrovirus

008.67 Enterovirus NEC
Coxsackie virus
Echovirus

[Excludes:] *poliovirus (045.0-045.9)*

008.69 Other viral enteritis
Torovirus

008.8 Other organism, not elsewhere classified
Viral:
enteritis NOS
gastroenteritis

[Excludes:] *influenza with involvement of gastrointestinal tract (487.8, 488.09, 488.19)*

009 Ill-defined intestinal infections

[Excludes:] *diarrheal disease or intestinal infection due to specified organism (001.0-008.8)*
diarrhea following gastrointestinal surgery (564.4)
intestinal malabsorption (579.0-579.9)
ischemic enteritis (557.0-557.9)
other noninfectious gastroenteritis and colitis (558.1-558.9)
regional enteritis (555.0-555.9)
ulcerative colitis (556)

009.0 Infectious colitis, enteritis, and gastroenteritis
Colitis, septic
Enteritis, septic
Gastroenteritis, septic
Dysentery:
NOS
catarrhal
hemorrhagic

009.1 Colitis, enteritis, and gastroenteritis of presumed infectious origin

[Excludes:] *colitis NOS (558.9)*
enteritis NOS (558.9)
gastroenteritis NOS (558.9)

009.2 Infectious diarrhea
Diarrhea:
dysenteric
epidemic
Infectious diarrheal disease NOS

009.3 Diarrhea of presumed infectious origin

[Excludes:] *diarrhea NOS (787.91)*

TUBERCULOSIS (010-018)

Includes: infection by Mycobacterium tuberculosis (human) (bovine)

[Excludes:] *congenital tuberculosis (771.2)*
late effects of tuberculosis (137.0-137.4)

DEFINITION Tuberculosis is a common and often deadly infectious disease caused by mycobacteria, in humans mainly mycobacterium tuberculosis. Tuberculosis usually attacks the lungs but can also affect the central nervous system, the lymphatic system, the circulatory system, the genitourinary system, the gastrointestinal system, bones, joints, and even the skin.

ALERT! For personal history of tuberculosis see V12.01

The following fifth-digit subclassification is for use with categories 010-018:

- **0 unspecified**
- **1 bacteriological or histological examination not done**
- **2 bacteriological or histological examination unknown (at present)**
- **3 tubercle bacilli found (in sputum) by microscopy**
- **4 tubercle bacilli not found (in sputum) by microscopy, but found by bacterial culture**
- **5 tubercle bacilli not found by bacteriological examination, but tuberculosis confirmed histologically**
- **6 tubercle bacilli not found by bacteriological or histological examination but tuberculosis confirmed by other methods [inoculation of animals]**

[5] **010 Primary tuberculous infection**

[Excludes:] *nonspecific reaction to test for tuberculosis without active tuberculosis (795.51-795.52)*
positive PPD (795.51)
positive tuberculin skin test without active tuberculosis (795.51)

[ALERT!] For coding late effects of tuberculosis see 137

[5] **010.0 Primary tuberculous complex**
[0-6]

[5] **010.1 Tuberculous pleurisy in primary progressive tuberculosis**
[0-6]

[5] **010.8 Other primary progressive tuberculosis**
[0-6]

[Excludes:] *tuberculous erythema nodosum (017.1)*

[5] **010.9 Primary tuberculous infection, unspecified**
[0-6]

[5] **011 Pulmonary tuberculosis**

Use additional code, if desired, to identify any associated silicosis (502)

[ALERT!] For coding late effects of respiratory or unspecified tuberculosis see 137.0

[5] **011.0 Tuberculosis of lung, infiltrative**
[0-6]

[5] **011.1 Tuberculosis of lung, nodular**
[0-6]

[5] **011.2 Tuberculosis of lung with cavitation**
[0-6]

[5] **011.3 Tuberculosis of bronchus**
[0-6]

[Excludes:] *isolated bronchial tuberculosis (012.2)*

[5] **011.4 Tuberculous fibrosis of lung**
[0-6]

[5] **011.5 Tuberculous bronchiectasis**
[0-6]

[5] **011.6 Tuberculous pneumonia [any form]**
[0-6]

[5] **011.7 Tuberculous pneumothorax**
[0-6]

[5] **011.8 Other specified pulmonary tuberculosis**
[0-6]

[5] **011.9 Pulmonary tuberculosis, unspecified**
[0-6]
Respiratory tuberculosis NOS
Tuberculosis of lung NOS

[5] **012 Other respiratory tuberculosis**

[Excludes:] *respiratory tuberculosis, unspecified (011.9)*

[ALERT!] For coding late effects of respiratory or unspecified tuberculosis see 137.0

[ALERT!] For personal history of other specified infectious and parasitic disease see V12.09

⑤ **012.0 Tuberculous pleurisy**
[0-6] Tuberculosis of pleura
Tuberculous empyema
Tuberculous hydrothorax

[Excludes:] *pleurisy with effusion without mention of cause (511.9)*
tuberculous pleurisy in primary progressive tuberculosis (010.1)

⑤ **012.1 Tuberculosis of intrathoracic lymph nodes**
[0-6] Tuberculosis of lymph nodes:
hilar
mediastinal
tracheobronchial
Tuberculous tracheobronchial adenopathy

[Excludes:] *that specified as primary (010.0-010.9)*

⑤ **012.2 Isolated tracheal or bronchial tuberculosis**
[0-6]

⑤ **012.3 Tuberculous laryngitis**
[0-6] Tuberculosis of glottis

⑤ **012.8 Other specified respiratory tuberculosis**
[0-6] Tuberculosis of:
mediastinum
nasopharynx
Tuberculosis of:
nose (septum)
sinus [any nasal]

⑤ **013 Tuberculosis of meninges and central nervous system**

[ALERT!] For coding late effects of central nervous system tuberculosis see 137.1

⑤ **013.0 Tuberculous meningitis**
[0-6] Tuberculosis of meninges (cerebral) (spinal)
Tuberculous:
leptomeningitis
meningoencephalitis

[Excludes:] *tuberculoma of meninges (013.1)*

⑤ **013.1 Tuberculoma of meninges**
[0-6]

⑤ **013.2 Tuberculoma of brain**
[0-6] Tuberculosis of brain (current disease)

⑤ **013.3 Tuberculous abscess of brain**
[0-6]

⑤ **013.4 Tuberculoma of spinal cord**
[0-6]

⑤ **013.5 Tuberculous abscess of spinal cord**
[0-6]

⑤ **013.6 Tuberculous encephalitis or myelitis**
[0-6]

⑤ **013.8 Other specified tuberculosis of central nervous system**
[0-6]

⑤ **013.9 Unspecified tuberculosis of central nervous system**
[0-6] Tuberculosis of central nervous system NOS

⑤ **014 Tuberculosis of intestines, peritoneum, and mesenteric glands**

⑤ **014.0 Tuberculous peritonitis**
[0-6] Tuberculous ascites

⑤ **014.8 Other**
[0-6] Tuberculosis (of):
anus
intestine (large) (small)
mesenteric glands
rectum
retroperitoneal (lymph nodes)
Tuberculous enteritis

[5] **015 Tuberculosis of bones and joints**

Use additional code, if desired, to identify manifestation, as:
tuberculous:
arthropathy (711.4)
necrosis of bone (730.8)
osteitis (730.8)
osteomyelitis (730.8)
synovitis (727.01)
tenosynovitis (727.01)

[ALERT!] For coding late effects of tuberculosis of bones and joints see 137.3

[5] **015.0 Vertebral column**
[0-6] Pott's disease
Use additional code, if desired, to identify manifestation, as:
curvature of spine [Pott's] (737.4)
kyphosis (737.4)
spondylitis (720.81)

[5] **015.1 Hip**
[0-6]

[5] **015.2 Knee**
[0-6]

[5] **015.5 Limb bones**
[0-6] Tuberculous dactylitis

[5] **015.6 Mastoid**
[0-6] Tuberculous mastoiditis

[5] **015.7 Other specified bone**
[0-6]

[5] **015.8 Other specified joint**
[0-6]

[5] **015.9 Tuberculosis of unspecified bones and joints**
[0-6]

[5] **016 Tuberculosis of genitourinary system**

[ALERT!] For coding late effects of genitourinary tuberculosis see 137.2

[5] **016.0 Kidney**
[0-6] Renal tuberculosis
Use additional code, if desired, to identify manifestation, as:
tuberculous:
nephropathy (583.81)
pyelitis (590.81)
pyelonephritis (590.81)

[5] **016.1 Bladder**
[0-6]

[5] **016.2 Ureter**
[0-6]

[5] **016.3 Other urinary organs**
[0-6]

[5] **016.4 Epididymis**
[0-6]

[5] **016.5 Other male genital organs**
[0-6]
Use additional code, if desired, to identify manifestation, as:
tuberculosis of:
prostate (601.4)
seminal vesicle (608.81)
testis (608.81)

[5] **016.6 Tuberculous oophoritis and salpingitis**
[0-6]

[5] **016.7 Other female genital organs**
[0-6] Tuberculous:
cervicitis
endometritis

[5] **016.9 Genitourinary tuberculosis, unspecified**
[0-6]

Add 4th or 5th digit | Nonspecific code | Unspecified code | Manifestation code

⑤ **017** **Tuberculosis of other organs**

    ALERT! For coding late effects of tuberculosis of other specified organs see 137.4

⑤ **017.0** **Skin and subcutaneous cellular tissue**
[0-6]

Lupus:	Tuberculosis:
exedens	colliquativa
vulgaris	cutis
Scrofuloderma	lichenoides
	papulonecrotica
	verrucosa cutis

    Excludes: *lupus erythematosus (695.4)*
          disseminated (710.0)
          lupus NOS (710.0)
          nonspecific reaction to test for tuberculosis without active tuberculosis
            (795.51-795.52)
          positive PPD (795.51)
          positive tuberculin skin test without active tuberculosis (795.51)

⑤ **017.1** **Erythema nodosum with hypersensitivity reaction in tuberculosis**
[0-6]

Bazin's disease	Tuberculosis indurativa
Erythema:	
induratum	
nodosum, tuberculous	

    Excludes: *erythema nodosum NOS (695.2)*

    DEFINITION Erythema nodosum is a type of skin inflammation located in a certain portion of the fatty layer of skin. Erythema nodosum results in reddish, painful, tender lumps most commonly located in the front of the legs below the knees.

⑤ **017.2** **Peripheral lymph nodes**
[0-6]

Scrofula	Tuberculous adenitis
Scrofulous abscess	

    Excludes: *tuberculosis of lymph nodes:*
          bronchial and mediastinal (012.1)
          mesenteric and retroperitoneal (014.8)
          tuberculous tracheobronchial adenopathy (012.1)

⑤ **017.3** **Eye**
[0-6]
Use additional code, if desired, to identify manifestation, as:
      tuberculous:
        chorioretinitis, disseminated (363.13)
        episcleritis (379.09)
        interstitial keratitis (370.59)
        iridocyclitis, chronic (364.11)
        keratoconjunctivitis (phlyctenular) (370.31)

⑤ **017.4** **Ear**
[0-6]
      Tuberculosis of ear
      Tuberculous otitis media

    Excludes: *tuberculous mastoiditis (015.6)*

⑤ **017.5** **Thyroid gland**
[0-6]

⑤ **017.6** **Adrenal glands**
[0-6]   Addison's disease, tuberculous

⑤ **017.7** **Spleen**
[0-6]

⑤ **017.8** **Esophagus**
[0-6]

⑤ **017.9** **Other specified organs**
[0-6]
Use additional code, if desired, to identify manifestation, as:
      tuberculosis of:
        endocardium [any valve] (424.91)
        myocardium (422.0)
        pericardium (420.0)

● Code new   ▲ Revision of   ④ ⑤ Fourth or fifth
      to 2012 edition   existing code   digit required

⑤ **018** **Miliary tuberculosis**
Includes: tuberculosis:
disseminated
generalized
miliary, whether of a single specified site, multiple sites, or unspecified site
polyserositis
DEFINITION Miliary tuberculosis acute tuberculosis characterized by the appearance of tiny tubercles on one or more organs of the body.

⑤ **018.0** **Acute miliary tuberculosis**
[0-6]

⑤ **018.8** **Other specified miliary tuberculosis**
[0-6]

⑤ **018.9** **Miliary tuberculosis, unspecified**
[0-6]

ZOONOTIC BACTERIAL DISEASES (020-027)

020 **Plague**
Includes: infection by Yersinia [Pasteurella] pestis
DEFINITION Plague is a deadly infectious disease caused by the enterobacteria yersinia pestis (pasteurella pestis).

020.0 **Bubonic**

020.1 **Cellulocutaneous**

020.2 **Septicemic**

020.3 **Primary pneumonic**

020.4 **Secondary pneumonic**

020.5 **Pneumonic, unspecified**

020.8 **Other specified types of plague**
Abortive plague   Pestis minor
Ambulatory plague

020.9 **Plague, unspecified**

021 **Tularemia**
Includes: deerfly fever
infection by Francisella [Pasteurella] tularensis
rabbit fever
DEFINITION Tularemia, aka rabbit fever, deer fly fever, O'Hara's fever is a serious infectious disease caused by the bacterium francisella tularensis.

021.0 **Ulceroglandular tularemia**

021.1 **Enteric tularemia**
Tularemia:
cryptogenic
intestinal
typhoidal

021.2 **Pulmonary tularemia**
Bronchopneumonic tularemia

021.3 **Oculoglandular tularemia**

021.8 **Other specified tularemia**
Tularemia:
generalized or disseminated
glandular

021.9 **Unspecified tularemia**

022 **Anthrax**
DEFINITION Anthrax is an acute disease in humans and animals caused by the bacterium bacillus anthracis which is highly lethal in some forms.

022.0 **Cutaneous anthrax**
Malignant pustule

022.1 **Pulmonary anthrax**
Respiratory anthrax
Wool-sorters' disease

022.2 **Gastrointestinal anthrax**

022.3 **Anthrax septicemia**

022.8 **Other specified manifestations of anthrax**

022.9 **Anthrax, unspecified**

Add 4th or   Nonspecific   Unspecified   Manifestation
5th digit   code   code   code

023 Brucellosis
    Includes: fever:
               Malta
               Mediterranean
               undulant

    DEFINITION Brucellosis, aka undulant fever, or malta fever is a highly contagious zoonosis caused by ingestion of unsterilized milk or meat from infected animals, or close contact with their secretions.

    023.0 Brucella melitensis

    023.1 Brucella abortus

    023.2 Brucella suis

    023.3 Brucella canis

    023.8 Other brucellosis
        Infection by more than one organism

    023.9 Brucellosis, unspecified

024 Glanders
    Infection by: Farcy
      Actinobacillus mallei   Malleus
      Malleomyces mallei
      Pseudomonas mallei

    DEFINITION Glanders is an infectious disease that occurs primarily in horses, mules, and donkeys and other animals such as dogs, cats and goats that can be transmitted to humans. It is caused by infection with the bacterium burkholderia mallei.

025 Melioidosis
    Infection by:
      Malleomyces pseudomallei
      Pseudomonas pseudomallei
      Whitmore's bacillus
    Pseudoglanders

    DEFINITION Melioidosis aka Whitmore disease or Nightcliff Gardener's disease, is an infectious disease caused by a gram-negative bacterium, burkholderia pseudomallei, found in soil and water.

026 Rat-bite fever
    DEFINITION Rat-bite fever is an acute, febrile human illness caused by bacteria transmitted by rodents, rats in most cases, which is passed from rodent to human via the rodent's urine or mucous secretions. Two types of gram-negative facultative anaerobic bacteria can cause the infection.

    026.0 Spirillary fever
        Rat-bite fever due to Spirillum minor [S. minus]
        Sodoku

    026.1 Streptobacillary fever
        Epidemic arthritic erythema
        Haverhill fever
        Rat-bite fever due to Streptobacillus moniliformis

    026.9 Unspecified rat-bite fever

027 Other zoonotic bacterial diseases
    DEFINITION Zoonotic refers to other diseases that can be passed from animals, whether wild or domesticated, to humans.

    ALERT! For personal history of other specified infectious and parasitic disease see V12.09

    027.0 Listeriosis
        Infection by Listeria monocytogenes
        Septicemia by Listeria monocytogenes
    Use additional code to identify manifestations, as meningitis (320.7)

        Excludes: congenital listeriosis (771.2)

    027.1 Erysipelothrix infection
        Erysipeloid (of Rosenbach)
        Infection by Erysipelothrix insidiosa [E. rhusiopathiae]
        Septicemia by Erysipelothrix insidiosa [E. rhusiopathiae]

    ● Code new   ▲ Revision of   ④ ⑤ Fourth or fifth
      to 2012 edition   existing code   digit required

027.2 Pasteurellosis
Pasteurella pseudotuberculosis infection
Mesenteric adenitis by Pasteurella multocida [P. septica]
Septic infection (cat bite) (dog bite) by Pasteurella multocida [P. septica]

[*Excludes:*] *infection by:*
Francisella [Pasteurella] tularensis (021.0-021.9)
Yersinia [Pasteurella] pestis (020.0-020.9)

027.8 Other specified zoonotic bacterial diseases

027.9 Unspecified zoonotic bacterial disease

OTHER BACTERIAL DISEASES (030-041)

[*Excludes:*] *bacterial venereal diseases (098.0-099.9)*
bartonellosis (088.0)

030 Leprosy
Includes: Hansen's disease
infection by Mycobacterium leprae

[DEFINITION] Leprosy is an infectious disease characterized by disfiguring skin sores, nerve damage, and progressive debilitation. Leprosy is caused by the organism mycobacterium leprae.

030.0 Lepromatous [type L]
Lepromatous leprosy (macular) (diffuse) (infiltrated) (nodular) (neuritic)

030.1 Tuberculoid [type T]
Tuberculoid leprosy (macular) (maculoanesthetic) (major) (minor) (neuritic)

030.2 Indeterminate [group I]
Indeterminate [uncharacteristic] leprosy (macular) (neuritic)

030.3 Borderline [group B]
Borderline or dimorphous leprosy (infiltrated) (neuritic)

030.8 Other specified leprosy

030.9 Leprosy, unspecified

031 Diseases due to other mycobacteria

031.0 Pulmonary
Infection by Mycobacterium:
avium
intracellulare [Battey bacillus]
kansasii
Battey disease

031.1 Cutaneous
Buruli ulcer
Infection by Mycobacterium:
marinum [M. balnei]
ulcerans

031.2 Disseminated
Disseminated mycobacterium avium-intracellulare complex (DMAC)
Mycobacterium avium-intracellulare complex (MAC) bacteremia

031.8 Other specified mycobacterial diseases

031.9 Unspecified diseases due to mycobacteria
Atypical mycobacterium infection NOS

032 Diphtheria
Includes: infection by Corynebacterium diphtheriae

[DEFINITION] Diphtheria is a highly infectious disease of the upper respiratory tract characterised by a sore throat, fever and causing difficulty in breathing.

032.0 Faucial diphtheria
Membranous angina, diphtheritic

032.1 Nasopharyngeal diphtheria

032.2 Anterior nasal diphtheria

032.3 Laryngeal diphtheria
Laryngotracheitis, diphtheritic

[5] **032.8 Other specified diphtheria**

032.81 Conjunctival diphtheria
Pseudomembranous diphtheritic conjunctivitis

032.82 Diphtheritic myocarditis

032.83 Diphtheritic peritonitis

032.84 Diphtheritic cystitis

032.85 Cutaneous diphtheria

032.89 Other

032.9 Diphtheria, unspecified

033 Whooping cough
Includes: pertussis

Use additional code, if desired, to identify any associated pneumonia (484.3)

DEFINITION Whooping cough, aka pertussis, is a highly contagious disease caused by bacteria. The most prominent symptom of whooping cough is a distinctive, uncontrollable cough, followed by a sharp, high-pitched intake of air.

033.0 Bordetella pertussis [B. pertussis]

033.1 Bordetella parapertussis [B. parapertussis]

033.8 Whooping cough due to other specified organism
Bordetella bronchiseptica [B. bronchiseptica]

033.9 Whooping cough, unspecified organism

034 Streptococcal sore throat and scarlet fever

DEFINITION Streptococcal sore throat is an infection of the oral pharynx and tonsils by streptococcus. Scarlet fever is an infection caused by a bacterium called streptococcus.

034.0 Streptococcal sore throat
Septic:
angina
sore throat
Streptococcal:
angina
laryngitis
pharyngitis
tonsillitis

034.1 Scarlet fever
Scarlatina

[Excludes:] *parascarlatina (057.8)*

035 Erysipelas

[Excludes:] *postpartum or puerperal erysipelas (670.8)*

DEFINITION Erysipelas is an acute febrile disease that is associated with intense often vesicular and edematous local inflammation of the skin and subcutaneous tissues and that is caused by a hemolytic streptococcus.

036 Meningococcal infection

DEFINITION Meningococcal infection is an infection with the bacterium neisseria meningitidis. Neisseria was formerly called meningococcus but the term meningococcal is still common.

036.0 Meningococcal meningitis
Cerebrospinal fever
(meningococcal)
Meningitis:
cerebrospinal
epidemic

036.1 Meningococcal encephalitis

036.2 Meningococcemia
Meningococcal septicemia

036.3 Waterhouse-Friderichsen syndrome, meningococcal
Meningococcal hemorrhagic adrenalitis
Meningococcic adrenal syndrome
Waterhouse-Friderichsen syndrome NOS

[5] **036.4 Meningococcal carditis**

036.40 Meningococcal carditis, unspecified

036.41 Meningococcal pericarditis

036.42 Meningococcal endocarditis

036.43 Meningococcal myocarditis

[5] **036.8 Other specified meningococcal infections**

036.81 Meningococcal optic neuritis

036.82 Meningococcal arthropathy

036.89 Other

036.9 Meningococcal infection, unspecified
Meningococcal infection NOS

037 Tetanus

[*Excludes:*] *tetanus:*
complicating:
abortion (634-638 with .0, 639.0)
ectopic or molar pregnancy (639.0)
neonatorum (771.3)
puerperal (670.8)

DEFINITION Tetanus is an often fatal infectious disease caused by the bacteria clostridium tetani (c. Tetani) which usually enters the body through a puncture, cut, or open wound.

038 Septicemia

[*Excludes:*] *bacteremia (790.7)*
during labor (659.3)
following ectopic or molar pregnancy (639.0)
following infusion, injection, transfusion, or vaccination (999.3)
postpartum, puerperal (670)
septicemia (sepsis) of newborn (771.81)
that complicating abortion (634-638 with .0, 639.0)

Use additional code for systemic inflammatory response syndrome (SIRS) (995.91-995.92)

DEFINITION Septicemia, aka blood poisoning, is a systemic illness with toxicity due to invasion of the bloodstream by virulent bacteria coming from a local seat of infection. The symptoms of chills, fever and exhaustion are caused by the bacteria and substances they produce.

038.0 Streptococcal septicemia

[5] **038.1 Staphylococcal septicemia**

038.10 Staphylococcal septicemia, unspecified

038.11 Methicillin susceptible Staphylococcus aureus septicemia
MSSA septicemia
Staphylococcus aureus septicemia NOS

038.12 Methicillin resistant Staphylococcus aureus septicemia

038.19 Other staphylococcal septicemia

038.2 Pneumococcal septicemia

038.3 Septicemia due to anaerobes
Septicemia due to bacteroides

[*Excludes:*] *gas gangrene (040.0)*
that due to anaerobic streptococci (038.0)

[5] **038.4 Septicemia due to other gram-negative organisms**

038.40 Gram-negative organism, unspecified
Gram-negative septicemia NOS

038.41 Hemophilus influenzae [H. influenzae]

038.42 Escherichia coli [E. coli]

038.43 Pseudomonas

038.44 Serratia

038.49 Other

038.8 Other specified septicemias

[*Excludes:*] *septicemia (due to):*
anthrax (022.3)
gonococcal (098.89)
herpetic (054.5)
meningococcal (036.2)
septicemic plague (020.2)

038.9 Unspecified septicemia
Septicemia NOS

[*Excludes:*] *bacteremia NOS (790.7)*

039 Actinomycotic infections
Includes: actinomycotic mycetoma
infection by Actinomycetales, such as species of Actinomyces, Actinomadura, Nocardia, Streptomyces
maduromycosis (actinomycotic)
schizomycetoma (actinomycotic)

[DEFINITION] Actinomycosis is an infection primarily caused by the bacterium actinomyces israelii. Infection most often occurs in the face and neck region and is characterized by the presence of a slowly enlarging, hard, red lump.

039.0 Cutaneous
Erythrasma
Trichomycosis axillaris

039.1 Pulmonary
Thoracic actinomycosis

039.2 Abdominal

039.3 Cervicofacial

039.4 Madura foot
[Excludes:] *madura foot due to mycotic infection (117.4)*

039.8 Of other specified sites

039.9 Of unspecified site
Actinomycosis NOS
Maduromycosis NOS
Nocardiosis NOS

040 Other bacterial diseases
[Excludes:] *bacteremia NOS (790.7)*
bacterial infection NOS (041.9)

[ALERT!] For personal history of other specified infectious and parasitic disease see V12.09

040.0 Gas gangrene
Gas bacillus infection or gangrene
Infection by Clostridium:
histolyticum
oedematiens
perfringens [welchii]
septicum
sordellii
Malignant edema
Myonecrosis, clostridial
Myositis, clostridial

040.1 Rhinoscleroma

040.2 Whipple's disease
Intestinal lipodystrophy

040.3 Necrobacillosis

⑤ **040.4 Other specified botulism**
Non-foodborne intoxication due to toxins of Clostridium botulinum [*C. botulinum*]
[Excludes:] *botulism NOS (005.1)*
food poisoning due to toxins of Clostridium botulinum (005.1)

040.41 Infant botulism

040.42 Wound botulism
Non-foodborne botulism NOS

Use additional code to identify complicated open wound

⑤ **040.8 Other specified bacterial diseases**

040.81 Tropical pyomyositis

040.82 Toxic shock syndrome
Use additional code to identify the organism

040.89 Other

041 Bacterial infection in conditions classified elsewhere and of unspecified site
Note: This category is provided to be used as an additional code where it is desired to identify the bacterial agent in diseases classified elsewhere. This category will also be used to classify bacterial infections of unspecified nature or site.
[Excludes:] *septicemia (038.0-038.9)*

⑤ **041.0 Streptococcus**

041.00 Streptococcus, unspecified

041.01 Group A

041.02 Group B

041.03 Group C

041.04 Group D [Enterococcus]

041.05 Group G

041.09 Other Streptococcus

[5] **041.1 Staphylococcus**

[ALERT!] For personal history of methicillin resistant staphylococcus aureus see V12.04

041.10 Staphylococcus, unspecified

041.11 Methicillin susceptible Staphylococcus aureus
MSSA
Staphylococcus aureus NOS

041.12 Methicillin resistant Staphylococcus aureus
Methicillin-resistant Staphylococcus aureus (MRSA)

041.19 Other Staphylococcus

041.2 Pneumococcus

041.3 Klebsiella pneumoniae

[5] **041.4 Escherichia coli [E. coli]**

● **041.41 Shiga toxin-producing Escherichia coli [E. coli] (STEC) O157**
E. coli O157:H- (nonmotile) with confirmation of Shiga toxin
E. coli O157 with confirmation of Shiga toxin when H antigen is unknown, or is not H7
O157:H7 Escherichia coli [E.coli] with or without confirmation of Shiga toxin-production
Shiga toxin-producing Escherichia coli [E.coli] O157:H7 with or without confirmation of Shiga toxin-production
STEC O157:H7 with or without confirmation of Shiga toxin-production

● **041.42 Other specified Shiga toxin-producing Escherichia coli [E. coli] (STEC)**
Non-O157 Shiga toxin-producing Escherichia coli [E.coli]
Non-O157 Shiga toxin-producing Escherichia coli [E.coli] with known O group

● **041.43 Shiga toxin-producing Escherichia coli [E. coli] (STEC), unspecified**
Shiga toxin-producing Escherichia coli [E. coli] with unspecified O group
STEC NOS

● **041.49 Other and unspecified Escherichia coli [E. coli]**
Escherichia coli [E. coli] NOS
Non-Shiga toxin-producing E. coli

041.5 Hemophilus influenzae [H. influenzae]

041.6 Proteus (mirabilis) (morganii)

041.7 Pseudomonas

[5] **041.8 Other specified bacterial infections**

041.81 Mycoplasma
Eaton's agent
Pleuropneumonia-like organisms [PPLO]

041.82 Bacteroides fragilis

041.83 Clostridium perfringens

041.84 Other anaerobes
Gram-negative anaerobes

[*Excludes:*] *Helicobacter pylori (041.86)*

041.85 Other Gram-negative organisms
Aerobacter aerogenes
Gram-negative bacteria NOS
Mima polymorpha
Serratia

[*Excludes:*] *Gram-negative anaerobes (041.84)*

041.86 Helicobacter pylori [H. pylori]

041.89 Other specified bacteria

041.9 Bacterial infection, unspecified

HUMAN IMMUNODEFICIENCY VIRUS (HIV) INFECTION (042)

042 Human immunodeficiency virus [HIV] disease
Acquired immune deficiency syndrome
Acquired immunodeficiency syndrome
AIDS
AIDS-like syndrome
AIDS-related complex
ARC
HIV infection, symptomatic

Use additional code(s) to identify all manifestations of HIV

Use additional code, if desired, to identify HIV-2 infection (079.53)

> *Excludes:* *asymptomatic HIV infection status (V08)*
> *exposure to HIV virus (V01.79)*
> *nonspecific serologic evidence of HIV (795.71)*

> **DEFINITION** Human immunodeficiency virus (HIV) disease is a virus that can lead to acquired immunodeficiency syndrome (AIDS), a condition in humans in which the immune system begins to fail, leading to life-threatening opportunistic infections.

POLIOMYELITIS AND OTHER NON-ARTHROPOD-BORNE VIRAL DISEASES AND PRION DISEASES OF CENTRAL NERVOUS SYSTEM (045-049)

⑤ **045** Acute poliomyelitis

> *Excludes:* *late effects of acute poliomyelitis (138)*

> **DEFINITION** Poliomyelitis, aka polio or infantile paralysis, is a highly infectious viral disease that may attack the central nervous system and is characterized by symptoms that range from a mild nonparalytic infection to total paralysis in a matter of hours.

> **ALERT!** For coding late effects of acute poliomyelitis see 138

> **ALERT!** For personal history of poliomyelitis see V12.02

The following fifth-digit subclassification is for use with category 045:

  0 **poliovirus, unspecified type**

  1 **poliovirus type I**

  2 **poliovirus type II**

  3 **poliovirus type III**

⑤ **045.0** **Acute paralytic poliomyelitis specified as bulbar**
[0-3]   Infantile paralysis (acute) specified as bulbar
    Poliomyelitis (acute) (anterior) specified as bulbar
    Polioencephalitis (acute) (bulbar)
    Polioencephalomyelitis (acute) (anterior) (bulbar)

⑤ **045.1** **Acute poliomyelitis with other paralysis**
[0-3]   Paralysis:
      acute atrophic, spinal
      infantile, paralytic
    Poliomyelitis (acute):
      anterior, with paralysis except bulbar
      epidemic, with paralysis except bulbar

⑤ **045.2** **Acute nonparalytic poliomyelitis**
[0-3]   Poliomyelitis (acute):
      anterior, specified as nonparalytic
      epidemic, specified as nonparalytic

⑤ **045.9** **Acute poliomyelitis, unspecified**
[0-3]   Infantile paralysis, unspecified whether paralytic or nonparalytic
    Poliomyelitis (acute):
      anterior, unspecified whether paralytic or nonparalytic
      epidemic, unspecified whether paralytic or nonparalytic

046 **Slow virus infections and prion diseases of central nervous system**

046.0 **Kuru**

⑤ **046.1** **Jakob-Creutzfeldt disease**
    Use additional code to identify dementia:
      with behavioral disturbance (294.11)
      without behavioral disturbance (294.10)

  046.11 **Variant Creutzfeldt-Jakob disease**
      vCJD

  046.19 **Other and unspecified Creutzfeldt-Jakob disease**
      CJD
      Familial Creutzfeldt-Jakob disease
      Iatrogenic Creutzfeldt-Jakob disease
      Jakob-Creutzfeldt disease, unspecified
      Sporadic Creutzfeldt-Jakob disease
      Subacute spongiform encephalopathy

  > *Excludes:* *variant Creutzfeldt-Jakob disease (vCJD) (046.11)*

  046.2 **Subacute sclerosing panencephalitis**
      Dawson's inclusion body encephalitis
      Van Bogaert's sclerosing leukoencephalitis

● Code new   ▲ Revision of   ④ ⑤ Fourth or fifth
    to 2012 edition   existing code   digit required

046.3 Progressive multifocal leukoencephalopathy
Multifocal leukoencephalopathy NOS

[5] **046.7 Other specified prion diseases of central nervous system**
[Excludes:] *Creutzfeldt-Jakob disease (046.11-046.19)*
Jakob-Creutzfeldt disease (046.11-046.19)
kuru (046.0)
variant Creutzfeldt-Jakob disease (vCJD) (046.11)

046.71 Gerstmann-Straussler-Scheinker syndrome
GSS syndrome

046.72 Fatal familial insomnia
FFI

046.79 Other and unspecified prion disease of central nervous system

046.8 Other specified slow virus infection of central nervous system

046.9 Unspecified slow virus infection of central nervous system

047 Meningitis due to enterovirus
Includes: meningitis:
abacterial
aseptic
viral

[Excludes:] *meningitis due to:*
adenovirus (049.1)
arthropod-borne virus (060.0-066.9)
leptospira (100.81)
virus of:
herpes simplex (054.72)
herpes zoster (053.0)
lymphocytic choriomeningitis (049.0)
mumps (072.1)
poliomyelitis (045.0-045.9)
any other infection specifically classified elsewhere

[DEFINITION] Meningitis due to enterovirus refers to any of a subgroup of picornaviruses, including polioviruses, coxsackie viruses, and echoviruses, that infect the gastrointestinal tract and often spread to other areas of the body, especially the nervous system.

047.0 Coxsackie virus

047.1 ECHO virus
Meningo-eruptive syndrome

047.8 Other specified viral meningitis

047.9 Unspecified viral meningitis
Viral meningitis NOS

048 Other enterovirus diseases of central nervous system
Boston exanthem

[ALERT!] For personal history of other specified infectious and parasitic disease see V12.09

049 Other non-arthropod-borne viral diseases of central nervous system
[Excludes:] *late effects of viral encephalitis (139.0)*

[DEFINITION] Non-arthropod-borne viral diseases refers to diseases caused by a virus that is not carried by insects, spiders, crustaceans, centipedes or millipedes.

[ALERT!] For coding late effects of viral encephalitis see 139.0

[ALERT!] For personal history of other specified infectious and parasitic disease see V12.09

049.0 Lymphocytic choriomeningitis
Lymphocytic:
meningitis (serous) (benign)
meningoencephalitis (serous) (benign)

049.1 Meningitis due to adenovirus

049.8 Other specified non-arthropod-borne viral diseases of central nervous system
Encephalitis:
acute:
inclusion body
necrotizing
epidemic

Encephalitis:
lethargica
Rio Bravo
von Economo's disease

[Excludes:] *human herpesvirus 6 encephalitis (058.21)*
other human herpesvirus encephalitis (058.29)

049.9 Unspecified non-arthropod-borne viral diseases of central nervous system
Viral encephalitis NOS

VIRAL DISEASES GENERALLY ACCOMPANIED BY EXANTHEM (050-059)

> Excludes: *arthropod-borne viral diseases (060.0-066.9)*
> *Boston exanthem (048)*

050 Smallpox

DEFINITION Smallpox, aka variola, a highly contagious and frequently fatal viral disease characterized by a biphasic fever and a distinctive skin rash that left pock marks in its wake. The disease is caused by the variola virus.

050.0 Variola major
Hemorrhagic (pustular)   Malignant smallpox
smallpox   Purpura variolosa

050.1 Alastrim
Variola minor

050.2 Modified smallpox
Varioloid

050.9 Smallpox, unspecified

051 Cowpox and paravaccinia

DEFINITION Cowpox and paravaccinia is a mild contagious skin disease of cattle, usually affecting the udder that is caused by a virus and characterized by the eruption of a pustular rash. When the virus is transmitted to humans, as by vaccination, it can confer immunity to smallpox.

⑤ **051.0 Cowpox and vaccinia not from vaccination**

051.01 Cowpox

051.02 Vaccinia not from vaccination

> Excludes: *vaccinia (generalized) (from vaccination) (999.0)*

051.1 Pseudocowpox
Milkers' node

051.2 Contagious pustular dermatitis
Ecthyma contagiosum   Orf

051.9 Paravaccinia, unspecified

052 Chickenpox

DEFINITION Chickenpox is an acute contagious disease caused by herpes varicella zoster virus; causes a rash of vesicles on the face and body.

052.0 Postvaricella encephalitis
Postchickenpox encephalitis

052.1 Varicella (hemorrhagic) pneumonitis

052.2 Postvaricella myelitis
Postchickenpox myelitis

052.7 With other specified complications

052.8 With unspecified complication

052.9 Varicella without mention of complication
Chickenpox NOS
Varicella NOS

053 Herpes zoster
Includes: shingles
zona

DEFINITION Herpes zoster is a viral disease characterized by a painful skin rash with blisters in a limited area on one side of the body, often in a stripe.

053.0 With meningitis

⑤ **053.1 With other nervous system complications**

053.10 With unspecified nervous system complication

053.11 Geniculate herpes zoster
Herpetic geniculate ganglionitis

053.12 Postherpetic trigeminal neuralgia

053.13 Postherpetic polyneuropathy

053.14 Herpes zoster myelitis

053.19 Other

● Code new   ▲ Revision of   ④ ⑤ Fourth or fifth
to 2012 edition   existing code   digit required

⑤ **053.2 With ophthalmic complications**

    053.20 Herpes zoster dermatitis of eyelid
        Herpes zoster ophthalmicus

    053.21 Herpes zoster keratoconjunctivitis

    053.22 Herpes zoster iridocyclitis

    053.29 Other

⑤ **053.7 With other specified complications**

    053.71 Otitis externa due to herpes zoster

    053.79 Other

053.8 With unspecified complication

053.9 Herpes zoster without mention of complication
    Herpes zoster NOS

054 Herpes simplex

> Excludes: *congenital herpes simplex (771.2)*

DEFINITION Herpes simplex is an infection caused by the herpes simplex virus; affects the skin and nervous system; produces small temporary blisters on the skin and mucous membranes.

054.0 Eczema herpeticum
    Kaposi's varicelliform eruption

⑤ **054.1 Genital herpes**

    054.10 Genital herpes, unspecified
        Herpes progenitalis

    054.11 Herpetic vulvovaginitis

    054.12 Herpetic ulceration of vulva

    054.13 Herpetic infection of penis

    054.19 Other

054.2 Herpetic gingivostomatitis

054.3 Herpetic meningoencephalitis
    Herpes encephalitis
    Simian B disease

> Excludes: *human herpesvirus 6 encephalitis (058.21)*
>   *other human herpesvirus encephalitis (058.29)*

⑤ **054.4 With ophthalmic complications**

    054.40 With unspecified ophthalmic complication

    054.41 Herpes simplex dermatitis of eyelid

    054.42 Dendritic keratitis

    054.43 Herpes simplex disciform keratitis

    054.44 Herpes simplex iridocyclitis

    054.49 Other

054.5 Herpetic septicemia

054.6 Herpetic whitlow
    Herpetic felon

⑤ **054.7 With other specified complications**

    054.71 Visceral herpes simplex

    054.72 Herpes simplex meningitis

    054.73 Herpes simplex otitis externa

    054.74 Herpes simplex myelitis

    054.79 Other

054.8 With unspecified complication

054.9 Herpes simplex without mention of complication

055 Measles
    Includes: morbilli
               rubeola

DEFINITION Measles is a viral infection which causes an illness displaying a characteristic skin rash. Measles is also sometimes called rubeola, 5-day measles, or hard measles.

▓ Add 4th or 5th digit	▓ Nonspecific code	▓ Unspecified code	▓ Manifestation code

055.0 Postmeasles encephalitis

055.1 Postmeasles pneumonia

055.2 Postmeasles otitis media

⑤ **055.7 With other specified complications**

055.71 Measles keratoconjunctivitis
Measles keratitis

055.79 Other

055.8 With unspecified complication

055.9 Measles without mention of complication

056 Rubella
Includes: German measles
[Excludes:] *congenital rubella (771.0)*

[DEFINITION] Rubella is a highly contagious viral disease, aka german measles. The symptoms include swollen glands, joint pain, low fever, and a fine red rash.

⑤ **056.0 With neurological complications**

056.00 With unspecified neurological complication

056.01 Encephalomyelitis due to rubella
Encephalitis due to rubella
Meningoencephalitis due to rubella

056.09 Other

⑤ **056.7 With other specified complications**

056.71 Arthritis due to rubella

056.79 Other

056.8 With unspecified complications

056.9 Rubella without mention of complication

057 Other viral exanthemata

[DEFINITION] Viral exanthemata refers to other skin eruptions occurring as a symptom of an acute viral or coccal disease.

[ALERT!] For personal history of other specified infectious and parasitic disease see V12.09

057.0 Erythema infectiosum [fifth disease]

057.8 Other specified viral exanthemata
Dukes (-Filatow) disease
Fourth disease
Parascarlatina
Pseudoscarlatina

[Excludes:] *exanthema subitum [sixth disease] (058.10-058.12)*
roseola infantum (058.10-058.12)

057.9 Viral exanthem, unspecified

⑤ **058 Other human herpesvirus**

[Excludes:] *congenital herpes (771.2)*
cytomegalovirus (078.5)
Epstein-Barr virus (075)
herpes NOS (054.0-054.9)
herpes simplex (054.0-054.9)
herpes zoster (053.0-053.9)
human herpesvirus NOS (054.0-054.9)
human herpesvirus 1 (054.0-054.9)
human herpesvirus 2 (054.0-054.9)
human herpesvirus 3 (052.0-053.9)
human herpesvirus 4 (075)
human herpesvirus 5 (078.5)
varicella (052.0-052.9)
varicella-zoster virus (052.0-053.9)

[DEFINITION] Human herpes viruses, refers to a family of viruses including herpes simplex, varicella zoster, and Epstein-Barr.

[ALERT!] For personal history of other specified infectious and parasitic disease see V12.09

⑤ **058.1 Roseola infantum**
Exanthema subitum [sixth disease]

058.10 Roseola infantum, unspecified
Exanthema subitum [sixth disease], unspecified

058.11 Roseola infantum due to human herpesvirus 6
Exanthema subitum [sixth disease] due to human herpesvirus 6

● Code new to 2012 edition ▲ Revision of existing code ④ ⑤ Fourth or fifth digit required

058.12 Roseola infantum due to human herpesvirus 7
Exanthema subitum [sixth disease] due to human herpesvirus 7

[5] **058.2 Other human herpesvirus encephalitis**
[Excludes:] *herpes encephalitis NOS (054.3)*
herpes simplex encephalitis (054.3)
human herpesvirus encephalitis NOS (054.3)
simian B herpes virus encephalitis (054.3)

058.21 Human herpesvirus 6 encephalitis

058.29 Other human herpesvirus encephalitis
Human herpesvirus 7 encephalitis

[5] **058.8 Other human herpesvirus infections**

058.81 Human herpesvirus 6 infection

058.82 Human herpesvirus 7 infection

058.89 Other human herpesvirus infection
Human herpesvirus 8 infection
Kaposi's sarcoma-associated herpesvirus infection

059 Other poxvirus infections
[Excludes:] *contagious pustular dermatitis (051.2)*
cowpox (051.01)
ecthyma contagiosum (051.2)
milker's nodule (051.1)
orf (051.2)
paravaccinia NOS (051.9)
pseudocowpox (051.1)
smallpox (050.0-050.9)
vaccinia (generalized) (from vaccination) (999.0)
vaccinia not from vaccination (051.02)

[DEFINITION] Poxvirus infections refers to a group of viruses that produce spreading vesicular lesions, including smallpox, vaccinia, and molluscum contagiosum.

[ALERT!] For personal history of other specified infectious and parasitic disease see V12.09

[5] **059.0 Other orthopoxvirus infections**

059.00 Orthopoxvirus infection, unspecified

059.01 Monkeypox

059.09 Other orthopoxvirus infection

[5] **059.1 Other parapoxvirus infections**

059.10 Parapoxvirus infection, unspecified

059.11 Bovine stomatitis

059.12 Sealpox

059.19 Other parapoxvirus infections

[5] **059.2 Yatapoxvirus infections**

059.20 Yatapoxvirus infection, unspecified

059.21 Tanapox

059.22 Yaba monkey tumor virus

059.8 Other poxvirus infections

059.9 Poxvirus infections, unspecified

ARTHROPOD-BORNE VIRAL DISEASES (060-066)

Use additional code, if desired, to identify any associated meningitis (321.2)
[Excludes:] *late effects of viral encephalitis (139.0)*

060 Yellow fever

[DEFINITION] Yellow fever is an acute systemic (body wide) illness caused by a virus called a flavivirus. In severe cases, the viral infection causes a high fever, bleeding into the skin, and necrosis (death) of cells in the kidney and liver.

[ALERT!] For coding late effects of viral encephalitis see 139.0

060.0 Sylvatic
Yellow fever:
jungle
sylvan

060.1 Urban

060.9 Yellow fever, unspecified

061 Dengue
Breakbone fever

> *Excludes:* hemorrhagic fever caused by dengue virus (065.4)

DEFINITION Dengue is an acute febrile and sometimes hemorrhagic disease endemic to the tropics, caused by any of four species of the virus genus flavivirus, and primarily transmitted to humans from mosquitoes, though human-to-human transmission is also well documented.

062 Mosquito-borne viral encephalitis
DEFINITION Mosquito-borne viral encephalitis is an inflammation of the brain, caused by a mosquito-bourne virus.
ALERT! For coding late effects of viral encephalitis see 139.0

062.0 Japanese encephalitis
Japanese B encephalitis

062.1 Western equine encephalitis

062.2 Eastern equine encephalitis

> *Excludes:* Venezuelan equine encephalitis (066.2)

062.3 St. Louis encephalitis

062.4 Australian encephalitis
Australian arboencephalitis
Australian X disease
Murray Valley encephalitis

062.5 California virus encephalitis
Encephalitis: Tahyna fever
  California
  La Crosse

062.8 Other specified mosquito-borne viral encephalitis
Encephalitis by Ilheus virus

> *Excludes:* West Nile virus (066.40-066.49)

062.9 Mosquito-borne viral encephalitis, unspecified

063 Tick-borne viral encephalitis
Includes: diphasic meningoencephalitis
DEFINITION Tick-borne viral encephalitis is an inflammation of the brain, caused by a tick-bourne virus.
ALERT! For coding late effects of viral encephalitis see 139.0

063.0 Russian spring-summer [taiga] encephalitis

063.1 Louping ill

063.2 Central European encephalitis

063.8 Other specified tick-borne viral encephalitis
Langat encephalitis
Powassan encephalitis

063.9 Tick-borne viral encephalitis, unspecified

064 Viral encephalitis transmitted by other and unspecified arthropods
Arthropod-borne viral encephalitis, vector unknown
Negishi virus encephalitis

> *Excludes:* viral encephalitis NOS (049.9)

DEFINITION Viral encephalitis is an inflammation of the brain.
ALERT! For coding late effects of viral encephalitis see 139.0

065 Arthropod-borne hemorrhagic fever
DEFINITION Hemorrhagic fever is a group of viral infections characterized by fever, chills, headache, malaise, and respiratory or gastrointestinal symptoms, followed by capillary hemorrhages and, in severe infection, by oliguria, kidney failure, hypotension, and possibly death.
ALERT! For coding late effects of viral encephalitis see 139.0

065.0 Crimean hemorrhagic fever [CHF Congo virus]
Central Asian hemorrhagic fever

065.1 Omsk hemorrhagic fever

065.2 Kyasanur Forest disease

065.3 Other tick-borne hemorrhagic fever

● Code new
  to 2012 edition
▲ Revision of
  existing code
④ ⑤ Fourth or fifth
     digit required

065.4 Mosquito-borne hemorrhagic fever
Chikungunya hemorrhagic fever
Dengue hemorrhagic fever

[Excludes:] *Chikungunya fever (066.3)*
dengue (061)
yellow fever (060.0-060.9)

065.8 Other specified arthropod-borne hemorrhagic fever
Mite-borne hemorrhagic fever

065.9 Arthropod-borne hemorrhagic fever, unspecified
Arbovirus hemorrhagic fever NOS

066 Other arthropod-borne viral diseases

[DEFINITION] Arthropod-borne viral diseases, refers to other viral diseases caused by insects.

[ALERT!] For coding late effects of viral encephalitis see 139.0

[ALERT!] For personal history of other specified infectious and parasitic disease see V12.09

066.0 Phlebotomus fever
Changuinola fever
Sandfly fever

066.1 Tick-borne fever
Nairobi sheep disease
Tick fever:
American mountain
Colorado
Tick fever:
Kemerovo
Quaranfil

066.2 Venezuelan equine fever
Venezuelan equine encephalitis

066.3 Other mosquito-borne fever
Fever (viral):
Bunyamwera
Bwamba
Chikungunya
GuamaR Mayaro
Mucambo
O'nyong-nyong
Fever (viral):
Oropouche
Pixuna
Rift valley
Ross river
Wesselsbron
Zika

[Excludes:] *dengue (061)*
yellow fever (060.0-060.9)

[5] **066.4 West Nile fever**

066.40 West Nile fever, unspecified
West Nile fever NOS
West Nile fever without complications
West Nile virus NOS

066.41 West Nile fever with encephalitis
West Nile encephalitis
West Nile encephalomyelitis

066.42 West Nile fever with other neurologic manifestation
Use additional code to specify the neurologic manifestation

066.49 West Nile fever with other complications
Use additional code to specify the other conditions

066.8 Other specified arthropod-borne viral diseases
Chandipura fever
Piry fever

066.9 Arthropod-borne viral disease, unspecified
Arbovirus infection NOS

OTHER DISEASES DUE TO VIRUSES AND CHLAMYDIAE (070-079)

070 Viral hepatitis
Includes: viral hepatitis (acute) (chronic)

[Excludes:] *cytomegalic inclusion virus hepatitis (078.5)*

The following fifth-digit subclassification is for use with categories 070.2 and 070.3:

0 acute or unspecified, without mention of hepatitis delta

1 acute or unspecified, with hepatitis delta

2 chronic, without mention of hepatitis delta

3 chronic, with hepatitis delta

DEFINITION Viral hepatitis is a liver inflammation due to a viral infection. It may present in acute or chronic forms. The most common causes of viral hepatitis are the five unrelated hepatotropic viruses hepatitis A, hepatitis B, hepatitis C, hepatitis D, and hepatitis E.

070.0 Viral hepatitis A with hepatic coma

070.1 Viral hepatitis A without mention of hepatic coma
Infectious hepatitis

⑤ **070.2 Viral hepatitis B with hepatic coma**
[0-3]

⑤ **070.3 Viral hepatitis B without mention of hepatic coma**
[0-3]   Serum hepatitis

⑤ **070.4 Other specified viral hepatitis with hepatic coma**

    070.41 Acute hepatitis C with hepatic coma

    070.42 Hepatitis delta without mention of active hepatitis B disease with hepatic coma
        Hepatitis delta with hepatitis B carrier state

    070.43 Hepatitis E with hepatic coma

    070.44 Chronic hepatitis C with hepatic coma

    070.49 Other specified viral hepatitis with hepatic coma

⑤ **070.5 Other specified viral hepatitis without mention of hepatic coma**

    070.51 Acute hepatitis C without mention of hepatic coma

    070.52 Hepatitis delta without mention of active hepatitis B disease or hepatic coma

    070.53 Hepatitis E without mention of hepatic coma

    070.54 Chronic hepatitis C without mention of hepatic coma

    070.59 Other specified viral hepatitis without mention of hepatic coma

070.6 Unspecified viral hepatitis with hepatic coma

    Excludes: *unspecified viral hepatitis C with hepatic coma (070.71)*

⑤ **070.7 Unspecified viral hepatitis C**

    070.70 Unspecified viral hepatitis C without hepatic coma
        Unspecified viral hepatitis C NOS

    070.71 Unspecified viral hepatitis C with hepatic coma

070.9 Unspecified viral hepatitis without mention of hepatic coma
Viral hepatitis NOS

    Excludes: *unspecified viral hepatitis C without hepatic coma (070.70)*

071 Rabies
Hydrophobia
Lyssa
    DEFINITION Rabies is a viral disease that causes acute encephalitis in warm-blooded animals and people, characterised by abnormal behaviour such as excitement, aggressiveness, and dementia, followed by paralysis and death.

072 Mumps
    DEFINITION Mumps, aka parotitis, is a viral disease of the human species, caused by the mumps virus. It is an acute contagious viral disease characterized by fever and by swelling of the parotid glands

072.0 Mumps orchitis

072.1 Mumps meningitis

072.2 Mumps encephalitis
Mumps meningoencephalitis

072.3 Mumps pancreatitis

⑤ **072.7 Mumps with other specified complications**

    072.71 Mumps hepatitis

    072.72 Mumps polyneuropathy

    072.79 Other

072.8 Mumps with unspecified complication

072.9 Mumps without mention of complication
Epidemic parotitis
Infectious parotitis

  ● Code new
    to 2012 edition
  ▲ Revision of
    existing code
  ④ ⑤ Fourth or fifth
    digit required

073 Ornithosis
Includes: parrot fever
psittacosis

[DEFINITION] Ornithosis is an atypical pneumonia caused by a rickettsia microorganism and transmitted to humans from infected birds.

073.0 With pneumonia
Lobular pneumonitis due to ornithosis

073.7 With other specified complications

073.8 With unspecified complication

073.9 Ornithosis, unspecified

074 Specific diseases due to Coxsackie virus

[Excludes:] *Coxsackie virus:*
infection NOS (079.2)
meningitis (047.0)

[DEFINITION] Coxsackie virus is any of a group of enteroviruses that are associated with a variety of diseases, including meningitis myocarditis and pericarditis and primarily affect children during the summer months.

074.0 Herpangina
Vesicular pharyngitis

074.1 Epidemic pleurodynia
Bornholm disease
Devil's grip
Epidemic:
myalgia
myositis

[5] **074.2 Coxsackie carditis**

074.20 Coxsackie carditis, unspecified

074.21 Coxsackie pericarditis

074.22 Coxsackie endocarditis

074.23 Coxsackie myocarditis
Aseptic myocarditis of newborn

074.3 Hand, foot, and mouth disease
Vesicular stomatitis and exanthem

074.8 Other specified diseases due to Coxsackie virus
Acute lymphonodular pharyngitis

075 Infectious mononucleosis
Glandular fever
Monocytic angina
Pfeiffer's disease

[DEFINITION] Infectious mononucleosis, aka mono, glandular fever, kissing disease is an acute disease characterized by fever and swollen lymph nodes and an abnormal increase of mononuclear leucocytes or monocytes in the bloodstream.

076 Trachoma

[Excludes:] *late effect of trachoma (139.1)*

[DEFINITION] Trachoma is a severe, chronic and contagious conjunctival eyelid and corneal infection caused by a virus that leads to corneal blood vessel formation, corneal clouding, conjunctival and eyelid scarring, and dry eyes.

[ALERT!] For coding late effects of trachoma see 139.1

076.0 Initial stage
Trachoma dubium

076.1 Active stage
Granular conjunctivitis (trachomatous)
Trachomatous:
follicular conjunctivitis
pannus

076.9 Trachoma, unspecified
Trachoma NOS

077 Other diseases of conjunctiva due to viruses and Chlamydiae

[Excludes:] *ophthalmic complications of viral diseases classified elsewhere*

[ALERT!] For personal history of other specified infectious and parasitic disease see V12.09

Add 4th or 5th digit | Nonspecific code | Unspecified code | Manifestation code

077.0 **Inclusion conjunctivitis**
Paratrachoma
Swimming pool conjunctivitis

Excludes: *inclusion blennorrhea (neonatal) (771.6)*

077.1 **Epidemic keratoconjunctivitis**
Shipyard eye

077.2 **Pharyngoconjunctival fever**
Viral pharyngoconjunctivitis

077.3 **Other adenoviral conjunctivitis**
Acute adenoviral follicular conjunctivitis

077.4 **Epidemic hemorrhagic conjunctivitis**
Apollo:
conjunctivitis
disease
Conjunctivitis due to enterovirus type 70
Hemorrhagic conjunctivitis (acute) (epidemic)

077.8 **Other viral conjunctivitis**
Newcastle conjunctivitis

⑤ **077.9** **Unspecified diseases of conjunctiva due to viruses and Chlamydiae**

077.98 **Due to Chlamydiae**

077.99 **Due to viruses**
Viral conjunctivitis NOS

078 **Other diseases due to viruses and Chlamydiae**

Excludes: *viral infection NOS (079.0-079.9)*
viremia NOS (790.8)

ALERT! For personal history of other specified infectious and parasitic disease see V12.09

078.0 **Molluscum contagiosum**

⑤ **078.1** **Viral warts**
Viral warts due to Human papillomavirus

078.10 **Viral warts, unspecified**
Verruca vulgaris
Warts (infectious)

078.11 **Condyloma acuminatum**
Condyloma NOS
Genital warts NOS

078.12 **Plantar wart**
Verruca plantaris

078.19 **Other specified viral warts**
Common wart
Flat wart
Verruca plana

078.2 **Sweating fever**
Miliary fever
Sweating disease

078.3 **Cat-scratch disease**
Benign lymphoreticulosis (of inoculation)
Cat-scratch fever

078.4 **Foot and mouth disease**
Aphthous fever
Epizootic:
aphthae
stomatitis

078.5 **Cytomegaloviral disease**
Cytomegalic inclusion disease
Salivary gland virus disease
Use additional code, if desired, to identify manifestation, as:
cytomegalic inclusion virus:
hepatitis (573.1)
pneumonia (484.1)

Excludes: *congenital cytomegalovirus infection (771.1)*

● Code new
to 2012 edition   ▲ Revision of
existing code   ④ ⑤ Fourth or fifth
digit required

078.6 Hemorrhagic nephrosonephritis

Hemorrhagic fever:
- epidemic
- Korean

Hemorrhagic fever:
- Russian
- with renal syndrome

078.7 Arenaviral hemorrhagic fever

Hemorrhagic fever:
- Argentine
- Bolivian

Hemorrhagic fever:
- Junin virus
- Machupo virus

[5] **078.8 Other specified diseases due to viruses and Chlamydiae**

[Excludes:] *epidemic diarrhea (009.2)*
lymphogranuloma venereum (099.1)

078.81 Epidemic vertigo

078.82 Epidemic vomiting syndrome
Winter vomiting disease

078.88 Other specified diseases due to Chlamydiae

078.89 Other specified diseases due to viruses
Epidemic cervical myalgia
Marburg disease

079 Viral and Chlamydial infection in conditions classified elsewhere and of unspecified site

Note: This category is provided to be used as an additional code where it is desired to identify the viral agent in diseases classifiable elsewhere. This category will also be used to classify virus infection of unspecified nature or site.

[ALERT!] For personal history of other specified infectious and parasitic disease see V12.09

079.0 Adenovirus

079.1 ECHO virus

079.2 Coxsackievirus

079.3 Rhinovirus

079.4 Human papillomavirus

[5] **079.5 Retrovirus**

[Excludes:] *human immunodeficiency virus, type 1 [HIV-1] (042)*
human T-cell lymphotrophic virus, type III [HTLV-III] (042)
lymphadenopathy-associated virus [LAV] (042)

[DEFINITION] Retrovirus refers to any of a group of viruses that contain two single-strand linear RNA molecules per virion and reverse transcriptase (RNA to DNA).

079.50 Retrovirus, unspecified

079.51 Human T-cell lymphotrophic virus, type I [HTLV-I]

079.52 Human T-cell lymphotrophic virus, type II [HTLV-II]

079.53 Human immunodeficiency virus, type 2 [HIV-2]

079.59 Other specified retrovirus

079.6 Respiratory syncytial virus (RSV)

[5] **079.8 Other specified viral and chlamydial infections**

079.81 Hantavirus

079.82 SARS-associated coronavirus

079.83 Parvovirus B19
Human parvovirus
Parvovirus NOS

[Excludes:] *erythema infectiosum [fifth disease] (057.0)*

079.88 Other specified chlamydial infection

079.89 Other specified viral infection

[5] **079.9 Unspecified viral and chlamydial infections**

[Excludes:] *viremia NOS (790.8)*

079.98 Unspecified chlamydial infection
Chlamydial infection NOS

079.99 Unspecified viral infection
Viral infection NOS

Add 4th or 5th digit | Nonspecific code | Unspecified code | Manifestation code

RICKETTSIOSES AND OTHER ARTHROPOD-BORNE DISEASES (080-088)

[Excludes:] *arthropod-borne viral diseases (060.0-066.9)*

080 Louse-borne [epidemic] typhus

Typhus (fever):
- classical
- epidemic
- exanthematic NOS
- louse-borne

[DEFINITION] Louse-borne typhus is any of several forms of infectious disease caused by rickettsia, especially those transmitted by fleas, lice, or mites, and characterized generally by severe headache, sustained high fever, depression, delirium, and the eruption of red rashes on the skin. Also called prison fever, ship fever, typhus fever.

081 Other typhus

[ALERT!] For personal history of other specified infectious and parasitic disease see V12.09

081.0 Murine [endemic] typhus

Typhus (fever):
- endemic
- flea-borne

081.1 Brill's disease

Brill-Zinsser disease
Recrudescent typhus (fever)

081.2 Scrub typhus

Japanese river fever
Kedani fever
Mite-borne typhus
Tsutsugamushi

081.9 Typhus, unspecified

Typhus (fever) NOS

082 Tick-borne rickettsioses

082.0 Spotted fevers

Rocky mountain spotted fever
São Paulo fever

082.1 Boutonneuse fever

African tick typhus
India tick typhus
Kenya tick typhus
Marseilles fever
Mediterranean tick fever

082.2 North Asian tick fever

Siberian tick typhus

082.3 Queensland tick typhus

⑤ **082.4 Ehrlichiosis**

082.40 Ehrlichiosis, unspecified

082.41 Ehrlichiosis chafeensis (E. chafeensis)

082.49 Other ehrlichiosis

082.8 Other specified tick-borne rickettsioses

Lone star fever

082.9 Tick-borne rickettsiosis, unspecified

Tick-borne typhus NOS

083 Other rickettsioses

[DEFINITION] Rickettsioses is a disease caused by intracellular bacteria. Examples of rickettsioses include typhus, Rocky Mountain spotted fever, and Rickettsialpox.

[ALERT!] For personal history of other specified infectious and parasitic disease see V12.09

083.0 Q fever

083.1 Trench fever

Quintan fever
Wolhynian fever

083.2 Rickettsialpox

Vesicular rickettsiosis

083.8 Other specified rickettsioses

083.9 Rickettsiosis, unspecified

084 Malaria

Note: Subcategories 084.0-084.6 exclude the listed conditions with mention of pernicious complications (084.8-084.9).

[Excludes:] *congenital malaria (771.2)*

● Code new to 2012 edition ▲ Revision of existing code ④ ⑤ Fourth or fifth digit required

DEFINITION Malaria is an infective disease caused by sporozoan parasites that are transmitted through the bite of an infected anopheles mosquito; marked by paroxysms of chills and fever.

ALERT! For personal history of malaria see V12.03

084.0 Falciparum malaria [malignant tertian]
> Malaria (fever):
>> by Plasmodium falciparum
>> subtertian

084.1 Vivax malaria [benign tertian]
> Malaria (fever) by Plasmodium vivax

084.2 Quartan malaria
> Malaria (fever) by Plasmodium malariae
> Malariae malaria

084.3 Ovale malaria
> Malaria (fever) by Plasmodium ovale

084.4 Other malaria
> Monkey malaria

084.5 Mixed malaria
> Malaria (fever) by more than one parasite

084.6 Malaria, unspecified
> Malaria (fever) NOS

084.7 Induced malaria
> Therapeutically induced malaria

> Excludes: *accidental infection from syringe, blood transfusion, etc. (084.0-084.6, above, according to parasite species)*
> *transmission from mother to child during delivery (771.2)*

084.8 Blackwater fever
> Hemoglobinuric: Malarial hemoglobinuria
>> fever (bilious)
>> malaria

084.9 Other pernicious complications of malaria
> Algid malaria
> Cerebral malaria
> Use additional code, if desired, to identify complication, as:
>> malarial:
>>> hepatitis (573.2)
>>> nephrosis (581.81)

085 Leishmaniasis

DEFINITION Leishmaniasis is a disease caused by protozoan parasites that belong to the genus leishmania and is transmitted by the bite of certain species of sand fly.

085.0 Visceral [kala-azar]
> Dumdum fever   Leishmaniasis:
> Infection by Leishmania: dermal, post-kala-azar
>> donovani   Mediterranean
>> infantum   visceral (Indian)

085.1 Cutaneous, urban
> Aleppo boil   Leishmaniasis, cutaneous:
> Baghdad boil   dry form
> Delhi boil   late
> Infection by Leishmania   recurrent
>> tropica (minor)   ulcerating
>>   Oriental sore

085.2 Cutaneous, Asian desert
> Infection by Leishmania tropica major
> Leishmaniasis, cutaneous:
>> acute necrotizing
>> rural
>> wet form
>> zoonotic form

085.3 Cutaneous, Ethiopian
> Infection by Leishmania ethiopica
> Leishmaniasis, cutaneous:
>> diffuse
>> lepromatous

	Add 4th or 5th digit		Nonspecific code		Unspecified code		Manifestation code

085.4 Cutaneous, American
Chiclero ulcer
Infection by Leishmania mexicana
Leishmaniasis tegumentaria diffusa

085.5 Mucocutaneous (American)
Espundia
Infection by Leishmania braziliensis
Uta

085.9 Leishmaniasis, unspecified

086 Trypanosomiasis
Use additional code, if desired, to identify manifestations, as:
trypanosomiasis:
encephalitis (323.2)
meningitis (321.3)
DEFINITION Trypanosomiasis is an infection caused by a type of protozoan parasite of the genus trypanosoma that causes sleeping sickness and other diseases in man and animals (usually transmitted by insects).

086.0 Chagas' disease with heart involvement
American trypanosomiasis with heart involvement
Infection by Trypanosoma cruzi with heart involvement
Any condition classifiable to 086.2 with heart involvement

086.1 Chagas' disease with other organ involvement
American trypanosomiasis with involvement of organ other than heart
Infection by Trypanosoma cruzi with involvement of organ other than heart
Any condition classifiable to 086.2 with involvement of organ other than heart

086.2 Chagas' disease without mention of organ involvement
American trypanosomiasis
Infection by Trypanosoma cruzi

086.3 Gambian trypanosomiasis
Gambian sleeping sickness
Infection by Trypanosoma gambiense

086.4 Rhodesian trypanosomiasis
Infection by Trypanosoma rhodesiense
Rhodesian sleeping sickness

086.5 African trypanosomiasis, unspecified
Sleeping sickness NOS

086.9 Trypanosomiasis, unspecified

087 Relapsing fever
Includes: recurrent fever
DEFINITION Relapsing fever is an infection caused by certain bacteria in the genus borrelia. It is a vector-borne disease that is transmitted through louse or soft-bodied tick bites.

087.0 Louse-borne

087.1 Tick-borne

087.9 Relapsing fever, unspecified

088 Other arthropod-borne diseases
DEFINITION Arthropod-borne diseases are transmitted by insects, spiders and crustaceans.
ALERT! For personal history of other specified infectious and parasitic disease see V12.09

088.0 Bartonellosis
Carrión's disease   Verruga peruana
Oroya fever

⑤ **088.8 Other specified arthropod-borne diseases**

088.81 Lyme Disease
Erythema chronicum migrans

088.82 Babesiosis
Babesiasis

088.89 Other

088.9 Arthropod-borne disease, unspecified

● Code new
   to 2012 edition
▲ Revision of
   existing code
④ ⑤ Fourth or fifth
   digit required

SYPHILIS AND OTHER VENEREAL DISEASES (090-099)

[*Excludes:*] *nonvenereal endemic syphilis (104.0)*
urogenital trichomoniasis (131.0)

090 Congenital syphilis

[DEFINITION] Congenital syphilis is syphilis present in utero and at birth, and occurs when a child is born to a mother with secondary or tertiary syphilis.

090.0 Early congenital syphilis, symptomatic

Congenital syphilitic:
- choroiditis
- coryza (chronic)
- hepatomegaly
- mucous patches
- periostitis
- splenomegaly

Syphilitic (congenital):
- epiphysitis
- osteochondritis
- pemphigus

Any congenital syphilitic condition specified as early or manifest less than two years after birth

090.1 Early congenital syphilis, latent

Congenital syphilis without clinical manifestations, with positive serological reaction and negative spinal fluid test, less than two years after birth

090.2 Early congenital syphilis, unspecified

Congenital syphilis NOS, less than two years after birth

090.3 Syphilitic interstitial keratitis

Syphilitic keratitis:
- parenchymatous
- punctata profunda

[*Excludes:*] *interstitial keratitis NOS (370.50)*

[5] **090.4 Juvenile neurosyphilis**

Use additional code, if desired, to identify any associated mental disorder

090.40 Juvenile neurosyphilis, unspecified

Congenital neurosyphilis
Dementia paralytica juvenilis
Juvenile:
- general paresis
- tabes
- taboparesis

090.41 Congenital syphilitic encephalitis

090.42 Congenital syphilitic meningitis

090.49 Other

090.5 Other late congenital syphilis, symptomatic

Gumma due to congenital syphilis
Hutchinson's teeth
Syphilitic saddle nose
Any congenital syphilitic condition specified as late or manifest two years or more after birth

090.6 Late congenital syphilis, latent

Congenital syphilis without clinical manifestations, with positive serological reaction and negative spinal fluid test, two years or more after birth

090.7 Late congenital syphilis, unspecified

Congenital syphilis NOS, two years or more after birth

090.9 Congenital syphilis, unspecified

091 Early syphilis, symptomatic

[*Excludes:*] *early cardiovascular syphilis (093.0-093.9)*
early neurosyphilis (094.0-094.9)

[DEFINITION] Early syphilis is defined as the stages of syphilis (primary, secondary, and early latent syphilis) that typically occur within the first year after acquisition of the infection.

091.0 Genital syphilis (primary)

Genital chancre

091.1 Primary anal syphilis

091.2 Other primary syphilis

Primary syphilis of:
- breast
- fingers

Primary syphilis of:
- lip
- tonsils

091.3 Secondary syphilis of skin or mucous membranes
    Condyloma latum   Secondary syphilis of:
    Secondary syphilis of: skin
      anus   tonsils
      mouth   vulva
      pharynx

091.4 Adenopathy due to secondary syphilis
    Syphilitic adenopathy (secondary)
    Syphilitic lymphadenitis (secondary)

⑤ **091.5 Uveitis due to secondary syphilis**

    091.50 Syphilitic uveitis, unspecified

    091.51 Syphilitic chorioretinitis (secondary)

    091.52 Syphilitic iridocyclitis (secondary)

⑤ **091.6 Secondary syphilis of viscera and bone**

    091.61 Secondary syphilitic periostitis

    091.62 Secondary syphilitic hepatitis
        Secondary syphilis of liver

    091.69 Other viscera

091.7 Secondary syphilis, relapse
    Secondary syphilis, relapse (treated) (untreated)

⑤ **091.8 Other forms of secondary syphilis**

    091.81 Acute syphilitic meningitis (secondary)

    091.82 Syphilitic alopecia

    091.89 Other

091.9 Unspecified secondary syphilis

092 Early syphilis, latent
    Includes: syphilis (acquired) without clinical manifestations, with positive serological
           reaction and negative spinal fluid test, less than two years after infection

092.0 Early syphilis, latent, serological relapse after treatment

092.9 Early syphilis, latent, unspecified

093 Cardiovascular syphilis
    DEFINITION Cardiovascular syphilis refers to the involvement of the cardiovascular system in
    late syphilis usually resulting in aortitis aneurysm formation, and aortic valvular insufficiency.

093.0 Aneurysm of aorta, specified as syphilitic
    Dilatation of aorta, specified as syphilitic

093.1 Syphilitic aortitis

⑤ **093.2 Syphilitic endocarditis**

    093.20 Valve, unspecified
        Syphilitic ostial coronary disease

    093.21 Mitral valve

    093.22 Aortic valve
        Syphilitic aortic incompetence or stenosis

    093.23 Tricuspid valve

    093.24 Pulmonary valve

⑤ **093.8 Other specified cardiovascular syphilis**

    093.81 Syphilitic pericarditis

    093.82 Syphilitic myocarditis

    093.89 Other

093.9 Cardiovascular syphilis, unspecified

094 Neurosyphilis
    Use additional code, if desired, to identify any associated mental disorder
    DEFINITION Neurosyphilis, aka tabes dorsalis, is the slowly progressive degeneration of the
    spinal cord that occurs in the late (tertiary) phase of syphilis a decade or more after
    contracting the infection.

  ● Code new   ▲ Revision of   ④ ⑤ Fourth or fifth
       to 2012 edition   existing code   digit required

094.0 Tabes dorsalis
Locomotor ataxia (progressive)
Posterior spinal sclerosis (syphilitic)
Tabetic neurosyphilis
Use additional code, if desired, to identify manifestation, as:
neurogenic arthropathy [Charcot's joint disease] (713.5)

094.1 General paresis
Dementia paralytica
General paralysis (of the insane) (progressive)
Paretic neurosyphilis
Taboparesis

094.2 Syphilitic meningitis
Meningovascular syphilis
[Excludes:] *acute syphilitic meningitis (secondary) (091.81)*

094.3 Asymptomatic neurosyphilis

[5] **094.8 Other specified neurosyphilis**

094.81 Syphilitic encephalitis

094.82 Syphilitic Parkinsonism

094.83 Syphilitic disseminated retinochoroiditis

094.84 Syphilitic optic atrophy

094.85 Syphilitic retrobulbar neuritis

094.86 Syphilitic acoustic neuritis

094.87 Syphilitic ruptured cerebral aneurysm

094.89 Other

094.9 Neurosyphilis, unspecified
Gumma (syphilitic) of central nervous system NOS
Syphilis (early) (late) of central nervous system NOS
Syphiloma of central nervous system NOS

095 Other forms of late syphilis, with symptoms
Includes: gumma (syphilitic)
syphilis, late, tertiary, or unspecified stage
[ALERT!] For personal history of other specified infectious and parasitic disease see V12.09

095.0 Syphilitic episcleritis

095.1 Syphilis of lung

095.2 Syphilitic peritonitis

095.3 Syphilis of liver

095.4 Syphilis of kidney

095.5 Syphilis of bone

095.6 Syphilis of muscle
Syphilitic myositis

095.7 Syphilis of synovium, tendon, and bursa
Syphilitic:
bursitis
synovitis

095.8 Other specified forms of late symptomatic syphilis
[Excludes:] *cardiovascular syphilis (093.0-093.9)*
neurosyphilis (094.0-094.9)

095.9 Late symptomatic syphilis, unspecified

096 Late syphilis, latent
Syphilis (acquired) without clinical manifestations, with positive serological reaction and negative spinal fluid test, two years or more after infection
[DEFINITION] Late syphilis is defined as involvement of the cardiovascular or central nervous system, or the development of a gumma in any organ, due to infection with treponema pallidum; usually several years to 2-3 decades after the initial infection. Also known as tertiary syphilis.

097 Other and unspecified syphilis
[ALERT!] For personal history of other specified infectious and parasitic disease see V12.09

097.0 Late syphilis, unspecified

097.1 Latent syphilis, unspecified
Positive serological reaction for syphilis

097.9 Syphilis, unspecified
Syphilis (acquired) NOS

Excludes: *syphilis NOS causing death under two years of age (090.9)*

098 Gonococcal infections
DEFINITION Gonococcal infection is a sexually transmitted disease caused by gonococcal bacteria that affects the mucous membrane chiefly of the genital and urinary tracts and is characterized by an acute purulent discharge and painful or difficult urination, though women often have no symptoms.

098.0 Acute, of lower genitourinary tract
Gonococcal: Gonorrhea (acute):
  Bartholinitis (acute)   NOS
  urethritis (acute)   genitourinary (tract) NOS
  vulvovaginitis (acute)

⑤ **098.1 Acute, of upper genitourinary tract**

098.10 Gonococcal infection (acute) of upper genitourinary tract, site unspecified

098.11 Gonococcal cystitis (acute)
Gonorrhea (acute) of bladder

098.12 Gonococcal prostatitis (acute)

098.13 Gonococcal epididymo-orchitis (acute)
Gonococcal orchitis (acute)

098.14 Gonococcal seminal vesiculitis (acute)
Gonorrhea (acute) of seminal vesicle

098.15 Gonococcal cervicitis (acute)
Gonorrhea (acute) of cervix

098.16 Gonococcal endometritis (acute)
Gonorrhea (acute) of uterus

098.17 Gonococcal salpingitis, specified as acute

098.19 Other

098.2 Chronic, of lower genitourinary tract
Gonococcal:
  Bartholinitis specified as chronic or with duration of two months or more
  urethritis specified as chronic or with duration of two months or more
  vulvovaginitis specified as chronic or with duration of two months or more
Gonorrhea:
  NOS specified as chronic or with duration of two months or more
  genitourinary (tract) specified as chronic or with duration of two months or more
Any condition classifiable to 098.0 specified as chronic or with duration of two months
  or more

⑤ **098.3 Chronic, of upper genitourinary tract**
Includes: any condition classifiable to 098.1 stated as chronic or with a duration of two
  months or more

098.30 Chronic gonococcal infection of upper genitourinary tract, site unspecified

098.31 Gonococcal cystitis, chronic
Any condition classifiable to 098.11, specified as chronic
Gonorrhea of bladder, chronic

098.32 Gonococcal prostatitis, chronic
Any condition classifiable to 098.12, specified as chronic

098.33 Gonococcal epididymo-orchitis, chronic
Any condition classifiable to 098.13, specified as chronic
Chronic gonococcal orchitis

098.34 Gonococcal seminal vesiculitis, chronic
Any condition classifiable to 098.14, specified as chronic
Gonorrhea of seminal vesicle, chronic

098.35 Gonococcal cervicitis, chronic
Any condition classifiable to 098.15, specified as chronic
Gonorrhea of cervix, chronic

098.36 Gonococcal endometritis, chronic
Any condition classifiable to 098.16, specified as chronic

098.37 Gonococcal salpingitis (chronic)

098.39 Other

⑤ **098.4 Gonococcal infection of eye**

098.40 Gonococcal conjunctivitis (neonatorum)
Gonococcal ophthalmia (neonatorum)

● Code new
  to 2012 edition

▲ Revision of
  existing code

④ ⑤ Fourth or fifth
   digit required

098.41 **Gonococcal iridocyclitis**

098.42 **Gonococcal endophthalmia**

098.43 **Gonococcal keratitis**

098.49 **Other**

⑤ **098.5 Gonococcal infection of joint**

098.50 **Gonococcal arthritis**
Gonococcal infection of joint NOS

098.51 **Gonococcal synovitis and tenosynovitis**

098.52 **Gonococcal bursitis**

098.53 **Gonococcal spondylitis**

098.59 **Other**
Gonococcal rheumatism

098.6 Gonococcal infection of pharynx

098.7 Gonococcal infection of anus and rectum
Gonococcal proctitis

⑤ **098.8 Gonococcal infection of other specified sites**

098.81 **Gonococcal keratosis (blennorrhagica)**

098.82 **Gonococcal meningitis**

098.83 **Gonococcal pericarditis**

098.84 **Gonococcal endocarditis**

098.85 **Other gonococcal heart disease**

098.86 **Gonococcal peritonitis**

098.89 **Other**
Gonococcemia

099 **Other venereal diseases**
DEFINITION Venereal disease is a disease that is contracted and transmitted by sexual contact, caused by microorganisms that survive on the skin or mucus membranes.

ALERT! For personal history of other specified infectious and parasitic disease see V12.09

099.0 Chancroid
Bubo (inguinal):	Chancre:
chancroidal	Ducrey's
due to Hemophilus ducreyi	simple
	soft
	Ulcus molle (cutis) (skin)

099.1 Lymphogranuloma venereum
Climatic or tropical bubo	Esthiomene
(Durand-) Nicolas- Favre	Lymphogranuloma inguinale
disease	

099.2 Granuloma inguinale
Donovanosis	Granuloma venereum
Granuloma pudendi	Pudendal ulcer
(ulcerating)	

099.3 Reiter's disease
Reactive arthritis
Reiter's syndrome
Use additional code for associated:
    arthropathy (711.1)
    conjunctivitis (372.33)

⑤ **099.4 Other nongonococcal urethritis [NGU]**

099.40 **Unspecified**
Nonspecific urethritis

099.41 **Chlamydia trachomatis**

099.49 **Other specified organism**

⑤ **099.5 Other venereal diseases due to Chlamydia trachomatis**

Excludes: *Chlamydia trachomatis infection of conjunctiva (076.0-076.9, 077.0, 077.9)*
Lymphogranuloma venereum (099.1)

099.50 **Unspecified site**

099.51 **Pharynx**

099.52 **Anus and rectum**

| | Add 4th or 5th digit | | Nonspecific code | | Unspecified code | | Manifestation code |

099.53 Lower genitourinary sites

[Excludes:] *urethra (099.41)*

Use additional code, if desired, to specify site of infection, such as:
bladder (595.4)
cervix (616.0)
vagina and vulva (616.11)

099.54 Other genitourinary sites

Use additional code, if desired, to specify site of infection, such as:
pelvic inflammatory disease NOS (614.9)
testis and epididymis (604.91)

099.55 Unspecified genitourinary site

099.56 Peritoneum
Perihepatitis

099.59 Other specified site

099.8 Other specified venereal diseases

099.9 Venereal disease, unspecified

OTHER SPIROCHETAL DISEASES (100-104)

100 Leptospirosis

DEFINITION Leptospirosis, aka swamp fever, is an acute, infectious, febrile disease of both humans and animals, caused by spirochetes of the genus leptospira.

100.0 Leptospirosis icterohemorrhagica
Leptospiral or spirochetal jaundice (hemorrhagic)
Weil's disease

⑤ **100.8 Other specified leptospiral infections**

100.81 Leptospiral meningitis (aseptic)

100.89 Other
Fever:
Fort Bragg
pretibial
swamp
Infection by Leptospira:
australis
bataviae
pyrogenes

100.9 Leptospirosis, unspecified

101 Vincent's angina
Acute necrotizing ulcerative:
gingivitis
stomatitis
Fusospirochetal pharyngitis
Spirochetal stomatitis
Trench mouth
Vincent's:
gingivitis
infection [any site]

DEFINITION Vincent's angina, aka trench mouth, is an acute communicable infection of the respiratory tract and mouth marked by ulceration of the mucous membrane.

102 Yaws
Includes: frambesia
pian

DEFINITION Yaws is a contagious tropical disease caused by the spirochete treponema pertenue, characterized by yellowish or reddish tumors, which often resemble currants, strawberries, or raspberries.

102.0 Initial lesions
Chancre of yaws
Frambesia, initial or primary
Initial frambesial ulcer
Mother yaw

102.1 Multiple papillomata and wet crab yaws
Butter yaws
Frambesioma
Pianoma
Planter or palmer papilloma of yaws

102.2 Other early skin lesions
Early yaws (cutaneous) (macular) (papular) (maculopapular) (micropapular)
Frambeside of early yaws
Cutaneous yaws, less than five years after infection

102.3 Hyperkeratosis
Ghoul hand
Hyperkeratosis, palmer or plantar (early) (late) due to yaws
Worm-eaten soles

102.4 Gummata and ulcers
Nodular late yaws (ulcerated)
Gummatous frambeside

● Code new to 2012 edition ▲ Revision of existing code ④ ⑤ Fourth or fifth digit required

102.5 Gangosa
Rhinopharyngitis mutilans

102.6 Bone and joint lesions
Goundou, of yaws (late)
Gumma, bone, of yaws (late)
Gummatous osteitis or periostitis, of yaws (late)
Hydrarthrosis, of yaws (early) (late)
Osteitis, of yaws (early) (late)
Periostitis (hypertrophic), of yaws (early) (late)

102.7 Other manifestations
Juxta-articular nodules of yaws
Mucosal yaws

102.8 Latent yaws
Yaws without clinical manifestations, with positive serology

102.9 Yaws, unspecified

103 Pinta

DEFINITION Pinta is a human skin disease endemic to Mexico, Central America, and South America caused by infection with a spirochete, treponema pallidum carateum, which is morphologically and serologically indistinguishable from the organism that causes syphilis.

103.0 Primary lesions
Chancre (primary) of pinta [carate]
Papule (primary) of pinta [carate]
Pintid of pinta [carate]

103.1 Intermediate lesions
Erythematous plaques of pinta [carate]
Hyperchromic lesions of pinta [carate]
Hyperkeratosis of pinta [carate]

103.2 Late lesions
Cardiovascular lesions, of pinta [carate]
Skin lesions:
    achromic of pinta [carate]
    cicatricial of pinta [carate]
    dyschromic of pinta [carate]
Vitiligo of pinta [carate]

103.3 Mixed lesions
Achromic and hyperchromic skin lesions of pinta [carate]

103.9 Pinta, unspecified

104 Other spirochetal infection

ALERT! For personal history of other specified infectious and parasitic disease see V12.09

104.0 Nonvenereal endemic syphilis
Bejel   Njovera

104.8 Other specified spirochetal infections

Excludes: relapsing fever (087.0-087.9)
                syphilis (090.0-097.9)

104.9 Spirochetal infection, unspecified

MYCOSES (110-118)

Use additional code, if desired, to identify manifestation, as:
arthropathy (711.6)
meningitis (321.0-321.1)
otitis externa (380.15)

Excludes: infection by Actinomycetales, such as species of Actinomyces, Actinomadura, Nocardia, Streptomyces (039.0-039.9)

110 Dermatophytosis
Includes: infection by species of Epidermophyton, Microsporum, and Trichophyton
                tinea, any type except those in 111

DEFINITION Dermatophytosis, aka tinea or ringworm, is a disease that can affect the scalp (tinea capitis), body (tinea corporis), nails (tinea unguium), feet (tinea pedis), groin (tinea cruris), and bearded skin (tinea harbae).

110.0 Of scalp and beard
Kerion
Sycosis, mycotic
Trichophytic tinea [black dot tinea], scalp

| | Add 4th or 5th digit | | Nonspecific code | | Unspecified code | | Manifestation code |

110.1 Of nail
Dermatophytic onychia   Tinea unguium
Onychomycosis

110.2 Of hand
Tinea manuum

110.3 Of groin and perianal area
Dhobie itch   Tinea cruris
Eczema marginatum

110.4 Of foot
Athlete's foot   Tinea pedis

110.5 Of the body
Herpes circinatus
Tinea imbricata [Tokelau]

110.6 Deep seated dermatophytosis
Granuloma trichophyticum
Majocchi's granuloma

110.8 Of other specified sites

110.9 Of unspecified site
Favus NOS   Ringworm NOS
Microsporic tinea NOS

111 Dermatomycosis, other and unspecified
DEFINITION Dermatomycosis is a superficial fungal infection of the skin or its appendages.

111.0 Pityriasis versicolor
Infection by Malassezia [Pityrosporum] furfur
Tinea flava
Tinea versicolor

111.1 Tinea nigra
Infection by   Microsporosis nigra
    Cladosporium species   Pityriasis nigra
Keratomycosis nigricans   Tinea palmaris nigra

111.2 Tinea blanca
Infection by Trichosporon (beigelii) cutaneum
White piedra

111.3 Black piedra
Infection by Piedraia hortai

111.8 Other specified dermatomycoses

111.9 Dermatomycosis, unspecified

112 Candidiasis
Includes: infection by Candida species
        moniliasis

Excludes: neonatal monilial infection (771.7)

DEFINITION Candidiasis is an infection caused by a species of the yeast candida, usually candida albicans. Candidiasis is a common cause of vaginal infections in women.

112.0 Of mouth
Thrush (oral)

112.1 Of vulva and vagina
Candidal vulvovaginitis   Monilial vulvovaginitis

112.2 Of other urogenital sites
Candidal balanitis

112.3 Of skin and nails
Candidal intertrigo   Candidal perionyxis [paronychia]
Candidal onychia

112.4 Of lung
Candidal pneumonia

112.5 Disseminated
Systemic candidiasis

⑤ **112.8 Of other specified sites**

    112.81 Candidal endocarditis

    112.82 Candidal otitis externa
        Otomycosis in moniliasis

● Code new   ▲ Revision of   ④ ⑤ Fourth or fifth
    to 2012 edition   existing code   digit required

112.83 Candidal meningitis

112.84 Candidal esophagitis

112.85 Candidal enteritis

112.89 Other

112.9 Of unspecified site

114 Coccidioidomycosis

Includes: infection by Coccidioides (immitis)
Posada-Wernicke disease

[DEFINITION] Coccidioidomycosis is an infection caused by inhaling the microscopic spores of the fungus coccidioides immitis. The chronic form can develop as many as 20 years after initial infection and, in the lungs, can produce inflamed, injured areas that can fill with pus.

114.0 Primary coccidioidomycosis (pulmonary)
Acute pulmonary coccidioidomycosis
Coccidioidomycotic pneumonitis
Desert rheumatism
Pulmonary coccidioidomycosis
San Joaquin Valley fever

114.1 Primary extrapulmonary coccidioidomycosis
Chancriform syndrome
Primary cutaneous coccidioidomycosis

114.2 Coccidioidal meningitis

114.3 Other forms of progressive coccidioidomycosis
Coccidioidal granuloma
Disseminated coccidioidomycosis

114.4 Chronic pulmonary coccidioidomycosis

114.5 Pulmonary coccidioidomycosis, unspecified

114.9 Coccidioidomycosis, unspecified

[5] **115 Histoplasmosis**

The following fifth-digit subclassification is for use with category 115:

0 without mention of manifestation
1 meningitis
2 retinitis
3 pericarditis
4 endocarditis
5 pneumonia
9 other

[DEFINITION] Histoplasmosis, aka Darling's disease, is a disease caused by the fungus histoplasma capsulatum. Symptoms vary greatly, but the disease primarily affects the lungs. Histoplasmosis is common among aids patients because of their lowered immune system.

[5] **115.0 Infection by Histoplasma capsulatum**
[0-5, 9] American histoplasmosis
Darling's disease
Reticuloendothelial cytomycosis
Small form histoplasmosis

[5] **115.1 Infection by Histoplasma duboisii**
[0-5, 9] African histoplasmosis
Large form histoplasmosis

[5] **115.9 Histoplasmosis, unspecified**
[0-5, 9] Histoplasmosis NOS

116 Blastomycotic infection

[DEFINITION] Blastomycotic infection, aka North American blastomycosis, blastomycetic dermatitis, and gilchrist's disease, is a fungal infection caused by the organism blastomyces dermatitidis. Endemic to portions of north america, blastomycosis causes clinical symptoms similar to histoplasmosis.

116.0 Blastomycosis
Blastomycotic dermatitis
Chicago disease
Cutaneous blastomycosis
Disseminated blastomycosis
Gilchrist's disease
Infection by Blastomyces [Ajellomyces] dermatitidis
North American blastomycosis
Primary pulmonary blastomycosis

116.1 Paracoccidioidomycosis
Brazilian blastomycosis
Infection by Paracoccidioides [Blastomyces] brasiliensis
Lutz-Splendore-Almeida disease
Mucocutaneous-lymphangitic paracoccidioidomycosis
Pulmonary paracoccidioidomycosis
South American blastomycosis
Visceral paracoccidioidomycosis

116.2 Lobomycosis
Infections by Loboa [Blastomyces] loboi
Keloidal blastomycosis
Lobo's disease

117 Other mycoses

DEFINITION Mycoses is a fungal infection in or on a part of the body.

ALERT! For personal history of other specified infectious and parasitic disease see V12.09

117.0 Rhinosporidiosis
Infection by Rhinosporidium seeberi

117.1 Sporotrichosis
Cutaneous sporotrichosis
Disseminated sporotrichosis
Infection by Sporothrix [Sporotrichum] schenckii
Lymphocutaneous sporotrichosis
Pulmonary sporotrichosis
Sporotrichosis of the bones

117.2 Chromoblastomycosis
Chromomycosis
Infection by Cladosporidium carrionii, Fonsecaea compactum, Fonsecaea pedrosoi, Phialophora verrucosa

117.3 Aspergillosis
Infection by Aspergillus species, mainly A. fumigatus, A. flavus group, A. terreus group

117.4 Mycotic mycetomas
Infection by various genera and species of Ascomycetes and Deuteromycetes, such as Acremonium [Cephalosporium] falciforme, Neotestudina rosatii, Madurella grisea, Madurella mycetomii, Pyrenochaeta romeroi, Zopfia [Leptosphaeria] senegalensis
Madura foot, mycotic
Maduromycosis, mycotic

Excludes: actinomycotic mycetomas (039.0-039.9)

117.5 Cryptococcosis

Busse-Buschke's disease	Pulmonary cryptococcosis
European cryptococcosis	Systemic cryptococcosis
Infection by Cryptococcus neoformans	Torula

117.6 Allescheriosis [Petriellidosis]
Infections by Allescheria [Petriellidium] boydii [Monosporium apiospermum]

Excludes: mycotic mycetoma (117.4)

117.7 Zygomycosis [Phycomycosis or Mucormycosis]
Infection by species of Absidia, Basidiobolus, Conidiobolus, Cunninghamella, Entomophthora, Mucor, Rhizopus, Saksenaea

117.8 Infection by dematiacious fungi, [Phaehyphomycosis]
Infection by dematiacious fungi, such as Cladosporium trichoides [bantianum], Dreschlera hawaiiensis, Phialophora gougerotii, Phialophora jeanselmi

117.9 Other and unspecified mycoses

118 Opportunistic mycoses
Infection of skin, subcutaneous tissues, and/or organs by a wide variety of fungi generally considered to be pathogenic to compromised hosts only (e.g., infection by species of Alternaria, Dreschlera, Fusarium)

Use additional code to identify manifestation, such as:
keratitis (370.8)

● Code new to 2012 edition   ▲ Revision of existing code   ④ ⑤ Fourth or fifth digit required

HELMINTHIASES (120-129)

120 **Schistosomiasis [bilharziasis]**

> **DEFINITION** Schistosomiasis [bilharziasis], aka bilharzia, bilharziosis or snail fever, is a parasitic disease caused by several species of fluke of the genus schistosoma. Schistosomiasis often is a chronic illness that can damage internal organs and, in children, impair growth and cognitive development.

120.0 Schistosoma haematobium
Vesical schistosomiasis NOS

120.1 Schistosoma mansoni
Intestinal schistosomiasis NOS

120.2 Schistosoma japonicum
Asiatic schistosomiasis NOS
Katayama disease or fever

120.3 Cutaneous
Cercarial dermatitis   Schistosome dermatitis
Infection by cercariae   Swimmers' itch
  of Schistosoma

120.8 Other specified schistosomiasis
Infection by Schistosoma: Infection by Schistosoma spindale
  bovis   Schistosomiasis chestermani
  intercalatum
  mattheii

120.9 Schistosomiasis, unspecified
Blood flukes NOS   Hemic distomiasis

121 **Other trematode infections**

> **DEFINITION** A trematode infection is the infection of the digestive tract by adult parasitic flatworms called cestodes or tapeworms.

> **ALERT!** For personal history of other specified infectious and parasitic disease see V12.09

121.0 Opisthorchiasis
Infection by:
  cat liver fluke
  Opisthorchis (felineus) (tenuicollis) (viverrini)

121.1 Clonorchiasis
Biliary cirrhosis due to clonorchiasis
Chinese liver fluke disease
Hepatic distomiasis due to Clonorchis sinensis
Oriental liver fluke disease

121.2 Paragonimiasis
Infection by Paragonimus   Pulmonary distomiasis
Lung fluke disease (oriental)

121.3 Fascioliasis
Infection by Fasciola: Liver flukes NOS
  gigantica   Sheep liver fluke infection
  hepatica

121.4 Fasciolopsiasis
Infection by Fasciolopsis [buski]
Intestinal distomiasis

121.5 Metagonimiasis
Infection by Metagonimus yokogawai

121.6 Heterophyiasis
Infection by:
  Heterophyes heterophyes
  Stellantchasmus falcatus

121.8 Other specified trematode infections
Infection by:
  Dicrocoelium dendriticum
  Echinostoma ilocanum
  Gastrodiscoides hominis

121.9 Trematode infection, unspecified
Distomiasis NOS
Fluke disease NOS

Add 4th or 5th digit   Nonspecific code   Unspecified code   Manifestation code

122 **Echinococcosis**
Includes: echinococciasis
hydatid disease
hydatidosis

DEFINITION Echinococcosis, aka hydatid disease, hydatid cyst, unilocular hydatid disease or cystic echinococcosis is a potentially fatal parasitic disease that can affect many animals, including wildlife, commercial livestock and humans. The disease results from infection by tapeworm larvae of the genus echinococcus.

122.0 **Echinococcus granulosus infection of liver**

122.1 **Echinococcus granulosus infection of lung**

122.2 **Echinococcus granulosus infection of thyroid**

122.3 **Echinococcus granulosus infection, other**

122.4 **Echinococcus granulosus infection, unspecified**

122.5 **Echinococcus multilocularis infection of liver**

122.6 **Echinococcus multilocularis infection, other**

122.7 **Echinococcus multilocularis infection, unspecified**

122.8 **Echinococcosis, unspecified, of liver**

122.9 **Echinococcosis, other and unspecified**

123 **Other cestode infection**
DEFINITION Cestode infection refers to infestation by any of various parasitic flatworms of the class cestoda, including the tapeworms.
ALERT! For personal history of other specified infectious and parasitic disease see V12.09

123.0 **Taenia solium infection, intestinal form**
Pork tapeworm (adult) (infection)

123.1 **Cysticercosis**
Cysticerciasis
Infection by Cysticercus cellulosae [larval form of Taenia solium]

123.2 **Taenia saginata infection**
Beef tapeworm (infection)
Infection by Taeniarhynchus saginatus

123.3 **Taeniasis, unspecified**

123.4 **Diphyllobothriasis, intestinal**
Diphyllobothrium (adult) (latum) (pacificum) infection
Fish tapeworm (infection)

123.5 **Sparganosis [larval diphyllobothriasis]**
Infection by:
Diphyllobothrium larvae
Sparganum (mansoni) (proliferum)
Spirometra larvae

123.6 **Hymenolepiasis**
Dwarf tapeworm (infection)
Hymenolepis (diminuta) (nana) infection
Rat tapeworm (infection)

123.8 **Other specified cestode infection**
Diplogonoporus (grandis) infection
Dipylidium (caninum) infection
Dog tapeworm (infection) infection

123.9 **Cestode infection, unspecified**
Tapeworm (infection) NOS

124 **Trichinosis**
Trichinella spiralis infection
Trichinellosis
Trichiniasis

DEFINITION Trichinosis, aka trichinellosis or trichiniasis, is a parasitic disease caused by eating raw or undercooked pork and wild game infected with the larvae of a species of roundworm trichinella spiralis commonly called the trichina worm.

● Code new
to 2012 edition
▲ Revision of
existing code
④ ⑤ Fourth or fifth
digit required

125 **Filarial infection and dracontiasis**

DEFINITION Filarial infection and dracontiasis is a group of tropical diseases caused by various thread-like parasitic round worms (nematodes) and their larvae transmitted to humans through a mosquito bite. Filariasis is characterized by fever, chills, headache, and skin lesions in the early stages and, if untreated, can progress to include gross enlargement of the limbs and genitalia in a condition called elephantiasis. Dracunculiasis more commonly known as guinea worm disease (GWD), dracontiasis or medina worm is a parasitic infection caused by the nematode dracunculus medinensis.

125.0 Bancroftian filariasis
Chyluria due to Wuchereria bancrofti
Elephantiasis due to Wuchereria bancrofti
Infection due to Wuchereria bancrofti
Lymphadenitis due to Wuchereria bancrofti
Lymphangitis due to Wuchereria bancrofti
Wuchereriasis

125.1 Malayan filariasis
Brugia filariasis due to Brugia [Wuchereria] malayi
Chyluria due to Brugia [Wuchereria] malayi
Elephantiasis due to Brugia [Wuchereria] malayi
Infection due to Brugia [Wuchereria] malayi
Lymphadenitis due to Brugia [Wuchereria] malayi
Lymphangitis due to Brugia [Wuchereria] malayi

125.2 Loiasis
Eyeworm disease of Africa
Loa loa infection

125.3 Onchocerciasis
Onchocerca volvulus infection
Onchocercosis

125.4 Dipetalonemiasis
Infection by:
  Acanthocheilonema perstans
  Dipetalonema perstans

125.5 Mansonella ozzardi infection
Filariasis ozzardi

125.6 **Other specified filariasis**
Dirofilaria infection
Infection by:
  Acanthocheilonema streptocerca
  Dipetalonema streptocerca

125.7 Dracontiasis
Guinea-worm infection
Infection by Dracunculus medinensis

125.9 Unspecified filariasis

126 **Ancylostomiasis and necatoriasis**
Includes: cutaneous larva migrans due to Ancylostoma
  hookworm (disease) (infection)
  uncinariasis

DEFINITION Ancylostomiasis and necatoriasis ancylostomiasis, aka hookworm disease or tunnel disease, is a disease caused by hookworm infestation and marked by progressive anemia. Necatoriasis is a hookworm disease caused by necator, the resulting anemia being usually less severe than that from ancylostomiasis.

126.0 Ancylostoma duodenale

126.1 Necator americanus

126.2 Ancylostoma braziliense

126.3 Ancylostoma ceylanicum

126.8 **Other specified Ancylostoma**

126.9 Ancylostomiasis and necatoriasis, unspecified
Creeping eruption NOS
Cutaneous larva migrans NOS

127 **Other intestinal helminthiases**

DEFINITION Helminthiases is a disease in which a part of the body is infested with worms such as pinworm, roundworm or tapeworm.

ALERT! For personal history of other specified infectious and parasitic disease see V12.09

| | Add 4th or 5th digit | | Nonspecific code | | Unspecified code | | Manifestation code |

127.0 Ascariasis
　　Ascaridiasis
　　Infection by Ascaris lumbricoides
　　Roundworm infection

127.1 Anisakiasis
　　Infection by Anisakis larva

127.2 Strongyloidiasis
　　Infection by Strongyloides stercoralis

　　| Excludes: | *trichostrongyliasis (127.6)*

127.3 Trichuriasis
　　Infection by Trichuris trichiuria
　　Trichocephaliasis
　　Whipworm (disease) (infection)

127.4 Enterobiasis
　　Infection by Enterobius vermicularis
　　Oxyuriasis
　　Oxyuris vermicularis infection
　　Pinworn (disease) (infection)
　　Threadworm infection

127.5 Capillariasis
　　Infection by Capillaria philippinensis

　　| Excludes: | *infection by Capillaria hepatica (128.8)*

127.6 Trichostrongyliasis
　　Infection by Trichostrongylus species

127.7 Other specified intestinal helminthiasis
　　Infection by:
　　　　Oesophagostomum apiostomum and related species
　　　　Ternidens diminutus
　　　　other specified intestinal helminth
　　Physalopteriasis

127.8 Mixed intestinal helminthiasis
　　Infection by intestinal helminths classified to more than one of the categories
　　　　120.0-127.7
　　Mixed helminthiasis NOS

127.9 Intestinal helminthiasis, unspecified

128 Other and unspecified helminthiases

　　ALERT! For personal history of other specified infectious and parasitic disease see V12.09

128.0 Toxocariasis
　　Larva migrans visceralis
　　Toxocara (canis) (cati) infection
　　Visceral larva migrans syndrome

128.1 Gnathostomiasis
　　Infection by Gnathostoma spinigerum and related species

128.8 Other specified helminthiasis
　　Infection by:
　　　　Angiostrongylus cantonensis
　　　　Capillaria hepatica
　　　　other specified helminth

128.9 Helminth infection, unspecified
　　Helminthiasis NOS
　　Worms NOS

129 Intestinal parasitism, unspecified

● Code new　　　　▲ Revision of　　　④ ⑤ Fourth or fifth
　to 2012 edition　　　existing code　　　　digit required

OTHER INFECTIOUS AND PARASITIC DISEASES (130-136)

[ALERT!] For coding late effects of other infectious and parasitic diseases see 139

130 Toxoplasmosis

Includes: infection by toxoplasma gondii
toxoplasmosis (acquired)

[Excludes:] *congenital toxoplasmosis (771.2)*

[DEFINITION] Toxoplasmosis is an infection caused by the parasite named toxoplasma gondii that can invade tissues and damage the brain, especially in a fetus and in a newborn baby. Symptoms include fever, fatigue, headache, swollen lymph glands, and muscle aches and pains.

130.0 Meningoencephalitis due to toxoplasmosis
Encephalitis due to acquired toxoplasmosis

130.1 Conjunctivitis due to toxoplasmosis

130.2 Chorioretinitis due to toxoplasmosis
Focal retinochoroiditis due to acquired toxoplasmosis

130.3 Myocarditis due to toxoplasmosis

130.4 Pneumonitis due to toxoplasmosis

130.5 Hepatitis due to toxoplasmosis

130.7 Toxoplasmosis of other specified sites

130.8 Multisystemic disseminated toxoplasmosis
Toxoplasmosis of multiple sites

130.9 Toxoplasmosis, unspecified

131 Trichomoniasis

Includes: infection due to Trichomonas (vaginalis)

[DEFINITION] Trichomoniasis is a common sexually transmitted disease caused by the parasite trichomonas vaginalis and infecting the urinary tract or vagina.

[ALERT!] For coding late effects of other infectious and parasitic diseases see 139

[5] **131.0 Urogenital trichomoniasis**

131.00 Urogenital trichomoniasis, unspecified
Fluor (vaginalis) trichomonal or due to Trichomonas (vaginalis)
Leukorrhea (vaginalis) trichomonal or due to Trichomonas (vaginalis)

131.01 Trichomonal vulvovaginitis
Vaginitis, trichomonal or due to Trichomonas (vaginalis)

131.02 Trichomonal urethritis

131.03 Trichomonal prostatitis

131.09 Other

131.8 Other specified sites

[Excludes:] *intestinal (007.3)*

131.9 Trichomoniasis, unspecified

132 Pediculosis and phthirus infestation

[DEFINITION] Pediculosis and phthirus infestation is an infestation with lice (pediculus humanus) or true lice or crab lice (phthirius) resulting in severe itching.

[ALERT!] For coding late effects of other infectious and parasitic diseases see 139

132.0 Pediculus capitis [head louse]

132.1 Pediculus corporis [body louse]

132.2 Phthirus pubis [pubic louse]
Pediculus pubis

132.3 Mixed infestation
Infestation classifiable to more than one of the categories 132.0-132.2

132.9 Pediculosis, unspecified

133 Acariasis

[DEFINITION] Acariasis is an infestation with arthropod parasites of the order acarina including the ticks and mites.

[ALERT!] For coding late effects of other infectious and parasitic diseases see 139

133.0 Scabies
Infestation by Sarcoptes scabiei
Norwegian scabies
Sarcoptic itch

133.8 Other acariasis
Chiggers
Infestation by:
Demodex folliculorum
Trombicula

133.9 Acariasis, unspecified
Infestation by mites NOS

134 Other infestation
[ALERT!] For coding late effects of other infectious and parasitic diseases see 139

134.0 Myiasis
Infestation by:
Dermatobia (hominis)
fly larvae
Gasterophilus (intestinalis)
Infestation by:
maggots
Oestrus ovis

134.1 Other arthropod infestation
Infestation by:
chigoe
sand flea
Tunga penetrans
Jigger disease
Scarabiasis
Tungiasis

134.2 Hirudiniasis
Hirudiniasis (external) (internal)
Leeches (aquatic) (land)

134.8 Other specified infestations

134.9 Infestation, unspecified
Infestation (skin) NOS
Skin parasites NOS

135 Sarcoidosis
Besnier-Boeck- Schaumann disease
Lupoid (miliary) of Boeck
Lupus pernio (Besnier)
Lymphogranulomatosis, benign (Schaumann's)
Sarcoid (any site):
NOS
Boeck
Darier-Roussy
Uveoparotid fever

[DEFINITION] Sarcoidosis is a disease of unknown origin that causes small lumps (granulomas) due to chronic inflammation to develop in a great range of body tissues. Sarcoidosis can appear in almost any body organ, but most often starts in the lungs or lymph nodes.

[ALERT!] For coding late effects of other infectious and parasitic diseases see 139

136 Other and unspecified infectious and parasitic diseases
[ALERT!] For coding late effects of other and unspecified infectious and parasitic diseases see 139.8

[ALERT!] For personal history of unspecified infectious and parasitic disease see V12.00

136.0 Ainhum
Dactylolysis spontanea

136.1 Behçet's syndrome

⑤ **136.2 Specific infections by free-living amebae**

136.21 Specific infection due to acanthamoeba
Use additional code to identify manifestation, such as:
keratitis (370.8)

136.29 Other specific infections by free-living amebae
Meningoencephalitis due to Naegleria

136.3 Pneumocystosis
Pneumonia due to Pneumocystis carinii
Pneumonia due to Pneumocystis jiroveci

136.4 Psorospermiasis

136.5 Sarcosporidiosis
Infection by Sarcocystis lindemanni

136.8 Other specified infectious and parasitic diseases
Candiru infestation

136.9 Unspecified infectious and parasitic diseases
Infectious disease NOS
Parasitic disease NOS

● Code new to 2012 edition
▲ Revision of existing code
④ ⑤ Fourth or fifth digit required

LATE EFFECTS OF INFECTIOUS AND PARASITIC DISEASES (137-139)

137 **Late effects of tuberculosis**

> Note: This category is to be used to indicate conditions classifiable to 010-018 as the cause of late effects, which are themselves classified elsewhere. The "late effects" include those specified as such, as sequelae, or as due to old or inactive tuberculosis, without evidence of active disease.
>
> **DEFINITION** Late effects of tuberculosis refers to condition that appears after the acute phase of tuberculosis has run its course.

137.0 **Late effects of respiratory or unspecified tuberculosis**

137.1 **Late effects of central nervous system tuberculosis**

137.2 **Late effects of genitourinary tuberculosis**

137.3 **Late effects of tuberculosis of bones and joints**

137.4 **Late effects of tuberculosis of other specified organs**

138 **Late effects of acute poliomyelitis**

> Note: This category is to be used to indicate conditions classifiable to 045 as the cause of late effects, which are themselves classified elsewhere. The "late effects" include conditions specified as such, or as sequelae, or as due to old or inactive poliomyelitis, without evidence of active disease.
>
> **DEFINITION** Late effects of acute poliomyelitis refers to condition that appears after the acute phase of poliomyelitis has run its course.

139 **Late effects of other infectious and parasitic diseases**

> Note: This category is to be used to indicate conditions classifiable to categories 001-009, 020-041, 046-136 as the cause of late effects, which are themselves classified elsewhere. The "late effects" include conditions specified as such; they also include sequela of diseases classifiable to the above categories if there is evidence that the disease itself is no longer present.
>
> **DEFINITION** Late effects of other infectious and parasitic diseases refers to condition that appears after the acute phase of other infectious and/or parasitic diseases has run its course.

139.0 **Late effects of viral encephalitis**
Late effects of conditions classifiable to 049.8-049.9, 062-064

139.1 **Late effects of trachoma**
Late effects of conditions classifiable to 076

139.8 **Late effects of other and unspecified infectious and parasitic diseases**

This page intentionally left blank.

● Code new
to 2012 edition

▲ Revision of
existing code

④ ⑤ Fourth or fifth
digit required

Chapter 2: Neoplasms (140-239)

GENERAL GUIDELINES

Chapter 2 of the ICD-9-CM contains the codes for most benign and all malignant neoplasms. Certain benign neoplasms, such as prostatic adenomas, may be found in the specific body system chapters. To properly code a neoplasm it is necessary to determine from the record if the neoplasm is benign, in-situ, malignant, or of uncertain histologic behavior. If malignant, any secondary (metastatic) sites should also be determined.

The neoplasm table in the Alphabetic Index should be referenced first. However, if the histological term is documented, that term should be referenced first, rather than going immediately to the Neoplasm Table, in order to determine which column in the Neoplasm Table is appropriate. For example, if the documentation indicates "adenoma," refer to the term in the Alphabetic Index to review the entries under this term and the instructional note to "see also neoplasm, by site, benign." The table provides the proper code based on the type of neoplasm and the site. It is important to select the proper column in the table that corresponds to the type of neoplasm. The tabular should then be referenced to verify that the correct code has been selected from the table and that a more specific site code does not exist.

See Chapter 18 "History (of)" for information regarding V codes for genetic susceptibility to cancer.

DEFINITIONS AND CODING ALERTS

This chapter includes definitions of selected key words, terms and phrases and coding alerts for adding points to the clinical domain, references to coding late effects where appropriate, and references to personal history V-codes in situations where the acute or chronic condition is no longer active. An example from this chapter is as follows:

⑤ **200** **Lymphosarcoma and reticulosarcoma and other specified malignant tumors of lymphatic tissue**

> **DEFINITION** Lymphosarcoma is a type of cancer that originates in lymphocytes of the immune system. The diseases often originates in lymph nodes, presenting as an enlargement of the node (a tumor). A reticulosarcoma is a malignant lymphoma, histiocytic or undifferentiated.
>
> **ALERT!** For personal history of other lymphatic and hematopoietic neoplasms see V10.7

MULTIPLE CODING FOR A SINGLE CONDITION

In addition to the etiology or manifestation convention that requires two codes to fully describe a single condition that affects multiple body systems, there are other single conditions that also require more than one code. "Use additional code" notes are found in the tabular at codes that are not part of an etiology or manifestation pair where a secondary code is useful to fully describe a condition. The sequencing rule is the same as the etiology or manifestation pair - , "use additional code" indicates that a secondary code should be added.

"Code first" notes are also under certain codes that are not specifically manifestation codes but may be due to an underlying cause. When a "code first" note is present and an underlying condition is present the underlying condition should be sequenced first.

"Code, if applicable, any causal condition first", notes indicate that this code may be assigned as a principal diagnosis when the causal condition is unknown or not applicable. If a causal condition is known, then the code for that condition should be sequenced as the principal or first-listed diagnosis. Multiple codes may be needed for late effects, complication codes and obstetric codes to more fully describe a condition. See the specific guidelines for these conditions for further instruction.

COMBINATION CODE

A combination code is a single code used to classify: two diagnoses, or a diagnosis with an associated secondary process (manifestation) A diagnosis with an associated complication Combination codes are identified by referring to subterm entries in the Alphabetic Index and by reading the inclusion and exclusion notes in the Tabular List.

Assign only the combination code when that code fully identifies the diagnostic conditions involved or when the Alphabetic Index so directs. Multiple coding should not be used when the classification provides a combination code that clearly identifies all of the elements documented in the diagnosis. When the combination code lacks necessary specificity in describing the manifestation or complication, an additional code should be used as a secondary code.

CODING LATE EFFECTS

A late effect is the residual effect (condition produced) after the acute phase of an illness or injury has terminated. There is no time limit on when a late effect code can be used. The residual may be apparent early, such as in cerebrovascular accident cases, or it may occur months or years later, such as that due to a previous injury. Coding of late effects generally requires two codes sequenced in the following order: The condition or nature of the late effect is sequenced first. The late effect code is sequenced second.

An exception to the above guidelines are those instances where the code for late effect is followed by a manifestation code identified in the Tabular List and title, or the late effect code has been expanded (at the fourth and fifth-digit levels) to include the manifestation(s). The code for the acute phase of an illness or injury that led to the late effect is never used with a code for the late effect.

TREATMENT DIRECTED AT THE MALIGNANCY

If the treatment is directed at the malignancy, designate the malignancy as the principal diagnosis.

The only exception to this guideline is if a patient admission or encounter is solely for the administration of chemotherapy, immunotherapy or radiation therapy, assign the appropriate V58.x code as the first-listed or principal diagnosis, and the diagnosis or problem for which the service is being performed as a secondary diagnosis.

TREATMENT OF SECONDARY SITE

When a patient is admitted because of a primary neoplasm with metastasis and treatment is directed toward the secondary site only, the secondary neoplasm is designated as the principal diagnosis even though the primary malignancy is still present.

CODING AND SEQUENCING OF COMPLICATIONS

Coding and sequencing of complications associated with the malignancies or with the therapy thereof are subject to the following guidelines:

Anemia associated with malignancy

When admission or encounter is for management of an anemia associated with the malignancy, and the treatment is only for anemia, the appropriate anemia code (such as code 285.22, Anemia in neoplastic disease) is designated as the principal diagnosis and is followed by the appropriate code(s) for the malignancy.

Code 285.22 may also be used as a secondary code if the patient suffers from anemia and is being treated for the malignancy.

Anemia associated with chemotherapy, immunotherapy and radiation therapy

When the admission or encounter is for management of an anemia associated with chemotherapy, immunotherapy or radiotherapy and the only treatment is for the anemia, the anemia is sequenced first followed by code E933.1. The appropriate neoplasm code should be assigned as an additional code.

Management of dehydration due to the malignancy

When the admission or encounter is for management of dehydration due to the malignancy or the therapy, or a combination of both, and only the dehydration is being treated (intravenous rehydration), the dehydration is sequenced first, followed by the code(s) for the malignancy.

Treatment of a complication resulting from a surgical procedure

When the admission or encounter is for treatment of a complication resulting from a surgical procedure, designate the complication as the principal or first-listed diagnosis if treatment is directed at resolving the complication.

Primary malignancy previously excised

When a primary malignancy has been previously excised or eradicated from its site and there is no further treatment directed to that site and there is no evidence of any existing primary malignancy, a code from category V10, Personal history of malignant neoplasm, should be used to indicate the former site of the malignancy. Any mention of extension, invasion, or metastasis to another site is coded as a secondary malignant neoplasm to that site. The secondary site may be the principal or first-listed with the V10 code used as a secondary code.

ADMISSIONS OR ENCOUNTERS INVOLVING CHEMOTHERAPY, IMMUNOTHERAPY AND RADIATION THERAPY

A. Episode of care involves surgical removal of neoplasm

When an episode of care involves the surgical removal of a neoplasm, primary or secondary site, followed by adjunct chemotherapy or radiation treatment during the same episode of care, the neoplasm code should be assigned as principal or first-listed diagnosis, using codes in the 140-198 series or where appropriate in the 200-203 series.

B. Patient admission or encounter solely for administration of chemotherapy, immunotherapy and radiation therapy

If a patient admission or encounter is solely for the administration of chemotherapy, immunotherapy or radiation therapy assign code V58.0, Encounter for radiation therapy, or V58.11, Encounter for antineoplastic chemotherapy, or V58.12, Encounter for antineoplastic immunotherapy as the first-listed or principal diagnosis. If a patient receives more than one of these therapies during the same admission more than one of these codes may be assigned, in any sequence.

The malignancy for which the therapy is being administered should be assigned as a secondary diagnosis.

C. Patient admitted for radiotherapy or chemotherapy and immunotherapy and develops complications

When a patient is admitted for the purpose of radiotherapy, immunotherapy or chemotherapy and develops complications such as uncontrolled nausea and vomiting or dehydration, the principal or first-listed diagnosis is V58.0, Encounter for radiotherapy, or V58.11, Encounter for antineoplastic chemotherapy, or V58.12, Encounter for antineoplastic immunotherapy followed by any codes for the complications.

ADMISSION OR ENCOUNTER TO DETERMINE EXTENT OF MALIGNANCY

When the reason for admission or encounter is to determine the extent of the malignancy, or for a procedure such as paracentesis or thoracentesis, the primary malignancy or appropriate metastatic site is designated as the principal or first-listed diagnosis, even though chemotherapy or radiotherapy is administered.

SYMPTOMS, SIGNS, AND ILL-DEFINED CONDITIONS LISTED IN CHAPTER 16 ASSOCIATED WITH NEOPLASMS

Symptoms, signs, and ill-defined conditions listed in Chapter 16 characteristic of, or associated with, an existing primary or secondary site malignancy cannot be used to replace the malignancy as principal or first-listed diagnosis, regardless of the number of admissions or encounters for treatment and care of the neoplasm.

See Chapter 18, "Prophylactic organ removal" for information regarding prophylactic organ removal..

ADMISSION OR ENCOUNTER FOR PAIN CONTROL OR MANAGEMENT

A malignant neoplasm of a transplanted organ should be coded as a transplant complication. Assign first the appropriate code from subcategory 996.8, Complications of transplanted organ, followed by code 199.2, Malignant neoplasm associated with transplanted organ. Use an additional code for the specific malignancy.

This page intentionally left blank.

● Code new
to 2012 edition

▲ Revision of
existing code

④ ⑤ Fourth or fifth
digit required

2. NEOPLASMS (140-239)

Notes:

1. Content
This chapter contains the following broad groups:

140-195	**Malignant neoplasms, stated or presumed to be primary, of specified sites, except of lymphatic and hematopoietic tissue**
196-198	**Malignant neoplasms, stated or presumed to be secondary, of specified sites**
199	**Malignant neoplasms, without specification of site**
200-208	**Malignant neoplasms, stated or presumed to be primary, of lymphatic and hematopoietic tissue**
209	**Neuroendocrine tumors**
210-229	**Benign neoplasms**
230-234	**Carcinoma in situ**
235-238	**Neoplasms of uncertain behavior**
239	**Neoplasms of unspecified nature**

2. Functional activity
All neoplasms are classified in this chapter, whether or not functionally active. An additional code from Chapter 3 may be used, if desired, to identify such functional activity associated with any neoplasm, e.g.:

> catecholamine-producing malignant pheochromocytoma of adrenal:
>> code 194.0, additional code 255.6
> basophil adenoma of pituitary with Cushing's syndrome:
>> code 227.3, additional code 255.0

3. Morphology [Histology]
For those wishing to identify the histological type of neoplasms, a comprehensive coded nomenclature, which comprises the morphology rubrics of the ICD-Oncology, is given in Appendix A.

4. Malignant neoplasms overlapping site boundaries
Categories 140-195 are for the classification of primary malignant neoplasms according to their point of origin. A malignant neoplasm that overlaps two or more subcategories within a three-digit rubric and whose point of origin cannot be determined should be classified to the subcategory .8 "Other." For example, "carcinoma involving tip and ventral surface of tongue" should be assigned to 141.8. On the other hand, "carcinoma of tip of tongue, extending to involve the ventral surface" should be coded to 141.2, as the point of origin, the tip, is known. Three subcategories (149.8, 159.8, 165.8) have been provided for malignant neoplasms that overlap the boundaries of three-digit rubrics within certain systems. Overlapping malignant neoplasms that cannot be classified as indicated above should be assigned to the appropriate subdivision of category 195 (Malignant neoplasm of other and ill-defined sites).

MALIGNANT NEOPLASM OF LIP, ORAL CAVITY, AND PHARYNX (140-149)

> *Excludes:* carcinoma in situ (230.0)

140 Malignant neoplasm of lip

> *Excludes:* malignant melanoma of skin of lip (172.0)
>
> malignant neoplasm of skin of lip (173.00-173.09)

> **DEFINITION** Malignant neoplasm refers to a tumor that tends to grow, invade, and metastasize. The tumor usually has an irregular shape and is composed of poorly differentiated cells. If untreated, it may result in death.

> **ALERT!** For personal history of malignant neoplasm see V10

140.0 Upper lip, vermilion border
Upper lip:
NOS
external
lipstick area

140.1 Lower lip, vermilion border
Lower lip:
NOS
external
lipstick area

140.3 Upper lip, inner aspect
Upper lip: Upper lip:
buccal aspect   mucosa
frenulum   oral aspect

140.4 Lower lip, inner aspect
Lower lip: Lower lip:
buccal aspect   mucosa
frenulum   oral aspect

Add 4th or 5th digit	Nonspecific code	Unspecified code	Manifestation code

140.5 Lip, unspecified, inner aspect
Lip, not specified whether upper or lower:
buccal aspect   frenulum
mucosa   oral aspect

140.6 Commissure of lip
Labial commissure

140.8 Other sites of lip
Malignant neoplasm of contiguous or overlapping sites of lip whose point of origin cannot be determined

140.9 Lip, unspecified, vermilion border
Lip, not specified as upper or lower:
NOS
external
lipstick area

141 Malignant neoplasm of tongue
ALERT! For personal history of malignant neoplasm of tongue see V10.01

141.0 Base of tongue
Dorsal surface of base of tongue
Fixed part of tongue NOS

141.1 Dorsal surface of tongue
Anterior two-thirds of tongue, dorsal surface
Dorsal tongue NOS
Midline of tongue

Excludes: *dorsal surface of base of tongue (141.0)*

141.2 Tip and lateral border of tongue

141.3 Ventral surface of tongue
Anterior two-thirds of tongue, ventral surface
Frenulum linguae

141.4 Anterior two-thirds of tongue, part unspecified
Mobile part of tongue NOS

141.5 Junctional zone
Border of tongue at junction of fixed and mobile parts at insertion of anterior tonsillar pillar

141.6 Lingual tonsil

141.8 Other sites of tongue
Malignant neoplasm of contiguous or overlapping sites of tongue whose point of origin cannot be determined

141.9 Tongue, unspecified
Tongue NOS

142 Malignant neoplasm of major salivary glands
Includes: salivary ducts

Excludes: *malignant neoplasm of minor salivary glands:*
    NOS (145.9)
    buccal mucosa (145.0)
    soft palate (145.3)
    tongue (141.0-141.9)
    tonsil, palatine (146.0)

142.0 Parotid gland

142.1 Submandibular gland
Submaxillary gland

142.2 Sublingual gland

142.8 Other major salivary glands
Malignant neoplasm of contiguous or overlapping sites of salivary glands and ducts whose point of origin cannot be determined

142.9 Salivary gland, unspecified
Salivary gland (major) NOS

143 Malignant neoplasm of gum
Includes: alveolar (ridge) mucosa
         gingiva (alveolar) (marginal)
         interdental papillae

Excludes: *malignant odontogenic neoplasms (170.0-170.1)*

● Code new to 2012 edition   ▲ Revision of existing code   ④ ⑤ Fourth or fifth digit required

143.0 Upper gum

143.1 Lower gum

143.8 Other sites of gum
Malignant neoplasm of contiguous or overlapping sites of gum whose point of origin cannot be determined

143.9 Gum, unspecified

144 Malignant neoplasm of floor of mouth

144.0 Anterior portion
Anterior to the premolar-canine junction

144.1 Lateral portion

144.8 Other sites of floor of mouth
Malignant neoplasm of contiguous or overlapping sites of floor of mouth whose point of origin cannot be determined

144.9 Floor of mouth, part unspecified

145 Malignant neoplasm of other and unspecified parts of mouth
Excludes: mucosa of lips (140.0-140.9)

145.0 Cheek mucosa
Buccal mucosa   Cheek, inner aspect

145.1 Vestibule of mouth
Buccal sulcus (upper) (lower)
Labial sulcus (upper) (lower)

145.2 Hard palate

145.3 Soft palate
Excludes: nasopharyngeal [posterior] [superior] surface of soft palate (147.3)

145.4 Uvula

145.5 Palate, unspecified
Junction of hard and soft palate
Roof of mouth

145.6 Retromolar area

145.8 Other specified parts of mouth
Malignant neoplasm of contiguous or overlapping sites of mouth whose point of origin cannot be determined

145.9 Mouth, unspecified
Buccal cavity NOS
Minor salivary gland, unspecified site
Oral cavity NOS

146 Malignant neoplasm of oropharynx

146.0 Tonsil
Tonsil:
NOS
faucial
palatine
Excludes: lingual tonsil (141.6)
pharyngeal tonsil (147.1)

146.1 Tonsillar fossa

146.2 Tonsillar pillars (anterior) (posterior)
Faucial pillar   Palatoglossal arch
Glossopalatine fold   Palatopharyngeal arch

146.3 Vallecula
Anterior and medial surface of the pharyngoepiglottic fold

146.4 Anterior aspect of epiglottis
Epiglottis, free border [margin]
Glossoepiglottic fold(s)
Excludes: epiglottis:
NOS (161.1)
suprahyoid portion (161.1)

146.5 Junctional region
Junction of the free margin of the epiglottis, the aryepiglottic fold, and the pharyngoepiglottic fold

	Add 4th or 5th digit		Nonspecific code		Unspecified code		Manifestation code	213

146.6 Lateral wall of oropharynx

146.7 Posterior wall of oropharynx

146.8 Other specified sites of oropharynx
Branchial cleft
Malignant neoplasm of contiguous or overlapping sites of oropharynx whose point of origin cannot be determined

146.9 Oropharynx, unspecified

147 Malignant neoplasm of nasopharynx

147.0 Superior wall
Roof of nasopharynx

147.1 Posterior wall
Adenoid
Pharyngeal tonsil

147.2 Lateral wall
Fossa of Rosenmüller
Opening of auditory tube
Pharyngeal recess

147.3 Anterior wall
Floor of nasopharynx
Nasopharyngeal [posterior] [superior] surface of soft palate
Posterior margin of nasal septum and choanae

147.8 Other specified sites of nasopharynx
Malignant neoplasm of contiguous or overlapping sites of nasopharynx whose point of origin cannot be determined

147.9 Nasopharynx, unspecified
Nasopharyngeal wall NOS

148 Malignant neoplasm of hypopharynx

148.0 Postcricoid region

148.1 Pyriform sinus
Pyriform fossa

148.2 Aryepiglottic fold, hypopharyngeal aspect
Aryepiglottic fold or interarytenoid fold:
NOS
marginal zone

[Excludes:] *aryepiglottic fold or interarytenoid fold, laryngeal aspect (161.1)*

148.3 Posterior hypopharyngeal wall

148.8 Other specified sites of hypopharynx
Malignant neoplasm of contiguous or overlapping sites of hypopharynx whose point of origin cannot be determined

148.9 Hypopharynx, unspecified
Hypopharyngeal wall NOS
Hypopharynx NOS

149 Malignant neoplasm of other and ill-defined sites within the lip, oral cavity, and pharynx

[ALERT!] For personal history of malignant neoplasm of other sites see V10.8

149.0 Pharynx, unspecified

149.1 Waldeyer's ring

149.8 Other
Malignant neoplasms of lip, oral cavity, and pharynx whose point of origin cannot be assigned to any one of the categories 140-148

[Excludes:] *"book leaf" neoplasm [ventral surface of tongue and floor of mouth] (145.8)*

149.9 Ill-defined

MALIGNANT NEOPLASM OF DIGESTIVE ORGANS AND PERITONEUM (150-159)

[Excludes:] *carcinoma in situ (230.1-230.9)*

[ALERT!] For personal history of malignant neoplasm of gastrointestinal tract see V10.0

150 Malignant neoplasm of esophagus

[ALERT!] For personal history of malignant neoplasm of esophagus see V10.03

150.0 Cervical esophagus

150.1 Thoracic esophagus

150.2 Abdominal esophagus

[Excludes:] *adenocarcinoma (151.0)*
cardio-esophageal junction (151.0)

● Code new to 2012 edition ▲ Revision of existing code ④ ⑤ Fourth or fifth digit required

150.3 Upper third of esophagus
Proximal third of esophagus

150.4 Middle third of esophagus

150.5 Lower third of esophagus
Distal third of esophagus

Excludes: *adenocarcinoma (151.0)*
cardio-esophageal junction (151.0)

150.8 Other specified part
Malignant neoplasm of contiguous or overlapping sites of esophagus whose point of origin cannot be determined

150.9 Esophagus, unspecified

151 Malignant neoplasm of stomach

Excludes: *benign carcinoid tumor of stomach (209.63)*
malignant carcinoid tumor of stomach (209.23)

ALERT! For personal history of malignant neoplasm of stomach see V10.04

151.0 Cardia
Cardiac orifice   Cardio-esophageal junction

Excludes: *squamous cell carcinoma (150.2, 150.5)*

151.1 Pylorus
Prepylorus   Pyloric canal

151.2 Pyloric antrum
Antrum of stomach NOS

151.3 Fundus of stomach

151.4 Body of stomach

151.5 Lesser curvature, unspecified
Lesser curvature, not classifiable to 151.1-151.4

151.6 Greater curvature, unspecified
Greater curvature, not classifiable to 151.0-151.4

151.8 Other specified sites of stomach
Anterior wall, not classifiable to 151.0-151.4
Posterior wall, not classifiable to 151.0-151.4
Malignant neoplasm of contiguous or overlapping sites of stomach whose point of origin cannot be determined

151.9 Stomach, unspecified
Carcinoma ventriculi   Gastric cancer

152 Malignant neoplasm of small intestine, including duodenum

Excludes: *benign carcinoid tumor of small intestine and duodenum (209.40-209.43)*
malignant carcinoid tumor of small intestine and duodenum (209.00-209.03)

152.0 Duodenum

152.1 Jejunum

152.2 Ileum

Excludes: *ileocecal valve (153.4)*

152.3 Meckel's diverticulum

152.8 Other specified sites of small intestine
Duodenojejunal junction
Malignant neoplasm of contiguous or overlapping sites of small intestine whose point of origin cannot be determined

152.9 Small intestine, unspecified

153 Malignant neoplasm of colon

Excludes: *benign carcinoid tumor of colon (209.50-209.56)*
malignant carcinoid tumor of colon (209.10-209.16)

ALERT! For personal history of colonic polyps see V12.72

153.0 Hepatic flexure

153.1 Transverse colon

153.2 Descending colon
Left colon

153.3 Sigmoid colon
Sigmoid (flexure)

Excludes: rectosigmoid junction (154.0)

153.4 Cecum
Ileocecal valve

153.5 Appendix

153.6 Ascending colon
Right colon

153.7 Splenic flexure

153.8 Other specified sites of large intestine
Malignant neoplasm of contiguous or overlapping sites of colon whose point of origin cannot be determined

Excludes: ileocecal valve (153.4)
rectosigmoid junction (154.0)

153.9 Colon, unspecified
Large intestine NOS

154 Malignant neoplasm of rectum, rectosigmoid junction, and anus

Excludes: benign carcinoid tumor of rectum (209.57)
malignant carcinoid tumor of rectum (209.17)

ALERT! For personal history of malignant neoplasm of rectum rectosigmoid junction and anus see V10.06

154.0 Rectosigmoid junction
Colon with rectum   Rectosigmoid (colon)

154.1 Rectum
Rectal ampulla

154.2 Anal canal
Anal sphincter

Excludes: malignant melanoma of skin of anus (172.5)
malignant neoplasm of skin of anus (173.50-173.59)

154.3 Anus, unspecified

Excludes: malignant melanoma of
anus:
margin (172.5)
skin (172.5)
perianal skin (172.5)
malignant neoplasm of
anus:
margin (173.50-173.59)
skin (173.50-173.59)
perianal skin (173.50-173.59)

154.8 Other
Anorectum
Cloacogenic zone
Malignant neoplasm of contiguous or overlapping sites of rectum, rectosigmoid junction, and anus whose point of origin cannot be determined

155 Malignant neoplasm of liver and intrahepatic bile ducts

ALERT! For personal history of malignant neoplasm of liver see V10.07

155.0 Liver, primary
Carcinoma:
liver, specified as primary
hepatocellular
liver cell
Hepatoblastoma

155.1 Intrahepatic bile ducts
Canaliculi biliferi   Intrahepatic:
Interlobular: biliary passages
bile ducts   canaliculi
biliary canals   gall duct

Excludes: hepatic duct (156.1)

155.2 Liver, not specified as primary or secondary

● Code new   ▲ Revision of   ④ ⑤ Fourth or fifth
to 2012 edition   existing code   digit required

156 Malignant neoplasm of gallbladder and extrahepatic bile ducts

156.0 **Gallbladder**

156.1 **Extrahepatic bile ducts**
Biliary duct or passage NOS   Cystic duct
Common bile duct   Hepatic duct
Sphincter of Oddi

156.2 **Ampulla of Vater**

156.8 **Other specified sites of gallbladder and extrahepatic bile ducts**
Malignant neoplasm of contiguous or overlapping sites of gallbladder and extrahepatic
bile ducts whose point of origin cannot be determined

156.9 **Biliary tract, part unspecified**
Malignant neoplasm involving both intrahepatic and extrahepatic bile ducts

157 Malignant neoplasm of pancreas

157.0 **Head of pancreas**

157.1 **Body of pancreas**

157.2 **Tail of pancreas**

157.3 **Pancreatic duct**
Duct of:
Santorini
Wirsung

157.4 **Islets of Langerhans**
Islets of Langerhans, any part of pancreas
Use additional code, if desired, to identify any functional activity

157.8 **Other specified sites of pancreas**
Ectopic pancreatic tissue
Malignant neoplasm of contiguous or overlapping sites of pancreas whose point of
origin cannot be determined

157.9 **Pancreas, part unspecified**

158 Malignant neoplasm of retroperitoneum and peritoneum

158.0 **Retroperitoneum**
Periadrenal tissue   Perirenal tissue
Perinephric tissue   Retrocecal tissue

158.8 **Specified parts of peritoneum**
Cul-de-sac (of Douglas)
Mesentery
Mesocolon
Omentum
Peritoneum:
parietal
pelvic
Rectouterine pouch
Malignant neoplasm of contiguous or overlapping sites of retroperitoneum and
peritoneum whose point of origin cannot be determined

158.9 **Peritoneum, unspecified**

159 Malignant neoplasm of other and ill-defined sites within the digestive organs and
peritoneum

ALERT! For personal history of malignant neoplasm of other sites in gastrointestinal tract see
V10.09

ALERT! For personal history of malignant neoplasm of other sites see V10.8

ALERT! For personal history of malignant neoplasm of unspecified site in gastrointestinal tract
see V10.00

159.0 **Intestinal tract, part unspecified**
Intestine NOS

159.1 **Spleen, not elsewhere classified**
Angiosarcoma of spleen
Fibrosarcoma of spleen

Excludes: *Hodgkin's disease (201.0-201.9)*
lymphosarcoma (200.1)
reticulosarcoma (200.0)

Add 4th or   Nonspecific   Unspecified   Manifestation
5th digit   code   code   code

159.8 Other sites of digestive system and intra-abdominal organs
> Malignant neoplasm of digestive organs and peritoneum whose point of origin cannot
> be assigned to any one of the categories 150-158

> Excludes: *anus and rectum (154.8)*
> > *cardio-esophageal junction (151.0)*
> > *colon and rectum ORANGE (154.0)*

159.9 Ill-defined
> Alimentary canal or tract NOS
> Gastrointestinal tract NOS

> Excludes: *abdominal NOS (195.2)*
> > *intra-abdominal NOS (195.2)*

MALIGNANT NEOPLASM OF RESPIRATORY AND INTRATHORACIC ORGANS (160-165)

> Excludes: *carcinoma in situ (231.0-231.9)*

160 Malignant neoplasm of nasal cavities, middle ear, and accessory sinuses
> ALERT! For personal history of malignant neoplasm of nasal cavities middle ear and accessory
> sinuses see V10.22

160.0 Nasal cavities

Cartilage of nose	Septum of nose
Conchae, nasal	Vestibule of nose
Internal nose	

> Excludes: *nasal bone (170.0)*
> > *nose NOS (195.0)*
> > *olfactory bulb (192.0)*
> > *posterior margin of septum and choanae (147.3)*
> > *malignant melanoma of skin of nose (172.3)*
> > *malignant neoplasm of skin of nose (173.30-173.39)*
> > *turbinates (170.0)*

160.1 Auditory tube, middle ear, and mastoid air cells

Antrum tympanicum	Tympanic cavity
Eustachian tube	

> Excludes: *bone of ear (meatus) (170.0)*
> > *cartilage of ear (171.0)*
> > *malignant melanoma of:*
> > > *auditory canal (external) (172.2)*
> > > *ear (external) (skin) (172.2)*
> > *malignant neoplasm of:*
> > > *auditory canal (external) (173.20-173.29)*
> > > *ear (external) (skin) (173.20-173.29)*

160.2 Maxillary sinus
> Antrum (Highmore) (maxillary)

160.3 Ethmoidal sinus

160.4 Frontal sinus

160.5 Sphenoidal sinus

160.8 Other
> Malignant neoplasm of contiguous or overlapping sites of nasal cavities, middle ear, and
> accessory sinuses whose point of origin cannot be determined

160.9 Accessory sinus, unspecified

161 Malignant neoplasm of larynx
> ALERT! For personal history of malignant neoplasm of larynx see V10.21

161.0 Glottis

Intrinsic larynx	True vocal cord
Laryngeal commissure	Vocal cord NOS
(anterior) (posterior)	

● Code new
to 2012 edition
▲ Revision of
existing code
④ ⑤ Fourth or fifth
digit required

161.1 Supraglottis
  Aryepiglottic fold or interarytenoid fold, laryngeal aspect
  Epiglottis (suprahyoid portion) NOS
  Extrinsic larynx
  False vocal cords
  Posterior (laryngeal) surface of epiglottis
  Ventricular bands

  Excludes: *anterior aspect of epiglottis (146.4)*
  aryepiglottic fold or interarytenoid fold:
    NOS (148.2)
    hypopharyngeal aspect (148.2)
    marginal zone (148.2)

161.2 Subglottis

161.3 Laryngeal cartilages
  Cartilage: Cartilage:
    arytenoid   cuneiform
    cricoid   thyroid

161.8 Other specified sites of larynx
  Malignant neoplasm of contiguous or overlapping sites of larynx whose point of origin cannot be determined

161.9 Larynx, unspecified

162 Malignant neoplasm of trachea, bronchus, and lung

  Excludes: *benign carcinoid tumor of bronchus (209.61)*
  malignant carcinoid tumor of bronchus (209.21)

  ALERT! For personal history of malignant neoplasm of bronchus and lung see V10.11
  ALERT! For personal history of malignant neoplasm of trachea see V10.12

162.0 Trachea
  Cartilage of trachea
  Mucosa of trachea

162.2 Main bronchus
  Carina   Hilus of lung

162.3 Upper lobe, bronchus or lung

162.4 Middle lobe, bronchus or lung

162.5 Lower lobe, bronchus or lung

162.8 Other parts of bronchus or lung
  Malignant neoplasm of contiguous or overlapping sites of bronchus or lung whose point of origin cannot be determined

162.9 Bronchus and lung, unspecified

163 Malignant neoplasm of pleura

163.0 Parietal pleura

163.1 Visceral pleura

163.8 Other specified sites of pleura
  Malignant neoplasm of contiguous or overlapping sites of pleura whose point of origin cannot be determined

163.9 Pleura, unspecified

164 Malignant neoplasm of thymus, heart, and mediastinum

164.0 Thymus

  Excludes: *benign carcinoid tumor of thymus (209.62)*
  malignant carcinoid tumor of thymus (209.22)

164.1 Heart
  Endocardium   Myocardium
  Epicardium   Pericardium

  Excludes: *great vessels (171.4)*

164.2 Anterior mediastinum

164.3 Posterior mediastinum

164.8 Other
  Malignant neoplasm of contiguous or overlapping sites of thymus, heart, and mediastinum whose point of origin cannot be determined

164.9 Mediastinum, part unspecified

	Add 4th or 5th digit		Nonspecific code		Unspecified code		Manifestation code

165 **Malignant neoplasm of other and ill-defined sites within the respiratory system and intrathoracic organs**

ALERT! For personal history of malignant neoplasm of other respiratory and intrathoracic organs see V10.29

ALERT! For personal history of malignant neoplasm of other sites see V10.8

ALERT! For personal history of malignant neoplasm of unspecified respiratory organ see V10.20

165.0 **Upper respiratory trace, part unspecified**

165.8 **Other**

Malignant neoplasm of respiratory and intrathoracic organs whose point of origin cannot be assigned to any one of the categories 160-164

ALERT! For personal history of malignant neoplasm of other respiratory and intrathoracic organs see V10.2

165.9 **Ill-defined sites within the respiratory system**

Respiratory tract NOS

Excludes: *intrathoracic NOS (195.1)*
thoracic NOS (195.1)

MALIGNANT NEOPLASM OF BONE, CONNECTIVE TISSUE, SKIN, AND BREAST (170-176)

Excludes: *carcinoma in situ:*
breast (233.0)
skin (232.0-232.9)

170 **Malignant neoplasm of bone and articular cartilage**

Includes: cartilage (articular) (joint)
periosteum

Excludes: *bone marrow NOS (202.9)*

cartilage:
ear (171.0)
eyelid (171.0)
larynx (161.3)
nose (160.0)
synovia (171.0-171.9)

ALERT! For personal history of malignant neoplasm of bone see V10.81

170.0 **Bones of skull and face, except mandible**

Bone:	Bone:
ethmoid	sphenoid
frontal	temporal
malar	zygomatic
nasal	Maxilla (superior)
occipital	Turbinate
orbital	Upper jaw bone
parietal	Vomer

Excludes: *carcinoma, any type except intraosseous or odontogenic:*
maxilla, maxillary (sinus) (160.2)
upper jaw bone (143.0)
jaw bone (lower) (170.1)

170.1 **Mandible**

Inferior maxilla   Lower jaw bone
Jaw bone NOS

Excludes: *carcinoma, any type except intraosseous or odontogenic:*
jaw bone NOS (143.9)
lower (143.1)
upper jaw bone (170.0)

170.2 **Vertebral column, excluding sacrum and coccyx**

Spinal column   Vertebra
Spine

Excludes: *sacrum and coccyx (170.6)*

170.3 **Ribs, sternum, and clavicle**

Costal cartilage   Xiphoid process
Costovertebral joint

● Code new
to 2012 edition

▲ Revision of
existing code

④ ⑤ Fourth or fifth
digit required

170.4 Scapula and long bones of upper limb

Acromion	Radius
Bones NOS of upper limb	Ulna
Humerus	

170.5 Short bones of upper limb

Carpal	Scaphoid (of hand)
Cuneiform, wrist	Semilunar or lunate
Metacarpal	Trapezium
Navicular, of hand	Trapezoid
Phalanges of hand	Unciform
Pisiform	

170.6 Pelvic bones, sacrum, and coccyx

Coccygeal vertebra	Pubic bone
Ilium	Sacral vertebra
Ischium	

170.7 Long bones of lower limb

Bones NOS of lower limb	Fibula
Femur	Tibia

170.8 Short bones of lower limb

Astragalus [talus]	Navicular (of ankle)
Calcaneus	Patella
Cuboid	Phalanges of foot
Cuneiform, ankle	Tarsal
Metatarsal	

170.9 Bone and articular cartilage, site unspecified

171 Malignant neoplasm of connective and other soft tissue

Includes: blood vessel
bursa
fascia
fat
ligament, except uterine
muscle
peripheral, sympathetic, and parasympathetic nerves and ganglia
synovia
tendon (sheath)

Excludes: *cartilage (of):*
articular (170.0-170.9)
larynx (161.3)
nose (160.0)
connective tissue:
breast (174.0-175.9)
internal organs—code to malignant neoplasm of the site [e.g., leiomyosarcoma
of stomach, 151.9]
heart (164.1)
uterine ligament (183.4)

171.0 Head, face, and neck

Cartilage of:
ear
eyelid

171.2 Upper limb, including shoulder

Arm	Forearm
Finger	Hand

171.3 Lower limb, including hip

Foot	Thigh
Leg	Toe
Popliteal space	

171.4 Thorax

Axilla	Great vessels
Diaphragm	

Excludes: *heart (164.1)*
mediastinum (164.2-164.9)
thymus (164.0)

■ Add 4th or 5th digit	■ Nonspecific code	Unspecified code	■ Manifestation code

171.5 Abdomen
Abdominal wall
Hypochondrium

Excludes: peritoneum (158.8)
retroperitoneum (158.0)

171.6 Pelvis

Buttock   Inguinal region
Groin   Perineum

Excludes: pelvic peritoneum (158.8)
retroperitoneum (158.0)
uterine ligament, any (183.3-183.5)

171.7 Trunk, unspecified
Back NOS
Flank NOS

171.8 Other specified sites of connective and other soft tissue
Malignant neoplasm of contiguous or overlapping sites of connective tissue whose point
of origin cannot be determined

171.9 Connective and other soft tissue, site unspecified

172 Malignant melanoma of skin
Includes: melanocarcinoma
melanoma in situ of skin
melanoma (skin) NOS

Excludes: skin of genital organs (184.0-184.9, 187.1-187.9)

sites other than skin—code to malignant neoplasm of the site

ALERT! For personal history of malignant melanoma of skin see V10.82

172.0 Lip

Excludes: vermilion border of lip (140.0-140.1, 140.9)

172.1 Eyelid, including canthus

172.2 Ear and external auditory canal
Auricle (ear)
Auricular canal, external
External [acoustic] meatus
Pinna

172.3 Other and unspecified parts of face

Cheek (external)   Forehead
Chin   Nose, external
Eyebrow   Temple

172.4 Scalp and neck

172.5 Trunk, except scrotum

Axilla   Perianal skin
Breast   Perineum
Buttock   Umbilicus
Groin

Excludes: anal canal (154.2)
anus NOS (154.3)
scrotum (187.7)

172.6 Upper limb, including shoulder
Arm   Forearm
Finger   Hand

172.7 Lower limb, including hip
Ankle   Leg
Foot   Popliteal area
Heel   Thigh
Knee   Toe

172.8 Other specified sites of skin
Malignant melanoma of contiguous or overlapping sites of skin whose point of origin
cannot be determined

172.9 Melanoma of skin, site unspecified

● Code new   ▲ Revision of   ④ ⑤ Fourth or fifth
   to 2012 edition   existing code   digit required

▲ **173** **Other and unspecified malignant neoplasm of skin**
　　Includes: malignant neoplasm of:
　　　　　　sebaceous glands
　　　　　　sudoriferous, sudoriparous glands
　　　　　　sweat glands

　　Excludes: *Kaposi's sarcoma (176.0-176.9)*
　　　　　　malignant melanoma of skin (172.0-172.9)
　　　　　　Merkel cell carcinoma of skin (209.31-209.36)
　　　　　　skin of genital organs (184.0-184.9, 187.1-187.9)

　　ALERT! For personal history of other malignant neoplasm of skin see V10.83

▲ **173.0** **Other and unspecified malignant neoplasm of skin of lip**
　　Excludes: *vermilion border of lip (140.0-140.1, 140.9)*

　　● **173.00** Unspecified malignant neoplasm of skin of lip
　　● **173.01** Basal cell carcinoma of skin of lip
　　● **173.02** Squamous cell carcinoma of skin of lip
　　● **173.09** Other specified malignant neoplasm of skin of lip

▲ **173.1** **Other and unspecified malignant neoplasm of eyelid, including canthus**
　　Excludes: *cartilage of eyelid (171.0)*

　　● **173.10** Unspecified malignant neoplasm of eyelid, including canthus
　　● **173.11** Basal cell carcinoma of eyelid, including canthus
　　● **173.12** Squamous cell carcinoma of eyelid, including canthus
　　● **173.19** Other specified malignant neoplasm of eyelid, including canthus

▲ **173.2** **Other and unspecified malignant neoplasm of skin of ear and external auditory canal**
　　Auricle (ear)　　　　　　　External meatus
　　Auricular canal, external　　Pinna

　　Excludes: *cartilage of ear (171.0)*

　　● **173.20** Unspecified malignant neoplasm of skin of ear and external auditory canal
　　● **173.21** Basal cell carcinoma of skin of ear and external auditory canal
　　● **173.22** Squamous cell carcinoma of skin of ear and external auditory canal
　　● **173.29** Other specified malignant neoplasm of skin of ear and external auditory canal

▲ **173.3** **Other and unspecified malignant neoplasm of skin of other and unspecified parts of face**
　　Cheek, external　　　　　Forehead
　　Chin　　　　　　　　　Nose, external
　　Eyebrow　　　　　　　Temple

　　● **173.30** Unspecified malignant neoplasm of skin of other and unspecified parts of face
　　● **173.31** Basal cell carcinoma of skin of other and unspecified parts of face
　　● **173.32** Squamous cell carcinoma of skin of other and unspecified parts of face
　　● **173.39** Other specified malignant neoplasm of skin of other and unspecified parts of face

▲ **173.4** **Other and unspecified malignant neoplasm of scalp and skin of neck**
　　● **173.40** Unspecified malignant neoplasm of scalp and skin of neck
　　● **173.41** Basal cell carcinoma of scalp and skin of neck
　　● **173.42** Squamous cell carcinoma of scalp and skin of neck
　　● **173.49** Other specified malignant neoplasm of scalp and skin of neck

	Add 4th or 5th digit		Nonspecific code		Unspecified code		Manifestation code

▲ **173.5** **Other and unspecified malignant neoplasm of skin of trunk, except scrotum**

Axillary fold
Perianal skin
Skin of:
  abdominal wall
  anus
  back
  breast

Skin of:
  buttock
  chest wall
  groin
  perineum
Umbilicus

Excludes: *anal canal (154.2)*
     anus NOS (154.3)
     skin of scrotum (187.7)

● **173.50** **Unspecified malignant neoplasm of skin of trunk, except scrotum**

● **173.51** **Basal cell carcinoma of skin of trunk, except scrotum**

● **173.52** **Squamous cell carcinoma of skin of trunk, except scrotum**

● **173.59** **Other specified malignant neoplasm of skin of trunk, except scrotum**

▲ **173.6** **Other and unspecified malignant neoplasm of skin of upper limb, including shoulder**

Arm
Finger

Forearm
Hand

● **173.60** **Unspecified malignant neoplasm of skin of upper limb, including shoulder**

● **173.61** **Basal cell carcinoma of skin of upper limb, including shoulder**

● **173.62** **Squamous cell carcinoma of skin of upper limb, including shoulder**

● **173.69** **Other specified malignant neoplasm of skin of upper limb, including shoulder**

▲ **173.7** **Other and unspecified malignant neoplasm of skin of lower limb, including hip**

Ankle
Foot
Heel
Knee

Leg
Popliteal area
Thigh
Toe

● **173.70** **Unspecified malignant neoplasm of skin of lower limb, including hip**

● **173.71** **Basal cell carcinoma of skin of lower limb, including hip**

● **173.72** **Squamous cell carcinoma of skin of lower limb, including hip**

● **173.79** **Other specified malignant neoplasm of skin of lower limb, including hip**

▲ **173.8** **Other and unspecified malignant neoplasm of other specified sites of skin**

Malignant neoplasm of contiguous or overlapping sites of skin whose point of origin cannot be determined

● **173.80** **Unspecified malignant neoplasm of other specified sites of skin**

● **173.81** **Basal cell carcinoma of other specified sites of skin**

● **173.82** **Squamous cell carcinoma of other specified sites of skin**

● **173.89** **Other specified malignant neoplasm of other specified sites of skin**

▲ **173.9** **Other and unspecified malignant neoplasm of skin, site unspecified**

● **173.90** **Unspecified malignant neoplasm of skin, site unspecified**

Malignant neoplasm of skin, NOS

● **173.91** **Basal cell carcinoma of skin, site unspecified**

● **173.92** **Squamous cell carcinoma of skin, site unspecified**

● **173.99** **Other specified malignant neoplasm of skin, site unspecified**

174 **Malignant neoplasm of female breast**

Use additional code to identify estrogen receptor status (V86.0,V86.1)

Includes: breast (female)
         connective tissue
         soft parts
         Paget's disease of:
           breast
           nipple

Excludes: *malignant melanoma of skin of breast (172.5)*
     malignant neoplasm of skin of breast (173.50-173.59)

ALERT! For personal history of malignant neoplasm of breast see V10.3

174.0 **Nipple and areola**

174.1 **Central portion**

174.2 **Upper-inner quadrant**

● Code new
  to 2012 edition
     ▲ Revision of
      existing code
        ④ ⑤ Fourth or fifth
           digit required

174.3 **Lower-inner quadrant**

174.4 **Upper-outer quadrant**

174.5 **Lower-outer quadrant**

174.6 **Axillary tail**

174.8 **Other specified sites of female breast**
Ectopic sites
Inner breast
Lower breast
Midline of breast
Outer breast
Upper breast
Malignant neoplasm of contiguous or overlapping sites of breast whose point of origin cannot be determined

174.9 **Breast (female), unspecified**

175 **Malignant neoplasm of male breast**
Use additional code to identify estrogen receptor status (V86.0,V86.1)

Excludes: *malignant melanoma of skin of breast (172.5)*
malignant neoplasm of skin of breast (173.50-173.59)

175.0 **Nipple and areola**

175.9 **Other and unspecified sites of male breast**
Ectopic breast tissue, male

176 **Kaposi's sarcoma**

DEFINITION Kaposi's sarcoma is a form of skin cancer that can involve internal organs. It is most often found in patients with acquired immunodeficiency syndrome (AIDS), and can be fatal.

176.0 **Skin**

176.1 **Soft tissue**
Includes: Blood vessel
Connective tissue
Fascia
Ligament
Lymphatic(s) NEC
Muscle

Excludes: *lymph glands and nodes (176.5)*

176.2 **Palate**

176.3 **Gastrointestinal sites**

176.4 **Lung**

176.5 **Lymph nodes**

176.8 **Other specified sites**
Includes: Oral cavity NEC

176.9 **Unspecified**
Viscera NOS

MALIGNANT NEOPLASM OF GENITOURINARY ORGANS (179-189)

Excludes: *carcinoma in situ (233.1-233.9)*

ALERT! For personal history of malignant neoplasm of genital organs see V10.4

179 **Malignant neoplasm of uterus, part unspecified**

180 **Malignant neoplasm of cervix uteri**
Includes: invasive malignancy [carcinoma]

Excludes: *carcinoma in situ (233.1)*

ALERT! For personal history of malignant neoplasm of cervix uteri see V10.41

180.0 **Endocervix**
Cervical canal NOS   Endocervical gland
Endocervical canal

180.1 **Exocervix**

180.8 **Other specified sites of cervix**
Cervical stump
Squamocolumnar junction of cervix
Malignant neoplasm of contiguous or overlapping sites of cervix uteri whose point of origin cannot be determined

| | Add 4th or 5th digit | | Nonspecific code | | Unspecified code | | Manifestation code |

180.9 Cervix uteri, unspecified

181 Malignant neoplasm of placenta
>>Choriocarcinoma NOS
>>Chorioepithelioma NOS

>*Excludes:* *chorioadenoma (destruens) (236.1)*
>>*hydatidiform mole (630)*
>>>*malignant (236.1)*
>>*invasive mole (236.1)*
>>*male choriocarcinoma NOS (186.0-186.9)*

182 Malignant neoplasm of body of uterus
>*Excludes:* *carcinoma in situ (233.2)*

182.0 Corpus uteri, except isthmus
>>Cornu   Fundus
>>Endometrium   Myometrium

182.1 Isthmus
>>Lower uterine segment

182.8 Other specified sites of body of uterus
>>Malignant neoplasm of contiguous or overlapping sites of body of uterus whose point of origin cannot be determined

>*Excludes:* *uterus NOS (179)*

>**ALERT!** For personal history of malignant neoplasm of other parts of uterus see V10.42

183 Malignant neoplasm of ovary and other uterine adnexa
>*Excludes:* *Douglas' cul-de-sac (158.8)*

>**ALERT!** For personal history of malignant neoplasm of ovary see V10.43

183.0 Ovary
Use additional code, if desired, to identify any functional activity

183.2 Fallopian tube
>>Oviduct
>>Uterine tube

183.3 Broad ligament
>>Mesovarium
>>Parovarian region

183.4 Parametrium
>>Uterine ligament NOS
>>Uterosacral ligament

183.5 Round ligament

183.8 Other specified sites of uterine adnexa
>>Tubo-ovarian
>>Utero-ovarian
>>Malignant neoplasm of contiguous or overlapping sites of ovary and other uterine adnexa whose point of origin cannot be determined

183.9 Uterine adnexa, unspecified

184 Malignant neoplasm of other and unspecified female genital organs
>*Excludes:* *carcinoma in situ (233.30-233.39)*

>**ALERT!** For personal history of malignant neoplasm of other female genital organs see V10.44
>**ALERT!** For personal history of malignant neoplasm of unspecified female genital organ see V10.40

184.0 Vagina
>>Gartner's duct
>>Vaginal vault

184.1 Labia majora
>>Greater vestibular [Bartholin's] gland

184.2 Labia minora

184.3 Clitoris

184.4 Vulva, unspecified
>>External female genitalia NOS
>>Pudendum

184.8 Other specified sites of female genital organs
>>Malignant neoplasm of contiguous or overlapping sites of female genital organs whose point of origin cannot be determined

● Code new   ▲ Revision of   ④ ⑤ Fourth or fifth
        to 2012 edition   existing code   digit required

184.9 Female genital organ, site unspecified
Female genitourinary tract NOS

185 Malignant neoplasm of prostate

Excludes: seminal vesicles (187.8)

ALERT! For personal history of malignant neoplasm of prostate see V10.46

186 Malignant neoplasm of testis
Use additional code, if desired, to identify any functional activity

ALERT! For personal history of malignant neoplasm of testis see V10.47

186.0 Undescended testis
Ectopic testis
Retained testis

186.9 Other and unspecified testis
Testis:
NOS
descended
scrotal

187 Malignant neoplasm of penis and other male genital organs

187.1 Prepuce
Foreskin

187.2 Glans penis

187.3 Body of penis
Corpus cavernosum

187.4 Penis, part unspecified
Skin of penis NOS

187.5 Epididymis

ALERT! For personal history of malignant neoplasm of epididymis see V10.48

187.6 Spermatic cord
Vas deferens

187.7 Scrotum
Skin of scrotum

187.8 Other specified sites of male genital organs
Seminal vesicle
Tunica vaginalis
Malignant neoplasm of contiguous or overlapping sites of penis and other male genital organs whose point of origin cannot be determined

ALERT! For personal history of malignant neoplasm of other male genital organs see V10.49

187.9 Male genital organ, site unspecified
Male genital organ or tract NOS

ALERT! For personal history of malignant neoplasm of other male genital organs see V10.49

ALERT! For personal history of malignant neoplasm of unspecified male genital organ see V10.45

188 Malignant neoplasm of bladder

Excludes: carcinoma in situ (233.7)

ALERT! For personal history of malignant neoplasm of bladder see V10.51

ALERT! For personal history of malignant neoplasm of urinary organs see V10.5

188.0 Trigone of urinary bladder

188.1 Dome of urinary bladder

188.2 Lateral wall of urinary bladder

188.3 Anterior wall of urinary bladder

188.4 Posterior wall of urinary bladder

188.5 Bladder neck
Internal urethral orifice

188.6 Ureteric orifice

188.7 Urachus

188.8 Other specified sites of bladder
Malignant neoplasm of contiguous or overlapping sites of bladder whose point of origin cannot be determined

188.9 Bladder, part unspecified
Bladder wall NOS

| | Add 4th or 5th digit | | Nonspecific code | | Unspecified code | | Manifestation code |

189 **Malignant neoplasm of kidney and other and unspecified urinary organs**

> *Excludes:* benign carcinoid tumor of kidney (209.64)
>
> malignant carcinoid tumor of kidney (209.24)

ALERT! For personal history of malignant neoplasm of kidney see V10.52

ALERT! For personal history of malignant neoplasm of unspecified urinary organ see V10.50

189.0 **Kidney, except pelvis**
Kidney NOS
Kidney parenchyma

189.1 **Renal pelvis**
Renal calyces
Ureteropelvic junction

ALERT! For personal history of malignant neoplasm of renal pelvis see V10.53

189.2 **Ureter**

> *Excludes:* ureteric orifice of bladder (188.6)

189.3 **Urethra**

> *Excludes:* urethral orifice of bladder (188.5)

189.4 **Paraurethral glands**

189.8 **Other specified sites of urinary organs**
Malignant neoplasm of contiguous or overlapping sites of kidney and other urinary
organs whose point of origin cannot be determined

ALERT! For personal history of malignant neoplasm of other urinary organs see V10.59

189.9 **Urinary organ, site unspecified**
Urinary system NOS

MALIGNANT NEOPLASM OF OTHER AND UNSPECIFIED SITES (190-199)

> *Excludes:* carcinoma in situ (234.0-234.9)

190 **Malignant neoplasm of eye**

> *Excludes:* carcinoma in situ (234.0)
>
> dark area on retina and choroid (239.81)
> malignant melanoma of eyelid (skin) (172.1)
>   cartilage (171.0)
> malignant neoplasm of eyelid (skin) (173.10-173.19)
> optic nerve (192.0)
> orbital bone (170.0)
> retinal freckle (239.81)

ALERT! For personal history of malignant neoplasm of eye see V10.84

190.0 **Eyeball, except conjunctiva, cornea, retina, and choroid**
Ciliary body   Sclera
Crystalline lens   Uveal tract
Iris

190.1 **Orbit**
Connective tissue of orbit
Extraocular muscle
Retrobulbar

> *Excludes:* bone of orbit (170.0)

190.2 **Lacrimal gland**

190.3 **Conjunctiva**

190.4 **Cornea**

190.5 **Retina**

190.6 **Choroid**

190.7 **Lacrimal duct**
Lacrimal sac
Nasolacrimal duct

190.8 **Other specified sites of eye**
Malignant neoplasm of contiguous or overlapping sites of eye whose point of origin
cannot be determined

190.9 **Eye, part unspecified**

● Code new   ▲ Revision of   ④ ⑤ Fourth or fifth
to 2012 edition   existing code   digit required

191 **Malignant neoplasm of brain**

> *Excludes:* cranial nerves (192.0)
> retrobulbar area (190.1)

> **ALERT!** For personal history of malignant neoplasm of brain see V10.85

191.0 **Cerebrum, except lobes and ventricles**
Basal ganglia   Globus pallidus
Cerebral cortex   Hypothalamus
Corpus striatum   Thalamus

191.1 **Frontal lobe**

191.2 **Temporal lobe**
Hippocampus
Uncus

191.3 **Parietal lobe**

191.4 **Occipital lobe**

191.5 **Ventricles**
Choroid plexus
Floor of ventricle

191.6 **Cerebellum NOS**
Cerebellopontine angle

191.7 **Brain stem**
Cerebral peduncle   Midbrain
Medulla oblongata   Pons

191.8 **Other parts of brain**
Corpus callosum
Tapetum
Malignant neoplasm of contiguous or overlapping sites of brain whose point of origin
cannot be determined

191.9 **Brain, unspecified**
Cranial fossa NOS

192 **Malignant neoplasm of other and unspecified parts of nervous system**

> *Excludes:* peripheral, sympathetic, and parasympathetic nerves and ganglia (171.0-171.9)

> **ALERT!** For personal history of malignant neoplasm of other parts of nervous system see
> V10.86

192.0 **Cranial nerves**
Olfactory bulb

192.1 **Cerebral meninges**
Dura (mater)   Meninges NOS
Falx (cerebelli) (cerebri)   Tentorium

192.2 **Spinal cord**
Cauda equina

192.3 **Spinal meninges**

192.8 **Other specified sites of nervous system**
Malignant neoplasm of contiguous or overlapping sites of other parts of nervous system
whose point of origin cannot be determined

192.9 **Nervous system, part unspecified**
Nervous system (central) NOS

> *Excludes:* meninges NOS (192.1)

193 **Malignant neoplasm of thyroid gland**
Thyroglossal duct

Use additional code, if desired, to identify any functional activity

> **ALERT!** For personal history of malignant neoplasm of thyroid see V10.87

194 **Malignant neoplasm of other endocrine glands and related structures**

> *Excludes:* islets of Langerhans (157.4)
> neuroendocrine tumors (209.00-209.69)
> ovary (183.0)
> testis (186.0-186.9)
> thymus (164.0)

> **ALERT!** For personal history of malignant neoplasm of other endocrine glands and related
> structures see V10.88

229

| | Add 4th or 5th digit | | Nonspecific code | | Unspecified code | | Manifestation code |

194.0 Adrenal gland
Adrenal cortex
Adrenal medulla
Suprarenal gland

194.1 Parathyroid gland

194.3 Pituitary gland and craniopharyngeal duct
Craniobuccal pouch
Hypophysis
Rathke's pouch
Sella turcica

194.4 Pineal gland

194.5 Carotid body

194.6 Aortic body and other paraganglia
Coccygeal body
Glomus jugulare
Para-aortic body

194.8 Other
Pluriglandular involvement NOS

Note: If the sites of multiple involvements are known, they should be coded separately.

194.9 Endocrine gland, site unspecified

195 Malignant neoplasm of other and ill-defined sites

Includes: malignant neoplasms of contiguous sites, not elsewhere classified, whose point of origin cannot be determined

[Excludes:] *malignant neoplasm:*
lymphatic and hematopoietic tissue (200.0-208.9)
secondary sites (196.0-198.8)
unspecified site (199.0-199.1)

[ALERT!] For personal history of malignant neoplasm of other sites see V10.89

195.0 Head, face, and neck
Cheek NOS
Jaw NOS
Nose NOS
Supraclavicular region NOS

195.1 Thorax
Axilla
Chest (wall) NOS
Intrathoracic NOS

195.2 Abdomen
Intra-abdominal NOS

195.3 Pelvis
Groin
Inguinal region NOS
Presacral region
Sacrococcygeal region
Sites overlapping systems within pelvis, as:
rectovaginal (septum)
rectovesical (septum)

195.4 Upper limb

195.5 Lower limb

195.8 Other specified sites
Back NOS
Flank NOS
Trunk NOS

196 Secondary and unspecified malignant neoplasm of lymph nodes

[Excludes:] *any malignant neoplasm of lymph nodes, specified as primary (200.0-202.9)*
Hodgkin's disease (201.0-201.9)
lymphosarcoma (200.1)
reticulosarcoma (200.0)
other forms of lymphoma (202.0-202.9)
secondary neuroendocrine tumor of (distant) lymph nodes (209.71)

[ALERT!] For personal history of unspecified type of malignant neoplasm see V10.90

196.0 Lymph nodes of head, face, and neck
Cervical
Cervicofacial
Scalene
Supraclavicular

196.1 Intrathoracic lymph nodes
Bronchopulmonary
Intercostal
Mediastinal
Tracheobronchial

196.2 Intra-abdominal lymph nodes
Intestinal
Mesenteric
Retroperitoneal

● Code new to 2012 edition ▲ Revision of existing code ④ ⑤ Fourth or fifth digit required

196.3 Lymph nodes of axilla and upper limb
Brachial
Epitrochlear
Infraclavicular
Pectoral

196.5 Lymph nodes of inguinal region and lower limb
Femoral
Groin
Popliteal
Tibial

196.6 Intrapelvic lymph nodes
Hypogastric
Iliac
Obturator
Parametrial

196.8 Lymph nodes of multiple sites

196.9 Site unspecified
Lymph nodes NOS

197 Secondary malignant neoplasm of respiratory and digestive systems

[Excludes:] *lymph node metastasis (196.0-196.9)*
secondary neuroendocrine tumor of liver (209.72)
secondary neuroendocrine tumor of respiratory organs (209.79)

ALERT! For personal history of unspecified type of malignant neoplasm see V10.90

197.0 Lung
Bronchus

197.1 Mediastinum

197.2 Pleura

197.3 Other respiratory organs
Trachea

ALERT! For personal history of malignant neoplasm of other respiratory and intrathoracic organs see V10.2

197.4 Small intestine, including duodenum

197.5 Large intestine and rectum

197.6 Retroperitoneum and peritoneum

197.7 Liver, specified as secondary

197.8 Other digestive organs and spleen

198 Secondary malignant neoplasm of other specified sites

[Excludes:] *lymph node metastasis (196.0-196.9)*
secondary neuroendocrine tumor of other specified sites (209.79)

ALERT! For personal history of malignant neoplasm of other sites see V10.8
ALERT! For personal history of unspecified type of malignant neoplasm see V10.90

198.0 Kidney

198.1 Other urinary organs

198.2 Skin
Skin of breast

198.3 Brain and spinal cord

198.4 Other parts of nervous system
Meninges (cerebral) (spinal)

198.5 Bone and bone marrow

198.6 Ovary

198.7 Adrenal gland
Suprarenal gland

[5] **198.8 Other specified sites**

198.81 Breast

[Excludes:] *skin of breast (198.2)*

198.82 Genital organs

198.89 Other

[Excludes:] *retroperitoneal lymph nodes (196.2)*

199 Malignant neoplasm without specification of site

[Excludes:] *malignant carcinoid tumor of unknown primary site (209.20)*
malignant (poorly differentiated) neuroendocrine carcinoma, any site (209.30)
malignant (poorly differentiated) neuroendocrine tumor, any site (209.30)
neuroendocrine carcinoma (high grade), any site (209.30)

Add 4th or 5th digit | Nonspecific code | Unspecified code | Manifestation code

[ALERT!] For personal history of unspecified type of malignant neoplasm see V10.90

199.0 Disseminated
Carcinomatosis unspecified site (primary) (secondary)
Generalized:
cancer unspecified site (primary) (secondary)
malignancy unspecified site (primary) (secondary)
Multiple cancer unspecified site (primary) (secondary)

199.1 Other
Cancer unspecified site (primary) (secondary)
Carcinoma unspecified site (primary) (secondary)
Malignancy unspecified site (primary) (secondary)

199.2 Malignant neoplasm associated with transplanted organ
Code first complication of transplanted organ (996.80-996.89)
Use additional code for specific malignancy

MALIGNANT NEOPLASM OF LYMPHATIC AND HEMATOPOIETIC TISSUE (200-208)

[Excludes:] *autoimmune lymphoproliferative syndrome (279.41)*
secondary neoplasm of:
bone marrow (198.5)
spleen (197.8)
secondary and unspecified neoplasm of lymph nodes (196.0-196.9)

The following fifth-digit subclassification is for use with categories 200-202:

0 unspecified site, extranodal and solid organ sites
1 lymph nodes of head, face, and neck
2 intrathoracic lymph nodes
3 intra-abdominal lymph nodes
4 lymph nodes of axilla and upper limb
5 lymph nodes of inguinal region and lower limb
6 intrapelvic lymph nodes
7 spleen
8 lymph nodes of multiple sites

[5] **200 Lymphosarcoma and reticulosarcoma and other specified malignant tumors of lymphatic tissue**
[DEFINITION] Lymphosarcoma is a type of cancer that originates in lymphocytes of the immune system. The diseases often originates in lymph nodes, presenting as an enlargement of the node (a tumor). A reticulosarcoma is a malignant lymphoma, histiocytic or undifferentiated.
[ALERT!] For personal history of other lymphatic and hematopoietic neoplasms see V10.7

[5] **200.0 Reticulosarcoma**
[0-8] Lymphoma (malignant):
histiocytic (diffuse):
nodular
pleomorphic cell type
reticulum cell type
Reticulum cell sarcoma:
NOS
pleomorphic cell type

[5] **200.1 Lymphosarcoma**
[0-8] Lymphoblastoma (diffuse)
Lymphoma (malignant):
lymphoblastic (diffuse)
lymphocytic (cell type) (diffuse)
lymphosarcoma type
Lymphosarcoma:
NOS
diffuse NOS
lymphoblastic (diffuse)
lymphocytic (diffuse)
prolymphocytic

[Excludes:] *lymphosarcoma:*
follicular or nodular (202.0)
mixed cell type (200.8)
lymphosarcoma cell leukemia (207.8)

[5] **200.2 Burkitt's tumor or lymphoma**
[0-8] Malignant lymphoma, Burkitt's type

● Code new to 2012 edition ▲ Revision of existing code [4] [5] Fourth or fifth digit required

[5] **200.3 Marginal zone lymphoma**
[0-8]
Extranodal marginal zone B-cell lymphoma
Mucosa associated lymphoid tissue [MALT]
Nodal marginal zone B-cell lymphoma
Splenic marginal zone B-cell lymphoma

[5] **200.4 Mantle cell lymphoma**
[0-8]

[5] **200.5 Primary central nervous system lymphoma**
[0-8]

[5] **200.6 Anaplastic large cell lymphoma**
[0-8]

[5] **200.7 Large cell lymphoma**
[0-8]

[5] **200.8 Other named variants**
[0-8]
Lymphoma (malignant):
  lymphoplasmacytoid type
  mixed lymphocytic-histiocytic (diffuse)
Lymphosarcoma, mixed cell type (diffuse)
Reticulolymphosarcoma (diffuse)

[5] **201 Hodgkin's disease**

DEFINITION Hodgkin's disease is a malignant disease of the lymphatic system is characterized by painless enlargement of lymph nodes, the spleen, or other lymphatic tissue. It is sometimes accompanied by symptoms such as fever, weight loss, fatigue and night sweats.

ALERT! For personal history of hodgkin's disease see V10.72

[5] **201.0 Hodgkin's paragranuloma**
[0-8]

[5] **201.1 Hodgkin's granuloma**
[0-8]

[5] **201.2 Hodgkin's sarcoma**
[0-8]

[5] **201.4 Lymphocytic-histiocytic predominance**
[0-8]

[5] **201.5 Nodular sclerosis**
[0-8]
Hodgkin's disease, nodular sclerosis:
  NOS
  cellular phase

[5] **201.6 Mixed cellularity**
[0-8]

[5] **201.7 Lymphocytic depletion**
[0-8]
Hodgkin's disease, lymphocytic depletion:
  NOS
  diffuse fibrosis
  reticular type

[5] **201.9 Hodgkin's disease, unspecified**
[0-8]
Hodgkin's:
  disease NOS
  lymphoma NOS
Malignant:
  lymphogranuloma
  lymphogranulomatosis

[5] **202 Other malignant neoplasms of lymphoid and histiocytic tissue**

ALERT! For personal history of other lymphatic and hematopoietic neoplasms see V10.79

[5] **202.0 Nodular lymphoma**
[0-8]
Brill-Symmers disease
Lymphoma:
  follicular (giant) (large cell)
  lymphocytic, nodular
Lymphosarcoma:
  follicular (giant)
  nodular

[5] **202.1 Mycosis fungoides**
[0-8]

[Excludes:] *peripheral T-cell lymphoma (202.7)*

[5] **202.2 Sézary's disease**
[0-8]

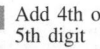

⑤ **202.3 Malignant histiocytosis**
[0-8]   Histiocytic medullary reticulosis
           Malignant:
             reticuloendotheliosis
             reticulosis

⑤ **202.4 Leukemic reticuloendotheliosis**
[0-8]   Hairy-cell leukemia

⑤ **202.5 Letterer-Siwe disease**
[0-8]   Acute:
             differentiated progressive histiocytosis
             histiocytosis X (progressive)
             infantile reticuloendotheliosis
             reticulosis of infancy

    Excludes: *adult pulmonary Langerhans cell histiocytic tissue (516.5)*
              Hand-Schüller-Christian disease (277.89)
              histiocytosis (acute) (chronic) (277.89)
              histiocytosis X (chronic) (277.89)

⑤ **202.6 Malignant mast cell tumors**
[0-8]   Malignant: Mast cell sarcoma
             mastocytoma   Systemic tissue mast cell disease
             mastocytosis

    Excludes: *mast cell leukemia (207.8)*

⑤ **202.7 Peripheral T-cell lymphoma**
[0-8]

⑤ **202.8 Other lymphomas**
[0-8]   Lymphoma (malignant):
             NOS
             diffuse

    Excludes: *benign lymphoma (229.0)*

⑤ **202.9 Other and unspecified malignant neoplasms of lymphoid and histiocytic tissue**
[0-8]   Follicular dendritic cell sarcoma
           Interdigitating dendritic cell sarcoma
           Langerhans cell sarcoma
           Malignant neoplasm of bone marrow NOS

⑤ **203 Multiple myeloma and immunoproliferative neoplasms**
    The following fifth-digit subclassification is for use with category 203

        **0 without mention of having achieved remission
             failed remission**

        1 in remission

        2 in relapse

    DEFINITION Multiple myeloma and immunoproliferative neoplasms is a cancer in which there
    is a uncontrolled proliferation and disordered function of cells called plasma cells in the bone
    marrow., aka a plasma cell neoplasm.

⑤ **203.0 Multiple myeloma**
[0-2]   Kahler's disease
           Myelomatosis

    Excludes: *solitary myeloma (238.6)*

⑤ **203.1 Plasma cell leukemia**
[0-2]   Plasmacytic leukemia

⑤ **203.8 Other immunoproliferative neoplasms**
[0-2]

● Code new   ▲ Revision of   ④ ⑤ Fourth or fifth
       to 2012 edition   existing code   digit required

⑤ **204 Lymphoid leukemia**
      Includes: leukemia:
                lymphatic
                lymphoblastic
                lymphocytic
                lymphogenous

The following fifth-digit subclassification is for use with category 204

    **0   without mention of having achieved remission
          failed remission**

    1   in remission

    2   in relapse

    DEFINITION Lymphoid leukemia is a form of leukemia associated with hyperplasia and overactivity of the lymphoid tissue, with increased levels of circulating malignant lymphocytes or lymphoblasts.

    ALERT! For personal history of leukemia see V10.6

⑤ **204.0 Acute**
    [0-2]

    Excludes: acute exacerbation of chronic lymphoid leukemia (204.1)

⑤ **204.1 Chronic**
    [0-2]

⑤ **204.2 Subacute**
    [0-2]

⑤ **204.8 Other lymphoid leukemia**
    [0-2]   Aleukemic leukemia:
            lymphatic
            lymphocytic
            lymphoid

⑤ **204.9 Unspecified lymphoid leukemia**
    [0-2]

⑤ **205 Myeloid leukemia**
      Includes: leukemia:
                granulocytic   myelomonocytic
                myeloblastic   myelosclerotic
                myelocytic   myelosis
                myelogenous

The following fifth-digit subclassification is for use with category 205

    **0   without mention of having achieved remission
          failed remission**

    1   in remission

    2   in relapse

    DEFINITION Myeloid leukemia is a type of leukemia affecting myeloid tissue (bone marrow).

    ALERT! For personal history of myeloid leukemia see V10.62

⑤ **205.0 Acute**
    [0-2]   Acute promyelocytic leukemia

    Excludes: acute exacerbation of chronic myeloid leukemia (205.1)

⑤ **205.1 Chronic**
    [0-2]   Eosinophilic leukemia   Neutrophilic leukemia

⑤ **205.2 Subacute**
    [0-2]

⑤ **205.3 Myeloid sarcoma**
    [0-2]   Chloroma
            Granulocytic sarcoma

⑤ **205.8 Other myeloid leukemia**
    [0-2]   Aleukemic leukemia:
            granulocytic
            myelogenous
            myeloid
        Aleukemic myelosis

⑤ **205.9 Unspecified myeloid leukemia**
    [0-2]

    ALERT! For personal history of unspecified leukemia see V10.60

	Add 4th or 5th digit		Nonspecific code		Unspecified code		Manifestation code

⑤ **206** **Monocytic leukemia**
      Includes: leukemia:
                  histiocytic
                  monoblastic
                  monocytoid

The following fifth-digit subclassification is for use with category 206

    0   **without mention of having achieved remission**
          failed remission

    1   **in remission**

    2   **in relapse**
    DEFINITION Monocytic leukemia is a type of leukemia characterized by the proliferation of monocytes and monoblasts in the blood .
    ALERT! ICD-9-CM codes in the Category 206 add points to the clinical domain as a Cancer & benign neoplasms diagnosis.
    ALERT! For personal history of monocytic leukemia see V10.63

⑤ **206.0** **Acute**
   [0-2]

    Excludes: *acute exacerbation of chronic monocytic leukemia (206.1)*

⑤ **206.1** **Chronic**
   [0-2]

⑤ **206.2** **Subacute**
   [0-2]

⑤ **206.8** **Other monocytic leukemia**
   [0-2]   Aleukemic:
        monocytic leukemia
        monocytoid leukemia

⑤ **206.9** **Unspecified monocytic leukemia**
   [0-2]
    ALERT! For personal history of unspecified leukemia see V10.60

⑤ **207** **Other specified leukemia**
    Excludes: *leukemic reticuloendotheliosis (202.4)*
              plasma cell leukemia (203.1)

The following fifth-digit subclassification is for use with category 207

    0   **without mention of having achieved remission**
          failed remission

    1   **in remission**

    2   **in relapse**
    ALERT! For personal history of other leukemia see V10.69

⑤ **207.0** **Acute erythremia and erythroleukemia**
   [0-2]   Acute erythremic myelosis
        Di Guglielmo's disease
        Erythremic myelosis

⑤ **207.1** **Chronic erythremia**
   [0-2]   Heilmeyer-Schöner disease

⑤ **207.2** **Megakaryocytic leukemia**
   [0-2]   Megakaryocytic myelosis   Thrombocytic leukemia

⑤ **207.8** **Other specified leukemia**
   [0-2]   Lymphosarcoma cell leukemia

⑤ **208** **Leukemia of unspecified cell type**
The following fifth-digit subclassification is for use with category 208

    0   **without mention of having achieved remission**
          failed remission

    1   **in remission**

    2   **in relapse**
    ALERT! For personal history of unspecified leukemia see V10.60

● Code new to 2012 edition   ▲ Revision of existing code   ④ ⑤ Fourth or fifth digit required

[5] **208.0 Acute**
[0-2] Acute leukemia NOS
Blast cell leukemia
Stem cell leukemia

[Excludes:] *acute exacerbation of chronic unspecified leukemia (208.1)*

[5] **208.1 Chronic**
[0-2] Chronic leukemia NOS

[5] **208.2 Subacute**
[0-2] Subacute leukemia NOS

[5] **208.8 Other leukemia of unspecified cell type**
[0-2]

[5] **208.9 Unspecified leukemia**
[0-2] Leukemia NOS

NEUROENDOCRINE TUMORS (209)

[5] **209 Neuroendocrine tumors**

Code first any associated multiple endocrine neoplasia syndrome (258.01-258.03)

Use additional code to identify associated endocrine syndrome, such as: carcinoid syndrome (259.2)

[Excludes:] *benign pancreatic islet cell tumors (211.7)*
malignant pancreatic islet cell tumors (157.4)

[DEFINITION] Neuroendocrine tumor is a tumor derived from cells that release a hormone in response to a signal from the nervous system. Examples of neuroendocrine tumors include carcinoid tumors islet cell tumors, medullary thyroid carcinoma, and pheochromocytoma.

[ALERT!] For personal history of malignant neuroendocrine tumor see V10.91

[5] **209.0 Malignant carcinoid tumors of the small intestine**

209.00 Malignant carcinoid tumor of the small intestine, unspecified portion

209.01 Malignant carcinoid tumor of the duodenum

209.02 Malignant carcinoid tumor of the jejunum

209.03 Malignant carcinoid tumor of the ileum

[5] **209.1 Malignant carcinoid tumors of the appendix, large intestine, and rectum**

209.10 Malignant carcinoid tumor of the large intestine, unspecified portion
Malignant carcinoid tumor of the colon NOS

209.11 Malignant carcinoid tumor of the appendix

209.12 Malignant carcinoid tumor of the cecum

209.13 Malignant carcinoid tumor of the ascending colon

209.14 Malignant carcinoid tumor of the transverse colon

209.15 Malignant carcinoid tumor of the descending colon

209.16 Malignant carcinoid tumor of the sigmoid colon

209.17 Malignant carcinoid tumor of the rectum

[5] **209.2 Malignant carcinoid tumors of other and unspecified sites**

209.20 Malignant carcinoid tumor of unknown primary site

209.21 Malignant carcinoid tumor of the bronchus and lung

209.22 Malignant carcinoid tumor of the thymus

209.23 Malignant carcinoid tumor of the stomach

209.24 Malignant carcinoid tumor of the kidney

209.25 Malignant carcinoid tumor of the foregut NOS

209.26 Malignant carcinoid tumor of the midgut NOS

209.27 Malignant carcinoid tumor of the hindgut NOS

209.29 Malignant carcinoid tumors of other sites

[5] **209.3 Malignant poorly differentiated neuroendocrine tumors**

209.30 Malignant poorly differentiated neuroendocrine carcinoma, any site
High grade neuroendocrine carcinoma, any site
Malignant poorly differentiated neuroendocrine tumor NOS

[Excludes:] *Merkel cell carcinoma (209.31-209.36)*

209.31 **Merkel cell carcinoma of the face**
Merkel cell carcinoma of the ear
Merkel cell carcinoma of the eyelid, including canthus
Merkel cell carcinoma of the lip

209.32 **Merkel cell carcinoma of the scalp and neck**

209.33 **Merkel cell carcinoma of the upper limb**

209.34 **Merkel cell carcinoma of the lower limb**

209.35 **Merkel cell carcinoma of the trunk**

209.36 **Merkel cell carcinoma of other sites**
Merkel cell carcinoma of the buttock
Merkel cell carcinoma of the genitals
Merkel cell carcinoma NOS

⑤ **209.4** **Benign carcinoid tumors of the small intestine**

209.40 **Benign carcinoid tumor of the small intestine, unspecified portion**

209.41 **Benign carcinoid tumor of the duodenum**

209.42 **Benign carcinoid tumor of the jejunum**

209.43 **Benign carcinoid tumor of the ileum**

⑤ **209.5** **Benign carcinoid tumors of the appendix, large intestine, and rectum**

209.50 **Benign carcinoid tumor of the large intestine, unspecified portion**
Benign carcinoid tumor of the colon NOS

209.51 **Benign carcinoid tumor of the appendix**

209.52 **Benign carcinoid tumor of the cecum**

209.53 **Benign carcinoid tumor of the ascending colon**

209.54 **Benign carcinoid tumor of the transverse colon**

209.55 **Benign carcinoid tumor of the descending colon**

209.56 **Benign carcinoid tumor of the sigmoid colon**

209.57 **Benign carcinoid tumor of the rectum**

⑤ **209.6** **Benign carcinoid tumors of other and unspecified sites**

209.60 **Benign carcinoid tumor of unknown primary site**
Carcinoid tumor NOS
Neuroendocrine tumor NOS

209.61 **Benign carcinoid tumor of the bronchus and lung**

209.62 **Benign carcinoid tumor of the thymus**

209.63 **Benign carcinoid tumor of the stomach**

209.64 **Benign carcinoid tumor of the kidney**

209.65 **Benign carcinoid tumor of the foregut NOS**

209.66 **Benign carcinoid tumor of the midgut NOS**

209.67 **Benign carcinoid tumor of the hindgut NOS**

209.69 **Benign carcinoid tumors of other sites**

⑤ **209.7** **Secondary neuroendocrine tumors**
Secondary carcinoid tumors

209.70 **Secondary neuroendocrine tumor, unspecified site**

209.71 **Secondary neuroendocrine tumor of distant lymph nodes**

209.72 **Secondary neuroendocrine tumor of liver**

209.73 **Secondary neuroendocrine tumor of bone**

209.74 **Secondary neuroendocrine tumor of peritoneum**
Mesentary metastasis of neuroendocrine tumor

209.75 **Secondary Merkel cell carcinoma**
Merkel cell carcinoma nodal presentation
Merkel cell carcinoma visceral metastatic presentation
Secondary Merkel cell carcinoma, any site

209.79 **Secondary neuroendocrine tumor of other sites**

● Code new
to 2012 edition
▲ Revision of
existing code
④ ⑤ Fourth or fifth
digit required

BENIGN NEOPLASMS (210-229)

210 **Benign neoplasm of lip, oral cavity, and pharynx**

Excludes: cyst (of):
> jaw (526.0-526.2, 526.89)
> oral soft tissue (528.4)
> radicular (522.8)

DEFINITION A benign neoplasm is a localized tumor that has a fibrous capsule, limited potential for growth, a regular shape, and cells that are well differentiated. A benign neoplasm does not invade surrounding tissue or metastasize to distant sites. Some kinds of benign neoplasms are adenoma, fibroma, hemangioma, and lipoma.

210.0 Lip
Frenulum labii
Lip (inner aspect) (mucosa) (vermilion border)

Excludes: labial commissure (210.4)
> skin of lip (216.0)

210.1 Tongue
Lingual tonsil

210.2 Major salivary glands
Gland:
> parotid
> sublingual
> submandibular

Excludes: benign neoplasms of minor salivary glands:
> NOS (210.4)
> buccal mucosa (210.4)
> lips (210.0)
> palate (hard) (soft) (210.4)
> tongue (210.1)
> tonsil, palatine (210.5)

210.3 Floor of mouth

210.4 **Other and unspecified parts of mouth**
Gingiva   Oral mucosa
Gum (upper) (lower)   Palate (hard) (soft)
Labial commissure   Uvula
Oral cavity NOS

Excludes: benign odontogenic neoplasms of bone (213.0-213.1)
> developmental odontogenic cysts (526.0)
> mucosa of lips (210.0)
> nasopharyngeal [posterior] [superior] surface of soft palate (210.7)

210.5 Tonsil
Tonsil (faucial) (palatine)

Excludes: lingual tonsil (210.1)
> pharyngeal tonsil (210.7)
> tonsillar:
> fossa (210.6)
> pillars (210.6)

210.6 **Other parts of oropharynx**
Branchial cleft or vestiges
Epiglottis, anterior aspect
Fauces NOS
Mesopharynx NOS
Tonsillar:
> fossa
> pillars
Vallecula

Excludes: epiglottis:
> NOS (212.1)
> suprahyoid portion (212.1)

210.7 Nasopharynx
Adenoid tissue   Pharyngeal tonsil
Lymphadenoid tissue   Posterior nasal septum

210.8 Hypopharynx
Arytenoid fold   Postcricoid region
Laryngopharynx   Pyriform fossa

210.9 Pharynx, unspecified
Throat NOS

211 Benign neoplasm of other parts of digestive system

Excludes: benign stromal tumors of digestive system (215.5)

211.0 Esophagus

211.1 Stomach
Body of stomach   Cardiac orifice
Cardia of stomach   Pylorus
Fundus of stomach

Excludes: benign carcinoid tumors of the stomach (209.63)

211.2 Duodenum, jejunum, and ileum
Small intestine NOS

Excludes: ampulla of Vater (211.5)
benign carcinoid tumors of the small intestine (209.40-209.43)
ileocecal valve (211.3)

211.3 Colon
Appendix   Ileocecal valve
Cecum   Large intestine NOS

Excludes: benign carcinoid tumors of the large intestine (209.50-209.56)
rectosigmoid junction (211.4)

ALERT! For personal history of colonic polyps see V12.72

211.4 Rectum and anal canal
Anal canal or sphincter Rectosigmoid junction
Anus NOS

Excludes: anus:
margin (216.5)
skin (216.5)
benign carcinoid tumors of the rectum (209.57)
perianal skin (216.5)

211.5 Liver and biliary passages
Ampulla of Vater   Gallbladder
Common bile duct   Hepatic duct
Cystic duct   Sphincter of Oddi

211.6 Pancreas, except islets of Langerhans

211.7 Islets of Langerhans
Islet cell tumor
Use additional code, if desired, to identify any functional activity

211.8 Retroperitoneum and peritoneum
Mesentery   Omentum
Mesocolon   Retroperitoneal tissue

211.9 Other and unspecified site
Alimentary tract NOS   Intestinal tract NOS
Digestive system NOS   Intestine NOS
Gastrointestinal tract NOS Spleen, not elsewhere classified

● Code new   ▲ Revision of   ④ ⑤ Fourth or fifth
to 2012 edition   existing code   digit required

212 **Benign neoplasm of respiratory and intrathoracic organs**

212.0 Nasal cavities, middle ear, and accessory sinuses

Cartilage of nose	Sinus:
Eustachian tube	ethmoidal
Nares	frontal
Septum of nose	maxillary
	sphenoidal

Excludes: *auditory canal (external) (216.2)*
bone of:
ear (213.0)
nose [turbinates] (213.0)
cartilage of ear (215.0)
ear (external) (skin) (216.2)
nose NOS (229.8)
skin (216.3)
olfactory bulb (225.1)
polyp of:
accessory sinus (471.8)
ear (385.30-385.35)
nasal cavity (471.0)
posterior margin of septum and choanae (210.7)

212.1 Larynx

Cartilage:	Epiglottis (suprahyoid portion) NOS
arytenoid	Glottis
cricoid	Vocal cords (false) (true)
cuneiform	
thyroid	

Excludes: *epiglottis, anterior aspect (210.6)*
polyp of vocal cord or larynx (478.4)

212.2 Trachea

212.3 Bronchus and lung
Carina
Hilus of lung

Excludes: *benign carcinoid tumors of bronchus and lung (209.61)*

212.4 Pleura

212.5 Mediastinum

212.6 Thymus

Excludes: *benign carcinoid tumors of thymus (209.62)*

212.7 Heart

Excludes: *great vessels (215.4)*

212.8 Other specified sites

212.9 Site unspecified
Respiratory organ NOS
Upper respiratory tract NOS

Excludes: *intrathoracic NOS (229.8)*
thoracic NOS (229.8)

213 **Benign neoplasm of bone and articular cartilage**
Includes: cartilage (articular) (joint)
periosteum

Excludes: *cartilage of:*
ear (215.0)
eyelid (215.0)
larynx (212.1)
nose (212.0)
exostosis NOS (726.91)
synovia (215.0-215.9)

213.0 Bones of skull and face

Excludes: *lower jaw bone (213.1)*

213.1 Lower jaw bone

213.2 Vertebral column, excluding sacrum and coccyx

213.3 Ribs, sternum, and clavicle

Add 4th or 5th digit	Nonspecific code	Unspecified code	Manifestation code

213.4 Scapula and long bones of upper limb

213.5 Short bones of upper limb

213.6 Pelvic bones, sacrum, and coccyx

213.7 Long bones of lower limb

213.8 Short bones of lower limb

213.9 Bone and articular cartilage, site unspecified

214 Lipoma

Includes: angiolipoma
fibrolipoma
hibernoma
lipoma (fetal) (infiltrating) (intramuscular)
myelolipoma
myxolipoma

DEFINITION Lipoma is a benign tumor composed chiefly of fat cells.

214.0 Skin and subcutaneous tissue of face

214.1 Other skin and subcutaneous tissue

214.2 Intrathoracic organs

214.3 Intra-abdominal organs

214.4 Spermatic cord

214.8 Other specified sites

214.9 Lipoma, unspecified site

215 Other benign neoplasm of connective and other soft tissue

Includes: blood vessel
bursa
fascia
ligament
muscle
peripheral, sympathetic, and parasympathetic nerves and ganglia
synovia
tendon (sheath)

Excludes: *cartilage:*
articular (213.0-213.9)
larynx (212.1)
nose (212.0)
connective tissue of:
breast (217)
internal organ, except lipoma and hemangioma — code to benign neoplasm of
the site
lipoma (214.0-214.9)

215.0 Head, face, and neck

215.2 Upper limb, including shoulder

215.3 Lower limb, including hip

215.4 Thorax

Excludes: *heart (212.7)*
mediastinum (212.5)
thymus (212.6)

215.5 Abdomen
Abdominal wall
Benign stromal tumors of abdomen
Hypochondrium

215.6 Pelvis
Buttock   Inguinal region
Groin   Perineum

Excludes: *uterine:*
leiomyoma (218.0-218.9)
ligament, any (221.0)

215.7 Trunk, unspecified
Back NOS
Flank NOS

215.8 Other specified sites

215.9 Site unspecified

● Code new   ▲ Revision of   ④ ⑤ Fourth or fifth
to 2012 edition   existing code   digit required

216 **Benign neoplasm of skin**
  Includes: blue nevus
        dermatofibroma
        hydrocystoma
        pigmented nevus
        syringoadenoma
        syringoma

  Excludes: *skin of genital organs (221.0-222.9)*

216.0 Skin of lip
  Excludes: *vermilion border of lip (210.0)*

216.1 Eyelid, including canthus
  Excludes: *cartilage of eyelid (215.0)*

216.2 Ear and external auditory canal
  Auricle (ear)   External meatus
  Auricular canal, external   Pinna
  Excludes: *cartilage of ear (215.0)*

216.3 Skin of other and unspecified parts of face
  Cheek, external   Nose, external
  Eyebrow   Temple

216.4 Scalp and skin of neck

216.5 Skin of trunk, except scrotum
  Axillary fold   Skin of:
  Perianal skin   buttock
  Skin of: chest wall
    abdominal wall   groin
    anus   perineum
    back   Umbilicus
    breast

  Excludes: *anal canal (211.4)*
         anus NOS (211.4)
         skin of scrotum (222.4)

216.6 Skin of upper limb, including shoulder

216.7 Skin of lower limb, including hip

216.8 Other specified sites of skin

216.9 Skin, site unspecified

217 **Benign neoplasm of breast**
  Breast (male) (female)
  connective tissue
  glandular tissue
  soft parts

  Excludes: *adenofibrosis (610.2)*
         benign cyst of breast (610.0)
         fibrocystic disease (610.1)
         skin of breast (216.5)

218 **Uterine leiomyoma**
  Includes: fibroid (bleeding) (uterine)
        uterine:
          fibromyoma
          myoma

  DEFINITION Uterine leiomyoma refers to one or more smooth, firm, painful, often waxy nodules arising from cutaneous or subcutaneous of the uterus.

218.0 Submucous leiomyoma of uterus

218.1 Intramural leiomyoma of uterus
  Interstitial leiomyoma of uterus

218.2 Subserous leiomyoma of uterus
  Subperitoneal leiomyoma of uterus

218.9 Leiomyoma of uterus, unspecified

219 **Other benign neoplasm of uterus**

219.0 Cervix uteri

Add 4th or   Nonspecific   Unspecified   Manifestation
5th digit   code   code   code

219.1 Corpus uteri
Endometrium
Fundus
Myometrium

219.8 Other specified parts of uterus

219.9 Uterus, part unspecified

220 Benign neoplasm of ovary
Use additional code, if desired, to identify any functional activity (256.0-256.1)

[Excludes:] *cyst:*
corpus albicans (620.2)
corpus luteum (620.1)
endometrial (617.1)
follicular (atretic) (620.0)
graafian follicle (620.0)
ovarian NOS (620.2)
retention (620.2)

221 Benign neoplasm of other female genital organs
Includes: adenomatous polyp
benign teratoma

[Excludes:] *cyst:*
epoophoron (752.11)
fimbrial (752.11)
Gartner's duct (752.11)
parovarian (752.11)

221.0 Fallopian tube and uterine ligaments
Oviduct
Parametrium
Uterine ligament (broad) (round) (uterosacral)
Uterine tube

221.1 Vagina

221.2 Vulva
Clitoris
External female genitalia NOS
Greater vestibular [Bartholin's] gland
Labia (majora) (minora)
Pudendum

[Excludes:] *Bartholin's (duct) (gland) cyst (616.2)*

221.8 Other specified sites of female genital organs

221.9 Female genital organ, site unspecified
Female genitourinary tract NOS

222 Benign neoplasm of male genital organs

222.0 Testis
Use additional code, if desired, to identify any functional activity

222.1 Penis
Corpus cavernosum
Glans penis
Prepuce

222.2 Prostate

[Excludes:] *adenomatous hyperplasia of prostate (600.20-600.21)*
prostatic:
adenoma (600.20-600.21)
enlargement (600.00-600.01)
hypertrophy (600.00-600.01)

222.3 Epididymis

222.4 Scrotum
Skin of scrotum

222.8 Other specified sites of male genital organs
Seminal vesicle
Spermatic cord

222.9 Male genital organ, site unspecified
Male genitourinary tract NOS

223 Benign neoplasm of kidney and other urinary organs

● Code new to 2012 edition ▲ Revision of existing code ④ ⑤ Fourth or fifth digit required

223.0 Kidney, except pelvis
Kidney NOS

[*Excludes:*] *benign carcinoid tumors of kidney (209.64)*
renal:
calyces (223.1)
pelvis (223.1)

223.1 Renal pelvis

223.2 Ureter

[*Excludes:*] *ureteric orifice of bladder (223.3)*

223.3 Bladder

[5] **223.8 Other specified sites of urinary organs**

223.81 Urethra

[*Excludes:*] *urethral orifice of bladder (223.3)*

223.89 Other
Paraurethral glands

223.9 Urinary organ, site unspecified
Urinary system NOS

224 Benign neoplasm of eye

[*Excludes:*] *cartilage of eyelid (215.0)*
eyelid (skin) (216.1)
optic nerve (225.1)
orbital bone (213.0)

224.0 Eyeball, except conjunctiva, cornea, retina, and choroid
Ciliary body
Iris
Sclera
Uveal tract

224.1 Orbit

[*Excludes:*] *bone of orbit (213.0)*

224.2 Lacrimal gland

224.3 Conjunctiva

224.4 Cornea

224.5 Retina

[*Excludes:*] *hemangioma of retina (228.03)*

224.6 Choroid

224.7 Lacrimal duct
Lacrimal sac
Nasolacrimal duct

224.8 Other specified parts of eye

224.9 Eye, part unspecified

225 Benign neoplasm of brain and other parts of nervous system

[*Excludes:*] *hemangioma (228.02)*
neurofibromatosis (237.70-237.79)
peripheral, sympathetic, and parasympathetic nerves and ganglia (215.0-215.9)
retrobulbar (224.1)

[ALERT!] For personal history of benign neoplasm of the brain see V12.41

225.0 Brain

225.1 Cranial nerves

225.2 Cerebral meninges
Meninges NOS
Meningioma (cerebral)

225.3 Spinal cord
Cauda equina

225.4 Spinal meninges
Spinal meningioma

225.8 Other specified sites of nervous system

225.9 Nervous system, part unspecified
Nervous system (central) NOS

[*Excludes:*] *meninges NOS (225.2)*

226 Benign neoplasm of thyroid glands
Use additional code, if desired, to identify any functional activity

227 Benign neoplasm of other endocrine glands and related structures
Use additional code, if desired, to identify any functional activity

> Excludes: *ovary (220)*
> *pancreas (211.6)*
> *testis (222.0)*

227.0 Adrenal gland
Suprarenal gland

227.1 Parathyroid gland

227.3 Pituitary gland and craniopharyngeal duct (pouch)
Craniobuccal pouch   Rathke's pouch
Hypophysis   Sella turcica

227.4 Pineal gland
Pineal body

227.5 Carotid body

227.6 Aortic body and other paraganglia
Coccygeal body   Para-aortic body
Glomus jugulare

227.8 Other

227.9 Endocrine gland, site unspecified

228 Hemangioma and lymphangioma, any site
Includes: angioma (benign) (cavernous) (congenital) NOS
cavernous nevus
glomus tumor
hemangioma (benign) (congenital)

> Excludes: *benign neoplasm of spleen, except hemangioma and lymphangioma (211.9)*
> *glomus jugulare (227.6)*
> *nevus:*
> *NOS (216.0-216.9)*
> *blue or pigmented (216.0-216.9)*
> *vascular (757.32)*

DEFINITION Hemangioma is a benign skin lesion consisting of dense, usually elevated masses of dilated blood vessels. Lymphangioma is a benign neoplasm characterized by lymph vessel proliferation.

⑤ **228.0 Hemangioma, any site**

228.00 Of unspecified site

228.01 Of skin and subcutaneous tissue

228.02 Of intracranial structures

228.03 Of retina

228.04 Of intra-abdominal structures
Peritoneum
Retroperitoneal tissue

228.09 Of other sites
Systemic angiomatosis

228.1 Lymphangioma, any site
Congenital lymphangioma
Lymphatic nevus

229 Benign neoplasm of other and unspecified sites

229.0 Lymph nodes

> Excludes: *lymphangioma (228.1)*

229.8 Other specified sites
Intrathoracic NOS
Thoracic NOS

229.9 Site unspecified

● Code new   ▲ Revision of   ④ ⑤ Fourth or fifth
to 2012 edition   existing code   digit required

CARCINOMA IN SITU (230-234)

Includes: Bowen's disease
erythroplasia
Queyrat's erythroplasia

Excludes: *leukoplakia—see Alphabetic Index*

230 Carcinoma in situ of digestive organs

DEFINITION Carcinoma in situ is a cluster of malignant cells that has not yet invaded the deeper epithelial tissue or spread to other parts of the body.

230.0 Lip, oral cavity, and pharynx

Gingiva	Oropharynx
Hypopharynx	Salivary gland or duct
Mouth [any part]	Tongue
Nasopharynx	

Excludes: *aryepiglottic fold or interarytenoid fold, laryngeal aspect (231.0)*
epiglottis:
NOS (231.0)
suprahyoid portion (231.0)
skin of lip (232.0)

230.1 Esophagus

230.2 Stomach

Body of stomach	Cardiac orifice
Cardia of stomach	Pylorus
Fundus of stomach	

230.3 Colon

Appendix	Ileocecal valve
Cecum	Large intestine NOS

Excludes: *rectosigmoid junction (230.4)*

230.4 Rectum
Rectosigmoid junction

230.5 Anal canal
Anal sphincter

230.6 Anus, unspecified

Excludes: *anus:*
margin (232.5)
skin (232.5)
perianal skin (232.5)

230.7 Other and unspecified parts of intestine

Duodenum	Jejunum
Ileum	Small intestine NOS

Excludes: *ampulla of Vater (230.8)*

230.8 Liver and biliary system

Ampulla of Vater	Gallbladder
Common bile duct	Hepatic duct
Cystic duct	Sphincter of Oddi

230.9 Other and unspecified digestive organs

Digestive organ NOS	Pancreas
Gastrointestinal tract NOS	Spleen

231 Carcinoma in situ of respiratory system

231.0 Larynx

Cartilage:	Epiglottis:
arytenoid	NOS
cricoid	posterior surface
cuneiform	suprahyoid portion
thyroid	Vocal cords (false) (true)

Excludes: *aryepiglottic fold or interarytenoid fold:*
NOS (230.0)
hypopharyngeal aspect (230.0)
marginal zone (230.0)

231.1 Trachea

231.2 Bronchus and lung
Carina
Hilus of lung

Add 4th or 5th digit	Nonspecific code
Unspecified code	Manifestation code

231.8 Other specified parts of respiratory system
Accessory sinuses
Middle ear
Nasal cavities
Pleura

[Excludes:] *ear (external) (skin) (232.2)*
nose NOS (234.8)
skin (232.3)

231.9 Respiratory system, part unspecified
Respiratory organ NOS

232 Carcinoma in situ of skin
Includes: pigment cells

[Excludes:] *melanoma in situ of skin (172.0-172.9)*

232.0 Skin of lip

[Excludes:] *vermilion border of lip (230.0)*

232.1 Eyelid, including canthus

232.2 Ear and external auditory canal

232.3 Skin of other and unspecified parts of face

232.4 Scalp and skin of neck

232.5 Skin of trunk, except scrotum
Anus, margin
Axillary fold
Perianal skin
Skin of:
abdominal wall
anus
back
Skin of:
breast
buttock
chest wall
groin
perineum
Umbilicus

[Excludes:] *anal canal (230.5)*
anus NOS (230.6)
skin of genital organs (233.30-233.39, 233.5-233.6)

232.6 Skin of upper limb, including shoulder

232.7 Skin of lower limb, including hip

232.8 Other specified sites of skin

232.9 Skin, site unspecified

233 Carcinoma in situ of breast and genitourinary system

233.0 Breast

[Excludes:] *Paget's disease (174.0-174.9)*
skin of breast (232.5)

233.1 Cervix uteri
Adenocarcinoma in situ of cervix
Cervical intraepithelial glandular neoplasia, grade III
Cervical intraepithelial neoplasia III [CIN III]
Severe dysplasia of cervix

[Excludes:] *cervical intraepithelial neoplasia II [CIN II] (622.12)*
cytologic evidence of malignancy without histologic confirmation (795.06)
high grade squamous intraepithelial lesion (HGSIL) (795.04)
moderate dysplasia of cervix (622.12)

233.2 Other and unspecified parts of uterus

[5] **233.3 Other and unspecified female genital organs**

233.30 Unspecified female genital organ

233.31 Vagina
Severe dysplasia of vagina
Vaginal intraepithelial neoplasia III [VAIN III]

233.32 Vulva
Severe dysplasia of vulva
Vulvar intraepithelial neoplasia III [VIN III]

233.39 Other female genital organ

233.4 Prostate

233.5 Penis

233.6 Other and unspecified male genital organs

233.7 Bladder

233.9 Other and unspecified urinary organs

234 Carcinoma in situ of other and unspecified sites

234.0 Eye

> *Excludes:* *cartilage of eyelid (234.8)*
> *eyelid (skin) (232.1)*
> *optic nerve (234.8)*
> *orbital bone (234.8)*

234.8 Other specified sites
Endocrine gland [any]

234.9 Site unspecified
Carcinoma in situ NOS

NEOPLASMS OF UNCERTAIN BEHAVIOR (235-238)

Note: Categories 235-238 classify by site certain histo-morphologically well-defined neoplasms, the subsequent behavior of which cannot be predicted from the present appearance.

235 Neoplasm of uncertain behavior of digestive and respiratory systems

> *Excludes:* *stromal tumors of uncertain behavior of digestive system (238.1)*

235.0 Major salivary glands
Gland:
parotid
sublingual
submandibular

> *Excludes:* *minor salivary glands (235.1)*

235.1 Lip, oral cavity, and pharynx

Gingiva	Nasopharynx
Hypopharynx	Oropharynx
Minor salivary glands	Tongue
Mouth	

> *Excludes:* *aryepiglottic fold or interarytenoid fold, laryngeal aspect (235.6)*
> *epiglottis:*
> *NOS (235.6)*
> *suprahyoid portion (235.6)*
> *skin of lip (238.2)*

235.2 Stomach, intestines, and rectum
ALERT! For personal history of colonic polyps see V12.72

235.3 Liver and biliary passages

Ampulla of Vater	Gallbladder
Bile ducts [any]	Liver

235.4 Retroperitoneum and peritoneum

235.5 Other and unspecified digestive organs

Anal:	Esophagus
canal	Pancreas
sphincter	Spleen
Anus NOS	

> *Excludes:* *anus:*
> *margin (238.2)*
> *skin (238.2)*
> *perianal skin (238.2)*

235.6 Larynx

> *Excludes:* *aryepiglottic fold or interarytenoid fold:*
> *NOS (235.1)*
> *hypopharyngeal aspect (235.1)*
> *marginal zone (235.1)*

235.7 Trachea, bronchus, and lung

235.8 Pleura, thymus, and mediastinum

Add 4th or 5th digit	Nonspecific code	Unspecified code	Manifestation code

235.9 **Other and unspecified respiratory organs**
Accessory sinuses   Nasal cavities
Middle ear   Respiratory organ NOS

> Excludes: *ear (external) (skin) (238.2)*
>   *nose (238.8)*
>   *skin (238.2)*

236   **Neoplasm of uncertain behavior of genitourinary organs**

236.0   **Uterus**

236.1   **Placenta**
Chorioadenoma (destruens)
Invasive mole
Malignant hydatid mole
Malignant hydatidiform mole

236.2   **Ovary**
Use additional code, if desired, to identify any functional activity

236.3   **Other and unspecified female genital organs**

236.4   **Testis**
Use additional code, if desired, to identify any functional activity

236.5   **Prostate**

236.6   **Other and unspecified male genital organs**

236.7   **Bladder**

⑤ **236.9**   **Other and unspecified urinary organs**

     236.90   **Urinary organ, unspecified**

     236.91   **Kidney and ureter**

     236.99   **Other**

237   **Neoplasm of uncertain behavior of endocrine glands and nervous system**

237.0   **Pituitary gland and craniopharyngeal duct**
Use additional code, if desired, to identify any functional activity

237.1   **Pineal gland**

237.2   **Adrenal gland**
Suprarenal gland
Use additional code, if desired, to identify any functional activity

237.3   **Paraganglia**
Aortic body
Carotid body
Coccygeal body
Glomus jugulare

237.4   **Other and unspecified endocrine glands**
Parathyroid gland
Thyroid gland

237.5   **Brain and spinal cord**

237.6   **Meninges**
Meninges:
   NOS
   cerebral
   spinal

⑤ **237.7**   **Neurofibromatosis**

     237.70   **Neurofibromatosis, unspecified**

     237.71   **Neurofibromatosis, Type I [von Recklinghausen's disease]**

     237.72   **Neurofibromatosis, Type II [acoustic neurofibromatosis]**

     237.73   **Schwannomatosis**

     237.79   **Other neurofibromatosis**

237.9   **Other and unspecified parts of nervous system**
Cranial nerves

> Excludes: *peripheral, sympathetic, and parasympathetic nerves and ganglia (238.1)*

● Code new   ▲ Revision of   ④ ⑤ Fourth or fifth
   to 2012 edition   existing code   digit required

238 Neoplasm of uncertain behavior of other and unspecified sites and tissues

238.0 Bone and articular cartilage

[Excludes:] *cartilage:*
ear (238.1)
eyelid (238.1)
larynx (235.6)
nose (235.9)
synovia (238.1)

238.1 Connective and other soft tissue
Peripheral, sympathetic, and parasympathetic nerves and ganglia
Stromal tumors of digestive system

[Excludes:] *cartilage (of):*
articular (238.0)
larynx (235.6)
nose (235.9)
connective tissue of breast (238.3)

238.2 Skin

[Excludes:] *anus NOS (235.5)*
skin of genital organs (236.3, 236.6)
vermilion border of lip (235.1)

238.3 Breast

[Excludes:] *skin of breast (238.2)*

238.4 Polycythemia vera

238.5 Histiocytic and mast cells
Mast cell tumor NOS
Mastocytoma NOS

238.6 Plasma cells
Plasmacytoma NOS
Solitary myeloma

[5] **238.7 Other lymphatic and hematopoietic tissues**

[Excludes:] *acute myelogenous leukemia (205.0)*
chronic myelomonocytic leukemia (205.1)
myelosclerosis NOS (289.89)
myelosis:
NOS (205.9)
megakaryocytic (207.2)

238.71 Essential thrombocythemia
Essential hemorrhagic thrombocythemia
Essential thrombocytosis
Idiopathic (hemorrhagic) thrombocythemia
Primary thrombocytosis

238.72 Low grade myelodysplastic syndrome lesions
Refractory anemia (RA)
Refractory anemia (RA) with excess blasts-1 (RAEB-1)
Refractory anemia with ringed sideroblasts (RARS)
Refractory cytopenia with multilineage dysplasia (RCMD)
Refractory cytopenia with multilineage dysplasia and ringed sideroblasts (RCMD-RS)

238.73 High grade myelodysplastic syndrome lesions
Refractory anemia with excess blasts-2 (RAEB-2)

238.74 Myelodysplastic syndrome with 5q deletion
5q minus syndrome NOS

[Excludes:] *constitutional 5q deletion (758.39)*
high grade myelodysplastic syndrome with 5q deletion (238.73)

238.75 Myelodysplastic syndrome, unspecified

238.76 Myelofibrosis with myeloid metaplasia
Agnogenic myeloid metaplasia
Idiopathic myelofibrosis (chronic)
Myelosclerosis with myeloid metaplasia
Primary myelofibrosis

Excludes: *myelofibrosis NOS (289.83)*
myelophthisic anemia (284.2)
myelophthisis (284.2)
secondary myelofibrosis (289.83)

238.77 Post-transplant lymphoproliferative disorder (PTLD)
Code first complications of transplant (996.80-996.89)

238.79 Other lymphatic and hematopoietic tissues
Lymphoproliferative disease (chronic) NOS
Megakaryocytic myelosclerosis
Myeloproliferative disease (chronic) NOS
Panmyelosis (acute)

238.8 Other specified sites
Eye
Heart

Excludes: *eyelid (skin) (238.2)*
cartilage (238.1)

238.9 Site unspecified

NEOPLASMS OF UNSPECIFIED NATURE (239)

239 Neoplasms of unspecified nature
Note: Category 239 classifies by site neoplasms of unspecified morphology and behavior. The term "mass," unless otherwise stated, is not to be regarded as a neoplastic growth.
Includes: "growth" NOS
neoplasm NOS
new growth NOS
tumor NOS

239.0 Digestive system
Excludes: *anus:*
margin (239.2)
skin (239.2)
perianal skin (239.2)

239.1 Respiratory system

239.2 Bone, soft tissue, and skin
Excludes: *anal canal (239.0)*
anus NOS (239.0)
bone marrow (202.9)
cartilage:
larynx (239.1)
nose (239.1)
connective tissue of breast (239.3)
skin of genital organs (239.5)
vermilion border of lip (239.0)

239.3 Breast
Excludes: *skin of breast (239.2)*

239.4 Bladder

239.5 Other genitourinary organs

239.6 Brain
Excludes: *cerebral meninges (239.7)*
cranial nerves (239.7)

239.7 Endocrine glands and other parts of nervous system
Excludes: *peripheral, sympathetic, and parasympathetic nerves and ganglia (239.2)*

⑤ **239.8 Other specified sites**
Excludes: *eyelids (skin) (239.2)*
cartilage (239.2)
great vessels (239.2)
optic nerve (239.7)

● Code new
to 2012 edition   ▲ Revision of
existing code   ④ ⑤ Fourth or fifth
digit required

239.81 **Retina and choroid**
  Dark area on retina
  Retinal freckle

239.89 **Other specified sites**

239.9 **Site unspecified**

This page intentionally left blank.

● Code new
  to 2012 edition

▲ Revision of
  existing code

④ ⑤ Fourth or fifth
    digit required

Chapter 3: Endocrine, Nutritional, and Metabolic Diseases and Immunity Disorders (240-279)

DEFINITIONS AND CODING ALERTS

This chapter includes definitions of selected key words, terms and phrases and coding alerts for adding points to the clinical domain, references to coding late effects where appropriate, and references to personal history V-codes in situations where the acute or chronic condition is no longer active. An example from this chapter is as follows:

240 **Simple and unspecified goiter**
> **DEFINITION** Simple and unspecified goiter is a simple enlargement of the thyroid gland, causing a swelling in the front part of the neck.
> **ALERT!** For personal history of endocrine metabolic and immunity disorders see V12.2

MULTIPLE CODING FOR A SINGLE CONDITION

In addition to the etiology or manifestation convention that requires two codes to fully describe a single condition that affects multiple body systems, there are other single conditions that also require more than one code. "Use additional code" notes are found in the tabular at codes that are not part of an etiology or manifestation pair where a secondary code is useful to fully describe a condition. The sequencing rule is the same as the etiology or manifestation pair - , "use additional code" indicates that a secondary code should be added.

"Code first" notes are also under certain codes that are not specifically manifestation codes but may be due to an underlying cause. When a "code first" note is present and an underlying condition is present the underlying condition should be sequenced first.

"Code, if applicable, any causal condition first", notes indicate that this code may be assigned as a principal diagnosis when the causal condition is unknown or not applicable. If a causal condition is known, then the code for that condition should be sequenced as the principal or first-listed diagnosis. Multiple codes may be needed for late effects, complication codes and obstetric codes to more fully describe a condition. See the specific guidelines for these conditions for further instruction.

COMBINATION CODE

A combination code is a single code used to classify: two diagnoses, or a diagnosis with an associated secondary process (manifestation) A diagnosis with an associated complication Combination codes are identified by referring to subterm entries in the Alphabetic Index and by reading the inclusion and exclusion notes in the Tabular List.

Assign only the combination code when that code fully identifies the diagnostic conditions involved or when the Alphabetic Index so directs. Multiple coding should not be used when the classification provides a combination code that clearly identifies all of the elements documented in the diagnosis. When the combination code lacks necessary specificity in describing the manifestation or complication, an additional code should be used as a secondary code.

CODING LATE EFFECTS

A late effect is the residual effect (condition produced) after the acute phase of an illness or injury has terminated. There is no time limit on when a late effect code can be used. The residual may be apparent early, such as in cerebrovascular accident cases, or it may occur months or years later, such as that due to a previous injury. Coding of late effects generally requires two codes sequenced in the following order: The condition or nature of the late effect is sequenced first. The late effect code is sequenced second.

An exception to the above guidelines are those instances where the code for late effect is followed by a manifestation code identified in the Tabular List and title, or the late effect code has been expanded (at the fourth and fifth-digit levels) to include the manifestation(s). The code for the acute phase of an illness or injury that led to the late effect is never used with a code for the late effect.

DIABETES MELLITUS

Codes under category 250, Diabetes mellitus, identify complications or manifestations associated with diabetes mellitus. A fifth-digit is required for all category 250 codes to identify the type of diabetes mellitus and whether the diabetes is controlled or uncontrolled.

	Add 4th or 5th digit		Nonspecific code		Unspecified code		Manifestation code

Fifth-digits for category 250:

The following are the fifth-digits for the codes under category 250:

0   **type II or unspecified type, not stated as uncontrolled**
1   **type I, [juvenile type], not stated as uncontrolled**
2   **type II or unspecified type, uncontrolled**
3   **type I, [juvenile type], uncontrolled**

The age of a patient is not the sole determining factor, though most type I diabetics develop the condition before reaching puberty. For this reason type I diabetes mellitus is also referred to as juvenile diabetes.

Type of diabetes mellitus not documented

If the type of diabetes mellitus is not documented in the medical record the default is type II.

Diabetes mellitus and the use of insulin

All type I diabetics must use insulin to replace what their bodies do not produce. However, the use of insulin does not mean that a patient is a type I diabetic. Some patients with type II diabetes mellitus are unable to control their blood sugar through diet and oral medication alone and do require insulin. If the documentation in a medical record does not indicate the type of diabetes but does indicate that the patient uses insulin, the appropriate fifth-digit for type II must be used. For type II patients who routinely use insulin, code V58.67, Long-term (current) use of insulin, should also be assigned to indicate that the patient uses insulin. Code V58.67 should not be assigned if insulin is given temporarily to bring a type II patient's blood sugar under control during an encounter.

Assigning and sequencing diabetes codes and associated conditions

When assigning codes for diabetes and its associated conditions, the code(s) from category 250 must be sequenced before the codes for the associated conditions. The diabetes codes and the secondary codes that correspond to them are paired codes that follow the etiology or manifestation convention of the classification (See Official Guidelines, Section I.A.6., Etiology or manifestation convention). Assign as many codes from category 250 as needed to identify all of the associated conditions that the patient has. The corresponding secondary codes are listed under each of the diabetes codes.

A.   Diabetic retinopathy or diabetic macular edema

    Diabetic macular edema, code 362.07, is only present with diabetic retinopathy. Another code from subcategory 362.0, Diabetic retinopathy, must be used with code 362.07. Codes under subcategory 362.0 are diabetes manifestation codes, so they must be used following the appropriate diabetes code.

Diabetes mellitus in pregnancy and gestational diabetes

A.   Diabetes mellitus in pregnancy

    Diabetes mellitus is a significant complicating factor in pregnancy. Pregnant women who are diabetic should be assigned code 648.0x, Diabetes mellitus complicating pregnancy, and a secondary code from category 250, Diabetes mellitus, or category 249, Secondary diabetes to identify the type of diabetes.

    Code V58.67, Long-term (current) use of insulin, should also be assigned if the diabetes mellitus is being treated with insulin.

B.   Gestational diabetes

    Gestational diabetes can occur during the second and third trimester of pregnancy in women who were not diabetic prior to pregnancy. Gestational diabetes can cause complications in the pregnancy similar to those of pre-existing diabetes mellitus. It also puts the woman at greater risk of developing diabetes after the pregnancy. Gestational diabetes is coded to 648.8x, Abnormal glucose tolerance. Codes 648.0x and 648.8x should never be used together on the same record.

    Code V58.67, Long-term (current) use of insulin, should also be assigned if the gestational diabetes is being treated with insulin.

● Code new
   to 2012 edition
▲ Revision of
   existing code
④ ⑤ Fourth or fifth
   digit required

Insulin pump malfunction

A. Underdose of insulin due insulin pump failure

An underdose of insulin due to an insulin pump failure should be assigned 996.57, Mechanical complication due to insulin pump, as the principal or first listed code, followed by the appropriate diabetes mellitus code based on documentation.

B. Overdose of insulin due to insulin pump failure

The principal or first listed code for an encounter due to an insulin pump malfunction resulting in an overdose of insulin, should also be 996.57, Mechanical complication due to insulin pump, followed by code 962.3, Poisoning by insulins and antidiabetic agents, and the appropriate diabetes mellitus code based on documentation.

Secondary Diabetes Mellitus

Codes under category 249, Secondary diabetes mellitus, identify complications or manifestations associated with secondary diabetes mellitus. Secondary diabetes is always caused by another condition or event (e.g., cystic fibrosis, malignant neoplasm of pancreas, pancreatectomy, adverse effect of drug, or poisoning).

A. Fifth-digits for category 249:

A fifth-digit is required for all category 249 codes to identify whether the diabetes is controlled or uncontrolled.

B. Secondary diabetes mellitus and the use of insulin

For patients who routinely use insulin, code V58.67, Long-term (current) use of insulin, should also be assigned. Code V58.67 should not be assigned if insulin is given temporarily to bring a patient's blood sugar under control during an encounter.

C. Assigning and sequencing secondary diabetes codes and associated conditions

When assigning codes for secondary diabetes and its associated conditions (e.g. renal manifestations), the code(s) from category 249 must be sequenced before the codes for the associated conditions. The secondary diabetes codes and the diabetic manifestation codes that correspond to them are paired codes that follow the etiology or manifestation convention of the classification. Assign as many codes from category 249 as needed to identify all of the associated conditions that the patient has. The corresponding codes for the associated conditions are listed under each of the secondary diabetes codes. For example, secondary diabetes with diabetic nephrosis is assigned to code 249.40, followed by 581.81.

D. Assigning and sequencing secondary diabetes codes and its causes

The sequencing of the secondary diabetes codes in relationship to codes for the cause of the diabetes is based on the reason for the encounter, applicable ICD-9-CM sequencing conventions, and chapter-specific guidelines.

If a patient is seen for treatment of the secondary diabetes or one of its associated conditions, a code from category 249 is sequenced as the principal or first-listed diagnosis, with the cause of the secondary diabetes (e.g. cystic fibrosis) sequenced as an additional diagnosis.

If, however, the patient is seen for the treatment of the condition causing the secondary diabetes (e.g., malignant neoplasm of pancreas), the code for the cause of the secondary diabetes should be sequenced as the principal or first-listed diagnosis followed by a code from category 249.

1) Secondary diabetes mellitus due to pancreatectomy

For postpancreatectomy diabetes mellitus (lack of insulin due to the surgical removal of all or part of the pancreas), assign code 251.3, Postsurgical hypoinsulinemia. A code from subcategory 249 should not be assigned for secondary diabetes mellitus due to pancreatectomy. Code also any diabetic manifestations (e.g. diabetic nephrosis 581.81).

2) Secondary diabetes due to drugs

Secondary diabetes may be caused by an adverse effect of correctly administered medications, poisoning or late effect of poisoning.

| | Add 4th or 5th digit | | Nonspecific code | | Unspecified code | | Manifestation code |

See Chapter 17 for coding of adverse effects and poisoning.

See Chapter 19 for reporting of E codes.

3. ENDOCRINE, NUTRITIONAL AND METABOLIC DISEASES, AND IMMUNITY DISORDERS (240-279)

[Excludes:] *endocrine and metabolic disturbances specific to the fetus and newborn (775.0-775.9)*

Note: All neoplasms, whether functionally active or not, are classified in Chapter 2. Codes in Chapter 3 (i.e., 242.8, 246.0, 251-253, 255-259) may be used, if desired, to identify such functional activity associated with any neoplasm, or by ectopic endocrine tissue.

DISORDERS OF THYROID GLAND (240-246)

240 Simple and unspecified goiter

[DEFINITION] Simple and unspecified goiter is a simple enlargement of the thyroid gland, causing a swelling in the front part of the neck.

[ALERT!] For personal history of endocrine metabolic and immunity disorders see V12.2

240.0 Goiter, specified as simple

Any condition classifiable to 240.9, specified as simple

240.9 Goiter, unspecified

Enlargement of thyroid
Goiter or struma:
  NOS
  diffuse colloid
  endemic
Goiter or struma:
  hyperplastic
  nontoxic (diffuse)
  parenchymatous
  sporadic

[Excludes:] *congenital (dyshormonogenic) goiter (246.1)*

241 Nontoxic nodular goiter

[Excludes:] *adenoma of thyroid (226)*
cystadenoma of thyroid (226)

[DEFINITION] Nontoxic nodular goiter is a type of simple goiter with enlargement caused by nodules, or lumps, on the thyroid.

241.0 Nontoxic uninodular goiter

Thyroid nodule
Uninodular goiter (nontoxic)

241.1 Nontoxic multinodular goiter

Multinodular goiter (nontoxic)

241.9 Unspecified nontoxic nodular goiter

Adenomatous goiter
Nodular goiter (nontoxic) NOS
Struma nodosa (simplex)

[5] **242 Thyrotoxicosis with or without goiter**

[Excludes:] *neonatal thyrotoxicosis (775.3)*

The following fifth-digit subclassification is for use with category 242:

0 without mention of thyrotoxic crisis or storm

1 with mention of thyrotoxic crisis or storm

[DEFINITION] Thyrotoxicosis with or without goiter is a condition resulting from excessive concentrations of thyroid hormones in the body, as in hyperthyroidism.

[5] **242.0 Toxic diffuse goiter**
[0-1]
Basedow's disease
Exophthalmic or toxic goiter NOS
Graves' disease
Primary thyroid hyperplasia

[5] **242.1 Toxic uninodular goiter**
[0-1]
Thyroid nodule, toxic or with hyperthyroidism
Uninodular goiter, toxic or with hyperthyroidism

[5] **242.2 Toxic multinodular goiter**
[0-1]
Secondary thyroid hyperplasia

[5] **242.3 Toxic nodular goiter, unspecified**
[0-1]
Adenomatous goiter, toxic or with hyperthyroidism
Nodular goiter, toxic or with hyperthyroidism
Struma nodosa, toxic or with hyperthyroidism
Any condition classifiable to 241.9 specified as toxic or with hyperthyroidism

[5] **242.4 Thyrotoxicosis from ectopic thyroid nodule**
[0-1]

Add 4th or 5th digit | Nonspecific code | Unspecified code | Manifestation code

⑤ **242.8 Thyrotoxicosis of other specified origin**
[0-1] Overproduction of thyroid-stimulating hormone [TSH]
Thyrotoxicosis:
factitia
from ingestion of excessive thyroid material

Use additional E code to identify cause, if drug-induced

⑤ **242.9 Thyrotoxicosis without mention of goiter or other cause**
[0-1] Hyperthyroidism NOS
Thyrotoxicosis NOS

243 Congenital hypothyroidism
Congenital thyroid insufficiency
Cretinism (athyrotic) (endemic)

Use additional code to identify associated intellectual disabilities

[Excludes:] *congenital (dyshormonogenic) goiter (246.1)*

[DEFINITION] Congenital hypothyroidism is a congenital glandular disorder resulting from insufficient production of thyroid hormones .

244 Acquired hypothyroidism
Includes: athyroidism (acquired)
hypothyroidism (acquired)
myxedema (adult) (juvenile)
thyroid (gland) insufficiency (acquired)

[DEFINITION] Acquired hypothyroidism is an acquired glandular disorder resulting from insufficient production of thyroid hormones .

244.0 Postsurgical hypothyroidism

244.1 Other postablative hypothyroidism
Hypothyroidism following therapy, such as irradiation

244.2 Iodine hypothyroidism
Hypothyroidism resulting from administration or ingestion of iodide

[Excludes:] *hypothyroidism resulting from administration of radioactive iodine (244.1)*

Use additional E code to identify drug

244.3 Other iatrogenic hypothyroidism
Hypothyroidism resulting from:
P-aminosalicylic acid [PAS]
Phenylbutazone
Resorcinol
Iatrogenic hypothyroidism NOS

Use additional E code to identify drug

244.8 Other specified acquired hypothyroidism
Secondary hypothyroidism NEC

244.9 Unspecified hypothyroidism
Hypothyroidism, primary or NOS
Myxedema, primary or NOS

245 Thyroiditis

[DEFINITION] Thyroiditis is an inflammation of the thyroid gland.

245.0 Acute thyroiditis
Abscess of thyroid
Thyroiditis:
nonsuppurative, acute
pyogenic
suppurative

Use additional code to identify organism

245.1 Subacute thyroiditis
Thyroiditis:
de Quervain's
giant cell
Thyroiditis:
granulomatous
viral

245.2 Chronic lymphocytic thyroiditis
Hashimoto's disease
Struma lymphomatosa
Thyroiditis:
autoimmune
lymphocytic (chronic)

245.3 Chronic fibrous thyroiditis
Struma fibrosa
Thyroiditis:
invasive (fibrous)
ligneous
Riedel's

245.4 Iatrogenic thyroiditis
Use additional code to identify cause

245.8 Other and unspecified chronic thyroiditis
Chronic thyroiditis:
NOS
nonspecific

245.9 Thyroiditis, unspecified
Thyroiditis NOS

246 Other disorders of thyroid

246.0 Disorders of thyrocalcitonin secretion
Hypersecretion of calcitonin or thyrocalcitonin

246.1 Dyshormonogenic goiter
Congenital (dyshormonogenic) goiter
Goiter due to enzyme defect in synthesis of thyroid hormone
Goitrous cretinism (sporadic)

246.2 Cyst of thyroid
Excludes: cystadenoma of thyroid (226)

246.3 Hemorrhage and infarction of thyroid

246.8 Other specified disorders of thyroid

Abnormality of	Hyper-TBG-nemia
thyroid-binding globulin	Hypo-TBG-nemia
Atrophy of thyroid	

246.9 Unspecified disorder of thyroid

DISEASES OF OTHER ENDOCRINE GLANDS (249-259)

⑤ **249 Secondary diabetes mellitus**
Includes: diabetes mellitus (due to) (in) (secondary) (with):
drug-induced or chemical induced
infection

Excludes: gestational diabetes (648.8)
hyperglycemia NOS (790.29)
neonatal diabetes mellitus (775.1)
nonclinical diabetes (790.29)
Type I diabetes - see category 250
Type II diabetes - see category 250

The following fifth-digit subclassification is for use with category 249:

0   not stated as uncontrolled, or unspecified

1   uncontrolled

Use additional code to identify any associated insulin use (V58.67)

DEFINITION Secondary diabetes is always caused by another condition or event, such as cystic fibrosis, malignant neoplasm of the pancreas, pancreatectomy, adverse effect or drug or poisoning

ALERT! Codes under this category identify complications or manifestations associated with secondary diabetes

ALERT! When assigning codes for secondary diabetes and its associated conditions (e.g., renal manifestations), the code(s) from category 249 must be sequenced before the codes for the associated conditions

⑤ **249.0 Secondary diabetes mellitus without mention of complication**
[0-1]   Secondary diabetes mellitus without mention of complication or manifestation classifiable to 249.1-249.9
Secondary diabetes mellitus NOS

⑤ **249.1 Secondary diabetes mellitus with ketoacidosis**
[0-1]   Secondary diabetes mellitus with diabetic acidosis without mention of coma
Secondary diabetes mellitus with diabetic ketosis without mention of coma

⑤ **249.2 Secondary diabetes mellitus with hyperosmolarity**
[0-1]   Secondary diabetes mellitus with hyperosmolar (nonketotic) coma

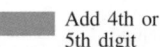 Add 4th or
5th digit

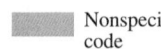 Nonspecific
code

Unspecified
code

Manifestation
code

⑤ **249.3 Secondary diabetes mellitus with other coma**
[0-1] Secondary diabetes mellitus with diabetic coma (with ketoacidosis)
Secondary diabetes mellitus with diabetic hypoglycemic coma
Secondary diabetes mellitus with insulin coma NOS

[Excludes:] *secondary diabetes mellitus with hyperosmolar coma (249.2)*

⑤ **249.4 Secondary diabetes mellitus with renal manifestations**
[0-1]
Use additional code to identify manifestation, as:
chronic kidney disease (585.1-585.9)
diabetic nephropathy NOS (583.81)
diabetic nephrosis (581.81)
intercapillary glomerulosclerosis (581.81)
Kimmelstiel-Wilson syndrome (581.81)

⑤ **249.5 Secondary diabetes mellitus with ophthalmic manifestations**
[0-1]
Use additional code to identify manifestation, as:
diabetic blindness (369.00-369.9)
diabetic cataract (366.41)
diabetic glaucoma (365.44)
diabetic macular edema (362.07)
diabetic retinal edema (362.07)
diabetic retinopathy (362.01-362.07)

⑤ **249.6 Secondary diabetes mellitus with neurological manifestations**
[0-1]
Use additional code to identify manifestation, as:
diabetic amyotrophy (353.5)
diabetic gastroparalysis (536.3)
diabetic gastroparesis (536.3)
diabetic mononeuropathy (354.0-355.9)
diabetic neurogenic arthropathy (713.5)
diabetic peripheral autonomic neuropathy (337.1)
diabetic polyneuropathy (357.2)

⑤ **249.7 Secondary diabetes mellitus with peripheral circulatory disorders**
[0-1]
Use additional code to identify manifestation, as:
diabetic gangrene (785.4)
diabetic peripheral angiopathy (443.81)

⑤ **249.8 Secondary diabetes mellitus with other specified manifestations**
[0-1] Secondary diabetic hypoglycemia in diabetes mellitus
Secondary hypoglycemic shock in diabetes mellitus

Use additional code to identify manifestation, as:
any associated ulceration (707.10-707.19, 707.8, 707.9)
diabetic bone changes (731.8)

⑤ **249.9 Secondary diabetes mellitus with unspecified complication**
[0-1]

⑤ **250 Diabetes mellitus**

[Excludes:] *gestational diabetes (648.8)*
hyperglycemia NOS (790.29)
neonatal diabetes mellitus (775.1)
nonclinical diabetes (790.29)
secondary diabetes (249.0-249.9)

The following fifth-digit subclassification is for use with category 250:

0 type II or unspecified type, not stated as uncontrolled
Fifth-digit 0 is for use with type II patients, even if the patient requires insulin
Use additional code, if applicable, for associated long-term (current) insulin use V58.67

1 type I [juvenile type], not stated as uncontrolled

2 type II or unspecified type, uncontrolled
Fifth-digit 2 is for use with type II patients, even if the patient requires insulin
Use additional code, if applicable, for associated long-term (current) insulin use V58.67

3 type I [juvenile type], uncontrolled

● Code new to 2012 edition ▲ Revision of existing code ④ ⑤ Fourth or fifth digit required

DEFINITION Diabetes mellitus is a condition in which the pancreas no longer produces enough insulin or cells stop responding to the insulin that is produced, so that glucose in the blood cannot be absorbed into the cells of the body. Symptoms include frequent urination, lethargy, excessive thirst, and hunger.

ALERT! A fifth-digit is required for all category 250 codes to identify the type of diabetes mellitus and whether the diabetes is controlled or uncontrolled

[5] **250.0 Diabetes mellitus without mention of complication**
[0-3] Diabetes mellitus without mention of complication or manifestation classifiable to 250.1-250.9
Diabetes (mellitus) NOS

[5] **250.1 Diabetes with ketoacidosis**
[0-3] Diabetic:
acidosis without mention of coma
ketosis without mention of coma

[5] **250.2 Diabetes with hyperosmolarity**
[0-3] Hyperosmolar (nonketotic) coma

[5] **250.3 Diabetes with other coma**
[0-3] Diabetic coma (with ketoacidosis)
Diabetic hypoglycemic coma
Insulin coma NOS

[*Excludes:*] *diabetes with hyperosmolar coma (250.2)*

[5] **250.4 Diabetes with renal manifestations**
[0-3]
Use additional code to identify manifestation, as:
chronic kidney disease (585.1-585.9)
diabetic:
nephropathy NOS (583.81)
nephrosis (581.81)
intercapillary glomerulosclerosis (581.81)
Kimmelstiel-Wilson syndrome (581.81)

[5] **250.5 Diabetes with ophthalmic manifestations**
[0-3]
Use additional code to identify manifestation, as:
diabetic:
blindness (369.00-369.9)
cataract (366.41)
glaucoma (365.44)
macular edema (362.07)
retinal edema (362.07)
retinopathy (362.01-362.07)

[5] **250.6 Diabetes with neurological manifestations**
[0-3]
Use additional code to identify manifestation, as:
diabetic:
amyotrophy (353.5)
gastroparalysis (536.3)
gastroparesis (536.3)
mononeuropathy (354.0-355.9)
neurogenic arthropathy (713.5)
peripheral autonomic neuropathy (337.1)
polyneuropathy (357.2)

[5] **250.7 Diabetes with peripheral circulatory disorders**
[0-3]
Use additional code to identify manifestation, as:
diabetic:
gangrene (785.4)
peripheral angiopathy (443.81)

[5] **250.8 Diabetes with other specified manifestations**
[0-3] Diabetic hypoglycemia NOS
Hypoglycemic shock NOS

Use additional code to identify manifestation, as:
any associated ulceration (707.10-707.19, 707.8, 707.9)
diabetic bone changes (731.8)

[5] **250.9 Diabetes with unspecified complication**
[0-3]

251 Other disorders of pancreatic internal secretion

Add 4th or 5th digit | Nonspecific code | Unspecified code | Manifestation code

251.0 Hypoglycemic coma
Iatrogenic hyperinsulinism
Non-diabetic insulin coma

Use additional E code to identify cause, if drug-induced

[Excludes:] *hypoglycemic coma in diabetes mellitus (249.3, 250.3)*

251.1 Other specified hypoglycemia
Hyperinsulinism:
NOS
ectopic
functional
Hyperplasia of pancreatic islet beta cells NOS

[Excludes:] *hypoglycemia in diabetes mellitus (249.8, 250.8)*
hypoglycemia in infant of diabetic mother (775.0)
hypoglycemic coma (251.0)
neonatal hypoglycemia (775.6)

Use additional E code to identify cause, if drug-induced

251.2 Hypoglycemia, unspecified
Hypoglycemia:
NOS
reactive
spontaneous

[Excludes:] *hypoglycemia:*
with coma (251.0)
in diabetes mellitus (249.8, 250.8)
leucine-induced (270.3)

[DEFINITION] Hypoglycemia is the medical term for abnormally low blood sugar usually resulting from excessive insulin or a poor diet.

251.3 Postsurgical hypoinsulinemia
Hypoinsulinemia following complete or partial pancreatectomy
Postpancreatectomy hyperglycemia

Use additional code to identify (any associated):
acquired absence of pancreas (V88.11-V88.12)
insulin use (V58.67)
secondary diabetes mellitus (249.00-249.91)

[Excludes:] *transient hyperglycemia post procedure (790.29)*
transient hypoglycemia post procedure (251.2)

251.4 Abnormality of secretion of glucagon
Hyperplasia of pancreatic islet alpha cells with glucagon excess

251.5 Abnormality of secretion of gastrin
Hyperplasia of pancreatic alpha cells with gastrin excess
Zollinger-Ellison syndrome

251.8 Other specified disorders of pancreatic internal secretion

251.9 Unspecified disorder of pancreatic internal secretion
Islet cell hyperplasia NOS

252 Disorders of parathyroid gland

[Excludes:] *hungry bone syndrome (275.5)*

[DEFINITION] Parathyroid glands are small endocrine glands in the neck that produce parathyroid hormone. Humans have four parathyroid glands, which are usually located behind the thyroid gland.

[DEFINITION] Disorders of parathyroid gland refers to disorders involving excessive or deficient blood levels of parathyroid hormone caused by abnormal functioning of the parathyroid gland.

⑤ **252.0 Hyperparathyroidism**

[Excludes:] *ectopic hyperparathyroidism (259.3)*

252.00 Hyperparathyroidism, unspecified

252.01 Primary hyperparathyroidism
Hyperplasia of parathyroid

252.02 Secondary hyperparathyroidism, non-renal

[Excludes:] *secondary hyperparathyroidism (of renal origin) (588.81)*

252.08 Other hyperparathyroidism
Tertiary hyperparathyroidism

● Code new to 2012 edition
▲ Revision of existing code
④ ⑤ Fourth or fifth digit required

252.1 Hypoparathyroidism
Parathyroiditis (autoimmune)
Tetany:
    parathyroid
    parathyroprival

Excludes: *pseudohypoparathyroidism (275.4)*
        pseudo-pseudohypoparathyroidism (275.4)
        tetany NOS (781.7)
        transitory neonatal hypoparathyroidism (775.4)

252.8 Other specified disorders of parathyroid gland
Cyst of parathyroid gland
Hemorrhage of parathyroid gland

252.9 Unspecified disorder of parathyroid gland

253 Disorders of the pituitary gland and its hypothalamic control
Includes: the listed conditions whether the disorder is in the pituitary or the hypothalamus

Excludes: *Cushing's syndrome (255.0)*

DEFINITION Disorders of the pituitary gland and its hypothalamic control refers to congenital or acquired abnormalities in the structure or function of the pituitary gland.

253.0 Acromegaly and gigantism
Overproduction of growth hormone

253.1 Other and unspecified anterior pituitary hyperfunction
Forbes-Albright syndrome

Excludes: *overproduction of:*
        ACTH (255.3)
        thyroid-stimulating hormone [TSH] (242.8)

253.2 Panhypopituitarism

Cachexia, pituitary	Sheehan's syndrome
Necrosis of pituitary	Simmonds' disease
(postpartum)	
Pituitary insufficiency NOS	

Excludes: *iatrogenic hypopituitarism (253.7)*

253.3 Pituitary dwarfism
Isolated deficiency of (human) growth hormone [HGH]
Lorain-Levi dwarfism

253.4 Other anterior pituitary disorders
Isolated or partial deficiency of an anterior pituitary hormone, other than growth
    hormone
Prolactin deficiency

253.5 Diabetes insipidus
Vasopressin deficiency

Excludes: *nephrogenic diabetes insipidus (588.1)*

253.6 Other disorders of neurohypophysis
Syndrome of inappropriate secretion of antidiuretic hormone [ADH]

Excludes: *ectopic antidiuretic hormone secretion (259.3)*

253.7 Iatrogenic pituitary disorders
Hypopituitarism:
    hormone-induced
    hypophysectomy-induced
    postablative
    radiotherapy-induced

Use additional E code to identify cause

**253.8 Other disorders of the pituitary and other syndromes of diencephalohypophyseal
    origin**

Abscess of pituitary	Cyst of Rathke's pouch
Adiposogenital dystrophy	Fröhlich's syndrome

Excludes: *craniopharyngioma (237.0)*

253.9 Unspecified
Dyspituitarism

Add 4th or	Nonspecific	Unspecified	Manifestation
5th digit	code	code	code

254 Diseases of thymus gland

[Excludes:] *aplasia or dysplasia with immunodeficiency (279.2)*
hypoplasia with immunodeficiency (279.2)
myasthenia gravis (358.00-358.01)

DEFINITION The thymus is a gland located behind the breastbone that functions in the development of the immune system. The thymus is large in infancy and early childhood but begins to atrophy between ages eight and ten.

254.0 Persistent hyperplasia of thymus
Hypertrophy of thymus

254.1 Abscess of thymus

254.8 Other specified diseases of thymus gland
Atrophy of thymus
Cyst of thymus

[Excludes] *thymoma (212.6)*

254.9 Unspecified disease of thymus gland

255 Disorders of adrenal glands
Includes: the listed conditions whether the basic disorder is in the adrenals or is pituitary-induced

DEFINITION The adrenal glands are located on each kidney and secrete hormones regulating metabolism, sexual function, water balance, and stress.

255.0 Cushing's syndrome
Adrenal hyperplasia due to excess ACTH
Cushing's syndrome:
NOS
iatrogenic
idiopathic
pituitary-dependent
Ectopic ACTH syndrome
Iatrogenic syndrome of excess cortisol
Overproduction of cortisol

[Excludes:] *congenital adrenal hyperplasia (255.2)*

Use additional E code to identify cause, if drug-induced

DEFINITION Cushing's syndrome is a condition due to tumors of the adrenal cortex or the anterior lobe of the pituitary gland.

⑤ **255.1 Hyperaldosteronism**

255.10 Hyperaldosteronism, unspecified
Aldosteronism NOS
Primary aldosteronism, unspecified

[Excludes:] *Conn's syndrome (255.12)*

255.11 Glucocorticoid-remediable aldosteronism
Familial aldosteronism type I

[Excludes:] *Conn's syndrome (255.12)*

255.12 Conn's syndrome

255.13 Bartter's syndrome

255.14 Other secondary aldosteronism

255.2 Adrenogenital disorders
Adrenogenital syndromes, virilizing or feminizing, whether acquired or associated with congenital adrenal hyperplasia consequent on inborn enzyme defects in hormone synthesis
Achard-Thiers syndrome
Congenital adrenal hyperplasia
Female adrenal pseudohermaphroditism
Male:
macrogenitosomia praecox
sexual precocity with adrenal hyperplasia
Virilization (female) (suprarenal)

[Excludes:] *adrenal hyperplasia due to excess ACTH (255.0)*
isosexual virilization (256.4)

255.3 Other corticoadrenal overactivity
Acquired benign adrenal androgenic overactivity
Overproduction of ACTH

⑤ **255.4 Corticoadrenal insufficiency**

[Excludes:] *tuberculous Addison's disease (017.6)*

● Code new to 2012 edition ▲ Revision of existing code ④ ⑤ Fourth or fifth digit required

255.41 Glucocorticoid deficiency
Addisonian crisis
Addison's disease NOS
Adrenal atrophy (autoimmune)
Adrenal calcification
Adrenal crisis
Adrenal hemorrhage
Adrenal infarction
Adrenal insufficiency NOS
Combined glucocorticoid and mineralocorticoid deficiency
Corticoadrenal insufficiency NOS

255.42 Mineralocorticoid deficiency
Hypoaldosteronism

Excludes: *combined glucocorticoid and mineralocorticoid deficiency (255.41)*

255.5 Other adrenal hypofunction
Adrenal medullary insufficiency

Excludes: *Waterhouse-Friderichsen syndrome (meningococcal) (036.3)*

255.6 Medulloadrenal hyperfunction
Catecholamine secretion by pheochromocytoma

255.8 Other specified disorders of adrenal glands
Abnormality of cortisol-binding globulin

255.9 Unspecified disorder of adrenal glands

256 Ovarian dysfunction
DEFINITION Ovarian dysfunction refers to improper functioning of the ovaries.

256.0 Hyperestrogenism

256.1 Other ovarian hyperfunction
Hypersecretion of ovarian androgens

256.2 Postablative ovarian failure
Use additional code for states associated with artifical menopause (627.4)
Ovarian failure:
iatrogenic
postirradiation
postsurgical

Excludes: *asymptomatic age-related (natural) postmenopausal status (V49.81)*
acquired absence of ovary (V45.77)

⑤ **256.3 Other ovarian failure**
Use additional code for states associated with natural menopause (627.2)
Excludes: *asymptomatic age-related (natural) postmenopausal status (V49.81)*

256.31 Premature menopause

256.39 Other ovarian failure
Delayed menarche
Ovarian hypofunction
Primary ovarian failure NOS

256.4 Polycystic ovaries
Isosexual virilization
Stein-Leventhal syndrome

256.8 Other ovarian dysfunction

256.9 Unspecified ovarian dysfunction

257 Testicular dysfunction
DEFINITION Testicular dysfunction refers to improper functioning of the testicles.

257.0 Testicular hyperfunction
Hypersecretion of testicular hormones

257.1 Postablative testicular hypofunction
Testicular hypofunction:
iatrogenic
postirradiation
postsurgical

	Add 4th or 5th digit		Nonspecific code		Unspecified code		Manifestation code

257.2 Other testicular hypofunction
Defective biosynthesis of testicular androgen
Eunuchoidism:
NOS
hypogonadotropic
Failure:
Leydig's cell, adult
seminiferous tubule, adult
Testicular hypogonadism

[Excludes:] *azoospermia (606.0)*

257.8 Other testicular dysfunction

[Excludes:] *androgen insensitivity syndromes (259.50-259.52)*

257.9 Unspecified testicular dysfunction

258 Polyglandular dysfunction and related disorders

DEFINITION Polyglandular dysfunction and related disorders refers to dysfunctional disorders involving multiple glands.

[5] **258.0 Polyglandular activity in multiple endocrine adenomatosis**
Multiple endocrine neoplasia [MEN] syndromes

Use additional codes to identify any malignancies and other conditions associated with the syndromes

258.01 Multiple endocrine neoplasia [MEN] type I
Wermer's syndrome

258.02 Multiple endocrine neoplasia [MEN] type IIA
Sipple's syndrome

258.03 Multiple endocrine neoplasia [MEN] type IIB

258.1 Other combinations of endocrine dysfunction
Lloyd's syndrome
Schmidt's syndrome

258.8 Other specified polyglandular dysfunction

258.9 Polyglandular dysfunction, unspecified

259 Other endocrine disorders

DEFINITION Endocrine disorders refers to disorders which involve the over-production or under-production of hormone substances from an endocrine gland. Examples include diabetes, hypothyroidism, hyperthyroidism, hyperparathyroidism, cushing's disease, cushing's syndrome and acromegaly.

259.0 Delay in sexual development and puberty, not elsewhere classified
Delayed puberty

259.1 Precocious sexual development and puberty, not elsewhere classified
Sexual precocity:
NOS
constitutional
cryptogenic
idiopathic

259.2 Carcinoid syndrome
Hormone secretion by carcinoid tumors

259.3 Ectopic hormone secretion, not elsewhere classified
Ectopic:
antidiuretic hormone secretion [ADH]
hyperparathyroidism

[Excludes:] *ectopic ACTH syndrome (255.0)*

259.4 Dwarfism, not elsewhere classified
Dwarfism:
NOS
constitutional

[Excludes:] *dwarfism:*
achondroplastic (756.4)
intrauterine (759.7)
nutritional (263.2)
pituitary (253.3)
renal (588.0)
progeria (259.8)

[5] **259.5 Androgen insensitivity syndrome**

259.50 Androgen insensitivity, unspecified

259.51 Androgen insensitivity syndrome
Complete androgen insensitivity
de Quervain's syndrome
Goldberg-Maxwell Syndrome

259.52 Partial androgen insensitivity
Partial androgen insensitivity syndrome
Reifenstein syndrome

259.8 Other specified endocrine disorders
Pineal gland dysfunction
Progeria

259.9 Unspecified endocrine disorder
Disturbance:
endocrine NOS
hormone NOS
Infantilism NOS

NUTRITIONAL DEFICIENCIES (260-269)

[Excludes:] *deficiency anemias (280.0-281.9)*

[ALERT!] For personal history of nutritional deficiency see V12.1

260 Kwashiorkor
Nutritional edema with dyspigmentation of skin and hair

[DEFINITION] Kwashiorkor is a virulent form of childhood malnutrition characterized by edema, irritability, anorexia, ulcerating dermatoses, and an enlarged liver with fatty infiltrates.

261 Nutritional marasmus
Nutritional atrophy
Severe calorie deficiency
Severe malnutrition NOS

[DEFINITION] Nutritional marasmus is extreme malnutrition and emaciation, especially in children; resulting from inadequate intake of food.

262 Other severe protein-calorie malnutrition
Nutritional edema without mention of dyspigmentation of skin and hair

263 Other and unspecified protein-calorie malnutrition

263.0 Malnutrition of moderate degree

263.1 Malnutrition of mild degree

263.2 Arrested development following protein-calorie malnutrition
Nutritional dwarfism
Physical retardation due to malnutrition

263.8 Other protein-calorie malnutrition

263.9 Unspecified protein-calorie malnutrition
Dystrophy due to malnutrition
Malnutrition (calorie) NOS

[Excludes:] *nutritional deficiency NOS (269.9)*

264 Vitamin A deficiency

[DEFINITION] Vitamin A deficiency may result in abnormal visual adaptation to darkness (night blindness), dry skin, dry hair, broken fingernails, and decreased resistance to infections .

264.0 With conjunctival xerosis

264.1 With conjunctival xerosis and Bitot's spot
Bitot's spot in the young child

264.2 With corneal xerosis

264.3 With corneal ulceration and xerosis

264.4 With keratomalacia

264.5 With night blindness

264.6 With xerophthalmic scars of cornea

264.7 Other ocular manifestations of vitamin A deficiency
Xerophthalmia due to vitamin A deficiency

264.8 Other manifestations of vitamin A deficiency
Follicular keratosis due to vitamin A deficiency
Xeroderma due to vitamin A deficiency

264.9 Unspecified vitamin A deficiency
Hypovitaminosis A NOS

265 **Thiamine and niacin deficiency states**

> DEFINITION Thiamine, aka vitamin B1, is a vitamin of the B complex, found in meat, yeast, and the bran coat of grains, necessary for carbohydrate metabolism and normal neural activity. Niacin, aka nicotinic acid, is a component of the vitamin b complex found in meat, wheat germ, dairy products, and yeast. .

265.0 **Beriberi**

265.1 **Other and unspecified manifestations of thiamine deficiency**

> Other vitamin B_1 deficiency states

265.2 **Pellagra**

> Deficiency:
>   niacin (-tryptophan)
>   nicotinamide
>   nicotinic acid
>   vitamin PP
> Pellagra (alcoholic)

266 **Deficiency of B-complex components**

266.0 **Ariboflavinosis**

> Riboflavin [vitamin B_2] deficiency

266.1 **Vitamin B_6 deficiency**

> Deficiency: Vitamin B_6 deficiency syndrome
>   pyridoxal
>   pyridoxamine
>   pyridoxine

> *Excludes:* *vitamin B_6-responsive sideroblastic anemia (285.0)*

266.2 **Other B-complex deficiencies**

> Deficiency:
>   cyanocobalamin
>   folic acid
>   vitamin B_{12}

> *Excludes:* *combined system disease with anemia (281.0-281.1)*
>   *deficiency anemias (281.0-281.9)*
>   *subacute degeneration of spinal cord with anemia (281.0-281.1)*

266.9 **Unspecified vitamin B deficiency**

267 **Ascorbic acid deficiency**

> Deficiency of vitamin C
> Scurvy

> *Excludes:* *scorbutic anemia (281.8)*

> DEFINITION Ascorbic acid deficiency, refers to a deficiency of ascorbic acid, aka vitamin c is found in citrus fruits, tomatoes, potatoes, and leafy green vegetables and used to prevent scurvy.

268 **Vitamin D deficiency**

> *Excludes:* *vitamin D-resistant:*
>   *osteomalacia (275.3)*
>   *rickets (275.3)*

> DEFINITION Vitamin D deficiency, refers to a deficiency of vitamin D2 or D3, required for normal growth of teeth and bones, and produced in general by ultraviolet irradiation of sterols found in milk, fish, and eggs.

268.0 **Rickets, active**

> *Excludes:* *celiac rickets (579.0)*
>   *renal rickets (588.0)*

268.1 **Rickets, late effect**

> Any condition specified as due to rickets and stated to be a late effect or sequela of rickets

> *Code first the nature of late effect*

268.2 **Osteomalacia, unspecified**

268.9 **Unspecified vitamin D deficiency**

> Avitaminosis D

269 **Other nutritional deficiencies**

> DEFINITION Nutritional deficiencies refers to a disease caused by a deficiency of a particular nutrient such as minerals, vitamins, carbohydrates, fats and proteins.

● Code new to 2012 edition   ▲ Revision of existing code   ④ ⑤ Fourth or fifth digit required

269.0 Deficiency of vitamin K

> *Excludes:* *deficiency of coagulation factor due to vitamin K deficiency (286.7)*
> *vitamin K deficiency of newborn (776.0)*

269.1 Deficiency of other vitamins
  Deficiency:
    vitamin E
    vitamin P

269.2 Unspecified vitamin deficiency
  Multiple vitamin deficiency NOS

269.3 Mineral deficiency, not elsewhere classified
  Deficiency:
    calcium, dietary
    iodine

> *Excludes:* *deficiency:*
> *calcium NOS (275.4)*
> *potassium (276.8)*
> *sodium (276.1)*

269.8 Other nutritional deficiency

> *Excludes:* *adult failure to thrive (783.7)*
> *failure to thrive in childhood (783.41)*
> *feeding problems (783.3)*
> *newborn (779.31-779.34)*

269.9 Unspecified nutritional deficiency

OTHER METABOLIC AND IMMUNITY DISORDERS (270-279)

Use additional code to identify any associated intellectual disabilities

270 Disorders of amino-acid transport and metabolism

> *Excludes:* *abnormal findings without manifest disease (790.0-796.9)*
> *disorders of purine and pyrimidine metabolism (277.1-277.2)*
> *gout (274.00-274.9)*

270.0 Disturbances of amino-acid transport
  Cystinosis
  Cystinuria
  Fanconi (-de Toni) (-Debré) syndrome
  Glycinuria (renal)
  Hartnup disease

270.1 Phenylketonuria [PKU]
  Hyperphenylalaninemia

270.2 Other disturbances of aromatic amino-acid metabolism

Albinism	Hypertyrosinemia
Alkaptonuria	Indicanuria
Alkaptonuric ochronosis	Kynureninase defects
Disturbances of metabolism	Oasthouse urine disease
of tyrosine and	Ochronosis
tryptophan	Tyrosinosis
Homogentisic acid defects	Tyrosinuria
Hydroxykynureninuria	Waardenburg syndrome

> *Excludes:* *vitamin B6-deficiency syndrome (266.1)*

270.3 Disturbances of branched-chain amino-acid metabolism
  Disturbances of metabolism of leucine, isoleucine, and valine
  Hypervalinemia
  Intermittent branched-chain ketonuria
  Leucine-induced hypoglycemia
  Leucinosis
  Maple syrup urine disease

270.4 Disturbances of sulphur-bearing amino-acid metabolism
  Cystathioninemia
  Cystathioninuria
  Disturbances of metabolism of methionine, homocystine, and cystathionine
  Homocystinuria
  Hypermethioninemia
  Methioninemia

Add 4th or 5th digit	Nonspecific code	Unspecified code	Manifestation code

270.5 Disturbances of histidine metabolism
Carnosinemia
Histidinemia
Hyperhistidinemia
Imidazole aminoaciduria

270.6 Disorders of urea cycle metabolism
Argininosuccinic aciduria
Citrullinemia
Disorders of metabolism of ornithine, citrulline, argininosuccinic acid, arginine, and ammonia
Hyperammonemia
Hyperornithinemia

270.7 Other disturbances of straight-chain amino-acid metabolism
Glucoglycinuria
Glycinemia (with methyl-malonic acidemia)
Hyperglycinemia
Hyperlysinemia
Pipecolic acidemia
Saccharopinuria
Other disturbances of metabolism of glycine, threonine, serine, glutamine, and lysine

270.8 Other specified disorders of amino-acid metabolism
Alaninemia
Ethanolaminuria
Glycoprolinuria
Hydroxyprolinemia
Hyperprolinemia
Iminoacidopathy
Prolinemia
Prolinuria
Sarcosinemia

270.9 Unspecified disorder of amino-acid metabolism

271 Disorders of carbohydrate transport and metabolism

Excludes: abnormality of secretion of glucagon (251.4)
diabetes mellitus (249.0-249.9, 250.0-250.9)
hypoglycemia NOS (251.2)
mucopolysaccharidosis (277.5)

271.0 Glycogenosis
Amylopectinosis
Glucose-6-phosphatase deficiency
Glycogen storage disease
McArdle's disease
Pompe's disease
von Gierke's disease

271.1 Galactosemia
Galactose-1-phosphate uridyl transferase deficiency
Galactosuria

271.2 Hereditary fructose intolerance
Essential benign fructosuria
Fructosemia

271.3 Intestinal disaccharidase deficiencies and disaccharide malabsorption
Intolerance or malabsorption (congenital) (of):
glucose-galactose
lactose
sucrose-isomaltose

271.4 Renal glycosuria
Renal diabetes

271.8 Other specified disorders of carbohydrate transport and metabolism
Essential benign pentosuria
Fucosidosis
Glycolic aciduria
Hyperoxaluria (primary)
Mannosidosis
Oxalosis
Xylosuria
Xylulosuria

271.9 Unspecified disorder of carbohydrate transport and metabolism

272 Disorders of lipoid metabolism

Excludes: localized cerebral lipidoses (330.1)

272.0 Pure hypercholesterolemia
Familial hypercholesterolemia
Fredrickson Type IIa hyperlipoproteinemia
Hyperbetalipoproteinemia
Hyperlipidemia, Group A
Low-density-lipoid-type [LDL] hyperlipoproteinemia

● Code new to 2012 edition   ▲ Revision of existing code   ④ ⑤ Fourth or fifth digit required

272.1 Pure hyperglyceridemia
Endogenous hyperglyceridemia
Frederickson Type IV hyperlipoproteinemia
Hyperlipidemia, Group B
Hyperprebetalipoproteinemia
Hypertriglyceridemia, essential
Very-low-density-lipoid-type [VLDL] hyperlipoproteinemia

272.2 Mixed hyperlipidemia
Broad- or floating-betalipoproteinemia
Combined hyperlipidemia
Elevated cholesterol with elevated triglycerides NEC
Fredrickson Type IIb or III hyperlipoproteinemia
Hypercholesterolemia with endogenous hyperglyceridemia
Hyperbetalipoproteinemia with prebetalipoproteinemia
Tubo-eruptive xanthoma
Xanthoma tuberosum

272.3 Hyperchylomicronemia
Bürger-Grütz syndrome
Fredrickson type I or V hyperlipoproteinemia
Hyperlipidemia, Group D
Mixed hyperglyceridemia

272.4 Other and unspecified hyperlipidemia
Alpha-lipoproteinemia
Hyperlipidemia NOS
Hyperlipoproteinemia NOS

272.5 Lipoprotein deficiencies
Abetalipoproteinemia
Bassen-Kornzweig syndrome
High-density lipoid deficiency
Hypoalphalipoproteinemia
Hypobetalipoproteinemia (familial)

272.6 Lipodystrophy
Barraquer-Simons disease
Progressive lipodystrophy
Use additional E code to identify cause, if iatrogenic

> Excludes: *intestinal lipodystrophy (040.2)*

272.7 Lipidoses

Chemically-induced lipidosis	Disease:
Disease:	triglyceride storage, Type I or II
Anderson's	Wolman's or triglyceride storage, Type III
Fabry's	Mucolipidosis II
Gaucher's	Primary familial xanthomatosis
I cell [mucolipidosis I]	
lipoid storage NOS	
Neimann-Pick	
pseudo-Hurler's or	
mucolipidosis III	

> Excludes: *cerebral lipidoses (330.1)*
> *Tay-Sachs disease (330.1)*

272.8 Other disorders of lipoid metabolism
Hoffa's disease or liposynovitis prepatellaris
Launois-Bensaude's lipomatosis
Lipoid dermatoarthritis

272.9 Unspecified disorder of lipoid metabolism

273 Disorders of plasma protein metabolism

> Excludes: *agammaglobulinemia and hypogammaglobulinemia (279.0 -279.2)*
> *coagulation defects (286.0-286.9)*
> *hereditary hemolytic anemias (282.0-282.9)*

273.0 Polyclonal hypergammaglobulinemia
Hypergammaglobulinemic purpura:
benign primary
Waldenström's

Add 4th or 5th digit	Nonspecific code	Unspecified code	Manifestation code

273.1 Monoclonal paraproteinemia
Benign monoclonal hypergammaglobulinemia [BMH]
Monoclonal gammopathy:
NOS
associated with lymphoplasmacytic dyscrasias
benign
Paraproteinemia:
benign (familial)
secondary to malignant or inflammatory disease

273.2 Other paraproteinemias
Cryoglobulinemic:
purpura
vasculitis
Mixed cryoglobulinemia

273.3 Macroglobulinemia
Macroglobulinemia (idiopathic) (primary)
Waldenström's macroglobulinemia

273.4 Alpha-1-antitrypsin deficiency
AAT deficiency

273.8 Other disorders of plasma protein metabolism
Abnormality of transport protein
Bisalbuminemia

273.9 Unspecified disorder of plasma protein metabolism

274 Gout

[Excludes:] *lead gout (984.0-984.9)*

[DEFINITION] Gout is a painful inflammation of the big toe and foot caused by defects in uric acid metabolism resulting in deposits of the acid and its salts in the blood and joints.

⑤ **274.0 Gouty arthropathy**

274.00 Gout arthropathy, unspecified

274.01 Acute gouty arthropathy
Acute gout
Gout attack
Gout flare
Podagra

274.02 Chronic gouty arthropathy without mention of tophus (tophi)
Chronic gout

274.03 Chronic gouty arthropathy with tophus (tophi)
Chronic tophaceous gout
Gout with tophi NOS

⑤ **274.1 Gouty nephropathy**

274.10 Gouty nephropathy, unspecified

274.11 Uric acid nephrolithiasis

274.19 Other

⑤ **274.8 Gout with other specified manifestations**

274.81 Gouty tophi of ear

274.82 Gouty tophi of other sites
Gouty tophi of heart

[Excludes:] *gout with tophi NOS (274.03)*
gouty arthropathy with tophi (274.03)

274.89 Other
Use additional code to identify manifestations, as:
gouty:
iritis (364.11)
neuritis (357.4)

274.9 Gout, unspecified

275 Disorders of mineral metabolism

[Excludes:] *abnormal findings without manifest disease (790.0-796.9)*

⑤ **275.0 Disorders of iron metabolism**

[Excludes:] *anemia:*
iron deficiency (280.0-280.9)
sideroblastic (285.0)

● Code new to 2012 edition ▲ Revision of existing code ④ ⑤ Fourth or fifth digit required

275.01 Hereditary hemochromatosis
Bronzed diabetes
Pigmentary cirrhosis (of liver)
Primary (hereditary) hemochromatosis

275.02 Hemochromatosis due to repeated red blood cell transfusions
Iron overload due to repeated red blood cell transfusions
Transfusion (red blood cell) associated hemochromatosis

275.03 Other hemochromatosis
Hemochromatosis NOS

275.09 Other disorders of iron metabolism

275.1 Disorders of copper metabolism
Hepatolenticular degeneration
Wilson's disease

275.2 Disorders of magnesium metabolism
Hypermagnesemia
Hypomagnesemia

275.3 Disorders of phosphorus metabolism
Familial hypophosphatemia
Hypophosphatasia
Vitamin D-resistant:
osteomalacia
rickets

[5] **275.4 Disorders of calcium metabolism**

[Excludes:] *hungry bone syndrome (275.5)*
parathyroid disorders (252.00-252.9)
vitamin D deficiency (268.0-268.9)

275.40 Unspecified disorder of calcium metabolism

275.41 Hypocalcemia

275.42 Hypercalcemia

275.49 Other disorders of calcium metabolism
Nephrocalcinosis
Pseudohypoparathyroidism
Pseudopseudohypoparathyroidism

275.5 Hungry bone syndrome

275.8 Other specified disorders of mineral metabolism

275.9 Unspecified disorder of mineral metabolism

276 Disorders of fluid, electrolyte, and acid-base balance

[Excludes:] *diabetes insipidus (253.5)*
familial periodic paralysis (359.3)

276.0 Hyperosmolality and/or hypernatremia
Sodium [Na] excess
Sodium [Na] overload

276.1 Hyposmolality and/or hyponatremia
Sodium [Na] deficiency

276.2 Acidosis
Acidosis:
NOS
lactic
metabolic
respiratory

[Excludes:] *diabetic acidosis (249.1, 250.1)*

276.3 Alkalosis
Alkalosis:
NOS
metabolic
respiratory

276.4 Mixed acid-base balance disorder
Hypercapnia with mixed acid-base disorder

[5] **276.5 Volume depletion**

[Excludes:] *hypovolemic shock:*
postoperative (998.09)

276.50 Volume depletion, unspecified

276.51 Dehydration

276.52 Hypovolemia
Depletion of volume of plasma

[5] **276.6 Fluid overload**

[Excludes:] *ascites (789.51-789.59)*
localized edema (782.3)

276.61 Transfusion associated circulatory overload
Fluid overload due to transfusion (blood) (blood components)
TACO

276.69 Other fluid overload
Fluid retention

276.7 Hyperpotassemia
Hyperkalemia
Potassium [K]:
excess
intoxication
overload

276.8 Hypopotassemia
Hypokalemia
Potassium [K] deficiency

276.9 Electrolyte and fluid disorders not elsewhere classified
Electrolyte imbalance
Hyperchloremia
Hypochloremia

[Excludes:] *electrolyte imbalance:*
associated with hyperemesis gravidarum (643.1)
complicating labor and delivery (669.0)
following abortion and ectopic or molar pregnancy (634-638 with .4, 639.4)

277 Other and unspecified disorders of metabolism

[5] **277.0 Cystic fibrosis**
Fibrocystic disease of the pancreas
Mucoviscidosis

277.00 Without mention of meconium ileus
Cystic fibrosis NOS

277.01 With meconium ileus
Meconium:
ileus (of newborn)
obstruction of intestine in mucoviscidosis

277.02 With pulmonary manifestations
Cystic fibrosis with pulmonary exacerbation

Use additional code to identify any infectious organism present, such as:
pseudomonas (041.7)

277.03 With gastrointestinal manifestations

[Excludes:] *with meconium ileus (277.01)*

277.09 With other manifestations

277.1 Disorders of porphyrin metabolism
Hematoporphyria
Hematoporphyrinuria
Hereditary coproporphyria
Porphyria
Porphyrinuria
Protocoproporphyria
Protoporphyria
Pyrroloporphyria

277.2 Other disorders of purine and pyrimidine metabolism
Hypoxanthine-guanine-phosphoribosyltransferase deficiency [HG-PRT deficiency]
Lesch-Nyhan syndrome
Xanthinuria

[Excludes:] *gout (274.00-274.9)*
orotic aciduric anemia (281.4)

[5] **277.3 Amyloidosis**

● Code new to 2012 edition ▲ Revision of existing code [4] [5] Fourth or fifth digit required

277.30 Amyloidosis, unspecified
Amyloidosis NOS

277.31 Familial Mediterranean fever
Benign paroxysmal peritonitis
Hereditary amyloid nephropathy
Periodic familial polyserositis
Recurrent polyserositis

277.39 Other amyloidosis
Hereditary cardiac amyloidosis
Inherited systemic amyloidosis
Neuropathic (Portuguese) (Swiss) amyloidosis
Secondary amyloidosis

277.4 Disorders of bilirubin excretion
Hyperbilirubinemia:
 congenital
 constitutional
Syndrome:
 Crigler-Najjar
 Dubin-Johnson
 Gilbert's
 Rotor's

Excludes: *hyperbilirubinemias specific to the perinatal period (774.0-774.7)*

277.5 Mucopolysaccharidosis

Gargoylism	Morquio-Brailsford disease
Hunter's syndrome	Osteochondrodystrophy
Hurler's syndrome	Sanfilippo's syndrome
Lipochondrodystrophy	Scheie's syndrome
Maroteaux-Lamy syndrome	

277.6 Other deficiencies of circulating enzymes
Hereditary angioedema

277.7 Dysmetabolic syndrome X
Use additional code for associated manifestation, such as:
 cardiovascular disease (414.00-414.07)
 obesity (278.00-278.03)

⑤ **277.8 Other specified disorders of metabolism**

277.81 Primary carnitine deficiency

277.82 Carnitine deficiency due to inborn errors of metabolism

277.83 Iatrogenic carnitine deficiency
Carnitine deficiency due to:
 hemodialysis
 valproic acid therapy

277.84 Other secondary carnitine deficiency

277.85 Disorders of fatty acid oxidation
Carnitine palmitoyltransferase deficiencies (CPT1, CPT2)
Glutaric aciduria type II (type IIA, IIB, IIC)
Long chain 3-hydroxyacyl CoA dehydrogenase deficiency (LCHAD)
Long chain/very long chain acyl CoA dehydrogenase deficiency (LCAD, VLCAD)
Medium chain acyl CoA dehydrogenase deficiency (MCAD)
Short chain acyl CoA dehydrogenase deficiency (SCAD)

Excludes: *primary carnitine deficiency (277.81)*

277.86 Peroxisomal disorders
Adrenomyeloneuropathy
Neonatal adrenoleukodystrophy
Rhizomelic chrondrodysplasia punctata
X-linked adrenoleukodystrophy
Zellweger syndrome

Excludes: *infantile Refsum disease (356.3)*

	Add 4th or 5th digit		Nonspecific code		Unspecified code		Manifestation code

277.87 Disorders of mitochondrial metabolism
Kearns-Sayre syndrome
Mitochondrial Encephalopathy, Lactic Acidosis and Stroke-like episodes
(MELAS syndrome)
Mitochondrial Neurogastrointestinal Encephalopathy syndrome (MNGIE)
Myoclonus with Epilepsy and with Ragged Red Fibers (MERRF syndrome)
Neuropathy, Ataxia and Retinitis Pigmentosa (NARP syndrome)

Use additional code for associated conditions

| Excludes: | *disorders of pyruvate metabolism (271.8)* |

Leber's optic atrophy (377.16)
Leigh's subacute necrotizing encephalopathy (330.8)
Reye's syndrome (331.81)

277.88 Tumor lysis syndrome
Spontaneous tumor lysis syndrome
Tumor lysis syndrome following antineoplastic drug therapy

Use additional E code to identify cause, if drug-induced

277.89 Other specified disorders of metabolism
Hand-Schuller-Christian disease
Histiocytosis (acute) (chronic)
Histiocytosis X (chronic)

| Excludes: | *histiocytosis:* |

acute differentiated progressive (202.5)
adult pulmonary Langerhans cell (516.5)
X, acute (progressive) (202.5)

277.9 Unspecified disorder of metabolism
Enzymopathy NOS

278 Overweight, obesity and other hyperalimentation

| Excludes: | *hyperalimentation NOS (783.6)* |

poisoning by vitamins NOS (963.5)
polyphagia (783.6)

Use additional code to identify Body Mass Index (BMI), if known (V85.21-V85.25,
V85.30-V85.39, V85.4, V85.53, V85.54)

DEFINITION Hyperalimentation refers to supplying total nutritional needs of patients who are
unable to eat normally by intravenous feeding or by tube through the nose into the stomach.

⑤ **278.0 Overweight and obesity**
Use additional code to identify Body Mass Index (BMI), if known (V85.0-V85.54)

| Excludes: | *adiposogenital dystrophy (253.8)* |

obesity of endocrine origin NOS (259.9)

278.00 Obesity, unspecified
Obesity NOS

278.01 Morbid obesity
Severe obesity

278.02 Overweight

278.03 Obesity hypoventilation syndrome
Pickwickian syndrome

278.1 Localized adiposity
Fat pad

278.2 Hypervitaminosis A

278.3 Hypercarotinemia

278.4 Hypervitaminosis D

278.8 Other hyperalimentation

279 Disorders involving the immune mechanism
Use additional code for associated manifestations

⑤ **279.0 Deficiency of humoral immunity**

279.00 Hypogammaglobulinemia, unspecified
Agammaglobulinemia NOS

279.01 Selective IgA immunodeficiency

279.02 Selective IgM immunodeficiency

279.03 Other selective immunoglobulin deficiencies
Selective deficiency of IgG

● Code new
to 2012 edition
▲ Revision of
existing code
④ ⑤ Fourth or fifth
digit required

279.04 Congenital hypogammaglobulinemia
Agammaglobulinemia:
Bruton's type
X-linked

279.05 Immunodeficiency with increased IgM
Immunodeficiency with hyper-IgM:
autosomal recessive
X-linked

279.06 Common variable immunodeficiency
Dysgammaglobulinemia (acquired) (congenital) (primary)
Hypogammaglobulinemia:
acquired primary
congenital non-sex-linked
sporadic

279.09 Other
Transient hypogammaglobulinemia of infancy

5 **279.1 Deficiency of cell-mediated immunity**

279.10 Immunodeficiency with predominant T-cell defect, unspecified

279.11 DiGeorge's syndrome
Pharyngeal pouch syndrome
Thymic hypoplasia

279.12 Wiskott-Aldrich syndrome

279.13 Nezelof's syndrome
Cellular immunodeficiency with abnormal immunoglobulin deficiency

279.19 Other

[Excludes:] *ataxia-telangiectasia (334.8)*

279.2 Combined immunity deficiency
Agammaglobulinemia:
autosomal recessive
Swiss-type
x-linked recessive
Severe combined immunodeficiency [SCID]
Thymic:
alymphoplasia
aplasia or dysplasia with immunodeficiency

[Excludes:] *thymic hypoplasia (279.11)*

279.3 Unspecified immunity deficiency

5 **279.4 Autoimmune disease, not elsewhere classified**

[Excludes:] *transplant failure or rejection (996.80-996.89)*

279.41 Autoimmune lymphoproliferative syndrome
ALPS

279.49 Autoimmune disease, not elsewhere classified
Autoimmune disease NOS

5 **279.5 Graft-versus-host disease**

Code first underlying cause, such as:
complication of blood transfusion (999.89)
complication of transplanted organ (996.80-996.89)

Use additional code to identify associated manifestations, such as:
desquamative dermatitis (695.89)
diarrhea (787.91)
elevated bilirubin (782.4)
hair loss (704.09)

279.50 Graft-versus-host disease, unspecified

279.51 Acute graft-versus-host disease

279.52 Chronic graft-versus-host disease

279.53 Acute on chronic graft-versus-host disease

279.8 Other specified disorders involving the immune mechanism
Single complement [C_1-C_9] deficiency or dysfunction

279.9 Unspecified disorder of immune mechanism

This page intentionally left blank.

● Code new
to 2012 edition

▲ Revision of
existing code

④ ⑤ Fourth or fifth
digit required

Chapter 4: Diseases of Blood and Blood Forming Organs (280-289)

DEFINITIONS AND CODING ALERTS

This chapter includes definitions of selected key words, terms and phrases and coding alerts for adding points to the clinical domain, references to coding late effects where appropriate, and references to personal history V-codes in situations where the acute or chronic condition is no longer active. An example from this chapter is as follows:

282 **Hereditary hemolytic anemias**

DEFINITION Hereditary hemolytic anemias are caused by the destruction of red blood cells by a disease process. Occurs in newborns as a result of blood- group incompatibility between mother and baby. It is also caused by abnormal red cell membranes or abnormal hemoglobin, ie, sickle cell anemia and thallassemia.

MULTIPLE CODING FOR A SINGLE CONDITION

In addition to the etiology or manifestation convention that requires two codes to fully describe a single condition that affects multiple body systems, there are other single conditions that also require more than one code. "Use additional code" notes are found in the tabular at codes that are not part of an etiology or manifestation pair where a secondary code is useful to fully describe a condition. The sequencing rule is the same as the etiology or manifestation pair - , "use additional code" indicates that a secondary code should be added.

"Code first" notes are also under certain codes that are not specifically manifestation codes but may be due to an underlying cause. When a "code first" note is present and an underlying condition is present the underlying condition should be sequenced first.

"Code, if applicable, any causal condition first", notes indicate that this code may be assigned as a principal diagnosis when the causal condition is unknown or not applicable. If a causal condition is known, then the code for that condition should be sequenced as the principal or first-listed diagnosis. Multiple codes may be needed for late effects, complication codes and obstetric codes to more fully describe a condition. See the specific guidelines for these conditions for further instruction.

COMBINATION CODE

A combination code is a single code used to classify: two diagnoses, or a diagnosis with an associated secondary process (manifestation) A diagnosis with an associated complication Combination codes are identified by referring to subterm entries in the Alphabetic Index and by reading the inclusion and exclusion notes in the Tabular List.

Assign only the combination code when that code fully identifies the diagnostic conditions involved or when the Alphabetic Index so directs. Multiple coding should not be used when the classification provides a combination code that clearly identifies all of the elements documented in the diagnosis. When the combination code lacks necessary specificity in describing the manifestation or complication, an additional code should be used as a secondary code.

CODING LATE EFFECTS

A late effect is the residual effect (condition produced) after the acute phase of an illness or injury has terminated. There is no time limit on when a late effect code can be used. The residual may be apparent early, such as in cerebrovascular accident cases, or it may occur months or years later, such as that due to a previous injury. Coding of late effects generally requires two codes sequenced in the following order: The condition or nature of the late effect is sequenced first. The late effect code is sequenced second.

An exception to the above guidelines are those instances where the code for late effect is followed by a manifestation code identified in the Tabular List and title, or the late effect code has been expanded (at the fourth and fifth-digit levels) to include the manifestation(s). The code for the acute phase of an illness or injury that led to the late effect is never used with a code for the late effect.

ANEMIA OF CHRONIC DISEASE

Subcategory 285.2, Anemia in chronic illness, has codes for anemia in chronic kidney disease, code 285.21; anemia in neoplastic disease, code 285.22; and anemia in other chronic illness, code 285.29. These codes can be used as the principal or first listed code if the reason for the encounter is to treat the anemia. They may also be used as secondary codes if treatment of the anemia is a component of an encounter, but not the primary reason for the encounter. When using a code from subcategory 285 it is also necessary to use the code for the chronic condition causing the anemia.

| | Add 4th or 5th digit | | Nonspecific code | | Unspecified code | | Manifestation code |

Anemia in chronic kidney disease

When assigning code 285.21, Anemia in chronic kidney disease, it is also necessary to assign a code from category 585, Chronic kidney disease, to indicate the stage of chronic kidney disease.

See Chapter 10 for information regarding. Chronic kidney disease (CKD).

Anemia in neoplastic disease

When assigning code 285.22, Anemia in neoplastic disease, it is also necessary to assign the neoplasm code that is responsible for the anemia. Code 285.22 is for use for anemia that is due to the malignancy, not for anemia due to antineoplastic chemotherapy drugs, which is an adverse effect.

See Chapter 2 for information regarding anemia associated with malignancy, chemotherapy, immunotherapy and radiation therapy.

See Chapter 17 for information regarding adverse effects.

● Code new
to 2012edition
▲ Revision of
existing code
④ ⑤ Fourth or fifth
digit required

4. DISEASES OF THE BLOOD AND BLOOD-FORMING ORGANS (280-289)

Excludes: anemia complicating pregnancy or the puerperium (648.2)

ALERT! For personal history of diseases of blood and blood-forming organs see V12.3

280 Iron deficiency anemias

Includes: anemia:
  asiderotic
  hypochromic-microcytic
  sideropenic

Excludes: familial microcytic anemia (282.49)

DEFINITION Iron deficiency anemia is a form of anemia due to lack of iron in the diet or to iron loss as a result of chronic bleeding.

280.0 Secondary to blood loss (chronic)
  Normocytic anemia due to blood loss

Excludes: acute posthemorrhagic anemia (285.1)

280.1 Secondary to inadequate dietary iron intake

280.8 Other specified iron deficiency anemias
  Paterson-Kelly syndrome
  Plummer-Vinson syndrome
  Sideropenic dysphagia

280.9 Iron deficiency anemia, unspecified
  Anemia:
  achlorhydric
  chlorotic
  idiopathic hypochromic
  iron [Fe] deficiency NOS

281 Other deficiency anemias

281.0 Pernicious anemia
  Anemia: Congenital intrinsic factor [Castle's] deficiency
  Addison's
  Biermer's
  congenital pernicious

Excludes: combined system disease without mention of anemia (266.2)
  subacute degeneration of spinal cord without mention of anemia (266.2)

281.1 Other vitamin B$_{12}$ deficiency anemia
  Anemia:
  vegan's
  vitamin B$_{12}$ deficiency (dietary)
  due to selective vitamin B$_{12}$ malabsorption with proteinuria
  Syndrome:
  Imerslund's
  Imerslund-Gräsbeck

Excludes: combined system disease without mention of anemia (266.2)
  subacute degeneration of spinal cord without mention of anemia (266.2)

281.2 Folate-deficiency anemia
  Congenital folate malabsorption
  Folate or folic acid deficiency anemia:
  NOS
  dietary
  drug-induced
  Goat's milk anemia
  Nutritional megaloblastic anemia (of infancy)

Use additional E code, if desired, to identify drug

281.3 Other specified megaloblastic anemias not elsewhere classified
  Combined B$_{12}$ and folate-deficiency anemia
  Refractory megaloblastic anemia

281.4 Protein-deficiency anemia
  Amino-acid-deficiency anemia

281.8 Anemia associated with other specified nutritional deficiency
  Scorbutic anemia

| | Add 4th or 5th digit | | Nonspecific code | | Unspecified code | | Manifestation code |

281.9 Unspecified deficiency anemia

Anemia:
- dimorphic
- macrocytic
- megaloblastic NOS

Anemia:
- nutritional NOS
- simple chronic

282 Hereditary hemolytic anemias

DEFINITION Hereditary hemolytic anemias are caused by the destruction of red blood cells by a disease process. Occurs in newborns as a result of blood- group incompatibility between mother and baby. It is also caused by abnormal red cell membranes or abnormal hemoglobin, ie, sickle cell anemia and thallassemia.

282.0 Hereditary spherocytosis

Acholuric (familial) jaundice
Congenital hemolytic anemia (spherocytic)
Congenital spherocytosis
Minkowski-Chauffard syndrome
Spherocytosis (familial)

[Excludes:] *hemolytic anemia of newborn (773.0-773.5)*

282.1 Hereditary elliptocytosis

Elliptocytosis (congenital)
Ovalocytosis (congenital) (hereditary)

282.2 Anemias due to disorders of glutathione metabolism

Anemia:
- 6-phosphogluconic dehydrogenase deficiency
- enzyme deficiency, drug-induced
- erythrocytic glutathione deficiency
- glucose-6-phosphate dehydrogenase [G-6-PD] deficiency
- glutathione-reductase deficiency
- hemolytic nonspherocytic (hereditary), type I

Disorder of pentose phosphate pathway
Favism

282.3 Other hemolytic anemias due to enzyme deficiency

Anemia:
- hemolytic nonspherocytic (hereditary), type II
- hexokinase deficiency
- pyruvate kinase [PK] deficiency
- triosephosphate isomerase deficiency

⑤ **282.4 Thalassemias**

[Excludes:] *sickle-cell:*
- *disease (282.60-282.69)*
- *trait (282.5)*

● **282.40 Thalassemia, unspecified**

Thalassemia NOS

282.41 Sickle-cell thalassemia without crisis

Sickle-cell thalassemia NOS
Microdrepanocytosis
Thalassemia Hb-S disease without crisis

282.42 Sickle-cell thalassemia with crisis

Sickle-cell thalassemia with vaso-occlusive pain
Thalassemia Hb-S disease with crisis

Use additional code for types of crisis, such as:
- acute chest syndrome (517.3)
- splenic sequestration (289.52)

● **282.43 Alpha thalassemia**

Alpha thalassemia major
Hemoglobin H Constant Spring
Hemoglobin H disease
Hydrops fetalis due to alpha thalassemia
Severe alpha thalassemia
Triple gene defect alpha thalassemia

[Excludes:] *alpha thalassemia trait or minor (282.46)*
hydrops fetalis due to isoimmunization (773.3)
hydrops fetalis not due to immune hemolysis (778.0)

● Code new to 2012edition ▲ Revision of existing code ④ ⑤ Fourth or fifth digit required

● **282.44   Beta thalassemia**
Beta thalassemia major
Cooley's anemia
Homozygous beta thalassemia
Severe beta thalassemia
Thalassemia intermedia
Thalassemia major

Excludes: *beta thalassemia minor (282.46)*
beta thalassemia trait (282.46)
delta-beta thalassemia (282.45)
hemoglobin E beta thalassemia (282.47)
sickle-cell beta thalassemia (282.41, 282.42)

● **282.45   Delta-beta thalassemia**
Homozygous delta-beta thalassemia

Excludes: *delta-beta thalassemia trait (282.46)*

● **282.46   Thalassemia minor**
Alpha thalassemia minor
Alpha thalassemia silent carrier
Alpha thalassemia trait
Beta thalassemia minor
Beta thalassemia trait
Delta-beta thalassemia trait
Thalassemia trait NOS

Excludes: *alpha thalassemia (282.43)*
beta thalassemia (282.44)
delta-beta thalassemia (282.45)
hemoglobin E-beta thalassemia (282.47)
sickle-cell trait (282.5)

● **282.47   Hemoglobin E-beta thalassemia**

Excludes: *beta thalassemia (282.44)*
beta thalassemia minor (282.46)
beta thalassemia trait (282.46)
delta-beta thalassemia (282.45)
delta-beta thalassemia trait (282.46)
hemoglobin E disease (282.7)
other hemoglobinopathies (282.7)
sickle-cell beta thalassemia (282.41, 282.42)

282.49   **Other thalassemia**
Dominant thalassemia
Hemoglobin C thalassemia
Hereditary leptocytosis
Mediterranean anemia (with other hemoglobinopathy)
Mixed thalassemia
Thalassemia with other hemoglobinopathy

Excludes: *hemoglobin C disease (282.7)*
hemoglobin E disease (282.7)
other hemoglobinopathies (282.7)
sickle-cell anemias (282.60-282.69)
sickle-cell beta thalassemia (282.41-282.42)

282.5   Sickle-cell trait

Hb-AS genotype	Heterozygous:
Hemoglobin S [Hb-S] trait	hemoglobin S
	Hb-S

Excludes: *that with other hemoglobinopathy (282.60-282.69)*
that with thalassemia (282.41-282.42)

⑤ **282.6   Sickle-cell disease**
Sickle-cell anemia

Excludes: *sickle-cell thalassemia (282.41-282.42)*
sickle-cell trait (282.5)

282.60   **Sickle-cell disease, unspecified**
Sickle-cell anemia NOS

282.61   Hb-SS disease without crisis

Add 4th or 5th digit	Nonspecific code	Unspecified code	Manifestation code

282.62 Hb-SS disease with crisis
Hb-SS disease with vaso-occlusive pain
Sickle-cell crisis NOS

Use additional code for type of crisis, such as:
acute chest syndrome (517.3)
splenic sequestration (289.52)

282.63 Sickle-cell/Hb-C disease without crisis
Hb-S/Hb-C disease without crisis

282.64 Sickle-cell/Hb-C disease with crisis
Hb-S/Hb-C disease with crisis
Sickle-cell/Hb-C disease with vaso-occlusive pain

Use additional code for type of crisis, such as:
acute chest syndrome (517.3)
splenic sequestration (289.52)

282.68 Other sickle-cell disease without crisis
Hb-S/Hb-D disease without crisis
Hb-S/Hb-E disease without crisis
Sickle-cell/Hb-D disease without crisis
Sickle-cell/Hb-E disease without crisis

282.69 Other sickle-cell disease with crisis
Hb-S/Hb-D disease with crisis
Hb-S/Hb-E disease with crisis
Other sickle-cell disease with vaso-occlusive pain
Sickle-cell/Hb-D disease with crisis
Sickle-cell/Hb-E disease with crisis

Use additional code for type of crisis, such as:
acute chest syndrome (517.3)
splenic sequestration (289.52)

282.7 Other hemoglobinopathies
Abnormal hemoglobin NOS
Congenital Heinz-body anemia
Disease:
hemoglobin C [Hb-C]
hemoglobin D [Hb-D]
hemoglobin E [Hb-E]
hemoglobin Zurich [Hb-Zurich]
Hemoglobinopathy NOS
Hereditary persistence of fetal hemoglobin [HPFH]
Unstable hemoglobin hemolytic disease

Excludes: *familial polycythemia (289.6)*
hemoglobin E-beta thalassemia (282.47)
hemoglobin M [Hb-M] disease (289.7)
high-oxygen-affinity hemoglobin (289.0)
other hemoglobinopathies with thalassemia (282.49)

282.8 Other specified hereditary hemolytic anemias
Stomatocytosis

282.9 Hereditary hemolytic anemia, unspecified
Hereditary hemolytic anemia NOS

283 Acquired hemolytic anemias
DEFINITION Hemolytic anemia is a condition in which there are not enough red blood cells in the blood, due to the premature destruction of red blood cells.

283.0 Autoimmune hemolytic anemias
Autoimmune hemolytic anemias (cold type) (warm type)
Chronic cold hemagglutinin disease
Cold agglutinin disease or hemoglobinuria
Hemolytic anemia:
cold type (secondary) (symptomatic)
drug-induced
warm type (secondary) (symptomatic)

Use additional E code, if desired, to identify cause, if drug-induced

Excludes: *Evans' syndrome (287.32)*
hemolytic disease of newborn (773.0-773.5)

⑤ **283.1 Non-autoimmune hemolytic anemias**

283.10 Non-autoimmune hemolytic anemia, unspecified

● Code new
to 2012edition

▲ Revision of
existing code

④ ⑤ Fourth or fifth
digit required

283.11 Hemolytic-uremic syndrome
Use additional code to identify associated:
E. coli infection (041.41-041.49)
Pneumococcal pnemonia (481)
Shigella dysenteriae (004.0)

283.19 Other non-autoimmune hemolytic anemias
Hemolytic anemia:
mechanical
microangiopathic
toxic
Use additional E code, if desired, to identify cause

283.2 Hemoglobinuria due to hemolysis from external causes
Acute intravascular hemolysis
Hemoglobinuria:
from exertion
march
paroxysmal (cold) (nocturnal)
due to other hemolysis
Marchiafava-Micheli syndrome
Use additional E code, if desired, to identify cause

283.9 Acquired hemolytic anemia, unspecified
Acquired hemolytic anemia NOS
Chronic idiopathic hemolytic anemia

284 Aplastic anemia and other bone marrow failure syndromes
[DEFINITION] Anemia is a condition where bone marrow does not produce sufficient new cells to replenish blood cells.

⑤ **284.0 Constitutional aplastic anemia**

284.01 Constitutional red blood cell aplasia
Aplasia, (pure) red cell:
congenital
of infants
primary
Blackfan-Diamond syndrome
Familial hypoplastic anemia

284.09 Other constitutional aplastic anemia
Fanconi's anemia
Pancytopenia with malformations

⑤ **284.1 Pancytopenia**
[Excludes:] *pancytopenia (due to) (with):*
aplastic anemia NOS (284.9)
bone marrow infiltration (284.2)
constitutional red blood cell aplasia (284.01)
hairy cell leukemia (202.4)
human immunodeficiency virus disease (042)
leukoerythroblastic anemia (284.2)
malformations (284.09)
myelodysplastic syndromes (238.72-238.75)
myeloproliferative disease (238.79)
other constitutional aplastic anemia (284.09)

● **284.11 Antineoplastic chemotherapy induced pancytopenia**
[Excludes:] *aplastic anemia due to antineoplastic chemotherapy (284.89)*

● **284.12 Other drug-induced pancytopenia**
[Excludes:] *aplastic anemia due to drugs (284.89)*

● **284.19 Other pancytopenia**

Add 4th or 5th digit | Nonspecific code | Unspecified code | Manifestation code

284.2 Myelophthisis
　　　Leukoerythroblastic anemia
　　　Myelophthisic anemia
Code first the underlying disorder, such as:
　　　malignant neoplasm of breast (174.0-174.9, 175.0-175.9)
　　　tuberculosis (015.0-015.9)

　　　| Excludes: | *idiopathic myelofibrosis (238.76)*

　　　　　myelofibrosis NOS (289.83)
　　　　　myelofibrosis with myeloid metaplasia (238.76)
　　　　　primary myelofibrosis (238.76)
　　　　　secondary myelofibrosis (289.83)

⑤ **284.8 Other specified aplastic anemias**

　　　284.81 Red cell aplasia (acquired) (adult) (with thymoma)
　　　　　Red cell aplasia NOS

　　　284.89 Other specified aplastic anemias
　　　　　Aplastic anemia (due to):
　　　　　　chronic systemic disease
　　　　　　drugs
　　　　　　infection
　　　　　　radiation
　　　　　　toxic (paralytic)

　　　Use additional E code to identify cause

284.9 Aplastic anemia, unspecified
　　　Anemia:　　　　　　　　　　Anemia:
　　　　aplastic (idiopathic) NOS　　　nonregenerative
　　　　aregenerative　　　　　　Medullary hypoplasia
　　　　hypoplastic NOS

　　　| Excludes: | *refractory anemia (238.72)*

285 Other and unspecified anemias
　　　ALERT! When using a code from this category it is also necessary to use the code for the chronic condition causing the anemia

285.0 Sideroblastic anemia
　　　Anemia:
　　　　hypochromic with iron loading
　　　　sideroachrestic
　　　　sideroblastic:
　　　　　acquired
　　　　　congenital
　　　　　hereditary
　　　　　primary
　　　　　secondary (drug-induced) (due to disease)
　　　　　sex-linked hypochromic
　　　　　vitamin B_6-responsive
　　　Pyridoxine-responsive (hypochromic) anemia
Use additional E code, if desired, to identify cause, if drug induced

　　　| Excludes: | *refractory sideroblastic anemia (238.72)*

285.1 Acute posthemorrhagic anemia
　　　Anemia due to acute blood loss

　　　| Excludes: | *anemia due to chronic blood loss (280.0)*
　　　　　blood loss anemia NOS (280.0)

⑤ **285.2 Anemia of chronic disease**
　　　Anemia in (due to) (with) chronic illness

　　　285.21 Anemia in chronic kidney disease
　　　　　Anemia in end stage renal disease
　　　　　Erythropoietin-resistant anemia (EPO resistant anemia)

　　　ALERT! When assigning this code it is also necessary to assign a code from Category 585 to indicate the stage of chronic kidney disease.

● Code new　　　　▲ Revision of　　　④ ⑤ Fourth or fifth
　to 2012edition　　　existing code　　　　digit required

285.22   Anemia in neoplastic disease

Excludes: *anemia due to antineoplastic chemotherapy (285.3)*

aplastic anemia due to antineoplastic chemotherapy (284.89)

ALERT! Code 285.22 is for use for anemia that is due to the malignancy, not for anemia due to antineoplastic chemotherapy drugs, which is an adverse effect. May be used as a secondary code if the patient suffers from anemia and is being treated for the malignancy. When assigning code 285.22, it is also necessary to assign the neoplasm code that is responsible for the anemia.

285.29   Anemia of other chronic disease
Anemia in other chronic illness

285.3   Antineoplastic chemotherapy induced anemia
Anemia due to antineoplastic chemotherapy

Excludes: *anemia due to drug NEC – code to type of anemia*

anemia in neoplastic disease (285.22)

aplastic anemia due to antineoplastic chemotherapy (284.89)

285.8   Other specified anemias
Anemia:
dyserythropoietic (congenital)
dyshematopoietic (congenital)
von Jaksch's
Infantile pseudoleukemia

285.9   Anemia, unspecified
Anemia:
NOS
essential
normocytic, not due to blood
loss

Anemia:
profound
progressive
secondary
Oligocythemia

Excludes: *anemia (due to):*

blood loss:
acute (285.1)
chronic or unspecified (280.0)
iron deficiency (280.0-280.9)

286   Coagulation defects
DEFINITION Coagulation defects, aka coagulopathy, clotting disorder, and bleeding disorder, refers to defect in the body's mechanism for blood clotting

286.0   Congenital factor VIII disorder
Antihemophilic globulin [AHG] deficiency
Factor VIII (functional) deficiency
Hemophilia:
NOS
A
classical
familial
hereditary
Subhemophilia

Excludes: *factor VIII deficiency with vascular defect (286.4)*

286.1   Congenital factor IX disorder
Christmas disease
Deficiency:
factor IX (functional)
plasma thromboplastin component [PTC]
Hemophilia B

286.2   Congenital factor XI deficiency
Hemophilia C
Plasma thromboplastin antecedent [PTA] deficiency
Rosenthal's disease

Add 4th or 5th digit	Nonspecific code	Unspecified code	Manifestation code

286.3 Congenital deficiency of other clotting factors

Congenital afibrinogenemia
Deficiency:
  AC globulin factor:
    I [fibrinogen]
    II [prothrombin]
    V [labile]
    VII [stable]
    X [Stuart-Prower]
    XII [Hageman]
    XIII [fibrin stabilizing]
Deficiency:
  Laki-Lorand factor
  proaccelerin
Disease:
  Owren's
  Stuart-Prower
Dysfibrinogenemia (congenital)
Dysprothrombinemia (constitutional)
Hypoproconvertinemia
Hypoprothrombinemia (hereditary)
Parahemophilia

286.4 von Willebrand's disease

Angiohemophilia (A) (B)
Constitutional thrombopathy
Factor VIII deficiency with vascular defect
Pseudohemophilia type B
Vascular hemophilia
von Willebrand's (-Jürgens') disease

[Excludes:] *factor VIII deficiency:*
  NOS (286.0)
  with functional defect (286.0)
hereditary capillary fragility (287.8)

▲ **286.5 Hemorrhagic disorder due to intrinsic circulating anticoagulants, antibodies or inhibitors**

● **286.52 Acquired hemophilia**

Autoimmune hemophilia
Autoimmune inhibitors to clotting factors
Secondary hemophilia

● **286.53 Antiphospholipid antibody with hemorrhagic disorder**

Lupus anticoagulant (LAC) with hemorrhagic disorder
Systemic lupus erythematosus [SLE] inhibitor with hemorrhagic disorder

[Excludes:] *antiphospholipid antibody, finding without diagnosis (795.79)*
antiphospholipid antibody syndrome (289.81)
antiphospholipid antibody with hypercoagulable state (289.81)
lupus anticoagulant (LAC) finding without diagnosis (795.79)
lupus anticoagulant (LAC) with hypercoagulable state (289.81)
systemic lupus erythematosus [SLE] inhibitor finding without diagnosis (795.79)
systemic lupus erythematosus [SLE] inhibitor with hypercoagulable state (289.81)

● **286.59 Other hemorrhagic disorder due to intrinsic circulating anticoagulants, antibodies, or inhibitors**

Antithrombinemia
Antithromboplastinemia
Antithromboplastinogenemia
Increase in:
  anti-II (prothrombin)
  anti-VIIIa
  anti-IXa
  anti-XIa

286.6 Defibrination syndrome

Afibrinogenemia, acquired
Consumption coagulopathy
Diffuse or disseminated intravascular coagulation [DIC syndrome]
Fibrinolytic hemorrhage, acquired
Hemorrhagic fibrinogenolysis
Pathologic fibrinolysis
Purpura:
  fibrinolytic
  fulminans

[Excludes:] *that complicating:*
  abortion (634-638 with .1, 639.1)
  pregnancy or the puerperium (641.3, 666.3)
disseminated intravascular coagulation in newborn (776.2)

● Code new to 2012edition   ▲ Revision of existing code   ④ ⑤ Fourth or fifth digit required

286.7 Acquired coagulation factor deficiency
Deficiency of coagulation factor due to:
liver disease
vitamin K deficiency
Hypoprothrombinemia, acquired

Excludes: *vitamin K deficiency of newborn (776.0)*

Use additional E-code, if desired, to identify cause, if drug induced

286.9 Other and unspecified coagulation defects
Defective coagulation NOS
Deficiency, coagulation factor NOS
Delay, coagulation
Disorder:
coagulation
hemostasis

Excludes: *abnormal coagulation profile (790.92)*
hemorrhagic disease of newborn (776.0)
that complicating:
abortion (634-638 with .1, 639.1)
pregnancy or the puerperium (641.3, 666.3)

287 Purpura and other hemorrhagic conditions

Excludes: *hemorrhagic thrombocythemia (238.79)*
purpura fulminans (286.6)

DEFINITION Purpura are purple-colored spots and patches that occur on the skin, organs, and in mucus membranes, including the lining of the mouth.

287.0 Allergic purpura
Peliosis rheumatica
Purpura:
anaphylactoid
autoimmune
Henoch's

Purpura:
nonthrombocytopenic:
hemorrhagic
idiopathic
rheumatica
Schönlein-Henoch
vascular
Vasculitis, allergic

Excludes: *hemorrhagic purpura (287.39)*
purpura annularis telangiectodes (709.1)

287.1 Qualitative platelet defects
Thrombasthenia (hemorrhagic) (hereditary)
Thrombocytasthenia
Thrombocytopathy (dystrophic)
Thrombopathy (Bernard-Soulier)

Excludes: *von Willebrand's disease (286.4)*

287.2 Other nonthrombocytopenic purpuras
Purpura:
NOS
senile
simplex

⑤ **287.3 Primary thrombocytopenia**

287.30 Primary thrombocytopenia, unspecified
Megakaryocytic hypoplasia

287.31 Immune thrombocytopenic purpura
Idiopathic thrombocytopenic purpura
Tidal platelet dysgenesis

287.32 Evans' syndrome

287.33 Congenital and hereditary thrombocytopenic purpura
Congenital and hereditary thrombocytopenia
Thrombocytopenia with absent radii (TAR) syndrome

Excludes: *Wiskott-Aldrich syndrome (279.12)*

287.39 Other primary thrombocytopenia

⑤ **287.4 Secondary thrombocytopenia**
Use additional E code, if desired, to identify cause

Excludes: *heparin-induced thrombocytopenia (HIT) (289.84)*
transient thrombocytopenia of newborn (776.1)

	Add 4th or 5th digit		Nonspecific code		Unspecified code		Manifestation code

287.41 Posttransfusion purpura
Posttransfusion purpura from whole blood (fresh) or blood products
PTP

287.49 Other secondary thrombocytopenia
Thrombocytopenia (due to):
dilutional
drugs
extracorporeal circulation of blood
massive blood transfusion
platelet alloimmunization
secondary NOS

287.5 Thrombocytopenia, unspecified

287.8 Other specified hemorrhagic conditions
Capillary fragility (hereditary)
Vascular pseudohemophilia

287.9 Unspecified hemorrhagic conditions
Hemorrhagic diathesis (familial)

288 Diseases of white blood cells

Excludes: *leukemia (204.0-208.9)*

DEFINITION White blood cells, aka leukocyte, refers to Any of various blood cells that help protect the body from infection and disease. White blood cells include neutrophils, eosinophils, basophils, lymphocytes, and monocytes.

⑤ **288.0 Neutropenia**
Decreased Absolute Neutrophil Count (ANC)
Use additional code for any associated:
fever (780.61)
mucositis (478.11, 528.00-528.09, 538, 616.81)

Excludes: *neutropenic splenomegaly (289.53)*
transitory neonatal neutropenia (776.7)

288.00 Neutropenia, unspecified

288.01 Congenital neutropenia
Congenital agranulocytosis
Infantile genetic agranulocytosis
Kostmann's syndrome

288.02 Cyclic neutropenia
Cyclic hematopoiesis
Periodic neutropenia

288.03 Drug induced neutropenia
Use additional E code to identify drug

288.04 Neutropenia due to infection

288.09 Other neutropenia
Agranulocytosis
Neutropenia:
immune
toxic

288.1 Functional disorders of polymorphonuclear neutrophils
Chronic (childhood) granulomatous disease
Congenital dysphagocytosis
Job's syndrome
Lipochrome histiocytosis (familial)
Progressive septic granulomatosis

288.2 Genetic anomalies of leukocytes
Anomaly (granulation) (granulocyte) or syndrome:
Alder's (-Reilly)
Chédiak-Steinbrinck (-Higashi)
Jordan's
May-Hegglin
Pelger-Huet
Hereditary:
hypersegmentation
hyposegmentation
leukomelanopathy

● Code new   ▲ Revision of   ④ ⑤ Fourth or fifth
to 2012edition   existing code   digit required

288.3 Eosinophilia
Eosinophilia
allergic
hereditary
idiopathic
secondary
Eosinophilic leukocytosis

[Excludes:] *Löffler's syndrome (518.3)*
pulmonary eosinophilia (518.3)

288.4 Hemophagocytic syndromes
Familial hemophagocytic lymphohistiocytosis
Familial hemophagocytic reticulosis
Hemophagocytic syndrome, infection-associated
Histiocytic syndromes
Macrophage activation syndrome

[5] **288.5 Decreased white blood cell count**

[Excludes:] *neutropenia (288.01-288.09)*

288.50 Leukocytopenia, unspecified
Decreased leukocytes, unspecified
Decreased white blood cell count, unspecified
Leukopenia NOS

288.51 Lymphocytopenia
Decreased lymphocytes

288.59 Other decreased white blood cell count
Basophilic leukopenia
Eosinophilic leukopenia
Monocytopenia
Plasmacytopenia

[5] **288.6 Elevated white blood cell count**

[Excludes:] *eosinophilia (288.3)*

288.60 Leukocytosis, unspecified
Elevated leukocytes, unspecified
Elevated white blood cell count, unspecified

288.61 Lymphocytosis (symptomatic)
Elevated lymphocytes

288.62 Leukemoid reaction
Basophilic leukemoid reaction
Lymphocytic leukemoid reaction
Monocytic leukemoid reaction
Myelocytic leukemoid reaction
Neutrophilic leukemoid reaction

288.63 Monocytosis (symptomatic)

[Excludes:] *infectious mononucleosis (075)*

288.64 Plasmacytosis

288.65 Basophilia

288.66 Bandemia
Bandemia without diagnosis of specific infection

[Excludes:] *confirmed infection – code to infection leukemia (204.00-208.9)*

288.69 Other elevated white blood cell count

288.8 Other specified disease of white blood cells

[Excludes:] *decreased white blood cell counts (288.50-288.59)*
elevated white blood cell counts (288.60-288.69)
immunity disorders (279.0-279.9)

288.9 Unspecified disease of white blood cells

Add 4th or 5th digit | Nonspecific code | Unspecified code | Manifestation code

289 Other diseases of blood and blood-forming organs

289.0 Polycythemia, secondary

High-oxygen-affinity
  hemoglobin
Polycythemia:
  acquired
  benign
  due to:
    fall in plasma volume
    high altitude
Polycythemia:
  emotional
  erythropoietin
  hypoxemic
  nephrogenous
  relative
  spurious
  stress

[Excludes:] *polycythemia:*
  neonatal (776.4)
  primary (238.4)
  vera (238.4)

289.1 Chronic lymphadenitis

Chronic:
  adenitis, any lymph node except mesenteric
  lymphadenitis, any lymph node except mesenteric

[Excludes:] *acute lymphadenitis (683)*
    mesenteric (289.2)
  enlarged glands NOS (785.6)

289.2 Nonspecific mesenteric lymphadenitis

Mesenteric lymphadenitis (acute) (chronic)

289.3 Lymphadenitis, unspecified, except mesenteric

289.4 Hypersplenism

"Big spleen" syndrome
Dyssplenism
Hypersplenia

[Excludes:] *primary splenic neutropenia (289.53)*

[5] **289.5 Other diseases of spleen**

289.50 Disease of spleen, unspecified

289.51 Chronic congestive splenomegaly

289.52 Splenic sequestration

Code first sickle-cell disease in crisis (282.42, 282.62, 282.64, 282.69)

289.53 Neutropenic splenomegaly

289.59 Other

Lien migrans
Perisplenitis
Splenic:
  abscess
  atrophy
  cyst
Splenic:
  fibrosis
  infarction
  rupture, nontraumatic
Splenitis
Wandering spleen

[Excludes:] *bilharzial splenic fibrosis (120.0-120.9)*
  hepatolienal fibrosis (571.5)
  splenomegaly NOS (789.2)

289.6 Familial polycythemia

Familial benign polycythemia
Familial erythrocytosis

289.7 Methemoglobinemia

Congenital NADH [DPNH]-methemoglobin-reductase deficiency
Hemoglobin M [Hb-M] disease
Methemoglobinemia:
  NOS
  acquired (with sulfhemoglobinemia)
  hereditary
  toxic
Stokvis' disease
Sulfhemoglobinemia

Use additional E code, if desired, to identify cause

⑤ **289.8** **Other specified diseases of blood and blood-forming organs**

    289.81 **Primary hypercoagulable state**
        Activated protein C resistance
        Antiphospholipid antibody syndrome
        Antithrombin III deficiency
        Factor V Leiden mutation
        Lupus anticoagulant with hypercoagulable state
        Protein C deficiency
        Protein S deficiency
        Prothrombin gene mutation
        Systemic lupus erythematosus [SLE] inhibitor with hypercoagulable state

    Excludes: *anti-phospholipid antibody, finding without diagnosis (795.79)*
        anti-phospholipid antibody with hemorrhagic disorder (286.53)
        lupus anticoagulant (LAC) finding without diagnosis (795.79)
        lupus anticoagulant (LAC) with hemorrhagic disorder (286.53)
        secondary activated protein C resistance (289.82)
        secondary antiphospholipid antibody syndrome (289.82)
        secondary lupus anticoagulant with hypercoagulable state (289.82)
        secondary systemic lupus erythematosus [SLE] inhibitor with hypercoagulable
          state (289.82)
        systemic lupus erythematosus [SLE] inhibitor finding without diagnosis (795.79)
        systemic lupus erythematosus [SLE] inhibitor with hemorrhagic disorder (286.53)

    289.82 **Secondary hypercoagulable state**

    Excludes: *heparin-induced thrombocytopenia (HIT) (289.84)*

    289.83 **Myelofibrosis**
        Myelofibrosis NOS
        Secondary myelofibrosis

    Code first the underlying disorder, such as:
        malignant neoplasm of breast (174.0-174.9, 175.0-175.9)

    Use additional code for associated therapy-related
        myelodysplastic syndrome, if applicable (238.72, 238.73)

    Use additional external cause code if due to anti-neoplastic chemotherapy (E933.1)

    Excludes: *idiopathic myelofibrosis (238.76)*
        leukoerythroblastic anemia (284.2)
        myelofibrosis with myeloid metaplasia (238.76)
        myelophthisic anemia (284.2)
        myelophthisis (284.2)
        primary myelofibrosis (238.76)

    289.84 **Heparin-induced thrombocytopenia (HIT)**

    289.89 **Other specified diseases of blood and blood-forming organs**
        Hypergammaglobulinemia
        Pseudocholinesterase deficiency

289.9 **Unspecified diseases of blood and blood-forming organs**
    Blood dyscrasia NOS
    Erythroid hyperplasia

	Add 4th or 5th digit		Nonspecific code		Unspecified code		Manifestation code

This page intentionally left blank.

● Code new
  to 2012edition
▲ Revision of
  existing code
④ ⑤ Fourth or fifth
  digit required

Chapter 5: Mental, Behavioral and Neurodevelopmental Disorders (290-319)

DEFINITIONS AND CODING ALERTS

This chapter includes definitions of selected key words, terms and phrases and coding alerts for adding points to the clinical domain, references to coding late effects where appropriate, and references to personal history V-codes in situations where the acute or chronic condition is no longer active. An example from this chapter is as follows:

⑤ **295** **Schizophrenic disorders**

> **DEFINITION** Schizophrenia is a psychotic disorder marked by severely impaired thinking, emotions, and behaviors. Schizophrenic patients are typically unable to filter sensory stimuli and may have enhanced perceptions of sounds, colors, and other features of their environment.
>
> **ALERT!** For personal history of schizophrenia see V11.0

MULTIPLE CODING FOR A SINGLE CONDITION

In addition to the etiology or manifestation convention that requires two codes to fully describe a single condition that affects multiple body systems, there are other single conditions that also require more than one code. "Use additional code" notes are found in the tabular at codes that are not part of an etiology or manifestation pair where a secondary code is useful to fully describe a condition. The sequencing rule is the same as the etiology or manifestation pair - , "use additional code" indicates that a secondary code should be added.

"Code first" notes are also under certain codes that are not specifically manifestation codes but may be due to an underlying cause. When a "code first" note is present and an underlying condition is present the underlying condition should be sequenced first.

"Code, if applicable, any causal condition first", notes indicate that this code may be assigned as a principal diagnosis when the causal condition is unknown or not applicable. If a causal condition is known, then the code for that condition should be sequenced as the principal or first-listed diagnosis. Multiple codes may be needed for late effects, complication codes and obstetric codes to more fully describe a condition. See the specific guidelines for these conditions for further instruction.

COMBINATION CODE

A combination code is a single code used to classify: two diagnoses, or a diagnosis with an associated secondary process (manifestation) A diagnosis with an associated complication Combination codes are identified by referring to subterm entries in the Alphabetic Index and by reading the inclusion and exclusion notes in the Tabular List.

Assign only the combination code when that code fully identifies the diagnostic conditions involved or when the Alphabetic Index so directs. Multiple coding should not be used when the classification provides a combination code that clearly identifies all of the elements documented in the diagnosis. When the combination code lacks necessary specificity in describing the manifestation or complication, an additional code should be used as a secondary code.

CODING LATE EFFECTS

A late effect is the residual effect (condition produced) after the acute phase of an illness or injury has terminated. There is no time limit on when a late effect code can be used. The residual may be apparent early, such as in cerebrovascular accident cases, or it may occur months or years later, such as that due to a previous injury. Coding of late effects generally requires two codes sequenced in the following order: The condition or nature of the late effect is sequenced first. The late effect code is sequenced second.

An exception to the above guidelines are those instances where the code for late effect is followed by a manifestation code identified in the Tabular List and title, or the late effect code has been expanded (at the fourth and fifth-digit levels) to include the manifestation(s). The code for the acute phase of an illness or injury that led to the late effect is never used with a code for the late effect.

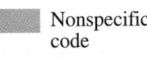

| | Add 4th or 5th digit | | Nonspecific code | | Unspecified code | | Manifestation code |

This page intentionally left blank.

● Code new
to 2012 edition

▲ Revision of
existing code

④ ⑤ Fourth or fifth
digit required

5. MENTAL, BEHAVIORAL AND NEURODEVELOPMENTAL DISORDERS (290-319)

PSYCHOSES (290-299)

[*Excludes:*] *intellectual disabilities (317-319)*

[DEFINITION] A severe mental disorder in which thought and emotions are so impaired that contact is lost with external reality.

ORGANIC PSYCHOTIC CONDITIONS (290-294)

Includes: psychotic organic brain syndrome

[*Excludes:*] *nonpsychotic syndromes of organic etiology (310.0-310.9)*
psychoses classifiable to 295-298 and without impairment of orientation, comprehension, calculation, learning capacity, and judgement, but associated with physical disease, injury, or condition affecting the brain [e.g., following childbirth] (295.0-298.8)

[DEFINITION] A severe mental illness produced by damage to the brain, as a result of poisoning, alcoholism, disease, etc.

[ALERT!] For personal history of mental disorder see V11.

290 Dementias

Code first the associated neurological condition

[*Excludes:*] *dementia due to alcohol (291.0-291.2)*
dementia due to drugs (292.82)
dementia not classified as senile, presenile, or arteriosclerotic (294.10-294.11)
psychoses classifiable to 295-298 occurring in the senium without dementia or delirium (295.0-298.8)
senility with mental changes of nonpsychotic severity (310.1)
transient organic psychotic conditions (293.0-293.9)

[DEFINITION] Dementia refers to a group of symptoms caused by disorders that affect the brain. It is not a specific disease.

290.0 Senile dementia, uncomplicated
Senile dementia:
NOS
simple type

[*Excludes:*] *mild memory disturbances, not amounting to dementia, associated with senile brain disease (310.89)*
senile dementia with:
delirium or confusion (290.3)
delusional [paranoid] features (290.20)
depressive features (290.21)

[5] **290.1 Presenile dementia**
Brain syndrome with presenile brain disease

[*Excludes:*] *arteriosclerotic dementia (290.40-290.43)*
dementia associated with other cerebral conditions (294.10-294.11)

290.10 Presenile dementia, uncomplicated
Presenile dementia:
NOS
simple type

290.11 Presenile dementia with delirium
Presenile dementia with acute confusional state

290.12 Presenile dementia with delusional features
Presenile dementia, paranoid type

290.13 Presenile dementia with depressive features
Presenile dementia, depressed type

[5] **290.2 Senile dementia with delusional or depressive features**

[*Excludes:*] *senile dementia:*
NOS (290.0)
with delirium and/or confusion (290.3)

290.20 Senile dementia with delusional features
Senile dementia, paranoid type
Senile psychosis NOS

290.21 Senile dementia with depressive features

Add 4th or 5th digit | Nonspecific code | Unspecified code | Manifestation code

290.3 Senile dementia with delirium
Senile dementia with acute confusional state

Excludes: *senile:*
dementia NOS (290.0)
psychosis NOS (290.20)

⑤ **290.4 Vascular dementia**
Multi-infarct dementia or psychosis

Use additional code to identify cerebral atherosclerosis (437.0)

Excludes: *suspected cases with no clear evidence of arteriosclerosis (290.9)*

290.40 Vascular dementia, uncomplicated
Arteriosclerotic dementia:
NOS
simple type

290.41 Vascular dementia with delirium
Arteriosclerotic dementia with acute confusional state

290.42 Vascular dementia with delusions
Arteriosclerotic dementia, paranoid type

290.43 Vascular dementia with depressed mood
Arteriosclerotic dementia, depressed type

290.8 Other specified senile psychotic conditions
Presbyophrenic psychosis

290.9 Unspecified senile psychotic condition

291 Alcohol-induced mental disorders

Excludes: *alcoholism without psychosis (303.0-303.9)*

DEFINITION Alcohol-induced mental disorders is an alcohol-induced psychological or behavioral pattern that occurs in an individual and is thought to cause distress or disability that is not expected as part of normal development or culture.

291.0 Alcohol withdrawal delirium
Alcoholic delirium
Delirium tremens

Excludes: *alcohol withdrawal (291.81)*

291.1 Alcohol-induced persisting amnestic disorder
Alcoholic polyneuritic psychosis
Korsakoff's psychosis, alcoholic
Wernicke-Korsakoff syndrome (alcoholic)

291.2 Alcohol-induced persisting dementia
Alcoholic dementia NOS
Alcoholism associated with dementia NOS
Chronic alcoholic brain syndrome

291.3 Alcohol-induced psychotic disorder with hallucinations
Alcoholic:
hallucinosis (acute)
psychosis with hallucinosis

Excludes: *alcohol withdrawal with delirium (291.0)*
schizophrenia (295.0-295.9) and paranoid states (297.0-297.9) taking the form of chronic hallucinosis with clear consciousness in an alcoholic

291.4 Idiosyncratic alcohol intoxication
Pathologic:
alcohol intoxication
drunkenness

Excludes: *acute alcohol intoxication (305.0)*
in alcoholism (303.0)
simple drunkenness (305.0)

291.5 Alcohol-induced psychotic disorder with delusions
Alcoholic:
paranoia
psychosis, paranoid type

Excludes: *nonalcoholic paranoid states (297.0-297.9)*
schizophrenia, paranoid type (295.3)

⑤ **291.8 Other specified alcohol induced mental disorders**
ALERT! For personal history of other mental disorders see V11.8

● Code new
to 2012 edition

▲ Revision of
existing code

④ ⑤ Fourth or fifth
digit required

291.81 Alcohol withdrawal
Alcohol:
withdrawal syndrome or symptoms
abstinence syndrome or symptoms

[Excludes:] *alcohol withdrawal:*
delirium (291.0)
hallucinosis (291.3)
delirium tremens (291.0)

291.82 Alcohol induced sleep disorders
Alcohol induced circadian rhythm sleep disorders
Alcohol induced hypersomnia
Alcohol induced insomnia
Alcohol induced parasomnia

291.89 Other
Alcohol induced anxiety disorder
Alcohol induced mood disorder
Alcohol induced sexual dysfunction

291.9 Unspecified alcohol-induced mental disorders
Alcohol-related disorder NOS
Alcoholic:
mania NOS
psychosis NOS
Alcoholism (chronic) with psychosis

292 Drug induced mental disorders
Includes: organic brain syndrome associated with consumption of drugs
Use additional code for any associated drug dependence (304.0-304.9)
Use additional E code, if desired, to identify drug

[DEFINITION] Drug-induced mental disorders is a drug-induced psychological or behavioral pattern that occurs in an individual and is thought to cause distress or disability that is not expected as part of normal development or culture.

292.0 Drug withdrawal
Drug:
abstinence syndrome or symptoms
withdrawal syndrome or symptoms

[5] **292.1 Drug-induced psychotic disorders**

292.11 Drug-induced psychotic disorder with delusions
Paranoid state induced by drugs

292.12 Drug-induced psychotic disorder with hallucinations
Hallucinatory state induced by drugs

[Excludes:] *states following LSD or other hallucinogens, lasting only a few days or less ["bad trips"] (305.3)*

292.2 Pathological drug intoxication
Drug reaction:
NOS resulting in brief psychotic states
idiosyncratic resulting in brief psychotic states
pathologic resulting in brief psychotic states

[Excludes:] *expected brief psychotic reactions to hallucinogens ["bad trips"] (305.3)*
physiological side-effects of drugs (e.g., dystonias)

[5] **292.8 Other specified drug induced mental disorders**
[ALERT!] For personal history of other mental disorders see V11.8

292.81 Drug induced delirium

292.82 Drug induced persisting dementia

292.83 Drug induced persisting amnestic disorder

292.84 Drug induced mood disorder
Depressive state induced by drugs

292.85 Drug induced sleep disorders
Drug induced circadian rhythm sleep disorder
Drug induced hypersomnia
Drug induced insomnia
Drug induced parasomnia

Add 4th or 5th digit | Nonspecific code | Unspecified code | Manifestation code

292.89 Other
Drug induced anxiety disorder
Drug induced organic personality syndrome
Drug induced sexual dysfunction
Drug intoxication

292.9 Unspecified drug-induced mental disorder
Drug-related disorder NOS
Organic psychosis NOS due to or associated with drugs

293 Transient mental disorders due to conditions classified elsewhere
Includes: transient organic mental disorders not associated with alcohol or drugs
Code first the associated physical or neurological condition

[Excludes:] *confusional state or delirium superimposed on senile dementia (290.3)*
dementia due to:
alcohol (291.0-291.9)
arteriosclerosis (290.40-290.43)
drugs (292.82)
senility (290.0)

293.0 Delirium due to conditions classified elsewhere
Acute:
confusional state
infective psychosis
organic reaction
posttraumatic organic psychosis
psycho-organic syndrome
Acute psychosis associated with endocrine, metabolic, or cerebrovascular disorder
Epileptic:
confusional state
twilight state

293.1 Subacute delirium
Subacute:
confusional state
infective psychosis
organic reaction
posttraumatic organic psychosis
psycho-organic syndrome
psychosis associated with endocrine or metabolic disorder

[5] ***293.8 Other specified transient mental disorders due to conditions classified elsewhere***
[ALERT!] For personal history of other mental disorders see V11.8

293.81 Psychotic disorder with delusions in conditions classified elsewhere
Transient organic psychotic condition, paranoid type

293.82 Psychotic disorder with hallucinations in conditions classified elsewhere
Transient organic psychotic condition, hallucinatory type

293.83 Mood disorder in conditions classified elsewhere
Transient organic psychotic condition, depressive type

293.84 Anxiety disorder in conditions classified elsewhere

293.89 Other
Catatonic disorder in conditions classified elsewhere

293.9 Unspecified transient mental disorder in conditions classified elsewhere
Organic psychosis:
infective NOS
posttraumatic NOS
transient NOS
Psycho-organic syndrome

294 Persistent mental disorders due to conditions classified elsewhere
Includes: organic psychotic brain syndromes (chronic), not elsewhere classified

294.0 Amnestic disorder in conditions classified elsewhere
Korsakoff's psychosis or syndrome (nonalcoholic)
Code first underlying condition

[Excludes:] *alcoholic:*
amnestic syndrome (291.1)
Korsakoff's psychosis (291.1)

[5] ***294.1 Dementia in conditions classified elsewhere***
Dementia of the Alzheimer's type

Code first any underlying physical condition, as:
Alzheimer's disease (331.0)
cerebral lipidoses (330.1)
dementia with Lewy bodies (331.82)
dementia with Parkinsonism (331.82)
epilepsy (345.0-345.9)
frontal dementia (331.19)
frontotemporal dementia (331.19)
general paresis [syphilis] (094.1)
hepatolenticular degeneration (275.1)
Huntington's chorea (333.4)
Jakob-Creutzfeldt disease (046.11-046.19)
multiple sclerosis (340)
Parkinson's disease (332.0)
Pick's disease of the brain (331.11)
polyarteritis nodosa (446.0)
syphilis (094.1)

[*Excludes:*] *dementia:*
arteriosclerotic (290.40-290.43)
presenile (290.10-290.13)
senile (290.0)
epileptic psychosis NOS (294.8)

294.10 Dementia in conditions classified elsewhere without behavioral disturbance
Dementia in conditions classified elsewhere NOS

294.11 Dementia in conditions classified elsewhere with behavioral disturbance
Aggressive behavior
Combative behavior
Violent behavior

Use additional code, where applicable, to identify:
wandering in conditions classified elsewhere (V40.31)

● **294.2 Dementia, unspecified**

[*Excludes:*] *mild memory disturbances, not amounting to dementia (310.89)*

● **294.20 Dementia, unspecified, without behavioral disturbance**
Dementia NOS

● **294.21 Dementia, unspecified, with behavioral disturbance**
Aggressive behavior
Combative behavior
Violent behavior

Use additional code, where applicable, to identify:
wandering in conditions classified elsewhere (V40.31)

294.8 Other persistent mental disorders due to conditions classified elsewhere
Amnestic disorder NOS
Epileptic psychosis NOS
Mixed paranoid and affective organic psychotic states

Use additional code for associated epilepsy (345.0-345.9)

[*Excludes:*] *mild memory disturbances, not amounting to dementia (310.89)*

[ALERT!] For personal history of other mental disorders see V11.8

294.9 Unspecified persistent mental disorders due to conditions classified elsewhere
Cognitive disorder NOS
Organic psychosis (chronic)

OTHER PSYCHOSES (295-299)

Use additional code to identify any associated physical disease, injury, or condition affecting the brain with psychoses classifiable to 295-298

⑤ **295 Schizophrenic disorders**

Includes: schizophrenia of the types described in 295.0-295.9 occurring in children

[Excludes:] *childhood type schizophrenia (299.9)*
infantile autism (299.0)

The following fifth-digit subclassification is for use with category 295:

0 unspecified
1 subchronic
2 chronic
3 subchronic with acute exacerbation
4 chronic with acute exacerbation
5 in remission

[DEFINITION] Schizophrenia is a psychotic disorder marked by severely impaired thinking, emotions, and behaviors. Schizophrenic patients are typically unable to filter sensory stimuli and may have enhanced perceptions of sounds, colors, and other features of their environment.

[ALERT!] For personal history of schizophrenia see V11.0

⑤ **295.0 Simple type**
[0-5] Schizophrenia simplex

[Excludes:] *latent schizophrenia (295.5)*

⑤ **295.1 Disorganized type**
[0-5] Hebephrenia
Hebephrenic type schizophrenia

⑤ **295.2 Catatonic type**
[0-5] Catatonic (schizophrenia):
agitation
excitation
excited type
stupor
withdrawn type
Schizophrenic:
catalepsy
catatonia
flexibilitas cerea

⑤ **295.3 Paranoid type**
[0-5] Paraphrenic schizophrenia

[Excludes:] *involutional paranoid state (297.2)*
paranoia (297.1)
paraphrenia (297.2)

⑤ **295.4 Schizophreniform disorder**
[0-5] Oneirophrenia
Schizophreniform:
attack
psychosis, confusional type

[Excludes:] *acute forms of schizophrenia of:*
catatonic type (295.2)
hebephrenic type (295.1)
paranoid type (295.3)
simple type (295.0)
undifferentiated type (295.8)

⑤ **295.5 Latent schizophrenia**
[0-5] Latent schizophrenic reaction
Schizophrenia:
borderline
incipient
Schizophrenia:
prepsychotic
prodromal
pseudoneurotic
pseudopsychopathic

[Excludes:] *schizoid personality (301.20-301.22)*

● Code new to 2012 edition ▲ Revision of existing code ④ ⑤ Fourth or fifth digit required

[5] **295.6 Residual type**
[0-5] Chronic undifferentiated schizophrenia
Restzustand (schizophrenic)
Schizophrenic residual state

[5] **295.7 Schizoaffective disorder**
[0-5] Cyclic schizophrenia
Mixed schizophrenic and affective psychosis
Schizoaffective psychosis
Schizophreniform psychosis, affective type

[5] **295.8 Other specified types of schizophrenia**
[0-5] Acute (undifferentiated) schizophrenia
Atypical schizophrenia
Cenesthopathic schizophrenia

[*Excludes:*] *infantile autism (299.0)*

[5] **295.9 Unspecified schizophrenia**
[0-5] Schizophrenia:
NOS
mixed NOS
undifferentiated NOS
undifferentiated type
Schizophrenic reaction NOS
Schizophreniform psychosis NOS

296 Episodic mood disorders
Includes: episodic affective disorders

[*Excludes:*] *neurotic depression (300.4)*
reactive depressive psychosis (298.0)
reactive excitation (298.1)

The following fifth-digit subclassification is for use with categories 296.0-296.6:

0 unspecified

1 mild

2 moderate

3 severe, without mention of psychotic behavior

4 severe, specified as with psychotic behavior

5 in partial or unspecified remission

6 in full remission

[DEFINITION] Episodic mood disorders are psychological disorders that may include depression, bipolar disorder (manic-depression), major depression, dysthymia, and cyclothymia.

[ALERT!] For personal history of affective disorders see V11.1

[5] **296.0 Bipolar I disorder, single manic episode**
[0-6] Hypomania (mild) NOS, single episode or unspecified
Hypomanic psychosis, single episode or unspecified
Mania (monopolar) NOS, single episode or unspecified
Manic-depressive psychosis or reaction:
hypomanic, single episode or unspecified
manic, single episode or unspecified

[*Excludes:*] *circular type, if there was a previous attack of depression (296.4)*

[5] **296.1 Manic disorder, recurrent episode**
[0-6] Any condition classifiable to 296.0, stated to be recurrent

[*Excludes:*] *circular type, if there was a previous attack of depression (296.4)*

[5] **296.2 Major depressive disorder, single episode**
[0-6] Depressive psychosis, single episode or unspecified
Endogenous depression, single episode or unspecified
Involutional melancholia, single episode or unspecified
Manic-depressive psychosis or reaction, depressed type, single episode or unspecified
Monopolar depression, single episode or unspecified
Psychotic depression, single episode or unspecified

[*Excludes:*] *circular type, if previous attack was of manic type (296.5)*
depression NOS (311)
reactive depression (neurotic) (300.4)
psychotic (298.0)

[5] **296.3 Major depressive disorder, recurrent episode**
[0-6] Any condition classifiable to 296.2, stated to be recurrent

[Excludes:] *circular type, if previous attack was of manic type (296.5)*
depression NOS (311)
reactive depression (neurotic) (300.4)
psychotic (298.0)

[5] **296.4 Bipolar I disorder, most recent episode (or current) manic**
[0-6] Bipolar disorder, now manic
Manic-depressive psychosis, circular type but currently manic

[Excludes:] *brief compensatory or rebound mood swings (296.99)*

[5] **296.5 Bipolar I disorder, most recent episode (or current) depressed**
[0-6] Bipolar disorder, now depressed
Manic-depressive psychosis, circular type but currently depressed

[Excludes:] *brief compensatory or rebound mood swings (296.99)*

[5] **296.6 Bipolar I disorder, most recent episode (or current) mixed**
[0-6] Manic-depressive psychosis, circular type, mixed

296.7 Bipolar I disorder, most recent episode (or current) unspecified
Atypical bipolar affective disorder NOS
Manic-depressive psychosis, circular type, current condition not specified as either manic or depressive

[5] **296.8 Other and unspecified bipolar disorders**

296.80 Bipolar disorder, unspecified
Bipolar disorder NOS
Manic-depressive:
reaction NOS
syndrome NOS

296.81 Atypical manic disorder

296.82 Atypical depressive disorder

296.89 Other
Bipolar II disorder
Manic-depressive psychosis, mixed type

[5] **296.9 Other and unspecified episodic mood disorder**

[Excludes:] *psychogenic affective psychoses (298.0-298.8)*

296.90 Unspecified episodic mood disorder
Affective psychosis NOS
Melancholia NOS
Mood disorder NOS

296.99 Other specified episodic mood disorder
Mood swings:
brief compensatory
rebound

297 Delusional disorders
Includes: paranoid disorders

[Excludes:] *acute paranoid reaction (298.3)*
alcoholic jealousy or paranoid state (291.5)
paranoid schizophrenia (295.3)

[DEFINITION] Delusional disorders refers to any mental disorder in which delusions play a significant role.

297.0 Paranoid state, simple

297.1 Delusional disorder
Chronic paranoid psychosis
Sander's disease
Systematized delusions

[Excludes:] *paranoid personality disorder (301.0)*

297.2 Paraphrenia
Involutional paranoid state
Late paraphrenia
Paraphrenia (involutional)

297.3 Shared psychotic disorder
Folie à deux
Induced psychosis or paranoid disorder

297.8 Other specified paranoid states
Paranoia querulans
Sensitiver Beziehungswahn

[Excludes:] *acute paranoid reaction or state (298.3)*
senile paranoid state (290.20)

297.9 Unspecified paranoid state
Paranoid:
disorder NOS
psychosis
Paranoid:
reaction NOS
state NOS

298 Other nonorganic psychoses
Includes: psychotic conditions due to or provoked by:
emotional stress
environmental factors as major part of etiology

298.0 Depressive type psychosis
Psychogenic depressive psychosis
Psychotic reactive depression
Reactive depressive psychosis

[Excludes:] *manic-depressive psychosis, depressed type (296.2-296.3)*
neurotic depression (300.4)
reactive depression NOS (300.4)

298.1 Excitative type psychosis
Acute hysterical psychosis
Psychogenic excitation
Reactive excitation

[Excludes:] *manic-depressive psychosis, manic type (296.0-296.1)*

298.2 Reactive confusion
Psychogenic confusion
Psychogenic twilight state

[Excludes:] *acute confusional state (293.0)*

298.3 Acute paranoid reaction
Acute psychogenic paranoid psychosis
Bouffée délirante

[Excludes:] *paranoid states (297.0-297.9)*

298.4 Psychogenic paranoid psychosis
Protracted reactive paranoid psychosis

298.8 Other and unspecified reactive psychosis
Brief psychotic disorder
Brief reactive psychosis NOS
Hysterical psychosis
Psychogenic psychosis NOS
Psychogenic stupor

[Excludes:] *acute hysterical psychosis (298.1)*

298.9 Unspecified psychosis
Atypical psychosis
Psychosis NOS
Psychotic disorder NOS

[5] **299 Pervasive developmental disorders**

[Excludes:] *adult type psychoses occurring in childhood, as:*
affective disorders (296.0-296.9)
manic-depressive disorders (296.0-296.9)
schizophrenia (295.0-295.9)

The following fifth-digit subclassification is for use with category 299:

0 current or active state

1 residual state

[5] **299.0 Autistic disorder**
[0-1]
Childhood autism
Infantile psychosis
Kanner's syndrome

[Excludes:] *disintegrative psychosis (299.1)*
Heller's syndrome (299.1)
schizophrenic syndrome of childhood (299.9)

Add 4th or 5th digit | Nonspecific code | Unspecified code | Manifestation code

⑤ **299.1   Childhood disintegrative disorder**
[0-1]   Heller's syndrome
Use additional code to identify any associated neurological disorder

> Excludes: *infantile autism (299.0)*
> *schizophrenic syndrome of childhood (299.9)*

⑤ **299.8   Other specified pervasive developmental disorders**
[0-1]   Asperger's disorder
         Atypical childhood psychosis
         Borderline psychosis of childhood

> Excludes: *simple stereotypies without psychotic disturbance (307.3)*

⑤ **299.9   Unspecified pervasive developmental disorder**
[0-1]   Child psychosis NOS
         Pervasive developmental disorder NOS
         Schizophrenia, childhood type NOS
         Schizophrenic syndrome of childhood NOS

> Excludes: *schizophrenia of adult type occurring in childhood (295.0-295.9)*

NEUROTIC DISORDERS, PERSONALITY DISORDERS, AND OTHER NONPSYCHOTIC MENTAL DISORDERS (300-316)

ALERT! For personal history of neurosis see V11.2

DEFINITION Neurotic disorders are a class of functional mental disorders involving distress but neither delusions nor hallucinations, whereby behavior is not outside socially acceptable norms.

DEFINITION Personality disorders are mental disorders characterized by inflexible, deeply ingrained, maladaptive patterns of adjustment to life that cause either subjective distress or significant impairment of adaptive functioning; manifestations are generally recognizable in adolescence or earlier.

300   Anxiety, dissociative and somatoform disorders

⑤ **300.0   Anxiety states**

> Excludes: *anxiety in:*
> *acute stress reaction (308.0)*
> *transient adjustment reaction (309.24)*
> *neurasthenia (300.5)*
> *psychophysiological disorders (306.0-306.9)*
> *separation anxiety (309.21)*

   300.00   Anxiety state, unspecified
           Anxiety:
             neurosis
             reaction
             state (neurotic)
           Atypical anxiety disorder

   300.01   Panic disorder without agoraphobia
           Panic attack
           Panic state

> Excludes: *panic disorder with agoraphobia (300.21)*

   300.02   Generalized anxiety disorder

   300.09   Other

⑤ **300.1   Dissociative, conversion and factitious disorders**

> Excludes: *adjustment reaction (309.0-309.9)*
> *anorexia nervosa (307.1)*
> *gross stress reaction (308.0-308.9)*
> *hysterical personality (301.50-301.59)*
> *psychophysiologic disorders (306.0-306.9)*

   300.10   Hysteria, unspecified

   300.11   Conversion disorder
           Astasia-abasia, hysterical
           Conversion hysteria or reaction
           Hysterical:
             blindness
             deafness
             paralysis

   300.12   Dissociative amnesia
           Hysterical amnesia

● Code new   ▲ Revision of   ④ ⑤ Fourth or fifth
         to 2012 edition   existing code   digit required

300.13 Dissociative fugue
Hysterical fugue

300.14 Dissociative identity disorder

300.15 Dissociative disorder or reaction, unspecified

300.16 Factitious disorder with predominantly psychological signs and symptoms
Compensation neurosis
Ganser's syndrome, hysterical

300.19 Other and unspecified factitious illness
Factitious disorder (with combined psychological and physical signs and symptoms) (with predominantly physical signs and symptoms) NOS

[Excludes:] *multiple operations or hospital addiction syndrome (301.51)*

[5] **300.2 Phobic disorders**

[Excludes:] *anxiety state not associated with a specific situation or object (300.0-300.09)*
obsessional phobias (300.3)

300.20 Phobia, unspecified
Anxiety-hysteria NOS
Phobia NOS

300.21 Agoraphobia with panic disorder
Fear of:
- open spaces with panic attacks
- streets with panic attacks
- travel with panic attacks

Panic disorder with agoraphobia

[Excludes:] *agoraphobia without panic disorder (300.22)*
panic disorder without agoraphobia (300.01)

300.22 Agoraphobia without mention of panic attacks
Any condition classifiable to 300.21 without mention of panic attacks

300.23 Social phobia
Fear of:
- eating in public
- public speaking
- washing in public

300.29 Other isolated or specific phobias
Acrophobia
Animal phobias
Claustrophobia
Fear of crowds

300.3 Obsessive-compulsive disorders
Anancastic neurosis
Compulsive neurosis
Obsessional phobia [any]

[Excludes:] *obsessive-compulsive symptoms occurring in:*
- *endogenous depression (296.2-296.3)*
- *organic states (e.g., encephalitis)*
- *schizophrenia (295.0-295.9)*

300.4 Dysthymic disorder
Anxiety depression
Depression with anxiety
Depressive reaction
Neurotic depressive state
Reactive depression

[Excludes:] *adjustment reaction with depressive symptoms (309.0-309.1)*
depression NOS (311)
manic-depressive psychosis, depressed type (296.2-296.3)
reactive depressive psychosis (298.0)

300.5 Neurasthenia
Fatigue neurosis
Nervous debility
Psychogenic:
- asthenia
- general fatigue

Use additional code to identify any associated physical disorder

[Excludes:] *anxiety state (300.00-300.09)*
neurotic depression (300.4)
psychophysiological disorders (306.0-306.9)
specific nonpsychotic mental disorders following organic brain damage (310.0-310.9)

300.6 Depersonalization disorder
Derealization (neurotic)
Neurotic state with depersonalization episode

Excludes: *depersonalization associated with:*
anxiety (300.00-300.09)
depression (300.4)
manic-depressive disorder or psychosis (296.0-296.9)
schizophrenia (295.0-295.9)

300.7 Hypochondriasis
Body dysmorphic disorder

Excludes: *hypochondriasis in:*
hysteria (300.10-300.19)
manic-depressive psychosis, depressed type (296.2-296.3)
neurasthenia (300.5)
obsessional disorder (300.3)
schizophrenia (295.0-295.9)

⑤ **300.8 Somatoform disorders**

300.81 Somatization disorder
Briquet's disorder
Severe somatoform disorder

300.82 Undifferentiated somatoform disorder
Atypical somatoform disorder
Somatoform disorder NOS

300.89 Other somatoform disorders
Occupational neurosis, including writers' cramp
Psychasthenia
Psychasthenic neurosis

300.9 Unspecified nonpsychotic mental disorder
Psychoneurosis NOS

301 Personality disorders
Includes: character neurosis

Use additional code to identify any associated neurosis or psychosis, or physical condition

Excludes: *nonpsychotic personality disorder associated with organic brain syndromes*
(310.0-310.9)

DEFINITION Personality disorders, formerly referred to as character disorders, are a class of personality types which deviate from the contemporary expectations of a society. Common types of personality disorders include paranoia, schizoid tendencies, antisocial behavior, narcissism, and obsessive-compulsive disorders.

301.0 Paranoid personality disorder
Fanatic personality
Paranoid personality (disorder)
Paranoid traits

Excludes: *acute paranoid reaction (298.3)*
alcoholic paranoia (291.5)
paranoid schizophrenia (295.3)
paranoid states (297.0-297.9)

⑤ **301.1 Affective personality disorder**

Excludes: *affective psychotic disorders (296.0-296.9)*
neurasthenia (300.5)
neurotic depression (300.4)

301.10 Affective personality disorder, unspecified

301.11 Chronic hypomanic personality disorder
Chronic hypomanic disorder
Hypomanic personality

301.12 Chronic depressive personality disorder
Chronic depressive disorder
Depressive character or personality

301.13 Cyclothymic disorder
Cycloid personality
Cyclothymia
Cyclothymic personality

● Code new
to 2012 edition
▲ Revision of
existing code
④ ⑤ Fourth or fifth
digit required

[5] **301.2 Schizoid personality disorder**

[Excludes:] *schizophrenia (295.0-295.9)*

301.20 Schizoid personality disorder, unspecified

301.21 Introverted personality

301.22 Schizotypal personality disorder

301.3 Explosive personality disorder

Aggressive:
 personality
 reaction
Aggressiveness
Emotional instability (excessive)
Pathological emotionality
Quarrelsomeness

[Excludes:] *dyssocial personality (301.7)*
hysterical neurosis (300.10-300.19)

301.4 Obsessive-compulsive personality disorder

Anancastic personality
Obsessional personality

[Excludes:] *obsessive-compulsive disorder (300.3)*
phobic state (300.20-300.29)

[5] **301.5 Histrionic personality disorder**

[Excludes:] *hysterical neurosis (300.10-300.19)*

301.50 Histrionic personality disorder, unspecified

Hysterical personality NOS

301.51 Chronic factitious illness with physical symptoms

Hospital addiction syndrome
Multiple operations syndrome
Munchausen syndrome

301.59 Other histrionic personality disorder

Personality:
 emotionally unstable
 labile
 psychoinfantile

301.6 Dependent personality disorder

Asthenic personality
Inadequate personality
Passive personality

[Excludes:] *neurasthenia (300.5)*
passive-aggressive personality (301.84)

301.7 Antisocial personality disorder

Amoral personality
Asocial personality
Dyssocial personality
Personality disorder with predominantly sociopathic or asocial manifestation

[Excludes:] *disturbance of conduct without specifiable personality disorder (312.0-312.9)*
explosive personality (301.3)

[5] **301.8 Other personality disorders**

301.81 Narcissistic personality disorder

301.82 Avoidant personality disorder

301.83 Borderline personality disorder

301.84 Passive-aggressive personality

301.89 Other

Personality:
 eccentric
 "haltlose" type
 immature
Personality:
 masochistic
 psychoneurotic

[Excludes:] *psychoinfantile personality (301.59)*

301.9 Unspecified personality disorder

Pathological personality NOS
Personality disorder NOS
Psychopathic:
 constitutional state
 personality (disorder)

302 Sexual and gender identity disorders

[Excludes:] *sexual disorder manifest in:*
organic brain syndrome (290.0-294.9, 310.0-310.9)
psychosis (295.0-298.9)

302.0 Ego-dystonic sexual orientation
Ego-dystonic lesbianism
Sexual orientation conflict disorder

[Excludes:] *homosexual pedophilia (302.2)*

302.1 Zoophilia
Bestiality

302.2 Pedophilia

302.3 Transvestic fetishism

[Excludes:] *trans-sexualism (302.5)*

302.4 Exhibitionism

[5] **302.5 Trans-sexualism**
Sex reassignment surgery status

[Excludes:] *transvestism (302.3)*

302.50 With unspecified sexual history

302.51 With asexual history

302.52 With homosexual history

302.53 With heterosexual history

302.6 Gender identity disorder in children
Feminism in boys
Gender identity disorder NOS

[Excludes:] *gender identity disorder in adult (302.85)*
trans-sexualism (302.50-302.53)
transvestism (302.3)

[5] **302.7 Psychosexual dysfunction**

[Excludes:] *impotence of organic origin (607.84)*
normal transient symptoms from ruptured hymen
transient or occasional failures of erection due to fatigue, anxiety, alcohol, or drugs

302.70 Psychosexual dysfunction, unspecified
Sexual dysfunction NOS

302.71 Hypoactive sexual desire disorder

[Excludes:] *decreased sexual desire NOS (799.81)*

302.72 With inhibited sexual excitement
Female sexual arousal disorder
Frigidity
Impotence
Male erectile disorder

302.73 Female orgasmic disorder

302.74 Male orgasmic disorder

302.75 Premature ejaculation

302.76 Dyspareunia, psychogenic

302.79 With other specified psychosexual dysfunctions
Sexual aversion disorder

[5] **302.8 Other specified psychosexual disorders**

302.81 Fetishism

302.82 Voyeurism

302.83 Sexual masochism

302.84 Sexual sadism

302.85 Gender identity disorder in adolescents or adults

Use additional code to identify sex reassignment surgery status (302.5)

[Excludes:] *gender identity disorder NOS (302.6)*
gender identity disorder in children (302.6)

● Code new to 2012 edition ▲ Revision of existing code [4] [5] Fourth or fifth digit required

302.89 Other
Frotteurism
Nymphomania
Satyriasis

302.9 Unspecified psychosexual disorder
Paraphilia NOS
Pathologic sexuality NOS
Sexual deviation NOS
Sexual disorder NOS

[5] **303 Alcohol dependence syndrome**
Use additional code to identify any associated condition, as:
alcoholic psychoses (291.0-291.9)
drug dependence (304.0-304.9)
physical complications of alcohol, such as:
cerebral degeneration (331.7)
cirrhosis of liver (571.2)
epilepsy (345.0-345.9)
gastritis (535.3)
hepatitis (571.1)
liver damage NOS (571.3)

[*Excludes:*] *drunkenness NOS (305.0)*

The following fifth-digit subclassification is for use with category 303:

0 unspecified
1 continuous
2 episodic
3 in remission

[DEFINITION] Alcohol dependence syndrome, aka, alcoholism, is the most severe stage of a group of drinking problems which begins with binge drinking and alcohol abuse.

[ALERT!] For personal history of alcoholism see V11.3

[5] **303.0 Acute alcoholic intoxication**
[0-3] Acute drunkenness in alcoholism

[5] **303.9 Other and unspecified alcohol dependence**
[0-3] Chronic alcoholism
Dipsomania

[5] **304 Drug dependence**
[*Excludes:*] *nondependent abuse of drugs (305.1-305.9)*

The following fifth-digit subclassification is for use with category 304:

0 unspecified
1 continuous
2 episodic
3 in remission

[5] **304.0 Opioid type dependence**
[0-3] Heroin
Meperidine
Methadone
Morphine
Opium
Opium alkaloids and their derivatives
Synthetics with morphine-like effects

[5] **304.1 Sedative, hypnotic or anxiolytic dependence**
[0-3] Barbiturates
Nonbarbiturate sedatives and tranquilizers with a similar effect:
chlordiazepoxide
diazepam
glutethimide
meprobamate
methaqualone

[5] **304.2 Cocaine dependence**
[0-3] Coca leaves and derivatives

[5] **304.3 Cannabis dependence**
[0-3] Hashish
Hemp
Marijuana

[5] **304.4 Amphetamine and other psychostimulant dependence**
[0-3] Methylphenidate
Phenmetrazine

[5] **304.5 Hallucinogen dependence**
[0-3] Dimethyltryptamine [DMT]
Lysergic acid diethylamide [LSD] and derivatives
Mescaline
Psilocybin

[5] **304.6 Other specified drug dependence**
[0-3] Absinthe addiction
Glue sniffing
Inhalant dependence
Phencyclidine dependence

[*Excludes:*] *tobacco dependence (305.1)*

[5] **304.7 Combinations of opioid type drug with any other**
[0-3]

[5] **304.8 Combinations of drug dependence excluding opioid type drug**
[0-3]

[5] **304.9 Unspecified drug dependence**
[0-3] Drug addiction NOS
Drug dependence NOS

305 Nondependent abuse of drugs

Note: Includes cases where a person, for whom no other diagnosis is possible, has come under medical care because of the maladaptive effect of a drug on which he is not dependent and that he has taken on his own initiative to the detriment of his health or social functioning.

[*Excludes:*] *alcohol dependence syndrome (303.0-303.9)*
drug dependence (304.0-304.9)
drug withdrawal syndrome (292.0)
poisoning by drugs or medicinal substances (960.0-979.9)

The following fifth-digit subclassification is for use with codes 305.0, 305.2-305.9:

0 unspecified

1 continuous

2 episodic

3 in remission

[5] **305.0 Alcohol abuse**
[0-3] Drunkenness NOS
Excessive drinking of alcohol NOS
"Hangover" (alcohol)
Inebriety NOS

[*Excludes:*] *acute alcohol intoxication in alcoholism (303.0)*
alcoholic psychoses (291.0-291.9)

305.1 Tobacco use disorder
Tobacco dependence

[*Excludes:*] *history of tobacco use (V15.82)*
smoking complicating pregnancy (649.0)
tobacco use disorder complicating pregnancy (649.0)

[ALERT!] For personal history of tobacco use see V15.82

[5] **305.2 Cannabis abuse**
[0-3]

[5] **305.3 Hallucinogen abuse**
[0-3] Acute intoxication from hallucinogens ["bad trips"]
LSD reaction

[5] **305.4 Sedative, hypnotic or anxiolytic abuse**
[0-3]

[5] **305.5 Opioid abuse**
[0-3]

[5] **305.6 Cocaine abuse**
[0-3]

[5] **305.7 Amphetamine or related acting sympathomimetic abuse**
[0-3]

[5] **305.8 Antidepressant type abuse**
[0-3]

[5] **305.9 Other, mixed, or unspecified drug abuse**
[0-3]
Caffeine intoxication
Inhalant abuse
"Laxative habit"
Misuse of drugs NOS
Nonprescribed use of drugs or patent medicinals
Phencyclidine abuse

306 Physiological malfunction arising from mental factors

Includes: psychogenic:
physical symptoms not involving tissue damage
physiological manifestation not involving tissue damage

[*Excludes:*] *hysteria (300.11-300.19)*
physical symptoms secondary to a psychiatric disorder classified elsewhere
psychic factors associated with physical conditions involving tissue damage classified elsewhere (316)
specific nonpsychotic mental disorders following organic brain damage (310.0-310.9)

306.0 Musculoskeletal
Psychogenic paralysis
Psychogenic torticollis

[*Excludes:*] *Gilles de la Tourette's syndrome (307.23)*
paralysis as hysterical or conversion reaction (300.11)
tics (307.20-307.22)

306.1 Respiratory
Psychogenic:
air hunger
cough
hiccough
hyperventilation
yawning

[*Excludes:*] *psychogenic asthma (316 and 493.9)*

306.2 Cardiovascular
Cardiac neurosis
Cardiovascular neurosis
Neurocirculatory asthenia
Psychogenic cardiovascular disorder

[*Excludes:*] *psychogenic paroxysmal tachycardia (316 and 427.2)*

306.3 Skin
Psychogenic pruritus

[*Excludes:*] *psychogenic:*
alopecia (316 and 704.00)
dermatitis (316 and 692.9)
eczema (316 and 691.8 or 692.9)
urticaria (316 and 708.0-708.9)

306.4 Gastrointestinal
Aerophagy
Cyclical vomiting, psychogenic
Diarrhea, psychogenic
Nervous gastritis
Psychogenic dyspepsia

[*Excludes:*] *cyclical vomiting NOS (536.2)*
associated with migraine (346.2)
globus hystericus (300.11)
mucous colitis (316 and 564.9)
psychogenic:
cardiospasm (316 and 530.0)
duodenal ulcer (316 and 532.0-532.9)
gastric ulcer (316 and 531.0-531.9)
peptic ulcer NOS (316 and 533.0-533.9)
vomiting NOS (307.54)

⑤ **306.5 Genitourinary**

[Excludes:] *enuresis, psychogenic (307.6)*
frigidity (302.72)
impotence (302.72)
psychogenic dyspareunia (302.76)

306.50 Psychogenic genitourinary malfunction, unspecified

306.51 Psychogenic vaginismus
Functional vaginismus

306.52 Psychogenic dysmenorrhea

306.53 Psychogenic dysuria

306.59 Other

306.6 Endocrine

306.7 Organs of special sense

[Excludes:] *hysterical blindness or deafness (300.11)*
psychophysical visual disturbances (368.16)

306.8 Other specified psychophysiological malfunction
Bruxism
Teeth grinding

306.9 Unspecified psychophysiological malfunction
Psychophysiologic disorder NOS
Psychosomatic disorder NOS

307 Special symptoms or syndromes, not elsewhere classified

Note: This category is intended for use if the psychopathology is manifested by a single specific symptom or group of symptoms which is not part of an organic illness or other mental disorder classifiable elsewhere.

[Excludes:] *those due to mental disorders classified elsewhere*
those of organic origin

307.0 Adult onset fluency disorder

[Excludes:] *childhood onset fluency disorder (315.35)*
dysphasia (784.59)
lisping or lalling (307.9)
retarded development of speech (315.31-315.39)
fluency disorder due to late effect of cerebrovascular accident (438.14)
fluency disorder in conditions classified elsewhere (784.52)

307.1 Anorexia nervosa

[Excludes:] *eating disturbance NOS (307.50)*
feeding problem (783.3)
of nonorganic origin (307.59)
loss of appetite (783.0)
of nonorganic origin (307.59)

⑤ **307.2 Tics**

[Excludes:] *nail-biting or thumb-sucking (307.9)*
stereotypies occurring in isolation (307.3)
tics of organic origin (333.3)

307.20 Tic disorder, unspecified
Tic disorder NOS

307.21 Transient tic disorder

307.22 Chronic motor or vocal tic disorder

307.23 Tourette's disorder
Motor-verbal tic disorder

307.3 Stereotypic movement disorder
Body-rocking
Head banging
Spasmus nutans
Stereotypies NOS

[Excludes:] *tics (307.20-307.23)*
of organic origin (333.3)

● Code new to 2012 edition ▲ Revision of existing code ④ ⑤ Fourth or fifth digit required

[5] **307.4 Specific disorders of sleep of nonorganic origin**

[Excludes:] *narcolepsy (347.00-347.11)*
organic hypersomnia (327.10-327.19)
organic insomnia (327.00-327.09)
those of unspecified cause (780.50-780.59)

307.40 Nonorganic sleep disorder, unspecified

307.41 Transient disorder of initiating or maintaining sleep
Adjustment insomnia
Hyposomnia associated with acute or intermittent emotional reactions or conflicts
Insomnia associated with acute or intermittent emotional reactions or conflicts
Sleeplessness associated with acute or intermittent emotional reactions or conflicts

307.42 Persistent disorder of initiating or maintaining sleep
Hyposomnia, insomnia, or sleeplessness associated with:
anxiety
conditioned arousal
depression (major) (minor)
psychosis
Idiopathic insomnia
Paradoxical insomnia
Primary insomnia
Psychophysiological insomnia

307.43 Transient disorder of initiating or maintaining wakefulness
Hypersomnia associated with acute or intermittent emotional reactions or conflicts

307.44 Persistent disorder of initiating or maintaining wakefulness
Hypersomnia associated with depression (major) (minor)
Insufficient sleep syndrome
Primary hypersomnia

[Excludes:] *sleep deprivation (V69.4)*

307.45 Circadian rhythm sleep disorder of nonorganic origin

307.46 Sleep arousal disorder
Night terror disorder
Night terrors
Sleep terror disorder
Sleepwalking
Somnambulism

307.47 Other dysfunctions of sleep stages or arousal from sleep
Dyssomnia NOS
Nightmare disorder
Nightmares:
NOS
REM-sleep type
Parasomnia NOS
Sleep drunkenness

307.48 Repetitive intrusions of sleep
Repetitive intrusion of sleep with:
atypical polysomnographic features
environmental disturbances
repeated REM-sleep interruptions

307.49 Other
"Short-sleeper"
Subjective insomnia complaint

[5] **307.5 Other and unspecified disorders of eating**

[Excludes:] *anorexia:*
nervosa (307.1)
of unspecified cause (783.0)
overeating, of unspecified cause (783.6)
vomiting:
NOS (787.03)
cyclical (536.2)
associated with migraine (346.2)
psychogenic (306.4)

307.50 Eating disorder, unspecified
Eating disorder NOS

307.51 Bulimia nervosa
Overeating of nonorganic origin

307.52 Pica
Perverted appetite of nonorganic origin

307.53 Rumination disorder
Regurgitation, of nonorganic origin, of food with reswallowing

[Excludes:] *obsessional rumination (300.3)*

307.54 Psychogenic vomiting

307.59 Other
Feeding disorder of infancy or early childhood of nonorganic origin
Infantile feeding disturbances of nonorganic origin
Loss of appetite of nonorganic origin

307.6 Enuresis
Enuresis (primary) (secondary) of nonorganic origin

[Excludes:] *enuresis of unspecified cause (788.3)*

307.7 Encopresis
Encopresis (continuous) (discontinuous) of nonorganic origin

[Excludes:] *encopresis of unspecified cause (787.60-787.63)*

[5] **307.8 Pain disorders related to psychological factors**

307.80 Psychogenic pain, site unspecified

307.81 Tension headache

[Excludes:] *headache:*
NOS (784.0)
migraine (346.0-346.9)
syndromes (339.00-339.89)
tension type (339.10-339.12)

307.89 Other
Code first to type or site of pain

[Excludes:] *pain disorder exclusively attributed to psychological factors (307.80)*
psychogenic pain (307.80)

307.9 Other and unspecified special symptoms or syndromes, not elsewhere classified
Communication disorder NOS
Hair plucking
Lalling
Lisping
Masturbation
Nail-biting
Thumb-sucking

308 Acute reaction to stress
Includes: catastrophic stress
combat and operational stress reaction
combat fatigue
gross stress reaction (acute)
transient disorders in response to exceptional physical or mental stress which usually subside within hours or days

[Excludes:] *adjustment reaction or disorder (309.0-309.9)*
chronic stress reaction (309.1-309.9)

308.0 Predominant disturbance of emotions
Anxiety as acute reaction to exceptional [gross] stress
Emotional crisis as acute reaction to exceptional [gross] stress
Panic state as acute reaction to exceptional [gross] stress

308.1 Predominant disturbance of consciousness
Fugues as acute reaction to exceptional [gross] stress

308.2 Predominant psychomotor disturbance
Agitation states as acute reaction to exceptional [gross] stress
Stupor as acute reaction to exceptional [gross] stress

308.3 Other acute reactions to stress
Acute situational disturbance
Acute stress disorder

[Excludes:] *prolonged posttraumatic emotional disturbance (309.81)*

308.4 Mixed disorders as reaction to stress

308.9 Unspecified acute reaction to stress

309 Adjustment reaction
Includes: adjustment disorders
reaction (adjustment) to chronic stress

[Excludes:] *acute reaction to major stress (308.0-308.9)*
neurotic disorders (300.0-300.9)

ALERT! For personal history of psychological trauma presenting hazards to health see V15.4

DEFINITION A person with an adjustment reaction has feelings of sadness, anxiety and anger following a stressful experience. The symptoms of adjustment reaction may last for a few months.

309.0 Adjustment disorder with depressed mood
Grief reaction

[Excludes:] *affective psychoses (296.0-296.9)*
neurotic depression (300.4)
prolonged depressive reaction (309.1)
psychogenic depressive psychosis (298.0)

309.1 Prolonged depressive reaction

[Excludes:] *affective psychoses (296.0-296.9)*
brief depressive reaction (309.0)
neurotic depression (300.4)
psychogenic depressive psychosis (298.0)

[5] **309.2 With predominant disturbance of other emotions**

309.21 Separation anxiety disorder

309.22 Emancipation disorder of adolescence and early adult life

309.23 Specific academic or work inhibition

309.24 Adjustment disorder with anxiety

309.28 Adjustment disorder with mixed anxiety and depressed mood
Adjustment reaction with anxiety and depression

309.29 Other
Culture shock

309.3 Adjustment disorder with disturbance of conduct
Conduct disturbance as adjustment reaction
Destructiveness as adjustment reaction

[Excludes:] *destructiveness in child (312.9)*
disturbance of conduct NOS (312.9)
dyssocial behavior without manifest psychiatric disorder (V71.01-V71.02)
personality disorder with predominantly sociopathic or asocial manifestations (301.7)

309.4 Adjustment disorder with mixed disturbance of emotions and conduct

[5] **309.8 Other specified adjustment reactions**

309.81 Posttraumatic stress disorder
Chronic posttraumatic stress disorder
Concentration camp syndrome
Posttraumatic stress disorder NOS
Post-Traumatic Stress Disorder (PTSD)

[Excludes:] *acute stress disorder (308.3)*
posttraumatic brain syndrome:
nonpsychotic (310.2)
psychotic (293.0-293.9)

309.82 Adjustment reaction with physical symptoms

309.83 Adjustment reaction with withdrawal
Elective mutism as adjustment reaction
Hospitalism (in children) NOS

309.89 Other

309.9 Unspecified adjustment reaction
Adaptation reaction NOS
Adjustment reaction NOS

310 Specific nonpsychotic mental disorders due to brain damage

Excludes: neuroses, personality disorders, or other nonpsychotic conditions occurring in a form similar to that seen with functional disorders but in association with a physical condition (300.0-300.9, 301.0-301.9)

ALERT! For personal history of unspecified mental disorder see V11.9

310.0 Frontal lobe syndrome
Lobotomy syndrome
Postleucotomy syndrome [state]

Excludes: postcontusion syndrome (310.2)

310.1 Personality change due to conditions classified elsewhere
Cognitive or personality change of other type, of nonpsychotic severity
Organic psychosyndrome of nonpsychotic severity
Presbyophrenia NOS
Senility with mental changes of nonpsychotic severity

Excludes: mild cognitive impairment (331.83)

postconcussion syndrome (310.2)
signs and symptoms involving emotional state (799.21-799.29)

310.2 Postconcussion syndrome
Postcontusion syndrome or encephalopathy
Posttraumatic brain syndrome, nonpsychotic
Status postcommotio cerebri

Use additional code to identify associated post-traumatic headache, if applicable (339.20-339.22)

Excludes: frontal lobe syndrome (310.0)

postencephalitic syndrome (310.89)
any organic psychotic conditions following head injury (293.0—294.0)

⑤ **310.8 Other specified nonpsychotic mental disorders following organic brain damage**

● **310.81 Pseudobulbar affect**
Involuntary emotional expression disorder

Code first underlying cause, if known, such as:
amyotrophic lateral sclerosis (335.20)
late effect of cerebrovascular accident (438.89)
late effect of traumatic brain injury (907.0)
multiple sclerosis (340)

● **310.89 Other specified nonpsychotic mental disorders following organic brain damage**
Mild memory disturbance
Other focal (partial) organic psychosyndromes
Postencephalitic syndrome

Excludes: memory loss of unknown cause (780.93)

310.9 Unspecified nonpsychotic mental disorder following organic brain damage

311 Depressive disorder, not elsewhere classified
Depressive disorder NOS
Depressive state NOS
Depression NOS

Excludes: acute reaction to major stress with depressive symptoms (308.0)

affective personality disorder (301.10-301.13)
affective psychoses (296.0-296.9)
brief depressive reaction (309.0)
depressive states associated with stressful events (309.0-309.1)
disturbance of emotions specific to childhood and adolescence, with misery and unhappiness (313.1)
mixed adjustment reaction with depressive symptoms (309.4)
neurotic depression (300.4)
prolonged depressive adjustment reaction (309.1)
psychogenic depressive psychosis (298.0)

ALERT! For personal history of unspecified mental disorder see V11.9

● Code new
to 2012 edition
▲ Revision of
existing code
④ ⑤ Fourth or fifth
digit required

312 **Disturbance of conduct, not elsewhere classified**

Excludes: *adjustment reaction with disturbance of conduct (309.3)*
drug dependence (304.0-304.9)
dyssocial behavior without manifest psychiatric disorder (V71.01-V71.02)
personality disorder with predominantly sociopathic or asocial manifestations (301.7)
sexual deviations (302.0-302.9)

The following fifth-digit subclassification is for use with categories 312.0-312.2:

0 **unspecified**

1 **mild**

2 **moderate**

3 **severe**

ALERT! For personal history of unspecified mental disorder see V11.9

⑤ **312.0** **Undersocialized conduct disorder, aggressive type**
[0-3]   Aggressive outburst
Anger reaction
Unsocialized aggressive disorder

⑤ **312.1** **Undersocialized conduct disorder, unaggressive type**
[0-3]   Childhood truancy,   Solitary stealing
unsocialized   Tantrums

⑤ **312.2** **Socialized conduct disorder**
[0-3]   Childhood truancy, socialized
Group delinquency

Excludes: *gang activity without manifest psychiatric disorder (V71.01)*

⑤ **312.3** **Disorders of impulse control, not elsewhere classified**

312.30 **Impulse control disorder, unspecified**

312.31 **Pathological gambling**

312.32 **Kleptomania**

312.33 **Pyromania**

312.34 **Intermittent explosive disorder**

312.35 **Isolated explosive disorder**

312.39 **Other**
Trichotillomania

312.4 **Mixed disturbance of conduct and emotions**
Neurotic delinquency

Excludes: *compulsive conduct disorder (312.3)*

⑤ **312.8** **Other specified disturbances of conduct, not elsewhere classified**

312.81 **Conduct disorder, childhood onset type**

312.82 **Conduct disorder, adolescent onset type**

312.89 **Other conduct disorder**
Conduct disorder of unspecified onset

312.9 **Unspecified disturbance of conduct**
Delinquency (juvenile)
Disruptive behavior disorder NOS

313 **Disturbance of emotions specific to childhood and adolescence**

Excludes: *adjustment reaction (309.0-309.9)*
emotional disorder of neurotic type (300.0-300.9)
masturbation, nail-biting, thumb-sucking, and other isolated symptoms (307.0-307.9)

313.0 **Overanxious disorder**
Anxiety and fearfulness of childhood and adolescence
Overanxious disorder of childhood and adolescence

Excludes: *abnormal separation anxiety (309.21)*
anxiety states (300.00-300.09)
hospitalism in children (309.83)
phobic state (300.20-300.29)

313.1 **Misery and unhappiness disorder**

Excludes: *depressive neurosis (300.4)*

| | Add 4th or 5th digit | | Nonspecific code | | Unspecified code | | Manifestation code |

⑤ **313.2 Sensitivity, shyness, and social withdrawal disorder**

> Excludes: *infantile autism (299.0)*
> *schizoid personality (301.20-301.22)*
> *schizophrenia (295.0-295.9)*

313.21 Shyness disorder of childhood
Sensitivity reaction of childhood or adolescence

313.22 Introverted disorder of childhood
Social withdrawal of childhood and adolescence
Withdrawal reaction of childhood and adolescence

313.23 Selective mutism

> Excludes: *elective mutism as adjustment reaction (309.83)*

313.3 Relationship problems
Sibling jealousy

> Excludes: *relationship problems associated with aggression, destruction, or other forms of*
> *conduct disturbance (312.0-312.9)*

⑤ **313.8 Other or mixed emotional disturbances of childhood or adolescence**

313.81 Oppositional defiant disorder

313.82 Identity disorder
Identity problem

313.83 Academic underachievement disorder

313.89 Other
Reactive attachment disorder of infancy or early childhood

313.9 Unspecified emotional disturbance of childhood or adolescence
Mental disorder of infancy, childhood or adolescence NOS

314 Hyperkinetic syndrome of childhood

> Excludes: *hyperkinesis as symptom of underlying disorder—code the underlying disorder*

DEFINITION Hyperkinetic syndrome of childhood is a childhood or adolescent disorder characterized by excessive activity, emotional instability, significantly reduced attention span, and an absence of shyness and fear, and that occasionally develops in individuals with brain injury, mental defect, or epilepsy.

⑤ **314.0 Attention deficit disorder**
Adult
Child

314.00 Without mention of hyperactivity
Predominantly inattentive type

314.01 With hyperactivity
Combined type
Overactivity NOS
Predominantly hyperactive/impulsive type
Simple disturbance of attention with overactivity

314.1 Hyperkinesis with developmental delay
Developmental disorder of hyperkinesis

Use additional code to identify any associated neurological disorder

314.2 Hyperkinetic conduct disorder
Hyperkinetic conduct disorder without developmental delay

> Excludes: *hyperkinesis with significant delays in specific skills (314.1)*

314.8 Other specified manifestations of hyperkinetic syndrome

314.9 Unspecified hyperkinetic syndrome
Hyperkinetic reaction of childhood or adolescence NOS
Hyperkinetic syndrome NOS

315 Specific delays in development

> Excludes: *that due to a neurological disorder (320.0-389.9)*

⑤ **315.0 Specific reading disorder**

315.00 Reading disorder, unspecified

315.01 Alexia

315.02 Developmental dyslexia

315.09 Other
Specific spelling difficulty

● Code new
to 2012 edition ▲ Revision of
existing code ④ ⑤ Fourth or fifth
digit required

315.1 **Mathematics disorder**
Dyscalculia

315.2 **Other specific learning difficulties**
Disorder of written expression

Excludes: *specific arithmetical disorder (315.1)*
specific reading disorder (315.00-315.09)

⑤ **315.3** **Developmental speech or language disorder**

315.31 **Expressive language disorder**
Developmental aphasia
Word deafness

Excludes: *acquired aphasia (784.3)*
elective mutism (309.83, 313.0, 313.23)

315.32 **Mixed receptive-expressive language disorder**
Central auditory processing disorder

Excludes: *acquired auditory processing disorder (388.45)*

315.34 **Speech and language developmental delay due to hearing loss**

315.35 **Childhood onset fluency disorder**
Cluttering NOS
Stuttering NOS

Excludes: *adult onset fluency disorder (307.0)*
fluency disorder due to late effect of cerebrovascular accident (438.14)
fluency disorder in conditions classified elsewhere (784.52)

315.39 **Other**
Developmental articulation disorder
Dyslalia
Phonological disorder

Excludes: *lisping and lalling (307.9)*

315.4 **Developmental coordination disorder**
Clumsiness syndrome
Dyspraxia syndrome
Specific motor development disorder

315.5 **Mixed development disorder**

315.8 **Other specified delays in development**

315.9 **Unspecified delay in development**
Developmental disorder NOS
Learning disorder NOS

316 **Psychic factors associated with diseases classified elsewhere**
Psychologic factors in physical conditions classified elsewhere

Use additional code to identify the associated physical condition, as:
psychogenic:
asthma (493.9)
dermatitis (692.9)
duodenal ulcer (532.0-532.9)
eczema (691.8, 692.9)
gastric ulcer (531.0-531.9)
mucous colitis (564.9)
paroxysmal tachycardia (427.2)
ulcerative colitis (556)
urticaria (708.0-708.9)
psychosocial dwarfism (259.4)

Excludes: *physical symptoms and physiological malfunctions, not involving tissue damage, of*
mental origin (306.0-306.9)

INTELLECTUAL DISABILITIES (317-319)

Use additional code(s) to identify any associated psychiatric or physical condition(s)

▲ **317** **Mild intellectual disabilities**
High-grade defect   Mild mental subnormality
IQ 50-70

DEFINITION Intellectual disabilities is a generalized disorder, characterized by sub average
cognitive functioning and deficits in two or more adaptive behaviors with onset before the
age of 18.

▲ **318** **Other specified intellectual disabilities**

| | Add 4th or 5th digit | | Nonspecific code | | Unspecified code | | Manifestation code |

▲ **318.0 Moderate intellectual disabilities**
IQ 35-49
Moderate mental subnormality

▲ **318.1 Severe intellectual disabilities**
IQ 20-34
Severe mental subnormality

▲ **318.2 Profound intellectual disabilities**
IQ under 20
Profound mental subnormality

▲ **319 Unspecified intellectual disabilities**
Mental deficiency NOS
Mental subnormality NOS

● Code new
to 2012 edition
▲ Revision of
existing code
④ ⑤ Fourth or fifth
digit required

Chapter 6: Diseases of Nervous System and Sense Organs (320-389)

DEFINITIONS AND CODING ALERTS

This chapter includes definitions of selected key words, terms and phrases and coding alerts for adding points to the clinical domain, references to coding late effects where appropriate, and references to personal history V-codes in situations where the acute or chronic condition is no longer active. An example from this chapter is as follows:

324 **Intracranial and intraspinal abscess**
DEFINITION Intracranial and intraspinal abscess refers to an abcess occuring inside the cranium or the spinal column
ALERT! For coding late effects of intracranial abscess or pyogenic infection see 326

MULTIPLE CODING FOR A SINGLE CONDITION

In addition to the etiology or manifestation convention that requires two codes to fully describe a single condition that affects multiple body systems, there are other single conditions that also require more than one code. "Use additional code" notes are found in the tabular at codes that are not part of an etiology or manifestation pair where a secondary code is useful to fully describe a condition. The sequencing rule is the same as the etiology or manifestation pair - , "use additional code" indicates that a secondary code should be added.

"Code first" notes are also under certain codes that are not specifically manifestation codes but may be due to an underlying cause. When a "code first" note is present and an underlying condition is present the underlying condition should be sequenced first.

"Code, if applicable, any causal condition first", notes indicate that this code may be assigned as a principal diagnosis when the causal condition is unknown or not applicable. If a causal condition is known, then the code for that condition should be sequenced as the principal or first-listed diagnosis. Multiple codes may be needed for late effects, complication codes and obstetric codes to more fully describe a condition. See the specific guidelines for these conditions for further instruction.

COMBINATION CODE

A combination code is a single code used to classify: two diagnoses, or a diagnosis with an associated secondary process (manifestation) A diagnosis with an associated complication Combination codes are identified by referring to subterm entries in the Alphabetic Index and by reading the inclusion and exclusion notes in the Tabular List.

Assign only the combination code when that code fully identifies the diagnostic conditions involved or when the Alphabetic Index so directs. Multiple coding should not be used when the classification provides a combination code that clearly identifies all of the elements documented in the diagnosis. When the combination code lacks necessary specificity in describing the manifestation or complication, an additional code should be used as a secondary code.

CODING LATE EFFECTS

A late effect is the residual effect (condition produced) after the acute phase of an illness or injury has terminated. There is no time limit on when a late effect code can be used. The residual may be apparent early, such as in cerebrovascular accident cases, or it may occur months or years later, such as that due to a previous injury. Coding of late effects generally requires two codes sequenced in the following order: The condition or nature of the late effect is sequenced first. The late effect code is sequenced second.

An exception to the above guidelines are those instances where the code for late effect is followed by a manifestation code identified in the Tabular List and title, or the late effect code has been expanded (at the fourth and fifth-digit levels) to include the manifestation(s). The code for the acute phase of an illness or injury that led to the late effect is never used with a code for the late effect.

PAIN - CATEGORY 338

General coding information

Codes in category 338 may be used in conjunction with codes from other categories and chapters to provide more detail about acute or chronic pain and neoplasm-related pain, unless otherwise indicated below.

| | Add 4th or 5th digit | | Nonspecific code | | Unspecified code | | Manifestation code |

If the pain is not specified as acute or chronic, do not assign codes from category 338, except for post-thoracotomy pain, postoperative pain, neoplasm related pain, or central pain syndrome.

A code from subcategories 338.1 and 338.2 should not be assigned if the underlying (definitive) diagnosis is known, unless the reason for the encounter is pain control or management and not management of the underlying condition.

A. Category 338 Codes as Principal or First-Listed Diagnosis

Category 338 codes are acceptable as principal diagnosis or the first-listed code:

1) When pain control or pain management is the reason for the admission or encounter (e.g., a patient with displaced intervertebral disc, nerve impingement and severe back pain presents for injection of steroid into the spinal canal). The underlying cause of the pain should be reported as an additional diagnosis, if known.

2) When an admission or encounter is for a procedure aimed at treating the underlying condition (e.g., spinal fusion, kyphoplasty), a code for the underlying condition (e.g., vertebral fracture, spinal stenosis) should be assigned as the principal diagnosis. No code from category 338 should be assigned.

3) When a patient is admitted for the insertion of a neurostimulator for pain control, assign the appropriate pain code as the principal or first listed diagnosis. When an admission or encounter is for a procedure aimed at treating the underlying condition and a neurostimulator is inserted for pain control during the same admission or encounter, a code for the underlying condition should be assigned as the principal diagnosis and the appropriate pain code should be assigned as a secondary diagnosis.

B. Use of Category 338 Codes in Conjunction with Site-Specific Pain Codes

1) Assigning Category 338 Codes and Site Specific Pain Codes

Codes from category 338 may be used in conjunction with codes that identify the site of pain including codes from chapter 16. If the category 338 code provides additional information. For example, if the code describes the site of the pain, but does not fully describe whether the pain is acute or chronic, then both codes should be assigned.

2) Sequencing of Category 338 Codes with Site Specific Pain Codes

The sequencing of category 338 codes with site specific pain codes (including chapter 16 codes), is dependent on the circumstances of the encounter or admission as follows:

a) If the encounter is for pain control or pain management, assign the code from category 338 followed by the code identifying the specific site of pain (e.g., encounter for pain management for acute neck pain from trauma is assigned code 338.11, Acute pain due to trauma, followed by code 723.1, Cervicalgia, to identify the site of pain).

b) If the encounter is for any other reason except pain control or pain management, and a related definitive diagnosis has not been established (confirmed) by the provider, assign the code for the specific site of pain first, followed by the appropriate code from category 338.

Pain due to devices, implants and grafts

Pain associated with devices, implants or grafts left in a surgical site (for example painful hip prosthesis) is assigned to the appropriate code(s) found in Chapter 17, Injury and Poisoning. Use additional code(s) from category 338 to identify acute or chronic pain due to presence of the device, implant or graft (338.18-338.19 or 338.28-338.29.

Postoperative Pain

Post-thoracotomy pain and other postoperative pain are classified to subcategories 338.1 and 338.2, depending on whether the pain is acute or chronic. The default for post-thoracotomy and other postoperative pain not specified as acute or chronic is the code for the acute form.

Routine or expected postoperative pain immediately after surgery should not be coded.

A. Postoperative pain not associated with specific postoperative complication

Postoperative pain not associated with a specific postoperative complication is assigned to the appropriate postoperative pain code in category 338.

● Code new
to 2012 edition

▲ Revision of
existing code

④ ⑤ Fourth or fifth
digit required

B. Postoperative pain associated with specific postoperative complication

Postoperative pain associated with a specific postoperative complication (such as painful wire sutures) is assigned to the appropriate code(s) found in Chapter 17, Injury and Poisoning. If appropriate, use additional code(s) from category 338 to identify acute or chronic pain (338.18 or 338.28). If pain control or management is the reason for the encounter, a code from category 338 should be assigned as the principal or first-listed diagnosis in accordance with Official Guidelines, Section I.C.6.a.1.a above.

C. Postoperative pain as principal or first-listed diagnosis

Postoperative pain may be reported as the principal or first-listed diagnosis when the stated reason for the admission or encounter is documented as postoperative pain control or management.

D. Postoperative pain as secondary diagnosis

Postoperative pain may be reported as a secondary diagnosis code when a patient presents for outpatient surgery and develops an unusual or inordinate amount of postoperative pain.

The provider's documentation should be used to guide the coding of postoperative pain, as well as Official Guidelines, Section III. Reporting Additional Diagnoses and Official Guidelines, Section IV. Diagnostic Coding and Reporting in the Outpatient Setting.

See Official Guidelines, Section II.I.2 for information on sequencing of diagnoses for patients admitted to hospital inpatient care following post-operative observation.

See Official Guidelines, Section II.J for information on sequencing of diagnoses for patients admitted to hospital inpatient care from outpatient surgery.

See Official Guidelines, Section IV.A.2 for information on sequencing of diagnoses for patients admitted for observation.

CHRONIC PAIN

Chronic pain is classified to subcategory 338.2. There is no time frame defining when pain becomes chronic pain. The provider's documentation should be used to guide use of these codes.

NEOPLASM RELATED PAIN

Code 338.3 is assigned to pain documented as being related, associated or due to cancer, primary or secondary malignancy, or tumor. This code is assigned regardless of whether the pain is acute or chronic.

This code may be assigned as the principal or first listed code when the stated reason for the admission or encounter is documented as pain control or pain management. The underlying neoplasm should be reported as an additional diagnosis.

When the reason for the admission or encounter is management of the neoplasm and the pain associated with the neoplasm is also documented, code 338.3 may be assigned as an additional diagnosis.

See Chapter 2 for instructions on the sequencing of neoplasms for all other stated reasons for the admission or encounter (except for pain control or pain management).

CHRONIC PAIN SYNDROME

This condition is different than the term "chronic pain," and therefore this code should only be used when the provider has specifically documented this condition.

Add 4th or 5th digit	Nonspecific code	Unspecified code	Manifestation code

This page intentionally left blank.

6. DISEASES OF THE NERVOUS SYSTEM AND SENSE ORGANS (320-389)

ALERT! For personal history of disorders of nervous system and sense organs see V12.4

INFLAMMATORY DISEASES OF THE CENTRAL NERVOUS SYSTEM (320-326)

ALERT! For personal history of infections of the central nervous system see V12.42

320 Bacterial meningitis

Includes: arachnoiditis, bacterial
leptomeningitis, bacterial
meningitis, bacterial
meningoencephalitis, bacterial
meningomyelitis, bacterial
pachymeningitis, bacterial

DEFINITION Meningitis is an infectious disease characterized by inflammation of the meninges (the tissues that surround the brain or spinal cord) usually caused by a bacterial infection; symptoms include headache and stiff neck and fever and nausea.

320.0 Hemophilus meningitis
Meningitis due to Hemophilus influenzae [H. influenzae]

320.1 Pneumococcal meningitis

320.2 Streptococcal meningitis

320.3 Staphylococcal meningitis

320.7 Meningitis in other bacterial diseases classified elsewhere

Code first underlying disease, as:
actinomycosis (039.8)
listeriosis (027.0)
typhoid fever (002.0)
whooping cough (033.0-033.9)

[Excludes:] *meningitis (in):*
epidemic (036.0)
gonococcal (098.82)
meningococcal (036.0)
salmonellosis (003.21)
syphilis:
NOS (094.2)
congenital (090.42)
meningovascular (094.2)
secondary (091.81)
tuberculous (013.0)

[5] **320.8 Meningitis due to other specified bacteria**

320.81 Anaerobic meningitis
Bacteroides (fragilis)
Gram-negative anaerobes

320.82 Meningitis due to Gram-negative bacteria, not elsewhere classified
Aerobacter aerogenes
Escherichia coli [E. coli]
Friedlander bacillus
Klebsiella pneumoniae
Proteus morganii
Pseudomonas

[Excludes:] *Gram-negative anaerobes (320.81)*

320.89 Meningitis due to other specified bacteria
Bacillus pyocyaneus

320.9 Meningitis due to unspecified bacterium

Meningitis:
bacterial NOS
purulent NOS

Meningitis:
pyogenic NOS
suppurative NOS

321 Meningitis due to other organisms

Includes: arachnoiditis due to organisms other than bacteria
leptomeningitis due to organisms other than bacteria
meningitis due to organisms other than bacteria
pachymeningitis due to organisms other than bacteria

321.0 Cryptococcal meningitis
Code first underlying disease (117.5)

Add 4th or 5th digit — Nonspecific code — Unspecified code — Manifestation code

321.1 ***Meningitis in other fungal diseases***
Code first underlying disease (110.0-118)
[Excludes:] *meningitis in:*
candidiasis (112.83)
coccidioidomycosis (114.2)
histoplasmosis (115.01, 115.11, 115.91)

321.2 ***Meningitis due to viruses not elsewhere classified***
Code first underlying disease, as:
meningitis due to arbovirus (060.0-066.9)
[Excludes:] *meningitis (due to):*
abacterial (047.0-047.9)
adenovirus (049.1)
aseptic NOS (047.9)
Coxsackie (virus) (047.0)
ECHO virus (047.1)
enterovirus (047.0-047.9)
herpes simplex virus (054.72)
herpes zoster virus (053.0)
lymphocytic choriomeningitis virus (049.0)
mumps (072.1)
viral NOS (047.9)
meningo-eruptive syndrome (047.1)

321.3 ***Meningitis due to trypanosomiasis***
Code first underlying disease (086.0-086.9)

321.4 ***Meningitis in sarcoidosis***
Code first underlying disease (135)

321.8 ***Meningitis due to other nonbacterial organisms classified elsewhere***
Code first underlying disease
[Excludes:] *leptospiral meningitis (100.81)*

322 Meningitis of unspecified cause
Includes: arachnoiditis with no organism specified as cause
leptomeningitis with no organism specified as cause
meningitis with no organism specified as cause
pachymeningitis with no organism specified as cause

322.0 Nonpyogenic meningitis
Meningitis with clear cerebrospinal fluid

322.1 Eosinophilic meningitis

322.2 Chronic meningitis

322.9 Meningitis, unspecified

323 Encephalitis, myelitis, and encephalomyelitis
Includes: acute disseminated encephalomyelitis
meningoencephalitis, except bacterial
meningomyelitis, except bacterial
myelitis:
ascending
transverse

[Excludes:] *acute transverse myelitis NOS (341.20)*
acute transverse myelitis in conditions classified elsewhere (341.21)
bacterial:
meningoencephalitis (320.0-320.9)
meningomyelitis (320.0-320.9)
idiopathic transverse myelitis (341.22)
idiopathic transverse myelitis (341.22)

DEFINITION Encephalitis is an inflammation of the brain, usually caused by a direct viral infection or a hypersensitivity reaction to a virus or foreign protein. Myelitis is an inflammation of the spinal column. Encephalomyelitis is an inflammation of the brain and spinal cord.

[5] **323.0** ***Encephalitis, myelitis,and encephalomyelitis in viral diseases classified elsewhere***
Code first underlying disease, as:
cat-scratch disease (078.3)
infectious mononucleosis (075)
human immunodeficiency virus [HIV] disease (042)
ornithosis (073.7)

323.01 ***Encephalitis and encephalomyelitis in viral diseases classified elsewhere***

[Excludes:] *encephalitis (in):*
arthropod-borne viral (062.0-064)
herpes simplex (054.3)
mumps (072.2)
other viral diseases of central nervous system (049.8-049.9)
poliomyelitis (045.0-045.9)
rubella (056.01)
slow virus infections of central nervous system (046.0-046.9)
viral NOS (049.9)
West Nile (066.41)

323.02 ***Myelitis in viral diseases classified elsewhere***

[Excludes:] *myelitis (in):*
herpes simplex (054.74)
herpes zoster (053.14)
poliomyelitis (045.0-045.9)
rubella (056.01)
other viral diseases of central nervous system (049.8-049.9)

323.1 ***Encephalitis, myelitis, and encephalomyelitis in rickettsial diseases classified elsewhere***
Code first underlying disease (080-083.9)

323.2 ***Encephalitis, myelitis, and encephalomyelitis in protozoal diseases classified elsewhere***
Code first underlying disease, as:
malaria (084.0-084.9)
trypanosomiasis (086.0-086.9)

▲ **323.4** ***Other encephalitis, myelitis, and encephalomyelitis due to other infections classified elsewhere***
Code first underlying disease

▲ **323.41** ***Other encephalitis and encephalomyelitis due to other infections classified elsewhere***

[Excludes:] *encephalitis (in):*
meningococcal (036.1)
syphilis:
NOS (094.81)
congenital (090.41)
toxoplasmosis (130.0)
tuberculosis (013.6)
meningoencephalitis due to free-living ameba [Naegleria] (136.29)

▲ **323.42** ***Other myelitis due to other infections classified elsewhere***

[Excludes:] *myelitis (in):*
syphilis (094.89)
tuberculosis (013.6)

[5] **323.5 Encephalitis, myelitis, and encephalomyelitis following immunization procedures**
Use additional E code, if desired, to identify vaccine

323.51 Encephalitis and encephalomyelitis following immunization procedures
Encephalitis postimmunization or postvaccinal
Encephalomyelitis postimmunization or postvaccinal

323.52 Myelitis following immunization procedures
Myelitis postimmunization or postvaccinal

[5] **323.6** ***Postinfectious encephalitis, myelitis, and encephalomyelitis***
Code first underlying disease

323.61 ***Infectious acute disseminated encephalomyelitis (ADEM)***
Acute necrotizing hemorrhagic encephalopathy

[Excludes:] *noninfectious acute disseminated encephalomyelitis (ADEM) (323.81)*

323.62 ***Other postinfectious encephalitis and encephalomyelitis***

[Excludes:] *encephalitis:*
postchickenpox (052.0)
postmeasles (055.0)

323.63 ***Postinfectious myelitis***

[Excludes:] *postchickenpox myelitis (052.2)*
herpes simplex myelitis (054.74)
herpes zoster myelitis (053.14)

⑤ **323.7** *Toxic encephalitis, myelitis, and encephalomyelitis*
  Code first underlying cause, as:
   carbon tetrachloride (982.1)
   hydroxyquinoline derivatives (961.3)
   lead (984.0-984.9)
   mercury (985.0)
   thallium (985.8)

  `323.71` *Toxic encephalitis and encephalomyelitis*

  `323.72` *Toxic myelitis*

⑤ **323.8** **Other causes of encephalitis, myelitis, and encephalomyelitis**

  `323.81` **Other causes of encephalitis and encephalomyelitis**
   Noninfectious acute disseminated encephalomyelitis (ADEM)

  `323.82` **Other causes of myelitis**
   Transverse myelitis NOS

 323.9 **Unspecified causes of encephalitis, myelitis, and encephalomyelitis**

`324` **Intracranial and intraspinal abscess**

 `DEFINITION` Intracranial and intraspinal abscess refers to an abcess occuring inside the cranium or the spinal column.

 `ALERT!` For coding late effects of intracranial abscess or pyogenic infection see 326

 324.0 **Intracranial abscess**
  Abscess (embolic):   Abscess (embolic) of brain [any part]:
   cerebellar   epidural
   cerebral   extradural
            otogenic
            subdural

Excludes:	tuberculous (013.3)

 324.1 **Intraspinal abscess**
  Abscess (embolic) of spinal cord [any part]:
   epidural
   extradural
   subdural

Excludes:	tuberculous (013.5)

 `324.9` **Of unspecified site**
  Extradural or subdural abscess NOS

325 **Phlebitis and thrombophlebitis of intracranial venous sinuses**
 Embolism, of cavernous, lateral, or other intracranial or unspecified intracranial venous sinus
 Endophlebitis, of cavernous, lateral, or other intracranial or unspecified intracranial venous sinus
 Phlebitis, septic or suppurative, of cavernous, lateral, or other intracranial or unspecified intracranial venous sinus
 Thrombophlebitis of cavernous, lateral, or other intracranial or unspecified intracranial venous sinus
 Thrombosis of cavernous, lateral, or other intracranial or unspecified intracranial venous sinus

Excludes:	that specified as:

   complicating pregnancy, childbirth, or the puerperium (671.5)
   of nonpyogenic origin (437.6)

 `DEFINITION` Phlebitis and thrombophlebitis of intracranial venous sinuses refers to the inflammation of a vein or phlebitis related to a blood clot of the intracranial venous sinuses.

 `ALERT!` For personal history of venous thrombosis and embolism see V12.51

326 **Late effects of intracranial abscess or pyogenic infection**
 Note: This category is to be used to indicate conditions whose primary classification is to 320-325 [excluding 320.7, 321.0-321.8, 323.01-323.42, 323.61-323.72] as the cause of late effects, themselves classifiable elsewhere. The "late effects" include conditions specified as such, or as sequelae, which may occur at any time after the resolution of the causal condition.

 Use additional code, if desired, to identify condition, as:
  hydrocephalus (331.4)
  paralysis (342.0-342.9, 344.0-344.9)

 `DEFINITION` Late effects of intracranial abscess or pyogenic infection refers to a condition that appears after the acute phase of an intracranial abscess or pyogenic infection ha run its course.

● Code new ▲ Revision of ④ ⑤ Fourth or fifth
  to 2012 edition   existing code   digit required

ORGANIC SLEEP DISORDERS (327)

327 Organic sleep disorders

DEFINITION Organic sleep disorders are sleep disorders that are the result of an anatomic or physiologic abnormality or disease process.

⑤ **327.0 Organic disorders of initiating and maintaining sleep [Organic insomnia]**

[Excludes:] *insomnia NOS (780.52)*
insomnia not due to a substance or known physiological condition (307.41-307.42)
insomnia with sleep apnea NOS (780.51)

327.00 Organic insomnia, unspecified

327.01 Insomnia due to medical condition classified elsewhere

Code first underlying condition

[Excludes:] *insomnia due to mental disorder (327.02)*

327.02 Insomnia due to mental disorder

Code first mental disorder

[Excludes:] *alcohol induced insomnia (291.82)*
drug induced insomnia (292.85)

327.09 Other organic insomnia

⑤ **327.1 Organic disorder of excessive somnolence [Organic hypersomnia]**

[Excludes:] *hypersomnia NOS (780.54)*
hypersomnia not due to a substance or known physiological condition (307.43-307.44)
hypersomnia with sleep apnea NOS (780.53)

327.10 Organic hypersomnia, unspecified

327.11 Idiopathic hypersomnia with long sleep time

327.12 Idiopathic hypersomnia without long sleep time

327.13 Recurrent hypersomnia
Kleine-Levin syndrome
Menstrual related hypersomnia

327.14 Hypersomnia due to medical condition classified elsewhere

Code first underlying condition

[Excludes:] *hypersomnia due to mental disorder (327.15)*

327.15 Hypersomnia due to mental disorder

Code first mental disorder

[Excludes:] *alcohol induced hypersomnia (291.82)*
drug induced hypersomnia (292.85)

327.19 Other organic hypersomnia

⑤ **327.2 Organic sleep apnea**

[Excludes:] *Cheyne-Stokes breathing (786.04)*
hypersomnia with sleep apnea NOS (780.53)
insomnia with sleep apnea NOS (780.51)
sleep apnea in newborn (770.81-770.82)
sleep apnea NOS (780.57)

327.20 Organic sleep apnea, unspecified

327.21 Primary central sleep apnea

327.22 High altitude periodic breathing

327.23 Obstructive sleep apnea (adult) (pediatric)

327.24 Idiopathic sleep related nonobstructive alveolar hypoventilation
Sleep related hypoxia

327.25 Congenital central alveolar hypoventilation syndrome

327.26 Sleep related hypoventilation/hypoxemia in conditions classifiable elsewhere

Code first underlying condition

327.27 Central sleep apnea in conditions classified elsewhere

Code first underlying condition

327.29 Other organic sleep apnea

Add 4th or 5th digit | Nonspecific code | Unspecified code | Manifestation code

⑤ **327.3 Circadian rhythm sleep disorder**
Organic disorder of sleep wake cycle
Organic disorder of sleep wake schedule

Excludes: *alcohol induced circadian rhythm sleep disorder (291.82)*
circadian rhythm sleep disorder of nonorganic origin (307.45)
disruption of 24 hour sleep wake cycle NOS (780.55)
drug induced circadian rhythm sleep disorder (292.85)

327.30 Circadian rhythm sleep disorder, unspecified

327.31 Circadian rhythm sleep disorder, delayed sleep phase type

327.32 Circadian rhythm sleep disorder, advanced sleep phase type

327.33 Circadian rhythm sleep disorder, irregular sleep-wake type

327.34 Circadian rhythm sleep disorder, free-running type

327.35 Circadian rhythm sleep disorder, jet lag type

327.36 Circadian rhythm sleep disorder, shift work type

327.37 Circadian rhythm sleep disorder in conditions classified elsewhere
Code first underlying condition

327.39 Other circadian rhythm sleep disorder

⑤ **327.4 Organic parasomnia**

Excludes: *alcohol induced parasomnia (291.82)*
drug induced parasomnia (292.85)
parasomnia not due to a known physiological condition (307.47)

327.40 Organic parasomnia, unspecified

327.41 Confusional arousals

327.42 REM sleep behavior disorder

327.43 Recurrent isolated sleep paralysis

327.44 Parasomnia in conditions classified elsewhere
Code first underlying condition

327.49 Other organic parasomnia

⑤ **327.5 Organic sleep related movement disorders**

Excludes: *restless legs syndrome (333.94)*
sleep related movement disorder NOS (780.58)

327.51 Periodic limb movement disorder
Periodic limb movement sleep disorder

327.52 Sleep related leg cramps

327.53 Sleep related bruxism

327.59 Other organic sleep related movement disorders

327.8 Other organic sleep disorders

HEREDITARY AND DEGENERATIVE DISEASES OF THE CENTRAL NERVOUS SYSTEM (330-337)

Excludes: *hepatolenticular degeneration (275.1)*
multiple sclerosis (340)
other demyelinating diseases of central nervous system (341.0-341.9)

330 Cerebral degenerations usually manifest in childhood
Use additional code, if desired, to identify associated intellectual disabilities

330.0 Leukodystrophy
Krabbe's disease
Leukodystrophy:
NOS
globoid cell
Leukodystrophy:
metachromatic
sudanophilic
Pelizaeus-Merzbacher disease
Sulfatide lipidosis

330.1 Cerebral lipidoses
Amaurotic (familial) idiocy
Disease:
Batten
Jansky-Bielschowsky
Disease:
Kufs'
Spielmeyer-Vogt
Tay-Sachs
Gangliosidosis

● Code new
to 2012 edition

▲ Revision of
existing code

④ ⑤ Fourth or fifth
digit required

330.2 Cerebral degeneration in generalized lipidoses
Code first underlying disease, as:
Fabry's disease (272.7)
Gaucher's disease (272.7)
Neimann-Pick disease (272.7)
sphingolipidosis (272.7)

330.3 Cerebral degeneration of childhood in other diseases classified elsewhere
Code first underlying disease, as:
Hunter's disease (277.5)
mucopolysaccharidosis (277.5)

330.8 Other specified cerebral degenerations in childhood
Alpers' disease or gray-matter degeneration
Infantile necrotizing encephalomyelopathy
Leigh's disease
Subacute necrotizing encephalopathy or encephalomyelopathy

330.9 Unspecified cerebral degeneration in childhood

331 Other cerebral degenerations
Use additional code, where applicable, to identify dementia:
with behavioral disturbance (294.11)
without behavioral disturbance (294.10)

> **ALERT!** For personal history of other disorders of nervous system and sense organs see V12.49

331.0 Alzheimer's disease

⑤ **331.1 Frontotemporal dementia**

    331.11 Pick's disease

    331.19 Other frontotemporal dementia
    Frontal dementia

331.2 Senile degeneration of brain

> Excludes: senility NOS (797)

331.3 Communicating hydrocephalus
Secondary normal pressure hydrocephalus

> Excludes: congenital hydrocephalus (742.3)
> idiopathic normal pressure hydrocephalus (331.5)
> normal pressure hydrocephalus (331.5)
> spina bifida with hydrocephalus (741.0)

331.4 Obstructive hydrocephalus
Acquired hydrocephalus NOS

> Excludes: congenital hydrocephalus (742.3)
> idiopathic normal pressure hydrocephalus (331.5)
> normal pressure hydrocephalus (331.5)
> spina bifida with hydrocephalus (741.0)

331.5 Idiopathic normal pressure hydrocephalus (INPH)
Normal pressure hydrocephalus NOS

> Excludes: congenital hydrocephalus (742.3)
> secondary normal pressure hydrocephalus (331.3)
> spina bifida with hydrocephalus (741.0)

● **331.6 Corticobasal degeneration**

331.7 Cerebral degeneration in diseases classified elsewhere
Code first underlying disease, as:
alcoholism (303.0-303.9)
beriberi (265.0)
cerebrovascular disease (430-438)
congenital hydrocephalus (741.0, 742.3)
neoplastic disease (140.0-239.9)
myxedema (244.0-244.9)
vitamin B_{12} deficiency (266.2)

> Excludes: cerebral degeneration in:
> Jakob-Creutzfeldt disease (046.11-046.19)
> progressive multifocal leukoencephalopathy (046.3)
> subacute spongiform encephalopathy (046.1)

⑤ **331.8 Other cerebral degeneration**

    331.81 Reye's syndrome

	Add 4th or 5th digit		Nonspecific code		Unspecified code		Manifestation code

331.82 Dementia with Lewy bodies
Dementia with Parkinsonism
Lewy body dementia
Lewy body disease

331.83 Mild cognitive impairment, so stated

Excludes: *altered mental status (780.97)*
cerebral degeneration (331.0-331.9)
change in mental status (780.97)
cognitive deficits following (late effects of) cerebral hemorrhage or infarction (438.0)
cognitive impairment due to intracranial or head injury (850-854, 959.01)
cognitive impairment due to late effect of intracranial injury (907.0)
cognitive impairment due to skull fracture (800-801, 803-804)
dementia (290.0-290.43, 294.20-294.21)
mild memory disturbance (310.89)
neurologic neglect syndrome (781.8)
personality change, nonpsychotic (310.1)

331.89 Other
Cerebral ataxia

331.9 Cerebral degeneration, unspecified

332 Parkinson's disease

Excludes: *dementia with Parkinsonism (331.82)*

DEFINITION Parkinson's disease is a degenerative disease of the brain (central nervous system) that often impairs motor skills, speech, and other functions.

332.0 Paralysis agitans
Parkinsonism or Parkinson's disease:
NOS
idiopathic
primary

332.1 Secondary Parkinsonism
Neuroleptic-induced Parkinsonism
Parkinsonism due to drugs

Use additional E code, if desired, to identify drug, if drug-induced

Excludes: *Parkinsonism (in):*
Huntington's disease (333.4)
progressive supranuclear palsy (333.0)
Shy-Drager syndrome (333.0)
syphilitic (094.82)

333 Other extrapyramidal disease and abnormal movement disorders
Includes: other forms of extrapyramidal, basal ganglia, or striatopallidal disease

Excludes: *abnormal movements of head NOS (781.0)*
sleep related movement disorders (327.51-327.59)

DEFINITION Extrapyramidal disease is a general term for a number of disorders caused by abnormalities of the basal ganglia or certain brain stem or thalamic nuclei; characterised by motor deficits, loss of postural reflexes, bradykinesia, tremor, rigidity, and various involuntary movements.

ALERT! For personal history of other disorders of nervous system and sense organs see V12.49

333.0 Other degenerative diseases of the basal ganglia
Atrophy or degeneration:
olivopontocerebellar [Déjérine-Thomas syndrome]
pigmentary pallidal [Hallervorden-Spatz disease]
striatonigral
Parkinsonian syndrome associated with:
idiopathic orthostatic hypotension
symptomatic orthostatic hypotension
Progressive supranuclear ophthalmoplegia
Shy-Drager syndrome

333.1 Essential and other specified forms of tremor
Benign essential tremor
Familial tremor
Medication-induced postural tremor

Use additional E code, if desired, to identify drug, if drug-induced

Excludes: *tremor NOS (781.0)*

● Code new
to 2012 edition

▲ Revision of
existing code

④ ⑤ Fourth or fifth
digit required

333.2 Myoclonus
Familial essential myoclonus
Palatal myoclonus

[Excludes:] *progressive myoclonic epilepsy (345.1)*
Unverricht-Lundborg disease (345.1)

Use additional E code, if desired, to identify drug, if drug-induced

333.3 Tics of organic origin

[Excludes:] *Gilles de la Tourette's syndrome (307.23)*
habit spasm (307.22)
tic NOS (307.20)

Use additional E code, if desired, to identify drug, if drug-induced

333.4 Huntington's chorea

333.5 Other choreas
Hemiballism(us)
Paroxysmal choreo-athetosis

[Excludes:] *Sydenham's or rheumatic chorea (392.0-392.9)*

Use additional E code, if desired, to identify drug, if drug-induced

333.6 Genetic torsion dystonia
Dystonia:
deformans progressiva
musculorum deformans
(Schwalbe-) Ziehen-Oppenheim disease

[5] **333.7 Acquired torsion dystonia**

333.71 Athetoid cerebral palsy
Double athetosis (syndrome)
Vogt's disease

[Excludes:] *infantile cerebral palsy (343.0-343.9)*

333.72 Acute dystonia due to drugs
Acute dystonic reaction due to drugs
Neuroleptic induced acute dystonia

Use additional E code to identify drug

[Excludes:] *blepharospasm due to drugs (333.85)*
orofacial dyskinesia due to drugs (333.85)
secondary Parkinsonism (332.1)
subacute dyskinesia due to drugs (333.85)
tardive dyskinesia (333.85)

333.79 Other acquired torsion dystonia

[5] **333.8 Fragments of torsion dystonia**
Use additional E code, if desired, to identify drug, if drug-induced

333.81 Blepharospasm

[Excludes:] *blepharospasm due to drugs (333.85)*

333.82 Orofacial dyskinesia

[Excludes:] *orofacial dyskinesia due to drugs (333.85)*

333.83 Spasmodic torticollis

[Excludes:] *torticollis:*
NOS (723.5)
hysterical (300.11)
psychogenic (306.0)

333.84 Organic writers' cramp

[Excludes:] *psychogenic (300.89)*

333.85 Subacute dyskinesia due to drugs
Blepharospasm due to drugs
Orofacial dyskinesia due to drugs
Tardive dyskinesia

Use additional E code to identify drug

[Excludes:] *acute dystonia due to drugs (333.72)*
acute dystonic reaction due to drugs (333.72)
secondary Parkinsonism (332.1)

333.89 Other

⑤ **333.9 Other and unspecified extrapyramidal diseases and abnormal movement disorders**

333.90 Unspecified extrapyramidal disease and abnormal movement disorder
Medication-induced movement disorders NOS
Use additional E code to identify drug, if drug-induced

333.91 Stiff-man syndrome

333.92 Neuroleptic malignant syndrome
Use additional E code to identify drug

Excludes: *neuroleptic induced Parkinsonism (332.1)*

333.93 Benign shuddering attacks

333.94 Restless legs syndrome (RLS)

333.99 Other
Neuroleptic-induced acute akathisia
Use additional E code to identify drug, if drug-induced

334 Spinocerebellar disease

Excludes: *olivopontocerebellar degeneration (333.0)*
peroneal muscular atrophy (356.1)

DEFINITION Spinocerebellar disease refers to a disease involving both the spinal cord and the cerebellum.

334.0 Friedreich's ataxia

334.1 Hereditary spastic paraplegia

334.2 Primary cerebellar degeneration
Cerebellar ataxia:
Marie's
Sanger-Brown
Dyssynergia cerebellaris myoclonica
Primary cerebellar degeneration:
NOS
hereditary
sporadic

334.3 Other cerebellar ataxia
Cerebellar ataxia NOS

Use additional E code, if desired, to identify drug, if drug-induced

334.4 *Cerebellar ataxia in diseases classified elsewhere*
Code first underlying disease, as:
alcoholism (303.0-303.9)
myxedema (244.0-244.9)
neoplastic disease (140.0-239.9)

334.8 Other spinocerebellar diseases
Ataxia-telangiectasia [Louis-Bar syndrome]
Corticostriatal-spinal degeneration

334.9 Spinocerebellar disease, unspecified

335 Anterior horn cell disease
DEFINITION Anterior horn cell disease refers to diseases characterized by a selective degeneration of the motor neurons of the spinal cord, brainstem, or motor cortex. Clinical subtypes are distinguished by the major site of degeneration

335.0 Werdnig-Hoffmann disease
Infantile spinal muscular atrophy
Progressive muscular atrophy of infancy

⑤ **335.1 Spinal muscular atrophy**

335.10 Spinal muscular atrophy, unspecified

335.11 Kugelberg-Welander disease
Spinal muscular atrophy:
familial
juvenile

335.19 Other
Adult spinal muscular atrophy

⑤ **335.2 Motor neuron disease**

335.20 Amyotrophic lateral sclerosis
Motor neuron disease (bulbar) (mixed type)

335.21 Progressive muscular atrophy
Duchenne-Aran muscular atrophy
Progressive muscular atrophy (pure)

● Code new
to 2012 edition

▲ Revision of
existing code

④ ⑤ Fourth or fifth
digit required

335.22 Progressive bulbar palsy

335.23 Pseudobulbar palsy

335.24 Primary lateral sclerosis

335.29 Other

335.8 Other anterior horn cell diseases

335.9 Anterior horn cell disease, unspecified

336 Other diseases of spinal cord

[ALERT!] For personal history of other disorders of nervous system and sense organs see V12.49

336.0 Syringomyelia and syringobulbia

336.1 Vascular myelopathies
Acute infarction of spinal cord (embolic) (nonembolic)
Arterial thrombosis of spinal cord
Edema of spinal cord
Hematomyelia
Subacute necrotic myelopathy

336.2 Subacute combined degeneration of spinal cord in diseases classified elsewhere
Code first underlying disease, as:
pernicious anemia (281.0)
other vitamin B_{12} deficiency anemia (281.1)
vitamin B_{12} deficiency (266.2)

336.3 Myelopathy in other diseases classified elsewhere
Code first underlying disease, as:
myelopathy in neoplastic disease (140.0-239.9)

[*Excludes:*] *myelopathy in:*
intervertebral disc disorder (722.70-722.73)
spondylosis (721.1, 721.41-721.42, 721.91)

336.8 Other myelopathy
Myelopathy:
drug-induced
radiation-induced

Use additional E code, if desired, to identify cause

336.9 Unspecified disease of spinal cord
Cord compression NOS
Myelopathy NOS

[*Excludes:*] *myelitis (323.02, 323.1, 323.2, 323.42, 323.52, 323.63, 323.72, 323.82, 323.9)*
spinal (canal) stenosis (723.0, 724.00-724.09)

337 Disorders of the autonomic nervous system
Includes: disorders of peripheral autonomic, sympathetic, parasympathetic, or vegetative system

[*Excludes:*] *familial dysautonomia [Riley-Day syndrome] (742.8)*

[DEFINITION] Disorders of the autonomic nervous system refers to disorders of the part of the nervous system that regulates involuntary action, as of the intestines, heart, and glands.

[5] **337.0 Idiopathic peripheral autonomic neuropathy**

337.00 Idiopathic peripheral autonomic neuropathy, unspecified

337.01 Carotid sinus syndrome
Carotid sinus syncope

337.09 Other idiopathic peripheral autonomic neuropathy
Cervical sympathetic dystrophy or paralysis

337.1 Peripheral autonomic neuropathy in disorders classified elsewhere
Code first underlying disease, as:
amyloidosis (277.30-277.39)
diabetes (249.6, 250.6)

[5] **337.2 Reflex sympathetic dystrophy**

337.20 Reflex sympathetic dystrophy, unspecified
Complex regional pain syndrome type I, unspecified

337.21 Reflex sympathetic dystrophy of the upper limb
Complex regional pain syndrome type I of the upper limb

337.22 Reflex sympathetic dystrophy of the lower limb
Complex regional pain syndrome type I of the lower limb

337.29 Reflex sympathetic dystrophy of other specified site
Complex regional pain syndrome type I of other specified site

Add 4th or 5th digit | Nonspecific code | Unspecified code | Manifestation code

337.3 Autonomic dysreflexia
Use additional code to identify the cause, such as:
    fecal impaction (560.32)
    pressure ulcer (707.00-707.09)
    urinary tract infection (599.0)

337.9 Unspecified disorder of autonomic nervous system

PAIN (338)

338 Pain, not elsewhere classified
Use additional code to identify:
    pain associated with psychological factors (307.89)

> Excludes: *generalized pain (780.96)*
>   *headache syndromes (339.00-339.89)*
>   *localized pain, unspecified type – code to pain by site*
>   *migraines (346.0-346.9)*
>   *pain disorder exclusively attributed to psychological factors (307.80)*
>   *vulvar vestibulitis (625.71)*
>   *vulvodynia (625.70-625.79)*

ALERT! Codes in category 338 may be used in conjunction with codes from other categories and chapters to provide more detail about acute or chronic pain and neoplasm-related pain, unless otherwise indicated.

338.0 Central pain syndrome
    Déjérine-Roussy syndrome
    Myelopathic pain syndrome
    Thalamic pain syndrome (hyperesthetic)

⑤ **338.1 Acute pain**

    338.11 Acute pain due to trauma

    338.12 Acute post-thoracotomy pain
        Post-thoracotomy pain NOS

    338.18 Other acute postoperative pain
        Postoperative pain NOS

    338.19 Other acute pain

> Excludes: *neoplasm related acute pain (338.3)*

⑤ **338.2 Chronic pain**

> Excludes: *causalgia (355.9)*
>   *lower limb (355.71)*
>   *upper limb (354.4)*
>   *chronic pain syndrome (338.4)*
>   *myofascial pain syndrome (729.1)*
>   *neoplasm related chronic pain (338.3)*
>   *reflex sympathetic dystrophy (337.20-337.29)*

ALERT! Chronic pain is classified to this subcategory. There is no time frame defining when pain becomes chronic pain. The provider's documentation should be used to guide use of these codes

    338.21 Chronic pain due to trauma

    338.22 Chronic post-thoracotomy pain

    338.28 Other chronic postoperative pain

    338.29 Other chronic pain

338.3 Neoplasm related pain (acute) (chronic)
    Cancer associated pain
    Pain due to malignancy (primary) (secondary)
    Tumor associated pain

338.4 Chronic pain syndrome
    Chronic pain associated with significant psychosocial dysfunction

OTHER HEADACHE SYNDROMES (339)

339 Other headache syndromes

> Excludes: *headache:*
>   *NOS (784.0)*
>   *due to lumbar puncture (349.0)*
>   *migraine (346.0-346.9)*

● Code new
    to 2012 edition
▲ Revision of
    existing code
④ ⑤ Fourth or fifth
    digit required

[5] **339.0 Cluster headaches and other trigeminal autonomic cephalgias**
TACS

339.00 Cluster headache syndrome, unspecified
Ciliary neuralgia
Cluster headache NOS
Histamine cephalgia
Lower half migraine
Migrainous neuralgia

339.01 Episodic cluster headache

339.02 Chronic cluster headache

339.03 Episodic paroxysmal hemicrania
Paroxysmal hemicrania NOS

339.04 Chronic paroxysmal hemicrania

339.05 Short lasting unilateral neuralgiform headache with conjunctival injection and tearing
SUNCT

339.09 Other trigeminal autonomic cephalgias

[5] **339.1 Tension type headache**
[*Excludes:*] *tension headache NOS (307.81)*
tension headache related to psychological factors (307.81)

339.10 Tension type headache, unspecified

339.11 Episodic tension type headache

339.12 Chronic tension type headache

[5] **339.2 Post-traumatic headache**

339.20 Post-traumatic headache, unspecified

339.21 Acute post-traumatic headache

339.22 Chronic post-traumatic headache

339.3 Drug induced headache not elsewhere classified
Medication overuse headache
Rebound headache

[5] **339.4 Complicated headache syndromes**

339.41 Hemicrania continua

339.42 New daily persistent headache
NDPH

339.43 Primary thunderclap headache

339.44 Other complicated headache syndrome

[5] **339.8 Other specified headache syndromes**

339.81 Hypnic headache

339.82 Headache associated with sexual activity
Orgasmic headache
Preorgasmic headache

339.83 Primary cough headache

339.84 Primary exertional headache

339.85 Primary stabbing headache

339.89 Other specified headache syndromes

OTHER DISORDERS OF THE CENTRAL NERVOUS SYSTEM (340-349)

340 Multiple sclerosis
Disseminated or multiple sclerosis:
NOS
brain stem
cord
generalized

[DEFINITION] Multiple sclerosis is a chronic autoimmune disorder affecting movement, sensation, and bodily functions. It is caused by destruction of the myelin insulation covering nerve fibers in the central nervous system.

Add 4th or 5th digit | Nonspecific code | Unspecified code | Manifestation code

341 **Other demyelinating diseases of central nervous system**

> **DEFINITION** Demyelinating diseases of the central nervous system is any disease of the nervous system in which the myelin sheath of neurons is damaged.

> **ALERT!** For personal history of other disorders of nervous system and sense organs see V12.49

341.0 Neuromyelitis optica

341.1 Schilder's disease
> Baló's concentric sclerosis
> Encephalitis periaxialis:
>   concentrica [Baló's]
>   diffusa [Schilder's]

⑤ **341.2 Acute (transverse) myelitis**

> Excludes: *acute (transverse)myelitis (in) (due to):*
> > *following immunization procedures (323.52)*
> > *infection classified elsewhere (323.42)*
> > *postinfectious (323.63)*
> > *protozoal diseases classified elsewhere (323.2)*
> > *rickettsial diseases classified elsewhere (323.1)*
> > *toxic (323.72)*
> > *viral diseases classified elsewhere (323.02)*
> > *transverse myelitis NOS (323.82)*

> **341.20 Acute (transverse) myelitis NOS**

> **341.21 Acute (transverse) myelitis in conditions classified elsewhere**
> *Code first underlying condition*

> **341.22 Idiopathic transverse myelitis**

341.8 Other demyelinating diseases of central nervous system
> Central demyelination of corpus callosum
> Central pontine myelinosis
> Marchiafava (-Bignami) disease

341.9 Demyelinating disease of central nervous system, unspecified

342 Hemiplegia and hemiparesis

> Excludes: *congenital (343.1)*
> > *hemiplegia due to late effect of cerebrovascular accident (438.20-438.22)*
> > *infantile NOS (343.4)*

Note: This category is to be used when hemiplegia (complete) (incomplete) is reported without further specification, or is stated to be old or long-standing but of unspecified cause. The category is also for use in multiple coding to identify these types of hemiplegia resulting from any cause.

The following fifth-digits are for use with codes 342.0-342.9

> **0 affecting unspecified side**

> **1 affecting dominant side**

> **2 affecting nondominant side**

> **DEFINITION** Hemiplegia is defined as paralysis or loss of voluntary motion, on one side of the body; may include head and neck, trunk and/or limbs. Hemiparesis is weakness on one side of the body.

⑤ **342.0 Flaccid hemiplegia**
[0-2]

⑤ **342.1 Spastic hemiplegia**
[0-2]

⑤ **342.8 Other specified hemiplegia**
[0-2]

⑤ **342.9 Hemiplegia, unspecified**
[0-2]

● Code new
to 2012 edition   ▲ Revision of
existing code   ④ ⑤ Fourth or fifth
digit required

343 Infantile cerebral palsy

Includes: cerebral:
palsy NOS
spastic infantile paralysis
congenital spastic paralysis (cerebral)
Little's disease
paralysis (spastic) due to birth injury:
intracranial
spinal

[Excludes:] *athetoid cerebral palsy (333.71)*
hereditary cerebral paralysis, such as:
hereditary spastic paraplegia (334.1)
Vogt's disease (333.71)
spastic paralysis specified as noncongenital or noninfantile (344.0-344.9)

DEFINITION Infantile cerebral palsy is the term used for a group of nonprogressive disorders of movement and posture caused by abnormal development of, or damage to, motor control centers of the brain. Cerebral palsy is caused by events before, during, or after birth. The abnormalities of muscle control that define cp are often accompanied by other neurological and physical abnormalities.

343.0 Diplegic
Congenital diplegia
Congenital paraplegia

343.1 Hemiplegic
Congenital hemiplegia

[Excludes:] *infantile hemiplegia NOS (343.4)*

343.2 Quadriplegic
Tetraplegic

343.3 Monoplegic

343.4 Infantile hemiplegia
Infantile hemiplegia (postnatal) NOS

343.8 Other specified infantile cerebral palsy

343.9 Infantile cerebral palsy, unspecified
Cerebral palsy NOS

344 Other paralytic syndromes

Note: This category is to be used when the listed conditions are reported without further specification or are stated to be old or long-standing but of unspecified cause. The category is also for use in multiple coding to identify these conditions resulting from any cause.

Includes: paralysis (complete) (incomplete), except as classifiable to 342 and 343

[Excludes:] *congenital or infantile cerebral palsy (343.0-343.9)*
hemiplegia (342.0-342.9)
congenital or infantile (343.1, 343.4)

DEFINITION Paralytic syndromes refers to other forms of paralysis resulting in the complete loss of muscle function for one or more muscle groups.

ALERT! For personal history of other disorders of nervous system and sense organs see V12.49

[5] **344.0 Quadriplegia and quadriparesis**

344.00 Quadriplegia, unspecified

344.01 C1-C4, complete

344.02 C1-C4, incomplete

344.03 C5-C7, complete

344.04 C5-C7, incomplete

344.09 Other

344.1 Paraplegia
Paralysis of both lower limbs
Paraplegia (lower)

344.2 Diplegia of upper limbs
Diplegia (upper)
Paralysis of both upper limbs

[5] **344.3 Monoplegia of lower limb**
Paralysis of lower limb

[Excludes:] *monoplegia of lower limb due to late effect of cerebrovascular accident (438.40-438.42)*

Add 4th or 5th digit | Nonspecific code | Unspecified code | Manifestation code

344.30 affecting unspecified side

344.31 affecting dominant side

344.32 affecting nondominant side

[5] **344.4 Monoplegia of upper limb**
Paralysis of upper limb

[Excludes:] *monoplegia of upper limb due to late effect of cerebrovascular accident (438.30-438.32)*

344.40 affecting unspecified side

344.41 affecting dominant side

344.42 affecting nondominant side

344.5 Unspecified monoplegia

[5] **344.6 Cauda equina syndrome**

344.60 Without mention of neurogenic bladder

344.61 With neurogenic bladder
Acontractile bladder
Autonomic hyperreflexia of bladder
Cord bladder
Detrusor hyperreflexia

[5] **344.8 Other specified paralytic syndromes**

344.81 Locked-in state

344.89 Other specified paralytic syndrome

344.9 Paralysis, unspecified

345 Epilepsy and recurrent seizures

The following fifth-digit subclassification is for use with categories 345.0, 345.1, 345.4-345.9:

0 without mention of intractable epilepsy

1 with intractable epilepsy
pharmacoresistant (pharmacologically resistant)
poorly controlled
refractory (medically)
treatment resistant

[Excludes:] *hippocampal sclerosis (348.81)*
mesial temporal sclerosis (348.81)
temporal sclerosis (348.81)

DEFINITION Epilepsy and recurrent seizures is a common chronic neurological disorder characterized by recurrent unprovoked seizures. These seizures are transient signs and/or symptoms of abnormal, excessive or synchronous neuronal activity in the brain.

[5] **345.0 Generalized nonconvulsive epilepsy**
[0-1]
Absences:
atonic
typical
Minor epilepsy
Petit mal
Pykno-epilepsy
Seizures:
akinetic
atonic

[5] **345.1 Generalized convulsive epilepsy**
[0-1]
Epileptic seizures:
clonic
myoclonic
tonic
tonic-clonic
Grand mal
Major epilepsy
Progressive myoclonic epilepsy
Unverricht-Lundborg disease

[Excludes:] *convulsions:*
NOS (780.39)
infantile (780.39)
newborn (779.0)
infantile spasms (345.6)

● Code new to 2012 edition   ▲ Revision of existing code   [4] [5] Fourth or fifth digit required

345.2 Petit mal status
Epileptic absence status

345.3 Grand mal status
Status epilepticus NOS

[Excludes:] *epilepsia partialis continua (345.7)*
status:
psychomotor (345.7)
temporal lobe (345.7)

⑤ **345.4 Localization-related (focal) (partial) epilepsy and epileptic syndromes with complex partial seizures**
[0-1] Epilepsy:
limbic system
partial:
secondarily generalized
with impairment of consciousness
with memory and ideational disturbances
psychomotor
psychosensory
temporal lobe
Epileptic automatism

⑤ **345.5 Localization-related (focal) (partial) epilepsy and epileptic syndromes with simple partial seizures**
[0-1]
Epilepsy:
Bravais-Jacksonian NOS
focal (motor) NOS
Jacksonian NOS
motor partial
partial NOS:
without impairment of consciousness
Epilepsy:
sensory-induced
somatomotor
somatosensory
visceral
visual

⑤ **345.6 Infantile spasms**
[0-1] Hypsarrhythmia
Lightning spasms
Salaam attacks

[Excludes:] *salaam tic (781.0)*

⑤ **345.7 Epilepsia partialis continua**
[0-1] Kojevnikov's epilepsy

⑤ **345.8 Other forms of epilepsy and recurrent seizures**
[0-1] Epilepsy:
cursive [running]
gelastic

⑤ **345.9 Epilepsy, unspecified**
[0-1] Epileptic convulsions, fits, or seizures NOS

[Excludes:] *convulsion (convulsive) disorder (780.39)*
convulsive seizure or fit NOS (780.39)
recurrent convulsions (780.39)

⑤ **346 Migraine**

[Excludes:] *headache:*
NOS (784.0)
syndromes (339.00-339.89)

The following fifth-digit subclassification is for use with category 346:

0 without mention of intractable migraine without mention of status migrainosus
without mention of refractory migraine without mention of status migrainosus

1 with intractable migraine, so stated, without mention of status migrainosus
with refractory migraine, so stated, without mention of status migrainosus

2 without mention of intractable migraine with status migrainosus
without mention of refractory migraine with status migrainosus

3 with intractable migraine, so stated, with status migrainosus
with refractory migraine, so stated, with status migrainosus

DEFINITION Migraine is a severe, disabling headache, usually affecting only one side of the head, and often accompanied by nausea, vomiting, photophobia and visual disturbances.

⑤ **346.0 Migraine with aura**
[0-3]   Basilar migraine
           Classic migraine
           Migraine preceded or accompanied by transient focal neurological phenomena
           Migraine triggered seizures
           Migraine with acute-onset aura
           Migraine with aura without headache (migraine equivalents)
           Migraine with prolonged aura
           Migraine with typical aura
           Retinal migraine

Excludes: *persistent migraine aura (346.5, 346.6)*

⑤ **346.1 Migraine without aura**
[0-3]   Common migraine

⑤ **346.2 Variants of migraine, not elsewhere classified**
[0-3]   Abdominal migraine
           Cyclical vomiting associated with migraine
           Ophthalmoplegic migraine
           Periodic headache syndromes in child or adolescent

Excludes: *cyclical vomiting NOS (536.2)*
          psychogenic cyclical vomiting (306.4)

⑤ **346.3 Hemiplegic migraine**
[0-3]   Familial migraine
           Sporadic migraine

⑤ **346.4 Menstrual migraine**
[0-3]   Menstrual headache
           Menstrually related migraine
           Premenstrual headache
           Premenstrual migraine
           Pure menstrual migraine

⑤ **346.5 Persistent migraine aura without cerebral infarction**
[0-3]   Persistent migraine aura NOS

⑤ **346.6 Persistent migraine aura with cerebral infarction**
[0-3]

⑤ **346.7 Chronic migraine without aura**
[0-3]   Transformed migraine without aura

⑤ **346.8 Other forms of migraine**
[0-3]

⑤ **346.9 Migraine, unspecified**
[0-3]

347 **Cataplexy and narcolepsy**

> **DEFINITION** Cataplexy is a sudden loss of muscle tone and reflexes that leads to muscle weakness, paralysis or postural collapse. Usually caused by an outburst of emotion such as laughter. Cataplexy is one of the first symptoms of narcolepsy, a chronic sleep disorder (a dyssomnia) which often causes sufferers to feel extreme tiredness, or spontaneously fall asleep.

⑤ **347.0 Narcolepsy**

 347.00 Without cataplexy
            Narcolepsy NOS

 347.01 With cataplexy

⑤ **347.1 Narcolepsy in conditions classified elsewhere**
Code first underlying condition

 347.10 *Without cataplexy*

 347.11 *With cataplexy*

348 **Other conditions of brain**

> **ALERT!** For personal history of other disorders of nervous system and sense organs see V12.49

348.0 Cerebral cysts
           Arachnoid cyst   Porencephaly, acquired
           Porencephalic cyst   Pseudoporencephaly

Excludes: *porencephaly (congenital) (742.4)*

● Code new   ▲ Revision of   ④ ⑤ Fourth or fifth
      to 2012 edition   existing code   digit required

348.1 Anoxic brain damage

[Excludes:] *that occurring in:*
abortion (634-638 with .7, 639.8)
ectopic or molar pregnancy (639.8)
labor or delivery (668.2, 669.4)
that of newborn (767.0, 768.0-768.9, 772.1-772.2)

Use additional E code, if desired, to identify cause

348.2 Benign intracranial hypertension
Pseudotumor cerebri

[Excludes:] *hypertensive encephalopathy (437.2)*

[5] **348.3 Encephalopathy, not elsewhere classified**

348.30 Encephalopathy, unspecified

348.31 Metabolic encephalopathy
Septic encephalopathy

[Excludes:] *toxic metabolic encephalopathy (349.82)*

348.39 Other encephalopathy

[Excludes:] *encephalopathy:*
alcoholic (291.2)
hepatic (572.2)
hypertensive (437.2)
toxic (349.82)

348.4 Compression of brain
Compression, brain (stem)
Herniation, brain (stem)
Posterior fossa compression syndrome

348.5 Cerebral edema

[5] **348.8 Other conditions of brain**

348.81 Temporal sclerosis
Hippocampal sclerosis
Mesial temporal sclerosis

● **348.82 Brain death**

348.89 Other conditions of brain
Cerebral:
calcification
fungus

[Excludes:] *brain death (348.82)*

348.9 Unspecified condition of brain

349 Other and unspecified disorders of the nervous system

[ALERT!] For personal history of other disorders of nervous system and sense organs see V12.49

[ALERT!] For personal history of unspecified disorder of nervous system and sense organs see V12.40

349.0 Reaction to spinal or lumbar puncture
Headache following lumbar puncture

349.1 Nervous system complications from surgically implanted device

349.2 Disorders of meninges, not elsewhere classified

[Excludes:] *immediate postoperative complications (997.00-997.09)*
mechanical complications of nervous system device (996.2)

Adhesions, meningeal (cerebral) (spinal)
Cyst, spinal meninges
Meningocele, acquired
Pseudomeningocele, acquired

[5] **349.3 Dural tear**

349.31 Accidental puncture or laceration of dura during a procedure
Incidental (inadvertent) durotomy

349.39 Other dural tear

[5] **349.8 Other specified disorders of nervous system**

349.81 Cerebrospinal fluid rhinorrhea

[Excludes:] *cerebrospinal fluid otorrhea (388.61)*

Add 4th or 5th digit | Nonspecific code | Unspecified code | Manifestation code

349.82   Toxic encephalopathy
Toxic metabolic encephalopathy

Use additional E code, if desired, to identify cause

349.89   Other

349.9   Unspecified disorders of nervous system
Disorder of nervous system (central) NOS

DISORDERS OF THE PERIPHERAL NERVOUS SYSTEM (350-359)

Excludes: *diseases of:*

acoustic [8th] nerve (388.5)
oculomotor [3rd, 4th, 6th] nerves (378.0-378.9)
optic [2nd] nerve (377.0-377.9)
peripheral autonomic nerves (337.0-337.9)
neuralgia NOS or "rheumatic" (729.2)
neuritis NOS or "rheumatic" (729.2)
radiculitis NOS or "rheumatic" (729.2)
peripheral neuritis in pregnancy (646.4)

350   Trigeminal nerve disorders
Includes: disorders of 5th cranial nerve
DEFINITION The trigeminal nerve is the main sensory nerve of the face and motor nerve for the muscles of chewing.

350.1   Trigeminal neuralgia
Tic douloureux   Trigeminal neuralgia NOS
Trifacial neuralgia

Excludes: *postherpetic (053.12)*

350.2   Atypical face pain

350.8   Other specified trigeminal nerve disorders

350.9   Trigeminal nerve disorder, unspecified

351   Facial nerve disorders
Includes: disorders of 7th cranial nerve

Excludes: *that in newborn (767.5)*

DEFINITION Facial nerve disorders refers to a disorder resulting from a weakness of the facial nerve. Bell's palsy is an example of a facial nerve disorder.

351.0   Bell's palsy
Facial palsy

351.1   Geniculate ganglionitis
Geniculate ganglionitis NOS

Excludes: *herpetic (053.11)*

351.8   Other facial nerve disorders
Facial myokymia
Melkersson's syndrome

351.9   Facial nerve disorder, unspecified

352   Disorders of other cranial nerves
DEFINITION Cranial nerves arise from the base of the brain or the brainstem that provide sensory and motor function to the eyes, nose, ears, tongue, and face.

352.0   Disorders of olfactory [1st] nerve

352.1   Glossopharyngeal neuralgia

352.2   Other disorders of glossopharyngeal [9th] nerve

352.3   Disorders of pneumogastric [10th] nerve
Disorders of vagal nerve

Excludes: *paralysis of vocal cords or larynx (478.30-478.34)*

352.4   Disorders of accessory [11th] nerve

352.5   Disorders of hypoglossal [12th] nerve

352.6   Multiple cranial nerve palsies
Collet-Sicard syndrome
Polyneuritis cranialis

352.9   Unspecified disorder of cranial nerves

● Code new
to 2012 edition   ▲ Revision of
existing code   ④ ⑤ Fourth or fifth
digit required

353 **Nerve root and plexus disorders**

> *Excludes:* *conditions due to:*
> > *intervertebral disc disorders (722.0-722.9)*
> > *spondylosis (720.0-721.9)*
> > *vertebrogenic disorders (723.0-724.9)*

DEFINITION A nerve root is the initial segment of a nerve leaving the central nervous system. Plexus refers to a network of intersecting nerves and blood vessels or of lymphatic vessels. The body contains many plexuses, such as the brachial plexus, the cardiac plexus, the cervical plexus, and the lumbar plexus.

353.0 Brachial plexus lesions
Cervical rib syndrome   Scalenus anticus syndrome
Costoclavicular syndrome   Thoracic outlet syndrome

> *Excludes:* *brachial neuritis or radiculitis NOS (723.4)*
> > *that in newborn (767.6)*

353.1 Lumbosacral plexus lesions

353.2 Cervical root lesions, not elsewhere classified

353.3 Thoracic root lesions, not elsewhere classified

353.4 Lumbosacral root lesions, not elsewhere classified

353.5 Neuralgic amyotrophy
Parsonage-Aldren-Turner syndrome

> *Code first any associated underlying disease, such as:*
> > diabetes mellitus (249.6, 250.6)

353.6 Phantom limb (syndrome)

353.8 **Other nerve root and plexus disorders**

353.9 **Unspecified nerve root and plexus disorder**

354 **Mononeuritis of upper limb and mononeuritis multiplex**

DEFINITION Mononeuritis is the inflammation of a single nerve of a upper limb. There are many causes of mononeuritis including diabetes mellitus, carpal tunnel syndrome, rheumatoid arthritis and lyme disease.

354.0 Carpal tunnel syndrome
Median nerve entrapment
Partial thenar atrophy

354.1 **Other lesion of median nerve**
Median nerve neuritis

354.2 Lesion of ulnar nerve
Cubital tunnel syndrome
Tardy ulnar nerve palsy

354.3 Lesion of radial nerve
Acute radial nerve palsy

354.4 Causalgia of upper limb
Complex regional pain syndrome type II of the upper limb

> *Excludes:* *causalgia:*
> > *NOS (355.9)*
> > *lower limb (355.71)*
> > *complex regional pain syndrome type II of the lower limb (355.71)*

354.5 Mononeuritis multiplex
Combinations of single conditions classifiable to 354 or 355

354.8 **Other mononeuritis of upper limb**

354.9 **Mononeuritis of upper limb, unspecified**

355 **Mononeuritis of lower limb and unspecified site**

355.0 Lesion of sciatic nerve

> *Excludes:* *sciatica NOS (724.3)*

355.1 Meralgia paresthetica
Lateral cutaneous femoral nerve of thigh compression or syndrome

355.2 **Other lesion of femoral nerve**

355.3 Lesion of lateral popliteal nerve
Lesion of common peroneal nerve

355.4 Lesion of medial popliteal nerve

355.5 Tarsal tunnel syndrome

| | Add 4th or 5th digit | | Nonspecific code | | Unspecified code | | Manifestation code |

355.6 Lesion of plantar nerve
Morton's metatarsalgia, neuralgia, or neuroma

⑤ **355.7 Other mononeuritis of lower limb**

355.71 Causalgia of lower limb

Excludes: *causalgia:*
NOS (355.9)
upper limb (354.4)
complex regional pain syndrome type II of upper limb (354.4)

355.79 Other mononeuritis of lower limb

355.8 Mononeuritis of lower limb, unspecified

355.9 Mononeuritis of unspecified site
Causalgia NOS
Complex regional pain syndrome NOS

Excludes: *causalgia:*
lower limb (355.71)
upper limb (354.4)
complex regional pain syndrome:
lower limb (355.71)
upper limb (354.4)

356 Hereditary and idiopathic peripheral neuropathy
DEFINITION Peripheral neuropathy refers to damage to nerves of the peripheral nervous system which may be caused either by diseases of the nerve or from the side-effects of systemic illness.

356.0 Hereditary peripheral neuropathy
Déjérine-Sottas disease

356.1 Peroneal muscular atrophy
Charcot-Marie-Tooth disease
Neuropathic muscular atrophy

356.2 Hereditary sensory neuropathy

356.3 Refsum's disease
Heredopathia atactica polyneuritiformis

356.4 Idiopathic progressive polyneuropathy

356.8 Other specified idiopathic peripheral neuropathy
Supranuclear paralysis

356.9 Unspecified

357 Inflammatory and toxic neuropathy
DEFINITION Inflammatory and toxic neuropathy refers to pathology of the peripheral nerves caused by inflammation or toxins

357.0 Acute infective polyneuritis
Guillain-Barré syndrome
Postinfectious polyneuritis

357.1 Polyneuropathy in collagen vascular disease
Code first underlying disease, as:
disseminated lupus erythematosus (710.0)
polyarteritis nodosa (446.0)
rheumatoid arthritis (714.0)

357.2 Polyneuropathy in diabetes
Code first underlying disease (249.6, 250.6)

357.3 Polyneuropathy in malignant disease
Code first underlying disease (140.0-208.9)

● Code new
to 2012 edition

▲ Revision of
existing code

④ ⑤ Fourth or fifth
digit required

357.4 Polyneuropathy in other diseases classified elsewhere

Code first underlying disease, as:
amyloidosis (277.30-277.39)
beriberi (265.0)
chronic uremia (585.9)
deficiency of B vitamins (266.0-266.9)
diphtheria (032.0-032.9)
hypoglycemia (251.2)
pellagra (265.2)
porphyria (277.1)
sarcoidosis (135)
uremia NOS (586)

[Excludes:] *polyneuropathy in:*
herpes zoster (053.13)
mumps (072.72)

357.5 Alcoholic polyneuropathy

357.6 Polyneuropathy due to drugs

Use additional E code, if desired, to identify drug

357.7 Polyneuropathy due to other toxic agents

Use additional E code, if desired, to identify toxic agent

[5] **357.8 Other**

357.81 Chronic inflammatory demyelinating polyneuritis

357.82 Critical illness polyneuropathy
Acute motor neuropathy

357.89 Other inflammatory and toxic neuropathy

357.9 Unspecified

358 Myoneural disorders

[DEFINITION] Myoneural disorders refers to disorders affecting both muscles and nerves, especially to nerve endings in muscle tissue

[5] **358.0 Myasthenia gravis**

358.00 Myasthenia gravis without (acute) exacerbation
Myasthenia gravis NOS

358.01 Myasthenia gravis with (acute) exacerbation
Myasthenia gravis in crisis

358.1 Myasthenic syndromes in diseases classified elsewhere

Code first underlying disease, as:
botulism (005.1, 040.41-040.42)
hypothyroidism (244.0-244.9)
malignant neoplasm (140.0-208.9)
pernicious anemia (281.0)
thyrotoxicosis (242.0-242.9)

358.2 Toxic myoneural disorders

Use additional E code, if desired, to identify toxic agent

● **358.3 Lambert-Eaton syndrome**
Eaton-Lambert syndrome

● **358.30 Lambert-Eaton syndrome, unspecified**
Lambert-Eaton syndrome NOS

● **358.31 Lambert-Eaton syndrome in neoplastic disease**
Code first the underlying neoplastic disease

● **358.39 Lambert-Eaton syndrome in other diseases classified elsewhere**
Code first the underlying condition

358.8 Other specified myoneural disorders

358.9 Myoneural disorders, unspecified

359 Muscular dystrophies and other myopathies

[Excludes:] *idiopathic polymyositis (710.4)*

[DEFINITION] Muscular dystrophy refers to a group of genetic, hereditary muscle diseases that weaken the muscles that move the human body. Muscular dystrophies are characterized by progressive skeletal muscle weakness, defects in muscle proteins, and the death of muscle cells and tissue.

359.0 Congenital hereditary muscular dystrophy
Benign congenital myopathy
Central core disease
Centronuclear myopathy
Myotubular myopathy
Nemaline body disease

[Excludes:] *arthrogryposis multiplex congenita (754.89)*

359.1 Hereditary progressive muscular dystrophy
Muscular dystrophy:
NOS
distal
Duchenne
Erb's
fascioscapulohumeral

Muscular dystrophy:
Gower's
Landouzy-Déjérine
limb-girdle
ocular
oculopharyngeal

[5] **359.2 Myotonic disorders**

[Excludes:] *periodic paralysis (359.3)*

359.21 Myotonic muscular dystrophy
Dystrophia myotonica
Myotonia atrophica
Myotonic dystrophy
Proximal myotonic myopathy (PROMM)
Steinert's disease

359.22 Myotonia congenita
Acetazolamide responsive myotonia congenita
Dominant form (Thomsen's disease)
Myotonia levior
Recessive form (Becker's disease)

359.23 Myotonic chondrodystrophy
Congenital myotonic chondrodystrophy
Schwartz-Jampel disease

359.24 Drug-induced myotonia
Use additional E code to identify drug

359.29 Other specified myotonic disorder
Myotonia fluctuans
Myotonia permanens
Paramyotonia congenita (of von Eulenburg)

359.3 Periodic paralysis
Familial periodic paralysis
Hyperkalemic periodic paralysis
Hypokalemic familial periodic paralysis
Hypokalemic periodic paralysis
Potassium sensitive periodic paralysis

[Excludes:] *paramyotonia congenita (of von Eulenburg) (359.29)*

359.4 Toxic myopathy
Use additional E code, if desired, to identify toxic agent

359.5 Myopathy in endocrine diseases classified elsewhere
Code first underlying disease, as:
Addison's disease (255.41)
Cushing's syndrome (255.0)
hypopituitarism (253.2)
myxedema (244.0-244.9)
thyrotoxicosis (242.0-242.9)

359.6 Symptomatic inflammatory myopathy in diseases classified elsewhere
Code first underlying disease, as:
amyloidosis (277.30-277.39)
disseminated lupus erythematosus (710.0)
malignant neoplasm (140.0-208.9)
polyarteritis nodosa (446.0)
rheumatoid arthritis (714.0)
sarcoidosis (135)
scleroderma (710.1)
Sjögren's disease (710.2)

[5] **359.7 Inflammatory and immune myopathies, NEC**

359.71 Inclusion body myositis
IBM

359.79 Other inflammatory and immune myopathies, NEC
Inflammatory myopathy NOS

[5] **359.8 Other myopathies**

359.81 Critical illness myopathy
Acute necrotizing myopathy
Acute quadriplegic myopathy
Intensive care (ICU) myopathy
Myopathy of critical illness

359.89 Other myopathies

359.9 Myopathy, unspecified

DISORDERS OF THE EYE AND ADNEXA (360-379)

Use additional external cause code, if applicable, to identify the cause of the eye condition

360 Disorders of the globe
Includes: disorders affecting multiple structures of eye
[DEFINITION] Disorders of the globe refers to disorders affecting the outer membranes of the eye.

[5] **360.0 Purulent endophthalmitis**
[Excludes:] *bleb associated endophthalmitis (379.63)*

360.00 Purulent endophthalmitis, unspecified

360.01 Acute endophthalmitis

360.02 Panophthalmitis

360.03 Chronic endophthalmitis

360.04 Vitreous abscess

[5] **360.1 Other endophthalmitis**
[Excludes:] *bleb associated endophthalmitis (379.63)*

360.11 Sympathetic uveitis

360.12 Panuveitis

360.13 Parasitic endophthalmitis NOS

360.14 Ophthalmia nodosa

360.19 Other
Phacoanaphylactic endophthalmitis

[5] **360.2 Degenerative disorders of globe**

360.20 Degenerative disorder of globe, unspecified

360.21 Progressive high (degenerative) myopia
Malignant myopia

360.23 Siderosis

360.24 Other metallosis
Chalcosis

360.29 Other
[Excludes:] *xerophthalmia (264.7)*

[5] **360.3 Hypotony of eye**

360.30 Hypotony, unspecified

360.31 Primary hypotony

360.32 Ocular fistula causing hypotony

360.33 Hypotony associated with other ocular disorders

360.34 Flat anterior chamber

[5] **360.4 Degenerated conditions of globe**

360.40 Degenerated globe or eye, unspecified

360.41 Blind hypotensive eye
Atrophy of globe
Phthisis bulbi

360.42 Blind hypertensive eye
Absolute glaucoma

360.43 Hemophthalmos, except current injury

[Excludes:] *traumatic (871.0-871.9, 921.0-921.9)*

360.44 Leucocoria

⑤ **360.5 Retained (old) intraocular foreign body, magnetic**
Use additional code to identify foreign body (V90.11)

[Excludes:] *current penetrating injury with magnetic foreign body (871.5)*
retained (old) foreign body of orbit (376.6)

360.50 Foreign body, magnetic, intraocular, unspecified

360.51 Foreign body, magnetic, in anterior chamber

360.52 Foreign body, magnetic, in iris or ciliary body

360.53 Foreign body, magnetic, in lens

360.54 Foreign body, magnetic, in vitreous

360.55 Foreign body, magnetic, in posterior wall

360.59 Foreign body, magnetic, in other or multiple sites

⑤ **360.6 Retained (old) intraocular foreign body, nonmagnetic**
Retained (old) foreign body:
NOS
nonmagnetic
Use additional code to identify foreign body (V90.01-V90.10, V90.12, V90.2-V90.9)

[Excludes:] *current penetrating injury with (nonmagnetic) foreign body (871.6)*
retained (old) foreign body in orbit (376.6)

360.60 Foreign body, intraocular, unspecified

360.61 Foreign body in anterior chamber

360.62 Foreign body in iris or ciliary body

360.63 Foreign body in lens

360.64 Foreign body in vitreous

360.65 Foreign body in posterior wall

360.69 Foreign body in other or multiple sites

⑤ **360.8 Other disorders of globe**

360.81 Luxation of globe

360.89 Other

360.9 Unspecified disorder of globe

361 Retinal detachments and defects

DEFINITION Retinal detachment is a disorder of the eye in which the retina peels away from its underlying layer of support tissue

⑤ **361.0 Retinal detachment with retinal defect**
Rhegmatogenous retinal detachment

[Excludes:] *detachment of retinal pigment epithelium (362.42-362.43)*
retinal detachment (serous) (without defect) (361.2)

361.00 Retinal detachment with retinal defect, unspecified

361.01 Recent detachment, partial, with single defect

361.02 Recent detachment, partial, with multiple defects

361.03 Recent detachment, partial, with giant tear

361.04 Recent detachment, partial, with retinal dialysis
Dialysis (juvenile) of retina (with detachment)

361.05 Recent detachment, total or subtotal

361.06 Old detachment, partial
Delimited old retinal detachment

361.07 Old detachment, total or subtotal

⑤ **361.1 Retinoschisis and retinal cysts**

[Excludes:] *juvenile retinoschisis (362.73)*
microcystoid degeneration of retina (362.62)
parasitic cyst of retina (360.13)

361.10 Retinoschisis, unspecified

361.11 Flat retinoschisis

361.12 Bullous retinoschisis

● Code new to 2012 edition ▲ Revision of existing code ④ ⑤ Fourth or fifth digit required

361.13 Primary retinal cysts

361.14 Secondary retinal cysts

361.19 Other
Pseudocyst of retina

361.2 Serous retinal detachment
Retinal detachment without retinal defect
[Excludes:] *central serous retinopathy (362.41)*
retinal pigment epithelium detachment (362.42-362.43)

[5] **361.3 Retinal defects without detachment**
[Excludes:] *chorioretinal scars after surgery for detachment (363.30-363.35)*
peripheral retinal degeneration without defect (362.60-362.66)

361.30 Retinal defect, unspecified
Retinal break(s) NOS

361.31 Round hole of retina without detachment

361.32 Horseshoe tear of retina without detachment
Operculum of retina without mention of detachment

361.33 Multiple defects of retina without detachment

[5] **361.8 Other forms of retinal detachment**

361.81 Traction detachment of retina
Traction detachment with vitreoretinal organization

361.89 Other

361.9 Unspecified retinal detachment

362 Other retinal disorders
[Excludes:] *chorioretinal scars (363.30-363.35)*
chorioretinitis (363.0-363.2)

[ALERT!] For personal history of other disorders of nervous system and sense organs see V12.49

[5] ***362.0 Diabetic retinopathy***
Code first diabetes (249.5, 250.5)

362.01 Background diabetic retinopathy
Diabetic retinal microaneurysms
Diabetic retinopathy NOS

362.02 Proliferative diabetic retinopathy

362.03 Nonproliferative diabetic retinopathy NOS

362.04 Mild nonproliferative diabetic retinopathy

362.05 Moderate nonproliferative diabetic retinopathy

362.06 Severe nonproliferative diabetic retinopathy

362.07 Diabetic macular edema
Diabetic retinal edema
Note: Code 362.07 must be used with a code for diabetic retinopathy (362.01-362.06)

[5] **362.1 Other background retinopathy and retinal vascular changes**

362.10 Background retinopathy, unspecified

362.11 Hypertensive retinopathy

362.12 Exudative retinopathy
Coats' syndrome

362.13 Changes in vascular appearance
Vascular sheathing of retina
Use additional code for any associated atherosclerosis (440.8)

362.14 Retinal microaneurysms NOS

362.15 Retinal telangiectasia

362.16 Retinal neovascularization NOS
Neovascularization:
choroidal
subretinal

362.17 Other intraretinal microvascular abnormalities
Retinal varices

362.18 Retinal vasculitis
　Eales' disease
　Retinal:　　　　　　　Retinal:
　　arteritis　　　　　　　perivasculitis
　　endarteritis　　　　　　phlebitis

⑤ **362.2 Other proliferative retinopathy**

362.20 Retinopathy of prematurity, unspecified
　Retinopathy of prematurity NOS

362.21 Retrolental fibroplasia
　Cicatricial retinopathy of prematurity

362.22 Retinopathy of prematurity, stage 0

362.23 Retinopathy of prematurity, stage 1

362.24 Retinopathy of prematurity, stage 2

362.25 Retinopathy of prematurity, stage 3

362.26 Retinopathy of prematurity, stage 4

362.27 Retinopathy of prematurity, stage 5

362.29 Other nondiabetic proliferative retinopathy

⑤ **362.3 Retinal vascular occlusion**

362.30 Retinal vascular occlusion, unspecified

362.31 Central retinal artery occlusion

362.32 Arterial branch occlusion

362.33 Partial arterial occlusion
　Hollenhorst plaque
　Retinal microembolism

362.34 Transient arterial occlusion
　Amaurosis fugax

362.35 Central retinal vein occlusion

362.36 Venous tributary (branch) occlusion

362.37 Venous engorgement
　Occlusion:
　　incipient of retinal vein
　　partial of retinal vein

⑤ **362.4 Separation of retinal layers**

Excludes: *retinal detachment (serous) (361.2)*
　　　　　rhegmatogenous (361.00-361.07)

362.40 Retinal layer separation, unspecified

362.41 Central serous retinopathy

362.42 Serous detachment of retinal pigment epithelium
　Exudative detachment of retinal pigment epithelium

362.43 Hemorrhagic detachment of retinal pigment epithelium

⑤ **362.5 Degeneration of macula and posterior pole**

Excludes: *degeneration of optic disc (377.21-377.24)*
　　　　　hereditary retinal degeneration [dystrophy] (362.70-362.77)

362.50 Macular degeneration (senile), unspecified

362.51 Nonexudative senile macular degeneration
　Senile macular degeneration:
　　atrophic
　　dry

362.52 Exudative senile macular degeneration
　Kuhnt-Junius degeneration
　Senile macular degeneration:
　　disciform
　　wet

362.53 Cystoid macular degeneration
　Cystoid macular edema

362.54 Macular cyst, hole, or pseudohole

362.55 Toxic maculopathy
Use additional E code, if desired, to identify drug, if drug induced

● Code new　　　　▲ Revision of　　　④ ⑤ Fourth or fifth
　to 2012 edition　　　existing code　　　　digit required

362.56 Macular puckering
Preretinal fibrosis

362.57 Drusen (degenerative)

⑤ **362.6 Peripheral retinal degenerations**

Excludes: *hereditary retinal degeneration [dystrophy] (362.70-362.77)*
retinal degeneration with retinal defect (361.00-361.07)

362.60 Peripheral retinal degeneration, unspecified

362.61 Paving stone degeneration

362.62 Microcystoid degeneration
Blessig's cysts   Iwanoff's cysts

362.63 Lattice degeneration
Palisade degeneration of retina

362.64 Senile reticular degeneration

362.65 Secondary pigmentary degeneration
Pseudoretinitis pigmentosa

362.66 Secondary vitreoretinal degenerations

⑤ **362.7 Hereditary retinal dystrophies**

362.70 Hereditary retinal dystrophy, unspecified

362.71 *Retinal dystrophy in systemic or cerebroretinal lipidoses*
Code first underlying disease, as:
cerebroretinal lipidoses (330.1)
systemic lipidoses (272.7)

362.72 *Retinal dystrophy in other systemic disorders and syndromes*
Code first underlying disease, as:
Bassen-Kornzweig syndrome (272.5)
Refsum's disease (356.3)

362.73 Vitreoretinal dystrophies
Juvenile retinoschisis

362.74 Pigmentary retinal dystrophy
Retinal dystrophy, albipunctate
Retinitis pigmentosa

362.75 Other dystrophies primarily involving the sensory retina
Progressive cone (-rod) dystrophy
Stargardt's disease

362.76 Dystrophies primarily involving the retinal pigment epithelium
Fundus flavimaculatus
Vitelliform dystrophy

362.77 Dystrophies primarily involving Bruch's membrane
Dystrophy:
hyaline
pseudoinflammatory foveal
Hereditary drusen

⑤ **362.8 Other retinal disorders**

Excludes: *chorioretinal inflammations (363.0-363.2)*
chorioretinal scars (363.30-363.35)

362.81 Retinal hemorrhage
Hemorrhage:
preretinal
retinal (deep) (superficial)
subretinal

362.82 Retinal exudates and deposits

362.83 Retinal edema
Retinal:
cotton wool spots
edema (localized) (macular) (peripheral)

362.84 Retinal ischemia

362.85 Retinal nerve fiber bundle defects

362.89 Other retinal disorders

362.9 Unspecified retinal disorder

| Add 4th or 5th digit | Nonspecific code | Unspecified code | Manifestation code |

363 Chorioretinal inflammations, scars, and other disorders of choroid

[DEFINITION] Chorioretinal inflammations, scars and other disorders of choroid is an inflammation affecting the choroid and the retina of the eye.

⑤ **363.0 Focal chorioretinitis and focal retinochoroiditis**

[Excludes:] *focal chorioretinitis or retinochoroiditis in:*
histoplasmosis (115.02, 115.12, 115.92)
toxoplasmosis (130.2)
congenital infection (771.2)

363.00 Focal chorioretinitis, unspecified
Focal:
choroiditis or chorioretinitis NOS
retinitis or retinochoroiditis NOS

363.01 Focal choroiditis and chorioretinitis, juxtapapillary

363.03 Focal choroiditis and chorioretinitis of other posterior pole

363.04 Focal choroiditis and chorioretinitis, peripheral

363.05 Focal retinitis and retinochoroiditis, juxtapapillary
Neuroretinitis

363.06 Focal retinitis and retinochoroiditis, macular or paramacular

363.07 Focal retinitis and retinochoroiditis of other posterior pole

363.08 Focal retinitis and retinochoroiditis, peripheral

⑤ **363.1 Disseminated chorioretinitis and disseminated retinochoroiditis**

[Excludes:] *disseminated choroiditis or chorioretinitis in secondary syphilis (091.51)*
neurosyphilitic disseminated retinitis or retinochoroiditis (094.83)
retinal (peri)vasculitis (362.18)

363.10 Disseminated chorioretinitis, unspecified
Disseminated:
choroiditis or chorioretinitis NOS
retinitis or retinochoroiditis NOS

363.11 Disseminated choroiditis and chorioretinitis, posterior pole

363.12 Disseminated choroiditis and chorioretinitis, peripheral

363.13 Disseminated choroiditis and chorioretinitis, generalized

Code first any underlying disease, as:
tuberculosis (017.3)

363.14 Disseminated retinitis and retinochoroiditis, metastatic

363.15 Disseminated retinitis and retinochoroiditis, pigment epitheliopathy
Acute posterior multifocal placoid pigment epitheliopathy

⑤ **363.2 Other and unspecified forms of chorioretinitis and retinochoroiditis**

[Excludes:] *panophthalmitis (360.02)*
sympathetic uveitis (360.11)
uveitis NOS (364.3)

363.20 Chorioretinitis, unspecified
Choroiditis NOS
Retinitis NOS
Uveitis, posterior NOS

363.21 Pars planitis
Posterior cyclitis

363.22 Harada's disease

⑤ **363.3 Chorioretinal scars**

Scar (postinflammatory) (postsurgical) (posttraumatic):
choroid
retina

363.30 Chorioretinal scar, unspecified

363.31 Solar retinopathy

363.32 Other macular scars

363.33 Other scars of posterior pole

363.34 Peripheral scars

363.35 Disseminated scars

⑤ **363.4 Choroidal degenerations**

● Code new to 2012 edition ▲ Revision of existing code ④ ⑤ Fourth or fifth digit required

363.40 Choroidal degeneration, unspecified
Choroidal sclerosis NOS

363.41 Senile atrophy of choroid

363.42 Diffuse secondary atrophy of choroid

363.43 Angioid streaks of choroid

[5] **363.5 Hereditary choroidal dystrophies**
Hereditary choroidal atrophy:
partial [choriocapillaris]
total [all vessels]

363.50 Hereditary choroidal dystrophy or atrophy, unspecified

363.51 Circumpapillary dystrophy of choroid, partial

363.52 Circumpapillary dystrophy of choroid, total
Helicoid dystrophy of choroid

363.53 Central dystrophy of choroid, partial
Dystrophy, choroidal:
central areolar
circinate

363.54 Central choroidal atrophy, total
Dystrophy, choroidal:
central gyrate
serpiginous

363.55 Choroideremia

363.56 Other diffuse or generalized dystrophy, partial
Diffuse choroidal sclerosis

363.57 Other diffuse or generalized dystrophy, total
Generalized gyrate atrophy, choroid

[5] **363.6 Choroidal hemorrhage and rupture**

363.61 Choroidal hemorrhage, unspecified

363.62 Expulsive choroidal hemorrhage

363.63 Choroidal rupture

[5] **363.7 Choroidal detachment**

363.70 Choroidal detachment, unspecified

363.71 Serous choroidal detachment

363.72 Hemorrhagic choroidal detachment

363.8 Other disorders of choroid

363.9 Unspecified disorder of choroid

364 Disorders of iris and ciliary body

[DEFINITION] The iris is a muscular diaphragm that controls the size of the pupil which in turn controls the amount of light that enters the eye. The ciliary body is part of the middle layer of the wall of the eye that includes the ring-shaped muscle that changes the size of the pupil and the shape of the lens when the eye focuses and also produces the fluid that fills the eye.

[5] **364.0 Acute and subacute iridocyclitis**
Anterior uveitis, acute, subacute
Cyclitis, acute, subacute
Iridocyclitis, acute, subacute
Iritis, acute, subacute

[Excludes:] *gonococcal (098.41)*
herpes simplex (054.44)
herpes zoster (053.22)

364.00 Acute and subacute iridocyclitis, unspecified

364.01 Primary iridocyclitis

364.02 Recurrent iridocyclitis

364.03 Secondary iridocyclitis, infectious

364.04 Secondary iridocyclitis, noninfectious
Aqueous:
cells
fibrin
flare

364.05 Hypopyon

⑤ **364.1 Chronic iridocyclitis**
     │Excludes:│ *posterior cyclitis (363.21)*

     364.10 Chronic iridocyclitis, unspecified
     364.11 Chronic iridocyclitis in diseases classified elsewhere
     Code first underlying disease, as:
         sarcoidosis (135)
         tuberculosis (017.3)
     │Excludes:│ *syphilitic iridocyclitis (091.52)*

⑤ **364.2 Certain types of iridocyclitis**
     │Excludes:│ *posterior cyclitis (363.21)*
               sympathetic uveitis (360.11)

     364.21 Fuchs' heterochromic cyclitis
     364.22 Glaucomatocyclitic crises
     364.23 Lens-induced iridocyclitis
     364.24 Vogt-Koyanagi syndrome

  364.3 Unspecified iridocyclitis
       Uveitis NOS

⑤ **364.4 Vascular disorders of iris and ciliary body**
     364.41 Hyphema
          Hemorrhage of iris or ciliary body
     364.42 Rubeosis iridis
          Neovascularization of iris or ciliary body

⑤ **364.5 Degenerations of iris and ciliary body**
     364.51 Essential or progressive iris atrophy
     364.52 Iridoschisis
     364.53 Pigmentary iris degeneration
          Acquired heterochromia of iris
          Pigment dispersion syndrome of iris
          Translucency of iris
     364.54 Degeneration of pupillary margin
          Atrophy of sphincter of iris
          Ectropion of pigment epithelium of iris
     364.55 Miotic cysts of pupillary margin
     364.56 Degenerative changes of chamber angle
     364.57 Degenerative changes of ciliary body
     364.59 Other iris atrophy
          Iris atrophy (generalized) (sector shaped)

⑤ **364.6 Cysts of iris, ciliary body, and anterior chamber**
     │Excludes:│ *miotic pupillary cyst (364.55)*
               parasitic cyst (360.13)

     364.60 Idiopathic cysts
     364.61 Implantation cysts
          Epithelial down-growth, anterior chamber
          Implantation cysts (surgical) (traumatic)
     364.62 Exudative cysts of iris or anterior chamber
     364.63 Primary cyst of pars plana
     364.64 Exudative cyst of pars plana

⑤ **364.7 Adhesions and disruptions of iris and ciliary body**
     │Excludes:│ *flat anterior chamber (360.34)*

     364.70 Adhesions of iris, unspecified
          Synechiae (iris) NOS
     364.71 Posterior synechiae
     364.72 Anterior synechiae
     364.73 Goniosynechiae
          Peripheral anterior synechiae

  ● Code new   ▲ Revision of   ④ ⑤ Fourth or fifth
       to 2012 edition   existing code   digit required

364.74 Pupillary membranes
Iris bombé
Pupillary:
occlusion
seclusion

364.75 Pupillary abnormalities
Deformed pupil
Ectopic pupil
Rupture of sphincter, pupil

364.76 Iridodialysis

364.77 Recession of chamber angle

[5] **364.8 Other disorders of iris and ciliary body**

364.81 Floppy iris syndrome
Intraoperative floppy iris syndrome (IFIS)

Use additional E code to identify cause, such as:
sympatholytics [antiadrenergics] causing adverse effect in therapeutic use (E941.3)

364.82 Plateau iris syndrome

364.89 Other disorders of iris and ciliary body
Prolapse of iris NOS

[Excludes:] *prolapse of iris in recent wound (871.1)*

364.9 Unspecified disorder of iris and ciliary body

365 Glaucoma

[Excludes:] *blind hypertensive eye [absolute glaucoma] (360.42)*
congenital glaucoma (743.20-743.22)

[DEFINITION] Glaucoma is a group of eye diseases characterized by damage to the optic nerve usually due to excessively high intraocular pressure.

[5] **365.0 Borderline glaucoma [glaucoma suspect]**

365.00 Preglaucoma, unspecified

▲ **365.01 Open angle with borderline findings, low risk**
Open angle, low risk

365.02 Anatomical narrow angle
Primary angle closure suspect

365.03 Steroid responders

365.04 Ocular hypertension

● **365.05 Open angle with borderline findings, high risk**
Open angle, high risk

● **365.06 Primary angle closure without glaucoma damage**

[5] **365.1 Open-angle glaucoma**

365.10 Open-angle glaucoma, unspecified
Wide-angle glaucoma NOS

Use additional code to identify glaucoma stage (365.70-365.74)

365.11 Primary open angle glaucoma
Chronic simple glaucoma

Use additional code to identify glaucoma stage (365.70-365.74)

365.12 Low tension glaucoma

Use additional code to identify glaucoma stage (365.70-365.74)

365.13 Pigmentary glaucoma

Use additional code to identify glaucoma stage (365.70-365.74)

365.14 Glaucoma of childhood
Infantile or juvenile glaucoma

365.15 Residual stage of open angle glaucoma

[5] **365.2 Primary angle-closure glaucoma**

365.20 Primary angle-closure glaucoma, unspecified

Use additional code to identify glaucoma stage (365.70-365.74)

365.21 Intermittent angle-closure glaucoma
Angle-closure glaucoma:
interval
subacute

365.22 **Acute angle-closure glaucoma**
Acute angle-closure glaucoma attack
Acute angle-closure glaucoma crisis

365.23 **Chronic angle-closure glaucoma**
Chronic primary angle closure glaucoma

Use additional code to identify glaucoma stage (365.70-365.74)

365.24 **Residual stage of angle-closure glaucoma**

⑤ **365.3** **Corticosteroid-induced glaucoma**

365.31 **Glaucomatous stage**
Use additional code to identify glaucoma stage (365.70-365.74)

365.32 **Residual stage**

⑤ **365.4** **Glaucoma associated with congenital anomalies, dystrophies, and systemic syndromes**

365.41 *Glaucoma associated with chamber angle anomalies*

365.42 *Glaucoma associated with anomalies of iris*

365.43 *Glaucoma associated with other anterior segment anomalies*

365.44 *Glaucoma associated with systemic syndromes*
Code first associated disease, as:
neurofibromatosis (237.70-237.79)
Sturge-Weber (-Dimitri) syndrome (759.6)

⑤ **365.5** **Glaucoma associated with disorders of the lens**

365.51 **Phacolytic glaucoma**

365.52 **Pseudoexfoliation glaucoma**
Use additional code to identify glaucoma stage (365.70-365.74)

365.59 **Glaucoma associated with other lens disorders**

⑤ **365.6** **Glaucoma associated with other ocular disorders**

365.60 **Glaucoma associated with unspecified ocular disorder**

365.61 **Glaucoma associated with pupillary block**

365.62 **Glaucoma associated with ocular inflammations**
Use additional code to identify glaucoma stage (365.70-365.74)

365.63 **Glaucoma associated with vascular disorders**
Use additional code to identify glaucoma stage (365.70-365.74)

365.64 **Glaucoma associated with tumors or cysts**

365.65 **Glaucoma associated with ocular trauma**
Use additional code to identify glaucoma stage (365.70-365.74)

● **365.7** **Glaucoma stage**
Code first associated type of glaucoma (365.10-365.13, 365.20, 365.23, 365.31, 365.52, 365.62-365.63, 365.65)

● **365.70** **Glaucoma stage, unspecified**
Glaucoma stage NOS

● **365.71** **Mild stage glaucoma**
Early stage glaucoma

● **365.72** **Moderate stage glaucoma**

● **365.73** **Severe stage glaucoma**
Advanced stage glaucoma
End-stage glaucoma

● **365.74** **Indeterminate stage glaucoma**

⑤ **365.8** **Other specified forms of glaucoma**

365.81 **Hypersecretion glaucoma**

365.82 **Glaucoma with increased episcleral venous pressure**

365.83 **Aqueous misdirection**
Malignant glaucoma

365.89 **Other specified glaucoma**

365.9 **Unspecified glaucoma**

● Code new
to 2012 edition
▲ Revision of
existing code
④ ⑤ Fourth or fifth
digit required

366 Cataract

> *Excludes:* congenital cataract *(743.30-743.34)*

> **DEFINITION** A cataract is a clouding that develops in the crystalline lens of the eye or in its envelope, varying in degree from slight to complete opacity and obstructing the passage of light.

⑤ **366.0** Infantile, juvenile, and presenile cataract

366.00 Nonsenile cataract, unspecified

366.01 Anterior subcapsular polar cataract

366.02 Posterior subcapsular polar cataract

366.03 Cortical, lamellar, or zonular cataract

366.04 Nuclear cataract

366.09 Other and combined forms of nonsenile cataract

⑤ **366.1** Senile cataract

366.10 Senile cataract, unspecified

366.11 Pseudoexfoliation of lens capsule

366.12 Incipient cataract
Cataract: Water clefts
   coronary
   immature NOS
   punctate

366.13 Anterior subcapsular polar senile cataract

366.14 Posterior subcapsular polar senile cataract

366.15 Cortical senile cataract

366.16 Nuclear sclerosis
Cataracta brunescens
Nuclear cataract

366.17 Total or mature cataract

366.18 Hypermature cataract
Morgagni cataract

366.19 Other and combined forms of senile cataract

⑤ **366.2** Traumatic cataract

366.20 Traumatic cataract, unspecified

366.21 Localized traumatic opacities
Vossius' ring

366.22 Total traumatic cataract

366.23 Partially resolved traumatic cataract

⑤ **366.3** Cataract secondary to ocular disorders

366.30 Cataracts complicata, unspecified

366.31 *Glaucomatous flecks (subcapsular)*
Code first underlying glaucoma (365.0-365.9)

366.32 *Cataract in inflammatory disorders*
Code first underlying condition, as:
   chronic choroiditis (363.0-363.2)

366.33 *Cataract with neovascularization*
Code first underlying condition, as:
   chronic iridocyclitis (364.10)

366.34 *Cataract in degenerative disorders*
Sunflower cataract

Code first underlying condition, as:
   chalcosis (360.24)
   degenerative myopia (360.21)
   pigmentary retinal dystrophy (362.74)

⑤ **366.4** Cataract associated with other disorders

366.41 *Diabetic cataract*
Code first diabetes (249.5, 250.5)

	Add 4th or 5th digit		Nonspecific code		Unspecified code		Manifestation code

366.42 *Tetanic cataract*
Code first underlying disease, as:
  calcinosis (275.4)
  hypoparathyroidism (252.1)

366.43 *Myotonic cataract*
Code first underlying disorder (359.21, 359.23)

366.44 *Cataract associated with other syndromes*
Code first underlying condition, as:
  craniofacial dysostosis (756.0)
  galactosemia (271.1)

366.45 Toxic cataract
  Drug-induced cataract

Use additional E code, if desired, to identify drug or other toxic substance

366.46 Cataract associated with radiation and other physical influences
Use additional E code, if desired, to identify cause

⑤ **366.5 After-cataract**

366.50 After-cataract, unspecified
  Secondary cataract NOS

366.51 Soemmering's ring

366.52 Other after-cataract, not obscuring vision

366.53 After-cataract, obscuring vision

366.8 Other cataract
  Calcification of lens

366.9 Unspecified cataract

367 Disorders of refraction and accommodation
  DEFINITION Refraction is the ability of the eye to bend light so that an image is focused on the retina. Accommodation is the automatic adjustment in focal length of the natural lens of the eye.

367.0 Hypermetropia
  Far-sightedness
  Hyperopia

367.1 Myopia
  Near-sightedness

⑤ **367.2 Astigmatism**

367.20 Astigmatism, unspecified

367.21 Regular astigmatism

367.22 Irregular astigmatism

⑤ **367.3 Anisometropia and aniseikonia**

367.31 Anisometropia

367.32 Aniseikonia

367.4 Presbyopia

⑤ **367.5 Disorders of accommodation**

367.51 Paresis of accommodation
  Cycloplegia

367.52 Total or complete internal ophthalmoplegia

367.53 Spasm of accommodation

⑤ **367.8 Other disorders of refraction and accommodation**

367.81 Transient refractive change

367.89 Other
  Drug-induced disorders of refraction and accommodation
  Toxic disorders of refraction and accommodation

367.9 Unspecified disorder of refraction and accommodation

368 Visual disturbances
  Excludes: *electrophysiological disturbances (794.11-794.14)*

⑤ **368.0 Amblyopia ex anopsia**
  DEFINITION Amblyopia refers to reduced vision in an eye that appears to be normal when examined with an ophthalmoscope.

368.00 Amblyopia, unspecified

● Code new
  to 2012 edition
▲ Revision of
  existing code
④ ⑤ Fourth or fifth
  digit required

368.01 Strabismic amblyopia
Suppression amblyopia

368.02 Deprivation amblyopia

368.03 Refractive amblyopia

[5] **368.1 Subjective visual disturbances**

368.10 Subjective visual disturbance, unspecified

368.11 Sudden visual loss

368.12 Transient visual loss
Concentric fading
Scintillating scotoma

368.13 Visual discomfort
Asthenopia
Eye strain
Photophobia

368.14 Visual distortions of shape and size
Macropsia
Metamorphopsia
Micropsia

368.15 Other visual distortions and entoptic phenomena
Photopsia
Refractive:
- diplopia
- polyopia

Visual halos

368.16 Psychophysical visual disturbances
Prosopagnosia
Visual:
- agnosia
- disorientation syndrome
- hallucinations
- object agnosia

368.2 Diplopia
Double vision

[5] **368.3 Other disorders of binocular vision**

368.30 Binocular vision disorder, unspecified

368.31 Suppression of binocular vision

368.32 Simultaneous visual perception without fusion

368.33 Fusion with defective stereopsis

368.34 Abnormal retinal correspondence

[5] **368.4 Visual field defects**

368.40 Visual field defect, unspecified

368.41 Scotoma involving central area
Scotoma:
- central
- centrocecal
- paracentral

368.42 Scotoma of blind spot area
Enlarged:
- angioscotoma
- blind spot

Paracecal scotoma

368.43 Sector or arcuate defects
Scotoma:
- arcuate
- Bjerrum
- Seidel

368.44 Other localized visual field defect
Scotoma:
- NOS
- ring

Visual field defect:
- nasal step
- peripheral

368.45 Generalized contraction or constriction

368.46 Homonymous bilateral field defects
Hemianopsia (altitudinal) (homonymous)
Quadrant anopia

368.47 Heteronymous bilateral field defects
Hemianopsia:
binasal
bitemporal

⑤ **368.5 Color vision deficiencies**
Color blindness

368.51 Protan defect
Protanomaly
Protanopia

368.52 Deutan defect
Deuteranomaly
Deuteranopia

368.53 Tritan defect
Tritanomaly
Tritanopia

368.54 Achromatopsia
Monochromatism (cone) (rod)

368.55 Acquired color vision deficiencies

368.59 Other color vision deficiencies

⑤ **368.6 Night blindness**
Nyctalopia

368.60 Night blindness, unspecified

368.61 Congenital night blindness
Hereditary night blindness
Oguchi's disease

368.62 Acquired night blindness

Excludes: *that due to vitamin A deficiency (264.5)*

368.63 Abnormal dark adaptation curve
Abnormal threshold of cones or rods
Delayed adaptation of cones or rods

368.69 Other night blindness

368.8 Other specified visual disturbances
Blurred vision NOS

368.9 Unspecified visual disturbance

● Code new
to 2012 edition
▲ Revision of
existing code
④ ⑤ Fourth or fifth
digit required

[369] Blindness and low vision

Note: Visual impairment refers to a functional limitation of the eye (e.g., limited visual acuity or visual field). It should be distinguished from visual disability, indicating a limitation of the abilities of the individual (e.g., limited reading skills, vocational skills), and from visual handicap, indicating a limitation of personal and socioeconomic independence (e.g., limited mobility, limited employability.)

The levels of impairment defined in the table in this section are based on the recommendations of the WHO Study Group on Prevention of Blindness (Geneva, November 6-10, 1972; WHO Technical Report Series 518), and of the International Council of Ophthalmology (1976).

Note that definitions of blindness vary in different settings.

For international reporting WHO defines blindness as profound impairment. This definition can be applied to blindness of one eye (369.1, 369.6) and to blindness of the individual (369.0).

For determination of benefits in the U.S.A., the definition of legal blindness as severe impairment is often used. This definition applies to blindness of the individual only.

[Excludes:] *correctable impaired vision due to refractive errors (367.0-367.9)*

Classification		LEVELS OF VISUAL IMPAIRMENT					Additional Descriptors which may be encountered
"legal"	WHO	Visual Acuity and/or Visual Field Limitation (whichever is worse)					
	(NEAR-) NORMAL VISION	**RANGE OF NORMAL VISION**					
		20/10	20/13	20/16	20/20	20/25	
		0.7	0.6	0.5	0.4	0.8	
		NEAR-NORMAL VISION					
			20/30	20/40	20/50	20/60	
		0.7	0.6	0.5	0.4	0.4	
	LOW VISION	**MODERATE VISUAL IMPAIRMENT**					Moderate low vision
		20/70	20/80	20/100	20/125	20/160	
			0.25	0.20	0.16	0.12	
LEGAL BLINDNESS		**SEVERE VISUAL IMPAIRMENT**					Severe low vision, "legal blindness"
			20/200	20/250	20/320	20/400	
			0.10	0.08	0.06	0.05	
		Visual Field:		20 degrees or less			
	BLINDNESS	**PROFOUND VISUAL IMPAIRMENT**					Profound low vision, moderate blindness
			20/500	20/630	20/800	20/1000	
			0.04	0.03	0.025	0.02	
		Count Fingers at:		less than 3 m (10ft)			
		Visual Field:		10 degrees or less			
		NEAR-TOTAL VISUAL IMPAIRMENT					Severe blindness
		Visual Acuity:		less than 0.02 (20/1000)			
		Count Fingers at:		1 m (3 ft) or less			
		Hand Movements:		5m (15ft) or less			Near-Total blindness
(USA) both eyes	(WHO) one or both eyes	Light projection, light perception					
		Visual Field:		5 degrees or less			
		TOTAL VISUAL IMPAIRMENT					Total blindness
		No light perception (NLP)					

Visual acuity refers to best achievable acuity with correction

Non-listed Snellen fractions may be classified by converting to the nearest decimal equivalent, e.g., 10/200=0.05, 6/30=0.20

CF (count fingers) without designation of distance, may be classified to profound impairment

HM (hand motion) without designation of distance, may be classified to near-total impairment.

Visual field measurements refer to the largest field diameter for a 1/100 white test object.

[5] **369.0 Profound impairment, both eyes**

[369.00] Impairment level not further specified
Blindness:
NOS according to WHO definition
both eyes

Add 4th or 5th digit | Nonspecific code | Unspecified code | Manifestation code

369.01 Better eye: total impairment;
　　　　 lesser eye: total impairment

369.02 Better eye: near-total impairment;
　　　　 lesser eye: not further specified

369.03 Better eye: near-total impairment;
　　　　 lesser eye: total impairment

369.04 Better eye: near-total impairment;
　　　　 lesser eye: near-total impairment

369.05 Better eye: profound impairment;
　　　　 lesser eye: not further specified

369.06 Better eye: profound impairment;
　　　　 lesser eye: total impairment

369.07 Better eye: profound impairment;
　　　　 lesser eye: near-total impairment

369.08 Better eye: profound impairment;
　　　　 lesser eye: profound impairment

⑤ **369.1 Moderate or severe impairment, better eye, profound impairment lesser eye**

369.10 Impairment level not further specified
　　　　 Blindness, one eye, low vision other eye

369.11 Better eye: severe impairment;
　　　　 lesser eye: blind, not further specified

369.12 Better eye: severe impairment;
　　　　 lesser eye: total impairment

369.13 Better eye: severe impairment;
　　　　 lesser eye: near-total impairment

369.14 Better eye: severe impairment;
　　　　 lesser eye: profound impairment

369.15 Better eye: moderate impairment;
　　　　 lesser eye: blind, not further specified

369.16 Better eye: moderate impairment;
　　　　 lesser eye: total impairment

369.17 Better eye: moderate impairment;
　　　　 lesser eye: near-total impairment

369.18 Better eye: moderate impairment;
　　　　 lesser eye: profound impairment

⑤ **369.2 Moderate or severe impairment, both eyes**

369.20 Impairment level not further specified
　　　　 Low vision, both eyes NOS

369.21 Better eye: severe impairment;
　　　　 lesser eye: not further specified

369.22 Better eye: severe impairment;
　　　　 lesser eye: severe impairment

369.23 Better eye: moderate impairment;
　　　　 lesser eye: not further specified

369.24 Better eye: moderate impairment;
　　　　 lesser eye: severe impairment

369.25 Better eye: moderate impairment;
　　　　 lesser eye: moderate impairment

369.3 Unqualified visual loss, both eyes

Excludes: *blindness NOS:*
　　　　　 legal [U.S.A. definition] (369.4)
　　　　　 WHO definition (369.00)

369.4 Legal blindness, as defined in U.S.A.
　　　　 Blindness NOS according to U.S.A. definition

Excludes: *legal blindness with specification of impairment level (369.01-369.08,*
　　　　　 369.11-369.14, 369.21-369.22)

⑤ **369.6 Profound impairment, one eye**

369.60 Impairment level not further specified
　　　　 Blindness, one eye

369.61 One eye: total impairment; other eye: not specified

● Code new
　 to 2012 edition
▲ Revision of
　 existing code
④ ⑤ Fourth or fifth
　　 digit required

369.62 **One eye: total impairment; other eye: near-normal vision**

369.63 **One eye: total impairment; other eye: normal vision**

369.64 **One eye: near-total impairment; other eye: not specified**

369.65 **One eye: near-total impairment; other eye: near-normal vision**

369.66 **One eye: near-total impairment; other eye: normal vision**

369.67 **One eye: profound impairment; other eye: not specified**

369.68 **One eye: profound impairment; other eye: near-normal vision**

369.69 **One eye: profound impairment; other eye: normal vision**

[5] **369.7** **Moderate or severe impairment, one eye**

369.70 **Impairment level not further specified**
Low vision, one eye

369.71 **One eye: severe impairment; other eye: not specified**

369.72 **One eye: severe impairment; other eye: near-normal vision**

369.73 **One eye: severe impairment; other eye: normal vision**

369.74 **One eye: moderate impairment; other eye: not specified**

369.75 **One eye: moderate impairment; other eye: near-normal vision**

369.76 **One eye: moderate impairment; other eye: normal vision**

369.8 **Unqualified visual loss, one eye**

369.9 **Unspecified visual loss**

370 **Keratitis**

DEFINITION Keratitis is an infection or inflammation of the cornea which can be caused by a variety of conditions, including infections, dry eyes, foreign objects, contact lenses, intense light, vitamin a deficiency or allergies.

[5] **370.0** **Corneal ulcer**

[Excludes:] *that due to vitamin A deficiency (264.3)*

370.00 **Corneal ulcer, unspecified**

370.01 **Marginal corneal ulcer**

370.02 **Ring corneal ulcer**

370.03 **Central corneal ulcer**

370.04 **Hypopyon ulcer**
Serpiginous ulcer

370.05 **Mycotic corneal ulcer**

370.06 **Perforated corneal ulcer**

370.07 **Mooren's ulcer**

[5] **370.2** **Superficial keratitis without conjunctivitis**

[Excludes:] *dendritic [herpes simplex] keratitis (054.42)*

370.20 **Superficial keratitis, unspecified**

370.21 **Punctate keratitis**
Thygeson's superficial punctate keratitis

370.22 **Macular keratitis**
Keratitis:
areolar
nummular

Keratitis:
stellate
striate

370.23 **Filamentary keratitis**

370.24 **Photokeratitis**
Snow blindness
Welders' keratitis

[5] **370.3** **Certain types of keratoconjunctivitis**

370.31 **Phlyctenular keratoconjunctivitis**
Phlyctenulosis

Use additional code for any associated tuberculosis (017.3)

370.32 **Limbar and corneal involvement in vernal conjunctivitis**

Use additional code for vernal conjunctivitis (372.13)

370.33 **Keratoconjunctivitis sicca, not specified as Sjögren's**

[Excludes:] *Sjögren's syndrome (710.2)*

370.34 **Exposure keratoconjunctivitis**

Add 4th or 5th digit | Nonspecific code | Unspecified code | Manifestation code

370.35 **Neurotrophic keratoconjunctivitis**

⑤ **370.4 Other and unspecified keratoconjunctivitis**

370.40 **Keratoconjunctivitis, unspecified**
Superficial keratitis with conjunctivitis NOS

370.44 *Keratitis or keratoconjunctivitis in exanthema*
Code first underlying condition (050.0-052.9)

Excludes: *herpes simplex (054.43)*
herpes zoster (053.21)
measles (055.71)

370.49 **Other**

Excludes: *epidemic keratoconjunctivitis (077.1)*

⑤ **370.5 Interstitial and deep keratitis**

370.50 **Interstitial keratitis, unspecified**

370.52 **Diffuse interstitial keratitis**
Cogan's syndrome

370.54 **Sclerosing keratitis**

370.55 **Corneal abscess**

370.59 **Other**

Excludes: *disciform herpes simplex keratitis (054.43)*
syphilitic keratitis (090.3)

⑤ **370.6 Corneal neovascularization**

370.60 **Corneal neovascularization, unspecified**

370.61 **Localized vascularization of cornea**

370.62 **Pannus (corneal)**

370.63 **Deep vascularization of cornea**

370.64 **Ghost vessels (corneal)**

370.8 Other forms of keratitis
Code first underlying condition, such as:
Acanthamoeba (136.21)
Fusarium (118)

370.9 Unspecified keratitis

371 **Corneal opacity and other disorders of cornea**

DEFINITION Corneal opacity is a cloudy spot in the cornea, which is normally transparent. Causes include corneal scar tissue and infection.

⑤ **371.0 Corneal scars and opacities**

Excludes: *that due to vitamin A deficiency (264.6)*

371.00 **Corneal opacity, unspecified**
Corneal scar NOS

371.01 **Minor opacity of cornea**
Corneal nebula

371.02 **Peripheral opacity of cornea**
Corneal macula not interfering with central vision

371.03 **Central opacity of cornea**
Corneal:
leucoma interfering with central vision
macula interfering with central vision

371.04 **Adherent leucoma**

371.05 *Phthisical cornea*
Code first underlying tuberculosis (017.3)

⑤ **371.1 Corneal pigmentations and deposits**

371.10 **Corneal deposit, unspecified**

371.11 **Anterior pigmentations**
Stähli's lines

371.12 **Stromal pigmentations**
Hematocornea

● Code new   ▲ Revision of   ④ ⑤ Fourth or fifth
to 2012 edition   existing code   digit required

371.13 Posterior pigmentations
Krukenberg spindle

371.14 Kayser-Fleischer ring

371.15 Other deposits associated with metabolic disorders

371.16 Argentous deposits

[5] **371.2 Corneal edema**

371.20 Corneal edema, unspecified

371.21 Idiopathic corneal edema

371.22 Secondary corneal edema

371.23 Bullous keratopathy

371.24 Corneal edema due to wearing of contact lenses

[5] **371.3 Changes of corneal membranes**

371.30 Corneal membrane change, unspecified

371.31 Folds and rupture of Bowman's membrane

371.32 Folds in Descemet's membrane

371.33 Rupture in Descemet's membrane

[5] **371.4 Corneal degenerations**

371.40 Corneal degeneration, unspecified

371.41 Senile corneal changes
Arcus senilis
Hassall-Henle bodies

371.42 Recurrent erosion of cornea
[*Excludes:*] *Mooren's ulcer (370.07)*

371.43 Band-shaped keratopathy

371.44 Other calcerous degenerations of cornea

371.45 Keratomalacia NOS
[*Excludes:*] *that due to vitamin A deficiency (264.4)*

371.46 Nodular degeneration of cornea
Salzmann's nodular dystrophy

371.48 Peripheral degenerations of cornea
Marginal degeneration of cornea [Terrien's]

371.49 Other
Discrete colliquative keratopathy

[5] **371.5 Hereditary corneal dystrophies**

371.50 Corneal dystrophy, unspecified

371.51 Juvenile epithelial corneal dystrophy

371.52 Other anterior corneal dystrophies
Corneal dystrophy:
- microscopic cystic
- ring-like

371.53 Granular corneal dystrophy

371.54 Lattice corneal dystrophy

371.55 Macular corneal dystrophy

371.56 Other stromal corneal dystrophies
Crystalline corneal dystrophy

371.57 Endothelial corneal dystrophy
Combined corneal dystrophy
Cornea guttata
Fuchs' endothelial dystrophy

371.58 Other posterior corneal dystrophies
Polymorphous corneal dystrophy

[5] **371.6 Keratoconus**

371.60 Keratoconus, unspecified

371.61 Keratoconus, stable condition

371.62 Keratoconus, acute hydrops

Add 4th or 5th digit | Nonspecific code | Unspecified code | Manifestation code

[5] **371.7 Other corneal deformities**

371.70 Corneal deformity, unspecified

371.71 Corneal ectasia

371.72 Descemetocele

371.73 Corneal staphyloma

[5] **371.8 Other corneal disorders**

371.81 Corneal anesthesia and hypoesthesia

371.82 Corneal disorder due to contact lens

[Excludes:] *corneal edema due to contact lens (371.24)*

371.89 Other

371.9 Unspecified corneal disorder

372 Disorders of conjunctiva

[Excludes:] *keratoconjunctivitis (370.3-370.4)*

[DEFINITION] Disorders of conjunctiva are disorders of the mucous membrane that lines the inner surface of the eyelid and the exposed surface of the eyeball.

[5] **372.0 Acute conjunctivitis**

372.00 Acute conjunctivitis, unspecified

372.01 Serous conjunctivitis, except viral

[Excludes:] *viral conjunctivitis NOS (077.9)*

372.02 Acute follicular conjunctivitis
Conjunctival folliculosis NOS

[Excludes:] *conjunctivitis:*
adenoviral (acute follicular) (077.3)
epidemic hemorrhagic (077.4)
inclusion (077.0)
Newcastle (077.8)
epidemic keratoconjunctivitis (077.1)
pharyngoconjunctival fever (077.2)

372.03 Other mucopurulent conjunctivitis
Catarrhal conjunctivitis

[Excludes:] *blennorrhea neonatorum (gonococcal) (098.40)*
neonatal conjunctivitis (771.6)
ophthalmia neonatorum NOS (771.6)

372.04 Pseudomembranous conjunctivitis
Membranous conjunctivitis

[Excludes:] *diphtheritic conjunctivitis (032.81)*

372.05 Acute atopic conjunctivitis

372.06 Acute chemical conjunctivitis
Acute toxic conjunctivitis

Use addtional E code to identify the chemical or toxic agent

[Excludes:] *burn of eye and adnexa (940.0-940.9)*
chemical corrosion injury of eye (940.2-940.3)

[5] **372.1 Chronic conjunctivitis**

372.10 Chronic conjunctivitis, unspecified

372.11 Simple chronic conjunctivitis

372.12 Chronic follicular conjunctivitis

372.13 Vernal conjunctivitis

372.14 Other chronic allergic conjunctivitis

372.15 Parasitic conjunctivitis

Code first underlying disease, as:
filariasis (125.0-125.9)
mucocutaneous leishmaniasis (085.5)

[5] **372.2 Blepharoconjunctivitis**

372.20 Blepharoconjunctivitis, unspecified

372.21 Angular blepharoconjunctivitis

372.22 Contact blepharoconjunctivitis

[5] **372.3 Other and unspecified conjunctivitis**

372.30 Conjunctivitis, unspecified

372.31 Rosacea conjunctivitis

Code first underlying rosacea dermatitis (695.3)

372.33 Conjunctivitis in mucocutaneous disease

Code first underlying disease, as:
erythema multiforme (695.10-695.19)
Reiter's disease (099.3)

[Excludes:] *ocular pemphigoid (694.61)*

372.34 Pingueculitis

[Excludes:] *pinguecula (372.51)*

372.39 Other

[5] **372.4 Pterygium**

[Excludes:] *pseudopterygium (372.52)*

372.40 Pterygium, unspecified

372.41 Peripheral pterygium, stationary

372.42 Peripheral pterygium, progressive

372.43 Central pterygium

372.44 Double pterygium

372.45 Recurrent pterygium

[5] **372.5 Conjunctival degenerations and deposits**

372.50 Conjunctival degeneration, unspecified

372.51 Pinguecula

[Excludes:] *pingueculitis (372.34)*

372.52 Pseudopterygium

372.53 Conjunctival xerosis

[Excludes:] *conjunctival xerosis due to vitamin A deficiency (264.0, 264.1, 264.7)*

372.54 Conjunctival concretions

372.55 Conjunctival pigmentations
Conjunctival argyrosis

372.56 Conjunctival deposits

[5] **372.6 Conjunctival scars**

372.61 Granuloma of conjunctiva

372.62 Localized adhesions and strands of conjunctiva

372.63 Symblepharon
Extensive adhesions of conjunctiva

372.64 Scarring of conjunctiva
Contraction of eye socket (after enucleation)

[5] **372.7 Conjunctival vascular disorders and cysts**

372.71 Hyperemia of conjunctiva

372.72 Conjunctival hemorrhage
Hyposphagma
Subconjunctival hemorrhage

372.73 Conjunctival edema
Chemosis of conjunctiva
Subconjunctival edema

372.74 Vascular abnormalities of conjunctiva
Aneurysm(ata) of conjunctiva

372.75 Conjunctival cysts

[5] **372.8 Other disorders of conjunctiva**

372.81 Conjunctivochalasis

372.89 Other disorders of conjunctiva

372.9 Unspecified disorder of conjunctiva

373 **Inflammation of eyelids**

> **DEFINITION** Inflammation of eyelids refers to swelling or redness of the eyelids caused by infection or injury.

⑤ **373.0** **Blepharitis**

> *Excludes:* blepharoconjunctivitis (372.20-372.22)

>> **373.00** **Blepharitis, unspecified**
>> **373.01** **Ulcerative blepharitis**
>> **373.02** **Squamous blepharitis**

⑤ **373.1** **Hordeolum and other deep inflammation of eyelid**

>> **373.11** **Hordeolum externum**
>> Hordeolum NOS
>> Stye

>> **373.12** **Hordeolum internum**
>> Infection of meibomian gland

>> **373.13** **Abscess of eyelid**
>> Furuncle of eyelid

373.2 **Chalazion**
> Meibomian (gland) cyst

> *Excludes:* infected meibomian gland (373.12)

⑤ **373.3** **Noninfectious dermatoses of eyelid**

>> **373.31** **Eczematous dermatitis of eyelid**
>> **373.32** **Contact and allergic dermatitis of eyelid**
>> **373.33** **Xeroderma of eyelid**
>> **373.34** **Discoid lupus erythematosus of eyelid**

373.4 *Infective dermatitis of eyelid of types resulting in deformity*
> *Code first underlying disease, as:*
> leprosy (030.0-030.9)
> lupus vulgaris (tuberculous) (017.0)
> yaws (102.0-102.9)

373.5 *Other infective dermatitis of eyelid*
> *Code first underlying disease, as:*
> actinomycosis (039.3)
> impetigo (684)
> mycotic dermatitis (110.0-111.9)
> vaccinia (051.0)
> postvaccination (999.0)

> *Excludes:* herpes:
>> simplex (054.41)
>> zoster (053.20)

373.6 *Parasitic infestation of eyelid*
> *Code first underlying disease, as:*
> leishmaniasis (085.0-085.9)
> loiasis (125.2)
> onchocerciasis (125.3)
> pediculosis (132.0)

373.8 **Other inflammations of eyelids**

373.9 **Unspecified inflammation of eyelid**

374 **Other disorders of eyelids**

> **ALERT!** For personal history of other disorders of nervous system and sense organs see V12.49

⑤ **374.0** **Entropion and trichiasis of eyelid**

>> **374.00** **Entropion, unspecified**
>> **374.01** **Senile entropion**
>> **374.02** **Mechanical entropion**
>> **374.03** **Spastic entropion**
>> **374.04** **Cicatricial entropion**
>> **374.05** **Trichiasis without entropion**

⑤ **374.1** **Ectropion**

● Code new to 2012 edition	▲ Revision of existing code	④ ⑤ Fourth or fifth digit required

374.10 Ectropion, unspecified

374.11 Senile ectropion

374.12 Mechanical ectropion

374.13 Spastic ectropion

374.14 Cicatricial ectropion

[5] **374.2 Lagophthalmos**

374.20 Lagophthalmos, unspecified

374.21 Paralytic lagophthalmos

374.22 Mechanical lagophthalmos

374.23 Cicatricial lagophthalmos

[5] **374.3 Ptosis of eyelid**

374.30 Ptosis of eyelid, unspecified

374.31 Paralytic ptosis

374.32 Myogenic ptosis

374.33 Mechanical ptosis

374.34 Blepharochalasis
Pseudoptosis

[5] **374.4 Other disorders affecting eyelid function**

[Excludes:] *blepharoclonus (333.81)*
blepharospasm (333.81)
facial nerve palsy (351.0)
third nerve palsy or paralysis (378.51-378.52)
tic (psychogenic) (307.20-307.23)
organic (333.3)

374.41 Lid retraction or lag

374.43 Abnormal innervation syndrome
Jaw-blinking
Paradoxical facial movements

374.44 Sensory disorders

374.45 Other sensorimotor disorders
Deficient blink reflex

374.46 Blepharophimosis
Ankyloblepharon

[5] **374.5 Degenerative disorders of eyelid and periocular area**

374.50 Degenerative disorder of eyelid, unspecified

374.51 Xanthelasma
Xanthoma (planum) (tuberosum) of eyelid

Code first underlying condition (272.0-272.9)

374.52 Hyperpigmentation of eyelid
Chloasma
Dyspigmentation

374.53 Hypopigmentation of eyelid
Vitiligo of eyelid

374.54 Hypertrichosis of eyelid

374.55 Hypotrichosis of eyelid
Madarosis of eyelid

374.56 Other degenerative disorders of skin affecting eyelid

[5] **374.8 Other disorders of eyelid**

374.81 Hemorrhage of eyelid

[Excludes:] *black eye (921.0)*

374.82 Edema of eyelid
Hyperemia of eyelid

374.83 Elephantiasis of eyelid

374.84 Cysts of eyelids
Sebaceous cyst of eyelid

374.85 Vascular anomalies of eyelid

374.86 Retained foreign body of eyelid
Use additional code to identify foreign body (V90.01-V90.9)

Add 4th or 5th digit | Nonspecific code | Unspecified code | Manifestation code

374.87 Dermatochalasis

374.89 Other disorders of eyelid

374.9 Unspecified disorder of eyelid

375 Disorders of lacrimal system

[DEFINITION] Disorders of lacrimal system refers to disorders of the lacrimal gland, lake, puncta, canaliculi, sac, and nasolacrimal duct.

[5] **375.0 Dacryoadenitis**

375.00 Dacryoadenitis, unspecified

375.01 Acute dacryoadenitis

375.02 Chronic dacryoadenitis

375.03 Chronic enlargement of lacrimal gland

[5] **375.1 Other disorders of lacrimal gland**

375.11 Dacryops

375.12 Other lacrimal cysts and cystic degeneration

375.13 Primary lacrimal atrophy

375.14 Secondary lacrimal atrophy

375.15 Tear film insufficiency, unspecified
Dry eye syndrome

375.16 Dislocation of lacrimal gland

[5] **375.2 Epiphora**

375.20 Epiphora, unspecified as to cause

375.21 Epiphora due to excess lacrimation

375.22 Epiphora due to insufficient drainage

[5] **375.3 Acute and unspecified inflammation of lacrimal passages**

[Excludes:] *neonatal dacryocystitis (771.6)*

375.30 Dacryocystitis, unspecified

375.31 Acute canaliculitis, lacrimal

375.32 Acute dacryocystitis
Acute peridacryocystitis

375.33 Phlegmonous dacryocystitis

[5] **375.4 Chronic inflammation of lacrimal passages**

375.41 Chronic canaliculitis

375.42 Chronic dacryocystitis

375.43 Lacrimal mucocele

[5] **375.5 Stenosis and insufficiency of lacrimal passages**

375.51 Eversion of lacrimal punctum

375.52 Stenosis of lacrimal punctum

375.53 Stenosis of lacrimal canaliculi

375.54 Stenosis of lacrimal sac

375.55 Obstruction of nasolacrimal duct, neonatal

[Excludes:] *congenital anomaly of nasolacrimal duct (743.65)*

375.56 Stenosis of nasolacrimal duct, acquired

375.57 Dacryolith

[5] **375.6 Other changes of lacrimal passages**

375.61 Lacrimal fistula

375.69 Other

[5] **375.8 Other disorders of lacrimal system**

375.81 Granuloma of lacrimal passages

375.89 Other

375.9 Unspecified disorder of lacrimal system

376 Disorders of the orbit

[DEFINITION] Disorders of the orbit refers to disorders of the eye socket.

[5] **376.0 Acute inflammation of orbit**

376.00 Acute inflammation of orbit, unspecified

376.01 Orbital cellulitis
Abscess of orbit

376.02 Orbital periostitis

376.03 Orbital osteomyelitis

376.04 Tenonitis

[5] **376.1 Chronic inflammatory disorders of orbit**

376.10 Chronic inflammation of orbit, unspecified

376.11 Orbital granuloma
Pseudotumor (inflammatory) of orbit

376.12 Orbital myositis

376.13 Parasitic infestation of orbit

Code first underlying disease, as:
hydatid infestation of orbit (122.3, 122.6, 122.9)
myiasis of orbit (134.0)

[5] ***376.2 Endocrine exophthalmos***

Code first underlying thyroid disorder (242.0-242.9)

376.21 Thyrotoxic exophthalmos

376.22 Exophthalmic ophthalmoplegia

[5] **376.3 Other exophthalmic conditions**

376.30 Exophthalmos, unspecified

376.31 Constant exophthalmos

376.32 Orbital hemorrhage

376.33 Orbital edema or congestion

376.34 Intermittent exophthalmos

376.35 Pulsating exophthalmos

376.36 Lateral displacement of globe

[5] **376.4 Deformity of orbit**

376.40 Deformity of orbit, unspecified

376.41 Hypertelorism of orbit

376.42 Exostosis of orbit

376.43 Local deformities due to bone disease

376.44 Orbital deformities associated with craniofacial deformities

376.45 Atrophy of orbit

376.46 Enlargement of orbit

376.47 Deformity due to trauma or surgery

[5] **376.5 Enophthalmos**

376.50 Enophthalmos, unspecified as to cause

376.51 Enophthalmos due to atrophy of orbital tissue

376.52 Enophthalmos due to trauma or surgery

376.6 Retained (old) foreign body following penetrating wound of orbit
Retrobulbar foreign body
Use additional code to identify foreign body (V90.01-V90.9)

[5] **376.8 Other orbital disorders**

376.81 Orbital cysts
Encephalocele of orbit

376.82 Myopathy of extraocular muscles

376.89 Other

376.9 Unspecified disorder of orbit

377 Disorders of optic nerve and visual pathways

[DEFINITION] The optic nerve transmits visual information from the retina to the brain.

[5] **377.0 Papilledema**

377.00 Papilledema, unspecified

377.01 Papilledema associated with increased intracranial pressure

Add 4th or 5th digit | Nonspecific code | Unspecified code | Manifestation code

377.02 Papilledema associated with decreased ocular pressure

377.03 Papilledema associated with retinal disorder

377.04 Foster-Kennedy syndrome

[5] **377.1 Optic atrophy**

377.10 Optic atrophy, unspecified

377.11 Primary optic atrophy

[Excludes:] *neurosyphilitic optic atrophy (094.84)*

377.12 Postinflammatory optic atrophy

377.13 Optic atrophy associated with retinal dystrophies

377.14 Glaucomatous atrophy [cupping] of optic disc

377.15 Partial optic atrophy
Temporal pallor of optic disc

377.16 Hereditary optic atrophy
Optic atrophy:
dominant hereditary
Leber's

[5] **377.2 Other disorders of optic disc**

377.21 Drusen of optic disc

377.22 Crater-like holes of optic disc

377.23 Coloboma of optic disc

377.24 Pseudopapilledema

[5] **377.3 Optic neuritis**

[Excludes:] *meningococcal optic neuritis (036.81)*

377.30 Optic neuritis, unspecified

377.31 Optic papillitis

377.32 Retrobulbar neuritis (acute)

[Excludes:] *syphilitic retrobulbar neuritis (094.85)*

377.33 Nutritional optic neuropathy

377.34 Toxic optic neuropathy
Toxic amblyopia

377.39 Other

[Excludes:] *ischemic optic neuropathy (377.41)*

[5] **377.4 Other disorders of optic nerve**

377.41 Ischemic optic neuropathy

377.42 Hemorrhage in optic nerve sheaths

377.43 Optic nerve hypoplasia

377.49 Other
Compression of optic nerve

[5] **377.5 Disorders of optic chiasm**

377.51 Associated with pituitary neoplasms and disorders

377.52 Associated with other neoplasms

377.53 Associated with vascular disorders

377.54 Associated with inflammatory disorders

[5] **377.6 Disorders of other visual pathways**

377.61 Associated with neoplasms

377.62 Associated with vascular disorders

377.63 Associated with inflammatory disorders

[5] **377.7 Disorders of visual cortex**

[Excludes:] *visual:*
agnosia (368.16)
hallucinations (368.16)
halos (368.15)

377.71 Associated with neoplasms

377.72 Associated with vascular disorders

377.73 Associated with inflammatory disorders

377.75 Cortical blindness

377.9 Unspecified disorder of optic nerve and visual pathways

378 Strabismus and other disorders of binocular eye movements

[Excludes:] *nystagmus and other irregular eye movements (379.50-379.59)*

DEFINITION Strabismus, aka crossed eyes, is a visual defect in which the eyes are misaligned and point in different directions. Strabismus usually occurs in childhood but can occur later in life.

[5] **378.0 Esotropia**
Convergent concomitant strabismus

[Excludes:] *intermittent esotropia (378.20-378.22)*

378.00 Esotropia, unspecified

378.01 Monocular esotropia

378.02 Monocular esotropia with A pattern

378.03 Monocular esotropia with V pattern

378.04 Monocular esotropia with other noncomitancies
Monocular esotropia with X or Y pattern

378.05 Alternating esotropia

378.06 Alternating esotropia with A pattern

378.07 Alternating esotropia with V pattern

378.08 Alternating esotropia with other noncomitancies
Alternating esotropia with X or Y pattern

[5] **378.1 Exotropia**
Divergent concomitant strabismus

[Excludes:] *intermittent exotropia (378.20, 378.23-378.24)*

378.10 Exotropia, unspecified

378.11 Monocular exotropia

378.12 Monocular exotropia with A pattern

378.13 Monocular exotropia with V pattern

378.14 Monocular exotropia with other noncomitancies
Monocular exotropia with X or Y pattern

378.15 Alternating exotropia

378.16 Alternating exotropia with A pattern

378.17 Alternating exotropia with V pattern

378.18 Alternating exotropia with other noncomitancies
Alternating exotropia with X or Y pattern

[5] **378.2 Intermittent heterotropia**

[Excludes:] *vertical heterotropia (intermittent) (378.31)*

378.20 Intermittent heterotropia, unspecified
Intermittent:
esotropia NOS
exotropia NOS

378.21 Intermittent esotropia, monocular

378.22 Intermittent esotropia, alternating

378.23 Intermittent exotropia, monocular

378.24 Intermittent exotropia, alternating

[5] **378.3 Other and unspecified heterotropia**

378.30 Heterotropia, unspecified

378.31 Hypertropia
Vertical heterotropia (constant) (intermittent)

378.32 Hypotropia

378.33 Cyclotropia

378.34 Monofixation syndrome
Microtropia

378.35 Accommodative component in esotropia

⑤ **378.4 Heterophoria**

    378.40 Heterophoria, unspecified

    378.41 Esophoria

    378.42 Exophoria

    378.43 Vertical heterophoria

    378.44 Cyclophoria

    378.45 Alternating hyperphoria

⑤ **378.5 Paralytic strabismus**

    378.50 Paralytic strabismus, unspecified

    378.51 Third or oculomotor nerve palsy, partial

    378.52 Third or oculomotor nerve palsy, total

    378.53 Fourth or trochlear nerve palsy

    378.54 Sixth or abducens nerve palsy

    378.55 External ophthalmoplegia

    378.56 Total ophthalmoplegia

⑤ **378.6 Mechanical strabismus**

    378.60 Mechanical strabismus, unspecified

    378.61 Brown's (tendon) sheath syndrome

    378.62 Mechanical strabismus from other musculofascial disorders

    378.63 Limited duction associated with other conditions

⑤ **378.7 Other specified strabismus**

    378.71 Duane's syndrome

    378.72 Progressive external ophthalmoplegia

    378.73 Strabismus in other neuromuscular disorders

⑤ **378.8 Other disorders of binocular eye movements**

    Excludes: nystagmus (379.50-379.56)

    378.81 Palsy of conjugate gaze

    378.82 Spasm of conjugate gaze

    378.83 Convergence insufficiency or palsy

    378.84 Convergence excess or spasm

    378.85 Anomalies of divergence

    378.86 Internuclear ophthalmoplegia

    378.87 Other dissociated deviation of eye movements
       Skew deviation

  378.9 Unspecified disorder of eye movements
    Ophthalmoplegia NOS
    Strabismus NOS

379 **Other disorders of eye**

    ALERT! For personal history of other disorders of nervous system and sense organs see V12.49

⑤ **379.0 Scleritis and episcleritis**

    Excludes: syphilitic episcleritis (095.0)

    379.00 Scleritis, unspecified
       Episcleritis NOS

    379.01 Episcleritis periodica fugax

    379.02 Nodular episcleritis

    379.03 Anterior scleritis

    379.04 Scleromalacia perforans

    379.05 Scleritis with corneal involvement
       Scleroperikeratitis

    379.06 Brawny scleritis

    379.07 Posterior scleritis
       Sclerotenonitis

● Code new to 2012 edition   ▲ Revision of existing code   ④ ⑤ Fourth or fifth digit required

379.09 **Other**
Scleral abscess

⑤ **379.1** **Other disorders of sclera**

Excludes: blue sclera (743.47)

379.11 **Scleral ectasia**
Scleral staphyloma NOS

379.12 **Staphyloma posticum**

379.13 **Equatorial staphyloma**

379.14 **Anterior staphyloma, localized**

379.15 **Ring staphyloma**

379.16 **Other degenerative disorders of sclera**

379.19 **Other**

⑤ **379.2** **Disorders of vitreous body**

379.21 **Vitreous degeneration**
Vitreous:
cavitation
detachment
liquefaction

379.22 **Crystalline deposits in vitreous**
Asteroid hyalitis
Synchysis scintillans

379.23 **Vitreous hemorrhage**

379.24 **Other vitreous opacities**
Vitreous floaters

379.25 **Vitreous membranes and strands**

379.26 **Vitreous prolapse**

● **379.27** **Vitreomacular adhesion**
Vitreomacular traction

Excludes: traction detachment with vitreoretinal organization (361.81)

379.29 **Other disorders of vitreous**

Excludes: vitreous abscess (360.04)

⑤ **379.3** **Aphakia and other disorders of lens**

Excludes: after-cataract (366.50-366.53)

379.31 **Aphakia**

Excludes: cataract extraction status (V45.61)

379.32 **Subluxation of lens**

379.33 **Anterior dislocation of lens**

379.34 **Posterior dislocation of lens**

379.39 **Other disorders of lens**

⑤ **379.4** **Anomalies of pupillary function**

379.40 **Abnormal pupillary function, unspecified**

379.41 **Anisocoria**

379.42 **Miosis (persistent), not due to miotics**

379.43 **Mydriasis (persistent) not due to mydriatics**

379.45 **Argyll Robertson pupil, atypical**
Argyll Robertson phenomenon or pupil, nonsyphilitic

Excludes: Argyll Robertson pupil (syphilitic) (094.89)

379.46 **Tonic pupillary reaction**
Adie's pupil or syndrome

379.49 **Other**
Hippus
Pupillary paralysis

⑤ **379.5** **Nystagmus and other irregular eye movements**

379.50 **Nystagmus, unspecified**

379.51 **Congenital nystagmus**

379.52 **Latent nystagmus**

	Add 4th or 5th digit		Nonspecific code		Unspecified code		Manifestation code

381

379.53 **Visual deprivation nystagmus**

379.54 **Nystagmus associated with disorders of the vestibular system**

379.55 **Dissociated nystagmus**

379.56 **Other forms of nystagmus**

379.57 **Deficiencies of saccadic eye movements**
Abnormal optokinetic response

379.58 **Deficiencies of smooth pursuit movements**

379.59 **Other irregularities of eye movements**
Opsoclonus

⑤ 379.6 **Inflammation (infection) of postprocedural bleb**
Postprocedural blebitis

379.60 **Inflammation (infection) of postprocedural bleb, unspecified**

379.61 **Inflammation (infection) of postprocedural bleb, stage 1**

379.62 **Inflammation (infection) of postprocedural bleb, stage 2**

379.63 **Inflammation (infection) of postprocedural bleb, stage 3**
Bleb associated endophthalmitis

379.8 **Other specified disorders of eye and adnexa**

⑤ 379.9 **Unspecified disorder of eye and adnexa**

379.90 **Disorder of eye, unspecified**

379.91 **Pain in or around eye**

379.92 **Swelling or mass of eye**

379.93 **Redness or discharge of eye**

379.99 **Other ill-defined disorders of eye**

Excludes: *blurred vision NOS (368.8)*

DISEASES OF THE EAR AND MASTOID PROCESS (380-389)

Use additional external cause code, if applicable, to identify the cause of the ear condition

380 **Disorders of external ear**

⑤ 380.0 **Perichondritis and chondritis of pinna**
Chondritis of auricle
Perichondritis of auricle

380.00 **Perichondritis of pinna, unspecified**

380.01 **Acute perichondritis of pinna**

380.02 **Chronic perichondritis of pinna**

380.03 **Chondritis of pinna**

⑤ 380.1 **Infective otitis externa**

380.10 **Infective otitis externa, unspecified**
Otitis externa (acute):
    NOS
    circumscribed
    diffuse
    hemorrhagica
    infective NOS

380.11 **Acute infection of pinna**

Excludes: *furuncular otitis externa (680.0)*

380.12 **Acute swimmers' ear**
Beach ear
Tank ear

380.13 *Other acute infections of external ear*
Code first underlying disease, as:
    erysipelas (035)
    impetigo (684)
    seborrheic dermatitis (690.10-690.18)

Excludes: *herpes simplex (054.73)*
    herpes zoster (053.71)

380.14 **Malignant otitis externa**

● Code new
to 2012 edition

▲ Revision of
existing code

④ ⑤ Fourth or fifth
digit required

380.15 *Chronic mycotic otitis externa*
Code first underlying disease, as:
aspergillosis (117.3)
otomycosis NOS (111.9)

Excludes: *candidal otitis externa (112.82)*

380.16 **Other chronic infective otitis externa**
Chronic infective otitis externa NOS

⑤ **380.2** **Other otitis externa**

380.21 **Cholesteatoma of external ear**
Keratosis obturans of external ear (canal)

Excludes: *cholesteatoma NOS (385.30-385.35)*
postmastoidectomy (383.32)

380.22 **Other acute otitis externa**
Acute otitis externa:
actinic
chemical
contact
eczematoid
reactive

380.23 **Other chronic otitis externa**
Chronic otitis externa NOS

⑤ **380.3** **Noninfectious disorders of pinna**

380.30 **Disorder of pinna, unspecified**

380.31 **Hematoma of auricle or pinna**

380.32 **Acquired deformities of auricle or pinna**

Excludes: *cauliflower ear (738.7)*

380.39 **Other**

Excludes: *gouty tophi of ear (274.81)*

380.4 **Impacted cerumen**
Wax in ear

⑤ **380.5** **Acquired stenosis of external ear canal**
Collapse of external ear canal

380.50 **Acquired stenosis of external ear canal, unspecified as to cause**

380.51 **Secondary to trauma**

380.52 **Secondary to surgery**

380.53 **Secondary to inflammation**

⑤ **380.8** **Other disorders of external ear**

380.81 **Exostosis of external ear canal**

380.89 **Other**

380.9 **Unspecified disorder of external ear**

381 **Nonsuppurative otitis media and Eustachian tube disorders**
DEFINITION Nonsuppurative otitis media and eustachian tube disorders, otitis media is an inflammation of the middle ear without the formation or discharge of pus.

⑤ **381.0** **Acute nonsuppurative otitis media**
Acute tubotympanic catarrh
Otitis media, acute or subacute:
catarrhal
exudative
transudative
with effusion

Excludes: *otitic barotrauma (993.0)*

381.00 **Acute nonsuppurative otitis media, unspecified**

381.01 **Acute serous otitis media**
Acute or subacute secretory otitis media

381.02 **Acute mucoid otitis media**
Acute or subacute seromucinous otitis media
Blue drum syndrome

381.03 **Acute sanguinous otitis media**

381.04 **Acute allergic serous otitis media**

| | Add 4th or 5th digit | | Nonspecific code | | Unspecified code | | Manifestation code |

381.05 Acute allergic mucoid otitis media

381.06 Acute allergic sanguinous otitis media

⑤ **381.1 Chronic serous otitis media**
Chronic tubotympanic catarrh

381.10 Chronic serous otitis media, simple or unspecified

381.19 Other
Serosanguinous chronic otitis media

⑤ **381.2 Chronic mucoid otitis media**
Glue ear

Excludes: *adhesive middle ear disease (385.10-385.19)*

381.20 Chronic mucoid otitis media, simple or unspecified

381.29 Other
Mucosanguinous chronic otitis media

381.3 Other and unspecified chronic nonsuppurative otitis media

Otitis media, chronic:	Otitis media, chronic:
allergic	seromucinous
exudative	transudative
secretory	with effusion

381.4 Nonsuppurative otitis media, not specified as acute or chronic

Otitis media:	Otitis media:
allergic	secretory
catarrhal	seromucinous
exudative	serous
mucoid	transudative
	with effusion

⑤ **381.5 Eustachian salpingitis**

381.50 Eustachian salpingitis, unspecified

381.51 Acute Eustachian salpingitis

381.52 Chronic Eustachian salpingitis

⑤ **381.6 Obstruction of Eustachian tube**
Stenosis of Eustachian tube
Stricture of Eustachian tube

381.60 Obstruction of Eustachian tube, unspecified

381.61 Osseous obstruction of Eustachian tube
Obstruction of Eustachian tube from cholesteatoma, polyp, or other osseous lesion

381.62 Intrinsic cartilagenous obstruction of Eustachian tube

381.63 Extrinsic cartilagenous obstruction of Eustachian tube
Compression of Eustachian tube

381.7 Patulous Eustachian tube

⑤ **381.8 Other disorders of Eustachian tube**

381.81 Dysfunction of Eustachian tube

381.89 Other

381.9 Unspecified Eustachian tube disorder

382 Suppurative and unspecified otitis media

DEFINITION Suppurative and unspecified otitis media is an inflammation of the middle ear including the formation or discharge of pus.

⑤ **382.0 Acute suppurative otitis media**
Otitis media, acute:
necrotizing NOS
purulent

382.00 Acute suppurative otitis media without spontaneous rupture of ear drum

382.01 Acute suppurative otitis media with spontaneous rupture of ear drum

382.02 *Acute suppurative otitis media in diseases classified elsewhere*
Code first underlying disease, as:
influenza (487.8, 488.09, 488.19)
scarlet fever (034.1)

Excludes: *postmeasles otitis (055.2)*

● Code new   ▲ Revision of   ④ ⑤ Fourth or fifth
to 2012 edition   existing code   digit required

382.1 Chronic tubotympanic suppurative otitis media
Benign chronic suppurative otitis media (with anterior perforation of ear drum)
Chronic tubotympanic disease (with anterior perforation of ear drum)

382.2 Chronic atticoantral suppurative otitis media
Chronic atticoantral disease (with posterior or superior marginal perforation of ear drum)
Persistent mucosal disease (with posterior or superior marginal perforation of ear drum)

382.3 Unspecified chronic suppurative otitis media
Chronic purulent otitis media

[Excludes:] *tuberculous otitis media (017.4)*

382.4 Unspecified suppurative otitis media
Purulent otitis media NOS

382.9 Unspecified otitis media
Otitis media:
NOS
acute NOS
chronic NOS

383 Mastoiditis and related conditions

[DEFINITION] Mastoiditis is an infection of the spaces within the mastoid bone. It is almost always associated with otitis media, an infection of the middle ear. In the most serious cases, the bone itself becomes infected.

[5] **383.0 Acute mastoiditis**
Abscess of mastoid
Empyema of mastoid

383.00 Acute mastoiditis without complications

383.01 Subperiosteal abscess of mastoid

383.02 Acute mastoiditis with other complications
Gradenigo's syndrome

383.1 Chronic mastoiditis
Caries of mastoid
Fistula of mastoid

[Excludes:] *tuberculous mastoiditis (015.6)*

[5] **383.2 Petrositis**
Coalescing osteitis of petrous bone
Inflammation of petrous bone
Osteomyelitis of petrous bone

383.20 Petrositis, unspecified

383.21 Acute petrositis

383.22 Chronic petrositis

[5] **383.3 Complications following mastoidectomy**

383.30 Postmastoidectomy complication, unspecified

383.31 Mucosal cyst of postmastoidectomy cavity

383.32 Recurrent cholesteatoma of postmastoidectomy cavity

383.33 Granulations of postmastoidectomy cavity
Chronic inflammation of postmastoidectomy cavity

[5] **383.8 Other disorders of mastoid**

383.81 Postauricular fistula

383.89 Other

383.9 Unspecified mastoiditis

384 Other disorders of tympanic membrane

[DEFINITION] The tympanic membrane is a thin membrane that separates the external ear from the middle ear.

[ALERT!] For personal history of other disorders of nervous system and sense organs see V12.49

[5] **384.0 Acute myringitis without mention of otitis media**

384.00 Acute myringitis, unspecified
Acute tympanitis NOS

384.01 Bullous myringitis
Myringitis bullosa hemorrhagica

Add 4th or 5th digit | Nonspecific code | Unspecified code | Manifestation code

384.09 Other

384.1 Chronic myringitis without mention of otitis media
Chronic tympanitis

⑤ **384.2 Perforation of tympanic membrane**
Perforation of ear drum:
NOS
persistent posttraumatic
postinflammatory

Excludes: *otitis media with perforation of tympanic membrane (382.00-382.9)*
traumatic perforation [current injury] (872.61)

384.20 Perforation of tympanic membrane, unspecified

384.21 Central perforation of tympanic membrane

384.22 Attic perforation of tympanic membrane
Pars flaccida

384.23 Other marginal perforation of tympanic membrane

384.24 Multiple perforations of tympanic membrane

384.25 Total perforation of tympanic membrane

⑤ **384.8 Other specified disorders of tympanic membrane**

384.81 Atrophic flaccid tympanic membrane
Healed perforation of ear drum

384.82 Atrophic nonflaccid tympanic membrane

384.9 Unspecified disorder of tympanic membrane

385 Other disorders of middle ear and mastoid

Excludes: *mastoiditis (383.0-383.9)*

DEFINITION The middle ear is the space between the eardrum and the inner ear that contains the three auditory ossicles, which convey vibrations through the oval window to the cochlea. The mastoid is the bone located directly behind the external ear.

ALERT! For personal history of other disorders of nervous system and sense organs see V12.49

⑤ **385.0 Tympanosclerosis**

385.00 Tympanosclerosis, unspecified as to involvement

385.01 Tympanosclerosis involving tympanic membrane only

385.02 Tympanosclerosis involving tympanic membrane and ear ossicles

385.03 Tympanosclerosis involving tympanic membrane, ear ossicles, and middle ear

385.09 Tympanosclerosis involving other combination of structures

⑤ **385.1 Adhesive middle ear disease**
Adhesive otitis
Otitis media:
chronic adhesive
fibrotic

Excludes: *glue ear (381.20-381.29)*

385.10 Adhesive middle ear disease, unspecified as to involvement

385.11 Adhesions of drum head to incus

385.12 Adhesions of drum head to stapes

385.13 Adhesions of drum head to promontorium

385.19 Other adhesions and combinations

⑤ **385.2 Other acquired abnormality of ear ossicles**

385.21 Impaired mobility of malleus
Ankylosis of malleus

385.22 Impaired mobility of other ear ossicles
Ankylosis of ear ossicles, except malleus

385.23 Discontinuity or dislocation of ear ossicles

385.24 Partial loss or necrosis of ear ossicles

● Code new
to 2012 edition
▲ Revision of
existing code
④ ⑤ Fourth or fifth
digit required

[5] **385.3 Cholesteatoma of middle ear and mastoid**
Cholesterosis of (middle) ear
Epidermosis of (middle) ear
Keratosis of (middle) ear
Polyp of (middle) ear

[*Excludes:*] *cholesteatoma:*
external ear canal (380.21)
recurrent of postmastoidectomy cavity (383.32)

385.30 Cholesteatoma, unspecified

385.31 Cholesteatoma of attic

385.32 Cholesteatoma of middle ear

385.33 Cholesteatoma of middle ear and mastoid

385.35 Diffuse cholesteatosis

[5] **385.8 Other disorders of middle ear and mastoid**

385.82 Cholesterin granuloma

385.83 Retained foreign body of middle ear
Use additional code to identify foreign body (V90.01-V90.9)

385.89 Other

385.9 Unspecified disorder of middle ear and mastoid

386 Vertiginous syndromes and other disorders of vestibular system

[*Excludes:*] *vertigo NOS (780.4)*

[DEFINITION] Vertiginous syndromes are disorders that cause vertigo (dizziness).

[5] **386.0 Ménière's disease**
Endolymphatic hydrops
Lermoyez's syndrome
Ménière's syndrome or vertigo

386.00 Ménière's disease, unspecified
Ménière's disease (active)

386.01 Active Ménière's disease, cochleovestibular

386.02 Active Ménière's disease, cochlear

386.03 Active Ménière's disease, vestibular

386.04 Inactive Ménière's disease
Ménière's disease in remission

[5] **386.1 Other and unspecified peripheral vertigo**

[*Excludes:*] *epidemic vertigo (078.81)*

386.10 Peripheral vertigo, unspecified

386.11 Benign paroxysmal positional vertigo
Benign paroxysmal positional nystagmus

386.12 Vestibular neuronitis
Acute (and recurrent) peripheral vestibulopathy

386.19 Other
Aural vertigo
Otogenic vertigo

386.2 Vertigo of central origin
Central positional nystagmus
Malignant positional vertigo

[5] **386.3 Labyrinthitis**

386.30 Labyrinthitis, unspecified

386.31 Serous labyrinthitis
Diffuse labyrinthitis

386.32 Circumscribed labyrinthitis
Focal labyrinthitis

386.33 Suppurative labyrinthitis
Purulent labyrinthitis

386.34 Toxic labyrinthitis

386.35 Viral labyrinthitis

[5] **386.4 Labyrinthine fistula**

386.40 Labyrinthine fistula, unspecified

386.41 Round window fistula

386.42   Oval window fistula

386.43   Semicircular canal fistula

386.48   Labyrinthine fistula of combined sites

⑤ **386.5   Labyrinthine dysfunction**

386.50   Labyrinthine dysfunction, unspecified

386.51   Hyperactive labyrinth, unilateral

386.52   Hyperactive labyrinth, bilateral

386.53   Hypoactive labyrinth, unilateral

386.54   Hypoactive labyrinth, bilateral

386.55   Loss of labyrinthine reactivity, unilateral

386.56   Loss of labyrinthine reactivity, bilateral

386.58   Other forms and combinations

386.8   Other disorders of labyrinth

386.9   Unspecified vertiginous syndromes and labyrinthine disorders

387   Otosclerosis
Includes: otospongiosis

DEFINITION Otosclerosis is a hereditary disorder in which ossification of the labyrinth of the inner ear causes tinnitus and eventual deafness .

387.0   Otosclerosis involving oval window, nonobliterative

387.1   Otosclerosis involving oval window, obliterative

387.2   Cochlear otosclerosis
Otosclerosis involving:
   otic capsule
   round window

387.8   Other otosclerosis

387.9   Otosclerosis, unspecified

388   Other disorders of ear

ALERT! For personal history of other disorders of nervous system and sense organs see V12.49

⑤ **388.0   Degenerative and vascular disorders of ear**

388.00   Degenerative and vascular disorders, unspecified

388.01   Presbyacusis

388.02   Transient ischemic deafness

⑤ **388.1   Noise effects on inner ear**

388.10   Noise effects on inner ear, unspecified

388.11   Acoustic trauma (explosive) to ear
Otitic blast injury

388.12   Noise-induced hearing loss

388.2   Sudden hearing loss, unspecified

⑤ **388.3   Tinnitus**

388.30   Tinnitus, unspecified

388.31   Subjective tinnitus

388.32   Objective tinnitus

⑤ **388.4   Other abnormal auditory perception**

388.40   Abnormal auditory perception, unspecified

388.41   Diplacusis

388.42   Hyperacusis

388.43   Impairment of auditory discrimination

388.44   Recruitment

388.45   Acquired auditory processing disorder
Auditory processing disorder NOS

Excludes: central auditory processing disorder (315.32)

● Code new   ▲ Revision of   ④ ⑤ Fourth or fifth
   to 2012 edition   existing code   digit required

388.5 Disorders of acoustic nerve
Acoustic neuritis
Degeneration of acoustic or eighth nerve
Disorder of acoustic or eighth nerve

[Excludes:] *acoustic neuroma (225.1)*
syphilitic acoustic neuritis (094.86)

[5] **388.6 Otorrhea**

388.60 Otorrhea, unspecified
Discharging ear NOS

388.61 Cerebrospinal fluid otorrhea

[Excludes:] *cerebrospinal fluid rhinorrhea (349.81)*

388.69 Other
Otorrhagia

[5] **388.7 Otalgia**

388.70 Otalgia, unspecified
Earache NOS

388.71 Otogenic pain

388.72 Referred pain

388.8 Other disorders of ear

388.9 Unspecified disorder of ear

389 Hearing loss

[DEFINITION] Hearing loss refers to the partial or complete loss of hearing

[5] **389.0 Conductive hearing loss**
Conductive deafness

[Excludes:] *mixed conductive and sensorineural hearing loss (389.20-389.22)*

389.00 Conductive hearing loss, unspecified

389.01 Conductive hearing loss, external ear

389.02 Conductive hearing loss, tympanic membrane

389.03 Conductive hearing loss, middle ear

389.04 Conductive hearing loss, inner ear

389.05 Conductive hearing loss, unilateral

389.06 Conductive hearing loss, bilateral

389.08 Conductive hearing loss of combined types

[5] **389.1 Sensorineural hearing loss**
Perceptive hearing loss or deafness

[Excludes:] *abnormal auditory perception (388.40-388.44)*
mixed conductive and sensorineural hearing loss (389.20-389.22)
psychogenic deafness (306.7)

389.10 Sensorineural hearing loss, unspecified

389.11 Sensory hearing loss, bilateral

389.12 Neural hearing loss, bilateral

389.13 Neural hearing loss, unilateral

389.14 Central hearing loss

389.15 Sensorineural hearing loss, unilateral

389.16 Sensorineural hearing loss, asymmetrical

389.17 Sensory hearing loss, unilateral

389.18 Sensorineural hearing loss, bilateral

[5] **389.2 Mixed conductive and sensorineural hearing loss**
Deafness or hearing loss of type classifiable to 389.00-389.08 with type classifiable to 389.10-389.18

389.20 Mixed hearing loss, unspecified

389.21 Mixed hearing loss, unilateral

389.22 Mixed hearing loss, bilateral

389.7 Deaf nonspeaking, not elsewhere classifiable

389.8 Other specified forms of hearing loss

389.9 **Unspecified hearing loss**
Deafness NOS

● Code new
to 2012 edition

▲ Revision of
existing code

④ ⑤ Fourth or fifth
digit required

Chapter 7: Diseases of Circulatory System (390-459)

DEFINITIONS AND CODING ALERTS

This chapter includes definitions of selected key words, terms and phrases and coding alerts for adding points to the clinical domain, references to coding late effects where appropriate, and references to personal history V-codes in situations where the acute or chronic condition is no longer active. An example from this chapter is as follows:

435 **Transient cerebral ischemia**

DEFINITION Transition cerebral ischemia is the reduction or loss of oxygen to the cerebrum; prolonged ischemia may lead to cerebral infarction.

ALERT For personal history of transient ischemic attack (tia), and cerebral infarction without residual deficits see v12.54.

MULTIPLE CODING FOR A SINGLE CONDITION

In addition to the etiology or manifestation convention that requires two codes to fully describe a single condition that affects multiple body systems, there are other single conditions that also require more than one code. "Use additional code" notes are found in the tabular at codes that are not part of an etiology or manifestation pair where a secondary code is useful to fully describe a condition. The sequencing rule is the same as the etiology or manifestation pair - , "use additional code" indicates that a secondary code should be added.

"Code first" notes are also under certain codes that are not specifically manifestation codes but may be due to an underlying cause. When a "code first" note is present and an underlying condition is present the underlying condition should be sequenced first.

"Code, if applicable, any causal condition first", notes indicate that this code may be assigned as a principal diagnosis when the causal condition is unknown or not applicable. If a causal condition is known, then the code for that condition should be sequenced as the principal or first-listed diagnosis. Multiple codes may be needed for late effects, complication codes and obstetric codes to more fully describe a condition. See the specific guidelines for these conditions for further instruction.

COMBINATION CODE

A combination code is a single code used to classify: two diagnoses, or a diagnosis with an associated secondary process (manifestation) A diagnosis with an associated complication Combination codes are identified by referring to subterm entries in the Alphabetic Index and by reading the inclusion and exclusion notes in the Tabular List.

Assign only the combination code when that code fully identifies the diagnostic conditions involved or when the Alphabetic Index so directs. Multiple coding should not be used when the classification provides a combination code that clearly identifies all of the elements documented in the diagnosis. When the combination code lacks necessary specificity in describing the manifestation or complication, an additional code should be used as a secondary code.

CODING LATE EFFECTS

A late effect is the residual effect (condition produced) after the acute phase of an illness or injury has terminated. There is no time limit on when a late effect code can be used. The residual may be apparent early, such as in cerebrovascular accident cases, or it may occur months or years later, such as that due to a previous injury. Coding of late effects generally requires two codes sequenced in the following order: The condition or nature of the late effect is sequenced first. The late effect code is sequenced second.

An exception to the above guidelines are those instances where the code for late effect is followed by a manifestation code identified in the Tabular List and title, or the late effect code has been expanded (at the fourth and fifth-digit levels) to include the manifestation(s). The code for the acute phase of an illness or injury that led to the late effect is never used with a code for the late effect.

HYPERTENSION

Hypertension Table

The Hypertension Table, found under the main term, "Hypertension", in the Alphabetic Index, contains a complete listing of all conditions due to or associated with hypertension and classifies them according to malignant, benign, and unspecified.

	Add 4th or 5th digit		Nonspecific code		Unspecified code		Manifestation code

Hypertension, Essential, or NOS

Assign hypertension (arterial) (essential) (primary) (systemic) (NOS) to category code 401 with the appropriate fourth digit to indicate malignant (.0), benign (.1), or unspecified (.9). Do not use either .0 malignant or .1 benign unless medical record documentation supports such a designation.

Hypertension with Heart Disease

Heart conditions (425.8, 429.0-429.3, 429.8, 429.9) are assigned to a code from category 402 when a causal relationship is stated (due to hypertension) or implied (hypertensive). Use an additional code from category 428 to identify the type of heart failure in those patients with heart failure. More than one code from category 428 may be assigned if the patient has systolic or diastolic failure and congestive heart failure.

The same heart conditions (425.8, 429.0-429.3, 429.8, 429.9) with hypertension, but without a stated causal relationship, are coded separately. Sequence according to the circumstances of the admission or encounter.

Hypertensive Chronic Kidney Disease

Assign codes from category 403, Hypertensive chronic kidney disease, when conditions classified to categories 585-587 are present. Unlike hypertension with heart disease, ICD-9-CM presumes a cause-and-effect relationship and classifies chronic kidney disease (CKD) with hypertension as hypertensive chronic kidney disease.

Fifth digits for category 403 should be assigned as follows:

0 with CKD stage I through stage IV, or unspecified.

1 with CKD stage V or end stage renal disease.

The appropriate code from category 585, Chronic kidney disease, should be used as a secondary code with a code from category 403 to identify the stage of chronic kidney disease.

See Chapter 10 for information on the coding of chronic kidney disease.

Hypertensive Heart And Chronic Kidney Disease

Assign codes from combination category 404, Hypertensive heart and chronic kidney disease, when both hypertensive kidney disease and hypertensive heart disease are stated in the diagnosis. Assume a relationship between the hypertension and the chronic kidney disease, whether or not the condition is so designated. Assign an additional code from category 428, to identify the type of heart failure. More than one code from category 428 may be assigned if the patient has systolic or diastolic failure and congestive heart failure.

Fifth digits for category 404 should be assigned as follows:

0 without heart failure and with chronic kidney disease (CKD) stage I through stage IV, or unspecified
1 with heart failure and with CKD stage I through stage IV, or unspecified
2 without heart failure and with CKD stage V or end stage renal disease
3 with heart failure and with CKD stage V or end stage renal disease

The appropriate code from category 585, Chronic kidney disease, should be used as a secondary code with a code from category 404 to identify the stage of kidney disease.

See Chapter 10 for information on the coding of chronic kidney disease.

Hypertensive Cerebrovascular Disease

First assign codes from 430-438, Cerebrovascular disease, then the appropriate hypertension code from categories 401-405.

Hypertensive Retinopathy

Two codes are necessary to identify the condition. First assign the code from subcategory 362.11, Hypertensive retinopathy, then the appropriate code from categories 401-405 to indicate the type of hypertension.

392 ● Code new
to 2012 edition   ▲ Revision of
existing code   ④ ⑤ Fourth or fifth
digit required

Hypertension, Secondary

Two codes are required: one to identify the underlying etiology and one from category 405 to identify the hypertension. Sequencing of codes is determined by the reason for admission or encounter.

Hypertension, Transient

Assign code 796.2, Elevated blood pressure reading without diagnosis of hypertension, unless patient has an established diagnosis of hypertension. Assign code 642.3x for transient hypertension of pregnancy.

Hypertension, Controlled

Assign appropriate code from categories 401-405. This diagnostic statement usually refers to an existing state of hypertension under control by therapy.

Hypertension, Uncontrolled

Uncontrolled hypertension may refer to untreated hypertension or hypertension not responding to current therapeutic regimen. In either case, assign the appropriate code from categories 401-405 to designate the stage and type of hypertension. Code to the type of hypertension.

Elevated Blood Pressure

For a statement of elevated blood pressure without further specificity, assign code 796.2, Elevated blood pressure reading without diagnosis of hypertension, rather than a code from category 401.

CEREBRAL INFARCTION OR STROKE OR CEREBROVASCULAR ACCIDENT (CVA)

The terms stroke and CVA are often used interchangeably to refer to a cerebral infarction. The terms stroke, CVA, and cerebral infarction NOS are all indexed to the default code 434.91, Cerebral artery occlusion, unspecified, with infarction. Code 436, Acute, but ill-defined, cerebrovascular disease, should not be used when the documentation states stroke or CVA.

See Chapter 18 for information on coding status post administration of tPA in a different facility within the last 24 hours.

POSTOPERATIVE CEREBROVASCULAR ACCIDENT

A cerebrovascular hemorrhage or infarction that occurs as a result of medical intervention is coded to 997.02, Iatrogenic cerebrovascular infarction or hemorrhage. Medical record documentation should clearly specify the cause- and-effect relationship between the medical intervention and the cerebrovascular accident in order to assign this code. A secondary code from the code range 430-432 or from a code from subcategories 433 or 434 with a fifth digit of "1" should also be used to identify the type of hemorrhage or infarct.

This guideline conforms to the use additional code note instruction at category 997. Code 436, Acute, but ill-defined, cerebrovascular disease, should not be used as a secondary code with code 997.02.

LATE EFFECTS OF CEREBROVASCULAR DISEASE

Category 438, Late Effects of Cerebrovascular disease

Category 438 is used to indicate conditions classifiable to categories 430-437 as the causes of late effects (neurologic deficits), themselves classified elsewhere. These "late effects" include neurologic deficits that persist after initial onset of conditions classifiable to 430-437. The neurologic deficits caused by cerebrovascular disease may be present from the onset or may arise at any time after the onset of the condition classifiable to 430-437.

Codes from category 438 with codes from 430-437

Codes from category 438 may be assigned on a health care record with codes from 430-437, if the patient has a current cerebrovascular accident (CVA) and deficits from an old CVA.

Code V12.54

Assign code V12.54, Transient ischemic attack (TIA), and cerebral infarction without residual deficits (and not a code from category 438 as an additional code for history of cerebrovascular disease when no neurologic deficits are present.

| | Add 4th or 5th digit | | Nonspecific code | | Unspecified code | | Manifestation code |

ACUTE MYOCARDIAL INFARCTION (AMI)

ST elevation myocardial infarction (STEMI) and non ST elevation myocardial infarction (NSTEMI)

The ICD-9-CM codes for acute myocardial infarction (AMI) identify the site, such as anterolateral wall or true posterior wall. Subcategories 410.0-410.6 and 410.8 are used for ST elevation myocardial infarction (STEMI). Subcategory 410.7, Subendocardial infarction, is used for non ST elevation myocardial infarction (NSTEMI) and nontransmural myocardial infarctions.

Acute myocardial infarction, unspecified

Subcategory 410.9 is the default for the unspecified term acute myocardial infarction. If only STEMI or transmural myocardial infarction without the site is documented, query the provider as to the site, or assign a code from subcategory 410.9.

AMI documented as nontransmural or subendocardial but site provided

If an AMI is documented as nontransmural or subendocardial, but the site is provided, it is still coded as a subendocardial AMI. If NSTEMI evolves to STEMI, assign the STEMI code. If STEMI converts to NSTEMI due to thrombolytic therapy, it is still coded as STEMI.

See Chapter 18 for information on coding status post administration of tPA in a different facility within the last 24 hours.

● Code new
  to 2012 edition

▲ Revision of
  existing code

④ ⑤ Fourth or fifth
  digit required

7. DISEASES OF THE CIRCULATORY SYSTEM (390-459)

ALERT! For personal history of diseases of circulatory system see V12.5

ACUTE RHEUMATIC FEVER (390-392)

390 Rheumatic fever without mention of heart involvement
Arthritis, rheumatic, acute or subacute
Rheumatic fever (active) (acute)
Rheumatism, articular, acute or subacute

Excludes: that with heart involvement (391.0-391.9)

DEFINITION Rheumatic fever is an illness which arises as a complication of untreated or inadequately treated strep throat infection. Rheumatic fever can seriously damage the valves of the heart.

391 Rheumatic fever with heart involvement

Excludes: chronic heart diseases of rheumatic origin (393-398.99) unless rheumatic fever is also present or there is evidence of recrudescence or activity of the rheumatic process

391.0 Acute rheumatic pericarditis
Rheumatic:
fever (active) (acute) with pericarditis
pericarditis (acute)
Any condition classifiable to 390 with pericarditis

Excludes: that not specified as rheumatic (420.0-420.9)

391.1 Acute rheumatic endocarditis
Rheumatic:
endocarditis, acute
fever (active) (acute) with endocarditis or valvulitis
valvulitis acute
Any condition classifiable to 390 with endocarditis or valvulitis

391.2 Acute rheumatic myocarditis
Rheumatic fever (active) (acute) with myocarditis
Any condition classifiable to 390 with myocarditis

391.8 Other acute rheumatic heart disease
Rheumatic:
fever (active) (acute) with other or multiple types of heart involvement
pancarditis, acute
Any condition classifiable to 390 with other or multiple types of heart involvement

391.9 Acute rheumatic heart disease, unspecified
Rheumatic:
carditis, acute
fever (active) (acute) with unspecified type of heart involvement
heart disease, active or acute
Any condition classifiable to 390 with unspecified type of heart involvement

392 Rheumatic chorea
Includes: Sydenham's chorea

Excludes: chorea:
NOS (333.5)
Huntington's (333.4)

DEFINITION Rheumatic chorea, aka Sydenham's chorea or Saint Vitus' Dance, is a disease characterized by rapid, uncoordinated jerking movements affecting primarily the face, feet and hands.

392.0 With heart involvement
Rheumatic chorea with heart involvement of any type classifiable to 391

392.9 Without mention of heart involvement

CHRONIC RHEUMATIC HEART DISEASE (393-398)

393 Chronic rheumatic pericarditis
Adherent pericardium, rheumatic
Chronic rheumatic:
mediastinopericarditis
myopericarditis

Excludes: pericarditis NOS or not specified as rheumatic (423.0-423.9)

DEFINITION Chronic rheumatic pericarditis is an inflammation of the pericardium resulting from rheumatic heart disease.

	Add 4th or 5th digit		Nonspecific code		Unspecified code		Manifestation code

394 Diseases of mitral valve

> *Excludes:* *that with aortic valve involvement (396.0-396.9)*

> **DEFINITION** The mitral valve is the valve that separates the two chambers on the left side of the heart. The mitral valve prevents blood from regurgitating backwards into the upper heart chambers during cardiac contractions.

394.0 Mitral stenosis
Mitral (valve):
    obstruction (rheumatic)
    stenosis NOS

394.1 Rheumatic mitral insufficiency
Rheumatic mitral:
    incompetence
    regurgitation

> *Excludes:* *that not specified as rheumatic (424.0)*

394.2 Mitral stenosis with insufficiency
Mitral stenosis with incompetence or regurgitation

394.9 Other and unspecified mitral valve diseases
Mitral (valve):
    disease (chronic)
    failure

395 Diseases of aortic valve

> *Excludes:* *that not specified as rheumatic (424.1)*
> *that with mitral valve involvement (396.0-396.9)*

> **DEFINITION** The aortic valve is a semilunar valve between the left ventricle and the aorta; prevents blood from flowing from the aorta back into the heart.

395.0 Rheumatic aortic stenosis
Rheumatic aortic (valve) obstruction

395.1 Rheumatic aortic insufficiency
Rheumatic aortic:
    incompetence
    regurgitation

395.2 Rheumatic aortic stenosis with insufficiency
Rheumatic aortic stenosis with incompetence or regurgitation

395.9 Other and unspecified rheumatic aortic diseases
Rheumatic aortic (valve) disease

396 Diseases of mitral and aortic valves
Includes: involvement of both mitral and aortic valves, whether specified as rheumatic or not

> **DEFINITION** The mitral valve is the valve that separates the two chambers on the left side of the heart. The aortic vale is a valve between the left ventricle and the aorta; prevents blood from flowing from the aorta back into the heart.

396.0 Mitral valve stenosis and aortic valve stenosis
Atypical aortic (valve) stenosis
Mitral and aortic (valve) obstruction (rheumatic)

396.1 Mitral valve stenosis and aortic valve insufficiency

396.2 Mitral valve insufficiency and aortic valve stenosis

396.3 Mitral valve insufficiency and aortic valve insufficiency
Mitral and aortic (valve):
    incompetence
    regurgitation

396.8 Multiple involvement of mitral and aortic valves
Stenosis and insufficiency of mitral or aortic valve with stenosis or insufficiency, or both, of the other valve

396.9 Mitral and aortic valve diseases, unspecified

397 Diseases of other endocardial structures

397.0 Diseases of tricuspid valve
Tricuspid (valve) (rheumatic):
    disease
    insufficiency
    obstruction
    regurgitation
    stenosis

397.1 Rheumatic diseases of pulmonary valve

Excludes: *that not specified as rheumatic (424.3)*

397.9 Rheumatic diseases of endocardium, valve unspecified
Rheumatic:
 endocarditis (chronic)
 valvulitis (chronic)

Excludes: *that not specified as rheumatic (424.90-424.99)*

398 Other rheumatic heart disease

DEFINITION Rheumatic heart disease refers to a thickening and stenosis of one or more of the heart valves and often requires surgery to repair or replace the involved valve(s).

398.0 Rheumatic myocarditis
Rheumatic degeneration of myocardium

Excludes: *myocarditis not specified as rheumatic (429.0)*

⑤ **398.9 Other and unspecified rheumatic heart diseases**

398.90 Rheumatic heart disease, unspecified
Rheumatic:
 carditis
 heart disease NOS

Excludes: *carditis not specified as rheumatic (429.89)*
 heart disease NOS not specified as rheumatic (429.9)

398.91 Rheumatic heart failure (congestive)
Rheumatic left ventricular failure

398.99 Other

HYPERTENSIVE DISEASE (401-405)

Excludes: *that complicating pregnancy, childbirth, or the puerperium (642.0-642.9)*
 that involving coronary vessels (410.00-414.9)

401 Essential hypertension
Includes: high blood pressure
 hyperpiesia
 hyperpiesis
 hypertension (arterial) (essential) (primary) (systemic)
 hypertensive vascular:
  degeneration
  disease

Excludes: *elevated blood pressure without diagnosis of hypertension (796.2)*
 pulmonary hypertension (416.0-416.9)
 that involving vessels of:
  brain (430-438)
  eye (362.11)

DEFINITION Essential hypertension is defined as hypertension without known cause.

401.0 Malignant

401.1 Benign

401.9 Unspecified

402 Hypertensive heart disease
Use additional code to specify type of heart failure (428.0-428.43), if known
Includes: hypertensive:
  cardiomegaly
  cardiopathy
  cardiovascular disease
  heart (disease) (failure)
  any condition classifiable to 429.0-429.3, 429.8, 429.9 due to hypertension
  any condition classifiable to 429.0-429.3, 429.8, 429.9 due to hypertension

DEFINITION Hypertensive heart disease refers to heart disease caused by high blood pressure, especially localised high blood pressure.

ALERT! Heart conditions (425.8, 429.0-429.3, 429.8, 429.9) are assigned to a code from category 402 when a causal relationship is stated (due to hypertension) or implied (hypertensive)

⑤ **402.0 Malignant**

402.00 Without heart failure

402.01 With heart failure

Add 4th or 5th digit	Nonspecific code	Unspecified code	Manifestation code	

⑤ **402.1 Benign**

    402.10   **Without heart failure**

    402.11   **With heart failure**

⑤ **402.9 Unspecified**

    402.90   **Without heart failure**

    402.91   **With heart failure**

⑤ **403** **Hypertensive chronic kidney disease**

The following fifth-digit subclassification is for use with category 403:

  0   **with chronic kidney disease stage I through stage IV, or unspecified**

    Use additional code to identify the stage of chronic kidney disease (585.1-585.4, 585.9)

  1   **with chronic kidney disease stage V or end stage renal disease**

    Use additional code to identify the stage of chronic kidney disease (585.5, 585.6)

Includes: arteriolar nephritis
            arteriosclerosis of:
              kidney
              renal arterioles
            arteriosclerotic nephritis (chronic) (interstitial)
            hypertensive:
              nephropathy
              renal failure
              uremia (chronic)
            nephrosclerosis
            renal sclerosis with hypertension
            any condition classifiable to 585 and 587 with any condition classifiable to 401

Excludes: *acute kidney failure (584.5-584.9)*
            renal disease stated as not due to hypertension
            renovascular hypertension (405.0-405.9 with fifth-digit 1)

DEFINITION Hypertensive chronic kidney disease, refers to diseases of the kidney caused by high blood pressure.

ALERT! The appropriate code from category 585, Chronic kidney disease, should be used as a secondary code with a code from category 403 to identify the stage of chronic kidney disease

⑤ **403.0 Malignant**
  [0-1]

⑤ **403.1 Benign**
  [0-1]

⑤ **403.9 Unspecified**
  [0-1]

⑤ **404** **Hypertensive heart and chronic kidney disease**

Use additional code to specify type of heart failure (428.0-428.43), if known

The following fifth-digit subclassification is for use with category 404:

  0   **without heart failure and with chronic kidney disease stage I through stage IV, or unspecified**

    Use additional code to identify the stage of chronic kidney disease (585.1-585.4, 585.9)

  1   **with heart failure and with chronic kidney disease stage I through stage IV, or unspecified**

    Use additional code to identify the stage of chronic kidney disease (585.1-585.4, 585.9)

  2   **without heart failure and with chronic kidney disease stage V or end stage renal disease**

    Use additional code to identify the stage of chronic kidney disease (585.5, 585.6)

  3   **with heart failure and chronic kidney disease stage V or end stage renal disease**

    Use additional code to identify the stage of chronic kidney disease (585.5-585.6)

Includes: disease:
           cardiornal
           cardiovascular renal
         any condition classifiable to 402 with any condition classifiable to 403

DEFINITION Hypertensive heart and chronic kidney disease, refers to diseases of the heart and kidneys cause by high blood pressure.

ALERT! The appropriate code from category 585, Chronic kidney disease, should be used as a secondary code with a code from category 404 to identify the stage of kidney disease

● Code new
to 2012 edition

▲ Revision of
existing code

④ ⑤ Fourth or fifth
digit required

[5] **404.0 Malignant**
[0-3]

[5] **404.1 Benign**
[0-3]

[5] **404.9 Unspecified**
[0-3]

405 Secondary hypertension

[DEFINITION] Secondary hypertension is a type of hypertension caused by an identifiable underlying secondary cause

[5] **405.0 Malignant**

405.01 Renovascular

405.09 Other

[5] **405.1 Benign**

405.11 Renovascular

405.19 Other

[5] **405.9 Unspecified**

405.91 Renovascular

405.99 Other

ISCHEMIC HEART DISEASE (410-414)

Includes: that with mention of hypertension

Use additional code, if desired, to identify presence of hypertension (401.0-405.9)

[DEFINITION] Ischemic heart disease is a condition caused by a reduced amount of blood supplying the heart muscle. It can be caused by cholesterol and other lipids building up on the inner walls of arteries that supply the heart, forming a thick plaque that can reduce the amount of blood carrying nutrients and oxygen to heart tissue.

[5] **410 Acute myocardial infarction**

ST elevation (STEMI) and non-ST elevation (NSTEMI) myocardial infarction

Includes: cardiac infarction
coronary (artery):
embolism
occlusion
rupture
thrombosis
infarction of heart, myocardium, or ventricle
rupture of heart, myocardium, or ventricle
any condition classifiable to 414.1-414.9 specified as acute or with a stated duration of 8 weeks or less

The following fifth-digit subclassification is for use with category 410:

0 episode of care unspecified
Use when the source document does not contain sufficient information for the assignment of fifth digit 1 or 2.

1 initial episode of care
Use fifth digit 1 to designate the first episode of care (regardless of facility site) for a newly diagnosed myocardial infarction. The fifth digit 1 is assigned regardless of the number of times a patient may be transferred during the initial episode of care

2 subsequent episode of care
Use fifth digit 2 to designate an episode of care following the initial episode when the patient is admitted for further observation, evaluation, or treatment for a myocardial infarction that has received initial treatment, but is still less than 8 weeks old.

[DEFINITION] Myocardial infarction, commonly known as a heart attack, occurs when the blood supply to part of the heart is interrupted causing some heart cells to die.

[5] **410.0 Of anterolateral wall**
[0-2] ST elevation myocardial infarction (STEMI) of anterolateral wall

[5] **410.1 Of other anterior wall**
[0-2] ST elevation myocardial infarction (STEMI) of other anterior wall
Infarction:
anterior (wall) NOS (with contiguous portion of intraventricular septum)
anteroapical (with contiguous portion of intraventricular septum)
anteroseptal (with contiguous portion of intraventricular septum)

[5] **410.2 Of inferolateral wall**
[0-2] ST elevation myocardial infarction (STEMI) of inferolateral wall

Add 4th or 5th digit | Nonspecific code | Unspecified code | Manifestation code

⑤ **410.3 Of inferoposterior wall**
[0-2]   ST elevation myocardial infarction (STEMI) of inferoposterior wall

⑤ **410.4 Of other inferior wall**
[0-2]   ST elevation myocardial infarction (STEMI) of other inferior wall
          Infarction:
              diaphragmatic wall NOS (with contiguous portion of intraventricular septum)
              inferior (wall) NOS (with contiguous portion of intraventricular septum)

⑤ **410.5 Of other lateral wall**
[0-2]   ST elevation myocardial infarction (STEMI) of other lateral wall
          Infarction: Infarction:
              apical-lateral   high lateral
              basal-lateral   posterolateral

⑤ **410.6 True posterior wall infarction**
[0-2]   ST elevation myocardial infarction (STEMI) of true posterior wall
          Infarction:
              posterobasal
              strictly posterior

⑤ **410.7 Subendocardial infarction**
[0-2]   Non-ST elevation myocardial infarction (NSTEMI)
          Nontransmural infarction

⑤ **410.8 Other specified sites**
[0-2]   ST elevation myocardial infarction (STEMI) of other specified sites
          Infarction of:
              atrium
              papillary muscle
              septum alone

⑤ **410.9 Unspecified site**
[0-2]   Acute myocardial infarction NOS
          Coronary occlusion NOS
          Myocardial infarction NOS
          ALERT! Subcategory 410.9 is the default for the unspecified term acute myocardial infarction.
          If only STEMI or transmural MI without the site is documented, query the provider as to the
          site, or assign a code from subcategory 410.9.

411 **Other acute and subacute forms of ischemic heart disease**
          DEFINITION Ischemic heart disease is caused by deposits of fat or plaque that occur in the
          walls of the coronary arteries.

     411.0 Postmyocardial infarction syndrome
              Dressler's syndrome

     411.1 Intermediate coronary syndrome
              Impending infarction   Preinfarction syndrome
              Preinfarction angina   Unstable angina

          Excludes: angina (pectoris) (413.9)
                          decubitus (413.0)

⑤ **411.8 Other**

          411.81 Acute coronary occlusion without myocardial infarction
                    Acute coronary (artery):
                        embolism without or not resulting in myocardial infarction
                        obstruction without or not resulting in myocardial infarction
                        occlusion without or not resulting in myocardial infarction
                        thrombosis without or not resulting in myocardial infarction

          Excludes: obstruction without infarction due to atherosclerosis (414.00-414.07)
                      occlusion without infarction due to atherosclerosis (414.00-414.07)

          411.89 Other
                    Coronary insufficiency (acute)
                    Subendocardial ischemia

412 **Old myocardial infarction**
          Healed myocardial infarction
          Past myocardial infarction diagnosed on ECG [EKG] or other special investigation, but
              currently presenting no symptoms
          DEFINITION Old myocardial infarction refers to an old occlusion or blockage of arteries
          supplying the muscles of the heart, resulting in injury or necrosis of the heart muscle.

413 **Angina pectoris**

● Code new   ▲ Revision of   ④ ⑤ Fourth or fifth
          to 2012 edition   existing code   digit required

[DEFINITION] Angina pectoris, commonly known as angina, is severe chest pain due to ischemia (a lack of blood and hence oxygen supply) of the heart muscle

413.0 Angina decubitus
Nocturnal angina

413.1 Prinzmetal angina
Variant angina pectoris

413.9 Other and unspecified angina pectoris

Angina:	Anginal syndrome
equivalent	Status anginosus
NOS	Stenocardia
cardiac	Syncope anginosa
of effort	

Use additional code(s) for symptoms associated with angina equivalent

[Excludes:] *preinfarction angina (411.1)*

414 Other forms of chronic ischemic heart disease

[Excludes:] *arteriosclerotic cardiovascular disease [ASCVD] (429.2)*
cardiovascular:
arteriosclerosis or sclerosis (429.2)
degeneration or disease (429.2)

[DEFINITION] Ischemic heart disease is a disease characterized by reduced blood supply to the heart muscle, usually due to coronary artery disease (atherosclerosis of the coronary arteries).

[5] **414.0 Coronary atherosclerosis**
Arteriosclerotic heart disease [ASHD]
Atherosclerotic heart disease
Coronary (artery):
arteriosclerosis
arteritis or endarteritis
atheroma
sclerosis
stricture

Use additional code, if applicable, to identify chronic total occlusion of coronary artery (414.2)

[Excludes:] *embolism of graft (996.72)*
occlusion NOS of graft (996.72)
thrombus of graft (996.72)

414.00 Of unspecified type of vessel, native or graft

414.01 Of native coronary artery

414.02 Of autologous vein bypass graft

414.03 Of nonautologous biological bypass graft

414.04 Of artery bypass graft
Internal mammary artery

414.05 Of unspecified type of bypass graft
Bypass graft NOS

414.06 Of native coronary artery of transplanted heart

414.07 Of bypass graft (artery) (vein) of transplanted heart

[5] **414.1 Aneurysm and dissection of heart**

414.10 Aneurysm of heart (wall)
Aneurysm (arteriovenous):
mural
ventricular

414.11 Aneurysm of coronary vessels
Aneurysm (arteriovenous) of coronary vessels

414.12 Dissection of coronary artery

414.19 Other aneurysm of heart
Arteriovenous fistula, acquired, of heart

414.2 Chronic total occlusion of coronary artery
Complete occlusion of coronary artery
Total occlusion of coronary artery

Code first coronary atherosclerosis (414.00-414.07)

[Excludes:] *acute coronary occlusion with myocardial infarction (410.00-410.92)*
acute coronary occlusion without myocardial infarction (411.81)

414.3 Coronary atherosclerosis due to lipid rich plaque

Code first coronary atherosclerosis (414.00-414.07)

● **414.4　Coronary atherosclerosis due to calcified coronary lesion**
　　　Coronary atherosclerosis due to severely calcified coronary lesion

Code first coronary atherosclerosis (414.00-414.07)

414.8　Other specified forms of chronic ischemic heart disease
　　　Chronic coronary insufficiency
　　　Ischemia, myocardial (chronic)
　　　Any condition classifiable to 410 specified as chronic, or presenting with symptoms
　　　　after 8 weeks from date of infarction

Excludes: *coronary insufficiency (acute) (411.89)*

414.9　Chronic ischemic heart disease, unspecified
　　　Ischemic heart disease NOS

DISEASES OF PULMONARY CIRCULATION (415-417)

415 **Acute pulmonary heart disease**
　　　DEFINITION Pulmonary heart disease is the enlargement and eventual failure of the right
　　　ventricle of the heart due to disorders of the lungs or their blood vessels or chest wall
　　　abnormalities.

415.0　Acute cor pulmonale

Excludes: *cor pulmonale NOS (416.9)*

⑤　**415.1　Pulmonary embolism and infarction**
　　　Pulmonary (artery) (vein):
　　　　apoplexy
　　　　embolism
　　　　infarction (hemorrhagic)
　　　　thrombosis

Excludes: *chronic pulmonary embolism (416.2)*
　　　　　personal history of pulmonary embolism (V12.55)
　　　　　that complicating:
　　　　　　abortion (634-638 with .6, 639.6)
　　　　　　ectopic or molar pregnancy (639.6)
　　　　　　pregnancy, childbirth, or the puerperium (673.0-673.8)

415.11　Iatrogenic pulmonary embolism and infarction
Use additional code for associated septic pulmonary embolism, if applicable, 415.12

415.12　Septic pulmonary embolism
　　　Septic embolism NOS

Code first underlying infection, such as:
　　septicemia (038.0-038.9)

Excludes: *septic arterial embolism (449)*

● **415.13　Saddle embolus of pulmonary artery**
415.19 **Other**

416 **Chronic pulmonary heart disease**

416.0　Primary pulmonary hypertension
　　　Idiopathic pulmonary arteriosclerosis
　　　Pulmonary hypertension (essential) (idiopathic) (primary)

Excludes: *pulmonary hypertension NOS (416.8)*
　　　　　secondary pulmonary hypertension (416.8)

416.1　Kyphoscoliotic heart disease

416.2　Chronic pulmonary embolism
Use additional code, if applicable, for associated long-term (current) use of anticoagulants
　　(V58.61)

Excludes: *personal history of pulmonary embolism (V12.55)*

416.8 **Other chronic pulmonary heart diseases**
　　　Pulmonary hypertension NOS
　　　Pulmonary hypertension, secondary

416.9　Chronic pulmonary heart disease, unspecified
　　　Chronic cardiopulmonary disease
　　　Cor pulmonale (chronic) NOS

417 **Other diseases of pulmonary circulation**
　　　DEFINITION Pulmonary circulation is the circulation of blood through the lungs for the
　　　purpose of oxygenation and the release of carbon dioxide. Also known as lesser circulation.

　● Code new　　　▲ Revision of　　　④ ⑤ Fourth or fifth
　　　to 2012 edition　　existing code　　　　digit required

417.0 Arteriovenous fistula of pulmonary vessels

[Excludes:] *congenital arteriovenous fistula (747.32)*

417.1 Aneurysm of pulmonary artery

[Excludes:] *congenital aneurysm (747.39)*
congenital arteriovenous aneurysm (747.32)

417.8 Other specified diseases of pulmonary circulation

Pulmonary:
  arteritis
  endarteritis
Rupture of pulmonary vessel
Stricture of pulmonary vessel

417.9 Unspecified disease of pulmonary circulation

OTHER FORMS OF HEART DISEASE (420-429)

420 Acute pericarditis

Includes: acute:
  mediastinopericarditis
  myopericarditis
  pericardial effusion
  pleuropericarditis
  pneumopericarditis

[Excludes:] *acute rheumatic pericarditis (391.0)*
postmyocardial infarction syndrome [Dressler's] (411.0)

DEFINITION Pericarditis is an inflammation of the two layers of the thin, sac-like membrane that surrounds the heart.

420.0 Acute pericarditis in diseases classified elsewhere

Code first underlying disease, as:
  actinomycosis (039.8)
  amebiasis (006.8)
  chronic uremia (585.9)
  nocardiosis (039.8)
  tuberculosis (017.9)
  uremia NOS (586)

[Excludes:] *pericarditis (acute) (in):*
  Coxsackie (virus) (074.21)
  gonococcal (098.83)
  histoplasmosis (115.0-115.9 with fifth-digit 3)
  meningococcal infection (036.41)
  syphilitic (093.81)

[5] **420.9 Other and unspecified acute pericarditis**

420.90 Acute pericarditis, unspecified

Pericarditis (acute):
  NOS
  infective NOS
  sicca

420.91 Acute idiopathic pericarditis

Pericarditis, acute:
  benign
  nonspecific
  viral

420.99 Other

Pericarditis (acute):
  pneumococcal
  purulent
  staphylococcal
Pericarditis (acute):
  streptococcal
  suppurative
Pneumopyopericardium
Pyopericardium

[Excludes:] *pericarditis in diseases classified elsewhere (420.0)*

421 Acute and subacute endocarditis

DEFINITION Endocarditis is an infection of the lining of the heart chambers and heart valves that is caused by bacteria, fungi, or other infectious substances.

Add 4th or 5th digit | Nonspecific code | Unspecified code | Manifestation code

421.0 Acute and subacute bacterial endocarditis

Endocarditis (acute)
(chronic) (subacute):
  bacterial
  infective NOS
  lenta
  malignant
  purulent

Endocarditis (acute) (chronic) (subacute):
  septic
  ulcerative
  vegetative
Infective aneurysm
Subacute bacterial endocarditis [SBE]

Use additional code, if desired, to identify infectious organism [e.g., Streptococcus 041.0, Staphylococcus 041.1]

421.1 *Acute and subacute infective endocarditis in diseases classified elsewhere*

Code first underlying disease, as:
  blastomycosis (116.0)
  Q fever (083.0)
  typhoid (fever) (002.0)

Excludes: *endocarditis (in):*
     Coxsackie (virus) (074.22)
     gonococcal (098.84)
     histoplasmosis (115.0-115.9 with fifth-digit 4)
     meningococcal infection (036.42)
     monilial (112.81)

421.9 Acute endocarditis, unspecified

Endocarditis, acute or subacute
Myoendocarditis, acute or subacute
Periendocarditis, acute or subacute

Excludes: *acute rheumatic endocarditis (391.1)*

422 Acute myocarditis

Excludes: *acute rheumatic myocarditis (391.2)*

DEFINITION Myocarditis is inflammation of the myocardium, the muscular tissue of the heart.

422.0 *Acute myocarditis in diseases classified elsewhere*

Code first underlying disease, as:
  myocarditis (acute):
    influenzal (487.8, 488.09, 488.19)
    tuberculous (017.9)

Excludes: *myocarditis (acute) (due to):*
     aseptic, of newborn (074.23)
     Coxsackie (virus) (074.23)
     diphtheritic (032.82)
     meningococcal infection (036.43)
     syphilitic (093.82)
     toxoplasmosis (130.3)

⑤ 422.9 Other and unspecified acute myocarditis

422.90 Acute myocarditis, unspecified
Acute or subacute (interstitial) myocarditis

422.91 Idiopathic myocarditis
Myocarditis (acute or subacute):
  Fiedler's
  giant cell
  isolated (diffuse) (granulomatous)
  nonspecific granulomatous

422.92 Septic myocarditis
Myocarditis, acute or subacute:
  pneumococcal
  staphylococcal

Use additional code, if desired, to identify infectious organism [e.g., Staphylococcus 041.1]

Excludes: *myocarditis, acute or subacute:*
    in bacterial diseases classified elsewhere (422.0)
    streptococcal (391.2)

422.93 Toxic myocarditis

422.99 Other

● Code new
to 2012 edition

▲ Revision of
existing code

④ ⑤ Fourth or fifth
digit required

423 Other diseases of pericardium

[Excludes:] *that specified as rheumatic (393)*

[DEFINITION] The pericardium is a double-walled sac that contains the heart and the roots of the great vessels

423.0 Hemopericardium

423.1 Adhesive pericarditis

Adherent pericardium
Fibrosis of pericardium
Milk spots
Pericarditis:
  adhesive
  obliterative
Soldiers' patches

423.2 Constrictive pericarditis

Concato's disease
Pick's disease of heart (and liver)

423.3 Cardiac tamponade

Code first the underlying cause

423.8 Other specified diseases of pericardium

Calcification of pericardium
Fistula of pericardium

423.9 Unspecified disease of pericardium

424 Other diseases of endocardium

[Excludes:] *bacterial endocarditis (421.0-421.9)*
rheumatic endocarditis (391.1, 394.0-397.9)
syphilitic endocarditis (093.20-093.24)

[DEFINITION] The endocardium is the membrane that lines the cavities of the heart and forms part of the heart valves .

424.0 Mitral valve disorders

Mitral (valve):
  incompetence NOS of specified cause, except rheumatic
  insufficiency NOS of specified cause, except rheumatic
  regurgitation NOS of specified cause, except rheumatic

[Excludes:] *mitral (valve):*
  disease (394.9)
  failure (394.9)
  stenosis (394.0)
the listed conditions:
  specified as rheumatic (394.1)
  unspecified as to cause but with mention of:
    diseases of aortic valve (396.0-396.9)
    mitral stenosis or obstruction (394.2)

424.1 Aortic valve disorders

Aortic (valve):
  incompetence NOS of specified cause, except rheumatic
  insufficiency NOS of specified cause, except rheumatic
  regurgitation NOS of specified cause, except rheumatic
  stenosis NOS of specified cause, except rheumatic

[Excludes:] *hypertrophic subaortic stenosis (425.11)*
that specified as rheumatic (395.0-395.9)
that of unspecified cause but with mention of diseases of mitral valve (396.0-396.9)

424.2 Tricuspid valve disorders, specified as nonrheumatic

Tricuspid valve:
  incompetence of specified cause, except rheumatic
  insufficiency of specified cause, except rheumatic
  regurgitation of specified cause, except rheumatic
  stenosis of specified cause, except rheumatic

[Excludes:] *rheumatic or of unspecified cause (397.0)*

424.3 Pulmonary valve disorders

Pulmonic:
  incompetence NOS
  insufficiency NOS
Pulmonic:
  regurgitation NOS
  stenosis NOS

[Excludes:] *that specified as rheumatic (397.1)*

[5] **424.9 Endocarditis, valve unspecified**

424.90 Endocarditis, valve unspecified, unspecified cause
Endocarditis (chronic):
NOS
nonbacterial thrombotic
Valvular:
incompetence of unspecified valve, unspecified cause
insufficiency of unspecified valve, unspecified cause
regurgitation of unspecified valve, unspecified cause
stenosis of unspecified valve, unspecified cause
Valvulitis (chronic)

424.91 Endocarditis in diseases classified elsewhere
Code first underlying disease, as:
atypical verrucous endocarditis [Libman-Sacks] (710.0)
disseminated lupus erythematosus (710.0)
tuberculosis (017.9)

Excludes: *syphilitic (093.20-093.24)*

424.99 Other
Any condition classifiable to 424.90 with specified cause, except rheumatic

Excludes: *endocardial fibroelastosis (425.3)*
that specified as rheumatic (397.9)

425 Cardiomyopathy
Includes: myocardiopathy
DEFINITION Cardiomyopathy is a weakening of the heart muscle or a change in heart muscle structure. It is often associated with inadequate heart pumping or other heart function problems.

425.0 Endomyocardial fibrosis

▲ **425.1 Hypertrophic cardiomyopathy**

Excludes: *ventricular hypertrophy (429.3)*

● **425.11   Hypertrophic obstructive cardiomyopathy**
Hypertrophic subaortic stenosis (idiopathic)

● **425.18   Other hypertrophic cardiomyopathy**
Nonobstructive hypertrophic cardiomyopathy

425.2 Obscure cardiomyopathy of Africa
Becker's disease
Idiopathic mural endomyocardial disease

425.3 Endocardial fibroelastosis
Elastomyofibrosis

425.4 Other primary cardiomyopathies

Cardiomyopathy:	Cardiomyopathy:
NOS	idiopathic
congestive	obstructive
constrictive	restrictive
familial	Cardiovascular collagenosis

425.5 Alcoholic cardiomyopathy

425.7 Nutritional and metabolic cardiomyopathy
Code first underlying disease, as:
amyloidosis (277.30-277.39)
beriberi (265.0)
cardiac glycogenosis (271.0)
mucopolysaccharidosis (277.5)
thyrotoxicosis (242.0-242.9)

Excludes: *gouty tophi of heart (274.82)*

425.8 Cardiomyopathy in other diseases classified elsewhere
Code first underlying disease, as:
Friedreich's ataxia (334.0)
myotonia atrophica (359.21)
progressive muscular dystrophy (359.1)
sarcoidosis (135)

Excludes: *cardiomyopathy in Chagas' disease (086.0)*

425.9 Secondary cardiomyopathy, unspecified

● Code new
to 2012 edition
▲ Revision of
existing code
④ ⑤ Fourth or fifth
digit required

426 Conduction disorders

[DEFINITION] Conduction disorders refers to interference with the normal electrical conduction in the heart

426.0 Atrioventricular block, complete
Third degree atrioventricular block

[5] **426.1 Atrioventricular block, other and unspecified**

426.10 Atrioventricular block, unspecified
Atrioventricular [AV] block (incomplete) (partial)

426.11 First degree atrioventricular block
Incomplete atrioventricular block, first degree
Prolonged P-R interval NOS

426.12 Mobitz (type) II atrioventricular block
Incomplete atrioventricular block:
Mobitz (type) II
second degree, Mobitz (type) II

426.13 Other second degree atrioventricular block
Incomplete atrioventricular block:
Mobitz (type) I [Wenckebach's]
second degree:
NOS
Mobitz (type) I
with 2:1 atrioventricular response [block]
Wenckebach's phenomenon

426.2 Left bundle branch hemiblock
Block:
left anterior fascicular
left posterior fascicular

426.3 Other left bundle branch block
Left bundle branch block:
NOS
anterior fascicular with posterior fascicular
complete
main stem

426.4 Right bundle branch block

[5] **426.5 Bundle branch block, other and unspecified**

426.50 Bundle branch block, unspecified

426.51 Right bundle branch block and left posterior fascicular block

426.52 Right bundle branch block and left anterior fascicular block

426.53 Other bilateral bundle branch block
Bifascicular block NOS
Bilateral bundle branch block NOS
Right bundle branch with left bundle branch block (incomplete) (main stem)

426.54 Trifascicular block

426.6 Other heart block
Intraventricular block:
NOS
diffuse
myofibrillar
Sinoatrial block
Sinoauricular block

426.7 Anomalous atrioventricular excitation
Atrioventricular conduction:
accelerated
accessory
pre-excitation
Ventricular pre-excitation
Wolff-Parkinson-White syndrome

[5] **426.8 Other specified conduction disorders**

426.81 Lown-Ganong-Levine syndrome
Syndrome of short P-R interval, normal QRS complexes, and supraventricular tachycardias

426.82 Long QT syndrome

426.89 Other
Dissociation:
atrioventricular [AV]
interference
isorhythmic
Nonparoxysmal AV nodal tachycardia

426.9 Conduction disorder, unspecified
Heart block NOS
Stokes-Adams syndrome

427 Cardiac dysrhythmias

[Excludes:] *that complicating:*
abortion (634-638 with .7, 639.8)
ectopic or molar pregnancy (639.8)
labor or delivery (668.1, 669.4)

[DEFINITION] Cardiac dysrhythmias is a term for any of a large and heterogeneous group of conditions in which there is abnormal electrical activity in the heart. The heart beat may be too fast or too slow, and may be regular or irregular.

427.0 Paroxysmal supraventricular tachycardia
Paroxysmal tachycardia:
atrial [PAT]
atrioventricular [AV]
junctional
nodal

427.1 Paroxysmal ventricular tachycardia
Ventricular tachycardia (paroxysmal)

427.2 Paroxysmal tachycardia, unspecified
Bouveret-Hoffmann syndrome
Paroxysmal tachycardia:
NOS
essential

[5] **427.3 Atrial fibrillation and flutter**

427.31 Atrial fibrillation

427.32 Atrial flutter

[5] **427.4 Ventricular fibrillation and flutter**

427.41 Ventricular fibrillation

427.42 Ventricular flutter

427.5 Cardiac arrest
Cardiorespiratory arrest

[ALERT!] For personal history of sudden cardiac arrest see V12.53

[5] **427.6 Premature beats**

427.60 Premature beats, unspecified
Ectopic beats
Extrasystoles
Extrasystolic arrhythmia
Premature contractions or systoles NOS

427.61 Supraventricular premature beats
Atrial premature beats, contractions, or systoles

427.69 Other
Ventricular premature beats, contractions, or systoles

[5] **427.8 Other specified cardiac dysrhythmias**

427.81 Sinoatrial node dysfunction
Sinus bradycardia:
persistent
severe
Syndrome:
sick sinus
tachycardia-bradycardia

[Excludes:] *sinus bradycardia NOS (427.89)*

427.89 Other

Rhythm disorder:
  coronary sinus
  ectopic

Rhythm disorder:
  nodal

Wandering (atrial) pacemaker

[Excludes:] *carotid sinus syncope (337.0)*
neonatal bradycardia (779.81)
neonatal tachycardia (779.82)
reflex bradycardia (337.0)
tachycardia (785.0)

427.9 Cardiac dysrhythmia, unspecified

Arrhythmia (cardiac) NOS

428 Heart failure

Code, if applicable, heart failure due to hypertension first (402.0-402.9, with fifth-digit 1 or 404.0-404.9 with fifth digit 1 or 3)

[Excludes:] *following cardiac surgery (429.4)*
rheumatic (398.91)
that complicating:
  abortion (634-638 with .7, 639.8)
  ectopic or molar pregnancy (639.8)
  labor or delivery (668.1, 669.4)

[DEFINITION] Heart failure is a condition where there is ineffective pumping of the heart leading to an accumulation of fluid in the lungs. Typical symptoms include shortness of breath with exertion, difficulty breathing when lying flat and leg or ankle swelling

428.0 Congestive heart failure, unspecified

Congestive heart disease
Right heart failure (secondary to left heart failure)

[Excludes:] *fluid overload NOS (276.69)*

428.1 Left heart failure

Acute edema of lung with heart disease NOS or heart failure
Acute pulmonary edema with heart disease NOS or heart failure
Cardiac asthma
Left ventricular failure

[5] **428.2 Systolic heart failure**

[Excludes:] *combined systolic and diastolic heart failure (428.40-428.43)*

428.20 Unspecified

428.21 Acute

428.22 Chronic

428.23 Acute on chronic

[5] **428.3 Diastolic heart failure**

[Excludes:] *combined systolic and diastolic heart failure (428.40-428.43)*

428.30 Unspecified

428.31 Acute

428.32 Chronic

428.33 Acute on chronic

[5] **428.4 Combined systolic and diastolic heart failure**

428.40 Unspecified

428.41 Acute

428.42 Chronic

428.43 Acute on chronic

428.9 Heart failure, unspecified

Cardiac failure NOS
Heart failure NOS
Myocardial failure NOS
Weak heart

429 Ill-defined descriptions and complications of heart disease

429.0 Myocarditis, unspecified
Myocarditis:
NOS (with mention of arteriosclerosis)
chronic (interstitial) (with mention of arteriosclerosis)
fibroid (with mention of arteriosclerosis)
senile (with mention of arteriosclerosis)
Use additional code, if desired, to identify presence of arteriosclerosis
[*Excludes:*] *acute or subacute (422.0-422.9)*
rheumatic (398.0)
acute (391.2)
that due to hypertension (402.0-402.9)

DEFINITION Myocarditis is inflammation of the heart muscle (myocardium) that usually occurs as a complication of underlying illness.

429.1 Myocardial degeneration
Degeneration of heart or myocardium:
fatty (with mention of arteriosclerosis)
mural (with mention of arteriosclerosis)
muscular (with mention of arteriosclerosis)
Myocardial:
degeneration (with mention of arteriosclerosis)
disease (with mention of arteriosclerosis)
Use additional code, if desired, to identify presence of arteriosclerosis
[*Excludes:*] *that due to hypertension (402.0-402.9)*

429.2 Cardiovascular disease, unspecified
Arteriosclerotic cardiovascular disease [ASCVD]
Cardiovascular arteriosclerosis
Cardiovascular:
degeneration (with mention of arteriosclerosis)
disease (with mention of arteriosclerosis)
sclerosis (with mention of arteriosclerosis)
Use additional code, if desired, to identify presence of arteriosclerosis
[*Excludes:*] *that due to hypertension (402.0-402.9)*

429.3 Cardiomegaly
Cardiac:
dilatation
hypertrophy
Ventricular dilatation
[*Excludes:*] *that due to hypertension (402.0-402.9)*

DEFINITION Cardiomegaly is an abnormal enlargement of the heart.

429.4 Functional disturbances following cardiac surgery
Cardiac insufficiency following cardiac surgery or due to prosthesis
Heart failure following cardiac surgery or due to prosthesis
Postcardiotomy syndrome
Postvalvulotomy syndrome
[*Excludes:*] *cardiac failure in the immediate postoperative period (997.1)*

429.5 Rupture of chordae tendineae

429.6 Rupture of papillary muscle

[5] **429.7 Certain sequelae of myocardial infarction, not elsewhere classified**
Use additional code to identify the associated myocardial infarction:
with onset of 8 weeks or less (410.00-410.92)
with onset of more than 8 weeks (414.8)
[*Excludes:*] *congenital defects of heart (745, 746)*
coronary aneurysm (414.11)
disorders of papillary muscle (429.6, 429.81)
postmyocardial infarction syndrome (411.0)
rupture of chordae tendineae (429.5)

429.71 Acquired cardiac septal defect
[*Excludes:*] *acute septal infarction (410.00-410.92)*

429.79 Other
Mural thrombus (atrial) (ventricular), acquired, following myocardial infarction

[5] **429.8 Other ill-defined heart diseases**

429.81 **Other disorders of papillary muscle**

Papillary muscle:
atrophy
degeneration
dysfunction

Papillary muscle:
incompetence
incoordination
scarring

429.82 **Hyperkinetic heart disease**

429.83 **Takotsubo syndrome**
Broken heart syndrome
Reversible left ventricular dysfunction following sudden emotional stress
Stress induced cardiomyopathy
Transient left ventricular apical ballooning syndrome

429.89 **Other**
Carditis

Excludes: *that due to hypertension (402.0-402.9)*

429.9 **Heart disease, unspecified**
Heart disease (organic) NOS
Morbus cordis NOS

Excludes: *that due to hypertension (402.0-402.9)*

CEREBROVASCULAR DISEASE (430-438)

Includes: with mention of hypertension (conditions classifiable to 401-405)

Use additional code, if desired, to identify presence of hypertension

Excludes: *any condition classifiable to 430-434, 436, 437 occurring during pregnancy,*
childbirth, or the puerperium, or specified as puerperal (674.0)
iatrogenic cerebrovascular infarction or hemorrhage (997.02)

DEFINITION Cerebrovascular disease is a disease of the blood vessels, especially the arteries that supply the brain.

430 **Subarachnoid hemorrhage**
Meningeal hemorrhage
Ruptured:
berry aneurysm
(congenital) cerebral aneurysm NOS

Excludes: *berry aneurysm, nonruptured (437.3)*
syphilitic ruptured cerebral aneurysm (094.87)

DEFINITION Subarachnoid hemorrhage refers to bleeding within the head into the space between two membranes that surround the brain.

ALERT! For coding late effects of cerebrovascular disease see 438

ALERT! For coding late effects of cerebrovascular disease, dysarthria see 438.13

ALERT! For coding late effects of cerebrovascular disease, fluency disorder see 438.14

431 **Intracerebral hemorrhage**

Hemorrhage (of):
basilar
bulbar
cerebellar
cerebral
cerebromeningeal
cortical
internal capsule

Hemorrhage (of):
intrapontine
pontine
subcortical
ventricular
Rupture of blood vessel in brain

DEFINITION Intracerebral hemorrhage is a medical condition indicated by the rupturing of a blood vessel in the brain and the subsequent bleeding into the tissues of the brain.

432 **Other and unspecified intracranial hemorrhage**
DEFINITION Intracranial hemorrhage is bleeding in the brain caused by the breaking (rupture) of a blood vessel in the head.

432.0 **Nontraumatic extradural hemorrhage**
Nontraumatic epidural hemorrhage

432.1 **Subdural hemorrhage**
Subdural hematoma, nontraumatic

432.9 **Unspecified intracranial hemorrhage**
Intracranial hemorrhage NOS

| | Add 4th or 5th digit | | Nonspecific code | | Unspecified code | | Manifestation code |

⑤ `433` **Occlusion and stenosis of precerebral arteries**

Use additional code, if applicable, to identify status post administration of tPA (rtPA) in a different facility within the last 24 hours prior to admission to current facility (V45.88)

The following fifth-digit subclassification is for use with category 433:

0   without mention of cerebral infarction

1   with cerebral infarction

Includes: embolism of basilar, carotid, and vertebral arteries
narrowing of basilar, carotid, and vertebral arteries
obstruction of basilar, carotid, and vertebral arteries
thrombosis of basilar, carotid, and vertebral arteries

Excludes: *insufficiency NOS of precerebral arteries (435.0-435.9)*

⑤ **433.0 Basilar artery**
[0-1]

⑤ **433.1 Carotid artery**
[0-1]

⑤ **433.2 Vertebral artery**
[0-1]

⑤ **433.3 Multiple and bilateral**
[0-1]

⑤ **433.8 Other specified precerebral artery**
[0-1]

⑤ **433.9 Unspecified precerebral artery**
[0-1]   Precerebral artery NOS

⑤ `434` **Occlusion of cerebral arteries**

Use additional code, if applicable, to identify status post administration of tPA (rtPA) in a different facility within the last 24 hours prior to admission to current facility (V45.88)

The following fifth-digit subclassification is for use with category 434:

0   without mention of cerebral infarction

1   with cerebral infarction

DEFINITION Occlusion of cerebral arteries, refers to any of the arteries supplying blood to the cerebral cortex.

⑤ **434.0 Cerebral thrombosis**
[0-1]   Thrombosis of cerebral arteries

⑤ **434.1 Cerebral embolism**
[0-1]

⑤ **434.9 Cerebral artery occlusion, unspecified**
[0-1]

ALERT! The terms stroke and CVA are often used interchangeably to refer to a cerebral infarction. The terms stroke, CVA, and cerebral infarction NOS are all indexed to the default code 434.91

`435` **Transient cerebral ischemia**

Includes: cerebrovascular insufficiency (acute) with transient focal neurological signs and symptoms
insufficiency of basilar, carotid, and vertebral arteries
spasm of cerebral arteries

Excludes: *acute cerebrovascular insufficiency NOS (437.1)*
that due to any condition classifiable to 433 (433.0-433.9)

DEFINITION Transient cerebral ischemia is the reduction or loss of oxygen to the cerebrum; prolonged ischemia may lead to cerebral infarction

ALERT! For personal history of transient ischemic attack (tia), and cerebral infarction without residual deficits see V12.54

435.0 Basilar artery syndrome

435.1 Vertebral artery syndrome

435.2 Subclavian steal syndrome

435.3 Vertebrobasilar artery syndrome

435.8 Other specified transient cerebral ischemias

435.9 Unspecified transient cerebral ischemia
Impending cerebrovascular accident
Intermittent cerebral ischemia
Transient ischemic attack [TIA]

● Code new   ▲ Revision of   ④ ⑤ Fourth or fifth
    to 2012 edition   existing code   digit required

436 Acute, but ill-defined, cerebrovascular disease

Apoplexy, apoplectic:
NOS
attack
cerebral
seizure
Cerebral seizure

[Excludes:] *any condition classifiable to categories 430-435*
cerebrovascular accident (434.91)
CVA (ischemic) (434.91)
embolic (434.11)
hemorrhagic (430, 431, 432.0-432.9)
thrombotic (434.01)
postoperative cerebrovascular accident (997.02)
stroke (ischemic) (434.91)
embolic (434.11)
hemorrhagic (430, 431, 432.0-432.9)
thrombotic (434.01)

DEFINITION Cerebrovascular disease is a disease of the blood vessels, especially, the arteries that supply the brain. Cerebrovascular disease is usually caused by atherosclerosis and can lead to a stroke.

ALERT! Code 436 should not be used when the documentation states stroke or CVA

ALERT! Code 436 should not be used as a secondary code with code 997.02.

437 Other and ill-defined cerebrovascular disease

437.0 Cerebral atherosclerosis
Atheroma of cerebral arteries
Cerebral arteriosclerosis

437.1 Other generalized ischemic cerebrovascular disease
Acute cerebrovascular insufficiency NOS
Cerebral ischemia (chronic)

437.2 Hypertensive encephalopathy

437.3 Cerebral aneurysm, nonruptured
Internal carotid artery, intracranial portion
Internal carotid artery NOS

[Excludes:] *congenital cerebral aneurysm, nonruptured (747.81)*
internal carotid artery, extracranial portion (442.81)

437.4 Cerebral arteritis

437.5 Moyamoya disease

437.6 Nonpyogenic thrombosis of intracranial venous sinus

[Excludes:] *pyogenic (325)*

437.7 Transient global amnesia

437.8 Other

437.9 Unspecified
Cerebrovascular disease or lesion NOS

438 Late effects of cerebrovascular disease

Note: This category is to be used to indicate conditions in 430-437 as the cause of late effects. The "late effects" include conditions specified as such, as sequelae, which may occur at any time after the onset of the causal condition.

[Excludes:] *personal history of:*
cerebral infarction without residual deficits (V12.54)
PRIND (Prolonged reversible ischemic neurologic deficit) (V12.54)
RIND (Reversible ischemic neurological deficit) (V12.54)
transient ischemic attack (TIA) (V12.54)

DEFINITION Late effects of cerebrovascular disease refers to a condition that appears after the acute phase of cerebral vascular disease has run its course

ALERT! Category 438 is used to indicate conditions classifiable to categories 430-437 as the causes of late effects (neurologic deficits), themselves classified elsewhere. These "late effects" include neurologic deficits that persist after initial onset of conditions classifiable to 430-437.

438.0 Cognitive deficits

[5] **438.1 Speech and language deficits**

438.10 Speech and language deficit, unspecified

Add 4th or 5th digit | Nonspecific code | Unspecified code | Manifestation code

438.11 **Aphasia**

438.12 **Dysphasia**

438.13 **Dysarthria**

438.14 **Fluency disorder**
Stuttering due to late effect of cerebrovascular accident

438.19 **Other speech and language deficits**

⑤ 438.2 **Hemiplegia/hemiparesis**

438.20 **Hemiplegia affecting unspecified side**

438.21 **Hemiplegia affecting dominant side**

438.22 **Hemiplegia affecting nondominant side**

⑤ 438.3 **Monoplegia of upper limb**

438.30 **Monoplegia of upper limb affecting unspecified side**

438.31 **Monoplegia of upper limb affecting dominant side**

438.32 **Monoplegia of upper limb affecting nondominant side**

⑤ 438.4 **Monoplegia of lower limb**

438.40 **Monoplegia of lower limb affecting unspecified side**

438.41 **Monoplegia of lower limb affecting dominant side**

438.42 **Monoplegia of lower limb affecting nondominant side**

⑤ 438.5 **Other paralytic syndrome**
Use additional code to identify type of paralytic syndrome, such as:
locked-in state (344.81)
quadriplegia (344.00-344.09)

Excludes: *late effects of cerebrovascular accident with:*
hemiplegia/hemiparesis (438.20-438.22)
monoplegia of lower limb (438.40-438.42)
monoplegia of upper limb (438.30-438.32)

438.50 **Other paralytic syndrome affecting unspecified side**

438.51 **Other paralytic syndrome affecting dominant side**

438.52 **Other paralytic syndrome affecting nondominant side**

438.53 **Other paralytic syndrome, bilateral**

438.6 **Alterations of sensations**
Use additional code to identify the altered sensation

438.7 **Disturbances of vision**
Use additional code to identify the visual disturbance

⑤ 438.8 **Other late effects of cerebrovascular disease**

438.81 **Apraxia**

438.82 **Dysphagia**
Use additional code to identify the type of dysphagia, if known (787.20-787.29)

438.83 **Facial weakness**
Facial droop

438.84 **Ataxia**

438.85 **Vertigo**

438.89 **Other late effects of cerebrovascular disease**
Use additional code to identify the late effect

438.9 **Unspecified late effects of cerebrovascular disease**

● Code new
to 2012 edition   ▲ Revision of
existing code   ④ ⑤ Fourth or fifth
digit required

DISEASES OF ARTERIES, ARTERIOLES, AND CAPILLARIES (440-449)

440 Atherosclerosis

Includes: arteriolosclerosis
arteriosclerosis (obliterans) (senile)
arteriosclerotic vascular disease
atheroma
degeneration:
arterial
arteriovascular
vascular
endarteritis deformans or obliterans
senile arteritis
senile endarteritis

[Excludes:] *atheroembolism (445.01-445.89)*
atherosclerosis of bypass graft of the extremities (440.30-440.32)

[DEFINITION] Atherosclerosis is a condition in which an artery wall thickens as the result of a build up of fatty materials such as cholesterol. It is a syndrome affecting arterial blood vessels.

440.0 Of aorta

440.1 Of renal artery

[Excludes:] *atherosclerosis of renal arterioles (403.00-403.91)*

[5] **440.2 Of native arteries of the extremities**

Use additional code, if applicable, to identify chronic total occlusion of artery of the extremities (440.4)

[Excludes:] *atherosclerosis of bypass graft of the extremities (440.30-440.32)*

440.20 Atherosclerosis of the extremities, unspecified

440.21 Atherosclerosis of the extremities with intermittent claudication

440.22 Atherosclerosis of the extremities with rest pain
Any condition classifiable to 440.21

440.23 Atherosclerosis of the extremities with ulceration
Any condition classifiable to 440.21 and 440.22

Use additional code for any associated ulceration (707.10-707.19, 707.8, 707.9)

440.24 Atherosclerosis of the extremities with gangrene
Any condition classifiable to 440.21, 440.22, and 440.23 with ischemic gangrene 785.4

Use additional code for any associated ulceration (707.10-707.19, 707.8, 707.9)

[Excludes:] *gas gangrene 040.0*

440.29 Other

[5] **440.3 Of bypass graft of the extremities**

[Excludes:] *atherosclerosis of native artery of the extremity (440.21-440.24)*
embolism [occlusion NOS] [thrombus]
of graft (996.74)

440.30 Of unspecified graft

440.31 Of autologous vein bypass graft

440.32 Of nonautologous biological bypass graft

440.4 Chronic total occlusion of artery of the extremities
Complete occlusion of artery of the extremities
Total occlusion of artery of the extremities

Code first atherosclerosis of arteries of the extremities (440.20-440.29, 440.30-440.32)

[Excludes:] *acute occlusion of artery of extremity (444.21- 444.22)*

440.8 Of other specified arteries

[Excludes:] *basilar (433.0)*
carotid (433.1)
cerebral (437.0)
coronary (414.00-414.07)
mesenteric (557.1)
precerebral (433.0-433.9)
pulmonary (416.0)
vertebral (433.2)

440.9 Generalized and unspecified atherosclerosis
Arteriosclerotic vascular disease NOS

Excludes: *arteriosclerotic cardiovascular disease [ASCVD] (429.2)*

441 Aortic aneurysm and dissection

Excludes: *aortic ectasia (447.70-447.73)*
syphilitic aortic aneurysm (093.0)
traumatic aortic aneurysm (901.0, 902.0)

DEFINITION Aortic aneurysm and dissection is a localized, abnormal and persistent dilation of a section of the aorta. This usually results from a weakness in the vessel wall. If severe enough, rupture of the aorta with severe hemorrhage is a potential hazard.

⑤ **441.0 Dissection of aorta**

441.00 Unspecified site

441.01 Thoracic

441.02 Abdominal

441.03 Thoracoabdominal

441.1 Thoracic aneurysm, ruptured

441.2 Thoracic aneurysm without mention of rupture

441.3 Abdominal aneurysm, ruptured

441.4 Abdominal aneurysm without mention of rupture

441.5 Aortic aneurysm of unspecified site, ruptured
Rupture of aorta NOS

441.6 Thoracoabdominal aneurysm, ruptured

441.7 Thoracoabdominal aneurysm, without mention of rupture

441.9 Aortic aneurysm of unspecified site without mention of rupture
Aneurysm
Dilatation of aorta
Hyaline necrosis of aorta

442 Other aneurysm
Includes: aneurysm (ruptured) (cirsoid) (false) (varicose)
aneurysmal varix

Excludes: *arteriovenous aneurysm or fistula:*
acquired (447.0)
congenital (747.60-747.69)
traumatic (900.0-904.9)

DEFINITION Aneurysm is a cardiovascular disease characterized by a saclike widening of an artery resulting from weakening of the artery wall.

442.0 Of artery of upper extremity

442.1 Of renal artery

442.2 Of iliac artery

442.3 Of artery of lower extremity
Aneurysm:
femoral artery
popliteal artery

⑤ **442.8 Of other specified artery**

442.81 Artery of neck
Aneurysm of carotid artery (common) (external) (internal, extracranial portion)

Excludes: *internal carotid artery, intracranial portion (437.3)*

442.82 Subclavian artery

442.83 Splenic artery

442.84 Other visceral artery
Aneurysm:
celiac artery
gastroduodenal artery
gastroepiploic artery
hepatic artery
pancreaticoduodenal artery
superior mesenteric artery

● Code new
to 2012 edition ▲ Revision of
existing code ④ ⑤ Fourth or fifth
digit required

442.89 **Other**
Aneurysm:
mediastinal artery
spinal artery

Excludes: *cerebral (nonruptured) (437.3)*
congenital (747.81)
ruptured (430)
coronary (414.11)
heart (414.10)
pulmonary (417.1)

442.9 **Of unspecified site**

443 **Other peripheral vascular disease**
DEFINITION Peripheral vascular disease (PVD), aka peripheral artery disease (PAD) or peripheral artery occlusive disease (PAOD), includes all diseases caused by the obstruction of large arteries in the arms and legs

443.0 **Raynaud's syndrome**
Raynaud's:
disease
phenomenon (secondary)

Use additional code, if desired, to identify gangrene (785.4)

443.1 **Thromboangiitis obliterans [Buerger's disease]**
Presenile gangrene

⑤ **443.2** **Other arterial dissection**

Excludes: *dissection of aorta (441.00-441.03)*
dissection of coronary arteries (414.12)

443.21 **Dissection of carotid artery**

443.22 **Dissection of iliac artery**

443.23 **Dissection of renal artery**

443.24 **Dissection of vertebral artery**

443.29 **Dissection of other artery**

⑤ **443.8** **Other specified peripheral vascular diseases**

443.81 *Peripheral angiopathy in diseases classified elsewhere*
Code first underlying disease, as:
diabetes mellitus (249.7, 250.7)

443.82 **Erythromelalgia**

443.89 **Other**
Acrocyanosis
Acroparesthesia:
simple [Schultze's type]
vasomotor [Nothnagel's type]
Erythrocyanosis

Excludes: *chilblains (991.5)*
frostbite (991.0-991.3)
immersion foot (991.4)

443.9 **Peripheral vascular disease, unspecified**
Intermittent claudication NOS
Peripheral:
angiopathy NOS
vascular disease NOS
Spasm of artery

Excludes: *atherosclerosis of the arteries of the extremities (440.20-440.22)*
spasm of cerebral artery (435.0-435.9)

Add 4th or 5th digit   Nonspecific code   Unspecified code   Manifestation code

444 **Arterial embolism and thrombosis**
Includes: infarction:
embolic
thrombotic
occlusion

Excludes: *atheroembolism (445.01-445.89)*
septic arterial embolism (449)
that complicating:
abortion (634-638 with .6, 639.6)
ectopic or molar pregnancy (639.6)
pregnancy, childbirth, or the puerperium (673.0-673.8)

DEFINITION An embolism is a sudden interruption in arterial blood flow to an organ or body extremity. The blockage is caused by a blood clot or foreign object. A Thrombosis is the formation or presence of a thrombus (a clot of coagulated blood) in a blood vessel.

⑤ **444.0** **Of abdominal aorta**

● **444.01** **Saddle embolus of abdominal aorta**

● **444.09** **Other arterial embolism and thrombosis of abdominal aorta**
Aortic bifurcation syndrome
Aortoiliac obstruction
Leriche's syndrome

444.1 **Of thoracic aorta**
Embolism or thrombosis of aorta (thoracic)

⑤ **444.2** **Of arteries of the extremities**

444.21 **Upper extremity**

444.22 **Lower extremity**
Arterial embolism or thrombosis:
femoral
peripheral NOS
popliteal

Excludes: *iliofemoral (444.81)*

⑤ **444.8** **Of other specified artery**

444.81 **Iliac artery**

444.89 **Other**

Excludes: *basilar (433.0)*
carotid (433.1)
cerebral (434.0-434.9)
coronary (410.00-410.92)
mesenteric (557.0)
ophthalmic (362.30-362.34)
precerebral (433.0-433.9)
pulmonary (415.11-415.19)
renal (593.81)
retinal (362.30-362.34)
vertebral (433.2)

444.9 **Of unspecified artery**

445 **Atheroembolism**
Includes: Atherothrombotic microembolism
Cholesterol embolism

DEFINITION Atheroembolism is the obstruction of a blood vessel by an atherosclerotic embolism originating from an atheroma in a major artery

⑤ **445.0** **Of extremities**

445.01 **Upper extremity**

445.02 **Lower extremity**

⑤ **445.8** **Of other sites**

445.81 **Kidney**
Use additional code for any associated acute kidney failure or chronic kidney disease (584, 585)

445.89 **Other site**

● Code new
to 2012 edition
▲ Revision of
existing code
④ ⑤ Fourth or fifth
digit required

446 **Polyarteritis nodosa and allied conditions**

> DEFINITION Polyarteritis nodosa is a progressive disease of connective tissue that is characterized by nodules along arteries; nodules may block the artery and result in inadequate circulation to the particular area

446.0 **Polyarteritis nodosa**
Disseminated necrotizing periarteritis
Necrotizing angiitis
Panarteritis (nodosa)
Periarteritis (nodosa)

446.1 **Acute febrile mucocutaneous lymph node syndrome [MLNS]**
Kawasaki disease

⑤ **446.2** **Hypersensitivity angiitis**

> Excludes: *antiglomerular basement membrane disease without pulmonary hemorrhage (583.89)*

446.20 **Hypersensitivity angiitis, unspecified**

446.21 **Goodpasture's syndrome**
Antiglomerular basement membrane antibody-mediated nephritis with pulmonary hemorrhage

Use additional code, if desired, to identify renal disease (583.81)

446.29 **Other specified hypersensitivity angiitis**

446.3 **Lethal midline granuloma**
Malignant granuloma of face

446.4 **Wegener's granulomatosis**
Necrotizing respiratory granulomatosis
Wegener's syndrome

446.5 **Giant cell arteritis**
Cranial arteritis   Temporal arteritis
Horton's disease

446.6 **Thrombotic microangiopathy**
Moschcowitz's syndrome
Thrombotic thrombocytopenic purpura

446.7 **Takayasu's disease**
Aortic arch arteritis
Pulseless disease

447 **Other disorders of arteries and arterioles**

> DEFINITION Arteries are blood vessels that carry blood away from the heart. An arteriole is a small diameter blood vessel that extends and branches out from an artery and leads to capillaries.

447.0 **Arteriovenous fistula, acquired**
Arteriovenous aneurysm, acquired

> Excludes: *cerebrovascular (437.3)*
>   *coronary (414.19)*
>   *pulmonary (417.0)*
>   *surgically created arteriovenous shunt or fistula:*
>   *complication (996.1, 996.61-996.62)*
>   *status or presence (V45.11)*
>   *traumatic (900.0-904.9)*

447.1 **Stricture of artery**

447.2 **Rupture of artery**
Erosion of artery
Fistula, except arteriovenous of artery
Ulcer of artery

> Excludes: *traumatic rupture of artery (900.0-904.9)*

447.3 **Hyperplasia of renal artery**
Fibromuscular hyperplasia of renal artery

447.4 **Celiac artery compression syndrome**
Celiac axis syndrome
Marable's syndrome

447.5 **Necrosis of artery**

447.6 Arteritis, unspecified
Aortitis NOS
Endarteritis NOS

Excludes: *arteritis, endarteritis:*
aortic arch (446.7)
cerebral (437.4)
coronary (414.00-414.07)
deformans (440.0-440.9)
obliterans (440.0-440.9)
pulmonary (417.8)
senile (440.0-440.9)
polyarteritis NOS (446.0)
syphilitic aortitis (093.1)

⑤ **447.7 Aortic ectasia**
Ectasis aorta

Excludes: *aortic aneurysm and dissection (441.00-441.9)*

447.70 Aortic ectasia, unspecified site

447.71 Thoracic aortic ectasia

447.72 Abdominal aortic ectasia

447.73 Thoracoabdominal aortic ectasia

447.8 Other specified disorders of arteries and arterioles
Fibromuscular hyperplasia of arteries, except renal

447.9 Unspecified disorders of arteries and arterioles

448 Disease of capillaries
DEFINITION Capillaries are the smallest of blood vessels. They serve to distribute oxygenated blood from arteries to the tissues of the body and to feed deoxygenated blood from the tissues back into the veins.

448.0 Hereditary hemorrhagic telangiectasia
Rendu-Osler-Weber disease

448.1 Nevus, non-neoplastic

Nevus:	Nevus:
araneus	spider
senile	stellar

Excludes: *neoplastic (216.0-216.9)*
port wine (757.32)
strawberry (757.32)

448.9 Other and unspecified capillary diseases
Capillary:
hemorrhage
hyperpermeability
thrombosis

Excludes: *capillary fragility (hereditary) (287.8)*

449 Septic arterial embolism
Code first underlying infection, such as:
infective endocarditis (421.0)
lung abscess (513.0)
Use additional code to identify the site of the embolism (433.0-433.9, 444.01-444.9)

Excludes: *septic pulmonary embolism (415.12)*

DEFINITION Septic arterial embolism is a sudden interruption in arterial blood flow to an organ or body extremity. The blockage is caused by a bacterial infection in the bloodstream.

● Code new
to 2012 edition

▲ Revision of
existing code

④ ⑤ Fourth or fifth
digit required

DISEASES OF VEINS AND LYMPHATICS, AND OTHER DISEASES OF CIRCULATORY SYSTEM (451-459)

451 Phlebitis and thrombophlebitis

Includes: endophlebitis
inflammation, vein
periphlebitis
suppurative phlebitis

Use additional E Code, if desired, to identify drug, if drug-induced

[Excludes:] *that complicating:*
abortion (634-638 with .7, 639.8)
ectopic or molar pregnancy (639.8)
pregnancy, childbirth, or the puerperium (671.0-671.9)
that due to or following:
implant or catheter device (996.61-996.62)
infusion, perfusion, or transfusion (999.2)

DEFINITION Phlebitis is the inflammation of a vein. Thrombophlebitis is a phlebitis related to a blood clot or thrombus.

ALERT! For personal history of thrombophlebitis see V12.52

451.0 Of superficial vessels of lower extremities
Saphenous vein (greater) (lesser)

[5] **451.1 Of deep vessels of lower extremities**

451.11 Femoral vein (deep) (superficial)

451.19 Other
Femoropopliteal vein
Popliteal vein
Tibial vein

451.2 Of lower extremities, unspecified

[5] **451.8 Of other sites**

[Excludes:] *intracranial venous sinus (325)*
nonpyogenic (437.6)
portal (vein) (572.1)

451.81 Iliac vein

451.82 Of superficial veins of upper extremities
Antecubital vein
Basilic vein
Cephalic vein

451.83 Of deep veins of upper extremities
Brachial vein
Radial vein
Ulnar vein

451.84 Of upper extremities, unspecified

451.89 Other
Axillary vein
Jugular vein
Subclavian vein
Thrombophlebitis of breast (Mondor's disease)

451.9 Of unspecified site

452 Portal vein thrombosis
Portal (vein) obstruction

[Excludes:] *hepatic vein thrombosis (453.0)*
phlebitis of portal vein (572.1)

DEFINITION Portal vein thrombosis is a form of venous thrombosis affecting the hepatic portal vein, which can lead to portal hypertension and reduction in the blood supply to the liver.

453 Other venous embolism and thrombosis

[Excludes:] *that complicating:*
abortion (634-638 with .7, 639.8)
ectopic or molar pregnancy (639.8)
pregnancy, childbirth, or the puerperium (671.0-671.9)

DEFINITION Venous embolism and thrombosis is a mass of clotted blood or other material moved by the blood from one vein and forced into a smaller one

ALERT! For personal history of venous thrombosis and embolism see V12.51

453.0 Budd-Chiari syndrome
Hepatic vein thrombosis

453.1 Thrombophlebitis migrans

453.2 Of inferior vena cava

453.3 Of renal vein

[5] **453.4 Acute venous embolism and thrombosis of deep vessels of lower extremity**

453.40 Acute venous embolism and thrombosis of unspecified deep vessels of lower extremity
Deep vein thrombosis NOS
DVT NOS

453.41 Acute venous embolism and thrombosis of deep vessels of proximal lower extremity
Femoral
Iliac
Popliteal
Thigh
Upper leg NOS

453.42 Acute venous embolism and thrombosis of deep vessels of distal lower extremity
Calf
Lower leg NOS
Peroneal
Tibial

[5] **453.5 Chronic venous embolism and thrombosis of deep vessels of lower extremity**
Use additional code, if applicable, for associated long-term (current) use of anticoagulants (V58.61)

[Excludes:] *personal history of venous thrombosis and embolism (V12.51)*

453.50 Chronic venous embolism and thrombosis of unspecified deep vessels of lower extremity

453.51 Chronic venous embolism and thrombosis of deep vessels of proximal lower extremity
Femoral
Iliac
Popliteal
Thigh
Upper leg NOS

453.52 Chronic venous embolism and thrombosis of deep vessels of distal lower extremity
Calf
Lower leg NOS
Peroneal
Tibial

453.6 Venous embolism and thrombosis of superficial vessels of lower extremity
Saphenous vein (greater) (lesser)

Use additional code, if applicable, for associated long-term (current) use of anticoagulants (V58.61)

[5] **453.7 Chronic venous embolism and thrombosis of other specified vessels**
Use additional code, if applicable, for associated long-term (current) use of anticoagulants (V58.61)

[Excludes:] *personal history of venous thrombosis and embolism (V12.51)*

453.71 Chronic venous embolism and thrombosis of superficial veins of upper extremity
Antecubital vein
Basilic vein
Cephalic vein

453.72 Chronic venous embolism and thrombosis of deep veins of upper extremity
Brachial vein
Radial vein
Ulnar vein

453.73 Chronic venous embolism and thrombosis of upper extremity, unspecified

453.74 Chronic venous embolism and thrombosis of axillary veins

453.75 Chronic venous embolism and thrombosis of subclavian veins

453.76 Chronic venous embolism and thrombosis of internal jugular veins

453.77 **Chronic venous embolism and thrombosis of other thoracic veins**
Brachiocephalic (innominate)
Superior vena cava

453.79 **Chronic venous embolism and thrombosis of other specified veins**

⑤ **453.8** **Acute venous embolism and thrombosis of other specified veins**

Excludes: *cerebral (434.0-434.9)*
coronary (410.00-410.92)
intracranial venous sinus (325)
  nonpyogenic (437.6)
mesenteric (557.0)
portal (452)
precerebral (433.0-433.9)
pulmonary (415.19)

453.81 **Acute venous embolism and thrombosis of superficial veins of upper extremity**
Antecubital vein
Basilic vein
Cephalic vein

453.82 **Acute venous embolism and thrombosis of deep veins of upper extremity**
Brachial vein
Radial vein
Ulnar vein

453.83 **Acute venous embolism and thrombosis of upper extremity, unspecified**

453.84 **Acute venous embolism and thrombosis of axillary veins**

453.85 **Acute venous embolism and thrombosis of subclavian veins**

453.86 **Acute venous embolism and thrombosis of internal jugular veins**

453.87 **Acute venous embolism and thrombosis of other thoracic veins**
Brachiocephalic (innominate)
Superior vena cava

453.89 **Acute venous embolism and thrombosis of other specified veins**

453.9 **Of unspecified site**
Embolism of vein
Thrombosis (vein)

454 **Varicose veins of lower extremities**

Excludes: *that complicating pregnancy, childbirth, or the puerperium (671.0)*

DEFINITION Varicose veins are dilated (widened) tortuous (twisting) veins, usually involving a superficial vein in the leg, often associated with incompetency of the valves in the vein.

454.0 **With ulcer**
Varicose ulcer (lower extremity, any part)
Varicose veins with ulcer of lower extremity [any part] or of unspecified site
Any condition classifiable to 454.9 with ulcer or specified as ulcerated

454.1 **With inflammation**
Stasis dermatitis
Varicose veins with inflammation of lower extremity [any part] or of unspecified site
Any condition classifiable to 454.9 with inflammation or specified as inflamed

454.2 **With ulcer and inflammation**
Varicose veins with ulcer and inflammation of lower extremity [any part] or of unspecified site
Any condition classifiable to 454.9 with ulcer and inflammation

454.8 **With other complications**
Edema
Pain
Swelling

454.9 **Asymptomatic varicose veins**
Phlebectasia of lower extremity [any part] or of unspecified site
Varicose veins NOS
Varicose veins of lower extremity [any part] or of unspecified site
Varix of lower extremity [any part] or of unspecified site

| | Add 4th or 5th digit | | Nonspecific code | | Unspecified code | | Manifestation code |

455 **Hemorrhoids**

Includes: hemorrhoids (anus) (rectum)
piles
varicose veins, anus or rectum

Excludes: *that complicating pregnancy, childbirth or the puerperium (671.8)*

DEFINITION Hemorrhoids are swollen blood vessels in and around the anus that cause itching, pain, and sometimes bleeding

455.0 **Internal hemorrhoids without mention of complication**

455.1 **Internal thrombosed hemorrhoids**

455.2 **Internal hemorrhoids with other complication**

Internal hemorrhoids:	Internal hemorrhoids:
bleeding	strangulated
prolapsed	ulcerated

455.3 **External hemorrhoids without mention of complication**

455.4 **External thrombosed hemorrhoids**

455.5 **External hemorrhoids with other complication**

External hemorrhoids:	External hemorrhoids:
bleeding	strangulated
prolapsed	ulcerated

455.6 **Unspecified hemorrhoids without mention of complication**
Hemorrhoids NOS

455.7 **Unspecified thrombosed hemorrhoids**
Thrombosed hemorrhoids, unspecified whether internal or external

455.8 **Unspecified hemorrhoids with other complication**
Hemorrhoids, unspecified whether internal or external:
bleeding
prolapsed
strangulated
ulcerated

455.9 **Residual hemorrhoidal skin tags**
Skin tags, anus or rectum

456 **Varicose veins of other sites**

DEFINITION Varicose veins are dilated (widened) tortuous (twisting) veins, often associated with incompetency of the valves in the vein.

456.0 **Esophageal varices with bleeding**

456.1 **Esophageal varices without mention of bleeding**

⑤ *456.2* *Esophageal varices in diseases classified elsewhere*
Code first underlying cause, as:
cirrhosis of liver (571.0-571.9)
portal hypertension (572.3)

456.20 *With bleeding*

456.21 *Without mention of bleeding*

456.3 **Sublingual varices**

456.4 **Scrotal varices**
Varicocele

456.5 **Pelvic varices**
Varices of broad ligament

456.6 **Vulval varices**
Varices of perineum

Excludes: *that complicating pregnancy, childbirth, or the puerperium (671.1)*

456.8 **Varices of other sites**
Varicose veins of nasal septum (with ulcer)

Excludes: *placental varices (656.7)*
retinal varices (362.17)
varicose ulcer of unspecified site (454.0)
varicose veins of unspecified site (454.9)

457 **Noninfectious disorders of lymphatic channels**

457.0 **Postmastectomy lymphedema syndrome**
Elephantiasis due to mastectomy
Obliteration of lymphatic vessel due to mastectomy

● Code new
to 2012 edition

▲ Revision of
existing code

④ ⑤ Fourth or fifth
digit required

457.1 Other lymphedema
Elephantiasis (nonfilarial) NOS
Lymphangiectasis
Lymphedema:
- acquired (chronic)
- praecox
- secondary

Obliteration, lymphatic vessel

[Excludes:] *elephantiasis (nonfilarial):*
- *congenital (757.0)*
- *eyelid (374.83)*
- *vulva (624.8)*

457.2 Lymphangitis
Lymphangitis:
- NOS
- chronic
- subacute

[Excludes:] *acute lymphangitis (682.0-682.9)*

457.8 Other noninfectious disorders of lymphatic channels
Chylocele (nonfilarial)
Chylous:
- ascites
- cyst

Lymph node or vessel:
- fistula
- infarction
- rupture

[Excludes:] *chylocele:*
- *filarial (125.0-125.9)*
- *tunica vaginalis (nonfilarial) (608.84)*

457.9 Unspecified noninfectious disorder of lymphatic channels

458 Hypotension
Includes: hypopiesis

[Excludes:] *cardiovascular collapse (785.50)*
maternal hypotension syndrome (669.2)
shock (785.50-785.59)
Shy-Drager syndrome (333.0)

[DEFINITION] Hypotension is the medical term for abnormally low blood pressure.

458.0 Orthostatic hypotension
Hypotension:
- orthostatic (chronic)
- postural

458.1 Chronic hypotension
Permanent idiopathic hypotension

[5] **458.2 Iatrogenic hypotension**

458.21 Hypotension of hemodialysis
Intra-dialytic hypotension

458.29 Other iatrogenic hypotension
Postoperative hypotension

458.8 Other specified hypotension

458.9 Hypotension, unspecified
Hypotension (arterial) NOS

459 Other disorders of circulatory system

[ALERT!] For personal history of other diseases of circulatory system not elsewhere classified see V12.59

459.0 Hemorrhage, unspecified
Rupture of blood vessel NOS
Spontaneous hemorrhage NEC

[Excludes:] *hemorrhage:*
- *gastrointestinal NOS (578.9)*
- *in newborn NOS (772.9)*
- *secondary or recurrent following trauma (958.2)*

nontraumatic hematoma of soft tissue (729.92)
traumatic rupture of blood vessel (900.0-904.9)

⑤ **459.1　Postphlebitic syndrome**
　　　　Chronic venous hypertension due to deep vein thrombosis

　　　　Excludes: *chronic venous hyptertension without deep vein thrombosis (459.30-459.39)*

　　　　459.10　Postphlebetic syndrome without complications
　　　　　　Asymptomatic postphlebetic syndrome
　　　　　　Postphlebetic syndrome NOS

　　　　459.11　Postphlebetic syndrome with ulcer

　　　　459.12　Postphlebetic syndrome with inflammation

　　　　459.13　Postphlebetic syndrome with ulcer and inflammation

　　　　459.19　Postphlebetic syndrome with other complication

　　459.2　Compression of vein
　　　　Stricture of vein
　　　　Vena cava syndrome (inferior) (superior)

⑤ **459.3　Chronic venous hypertension (idiopathic)**
　　　　Statis edema

　　　　Excludes: *chronic venous hypertension due to deep vein thrombosis (459.10-459.19)*
　　　　　　　　　　varicose veins (454.0-454.9)

　　　　459.30　Chronic venous hypertension without complications
　　　　　　Asymptomatic chronic venous hypertension
　　　　　　Chronic venous hypertension NOS

　　　　459.31　Chronic venous hypertension with ulcer

　　　　459.32　Chronic venous hypertension with inflammation

　　　　459.33　Chronic venous hypertension with ulcer and inflammation

　　　　459.39　Chronic venous hypertension with other complication

⑤ **459.8　Other specified disorders of circulatory system**

　　　　459.81　Venous (peripheral) insufficiency, unspecified
　　　　　　Chronic venous insufficiency NOS

　　　　Use additional code for any associated ulceration (707.10-707.19, 707.8, 707.9)

　　　　459.89　Other
　　　　　　Collateral circulation (venous), any site
　　　　　　Phlebosclerosis
　　　　　　Venofibrosis

　　459.9　Unspecified circulatory system disorder

● Code new
　to 2012 edition
▲ Revision of
　existing code
④ ⑤ Fourth or fifth
　　digit required

Chapter 8: Diseases of Respiratory System (460-519)

DEFINITIONS AND CODING ALERTS

This chapter includes definitions of selected key words, terms and phrases and coding alerts for adding points to the clinical domain, references to coding late effects where appropriate, and references to personal history V-codes in situations where the acute or chronic condition is no longer active. An example from this chapter is as follows:

501 Asbestosis

> **DEFINITION** Asbestosis is a condition featuring scarring of the lungs caused by inhaled asbestos fibers.
>
> **ALERT!** For personal history of contact with and (suspected) exposure to asbestos see V15.84

MULTIPLE CODING FOR A SINGLE CONDITION

In addition to the etiology or manifestation convention that requires two codes to fully describe a single condition that affects multiple body systems, there are other single conditions that also require more than one code. "Use additional code" notes are found in the tabular at codes that are not part of an etiology or manifestation pair where a secondary code is useful to fully describe a condition. The sequencing rule is the same as the etiology or manifestation pair - , "use additional code" indicates that a secondary code should be added.

"Code first" notes are also under certain codes that are not specifically manifestation codes but may be due to an underlying cause. When a "code first" note is present and an underlying condition is present the underlying condition should be sequenced first.

"Code, if applicable, any causal condition first", notes indicate that this code may be assigned as a principal diagnosis when the causal condition is unknown or not applicable. If a causal condition is known, then the code for that condition should be sequenced as the principal or first-listed diagnosis. Multiple codes may be needed for late effects, complication codes and obstetric codes to more fully describe a condition. See the specific guidelines for these conditions for further instruction.

COMBINATION CODE

A combination code is a single code used to classify: two diagnoses, or a diagnosis with an associated secondary process (manifestation) A diagnosis with an associated complication Combination codes are identified by referring to subterm entries in the Alphabetic Index and by reading the inclusion and exclusion notes in the Tabular List.

Assign only the combination code when that code fully identifies the diagnostic conditions involved or when the Alphabetic Index so directs. Multiple coding should not be used when the classification provides a combination code that clearly identifies all of the elements documented in the diagnosis. When the combination code lacks necessary specificity in describing the manifestation or complication, an additional code should be used as a secondary code.

CODING LATE EFFECTS

A late effect is the residual effect (condition produced) after the acute phase of an illness or injury has terminated. There is no time limit on when a late effect code can be used. The residual may be apparent early, such as in cerebrovascular accident cases, or it may occur months or years later, such as that due to a previous injury. Coding of late effects generally requires two codes sequenced in the following order: The condition or nature of the late effect is sequenced first. The late effect code is sequenced second.

An exception to the above guidelines are those instances where the code for late effect is followed by a manifestation code identified in the Tabular List and title, or the late effect code has been expanded (at the fourth and fifth-digit levels) to include the manifestation(s). The code for the acute phase of an illness or injury that led to the late effect is never used with a code for the late effect.

CHRONIC OBSTRUCTIVE PULMONARY DISEASE [COPD] AND ASTHMA

Conditions that comprise COPD and Asthma

The conditions that comprise COPD are obstructive chronic bronchitis, subcategory 491.2, and emphysema, category 492. All asthma codes are under category 493, Asthma. Code 496, Chronic airway obstruction, not elsewhere classified, is a nonspecific code that should only be used when the documentation in a medical record does not specify the type of COPD being treated.

| | Add 4th or 5th digit | | Nonspecific code | | Unspecified code | | Manifestation code |

Acute exacerbation of chronic obstructive bronchitis and asthma

The codes for chronic obstructive bronchitis and asthma distinguish between uncomplicated cases and those in acute exacerbation. An acute exacerbation is a worsening or a decompensation of a chronic condition. An acute exacerbation is not equivalent to an infection superimposed on a chronic condition, though an exacerbation may be triggered by an infection.

Overlapping nature of the conditions that comprise COPD and asthma

Due to the overlapping nature of the conditions that make up COPD and asthma, there are many variations in the way these conditions are documented. Code selection must be based on the terms as documented. When selecting the correct code for the documented type of COPD and asthma, it is essential to first review the index, and then verify the code in the tabular list. There are many instructional notes under the different COPD subcategories and codes. It is important that all such notes be reviewed to assure correct code assignment.

Acute exacerbation of asthma and status asthmaticus

An acute exacerbation of asthma is an increased severity of the asthma symptoms, such as wheezing and shortness of breath. Status asthmaticus refers to a patient's failure to respond to therapy administered during an asthmatic episode and is a life threatening complication that requires emergency care. If status asthmaticus is documented by the provider with any type of COPD or with acute bronchitis, the status asthmaticus should be sequenced first. It supersedes any type of COPD including that with acute exacerbation or acute bronchitis. It is inappropriate to assign an asthma code with 5th digit 2, with acute exacerbation, together with an asthma code with 5th digit 1, with status asthmatics. Only the 5th digit 1 should be assigned.

CHRONIC OBSTRUCTIVE PULMONARY DISEASE [COPD] AND BRONCHITIS

Acute bronchitis with COPD

Acute bronchitis, code 466.0, is due to an infectious organism. When acute bronchitis is documented with COPD, code 491.22, Obstructive chronic bronchitis with acute bronchitis, should be assigned. It is not necessary to also assign code 466.0. If a medical record documents acute bronchitis with COPD with acute exacerbation, only code 491.22 should be assigned. The acute bronchitis included in code 491.22 supersedes the acute exacerbation. If a medical record documents COPD with acute exacerbation without mention of acute bronchitis, only code 491.21 should be assigned.

ACUTE RESPIRATORY FAILURE

Acute respiratory failure as principal diagnosis

Code 518.81, Acute respiratory failure, may be assigned as a principal diagnosis when it is the condition established after study to be chiefly responsible for occasioning the admission to the hospital, and the selection is supported by the Alphabetic Index and Tabular List. However, chapter-specific coding guidelines (such as obstetrics, poisoning, HIV, newborn) that provide sequencing direction take precedence.

Acute respiratory failure as secondary diagnosis

Respiratory failure may be listed as a secondary diagnosis if it occurs after admission, or if it is present on admission, but does not meet the definition of principal diagnosis.

Sequencing of acute respiratory failure and another acute condition

When a patient is admitted with respiratory failure and another acute condition, (e.g., myocardial infarction, cerebrovascular accident, aspiration pneumonia), the principal diagnosis will not be the same in every situation. This applies whether the other acute condition is a respiratory or nonrespiratory condition. Selection of the principal diagnosis will be dependent on the circumstances of admission. If both the respiratory failure and the other acute condition are equally responsible for occasioning the admission to the hospital, and there are no chapter-specific sequencing rules, the guideline regarding two or more diagnoses that equally meet the definition for principal diagnosis (Official Guidelines, Section II) may be applied in these situations.

If the documentation is not clear as to whether acute respiratory failure and another condition are equally responsible for occasioning the admission, query the provider for clarification.

● Code new
to 2012 edition

▲ Revision of
existing code

④ ⑤ Fourth or fifth
digit required

INFLUENZA DUE TO IDENTIFIED AVIAN INFLUENZA VIRUS (AVIAN INFLUENZA)

Code only confirmed cases of avian influenza. This is an exception to the hospital inpatient guideline Official Guidelines, Section II, H. (Uncertain Diagnosis).

In this context, "confirmation" does not require documentation of positive laboratory testing specific for avian influenza. However, coding should be based on the provider's diagnostic statement that the patient has avian influenza.

If the provider records "suspected or possible or probable avian influenza," the appropriate influenza code from category 487 should be assigned. Code 488, Influenza due to identified avian influenza virus, should not be assigned.

| | Add 4th or 5th digit | | Nonspecific code | | Unspecified code | | Manifestation code |

This page intentionally left blank.

● Code new
to 2012 edition

▲ Revision of
existing code

④ ⑤ Fourth or fifth
digit required

8. DISEASES OF THE RESPIRATORY SYSTEM (460-519)

Use additional code, if desired, to identify infectious organism

ALERT! For personal history of diseases of respiratory system see V12.6

ACUTE RESPIRATORY INFECTIONS (460-466)

Excludes: *pneumonia and influenza (480.0-488.19)*

460 Acute nasopharyngitis [common cold]
Coryza (acute)
Nasal catarrh, acute
Nasopharyngitis:
  NOS
  acute
  infective NOS
Rhinitis:
  acute
  infective

Excludes: *nasopharyngitis, chronic (472.2)*
  pharyngitis:
    acute or unspecified (462)
    chronic (472.1)
  rhinitis:
    allergic (477.0-477.9)
    chronic or unspecified (472.0)
  sore throat:
    acute or unspecified (462)
    chronic (472.1)

DEFINITION Nasopharyngitis, usually known as the common cold, is a viral infectious disease of the upper respiratory system.

461 Acute sinusitis
Includes: abscess acute, of sinus (accessory) (nasal)
  empyema acute, of sinus (accessory) (nasal)
  infection acute, of sinus (accessory) (nasal)
  inflammation acute, of sinus (accessory) (nasal)
  suppuration acute, of sinus (accessory) (nasal)

Excludes: *chronic or unspecified sinusitis (473.0-473.9)*

DEFINITION Sinusitis is an infection of the small, air-filled cavities inside the cheekbones and forehead.

461.0 Maxillary
Acute antritis

461.1 Frontal

461.2 Ethmoidal

461.3 Sphenoidal

461.8 Other acute sinusitis
Acute pansinusitis

461.9 Acute sinusitis, unspecified
Acute sinusitis NOS

462 Acute pharyngitis

> Acute sore throat NOS
> Pharyngitis (acute):
>> NOS
>> gangrenous
>> infective
>> phlegmonous
>> pneumococcal
>> staphylococcal
>> suppurative
>> ulcerative
> Sore throat (viral) NOS
> Viral pharyngitis

> Excludes: *abscess:*
>> *peritonsillar [quinsy] (475)*
>> *pharyngeal NOS (478.29)*
>> *retropharyngeal (478.24)*
>> *chronic pharyngitis (472.1)*
>> *infectious mononucleosis (075)*
>> *that specified as (due to):*
>>> *Coxsackie (virus) (074.0)*
>>> *gonococcus (098.6)*
>>> *herpes simplex (054.79)*
>>> *influenza (487.1, 488.02, 488.12)*
>>> *septic (034.0)*
>>> *streptococcal (034.0)*

DEFINITION Pharyngitis, aka sore throat, is an inflammation of the pharynx. Most sore throats are viral and will not respond to antibiotics. Bacterial causes include group a streptococcus.

463 Acute tonsillitis

> Tonsillitis (acute):   Tonsillitis (acute):
>> NOS   septic
>> follicular   staphylococcal
>> gangrenous   suppurative
>> infective   ulcerative
>> pneumococcal   viral

> Excludes: *chronic tonsillitis (474.0)*
>> *hypertrophy of tonsils (474.1)*
>> *peritonsillar abscess [quinsy] (475)*
>> *sore throat:*
>>> *acute or NOS (462)*
>>> *septic (034.0)*
>> *streptococcal tonsillitis (034.0)*

DEFINITION Tonsillitis is an infection and swelling of the tonsils.

464 Acute laryngitis and tracheitis

> Excludes: *that associated with influenza (487.1, 488.02, 488.12)*
>> *that due to Streptococcus (034.0)*

DEFINITION Laryngitis and tracheitis is an inflammation of the mucous membrane of the larynx and trachea; characterized by hoarseness or loss of voice and coughing .

⑤ **464.0 Acute laryngitis**

> Laryngitis (acute):   Laryngitis (acute):
>> NOS   pneumococcal
>> edematous   septic
>> Hemophilus influenza   suppurative
>> [H. influenzae]   ulcerative

> Excludes: *chronic laryngitis (476.0-476.1)*
>> *influenzal laryngitis (487.1, 488.02, 488.12)*

> **464.00 Without mention of obstruction**

> **464.01 With obstruction**

⑤ **464.1 Acute tracheitis**

> Tracheitis (acute):
>> NOS
>> catarrhal
>> viral

> Excludes: *chronic tracheitis (491.8)*

> **464.10 Without mention of obstruction**

● Code new to 2012 edition ▲ Revision of existing code ④ ⑤ Fourth or fifth digit required

464.11 **With obstruction**

⑤ **464.2** **Acute laryngotracheitis**
Laryngotracheitis (acute)
Tracheitis (acute) with laryngitis (acute)

Excludes: chronic laryngotracheitis (476.1)

464.20 **Without mention of obstruction**

464.21 **With obstruction**

⑤ **464.3** **Acute epiglottitis**
Viral epiglottitis

Excludes: epiglottitis, chronic (476.1)

464.30 **Without mention of obstruction**

464.31 **With obstruction**

464.4 **Croup**
Croup syndrome

⑤ **464.5** **Supraglottitis, unspecified**

464.50 **Without mention of obstruction**

464.51 **With obstruction**

465 **Acute upper respiratory infections of multiple or unspecified sites**

Excludes: upper respiratory infection due to:
influenza (487.1, 488.02, 488.12)
Streptococcus (034.0)

DEFINITION Upper respiratory infection is an inflammation of the nose, sinuses, ears or throat, caused by a viral infection.

465.0 **Acute laryngopharyngitis**

465.8 **Other multiple sites**
Multiple URI

465.9 **Unspecified site**
Acute URI NOS
Upper respiratory infection (acute)

466 **Acute bronchitis and bronchiolitis**
Includes: that with:
bronchospasm
obstruction

DEFINITION Bronchitis and bronchiolitis is an inflammation of the membranes lining the bronchial tubes

466.0 **Acute bronchitis**
Bronchitis, acute or subacute:
fibrinous
membranous
pneumococcal
purulent
septic
viral
with tracheitis
Croupous bronchitis
Tracheobronchitis, acute

Excludes: acute bronchitis with chronic obstructive pulmonary disease (491.22)

⑤ **466.1** **Acute bronchiolitis**
Bronchiolitis (acute)
Capillary pneumonia

Excludes: respiratory bronchiolitis interstitial lung disease (516.34)

466.11 **Acute bronchiolitis due to respiratory syncytial virus (RSV)**

466.19 **Acute bronchiolitis due to other infectious organisms**
Use additional code to identify organism

OTHER DISEASES OF THE UPPER RESPIRATORY TRACT (470-478)

470 Deviated nasal septum
Deflected septum (nasal) (acquired)

[Excludes:] *congenital (754.0)*

[DEFINITION] A Deviated nasal septum is an abnormal shift in location of the nasal septum; a common condition causing obstruction of the nasal passages and difficulty in breathing and recurrent nosebleeds.

471 Nasal polyps

[Excludes:] *adenomatous polyps (212.0)*

[DEFINITION] Nasal polyps are small, sac-like growths made up of inflamed tissue lining the nose (nasal mucosa).

471.0 Polyp of nasal cavity
Polyp:
choanal
nasopharyngeal

471.1 Polypoid sinus degeneration
Woakes' syndrome or ethmoiditis

471.8 Other polyp of sinus
Polyp of sinus:
accessory
ethmoidal
Polyp of sinus:
maxillary
sphenoidal

471.9 Unspecified nasal polyp
Nasal polyp NOS

472 Chronic pharyngitis and nasopharyngitis

[DEFINITION] Pharyngitis and nasopharyngitis, aka sore throat, is an inflammation of the pharynx. Most sore throats are viral and will not respond to antibiotics. Bacterial causes include group a streptococcus.

472.0 Chronic rhinitis
Ozena
Rhinitis:
NOS
atrophic
granulomatous
Rhinitis:
hypertrophic
obstructive
purulent
ulcerative

[Excludes:] *allergic rhinitis (477.0-477.9)*

472.1 Chronic pharyngitis
Chronic sore throat
Pharyngitis:
atrophic
granular (chronic)
hypertrophic

472.2 Chronic nasopharyngitis

[Excludes:] *acute or unspecified nasopharyngitis (460)*

473 Chronic sinusitis
Includes: abscess (chronic) of sinus (accessory) (nasal)
empyema (chronic) of sinus (accessory) (nasal)
infection (chronic) of sinus (accessory) (nasal)
suppuration (chronic) of sinus (accessory) (nasal)

[Excludes:] *acute sinusitis (461.0-461.9)*

[DEFINITION] Sinusitis is an infection of the small, air-filled cavities inside the cheekbones and forehead.

473.0 Maxillary
Antritis (chronic)

473.1 Frontal

473.2 Ethmoidal

[Excludes:] *Woakes' ethmoiditis (471.1)*

473.3 Sphenoidal

473.8 Other chronic sinusitis
Pansinusitis (chronic)

473.9 Unspecified sinusitis (chronic)
Sinusitis (chronic) NOS

474 Chronic disease of tonsils and adenoids

⑤ **474.0 Chronic tonsillitis and adenoiditis**

Excludes: *acute or unspecified tonsillitis (463)*

474.00   Chronic tonsillitis

474.01   Chronic adenoiditis

474.02   Chronic tonsillitis and adenoiditis

⑤ **474.1 Hypertrophy of tonsils and adenoids**
Enlargement of tonsils or adenoids
Hyperplasia of tonsils or adenoids
Hypertrophy of tonsils or adenoids

Excludes: *that with adenoiditis (474.01)*

that with adenoiditis and tonsillitis (474.02)
that with tonsillitis (474.00)

474.10   Tonsils with adenoids

474.11   Tonsils alone

474.12   Adenoids alone

474.2 Adenoid vegetations

474.8 Other chronic disease of tonsils and adenoids
Amygdalolith
Calculus, tonsil
Cicatrix of tonsil (and adenoid)
Tonsillar tag
Ulcer, tonsil

474.9 Unspecified chronic disease of tonsils and adenoids
Disease (chronic) of tonsils (and adenoids)

475 Peritonsillar abscess
Abscess of tonsil
Peritonsillar cellulitis
Quinsy

Excludes: *tonsillitis:*

acute or NOS (463)
chronic (474.0)

DEFINITION A Peritonsillar abscess is an abscess forming in acute tonsillitis around one or both tonsils.

476 Chronic laryngitis and laryngotracheitis

DEFINITION Chronic laryngitis and laryngotracheitis refer to an inflammation of the mucous membrane of the larynx and trachea; characterized by hoarseness or loss of voice and coughing .

476.0 Chronic laryngitis
Laryngitis:
catarrhal
hypertrophic
Sicca

476.1 Chronic laryngotracheitis
Laryngitis, chronic, with tracheitis (chronic)
Tracheitis, chronic, with laryngitis

Excludes: *chronic tracheitis (491.8)*

laryngitis and tracheitis, acute or unspecified (464.00-464.51)

477 Allergic rhinitis
Includes: allergic rhinitis (nonseasonal) (seasonal)
hay fever
spasmodic rhinorrhea

Excludes: *allergic rhinitis with asthma (bronchial) (493.0)*

DEFINITION Allergic rhinitis refers to a group of symptoms similar to those of a cold such as runny nose and sore throat, caused by an allergic reaction to an allergen such as dust, plant pollens or animal dander.

477.0 Due to pollen
Pollinosis

477.1 Due to food

477.2 Due to animal (cat) (dog) hair and dander

477.8 Due to other allergen

477.9 Cause unspecified

478 Other diseases of upper respiratory tract

DEFINITION Diseases of upper respiratory tract refers to the part of the respiratory system including the nose, nasal passages, and nasopharynx.

478.0 **Hypertrophy of nasal turbinates**

⑤ **478.1** **Other diseases of nasal cavity and sinuses**

Excludes: *varicose ulcer of nasal septum (456.8)*

478.11 **Nasal mucositis (ulcerative)**

Use additional E code to identify adverse effects of therapy, such as:
antineoplastic and immunosuppressive drugs (E930.7, E933.1)
radiation therapy (E879.2)

478.19 **Other disease of nasal cavity and sinuses**
Abscess of nose (septum)
Necrosis of nose (septum)
Ulcer of nose (septum)
Cyst or mucocele of sinus (nasal)
Rhinolith

⑤ **478.2** **Other diseases of pharynx, not elsewhere classified**

478.20 **Unspecified disease of pharynx**

478.21 **Cellulitis of pharynx or nasopharynx**

478.22 **Parapharyngeal abscess**

478.24 **Retropharyngeal abscess**

478.25 **Edema of pharynx or nasopharynx**

478.26 **Cyst of pharynx or nasopharynx**

478.29 **Other**
Abscess of pharynx or nasopharynx

Excludes: *ulcerative pharyngitis (462)*

⑤ **478.3** **Paralysis of vocal cords or larynx**

478.30 **Paralysis, unspecified**
Laryngoplegia
Paralysis of glottis

478.31 **Unilateral, partial**

478.32 **Unilateral, complete**

478.33 **Bilateral, partial**

478.34 **Bilateral, complete**

478.4 **Polyp of vocal cord or larynx**

Excludes: *adenomatous polyps (212.1)*

478.5 **Other diseases of vocal cords**
Abscess of vocal cords
Cellulitis of vocal cords
Granuloma of vocal cords
Leukoplakia of vocal cords
Chorditis (fibrinous) (nodosa) (tuberosa)
Singers' nodes

478.6 **Edema of larynx**
Edema (of):
glottis
subglottic
supraglottic

⑤ **478.7** **Other diseases of larynx, not elsewhere classified**

478.70 **Unspecified disease of larynx**

478.71 **Cellulitis and perichondritis of larynx**

478.74 **Stenosis of larynx**

478.75 **Laryngeal spasm**
Laryngismus (stridulus)

478.79 **Other**
Abscess of larynx
Necrosis of larynx
Obstruction of larynx
Pachyderma of larynx
Ulcer of larynx

● Code new
to 2012 edition
▲ Revision of
existing code
④ ⑤ Fourth or fifth
digit required

[Excludes:] *ulcerative laryngitis (464.00-464.01)*

478.8 Upper respiratory tract hypersensitivity reaction, site unspecified

[Excludes:] *hypersensitivity reaction of lower respiratory tract, as:*
extrinsic allergic alveolitis (495.0-495.9)
pneumoconiosis (500-505)

478.9 Other and unspecified diseases of upper respiratory tract
Abscess of trachea
Cicatrix of trachea

PNEUMONIA AND INFLUENZA (480-488)

[Excludes:] *pneumonia:*
allergic or eosinophilic (518.3)
aspiration:
NOS (507.0)
newborn (770.18)
solids and liquids (507.0-507.8)
congenital (770.0)
lipoid (507.1)
passive (514)
rheumatic (390)
ventilator-associated (997.31)

ALERT! For personal history of pneumonia (recurrent) see V12.61

480 Viral pneumonia

DEFINITION Viral pneumonia is an inflammation of the lungs caused by infection with a virus.

480.0 Pneumonia due to adenovirus

480.1 Pneumonia due to respiratory syncytial virus

480.2 Pneumonia due to parainfluenza virus

480.3 Pneumonia due to SARS-associated coronavirus

480.8 Pneumonia due to other virus not elsewhere classified

[Excludes:] *congenital rubella pneumonitis (771.0)*
pneumonia complicating viral diseases classified elsewhere (484.1-484.8)

480.9 Viral pneumonia, unspecified

481 Pneumococcal pneumonia [*Streptococcus pneumoniae* pneumonia]
Lobar pneumonia, organism unspecified

482 Other bacterial pneumonia

DEFINITION Bacterial pneumonia is an acute inflammation of lung tissue caused by bacteria.

482.0 Pneumonia due to Klebsiella pneumoniae

482.1 Pneumonia due to Pseudomonas

482.2 Pneumonia due to Hemophilus influenzae [H. influenzae]

[5] **482.3 Pneumonia due to Streptococcus**

[Excludes:] *Streptococcus pneumoniae pneumonia (481)*

482.30 Streptococcus, unspecified

482.31 Group A

482.32 Group B

482.39 Other Streptococcus

[5] **482.4 Pneumonia due to Staphylococcus**

482.40 Pneumonia due to Staphylococcus, unspecified

482.41 Methicillin susceptible pneumonia due to Staphylococcus aureus
MSSA pneumonia
Pneumonia due to Staphylococcus aureus NOS

482.42 Methicillin resistant pneumonia due to Staphylococcus aureus

482.49 Other Staphylococcus pneumonia

[5] **482.8 Pneumonia due to other specified bacteria**

[Excludes:] *pneumonia complicating infectious disease classified elsewhere (484.1-484.8)*

482.81 Anaerobes
Bacteroides (melaninogenicus)
Gram-negative anaerobes

482.82 Escherichia coli [E. coli]

Add 4th or 5th digit | Nonspecific code | Unspecified code | Manifestation code

482.83 Other gram-negative bacteria
Gram-negative pneumonia NOS
Proteus
Serratia marcescens

Excludes: *Gram-negative anaerobes (482.81)*
Legionnaires' disease (482.84)

482.84 Legionnaires' disease

482.89 Other specified bacteria

482.9 Bacterial pneumonia unspecified

483 Pneumonia due to other specified organism

483.0 Mycoplasma pneumoniae
Eaton's agent
Pleuropneumonia-like organism [PPLO]

483.1 Chlamydia

483.8 Other specified organism

484 Pneumonia in infectious diseases classified elsewhere

484.1 Pneumonia in cytomegalic inclusion disease
Code first underlying disease (078.5)

484.3 Pneumonia in whooping cough
Code first underlying disease (033.0-033.9)

484.5 Pneumonia in anthrax
Code first underlying disease (022.1)

484.6 Pneumonia in aspergillosis
Code first underlying disease (117.3)

484.7 Pneumonia in other systemic mycoses
Code first underlying disease

Excludes: *pneumonia in:*
candidiasis (112.4)
coccidioidomycosis (114.0)
histoplasmosis (115.0-115.9 with fifth-digit 5)

484.8 Pneumonia in other infectious diseases classified elsewhere
Code first underlying disease, as:
Q fever (083.0)
typhoid fever (002.0)

Excludes: *pneumonia in:*
actinomycosis (039.1)
measles (055.1)
nocardiosis (039.1)
ornithosis (073.0)
Pneumocystis carinii (136.3)
salmonellosis (003.22)
toxoplasmosis (130.4)
tuberculosis (011.6)
tularemia (021.2)
varicella (052.1)

485 Bronchopneumonia, organism unspecified

Bronchopneumonia:	Pneumonia:
hemorrhagic	lobular
terminal	segmental

Pleurobronchopneumonia

Excludes: *bronchiolitis (acute) (466.11-466.19)*
chronic (491.8)
lipoid pneumonia (507.1)

DEFINITION Bronchopneumonia is a pneumonia characterized by acute inflammation of the walls of the bronchioles

486 Pneumonia, organism unspecified

Excludes: *hypostatic or passive pneumonia (514)*
inhalation or aspiration pneumonia due to foreign materials (507.0-507.8)
pneumonitis due to fumes and vapors (506.0)

● Code new
to 2012 edition
▲ Revision of
existing code
④ ⑤ Fourth or fifth
digit required

487 Influenza

Influenza caused by unspecified influenza virus

[Excludes:] *Hemophilus influenzae [H. influenzae]:*
infection NOS (041.5)
laryngitis (464.00-464.01)
meningitis (320.0)
influenza due to 2009 H1N1 [swine] influenza virus (488.11-488.19)
influenza due to identified avian influenza virus (488.01-488.09)
influenza due to identified (novel) 2009 H1N1 influenza virus (488.11-488.19)

DEFINITION Influenza, usually referred to as the flu, is a highly infectious respiratory disease. The disease is caused by certain strains of the influenza virus.

487.0 With pneumonia

Influenza with pneumonia, any form
Influenzal:
bronchopneumonia
pneumonia
Use additional code to identify the type of pneumonia (480.0-480.9, 481, 482.0-482.9, 483.0-483.8, 485)

487.1 With other respiratory manifestations

Influenza NEC
Influenza NOS
Influenzal:
laryngitis
pharyngitis
respiratory infection (upper) (acute)

487.8 With other manifestations

Encephalopathy due to influenza
Influenza with involvement of gastrointestinal tract

[Excludes:] *"intestinal flu" [viral gastroenteritis] (008.8)*

488 Influenza due to certain identified influenza viruses

[Excludes:] *influenza caused by unspecified or seasonal influenza viruses (487.0-487.8)*

[5] **488.0 Influenza due to identified avian influenza virus**

Avian influenza
Bird flu
Influenza A/H5N1

488.01 Influenza due to identified avian influenza virus with pneumonia

Avian influenzal:
bronchopneumonia
pneumonia
Influenza due to identified avian influenza virus with pneumonia, any form

Use additional code to identify the type of pneumonia (480.0-480.9, 481, 482.0-482.9, 483.0-483.8, 485)

488.02 Influenza due to identified avian influenza virus with other respiratory manifestations

Avian influenzal:
laryngitis
pharyngitis
respiratory infection (acute) (upper)
Identified avian influenza NOS

488.09 Influenza due to identified avian influenza virus with other manifestations

Avian influenza with involvement of gastrointestinal tract
Encephalopathy due to identified avian influenza

[Excludes:] *"intestinal flu" [viral gastroenteritis] (008.8)*

▲ **488.1 Influenza due to identified 2009 H1N1 influenza virus**

2009 H1N1 swine influenza virus
(Novel) 2009 influenza H1N1
Novel H1N1 influenza
Novel influenza A/H1N1

[Excludes:] *bird influenza virus infection (488.01-488.09)*
influenza A/H5N1 (488.01-488.09)
other human infection with influenza virus of animal origin (488.81-488.89)
swine influenza virus infection (488.81-488.89)

Add 4th or 5th digit | Nonspecific code | Unspecified code | Manifestation code

▲ 488.11 **Influenza due to identified 2009 H1N1 influenza virus with pneumonia**
Influenza due to identified (novel) 2009 H1N1 with pneumonia, any form
(Novel) 2009 H1N1 influenzal:
bronchopneumonia
pneumonia

Use additional code to identify the type of pneumonia (480.0-480.9, 481, 482.0-482.9, 483.0-483.8, 485)

▲ 488.12 **Influenza due to identified 2009 H1N1 influenza virus with other respiratory manifestations**
(Novel) 2009 H1N1 influenza NOS
(Novel) 2009 H1N1 influenzal:
laryngitis
pharyngitis
respiratory infection (acute) (upper)

▲ 488.19 **Influenza due to identified 2009 H1N1 influenza virus with other manifestations**
Encephalopathy due to identified (novel) 2009 H1N1 influenza
(Novel) 2009 H1N1 influenza with involvement of gastrointestinal tract

[Excludes:] *"intestinal flu" [viral gastroenteritis] (008.8)*

● 488.8 **Influenza due to novel influenza A**
Influenza due to animal origin influenza virus
Infection with influenza viruses occurring in pigs or other animals
Other novel influenza A viruses not previously found in humans

[Excludes:] *bird influenza virus infection (488.01-488.09)*
influenza A/H5N1 (488.01-488.09)
influenza due to identified 2009 H1N1 influenza virus (488.11- 488.19)

● 488.81 **Influenza due to identified novel influenza A virus with pneumonia**
Influenza due to animal origin influenza virus with pneumonia, any form
Novel influenza A:
bronchopneumonia
pneumonia

Use additional code to identify the type of pneumonia (480.0-480.9, 481, 482.0-482.9, 483.0-483.8, 485)

● 488.82 **Influenza due to identified novel influenza A virus with other respiratory manifestations**
Influenza due to animal origin influenza A virus with other respiratory manifestations
Novel influenza A:
laryngitis
pharyngitis
respiratory infection (acute) (upper)

● 488.89 **Influenza due to identified novel influenza A virus with other manifestations**
Encephalopathy due to novel influenza A
Influenza due to animal origin influenza virus with encephalopathy
Influenza due to animal origin influenza virus with involvement of gastrointestinal tract
Novel influenza A with involvement of gastrointestinal tract

[Excludes:] *"intestinal flu" [viral gastroenteritis] (008.8)*

CHRONIC OBSTRUCTIVE PULMONARY DISEASE AND ALLIED CONDITIONS (490-496)

490 **Bronchitis, not specified as acute or chronic**
Bro nchitis NOS:
catarrhal
with tracheitis NOS
Tracheobronchitis NOS

[Excludes:] *bronchitis:*
allergic NOS (493.9)
asthmatic NOS (493.9)
due to fumes and vapors (506.0)

DEFINITION Bronchitis is an inflammation of the membranes lining the bronchial tubes.

491 **Chronic bronchitis**

[Excludes:] *chronic obstructive asthma (493.2)*

DEFINITION Chronic bronchitis is an inflammation of the membranes lining the bronchial tubes.

● Code new to 2012 edition ▲ Revision of existing code ④ ⑤ Fourth or fifth digit required

491.0 Simple chronic bronchitis
Catarrhal bronchitis, chronic
Smokers' cough

491.1 Mucopurulent chronic bronchitis
Bronchitis (chronic) (recurrent):
fetid
mucopurulent
purulent

[5] **491.2 Obstructive chronic bronchitis**
Bronchitis:
emphysematous
obstructive (chronic) (diffuse)
Bronchitis with:
chronic airway obstruction
emphysema

[Excludes:] asthmatic bronchitis (acute) NOS (493.9)
chronic obstructive asthma (493.2)

491.20 Without exacerbation
Emphysema with chronic bronchitis

491.21 With (acute) exacerbation
Acute exacerbation of chronic obstructive pulmonary disease [COPD]
Decompensated chronic obstructive pulmonary disease [COPD]
Decompensated chronic obstructive pulmonary disease [COPD] with exacerbation

[Excludes:] chronic obstructive asthma with acute exacerbation (493.22)

491.22 With acute bronchitis

491.8 Other chronic bronchitis
Chronic:
tracheitis
tracheobronchitis

491.9 Unspecified chronic bronchitis

492 Emphysema

[DEFINITION] Emphysema is a chronic respiratory disease where there is over-inflation of the air sacs (alveoli) in the lungs, causing a decrease in lung function, and often, breathlessness.

492.0 Emphysematous bleb
Giant bullous emphysema
Ruptured emphysematous bleb
Tension pneumatocele
Vanishing lung

492.8 Other emphysema
Emphysema (lung or pulmonary):
NOS
centriacinar
centrilobular
obstructive
panacinar
Emphysema (lung or pulmonary):
panlobular
unilateral
vesicular
MacLeod's syndrome
Swyer-James syndrome
Unilateral hyperlucent lung

[Excludes:] emphysema:
compensatory (518.2)
due to fumes and vapors (506.4)
interstitial (518.1)
newborn (770.2)
mediastinal (518.1)
surgical (subcutaneous) (998.81)
traumatic (958.7)
with chronic bronchitis (491.20-491.22)

493 Asthma

[Excludes:] wheezing NOS (786.07)

The following fifth-digit subclassification is for use with codes 493.0-493.2, 493.9:

0 unspecified

1 with status asthmaticus

2 with (acute) exacerbation

[DEFINITION] Asthma is a condition often of allergic origin that is marked by labored breathing accompanied by wheezing and a sense of constriction in the chest, and often by attacks of coughing or gasping

⑤ **493.0 extrinsic asthma**
[0-2] Asthma:
allergic with stated cause
atopic
childhood
hay
platinum
Hay fever with asthma

> Excludes: *asthma:*
> *allergic NOS (493.9)*
> *detergent (507.8)*
> *miners' (500)*
> *wood (495.8)*

⑤ **493.1 Intrinsic asthma**
[0-2] Late-onset asthma

⑤ **493.2 Chronic obstructive asthma**
[0-2] Asthma with chronic obstructive pulmonary disease [COPD]
Chronic asthmatic bronchitis

> Excludes: *chronic obstructive bronchitis (491.20-491.22)*
> *acute bronchitis (466.0)*

⑤ **493.8 Other forms of asthma**

493.81 Exercise induced bronchospasm

493.82 Cough variant asthma

⑤ **493.9 Asthma, unspecified**
[0-2] Asthma (bronchial) (allergic NOS)
Bronchitis:
allergic
asthmatic

494 Bronchiectasis
Bronchiectasis (fusiform) (postinfectious) (recurrent)
Bronchiolectasis

> Excludes: *congenital (748.61)*
> *tuberculous bronchiectasis (current disease) (011.5)*

DEFINITION Bronchiectasis is a condition characterized by abnormal dilatation of the bronchi (airways) and excessive mucus production. The mucus accumulation may obstruct the bronchi. Is often associated with repeated bronchial infections.

494.0 Bronchiectasis without acute exacerbation

494.1 Bronchiectasis with acute exacerbation

495 Extrinsic allergic alveolitis
Includes: allergic alveolitis and pneumonitis due to inhaled organic dust particles of fungal, thermophilic actinomycete, or other origin

DEFINITION Extrinsic allergic alveolitis is an inflammation of the alveoli in the lungs caused by inhaling dust.

495.0 Farmers' lung

495.1 Bagassosis

495.2 Bird-fanciers' lung
Budgerigar-fanciers' disease or lung
Pigeon-fanciers' disease or lung

495.3 Suberosis
Cork-handlers' disease or lung

495.4 Malt workers' lung
Alveolitis due to Aspergillus clavatus

495.5 Mushroom workers' lung

495.6 Maple bark-strippers' lung
Alveolitis due to Cryptostroma corticale

495.7 "Ventilation" pneumonitis
Allergic alveolitis due to fungal, thermophilic actinomycete, and other organisms growing in ventilation [air conditioning] systems

● Code new
to 2012 edition
▲ Revision of
existing code
④ ⑤ Fourth or fifth
digit required

495.8 Other specified allergic alveolitis and pneumonitis
Cheese-washers' lung
Coffee workers' lung
Fish-meal workers' lung
Furriers' lung
Grain-handlers' disease or lung
Pituitary snuff-takers' disease
Sequoiosis or red-cedar asthma
Wood asthma

495.9 Unspecified allergic alveolitis and pneumonitis
Alveolitis, allergic (extrinsic)
Hypersensitivity pneumonitis

496 Chronic airway obstruction, not elsewhere classified
Note: This code is not to be used with any code from categories 491-493
Chronic:
nonspecific lung disease
obstructive lung disease
obstructive pulmonary disease [COPD] NOS

> Excludes: *chronic obstructive lung disease [COPD] specified (as) (with):*
> *allergic alveolitis (495.0-495.9)*
> *asthma (493.2)*
> *bronchiectasis (494.0-494.1)*
> *bronchitis (491.20-491.22)*
> *with emphysema (491.20-491.22)*
> *decompensated (491.21)*
> *emphysema (492.0-492.8)*

DEFINITION Chronic airway obstruction is a pulmonary disorder, such as emphysema or chronic bronchitis, in which the upper or lower airway is chronically obstructed.

ALERT! Code 496 is a nonspecific code that should only be used when the documentation in a medical record does not specify the type of COPD being treated.

PNEUMOCONIOSES AND OTHER LUNG DISEASES DUE TO EXTERNAL AGENTS (500-508)

500 Coal workers' pneumoconiosis
Anthracosilicosis
Anthracosis
Black lung disease
Coal workers' lung
Miner's asthma

DEFINITION Coal workers' pneumoconiosis is a diseases characterized by fibrosis and scarring of the lungs caused by repeated inhalation of occupationally associated dust, such as silica, asbestos, and coal dust.

501 Asbestosis

DEFINITION Asbestosis is a condition featuring scarring of the lungs caused by inhaled asbestos fibers.

ALERT! For personal history of contact with and (suspected) exposure to asbestos see V15.84

502 Pneumoconiosis due to other silica or silicates
Pneumoconiosis due to talc
Silicotic fibrosis (massive) of lung
Silicosis (simple) (complicated)

DEFINITION Pneumoconiosis is a fibrosis and scarring of the lungs caused by repeated inhalation of occupationally associated dust, such as silica, asbestos, and coal dust.

503 Pneumoconiosis due to other inorganic dust
Aluminosis (of lung)
Bauxite fibrosis (of lung)
Berylliosis
Graphite fibrosis (of lung)
Siderosis
Stannosis

504 Pneumonopathy due to inhalation of other dust
Byssinosis
Cannabinosis
Flax-dressers' disease

> Excludes: *allergic alveolitis (495.0-495.9)*
> *asbestosis (501)*
> *bagassosis (495.1)*
> *farmers' lung (495.0)*

DEFINITION Pneumopathy due to inhalation of other dust is any disease of the lungs caused by dust inhalation

505 Pneumoconiosis, unspecified

DEFINITION Pneumoconiosis is fibrosis and scarring of the lungs as a result of repeated inhalation of occupationally associated dust, such as silica, asbestos, and coal dust.

Add 4th or 5th digit   Nonspecific code   Unspecified code   Manifestation code

506 **Respiratory conditions due to chemical fumes and vapors**
Use additional E code, if desired, to identify cause
Use additional code to identify associated respiratory conditions, such as:
acute respiratory failure (518.81)

506.0 **Bronchitis and pneumonitis due to fumes and vapors**
Chemical bronchitis (acute)

506.1 **Acute pulmonary edema due to fumes and vapors**
Chemical pulmonary edema (acute)

Excludes: *acute pulmonary edema NOS (518.4)*
chronic or unspecified pulmonary edema (514)

506.2 **Upper respiratory inflammation due to fumes and vapors**

506.3 **Other acute and subacute respiratory conditions due to fumes and vapors**

506.4 **Chronic respiratory conditions due to fumes and vapors**
Emphysema (diffuse) (chronic) due to inhalation of chemical fumes and vapors
Obliterative bronchiolitis (chronic) (subacute) due to inhalation of chemical fumes and vapors
Pulmonary fibrosis (chronic) due to inhalation of chemical fumes and vapors

506.9 **Unspecified respiratory conditions due to fumes and vapors**
Silo-fillers' disease

507 **Pneumonitis due to solids and liquids**

Excludes: *fetal aspiration pneumonitis (770.18)*
postprocedural pneumonitis (997.32)

507.0 **Due to inhalation of food or vomitus**
Aspiration pneumonia (due to):
NOS
food (regurgitated)
gastric secretions
milk
saliva
vomitus

507.1 **Due to inhalation of oils and essences**
Lipoid pneumonia (exogenous)

Excludes: *endogenous lipoid pneumonia (516.8)*

507.8 **Due to other solids and liquids**
Detergent asthma

508 **Respiratory conditions due to other and unspecified external agents**
Use additional E code, if desired, to identify cause
Use additional code to identify associated respiratory conditions, such as:
acute respiratory failure (518.81)

508.0 **Acute pulmonary manifestations due to radiation**
Radiation pneumonitis

508.1 **Chronic and other pulmonary manifestations due to radiation**
Fibrosis of lung following radiation

● **508.2** **Respiratory conditions due to smoke inhalation**
Smoke inhalation NOS

Excludes: *smoke inhalation due to chemical fumes and vapors (506.9)*

508.8 **Respiratory conditions due to other specified external agents**

508.9 **Respiratory conditions due to unspecified external agent**

OTHER DISEASES OF RESPIRATORY SYSTEM (510-519)

510 **Empyema**
Use additional code, if desired, to identify infectious organism (041.0-041.9)

Excludes: *abscess of lung (513.0)*

DEFINITION Empyema is a collection of pus within a naturally existing anatomical cavity

510.0 **With fistula**

Fistula:	Fistula:
bronchocutaneous	mediastinal
bronchopleural	pleural
hepatopleural	thoracic

Any condition classifiable to 510.9 with fistula

● Code new   ▲ Revision of   ④ ⑤ Fourth or fifth
         to 2012 edition   existing code   digit required

510.9 Without mention of fistula

Abscess:
  pleura
  thorax
Empyema (chest) (lung) (pleura)
Fibrinopurulent pleurisy
Pleurisy:
  purulent
  septic
  seropurulent
  suppurative
Pyopneumothorax
Pyothorax

511 Pleurisy

[Excludes:] *pleurisy with mention of tuberculosis, current disease (012.0)*

[DEFINITION] Pleurisy is an inflammation of the membrane that surrounds and protects the lungs (the pleura). Inflammation occurs when an infection or damaging agent irritates the pleural surface.

511.0 Without mention of effusion or current tuberculosis

Adhesion, lung or pleura
Calcification of pleura
Pleurisy (acute) (sterile):
  diaphragmatic
  fibrinous
  interlobar
Pleurisy:
  NOS
  pneumococcal
  staphylococcal
  streptococcal
Thickening of pleura

511.1 With effusion, with mention of a bacterial cause other than tuberculosis

Pleurisy with effusion (exudative) (serous):
  pneumococcal
  staphylococcal
  streptococcal
  other specified nontuberculous bacterial cause

[5] **511.8 Other specified forms of effusion, except tuberculous**

[Excludes:] *traumatic (860.2-860.5, 862.29, 862.39)*

511.81 Malignant pleural effusion

Code first malignant neoplasm, if known

511.89 Other specified forms of effusion, except tuberculous

Encysted pleurisy
Hemopneumothorax
Hemothorax
Hydropneumothorax
Hydrothorax

511.9 Unspecified pleural effusion

Pleural effusion NOS
Pleurisy:
  exudative
  serofibrinous
Pleurisy:
  serous
  with effusion NOS

▲ **512 Pneumothorax and air leak**

[DEFINITION] Pneumothorax is a collection of air or gas in the chest or pleural space that causes part or all of a lung to collapse

512.0 Spontaneous tension pneumothorax

512.1 Iatrogenic pneumothorax

Postoperative pneumothorax

● **512.2 Postoperative air leak**

▲ **512.8 Other pneumothorax and air leak**

[Excludes:] *pneumothorax:*
  congenital (770.2)
  traumatic (860.0-860.1, 860.4-860.5)
  tuberculous, current disease (011.7)

● **512.81 Primary spontaneous pneumothorax**

● *512.82* **Secondary spontaneous pneumothorax**

Code first underlying condition, such as:
 cancer metastatic to lung (197.0)
 catamenial pneumothorax due to endometriosis (617.8)
 cystic fibrosis (277.02)
 eosinophilic pneumonia (518.3)
 lymphangioleiomyomatosis (516.4)
 Marfan syndrome (759.82)
 pneumocystis carinii pneumonia (136.3)
 primary lung cancer (162.3-162.9)
 spontaneous rupture of the esophagus (530.4)

● **512.83** **Chronic pneumothorax**

● **512.84** **Other air leak**
 Persistent air leak

● **512.89** **Other pneumothorax**
 Acute pneumothorax
 Pneumothorax NOS
 Spontaneous pneumothorax NOS

513 **Abscess of lung and mediastinum**

DEFINITION The mediastinum refers to the area in the middle of the chest containing the heart, great vessels, esophagus and other structures.

513.0 **Abscess of lung**
 Abscess (multiple) of lung
 Gangrenous or necrotic pneumonia
 Pulmonary gangrene or necrosis

513.1 **Abscess of mediastinum**

514 **Pulmonary congestion and hypostasis**
 Hypostatic:
  bronchopneumonia
  pneumonia
 Passive pneumonia
 Pulmonary congestion (chronic) (passive)
 Pulmonary edema:
  NOS
  chronic

 Excludes: acute pulmonary edema:
  NOS (518.4)
  with mention of heart disease or failure (428.1)
  hypostatic pneumonia due to or specified as a specific type of pneumonia – code
   to the type of pneumonia (480.0-480.9, 481, 482.0-482.9, 483.0-483.8, 487.0,
   488.01, 488.11)

DEFINITION Pulmonary congestion and hypostasis refers to excess fluid or blood in the lungs

515 **Postinflammatory pulmonary fibrosis**
 Cirrhosis of lung, chronic or unspecified
 Fibrosis of lung (atrophic) (confluent) (massive) (perialveolar) (peribronchial), chronic or
  unspecified
 Induration of lung, chronic or unspecified

DEFINITION Pulmonary fibrosis is a condition characterized by deposition of fibrous tissue in the lung. It decreases lung compliance and results in a restrictive ventilatory defect as seen on pulmonary function testing.

516 **Other alveolar and parietoalveolar pneumonopathy**

516.0 **Pulmonary alveolar proteinosis**

516.1 **Idiopathic pulmonary hemosiderosis**
 Essential brown induration of lung

 Code first underlying disease (275.01-275.09)

 Excludes: acute idiopathic pulmonary hemorrhage in infants [AIPHI] (786.31)

516.2 **Pulmonary alveolar microlithiasis**

▲ **516.3** **Idiopathic interstitial pneumonia**

● **516.30** **Idiopathic interstitial pneumonia, not otherwise specified**
 Idiopathic fibrosing alveolitis

● **516.31** **Idiopathic pulmonary fibrosis**
 Cryptogenic fibrosing alveolitis

● Code new
 to 2012 edition
▲ Revision of
 existing code
④ ⑤ Fourth or fifth
 digit required

● **516.32 Idiopathic non-specific interstitial pneumonitis**

Excludes: *non-specific interstitial pneumonia NOS, or due to known underlying cause (516.8)*

● **516.33 Acute interstitial pneumonitis**
Hamman-Rich syndrome

Excludes: *pneumocystis pneumonia (136.3)*

● **516.34 Respiratory bronchiolitis interstitial lung disease**

● **516.35 Idiopathic lymphoid interstitial pneumonia**
Idiopathic lymphocytic interstitial pneumonitis

Excludes: *lymphoid interstitial pneumonia NOS, or due to known underlying cause (516.8)*
pneumocystis pneumonia (136.3)

● **516.36 Cryptogenic organizing pneumonia**

Excludes: *organizing pneumonia NOS, or due to known underlying cause (516.8)*

● **516.37 Desquamative interstitial pneumonia**

● **516.4 Lymphangioleiomyomatosis**
Lymphangiomyomatosis

● **516.5 Adult pulmonary Langerhans cell histiocytosis**
Adult PLCH

● **516.6 Interstitial lung diseases of childhood**

● **516.61 Neuroendocrine cell hyperplasia of infancy**

● **516.62 Pulmonary interstitial glycogenosis**

● **516.63 Surfactant mutations of the lung**

● **516.64 Alveolar capillary dysplasia with vein misalignment**

● **516.69 Other interstitial lung diseases of childhood**

516.8 Other specified alveolar and parietoalveolar pneumonopathies
Endogenous lipoid pneumonia
Interstitial pneumonia
Lymphoid interstitial pneumonia due to known underlying cause
Lymphoid interstitial pneumonia NOS
Non-specific interstitial pneumonia due to known underlying cause
Non-specific interstitial pneumonia NOS
Organizing pneumonia due to known underlying cause
Organizing pneumonia NOS

Code first, if applicable, underlying cause of pneumonopathy, if known
Use additional E code, if applicable, for drug-induced or toxic pneumonopathy

Excludes: *cryptogenic organizing pneumonia (516.36)*
idiopathic lymphoid interstitial pneumonia (516.35)
idiopathic non-specific interstitial pneumonitis (516.32)
lipoid pneumonia, exogenous or unspecified (507.1)

516.9 Unspecified alveolar and parietoalveolar pneumonopathy

517 Lung involvement in conditions classified elsewhere

Excludes: *rheumatoid lung (714.81)*

517.1 *Rheumatic pneumonia*
Code first underlying disease (390)

517.2 *Lung involvement in systemic sclerosis*
Code first underlying disease (710.1)

517.3 *Acute chest syndrome*
Code first sickle-cell disease in crisis (282.42, 282.62, 282.64, 282.69)

517.8 *Lung involvement in other diseases classified elsewhere*
Code first underlying disease, as:
amyloidosis (277.30-277.39)
polymyositis (710.4)
sarcoidosis (135)
Sjögren's disease (710.2)
systemic lupus erythematosus (710.0)

Excludes: *syphilis (095.1)*

518 Other diseases of lung

Add 4th or 5th digit Nonspecific code Unspecified code Manifestation code

518.0 Pulmonary collapse
  Atelectasis
  Collapse of lung
  Middle lobe syndrome

Excludes: *atelectasis:*
      congenital (partial) (770.5)
        primary (770.4)
      tuberculous, current disease (011.8)

518.1 Interstitial emphysema
  Mediastinal emphysema

Excludes: *surgical (subcutaneous) emphysema (998.81)*
      that in fetus or newborn (770.2)
      traumatic emphysema (958.7)

518.2 Compensatory emphysema

518.3 Pulmonary eosinophilia
  Eosinophilic asthma   Tropical eosinophilia
  Löffler's syndrome
  Pneumonia:
   allergic
   eosinophilic

Excludes: *pulmonary infiltrate NOS (793.19)*

518.4 Acute edema of lung, unspecified
  Acute pulmonary edema NOS
  Pulmonary edema, postoperative

Excludes: *pulmonary edema:*
      acute, with mention of heart disease or failure (428.1)
      chronic or unspecified (514)
      due to external agents (506.0-508.9)

⑤ **518.5 Pulmonary insufficiency following trauma and surgery**

Excludes: *adult respiratory distress syndrome associated with other conditions (518.82)*
      pneumonia:
       aspiration (507.0)
       hypostatic (514)
      respiratory failure in other conditions (518.81, 518.83-518.84)

● **518.51 Acute respiratory failure following trauma and surgery**
      Respiratory failure, not otherwise specified, following trauma and surgery

Excludes: *acute respiratory failure in other conditions (518.81)*

● **518.52 Other pulmonary insufficiency, not elsewhere classified, following trauma and surgery**
      Adult respiratory distress syndrome
      Pulmonary insufficiency following surgery
      Pulmonary insufficiency following trauma
      Shock lung related to trauma and surgery

Excludes: *adult respiratory distress syndrome associated with other conditions (518.82)*
      aspiration pneumonia (507.0)
      hypostatic pneumonia (514)
      shock lung, not related to trauma or surgery (518.82)

● **518.53 Acute and chronic respiratory failure following trauma and surgery**

Excludes: *acute and chronic respiratory failure in other conditions (518.84)*

518.6 Allergic bronchopulmonary aspergillosis

518.7 Transfusion related acute lung injury (TRALI)

⑤ **518.8 Other diseases of lung**

● Code new   ▲ Revision of   ④ ⑤ Fourth or fifth
        to 2012 edition   existing code   digit required

518.81   Acute respiratory failure
Respiratory failure NOS

Excludes: *acute and chronic respiratory failure (518.84)*
acute respiratory distress (518.82)
acute respiratory failure following trauma and surgery (518.51)
chronic respiratory failure (518.83)
respiratory arrest (799.1)
respiratory failure, newborn (770.84)

ALERT! Code 518.81 may be assigned as a principal diagnosis when it is the condition established after study to be chiefly responsible for occasioning the admission to the hospital, and the selection is supported by the Alphabetic Index and Tabular List

518.82   Other pulmonary insufficiency, not elsewhere classified
Acute respiratory distress
Acute respiratory insufficiency
Adult respiratory distress syndrome NEC

Excludes: *acute interstitial pneumonitis (516.33)*
adult respiratory distress syndrome associated with trauma or surgery (518.52)
pulmonary insufficiency following trauma or surgery (518.52)
respiratory distress:
NOS (786.09)
newborn (770.89)
syndrome, newborn (769)

518.83   Chronic respiratory failure

518.84   Acute and chronic respiratory failure
Acute or chronic respiratory failure

Excludes: *acute and chronic respiratory failure following trauma or surgery (518.53)*

518.89   Other diseases of lung, not elsewhere classified

Broncholithiasis	Lung disease NOS
Calcification of lung	Pulmolithiasis

519   Other diseases of respiratory system
ALERT! For personal history of other diseases of respiratory system see V12.69

⑤ **519.0   Tracheostomy complications**

519.00   Tracheostomy complication, unspecified

519.01   Infection of tracheostomy
Use additional code to identify type of infection, such as:
abscess or cellulitis of neck (682.1)
septicemia (038.0-038.9)

Use additional code to identify organism (041.00-041.9)

519.02   Mechanical complication of tracheostomy
Tracheal stenosis due to tracheostomy

519.09   Other tracheostomy complications
Hemorrhage due to tracheostomy
Tracheoesophageal fistula due to tracheostomy

⑤ **519.1   Other diseases of trachea and bronchus, not elsewhere classified**

519.11   Acute bronchospasm
Bronchospasm NOS

Excludes: *acute bronchitis with bronchospasm (466.0)*
asthma (493.00-493.92)
exercise induced bronchospasm (493.81)

519.19   Other diseases of trachea and bronchus
Calcification of bronchus or trachea
Stenosis of bronchus or trachea
Ulcer of bronchus or trachea

519.2   Mediastinitis

519.3   Other diseases of mediastinum, not elsewhere classified
Fibrosis of mediastinum
Hernia of mediastinum
Retraction of mediastinum

▰ Add 4th or 5th digit	▨ Nonspecific code	▱ Unspecified code	▤ Manifestation code

519.4 Disorders of diaphragm
Diaphragmitis
Paralysis of diaphragm
Relaxation of diaphragm

Excludes: *congenital defect of diaphragm (756.6)*
diaphragmatic hernia (551-553 with .3)
congenital (756.6)

519.8 Other diseases of respiratory system, not elsewhere classified

519.9 Unspecified disease of respiratory system
Respiratory disease (chronic) NOS

ALERT! For personal history of unspecified disease of respiratory system see V12.60

● Code new   ▲ Revision of   ④ ⑤ Fourth or fifth
         to 2012 edition   existing code   digit required

Chapter 9: Diseases of Digestive System (520-579)

DEFINITIONS AND CODING ALERTS

This chapter includes definitions of selected key words, terms and phrases and coding alerts for adding points to the clinical domain, references to coding late effects where appropriate, and references to personal history V-codes in situations where the acute or chronic condition is no longer active. An example from this chapter is as follows:

⑤ **533** **Peptic ulcer, site unspecified**

> **DEFINITION** A Peptic ulcer is an ulcer of the mucous membrane lining of the alimentary tract.
>
> **ALERT!** For personal history of peptic ulcer disease see V12.71

MULTIPLE CODING FOR A SINGLE CONDITION

In addition to the etiology or manifestation convention that requires two codes to fully describe a single condition that affects multiple body systems, there are other single conditions that also require more than one code. "Use additional code" notes are found in the tabular at codes that are not part of an etiology or manifestation pair where a secondary code is useful to fully describe a condition. The sequencing rule is the same as the etiology or manifestation pair - , "use additional code" indicates that a secondary code should be added.

"Code first" notes are also under certain codes that are not specifically manifestation codes but may be due to an underlying cause. When a "code first" note is present and an underlying condition is present the underlying condition should be sequenced first.

"Code, if applicable, any causal condition first", notes indicate that this code may be assigned as a principal diagnosis when the causal condition is unknown or not applicable. If a causal condition is known, then the code for that condition should be sequenced as the principal or first-listed diagnosis. Multiple codes may be needed for late effects, complication codes and obstetric codes to more fully describe a condition. See the specific guidelines for these conditions for further instruction.

COMBINATION CODE

A combination code is a single code used to classify: two diagnoses, or a diagnosis with an associated secondary process (manifestation) A diagnosis with an associated complication Combination codes are identified by referring to subterm entries in the Alphabetic Index and by reading the inclusion and exclusion notes in the Tabular List.

Assign only the combination code when that code fully identifies the diagnostic conditions involved or when the Alphabetic Index so directs. Multiple coding should not be used when the classification provides a combination code that clearly identifies all of the elements documented in the diagnosis. When the combination code lacks necessary specificity in describing the manifestation or complication, an additional code should be used as a secondary code.

CODING LATE EFFECTS

A late effect is the residual effect (condition produced) after the acute phase of an illness or injury has terminated. There is no time limit on when a late effect code can be used. The residual may be apparent early, such as in cerebrovascular accident cases, or it may occur months or years later, such as that due to a previous injury. Coding of late effects generally requires two codes sequenced in the following order: The condition or nature of the late effect is sequenced first. The late effect code is sequenced second.

An exception to the above guidelines are those instances where the code for late effect is followed by a manifestation code identified in the Tabular List and title, or the late effect code has been expanded (at the fourth and fifth-digit levels) to include the manifestation(s). The code for the acute phase of an illness or injury that led to the late effect is never used with a code for the late effect.

	Add 4th or 5th digit		Nonspecific code		Unspecified code		Manifestation code

This page intentionally left blank.

● Code new
to 2012 edition
▲ Revision of
existing code
④ ⑤ Fourth or fifth
digit required

9. DISEASES OF THE DIGESTIVE SYSTEM (520-579)

[ALERT!] For personal history of digestive disease see V12.7

DISEASES OF ORAL CAVITY, SALIVARY GLANDS, AND JAWS (520-529)

520 Disorders of tooth development and eruption

520.0 Anodontia
Absence of teeth (complete) (congenital) (partial)
Hypodontia
Oligodontia

[Excludes:] *acquired absence of teeth (525.10-525.19)*

520.1 Supernumerary teeth
Distomolar
Fourth molar
Mesiodens
Paramolar
Supplemental teeth

[Excludes:] *supernumerary roots (520.2)*

520.2 Abnormalities of size and form
Concrescence of teeth
Fusion of teeth
Gemination of teeth
Dens evaginatus
Dens in dente
Dens invaginatus
Enamel pearls
Macrodontia
Microdontia
Peg-shaped [conical] teeth
Supernumerary roots
Taurodontism
Tuberculum paramolare

[Excludes:] *that due to congenital syphilis (090.5)*
tuberculum Carabelli, which is regarded as a normal variation

520.3 Mottled teeth
Dental fluorosis
Mottling of enamel
Nonfluoride enamel opacities

520.4 Disturbances of tooth formation
Aplasia and hypoplasia of cementum
Dilaceration of tooth
Enamel hypoplasia (neonatal) (postnatal) (prenatal)
Horner's teeth
Hypocalcification of teeth
Regional odontodysplasia
Turner's tooth

[Excludes:] *Hutchinson's teeth and mulberry molars in congenital syphilis (090.5)*
mottled teeth (520.3)

520.5 Hereditary disturbances in tooth structure, not elsewhere classified
Amelogenesis imperfecta
Dentinogenesis imperfecta
Odontogenesis imperfecta
Dentinal dysplasia
Shell teeth

520.6 Disturbances of tooth eruption
Teeth:
- embedded
- impacted
- natal
- neonatal
- prenatal
- primary [deciduous]:
  - persistent
  - shedding, premature

Tooth eruption:
- late
- obstructed
- premature

[Excludes:] *exfoliation of teeth (attributable to disease of surrounding tissues) (525.0-525.19)*

520.7 Teething syndrome

520.8 Other specified disorders of tooth development and eruption
Color changes during tooth formation
Pre-eruptive color changes

[Excludes:] *posteruptive color changes (521.7)*

520.9 Unspecified disorder of tooth development and eruption

521 Diseases of hard tissue of teeth

[5] **521.0 Dental caries**

521.00 Dental caries, unspecified

Add 4th or 5th digit | Nonspecific code | Unspecified code | Manifestation code

521.01 Dental caries limited to enamel
Initial caries
White spot lesion

521.02 Dental caries extending into dentine

521.03 Dental caries extending into pulp

521.04 Arrested dental caries

521.05 Odontoclasia
Infantile melanodontia
Melanodontoclasia

[Excludes:] *internal and external resorption of teeth (521.40-521.49)*

521.06 Dental caries pit and fissure
Primary dental caries, pit and fissure origin

521.07 Dental caries of smooth surface
Primary dental caries, smooth surface origin

521.08 Dental caries of root surface
Primary dental caries, root surface

521.09 Other dental caries

[5] **521.1 Excessive attrition (approximal wear) (occlusal wear)**

521.10 Excessive attrition, unspecified

521.11 Excessive attrition, limited to enamel

521.12 Excessive attrition, extending into dentine

521.13 Excessive attrition, extending into pulp

521.14 Excessive attrition, localized

521.15 Excessive attrition, generalized

[5] **521.2 Abrasion**
Abrasion of teeth:
dentifrice
habitual
occupational
ritual
traditional
Wedge defect NOS of teeth

521.20 Abrasion, unspecified

521.21 Abrasion, limited to enamal

521.22 Abrasion, extending into dentine

521.23 Abrasion, extending into pulp

521.24 Abrasion, localized

521.25 Abrasion, generalized

[5] **521.3 Erosion**
Erosion of teeth:
NOS
due to:
medicine
persistent vomiting
Erosion of teeth:
idiopathic
occupational

521.30 Erosion, unspecified

521.31 Erosion, limited to enamal

521.32 Erosion, extending into dentine

521.33 Erosion, extending into pulp

521.34 Erosion, localized

521.35 Erosion, generalized

[5] **521.4 Pathological resorption**

521.40 Pathological resorption, unspecified

521.41 Pathological resorption, internal

521.42 Pathological resorption, external

521.49 Other pathological resorption
Internal granuloma of pulp

521.5 Hypercementosis
Cementation hyperplasia

521.6 Ankylosis of teeth

521.7 Intrinsic posteruptive color changes
Staining [discoloration] of teeth:
 NOS
 due to:
  drugs
  metals
  pulpal bleeding

Excludes: *accretions [deposits] on teeth (523.6)*
      extrinsic color changes (523.6)
      pre-eruptive color changes (520.8)

⑤ **521.8 Other specific diseases of hard tissues of teeth**

521.81 Cracked tooth

Excludes: *asymptomatic craze lines in enamel – omit code*
      broken tooth due to trauma (873.63, 873.73)
      fractured tooth due to trauma (873.63, 873.73)

521.89 Other specific diseases of hard tissues of teeth
Irradiated enamel
Sensitive dentin

521.9 Unspecified disease of hard tissues of teeth

522 Diseases of pulp and periapical tissues
DEFINITION Pulp is the part in the center of a tooth made up of living soft tissue and cells called odontoblasts.

522.0 Pulpitis

Pulpal:	Pulpitis:
abscess	acute
polyp	chronic (hyperplastic) (ulcerative)
	suppurative

522.1 Necrosis of the pulp
Pulp gangrene

522.2 Pulp degeneration
Denticles
Pulp calcifications
Pulp stones

522.3 Abnormal hard tissue formation in pulp
Secondary or irregular dentin

522.4 Acute apical periodontitis of pulpal origin

522.5 Periapical abscess without sinus
Abscess:
 dental
 dentoalveolar

Excludes: *periapical abscess with sinus (522.7)*

522.6 Chronic apical periodontitis
Apical or periapical granuloma
Apical periodontitis NOS

522.7 Periapical abscess with sinus
Fistula:
 alveolar process
 dental

522.8 Radicular cyst
Cyst:
 apical (periodontal)
 periapical
 radiculodental
 residual radicular

Excludes: *lateral developmental or lateral periodontal cyst (526.0)*

522.9 Other and unspecified diseases of pulp and periapical tissues

523 Gingival and periodontal diseases
DEFINITION Gingival and periodontal diseases are diseases of the gums and/or tissue and bones that support the teeth

Add 4th or 5th digit	Nonspecific code	Unspecified code	Manifestation code

⑤ **523.0 Acute gingivitis**

[Excludes:] *acute necrotizing ulcerative gingivitis (101)*
herpetic gingivostomatitis (054.2)

523.00 Acute gingivitis, plaque induced
Acute gingivitis NOS

523.01 Acute gingivitis, non-plaque induced

⑤ **523.1 Chronic gingivitis**
Gingivitis (chronic):
desquamative
hyperplastic
Gingivitis (chronic):
simple marginal
ulcerative

[Excludes:] *herpetic gingivostomatitis (054.2)*

523.10 Chronic gingivitis, plaque induced
Chronic gingivitis NOS
Gingivitis NOS

523.11 Chronic gingivitis, non-plaque induced

⑤ **523.2 Gingival recession**
Gingival recession (postinfective) (postoperative)

523.20 Gingival recession, unspecified

523.21 Gingival recession, minimal

523.22 Gingival recession, moderate

523.23 Gingival recession, severe

523.24 Gingival recession, localized

523.25 Gingival recession, generalized

⑤ **523.3 Aggressive and acute periodontitis**
Acute:
pericementitis
pericoronitis

[Excludes:] *acute apical periodontitis (522.4)*
periapical abscess (522.5, 522.7)

523.30 Aggressive periodontitis, unspecified

523.31 Aggressive periodontitis, localized
Periodontal abscess

523.32 Aggressive periodontitis, generalized

523.33 Aggressive periodontitis

⑤ **523.4 Chronic periodontitis**
Chronic pericoronitis
Pericementitis (chronic)
Periodontitis:
NOS
complex
simplex

[Excludes:] *chronic apical periodontitis (522.6)*

523.40 Chronic periodontitis, unspecified

523.41 Chronic periodontitis, localized

523.42 Chronic periodontitis, generalized

523.5 Periodontosis

523.6 Accretions on teeth
Dental calculus:
subgingival
supragingival
Deposits on teeth:
betel
materia alba
soft
tartar
tobacco
Extrinsic discoloration of teeth

[Excludes:] *intrinsic discoloration of teeth (521.7)*

● Code new to 2012 edition ▲ Revision of existing code ④ ⑤ Fourth or fifth digit required

523.8 Other specified periodontal diseases

Giant cell:
- epulis
- peripheral granuloma

Gingival:
- cysts
- enlargement NOS
- fibromatosis

Gingival polyp
Periodontal lesions due to traumatic occlusion
Peripheral giant cell granuloma

[Excludes:] *leukoplakia of gingiva (528.6)*

523.9 Unspecified gingival and periodontal disease

524 Dentofacial anomalies, including malocclusion

DEFINITION Dentofacial anomalies, including malocclusion, malocclusion is a misalignment of teeth and/or incorrect relation between the teeth of the two dental arches.

[5] **524.0 Major anomalies of jaw size**

[Excludes:] *hemifacial atrophy or hypertrophy (754.0)*
unilateral condylar hyperplasia or hypoplasia of mandible (526.89)

524.00 Unspecified anomaly

524.01 Maxillary hyperplasia

524.02 Mandibular hyperplasia

524.03 Maxillary hypoplasia

524.04 Mandibular hypoplasia

524.05 Macrogenia

524.06 Microgenia

524.07 Excessive tuberosity of jaw
Entire maxillary tuberosity

524.09 Other specified anomaly

[5] **524.1 Anomalies of relationship of jaw to cranial base**

524.10 Unspecified anomaly
prognathism
retrognathism

524.11 Maxillary asymmetry

524.12 Other jaw asymmetry

524.19 Other specified anomaly

[5] **524.2 Anomalies of dental arch relationship**
Anomaly of dental arch

[Excludes:] *hemifacial atrophy or hypertrophy (754.0)*
soft tissue impingement (524.81-524.82)
unilateral condylar hyperplasia or hypoplasia of mandible (526.89)

524.20 Unspecified anomaly of dental arch relationship

524.21 Malocclusion, Angle's class I
Neutro-occlusion

524.22 Malocclusion, Angle's class II
Disto-occlusion Division I
Disto-occlusion Division II

524.23 Malocclusion, Angle's class III
Mesio-occlusion

524.24 Open anterior occlusal relationship
Anterior open bite

524.25 Open posterior occlusal relationship
Posterior open bite

524.26 Excessive horizontal overlap
Excessive horizontal overjet

524.27 Reverse articulation
Anterior articulation
Crossbite
Posterior articulation

524.28 Anomalies of interarch distance
Excessive interarch distance
Inadequate interarch distance

524.29 **Other anomalies of dental arch relationship**
Other anomalies of dental arch

⑤ **524.3** **Anomalies of tooth position of fully erupted teeth**

Excludes: *impacted or embedded teeth with abnormal position of such teeth or adjacent teeth (520.6)*

524.30 **Unspecified anomaly of tooth position**
Diastema of teeth NOS
Displacement of teeth NOS
Transposition of teeth NOS

524.31 **Crowding of teeth**

524.32 **Excessive spacing of teeth**

524.33 **Horizontal displacement of teeth**
Tipped teeth
Tipping of teeth

524.34 **Vertical displacement of teeth**
Extruded tooth
Infraeruption of teeth
Intruded tooth
Supraeruption of teeth

524.35 **Rotation of tooth/teeth**

524.36 **Insufficient interocclusal distance of teeth (ridge)**
Lack of adequate intermaxillary vertical dimension

524.37 **Excessive interocclusal distance of teeth**
Excessive intermaxillary vertical dimension
Loss of occlusal vertical dimension

524.39 **Other anomalies of tooth position**

524.4 **Malocclusion, unspecified**

⑤ **524.5** **Dentofacial functional abnormalities**

524.50 **Dentofacial functional abnormality, unspecified**

524.51 **Abnormal jaw closure**

524.52 **Limited mandibular range of motion**

524.53 **Deviation in opening and closing of the mandible**

524.54 **Insufficient anterior guidance**
Insufficient anterior occlusal guidance

524.55 **Centric occlusion maximum intercuspation discrepancy**
Centric occlusion of teeth discrepancy

524.56 **Non-working side interference**
Balancing side interference

524.57 **Lack of posterior occlusal support**

524.59 **Other dentofacial functional abnormalities**
Abnormal swallowing
Mouth breathing
Sleep postures
Tongue, lip, or finger habits

⑤ **524.6** **Temporomandibular joint disorders**

Excludes: *current temporomandibular joint:*
dislocation (830.0-830.1)
strain (848.1)

524.60 **Temporomandibular joint disorders, unspecified**
Temporomandibular joint-pain-dysfunction syndrome [TMJ]

524.61 **Adhesions and ankylosis (bony or fibrous)**

524.62 **Arthralgia of temporomandibular joint**

524.63 **Articular disc disorder (reducing or non-reducing)**

524.64 **Temporomandibular joint sounds on opening and/or closing the jaw**

524.69 **Other specified temporomandibular joint disorders**

⑤ **524.7** **Dental alveolar anomalies**

524.70 **Unspecified alveolar anomaly**

524.71 **Alveolar maxillary hyperplasia**

524.72 **Alveolar mandibular hyperplasia**

● Code new
to 2012 edition

▲ Revision of
existing code

④ ⑤ Fourth or fifth
digit required

524.73 Alveolar maxillary hypoplasia

524.74 Alveolar mandibular hypoplasia

524.75 Vertical displacement of alveolus and teeth
Extrusion of alveolus and teeth

524.76 Occlusal plane deviation

524.79 Other specified alveolar anomaly

[5] **524.8 Other specified dentofacial anomalies**

524.81 Anterior soft tissue impingement

524.82 Posterior soft tissue impingement

524.89 Other specified dentofacial anomalies

524.9 Unspecified dentofacial anomalies

525 Other diseases and conditions of the teeth and supporting structures
[ALERT!] For personal history of other specified digestive system diseases see V12.79

525.0 Exfoliation of teeth due to systemic causes

[5] **525.1 Loss of teeth due to trauma, extraction, or periodontal disease**
Code first class of edentulism (525.40-525.44, 525.50-525.54)

525.10 Acquired absence of teeth, unspecified
Tooth extraction status, NOS

525.11 Loss of teeth due to trauma

525.12 Loss of teeth due to periodontal disease

525.13 Loss of teeth due to caries

525.19 Other loss of teeth

[5] **525.2 Atrophy of edentulous alveolar ridge**

525.20 Unspecified atrophy of edentulous alveolar ridge
Atrophy of the mandible NOS
Atrophy of the maxilla NOS

525.21 Minimal atrophy of the mandible

525.22 Moderate atrophy of the mandible

525.23 Severe atrophy of the mandible

525.24 Minimal atrophy of the maxilla

525.25 Moderate atrophy of the maxilla

525.26 Severe atrophy of the maxilla

525.3 Retained dental root

[5] **525.4 Complete edentulism**
Use additional code to identify cause of edentulism (525.10-525.19)

525.40 Complete edentulism, unspecified
Edentulism NOS

525.41 Complete edentulism, class I

525.42 Complete edentulism, class II

525.43 Complete edentulism, class III

525.44 Complete edentulism, class IV

[5] **525.5 Partial edentulism**
Use additional code to identify cause of edentulism (525.10-525.19)

525.50 Partial edentulism, unspecified

525.51 Partial edentulism, class I

525.52 Partial edentulism, class II

525.53 Partial edentulism, class III

525.54 Partial edentulism, class IV

[5] **525.6 Unsatisfactory restoration of tooth**
Defective bridge, crown, fillings
Defective dental restoration

[Excludes:] dental restoration status (V45.84)
unsatisfactory endodontic treatment (526.61-526.69)

525.60 Unspecified unsatisfactory restoration of tooth
Unspecified defective dental restoration

525.61 Open restoration margins
Dental restoration failure of marginal integrity
Open margin on tooth restoration

525.62 Unrepairable overhanging of dental restorative materials
Overhanging of tooth restoration

525.63 Fractured dental restorative material without loss of material

Excludes: *cracked tooth (521.81)*
fractured tooth (873.63, 873.73)

525.64 Fractured dental restorative material with loss of material

Excludes: *cracked tooth (521.81)*
fractured tooth (873.63, 873.73)

525.65 Contour of existing restoration of tooth biologically incompatible with oral health
Dental restoration failure of periodontal anatomical integrity
Unacceptable contours of existing restoration
Unacceptable morphology of existing restoration

525.66 Allergy to existing dental restorative material
Use additional code to identify the specific type of allergy

525.67 Poor aesthetics of existing restoration
Dental restoration aesthetically inadequate or displeasing

525.69 Other unsatisfactory restoration of existing tooth

⑤ **525.7 Endosseous dental implant failure**

525.71 Osseointegration failure of dental implant
Failure of dental implant due to infection
Failure of dental implant due to unintentional loading
Failure of dental implant osseointegration due to premature loading
Failure of dental implant to osseointegrate prior to intentional prosthetic loading
Hemorrhagic complications of dental implant placement
Iatrogenic osseointegration failure of dental implant
Osseointegration failure of dental implant due to complications of systemic disease
Osseointegration failure of dental implant due to poor bone quality
Pre-integration failure of dental implant NOS
Pre-osseointegration failure of dental implant

525.72 Post-osseointegration biological failure of dental implant
Failure of dental implant due to lack of attached gingiva
Failure of dental implant due to occlusal trauma (caused by poor prosthetic design)
Failure of dental implant to osseointegrate following intentional prosthetic loading
Failure of dental implant due to parafunctional habits
Failure of dental implant due to periodontal infection (peri-implantitis)
Failure of dental implant due to poor oral hygiene
Iatrogenic post-osseointegration failure of dental implant
Post-osseointegration failure of dental implant due to complications of systemic disease

525.73 Post-osseointegration mechanical failure of dental implant
Failure of dental prosthesis causing loss of dental implant
Fracture of dental implant
Mechanical failure of dental implant NOS

Excludes: *cracked tooth (521.81)*
fractured dental restorative material with loss of material (525.64)
fractured dental restorative material without loss of material (525.63)
fractured tooth (873.63, 873.73)

525.79 Other endosseous dental implant failure
Dental implant failure NOS

525.8 Other specified disorders of the teeth and supporting structures
Enlargement of alveolar ridge NOS
Irregular alveolar process

525.9 Unspecified disorder of the teeth and supporting structures

● Code new to 2012 edition   ▲ Revision of existing code   ④ ⑤ Fourth or fifth digit required

<u>526</u> **Diseases of the jaws**

526.0 Developmental odontogenic cysts
Cyst:
  dentigerous
  eruption
  follicular
  lateral developmental
Cyst:
  lateral periodontal
  primordial
  Keratocyst

Excludes: radicular cyst (522.8)

526.1 Fissural cysts of jaw
Cyst:
  globulomaxillary
  incisor canal
  median anterior maxillary
  median palatal
  nasopalatine
  palatine of papilla

Excludes: cysts of oral soft tissues (528.4)

526.2 Other cysts of jaws
Cyst of jaw:
  NOS
  aneurysmal
Cyst of jaw:
  hemorrhagic
  traumatic

526.3 Central giant cell (reparative) granuloma

Excludes: peripheral giant cell granuloma (523.8)

526.4 Inflammatory conditions
Abscess of jaw (acute) (chronic) (suppurative)
Osteitis of jaw (acute) (chronic) (suppurative)
Osteomyelitis (neonatal) of jaw (acute) (chronic) (suppurative)
Periostitis of jaw (acute) (chronic) (suppurative)
Sequestrum of jaw bone

Excludes: alveolar osteitis (526.5)
  osteonecrosis of jaw (733.45)

526.5 Alveolitis of jaw
Alveolar osteitis
Dry socket

⑤ **526.6 Periradicular pathology associated with previous endodontic treatment**

526.61 Perforation of root canal space

526.62 Endodontic overfill

526.63 Endodontic underfill

526.69 Other periradicular pathology associated with previous endodontic treatment

⑤ **526.8 Other specified diseases of the jaws**

526.81 Exostosis of jaw
Torus mandibularis
Torus palatinus

526.89 Other
Cherubism of jaw(s)
Fibrous dysplasia of jaw(s)
Latent bone cyst of jaw(s)
Osteoradionecrosis of jaw(s)
Unilateral condylar hyperplasia or hypoplasia of mandible

526.9 Unspecified disease of the jaws

<u>527</u> **Diseases of the salivary glands**
DEFINITION The salivary gland is a gland that secretes saliva, especially any of three pairs of large glands, the parotid, submaxillary, and sublingual, whose secretions enter the mouth and mingle in saliva

527.0 Atrophy

527.1 Hypertrophy

	Add 4th or 5th digit		Nonspecific code		Unspecified code		Manifestation code

527.2 Sialoadenitis
Parotitis: Sialoangitis
   NOS   Sialodochitis
   allergic
   toxic

Excludes: epidemic or infectious parotitis (072.0-072.9)
        uveoparotid fever (135)

527.3 Abscess

527.4 Fistula

Excludes: congenital fistula of salivary glands (750.24)

527.5 Sialolithiasis
Calculus of salivary gland or duct
Stone of salivary gland or duct
Sialodocholithiasis

527.6 Mucocele
Mucous:
  extravasation cyst of salivary gland
  retention cyst of salivary gland
Ranula

527.7 Disturbance of salivary secretion
Hyposecretion   Sialorrhea
Ptyalism   Xerostomia

527.8 Other specified diseases of the salivary glands
Benign lymphoepithelial lesion of salivary gland
Sialectasia
Sialosis
Stenosis of salivary duct
Stricture of salivary duct

527.9 Unspecified disease of the salivary glands

528 Diseases of the oral soft tissues, excluding lesions specific for gingiva and tongue

⑤ **528.0 Stomatitis and mucositis (ulcerative)**

Excludes: cellulitis and abscess of mouth (528.3)
    diphtheritic stomatitis (032.0)
    epizootic stomatitis (078.4)
    gingivitis (523.0-523.1)
    oral thrush (112.0)
    Stevens-Johnson syndrome (695.13)
    stomatitis:
      acute necrotizing ulcerative (101)
      aphthous (528.2)
      gangrenous (528.1)
      herpetic (054.2)
      Vincent's (101)

528.00 Stomatitis and mucositis, unspecified
Mucositis NOS
Ulcerative mucositis NOS
Ulcerative stomatitis NOS
Vesicular stomatitis NOS

528.01 Mucositis (ulcerative) due to antineoplastic therapy
Use additional E code to identify adverse effects of therapy, such as:
    antineoplastic and immunosuppressive drugs (E930.7, E933.1)
    radiation therapy (E879.2)
ALERT! For personal history of antineoplastic chemotherapy see V87.41

528.02 Mucositis (ulcerative) due to other drugs
Use additional E code to identify drug

528.09 Other stomatitis and mucositis (ulcerative)

528.1 Cancrum oris
Gangrenous stomatitis
Noma

● Code new to 2012 edition ▲ Revision of existing code ④ ⑤ Fourth or fifth digit required

528.2 Oral aphthae
Aphthous stomatitis
Canker sore
Periadenitis mucosa necrotica recurrens
Recurrent aphthous ulcer
Stomatitis herpetiformis

[Excludes:] *herpetic stomatitis (054.2)*

528.3 Cellulitis and abscess
Cellulitis of mouth (floor)
Ludwig's angina
Oral fistula

[Excludes:] *abscess of tongue (529.0)*
cellulitis or abscess of lip (528.5)
fistula (of):
  dental (522.7)
  lip (528.5)
gingivitis (523.00-523.11)

528.4 Cysts
Dermoid cyst of mouth
Epidermoid cyst of mouth
Epstein's pearl of mouth
Lymphoepithelial cyst of mouth
Nasoalveolar cyst of mouth
Nasolabial cyst of mouth

[Excludes:] *cyst:*
  gingiva (523.8)
  tongue (529.8)

528.5 Diseases of lips
Abscess of lip(s)
Cellulitis of lip(s)
Fistula of lip(s)
Hypertrophy of lip(s)
Cheilitis:
  NOS
  angular
Cheilodynia
Cheilosis

[Excludes:] *actinic cheilitis (692.79)*
congenital fistula of lip (750.25)
leukoplakia of lips (528.6)

528.6 Leukoplakia of oral mucosa, including tongue
Leukokeratosis of oral mucosa
Leukoplakia of:
  gingiva
  lips
  tongue

[Excludes:] *carcinoma in situ (230.0, 232.0)*
leukokeratosis nicotina palati (528.79)

[5] **528.7 Other disturbances of oral epithelium, including tongue**

[Excludes:] *carcinoma in situ (230.0, 232.0)*
leukokeratosis NOS (702.8)

528.71 Minimal keratinized residual ridge mucosa
Minimal keratinization of alveolar ridge mucosa

528.72 Excessive keratinized residual ridge mucosa
Excessive keratinization of alveolar ridge mucosa

528.79 Other disturbances of oral epithelium, including tongue
Erythroplakia of mouth or tongue
Focal epithelial hyperplasia of mouth or tongue
Leukoedema of mouth or tongue
Leukokeratosis nicotina palate
Other oral epithelium disturbances

528.8 Oral submucosal fibrosis, including of tongue

Add 4th or 5th digit
Nonspecific code
Unspecified code
Manifestation code

528.9 Other and unspecified diseases of the oral soft tissues
Cheek and lip biting
Denture sore mouth
Denture stomatitis
Melanoplakia
Papillary hyperplasia of palate
Eosinophilic granuloma of oral mucosa
Irritative hyperplasia of oral mucosa
Pyogenic granuloma of oral mucosa
Ulcer (traumatic) of oral mucosa

529 Diseases and other conditions of the tongue

529.0 Glossitis
Abscess of tongue
Ulceration (traumatic) of tongue

Excludes: *glossitis:*
> *benign migratory (529.1)*
> *Hunter's (529.4)*
> *median rhomboid (529.2)*
> *Moeller's (529.4)*

529.1 Geographic tongue
Benign migratory glossitis
Glossitis areata exfoliativa

529.2 Median rhomboid glossitis

529.3 Hypertrophy of tongue papillae
Black hairy tongue
Coated tongue
Hypertrophy of foliate papillae
Lingua villosa nigra

529.4 Atrophy of tongue papillae
Bald tongue   Glossodynia exfoliativa
Glazed tongue   Smooth atrophic tongue
Glossitis:
   Hunter's
   Moeller's

529.5 Plicated tongue
Fissured tongue
Furrowed tongue
Scrotal tongue

Excludes: *fissure of tongue, congenital (750.13)*

529.6 Glossodynia
Glossopyrosis
Painful tongue

Excludes: *glossodynia exfoliativa (529.4)*

529.8 Other specified conditions of the tongue
Atrophy (of) tongue
Crenated (of) tongue
Enlargement (of) tongue
Hypertrophy (of) tongue
Glossocele
Glossoptosis

Excludes: *erythroplasia of tongue (528.79)*
> *leukoplakia of tongue (528.6)*
> *macroglossia (congenital) (750.15)*
> *microglossia (congenital) (750.16)*
> *oral submucosal fibrosis (528.8)*

529.9 Unspecified condition of the tongue

DISEASES OF ESOPHAGUS, STOMACH, AND DUODENUM (530-539)

530 Diseases of esophagus

Excludes: *esophageal varices (456.0-456.2)*

DEFINITION The esophagus, the muscular membranous tube for the passage of food from the pharynx to the stomach; the gullet.

● Code new   ▲ Revision of   ④ ⑤ Fourth or fifth
    to 2012 edition   existing code   digit required

530.0 Achalasia and cardiospasm
Achalasia (of cardia)
Aperistalsis of esophagus
Megaesophagus

[Excludes:] *congenital cardiospasm (750.7)*

[5] **530.1 Esophagitis**
Esophagitis:
- chemical
- peptic
- postoperative
- regurgitant

Use additional E code, if desired, to identify cause, if induced by chemical

[Excludes:] *tuberculous esophagitis (017.8)*

530.10 Esophagitis, unspecified
Esophagitis NOS

530.11 Reflux esophagitis

530.12 Acute esophagitis

530.13 Eosinophilic esophagitis

530.19 Other esophagitis
Abscess of esophagus

[5] **530.2 Ulcer of esophagus**
Ulcer of esophagus
- fungal
- peptic

Ulcer of esophagus due to ingestion of:
- aspirin
- chemicals
- medicines

Use additional E code, if desired, to identify cause, if induced by chemical or drug

530.20 Ulcer of esophagus without bleeding
Ulcer of esophagus NOS

530.21 Ulcer of esophagus with bleeding

[Excludes:] *bleeding esophageal varices (456.0, 456.20)*

530.3 Stricture and stenosis of esophagus
Compression of esophagus
Obstruction of esophagus

[Excludes:] *congenital stricture of esophagus (750.3)*

530.4 Perforation of esophagus
Rupture of esophagus

[Excludes:] *traumatic perforation of esophagus (862.22, 862.32, 874.4-874.5)*

530.5 Dyskinesia of esophagus
Corkscrew esophagus
Curling esophagus
Esophagospasm
Spasm of esophagus

[Excludes:] *cardiospasm (530.0)*

530.6 Diverticulum of esophagus, acquired
Diverticulum, acquired:
- epiphrenic
- pharyngoesophageal
- pulsion
- subdiaphragmatic
- traction
- Zenker's (hypopharyngeal)

Esophageal pouch, acquired
Esophagocele, acquired

[Excludes:] *congenital diverticulum of esophagus (750.4)*

530.7 Gastroesophageal laceration-hemorrhage syndrome
Mallory-Weiss syndrome

[5] **530.8 Other specified disorders of esophagus**

530.81 Esophageal reflux
Gastroesophageal reflux

[Excludes:] *reflux esophagitis (530.11)*

Add 4th or 5th digit | Nonspecific code | Unspecified code | Manifestation code

530.82 Esophageal hemorrhage

[Excludes:] *hemorrhage due to esophageal varices (456.0-456.2)*

530.83 Esophageal leukoplakia

530.84 Tracheoesophageal fistula

[Excludes:] *congenital tracheoesophageal fistula (750.3)*

530.85 Barrett's esophagus

530.86 Infection of esophagostomy

Use additional code to specify infection

530.87 Mechanical complication of esophagostomy
Malfunction of esophagostomy

530.89 Other

[Excludes:] *Paterson-Kelly syndrome (280.8)*

530.9 Unspecified disorder of esophagus

[ALERT!] For personal history of unspecified digestive disease see V12.70

[5] **531 Gastric ulcer**

Includes: ulcer (peptic):
- prepyloric
- pylorus
- stomach

Use additional E code, if desired, to identify drug, if drug-induced

[Excludes:] *peptic ulcer NOS (533.0-533.9)*

The following fifth-digit subclassification is for use with category 531:

0 without mention of obstruction

1 with obstruction

[DEFINITION] A Gastric ulcer is a hole in the lining of the stomach corroded by the acidic digestive juices which are secreted by the stomach cells.

[5] **531.0 Acute with hemorrhage**
[0-1]

[5] **531.1 Acute with perforation**
[0-1]

[5] **531.2 Acute with hemorrhage and perforation**
[0-1]

[5] **531.3 Acute without mention of hemorrhage or perforation**
[0-1]

[5] **531.4 Chronic or unspecified with hemorrhage**
[0-1]

[5] **531.5 Chronic or unspecified with perforation**
[0-1]

[5] **531.6 Chronic or unspecified with hemorrhage and perforation**
[0-1]

[5] **531.7 Chronic without mention of hemorrhage or perforation**
[0-1]

[5] **531.9 Unspecified as acute or chronic, without mention of hemorrhage or perforation**
[0-1]

[5] **532 Duodenal ulcer**

Includes: erosion (acute) of duodenum
ulcer (peptic):
- duodenum
- postpyloric

Use additional E code, if desired, to identify drug, if drug-induced

[Excludes:] *peptic ulcer NOS (533.0-533.9)*

The following fifth-digit subclassification is for use with category 532:

0 without mention of obstruction

1 with obstruction

[DEFINITION] A Duodenal ulcer is a ulcer in the lining of the first part of the small intestine (duodenum)

⑤ **532.0 Acute with hemorrhage**
[0-1]

⑤ **532.1 Acute with perforation**
[0-1]

⑤ **532.2 Acute with hemorrhage and perforation**
[0-1]

⑤ **532.3 Acute without mention of hemorrhage or perforation**
[0-1]

⑤ **532.4 Chronic or unspecified with hemorrhage**
[0-1]

⑤ **532.5 Chronic or unspecified with perforation**
[0-1]

⑤ **532.6 Chronic or unspecified with hemorrhage and perforation**
[0-1]

⑤ **532.7 Chronic without mention of hemorrhage or perforation**
[0-1]

⑤ **532.9 Unspecified as acute or chronic, without mention of hemorrhage or perforation**
[0-1]

⑤ **533 Peptic ulcer, site unspecified**
Includes: gastroduodenal ulcer NOS
peptic ulcer NOS
stress ulcer NOS

Use additional E code, if desired, to identify drug, if drug-induced

Excludes: *peptic ulcer:*
duodenal (532.0-532.9)
gastric (531.0-531.9)

The following fifth-digit subclassification is for use with category 533:

0   without mention of obstruction

1   with obstruction

DEFINITION A Peptic ulcer is an ulcer of the mucous membrane lining of the alimentary tract.

ALERT! For personal history of peptic ulcer disease see V12.71

⑤ **533.0 Acute with hemorrhage**
[0-1]

⑤ **533.1 Acute with perforation**
[0-1]

⑤ **533.2 Acute with hemorrhage and perforation**
[0-1]

⑤ **533.3 Acute without mention of hemorrhage and perforation**
[0-1]

⑤ **533.4 Chronic or unspecified with hemorrhage**
[0-1]

⑤ **533.5 Chronic or unspecified with perforation**
[0-1]

⑤ **533.6 Chronic or unspecified with hemorrhage and perforation**
[0-1]

⑤ **533.7 Chronic without mention of hemorrhage or perforation**
[0-1]

⑤ **533.9 Unspecified as acute or chronic, without mention of hemorrhage or perforation**
[0-1]

ALERT! For personal history of unspecified digestive disease see V12.70

	Add 4th or 5th digit		Nonspecific code		Unspecified code		Manifestation code

[5] **534 Gastrojejunal ulcer**

Includes: ulcer (peptic) or erosion:
- anastomotic
- gastrocolic
- gastrointestinal
- gastrojejunal
- jejunal
- marginal
- stomal

[Excludes:] *primary ulcer of small intestine (569.82)*

The following fifth-digit subclassification is for use with category 534:

0 without mention of obstruction

1 with obstruction

[DEFINITION] A gastrojejunal ulcer is an ulcer that forms in the area between the stomach and the part of the small intestine known as the jejunum.

[5] **534.0 Acute with hemorrhage**
[0-1]

[5] **534.1 Acute with perforation**
[0-1]

[5] **534.2 Acute with hemorrhage and perforation**
[0-1]

[5] **534.3 Acute without mention of hemorrhage or perforation**
[0-1]

[5] **534.4 Chronic or unspecified with hemorrhage**
[0-1]

[5] **534.5 Chronic or unspecified with perforation**
[0-1]

[5] **534.6 Chronic or unspecified with hemorrhage and perforation**
[0-1]

[5] **534.7 Chronic without mention of hemorrhage or perforation**
[0-1]

[5] **534.9 Unspecified as acute or chronic, without mention of hemorrhage or perforation**
[0-1]

[ALERT!] For personal history of unspecified digestive disease see V12.70

[5] **535 Gastritis and duodenitis**

The following fifth-digit subclassification is for use with category 535

0 without mention of hemorrhage

1 with hemorrhage

[DEFINITION] Gastritis is an inflammation of the lining of the stomach; nausea and loss of appetite and discomfort after eating. Duodenitis is an inflammation of the duodenum. It may persist acutely or chronically

[5] **535.0 Acute gastritis**
[0-1]

[5] **535.1 Atrophic gastritis**
[0-1] Gastritis:
- atrophic-hyperplastic
- chronic (atrophic)

[5] **535.2 Gastric mucosal hypertrophy**
[0-1] Hypertrophic gastritis

[5] **535.3 Alcoholic gastritis**
[0-1]

[5] **535.4 Other specified gastritis**
[0-1] Gastritis:
- allergic
- bile induced
- irritant
- superficial
- toxic

[Excludes:] *eosinophilic gastritis (535.7)*

[5] **535.5 Unspecified gastritis and gastroduodenitis**
[0-1]

[ALERT!] For personal history of unspecified digestive disease see V12.70

[5] **535.6 Duodenitis**
[0-1]

[5] **535.7 Eosinophilic gastritis**
[0-1]

536 Disorders of function of stomach

[Excludes:] *functional disorders of stomach specified as psychogenic (306.4)*

536.0 Achlorhydria

536.1 Acute dilatation of stomach
Acute distention of stomach

536.2 Persistent vomiting
Cyclical vomiting
Habit vomiting
Persistent vomiting [not of pregnancy]
Uncontrollable vomiting

[Excludes:] *bilious emesis (vomiting) (787.04)*
excessive vomiting in pregnancy (643.0-643.9)
vomiting NOS (787.03)
cyclical, associated with migraine (346.2)
vomiting of fecal matter (569.87)

536.3 Gastroparesis
Gastroparalysis

Code first underlying disease, if known, such as:
diabetes mellitus (249.6, 250.6)

[5] **536.4 Gastrostomy complications**

536.40 Gastrostomy complications, unspecified

536.41 Infection of gastrostomy

Use additional code to specify type of infection, such as:
abscess or cellulitis of abdomen (682.2)
septicemia (038.0-038.9)

Use additional code to identify organism (041.00-041.9)

536.42 Mechanical complication of gastrostomy

536.49 Other gastrostomy complications

536.8 Dyspepsia and other specified disorders of function of stomach
Achylia gastrica
Hourglass contraction of stomach
Hyperacidity
Hyperchlorhydria
Hypochlorhydria
Indigestion
Tachygastria

[Excludes:] *achlorhydria (536.0)*
heartburn (787.1)

536.9 Unspecified functional disorder of stomach
Functional gastrointestinal:
disorder
disturbance
irritation

[ALERT!] For personal history of unspecified digestive disease see V12.70

537 Other disorders of stomach and duodenum

[DEFINITION] The duodenum is the beginning portion of the small intestine, starting at the lower end of the stomach and extending to the jejunum

[ALERT!] For personal history of other specified digestive system diseases see V12.79

537.0 Acquired hypertrophic pyloric stenosis
Constriction of pylorus, acquired or adult
Obstruction of pylorus, acquired or adult
Stricture of pylorus, acquired or adult

[Excludes:] *congenital or infantile pyloric stenosis (750.5)*

537.1 Gastric diverticulum

[Excludes:] *congenital diverticulum of stomach (750.7)*

537.2 Chronic duodenal ileus

537.3 Other obstruction of duodenum
Cicatrix of duodenum
Stenosis of duodenum
Stricture of duodenum
Volvulus of duodenum

Excludes: *congenital obstruction of duodenum (751.1)*

537.4 Fistula of stomach or duodenum
Gastrocolic fistula
Gastrojejunocolic fistula

537.5 Gastroptosis

537.6 Hourglass stricture or stenosis of stomach
Cascade stomach

Excludes: *congenital hourglass stomach (750.7)*
hourglass contraction of stomach (536.8)

⑤ **537.8 Other specified disorders of stomach and duodenum**

537.81 Pylorospasm

Excludes: *congenital pylorospasm (750.5)*

537.82 Angiodysplasia of stomach and duodenum without mention of hemorrhage

537.83 Angiodysplasia of stomach and duodenum with hemorrhage

537.84 Dieulafoy lesion (hemorrhagic) of stomach and duodenum

537.89 Other
Gastric or duodenal:
prolapse
rupture
Intestinal metaplasia of gastric mucosa
Passive congestion of stomach

Excludes: *diverticula of duodenum (562.00-562.01)*
gastrointestinal hemorrhage (578.0-578.9)

537.9 Unspecified disorder of stomach and duodenum
ALERT! For personal history of unspecified digestive disease see V12.70

538 Gastrointestinal mucositis (ulcerative)
Use additional E code to identify adverse effects of therapy, such as:
antineoplastic and immunosuppressive drugs (E930.7, E933.1)
radiation therapy (E879.2)

Excludes: *mucositis (ulcerative) of mouth and oral soft tissue (528.00-528.09)*

DEFINITION Gastrointestinal mucositis (ulcerative) is the inflammation of a mucous membrane of the gastrointestinal system

● **539 Complications of bariatric procedures**
DEFINITION Bariatric procedures, aka bariatric surgery, refers to surgery to reduce the volume of the stomach.

● **539.0 Complications of gastric band procedure**

● **539.01 Infection due to gastric band procedure**
Use additional code to specify type of infection, such as:
abscess or cellulitis of abdomen (682.2)
septicemia (038.0-038.9)

Use additional code to identify organism (041.00-041.9)

● **539.09 Other complications of gastric band procedure**
Use additional code(s) to further specify complication

● **539.8 Complications of other bariatric procedure**

Excludes: *complications of gastric band surgery (539.01-539.09)*

● **539.81 Infection due to other bariatric procedure**
Use additional code to specify type of infection, such as:
abscess or cellulitis of abdomen (682.2)
septicemia (038.0-038.9)

Use additional code to identify organism (041.00-041.9)

● **539.89 Other complications of other bariatric procedure**
Use additional code(s) to further specify complication

● Code new   ▲ Revision of   ④ ⑤ Fourth or fifth
to 2012 edition   existing code   digit required

APPENDICITIS (540-543)

540 Acute appendicitis

[DEFINITION] Appendicitis is an inflammation of the appendix, which is the worm-shaped pouch attached to the cecum, the beginning of the large intestine

540.0 With generalized peritonitis
Appendicitis (acute):
fulminating with: perforation, peritonitis (generalized), rupture
gangrenous with: perforation, peritonitis (generalized), rupture
obstructive with: perforation, peritonitis (generalized), rupture
Cecitis (acute) with: perforation peritonitis (generalized) rupture
Rupture of appendix

[Excludes:] *acute appendicitis with peritoneal abscess (540.1)*

540.1 With peritoneal abscess
Abscess of appendix
With generalized peritonitis

540.9 Without mention of peritonitis
Acute:
appendicitis:
fulminating without mention of perforation, peritonitis, or rupture
gangrenous without mention of perforation, peritonitis, or rupture
inflamed without mention of perforation, peritonitis, or rupture
obstructive without mention of perforation, peritonitis, or rupture
cecitis without mention of perforation, peritonitis, or rupture

541 Appendicitis, unqualified

542 Other appendicitis
Appendicitis:
chronic
recurrent
Appendicitis:
relapsing
subacute

[Excludes:] *hyperplasia (lymphoid) of appendix (543.0)*

[ALERT!] For personal history of other specified digestive system diseases see V12.79

543 Other diseases of appendix

[ALERT!] For personal history of other specified digestive system diseases see V12.79

543.0 Hyperplasia of appendix (lymphoid)

543.9 Other and unspecified diseases of appendix
Appendicular or appendiceal:
colic
concretion
fistula
Diverticulum of appendix
Fecalith of appendix
Intussusception of appendix
Mucocele of appendix
Stercolith of appendix

HERNIA OF ABDOMINAL CAVITY (550-553)

Includes: hernia:
acquired
congenital, except diaphragmatic or hiatal

[5] **550 Inguinal hernia**
Includes: bubonocele
inguinal hernia (direct) (double) (indirect) (oblique) (sliding)
scrotal hernia

The following fifth-digit subclassification is for use with category 550:

0 unilateral or unspecified (not specified as recurrent)
Unilateral NOS

1 unilateral or unspecified, recurrent

2 bilateral (not specified as recurrent)
Bilateral NOS

3 bilateral, recurrent

[DEFINITION] Inguinal hernia, protrusion of the abdominal viscera through the inguinal canal.

[5] **550.0 Inguinal hernia, with gangrene**
[0-3] Inguinal hernia with gangrene (and obstruction)

[5] **550.1 Inguinal hernia, with obstruction, without mention of gangrene**
[0-3] Inguinal hernia with mention of incarceration, irreducibility, or strangulation

[5] **550.9 Inguinal hernia, without mention of obstruction or gangrene**
[0-3] Inguinal hernia NOS

551 Other hernia of abdominal cavity, with gangrene
Includes: that with gangrene (and obstruction)

[DEFINITION] Gangrene is the decay or death of an organ or tissue caused by a lack of blood supply. It is a complication resulting from infectious or inflammatory processes, injury, or degenerative changes associated with chronic diseases, such as diabetes mellitus.

[ALERT!] For personal history of other specified digestive system diseases see V12.79

[5] **551.0 Femoral hernia with gangrene**

551.00 Unilateral or unspecified (not specified as recurrent)
Femoral hernia NOS with gangrene

551.01 Unilateral or unspecified, recurrent

551.02 Bilateral (not specified as recurrent)

551.03 Bilateral, recurrent

551.1 Umbilical hernia with gangrene
Parumbilical hernia specified as gangrenous

[5] **551.2 Ventral hernia with gangrene**

551.20 Ventral, unspecified, with gangrene

551.21 Incisional, with gangrene
Hernia:
postoperative specified as gangrenous
recurrent, ventral specified as gangrenous

551.29 Other
Epigastric hernia specified as gangrenous

551.3 Diaphragmatic hernia with gangrene
Hernia:
hiatal (esophageal) (sliding) specified as gangrenous
paraesophageal specified as gangrenous
Thoracic stomach specified as gangrenous
[Excludes:] *congenital diaphragmatic hernia (756.6)*

551.8 Hernia of other specified sites, with gangrene
Any condition classifiable to 553.8 if specified as gangrenous

551.9 Hernia of unspecified site, with gangrene
Any condition classifiable to 553.9 if specified as gangrenous

552 Other hernia of abdominal cavity, with obstruction, but without mention of gangrene
[Excludes:] *that with mention of gangrene (551.0-551.9)*

[ALERT!] For personal history of other specified digestive system diseases see V12.79

[5] **552.0 Femoral hernia with obstruction**
Femoral hernia specified as incarcerated, irreducible, strangulated, or causing obstruction

552.00 Unilateral or unspecified (not specified as recurrent)

552.01 Unilateral or unspecified, recurrent

552.02 Bilateral (not specified as recurrent)

552.03 Bilateral, recurrent

552.1 Umbilical hernia with obstruction
Parumbilical hernia specified as incarcerated, irreducible, strangulated, or causing obstruction

[5] **552.2 Ventral hernia with obstruction**
Ventral hernia specified as incarcerated, irreducible, strangulated, or causing obstruction

552.20 Ventral, unspecified, with obstruction

552.21 Incisional, with obstruction
Hernia:
postoperative specified as incarcerated, irreducible, strangulated, or causing obstruction
recurrent, ventral specified as incarcerated, irreducible, strangulated, or causing obstruction

552.29 Other
Epigastric hernia specified as incarcerated, irreducible, strangulated, or causing obstruction

552.3 Diaphragmatic hernia with obstruction
Hernia:
hiatal (esophageal) (sliding), specified as incarcerated, irreducible, strangulated, or causing obstruction
paraesophageal, specified as incarcerated, irreducible, strangulated, or causing obstruction
Thoracic stomach, specified as incarcerated, irreducible, strangulated, or causing obstruction

Excludes: congenital diaphragmatic hernia (756.6)

552.8 Hernia of other specified sites, with obstruction
Any condition classifiable to 553.8 if specified as incarcerated, irreducible, strangulated, or causing obstruction

552.9 Hernia of unspecified site, with obstruction
Any condition classifiable to 553.9 if specified as incarcerated, irreducible, strangulated, or causing obstruction

553 Other hernia of abdominal cavity without mention of obstruction or gangrene

Excludes: the listed conditions with mention of:
gangrene (and obstruction) (551.0-551.9)
obstruction (552.0-552.9)

ALERT! For personal history of other specified digestive system diseases see V12.79

⑤ **553.0 Femoral hernia**

553.00 Unilateral or unspecified (not specified as recurrent)
Femoral hernia NOS

553.01 Unilateral or unspecified, recurrent

553.02 Bilateral (not specified as recurrent)

553.03 Bilateral, recurrent

553.1 Umbilical hernia
Parumbilical hernia

⑤ **553.2 Ventral hernia**

553.20 Ventral, unspecified

553.21 Incisional
Hernia:
postoperative
recurrent, ventral

553.29 Other
Hernia:
epigastric
spigelian

553.3 Diaphragmatic hernia
Hernia:
hiatal (esophageal) (sliding)
paraesophageal
Thoracic stomach

Excludes: congenital:
diaphragmatic hernia (756.6)
hiatal hernia (750.6)
esophagocele (530.6)

553.8 Hernia of other specified sites
Hernia:
ischiatic
ischiorectal
lumbar
obturator
pudendal

Hernia:
retroperitoneal
sciatic
Other abdominal hernia of specified site

Excludes: vaginal enterocele (618.6)

553.9 Hernia of unspecified site
Enterocele
Epiplocele
Hernia:
NOS
interstitial

Hernia:
intestinal
intra-abdominal
Rupture (nontraumatic)
Sarcoepiplocele

| | Add 4th or 5th digit | | Nonspecific code | | Unspecified code | | Manifestation code |

NONINFECTIOUS ENTERITIS AND COLITIS (555-558)

555 Regional enteritis

Includes: Crohn's disease
Granulomatous enteritis

[Excludes:] *ulcerative colitis (556)*

DEFINITION Regional enteritis refers to inflammation of the intestinal tract, especially of the small intestine

555.0 Small intestine

Ileitis:
regional
segmental
terminal

Regional enteritis or Crohn's disease of:
duodenum
ileum
jejunum

555.1 Large intestine

Colitis:
granulomatous
regional
transmural

Regional enteritis or Crohn's disease of:
colon
large bowel
rectum

555.2 Small intestine with large intestine

Regional ileocolitis

555.9 Unspecified site

Crohn's disease NOS
Regional enteritis NOS

556 Ulcerative colitis

DEFINITION Ulcerative colitis ulcerative colitis is a form of inflammatory bowel disease (ibd). It causes swelling, ulcerations, and loss of function of the large intestine

556.0 Ulcerative (chronic) enterocolitis

556.1 Ulcerative (chronic) ileocolitis

556.2 Ulcerative (chronic) proctitis

556.3 Ulcerative (chronic) proctosigmoiditis

556.4 Pseudopolyposis of colon

556.5 Left-sided ulcerative (chronic) colitis

556.6 Universal ulcerative (chronic) colitis

Pancolitis

556.8 Other ulcerative colitis

556.9 Ulcerative colitis, unspecified

Ulcerative enteritis NOS

ALERT! For personal history of unspecified digestive disease see V12.70

557 Vascular insufficiency of intestine

[Excludes:] *necrotizing enterocolitis of the newborn (777.50-777.53)*

DEFINITION Vascular insufficiency of intestine, refers to inadequate peripheral blood flow to the intestines

557.0 Acute vascular insufficiency of intestine

Acute:
hemorrhagic enterocolitis
ischemic colitis, enteritis, or enterocolitis
massive necrosis of intestine
Bowel infarction
Embolism of mesenteric artery
Fulminant enterocolitis
Hemorrhagic necrosis of intestine
Infarction of appendices epiploicae
Intestinal gangrene
Intestinal infarction (acute) (agnogenic) (hemorrhagic) (nonocclusive)
Mesenteric infarction (embolic) (thrombotic)
Necrosis of intestine
Terminal hemorrhagic enteropathy
Thrombosis of mesenteric artery

557.1 Chronic vascular insufficiency of intestine
Angina, abdominal
Chronic ischemic colitis, enteritis, or enterocolitis
Ischemic stricture of intestine
Mesenteric:
angina
artery syndrome (superior)
vascular insufficiency

557.9 Unspecified vascular insufficiency of intestine
Alimentary pain due to vascular insufficiency
Ischemic colitis, enteritis, or enterocolitis NOS

ALERT! For personal history of unspecified digestive disease see V12.70

558 Other and unspecified noninfectious gastroenteritis and colitis

[Excludes:] *infectious:*
colitis, enteritis, or gastroenteritis (009.0-009.1)
diarrhea (009.2-009.3)

ALERT! For personal history of other specified digestive system diseases see V12.79

558.1 Gastroenteritis and colitis due to radiation
Radiation enterocolitis

558.2 Toxic gastroenteritis and colitis
Use additional E code, if desired, to identify cause

558.3 Allergic gastroenteritis and colitis
Use additional code to identify type of food allergy (V15.01-V15.05)

[5] **558.4 Eosinophilic gastroenteritis and colitis**

558.41 Eosinophilic gastroenteritis
Eosinophilic enteritis

558.42 Eosinophilic colitis

558.9 Other and unspecified noninfectious gastroenteritis and colitis
Colitis NOS, dietetic, or noninfectious
Enteritis NOS, dietetic, or noninfectious
Gastroenteritis NOS, dietetic, or noninfectious
Ileitis NOS, dietetic, or noninfectious
Jejunitis NOS, dietetic, or noninfectious
Sigmoiditis NOS, dietetic, or noninfectious

OTHER DISEASES OF INTESTINES AND PERITONEUM (560-569)

560 Intestinal obstruction without mention of hernia

[Excludes:] *duodenum (537.2-537.3)*
inguinal hernia with obstruction (550.1)
intestinal obstruction complicating hernia (552.0-552.9)
mesenteric:
embolism (557.0)
infarction (557.0)
thrombosis (557.0)
neonatal intestinal obstruction (277.01, 777.1-777.2, 777.4)

DEFINITION Intestinal obstruction without mention of hernia, a blockage in the intestine which prevents the normal flow of waste down the length of the intestine

560.0 Intussusception
Intussusception (colon) (intestine) (rectum)
Invagination of intestine or colon

[Excludes:] *intussusception of appendix (543.9)*

560.1 Paralytic ileus
Adynamic ileus
Ileus (of intestine) (of bowel) (of colon)
Paralysis of intestine or colon

[Excludes:] *gallstone ileus (560.31)*

560.2 Volvulus
Knotting of intestine, bowel, or colon
Strangulation of intestine, bowel, or colon
Torsion of intestine, bowel, or colon
Twist of intestine, bowel, or colon

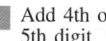

Add 4th or 5th digit | Nonspecific code | Unspecified code | Manifestation code

⑤ **560.3** **Impaction of intestine**

> **560.30** **Impaction of intestine, unspecified**
> Impaction of colon

> **560.31** **Gallstone ileus**
> Obstruction of intestine by gallstone

> **560.32** **Fecal impaction**

Excludes: *constipation (564.00-564.09)*

incomplete defecation (787.61)

> **560.39** **Other**
> Concretion of intestine
> Enterolith

⑤ **560.8** **Other specified intestinal obstruction**

> **560.81** **Intestinal or peritoneal adhesions with obstruction (postoperative) (postinfection)**

Excludes: *adhesions without obstruction (568.0)*

> **560.89** **Other**
> Acute pseudo-obstruction of intestine
> Mural thickening causing obstruction

Excludes: *ischemic stricture of intestine (557.1)*

560.9 **Unspecified intestinal obstruction**
Enterostenosis
Obstruction of intestine or colon
Occlusion of intestine or colon
Stenosis of intestine or colon
Stricture of intestine or colon

Excludes: *congenital stricture or stenosis of intestine (751.1-751.2)*

ALERT! For personal history of unspecified digestive disease see V12.70

562 **Diverticula of intestine**
Use additional code, if desired, to identify any associated:
peritonitis (567.0-567.9)

Excludes: *congenital diverticulum of colon (751.5)*

diverticulum of appendix (543.9)
Meckel's diverticulum (751.0)

DEFINITION A diverticulum of the colon is a sac or pouch in the colon walls which is usually asymptomatic (without symptoms) but may cause difficulty if it becomes inflamed

⑤ **562.0** **Small intestine**

> **562.00** **Diverticulosis of small intestine (without mention of hemorrhage)**
> Diverticulosis:
> duodenum without mention of diverticulitis
> ileum without mention of diverticulitis
> jejunum without mention of diverticulitis

> **562.01** **Diverticulitis of small intestine (without mention of hemorrhage)**
> Diverticulitis (with diverticulosis):
> duodenum
> ileum
> jejunum
> small intestine

> **562.02** **Diverticulosis of small intestine with hemorrhage**

> **562.03** **Diverticulitis of small intestine with hemorrhage**

⑤ **562.1** **Colon**

> **562.10** **Diverticulosis of colon (without mention of hemorrhage)**
> Diverticulosis:
> NOS without mention of diverticulitis
> intestine (large) without mention of diverticulitis
> Diverticular disease (colon) without mention of diverticulitis

> **562.11** **Diverticulitis of colon (without mention of hemorrhage)**
> Diverticulitis (with diverticulosis):
> NOS
> colon
> intestine (large)

> **562.12** **Diverticulosis of colon with hemorrhage**

> **562.13** **Diverticulitis of colon with hemorrhage**

● Code new
to 2012 edition
▲ Revision of
existing code
④ ⑤ Fourth or fifth
digit required

564 **Functional digestive disorders, not elsewhere classified**

Excludes: *functional disorders of stomach (536.0-536.9)*
those specified as psychogenic (306.4)

DEFINITION Functional digestive disorders are a group of disorders, which include irritable bowel syndrome or ibs, dyspepsia, gerd, and chronic constipation or diarrhea

⑤ **564.0 Constipation**

Excludes: *fecal impaction (560.32)*
incomplete defecation (787.61)

564.00 Constipation, unspecified

564.01 Slow transit constipation

564.02 Outlet dysfunction constipation

564.09 Other constipation

564.1 Irritable bowel syndrome
Irritable colon   Spastic colon

564.2 Postgastric surgery syndromes
Dumping syndrome   Postgastrectomy syndrome
Jejunal syndrome   Postvagotomy syndrome

Excludes: *malnutrition following gastrointestinal surgery (579.3)*
postgastrojejunostomy ulcer (534.0-534.9)

564.3 Vomiting following gastrointestinal surgery
Vomiting (bilious) following gastrointestinal surgery

564.4 Other postoperative functional disorders
Diarrhea following gastrointestinal surgery

Excludes: *colostomy and enterostomy complications (569.60-569.69)*

564.5 Functional diarrhea

Excludes: *diarrhea:*
NOS (787.91)
psychogenic (306.4)

564.6 Anal spasm
Proctalgia fugax

564.7 Megacolon, other than Hirschsprung's
Dilatation of colon

Excludes: *megacolon:*
congenital [Hirschsprung's] (751.3)
toxic (556)

⑤ **564.8 Other specified functional disorders of intestine**

Excludes: *malabsorption (579.0-579.9)*

564.81 Neurogenic bowel

564.89 Other functional disorders of intestine
Atony of colon

564.9 Unspecified functional disorder of intestine

ALERT! For personal history of unspecified digestive disease see V12.70

565 **Anal fissure and fistula**

DEFINITION An anal fissure is a crack-like sore in the anal region. It is the commonest reason for pain in this area. An anal fistula is a channel that develops between the anus and the skin. Most fistulas are the result of an abscess that spreads to the skin

565.0 Anal fissure

Excludes: *anal sphincter tear (healed) (non-traumatic) (old) (569.43)*
traumatic (863.89, 863.99)

565.1 Anal fistula
Fistula:
anorectal
rectal
rectum to skin

Excludes: *fistula of rectum to internal organs—see Alphabetic Index*
ischiorectal fistula (566)
rectovaginal fistula (619.1)

| | Add 4th or 5th digit | | Nonspecific code | | Unspecified code | | Manifestation code |

566 Abscess of anal and rectal regions
Abscess:
ischiorectal
perianal
perirectal
Cellulitis:
anal
perirectal
rectal
Ischiorectal fistula

ALERT! ICD-9-CM codes in the Category 566 add points to the clinical domain as a Skin 2 diagnosis

567 Peritonitis and retroperitoneal infections

Excludes: peritonitis:
benign paroxysmal (277.31)
pelvic, female (614.5, 614.7)
periodic familial (277.31)
puerperal (670.8)
with or following:
abortion (634-638 with .0, 639.0)
appendicitis (540.0-540.1)
ectopic or molar pregnancy (639.0)

DEFINITION Peritonitis is an inflammation of the membrane which lines the inside of the abdomen and all of the internal organs.

567.0 Peritonitis in infectious diseases classified elsewhere
Code first underlying disease

Excludes: peritonitis:
gonococcal (098.86)
syphilitic (095.2)
tuberculous (014.0)

567.1 Pneumococcal peritonitis

⑤ **567.2 Other suppurative peritonitis**

567.21 Peritonitis (acute) generalized
Pelvic peritonitis, male

567.22 Peritoneal abscess
Abscess (of):   Abscess (of):
abdominopelvic   retrocecal
mesenteric   subdiaphragmatic
omentum   subhepatic
peritoneum   subphrenic

567.23 Spontaneous bacterial peritonitis

Excludes: bacterial peritonitis NOS (567.29)

567.29 Other suppurative peritonitis
Subphrenic peritonitis

⑤ **567.3 Retroperitoneal infections**

567.31 Psoas muscle abscess

567.38 Other retroperitoneal abscess

567.39 Other retroperitoneal infections

⑤ **567.8 Other specified peritonitis**

567.81 Choleperitonitis
Peritonitis due to bile

567.82 Sclerosing mesenteritis
Fat necrosis of peritoneum
(Idiopathic) sclerosing mesenteric fibrosis
Mesenteric lipodystrophy
Mesenteric panniculitis
Retractile mesenteritis

567.89 Other specified peritonitis
Chronic proliferative peritonitis
Mesenteric saponification
Peritonitis due to urine

● Code new   ▲ Revision of   ④ ⑤ Fourth or fifth
     to 2012 edition   existing code   digit required

567.9 Unspecified peritonitis
Peritonitis:
NOS
of unspecified cause
ALERT! For personal history of unspecified digestive disease see V12.70

568 Other disorders of peritoneum
DEFINITION The peritoneum is the membrane that lines the abdominal cavity and covers most of the abdominal organs
ALERT! For personal history of other specified digestive system diseases see V12.79

568.0 Peritoneal adhesions (postoperative) (postinfection)

Adhesions (of):   Adhesions (of):
  abdominal (wall)   mesenteric
  diaphragm   omentum
  intestine   stomach
  male pelvis   Adhesive bands

Excludes: *adhesions:*
         pelvic, female (614.6)
         with obstruction:
           duodenum (537.3)
           intestine (560.81)

⑤ **568.8 Other specified disorders of peritoneum**

568.81   Hemoperitoneum (nontraumatic)

568.82   Peritoneal effusion (chronic)

Excludes: *ascites NOS (789.51-789.59)*

568.89   Other
Peritoneal:
  cyst
  granuloma

568.9 Unspecified disorder of peritoneum
ALERT! For personal history of unspecified digestive disease see V12.70

569 Other disorders of intestine
ALERT! For personal history of other specified digestive system diseases see V12.79

569.0 Anal and rectal polyp
Anal and rectal polyp NOS

Excludes: *adenomatous anal and rectal polyp (211.4)*

569.1 Rectal prolapse
Procidentia: Prolapse:
  anus (sphincter)   anal canal
  rectum (sphincter)   rectal mucosa
Proctoptosis

Excludes: *prolapsed hemorrhoids (455.2, 455.5)*

569.2 Stenosis of rectum and anus
Stricture of anus (sphincter)

569.3 Hemorrhage of rectum and anus

Excludes: *gastrointestinal bleeding NOS (578.9)*
         melena (578.1)

⑤ **569.4 Other specified disorders of rectum and anus**

569.41   Ulcer of anus and rectum
Solitary ulcer of anus (sphincter) or rectum (sphincter)
Stercoral ulcer of anus (sphincter) or rectum (sphincter)

569.42   Anal or rectal pain

569.43   Anal sphincter tear (healed) (old)
Tear of anus, nontraumatic

Use additional code for any associated fecal incontinence (787.60-787.63)

Excludes: *anal fissure (565.0)*
         anal sphincter tear (healed) (old) complicating delivery (654.8)

| | Add 4th or 5th digit | | Nonspecific code | | Unspecified code | | Manifestation code |

569.44 Dysplasia of anus
Anal intraepithelial neoplasia I and II (AIN I and II) (histologically confirmed)
Dysplasia of anus NOS
Mild and moderate dysplasia of anus (histologically confirmed)

[Excludes:] *abnormal results from anal cytologic examination without histologic confirmation (796.70-796.79)*
anal intraepithelial neoplasia III (230.5, 230.6)
carcinoma in situ of anus (230.5, 230.6)
HGSIL of anus (796.74)
severe dysplasia of anus (230.5, 230.6)

569.49 Other
Granuloma of rectum (sphincter)
Rupture of rectum (sphincter)
Hypertrophy of anal papillae
Proctitis NOS

Use additional code for any associated fecal incontinence (787.60-787.63)

[Excludes:] *fistula of rectum to:*
internal organs—see Alphabetic Index
skin (565.1)
hemorrhoids (455.0-455.9)

569.5 Abscess of intestine

[Excludes:] *appendiceal abscess (540.1)*

[5] **569.6 Colostomy and enterostomy complications**

569.60 Colostomy and enterostomy complication, unspecified

569.61 Infection of colostomy or enterostomy

Use additional code to specify type of infection, such as:
abscess or cellulitis of abdomen (682.2)
septicemia (038.0-038.9)

Use additional code to identify organism (041.00-041.9)

569.62 Mechanical complication of colostomy and enterostomy
Malfunction of colostomy and enterostomy

569.69 Other complication
Fistula
Hernia
Prolapse

[5] **569.7 Complications of intestinal pouch**

569.71 Pouchitis
Inflammation of internal ileoanal pouch

569.79 Other complications of intestinal pouch

[5] **569.8 Other specified disorders of intestine**

569.81 Fistula of intestine, excluding rectum and anus
Fistula:
abdominal wall
enterocolic
Fistula:
enteroenteric
ileorectal

[Excludes:] *fistula of intestine to internal organs —see Alphabetic Index*
persistent postoperative fistula (998.6)

569.82 Ulceration of intestine
Primary ulcer of intestine
Ulceration of colon

[Excludes:] *that with perforation (569.83)*

569.83 Perforation of intestine

569.84 Angiodysplasia of intestine (without mention of hemorrhage)

569.85 Angiodysplasia of intestine with hemorrhage

569.86 Dieulafoy lesion (hemorrhagic) of intestine

569.87 Vomiting of fecal matter

569.89 Other
Enteroptosis
Granuloma of intestine
Prolapse of intestine
Pericolitis
Perisigmoiditis
Visceroptosis

[Excludes:] *gangrene of intestine, mesentery, or omentum (557.0)*
hemorrhage of intestine NOS (578.9)
obstruction of intestine (560.0-560.9)

569.9 Unspecified disorder of intestine
[ALERT!] For personal history of unspecified digestive disease see V12.70

OTHER DISEASES OF DIGESTIVE SYSTEM (570-579)

570 Acute and subacute necrosis of liver
Acute hepatic failure
Acute or subacute hepatitis, not specified as infective
Necrosis of liver (acute) (diffuse) (massive) (subacute)
Parenchymatous degeneration of liver
Yellow atrophy (liver) (acute) (subacute)

[Excludes:] *icterus gravis of newborn (773.0-773.2)*
serum hepatitis (070.2-070.3)
that with:
abortion (634-638 with .7, 639.8)
ectopic or molar pregnancy (639.8)
pregnancy, childbirth, or the puerperium (646.7)
viral hepatitis (070.0-070.9)

571 Chronic liver disease and cirrhosis
[DEFINITION] Cirrhosis is the chronic scarring of the liver, leading to loss of normal liver function.

571.0 Alcoholic fatty liver

571.1 Acute alcoholic hepatitis
Acute alcoholic liver disease

571.2 Alcoholic cirrhosis of liver
Florid cirrhosis
Laennec's cirrhosis (alcoholic)

571.3 Alcoholic liver damage, unspecified

[5] **571.4 Chronic hepatitis**
[Excludes:] *viral hepatitis (acute) (chronic) (070.0-070.9)*

571.40 Chronic hepatitis, unspecified

571.41 Chronic persistent hepatitis

571.42 Autoimmune hepatitis

571.49 Other
Chronic hepatitis:
active
aggressive
Recurrent hepatitis

571.5 Cirrhosis of liver without mention of alcohol
Cirrhosis of liver:
NOS
cryptogenic
macronodular
micronodular
Cirrhosis of liver:
posthepatitic
postnecrotic
Healed yellow atrophy (liver)
Portal cirrhosis

Code first, if applicable, viral hepatitis (acute) (chronic) (070.0-070.9)

571.6 Biliary cirrhosis
Chronic nonsuppurative destructive cholangitis
Cirrhosis:
cholangitic
cholestatic

571.8 Other chronic nonalcoholic liver disease
Chronic yellow atrophy (liver)
Fatty liver, without mention of alcohol

571.9 Unspecified chronic liver disease without mention of alcohol

> **ALERT!** For personal history of unspecified digestive disease see V12.70

572 Liver abscess and sequelae of chronic liver disease

> **DEFINITION** A liver abscess is an abscess in the liver cells, usually caused by an amebic infection, bacterial infection, or trauma.

572.0 Abscess of liver

> *Excludes:* amebic liver abscess (006.3)

572.1 Portal pyemia
   Phlebitis of portal vein   Pylephlebitis
   Portal thrombophlebitis   Pylethrombophlebitis

572.2 Hepatic encephalopathy
   Hepatic coma
   Hepatocerebral intoxication
   Portal-systemic encephalopathy

> *Excludes:* hepatic coma associated with viral hepatitis – see category 070

572.3 Portal hypertension
   Use additional code for any associated complications, such as:
      portal hypertensive gastropathy (537.89)

572.4 Hepatorenal syndrome

> *Excludes:* that following delivery (674.8)

572.8 Other sequelae of chronic liver disease

> *Excludes:* hepatopulmonary syndrome (573.5)

573 Other disorders of liver

> *Excludes:* amyloid or lardaceous degeneration of liver (277.39)
>   congenital cystic disease of liver (751.62)
>   glycogen infiltration of liver (271.0)
>   hepatomegaly NOS (789.1)
>   portal vein obstruction (452)

> **ALERT!** For personal history of other specified digestive system diseases see V12.79

573.0 Chronic passive congestion of liver

573.1 Hepatitis in viral diseases classified elsewhere
   Code first underlying disease as:
      Coxsackie virus disease (074.8)
      cytomegalic inclusion virus disease (078.5)
      infectious mononucleosis (075)

> *Excludes:* hepatitis (in):
>   mumps (072.71)
>   viral (070.0-070.9)
>   yellow fever (060.0-060.9)

573.2 Hepatitis in other infectious diseases classified elsewhere
   Code first underlying disease, as:
      malaria (084.9)

> *Excludes:* hepatitis in:
>   late syphilis (095.3)
>   secondary syphilis (091.62)
>   toxoplasmosis (130.5)

573.3 Hepatitis, unspecified
   Toxic (noninfectious) hepatitis
Use additional E code, if desired, to identify cause

573.4 Hepatic infarction

● **573.5 Hepatopulmonary syndrome**
   Code first underlying liver disease, such as:
      alcoholic cirrhosis of liver (571.2)
      cirrhosis of liver without mention of alcohol (571.5)

573.8 Other specified disorders of liver
   Hepatoptosis

573.9 Unspecified disorder of liver

● Code new   ▲ Revision of   ④ ⑤ Fourth or fifth
  to 2012 edition   existing code   digit required

⑤ **574** **Cholelithiasis**

The following fifth-digit subclassification is for use with category 574:

0 **without mention of obstruction**

1 **with obstruction**

DEFINITION Cholelithiasis the presence or formation of gallstones in the gallbladder or bile ducts

Excludes: retained cholelithiasis following cholecystecomy (997.41)

⑤ **574.0** **Calculus of gallbladder with acute cholecystitis**
[0-1] Biliary calculus with acute cholecystitis
Calculus of cystic duct with acute cholecystitis
Cholelithiasis with acute cholecystitis
Any condition classifiable to 574.2 with acute cholecystitis

⑤ **574.1** **Calculus of gallbladder with other cholecystitis**
[0-1] Biliary calculus with cholecystitis
Calculus of cystic duct with cholecystitis
Cholelithiasis with cholecystitis
Cholecystitis with cholelithiasis NOS
Any condition classifiable to 574.2 with cholecystitis (chronic)

⑤ **574.2** **Calculus of gallbladder without mention of cholecystitis**
[0-1] Biliary:
calculus NOS
colic NOS
Calculus of cystic duct
Cholelithiasis NOS
Colic (recurrent) of
gallbladder
Gallstone (impacted)

⑤ **574.3** **Calculus of bile duct with acute cholecystitis**
[0-1] Calculus of bile duct [any] with acute cholecystitis
Choledocholithiasis with acute cholecystitis
Any condition classifiable to 574.5 with acute cholecystitis

⑤ **574.4** **Calculus of bile duct with other cholecystitis**
[0-1] Calculus of bile duct [any] with cholecystitis (chronic)
Choledocholithiasis with cholecystitis (chronic)
Any condition classifiable to 574.5 with cholecystitis (chronic)

⑤ **574.5** **Calculus of bile duct without mention of cholecystitis**
[0-1] Calculus of:
bile duct [any]
common duct
hepatic duct
Choledocholithiasis
Hepatic:
colic (recurrent)
lithiasis

⑤ **574.6** **Calculus of gallbladder and bile duct with acute cholecystitis**
[0-1] Any condition classifiable to 574.0 and 574.3

⑤ **574.7** **Calculus of gallbladder and bile duct with other cholecystitis**
[0-1] Any condition classifiable to 574.1 and 574.4

⑤ **574.8** **Calculus of gallbladder and bile duct with acute and chronic cholecystitis**
[0-1] Any condition classifiable to 574.6 and 574.7

⑤ **574.9** **Calculus of gallbladder and bile duct without cholecystitis**
[0-1] Any condition classifiable to 574.2 and 574.5

575 **Other disorders of gallbladder**

DEFINITION The gallbladder is a small, pear-shaped muscular sac, located under the right lobe of the liver, in which bile secreted by the liver is stored until needed by the body for digestion.

ALERT! For personal history of other specified digestive system diseases see V12.79

| | Add 4th or 5th digit | | Nonspecific code | | Unspecified code | | Manifestation code |

575.0 Acute cholecystitis
Abscess of gallbladder without mention of calculus
Angiocholecystitis without mention of calculus
Cholecystitis without mention of calculus:
emphysematous (acute)
gangrenous
suppurative
Empyema of gallbladder without mention of calculus
Gangrene of gallbladder without mention of calculus

[*Excludes:*] *that with:*
acute and chronic cholecystitis (575.12)
choledocholithiasis (574.3)
choledocholithiasis and cholelithiasis (574.6)
cholelithiasis (574.0)

⑤ **575.1 Other cholecystitis**
Cholecystitis:
NOS without mention of calculus
chronic without mention of calculus

[*Excludes:*] *that with:*
choledocholithiasis (574.4)
choledocholithiasis and cholelithiasis (574.8)
cholelithiasis (574.1)

575.10 Cholecystitis, unspecified
Cholecystitis NOS

575.11 Chronic cholecystitis

575.12 Acute and chronic cholecystits

575.2 Obstruction of gallbladder
Occlusion of cystic duct or gallbladder without mention of calculus
Stenosis of cystic duct or gallbladder without mention of calculus
Stricture of cystic duct or gallbladder without mention of calculus

[*Excludes:*] *that with calculus (574.0-574.2 with fifth-digit 1)*

575.3 Hydrops of gallbladder
Mucocele of gallbladder

575.4 Perforation of gallbladder
Rupture of cystic duct or gallbladder

575.5 Fistula of gallbladder
Fistula:
cholecystoduodenal
cholecystoenteric

575.6 Cholesterolosis of gallbladder
Strawberry gallbladder

575.8 Other specified disorders of gallbladder
Adhesions (of) cystic duct or gallbladder
Atrophy (of) cystic duct or gallbladder
Cyst (of) cystic duct or gallbladder
Hypertrophy (of) cystic duct or gallbladder
Nonfunctioning (of) cystic duct or gallbladder
Ulcer (of) cystic duct or gallbladder
Biliary dyskinesia

[*Excludes:*] *nonvisualization of gallbladder (793.3)*
Hartmann's pouch of intestine (V44.3)

575.9 Unspecified disorder of gallbladder

576 Other disorders of biliary tract

[*Excludes:*] *that involving the:*
cystic duct (575.0-575.9)
gallbladder (575.0-575.9)

[DEFINITION] The biliary tract is the system of organs and ducts through which bile is made and transported from the liver. Bile is a liquid produced in the liver whose function is to remove waste from the liver and break down fats as food is digested

[ALERT!] For personal history of other specified digestive system diseases see V12.79

576.0 Postcholecystectomy syndrome

● Code new to 2012 edition ▲ Revision of existing code ④ ⑤ Fourth or fifth digit required

576.1 Cholangitis

Cholangitis:
  NOS
  acute
  ascending
  chronic
  primary

Cholangitis:
  recurrent
  sclerosing
  secondary
  stenosing
  suppurative

576.2 Obstruction of bile duct

Occlusion of bile duct, except cystic duct, without mention of calculus
Stenosis of bile duct, except cystic duct, without mention of calculus
Stricture of bile duct, except cystic duct, without mention of calculus

Excludes: *congenital (751.61)*
    that with calculus (574.3-574.5 with fifth-digit 1)

576.3 Perforation of bile duct

Rupture of bile duct, except cystic duct

576.4 Fistula of bile duct

Choledochoduodenal fistula

576.5 Spasm of sphincter of Oddi

576.8 Other specified disorders of biliary tract

Adhesions of bile duct [any]
Atrophy of bile duct [any]
Cyst of bile duct [any]
Hypertrophy of bile duct [any]
Stasis of bile duct [any]
Ulcer of bile duct [any]

Excludes: *congenital choledochal cyst (751.69)*

576.9 Unspecified disorder of biliary tract

ALERT! For personal history of unspecified digestive disease see V12.70

577 Diseases of pancreas

DEFINITION The pancreas is gland that lies in the abdomen behind the stomach. It produces enzymes that are released into the small intestine to help with digestion. It also contains clusters of cells called islets that produce hormones such as insulin and glucagon, which help control the level of glucose in the blood.

577.0 Acute pancreatitis

Abscess of pancreas
Necrosis of pancreas:
  acute
  infective

Pancreatitis:
  NOS
  acute (recurrent)
  apoplectic
  hemorrhagic
  subacute
  suppurative

Excludes: *mumps pancreatitis (072.3)*

577.1 Chronic pancreatitis

Chronic pancreatitis:
  NOS
  infectious
  interstitial

Pancreatitis:
  painless
  recurrent
  relapsing

577.2 Cyst and pseudocyst of pancreas

577.8 Other specified diseases of pancreas

Atrophy of pancreas
Calculus of pancreas
Cirrhosis of pancreas
Fibrosis of pancreas

Pancreatic:
  infantilism
  necrosis:
    NOS
    aseptic
    fat
Pancreatolithiasis

Excludes: *fibrocystic disease of pancreas (277.00-277.09)*
    islet cell tumor of pancreas (211.7)
    pancreatic steatorrhea (579.4)

577.9 Unspecified disease of pancreas

ALERT! For personal history of unspecified digestive disease see V12.70

| | Add 4th or 5th digit | | Nonspecific code | | Unspecified code | | Manifestation code |

578 **Gastrointestinal hemorrhage**

> *Excludes:* *that with mention of:*
>> *angiodysplasia of stomach and duodenum (537.83)*
>> *angiodysplasia of intestine (569.85)*
>> *diverticulitis, intestine:*
>>> *large (562.13)*
>>> *small (562.03)*
>> *diverticulosis, intestine:*
>>> *large (562.12)*
>>> *small (562.02)*
>> *gastritis and duodenitis (535.0-535.6)*
>> *ulcer:*
>>> *duodenal (532.0-532.9)*
>>> *gastric (531.0-531.9)*
>>> *gastrojejunal (534.0-534.9)*
>>> *peptic (533.0-533.9)*

DEFINITION Gastrointestinal hemorrhage refers to bleeding in any segment of the gastrointestinal tract from esophagus to rectum

578.0 **Hematemesis**
Vomiting of blood

578.1 **Blood in stool**
Melena

> *Excludes:* *occult blood (792.1)*

578.9 **Hemorrhage of gastrointestinal tract, unspecified**
Gastric hemorrhage
Intestinal hemorrhage

ALERT! For personal history of unspecified digestive disease see V12.70

579 **Intestinal malabsorption**

DEFINITION Intestinal malabsorption is a state arising from abnormality in digestion or absorption of food nutrients across the gastrointestinal(GI) tract.

579.0 **Celiac disease**
Celiac:	Gee (-Herter) disease
crisis	Gluten enteropathy
infantilism	Idiopathic steatorrhea
rickets	Nontropical sprue

579.1 **Tropical sprue**
Sprue:	Tropical steatorrhea
NOS	
tropical	

579.2 **Blind loop syndrome**
Postoperative blind loop syndrome

579.3 **Other and unspecified postsurgical nonabsorption**
Hypoglycemia following gastrointestinal surgery
Malnutrition following gastrointestinal surgery

579.4 **Pancreatic steatorrhea**

579.8 **Other specified intestinal malabsorption**
Enteropathy:	Steatorrhea (chronic)
exudative	
protein-losing	

579.9 **Unspecified intestinal malabsorption**
Malabsorption syndrome NOS

ALERT! For personal history of unspecified digestive disease see V12.70

● Code new to 2012 edition   ▲ Revision of existing code   ④ ⑤ Fourth or fifth digit required

Chapter 10: Diseases of Genitourinary System (580-629)

DEFINITIONS AND CODING ALERTS

This chapter includes definitions of selected key words, terms and phrases and coding alerts for adding points to the clinical domain, references to coding late effects where appropriate, and references to personal history V-codes in situations where the acute or chronic condition is no longer active. An example from this chapter is as follows:

581 **Nephrotic syndrome**

> **DEFINITION** Nephrotic syndrome is a collection of symptoms which occur because the glomeruli (tiny blood vessels) in the kidney become leaky. This allows protein, normally never passed out in the urine, to leave the body in large amounts.
>
> **ALERT!** For personal history of nephrotic syndrome see V13.03

MULTIPLE CODING FOR A SINGLE CONDITION

In addition to the etiology or manifestation convention that requires two codes to fully describe a single condition that affects multiple body systems, there are other single conditions that also require more than one code. "Use additional code" notes are found in the tabular at codes that are not part of an etiology or manifestation pair where a secondary code is useful to fully describe a condition. The sequencing rule is the same as the etiology or manifestation pair - , "use additional code" indicates that a secondary code should be added.

"Code first" notes are also under certain codes that are not specifically manifestation codes but may be due to an underlying cause. When a "code first" note is present and an underlying condition is present the underlying condition should be sequenced first.

"Code, if applicable, any causal condition first", notes indicate that this code may be assigned as a principal diagnosis when the causal condition is unknown or not applicable. If a causal condition is known, then the code for that condition should be sequenced as the principal or first-listed diagnosis. Multiple codes may be needed for late effects, complication codes and obstetric codes to more fully describe a condition. See the specific guidelines for these conditions for further instruction.

COMBINATION CODE

A combination code is a single code used to classify: two diagnoses, or a diagnosis with an associated secondary process (manifestation) A diagnosis with an associated complication Combination codes are identified by referring to subterm entries in the Alphabetic Index and by reading the inclusion and exclusion notes in the Tabular List.

Assign only the combination code when that code fully identifies the diagnostic conditions involved or when the Alphabetic Index so directs. Multiple coding should not be used when the classification provides a combination code that clearly identifies all of the elements documented in the diagnosis. When the combination code lacks necessary specificity in describing the manifestation or complication, an additional code should be
used as a secondary code.

CODING LATE EFFECTS

A late effect is the residual effect (condition produced) after the acute phase of an illness or injury has terminated. There is no time limit on when a late effect code can be used. The residual may be apparent early, such as in cerebrovascular accident cases, or it may occur months or years later, such as that due to a previous injury. Coding of late effects generally requires two codes sequenced in the following order: The condition or nature of the late effect is sequenced first. The late effect code is sequenced second.

An exception to the above guidelines are those instances where the code for late effect is followed by a manifestation code identified in the Tabular List and title, or the late effect code has been expanded (at the fourth and fifth-digit levels) to include the manifestation(s). The code for the acute phase of an illness or injury that led to the late effect is never used with a code for the late effect.

CHRONIC KIDNEY DISEASE

Stages of chronic kidney disease (CKD)

The ICD-9-CM classifies CKD based on severity. The severity of CKD is designated by stages I-V. Stage II, code 585.2, equates to mild CKD; stage III, code 585.3, equates to moderate CKD; and stage IV, code

	Add 4th or 5th digit		Nonspecific code		Unspecified code		Manifestation code

585.4, equates to severe CKD. Code 585.6, End stage renal disease (ESRD), is assigned when the provider has documented end-stage-renal disease (ESRD).

If both a stage of CKD and ESRD are documented, assign code 585.6 only.

Chronic kidney disease and kidney transplant status

Patients who have undergone kidney transplant may still have some form of CKD, because the kidney transplant may not fully restore kidney function. Therefore, the presence of CKD alone does not constitute a transplant complication. Assign the appropriate 585 code for the patient's stage of CKD and code V42.0. If a transplant complication such as failure or rejection is documented, see Official Guidelines, Section I.C.17.f.1.b for information on coding complications of a kidney transplant. If the documentation is unclear as to whether the patient has a complication of the transplant, query the provider.

Chronic kidney disease with other conditions

Patients with CKD may also suffer from other serious conditions, most commonly diabetes mellitus and hypertension. The sequencing of the CKD code in relationship to codes for other contributing conditions is based on the conventions in the tabular list.

See Chapter 3 for sequencing instructions for diabetes.
See Chapter 4 for anemia in CKD.
See Chapter 7 for hypertensive chronic kidney disease.
See Chapter 17 for instructions on coding of documented rejection or failure of kidney transplant.

● Code new
to 2012 edition
▲ Revision of
existing code
④ ⑤ Fourth or fifth
digit required

10. DISEASES OF THE GENITOURINARY SYSTEM (580-629)

NEPHRITIS, NEPHROTIC SYNDROME, AND NEPHROSIS (580-589)

Excludes: hypertensive chronic kidney disease (403.00-403.91, 404.00-404.93)

ALERT! For personal history of disorders of the urinary system see V13.0

580 Acute glomerulonephritis
Includes: acute nephritis

DEFINITION Glomerulonephritis is a form of nephritis with inflammation of the capillary loops in the renal glomeruli. The acute form is characterized by proteinuria, edema, hematuria, renal failure, and hypertension, sometimes preceded by tonsillitis or febrile pharyngitis

580.0 **With lesion of proliferative glomerulonephritis**
Acute (diffuse) proliferative glomerulonephritis
Acute poststreptococcal glomerulonephritis

580.4 **With lesion of rapidly progressive glomerulonephritis**
Acute nephritis with lesion of necrotizing glomerulitis

⑤ **580.8** **With other specified pathological lesion in kidney**

580.81 *Acute glomerulonephritis in diseases classified elsewhere*
Code first underlying disease, as:
infectious hepatitis (070.0-070.9)
mumps (072.79)
subacute bacterial endocarditis (421.0)
typhoid fever (002.0)

580.89 **Other**
Glomerulonephritis, acute, with lesion of:
exudative nephritis
interstitial (diffuse) (focal) nephritis

580.9 **Acute glomerulonephritis with unspecified pathological lesion in kidney**
Glomerulonephritis:
NOS specified as acute
hemorrhagic specified as acute
Nephritis specified as acute
Nephropathy specified as acute

581 Nephrotic syndrome

DEFINITION Nephrotic syndrome is a collection of symptoms which occur because the glomeruli (tiny blood vessels) in the kidney become leaky. This allows protein, normally never passed out in the urine, to leave the body in large amounts

ALERT! For personal history of nephrotic syndrome see V13.03

581.0 **With lesion of proliferative glomerulonephritis**

581.1 **With lesion of membranous glomerulonephritis**
Epimembranous nephritis
Idiopathic membranous glomerular disease
Nephrotic syndrome with lesion of:
focal glomerulosclerosis
sclerosing membranous glomerulonephritis
segmental hyalinosis

581.2 **With lesion of membranoproliferative glomerulonephritis**
Nephrotic syndrome with lesion (of):
endothelial glomerulonephritis
hypocomplementemic persistent glomerulonephritis
lobular glomerulonephritis
mesangiocapillary glomerulonephritis
mixed membranous and proliferative glomerulonephritis

581.3 **With lesion of minimal change glomerulonephritis**
Foot process disease
Lipoid nephrosis
Minimal change:
glomerular disease
glomerulitis
nephrotic syndrome

⑤ **581.8** **With other specified pathological lesion in kidney**

581.81 *Nephrotic syndrome in diseases classified elsewhere*
Code first underlying disease, as:
amyloidosis (277.30-277.39)
diabetes mellitus (249.4, 250.4)
malaria (084.9)
polyarteritis (446.0)
systemic lupus erythematosus (710.0)

				489
Add 4th or 5th digit	Nonspecific code	Unspecified code	Manifestation code	

Excludes: *nephrosis in epidemic hemorrhagic fever (078.6)*

581.89 Other
Glomerulonephritis with edema and lesion of:
exudative nephritis
interstitial (diffuse) (focal) nephritis

581.9 Nephrotic syndrome with unspecified pathological lesion in kidney
Glomerulonephritis with edema NOS
Nephritis:
nephrotic NOS
with edema NOS
Nephrosis NOS
Renal disease with edema NOS

582 Chronic glomerulonephritis
Includes: chronic nephritis

DEFINITION Glomerulonephritis is a form of nephritis with inflammation of the capillary loops in the renal glomeruli.

582.0 With lesion of proliferative glomerulonephritis
Chronic (diffuse) proliferative glomerulonephritis

582.1 With lesion of membranous glomerulonephritis
Chronic glomerulonephritis:
membranous
sclerosing
Focal glomerulosclerosis
Segmental hyalinosis

582.2 With lesion of membranoproliferative glomerulonephritis
Chronic glomerulonephritis:
endothelial
hypocomplementemic persistent
lobular
membranoproliferative
mesangiocapillary
mixed membranous and proliferative

582.4 With lesion of rapidly progressive glomerulonephritis
Chronic nephritis with lesion of necrotizing glomerulitis

⑤ **582.8 With other specified pathological lesion in kidney**

582.81 *Chronic glomerulonephritis in diseases classified elsewhere*
Code first underlying disease, as:
amyloidosis (277.30-277.39)
systemic lupus erythematosus (710.0)

582.89 Other
Chronic glomerulonephritis with lesion of:
exudative nephritis
interstitial (diffuse) (focal) nephritis

582.9 Chronic glomerulonephritis with unspecified pathological lesion in kidney
Glomerulonephritis:
NOS specified as chronic
hemorrhagic specified as chronic
Nephritis specified as chronic
Nephropathy specified as chronic

583 Nephritis and nephropathy, not specified as acute or chronic
Includes: "renal disease" so stated, not specified as acute or chronic but with stated pathology or cause

DEFINITION Nephritis and nephropathy refers to inflammation or other damage to the kidney

583.0 With lesion of proliferative glomerulonephritis
Proliferative:
glomerulonephritis (diffuse) NOS
nephritis NOS
nephropathy NOS

583.1 With lesion of membranous glomerulonephritis
Membranous: Membranous nephropathy NOS
glomerulonephritis NOS
nephritis NOS

● Code new
to 2012 edition

▲ Revision of
existing code

④ ⑤ Fourth or fifth
digit required

583.2 With lesion of membranoproliferative glomerulonephritis
Membranoproliferative:
  glomerulonephritis NOS
  nephritis NOS
  nephropathy NOS
Nephritis NOS, with lesion of:
  hypocomplementemic persistent glomerulonephritis
  lobular glomerulonephritis
  mesangiocapillary glomerulonephritis
  mixed membranous and proliferative glomerulonephritis

583.4 With lesion of rapidly progressive glomerulonephritis
Necrotizing or rapidly progressive:
  glomerulitis NOS
  glomerulonephritis NOS
  nephritis NOS
  nephropathy NOS
Nephritis, unspecified, with lesion of necrotizing glomerulitis

583.6 With lesion of renal cortical necrosis
Nephritis NOS with (renal) cortical necrosis
Nephropathy NOS with (renal) cortical necrosis
Renal cortical necrosis NOS

583.7 With lesion of renal medullary necrosis
Nephritis NOS with (renal) medullary [papillary] necrosis
Nephropathy NOS with (renal) medullary [papillary] necrosis

[5] **583.8 With other specified pathological lesion in kidney**

583.81 Nephritis and nephropathy, not specified as acute or chronic, in diseases classified elsewhere

Code first underlying disease, as:
  amyloidosis (277.30-277.39)
  diabetes mellitus (249.4, 250.4)
  gonococcal infection (098.19)
  Goodpasture's syndrome (446.21)
  systemic lupus erythematosus (710.0)
  tuberculosis (016.0)

[*Excludes:*] *gouty nephropathy (274.10)*
syphilitic nephritis (095.4)

583.89 Other
Glomerulitis with lesion of:
  exudative nephritis
  interstitial nephritis
Glomerulonephritis with lesion of:
  exudative nephritis
  interstitial nephritis
Nephritis with lesion of:
  exudative nephritis
  interstitial nephritis
Nephropathy with lesion of:
  exudative nephritis
  interstitial nephritis
Renal disease with lesion of:
  exudative nephritis
  interstitial nephritis

583.9 With unspecified pathological lesion in kidney
Glomerulitis NOS
Glomerulonephritis NOS
Nephritis NOS
Nephropathy NOS

[*Excludes:*] *nephropathy complicating pregnancy, labor, or the puerperium (642.0-642.9, 646.2)*
renal disease NOS with no stated cause (593.9)

584 Acute kidney failure
    Includes: Acute renal failure

    Excludes: *following labor and delivery (669.3)*
        posttraumatic (958.5)
        that complicating:
            abortion (634-638 with .3, 639.3)
            ectopic or molar pregnancy (639.3)

    DEFINITION Kidney failure is the sudden loss of the kidneys' ability to eliminate excess fluid and electrolytes as well as waste material from the blood

584.5 Acute kidney failure with lesion of tubular necrosis
    Lower nephron nephrosis
    Renal failure with (acute) tubular necrosis
    Tubular necrosis:
        NOS
        acute

584.6 Acute kidney failure with lesion of renal cortical necrosis

584.7 Acute kidney failure with lesion of renal medullary [papillary] necrosis
    Necrotizing renal papillitis

584.8 Acute kidney failure with other specified pathological lesion in kidney

584.9 Acute kidney failure, unspecified
    Acute kidney injury (nontraumatic)

    Excludes: *traumatic kidney injury (866.00-866.13)*

585 Chronic kidney disease (CKD)
    Code first hypertensive chronic kidney disease, if applicable, (403.00-403.91, 404.00-404.93)

    Use additional code to identify kidney transplant status, if applicable (V42.0)

    DEFINITION Chronic kidney disease (CKD), aka chronic renal disease, is a progressive loss of renal function over a period of months or years

585.1 Chronic kidney disease, Stage I

585.2 Chronic kidney disease, Stage II (mild)

585.3 Chronic kidney disease, Stage III (moderate)

585.4 Chronic kidney disease, Stage IV (severe)

585.5 Chronic kidney disease, Stage V

    Excludes: *chronic kidney disease, stage V requiring chronic dialysis (585.6)*

585.6 End stage renal disease
    Chronic kidney disease requiring chronic dialysis

585.9 Chronic kidney disease, unspecified
    Chronic renal disease
    Chronic renal failure NOS
    Chronic renal insufficiency

586 Renal failure, unspecified
    Uremia NOS

    Excludes: *following labor and delivery (669.3)*
        posttraumatic renal failure (958.5)
        that complicating:
            abortion (634-638 with .3, 639.3)
            ectopic or molar pregnancy (639.3)
        uremia:
            extrarenal (788.9)
            prerenal (788.9)

    DEFINITION Renal failure refers to severe malfunction of the kidneys, producing uremia and the resulting constitutional symptoms

587 Renal sclerosis, unspecified
    Includes: Atrophy of kidney
    Contracted kidney
    Renal:
        cirrhosis
        fibrosis

    DEFINITION Renal sclerosis is a sclerosis or hardening of the kidney due to renovascular disease

● Code new   ▲ Revision of   ④ ⑤ Fourth or fifth
        to 2012 edition   existing code   digit required

588 **Disorders resulting from impaired renal function**

588.0 Renal osteodystrophy
Azotemic osteodystrophy
Phosphate-losing tubular
disorders

Renal:
dwarfism
infantilism
rickets

588.1 Nephrogenic diabetes insipidus
Excludes: *diabetes insipidus NOS (253.5)*

⑤ **588.8 Other specified disorders resulting from impaired renal function**
Excludes: *secondary hypertension (405.0-405.9)*

588.81 Secondary hyperparathyroidism (of renal origin)
Secondary hyperparathyroidism NOS

588.89 Other specified disorders resulting from impaired renal function
Hypokalemic nephropathy

588.9 Unspecified disorder resulting from impaired renal function

589 **Small kidney of unknown cause**

589.0 Unilateral small kidney

589.1 Bilateral small kidneys

589.9 Small kidney, unspecified

OTHER DISEASES OF URINARY SYSTEM (590-599)

590 **Infections of kidney**
Use additional code to identify organism, such as Escherichia coli [E. coli] (041.41-041.49)

⑤ **590.0 Chronic pyelonephritis**
Chronic pyelitis
Chronic pyonephrosis

Code, if applicable, any causal condition first

590.00 Without lesion of renal medullary necrosis

590.01 With lesion of renal medullary necrosis

⑤ **590.1 Acute pyelonephritis**
Acute pyelitis
Acute pyonephrosis

590.10 Without lesion of renal medullary necrosis

590.11 With lesion of renal medullary necrosis

590.2 Renal and perinephric abscess
Abscess:
kidney
nephritic
perirenal

Carbuncle of kidney

590.3 Pyeloureteritis cystica
Infection of renal pelvis and ureter
Ureteritis cystica

⑤ **590.8 Other pyelonephritis or pyonephrosis, not specified as acute or chronic**

590.80 Pyelonephritis, unspecified
Pyelitis NOS
Pyelonephritis NOS

590.81 *Pyelitis or pyelonephritis in diseases classified elsewhere*
Code first underlying disease, as:
tuberculosis (016.0)

590.9 Infection of kidney, unspecified
Excludes: *urinary tract infection NOS (599.0)*

591 **Hydronephrosis**
Hydrocalycosis
Hydronephrosis

Hydroureteronephrosis

Excludes: *congenital hydronephrosis (753.29)*
hydroureter (593.5)

DEFINITION Hydronephrosis is a condition that occurs as a result of urine accumulation in the upper urinary tract. This usually occurs from a blockage somewhere along the urinary tract.

	Add 4th or 5th digit		Nonspecific code		Unspecified code		Manifestation code

493

592 Calculus of kidney and ureter

[Excludes:] *nephrocalcinosis (275.4)*

[ALERT!] For personal history of urinary calculi see V13.01

592.0 Calculus of kidney

Nephrolithiasis NOS
Renal calculus or stone
Staghorn calculus
Stone in kidney

[Excludes:] *uric acid nephrolithiasis (274.11)*

592.1 Calculus of ureter

Ureteric stone
Ureterolithiasis

592.9 Urinary calculus, unspecified

593 Other disorders of kidney and ureter

[ALERT!] For personal history of other specified urinary system disorders see V13.09

593.0 Nephroptosis

Floating kidney
Mobile kidney

593.1 Hypertrophy of kidney

593.2 Cyst of kidney, acquired

Cyst (multiple) (solitary) of kidney, not congenital
Peripelvic (lymphatic) cyst

[Excludes:] *calyceal or pyelogenic cyst of kidney (591)*
congenital cyst of kidney (753.1)
polycystic (disease of) kidney (753.1)

593.3 Stricture or kinking of ureter

Angulation of ureter (postoperative)
Constriction of ureter (postoperative)
Stricture of pelviureteric junction

593.4 Other ureteric obstruction

Idiopathic retroperitoneal fibrosis
Occlusion NOS of ureter

[Excludes:] *that due to calculus (592.1)*

593.5 Hydroureter

[Excludes:] *congenital hydroureter (753.22)*
hydroureteronephrosis (591)

593.6 Postural proteinuria

Benign postural proteinuria
Orthostatic proteinuria

[Excludes:] *proteinuria NOS (791.0)*

[5] **593.7 Vesicoureteral reflux**

593.70 Unspecified or without reflux nephropathy

593.71 With reflux nephropathy, unilateral

593.72 With reflux nephropathy, bilateral

593.73 With reflux nephropathy NOS

[5] **593.8 Other specified disorders of kidney and ureter**

593.81 Vascular disorders of kidney

Renal (artery):
embolism
hemorrhage
thrombosis
Renal infarction

593.82 Ureteral fistula

Intestinoureteral fistula

[Excludes:] *fistula between ureter and female genital tract (619.0)*

593.89 Other
    Adhesions, kidney or ureter
    Periureteritis
    Polyp of ureter
    Pyelectasia
    Ureterocele

Excludes: tuberculosis of ureter (016.2)
       ureteritis cystica (590.3)

593.9 Unspecified disorder of kidney and ureter
    Acute renal disease
    Acute renal insufficiency
    Renal disease NOS
    Salt-losing nephritis or syndrome

Excludes: chronic renal insufficiency (585.9)
       cystic kidney disease (753.1)
       nephropathy, so stated (583.0-583.9)
       renal disease:
         arising in pregnancy or the puerperium (642.1-642.2, 642.4-642.7, 646.2)
         not specified as acute or chronic, but with stated pathology or cause
           (583.0-583.9)

594 Calculus of lower urinary tract
    DEFINITION A Calculus of lower urinary tract is a stone (calculus) located in the lower urinary tract.

594.0 Calculus in diverticulum of bladder

594.1 Other calculus in bladder
    Urinary bladder stone

Excludes: staghorn calculus (592.0)

594.2 Calculus in urethra

594.8 Other lower urinary tract calculus

594.9 Calculus of lower urinary tract, unspecified

Excludes: calculus of urinary tract NOS (592.9)

595 Cystitis

Excludes: prostatocystitis (601.3)

Use additional code to identify organism, such as Escherichia coli [E. coli] (041.41-041.49)
    DEFINITION Cystitis is an inflammation of the urinary bladder and ureters

595.0 Acute cystitis

Excludes: trigonitis (595.3)

595.1 Chronic interstitial cystitis
    Hunner's ulcer   Submucous cystitis
    Panmural fibrosis of bladder

595.2 Other chronic cystitis
    Chronic cystitis NOS
    Subacute cystitis

Excludes: trigonitis (595.3)

595.3 Trigonitis
    Follicular cystitis
    Trigonitis (acute) (chronic)
    Urethrotrigonitis

595.4 *Cystitis in diseases classified elsewhere*
Code first underlying disease, as:
    actinomycosis (039.8)
    amebiasis (006.8)
    bilharziasis (120.0-120.9)
    Echinococcus infestation (122.3, 122.6)

Excludes: cystitis:
        diphtheritic (032.84)
        gonococcal (098.11, 098.31)
        monilial (112.2)
        trichomonal (131.09)
        tuberculous (016.1)

⑤ **595.8 Other specified types of cystitis**

    595.81   Cystitis cystica

    595.82   Irradiation cystitis
    Use additional E code, if desired, to identify cause

    595.89 **Other**
        Abscess of bladder
        Cystitis:
          bullous
          emphysematous
          glandularis

595.9 Cystitis, unspecified

596 **Other disorders of bladder**
Use additional code, if desired, to identify urinary incontinence (625.6, 788.30-788.39)
    ALERT! For personal history of other specified urinary system disorders see V13.09

596.0 Bladder neck obstruction
    Contracture (acquired) of bladder neck or vesicourethral orifice
    Obstruction (acquired) of bladder neck or vesicourethral orifice
    Stenosis (acquired) of bladder neck or vesicourethral orifice

    Excludes: *congenital (753.6)*

596.1 Intestinovesical fistula
    Fistula: Fistula:
      enterovesical   vesicoenteric
      vesicocolic   vesicorectal

596.2 Vesical fistula, not elsewhere classified
    Fistula: Fistula:
      bladder NOS   vesicocutaneous
      urethrovesical   vesicoperineal

    Excludes: *fistula between bladder and female genital tract (619.0)*

596.3 Diverticulum of bladder
    Diverticulitis of bladder
    Diverticulum (acquired) (false) of bladder

    Excludes: *that with calculus in diverticulum of bladder (594.0)*

596.4 Atony of bladder
    High compliance bladder, of bladder
    Hypotonicity of bladder
    Inertia of bladder

    Excludes: *neurogenic bladder (596.54)*

⑤ **596.5 Other functional disorders of bladder**

    Excludes: *cauda equina syndrome*
                  with neurogenic bladder (344.61)

    596.51   Hypertonicity of bladder
        Hyperactivity
        Overactive bladder

    596.52   Low bladder compliance

    596.53   Paralysis of bladder

    596.54   Neurogenic bladder NOS

    596.55   Detrusor sphincter dyssynergia

    596.59 **Other functional disorder of bladder**
        Detrusor instability

596.6 Rupture of bladder, nontraumatic

596.7 Hemorrhage into bladder wall
    Hyperemia of bladder

    Excludes: *acute hemorrhagic cystitis (595.0)*

⑤ **596.8 Other specified disorders of bladder**

    Excludes: *cystocele, female (618.01-618.02, 618.09, 618.2-618.4)*
              hernia or prolapse of bladder, female (618.01-618.02, 618.09, 618.2-618.4)

● Code new   ▲ Revision of   ④ ⑤ Fourth or fifth
   to 2012 edition   existing code   digit required

● **596.81 Infection of cystostomy**

Use additional code to specify type of infection, such as:
abscess or cellulitis of abdomen (682.2)
septicemia (038.0-038.9)

Use additional code to identify organism (041.00-041.9)

● **596.82 Mechanical complication of cystostomy**
Malfunction of cystostomy

● **596.83 Other complication of cystostomy**
Fistula
Hernia
Prolapse

● **596.89 Other specified disorders of bladder**
Bladder hemorrhage
Bladder hypertrophy
Calcified bladder
Contracted bladder

596.9 Unspecified disorder of bladder

597 Urethritis, not sexually transmitted, and urethral syndrome

[Excludes:] *nonspecific urethritis, so stated (099.4)*

DEFINITION Urethritis is inflammation of the urethra; resulting in painful urination. Urethral syndrome is a term used to describe symptoms of urethritis , without any evidence of bacterial or viral infection as a cause.

597.0 Urethral abscess

Abscess of:
bulbourethral gland
Cowper's gland
Littré's gland

Abscess:
periurethral
urethral (gland)
Periurethral cellulitis

[Excludes:] *urethral caruncle (599.3)*

⑤ **597.8 Other urethritis**

597.80 Urethritis, unspecified

597.81 Urethral syndrome NOS

597.89 Other

Adenitis, Skene's glands
Cowperitis
Meatitis, urethral
Ulcer, urethra (meatus)
Verumontanitis

[Excludes:] *trichomonal (131.02)*

598 Urethral stricture

Includes: pinhole meatus
stricture of urinary meatus

[Excludes:] *congenital stricture of urethra and urinary meatus (753.6)*

Use additional code to identify urinary incontinence (625.6, 788.30-788.39)

DEFINITION Urethral stricture is a narrowing of the urethra caused by injury or disease such as urinary tract infections or other forms of urethritis

⑤ **598.0 Urethral stricture due to infection**

598.00 Due to unspecified infection

598.01 Due to infective diseases classified elsewhere

Code first underlying disease, as:
gonococcal infection (098.2)
schistosomiasis (120.0-120.9)
syphilis (095.8)

598.1 Traumatic urethral stricture

Stricture of urethra:
late effect of injury
postobstetric

[Excludes:] *postoperative following surgery on genitourinary tract (598.2)*

598.2 Postoperative urethral stricture
Postcatheterization stricture of urethra

598.8 Other specified causes of urethral stricture

598.9 Urethral stricture, unspecified

Add 4th or 5th digit | Nonspecific code | Unspecified code | Manifestation code

599 Other disorders of urethra and urinary tract

[ALERT!] For personal history of other specified urinary system disorders see V13.09

[ALERT!] For personal history of urinary (tract) infection see V13.02

599.0 Urinary tract infection, site not specified
Pyuria

[Excludes:] *candidiasis of urinary tract (112.2)*
urinary tract infection of newborn (771.82)

Use additional code to identify organism, such as Escherichia coli [E. coli] (041.41-041.49)

599.1 Urethral fistula
Fistula:
urethroperineal
urethrorectal
Urinary fistula NOS

[Excludes:] *fistula:*
urethroscrotal (608.89)
urethrovaginal (619.0)
urethrovesicovaginal (619.0)

599.2 Urethral diverticulum

599.3 Urethral caruncle
Polyp of urethra

599.4 Urethral false passage

599.5 Prolapsed urethral mucosa
Prolapse of urethra
Urethrocele

[Excludes:] *urethrocele, female (618.03, 618.09, 618.2-618.4)*

[5] **599.6 Urinary obstruction**

599.60 Urinary obstruction, unspecified
Obstructive uropathy NOS
Urinary (tract) obstruction NOS

599.69 Urinary obstruction, not elsewhere classified

Code, if applicable, any causal condition first, such as:
hyperplasia of prostate (600.0-600.9 with fifth-digit 1)

[5] **599.7 Hematuria**
Hematuria (benign) (essential)

[Excludes:] *hemoglobinuria (791.2)*

599.70 Hematuria, unspecified

599.71 Gross hematuria

599.72 Microscopic hematuria

[5] **599.8 Other specified disorders of urethra and urinary tract**

[Excludes:] *symptoms and other conditions classifiable to 788.0-788.9, 791.0-791.9*

Use additional code, if desired, to identify urinary incontinence (625.6, 788.30-788.39)

599.81 Urethral hypermobility

599.82 Intrinsic (urethral) sphincter deficiency [ISD]

599.83 Urethral instability

599.84 Other specified disorders of urethra
Rupture of urethra (nontraumatic)
Urethral:
cyst
granuloma

599.89 Other specified disorders of urinary tract

599.9 Unspecified disorder of urethra and urinary tract

[ALERT!] For personal history of unspecified urinary disorder see V13.00

DISEASES OF MALE GENITAL ORGANS (600-608)

600 Hyperplasia of prostate
Includes: enlarged prostate

[DEFINITION] Hyperplasia of prostate is a nonmalignant enlargement of the prostate gland commonly occurring in men after the age of 50, and sometimes leading to compression of the urethra and obstruction of the flow of urine

[5] **600.0 Hypertrophy (benign) of prostate**
Benign prostatic hypertrophy
Enlargement of prostate
Smooth enlarged prostate
Soft enlarged prostate

600.00 Hypertrophy (benign) of prostate without urinary obstruction and other lower urinary tract symptoms (LUTS)
Hypertrophy (benign) of prostate NOS

600.01 Hypertrophy (benign) of prostate with urinary obstruction and other lower urinary tract symptoms (LUTS)
Hypertrophy (benign) of prostate with urinary retention

Use additional code to identify symptoms:
incomplete bladder emptying (788.21)
nocturia (788.43)
straining on urination (788.65)
urinary frequency (788.41)
urinary hesitancy (788.64)
urinary incontinence (788.30-788.39)
urinary obstruction (599.69)
urinary retention (788.20)
urinary urgency (788.63)
weak urinary stream (788.62)

[5] **600.1 Nodular prostate**
Hard, firm prostate
Multinodular prostate

[Excludes:] *malignant neoplasm of prostate (185)*

600.10 Nodular prostate without urinary obstruction
Nodular prostate NOS

600.11 Nodular prostate with urinary obstruction
Nodular prostate with urinary retention

[5] **600.2 Benign localized hyperplasia of prostate**
Adenofibromatous hypertrophy of prostate
Adenoma of prostate
Fibroadenoma of prostate
Fibroma of prostate
Myoma of prostate
Polyp of prostate

[Excludes:] *benign neoplasms of prostate (222.2)*
hypertrophy of prostate (600.00-600.01)
malignant neoplasm of prostate (185)

600.20 Benign localized hyperplasia of prostate without urinary obstruction and other lower urinary tract symptoms (LUTS)
Benign localized hyperplasia of prostate NOS

600.21 Benign localized hyperplasia of prostate with urinary obstruction and other lower urinary tract symptoms (LUTS)
Benign localized hyperplasia of prostate with urinary retention

Use additional code to identify symptoms:
incomplete bladder emptying (788.21)
nocturia (788.43)
straining on urination (788.65)
urinary frequency (788.41)
urinary hesitancy (788.64)
urinary incontinence (788.30-788.39)
urinary obstruction (599.69)
urinary retention (788.20)
urinary urgency (788.63)
weak urinary stream (788.62)

600.3 Cyst of prostate

[5] **600.9 Hyperplasia of prostate, unspecified**
Median bar
Prostatic obstruction NOS

600.90 Hyperplasia of prostate, unspecified, without urinary obstruction and other lower urinary symptoms (LUTS)
Hyperplasia of prostate NOS

600.91 Hyperplasia of prostate, unspecified, with urinary obstruction and other lower urinary symptoms (LUTS)
Hyperplasia of prostate, unspecified, with urinary retention

Use additional code to identify symptoms:
> incomplete bladder emptying (788.21)
> nocturia (788.43)
> straining on urination (788.65)
> urinary frequency (788.41)
> urinary hesitancy (788.64)
> urinary incontinence (788.30-788.39)
> urinary obstruction (599.69)
> urinary retention (788.20)
> urinary urgency (788.63)
> weak urinary stream (788.62)

601 Inflammatory diseases of prostate
Use additional code, if desired, to identify organism, such as Staphylococcus (041.1), or Streptococcus (041.0)

601.0 Acute prostatitis

601.1 Chronic prostatitis

601.2 Abscess of prostate

601.3 Prostatocystitis

601.4 Prostatitis in diseases classified elsewhere
Code first underlying disease, as:
> actinomycosis (039.8)
> blastomycosis (116.0)
> syphilis (095.8)
> tuberculosis (016.5)

> Excludes: *prostatitis:*
>> *gonococcal (098.12, 098.32)*
>> *monilial (112.2)*
>> *trichomonal (131.03)*

601.8 Other specified inflammatory diseases of prostate
Prostatitis:
> cavitary
> diverticular
> granulomatous

601.9 Prostatitis, unspecified
Prostatitis NOS

602 Other disorders of prostate

602.0 Calculus of prostate
Prostatic stone

602.1 Congestion or hemorrhage of prostate

602.2 Atrophy of prostate

602.3 Dysplasia of prostate
Prostatic intraepithelial neoplasia I (PIN I)
Prostatic intraepithelial neoplasia II (PIN II)

> Excludes: *Prostatic intraepithelial neoplasia III (PIN III) (233.4)*

602.8 Other specified disorders of prostate
Fistula of prostate
Infarction of prostate
Stricture of prostate
Periprostatic adhesions

602.9 Unspecified disorder of prostate

603 Hydrocele
Includes: hydrocele of spermatic cord, testis, or tunica vaginalis

> Excludes: *congenital (778.6)*

> **DEFINITION** A Hydrocele is a painless swelling of the scrotum, caused by a collection of fluid around the testicle; commonly occurs in middle-aged men

603.0 Encysted hydrocele

603.1 Infected hydrocele
Use additional code, if desired, to identify organism

● Code new to 2012 edition   ▲ Revision of existing code   ④ ⑤ Fourth or fifth digit required

603.8 Other specified types of hydrocele

603.9 Hydrocele, unspecified

604 Orchitis and epididymitis

Use additional code to identify organism, such as:
Escherichia coli [E. coli] (041.41-041.49)
Staphylococcus (041.10-041.19)
Streptococcus (041.00-041.09)

DEFINITION Orchitis is the inflammation and swelling of the testes as a result of infection or physical injury. Epididymitis is an inflammation of the epididymis which is located along the posterior aspect of the testicle.

604.0 Orchitis, epididymitis, and epididymo-orchitis, with abscess
Abscess of epididymis or testis

[5] **604.9 Other orchitis, epididymitis, and epididymo-orchitis, without mention of abscess**

604.90 Orchitis and epididymitis, unspecified

604.91 Orchitis and epididymitis in diseases classified elsewhere

Code first underlying disease, as:
diphtheria (032.89)
filariasis (125.0-125.9)
syphilis (095.8)

[Excludes:] orchitis:
gonococcal (098.13, 098.33)
mumps (072.0)
tuberculous (016.5)
tuberculous epididymitis (016.4)

604.99 Other

605 Redundant prepuce and phimosis

Adherent prepuce
Paraphimosis
Phimosis (congenital)
Tight foreskin

DEFINITION Redundant prepuce is a condition where the foreskin of the penis more than covers the glans when not erect and does not automatically fully retract upon erection. Phimosis is a constriction of the foreskin of the penis resulting in the inability to retract the prepuce over the glans

606 Infertility, male

DEFINITION Male Infertility refers to the biological inability of the male to contribute to conception

606.0 Azoospermia
Absolute infertility
Infertility due to:
germinal (cell) aplasia
spermatogenic arrest (complete)

606.1 Oligospermia
Infertility due to:
germinal cell desquamation
hypospermatogenesis
incomplete spermatogenic arrest

606.8 Infertility due to extratesticular causes
Infertility due to:
drug therapy
infection
obstruction of efferent ducts
radiation
systemic disease

ALERT! For personal history of drug therapy see V87.4

606.9 Male infertility, unspecified

607 Disorders of penis

[Excludes:] phimosis (605)

607.0 Leukoplakia of penis
Kraurosis of penis

[Excludes:] carcinoma in situ of penis (233.5)
erythroplasia of Queyrat (233.5)

607.1 Balanoposthitis
Balanitis

Use additional code, if desired, to identify organism

Add 4th or 5th digit | Nonspecific code | Unspecified code | Manifestation code

607.2 Other inflammatory disorders of penis
Abscess of corpus cavernosum or penis
Boil of corpus cavernosum or penis
Carbuncle of corpus cavernosum or penis
Cellulitis of corpus cavernosum or penis
Cavernitis (penis)

Use additional code, if desired, to identify organism

Excludes: herpetic infection (054.13)

607.3 Priapism
Painful erection

⑤ **607.8 Other specified disorders of penis**

607.81 Balanitis xerotica obliterans
Induratio penis plastica

607.82 Vascular disorders of penis
Embolism of corpus cavernosum or penis
Hematoma (nontraumatic) of corpus cavernosum or penis
Hemorrhage of corpus cavernosum or penis
Thrombosis of corpus cavernosum or penis

607.83 Edema of penis

607.84 Impotence of organic origin

Excludes: nonorganic (302.72)

607.85 Peyronie's disease

607.89 Other
Atrophy of corpus cavernosum or penis
Fibrosis of corpus cavernosum or penis
Hypertrophy of corpus cavernosum or penis
Ulcer (chronic) of corpus cavernosum or penis

607.9 Unspecified disorder of penis

608 Other disorders of male genital organs
ALERT! For personal history of other genital system and obstetric disorders see V13.2

608.0 Seminal vesiculitis
Abscess of seminal vesicle
Cellulitis of seminal vesicle
Vesiculitis (seminal)

Use additional code, if desired, to identify organism

Excludes: gonococcal infection (098.14, 098.34)

608.1 Spermatocele

⑤ **608.2 Torsion of testis**

608.20 Torsion of testis, unspecified

608.21 Extravaginal torsion of spermatic cord

608.22 Intravaginal torsion of spermatic cord
Torsion of spermatic cord NOS

608.23 Torsion of appendix testis

608.24 Torsion of appendix epididymis

608.3 Atrophy of testis

608.4 Other inflammatory disorders of male genital organs
Abscess of scrotum, spermatic cord, testis [except abscess], tunica vaginalis, or vas deferens
Boil of scrotum, spermatic cord, testis [except abscess], tunica vaginalis, or vas deferens
Carbuncle of scrotum, spermatic cord, testis [except abscess], tunica vaginalis, or vas deferens
Cellulitis of scrotum, spermatic cord, testis [except abscess], tunica vaginalis, or vas deferens
Vasitis

Use additional code, if desired, to identify organism

Excludes: abscess of testis (604.0)

⑤ **608.8 Other specified disorders of male genital organs**

608.81 Disorders of male genital organs in diseases classified elsewhere
Code first underlying disease, as:
filariasis (125.0-125.9)
tuberculosis (016.5)

608.82 Hematospermia

● Code new
to 2012 edition
▲ Revision of
existing code
④ ⑤ Fourth or fifth
digit required

608.83 Vascular disorders
Hematoma (nontraumatic) of seminal vesicle, spermatic cord, testis, scrotum, tunica vaginalis, or vas deferens
Hemorrhage of seminal vesicle, spermatic cord, testis, scrotum, tunica vaginalis, or vas deferens
Thrombosis of seminal vesicle, spermatic cord, testis, scrotum, tunica vaginalis, or vas deferens
Hematocele NOS, male

608.84 Chylocele of tunica vaginalis

608.85 Stricture
Stricture of:
   spermatic cord
   tunica vaginalis
   vas deferens

608.86 Edema

608.87 Retrograde ejaculation

608.89 Other
Atrophy of seminal vesicle, spermatic cord, testis, scrotum, tunica vaginalis, or vas deferens
Fibrosis of seminal vesicle, spermatic cord, testis, scrotum, tunica vaginalis, or vas deferens
Hypertrophy of seminal vesicle, spermatic cord, testis, scrotum, tunica vaginalis, or vas deferens
Ulcer of seminal vesicle, spermatic cord, testis, scrotum, tunica vaginalis, or vas deferens

Excludes: atrophy of testis (608.3)

608.9 Unspecified disorder of male genital organs

DISORDERS OF BREAST (610-612)

610 Benign mammary dysplasias
DEFINITION Mammary dysplasia is a common condition marked by benign (noncancerous) changes in breast tissue. These changes may include irregular lumps or cysts, breast discomfort, sensitive nipples, and itching.

610.0 Solitary cyst of breast
Cyst (solitary) of breast

610.1 Diffuse cystic mastopathy
Chronic cystic mastitis   Fibrocystic disease of breast
Cystic breast

610.2 Fibroadenosis of breast
Fibroadenosis of breast: Fibroadenosis of breast:
   NOS   diffuse
   chronic   periodic
   cystic   segmental

610.3 Fibrosclerosis of breast

610.4 Mammary duct ectasia
Comedomastitis   Mastitis:
Dust ectasia   periductal
                                     plasma cell

610.8 Other specified benign mammary dysplasias
Mazoplasia
Sebaceous cyst of breast

610.9 Benign mammary dysplasia, unspecified

611 Other disorders of breast

Excludes: that associated with lactation or the puerperium (675.0-676.9)

611.0 Inflammatory disease of breast
Abscess (acute) (chronic) (nonpuerperal) of:
areola
breast
Mammillary fistula
Mastitis (acute) (subacute) (nonpuerperal):
NOS
infective
retromammary
submammary

[Excludes:] *carbuncle of breast (680.2)*
chronic cystic mastitis (610.1)
neonatal infective mastitis (771.5)
thrombophlebitis of breast [Mondor's disease] (451.89)

611.1 Hypertrophy of breast
Gynecomastia
Hypertrophy of breast:
NOS
massive pubertal

[Excludes:] *breast engorgement in newborn (778.7)*
disproportion of reconstructed breast (612.1)

611.2 Fissure of nipple

611.3 Fat necrosis of breast
Fat necrosis (segmental) of breast

Code first breast necrosis due to breast graft (996.79)

611.4 Atrophy of breast

611.5 Galactocele

611.6 Galactorrhea not associated with childbirth

[5] **611.7 Signs and symptoms in breast**

611.71 Mastodynia
Pain in breast

611.72 Lump or mass in breast

611.79 Other
Induration of breast
Inversion of nipple
Nipple discharge
Retraction of nipple

[5] **611.8 Other specified disorders of breast**

611.81 Ptosis of breast

[Excludes:] *ptosis of native breast in relation to reconstructed breast (612.1)*

611.82 Hypoplasia of breast
Micromastia

[Excludes:] *congenital absence of breast (757.6)*
hypoplasia of native breast in relation to reconstructed breast (612.1)

611.83 Capsular contracture of breast implant

611.89 Other specified disorders of breast
Hematoma (nontraumatic) of breast
Infarction of breast
Occlusion of breast duct
Subinvolution of breast (postlactational) (postpartum)

611.9 Unspecified breast disorder

612 Deformity and disproportion of reconstructed breast

612.0 Deformity of reconstructed breast
Contour irregularity in reconstructed breast
Excess tissue in reconstructed breast
Misshapen reconstructed breast

612.1 Disproportion of reconstructed breast
Breast asymmetry between native breast and reconstructed breast
Disproportion between native breast and reconstructed breast

INFLAMMATORY DISEASE OF FEMALE PELVIC ORGANS (614-616)

> Use additional code, if desired, to identify organism, such as Staphylococcus (041.1), or Streptococcus (041.0)
>
> *Excludes:* *that associated with pregnancy, abortion, childbirth, or the puerperium (630-676.9)*

614 **Inflammatory disease of ovary, fallopian tube, pelvic cellular tissue, and peritoneum**

> *Excludes:* *endometritis (615.0-615.9)*
>> *major infection following delivery (670.0-670.8)*
>> *that complicating:*
>> *abortion (634-638 with .0, 639.0)*
>> *ectopic or molar pregnancy (639.0)*
>> *pregnancy or labor (646.6)*

DEFINITION Inflammatory disease is a general term for infection of the uterus lining, fallopian tubes, or ovaries.

614.0 Acute salpingitis and oophoritis
> Any condition classifiable to 614.2, specified as acute or subacute

614.1 Chronic salpingitis and oophoritis
> Hydrosalpinx
> Salpingitis:
> follicularis
> isthmica nodosa
> Any condition classifiable to 614.2, specified as chronic

614.2 Salpingitis and oophoritis not specified as acute, subacute, or chronic
> Abscess (of):   Perisalpingitis
> fallopian tube   Pyosalpinx
> ovary   Salpingitis
> tubo-ovarian   Salpingo-oophoritisRTubo-ovarian inflammatory disease
> Oophoritis
> Perioophoritis

> *Excludes:* *gonococcal infection (chronic) (098.37)*
>> *acute (098.17)*
>> *tuberculous (016.6)*

614.3 Acute parametritis and pelvic cellulitis
> Acute inflammatory pelvic disease
> Any condition classifiable to 614.4, specified as acute

614.4 Chronic or unspecified parametritis and pelvic cellulitis
> Abscess (of):
> broad ligament, chronic or NOS
> parametrium, chronic or NOS
> pelvis, female, chronic or NOS
> pouch of Douglas, chronic or NOS
> Chronic inflammatory pelvic disease
> Pelvic cellulitis, female

> *Excludes:* *tuberculous (016.7)*

614.5 Acute or unspecified pelvic peritonitis, female

614.6 Pelvic peritoneal adhesions, female (postoperative) (postinfection)
> Adhesions:
> peritubal
> tubo-ovarian

Use additional code, if desired, to identify any associated infertility (628.2)

614.7 **Other chronic pelvic peritonitis, female**
> *Excludes:* *tuberculous (016.7)*

614.8 **Other specified inflammatory disease of female pelvic organs and tissues**

614.9 **Unspecified inflammatory disease of female pelvic organs and tissues**
> Pelvic infection or inflammation, female NOS
> Pelvic inflammatory disease [PID]

615 **Inflammatory diseases of uterus, except cervix**

> *Excludes:* *following delivery (670.0-670.8)*
>> *hyperplastic endometritis (621.30-621.35)*
>> *that complicating:*
>> *abortion (634-638 with .0, 639.0)*
>> *ectopic or molar pregnancy (639.0)*
>> *pregnancy or labor (646.6)*

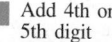 Add 4th or 5th digit
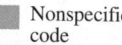 Nonspecific code
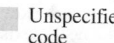 Unspecified code
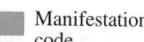 Manifestation code

615.0 Acute
Any condition classifiable to 615.9, specified as acute or subacute

615.1 Chronic
Any condition classifiable to 615.9, specified as chronic

615.9 Unspecified inflammatory disease of uterus
Endometritis
Endomyometritis
Metritis
Myometritis
Perimetritis
Pyometra
Uterine abscess

616 Inflammatory disease of cervix, vagina, and vulva

[Excludes:] *that complicating:*
abortion (634-638 with .0, 639.0)
ectopic or molar pregnancy (639.0)
pregnancy, childbirth, or the puerperium (646.6)

616.0 Cervicitis and endocervicitis
Cervicitis with or without mention of erosion or ectropion
Endocervicitis with or without mention of erosion or ectropion
Nabothian (gland) cyst or follicle

[Excludes:] *erosion or ectropion without mention of cervicitis (622.0)*

[5] **616.1 Vaginitis and vulvovaginitis**

[Excludes:] *vulvar vestibulitis (625.71)*

616.10 Vaginitis and vulvovaginitis, unspecified
Vaginitis:
NOS
postirradiation
Vulvitis NOS
Vulvovaginitis NOS

Use additional code to identify organism, such as:
Escherichia coli [E. coli] (041.41-041.49)
Staphylococcus (041.10-041.19)
Streptococcus (041.00-041.09)

[Excludes:] *noninfective leukorrhea (623.5)*
postmenopausal or senile vaginitis (627.3)

616.11 Vaginitis and vulvovaginitis in diseases classified elsewhere
Code first underlying disease, as:
pinworm vaginitis (127.4)

[Excludes:] *herpetic vulvovaginitis (054.11)*
monilial vulvovaginitis (112.1)
trichomonal vaginitis or vulvovaginitis (131.01)

616.2 Cyst of Bartholin's gland
Bartholin's duct cyst

616.3 Abscess of Bartholin's gland
Vulvovaginal gland abscess

616.4 Other abscess of vulva
Abscess of vulva
Carbuncle of vulva
Furuncle of vulva

[5] **616.5 Ulceration of vulva**

616.50 Ulceration of vulva, unspecified
Ulcer NOS of vulva

616.51 Ulceration of vulva in diseases classified elsewhere
Code first underlying disease, as:
Behçet's syndrome (136.1)
tuberculosis (016.7)

[Excludes:] *vulvar ulcer (in):*
gonococcal (098.0)
herpes simplex (054.12)
syphilitic (091.0)

⑤ **616.8 Other specified inflammatory diseases of cervix, vagina, and vulva**

Excludes: noninflammatory disorders of:
> cervix (622.0-622.9)
> vagina (623.0-623.9)
> vulva (624.0-624.9)

616.81 Mucositis (ulcerative) of cervix, vagina, and vulva
Use additional E code to identify adverse effects of therapy, such as:
> antineoplastic and immunosuppressive drugs (E930.7, E933.1)
> radiation therapy (E879.2)

616.89 Other inflammatory disease of cervix, vagina and vulva
Caruncle, vagina or labium
Ulcer, vagina

616.9 Unspecified inflammatory disease of cervix, vagina, and vulva

OTHER DISORDERS OF FEMALE GENITAL TRACT (617-629)

617 Endometriosis

> **DEFINITION** Endometriosis is a condition where tissue that normally lines the uterus grows in other areas of the body. This can cause pain, irregular menstrual bleeding, and infertility for some women.

617.0 Endometriosis of uterus
Adenomyosis
Endometriosis:
> cervix
> internal
> myometrium

Excludes: stromal endometriosis (236.0)

617.1 Endometriosis of ovary
Chocolate cyst of ovary
Endometrial cystoma of ovary

617.2 Endometriosis of fallopian tube

617.3 Endometriosis of pelvic peritoneum

Endometriosis:
> broad ligament
> cul-de-sac (Douglas')

Endometriosis:
> parametrium
> round ligament

617.4 Endometriosis of rectovaginal septum and vagina

617.5 Endometriosis of intestine
Endometriosis:
> appendix
> colon
> rectum

617.6 Endometriosis in scar of skin

617.8 Endometriosis of other specified sites

Endometriosis:
> bladder
> lung

Endometriosis:
> umbilicus
> vulva

617.9 Endometriosis, site unspecified

618 Genital prolapse
Use additional code, if desired, to identify urinary incontinence (625.6, 788.31, 788.33-788.39)

Excludes: that complicating pregnancy, labor, or delivery (654.4)

> **DEFINITION** Genital prolapse is a condition in which the vaginal wall or uterus descend below their normal positions; part of the bladder or rectum may protrude from the vagina

⑤ **618.0 Prolapse of vaginal walls without mention of uterine prolapse**

Excludes: that with uterine prolapse (618.2-618.4)
> enterocele (618.6)
> vaginal vault prolapse following hysterectomy (618.5)

618.00 Unspecified prolapse of vaginal walls
Vaginal prolapse NOS

618.01 Cystocele, midline
Cystocele NOS

618.02 Cystocele, lateral
Paravaginal

618.03 Urethrocele

Add 4th or 5th digit	Nonspecific code	Unspecified code	Manifestation code

507

618.04 Rectocele
Proctocele

Use additional code for any associated fecal incontinence (787.60-787.63)

618.05 Perineocele

618.09 **Other prolapse of vaginal walls without mention of uterine prolapse**
Cystourethrocele

618.1 Uterine prolapse without mention of vaginal wall prolapse

Descensus uteri
Uterine prolapse:
  NOS
  complete

Uterine prolapse:
  first degree
  second degree
  third degree

Excludes: that with mention of cystocele, urethrocele, or rectocele (618.2-618.4)

618.2 Uterovaginal prolapse, incomplete

618.3 Uterovaginal prolapse, complete

618.4 Uterovaginal prolapse, unspecified

618.5 Prolapse of vaginal vault after hysterectomy

618.6 Vaginal enterocele, congenital or acquired
Pelvic enterocele, congenital or acquired

618.7 Old laceration of muscles of pelvic floor

⑤ **618.8 Other specified genital prolapse**

  618.81 Incompetence or weakening of pubocervical tissue

  618.82 Incompetence or weakening of rectovaginal tissue

  618.83 Pelvic muscle wasting
    Disuse atrophy of pelvic muscles and anal sphincter

  618.84 Cervical stump prolapse

  618.89 **Other specified genital prolapse**

618.9 Unspecified genital prolapse

619 Fistula involving female genital tract

Excludes: vesicorectal and intestinovesical fistula (596.1)

DEFINITION A fistula involving female genital tract is a fistula that has formed in the wall of the vagina. A vaginal fistula may open into the urinary tract, the rectum, the colon, or the small bowel

619.0 Urinary-genital tract fistula, female

Fistula:
  cervicovesical
  ureterovaginal
  urethrovaginal
  urethrovesicovaginal

Fistula:
  uteroureteric
  uterovesical
  vesicocervicovaginal
  vesicovaginal

619.1 Digestive-genital tract fistula, female

Fistula:
  intestinouterine
  intestinovaginal
  rectovaginal

Fistula:
  rectovulval
  sigmoidovaginal
  uterorectal

619.2 Genital tract-skin fistula, female

Fistula:
  uterus to abdominal wall
  vaginoperinea

619.8 **Other specified fistulas involving female genital tract**

Fistula:
  cervix
  cul-de-sac (Douglas')

Fistula:
  uterus
  vagina

619.9 **Unspecified fistula involving female genital tract**

620 Noninflammatory disorders of ovary, fallopian tube, and broad ligament

Excludes: hydrosalpinx (614.1)

DEFINITION Noninflammatory disorders of ovary, fallopian tube, and broad ligament, noninflammatory refer to degenerative and/or neoplastic disorders of the ovary, fallopian tube, and broad ligament.

620.0 Follicular cyst of ovary
Cyst of graafian follicle

● Code new
to 2012 edition

▲ Revision of
existing code

④ ⑤ Fourth or fifth
digit required

620.1 Corpus luteum cyst or hematoma
Corpus luteum hemorrhage or rupture
Lutein cyst

620.2 Other and unspecified ovarian cyst
Cyst of ovary:
  NOS
  corpus albicans
  retention NOS
  serous
  theca-lutein
Simple cystoma of ovary

Excludes: *cystadenoma (benign) (serous) (220)*
developmental cysts (752.0)
neoplastic cysts (220)
polycystic ovaries (256.4)
Stein-Leventhal syndrome (256.4)

620.3 Acquired atrophy of ovary and fallopian tube
Senile involution of ovary

620.4 Prolapse or hernia of ovary and fallopian tube
Displacement of ovary and fallopian tube
Salpingocele

620.5 Torsion of ovary, ovarian pedicle, or fallopian tube
Torsion:
  accessory tube
  hydatid of Morgagni

620.6 Broad ligament laceration syndrome
Masters-Allen syndrome

620.7 Hematoma of broad ligament
Hematocele, broad ligament

620.8 Other noninflammatory disorders of ovary, fallopian tube, and broad ligament
Cyst of broad ligament or fallopian tube
Polyp of broad ligament or fallopian tube
Infarction of ovary or fallopian tube
Rupture of ovary or fallopian tube
Hematosalpinx of ovary or fallopian tube

Excludes: *hematosalpinx in ectopic pregnancy (639.2)*
peritubal adhesions (614.6)
torsion of ovary, ovarian pedicle, or fallopian tube (620.5)

620.9 Unspecified noninflammatory disorder of ovary, fallopian tube, and broad ligament

621 Disorders of uterus, not elsewhere classified

621.0 Polyp of corpus uteri
Polyp:
  endometrium
  uterus NOS

Excludes: *cervical polyp NOS (622.7)*

621.1 Chronic subinvolution of uterus

Excludes: *puerperal (674.8)*

621.2 Hypertrophy of uterus
Bulky or enlarged uterus

Excludes: *puerperal (674.8)*

⑤ **621.3 Endometrial hyperplasia**

621.30 Endometrial hyperplasia, unspecified
Endometrial hyperplasia NOS
Hyperplasia (adenomatous) (cystic) (glandular) of endometrium
Hyperplastic endometritis

621.31 Simple endometrial hyperplasia without atypia

Excludes: *benign endometrial hyperplasia (621.34)*

621.32 Complex endometrial hyperplasia without atypia

Excludes: *benign endometrial hyperplasia (621.34)*

621.33 Endometrial hyperplasia with atypia

Excludes: *endometrial intraepithelial neoplasia [EIN] (621.35)*

| Add 4th or 5th digit | Nonspecific code | Unspecified code | Manifestation code |

621.34 Benign endometrial hyperplasia

621.35 Endometrial intraepithelial neoplasia [EIN]

Excludes: *malignant neoplasm of endometrium with endometrial intraepithelial neoplasia [EIN] (182.0)*

621.4 Hematometra
Hemometra

Excludes: *that in congenital anomaly (752.2-752.39)*

621.5 Intrauterine synechiae
Adhesions of uterus
Band(s) of uterus

621.6 Malposition of uterus
Anteversion of uterus
Retroflexion of uterus
Retroversion of uterus

Excludes: *malposition complicating pregnancy, labor, or delivery (654.3-654.4)*
prolapse of uterus (618.1-618.4)

621.7 Chronic inversion of uterus

Excludes: *current obstetrical trauma (665.2)*
prolapse of uterus (618.1-618.4)

621.8 Other specified disorders of uterus, not elsewhere classified
Atrophy, acquired of uterus
Cyst of uterus
Fibrosis NOS of uterus
Old laceration (postpartum) of uterus
Ulcer of uterus

Excludes: *bilharzial fibrosis (120.0-120.9)*
endometriosis (617.0)
fistulas (619.0-619.8)
inflammatory diseases (615.0-615.9)

621.9 Unspecified disorder of uterus

622 Noninflammatory disorders of cervix

Excludes: *abnormality of cervix complicating pregnancy, labor, or delivery (654.5-654.6)*
fistula (619.0-619.8)

622.0 Erosion and ectropion of cervix
Eversion of cervix
Ulcer of cervix

Excludes: *that in chronic cervicitis (616.0)*

⑤ **622.1 Dysplasia of cervix (uteri)**

Excludes: *abnormal results from cervical cytologic examination without histologic confirmation (795.00-795.09)*
carcinoma in situ of cervix (233.1)
cervical intraepithelial neoplasia III [CIN III] (233.1)
HGSIL of cervix (795.04)

ALERT! For personal history of cervical dysplasia see V13.22

622.10 Dysplasia of cervix, unspecified
Anaplasia of cervix
Cervical atypism
Cervical dysplasia NOS

622.11 Mild dysplasia of cervix
Cervical intraepithelial neoplasia I [CIN I]

622.12 Moderate dysplasia of cervix
Cervical intraepithelial neoplasia II [CIN II]

Excludes: *carcinoma in situ of cervix (233.1)*
cervical intraepithelial neoplasia III [CIN III] (233.1)
severe dysplasia (233.1)

622.2 Leukoplakia of cervix (uteri)

Excludes: *carcinoma in situ of cervix (233.1)*

● Code new
to 2012 edition

▲ Revision of
existing code

④ ⑤ Fourth or fifth
digit required

622.3 Old laceration of cervix
　　　　Adhesions of cervix
　　　　Band(s) of cervix
　　　　Cicatrix (postpartum) of cervix

　　Excludes: *current obstetrical trauma (665.3)*

622.4 Stricture and stenosis of cervix
　　　　Atresia (acquired) of cervix
　　　　Contracture of cervix
　　　　Occlusion of cervix
　　　　Pinpoint os uteri

　　Excludes: *congenital (752.49)*
　　　　　　　that complicating labor (654.6)

622.5 Incompetence of cervix

　　Excludes: *complicating pregnancy (654.5)*
　　　　　　　that affecting fetus or newborn (761.0)

622.6 Hypertrophic elongation of cervix

622.7 Mucous polyp of cervix
　　　　Polyp NOS of cervix

　　Excludes: *adenomatous polyp of cervix (219.0)*

622.8 Other specified noninflammatory disorders of cervix
　　　　Atrophy (senile) of cervix
　　　　Cyst of cervix
　　　　Fibrosis of cervix
　　　　Hemorrhage of cervix

　　Excludes: *endometriosis (617.0)*
　　　　　　　fistula (619.0-619.8)
　　　　　　　inflammatory diseases (616.0)

622.9 Unspecified noninflammatory disorder of cervix

623 Noninflammatory disorders of vagina

　　Excludes: *abnormality of vagina complicating pregnancy, labor, or delivery (654.7)*
　　　　　　　congenital absence of vagina (752.49)
　　　　　　　congenital diaphragm or bands (752.49)
　　　　　　　fistulas involving vagina (619.0-619.8)

623.0 Dysplasia of vagina
　　　　Mild and moderate dysplasia of vagina
　　　　Vaginal intraepithelial neoplasia I and II [VAIN I and II]

　　Excludes: *abnormal results from vaginal cytological examination without histologic*
　　　　　　　confirmation (795.10-795.19)
　　　　　　　carcinoma in situ of vagina (233.31)
　　　　　　　HGSIL of vagina (795.14)
　　　　　　　severe dysplasia of vagina (233.31)
　　　　　　　vaginal intraepithelial neoplasia III [VAIN III] (233.31)

623.1 Leukoplakia of vagina

623.2 Stricture or atresia of vagina
　　　　Adhesions (postoperative) (postradiation) of vagina
　　　　Occlusion of vagina
　　　　Stenosis, vagina

Use additional E code, if desired, to identify any external cause

　　Excludes: *congenital atresia or stricture (752.49)*

623.3 Tight hymenal ring
　　　　Rigid hymen acquired or congenital
　　　　Tight hymenal ring acquired or congenital
　　　　Tight introitus acquired or congenital

　　Excludes: *imperforate hymen (752.42)*

623.4 Old vaginal laceration

　　Excludes: *old laceration involving muscles of pelvic floor (618.7)*

623.5 Leukorrhea, not specified as infective
　　　　Leukorrhea NOS of vagina
　　　　Vaginal discharge NOS

　　Excludes: *trichomonal (131.00)*

Add 4th or　　　　Nonspecific　　　　Unspecified　　　　Manifestation
5th digit　　　　　code　　　　　　code　　　　　　code

623.6 Vaginal hematoma
[Excludes:] *current obstetrical trauma (665.7)*

623.7 Polyp of vagina

623.8 Other specified noninflammatory disorders of vagina
Cyst of vagina
Hemorrhage of vagina

623.9 Unspecified noninflammatory disorder of vagina

624 Noninflammatory disorders of vulva and perineum
[Excludes:] *abnormality of vulva and perineum complicating pregnancy, labor, or delivery (654.8)*
condyloma acuminatum (078.11)
fistulas involving:
perineum—see Alphabetic Index
vulva (619.0-619.8)
vulval varices (456.6)
vulvar involvement in skin conditions (690-709.9)

[5] **624.0 Dystrophy of vulva**
[Excludes:] *carcinoma in situ of vulva (233.32)*
severe dysplasia of vulva (233.32)
vulvar intraepithelial neoplasia III [VIN III] (233.32)

624.01 Vulvar intraepithelial neoplasia I [VIN I]
Mild dysplasia of vulva

624.02 Vulvar intraepithelial neoplasia II [VIN II]
Moderate dysplasia of vulva

624.09 Other dystrophy of vulva
Kraurosis of vulva
Leukoplakia of vulva

624.1 Atrophy of vulva

624.2 Hypertrophy of clitoris
[Excludes:] *that in endocrine disorders (255.2, 256.1)*

624.3 Hypertrophy of labia
Hypertrophy of vulva NOS

624.4 Old laceration or scarring of vulva

624.5 Hematoma of vulva
[Excludes:] *that complicating delivery (664.5)*

624.6 Polyp of labia and vulva

624.8 Other specified noninflammatory disorders of vulva and perineum
Cyst of vulva
Edema of vulva
Stricture of vulva

624.9 Unspecified noninflammatory disorder of vulva and perineum

625 Pain and other symptoms associated with female genital organs

625.0 Dyspareunia
[Excludes:] *psychogenic dyspareunia (302.76)*

625.1 Vaginismus
Colpospasm
Vulvismus

[Excludes:] *psychogenic vaginismus (306.51)*

625.2 Mittelschmerz
Intermenstrual pain
Ovulation pain

625.3 Dysmenorrhea
Painful menstruation

[Excludes:] *psychogenic dysmenorrhea (306.52)*

625.4 Premenstrual tension syndromes
Menstrual molimen
Premenstrual dysphoric disorder
Premenstrual syndrome
Premenstrual tension NOS

Excludes: menstrual migraine (346.4)

625.5 Pelvic congestion syndrome
Congestion-fibrosis syndrome
Taylor's syndrome

625.6 Stress incontinence, female

Excludes: mixed incontinence (788.33)
stress incontinence, male (788.32)

⑤ **625.7 Vulvodynia**

625.70 Vulvodynia, unspecified
Vulvodynia NOS

625.71 Vulvar vestibulitis

625.79 Other vulvodynia

625.8 Other specified symptoms associated with female genital organs

625.9 Unspecified symptom associated with female genital organs

626 Disorders of menstruation and other abnormal bleeding from female genital tract

Excludes: menopausal and premenopausal bleeding (627.0)
pain and other symptoms associated with menstrual cycle (625.2-625.4)
postmenopausal bleeding (627.1)
precocious puberty (259.1)

626.0 Absence of menstruation
Amenorrhea (primary) (secondary)

626.1 Scanty or infrequent menstruation
Hypomenorrhea
Oligomenorrhea

626.2 Excessive or frequent menstruation
Heavy periods   Menorrhagia
Menometrorrhagia   Polymenorrhea

Excludes: premenopausal (627.0)
that in puberty (626.3)

626.3 Puberty bleeding
Excessive bleeding associated with onset of menstrual periods
Pubertal menorrhagia

626.4 Irregular menstrual cycle
Irregular:
bleeding NOS
menstruation
periods

626.5 Ovulation bleeding
Regular intermenstrual bleeding

626.6 Metrorrhagia
Bleeding unrelated to menstrual cycle
Irregular intermenstrual bleeding

626.7 Postcoital bleeding

626.8 Other
Dysfunctional or functional uterine hemorrhage NOS
Menstruation:
retained
suppression of

626.9 Unspecified

627 Menopausal and postmenopausal disorders

Excludes: asymptomatic age-related (natural) postmenopausal status (V49.81)

DEFINITION Menopausal and postmenopausal disorders refer to disorders occuring during and after the menopausal period.

Add 4th or 5th digit	Nonspecific code	Unspecified code	Manifestation code	

627.0 Premenopausal menorrhagia
Excessive bleeding associated with onset of menopause
Menorrhagia:
  climacteric
  menopausal
  preclimacteric

627.1 Postmenopausal bleeding

627.2 Symptomatic menopausal or female climacteric states
Symptoms, such as flushing, sleeplessness, headache, lack of concentration, associated with the menopause

627.3 Postmenopausal atrophic vaginitis
Senile (atrophic) vaginitis

627.4 Symptomatic states associated with artificial menopause
Postartificial menopause syndromes
Any condition classifiable to 627.1, 627.2, or 627.3 which follows induced menopause

627.8 Other specified menopausal and postmenopausal disorders

Excludes: *premature menopause NOS (256.31)*

627.9 Unspecified menopausal and postmenopausal disorder

628 Infertility, female
Includes: primary and secondary sterility
DEFINITION Female Infertility refers to the biological inability of the female to contribute to conception.

628.0 Associated with anovulation
Anovulatory cycle
Use additional code for any associated Stein-Leventhal syndrome (256.4)

628.1 *Of pituitary-hypothalamic origin*
Code first underlying cause, as:
  adiposogenital dystrophy (253.8)
  anterior pituitary disorder (253.0-253.4)

628.2 Of tubal origin
Infertility associated with congenital anomaly of tube
Tubal:
  block
  occlusion
  stenosis
Use additional code for any associated peritubal adhesions (614.6)

628.3 Of uterine origin
Infertility associated with congenital anomaly of uterus
Nonimplantation
Use additional code for any associated tuberculous endometritis (016.7)

628.4 Of cervical or vaginal origin
Infertility associated with:
  anomaly of cervical mucus
  congenital structural anomaly
  dysmucorrhea

628.8 Of other specified origin

628.9 Of unspecified origin

629 Other disorders of female genital organs
ALERT! For personal history of other genital system and obstetric disorders see V13.2

629.0 Hematocele, female, not elsewhere classified

Excludes: *hematocele or hematoma:*
  broad ligament (620.7)
  fallopian tube (620.8)
  that associated with ectopic pregnancy (633.00-633.91)
  uterus (621.4)
  vagina (623.6)
  vulva (624.5)

629.1 Hydrocele, canal of Nuck
Cyst of canal of Nuck (acquired)

Excludes: *congenital (752.41)*

● Code new to 2012 edition   ▲ Revision of existing code   ④ ⑤ Fourth or fifth digit required

[5] **629.2 Female genital mutilation status**
Female circumcision status
Female genital cutting

629.20 Female genital mutilation status, unspecified
Female genital cutting status, unspecified
Female genital mutilation status NOS
Female genital mutilation status, type 4

629.21 Female genital mutilation Type I status
Clitorectomy status
Female genital cutting Type I status

629.22 Female genital mutilation Type II status
Clitorectomy with excision of labia minor status
Female genital cutting Type II status

629.23 Female genital mutilation Type III status
Female genital cutting Type III status
Infibulation status

629.29 Other female genital mutilation status
Female genital cutting Type IV status
Female genital mutilation Type IV status
Other female genital cutting status

● **629.3 Complication of implanted vaginal mesh and other prosthetic materials**

● **629.31 Erosion of implanted vaginal mesh and other prosthetic materials to surrounding organ or tissue**
Erosion of implanted vaginal mesh and other prosthetic materials into pelvic floor muscles

● **629.32 Exposure of implanted vaginal mesh and other prosthetic materials into vagina**
Exposure of vaginal mesh and other prosthetic materials through vaginal wall

[5] **629.8 Other specified disorders of female genital organs**

629.81 Recurrent pregnancy loss without current pregnancy
[*Excludes:*] *recurrent pregnancy loss with current pregnancy (646.3)*

629.89 Other specified disorders of female genital organs

629.9 Unspecified disorder of female genital organs

This page intentionally left blank

● Code new
  to 2012 edition

▲ Revision of
  existing code

④ ⑤ Fourth or fifth
    digit required

Chapter 11: Complications of Pregnancy, Childbirth, and the Puerperium (630-679)

DEFINITIONS AND CODING ALERTS

This chapter includes definitions of selected key words, terms and phrases and coding alerts for adding points to the clinical domain, references to coding late effects where appropriate, and references to personal history V-codes in situations where the acute or chronic condition is no longer active. An example from this chapter is as follows:

⑤ **679** **Complications of in utero procedures**

> **DEFINITION** Complications of in utero procedures, refers to problems caused by procedures performed on the unborn fetus.
>
> **ALERT!** For personal history of undergoing in utero procedure during pregnancy see V15.21
>
> **ALERT!** For personal history of undergoing in utero procedure while a fetus see V15.22

MULTIPLE CODING FOR A SINGLE CONDITION

In addition to the etiology or manifestation convention that requires two codes to fully describe a single condition that affects multiple body systems, there are other single conditions that also require more than one code. "Use additional code" notes are found in the tabular at codes that are not part of an etiology or manifestation pair where a secondary code is useful to fully describe a condition. The sequencing rule is the same as the etiology or manifestation pair - , "use additional code" indicates that a secondary code should be added.

"Code first" notes are also under certain codes that are not specifically manifestation codes but may be due to an underlying cause. When a "code first" note is present and an underlying condition is present the underlying condition should be sequenced first.

"Code, if applicable, any causal condition first", notes indicate that this code may be assigned as a principal diagnosis when the causal condition is unknown or not applicable. If a causal condition is known, then the code for that condition should be sequenced as the principal or first-listed diagnosis. Multiple codes may be needed for late effects, complication codes and obstetric codes to more fully describe a condition. See the specific guidelines for these conditions for further instruction.

COMBINATION CODE

A combination code is a single code used to classify: two diagnoses, or a diagnosis with an associated secondary process (manifestation) A diagnosis with an associated complication Combination codes are identified by referring to subterm entries in the Alphabetic Index and by reading the inclusion and exclusion notes in the Tabular List.

Assign only the combination code when that code fully identifies the diagnostic conditions involved or when the Alphabetic Index so directs. Multiple coding should not be used when the classification provides a combination code that clearly identifies all of the elements documented in the diagnosis. When the combination code lacks necessary specificity in describing the manifestation or complication, an additional code should be used as a secondary code.

CODING LATE EFFECTS

A late effect is the residual effect (condition produced) after the acute phase of an illness or injury has terminated. There is no time limit on when a late effect code can be used. The residual may be apparent early, such as in cerebrovascular accident cases, or it may occur months or years later, such as that due to a previous injury. Coding of late effects generally requires two codes sequenced in the following order: The condition or nature of the late effect is sequenced first. The late effect code is sequenced second.

An exception to the above guidelines are those instances where the code for late effect is followed by a manifestation code identified in the Tabular List and title, or the late effect code has been expanded (at the fourth and fifth-digit levels) to include the manifestation(s). The code for the acute phase of an illness or injury that led to the late effect is never used with a code for the late effect.

GENERAL RULES FOR OBSTETRIC CASES

Codes from chapter 11 and sequencing priority

Obstetric cases require codes from chapter 11, codes in the range 630-677, Complications of Pregnancy, Childbirth, and the Puerperium. Chapter 11 codes have sequencing priority over codes from other chapters. Additional codes from other chapters may be used in conjunction with chapter 11 codes to further specify

	Add 4th or 5th digit		Nonspecific code		Unspecified code		Manifestation code

conditions. Should the provider document that the pregnancy is incidental to the encounter, then code V22.2 should be used in place of any chapter 11 codes. It is the provider's responsibility to state that the condition being treated is not affecting the pregnancy.

Chapter 11 codes are to be used only on the maternal record, never on the record of the newborn.

Chapter 11 fifth-digits

Categories 640-648, 651-676 have required fifth-digits, which indicate whether the encounter is antepartum, postpartum and whether a delivery has also occurred.

The fifth-digits, which are appropriate for each code number, are listed in brackets under each code. The fifth-digits on each code should all be consistent with each other. That is, should a delivery occur all of the fifth-digits should indicate the delivery.

SELECTION OF OB PRINCIPAL OR FIRST-LISTED DIAGNOSIS

Routine outpatient prenatal visits

For routine outpatient prenatal visits when no complications are present codes V22.0, Supervision of normal first pregnancy, and V22.1, Supervision of other normal pregnancy, should be used as the first-listed diagnoses. These codes should not be used in conjunction with chapter 11 codes.

Prenatal outpatient visits for high-risk patients

For prenatal outpatient visits for patients with high-risk pregnancies, a code from category V23, Supervision of high-risk pregnancy, should be used as the first-listed diagnosis. Secondary chapter 11 codes may be used in conjunction with these codes if appropriate.

Episodes when no delivery occurs

In episodes when no delivery occurs, the principal diagnosis should correspond to the principal complication of the pregnancy, which necessitated the encounter. Should more than one complication exist, all of which are treated or monitored, any of the complications codes may be sequenced first.

When a delivery occurs

When a delivery occurs, the principal diagnosis should correspond to the main circumstances or complication of the delivery. In cases of cesarean delivery, the selection of the principal diagnosis should correspond to the reason the cesarean delivery was performed unless the reason for admission or encounter was unrelated to the condition resulting in the cesarean delivery.

Outcome of delivery

An outcome of delivery code, V27.0-V27.9, should be included on every maternal record when a delivery has occurred. These codes are not to be used on subsequent records or on the newborn record.

FETAL CONDITIONS AFFECTING THE MANAGEMENT OF THE MOTHER

Codes from category 655

Known or suspected fetal abnormality affecting management of the mother, and category 656, Other fetal and placental problems affecting the management of the mother, are assigned only when the fetal condition is actually responsible for modifying the management of the mother, i.e., by requiring diagnostic studies, additional observation, special care, or termination of pregnancy. The fact that the fetal condition exists does not justify assigning a code from this series to the mother's record.

See Chapter 18 for suspected maternal and fetal conditions not found.

In utero surgery

In cases when surgery is performed on the fetus, a diagnosis code from category 655, Known or suspected fetal abnormalities affecting management of the mother, should be assigned identifying the fetal condition. Procedure code 75.36, Correction of fetal defect, should be assigned on the hospital inpatient record.

No code from Chapter 15, the perinatal codes, should be used on the mother's record to identify fetal conditions. Surgery performed in utero on a fetus is still to be coded as an obstetric encounter.

● Code new to 2012 edition   ▲ Revision of existing code   ④ ⑤ Fourth or fifth digit required

HIV INFECTION IN PREGNANCY, CHILDBIRTH AND THE PUERPERIUM

During pregnancy, childbirth or the puerperium, a patient admitted because of an HIV-related illness should receive a principal diagnosis of 647.6X, Other specified infectious and parasitic diseases in the mother classifiable elsewhere, but complicating the pregnancy, childbirth or the puerperium, followed by 042 and the code(s) for the HIV-related illness(es).

Patients with asymptomatic HIV infection status admitted during pregnancy, childbirth, or the puerperium should receive codes of 647.6X and V08.

CURRENT CONDITIONS COMPLICATING PREGNANCY

Assign a code from subcategory 648.x for patients that have current conditions when the condition affects the management of the pregnancy, childbirth, or the puerperium. Use additional secondary codes from other chapters to identify the conditions, as appropriate.

DIABETES MELLITUS IN PREGNANCY

Diabetes mellitus is a significant complicating factor in pregnancy. Pregnant women who are diabetic should be assigned code 648.0x, Diabetes mellitus complicating pregnancy, and a secondary code from category 250, Diabetes mellitus, or category 249, Secondary diabetes, to identify the type of diabetes.

Code V58.67, Long-term (current) use of insulin, should also be assigned if the diabetes mellitus is being treated with insulin.

GESTATIONAL DIABETES

Gestational diabetes can occur during the second and third trimester of pregnancy in women who were not diabetic prior to pregnancy. Gestational diabetes can cause complications in the pregnancy similar to those of pre-existing diabetes mellitus. It also puts the woman at greater risk of developing diabetes after the pregnancy. Gestational diabetes is coded to 648.8x, Abnormal glucose tolerance. Codes 648.0x and 648.8x should never be used together on the same record.

Code V58.67, Long-term (current) use of insulin, should also be assigned if the gestational diabetes is being treated with insulin.

NORMAL DELIVERY, CODE 650

Normal delivery

Code 650 is for use in cases when a woman is admitted for a full-term normal delivery and delivers a single, healthy infant without any complications antepartum, during the delivery, or postpartum during the delivery episode. Code 650 is always a principal diagnosis. It is not to be used if any other code from chapter 11 is needed to describe a current complication of the antenatal, delivery, or perinatal period. Additional codes from other chapters may be used with code 650 if they are not related to or are in any way complicating the pregnancy.

Normal delivery with resolved antepartum complication

Code 650 may be used if the patient had a complication at some point during her pregnancy, but the complication is not present at the time of the admission for delivery.

V27.0, Single liveborn, outcome of delivery

V27.0, Single liveborn, is the only outcome of delivery code appropriate for use with 650.

THE POSTPARTUM AND PERIPARTUM PERIODS

Postpartum and peripartum periods

The postpartum period begins immediately after delivery and continues for six weeks following delivery. The peripartum period is defined as the last month of pregnancy to five months postpartum.

Complications

A postpartum complication is any complication occurring within the six-week period.

| | Add 4th or 5th digit | | Nonspecific code | | Unspecified code | | Manifestation code |

Chapter 11 codes may also be used to describe pregnancy-related complications after the six-week period should the provider document that a condition is pregnancy related.

Postpartum complications that occur during the same admission as the delivery are identified with a fifth digit of "2." Subsequent admissions or encounters for postpartum complications should be identified with a fifth digit of "4."

Admission for routine postpartum care following delivery outside hospital

When the mother delivers outside the hospital prior to admission and is admitted for routine postpartum care and no complications are noted, code V24.0, Postpartum care and examination immediately after delivery, should be assigned as the principal diagnosis.

Admission following delivery outside hospital with postpartum conditions

A delivery diagnosis code should not be used for a woman who has delivered prior to admission to the hospital. Any postpartum conditions and/or postpartum procedures should be coded.

CODE 677, LATE EFFECT OF COMPLICATION OF PREGNANCY

Code 677, Late effect of complication of pregnancy, childbirth, and the puerperium is for use in those cases when an initial complication of a pregnancy develops a sequelae requiring care or treatment at a future date.

This code may be used at any time after the initial postpartum period.

This code, like all late effect codes, is to be sequenced following the code describing the sequelae of the complication.

ABORTIONS

Fifth-digits required for abortion categories

Fifth-digits are required for abortion categories 634-637. Fifth-digit 1, incomplete, indicates that all of the products of conception have not been expelled from the uterus. Fifth-digit 2, complete, indicates that all products of conception have been expelled from the uterus prior to the episode of care.

Code from categories 640-648 and 651-659

A code from categories 640-648 and 651-659 may be used as additional codes with an abortion code to indicate the complication leading to the abortion.
Fifth digit 3 is assigned with codes from these categories when used with an abortion code because the other fifth digits will not apply. Codes from the 660-669 series are not to be used for complications of abortion.

Code 639 for complications

Code 639 is to be used for all complications following abortion. Code 639 cannot be assigned with codes from categories 634-638.

Abortion with Liveborn Fetus

When an attempted termination of pregnancy results in a liveborn fetus assign code 644.21, Early onset of delivery, with an appropriate code from category V27, Outcome of Delivery. The procedure code for the attempted termination of pregnancy should also be assigned.

Retained Products of Conception following an abortion

Subsequent admissions for retained products of conception following a spontaneous or legally induced abortion are assigned the appropriate code from category 634, Spontaneous abortion, or 635 Legally induced abortion, with a fifth digit of "1" (incomplete). This advice is appropriate even when the patient was discharged previously with a discharge diagnosis of complete abortion.

● Code new
to 2012 edition
▲ Revision of
existing code
④ ⑤ Fourth or fifth
digit required

11. COMPLICATIONS OF PREGNANCY, CHILDBIRTH, AND THE PUERPERIUM (630-679)

ECTOPIC AND MOLAR PREGNANCY (630-633)

Use additional code from category 639 to identify any complications

630 Hydatidiform mole
Trophoblastic disease NOS
Vesicular mole

[Excludes:] *chorioadenoma (destruens) (236.1)*
chorionepithelioma (181)
malignant hydatidiform mole (236.1)

[DEFINITION] A Hydatidiform mole is a rare mass or growth that forms inside the uterus at the beginning of a pregnancy. It is a type of gestational trophoblastic disease (GTD)

[ALERT!] For personal history of trophoblastic disease see V13.1

631 Other abnormal product of conception

● **631.0 Inappropriate change in quantitative human chorionic gonadotropin (hCG) in early pregnancy**
Biochemical pregnancy
Chemical pregnancy
Inappropriate level of quantitative human chorionic gonadotropin (hCG) for gestational age in early pregnancy

[Excludes:] *blighted ovum (631.8)*
molar pregnancy (631.8)

● **631.8 Other abnormal products of conception**
Blighted ovum

632 Missed abortion
Early fetal death before completion of 22 weeks' gestation with retention of dead fetus
Retained products of conception, not following spontaneous or induced abortion or delivery

[Excludes:] *failed induced abortion (638.0-638.9)*
fetal death (intrauterine) (late) (656.4)
missed delivery (656.4)
that with hydatiform mole (630)
that with other abnormal products of conception (631.8)

[DEFINITION] Missed abortion refers to retention in the uterus of an fetus that has been dead for at least eight weeks.

633 Ectopic pregnancy
Includes: ruptured ectopic pregnancy

[DEFINITION] Ectopic pregnancy occurs with the implantation and subsequent development of a fertilized ovum outside the uterus, as in a fallopian tube.

[5] **633.0 Abdominal pregnancy**
Intraperitoneal pregnancy

633.00 Abdominal pregnancy without intrauterine pregnancy

633.01 Abdominal pregnancy with intrauterine pregnancy

[5] **633.1 Tubal pregnancy**
Fallopian pregnancy
Rupture of (fallopian) tube due to pregnancy
Tubal abortion

633.10 Tubal pregnancy without intrauterine pregnancy

633.11 Tubal pregnancy with intrauterine pregnancy

[5] **633.2 Ovarian pregnancy**

633.20 Ovarian pregnancy without intrauterine pregnancy

633.21 Ovarian pregnancy with intrauterine pregnancy

[5] **633.8 Other ectopic pregnancy**
Pregnancy:
cervical
combined
cornual
Pregnancy:
intraligamentous
mesometric
mural

633.80 Other ectopic pregnancy without intrauterine pregnancy

633.81 Other ectopic pregnancy with intrauterine pregnancy

[5] **633.9 Unspecified ectopic pregnancy**

633.90 Unspecified ectopic pregnancy without intrauterine pregnancy

Add 4th or 5th digit | Nonspecific code | Unspecified code | Manifestation code

633.91 Unspecified ectopic pregnancy with intrauterine pregnancy

OTHER PREGNANCY WITH ABORTIVE OUTCOME (634-639)

Note: Use the following fifth-digit subclassification with categories 634-637:

0 Unspecified

1 Incomplete

2 Complete

The following fourth-digit subdivisions are for use with categories 634-638:

.0 Complicated by genital tract and pelvic infection
Endometritis
Salpingo-oophoritis
Sepsis NOS
Septicemia NOS
Any condition classifiable to 639.0, with condition classifiable to 634-638

[Excludes:] *urinary tract infection (634-638 with .7)*

.1 Complicated by delayed or excessive hemorrhage
Afibrinogenemia
Defibrination syndrome
Intravascular hemolysis
Any condition classifiable to 639.1, with condition classifiable to 634-638

.2 Complicated by damage to pelvic organs and tissues
Laceration, perforation, or tear of:
 bladder
 uterus
Any condition classifiable to 639.2, with condition classifiable to 634-638

.3 Complicated by renal failure
Oliguria
Uremia
Any condition classifiable to 639.3, with condition classifiable to 634-638

.4 Complicated by metabolic disorder
Electrolyte imbalance with conditions classifiable to 634-638

.5 Complicated by shock
Circulatory collapse
Shock (postoperative) (septic)
Any condition classifiable to 639.5, with condition classifiable to 634-638

.6 Complicated by embolism
Embolism:
 NOS
 amniotic fluid
 pulmonary
Any condition classifiable to 639.6, with condition classifiable to 634-638

.7 With other specified complications
Cardiac arrest or failure
Urinary tract infection
Any condition classifiable to 639.8, with condition classifiable to 634-638

.8 With unspecified complication

.9 Without mention of complication

[5] **634 Spontaneous abortion**
Includes: miscarriage
 spontaneous abortion

DEFINITION An abortion is the termination of a pregnancy by the removal or expulsion from the uterus of a fetus/embryo, resulting in or caused by its death. An abortion can occur spontaneously due to complications during pregnancy or can be induced.

[5] **634.0 Complicated by genital tract and pelvic infection**
[0-2]

[5] **634.1 Complicated by delayed or excessive hemorrhage**
[0-2]

[5] **634.2 Complicated by damage to pelvic organs or tissues**
[0-2]

[5] **634.3 Complicated by renal failure**
[0-2]

[5] **634.4 Complicated by metabolic disorder**
[0-2]

[5] **634.5 Complicated by shock**
[0-2]

[5] **634.6 Complicated by embolism**
[0-2]

[5] **634.7 With other specified complications**
[0-2]

[5] **634.8 With unspecified complication**
[0-2]

[5] **634.9 Without mention of complication**
[0-2]

[5] **635 Legally induced abortion**

Includes: abortion or termination of pregnancy:
- elective
- legal
- therapeutic

[Excludes:] *menstrual extraction or regulation (V25.3)*

DEFINITION Legally induced abortion refers to an abortion performed by medical professionals conforming to the legal guidelines of the state where the abortion is performed.

[5] **635.0 Complicated by genital tract and pelvic infection**
[0-2]

[5] **635.1 Complicated by delayed or excessive hemorrhage**
[0-2]

[5] **635.2 Complicated by damage to pelvic organs or tissues**
[0-2]

[5] **635.3 Complicated by renal failure**
[0-2]

[5] **635.4 Complicated by metabolic disorder**
[0-2]

[5] **635.5 Complicated by shock**
[0-2]

[5] **635.6 Complicated by embolism**
[0-2]

[5] **635.7 With other specified complications**
[0-2]

[5] **635.8 With unspecified complication**
[0-2]

[5] **635.9 Without mention of complication**
[0-2]

[5] **636 Illegally induced abortion**

Includes: abortion:
- criminal
- illegal
- self-induced

DEFINITION Illegally induced abortion refers to an abortion performed by medical professionals or non-medical persons outside the legal guidelines of the state where the abortion is performed.

[5] **636.0 Complicated by genital tract and pelvic infection**
[0-2]

[5] **636.1 Complicated by delayed or excessive hemorrhage**
[0-2]

[5] **636.2 Complicated by damage to pelvic organs or tissues**
[0-2]

[5] **636.3 Complicated by renal failure**
[0-2]

[5] **636.4 Complicated by metabolic disorder**
[0-2]

[5] **636.5 Complicated by shock**
[0-2]

[5] **636.6 Complicated by embolism**
[0-2]

[5] **636.7 With other specified complications**
[0-2]

⑤ **636.8 With unspecified complication**
[0-2]

⑤ **636.9 Without mention of complication**
[0-2]

⑤ **637 Unspecified abortion**
Includes: abortion NOS
retained products of conception following abortion, not classifiable elsewhere

⑤ **637.0 Complicated by genital tract and pelvic infection**
[0-2]

⑤ **637.1 Complicated by delayed or excessive hemorrhage**
[0-2]

⑤ **637.2 Complicated by damage to pelvic organs or tissues**
[0-2]

⑤ **637.3 Complicated by renal failure**
[0-2]

⑤ **637.4 Complicated by metabolic disorder**
[0-2]

⑤ **637.5 Complicated by shock**
[0-2]

⑤ **637.6 Complicated by embolism**
[0-2]

⑤ **637.7 With other specified complications**
[0-2]

⑤ **637.8 With unspecified complication**
[0-2]

⑤ **637.9 Without mention of complication**
[0-2]

638 Failed attempted abortion
Includes: failure of attempted induction of (legal) abortion

Excludes: incomplete abortion (634.0-637.9)

DEFINITION Failed attempted abortion refers to an attempted abortion that is incomplete.

638.0 Complicated by genital tract and pelvic infection

638.1 Complicated by delayed or excessive hemorrhage

638.2 Complicated by damage to pelvic organs or tissues

638.3 Complicated by renal failure

638.4 Complicated by metabolic disorder

638.5 Complicated by shock

638.6 Complicated by embolism

638.7 With other specified complications

638.8 With unspecified complication

638.9 Without mention of complication

639 Complications following abortion and ectopic and molar pregnancies
Note: This category is provided for use when it is required to classify separately the
complications classifiable to the fourth-digit level in categories 634-638; for example:
    a) when the complication itself was responsible for an episode of medical care, the
abortion, ectopic or molar pregnancy itself having been dealt with at a previous
episode
    b) when these conditions are immediate complications of ectopic or molar pregnancies
classifiable to 630-633 where they cannot be identified at fourth-digit level.

DEFINITION Ectopic pregnancy is the implantation and subsequent development of a fertilized
ovum outside the uterus, as in a fallopian tube. Molar pregnancy is the conversion of the
early embryo into a mole.

ALERT! Code 639 is to be used for all complications following abortion. Code 639 cannot be
assigned with codes from categories 634-638

639.0 Genital tract and pelvic infection
Endometritis following conditions classifiable to 630-638
Parametritis following conditions classifiable to 630-638
Pelvic peritonitis following conditions classifiable to 630-638
Salpingitis following conditions classifiable to 630-638
Salpingo-oophoritis following conditions classifiable to 630-638
Sepsis NOS following conditions classifiable to 630-638

● Code new   ▲ Revision of   ④ ⑤ Fourth or fifth
  to 2012 edition   existing code   digit required

Septicemia NOS following conditions classifiable to 630-638

Excludes: urinary tract infection (639.8)

639.1 Delayed or excessive hemorrhage
Afibrinogenemia following conditions classifiable to 630-638
Defibrination syndrome following conditions classifiable to 630-638
Intravascular hemolysis following conditions classifiable to 630-638

639.2 Damage to pelvic organs and tissues
Laceration, perforation, or tear of:
bladder following conditions classifiable to 630-638
bowel following conditions classifiable to 630-638
broad ligament following conditions classifiable to 630-638
cervix following conditions classifiable to 630-638
periurethral tissue following conditions classifiable to 630-638
uterus following conditions classifiable to 630-638
vagina following conditions classifiable to 630-638

639.3 Kidney failure
Oliguria following conditions classifiable to 630-638
Renal (kidney):
failure (acute) following conditions classifiable to 630-638
shutdown following conditions classifiable to 630-638
tubular necrosis following conditions classifiable to 630-638
Uremia following conditions classifiable to 630-638

639.4 Metabolic disorders
Electrolyte imbalance following conditions classifiable to 630-638

639.5 Shock
Circulatory collapse following conditions classifiable to 630-638
Shock (postoperative) (septic) following conditions classifiable to 630-638

639.6 Embolism
Embolism:
NOS following conditions classifiable to 630-638
air following conditions classifiable to 630-638
amniotic fluid following conditions classifiable to 630-638
blood-clot following conditions classifiable to 630-638
fat following conditions classifiable to 630-638
pulmonary following conditions classifiable to 630-638
pyemic following conditions classifiable to 630-638
septic following conditions classifiable to 630-638
soap following conditions classifiable to 630-638

`639.8` Other specified complications following abortion or ectopic and molar pregnancy
Acute yellow atrophy or necrosis of liver following conditions classifiable to 630-638
Cardiac arrest or failure following conditions classifiable to 630-638
Cerebral anoxia following conditions classifiable to 630-638
Urinary tract infection following conditions classifiable to 630-638

`639.9` Unspecified complication following abortion or ectopic and molar pregnancy
Complication(s) not further specified following conditions classifiable to 630-638

COMPLICATIONS MAINLY RELATED TO PREGNANCY (640-649)

Includes: the listed conditions even if they arose or were present during labor, delivery, or the puerperium

The following fifth-digit subclassification is for use with categories 640-649 to denote the current episode of care:

`0` unspecified as to episode of care or not applicable

`1` delivered, with or without mention of antepartum condition
Antepartum condition with delivery
Delivery NOS (with mention of antepartum complication during current episode of care)
Intrapartum obstetric condition (with mention of antepartum complication during current episode of care)
Pregnancy, delivered (with mention of antepartum complication during current episode of care)

`2` delivered, with mention of postpartum complication
Delivery with mention of puerperal complication during current episode of care

`3` antepartum condition or complication
Antepartum obstetric condition, not delivered during the current episode of care

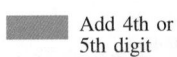 Add 4th or 5th digit   Nonspecific code   Unspecified code   Manifestation code

4   postpartum condition or complication
>   Postpartum or puerperal obstetric condition or complication following delivery that occurred:
>   during previous episode of care
>   outside hospital, with subsequent admission for observation or care

⑤ **640** **Hemorrhage in early pregnancy**
>   Includes: hemorrhage before completion of 22 weeks' gestation

>   Requires fifth digit; valid digits are in [brackets] under each code. See beginning of section 640-649 for definitions.

>   **ALERT!** For coding late effect of complication of pregnancy childbirth the puerperium see 677

⑤ **640.0   Threatened abortion**
[0,1,3]

⑤ **640.8   Other specified hemorrhage in early pregnancy**
[0,1,3]

⑤ **640.9   Unspecified hemorrhage in early pregnancy**
[0,1,3]

⑤ **641** **Antepartum hemorrhage, abruptio placentae, and placenta previa**
>   Requires fifth digit; valid digits are in [brackets] under each code. See beginning of section 640-649 for definitions.

>   **DEFINITION** Antepartum hemorrhage refers to bleeding before delivery. Abruptio placentae is the premature separation of the placenta from the wall of the uterus. Placenta previa is a pregnancy in which the placenta is implanted in the lower uterine segment instead of the upper segmen

⑤ **641.0   Placenta previa without hemorrhage**
[0,1,3]   Low implantation of placenta without hemorrhage
>   Placenta previa noted:
>   during pregnancy without hemorrhage
>   before labor (and delivered by cesarean delivery) without hemorrhage

⑤ **641.1   Hemorrhage from placenta previa**
[0,1,3]   Low-lying placenta NOS or with hemorrhage (intrapartum)
>   Placenta previa:
>   incomplete NOS or with hemorrhage (intrapartum)
>   marginal NOS or with hemorrhage (intrapartum)
>   partial NOS or with hemorrhage (intrapartum)
>   total NOS or with hemorrhage (intrapartum)

>   *Excludes:* hemorrhage from vasa previa (663.5)

⑤ **641.2   Premature separation of placenta**
[0,1,3]   Ablatio placentae
>   Abruptio placentae
>   Accidental antepartum hemorrhage
>   Couvelaire uterus
>   Detachment of placenta (premature)
>   Premature separation of normally implanted placenta

⑤ **641.3   Antepartum hemorrhage associated with coagulation defects**
[0,1,3]   Antepartum or intrapartum hemorrhage associated with:
>   afibrinogenemia
>   hyperfibrinolysis
>   hypofibrinogenemia

>   *Excludes:* coagulation defects not associated with antepartum hemorrhage (649.3)

⑤ **641.8   Other antepartum hemorrhage**
[0,1,3]   Antepartum or intrapartum hemorrhage associated with:
>   trauma
>   uterine leiomyoma

⑤ **641.9   Unspecified antepartum hemorrhage**
[0,1,3]   Hemorrhage:
>   antepartum NOS
>   intrapartum NOS
>   of pregnancy NOS

⑤ **642** **Hypertension complicating pregnancy, childbirth, and the puerperium**
>   Requires fifth digit; valid digits are in [brackets] under each code. See beginning of section 640-649 for definitions.

● Code new
to 2012 edition
▲ Revision of
existing code
④ ⑤ Fourth or fifth
digit required

DEFINITION Pregnancy-induced hypertension is a rise in blood pressure, without proteinuria, during the second half of pregnancy. Pre-eclampsia is a multisystem disorder, unique to pregnancy, that is usually associated with raised blood pressure and proteinuria. Eclampsia is one or more convulsions in association with the syndrome of pre-eclampsia.

⑤ **642.0 Benign essential hypertension complicating pregnancy, childbirth, and the puerperium**
[0-4] Hypertension:
benign essential specified as complicating, or as a reason for obstetric care during pregnancy, childbirth, or the puerperium
chronic NOS specified as complicating, or as a reason for obstetric care during pregnancy, childbirth, or the puerperium
essential specified as complicating, or as a reason for obstetric care during pregnancy, childbirth, or the puerperium
pre-existing NOS specified as complicating, or as a reason for obstetric care during pregnancy, childbirth, or the puerperium

⑤ **642.1 Hypertension secondary to renal disease, complicating pregnancy, childbirth, and the puerperium**
[0-4] Hypertension secondary to renal disease, specified as complicating, or as a reason for obstetric care during pregnancy, childbirth, or the puerperium

⑤ **642.2 Other pre-existing hypertension complicating pregnancy, childbirth, and the puerperium**
[0-4] Hypertensive:
chronic kidney disease specified as complicating, or as a reason for obstetric care during pregnancy, childbirth, or the puerperium
heart and chronic kidney disease specified as complicating, or as a reason for obstetric care during pregnancy, childbirth, or the puerperium
heart disease specified as complicating, or as a reason for obstetric care during pregnancy, childbirth, or the puerperium
Malignant hypertension specified as complicating, or as a reason for obstetric care during pregnancy, childbirth, or the puerperium

⑤ **642.3 Transient hypertension of pregnancy**
[0-4] Gestational hypertension
Transient hypertension, so described, in pregnancy, childbirth, or the puerperium

⑤ **642.4 Mild or unspecified pre-eclampsia**
[0-4] Hypertension in pregnancy, childbirth, or the puerperium, not specified as pre-existing, with either albuminuria or edema, or both; mild or unspecified
Pre-eclampsia:
NOS
mild
Toxemia (pre-eclamptic):
NOS
mild

[Excludes:] *albuminuria in pregnancy, without mention of hypertension (646.2)*
edema in pregnancy, without mention of hypertension (646.1)

⑤ **642.5 Severe pre-eclampsia**
[0-4] Hypertension in pregnancy, childbirth, or the puerperium, not specified as pre-existing, with either albuminuria or edema, or both; specified as severe
Pre-eclampsia, severe
Toxemia (pre-eclamptic), severe

⑤ **642.6 Eclampsia**
[0-4] Toxemia:
eclamptic
with convulsions

⑤ **642.7 Pre-eclampsia or eclampsia superimposed on pre-existing hypertension**
[0-4] Conditions classifiable to 642.4-642.6, with conditions classifiable to 642.0-642.2

⑤ **642.9 Unspecified hypertension complicating pregnancy, childbirth, or the puerperium**
[0-4] Hypertension NOS, without mention of albuminuria or edema, complicating pregnancy, childbirth, or the puerperium

⑤ **643 Excessive vomiting in pregnancy**
Includes: hyperemesis arising during pregnancy
vomiting:
persistent arising during pregnancy
vicious arising during pregnancy
hyperemesis gravidarum

Requires fifth digit; valid digits are in [brackets] under each code. See beginning of section 640-649 for definitions.

DEFINITION Excessive vomiting in pregnancy, aka hyperemesis gravidarum, refers to excessive vomiting in early pregnancy.

⑤ **643.0 Mild hyperemesis gravidarum**
[0,1,3] Hyperemesis gravidarum, mild or unspecified, starting before the end of the 22nd week of gestation

Add 4th or 5th digit | Nonspecific code | Unspecified code | Manifestation code

[5] **643.1 Hyperemesis gravidarum with metabolic disturbance**
[0,1,3] Hyperemesis gravidarum, starting before the end of the 22nd week of gestation, with metabolic disturbance, such as:
carbohydrate depletion
dehydration
electrolyte imbalance

[5] **643.2 Late vomiting of pregnancy**
[0,1,3] Excessive vomiting starting after 22 completed weeks of gestation

[5] **643.8 Other vomiting complicating pregnancy**
[0,1,3] Vomiting due to organic disease or other cause, specified as complicating pregnancy, or as a reason for obstetric care during pregnancy

Use additional code, if desired, to specify cause

[5] **643.9 Unspecified vomiting of pregnancy**
[0,1,3] Vomiting as a reason for care during pregnancy, length of gestation unspecified

[5] **644 Early or threatened labor**
Requires fifth digit; valid digits are in [brackets] under each code. See beginning of section 640-649 for definitions.

[ALERT!] For personal history of pre-term labor see V13.21

[5] **644.0 Threatened premature labor**
[0,3] Premature labor after 22 weeks, but before 37 completed weeks of gestation without delivery

[Excludes:] *that occurring before 22 completed weeks of gestation (640.0)*

[5] **644.1 Other threatened labor**
[0,3] False labor:
NOS without delivery
after 37 completed weeks of gestation without delivery
Threatened labor NOS without delivery

[5] **644.2 Early onset of delivery**
[0,1] Onset (spontaneous) of delivery before 37 completed weeks of gestation
Premature labor with onset of delivery before 37 completed weeks of gestation

[ALERT!] Assign code 644.21 with an appropriate code from category V27 when an attempted termination of pregnancy results in a liveborn fetus. The procedure code for the attempted termination of pregnancy should also be assigned

[5] **645 Late pregnancy**
Requires fifth digit; valid digits are in [brackets] under each code. See beginning of section 640-649 for definitions.

[5] **645.1 Post term pregnancy**
[0,1,3] Pregnancy over 40 completed weeks to 42 completed weeks gestation

[5] **645.2 Prolonged pregnancy**
[0,1,3] Pregnancy which has advanced beyond 42 completed weeks gestation

[5] **646 Other complications of pregnancy, not elsewhere classified**
Requires fifth digit; valid digits are in [brackets] under each code. See beginning of section 640-649 for definitions.

Use additional code(s) to further specify complication

[ALERT!] For personal history of other genital system and obstetric disorders see V13.2

[5] **646.0 Papyraceous fetus**
[0,1,3]

[5] **646.1 Edema or excessive weight gain in pregnancy, without mention of hypertension**
[0-4] Gestational edema
Maternal obesity syndrome

[Excludes:] *that with mention of hypertension (642.0-642.9)*

[5] **646.2 Unspecified renal disease in pregnancy, without mention of hypertension**
[0-4] Albuminuria in pregnancy or the puerperium, without mention of hypertension
Nephropathy NOS in pregnancy or the puerperium, without mention of hypertension
Renal disease NOS in pregnancy or the puerperium, without mention of hypertension
Uremia in pregnancy or the puerperium, without mention of hypertension
Gestational proteinuria in pregnancy or the puerperium, without mention of hypertension

[Excludes:] *that with mention of hypertension (642.0-642.9)*

[5] **646.3 Recurrent pregnancy loss**
[0,1,3]

[Excludes:] *with current abortion (634.0-634.9)*
without current pregnancy (629.81)

⑤ **646.4 Peripheral neuritis in pregnancy**
[0-4]

⑤ **646.5 Asymptomatic bacteriuria in pregnancy**
[0-4]

⑤ **646.6 Infections of genitourinary tract in pregnancy**
[0-4]   Conditions classifiable to 590, 595, 597, 599.0, 616 complicating pregnancy, childbirth,
or the puerperium
Conditions classifiable to (614.0-614.5, 617.7-614.9, 615) complicating pregnancy or
labor

Excludes: *major puerperal infection (670.0-670.8)*

▲ **646.7 Liver and biliary tract disorders in pregnancy**
[0,1,3]   Acute yellow atrophy of liver (obstetric) (true) of pregnancy
Icterus gravis of pregnancy
Necrosis of liver of pregnancy

Excludes: *hepatorenal syndrome following delivery (674.8)*
        viral hepatitis (647.6)

⑤ **646.8 Other specified complications of pregnancy**
[0-4]   Fatigue during pregnancy
Herpes gestationis
Insufficient weight gain of pregnancy

⑤ **646.9 Unspecified complication of pregnancy**
[0,1,3]

⑤ **647 Infectious and parasitic conditions in the mother classifiable elsewhere, but complicating
pregnancy, childbirth, or the puerperium**
Includes: the listed conditions when complicating the pregnant state, aggravated by the
pregnancy, or when a main reason for obstetric care

Excludes: *those conditions in the mother known or suspected to have affected the fetus
(655.0-655.9)*

Requires fifth digit; valid digits are in [brackets] under each code. See beginning of section
640-649 for definitions.

Use additional code(s) to further specify complication

⑤ **647.0 Syphilis**
[0-4]   Conditions classifiable to 090-097

⑤ **647.1 Gonorrhea**
[0-4]   Conditions classifiable to 098

⑤ **647.2 Other venereal diseases**
[0-4]   Conditions classifiable to 099

⑤ **647.3 Tuberculosis**
[0-4]   Conditions classifiable to 010-018

⑤ **647.4 Malaria**
[0-4]   Conditions classifiable to 084

⑤ **647.5 Rubella**
[0-4]   Conditions classifiable to 056

⑤ **647.6 Other viral diseases**
[0-4]   Conditions classifiable to 042, 050-055, 057-079, 795.05, 795.15, 795.75

⑤ **647.8 Other specified infectious and parasitic diseases**
[0-4]

⑤ **647.9 Unspecified infection or infestation**
[0-4]

⑤ **648 Other current conditions in the mother classifiable elsewhere, but complicating pregnancy,
childbirth, or the puerperium**
Includes: the listed conditions when complicating the pregnant state, aggravated by the
pregnancy, or when a main reason for obstetric care

Excludes: *those conditions in the mother known or suspected to have affected the fetus
(655.0-655.9)*

Requires fifth digit; valid digits are in [brackets] under each code. See beginning of section
640-649 for definitions.

Use additional code(s) to identify the condition

⑤ **648.0 Diabetes mellitus**
[0-4]   Conditions classifiable to 249, 250

Excludes: *gestational diabetes (648.8)*

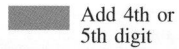

	Add 4th or		Nonspecific		Unspecified		Manifestation
	5th digit		code		code		code

529

⑤ **648.1 Thyroid dysfunction**
[0-4]   Conditions classifiable to 240-246

⑤ **648.2 Anemia**
[0-4]   Conditions classifiable to 280-285

⑤ **648.3 Drug dependence**
[0-4]   Conditions classifiable to 304

⑤ **648.4 Mental disorders**
[0-4]   Conditions classifiable to 290-303, 305.0, 305.2-305.9, 306-316, 317-319

⑤ **648.5 Congenital cardiovascular disorders**
[0-4]   Conditions classifiable to 745-747

⑤ **648.6 Other cardiovascular diseases**
[0-4]   Conditions classifiable to 390-398, 410-429

> Excludes: *cerebrovascular disorders in the puerperium (674.0)*
> *peripartum cardiomyopathy (674.5)*
> *venous complications (671.0-671.9)*

⑤ **648.7 Bone and joint disorders of back, pelvis, and lower limbs**
[0-4]   Conditions classifiable to 720-724, and those classifiable to 711-719 or 725-738,
           specified as affecting the lower limbs

⑤ **648.8 Abnormal glucose tolerance**
[0-4]   Conditions classifiable to 790.21-790.29
           Gestational diabetes
           Use additional code, if applicable, for associated long-term (current) insulin use
           (V58.67)

⑤ **648.9 Other current conditions classifiable elsewhere**
[0-4]   Conditions classifiable to 440-459, 795.01-795.04, 795.06, 795.10-795.14, 795.16,
           796.70-796.74, 796.76
           Nutritional deficiencies [conditions classifiable to 260-269]

649 **Other conditions or status of the mother complicating pregnancy, childbirth, or the puerperium**

The following fifth-digit subclassification is for use with categories 640-649 to denote the current episode of care:

0 **unspecified as to episode of care or not applicable**

1 **delivered, with or without mention of antepartum condition**
       Antepartum condition with delivery
       Delivery NOS (with mention of antepartum complication during current episode of care)
       Intrapartum obstetric condition (with mention of antepartum complication during current episode of care)
       Pregnancy, delivered (with mention of antepartum complication during current episode of care)

2 **delivered, with mention of postpartum complication**
       Delivery with mention of puerperal complication during current episode of care

3 **antepartum condition or complication**
       Antepartum obstetric condition, not delivered during the current episode of care

4 **postpartum condition or complication**
       Postpartum or puerperal obstetric condition or complication following delivery that occurred:
       during previous episode of care
       outside hospital, with subsequent admission for observation or care

ALERT! For personal history of tobacco use see V15.82

⑤ **649.0 Tobacco use disorder complicating pregnancy, childbirth, or the puerperium**
[0-4]   Smoking complicating pregnancy, childbirth, or the puerperium

⑤ **649.1 Obesity complicating pregnancy, childbirth, or the puerperium**
[0-4]
Use additional code to identify the obesity (278.00-278.03)

⑤ **649.2 Bariatric surgery status complicating pregnancy, childbirth, or the puerperium**
[0-4]   Gastric banding status complicating pregnancy, childbirth, or the puerperium
           Gastric bypass status for obesity complicating pregnancy, childbirth, or the puerperium
           Obesity surgery status complicating pregnancy, childbirth, or the puerperium

⑤ **649.3 Coagulation defects complicating pregnancy, childbirth, or the puerperium**
[0-4]   Conditions classifiable to 286, 287, 289
Use additional code to identify the specific coagulation defect (286.0-286.9, 287.0-287.9, 289.0-289.9)

● Code new   ▲ Revision of   ④ ⑤ Fourth or fifth
         to 2012 edition   existing code   digit required

[Excludes:] *coagulation defects causing antepartum hemorrhage (641.3)*
postpartum coagulation defects (666.3)

[5] **649.4 Epilepsy complicating pregnancy, childbirth, or the puerperium**
[0-4] Conditions classifiable to 345

Use additional code to identify the specific type of epilepsy (345.00-345.91)

[Excludes:] *eclampsia (642.6)*

[5] **649.5 Spotting complicating pregnancy**
[0,1,3]

[Excludes:] *antepartum hemorrhage (641.0-641.9)*
hemorrhage in early pregnancy (640.0-640.9)

[5] **649.6 Uterine size date discrepancy**
[0-4]

[Excludes:] *suspected problem with fetal growth not found (V89.04)*

[5] **649.7 Cervical shortening**
[0,1,3]

[Excludes:] *suspected cervical shortening not found (V89.05)*

● **649.8 Onset (spontaneous) of labor after 37 completed weeks of gestation but before 39 completed weeks gestation, with delivery by (planned) cesarean section**
[1-2]
Delivery by (planned) cesarean section occurring after 37 completed weeks of gestation but before 39 completed weeks gestation due to (spontaneous) onset of labor

Use additional code to specify reason for planned cesarean section such as:
cephalopelvic disproportion (normally formed fetus) (653.4)
previous cesarean delivery (654.2)

NORMAL DELIVERY, AND OTHER INDICATIONS FOR CARE IN PREGNANCY, LABOR, AND DELIVERY (650-659)

650 Normal delivery

Delivery requiring minimal or no assistance, with or without episiotomy, without fetal manipulation [e.g., rotation version] or instrumentation [forceps] of spontaneous, cephalic, vaginal, full-term, single, live born infant. This code is for use as a single diagnosis code and is not to be used with any other code in the range 630-676.

[Excludes:] *breech delivery (assisted) (spontaneous) NOS (652.2)*
delivery by vacuum extractor, forceps, cesarean section, or breech extraction, without specified complication (669.5-669.7)

Use additional code to indicate outcome of delivery (V27.0)

[ALERT!] Code 650 is for use in cases when a woman is admitted for a full-term normal delivery and delivers a single, healthy infant without any complications antepartum, during the delivery, or postpartum during the delivery episode. Code 650 is always a principal diagnosis

[ALERT!] V27.0, Single liveborn, is the only outcome of delivery code appropriate for use with 650.

The following fifth-digit subclassification is for use with categories 651-659 to denote the current episode of care:

0 unspecified as to episode of care or not applicable
1 delivered, with or without mention of antepartum condition
2 delivered, with mention of postpartum complication
3 antepartum condition or complication
4 postpartum condition or complication

[5] **651 Multiple gestation**

Use additional code to specify placenta status (V91.00-V91.99)

[DEFINITION] Multiple gestation is a multiple birth occurs when more than one fetus is carried to term in a single pregnancy

[5] **651.0 Twin pregnancy**
[0,1,3]

[Excludes:] *fetal conjoined twins (678.1)*

[5] **651.1 Triplet pregnancy**
[0,1,3]

[5] **651.2 Quadruplet pregnancy**
[0,1,3]

⑤ **651.3** **Twin pregnancy with fetal loss and retention of one fetus**
[0,1,3]

⑤ **651.4** **Triplet pregnancy with fetal loss and retention of one or more fetus(es)**
[0,1,3]

⑤ **651.5** **Quadruplet pregnancy with fetal loss and retention of one or more fetus(es)**
[0,1,3]

⑤ **651.6** **Other multiple pregnancy with fetal loss and retention of one or more fetus(es)**
[0,1,3]

⑤ **651.7** **Multiple gestation following (elective) fetal reduction**
Fetal reduction of multiple fetuses reduced to single fetus

    651.70 **Multiple gestation following (elective) fetal reduction, unspecified as to episode of care or not applicable**

    651.71 **Multiple gestation following (elective) fetal reduction, delivered, with or without mention of antepartum condition**

    651.73 **Multiple gestation following (elective) fetal reduction, antepartum condition or complication**

⑤ **651.8** **Other specified multiple gestation**
[0,1,3]

⑤ **651.9** **Unspecified multiple gestation**
[0,1,3]

⑤ **652** **Malposition and malpresentation of fetus**
Code first any associated obstructed labor (660.0)
DEFINITION Malposition and malpresentation of fetus refers to presentation of the fetal parts in inappropriate positions for the easiest passage through the cervix, e.g. Retention of the head, breech presentation.

⑤ **652.0** **Unstable lie**
[0,1,3]

⑤ **652.1** **Breech or other malpresentation successfully converted to cephalic presentation**
[0,1,3]   Cephalic version NOS

⑤ **652.2** **Breech presentation without mention of version**
[0,1,3]   Breech delivery (assisted) (spontaneous) NOS
Buttocks presentation
Complete breech
Frank breech

Excludes: *footling presentation (652.8)*
        incomplete breech (652.8)

⑤ **652.3** **Transverse or oblique presentation**
[0,1,3]   Oblique lie   Transverse lie

Excludes: *transverse arrest of fetal head (660.3)*

⑤ **652.4** **Face or brow presentation**
[0,1,3]   Mentum presentation

⑤ **652.5** **High head at term**
[0,1,3]   Failure of head to enter pelvic brim

⑤ **652.6** **Multiple gestation with malpresentation of one fetus or more**
[0,1,3]

⑤ **652.7** **Prolapsed arm**
[0,1,3]

⑤ **652.8** **Other specified malposition or malpresentation**
[0,1,3]   Compound presentation

⑤ **652.9** **Unspecified malposition or malpresentation**
[0,1,3]

⑤ **653** **Disproportion**
Code first any associated obstructed labor (660.1)

⑤ **653.0** **Major abnormality of bony pelvis, not further specified**
[0,1,3]   Pelvic deformity NOS

⑤ **653.1** **Generally contracted pelvis**
[0,1,3]   Contracted pelvis NOS

⑤ **653.2** **Inlet contraction of pelvis**
[0,1,3]   Inlet contraction (pelvis)

⑤ **653.3** **Outlet contraction of pelvis**
[0,1,3]   Outlet contraction (pelvis)

    ● Code new   ▲ Revision of   ④ ⑤ Fourth or fifth
          to 2012 edition   existing code   digit required

[5] **653.4 Fetopelvic disproportion**
[0,1,3] Cephalopelvic disproportion NOS
Disproportion of mixed maternal and fetal origin, with normally formed fetus

[5] **653.5 Unusually large fetus causing disproportion**
[0,1,3] Disproportion of fetal origin with normally formed fetus
Fetal disproportion NOS

[*Excludes:*] *that when the reason for medical care was concern for the fetus (656.6)*

[5] **653.6 Hydrocephalic fetus causing disproportion**
[0,1,3]

[*Excludes:*] *that when the reason for medical care was concern for the fetus (655.0)*

[5] **653.7 Other fetal abnormality causing disproportion**
[0,1,3] Fetal:
- ascites
- hydrops
- myelomeningocele
- sacral teratoma
- tumor

[*Excludes:*] *conjoined twins causing disproportion (678.1)*

[5] **653.8 Disproportion of other origin**
[0,1,3]

[*Excludes:*] *shoulder (girdle) dystocia (660.4)*

[5] **653.9 Unspecified disproportion**
[0,1,3]

[5] **654 Abnormality of organs and soft tissues of pelvis**
Includes: the listed conditions during pregnancy, childbirth, or the puerperium
Code first any associated obstructed labor (660.2)

[*Excludes:*] *trauma to perineum and vulva complicating current delivery (664.0-664.9)*

[5] **654.0 Congenital abnormalities of uterus**
[0-4] Double uterus
Uterus bicornis

[5] **654.1 Tumors of body of uterus**
[0-4] Uterine fibroids

[5] **654.2 Previous cesarean delivery NOS**
[0,1,3] Uterine scar from previous cesarean delivery

[5] **654.3 Retroverted and incarcerated gravid uterus**
[0-4]

[5] **654.4 Other abnormalities in shape or position of gravid uterus and of neighboring structures**
[0-4] Cystocele
Pelvic floor repair
Pendulous abdomen
Prolapse of gravid uterus
Rectocele
Rigid pelvic floor

[5] **654.5 Cervical incompetence**
[0-4] Presence of Shirodkar suture with or without mention of cervical incompetence

[5] **654.6 Other congenital or acquired abnormality of cervix**
[0-4] Cicatricial cervix
Polyp of cervix
Previous surgery to cervix
Rigid cervix (uteri)
Stenosis or stricture of cervix
Tumor of cervix

[5] **654.7 Congenital or acquired abnormality of vagina**
[0-4] Previous surgery to vagina
Septate vagina
Stenosis of vagina (acquired) (congenital)
Stricture of vagina
Tumor of vagina

⑤ **654.8 Congenital or acquired abnormality of vulva**
[0-4] Anal sphincter tear (healed) (old) complicating delivery
Fibrosis of perineum
Persistent hymen
Previous surgery to perineum or vulva
Rigid perineum
Tumor of vulva

[Excludes:] *anal sphincter tear (healed) (old) not associated with delivery (569.43)*
varicose veins of vulva (671.1)

⑤ **654.9 Other and unspecified**
[0-4] Uterine scar NEC

⑤ **655 Known or suspected fetal abnormality affecting management of mother**
Includes: the listed conditions in the fetus as a reason for observation or obstetrical care of the mother, or for termination of pregnancy

[ALERT!] In cases where surgery is performed on the fetus a diagnosis code from this category should be assigned to identify the fetal condition

⑤ **655.0 Central nervous system malformation in fetus**
[0,1,3] Fetal or suspected fetal:
anencephaly
hydrocephalus
spina bifida (with myelomeningocele)

⑤ **655.1 Chromosomal abnormality in fetus**
[0,1,3]

⑤ **655.2 Hereditary disease in family possibly affecting fetus**
[0,1,3]

⑤ **655.3 Suspected damage to fetus from viral disease in the mother**
[0,1,3] Suspected damage to fetus from maternal rubella

⑤ **655.4 Suspected damage to fetus from other disease in the mother**
[0,1,3] Suspected damage to fetus from maternal:
alcohol addiction
listeriosis
toxoplasmosis

⑤ **655.5 Suspected damage to fetus from drugs**
[0,1,3]

⑤ **655.6 Suspected damage to fetus from radiation**
[0,1,3]

⑤ **655.7 Decreased fetal movements**
[0,1,3]

⑤ **655.8 Other known or suspected fetal abnormality, not elsewhere classified**
[0,1,3] Suspected damage to fetus from:
environmental toxins
intrauterine contraceptive device

⑤ **655.9 Unspecified**
[0,1,3]

⑤ **656 Other known or suspected fetal and placental problems affecting management of mother**
[Excludes:] *fetal hematologic conditions (678.0)*
suspected placental problems not found (V89.02)

⑤ **656.0 Fetal-maternal hemorrhage**
[0,1,3] Leakage (microscopic) of fetal blood into maternal circulation

⑤ **656.1 Rhesus isoimmunization**
[0,1,3] Anti-D [Rh] antibodies
Rh incompatibility

⑤ **656.2 Isoimmunization from other and unspecified blood-group incompatibility**
[0,1,3] ABO isoimmunization

⑤ **656.3 Fetal distress**
[0,1,3] Fetal metabolic acidemia

[Excludes:] *abnormal fetal acid-base balance (656.8)*
abnormality in fetal heart rate or rhythm (659.7)
fetal bradycardia (659.7)
fetal tachycardia (659.7)
meconium in liquor (656.8)

● Code new to 2012 edition ▲ Revision of existing code ④ ⑤ Fourth or fifth digit required

[5] **656.4 Intrauterine death**
[0,1,3] Fetal death:
NOS
after completion of 22 weeks' gestation
late
Missed delivery
[Excludes:] *missed abortion (632)*

[5] **656.5 Poor fetal growth**
[0,1,3] "Light-for-dates"
"Placental insufficiency"
"Small-for-dates"

[5] **656.6 Excessive fetal growth**
[0,1,3] "Large-for-dates"

[5] **656.7 Other placental conditions**
[0,1,3] Abnormal placenta
Placental infarct
[Excludes:] *placental polyp (674.4)*
placentitis (658.4)

[5] **656.8 Other specified fetal and placental problems**
[0,1,3] Abnormal acid-base balance
Intrauterine acidosis
Lithopedian
Meconium in liquor
Subchorionic hematoma

[5] **656.9 Unspecified fetal and placental problem**
[0,1,3]

[5] **657 Polyhydramnios**
[0,1,3] Hydramnios
[Excludes:] *suspected polyhydramnios not found (V89.01)*
DEFINITION Polyhydramnios is a condition that exists when there is too much amniotic fluid in the uterus.
Use 0 as fourth-digit for this category

[5] **658 Other problems associated with amniotic cavity and membranes**
[Excludes:] *amniotic fluid embolism (673.1)*
suspected problems with amniotic cavity and membranes not found (V89.01)
DEFINITION The amniotic cavity is the fluid-filled cavity that surrounds the developing embryo

[5] **658.0 Oligohydramnios**
[0,1,3] Oligohydramnios without mention of rupture of membranes

[5] **658.1 Premature rupture of membranes**
[0,1,3] Rupture of amniotic sac less than 24 hours prior to the onset of labor

[5] **658.2 Delayed delivery after spontaneous or unspecified rupture of membranes**
[0,1,3] Prolonged rupture of membranes NOS
Rupture of amniotic sac 24 hours or more prior to the onset of labor

[5] **658.3 Delayed delivery after artificial rupture of membranes**
[0,1,3]

[5] **658.4 Infection of amniotic cavity**
[0,1,3] Amnionitis
Chorioamnionitis
Membranitis
Placentitis

[5] **658.8 Other**
[0,1,3] Amnion nodosum
Amniotic cyst

[5] **658.9 Unspecified**
[0,1,3]

[5] **659 Other indications for care or intervention related to labor and delivery, not elsewhere classified**

[5] **659.0 Failed mechanical induction**
[0,1,3] Failure of induction of labor by surgical or other instrumental methods

[5] **659.1 Failed medical or unspecified induction**
[0,1,3] Failed induction NOS
Failure of induction of labor by medical methods, such as oxytocic drugs

⑤ **659.2** **Maternal pyrexia during labor, unspecified**
[0,1,3]

⑤ **659.3** **Generalized infection during labor**
[0,1,3]   Septicemia during labor

⑤ **659.4** **Grand multiparity**
[0,1,3]

Excludes: *supervision only, in pregnancy (V23.3)*
without current pregnancy (V61.5)

⑤ **659.5** **Elderly primigravida**
[0,1,3]   First pregnancy in a woman who will be 35 years of age or older at expected date of
delivery

Excludes: *supervision only, in pregnancy (V23.81)*

⑤ **659.6** **Elderly multigravida**
[0,1,3]   Second or more pregnancy in a woman who will be 35 years of age or older at
expected date of delivery

Excludes: *elderly primigravida 659.5*
supervision only, in pregnancy (V23.82)

⑤ **659.7** **Abnormality in fetal heart rate or rhythm**
[0,1,3]   Depressed fetal heart tones
Fetal:
bradycardia
tachycardia
Fetal heart rate decelerations
Non-reassuring fetal heart rate or rhythm

⑤ **659.8** **Other specified indications for care or intervention related to labor and delivery**
[0,1,3]   Pregnancy in female less than 16 years old at expected date of delivery
Very young maternal age

⑤ **659.9** **Unspecified indication for care or intervention related to labor and delivery**
[0,1,3]

COMPLICATIONS OCCURRING MAINLY IN THE COURSE OF LABOR AND DELIVERY (660-669)

The following fifth-digit subclassification is for use with categories 660-669 to denote the
current episode of care:

0 **unspecified as to episode of care or not applicable**

1 **delivered, with or without mention of antepartum condition**

2 **delivered, with mention of postpartum complication**

3 **antepartum condition or complication**

4 **postpartum condition or complication**

⑤ **660** **Obstructed labor**
DEFINITION Obstructed labor is a labor in which delivery is prevented by mechanical factors;
delivery often requires cesarean section.

⑤ **660.0** **Obstruction caused by malposition of fetus at onset of labor**
[0,1,3]   Any condition classifiable to 652, causing obstruction during labor
Use additional code from 652.0-652.9, if desired, to identify condition

⑤ **660.1** **Obstruction by bony pelvis**
[0,1,3]   Any condition classifiable to 653, causing obstruction during labor
Use additional code from 653.0-653.9, if desired, to identify condition

⑤ **660.2** **Obstruction by abnormal pelvic soft tissues**
[0,1,3]   Prolapse of anterior lip of cervix
Any condition classifiable to 654, causing obstruction during labor
Use additional code from 654.0-654.9, if desired, to identify condition

⑤ **660.3** **Deep transverse arrest and persistent occipitoposterior position**
[0,1,3]

⑤ **660.4** **Shoulder (girdle) dystocia**
[0,1,3]   Impacted shoulders

⑤ **660.5** **Locked twins**
[0,1,3]

⑤ **660.6** **Failed trial of labor, unspecified**
[0,1,3]   Failed trial of labor, without mention of condition or suspected condition

● Code new
to 2012 edition
▲ Revision of
existing code
④ ⑤ Fourth or fifth
digit required

[5] **660.7 Failed forceps or vacuum extractor, unspecified**
[0,1,3] Application of ventouse or forceps, without mention of condition

[5] **660.8 Other causes of obstructed labor**
[0,1,3] Use additional code to identify condition

[5] **660.9 Unspecified obstructed labor**
[0,1,3] Dystocia:
NOS
fetal NOS
maternal NOS

[5] **661 Abnormality of forces of labor**

[5] **661.0 Primary uterine inertia**
[0,1,3] Failure of cervical dilation
Hypotonic uterine dysfunction, primary
Prolonged latent phase of labor

[5] **661.1 Secondary uterine inertia**
[0,1,3] Arrested active phase of labor
Hypotonic uterine dysfunction, secondary

[5] **661.2 Other and unspecified uterine inertia**
[0,1,3] Atony of uterus without hemorrhage
Desultory labor
Irregular labor
Poor contractions
Slow slope active phase of labor

[Excludes:] *atony of uterus with hemorrhage (666.1)*
postpartum atony of uterus without hemorrhage (669.8)

[5] **661.3 Precipitate labor**
[0,1,3]

[5] **661.4 Hypertonic, incoordinate, or prolonged uterine contractions**
[0,1,3] Cervical spasm
Contraction ring (dystocia)
Dyscoordinate labor
Hourglass contraction of uterus
Hypertonic uterine dysfunction
Incoordinate uterine action
Retraction ring (Bandl's) (pathological)
Tetanic contractions
Uterine dystocia NOS
Uterine spasm

[5] **661.9 Unspecified abnormality of labor**
[0,1,3]

[5] **662 Long labor**

[5] **662.0 Prolonged first stage**
[0,1,3]

[5] **662.1 Prolonged labor, unspecified**
[0,1,3]

[5] **662.2 Prolonged second stage**
[0,1,3]

[5] **662.3 Delayed delivery of second twin, triplet, etc.**
[0,1,3]

[5] **663 Umbilical cord complications**

[DEFINITION] The Umbilical cord is the cord that transports blood, oxygen and nutrients to the baby from the placenta.

[5] **663.0 Prolapse of cord**
[0,1,3] Presentation of cord

[5] **663.1 Cord around neck, with compression**
[0,1,3] Cord tightly around neck

[5] **663.2 Other and unspecified cord entanglement, with compression**
[0,1,3] Entanglement of cords of twins in mono-amniotic sac
Knot in cord (with compression)

[5] **663.3 Other and unspecified cord entanglement, without mention of compression**
[0,1,3]

[5] **663.4 Short cord**
[0,1,3]

[5] **663.5 Vasa previa**
[0,1,3]

⑤ **663.6 Vascular lesions of cord**
[0,1,3] Bruising of cord
Hematoma of cord
Thrombosis of vessels of cord

⑤ **663.8 Other umbilical cord complications**
[0,1,3] Velamentous insertion of umbilical cord

⑤ **663.9 Unspecified umbilical cord complication**
[0,1,3]

⑤ **664 Trauma to perineum and vulva during delivery**
Includes: damage from instruments
that from extension of episiotomy

[DEFINITION] The perineum is the area between the vagina and the rectum.

⑤ **664.0 First-degree perineal laceration**
[0,1,4] Perineal laceration, rupture, or tear involving:
fourchette
hymen
labia
skin
vagina
vulva

⑤ **664.1 Second-degree perineal laceration**
[0,1,4] Perineal laceration, rupture, or tear (following episiotomy) involving:
pelvic floor
perineal muscles
vaginal muscles

[Excludes:] *that involving anal sphincter (664.2)*

⑤ **664.2 Third-degree perineal laceration**
[0,1,4] Perineal laceration, rupture, or tear (following episiotomy) involving:
anal sphincter
rectovaginal septum
sphincter NOS

[Excludes:] *anal sphincter tear during delivery not associated with third-degree perineal laceration (664.6)*
that with anal or rectal mucosal laceration (664.3)

⑤ **664.3 Fourth-degree perineal laceration**
[0,1,4] Perineal laceration, rupture, or tear as classifiable to 664.2 and involving also:
anal mucosa
rectal mucosa

⑤ **664.4 Unspecified perineal laceration**
[0,1,4] Central laceration

⑤ **664.6 Anal sphincter tear complicating delivery, not associated with third-degree perineal laceration**
[0,1,4]

[Excludes:] *third-degree perineal laceration (664.2)*

⑤ **664.5 Vulval and perineal hematoma**
[0,1,4]

⑤ **664.8 Other specified trauma to perineum and vulva**
[0,1,4] Periurethral trauma

⑤ **664.9 Unspecified trauma to perineum and vulva**
[0,1,4]

⑤ **665 Other obstetrical trauma**
Includes: damage from instruments

[ALERT!] For personal history of other genital system and obstetric disorders see V13.2

⑤ **665.0 Rupture of uterus before onset of labor**
[0,1,3]

⑤ **665.1 Rupture of uterus during labor**
[0,1] Rupture of uterus NOS

⑤ **665.2 Inversion of uterus**
[0,2,4]

⑤ **665.3 Laceration of cervix**
[0,1,4]

⑤ **665.4 High vaginal laceration**
[0,1,4] Laceration of vaginal wall or sulcus without mention of perineal laceration

● Code new to 2012 edition ▲ Revision of existing code ④ ⑤ Fourth or fifth digit required

[5] **665.5 Other injury to pelvic organs**
[0,1,4] Injury to:
bladder
urethra
[Excludes:] *periurethral trauma (664.8)*

[5] **665.6 Damage to pelvic joints and ligaments**
[0,1,4] Avulsion of inner symphyseal cartilage
Damage to coccyx
Separation of symphysis (pubis)

[5] **665.7 Pelvic hematoma**
[0,1,2,4] Hematoma of vagina

[5] **665.8 Other specified obstetrical trauma**
[0-4]

[5] **665.9 Unspecified obstetrical trauma**
[0-4]

[5] **666 Postpartum hemorrhage**
[DEFINITION] Postpartum hemorrhage refers to abnormal bleeding after delivery.

[5] **666.0 Third-stage hemorrhage**
[0,2,4] Hemorrhage associated with retained, trapped, or adherent placenta
Retained placenta NOS

[5] **666.1 Other immediate postpartum hemorrhage**
[0,2,4] Atony of uterus with hemorrhage
Hemorrhage within the first 24 hours following delivery of placenta
Postpartum atony of uterus with hemorrhage
Postpartum hemorrhage (atonic) NOS
[Excludes:] *atony of uterus without hemorrhage (661.2)*
postpartum atony of uterus without hemorrhage (669.8)

[5] **666.2 Delayed and secondary postpartum hemorrhage**
[0,2,4] Hemorrhage:
after the first 24 hours following delivery
associated with retained portions of placenta or membranes
Postpartum hemorrhage specified as delayed or secondary
Retained products of conception NOS, following delivery

[5] **666.3 Postpartum coagulation defects**
[0,2,4] Postpartum afibrinogenemia
Postpartum fibrinolysis

[5] **667 Retained placenta or membranes, without hemorrhage**
[DEFINITION] A Retained placenta is a placenta that remains inside the womb after the birth of the baby.

[5] **667.0 Retained placenta without hemorrhage**
[0,2,4] Placenta accreta without hemorrhage
Retained placenta: without hemorrhage
NOS without hemorrhage
total without hemorrhage

[5] **667.1 Retained portions of placenta or membranes, without hemorrhage**
[0,2,4] Retained products of conception following delivery, without hemorrhage

[5] **668 Complications of the administration of anesthetic or other sedation in labor and delivery**
Includes: complications arising from the administration of a general or local anesthetic, analgesic, or other sedation in labor and delivery
[Excludes:] *reaction to spinal or lumbar puncture (349.0)*
spinal headache (349.0)

Use additional code(s) to further specify complication
[ALERT!] For personal history of failed moderate sedation see V15.80

[5] **668.0 Pulmonary complications**
[0-4] Inhalation [aspiration] of stomach contents or secretions following anesthesia or other sedation in labor or delivery
Mendelson's syndrome following anesthesia or other sedation in labor or delivery
Pressure collapse of lung following anesthesia or other sedation in labor or delivery

[5] **668.1 Cardiac complications**
[0-4] Cardiac arrest or failure following anesthesia or other sedation in labor and delivery

[5] **668.2 Central nervous system complications**
[0-4] Cerebral anoxia following anesthesia or other sedation in labor and delivery

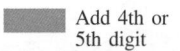

⑤ **668.8** Other complications of anesthesia or other sedation in labor and delivery
[0-4]

⑤ **668.9** Unspecified complication of anesthesia and other sedation
[0-4]

⑤ **669** Other complications of labor and delivery, not elsewhere classified

ALERT! For personal history of other genital system and obstetric disorders see V13.2

⑤ **669.0** Maternal distress
[0-4]   Metabolic disturbance in labor and delivery

⑤ **669.1** Shock during or following labor and delivery
[0-4]   Obstetric shock

⑤ **669.2** Maternal hypotension syndrome
[0-4]

⑤ **669.3** Acute kidney failure following labor and delivery
[0,2,4]

⑤ **669.4** Other complications of obstetrical surgery and procedures
[0-4]   Cardiac:
          arrest following cesarean or other obstetrical surgery or procedure, including delivery NOS
          failure following cesarean or other obstetrical surgery or procedure, including delivery NOS
          Cerebral anoxia following cesarean or other obstetrical surgery or procedure, including
          delivery NOS

Excludes: complications of obstetrical surgical wounds (674.1-674.3)

⑤ **669.5** Forceps or vacuum extractor delivery without mention of indication
[0,1]   Delivery by ventouse, without mention of indication

⑤ **669.6** Breech extraction, without mention of indication
[0,1]

Excludes: breech delivery NOS (652.2)

⑤ **669.7** Cesarean delivery, without mention of indication
[0,1]

⑤ **669.8** Other complications of labor and delivery
[0-4]

⑤ **669.9** Unspecified complication of labor and delivery
[0-4]

COMPLICATIONS OF THE PUERPERIUM (670-677)

Note: Categories 671 and 673-676 include the listed conditions even if they occur during pregnancy or childbirth.

The following fifth-digit subclassification is for use with categories 670-676 to denote the current episode of care:

0 unspecified as to episode of care or not applicable

1 delivered, with or without mention of antepartum condition

2 delivered, with mention of postpartum complication

3 antepartum condition or complication

4 postpartum condition or complication

DEFINITION The puerperium is the time period after childbirth (about 6 weeks) during which a woman's body returns to its normal physical state.

⑤ **670** Major puerperal infection

Excludes: infection following abortion (639.0)
          minor genital tract infection following delivery (646.6)
          puerperal pyrexia NOS (672)
          puerperal fever NOS (672)
          puerperal pyrexia of unknown origin (672)
          urinary tract infection following delivery (646.6)

DEFINITION Major puerperal infection refers to a bacterial infection following childbirth. The infection may also be referred to as puerperal or postpartum fever.

⑤ **670.0** Major puerperal infection, unspecified
[0,2,4]

⑤ **670.1** Puerperal endometritis
[0,2,4]

⑤ **670.2** Puerperal sepsis
[0,2,4]   Puerperal pyemia

● Code new   ▲ Revision of   ④ ⑤ Fourth or fifth
     to 2012 edition   existing code   digit required

Use additional code to identify severe sepsis (995.92) and any associated acute organ dysfunction, if applicable

[5] **670.3 Puerperal septic thrombophlebitis**
[0,2,4]

[5] **670.8 Other major puerperal infection**
[0,2,4] Puerperal:
pelvic cellulitis
peritonitis
salpingitis

[5] **671 Venous complications in pregnancy and the puerperium**

[Excludes:] *personal history of venous complications prior to pregnancy, such as:*
thrombophlebitis (V12.52)
thrombosis and embolism (V12.51)

[5] **671.0 Varicose veins of legs**
[0-4] Varicose veins NOS

[5] **671.1 Varicose veins of vulva and perineum**
[0-4]

[5] **671.2 Superficial thrombophlebitis**
[0-4] Phlebitis NOS
Thrombophlebitis (superficial)
Thrombosis NOS

Use additional code to identify the superficial thrombophlebitis (453.6, 453.71, 453.81)

[5] **671.3 Deep phlebothrombosis, antepartum**
[0,1,3] Deep-vein thrombosis, antepartum

Use additional code to identify the deep vein thrombosis (453.40-453.42, 453.50-453.52, 453.72-453.79, 453.82-453.89)

Use additional code for long term (current) use of anticoagulants, if applicable (V58.61)

[5] **671.4 Deep phlebothrombosis, postpartum**
[0,2,4] Deep-vein thrombosis, postpartum
Pelvic thrombophlebitis, postpartum
Phlegmasia alba dolens (puerperal)

Use additional code to identify the deep vein thrombosis (453.40-453.42, 453.50-453.52, 453.72-453.79, 453.82-453.89)

Use additional code for long term (current) use of anticoagulants, if applicable (V58.61)

[5] **671.5 Other phlebitis and thrombosis**
[0-4] Cerebral venous thrombosis
Thrombosis of intracranial venous sinus

ALERT! For personal history of venous thrombosis and embolism see V12.51

[5] **671.8 Other venous complications**
[0-4] Hemorrhoids

[5] **671.9 Unspecified venous complication**
[0-4]

[5] **672 Pyrexia of unknown origin during the puerperium**
[0,2,4] Puerperal fever NOS
Postpartum fever NOS

Use 0 as fourth-digit for this category

DEFINITION Pyrexia of unknown origin during the puerperium, refers to a fever or febrile condition during the period following childbirth.

[5] **673 Obstetrical pulmonary embolism**

Includes: pulmonary emboli in pregnancy, childbirth, or the puerperium, or specified as puerperal

[Excludes:] *embolism following abortion (639.6)*

DEFINITION Obstetrical pulmonary embolism is a blood clot that lodges in the lungs and blocks the lung arteries during pregnancy so the flow of blood to the lungs and heart is reduced

[5] **673.0 Obstetrical air embolism**
[0-4]

[5] **673.1 Amniotic fluid embolism**
[0-4]

[5] **673.2 Obstetrical blood-clot embolism**
[0-4] Puerperal pulmonary embolism NOS

⑤ **673.3 Obstetrical pyemic and septic embolism**
[0-4]

⑤ **673.8 Other pulmonary embolism**
[0-4]   Fat embolism

⑤ **674 Other and unspecified complications of the puerperium, not elsewhere classified**
ALERT! For personal history of other genital system and obstetric disorders see V13.2

⑤ **674.0 Cerebrovascular disorders in the puerperium**
[0-4]   Any condition classifiable to 430-434, 436-437 occurring during pregnancy, childbirth, or the puerperium, or specified as puerperal

    Excludes: *intracranial venous sinus thrombosis (671.5)*

⑤ **674.1 Disruption of cesarean wound**
[0,2,4]   Dehiscence or disruption of uterine wound

    Excludes: *uterine rupture before onset of labor (665.0)*
                   uterine rupture during labor (665.1)

⑤ **674.2 Disruption of perineal wound**
[0,2,4]   Breakdown of perineum
    Disruption of wound of:
      episiotomy
      perineal laceration
    Secondary perineal tear

⑤ **674.3 Other complications of obstetrical surgical wounds**
[0,2,4]   Hematoma of cesarean section or perineal wound
    Hemorrhage of cesarean section or perineal wound
    Infection of cesarean section or perineal wound

    Excludes: *damage from instruments in delivery (664.0-665.9)*

⑤ **674.4 Placental polyp**
[0,2,4]

⑤ **674.5 Peripartum cardiomyopathy**
[0-4]   Postpartum cardiomyopathy

⑤ **674.8 Other**
[0,2,4]   Hepatorenal syndrome, following delivery
    Postpartum:
      subinvolution of uterus
      uterine hypertrophy

⑤ **674.9 Unspecified**
[0,2,4]   Sudden death of unknown cause during the puerperium

⑤ **675 Infections of the breast and nipple associated with childbirth**
    Includes: the listed conditions during pregnancy, childbirth, or the puerperium

⑤ **675.0 Infections of nipple**
[0-4]   Abscess of nipple

⑤ **675.1 Abscess of breast**
[0-4]   Abscess:
      mammary
      subareolar
      submammary
    Mastitis:
      purulent
      retromammary
      submammary

⑤ **675.2 Nonpurulent mastitis**
[0-4]   Lymphangitis of breast
    Mastitis:
      NOS
      interstitial
      parenchymatous

⑤ **675.8 Other specified infections of the breast and nipple**
[0-4]

⑤ **675.9 Unspecified infection of the breast and nipple**
[0-4]

⑤ **676 Other disorders of the breast associated with childbirth and disorders of lactation**
    Includes: the listed conditions during pregnancy, the puerperium, or lactation

⑤ **676.0 Retracted nipple**
[0-4]

● Code new to 2012 edition   ▲ Revision of existing code   ④ ⑤ Fourth or fifth digit required

[5] **676.1 Cracked nipple**
[0-4] Fissure of nipple

[5] **676.2 Engorgement of breasts**
[0-4]

[5] **676.3 Other and unspecified disorder of breast**
[0-4]

[5] **676.4 Failure of lactation**
[0-4] Agalactia

[5] **676.5 Suppressed lactation**
[0-4]

[5] **676.6 Galactorrhea**
[0-4]

[Excludes:] *galactorrhea not associated with childbirth (611.6)*

[5] **676.8 Other disorders of lactation**
[0-4] Galactocele

[5] **676.9 Unspecified disorder of lactation**
[0-4]

677 Late effect of complication of pregnancy, childbirth, and the puerperium

Note: This category is to be used to indicate conditions in 632-648.9 and 651-676.9 as the cause of the late effect, themselves classifiable elsewhere. The "late effects" include conditions specified as such, or as sequelae, which may occur at any time after the puerperium.

Code first any sequelae

[DEFINITION] Late effect of complication of pregnancy, childbirth, and the puerperium is a condition that appears after the acute phase of the pregnancy complication has run its course

[ALERT!] Code 677 is for use in those cases when an initial complication of a pregnancy develops a sequelae requiring care or treatment at a future date. This code, like all late effect codes, is to be sequenced following the code describing the sequelae of the complication.

OTHER MATERNAL AND FETAL COMPLICATIONS (678-679)

The following fifth-digit subclassification is for use with categories 678-679 to denote the current episode of care:

0 unspecified as to episode of care or not applicable

1 delivered, with or without mention of antepartum condition

2 delivered, with mention of postpartum complication

3 antepartum condition or complication

4 postpartum condition or complication

[5] **678 Other fetal conditions**

Requires fifth digit; valid digits are in [brackets] under each code. See beginning of section 678-679 for definitions.

[5] **678.0 Fetal hematologic conditions**
[0,1,3] Fetal anemia
Fetal thrombocytopenia
Fetal twin to twin transfusion

[Excludes:] *fetal and neonatal hemorrhage (772.0-772.9)*
fetal hematologic disorders affecting newborn (776.0-776.9)
fetal-maternal hemorrhage (656.00-656.03)
isoimmunization incompatibility (656.10-656.13, 656.20-656.23)

[5] **678.1 Fetal conjoined twins**
[0,1,3]

[5] **679 Complications of in utero procedures**

Requires fifth digit; valid digits are in [brackets] under each code. See beginning of section 678-679 for definitions.

[DEFINITION] Complications of in utero procedures, refers to problems caused by procedures performed on the unborn fetus.

[ALERT!] For personal history of undergoing in utero procedure during pregnancy see V15.21

[ALERT!] For personal history of undergoing in utero procedure while a fetus see V15.22

[5] **679.0 Maternal complications from in utero procedure**
[0-4]

[Excludes:] *maternal history of in utero procedure during previous pregnancy (V23.86)*

⑤ **679.1   Fetal complications from in utero procedure**
[0-4]   Fetal complications from amniocentesis

   Excludes: *newborn affected by in utero procedure (760.61-760.64)*

● Code new   ▲ Revision of   ④ ⑤ Fourth or fifth
        to 2012 edition   existing code   digit required

Chapter 12: Diseases Skin and Subcutaneous Tissue (680-709)

DEFINITIONS AND CODING ALERTS

This chapter includes definitions of selected key words, terms and phrases and coding alerts for adding points to the clinical domain, references to coding late effects where appropriate, and references to personal history V-codes in situations where the acute or chronic condition is no longer active. An example from this chapter is as follows:

706 Diseases of sebaceous glands

[DEFINITION] Sebaceous glands are microscopic glands in the skin which secrete an oily matter (sebum) in the hair follicles to lubricate the skin and hair.

[5] **707.2 Pressure ulcer stages**

[ALERT!] Two codes are needed to completely describe a pressure ulcer: a code from subcategory 707.0 to identify the site of the pressure ulcer, and a code from subcategory 707.2

MULTIPLE CODING FOR A SINGLE CONDITION

In addition to the etiology or manifestation convention that requires two codes to fully describe a single condition that affects multiple body systems, there are other single conditions that also require more than one code. "Use additional code" notes are found in the tabular at codes that are not part of an etiology or manifestation pair where a secondary code is useful to fully describe a condition. The sequencing rule is the same as the etiology or manifestation pair - , "use additional code" indicates that a secondary code should be added.

"Code first" notes are also under certain codes that are not specifically manifestation codes but may be due to an underlying cause. When a "code first" note is present and an underlying condition is present the underlying condition should be sequenced first.

"Code, if applicable, any causal condition first", notes indicate that this code may be assigned as a principal diagnosis when the causal condition is unknown or not applicable. If a causal condition is known, then the code for that condition should be sequenced as the principal or first-listed diagnosis. Multiple codes may be needed for late effects, complication codes and obstetric codes to more fully describe a condition. See the specific guidelines for these conditions for further instruction.

COMBINATION CODE

A combination code is a single code used to classify: two diagnoses, or a diagnosis with an associated secondary process (manifestation) A diagnosis with an associated complication Combination codes are identified by referring to subterm entries in the Alphabetic Index and by reading the inclusion and exclusion notes in the Tabular List.

Assign only the combination code when that code fully identifies the diagnostic conditions involved or when the Alphabetic Index so directs. Multiple coding should not be used when the classification provides a combination code that clearly identifies all of the elements documented in the diagnosis. When the combination code lacks necessary specificity in describing the manifestation or complication, an additional code should be used as a secondary code.

CODING LATE EFFECTS

A late effect is the residual effect (condition produced) after the acute phase of an illness or injury has terminated. There is no time limit on when a late effect code can be used. The residual may be apparent early, such as in cerebrovascular accident cases, or it may occur months or years later, such as that due to a previous injury. Coding of late effects generally requires two codes sequenced in the following order: The condition or nature of the late effect is sequenced first. The late effect code is sequenced second.

An exception to the above guidelines are those instances where the code for late effect is followed by a manifestation code identified in the Tabular List and title, or the late effect code has been expanded (at the fourth and fifth-digit levels) to include the manifestation(s). The code for the acute phase of an illness or injury that led to the late effect is never used with a code for the late effect.

PRESSURE ULCER STAGE CODES

Pressure ulcer stages

Two codes are needed to completely describe a pressure ulcer: A code from subcategory 707.0, Pressure ulcer, to identify the site of the pressure ulcer and a code from subcategory 707.2, Pressure ulcer stages.

The codes in subcategory 707.2, Pressure ulcer stages, are to be used as an additional diagnosis with a code(s) from subcategory 707.0, Pressure Ulcer. Codes from 707.2, Pressure ulcer stages, may not be assigned as a principal or first-listed diagnosis. The pressure ulcer stage codes should only be used with pressure ulcers and not with other types of ulcers (e.g., stasis ulcer).

The ICD-9-CM classifies pressure ulcer stages based on severity, which is designated by stages I-IV and unstageable.

Unstageable pressure ulcers

Assignment of code 707.25, Pressure ulcer, unstageable, should be based on the clinical documentation. Code 707.25 is used for pressure ulcers whose stage cannot be clinically determined (e.g., the ulcer is covered by eschar or has been treated with a skin or muscle graft) and pressure ulcers that are documented as deep tissue injury but not documented as due to trauma. This code should not be confused with code 707.20, Pressure ulcer, stage unspecified. Code 707.20 should be assigned when there is no documentation regarding the stage of the pressure ulcer.

Documented pressure ulcer stage

Assignment of the pressure ulcer stage code should be guided by clinical documentation of the stage or documentation of the terms found in the index. For clinical terms describing the stage that are not found in the index, and there is no documentation of the stage, the provider should be queried.

Bilateral pressure ulcers with same stage

When a patient has bilateral pressure ulcers (e.g., both buttocks) and both pressure ulcers are documented as being the same stage, only the code for the site and one code for the stage should be reported.

Bilateral pressure ulcers with different stages

When a patient has bilateral pressure ulcers at the same site (e.g., both buttocks) and each pressure ulcer is documented as being at a different stage, assign one code for the site and the appropriate codes for the pressure ulcer stage.

Multiple pressure ulcers of different sites and stages

When a patient has multiple pressure ulcers at different sites (e.g., buttock, heel, shoulder) and each pressure ulcer is documented as being at different stages (e.g., stage 3 and stage 4), assign the appropriate codes for each different site and a code for each different pressure ulcer stage.

No code is assigned if the documentation states that the pressure ulcer is completely healed.

Pressure ulcers described as healing should be assigned the appropriate pressure ulcer stage code based on the documentation in the medical record. If the documentation does not provide information about the stage of the healing pressure ulcer, assign code 707.20, Pressure ulcer stage, unspecified.

If the documentation is unclear as to whether the patient has a current (new) pressure ulcer or if the patient is being treated for a healing pressure ulcer, query the provider.

If a patient is admitted with a pressure ulcer at one stage and it progresses to a higher stage, assign the code for highest stage reported for that site.

12. DISEASES OF THE SKIN AND SUBCUTANEOUS TISSUE (680-709)

INFECTIONS OF SKIN AND SUBCUTANEOUS TISSUE (680-686)

Excludes: *certain infections of skin classified under "Infectious and Parasitic Diseases," such as:*
erysipelas (035)
erysipeloid of Rosenbach (027.1)
herpes:
   simplex (054.0-054.9)
   zoster (053.0-053.9)
molluscum contagiosum (078.0)
viral warts (078.10-078.19)

ALERT! For personal history of diseases of skin and subcutaneous tissue see V13.3

680 Carbuncle and furuncle
Includes: boil
   furunculosis

DEFINITION A carbuncle is an abscess larger than a boil, usually with one or more openings draining pus onto the skin. It is usually caused by bacterial infection, most commonly staphylococcus aureus. A furuncle is a skin disease caused by the infection of hair follicles, resulting in the localized accumulation of pus and dead tissue

680.0 Face
Ear [any part]
Face [any part, except eye]
Nose (septum)
Temple (region)

Excludes: *eyelid (373.13)*
   lacrimal apparatus (375.31)
   orbit (376.01)

680.1 Neck

680.2 Trunk
Abdominal wall	Flank
Back [any part, except buttocks]	Groin
	Pectoral region
Breast	Perineum
Chest wall	Umbilicus

Excludes: *buttocks (680.5)*
   external genital organs:
   female (616.4)
   male (607.2, 608.4)

680.3 Upper arm and forearm
Arm [any part, except hand]
Axilla
Shoulder

680.4 Hand
Finger [any]   Wrist
Thumb

680.5 Buttock
Anus
Gluteal region

680.6 Leg, except foot
Ankle   Knee
Hip   Thigh

680.7 Foot
Heel
Toe

680.8 Other specified sites
Head [any part, except face]
Scalp

Excludes: *external genital organs:*
   female (616.4)
   male (607.2, 608.4)

680.9 Unspecified site
Boil NOS   Furuncle NOS
Carbuncle NOS

Add 4th or 5th digit	Nonspecific code	Unspecified code	Manifestation code

681 **Cellulitis and abscess of finger and toe**
Includes: that with lymphangitis

Use additional code, if desired, to identify organism, such as Staphylococcus (041.1)

DEFINITION Cellulitis is an infection of the finger or toe, usually caused by normal skin bacteria that get under the top layer of skin. Signs of infection include red, warm, tender skin, swelling, fever, and/or chills.

⑤ **681.0 Finger**

681.00 **Cellulitis and abscess, unspecified**

681.01 Felon
Pulp abscess
Whitlow

Excludes: herpetic whitlow (054.6)

681.02 Onychia and paronychia of finger
Panaritium of finger
Perionychia of finger

⑤ **681.1 Toe**

681.10 **Cellulitis and abscess, unspecified**

681.11 Onychia and paronychia of toe
Panaritium of toe
Perionychia of toe

681.9 Cellulitis and abscess of unspecified digit
Infection of nail NOS

682 **Other cellulitis and abscess**
Includes: abscess (acute) (with lymphangitis) except of finger or toe
cellulitis (diffuse) (with lymphangitis) except of finger or toe
lymphangitis, acute (with lymphangitis) except of finger or toe

Use additional code, if desired, to identify organism, such as Staphylococcus (041.1)

Excludes: lymphangitis (chronic) (subacute) (457.2)

682.0 Face

Cheek, external	Nose, external
Chin	Submandibular
Forehead	Temple (region)

Excludes: ear [any part] (380.10-380.16)
eyelid (373.13)
lacrimal apparatus (375.31)
lip (528.5)
mouth (528.3)
nose (internal) (478.1)
orbit (376.01)

682.1 Neck

682.2 Trunk

Abdominal wall	Groin
Back [any part, except buttock]	Pectoral region
	Perineum
Chest wall	Umbilicus, except newborn
Flank	

Excludes: anal and rectal regions (566)
breast:
NOS (611.0)
puerperal (675.1)
external genital organs:
female (616.3-616.4)
male (604.0, 607.2, 608.4)
umbilicus, newborn (771.4)

682.3 Upper arm and forearm
Arm [any part, except hand]
Axilla
Shoulder

Excludes: hand (682.4)

682.4 Hand, except fingers and thumb
Wrist

Excludes: finger and thumb (681.00-681.02)

● Code new
to 2012 edition
▲ Revision of
existing code
④ ⑤ Fourth or fifth
digit required

682.5 Buttock
Gluteal region

[Excludes:] *anal and rectal regions (566)*

682.6 Leg, except foot
Ankle
Hip
Knee
Thigh

682.7 Foot, except toes
Heel

[Excludes:] *toe (681.10-681.11)*

682.8 Other specified sites
Head [except face]
Scalp

[Excludes:] *face (682.0)*

682.9 Unspecified site
Abscess NOS
Cellulitis NOS
Lymphangitis, acute NOS

[Excludes:] *lymphangitis NOS (457.2)*

683 Acute lymphadenitis
Abscess (acute), lymph gland or node, except mesenteric
Adenitis, acute, lymph gland or node, except mesenteric
Lymphadenitis, acute, lymph gland or node, except mesenteric

Use additional code, if desired, to identify organism, such as Staphylococcus (041.1)

[Excludes:] *enlarged glands NOS (785.6)*
lymphadenitis:
chronic or subacute, except mesenteric (289.1)
mesenteric (acute) (chronic) (subacute) (289.2)
unspecified (289.3)

DEFINITION Lymphadenitis is an inflammation of a lymph node. It is often a complication of a bacterial infection of a wound, although it can also be caused by viruses or other disease agents

684 Impetigo
Impetiginization of other dermatoses
Impetigo (contagiosa) [any site] [any organism]:
bullous
circinate
neonatorum
simplex
Pemphigus neonatorum

[Excludes:] *impetigo herpetiformis (694.3)*

DEFINITION Impetigo is a contagious bacterial skin disease forming pustules and yellow crusty sores, chiefly on the face and hands.

685 Pilonidal cyst
Includes:
fistula, coccygeal or pilonidal
sinus, coccygeal or pilonidal

DEFINITION Pilonidal cyst is a special kind of abscess that occurs in the cleft between the buttocks. Forms frequently in adolescence after long trips that involve sitting.

685.0 With abscess

685.1 Without mention of abscess

686 Other local infections of skin and subcutaneous tissue

Use additional code, if desired, to identify any infectious organism (041.0-041.8)

DEFINITION Subcutaneous tissue is the bottom layer of he skin and is composed of fat cells, connective tissue, blood vessels and nerves.

[5] **686.0 Pyoderma**
Dermatitis:
purulent
septic
suppurative

686.00 Pyoderma, unspecified

686.01 Pyoderma gangrenosum

686.09 Other pyoderma

686.1 Pyogenic granuloma
Granuloma:
septic
suppurative
telangiectaticum

[Excludes:] *pyogenic granuloma of oral mucosa (528.9)*

686.8 Other specified local infections of skin and subcutaneous tissue
Bacterid (pustular)
Dermatitis vegetans
Ecthyma
Perlèche

[Excludes:] *dermatitis infectiosa eczematoides (690.8)*
panniculitis (729.30-729.39)

686.9 Unspecified local infection of skin and subcutaneous tissue
Fistula of skin NOS
Skin infection NOS

[Excludes:] *fistula to skin from internal organs—see Alphabetic Index*

OTHER INFLAMMATORY CONDITIONS OF SKIN AND SUBCUTANEOUS TISSUE (690-698)

[Excludes:] *panniculitis (729.30-729.39)*

690 Erythematosquamous dermatosis

[Excludes:] *eczematous dermatitis of eyelid (373.31)*
parakeratosis variegata (696.2)
psoriasis (696.0-696.1)
seborrheic keratosis (702.11-702.19)

[DEFINITION] Erythematosquamous dermatosis is a skin disease, especially one that is not accompanied by inflammation.

⑤ **690.1 Seborrheic dermatitis**

690.10 Seborrheic dermatitis, unspecified
Seborrheic dermatitis NOS

690.11 Seborrhea capitis
Cradle cap

690.12 Seborrheic infantile dermatitis

690.18 Other seborrheic dermatitis

690.8 Other erythematosquamous dermatosis

691 Atopic dermatitis and related conditions

[DEFINITION] Atopic dermatitis and related conditions, aka eczema, is a chronic, recurring inflammatory skin disorder that usually first appears in babies or very young children and may last through adulthood. Eczema causes the skin to itch and develop a red, scaly, patchy rash.

691.0 Diaper or napkin rash
Ammonia dermatitis
Diaper or napkin:
dermatitis
erythema
rash
Psoriasiform napkin eruption

691.8 Other atopic dermatitis and related conditions
Atopic dermatitis
Besnier's prurigo
Eczema:
atopic
flexural
intrinsic (allergic)
Neurodermatitis:
atopic
diffuse (of Brocq)

● Code new to 2012 edition ▲ Revision of existing code ④ ⑤ Fourth or fifth digit required

692 **Contact dermatitis and other eczema**
Includes:

dermatitis:	eczema (acute) (chronic):
NOS	NOS
contact	allergic
occupational	erythematous
venenata	occupational

Excludes: *allergy NOS (995.3)*

contact dermatitis of eyelids (373.32)
dermatitis due to substances taken internally (693.0-693.9)
eczema of external ear (380.22)
perioral dermatitis (695.3)
urticarial reactions (708.0-708.9, 995.1)

DEFINITION Contact dermatitis refers to a skin reaction resulting from exposure to allergens (allergic contact dermatitis) or irritants (irritant contact dermatitis). Phototoxic dermatitis occurs when the allergen or irritant is activated by sunlight.

692.0 Due to detergents

692.1 Due to oils and greases

692.2 Due to solvents
Dermatitis due to solvents of:
chlorocompound group
cyclohexane group
ester group
glycol group
hydrocarbon group
ketone group

692.3 Due to drugs and medicines in contact with skin
Dermatitis (allergic) (contact) due to:
arnica
fungicides
iodine
keratolytics
mercurials
neomycin
pediculocides
phenols
scabicides
any drug applied to skin
Dermatitis medicamentosa due to drug applied to skin

Use additional E code, if desired, to identify drug

Excludes: *allergy NOS due to drugs (995.27)*

dermatitis due to ingested drugs (693.0)
dermatitis medicamentosa NOS (693.0)

692.4 Due to other chemical products

Dermatitis due to:	Dermatitis due to:
acids	insecticide
adhesive plaster	nylon
alkalis	plastic
caustics	rubber
dichromate	

692.5 Due to food in contact with skin

Dermatitis, contact, due to:	Dermatitis, contact, due to:
cereals	fruit
fish	meat
flour	milk

Excludes: *dermatitis due to:*

dyes (692.89)
ingested foods (693.1)
preservatives (692.89)

Add 4th or 5th digit	Nonspecific code	Unspecified code	Manifestation code

692.6 Due to plants [except food]
Dermatitis due to:
lacquer tree [Rhus verniciflua]
poison ivy [Rhus toxicodendron]
poison oak [Rhus diversiloba]
poison sumac [Rhus venenata]
poison vine [Rhus radicans]
primrose [Primula]
ragweed [Senecio jacobae]
other plants in contact with the skin

[Excludes:] *allergy NOS due to pollen (477.0)*
nettle rash (708.8)

⑤ **692.7 Due to solar radiation**

[Excludes:] *sunburn due to other ultraviolet radiation exposure (692.82)*

692.70 Unspecified dermatitis due to sun

692.71 Sunburn
First degree sunburn
Sunburn NOS

692.72 Acute dermatitis due to solar radiation
Berloque dermatitis
Photoallergic response
Phototoxic response
Polymorphus light eruption
Acute solar skin damage NOS

[Excludes:] *sunburn (692.71, 692.76-692.77)*

Use additional E code, if desired, to identify drug, if drug induced

692.73 Actinic reticuloid and actinic granuloma

692.74 Other chronic dermatitis due to solar radiation
Solar elastosis
Chronic solar skin damage NOS

[Excludes:] *actinic [solar] keratosis (702.0)*

692.75 Disseminated superficial actinic porokeratosis (DSAP)

692.76 Sunburn of second degree

692.77 Sunburn of third degree

692.79 Other dermatitis due to solar radiation
Hydroa aestivale
Photodermatitis due to sun
Photosensitiveness due to sun
Solar skin damage NOS

⑤ **692.8 Due to other specified agents**

692.81 Dermatitis due to cosmetics

692.82 Dermatitis due to other radiation
Infrared rays
Light, except from sun
Radiation NOS
Ultraviolet rays, except from sun
X-rays
Tanning bed

[Excludes:] *that due to solar radiation (692.70-692.79)*

692.83 Dermatitis due to metals
Jewelry

692.84 Due to animal (cat) (dog) dander
Due to animal (cat) (dog) hair

692.89 Other
Dermatitis due to:
cold weather
dyes
hot weather
preservatives

[Excludes:] *allergy (NOS) (rhinitis) due to animal hair or dander (477.2)*
allergy to dust (477.8)
sunburn (692.71, 692.76-692.77)

● Code new to 2012 edition ▲ Revision of existing code ④ ⑤ Fourth or fifth digit required

692.9 Unspecified cause

Dermatitis:
  NOS
  contact NOS
  venenata NOS

Eczema NOS

693 Dermatitis due to substances taken internally

[Excludes:] *adverse effect NOS of drugs and medicines (995.20)*
allergy NOS (995.3)
contact dermatitis (692.0-692.9)
urticarial reactions (708.0-708.9, 995.1)

693.0 Due to drugs and medicines

Dermatitis medicamentosa NOS

Use additional E code, if desired, to identify drug

[Excludes:] *that due to drugs in contact with skin (692.3)*

693.1 Due to food

693.8 Due to other specified substances taken internally

693.9 Due to unspecified substance taken internally

[Excludes:] *dermatitis NOS (692.9)*

694 Bullous dermatoses

[DEFINITION] Bullous dermatoses is a skin disease, especially one that is not accompanied by inflammation

694.0 Dermatitis herpetiformis

Dermatosis herpetiformis
Duhring's disease
Hydroa herpetiformis

[Excludes:] *herpes gestationis (646.8)*
dermatitis herpetiformis:
  juvenile (694.2)
  senile (694.5)

694.1 Subcorneal pustular dermatosis

Sneddon-Wilkinson disease or syndrome

694.2 Juvenile dermatitis herpetiformis

Juvenile pemphigoid

694.3 Impetigo herpetiformis

694.4 Pemphigus

Pemphigus:
  NOS
  erythematosus
  foliaceus

Pemphigus:
  malignant
  vegetans
  vulgaris

[Excludes:] *pemphigus neonatorum (684)*

694.5 Pemphigoid

Benign pemphigus NOS
Bullous pemphigoid
Herpes circinatus bullosus
Senile dermatitis herpetiformis

[5] **694.6 Benign mucous membrane pemphigoid**

Cicatricial pemphigoid
Mucosynechial atrophic bullous dermatitis

694.60 Without mention of ocular involvement

694.61 With ocular involvement

Ocular pemphigus

694.8 Other specified bullous dermatoses

[Excludes:] *herpes gestationis (646.8)*

694.9 Unspecified bullous dermatoses

695 Erythematous conditions

[DEFINITION] Erythematous conditions refers to conditions causing diffuse or patchy redness of skin

695.0 Toxic erythema

Erythema venenatum

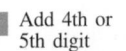

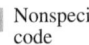

⑤ **695.1 Erythema multiforme**
Use additional code to identify associated manifestations, such as:
arthropathy associated with dermatological disorders (713.3)
conjunctival edema (372.73)
conjunctivitis (372.04, 372.33)
corneal scars and opacities (371.00-371.05)
corneal ulcer (370.00-370.07)
edema of eyelid (374.82)
inflammation of eyelid (373.8)
keratoconjunctivitis sicca (370.33)
mechanical lagophthalmos (374.22)
mucositis (478.11, 528.00, 538, 616.81)
stomatitis (528.00)
symblepharon (372.63)
Use additional E-code to identify drug, if drug-induced
Use additional code to identify percentage of skin exfoliation (695.50-695.59)
Excludes: (staphylococcal) scalded skin syndrome (695.81)

695.10   Erythema multiforme, unspecified
Erythema iris
Herpes iris

695.11   Erythema multiforme minor

695.12   Erythema multiforme major

695.13   Stevens-Johnson syndrome

695.14   Stevens-Johnson syndrome-toxic epidermal
necrolysis overlap syndrome
SJS-TEN overlap syndrome

695.15   Toxic epidermal necrolysis
Lyell's syndrome

695.19   Other erythema multiforme

695.2 Erythema nodosum
Excludes: tuberculous erythema nodosum (017.1)

695.3 Rosacea
Acne: Perioral dermatitis
  erythematosa   Rhinophyma
  rosacea

695.4 Lupus erythematosus
Lupus:
  erythematodes (discoid)
  erythematosus (discoid), not disseminated
Excludes: lupus (vulgaris) NOS (017.0)
          systemic [disseminated] lupus erythematosus (710.0)

⑤ **695.5 Exfoliation due to erythematous conditions according to extent of body surface involved**
Code first erythematous condition causing exfoliation, such as:
Ritter's disease (695.81)
(Staphylococcal) scalded skin syndrome (695.81)
Stevens-Johnson syndrome (695.13)
Stevens-Johnson syndrome-toxic epidermal necrolysis overlap syndrome (695.14)
Toxic epidermal necrolysis (695.15)

695.50   *Exfoliation due to erythematous condition involving less than 10 percent of body surface*
Exfoliation due to erythematous condition NOS

695.51   *Exfoliation due to erythematous condition involving 10-19 percent of body surface*

695.52   *Exfoliation due to erythematous condition involving 20-29 percent of body surface*

695.53   *Exfoliation due to erythematous condition involving 30-39 percent of body surface*

695.54   *Exfoliation due to erythematous condition involving 40-49 percent of body surface*

695.55   *Exfoliation due to erythematous condition involving 50-59 percent of body surface*

● Code new   ▲ Revision of   ④ ⑤ Fourth or fifth
     to 2012 edition   existing code   digit required

695.56 *Exfoliation due to erythematous condition involving 60-69 percent of body surface*

695.57 *Exfoliation due to erythematous condition involving 70-79 percent of body surface*

695.58 *Exfoliation due to erythematous condition involving 80-89 percent of body surface*

695.59 *Exfoliation due to erythematous condition involving 90 percent or more of body surface*

⑤ **695.8 Other specified erythematous conditions**

695.81 Ritter's disease
Dermatitis exfoliativa neonatorum
(Staphylococcal) Scalded skin syndrome

Use additional code to identify percentage of skin exfoliation (695.50-695.59)

695.89 Other
Erythema intertrigo
Intertrigo
Pityriasis rubra (Hebra)

Excludes: mycotic intertrigo (111.0-111.9)

695.9 Unspecified erythematous condition
Erythema NOS
Erythroderma (secondary)

696 Psoriasis and similar disorders
DEFINITION Psoriasis is a chronic, noncontagious genetic disease of the immune system that prompts skin cells to regenerate too quickly, causing red, scaly lesions that crack and bleed. .

696.0 Psoriatic arthropathy

696.1 Other psoriasis
Acrodermatitis continua
Dermatitis repens
Psoriasis:
  NOS
  any type, except arthropathic

Excludes: psoriatic arthropathy (696.0)

696.2 Parapsoriasis
Parakeratosis variegata
Parapsoriasis lichenoides chronica
Pityriasis lichenoides et varioliformis

696.3 Pityriasis rosea
Pityriasis circinata (et maculata)

696.4 Pityriasis rubra pilaris
Devergie's disease
Lichen ruber acuminatus

Excludes: pityriasis rubra (Hebra) (695.89)

696.5 Other and unspecified pityriasis
Pityriasis:
  NOS
  alba
  streptogenes

Excludes: pityriasis simplex (690.18)
  pityriasis versicolor (111.0)

696.8 Other

697 Lichen

Excludes: lichen:
  obtusus corneus (698.3)
  pilaris (congenital) (757.39)
  ruber acuminatus (696.4)
  sclerosus et atrophicus (701.0)
  scrofulosus (017.0)
  simplex chronicus (698.3)
  spinulosus (congenital) (757.39)
  urticatus (698.2)

DEFINITION Lichen refers to any of several eruptive skin diseases characterized by hard thick lesions grouped together and resembling lichens growing on rocks.

Add 4th or 5th digit		Nonspecific code		Unspecified code		Manifestation code	

697.0 Lichen planus
Lichen:
planopilaris
ruber planus

697.1 Lichen nitidus
Pinkus' disease

697.8 Other lichen, not elsewhere classified
Lichen:
ruber moniliforme
striata

697.9 Lichen, unspecified

698 Pruritus and related conditions

[Excludes:] *pruritus specified as psychogenic (306.3)*

DEFINITION Pruritus is the medical term for itching. Pruritus can result from drug reaction, food allergy, kidney or liver disease, cancers, parasites, aging or dry skin, contact skin reaction, such as poison ivy, and for unknown reasons.

698.0 Pruritus ani
Perianal itch

698.1 Pruritus of genital organs

698.2 Prurigo
Lichen urticatus
Prurigo:
NOS
Hebra's
mitis
simplex
Urticaria papulosa (Hebra)

[Excludes:] *prurigo nodularis (698.3)*

698.3 Lichenification and lichen simplex chronicus
Hyde's disease
Neurodermatitis (circumscripta) (local)
Prurigo nodularis

[Excludes:] *neurodermatitis, diffuse (of Brocq) (691.8)*

698.4 Dermatitis factitia [artefacta]
Dermatitis ficta
Neurotic excoriation

Use additional code, if desired, to identify any associated mental disorder

698.8 Other specified pruritic conditions
Pruritus:
hiemalis
senilis
Winter itch

698.9 Unspecified pruritic disorder
Itch NOS
Pruritus NOS

OTHER DISEASES OF SKIN AND SUBCUTANEOUS TISSUE (700-709)

[Excludes:] *conditions confined to eyelids (373.0-374.9)*
congenital conditions of skin, hair, and nails (757.0-757.9)

700 Corns and callosities
Callus
Clavus

DEFINITION Corns and callosities is an especially toughened area of skin which has become relatively thick and hard in response to repeated friction, pressure or other irritation.

701 Other hypertrophic and atrophic conditions of skin

[Excludes:] *dermatomyositis (710.3)*
hereditary edema of legs (757.0)
scleroderma (generalized) (710.1)

DEFINITION Hypertrophic and atrophic conditions of skin, are conditions that cause enlargement or wasting away of the skin.

● Code new to 2012 edition ▲ Revision of existing code ④ ⑤ Fourth or fifth digit required

701.0 Circumscribed scleroderma
Addison's keloid
Dermatosclerosis, localized
Lichen sclerosus et atrophicus
Morphea
Scleroderma, circumscribed or localized

701.1 Keratoderma, acquired
Acquired:
- ichthyosis
- keratoderma palmaris et plantaris

Elastosis perforans serpiginosa
Hyperkeratosis:
- NOS
- follicularis in cutem penetrans
- palmoplantaris climacterica

Keratoderma:
- climactericum
- tylodes, progressive

Keratosis (blennorrhagica)

[Excludes:] *Darier's disease [keratosis follicularis] (congenital) (757.39)*
keratosis:
- *arsenical (692.4)*
- *gonococcal (098.81)*

701.2 Acquired acanthosis nigricans
Keratosis nigricans

701.3 Striae atrophicae
Atrophic spots of skin
Atrophoderma maculatum
Atrophy blanche (of Milian)
Degenerative colloid atrophy
Senile degenerative atrophy
Striae distensae

701.4 Keloid scar
Cheloid
Hypertrophic scar
Keloid

701.5 Other abnormal granulation tissue
Excessive granulation

701.8 Other specified hypertrophic and atrophic conditions of skin
Acrodermatitis atrophicans chronica
Atrophia cutis senilis
Atrophoderma neuriticum
Confluent and reticulate papillomatosis
Cutis laxa senilis
Elastosis senilis
Folliculitis ulerythematosa reticulata
Gougerot-Carteaud syndrome or disease

701.9 Unspecified hypertrophic and atrophic conditions of skin
Atrophoderma

702 Other dermatoses

[Excludes:] *carcinoma in situ (232.0-232.9)*

[DEFINITION] Dermatoses are other skin diseases, especially those not accompanied by inflammation.

702.0 Actinic keratosis

[5] **702.1 Seborrheic keratosis**

702.11 Inflamed seborrheic keratosis

702.19 Other seborrheic keratosis
Seborrheic keratosis NOS

702.8 Other specified dermatoses

703 Diseases of nail

[Excludes:] *congenital anomalies (757.5)*
onychia and paronychia (681.02, 681.11)

703.0 Ingrowing nail
Ingrowing nail with infection
Unguis incarnatus

Excludes: infection, nail NOS (681.9)

703.8 Other specified diseases of nail
Dystrophia unguium
Hypertrophy of nail
Koilonychia
Leukonychia (punctata) (striata)
Onychauxis
Onychogryposis
Onycholysis

703.9 Unspecified disease of nail

704 Diseases of hair and hair follicles

Excludes: congenital anomalies (757.4)

DEFINITION A hair follicle is part of the skin that grows hair by packing old cells together. Attached to the follicle is a sebaceous gland,

⑤ **704.0 Alopecia**

Excludes: madarosis (374.55)
syphilitic alopecia (091.82)

704.00 Alopecia, unspecified
Baldness
Loss of hair

704.01 Alopecia areata
Ophiasis

704.02 Telogen effluvim

704.09 Other
Folliculitis decalvans
Hypotrichosis:
NOS
postinfectional NOS
Pseudopelade

704.1 Hirsutism
Hypertrichosis:
NOS
lanuginosa, acquired
Polytrichia

Excludes: hypertrichosis of eyelid (374.54)

704.2 Abnormalities of the hair
Atrophic hair
Clastothrix
Fragilitas crinium
Trichiasis:
NOS
cicatrical
Trichorrhexis (nodosa)

Excludes: trichiasis of eyelid (374.05)

704.3 Variations in hair color
Canities (premature)
Grayness, hair (premature)
Heterochromia of hair
Poliosis:
NOS
circumscripta, acquired

● **704.4 Pilar and trichilemmal cysts**

● **704.41 Pilar cyst**

● **704.42 Trichilemmal cyst**
Trichilemmal proliferating cyst

704.8 Other specified diseases of hair and hair follicles
Folliculitis:
NOS
abscedens et suffodiens
pustular
Perifolliculitis:
NOS
capitis abscedens et suffodiens
scalp
Sycosis:
NOS
barbae [not parasitic]
lupoid
vulgaris

704.9 Unspecified disease of hair and hair follicles

● Code new
to 2012 edition
▲ Revision of
existing code
④ ⑤ Fourth or fifth
digit required

705 Disorders of sweat glands

[DEFINITION] Sweat glands are numerous small, tubular glands that are found nearly everywhere in the skin of humans and that secrete perspiration externally through pores to help regulate body temperature.

705.0 Anhidrosis
Hypohidrosis
Oligohidrosis

705.1 Prickly heat
Heat rash
Miliaria rubra (tropicalis)
Sudamina

[5] **705.2 Focal hyperhidrosis**
[Excludes:] *generalized (secondary) hyperhidrosis (780.8)*

705.21 Primary focal hyperhidrosis
Focal hyperhidrosis NOS
Hyperhidrosis NOS
Hyperhidrosis of:
axilla
face
palms
soles

705.22 Secondary focal hyperhidrosis
Frey's syndrome

[5] **705.8 Other specified disorders of sweat glands**

705.81 Dyshidrosis
Cheiropompholyx
Pompholyx

705.82 Fox-Fordyce disease

705.83 Hidradenitis
Hidradenitis suppurativa

705.89 Other
Bromhidrosis
Chromhidrosis
Granulosis rubra nasi
Urhidrosis

[Excludes:] *generalized hyperhidrosis (780.8)*
hidrocystoma (216.0-216.9)

705.9 Unspecified disorder of sweat glands
Disorder of sweat glands NOS

706 Diseases of sebaceous glands

[DEFINITION] Sebaceous glands are microscopic glands in the skin which secrete an oily matter (sebum) in the hair follicles to lubricate the skin and hair.

706.0 Acne varioliformis
Acne:
frontalis
necrotica

706.1 Other acne
Acne:
NOS
conglobata
cystic
pustular
vulgaris
Blackhead
Comedo

[Excludes:] *acne rosacea (695.3)*

706.2 Sebaceous cyst
Atheroma, skin
Keratin cyst
Wen

[Excludes:] *pilar cyst (704.41)*
trichilemmal (proliferating) cyst (704.42)

706.3 Seborrhea

[*Excludes:*] *seborrhea:*
capitis (690.11)
sicca (690.18)
seborrheic dermatitis (690.11)
seborrheic keratosis (702.11-702.19)

706.8 Other specified diseases of sebaceous glands
Asteatosis (cutis)
Xerosis cutis

706.9 Unspecified disease of sebaceous glands

707 Chronic ulcer of skin
Includes: non-infected sinus of skin
non-healing ulcer

[*Excludes:*] *varicose ulcer (454.0, 454.2)*

[5] **707.0 Pressure ulcer**
Bed sore
Decubitus ulcer
Plaster ulcer

Use additional code to identify pressure ulcer stage (707.20 -707.25)

[ALERT!] Two codes are needed to completely describe a pressure ulcer: a code from subcategory 707.0 to identify the site of the pressure ulcer, and a code from subcategory 707.2

707.00 Unspecified site

707.01 Elbow

707.02 Upper back
Shoulder blades

707.03 Lower back
Coccyx
Sacrum

707.04 Hip

707.05 Buttock

707.06 Ankle

707.07 Heel

707.09 Other site
Head

[5] **707.1 Ulcer of lower limbs, except pressure ulcer**
Ulcer, chronic, of lower limb:
neurogenic of lower limb
trophic of lower limb

Code, if applicable, any causal condition first:
atherosclerosis of the extremities with ulceration (440.23)
chronic venous hypertension with ulcer (459.31)
chronic venous hypertension with ulcer and inflammation (459.33)
diabetes mellitus (249.80-249.81, 250.80-250.83)
postphlebetic syndrome with ulcer (459.11)
postphlebetic syndrome with ulcer and inflammation (459.13)

707.10 Ulcer of lower limb, unspecified

707.11 Ulcer of thigh

707.12 Ulcer of calf

707.13 Ulcer of ankle

707.14 Ulcer of heel and midfoot
Plantar surface of midfoot

707.15 Ulcer of other part of foot
Toes

707.19 Ulcer of other part of lower limb

[5] **707.2 Pressure ulcer stages**
Code first site of pressure ulcer (707.00-707.09)

[ALERT!] Two codes are needed to completely describe a pressure ulcer: a code from subcategory 707.0 to identify the site of the pressure ulcer, and a code from subcategory 707.2

707.20 Pressure ulcer, unspecified stage
Healing pressure ulcer NOS
Healing pressure ulcer, unspecified stage

707.21 Pressure ulcer stage I
Healing pressure ulcer, stage I
Pressure pre-ulcer skin changes limited to persistent focal erythema

707.22 Pressure ulcer stage II
Healing pressure ulcer, stage II
Pressure ulcer with abrasion, blister, partial thickness skin loss involving epidermis and/or dermis

707.23 Pressure ulcer stage III
Healing pressure ulcer, stage III
Pressure ulcer with full thickness skin loss involving damage or necrosis of subcutaneous tissue

707.24 Pressure ulcer stage IV
Healing pressure ulcer, stage IV
Pressure ulcer with necrosis of soft tissues through to underlying muscle, tendon, or bone

707.25 Pressure ulcer, unstageable

ALERT! Code 707.25 is used for pressure ulcers whose stage cannot be clinically determined (e.g., the ulcer is covered by eschar or has been treated with a skin or muscle graft) and pressure ulcers that are documented as deep tissue injury but not documented as due to trauma. This code should not be confused with code 707.20, Pressure ulcer, stage unspecified

707.8 Chronic ulcer of other specified sites
Ulcer, chronic, of other specified sites:
neurogenic of other specified sites
trophic of other specified sites

707.9 Chronic ulcer of unspecified site
Chronic ulcer NOS
Trophic ulcer NOS
Tropical ulcer NOS
Ulcer of skin NOS

708 Urticaria

[Excludes:] *edema:*
angioneurotic (995.1)
Quincke's (995.1)
hereditary angioedema (277.6)
urticaria:
giant (995.1)
papulosa (Hebra) (698.2)
pigmentosa (juvenile) (congenital) (757.33)

DEFINITION Urticaria, aka hives, is the transient appearance of slightly raised patches of skin which are redder or paler than the surrounding skin and often attended by severe itching.

708.0 Allergic urticaria

708.1 Idiopathic urticaria

708.2 Urticaria due to cold and heat
Thermal urticaria

708.3 Dermatographic urticaria
Dermatographia
Factitial urticaria

708.4 Vibratory urticaria

708.5 Cholinergic urticaria

708.8 Other specified urticaria
Nettle rash
Urticaria:
chronic
recurrent periodic

708.9 Urticaria, unspecified
Hives NOS

709 Other disorders of skin and subcutaneous tissue

[5] **709.0 Dyschromia**

[Excludes:] *albinism (270.2)*
pigmented nevus (216.0-216.9)
that of eyelid (374.52-374.53)

709.00 **Dyschromia, unspecified**

709.01 **Vitiligo**

709.09 **Other**

709.1 **Vascular disorders of skin**
Angioma serpiginosum
Purpura (primary) annularis telangiectodes

709.2 **Scar conditions and fibrosis of skin**
Adherent scar (skin)
Cicatrix
Disfigurement (due to scar)
Fibrosis, skin NOS
Scar NOS

Excludes: keloid scar (701.4)

709.3 **Degenerative skin disorders**
Calcinosis: Degeneration, skin
  circumscripta   Deposits, skin
  cutis   Senile dermatosis NOS
Colloid milium   Subcutaneous calcification

709.4 **Foreign body granuloma of skin and subcutaneous tissue**

Excludes: residual foreign body without granuloma of skin and subcutaneous tissue (729.6)
that of muscle (728.82)

Use additional code to identify foreign body (V90.01-V90.9)

709.8 **Other specified disorders of skin**
Epithelial hyperplasia
Menstrual dermatosis
Vesicular eruption

709.9 **Unspecified disorder of skin and subcutaneous tissue**
Dermatosis NOS

● Code new
  to 2012 edition

▲ Revision of
  existing code

④ ⑤ Fourth or fifth
    digit required

Chapter 13: Diseases of Musculoskeletal and Connective Tissue (710-739)

DEFINITIONS AND CODING ALERTS

This chapter includes definitions of selected key words, terms and phrases and coding alerts for adding points to the clinical domain, references to coding late effects where appropriate, and references to personal history V-codes in situations where the acute or chronic condition is no longer active. An example from this chapter is as follows:

710 **Diffuse diseases of connective tissue**
> **DEFINITION** Connective tissue is a type of tissue made up of fibers forming a framework and support structure for body tissues and organs.
> **ALERT!** For personal history of arthritis see V13.4

MULTIPLE CODING FOR A SINGLE CONDITION

In addition to the etiology or manifestation convention that requires two codes to fully describe a single condition that affects multiple body systems, there are other single conditions that also require more than one code. "Use additional code" notes are found in the tabular at codes that are not part of an etiology or manifestation pair where a secondary code is useful to fully describe a condition. The sequencing rule is the same as the etiology or manifestation pair - , "use additional code" indicates that a secondary code should be added.

"Code first" notes are also under certain codes that are not specifically manifestation codes but may be due to an underlying cause. When a "code first" note is present and an underlying condition is present the underlying condition should be sequenced first.

"Code, if applicable, any causal condition first", notes indicate that this code may be assigned as a principal diagnosis when the causal condition is unknown or not applicable. If a causal condition is known, then the code for that condition should be sequenced as the principal or first-listed diagnosis. Multiple codes may be needed for late effects, complication codes and obstetric codes to more fully describe a condition. See the specific guidelines for these conditions for further instruction.

COMBINATION CODE

A combination code is a single code used to classify: two diagnoses, or a diagnosis with an associated secondary process (manifestation) A diagnosis with an associated complication Combination codes are identified by referring to subterm entries in the Alphabetic Index and by reading the inclusion and exclusion notes in the Tabular List.

Assign only the combination code when that code fully identifies the diagnostic conditions involved or when the Alphabetic Index so directs. Multiple coding should not be used when the classification provides a combination code that clearly identifies all of the elements documented in the diagnosis. When the combination code lacks necessary specificity in describing the manifestation or complication, an additional code should be used as a secondary code.

CODING LATE EFFECTS

A late effect is the residual effect (condition produced) after the acute phase of an illness or injury has terminated. There is no time limit on when a late effect code can be used. The residual may be apparent early, such as in cerebrovascular accident cases, or it may occur months or years later, such as that due to a previous injury. Coding of late effects generally requires two codes sequenced in the following order: The condition or nature of the late effect is sequenced first. The late effect code is sequenced second.

An exception to the above guidelines are those instances where the code for late effect is followed by a manifestation code identified in the Tabular List and title, or the late effect code has been expanded (at the fourth and fifth-digit levels) to include the manifestation(s). The code for the acute phase of an illness or injury that led to the late effect is never used with a code for the late effect.

CODING OF PATHOLOGIC FRACTURES

Acute Fractures vs. Aftercare

Pathologic fractures are reported using subcategory 733.1, when the fracture is newly diagnosed. Subcategory 733.1 may be used while the patient is receiving active treatment for the fracture. Examples of active treatment are: surgical treatment, emergency department encounter, evaluation and treatment by a new physician.

	Add 4th or 5th digit		Nonspecific code		Unspecified code		Manifestation code

Fractures are coded using the aftercare codes (subcategories V54.0, V54.2, V54.8 or V54.9) for encounters after the patient has completed active treatment of the fracture and is receiving routine care for the fracture during the healing or recovery phase. Examples of fracture aftercare are: cast change or removal, removal of external or internal fixation device, medication adjustment, and follow up visits following fracture treatment.

Care for complications of surgical treatment for fracture repairs during the healing or recovery phase should be coded with the appropriate complication codes.

Care of complications of fractures, such as malunion and nonunion, should be reported with the appropriate codes. See Official Guidelines, Section I. C. 17.b for information on the coding of traumatic fractures.

13. DISEASES OF THE MUSCULOSKELETAL SYSTEM AND CONNECTIVE TISSUE (710-739)

Use additional external cause code, if applicable, to identify the cause of the musculoskeletal condition

The following fifth-digit subclassification is for use with categories 711-712, 715-716, 718-719, and 730:

0 site unspecified

1 shoulder region
Acromioclavicular joint(s)
Glenohumeral joint(s)
Sternoclavicular joint(s)
Clavicle
Scapula

2 upper arm
Elbow joint   Humerus

3 forearm
Radius   Wrist joint
Ulna

4 hand
Carpus   Phalanges [fingers]
Metacarpus

5 pelvic region and thigh
Buttock   Hip (joint)
Femur

6 lower leg
Fibula   Patella
Knee joint   Tibia

7 ankle and foot
Ankle joint   Phalanges, foot
Digits [toes]   Tarsus
Metatarsus   Other joints in foot

8 other specified sites
Head   Skull
Neck   Trunk
Ribs   Vertebral column

9 multiple sites

ARTHROPATHIES AND RELATED DISORDERS (710-719)

Excludes: *disorders of spine (720.0-724.9)*

DEFINITION Arthropathy refers to any disease or abnormal condition affecting a joint.

710 Diffuse diseases of connective tissue
Includes: all collagen diseases whose effects are not mainly confined to a single system

Excludes: *those affecting mainly the cardiovascular system, i.e., polyarteritis nodosa and allied conditions (446.0-446.7)*

DEFINITION Connective tissue is a type of tissue made up of fibers forming a framework and support structure for body tissues and organs.

ALERT! For personal history of arthritis see V13.4

710.0 Systemic lupus erythematosus
Disseminated lupus erythematosus
Libman-Sacks disease

Use additional code, if desired, to identify manifestation, as:
endocarditis (424.91)
nephritis (583.81)
chronic (582.81)
nephrotic syndrome (581.81)

Excludes: *lupus erythematosus (discoid) NOS (695.4)*

| | Add 4th or 5th digit | | Nonspecific code | | Unspecified code | | Manifestation code |

710.1 Systemic sclerosis
   Acrosclerosis
   CRST syndrome
   Progressive systemic sclerosis
   Scleroderma

Use additional code, if desired, to identify manifestation, as:
   lung involvement (517.2)
   myopathy (359.6)

   Excludes: *circumscribed scleroderma (701.0)*

710.2 Sicca syndrome
   Keratoconjunctivitis sicca
   Sjögren's disease

710.3 Dermatomyositis
   Poikilodermatomyositis
   Polymyositis with skin involvement

710.4 Polymyositis

710.5 Eosinophilia myalgia syndrome
   Toxic oil syndrome

Use additional E code, if desired, to identify drug, if drug induced

710.8 Other specified diffuse diseases of connective tissue
   Multifocal fibrosclerosis (idiopathic) NEC
   Systemic fibrosclerosing syndrome

710.9 Unspecified diffuse connective tissue disease
   Collagen disease NOS

⑤ **711 Arthropathy associated with infections**
   Includes: arthritis associated with conditions classifiable below
         arthropathy associated with conditions classifiable below
         polyarthritis associated with conditions classifiable below
         polyarthropathy associated with conditions classifiable below

   Excludes: *rheumatic fever (390)*
The following fifth-digit subclassification is for use with category 711; valid digits are in
   [brackets] under each code. For definitions, see the beginning of this chapter:

   0   site unspecified

   1   shoulder region

   2   upper arm

   3   forearm

   4   hand

   5   pelvic region and thigh

   6   lower leg

   7   ankle and foot

   8   other specified sites

   9   multiple sites
   DEFINITION Arthropathy is any disease or abnormal condition affecting a joint

⑤ **711.0 Pyogenic arthritis**
   [0-9]   Arthritis or polyarthritis (due to):
         coliform [Escherichia coli]
         Hemophilus influenzae [H. influenzae]
         pneumococcal
         Pseudomonas
         staphylococcal
         streptococcal
      Pyarthrosis

Use additional code, if desired, to identify infectious organism (041.0-041.8)

⑤ **711.1 *Arthropathy associated with Reiter's disease and nonspecific urethritis***
   [0-9]   *Code first underlying disease, as:*
         nonspecific urethritis (099.4)
         Reiter's disease (099.3)

⑤ **711.2 *Arthropathy in Behçet's syndrome***
   [0-9]   *Code first underlying disease (136.1)*

● Code new   ▲ Revision of   ④ ⑤ Fourth or fifth
         to 2012 edition   existing code   digit required

⑤ **711.3** *Postdysenteric arthropathy*
[0-9]   *Code first underlying disease, as:*
          dysentery (009.0)
          enteritis, infectious (008.0-009.3)
          paratyphoid fever (002.1-002.9)
          typhoid fever (002.0)

Excludes: salmonella arthritis (003.23)

⑤ **711.4** *Arthropathy associated with other bacterial diseases*
[0-9]   *Code first underlying disease, as:*
          diseases classifiable to 010-040, 090-099, except as in 711.1, 711.3, and 713.5
          leprosy (030.0-030.9)
          tuberculosis (015.0-015.9)

Excludes: gonococcal arthritis (098.50)
          meningococcal arthritis (036.82)

⑤ **711.5** *Arthropathy associated with other viral diseases*
[0-9]   *Code first underlying disease, as:*
          diseases classifiable to 045-049, 050-079, 480, 487
          O'nyong nyong (066.3)

Excludes: that due to rubella (056.71)

⑤ **711.6** *Arthropathy associated with mycoses*
[0-9]   *Code first underlying disease (110.0-118)*

⑤ **711.7** *Arthropathy associated with helminthiasis*
[0-9]   *Code first underlying disease, as:*
          filariasis (125.0-125.9)

⑤ **711.8** *Arthropathy associated with other infectious and parasitic diseases*
[0-9]   *Code first underlying disease, as:*
          diseases classifiable to 080-088, 100-104, 130-136

Excludes: arthropathy associated with sarcoidosis (713.7)

⑤ **711.9** **Unspecified infective arthritis**
[0-9]   Infective arthritis or polyarthritis (acute) (chronic) (subacute) NOS

⑤ **712** **Crystal arthropathies**
          Includes: crystal-induced arthritis and synovitis

Excludes: gouty arthropathy (274.00-274.03)

The following fifth-digit subclassification is for use with category 712; valid digits are in
[brackets] under each code. See beginning of this chapter for definitions:

0 **site unspecified**

1 **shoulder region**

2 **upper arm**

3 **forearm**

4 **hand**

5 **pelvic region and thigh**

6 **lower leg**

7 **ankle and foot**

8 **other specified sites**

9 **multiple sites**

DEFINITION Crystal arthropathies refers to a type of arthropathy characterized by accumulation
of crystals in joints.

⑤ **712.1** *Chondrocalcinosis due to dicalcium phosphate crystals*
[0-9]   Chondrocalcinosis due to dicalcium phosphate crystals (with other crystals)
          Code first underlying disease (275.4)

⑤ **712.2** *Chondrocalcinosis due to pyrophosphate crystals*
[0-9]   *Code first underlying disease (275.4)*

⑤ **712.3** *Chondrocalcinosis, unspecified*
[0-9]   *Code first underlying disease (275.4)*

⑤ **712.8** **Other specified crystal arthropathies**
[0-9]

⑤ **712.9** **Unspecified crystal arthropathy**
[0-9]

	Add 4th or 5th digit		Nonspecific code		Unspecified code		Manifestation code

713 **Arthropathy associated with other disorders classified elsewhere**
Includes: arthritis associated with conditions classifiable below
arthropathy associated with conditions classifiable below
polyarthritis associated with conditions classifiable below
polyarthropathy associated with conditions classifiable below

DEFINITION Arthropathy is any disease or abnormal condition affecting a joint

713.0 *Arthropathy associated with other endocrine and metabolic disorders*
Code first underlying disease, as:
acromegaly (253.0)
hemochromatosis (275.01-275.09)
hyperparathyroidism (252.00-252.08)
hypogammaglobulinemia (279.00-279.09)
hypothyroidism (243-244.9)
lipoid metabolism disorder (272.0-272.9)
ochronosis (270.2)

Excludes: *arthropathy associated with:*
amyloidosis (713.7)
crystal deposition disorders, except gout (712.1-712.9)
diabetic neuropathy (713.5)
gout (274.00-274.03)

713.1 *Arthropathy associated with gastrointestinal conditions other than infections*
Code first underlying disease, as:
regional enteritis (555.0-555.9)
ulcerative colitis (556)

713.2 *Arthropathy associated with hematological disorders*
Code first underlying disease, as:
hemoglobinopathy (282.4-282.7)
hemophilia (286.0-286.2)
leukemia (204.0-208.9)
malignant reticulosis (202.3)
multiple myelomatosis (203.0)

Excludes: *arthropathy associated with Henoch-Schönlein purpura (713.6)*

713.3 *Arthropathy associated with dermatological disorders*
Code first underlying disease, as:
erythema multiforme (695.10-695.19)
erythema nodosum (695.2)

Excludes: *psoriatic arthropathy (696.0)*

713.4 *Arthropathy associated with respiratory disorders*
Code first underlying disease, as:
diseases classifiable to 490-519

Excludes: *arthropathy associated with respiratory infections (711.0, 711.4-711.8)*

713.5 *Arthropathy associated with neurological disorders*
Charcot's arthropathy associated with diseases classifiable elsewhere
Neuropathic arthritis associated with diseases classifiable elsewhere

Code first underlying disease, as:
neuropathic joint disease [Charcot's joints]:
NOS (094.0)
diabetic (249.6, 250.6)
syringomyelic (336.0)
tabetic [syphilitic] (094.0)

713.6 *Arthropathy associated with hypersensitivity reaction*
Code first underlying disease, as:
Henoch (-Schönlein) purpura (287.0)
serum sickness (999.51-999.59)

Excludes: *allergic arthritis NOS (716.2)*

713.7 *Other general diseases with articular involvement*
Code first underlying disease, as:
amyloidosis (277.30-277.39)
familial Mediterranean fever (277.31)
sarcoidosis (135)

713.8 *Arthropathy associated with other conditions classifiable elsewhere*
Code first underlying disease, as:
conditions classifiable elsewhere except as in 711.1-711.8, 712, and 713.0-713.7

● Code new
to 2012 edition   ▲ Revision of
existing code   ④ ⑤ Fourth or fifth
digit required

714 Rheumatoid arthritis and other inflammatory polyarthropathies

[Excludes:] *rheumatic fever (390)*
rheumatoid arthritis of spine NOS (720.0)

[DEFINITION] Rheumatoid arthritis is a chronic, systemic inflammatory disorder that may affect many tissues and organs, but principally attacks the joints producing a inflammatory synovitis that often progresses to destruction of the articular cartilage and ankylosis of the joints.

714.0 Rheumatoid arthritis
Arthritis or polyarthritis:
atrophic
rheumatic (chronic)

Use additional code, if desired, to identify manifestation, as:
myopathy (359.6)
polyneuropathy (357.1)

[Excludes:] *juvenile rheumatoid arthritis NOS (714.30)*

714.1 Felty's syndrome
Rheumatoid arthritis with splenoadenomegaly and leukopenia

714.2 Other rheumatoid arthritis with visceral or systemic involvement
Rheumatoid carditis

[5] **714.3 Juvenile chronic polyarthritis**

714.30 Polyarticular juvenile rheumatoid arthritis, chronic or unspecified
Juvenile rheumatoid arthritis NOS
Still's disease

714.31 Polyarticular juvenile rheumatoid arthritis, acute

714.32 Pauciarticular juvenile rheumatoid arthritis

714.33 Monoarticular juvenile rheumatoid arthritis

714.4 Chronic postrheumatic arthropathy
Chronic rheumatoid nodular fibrositis
Jaccoud's syndrome

[5] **714.8 Other specified inflammatory polyarthropathies**

714.81 Rheumatoid lung
Caplan's syndrome
Diffuse interstitial rheumatoid disease of lung
Fibrosing alveolitis, rheumatoid

714.89 Other

714.9 Unspecified inflammatory polyarthropathy
Inflammatory polyarthropathy or polyarthritis NOS

[Excludes:] *polyarthropathy NOS (716.5)*

[5] **715 Osteoarthrosis and allied disorders**

Note: Localized, in the subcategories below, includes bilateral involvement of the same site.

Includes: arthritis or polyarthritis:
degenerative
hypertrophic
degenerative joint disease
osteoarthritis

[Excludes:] *Marie-Strümpell spondylitis (720.0)*
osteoarthrosis [osteoarthritis] of spine (721.0-721.9)

The following fifth-digit subclassification is for use with category 715; valid digits are in [brackets] under each code. See beginning of this chapter for definitions:

0 site unspecified
1 shoulder region
2 upper arm
3 forearm
4 hand
5 pelvic region and thigh
6 lower leg
7 ankle and foot
8 other specified sites
9 multiple sites

Add 4th or 5th digit | Nonspecific code | Unspecified code | Manifestation code

DEFINITION Osteoarthrosis is the degeneration of cartilage at a joint and growth of bone spurs that inflame surrounding tissue.

⑤ **715.0 Osteoarthrosis, generalized**
[0,4,9] Degenerative joint disease, involving multiple joints
Primary generalized hypertrophic osteoarthrosis

⑤ **715.1 Osteoarthrosis, localized, primary**
[0-8] Localized osteoarthropathy, idiopathic

⑤ **715.2 Osteoarthrosis, localized, secondary**
[0-8] Coxae malum senilis

⑤ **715.3 Osteoarthrosis, localized, not specified whether primary or secondary**
[0-8] Otto's pelvis

⑤ **715.8 Osteoarthrosis involving, or with mention of more than one site, but not specified as**
[0,9] **generalized**

⑤ **715.9 Osteoarthrosis, unspecified whether generalized or localized**
[0-8]

⑤ **716 Other and unspecified arthropathies**

Excludes: cricoarytenoid arthropathy (478.79)

The following fifth-digit subclassification is for use with category 716; valid digits are in [brackets] under each code. See beginning of this chapter for definitions:

0 **site unspecified**

1 **shoulder region**

2 **upper arm**

3 **forearm**

4 **hand**

5 **pelvic region and thigh**

6 **lower leg**

7 **ankle and foot**

8 **other specified sites**

9 **multiple sites**

DEFINITION Arthropathy refers to any disease or abnormal condition affecting a joint.

ALERT! For personal history of other musculoskeletal disorders see V13.5

⑤ **716.0 Kaschin-Beck disease**
[0-9] Endemic polyarthritis

⑤ **716.1 Traumatic arthropathy**
[0-9]

⑤ **716.2 Allergic arthritis**
[0-9]

Excludes: arthritis associated with Henoch-Schönlein purpura or serum sickness (713.6)

⑤ **716.3 Climacteric arthritis**
[0-9] Menopausal arthritis

⑤ **716.4 Transient arthropathy**
[0-9]

Excludes: palindromic rheumatism (719.3)

⑤ **716.5 Unspecified polyarthropathy or polyarthritis**
[0-9]

⑤ **716.6 Unspecified monoarthritis**
[0-8] Coxitis

⑤ **716.8 Other specified arthropathy**
[0-9]

⑤ **716.9 Arthropathy, unspecified**
[0-9] Arthritis (acute) (chronic) (subacute)
Arthropathy (acute) (chronic) (subacute)
Articular rheumatism (chronic)
Inflammation of joint NOS

● Code new to 2012 edition   ▲ Revision of existing code   ④ ⑤ Fourth or fifth digit required

717 Internal derangement of knee

Includes: degeneration of articular cartilage or meniscus of knee
rupture, old, of articular cartilage or meniscus of knee
tear, old, of articular cartilage or meniscus of knee

[*Excludes:*] *acute derangement of knee (836.0-836.6)*
ankylosis (718.5)
contracture (718.4)
current injury (836.0-836.6)
deformity (736.4-736.6)
recurrent dislocation (718.3)

[DEFINITION] Internal derangement of knee is a term that describes internal damage to the knee joint, generally caused by trauma. It is a nonspecific term that usually must be further refined by history, physical exam, x-rays, and frequently mri studies.

717.0 Old bucket handle tear of medial meniscus
Old bucket handle tear of unspecified cartilage

717.1 Derangement of anterior horn of medial meniscus

717.2 Derangement of posterior horn of medial meniscus

717.3 Other and unspecified derangement of medial meniscus
Degeneration of internal semilunar cartilage

[5] **717.4 Derangement of lateral meniscus**

717.40 Derangement of lateral meniscus, unspecified

717.41 Bucket handle tear of lateral meniscus

717.42 Derangement of anterior horn of lateral meniscus

717.43 Derangement of posterior horn of lateral meniscus

717.49 Other

717.5 Derangement of meniscus, not elsewhere classified
Congenital discoid meniscus
Cyst of semilunar cartilage
Derangement of semilunar cartilage NOS

717.6 Loose body in knee
Joint mice, knee
Rice bodies, knee (joint)

717.7 Chondromalacia of patella
Chondromalacia patellae
Degeneration [softening] of articular cartilage of patella

[5] **717.8 Other internal derangement of knee**

717.81 Old disruption of lateral collateral ligament

717.82 Old disruption of medial collateral ligament

717.83 Old disruption of anterior cruciate ligament

717.84 Old disruption of posterior cruciate ligament

717.85 Old disruption of other ligaments of knee
Capsular ligament of knee

717.89 Other
Old disruption of ligaments of knee NOS

717.9 Unspecified internal derangement of knee
Derangement NOS of knee

[5] **718 Other derangement of joint**

[*Excludes:*] *current injury (830.0-848.9)*
jaw (524.60-524.69)

The following fifth-digit subclassification is for use with category 718; valid digits are in [brackets] under each code. See beginning of this chapter for definitions:

0 site unspecified

1 shoulder region

2 upper arm

3 forearm

4 hand

5 pelvic region and thigh

6 lower leg

7 ankle and foot

Add 4th or 5th digit | Nonspecific code | Unspecified code | Manifestation code

8 other specified sites

9 multiple sites

ALERT! For personal history of other musculoskeletal disorders see V13.5

⑤ **718.0 Articular cartilage disorder**
[0-5, 7-9] Meniscus:
disorder
rupture, old
tear, old
Old rupture of ligament(s) of joint NOS

Excludes: *articular cartilage disorder:*
in ochronosis (270.2)
knee (717.0-717.9)
chondrocalcinosis (275.4)
metastatic calcification (275.4)

⑤ **718.1 Loose body in joint**
[0-5, 7-9] Joint mice

Excludes: *knee (717.6)*

⑤ **718.2 Pathological dislocation**
[0-9] Dislocation or displacement of joint, not recurrent and not current injury
Spontaneous dislocation (joint)

⑤ **718.3 Recurrent dislocation of joint**
[0-9]

⑤ **718.4 Contracture of joint**
[0-9]

⑤ **718.5 Ankylosis of joint**
[0-9] Ankylosis of joint (fibrous) (osseous)

Excludes: *spine (724.9)*
stiffness of joint without mention of ankylosis (719.5)

⑤ **718.6 Unspecified intrapelvic protrusion of acetabulum**
[5] Protrusio acetabuli, unspecified

⑤ **718.7 Developmental dislocation of joint**
[0-9]

Excludes: *congenital dislocation of joint (754.0-755.8)*
traumatic dislocation of joint (830-839)

⑤ **718.8 Other joint derangement, not elsewhere classified**
[0-9] Flail joint (paralytic)   Instability of joint

Excludes: *deformities classifiable to 736 (736.0-736.9)*

⑤ **718.9 Unspecified derangement of joint**
[0-5, 7-9]

Excludes: *knee (717.9)*

719 Other and unspecified disorders of joint

Excludes: *jaw (524.60-524.69)*

The following fifth-digit subclassification is for use with codes 719.0-719.6, 719.8-719.9; valid digits are in [brackets] under each code. See list at beginning of chapter for definitions:

0 site unspecified

1 shoulder region

2 upper arm

3 forearm

4 hand

5 pelvic region and thigh

6 lower leg

7 ankle and foot

8 other specified sites

9 multiple sites

ALERT! For personal history of other musculoskeletal disorders see V13.5

● Code new   ▲ Revision of   ④ ⑤ Fourth or fifth
to 2012 edition   existing code   digit required

⑤ **719.0 Effusion of joint**
[0-9]   Hydrarthrosis
           Swelling of joint, with or without pain

Excludes: intermittent hydrarthrosis (719.3)

⑤ **719.1 Hemarthrosis**
[0-9]

Excludes: current injury (840.0-848.9)

⑤ **719.2 Villonodular synovitis**
[0-9]

⑤ **719.3 Palindromic rheumatism**
[0-9]   Hench-Rosenberg syndrome
           Intermittent hydrarthrosis

⑤ **719.4 Pain in joint**
[0-9]   Arthralgia

⑤ **719.5 Stiffness of joint, not elsewhere classified**
[0-9]

⑤ **719.6 Other symptoms referable to joint**
[0-9]   Joint crepitus   Snapping hip

719.7 Difficulty in walking

Excludes: abnormality of gait (781.2)

⑤ **719.8 Other specified disorders of joint**
[0-9]   Calcification of joint   Fistula of joint

Excludes: temporomandibular joint-pain-dysfunction syndrome [Costen's syndrome] (524.60)

⑤ **719.9 Unspecified disorder of joint**
[0-9]

DORSOPATHIES (720-724)

Excludes: curvature of spine (737.0-737.9)
           osteochondrosis of spine (juvenile) (732.0)
             adult (732.8)

DEFINITION Dorsopathy is a term used to describe various diseases of the back and or spine.

720 Ankylosing spondylitis and other inflammatory spondylopathies
DEFINITION Ankylosing spondylitis is a long-term disease that causes inflammation of the joints between the spinal bones and the joints between the spine and the pelvis. It eventually causes the affected spinal bones to join together.

720.0 Ankylosing spondylitis
       Rheumatoid arthritis of spine NOS
       Spondylitis:
         Marie-Strümpell
         rheumatoid

720.1 Spinal enthesopathy
       Disorder of peripheral ligamentous or muscular attachments of spine
       Romanus lesion

720.2 Sacroiliitis, not elsewhere classified
       Inflammation of sacroiliac joint NOS

⑤ **720.8 Other inflammatory spondylopathies**

720.81 Inflammatory spondylopathies in diseases classified elsewhere
Code first underlying disease, as:
       tuberculosis (015.0)

720.89 Other

720.9 Unspecified inflammatory spondylopathy
       Spondylitis NOS

721 Spondylosis and allied disorders
DEFINITION Spondylosis is degenerative arthritis (osteoarthritis) of the spinal vertebra and related tissue.

721.0 Cervical spondylosis without myelopathy
       Cervical or cervicodorsal:
         arthritis
         osteoarthritis
         spondylarthritis

	Add 4th or 5th digit		Nonspecific code		Unspecified code		Manifestation code

721.1 Cervical spondylosis with myelopathy
Anterior spinal artery compression syndrome
Spondylogenic compression of cervical spinal cord
Vertebral artery compression syndrome

721.2 Thoracic spondylosis without myelopathy
Thoracic:
arthritis
osteoarthritis
spondylarthritis

721.3 Lumbosacral spondylosis without myelopathy
Lumbar or lumbosacral:
arthritis
osteoarthritis
spondylarthritis

⑤ **721.4 Thoracic or lumbar spondylosis with myelopathy**

    721.41 Thoracic region
        Spondylogenic compression of thoracic spinal cord

    721.42 Lumbar region

721.5 Kissing spine
Baastrup's syndrome

721.6 Ankylosing vertebral hyperostosis

721.7 Traumatic spondylopathy
Kümmell's disease or spondylitis

721.8 Other allied disorders of spine

⑤ **721.9 Spondylosis of unspecified site**

    721.90 Without mention of myelopathy
        Spinal:
          arthritis (deformans) (degenerative) (hypertrophic)
          osteoarthritis NOS
        Spondylarthrosis NOS

    721.91 With myelopathy
        Spondylogenic compression of spinal cord NOS

722 Intervertebral disc disorders

    DEFINITION Intervertebral disc disorders result from a protrusion or herniation of one of the gel-like cushions (discs) that separate the vertebrae of the spine.

722.0 Displacement of cervical intervertebral disc without myelopathy
Neuritis (brachial) or radiculitis due to displacement or rupture of cervical intervertebral disc
Any condition classifiable to 722.2 of the cervical or cervicothoracic intervertebral disc

⑤ **722.1 Displacement of thoracic or lumbar intervertebral disc without myelopathy**

    722.10 Lumbar intervertebral disc without myelopathy
        Lumbago or sciatica due to displacement of intervertebral disc
        Neuritis or radiculitis due to displacement or rupture of lumbar intervertebral disc
        Any condition classifiable to 722.2 of the lumbar or lumbosacral intervertebral disc

    722.11 Thoracic intervertebral disc without myelopathy
        Any condition classifiable to 722.2 of thoracic intervertebral disc

722.2 Displacement of intervertebral disc, site unspecified, without myelopathy
Discogenic syndrome NOS
Herniation of nucleus pulposus NOS
Intervertebral disc NOS:
extrusion
prolapse
protrusion
rupture
Neuritis or radiculitis due to displacement or rupture of intervertebral disc

⑤ **722.3 Schmorl's nodes**

    722.30 Unspecified region

    722.31 Thoracic region

    722.32 Lumbar region

    722.39 Other

● Code new
  to 2012 edition
▲ Revision of
  existing code
④ ⑤ Fourth or fifth
  digit required

722.4 **Degeneration of cervical intervertebral disc**
Degeneration of cervicothoracic intervertebral disc

[5] 722.5 **Degeneration of thoracic or lumbar intervertebral disc**

722.51 **Thoracic or thoracolumbar intervertebral disc**

722.52 **Lumbar or lumbosacral intervertebral disc**

722.6 **Degeneration of intervertebral disc, site unspecified**
Degenerative disc disease NOS
Narrowing of intervertebral disc or space NOS

[5] 722.7 **Intervertebral disc disorder with myelopathy**

722.70 **Unspecified region**

722.71 **Cervical region**

722.72 **Thoracic region**

722.73 **Lumbar region**

[5] 722.8 **Postlaminectomy syndrome**

722.80 **Unspecified region**

722.81 **Cervical region**

722.82 **Thoracic region**

722.83 **Lumbar region**

[5] 722.9 **Other and unspecified disc disorder**
Calcification of intervertebral cartilage or disc
Discitis

722.90 **Unspecified region**

722.91 **Cervical region**

722.92 **Thoracic region**

722.93 **Lumbar region**

723 Other disorders of cervical region

[*Excludes:*] *conditions due to:*
intervertebral disc disorders (722.0-722.9)
spondylosis (721.0-721.9)

[ALERT!] For personal history of other musculoskeletal disorders see V13.5

723.0 **Spinal stenosis in cervical region**

723.1 **Cervicalgia**
Pain in neck

723.2 **Cervicocranial syndrome**
Barré-Liéou syndrome
Posterior cervical sympathetic syndrome

723.3 **Cervicobrachial syndrome (diffuse)**

723.4 **Brachial neuritis or radiculitis NOS**
Cervical radiculitis
Radicular syndrome of upper limbs

723.5 **Torticollis, unspecified**
Contracture of neck

[*Excludes:*] *congenital (754.1)*
due to birth injury (767.8)
hysterical (300.11)
ocular torticollis (781.93)
psychogenic (306.0)
spasmodic (333.83)
traumatic, current (847.0)

723.6 **Panniculitis specified as affecting neck**

723.7 **Ossification of posterior longitudinal ligament in cervical region**

723.8 **Other syndromes affecting cervical region**
Cervical syndrome NEC
Klippel's disease
Occipital neuralgia

723.9 **Unspecified musculoskeletal disorders and symptoms referable to neck**
Cervical (region) disorder NOS

724 **Other and unspecified disorders of back**

> *Excludes:* collapsed vertebra (code to cause, e.g., osteoporosis, 733.00-733.09)
>> conditions due to:
>>> intervertebral disc disorders (722.0-722.9)
>>> spondylosis (721.0-721.9)

> **ALERT!** For personal history of other musculoskeletal disorders see V13.5

⑤ **724.0** **Spinal stenosis, other than cervical**

> **724.00** **Spinal stenosis, unspecified region**

> **724.01** **Thoracic region**

> **724.02** **Lumbar region, without neurogenic claudication**
>> Lumbar region NOS

> **724.03** **Lumbar region, with neurogenic claudication**

> **724.09** **Other**

724.1 **Pain in thoracic spine**

724.2 **Lumbago**
> Low back pain
> Low back syndrome
> Lumbalgia

724.3 **Sciatica**
> Neuralgia or neuritis of sciatic nerve

> *Excludes:* specified lesion of sciatic nerve (355.0)

724.4 **Thoracic or lumbosacral neuritis or radiculitis, unspecified**
> Radicular syndrome of lower limbs

724.5 **Backache, unspecified**
> Vertebrogenic (pain) syndrome NOS

724.6 **Disorders of sacrum**
> Ankylosis, lumbosacral or sacroiliac (joint)
> Instability, lumbosacral or sacroiliac (joint)

⑤ **724.7** **Disorders of coccyx**

> **724.70** **Unspecified disorder of coccyx**

> **724.71** **Hypermobility of coccyx**

> **724.79** **Other**
>> Coccygodynia

724.8 **Other symptoms referable to back**
> Ossification of posterior longitudinal ligament NOS
> Panniculitis specified as sacral or affecting back

724.9 **Other unspecified back disorders**
> Ankylosis of spine NOS
> Compression of spinal nerve root NEC
> Spinal disorder NOS

> *Excludes:* sacroiliitis (720.2)

RHEUMATISM, EXCLUDING THE BACK (725-729)

> Includes: disorders of muscles and tendons and their attachments, and of other soft tissues
> **DEFINITION** Rheumatism refers to 1) any painful disorder of the joints or muscles or connective tissues or 2) a chronic autoimmune disease with inflammation of the joints and marked deformities.

725 **Polymyalgia rheumatica**
> **DEFINITION** Polymyalgia rheumatica is a rheumatic disorder that is associated with moderate to severe muscle pain and stiffness in the neck, shoulder and hip areas.

726 **Peripheral enthesopathies and allied syndromes**
> Note: Enthesopathies are disorders of peripheral ligamentous or muscular attachments.

> *Excludes:* spinal enthesopathy (720.1)

> **DEFINITION** Peripheral enthesopathies and allied syndromes refers to any pathological condition of the enthesis (teno-osseous junction), for example tennis elbow, and jumper's knee

726.0 **Adhesive capsulitis of shoulder**

⑤ **726.1** **Rotator cuff syndrome of shoulder and allied disorders**

● Code new ▲ Revision of ④ ⑤ Fourth or fifth
   to 2012 edition   existing code   digit required

726.10 **Disorders of bursae and tendons in shoulder region, unspecified**
Rotator cuff syndrome NOS
Supraspinatus syndrome NOS

726.11 **Calcifying tendinitis of shoulder**

726.12 **Bicipital tenosynovitis**

● **726.13** **Partial tear of rotator cuff**

Excludes: complete rupture of rotator cuff, nontraumatic (727.61)

726.19 **Other specified disorders**

Excludes: complete rupture of rotator cuff, nontraumatic (727.61)

726.2 **Other affections of shoulder region, not elsewhere classified**
Periarthritis of shoulder
Scapulohumeral fibrositis

⑤ **726.3** **Enthesopathy of elbow region**

726.30 **Enthesopathy of elbow, unspecified**

726.31 **Medial epicondylitis**

726.32 **Lateral epicondylitis**
Epicondylitis NOS
Golfers' elbow
Tennis elbow

726.33 **Olecranon bursitis**
Bursitis of elbow

726.39 **Other**

726.4 **Enthesopathy of wrist and carpus**
Bursitis of hand or wrist
Periarthritis of wrist

726.5 **Enthesopathy of hip region**
Bursitis of hip   Psoas tendinitis
Gluteal tendinitis   Trochanteric tendinitis
Iliac crest spur

⑤ **726.6** **Enthesopathy of knee**

726.60 **Enthesopathy of knee, unspecified**
Bursitis of knee NOS

726.61 **Pes anserinus tendinitis or bursitis**

726.62 **Tibial collateral ligament bursitis**
Pellegrini-Stieda syndrome

726.63 **Fibular collateral ligament bursitis**

726.64 **Patellar tendinitis**

726.65 **Prepatellar bursitis**

726.69 **Other**
Bursitis infrapatellar
Bursitis subpatellar

⑤ **726.7** **Enthesopathy of ankle and tarsus**

726.70 **Enthesopathy of ankle and tarsus, unspecified**
Metatarsalgia NOS

Excludes: Morton's metatarsalgia (355.6)

726.71 **Achilles bursitis or tendinitis**

726.72 **Tibialis tendinitis**
Tibialis (anterior) (posterior) tendinitis

726.73 **Calcaneal spur**

726.79 **Other**
Peroneal tendinitis

726.8 **Other peripheral enthesopathies**

⑤ **726.9** **Unspecified enthesopathy**

726.90 **Enthesopathy of unspecified site**
Capsulitis NOS
Periarthritis NOS
Tendinitis NOS

726.91 **Exostosis of unspecified site**
Bone spur NOS

| | Add 4th or 5th digit | | Nonspecific code | | Unspecified code | | Manifestation code |

727 **Other disorders of synovium, tendon, and bursa**

DEFINITION Synovium is a tissue that surrounds and protects the joints. It produces synovial fluid that nourishes and lubricates the joints

ALERT! For personal history of other musculoskeletal disorders see V13.5

⑤ **727.0 Synovitis and tenosynovitis**

727.00 Synovitis and tenosynovitis, unspecified
Synovitis NOS
Tenosynovitis NOS

727.01 Synovitis and tenosynovitis in diseases classified elsewhere
Code first underlying disease, as:
tuberculosis (015.0-015.9)

Excludes: crystal-induced (275.4)
gonococcal (098.51)
gout (274.00-274.03)
syphilitic (095.7)

727.02 Giant cell tumor of tendon sheath

727.03 Trigger finger (acquired)

727.04 Radial styloid tenosynovitis
de Quervain's disease

727.05 Other tenosynovitis of hand and wrist

727.06 Tenosynovitis of foot and ankle

727.09 Other

727.1 Bunion

727.2 Specific bursitides often of occupational origin
Beat:
elbow
hand
knee
Chronic crepitant synovitis of wrist
Miners':
elbow
knee

727.3 Other bursitis
Bursitis NOS

Excludes: bursitis:
gonococcal (098.52)
subacromial (726.19)
subcoracoid (726.19)
subdeltoid (726.19)
syphilitic (095.7)
"frozen shoulder" (726.0)

⑤ **727.4 Ganglion and cyst of synovium, tendon, and bursa**

727.40 Synovial cyst, unspecified

Excludes: that of popliteal space (727.51)

727.41 Ganglion of joint

727.42 Ganglion of tendon sheath

727.43 Ganglion, unspecified

727.49 Other
Cyst of bursa

⑤ **727.5 Rupture of synovium**

727.50 Rupture of synovium, unspecified

727.51 Synovial cyst of popliteal space
Baker's cyst (knee)

727.59 Other

⑤ **727.6 Rupture of tendon, nontraumatic**

727.60 Nontraumatic rupture of unspecified tendon

727.61 Complete rupture of rotator cuff

Excludes: partial tear of rotator cuff (726.13)

727.62 Tendons of biceps (long head)

● Code new
to 2012 edition

▲ Revision of
existing code

④ ⑤ Fourth or fifth
digit required

727.63 Extensor tendons of hand and wrist

727.64 Flexor tendons of hand and wrist

727.65 Quadriceps tendon

727.66 Patellar tendon

727.67 Achilles tendon

727.68 Other tendons of foot and ankle

727.69 Other

[5] **727.8 Other disorders of synovium, tendon, and bursa**

727.81 Contracture of tendon (sheath)
Short Achilles tendon (acquired)

727.82 Calcium deposits in tendon and bursa
Calcification of tendon NOS
Calcific tendinitis NOS

[Excludes:] *peripheral ligamentous or muscular attachments (726.0-726.9)*

727.83 Plica syndrome
Plica knee

727.89 Other
Abscess of bursa or tendon

[Excludes:] *xanthomatosis localized to tendons (272.7)*

727.9 Unspecified disorder of synovium, tendon, and bursa

728 Disorders of muscle, ligament, and fascia

[Excludes:] *enthesopathies (726.0-726.9)*
muscular dystrophies (359.0-359.1)
myoneural disorders (358.00-358.9)
myopathies (359.2-359.9)
nontraumatic hematoma of muscle (729.92)
old disruption of ligaments of knee (717.81-717.89)

DEFINITION Disorders of muscle, ligament, and fascia, fascia is a flat band of tissue below the skin that covers the underlying tissues and separates different layers of tissue.

728.0 Infective myositis
Myositis:
purulent
suppurative

[Excludes:] *myositis:*
epidemic (074.1)
interstitial (728.81)
syphilitic (095.6)
tropical (040.81)

[5] **728.1 Muscular calcification and ossification**

728.10 Calcification and ossification, unspecified
Massive calcification (paraplegic)

728.11 Progressive myositis ossificans

728.12 Traumatic myositis ossificans
Myositis ossificans (circumscripta)

728.13 Postoperative heterotopic calcification

728.19 Other
Polymyositis ossificans

728.2 Muscular wasting and disuse atrophy, not elsewhere classified
Amyotrophia NOS
Myofibrosis

[Excludes:] *neuralgic amyotrophy (353.5)*
pelvic muscle wasting and disuse atrophy (618.83)
progressive muscular atrophy (335.0-335.9)

728.3 Other specific muscle disorders
Arthrogryposis
Immobility syndrome (paraplegic)

[Excludes:] *arthrogryposis multiplex congenita (754.89)*
stiff-man syndrome (333.91)

728.4 Laxity of ligament

728.5 Hypermobility syndrome

728.6 Contracture of palmar fascia
Dupuytren's contracture

⑤ **728.7 Other fibromatoses**

728.71 Plantar fascial fibromatosis
Contracture of plantar fascia
Plantar fasciitis (traumatic)

728.79 Other
Garrod's or knuckle pads
Nodular fasciitis
Pseudosarcomatous fibromatosis (proliferative) (subcutaneous)

⑤ **728.8 Other disorders of muscle, ligament, and fascia**

728.81 Interstitial myositis

728.82 Foreign body granuloma of muscle
Talc granuloma of muscle

Use additional code to identify foreign body (V90.01-V90.9)

728.83 Rupture of muscle, nontraumatic

728.84 Diastasis of muscle
Diastasis recti (abdomen)

Excludes: *diastasis recti complicating pregnancy, labor, and delivery (665.8)*

728.85 Spasm of muscle

728.86 Necrotizing fasciitis
Use additional code to identify:
infectious organism (041.00 - 041.89)
gangrene (785.4), if applicable

728.87 Muscle weakness (generalized)

Excludes: *generalized weakness (780.79)*

728.88 Rhabdomyolysis

728.89 Other
Eosinophilic fasciitis

Use additional E code, if desired, to identify drug, if drug induced

728.9 Unspecified disorder of muscle, ligament, and fascia

729 Other disorders of soft tissues

Excludes: *acroparesthesia (443.89)*
carpal tunnel syndrome (354.0)
disorders of the back (720.0-724.9)
entrapment syndromes (354.0-355.9)
palindromic rheumatism (719.3)
periarthritis (726.0-726.9)
psychogenic rheumatism (306.0)

DEFINITION Disorders of soft tissues, refers to tissues that connect, support, or surround other structures and organs of the body.

ALERT! For personal history of other musculoskeletal disorders see V13.5

729.0 Rheumatism, unspecified and fibrositis

729.1 Myalgia and myositis, unspecified
Fibromyositis NOS

729.2 Neuralgia, neuritis, and radiculitis, unspecified

Excludes: *brachial radiculitis (723.4)*
cervical radiculitis (723.4)
lumbosacral radiculitis (724.4)
mononeuritis (354.0-355.9)
radiculitis due to intervertebral disc involvement (722.0-722.2, 722.7)
sciatica (724.3)

⑤ **729.3 Panniculitis, unspecified**

729.30 Panniculitis, unspecified site
Weber-Christian disease

729.31 Hypertrophy of fat pad, knee
Hypertrophy of infrapatellar fat pad

● Code new
to 2012 edition   ▲ Revision of
existing code   ④ ⑤ Fourth or fifth
digit required

729.39   Other site

Excludes: *panniculitis specified as (affecting):*
    back (724.8)
    neck (723.6)
    sacral (724.8)

729.4   **Fasciitis, unspecified**

Excludes: *necrotizing fasciitis (728.86)*
    nodular fasciitis (728.79)

729.5   **Pain in limb**

729.6   **Residual foreign body in soft tissue**

Use additional code to identify foreign body (V90.01-V90.9)

Excludes: *foreign body granuloma:*
    muscle (728.82)
    skin and subcutaneous tissue (709.4)

⑤ **729.7**   **Nontraumatic compartment syndrome**

Code first, if applicable, postprocedural complication (998.89)

Excludes: *compartment syndrome NOS (958.90)*
    traumatic compartment syndrome (958.90-958.99)

729.71   **Nontraumatic compartment syndrome of upper extremity**
Nontraumatic compartment syndrome of shoulder, arm, forearm, wrist, hand and fingers

729.72   **Nontraumatic compartment syndrome of lower extremity**
Nontraumatic compartment syndrome of hip, buttock, thigh, leg, foot and toes

729.73   **Nontraumatic compartment syndrome of abdomen**

729.79   **Nontraumatic compartment syndrome of other sites**

⑤ **729.8**   **Other musculoskeletal symptoms referable to limbs**

729.81   **Swelling of limb**

729.82   **Cramp**

729.89   **Other**

Excludes: *abnormality of gait (781.2)*
    tetany (781.7)
    transient paralysis of limb (781.4)

⑤ **729.9**   **Other and unspecified disorders of soft tissue**

729.90   **Disorders of soft tissue, unspecified**

729.91   **Post-traumatic seroma**

Excludes: *seroma complicating a procedure (998.13)*

729.92   **Nontraumatic hematoma of soft tissue**
Nontraumatic hematoma of muscle

729.99   **Other disorders of soft tissue**
Polyalgia

OSTEOPATHIES, CHONDROPATHIES, AND ACQUIRED MUSCULOSKELETAL DEFORMITIES (730-739)

DEFINITION Chondropathy refers to a disease of the cartilage.

⑤ **730**   **Osteomyelitis, periostitis, and other infections involving bone**

Excludes: *jaw (526.4-526.5)*
    petrous bone (383.2)

Use additional code, if desired, to identify organism, such as Staphylococcus (041.1)

The following fifth-digit subclassification is for use with category 730; valid digits are in [brackets] under each code. See beginning of this chapter for definitions:

0   **site unspecified**

1   **shoulder region**

2   **upper arm**

3   **forearm**

4   **hand**

5   **pelvic region and thigh**

6   **lower leg**

■ Add 4th or 5th digit   ■ Nonspecific code   ■ Unspecified code   ■ Manifestation code

   7   ankle and foot

   8   other specified sites

   9   multiple sites

   DEFINITION Osteomyelitis is an inflammation of bone and bone marrow (usually caused by bacterial infection). Periostitis is an inflammation of the membrane which covers bones .

⑤ **730.0   Acute osteomyelitis**
   [0-9]   Abscess of any bone except accessory sinus, jaw, or mastoid
              Acute or subacute osteomyelitis, with or without mention of periostitis
   Use additional code to identify major osseous defect, if applicable (731.3)

⑤ **730.1   Chronic osteomyelitis**
   [0-9]   Brodie's abscess
              Chronic or old osteomyelitis, with or without mention of periostitis
              Sequestrum of bone
              Sclerosing osteomyelitis of Garré
   Use additional code to identify major osseous defect, if applicable (731.3)

   Excludes: *aseptic necrosis of bone (733.40-733.49)*

⑤ **730.2   Unspecified osteomyelitis**
   [0-9]   Osteitis or osteomyelitis NOS, with or without mention of periostitis
   Use additional code to identify major osseous defect, if applicable (731.3)

⑤ **730.3   Periostitis without mention of osteomyelitis**
   [0-9]   Abscess of periosteum without mention of osteomyelitis
              Periostosis without mention of osteomyelitis

   Excludes: *that in secondary syphilis (091.61)*

⑤ **730.7   *Osteopathy resulting from poliomyelitis***
   [0-9]   *Code first underlying disease (045.0-045.9)*

⑤ **730.8   *Other infections involving bone in diseases classified elsewhere***
   [0-9]   *Code first underlying disease, as:*
                 tuberculosis (015.0-015.9)
                 typhoid fever (002.0)

   Excludes: *syphilis of bone NOS (095.5)*

⑤ **730.9   Unspecified infection of bone**
   [0-9]

731 Osteitis deformans and osteopathies associated with other disorders classified elsewhere
   DEFINITION Osteitis deformans, aka paget's disease, is a disease of bone occurring in the middle aged and elderly; excessive bone destruction sometimes leading to bone pain and fractures and skeletal deformities.

   731.0   Osteitis deformans without mention of bone tumor
              Paget's disease of bone

   731.1   *Osteitis deformans in diseases classified elsewhere*
              Code first underlying disease, as:
                 malignant neoplasm of bone (170.0-170.9)

   731.2   Hypertrophic pulmonary osteoarthropathy
              Bamberger-Marie disease

   731.3   Major osseous defects
              Code first underlying disease, if known, such as:
                 aseptic necrosis (733.40-733.49)
                 malignant neoplasm of bone (170.0-170.9)
                 osteomyelitis (730.00-730.29)
                 osteoporosis (733.00-733.09)
                 peri-prosthetic osteolysis (996.45)

   731.8   *Other bone involvement in diseases classified elsewhere*
              Code first underlying disease, as:
                 diabetes mellitus (249.8, 250.8)

              Use additional code to specify bone condition, such as:
                 acute osteomyelitis (730.00-730.09)

732 Osteochondropathies
   DEFINITION Osteochondropathies refers to diseases involving both bone and cartilage

● Code new   ▲ Revision of   ④ ⑤ Fourth or fifth
           to 2012 edition   existing code   digit required

732.0 Juvenile osteochondrosis of spine

Juvenile osteochondrosis (of):
marginal or vertebral epiphysis (of Scheuermann)
spine NOS
Vertebral epiphysitis

Excludes: *adolescent postural kyphosis (737.0)*

732.1 Juvenile osteochondrosis of hip and pelvis

Coxa plana
Ischiopubic synchondrosis (of van Neck)
Osteochondrosis (juvenile) of:
acetabulum
head of femur (of Legg-Calvé-Perthes)
iliac crest (of Buchanan)
symphysis pubis (of Pierson)
Pseudocoxalgia

732.2 Nontraumatic slipped upper femoral epiphysis

Slipped upper femoral epiphysis NOS

732.3 Juvenile osteochondrosis of upper extremity

Osteochondrosis (juvenile) of:
capitulum of humerus (of Panner)
carpal lunate (of Kienbock)
hand NOS
head of humerus (of Haas)
heads of metacarpals (of Mauclaire)
lower ulna (of Burns)
radial head (of Brailsford)
upper extremity NOS

732.4 Juvenile osteochondrosis of lower extremity, excluding foot

Osteochondrosis (juvenile) of:
lower extremity NOS
primary patellar center (of Köhler)
proximal tibia (of Blount)
secondary patellar center (of Sinding-Larsen)
tibial tubercle (of Osgood-Schlatter)
Tibia vara

732.5 Juvenile osteochondrosis of foot

Calcaneal apophysitis
Epiphysitis, os calcis
Osteochondrosis (juvenile) of:
astragalus (of Diaz)
calcaneum (of Sever)
foot NOS
metatarsal
second (of Freiberg)
fifth (of Iselin)
os tibiale externum (Haglund)
tarsal navicular (of Köhler)

732.6 Other juvenile osteochondrosis

Apophysitis specified as juvenile, of other site, or site NOS
Epiphysitis specified as juvenile, of other site, or site NOS
Osteochondritis specified as juvenile, of other site, or site NOS
Osteochondrosis specified as juvenile, of other site, or site NOS

732.7 Osteochondritis dissecans

732.8 Other specified forms of osteochondropathy

Adult osteochondrosis of spine

732.9 Unspecified osteochondropathy

Apophysitis
NOS
not specified as adult or juvenile, of unspecified site
Epiphysitis
NOS
not specified as adult or juvenile, of unspecified site
Osteochondritis
NOS
not specified as adult or juvenile, of unspecified site
Osteochondrosis
NOS
not specified as adult or juvenile, of unspecified site

| Add 4th or 5th digit | Nonspecific code | Unspecified code | Manifestation code |

733 **Other disorders of bone and cartilage**

Excludes: *bone spur (726.91)*
cartilage of, or loose body in, joint (717.0-717.9, 718.0-718.9)
giant cell granuloma of jaw (526.3)
osteitis fibrosa cystica generalisata (252.01)
osteomalacia (268.2)
polyostotic fibrous dysplasia of bone (756.54)
prognathism, retrognathism (524.1)
xanthomatosis localized to bone (272.7)

DEFINITION Bone cartilage is a tough, elastic, fibrous connective tissue found in various parts of the body, such as the joints, outer ear, and larynx

ALERT! For personal history of other musculoskeletal disorders see V13.5

⑤ **733.0** **Osteoporosis**

Use additional code to identify major osseous defect, if applicable (731.3)

Use additional code to identify personal history of pathologic (healed) fracture (V13.51)

733.00 **Osteoporosis, unspecified**
Wedging of vertebra NOS

733.01 **Senile osteoporosis**
Postmenopausal osteoporosis

733.02 **Idiopathic osteoporosis**

733.03 **Disuse osteoporosis**

733.09 **Other**
Drug-induced osteoporosis
Use additional E code, if desired, to identify drug

⑤ **733.1** **Pathologic fracture**
Chronic fracture
Spontaneous fracture

Excludes: *traumatic fracture (800-829)*
stress fracture (733.93-733.95)

ALERT! Code 733.1 is used to report pathologic fractures when the fracture is newly diagnosed. Subcategory 733.1 may be used while the patient is receiving active treatment for the fracture

ALERT! For personal history of pathologic fracture see V13.51

733.10 **Pathologic fracture, unspecified site**

733.11 **Pathologic fracture of humerus**

733.12 **Pathologic fracture of distal radius and ulna**
Wrist NOS

733.13 **Pathologic fracture of vertebrae**
Collapse of vertebra NOS

733.14 **Pathologic fracture of neck of femur**
Femur NOS
Hip NOS

733.15 **Pathologic fracture of other specified part of femur**

733.16 **Pathologic fracture of tibia or fibula**
Ankle NOS

733.19 **Pathologic fracture of other specified site**

⑤ **733.2** **Cyst of bone**

733.20 **Cyst of bone (localized), unspecified**

733.21 **Solitary bone cyst**
Unicameral bone cyst

733.22 **Aneurysmal bone cyst**

733.29 **Other**
Fibrous dysplasia (monostotic)

Excludes: *cyst of jaw (526.0-526.2, 526.89)*
osteitis fibrosa cystica (252.01)
polyostotic fibrous dysplasia of bone (756.54)

733.3 **Hyperostosis of skull**
Hyperostosis interna frontalis
Leontiasis ossium

● Code new
to 2012 edition
▲ Revision of
existing code
④ ⑤ Fourth or fifth
digit required

⑤ **733.4 Aseptic necrosis of bone**
Use additional code to identify major osseous defect, if applicable (731.3)

> *Excludes:* *osteochondropathies (732.0-732.9)*

>> **733.40 Aseptic necrosis of bone, site unspecified**

>> **733.41 Head of humerus**

>> **733.42 Head and neck of femur**
>> Femur NOS

> *Excludes:* *Legg-Calvé-Perthes disease (732.1)*

>> **733.43 Medial femoral condyle**

>> **733.44 Talus**

>> **733.45 Jaw**
>> Use additional E code to identify drug, if drug-induced

> *Excludes:* *osteoradionecrosis of jaw (526.89)*

>> **733.49 Other**

733.5 Osteitis condensans
Piriform sclerosis of ilium

733.6 Tietze's disease
Costochondral junction syndrome
Costochondritis

733.7 Algoneurodystrophy
Disuse atrophy of bone   Sudeck's atrophy

⑤ **733.8 Malunion and nonunion of fracture**

>> **733.81 Malunion of fracture**

>> **733.82 Nonunion of fracture**
>> Pseudoarthrosis (bone)

⑤ **733.9 Other and unspecified disorders of bone and cartilage**
ALERT! For personal history of stress fracture see V13.52

>> **733.90 Disorder of bone and cartilage, unspecified**

>> **733.91 Arrest of bone development or growth**
>> Epiphyseal arrest

>> **733.92 Chondromalacia**
>> Chondromalacia:
>> NOS
>> localized, except patella
>> systemic
>> tibial plateau

> *Excludes:* *chondromalacia of patella (717.7)*

>> **733.93 Stress fracture of tibia or fibula**
>> Stress reaction of tibia or fibula

> Use additional external cause code(s) to identify the cause of the stress fracture

>> **733.94 Stress fracture of the metatarsals**
>> Stress reaction of metatarsals

> Use additional external cause code(s) to identify the cause of the stress fracture

>> **733.95 Stress fracture of other bone**
>> Stress reaction of other bone

> Use additional external cause code(s) to identify the cause of the stress fracture

> *Excludes:* *stress fracture of:*
> *femoral neck (733.96)*
> *fibula (733.93)*
> *metatarsals (733.94)*
> *pelvis (733.98)*
> *shaft of femur (733.97)*
> *tibia (733.93)*

>> **733.96 Stress fracture of femoral neck**
>> Stress reaction of femoral neck

> Use additional external cause code(s) to identify the cause of the stress fracture

>> **733.97 Stress fracture of shaft of femur**
>> Stress reaction of shaft of femur

> Use additional external cause code(s) to identify the cause of the stress fracture

| | Add 4th or 5th digit | | Nonspecific code | | Unspecified code | | Manifestation code |

733.98 Stress fracture of pelvis
Stress reaction of pelvis

Use additional external cause code(s) to identify the cause of the stress fracture

733.99 Other
Diaphysitis
Hypertrophy of bone
Relapsing polychondritis

734 Flat foot
Pes planus (acquired)
Talipes planus (acquired)

Excludes: congenital (754.61)
rigid flat foot (754.61)
spastic (everted) flat foot (754.61)

DEFINITION Flat foot, aka pes planus or fallen arches, is an informal reference to a medical condition in which the arch of the foot collapses.

735 Acquired deformities of toe

Excludes: congenital (754.60-754.69, 755.65-755.66)

DEFINITION Acquired deformities of toe is a deformity of the toe acquired after birth resulting from injury or disease.

735.0 Hallux valgus (acquired)

735.1 Hallux varus (acquired)

735.2 Hallux rigidus

735.3 Hallux malleus

735.4 Other hammer toe (acquired)

735.5 Claw toe (acquired)

735.8 Other acquired deformities of toe

735.9 Unspecified acquired deformity of toe

736 Other acquired deformities of limbs

Excludes: congenital (754.3-755.9)

DEFINITION Acquired deformities of limbs, refers to other deformities of the limbs acquired after birth resulting from injury or disease

ALERT! For personal history of other musculoskeletal disorders see V13.5

⑤ **736.0 Acquired deformities of forearm, excluding fingers**

736.00 Unspecified deformity
Deformity of elbow, forearm, hand, or wrist (acquired) NOS

736.01 Cubitus valgus (acquired)

736.02 Cubitus varus (acquired)

736.03 Valgus deformity of wrist (acquired)

736.04 Varus deformity of wrist (acquired)

736.05 Wrist drop (acquired)

736.06 Claw hand (acquired)

736.07 Club hand, acquired

736.09 Other

736.1 Mallet finger

⑤ **736.2 Other acquired deformities of finger**

736.20 Unspecified deformity
Deformity of finger (acquired) NOS

736.21 Boutonniere deformity

736.22 Swan-neck deformity

736.29 Other

Excludes: trigger finger (727.03)

⑤ **736.3 Acquired deformities of hip**

736.30 Unspecified deformity
Deformity of hip (acquired) NOS

736.31 Coxa valga (acquired)

736.32 Coxa vara (acquired)

● Code new
  to 2012 edition

▲ Revision of
  existing code

④ ⑤ Fourth or fifth
    digit required

736.39 Other

[5] **736.4 Genu valgum or varum (acquired)**

736.41 Genu valgum (acquired)

736.42 Genu varum (acquired)

736.5 Genu recurvatum (acquired)

736.6 Other acquired deformities of knee
Deformity of knee (acquired) NOS

[5] **736.7 Other acquired deformities of ankle and foot**

[Excludes:] *deformities of toe (acquired) (735.0-735.9)*
pes planus (acquired) (734)

736.70 Unspecified deformity of ankle and foot, acquired

736.71 Acquired equinovarus deformity
Clubfoot, acquired

[Excludes:] *clubfoot not specified as acquired (754.5-754.7)*

736.72 Equinus deformity of foot, acquired

736.73 Cavus deformity of foot

[Excludes:] *that with claw foot (736.74)*

736.74 Claw foot, acquired

736.75 Cavovarus deformity of foot, acquired

736.76 Other calcaneus deformity

736.79 Other
Acquired:
pes not elsewhere classified
talipes not elsewhere classified

[5] **736.8 Acquired deformities of other parts of limbs**

736.81 Unequal leg length (acquired)

736.89 Other
Deformity (acquired):
arm or leg, not elsewhere classified
shoulder

736.9 Acquired deformity of limb, site unspecified

737 Curvature of spine

[Excludes:] *congenital (754.2)*

[DEFINITION] Curvature of spine, aka scoliosis, is an abnormal curving of the spine, especially in a lateral direction.

737.0 Adolescent postural kyphosis

[Excludes:] *osteochondrosis of spine (juvenile) (732.0)*
adult (732.8)

[5] **737.1 Kyphosis (acquired)**

737.10 Kyphosis (acquired) (postural)

737.11 Kyphosis due to radiation

737.12 Kyphosis, postlaminectomy

737.19 Other

[Excludes:] *that associated with conditions classifiable elsewhere (737.41)*

[5] **737.2 Lordosis (acquired)**

737.20 Lordosis (acquired) (postural)

737.21 Lordosis, postlaminectomy

737.22 Other postsurgical lordosis

737.29 Other

[Excludes:] *that associated with conditions classifiable elsewhere (737.42)*

[5] **737.3 Kyphoscoliosis and scoliosis**

737.30 Scoliosis [and kyphoscoliosis], idiopathic

737.31 Resolving infantile idiopathic scoliosis

737.32 Progressive infantile idiopathic scoliosis

737.33 Scoliosis due to radiation

737.34 Thoracogenic scoliosis

737.39 Other

[Excludes:] *that associated with conditions classifiable elsewhere (737.43)*
that in kyphoscoliotic heart disease (416.1)

⑤ ***737.4 Curvature of spine associated with other conditions***

Code first associated condition, as:
Charcot-Marie-Tooth disease (356.1)
mucopolysaccharidosis (277.5)
neurofibromatosis (237.70-237.79)
osteitis deformans (731.0)
osteitis fibrosa cystica (252.01)
osteoporosis (733.00-733.09)
poliomyelitis (138)
tuberculosis [Pott's curvature] (015.0)

737.40 Curvature of spine, unspecified

737.41 Kyphosis

737.42 Lordosis

737.43 Scoliosis

737.8 Other curvatures of spine

737.9 Unspecified curvature of spine
Curvature of spine (acquired) (idiopathic) NOS
Hunchback, acquired

[Excludes:] *deformity of spine NOS (738.5)*

738 Other acquired deformity

[Excludes:] *congenital (754.0-756.9, 758.0-759.9)*
dentofacial anomalies (524.0-524.9)

[DEFINITION] An Acquired deformity is a deformity acquired after birth from injury or disease.

[ALERT!] For personal history of other musculoskeletal disorders see V13.5

738.0 Acquired deformity of nose
Deformity of nose (acquired)
Overdevelopment of nasal bones

[Excludes:] *deflected or deviated nasal septum (470)*

⑤ **738.1 Other acquired deformity of head**

738.10 Unspecified deformity

738.11 Zygomatic hyperplasia

738.12 Zygomatic hypoplasia

738.19 Other specified deformity

738.2 Acquired deformity of neck

738.3 Acquired deformity of chest and rib
Deformity:
chest (acquired)
rib (acquired)
Pectus:
carinatum, acquired
excavatum, acquired

738.4 Acquired spondylolisthesis
Degenerative spondylolisthesis
Spondylolysis, acquired

[Excludes:] *congenital (756.12)*

738.5 Other acquired deformity of back or spine
Deformity of spine NOS

[Excludes:] *curvature of spine (737.0-737.9)*

738.6 Acquired deformity of pelvis
Pelvic obliquity

[Excludes:] *intrapelvic protrusion of acetabulum (718.6)*
that in relation to labor and delivery (653.0-653.4, 653.8-653.9)

738.7 Cauliflower ear

738.8 Acquired deformity of other specified site
Deformity of clavicle

738.9 Acquired deformity of unspecified site

● Code new to 2012 edition ▲ Revision of existing code ④ ⑤ Fourth or fifth digit required

739 **Nonallopathic lesions, not elsewhere classified**
  Includes: segmental dysfunction
        somatic dysfunction

  DEFINITION In the United States and Canada the term "nonallopathic lesion" is commonly used in place of subluxation as a diagnosis, and is considered a more accurate descriptor of lesions that chiropractors treat most commonly.

739.0 Head region
    Occipitocervical region

739.1 Cervical region
    Cervicothoracic region

739.2 Thoracic region
    Thoracolumbar region

739.3 Lumbar region
    Lumbosacral region

739.4 Sacral region
    Sacrococcygeal region
    Sacroiliac region

739.5 Pelvic region
    Hip region
    Pubic region

739.6 Lower extremities

739.7 Upper extremities
    Acromioclavicular region
    Sternoclavicular region

739.8 Rib cage
    Costochondral region   Sternochondral region
    Costovertebral region

739.9 Abdomen and other

■ Add 4th or   ■ Nonspecific   ■ Unspecified   ■ Manifestation
  5th digit   code   code   code

This page intentionally left blank.

● Code new
to 2012 edition

▲ Revision of
existing code

④ ⑤ Fourth or fifth
digit required

Chapter 14: Congenital Anomalies (740-759)

DEFINITIONS AND CODING ALERTS

This chapter includes definitions of selected key words, terms and phrases and coding alerts for adding points to the clinical domain, references to coding late effects where appropriate, and references to personal history V-codes in situations where the acute or chronic condition is no longer active. An example from this chapter is as follows:

746 **Other congenital anomalies of heart**

> **DEFINITION** Congenital anomalies of heart refers to other defects of the heart that are present at birth.
>
> **ALERT!** For personal history of other congenital malformations see V13.69

MULTIPLE CODING FOR A SINGLE CONDITION

In addition to the etiology or manifestation convention that requires two codes to fully describe a single condition that affects multiple body systems, there are other single conditions that also require more than one code. "Use additional code" notes are found in the tabular at codes that are not part of an etiology or manifestation pair where a secondary code is useful to fully describe a condition. The sequencing rule is the same as the etiology or manifestation pair - , "use additional code" indicates that a secondary code should be added.

"Code first" notes are also under certain codes that are not specifically manifestation codes but may be due to an underlying cause. When a "code first" note is present and an underlying condition is present the underlying condition should be sequenced first.

"Code, if applicable, any causal condition first", notes indicate that this code may be assigned as a principal diagnosis when the causal condition is unknown or not applicable. If a causal condition is known, then the code for that condition should be sequenced as the principal or first-listed diagnosis. Multiple codes may be needed for late effects, complication codes and obstetric codes to more fully describe a condition. See the specific guidelines for these conditions for further instruction.

COMBINATION CODE

A combination code is a single code used to classify: two diagnoses, or a diagnosis with an associated secondary process (manifestation) A diagnosis with an associated complication Combination codes are identified by referring to subterm entries in the Alphabetic Index and by reading the inclusion and exclusion notes in the Tabular List.

Assign only the combination code when that code fully identifies the diagnostic conditions involved or when the Alphabetic Index so directs. Multiple coding should not be used when the classification provides a combination code that clearly identifies all of the elements documented in the diagnosis. When the combination code lacks necessary specificity in describing the manifestation or complication, an additional code should be used as a secondary code.

CODING LATE EFFECTS

A late effect is the residual effect (condition produced) after the acute phase of an illness or injury has terminated. There is no time limit on when a late effect code can be used. The residual may be apparent early, such as in cerebrovascular accident cases, or it may occur months or years later, such as that due to a previous injury. Coding of late effects generally requires two codes sequenced in the following order: The condition or nature of the late effect is sequenced first. The late effect code is sequenced second.

An exception to the above guidelines are those instances where the code for late effect is followed by a manifestation code identified in the Tabular List and title, or the late effect code has been expanded (at the fourth and fifth-digit levels) to include the manifestation(s). The code for the acute phase of an illness or injury that led to the late effect is never used with a code for the late effect.

CODES IN CATEGORIES 740-759, CONGENITAL ANOMALIES

Assign an appropriate code(s) from categories 740-759, Congenital Anomalies, when an anomaly is documented. A congenital anomaly may be the principal or first listed diagnosis on a record or a secondary diagnosis.

When a congenital anomaly does not have a unique code assignment, assign additional code(s) for any manifestations that may be present.

| | Add 4th or 5th digit | | Nonspecific code | | Unspecified code | | Manifestation code |

When the code assignment specifically identifies the congenital anomaly, manifestations that are an inherent component of the anomaly should not be coded separately. Additional codes should be assigned for manifestations that are not an inherent component.

Codes from Chapter 14 may be used throughout the life of the patient. If a congenital anomaly has been corrected, a personal history code should be used to identify the history of the anomaly. Although present at birth, a congenital anomaly may not be identified until later in life. Whenever the condition is diagnosed by the physician, it is appropriate to assign a code from codes 740-759.

For the birth admission, the appropriate code from category V30, Liveborn infants, according to type of birth should be sequenced as the principal diagnosis, followed by any congenital anomaly codes, 740-759.

● Code new
to 2012 edition

▲ Revision of
existing code

④ ⑤ Fourth or fifth
digit required

14. CONGENITAL ANOMALIES (740-759)

ALERT! For personal history of congenital malformations see V13.6

740 Anencephalus and similar anomalies

DEFINITION Anencephalus and similar anomalies, refers to the congenital absence of most of the brain and spinal cord

740.0 Anencephalus

Acrania	Hemianencephaly
Amyelencephalus	Hemicephaly

740.1 Craniorachischisis

740.2 Iniencephaly

⑤ **741 Spina bifida**

Excludes: spina bifida occulta (756.17)

The following fifth-digit subclassification is for use with category 741:

0 unspecified region

1 cervical region

2 dorsal [thoracic] region

3 lumbar region

DEFINITION Spina bifida is a serious birth abnormality in which the spinal cord is malformed and lacks its usual protective skeletal and soft tissue coverings

⑤ **741.0 With hydrocephalus**

[0-3]   Arnold-Chiari syndrome, type II
Any condition classifiable to 741.9 with any condition classifiable to 742.3
Chiari malformation, type II

⑤ **741.9 Without mention of hydrocephalus**

[0-3]   Hydromeningocele (spinal)

Hydromyelocele	Myelocystocele
Meningocele (spinal)	Rachischisis
Meningomyelocele	Spina bifida (aperta)
Myelocele	Syringomyelocele

742 Other congenital anomalies of nervous system

Excludes: congenital central alveolar hypoventilation syndrome (327.25)

DEFINITION Congenital anomalies of nervous system refers to defects of the nervous system that are present at birth.

ALERT! For personal history of other congenital malformations see V13.69

742.0 Encephalocele

Encephalocystocele	Meningocele, cerebral
Encephalomyelocele	Meningoencephalocele
Hydroencephalocele	
Hydromeningocele, cranial	

742.1 Microcephalus

Hydromicrocephaly
Micrencephaly

742.2 Reduction deformities of brain

Absence of part of brain
Agenesis of part of brain
Agyria
Aplasia of part of brain
Arhinencephaly
Hypoplasia of part of brain
Holoprosencephaly
Microgyria

▮ Add 4th or 5th digit	▮ Nonspecific code	▯ Unspecified code	▮ Manifestation code

742.3 Congenital hydrocephalus
Aqueduct of Sylvius:
anomaly
obstruction, congenital
stenosis
Atresia of foramina of Magendie and Luschka
Hydrocephalus in newborn

Excludes: *hydrocephalus:*
acquired (331.3-331.4)
due to congenital toxoplasmosis (771.2)
with any condition classifiable to 741.9 (741.0)

742.4 Other specified anomalies of brain
Congenital cerebral cyst	Multiple anomalies of brain NOS
Macroencephaly	Porencephaly
Macrogyria	Ulegyria
Megalencephaly	

⑤ **742.5 Other specified anomalies of spinal cord**

742.51 Diastematomyelia

742.53 Hydromyelia
Hydrorhachis

742.59 Other
Amyelia
Atelomyelia
Congenital anomaly of spinal meninges
Defective development of cauda equina
Hypoplasia of spinal cord
Myelatelia
Myelodysplasia

742.8 Other specified anomalies of nervous system
Agenesis of nerve	Jaw-winking syndrome
Displacement of brachial	Marcus-Gunn syndrome
plexus	Riley-Day syndrome
Familial dysautonomia	

Excludes: *neurofibromatosis (237.70-237.79)*

742.9 Unspecified anomaly of brain, spinal cord, and nervous system
Anomaly of brain, nervous system, and spinal cord
Congenital:
disease of brain, nervous system, and spinal cord
lesion of brain, nervous system, and spinal cord
Deformity of brain, nervous system, and spinal cord

743 Congenital anomalies of eye
DEFINITION Congenital anomalies of eye, refers to defects of the eye and ocular adnexa that are present at birth.

⑤ **743.0 Anophthalmos**

743.00 Clinical anophthalmos, unspecified
Agenesis of eye
Congenital absence of eye
Anophthalmos NOS

743.03 Cystic eyeball, congenital

743.06 Cryptophthalmos

⑤ **743.1 Microphthalmos**
Dysplasia of eye
Hypoplasia of eye
Rudimentary eye

743.10 Microphthalmos, unspecified

743.11 Simple microphthalmos

743.12 Microphthalmos associated with other anomalies of eye and adnexa

⑤ **743.2 Buphthalmos**
Glaucoma:	Hydrophthalmos
congenital	
newborn	

Excludes: *glaucoma of childhood (365.14)*
traumatic glaucoma due to birth injury (767.8)

● Code new
to 2012 edition

▲ Revision of
existing code

④ ⑤ Fourth or fifth
digit required

743.20   Buphthalmos, unspecified

743.21   Simple buphthalmos

743.22   Buphthalmos associated with other ocular anomalies
Keratoglobus, congenital associated with buphthalmos
Megalocornea associated with buphthalmos

⑤ 743.3   Congenital cataract and lens anomalies

Excludes: *infantile cataract (366.00-366.09)*

743.30   Congenital cataract, unspecified

743.31   Capsular and subcapsular cataract

743.32   Cortical and zonular cataract

743.33   Nuclear cataract

743.34   Total and subtotal cataract, congenital

743.35   Congenital aphakia
Congenital absence of lens

743.36   Anomalies of lens shape
Microphakia
Spherophakia

743.37   Congenital ectopic lens

743.39   Other

⑤ 743.4   Coloboma and other anomalies of anterior segment

743.41   Anomalies of corneal size and shape
Microcornea

Excludes: *that associated with buphthalmos (743.22)*

743.42   Corneal opacities, interfering with vision, congenital

743.43   Other corneal opacities, congenital

743.44   Specified anomalies of anterior chamber, chamber angle, and related
structures
Anomaly:
Axenfeld's
Peters'
Rieger's

743.45   Aniridia

743.46   Other specified anomalies of iris and ciliary body
Anisocoria, congenital
Atresia of pupil
Coloboma of iris
Corectopia

743.47   Specified anomalies of sclera

743.48   Multiple and combined anomalies of anterior segment

743.49   Other

⑤ 743.5   Congenital anomalies of posterior segment

743.51   Vitreous anomalies
Congenital vitreous opacity

743.52   Fundus coloboma

743.53   Chorioretinal degeneration, congenital

743.54   Congenital folds and cysts of posterior segment

743.55   Congenital macular changes

743.56   Other retinal changes, congenital

743.57   Specified anomalies of optic disc
Coloboma of optic disc (congenital)

743.58   Vascular anomalies
Congenital retinal aneurysm

743.59   Other

⑤ 743.6   Congenital anomalies of eyelids, lacrimal system, and orbit

743.61   Congenital ptosis

	Add 4th or 5th digit		Nonspecific code		Unspecified code		Manifestation code

743.62 Congenital deformities of eyelids
Ablepharon   Congenital:
Absence of eyelid   ectropion
Accessory eyelid   entropion

743.63 Other specified congenital anomalies of eyelid
Absence, agenesis, of cilia

743.64 Specified congenital anomalies of lacrimal gland

743.65 Specified congenital anomalies of lacrimal passages
Absence, agenesis of:
lacrimal apparatus
punctum lacrimale
Accessory lacrimal canal

743.66 Specified congenital anomalies of orbit

743.69 Other
Accessory eye muscles

743.8 Other specified anomalies of eye

Excludes: *congenital nystagmus (379.51)*
ocular albinism (270.2)
optic nerve hypoplasia (377.43)
retinitis pigmentosa (362.74)

743.9 Unspecified anomaly of eye
Congenital:
anomaly NOS of eye [any part]
deformity NOS of eye [any part]

744 Congenital anomalies of ear, face, and neck

Excludes: *anomaly of:*
cervical spine (754.2, 756.10-756.19)
larynx (748.2-748.3)
nose (748.0-748.1)
parathyroid gland (759.2)
thyroid gland (759.2)
cleft lip (749.10-749.25)

DEFINITION Congenital anomalies of ear, face, and neck, refers to defects of the ear, face and/or neck that are present at birth.

⑤ **744.0 Anomalies of ear causing impairment of hearing**

Excludes: *congenital deafness without mention of cause (389.0-389.9)*

744.00 Unspecified anomaly of ear with impairment of hearing

744.01 Absence of external ear
Absence of:
auditory canal (external)
auricle (ear) (with stenosis or atresia of auditory canal)

744.02 Other anomalies of external ear with impairment of hearing
Atresia or stricture of auditory canal (external)

744.03 Anomaly of middle ear, except ossicles
Atresia or stricture of osseous meatus (ear)

744.04 Anomalies of ear ossicles
Fusion of ear ossicles

744.05 Anomalies of inner ear
Congenital anomaly of:
membranous labyrinth
organ of Corti

744.09 Other
Absence of ear, congenital

744.1 Accessory auricle
Accessory tragus   Supernumerary:
Polyotia   ear
Preauricular appendage   lobule

⑤ **744.2 Other specified anomalies of ear**

Excludes: *that with impairment of hearing (744.00-744.09)*

744.21 Absence of ear lobe, congenital

744.22 Macrotia

744.23 Microtia

● Code new
to 2012 edition
▲ Revision of
existing code
④ ⑤ Fourth or fifth
digit required

744.24 Specified anomalies of Eustachian tube
Absence of Eustachian tube

744.29 Other
Bat ear
Darwin's tubercle
Pointed ear
Prominence of auricle
Ridge ear

[Excludes:] *preauricular sinus (744.46)*

744.3 Unspecified anomaly of ear
Congenital:
anomaly NOS of ear, not elsewhere classified
deformity NOS of ear, not elsewhere classified

[5] **744.4 Branchial cleft cyst or fistula; preauricular sinus**

744.41 Branchial cleft sinus or fistula
Branchial:
sinus (external) (internal)
vestige

744.42 Branchial cleft cyst

744.43 Cervical auricle

744.46 Preauricular sinus or fistula

744.47 Preauricular cyst

744.49 Other
Fistula (of):
auricle, congenital
cervicoaural

744.5 Webbing of neck
Pterygium colli

[5] **744.8 Other specified anomalies of face and neck**

744.81 Macrocheilia
Hypertrophy of lip, congenital

744.82 Microcheilia

744.83 Macrostomia

744.84 Microstomia

744.89 Other

[Excludes:] *congenital fistula of lip (750.25)*
musculoskeletal anomalies (754.0-754.1, 756.0)

744.9 Unspecified anomalies of face and neck
Congenital:
anomaly NOS of face [any part] or neck [any part]
deformity NOS of face [any part] or neck [any part]

745 Bulbus cordis anomalies and anomalies of cardiac septal closure

DEFINITION Bulbus cordis anomalies and anomalies of cardiac septal closure, bulbus cordis is a transitory dilation in the embryonic heart where the arterial trunk joins the ventral roots of the aortic arches

745.0 Common truncus
Absent septum between aorta and pulmonary artery
Communication (abnormal) between aorta and pulmonary artery
Aortic septal defect
Common aortopulmonary trunk
Persistent truncus arteriosus

[5] **745.1 Transposition of great vessels**

745.10 Complete transposition of great vessels
Transposition of great vessels:
NOS
classical

745.11 Double outlet right ventricle
Dextratransposition of aorta
Incomplete transposition of great vessels
Origin of both great vessels from right ventricle
Taussig-Bing syndrome or defect

745.12 Corrected transposition of great vessels

745.19 Other

Add 4th or 5th digit — Nonspecific code — Unspecified code — Manifestation code

745.2 Tetralogy of Fallot
Fallot's pentalogy
Ventricular septal defect with pulmonary stenosis or atresia, dextraposition of aorta, and hypertrophy of right ventricle

[Excludes:] *Fallot's triad (746.09)*

745.3 Common ventricle
Cor triloculare biatriatum
Single ventricle

745.4 Ventricular septal defect
Eisenmenger's defect or complex
Gerbode defect
Interventricular septal defect
Left ventricular-right atrial communication
Roger's disease

[Excludes:] *common atrioventricular canal type (745.69)*
single ventricle (745.3)

745.5 Ostium secundum type atrial septal defect
Defect:
atrium secundum
fossa ovalis
Patent or persistent:
foramen ovale
ostium secundum
Lutembacher's syndrome

⑤ **745.6 Endocardial cushion defects**

745.60 Endocardial cushion defect, unspecified type

745.61 Ostium primum defect
Persistent ostium primum

745.69 Other
Absence of atrial septum
Atrioventricular canal type ventricular septal defect
Common atrioventricular canal
Common atrium

745.7 Cor biloculare
Absence of atrial and ventricular septa

745.8 Other

745.9 Unspecified defect of septal closure
Septal defect NOS

746 Other congenital anomalies of heart

[Excludes:] *endocardial fibroelastosis (425.3)*

[DEFINITION] Congenital anomalies of heart refers to other defects of the heart that are present at birth.

[ALERT!] For personal history of other congenital malformations see V13.69

⑤ **746.0 Anomalies of pulmonary valve**

[Excludes:] *infundibular or subvalvular pulmonic stenosis (746.83)*
tetralogy of Fallot (745.2)

746.00 Pulmonary valve anomaly, unspecified

746.01 Atresia, congenital
Congenital absence of pulmonary valve

746.02 Stenosis, congenital

746.09 Other
Congenital insufficiency of pulmonary valve
Fallot's triad or trilogy

746.1 Tricuspid atresia and stenosis, congenital
Absence of tricuspid valve

746.2 Ebstein's anomaly

746.3 Congenital stenosis of aortic valve
Congenital aortic stenosis

[Excludes:] *congenital:*
subaortic stenosis (746.81)
supravalvular aortic stenosis (747.22)

746.4 Congenital insufficiency of aortic valve
Bicuspid aortic valve
Congenital aortic insufficiency

● Code new to 2012 edition ▲ Revision of existing code ④ ⑤ Fourth or fifth digit required

746.5 Congenital mitral stenosis
Fused commissure of mitral valve
Parachute deformity of mitral valve
Supernumerary cusps of mitral valve

746.6 Congenital mitral insufficiency

746.7 Hypoplastic left heart syndrome
Atresia, or marked hypoplasia, of aortic orifice or valve, with hypoplasia of ascending aorta and defective development of left ventricle (with mitral valve atresia)

[5] **746.8 Other specified anomalies of heart**

746.81 Subaortic stenosis

746.82 Cor triatriatum

746.83 Infundibular pulmonic stenosis
Subvalvular pulmonic stenosis

746.84 Obstructive anomalies of heart, not elsewhere classified
Shone's syndrome
Uhl's disease

Use additional code for associated anomalies, such as:
coarctation of aorta (747.10)
congenital mitral stenosis (746.5)
subaortic stenosis (746.81)

746.85 Coronary artery anomaly
Anomalous origin or communication of coronary artery
Arteriovenous malformation of coronary artery
Coronary artery:
absence
arising from aorta or pulmonary trunk
single

746.86 Congenital heart block
Complete or incomplete atrioventricular [AV] block

746.87 Malposition of heart and cardiac apex
Abdominal heart
Dextrocardia
Ectopia cordis
Levocardia (isolated)
Mesocardia

[*Excludes:*] *dextrocardia with complete transposition of viscera (759.3)*

746.89 Other
Atresia of cardiac vein
Hypoplasia of cardiac vein
Congenital:
cardiomegaly
diverticulum, left ventricle
pericardial defect

746.9 Unspecified anomaly of heart
Congenital:
anomaly of heart NOS
heart disease NOS

747 Other congenital anomalies of circulatory system

[DEFINITION] Congenital anomalies of circulatory system refers to other defects of the circulatory system that are present at birth.

[ALERT!] For personal history of other congenital malformations see V13.69

747.0 Patent ductus arteriosus
Patent ductus Botalli
Persistent ductus arteriosus

[5] **747.1 Coarctation of aorta**

747.10 Coarctation of aorta (preductal) (postductal)
Hypoplasia of aortic arch

747.11 Interruption of aortic arch

[5] **747.2 Other anomalies of aorta**

747.20 Anomaly of aorta, unspecified

747.21 Anomalies of aortic arch
  Anomalous origin, right subclavian artery
  Dextraposition of aorta
  Double aortic arch
  Kommerell's diverticulum
  Overriding aorta
  Persistent:
    convolutions, aortic arch
    right aortic arch
  Vascular ring

Excludes: *hypoplasia of aortic arch (747.10)*

747.22 Atresia and stenosis of aorta
  Absence of aorta
  Aplasia of aorta
  Hypoplasia of aorta
  Stricture of aorta
  Supra (valvular)-aortic stenosis

Excludes: *congenital aortic (valvular) stenosis or stricture, so stated (746.3)*
         hypoplasia of aorta in hypoplastic left heart syndrome (746.7)

747.29 Other
  Aneurysm of sinus of Valsalva
  Congenital:
    aneurysm of aorta
    dilation of aorta

⑤ **747.3 Anomalies of pulmonary artery**

● **747.31 Pulmonary artery coarctation and atresia**
  Agenesis of pulmonary artery
  Atresia of pulmonary artery
  Coarctation of pulmonary artery
  Hypoplasia of pulmonary artery
  Stenosis of pulmonary artery

● **747.32 Pulmonary arteriovenous malformation**
  Pulmonary arteriovenous aneurysm

Excludes: *acquired pulmonary arteriovenous fistula (417.0)*

● **747.39 Other anomalies of pulmonary artery and pulmonary circulation**
  Anomaly of pulmonary artery

⑤ **747.4 Anomalies of great veins**

747.40 Anomaly of great veins, unspecified
  Anomaly NOS of:
    pulmonary veins
    vena cava

747.41 Total anomalous pulmonary venous connection
  Total anomalous pulmonary venous return [TAPVR]:
    subdiaphragmatic
    supradiaphragmatic

747.42 Partial anomalous pulmonary venous connection
  Partial anomalous pulmonary venous return

747.49 Other anomalies of great veins
  Absence of vena cava (inferior) (superior)
  Congenital stenosis of vena cava (inferior) (superior)
  Persistent:
    left posterior cardinal vein
    left superior vena cava
  Scimitar syndrome
  Transposition of pulmonary veins NOS

747.5 Absence or hypoplasia of umbilical artery
  Single umbilical artery

[5] **747.6 Other anomalies of peripheral vascular system**
Absence of artery or vein, not elsewhere classified
Anomaly of artery or vein, not elsewhere classified
Atresia of artery or vein, not elsewhere classified
Arteriovenous aneurysm (peripheral)
Arteriovenous malformation of the peripheral vascular system
Congenital:
  aneurysm (peripheral)
  phlebectasia
  stricture, artery
  varix
Multiple renal arteries

[Excludes:] *anomalies of:*
  cerebral vessels (747.81)
  pulmonary artery (747.39)
congenital retinal aneurysm (743.58)
hemangioma (228.00-228.09)
lymphangioma (228.1)

747.60 Anomaly of the peripheral vascular system, unspecified site

747.61 Gastrointestinal vessel anomaly

747.62 Renal vessel anomaly

747.63 Upper limb vessel anomaly

747.64 Lower limb vessel anomaly

747.69 Anomalies of other specified sites of peripheral vascular system

[5] **747.8 Other specified anomalies of circulatory system**

747.81 Anomalies of cerebrovascular system
Arteriovenous malformation of brain
Cerebral arteriovenous aneurysm, congenital
Congenital anomalies of cerebral vessels

[Excludes:] *ruptured cerebral (arteriovenous) aneurysm (430)*

747.82 Spinal vessel anomaly
Arteriovenous malformation of spinal vessel

747.83 Persistent fetal circulation
Persistent pulmonary hypertension
Primary pulmonary hypertension of newborn

747.89 Other
Aneurysm, congenital, specified site not elsewhere classified

[Excludes:] *congenital aneurysm:*
  coronary (746.85)
  peripheral (747.6)
  pulmonary (747.39)
    arteriovenous (747.32)
  retinal (743.58)

747.9 Unspecified anomaly of circulatory system

748 Congenital anomalies of respiratory system

[Excludes:] *congenital central alveolar hypoventilation syndrome (327.25)*
congenital defect of diaphragm (756.6)

DEFINITION Congenital anomalies of respiratory system refers to other defects of the respiratory system that are present at birth.

748.0 Choanal atresia
Atresia of nares (anterior) (posterior)
Congenital stenosis of nares (anterior) (posterior)

748.1 Other anomalies of nose
Absent nose
Accessory nose
Cleft nose
Deformity of wall of nasal sinus
Congenital:
  deformity of nose
  notching of tip of nose
  perforation of wall of nasal sinus

[Excludes:] *congenital deviation of nasal septum (754.0)*

748.2 Web of larynx
Web of larynx:
NOS
glottic
subglottic

748.3 Other anomalies of larynx, trachea, and bronchus
Absence or agenesis of:
bronchus
larynx
trachea
Anomaly (of):
cricoid cartilage
epiglottis
thyroid cartilage
tracheal cartilage
Atresia (of):
epiglottis
glottis
larynx
trachea
Cleft thyroid, cartilage, congenital
Congenital:
dilation, trachea
stenosis:
larynx
trachea
tracheocele
Diverticulum:
bronchus
trachea
Fissure of epiglottis
Laryngocele
Posterior cleft of cricoid cartilage (congenital)
Rudimentary tracheal bronchus
Stridor, laryngeal, congenital

748.4 Congenital cystic lung
Disease, lung:
cystic, congenital
polycystic, congenital
Honeycomb lung, congenital

[Excludes:] *acquired or unspecified cystic lung (518.89)*

748.5 Agenesis, hypoplasia, and dysplasia of lung
Absence of lung (fissures) (lobe)
Aplasia of lung
Hypoplasia of lung (lobe)
Sequestration of lung

[5] **748.6 Other anomalies of lung**

748.60 Anomaly of lung, unspecified

748.61 Congenital bronchiectasis

748.69 Other
Accessory lung (lobe)
Azygos lobe (fissure), lung

748.8 Other specified anomalies of respiratory system
Abnormal communication between pericardial and pleural sacs
Anomaly, pleural folds
Atresia of nasopharynx
Congenital cyst of mediastinum

748.9 Unspecified anomaly of respiratory system
Anomaly of respiratory system NOS

749 Cleft palate and cleft lip

[DEFINITION] Cleft palate is a congenital fissure in the roof of the mouth, resulting from incomplete fusion of the palate during embryonic development. Cleft lip is a congenital deformity characterized by a vertical cleft or pair of clefts in the upper lip, with or without involvement of the palate.

[5] **749.0 Cleft palate**

749.00 Cleft palate, unspecified

749.01 Unilateral, complete

749.02 Unilateral, incomplete
Cleft uvula

749.03 Bilateral, complete

749.04 Bilateral, incomplete

[5] **749.1 Cleft lip**
Cheiloschisis
Congenital fissure of lip
Harelip
Labium leporinum

749.10 Cleft lip, unspecified

749.11 Unilateral, complete

749.12 Unilateral, incomplete

749.13 Bilateral, complete

749.14 Bilateral, incomplete

⑤ **749.2 Cleft palate with cleft lip**
Cheilopalatoschisis

749.20 Cleft palate with cleft lip, unspecified

749.21 Unilateral, complete

749.22 Unilateral, incomplete

749.23 Bilateral, complete

749.24 Bilateral, incomplete

749.25 Other combinations

750 Other congenital anomalies of upper alimentary tract

[Excludes:] *dentofacial anomalies (524.0-524.9)*

[DEFINITION] Congenital anomalies of upper alimentary tract refers to other defects of the upper alimentary tract that are present at birth.

[ALERT!] For personal history of other congenital malformations see V13.69

750.0 Tongue tie
Ankyloglossia

⑤ **750.1 Other anomalies of tongue**

750.10 Anomaly of tongue, unspecified

750.11 Aglossia

750.12 Congenital adhesions of tongue

750.13 Fissure of tongue
Bifid tongue
Double tongue

750.15 Macroglossia
Congenital hypertrophy of tongue

750.16 Microglossia
Hypoplasia of tongue

750.19 Other

⑤ **750.2 Other specified anomalies of mouth and pharynx**

750.21 Absence of salivary gland

750.22 Accessory salivary gland

750.23 Atresia, salivary duct
Imperforate salivary duct

750.24 Congenital fistula of salivary gland

750.25 Congenital fistula of lip
Congenital (mucus) lip pits

750.26 Other specified anomalies of mouth
Absence of uvula

750.27 Diverticulum of pharynx
Pharyngeal pouch

750.29 Other specified anomalies of pharynx
Imperforate pharynx

750.3 Tracheoesophageal fistula, esophageal atresia and stenosis
Absent esophagus
Atresia of esophagus
Congenital:
  esophageal ring
  stenosis of esophagus
  stricture of esophagus
Congenital fistula:
  esophagobronchial
  esophagotracheal
Imperforate esophagus
Webbed esophagus

750.4 Other specified anomalies of esophagus
Dilatation, congenital (of) esophagus
Displacement, congenital (of) esophagus
Diverticulum (of) esophagus
Duplication (of) esophagus
Giant esophagus
Esophageal pouch

Excludes: *congenital hiatus hernia (750.6)*

750.5 Congenital hypertrophic pyloric stenosis
Congenital or infantile:
constriction of pylorus
hypertrophy of pylorus
spasm of pylorus
stenosis of pylorus
stricture of pylorus

750.6 Congenital hiatus hernia
Displacement of cardia through esophageal hiatus

Excludes: *congenital diaphragmatic hernia (756.6)*

750.7 Other specified anomalies of stomach
Congenital: Duplication of stomach
cardiospasm   Megalogastria
hourglass stomach   Microgastria
Displacement of stomach   Transposition of stomach
Diverticulum of stomach,
congenital

750.8 Other specified anomalies of upper alimentary tract

750.9 Unspecified anomaly of upper alimentary tract
Congenital:
anomaly NOS of upper alimentary tract [any part, except tongue]
deformity NOS of upper alimentary tract [any part, except tongue]

751 Other congenital anomalies of digestive system
DEFINITION Congenital anomalies of digestive system refers to other defects of the digestive system that are present at birth.
ALERT! For personal history of other congenital malformations see V13.69

751.0 Meckel's diverticulum
Meckel's diverticulum (displaced) (hypertrophic)
Persistent:
omphalomesenteric duct
vitelline duct

751.1 Atresia and stenosis of small intestine
Atresia of:
duodenum
ileum
intestine NOS
Congenital:
absence of small intestine or intestine NOS
obstruction of small intestine or intestine NOS
stenosis of small intestine or intestine NOS
stricture of small intestine or intestine NOS
Imperforate jejunum

751.2 Atresia and stenosis of large intestine, rectum, and anal canal
Absence: Congenital or infantile:
anus (congenital)   obstruction of large intestine
appendix, congenital   occlusion of anus
large intestine, congenital   stricture of anus
rectum   Imperforate:
Atresia of: anus
anus   rectum
colon   Stricture of rectum, congenital
rectum

751.3 Hirschsprung's disease and other congenital functional disorders of colon
Aganglionosis   Congenital megacolon
Congenital dilation of colon   Macrocolon

751.4 Anomalies of intestinal fixation

Congenital adhesions:
- omental, anomalous
- peritoneal

Jackson's membrane
Malrotation of colon
Rotation of cecum or colon:
- failure of
- incomplete
- insufficient

Universal mesentery

751.5 Other anomalies of intestine

Congenital diverticulum, colon
Dolichocolon
Duplication of:
- anus
- appendix
- cecum
- intestine

Ectopic anus
Megaloappendix
Megaloduodenum
Microcolon
Persistent cloaca
Transposition of:
- appendix
- colon
- intestine

[5] **751.6 Anomalies of gallbladder, bile ducts, and liver**

751.60 Unspecified anomaly of gallbladder, bile ducts, and liver

751.61 Biliary atresia

Congenital:
- absence of bile duct (common) or passage
- hypoplasia of bile duct (common) or passage
- obstruction of bile duct (common) or passage
- stricture of bile duct (common) or passage

751.62 Congenital cystic disease of liver

Congenital polycystic disease of liver
Fibrocystic disease of liver

751.69 Other anomalies of gallbladder, bile ducts, and liver

Absence of:
- gallbladder, congenital
- liver (lobe)

Accessory:
- hepatic ducts
- liver

Congenital:
- choledochal cyst
- hepatomegaly

Duplication of:
- biliary duct
- cystic duct
- gallbladder
- liver

Floating:
- gallbladder
- liver

Intrahepatic gallbladder

751.7 Anomalies of pancreas

Absence of pancreas
Accessory pancreas
Agenesis of pancreas
Annular pancreas
Ectopic pancreatic tissue
Hypoplasia of pancreas
Pancreatic heterotopia

[Excludes:] *diabetes mellitus (249.0-249.9, 250.0-250.9)*
fibrocystic disease of pancreas (277.00-277.09)
neonatal diabetes mellitus (775.1)

751.8 Other specified anomalies of digestive system

Absence (complete) (partial) of alimentary tract NOS
Duplication of digestive organs NOS
Malposition, congenital of digestive organs NOS

[Excludes:] *congenital diaphragmatic hernia (756.6)*
congenital hiatus hernia (750.6)

751.9 Unspecified anomaly of digestive system

Congenital:
- anomaly NOS of digestive system NOS
- deformity NOS of digestive system NOS

752 Congenital anomalies of genital organs

[Excludes:] *syndromes associated with anomalies in the number and form of chromosomes (758.0-758.9)*

[DEFINITION] Congenital anomalies of genital organs refers to defects of the genital organs that are present at birth.

752.0 Anomalies of ovaries
Absence, congenital (of) ovary
Accessory ovary
Ectopic ovary
Streak of ovary

[5] **752.1 Anomalies of fallopian tubes and broad ligaments**

752.10 Unspecified anomaly of fallopian tubes and broad ligaments

752.11 Embryonic cyst of fallopian tubes and broad ligaments
Cyst:
epoophoron
fimbrial
parovarian

752.19 Other
Absence of fallopian tube or broad ligament
Accessory fallopian tube or broad ligament
Atresia of fallopian tube or broad ligament

752.2 Doubling of uterus
Didelphic uterus
Doubling of uterus [any degree] (associated with doubling of cervix and vagina)

[5] **752.3 Other anomalies of uterus**

752.31 Agenesis of uterus
Congenital absence of uterus

752.32 Hypoplasia of uterus

752.33 Unicornuate uterus
Unicornate uterus with or without a separate uterine horn
Uterus with only one functioning horn

752.34 Bicornuate uterus
Bicornuate uterus, complete or partial

752.35 Septate uterus
Septate uterus, complete or partial

752.36 Arcuate uterus

752.39 Other anomalies of uterus
Aplasia of uterus NOS
Müllerian anomaly of the uterus, NEC

[Excludes:] *anomaly of uterus due to exposure to diethylstilbestrol [DES] in utero (760.76)*
didelphic uterus (752.2)
doubling of uterus (752.2)

[5] **752.4 Anomalies of cervix, vagina, and external female genitalia**

752.40 Unspecified anomaly of cervix, vagina, and external female genitalia

752.41 Embryonic cyst of cervix, vagina, and external female genitalia
Cyst of:
canal of Nuck, congenital
Gartner's duct
Cyst of:
vagina, embryonal
vulva, congenital

752.42 Imperforate hymen

752.43 Cervical agenesis
Cervical hypoplasia

752.44 Cervical duplication

752.45 Vaginal agenesis
Agenesis of vagina, total or partial

752.46 Transverse vaginal septum

752.47 Longitudinal vaginal septum
Longitudinal vaginal septum with or without obstruction

752.49 Other anomalies of cervix, vagina, and external female genitalia
Absence of clitoris or vulva
Agenesis of clitoris or vulva
Anomalies of cervix, NEC
Anomalies of hymen, NEC
Congenital stenosis or stricture of:
cervical canal
vagina
Müllerian anomalies of the cervix and vagina, NEC

[Excludes:] *double vagina associated with total duplication (752.2)*

⑤ **752.5 Undescribed and retractile testicle**

    752.51 Undescended testis
        Cryptorchism
        Ectopic testis

    752.52 Retractile testis

⑤ **752.6 Hypospadias and epispadias and other penile anomalies**
    ALERT! For personal history of hypospadias see V13.61

    752.61 Hypospadias

    752.62 Epispadias
        Anaspadias

    752.63 Congenital chordee

    752.64 Micropenis

    752.65 Hidden penis

    752.69 Other penile anomalies

752.7 Indeterminate sex and pseudohermaphroditism
    Gynandrism   Pseudohermaphroditism (male) (female)
    Hermaphroditism   Pure gonadal dysgenesis
    Ovotestis

    Excludes: *androgen insensitivity (259.50-259.52)*

        pseudohermaphroditism:
          female, with adrenocortical disorder (255.2)
          male, with gonadal disorder (257.8)
          with specified chromosomal anomaly (758.0-758.9)
        testicular feminization syndrome (259.50-259.72)

⑤ **752.8 Other specified anomalies of genital organs**

    Excludes: *congenital hydrocele (778.6)*

        penile anomalies (752.61-752.69)
        phimosis or paraphimosis (605)

    752.81 Scrotal transposition

    752.89 Other specified anomalies of genital organs
        Absence of:
          prostate
          spermatic cord
          vas deferens
        Anorchism
        Aplasia (congenital) of:
          prostate
          round ligament
          testicle
        Atresia of:
          ejaculatory duct
          vas deferens
        Fusion of testes
        Hypoplasia of testes
        Monorchism
        Polyorchism

752.9 Unspecified anomaly of genital organs
    Congenital:
        anomaly NOS of genital organ, NEC
        deformity NOS of genital organ, NEC

753 Congenital anomalies of urinary system
    DEFINITION Congenital anomalies of urinary system refers to defects of the urinary system that are present at birth

753.0 Renal agenesis and dysgenesis
    Atrophy of kidney: Congenital absence of kidney(s)
      congenital   Hypoplasia of kidney(s)
      infantile

⑤ **753.1 Cystic kidney disease**

    Excludes: *acquired cyst of kidney (593.2)*

    753.10 Cystic kidney disease, unspecified

    753.11 Congenital single renal cyst

    753.12 Polycystic kidney, unspecified type

	Add 4th or 5th digit		Nonspecific code		Unspecified code		Manifestation code

753.13 Polycystic kidney, autosomal dominant

753.14 Polycystic kidney, autosomal recessive

753.15 Renal dysplasia

753.16 Medullary cystic kidney
Nephronopthisis

753.17 Medullary sponge kidney

753.19 Other specified cystic kidney disease
Multicystic kidney

⑤ **753.2 Obstructive defects of renal pelvis and ureter**

753.20 Unspecified obstructive defect of renal pelvis and ureter

753.21 Congenital obstruction of ureteropelvic junction

753.22 Congenital obstruction of ureterovesical junction
Adynamic ureter
Congenital hydroureter

753.23 Congenital ureterocele

753.29 Other

753.3 Other specified anomalies of kidney
Accessory kidney
Congenital:
  calculus of kidney
  displaced kidney
Discoid kidney
Double kidney with double pelvis
Ectopic kidney
Fusion of kidneys
Giant kidney
Horseshoe kidney
Hyperplasia of kidney
Lobulation of kidney
Malrotation of kidney
Trifid kidney (pelvis)

753.4 Other specified anomalies of ureter
Absent ureter
Accessory ureter
Deviation of ureter
Displaced ureteric orifice
Double ureter
Ectopic ureter
Implantation, anomalous of ureter

753.5 Exstrophy of urinary bladder
Ectopia vesicae
Extroversion of bladder

753.6 Atresia and stenosis of urethra and bladder neck
Congenital obstruction:
  bladder neck
  urethra
Congenital stricture of:
  urethra (valvular)
  urinary meatus
  vesicourethral orifice
Imperforate urinary meatus
Impervious urethra
Urethral valve formation

753.7 Anomalies of urachus
Cyst (of) urachus
Fistula (of) urachus
Patent (of) urachus
Persistent umbilical sinus

753.8 Other specified anomalies of bladder and urethra
Absence, congenital of:
  bladder
  urethra
Accessory:
  bladder
  urethra
Congenital:
  diverticulum of bladder
  hernia of bladder
Congenital urethrorectal fistula
Congenital prolapse of:
  bladder (mucosa)
  urethra
Double:
  urethra
  urinary meatus

753.9 Unspecified anomaly of urinary system
Congenital:
  anomaly NOS of urinary system [any part, except urachus]
  deformity NOS of urinary system [any part, except urachus]

754 Certain congenital musculoskeletal deformities
Includes: nonteratogenic deformities which are considered to be due to intrauterine malposition and pressure

[DEFINITION] Certain congenital musculoskeletal deformities refers to defects of the musculoskeletal system that are present at birth.

● Code new to 2012 edition ▲ Revision of existing code ④ ⑤ Fourth or fifth digit required

754.0 Of skull, face, and jaw

Asymmetry of face
Compression facies
Depressions in skull
Deviation of nasal septum, congenital
Dolichocephaly
Plagiocephaly
Potter's facies
Squashed or bent nose, congenital

[Excludes:] *dentofacial anomalies (524.0-524.9)*
syphilitic saddle nose (090.5)

754.1 Of sternocleidomastoid muscle

Congenital sternomastoid torticollis
Congenital wryneck
Contracture of sternocleidomastoid (muscle)
Sternomastoid tumor

754.2 Of spine

Congenital postural:
- lordosis
- scoliosis

[5] **754.3 Congenital dislocation of hip**

754.30 Congenital dislocation of hip, unilateral
Congenital dislocation of hip NOS

754.31 Congenital dislocation of hip, bilateral

754.32 Congenital subluxation of hip, unilateral
Congenital flexion deformity, hip or thigh
Predislocation status of hip at birth
Preluxation of hip, congenital

754.33 Congenital subluxation of hip, bilateral

754.35 Congenital dislocation of one hip with subluxation of other hip

[5] **754.4 Congenital genu recurvatum and bowing of long bones of leg**

754.40 Genu recurvatum

754.41 Congenital dislocation of knee (with genu recurvatum)

754.42 Congenital bowing of femur

754.43 Congenital bowing of tibia and fibula

754.44 Congenital bowing of unspecified long bones of leg

[5] **754.5 Varus deformities of feet**

[Excludes:] *acquired (736.71, 736.75, 736.79)*

754.50 Talipes varus
Congenital varus deformity of foot, unspecified
Pes varus

754.51 Talipes equinovarus
Equinovarus (congenital)

754.52 Metatarsus primus varus

754.53 Metatarsus varus

754.59 Other
Talipes calcaneovarus

[5] **754.6 Valgus deformities of feet**

[Excludes:] *valgus deformity of foot (acquired) (736.79)*

754.60 Talipes valgus
Congenital valgus deformity of foot, unspecified

754.61 Congenital pes planus
Congenital rocker bottom flat foot
Flat foot, congenital

[Excludes:] *pes planus (acquired) (734)*

754.62 Talipes calcaneovalgus

754.69 Other
Talipes:
- equinovalgus
- planovalgus

[5] **754.7 Other deformities of feet**

[Excludes:] *acquired (736.70-736.79)*

754.70 Talipes, unspecified
Congenital deformity of foot NOS

754.71 Talipes cavus
Cavus foot (congenital)

754.79 Other
Asymmetric talipes
Talipes:
  calcaneus
  equinus

⑤ **754.8 Other specified nonteratogenic anomalies**

754.81 Pectus excavatum
Congenital funnel chest

754.82 Pectus carinatum
Congenital pigeon chest [breast]

754.89 Other
Club hand (congenital)
Congenital:
  deformity of chest wall
  dislocation of elbow
Generalized flexion contractures of lower limb joints, congenital
Spade-like hand (congenital)

755 Other congenital anomalies of limbs

Excludes: *those deformities classifiable to 754.0-754.8*

DEFINITION Congenital anomalies of limbs refers to other defects of the limbs that are present at birth

ALERT! For personal history of other congenital malformations see V13.69

⑤ **755.0 Polydactyly**

755.00 Polydactyly, unspecified digits
Supernumerary digits

755.01 Of fingers
Accessory fingers

755.02 Of toes
Accessory toes

⑤ **755.1 Syndactyly**
Symphalangy
Webbing of digits

755.10 Of multiple and unspecified sites

755.11 Of fingers without fusion of bone

755.12 Of fingers with fusion of bone

755.13 Of toes without fusion of bone

755.14 Of toes with fusion of bone

⑤ **755.2 Reduction deformities of upper limb**

DEFINITION A reduction deformity is a congenital deformity in which a body part, especially a limb, is shorter than normal or missing.

755.20 Unspecified reduction deformity of upper limb
Ectromelia NOS of upper limb
Hemimelia NOS of upper limb
Shortening of arm, congenital

755.21 Transverse deficiency of upper limb
Amelia of upper limb
Congenital absence of:
  fingers, all (complete or partial)
  forearm, including hand and fingers
  upper limb, complete
Congenital amputation of upper limb
Transverse hemimelia of upper limb

755.22 Longitudinal deficiency of upper limb, not elsewhere classified
Phocomelia NOS of upper limb
Rudimentary arm

● Code new
to 2012 edition

▲ Revision of
existing code

④ ⑤ Fourth or fifth
digit required

755.23 Longitudinal deficiency, combined, involving humerus, radius, and ulna (complete or incomplete)

Congenital absence of arm and forearm (complete or incomplete) with or without metacarpal deficiency and/or phalangeal deficiency, incomplete

Phocomelia, complete, of upper limb

755.24 Longitudinal deficiency, humeral, complete or partial (with or without distal deficiencies, incomplete)

Congenital absence of humerus (with or without absence of some [but not all] distal elements)

Proximal phocomelia of upper limb

755.25 Longitudinal deficiency, radioulnar, complete or partial (with or without distal deficiencies, incomplete)

Congenital absence of radius and ulna (with or without absence of some [but not all] distal elements)

Distal phocomelia of upper limb

755.26 Longitudinal deficiency, radial, complete or partial (with or without distal deficiencies, incomplete)

Agenesis of radius

Congenital absence of radius (with or without absence of some [but not all] distal elements)

755.27 Longitudinal deficiency, ulnar, complete or partial (with or without distal deficiencies, incomplete)

Agenesis of ulna

Congenital absence of ulna (with or without absence of some [but not all] distal elements)

755.28 Longitudinal deficiency, carpals or metacarpals, complete or partial (with or without incomplete phalangeal deficiency)

755.29 Longitudinal deficiency, phalanges, complete or partial

Absence of finger, congenital

Aphalangia of upper limb, terminal, complete or partial

Excludes: *terminal deficiency of all five digits (755.21)*

transverse deficiency of phalanges (755.21)

⑤ **755.3 Reduction deformities of lower limb**

DEFINITION A reduction deformity is a congenital deformity in which a body part, especially a limb, is shorter than normal or missing.

755.30 Unspecified reduction deformity of lower limb

Ectromelia NOS of lower limb

Hemimelia NOS of lower limb

Shortening of leg, congenital

755.31 Transverse deficiency of lower limb

Amelia of lower limb

Congenital absence of:

foot

leg, including foot and toes

lower limb, complete

toes, all, complete

Transverse hemimelia of lower limb

755.32 Longitudinal deficiency of lower limb, not elsewhere classified

Phocomelia NOS of lower limb

755.33 Longitudinal deficiency, combined, involving femur, tibia, and fibula (complete or incomplete)

Congenital absence of thigh and (lower) leg (complete or incomplete) with or without metacarpal deficiency and/or phalangeal deficiency, incomplete

Phocomelia, complete, of lower limb

755.34 Longitudinal deficiency, femoral, complete or partial (with or without distal deficiencies, incomplete)

Congenital absence of femur (with or without absence of some [but not all] distal elements)

Proximal phocomelia of lower limb

755.35 Longitudinal deficiency, tibiofibular, complete or partial (with or without distal deficiencies, incomplete)

Congenital absence of tibia and fibula (with or without absence of some [but not all] distal elements)

Distal phocomelia of lower limb

755.36 Longitudinal deficiency, tibia, complete or partial (with or without distal deficiencies, incomplete)
Agenesis of tibia
Congenital absence of tibia (with or without absence of some [but not all] distal elements)

755.37 Longitudinal deficiency, fibular, complete or partial (with or without distal deficiencies, incomplete)
Agenesis of fibula
Congenital absence of fibula (with or without absence of some [but not all] distal elements)

755.38 Longitudinal deficiency, tarsals or metatarsals, complete or partial (with or without incomplete phalangeal deficiency)

755.39 Longitudinal deficiency, phalanges, complete or partial
Absence of toe, congenital
Aphalangia of lower limb, terminal, complete or partial

[Excludes:] *terminal deficiency of all five digits (755.31)*
transverse deficiency of phalanges (755.31)

755.4 Reduction deformities, unspecified limb
Absence, congenital (complete or partial) of limb NOS
Amelia of unspecified limb
Ectromelia of unspecified limb
Hemimelia of unspecified limb
Phocomelia of unspecified limb

[5] **755.5 Other anomalies of upper limb, including shoulder girdle**

755.50 Unspecified anomaly of upper limb

755.51 Congenital deformity of clavicle

755.52 Congenital elevation of scapula
Sprengel's deformity

755.53 Radioulnar synostosis

755.54 Madelung's deformity

755.55 Acrocephalosyndactyly
Apert's syndrome

755.56 Accessory carpal bones

755.57 Macrodactylia (fingers)

755.58 Cleft hand, congenital
Lobster-claw hand

755.59 Other
Cleidocranial dysostosis
Cubitus:
valgus, congenital
varus, congenital

[Excludes:] *club hand (congenital) (754.89)*
congenital dislocation of elbow (754.89)

[5] **755.6 Other anomalies of lower limb, including pelvic girdle**

755.60 Unspecified anomaly of lower limb

755.61 Coxa valga, congenital

755.62 Coxa vara, congenital

755.63 Other congenital deformity of hip (joint)
Congenital anteversion of femur (neck)

[Excludes:] *congenital dislocation of hip (754.30-754.35)*

755.64 Congenital deformity of knee (joint)
Congenital:
absence of patella
genu valgum [knock-knee]
genu varum [bowleg]
Rudimentary patella

755.65 Macrodactylia of toes

755.66 Other anomalies of toes
Congenital:
hallux valgus
hallux varus
hammer toe

755.67 Anomalies of foot, not elsewhere classified
Astragaloscaphoid synostosis
Calcaneonavicular bar
Coalition of calcaneus
Talonavicular synostosis
Tarsal coalitions

755.69 Other
Congenital:
  angulation of tibia
  deformity (of):
    ankle (joint)
    sacroiliac (joint)
  fusion of sacroiliac joint

755.8 Other specified anomalies of unspecified limb

755.9 Unspecified anomaly of unspecified limb
Congenital:
  anomaly NOS of unspecified limb
  deformity NOS of unspecified limb

[Excludes:] *reduction deformity of unspecified limb (755.4)*

756 Other congenital musculoskeletal anomalies

[Excludes:] *congenital myotonic chondrodystrophy (359.23)*
those deformities classifiable to 754.0-754.8

DEFINITION Congenital musculoskeletal anomalies refers to other defects of the musculoskeletal system that are present at birth.

ALERT! For personal history of other congenital malformations see V13.69

756.0 Anomalies of skull and face bones
Absence of skull bones
Acrocephaly
Congenital deformity of forehead
Craniosynostosis
Crouzon's disease
Hypertelorism
Imperfect fusion of skull
Oxycephaly
Platybasia
Premature closure of cranial sutures
Tower skull
Trigonocephaly

[Excludes:] *acrocephalosyndactyly [Apert's syndrome] (755.55)*
dentofacial anomalies (524.0-524.9)
skull defects associated with brain anomalies, such as:
  anencephalus (740.0)
  encephalocele (742.0)
  hydrocephalus (742.3)
  microcephalus (742.1)

[5] **756.1 Anomalies of spine**

756.10 Anomaly of spine, unspecified

756.11 Spondylolysis, lumbosacral region
Prespondylolisthesis (lumbosacral)

756.12 Spondylolisthesis

756.13 Absence of vertebra, congenital

756.14 Hemivertebra

756.15 Fusion of spine [vertebra], congenital

756.16 Klippel-Feil syndrome

756.17 Spina bifida occulta

[Excludes:] *spina bifida (aperta) (741.0-741.9)*

756.19 Other
Platyspondylia
Supernumerary vertebra

756.2 Cervical rib
Supernumerary rib in the cervical region

756.3 **Other anomalies of ribs and sternum**
Congenital absence of:
rib
sternum
Congenital:
fissure of sternum
fusion of ribs
Sternum bifidum
Excludes: *nonteratogenic deformity of chest wall (754.81-754.89)*

756.4 **Chondrodystrophy**
Achondroplasia
Chondrodystrophia (fetalis)
Dyschondroplasia
Enchondromatosis
Ollier's disease
Excludes: *congenital myotonic chondrodystrophy (359.23)*
lipochondrodystrophy [Hurler's syndrome] (277.5)
Morquio's disease (277.5)

⑤ **756.5** **Osteodystrophies**

756.50 **Osteodystrophy, unspecified**

756.51 **Osteogenesis imperfecta**
Fragilitas ossium
Osteopsathyrosis

756.52 **Osteopetrosis**

756.53 **Osteopoikilosis**

756.54 **Polyostotic fibrous dysplasia of bone**

756.55 **Chondroectodermal dysplasia**
Ellis-van Creveld syndrome

756.56 **Multiple epiphyseal dysplasia**

756.59 **Other**
Albright (-McCune)-Sternberg syndrome

756.6 **Anomalies of diaphragm**
Absence of diaphragm
Congenital hernia:
diaphragmatic
foramen of Morgagni
Eventration of diaphragm
Excludes: *congenital hiatus hernia (750.6)*

⑤ **756.7** **Anomalies of abdominal wall**

756.70 **Anomaly of abdominal wall, unspecified**

756.71 **Prune belly syndrome**
Eagle-Barrett syndrome
Prolapse of bladder mucosa

756.72 **Omphalocele**
Exomphalos

756.73 **Gastroschisis**

756.79 **Other congenital anomalies of abdominal wall**
Excludes: *umbilical hernia (551-553 with .1)*

⑤ **756.8** **Other specified anomalies of muscle, tendon, fascia, and connective tissue**

756.81 **Absence of muscle and tendon**
Absence of muscle (pectoral)

756.82 **Accessory muscle**

756.83 **Ehlers-Danlos syndrome**

756.89 **Other**
Amyotrophia congenita
Congenital shortening of tendon

756.9 **Other and unspecified anomalies of musculoskeletal system**
Congenital:
anomaly NOS of musculoskeletal system, not elsewhere classified
deformity NOS of musculoskeletal system, not elsewhere classified

● Code new
to 2012 edition
▲ Revision of
existing code
④ ⑤ Fourth or fifth
digit required

757 Congenital anomalies of the integument

Includes: anomalies of skin, subcutaneous tissue, hair, nails, and breast

[Excludes:] *hemangioma (228.00-228.09)*
pigmented nevus (216.0-216.9)

DEFINITION Congenital anomalies of the integument refers to defects of the integumentary system that are present at birth.

757.0 Hereditary edema of legs
Congenital lymphedema
Hereditary trophedema
Milroy's disease

757.1 Ichthyosis congenita
Congenital ichthyosis
Harlequin fetus
Ichthyosiform erythroderma

757.2 Dermatoglyphic anomalies
Abnormal palmar creases

[5] **757.3 Other specified anomalies of skin**

757.31 Congenital ectodermal dysplasia

757.32 Vascular hamartomas
Birthmarks
Port-wine stain
Strawberry nevus

757.33 Congenital pigmentary anomalies of skin
Congenital poikiloderma
Urticaria pigmentosa
Xeroderma pigmentosum

[Excludes:] *albinism (270.2)*

757.39 Other
Accessory skin tags, congenital
Congenital scar
Epidermolysis bullosa
Keratoderma (congenital)

[Excludes:] *pilonidal cyst (685.0-685.1)*

757.4 Specified anomalies of hair
Congenital:
alopecia
atrichosis
beaded hair
Congenital:
hypertrichosis
monilethrix
Persistent lanugo

757.5 Specified anomalies of nails
Anonychia
Congenital:
clubnail
koilonychia
Congenital:
leukonychia
onychauxis
pachyonychia

757.6 Specified congenital anomalies of breast
Congenital absent breast or nipple
Accessory breast or nipple
Supernumerary breast or nipple

[Excludes:] *absence of pectoral muscle (756.81)*
hypoplasia of breast (611.82)
micromastia (611.82)

757.8 Other specified anomalies of the integument

757.9 Unspecified anomaly of the integument
Congenital:
anomaly NOS of integument
deformity NOS of integument

758 Chromosomal anomalies

Includes: syndromes associated with anomalies in the number and form of chromosomes

Use additional codes for conditions associated with the chromosomal anomalies

DEFINITION Chromosomal anomalies refer to changes in the normal structure or number of chromosomes; often resulting in physical or mental abnormalities

758.0 Down's syndrome
Mongolism
Translocation Down's syndrome
Trisomy:
21 or 22
G

Add 4th or 5th digit
Nonspecific code
Unspecified code
Manifestation code

758.1 Patau's syndrome
  Trisomy:
    13
    D_1

758.2 Edwards' syndrome
  Trisomy:
    18
    E_3

⑤ **758.3 Autosomal deletion syndromes**

  758.31 Cri-du-chat syndrome
    Deletion 5p

  758.32 Velo-cardio-facial syndrome
    Deletion 22q11.2

  758.33 Other microdeletions
    Miller-Dieker syndrome
    Smith-Magenis syndrome

  758.39 Other autosomal deletions

758.4 Balanced autosomal translocation in normal individual

758.5 Other conditions due to autosomal anomalies
  Accessory autosomes NEC

758.6 Gonadal dysgenesis
  Ovarian dysgenesis
  Turner's syndrome
  XO syndrome

  Excludes: pure gonadal dysgenesis (752.7)

758.7 Klinefelter's syndrome
  XXY syndrome

⑤ **758.8 Other conditions due to chromosome anomalies**

  758.81 Other conditions due to sex chromosome anomalies

  758.89 Other

758.9 Conditions due to anomaly of unspecified chromosome

759 Other and unspecified congenital anomalies

759.0 Anomalies of spleen
  Aberrant spleen   Congenital splenomegaly
  Absent spleen   Ectopic spleen
  Accessory spleen   Lobulation of spleen

759.1 Anomalies of adrenal gland
  Aberrant adrenal gland
  Absent adrenal gland
  Accessory adrenal gland

  Excludes: adrenogenital disorders (255.2)
            congenital disorders of steroid metabolism (255.2)

759.2 Anomalies of other endocrine glands
  Absent parathyroid gland
  Accessory thyroid gland
  Persistent thyroglossal or thyrolingual duct
  Thyroglossal (duct) cyst

  Excludes: congenital:
              goiter (246.1)
              hypothyroidism (243)

759.3 Situs inversus
  Situs inversus or transversus:
    abdominalis
    thoracis
  Transposition of viscera:
    abdominal
    thoracic

  Excludes: dextrocardia without mention of complete transposition (746.87)

759.4 Conjoined twins
  Craniopagus   Thoracopagus
  Dicephalus   Xiphopagus
  Pygopagus

● Code new   ▲ Revision of   ④ ⑤ Fourth or fifth
  to 2012 edition   existing code   digit required

759.5 Tuberous sclerosis
Bourneville's disease
Epiloia

759.6 Other hamartoses, not elsewhere classified
Syndrome:
Peutz-Jeghers
Sturge-Weber (-Dimitri)
von Hippel-Lindau

[Excludes:] *neurofibromatosis (237.70-237.79)*

759.7 Multiple congenital anomalies, so described
Congenital:
anomaly, multiple NOS
deformity, multiple NOS

[5] **759.8 Other specified anomalies**

759.81 Prader-Willi syndrome

759.82 Marfan syndrome

759.83 Fragile X syndrome

759.89 Other
Congenital malformation syndromes affecting multiple systems, not elsewhere classified
Laurence-Moon-Biedl syndrome

759.9 Congenital anomaly, unspecified

Add 4th or 5th digit | Nonspecific code | Unspecified code | Manifestation code

This page intentionally left blank.

● Code new
  to 2012 edition

▲ Revision of
  existing code

④ ⑤ Fourth or fifth
    digit required

Chapter 15: Newborn (Perinatal) Guidelines (760-779)

DEFINITIONS AND CODING ALERTS

This chapter includes definitions of selected key words, terms and phrases and coding alerts for adding points to the clinical domain, references to coding late effects where appropriate, and references to personal history V-codes in situations where the acute or chronic condition is no longer active. An example from this chapter is as follows:

771.81   Septicemia [sepsis] of newborn

ALERT This code should be assigned with a secondary code from category 041, Bacterial infections in conditions classified elsewhere and of unspecified site, to identify the organism. A code from 038, Septicemia should not be used on a newborn record. Do not assign code 995.91, Sepsis, as code 771.81 describes the sepsis.

ALERT If applicable, use additional codes to identify severe sepsis (995.92) and any associated acute organ dysfunction.

MULTIPLE CODING FOR A SINGLE CONDITION

In addition to the etiology or manifestation convention that requires two codes to fully describe a single condition that affects multiple body systems, there are other single conditions that also require more than one code. "Use additional code" notes are found in the tabular at codes that are not part of an etiology or manifestation pair where a secondary code is useful to fully describe a condition. The sequencing rule is the same as the etiology or manifestation pair - , "use additional code" indicates that a secondary code should be added.

"Code first" notes are also under certain codes that are not specifically manifestation codes but may be due to an underlying cause. When a "code first" note is present and an underlying condition is present the underlying condition should be sequenced first.

"Code, if applicable, any causal condition first", notes indicate that this code may be assigned as a principal diagnosis when the causal condition is unknown or not applicable. If a causal condition is known, then the code for that condition should be sequenced as the principal or first-listed diagnosis. Multiple codes may be needed for late effects, complication codes and obstetric codes to more fully describe a condition. See the specific guidelines for these conditions for further instruction.

COMBINATION CODE

A combination code is a single code used to classify: two diagnoses, or a diagnosis with an associated secondary process (manifestation) A diagnosis with an associated complication Combination codes are identified by referring to subterm entries in the Alphabetic Index and by reading the inclusion and exclusion notes in the Tabular List.

Assign only the combination code when that code fully identifies the diagnostic conditions involved or when the Alphabetic Index so directs. Multiple coding should not be used when the classification provides a combination code that clearly identifies all of the elements documented in the diagnosis. When the combination code lacks necessary specificity in describing the manifestation or complication, an additional code should be used as a secondary code.

CODING LATE EFFECTS

A late effect is the residual effect (condition produced) after the acute phase of an illness or injury has terminated. There is no time limit on when a late effect code can be used. The residual may be apparent early, such as in cerebrovascular accident cases, or it may occur months or years later, such as that due to a previous injury. Coding of late effects generally requires two codes sequenced in the following order: The condition or nature of the late effect is sequenced first. The late effect code is sequenced second.

An exception to the above guidelines are those instances where the code for late effect is followed by a manifestation code identified in the Tabular List and title, or the late effect code has been expanded (at the fourth and fifth-digit levels) to include the manifestation(s). The code for the acute phase of an illness or injury that led to the late effect is never used with a code for the late effect.

For coding and reporting purposes the perinatal period is defined as before birth through the 28th day following birth. The following guidelines are provided for reporting purposes. Hospitals may record other diagnoses as needed for internal data use.

| | Add 4th or 5th digit | | Nonspecific code | | Unspecified code | | Manifestation code |

GENERAL PERINATAL RULES

Chapter 15 Codes

They are never for use on the maternal record. Codes from Chapter 11, the obstetric chapter, are never permitted on the newborn record. Chapter 15 code may be used throughout the life of the patient if the condition is still present.

Sequencing of perinatal codes

Generally, codes from Chapter 15 should be sequenced as the principal or first-listed diagnosis on the newborn record, with the exception of the appropriate V30 code for the birth episode, followed by codes from any other chapter that provide additional detail. The "use additional code" note at the beginning of the chapter supports this guideline. If the index does not provide a specific code for a perinatal condition, assign code 779.89, Other specified conditions originating in the perinatal period, followed by the code from another chapter that specifies the condition. Codes for signs and symptoms may be assigned when a definitive diagnosis has not been established.

Birth process or community acquired conditions

If a newborn has a condition that may be either due to the birth process or community acquired and the documentation does not indicate which it is, the default is due to the birth process and the code from Chapter 15 should be used. If the condition is community-acquired, a code from Chapter 15 should not be assigned.

Code all clinically significant conditions

All clinically significant conditions noted on routine newborn examination should be coded. A condition is clinically significant if it requires:

- clinical evaluation; or
- therapeutic treatment; or
- diagnostic procedures; or
- extended length of hospital stay; or
- increased nursing care and/or monitoring; or
- has implications for future health care needs

Note: The perinatal guidelines listed above are the same as the general coding guidelines for "additional diagnoses", except for the final point regarding implications for future health care needs. Codes should be assigned for conditions that have been specified by the provider as having implications for future health care needs. Codes from the perinatal chapter should not be assigned unless the provider has established a definitive diagnosis.

USE OF CODES V30-V39

When coding the birth of an infant, assign a code from categories V30-V39, according to the type of birth. A code from this series is assigned as a principal diagnosis, and assigned only once to a newborn at the time of birth.

NEWBORN TRANSFERS

If the newborn is transferred to another institution, the V30 series is not used at the receiving hospital.

USE OF CATEGORY V29

Assigning a code from category V29

Assign a code from category V29, Observation and evaluation of newborns and infants for suspected conditions not found, to identify those instances when a healthy newborn is evaluated for a suspected condition that is determined after study not to be present. Do not use a code from category V29 when the patient has identified signs or symptoms of a suspected problem; in such cases, code the sign or symptom.

A code from category V29 may also be assigned as a principal code for readmissions or encounters when the V30 code no longer applies. Codes from category V29 are for use only for healthy newborns and infants for which no condition after study is found to be present.

A V29 code is to be used as a secondary code after the V30, Outcome of delivery, code.

● Code new
  to 2012 edition

▲ Revision of
  existing code

④ ⑤ Fourth or fifth
  digit required

USE OF OTHER V CODES ON PERINATAL RECORDS

V codes other than V30 and V29 may be assigned on a perinatal or newborn record code. The codes may be used as a principal or first listed diagnosis for specific types of encounters or for readmissions or encounters when the V30 code no longer applies.

See Official Guidelines, Section I.C.18 for information regarding the assignment of V codes.

MATERNAL CAUSES OF PERINATAL MORBIDITY

Codes from categories 760-763, Maternal causes of perinatal morbidity and mortality, are assigned only when the maternal condition has actually affected the fetus or newborn. The fact that the mother has an associated medical condition or experiences some complication of pregnancy, labor or delivery does not justify the routine assignment of codes from these categories to the newborn record.

CONGENITAL ANOMALIES IN NEWBORNS

For the birth admission, the appropriate code from category V30, Liveborn infants according to type of birth, should be used, followed by any congenital anomaly codes, categories 740-759. Use additional secondary codes from other chapters to specify conditions associated with the anomaly, if applicable.

Also, see Official Guidelines, Section I.C.14 for information on the coding of congenital anomalies.

CODING ADDITIONAL PERINATAL DIAGNOSES

Assigning codes for conditions that require treatment

Assign codes for conditions that require treatment or further investigation, prolong the length of stay, or require resource utilization.

Codes for conditions specified as having implications for future health care needs

Assign codes for conditions that have been specified by the provider as having implications for future health care needs. This guideline should not be used for adult patients.

Codes for newborn conditions originating in the perinatal period

Assign a code for newborn conditions originating in the perinatal period (categories 760-779, as well as complications arising during the current episode of care classified in other chapters, only if the diagnoses have been documented by the responsible provider at the time of transfer or discharge as having affected the fetus or newborn.

PREMATURITY AND FETAL GROWTH RETARDATION

Providers utilize different criteria in determining prematurity. A code for prematurity should not be assigned unless it is documented. The 5th digit assignment for codes from category 764 and subcategories 765.0 and 765.1 should be based on the recorded birth weight and estimated gestational age.

A code from subcategory 765.2, Weeks of gestation, should be assigned as an additional code with category 764 and codes from 765.0 and 765.1 to specify weeks of gestation as documented by the provider in the record.

NEWBORN SEPSIS

Code 771.81, Septicemia [sepsis] of newborn, should be assigned with a secondary code from category 041, Bacterial infections in conditions classified elsewhere and of unspecified site, to identify the organism.

A code from category 038, Septicemia, should not be used on a newborn record. Do not assign code 995.91, Sepsis, as code 771.81 describes the sepsis. If applicable, use additional codes to identify severe sepsis (995.92) and any associated acute organ dysfunction.

Add 4th or 5th digit   Nonspecific code   Unspecified code   Manifestation code

This page intentionally left blank.

● Code new
to 2012 edition

▲ Revision of
existing code

④ ⑤ Fourth or fifth
digit required

15. CERTAIN CONDITIONS ORIGINATING IN THE PERINATAL PERIOD (760-779)

Includes: conditions which have their origin in the perinatal period, before birth through the first 28 days after birth, even though death or morbidity occurs later

Use additional code(s) to further specify condition

MATERNAL CAUSES OF PERINATAL MORBIDITY AND MORTALITY (760-763)

ALERT! For personal history of perinatal problems see V13.7

760 **Fetus or newborn affected by maternal conditions which may be unrelated to present pregnancy**
Includes: the listed maternal conditions only when specified as a cause of mortality or morbidity of the fetus or newborn

Excludes: *maternal endocrine and metabolic disorders affecting fetus or newborn (775.0-775.9)*

760.0 Maternal hypertensive disorders
Fetus or newborn affected by maternal conditions classifiable to 642

760.1 Maternal renal and urinary tract diseases
Fetus or newborn affected by maternal conditions classifiable to 580-599

760.2 Maternal infections
Fetus or newborn affected by maternal infectious disease classifiable to 001-136 and 487, but fetus or newborn not manifesting that disease

Excludes: *congenital infectious diseases (771.0-771.8)*
maternal genital tract and other localized infections (760.8)

760.3 Other chronic maternal circulatory and respiratory diseases
Fetus or newborn affected by chronic maternal conditions classifiable to 390-459, 490-519, 745-748

760.4 Maternal nutritional disorders
Fetus or newborn affected by:
maternal disorders classifiable to 260-269
maternal malnutrition NOS

Excludes: *fetal malnutrition (764.10-764.29)*

760.5 Maternal injury
Fetus or newborn affected by maternal conditions classifiable to 800-995

⑤ **760.6 Surgical operation on mother and fetus**

Excludes: *cesarean section for present delivery (763.4)*
damage to placenta from amniocentesis, cesarean section, or surgical induction (762.1)

760.61 Newborn affected by amniocentesis

Excludes: *fetal complications from amniocentesis (679.1)*

760.62 Newborn affected by other in utero procedure

Excludes: *fetal complications of in utero procedure (679.1)*

760.63 Newborn affected by other surgical operations on mother during pregnancy

Excludes: *newborn affected by previous surgical procedure on mother not associated with pregnancy (760.64)*

760.64 Newborn affected by previous surgical procedure on mother not associated with pregnancy

⑤ **760.7 Noxious influences affecting fetus or newborn via placenta or breast milk**
Fetus or newborn affected by noxious substance transmitted via placenta or breast milk

Excludes: *anesthetic and analgesic drugs administered during labor and delivery (763.5)*
drug withdrawal syndrome in newborn (779.5)

760.70 Unspecified noxious substance
Fetus or newborn affected by:
Drug NEC

760.71 Alcohol
Fetal alcohol syndrome

760.72 Narcotics

760.73 Hallucinogenic agents

760.74 Anti-infectives
Antibiotics
Antifungals

760.75 Cocaine

| ▮ | Add 4th or 5th digit | ▮ | Nonspecific code | ▮ | Unspecified code | ▮ | Manifestation code |

760.76 **Diethylstilbestrol (DES)**

760.77 **Anticonvulsants**
Carbamazepine
Phenobarbital
Phenytoin
Valproic acid

760.78 **Antimetabolic agents**
Methotrexate
Retinoic acid
Statins

760.79 **Other**
Fetus or newborn affected by:
immune sera transmitted via placenta or breast milk
medicinal agents NEC transmitted via placenta or breast milk
toxic substance NEC transmitted via placenta or breast milk

760.8 **Other specified maternal conditions affecting fetus or newborn**
Maternal genital tract and other localized infection affecting fetus or newborn, but fetus or newborn not manifesting that disease

Excludes: *maternal urinary tract infection affecting fetus or newborn (760.1)*

760.9 **Unspecified maternal condition affecting fetus or newborn**

761 **Fetus or newborn affected by maternal complications of pregnancy**
Includes: the listed maternal conditions only when specified as a cause of mortality or morbidity of the fetus or newborn

761.0 **Incompetent cervix**

761.1 **Premature rupture of membranes**

761.2 **Oligohydramnios**

Excludes: *that due to premature rupture of membranes (761.1)*

761.3 **Polyhydramnios**
Hydramnios (acute) (chronic)

761.4 **Ectopic pregnancy**
Pregnancy:
abdominal
intraperitoneal
tubal

761.5 **Multiple pregnancy**
Triplet (pregnancy)
Twin (pregnancy)

761.6 **Maternal death**

761.7 **Malpresentation before labor**
Breech presentation before labor
External version before labor
Oblique lie before labor
Transverse lie before labor
Unstable lie before labor

761.8 **Other specified maternal complications of pregnancy affecting fetus or newborn**
Spontaneous abortion, fetus

761.9 **Unspecified maternal complication of pregnancy affecting fetus or newborn**

762 **Fetus or newborn affected by complications of placenta, cord, and membranes**
Includes: the listed maternal conditions only when specified as a cause of mortality or morbidity in the fetus or newborn

762.0 **Placenta previa**

762.1 **Other forms of placental separation and hemorrhage**
Abruptio placentae
Antepartum hemorrhage
Damage to placenta from amniocentesis, cesarean section, or surgical induction
Maternal blood loss
Premature separation of placenta
Rupture of marginal sinus

762.2 **Other and unspecified morphological and functional abnormalities of placenta**
Placental:
dysfunction
infarction
insufficiency

● Code new to 2012 edition ▲ Revision of existing code ④ ⑤ Fourth or fifth digit required

762.3 Placental transfusion syndromes
Placental and cord abnormality resulting in twin-to-twin or other transplacental transfusion

Use additional code to indicate resultant condition in newborn:
fetal blood loss (772.0)
polycythemia neonatorum (776.4)

762.4 Prolapsed cord
Cord presentation

762.5 Other compression of umbilical cord
Cord around neck
Entanglement of cord
Knot in cord
Torsion of cord

762.6 Other and unspecified conditions of umbilical cord
Short umbilical cord
Thrombosis of umbilical cord
Varices of umbilical cord
Velamentous insertion of umbilical cord
Vasa previa

[Excludes:] *infection of umbilical cord (771.4)*
single umbilical artery (747.5)

762.7 Chorioamnionitis
Amnionitis
Membranitis
Placentitis

762.8 Other specified abnormalities of chorion and amnion

762.9 Unspecified abnormality of chorion and amnion

763 Fetus or newborn affected by other complications of labor and delivery
Includes: the listed conditions only when specified as a cause of mortality or morbidity in the fetus or newborn

[Excludes:] *newborn affected by surgical procedures on mother (760.61-760.64)*

763.0 Breech delivery and extraction

763.1 Other malpresentation, malposition, and disproportion during labor and delivery
Fetus or newborn affected by:
abnormality of bony pelvis
contracted pelvis
persistent occipitoposterior position
shoulder presentation
transverse lie
conditions classifiable to 652, 653, and 660

763.2 Forceps delivery
Fetus or newborn affected by forceps extraction

763.3 Delivery by vacuum extractor

763.4 Cesarean delivery

[Excludes:] *placental separation or hemorrhage from cesarean section (762.1)*

763.5 Maternal anesthesia and analgesia
Reactions and intoxications from maternal opiates and tranquilizers during labor and delivery

[Excludes:] *drug withdrawal syndrome in newborn (779.5)*

763.6 Precipitate delivery
Rapid second stage

763.7 Abnormal uterine contractions
Fetus or newborn affected by:
contraction ring
hypertonic labor
hypotonic uterine dysfunction
uterine inertia or dysfunction
conditions classifiable to 661, except 661.3

[5] **763.8 Other specified complications of labor and delivery affecting fetus or newborn**

763.81 Abnormality in fetal heart rate or rhythm before the onset of labor

763.82 Abnormality in fetal heart rate or rhythm during labor

763.83 Abnormality in fetal heart rate or rhythm, unspecified as to time of onset

Add 4th or 5th digit | Nonspecific code | Unspecified code | Manifestation code

763.84 Meconium passage during delivery

<u>Excludes:</u> *meconium aspiration (770.11, 770.12)*
meconium staining (779.84)

763.89 Other specified complications of labor and delivery affecting fetus or newborn
Fetus or newborn affected by:
abnormality of maternal soft tissues
destructive operation on live fetus to facilitate delivery
induction of labor (medical)
other conditions classifiable to 650-669
other procedures used in labor and delivery

763.9 Unspecified complication of labor and delivery affecting fetus or newborn

OTHER CONDITIONS ORIGINATING IN THE PERINATAL PERIOD (764-779)

The following fifth-digit subclassification is for use with categories 764 and codes 765.0 and 765.1 to denote birthweight:

0 unspecified [weight]
1 less than 500 grams
2 500-749 grams
3 750-999 grams
4 1,000- 1,249 grams
5 1,250-1,499 grams
6 1,500-1,749 grams
7 1,750-1,999 grams
8 2,000-2,499 grams
9 2,500 grams and over

⑤ **764 Slow fetal growth and fetal malnutrition**

⑤ **764.0 "Light-for-dates" without mention of fetal malnutrition**
[0-9] Infants underweight for gestational age
"Small-for-dates"

⑤ **764.1 "Light-for-dates" with signs of fetal malnutrition**
[0-9] Infants "light-for-dates" classifiable to 764.0, who in addition show signs of fetal malnutrition, such as dry peeling skin and loss of subcutaneous tissue

⑤ **764.2 Fetal malnutrition without mention of "light-for-dates"**
[0-9] Infants, not underweight for gestational age, showing signs of fetal malnutrition, such as dry peeling skin and loss of subcutaneous tissue
Intrauterine malnutrition

⑤ **764.9 Fetal growth retardation, unspecified**
[0-9] Intrauterine growth retardation

765 Disorders relating to short gestation and low birthweight
Includes: the listed conditions, without further specification, as causes of mortality, morbidity, or additional care, in fetus or newborn

⑤ **765.0 Extreme immaturity**
[0-9]
Note: Usually implies a birthweight of less than 1000 grams
Use additional code for weeks of gestation (765.20-765.29)

⑤ **765.1 Other preterm infants**
[0-9] Prematurity NOS
Prematurity or small size, not classifiable to 765.0 or as "light-for-dates" in 764
Note: Usually implies a birthweight of 1000-2499 grams
Use additional code for weeks of gestation (765.20-765.29)

⑤ **765.2 Weeks of gestation**

765.20 Unspecified weeks of gestation
765.21 Less than 24 completed weeks of gestation
765.22 24 completed weeks of gestation
765.23 25-26 completed weeks of gestation
765.24 27-28 completed weeks of gestation
765.25 29-30 completed weeks of gestation
765.26 31-32 completed weeks of gestation

● Code new to 2012 edition   ▲ Revision of existing code   ④ ⑤ Fourth or fifth digit required

765.27 33-34 completed weeks of gestation

765.28 35-36 completed weeks of gestation

765.29 37 or more completed weeks of gestation

766 Disorders relating to long gestation and high birthweight

Includes: the listed conditions, without further specification, as causes of mortality, morbidity, or additional care, in fetus or newborn

766.0 Exceptionally large baby

Note: Usually implies a birthweight of 4500 grams or more.

766.1 Other "heavy-for-dates" infants

Other fetus or infant "heavy-" or "large-for-dates" regardless of period of gestation

[5] **766.2 Late infant, not "heavy-for-dates"**

766.21 Post-term infant

Infant with gestation period over 40 completed weeks to 42 completed weeks

766.22 Prolonged gestation of infant

Infant with gestation period over 42 completed weeks

Postmaturity NOS

767 Birth trauma

DEFINITION Birth trauma refers to: 1) a physical injury sustained by an infant during birth; or 2) the psychological shock said to be experienced by an infant during birth.

767.0 Subdural and cerebral hemorrhage

Subdural and cerebral hemorrhage, whether described as due to birth trauma or to intrapartum anoxia or hypoxia

Subdural hematoma (localized)

Tentorial tear

Use additional code, if desired, to identify cause

[Excludes:] *intraventricular hemorrhage (772.10-772.14)*

subarachnoid hemorrhage (772.2)

[5] **767.1 Injuries to scalp**

767.11 Epicranial subaponeurotic hemorrhage (massive)

Subgaleal hemorrhage

767.19 Other injuries to scalp

Caput succedaneum

Cephalhematoma

Chignon (from vacuum extraction)

767.2 Fracture of clavicle

767.3 Other injuries to skeleton

Fracture of:

- long bones
- skull

[Excludes:] *congenital dislocation of hip (754.30-754.35)*

fracture of spine, congenital (767.4)

767.4 Injury to spine and spinal cord

Dislocation of spine or spinal cord due to birth trauma

Fracture of spine or spinal cord due to birth trauma

Laceration of spine or spinal cord due to birth trauma

Rupture of spine or spinal cord due to birth trauma

767.5 Facial nerve injury

Facial palsy

767.6 Injury to brachial plexus

Palsy or paralysis:

- brachial
- Erb (-Duchenne)
- Klumpke (-Déjérine)

767.7 Other cranial and peripheral nerve injuries

Phrenic nerve paralysis

767.8 Other specified birth trauma

Eye damage

Hematoma of:

- liver (subcapsular)
- testes
- vulva

Rupture of:

- liver
- spleen

Scalpel wound

Traumatic glaucoma

[Excludes:] *hemorrhage classifiable to 772.0-772.9*

767.9 Birth trauma, unspecified
Birth injury NOS

768 Intrauterine hypoxia and birth asphyxia
Use only when associated with newborn morbidity classifiable elsewhere

[Excludes:] *acidemia NOS of newborn (775.81)*
acidosis NOS of newborn (775.81)
cerebral ischemia NOS (779.2)
hypoxia NOS of newborn (770.88)
mixed metabolic and respiratory acidosis of newborn (775.81)
respiratory arrest of newborn (770.87)

[DEFINITION] Intrauterine hypoxia (IH) occurs when the fetus is deprived of an adequate supply of oxygen.

768.0 Fetal death from asphyxia or anoxia before onset of labor or at unspecified time

768.1 Fetal death from asphyxia or anoxia during labor

768.2 Fetal distress before onset of labor, in liveborn infant
Fetal metabolic acidemia before onset of labor, in liveborn infant

768.3 Fetal distress first noted during labor and delivery, in liveborn infant
Fetal metabolic acidemia first noted during labor and delivery, in liveborn infant

768.4 Fetal distress, unspecified as to time of onset, in liveborn infant
Fetal metabolic acidemia unspecified as to time of onset, in liveborn infant

768.5 Severe birth asphyxia
Birth asphyxia with neurologic involvement

[Excludes:] *hypoxic-ischemic encephalopathy (HIE) (768.70-768.73)*

768.6 Mild or moderate birth asphyxia
Other specified birth asphyxia (without mention of neurologic involvement)

[Excludes:] *hypoxic-ischemic encephalopathy (HIE) (768.70-768.73)*

[5] **768.7 Hypoxic-ischemic encephalopathy (HIE)**

768.70 Hypoxic-ischemic encephalopathy, unspecified

768.71 Mild hypoxic-ischemic encephalopathy

768.72 Moderate hypoxic-ischemic encephalopathy

768.73 Severe hypoxic-ischemic encephalopathy

768.9 Unspecified birth asphyxia in liveborn infant
Anoxia NOS, in liveborn infant
Asphyxia NOS, in liveborn infant

769 Respiratory distress syndrome
Cardiorespiratory distress syndrome of newborn
Hyaline membrane disease (pulmonary)
Idiopathic respiratory distress syndrome [IRDS or RDS] of newborn
Pulmonary hypoperfusion syndrome

[Excludes:] *transient tachypnea of newborn (770.6)*

770 Other respiratory conditions of fetus and newborn

770.0 Congenital pneumonia
Infective pneumonia acquired prenatally

[Excludes:] *pneumonia from infection acquired after birth (480.0-486)*

[5] **770.1 Fetal and newborn aspiration**

[Excludes:] *aspiration of postnatal stomach contents (770.85, 770.86)*
meconium passage during delivery (763.84)
meconium staining (779.84)

770.10 Fetal and newborn aspiration, unspecified

770.11 Meconium aspiration without respiratory symptoms
Meconium aspiration NOS

770.12 Meconium aspiration with respiratory symptoms
Meconium aspiration pneumonia
Meconium aspiration pneumonitis
Meconium aspiration syndrome NOS

Use additional code to identify any secondary pulmonary hypertension (416.8), if applicable

770.13 Aspiration of clear amniotic fluid without respiratory symptoms
Aspiration of clear amniotic fluid NOS

770.14 Aspiration of clear amniotic fluid with respiratory symptoms
Aspiration of clear amniotic fluid with pneumonia
Aspiration of clear amniotic fluid with pneumonitis
Use additional code to identify any secondary pulmonary hypertension (416.8), if applicable

770.15 Aspiration of blood without respiratory symptoms
Aspiration of blood NOS

770.16 Aspiration of blood with respiratory symptoms
Aspiration of blood with pneumonia
Aspiration of blood with pneumonitis
Use additional code to identify any secondary pulmonary hypertension (416.8), if applicable

770.17 Other fetal and newborn aspiration without respiratory symptoms

770.18 Other fetal and newborn aspiration with respiratory symptoms
Other aspiration pneumonia
Other aspiration pneumonitis
Use additional code to identify any secondary pulmonary hypertension (416.8), if applicable

770.2 Interstitial emphysema and related conditions
Pneumomediastinum originating in the perinatal period
Pneumopericardium originating in the perinatal period
Pneumothorax originating in the perinatal period

770.3 Pulmonary hemorrhage
Hemorrhage:
alveolar (lung) originating in the perinatal period
intra-alveolar (lung) originating in the perinatal period
massive pulmonary originating in the perinatal period

770.4 Primary atelectasis
Pulmonary immaturity NOS

770.5 Other and unspecified atelectasis
Atelectasis:
NOS, originating in the perinatal period
partial, originating in the perinatal period
secondary, originating in the perinatal period
Pulmonary collapse, originating in the perinatal period

770.6 Transitory tachypnea of newborn
Idiopathic tachypnea of newborn
Wet lung syndrome
[*Excludes:*] *respiratory distress syndrome (769)*

770.7 Chronic respiratory disease arising in the perinatal period
Bronchopulmonary dysplasia
Interstitial pulmonary fibrosis of prematurity
Wilson-Mikity syndrome

[5] **770.8 Other respiratory problems after birth**
[*Excludes:*] *mixed metabolic and respiratory acidosis of newborn (775.81)*

770.81 Primary apnea of newborn
Apneic spells of newborn NOS
Essential apnea of newborn
Sleep apnea of newborn

770.82 Other apnea of newborn
Obstructure apnea of newborn

770.83 Cyanotic attacks of newborn

770.84 Respiratory failure of newborn
[*Excludes:*] *respiratory distress syndrome (769)*

770.85 Aspiration of postnatal stomach contents without respiratory symptoms
Aspiration of postnatal stomach contents NOS

770.86 Aspiration of postnatal stomach contents with respiratory symptoms
Aspiration of postnatal stomach contents with pneumonia
Aspiration of postnatal stomach contents with pneumonitis
Use additional code to identify any secondary pulmonary hypertension (416.8), if applicable

770.87 Respiratory arrest of newborn

770.88 Hypoxemia of newborn
Hypoxia NOS of newborn

770.89 Other respiratory problems after birth

770.9 Unspecified respiratory condition of fetus and newborn

771 Infections specific to the perinatal period
Includes: infections acquired before or during birth via the umbilicus or during the first 28 days after birth

Excludes: *congenital pneumonia (770.0)*
congenital syphilis (090.0-090.9)
infant botulism (040.41)
maternal infectious disease as a cause of mortality or morbidity in fetus or newborn, but fetus or newborn not manifesting the disease (760.2)
ophthalmia neonatorum due to gonococcus (098.40)
other infections not specifically classified to this category

771.0 Congenital rubella
Congenital rubella pneumonitis

771.1 Congenital cytomegalovirus infection
Congenital cytomegalic inclusion disease

771.2 Other congenital infections
Congenital:
  herpes simplex
  listeriosis
  malaria
Congenital:
  toxoplasmosis
  tuberculosis

771.3 Tetanus neonatorum
Tetanus omphalitis

Excludes: *hypocalcemic tetany (775.4)*

771.4 Omphalitis of the newborn
Infection:
  navel cord
  umbilical stump

Excludes: *tetanus omphalitis (771.3)*

771.5 Neonatal infective mastitis

Excludes: *noninfective neonatal mastitis (778.7)*

771.6 Neonatal conjunctivitis and dacryocystitis
Ophthalmia neonatorum NOS

Excludes: *ophthalmia neonatorum due to gonococcus (098.40)*

771.7 Neonatal Candida infection
Neonatal moniliasis
Thrush in newborn

⑤ **771.8** Other infections specific to the perinatal period
Use additional code to identify organism or specific infection

771.81 Septicemia [sepsis] of newborn
Use additional code(s) to identify severe sepsis (995.92) and any associated acute organ dysfunction, if applicable

ALERT This code should be assigned with a secondary code from category 041, Bacterial infections in conditions classified elsewhere and of unspecified site, to identify the organism. A code from 038, Septicemia should not be used on a newborn record. Do not assign code 995.91, Sepsis, as code 771.81 describes the sepsis.

ALERT If applicable, use additional codes to identify severe sepsis (995.92) and any associated acute organ dysfunction.

771.82 Urinary tract infection of newborn

771.83 Bacteremia of newborn

771.89 Other infections specific to the perinatal period
Intra-amniotic infection of fetus NOS
Infection of newborn NOS

772 Fetal and neonatal hemorrhage

Excludes: *fetal hematologic conditions complicating pregnancy (678.0)*
hematological disorders of fetus and newborn (776.0-776.9)

● Code new
  to 2012 edition
▲ Revision of
  existing code
④ ⑤ Fourth or fifth
  digit required

772.0 Fetal blood loss affecting newborn

Fetal blood loss from:
 cut end of co-twin's cord
 placenta
 ruptured cord
 vasa previa

Fetal exsanguination
Fetal hemorrhage into:
 co-twin
 mother's circulation

[5] **772.1 Intraventricular hemorrhage**

Intraventricular hemorrhage from any perinatal cause

772.10 Unspecified grade

772.11 Grade I
Bleeding into germinal matrix

772.12 Grade II
Bleeding into ventricle

772.13 Grade III
Bleeding with enlargement of ventricle

772.14 Grade IV
Bleeding into cerebral cortex

772.2 Subarachnoid hemorrhage

Subarachnoid hemorrhage from any perinatal cause

[*Excludes:*] *subdural and cerebral hemorrhage (767.0)*

772.3 Umbilical hemorrhage after birth

Slipped umbilical ligature

772.4 Gastrointestinal hemorrhage

[*Excludes:*] *swallowed maternal blood (777.3)*

772.5 Adrenal hemorrhage

772.6 Cutaneous hemorrhage

Bruising in fetus or newborn
Ecchymoses in fetus or newborn
Petechiae in fetus or newborn
Superficial hematoma in fetus or newborn

772.8 Other specified hemorrhage of fetus or newborn

[*Excludes:*] *hemorrhagic disease of newborn (776.0)*
pulmonary hemorrhage (770.3)

772.9 Unspecified hemorrhage of newborn

773 Hemolytic disease of fetus or newborn, due to isoimmunization

773.0 Hemolytic disease due to Rh isoimmunization

Anemia due to RH:
 antibodies
 isoimmunization
 maternal/fetal incompatibility
Erythroblastosis (fetalis) due to RH:
 antibodies
 isoimmunization
 maternal/fetal incompatibility
Hemolytic disease (fetus) (newborn) due to RH:
 antibodies
 isoimmunization
 maternal/fetal incompatibility
Jaundice due to RH:
 antibodies
 isoimmunization
 maternal/fetal incompatibility
Rh hemolytic disease
Rh isoimmunization

773.1 Hemolytic disease due to ABO isoimmunization
ABO hemolytic disease
ABO isoimmunization
Anemia due to ABO: antibodies, isoimmunization, or maternal/fetal incompatibility
Erythroblastosis (fetalis) due to ABO:
  antibodies
  isoimmunization
  maternal/fetal incompatibility
Hemolytic disease (fetus) (newborn) due to ABO:
  antibodies
  isoimmunization
  maternal/fetal incompatibility
Jaundice due to ABO:
  antibodies
  isoimmunization
  maternal/fetal incompatibility

773.2 Hemolytic disease due to other and unspecified isoimmunization
Erythroblastosis (fetalis) (neonatorum) NOS
Hemolytic disease (fetus) (newborn) NOS
Jaundice or anemia due to other and unspecified blood-group incompatibility

773.3 Hydrops fetalis due to isoimmunization
Use additional code, if desired, to identify type of isoimmunization (773.0-773.2)

773.4 Kernicterus due to isoimmunization
Use additional code, if desired, to identify type of isoimmunization (773.0-773.2)

773.5 Late anemia due to isoimmunization

774 **Other perinatal jaundice**
> **DEFINITION** Jaundice is a condition in which a person's skin and the whites of the eyes are discolored yellow due to an increased level of bile pigments in the blood.

774.0 *Perinatal jaundice from hereditary hemolytic anemias*
Code first underlying disease (282.0-282.9)

774.1 **Perinatal jaundice from other excessive hemolysis**
Fetal or neonatal jaundice from:
  bruising
  drugs or toxins transmitted from mother
  infection
  polycythemia
  swallowed maternal blood
Use additional code, if desired, to identify cause

> Excludes: *jaundice due to isoimmunization (773.0-773.2)*

774.2 Neonatal jaundice associated with preterm delivery
Hyperbilirubinemia of prematurity
Jaundice due to delayed conjugation associated with preterm delivery

⑤ **774.3 Neonatal jaundice due to delayed conjugation from other causes**

  774.30 **Neonatal jaundice due to delayed conjugation, cause unspecified**

  774.31 *Neonatal jaundice due to delayed conjugation in diseases classified elsewhere*
Code first underlying diseases, as:
  congenital hypothyroidism (243)
  Crigler-Najjar syndrome (277.4)
  Gilbert's syndrome (277.4)

  774.39 **Other**
    Jaundice due to delayed conjugation from causes, such as:
      breast milk inhibitors
      delayed development of conjugating system

774.4 Perinatal jaundice due to hepatocellular damage
Fetal or neonatal hepatitis
Giant cell hepatitis
Inspissated bile syndrome

774.5 *Perinatal jaundice from other causes*
Code first underlying cause, as:
  congenital obstruction of bile duct (751.61)
  galactosemia (271.1)
  mucoviscidosis (277.00-277.09)

● Code new
  to 2012 edition
▲ Revision of
  existing code
④ ⑤ Fourth or fifth
    digit required

774.6 **Unspecified fetal and neonatal jaundice**
Icterus neonatorum
Neonatal hyperbilirubinemia (transient)
Physiologic jaundice NOS in newborn

Excludes: *that in preterm infants (774.2)*

774.7 **Kernicterus not due to isoimmunization**
Bilirubin encephalopathy
Kernicterus of newborn NOS

Excludes: *kernicterus due to isoimmunization (773.4)*

775 **Endocrine and metabolic disturbances specific to the fetus and newborn**
Includes: transitory endocrine and metabolic disturbances caused by the infant's response to maternal endocrine and metabolic factors, its removal from them, or its adjustment to extrauterine existence

ALERT! For personal history of endocrine metabolic and immunity disorders see V12.2

775.0 **Syndrome of "infant of a diabetic mother"**
Maternal diabetes mellitus affecting fetus or newborn (with hypoglycemia)

775.1 **Neonatal diabetes mellitus**
Diabetes mellitus syndrome in newborn infant

775.2 **Neonatal myasthenia gravis**

775.3 **Neonatal thyrotoxicosis**
Neonatal hyperthyroidism (transient)

775.4 **Hypocalcemia and hypomagnesemia of newborn**
Cow's milk hypocalcemia
Hypocalcemic tetany, neonatal
Neonatal hypoparathyroidism
Phosphate-loading hypocalcemia

775.5 **Other transitory neonatal electrolyte disturbances**
Dehydration, neonatal

775.6 **Neonatal hypoglycemia**

Excludes: *infant of mother with diabetes mellitus (775.0)*

775.7 **Late metabolic acidosis of newborn**

⑤ **775.8** **Other neonatal endocrine and metabolic disturbances**

775.81 **Other acidosis of newborn**
Acidemia NOS of newborn
Acidosis of newborn NOS
Mixed metabolic and respiratory acidosis of newborn

775.89 **Other neonatal endocrine and metabolic disturbances**
Amino-acid metabolic disorders described as transitory

775.9 **Unspecified endocrine and metabolic disturbances specific to the fetus and newborn**

776 **Hematological disorders of newborn**
Includes: disorders specific to the newborn though possibly originating in utero

Excludes: *fetal hematologic conditions (678.0)*

776.0 **Hemorrhagic disease of newborn**
Hemorrhagic diathesis of newborn
Vitamin K deficiency of newborn

Excludes: *fetal or neonatal hemorrhage (772.0-772.9)*

776.1 **Transient neonatal thrombocytopenia**
Neonatal thrombocytopenia due to:
exchange transfusion
idiopathic maternal thrombocytopenia
isoimmunization

776.2 **Disseminated intravascular coagulation in newborn**

776.3 **Other transient neonatal disorders of coagulation**
Transient coagulation defect, newborn

776.4 **Polycythemia neonatorum**
Plethora of newborn
Polycythemia due to:
donor twin transfusion
maternal-fetal transfusion

Add 4th or
5th digit

Nonspecific
code

Unspecified
code

Manifestation
code

776.5 Congenital anemia
Anemia following fetal blood loss

Excludes: *anemia due to isoimmunization (773.0-773.2, 773.5)*
hereditary hemolytic anemias (282.0-282.9)

776.6 Anemia of prematurity

776.7 Transient neonatal neutropenia
Isoimmune neutropenia
Maternal transfer neutropenia

Excludes: *congenital neutropenia (nontransient) (288.01)*

776.8 Other specified transient hematological disorders

776.9 Unspecified hematological disorder specific to newborn

777 Perinatal disorders of digestive system
Includes: disorders specific to the fetus and newborn

Excludes: *intestinal obstruction classifiable to 560.0-560.9*

777.1 Meconium obstruction
Congenital fecaliths
Delayed passage of meconium
Meconium ileus NOS
Meconium plug syndrome

Excludes: *meconium ileus in cystic fibrosis (277.01)*

777.2 Intestinal obstruction due to inspissated milk

777.3 Hematemesis and melena due to swallowed maternal blood
Swallowed blood syndrome in newborn

Excludes: *that not due to swallowed maternal blood (772.4)*

777.4 Transitory ileus of newborn

Excludes: *Hirschsprung's disease (751.3)*

⑤ **777.5 Necrotizing enterocolitis in newborn**

777.50 Necrotizing enterocolitis in newborn, unspecified
Necrotizing enterocolitis in newborn, NOS

777.51 Stage I necrotizing enterocolitis in newborn
Necrotizing enterocolitis without pneumatosis, without perforation

777.52 Stage II necrotizing enterocolitis in newborn
Necrotizing enterocolitis with pneumatosis, without perforation

777.53 Stage III necrotizing enterocolitis in newborn
Necrotizing enterocolitis with perforation
Necrotizing enterocolitis with pneumatosis and perforation

777.6 Perinatal intestinal perforation
Meconium peritonitis

777.8 Other specified perinatal disorders of digestive system

777.9 Unspecified perinatal disorder of digestive system

778 Conditions involving the integument and temperature regulation of fetus and newborn

778.0 Hydrops fetalis not due to isoimmunization
Idiopathic hydrops

Excludes: *hydrops fetalis due to isoimmunization (773.3)*

778.1 Sclerema neonatorum
Subcutaneous fat necrosis

778.2 Cold injury syndrome of newborn

778.3 Other hypothermia of newborn

778.4 Other disturbances of temperature regulation of newborn
Dehydration fever in newborn
Environmentally-induced pyrexia
Hyperthermia in newborn
Transitory fever of newborn

778.5 Other and unspecified edema of newborn
Edema neonatorum

778.6 Congenital hydrocele
Congenital hydrocele of tunica vaginalis

● Code new
 to 2012 edition
▲ Revision of
 existing code
④ ⑤ Fourth or fifth
 digit required

778.7 Breast engorgement in newborn
Noninfective mastitis of newborn

[Excludes:] *infective mastitis of newborn (771.5)*

778.8 Other specified conditions involving the integument of fetus and newborn
Urticaria neonatorum

[Excludes:] *impetigo neonatorum (684)*
pemphigus neonatorum (684)

778.9 Unspecified condition involving the integument and temperature regulation of fetus and newborn

779 Other and ill-defined conditions originating in the perinatal period

779.0 Convulsions in newborn
Fits in newborn
Seizures in newborn

779.1 Other and unspecified cerebral irritability in newborn

779.2 Cerebral depression, coma, and other abnormal cerebral signs
Cerebral ischemia NOS of newborn
CNS dysfunction in newborn NOS

[Excludes:] *cerebral ischemia due to birth trauma (767.0)*
intrauterine cerebral ischemia (768.2-768.9)
intraventricular hemorrhage (772.10-772.14)

[5] **779.3 Disorder of stomach function and feeding problems in newborn**

779.31 Feeding problems in newborn
Slow feeding in newborn

[Excludes:] *feeding problem in child over 28 days old (783.3)*

779.32 Bilious vomiting in newborn

[Excludes:] *bilious vomiting in child over 28 days old (787.04)*

779.33 Other vomiting in newborn
Regurgitation of food in newborn

[Excludes:] *vomiting in child over 28 days old (536.2,787.01-787.03, 787.04)*

779.34 Failure to thrive in newborn

[Excludes:] *failure to thrive in child over 28 days old (783.41)*

779.4 Drug reactions and intoxications specific to newborn
Gray syndrome from chloramphenicol administration in newborn

[Excludes:] *fetal alcohol syndrome (760.71)*
reactions and intoxications from maternal opiates and tranquilizers (763.5)

779.5 Drug withdrawal syndrome in newborn
Drug withdrawal syndrome in infant of dependent mother

[Excludes:] *fetal alcohol syndrome (760.71)*

779.6 Termination of pregnancy (fetus)
Fetus death due to:
induced abortion
termination of pregnancy

[Excludes:] *spontaneous abortion (fetus) (761.8)*

779.7 Periventricular leukomalacia

[5] **779.8 Other specified conditions originating in the perinatal period**

779.81 Neonatal bradycardia

[Excludes:] *abnormality in fetal heart rate or rhythm complicating labor and delivery (763.81-763.83)*
bradycardia due to birth asphyxia (768.5-768.9)

779.82 Neonatal tachycardia

[Excludes:] *abnormality in fetal heart rate or rhythm complicating labor and delivery (763.81-763.83)*

779.83 Delayed separation of umbilical cord

779.84 Meconium staining

[Excludes:] *meconium aspiration (770.11, 770.12)*
meconium passage during delivery (763.84)

779.85 Cardiac arrest of newborn

779.89 Other specified conditions originating in the perinatal period
Use additional code to specify condition

779.9 Unspecified condition originating in the perinatal period
Congenital debility NOS
Stillbirth NEC

● Code new   ▲ Revision of   ④ ⑤ Fourth or fifth
      to 2012 edition   existing code   digit required

Chapter 16: Symptoms, Signs and Ill-Defined Conditions (780-799)

DEFINITIONS AND CODING ALERTS

This chapter includes definitions of selected key words, terms and phrases and coding alerts for adding points to the clinical domain, references to coding late effects where appropriate, and references to personal history V-codes in situations where the acute or chronic condition is no longer active. An example from this chapter is as follows:

780.5 Sleep disturbances
> **DEFINITION** A sleep disorder (somnipathy) is a medical disorder of the sleep patterns. Some sleep disorders are serious enough to interfere with normal physical, mental and emotional functioning..

MULTIPLE CODING FOR A SINGLE CONDITION

In addition to the etiology or manifestation convention that requires two codes to fully describe a single condition that affects multiple body systems, there are other single conditions that also require more than one code. "Use additional code" notes are found in the tabular at codes that are not part of an etiology or manifestation pair where a secondary code is useful to fully describe a condition. The sequencing rule is the same as the etiology or manifestation pair - , "use additional code" indicates that a secondary code should be added. For example, for infections that are not included in chapter 1, a secondary code from category 041, Bacterial infection in conditions classified elsewhere and of unspecified site, may be required to identify the bacterial organism causing the infection. A "use additional code" note will normally be found at the infectious disease code, indicating a need for the organism code to be added as a secondary code.

"Code first" notes are also under certain codes that are not specifically manifestation codes but may be due to an underlying cause. When a "code first" note is present and an underlying condition is present the underlying condition should be sequenced first.

"Code, if applicable, any causal condition first", notes indicate that this code may be assigned as a principal diagnosis when the causal condition is unknown or not applicable. If a causal condition is known, then the code for that condition should be sequenced as the principal or first-listed diagnosis. Multiple codes may be needed for late effects, complication codes and obstetric codes to more fully describe a condition. See the specific guidelines for these conditions for further instruction.

COMBINATION CODE

A combination code is a single code used to classify: two diagnoses, or a diagnosis with an associated secondary process (manifestation) A diagnosis with an associated complication Combination codes are identified by referring to subterm entries in the Alphabetic Index and by reading the inclusion and exclusion notes in the Tabular List.

Assign only the combination code when that code fully identifies the diagnostic conditions involved or when the Alphabetic Index so directs. Multiple coding should not be used when the classification provides a combination code that clearly identifies all of the elements documented in the diagnosis. When the combination code lacks necessary specificity in describing the manifestation or complication, an additional code should be used as a secondary code.

CODING LATE EFFECTS

A late effect is the residual effect (condition produced) after the acute phase of an illness or injury has terminated. There is no time limit on when a late effect code can be used. The residual may be apparent early, such as in cerebrovascular accident cases, or it may occur months or years later, such as that due to a previous injury. Coding of late effects generally requires two codes sequenced in the following order: The condition or nature of the late effect is sequenced first. The late effect code is sequenced second.

An exception to the above guidelines are those instances where the code for late effect is followed by a manifestation code identified in the Tabular List and title, or the late effect code has been expanded (at the fourth and fifth-digit levels) to include the manifestation(s). The code for the acute phase of an illness or injury that led to the late effect is never used with a code for the late effect.

| | Add 4th or 5th digit | | Nonspecific code | | Unspecified code | | Manifestation code |

This page intentionally left blank.

● Code new
   to 2012 edition

▲ Revision of
   existing code

④ ⑤ Fourth or fifth
      digit required

16. SYMPTOMS, SIGNS, AND ILL-DEFINED CONDITIONS (780-799)

This section includes symptoms, signs, abnormal results of laboratory or other investigative procedures, and ill-defined conditions regarding which no diagnosis classifiable elsewhere is recorded.

Signs and symptoms that point rather definitely to a given diagnosis are assigned to some category in the preceding part of the classification. In general, categories 780-796 include the more ill-defined conditions and symptoms that point with perhaps equal suspicion to two or more diseases or to two or more systems of the body, and without the necessary study of the case to make a final diagnosis. Practically all categories in this group could be designated as "not otherwise specified," or as "unknown etiology," or as "transient." The Alphabetic Index should be consulted to determine which symptoms and signs are to be allocated here and which to more specific sections of the classification; the residual subcategories numbered .9 are provided for other relevant symptoms which cannot be allocated elsewhere in the classification.

The conditions and signs or symptoms included in categories 780-796 consist of: (a) cases for which no more specific diagnosis can be made even after all facts bearing on the case have been investigated; (b) signs or symptoms existing at the time of initial encounter that proved to be transient and whose causes could not be determined; (c) provisional diagnoses in a patient who failed to return for further investigation or care; (d) cases referred elsewhere for investigation or treatment before the diagnosis was made; (e) cases in which a more precise diagnosis was not available for any other reason; (f) certain symptoms which represent important problems in medical care and which it might be desired to classify in addition to a known cause.

SYMPTOMS (780-789)

780 General symptoms

[5] **780.0 Alteration of consciousness**

[Excludes:] *alteration of consciousness due to:*
intracranial injuries (850.0-854.19)
skull fractures (800.00-801.99, 803.00-804.99)
coma:
diabetic (249.2-249.3, 250.2-250.3)
hepatic (572.2)
originating in the perinatal period (779.2)

780.01 Coma

780.02 Transient alteration of awareness

780.03 Persistent vegetative state

780.09 Other
Drowsiness
Semicoma
Unconsciousness
Somnolence
Stupor

780.1 Hallucinations
Hallucinations:
NOS
auditory
gustatory
olfactory
tactile

[Excludes:] *those associated with mental disorders, as functional psychoses (295.0-298.9)*
organic brain syndromes (290.0-294.9, 310.0-310.9)
visual hallucinations (368.16)

780.2 Syncope and collapse
Blackout
Fainting
(Near) (Pre) syncope
Vasovagal attack

[Excludes:] *carotid sinus syncope (337.0)*
heat syncope (992.1)
neurocirculatory asthenia (306.2)
orthostatic hypotension (458.0)
shock NOS (785.50)

[5] **780.3 Convulsions**

[Excludes:] *convulsions:*
epileptic (345.10-345.91)
in newborn (779.0)

780.31 Febrile convulsions (simple), unspecified
Febrile seizure NOS

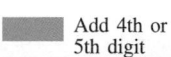

780.32 Complex febrile convulsions
Febrile seizure:
atypical
complex
complicated

[Excludes:] *status epilepticus (345.3)*

780.33 Post traumatic seizures

[Excludes:] *post traumatic epilepsy (345.00-345.91)*

780.39 Other convulsions
Convulsive disorder NOS
Fit NOS
Recurrent convulsions NOS
Seizure NOS

780.4 Dizziness and giddiness
Light-headedness
Vertigo NOS

[Excludes:] *Ménière's disease and other specified vertiginous syndromes (386.0-386.9)*

⑤ **780.5 Sleep disturbances**

[Excludes:] *circadian rhythm sleep disorders (327.30-327.39)*
organic hypersomnia (327.10-327.19)
organic insomnia (327.00-327.09)
organic sleep apnea (327.20-327.29)
organic sleep related movement disorders (327.51-327.59)
parasomnias (327.40-327.49)
that of nonorganic origin (307.40-307.49)

DEFINITION A sleep disorder (somnipathy) is a medical disorder of the sleep patterns. Some sleep disorders are serious enough to interfere with normal physical, mental and emotional functioning.

780.50 Sleep disturbance, unspecified

780.51 Insomnia with sleep apnea, unspecified

780.52 Insomnia, unspecified

780.53 Hypersomnia with sleep apnea, unspecified

780.54 Hypersomnia, unspecified

780.55 Disruption of 24 hour sleep wake cycle, unspecified

780.56 Dysfunctions associated with sleep stages or arousal from sleep

780.57 Unspecified sleep apnea

780.58 Sleep related movement disorder, unspecified

[Excludes:] *restless legs syndrome (333.94)*

780.59 Other

⑤ **780.6 Fever and other physiologic disturbances of temperature regulation**

[Excludes:] *effects of reduced environmental temperature (991.0-991.9)*
effects of heat and light (992.0-992.9)
fever, chills or hypothermia associated with confirmed infection - code to infection

780.60 Fever, unspecified
Chills with fever
Fever NOS
Fever of unknown origin (FUO)
Hyperpyrexia NOS
Pyrexia NOS
Pyrexia of unknown origin

[Excludes:] *chills without fever (780.64)*
neonatal fever (778.4)
pyrexia of unknown origin (during):
in newborn (778.4)
labor (659.2)
the puerperium (672)

780.61 Fever presenting with conditions classified elsewhere

Code first underlying condition when associated fever is present, such as with:
leukemia (conditions classifiable to 204-208)
neutropenia (288.00-288.09)
sickle-cell disease (282.60-282.69)

● Code new to 2012 edition ▲ Revision of existing code ④ ⑤ Fourth or fifth digit required

780.62 Postprocedural fever

[Excludes:] *posttransfusion fever (780.66)*
postvaccination fever (780.63)

780.63 Postvaccination fever
Postimmunization fever

780.64 Chills (without fever)
Chills NOS

[Excludes:] *chills with fever (780.60)*

780.65 Hypothermia not associated with low environmental temperature

[Excludes:] *hypothermia:*
associated with low environmental temperature (991.6)
due to anesthesia (995.89)
of newborn (778.2, 778.3)

780.66 Febrile nonhemolytic transfusion reaction
FNHTR
Posttransfusion fever

[5] **780.7 Malaise and fatigue**

[Excludes:] *debility, unspecified (799.3)*
fatigue (during):
combat (308.0-308.9)
heat (992.6)
pregnancy (646.8)
neurasthenia (300.5)
senile asthenia (797.5)

780.71 Chronic fatigue syndrome

780.72 Functional quadriplegia
Complete immobility due to severe physical disability or frailty

[Excludes:] *hysterical paralysis (300.11)*
immobility syndrome (728.3)
neurologic quadriplegia (344.00-344.09)
quadriplegia NOS (344.00)

780.79 Other malaise and fatigue
Asthenia NOS
Lethargy
Postviral (asthenic) syndrome
Tiredness

780.8 Generalized hyperhidrosis
Diaphoresis
Excessive sweating
Secondary hyperhidrosis

[Excludes:] *focal (localized) (primary) (secondary) hyperhidrosis (705.21-705.22)*
Frey's syndrome (705.22)

[5] **780.9 Other general symptoms**

[Excludes:] *hypothermia:*
NOS (accidental) (991.6)
due to anesthesia (995.89)
of newborn (778.2-778.3)
memory disturbance as part of a pattern of mental disorder

780.91 Fussy infant (baby)

780.92 Excessive crying of infant (baby)

[Excludes:] *excessive crying of child, adolescent or adult (780.95)*

780.93 Memory loss
Amnesia (retrograde)
Memory loss NOS

[Excludes:] *memory loss due to:*
intracranial injuries (850.0-854.19)
skull fractures (800.00-801.99, 803.00-804.99)
mild memory disturbance due to organic brain damage (310.89)
transient global amnesia (437.7)

780.94 Early satiety

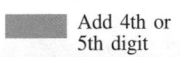

780.95   Excessive crying of child, adolescent, or adult

Excludes: *excessive crying of infant (baby) (780.92)*

780.96   Generalized pain
Pain NOS

780.97   Altered mental status
Change in mental status

Excludes: *altered level of consciousness (780.01-780.09)*

altered mental status due to known condition — code to condition
delirium NOS (780.09)

780.99   Other general symptoms

781   Symptoms involving nervous and musculoskeletal systems

Excludes: *depression NOS (311)*

disorders specifically relating to:
back (724.0-724.9)
hearing (388.0-389.9)
joint (718.0-719.9)
limb (729.0-729.9)
neck (723.0-723.9)
vision (368.0-369.9)
pain in limb (729.5)

781.0   Abnormal involuntary movements
Abnormal head movements
Fasciculation
Spasms NOS
Tremor NOS

Excludes: *abnormal reflex (796.1)*

chorea NOS (333.5)
infantile spasms (345.60-345.61)
spastic paralysis (342.1, 343.0-344.9)
specified movement disorders classifiable to 333 (333.0-333.9)
that of nonorganic origin (307.2-307.3)

781.1   Disturbances of sensation of smell and taste
Anosmia   Parosmia
Parageusia

781.2   Abnormality of gait
Gait: Gait:
  ataxic   spastic
  paralytic   staggering

Excludes: *ataxia:*

NOS (781.3)
locomotor (progressive) (094.0)
difficulty in walking (719.7)

781.3   Lack of coordination
Ataxia NOS
Muscular incoordination

Excludes: *ataxic gait (781.2)*

cerebellar ataxia (334.0-334.9)
difficulty in walking (719.7)
vertigo NOS (780.4)

781.4   Transient paralysis of limb
Monoplegia, transient NOS

Excludes: *paralysis (342.0-344.9)*

781.5   Clubbing of fingers

781.6   Meningismus
Dupré's syndrome
Meningism

● Code new
  to 2012 edition

▲ Revision of
  existing code

④ ⑤ Fourth or fifth
    digit required

781.7 Tetany
Carpopedal spasm

Excludes: *tetanus neonatorum (771.3)*
tetany:
hysterical (300.11)
newborn (hypocalcemic) (775.4)
parathyroid (252.1)
psychogenic (306.0)

781.8 Neurologic neglect syndrome

Asomatognosia	Left-sided neglect
Hemi-akinesia	Sensory extinction
Hemi-inattention	Sensory neglect
Hemispatial neglect	Visuospatial neglect

Excludes: *visuospatial deficit (799.53)*

⑤ **781.9 Other symptoms involving nervous and musculoskeletal systems**

    781.91 Loss of height

Excludes: *osteoporosis (733.00-733.09)*

    781.92 Abnormal posture

    781.93 Ocular torticollis

    781.94 Facial weakness
      Facial droop

Excludes: *facial weakness due to late effect of cerebrovascular accident (438.83)*

    781.99 Other symptoms involving nervous and musculoskeletal systems

782 Symptoms involving skin and other integumentary tissue

Excludes: *symptoms relating to breast (611.71-611.79)*

782.0 Disturbance of skin sensation

Anesthesia of skin	Hypoesthesia
Burning or prickling	Numbness
sensation	Paresthesia
Hyperesthesia	Tingling

782.1 Rash and other nonspecific skin eruption
Exanthem

Excludes: *vesicular eruption (709.8)*

782.2 Localized superficial swelling, mass, or lump
Subcutaneous nodules

Excludes: *localized adiposity (278.1)*

782.3 Edema

Anasarca	Localized edema NOS
Dropsy	

Excludes: *ascites (789.51-789.59)*
edema of:
newborn NOS (778.5)
pregnancy (642.0-642.9, 646.1)
fluid retention (276.69)
hydrops fetalis (773.3, 778.0)
hydrothorax (511.81-511.89)
nutritional edema (260, 262)

782.4 Jaundice, unspecified, not of newborn
Cholemia NOS
Icterus NOS

Excludes: *jaundice in newborn (774.0-774.7)*
due to isoimmunization (773.0-773.2, 773.4)

782.5 Cyanosis

Excludes: *newborn (770.83)*

⑤ **782.6 Pallor and flushing**

    782.61 Pallor

    782.62 Flushing
      Excessive blushing

	Add 4th or 5th digit		Nonspecific code		Unspecified code		Manifestation code

782.7 Spontaneous ecchymoses
Petechiae

Excludes: *ecchymosis in fetus or newborn (772.6)*
purpura (287.0-287.9)

782.8 Changes in skin texture
Induration of skin
Thickening of skin

782.9 Other symptoms involving skin and integumentary tissues

783 Symptoms concerning nutrition, metabolism, and development

783.0 Anorexia
Loss of appetite

Excludes: *anorexia nervosa (307.1)*
loss of appetite of nonorganic origin (307.59)

783.1 Abnormal weight gain

Excludes: *excessive weight gain in pregnancy (646.1)*
obesity (278.00)
morbid (278.01)

⑤ **783.2 Abnormal loss of weight and underweight**
Use additional code to identify Body Mass Index (BMI), if known (V85.0-V85.54)

783.21 Loss of weight

783.22 Underweight

783.3 Feeding difficulties and mismanagement
Feeding problem (elderly) (infant)

Excludes: *feeding disturbance or problems:*
in newborn (779.31-779.34)
of nonorganic origin (307.50-307.59)

⑤ **783.4 Lack of expected normal physiological development in childhood**

Excludes: *delay in sexual development and puberty (259.0)*
gonadal dysgenesis (758.6)
pituitary dwarfism (253.3)
slow fetal growth and fetal malnutrition (764.00-764.99)
specific delays in mental development (315.0-315.9)

783.40 Lack of normal physiological development, unspecified
Inadequate development
Lack of development

783.41 Failure to thrive
Failure to gain weight

Excludes: *failure to thrive in newborn (779.34)*

783.42 Delayed milestones
Late talker
Late walker

783.43 Short stature
Growth failure
Growth retardation
Lack of growth
Physical retardation

783.5 Polydipsia
Excessive thirst

783.6 Polyphagia
Excessive eating
Hyperalimentation NOS

Excludes: *disorders of eating of nonorganic origin (307.50-307.59)*

783.7 Adult failure to thrive

783.9 Other symptoms concerning nutrition, metabolism, and development
Hypometabolism

Excludes: *abnormal basal metabolic rate (794.7)*
dehydration (276.51)
other disorders of fluid, electrolyte, and acid-base balance (276.0-276.9)

● Code new
to 2012 edition   ▲ Revision of
existing code   ④ ⑤ Fourth or fifth
digit required

784 **Symptoms involving head and neck**

> *Excludes:* *encephalopathy NOS (348.30)*
>
> *specific symptoms involving neck classifiable to 723 (723.0-723.9)*

784.0 **Headache**
Facial pain
Pain in head NOS

> *Excludes:* *atypical face pain (350.2)*
>
> *migraine (346.0-346.9)*
>
> *tension headache (307.81)*

784.1 **Throat pain**

> *Excludes:* *dysphagia (787.20-787.29)*
>
> *neck pain (723.1)*
>
> *sore throat (462)*
>
> *chronic (472.1)*

784.2 **Swelling, mass, or lump in head and neck**
Space-occupying lesion, intracranial NOS

784.3 **Aphasia**

> *Excludes:* *aphasia due to late effects of cerebrovascular disease (438.11)*
>
> *developmental aphasia (315.31)*

⑤ **784.4** **Voice and resonance disorders**

784.40 **Voice and resonance disorder, unspecified**

784.41 **Aphonia**
Loss of voice

784.42 **Dysphonia**
Hoarseness

784.43 **Hypernasality**

784.44 **Hyponasality**

784.49 **Other voice and resonance disorders**
Change in voice

⑤ **784.5** **Other speech disturbance**

> *Excludes:* *speech disorder due to late effect of cerebrovascular accident (438.10 - 438.19)*
>
> *stuttering (315.35)*

784.51 **Dysarthria**

> *Excludes:* *dysarthria due to late effect of cerebrovascular accident (438.13)*

784.52 **Fluency disorder in conditions classified elsewhere**
Stuttering in conditions classified elsewhere

Code first underlying disease or condition, such as:
Parkinson's disease (332.0)

> *Excludes:* *adult onset fluency disorder (307.0)*
>
> *childhood onset fluency disorder (315.35)*
>
> *fluency disorder due to late effect of cerebrovascular accident (438.14)*

784.59 **Other speech disturbance**
Dysphasia
Slurred speech
Speech disturbance NOS

⑤ **784.6** **Other symbolic dysfunction**

> *Excludes:* *developmental learning delays (315.0-315.9)*

784.60 **Symbolic dysfunction, unspecified**

784.61 **Alexia and dyslexia**
Alexia (with agraphia)

784.69 **Other**
Acalculia   Agraphia NOS
Agnosia   Apraxia

784.7 **Epistaxis**
Hemorrhage from nose
Nosebleed

784.8 **Hemorrhage from throat**

> *Excludes:* *hemoptysis (786.30-786.39)*

[5] **784.9 Other symptoms involving head and neck**

784.91 Postnasal drip

784.92 Jaw pain
Mandibular pain
Maxilla pain

[Excludes:] *temporomandibular joint arthralgia (524.62)*

784.99 Other symptoms involving head and neck
Choking sensation
Feeling of foreign body in throat
Halitosis
Mouth breathing
Sneezing

[Excludes:] *foreign body in throat (933.0)*

785 Symptoms involving cardiovascular system

[Excludes:] *heart failure NOS (428.9)*

785.0 Tachycardia, unspecified
Rapid heart beat

[Excludes:] *neonatal tachycardia (779.82)*
paroxysmal tachycardia (427.0-427.2)

785.1 Palpitations
Awareness of heart beat

[Excludes:] *specified dysrhythmias (427.0-427.9)*

785.2 Undiagnosed cardiac murmurs
Heart murmur NOS

785.3 Other abnormal heart sounds
Cardiac dullness, increased or decreased
Friction fremitus, cardiac
Precordial friction

785.4 Gangrene
Gangrene NOS
Gangrene spreading cutaneous
Gangrenous cellulitis
Phagedena

Code first any associated underlying condition, as:
diabetes (250.7)
Raynaud's syndrome (443.0)

[Excludes:] *gangrene of certain sites—see Alphabetic Index*
gangrene with atherosclerosis of the extremities (440.24)
gas gangrene (040.0)

[5] **785.5 Shock without mention of trauma**

785.50 Shock, unspecified
Failure of peripheral circulation

785.51 Cardiogenic shock

785.52 Septic shock
endotoxic
gram-negative

Code first underlying infection

Use additional code, if applicable, to identify systemic inflammatory response syndrome due to infectious process with organ dysfunction (995.92)

785.59 Other
Shock:
hypovolemic

[Excludes:] *shock (due to):*
anesthetic (995.4)
anaphylactic (995.0)
due to serum (999.41-999.49)
electric (994.8)
following abortion (639.5)
lightning (994.0)
obstetrical (669.1)
postoperative (998.00-998.09)
traumatic (958.4)

785.6 Enlargement of lymph nodes
Lymphadenopathy
"Swollen glands"

[Excludes:] *lymphadenitis (chronic) (289.1-289.3)*
acute (683)

785.9 Other symptoms involving cardiovascular system
Bruit (arterial)
Weak pulse

786 Symptoms involving respiratory system and other chest symptoms

[5] **786.0 Dyspnea and respiratory abnormalities**

786.00 Respiratory abnormality, unspecified

786.01 Hyperventilation

[Excludes:] *hyperventilation, psychogenic (306.1)*

786.02 Orthopnea

786.03 Apnea

[Excludes:] *apnea of newborn (770.81, 770.82)*
sleep apnea (780.51, 780.53, 780.57)

786.04 Cheyne-Stokes respiration

786.05 Shortness of breath

786.06 Tachypnea

[Excludes:] *transitory tachypnea of newborn (770.6)*

786.07 Wheezing

[Excludes:] *asthma (493.00-493.92)*

786.09 Other
Respiratory:
distress
insufficiency

[Excludes:] *respiratory distress:*
following trauma and surgery (518.52)
newborn (770.89)
syndrome (newborn) (769)
adult (518.52)
respiratory failure (518.81, 518.83-518.84)
newborn (770.84)

786.1 Stridor

[Excludes:] *congenital laryngeal stridor (748.3)*

786.2 Cough

[Excludes:] *cough:*
psychogenic (306.1)
smokers' (491.0)
with hemorrhage (786.39)

[5] **786.3 Hemoptysis**

786.30 Hemoptysis, unspecified
Pulmonary hemorrhage NOS

Add 4th or 5th digit | Nonspecific code | Unspecified code | Manifestation code

786.31 Acute idiopathic pulmonary hemorrhage in infants [AIPHI]
Acute idiopathic pulmonary hemorrhage in infant over 28 days old

Excludes: *pulmonary hemorrhage of newborn under 28 days old (770.3)*
von Willebrand's disease (286.4)

786.39 Other hemoptysis
Cough with hemorrhage

786.4 Abnormal sputum
Abnormal:
amount (of) sputum
color (of) sputum
odor (of) sputum
Excessive sputum

⑤ **786.5 Chest pain**

786.50 Chest pain, unspecified

786.51 Precordial pain

786.52 Painful respiration
Pain:
anterior chest wall
pleuritic
Pleurodynia

Excludes: *epidemic pleurodynia (074.1)*

786.59 Other
Discomfort in chest
Pressure in chest
Tightness in chest

Excludes: *pain in breast (611.71)*

786.6 Swelling, mass, or lump in chest

Excludes: *lump in breast (611.72)*

786.7 Abnormal chest sounds
Abnormal percussion, chest   Rales
Friction sounds, chest   Tympany, chest

Excludes: *wheezing (786.07)*

786.8 Hiccough

Excludes: *psychogenic hiccough (306.1)*

786.9 Other symptoms involving respiratory system and chest
Breath-holding spell

787 Symptoms involving digestive system

Excludes: *constipation (564.00-564.09)*
pylorospasm (537.81)
congenital (750.5)

⑤ **787.0 Nausea and vomiting**
Emesis

Excludes: *hematemesis NOS (578.0)*
vomiting:
bilious, following gastrointestinal surgery (564.3)
cyclical (536.2)
associated with migraine (346.2)
psychogenic (306.4)
excessive, in pregnancy (643.0-643.9)
fecal matter (569.87)
habit (536.2)
of newborn (779.32, 779.33)
persistent (536.2)
psychogenic NOS (307.54)

787.01 Nausea with vomiting

787.02 Nausea alone

787.03 Vomiting alone

787.04 Bilious emesis
Bilious vomiting

Excludes: *bilious emesis (vomiting) in newborn (779.32)*

● Code new   ▲ Revision of   ④ ⑤ Fourth or fifth
to 2012 edition   existing code   digit required

787.1 Heartburn
Pyrosis
Waterbrash

[Excludes:] *dyspepsia or indigestion (536.8)*

[5] **787.2 Dysphagia**

Code first, if applicable, dysphagia due to late effect of cerebrovascular accident (438.82)

787.20 Dysphagia, unspecified
Difficulty in swallowing NOS

787.21 Dysphagia, oral phase

787.22 Dysphagia, oropharyngeal phase

787.23 Dysphagia, pharyngeal phase

787.24 Dysphagia, pharyngoesophageal phase

787.29 Other dysphagia
Cervical dysphagia
Neurogenic dysphagia

787.3 Flatulence, eructation, and gas pain
Abdominal distention (gaseous)
Bloating
Tympanites (abdominal) (intestinal)

[Excludes:] *aerophagy (306.4)*

787.4 Visible peristalsis
Hyperperistalsis

787.5 Abnormal bowel sounds
Absent bowel sounds
Hyperactive bowel sounds

[5] **787.6 Incontinence of feces**
Encopresis NOS
Incontinence of sphincter ani

[Excludes:] *that of nonorganic origin (307.7)*

787.60 Full incontinence of feces
Fecal incontinence NOS

787.61 Incomplete defecation

[Excludes:] *constipation (564.00-564.09)*
fecal impaction (560.32)

787.62 Fecal smearing
Fecal soiling

787.63 Fecal urgency

787.7 Abnormal feces
Bulky stools

[Excludes:] *abnormal stool content (792.1)*
melena:
NOS (578.1)
newborn (772.4, 777.3)

[5] **787.9 Other symptoms involving digestive system**

[Excludes:] *gastrointestinal hemorrhage (578.0-578.9)*
intestinal obstruction (560.0-560.9)
specific functional digestive disorders:
esophagus (530.0-530.9)
stomach and duodenum (536.0-536.9)
those not elsewhere classified (564.00-564.9)

787.91 Diarrhea
Diarrhea NOS

787.99 Other
Change in bowel habitsTenesmus (rectal)

788 Symptoms involving urinary system

[Excludes:] *hematuria (599.70-599.72)*
nonspecific findings on examination of the urine (791.0-791.9)
small kidney of unknown cause (589.0-589.9)
uremia NOS (586)
urinary obstruction (599.60, 599.69)

Add 4th or 5th digit | Nonspecific code | Unspecified code | Manifestation code

788.0 Renal colic
Colic (recurrent) of:
kidney
ureter

788.1 Dysuria
Painful urination
Strangury

5 **788.2 Retention of urine**
Code, if applicable, any causal condition first, such as:
hyperplasia of prostate (600.0-600.9 with fifth-digit 1)

788.20 Retention of urine, unspecified

788.21 Incomplete bladder emptying

788.29 Other specified retention of urine

5 **788.*3* Urinary incontinence**
[Excludes:] *functional urinary incontinence (788.91)*
that of nonorganic origin (307.6)
urinary incontinence associated with cognitive impairment (788.91)
Code, if applicable, any causal condition first, such as:
congenital ureterocele (753.23)
genital prolapse (618.00-618.9)
hyperplasia of prostate (600.0-600.9 with fifth-digit 1)

788.30 Urinary incontinence, unspecified
Enuresis NOS

788.31 Urge incontinence

788.32 Stress incontinence, male
[Excludes:] *stress incontinence (female) (625.6)*

788.33 Mixed incontinence (male) (female)
Urge and stress

788.34 Incontinence without sensory awareness

788.35 Post-void dribbling

788.36 Nocturnal enuresis

788.37 Continuous leakage

788.38 Overflow incontinence

788.39 Other urinary incontinence

5 **788.4 Frequency of urination and polyuria**
Code, if applicable, any causal condition first, such as:
hyperplasia of prostate (600.0-600.9 with fifth-digit 1)

788.41 Urinary frequency
Frequency of micturition

788.42 Polyuria

788.43 Nocturia

788.5 Oliguria and anuria
Deficient secretion of urine
Suppression of urinary secretion
[Excludes:] *that complicating:*
abortion (634-638 with .3, 639.3)
ectopic or molar pregnancy (639.3)
pregnancy, childbirth, or the puerperium (642.0-642.9, 646.2)

5 **788.6 Other abnormality of urination**
Code, if applicable, any causal condition first, such as:
hyperplasia of prostate (600.0-600.9 with fifth-digit 1)

788.61 Splitting of urinary stream
Intermittent urinary stream

788.62 Slowing of urinary stream
Weak stream

788.63 Urgency of urination
[Excludes:] *urge incontinence (788.31, 788.33)*

788.64 Urinary hesitancy

788.65 Straining on urination

788.69 **Other**

788.7 Urethral discharge
Penile discharge
Urethrorrhea

788.8 Extravasation of urine

[5] **788.9 Other symptoms involving urinary system**

788.91 Functional urinary incontinence
Urinary incontinence due to cognitive impairment, or severe physical disability or immobility

[Excludes:] *urinary incontinence due to physiologic condition (788.30-788.39)*

788.99 **Other symptoms involving urinary system**
Extrarenal uremia
Vesical:
pain
tenesmus

789 **Other symptoms involving abdomen and pelvis**

The following fifth-digit subclassification is to be used for codes 789.0, 789.3, 789.4, 789.6

0 **unspecified site**
1 **right upper quadrant**
2 **left upper quadrant**
3 **right lower quadrant**
4 **left lower quadrant**
5 **periumbilic**
6 **epigastric**
7 **generalized**
9 **other specified site**
multiple sites

[Excludes:] *symptoms referable to genital organs:*
female (625.0-625.9)
male (607.0-608.9)
psychogenic (302.70-302.79)

[5] **789.0 Abdominal pain**
[0-7,9] Cramps, abdominal

789.1 Hepatomegaly
Enlargement of liver

789.2 Splenomegaly
Enlargement of spleen

[5] **789.3 Abdominal or pelvic swelling, mass, or lump**
[0-7,9] Diffuse or generalized swelling or mass:
abdominal NOS
umbilical

[Excludes:] *abdominal distention (gaseous) (787.3)*
ascites (789.51-789.59)

[5] **789.4 Abdominal rigidity**
[0-7,9]

[5] **789.5 Ascites**
Fluid in peritoneal cavity

789.51 Malignant ascites
Code first malignancy, such as:
malignant neoplasm of ovary (183.0)
secondary malignant neoplasm of retroperitoneum and peritoneum (197.6)

789.59 **Other ascites**

[5] **789.6 Abdominal tenderness**
[0-7,9] Rebound tenderness

789.7 Colic
Colic NOS
Infantile colic

[Excludes:] *colic in adult and child over 12 months old (789.0)*
renal colic (788.0)

789.9 Other symptoms involving abdomen and pelvis
Umbilical:
bleeding
discharge

NONSPECIFIC ABNORMAL FINDINGS (790-796)

790 Nonspecific findings on examination of blood

[Excludes:] *abnormalities of:*
platelets (287.0-287.9)
thrombocytes (287.0-287.9)
white blood cells (288.00-288.9)

[5] **790.0 Abnormality of red blood cells**

[Excludes:] *anemia:*
congenital (776.5)
newborn, due to isoimmunization (773.0-773.2, 773.5)
of premature infant (776.6)
other specified types (280.0-285.9)
hemoglobin disorders (282.5-282.7)
polycythemia:
familial (289.6)
neonatorum (776.4)
secondary (289.0)
vera (238.4)

790.01 Precipitous drop in hematocrit
Drop in hematocrit
Drop in hemoglobin

790.09 Other abnormality of red blood cells
Abnormal red cell morphology NOS
Abnormal red cell volume NOS
Anisocytosis
Poikilocytosis

790.1 Elevated sedimentation rate

[5] **790.2 Abnormal glucose**

[Excludes:] *diabetes mellitus (249.00-249.91, 250.00-250.93)*
dysmetabolic syndrome X (277.7)
gestational diabetes (648.8)
glycosuria (791.5)
hypoglycemia (251.2)
that complicating pregnancy, childbirth, or the puerperium (648.8)

790.21 Impaired fasting glucose
Elevated fasting glucose

790.22 Impaired glucose tolerance test (oral)
Elevated glucose tolerance test

790.29 Other abnormal glucose
Abnormal glucose NOS
Abnormal non-fasting glucose
Hyperglycemia NOS
Pre-diabetes NOS

790.3 Excessive blood level of alcohol
Elevated blood-alcohol

790.4 Nonspecific elevation of levels of transaminase or lactic acid dehydrogenase [LDH]

790.5 Other nonspecific abnormal serum enzyme levels
Abnormal serum level of:
acid phosphatase
alkaline phosphatase
Abnormal serum level of:
amylase
lipase

[Excludes:] *deficiency of circulating enzymes (277.6)*

790.6 Other abnormal blood chemistry

Abnormal blood level of:
- cobalt
- copper
- iron
- lead

Abnormal blood level of:
- lithium
- magnesium
- mineral
- zinc

[Excludes:] *abnormality of electrolyte or acid-base balance (276.0-276.9)*
hypoglycemia NOS (251.2)
lead poisoning (984.0-984.9)
specific finding indicating abnormality of:
amino-acid transport and metabolism (270.0-270.9)
carbohydrate transport and metabolism (271.0-271.9)
lipid metabolism (272.0-272.9)
uremia NOS (586)

790.7 Bacteremia

[Excludes:] *bacteremia of newborn (771.83)*
septicemia (038)

Use additional code, if desired, to identify organism (041)

790.8 Viremia, unspecified

[5] **790.9 Other nonspecific findings on examination of blood**

790.91 Abnormal arterial blood gases

790.92 Abnormal coagulation profile

Abnormal or prolonged:
- bleeding time
- coagulation time
- partial thromboplastin time [PTT]
- prothrombin time [PT]

[Excludes:] *coagulation (hemorrhagic) disorders (286.0-286.9)*

790.93 Elevated prostate specific antigen (PSA)

790.94 Euthyroid sick syndrome

790.95 Elevated C-reactive protein (CRP)

790.99 Other

791 Nonspecific findings on examination of urine

[Excludes:] *hematuria NOS (599.70-599.72)*
specific findings indicating abnormality of:
amino-acid transport and metabolism (270.0-270.9)
carbohydrate transport and metabolism (271.0-271.9)

791.0 Proteinuria

Albuminuria
Bence-Jones proteinuria

[Excludes:] *postural proteinuria (593.6)*
that arising during pregnancy or the puerperium (642.0-642.9, 646.2)

791.1 Chyluria

[Excludes:] *filarial (125.0-125.9)*

791.2 Hemoglobinuria

791.3 Myoglobinuria

791.4 Biliuria

791.5 Glycosuria

[Excludes:] *renal glycosuria (271.4)*

791.6 Acetonuria

Ketonuria

791.7 Other cells and casts in urine

791.9 Other nonspecific findings on examination of urine
Crystalluria
Elevated urine levels of:
17-ketosteroids
catecholamines
indolacetic acid
vanillylmandelic acid [VMA]
Melanuria

792 Nonspecific abnormal findings in other body substances

[Excludes:] *that in chromosomal analysis (795.2)*

792.0 Cerebrospinal fluid

792.1 Stool contents
Abnormal stool color
Fat in stool
Mucus in stool
Occult blood
Pus in stool

[Excludes:] *blood in stool [melena] (578.1)*
newborn (772.4, 777.3)

792.2 Semen
Abnormal spermatozoa

[Excludes:] *azoospermia (606.0)*
oligospermia (606.1)

792.3 Amniotic fluid

792.4 Saliva

[Excludes:] *that in chromosomal analysis (795.2)*

792.5 Cloudy (hemodialysis) (peritoneal) dialysis effluent

792.9 Other nonspecific abnormal findings in body substances
Peritoneal fluid
Pleural fluid
Synovial fluid
Vaginal fluids

793 Nonspecific (abnormal) findings on radiological and other examinations of body structure

Includes: nonspecific abnormal findings of:
thermography
ultrasound examination [echogram]
x-ray examination

[Excludes:] *abnormal results of function studies and radioisotope scans (794.0-794.9)*

793.0 Skull and head

[Excludes:] *nonspecific abnormal echoencephalogram (794.01)*

[5] **793.1 Lung field**

● **793.11 Solitary pulmonary nodule**
Coin lesion lung
Solitary pulmonary nodule, subsegmental branch of the bronchial tree

● **793.19 Other nonspecific abnormal finding of lung field**
Pulmonary infiltrate NOS
Shadow, lung

793.2 Other intrathoracic organ
Abnormal:
echocardiogram
heart shadow
ultrasound cardiogram
Mediastinal shift

793.3 Biliary tract
Nonvisualization of gallbladder

793.4 Gastrointestinal tract

793.5 Genitourinary organs
Filling defect:
bladder
kidney
ureter

793.6 Abdominal area, including retroperitoneum

793.7 Musculoskeletal system

[5] **793.8 Breast**

793.80 Abnormal mammogram, unspecified

793.81 Mammographic microcalcification
Excludes: *mammographic calcification (793.89)*
mammographic calculus (793.89)

793.82 Inconclusive mammogram
Dense breasts NOS
Inconclusive mammogram NEC
Inconclusive mammography due to dense breasts
Inconclusive mammography NEC

793.89 Other (abnormal) findings on radiological examination of breast
Mammographic calcification
Mammographic calculus

⑤ **793.9 Other**
Excludes: *abnormal finding by radioisotope localization of placenta (794.9)*

793.91 Image test inconclusive due to excess body fat
Use additional code to identify Body Mass Index (BMI), if known (V85.0-V85.54)

793.99 Other nonspecific (abnormal) findings on radiological and other examinations of body structure
Abnormal:
placental finding by x-ray or ultrasound method
radiological findings in skin and subcutaneous tissue

794 Nonspecific abnormal results of function studies
Includes: radioisotope:
scans
uptake studies
scintiphotography

⑤ **794.0 Brain and central nervous system**

794.00 Abnormal function study, unspecified

794.01 Abnormal echoencephalogram

794.02 Abnormal electroencephalogram [EEG]

794.09 Other
Abnormal brain scan

⑤ **794.1 Peripheral nervous system and special senses**

794.10 Abnormal response to nerve stimulation, unspecified

794.11 Abnormal retinal function studies
Abnormal electroretinogram [ERG]

794.12 Abnormal electro-oculogram [EOG]

794.13 Abnormal visually evoked potential

794.14 Abnormal oculomotor studies

794.15 Abnormal auditory function studies

794.16 Abnormal vestibular function studies

794.17 Abnormal electromyogram [EMG]
Excludes: *that of eye (794.14)*

794.19 Other

794.2 Pulmonary
Abnormal lung scan
Reduced:
ventilatory capacity
vital capacity

⑤ **794.3 Cardiovascular**

794.30 Abnormal function study, unspecified

794.31 Abnormal electrocardiogram [ECG] [EKG]
Excludes: *long QT syndrome (426.82)*

794.39 Other
Abnormal:
ballistocardiogram
phonocardiogram
vectorcardiogram

794.4 Kidney
Abnormal renal function test

| | Add 4th or 5th digit | | Nonspecific code | | Unspecified code | | Manifestation code |

794.5 Thyroid
Abnormal thyroid:
scan
uptake

794.6 Other endocrine function study

794.7 Basal metabolism
Abnormal basal metabolic rate [BMR]

794.8 Liver
Abnormal liver scan

794.9 Other
Bladder
Pancreas
Placenta
Spleen

795 Other and nonspecific abnormal cytological, histological, immunological and DNA test findings

Excludes: *abnormal cytologic smear of anus and anal HPV (796.70-796.79)*
nonspecific abnormalities of red blood cells (790.01-790.09)

⑤ **795.0 Abnormal Papanicolaou smear of cervix and cervical HPV**
Abnormal thin preparation smear of cervix
Abnormal cervical cytology

Excludes: *abnormal cytologic smear of vagina and vaginal HPV (795.10-795.19)*
carcinoma in situ of cervix (233.1)
cervical intraepithelial neoplasia I [CIN I] (622.11)
cervical intraepithelial neoplasia II [CIN II] (622.12)
cervical intraepithelial neoplasia III [CIN III] (233.1)
dysplasia (histologically confirmed) of cervix (uteri) NOS (622.10)
mild cervical dysplasia (histologically confirmed) (622.11)
moderate cervical dysplasia (histologically confirmed) (622.12)
severe cervical dysplasia (histologically confirmed) (233.1)

795.00 Abnormal glandular Papanicolaou smear of cervix
Atypical cervical glandular cells NOS
Atypical endocervical cells NOS
Atypical endometrial cells NOS

795.01 Papanicolaou smear of cervix with atypical squamous cells of undetermined significance (ASC-US)

795.02 Papanicolaou smear of cervix with atypical squamous cells cannot exclude high grade squamous intraepithelial lesion (ASC-H)

795.03 Papanicolaou smear of cervix with low grade squamous intraepithelial lesion (LGSIL)

795.04 Papanicolaou smear of cervix with high grade squamous intraepithelial lesion (HGSIL)

795.05 Cervical high risk human papillomavirus (HPV) DNA test positive

795.06 Papanicolaou smear of cervix with cytologic evidence of malignancy

795.07 Satisfactory cervical smear but lacking transformation zone

795.08 Unsatisfactory cervical cytology smear
Inadequate cervical cytology sample

795.09 Other abnormal Papanicolaou smear of cervix and cervical HPV
Cervical low risk human papillomavirus (HPV) DNA test positive
Papanicolaou smear of cervix with low risk human papillomavirus (HPV) DNA test positive
Use additional code for associated human papillomavirus (HPV) (079.4)

Excludes: *encounter for Papanicolaou cervical smear to confirm findings of recent normal smear following initial abnormal smear (V72.32)*

● Code new
to 2012 edition
▲ Revision of
existing code
④ ⑤ Fourth or fifth
digit required

[5] **795.1 Abnormal Papanicolaou smear of vagina and vaginal HPV**
Abnormal thin preparation smear of vagina NOS
Abnormal vaginal cytology NOS

Use additional code to identify acquired absence of uterus and cervix, if applicable (V88.01-V88.03)

[Excludes:] *abnormal cytologic smear of cervix and cervical HPV (795.00-795.09)*
carcinoma in situ of vagina (233.31)
carcinoma in situ of vulva (233.32)
dysplasia (histologically confirmed) of vagina NOS (623.0, 233.31)
dysplasia (histologically confirmed) of vulva NOS (624.01, 624.02, 233.32)
mild vaginal dysplasia (histologically confirmed) (623.0)
mild vulvar dysplasia (histologically confirmed) (624.01)
moderate vaginal dysplasia (histologically confirmed) (623.0)
moderate vulvar dysplasia (histologically confirmed) (624.02)
severe vaginal dysplasia (histologically confirmed) (233.31)
severe vulvar dysplasia (histologically confirmed) (233.32)
vaginal intraepithelial neoplasia I (VAIN I) (623.0)
vaginal intraepithelial neoplasia II (VAIN II) (623.0)
vaginal intraepithelial neoplasia III (VAIN III) (233.31)
vulvar intraepithelial neoplasia I (VIN I) (624.01)
vulvar intraepithelial neoplasia II (VIN II) (624.02)
vulvar intraepithelial neoplasia III (VIN III) (233.32)

795.10 Abnormal glandular Papanicolaou smear of vagina
Atypical vaginal glandular cells NOS

795.11 Papanicolaou smear of vagina with atypical squamous cells of undetermined significance (ASC-US)

795.12 Papanicolaou smear of vagina with atypical squamous cells cannot exclude high grade squamous intraepithelial lesion (ASC-H)

795.13 Papanicolaou smear of vagina with low grade squamous intraepithelial lesion (LGSIL)

795.14 Papanicolaou smear of vagina with high grade squamous intraepithelial lesion (HGSIL)

795.15 Vaginal high risk human papillomavirus (HPV) DNA test positive

[Excludes:] *condyloma acuminatum (078.11)*
genital warts (078.11)

795.16 Papanicolaou smear of vagina with cytologic evidence of malignancy

795.18 Unsatisfactory vaginal cytology smear
Inadequate vaginal cytology sample

795.19 Other abnormal Papanicolaou smear of vagina and vaginal HPV
Vaginal low risk human papillomavirus (HPV) DNA test positive

Use additional code for associated human papillomavirus (079.4)

795.2 Nonspecific abnormal findings on chromosomal analysis
Abnormal karyotype

[5] **795.3 Nonspecific positive culture findings**
Positive culture findings in:
nose
sputum
throat
wound

[Excludes:] *that of:*
blood (790.7-790.8)
urine (791.9)

795.31 Nonspecific positive findings for anthrax
Positive findings by nasal swab

795.39 Other nonspecific positive culture findings

[Excludes:] *colonization status (V02.0-V02.9)*

795.4 Other nonspecific abnormal histological findings

▲ **795.5 Nonspecific reaction to test for tuberculosis**

● **795.51 Nonspecific reaction to tuberculin skin test without active tuberculosis**
Abnormal result of Mantoux test
PPD positive
Tuberculin (skin test) positive
Tuberculin (skin test) reactor

[Excludes:] *nonspecific reaction to cell mediated immunity measurement of gamma interferon antigen response without active tuberculosis (795.52)*

● **795.52 Nonspecific reaction to cell mediated immunity measurement of gamma interferon antigen response without active tuberculosis**
Nonspecific reaction to QuantiFERON-TB test (QFT) without active tuberculosis

[Excludes:] *nonspecific reaction to tuberculin skin test without active tuberculosis (795.51)*
positive tuberculin skin test (795.51)

795.6 False positive serological test for syphilis
False positive Wassermann reaction

⑤ **795.7 Other nonspecific immunological findings**

[Excludes:] *abnormal tumor markers (795.81-795.89)*
elevated prostate specific antigen [PSA] (790.93)
elevated tumor associated antigens (795.81-795.89)
isoimmunization, in pregnancy (656.1-656.2)
affecting fetus or newborn (773.0-773.2)

795.71 Nonspecific serologic evidence of human immunodeficiency virus [HIV]
Inconclusive human immunodeficiency virus [HIV] test (adult) (infant)

Note: This code is ONLY to be used when a test finding is reported as nonspecific. Asymptomatic positive findings are coded to V08. If any HIV infection symptom or condition is present, see code 042. Negative findings are not coded.

[Excludes:] *acquired immunodeficiency syndrome [AIDS] (042)*
asymptomatic human immunodeficiency virus, [HIV] infection status (V08)
HIV infection, symptomatic (042)
human immunodeficiency virus [HIV] disease (042)
positive (status) NOS (V08)

795.79 Other and unspecified nonspecific immunological findings
Raised antibody titer
Raised level of immunoglobulins

⑤ **795.8 Abnormal tumor markers**
Elevated tumor associated antigens [TAA]
Elevated tumor specific antigens [TSA]

[Excludes:] *elevated prostate specific antigen [PSA] (790.93)*

795.81 Elevated carcinoembryonic antigen (CEA)

795.82 Elevated cancer antigen 125 (CA 125)

795.89 Other abnormal tumor markers

796 Other nonspecific abnormal findings

796.0 Nonspecific abnormal toxicological findings
Abnormal levels of heavy metals or drugs in blood, urine, or other tissue

Use additional code for retained foreign body, if applicable, (V90.01-V90.9)

[Excludes:] *excessive blood level of alcohol (790.3)*

796.1 Abnormal reflex

796.2 Elevated blood pressure reading without diagnosis of hypertension

Note: This category is to be used to record an episode of elevated blood pressure in a patient in whom no formal diagnosis of hypertension has been made, or as an incidental finding.

796.3 Nonspecific low blood pressure reading

796.4 Other abnormal clinical findings

796.5 Abnormal finding on antenatal screening

796.6 Abnormal findings on neonatal screening

[Excludes:] *nonspecific serologic evidence of human immunodeficiency virus [HIV] (795.71)*

● Code new to 2012 edition ▲ Revision of existing code ④ ⑤ Fourth or fifth digit required

[5] **796.7 Abnormal cytologic smear of anus and anal HPV**

[Excludes:] *abnormal cytologic smear of cervix and cervical HPV (795.00-795.09)*
abnormal cytologic smear of vagina and vaginal HPV (795.10-795.19)
anal intraepithelial neoplasia I (AIN I) (569.44)
anal intraepithelial neoplasia II (AIN II) (569.44)
anal intraepithelial neoplasia III (AIN III) (230.5, 230.6)
carcinoma in situ of anus (230.5, 230.6)
dysplasia (histologically confirmed) of anus NOS (569.44)
mild anal dysplasia (histologically confirmed) (569.44)
moderate anal dysplasia (histologically confirmed) (569.44)
severe anal dysplasia (histologically confirmed) (230.5, 230.6)

796.70 Abnormal glandular Papanicolaou smear of anus
Atypical anal glandular cells NOS

796.71 Papanicolaou smear of anus with atypical squamous cells of undetermined significance (ASC-US)

796.72 Papanicolaou smear of anus with atypical squamous cells cannot exclude high grade squamous intraepithelial lesion (ASC-H)

796.73 Papanicolaou smear of anus with low grade squamous intraepithelial lesion (LGSIL)

796.74 Papanicolaou smear of anus with high grade squamous intraepithelial lesion (HGSIL)

796.75 Anal high risk human papillomavirus (HPV) DNA test positive

796.76 Papanicolaou smear of anus with cytologic evidence of malignancy

796.77 Satisfactory anal smear but lacking transformation zone

796.78 Unsatisfactory anal cytology smear
Inadequate anal cytology sample

796.79 Other abnormal Papanicolaou smear of anus and anal HPV
Anal low risk human papillomavirus (HPV)
DNA test positive

Use additional code for associated human papillomavirus (079.4)

796.9 Other

ILL-DEFINED AND UNKNOWN CAUSES OF MORBIDITY AND MORTALITY (797-799)

797 Senility without mention of psychosis
Frailty
Old age
Senescence
Senile asthenia
Senile debility
Senile exhaustion

[Excludes:] *senile psychoses (290.0-290.9)*

[DEFINITION] Senility is a progressive decline in mental functioning that is a part of the aging process.

798 Sudden death, cause unknown

798.0 Sudden infant death syndrome
Cot death
Crib death
Sudden death of nonspecific cause in infancy

798.1 Instantaneous death

798.2 Death occurring in less than 24 hours from onset of symptoms, not otherwise explained
Death known not to be violent or instantaneous, for which no cause could be discovered
Died without sign of disease

798.9 Unattended death
Death in circumstances where the body of the deceased was found and no cause could be discovered
Found dead

799 Other ill-defined and unknown causes of morbidity and mortality

[5] **799.0 Asphyxia and hypoxemia**

[Excludes:] *asphyxia and hypoxemia (due to)*
hypercapnia (786.09)

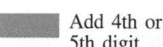

799.01 Asphyxia

799.02 Hypoxemia

799.1 Respiratory arrest
Cardiorespiratory failure

Excludes: *cardiac arrest (427.5)*
failure of peripheral circulation (785.50)
respiratory distress:
    NOS (786.09)
    acute (518.82)
    following trauma or surgery (518.52)
    newborn (770.89)
    syndrome (newborn) (769)
        adult (following trauma or surgery) (518.52)
        other (518.82)
respiratory failure (518.81, 518.83-518.84)
    newborn (770.84)
respiratory insufficiency (786.09)
    acute (518.82)

⑤ **799.2 Signs and symptoms involving emotional state**

Excludes: *anxiety (293.84, 300.00-300.09)*
depression (311)

799.21 Nervousness
Nervous

799.22 Irritability
Irritable

799.23 Impulsiveness
Impulsive

Excludes: *impulsive neurosis (300.3)*

799.24 Emotional lability

799.25 Demoralization and apathy
Apathetic

799.29 Other signs and symptoms involving emotional state

799.3 Debility, unspecified

Excludes: *asthenia (780.79)*
nervous debility (300.5)
neurasthenia (300.5)
senile asthenia (797)

799.4 Cachexia
Wasting disease
Code first underlying condition, if known

⑤ **799.5 Signs and symptoms involving cognition**

Excludes: *amnesia (780.93)*
amnestic syndrome (294.0)
attention deficit disorder (314.00-314.01)
late effects of cerebrovascular disease (438)
memory loss (780.93)
mild cognitive impairment, so stated (331.83)
specific problems in developmental delay (315.00-315.9)
transient global amnesia (437.7)
visuospatial neglect (781.8)

799.51 Attention or concentration deficit

799.52 Cognitive communication deficit

799.53 Visuospatial deficit

799.54 Psychomotor deficit

799.55 Frontal lobe and executive function deficit

799.59 Other signs and symptoms involving cognition

⑤ **799.8 Other ill-defined conditions**

799.81 Decreased libido
Decreased sexual desire

Excludes: *psychosexual dysfunction with inhibited sexual desire (302.71)*

● Code new
to 2012 edition   ▲ Revision of
existing code   ④ ⑤ Fourth or fifth
digit required

799.82   Apparent life threatening event in infant
ALTE
Apparent life threatening event in newborn and infant

Code first confirmed diagnosis, if known

Use additional code(s) for associated signs and symptoms if no confirmed diagnosis established, or if signs and symptoms are not associated routinely with confirmed diagnosis, or provide additional information for cause of ALTE

799.89   Other ill-defined conditions

799.9   Other unknown and unspecified cause
Undiagnosed disease, not specified as to site or system involved
Unknown cause of morbidity or mortality

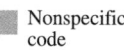

This page intentionally left blank.

● Code new
to 2012 edition

▲ Revision of
existing code

④ ⑤ Fourth or fifth
digit required

Chapter 17: Injury and Poisoning (800-999)

DEFINITIONS AND CODING ALERTS

This chapter includes definitions of selected key words, terms and phrases and coding alerts for adding points to the clinical domain, references to coding late effects where appropriate, and references to personal history V-codes in situations where the acute or chronic condition is no longer active. An example from this chapter is as follows:

⑤ **800** **Fracture of vault of skull**

DEFINITION A fracture is a complete or incomplete break in a bone resulting from the application of excessive force

ALERT! For coding late effect of fracture of skull and face bones see 905.0

MULTIPLE CODING FOR A SINGLE CONDITION

In addition to the etiology or manifestation convention that requires two codes to fully describe a single condition that affects multiple body systems, there are other single conditions that also require more than one code. "Use additional code" notes are found in the tabular at codes that are not part of an etiology or manifestation pair where a secondary code is useful to fully describe a condition. The sequencing rule is the same as the etiology or manifestation pair - , "use additional code" indicates that a secondary code should be added.

"Code first" notes are also under certain codes that are not specifically manifestation codes but may be due to an underlying cause. When a "code first" note is present and an underlying condition is present the underlying condition should be sequenced first.

"Code, if applicable, any causal condition first", notes indicate that this code may be assigned as a principal diagnosis when the causal condition is unknown or not applicable. If a causal condition is known, then the code for that condition should be sequenced as the principal or first-listed diagnosis. Multiple codes may be needed for late effects, complication codes and obstetric codes to more fully describe a condition. See the specific guidelines for these conditions for further instruction.

COMBINATION CODE

A combination code is a single code used to classify: two diagnoses, or a diagnosis with an associated secondary process (manifestation) A diagnosis with an associated complication Combination codes are identified by referring to subterm entries in the Alphabetic Index and by reading the inclusion and exclusion notes in the Tabular List.

Assign only the combination code when that code fully identifies the diagnostic conditions involved or when the Alphabetic Index so directs. Multiple coding should not be used when the classification provides a combination code that clearly identifies all of the elements documented in the diagnosis. When the combination code lacks necessary specificity in describing the manifestation or complication, an additional code should be used as a secondary code.

CODING LATE EFFECTS

A late effect is the residual effect (condition produced) after the acute phase of an illness or injury has terminated. There is no time limit on when a late effect code can be used. The residual may be apparent early, such as in cerebrovascular accident cases, or it may occur months or years later, such as that due to a previous injury. Coding of late effects generally requires two codes sequenced in the following order: The condition or nature of the late effect is sequenced first. The late effect code is sequenced second.

An exception to the above guidelines are those instances where the code for late effect is followed by a manifestation code identified in the Tabular List and title, or the late effect code has been expanded (at the fourth and fifth-digit levels) to include the manifestation(s). The code for the acute phase of an illness or injury that led to the late effect is never used with a code for the late effect.

CODING OF INJURIES

When coding injuries, assign separate codes for each injury unless a combination code is provided, in which case the combination code is assigned. Multiple injury codes are provided in ICD-9-CM, but should not be assigned unless information for a more specific code is not available. These codes are not to be used for normal, healing surgical wounds or to identify complications of surgical wounds.

The code for the most serious injury, as determined by the provider and the focus of treatment, is sequenced first.

| | Add 4th or 5th digit | | Nonspecific code | | Unspecified code | | Medicare secondary payer (MSP) alert |

Superficial injuries

Superficial injuries such as abrasions or contusions are not coded when associated with more severe injuries of the same site.

Primary injury with damage to nerves or blood vessels

When a primary injury results in minor damage to peripheral nerves or blood vessels, the primary injury is sequenced first with additional code(s) from categories 950-957, Injury to nerves and spinal cord, and/or 900-904, Injury to blood vessels. When the primary injury is to the blood vessels or nerves, that injury should be sequenced first.

CODING OF TRAUMATIC FRACTURES

The principles of multiple coding of injuries should be followed in coding fractures. Fractures of specified sites are coded individually by site in accordance with both the provisions within categories 800-829 and the level of detail furnished by medical record content.

Combination categories for multiple fractures are provided for use when there is insufficient detail in the medical record (such as trauma cases transferred to another hospital), when the reporting form limits the number of codes that can be used in reporting pertinent clinical data, or when there is insufficient specificity at the fourth-digit or fifth-digit level. More specific guidelines are as follows:

Acute Fractures vs. Aftercare

Traumatic fractures are coded using the acute fracture codes (800-829) while the patient is receiving active treatment for the fracture. Examples of active treatment are: surgical treatment, emergency department encounter, and evaluation and treatment by a new physician.

Fractures are coded using the aftercare codes (subcategories V54.0, V54.1, V54.8, or V54.9) for encounters after the patient has completed active treatment of the fracture and is receiving routine care for the fracture during the healing or recovery phase. Examples of fracture aftercare are: cast change or removal, removal of external or internal fixation device, medication adjustment, and follow up visits following fracture treatment.

Care for complications of surgical treatment for fracture repairs during the healing or recovery phase should be coded with the appropriate complication codes.

Care of complications of fractures, such as malunion and nonunion, should be reported with the appropriate codes.

Pathologic fractures are not coded in the 800-829 range, but instead are assigned to subcategory 733.1. See Official Guidelines, Section I.C.13.a for additional information.

Multiple fractures

Multiple fractures of same limb classifiable to the same three-digit or four-digit category are coded to that category.

Multiple unilateral or bilateral fractures of same bone(s) but classified to different fourth-digit subdivisions (bone part) within the same three-digit category are coded individually by site.

Multiple fracture categories 819 and 828 classify bilateral fractures of both upper limbs (819) and both lower limbs (828), but without any detail at the fourth-digit level other than open and closed type of fractures.

Multiple fractures sequencing

Multiple fractures are sequenced in accordance with the severity of the fracture. The provider should be asked to list the fracture diagnoses in the order of severity.

CODING OF BURNS

Current burns (940-948) are classified by depth, extent and by agent (E code). Burns are classified by depth as first degree (erythema), second degree (blistering), and third degree (full-thickness involvement).

Sequencing of burn and related condition codes

Sequence first the code that reflects the highest degree of burn when more than one burn is present.

● Code new
to 2012 edition
   ▲ Revision of
existing code
   ④ ⑤ Fourth or fifth
digit required

When the reason for the admission or encounter is for treatment of external multiple burns, sequence first the code that reflects the burn of the highest degree.

When a patient has both internal and external burns, the circumstances of admission govern the selection of the principal diagnosis or first-listed diagnosis.

When a patient is admitted for burn injuries and other related conditions such as smoke inhalation and/or respiratory failure, the circumstances of admission govern the selection of the principal or first-listed diagnosis.

Burns of the same local site

Classify burns of the same local site (three-digit category level, 940-947). but of different degrees to the subcategory identifying the highest degree recorded in the diagnosis.

Non-healing burns

Non-healing burns are coded as acute burns. Necrosis of burned skin should be coded as a non-healed burn.

Code 958.3, Posttraumatic wound infection

Assign code 958.3, Posttraumatic wound infection, not elsewhere classified, as an additional code for any documented infected burn site.

Assign separate codes for each burn site

When coding burns, assign separate codes for each burn site. Category 946 Burns of Multiple specified sites, should only be used if the location of the burns are not documented.

Category 949, Burn, unspecified, is extremely vague and should rarely be used.

Assign codes from category 948, Burns

Burns classified according to extent of body surface involved, when the site of the burn is not specified or when there is a need for additional data. It is advisable to use category 948 as additional coding when needed to provide data for evaluating burn mortality, such as that needed by burn units. It is also advisable to use category 948 as an additional code for reporting purposes when there is mention of a third-degree burn involving 20 percent or more of the body surface.

In assigning a code from category 948:

> Fourth-digit codes are used to identify the percentage of total body surface involved in a burn (all degree).

> Fifth-digits are assigned to identify the percentage of body surface involved in third-degree burn.

> Fifth-digit zero (0) is assigned when less than 10 percent or when no body surface is involved in a third-degree burn.

Category 948 is based on the classic "rule of nines" in estimating body surface involved: head and neck are assigned nine percent, each arm nine percent, each leg 18 percent, the anterior trunk 18 percent, posterior trunk 18 percent, and genitalia one percent. Providers may change these percentage assignments where necessary to accommodate infants and children who have proportionately larger heads than adults and patients who have large buttocks, thighs, or abdomen that involve burns.

Encounters for treatment of late effects of burns

Encounters for the treatment of the late effects of burns (i.e., scars or joint contractures) should be coded to the residual condition (sequelae) followed by the appropriate late effect code (906.5-906.9). A late effect E code may also be used, if desired.

Sequelae with a late effect code and current burn

When appropriate, both a sequelae with a late effect code, and a current burn code may be assigned on the same record (when both a current burn and sequelae of an old burn exist).

Add 4th or 5th digit | Nonspecific code | Unspecified code | Medicare secondary payer (MSP) alert

CODING OF DEBRIDEMENT OF WOUND, INFECTION, OR BURN

Excisional debridement involves surgical removal or cutting away, as opposed to a mechanical (brushing, scrubbing, washing) debridement.

For coding purposes, excisional debridement is assigned to code 86.22. Nonexcisional debridement is assigned to code 86.28.

ADVERSE EFFECTS, POISONING AND TOXIC EFFECTS

The properties of certain drugs, medicinal and biological substances or combinations of such substances, may cause toxic reactions. The occurrence of drug toxicity is classified in ICD-9-CM as follows:

Adverse Effect

When the drug was correctly prescribed and properly administered, code the reaction plus the appropriate code from the E930-E949 series. Codes from the E930-E949 series must be used to identify the causative substance for an adverse effect of drug, medicinal and biological substances, correctly prescribed and properly administered. The effect, such as tachycardia, delirium, gastrointestinal hemorrhaging, vomiting, hypokalemia, hepatitis, renal failure, or respiratory failure, is coded and followed by the appropriate code from the E930-E949 series.

Adverse effects of therapeutic substances correctly prescribed and properly administered (toxicity, synergistic reaction, side effect, and idiosyncratic reaction) may be due to (1) differences among patients, such as age, sex, disease, and genetic factors, and (2) drug-related factors, such as type of drug, route of administration, duration of therapy, dosage, and bioavailability.

Poisoning

A. Error was made in drug prescription

Errors made in drug prescription or in the administration of the drug by provider, nurse, patient, or other person, use the appropriate poisoning code from the 960-979 series.

B. Overdose of a drug intentionally taken

If an overdose of a drug was intentionally taken or administered and resulted in drug toxicity, it would be coded as a poisoning (960-979 series).

C. Nonprescribed drug taken with correctly prescribed and properly administered drug

If a nonprescribed drug or medicinal agent was taken in combination with a correctly prescribed and properly administered drug, any drug toxicity or other reaction resulting from the interaction of the two drugs would be classified as a poisoning.

D. Interaction of drug(s) and alcohol

When a reaction results from the interaction of a drug(s) and alcohol, this would be classified as poisoning.

E. Sequencing of poisoning

When coding a poisoning or reaction to the improper use of a medication (e.g., wrong dose, wrong substance, wrong route of administration) the poisoning code is sequenced first, followed by a code for the manifestation. If there is also a diagnosis of drug abuse or dependence to the substance, the abuse or dependence is coded as an additional code.

See Official Guidelines, Section I.C.3.a.6.b. if poisoning is the result of insulin pump malfunctions and Official Guidelines, Section I.C.19 for general use of E-codes.

Toxic Effects

A. Toxic effect codes

When a harmful substance is ingested or comes in contact with a person, this is classified as a toxic effect. The toxic effect codes are in categories 980-989.

B. Sequencing toxic effect codes

A toxic effect code should be sequenced first, followed by the code(s) that identify the result of the toxic effect.

● Code new
to 2012 edition

▲ Revision of
existing code

④ ⑤ Fourth or fifth
digit required

C.   External cause codes for toxic effects

An external cause code from categories E860-E869 for accidental exposure, codes E950.6 or E950.7 for intentional self-harm, category E962 for assault, or categories E980-E982, for undetermined, should also be assigned to indicate intent.

COMPLICATIONS OF CARE

Documentation of complications of care

As with all procedural or postprocedural complications, code assignment is based on the provider's documentation of the relationship between the condition and the procedure.

Transplant complications

A.   Transplant complications other than kidney

Codes under subcategory 996.8, Complications of transplanted organ, are for use for both complications and rejection of transplanted organs. A transplant complication code is only assigned if the complication affects the function of the transplanted organ. Two codes are required to fully describe a transplant complication, the appropriate code from subcategory 996.8 and a secondary code that identifies the complication.

Pre-existing conditions or conditions that develop after the transplant are not coded as complications unless they affect the function of the transplanted organs.

See I.C.18.d.3.for transplant organ removal status. See I.C.2.i for malignant neoplasm associated with transplanted organ.

B.   Chronic kidney disease and kidney transplant complications

Patients who have undergone kidney transplant may still have some form of chronic kidney disease (CKD) because the kidney transplant may not fully restore kidney function. Code 996.81 should be assigned for documented complications of a kidney transplant, such as transplant failure or rejection or other transplant complication. Code 996.81 should not be assigned for post kidney transplant patients who have chronic kidney (CKD) unless a transplant complication such as transplant failure or rejection is documented. If the documentation is unclear as to whether the patient has a complication of the transplant, query the provider.

For patients with CKD following a kidney transplant, but who do not have a complication such as failure or rejection, see Chapter 10.

Ventilator associated pneumonia

A.   Documentation of Ventilator associated pneumonia

As with all procedural or postprocedural complications, code assignment is based on the provider's documentation of the relationship between the condition and the procedure.

Code 997.31, Ventilator associated pneumonia, should be assigned only when the provider has documented ventilator associated pneumonia (VAP). An additional code to identify the organism (e.g., Pseudomonas aeruginosa, code 041.7) should also be assigned. Do not assign an additional code from categories 480-484 to identify the type of pneumonia.

Code 997.31 should not be assigned for cases where the patient has pneumonia and is on a mechanical ventilator but the provider has not specifically stated that the pneumonia is ventilator-associated pneumonia.

If the documentation is unclear as to whether the patient has a pneumonia that is a complication attributable to the mechanical ventilator, query the provider.

B.   Patient admitted with pneumonia and develops VAP

A patient may be admitted with one type of pneumonia (e.g., code 481, Pneumococcal pneumonia) and subsequently develop VAP. In this instance, the principal diagnosis would be the appropriate code from categories 480-484 for the pneumonia diagnosed at the time of admission. Code 997.31, Ventilator associated pneumonia, would be assigned as an additional diagnosis when the provider has also documented the presence of ventilator associated pneumonia.

| | Add 4th or 5th digit | | Nonspecific code | | Unspecified code | | Medicare secondary payer (MSP) alert |

SIRS DUE TO NON-INFECTIOUS PROCESS

The systemic inflammatory response syndrome (SIRS) can develop as a result of certain non-infectious disease processes, such as trauma, malignant neoplasm, or pancreatitis. When SIRS is documented with a noninfectious condition, and no subsequent infection is documented, the code for the underlying condition, such as an injury, should be assigned, followed by code 995.93, Systemic inflammatory response syndrome due to noninfectious process without acute organ dysfunction, or 995.94, Systemic inflammatory response syndrome due to non-infectious process with acute organ dysfunction. If an acute organ dysfunction is documented, the appropriate code(s) for the associated acute organ dysfunction(s) should be assigned in addition to code 995.94. If acute organ dysfunction is documented, but it cannot be determined if the acute organ dysfunction is associated with SIRS or due to another condition (e.g., directly due to the trauma), the provider should be queried.

Sepsis and Severe Sepsis Associated with Non-infectious Process

In some cases, a non-infectious process, such as trauma, may lead to an infection which can result in sepsis or severe sepsis. If sepsis or severe sepsis is documented as associated with a non-infectious condition, such as a burn or serious injury, and this condition meets the definition for principal diagnosis, the code for the non-infectious condition should be sequenced first, followed by the code for the systemic infection and either code 995.91, Sepsis, or 995.92, Severe sepsis. Additional codes for any associated acute organ dysfunction(s) should also be assigned for cases of severe sepsis. If the sepsis or severe sepsis meets the definition of principal diagnosis, the systemic infection and sepsis codes should be sequenced before the non-infectious condition. When both the associated non-infectious condition and the sepsis or severe sepsis meet the definition of principal diagnosis, either may be assigned as principal diagnosis.

668 ● Code new
to 2012 edition   ▲ Revision of
existing code   ④ ⑤ Fourth or fifth
digit required

17. INJURY AND POISONING (800-999)

Use E code(s) to identify the cause and intent of the injury or poisoning (E800-E999)

Use additional code for retained foreign body, if applicable, V90.01- V90.9)

Note:

1. The principle of multiple coding of injuries should be followed wherever possible. Combination categories for multiple injuries are provided for use when there is insufficient detail as to the nature of the individual conditions, or for primary tabulation purposes when it is more convenient to record a single code; otherwise, the component injuries should be coded separately.

   Where multiple sites of injury are specified in the titles, the word "with" indicates involvement of both sites, and the word "and" indicates involvement of either or both sites. The word "finger" includes thumb.
2. Categories for "late effect" of injuries are to be found at 905-909.

FRACTURES (800-829)

[Excludes:] *malunion (733.81)*
nonunion (733.82)
pathologic or spontaneous fracture (733.10-733.19)
stress fractures (733.93-733.95)

The terms "condyle," "coronoid process," "ramus," and "symphysis" indicate the portion of the bone fractured, not the name of the bone involved.

The descriptions "closed" and "open" used in the fourth-digit subdivisions include the following terms:

closed (with or without delayed healing):
comminuted
depressed
elevated
fissured
fracture NOS
greenstick
impacted
linear
simple
slipped epiphysis
spiral

open (with or without delayed healing):
compound
infected
missile
puncture
with foreign body

A fracture not indicated as closed or open should be classified as closed.

[DEFINITION] A fracture is a complete or incomplete break in a bone resulting from the application of excessive force.

[ALERT!] For coding late effects of musculoskeletal and connective tissue injuries see 905

[ALERT!] For personal history of traumatic fracture see V15.51

FRACTURE OF SKULL (800-804)

Includes: traumatic brain injury due to fracture of skull

The following fifth-digit subclassification is for use with the appropriate codes in categories 800, 801, 803, and 804:

0 unspecified state of consciousness

1 with no loss of consciousness

2 with brief [less than one hour] loss of consciousness

3 with moderate [1-24 hours] loss of consciousness and return to pre-existing conscious level

4 with prolonged [more than 24 hours] loss of consciousness and return to pre-existing conscious level

5 with prolonged [more than 24 hours] loss of consciousness, without return to pre-existing conscious level
Use fifth-digit 5 to designate when a patient is unconscious and dies before regaining consciousness, regardless of the duration of the loss of consciousness

6 with loss of consciousness of unspecified duration

9 with concussion, unspecified

[5] **800 Fracture of vault of skull**

Includes: frontal bone
parietal bone

[DEFINITION] A fracture is a complete or incomplete break in a bone resulting from the application of excessive force

[ALERT!] For coding late effect of fracture of skull and face bones see 905.0

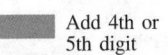

Add 4th or 5th digit | Nonspecific code | Unspecified code | Medicare secondary payer (MSP) alert

⑤ **800.0** Closed without mention of intracranial injury
[0-6,9]

⑤ **800.1** Closed with cerebral laceration and contusion
[0-6,9]

⑤ **800.2** Closed with subarachnoid, subdural, and extradural hemorrhage
[0-6,9]

⑤ **800.3** Closed with other and unspecified intracranial hemorrhage
[0-6,9]

⑤ **800.4** Closed with intracranial injury of other and unspecified nature
[0-6,9]

⑤ **800.5** Open without mention of intracranial injury
[0-6,9]

⑤ **800.6** Open with cerebral laceration and contusion
[0-6,9]

⑤ **800.7** Open with subarachnoid, subdural, and extradural hemorrhage
[0-6,9]

⑤ **800.8** Open with other and unspecified intracranial hemorrhage
[0-6,9]

⑤ **800.9** Open with intracranial injury of other and unspecified nature
[0-6,9]

⑤ **801** Fracture of base of skull
Includes:

fossa:	sinus:
anterior	ethmoid
middle	frontal
posterior	sphenoid bone
occiput bone	temporal bone
orbital roof	

ALERT! For coding late effect of fracture of skull and face bones see 905.0

⑤ **801.0** Closed without mention of intracranial injury
[0-6,9]

⑤ **801.1** Closed with cerebral laceration and contusion
[0-6,9]

⑤ **801.2** Closed with subarachnoid, subdural, and extradural hemorrhage
[0-6,9]

⑤ **801.3** Closed with other and unspecified intracranial hemorrhage
[0-6,9]

⑤ **801.4** Closed with intracranial injury of other and unspecified nature
[0-6,9]

⑤ **801.5** Open without mention of intracranial injury
[0-6,9]

⑤ **801.6** Open with cerebral laceration and contusion
[0-6,9]

⑤ **801.7** Open with subarachnoid, subdural, and extradural hemorrhage
[0-6,9]

⑤ **801.8** Open with other and unspecified intracranial hemorrhage
[0-6,9]

⑤ **801.9** Open with intracranial injury of other and unspecified nature
[0-6,9]

802 Fracture of face bones
ALERT! For coding late effect of fracture of skull and face bones see 905.0

802.0 Nasal bones, closed

802.1 Nasal bones, open

⑤ **802.2** Mandible, closed
Inferior maxilla
Lower jaw (bone)

802.20 Unspecified site

802.21 Condylar process

802.22 Subcondylar

802.23 Coronoid process

● Code new
to 2012 edition

▲ Revision of
existing code

④ ⑤ Fourth or fifth
digit required

	802.24	Ramus, unspecified
	802.25	Angle of jaw
	802.26	Symphysis of body
	802.27	Alveolar border of body
	802.28	Body, other and unspecified
	802.29	Multiple sites

⑤ **802.3 Mandible, open**

	802.30	Unspecified site
	802.31	Condylar process
	802.32	Subcondylar
	802.33	Coronoid process
	802.34	Ramus, unspecified
	802.35	Angle of jaw
	802.36	Symphysis of body
	802.37	Alveolar border of body
	802.38	Body, other and unspecified
	802.39	Multiple sites

802.4 Malar and maxillary bones, closed
Superior maxilla   Zygoma
Upper jaw (bone)   Zygomatic arch

802.5 Malar and maxillary bones, open

802.6 Orbital floor (blow-out), closed

802.7 Orbital floor (blow-out), open

802.8 Other facial bones, closed
Alveolus
Orbit:
  NOS
  part other than roof or floor
Palate

Excludes: orbital:
  floor (802.6)
  roof (801.0-801.9)

802.9 Other facial bones, open

⑤ **803 Other and unqualified skull fractures**
Includes: skull NOS
                skull multiple NOS

ALERT! For coding late effect of fracture of skull and face bones see 905.0

⑤ **803.0 Closed without mention of intracranial injury**
[0-6,9]

⑤ **803.1 Closed with cerebral laceration and contusion**
[0-6,9]

⑤ **803.2 Closed with subarachnoid, subdural, and extradural hemorrhage**
[0-6,9]

⑤ **803.3 Closed with other and unspecified intracranial hemorrhage**
[0-6,9]

⑤ **803.4 Closed with intracranial injury of other and unspecified nature**
[0-6,9]

⑤ **803.5 Open without mention of intracranial injury**
[0-6,9]

⑤ **803.6 Open with cerebral laceration and contusion**
[0-6,9]

⑤ **803.7 Open with subarachnoid, subdural, and extradural hemorrhage**
[0-6,9]

⑤ **803.8 Open with other and unspecified intracranial hemorrhage**
[0-6,9]

⑤ **803.9 Open with intracranial injury of other and unspecified nature**
[0-6,9]

671

Add 4th or 5th digit	Nonspecific code	Unspecified code	Medicare secondary payer (MSP) alert

⑤ **804** **Multiple fractures involving skull or face with other bones**
> **ALERT!** For coding late effect of fracture of skull and face bones see 905.0

 ⑤ **804.0** **Closed without mention of intracranial injury**
  [0-6,9]

 ⑤ **804.1** **Closed with cerebral laceration and contusion**
  [0-6,9]

 ⑤ **804.2** **Closed with subarachnoid, subdural, and extradural hemorrhage**
  [0-6,9]

 ⑤ **804.3** **Closed with other and unspecified intracranial hemorrhage**
  [0-6,9]

 ⑤ **804.4** **Closed with intracranial injury of other and unspecified nature**
  [0-6,9]

 ⑤ **804.5** **Open without mention of intracranial injury**
  [0-6,9]

 ⑤ **804.6** **Open with cerebral laceration and contusion**
  [0-6,9]

 ⑤ **804.7** **Open with subarachnoid, subdural, and extradural hemorrhage**
  [0-6,9]

 ⑤ **804.8** **Open with other and unspecified intracranial hemorrhage**
  [0-6,9]

 ⑤ **804.9** **Open with intracranial injury of other and unspecified nature**
  [0-6,9]

FRACTURE OF NECK AND TRUNK (805-809)

805 **Fracture of vertebral column without mention of spinal cord injury**
> Includes: neural arch
>   spine
>   spinous process
>   transverse process
>   vertebra

The following fifth-digit subclassification is for use with codes 805.0-805.1:

 0 cervical vertebra, unspecified level
 1 first cervical vertebra
 2 second cervical vertebra
 3 third cervical vertebra
 4 fourth cervical vertebra
 5 fifth cervical vertebra
 6 sixth cervical vertebra
 7 seventh cervical vertebra
 8 multiple cervical vertebrae

> **ALERT!** For coding late effect of fracture of spine and trunk without spinal cord lesion see 905.1

 ⑤ **805.0** **Cervical, closed**
  [0-8] Atlas
     Axis

 ⑤ **805.1** **Cervical, open**
  [0-8]

 805.2 **Dorsal [thoracic], closed**

 805.3 **Dorsal [thoracic], open**

 805.4 **Lumbar, closed**

 805.5 **Lumbar, open**

 805.6 **Sacrum and coccyx, closed**

 805.7 **Sacrum and coccyx, open**

 805.8 **Unspecified, closed**

 805.9 **Unspecified, open**

● Code new   ▲ Revision of   ④ ⑤ Fourth or fifth
   to 2012 edition   existing code   digit required

806 Fracture of vertebral column with spinal cord injury

Includes: any condition classifiable to 805 with:
- complete or incomplete transverse lesion (of cord)
- hematomyelia
- injury to:
  - cauda equina
  - nerve
- paralysis
- paraplegia
- quadriplegia
- spinal concussion

[ALERT!] For coding late effect of fracture of spine and trunk without spinal cord lesion see 905.1

[5] **806.0 Cervical, closed**

806.00 C_1-C_4 level with unspecified spinal cord injury
Cervical region NOS with spinal cord injury NOS

806.01 C_1-C_4 level with complete lesion of cord

806.02 C_1-C_4 level with anterior cord syndrome

806.03 C_1-C_4 level with central cord syndrome

806.04 C_1-C_4 level with other specified spinal cord injury
C_1-C_4 level with:
- incomplete spinal cord lesion NOS
- posterior cord syndrome

806.05 C_5-C_7 level with unspecified spinal cord injury

806.06 C_5-C_7 level with complete lesion of cord

806.07 C_5-C_7 level with anterior cord syndrome

806.08 C_5-C_7 level with central cord syndrome

806.09 C_5-C_7 level with other specified spinal cord injury
C_5-C_7 level with:
- incomplete spinal cord lesion NOS
- posterior cord syndrome

[5] **806.1 Cervical, open**

806.10 C_1-C_4 level with unspecified spinal cord injury

806.11 C_1-C_4 level with complete lesion of cord

806.12 C_1-C_4 level with anterior cord syndrome

806.13 C_1-C_4 level with central cord syndrome

806.14 C_1-C_4 level with other specified spinal cord injury
C_1-C_4 level with:
- incomplete spinal cord lesion NOS
- posterior cord syndrome

806.15 C_5-C_7 level with unspecified spinal cord injury

806.16 C_5-C_7 level with complete lesion of cord

806.17 C_5-C_7 level with anterior cord syndrome

806.18 C_5-C_7 level with central cord syndrome

806.19 C_5-C_7 level with other specified spinal cord injury
C_5-C_7 level with:
- incomplete spinal cord lesion NOS
- posterior cord syndrome

[5] **806.2 Dorsal [thoracic], closed**

806.20 T_1-T_6 level with unspecified spinal cord injury
Thoracic region NOS with spinal cord injury NOS

806.21 T_1-T_6 level with complete lesion of cord

806.22 T_1-T_6 level with anterior cord syndrome

806.23 T_1-T_6 level with central cord syndrome

806.24 T_1-T_6 level with other specified spinal cord injury
T_1-T_6 level with:
- incomplete spinal cord lesion NOS
- posterior cord syndrome

806.25 T_7-T_{12} level with unspecified spinal cord injury

806.26 T_7-T_{12} level with complete lesion of cord

806.27 **T_7-T_{12} level with anterior cord syndrome**

806.28 **T_7-T_{12} level with central cord syndrome**

806.29 **T_7-T_{12} level with other specified spinal cord injury**
T_7-T_{12} level with:
incomplete spinal cord lesion NOS
posterior cord syndrome

[5] **806.3 Dorsal [thoracic], open**

806.30 **T_1-T_6 level with unspecified spinal cord injury**

806.31 **T_1-T_6 level with complete lesion of cord**

806.32 **T_1-T_6 level with anterior cord syndrome**

806.33 **T_1-T_6 level with central cord syndrome**

806.34 **T_1-T_6 level with other specified spinal cord injury**
T_1-T_6 level with:
incomplete spinal cord lesion NOS
posterior cord syndrome

806.35 **T_7-T_{12} level with unspecified spinal cord injury**

806.36 **T_7-T_{12} level with complete lesion of cord**

806.37 **T_7-T_{12} level with anterior cord syndrome**

806.38 **T_7-T_{12} level with central cord syndrome**

806.39 **T_7-T_{12} level with other specified spinal cord injury**
T_7-T_{12} level with:
incomplete spinal cord lesion NOS
posterior cord syndrome

806.4 Lumbar, closed

806.5 Lumbar, open

[5] **806.6 Sacrum and coccyx, closed**

806.60 **With unspecified spinal cord injury**

806.61 **With complete cauda equina lesion**

806.62 **With other cauda equina injury**

806.69 **With other spinal cord injury**

[5] **806.7 Sacrum and coccyx, open**

806.70 **With unspecified spinal cord injury**

806.71 **With complete cauda equina lesion**

806.72 **With other cauda equina injury**

806.79 **With other spinal cord injury**

806.8 Unspecified, closed

806.9 Unspecified, open

807 Fracture of rib(s), sternum, larynx, and trachea

The following fifth-digit subclassification is for use with codes 807.0-807.1:

0 **rib(s), unspecified**
1 **one rib**
2 **two ribs**
3 **three ribs**
4 **four ribs**
5 **five ribs**
6 **six ribs**
7 **seven ribs**
8 **eight or more ribs**
9 **multiple ribs, unspecified**

[ALERT!] For coding late effect of fracture of spine and trunk without spinal cord lesion see 905.1

[5] **807.0 Rib(s), closed**
[0-9]

[5] **807.1 Rib(s), open**
[0-9]

807.2 Sternum, closed

807.3 Sternum, open

807.4 Flail chest

807.5 Larynx and trachea, closed
    Hyoid bone   Trachea
    Thyroid cartilage

807.6 Larynx and trachea, open

808 Fracture of pelvis
    ALERT! For coding late effect of fracture of spine and trunk without spinal cord lesion see 905.1

808.0 Acetabulum, closed

808.1 Acetabulum, open

808.2 Pubis, closed

808.3 Pubis, open

⑤ **808.4** Other specified part, closed

    808.41 Ilium

    808.42 Ischium

▲   **808.43** Multiple closed pelvic fractures with disruption of pelvic circle
        Multiple closed pelvic fractures with disruption of pelvic ring

●   **808.44** Multiple closed pelvic fractures without disruption of pelvic circle
        Multiple closed pelvic fractures without disruption of pelvic ring

    808.49 Other
        Innominate bone
        Pelvic rim

⑤ **808.5** Other specified part, open

    808.51 Ilium

    808.52 Ischium

    808.53 Multiple open pelvic fractures with disruption of pelvic circle
        Multiple open pelvic fractures with disruption of pelvic ring

●   **808.54** Multiple open pelvic fractures without disruption of pelvic circle
        Multiple open pelvic fractures without disruption of pelvic ring

    808.59 Other

808.8 Unspecified, closed

808.9 Unspecified, open

809 Ill-defined fractures of bones of trunk
    Includes: bones of trunk with other bones except those of skull and face
               multiple bones of trunk

    Excludes: *multiple fractures of:*
            pelvic bones alone (808.0-808.9)
            ribs alone (807.0-807.1, 807.4)
            ribs or sternum with limb bones (819.0-819.1, 828.0-828.1)
            skull or face with other bones (804.0-804.9)

    ALERT! For coding late effect of fracture of spine and trunk without spinal cord lesion see 905.1

809.0 Fracture of bones of trunk, closed

809.1 Fracture of bones of trunk, open

FRACTURE OF UPPER LIMB (810-819)

⑤ **810** Fracture of clavicle
    Includes: collar bone
            interligamentous part of clavicle

The following fifth-digit subclassification is for use with category 810:

    0 unspecified part
        Clavicle NOS

    1 sternal end of clavicle

    2 shaft of clavicle

    3 acromial end of clavicle

    ALERT! For coding late effect of fracture of upper extremities see 905.2

Add 4th or 5th digit	Nonspecific code	Unspecified code	Medicare secondary payer (MSP) alert

⑤ **810.0** **Closed**
[0-3]

⑤ **810.1** **Open**
[0-3]

⑤ **811** **Fracture of scapula**
Includes: shoulder blade

The following fifth-digit subclassification is for use with category 811:

0 **unspecified part**

1 **acromial process**
Acromion (process)

2 **coracoid process**

3 **glenoid cavity and neck of scapula**

9 **other**
Scapula body

ALERT! For coding late effect of fracture of upper extremities see 905.2

⑤ **811.0** **Closed**
[0-3,9]

⑤ **811.1** **Open**
[0-3,9]

812 **Fracture of humerus**
ALERT! For coding late effect of fracture of upper extremities see 905.2

⑤ **812.0** **Upper end, closed**

812.00 **Upper end, unspecified part**
Proximal end
Shoulder

812.01 **Surgical neck**
Neck of humerus NOS

812.02 **Anatomical neck**

812.03 **Greater tuberosity**

812.09 **Other**
Head
Upper epiphysis

⑤ **812.1** **Upper end, open**

812.10 **Upper end, unspecified part**

812.11 **Surgical neck**

812.12 **Anatomical neck**

812.13 **Greater tuberosity**

812.19 **Other**

⑤ **812.2** **Shaft or unspecified part, closed**

812.20 **Unspecified part of humerus**
Humerus NOS
Upper arm NOS

812.21 **Shaft of humerus**

⑤ **812.3** **Shaft or unspecified part, open**

812.30 **Unspecified part of humerus**

812.31 **Shaft of humerus**

⑤ **812.4** **Lower end, closed**
Distal end of humerus
Elbow

812.40 **Lower end, unspecified part**

812.41 **Supracondylar fracture of humerus**

812.42 **Lateral condyle**
External condyle

812.43 **Medial condyle**
Internal epicondyle

812.44 **Condyle(s), unspecified**
Articular process NOS
Lower epiphysis NOS

● Code new
to 2012 edition ▲ Revision of
existing code ④ ⑤ Fourth or fifth
digit required

812.49 Other
Multiple fractures of lower end
Trochlea

[5] **812.5 Lower end, open**

812.50 Lower end, unspecified part

812.51 Supracondylar fracture of humerus

812.52 Lateral condyle

812.53 Medial condyle

812.54 Condyle(s), unspecified

812.59 Other

813 Fracture of radius and ulna

[ALERT!] For coding late effect of fracture of upper extremities see 905.2

[5] **813.0 Upper end, closed**
Proximal end

813.00 Upper end of forearm, unspecified

813.01 Olecranon process of ulna

813.02 Coronoid process of ulna

813.03 Monteggia's fracture

813.04 Other and unspecified fractures of proximal end of ulna (alone)
Multiple fractures of ulna, upper end

813.05 Head of radius

813.06 Neck of radius

813.07 Other and unspecified fractures of proximal end of radius (alone)
Multiple fractures of radius, upper end

813.08 Radius with ulna, upper end [any part]

[5] **813.1 Upper end, open**

813.10 Upper end of forearm, unspecified

813.11 Olecranon process of ulna

813.12 Coronoid process of ulna

813.13 Monteggia's fracture

813.14 Other and unspecified fractures of proximal end of ulna (alone)

813.15 Head of radius

813.16 Neck of radius

813.17 Other and unspecified fractures of proximal end of radius (alone)

813.18 Radius with ulna, upper end [any part]

[5] **813.2 Shaft, closed**

813.20 Shaft, unspecified

813.21 Radius (alone)

813.22 Ulna (alone)

813.23 Radius with ulna

[5] **813.3 Shaft, open**

813.30 Shaft, unspecified

813.31 Radius (alone)

813.32 Ulna (alone)

813.33 Radius with ulna

[5] **813.4 Lower end, closed**
Distal end

813.40 Lower end of forearm, unspecified

813.41 Colles' fracture
Smith's fracture

813.42 Other fractures of distal end of radius (alone)
Dupuytren's fracture, radius
Radius, lower end

813.43 Distal end of ulna (alone)
    Ulna: Ulna:
      head   lower epiphysis
      lower end   styloid process

813.44 Radius with ulna, lower end

813.45 Torus fracture of radius (alone)

Excludes:	*Torus fracture of radius and ulna (813.47)*

813.46 Torus fracture of ulna (alone)

Excludes:	*Torus fracture of radius and ulna (813.47)*

813.47 Torus fracture of radius and ulna

⑤ **813.5 Lower end, open**

813.50 Lower end of forearm, unspecified

813.51 Colles' fracture

813.52 Other fractures of distal end of radius (alone)

813.53 Distal end of ulna (alone)

813.54 Radius with ulna, lower end

⑤ **813.8 Unspecified part, closed**

813.80 Forearm, unspecified

813.81 Radius (alone)

813.82 Ulna (alone)

813.83 Radius with ulna

⑤ **813.9 Unspecified part, open**

813.90 Forearm, unspecified

813.91 Radius (alone)

813.92 Ulna (alone)

813.93 Radius with ulna

⑤ **814 Fracture of carpal bone(s)**
The following fifth-digit subclassification is for use with category 814:

0 carpal bone, unspecified
    Wrist NOS

1 navicular [scaphoid] of wrist

2 lunate [semilunar] bone of wrist

3 triquetral [cuneiform] bone of wrist

4 pisiform

5 trapezium bone [larger multangular]

6 trapezoid bone [smaller multangular]

7 capitate bone [os magnum]

8 hamate [unciform] bone

9 other

ALERT! For coding late effect of fracture of upper extremities see 905.2

⑤ **814.0 Closed**
[0-9]

⑤ **814.1 Open**
[0-9]

⑤ **815 Fracture of metacarpal bone(s)**
    Includes: hand [except finger]
              metacarpus
The following fifth-digit subclassification is for use with category 815:

0 metacarpal bone(s), site unspecified

1 base of thumb [first] metacarpal
    Bennett's fracture

2 base of other metacarpal bone(s)

3 shaft of metacarpal bone(s)

4 neck of metacarpal bone(s)

9 multiple sites of metacarpus

   ● Code new   ▲ Revision of   ④ ⑤ Fourth or fifth
      to 2012 edition   existing code   digit required

ALERT! For coding late effect of fracture of upper extremities see 905.2

[5] **815.0 Closed**
[0-4,9]

[5] **815.1 Open**
[0-4,9]

[5] **816 Fracture of one or more phalanges of hand**
Includes: finger(s)
thumb

The following fifth-digit subclassification is for use with category 816:

0 phalanx or phalanges, unspecified
1 middle or proximal phalanx or phalanges
2 distal phalanx or phalanges
3 multiple sites

ALERT! For coding late effect of fracture of upper extremities see 905.2

[5] **816.0 Closed**
[0-3]

[5] **816.1 Open**
[0-3]

817 Multiple fractures of hand bones
Includes: metacarpal bone(s) with phalanx or phalanges of same hand

ALERT! For coding late effect of fracture of upper extremities see 905.2

817.0 Closed

817.1 Open

818 Ill-defined fractures of upper limb
Includes: arm NOS
multiple bones of same upper limb

[*Excludes:*] *multiple fractures of:*
metacarpal bone(s) with phalanx or phalanges (817.0-817.1)
phalanges of hand alone (816.0-816.1)
radius with ulna (813.0-813.9)

ALERT! For coding late effect of fracture of upper extremities see 905.2

818.0 Closed

818.1 Open

819 Multiple fractures involving both upper limbs, and upper limb with rib(s) and sternum
Includes: arm(s) with rib(s) or sternum
both arms [any bones]

ALERT! For coding late effect of fracture of upper extremities see 905.2

819.0 Closed

819.1 Open

FRACTURE OF LOWER LIMB (820-829)

820 Fracture of neck of femur

ALERT! For coding late effect of fracture of neck of femur see 905.3

[5] **820.0 Transcervical fracture, closed**

820.00 Intracapsular section, unspecified

820.01 Epiphysis (separation) (upper)
Transepiphyseal

820.02 Midcervical section
Transcervical NOS

820.03 Base of neck
Cervicotrochanteric section

820.09 Other
Head of femur
Subcapital

[5] **820.1 Transcervical fracture, open**

820.10 Intracapsular section, unspecified

820.11 Epiphysis (separation) (upper)

820.12 Midcervical section

820.13 Base of neck

820.19 Other

⑤ **820.2** Pertrochanteric fracture, closed

820.20 Trochanteric section, unspecified
Trochanter:
NOS
greater
lesser

820.21 Intertrochanteric section

820.22 Subtrochanteric section

⑤ **820.3** Pertrochanteric fracture, open

820.30 Trochanteric section, unspecified

820.31 Intertrochanteric section

820.32 Subtrochanteric section

820.8 Unspecified part of neck of femur, closed
Hip NOS
Neck of femur NOS

820.9 Unspecified part of neck of femur, open

821 Fracture of other and unspecified parts of femur
ALERT! For coding late effect of fracture of lower extremities see 905.4

⑤ **821.0** Shaft or unspecified part, closed

821.00 Unspecified part of femur
Thigh
Upper leg

Excludes: hip NOS (820.8)

821.01 Shaft

⑤ **821.1** Shaft or unspecified part, open

821.10 Unspecified part of femur

821.11 Shaft

⑤ **821.2** Lower end, closed
Distal end

821.20 Lower end, unspecified part

821.21 Condyle, femoral

821.22 Epiphysis, lower (separation)

821.23 Supracondylar fracture of femur

821.29 Other
Multiple fractures of lower end

⑤ **821.3** Lower end, open

821.30 Lower end, unspecified part

821.31 Condyle, femoral

821.32 Epiphysis, lower (separation)

821.33 Supracondylar fracture of femur

821.39 Other

822 Fracture of patella
ALERT! For coding late effect of fracture of lower extremities see 905.4

822.0 Closed

822.1 Open

⑤ **823** Fracture of tibia and fibula
Excludes: Dupuytren's fracture (824.4-824.5)
ankle (824.4-824.5)
radius (813.42, 813.52)
Pott's fracture (824.4-824.5)
that involving ankle (824.0-824.9)

The following fifth-digit subclassification is for use with category 823:

0 tibia alone

1 fibula alone

2 fibula with tibia

● Code new
to 2012 edition
▲ Revision of
existing code
④ ⑤ Fourth or fifth
digit required

[ALERT!] For coding late effect of fracture of lower extremities see 905.4

[5] **823.0** **Upper end, closed**
[0-2]
Head
Proximal end
Tibia:
  condyles
  tuberosity

[5] **823.1** **Upper end, open**
[0-2]

[5] **823.2** **Shaft, closed**
[0-2]

[5] **823.3** **Shaft, open**
[0-2]

[5] **823.4** **Torus fracture**
[0-2]

[5] **823.8** **Unspecified part, closed**
[0-2]
Lower leg NOS

[5] **823.9** **Unspecified part, open**
[0-2]

824 **Fracture of ankle**

[ALERT!] For coding late effect of fracture of lower extremities see 905.4

824.0 **Medial malleolus, closed**
Tibia involving:
  ankle
  malleolus

824.1 **Medial malleolus, open**

824.2 **Lateral malleolus, closed**
Fibula involving:
  ankle
  malleolus

824.3 **Lateral malleolus, open**

824.4 **Bimalleolar, closed**
Dupuytren's fracture, fibula
Pott's fracture

824.5 **Bimalleolar, open**

824.6 **Trimalleolar, closed**
Lateral and medial malleolus with anterior or posterior lip of tibia

824.7 **Trimalleolar, open**

824.8 **Unspecified, closed**
Ankle NOS

824.9 **Unspecified, open**

825 **Fracture of one or more tarsal and metatarsal bones**

[ALERT!] For coding late effect of fracture of lower extremities see 905.4

825.0 **Fracture of calcaneus, closed**
Heel bone
Os calcis

825.1 **Fracture of calcaneus, open**

[5] **825.2** **Fracture of other tarsal and metatarsal bones, closed**

825.20 **Unspecified bone(s) of foot [except toes]**
Instep

825.21 **Astragalus**
Talus

825.22 **Navicular [scaphoid], foot**

825.23 **Cuboid**

825.24 **Cuneiform, foot**

825.25 **Metatarsal bone(s)**

825.29 **Other**
Tarsal with metatarsal bone(s) only

[*Excludes:*] *calcaneus (825.0)*

[5] **825.3** **Fracture of other tarsal and metatarsal bones, open**

825.30 **Unspecified bone(s) of foot [except toes]**

825.31 **Astragalus**

825.32 **Navicular [scaphoid], foot**

825.33 **Cuboid**

825.34 **Cuneiform, foot**

825.35 **Metatarsal bone(s)**

825.39 **Other**

826 Fracture of one or more phalanges of foot
Includes: toe(s)

ALERT! For coding late effect of fracture of lower extremities see 905.4

826.0 **Closed**

826.1 **Open**

827 Other, multiple, and ill-defined fractures of lower limb
Includes: leg NOS
multiple bones of same lower limb

Excludes: *multiple fractures of:*
ankle bones alone (824.4-824.9)
phalanges of foot alone (826.0-826.1)
tarsal with metatarsal bones (825.29, 825.39)
tibia with fibula (823.0-823.9 with fifth-digit 2)

ALERT! For coding late effect of fracture of lower extremities see 905.4

827.0 **Closed**

827.1 **Open**

828 Multiple fractures involving both lower limbs, lower with upper limb, and lower limb(s) with rib(s) and sternum
Includes: arm(s) with leg(s) [any bones]
both legs [any bones]
leg(s) with rib(s) or sternum

ALERT! For coding late effect of fracture of lower extremities see 905.4

828.0 **Closed**

828.1 **Open**

829 Fracture of unspecified bones

ALERT! For coding late effect of fracture of multiple and unspecified bones see 905.5

829.0 **Unspecified bone, closed**

829.1 **Unspecified bone, open**

DISLOCATION (830-839)

Includes: displacement
subluxation

Excludes: *congenital dislocation (754.0-755.8)*
pathological dislocation (718.2)
recurrent dislocation (718.3)

The descriptions "closed" and "open", used in the fourth-digit subdivisions, include the following terms:

closed: open:
  complete   compound
  dislocation NOS   infected
  partial   with foreign body
  simple
  uncomplicated

A dislocation not indicated as closed or open should be classified as closed.

830 Dislocation of jaw
Includes: jaw (cartilage) (meniscus)
mandible
maxilla (inferior)
temporomandibular (joint)

DEFINITION Dislocation refers to the displacement of bones that form a joint, often resulting from trauma.

ALERT! For coding late effect of dislocation see 905.6

830.0 **Closed dislocation**

830.1 **Open dislocation**

● Code new
to 2012 edition ▲ Revision of
existing code ④ ⑤ Fourth or fifth
digit required

⑤ **831** **Dislocation of shoulder**

     Excludes: *sternoclavicular joint (839.61, 839.71)*
               sternum (839.61, 839.71)

    The following fifth-digit subclassification is for use with category 831:

    0 **shoulder, unspecified**
        Humerus NOS

    1 **anterior dislocation of humerus**

    2 **posterior dislocation of humerus**

    3 **inferior dislocation of humerus**

    4 **acromioclavicular (joint)**
        Clavicle

    9 **other**
        Scapula

    ALERT! For coding late effect of dislocation see 905.6

⑤ **831.0** **Closed dislocation**
    [0-4,9]

⑤ **831.1** **Open dislocation**
    [0-4,9]

832 **Dislocation of elbow**

    The following fifth-digit subclassification is for use with subcategories 832.0 and 832.1:

    0 **elbow unspecified**

    1 **anterior dislocation of elbow**

    2 **posterior dislocation of elbow**

    3 **medial dislocation of elbow**

    4 **lateral dislocation of elbow**

    9 **other**

    ALERT! For coding late effect of dislocation see 905.6

⑤ **832.0** **Closed dislocation**
    [0-4,9]

⑤ **832.1** **Open dislocation**
    [0-4,9]

    832.2 Nursemaid's elbow
        Subluxation of radial head

⑤ **833** **Dislocation of wrist**

    The following fifth-digit subclassification is for use with category 833:

    0 **wrist, unspecified part**
        Carpal (bone)   Radius, distal end

    1 **radioulnar (joint), distal**

    2 **radiocarpal (joint)**

    3 **midcarpal (joint)**

    4 **carpometacarpal (joint)**

    5 **metacarpal (bone), proximal end**

    9 **other**
        Ulna, distal end

    ALERT! For coding late effect of dislocation see 905.6

⑤ **833.0** **Closed dislocation**
    [0-5,9]

⑤ **833.1** **Open dislocation**
    [0-5,9]

⑤ **834** **Dislocation of finger**
    Includes: finger(s)
               phalanx of hand
               thumb

The following fifth-digit subclassification is for use with category 834:

  0 **finger, unspecified part**

  1 **metacarpophalangeal (joint)**
     Metacarpal (bone), distal end

  2 **interphalangeal (joint), hand**
  ALERT! For coding late effect of dislocation see 905.6

⑤ **834.0** **Closed dislocation**
   [0-2]

⑤ **834.1** **Open dislocation**
   [0-2]

⑤ **835** **Dislocation of hip**
The following fifth-digit subclassification is for use with category 835:

  0 **dislocation of hip, unspecified**

  1 **posterior dislocation**

  2 **obturator dislocation**

  3 **other anterior dislocation**
  ALERT! For coding late effect of dislocation see 905.6

⑤ **835.0** **Closed dislocation**
   [0-3]

⑤ **835.1** **Open dislocation**
   [0-3]

836 **Dislocation of knee**

   Excludes: *dislocation of knee:*
                  old or pathological (718.2)
                  recurrent (718.3)
              internal derangement of knee joint (717.0-717.5, 717.8-717.9)
              old tear of cartilage or meniscus of knee (717.0-717.5, 717.8-717.9)

   ALERT! For coding late effect of dislocation see 905.6

  836.0 **Tear of medial cartilage or meniscus of knee, current**
     Bucket handle tear:
        NOS current injury
     medial meniscus current injury

  836.1 **Tear of lateral cartilage or meniscus of knee, current**

  836.2 **Other tear of cartilage or meniscus of knee, current**
     Tear of:
        cartilage (semilunar) current injury, not specified as medial or lateral
        meniscus current injury, not specified as medial or lateral

  836.3 **Dislocation of patella, closed**

  836.4 **Dislocation of patella, open**

⑤ **836.5** **Other dislocation of knee, closed**

    836.50 **Dislocation of knee, unspecified**

    836.51 **Anterior dislocation of tibia, proximal end**
       Posterior dislocation of femur, distal end, closed

    836.52 **Posterior dislocation of tibia, proximal end**
       Anterior dislocation of femur, distal end, closed

    836.53 **Medial dislocation of tibia, proximal end**

    836.54 **Lateral dislocation of tibia, proximal end**

    836.59 **Other**

⑤ **836.6** **Other dislocation of knee, open**

    836.60 **Dislocation of knee, unspecified**

    836.61 **Anterior dislocation of tibia, proximal end**
       Posterior dislocation of femur, distal end, open

    836.62 **Posterior dislocation of tibia, proximal end**
       Anterior dislocation of femur, distal end, open

    836.63 **Medial dislocation of tibia, proximal end**

● Code new   ▲ Revision of   ④ ⑤ Fourth or fifth
                 to 2012 edition   existing code   digit required

836.64 Lateral dislocation of tibia, proximal end

836.69 Other

837 Dislocation of ankle

Includes: astragalus
fibula, distal end
navicular, foot
scaphoid, foot
tibia, distal end

[ALERT!] For coding late effect of dislocation see 905.6

837.0 Closed dislocation

837.1 Open dislocation

[5] **838 Dislocation of foot**

The following fifth-digit subclassification is for use with category 838:

0 foot, unspecified

1 tarsal (bone), joint unspecified

2 midtarsal (joint)

3 tarsometatarsal (joint)

4 metatarsal (bone), joint unspecified

5 metatarsophalangeal (joint)

6 interphalangeal (joint), foot

9 other
Phalanx of foot
Toe(s)

[ALERT!] For coding late effect of dislocation see 905.6

[5] **838.0 Closed dislocation**
[0-6,9]

[5] **838.1 Open dislocation**
[0-6,9]

839 Other, multiple, and ill-defined dislocations

[ALERT!] For coding late effect of dislocation see 905.6

[5] **839.0 Cervical vertebra, closed**
Cervical spine
Neck

839.00 Cervical vertebra, unspecified

839.01 First cervical vertebra

839.02 Second cervical vertebra

839.03 Third cervical vertebra

839.04 Fourth cervical vertebra

839.05 Fifth cervical vertebra

839.06 Sixth cervical vertebra

839.07 Seventh cervical vertebra

839.08 Multiple cervical vertebrae

[5] **839.1 Cervical vertebra, open**

839.10 Cervical vertebra, unspecified

839.11 First cervical vertebra

839.12 Second cervical vertebra

839.13 Third cervical vertebra

839.14 Fourth cervical vertebra

839.15 Fifth cervical vertebra

839.16 Sixth cervical vertebra

839.17 Seventh cervical vertebra

839.18 Multiple cervical vertebrae

[5] **839.2 Thoracic and lumbar vertebra, closed**

839.20 Lumbar vertebra

839.21 Thoracic vertebra
Dorsal [thoracic] vertebra

⑤ **839.3 Thoracic and lumbar vertebra, open**

　　839.30 Lumbar vertebra

　　839.31 Thoracic vertebra

⑤ **839.4 Other vertebra, closed**

　　839.40 Vertebra, unspecified site
　　　　Spine NOS

　　839.41 Coccyx

　　839.42 Sacrum
　　　　Sacroiliac (joint)

　　839.49 Other

⑤ **839.5 Other vertebra, open**

　　839.50 Vertebra, unspecified site

　　839.51 Coccyx

　　839.52 Sacrum

　　839.59 Other

⑤ **839.6 Other location, closed**

　　839.61 Sternum
　　　　Sternoclavicular joint

　　839.69 Other
　　　　Pelvis

⑤ **839.7 Other location, open**

　　839.71 Sternum

　　839.79 Other

839.8 Multiple and ill-defined, closed
　　Arm
　　Back
　　Hand
　　Multiple locations, except fingers or toes alone
　　Other ill-defined locations
　　Unspecified location

839.9 Multiple and ill-defined, open

SPRAINS AND STRAINS OF JOINTS AND ADJACENT MUSCLES (840-848)

　　Includes: avulsion of: joint capsule, ligament, muscle, tendon
　　　　　　hemarthrosis of: joint capsule, ligament, muscle, tendon
　　　　　　laceration of: joint capsule, ligament, muscle, tendon
　　　　　　rupture of: joint capsule, ligament, muscle, tendon
　　　　　　sprain of: joint capsule, ligament, muscle, tendon
　　　　　　strain of: joint capsule, ligament, muscle, tendon
　　　　　　tear of: joint capsule, ligament, muscle, tendon

　　Excludes: *laceration of tendon in open wounds (880-884 and 890-894 with .2)*

840 Sprains and strains of shoulder and upper arm
　　DEFINITION Sprain refers to damage or tearing of ligaments or a joint capsule
　　ALERT! For coding late effect of sprain and strain without tendon injury see 905.7
　　ALERT! For coding late effect of tendon injury see 905.8

　　840.0 Acromioclavicular (joint) (ligament)

　　840.1 Coracoclavicular (ligament)

　　840.2 Coracohumeral (ligament)

　　840.3 Infraspinatus (muscle) (tendon)

　　840.4 Rotator cuff (capsule)

　　Excludes: *complete rupture of rotator cuff, nontraumatic (727.61)*

　　840.5 Subscapularis (muscle)

　　840.6 Supraspinatus (muscle) (tendon)

　　840.7 Superior glenoid labrum lesion
　　　　SLAP lesion

　　840.8 Other specified sites of shoulder and upper arm

● Code new
　to 2012 edition
▲ Revision of
　existing code
④ ⑤ Fourth or fifth
　　digit required

840.9 Unspecified site of shoulder and upper arm
Arm NOS
Shoulder NOS

841 Sprains and strains of elbow and forearm
ALERT! For coding late effect of sprain and strain without tendon injury see 905.7
ALERT! For coding late effect of tendon injury see 905.8

841.0 Radial collateral ligament

841.1 Ulnar collateral ligament

841.2 Radiohumeral (joint)

841.3 Ulnohumeral (joint)

841.8 Other specified sites of elbow and forearm

841.9 Unspecified site of elbow and forearm
Elbow NOS

842 Sprains and strains of wrist and hand
ALERT! For coding late effect of sprain and strain without tendon injury see 905.7
ALERT! For coding late effect of tendon injury see 905.8

⑤ **842.0 Wrist**

   842.00 Unspecified site

   842.01 Carpal (joint)

   842.02 Radiocarpal (joint) (ligament)

   842.09 Other
   Radioulnar joint, distal

⑤ **842.1 Hand**

   842.10 Unspecified site

   842.11 Carpometacarpal (joint)

   842.12 Metacarpophalangeal (joint)

   842.13 Interphalangeal (joint)

   842.19 Other
   Midcarpal (joint)

843 Sprains and strains of hip and thigh
ALERT! For coding late effect of sprain and strain without tendon injury see 905.7
ALERT! For coding late effect of tendon injury see 905.8

843.0 Iliofemoral (ligament)

843.1 Ischiocapsular (ligament)

843.8 Other specified sites of hip and thigh

843.9 Unspecified site of hip and thigh
Hip NOS
Thigh NOS

844 Sprains and strains of knee and leg
ALERT! For coding late effect of sprain and strain without tendon injury see 905.7
ALERT! For coding late effect of tendon injury see 905.8

844.0 Lateral collateral ligament of knee

844.1 Medial collateral ligament of knee

844.2 Cruciate ligament of knee

844.3 Tibiofibular (joint) (ligament), superior

844.8 Other specified sites of knee and leg

844.9 Unspecified site of knee and leg
Knee NOS
Leg NOS

845 Sprains and strains of ankle and foot
ALERT! For coding late effect of sprain and strain without tendon injury see 905.7
ALERT! For coding late effect of tendon injury see 905.8

⑤ **845.0 Ankle**

   845.00 Unspecified site

   845.01 Deltoid (ligament), ankle
   Internal collateral (ligament), ankle

	Add 4th or 5th digit		Nonspecific code		Unspecified code		Medicare secondary payer (MSP) alert

845.02 Calcaneofibular (ligament)

845.03 Tibiofibular (ligament), distal

845.09 Other
Achilles tendon

[5] **845.1 Foot**

845.10 Unspecified site

845.11 Tarsometatarsal (joint) (ligament)

845.12 Metatarsophalangeal (joint)

845.13 Interphalangeal (joint), toe

845.19 Other

846 Sprains and strains of sacroiliac region

[ALERT!] For coding late effect of sprain and strain without tendon injury see 905.7

[ALERT!] For coding late effect of tendon injury see 905.8

846.0 Lumbosacral (joint) (ligament)

846.1 Sacroiliac ligament

846.2 Sacrospinatus (ligament)

846.3 Sacrotuberous (ligament)

846.8 Other specified sites of sacroiliac region

846.9 Unspecified site of sacroiliac region

847 Sprains and strains of other and unspecified parts of back

[*Excludes:*] *lumbosacral (846.0)*

[ALERT!] For coding late effect of sprain and strain without tendon injury see 905.7

[ALERT!] For coding late effect of tendon injury see 905.8

847.0 Neck
Anterior longitudinal (ligament), cervical
Atlanto-axial (joints)
Atlanto-occipital (joints)
Whiplash injury

[*Excludes:*] *neck injury NOS (959.0)*
thyroid region (848.2)

847.1 Thoracic

847.2 Lumbar

847.3 Sacrum
Sacrococcygeal (ligament)

847.4 Coccyx

847.9 Unspecified site of back
Back NOS

848 Other and ill-defined sprains and strains

[ALERT!] For coding late effect of sprain and strain without tendon injury see 905.7

[ALERT!] For coding late effect of tendon injury see 905.8

848.0 Septal cartilage of nose

848.1 Jaw
Temporomandibular (joint) (ligament)

848.2 Thyroid region
Cricoarytenoid (joint) (ligament)
Cricothyroid (joint) (ligament)
Thyroid cartilage

848.3 Ribs
Chondrocostal (joint) without mention of injury to sternum
Costal cartilage without mention of injury to sternum

[5] **848.4 Sternum**

848.40 Unspecified site

848.41 Sternoclavicular (joint) (ligament)

848.42 Chondrosternal (joint)

848.49 Other
Xiphoid cartilage

● Code new to 2012 edition ▲ Revision of existing code [4] [5] Fourth or fifth digit required

848.5 Pelvis
Symphysis pubis
[Excludes:] *that in childbirth (665.6)*

848.8 Other specified sites of sprains and strains

848.9 Unspecified site of sprain and strain

INTRACRANIAL INJURY, EXCLUDING THOSE WITH SKULL FRACTURE (850-854)

[Excludes:] *intracranial injury with skull fracture (800-801 and 803-804, except .0 and .5)*
open wound of head without intracranial injury (870.0-873.9)
skull fracture alone (800-801 and 803-804 with .0, .5)

Includes: traumatic brain injury without skull fracture

The description "with open intracranial wound," used in the fourth-digit subdivisions, includes those specified as open or with mention of infection or foreign body.

The following fifth-digit subclassification is for use with categories 851-854:

0 unspecified state of consciousness

1 with no loss of consciousness

2 with brief [less than one hour] loss of consciousness

3 with moderate [1-24 hours] loss of consciousness

4 with prolonged [more than 24 hours] loss of consciousness and return to pre-existing conscious level

5 with prolonged [more than 24 hours] loss of consciousness, without return to pre-existing conscious level
Use fifth-digit 5 to designate when a patient is unconscious and dies before regaining consciousness, regardless of the duration of the loss of consciousness

6 with loss of consciousness of unspecified duration

9 with concussion, unspecified

[ALERT!] For coding late effect of intracranial injury without skull fracture see 907.0

850 Concussion
Includes: commotio cerebri
[Excludes:] *concussion with:*
cerebral laceration or contusion (851.0-851.9)
cerebral hemorrhage (852-853)
head injury NOS (959.01)

[DEFINITION] Concussion is a trauma-induced change in mental status, with confusion and amnesia, and with or without a brief loss of consciousness

[ALERT!] For personal history of traumatic brain injury see V15.52

850.0 With no loss of consciousness
Concussion with mental confusion or disorientation, without loss of consciousness

[5] **850.1 With brief loss of consciousness**
Loss of consciousness for less than one hour

850.11 With loss of consciousness of 30 minutes or less

850.12 With loss of consciousness from 31 to 59 minutes

850.2 With moderate loss of consciousness
Loss of consciousness for 1-24 hours

850.3 With prolonged loss of consciousness and return to pre-existing conscious level
Loss of consciousness for more than 24 hours with complete recovery

850.4 With prolonged loss of consciousness, without return to pre-existing conscious level

850.5 With loss of consciousness of unspecified duration

850.9 Concussion, unspecified

[5] **851 Cerebral laceration and contusion**

[DEFINITION] Cerebral laceration and contusion is a type of traumatic brain injury that occurs when the tissue of the brain is mechanically cut or torn.

[ALERT!] For personal history of traumatic brain injury see V15.52

[5] **851.0 Cortex (cerebral) contusion without mention of open intracranial wound**
[0-6,9]

[5] **851.1 Cortex (cerebral) contusion with open intracranial wound**
[0-6,9]

[5] **851.2 Cortex (cerebral) laceration without mention of open intracranial wound**
[0-6,9]

Add 4th or 5th digit | Nonspecific code | Unspecified code | Medicare secondary payer (MSP) alert

[5] **851.3** **Cortex (cerebral) laceration with open intracranial wound**
[0-6,9]

[5] **851.4** **Cerebellar or brain stem contusion without mention of open intracranial wound**
[0-6,9]

[5] **851.5** **Cerebellar or brain stem contusion with open intracranial wound**
[0-6,9]

[5] **851.6** **Cerebellar or brain stem laceration without mention of open intracranial wound**
[0-6,9]

[5] **851.7** **Cerebellar or brain stem laceration with open intracranial wound**
[0-6,9]

[5] **851.8** **Other and unspecified cerebral laceration and contusion, without mention of open intracranial wound**
[0-6,9] Brain (membrane) NOS

[5] **851.9** **Other and unspecified cerebral laceration and contusion, with open intracranial wound**
[0-6,9]

[5] **852** **Subarachnoid, subdural, and extradural hemorrhage, following injury**

[Excludes:] *Cerebral contusion or laceration (with hemorrhage) (851.0-851.9)*

[DEFINITION] Subarachnoid, subdural, and extradural hemorrhage, following injury, refers to an abnormal condition in which blood collects beneath the arachnoid mater or the dura mater or outside the dura mater

[ALERT!] For personal history of traumatic brain injury see V15.52

[5] **852.0** **Subarachnoid hemorrhage following injury without mention of open intracranial wound**
[0-6,9] Middle meningeal hemorrhage following injury

[5] **852.1** **Subarachnoid hemorrhage following injury with open intracranial wound**
[0-6,9]

[5] **852.2** **Subdural hemorrhage following injury without mention of open intracranial wound**
[0-6,9]

[5] **852.3** **Subdural hemorrhage following injury with open intracranial wound**
[0-6,9]

[5] **852.4** **Extradural hemorrhage following injury without mention of open intracranial wound**
[0-6,9] Epidural hematoma following injury

[5] **852.5** **Extradural hemorrhage following injury with open intracranial wound**
[0-6,9]

[5] **853** **Other and unspecified intracranial hemorrhage following injury**

[DEFINITION] Intracranial hemorrhage refers to bleeding within the cranium due to the loss of integrity of vascular channels and frequently leading to formation of a hematoma.

[ALERT!] For personal history of traumatic brain injury see V15.52

[5] **853.0** **Without mention of open intracranial wound**
[0-6,9] Cerebral compression due to injury
Intracranial hematoma following injury
Traumatic cerebral hemorrhage

[5] **853.1** **With open intracranial wound**
[0-6,9]

[5] **854** **Intracranial injury of other and unspecified nature**

Includes: injury
- brain NOS
- intracranial
- traumatic brain NOS

cavernous sinus

[Excludes:] *any condition classifiable to 850-853*
head injury NOS (959.01)

[ALERT!] For personal history of traumatic brain injury see V15.52

[5] **854.0** **Without mention of open intracranial wound**
[0-6,9]

[5] **854.1** **With open intracranial wound**
[0-6,9]

INTERNAL INJURY OF THORAX, ABDOMEN, AND PELVIS (860-869)

Includes:
>
> blast injuries of internal organs
> blunt trauma of internal organs
> bruise of internal organs
> concussion injuries (except cerebral) of internal organs
> crushing of internal organs
> hematoma of internal organs
> laceration of internal organs
> puncture of internal organs
> tear of internal organs
> traumatic rupture of internal organs

> Excludes: *concussion NOS (850.0-850.9)*
> *flail chest (807.4)*
> *foreign body entering through orifice (930.0-939.9)*
> *injury to blood vessels (901.0-902.9)*

The description "with open wound," used in the fourth-digit subdivisions, includes those with mention of infection or foreign body.

860 **Traumatic pneumothorax and hemothorax**

> **DEFINITION** Pneumothorax is a collection of air or gas in the chest or pleural space that causes part or all of a lung to collapse. Hemothorax is the accumulation of blood in the pleural cavity.

860.0 **Pneumothorax without mention of open wound into thorax**

860.1 **Pneumothorax with open wound into thorax**

860.2 **Hemothorax without mention of open wound into thorax**

860.3 **Hemothorax with open wound into thorax**

860.4 **Pneumohemothorax without mention of open wound into thorax**

860.5 **Pneumohemothorax with open wound into thorax**

861 **Injury to heart and lung**

> Excludes: *injury to blood vessels of thorax (901.0-901.9)*

⑤ **861.0** **Heart, without mention of open wound into thorax**

861.00 **Unspecified injury**

861.01 **Contusion**
Cardiac contusion
Myocardial contusion

861.02 **Laceration without penetration of heart chambers**

861.03 **Laceration with penetration of heart chambers**

⑤ **861.1** **Heart, with open wound into thorax**

861.10 **Unspecified injury**

861.11 **Contusion**

861.12 **Laceration without penetration of heart chambers**

861.13 **Laceration with penetration of heart chambers**

⑤ **861.2** **Lung, without mention of open wound into thorax**

861.20 **Unspecified injury**

861.21 **Contusion**

861.22 **Laceration**

⑤ **861.3** **Lung, with open wound into thorax**

861.30 **Unspecified injury**

861.31 **Contusion**

861.32 **Laceration**

862 **Injury to other and unspecified intrathoracic organs**

> Excludes: *injury to blood vessels of thorax (901.0-901.9)*

862.0 **Diaphragm, without mention of open wound into cavity**

862.1 **Diaphragm, with open wound into cavity**

⑤ **862.2** **Other specified intrathoracic organs, without mention of open wound into cavity**

862.21 **Bronchus**

862.22 **Esophagus**

	Add 4th or 5th digit		Nonspecific code		Unspecified code		Medicare secondary payer (MSP) alert

862.29 Other
Pleura
Thymus gland

⑤ **862.3 Other specified intrathoracic organs, with open wound into cavity**

862.31 Bronchus

862.32 Esophagus

862.39 Other

862.8 Multiple and unspecified intrathoracic organs, without mention of open wound into cavity
Crushed chest
Multiple intrathoracic organs

862.9 Multiple and unspecified intrathoracic organs, with open wound into cavity

863 Injury to gastrointestinal tract

[Excludes:] *anal sphincter laceration during delivery (664.2)*
bile duct (868.0-868.1 with fifth-digit 2)
gallbladder (868.0-868.1 with fifth-digit 2)

863.0 Stomach, without mention of open wound into cavity

863.1 Stomach, with open wound into cavity

⑤ **863.2 Small intestine, without mention of open wound into cavity**

863.20 Small intestine, unspecified site

863.21 Duodenum

863.29 Other

⑤ **863.3 Small intestine, with open wound into cavity**

863.30 Small intestine, unspecified site

863.31 Duodenum

863.39 Other

⑤ **863.4 Colon or rectum, without mention of open wound into cavity**

863.40 Colon, unspecified site

863.41 Ascending [right] colon

863.42 Transverse colon

863.43 Descending [left] colon

863.44 Sigmoid colon

863.45 Rectum

863.46 Multiple sites in colon and rectum

863.49 Other

⑤ **863.5 Colon or rectum, with open wound into cavity**

863.50 Colon, unspecified site

863.51 Ascending [right] colon

863.52 Transverse colon

863.53 Descending [left] colon

863.54 Sigmoid colon

863.55 Rectum

863.56 Multiple sites in colon and rectum

863.59 Other

⑤ **863.8 Other and unspecified gastrointestinal sites, without mention of open wound into cavity**

863.80 Gastrointestinal tract, unspecified site

863.81 Pancreas, head

863.82 Pancreas, body

863.83 Pancreas, tail

863.84 Pancreas, multiple and unspecified sites

863.85 Appendix

863.89 Other
Intestine NOS

● Code new to 2012 edition ▲ Revision of existing code ④ ⑤ Fourth or fifth digit required

[5] **863.9 Other and unspecified gastrointestinal sites, with open wound into cavity**

863.90 Gastrointestinal tract, unspecified site

863.91 Pancreas, head

863.92 Pancreas, body

863.93 Pancreas, tail

863.94 Pancreas, multiple and unspecified sites

863.95 Appendix

863.99 Other

[5] **864 Injury to liver**

The following fifth-digit subclassification is for use with category 864:

0 unspecified injury

1 hematoma and contusion

2 laceration, minor

Laceration involving capsule only, or without significant involvement of hepatic parenchyma [i.e., less than 1 cm deep]

3 laceration, moderate

Laceration involving parenchyma but without major disruption of parenchyma [i.e., less than 10 cm long and less than 3 cm deep]

4 laceration, major

Laceration with significant disruption of hepatic parenchyma [i.e., 10 cm long and 3 cm deep]

Multiple moderate lacerations, with or without hematoma

Stellate lacerations of liver

5 laceration, unspecified

9 other

[5] **864.0 Without mention of open wound into cavity**

[0-5,9]

[5] **864.1 With open wound into cavity**

[0-5,9]

[5] **865 Injury to spleen**

The following fifth-digit subclassification is for use with category 865:

0 unspecified injury

1 hematoma without rupture of capsule

2 capsular tears, without major disruption of parenchyma

3 laceration extending into parenchyma

4 massive parenchymal disruption

9 other

[5] **865.0 Without mention of open wound into cavity**

[0-4,9]

[5] **865.1 With open wound into cavity**

[0-4,9]

[5] **866 Injury to kidney**

[Excludes:] *acute kidney injury (nontraumatic) (584.9)*

The following fifth-digit subclassification is for use with category 866:

0 unspecified injury

1 hematoma without rupture of capsule

2 laceration

3 complete disruption of kidney parenchyma

[5] **866.0 Without mention of open wound into cavity**

[0-3]

[5] **866.1 With open wound into cavity**

[0-3]

867 Injury to pelvic organs

[Excludes:] *injury during delivery (664.0-665.9)*

867.0 Bladder and urethra, without mention of open wound into cavity

867.1 Bladder and urethra, with open wound into cavity

867.2 Ureter, without mention of open wound into cavity

867.3 Ureter, with open wound into cavity

867.4 Uterus, without mention of open wound into cavity

867.5 Uterus, with open wound into cavity

867.6 Other specified pelvic organs, without mention of open wound into cavity
Fallopian tube	Seminal vesicle
Ovary	Vas deferens
Prostate	

867.7 Other specified pelvic organs, with open wound into cavity

867.8 Unspecified pelvic organs, without mention of open wound into cavity

867.9 Unspecified pelvic organ, with open wound into cavity

⑤ **868** Injury to other intra-abdominal organs

The following fifth-digit subclassification is for use with category 868:

   0 unspecified intra-abdominal organ

   1 adrenal gland

   2 bile duct and gallbladder

   3 peritoneum

   4 retroperitoneum

   9 other and multiple intra-abdominal organs

⑤ **868.0** Without mention of open wound into cavity
[0-4,9]

⑤ **868.1** With open wound into cavity
[0-4,9]

869 Internal injury to unspecified or ill-defined organs
Includes: internal injury NOS
           multiple internal injury NOS

869.0 Without mention of open wound into cavity

869.1 With open wound into cavity

OPEN WOUNDS (870-897)

Includes: animal bite
        avulsion
        cut
        laceration
        puncture wound
        traumatic amputation

Excludes: *burn (940.0-949.5)*
crushing (925-929.9)
puncture of internal organs (860.0-869.1)
superficial injury (910.0-919.9)
that incidental to:
  dislocation (830.0-839.9)
  fracture (800.0-829.1)
  internal injury (860.0-869.1)
  intracranial injury (851.0-854.1)

Note: The description "complicated" used in the fourth-digit subdivisions includes those with mention of delayed healing, delayed treatment, foreign body, or infection.

OPEN WOUND OF HEAD, NECK, AND TRUNK (870-879)

870 Open wound of ocular adnexa

ALERT! For coding late effect of open wound of head neck and trunk see 906.0

870.0 Laceration of skin of eyelid and periocular area

870.1 Laceration of eyelid, full-thickness, not involving lacrimal passages

870.2 Laceration of eyelid involving lacrimal passages

870.3 Penetrating wound of orbit, without mention of foreign body

870.4 Penetrating wound of orbit with foreign body

Excludes: *retained (old) foreign body in orbit (376.6)*

870.8 Other specified open wounds of ocular adnexa

870.9 Unspecified open wound of ocular adnexa

● Code new to 2012 edition   ▲ Revision of existing code   ④ ⑤ Fourth or fifth digit required

871 Open wound of eyeball

[Excludes:] *2nd cranial nerve [optic] injury (950.0-950.9)*
3rd cranial nerve [oculomotor] injury (951.0)

[ALERT!] For coding late effect of open wound of head neck and trunk see 906.0

871.0 Ocular laceration without prolapse of intraocular tissue

871.1 Ocular laceration with prolapse or exposure of intraocular tissue

871.2 Rupture of eye with partial loss of intraocular tissue

871.3 Avulsion of eye
Traumatic enucleation

871.4 Unspecified laceration of eye

871.5 Penetration of eyeball with magnetic foreign body

[Excludes:] *retained (old) magnetic foreign body in globe (360.50-360.59)*

871.6 Penetration of eyeball with (nonmagnetic) foreign body

[Excludes:] *retained (old) (nonmagnetic) foreign body in globe (360.60-360.69)*

871.7 Unspecified ocular penetration

871.9 Unspecified open wound of eyeball

872 Open wound of ear

[ALERT!] For coding late effect of open wound of head neck and trunk see 906.0

[5] **872.0 External ear, without mention of complication**

872.00 External ear, unspecified site

872.01 Auricle, ear
Pinna

872.02 Auditory canal

[5] **872.1 External ear, complicated**

872.10 External ear, unspecified site

872.11 Auricle, ear

872.12 Auditory canal

[5] **872.6 Other specified parts of ear, without mention of complication**

872.61 Ear drum
Drumhead
Tympanic membrane

872.62 Ossicles

872.63 Eustachian tube

872.64 Cochlea

872.69 Other and multiple sites

[5] **872.7 Other specified parts of ear, complicated**

872.71 Ear drum

872.72 Ossicles

872.73 Eustachian tube

872.74 Cochlea

872.79 Other and multiple sites

872.8 Ear, part unspecified, without mention of complication
Ear NOS

872.9 Ear, part unspecified, complicated

873 Other open wound of head

[ALERT!] For coding late effect of open wound of head neck and trunk see 906.0

873.0 Scalp, without mention of complication

873.1 Scalp, complicated

[5] **873.2 Nose, without mention of complication**

873.20 Nose, unspecified site

873.21 Nasal septum

873.22 Nasal cavity

873.23 Nasal sinus

873.29 Multiple sites

Add 4th or 5th digit | Nonspecific code | Unspecified code | Medicare secondary payer (MSP) alert

⑤ **873.3 Nose, complicated**

    873.30   Nose, unspecified site

    873.31   Nasal septum

    873.32   Nasal cavity

    873.33   Nasal sinus

    873.39   Multiple sites

⑤ **873.4 Face, without mention of complication**

    873.40   Face, unspecified site

    873.41   Cheek

    873.42   Forehead
            Eyebrow

    873.43   Lip

    873.44   Jaw

    873.49   Other and multiple sites

⑤ **873.5 Face, complicated**

    873.50   Face, unspecified site

    873.51   Cheek

    873.52   Forehead

    873.53   Lip

    873.54   Jaw

    873.59   Other and multiple sites

⑤ **873.6 Internal structures of mouth, without mention of complication**

    873.60   Mouth, unspecified site

    873.61   Buccal mucosa

    873.62   Gum (alveolar process)

    873.63   Tooth (broken) (fractured) (due to trauma)

    Excludes: *cracked tooth (521.81)*

    873.64   Tongue and floor of mouth

    873.65   Palate

    873.69   Other and multiple sites

⑤ **873.7 Internal structures of mouth, complicated**

    873.70   Mouth, unspecified site

    873.71   Buccal mucosa

    873.72   Gum (alveolar process)

    873.73   Tooth (broken) (fractured) (due to trauma)

    Excludes: *cracked tooth (521.81)*

    873.74   Tongue and floor of mouth

    873.75   Palate

    873.79   Other and multiple sites

873.8 Other and unspecified open wound of head without mention of complication
    Head NOS

873.9 Other and unspecified open wound of head, complicated

874 Open wound of neck

    ALERT! For coding late effect of open wound of head neck and trunk see 906.0

⑤ **874.0 Larynx and trachea, without mention of complication**

    874.00   Larynx with trachea

    874.01   Larynx

    874.02   Trachea

⑤ **874.1 Larynx and trachea, complicated**

    874.10   Larynx with trachea

    874.11   Larynx

    874.12   Trachea

| ● Code new to 2012 edition | ▲ Revision of existing code | ④ ⑤ Fourth or fifth digit required |

874.2 Thyroid gland, without mention of complication

874.3 Thyroid gland, complicated

874.4 Pharynx, without mention of complication
Cervical esophagus

874.5 Pharynx, complicated

874.8 Other and unspecified parts, without mention of complication
Nape of neck   Throat NOS
Supraclavicular region

874.9 Other and unspecified parts, complicated

875 Open wound of chest (wall)

Excludes: *open wound into thoracic cavity (860.0-862.9)*
traumatic pneumothorax and hemothorax (860.1, 860.3, 860.5)

ALERT! For coding late effect of open wound of head neck and trunk see 906.0

875.0 Without mention of complication

875.1 Complicated

876 Open wound of back
Includes: loin
lumbar region

Excludes: *open wound into thoracic cavity (860.0-862.9)*
traumatic pneumothorax and hemothorax (860.1, 860.3, 860.5)

ALERT! For coding late effect of open wound of head neck and trunk see 906.0

876.0 Without mention of complication

876.1 Complicated

877 Open wound of buttock
Includes: sacroiliac region

ALERT! For coding late effect of open wound of head neck and trunk see 906.0

877.0 Without mention of complication

877.1 Complicated

878 Open wound of genital organs (external), including traumatic amputation

Excludes: *injury during delivery (664.0-665.9)*
internal genital organs (867.0-867.9)

ALERT! For coding late effect of open wound of head neck and trunk see 906.0
ALERT! For coding late effect of traumatic amputation see 905.9

878.0 Penis, without mention of complication

878.1 Penis, complicated

878.2 Scrotum and testes, without mention of complication

878.3 Scrotum and testes, complicated

878.4 Vulva, without mention of complication
Labium (majus) (minus)

878.5 Vulva, complicated

878.6 Vagina, without mention of complication

878.7 Vagina, complicated

878.8 Other and unspecified parts, without mention of complication

878.9 Other and unspecified parts, complicated

879 Open wound of other and unspecified sites, except limbs

ALERT! For coding late effect of open wound of head neck and trunk see 906.0

879.0 Breast, without mention of complication

879.1 Breast, complicated

879.2 Abdominal wall, anterior, without mention of complication
Abdominal wall NOS   Pubic region
Epigastric region   Umbilical region
Hypogastric region

879.3 Abdominal wall, anterior, complicated

879.4 Abdominal wall, lateral, without mention of complication
Flank   Iliac (region)
Groin   Inguinal region
Hypochondrium

| | Add 4th or 5th digit | | Nonspecific code | | Unspecified code | | Medicare secondary payer (MSP) alert |

879.5 **Abdominal wall, lateral, complicated**

879.6 **Other and unspecified parts of trunk, without mention of complication**
Pelvic region   Trunk NOS
Perineum

879.7 **Other and unspecified parts of trunk, complicated**

879.8 **Open wound(s) (multiple) of unspecified site(s) without mention of complication**
Multiple open wounds NOS
Open wound NOS

879.9 **Open wound(s) (multiple) of unspecified site(s), complicated**

OPEN WOUND OF UPPER LIMB (880-887)

⑤ **880** **Open wound of shoulder and upper arm**
The following fifth-digit subclassification is for use with category 880:

 0 **shoulder region**

 1 **scapular region**

 2 **axillary region**

 3 **upper arm**

 9 **multiple sites**

 ALERT! For coding late effect of open wound of extremities without tendon injury see 906.1

⑤ **880.0** **Without mention of complication**

⑤ **880.1** **Complicated**

⑤ **880.2** **With tendon involvement**

⑤ **881** **Open wound of elbow, forearm, and wrist**
The following fifth-digit subclassification is for use with category 881:

 0 **forearm**

 1 **elbow**

 2 **wrist**

 ALERT! For coding late effect of open wound of extremities without tendon injury see 906.1

⑤ **881.0** **Without mention of complication**

⑤ **881.1** **Complicated**

⑤ **881.2** **With tendon involvement**

882 **Open wound of hand except finger(s) alone**
 ALERT! For coding late effect of open wound of extremities without tendon injury see 906.1

882.0 **Without mention of complication**

882.1 **Complicated**

882.2 **With tendon involvement**

883 **Open wound of finger(s)**
Includes: fingernail
   thumb (nail)
 ALERT! For coding late effect of open wound of extremities without tendon injury see 906.1

883.0 **Without mention of complication**

883.1 **Complicated**

883.2 **With tendon involvement**

884 **Multiple and unspecified open wound of upper limb**
Includes: arm NOS
   multiple sites of one upper limb
   upper limb NOS
 ALERT! For coding late effect of open wound of extremities without tendon injury see 906.1

884.0 **Without mention of complication**

884.1 **Complicated**

884.2 **With tendon involvement**

885 **Traumatic amputation of thumb (complete) (partial)**
Includes: thumb(s) (with finger(s) of either hand)
 ALERT! For coding late effect of traumatic amputation see 905.9

885.0 **Without mention of complication**

885.1 **Complicated**

● Code new   ▲ Revision of   ④ ⑤ Fourth or fifth
 to 2012 edition   existing code   digit required

886 Traumatic amputation of other finger(s) (complete) (partial)
Includes: finger(s) of one or both hands, without mention of thumb(s)
ALERT! For coding late effect of traumatic amputation see 905.9

886.0 **Without mention of complication**

886.1 **Complicated**

887 Traumatic amputation of arm and hand (complete) (partial)
ALERT! For coding late effect of traumatic amputation see 905.9

887.0 **Unilateral, below elbow, without mention of complication**

887.1 **Unilateral, below elbow, complicated**

887.2 **Unilateral, at or above elbow, without mention of complication**

887.3 **Unilateral, at or above elbow, complicated**

887.4 **Unilateral, level not specified, without mention of complication**

887.5 **Unilateral, level not specified, complicated**

887.6 **Bilateral [any level], without mention of complication**
One hand and other arm

887.7 **Bilateral [any level], complicated**

OPEN WOUND OF LOWER LIMB (890-897)

890 Open wound of hip and thigh
ALERT! For coding late effect of open wound of extremities without tendon injury see 906.1

890.0 **Without mention of complication**

890.1 **Complicated**

890.2 **With tendon involvement**

891 Open wound of knee, leg [except thigh], and ankle
Includes: leg NOS
multiple sites of leg, except thigh
Excludes: *that of thigh (890.0-890.2)*
with multiple sites of lower limb (894.0-894.2)
ALERT! For coding late effect of open wound of extremities without tendon injury see 906.1

891.0 **Without mention of complication**

891.1 **Complicated**

891.2 **With tendon involvement**

892 Open wound of foot except toe(s) alone
Includes: heel
ALERT! For coding late effect of open wound of extremities without tendon injury see 906.1

892.0 **Without mention of complication**

892.1 **Complicated**

892.2 **With tendon involvement**

893 Open wound of toe(s)
Includes: toenail
ALERT! For coding late effect of open wound of extremities without tendon injury see 906.1

893.0 **Without mention of complication**

893.1 **Complicated**

893.2 **With tendon involvement**

894 Multiple and unspecified open wound of lower limb
Includes: lower limb NOS
multiple sites of one lower limb, with thigh
ALERT! For coding late effect of open wound of extremities without tendon injury see 906.1

894.0 **Without mention of complication**

894.1 **Complicated**

894.2 **With tendon involvement**

895 Traumatic amputation of toe(s) (complete) (partial)
Includes: toe(s) of one or both feet
ALERT! For coding late effect of traumatic amputation see 905.9

895.0 **Without mention of complication**

895.1 **Complicated**

Add 4th or 5th digit	Nonspecific code	Unspecified code	Medicare secondary payer (MSP) alert

896 Traumatic amputation of foot (complete) (partial)

[ALERT!] For coding late effect of traumatic amputation see 905.9

896.0 Unilateral, without mention of complication

896.1 Unilateral, complicated

896.2 Bilateral, without mention of complication

[Excludes:] *one foot and other leg (897.6-897.7)*

896.3 Bilateral, complicated

897 Traumatic amputation of leg(s) (complete) (partial)

[ALERT!] For coding late effect of traumatic amputation see 905.9

897.0 Unilateral, below knee, without mention of complication

897.1 Unilateral, below knee, complicated

897.2 Unilateral, at or above knee, without mention of complication

897.3 Unilateral, at or above knee, complicated

897.4 Unilateral, level not specified, without mention of complication

897.5 Unilateral, level not specified, complicated

897.6 Bilateral [any level], without mention of complication

One foot and other leg

897.7 Bilateral [any level], complicated

INJURY TO BLOOD VESSELS (900-904)

Includes: arterial hematoma of blood vessel, secondary to other injuries e.g., fracture or open wound
avulsion of blood vessel, secondary to other injuries e.g., fracture or open wound
cut of blood vessel, secondary to other injuries e.g., fracture or open wound
laceration of blood vessel, secondary to other injuries e.g., fracture or open wound
rupture of blood vessel, secondary to other injuries e.g., fracture or open wound
traumatic aneurysm or fistula (arteriovenous) of blood vessel, secondary to other injuries e.g., fracture or open wound

[Excludes:] *accidental puncture or laceration during medical procedure (998.2)*
intracranial hemorrhage following injury (851.0-854.1)

900 Injury to blood vessels of head and neck

[ALERT!] For coding late effect of injury to blood vessel of head neck and extremities see 908.3

[5] **900.0 Carotid artery**

900.00 Carotid artery, unspecified

900.01 Common carotid artery

900.02 External carotid artery

900.03 Internal carotid artery

900.1 Internal jugular vein

[5] **900.8 Other specified blood vessels of head and neck**

900.81 External jugular vein

Jugular vein NOS

900.82 Multiple blood vessels of head and neck

900.89 Other

900.9 Unspecified blood vessel of head and neck

901 Injury to blood vessels of thorax

[Excludes:] *traumatic hemothorax (860.2-860.5)*

[ALERT!] For coding late effect of injury to blood vessel of thorax abdomen and pelvis see 908.4

901.0 Thoracic aorta

901.1 Innominate and subclavian arteries

901.2 Superior vena cava

901.3 Innominate and subclavian veins

[5] **901.4 Pulmonary blood vessels**

901.40 Pulmonary vessel(s), unspecified

901.41 Pulmonary artery

● Code new to 2012 edition ▲ Revision of existing code [4] [5] Fourth or fifth digit required

901.42 Pulmonary vein

[5] **901.8 Other specified blood vessels of thorax**

901.81 Intercostal artery or vein

901.82 Internal mammary artery or vein

901.83 Multiple blood vessels of thorax

901.89 Other
Azygos vein
Hemiazygos vein

901.9 Unspecified blood vessel of thorax

902 Injury to blood vessels of abdomen and pelvis
ALERT! For coding late effect of injury to blood vessel of thorax abdomen and pelvis see 908.4

902.0 Abdominal aorta

[5] **902.1 Inferior vena cava**

902.10 Inferior vena cava, unspecified

902.11 Hepatic veins

902.19 Other

[5] **902.2 Celiac and mesenteric arteries**

902.20 Celiac and mesenteric arteries, unspecified

902.21 Gastric artery

902.22 Hepatic artery

902.23 Splenic artery

902.24 Other specified branches of celiac axis

902.25 Superior mesenteric artery (trunk)

902.26 Primary branches of superior mesenteric artery
Ileo-colic artery

902.27 Inferior mesenteric artery

902.29 Other

[5] **902.3 Portal and splenic veins**

902.31 Superior mesenteric vein and primary subdivisions
Ileo-colic vein

902.32 Inferior mesenteric vein

902.33 Portal vein

902.34 Splenic vein

902.39 Other
Cystic vein
Gastric vein

[5] **902.4 Renal blood vessels**

902.40 Renal vessel(s), unspecified

902.41 Renal artery

902.42 Renal vein

902.49 Other
Suprarenal arteries

[5] **902.5 Iliac blood vessels**

902.50 Iliac vessel(s), unspecified

902.51 Hypogastric artery

902.52 Hypogastric vein

902.53 Iliac artery

902.54 Iliac vein

902.55 Uterine artery

902.56 Uterine vein

902.59 Other

[5] **902.8 Other specified blood vessels of abdomen and pelvis**

902.81 Ovarian artery

902.82 Ovarian vein

902.87   **Multiple blood vessels of abdomen and pelvis**

902.89   **Other**

902.9 Unspecified blood vessel of abdomen and pelvis

903 Injury to blood vessels of upper extremity

    ALERT! For coding late effect of injury to blood vessel of head neck and extremities see 908.3

⑤ **903.0 Axillary blood vessels**

    903.00   **Axillary vessel(s), unspecified**

    903.01   **Axillary artery**

    903.02   **Axillary vein**

903.1 Brachial blood vessels

903.2 Radial blood vessels

903.3 Ulnar blood vessels

903.4 Palmar artery

903.5 Digital blood vessels

903.8 Other specified blood vessels of upper extremity
    Multiple blood vessels of upper extremity

903.9 Unspecified blood vessel of upper extremity

904 Injury to blood vessels of lower extremity and unspecified sites

    ALERT! For coding late effect of injury to blood vessel of head neck and extremities see 908.3

904.0 Common femoral artery
    Femoral artery above profunda origin

904.1 Superficial femoral artery

904.2 Femoral veins

904.3 Saphenous veins
    Saphenous vein (greater) (lesser)

⑤ **904.4 Popliteal blood vessels**

    904.40   **Popliteal vessel(s), unspecified**

    904.41   **Popliteal artery**

    904.42   **Popliteal vein**

⑤ **904.5 Tibial blood vessels**

    904.50   **Tibial vessel(s), unspecified**

    904.51   **Anterior tibial artery**

    904.52   **Anterior tibial vein**

    904.53   **Posterior tibial artery**

    904.54   **Posterior tibial vein**

904.6 Deep plantar blood vessels

904.7 Other specified blood vessels of lower extremity
    Multiple blood vessels of lower extremity

904.8 Unspecified blood vessel of lower extremity

904.9 Unspecified site
    Injury to blood vessel NOS

LATE EFFECTS OF INJURIES, POISONINGS, TOXIC EFFECTS, AND OTHER EXTERNAL CAUSES (905-909)

Note: These categories are to be used to indicate conditions classifiable to 800-999 as the cause of late effects, which are themselves classified elsewhere. The "late effects" include those specified as such, or as sequelae, which may occur at any time after the acute injury.

905 Late effects of musculoskeletal and connective tissue injuries

    DEFINITION Late effects of musculoskeletal and connective tissue injuries refers to a condition that appears after the acute phase of the musculoskeletal and connective tissue injuries has run its course

905.0 Late effect of fracture of skull and face bones
    Late effect of injury classifiable to 800-804

905.1 Late effect of fracture of spine and trunk without mention of spinal cord lesion
    Late effect of injury classifiable to 805, 807-809

905.2 Late effect of fracture of upper extremities
    Late effect of injury classifiable to 810-819

● Code new to 2012 edition   ▲ Revision of existing code   ④ ⑤ Fourth or fifth digit required

905.3 Late effect of fracture of neck of femur
Late effect of injury classifiable to 820

905.4 Late effect of fracture of lower extremities
Late effect of injury classifiable to 821-827

905.5 Late effect of fracture of multiple and unspecified bones
Late effect of injury classifiable to 828-829

905.6 Late effect of dislocation
Late effect of injury classifiable to 830-839

905.7 Late effect of sprain and strain without mention of tendon injury
Late effect of injury classifiable to 840-848, except tendon injury

905.8 Late effect of tendon injury
Late effect of tendon injury due to:
open wound [injury classifiable to 880-884 with .2, 890-894 with .2]
sprain and strain [injury classifiable to 840-848]

905.9 Late effect of traumatic amputation
Late effect of injury classifiable to 885-887, 895-897

> *Excludes:* late amputation stump complication (997.60-997.69)

906 Late effects of injuries to skin and subcutaneous tissues
> **DEFINITION** Late effects of injuries to skin and subcutaneous tissues refers to a condition that appears after the acute phase of the skin and subcutaneous tissues injuries has run its course

906.0 Late effect of open wound of head, neck, and trunk
Late effect of injury classifiable to 870-879

906.1 Late effect of open wound of extremities without mention of tendon injury
Late effect of injury classifiable to 880-884, 890-894 except .2

906.2 Late effect of superficial injury
Late effect of injury classifiable to 910-919

906.3 Late effect of contusion
Late effect of injury classifiable to 920-924

906.4 Late effect of crushing
Late effect of injury classifiable to 925-929

906.5 Late effect of burn of eye, face, head, and neck
Late effect of injury classifiable to 940-941

906.6 Late effect of burn of wrist and hand
Late effect of injury classifiable to 944

906.7 Late effect of burn of other extremities
Late effect of injury classifiable to 943 or 945

906.8 Late effect of burns of other specified sites
Late effect of injury classifiable to 942, 946-947

906.9 Late effect of burn of unspecified site
Late effect of injury classifiable to 948-949

907 Late effects of injuries to the nervous system
> **DEFINITION** Late effects of injuries to the nervous system refers to a condition that appears after the acute phase of the nervous system has run its course.

907.0 Late effect of intracranial injury without mention of skull fracture
Late effect of injury classifiable to 850-854

907.1 Late effect of injury to cranial nerve
Late effect of injury classifiable to 950-951

907.2 Late effect of spinal cord injury
Late effect of injury classifiable to 806, 952

907.3 Late effect of injury to nerve root(s), spinal plexus(es), and other nerves of trunk
Late effect of injury classifiable to 953-954

907.4 Late effect of injury to peripheral nerve of shoulder girdle and upper limb
Late effect of injury classifiable to 955

907.5 Late effect of injury to peripheral nerve of pelvic girdle and lower limb
Late effect of injury classifiable to 956

907.9 Late effect of injury to other and unspecified nerve
Late effect of injury classifiable to 957

908 Late effects of other and unspecified injuries

908.0 Late effect of internal injury to chest
Late effect of injury classifiable to 860-862

Add 4th or 5th digit	Nonspecific code	Unspecified code	Medicare secondary payer (MSP) alert

908.1 Late effect of internal injury to intra-abdominal organs
Late effect of injury classifiable to 863-866, 868

908.2 Late effect of internal injury to other internal organs
Late effect of injury classifiable to 867 or 869

908.3 Late effect of injury to blood vessel of head, neck, and extremities
Late effect of injury classifiable to 900, 903-904

908.4 Late effect of injury to blood vessel of thorax, abdomen, and pelvis
Late effect of injury classifiable to 901-902

908.5 Late effect of foreign body in orifice
Late effect of injury classifiable to 930-939

908.6 Late effect of certain complications of trauma
Late effect of complications classifiable to 958

908.9 Late effect of unspecified injury
Late effect of injury classifiable to 959

909 Late effects of other and unspecified external causes

909.0 Late effect of poisoning due to drug, medicinal or biological substance
Late effect of conditions classifiable to 960-979

Excludes: late effect of adverse effect of drug, medicinal or biological substance (909.5)

909.1 Late effect of toxic effects of nonmedical substances
Late effect of conditions classifiable to 980-989

909.2 Late effect of radiation
Late effect of conditions classifiable to 990

909.3 Late effect of complications of surgical and medical care
Late effect of conditions classifiable to 996-999

909.4 Late effect of certain other external causes
Late effect of conditions classifiable to 991-994

909.5 Late effect of adverse effect of drug, medicinal or biological substance

Excludes: late effect of poisoning due to drug, medicinal or biological substance (909.0)

909.9 Late effect of other and unspecified external causes

SUPERFICIAL INJURY (910-919)

Excludes: burn (blisters) (940.0-949.5)
contusion (920-924.9)
foreign body:
  granuloma (728.82)
  inadvertently left in operative wound (998.4)
  residual, in soft tissue (729.6)
insect bite, venomous (989.5)
open wound with incidental foreign body (870.0-897.7)

910 Superficial injury of face, neck, and scalp except eye
Includes: cheek
            ear
            gum
            lip
            nose
            throat

Excludes: eye and adnexa (918.0-918.9)

ALERT! For coding late effect of superficial injury see 906.2

910.0 Abrasion or friction burn without mention of infection

910.1 Abrasion or friction burn, infected

910.2 Blister without mention of infection

910.3 Blister, infected

910.4 Insect bite, nonvenomous, without mention of infection

910.5 Insect bite, nonvenomous, infected

910.6 Superficial foreign body (splinter) without major open wound and without mention of infection

910.7 Superficial foreign body (splinter) without major open wound, infected

910.8 Other and unspecified superficial injury of face, neck, and scalp without mention of infection

910.9 Other and unspecified superficial injury of face, neck, and scalp, infected

● Code new
to 2012 edition

▲ Revision of
existing code

④ ⑤ Fourth or fifth
digit required

911 **Superficial injury of trunk**
　　Includes:

abdominal wall	interscapular region
anus	labium (majus) (minus)
back	penis
breast	perineum
buttock	scrotum
chest wall	testis
flank	vagina
groin	vulva

　　Excludes: *hip (916.0-916.9)*
　　　　　　　scapular region (912.0-912.9)

　　ALERT! For coding late effect of superficial injury see 906.2

911.0 **Abrasion or friction burn without mention of infection**

911.1 **Abrasion or friction burn, infected**

911.2 **Blister without mention of infection**

911.3 **Blister, infected**

911.4 **Insect bite, nonvenomous, without mention of infection**

911.5 **Insect bite, nonvenomous, infected**

911.6 **Superficial foreign body (splinter) without major open wound and without mention of infection**

911.7 **Superficial foreign body (splinter) without major open wound, infected**

911.8 **Other and unspecified superficial injury of trunk without mention of infection**

911.9 **Other and unspecified superficial injury of trunk, infected**

912 **Superficial injury of shoulder and upper arm**
　　Includes:　axilla　　　　scapular region

　　ALERT! For coding late effect of superficial injury see 906.2

912.0 **Abrasion or friction burn without mention of infection**

912.1 **Abrasion or friction burn, infected**

912.2 **Blister without mention of infection**

912.3 **Blister, infected**

912.4 **Insect bite, nonvenomous, without mention of infection**

912.5 **Insect bite, nonvenomous, infected**

912.6 **Superficial foreign body (splinter) without major open wound and without mention of infection**

912.7 **Superficial foreign body (splinter) without major open wound, infected**

912.8 **Other and unspecified superficial injury of shoulder and upper arm without mention of infection**

912.9 **Other and unspecified superficial injury of shoulder and upper arm, infected**

913 **Superficial injury of elbow, forearm, and wrist**

　　ALERT! For coding late effect of superficial injury see 906.2

913.0 **Abrasion or friction burn without mention of infection**

913.1 **Abrasion or friction burn, infected**

913.2 **Blister without mention of infection**

913.3 **Blister, infected**

913.4 **Insect bite, nonvenomous, without mention of infection**

913.5 **Insect bite, nonvenomous, infected**

913.6 **Superficial foreign body (splinter) without major open wound and without mention of infection**

913.7 **Superficial foreign body (splinter) without major open wound, infected**

913.8 **Other and unspecified superficial injury of elbow, forearm, and wrist without mention of infection**

913.9 **Other and unspecified superficial injury of elbow, forearm, and wrist, infected**

914 **Superficial injury of hand(s) except finger(s) alone**

　　ALERT! For coding late effect of superficial injury see 906.2

914.0 **Abrasion or friction burn without mention of infection**

914.1 **Abrasion or friction burn, infected**

▓ Add 4th or 5th digit	▓ Nonspecific code	░ Unspecified code	▒ Medicare secondary payer (MSP) alert

914.2 Blister without mention of infection

914.3 Blister, infected

914.4 Insect bite, nonvenomous, without mention of infection

914.5 Insect bite, nonvenomous, infected

914.6 Superficial foreign body (splinter) without major open wound and without mention of infection

914.7 Superficial foreign body (splinter) without major open wound, infected

914.8 Other and unspecified superficial injury of hand without mention of infection

914.9 Other and unspecified superficial injury of hand, infected

915 Superficial injury of finger(s)

Includes: fingernail   thumb (nail)

ALERT! For coding late effect of superficial injury see 906.2

915.0 Abrasion or friction burn without mention of infection

915.1 Abrasion or friction burn, infected

915.2 Blister without mention of infection

915.3 Blister, infected

915.4 Insect bite, nonvenomous, without mention of infection

915.5 Insect bite, nonvenomous, infected

915.6 Superficial foreign body (splinter) without major open wound and without mention of infection

915.7 Superficial foreign body (splinter) without major open wound, infected

915.8 Other and unspecified superficial injury of fingers without mention of infection

915.9 Other and unspecified superficial injury of fingers, infected

916 Superficial injury of hip, thigh, leg, and ankle

ALERT! For coding late effect of superficial injury see 906.2

916.0 Abrasion or friction burn without mention of infection

916.1 Abrasion or friction burn, infected

916.2 Blister without mention of infection

916.3 Blister, infected

916.4 Insect bite, nonvenomous, without mention of infection

916.5 Insect bite, nonvenomous, infected

916.6 Superficial foreign body (splinter) without major open wound and without mention of infection

916.7 Superficial foreign body (splinter) without major open wound, infected

916.8 Other and unspecified superficial injury of hip, thigh, leg, and ankle without mention of infection

916.9 Other and unspecified superficial injury of hip, thigh, leg, and ankle, infected

917 Superficial injury of foot and toe(s)

Includes: heel   toenail

ALERT! For coding late effect of superficial injury see 906.2

917.0 Abrasion or friction burn without mention of infection

917.1 Abrasion or friction burn, infected

917.2 Blister without mention of infection

917.3 Blister, infected

917.4 Insect bite, nonvenomous, without mention of infection

917.5 Insect bite, nonvenomous, infected

917.6 Superficial foreign body (splinter) without major open wound and without mention of infection

917.7 Superficial foreign body (splinter) without major open wound, infected

917.8 Other and unspecified superficial injury of foot and toes without mention of infection

917.9 Other and unspecified superficial injury of foot and toes, infected

● Code new
to 2012 edition   ▲ Revision of
existing code   ④ ⑤ Fourth or fifth
digit required

918 **Superficial injury of eye and adnexa**

Excludes: burn (940.0-940.9)

foreign body on external eye (930.0-930.9)

ALERT! For coding late effect of superficial injury see 906.2

918.0 Eyelids and periocular area
Abrasion   Superficial foreign body (splinter)
Insect bite

918.1 Cornea
Corneal abrasion
Superficial laceration

Excludes: corneal injury due to contact lens (371.82)

918.2 Conjunctiva

918.9 Other and unspecified superficial injuries of eye
Eye (ball) NOS

919 **Superficial injury of other, multiple, and unspecified sites**

Excludes: multiple sites classifiable to the same three-digit category (910.0-918.9)

ALERT! For coding late effect of superficial injury see 906.2

919.0 Abrasion or friction burn without mention of infection

919.1 Abrasion or friction burn, infected

919.2 Blister without mention of infection

919.3 Blister, infected

919.4 Insect bite, nonvenomous, without mention of infection

919.5 Insect bite, nonvenomous, infected

919.6 Superficial foreign body (splinter) without major open wound and without mention of infection

919.7 Superficial foreign body (splinter) without major open wound, infected

919.8 Other and unspecified superficial injury without mention of infection

919.9 Other and unspecified superficial injury, infected

CONTUSION WITH INTACT SKIN SURFACE (920-924)

Includes: bruise without fracture or open wound
hematoma without fracture or open wound

Excludes: concussion (850.0-850.9)

hemarthrosis (840.0-848.9)
internal organs (860.0-869.1)
that incidental to:
crushing injury (925-929.9)
dislocation (830.0-839.9)
fracture (800.0-829.1)
internal injury (860.0-869.1)
intracranial injury (850.0-854.1)
nerve injury (950.0-957.9)
open wound (870.0-897.7)

920 Contusion of face, scalp, and neck except eye(s)
Cheek   Mandibular joint area
Ear (auricle)   Nose
Gum   Throat
Lip

DEFINITION A Contusion, aka bruise, is an injury caused by a blow to the muscle, tendon or ligament; occurs when blood pools around the injury and discolors the skin.

ALERT! For coding late effect of contusion see 906.3

921 **Contusion of eye and adnexa**

ALERT! For coding late effect of contusion see 906.3

921.0 Black eye, not otherwise specified

921.1 Contusion of eyelids and periocular area

921.2 Contusion of orbital tissues

921.3 Contusion of eyeball

921.9 Unspecified contusion of eye
Injury of eye NOS

| Add 4th or 5th digit | Nonspecific code | Unspecified code | Medicare secondary payer (MSP) alert |

922 Contusion of trunk

[ALERT!] For coding late effect of contusion see 906.3

922.0 Breast

922.1 Chest wall

922.2 Abdominal wall
Flank
Groin

⑤ **922.3 Back**

[Excludes:] scapular region (923.01)

922.31 Back

[Excludes:] interscapular region (922.33)

922.32 Buttock

922.33 Interscapular region

922.4 Genital organs
Labium (majus) (minus)
Penis
Perineum
Scrotum
Testis
Vagina
Vulva

922.8 Multiple sites of trunk

922.9 Unspecified part
Trunk NOS

923 Contusion of upper limb

[ALERT!] For coding late effect of contusion see 906.3

⑤ **923.0 Shoulder and upper arm**

923.00 Shoulder region

923.01 Scapular region

923.02 Axillary region

923.03 Upper arm

923.09 Multiple sites

⑤ **923.1 Elbow and forearm**

923.10 Forearm

923.11 Elbow

⑤ **923.2 Wrist and hand(s), except finger(s) alone**

923.20 Hand(s)

923.21 Wrist

923.3 Finger
Fingernail
Thumb (nail)

923.8 Multiple sites of upper limb

923.9 Unspecified part of upper limb
Arm NOS

924 Contusion of lower limb and of other and unspecified sites

[ALERT!] For coding late effect of contusion see 906.3

⑤ **924.0 Hip and thigh**

924.00 Thigh

924.01 Hip

⑤ **924.1 Knee and lower leg**

924.10 Lower leg

924.11 Knee

⑤ **924.2 Ankle and foot, excluding toe(s)**

924.20 Foot
Heel

924.21 Ankle

924.3 Toe
Toenail

● Code new to 2012 edition ▲ Revision of existing code ④ ⑤ Fourth or fifth digit required

924.4 Multiple sites of lower limb

924.5 Unspecified part of lower limb
Leg NOS

924.8 Multiple sites, not elsewhere classified

924.9 Unspecified site

CRUSHING INJURY (925-929)

Use additional code to identify any associated injuries, such as:
fractures (800-829)
internal injuries (860.0-869.1)
intracranial injury (850.0-854.1)

925 Crushing injury of face, scalp, and neck
Cheek
Ear
Larynx
Pharynx
Throat

[ALERT!] For coding late effect of crushing see 906.4

925.1 Crushing injury of face and scalp
Cheek
Ear

925.2 Crushing injury of neck
Larynx
Pharynx
Throat

926 Crushing injury of trunk

[DEFINITION] A crushing injury occurs when a body part is subjected to a high degree of force or pressure, usually after being squeezed between two heavy objects

[ALERT!] For coding late effect of crushing see 906.4

926.0 External genitalia
Labium (majus) (minus)
Penis
Scrotum
Testis
Vulva

[5] **926.1 Other specified sites**

926.11 Back

926.12 Buttock

926.19 Other
Breast

926.8 Multiple sites of trunk

926.9 Unspecified site
Trunk NOS

927 Crushing injury of upper limb

[ALERT!] For coding late effect of crushing see 906.4

[5] **927.0 Shoulder and upper arm**

927.00 Shoulder region

927.01 Scapular region

927.02 Axillary region

927.03 Upper arm

927.09 Multiple sites

[5] **927.1 Elbow and forearm**

927.10 Forearm

927.11 Elbow

[5] **927.2 Wrist and hand(s), except finger(s) alone**

927.20 Hand(s)

927.21 Wrist

927.3 Finger(s)

927.8 Multiple sites of upper limb

927.9 Unspecified site
Arm NOS

928 Crushing injury of lower limb

[ALERT!] For coding late effect of crushing see 906.4

[5] **928.0 Hip and thigh**

Add 4th or 5th digit | Nonspecific code | Unspecified code | Medicare secondary payer (MSP) alert

928.00 Thigh

928.01 Hip

[5] **928.1 Knee and lower leg**

928.10 Lower leg

928.11 Knee

[5] **928.2 Ankle and foot, excluding toe(s) alone**

928.20 Foot
Heel

928.21 Ankle

928.3 Toe(s)

928.8 Multiple sites of lower limb

928.9 Unspecified site
Leg NOS

929 Crushing injury of multiple and unspecified sites
[ALERT!] For coding late effect of crushing see 906.4

929.0 Multiple sites, not elsewhere classified

929.9 Unspecified site

EFFECTS OF FOREIGN BODY ENTERING THROUGH ORIFICE (930-939)

[*Excludes:*] *foreign body:*
granuloma (728.82)
inadvertently left in operative wound (998.4, 998.7)
in open wound (800-839, 851-897)
residual, in soft tissues (729.6)
superficial without major open wound (910-919 with .6 or .7)

930 Foreign body on external eye
[*Excludes:*] *foreign body in penetrating wound of:*
eyeball (871.5-871.6)
retained (old) (360.5-360.6)
ocular adnexa (870.4)
retained (old) (376.6)
[ALERT!] For coding late effect of foreign body in orifice see 908.5

930.0 Corneal foreign body

930.1 Foreign body in conjunctival sac

930.2 Foreign body in lacrimal punctum

930.8 Other and combined sites

930.9 Unspecified site
External eye NOS

931 Foreign body in ear
Auditory canal
Auricle
[ALERT!] For coding late effect of foreign body in orifice see 908.5

932 Foreign body in nose
Nasal sinus
Nostril
[ALERT!] For coding late effect of foreign body in orifice see 908.5

933 Foreign body in pharynx and larynx
[ALERT!] For coding late effect of foreign body in orifice see 908.5

933.0 Pharynx
Nasopharynx
Throat NOS

933.1 Larynx
Asphyxia due to foreign body
Choking due to:
food (regurgitated)
phlegm

934 Foreign body in trachea, bronchus, and lung
[ALERT!] For coding late effect of foreign body in orifice see 908.5

934.0 Trachea

934.1 Main bronchus

934.8 Other specified parts
Bronchioles
Lung

934.9 Respiratory tree, unspecified
Inhalation of liquid or vomitus, lower respiratory tract NOS

935 Foreign body in mouth, esophagus, and stomach
[ALERT!] For coding late effect of foreign body in orifice see 908.5

935.0 Mouth

935.1 Esophagus

935.2 Stomach

936 Foreign body in intestine and colon
[ALERT!] For coding late effect of foreign body in orifice see 908.5

937 Foreign body in anus and rectum
Rectosigmoid (junction)
[ALERT!] For coding late effect of foreign body in orifice see 908.5

938 Foreign body in digestive system, unspecified
Alimentary tract NOS
Swallowed foreign body
[ALERT!] For coding late effect of foreign body in orifice see 908.5

939 Foreign body in genitourinary tract
[ALERT!] For coding late effect of foreign body in orifice see 908.5

939.0 Bladder and urethra

939.1 Uterus, any part
[*Excludes:*] *intrauterine contraceptive device:*
complications from (996.32, 996.65)
presence of (V45.51)

939.2 Vulva and vagina

939.3 Penis

939.9 Unspecified site

BURNS (940-949)

Includes: burns from:
electrical heating appliance
electricity
flame
hot object
lightning
radiation
chemical burns (external) (internal)
scalds

[*Excludes:*] *friction burns (910-919 with .0, .1)*
sunburn (692.71, 692.76-692.77)

940 Burn confined to eye and adnexa
[ALERT!] For coding late effect of burn of eye face head and neck see 906.5

940.0 Chemical burn of eyelids and periocular area

940.1 Other burns of eyelids and periocular area

940.2 Alkaline chemical burn of cornea and conjunctival sac

940.3 Acid chemical burn of cornea and conjunctival sac

940.4 Other burn of cornea and conjunctival sac

940.5 Burn with resulting rupture and destruction of eyeball

940.9 Unspecified burn of eye and adnexa

[5] **941 Burn of face, head, and neck**
[*Excludes:*] *mouth (947.0)*
The following fifth-digit subclassification is for use with category 941:

0 face and head, unspecified site
1 ear [any part]
2 eye (with other parts of face, head, and neck)

    3   lip(s)

    4   chin

    5   nose (septum)

    6   scalp [any part]
          Temple (region)

    7   forehead and cheek

    8   neck

    9   multiple sites [except with eye] of face, head, and neck

    ALERT! For coding late effect of burn of eye face head and neck see 906.5

⑤ **941.0** Unspecified degree
    [0-9]

⑤ **941.1** Erythema [first degree]
    [0-9]

⑤ **941.2** Blisters, epidermal loss [second degree]
    [0-9]

⑤ **941.3** Full-thickness skin loss [third degree NOS]
    [0-9]

⑤ **941.4** Deep necrosis of underlying tissues [deep third degree] without mention of loss of a
          body part
    [0-9]

⑤ **941.5** Deep necrosis of underlying tissues [deep third degree] with loss of a body part
    [0-9]

⑤ **942** Burn of trunk

    Excludes: scapular region (943.0-943.5 with fifth-digit 6)
    The following fifth-digit subclassification is for use with category 942:

    0   trunk, unspecified site

    1   breast

    2   chest wall, excluding breast and nipple

    3   abdominal wall
          Flank   Groin

    4   back [any part]
          Buttock   Interscapular region

    5   genitalia
          Labium (majus) (minus)   Scrotum
          Penis   Testis
          Perineum   Vulva

    9   other and multiple sites of trunk

    ALERT! For coding late effect of burn of eye face head and neck see 906.5

⑤ **942.0** Unspecified degree
    [0-5,9]

⑤ **942.1** Erythema [first degree]
    [0-5,9]

⑤ **942.2** Blisters, epidermal loss [second degree]
    [0-5,9]

⑤ **942.3** Full-thickness skin loss [third degree NOS]
    [0-5,9]

⑤ **942.4** Deep necrosis of underlying tissues [deep third degree] without mention of loss of a
          body part
    [0-5,9]

⑤ **942.5** Deep necrosis of underlying tissues [deep third degree] with loss of a body part
    [0-5,9]

⑤ **943** Burn of upper limb, except wrist and hand

    The following fifth-digit subclassification is for use with category 943:

    0   upper limb, unspecified site

    1   forearm

    2   elbow

    3   upper arm

    4   axilla

  ● Code new   ▲ Revision of   ④ ⑤ Fourth or fifth
       to 2012 edition   existing code   digit required

    5 shoulder

    6 scapular region

    9 multiple sites of upper limb, except wrist and hand

⑤ **943.0** Unspecified degree
[0-6,9]

⑤ **943.1** Erythema [first degree]
[0-6,9]

⑤ **943.2** Blisters, epidermal loss [second degree]
[0-6,9]

⑤ **943.3** Full-thickness skin loss [third degree NOS]
[0-6,9]

⑤ **943.4** Deep necrosis of underlying tissues [deep third degree] without mention of loss of a
       body part
[0-6,9]

⑤ **943.5** Deep necrosis of underlying tissues [deep third degree] with loss of a body part
[0-6,9]

⑤ **944** Burn of wrist(s) and hand(s)
The following fifth-digit subclassification is for use with category 944:

    0 hand, unspecified site

    1 single digit [finger (nail)] other than thumb

    2 thumb (nail)

    3 two or more digits, not including thumb

    4 two or more digits including thumb

    5 palm

    6 back of hand

    7 wrist

    8 multiple sites of wrist(s) and hand(s)
    ALERT! For coding late effect of burn of wrist and hand see 906.6

⑤ **944.0** Unspecified degree
[0-8]

⑤ **944.1** Erythema [first degree]
[0-8]

⑤ **944.2** Blisters, epidermal loss [second degree]
[0-8]

⑤ **944.3** Full-thickness skin loss [third degree NOS]
[0-8]

⑤ **944.4** Deep necrosis of underlying tissues [deep third degree] without mention of loss of a
       body part
[0-8]

⑤ **944.5** Deep necrosis of underlying tissues [deep third degree] with loss of a body part
[0-8]

⑤ **945** Burn of lower limb(s)
The following fifth-digit subclassification is for use with category 945:

    0 lower limb [leg], unspecified site

    1 toe(s) (nail)

    2 foot

    3 ankle

    4 lower leg

    5 knee

    6 thigh [any part]

    9 multiple sites of lower limb(s)
    ALERT! For coding late effect of burn of other extremities see 906.7

⑤ **945.0** Unspecified degree
[0-6,9]

⑤ **945.1** Erythema [first degree]
[0-6,9]

⑤ **945.2** Blisters, epidermal loss [second degree]
[0-6,9]

713

| Add 4th or 5th digit | Nonspecific code | Unspecified code | Medicare secondary payer (MSP) alert |

⑤ **945.3 Full-thickness skin loss [third degree NOS]**
[0-6,9]

⑤ **945.4 Deep necrosis of underlying tissues [deep third degree] without mention of loss of a body part**
[0-6,9]

⑤ **945.5 Deep necrosis of underlying tissues [deep third degree] with loss of a body part**
[0-6,9]

946 Burns of multiple specified sites
Includes: burns of sites classifiable to more than one three-digit category in 940-945

Excludes: multiple burns NOS (949.0-949.5)

ALERT! For coding late effect of burns of other specified sites see 906.8

946.0 Unspecified degree

946.1 Erythema [first degree]

946.2 Blisters, epidermal loss [second degree]

946.3 Full-thickness skin loss [third degree NOS]

946.4 Deep necrosis of underlying tissues [deep third degree] without mention of loss of a body part

946.5 Deep necrosis of underlying tissues [deep third degree] with loss of a body part

947 Burn of internal organs
Includes: burns from chemical agents (ingested)

947.0 Mouth and pharynx
Gum
Tongue

947.1 Larynx, trachea, and lung

947.2 Esophagus

947.3 Gastrointestinal tract
Colon   Small intestine
Rectum   Stomach

947.4 Vagina and uterus

947.8 Other specified sites

947.9 Unspecified site

⑤ **948 Burns classified according to extent of body surface involved**

Excludes: sunburn (692.71, 692.76-692.77)

Note: This category is to be used when the site of the burn is unspecified, or with categories 940-947 when the site is specified.

The following fifth-digit subclassification is for use with category 948 to indicate the percent of *body surface* with *third degree burn*; valid digits are in [brackets] under each code:

0 less than 10 percent or unspecified

1 10-19%

2 20-29%

3 30-39%

4 40-49%

5 50-59%

6 60-69%

7 70-79%

8 80-89%

9 90% or more of body surface

ALERT! It is advisable to use category 948 as additional coding when needed to provide data for evaluating burn mortality, such as that needed by burn units. It is also advisable to use category 948 as an additional code for reporting purposes when there is mention of a third-degree burn involving 20 percent or more of the body surface.

⑤ **948.0 Burn [any degree] involving less than 10 percent of body surface**
[0]

⑤ **948.1 10-19 percent of body surface**
[0-1]

⑤ **948.2 20-29 percent of body surface**
[0-2]

● Code new
to 2012 edition
▲ Revision of
existing code
④ ⑤ Fourth or fifth
digit required

[5] **948.3 30-39 percent of body surface**
[0-3]

[5] **948.4 40-49 percent of body surface**
[0-4]

[5] **948.5 50-59 percent of body surface**
[0-5]

[5] **948.6 60-69 percent of body surface**
[0-6]

[5] **948.7 70-79 percent of body surface**
[0-7]

[5] **948.8 80-89 percent of body surface**
[0-8]

[5] **948.9 90 percent or more of body surface**
[0-9]

949 Burn, unspecified

Includes: burn NOS
multiple burns NOS

[Excludes:] *burn of unspecified site but with statement of the extent of body surface involved (948.0-948.9)*

[ALERT!] For coding late effect of burn of unspecified site see 906.9

949.0 Unspecified degree

949.1 Erythema [first degree]

949.2 Blisters, epidermal loss [second degree]

949.3 Full-thickness skin loss [third degree NOS]

949.4 Deep necrosis of underlying tissues [deep third degree] without mention of loss of a body part

949.5 Deep necrosis of underlying tissues [deep third degree] with loss of a body part

INJURY TO NERVES AND SPINAL CORD (950-957)

Includes:
division of nerve (with open wound)
lesion in continuity (with open wound)
traumatic neuroma (with open wound)
traumatic transient paralysis (with open wound)

[Excludes:] *accidental puncture or laceration during medical procedure (998.2)*

950 Injury to optic nerve and pathways

[ALERT!] For coding late effects of injuries to the nervous system see 907

950.0 Optic nerve injury
Second cranial nerve

950.1 Injury to optic chiasm

950.2 Injury to optic pathways

950.3 Injury to visual cortex

950.9 Unspecified
Traumatic blindness NOS

951 Injury to other cranial nerve(s)

[ALERT!] For coding late effect of injury to cranial nerve see 907.1

[ALERT!] For coding late effects of injuries to the nervous system see 907

951.0 Injury to oculomotor nerve
Third cranial nerve

951.1 Injury to trochlear nerve
Fourth cranial nerve

951.2 Injury to trigeminal nerve
Fifth cranial nerve

951.3 Injury to abducens nerve
Sixth cranial nerve

951.4 Injury to facial nerve
Seventh cranial nerve

951.5 Injury to acoustic nerve
Auditory nerve
Eighth cranial nerve
Traumatic deafness NOS

951.6 Injury to accessory nerve
Eleventh cranial nerve

951.7 Injury to hypoglossal nerve
Twelfth cranial nerve

951.8 Injury to other specified cranial nerves
Glossopharyngeal [9th cranial] nerve
Olfactory [1st cranial] nerve
Pneumogastric [10th cranial] nerve
Traumatic anosmia NOS
Vagus [10th cranial] nerve

951.9 Injury to unspecified cranial nerve

952 Spinal cord injury without evidence of spinal bone injury

> **ALERT!** For coding late effect of spinal cord injury see 907.2

> **ALERT!** For coding late effects of injuries to the nervous system see 907

⑤ **952.0 Cervical**

952.00 C_1-C_4 level with unspecified spinal cord injury
Spinal cord injury, cervical region NOS

952.01 C_1-C_4 level with complete lesion of spinal cord

952.02 C_1-C_4 level with anterior cord syndrome

952.03 C_1-C_4 level with central cord syndrome

952.04 C_1-C_4 level with other specified spinal cord injury
Incomplete spinal cord lesion at C_1-C_4 level:
NOS
with posterior cord syndrome

952.05 C_5-C_7 level with unspecified spinal cord injury

952.06 C_5-C_7 level with complete lesion of spinal cord

952.07 C_5-C_7 level with anterior cord syndrome

952.08 C_5-C_7 level with central cord syndrome

952.09 C_5-C_7 level with other specified spinal cord injury
Incomplete spinal cord lesion at C_5-C_7 level:
NOS
with posterior cord syndrome

⑤ **952.1 Dorsal [thoracic]**

952.10 T_1-T_6 level with unspecified spinal cord injury
Spinal cord injury, thoracic region NOS

952.11 T_1-T_6 level with complete lesion of spinal cord

952.12 T_1-T_6 level with anterior cord syndrome

952.13 T_1-T_6 level with central cord syndrome

952.14 T_1-T_6 level with other specified spinal cord injury
Incomplete spinal cord lesion at T_1-T_6 level:
NOS
with posterior cord syndrome

952.15 T_7-T_{12} level with unspecified spinal cord injury

952.16 T_7-T_{12} level with complete lesion of spinal cord

952.17 T_7-T_{12} level with anterior cord syndrome

952.18 T_7-T_{12} level with central cord syndrome

952.19 T_7-T_{12} level with other specified spinal cord injury
Incomplete spinal cord lesion at T_7-T_{12} level:
NOS
with posterior cord syndrome

952.2 Lumbar

952.3 Sacral

952.4 Cauda equina

952.8 Multiple sites of spinal cord

952.9 Unspecified site of spinal cord

953 Injury to nerve roots and spinal plexus

> **ALERT!** For coding late effect of injury to nerve root(s) spinal plexus(es) and other nerves of trunk see 907.3

> **ALERT!** For coding late effects of injuries to the nervous system see 907

● Code new   ▲ Revision of   ④ ⑤ Fourth or fifth
to 2012 edition   existing code   digit required

953.0 Cervical root

953.1 Dorsal root

953.2 Lumbar root

953.3 Sacral root

953.4 Brachial plexus

953.5 Lumbosacral plexus

953.8 Multiple sites

953.9 Unspecified site

954 Injury to other nerve(s) of trunk, excluding shoulder and pelvic girdles

ALERT! For coding late effects of injuries to the nervous system see 907

954.0 Cervical sympathetic

954.1 Other sympathetic
| Celiac ganglion or plexus | Splanchnic nerve(s) |
| Inferior mesenteric plexus | Stellate ganglion |

954.8 Other specified nerve(s) of trunk

954.9 Unspecified nerve of trunk

955 Injury to peripheral nerve(s) of shoulder girdle and upper limb

ALERT! For coding late effect of injury to peripheral nerve of shoulder girdle and upper limb see 907.4

ALERT! For coding late effects of injuries to the nervous system see 907

955.0 Axillary nerve

955.1 Median nerve

955.2 Ulnar nerve

955.3 Radial nerve

955.4 Musculocutaneous nerve

955.5 Cutaneous sensory nerve, upper limb

955.6 Digital nerve

955.7 Other specified nerve(s) of shoulder girdle and upper limb

955.8 Multiple nerves of shoulder girdle and upper limb

955.9 Unspecified nerve of shoulder girdle and upper limb

956 Injury to peripheral nerve(s) of pelvic girdle and lower limb

ALERT! For coding late effect of injury to peripheral nerve of pelvic girdle and lower limb see 907.5

ALERT! For coding late effects of injuries to the nervous system see 907

956.0 Sciatic nerve

956.1 Femoral nerve

956.2 Posterior tibial nerve

956.3 Peroneal nerve

956.4 Cutaneous sensory nerve, lower limb

956.5 Other specified nerve(s) of pelvic girdle and lower limb

956.8 Multiple nerves of pelvic girdle and lower limb

956.9 Unspecified nerve of pelvic girdle and lower limb

957 Injury to other and unspecified nerves

ALERT! For coding late effect of injury to other and unspecified nerve see 907.9

ALERT! For coding late effects of injuries to the nervous system see 907

957.0 Superficial nerves of head and neck

957.1 Other specified nerve(s)

957.8 Multiple nerves in several parts
Multiple nerve injury NOS

957.9 Unspecified site
Nerve injury NOS

| ▓ | Add 4th or 5th digit | ▓ | Nonspecific code | ░ | Unspecified code | ▒ | Medicare secondary payer (MSP) alert |

CERTAIN TRAUMATIC COMPLICATIONS AND UNSPECIFIED INJURIES (958-959)

958 Certain early complications of trauma

Excludes: adult respiratory distress syndrome (518.52)
flail chest (807.4)
post-traumatic seroma (729.91)
shock lung related to trauma and surgery (518.52)
that occurring during or following medical procedures (996.0-999.9)

ALERT! For coding late effect of certain complications of trauma see 908.6

ALERT! For coding late effects of other and unspecified injuries see 908

958.0 Air embolism
Pneumathemia

Excludes: that complicating:
abortion (634-638 with .6, 639.6)
ectopic or molar pregnancy (639.6)
pregnancy, childbirth, or the puerperium (673.0)

958.1 Fat embolism

Excludes: that complicating:
abortion (634-638 with .6, 639.6)
pregnancy, childbirth, or the puerperium (673.8)

958.2 Secondary and recurrent hemorrhage

958.3 Posttraumatic wound infection, not elsewhere classified

Excludes: infected open wounds—code to complicated open wound of site

ALERT! Assign code 958.3 as an additional code for any documented infected burn site

958.4 Traumatic shock
Shock (immediate) (delayed) following injury

Excludes: shock:
anaphylactic (995.0)
due to serum (999.41-999.49)
anesthetic (995.4)
electric (994.8)
following abortion (639.5)
lightning (994.0)
nontraumatic NOS (785.50)
obstetric (669.1)
postoperative (998.00-998.09)

958.5 Traumatic anuria
Crush syndrome
Renal failure following crushing

Excludes: that due to a medical procedure (997.5)

958.6 Volkmann's ischemic contracture
Posttraumatic muscle contracture

958.7 Traumatic subcutaneous emphysema

Excludes: subcutaneous emphysema resulting from a procedure (998.81)

958.8 Other early complications of trauma

⑤ **958.9 Traumatic compartment syndrome**

Excludes: nontraumatic compartment syndrome (729.71-729.79)

958.90 Compartment syndrome, unspecified

958.91 Traumatic compartment syndrome of upper extremity
Traumatic compartment syndrome of shoulder, arm, forearm, wrist, hand, and fingers

958.92 Traumatic compartment syndrome of lower extremity
Traumatic compartment syndrome of hip, buttock, thigh, leg, foot, and toes

958.93 Traumatic compartment syndrome of abdomen

958.99 Traumatic compartment syndrome of other sites

● Code new   ▲ Revision of   ④ ⑤ Fourth or fifth
to 2012 edition   existing code   digit required

959 Injury, other and unspecified
Includes: injury NOS
[Excludes:] *injury NOS of:*
blood vessels (900.0-904.9)
eye (921.0-921.9)
internal organs (860.0-869.1)
intracranial sites (854.0-854.1)
nerves (950.0-951.9, 953.0-957.9)
spinal cord (952.0-952.9)

ALERT! For coding late effect of unspecified injury see 908.9

ALERT! For coding late effects of other and unspecified injuries see 908

[5] **959.0 Head, face and neck**
Cheek
Ear
Eyebrow
Lip
Mouth
Nose
Throat

959.01 Head injury, unspecified
[Excludes:] *concussion (850.1-850.9)*
with head injury NOS (850.1-850.9)
head injury NOS with loss of consciousness (850.1-850.5)
specified intracranial injuries (850.0-854.1)

959.09 Injury of face and neck

[5] **959.1 Trunk**
[Excludes:] *scapular region (959.2)*

959.11 Other injury of chest wall

959.12 Other injury of abdomen

959.13 Fracture of corpus cavernosum penis

959.14 Other injury of external genitals

959.19 Other injury of other sites of trunk
Injury of trunk NOS

959.2 Shoulder and upper arm
Axilla
Scapular region

959.3 Elbow, forearm, and wrist

959.4 Hand, except finger

959.5 Finger
Fingernail
Thumb (nail)

959.6 Hip and thigh
Upper leg

959.7 Knee, leg, ankle, and foot

959.8 Other specified sites, including multiple
[Excludes:] *multiple sites classifiable to the same four-digit category (959.0-959.7)*

959.9 Unspecified site

POISONING BY DRUGS, MEDICINAL AND BIOLOGICAL SUBSTANCES (960-979)

Includes: overdose of these substances
wrong substances given or taken in error

Excludes: *adverse effects ["hypersensitivity," "reaction," etc.] of correct substance properly administered. Such cases are to be classified according to the nature of the adverse effect, such as:*
adverse effect NOS (995.20)
allergic lymphadenitis (289.3)
aspirin gastritis (535.4)
blood disorders (280.0-289.9)
dermatitis:
contact (692.0-692.9)
due to ingestion (693.0-693.9)
nephropathy (583.9)
[The drug giving rise to the adverse effect may be identified by use of categories E930-E949]
drug dependence (304.0-304.9)
drug reaction and poisoning affecting the newborn (760.0-779.9)
nondependent abuse of drugs (305.0-305.9)
pathological drug intoxication (292.2)

Use additional code to specify the effects of the poisoning

ALERT! For coding late effect of poisoning due to drug medicinal or biological substance see 909.0

ALERT! For personal history of poisoning presenting hazards to health see V15.6

960 Poisoning by antibiotics

Excludes: *antibiotics:*
ear, nose, and throat (976.6)
eye (976.5)
local (976.0)

960.0 Penicillins
Ampicillin   Cloxacillin
Carbenicillin   Penicillin G

960.1 Antifungal antibiotics
Amphotericin B   Nystatin
Griseofulvin   Trichomycin

Excludes: *preparations intended for topical use (976.0-976.9)*

960.2 Chloramphenicol group
Chloramphenicol
Thiamphenicol

960.3 Erythromycin and other macrolides
Oleandomycin
Spiramycin

960.4 Tetracycline group
Doxycycline   Oxytetracycline
Minocycline

960.5 Cephalosporin group
Cephalexin   Cephaloridine
Cephaloglycin   Cephalothin

960.6 Antimycobacterial antibiotics
Cycloserine   Rifampin
Kanamycin   Streptomycin

960.7 Antineoplastic antibiotics
Actinomycin such as: Bleomycin
Cactinomycin   Daunorubicin
Dactinomycin   Mitomycin

960.8 Other specified antibiotics

960.9 Unspecified antibiotic

● Code new
to 2012 edition

▲ Revision of
existing code

④ ⑤ Fourth or fifth
digit required

961 **Poisoning by other anti-infectives**

> *Excludes:* anti-infectives:
>> ear, nose, and throat (976.6)
>> eye (976.5)
>> local (976.0)

ALERT! For coding late effect of poisoning due to drug medicinal or biological substance see 909.0

961.0 Sulfonamides
  Sulfadiazine   Sulfamethoxazole
  Sulfafurazole

961.1 Arsenical anti-infectives

961.2 Heavy metal anti-infectives
  Compounds of: Compounds of:
    antimony   lead
    bismuth   mercury

> *Excludes:* mercurial diuretics (974.0)

ALERT! For personal history of contact with and (suspected) exposure to lead see V15.86

961.3 Quinoline and hydroxyquinoline derivatives
  Chiniofon
  Diiodohydroxyquin

> *Excludes:* antimalarial drugs (961.4)

961.4 Antimalarials and drugs acting on other blood protozoa
  Chloroquine   Proguanil [chloroguanide]
  Cycloguanil   Pyrimethamine
  Primaquine   Quinine

961.5 Other antiprotozoal drugs
  Emetine

961.6 Anthelmintics
  Hexylresorcinol   Thiabendazole
  Piperazine

961.7 Antiviral drugs
  Methisazone

> *Excludes:* amantadine (966.4)
>> cytarabine (963.1)
>> idoxuridine (976.5)

961.8 Other antimycobacterial drugs
  Ethambutol   Para-aminosalicylic acid derivatives
  Ethionamide   Sulfones
  Isoniazid

961.9 Other and unspecified anti-infectives
  Flucytosine
  Nitrofuran derivatives

962 **Poisoning by hormones and synthetic substitutes**

> *Excludes:* oxytocic hormones (975.0)

ALERT! For coding late effect of poisoning due to drug medicinal or biological substance see 909.0

ALERT! For personal history of inhaled steroid therapy see V87.44

ALERT! For personal history of systemic steroid therapy see V87.45

962.0 Adrenal cortical steroids
  Cortisone derivatives
  Desoxycorticosterone derivatives
  Fluorinated corticosteroids

962.1 Androgens and anabolic congeners
  Methandriol   Oxymetholone
  Nandrolone   Testosterone

962.2 Ovarian hormones and synthetic substitutes
  Contraceptives, oral
  Estrogens
  Estrogens and progestogens, combined
  Progestogens

ALERT! For personal history of estrogen therapy see V87.43

| | Add 4th or 5th digit | | Nonspecific code | | Unspecified code | | Medicare secondary payer (MSP) alert |

962.3 Insulins and antidiabetic agents
Acetohexamide
Biguanide derivatives, oral
Chlorpropamide
Glucagon
Insulin
Phenformin
Sulfonylurea derivatives, oral
Tolbutamide

962.4 Anterior pituitary hormones
Corticotropin
Gonadotropin
Somatotropin [growth hormone]

962.5 Posterior pituitary hormones
Vasopressin

Excludes: oxytocic hormones (975.0)

962.6 Parathyroid and parathyroid derivatives

962.7 Thyroid and thyroid derivatives
Dextrothyroxin
Levothyroxine sodium
Liothyronine
Thyroglobulin

962.8 Antithyroid agents
Iodides
Thiouracil
Thiourea

962.9 Other and unspecified hormones and synthetic substitutes

963 Poisoning by primarily systemic agents
ALERT! For coding late effect of poisoning due to drug medicinal or biological substance see 909.0

963.0 Antiallergic and antiemetic drugs
Antihistamines
Chlorpheniramine
Diphenhydramine
Diphenylpyraline
Thonzylamine
Tripelennamine

Excludes: phenothiazine-based tranquilizers (969.1)

963.1 Antineoplastic and immunosuppressive drugs
Azathioprine
Busulfan
Chlorambucil
Cyclophosphamide
Cytarabine
Fluorouracil
Mercaptopurine
thio-TEPA

Excludes: antineoplastic antibiotics (960.7)

ALERT! For personal history of antineoplastic chemotherapy see V87.41
ALERT! For personal history of immunosuppressive therapy see V87.46

963.2 Acidifying agents

963.3 Alkalizing agents

963.4 Enzymes, not elsewhere classified
Penicillinase

963.5 Vitamins, not elsewhere classified
Vitamin A
Vitamin D

Excludes: nicotinic acid (972.2)
vitamin K (964.3)

963.8 Other specified systemic agents
Heavy metal antagonists

963.9 Unspecified systemic agent

964 Poisoning by agents primarily affecting blood constituents
ALERT! For coding late effect of poisoning due to drug medicinal or biological substance see 909.0

964.0 Iron and its compounds
Ferric salts
Ferrous sulfate and other ferrous salts

964.1 Liver preparations and other antianemic agents
Folic acid

964.2 Anticoagulants
Coumarin
Heparin
Phenindione
Warfarin sodium

964.3 Vitamin K [phytonadione]

● Code new
to 2012 edition
▲ Revision of
existing code
④ ⑤ Fourth or fifth
digit required

964.4 Fibrinolysis-affecting drugs
Aminocaproic acid   Streptokinase
Streptodornase   Urokinase

964.5 Anticoagulant antagonists and other coagulants
Hexadimethrine
Protamine sulfate

964.6 Gamma globulin

964.7 Natural blood and blood products
Blood plasma   Packed red cells
Human fibrinogen   Whole blood

Excludes: transfusion reactions (999.41-999.8)

964.8 Other specified agents affecting blood constituents
Macromolecular blood substitutes
Plasma expanders

964.9 Unspecified agent affecting blood constituents

965 Poisoning by analgesics, antipyretics, and antirheumatics

Excludes: drug dependence (304.0-304.9)
         nondependent abuse (305.0-305.9)

ALERT! For coding late effect of poisoning due to drug medicinal or biological substance see 909.0

⑤ **965.0 Opiates and related narcotics**

965.00 Opium (alkaloids), unspecified

965.01 Heroin
Diacetylmorphine

965.02 Methadone

965.09 Other
Codeine [methylmorphine]
Meperidine [pethidine]
Morphine

965.1 Salicylates
Acetylsalicylic acid [aspirin]
Salicylic acid salts

965.4 Aromatic analgesics, not elsewhere classified
Acetanilid
Paracetamol [acetaminophen]
Phenacetin [acetophenetidin]

965.5 Pyrazole derivatives
Aminophenazone [aminopyrine]
Phenylbutazone

⑤ **965.6 Antirheumatics [antiphlogistics]**

Excludes: salicylates (965.1)
         steroids (962.0-962.9)

965.61 Propionic acid derivatives
Fenoprofen   Ketoprofen
Flurbiprofen   Naproxen
Ibuprofen   Oxaprozin

965.69 Other antirheumatics
Gold salts
Indomethacin

965.7 Other non-narcotic analgesics
Pyrabital

965.8 Other specified analgesics and antipyretics
Pentazocine

965.9 Unspecified analgesic and antipyretic

966 Poisoning by anticonvulsants and anti-Parkinsonism drugs

ALERT! For coding late effect of poisoning due to drug medicinal or biological substance see 909.0

966.0 Oxazolidine derivatives
Paramethadione
Trimethadione

Add 4th or 5th digit	Nonspecific code	Unspecified code	Medicare secondary payer (MSP) alert

966.1 Hydantoin derivatives
Phenytoin

966.2 Succinimides
Ethosuximide
Phensuximide

966.3 Other and unspecified anticonvulsants
Primidone

Excludes: *barbiturates (967.0)*
sulfonamides (961.0)

966.4 Anti-Parkinsonism drugs
Amantadine
Ethopropazine [profenamine]
Levodopa [L-dopa]

967 Poisoning by sedatives and hypnotics

Excludes: *drug dependence (304.0-304.9)*
nondependent abuse (305.0-305.9)

ALERT! For coding late effect of poisoning due to drug medicinal or biological substance see 909.0

967.0 Barbiturates
Amobarbital [amylobarbitone]
Barbital [barbitone]
Butabarbital [butabarbitone]
Pentobarbital [pentobarbitone]
Phenobarbital [phenobarbitone]
Secobarbital [quinalbarbitone]

Excludes: *thiobarbiturate anesthetics (968.3)*

967.1 Chloral hydrate group

967.2 Paraldehyde

967.3 Bromine compounds
Bromide
Carbromal (derivatives)

967.4 Methaqualone compounds

967.5 Glutethimide group

967.6 Mixed sedatives, not elsewhere classified

967.8 Other sedatives and hypnotics

967.9 Unspecified sedative or hypnotic
Sleeping:
drug NOS
pill NOS
tablet NOS

968 Poisoning by other central nervous system depressants and anesthetics

Excludes: *drug dependence (304.0-304.9)*
nondependent abuse (305.0-305.9)

ALERT! For coding late effect of poisoning due to drug medicinal or biological substance see 909.0

968.0 Central nervous system muscle-tone depressants
Chlorphenesin (carbamate)   Methocarbamol
Mephenesin

968.1 Halothane

968.2 Other gaseous anesthetics
Ether
Halogenated hydrocarbon derivatives, except halothane
Nitrous oxide

968.3 Intravenous anesthetics

Excludes: *Methohexital [methohexitone]*
Thiobarbiturates, such as thiopental sodium

968.4 Other and unspecified general anesthetics

▲ **968.5 Surface (topical) and infiltration anesthetics**
Cocaine (topical) | Procaine
Lidocaine [lignocaine] | Tetracaine

[Excludes:] *poisoning by cocaine used as a central nervous system stimulant (970.81)*

968.6 Peripheral nerve and plexus-blocking anesthetics

968.7 Spinal anesthetics

968.9 Other and unspecified local anesthetics

969 Poisoning by psychotropic agents

[Excludes:] *drug dependence (304.0-304.9)*
nondependent abuse (305.0-305.9)

ALERT! For coding late effect of poisoning due to drug medicinal or biological substance see 909.0

[5] **969.0 Antidepressants**

969.00 Antidepressant, unspecified

969.01 Monoamine oxidase inhibitors
MAOI

969.02 Selective serotonin and norepinephrine reuptake inhibitors
SSNRI antidepressants

969.03 Selective serotonin reuptake inhibitors
SSRI antidepressants

969.04 Tetracyclic antidepressants

969.05 Tricyclic antidepressants

969.09 Other antidepressants

969.1 Phenothiazine-based tranquilizers
Chlorpromazine | Prochlorperazine
Fluphenazine | Promazine

969.2 Butyrophenone-based tranquilizers
Haloperidol | Trifluperidol
Spiperone

969.3 Other antipsychotics, neuroleptics, and major tranquilizers

969.4 Benzodiazepine-based tranquilizers
Chlordiazepoxide | Lorazepam
Diazepam | Medazepam
Flurazepam | Nitrazepam

969.5 Other tranquilizers
Hydroxyzine
Meprobamate

969.6 Psychodysleptics [hallucinogens]
Cannabis (derivatives) | Mescaline
Lysergide [LSD] | Psilocin
Marijuana (derivatives) | Psilocybin

[5] **969.7 Psychostimulants**

[Excludes:] *central appetite depressants (977.0)*

969.70 Psychostimulant, unspecified

969.71 Caffeine

969.72 Amphetamines
Methamphetamines

969.73 Methylphenidate

969.79 Other psychostimulants

969.8 Other specified psychotropic agents

969.9 Unspecified psychotropic agent

970 Poisoning by central nervous system stimulants

ALERT! For coding late effect of poisoning due to drug medicinal or biological substance see 909.0

970.0 Analeptics
Lobeline
Nikethamide

970.1 Opiate antagonists
Levallorphan   Naloxone
Nalorphine

⑤ **970.8 Other specified central nervous system stimulants**

970.81 Cocaine
Crack

970.89 Other central nervous system stimulants

970.9 Unspecified central nervous system stimulant

971 Poisoning by drugs primarily affecting the autonomic nervous system
ALERT! For coding late effect of poisoning due to drug medicinal or biological substance see 909.0

971.0 Parasympathomimetics [cholinergics]
Acetylcholine   Pilocarpine
Anticholinesterase:
   organophosphorus
   reversible

971.1 Parasympatholytics [anticholinergics and antimuscarinics] and spasmolytics
Atropine   Hyoscine [scopolamine]
Homatropine   Quaternary ammonium derivatives

Excludes: papaverine (972.5)

971.2 Sympathomimetics [adrenergics]
Epinephrine [adrenalin]
Levarterenol [noradrenalin]

971.3 Sympatholytics [antiadrenergics]
Phenoxybenzamine
Tolazoline hydrochloride

971.9 Unspecified drug primarily affecting autonomic nervous system

972 Poisoning by agents primarily affecting the cardiovascular system
ALERT! For coding late effect of poisoning due to drug medicinal or biological substance see 909.0

972.0 Cardiac rhythm regulators
Practolol   Propranolol
Procainamide   Quinidine

Excludes: lidocaine (968.5)

972.1 Cardiotonic glycosides and drugs of similar action
Digitalis glycosides   Strophanthins
Digoxin

972.2 Antilipemic and antiarteriosclerotic drugs
Clofibrate
Nicotinic acid derivatives

972.3 Ganglion-blocking agents
Pentamethonium bromide

972.4 Coronary vasodilators
Dipyridamole   Nitrites
Nitrates [nitroglycerin]

972.5 Other vasodilators
Cyclandelate   Papaverine
Diazoxide

Excludes: nicotinic acid (972.2)

972.6 Other antihypertensive agents
Clonidine   Rauwolfia alkaloids
Guanethidine   Reserpine

972.7 Antivaricose drugs, including sclerosing agents
Sodium morrhuate
Zinc salts

972.8 Capillary-active drugs
Adrenochrome derivatives
Metaraminol

972.9 Other and unspecified agents primarily affecting the cardiovascular system

● Code new   ▲ Revision of   ④ ⑤ Fourth or fifth
to 2012 edition   existing code   digit required

973 **Poisoning by agents primarily affecting the gastrointestinal system**

> **ALERT!** For coding late effect of poisoning due to drug medicinal or biological substance see 909.0

973.0 **Antacids and antigastric secretion drugs**
Aluminum hydroxide
Magnesium trisilicate

973.1 **Irritant cathartics**
Bisacodyl   Phenolphthalein
Castor oil

973.2 **Emollient cathartics**
Dioctyl sulfosuccinates

973.3 **Other cathartics, including intestinal atonia drugs**
Magnesium sulfate

973.4 **Digestants**
Pancreatin   Pepsin
Papain

973.5 **Antidiarrheal drugs**
Kaolin
Pectin

> *Excludes:* *anti-infectives (960.0-961.9)*

973.6 **Emetics**

973.8 **Other specified agents primarily affecting the gastrointestinal system**

973.9 **Unspecified agent primarily affecting the gastrointestinal system**

974 **Poisoning by water, mineral, and uric acid metabolism drugs**

> **ALERT!** For coding late effect of poisoning due to drug medicinal or biological substance see 909.0

974.0 **Mercurial diuretics**
Chlormerodrin
Mercaptomerin
Mersalyl

974.1 **Purine derivative diuretics**
Theobromine
Theophylline

> *Excludes:* *aminophylline [theophylline ethylenediamine] (975.7)*
> *caffeine (969.71)*

974.2 **Carbonic acid anhydrase inhibitors**
Acetazolamide

974.3 **Saluretics**
Benzothiadiazides
Chlorothiazide group

974.4 **Other diuretics**
Ethacrynic acid
Furosemide

974.5 **Electrolytic, caloric, and water-balance agents**

974.6 **Other mineral salts, not elsewhere classified**

974.7 **Uric acid metabolism drugs**
Allopurinol   Probenecid
Colchicine

975 **Poisoning by agents primarily acting on the smooth and skeletal muscles and respiratory system**

> **ALERT!** For coding late effect of poisoning due to drug medicinal or biological substance see 909.0

975.0 **Oxytocic agents**
Ergot alkaloids   Prostaglandins
Oxytocin

975.1 **Smooth muscle relaxants**
Adiphenine
Metaproterenol [orciprenaline]

> *Excludes:* *papaverine (972.5)*

975.2 Skeletal muscle relaxants

975.3 Other and unspecified drugs acting on muscles

975.4 Antitussives
Dextromethorphan
Pipazethate

975.5 Expectorants
Acetylcysteine   Terpin hydrate
Guaifenesin

975.6 Anti-common cold drugs

975.7 Antiasthmatics
Aminophylline [theophylline ethylenediamine]

975.8 Other and unspecified respiratory drugs

976 Poisoning by agents primarily affecting skin and mucous membrane, ophthalmological, otorhinolaryngological, and dental drugs
ALERT! For coding late effect of poisoning due to drug medicinal or biological substance see 909.0

976.0 Local anti-infectives and anti-inflammatory drugs

976.1 Antipruritics

976.2 Local astringents and local detergents

976.3 Emollients, demulcents, and protectants

976.4 Keratolytics, keratoplastics, other hair treatment drugs and preparations

976.5 Eye anti-infectives and other eye drugs
Idoxuridine

976.6 Anti-infectives and other drugs and preparations for ear, nose, and throat

976.7 Dental drugs topically applied

Excludes: anti-infectives (976.0)
local anesthetics (968.5)

976.8 Other agents primarily affecting skin and mucous membrane
Spermicides [vaginal contraceptives]

976.9 Unspecified agent primarily affecting skin and mucous membrane

977 Poisoning by other and unspecified drugs and medicinal substances
ALERT! For coding late effect of poisoning due to drug medicinal or biological substance see 909.0

977.0 Dietetics
Central appetite depressants

977.1 Lipotropic drugs

977.2 Antidotes and chelating agents, not elsewhere classified

977.3 Alcohol deterrents

977.4 Pharmaceutical excipients
Pharmaceutical adjuncts

977.8 Other specified drugs and medicinal substances
Contrast media used for diagnostic x-ray procedures
Diagnostic agents and kits

977.9 Unspecified drug or medicinal substance

978 Poisoning by bacterial vaccines
ALERT! For coding late effect of poisoning due to drug medicinal or biological substance see 909.0

978.0 BCG

978.1 Typhoid and paratyphoid

978.2 Cholera

978.3 Plague

978.4 Tetanus

978.5 Diphtheria

978.6 Pertussis vaccine, including combinations with a pertussis component

978.8 Other and unspecified bacterial vaccines

978.9 Mixed bacterial vaccines, except combinations with a pertussis component

● Code new
to 2012 edition   ▲ Revision of
existing code   ④ ⑤ Fourth or fifth
digit required

979 **Poisoning by other vaccines and biological substances**

Excludes: *gamma globulin (964.6)*

ALERT! For coding late effect of poisoning due to drug medicinal or biological substance see 909.0

979.0 **Smallpox vaccine**

979.1 **Rabies vaccine**

979.2 **Typhus vaccine**

979.3 **Yellow fever vaccine**

979.4 **Measles vaccine**

979.5 **Poliomyelitis vaccine**

979.6 **Other and unspecified viral and rickettsial vaccines**
Mumps vaccine

979.7 **Mixed viral-rickettsial and bacterial vaccines, except combinations with a pertussis component**

Excludes: *combinations with a pertussis component (978.6)*

979.9 **Other and unspecified vaccines and biological substances**

TOXIC EFFECTS OF SUBSTANCES CHIEFLY NONMEDICINAL AS TO SOURCE (980-989)

Excludes: *burns from chemical agents (ingested) (947.0-947.9)*
localized toxic effects indexed elsewhere (001.0-799.9)
respiratory conditions due to external agents (506.0-508.9)
respiratory conditions due to smoke inhalation NOS (508.2)

Use additional code to specify the nature of the toxic effect

Use additional code to identify:
personal history of retained foreign body fully removed (V15.53)
retained foreign body status, if applicable (V90.01-V90.9)

980 **Toxic effect of alcohol**

ALERT! For coding late effect of toxic effects of nonmedical substances see 909.1

DEFINITION Toxic effect is a reaction to a biological toxin; may involve death or dysfunction of specific organs or organ systems such as the liver, kidney, brain or immune suppression.

980.0 **Ethyl alcohol**
Denatured alcohol
Ethanol
Grain alcohol

Use additional code to identify any associated:
acute alcohol intoxication (305.0)
in alcoholism (303.0)
drunkenness (simple) (305.0)
pathological (291.4)

980.1 **Methyl alcohol**
Methanol
Wood alcohol

980.2 **Isopropyl alcohol**
Dimethyl carbinol
Isopropanol
Rubbing alcohol

980.3 **Fusel oil**
Alcohol:
amyl
butyl
propyl

980.8 **Other specified alcohols**

980.9 **Unspecified alcohol**

981 **Toxic effect of petroleum products**

Benzine	Petroleum:
Gasoline	ether
Kerosene	naphtha
Paraffin wax	spirit

ALERT! For coding late effect of toxic effects of nonmedical substances see 909.1

982 **Toxic effect of solvents other than petroleum-based**

ALERT! For coding late effect of toxic effects of nonmedical substances see 909.1

| Add 4th or 5th digit | Nonspecific code | Unspecified code | Medicare secondary payer (MSP) alert |

982.0 **Benzene and homologues**

982.1 **Carbon tetrachloride**

982.2 **Carbon disulfide**
Carbon bisulfide

982.3 **Other chlorinated hydrocarbon solvents**
Tetrachloroethylene
Trichloroethylene

Excludes: chlorinated hydrocarbon preparations other than solvents (989.2)

982.4 **Nitroglycol**

982.8 **Other nonpetroleum-based solvents**
Acetone

983 **Toxic effect of corrosive aromatics, acids, and caustic alkalis**
ALERT! For coding late effect of toxic effects of nonmedical substances see 909.1

983.0 **Corrosive aromatics**
Carbolic acid or phenol
Cresol

983.1 **Acids**
Acid:
hydrochloric
nitric
sulfuric

983.2 **Caustic alkalis**
Lye
Potassium hydroxide
Sodium hydroxide

983.9 **Caustic, unspecified**

984 **Toxic effect of lead and its compounds (including fumes)**
Includes: that from all sources except medicinal substances
ALERT! For coding late effect of toxic effects of nonmedical substances see 909.1
ALERT! For personal history of contact with and (suspected) exposure to lead see V15.86

984.0 **Inorganic lead compounds**
Lead dioxide   Lead salts

984.1 **Organic lead compounds**
Lead acetate   Tetraethyl lead

984.8 **Other lead compounds**

984.9 **Unspecified lead compound**

985 **Toxic effect of other metals**
Includes: that from all sources except medicinal substances
ALERT! For coding late effect of toxic effects of nonmedical substances see 909.1

985.0 **Mercury and its compounds**
Minamata disease

985.1 **Arsenic and its compounds**

985.2 **Manganese and its compounds**

985.3 **Beryllium and its compounds**

985.4 **Antimony and its compounds**

985.5 **Cadmium and its compounds**

985.6 **Chromium**

985.8 **Other specified metals**
Brass fumes   Iron compounds
Copper salts   Nickel compounds

985.9 **Unspecified metal**

986 **Toxic effect of carbon monoxide**
Carbon monoxide from any source
ALERT! For coding late effect of toxic effects of nonmedical substances see 909.1

987 **Toxic effect of other gases, fumes, or vapors**
ALERT! For coding late effect of toxic effects of nonmedical substances see 909.1

987.0 **Liquefied petroleum gases**
Butane
Propane

● Code new   ▲ Revision of   ④ ⑤ Fourth or fifth
    to 2012 edition   existing code   digit required

987.1 Other hydrocarbon gas

987.2 Nitrogen oxides
Nitrogen dioxide
Nitrous fumes

987.3 Sulfur dioxide

987.4 Freon
Dichloromonofluoromethane

987.5 Lacrimogenic gas
Bromobenzyl cyanide
Chloroacetophenone
Ethyliodoacetate

987.6 Chlorine gas

987.7 Hydrocyanic acid gas

987.8 Other specified gases, fumes, or vapors
Phosgene
Polyester fumes

987.9 Unspecified gas, fume, or vapor

988 Toxic effect of noxious substances eaten as food

[Excludes:] *allergic reaction to food, such as:*
gastroenteritis (558.3)
rash (692.5, 693.1)
food poisoning (bacterial) (005.0-005.9)
toxic effects of food contaminants, such as:
aflatoxin and other mycotoxin (989.7)
mercury (985.0)

ALERT! For coding late effect of toxic effects of nonmedical substances see 909.1

988.0 Fish and shellfish

988.1 Mushrooms

988.2 Berries and other plants

988.8 Other specified noxious substances eaten as food

988.9 Unspecified noxious substance eaten as food

989 Toxic effect of other substances, chiefly nonmedicinal as to source

ALERT! For coding late effect of toxic effects of nonmedical substances see 909.1

989.0 Hydrocyanic acid and cyanides
Potassium cyanide
Sodium cyanide

[Excludes:] *gas and fumes (987.7)*

989.1 Strychnine and salts

989.2 Chlorinated hydrocarbons
Aldrin
Chlordane
DDT
Dieldrin

[Excludes:] *chlorinated hydrocarbon solvents (982.0-982.3)*

989.3 Organophosphate and carbamate
Carbaryl
Dichlorvos
Malathion
Parathion
Phorate
Phosdrin

989.4 Other pesticides, not elsewhere classified
Mixtures of insecticides

989.5 Venom
Bites of venomous snakes, lizards, and spiders
Tick paralysis

989.6 Soaps and detergents

989.7 Aflatoxin and other mycotoxin [food contaminants]

[5] **989.8 Other substances, chiefly nonmedicinal as to source**

ALERT! For personal history of contact with and (suspected) exposure to asbestos see V15.84

989.81 Asbestos

[Excludes:] *asbestosis (501)*
exposure to asbestos (V15.84)

989.82 Latex

Add 4th or 5th digit | Nonspecific code | Unspecified code | Medicare secondary payer (MSP) alert

989.83 **Silicone**

Excludes: silicone used in medical devices, implants and grafts (996.00-996.79)

989.84 **Tobacco**

989.89 **Other**

989.9 **Unspecified substance, chiefly nonmedicinal as to source**

OTHER AND UNSPECIFIED EFFECTS OF EXTERNAL CAUSES (990-995)

990 **Effects of radiation, unspecified**
Complication of phototherapy   Radiation sickness
Complication of radiation therapy

Excludes: specified adverse effects of radiation
    Such conditions are to be classified according to the nature of the adverse effect, as:
    burns (940.0-949.5)
    dermatitis (692.7-692.8)
    leukemia (204.0-208.9)
    pneumonia (508.0)
    sunburn (692.71, 692.76-692.77)
    [The type of radiation giving rise to the adverse effect may be identified by use of the E codes.]

ALERT! For coding late effect of radiation see 909.2

ALERT! For personal history of irradiation presenting hazards to health see V15.3

991 **Effects of reduced temperature**

991.0 **Frostbite of face**

991.1 **Frostbite of hand**

991.2 **Frostbite of foot**

991.3 **Frostbite of other and unspecified sites**

991.4 **Immersion foot**
Trench foot

991.5 **Chilblains**
Erythema pernio
Perniosis

991.6 **Hypothermia**
Hypothermia (accidental)

Excludes: hypothermia following anesthesia (995.89)
    hypothermia not associated with low environmental temperature (780.65)

991.8 **Other specified effects of reduced temperature**

991.9 **Unspecified effect of reduced temperature**
Effects of freezing or excessive cold NOS

992 **Effects of heat and light**

Excludes: burns (940.0-949.5)
    diseases of sweat glands due to heat (705.0-705.9)
    malignant hyperpyrexia following anesthesia (995.86)
    sunburn (692.71, 692.76-692.77)

992.0 **Heat stroke and sunstroke**
Heat apoplexy
Heat pyrexia
Ictus solaris
Siriasis
Thermoplegia

Use additional code(s) to identify any associated complications of heat stroke, such as:
alterations of consciousness (780.01-780.09)
systemic inflammatory response syndrome (995.93-995.94)

992.1 **Heat syncope**
Heat collapse

992.2 **Heat cramps**

992.3 **Heat exhaustion, anhydrotic**
Heat prostration due to water depletion

Excludes: that associated with salt depletion (992.4)

992.4 **Heat exhaustion due to salt depletion**
Heat prostration due to salt (and water) depletion

  ● Code new
    to 2012 edition
    ▲ Revision of
      existing code
    ④ ⑤ Fourth or fifth
      digit required

992.5 Heat exhaustion, unspecified
Heat prostration NOS

992.6 Heat fatigue, transient

992.7 Heat edema

992.8 Other specified heat effects

992.9 Unspecified

993 Effects of air pressure

993.0 Barotrauma, otitic
Aero-otitis media
Effects of high altitude on ears

993.1 Barotrauma, sinus
Aerosinusitis
Effects of high altitude on sinuses

993.2 Other and unspecified effects of high altitude
Alpine sickness
Andes disease
Anoxia due to high altitude
Hypobaropathy
Mountain sickness

993.3 Caisson disease
Bends
Compressed-air disease
Decompression sickness
Divers' palsy or paralysis

993.4 Effects of air pressure caused by explosion

993.8 Other specified effects of air pressure

993.9 Unspecified effect of air pressure

994 Effects of other external causes

Excludes: *certain adverse effects not elsewhere classified (995.0-995.8)*

994.0 Effects of lightning
Shock from lightning
Struck by lightning NOS

Excludes: *burns (940.0-949.5)*

994.1 Drowning and nonfatal submersion
Bathing cramp
Immersion

994.2 Effects of hunger
Deprivation of food
Starvation

994.3 Effects of thirst
Deprivation of water

994.4 Exhaustion due to exposure

994.5 Exhaustion due to excessive exertion
Exhaustion due to overexertion

994.6 Motion sickness
Air sickness
Seasickness
Travel sickness

994.7 Asphyxiation and strangulation

Suffocation (by):	Suffocation (by):
bedclothes	plastic bag
cave-in	pressure
constriction	strangulation
mechanical	

Excludes: *asphyxia from:*
carbon monoxide (986)
inhalation of food or foreign body (932-934.9)
other gases, fumes, and vapors (987.0-987.9)

▓ Add 4th or	▓ Nonspecific	░ Unspecified	▒ Medicare secondary
5th digit	code	code	payer (MSP) alert

994.8 Electrocution and nonfatal effects of electric current
Shock from electric current
Shock from electroshock gun (taser)

[Excludes:] *electric burns (940.0-949.5)*

994.9 Other effects of external causes
Effects of:
abnormal gravitational [G] forces or states
weightlessness

995 Certain adverse effects not elsewhere classified

[Excludes:] *complications of surgical and medical care (996.0-999.9)*

[ALERT!] For personal history of allergy other than to medicinal agents see V15.0

▲ **995.0 Other anaphylactic reaction**
Allergic shock NOS or due to adverse effect of correct medicinal substance properly administered
Anaphylactic reaction NOS or due to adverse effect of correct medicinal substance properly administered
Anaphylactic shock NOS or due to adverse effect of correct medicinal substance properly administered
Anaphylactoid reaction NOS
Anaphylaxis NOS or due to adverse effect of correct medicinal substance properly administered

[Excludes:] *anaphylactic reaction to serum (999.41-999.49)*
anaphylactic shock or reaction due to adverse food reaction (995.60-995.69)

Use additional E code, if desired, to identify external cause, such as:
adverse effects of correct medicinal substance properly administered (E930-E949)

995.1 Angioneurotic edema
Allergic angioedema
Giant urticaria

[Excludes:] *Urticaria:*
due to serum (999.51-999.59)
other specified (698.2, 708.0-708.9, 757.33)

[5] **995.2 Other and unspecified adverse effect of drug, medicinal and biological substance**

[Excludes:] *pathological drug intoxication (292.2)*

[ALERT!] For coding late effect of adverse effect of drug medicinal or biological substance see 909.5

995.20 Unspecified adverse effect of unspecified drug, medicinal and biological substance
Unspecified adverse effect of unspecified medicinal substance properly administered

995.21 Arthus phenomenon
Arthus reaction

995.22 Unspecified adverse effect of anesthesia

995.23 Unspecified adverse effect of insulin

995.24 Failed moderate sedation during procedure
Failed conscious sedation during procedure

995.27 Other drug allergy
Allergic reaction NEC (due) to correct medical substance properly administered
Drug allergy NOS
Drug hypersensitivity NOS
Hypersensitivity (due) to correct medical substance properly administered

995.29 Unspecified adverse effect of other drug, medicinal and biological substance
Unspecified adverse effect of medicinal substance NEC properly administered

995.3 Allergy, unspecified
Allergic reaction NOS
Hypersensitivity NOS
Idiosyncrasy NOS

[Excludes:] *allergic reaction NOS to correct medicinal substance properly administered (995.27)*
allergy to existing dental restorative materials (525.66)
specific types of allergic reaction, such as:
allergic diarrhea (558.3)
dermatitis (691.0-693.9)
hay fever (477.0-477.9)

995.4 Shock due to anesthesia
Shock due to anesthesia in which the correct substance was properly administered

[Excludes:] *complications of anesthesia in labor or delivery (668.0-668.9)*
overdose or wrong substance given (968.0-969.9)
postoperative shock NOS (998.00)
specified adverse effects of anesthesia classified elsewhere, such as:
anoxic brain damage (348.1)
hepatitis (070.0-070.9), etc.
unspecified adverse effect of anesthesia (995.22)

⑤ **995.5 Child maltreatment syndrome**
Use additional code(s), if applicable, to identify any associated injuries
Use additional E code to identify:
nature of abuse (E960-E968)
perpetrator (E967.0-E967.9)

995.50 Child abuse, unspecified

995.51 Child emotional/psychological abuse

[ALERT!] For personal history of emotional abuse see V15.42

995.52 Child neglect (nutritional)

995.53 Child sexual abuse

995.54 Child physical abuse
Battered baby or child syndrome

[Excludes:] *Shaken infant syndrome (995.55)*

[ALERT!] For personal history of physical abuse see V15.41

995.55 Shaken infant syndrome
Use additional code(s) to identify any associated injuries

995.59 Other child abuse and neglect
Multiple forms of abuse

▲ **995.6 Anaphylactic reaction due to food**
Anaphylactic reaction due to adverse food reaction
Anaphylactic shock or reaction due to nonpoisonous foods
Anaphylactoid reaction due to food

[DEFINITION] Anaphylactic shock is a sudden, severe, potentially life-threatening allergic reaction caused by food allergy, insect stings or medications.

▲ **995.60 Anaphylactic reaction due to unspecified food**

▲ **995.61 Anaphylactic reaction due to peanuts**

▲ **995.62 Anaphylactic reaction due to crustaceans**

▲ **995.63 Anaphylactic reaction due to fruits and vegetables**

▲ **995.64 Anaphylactic reaction due to tree nuts and seeds**

▲ **995.65 Anaphylactic reaction due to fish**

▲ **995.66 Anaphylactic reaction due to food additives**

▲ **995.67 Anaphylactic reaction due to milk products**

▲ **995.68 Anaphylactic reaction due to eggs**

▲ **995.69 Anaphylactic reaction due to other specified food**

995.7 Other adverse food reactions, not elsewhere classified
Use additional code to identify the type of reaction, such as:
hives (708.0)
wheezing (786.07)

[Excludes:] *anaphylactic reaction or shock due to adverse food reaction (995.60-995.69)*
asthma (493.0, 493.9)
dermatitis due to food (693.1)
in contact with the skin (692.5)
gastroenteritis and colitis due to food (558.3)
rhinitis due to food (477.1)

⑤ **995.8 Other specified adverse effects, not elsewhere classified**

995.80 Adult maltreatment, unspecified
Abused person NOS

Use additional code to identify:
any associated injury
perpetrator (E967.0-E967.9)

Add 4th or 5th digit | Nonspecific code | Unspecified code | Medicare secondary payer (MSP) alert

995.81   Adult physical abuse
Battered:
person syndrome NEC
man
spouse
woman

Use additional code to identify:
any associated injury
nature of abuse (E960-E968)
perpetrator (E967.0-E967.9)

ALERT! For personal history of physical abuse see V15.41

995.82   Adult emotional/psychological abuse
Use additional E code to identify perpetrator (E967.0-E967.9)

ALERT! For personal history of emotional abuse see V15.42

995.83   Adult sexual abuse
Use additional code to identify:
any associated injury
perpetrator (E967.0-E967.9)

995.84   Adult neglect (nutritional)
Use additional code to identify:
intent of neglect (E904.0, E968.4)
perpetrator (E967.0-967.9)

995.85   Other adult abuse and neglect
Multiple forms of abuse and neglect

Use additional code to identify:
any associated injury
intent of neglect (E904.0, E968.4)
nature of abuse (E960-E968)
perpetrator (E967.0-E967.9)

995.86   Malignant hyperthermia
Malignant hyperpyrexia due to anesthesia

995.89   Other
Hypothermia due to anesthesia

⑤ **995.9   Systemic inflammatory response syndrome (SIRS)**

995.90   Systemic inflammatory response syndrome, unspecified
SIRS NOS

995.91   Sepsis
Systemic inflammatory response syndrome due to infectious process without acute organ dysfunction

Code first underlying infection

Excludes: *sepsis with acute organ dysfunction (995.92)*
sepsis with multiple organ dysfunction (995.92)
severe sepsis (995.92)

995.92   Severe sepsis
Sepsis with acute organ dysfunction
Sepsis with multiple organ dysfunction (MOD)
Systemic inflammatory response syndrome due to infectious process with acute organ dysfunction

Code first underlying infection

Use additional code to specify acute organ dysfunction, such as:
acute kidney failure (584.5-584.9)
acute respiratory failure (518.81)
critical illness myopathy (359.81)
critical illness polyneuropathy (357.82)
disseminated intravascular coagulopathy (DIC) syndrome (286.6)
encephalopathy (348.31)
hepatic failure (570)
septic shock (785.52)

995.93   Systemic inflammatory response syndrome due to noninfectious process without acute organ dysfunction

Code first underlying conditions, such as:
acute pancreatitis (577.0)
trauma

Excludes: *systemic inflammatory response syndrome due to noninfectious process with acute organ dysfunction (995.94)*

◗ Code new   ▲ Revision of   ④ ⑤ Fourth or fifth
to 2012 edition   existing code   digit required

995.94 Systemic inflammatory response syndrome due to non-infectious process with acute organ dysfunction

Code first underlying condition, such as:
acute pancreatitis (577.0)
heat stroke (992.0)
trauma

Use additional code to specify acute organ dysfunction, such as:
acute kidney failure (584.5-584.9)
acute respiratory failure (518.81)
critical illness myopathy (359.81)
critical illness polyneuropathy (357.82)
disseminated intravascular coagulopathy (DIC) syndrome (286.6)
encephalopathy (348.31)
hepatic failure (570)

[Excludes:] *severe sepsis (995.92)*

COMPLICATIONS OF SURGICAL AND MEDICAL CARE, NOT ELSEWHERE CLASSIFIED (996-999)

[Excludes:] *adverse effects of medicinal agents (001.0-799.9, 995.0-995.8)*
burns from local applications and irradiation (940.0-949.5)
complications of:
conditions for which the procedure was performed
surgical procedures during abortion, labor, and delivery (630-676.9)
poisoning and toxic effects of drugs and chemicals (960.0-989.9)
postoperative conditions in which no complications are present, such as:
artificial opening status (V44.0-V44.9)
closure of external stoma (V55.0-V55.9)
fitting of prosthetic device (V52.0-V52.9)
specified complications classified elsewhere
anesthetic shock (995.4)
electrolyte imbalance (276.0-276.9)
postlaminectomy syndrome (772.80-722.83)
postmastectomy lymphedema syndrome (457.0)
postoperative psychosis (293.0-293.9)
any other condition classified elsewhere in the Alphabetic Index when described as due to a procedure

996 Complications peculiar to certain specified procedures

Includes: complications, not elsewhere classified, in the use of artificial substitutes [e.g., Dacron, metal, Silastic, Teflon] or natural sources [e.g., bone] involving:
anastomosis (internal)
graft (bypass) (patch)
implant
internal device:
catheter
electronic
fixation
prosthetic
reimplant
transplant

[Excludes:] *accidental puncture or laceration during procedure (998.2)*
capsular contracture of breast implant (611.83)
complications of internal anastomosis of:
gastrointestinal tract (997.49)
urinary tract (997.5)
endosseous dental implant failures (525.71-525.79)
intraoperative floppy iris syndrome (IFIS) (364.81)
mechanical complication of respirator (V46.14)
other specified complications classified elsewhere, such as:
hemolytic anemia (283.1)
functional cardiac disturbances (429.4)
serum hepatitis (070.2-070.3)

[ALERT!] For coding late effect of complications of surgical and medical care see 909.3

[ALERT!] For personal history of surgery to other organs see V15.29

[5] **996.0 Mechanical complication of cardiac device, implant, and graft**

Breakdown (mechanical)	Obstruction, mechanical
Displacement	Perforation
Leakage	Protrusion

996.00 Unspecified device, implant, and graft

Add 4th or 5th digit — Nonspecific code — Unspecified code — Medicare secondary payer (MSP) alert

996.01 Due to cardiac pacemaker (electrode)

996.02 Due to heart valve prosthesis

996.03 Due to coronary bypass graft

[Excludes:] *atherosclerosis of graft (414.02, 414.03)*
embolism [occlusion NOS] [thrombus] of graft (996.72)

996.04 Due to automatic implantable cardiac defibrillator

996.09 Other

996.1 Mechanical complication of other vascular device, implant, and graft
Mechanical complications involving:
aortic (bifurcation) graft (replacement)
arteriovenous:
dialysis catheter
fistula surgically created
shunt surgicall created
balloon (counterpulsation) device, intra-aortic
carotid artery bypass graft
femoral-popliteal bypass graft
umbrella device, vena cava

[Excludes:] *atherosclerosis of biological graft (440.30-440.32)*
embolism [occlusion NOS] [thrombus] of (biological) (synthetic) graft (996.74)
peritoneal dialysis catheter (996.56)

996.2 Mechanical complication of nervous system device, implant, and graft
Mechanical complications involving:
dorsal column stimulator
electrodes implanted in brain [brain "pacemaker"]
peripheral nerve graft
ventricular (communicating) shunt

[5] **996.3 Mechanical complication of genitourinary device, implant, and graft**

996.30 Unspecified device, implant, and graft

996.31 Due to urethral [indwelling] catheter

996.32 Due to intrauterine contraceptive device

996.39 Other
Prosthetic reconstruction of vas deferens
Repair (graft) of ureter without mention of resection

[Excludes:] *complications due to:*
external stoma of urinary tract (596.81-596.83)
internal anastomosis of urinary tract (997.5)

[5] **996.4 Mechanical complication of internal orthopedic device, implant, and graft**
Use additional code to identify prosthetic joint with mechanical complication (V43.60-V43.69)

996.40 Unspecified mechanical complication of internal orthopedic device, implant, and graft

996.41 Mechanical loosening of prosthetic joint
Aseptic loosening

996.42 Dislocation of prosthetic joint
Instability of prosthetic joint
Subluxation of prosthetic joint

996.43 Broken prosthetic joint implant
Breakage (fracture) of prosthetic joint

996.44 Peri-prosthetic fracture around prosthetic joint

996.45 Peri-prosthetic osteolysis
Use additional code to identify major osseous defect, if applicable (731.3)

996.46 Articular bearing surface wear of prosthetic joint

996.47 Other mechanical complication of prosthetic joint implant
Mechanical complication of prosthetic joint NOS
Prosthetic joint implant failure NOS

996.49 Other mechanical complication of other internal orthopedic device, implant, and graft
Breakage of internal fixation device in bone
Dislocation of internal fixation device in bone

[Excludes:] *mechanical complication of prosthetic joint implant (996.41-996.47)*

⑤ **996.5   Mechanical complication of other specified prosthetic device, implant, and graft**
Mechanical complications involving:
   prosthetic implant in:
      bile duct
      breast
      chin
      orbit of eye
   nonabsorbable surgical material NOS
   other graft, implant, and internal device, not elsewhere classified

996.51   Due to corneal graft

996.52   Due to graft of other tissue, not elsewhere classified
   Skin graft failure or rejection

Excludes: *failure of artificial skin graft (996.55)*
         failure of decellularized allodermis (996.55)
         sloughing of temporary skin allografts or xenografts (pigskin)—omit code

996.53   Due to ocular lens prosthesis

Excludes: *contact lenses—code to condition*

996.54   Due to breast prosthesis
   Breast capsule (prosthesis)
   Mammary implant

996.55   Due to artificial skin graft and decellularized allodermis
   Dislodgement   Displacement
   Failure   Non-adherence
   Poor incorporation   Shearing

996.56   Due to peritoneal dialysis catheter

Excludes: *mechanical complication of arteriovenous dialysis catheter (996.1)*

996.57   Due to insulin pump

996.59   Due to other implant and internal device, not elsewhere classified
   Nonabsorbable surgical material NOS
   Prosthetic implant in:
      bile duct
      chin
      orbit of eye

⑤ **996.6   Infection and inflammatory reaction due to internal prosthetic device, implant, and graft**
   Infection (causing obstruction) due to (presence of) any device, implant and graft classifiable to 996.0-996.5
   Inflammation due to (presence of) any device, implant and graft classifiable to 996.0-996.5
   Use additional code to identify specified infections

996.60   Due to unspecified device, implant, and graft

996.61   Due to cardiac device, implant, and graft
   Cardiac pacemaker or defibrillator:
      electrode(s), lead(s)
      pulse generator
      subcutaneous pocket
   Coronary artery bypass graft
   Heart valve prosthesis

996.62   Due to other vascular device, implant, and graft
   Arterial graft
   Arteriovenous fistula or shunt
   Infusion pump
   Vascular catheter (arterial) (dialysis) (peripheral venous)

Excludes: *infection due to:*
         central venous catheter (999.31-999.32)
         Hickman catheter (999.31-999.32)
         peripherally inserted central catheter (PICC) (999.31-999.32)
         portacath (port-a-cath) (999.31999.32)
         triple lumen catheter (999.31-999.32)
         umbilical venous catheter (999.31-999.32)

996.63   Due to nervous system device, implant, and graft
   Electrodes implanted in brain
   Peripheral nerve graft
   Spinal canal catheter
   Ventricular (communicating) shunt (catheter)

| Add 4th or 5th digit | Nonspecific code | Unspecified code | Medicare secondary payer (MSP) alert |

996.64 Due to indwelling urinary catheter
Use additional code to identify specified infections, such as:
    Cystitis (595.0-595.9)
    Sepsis (038.0-038.9)

Excludes: *complications due to:*
    external stoma of urinary tract (596.81-596.83)

996.65 Due to other genitourinary device, implant, and graft
    Intrauterine contraceptive device

996.66 Due to internal joint prosthesis
Use additional code to identify infected prosthetic joint (V43.60-V43.69)

996.67 Due to other internal orthopedic device, implant, and graft
    Bone growth stimulator (electrode)
    Internal fixation device (pin) (rod) (screw)

996.68 Due to peritoneal dialysis catheter
    Exit-site infection or inflammation

996.69 Due to other internal prosthetic device, implant, and graft
    Breast prosthesis
    Ocular lens prosthesis
    Prosthetic orbital implant

⑤ **996.7 Other complications of internal (biological) (synthetic) prosthetic device, implant, and graft**
    Complication NOS due to (presence of) any device, implant, and graft classifiable to 996.0-996.5
    occlusion NOS
    Embolism due to (presence of) any device, implant, and graft classifiable to 996.0-996.5
    Fibrosis due to (presence of) any device, implant, and graft classifiable to 996.0-996.5
    Hemorrhage due to (presence of) any device, implant, and graft classifiable to 996.0-996.5
    Pain due to (presence of) any device, implant, and graft classifiable to 996.0-996.5
    Stenosis due to (presence of) any device, implant, and graft classifiable to 996.0-996.5
    Thrombus due to (presence of) any device, implant, and graft classifiable to 996.0-996.5
Use additional code to identify complication, such as:
    pain due to presence of device, implant or graft (338.18-338.19,338.28-338.29)
    venous embolism and thrombosis (453.2-453.9)

Excludes: *disruption (dehiscence) of internal suture material (998.31)*
    transplant rejection (996.80-996.89)

996.70 Due to unspecified device, implant, and graft

996.71 Due to heart valve prosthesis

996.72 Due to other cardiac device, implant, and graft
    Cardiac pacemaker or defibrillator:
      electrode(s), lead(s)
      subcutaneous pocket
    Coronary artery bypass (graft)

Excludes: *occlusion due to atherosclerosis (414.02-414.06)*

996.73 Due to renal dialysis device, implant, and graft

996.74 Due to other vascular device, implant, and graft

Excludes: *occlusion of biological graft due to atherosclerosis (440.30-440.32)*

996.75 Due to nervous system device, implant, and graft

996.76 Due to genitourinary device, implant, and graft

Excludes: *complications of implanted vaginal mesh (629.31-629.32)*

996.77 Due to internal joint prosthesis
Use additional code to identify prosthetic joint (V43.60 - V43.69)

996.78 Due to other internal orthopedic device, implant, and graft

996.79 Due to other internal prosthetic device, implant, and graft

● Code new
   to 2012 edition
▲ Revision of
   existing code
④ ⑤ Fourth or fifth
     digit required

⑤ **996.8   Complications of transplanted organ**

Use additional code, if desired, to identify nature of complication, such as:
> cytomegalovirus (CMV) infection (078.5)
> graft-versus-host disease (279.50-279.53)
> malignancy associated with organ transplant (199.2)
> post-transplant lymphoproliferative disorder (PTLD) (238.77)
> transplant failure or rejection

ALERT! Codes under subcategory 996.8 are for use for both complications and rejection of transplanted organs. A transplant complication code is only assigned if the complication affects the function of the transplanted organ. Two codes are required to fully describe a transplant complication, the appropriate code from subcategory 996.8 and a secondary code that identifies the complication.

996.80   Transplanted organ, unspecified

996.81   Kidney

ALERT! Code 996.81 should be assigned for documented complications of a kidney transplant, such as transplant failure or rejection or other transplant complication

ALERT! Code 996.81 should not be assigned for post kidney transplant patients who have chronic kidney (CKD) unless a transplant complication such as transplant failure or rejection is documented. If the documentation is unclear as to whether the patient has a complication of the transplant, query the provider

996.82   Liver

996.83   Heart

996.84   Lung

996.85   Bone Marrow

996.86   Pancreas

996.87   Intestine

● **996.88   Stem cell**
> Complications from stem cells from:
> peripheral blood
> umbilical cord

996.89   Other specified transplanted organ

⑤ **996.9   Complications of reattached extremity or body part**

996.90   Unspecified extremity

996.91   Forearm

996.92   Hand

996.93   Finger(s)

996.94   Upper extremity, other and unspecified

996.95   Foot and toe(s)

996.96   Lower extremity, other and unspecified

996.99   Other specified body part

997   **Complications affecting specified body systems, not elsewhere classified**

Use additional code to identify complication

> Excludes: *the listed conditions when specified as:*
> *causing shock (998.00-998.09)*
> *complications of:*
> *anesthesia:*
> *adverse effect (001.0-799.9, 995.0-995.8)*
> *in labor or delivery (668.0-668.9)*
> *poisoning (968.0-969.9)*
> *implanted device or graft (996.0-996.9)*
> *obstetrical procedures (669.0-669.4)*
> *reattached extremity (996.90-996.96)*
> *transplanted organ (996.80-996.89)*

ALERT! For coding late effect of complications of surgical and medical care see 909.3

⑤ **997.0   Nervous system complications**

997.00   Nervous system complication, unspecified

997.01   Central nervous system complication
> Anoxic brain damage   Cerebral hypoxia

> Excludes: *cerebrovascular hemorrhage or infarction (997.02)*

997.02   Iatrogenic cerebrovascular infarction or hemorrhage
> Postoperative stroke

	Add 4th or 5th digit		Nonspecific code		Unspecified code		Medicare secondary payer (MSP) alert

997.09 Other nervous system complications

997.1 Cardiac complications
Cardiac arrest during or resulting from a procedure
Cardiac insufficiency during or resulting from a procedure
Cardiorespiratory failure during or resulting from a procedure
Heart failure during or resulting from a procedure

Excludes: *the listed conditions as long-term effects of cardiac surgery or due to the presence of cardiac prosthetic device (429.4)*

997.2 Peripheral vascular complications
Phlebitis or thrombophlebitis during or resulting from a procedure

Excludes: *the listed conditions due to:*
implant or catheter device (996.62)
infusion, perfusion, or transfusion (999.2)
complications affecting blood vessels (997.71-997.79)

⑤ **997.3 Respiratory complications**

Excludes: *iatrogenic [postoperative] pneumothorax (512.1)*
iatrogenic pulmonary embolism (415.11)
specified complications classified elsewhere, such as:
adult respiratory distress syndrome (518.52)
pulmonary edema, postoperative (518.4)
respiratory insufficiency, acute, postoperative (518.52)
shock lung related to trauma and surgery (518.52)
tracheostomy complications (519.00-519.09)
transfusion related acute lung injury (TRALI) (518.7)

997.31 Ventilator associated pneumonia
Ventilator associated pneumonitis

Use additional code to identify organism

ALERT! Code 997.31 should be assigned only when the provider has documented ventilator associated pneumonia (VAP). An additional code to identify the organism (e.g., Pseudomonas aeruginosa, code 041.7) should also be assigned.

ALERT! Code 997.31 should not be assigned for cases where the patient has pneumonia and is on a mechanical ventilator but the provider has not specifically stated that the pneumonia is ventilator-associated pneumonia

● **997.32 Postprocedural aspiration pneumonia**
Chemical pneumonitis resulting from a procedure
Mendelson's syndrome resulting from a procedure

Excludes: *aspiration pneumonia during labor and delivery (668.0)*

997.39 Other respiratory complications

⑤ **997.4 Digestive system complications**
Complications of intestinal (internal) anastomosis and bypass, not elsewhere classified, except that involving urinary tract
Hepatic failure specified as due to a procedure
Hepatorenal syndrome specified as due to a procedure
Intestinal obstruction NOS specified as due to a procedure

Excludes: *complications of gastric band procedure (539.01-539.09)*
complications of other bariatric procedure (539.81-539.89)
specified gastrointestinal complications classified elsewhere, such as:
blind loop syndrome (579.2)
colostomy or enterostomy complications (569.60-569.69)
complications of intestinal pouch (569.71-569.79)
gastrostomy complications (536.40-536.49)
gastrojejunal ulcer (534.0-534.9)
infection of esophagostomy (530.86)
infection of external stoma (569.61)
mechanical complication of esophagostomy (530.87)
pelvic peritoneal adhesions, female (614.6)
peritoneal adhesions (568.0)
peritoneal adhesions with obstruction (560.81)
postcholecystectomy syndrome (576.0)
postgastric surgery syndromes (564.2)
pouchitis (569.71)
vomiting following gastrointestinal surgery (564.3)

● **997.41 Retained cholelithiasis following cholecystectomy**

● **997.49** Other digestive system complications

● Code new
to 2012 edition
▲ Revision of
existing code
④ ⑤ Fourth or fifth
digit required

997.5 Urinary complications
Complications of:
internal anastomosis and bypass of urinary tract, including that involving intestinal tract
Oliguria or anuria specified as due to procedure
Renal (kidney):
failure (acute) specified as due to procedure
insufficiency (acute) specified as due to procedure
Tubular necrosis (acute) specified as due to procedure

Excludes: *complications of cystostomy (596.81-596.83)*
complications of external stoma of urinary tract (596.81-596.83)
specified complications classified elsewhere, such as:
postoperative stricture of:
ureter (593.3)
urethra (598.2)

⑤ **997.6 Amputation stump complication**

Excludes: *admission for treatment for a current traumatic amputation; code to complicated*
traumatic amputation
phantom limb (syndrome) (353.6)

997.60 Unspecified complication

997.61 Neuroma of amputation stump

997.62 Infection (chronic)
Use additional code to identify the organism

997.69 Other

⑤ **997.7 Vascular complications of other vessels**

Excludes: *peripheral vascular complications (997.2)*

997.71 Vascular complications of mesenteric artery

997.72 Vascular complications of renal artery

997.79 Vascular complications of other vessels

⑤ **997.9 Complications affecting other specified body systems, not elsewhere classified**

Excludes: *specified complications classified elsewhere, such as:*
broad ligament laceration syndrome (620.6)
postartificial menopause syndrome (627.4)
postoperative stricture of vagina (623.2)

997.91 Hypertension
Excludes: *essential hypertension (401.0-401.9)*

997.99 Other
Vitreous touch syndrome

998 Other complications of procedures, not elsewhere classified

Excludes: *fluid overload due to transfusion (blood) (276.61)*
TACO (276.61)
transfusion associated circulatory overload (276.61)

ALERT! For coding late effect of complications of surgical and medical care see 909.3

⑤ **998.0 Postoperative shock**
Shock during or resulting from a surgical procedure

Excludes: *shock:*
anaphylactic due to serum (999.41-999.49)
anesthetic (995.4)
electric (994.8)
following abortion (639.5)
obstetric (669.1)
traumatic (958.4)

● **998.00 Postoperative shock, unspecified**
Collapse, not otherwise specified, during or resulting from a surgical procedure
Failure of peripheral circulation, postoperative

● **998.01 Postoperative shock, cardiogenic**

Add 4th or 5th digit   Nonspecific code   Unspecified code   Medicare secondary payer (MSP) alert

● **998.02 Postoperative shock, septic**
　　　　Postoperative endotoxic shock
　　　　Postoperative gram-negative shock

Code first underlying infection

Use additional code, to identify severe sepsis (995.92) and any associated acute organ
　　dysfunction, if applicable

● **998.09 Postoperative shock, other**
　　　　Postoperative hypovolemic shock

⑤ **998.1 Hemorrhage or hematoma or seroma complicating a procedure**

Excludes: *hemorrhage due to implanted device or graft (996.70-996.79)*

*hemorrhage, hematoma or seroma complicating cesarean section or puerperal
　　perineal wound (674.3)*

998.11 Hemorrhage complicating a procedure

998.12 Hematoma complicating a procedure

998.13 Seroma complicating a procedure

998.2 Accidental puncture or laceration during a procedure
　　　　Accidental perforation by catheter or other instrument during a procedure on:
　　　　blood vessel
　　　　nerve
　　　　organ

Excludes: *iatrogenic [postoperative] pneumothorax (512.1)*

*puncture or laceration caused by implanted device intentionally left in operation
　　wound (996.0-996.5)*
specified complications classified elsewhere, such as:
　　broad ligament laceration syndrome (620.6)
　　dural tear (349.31)
　　incidental durotomy (349.31)
　　trauma from instruments during delivery (664.0-665.9)

⑤ **998.3 Disruption of wound**
　　　　Dehiscence of operation wound
　　　　Disruption of any suture materials or other closure method
　　　　Rupture of operation wound

Excludes: *disruption of:*
　　cesarean wound (674.1)
　　perineal wound, puerperal (674.2)

998.30 Disruption of wound, unspecified
　　　　Disruption of wound NOS

998.31 Disruption of internal operation (surgical) wound
　　　　Disruption or dehiscence of closure of:
　　　　　　fascia, superficial or muscular
　　　　　　internal organ
　　　　　　muscle or muscle flap
　　　　　　ribs or rib cage
　　　　　　skull or craniotomy
　　　　　　sternum or sternotomy
　　　　　　tendon or ligament
　　　　Deep disruption or dehiscence of operation wound NOS

Excludes: *complications of internal anastomosis of:*
　　gastrointestinal tract (997.49)
　　urinary tract (997.5)

998.32 Disruption of external operation (surgical) wound
　　　　Disruption or dehiscence of closure of:
　　　　　　cornea
　　　　　　mucosa
　　　　　　skin
　　　　　　subcutaneous tissue
　　　　Disruption of operation wound NOS
　　　　Full-thickness skin disruption or dehiscence
　　　　Superficial disruption or dehiscence of operation wound

998.33 Disruption of traumatic injury wound repair
　　　　Disruption or dehiscence of closure of traumatic laceration (external) (internal)

● Code new
　to 2012 edition　　　　▲ Revision of
　　　　　　　　　　　　existing code　　　　④ ⑤ Fourth or fifth
　　　　　　　　　　　　　　　　　　　　　　digit required

998.4 Foreign body accidentally left during a procedure
  Adhesions due to foreign body accidentally left in operative wound or body cavity
   during a procedure
  Obstruction due to foreign body accidentally left in operative wound or body cavity
   during a procedure
  Perforation due to foreign body accidentally left in operative wound or body cavity
   during a procedure

  | Excludes: | *obstruction or perforation caused by implanted device intentionally left in body*
   (996.0-996.5)

⑤ **998.5 Postoperative infection**

  | Excludes: | *bleb associated endophthalmitis (379.63)*
    infection due to:
     implanted device (996.60-996.69)
     infusion, perfusion, or transfusion (999.31-999.39)
     postoperative obstetrical wound infection (674.3)

  998.51 Infected postoperative seroma
  Use additional code to identify organism

  998.59 Other postoperative infection
   Abscess: postoperative
    intra-abdominal postoperative
    stitch postoperative
    subphrenic postoperative
    wound postoperative
   Septicemia postoperative
  Use additional code to identify infection

998.6 Persistent postoperative fistula

998.7 Acute reaction to foreign substance accidentally left during a procedure
  Peritonitis:
   aseptic
   chemical

⑤ **998.8 Other specified complications of procedures, not elsewhere classified**

  998.81 Emphysema (subcutaneous) (surgical) resulting from a procedure

  998.82 Cataract fragments in eye following cataract surgery

  998.83 Non-healing surgical wound

  998.89 Other specified complications

998.9 Unspecified complication of procedure, not elsewhere classified
  Postoperative complication NOS

  | Excludes: | *complication NOS of obstetrical surgery or procedure (669.4)*

Add 4th or 5th digit   Nonspecific code   Unspecified code   Medicare secondary payer (MSP) alert

999 **Complications of medical care, not elsewhere classified**

Use additional code, where applicable, to identify specific complication

Includes: complications, not elsewhere classified, of:
> dialysis (hemodialysis) (peritoneal) (renal)
> extracorporeal circulation
> hyperalimentation therapy
> immunization
> infusion
> inhalation therapy
> injection
> inoculation
> perfusion
> transfusion
> vaccination
> ventilation therapy

Excludes: *specified complications classified elsewhere such as:*
> *complications of implanted device (996.0-996.9)*
> *contact dermatitis due to drugs (692.3)*
> *dementia dialysis (294.8)*
> *transient (293.9)*
> *dialysis disequilibrium syndrome (276.0-276.9)*
> *poisoning and toxic effects of drugs and chemicals (960.0-989.9)*
> *postvaccinal encephalitis (323.51)*
> *water and electrolyte imbalance (276.0-276.9)*

ALERT! For coding late effect of complications of surgical and medical care see 909.3

DEFINITION Complications of medical care, also known as iatrogenesis, is an inadvertent adverse effect or complication resulting from medical treatment or advice.

999.0 Generalized vaccinia

Excludes: *vaccinia not from vaccine (051.02)*

999.1 Air embolism

Air embolism to any site following infusion, perfusion, or transfusion

Excludes: *embolism specified as:*
> *complicating:*
> *abortion (634-638 with .6, 639.6)*
> *ectopic or molar pregnancy (639.6)*
> *pregnancy, childbirth, or the puerperium (673.0)*
> *due to implanted device (996.7)*
> *traumatic (958.0)*

999.2 **Other vascular complications**

Phlebitis following infusion, perfusion, or transfusion
Thromboembolism following infusion, perfusion, or transfusion
Thrombophlebitis following infusion, perfusion, or transfusion

Excludes: *extravasation of vesicant drugs (999.81, 999.82)*

> *the listed conditions when specified as:*
> *due to implanted device (996.61-996.62, 996.72-996.74)*
> *postoperative NOS (997.2, 997.71-997.79)*

⑤ **999.3 Other infection**

Infection following infusion, injection, transfusion, or vaccination
Sepsis following infusion, injection, transfusion, or vaccination
Septicemia following infusion, injection, transfusion, or vaccination

Use additional code to identify the specified infection, such as:
> septicemia (038.0-038.9)

Excludes: *the listed conditions when specified as:*
> *due to implanted device (996.60-996.69)*
> *postoperative NOS (998.51-998.59)*

● Code new to 2012 edition   ▲ Revision of existing code   ④ ⑤ Fourth or fifth digit required

▲ **999.31 Other and unspecified infection due to central venous catheter**
Central line-associated infection
Infection due to:
central venous catheter NOS
Hickman catheter
peripherally inserted central catheter (PICC)
triple lumen catheter
umbilical venous catheter

[Excludes:] *infection due to:*
arterial catheter (996.62)
catheter NOS (996.69)
peripheral venous catheter (996.62)
urinary catheter (996.64)

● **999.32 Bloodstream infection due to central venous catheter**
Bloodstream infection due to:
Hickman catheter
peripherally inserted central catheter (PICC)
portacath (port-a-cath)
triple lumen catheter
umbilical venous catheter
Catheter-related bloodstream infection (CRBSI) NOS
Central line-associated bloodstream infection (CLABSI)

● **999.33 Local infection due to central venous catheter**
Exit or insertion site infection
Local infection due to:
Hickman catheter
peripherally inserted central catheter (PICC)
portacath (port-a-cath)
triple lumen catheter
umbilical venous catheter
Port or reservoir infection
Tunnel infection

● **999.34 Acute infection following transfusion, infusion, or injection of blood and blood products**

999.39 Infection following other infusion, injection, transfusion, or vaccination

▲ **999.4 Anaphylactic reaction due to serum**
Allergic shock
Anaphylactic shock due to serum
Anaphylactoid reaction due to serum
Anaphylaxis

[Excludes:] *ABO incompatibility reaction due to transfusion of blood or blood products (999.60-999.69)*
reaction:
allergic NOS (995.0)
anaphylactic:
NOS (995.0)
due to drugs and chemicals (995.0)
other serum (999.51-999.59)
shock:
allergic NOS (995.0)
anaphylactic:
NOS (995.0)
due to drugs and chemicals (995.0)

● **999.41 Anaphylactic reaction due to administration of blood and blood products**

● **999.42 Anaphylactic reaction due to vaccination**

● **999.49 Anaphylactic reaction due to other serum**

[5] **999.5 Other serum reaction**
Intoxication by serum
Protein sickness
Serum rash
Serum sickness
Urticaria due to serum

[Excludes:] *serum hepatitis (070.2-070.3)*

● **999.51 Other serum reaction due to administration of blood and blood products**

● **999.52 Other serum reaction due to vaccination**

● **999.59 Other serum reaction**

⑤ **999.6 ABO incompatibility reaction due to transfusion of blood or blood products**

> Excludes: *minor blood group antigens reactions (Duffy) (E) (K(ell)) (Kidd) (Lewis) (M) (N)*
> *(P) (S) (999.75-999.79)*

999.60 ABO incompatibility reaction, unspecified
ABO incompatible blood transfusion NOS
Reaction to ABO incompatibility from transfusion NOS

999.61 ABO incompatibility with hemolytic transfusion reaction not specified as acute or delayed
ABO incompatibility with hemolytic transfusion reaction at unspecified time after transfusion
Hemolytic transfusion reaction (HTR) due to ABO incompatibility

999.62 ABO incompatibility with acute hemolytic transfusion reaction
ABO incompatibility with hemolytic transfusion reaction less than 24 hours after transfusion
Acute hemolytic transfusion reaction (AHTR) due to ABO incompatibility

999.63 ABO incompatibility with delayed hemolytic transfusion reaction
ABO incompatibility with hemolytic transfusion reaction 24 hours or more after transfusion
Delayed hemolytic transfusion reaction (DHTR) due to ABO incompatibility

999.69 Other ABO incompatibility reaction
Delayed serologic transfusion reaction (DSTR) from ABO incompatibility
Other ABO incompatible blood transfusion
Other reaction to ABO incompatibility from transfusion

⑤ **999.7 Rh and other non-ABO incompatibility reaction due to transfusion of blood or blood products**

999.70 Rh incompatibility reaction, unspecified
Reaction due to Rh factor in transfusion NOS
Rh incompatible blood transfusion NOS
Unspecified reaction due to incompatibility related to Rh antigens (C) (c) (D) (E) (e)
Unspecified reaction to Rh incompatibility

999.71 Rh incompatibility with hemolytic transfusion reaction not specified as acute or delayed
Hemolytic transfusion reaction (HTR) due to Rh incompatibility
HTR due to incompatibility related to Rh antigens (C) (c) (D) (E) (e), not specified as acute or delayed
Rh incompatibility with hemolytic transfusion reaction at unspecified time after transfusion

999.72 Rh incompatibility with acute hemolytic transfusion reaction
Acute hemolytic transfusion reaction (AHTR) due to Rh incompatibility
AHTR due to incompatibility related to Rh antigens (C) (c) (D) (E) (e)
Rh incompatibility with hemolytic transfusion reaction less than 24 hours after transfusion

999.73 Rh incompatibility with delayed hemolytic transfusion reaction
Delayed hemolytic transfusion reaction (DHTR) due to Rh incompatibility
DHTR due to incompatibility related to Rh antigens (C) (c) (D) (E) (e)
Rh incompatibility with hemolytic transfusion reaction 24 hours or more after transfusion

999.74 Other Rh incompatibility reaction
Delayed serologic transfusion reaction (DSTR) from Rh incompatibility
Other reaction due to incompatibility related to Rh antigens (C) (c) (D) (E) (e)
Other reaction to Rh incompatible blood transfusion

999.75 Non-ABO incompatibility reaction, unspecified
Non-ABO incompatible blood transfusion NOS
Reaction to non-ABO antigen incompatibility from transfusion NOS
Unspecified reaction due to incompatibility related to minor antigens (Duffy) (Kell) (Kidd) (Lewis) (M) (N) (P) (S)

999.76 Non-ABO incompatibility with hemolytic transfusion reaction not specified as acute or delayed
Hemolytic transfusion reaction (HTR) due to non-ABO incompatibility
HTR from incompatibility related to minor antigens (Duffy) (Kell) (Kidd) (Lewis) (M) (N) (P) (S)
Non-ABO incompatibility with hemolytic transfusion reaction at unspecified time after transfusion

● Code new to 2012 edition ▲ Revision of existing code ④ ⑤ Fourth or fifth digit required

999.77 Non-ABO incompatibility with acute hemolytic transfusion reaction
Acute hemolytic transfusion reaction (AHTR) due to non-ABO incompatibility
AHTR from incompatibility related to minor antigens (Duffy) (Kell) (Kidd) (Lewis) (M) (N) (P) (S)
Non-ABO incompatibility with hemolytic transfusion reaction less than 24 hours after transfusion

999.78 Non-ABO incompatibility with delayed hemolytic transfusion reaction
Delayed hemolytic transfusion reaction (DHTR) due to non-ABO incompatibility
DHTR from incompatibility related to minor antigens (Duffy) (Kell) (Kidd) (Lewis) (M) (N) (P) (S)
Non-ABO incompatibility with hemolytic transfusion reaction 24 hours or more after transfusion

999.79 Other non-ABO incompatibility reaction
Delayed serologic transfusion reaction (DSTR) from non-ABO incompatibility
Other non-ABO incompatible blood transfusion
Other reaction due to incompatibility related to minor antigens (Duffy) (Kell) (Kidd) (Lewis) (M) (N) (P) (S)
Other reaction to non-ABO incompatibility from transfusion

[5] **999.8 Other and unspecified infusion and transfusion reaction**

[Excludes:] *ABO incompatibility reactions (999.60-999.69)*
febrile nonhemolytic transfusion reaction (FNHTR) (780.66)
hemochromatosis due to repeated red blood cell transfusions (275.02)
non-ABO incompatibility reactions (999.70-999.79)
postoperative shock (998.00-998.09)
posttransfusion purpura (287.41)
Rh incompatibility reactions (999.70-999.74)
transfusion associated circulatory overload (TACO) (276.61)
transfusion related acute lung injury (TRALI) (518.7)

999.80 Transfusion reaction, unspecified
Incompatible blood transfusion NOS
Reaction to blood group incompatibility in infusion or transfusion NOS

999.81 Extravasation of vesicant chemotherapy
Infiltration of vesicant chemotherapy

999.82 Extravasation of other vesicant agent
Infiltration of other vesicant agent

999.83 Hemolytic transfusion reaction, incompatibility unspecified
Hemolytic transfusion reaction (HTR) with antigen incompatibility unspecified, not specified as acute or delayed
HTR with incompatibility unspecified at unspecified time after transfusion

999.84 Acute hemolytic transfusion reaction, incompatibility unspecified
Acute hemolytic transfusion reaction (AHTR) with antigen incompatibility unspecified
AHTR, incompatibility unspecified

999.85 Delayed hemolytic transfusion reaction, incompatibility unspecified
Delayed hemolytic transfusion reaction (DHTR) with antigen incompatibility unspecified
DHTR, incompatibility unspecified

999.88 Other infusion reaction

999.89 Other transfusion reaction
Delayed serologic transfusion reaction (DSTR), incompatibility unspecified

Use additional code to identify graft-versus-host reaction (279.5)

999.9 Other and unspecified complications of medical care, not elsewhere classified
Complications, not elsewhere classified, of:
electroshock therapy
inhalation therapy
ultrasound therapy
ventilation therapy
Unspecified misadventure of medical care

[Excludes:] *unspecified complication of:*
phototherapy (990)
radiation therapy (990)
ventilator associated pneumonia (997.31)

Add 4th or 5th digit
Nonspecific code
Unspecified code
Medicare secondary payer (MSP) alert

This page intentionally left blank

Chapter 18: Classification of Factors Influencing Health Status and Contact with Health Service (Supplemental V01-V91)

DEFINITIONS AND CODING ALERTS

This chapter includes definitions of selected key words, terms and phrases and coding alerts for adding points to the clinical domain, references to coding late effects where appropriate, and references to personal history V-codes in situations where the acute or chronic condition is no longer active. An example from this chapter is as follows:

V22.0 Supervision of normal first pregnancy
> **ALERT!** Codes V22.0 and V22.1 are always first listed and are not to be used with any other code from the OB chapter.

V23 Supervision of high-risk pregnancy
> **DEFINITION** A high risk pregnancy is one in which some condition puts the mother, the developing fetus, or both at higher-than-normal risk for complications during or after the pregnancy and birth.

MULTIPLE CODING FOR A SINGLE CONDITION

In addition to the etiology or manifestation convention that requires two codes to fully describe a single condition that affects multiple body systems, there are other single conditions that also require more than one code. "Use additional code" notes are found in the tabular at codes that are not part of an etiology or manifestation pair where a secondary code is useful to fully describe a condition. The sequencing rule is the same as the etiology or manifestation pair - , "use additional code" indicates that a secondary code should be added.

"Code first" notes are also under certain codes that are not specifically manifestation codes but may be due to an underlying cause. When a "code first" note is present and an underlying condition is present the underlying condition should be sequenced first.

"Code, if applicable, any causal condition first", notes indicate that this code may be assigned as a principal diagnosis when the causal condition is unknown or not applicable. If a causal condition is known, then the code for that condition should be sequenced as the principal or first-listed diagnosis. Multiple codes may be needed for late effects, complication codes and obstetric codes to more fully describe a condition. See the specific guidelines for these conditions for further instruction.

COMBINATION CODE

A combination code is a single code used to classify: two diagnoses, or a diagnosis with an associated secondary process (manifestation) A diagnosis with an associated complication Combination codes are identified by referring to subterm entries in the Alphabetic Index and by reading the inclusion and exclusion notes in the Tabular List.

Assign only the combination code when that code fully identifies the diagnostic conditions involved or when the Alphabetic Index so directs. Multiple coding should not be used when the classification provides a combination code that clearly identifies all of the elements documented in the diagnosis. When the combination code lacks necessary specificity in describing the manifestation or complication, an additional code should be used as a secondary code.

CODING LATE EFFECTS

A late effect is the residual effect (condition produced) after the acute phase of an illness or injury has terminated. There is no time limit on when a late effect code can be used. The residual may be apparent early, such as in cerebrovascular accident cases, or it may occur months or years later, such as that due to a previous injury. Coding of late effects generally requires two codes sequenced in the following order: The condition or nature of the late effect is sequenced first. The late effect code is sequenced second.

An exception to the above guidelines are those instances where the code for late effect is followed by a manifestation code identified in the Tabular List and title, or the late effect code has been expanded (at the fourth and fifth-digit levels) to include the manifestation(s). The code for the acute phase of an illness or injury that led to the late effect is never used with a code for the late effect.

V CODES

| | Add 4th or 5th digit | | Nonspecific code | | Unspecific code | | Secondary Dx Only | | Primary Dx Only |

INTRODUCTION

ICD-9-CM provides codes to deal with encounters for circumstances other than a disease or injury. The Supplementary Classification of Factors Influencing Health Status and Contact with Health Services (V01.0 - V89.09) is provided to deal with occasions when circumstances other than a disease or injury (codes 001-999) are recorded as a diagnosis or problem.

There are four primary circumstances for the use of V codes:

1. A person who is not currently sick encounters the health services for some specific reason, such as to act as an organ donor, to receive prophylactic care, such as inoculations or health screenings, or to receive counseling on health related issues.

2. A person with a resolving disease or injury, or a chronic, long term condition requiring continuous care, encounters the health care system for specific aftercare of that disease or injury (e.g., dialysis for renal disease; chemotherapy for malignancy; cast change). A diagnosis or symptom code should be used whenever a current, acute, diagnosis is being treated or a sign or symptom is being studied.

3. Circumstances or problems influence a person's health status but are not in themselves a current illness or injury.

4. Newborns, to indicate birth status

V CODES USE IN ANY HEALTH CARE SETTING

V codes are for use in any health care setting. V codes may be used as either a first listed (principal diagnosis code in the inpatient setting) or secondary code, depending on the circumstances of the encounter. Certain V codes may only be used as first listed, others only as secondary codes.

V CODES INDICATE A REASON FOR AN ENCOUNTER

They are not procedure codes. A corresponding procedure code must accompany a V code to describe the procedure performed.

CATEGORIES OF V CODES

Contact or Exposure

Category V01 indicates contact with or exposure to communicable diseases. These codes are for patients who do not show any sign or symptom of a disease but have been exposed to it by close personal contact with an infected individual or are in an area where a disease is epidemic. These codes may be used as a first listed code to explain an encounter for testing, or, more commonly, as a secondary code to identify a potential risk.

Inoculations and vaccinations

Categories V03-V06 are for encounters for inoculations and vaccinations. They indicate that a patient is being seen to receive a prophylactic inoculation against a disease. The injection itself must be represented by the appropriate procedure code. A code from V03-V06 may be used as a secondary code if the inoculation is given as a routine part of preventive health care, such as a well-baby visit.

Status

Status codes indicate that a patient is either a carrier of a disease or has the sequelae or residual of a past disease or condition. This includes such things as the presence of prosthetic or mechanical devices resulting from past treatment. A status code is informative, because the status may affect the course of treatment and its outcome. A status code is distinct from a history code. The history code indicates that the patient no longer has the condition.

A status code should not be used with a diagnosis code from one of the body system chapters, if the diagnosis code includes the information provided by the status code. For example, code V42.1, Heart transplant status, should not be used with code 996.83, Complications of transplanted heart. The status code does not provide additional information. The complication code indicates that the patient is a heart transplant patient.

● Code new
to 2012 edition

▲ Revision of
existing code

④ ⑤ Fourth or fifth
digit required

History (of)

There are two types of history V codes, personal and family. Personal history codes explain a patient's past medical condition that no longer exists and is not receiving any treatment, but that has the potential for recurrence, and therefore may require continued monitoring. The exceptions to this general rule are category V14, Personal history of allergy to medicinal agents, and subcategory V15.0, Allergy, other than to medicinal agents. A person who has had an allergic episode to a substance or food in the past should always be considered allergic to the substance.

Family history codes are for use when a patient has a family member(s) who has had a particular disease that causes the patient to be at higher risk of also contracting the disease.

Personal history codes may be used in conjunction with followup codes and family history codes may be used in conjunction with screening codes to explain the need for a test or procedure. History codes are also acceptable on any medical record regardless of the reason for visit. A history of an illness, even if no longer present, is important information that may alter the type of treatment ordered.

Screening

Screening is the testing for disease or disease precursors in seemingly well individuals so that early detection and treatment can be provided for those who test positive for the disease. Screenings that are recommended for many subgroups in a population include: routine mammograms for women over 40, a fecal occult blood test for everyone over 50, an amniocentesis to rule out a fetal anomaly for pregnant women over 35, because the incidence of breast cancer and colon cancer in these subgroups is higher than in the general population, as is the incidence of Down's syndrome in older mothers.

The testing of a person to rule out or confirm a suspected diagnosis because the patient has some sign or symptom is a diagnostic examination, not a screening. In these cases, the sign or symptom is used to explain the reason for the test. A screening code may be a first listed code if the reason for the visit is specifically the screening exam. It may also be used as an additional code if the screening is done during an office visit for other health problems. A screening code is not necessary if the screening is inherent to a routine examination, such as a pap smear done during a routine pelvic examination.

Should a condition be discovered during the screening then the code for the condition may be assigned as an additional diagnosis.

The V code indicates that a screening exam is planned. A procedure code is required to confirm that the screening was performed.

Observation

There are three observation V code categories. They are for use in very limited circumstances when a person is being observed for a suspected condition that is ruled out. The observation codes are not for use if an injury or illness or any signs or symptoms related to the suspected condition are present. In such cases the diagnosis or symptom code is used with the corresponding E code to identify any external cause.

The observation codes are to be used as principal diagnosis only. The only exception to this is when the principal diagnosis is required to be a code from the V30, Live born infant, category. Then the V29 observation code is sequenced after the V30 code. Additional codes may be used in addition to the observation code but only if they are unrelated to the suspected condition being observed.

Codes from subcategory V89.0, Suspected maternal and fetal conditions not found, may either be used as a first listed or as an additional code assignment depending on the case. They are for use in very limited circumstances on a maternal record when an encounter is for a suspected maternal or fetal condition that is ruled out during that encounter (for example, a maternal or fetal condition may be suspected due to an abnormal test result). These codes should not be used when the condition is confirmed. In those cases, the confirmed condition should be coded. In addition, these codes are not for use if an illness or any signs or symptoms related to the suspected condition or problem are present. In such cases the diagnosis or symptom code is used.

Additional codes may be used in addition to the code from subcategory V89.0, but only if they are unrelated to the suspected condition being evaluated.

Codes from subcategory V89.0 may not be used for encounters for antenatal screening of mother. See Official Guidelines, Section I.C.18.d., Screening).

For encounters for suspected fetal condition that are inconclusive following testing and evaluation, assign the appropriate code from category 655, 656, 657 or 658.

| ■ Add 4th or 5th digit | ■ Nonspecific code | ■ Unspecific code | ■ Secondary Dx Only | ■ Primary Dx Only |

Aftercare

Aftercare visit codes cover situations when the initial treatment of a disease or injury has been performed and the patient requires continued care during the healing or recovery phase, or for the long-term consequences of the disease. The aftercare V code should not be used if treatment is directed at a current, acute disease or injury. The diagnosis code is to be used in these cases. Exceptions to this rule are codes V58.0, Radiotherapy, and codes from subcategory V58.1, Encounter for chemotherapy and immunotherapy for neoplastic conditions. These codes are to be first listed, followed by the diagnosis code when a patient's encounter is solely to receive radiation therapy or chemotherapy for the treatment of a neoplasm. Should a patient receive both chemotherapy and radiation therapy during the same encounter code V58.0 and V58.1 may be used together on a record with either one being sequenced first.

The aftercare codes are generally first listed to explain the specific reason for the encounter. An aftercare code may be used as an additional code when some type of aftercare is provided in addition to the reason for admission and no diagnosis code is applicable. An example of this would be the closure of a colostomy during an encounter for treatment of another condition.

Aftercare codes should be used in conjunction with any other aftercare codes or other diagnosis codes to provide better detail on the specifics of an aftercare encounter visit, unless otherwise directed by the classification. The sequencing of multiple aftercare codes is discretionary.

Certain aftercare V code categories need a secondary diagnosis code to describe the resolving condition or sequelae, for others, the condition is inherent in the code title.

Additional V code aftercare category terms include, fitting and adjustment, and attention to artificial openings. Status V codes may be used with aftercare V codes to indicate the nature of the aftercare. For example code V45.81, Aortocoronary bypass status, may be used with code V58.73, Aftercare following surgery of the circulatory system, NEC, to indicate the surgery for which the aftercare is being performed. Also, a transplant status code may be used following code V58.44, Aftercare following organ transplant, to identify the organ transplanted. A status code should not be used when the aftercare code indicates the type of status, such as using V55.0, Attention to tracheostomy with V44.0, Tracheostomy status.

See Chapter 16 for admissions or encounter for rehabilitation.

Follow-up

The follow-up codes are used to explain continuing surveillance following completed treatment of a disease, condition, or injury. They imply that the condition has been fully treated and no longer exists. They should not be confused with aftercare codes that explain current treatment for a healing condition or its sequelae. Follow-up codes may be used in conjunction with history codes to provide the full picture of the healed condition and its treatment. The follow-up code is sequenced first, followed by the history code.

A follow-up code may be used to explain repeated visits.

Should a condition be found to have recurred on the follow-up visit, then the diagnosis code should be used in place of the follow-up code.

Donor

Category V59 is the donor codes. They are used for living individuals who are donating blood or other body tissue. These codes are only for individuals donating for others, not for self donations. They are not for use to identify cadaveric donations.

Counseling

Counseling V codes are used when a patient or family member receives assistance in the aftermath of an illness or injury, or when support is required in coping with family or social problems. They are not necessary for use in conjunction with a diagnosis code when the counseling component of care is considered integral to standard treatment.

Obstetrics and related conditions

See Chapter 11, obstetrics guidelines for further instruction on the use of these codes.

V codes for pregnancy are for use in those circumstances when none of the problems or complications included in the codes from the Obstetrics chapter exist (a routine prenatal visit or postpartum care). Codes V22.0, Supervision of normal first pregnancy, and V22.1, Supervision of other normal pregnancy, are always first listed and are not to be used with any other code from the OB chapter.

● Code new
to 2012 edition ▲ Revision of
existing code ④ ⑤ Fourth or fifth
digit required

The outcome of delivery, category V27, should be included on all maternal delivery records. It is always a secondary code.

V codes for family planning (contraceptive) or procreative management and counseling should be included on an obstetric record either during the pregnancy or the postpartum stage, if applicable.

Routine and administrative examinations

The V codes allow for the description of encounters for routine examinations, such as, a general check-up, or, examinations for administrative purposes, such as, a pre-employment physical. The codes are not to be used if the examination is for diagnosis of a suspected condition or for treatment purposes. In such cases the diagnosis code is used. During a routine exam, should a diagnosis or condition be discovered, it should be coded as an additional code. Pre-existing and chronic conditions and history codes may also be included as additional codes as long as the examination is for administrative purposes and not focused on any particular condition.

Pre-operative examination V codes are for use only in those situations when a patient is being cleared for surgery and no treatment is given.

Miscellaneous V codes

The miscellaneous V codes capture a number of other health care encounters that do not fall into one of the other categories. Certain of these codes identify the reason for the encounter, others are for use as additional codes that provide useful information on circumstances that may affect a patient's care and treatment.

PROPHYLACTIC ORGAN REMOVAL

For encounters specifically for prophylactic removal of breasts, ovaries, or another organ due to a genetic susceptibility to cancer or a family history of cancer, the principal or first listed code should be a code from subcategory V50.4, Prophylactic organ removal, followed by the appropriate genetic susceptibility code and the appropriate family history code.

If the patient has a malignancy of one site and is having prophylactic removal at another site to prevent either a new primary malignancy or metastatic disease, a code for the malignancy should also be assigned in addition to a code from subcategory V50.4. A V50.4 code should not be assigned if the patient is having organ removal for treatment of a malignancy, such as the removal of the testes for the treatment of prostate cancer.

Nonspecific V codes

Certain V codes are so non-specific, or potentially redundant with other codes in the classification, that there can be little justification for their use in the inpatient setting. Their use in the outpatient setting should be limited to those instances when there is no further documentation to permit more precise coding. Otherwise, any sign or symptom or any other reason for visit that is captured in another code should be used.

See Official Guidelines, Section IV, .K. and Official Guidelines, Section IV.L. of the Outpatient guidelines.

V CODE TABLE

The V code table in the Official Coding Guidelines contains columns for 1st listed, 1st or additional, additional only, and non-specific. Each code or category is listed on the left hand column and the allowable sequencing of the code or codes within the category is noted under the appropriate column.

The V codes designated as first-listed only are generally intended to be limited for use as a first-listed only diagnosis, but may be reported as an additional diagnosis in those situations when the patient has more than one encounter on a single day and the codes for the multiple encounters are combined, or when there is more than one V code that meets the definition of principal diagnosis (e.g., a patient is admitted to home healthcare for both aftercare and rehabilitation and they equally meet the definition of principal diagnosis). The V codes designated as first-listed only should not be reported if they do not meet the definition of principal or first-listed diagnosis.

See Official Guidelines, Section II and Official Guidelines, Section IV,.A for information on selection of principal and first-listed diagnosis.

See Official Guidelines, Section II.C for information on two or more diagnoses that equally meet the definition for principal diagnosis.

| ▮ Add 4th or 5th digit | ▮ Nonspecific code | ▮ Unspecific code | ▮ Secondary Dx Only | ▮ Primary Dx Only |

This page intentionally left blank.

SUPPLEMENTARY CLASSIFICATION OF FACTORS INFLUENCING HEALTH STATUS AND CONTACT WITH HEALTH SERVICES (V01-V91)

This classification is provided to deal with occasions when circumstances other than a disease or injury classifiable to categories 001-999 (the main part of ICD) are recorded as "diagnoses" or "problems." This can arise mainly in three ways:

a) When a person who is not currently sick encounters the health services for some specific purpose, such as to act as a donor of an organ or tissue, to receive prophylactic vaccination, or to discuss a problem which is in itself not a disease or injury. This will be a fairly rare occurrence among hospital inpatients, but will be relatively more common among hospital outpatients and patients of family practitioners, health clinics, etc.

b) When a person with a known disease or injury, whether it is current or resolving, encounters the health care system for a specific treatment of that disease or injury (e.g., dialysis for renal disease; chemotherapy for malignancy; cast change).

c) When some circumstance or problem is present which influences the person's health status but is not in itself a current illness or injury. Such factors may be elicited during population surveys, when the person may or may not be currently sick, or be recorded as an additional factor to be borne in mind when the person is receiving care for some current illness or injury classifiable to categories 001-999.

In the latter circumstances the V code should be used only as a supplementary code and should not be the one selected for use in primary, single cause tabulations. Examples of these circumstances are a personal history of certain diseases, or a person with an artificial heart valve in situ.

PERSONS WITH POTENTIAL HEALTH HAZARDS RELATED TO COMMUNICABLE DISEASES (V01-V06)

> Excludes: family history of infectious and parasitic diseases (V18.8)
> personal history of infectious and parasitic diseases (V12.0)

V01 **Contact with or exposure to communicable diseases**

> **ALERT!** Category V01 indicates contact with or exposure to communicable diseases. These codes are for patients who do not show any sign or symptom of a disease but have been exposed to it by close personal contact with an infected individual or are in an area where a disease is epidemic. These codes may be used as a first listed code to explain an encounter for testing, or, more commonly, as a secondary code to identify a potential risk

V01.0 Cholera
Conditions classifiable to 001

V01.1 Tuberculosis
Conditions classifiable to 010-018

V01.2 Poliomyelitis
Conditions classifiable to 045

V01.3 Smallpox
Conditions classifiable to 050

V01.4 Rubella
Conditions classifiable to 056

V01.5 Rabies
Conditions classifiable to 071

V01.6 Venereal diseases
Conditions classifiable to 090-099

⑤ **V01.7 Other viral diseases**
Conditions classifiable to 042-078 and V08, except as above

    V01.71 Varicella

    V01.79 Other viral diseases

⑤ **V01.8 Other communicable diseases**
Conditions classifiable to 001-136, except as above

    V01.81 Anthrax

    V01.82 Exposure to SARS-associated coronavirus

    V01.83 Escherichia coli (E. coli)

    V01.84 Meningococcus

    V01.89 Other communicable diseases

V01.9 Unspecified communicable disease

V02 **Carrier or suspected carrier of infectious diseases**
Includes: Colonization status

V02.0 Cholera

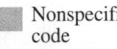 Add 4th or 5th digit   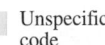 Nonspecific code   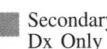 Unspecific code   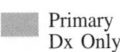 Secondary Dx Only   Primary Dx Only

V02.1 **Typhoid**

V02.2 **Amebiasis**

`V02.3` **Other gastrointestinal pathogens**

V02.4 **Diphtheria**

⑤ V02.5 **Other specified bacterial diseases**

    V02.51 **Group B streptococcus**

    `V02.52` **Other streptococcus**

    V02.53 **Methicillin susceptible Staphylococcus aureus**
        MSSA colonization

`ALERT!` Assign this code for patients documented as having MSRA colonization

    V02.54 **Methicillin resistant Staphylococcus aureus**
        MRSA colonization

`ALERT!` Assign this code for patients documented as having MSRA colonization

    `V02.59` **Other specified bacterial diseases**
        Meningococcal
        Staphylococcal

⑤ V02.6 **Viral hepatitis**
      Hepatitis Australian-antigen [HAA] [SH] carrier
      Serum hepatitis carrier

    V02.60 **Viral hepatitis carrier, unspecified**

    V02.61 **Hepatitis B carrier**

    V02.62 **Hepatitis C carrier**

    `V02.69` **Other viral hepatitis carrier**

V02.7 **Gonorrhea**

`V02.8` **Other venereal diseases**

`V02.9` **Other specified infectious organism**

`V03` **Need for prophylactic vaccination and inoculation against bacterial diseases**

    Excludes: *vaccination not carried out (V64.00-V64.09)*
              vaccines against combinations of diseases (V06.0-V06.9)

    `DEFINITION` Prophylactic vaccination performed to prevent infectious diseases. Suspension of attenuated or killed viruses or bacteria or parts thereof that is capable of producing a protective immune response to such infectious agents.

V03.0 **Cholera alone**

V03.1 **Typhoid-paratyphoid alone [TAB]**

V03.2 **Tuberculosis [BCG]**

V03.3 **Plague**

V03.4 **Tularemia**

V03.5 **Diphtheria alone**

V03.6 **Pertussis alone**

V03.7 **Tetanus toxoid alone**

⑤ V03.8 **Other specified vaccinations against single bacterial diseases**

    V03.81 **Hemophilus influenza, type B [Hib]**

    V03.82 **Streptococcus pneumoniae [pneumococcus]**

    `V03.89` **Other specified vaccination**

`V03.9` **Unspecified single bacterial disease**

`V04` **Need for prophylactic vaccination and inoculation against certain viral diseases**

    Excludes: *vaccines against combinations of diseases (V06.0-V06.9)*

V04.0 **Poliomyelitis**

V04.1 **Smallpox**

V04.2 **Measles alone**

V04.3 **Rubella alone**

V04.4 **Yellow fever**

V04.5 **Rabies**

V04.6 **Mumps alone**

V04.7 **Common cold**

● Code new
   to 2012 edition
▲ Revision of
   existing code
④ ⑤ Fourth or fifth
      digit required

⑤ **V04.8 Other viral diseases**

V04.81 Influenza

V04.82 Respiratory syncytial virus (RSV)

V04.89 Other viral diseases

V05 Need for other prophylactic vaccination and inoculation against single diseases

[Excludes:] *vaccines against combinations of diseases (V06.0-V06.9)*

V05.0 Arthropod-borne viral encephalitis

V05.1 Other arthropod-borne viral diseases

V05.2 Leishmaniasis

V05.3 Viral hepatitis

V05.4 Varicella
Chickenpox

V05.8 Other specified disease

V05.9 Unspecified single disease

V06 Need for prophylactic vaccination and inoculation against combinations of diseases

Note: Use additional single vaccination codes from categories V03-V05 to identify any vaccinations not included in a combination code.

V06.0 Cholera with typhoid-paratyphoid [cholera + TAB]

V06.1 Diphtheria-tetanus-pertussis, combined [DTP] [DTaP]

V06.2 Diphtheria-tetanus-pertussis with typhoid-paratyphoid [DTP + TAB]

V06.3 Diphtheria-tetanus-pertussis with poliomyelitis [DTP + polio]

V06.4 Measles-mumps-rubella [MMR]

V06.5 Tetanus-diphtheria [Td] [DT]

V06.6 Streptococcus pneumoniae [pneumococcus] and influenza

V06.8 Other combinations

[Excludes:] *multiple single vaccination codes (V03.0-V05.9)*

V06.9 Unspecified combined vaccine

PERSONS WITH NEED FOR ISOLATION, OTHER POTENTIAL HEALTH HAZARDS AND PROPHYLACTIC MEASURES (V07-V09)

V07 Need for isolation and other prophylactic or treatment measures

[Excludes:] *long-term (current) (prophylactic) use of certain specific drugs (V58.61-V58.69)*
prophylactic organ removal (V50.41-V50.49)

V07.0 Isolation
Admission to protect the individual from his surroundings or for isolation of individual after contact with infectious diseases

V07.1 Desensitization to allergens

V07.2 Prophylactic immunotherapy
Administration of:
- antivenin
- immune sera [gamma globulin]
- RhoGAM
- tetanus antitoxin

⑤ **V07.3 Other prophylactic chemotherapy**

V07.31 Prophylactic fluoride administration

V07.39 Other prophylactic chemotherapy

[Excludes:] *maintenance chemotherapy following disease (V58.11)*

V07.4 Hormone replacement therapy (postmenopausal)

Add 4th or 5th digit | Nonspecific code | Unspecific code | Secondary Dx Only | Primary Dx Only

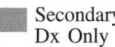

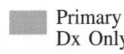

⑤ **V07.5 Use of agents affecting estrogen receptors and estrogen levels**

Code first, if applicable:
malignant neoplasm of breast (174.0-174.9, 175.0-175.9)
malignant neoplasm of prostate (185)

Use additional code, if applicable, to identify:
estrogen receptor positive status (V86.0)
family history of breast cancer (V16.3)
genetic susceptibility to cancer (V84.01-V84.09)
personal history of breast cancer (V10.3)
personal history of prostate cancer (V10.46)
postmenopausal status (V49.81)

Excludes: *hormone replacement therapy (postmenopausal) (V07.4)*

V07.51   Use of selective estrogen receptor modulators (SERMs)
Use of:
raloxifene (Evista)
tamoxifen (Nolvadex)
toremifene (Fareston)

V07.52   Use of aromatase inhibitors
Use of:
anastrozole (Arimidex)
exemestane (Aromasin)
letrozole (Femara)

V07.59   Use of other agents affecting estrogen receptors and estrogen levels
Use of:
estrogen receptor downregulators
fulvestrant (Faslodex)
gonadotropin-releasing hormone (GnRH) agonist
goserelin acetate (Zoladex)
leuprolide acetate (leuprorelin) (Lupron)
megestrol acetate (Megace)

V07.8 Other specified prophylactic or treatment measure

V07.9 Unspecified prophylactic or treatment measure

V08 Asymptomatic human immunodeficiency virus [HIV] infection status
HIV positive NOS

Note: This code is ONLY to be used when NO HIV infection symptoms or conditions are present. If any HIV infection symptoms or conditions are present, see code 042.

Excludes: *AIDS (042)*
human immunodeficiency virus [HIV] disease (042)
exposure to HIV (V01.79)
nonspecific serologic evidence of HIV (795.71)
symptomatic human immunodeficiency virus [HIV] infection (042)

V09 Infection with drug-resistant microorganisms
Note: This category is intended for use as an additional code for infectious conditions classified elsewhere to indicate the presence of drug-resistance of the infectious organism.

V09.0 Infection with microorganisms resistant to penicillins

V09.1 Infection with microorganisms resistant to cephalosporins and other B-lactam antibiotics

V09.2 Infection with microorganisms resistant to macrolides

V09.3 Infection with microorganisms resistant to tetracyclines

V09.4 Infection with microorganisms resistant to aminoglycosides

⑤ **V09.5 Infection with microorganisms resistant to quinolones and fluoroquinolones**

V09.50   Without mention of resistance to multiple quinolones and fluoroquinolones

V09.51   With resistance to multiple quinolones and fluoroquinolones

V09.6 Infection with microorganisms resistant to sulfonamides

⑤ **V09.7 Infection with microorganisms resistant to other specified antimycobacterial agents**

Excludes: *Amikacin (V09.4)*
Kanamycin (V09.4)
Streptomycin [SM] (V09.4)

V09.70   Without mention of resistance to multiple antimycobacterial agents

V09.71   With resistance to multiple antimycobacterial agents

● Code new
to 2012 edition
▲ Revision of
existing code
④ ⑤ Fourth or fifth
digit required

⑤ **V09.8 Infection with microorganisms resistant to other specified drugs**
Vancomycin (glycopeptide) intermediate staphylococcus aureus (VISA/GISA)
Vancomycin (glycopeptide) resistant enterococcus (VRE)
Vancomycin (glycopeptide) resistant staphylococcus aureus (VRSA/GRSA)

V09.80 **Without mention of resistance to multiple drugs**

V09.81 **With resistance to multiple drugs**

⑤ **V09.9 Infection with drug-resistant microorganisms, unspecified**
Drug resistance NOS

V09.90 **Without mention of multiple drug resistance**

V09.91 **With multiple drug resistance**
Multiple drug resistance NOS

PERSONS WITH POTENTIAL HEALTH HAZARDS RELATED TO PERSONAL AND FAMILY HISTORY (V10-V19)

Excludes: *obstetric patients where the possibility that the fetus might be affected is the reason for observation or management during pregnancy (655.0-655.9)*

V10 **Personal history of malignant neoplasm**

⑤ **V10.0 Gastrointestinal tract**
History of conditions classifiable to 140-159

Excludes: *personal history of malignant carcinoid tumor (V10.91)*
personal history of malignant neuroendocrine tumor (V10.91)

V10.00 **Gastrointestinal tract, unspecified**

V10.01 **Tongue**

V10.02 **Other and unspecified oral cavity and pharynx**

V10.03 **Esophagus**

V10.04 **Stomach**

V10.05 **Large intestine**

V10.06 **Rectum, rectosigmoid junction, and anus**

V10.07 **Liver**

V10.09 **Other**

⑤ **V10.1 Trachea, bronchus, and lung**
History of conditions classifiable to 162

Excludes: *personal history of malignant carcinoid tumor (V10.91)*
personal history of malignant neuroendocrine tumor (V10.91)

V10.11 **Bronchus and lung**

V10.12 **Trachea**

⑤ **V10.2 Other respiratory and intrathoracic organs**
History of conditions classifiable to 160, 161, 163-165

V10.20 **Respiratory organ, unspecified**

V10.21 **Larynx**

V10.22 **Nasal cavities, middle ear, and accessory sinuses**

V10.29 **Other**

V10.3 Breast
History of conditions classifiable to 174 and 175

⑤ **V10.4 Genital organs**
History of conditions classifiable to 179-187

V10.40 **Female genital organ, unspecified**

V10.41 **Cervix uteri**

V10.42 **Other parts of uterus**

V10.43 **Ovary**

V10.44 **Other female genital organs**

V10.45 **Male genital organ, unspecified**

V10.46 **Prostate**

V10.47 **Testis**

V10.48 **Epididymis**

V10.49 **Other male genital organs**

	Add 4th or 5th digit		Nonspecific code		Unspecific code		Secondary Dx Only		Primary Dx Only

⑤ **V10.5 Urinary organs**
　　　　History of conditions classifiable to 188 and 189

　　Excludes: *personal history of malignant carcinoid tumor (V10.91)*
　　　　　　　personal history of malignant neuroendocrine tumor (V10.91)

　　　　V10.50 Urinary organ, unspecified

　　　　V10.51 Bladder

　　　　V10.52 Kidney

　　Excludes: *renal pelvis (V10.53)*

　　　　V10.53 Renal pelvis

　　　　V10.59 Other

⑤ **V10.6 Leukemia**
　　　　Conditions classifiable to 204-208

　　Excludes: *leukemia in remission (204-208)*

　　　　V10.60 Leukemia, unspecified

　　　　V10.61 Lymphoid leukemia

　　　　V10.62 Myeloid leukemia

　　　　V10.63 Monocytic leukemia

　　　　V10.69 Other

⑤ **V10.7 Other lymphatic and hematopoietic neoplasms**
　　　　Conditions classifiable to 200-203

　　Excludes: *listed conditions in 200-203 in remission*

　　　　V10.71 Lymphosarcoma and reticulosarcoma

　　　　V10.72 Hodgkin's disease

　　　　V10.79 Other

⑤ **V10.8 Personal history of malignant neoplasm of other sites**
　　　　History of conditions classifiable to 170-173, 190-195

　　Excludes: *personal history of malignant carcinoid tumor (V10.91)*
　　　　　　　personal history of malignant neuroendocrine tumor (V10.91)

　　　　V10.81 Bone

　　　　V10.82 Malignant melanoma of skin

　　　　V10.83 Other malignant neoplasm of skin

　　　　V10.84 Eye

　　　　V10.85 Brain

　　　　V10.86 Other parts of nervous system

　　Excludes: *peripheral, sympathetic, and parasympathetic nerves (V10.89)*

　　　　V10.87 Thyroid

　　　　V10.88 Other endocrine glands and related structures

　　　　V10.89 Other

⑤ **V10.9 Other and unspecified personal history of malignant neoplasm**

　　　　V10.90 Personal history of unspecified malignant neoplasm
　　　　　　　Personal history of malignant neoplasm NOS

　　Excludes: *personal history of malignant carcinoid tumor (V10.91)*
　　　　　　　personal history of malignant neuroendocrine tumor (V10.91)
　　　　　　　personal history of Merkel cell carcinoma (V10.91)

　　　　V10.91 Personal history of malignant neuroendocrine tumor
　　　　　　　Personal history of malignant carcinoid tumor NOS
　　　　　　　Personal history of malignant neuroendocrine tumor NOS
　　　　　　　Personal history of Merkel cell carcinoma NOS

　　　　Code first any continuing functional activity, such as: carcinoid syndrome (259.2)

V11 Personal history of mental disorder

　　V11.0 Schizophrenia

　　Excludes: *that in remission (295.0-295.9 with fifth-digit 5)*

762　　● Code new　　　　▲ Revision of　　　④ ⑤ Fourth or fifth
　　　　　to 2012 edition　　　　existing code　　　　digit required

V11.1 **Affective disorders**
Personal history of manic-depressive psychosis
Excludes: *that in remission (296.0-296.6 with fifth-digit 5, 6)*

V11.2 **Neurosis**

V11.3 **Alcoholism**

V11.4 **Combat and operational stress reaction**

V11.8 **Other mental disorders**

V11.9 **Unspecified mental disorder**

V12 **Personal history of certain other diseases**

⑤ **V12.0** **Infectious and parasitic diseases**
Excludes: *personal history of infectious diseases specific to a body system*

    V12.00 **Unspecified infectious and parasitic disease**

    V12.01 **Tuberculosis**

    V12.02 **Poliomyelitis**

    V12.03 **Malaria**

    V12.04 **Methicillin resistant Staphylococcus aureus**
      MRSA

    V12.09 **Other**

V12.1 **Nutritional deficiency**

⑤ **V12.2** **Endocrine, metabolic, and immunity disorders**
Excludes: *history of allergy (V14.0-V14.9, V15.01-V15.09)*

  ● **V12.21** **Gestational diabetes**

  ● **V12.29** **Other endocrine, metabolic, and immunity disorders**

V12.3 **Diseases of blood and blood-forming organs**

⑤ **V12.4** **Disorders of nervous system and sense organs**

    V12.40 **Unspecified disorder of nervous system and sense organs**

    V12.41 **Benign neoplasm of the brain**

    V12.42 **Infections of the central nervous system**
      Encephalitis
      Meningitis

    V12.49 **Other disorders of nervous system and sense organs**

⑤ **V12.5** **Diseases of circulatory system**
Excludes: *history of anaphylactic shcok (V13.81)*
      old myocardial infarction (412)
      postmyocardial infarction syndrome (411.0)

    V12.50 **Unspecified circulatory disease**

    V12.51 **Venous thrombosis and embolism**
Excludes: *pulmonary embolism V12.55*

    V12.52 **Thrombophlebitis**

    V12.53 **Sudden cardiac arrest**
      Sudden cardiac death successfully resuscitated

    V12.54 **Transient ischemic attack (TIA), and cerebral infarction without residual deficits**
      Prolonged reversible ischemic neurological deficit (PRIND)
      Reversible ischemic neurologic deficit (RIND)
      Stroke NOS without residual deficits
Excludes: *history of traumatic brain injury (V15.52)*
      late effects of cerebrovascular disease (438.0-438.9)

ALERT! Assign code V12.54, not a code from category 438 as an additional code for history of cerebrovascular disease when no neurologic deficits are present

  ● **V12.55** **Pulmonary embolism**

    V12.59 **Other**
      Note: Assign code V12.59 (and not a code from category 438) as an additional code for history of cerebrovascular disease when no neurologic deficits are present.

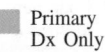

| | Add 4th or 5th digit | | Nonspecific code | | Unspecific code | | Secondary Dx Only | | Primary Dx Only |

⑤ **V12.6 Diseases of respiratory system**

Excludes: *tuberculosis (V12.01)*

    V12.60 Unspecified disease of respiratory system

    V12.61 Pneumonia (recurrent)

    V12.69 Other diseases of respiratory system

⑤ **V12.7 Diseases of digestive system**

    V12.70 Unspecified digestive disease

    V12.71 Peptic ulcer disease

    V12.72 Colonic polyps

    V12.79 Other

V13 Personal history of other diseases

⑤ **V13.0 Disorders of urinary system**

    V13.00 Unspecified urinary disorder

    V13.01 Urinary calculi

    V13.02 Urinary (tract) infection

    V13.03 Nephrotic syndrome

    V13.09 Other

V13.1 Trophoblastic disease

Excludes: *supervision during a current pregnancy (V23.1)*

⑤ **V13.2 Other genital system and obstetric disorders**

Excludes: *supervision during a current pregnancy of a woman with poor obstetric history*
    (V23.0-V23.9)
    recurrent pregnancy loss (646.3)
    without current pregnancy (629.81)

    V13.21 Personal history of pre-term labor

Excludes: *current pregnancy with history of pre-term labor (V23.41)*

    V13.22 Personal history of cervical dysplasia
        Personal history of conditions classifiable to 622.10-622.12

Excludes: *personal history of malignant neoplasm of cervix uteri (V10.41)*

    V13.23 Personal history of vaginal dysplasia
        Personal history of conditions classifiable to 623.0

Excludes: *personal history of malignant neoplasm of vagina (V10.44)*

    V13.24 Personal history of vulvar dysplasia
        Personal history of conditions classifiable to 624.01-624.02

Excludes: *personal history of malignant neoplasm of vulva (V10.44)*

    V13.29 Other genital system and obstetric disorders

V13.3 Diseases of skin and subcutaneous tissue

V13.4 Arthritis

⑤ **V13.5 Other musculoskeletal disorders**

    V13.51 Pathologic fracture
        Healed pathologic fracture

Excludes: *personal history of traumatic fracture (V15.51)*

    V13.52 Stress fracture
        Healed stress fracture

Excludes: *personal history of traumatic fracture (V15.51)*

    V13.59 Other musculoskeletal disorders

⑤ **V13.6 Congenital (corrected) malformations**

    V13.61 Personal history of (corrected) hypospadias

    V13.62 Personal history of other (corrected) congenital malformations of genitourinary system

    V13.63 Personal history of (corrected) congenital malformations of nervous system

    V13.64 Personal history of (corrected) congenital malformations of eye, ear, face and neck
        Corrected cleft lip and palate

● Code new
  to 2012 edition
▲ Revision of
  existing code
④ ⑤ Fourth or fifth
    digit required

V13.65 Personal history of (corrected) congenital malformations of heart and circulatory system

V13.66 Personal history of (corrected) congenital malformations of respiratory system

V13.67 Personal history of (corrected) congenital malformations of digestive system

V13.68 Personal history of (corrected) congenital malformations of integument, limbs, and musculoskeletal systems

V13.69 Personal history of other (corrected) congenital malformations

V13.7 Perinatal problems

[Excludes:] *low birth weight status (V21.30-V21.35)*

[5] **V13.8 Other specified diseases**

● **V13.81 Anaphylaxis**

● **V13.89 Other specified diseases**

V13.9 Unspecified disease

V14 Personal history of allergy to medicinal agents

V14.0 Penicillin

V14.1 Other antibiotic agent

V14.2 Sulfonamides

V14.3 Other anti-infective agent

V14.4 Anesthetic agent

V14.5 Narcotic agent

V14.6 Analgesic agent

V14.7 Serum or vaccine

V14.8 Other specified medicinal agents

V14.9 Unspecified medicinal agent

V15 Other personal history presenting hazards to health

[Excludes:] *personal history of drug therapy (V87.41-V87.49)*

[5] **V15.0 Allergy, other than to medicinal agents**

[Excludes:] *allergy to food substance used as base for medicinal agent (V14.0-V14.9)*

V15.01 Allergy to peanuts

V15.02 Allergy to milk products

[Excludes:] *lactose intolerance (271.3)*

V15.03 Allergy to eggs

V15.04 Allergy to seafood
Seafood (octopus) (squid) ink
Shellfish

V15.05 Allergy to other foods
Food additives
Nuts other than peanuts

V15.06 Allergy to insects and arachnids
Bugs
Insect bites and stings
Spiders

V15.07 Allergy to latex
Latex sensitivity

V15.08 Allergy to radiographic dye
Contrast media used for diagnostic x-ray procedures

V15.09 Other allergy, other than to medicinal agents

V15.1 Surgery to heart and great vessels

[Excludes:] *replacement by transplant or other means (V42.1-V42.2, V43.2-V43.4)*

[5] **V15.2 Surgery to other organs**

[Excludes:] *replacement by transplant or other means (V42.0-V43.8)*

V15.21 Personal history of undergoing in utero procedure during pregnancy

V15.22 Personal history of undergoing in utero procedure while a fetus

V15.29 Surgery to other organs

V15.3 Irradiation
Previous exposure to therapeutic or other ionizing radiation

⑤ **V15.4 Psychological trauma**
Excludes: history of condition classifiable to 290-316 (V11.0-V11.9)

V15.41 History of physical abuse
Rape

V15.42 History of emotional abuse
Neglect

V15.49 Other

⑤ **V15.5 Injury**

V15.51 Traumatic fracture
Healed traumatic fracture

Excludes: personal history of pathologic and stress fracture (V13.51, V13.52)

V15.52 History of traumatic brain injury

Excludes: personal history of cerebrovascular accident (cerebral infarction) without residual deficits (V12.54)

V15.53 Personal history of retained foreign body fully removed

V15.59 Other injury

V15.6 Poisoning

V15.7 Contraception
Excludes: current contraceptive management (V25.0-V25.4)
presence of intrauterine contraceptive device as incidental finding (V45.5)

⑤ **V15.8 Other specified personal history presenting hazards to health**
Excludes: contact with and (suspected) exposure to:
aromatic compounds and dyes (V87.11-V87.19)
arsenic and other metals (V87.01-V87.09)
molds (V87.31)

V15.80 History of failed moderate sedation
History of failed conscious sedation

V15.81 Noncompliance with medical treatment
Excludes: noncompliance with renal dialysis (V45.12)

V15.82 History of tobacco use
Excludes: tobacco dependence (305.1)

V15.83 Underimmunization status
Delinquent immunization status
Lapsed immunization schedule status

V15.84 Contact with and (suspected) exposure to asbestos

V15.85 Contact with and (suspected) exposure to potentially hazardous body fluids

V15.86 Contact with and (suspected) exposure to lead

V15.87 History of extracorporeal membrane oxygenation [ECMO]

V15.88 History of fall
At risk for falling

V15.89 Other
Excludes: contact with and (suspected) exposure to other potentially hazardous chemicals (V87.2)
contact with and (suspected) exposure to other potentially hazardous substances (V87.39)

V15.9 Unspecified personal history presenting hazards to health

V16 Family history of malignant neoplasm

V16.0 Gastrointestinal tract
Family history of condition classifiable to 140-159

V16.1 Trachea, bronchus, and lung
Family history of condition classifiable to 162

V16.2 Other respiratory and intrathoracic organs
Family history of condition classifiable to 160-161, 163-165

V16.3 Breast
Family history of condition classifiable to 174

● Code new to 2012 edition ▲ Revision of existing code ④ ⑤ Fourth or fifth digit required

[5] **V16.4 Genital organs**
Family history of condition classifiable to 179-187

V16.40 Genital organ, unspecified

V16.41 Ovary

V16.42 Prostate

V16.43 Testis

V16.49 Other

[5] **V16.5 Urinary organs**
Family history of condition classifiable to 188-189

V16.51 Kidney

V16.52 Bladder

V16.59 Other

V16.6 Leukemia
Family history of condition classifiable to 204-208

V16.7 Other lymphatic and hematopoietic neoplasms
Family history of condition classifiable to 200-203

V16.8 Other specified malignant neoplasm
Family history of other condition classifiable to 140-199

V16.9 Unspecified malignant neoplasm

V17 Family history of certain chronic disabling diseases

V17.0 Psychiatric condition
[Excludes:] *family history of intellectual disabilities (V18.4)*

V17.1 Stroke (cerebrovascular)

V17.2 Other neurological diseases
Epilepsy
Huntington's chorea

V17.3 Ischemic heart disease

[5] **V17.4 Other cardiovascular diseases**

V17.41 Family history of sudden cardiac death (SCD)
[Excludes:] *family history of ischemic heart disease (V17.3)*
family history of myocardial infarction (V17.3)

V17.49 Family history of other cardiovascular diseases
Family history of cardiovascular disease NOS

V17.5 Asthma

V17.6 Other chronic respiratory conditions

V17.7 Arthritis

[5] **V17.8 Other musculoskeletal diseases**

V17.81 Osteoporosis

V17.89 Other musculoskeletal diseases

V18 Family history of certain other specific conditions

V18.0 Diabetes mellitus

[5] **V18.1 Other endocrine and metabolic diseases**

V18.11 Multiple endocrine neoplasia [MEN] syndrome

V18.19 Other endocrine and metabolic diseases

V18.2 Anemia

V18.3 Other blood disorders

▲ **V18.4 Intellectual disabilities**

[5] **V18.5 Digestive disorders**

V18.51 Colonic polyps
[Excludes:] *family history of malignant neoplasm of gastrointestinal tract (V16.0)*

V18.59 Other digestive disorders

[5] **V18.6 Kidney diseases**

V18.61 Polycystic kidney

V18.69 Other kidney diseases

Add 4th or 5th digit | Nonspecific code | Unspecific code | Secondary Dx Only | Primary Dx Only

V18.7 Other genitourinary diseases

V18.8 Infectious and parasitic diseases

V18.9 Genetic disease carrier

V19 Family history of other conditions

V19.0 Blindness or visual loss

⑤ V19.1 Other eye disorders

● V19.11 Glaucoma

● V19.19 Other specified eye disorder

V19.2 Deafness or hearing loss

V19.3 Other ear disorders

V19.4 Skin conditions

V19.5 Congenital anomalies

V19.6 Allergic disorders

V19.7 Consanguinity

V19.8 Other condition

PERSONS ENCOUNTERING HEALTH SERVICES IN CIRCUMSTANCES RELATED TO REPRODUCTION AND DEVELOPMENT (V20-V29)

V20 Health supervision of infant or child

V20.0 Foundling

V20.1 Other healthy infant or child receiving care
Medical or nursing care supervision of healthy infant in cases of:
maternal illness, physical or psychiatric
socioeconomic adverse condition at home
too many children at home preventing or interfering with normal care

V20.2 Routine infant or child health check
Developmental testing of infant or child
Health check for child over 28 days old
Immunizations appropriate for age
Routine vision and hearing testing

Excludes: health check for child under 29 days old (V20.31-V20.32)
newborn health supervision (V20.31-V20.32)
special screening for developmental handicaps (V79.3)

Use additional code(s) to identify:
Special screening examination(s) performed (V73.0-V82.9)

⑤ V20.3 Newborn health supervision
Health check for child under 29 days old

Excludes: health check for child over 28 days old (V20.2)

V20.31 Health supervision for newborn under 8 days old
Health check for newborn under 8 days old

V20.32 Health supervision for newborn 8 to 28 days old
Health check for newborn 8 to 28 days old
Newborn weight check

V21 Constitutional states in development

V21.0 Period of rapid growth in childhood

V21.1 Puberty

V21.2 Other adolescence

⑤ V21.3 Low birth weight status

Excludes: history of perinatal problems (V13.7)

V21.30 Low birth weight status, unspecified

V21.31 Low birth weight status, less than 500 grams

V21.32 Low birth weight status, 500-999 grams

V21.33 Low birth weight status, 1000-1499 grams

V21.34 Low birth weight status, 1500-1999 grams

V21.35 Low birth weight status, 2000-2500 grams

V21.8 Other specified constitutional states in development

V21.9 Unspecified constitutional state in development

● Code new
to 2012 edition   ▲ Revision of
existing code   ④ ⑤ Fourth or fifth
digit required

V22 Normal pregnancy

Excludes: pregnancy examination or test, pregnancy unconfirmed (V72.40)

V22.0 Supervision of normal first pregnancy

[ALERT!] Codes V22.0 and V22.1 are always first listed and are not to be used with any other code from the OB chapter.

V22.1 Supervision of other normal pregnancy

[ALERT!] Codes V22.0 and V22.1 are always first listed and are not to be used with any other code from the OB chapter.

V22.2 Pregnant state, incidental
Pregnant state NOS

V23 Supervision of high-risk pregnancy

[DEFINITION] A high-risk pregnancy is one in which some condition puts the mother, the developing fetus, or both at higher-than-normal risk for complications during or after the pregnancy and birth.

V23.0 Pregnancy with history of infertility

V23.1 Pregnancy with history of trophoblastic disease
Pregnancy with history of:
hydatidiform mole
vesicular mole

Excludes: that without current pregnancy (V13.1)

V23.2 Pregnancy with history of abortion
Pregnancy with history of conditions classifiable to 634-638

Excludes: recurrent pregnancy loss:
care during pregnancy (646.3)
that without current pregnancy (629.81)

V23.3 Grand multiparity

Excludes: care in relation to labor and delivery (659.4)
that without current pregnancy (V61.5)

[5] **V23.4 Pregnancy with other poor obstetric history**
Pregnancy with history of other conditions classifiable to 630-676

V23.41 Pregnancy with history of pre-term labor

● **V23.42 Pregnancy with history of ectopic pregnancy**

V23.49 Pregnancy with other poor obstetric history

V23.5 Pregnancy with other poor reproductive history
Pregnancy with history of stillbirth or neonatal death

V23.7 Insufficient prenatal care
History of little or no prenatal care

[5] **V23.8 Other high-risk pregnancy**

V23.81 Elderly primigravida
First pregnancy in a woman who will be 35 years of age or older at expected date of delivery

Excludes: elderly primigravida complicating pregnancy (659.5)

V23.82 Elderly multigravida
Second or more pregnancy in a woman who will be 35 years of age or older at expected date of delivery

Excludes: elderly multigravida complicating pregnancy (659.6)

V23.83 Young primigravida
First pregnancy in a female less than 16 years old at expected date of delivery

Excludes: young primigravida complicating pregnancy (659.8)

V23.84 Young multigravida
Second or more pregnancy in a female less than 16 years old at expected date of delivery

Excludes: young multigravida complicating pregnancy (659.8)

V23.85 Pregnancy resulting from assisted reproductive technology
Pregnancy resulting from in vitro fertilization

V23.86 Pregnancy with history of in utero procedure during previous pregnancy

Excludes: management of pregnancy affected by in utero procedure during current pregnancy (679.0-679.1)

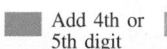

● **V23.87 Pregnancy with inconclusive fetal viability**
Encounter to determine fetal viability of pregnancy

V23.89 Other high-risk pregnancy

V23.9 Unspecified high-risk pregnancy

V24 Postpartum care and examination

[DEFINITION] A high risk pregnancy is one in which some condition puts the mother, the developing fetus, or both at higher-than-normal risk for complications during or after the pregnancy and birth.

V24.0 Immediately after delivery
Care and observation in uncomplicated cases

V24.1 Lactating mother
Supervision of lactation

V24.2 Routine postpartum follow-up

V25 Encounter for contraceptive management

[DEFINITION] Contraceptive management refers to the process of reviewing contraceptive options as well as dispensing contraceptive devices or medications.

[5] **V25.0 General counseling and advice**

V25.01 Prescription of oral contraceptives

V25.02 Initiation of other contraceptive measures
Fitting of diaphragm
Prescription of foams, creams, or other agents

V25.03 Encounter for emergency contraceptive counseling and prescription
Encounter for postcoital contraceptive counseling and prescription

V25.04 Counseling and instruction in natural family planning to avoid pregnancy

V25.09 Other
Family planning advice

[5] **V25.1 Encounter for insertion or removal of intrauterine contraceptive device**

[Excludes:] *encounter for routine checking of intrauterine contraceptive device (V25.42)*

V25.11 Encounter for insertion of intrauterine contraceptive device

V25.12 Encounter for removal of intrauterine contraceptive device

V25.13 Encounter for removal and reinsertion of intrauterine contraceptive device
Encounter for replacement of intrauterine contraceptive device

V25.2 Sterilization
Admission for interruption of fallopian tubes or vas deferens

V25.3 Menstrual extraction
Menstrual regulation

[5] **V25.4 Surveillance of previously prescribed contraceptive methods**
Checking, reinsertion, or removal of contraceptive device
Repeat prescription for contraceptive method
Routine examination in connection with contraceptive maintenance

V25.40 Contraceptive surveillance, unspecified

V25.41 Contraceptive pill

V25.42 Intrauterine contraceptive device
Checking of intrauterine device

[Excludes:] *insertion or removal of intrauterine contraceptive device (V25.11-V25.13)*
presence of intrauterine contraceptive device as incidental finding (V45.5)

V25.43 Implantable subdermal contraceptive

V25.49 Other contraceptive method

V25.5 Insertion of implantable subdermal contraceptive

V25.8 Other specified contraceptive management
Postvasectomy sperm count

[Excludes:] *sperm count following sterilization reversal (V26.22)*
sperm count for fertility testing (V26.21)

V25.9 Unspecified contraceptive management

V26 Procreative management

[DEFINITION] Procreative management may include fertility testing, genetic counseling, procreative counseling, and status of tubal ligation or vasectomy.

V26.0 Tuboplasty or vasoplasty after previous sterilization

● Code new to 2012 edition ▲ Revision of existing code [4] [5] Fourth or fifth digit required

V26.1 Artificial insemination

⑤ **V26.2 Investigation and testing**
> Excludes: *postvasectomy sperm count (V25.8)*

> **V26.21 Fertility testing**
> Fallopian insufflation
> Sperm count for fertility testing

> Excludes: *genetic counseling and testing (V26.31-V26.39)*

> **V26.22 Aftercare following sterilization reversal**
> Fallopian insufflation following sterilization reversal
> Sperm count following sterilization reversal

> **V26.29 Other investigation and testing**

⑤ **V26.3 Genetic counseling and testing**
> Excludes: *fertility testing (V26.21)*
> *nonprocreative genetic screening (V82.71, V82.79)*

> **V26.31 Testing of female for genetic disease carrier status**

> **V26.32 Other genetic testing of female**
> Use additional code to identify recurrent pregnancy loss (629.81, 646.3)

> **V26.33 Genetic counseling**

> **V26.34 Testing of male for genetic disease carrier status**

> **V26.35 Encounter for testing of male partner of female with recurrent pregnancy loss**

> **V26.39 Other genetic testing of male**

⑤ **V26.4 General counseling and advice**

> **V26.41 Procreative counseling and advice using natural family planning**

> **V26.42 Encounter for fertility preservation counseling**
> Encounter for fertility preservation counseling prior to cancer therapy
> Encounter for fertility preservation counseling prior to surgical removal of gonads

> **V26.49 Other procreative management counseling and advice**

⑤ **V26.5 Sterilization status**

> **V26.51 Tubal ligation status**

> Excludes: *infertility not due to previous tubal ligation (628.0-628.9)*

> **V26.52 Vasectomy status**

⑤ **V26.8 Other specified procreative management**

> **V26.81 Encounter for assisted reproductive fertility procedure cycle**
> Patient undergoing in vitro fertilization cycle
> Use additional code to identify the type of infertility

> Excludes: *pre-cycle diagnosis and testing – code to reason for encounter*

> **V26.82 Encounter for fertility preservation procedure**
> Encounter for fertility preservation procedure prior to cancer therapy
> Encounter for fertility preservation procedure prior to surgical removal of gonads

> **V26.89 Other specified procreative management**

V26.9 Unspecified procreative management

V27 Outcome of delivery
> Note: This category is intended for the coding of the outcome of delivery on the mother's record.

> **ALERT!** The outcome of delivery, category V27, should be included on all maternal delivery records. It is always a secondary code.

V27.0 Single liveborn

V27.1 Single stillborn

V27.2 Twins, both liveborn

V27.3 Twins, one liveborn and one stillborn

V27.4 Twins, both stillborn

V27.5 Other multiple birth, all liveborn

V27.6 Other multiple birth, some liveborn

▮	Add 4th or 5th digit	▮	Nonspecific code	▮	Unspecific code	▮	Secondary Dx Only	▮	Primary Dx Only

V27.7 Other multiple birth, all stillborn

V27.9 Unspecified outcome of delivery
Single birth, outcome to infant unspecified
Multiple birth, outcome to infant unspecified

V28 Encounter for antenatal screening of mother

[Excludes:] *abnormal findings on screening—code to findings*
routine prenatal care (V22.0-V23.9)
suspected fetal conditions affecting management of pregnancy (655.00-655.93, 656.00-656.93, 657.00-657.03, 658.00 -658.93)
suspected fetal conditions not found (V89.01-V89.09)

DEFINITION Antenatal screening refers to any of various diagnostic techniques to determine whether a developing fetus is affected with a genetic disorder or other abnormality.

V28.0 Screening for chromosomal anomalies by amniocentesis

V28.1 Screening for raised alpha-fetoprotein levels in amniotic fluid

V28.2 Other screening based on amniocentesis

V28.3 Encounter for routine screening for malformation using ultrasonics
Encounter for routine fetal ultrasound NOS

[Excludes:] *encounter for feal anatomic survey (V28.81)*
genetic counseling and testing (V26.31-V26.39)

V28.4 Screening for fetal growth retardation using ultrasonics

V28.5 Screening for isoimmunization

V28.6 Screening for Streptococcus B

[5] **V28.8 Other specified antenatal screening**

V28.81 Encounter for fetal anatomic survey

V28.82 Encounter for screening for risk of pre-term labor

V28.89 Other specified antenatal screening
Chorionic villus sampling
Genomic screening
Nuchal translucency testing
Proteomic screening

V28.9 Unspecified antenatal screening

V29 Observation and evaluation of newborns for suspected condition not found

Note: This category is to be used for newborns, within the neonatal period, (the first 28 days of life) who are suspected of having an abnormal condition resulting from exposure from the mother or the birth process, but without signs or symptoms, and, which after examination and observation, is found not to exist.

[Excludes:] *suspected fetal conditions not found (V89.01-V89.09)*

ALERT! Assign a code from category V29 to identify those instances when a healthy newborn is evaluated for a suspected condition that is determined after study not to be present.

ALERT! Do not use a code from category V29 when the patient has identified signs or symptoms of a suspected problem; in such cases, code the sign or symptom.

V29.0 Observation for suspected infectious condition

V29.1 Observation for suspected neurological condition

V29.2 Observation for suspected respiratory condition

V29.3 Observation for suspected genetic or metabolic condition

V29.8 Observation for other specified suspected condition

V29.9 Observation for unspecified suspected condition

LIVEBORN INFANTS ACCORDING TO TYPE OF BIRTH (V30-V39)

Note: These categories are intended for the coding of liveborn infants who are consuming health care [e.g., crib or bassinet occupancy].

The following fourth-digit subdivisions are for use with categories V30-V39:

[5] **.0 Born in hospital**

.1 Born before admission to hospital

.2 Born outside hospital and not hospitalized

The following two fifth-digits are for use with the fourth-digit .0, Born in hospital:

0 delivered without mention of cesarean delivery

1 delivered by cesarean delivery

④ **V30** Single liveborn

④ **V31** Twin, mate liveborn

④ **V32** Twin, mate stillborn

④ **V33** Twin, unspecified

④ **V34** Other multiple, mates all liveborn

④ **V35** Other multiple, mates all stillborn

④ **V36** Other multiple, mates live- and stillborn

④ **V37** Other multiple, unspecified

④ **V39** Unspecified

PERSONS WITH A CONDITION INFLUENCING THEIR HEALTH STATUS (V40-V49)

Note: These categories are intended for use when these conditions are recorded as "diagnoses" or "problems."

V40 Mental and behavioral problems

V40.0 Problems with learning

V40.1 Problems with communication [including speech]

V40.2 Other mental problems

⑤ V40.3 Other behavioral problems

● V40.31 Wandering in diseases classified elsewhere
Code first underlying disorder such as:
Alzheimer's disease (331.0)
autism or pervasive developmental disorder (299.0-299.9)
dementia, unspecified, with behavioral disturbance (294.21)
intellectual disabilities (317-319)

● **V40.39** Other specified behavioral problem

V40.9 Unspecified mental or behavioral problem

V41 Problems with special senses and other special functions

V41.0 Problems with sight

V41.1 Other eye problems

V41.2 Problems with hearing

V41.3 Other ear problems

V41.4 Problems with voice production

V41.5 Problems with smell and taste

V41.6 Problems with swallowing and mastication

V41.7 Problems with sexual function
Excludes: *marital problems (V61.10)*
psychosexual disorders (302.0-302.9)

V41.8 Other problems with special functions

V41.9 Unspecified problem with special function

V42 Organ or tissue replaced by transplant
Includes: homologous or heterologous (animal) (human) transplant organ status

V42.0 Kidney

V42.1 Heart

V42.2 Heart valve

V42.3 Skin

V42.4 Bone

V42.5 Cornea

V42.6 Lung

V42.7 Liver

⑤ V42.8 Other specified organ or tissue

V42.81 Bone marrow

V42.82 Peripheral stem cells

V42.83 Pancreas

V42.84 Intestines

V42.89 Other

| | Add 4th or 5th digit | | Nonspecific code | | Unspecific code | | Secondary Dx Only | | Primary Dx Only |

V42.9 Unspecified organ or tissue

V43 Organ or tissue replaced by other means

Includes: organ or tissue assisted by other means
replacement of organ by:
artificial device
mechanical device
prosthesis

Excludes: *cardiac pacemaker in situ (V45.01)*
fitting and adjustment of prosthetic device (V52.0-V52.9)
renal dialysis status (V45.11)

V43.0 Eye globe

V43.1 Lens
Pseudophakos

⑤ **V43.2** Heart

V43.21 Heart assist device

V43.22 Fully implantable artificial heart

V43.3 Heart valve

V43.4 Blood vessel

V43.5 Bladder

⑤ **V43.6** Joint

V43.60 Unspecified joint

V43.61 Shoulder

V43.62 Elbow

V43.63 Wrist

V43.64 Hip

V43.65 Knee

V43.66 Ankle

V43.69 Other

V43.7 Limb

⑤ **V43.8** Other organ or tissue

V43.81 Larynx

V43.82 Breast

V43.83 Artificial skin

V43.89 Other

V44 Artificial opening status

Excludes: *artificial openings requiring attention or management (V55.0-V55.9)*

V44.0 Tracheostomy

V44.1 Gastrostomy

V44.2 Ileostomy

V44.3 Colostomy

V44.4 Other artificial opening of gastrointestinal tract

⑤ **V44.5** Cystostomy

V44.50 Cystostomy, unspecified

V44.51 Cutaneous-vesicostomy

V44.52 Appendico-vesicostomy

V44.59 Other cystostomy

V44.6 Other artificial opening of urinary tract
Nephrostomy
Ureterostomy
Urethrostomy

V44.7 Artificial vagina

V44.8 Other artificial opening status

V44.9 Unspecified artificial opening status

● Code new
to 2012 edition

▲ Revision of
existing code

④ ⑤ Fourth or fifth
digit required

V45 Other postprocedural states

[Excludes:] *aftercare management (V51-V58.9)*
malfunction or other complication—code to condition

[5] **V45.0 Cardiac device in situ**

[Excludes:] *artificial heart (V43.22)*
heart assist device (V43.21)

V45.00 Unspecified cardiac device

V45.01 Cardiac pacemaker

[Excludes:] *cardiac defibrillator with synchronous cardiac pacemaker (V45.02)*

V45.02 Automatic implantable cardiac defibrillator
With synchronous cardiac pacemaker

V45.09 Other specified cardiac device
Carotid sinus pacemaker in situ

[5] **V45.1 Renal dialysis status**

[Excludes:] *admission for dialysis treatment, or session (V56.0)*

V45.11 Renal dialysis status
Hemodialysis status
Patient requiring intermittent renal dialysis
Peritoneal dialysis status
Presence of arterial-venous shunt (for dialysis)

V45.12 Noncompliance with renal dialysis

V45.2 Presence of cerebrospinal fluid drainage device
Cerebral ventricle (communicating) shunt, valve, or device in situ

[Excludes:] *malfunction (996.2)*

V45.3 Intestinal bypass or anastomosis status

[Excludes:] *bariatric surgery status (V45.86)*
gastric bypass status (V45.86)
obesity surgery status (V45.86)

V45.4 Arthrodesis status

[5] **V45.5 Presence of contraceptive device**

V45.51 Intrauterine contraceptive device

[Excludes:] *checking of device (V25.42)*
complication from device (996.32)
insertion and removal of device (V25.11-V25.13)

V45.52 Subdermal contraceptive implant

V45.59 Other

[5] **V45.6 States following surgery of eye and adnexa**
Cataract extraction state following eye surgery
Filtering bleb state following eye surgery
Surgical eyelid adhesion state following eye surgery

[Excludes:] *aphakia (379.31)*
artificial eye globe (V43.0)

V45.61 Cataract extraction status
Use additional code for associated artificial lens status (V43.1)

V45.69 Other states following surgery of eye and adnexa

[5] **V45.7 Acquired absence of organ**

V45.71 Acquired absence of breast and nipple

[Excludes:] *congenital absence of breast and nipple (757.6)*

V45.72 Acquired absence of intestine (large) (small)

V45.73 Acquired absence of kidney

V45.74 Other parts of urinary tract
Bladder

V45.75 Stomach

V45.76 Lung

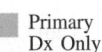

Add 4th or 5th digit | Nonspecific code | Unspecific code | Secondary Dx Only | Primary Dx Only

V45.77 Genital organs

Excludes: *acquired absence of cervix and uterus (V88.01-V88.03)*
female genital mutilation status (629.20-629.29)

V45.78 Eye

V45.79 Other acquired absence of organ

Excludes: *acquired absence of pancreas (V88.11-V88.12)*

⑤ **V45.8 Other postprocedural status**

V45.81 Aortocoronary bypass status

V45.82 Percutaneous transluminal coronary angioplasty status

V45.83 Breast implant removal status

V45.84 Dental restoration status
Dental crowns status
Dental fillings status

V45.85 Insulin pump status

V45.86 Bariatric surgery status
Gastric banding status
Gastric bypass status for obesity
Obesity surgery status

Excludes: *bariatric surgery status complicating pregnancy, childbirth or the puerperium (649.2)*
intestinal bypass or anastomosis status (V45.3)

V45.87 Transplanted organ removal status
Transplanted organ previously removed due to complication, failure, rejection or infection

Excludes: *encounter for removal of transplanted organ - code to complication of transplanted organ (996.80-996.89)*

V45.88 Status post administration of tPA (rtPA) in a different facility within the last 24 hours prior to admission to current facility
Code first condition requiring tPA administration, such as:
acute cerebral infarction (433.0-433.9 with fifth-digit 1, 434.0-434.9 with fifth digit 1)
acute myocardial infarction (410.00-410.92)

ALERT! Assign code V45.88 as a secondary diagnosis when a patient is received by transfer into a facility and documentation indicates they were administered tissue plasminogen activator (tPA) within the last 24 hours prior to admission to the current facility.

V45.89 Other
Presence of neuropacemaker or other electronic device

Excludes: *artificial heart valve in situ (V43.3)*
vascular prosthesis in situ (V43.4)

V46 Other dependence on machines and devices

V46.0 Aspirator

⑤ **V46.1 Respirator [Ventilator]**
Iron lung

V46.11 Dependence on respirator, status

V46.12 Encounter for respirator dependence during power failure

V46.13 Encounter for weaning from respirator [ventilator]

V46.14 Mechanical complication of respirator [ventilator]
Mechanical failure of respirator [ventilator]

V46.2 Supplemental oxygen
Long-term oxygen therapy

V46.3 Wheelchair dependence
Wheelchair confinement status

Code first cause of dependence, such as:
muscular dystrophy (359.1)
obesity (278.00-278.03)

V46.8 Other enabling machines
Hyperbaric chamber
Possum [Patient-Operated-Selector-Mechanism]

Excludes: *cardiac pacemaker (V45.0)*
kidney dialysis machine (V45.11)

● Code new
to 2012 edition ▲ Revision of
existing code ④ ⑤ Fourth or fifth
digit required

V46.9 Unspecified machine dependence

V47 Other problems with internal organs

V47.0 Deficiencies of internal organs

V47.1 Mechanical and motor problems with internal organs

V47.2 Other cardiorespiratory problems

Cardiovascular exercise intolerance with pain (with):
at rest
less than ordinary activity
ordinary activity

V47.3 Other digestive problems

V47.4 Other urinary problems

V47.5 Other genital problems

V47.9 Unspecified

V48 Problems with head, neck, and trunk

V48.0 Deficiencies of head

[Excludes:] *deficiencies of ears, eyelids, and nose (V48.8)*

V48.1 Deficiencies of neck and trunk

V48.2 Mechanical and motor problems with head

V48.3 Mechanical and motor problems with neck and trunk

V48.4 Sensory problem with head

V48.5 Sensory problem with neck and trunk

V48.6 Disfigurements of head

V48.7 Disfigurements of neck and trunk

V48.8 Other problems with head, neck, and trunk

V48.9 Unspecified problem with head, neck, or trunk

V49 Other conditions influencing health status

V49.0 Deficiencies of limbs

V49.1 Mechanical problems with limbs

V49.2 Motor problems with limbs

V49.3 Sensory problems with limbs

V49.4 Disfigurements of limbs

V49.5 Other problems of limbs

[5] **V49.6 Upper limb amputation status**

V49.60 Unspecified level

V49.61 Thumb

V49.62 Other finger(s)

V49.63 Hand

V49.64 Wrist
Disarticulation of wrist

V49.65 Below elbow

V49.66 Above elbow
Disarticulation of elbow

V49.67 Shoulder
Disarticulation of shoulder

[5] **V49.7 Lower limb amputation status**

V49.70 Unspecified level

V49.71 Great toe

V49.72 Other toe(s)

V49.73 Foot

V49.74 Ankle
Disarticulation of ankle

V49.75 Below knee

V49.76 Above knee
Disarticulation of knee

V49.77 Hip
Disarticulation of hip

⑤ **V49.8 Other specified conditions influencing health status**

V49.81 Asymptomatic postmenopausal status (age-related) (natural)

Excludes: menopausal and premenopausal disorders (627.0-627.9)
postsurgical menopause (256.2)
premature menopause (256.31)
symptomatic menopause (627.0-627.9)

V49.82 Dental sealant status

V49.83 Awaiting organ transplant status

V49.84 Bed confinement status

V49.85 Dual sensory impairment
Blindness with deafness
Combined visual hearing impairment

Code first:
hearing impairment (389.00-389.9)
visual impairment (369.00-369.9)

V49.86 Do not resuscitate status

V49.87 Physical restraints status

Excludes: restraint due to a procedure – omit code

V49.89 Other specified conditions influencing health status

V49.9 Unspecified

PERSONS ENCOUNTERING HEALTH SERVICES FOR SPECIFIC PROCEDURES AND AFTERCARE (V50-V59)

Note: Categories V51-V58 are intended for use to indicate a reason for care in patients who may have already been treated for some disease or injury not now present, but who are receiving care to consolidate the treatment, to deal with residual states, or to prevent recurrence.

Excludes: follow-up examination for medical surveillance following treatment (V67.0-V67.9)

V50 Elective surgery for purposes other than remedying health states

V50.0 Hair transplant

V50.1 Other plastic surgery for unacceptable cosmetic appearance
Breast augmentation or reduction
Face-lift

Excludes: encounter for breast reduction (611.1)
plastic surgery following healed injury or operation (V51.0-V51.8)

V50.2 Routine or ritual circumcision
Circumcision in the absence of significant medical indication

V50.3 Ear piercing

⑤ **V50.4 Prophylactic organ removal**

Excludes: organ donations (V59.0-V59.9)
therapeutic organ removal—code to condition

V50.41 Breast

V50.42 Ovary

V50.49 Other

V50.8 Other

V50.9 Unspecified

V51 Aftercare involving the use of plastic surgery
Plastic surgery following healed injury or operation

Excludes: cosmetic plastic surgery (V50.1)
plastic surgery as treatment for current condition or injury—code to condition or injury
repair of scarred tissue—code to scar

V51.0 Encounter for breast reconstruction following mastectomy

Excludes: deformity and disproportion of reconstructed breast (612.0-612.1)

V51.8 Other aftercare involving the use of plastic surgery

● Code new
to 2012 edition
▲ Revision of
existing code
④ ⑤ Fourth or fifth
digit required

V52 Fitting and adjustment of prosthetic device and implant
Includes: removal of device
[Excludes:] *malfunction or complication of prosthetic device (996.0-996.7)*
status only, without need for care (V43.0-V43.8)

V52.0 Artificial arm (complete) (partial)

V52.1 Artificial leg (complete) (partial)

V52.2 Artificial eye

V52.3 Dental prosthetic device

V52.4 Breast prosthesis and implant
Elective implant exchange (different material) (different size)
Removal of tissue expander without synchronous insertion of permanent implant
[Excludes:] *admission for initial breast implant insertion for breast augmentation (V50.1)*
complications of breast implant (996.54, 996.69, 996.79)
encounter for breast reconstruction following mastectomy (V51.0)

V52.8 Other specified prosthetic device

V52.9 Unspecified prosthetic device

V53 Fitting and adjustment of other device
Includes: removal of device
replacement of device
[Excludes:] *status only, without need for care (V45.0-V45.8)*

[5] **V53.0 Devices related to nervous system and special senses**

V53.01 Fitting and adjustment of cerebral ventricular (communicating) shunt

V53.02 Neuropacemaker (brain) (peripheral nerve) (spinal cord)

V53.09 Fitting and adjustment of other devices related to nervous system and special senses
Auditory substitution device
Visual substitution device

V53.1 Spectacles and contact lenses

V53.2 Hearing aid

[5] **V53.3 Cardiac device**
Reprogramming

V53.31 Cardiac pacemaker
[Excludes:] *automatic implantable cardiac defibrillator with synchronous cardiac pacemaker (V53.32)*
mechanical complication of cardiac pacemaker (996.01)

V53.32 Automatic implantable cardiac defibrillator
With synchronous cardiac pacemaker

V53.39 Other cardiac device

V53.4 Orthodontic devices

[5] **V53.5 Other gastrointestinal appliance and device**
[Excludes:] *colostomy (V55.3)*
ileostomy (V55.2)
other artificial opening of digestive tract (V55.4)

V53.50 Fitting and adjustment of intestinal appliance and device

V53.51 Fitting and adjustment of gastric lap band

V53.59 Fitting and adjustment of other gastrointestinal appliance and device

V53.6 Urinary devices
Urinary catheter
[Excludes:] *cystostomy (V55.5)*
nephrostomy (V55.6)
ureterostomy (V55.6)
urethrostomy (V55.6)

V53.7 Orthopedic devices
Orthopedic:
brace
cast

Orthopedic:
corset
shoes

[Excludes:] *other orthopedic aftercare (V54)*

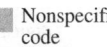

Add 4th or 5th digit | Nonspecific code | Unspecific code | Secondary Dx Only | Primary Dx Only

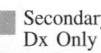

V53.8 **Wheelchair**

⑤ **V53.9 Other and unspecified device**

   V53.90 **Unspecified device**

   V53.91 **Fitting and adjustment of insulin pump**
   Insulin pump titration

   V53.99 **Other device**

V54 **Other orthopedic aftercare**

   Excludes: *fitting and adjustment of orthopedic devices (V53.7)*
         malfunction of internal orthopedic device (996.40-996.49)
         other complication of nonmechanical nature (996.60-996.79)

⑤ **V54.0 Aftercare involving internal fixation device**

   Excludes: *malfunction of internal orthopedic device (996.40-996.49)*
         removal of external fixation device (V54.89)

   V54.01 **Encounter for removal of internal fixation device**

   V54.02 **Encounter for lengthening/adjustment of growth rod**

   V54.09 **Other aftercare involving internal fixation device**

⑤ **V54.1 Aftercare for healing traumatic fracture**

   Excludes: *aftercare following joint replacement (V54.81)*
         aftercare for amputation stump (V54.89)

   V54.10 **Aftercare for healing traumatic fracture of arm, unspecified**

   V54.11 **Aftercare for healing traumatic fracture of upper arm**

   V54.12 **Aftercare for healing traumatic fracture of lower arm**

   V54.13 **Aftercare for healing traumatic fracture of hip**

   V54.14 **Aftercare for healing traumatic fracture of leg, unspecified**

   V54.15 **Aftercare for healing traumatic fracture of upper leg**

   Excludes: *aftercare for healing traumatic fracture of hip (V54.13)*

   V54.16 **Aftercare for healing traumatic fracture of lower leg**

   V54.17 **Aftercare for healing traumatic fracture of vertebrae**

   V54.19 **Aftercare for healing traumatic fracture of other bone**

⑤ **V54.2 Aftercare for healing pathologic fracture**

   Excludes: *aftercare following joint replacement (V54.81)*

   V54.20 **Aftercare for healing pathologic fracture of arm, unspecified**

   V54.21 **Aftercare for healing pathologic fracture of upper arm**

   V54.22 **Aftercare for healing pathologic fracture of lower arm**

   V54.23 **Aftercare for healing pathologic fracture of hip**

   V54.24 **Aftercare for healing pathologic fracture of leg, unspecified**

   V54.25 **Aftercare for healing pathologic fracture of upper leg**

   Excludes: *aftercare for healing pathologic fracture of hip (V54.23)*

   V54.26 **Aftercare for healing pathologic fracture of lower leg**

   V54.27 **Aftercare for healing pathologic fracture of vertebrae**

   V54.29 **Aftercare for healing pathologic fracture of other bone**

⑤ **V54.8 Other orthopedic aftercare**

   V54.81 **Aftercare following joint replacement**
   Use additional code to identify joint replacement site (V43.60-V43.69)

● V54.82 **Aftercare following explantation of joint prosthesis**
   Aftercare following explantation of joint prosthesis, staged procedure
   Encounter for joint prosthesis insertion following prior explantation of joint
   prosthesis

   V54.89 **Other orthopedic aftercare**
   Aftercare for healing fracture NOS

   V54.9 **Unspecified orthopedic aftercare**

V55 Attention to artificial openings
Includes: adjustment or repositioning of catheter
closure
passage of sounds or bougies
reforming
removal or replacement of catheter
toilet or cleansing

[Excludes:] *complications of external stoma (519.00-519.09, 569.60-569.69, 596.81-596.83, 997.49)*
status only, without need for care (V44.0-V44.9)

V55.0 Tracheostomy

V55.1 Gastrostomy

V55.2 Ileostomy

V55.3 Colostomy

V55.4 Other artificial opening of digestive tract

V55.5 Cystostomy

V55.6 Other artificial opening of urinary tract
Nephrostomy
Urethrostomy
Ureterostomy

V55.7 Artificial vagina

V55.8 Other specified artificial opening

V55.9 Unspecified artificial opening

V56 Encounter for dialysis and dialysis catheter care
Use additional code to identify the associated condition

[Excludes:] *dialysis preparation—code to condition*

DEFINITION Dialysis is a medical procedure to remove wastes and additional fluid from the blood after the kidneys have stopped functioning.

V56.0 Extracorporeal dialysis
Dialysis (renal) NOS

[Excludes:] *dialysis status (V45.11)*

V56.1 Fitting and adjustment of extracorporeal dialysis catheter
Removal or replacement of catheter
Toilet or cleansing

Use additional code for any concurrent extracorporeal dialysis (V56.0)

V56.2 Fitting and adjustment of peritoneal dialysis catheter
Use additional code for any concurrent peritoneal dialysis (V56.8)

[5] **V56.3 Encounter for adequacy testing for dialysis**

V56.31 Encounter for adequacy testing for hemodialysis

V56.32 Encounter for adequacy testing for peritoneal dialysis
Peritoneal equilibration test

V56.8 Other dialysis
Peritoneal dialysis

V57 Care involving use of rehabilitation procedures
Use additional code to identify underlying condition

V57.0 Breathing exercises

V57.1 Other physical therapy
Therapeutic and remedial exercises, except breathing

[5] **V57.2 Occupational therapy and vocational rehabilitation**

V57.21 Encounter for occupational therapy

V57.22 Encounter for vocational therapy

V57.3 Speech-language therapy

V57.4 Orthoptic training

[5] **V57.8 Other specified rehabilitation procedure**

V57.81 Orthotic training
Gait training in the use of artificial limbs

V57.89 Other
Multiple training or therapy

V57.9 Unspecified rehabilitation procedure

V58 Encounter for other and unspecified procedures and aftercare

[Excludes:] *convalescence and palliative care (V66)*

V58.0 Radiotherapy

Encounter or admission for radiotherapy

[Excludes:] *encounter for radioactive implant—code to condition*
radioactive iodine therapy—code to condition

[5] **V58.1 Encounter for chemotherapy and immunotherapy for neoplastic conditions**

Encounter or admission for chemotherapy

[Excludes:] *chemotherapy and immunotherapy for nonneoplastic conditions—code to condition*

V58.11 Encounter for antineoplastic chemotherapy

V58.12 Encounter for antineoplastic immunotherapy

V58.2 Blood transfusion, without reported diagnosis

[5] **V58.3 Attention to dressings and sutures**

Change or removal of wound packing

[Excludes:] *attention to drains (V58.49)*
planned postoperative wound closure (V58.41)

V58.30 Encounter for change or removal of nonsurgical wound dressing

Encounter for change or removal of wound dressing NOS

V58.31 Encounter for change or removal of surgical wound dressing

V58.32 Encounter for removal of sutures

Encounter for removal of staples

[5] **V58.4 Other aftercare following surgery**

Note: Codes from this subcategory should be used in conjunction with other aftercare codes to fully identify the reason for the aftercare encounter

[Excludes:] *aftercare following sterilization reversal surgery (V26.22)*
attention to artificial openings (V55.0-V55.9)
orthopedic aftercare (V54.0-V54.9)

V58.41 Encounter for planned postoperative wound closure

[Excludes:] *disruption of operative wound (998.31-998.32)*
encounter for dressings and suture aftercare (V58.30-V58.32)

V58.42 Aftercare following surgery for neoplasm

Conditions classifiable to 140-239

V58.43 Aftercare following surgery for injury and trauma

Conditions classifiable to 800-999

[Excludes:] *aftercare for healing traumatic fracture (V54.10-V54.19)*

V58.44 Aftercare following organ transplant

Use additional code to identify the organ transplanted (V42.0-V42.9)

V58.49 Other specified aftercare following surgery

Change or removal of drains

V58.5 Orthodontics

[Excludes:] *fitting and adjustment of orthodontic device (V53.4)*

[5] **V58.6 Long-term (current) drug use**

Long-term (current) prophylactic drug use

[Excludes:] *drug abuse (305.00-305.93)*
drug abuse and dependence complicating pregnancy (648.3-648.4)
drug dependence (304.00-304.93)
hormone replacement therapy (postmenopausal) (V07.4)
use of agents affecting estrogen receptors and estrogen levels (V07.51-V07.59)

[ALERT!] Assign a code from subcategory V58.6 if the patient is receiving a medication for an extended period as a prophylactic measure (such as for the prevention of deep vein thrombosis) or as treatment of a chronic condition (such as arthritis) or a disease requiring a lengthy course of treatment (such as cancer).

[ALERT!] Do not assign a code from subcategory V58.6 for medication being administered for a brief period of time to treat an acute illness or injury (such as a course of antibiotics to treat acute bronchitis).

V58.61 Long-term (current) use of anticoagulants

[Excludes:] *long-term (current) use of aspirin (V58.66)*

V58.62 Long-term (current) use of antibiotics

V58.63 Long-term (current) use of antiplatelets/antithrombotics
[Excludes:] *long-term (current) use of aspirin (V58.66)*

V58.64 Long-term (current) use of non-steroidal anti-inflammatories (NSAID)
[Excludes:] *long-term (current) use of aspirin (V58.66)*

V58.65 Long-term (current) use of steroids

V58.66 Long-term (current) use of aspirin

V58.67 Long-term (current) use of insulin

● **V58.68 Long term (current) use of bisphosphonates**

V58.69 Long-term (current) use of other medications
Long term current use of methadone for pain control
Long term current use of opiate analgesic
Other high-risk medications

[Excludes:] *methadone maintenance NOS (304.00)*
methadone use NOS (304.00)

[5] **V58.7 Aftercare following surgery to specified body systems, not elsewhere classified**
Note: Codes from this subcategory should be used in conjunction with other aftercare codes to fully identify the reason for the aftercare encounter

[Excludes:] *aftercare following organ transplant (V58.44)*
aftercare following surgery for neoplasm (V58.42)

V58.71 Aftercare following surgery of the sense organs, NEC
Conditions classifiable to 360-379, 380-389

V58.72 Aftercare following surgery of the nervous system, NEC
Conditions classifiable to 320-359

[Excludes:] *aftercare following surgery of the sense organs, NEC (V58.71)*

V58.73 Aftercare following surgery of the circulatory system, NEC
Conditions classifiable to 390-459

V58.74 Aftercare following surgery of the respiratory system, NEC
Conditions classifiable to 460-519

V58.75 Aftercare following surgery of the teeth, oral cavity and digestive system, NEC
Conditions classifiable to 520-579

V58.76 Aftercare following surgery of the genitourinary system, NEC
Conditions classifiable to 580-629

[Excludes:] *aftercare following sterilization reversal (V26.22)*

V58.77 Aftercare following surgery of the skin and subcutaneous tissue, NEC
Conditions classifiable to 680-709

V58.78 Aftercare following surgery of the musculoskeletal system, NEC
Conditions classifiable to 710-739

[Excludes:] *orthopedic aftercare (V54.01-V54.9)*

[5] **V58.8 Other specified procedures and aftercare**

V58.81 Fitting and adjustment of vascular catheter
Removal or replacement of catheter
Toilet or cleansing

[Excludes:] *complication of renal dialysis catheter (996.73)*
complication of vascular catheter (996.74)
dialysis preparation — code to condition
encounter for dialysis (V56.0-V56.8)
fitting and adjustment of dialysis catheter (V56.1)

V58.82 Fitting and adjustment of non-vascular catheter NEC
Removal or replacement of catheter
Toilet or cleansing

[Excludes:] *fitting and adjustment of peritoneal dialysis catheter (V56.2)*
fitting and adjustment of urinary catheter (V53.6)

V58.83 Encounter for therapeutic drug monitoring
Use additional code for any associated long-term (current) drug use (V58.61-V58.69)
[Excludes:] *blood-drug testing for medicolegal reasons (V70.4)*

V58.89 Other specified aftercare

V58.9 Unspecified aftercare

V59 Donors

> Excludes: examination of potential donor (V70.8)
> self-donation of organ or tissue—code to condition

ALERT! Category V59 donor codes are are used for living individuals who are donating blood or other body tissue. These codes are only for individuals donating for others, not for self donations. They are not for use to identify cadaveric donations

⑤ **V59.0 Blood**

V59.01 Whole blood

V59.02 Stem cells

V59.09 Other

V59.1 Skin

V59.2 Bone

V59.3 Bone marrow

V59.4 Kidney

V59.5 Cornea

V59.6 Liver

⑤ **V59.7 Egg (oocyte) (ovum)**

V59.70 Egg (oocyte) (ovum) donor, unspecified

V59.71 Egg (oocyte) (ovum) donor, under age 35, anonymous recipient
Egg donor, under age 35 NOS

V59.72 Egg (oocyte) (ovum) donor, under age 35, designated recipient

V59.73 Egg (oocyte) (ovum) donor, age 35 and over, anonymous recipient
Egg donor, age 35 and over NOS

V59.74 Egg (oocyte) (ovum) donor, age 35 and over, designated recipient

V59.8 Other specified organ or tissue

V59.9 Unspecified organ or tissue

PERSONS ENCOUNTERING HEALTH SERVICES IN OTHER CIRCUMSTANCES (V60-V69)

V60 Housing, household, and economic circumstances

V60.0 Lack of housing

Hobos	Transients
Social migrants	Vagabonds
Tramps	

V60.1 Inadequate housing
Lack of heating
Restriction of space
Technical defects in home preventing adequate care

V60.2 Inadequate material resources

Economic problem	Poverty NOS

V60.3 Person living alone

V60.4 No other household member able to render care
Person requiring care (has) (is):
family member too handicapped, ill, or otherwise unsuited to render care
partner temporarily away from home
temporarily away from usual place of abode

> Excludes: holiday relief care (V60.5)

V60.5 Holiday relief care
Provision of health care facilities to a person normally cared for at home, to enable relatives to take a vacation

V60.6 Person living in residential institution
Boarding school resident

⑤ **V60.8 Other specified housing or economic circumstances**

V60.81 Foster care (status)

V60.89 Other specified housing or economic circumstances

V60.9 Unspecified housing or economic circumstance

V61 Other family circumstances
Includes: when these circumstances or fear of them, affecting the person directly involved or others, are mentioned as the reason, justified or not, for seeking or receiving medical advice or care

---

● Code new
to 2012 edition   ▲ Revision of
existing code   ④ ⑤ Fourth or fifth
digit required

⑤ **V61.0 Family disruption**

    V61.01 Family disruption due to family member on military deployment
Individual or family affected by other family member being on deployment

    Excludes: *family disruption due to family member on non-military extended absence from home (V61.08)*

    V61.02 Family disruption due to return of family member from military deployment
Individual or family affected by other family member having returned from deployment (current or past conflict)

    V61.03 Family disruption due to divorce or legal separation

    V61.04 Family disruption due to parent-child estrangement

    Excludes: *other family estrangement (V61.09)*

    V61.05 Family disruption due to child in welfare custody

    V61.06 Family disruption due to child in foster care or in care of non-parental family member

    V61.07 Family disruption due to death of family member

    Excludes: *bereavement (V62.82)*

    V61.08 Family disruption due to other extended absence of family member

    Excludes: *family disruption due to family member on military deployment (V61.01)*

    V61.09 Other family disruption
Family estrangement NOS

⑤ **V61.1 Counseling for marital and partner problems**

    Excludes: *problems related to:*
        psychosexual disorders (302.0-302.9)
        sexual function (V41.7)

    V61.10 Counseling for marital and partner problems, unspecified
Marital conflict
Marital relationship problem
Partner conflict
Partner relationship problem

    V61.11 Counseling for victim of spousal and partner abuse

    Excludes: *encounter for treatment of current injuries due to abuse (995.80-995.85)*

    V61.12 Counseling for perpetrator of spousal and partner abuse

⑤ **V61.2 Parent-child problems**

    V61.20 Counseling for parent-child problem, unspecified
Concern about behavior of child
Parent-child conflict
Parent-child relationship problem

    V61.21 Counseling for victim of child abuse
Child battering
Child neglect

    Excludes: *current injuries due to abuse (995.50-995.59)*

    V61.22 Counseling for perpetrator of parental child abuse

    Excludes: *counseling for non-parental abuser (V62.83)*

    V61.23 Counseling for parent-biological child problem
Concern about behavior of biological child
Parent-biological child conflict
Parent-biological child relationship problem

    V61.24 Counseling for parent-adopted child problem
Concern about behavior of adopted child
Parent-adopted child conflict
Parent-adopted child relationship problem

    V61.25 Counseling for parent (guardian)-foster child problem
Concern about behavior of foster child
Parent (guardian)-foster child conflict
Parent (guardian)-foster child relationship problem

    V61.29 Other parent-child problems

  V61.3 Problems with aged parents or in-laws

⑤ **V61.4 Health problems within family**

| ▨ Add 4th or 5th digit | ▨ Nonspecific code | ▨ Unspecific code | ▨ Secondary Dx Only | ▨ Primary Dx Only |

V61.41 Alcoholism in family

V61.42 Substance abuse in family

V61.49 Other

Care of sick or handicapped person in family or household

Presence of sick or handicapped person in family or household

V61.5 Multiparity

V61.6 Illegitimacy or illegitimate pregnancy

V61.7 Other unwanted pregnancy

V61.8 Other specified family circumstances

Problems with family members NEC

Sibling relationship problem

V61.9 Unspecified family circumstance

V62 Other psychosocial circumstances

Includes: those circumstances or fear of them, affecting the person directly involved or others, mentioned as the reason, justified or not, for seeking or receiving medical advice or care

Excludes: previous psychological trauma (V15.41-V15.49)

V62.0 Unemployment

Excludes: circumstances when main problem is economic inadequacy or poverty (V60.2)

V62.1 Adverse effects of work environment

⑤ **V62.2** Other occupational circumstances or maladjustment

V62.21 Personal current military deployment status

Individual (civilian or military) currently deployed in theater or in support of military war, peacekeeping and humanitarian operations

V62.22 Personal history of return from military deployment

Individual (civilian or military) with past history of military war, peacekeeping and humanitarian deployment (current or past conflict)

V62.29 Other occupational circumstances or maladjustment

Career choice problem

Dissatisfaction with employment

Occupational problem

V62.3 Educational circumstances

Academic problem

Dissatisfaction with school environment

Educational handicap

V62.4 Social maladjustment

Acculturation problem

Cultural deprivation

Political, religious, or sex discrimination

Social:

isolation

persecution

V62.5 Legal circumstances

Imprisonment

Legal investigation

Litigation

Prosecution

V62.6 Refusal of treatment for reasons of religion or conscience

⑤ **V62.8** Other psychological or physical stress, not elsewhere classified

V62.81 Interpersonal problems, not elsewhere classified

Relational problem NOS

V62.82 Bereavement, uncomplicated

Excludes: bereavement as adjustment reaction (309.0)

family disruption due to death of family member (V61.07)

V62.83 Counseling for perpetrator of physical/sexual abuse

Excludes: counseling for perpetrator of parental child abuse (V61.22)

counseling for perpetrator of spousal and partner abuse (V61.12)

V62.84 Suicidal ideation

Excludes: suicidal tendencies (300.9)

V62.85 Homicidal ideation

● Code new to 2012 edition   ▲ Revision of existing code   ④ ⑤ Fourth or fifth digit required

V62.89 Other
Borderline intellectual functioning
Life circumstance problems
Phase of life problems
Religious or spiritual problem

V62.9 Unspecified psychosocial circumstance

V63 Unavailability of other medical facilities for care

V63.0 Residence remote from hospital or other health care facility

V63.1 Medical services in home not available

[Excludes:] *no other household member able to render care (V60.4)*

V63.2 Person awaiting admission to adequate facility elsewhere

V63.8 Other specified reasons for unavailability of medical facilities
Person on waiting list undergoing social agency investigation

V63.9 Unspecified reason for unavailability of medical facilities

V64 Persons encountering health services for specific procedures, not carried out

[5] **V64.0 Vaccination not carried out**

V64.00 Vaccination not carried out, unspecified reason

V64.01 Vaccination not carried out because of acute illness

V64.02 Vaccination not carried out because of chronic illness or condition

V64.03 Vaccination not carried out because of immune compromised state

V64.04 Vaccination not carried out because of allergy to vaccine or component

V64.05 Vaccination not carried out because of caregiver refusal
Guardian refusal — Parent refusal

[Excludes:] *vaccination not carried out because of caregiver refusal for religious reasons (V64.07)*

V64.06 Vaccination not carried out because of patient refusal

V64.07 Vaccination not carried out for religious reasons

V64.08 Vaccination not carried out because patient had disease being vaccinated against

V64.09 Vaccination not carried out for other reason

V64.1 Surgical or other procedure not carried out because of contraindication

V64.2 Surgical or other procedure not carried out because of patient's decision

V64.3 Procedure not carried out for other reasons

[5] **V64.4 Closed surgical procedure converted to open procedure**

V64.41 Laparoscopic surgical procedure converted to open procedure

V64.42 Thoracoscopic surgical procedure converted to open procedure

V64.43 Arthroscopic surgical procedure converted to open procedure

V65 Other persons seeking consultation

V65.0 Healthy person accompanying sick person
Boarder

[5] **V65.1 Person consulting on behalf of another person**
Advice or treatment for nonattending third party

[Excludes:] *concern (normal) about sick person in family (V61.41-V61.49)*

V65.11 Pediatric pre-birth visit for expectant parent(s)
Pre-adoption visit for adoptive parent(s)

V65.19 Other person consulting on behalf of another person

V65.2 Person feigning illness
Malingerer — Peregrinating patient

V65.3 Dietary surveillance and counseling
Dietary surveillance and counseling (in):
NOS
colitis
diabetes mellitus
food allergies or intolerance
gastritis
hypercholesterolemia
hypoglycemia
obesity

Use additional code to identify Body Mass Index (BMI), if known (V85.0-V85.54)

Add 4th or 5th digit | Nonspecific code | Unspecific code | Secondary Dx Only | Primary Dx Only

⑤ **V65.4 Other counseling, not elsewhere classified**
Health:
   advice
   education
   instruction

Excludes: counseling (for):
   contraception (V25.40-V25.49)
   genetic (V26.31-V26.39)
   on behalf of third party (V65.11, V65.19)
   procreative management (V26.41-V26.49)

V65.40 Counseling NOS

V65.41 Exercise counseling

V65.42 Counseling on substance use and abuse

V65.43 Counseling on injury prevention

V65.44 Human immunodeficiency virus [HIV] counseling

V65.45 Counseling on other sexually transmitted diseases

V65.46 Encounter for insulin pump training

V65.49 Other specified counseling

V65.5 Person with feared complaint in whom no diagnosis was made
Feared condition not demonstrated
Problem was normal state
"Worried well"

V65.8 Other reasons for seeking consultation

Excludes: specified symptoms

V65.9 Unspecified reason for consultation

V66 Convalescence and palliative care
DEFINITION Palliative care is patient care provided to relieve pain rather than provide a cure. Also called "comfort care."

V66.0 Following surgery

V66.1 Following radiotherapy

V66.2 Following chemotherapy

V66.3 Following psychotherapy and other treatment for mental disorder

V66.4 Following treatment of fracture

V66.5 Following other treatment

V66.6 Following combined treatment

V66.7 Encounter for palliative care
End-of-life care
Hospice care
Terminal care

Code first underlying disease

V66.9 Unspecified convalescence

V67 Follow-up examination
Includes: surveillance only following completed treatment

Excludes: surveillance of contraception (V25.40-V25.49)

⑤ **V67.0 Following surgery**

V67.00 Following surgery, unspecified

V67.01 Follow-up vaginal pap smear
Vaginal pap smear, status-post hysterectomy for malignant condition

Use additional code to identify:
   acquired absence of uterus (V88.01-88.03)
   personal history of malignant neoplasm (V10.40-V10.44)

Excludes: vaginal pap smear status-post hysterectomy for non-malignant condition (V76.47)

V67.09 Following other surgery

Excludes: sperm count following sterilization reversal (V26.22)
   sperm count for fertility testing (V26.21)

V67.1 Following radiotherapy

V67.2 Following chemotherapy
Cancer chemotherapy follow-up

● Code new
to 2012 edition   ▲ Revision of
existing code   ④ ⑤ Fourth or fifth
digit required

V67.3　**Following psychotherapy and other treatment for mental disorder**

V67.4　**Following treatment of healed fracture**

　　Excludes: *current (healing) fracture aftercare (V54.0-V54.9)*

⑤　V67.5　**Following other treatment**

　　　　V67.51　**Following completed treatment with high-risk medication, NEC**

　　Excludes: *long-term (current) drug use (V58.61-V58.69)*

　　　　V67.59　**Other**

V67.6　**Following combined treatment**

V67.9　**Unspecified follow-up examination**

V68　**Encounters for administrative purposes**

⑤　**V68.0**　**Issue of medical certificates**

　　Excludes: *encounter for general medical examination (V70.0-V70.9)*

　　　　V68.01　**Disability examination**

　　Use additional code(s) to identify:
　　　　specific examination(s), screening and testing performed (V72.0-V82.9)

　　　　V68.09　**Other issue of medical certificates**

V68.1　**Issue of repeat prescriptions**

　　Issue of repeat prescription for:
　　　　appliance
　　　　glasses
　　　　medications

　　Excludes: *repeat prescription for contraceptives (V25.41-V25.49)*

V68.2　**Request for expert evidence**

⑤　**V68.8**　**Other specified administrative purpose**

　　　　V68.81　**Referral of patient without examination or treatment**

　　　　V68.89　**Other**

V68.9　**Unspecified administrative purpose**

V69　**Problems related to lifestyle**

V69.0　**Lack of physical exercise**

V69.1　**Inappropriate diet and eating habits**

　　Excludes: *anorexia nervosa (307.1)*
　　　　bulimia (783.6)
　　　　malnutrition and other nutritional deficiencies (260-269.9)
　　　　other and unspecified eating disorders (307.50-307.59)

V69.2　**High-risk sexual behavior**

V69.3　**Gambling and betting**

　　Excludes: *pathological gambling (312.31)*

V69.4　**Lack of adequate sleep**

　　Sleep deprivation

　　Excludes: *insomnia (780.52)*

V69.5　**Behavioral insomnia of childhood**

V69.8　**Other problems related to lifestyle**

　　Self-damaging behavior

　　ALERT! Use this code as a secondary code if an asymptomatic patient is in a known high risk group for HIV

V69.9　**Problem related to lifestyle, unspecified**

PERSONS WITHOUT REPORTED DIAGNOSIS ENCOUNTERED DURING EXAMINATION AND INVESTIGATION OF INDIVIDUALS AND POPULATIONS (V70-V82)

　　Note: Nonspecific abnormal findings disclosed at the time of these examinations are classifiable to categories 790-796.

V70　**General medical examination**

　　Use additional code(s) to identify any special screening examination(s) performed (V73.0-V82.9)

| ■ | Add 4th or 5th digit | ■ | Nonspecific code | ■ | Unspecific code | ■ | Secondary Dx Only | ■ | Primary Dx Only |

V70.0 Routine general medical examination at a health care facility
Health checkup

[Excludes:] *health checkup of infant or child over 28 days old (V20.2)*
health supervision of newborn 8 to 28 days old (V20.32)
health supervision of newborn under 8 days old (V20.31)
pre-procedural general physical examination (V72.83)

V70.1 General psychiatric examination, requested by the authority

V70.2 General psychiatric examination, other and unspecified

V70.3 Other medical examination for administrative purposes
General medical examination for:
admission to old age home
adoption
camp
driving license
immigration and naturalization
insurance certification
marriage
prison
school admission
sports competition

[Excludes:] *attendance for issue of medical certificates (V68.0)*
pre-employment screening (V70.5)

V70.4 Examination for medicolegal reasons
Blood-alcohol tests
Blood-drug tests
Paternity testing

[Excludes:] *examination and observation following:*
accidents (V71.3, V71.4)
assault (V71.6)
rape (V71.5)

V70.5 Health examination of defined subpopulations
Armed forces personnel
Inhabitants of institutions
Occupational health examinations
Pre-employment screening
Preschool children
Prisoners
Prostitutes
Refugees
School children
Students

V70.6 Health examination in population surveys
[Excludes:] *special screening (V73.0-V82.9)*

V70.7 Examination of participant in clinical trial
Examination of participant or control in clinical research

V70.8 Other specified general medical examinations
Examination of potential donor of organ or tissue

V70.9 Unspecified general medical examination

V71 Observation and evaluation for suspected conditions not found
Note: This category is to be used when persons without a diagnosis are suspected of having an abnormal condition, without signs or symptoms, which requires study, but after examination and observation, is found not to exist. This category is also for use for administrative and legal observation status.

[Excludes:] *suspected maternal and fetal conditions not found (V89.01-V89.09)*

[5] **V71.0 Observation for suspected mental condition**

V71.01 Adult antisocial behavior
Dyssocial behavior or gang activity in adult without manifest psychiatric disorder

V71.02 Childhood or adolescent antisocial behavior
Dyssocial behavior or gang activity in child or adolescent without manifest psychiatric disorder

V71.09 Other suspected mental condition

V71.1 Observation for suspected malignant neoplasm

V71.2 Observation for suspected tuberculosis

V71.3 Observation following accident at work

V71.4 Observation following other accident
Examination of individual involved in motor vehicle traffic accident

V71.5 Observation following alleged rape or seduction
Examination of victim or culprit

V71.6 Observation following other inflicted injury
Examination of victim or culprit

V71.7 Observation for suspected cardiovascular disease

[5] **V71.8 Observation and evaluation for other specified suspected conditions**
[Excludes:] *contact with and (suspected) exposure to (potentially) hazardous substances (V15.84-V15.86, V87.0- V87.31)*

V71.81 Abuse and neglect
[Excludes:] *adult abuse and neglect (995.80-995.85)*
child abuse and neglect (995.50-995.59)

V71.82 Observation and evaluation for suspected exposure to anthrax

V71.83 Observation and evaluation for suspected exposure to other biological agent

V71.89 Other specified suspected conditions

V71.9 Observation for unspecified suspected condition

V72 Special investigations and examinations
Includes: routine examination of specific system
[Excludes:] *general medical examination (V70.0-V70.4)*
general screening examination of defined population groups (V70.5, V70.6, V70.7)
health supervision of newborn 8 to 28 days old (V20.32)
health supervision of newborn under 8 days old (V20.31)
routine examination of infant or child over 28 days old (V20.2)
Use additional code(s) to identify any special screening examination(s) performed (V73.0-V82.9)

V72.0 Examination of eyes and vision

[5] **V72.1 Examination of ears and hearing**

V72.11 Encounter for hearing examination following failed hearing screening

V72.12 Encounter for hearing conservation and treatment

V72.19 Other examination of ears and hearing

V72.2 Dental examination

[5] **V72.3 Gynecological examination**
[Excludes:] *cervical Papanicolaou smear without general gynecological examination (V76.2)*
routine examination in contraceptive management (V25.40-V25.49)

V72.31 Routine gynecological examination
General gynecological examination with or without Papanicolaou cervical smear
Pelvic examination (annual) (periodic)
Use additional code to identify routine:
human papillomavirus (HPV) screening (V73.81)
routine vaginal Papanicolaou smear (V76.47)

V72.32 Encounter for Papanicolaou cervical smear to confirm findings of recent normal smear following initial abnormal smear

[5] **V72.4 Pregnancy examination or test**

V72.40 Pregnancy examination or test, pregnancy unconfirmed
Possible pregnancy, not (yet) confirmed

V72.41 Pregnancy examination or test, negative result

V72.42 Pregnancy examination or test, positive result

V72.5 Radiological examination, not elsewhere classified
Routine chest x-ray
[Excludes:] *radiologic examinations as part of pre-procedural testing (V72.81-V72.84)*

[5] **V72.6 Laboratory examination**
Encounters for blood and urine testing

V72.60 Laboratory examination, unspecified

V72.61 Antibody response examination
Immunity status testing
[Excludes:] *encounter for allergy testing (V72.7)*

V72.62 Laboratory examination ordered as part of a routine general medical examination
Blood tests for routine general physical examination

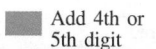

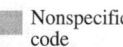

V72.63 Pre-procedural laboratory examination
Blood tests prior to treatment or procedure
Pre-operative laboratory examination

V72.69 Other laboratory examination

V72.7 Diagnostic skin and sensitization tests
Allergy tests
Skin tests for hypersensitivity

Excludes: *diagnostic skin tests for bacterial diseases (V74.0-V74.9)*

⑤ **V72.8 Other specified examinations**

Excludes: *pre-procedural laboratory examinations (V72.63)*

V72.81 Pre-operative cardiovascular examination
Pre-procedural cardiovascular examination

V72.82 Pre-operative respiratory examination
Pre-procedural respiratory examination

V72.83 Other specified pre-operative examination
Examination prior to chemotherapy
Other pre-procedural examination
Pre-procedural general physical examination

Excludes: *routine general medical examination (V70.0)*

V72.84 Pre-operative examination, unspecified
Pre-procedural examination, unspecified

V72.85 Other specified examination

V72.86 Encounter for blood typing

V72.9 Unspecified examination

V73 Special screening examination for viral and chlamydial diseases
DEFINITION Chlamydia is a type of bacteria one species of which causes an infection very similar to gonorrhea in the way that it is spread, the symptoms it produces, and the long-term consequences.

V73.0 Poliomyelitis

V73.1 Smallpox

V73.2 Measles

V73.3 Rubella

V73.4 Yellow fever

V73.5 Other arthropod-borne viral diseases
Dengue fever   Viral encephalitis:
Hemorrhagic fever   mosquito-borne
                                    tick-borne

V73.6 Trachoma

⑤ **V73.8 Other specified viral and chlamydial diseases**

V73.81 Human papillomavirus (HPV)

V73.88 Other specified chlamydial diseases

V73.89 Other specified viral diseases
ALERT! Use this code if a patient is being seen to determine his or her HIV status

⑤ **V73.9 Unspecified viral and chlamydial disease**

V73.98 Unspecified chlamydial disease

V73.99 Unspecified viral disease

V74 Special screening examination for bacterial and spirochetal diseases
Includes: diagnostic skin tests for these diseases

V74.0 Cholera

V74.1 Pulmonary tuberculosis

V74.2 Leprosy [Hansen's disease]

V74.3 Diphtheria

V74.4 Bacterial conjunctivitis

● Code new
to 2012 edition
▲ Revision of
existing code
④ ⑤ Fourth or fifth
digit required

V74.5 Venereal disease
Screening for bacterial and spirochetal sexually transmitted diseases
Screening for sexually transmitted diseases NOS

[Excludes:] *special screening for nonbacterial sexually transmitted diseases (V73.81-V73.89, V75.4, V75.8)*

V74.6 Yaws

V74.8 Other specified bacterial and spirochetal diseases
Brucellosis
Leptospirosis
Plague
Tetanus
Whooping cough

V74.9 Unspecified bacterial and spirochetal disease

V75 Special screening examination for other infectious diseases

V75.0 Rickettsial diseases

V75.1 Malaria

V75.2 Leishmaniasis

V75.3 Trypanosomiasis
Chagas' disease
Sleeping sickness

V75.4 Mycotic infections

V75.5 Schistosomiasis

V75.6 Filariasis

V75.7 Intestinal helminthiasis

V75.8 Other specified parasitic infections

V75.9 Unspecified infectious disease

V76 Special screening for malignant neoplasms

V76.0 Respiratory organs

[5] **V76.1 Breast**

V76.10 Breast screening, unspecified

V76.11 Screening mammogram for high-risk patient

V76.12 Other screening mammogram

V76.19 Other screening breast examination

V76.2 Cervix
Routine cervical Papanicolaou smear

[Excludes:] *special screening for human papillomavirus (V73.81)*
that as part of a general gynecological examination (V72.31)

V76.3 Bladder

[5] **V76.4 Other sites**

V76.41 Rectum

V76.42 Oral cavity

V76.43 Skin

V76.44 Prostate

V76.45 Testis

V76.46 Ovary

V76.47 Vagina
Vaginal pap smear status-post hysterectomy for non-malignant condition

Use additional code to identify acquired absence of uterus (V88.01-V88.03)

[Excludes:] *vaginal pap smear status-post hysterectomy for malignant condition (V67.01)*

V76.49 Other sites

[5] **V76.5 Intestine**

V76.50 Intestine, unspecified

V76.51 Colon
Screening colonoscopy NOS

[Excludes:] *rectum (V76.41)*

V76.52 Small intestine

[5] **V76.8 Other neoplasm**

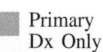

Add 4th or 5th digit | Nonspecific code | Unspecific code | Secondary Dx Only | Primary Dx Only

V76.81 Nervous system

V76.89 Other neoplasm

V76.9 Unspecified

V77 Special screening for endocrine, nutritional, metabolic, and immunity disorders

V77.0 Thyroid disorders

V77.1 Diabetes mellitus

V77.2 Malnutrition

V77.3 Phenylketonuria [PKU]

V77.4 Galactosemia

V77.5 Gout

V77.6 Cystic fibrosis
> Screening for mucoviscidosis

V77.7 Other inborn errors of metabolism

V77.8 Obesity

⑤ V77.9 Other and unspecified endocrine, nutritional, metabolic, and immunity disorders

V77.91 Screening for lipoid disorders
> Screening cholesterol level
> Screening for hypercholesterolemia
> Screening for hyperlipidemia

V77.99 Other and unspecified endocrine, nutritional, metabolic, and immunity disorders

V78 Special screening for disorders of blood and blood-forming organs

V78.0 Iron deficiency anemia

V78.1 Other and unspecified deficiency anemia

V78.2 Sickle-cell disease or trait

V78.3 Other hemoglobinopathies

V78.8 Other disorders of blood and blood-forming organs

V78.9 Unspecified disorder of blood and blood-forming organs

V79 Special screening for mental disorders and developmental handicaps

V79.0 Depression

V79.1 Alcoholism

▲ V79.2 Intellectual disabilities

V79.3 Developmental handicaps in early childhood

V79.8 Other specified mental disorders and developmental handicaps

V79.9 Unspecified mental disorder and developmental handicap

V80 Special screening for neurological, eye, and ear diseases

⑤ V80.0 Neurological conditions

V80.01 Traumatic brain injury

V80.09 Other neurological conditions

V80.1 Glaucoma

V80.2 Other eye conditions
> Screening for:
>   cataract
>   congenital anomaly of eye
>   senile macular lesions

Excludes: general vision examination (V72.0)

V80.3 Ear diseases

Excludes: general hearing examination (V72.11-V72.19)

V81 Special screening for cardiovascular, respiratory, and genitourinary diseases

V81.0 Ischemic heart disease

V81.1 Hypertension

V81.2 Other and unspecified cardiovascular conditions

V81.3 Chronic bronchitis and emphysema

● Code new
to 2012 edition
▲ Revision of
existing code
④ ⑤ Fourth or fifth
digit required

V81.4 Other and unspecified respiratory conditions
[Excludes:] *screening for:*
lung neoplasm (V76.0)
pulmonary tuberculosis (V74.1)

V81.5 Nephropathy
Screening for asymptomatic bacteriuria

V81.6 Other and unspecified genitourinary conditions

V82 Special screening for other conditions

V82.0 Skin conditions

V82.1 Rheumatoid arthritis

V82.2 Other rheumatic disorders

V82.3 Congenital dislocation of hip

V82.4 Maternal postnatal screening for chromosomal anomalies
[Excludes:] *antenatal screening by amniocentesis (V28.0)*

V82.5 Chemical poisoning and other contamination
Screening for:
heavy metal poisoning
ingestion of radioactive substance
poisoning from contaminated water supply
radiation exposure

V82.6 Multiphasic screening

[5] **V82.7 Genetic screening**
[Excludes:] *genetic testing for procreative management (V26.31-V26.39)*

V82.71 Screening for genetic disease carrier status

V82.79 Other genetic screening

[5] **V82.8 Other specified conditions**

V82.81 Osteoporosis
Use additional code to identify:
hormone replacement therapy (postmenopausal) status (V07.4)
postmenopausal (natural) status (V49.81)

V82.89 Other specified conditions

V82.9 Unspecified condition

GENETICS (V83-V84)

V83 Genetic carrier status

[DEFINITION] A genetic carrier is a person who has inherited a genetic trait or mutation, but who does not display that trait or show symptoms of the disease. They are able to pass the gene to their offspring, who may then express the gene.

[5] **V83.0 Hemophilia A carrier**

V83.01 Asymptomatic hemophilia A carrier

V83.02 Symptomatic hemophilia A carrier

[5] **V83.8 Other genetic carrier status**

V83.81 Cystic fibrosis gene carrier

V83.89 Other genetic carrier status

V84 Genetic susceptibility to disease
Includes: Confirmed abnormal gene
[Excludes:] *chromosomal anomalies (758.0-758.9)*
Use additional code, if applicable, for any associated family history of the disease (V16-V19)

[ALERT!] Codes from category V84 should not be used as principal or first listed codes. If the patient has the condition to which he or she is susceptible, and that condition is the reason for the encounter, the code for the current condition should be sequenced first.

[5] **V84.0 Genetic susceptibility to malignant neoplasm**
Code first, if applicable, any current malignant neoplasms (140.0-195.8, 200.0-208.9, 230.0-234.9)
Use additional code, if applicable, for any personal history of malignant neoplasm (V10.0-V10.9)

V84.01 Genetic susceptibility to malignant neoplasm of breast

V84.02 Genetic susceptibility to malignant neoplasm of ovary

V84.03 Genetic susceptibility to malignant neoplasm of prostate

V84.04 **Genetic susceptibility to malignant neoplasm of endometrium**

V84.09 **Genetic susceptibility to other malignant neoplasm**

⑤ **V84.8 Genetic susceptibility to other disease**

V84.81 **Genetic susceptibility to multiple endocrine neoplasia [MEN]**

[Excludes:] *multiple endocrine neoplasia [MEN] syndromes (258.01-258.03)*

V84.89 **Genetic susceptibility to other disease**

BODY MASS INDEX (V85)

V85 **Body Mass Index [BMI]**

Kilograms per meters squared

Note: BMI adult codes are for use for persons over 20 years old

[DEFINITION] Body mass index (BMI) is a measurement of the relative percentages of fat and muscle mass in the human body

V85.0 **Body Mass Index less than 19, adult**

V85.1 **Body Mass Index between 19-24, adult**

⑤ **V85.2 Body Mass Index between 25-29, adult**

V85.21 **Body Mass Index 25.0-25.9, adult**

V85.22 **Body Mass Index 26.0-26.9, adult**

V85.23 **Body Mass Index 27.0-27.9, adult**

V85.24 **Body Mass Index 28.0-28.9, adult**

V85.25 **Body Mass Index 29.0-29.9, adult**

⑤ **V85.3 Body Mass Index between 30-39, adult**

V85.30 **Body Mass Index 30.0-30.9, adult**

V85.31 **Body Mass Index 31.0-31.9, adult**

V85.32 **Body Mass Index 32.0-32.9, adult**

V85.33 **Body Mass Index 33.0-33.9, adult**

V85.34 **Body Mass Index 34.0-34.9, adult**

V85.35 **Body Mass Index 35.0-35.9, adult**

V85.36 **Body Mass Index 36.0-36.9, adult**

V85.37 **Body Mass Index 37.0-37.9, adult**

V85.38 **Body Mass Index 38.0-38.9, adult**

V85.39 **Body Mass Index 39.0-39.9, adult**

⑤ **V85.4 Body Mass Index 40 and over, adult**

V85.41 **Body Mass Index 40.0-44.9, adult**

V85.42 **Body Mass Index 45.0-49.9, adult**

V85.43 **Body Mass Index 50.0-59.9, adult**

V85.44 **Body Mass Index 60.0-69.9, adult**

V85.45 **Body Mass Index 70 and over, adult**

⑤ **V85.5 Body Mass Index, pediatric**

Note:BMI pediatric codes are for use for persons age 2-20 years old. These percentiles are based on the growth charts published by the Centers for Disease Control and Prevention (CDC)

V85.51 **Body Mass Index, pediatric, less than 5th percentile for age**

V85.52 **Body Mass Index, pediatric, 5th percentile to less than 85th percentile for age**

V85.53 **Body Mass Index, pediatric, 85th percentile to less than 95th percentile for age**

V85.54 **Body Mass Index, pediatric, greater than or equal to 95th percentile for age**

ESTROGEN RECEPTOR STATUS (V86)

V86 **Estrogen receptor status**

Code first malignant neoplasm of breast (174.0-174.9, 175.0-175.9)

V86.0 **Estrogen receptor positive status (ER+)**

V86.1 **Estrogen receptor negative status (ER–)**

● Code new to 2012 edition ▲ Revision of existing code ④ ⑤ Fourth or fifth digit required

OTHER SPECIFIED PERSONAL EXPOSURES AND HISTORY PRESENTING HAZARDS TO HEALTH (V87)

V87 Other specified personal exposures and history presenting hazards to health

⑤ **V87.0** Contact with and (suspected) exposure to hazardous metals

Excludes: exposure to lead (V15.86)
toxic effect of metals (984.0-985.9)

V87.01 Arsenic

● **V87.02** Contact with and (suspected) exposure to uranium

Excludes: retained depleted uranium fragments (V90.01)

V87.09 Other hazardous metals
Chromium compounds
Nickel dust

⑤ **V87.1** Contact with and (suspected) exposure to hazardous aromatic compounds

Excludes: toxic effects of aromatic compounds (982.0, 983.0)

V87.11 Aromatic amines

V87.12 Benzene

V87.19 Other hazardous aromatic compounds
Aromatic dyes NOS
Polycyclic aromatic hydrocarbons

V87.2 Contact with and (suspected) exposure to other potentially hazardous chemicals
Dyes NOS

Excludes: exposure to asbestos (V15.84)
toxic effect of chemicals (980-989)

⑤ **V87.3** Contact with and (suspected) exposure to other potentially hazardous substances

Excludes: contact with and (suspected) exposure to potentially hazardous body fluids
(V15.85)
personal history of retained foreign body fully removed (V15.53)
toxic effect of substances (980-989)

V87.31 Exposure to mold

V87.32 Contact with and (suspected) exposure to algae bloom

V87.39 Contact with and (suspected) exposure to other potentially hazardous
substances

⑤ **V87.4** Personal history of drug therapy

Excludes: long-term (current) drug use (V58.61-V58.69)

V87.41 Personal history of antineoplastic chemotherapy

V87.42 Personal history of monoclonal drug therapy

V87.43 Personal history of estrogen therapy

V87.44 Personal history of inhaled steroid therapy

V87.45 Personal history of systemic steroid therapy
Personal history of steroid therapy NOS

V87.46 Personal history of immunosuppression therapy

Excludes: personal history of steroid therapy (V87.44, V87.45)

V87.49 Personal history of other drug therapy

ACQUIRED ABSENCE OF OTHER ORGANS AND TISSUE (V88)

⑤ **V88** Acquired absence of other organs and tissue

⑤ **V88.0** Acquired absence of cervix and uterus

V88.01 Acquired absence of both cervix and uterus
Acquired absence of uterus NOS
Status post total hysterectomy

V88.02 Acquired absence of uterus with remaining cervical stump
Status post partial hysterectomy with remaining cervical stump

V88.03 Acquired absence of cervix with remaining uterus

⑤ **V88.1** Acquired absence of pancreas
Use additional code to identify any associated:
insulin use (V58.67)
secondary diabetes mellitus (249.00-249.91)

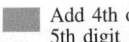

| | Add 4th or | | Nonspecific | | Unspecific | | Secondary | | Primary |
| | 5th digit | | code | | code | | Dx Only | | Dx Only |

V88.11 **Acquired total absence of pancreas**
Acquired absence of pancreas NOS

V88.12 **Acquired partial absence of pancreas**

● **V88.2** **Acquired absence of joint**
Acquired absence of joint following prior explantation of joint prosthesis
Joint prosthesis explantation status

● **V88.21** **Acquired absence of hip joint**
Acquired absence of hip joint following explantation of joint prosthesis, with
or without presence of antibiotic-impregnated cement spacer

● **V88.22** **Acquired absence of knee joint**
Acquired absence of knee joint following explantation of joint prosthesis, with
or without presence of antibiotic-impregnated cement spacer

● **V88.29** **Acquired absence of other joint**
Acquired absence of other joint following explantation of joint prosthesis, with
or without presence of antibiotic-impregnated cement spacer

OTHER SUSPECTED CONDITIONS NOT FOUND (V89)

⑤ **V89** **Other suspected conditions not found**

⑤ **V89.0** **Suspected maternal and fetal conditions not found**

Excludes: *known or suspected fetal anomalies affecting management of mother, not ruled out*
(655.00, 655.93, 656.00-656.93, 657.00-657.03, 658.00-658.93)
newborn and perinatal conditions - code to condition

V89.01 **Suspected problem with amniotic cavity and membrane not found**
Suspected oligohydramnios not found
Suspected polyhydramnios not found

V89.02 **Suspected placental problem not found**

V89.03 **Suspected fetal anomaly not found**

V89.04 **Suspected problem with fetal growth not found**

V89.05 **Suspected cervical shortening not found**

V89.09 **Other suspected maternal and fetal condition not found**

RETAINED FOREIGN BODY (V90)

V90 **Retained foreign body**
Embedded fragment (status)
Embedded splinter (status)
Retained foreign body status

Excludes: *artificial joint prosthesis status (V43.60-V43.69)*
foreign body accidentally left during a procedure (998.4)
foreign body entering through orifice (930.0-939.9)
in situ cardiac devices (V45.00-V45.09)
organ or tissue replaced by other means (V43.0-V43.89)
organ or tissue replaced by transplant (V42.0-V42.9)
personal history of retained foreign body removed (V15.53)
superficial foreign body (splinter) (categories 910-917 and 919 with 4th character
6 or 7, 918.0)

⑤ **V90.0** **Retained radioactive fragment**

V90.01 **Retained depleted uranium fragments**

V90.09 **Other retained radioactive fragments**
Other retained depleted isotope fragments
Retained nontherapeutic radioactive fragments

⑤ **V90.1** **Retained metal fragments**

Excludes: *retained radioactive metal fragments (V90.01-V90.09)*

V90.10 **Retained metal fragments, unspecified**
Retained metal fragment NOS

V90.11 **Retained magnetic metal fragments**

V90.12 **Retained nonmagnetic metal fragments**

V90.2 **Retained plastic fragments**
Acrylics fragments
Diethylhexylphthalates fragments
Isocyanate fragments

⑤ **V90.3** **Retained organic fragments**

V90.31 **Retained animal quills or spines**

● Code new
to 2012 edition
▲ Revision of
existing code
④ ⑤ Fourth or fifth
digit required

V90.32 **Retained tooth**

V90.33 **Retained wood fragments**

V90.39 **Other retained organic fragments**

⑤ **V90.8 Other specified retained foreign body**

V90.81 **Retained glass fragments**

V90.83 **Retained stone or crystalline fragments**
Retained concrete or cement fragments

V90.89 **Other specified retained foreign body**

V90.9 **Retained foreign body, unspecified material**

MULTIPLE GESTATION PLACENTA STATUS (V91)

V91 Multiple gestation placenta status

Code first multiple gestation (651.0-651.9)

DEFINITION Multiple gestation refers to more than one fetus being carried to term in a single pregnancy.

⑤ **V91.0 Twin gestation placenta status**

V91.00 **Twin gestation, unspecified number of placenta, unspecified number of amniotic sacs**

V91.01 **Twin gestation, monochorionic/monoamniotic (one placenta, one amniotic sac)**

V91.02 **Twin gestation, monochorionic/diamniotic (one placenta, two amniotic sacs)**

V91.03 **Twin gestation, dichorionic/diamniotic (two placentae, two amniotic sacs)**

V91.09 **Twin gestation, unable to determine number of placenta and number of amniotic sacs**

⑤ **V91.1 Triplet gestation placenta status**

V91.10 **Triplet gestation, unspecified number of placenta and unspecified number of amniotic sacs**

V91.11 **Triplet gestation, with two or more monochorionic fetuses**

V91.12 **Triplet gestation, with two or more monoamniotic fetuses**

V91.19 **Triplet gestation, unable to determine number of placenta and number of amniotic sacs**

⑤ **V91.2 Quadruplet gestation placenta status**

V91.20 **Quadruplet gestation, unspecified number of placenta and unspecified number of amniotic sacs**

V91.21 **Quadruplet gestation, with two or more monochorionic fetuses**

V91.22 **Quadruplet gestation, with two or more monoamniotic fetuses**

V91.29 **Quadruplet gestation, unable to determine number of placenta and number of amniotic sacs**

⑤ **V91.9 Other specified multiple gestation placenta status**
Placenta status for multiple gestations greater than quadruplets

V91.90 **Other specified multiple gestation, unspecified number of placenta and unspecified number of amniotic sacs**

V91.91 **Other specified multiple gestation, with two or more monochorionic fetuses**

V91.92 **Other specified multiple gestation, with two or more monoamniotic fetuses**

V91.99 **Other specified multiple gestation, unable to determine number of placenta and number of amniotic sacs**

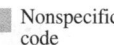 Add 4th or 5th digit   Nonspecific code   Unspecific code   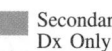 Secondary Dx Only   Primary Dx Only

This page intentionally left blank.

● Code new
to 2012 edition

▲ Revision of
existing code

④ ⑤ Fourth or fifth
digit required

Chapter 19: Supplemental Classification of External Causes of Injury and Poisoning (E-codes, E800-E999)

DEFINITIONS AND CODING ALERTS

This chapter includes definitions of selected key words, terms and phrases and coding alerts for adding points to the clinical domain, references to coding late effects where appropriate, and references to personal history V-codes in situations where the acute or chronic condition is no longer active. An example from this chapter is as follows:

ACCIDENTAL FALLS (E880-E888)

> **ALERT!** For coding late effects of accidental fall see E929.3
> **ALERT!** For personal history of fall see V15.88

MULTIPLE CODING FOR A SINGLE CONDITION

In addition to the etiology or manifestation convention that requires two codes to fully describe a single condition that affects multiple body systems, there are other single conditions that also require more than one code. "Use additional code" notes are found in the tabular at codes that are not part of an etiology or manifestation pair where a secondary code is useful to fully describe a condition. The sequencing rule is the same as the etiology or manifestation pair - , "use additional code" indicates that a secondary code should be added.

"Code first" notes are also under certain codes that are not specifically manifestation codes but may be due to an underlying cause. When a "code first" note is present and an underlying condition is present the underlying condition should be sequenced first.

"Code, if applicable, any causal condition first", notes indicate that this code may be assigned as a principal diagnosis when the causal condition is unknown or not applicable. If a causal condition is known, then the code for that condition should be sequenced as the principal or first-listed diagnosis. Multiple codes may be needed for late effects, complication codes and obstetric codes to more fully describe a condition. See the specific guidelines for these conditions for further instruction.

COMBINATION CODE

A combination code is a single code used to classify: two diagnoses, or a diagnosis with an associated secondary process (manifestation) A diagnosis with an associated complication Combination codes are identified by referring to subterm entries in the Alphabetic Index and by reading the inclusion and exclusion notes in the Tabular List.

Assign only the combination code when that code fully identifies the diagnostic conditions involved or when the Alphabetic Index so directs. Multiple coding should not be used when the classification provides a combination code that clearly identifies all of the elements documented in the diagnosis. When the combination code lacks necessary specificity in describing the manifestation or complication, an additional code should be used as a secondary code.

CODING LATE EFFECTS

A late effect is the residual effect (condition produced) after the acute phase of an illness or injury has terminated. There is no time limit on when a late effect code can be used. The residual may be apparent early, such as in cerebrovascular accident cases, or it may occur months or years later, such as that due to a previous injury. Coding of late effects generally requires two codes sequenced in the following order: The condition or nature of the late effect is sequenced first. The late effect code is sequenced second.

An exception to the above guidelines are those instances where the code for late effect is followed by a manifestation code identified in the Tabular List and title, or the late effect code has been expanded (at the fourth and fifth-digit levels) to include the manifestation(s). The code for the acute phase of an illness or injury that led to the late effect is never used with a code for the late effect.

| | Add 4th or 5th digit | | Nonspecific code | | Unspecified code | | Manifestation code |

INTRODUCTION

These guidelines are provided for those who are currently collecting E codes in order that there will be standardization in the process. If your institution plans to begin collecting E codes, these guidelines are to be applied. The use of E codes is supplemental to the application of ICD-9-CM diagnosis codes. E codes are never to be recorded as principal diagnoses (first-listed in non-inpatient setting) and are not required for reporting to CMS.

External causes of injury and poisoning codes (E codes) are intended to provide data for injury research and evaluation of injury prevention strategies. E codes capture how the injury or poisoning happened (cause), the intent (unintentional or accidental; or intentional, such as suicide or assault), and the place where the event occurred.

Some major categories of E codes include:

transport accidents poisoning and adverse effects of drugs, medicinal substances and biologicals accidental falls accidents caused by fire and flames accidents due to natural and environmental factors late effects of accidents, assaults or self injury assaults or purposely inflicted injury suicide or self inflicted injury

These guidelines apply for the coding and collection of E codes from records in hospitals, outpatient clinics, emergency departments, other ambulatory care settings and provider offices, and nonacute care settings, except when other specific guidelines apply.

GENERAL E CODE CODING GUIDELINES

An E code may be used with any code in the range of 001-V84.8, which indicates an injury, poisoning, or adverse effect due to an external cause.

Assign the appropriate E code for the initial encounter of an injury, poisoning, or adverse effect of drugs, not for subsequent treatment. External cause of injury codes (E-codes) may be assigned while the acute fracture codes are still applicable.

See Official Guidelines, Section I.C.17.b.1 for coding of acute fractures.

Use the full range of E codes to completely describe the cause, the intent and the place of occurrence, if applicable, for all injuries, poisonings, and adverse effects of drugs.

Assign as many E codes as necessary to fully explain each cause. If only one E code can be recorded, assign the E code most related to the principal diagnosis.

The selection of the appropriate E code is guided by the Index to External Causes, which is located after the alphabetical index to diseases and by Inclusion and Exclusion notes in the Tabular List.

An E code can never be a principal (first listed) diagnosis.

An external cause code is not appropriate with a code from subcategory 995.9, unless the patient also has an injury, poisoning, or adverse effect of drugs.

PLACE OF OCCURRENCE GUIDELINE

Use an additional code from category E849 to indicate the Place of Occurrence for injuries and poisonings. The Place of Occurrence describes the place where the event occurred and not the patient's activity at the time of the event.

Do not use E849.9 if the place of occurrence is not stated.

ADVERSE EFFECTS OF DRUGS, MEDICINAL AND BIOLOGICAL SUBSTANCES GUIDELINES

Do not code directly from the Table of Drugs and Chemicals. Always refer back to the Tabular List.

Use as many codes as necessary to describe completely all drugs, medicinal or biological substances.

If the same E code would describe the causative agent for more than one adverse reaction, assign the code only once.

If two or more drugs, medicinal or biological substances are reported, code each individually unless the combination code is listed in the Table of Drugs and Chemicals. In that case, assign the E code for the combination.

● Code new to 2012 edition　　▲ Revision of existing code　　④ ⑤ Fourth or fifth digit required

When a reaction results from the interaction of a drug(s) and alcohol, use poisoning codes and E codes for both.

If the reporting format limits the number of E codes that can be used in reporting clinical data, code the one most related to the principal diagnosis. Include at least one from each category (cause, intent, place) if possible.

If there are different fourth digit codes in the same three digit category, use the code for "Other specified" of that category. If there is no "Other specified" code in that category, use the appropriate "Unspecified" code in that category.

If the codes are in different three digit categories, assign the appropriate E code for other multiple drugs and medicinal substances.

Codes from the E930-E949 series must be used to identify the causative substance for an adverse effect of drug, medicinal and biological substances, correctly prescribed and properly administered. The effect, such as tachycardia, delirium, gastrointestinal hemorrhaging, vomiting, hypokalemia, hepatitis, renal failure, or respiratory failure, is coded and followed by the appropriate code from the E930-E949 series.

MULTIPLE CAUSE E CODE CODING GUIDELINES

If two or more events cause separate injuries, an E code should be assigned for each cause. The first listed E code will be selected in the following order:

1. E codes for child and adult abuse take priority over all other E codes.

2. E codes for terrorism events take priority over all other E codes except child and adult abuse

3. E codes for cataclysmic events take priority over all other E codes except child and adult abuse and terrorism.

4. E codes for transport accidents take priority over all other E codes except cataclysmic events and child and adult abuse and terrorism.

5. The first-listed E code should correspond to the cause of the most serious diagnosis due to an assault, accident, or self-harm, following the order of hierarchy listed above.

CHILD AND ADULT ABUSE GUIDELINE

Intentional injury

When the cause of an injury or neglect is intentional child or adult abuse, the first listed E code should be assigned from categories E960-E968, Homicide and injury purposely inflicted by other persons, (except category E967.. An E code from category E967, Child and adult battering and other maltreatment, should be added as an additional code to identify the perpetrator, if known.

Accidental intent

In cases of neglect when the intent is determined to be accidental E code E904.0, Abandonment or neglect of infant and helpless person, should be the first listed E code.

UNKNOWN OR SUSPECTED INTENT GUIDELINE

If the intent (accident, self-harm, assault) of the cause of an injury or poisoning is unknown or unspecified, code the intent as undetermined E980-E989.

If the intent (accident, self-harm, assault) of the cause of an injury or poisoning is questionable, probable or suspected, code the intent as undetermined E980-E989.

UNDETERMINED CAUSE

When the intent of an injury or poisoning is known, but the cause is unknown, use codes: E928.9, Unspecified accident, E958.9, Suicide and self-inflicted injury by unspecified means, and E968.9, Assault by unspecified means.

These E codes should rarely be used, as the documentation in the medical record, in both the inpatient outpatient and other settings, should normally provide sufficient detail to determine the cause of the injury.

| | Add 4th or 5th digit | | Nonspecific code | | Unspecified code | | Manifestation code |

LATE EFFECTS OF EXTERNAL CAUSE GUIDELINES

Late effect E codes exist for injuries and poisonings but not for adverse effects of drugs, misadventures and surgical complications.

A late effect E code (E929, E959, E969, E977, E989, or E999.1), should be used with any report of a late effect or sequela resulting from a previous injury or poisoning (905-909..

A late effect E code should never be used with a related current nature of injury code.

Use a late effect E code for subsequent visits when a late effect of the initial injury or poisoning is being treated. There is no late effect E code for adverse effects of drugs.
Do not use a late effect E code for subsequent visits for followup care (e.g., to assess healing, to receive rehabilitative therapy) of the injury or poisoning when no late effect of the injury has been documented.

MISADVENTURES AND COMPLICATIONS OF CARE GUIDELINES

Assign a code in the range of E870-E876 if misadventures are stated by the provider.

Assign a code in the range of E878-E879 if the provider attributes an abnormal reaction or later complication to a surgical or medical procedure, but does not mention misadventure at the time of the procedure as the cause of the reaction.

TERRORISM GUIDELINES

Cause of injury identified by the Federal Government (FBI) as terrorism

When the cause of an injury is identified by the Federal Government (FBI) as terrorism, the first-listed E-code should be a code from category E979, Terrorism. The definition of terrorism employed by the FBI is found at the inclusion note at E979. The terrorism E-code is the only E-code that should be assigned. Additional E codes from the assault categories should not be assigned.

Cause of an injury is suspected to be the result of terrorism

When the cause of an injury is suspected to be the result of terrorism a code from category E979 should not be assigned. Assign a code in the range of E codes based circumstances on the documentation of intent and mechanism.

Code E979.9, Terrorism, secondary effects

Assign code E979.9, Terrorism, secondary effects, for conditions occurring subsequent to the terrorist event. This code should not be assigned for conditions that are due to the initial terrorist act.

● Code new
to 2012 edition   ▲ Revision of
existing code   ④ ⑤ Fourth or fifth
digit required

SUPPLEMENTARY CLASSIFICATION OF EXTERNAL CAUSES OF INJURY AND POISONING (E000-E999)

This section is provided to permit the classification of environmental events, circumstances, and conditions as the cause of injury, poisoning, and other adverse effects. Where a code from this section is applicable, it is intended that it shall be used in addition to a code from one of the main chapters of *ICD-9-CM*, indicating the nature of the condition. Certain other conditions which may be stated to be due to external causes are classified in Chapters 1 to 16 of *ICD-9-CM*. For these, the "E" code classification should be used for more detailed analysis.

Machinery accidents [other than those connected with transport] are classifiable to category E919, in which the fourth-digit allows a broad classification of the type of machinery involved.

Categories for "late effects" of accidents and other external causes are to be found at E929, E959, E969, E977, E989, and E999.

EXTERNAL CAUSE STATUS (E000)

> Note: A code from category E000 should be used in conjunction with the external cause code(s) assigned to a record to indicate the status of the person at the time the event occurred. A single code from category E000 should be assigned for an encounter.

E000 **External cause status**

E000.0 **Civilian activity done for income or pay**
Civilian activity done for financial or other compensation

[Excludes:] *military activity (E000.1)*

E000.1 **Military activity**

[Excludes:] *activity of off duty military personnel (E000.8)*

E000.2 **Volunteer activity**

[Excludes:] *activity of child or other family member assisting in compensated work of other family member (E000.8)*

E000.8 **Other external cause status**
Activity NEC
Activity of child or other family member assisting in compensated work of other family member
Hobby not done for income
Leisure activity
Off-duty activity of military personnel
Recreation or sport not for income or while a student
Student activity

E000.9 **Unspecified external cause status**

ACTIVITY (E001-E030)

> Note: Categories E001 to E030 are provided for use to indicate the activity of the person seeking healthcare for an injury or health condition, such as a heart attack while shoveling snow, which resulted from, or was contributed to, by the activity. These codes are appropriate for use for both acute injuries, such as those from chapter 17, and conditions that are due to the long-term, cumulative effects of an activity, such as those from chapter 13. They are also appropriate for use with external cause codes for cause and intent if identifying the activity provides additional information on the event.

These codes should be used in conjunction with other external cause codes for external cause status (E000) and place of occurrence (E849).

This section contains the following broad activity categories:
E001 Activities involving walking and running
E002 Activities involving water and water craft
E003 Activities involving ice and snow
E004 Activities involving climbing, rappelling, and jumping off
E005 Activities involving dancing and other rhythmic movement
E006 Activities involving other sports and athletics played individually
E007 Activities involving other sports and athletics played as a team or group
E008 Activities involving other specified sports and athletics
E009 Activity involving other cardiorespiratory exercise
E010 Activity involving other muscle strengthening exercises
E011 Activities involving computer technology and electronic devices
E012 Activities involving arts and handcrafts
E013 Activities involving personal hygiene and household maintenance
E014 Activities involving person providing caregiving
E015 Activities involving food preparation, cooking and grilling

| ▨ | Add 4th or 5th digit | ▨ | Nonspecific code | ▨ | Unspecified code | ▨ | Manifestation code |

E016 Activities involving property and land maintenance, building and construction
E017 Activities involving roller coasters and other types of external motion
E018 Activities involving playing musical instrument
E019 Activities involving animal care
E029 Other activity
E030 Unspecified activity

E001 Activities involving walking and running
> *Excludes:* *walking an animal (E019.0)*
> *walking or running on a treadmill (E009.0)*

E001.0 Walking, marching and hiking
Walking, marching and hiking on level or elevated terrain
> *Excludes:* *mountain climbing (E004.0)*

E001.1 Running

E002 Activities involving water and water craft
> *Excludes:* *activities involving ice (E003.0-E003.9)*
> *boating and other watercraft transport accidents (E830-E838)*

E002.0 Swimming

E002.1 Springboard and platform diving

E002.2 Water polo

E002.3 Water aerobics and water exercise

E002.4 Underwater diving and snorkeling
SCUBA diving

E002.5 Rowing, canoeing, kayaking, rafting and tubing
Canoeing, kayaking, rafting and tubing in calm and turbulent water

E002.6 Water skiing and wake boarding

E002.7 Surfing, windsurfing and boogie boarding

E002.8 Water sliding

E002.9 Other activity involving water and watercraft
Activity involving water NOS
Parasailing
Water survival training and testing

E003 Activities involving ice and snow
> *Excludes:* *shoveling ice and snow (E016.0)*

E003.0 Ice skating
Figure skating (singles) (pairs)
Ice dancing
> *Excludes:* *ice hockey (E003.1)*

E003.1 Ice hockey

E003.2 Snow (alpine) (downhill) skiing, snow boarding, sledding, tobogganing and snow tubing
> *Excludes:* *cross country skiing (E003.3)*

E003.3 Cross country skiing
Nordic skiing

E003.9 Other activity involving ice and snow
Activity involving ice and snow NOS

E004 Activities involving climbing, rappelling and jumping off
> *Excludes:* *hiking on level or elevated terrain (E001.0)*
> *jumping rope (E006.5)*
> *sky diving (E840-E844)*
> *trampoline jumping (E005.3)*

E004.0 Mountain climbing, rock climbing and wall climbing

E004.1 Rappelling

E004.2 BASE jumping
Building, Antenna, Span, Earth jumping

E004.3 Bungee jumping

E004.4 Hang gliding

● Code new to 2012 edition ▲ Revision of existing code ④ ⑤ Fourth or fifth digit required

E004.9 Other activity involving climbing, rappelling and jumping off

E005 Activities involving dancing and other rhythmic movement

> *Excludes:* martial arts (E008.4)

E005.0 Dancing

E005.1 Yoga

E005.2 Gymnastics
Rhythmic gymnastics

> *Excludes:* trampoline (E005.3)

E005.3 Trampoline

E005.4 Cheerleading

E005.9 Other activity involving dancing and other rhythmic movements

E006 Activities involving other sports and athletics played individually

> *Excludes:* dancing (E005.0)
> gymnastic (E005.2)
> trampoline (E005.3)
> yoga (E005.1)

E006.0 Roller skating (inline) and skateboarding

E006.1 Horseback riding

E006.2 Golf

E006.3 Bowling

E006.4 Bike riding

> *Excludes:* transport accident involving bike riding (E800-E829)

E006.5 Jumping rope

E006.6 Non-running track and field events

> *Excludes:* running (any form) (E001.1)

E006.9 Other activity involving other sports and athletics played individually

> *Excludes:* activities involving climbing, rappelling, and jumping (E004.0-E004.9)
> activities involving ice and snow (E003.0-E003.9)
> activities involving walking and running (E001.0-E001.9)
> activities involving water and watercraft (E002.0-E002.9)

E007 Activities involving other sports and athletics played as a team or group

> *Excludes:* ice hockey (E003.1)
> water polo (E002.2)

E007.0 American tackle football
Football NOS

E007.1 American flag or touch football

E007.2 Rugby

E007.3 Baseball
Softball

E007.4 Lacrosse and field hockey

E007.5 Soccer

E007.6 Basketball

E007.7 Volleyball (beach) (court)

E007.8 Physical games generally associated with school recess, summer camp and children
Capture the flag
Dodge ball
Four square
Kickball

E007.9 Other activity involving other sports and athletics played as a team or group
Cricket

E008 Activities involving other specified sports and athletics

E008.0 Boxing

E008.1 Wrestling

807

	Add 4th or 5th digit		Nonspecific code		Unspecified code		Manifestation code

E008.2 **Racquet and hand sports**
 Handball
 Racquetball
 Squash
 Tennis

E008.3 **Frisbee**
 Ultimate frisbee

E008.4 **Martial arts**
 Combatives

E008.9 **Other specified sports and athletics activity**

> *Excludes:* sports and athletics activities specified in categories E001-E007

E009 **Activity involving other cardiorespiratory exercise**
 Activity involving physical training

E009.0 **Exercise machines primarily for cardiorespiratory conditioning**
 Elliptical and stepper machines
 Stationary bike
 Treadmill

E009.1 **Calisthenics**
 Jumping jacks
 Warm up and cool down

E009.2 **Aerobic and step exercise**

E009.3 **Circuit training**

E009.4 **Obstacle course**
 Challenge course
 Confidence course

E009.5 **Grass drills**
 Guerilla drills

E009.9 **Other activity involving other cardiorespiratory exercise**

> *Excludes:* activities involving cardiorespiratory exercise specified in categories E001-E008

E010 **Activity involving other muscle strengthening exercises**

E010.0 **Exercise machines primarily for muscle strengthening**

E010.1 **Push-ups, pull-ups, sit-ups**

E010.2 **Free weights**
 Barbells
 Dumbbells

E010.3 **Pilates**

E010.9 **Other activity involving other muscle strengthening exercises**

> *Excludes:* activities involving muscle strengthening specified in categories E001-E009

E011 **Activities involving computer technology and electronic devices**

> *Excludes:* electronic musical keyboard or instruments (E018.0)

E011.0 **Computer keyboarding**
 Electronic game playing using keyboard or other stationary device

E011.1 **Hand held interactive electronic device**
 Cellular telephone and communication device
 Electronic game playing using interactive device

> *Excludes:* electronic game playing using keyboard or other stationary device (E011.0)

E011.9 **Other activity involving computer technology and electronic devices**

E012 **Activities involving arts and handcrafts**

> *Excludes:* activities involving playing musical instrument (E018.0-E018.3)

E012.0 **Knitting and crocheting**

E012.1 **Sewing**

E012.2 **Furniture building and finishing**
 Furniture repair

E012.9 **Activity involving other arts and handcrafts**

  ● Code new   ▲ Revision of   ④ ⑤ Fourth or fifth
    to 2012 edition   existing code   digit required

E013 **Activities involving personal hygiene and household maintenance**

> *Excludes:* activities involving cooking and grilling (E015.0-E015.9)
>
> > activities involving property and land maintenance, building and construction (E016.0-E016.9)
> > activity involving persons providing caregiving (E014.0-E014.9)
> > dishwashing (E015.0)
> > food preparation (E015.0)
> > gardening (E016.1)

E013.0 **Personal bathing and showering**

E013.1 **Laundry**

E013.2 **Vacuuming**

E013.3 **Ironing**

E013.4 **Floor mopping and cleaning**

E013.5 **Residential relocation**
Packing up and unpacking involved in moving to a new residence

E013.8 **Other personal hygiene activity**

E013.9 **Other household maintenance**

E014 **Activities involving person providing caregiving**

E014.0 **Caregiving involving bathing**

E014.1 **Caregiving involving lifting**

E014.9 **Other activity involving person providing caregiving**

E015 **Activities involving food preparation, cooking and grilling**

E015.0 **Food preparation and clean up**
Dishwashing

E015.1 **Grilling and smoking food**

E015.2 **Cooking and baking**
Use of stove, oven and microwave oven

E015.9 **Other activity involving cooking and grilling**

E016 **Activities involving property and land maintenance, building and construction**

E016.0 **Digging, shoveling and raking**
Dirt digging
Raking leaves
Snow shoveling

E016.1 **Gardening and landscaping**
Pruning, trimming shrubs, weeding

E016.2 **Building and construction**

E016.9 **Other activity involving property and land maintenance, building and construction**

E017 **Activities involving roller coasters and other types of external motion**

E017.0 **Roller coaster riding**

E017.9 **Other activity involving external motion**

E018 **Activities involving playing musical instrument**
Activity involving playing electric musical instrument

E018.0 **Piano playing**
Musical keyboard (electronic) playing

E018.1 **Drum and other percussion instrument playing**

E018.2 **String instrument playing**

E018.3 **Wind and brass instrument playing**

E019 **Activities involving animal care**

> *Excludes:* horseback riding (E006.1)

E019.0 **Walking an animal**

E019.1 **Milking an animal**

E019.2 **Grooming and shearing an animal**

E019.9 **Other activity involving animal care**

E029 **Other activity**

E029.0 **Refereeing a sports activity**

E029.1 **Spectator at an event**

	Add 4th or 5th digit		Nonspecific code		Unspecified code		Manifestation code

> E029.2 **Rough housing and horseplay**
>
> E029.9 **Other activity**

E030 Unspecified activity

TRANSPORT ACCIDENTS (E800-E848)

Definitions and examples related to transport accidents

(a) A **transport accident** (E800-E848) is any accident involving a device designed primarily for, or being used at the time primarily for, conveying persons or goods from one place to another.

> Includes: accidents involving:
>> aircraft and spacecraft (E840-E845)
>> watercraft (E830-E838)
>> motor vehicle (E810-E825)
>> railway (E800-E807)
>> other road vehicles (E826-E829)

In classifying accidents which involve more than one kind of transport, the above order of precedence of transport accidents should be used.

Accidents involving agriculture and construction machines, such as tractors, cranes, and bulldozers, are regarded as transport accidents only when these vehicles are under their own power on a highway [otherwise the vehicles are regarded as machinery]. Vehicles which can travel on land or water, such as hovercraft and other amphibious vehicles, are regarded as watercraft when on the water, as motor vehicles when on the highway, and as off-road motor vehicles when on land, but off the highway.

> *Excludes:* *accidents:*
>> *in sports which involve the use of transport but where the transport vehicle itself was not involved in the accident*
>> *involving vehicles which are part of industrial equipment used entirely on industrial premises*
>> *occurring during transportation but unrelated to the hazards associated with the means of transportation [e.g., injuries received in a fight on board ship; transport vehicle involved in a cataclysm such as an earthquake]*
>> *to persons engaged in the maintenance or repair of transport equipment or vehicle not in motion, unless injured by another vehicle in motion*

(b) A **railway accident** is a transport accident involving a railway train or other railway vehicle operated on rails, whether in motion or not.

> *Excludes:* *accidents:*
>> *in repair shops*
>> *in roundhouse or on turntable*
>> *on railway premises but not involving a train or other railway vehicle*

(c) A **railway train** or **railway vehicle** is any device with or without cars coupled to it, designed for traffic on a railway.

> Includes: interurban:
>> electric car (operated chiefly on its own right-of-way, not open to other traffic)
>> streetcar (operated chiefly on its own right-of-way, not open to other traffic)
>> railway train, any power [diesel] [electric] [steam]
>>> funicular
>>> monorail or two-rail
>>> subterranean or elevated
>> other vehicle designed to run on a railway track

> *Excludes:* *interurban electric cars [streetcars] specified to be operating on a right-of-way that forms part of the public street or highway [definition (n)]*

(d) A **railway** or **railroad** is a right-of-way designed for traffic on rails, which is used by carriages or wagons transporting passengers or freight, and by other rolling stock, and which is not open to other public vehicular traffic.

(e) A **motor vehicle accident** is a transport accident involving a motor vehicle. It is defined as a motor vehicle traffic accident or as a motor vehicle nontraffic accident according to whether the accident occurs on a public highway or elsewhere.

> *Excludes:* *injury or damage due to cataclysm*
>> *injury or damage while a motor vehicle, not under its own power, is being loaded on, or unloaded from, another conveyance*

(f) A **motor vehicle traffic accident** is any motor vehicle accident occurring on a public highway [i.e., originating, terminating, or involving a vehicle partially on the highway]. A motor vehicle accident is assumed to have occurred on the highway unless another place is specified, except in the case of accidents involving only off-road motor vehicles which are classified as nontraffic accidents unless the contrary is stated.

(g) A **motor vehicle nontraffic accident** is any motor vehicle accident which occurs entirely in any place other than a public highway.

---

810   ● Code new   ▲ Revision of   ④ ⑤ Fourth or fifth
to 2012 edition   existing code   digit required

(h) A **public highway [trafficway]** or **street** is the entire width between property lines [or other boundary lines] of every way or place, of which any part is open to the use of the public for purposes of vehicular traffic as a matter of right or custom. A roadway is that part of the public highway designed, improved, and ordinarily used, for vehicular travel.

Includes: approaches (public) to:
    docks
    public building
    station

Excludes: *driveway (private)*
    parking lot
    ramp
    roads in:
    airfield
    farm
    industrial premises
    mine
    private grounds
    quarry

(i) A **motor vehicle** is any mechanically or electrically powered device, not operated on rails, upon which any person or property may be transported or drawn upon a highway. Any object such as a trailer, coaster, sled, or wagon being towed by a motor vehicle is considered a part of the motor vehicle.

Includes: automobile [any type]
    bus
    construction machinery, farm and industrial machinery, steam roller, tractor, army tank, highway grader, or similar vehicle on wheels or treads, while in transport under own power
    fire engine (motorized)
    motorcycle
    motorized bicycle [moped] or scooter
    trolley bus not operating on rails
    truck
    van

Excludes: *devices used solely to move persons or materials within the confines of a building and its premises, such as:*
    building elevator
    coal car in mine
    electric baggage or mail truck used solely within a railroad station
    electric truck used solely within an industrial plant
    moving overhead crane

(j) A **motorcycle** is a two-wheeled motor vehicle having one or two riding saddles and sometimes having a third wheel for the support of a sidecar. The sidecar is considered part of the motorcycle.

Includes: motorized:
    bicycle [moped]
    scooter
    tricycle

(k) An **off-road motor vehicle** is a motor vehicle of special design, to enable it to negotiate rough or soft terrain or snow. Examples of special design are high construction, special wheels and tires, driven by treads, or support on a cushion of air.

Includes: all terrain vehicle [ATV]
    army tank
    hovercraft, on land or swamp
    snowmobile

(l) A **driver** of a motor vehicle is the occupant of the motor vehicle operating it or intending to operate it. A **motorcyclist** is the driver of a motorcycle. Other authorized occupants of a motor vehicle are **passengers.**

(m) An **other road vehicle** is any device, except a motor vehicle, in, on, or by which any person or property may be transported on a highway.

Includes: animal carrying a person or goods
    animal-drawn vehicle
    animal harnessed to conveyance
    bicycle [pedal cycle]
    streetcar
    tricycle (pedal)

Excludes: *pedestrian conveyance [definition (q)]*

| | Add 4th or 5th digit | | Nonspecific code | | Unspecified code | | Manifestation code |

(n) A **streetcar** is a device designed and used primarily for transporting persons within a municipality, running on rails, usually subject to normal traffic control signals, and operated principally on a right-of-way that forms part of the traffic way. A trailer being towed by a streetcar is considered a part of the streetcar.

Includes: interurban or intraurban electric or streetcar, when specified to be operating on a street or public highway

tram (car)

trolley (car)

(o) A **pedal cycle** is any road transport vehicle operated solely by pedals.

Includes: bicycle

pedal cycle

tricycle

Excludes: *motorized bicycle [definition (i)]*

(p) A **pedal cyclist** is any person riding on a pedal cycle or in a sidecar attached to such a vehicle.

(q) A **pedestrian conveyance** is any human powered device by which a pedestrian may move other than by walking or by which a walking person may move another pedestrian.

Includes:

baby carriage	pushchair
coaster wagon	roller skates
heelies	scooter
ice skates	skateboard
motorized mobility	skis
scooter	sled
perambulator	wheelchair (electric)
pushcart	wheelies

(r) A **pedestrian** is any person involved in an accident who was not at the time of the accident riding in or on a motor vehicle, railroad train, streetcar, animal-drawn or other vehicle, or on a bicycle or animal.

Includes: person:

changing tire of vehicle

in or operating a pedestrian conveyance

making adjustment to motor of vehicle

on foot

(s) A **watercraft** is any device for transporting passengers or goods on the water.

(t) A **small boat** is any watercraft propelled by paddle, oars, or small motor, with a passenger capacity of less than ten.

Includes:

boat NOS	rowboat
canoe	rowing shell
coble	scull
dinghy	skiff
punt	small motorboat
raft	

Excludes: *barge*

lifeboat (used after abandoning ship)

raft (anchored) being used as diving platform

yacht

(u) An **aircraft** is any device for transporting passengers or goods in the air.

Includes: airplane [any type]

balloon

bomber

dirigible

glider (hang)

military aircraft

parachute

(v) A **commercial transport aircraft** is any device for collective passenger or freight transportation by air, whether run on commercial lines for profit or by government authorities, with the exception of military craft.

● Code new to 2012 edition   ▲ Revision of existing code   ④ ⑤ Fourth or fifth digit required

RAILWAY ACCIDENTS (E800-E807)

Note: For definitions of railway accident and related terms see definitions (a) to (d).

Excludes: *accidents involving railway train and:*
        aircraft (E840.0-E845.9)
        motor vehicle (E810.0-E825.9)
        watercraft (E830.0-E838.9)

The following fourth-digit subdivisions are for use with categories E800-E807 to identify the injured person:

.0 Railway employee
Any person who by virtue of his employment in connection with a railway, whether by the railway company or not, is at increased risk of involvement in a railway accident, such as:
catering staff of train
driver
guard
porter
postal staff on train
railway fireman
shunter
sleeping car attendant

.1 Passenger on railway
Any authorized person traveling on a train, except a railway employee.

Excludes: *intending passenger waiting at station (.8)*
        unauthorized rider on railway vehicle (.8)

.2 Pedestrian
See definition (r)

.3 Pedal cyclist
See definition (p)

.8 Other specified person
Intending passenger or bystander waiting at station
Unauthorized rider on railway vehicle

.9 Unspecified person

④**E800** **Railway accident involving collision with rolling stock**
Includes: collision between railway trains or railway vehicles, any kind
collision NOS on railway
derailment with antecedent collision with rolling stock or NOS

④**E801** **Railway accident involving collision with other object**
Includes: collision of railway train with:
      buffers
      fallen tree on railway
      gates
      platform
      rock on railway
      streetcar
      other nonmotor vehicle
      other object

Excludes: *collision with:*
        aircraft (E840.0-E842.9)
        motor vehicle (E810.0-E810.9, E820.0-E822.9)

④**E802** **Railway accident involving derailment without antecedent collision**

④**E803** **Railway accident involving explosion, fire, or burning**

Excludes: *explosion or fire, with antecedent derailment (E802.0-E802.9)*
        explosion or fire, with mention of antecedent collision (E800.0-E801.9)

④**E804** **Fall in, on, or from railway train**
Includes: fall while alighting from or boarding railway train

Excludes: *fall related to collision, derailment, or explosion of railway train (E800.0-E803.9)*

| | Add 4th or 5th digit | | Nonspecific code | | Unspecified code | | Manifestation code |

④ **E805** **Hit by rolling stock**
    Includes: crushed by railway train or part
              injured by railway train or part
              killed by railway train or part
              knocked down by railway train or part
              run over by railway train or part

    Excludes: *pedestrian hit by object set in motion by railway train (E806.0-E806.9)*

④ **E806** **Other specified railway accident**
    Includes: hit by object falling in railway train
              injured by door or window on railway train
              nonmotor road vehicle or pedestrian hit by object set in motion by railway train
              railway train hit by falling:
              earth NOS
              rock
              tree
              other object

    Excludes: *railway accident due to cataclysm (E908-E909)*

④ **E807** **Railway accident of unspecified nature**
    Includes:
              found dead on railway right-of-way NOS
              injured on railway right-of-way NOS
              railway accident NOS

MOTOR VEHICLE TRAFFIC ACCIDENTS (E810-E819)

Note: For definitions of motor vehicle traffic accident, and related terms, see definitions (e) to (k).

    Excludes: *accidents involving motor vehicle and aircraft (E840.0-E845.9)*

The following fourth-digit subdivisions are for use with categories E810-E819 to identify the injured person:

  .0 **Driver of motor vehicle other than motorcycle**
    See definition (l)

  .1 **Passenger in motor vehicle other than motorcycle**
    See definition (l)

  .2 **Motorcyclist**
    See definition (l)

  .3 **Passenger on motorcycle**
    See definition (l)

  .4 **Occupant of streetcar**

  .5 **Rider of animal; occupant of animal-drawn vehicle**

  .6 **Pedal cyclist**
    See definition (p)

  .7 **Pedestrian**
    See definition (r)

  .8 **Other specified person**
    Occupant of vehicle other than above
    Person in railway train involved in accident
    Unauthorized rider of motor vehicle

  .9 **Unspecified person**

  ALERT! For coding late effects of motor vehicle accident see E929.0

④ **E810** **Motor vehicle traffic accident involving collision with train**

    Excludes: *motor vehicle collision with object set in motion by railway train (E815.0-E815.9)*
             railway train hit by object set in motion by motor vehicle (E818.0-E818.9)

④ **E811** **Motor vehicle traffic accident involving re-entrant collision with another motor vehicle**
    Includes: collision between motor vehicle which accidentally leaves the roadway then re-enters the same roadway, or the opposite roadway on a divided highway, and another motor vehicle

    Excludes: *collision on the same roadway when none of the motor vehicles involved have left and re-entered the roadway (E812.0-E812.9)*

④ **E812** **Other motor vehicle traffic accident involving collision with motor vehicle**
    Includes: collision with another motor vehicle parked, stopped, stalled, disabled, or abandoned on the highway
              motor vehicle collision NOS

    Excludes: *collision with object set in motion by another motor vehicle (E815.0-E815.9)*
             re-entrant collision with another motor vehicle (E811.0-E811.9)

  ● Code new   ▲ Revision of   ④ ⑤ Fourth or fifth
     to 2012 edition   existing code   digit required

④ **E813** **Motor vehicle traffic accident involving collision with other vehicle**
　　　　Includes: collision between motor vehicle, any kind, and:
　　　　　　　　other road (nonmotor transport) vehicle, such as:
　　　　　　　　　animal carrying a person
　　　　　　　　　animal-drawn vehicle
　　　　　　　　　pedal cycle
　　　　　　　　　streetcar

　　　Excludes: *collision with:*
　　　　　　object set in motion by nonmotor road vehicle (E815.0-E815.9)
　　　　　　pedestrian (E814.0-E814.9)
　　　　　　nonmotor road vehicle hit by object set in motion by motor vehicle
　　　　　　　(E818.0-E818.9)

④ **E814** **Motor vehicle traffic accident involving collision with pedestrian**
　　　　Includes: collision between motor vehicle, any kind, and pedestrian
　　　　　　　　pedestrian dragged, hit, or run over by motor vehicle, any kind

　　　Excludes: *pedestrian hit by object set in motion by motor vehicle (E818.0-E818.9)*

④ **E815** **Other motor vehicle traffic accident involving collision on the highway**
　　　　Includes: collision (due to loss of control) (on highway) between motor vehicle, any kind, and:
　　　　　　　　abutment (bridge) (overpass)
　　　　　　　　animal (herded) (unattended)
　　　　　　　　fallen stone, traffic sign, tree, utility pole
　　　　　　　　guard rail or boundary fence
　　　　　　　　interhighway divider
　　　　　　　　landslide (not moving)
　　　　　　　　object set in motion by railway train or road vehicle (motor) (nonmotor)
　　　　　　　　object thrown in front of motor vehicle
　　　　　　　　safety island
　　　　　　　　temporary traffic sign or marker
　　　　　　　　wall of cut made for road
　　　　　　　　other object, fixed, movable, or moving

　　　Excludes: *collision with:*
　　　　　　any object off the highway (resulting from loss of control) (E816.0-E816.9)
　　　　　　any object which normally would have been off the highway and is not stated to
　　　　　　　have been on it (E816.0-E816.9)
　　　　　　motor vehicle parked, stopped, stalled, disabled, or abandoned on highway
　　　　　　　(E812.0-E812.9)
　　　　　　moving landslide (E909)
　　　　　motor vehicle hit by object:
　　　　　　set in motion by railway train or road vehicle (motor) (nonmotor)
　　　　　　　(E818.0-E818.9)
　　　　　　thrown into or on vehicle (E818.0-E818.9)

④ **E816** **Motor vehicle traffic accident due to loss of control, without collision on the highway**
    Includes: motor vehicle:
                failing to make curve and:
                    colliding with object off the highway
                    overturning
                    stopping abruptly off the highway
                going out of control (due to):
                    blowout and:
                        colliding with object off the highway
                        overturning
                        stopping abruptly off the highway
                    burst tire and:
                        colliding with object off the highway
                        overturning
                        stopping abruptly off the highway
                    driver falling asleep and:
                        colliding with object off the highway
                        overturning
                        stopping abruptly off the highway
                    driver inattention and:
                        colliding with object off the highway
                        overturning
                        stopping abruptly off the highway
                    excessive speed and:
                        colliding with object off the highway
                        overturning
                        stopping abruptly off the highway
                    failure of mechanical part and:
                        colliding with object off the highway
                        overturning
                        stopping abruptly off the highway

    Excludes: *collision on highway following loss of control (E810.0-E815.9)*
            loss of control of motor vehicle following collision on the highway
              (E810.0-E815.9)

④ **E817** **Noncollision motor vehicle traffic accident while boarding or alighting**
    Includes: fall down stairs of motor bus while boarding or alighting
                fall from car in street while boarding or alighting
                injured by moving part of the vehicle while boarding or alighting
                trapped by door of motor bus while boarding or alighting

④ **E818** **Other noncollision motor vehicle traffic accident**
    Includes: accidental poisoning from exhaust gas generated by motor vehicle while in motion
                breakage of any part of motor vehicle while in motion
                explosion of any part of motor vehicle while in motion
                fall, jump, or being accidentally pushed from motor vehicle while in motion
                fire starting in motor vehicle while in motion
                hit by object thrown into or on motor vehicle while in motion
                injured by being thrown against some part of, or object in motor vehicle while in
                    motion
                injury from moving part of motor vehicle while in motion
                object falling in or on motor vehicle while in motion
                object thrown on motor vehicle while in motion
                collision of railway train or road vehicle except motor vehicle, with object set in
                    motion by motor vehicle
                motor vehicle hit by object set in motion by railway train or road vehicle (motor)
                    (nonmotor)
                pedestrian, railway train, or road vehicle (motor) (nonmotor) hit by object set in
                    motion by motor vehicle

    Excludes: *collision between motor vehicle and:*

        object set in motion by railway train or road vehicle (motor) (nonmotor)
            (E815.0-E815.9)
        object thrown towards the motor vehicle (E815.0-E815.9)
        person overcome by carbon monoxide generated by stationary motor vehicle off
            the roadway with motor running (E868.2)

④ **E819** **Motor vehicle traffic accident of unspecified nature**
    Includes: motor vehicle traffic accident NOS
                traffic accident NOS

   ● Code new   ▲ Revision of   ④ ⑤ Fourth or fifth
          to 2012 edition   existing code   digit required

MOTOR VEHICLE NONTRAFFIC ACCIDENTS (E820-E825)

Note: For definitions of motor vehicle nontraffic accident and related terms see definitions (a) to (k).

Includes: accidents involving motor vehicles being used in recreational or sporting activities off the highway

collision and noncollision motor vehicle accidents occurring entirely off the highway

Excludes: *accidents involving motor vehicle and:*
> *aircraft (E840.0-E845.9)*
> *watercraft (E830.0-E838.9)*
> *accidents, not on the public highway, involving agricultural and construction machinery but not involving another motor vehicle (E919.0, E919.2, E919.7)*

The following fourth-digit subdivisions are for use with categories E820-E825 to identify the injured person:

.0 Driver of motor vehicle other than motorcycle
See definition (l)

.1 Passenger in motor vehicle other than motorcycle
See definition (l)

.2 Motorcyclist
See definition (l)

.3 Passenger on motorcycle
See definition (l)

.4 Occupant of streetcar

.5 Rider of animal; occupant of animal-drawn vehicle

.6 Pedal cyclist
See definition (p)

.7 Pedestrian
See definition (r)

.8 Other specified person
Occupant of vehicle other than above
Person on railway train involved in accident
Unauthorized rider of motor vehicle

.9 Unspecified person

ALERT! For coding late effects of motor vehicle accident see E929.0

ALERT! For coding late effects of other transport accident see E929.1

④ **E820 Nontraffic accident involving motor-driven snow vehicle**
Includes: breakage of part of motor-driven snow vehicle (not on public highway)
fall from motor-driven snow vehicle (not on public highway)
hit by motor-driven snow vehicle (not on public highway)
overturning of motor-driven snow vehicle (not on public highway)
run over or dragged by motor-driven snow vehicle (not on public highway)
collision of motor-driven snow vehicle with:
animal (being ridden) (-drawn vehicle)
another off-road motor vehicle
other motor vehicle, not on public highway
railway train
other object, fixed or movable
injury caused by rough landing of motor-driven snow vehicle (after leaving ground on rough terrain)

Excludes: *accident on the public highway involving motor driven snow vehicle (E810.0-E819.9)*

▓ Add 4th or 5th digit	▓ Nonspecific code	▓ Unspecified code	▓ Manifestation code

④ **E821** **Nontraffic accident involving other off-road motor vehicle**

Includes: breakage of part of off-road motor vehicle, except snow vehicle (not on public highway)

fall from off-road motor vehicle, except snow vehicle (not on public highway)

hit by off-road motor vehicle, except snow vehicle (not on public highway)

overturning of off-road motor vehicle, except snow vehicle (not on public highway)

run over or dragged by off-road motor vehicle, except snow vehicle (not on public highway)

thrown against some part of or object in off-road motor vehicle, except snow vehicle (not on public highway)

collision with:

animal (being ridden) (-drawn vehicle)

another off-road motor vehicle, except snow vehicle

other motor vehicle, not on public highway

other object, fixed or movable

Excludes: *accident on public highway involving off-road motor vehicle (E810.0-E819.9)*

collision between motor driven snow vehicle and other off-road motor vehicle (E820.0-E820.9)

hovercraft accident on water (E830.0-E838.9)

④ **E822** **Other motor vehicle nontraffic accident involving collision with moving object**

Includes: collision, not on public highway, between motor vehicle, except off-road motor vehicle and:

animal

nonmotor vehicle

other motor vehicle, except off-road motor vehicle

pedestrian

railway train

other moving object

Excludes: *collision with:*

motor-driven snow vehicle (E820.0-E820.9)

other off-road motor vehicle (E821.0-E821.9)

④ **E823** **Other motor vehicle nontraffic accident involving collision with stationary object**

Includes: collision, not on public highway, between motor vehicle, except off-road motor vehicle, and any object, fixed or movable, but not in motion

④ **E824** **Other motor vehicle nontraffic accident while boarding and alighting**

Includes: fall while boarding or alighting from motor vehicle, except off-road motor vehicle, not on public highway

injury from moving part of motor vehicle while boarding or alighting from motor vehicle, except off-road motor vehicle, not on public highway

trapped by door of motor vehicle while boarding or alighting from motor vehicle, except off-road motor vehicle, not on public highway

④ **E825** **Other motor vehicle nontraffic accident of other and unspecified nature**

Includes: accidental poisoning from carbon monoxide generated by motor vehicle while in motion, not on public highway

breakage of any part of motor vehicle while in motion, not on public highway

explosion of any part of motor vehicle while in motion, not on public highway

fall, jump, or being accidentally pushed from motor vehicle while in motion, not on public highway

fire starting in motor vehicle while in motion, not on public highway

hit by object thrown into, towards, or on motor vehicle while in motion, not on public highway

injured by being thrown against some part of, or object in motor vehicle while in motion, not on public highway

injury from moving part of motor vehicle while in motion, not on public highway

object falling in or on motor vehicle while in motion, not on public highway

motor vehicle nontraffic accident NOS

Excludes: *fall from or in stationary motor vehicle (E884.9, E885.9)*

overcome by carbon monoxide or exhaust gas generated by stationary motor vehicle off the roadway with motor running (E868.2)

struck by falling object from or in stationary motor vehicle (E916)

● Code new to 2012 edition   ▲ Revision of existing code   ④ ⑤ Fourth or fifth digit required

OTHER ROAD VEHICLE ACCIDENTS (E826-E829)

Note: Other road vehicle accidents are transport accidents involving road vehicles other than motor vehicles. For definitions of other road vehicle and related terms see definitions (m) to (o).

Includes: accidents involving other road vehicles being used in recreational or sporting activities

Excludes: *collision of other road vehicle [any] with:*
aircraft (E840.0-E845.9)
motor vehicle (E813.0-E813.9, E820.0-E822.9)
railway train (E801.0-E801.9)

The following fourth-digit subdivisions are for use with categories E826-E829 to identify the injured person:

.0 Pedestrian
See definition (r)

.1 Pedal cyclist
See definition (p)

.2 Rider of animal

.3 Occupant of animal-drawn vehicle

.4 Occupant of streetcar

.8 Other specified person

.9 Unspecified person

④ **E826 Pedal cycle accident**
[0-9]

Includes: breakage of any part of pedal cycle
collision between pedal cycle and:
animal (being ridden) (herded) (unattended)
another pedal cycle
nonmotor road vehicle, any
pedestrian
other object, fixed, movable, or moving, not set in motion by motor vehicle, railway train, or aircraft
entanglement in wheel of pedal cycle
fall from pedal cycle
hit by object falling or thrown on the pedal cycle
pedal cycle accident NOS
pedal cycle overturned

④ **E827 Animal-drawn vehicle accident**
[0,2-4,8,9]

Includes: breakage of any part of vehicle
collision between animal-drawn vehicle and:
animal (being ridden) (herded) (unattended)
nonmotor road vehicle, except pedal cycle
pedestrian, pedestrian conveyance, or pedestrian vehicle
other object, fixed, movable, or moving, not set in motion by motor vehicle, railway train, or aircraft
fall from animal-drawn vehicle
knocked down by animal-drawn vehicle
overturning of animal-drawn vehicle
run over by animal-drawn vehicle
thrown from animal-drawn vehicle

Excludes: *collision of animal-drawn vehicle with pedal cycle (E826.0-E826.9)*

	Add 4th or 5th digit		Nonspecific code		Unspecified code		Manifestation code

④ **E828** **Accident involving animal being ridden**
[0,2,4,8,9]

     Includes: collision between animal being ridden and:
          another animal
          nonmotor road vehicle, except pedal cycle, and animal-drawn vehicle
          pedestrian, pedestrian conveyance, or pedestrian vehicle
          other object, fixed, movable, or moving, not set in motion by motor vehicle,
             railway train, or aircraft
          fall from animal being ridden
          knocked down by animal being ridden
          thrown from animal being ridden
          trampled by animal being ridden
          ridden animal stumbled and fell

     Excludes: *collision of animal being ridden with:*
          animal-drawn vehicle (E827.0-E827.9)
          pedal cycle (E826.0-E826.9)

④ **E829** **Other road vehicle accidents**
[0,4,8,9]

     Includes: accident while boarding or alighting from:
          streetcar
          nonmotor road vehicle not classifiable to E826-E828
          blow from object in:
          streetcar
          nonmotor road vehicle not classifiable to E826-E828
          breakage of any part of:
          streetcar
          nonmotor road vehicle not classifiable to E826-E828
          caught in door of:
          streetcar
          nonmotor road vehicle not classifiable to E826-E828
          derailment of:
          streetcar
          nonmotor road vehicle not classifiable to E826-E828
          fall in, on, or from:
          streetcar
          nonmotor road vehicle not classifiable to E826-E828
          fire in:
          streetcar
          nonmotor road vehicle not classifiable to E826-E828
          collision between streetcar or nonmotor road vehicle, except as in E826-E828, and:
          animal (not being ridden)
          another nonmotor road vehicle not classifiable to E826-E828
          pedestrian
          other object, fixed, movable, or moving, not set in motion by motor vehicle,
             railway train, or aircraft
          nonmotor road vehicle accident NOS
          streetcar accident NOS

     Excludes: *collision with:*
          animal being ridden (E828.0-E828.9)
          animal-drawn vehicle (E827.0-E827.9)
          pedal cycle (E826.0-E826.9)

● Code new   ▲ Revision of   ④ ⑤ Fourth or fifth
       to 2012 edition   existing code   digit required

WATER TRANSPORT ACCIDENTS (E830-E838)

Note: For definitions of water transport accident and related terms see definitions (a), (s), and (t).

Includes: watercraft accidents in the course of recreational activities

Excludes: *accidents involving both aircraft, including objects set in motion by aircraft, and watercraft (E840.0-E845.9)*

The following fourth-digit subdivisions are for use with categories E830-E838 to identify the injured person:

.0 Occupant of small boat, unpowered

.1 Occupant of small boat, powered
See definition (t)

Excludes: *water skier (.4)*

.2 Occupant of other watercraft—crew
Persons:
engaged in operation of watercraft
providing passenger services [cabin attendants, ship's physician, catering personnel]
working on ship during voyage in other capacity [musician in band, operators of shops and beauty parlors]

.3 Occupant of other watercraft—other than crew
Passenger
Occupant of lifeboat, other than crew, after abandoning ship

.4 Water skier

.5 Swimmer

.6 Dockers, stevedores
Longshoreman employed on the dock in loading and unloading ships

.7 Occupant of military watercraft, any type

.8 Other specified person
Immigration and custom officials on board ship
Person:
accompanying passenger or member of crew
visiting boat
Pilot (guiding ship into port)

.9 Unspecified person

④ **E830 Accident to watercraft causing submersion**
Includes: submersion and drowning due to:
boat overturning
boat submerging
falling or jumping from burning ship
falling or jumping from crushed watercraft
ship sinking
other accident to watercraft

④ **E831 Accident to watercraft causing other injury**
Includes: any injury, except submersion and drowning, as a result of an accident to watercraft
burned while ship on fire
crushed between ships in collision
crushed by lifeboat after abandoning ship
fall due to collision or other accident to watercraft
hit by falling object due to accident to watercraft
injured in watercraft accident involving collision
struck by boat or part thereof after fall or jump from damaged boat

Excludes: *burns from localized fire or explosion on board ship (E837.0-E837.9)*

④ **E832 Other accidental submersion or drowning in water transport accident**
Includes: submersion or drowning as a result of an accident other than accident to the watercraft, such as:
fall:
from gangplank
from ship
overboard
thrown overboard by motion of ship
washed overboard

Excludes: *submersion or drowning of swimmer or diver who voluntarily jumps from boat not involved in an accident (E910.0-E910.9)*

Add 4th or 5th digit	Nonspecific code	Unspecified code	Manifestation code

④ **E833** **Fall on stairs or ladders in water transport**
> *Excludes:* *fall due to accident to watercraft (E831.0-E831.9)*

④ **E834** **Other fall from one level to another in water transport**
> *Excludes:* *fall due to accident to watercraft (E831.0-E831.9)*

④ **E835** **Other and unspecified fall in water transport**
> *Excludes:* *fall due to accident to watercraft (E831.0-E831.9)*

④ **E836** **Machinery accident in water transport**
Includes: injuries in water transport caused by:
>> deck machinery
>> engine room machinery
>> galley machinery
>> laundry machinery
>> loading machinery

④ **E837** **Explosion, fire, or burning in watercraft**
Includes: explosion of boiler on steamship
> localized fire on ship

> *Excludes:* *burning ship (due to collision or explosion) resulting in:*
>> *submersion or drowning (E830.0-E830.9)*
>> *other injury (E831.0-E831.9)*

④ **E838** **Other and unspecified water transport accident**
Includes: accidental poisoning by gases or fumes on ship
> atomic power plant malfunction in watercraft
> crushed between ship and stationary object [wharf]
> crushed between ships without accident to watercraft
> crushed by falling object on ship or while loading or unloading
> hit by boat while water skiing
> struck by boat or part thereof (after fall from boat)
> watercraft accident NOS

AIR AND SPACE TRANSPORT ACCIDENTS (E840-E845)

Note: For definition of aircraft and related terms see definitions (u) and (v).

The following fourth-digit subdivisions are for use with categories E840-E845 to identify the injured person:

.0 Occupant of spacecraft

.1 Occupant of military aircraft, any
Crew in military aircraft [air force] [army] [national guard] [navy]
Passenger (civilian) (military) in military aircraft [air force] [army] [national guard] [navy]
Troops in military aircraft [air force] [army] [national guard] [navy]

> *Excludes:* *occupants of aircraft operated under jurisdiction of police departments (.5)*
>> *parachutist (.7)*

.2 Crew of commercial aircraft (powered) in surface to surface transport

.3 Other occupant of commercial aircraft (powered) in surface to surface transport
Flight personnel:
 not part of crew
 on familiarization flight
Passenger on aircraft (powered) NOS

.4 Occupant of commercial aircraft (powered) in surface to air transport
Occupant [crew] [passenger] of aircraft (powered) engaged in activities, such as:
 aerial spraying (crops) (fire retardants)
 air drops of emergency supplies
 air drops of parachutists, except from military craft
 crop dusting
 lowering of construction material [bridge or telephone pole]
 sky writing

.5 Occupant of other powered aircraft
Occupant [crew] [passenger] of aircraft [powered] engaged in activities, such as:
 aerobatic flying
 aircraft racing
 rescue operation
 storm surveillance
 traffic surveillance
Occupant of private plane NOS

● Code new
to 2012 edition
▲ Revision of
existing code
④ ⑤ Fourth or fifth
digit required

.6 Occupant of unpowered aircraft, except parachutist
Occupant of aircraft classifiable to E842

.7 Parachutist (military) (other)
Person making voluntary descent

Excludes: *person making descent after accident to aircraft (.1-.6)*

.8 Ground crew, airline employee
Persons employed at airfields (civil) (military) or launching pads, not occupants of aircraft

.9 Other person

④ **E840 Accident to powered aircraft at takeoff or landing**
Includes: collision of aircraft with any object, fixed, movable, or moving while taking off or landing
crash while taking off or landing
explosion on aircraft while taking off or landing
fire on aircraft while taking off or landing
forced landing

④ **E841 Accident to powered aircraft, other and unspecified**
Includes: aircraft accident NOS
aircraft crash or wreck NOS
any accident to powered aircraft while in transit or when not specified whether in transit, taking off, or landing
collision of aircraft with another aircraft, bird, or any object, while in transit
explosion on aircraft while in transit
fire on aircraft while in transit

④ **E842 Accident to unpowered aircraft**
[6-9]
Includes: any accident, except collision with powered aircraft, to:
balloon
glider
hang glider
kite carrying a person
hit by object falling from unpowered aircraft

④ **E843 Fall in, on, or from aircraft**
[0-9]
Includes: accident in boarding or alighting from aircraft, any kind
fall in, on, or from aircraft [any kind], while in transit, taking off, or landing, except when as a result of an accident to aircraft

④ **E844 Other specified air transport accidents**
[0-9]
Includes: hit by:
aircraft without accident to aircraft
object falling from aircraft without accident to aircraft
injury by or from:
machinery on aircraft without accident to aircraft
rotating propeller without accident to aircraft
voluntary parachute descent without accident to aircraft
poisoning by carbon monoxide from aircraft while in transit without accident to aircraft
sucked into jet without accident to aircraft
any accident involving other transport vehicle (motor) (nonmotor) due to being hit by object set in motion by aircraft (powered)

Excludes: *air sickness (E903)*
effects of:
high altitude (E902.0-E902.1)
pressure change (E902.0-E902.1)
injury in parachute descent due to accident to aircraft (840.0-E842.9)

④ **E845 Accident involving spacecraft**
[0,8,9]
Includes: launching pad accident
Excludes: *effects of weightlessness in spacecraft (E928.0)*

VEHICLE ACCIDENTS NOT ELSEWHERE CLASSIFIABLE (E846-E848)

E846 Accidents involving powered vehicles used solely within the buildings and premises of industrial or commercial establishment

Accident to, on, or involving:
- battery powered airport passenger vehicle
- battery powered trucks (baggage) (mail)
- coal car in mine
- logging car
- self propelled truck, industrial
- station baggage truck (powered)
- tram, truck, or tub (powered) in mine or quarry

Breakage of any part of vehicle

Collision with:
- pedestrian
- other vehicle or object within premises

Explosion of powered vehicle, industrial or commercial

Fall from powered vehicle, industrial or commercial

Overturning of powered vehicle, industrial or commercial

Struck by powered vehicle, industrial or commercial

[Excludes:] *accidental poisoning by exhaust gas from vehicle not elsewhere classifiable (E868.2)*
injury by crane, lift (fork), or elevator (E919.2)

E847 Accidents involving cable cars not running on rails

Accident to, on, or involving:
- cable car, not on rails
- ski chair-lift
- ski-lift with gondola
- téléférique

Breakage of cable

Caught or dragged by cable car, not on rails

Fall or jump from cable car, not on rails

Object thrown from or in cable car, not on rails

E848 Accidents involving other vehicles, not elsewhere classifiable

Accident to, on, or involving:
- ice yacht
- land yacht
- nonmotor, nonroad vehicle NOS

PLACE OF OCCURRENCE (E849)

E849 Place of occurrence

The following category is for use to denote the place where the injury or poisoning occurred.

E849.0 Home

Apartment
Boarding house
Farm house
Home premises
House (residential)
Noninstitutional place of residence

Private:
- driveway
- garage
- garden
- home
- walk

Swimming pool in private house or garden
Yard of home

[Excludes:] *home under construction but not yet occupied (E849.3)*
institutional place of residence (E849.7)

E849.1 Farm

Farm:
- buildings
- land under cultivation

[Excludes:] *farm house and home premises of farm (E849.0)*

E849.2 Mine and quarry

Gravel pit
Sand pit
Tunnel under construction

● Code new to 2012 edition ▲ Revision of existing code ④ ⑤ Fourth or fifth digit required

E849.3 Industrial place and premises

Building under
  construction
Dockyard
Dry dock
Factory
  building
  premises
Garage (place of work)

Industrial yard
Loading platform (factory) (store)
Plant, industrial
Railway yard
Shop (place of work)
Warehouse
Workhouse

E849.4 Place for recreation and sport

Amusement park
Baseball field
Basketball court
Beach resort
Cricket ground
Fives court
Football field
Golf course
Gymnasium
Hockey field
Holiday camp
Ice palace
Lake resort
Mountain resort
Playground, including
  school playground

Public park
Racecourse
Resort NOS
Riding school
Rifle range
Seashore resort
Skating rink
Sports ground
Sports palace
Stadium
Swimming pool, public
Tennis court
Vacation resort

Excludes: *that in private house or garden (E849.0)*

E849.5 Street and highway

E849.6 Public building

Building (including adjacent grounds) used by the general public or by a particular
  group of the public, such as:

airport
bank
café
casino
church
cinema
clubhouse
courthouse
dance hall
garage building (for car
  storage)
hotel
market (grocery or other
  commodity)
movie house
music hall

nightclub
office
office building
opera house
post office
public hall
radio broadcasting station
restaurant
school (state) (public) (private)
shop, commercial
station (bus) (railway)
store
theater

Excludes: *home garage (E849.0)*
           industrial building or workplace (E849.3)

E849.7 Residential institution

Children's home
Dormitory
Hospital
Jail

Old people's home
Orphanage
Prison
Reform school

E849.8 Other specified places

Beach NOS
Canal
Caravan site NOS
Derelict house
Desert
Dock
Forest
Harbor
Hill
Lake NOS
Mountain
Parking lot
Parking place

Pond or pool (natural)
Prairie
Public place NOS
Railway line
Reservoir
River
Sea
Seashore NOS
Stream
Swamp
Trailer court
Woods

Add 4th or
5th digit

Nonspecific
code

Unspecified
code

Manifestation
code

E849.9 **Unspecified place**

ACCIDENTAL POISONING BY DRUGS, MEDICINAL SUBSTANCES, AND BIOLOGICALS (E850-E858)

Includes: accidental overdose of drug, wrong drug given or taken in error, and drug taken inadvertently

accidents in the use of drugs and biologicals in medical and surgical procedures

Excludes: *administration with suicidal or homicidal intent or intent to harm, or in circumstances classifiable to E980-E989 (E950.0-E950.5, E962.0, E980.0-E980.5)*

correct drug properly administered in therapeutic or prophylactic dosage, as the cause of adverse effect (E930.0-E949.9)

See Alphabetic Index for more complete list of specific drugs to be classified under the fourth-digit subdivisions. The American Hospital Formulary numbers can be used to classify new drugs listed by the American Hospital Formulary Service (AHFS). See appendix C.

ALERT! For coding late effects of accidental poisoning see E929.2

E850 **Accidental poisoning by analgesics, antipyretics, and antirheumatics**

E850.0 **Heroin**
Diacetylmorphine

E850.1 **Methadone**

E850.2 **Other opiates and related narcotics**
Codeine [methylmorphine]   Morphine
Meperidine [pethidine]   Opium (alkaloids)

E850.3 **Salicylates**
Acetylsalicylic acid [aspirin]
Amino derivatives of salicylic acid
Salicylic acid salts

E850.4 **Aromatic analgesics, not elsewhere classified**
Acetanilid
Paracetamol [acetaminophen]
Phenacetin [acetophenetidin]

E850.5 **Pyrazole derivatives**
Aminophenazone [amidopyrine]
Phenylbutazone

E850.6 **Antirheumatics [antiphlogistics]**
Gold salts   Indomethacin
Excludes: *salicylates (E850.3)*
steroids (E858.0)

E850.7 **Other non-narcotic analgesics**
Pyrabital

E850.8 **Other specified analgesics and antipyretics**
Pentazocine

E850.9 **Unspecified analgesic or antipyretic**

E851 **Accidental poisoning by barbiturates**
Amobarbital [amylobarbitone]
Barbital [barbitone]
Butabarbital [butabarbitone]
Pentobarbital [pentobarbitone]
Phenobarbital [phenobarbitone]
Secobarbital [quinalbarbitone]
Excludes: *thiobarbiturates (E855.1)*

E852 **Accidental poisoning by other sedatives and hypnotics**

E852.0 **Chloral hydrate group**

E852.1 **Paraldehyde**

E852.2 **Bromine compounds**
Bromides   Carbromal (derivatives)

E852.3 **Methaqualone compounds**

E852.4 **Glutethimide group**

E852.5 **Mixed sedatives, not elsewhere classified**

E852.8 **Other specified sedatives and hypnotics**

E852.9 **Unspecified sedative or hypnotic**
Sleeping:
   drug NOS
   pill NOS
   tablet NOS

E853 **Accidental poisoning by tranquilizers**

E853.0 **Phenothiazine-based tranquilizers**
Chlorpromazine   Prochlorperazine
Fluphenazine   Promazine

E853.1 **Butyrophenone-based tranquilizers**
Haloperidol   Trifluperidol
Spiperone

E853.2 **Benzodiazepine-based tranquilizers**
Chlordiazepoxide   Lorazepam
Diazepam   Medazepam
Flurazepam   Nitrazepam

E853.8 **Other specified tranquilizers**
Hydroxyzine   Meprobamate

E853.9 **Unspecified tranquilizer**

E854 **Accidental poisoning by other psychotropic agents**

E854.0 **Antidepressants**
Amitriptyline   Monoamine oxidase [MAO] inhibitors
Imipramine

E854.1 **Psychodysleptics [hallucinogens]**
Cannabis derivatives   Mescaline
Lysergide [LSD]   Psilocin
marijuana (derivatives) Psilocybin

E854.2 **Psychostimulants**
Amphetamine   Caffeine

> Excludes: central appetite depressants (E858.8)

E854.3 **Central nervous system stimulants**
Analeptics   Opiate antagonists

E854.8 **Other psychotropic agents**

E855 **Accidental poisoning by other drugs acting on central and autonomic nervous system**

E855.0 **Anticonvulsant and anti-Parkinsonism drugs**
Amantadine
Hydantoin derivatives
Levodopa [L-dopa]
Oxazolidine derivatives [paramethadione] [trimethadione]
Succinimides

E855.1 **Other central nervous system depressants**
Ether   Intravenous anesthetics
Gaseous anesthetics   Thiobarbiturates, such as thiopental sodium
Halogenated hydrocarbon
   derivatives

E855.2 **Local anesthetics**
Cocaine   Procaine
Lidocaine [lignocaine] Tetracaine

E855.3 **Parasympathomimetics [cholinergics]**
Acetylcholine   Pilocarpine
Anticholinesterase:
   organophosphorus
   reversible

E855.4 **Parasympatholytics [anticholinergics and antimuscarinics] and spasmolytics**
Atropine   Hyoscine [scopolamine]
Homatropine   Quaternary ammonium derivatives

E855.5 **Sympathomimetics [adrenergics]**
Epinephrine [adrenalin]
Levarterenol [noradrenalin]

E855.6 **Sympatholytics [antiadrenergics]**
Phenoxybenzamine   Tolazoline hydrochloride

Add 4th or 5th digit   Nonspecific code   Unspecified code   Manifestation code

E855.8　Other specified drugs acting on central and autonomic nervous systems

E855.9　Unspecified drug acting on central and autonomic nervous systems

E856　Accidental poisoning by antibiotics

E857　Accidental poisoning by other anti-infectives

E858　Accidental poisoning by other drugs

E858.0　Hormones and synthetic substitutes

E858.1　Primarily systemic agents

E858.2　Agents primarily affecting blood constituents

E858.3　Agents primarily affecting cardiovascular system

E858.4　Agents primarily affecting gastrointestinal system

E858.5　Water, mineral, and uric acid metabolism drugs

E858.6　Agents primarily acting on the smooth and skeletal muscles and respiratory system

E858.7　Agents primarily affecting skin and mucous membrane, ophthalmological, otorhinolaryngological, and dental drugs

E858.8　Other specified drugs
　　　　Central appetite depressants

E858.9　Unspecified drug

ACCIDENTAL POISONING BY OTHER SOLID AND LIQUID SUBSTANCES, GASES, AND VAPORS (E860-E869)

Note: Categories in this section are intended primarily to indicate the external cause of poisoning states classifiable to 980-989. They may also be used to indicate external causes of localized effects classifiable to 001-799.

　　　ALERT! For coding late effects of accidental poisoning see E929.2

E860　Accidental poisoning by alcohol, not elsewhere classified

E860.0　Alcoholic beverages
　　　　Alcohol in preparations intended for consumption

E860.1　Other and unspecified ethyl alcohol and its products
　　　　Denatured alcohol　　　　Grain alcohol NOS
　　　　Ethanol NOS　　　　　　Methylated spirit

E860.2　Methyl alcohol
　　　　Methanol　　　　　　　Wood alcohol

E860.3　Isopropyl alcohol
　　　　Dimethyl carbinol　　　　Secondary propyl alcohol
　　　　Isopropanol
　　　　Rubbing alcohol substitute

E860.4　Fusel oil
　　　　Alcohol:
　　　　　amyl
　　　　　butyl
　　　　　propyl

E860.8　Other specified alcohols

E860.9　Unspecified alcohol

E861　Accidental poisoning by cleansing and polishing agents, disinfectants, paints, and varnishes

E861.0　Synthetic detergents and shampoos

E861.1　Soap products

E861.2　Polishes

E861.3　Other cleansing and polishing agents
　　　　Scouring powders

E861.4　Disinfectants
　　　　Household and other disinfectants not ordinarily used on the person

　　　　Excludes: carbolic acid or phenol (E864.0)

E861.5　Lead paints
　　　　ALERT! For personal history of contact with and (suspected) exposure to lead see V15.86

E861.6　Other paints and varnishes
　　　　Lacquers　　　　　　　Paints, other than lead
　　　　Oil colors　　　　　　　White washes

E861.9   Unspecified

E862   Accidental poisoning by petroleum products, other solvents and their vapors, not elsewhere classified

E862.0   **Petroleum solvents**
Petroleum:
  ether
  benzine
  naphtha

E862.1   **Petroleum fuels and cleaners**
Antiknock additives to petroleum fuels
Gas oils
Gasoline or petrol
Kerosene

> Excludes: kerosene insecticides (E863.4)

E862.2   **Lubricating oils**

E862.3   **Petroleum solids**
Paraffin wax

E862.4   **Other specified solvents**
Benzene

E862.9   **Unspecified solvent**

E863   Accidental poisoning by agricultural and horticultural chemical and pharmaceutical preparations other than plant foods and fertilizers

> Excludes: plant foods and fertilizers (E866.5)

E863.0   **Insecticides of organochlorine compounds**
Benzene hexachloride	Dieldrin
Chlordane	Endrine
DDT	Toxaphene

E863.1   **Insecticides of organophosphorus compounds**
Demeton	Parathion
Diazinon	Phenylsulphthion
Dichlorvos	Phorate
Malathion	Phosdrin
Methyl parathion	

E863.2   **Carbamates**
Aldicarb	Propoxur
Carbaryl	

E863.3   **Mixtures of insecticides**

E863.4   **Other and unspecified insecticides**
Kerosene insecticides

E863.5   **Herbicides**
2, 4-Dichlorophenoxyacetic acid [2, 4-D]
2, 4, 5-Trichlorophenoxyacetic acid [2, 4, 5-T]
Chlorates
Diquat
Mixtures of plant food and fertilizers with herbicides
Paraquat

E863.6   **Fungicides**
Organic mercurials (used in seed dressing)
Pentachlorophenols

E863.7   **Rodenticides**
Fluoroacetates	Warfarin
Squill and derivatives	Zinc phosphide
Thallium	

E863.8   **Fumigants**
Cyanides	Phosphine
Methyl bromide	

E863.9   **Other and unspecified**

E864   Accidental poisoning by corrosives and caustics, not elsewhere classified

> Excludes: those as components of disinfectants (E861.4)

E864.0   **Corrosive aromatics**
Carbolic acid or phenol

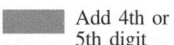 Add 4th or 5th digit   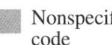 Nonspecific code   Unspecified code   Manifestation code

E864.1 **Acids**
    Acid:
      hydrochloric
      nitric
      sulfuric

E864.2 **Caustic alkalis**
    Lye

E864.3 **Other specified corrosives and caustics**

E864.4 **Unspecified corrosives and caustics**

E865 **Accidental poisoning from poisonous foodstuffs and poisonous plants**
    Includes: any meat, fish, or shellfish
               plants, berries, and fungi eaten as, or in mistake for, food, or by a child

    Excludes: *anaphylactic shock due to adverse food reaction (995.60-995.69)*
            food poisoning (bacterial) (005.0-005.9)
            poisoning and toxic reactions to venomous plants (E905.6-E905.7)

E865.0 **Meat**

E865.1 **Shellfish**

E865.2 **Other fish**

E865.3 **Berries and seeds**

E865.4 **Other specified plants**

E865.5 **Mushrooms and other fungi**

E865.8 **Other specified foods**

E865.9 **Unspecified foodstuff or poisonous plant**

E866 **Accidental poisoning by other and unspecified solid and liquid substances**
    Excludes: *these substances as a component of:*
            medicines (E850.0-E858.9)
            paints (E861.5-E861.6)
            pesticides (E863.0-E863.9)
            petroleum fuels (E862.1)

E866.0 **Lead and its compounds and fumes**
    ALERT! For personal history of contact with and (suspected) exposure to lead see V15.86

E866.1 **Mercury and its compounds and fumes**

E866.2 **Antimony and its compounds and fumes**

E866.3 **Arsenic and its compounds and fumes**

E866.4 **Other metals and their compounds and fumes**

Beryllium (compounds)	Iron (compounds)
Brass fumes	Manganese (compounds)
Cadmium (compounds)	Nickel (compounds)
Copper salts	Thallium (compounds)

E866.5 **Plant foods and fertilizers**
    Excludes: *mixtures with herbicides (E863.5)*

E866.6 **Glues and adhesives**

E866.7 **Cosmetics**

E866.8 **Other specified solid or liquid substances**

E866.9 **Unspecified solid or liquid substance**

E867 **Accidental poisoning by gas distributed by pipeline**
    Carbon monoxide from incomplete combustion of piped gas
    Coal gas NOS
    Liquefied petroleum gas distributed through pipes (pure or mixed with air)
    Piped gas (natural) (manufactured)

E868 **Accidental poisoning by other utility gas and other carbon monoxide**

E868.0 **Liquefied petroleum gas distributed in mobile containers**
    Butane or carbon monoxide from incomplete combustion of this gas
    Liquefied hydrocarbon gas NOS or carbon monoxide from incomplete combustion of
        this gas
    Propane or carbon monoxide from incomplete combustion of this gas

  ● Code new
     to 2012 edition
  ▲ Revision of
     existing code
  ④ ⑤ Fourth or fifth
      digit required

E868.1 **Other and unspecified utility gas**
Acetylene or or carbon monoxide from incomplete combustion of these gases
Gas NOS used for lighting, heating, cooking, or carbon monoxide from incomplete combustion of these gases
Water gas or carbon monoxide from incomplete combustion of these gases

E868.2 **Motor vehicle exhaust gas**
Exhaust gas from:
farm tractor, not in transit
gas engine
motor pump
motor vehicle, not in transit
any type of combustion engine not in watercraft

Excludes: *poisoning by carbon monoxide from:*
  aircraft while in transit (E844.0-E844.9)
  motor vehicle while in transit (E818.0-E818.9)
  watercraft whether or not in transit (E838.0-E838.9)

E868.3 **Carbon monoxide from incomplete combustion of other domestic fuels**
Carbon monoxide from incomplete combustion of:
coal in domestic stove or fireplace
coke in domestic stove or fireplace
kerosene in domestic stove or fireplace
wood in domestic stove or fireplace

Excludes: *carbon monoxide from smoke and fumes due to conflagration (E890.0-E893.9)*

E868.8 **Carbon monoxide from other sources**
Carbon monoxide from:
blast furnace gas
incomplete combustion of fuels in industrial use
kiln vapor

E868.9 **Unspecified carbon monoxide**

E869 **Accidental poisoning by other gases and vapors**

Excludes: *effects of gases used as anesthetics (E855.1, E938.2)*
  fumes from heavy metals (E866.0-E866.4)
  smoke and fumes due to conflagration or explosion (E890.0-E899)

E869.0 **Nitrogen oxides**

E869.1 **Sulfur dioxide**

E869.2 **Freon**

E869.3 **Lacrimogenic gas [tear gas]**
Bromobenzyl cyanide   Ethyliodoacetate
Chloroacetophenone

E869.4 **Second-hand tobacco smoke**

E869.8 **Other specified gases and vapors**
Chlorine   Hydrocyanic acid gas

E869.9 **Unspecified gases and vapors**

MISADVENTURES TO PATIENTS DURING SURGICAL AND MEDICAL CARE (E870-E876)

Excludes: *accidental overdose of drug and wrong drug given in error (E850.0-E858.9)*
  surgical and medical procedures as the cause of abnormal reaction by the patient, without mention of misadventure at the time of procedure (E878.0-E879.9)

E870 **Accidental cut, puncture, perforation, or hemorrhage during medical care**

E870.0 **Surgical operation**

E870.1 **Infusion or transfusion**

E870.2 **Kidney dialysis or other perfusion**

E870.3 **Injection or vaccination**

E870.4 **Endoscopic examination**

E870.5 **Aspiration of fluid or tissue, puncture, and catheterization**
Abdominal paracentesis   Lumbar puncture
Aspirating needle biopsy   Thoracentesis
Blood sampling

Excludes: *heart catheterization (E870.6)*

E870.6 **Heart catheterization**

E870.7 **Administration of enema**

Add 4th or   Nonspecific   Unspecified   Manifestation
5th digit   code   code   code

E870.8 Other specified medical care

E870.9 Unspecified medical care

E871 Foreign object left in body during procedure

E871.0 Surgical operation

E871.1 Infusion or transfusion

E871.2 Kidney dialysis or other perfusion

E871.3 Injection or vaccination

E871.4 Endoscopic examination

E871.5 Aspiration of fluid or tissue, puncture, and catheterization
Abdominal paracentesis   Lumbar puncture
Aspiration needle biopsy   Thoracentesis
Blood sampling

> *Excludes:* heart catheterization (E871.6)

E871.6 Heart catheterization

E871.7 Removal of catheter or packing

E871.8 Other specified procedures

E871.9 Unspecified procedure

E872 Failure of sterile precautions during procedure

E872.0 Surgical operation

E872.1 Infusion or transfusion

E872.2 Kidney dialysis and other perfusion

E872.3 Injection or vaccination

E872.4 Endoscopic examination

E872.5 Aspiration of fluid or tissue, puncture, and catheterization
Abdominal paracentesis   Lumbar puncture
Aspirating needle biopsy   Thoracentesis
Blood sampling

> *Excludes:* heart catheterization (E872.6)

E872.6 Heart catheterization

E872.8 Other specified procedures

E872.9 Unspecified procedure

E873 Failure in dosage

> *Excludes:* accidental overdose of drug, medicinal or biological substance (E850.0-E858.9)

E873.0 Excessive amount of blood or other fluid during transfusion or infusion

E873.1 Incorrect dilution of fluid during infusion

E873.2 Overdose of radiation in therapy

E873.3 Inadvertent exposure of patient to radiation during medical care

E873.4 Failure in dosage in electroshock or insulin-shock therapy

E873.5 Inappropriate [too hot or too cold] temperature in local application and packing

E873.6 Nonadministration of necessary drug or medicinal substance

E873.8 Other specified failure in dosage

E873.9 Unspecified failure in dosage

E874 Mechanical failure of instrument or apparatus during procedure

E874.0 Surgical operation

E874.1 Infusion and transfusion
Air in system

E874.2 Kidney dialysis and other perfusion

E874.3 Endoscopic examination

E874.4 Aspiration of fluid or tissue, puncture, and catheterization
Abdominal paracentesis   Lumbar puncture
Aspirating needle biopsy   Thoracentesis
Blood sampling

> *Excludes:* heart catheterization (E874.5)

E874.5 Heart catheterization

● Code new   ▲ Revision of   ④ ⑤ Fourth or fifth
      to 2012 edition   existing code   digit required

E874.8 Other specified procedures

E874.9 Unspecified procedure

E875 Contaminated or infected blood, other fluid, drug, or biological substance
Includes: presence of:
bacterial pyrogens
endotoxin-producing bacteria
serum hepatitis-producing agent

E875.0 Contaminated substance transfused or infused

E875.1 Contaminated substance injected or used for vaccination

E875.2 Contaminated drug or biological substance administered by other means

E875.8 Other

E875.9 Unspecified

E876 Other and unspecified misadventures during medical care

E876.0 Mismatched blood in transfusion

E876.1 Wrong fluid in infusion

E876.2 Failure in suture and ligature during surgical operation

E876.3 Endotracheal tube wrongly placed during anesthetic procedure

E876.4 Failure to introduce or to remove other tube or instrument

Excludes: *foreign object left in body during procedure (E871.0-E871.9)*

E876.5 Performance of wrong operation (procedure) on correct patient
Wrong device implanted into correct surgical site

Excludes: *correct operation (procedure) performed on wrong body part (E876.7)*

E876.6 Performance of operation (procedure) on patient not scheduled for surgery
Performance of operation (procedure) intended for another patient
Performance of operation (procedure) on wrong patient

E876.7 Performance of correct operation (procedure) on wrong side/body part
Performance of correct operation (procedure) on wrong side
Performance of correct operation (procedure) on wrong site

E876.8 Other specified misadventures during medical care
Performance of inappropriate treatment NEC

E876.9 Unspecified misadventure during medical care

SURGICAL AND MEDICAL PROCEDURES AS THE CAUSE OF ABNORMAL REACTION OF PATIENT OR LATER COMPLICATION, WITHOUT MENTION OF MISADVENTURE AT THE TIME OF PROCEDURE (E878-E879)

Includes: procedures as the cause of abnormal reaction, such as:
displacement or malfunction of prosthetic device
hepatorenal failure, postoperative
malfunction of external stoma
postoperative intestinal obstruction
rejection of transplanted organ

Excludes: *anesthetic management properly carried out as the cause of adverse effect*
(E937.0-E938.9)
infusion and transfusion, without mention of misadventure in the technique of
procedure (E930.0-E949.9)

E878 Surgical operation and other surgical procedures as the cause of abnormal reaction of
patient, or of later complication, without mention of misadventure at the time of
operation

E878.0 Surgical operation with transplant of whole organ
Transplantation of:
heart
kidney
liver

E878.1 Surgical operation with implant of artificial internal device
Cardiac pacemaker   Heart valve prosthesis
Electrodes implanted in brain   Internal orthopedic device

Add 4th or
5th digit

Nonspecific
code

Unspecified
code

Manifestation
code

E878.2 Surgical operation with anastomosis, bypass, or graft, with natural or artificial tissues used as implant
Anastomosis: Graft of blood vessel, tendon, or skin
  arteriovenous
  gastrojejunal
Excludes: external stoma (E878.3)

E878.3 Surgical operation with formation of external stoma
Colostomy   Gastrostomy
Cystostomy   Ureterostomy
Duodenostomy

E878.4 Other restorative surgery

E878.5 Amputation of limb(s)

E878.6 Removal of other organ (partial) (total)

E878.8 Other specified surgical operations and procedures

E878.9 Unspecified surgical operations and procedures

E879 Other procedures, without mention of misadventure at the time of procedure, as the cause of abnormal reaction of patient, or of later complication

E879.0 Cardiac catheterization

E879.1 Kidney dialysis

E879.2 Radiological procedure and radiotherapy
Excludes: radio-opaque dyes for diagnostic x-ray procedures (E947.8)

E879.3 Shock therapy
Electroshock therapy   Insulin-shock therapy

E879.4 Aspiration of fluid
Lumbar puncture   Thoracentesis

E879.5 Insertion of gastric or duodenal sound

E879.6 Urinary catheterization

E879.7 Blood sampling

E879.8 Other specified procedures
Blood transfusion

E879.9 Unspecified procedure

ACCIDENTAL FALLS (E880-E888)

Excludes: falls (in or from):
  burning building (E890.8, E891.8)
  into fire (E890.0-E899)
  into water (with submersion or drowning) (E910.0-E910.9)
  machinery (in operation) (E919.0-E919.9)
  on edged, pointed, or sharp object (E920.0-E920.9)
  transport vehicle (E800.0-E845.9)
  vehicle not elsewhere classifiable (E846-E848)
ALERT! For coding late effects of accidental fall see E929.3
ALERT! For personal history of fall see V15.88

E880 Fall on or from stairs or steps

E880.0 Escalator

E880.1 Fall on or from sidewalk curb
Excludes: fall from moving sidewalk (E885.9)

E880.9 Other stairs or steps

E881 Fall on or from ladders or scaffolding

E881.0 Fall from ladder

E881.1 Fall from scaffolding

● Code new to 2012 edition   ▲ Revision of existing code   ④ ⑤ Fourth or fifth digit required

E882 Fall from or out of building or other structure

Fall from:	Fall from:
balcony	turret
bridge	viaduct
building	wall
flagpole	window
tower	Fall through roof

Excludes: collapse of a building or structure (E916)
fall or jump from burning building (E890.8, E891.8)

E883 Fall into hole or other opening in surface

Includes:

fall into:	fall into:
cavity	shaft
dock	swimming pool
hole	tank
pit	well
quarry	

Excludes: fall into water NOS (E910.9)
that resulting in drowning or submersion without mention of injury (E910.0-E910.9)

E883.0 Accident from diving or jumping into water [swimming pool]

Strike or hit:
against bottom when jumping or diving into water
wall or board of swimming pool
water surface

Excludes: diving with insufficient air supply (E913.2)
effects of air pressure from diving (E902.2)

E883.1 Accidental fall into well

E883.2 Accidental fall into storm drain or manhole

E883.9 Fall into other hole or other opening in surface

E884 Other fall from one level to another

E884.0 Fall from playground equipment

Excludes: recreational machinery (E919.8)

E884.1 Fall from cliff

E884.2 Fall from chair

E884.3 Fall from wheelchair

Fall from motorized mobility scooter
Fall from motorized wheelchair

E884.4 Fall from bed

E884.5 Fall from other furniture

E884.6 Fall from commode

Toilet

E884.9 Other fall from one level to another

Fall from:	Fall from:
embankment	stationary vehicle
haystack	tree

E885 Fall on same level from slipping, tripping, or stumbling

E885.0 Fall from (nonmotorized) scooter

Excludes: fall from motorized mobility scooter (E884.3)

E885.1 Fall from roller skates

Heelies
In-line skates
Wheelies

E885.2 Fall from skateboard

E885.3 Fall from skis

E885.4 Fall from snowboard

E885.9 Fall from other slipping, tripping or stumbling

Fall on moving sidewalk

E886 Fall on same level from collision, pushing, or shoving, by or with other person

Excludes: crushed or pushed by a crowd or human stampede (E917.1, E917.6)

	Add 4th or 5th digit		Nonspecific code		Unspecified code		Manifestation code

E886.0 In sports
Tackles in sports

Excludes: kicked, stepped on, struck by object, in sports (E917.0, E917.5)

E886.9 Other and unspecified
Fall from collision of pedestrian (conveyance) with another pedestrian (conveyance)

E887 Fracture, cause unspecified

E888 Other and unspecified fall
Accidental fall NOS
Fall on same level NOS

E888.0 Fall resulting in striking against sharp object
Use additional external cause code to identify object (E920)

E888.1 Fall resulting in striking against other object

E888.8 Other fall

E888.9 Unspecified fall
Fall NOS

ACCIDENTS CAUSED BY FIRE AND FLAMES (E890-E899)

Includes: asphyxia or poisoning due to conflagration or ignition
burning by fire
secondary fires resulting from explosion

Excludes: arson (E968.0)

fire in or on:
machinery (in operation) (E919.0-E919.9)
transport vehicle other than stationary vehicle (E800.0-E845.9)
vehicle not elsewhere classifiable (E846-E848)

ALERT! For coding late effects of accident caused by fire see E929.4

E890 Conflagration in private dwelling
Includes: conflagration in:
apartment
boarding house
camping place
caravan
farmhouse
house
lodging house
mobile home
private garage
rooming house
tenement
conflagration originating from sources classifiable to E893-E898 in the above
buildings

E890.0 Explosion caused by conflagration

E890.1 Fumes from combustion of polyvinylchloride [PVC] and similar material in conflagration

E890.2 Other smoke and fumes from conflagration
Carbon monoxide from conflagration in private building
Fumes NOS from conflagration in private building
Smoke NOS from conflagration in private building

E890.3 Burning caused by conflagration

E890.8 Other accident resulting from conflagration
Collapse of burning private building
Fall from burning private building
Hit by object falling from burning private building
Jump from burning private building

E890.9 Unspecified accident resulting from conflagration in private dwelling
ALERT! For coding late effects of unspecified accident see E929.9

● Code new
to 2012 edition
▲ Revision of
existing code
④ ⑤ Fourth or fifth
digit required

E891 **Conflagration in other and unspecified building or structure**

Conflagration in:

barn
church
convalescent and other
   residential home
dormitory of educational
   institution
factory

Conflagration in:

farm outbuildings
hospital
hotel
school
store
theater

Conflagration originating from sources classifiable to E893-E898, in the above buildings

E891.0 **Explosion caused by conflagration**

E891.1 **Fumes from combustion of polyvinylchloride [PVC] and similar material in conflagration**

E891.2 **Other smoke and fumes from conflagration**

Carbon monoxide from conflagration in building or structure
Fumes NOS from conflagration in building or structure
Smoke NOS from conflagration in building or structure

E891.3 **Burning caused by conflagration**

E891.8 **Other accident resulting from conflagration**

Collapse of burning building or structure
Fall from burning building or structure
Hit by object falling from burning building or structure
Jump from burning building or structure

E891.9 **Unspecified accident resulting from conflagration of other and unspecified building or structure**

ALERT! For coding late effects of unspecified accident see E929.9

E892 **Conflagration not in building or structure**

Fire (uncontrolled) (in) (of):

forest
grass
hay
lumber
mine
prairie
transport vehicle [any], except while in transit
tunnel

E893 **Accident caused by ignition of clothing**

Excludes: ignition of clothing:
    from highly inflammable material (E894)
    with conflagration (E890.0-E892)

E893.0 **From controlled fire in private dwelling**

Ignition of clothing from:
   normal fire (charcoal) (coal) (electric) (gas) (wood) in:
     brazier in private dwelling (as listed in E890)
     fireplace in private dwelling (as listed in E890)
     furnace in private dwelling (as listed in E890)
     stove in private dwelling (as listed in E890)

E893.1 **From controlled fire in other building or structure**

Ignition of clothing from:
   normal fire (charcoal) (coal) (electric) (gas) (wood) in:
     brazier in other building or structure (as listed in E891)
     fireplace in other building or structure (as listed in E891)
     furnace in other building or structure (as listed in E891)
     stove in other building or structure (as listed in E891)

E893.2 **From controlled fire not in building or structure**

Ignition of clothing from:
   bonfire (controlled)
   brazier fire (controlled), not in building or structure
   trash fire (controlled)

Excludes: conflagration not in building (E892)
    trash fire out of control (E892)

▓	Add 4th or 5th digit	▒	Nonspecific code	░	Unspecified code	▓ Manifestation code

E893.8 From other specified sources

Ignition of clothing from: Ignition of clothing from:
- blowlamp
- blowtorch
- burning bedspread
- candle
- cigar

- cigarette
- lighter
- matches
- pipe
- welding torch

E893.9 Unspecified source

Ignition of clothing (from controlled fire NOS) (in building NOS) NOS

E894 Ignition of highly inflammable material

Ignition of:
- benzine (with ignition of clothing)
- gasoline (with ignition of clothing)
- fat (with ignition of clothing)
- kerosene (with ignition of clothing)
- paraffin (with ignition of clothing)
- petrol (with ignition of clothing)

Excludes: *ignition of highly inflammable material with:*
> *conflagration (E890.0-E892)*
> *explosion (E923.0-E923.9)*

E895 Accident caused by controlled fire in private dwelling

Burning by (flame of) normal fire (charcoal) (coal) (electric) (gas) (wood) in:
- brazier in private dwelling (as listed in E890)
- fireplace in private dwelling (as listed in E890)
- furnace in private dwelling (as listed in E890)
- stove in private dwelling (as listed in E890)

Excludes: *burning by hot objects not producing fire or flames (E924.0-E924.9)*
> *ignition of clothing from these sources (E893.0)*
> *poisoning by carbon monoxide from incomplete combustion of fuel (E867-E868.9)*
> *that with conflagration (E890.0-E890.9)*

E896 Accident caused by controlled fire in other and unspecified building or structure

Burning by (flame of) normal fire (charcoal) (coal) (electric) (gas) (wood) in:
- brazier in other building or structure (as listed in E891)
- fireplace in other building or structure (as listed in E891)
- furnace in other building or structure (as listed in E891)
- stove in other building or structure (as listed in E891)

Excludes: *burning by hot objects not producing fire or flames (E924.0-E924.9)*
> *ignition of clothing from these sources (E893.1)*
> *poisoning by carbon monoxide from incomplete combustion of fuel (E867-E868.9)*
> *that with conflagration (E891.0-E891.9)*

E897 Accident caused by controlled fire not in building or structure

Burns from flame of:
- bonfire (controlled)
- brazier fire (controlled), not in building or structure
- trash fire (controlled)

Excludes: *ignition of clothing from these sources (E893.2)*
> *trash fire out of control (E892)*
> *that with conflagration (E892)*

E898 Accident caused by other specified fire and flames

Excludes: *conflagration (E890.0-E892)*
> *that with ignition of:*
> *clothing (E893.0-E893.9)*
> *highly inflammable material (E894)*

E898.0 Burning bedclothes

Bed set on fire NOS

E898.1 Other

Burning by: Burning by:
- blowlamp
- blowtorch
- candle
- cigar
- cigarette
- fire in room NOS

- lamp
- lighter
- matches
- pipe
- welding torch

E899 Accident caused by unspecified fire

Burning NOS

● Code new
  to 2012 edition
▲ Revision of
  existing code
④ ⑤ Fourth or fifth
    digit required

ACCIDENTS DUE TO NATURAL AND ENVIRONMENTAL FACTORS (E900-E909)

ALERT! For coding late effects of accident due to natural and environmental factors see E929.5

E900 **Excessive heat**

E900.0 **Due to weather conditions**
Excessive heat as the external cause of:
ictus solaris
siriasis
sunstroke

E900.1 **Of man-made origin**
Heat (in):   Heat (in):
boiler room   generated in transport vehicle
drying room   kitchen
factory
furnace room

E900.9 **Of unspecified origin**

E901 **Excessive cold**

E901.0 **Due to weather conditions**
Excessive cold as the cause of:
chilblains NOS
immersion foot

E901.1 **Of man-made origin**
Contact with or inhalation of:
dry ice
liquid air
liquid hydrogen
liquid nitrogen
Prolonged exposure in:
deep freeze unit
refrigerator

E901.8 **Other specified origin**

E901.9 **Of unspecified origin**

E902 **High and low air pressure and changes in air pressure**

E902.0 **Residence or prolonged visit at high altitude**
Residence or prolonged visit at high altitude as the cause of:
Acosta syndrome
Alpine sickness
altitude sickness
Andes disease
anoxia, hypoxia
barotitis, barodontalgia, barosinusitis, otitic barotrauma
hypobarism, hypobaropathy
mountain sickness
range disease

E902.1 **In aircraft**
Sudden change in air pressure in aircraft during ascent or descent as the cause of:
aeroneurosis
aviators' disease

E902.2 **Due to diving**
High air pressure from rapid descent in water as the cause of:
caisson disease
divers' disease
divers' palsy or paralysis
Reduction in atmospheric pressure while surfacing from deep water diving as the cause of:
caisson disease
divers' disease
divers' palsy or paralysis

E902.8 **Due to other specified causes**
Reduction in atmospheric pressure while surfacing from underground

E902.9 **Unspecified cause**

E903 Travel and motion

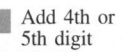 Add 4th or 5th digit   Nonspecific code   Unspecified code   Manifestation code

E904 Hunger, thirst, exposure, and neglect

Excludes: *any condition resulting from homicidal intent (E968.0-E968.9)*

hunger, thirst, and exposure resulting from accidents connected with transport (E800.0-E848)

E904.0 Abandonment or neglect of infants and helpless persons
Exposure to weather conditions resulting from abandonment or neglect
Hunger or thirst resulting from abandonment or neglect
Desertion of newborn
Inattention at or after birth
Lack of care (helpless person) (infant)

Excludes: *criminal [purposeful] neglect (E968.4)*

E904.1 Lack of food
Lack of food as the cause of:
  inanition
  insufficient nourishment
  starvation

Excludes: *hunger resulting from abandonment or neglect (E904.0)*

E904.2 Lack of water
Lack of water as the cause of:
  dehydration
  inanition

Excludes: *dehydration due to acute fluid loss (276.51)*

E904.3 Exposure (to weather conditions), not elsewhere classifiable
Exposure NOS   Struck by hailstones
Humidity

Excludes: *struck by lightning (E907)*

E904.9 Privation, unqualified
Destitution

E905 Venomous animals and plants as the cause of poisoning and toxic reactions
Includes: chemical released by animal
          insects
          release of venom through fangs, hairs, spines, tentacles, and other venom
            apparatus

Excludes: *eating of poisonous animals or plants (E865.0-E865.9)*

E905.0 Venomous snakes and lizards
Cobra   Mamba
Copperhead snake   Rattlesnake
Coral snake   Sea snake
Fer de lance   Snake (venomous)
Gila monster   Viper
Krait   Water moccasin

Excludes: *bites of snakes and lizards known to be nonvenomous (E906.2)*

E905.1 Venomous spiders
Black widow spider   Tarantula (venomous)
Brown spider

E905.2 Scorpion

E905.3 Hornets, wasps, and bees
Yellow jacket

E905.4 Centipede and venomous millipede (tropical)

E905.5 Other venomous arthropods
Sting of:
  ant
  caterpillar

E905.6 Venomous marine animals and plants
Puncture by sea urchin spine   Sting of:
Sting of: nematocysts
  coral   sea anemone
  jelly fish   sea cucumber
                                  other marine animal or plant

Excludes: *bites and other injuries caused by nonvenomous marine animal (E906.2-E906.8)*

bite of sea snake (venomous) (E905.0)

● Code new   ▲ Revision of   ④ ⑤ Fourth or fifth
    to 2012 edition   existing code   digit required

E905.7 **Poisoning and toxic reactions caused by other plants**
Injection of poisons or toxins into or through skin by plant thorns, spines, or other mechanisms

Excludes: *puncture wound NOS by plant thorns or spines (E920.8)*

E905.8 **Other specified**

E905.9 **Unspecified**
Sting NOS   Venomous bite NOS

E906 **Other injury caused by animals**

Excludes: *poisoning and toxic reactions caused by venomous animals and insects (E905.0-E905.9)*
road vehicle accident involving animals (E827.0-E828.9)
tripping or falling over an animal (E885.9)

E906.0 **Dog bite**

E906.1 **Rat bite**

E906.2 **Bite of nonvenomous snakes and lizards**

E906.3 **Bite of other animal except arthropod**
Cats   Rodents, except rats
Moray eel   Shark

E906.4 **Bite of nonvenomous arthropod**
Insect bite NOS

E906.5 **Bite by unspecified animal**
Animal bite NOS

E906.8 **Other specified injury caused by animal**
Butted by animal
Fallen on by horse or other animal, not being ridden
Gored by animal
Implantation of quills of porcupine
Pecked by bird
Run over by animal, not being ridden
Stepped on by animal, not being ridden

Excludes: *injury by animal being ridden (E828.0-E828.9)*

E906.9 **Unspecified injury caused by animal**

E907 **Lightning**

Excludes: *injury from:*
fall of tree or other object caused by lightning (E916)
fire caused by lightning (E890.0-E892)

E908 **Cataclysmic storms, and floods resulting from storms**

Excludes: *collapse of dam or man-made structure causing flood (E909.3)*

E908.0 **Hurricane**
Storm surge
"Tidal wave" caused by storm action
Typhoon

E908.1 **Tornado**
Cyclone
Twisters

E908.2 **Floods**
Torrential rainfall
Flash flood

Excludes: *collapse of dam or man-made structure causing flood (909.3)*

E908.3 **Blizzard (snow) (ice)**

E908.4 **Dust storm**

E908.8 **Other cataclysmic storms**

E908.9 **Unspecified cataclysmic storms, and floods resulting from storms**
Storm NOS

E909 **Cataclysmic earth surface movements and eruptions**

Excludes: *"tidal wave" caused by storm action (E908.0)*
transport accident involving collision with avalanche or landslide not in motion (E800.0-E848)

Add 4th or   Nonspecific   Unspecified   Manifestation
5th digit   code   code   code

E909.0 **Earthquakes**

E909.1 **Volcanic eruptions**
Burns from lava
Ash inhalation

E909.2 **Avalanche, landslide, or mudslide**

E909.3 **Collapse of dam or man-made structure**

E909.4 **Tidal wave caused by earthquake**
Tidal wave NOS
Tsunami

Excludes: *tidal wave caused by tropical storm (E908.0)*

E909.8 **Other cataclysmic earth surface movements and eruptions**

E909.9 **Unspecified cataclysmic earth surface movements and eruptions**

ACCIDENTS CAUSED BY SUBMERSION, SUFFOCATION, AND FOREIGN BODIES (E910-E915)

E910 **Accidental drowning and submersion**
Includes: immersion
swimmers' cramp

Excludes: *diving accident (NOS) (resulting in injury except drowning) (E883.0)*
diving with insufficient air supply (E913.2)
drowning and submersion due to:
cataclysm (E908-E909)
machinery accident (E919.0-E919.9)
transport accident (E800.0-E845.9)
effect of high and low air pressure (E902.2)
injury from striking against objects while in running water (E917.2)

E910.0 **While water-skiing**
Fall from water skis with submersion or drowning

Excludes: *accident to water-skier involving a watercraft and resulting in submersion or other injury (E830.4, E831.4)*

E910.1 **While engaged in other sport or recreational activity with diving equipment**
Scuba diving NOS
Skin diving NOS
Underwater spear fishing NOS

E910.2 **While engaged in other sport or recreational activity without diving equipment**
Fishing or hunting, except from boat or with diving equipment
Ice skating
Playing in water
Surfboarding
Swimming NOS
Voluntarily jumping from boat, not involved in accident, for swim NOS
Wading in water

Excludes: *jumping into water to rescue another person (E910.3)*

E910.3 **While swimming or diving for purposes other than recreation or sport**
Marine salvage (with diving equipment)
Pearl diving (with diving equipment)
Placement of fishing nets (with diving equipment)
Rescue (attempt) of another person (with diving equipment)
Underwater construction or repairs (with diving equipment)

E910.4 **In bathtub**

E910.8 **Other accidental drowning or submersion**
Drowning in:
quenching tank
swimming pool

E910.9 **Unspecified accidental drowning or submersion**
Accidental fall into water NOS
Drowning NOS

● Code new
to 2012 edition
▲ Revision of
existing code
④ ⑤ Fourth or fifth
digit required

E911 Inhalation and ingestion of food causing obstruction of respiratory tract or suffocation
    Aspiration and inhalation of food [any] (into respiratory tract) NOS
    Asphyxia by food [including bone, seed in food, regurgitated food]
    Choked on food [including bone, seed in food, regurgitated food]
    Suffocation by food [including bone, seed in food, regurgitated food]
    Compression of trachea by food lodged in esophagus
    Interruption of respiration by food lodged in esophagus
    Obstruction of respiration by food lodged in esophagus
    Obstruction of pharynx by food (bolus)

> *Excludes:* *injury, except asphyxia and obstruction of respiratory passage, caused by food (E915)*
>   *obstruction of esophagus by food without mention of asphyxia or obstruction of respiratory passage (E915)*

E912 Inhalation and ingestion of other object causing obstruction of respiratory tract or suffocation
    Aspiration and inhalation of foreign body except food (into respiratory tract) NOS
    Foreign object [bean] [marble] in nose
    Obstruction of pharynx by foreign body
    Compression by foreign body in esophagus
    Interruption of respiration by foreign body in esophagus
    Obstruction of respiration by foreign body in esophagus

> *Excludes:* *injury, except asphyxia and obstruction of respiratory passage, caused by foreign body (E915)*
>   *obstruction of esophagus by foreign body without mention of asphyxia or obstruction in respiratory passage (E915)*

E913 Accidental mechanical suffocation

> *Excludes:* *mechanical suffocation from or by:*
>   *accidental inhalation or ingestion of:*
>   *food (E911)*
>   *foreign object (E912)*
>   *cataclysm (E908-E909)*
>   *explosion (E921.0-E921.9, E923.0-E923.9)*
>   *machinery accident (E919.0-E919.9)*

E913.0 In bed or cradle

> *Excludes:* *suffocation by plastic bag (E913.1)*

E913.1 By plastic bag

E913.2 Due to lack of air (in closed place)
    Accidentally closed up in refrigerator or other airtight enclosed space
    Diving with insufficient air supply

> *Excludes:* *suffocation by plastic bag (E913.1)*

E913.3 By falling earth or other substance
    Cave-in NOS

> *Excludes:* *cave-in caused by cataclysmic earth surface movements and eruptions (E909)*
>   *struck by cave-in without asphyxiation or suffocation (E916)*

E913.8 Other specified means
    Accidental hanging, except in bed or cradle

E913.9 Unspecified means
    Asphyxia, mechanical NOS
    Strangulation NOS
    Suffocation NOS

E914 Foreign body accidentally entering eye and adnexa

> *Excludes:* *corrosive liquid (E924.1)*

E915 Foreign body accidentally entering other orifice

> *Excludes:* *aspiration and inhalation of foreign body, any, (into respiratory tract) NOS (E911-E912)*

	Add 4th or 5th digit		Nonspecific code		Unspecified code		Manifestation code

OTHER ACCIDENTS (E916-E928)

E916 Struck accidentally by falling object

Collapse of building, except on fire
Falling:
  rock
  snowslide NOS
  stone
  tree

Object falling from:
  machine, not in operation
  stationary vehicle

Code first: collapse of building on fire (E890.0-E891.9)
falling object in:
  cataclysm (E908-E909)
  machinery accidents (E919.0-E919.9)
  transport accidents (E800.0-E845.9)
  vehicle accidents not elsewhere classifiable (E846-E848)
object set in motion by:
  explosion (E921.0-E921.9, E923.0-E923.9)
  firearm (E922.0-E922.9)
projected object (E917.0-E917.9)

ALERT! For coding late effects of other accidents see E929.8

E917 Striking against or struck accidentally by objects or persons

Includes: bumping into or against:
  object (moving) (projected) (stationary)
  pedestrian conveyance
  person
colliding with:
  object (moving) (projected) (stationary)
  pedestrian conveyance
  person
kicking against:
  object (moving) (projected) (stationary)
  pedestrian conveyance
  person
stepping on:
  object (moving) (projected) (stationary)
  pedestrian conveyance
  person
struck by:
  object (moving) (projected) (stationary)
  pedestrian conveyance
  person

[Excludes:] *fall from collision with another person, except when caused by a crowd (E886.0-E886.9)*
fall from stumbling over object (E885.9)
fall resulting in striking against object (E888.0, E888.1)
injury caused by:
  assault (E960.0-E960.1, E967.0-E967.9)
  cutting or piercing instrument (E920.0-E920.9)
  explosion (E921.0-E921.9, E923.0-E923.9)
  firearm (E922.0-E922.9)
  machinery (E919.0-E919.9)
  transport vehicle (E800.0-E845.9)
  vehicle not elsewhere classifiable (E846-E848)

E917.0 In sports without subsequent fall

Kicked or stepped on during game (football) (rugby)
Struck by hit or thrown ball
Struck by hockey stick or puck

E917.1 Caused by a crowd, by collective fear or panic without subsequent fall

Crushed by crown or human stampede
Pushed by crown or human stampede
Stepped on by crown or human stampede

E917.2 In running water without subsequent fall

[Excludes:] *drowning or submersion (E910.0-E910.9)*
that in sports (E917.0, E917.5)

E917.3 Furniture without subsequent fall

[Excludes:] *fall from furniture (E884.2, E884.4-E884.5)*

E917.4   Other stationary object without subsequent fall
Bath tub
Fence
Lamp-post

E917.5   Object in sports with subsequent fall
Knocked down while boxing

E917.6   Caused by a crowd, by collective fear or panic with subsequent fall

E917.7   Furniture with subsequent fall

Excludes: fall from furniture (E884.2, E884.4-E884.5)

E917.8   Other stationary object with subsequent fall
Bath tub
Fence
Lamp-post

E917.9   Other striking against with or without subsequent fall

E918   Caught accidentally in or between objects
Caught, crushed, jammed, or pinched in or between moving or stationary objects, such as:
escalator
folding object
hand tools, appliances, or implements
sliding door and door frame
under packing crate
washing machine wringer

Excludes: injury caused by:
    cutting or piercing instrument (E920.0-E920.9)
    machinery (E919.0-E919.9)
    mechanism or component of firearm and air gun (E928.7)
    transport vehicle (E800.0-E845.9)
    vehicle not elsewhere classifiable (E846-E848)
    struck accidentally by:
      falling object (E916)
      object (moving) (projected) (E917.0-E917.9)

E919   Accidents caused by machinery
Includes:
    burned by machinery (accident)
    caught in (moving parts of) machinery (accident)
    collapse of machinery (accident)
    crushed by machinery (accident)
    cut or pierced by machinery (accident)
    drowning or submersion caused by machinery (accident)
    explosion of, on, in machinery (accident)
    fall from or into moving part of machinery (accident)
    fire starting in or on machinery (accident)
    mechanical suffocation caused by machinery (accident)
    object falling from, on, in motion by machinery (accident)
    overturning of machinery (accident)
    pinned under machinery (accident)
    run over by machinery (accident)
    struck by machinery (accident)
    thrown from machinery (accident)
    caught between machinery and other object
    machinery accident NOS

Excludes: accidents involving machinery, not in operation (E884.9, E916-E918)
    injury caused by:
      electric current in connection with machinery (E925.0-E925.9)
      escalator (E880.0, E918)
      explosion of pressure vessel in connection with machinery (E921.0-E921.9)
      mechanism or component of firearm and air gun (E928.7)
      moving sidewalk (E885.9)
      powered hand tools, appliances, and implements (E916-E918, E920.0-E921.9,
        E923.0-E926.9)
      transport vehicle accidents involving machinery (E800.0-E848.9)
    poisoning by carbon monoxide generated by machine (E868.8)

Add 4th or   Nonspecific   Unspecified   Manifestation
5th digit   code   code   code

E919.0 Agriculture machines

Animal-powered agricultural machine	Farm tractor
	Harvester
Combine	Hay mower or rake
Derrick, hay	Reaper
Farm machinery NOS	Thresher

Excludes: *that in transport under own power on the highway (E810.0-E819.9)*
that being towed by another vehicle on the highway (E810.0-E819.9, E827.0-E827.9, E829.0-E829.9)
that involved in accident classifiable to E820-E829 (E820.0-E829.9)

E919.1 Mining and earth-drilling machinery

Bore or drill (land)	Shaft lift
(seabed)	Under-cutter
Shaft hoist	

Excludes: *coal car, tram, truck, and tub in mine (E846)*

E919.2 Lifting machines and appliances

Chain hoist except in agricultural or mining operations
Crane except in agricultural or mining operations
Derrick except in agricultural or mining operations
Elevator (building) (grain) except in agricultural or mining operations
Forklift truck except in agricultural or mining operations
Lift except in agricultural or mining operations
Pulley block except in agricultural or mining operations
Winch except in agricultural or mining operations

Excludes: *that being towed by another vehicle on the highway (E810.0-E819.9, E827.0-E827.9, E829.0-E829.9)*
that in transport under own power on the highway (E810.0-E819.9)
that involved in accident classifiable to E820-E829 (E820.0-E829.9)

E919.3 Metalworking machines

Abrasive wheel	Metal:
Forging machine	drilling machine
Lathe	milling machine
Mechanical shears	power press
	rolling-mill
	sawing machine

E919.4 Woodworking and forming machines

Band saw	Powered saw
Bench saw	Radial saw
Circular saw	Sander
Molding machine	
Overhead plane	

Excludes: *hand saw (E920.1)*

E919.5 Prime movers, except electrical motors

Gas turbine	Steam engine
Internal combustion engine	Water driven turbine

Excludes: *that being towed by other vehicle on the highway (E810.0-E819.9, E827.0-E827.9, E829.0-E829.9)*
that in transport under own power on the highway (E810.0-E819.9)

E919.6 Transmission machinery

Transmission:	Transmission:
belt	pinion
cable	pulley
chain	shaft
gear	

E919.7 Earth moving, scraping, and other excavating machines

Bulldozer	Steam shovel
Road scraper	

Excludes: *that being towed by other vehicle on the highway (E810.0-E819.9, E827.0-E827.9, E829.0-E829.9)*
that in transport under own power on the highway (E810.0-E819.9)

● Code new to 2012 edition   ▲ Revision of existing code   ④ ⑤ Fourth or fifth digit required

E919.8 **Other specified machinery**

Machines for manufacture of:	Printing machine
clothing	Recreational machinery
foodstuffs and beverages	Spinning, weaving, and textile machines
paper	

E919.9 **Unspecified machinery**

E920 **Accidents caused by cutting and piercing instruments or objects**
Includes: accidental injury (by) object:
   edged
   pointed
   sharp

Excludes: *injury caused by mechanism or component of firearm and air gun (E928.7)*

E920.0 **Powered lawn mower**

E920.1 **Other powered hand tools**
Any powered hand tool [compressed air] [electric] [explosive cartridge] [hydraulic power], such as:

drill	rivet gun
hand saw	snow blower
hedge clipper	staple gun

Excludes: *band saw (E919.4)*
   bench saw (E919.4)

E920.2 **Powered household appliances and implements**

Blender	Electric:
Electric:	knife
beater or mixer	sewing machine
can opener	Garbage disposal appliance
fan	

E920.3 **Knives, swords, and daggers**

E920.4 **Other hand tools and implements**

Axe	Paper cutter
Can opener NOS	Pitchfork
Chisel	Rake
Fork	Scissors
Hand saw	Screwdriver
Hoe	Sewing machine, not powered
Ice pick	Shovel
Needle (sewing)	

E920.5 **Hypodermic needle**
Contaminated needle
Needle stick

E920.8 **Other specified cutting and piercing instruments or objects**

Arrow	Nail
Broken glass	Plant thorn
Dart	Splinter
Edge of stiff paper	Tin can lid
Lathe turnings	

Excludes: *animal spines or quills (E906.8)*
   flying glass due to explosion (E921.0-E923.9)

E920.9 **Unspecified cutting and piercing instrument or object**

E921 **Accident caused by explosion of pressure vessel**
Includes: accidental explosion of pressure vessels, whether or not part of machinery
Excludes: *explosion of pressure vessel on transport vehicle (E800.0-E845.9)*

E921.0 **Boilers**

E921.1 **Gas cylinders**

| Air tank | Pressure gas tank |

E921.8 **Other specified pressure vessels**

| Aerosol can | Pressure cooker |
| Automobile tire | |

E921.9 **Unspecified pressure vessel**

| ▮ Add 4th or 5th digit | ▮ Nonspecific code | ▮ Unspecified code | ▮ Manifestation code |

E922 Accident caused by firearm and air gun missile

> Excludes: *injury caused by mechanism or component of firearm and air gun (E928.7)*

E922.0 **Handgun**

Pistol   Revolver

> Excludes: *Verey pistol (E922.8)*

E922.1 **Shotgun (automatic)**

E922.2 **Hunting rifle**

E922.3 **Military firearms**

Army rifle   Machine gun

E922.4 **Air gun**

BB gun   Pellet gun

E922.5 **Paintball gun**

E922.8 Other specified firearm missile

Verey pistol [flare]

E922.9 Unspecified firearm missile

Gunshot wound NOS   Shot NOS

E923 Accident caused by explosive material

Includes: flash burns and other injuries resulting from explosion of explosive material
ignition of highly explosive material with explosion

> Excludes: *explosion:*
>
> *in or on machinery (E919.0-E919.9)*
> *on any transport vehicle, except stationary motor vehicle (E800.0-E848)*
> *with conflagration (E890.0, E891.0, E892)*
> *injury caused by mechanism or component of firearm and air gun (E928.7)*
> *secondary fires resulting from explosion (E890.0-E899)*

E923.0 **Fireworks**

E923.1 **Blasting materials**

Blasting cap   Explosive [any] used in blasting operations
Detonator
Dynamite

E923.2 **Explosive gases**

Acetylene   Fire damp
Butane   Gasoline fumes
Coal gas   Methane
Explosion in mine NOS   Propane

E923.8 Other explosive materials

Bomb   Torpedo
Explosive missile   Explosion in munitions:
Grenade   dump
Mine   factory
Shell

E923.9 Unspecified explosive material

Explosion NOS

E924 Accident caused by hot substance or object, caustic or corrosive material, and steam

> Excludes: *burning NOS (E899)*
>
> *chemical burn resulting from swallowing a corrosive substance (E860.0-E864.4)*
> *fire caused by these substances and objects (E890.0-E894)*
> *radiation burns (E926.0-E926.9)*
> *therapeutic misadventures (E870.0-E876.9)*

E924.0 **Hot liquids and vapors, including steam**

Burning or scalding by:
boiling water
hot or boiling liquids not primarily caustic or corrosive
liquid metal
steam
other hot vapor

> Excludes: *hot (boiling) tap water (E924.2)*

● Code new   ▲ Revision of   ④ ⑤ Fourth or fifth
to 2012 edition   existing code   digit required

E924.1 **Caustic and corrosive substances**
Burning by:
acid [any kind]
ammonia
caustic oven cleaner or other substance
corrosive substance
lye
vitriol

E924.2 **Hot (boiling) tap water**

E924.8 **Other**
Burning by:
heat from electric heating appliance
hot object NOS
light bulb
steam pipe

E924.9 **Unspecified**

E925 **Accident caused by electric current**
Includes: electric current from exposed wire, faulty appliance, high voltage cable, live rail,
or open electric socket as the cause of:
burn
cardiac fibrillation
convulsion
electric shock
electrocution
puncture wound
respiratory paralysis

Excludes: *burn by heat from electrical appliance (E924.8)*
lightning (E907)

E925.0 **Domestic wiring and appliances**

E925.1 **Electric power generating plants, distribution stations, transmission lines**
Broken power line

E925.2 **Industrial wiring, appliances, and electrical machinery**
Conductors
Control apparatus
Electrical equipment and machinery
Transformers

E925.8 **Other electric current**
Wiring and appliances in or on:
farm [not farmhouse]
outdoors
public building
residential institutions
schools

E925.9 **Unspecified electric current**
Burns or other injury from electric current NOS
Electric shock NOS
Electrocution NOS

E926 **Exposure to radiation**

Excludes: *abnormal reaction to or complication of treatment without mention of*
misadventure (E879.2)
atomic power plant malfunction in water transport (E838.0-E838.9)
misadventure to patient in surgical and medical procedures (E873.2-E873.3)
use of radiation in war operations (E996-E997.9)

| | Add 4th or 5th digit | | Nonspecific code | | Unspecified code | | Manifestation code |

E926.0   Radiofrequency radiation
Overexposure to:
microwave radiation from:
high-powered radio and television transmitters
industrial radiofrequency induction heaters
radar installations
radar radiation from:
high-powered radio and television transmitters
industrial radiofrequency induction heaters
radar installations
radiofrequency from:
high-powered radio and television transmitters
industrial radiofrequency induction heaters
radar installations
radiofrequency radiation [any] from:
high-powered radio and television transmitters
industrial radiofrequency induction heaters
radar installations

E926.1   Infra-red heaters and lamps
Exposure to infra-red radiation from heaters and lamps as the cause of:
blistering
burning
charring
inflammatory change

Excludes: *physical contact with heater or lamp (E924.8)*

E926.2   Visible and ultraviolet light sources
Arc lamps
Black light sources
Electrical welding arc
Oxygas welding torch
Sun rays
Tanning bed

Excludes: *excessive heat from these sources (E900.1-E900.9)*

E926.3   X-rays and other electromagnetic ionizing radiation
Gamma rays   X-rays (hard) (soft)

E926.4   Lasers

E926.5   Radioactive isotopes
Radiobiologicals   Radiopharmaceuticals

E926.8   Other specified radiation
Artificially accelerated beams of ionized particles generated by:
betatrons
synchrotrons

E926.9   Unspecified radiation
Radiation NOS

E927   Overexertion and strenuous and repetitive movements or loads
Use additional code to identify activity (E001-E030)

E927.0   Overexertion from sudden strenuous movement
Sudden trauma from strenuous movement

E927.1   Overexertion from prolonged static position
Overexertion from maintaining prolonged positions, such as:
holding
sitting
standing

E927.2   Excessive physical exertion from prolonged activity

E927.3   Cumulative trauma from repetitive motion
Cumulative trauma from repetitive movements

E927.4   Cumulative trauma from repetitive impact

E927.8   Other overexertion and strenuous and repetitive movements or loads

E927.9   Unspecified overexertion and strenuous and repetitive movements or loads

E928   Other and unspecified environmental and accidental causes

E928.0   Prolonged stay in weightless environment
Weightlessness in spacecraft (simulator)

● Code new   ▲ Revision of   ④ ⑤ Fourth or fifth
to 2012 edition   existing code   digit required

E928.1 Exposure to noise
Noise (pollution)
Sound waves
Supersonic waves

E928.2 Vibration

E928.3 Human bite

E928.4 External constriction caused by hair

E928.5 External constriction caused by other object

E928.6 Environmental exposure to harmful algae and toxins
Algae bloom NOS
Blue-green algae bloom
Brown tide
Cyanobacteria bloom
Florida red tide
Harmful algae bloom
Pfiesteria piscicida
Red tide

E928.7 Mechanism or component of firearm and air gun
Injury due to:
 explosion of gun parts
 recoil
Pierced, cut, crushed, or pinched by slide trigger mechanism, scope or other gun part
Powder burn from firearm or air gun

Excludes: *accident caused by firearm and air gun missile (E922.0-E922.9)*

E928.8 Other

E928.9 Unspecified accident
Accident NOS stated as accidentally inflicted
Blow NOS stated as accidentally inflicted
Casualty (not due to war), stated as accidentally inflicted, but not otherwise specified
Decapitation, stated as accidentally inflicted, but not otherwise specified
Injury [any part of body, or unspecified], stated as accidentally inflicted, but not
 otherwise specified
Killed, stated as accidentally inflicted, but not otherwise specified
Knocked down, stated as accidentally inflicted, but not otherwise specified
Mangled, stated as accidentally inflicted, but not otherwise specified
Wound, stated as accidentally inflicted, but not otherwise specified

Excludes: *fracture, cause unspecified (E887)*
 injuries undetermined whether accidentally or purposely inflicted (E980.0-E989)

ALERT! For coding late effects of unspecified accident see E929.9

LATE EFFECTS OF ACCIDENTAL INJURY (E929)

Note: This category is to be used to indicate accidental injury as the cause of death or disability from late effects, which are themselves classifiable elsewhere. The "late effects" include conditions reported as such or as sequelae which may occur at any time after the acute injury.

E929 Late effects of accidental injury
Excludes: *late effects of:*
 surgical and medical procedures (E870.0-E879.9)
 therapeutic use of drugs and medicines (E930.0-E949.9)

E929.0 Late effects of motor vehicle accident
Late effects of accidents classifiable to E810-E825

E929.1 Late effects of other transport accident
Late effects of accidents classifiable to E800-E807, E826-E838, E840-E848

E929.2 Late effects of accidental poisoning
Late effects of accidents classifiable to E850-E858, E860-E869

E929.3 Late effects of accidental fall
Late effects of accidents classifiable to E880-E888

E929.4 Late effects of accident caused by fire
Late effects of accidents classifiable to E890-E899

E929.5 Late effects of accident due to natural and environmental factors
Late effects of accidents classifiable to E900-E909

E929.8 Late effects of other accidents
Late effects of accidents classifiable to E910-E928.8

	Add 4th or 5th digit		Nonspecific code		Unspecified code		Manifestation code

E929.9 Late effects of unspecified accident
Late effects of accidents classifiable to E928.9

DRUGS, MEDICINAL AND BIOLOGICAL SUBSTANCES CAUSING ADVERSE EFFECTS IN THERAPEUTIC USE (E930-E949)

Includes: correct drug properly administered in therapeutic or prophylactic dosage, as the cause of any adverse effect including allergic or hypersensitivity reactions

Excludes: *accidental overdose of drug and wrong drug given or taken in error (E850.0-E858.9)*
accidents in the technique of administration of drug or biological substance, such as accidental puncture during injection, or contamination of drug (E870.0-E876.9)
administration with suicidal or homicidal intent or intent to harm, or in circumstances classifiable to E950.0-E950.5, E962.0, E980.0-E980.5

See Alphabetic Index for more complete list of specific drugs to be classified under the fourth-digit subdivisions. The American Hospital Formulary numbers can be used to classify new drugs listed by the American Hospital Formulary Service (AHFS). See appendix C.

E930 Antibiotics

Excludes: *that used as eye, ear, nose, and throat [ENT], and local anti-infectives (E946.0-E946.9)*

DEFINITION An antibiotic is any substance that can destroy or inhibit the growth of bacteria and similar microorganisms

E930.0 Penicillins
Natural
Synthetic
Semisynthetic, such as:
ampicillin
cloxacillin
nafcillin
oxacillin

E930.1 Antifungal antibiotics
Amphotericin B
Griseofulvin
Hachimycin [trichomycin]
Nystatin

E930.2 Chloramphenicol group
Chloramphenicol
Thiamphenicol

E930.3 Erythromycin and other macrolides
Oleandomycin
Spiramycin

E930.4 Tetracycline group
Doxycycline
Minocycline
Oxytetracycline

E930.5 Cephalosporin group
Cephalexin
Cephaloglycin
Cephaloridine
Cephalothin

E930.6 Antimycobacterial antibiotics
Cycloserine
Kanamycin
Rifampin
Streptomycin

E930.7 Antineoplastic antibiotics
Actinomycins, such as:
Cactinomycin
Dactinomycin
Bleomycin
Daunorubicin
Mitomycin

Excludes: *other antineoplastic drugs (E933.1)*

● Code new
to 2012 edition
▲ Revision of
existing code
④ ⑤ Fourth or fifth
digit required

E930.8 Other specified antibiotics

E930.9 Unspecified antibiotic

E931 Other anti-infectives

> *Excludes:* ENT, and local anti-infectives (E946.0-E946.9)

E931.0 **Sulfonamides**
Sulfadiazine
Sulfafurazole
Sulfamethoxazole

E931.1 **Arsenical anti-infectives**

E931.2 **Heavy metal anti-infectives**
Compounds of:
antimony
bismuth
lead
mercury

> *Excludes:* mercurial diuretics (E944.0)

> **ALERT!** For personal history of contact with and (suspected) exposure to lead see V15.86

E931.3 **Quinoline and hydroxyquinoline derivatives**
Chiniofon
Diiodohydroxyquin

> *Excludes:* antimalarial drugs (E931.4)

E931.4 **Antimalarials and drugs acting on other blood protozoa**
Chloroquine phosphate   Proguanil [chloroguanide]
Cycloguanil   Pyrimethamine
Primaquine   Quinine (sulphate)

E931.5 **Other antiprotozoal drugs**
Emetine

E931.6 **Anthelmintics**
Hexylresorcinol   Piperazine
Male fern oleoresin Thiabendazole

E931.7 **Antiviral drugs**
Methisazone

> *Excludes:* amantadine (E936.4)
> cytarabine (E933.1)
> idoxuridine (E946.5)

E931.8 **Other antimycobacterial drugs**
Ethambutol   Para-aminosalicylic acid derivatives
Ethionamide   Sulfones
Isoniazid

E931.9 **Other and unspecified anti-infectives**
Flucytosine   Nitrofuran derivatives

E932 Hormones and synthetic substitutes

> **DEFINITION** Hormones are chemical substances having a specific regulatory effect on the activity of a certain organ or organs.

E932.0 **Adrenal cortical steroids**
Cortisone derivatives
Desoxycorticosterone derivatives
Fluorinated corticosteroids

> **ALERT!** For personal history of inhaled steroid therapy see V87.44

> **ALERT!** For personal history of systemic steroid therapy see V87.45

E932.1 **Androgens and anabolic congeners**
Nandrolone phenpropionate
Oxymetholone
Testosterone and preparations

E932.2 **Ovarian hormones and synthetic substitutes**
Contraceptives, oral
Estrogens
Estrogens and progestogens combined
Progestogens

> **ALERT!** For personal history of estrogen therapy see V87.43

	Add 4th or 5th digit		Nonspecific code		Unspecified code		Manifestation code

E932.3 Insulins and antidiabetic agents

Acetohexamide	Insulin
Biguanide derivatives, oral	Phenformin
Chlorpropamide	Sulfonylurea derivatives, oral
Glucagon	Tolbutamide

Excludes: adverse effect of insulin administered for shock therapy (E879.3)

E932.4 Anterior pituitary hormones

Corticotropin	Somatotropin [growth hormone]
Gonadotropin	

E932.5 Posterior pituitary hormones
Vasopressin

Excludes: oxytocic agents (E945.0)

E932.6 Parathyroid and parathyroid derivatives

E932.7 Thyroid and thyroid derivatives

Dextrothyroxine	Liothyronine
Levothyroxine sodium	Thyroglobulin

E932.8 Antithyroid agents

Iodides	Thiourea
Thiouracil	

E932.9 Other and unspecified hormones and synthetic substitutes

E933 Primarily systemic agents

E933.0 Antiallergic and antiemetic drugs

Antihistamines	Diphenylpyraline
Chlorpheniramine	Thonzylamine
Diphenhydramine	Tripelennamine

Excludes: phenothiazine-based tranquilizers (E939.1)

E933.1 Antineoplastic and immunosuppressive drugs

Azathioprine	Mechlorethamine hydrochloride
Busulfan	Mercaptopurine
Chlorambucil	Triethylenethiophosphoramide [thio-TEPA]
Cyclophosphamide	
Cytarabine	
Fluorouracil	

Excludes: antineoplastic antibiotics (E930.7)

ALERT! For personal history of antineoplastic chemotherapy see V87.41

ALERT! For personal history of immunosuppressive therapy see V87.46

E933.2 Acidifying agents

E933.3 Alkalizing agents

E933.4 Enzymes, not elsewhere classified
Penicillinase

E933.5 Vitamins, not elsewhere classified
Vitamin A
Vitamin D

Excludes: nicotinic acid (E942.2)
vitamin K (E934.3)

E933.6 Oral bisphosphonates

E933.7 Intravenous bisphosphonates

E933.8 Other systemic agents, not elsewhere classified
Heavy metal antagonists

E933.9 Unspecified systemic agent

E934 Agents primarily affecting blood constituents

E934.0 Iron and its compounds
Ferric salts
Ferrous sulphate and other ferrous salts

E934.1 Liver preparations and other antianemic agents
Folic acid

E934.2 Anticoagulants

Coumarin	Prothrombin synthesis inhibitor
Heparin	Warfarin sodium
Phenindione	

● Code new
to 2012 edition

▲ Revision of
existing code

④ ⑤ Fourth or fifth
digit required

E934.3 Vitamin K [phytonadione]

E934.4 Fibrinolysis-affecting drugs
Aminocaproic acid   Streptokinase
Streptodornase   Urokinase

E934.5 Anticoagulant antagonists and other coagulants
Hexadimethrine bromide   Protamine sulfate

E934.6 Gamma globulin

E934.7 Natural blood and blood products
Blood plasma   Packed red cells
Human fibrinogen   Whole blood

E934.8 Other agents affecting blood constituents
Macromolecular blood substitutes

E934.9 Unspecified agent affecting blood constituents

E935 Analgesics, antipyretics, and antirheumatics
DEFINITION Analgesics are drugs that reduce or eliminate pain. Antipyretics are drugs that reduce body temperature in situations such as fever. Antirheumatics are drugs that act against diseases with inflammation or pain in muscles or joints.

E935.0 Heroin
Diacetylmorphine

E935.1 Methadone

E935.2 Other opiates and related narcotics
Codeine [methylmorphine]   Opium (alkaloids)
Morphine   Meperidine [pethidine]

E935.3 Salicylates
Acetylsalicylic acid [aspirin]
Amino derivatives of salicylic acid
Salicylic acid salts

E935.4 Aromatic analgesics, not elsewhere classified
Acetanilid
Paracetamol [acetaminophen]
Phenacetin [acetophenetidin]

E935.5 Pyrazole derivatives
Aminophenazone [aminopyrine]
Phenylbutazone

E935.6 Antirheumatics [antiphlogistics]
Gold salts   Indomethacin

Excludes: salicylates (E935.3)
steroids (E932.0)

E935.7 Other non-narcotic analgesics
Pyrabital

E935.8 Other specified analgesics and antipyretics
Pentazocine

E935.9 Unspecified analgesic and antipyretic

E936 Anticonvulsants and anti-Parkinsonism drugs
DEFINITION Anticonvulsants are drugs used to prevent or treat seizures.

E936.0 Oxazolidine derivatives
Paramethadione
Trimethadione

E936.1 Hydantoin derivatives
Phenytoin

E936.2 Succinimides
Ethosuximide
Phensuximide

E936.3 Other and unspecified anticonvulsants
Beclamide
Primidone

E936.4 Anti-Parkinsonism drugs
Amantadine
Ethopropazine [profenamine]
Levodopa [L-dopa]

Add 4th or 5th digit   Nonspecific code   Unspecified code   Manifestation code

E937 **Sedatives and hypnotics**

E937.0 **Barbiturates**
Amobarbital [amylobarbitone]
Barbital [barbitone]
Butabarbital [butabarbitone]
Pentobarbital [pentobarbitone]
Phenobarbital [phenobarbitone]
Secobarbital [quinalbarbitone]

Excludes: thiobarbiturates (E938.3)

E937.1 **Chloral hydrate group**

E937.2 **Paraldehyde**

E937.3 **Bromine compounds**
Bromide
Carbromal (derivatives)

E937.4 **Methaqualone compounds**

E937.5 **Glutethimide group**

E937.6 **Mixed sedatives, not elsewhere classified**

E937.8 **Other sedatives and hypnotics**

E937.9 **Unspecified**
Sleeping:
drug NOS
pill NOS
tablet NOS

E938 **Other central nervous system depressants and anesthetics**

E938.0 **Central nervous system muscle-tone depressants**
Chlorphenesin (carbamate)   Methocarbamol
Mephenesin

E938.1 **Halothane**

E938.2 **Other gaseous anesthetics**
Ether
Halogenated hydrocarbon derivatives, except halothane
Nitrous oxide

E938.3 **Intravenous anesthetics**
Ketamine   Thiobarbiturates, such as thiopental sodium
Methohexital
[methohexitone]

E938.4 **Other and unspecified general anesthetics**

E938.5 **Surface and infiltration anesthetics**
Cocaine   Procaine
Lidocaine [lignocaine]   Tetracaine

E938.6 **Peripheral nerve- and plexus-blocking anesthetics**

E938.7 **Spinal anesthetics**

E938.9 **Other and unspecified local anesthetics**

E939 **Psychotropic agents**
DEFINITION Psychotropic agents are drugs that act primarily upon the central nervous system resulting in altered brain function, changes in perception, mood, consciousness and behavior.

E939.0 **Antidepressants**
Amitriptyline   Monoamine oxidase [MAO] inhibitors
Imipramine

E939.1 **Phenothiazine-based tranquilizers**
Chlorpromazine   Prochlorperazine
Fluphenazine   Promazine
Phenothiazine

E939.2 **Butyrophenone-based tranquilizers**
Haloperidol   Trifluperidol
Spiperone

E939.3 **Other antipsychotics, neuroleptics, and major tranquilizers**

E939.4 **Benzodiazepine-based tranquilizers**
Chlordiazepoxide   Lorazepam
Diazepam   Medazepam
Flurazepam   Nitrazepam

● Code new   ▲ Revision of   ④ ⑤ Fourth or fifth
      to 2012 edition   existing code   digit required

E939.5 **Other tranquilizers**
Hydroxyzine   Meprobamate

E939.6 **Psychodysleptics [hallucinogens]**
Cannabis (derivatives)   Mescaline
Lysergide [LSD]   Psilocin
Marijuana (derivatives)   Psilocybin

E939.7 **Psychostimulants**
Amphetamine   Caffeine

Excludes: central appetite depressants (E947.0)

E939.8 **Other psychotropic agents**

E939.9 **Unspecified psychotropic agent**

E940 **Central nervous system stimulants**

E940.0 **Analeptics**
Lobeline
Nikethamide

E940.1 **Opiate antagonists**
Levallorphan
Nalorphine
Naloxone

E940.8 **Other specified central nervous system stimulants**

E940.9 **Unspecified central nervous system stimulant**

E941 **Drugs primarily affecting the autonomic nervous system**

E941.0 **Parasympathomimetics [cholinergics]**
Acetylcholine   Pilocarpine
Anticholinesterase:
  organophosphorus
  reversible

E941.1 **Parasympatholytics [anticholinergics and antimuscarinics] and spasmolytics**
Atropine   Hyoscine [scopolamine]
Homatropine   Quaternary ammonium derivatives

Excludes: papaverine (E942.5)

E941.2 **Sympathomimetics [adrenergics]**
Epinephrine [adrenalin]
Levarterenol [noradrenalin]

E941.3 **Sympatholytics [antiadrenergics]**
Phenoxybenzamine
Tolazoline hydrochloride

E941.9 **Unspecified drug primarily affecting the autonomic nervous system**

E942 **Agents primarily affecting the cardiovascular system**

E942.0 **Cardiac rhythm regulators**
Practolol   Propranolol
Procainamide   Quinidine

E942.1 **Cardiotonic glycosides and drugs of similar action**
Digitalis glycosides   Strophanthins
Digoxin

E942.2 **Antilipemic and antiarteriosclerotic drugs**
Cholestyramine   Nicotinic acid derivatives
Clofibrate   Sitosterols

Excludes: dextrothyroxine (E932.7)

E942.3 **Ganglion-blocking agents**
Pentamethonium bromide

E942.4 **Coronary vasodilators**
Dipyridamole   Nitrites
Nitrates [nitroglycerin]   Prenylamine

E942.5 **Other vasodilators**
Cyclandelate   Hydralazine
Diazoxide   Papaverine

E942.6 **Other antihypertensive agents**
Clonidine   Rauwolfia alkaloids
Guanethidine   Reserpine

Add 4th or 5th digit   Nonspecific code   Unspecified code   Manifestation code

E942.7   Antivaricose drugs, including sclerosing agents
Monoethanolamine   Zinc salts

E942.8   Capillary-active drugs
Adrenochrome derivatives   Metaraminol
Bioflavonoids

E942.9   Other and unspecified agents primarily affecting the cardiovascular system

E943   Agents primarily affecting gastrointestinal system

E943.0   Antacids and antigastric secretion drugs
Aluminum hydroxide   Magnesium trisilicate

E943.1   Irritant cathartics
Bisacodyl   Phenolphthalein
Castor oil

E943.2   Emollient cathartics
Sodium dioctyl sulfosuccinate

E943.3   Other cathartics, including intestinal atonia drugs
Magnesium sulfate

E943.4   Digestants
Pancreatin   Pepsin
Papain

E943.5   Antidiarrheal drugs
Bismuth subcarbonate   Pectin
Kaolin

    Excludes: anti-infectives (E930.0-E931.9)

E943.6   Emetics

E943.8   Other specified agents primarily affecting the gastrointestinal system

E943.9   Unspecified agent primarily affecting the gastrointestinal system

E944   Water, mineral, and uric acid metabolism drugs

E944.0   Mercurial diuretics
Chlormerodrin   Mercurophylline
Mercaptomerin   Mersalyl

E944.1   Purine derivative diuretics
Theobromine   Theophylline

    Excludes: aminophylline [theophylline ethylenediamine] (E945.7)

E944.2   Carbonic acid anhydrase inhibitors
Acetazolamide

E944.3   Saluretics
Benzothiadiazides
Chlorothiazide group

E944.4   Other diuretics
Ethacrynic acid
Furosemide

E944.5   Electrolytic, caloric, and water-balance agents

E944.6   Other mineral salts, not elsewhere classified

E944.7   Uric acid metabolism drugs
Cinchophen and congeners   Phenoquin
Colchicine   Probenecid

E945   Agents primarily acting on the smooth and skeletal muscles and respiratory system

E945.0   Oxytocic agents
Ergot alkaloids
Prostaglandins

E945.1   Smooth muscle relaxants
Adiphenine
Metaproterenol [orciprenaline]

    Excludes: papaverine (E942.5)

E945.2   Skeletal muscle relaxants
Alcuronium chloride
Suxamethonium chloride

E945.3   Other and unspecified drugs acting on muscles

● Code new   ▲ Revision of   ④ ⑤ Fourth or fifth
        to 2012 edition   existing code   digit required

E945.4 **Antitussives**
Dextromethorphan
Pipazethate hydrochloride

E945.5 **Expectorants**
Acetylcysteine Ipecacuanha
Cocillana Terpin hydrate
Guaifenesin [glyceryl guaiacolate]

E945.6 **Anti-common cold drugs**

E945.7 **Antiasthmatics**
Aminophylline [theophylline ethylenediamine]

E945.8 **Other and unspecified respiratory drugs**

E946 **Agents primarily affecting skin and mucous membrane, ophthalmological, otorhinolaryngological, and dental drugs**

E946.0 **Local anti-infectives and anti-inflammatory drugs**

E946.1 **Antipruritics**

E946.2 **Local astringents and local detergents**

E946.3 **Emollients, demulcents, and protectants**

E946.4 **Keratolytics, keratoplastics, other hair treatment drugs and preparations**

E946.5 **Eye anti-infectives and other eye drugs**
Idoxuridine

E946.6 **Anti-infectives and other drugs and preparations for ear, nose, and throat**

E946.7 **Dental drugs topically applied**

E946.8 **Other agents primarily affecting skin and mucous membrane**
Spermicides

E946.9 **Unspecified agent primarily affecting skin and mucous membrane**

E947 **Other and unspecified drugs and medicinal substances**

E947.0 **Dietetics**

E947.1 **Lipotropic drugs**

E947.2 **Antidotes and chelating agents, not elsewhere classified**

E947.3 **Alcohol deterrents**

E947.4 **Pharmaceutical excipients**

E947.8 **Other drugs and medicinal substances**
Contrast media used for diagnostic x-ray procedures
Diagnostic agents and kits

ALERT! For personal history of allergy to radiographic dye see V15.08

E947.9 **Unspecified drug or medicinal substance**

E948 **Bacterial vaccines**

E948.0 **BCG vaccine**

E948.1 **Typhoid and paratyphoid**

E948.2 **Cholera**

E948.3 **Plague**

E948.4 **Tetanus**

E948.5 **Diphtheria**

E948.6 **Pertussis vaccine, including combinations with a pertussis component**

E948.8 **Other and unspecified bacterial vaccines**

E948.9 **Mixed bacterial vaccines, except combinations with a pertussis component**

E949 **Other vaccines and biological substances**

Excludes: gamma globulin (E934.6)

E949.0 **Smallpox vaccine**

E949.1 **Rabies vaccine**

E949.2 **Typhus vaccine**

E949.3 **Yellow fever vaccine**

E949.4 **Measles vaccine**

E949.5 **Poliomyelitis vaccine**

E949.6 **Other and unspecified viral and rickettsial vaccines**
Mumps vaccine

| | Add 4th or 5th digit | | Nonspecific code | | Unspecified code | | Manifestation code |

E949.7 Mixed viral-rickettsial and bacterial vaccines, except combinations with a pertussis component

Excludes: combinations with a pertussis component (E948.6)

E949.9 Other and unspecified vaccines and biological substances

SUICIDE AND SELF-INFLICTED INJURY (E950-E959)

Includes: injuries in suicide and attempted suicide
self-inflicted injuries specified as intentional

ALERT! For coding late effects of self-inflicted injury see E959

E950 Suicide and self-inflicted poisoning by solid or liquid substances

E950.0 Analgesics, antipyretics, and antirheumatics

E950.1 Barbiturates

E950.2 Other sedatives and hypnotics

E950.3 Tranquilizers and other psychotropic agents

E950.4 Other specified drugs and medicinal substances

E950.5 Unspecified drug or medicinal substances

E950.6 Agricultural and horticultural chemical and pharmaceutical preparations other than plant foods and fertilizers

E950.7 Corrosive and caustic substances
Suicide and self-inflicted poisoning by substances classifiable to E864

E950.8 Arsenic and its compounds

E950.9 Other and unspecified solid and liquid substances

E951 Suicide and self-inflicted poisoning by gases in domestic use

E951.0 Gas distributed by pipeline

E951.1 Liquefied petroleum gas distributed in mobile containers

E951.8 Other utility gas

E952 Suicide and self-inflicted poisoning by other gases and vapors

E952.0 Motor vehicle exhaust gas

E952.1 Other carbon monoxide

E952.8 Other specified gases and vapors

E952.9 Unspecified gases and vapors

E953 Suicide and self-inflicted injury by hanging, strangulation, and suffocation

E953.0 Hanging

E953.1 Suffocation by plastic bag

E953.8 Other specified means

E953.9 Unspecified means

E954 Suicide and self-inflicted injury by submersion [drowning]

E955 Suicide and self-inflicted injury by firearms, air guns and explosives

E955.0 Handgun

E955.1 Shotgun

E955.2 Hunting rifle

E955.3 Military firearms

E955.4 Other and unspecified firearm
Gunshot NOS
Shot NOS

E955.5 Explosives

E955.6 Air gun
BB gun
Pellet gun

E955.7 Paintball gun

E955.9 Unspecified

E956 Suicide and self-inflicted injury by cutting and piercing instrument

E957 Suicide and self-inflicted injuries by jumping from high place

E957.0 Residential premises

E957.1 Other man-made structures

● Code new
to 2012 edition
▲ Revision of
existing code
④ ⑤ Fourth or fifth
digit required

E957.2 Natural sites

E957.9 Unspecified

E958 Suicide and self-inflicted injury by other and unspecified means

  E958.0 Jumping or lying before moving object

  E958.1 Burns, fire

  E958.2 Scald

  E958.3 Extremes of cold

  E958.4 Electrocution

  E958.5 Crashing of motor vehicle

  E958.6 Crashing of aircraft

  E958.7 Caustic substances, except poisoning

     Excludes: *poisoning by caustic substance (E950.7)*

  E958.8 Other specified means

  E958.9 Unspecified means

E959 Late effects of self-inflicted injury

  Note: This category is to be used to indicate circumstances classifiable to E950-E958 as the cause of death or disability from late effects, which are themselves classifiable elsewhere. The "late effects" include conditions reported as such or as sequelae which may occur at any time after the attempted suicide or self-inflicted injury.

HOMICIDE AND INJURY PURPOSELY INFLICTED BY OTHER PERSONS (E960-E969)

  Includes: injuries inflicted by another person with intent to injure or kill, by any means

  Excludes: *injuries due to:*

      legal intervention (E970-E978)
      operations of war (E990-E999)
      terrorism (E979)

  ALERT! For coding late effects of injury purposely inflicted by other person see E969

E960 Fight, brawl, rape

  E960.0 Unarmed fight or brawl
     Beatings NOS
     Brawl or fight with hands, fists, feet
     Injured or killed in fight NOS

  Excludes: *homicidal:*

      injury by weapons (E965.0-E966, E969)
      strangulation (E963)
      submersion (E964)

  E960.1 Rape

E961 Assault by corrosive or caustic substance, except poisoning
  Injury or death purposely caused by corrosive or caustic substance, such as:
    acid [any]
    corrosive substance
    vitriol

  Excludes: *burns from hot liquid (E968.3)*

      chemical burns from swallowing a corrosive substance (E962.0-E962.9)

E962 Assault by poisoning

  E962.0 Drugs and medicinal substances
     Homicidal poisoning by any drug or medicinal substance

  E962.1 Other solid and liquid substances

  E962.2 Other gases and vapors

  E962.9 Unspecified poisoning

E963 Assault by hanging and strangulation
  Homicidal (attempt):
    garrotting or ligature
    hanging
    strangulation
    suffocation

E964 Assault by submersion [drowning]

E965 Assault by firearms and explosives

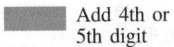 Add 4th or 5th digit   Nonspecific code   Unspecified code   Manifestation code

E965.0 Handgun
Pistol
Revolver

E965.1 Shotgun

E965.2 Hunting rifle

E965.3 Military firearms

E965.4 Other and unspecified firearm

E965.5 Antipersonnel bomb

E965.6 Gasoline bomb

E965.7 Letter bomb

E965.8 Other specified explosive
Bomb NOS (placed in) car
Bomb NOS (placed in) house
Dynamite

E965.9 Unspecified explosive

E966 Assault by cutting and piercing instrument
Assassination (attempt), homicide (attempt) by any instrument classifiable under E920
Homicidal cut, any part of the body
Homicidal puncture, any part of the body
Homicidal stab, any part of the body
Stabbed, any part of the body

E967 Perpetrator of child and adult abuse
Note: selection of the correct perpetrator code is based on the relationship between the
perpetrator and the victim

E967.0 By father, stepfather or boyfriend
Male partner of child's parent or guardian

E967.1 By other specified person

E967.2 By mother, stepmother or girlfriend
Female partner of child's parent or guardian

E967.3 By spouse or partner
Abuse of spouse or partner by ex-spouse or ex-partner

E967.4 By child

E967.5 By sibling

E967.6 By grandparent

E967.7 By other relative

E967.8 By non-related caregiver

E967.9 By unspecified person

E968 Assault by other and unspecified means

E968.0 Fire
Arson
Homicidal burns NOS

Excludes: burns from hot liquid (E968.3)

E968.1 Pushing from a high place

E968.2 Striking by blunt or thrown object

E968.3 Hot liquid
Homicidal burns by scalding

E968.4 Criminal neglect
Abandonment of child, infant, or other helpless person with intent to injure or kill

E968.5 Transport vehicle
Being struck by other vehicle or run down with intent to injure
Pushed in front of, thrown from, or dragged by moving vehicle with intent to injure

E968.6 Air gun
BB gun
Pellet gun

E968.7 Human bite

E968.8 Other specified means

● Code new
to 2012 edition
▲ Revision of
existing code
④ ⑤ Fourth or fifth
digit required

E968.9 Unspecified means
Assassination (attempt) NOS
Homicidal (attempt):
  injury NOS
  wound NOS
Manslaughter (nonaccidental)
Murder (attempt) NOS
Violence, non-accidental

E969 Late effects of injury purposely inflicted by other person
Note: This category is to be used to indicate circumstances classifiable to E960-E968 as the cause of death or disability from late effects, which are themselves classifiable elsewhere. The "late effects" include conditions reported as such, or as sequelae which may occur at any time after the acute injury.

LEGAL INTERVENTION (E970-E978)
Includes: injuries inflicted by the police or other law-enforcing agents, including military on duty, in the course of arresting or attempting to arrest lawbreakers, suppressing disturbances, maintaining order, and other legal action
            legal execution

Excludes: *injuries caused by civil insurrections (E990.0-E999)*

ALERT! For coding late effects of injuries due to legal intervention see E977

E970 Injury due to legal intervention by firearms
Gunshot wound
Injury by:
  machine gun
  revolver
  rifle pellet or rubber bullet
  shot NOS

E971 Injury due to legal intervention by explosives
Injury by:
  dynamite
  explosive shell
  grenade
  mortar bomb

E972 Injury due to legal intervention by gas
Asphyxiation by gas
Injury by tear gas
Poisoning by gas

E973 Injury due to legal intervention by blunt object
Hit, struck by:
  baton (nightstick)
  blunt object
  stave

E974 Injury due to legal intervention by cutting and piercing instrument
Cut
Incised wound
Injured by bayonet
Stab wound

E975 Injury due to legal intervention by other specified means
Blow
Manhandling

E976 Injury due to legal intervention by unspecified means

E977 Late effects of injuries due to legal intervention
Note: This category is to be used to indicate circumstances classifiable to E970-E976 as the cause of death or disability from late effects, which are themselves classifiable elsewhere. The "late effects" include conditions reported as such, or as sequelae which may occur at any time after the acute injury due to legal intervention.

E978 Legal execution
All executions performed at the behest of the judiciary or ruling authority [whether permanent or temporary] as:
asphyxiation by gas
beheading, decapitation
  (by guillotine)
capital punishment
electrocution
hanging
poisoning
shooting
other specified means

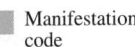

■ Add 4th or 5th digit   ■ Nonspecific code   ■ Unspecified code   ■ Manifestation code

TERRORISM (E979)

E979 Terrorism
Injuries resulting from the unlawful use of force or violence against persons or property to intimidate or coerce a Government, the civilian population, or any segment thereof, in furtherance of political or social objective

ALERT! For coding late effect of injury due to terrorism see E999.1

E979.0 Terrorism involving explosion of marine weapons
Depth-charge
Marine mine
Mine NOS, at sea or in harbor
Sea-based artillery shell
Torpedo
Underwater blast

E979.1 Terrorism involving destruction of aircraft
Aircraft used as a weapon
Aircraft:
  burned
  exploded
  shot down
Crushed by falling aircraft

E979.2 Terrorism involving other explosions and fragments
Antipersonnel bomb (fragments)
Blast NOS
Explosion (of):
  artillery shell
  breech-block
  cannon block
  mortar bomb
  munitions being used in terrorism
  NOS
Fragments from:
  artillery shell
  bomb
  grenade
  guided missile
  land-mine
  rocket
  shell
  shrapnel
Mine NOS

E979.3 Terrorism involving fires, conflagration and hot substances
Burning building or structure:
  collapse of
  fall from
  hit by falling object in
  jump from
Conflagration NOS
Fire (causing):
  asphyxia
  burns
  NOS
  other injury
Melting of fittings and furniture in burning
Petrol bomb
Smouldering building or structure

E979.4 Terrorism involving firearms
Bullet:
  carbine
  machine gun
  pistol
  rifle
  rubber (rifle)
Pellets (shotgun)

E979.5 Terrorism involving nuclear weapons
Blast effects
Exposure to ionizing radiation from nuclear weapon
Fireball effects
Heat from nuclear weapon
Other direct and secondary effects of nuclear weapons

● Code new to 2012 edition   ▲ Revision of existing code   ④ ⑤ Fourth or fifth digit required

E979.6 **Terrorism involving biological weapons**
    Anthrax
    Cholera
    Smallpox

E979.7 **Terrorism involving chemical weapons**
    Gases, fumes, chemicals
    Hydrogen cyanide
    Phosgene
    Sarin

E979.8 **Terrorism involving other means**
    Drowning and submersion
    Lasers
    Piercing or stabbing instruments
    Terrorism NOS

E979.9 **Terrorism, secondary effects**
Note: This code is for use to identify conditions occuring subsequent to a terrorist attack not those that are due to the intial terrorist act

> *Excludes:* *late effect of terroist attack (E999.1)*

INJURY UNDETERMINED WHETHER ACCIDENTALLY OR PURPOSELY INFLICTED (E980-E989)

Note: Categories E980-E989 are for use when it is unspecified or it cannot be determined whether the injuries are accidental (unintentional), suicide (attempted), or assault.

ALERT! For coding late effects of injury undetermined whether accidentally or purposely inflicted see E989

E980 **Poisoning by solid or liquid substances, undetermined whether accidentally or purposely inflicted**

E980.0 **Analgesics, antipyretics, and antirheumatics**

E980.1 **Barbiturates**

E980.2 **Other sedatives and hypnotics**

E980.3 **Tranquilizers and other psychotropic agents**

E980.4 **Other specified drugs and medicinal substances**

E980.5 **Unspecified drug or medicinal substance**

E980.6 **Corrosive and caustic substances**
    Poisoning, undetermined whether accidental or purposeful, by substances classifiable to E864

E980.7 **Agricultural and horticultural chemical and pharmaceutical preparations other than plant foods and fertilizers**

E980.8 **Arsenic and its compounds**

E980.9 **Other and unspecified solid and liquid substances**

E981 **Poisoning by gases in domestic use, undetermined whether accidentally or purposely inflicted**

E981.0 **Gas distributed by pipeline**

E981.1 **Liquefied petroleum gas distributed in mobile containers**

E981.8 **Other utility gas**

E982 **Poisoning by other gases, undetermined whether accidentally or purposely inflicted**

E982.0 **Motor vehicle exhaust gas**

E982.1 **Other carbon monoxide**

E982.8 **Other specified gases and vapors**

E982.9 **Unspecified gases and vapors**

E983 **Hanging, strangulation, or suffocation, undetermined whether accidentally or purposely inflicted**

E983.0 **Hanging**

E983.1 **Suffocation by plastic bag**

E983.8 **Other specified means**

E983.9 **Unspecified means**

E984 **Submersion [drowning], undetermined whether accidentally or purposely inflicted**

E985 **Injury by firearms, air guns and explosives, undetermined whether accidentally or purposely inflicted**

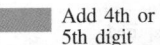
Add 4th or 5th digit   Nonspecific code   Unspecified code   Manifestation code

E985.0	Handgun
E985.1	Shotgun
E985.2	Hunting rifle
E985.3	Military firearms
E985.4	Other and unspecified firearm
E985.5	Explosives
E985.6	Air gun

        BB gun
        Pellet gun

| E985.7 | Paintball gun |

E986 **Injury by cutting and piercing instruments, undetermined whether accidentally or purposely inflicted**

E987	**Falling from high place, undetermined whether accidentally or purposely inflicted**
E987.0	Residential premises
E987.1	Other man-made structures
E987.2	Natural sites
E987.9	Unspecified site

E988 **Injury by other and unspecified means, undetermined whether accidentally or purposely inflicted**

E988.0	Jumping or lying before moving object
E988.1	Burns, fire
E988.2	Scald
E988.3	Extremes of cold
E988.4	Electrocution
E988.5	Crashing of motor vehicle
E988.6	Crashing of aircraft
E988.7	Caustic substances, except poisoning
E988.8	Other specified means
E988.9	Unspecified means

E989 **Late effects of injury, undetermined whether accidentally or purposely inflicted**

Note: This category is to be used to indicate circumstances classifiable to E980-E988 as the cause of death or disability from late effects, which are themselves classifiable elsewhere. The "late effects" include conditions reported as such or as sequelae which may occur at any time after the acute injury, undetermined whether accidentally or purposely inflicted.

INJURY RESULTING FROM OPERATIONS OF WAR (E990-E999)

Includes: injuries to military personnel and civilians caused by war and civil insurrections and occurring during the time of war and insurrection, and peacekeeping missions.

Excludes: *accidents during training of military personnel, manufacture of war material and transport, unless attributable to enemy action*

ALERT! For coding late effect of injury due to war operations see E999.0

E990 **Injury due to war operations by fires and conflagrations**
Includes: asphyxia, burns, or other injury originating from fire caused by a fire-producing device or indirectly by any conventional weapon

E990.0	From gasoline bomb

        Incendiary bomb

E990.1	From flamethrower
E990.2	From incendiary bullet
E990.3	From fire caused indirectly from conventional weapon

Excludes: *fire aboard military aircraft (E994.3)*

| **E990.9** | From other and unspecified source |

E991 **Injury due to war operations by bullets and fragments**

Excludes: *injury due to bullets and fragments due to war operations, but occurring after cessation of hostilities (E998.0)*
injury due to explosion of artillery shells and mortars (E993.2)
injury due to explosion of improvised explosive device [IED] (E993.3-E993.5)
injury due to sea-based artillery shell (E992.3)

● Code new
to 2012 edition

▲ Revision of
existing code

④ ⑤ Fourth or fifth
digit required

E991.0 **Rubber bullets (rifle)**

E991.1 **Pellets (rifle)**

E991.2 **Other bullets**
Bullet [any, except rubber bullets and pellets]
carbine
machine gun
pistol
rifle
shotgun

E991.3 **Antipersonnel bomb (fragments)**

E991.4 **Fragments from munitions**
Fragments from:
artillery shell
bombs, except antipersonnel
detonation of unexploded ordnance [UXO]
grenade
guided missile
land mine
rockets
shell

E991.5 **Fragments from person-borne improvised explosive device [IED]**

E991.6 **Fragments from vehicle-borne improvised explosive device [IED]**
IED borne by land, air, or water transport vehicle

E991.7 **Fragments from other improvised explosive device [IED]**
Roadside IED

E991.8 **Fragments from weapons**
Fragments from:
artillery
autocannons
automatic grenade launchers
missile launchers
mortars
small arms

E991.9 **Other and unspecified fragments**
Shrapnel NOS

E992 **Injury due to war operations by explosion of marine weapons**

E992.0 **Torpedo**

E992.1 **Depth charge**

E992.2 **Marine mines**
Marine mines at sea or in harbor

E992.3 **Sea-based artillery shell**

E992.8 **Other by other marine weapons**

E992.9 **Unspecified marine weapon**
Underwater blast NOS

E993 **Injury due to war operations by other explosion**
Injuries due to direct or indirect pressure or air blast of an explosion occurring during war operations

> Excludes: *injury due to fragments resulting from an explosion (E991.0-E991.9)*
> *injury due to detonation of unexploded ordnance but occurring after cessation of hostilities (E998.0-E998.9)*
> *injury due to nuclear weapons (E996.0-E996.9)*

E993.0 **Aerial bomb**

E993.1 **Guided missile**

E993.2 **Mortar**
Artillery shell

E993.3 **Person-borne improvised explosive device [IED]**

E993.4 **Vehicle-borne improvised explosive device [IED]**
IED borne by land, air, or water transport vehicle

E993.5 **Other improvised explosive device [IED]**
Roadside IED

E993.6 **Unintentional detonation of own munitions**
Unintentional detonation of own ammunition (artillery) (mortars)

	Add 4th or 5th digit		Nonspecific code		Unspecified code		Manifestation code

E993.7 Unintentional discharge of own munitions launch device
Unintentional explosion of own:
Autocannons
Automatic grenade launchers
Missile launchers
Small arms

E993.8 Other specified explosion
Bomb
Grenade
Land mine

E993.9 Unspecified explosion
Air blast NOS
Blast NOS
Blast wave NOS
Blast wind NOS
Explosion NOS

E994 Injury due to war operations by destruction of aircraft

E994.0 Destruction of aircraft due to enemy fire or explosives
Air to air missile
Explosive device placed on aircraft
Rocket propelled grenade [RPG]
Small arms fire
Surface to air missile

E994.1 Unintentional destruction of aircraft due to own onboard explosives

E994.2 Destruction of aircraft due to collision with other aircraft

E994.3 Destruction of aircraft due to onboard fire

E994.8 Other destruction of aircraft

E994.9 Unspecified destruction of aircraft

E995 Injury due to war operations by other and unspecified forms of conventional warfare

E995.0 Unarmed hand-to-hand combat
Excludes: intentional restriction of airway (E995.3)

E995.1 Struck by blunt object
Baton (nightstick)
Stave

E995.2 Piercing object
Bayonet
Knife
Sword

E995.3 Intentional restriction of air and airway
Intentional submersion
Strangulation
Suffocation

E995.4 Unintentional drowning due to inability to surface or obtain air
Submersion

E995.8 Other forms of conventional warfare

E995.9 Unspecified form of conventional warfare

E996 Injury due to war operations by nuclear weapons
Dirty bomb NOS
Excludes: late effects of injury due to nuclear weapons (E999.1, E999.0)

E996.0 Direct blast effect of nuclear weapon
Injury to bodily organs due to blast pressure

E996.1 Indirect blast effect of nuclear weapon
Injury due to being thrown by blast
Injury due to being struck or crushed by blast debris

E996.2 Thermal radiation effect of nuclear weapon
Burns due to thermal radiation
Fireball effects
Flash burns
Heat effects

● Code new
to 2012 edition ▲ Revision of
existing code ④ ⑤ Fourth or fifth
digit required

E996.3 **Nuclear radiation effects**
Acute radiation exposure
Beta burns
Fallout exposure
Radiation sickness
Secondary effects of nuclear weapons

E996.8 **Other effects of nuclear weapons**

E996.9 **Unspecified effect of nuclear weapon**

E997 **Injury due to war operations by other forms of unconventional warfare**

E997.0 **Lasers**

E997.1 **Biological warfare**

E997.2 **Gases, fumes, and chemicals**

E997.3 **Weapon of mass destruction [WMD], unspecified**

E997.8 **Other specified forms of unconventional warfare**

E997.9 **Unspecified form of unconventional warfare**

E998 **Injury due to war operations but occurring after cessation of hostilities**
Injuries due to operations of war but occurring after cessation of hostilities by any means
classifiable under E990-E997
Injuries by explosion of bombs or mines placed in the course of operations of war, if the
explosion occurred after cessation of hostilities

E998.0 **Explosion of mines**

E998.1 **Explosion of bombs**

E998.8 **Injury due to other war operations but occurring after cessation of hostilities**

E998.9 **Injury due to unspecified war operations but occurring after cessation of hostilities**

E999 **Late effect of injury due to war operations and terrorism**
Note: This category is to be used to indicate circumstances classifiable to E979, E990-E998 as
the cause of death or disability from late effects, which are themselves classifiable
elsewhere. The "late effects" include conditions reported as such or as sequelae which
may occur at any time after the acute injury, resulting from operations of war or terrorism.

E999.0 **Late effect of injury due to war operations**

E999.1 **Late effect of injury due to terrorism**

| | Add 4th or 5th digit | | Nonspecific code | | Unspecified code | | Manifestation code |

This page intentionally left blank.

APPENDIX A:
MORPHOLOGY OF NEOPLASMS

The World Health Organization has published an adaptation of the International Classification of Diseases for oncology (ICD-O). It contains a coded nomenclature for the morphology of neoplasms, which is reproduced here for those who wish to use it in conjunction with Chapter 2 of the *International Classification of Diseases, 9th Revision, Clinical Modification.*

The morphology code numbers consist of five digits; the first four identify the histological type of the neoplasm and the fifth indicates its behavior. The one-digit behavior code is as follows:

/0 Benign

/1 Uncertain whether benign or malignant
  Borderline malignancy

/2 Carcinoma in situ
  Intraepithelial
  Noninfiltrating
  Noninvasive

/3 Malignant, primary site

/6 Malignant, metastatic site
  Secondary site

/9 Malignant, uncertain whether primary or metastatic site

In the nomenclature below, the morphology code numbers include the behavior code appropriate to the histological type of neoplasm, but this behavior code should be changed if other reported information makes this necessary. For example, "chordoma (M9370/3)" is assumed to be malignant; the term "benign chordoma" should be coded M9370/0. Similarly, "superficial spreading adenocarcinoma (M8143/3)" described as "noninvasive" should be coded M8143/2 and "melanoma (M8720/3)" described as "secondary" should be coded M8720/6.

The following table shows the correspondence between the morphology code and the different sections of Chapter 2:

Morphology code Histology/Behavior			ICD-9-CM Chapter 2
Any	0	210-229	Benign neoplasms
M8000-M8004	1	239	Neoplasms of unspecified nature
M8010+	1	235-238	Neoplasms of uncertain behavior
Any	2	230-234	Carcinoma in situ
Any	3	140-195	Malignant neoplasms, stated or presumed to be primary
		200-208	
Any	6	196-198	Malignant neoplasms, stated or presumed to be secondary

The ICD-O behavior digit /9 is inapplicable in an ICD context, since all malignant neoplasms are presumed to be primary (/3) or secondary (/6) according to other information on the medical record.

Only the first-listed term of the full ICD-O morphology nomenclature appears against each code number in the list below. The ICD-9-CM Alphabetical Index (Volume 2), however, includes all the ICD-O synonyms as well as a number of other morphological names still likely to be encountered on medical records but omitted from ICD-O as outdated or otherwise undesirable.

A coding difficulty sometimes arises where a morphological diagnosis contains two qualifying adjectives that have different code numbers. An example is "transitional cell epidermoid carcinoma." "Transitional cell carcinoma NOS" is M8120/3 and "epidermoid carcinoma NOS" is M8070/3. In such circumstances, the higher number (M8120/3 in this example) should be used, as it is usually more specific.

CODED NOMENCLATURE FOR MORPHOLOGY OF NEOPLASMS

M800   **Neoplasms NOS**
M8000/0   *Neoplasm, benign*
M8000/1   *Neoplasm, uncertain whether benign or malignant*
M8000/3   *Neoplasm, malignant*
M8000/6   *Neoplasm, metastatic*
M8000/9   *Neoplasm, malignant, uncertain whether primary or metastatic*
M8001/0   *Tumor cells, benign*
M8001/1   *Tumor cells, uncertain whether benign or malignant*
M8001/3   *Tumor cells, malignant*
M8002/3   *Malignant tumor, small cell type*
M8003/3   *Malignant tumor, giant cell type*
M8004/3   *Malignant tumor, fusiform cell type*

M801-M804   **Epithelial neoplasms NOS**
M8010/0   *Epithelial tumor, benign*
M8010/2   *Carcinoma in situ NOS*
M8010/3   *Carcinoma NOS*
M8010/6   *Carcinoma, metastatic NOS*
M8010/9   *Carcinomatosis*
M8011/0   *Epithelioma, benign*
M8011/3   *Epithelioma, malignant*
M8012/3   *Large cell carcinoma NOS*
M8020/3   *Carcinoma, undifferentiated type NOS*
M8021/3   *Carcinoma, anaplastic type NOS*
M8022/3   *Pleomorphic carcinoma*
M8030/3   *Giant cell and spindle cell carcinoma*
M8031/3   *Giant cell carcinoma*
M8032/3   *Spindle cell carcinoma*
M8033/3   *Pseudosarcomatous carcinoma*
M8034/3   *Polygonal cell carcinoma*
M8035/3   *Spheroidal cell carcinoma*
M8040/1   *Tumorlet*
M8041/3   *Small cell carcinoma NOS*
M8042/3   *Oat cell carcinoma*
M8043/3   *Small cell carcinoma, fusiform cell type*

M805-M808   **Papillary and squamous cell neoplasms**
M8050/0   *Papilloma NOS (except Papilloma of urinary bladder M8120/1)*
M8050/2   *Papillary carcinoma in situ*
M8050/3   *Papillary carcinoma NOS*
M8051/0   *Verrucous papilloma*
M8051/3   *Verrucous carcinoma NOS*
M8052/0   *Squamous cell papilloma*
M8052/3   *Papillary squamous cell carcinoma*
M8053/0   *Inverted papilloma*
M8060/0   *Papillomatosis NOS*
M8070/2   *Squamous cell carcinoma in situ NOS*
M8070/3   *Squamous cell carcinoma NOS*
M8070/6   *Squamous cell carcinoma, metastatic NOS*
M8071/3   *Squamous cell carcinoma, keratinizing type NOS*
M8072/3   *Squamous cell carcinoma, large cell, nonkeratinizing type*
M8073/3   *Squamous cell carcinoma, small cell, nonkeratinizing type*
M8074/3   *Squamous cell carcinoma, spindle cell type*
M8075/3   *Adenoid squamous cell carcinoma*
M8076/2   *Squamous cell carcinoma in situ with questionable stromal invasion*
M8076/3   *Squamous cell carcinoma, microinvasive*
M8080/2   *Queyrat's erythroplasia*
M8081/2   *Bowen's disease*
M8082/3   *Lymphoepithelial carcinoma*

M809-M811   **Basal cell neoplasms**
M8090/1   *Basal cell tumor*
M8090/3   *Basal cell carcinoma NOS*
M8091/3   *Multicentric basal cell carcinoma*
M8092/3   *Basal cell carcinoma, morphea type*
M8093/3   *Basal cell carcinoma, fibroepithelial type*
M8094/3   *Basosquamous carcinoma*
M8095/3   *Metatypical carcinoma*
M8096/0   *Intraepidermal epithelioma of Jadassohn*
M8100/0   *Trichoepithelioma*
M8101/0   *Trichofolliculoma*

| M8102/0 | *Tricholemmoma* |
| M8110/0 | *Pilomatrixoma* |

M812-M813 Transitional cell papillomas and carcinomas

M8120/0	*Transitional cell papilloma NOS*
M8120/1	*Urothelial papilloma*
M8120/2	*Transitional cell carcinoma in situ*
M8120/3	*Transitional cell carcinoma NOS*
M8121/0	*Schneiderian papilloma*
M8121/1	*Transitional cell papilloma, inverted type*
M8121/3	*Schneiderian carcinoma*
M8122/3	*Transitional cell carcinoma, spindle cell type*
M8123/3	*Basaloid carcinoma*
M8124/3	*Cloacogenic carcinoma*
M8130/3	*Papillary transitional cell carcinoma*

M814-M838 Adenomas and adenocarcinomas

M8140/0	*Adenoma NOS*
M8140/1	*Bronchial adenoma NOS*
M8140/2	*Adenocarcinoma in situ*
M8140/3	*Adenocarcinoma NOS*
M8140/6	*Adenocarcinoma, metastatic NOS*
M8141/3	*Scirrhous adenocarcinoma*
M8142/3	*Linitis plastica*
M8143/3	*Superficial spreading adenocarcinoma*
M8144/3	*Adenocarcinoma, intestinal type*
M8145/3	*Carcinoma, diffuse type*
M8146/0	*Monomorphic adenoma*
M8147/0	*Basal cell adenoma*
M8150/0	*Islet cell adenoma*
M8150/3	*Islet cell carcinoma*
M8151/0	*Insulinoma NOS*
M8151/3	*Insulinoma, malignant*
M8152/0	*Glucagonoma NOS*
M8152/3	*Glucagonoma, malignant*
M8153/1	*Gastrinoma NOS*
M8153/3	*Gastrinoma, malignant*
M8154/3	*Mixed islet cell and exocrine adenocarcinoma*
M8160/0	*Bile duct adenoma*
M8160/3	*Cholangiocarcinoma*
M8161/0	*Bile duct cystadenoma*
M8161/3	*Bile duct cystadenocarcinoma*
M8170/0	*Liver cell adenoma*
M8170/3	*Hepatocellular carcinoma NOS*
M8180/0	*Hepatocholangioma, benign*
M8180/3	*Combined hepatocellular carcinoma and cholangiocarcinoma*
M8190/0	*Trabecular adenoma*
M8190/3	*Trabecular adenocarcinoma*
M8191/0	*Embryonal adenoma*
M8200/0	*Eccrine dermal cylindroma*
M8200/3	*Adenoid cystic carcinoma*
M8201/3	*Cribriform carcinoma*
M8210/0	*Adenomatous polyp NOS*
M8210/3	*Adenocarcinoma in adenomatous polyp*
M8211/0	*Tubular adenoma NOS*
M8211/3	*Tubular adenocarcinoma*
M8220/0	*Adenomatous polyposis coli*
M8220/3	*Adenocarcinoma in adenomatous polyposis coli*
M8221/0	*Multiple adenomatous polyps*
M8230/3	*Solid carcinoma NOS*
M8231/3	*Carcinoma simplex*
M8240/1	*Carcinoid tumor NOS*
M8240/3	*Carcinoid tumor, malignant*
M8241/1	*Carcinoid tumor, argentaffin NOS*
M8241/3	*Carcinoid tumor, argentaffin, malignant*
M8242/1	*Carcinoid tumor, nonargentaffin NOS*
M8242/3	*Carcinoid tumor, nonargentaffin, malignant*
M8243/3	*Mucocarcinoid tumor, malignant*
M8244/3	*Composite carcinoid*
M8250/1	*Pulmonary adenomatosis*
M8250/3	*Bronchiolo-alveolar adenocarcinoma*
M8251/0	*Alveolar adenoma*

M8251/3	*Alveolar adenocarcinoma*
M8260/0	*Papillary adenoma NOS*
M8260/3	*Papillary adenocarcinoma NOS*
M8261/1	*Villous adenoma NOS*
M8261/3	*Adenocarcinoma in villous adenoma*
M8262/3	*Villous adenocarcinoma*
M8263/0	*Tubulovillous adenoma*
M8270/0	*Chromophobe adenoma*
M8270/3	*Chromophobe carcinoma*
M8280/0	*Acidophil adenoma*
M8280/3	*Acidophil carcinoma*
M8281/0	*Mixed acidophil-basophil adenoma*
M8281/3	*Mixed acidophil-basophil carcinoma*
M8290/0	*Oxyphilic adenoma*
M8290/3	*Oxyphilic adenocarcinoma*
M8300/0	*Basophil adenoma*
M8300/3	*Basophil carcinoma*
M8310/0	*Clear cell adenoma*
M8310/3	*Clear cell adenocarcinoma NOS*
M8311/1	*Hypernephroid tumor*
M8312/3	*Renal cell carcinoma*
M8313/0	*Clear cell adenofibroma*
M8320/3	*Granular cell carcinoma*
M8321/0	*Chief cell adenoma*
M8322/0	*Water-clear cell adenoma*
M8322/3	*Water-clear cell adenocarcinoma*
M8323/0	*Mixed cell adenoma*
M8323/3	*Mixed cell adenocarcinoma*
M8324/0	*Lipoadenoma*
M8330/0	*Follicular adenoma*
M8330/3	*Follicular adenocarcinoma NOS*
M8331/3	*Follicular adenocarcinoma, well differentiated type*
M8332/3	*Follicular adenocarcinoma, trabecular type*
M8333/0	*Microfollicular adenoma*
M8334/0	*Macrofollicular adenoma*
M8340/3	*Papillary and follicular adenocarcinoma*
M8350/3	*Nonencapsulated sclerosing carcinoma*
M8360/1	*Multiple endocrine adenomas*
M8361/1	*Juxtaglomerular tumor*
M8370/0	*Adrenal cortical adenoma NOS*
M8370/3	*Adrenal cortical carcinoma*
M8371/0	*Adrenal cortical adenoma, compact cell type*
M8372/0	*Adrenal cortical adenoma, heavily pigmented variant*
M8373/0	*Adrenal cortical adenoma, clear cell type*
M8374/0	*Adrenal cortical adenoma, glomerulosa cell type*
M8375/0	*Adrenal cortical adenoma, mixed cell type*
M8380/0	*Endometrioid adenoma NOS*
M8380/1	*Endometrioid adenoma, borderline malignancy*
M8380/3	*Endometrioid carcinoma*
M8381/0	*Endometrioid adenofibroma NOS*
M8381/1	*Endometrioid adenofibroma, borderline malignancy*
M8381/3	*Endometrioid adenofibroma, malignant*
M839-M842	**Adnexal and skin appendage neoplasms**
M8390/0	*Skin appendage adenoma*
M8390/3	*Skin appendage carcinoma*
M8400/0	*Sweat gland adenoma*
M8400/1	*Sweat gland tumor NOS*
M8400/3	*Sweat gland adenocarcinoma*
M8401/0	*Apocrine adenoma*
M8401/3	*Apocrine adenocarcinoma*
M8402/0	*Eccrine acrospiroma*
M8403/0	*Eccrine spiradenoma*
M8404/0	*Hidrocystoma*
M8405/0	*Papillary hydradenoma*
M8406/0	*Papillary syringadenoma*
M8407/0	*Syringoma NOS*
M8410/0	*Sebaceous adenoma*
M8410/3	*Sebaceous adenocarcinoma*
M8420/0	*Ceruminous adenoma*
M8420/3	*Ceruminous adenocarcinoma*

M843 **Mucoepidermoid neoplasms**
M8430/1 *Mucoepidermoid tumor*
M8430/3 *Mucoepidermoid carcinoma*

M844-M849 **Cystic, mucinous, and serous neoplasms**
M8440/0 *Cystadenoma NOS*
M8440/3 *Cystadenocarcinoma NOS*
M8441/0 *Serous cystadenoma NOS*
M8441/1 *Serous cystadenoma, borderline malignancy*
M8441/3 *Serous cystadenocarcinoma NOS*
M8450/0 *Papillary cystadenoma NOS*
M8450/1 *Papillary cystadenoma, borderline malignancy*
M8450/3 *Papillary cystadenocarcinoma NOS*
M8460/0 *Papillary serous cystadenoma NOS*
M8460/1 *Papillary serous cystadenoma, borderline malignancy*
M8460/3 *Papillary serous cystadenocarcinoma*
M8461/0 *Serous surface papilloma NOS*
M8461/1 *Serous surface papilloma, borderline malignancy*
M8461/3 *Serous surface papillary carcinoma*
M8470/0 *Mucinous cystadenoma NOS*
M8470/1 *Mucinous cystadenoma, borderline malignancy*
M8470/3 *Mucinous cystadenocarcinoma NOS*
M8471/0 *Papillary mucinous cystadenoma NOS*
M8471/1 *Papillary mucinous cystadenoma, borderline malignancy*
M8471/3 *Papillary mucinous cystadenocarcinoma*
M8480/0 *Mucinous adenoma*
M8480/3 *Mucinous adenocarcinoma*
M8480/6 *Pseudomyxoma peritonei*
M8481/3 *Mucin-producing adenocarcinoma*
M8490/3 *Signet ring cell carcinoma*
M8490/6 *Metastatic signet ring cell carcinoma*

M850-M854 **Ductal, lobular, and medullary neoplasms**
M8500/2 *Intraductal carcinoma, noninfiltrating NOS*
M8500/3 *Infiltrating duct carcinoma*
M8501/2 *Comedocarcinoma, noninfiltrating*
M8501/3 *Comedocarcinoma NOS*
M8502/3 *Juvenile carcinoma of the breast*
M8503/0 *Intraductal papilloma*
M8503/2 *Noninfiltrating intraductal papillary adenocarcinoma*
M8504/0 *Intracystic papillary adenoma*
M8504/2 *Noninfiltrating intracystic carcinoma*
M8505/0 *Intraductal papillomatosis NOS*
M8506/0 *Subareolar duct papillomatosis*
M8510/3 *Medullary carcinoma NOS*
M8511/3 *Medullary carcinoma with amyloid stroma*
M8512/3 *Medullary carcinoma with lymphoid stroma*
M8520/2 *Lobular carcinoma in situ*
M8520/3 *Lobular carcinoma NOS*
M8521/3 *Infiltrating ductular carcinoma*
M8530/3 *Inflammatory carcinoma*
M8540/3 *Paget's disease, mammary*
M8541/3 *Paget's disease and infiltrating duct carcinoma of breast*
M8542/3 *Paget's disease, extramammary (except Paget's disease of bone)*

M855 **Acinar cell neoplasms**
M8550/0 *Acinar cell adenoma*
M8550/1 *Acinar cell tumor*
M8550/3 *Acinar cell carcinoma*

M856-M858 **Complex epithelial neoplasms**
M8560/3 *Adenosquamous carcinoma*
M8561/0 *Adenolymphoma*
M8570/3 *Adenocarcinoma with squamous metaplasia*
M8571/3 *Adenocarcinoma with cartilaginous and osseous metaplasia*
M8572/3 *Adenocarcinoma with spindle cell metaplasia*
M8573/3 *Adenocarcinoma with apocrine metaplasia*
M8580/0 *Thymoma, benign*
M8580/3 *Thymoma, malignant*

M859-M867 **Specialized gonadal neoplasms**
M8590/1 *Sex cord-stromal tumor*
M8600/0 *Thecoma NOS*
M8600/3 *Theca cell carcinoma*

M8610/0	*Luteoma NOS*
M8620/1	*Granulosa cell tumor NOS*
M8620/3	*Granulosa cell tumor, malignant*
M8621/1	*Granulosa cell-theca cell tumor*
M8630/0	*Androblastoma, benign*
M8630/1	*Androblastoma NOS*
M8630/3	*Androblastoma, malignant*
M8631/0	*Sertoli-Leydig cell tumor*
M8632/1	*Gynandroblastoma*
M8640/0	*Tubular androblastoma NOS*
M8640/3	*Sertoli cell carcinoma*
M8641/0	*Tubular androblastoma with lipid storage*
M8650/0	*Leydig cell tumor, benign*
M8650/1	*Leydig cell tumor NOS*
M8650/3	*Leydig cell tumor, malignant*
M8660/0	*Hilar cell tumor*
M8670/0	*Lipid cell tumor of ovary*
M8671/0	*Adrenal rest tumor*

M868-M871	**Paragangliomas and glomus tumors**
M8680/1	*Paraganglioma NOS*
M8680/3	*Paraganglioma, malignant*
M8681/1	*Sympathetic paraganglioma*
M8682/1	*Parasympathetic paraganglioma*
M8690/1	*Glomus jugulare tumor*
M8691/1	*Aortic body tumor*
M8692/1	*Carotid body tumor*
M8693/1	*Extra-adrenal paraganglioma NOS*
M8693/3	*Extra-adrenal paraganglioma, malignant*
M8700/0	*Pheochromocytoma NOS*
M8700/3	*Pheochromocytoma, malignant*
M8710/3	*Glomangiosarcoma*
M8711/0	*Glomus tumor*
M8712/0	*Glomangioma*

M872-M879	**Nevi and melanomas**
M8720/0	*Pigmented nevus NOS*
M8720/3	*Malignant melanoma NOS*
M8721/3	*Nodular melanoma*
M8722/0	*Balloon cell nevus*
M8722/3	*Balloon cell melanoma*
M8723/0	*Halo nevus*
M8724/0	*Fibrous papule of the nose*
M8725/0	*Neuronevus*
M8726/0	*Magnocellular nevus*
M8730/0	*Nonpigmented nevus*
M8730/3	*Amelanotic melanoma*
M8740/0	*Junctional nevus*
M8740/3	*Malignant melanoma in junctional nevus*
M8741/2	*Precancerous melanosis NOS*
M8741/3	*Malignant melanoma in precancerous melanosis*
M8742/2	*Hutchinson's melanotic freckle*
M8742/3	*Malignant melanoma in Hutchinson's melanotic freckle*
M8743/3	*Superficial spreading melanoma*
M8750/0	*Intradermal nevus*
M8760/0	*Compound nevus*
M8761/1	*Giant pigmented nevus*
M8761/3	*Malignant melanoma in giant pigmented nevus*
M8770/0	*Epithelioid and spindle cell nevus*
M8771/3	*Epithelioid cell melanoma*
M8772/3	*Spindle cell melanoma NOS*
M8773/3	*Spindle cell melanoma, type A*
M8774/3	*Spindle cell melanoma, type B*
M8775/3	*Mixed epithelioid and spindle cell melanoma*
M8780/0	*Blue nevus NOS*
M8780/3	*Blue nevus, malignant*
M8790/0	*Cellular blue nevus*

M880	**Soft tissue tumors and sarcomas NOS**
M8800/0	*Soft tissue tumor, benign*
M8800/3	*Sarcoma NOS*
M8800/9	*Sarcomatosis NOS*
M8801/3	*Spindle cell sarcoma*

M8802/3	*Giant cell sarcoma (except of bone M9250/3)*
M8803/3	*Small cell sarcoma*
M8804/3	*Epithelioid cell sarcoma*

M881-M883 Fibromatous neoplasms

M8810/0	*Fibroma NOS*
M8810/3	*Fibrosarcoma NOS*
M8811/0	*Fibromyxoma*
M8811/3	*Fibromyxosarcoma*
M8812/0	*Periosteal fibroma*
M8812/3	*Periosteal fibrosarcoma*
M8813/0	*Fascial fibroma*
M8813/3	*Fascial fibrosarcoma*
M8814/3	*Infantile fibrosarcoma*
M8820/0	*Elastofibroma*
M8821/1	*Aggressive fibromatosis*
M8822/1	*Abdominal fibromatosis*
M8823/1	*Desmoplastic fibroma*
M8830/0	*Fibrous histiocytoma NOS*
M8830/1	*Atypical fibrous histiocytoma*
M8830/3	*Fibrous histiocytoma, malignant*
M8831/0	*Fibroxanthoma NOS*
M8831/1	*Atypical fibroxanthoma*
M8831/3	*Fibroxanthoma, malignant*
M8832/0	*Dermatofibroma NOS*
M8832/1	*Dermatofibroma protuberans*
M8832/3	*Dermatofibrosarcoma NOS*

M884 Myxomatous neoplasms

| M8840/0 | *Myxoma NOS* |
| M8840/3 | *Myxosarcoma* |

M885-M888 Lipomatous neoplasms

M8850/0	*Lipoma NOS*
M8850/3	*Liposarcoma NOS*
M8851/0	*Fibrolipoma*
M8851/3	*Liposarcoma, well differentiated type*
M8852/0	*Fibromyxolipoma*
M8852/3	*Myxoid liposarcoma*
M8853/3	*Round cell liposarcoma*
M8854/3	*Pleomorphic liposarcoma*
M8855/3	*Mixed type liposarcoma*
M8856/0	*Intramuscular lipoma*
M8857/0	*Spindle cell lipoma*
M8860/0	*Angiomyolipoma*
M8860/3	*Angiomyoliposarcoma*
M8861/0	*Angiolipoma NOS*
M8861/1	*Angiolipoma, infiltrating*
M8870/0	*Myelolipoma*
M8880/0	*Hibernoma*
M8881/0	*Lipoblastomatosis*

M889-M892 Myomatous neoplasms

M8890/0	*Leiomyoma NOS*
M8890/1	*Intravascular leiomyomatosis*
M8890/3	*Leiomyosarcoma NOS*
M8891/1	*Epithelioid leiomyoma*
M8891/3	*Epithelioid leiomyosarcoma*
M8892/1	*Cellular leiomyoma*
M8893/0	*Bizarre leiomyoma*
M8894/0	*Angiomyoma*
M8894/3	*Angiomyosarcoma*
M8895/0	*Myoma*
M8895/3	*Myosarcoma*
M8900/0	*Rhabdomyoma NOS*
M8900/3	*Rhabdomyosarcoma NOS*
M8901/3	*Pleomorphic rhabdomyosarcoma*
M8902/3	*Mixed type rhabdomyosarcoma*
M8903/0	*Fetal rhabdomyoma*
M8904/0	*Adult rhabdomyoma*
M8910/3	*Embryonal rhabdomyosarcoma*
M8920/3	*Alveolar rhabdomyosarcoma*

M893-M899 Complex mixed and stromal neoplasms

M8930/3	*Endometrial stromal sarcoma*
M8931/1	*Endolymphatic stromal myosis*
M8932/0	*Adenomyoma*
M8940/0	*Pleomorphic adenoma*
M8940/3	*Mixed tumor, malignant NOS*
M8950/3	*Mullerian mixed tumor*
M8951/3	*Mesodermal mixed tumor*
M8960/1	*Mesoblastic nephroma*
M8960/3	*Nephroblastoma NOS*
M8961/3	*Epithelial nephroblastoma*
M8962/3	*Mesenchymal nephroblastoma*
M8970/3	*Hepatoblastoma*
M8980/3	*Carcinosarcoma NOS*
M8981/3	*Carcinosarcoma, embryonal type*
M8982/0	*Myoepithelioma*
M8990/0	*Mesenchymoma, benign*
M8990/1	*Mesenchymoma, NOS*
M8990/3	*Mesenchymoma, malignant*
M8991/3	*Embryonal sarcoma*

M900-M903 Fibroepithelial neoplasms

M9000/0	*Brenner tumor NOS*
M9000/1	*Brenner tumor, borderline malignancy*
M9000/3	*Brenner tumor, malignant*
M9010/0	*Fibroadenoma NOS*
M9011/0	*Intracanalicular fibroadenoma NOS*
M9012/0	*Pericanalicular fibroadenoma*
M9013/0	*Adenofibroma NOS*
M9014/0	*Serous adenofibroma*
M9015/0	*Mucinous adenofibroma*
M9020/0	*Cellular intracanalicular fibroadenoma*
M9020/1	*Cystosarcoma phyllodes NOS*
M9020/3	*Cystosarcoma phyllodes, malignant*
M9030/0	*Juvenile fibroadenoma*

M904 Synovial neoplasms

M9040/0	*Synovioma, benign*
M9040/3	*Synovial sarcoma NOS*
M9041/3	*Synovial sarcoma, spindle cell type*
M9042/3	*Synovial sarcoma, epithelioid cell type*
M9043/3	*Synovial sarcoma, biphasic type*
M9044/3	*Clear cell sarcoma of tendons and aponeuroses*

M905 Mesothelial neoplasms

M9050/0	*Mesothelioma, benign*
M9050/3	*Mesothelioma, malignant*
M9051/0	*Fibrous mesothelioma, benign*
M9051/3	*Fibrous mesothelioma, malignant*
M9052/0	*Epithelioid mesothelioma, benign*
M9052/3	*Epithelioid mesothelioma, malignant*
M9053/0	*Mesothelioma, biphasic type, benign*
M9053/3	*Mesothelioma, biphasic type, malignant*
M9054/0	*Adenomatoid tumor NOS*

M906-M909 Germ cell neoplasms

M9060/3	*Dysgerminoma*
M9061/3	*Seminoma NOS*
M9062/3	*Seminoma, anaplastic type*
M9063/3	*Spermatocytic seminoma*
M9064/3	*Germinoma*
M9070/3	*Embryonal carcinoma NOS*
M9071/3	*Endodermal sinus tumor*
M9072/3	*Polyembryoma*
M9073/1	*Gonadoblastoma*
M9080/0	*Teratoma, benign*
M9080/1	*Teratoma NOS*
M9080/3	*Teratoma, malignant NOS*
M9081/3	*Teratocarcinoma*
M9082/3	*Malignant teratoma, undifferentiated type*
M9083/3	*Malignant teratoma, intermediate type*
M9084/0	*Dermoid cyst*
M9084/3	*Dermoid cyst with malignant transformation*

M9090/0	*Struma ovarii NOS*
M9090/3	*Struma ovarii, malignant*
M9091/1	*Strumal carcinoid*

M910 **Trophoblastic neoplasms**
M9100/0	*Hydatidiform mole NOS*
M9100/1	*Invasive hydatidiform mole*
M9100/3	*Choriocarcinoma*
M9101/3	*Choriocarcinoma combined with teratoma*
M9102/3	*Malignant teratoma, trophoblastic*

M911 **Mesonephromas**
M9110/0	*Mesonephroma, benign*
M9110/1	*Mesonephric tumor*
M9110/3	*Mesonephroma, malignant*
M9111/1	*Endosalpingioma*

M912-M916 Blood vessel tumors
M9120/0	*Hemangioma NOS*
M9120/3	*Hemangiosarcoma*
M9121/0	*Cavernous hemangioma*
M9122/0	*Venous hemangioma*
M9123/0	*Racemose hemangioma*
M9124/3	*Kupffer cell sarcoma*
M9130/0	*Hemangioendothelioma, benign*
M9130/1	*Hemangioendothelioma NOS*
M9130/3	*Hemangioendothelioma, malignant*
M9131/0	*Capillary hemangioma*
M9132/0	*Intramuscular hemangioma*
M9140/3	*Kaposi's sarcoma*
M9141/0	*Angiokeratoma*
M9142/0	*Verrucous keratotic hemangioma*
M9150/0	*Hemangiopericytoma, benign*
M9150/1	*Hemangiopericytoma NOS*
M9150/3	*Hemangiopericytoma, malignant*
M9160/0	*Angiofibroma NOS*
M9161/1	*Hemangioblastoma*

M917 **Lymphatic vessel tumors**
M9170/0	*Lymphangioma NOS*
M9170/3	*Lymphangiosarcoma*
M9171/0	*Capillary lymphangioma*
M9172/0	*Cavernous lymphangioma*
M9173/0	*Cystic lymphangioma*
M9174/0	*Lymphangiomyoma*
M9174/1	*Lymphangiomyomatosis*
M9175/0	*Hemolymphangioma*

M918-M920 Osteomas and osteosarcomas
M9180/0	*Osteoma NOS*
M9180/3	*Osteosarcoma NOS*
M9181/3	*Chondroblastic osteosarcoma*
M9182/3	*Fibroblastic osteosarcoma*
M9183/3	*Telangiectatic osteosarcoma*
M9184/3	*Osteosarcoma in Paget's disease of bone*
M9190/3	*Juxtacortical osteosarcoma*
M9191/0	*Osteoid osteoma NOS*
M9200/0	*Osteoblastoma*

M921-M924 Chondromatous neoplasms
M9210/0	*Osteochondroma*
M9210/1	*Osteochondromatosis NOS*
M9220/0	*Chondroma NOS*
M9220/1	*Chondromatosis NOS*
M9220/3	*Chondrosarcoma NOS*
M9221/0	*Juxtacortical chondroma*
M9221/3	*Juxtacortical chondrosarcoma*
M9230/0	*Chondroblastoma NOS*
M9230/3	*Chondroblastoma, malignant*
M9240/3	*Mesenchymal chondrosarcoma*
M9241/0	*Chondromyxoid fibroma*

M925 **Giant cell tumors**
| M9250/1 | *Giant cell tumor of bone NOS* |
| M9250/3 | *Giant cell tumor of bone, malignant* |

M9251/1	*Giant cell tumor of soft parts NOS*
M9251/3	*Malignant giant cell tumor of soft parts*

M926   **Miscellaneous bone tumors**
M9260/3	*Ewing's sarcoma*
M9261/3	*Adamantinoma of long bones*
M9262/0	*Ossifying fibroma*

M927-M934 Odontogenic tumors
M9270/0	*Odontogenic tumor, benign*
M9270/1	*Odontogenic tumor NOS*
M9270/3	*Odontogenic tumor, malignant*
M9271/0	*Dentinoma*
M9272/0	*Cementoma NOS*
M9273/0	*Cementoblastoma, benign*
M9274/0	*Cementifying fibroma*
M9275/0	*Gigantiform cementoma*
M9280/0	*Odontoma NOS*
M9281/0	*Compound odontoma*
M9282/0	*Complex odontoma*
M9290/0	*Ameloblastic fibro-odontoma*
M9290/3	*Ameloblastic odontosarcoma*
M9300/0	*Adenomatoid odontogenic tumor*
M9301/0	*Calcifying odontogenic cyst*
M9310/0	*Ameloblastoma NOS*
M9310/3	*Ameloblastoma, malignant*
M9311/0	*Odontoameloblastoma*
M9312/0	*Squamous odontogenic tumor*
M9320/0	*Odontogenic myxoma*
M9321/0	*Odontogenic fibroma NOS*
M9330/0	*Ameloblastic fibroma*
M9330/3	*Ameloblastic fibrosarcoma*
M9340/0	*Calcifying epithelial odontogenic tumor*

M935-M937 Miscellaneous tumors
M9350/1	*Craniopharyngioma*
M9360/1	*Pinealoma*
M9361/1	*Pineocytoma*
M9362/3	*Pineoblastoma*
M9363/0	*Melanotic neuroectodermal tumor*
M9370/3	*Chordoma*

M938-M948 Gliomas
M9380/3	*Glioma, malignant*
M9381/3	*Gliomatosis cerebri*
M9382/3	*Mixed glioma*
M9383/1	*Subependymal glioma*
M9384/1	*Subependymal giant cell astrocytoma*
M9390/0	*Choroid plexus papilloma NOS*
M9390/3	*Choroid plexus papilloma, malignant*
M9391/3	*Ependymoma NOS*
M9392/3	*Ependymoma, anaplastic type*
M9393/1	*Papillary ependymoma*
M9394/1	*Myxopapillary ependymoma*
M9400/3	*Astrocytoma NOS*
M9401/3	*Astrocytoma, anaplastic type*
M9410/3	*Protoplasmic astrocytoma*
M9411/3	*Gemistocytic astrocytoma*
M9420/3	*Fibrillary astrocytoma*
M9421/3	*Pilocytic astrocytoma*
M9422/3	*Spongioblastoma NOS*
M9423/3	*Spongioblastoma polare*
M9430/3	*Astroblastoma*
M9440/3	*Glioblastoma NOS*
M9441/3	*Giant cell glioblastoma*
M9442/3	*Glioblastoma with sarcomatous component*
M9443/3	*Primitive polar spongioblastoma*
M9450/3	*Oligodendroglioma NOS*
M9451/3	*Oligodendroglioma, anaplastic type*
M9460/3	*Oligodendroblastoma*
M9470/3	*Medulloblastoma NOS*
M9471/3	*Desmoplastic medulloblastoma*
M9472/3	*Medullomyoblastoma*

M9480/3	*Cerebellar sarcoma NOS*
M9481/3	*Monstrocellular sarcoma*

M949-M952 Neuroepitheliomatous neoplasms

M9490/0	*Ganglioneuroma*
M9490/3	*Ganglioneuroblastoma*
M9491/0	*Ganglioneuromatosis*
M9500/3	*Neuroblastoma NOS*
M9501/3	*Medulloepithelioma NOS*
M9502/3	*Teratoid medulloepithelioma*
M9503/3	*Neuroepithelioma NOS*
M9504/3	*Spongioneuroblastoma*
M9505/1	*Ganglioglioma*
M9506/0	*Neurocytoma*
M9507/0	*Pacinian tumor*
M9510/3	*Retinoblastoma NOS*
M9511/3	*Retinoblastoma, differentiated type*
M9512/3	*Retinoblastoma, undifferentiated type*
M9520/3	*Olfactory neurogenic tumor*
M9521/3	*Esthesioneurocytoma*
M9522/3	*Esthesioneuroblastoma*
M9523/3	*Esthesioneuroepithelioma*

M953   **Meningiomas**

M9530/0	*Meningioma NOS*
M9530/1	*Meningiomatosis NOS*
M9530/3	*Meningioma, malignant*
M9531/0	*Meningotheliomatous meningioma*
M9532/0	*Fibrous meningioma*
M9533/0	*Psammomatous meningioma*
M9534/0	*Angiomatous meningioma*
M9535/0	*Hemangioblastic meningioma*
M9536/0	*Hemangiopericytic meningioma*
M9537/0	*Transitional meningioma*
M9538/1	*Papillary meningioma*
M9539/3	*Meningeal sarcomatosis*

M954-M957 Nerve sheath tumor

M9540/0	*Neurofibroma NOS*
M9540/1	*Neurofibromatosis NOS*
M9540/3	*Neurofibrosarcoma*
M9541/0	*Melanotic neurofibroma*
M9550/0	*Plexiform neurofibroma*
M9560/0	*Neurilemmoma NOS*
M9560/1	*Neurinomatosis*
M9560/3	*Neurilemmoma, malignant*
M9570/0	*Neuroma NOS*

M958   **Granular cell tumors and alveolar soft part sarcoma**

M9580/0	*Granular cell tumor NOS*
M9580/3	*Granular cell tumor, malignant*
M9581/3	*Alveolar soft part sarcoma*

M959-M963 Lymphomas, NOS or diffuse

M9590/0	*Lymphomatous tumor, benign*
M9590/3	*Malignant lymphoma NOS*
M9591/3	*Malignant lymphoma, non Hodgkin's type*
M9600/3	*Malignant lymphoma, undifferentiated cell type NOS*
M9601/3	*Malignant lymphoma, stem cell type*
M9602/3	*Malignant lymphoma, convoluted cell type NOS*
M9610/3	*Lymphosarcoma NOS*
M9611/3	*Malignant lymphoma, lymphoplasmacytoid type*
M9612/3	*Malignant lymphoma, immunoblastic type*
M9613/3	*Malignant lymphoma, mixed lymphocytic-histiocytic NOS*
M9614/3	*Malignant lymphoma, centroblastic-centrocytic, diffuse*
M9615/3	*Malignant lymphoma, follicular center cell NOS*
M9620/3	*Malignant lymphoma, lymphocytic, well differentiated NOS*
M9621/3	*Malignant lymphoma, lymphocytic, intermediate differentiation NOS*
M9622/3	*Malignant lymphoma, centrocytic*
M9623/3	*Malignant lymphoma, follicular center cell, cleaved NOS*
M9630/3	*Malignant lymphoma, lymphocytic, poorly differentiated NOS*
M9631/3	*Prolymphocytic lymphosarcoma*
M9632/3	*Malignant lymphoma, centroblastic type NOS*
M9633/3	*Malignant lymphoma, follicular center cell, noncleaved NOS*

M964   **Reticulosarcomas**
M9640/3   *Reticulosarcoma NOS*
M9641/3   *Reticulosarcoma, pleomorphic cell type*
M9642/3   *Reticulosarcoma, nodular*

M965-M966 Hodgkin's disease
M9650/3   *Hodgkin's disease NOS*
M9651/3   *Hodgkin's disease, lymphocytic predominance*
M9652/3   *Hodgkin's disease, mixed cellularity*
M9653/3   *Hodgkin's disease, lymphocytic depletion NOS*
M9654/3   *Hodgkin's disease, lymphocytic depletion, diffuse fibrosis*
M9655/3   *Hodgkin's disease, lymphocytic depletion, reticular type*
M9656/3   *Hodgkin's disease, nodular sclerosis NOS*
M9657/3   *Hodgkin's disease, nodular sclerosis, cellular phase*
M9660/3   *Hodgkin's paragranuloma*
M9661/3   *Hodgkin's granuloma*
M9662/3   *Hodgkin's sarcoma*

M969   **Lymphomas, nodular or follicular**
M9690/3   *Malignant lymphoma, nodular NOS*
M9691/3   *Malignant lymphoma, mixed lymphocytic-histiocytic, nodular*
M9692/3   *Malignant lymphoma, centroblastic-centrocytic, follicular*
M9693/3   *Malignant lymphoma, lymphocytic, well differentiated, nodular*
M9694/3   *Malignant lymphoma, lymphocytic, intermediate differentiation, nodular*
M9695/3   *Malignant lymphoma, follicular center cell, cleaved, follicular*
M9696/3   *Malignant lymphoma, lymphocytic, poorly differentiated, nodular*
M9697/3   *Malignant lymphoma, centroblastic type, follicular*
M9698/3   *Malignant lymphoma, follicular center cell, noncleaved, follicular*

M970   **Mycosis fungoides**
M9700/3   *Mycosis fungoides*
M9701/3   *Sezary's disease*

M971-M972 Miscellaneous reticuloendothelial neoplasms
M9710/3   *Microglioma*
M9720/3   *Malignant histiocytosis*
M9721/3   *Histiocytic medullary reticulosis*
M9722/3   *Letterer-Siwe's disease*

M973   **Plasma cell tumors**
M9730/3   *Plasma cell myeloma*
M9731/0   *Plasma cell tumor, benign*
M9731/1   *Plasmacytoma NOS*
M9731/3   *Plasma cell tumor, malignant*

M974   **Mast cell tumors**
M9740/1   *Mastocytoma NOS*
M9740/3   *Mast cell sarcoma*
M9741/3   *Malignant mastocytosis*

M975   **Burkitt's tumor**
M9750/3   *Burkitt's tumor*

M980-M994 Leukemias

M980   **Leukemias NOS**
M9800/3   *Leukemia NOS*
M9801/3   *Acute leukemia NOS*
M9802/3   *Subacute leukemia NOS*
M9803/3   *Chronic leukemia NOS*
M9804/3   *Aleukemic leukemia NOS*

M981   **Compound leukemias**
M9810/3   *Compound leukemia*

M982   **Lymphoid leukemias**
M9820/3   *Lymphoid leukemia NOS*
M9821/3   *Acute lymphoid leukemia*
M9822/3   *Subacute lymphoid leukemia*
M9823/3   *Chronic lymphoid leukemia*
M9824/3   *Aleukemic lymphoid leukemia*
M9825/3   *Prolymphocytic leukemia*

M983   **Plasma cell leukemias**
M9830/3   *Plasma cell leukemia*

M984   **Erythroleukemias**
M9840/3   *Erythroleukemia*
M9841/3   *Acute erythremia*

M9842/3	*Chronic erythremia*
M985	**Lymphosarcoma cell leukemias**
M9850/3	*Lymphosarcoma cell leukemia*
M986	**Myeloid leukemias**
M9860/3	*Myeloid leukemia NOS*
M9861/3	*Acute myeloid leukemia*
M9862/3	*Subacute myeloid leukemia*
M9863/3	*Chronic myeloid leukemia*
M9864/3	*Aleukemic myeloid leukemia*
M9865/3	*Neutrophilic leukemia*
M9866/3	*Acute promyelocytic leukemia*
M987	**Basophilic leukemias**
M9870/3	*Basophilic leukemia*
M988	**Eosinophilic leukemias**
M9880/3	*Eosinophilic leukemia*
M989	**Monocytic leukemias**
M9890/3	*Monocytic leukemia NOS*
M9891/3	*Acute monocytic leukemia*
M9892/3	*Subacute monocytic leukemia*
M9893/3	*Chronic monocytic leukemia*
M9894/3	*Aleukemic monocytic leukemia*
M990-M994	**Miscellaneous leukemias**
M9900/3	*Mast cell leukemia*
M9910/3	*Megakaryocytic leukemia*
M9920/3	*Megakaryocytic myelosis*
M9930/3	*Myeloid sarcoma*
M9940/3	*Hairy cell leukemia*
M995-M997	**Miscellaneous myeloproliferative and lymphoproliferative disorders**
M9950/1	*Polycythemia vera*
M9951/1	*Acute panmyelosis*
M9960/1	*Chronic myeloproliferative disease*
M9961/1	*Myelosclerosis with myeloid metaplasia*
M9962/1	*Idiopathic thrombocythemia*
M9970/1	*Chronic lymphoproliferative disease*

This page intentionally left blank.

APPENDIX B:
GLOSSARY OF MENTAL DISORDERS

Note: *Appendix B Glossary of Mental Disorders* has been removed from the official ICD-9-CM CD-Rom effective with the FY2005 update.

This page intentionally left blank.

APPENDIX C:
CLASSIFICATION OF DRUGS BY AMERICAN HOSPITAL FORMULARY SERVICE LIST NUMBER AND THEIR ICD-9-CM EQUIVALENTS

The coding of adverse effects of drugs is keyed to the continually revised Hospital Formulary of the American Hospital Formulary Service (AHFS) published under the direction of the American Society of Hospital Pharmacists.

AHFS*LIST	ICD-9-CM Diagnosis Code

The following section gives the ICD-9-CM diagnosis code for each AHFS list.

4:00	**ANTIHISTAMINE DRUGS**	963.0
8:00	**ANTI-INFECTIVE AGENTS**	
8:04	Amebacides	961.5
	hydroxyquinoline derivatives	961.3
	arsenical anti-infectives	961.1
8:08	Anthelmintics	961.6
	quinoline derivatives	961.3
8:12.04	Antifungal Antibiotics	960.1
	nonantibiotics	961.9
8:12.06	Cephalosporins	960.5
8:12.08	Chloramphenicol	960.2
8:12.12	The Erythromycins	960.3
8:12.16	The Penicillins	960.0
8:12.20	The Streptomycins	960.6
8:12.24	The Tetracyclines	960.4
8:12.28	Other Antibiotics	960.8
	antimycobacterial antibiotics	960.6
	macrolides	960.3
8:16	Antituberculars	961.8
	antibiotics	960.6
8:18	Antivirals	961.7
8:20	Plasmodicides (antimalarials)	961.4
8:24	Sulfonamides	961.0
8:26	The Sulfones	961.8
8:28	Treponemicides	961.2
8:32	Trichomonacides	961.5
	hydroxyquinoline derivatives	961.3
	nitrofuran derivatives	961.9
8:36	Urinary Germicides	961.9
	quinoline derivatives	961.3
8:40	Other Anti-Infectives	961.9
10:00	**ANTINEOPLASTIC AGENTS**	963.1
	antibiotics	960.7
	progestogens	962.2
12:00	**AUTONOMIC DRUGS**	
12:04	Parasympathomimetic (Cholinergic) Agents	971.0
12:08	Parasympatholytic (Cholinergic Blocking) Agents	971.1
12:12	Sympathomimetic (Adrenergic) Agents	971.2
12:16	Sympatholytic (Adrenergic Blocking) Agents	971.3

	AHFS*LIST	ICD-9-CM Diagnosis Code
12:20	Skeletal Muscle Relaxants	975.2
	central nervous system muscle-tone depressants	968.0
16:00	**BLOOD DERIVATIVES**	964.7
20:00	**BLOOD FORMATION AND COAGULATION**	
20:04	Antianemia Drugs	964.1
20:04.04	Iron Preparations	964.0
20:04.08	Liver and Stomach Preparations	964.1
20:12.04	Anticoagulants	964.2
20:12.08	Antiheparin agents	964.5
20:12.12	Coagulants	964.5
20:12.16	Hemostatics	964.5
	capillary-active drugs	972.8
	fibrinolysis-affecting agents	964.4
	natural products	964.7
24:00	**CARDIOVASCULAR DRUGS**	
24:04	Cardiac Drugs	972.9
	cardiotonic agents	972.1
	rhythm regulators	972.0
24:06	Antilipemic Agents	972.2
	thyroid derivatives	962.7
24:08	Hypotensive Agents	972.6
	adrenergic blocking agents	971.3
	ganglion-blocking agents	972.3
	vasodilators	972.5
24:12	Vasodilating Agents	972.5
	coronary	972.4
	nicotinic acid derivatives	972.2
24:16	Sclerosing Agents	972.7
28:00	**CENTRAL NERVOUS SYSTEM DRUGS**	
28:04	General Anesthetics	968.4
	gaseous anesthetics	968.2
	halothane	968.1
	intravenous anesthetics	968.3
28:08	Analgesics and Antipyretics	965.9
	antirheumatics	965.6
	aromatic analgesics	965.4
	non-narcotics NEC	965.7
	opium alkaloids	965.00
	heroin	965.01
	methadone	965.02
	specified type NEC	965.09
	pyrazole derivatives	965.5
	salicylates	965.1
	specified type NEC	965.8
28:10	Narcotic Antagonists	970.1
28:12	Anticonvulsants	966.3
	barbiturates	967.0
	benzodiazepine-based tranquilizers	969.4
	bromides	967.3
	hydantoin derivatives	966.1
	oxazolidine derivative	966.0
	succinimides	966.2
28:16.04	Antidepressants	969.0

	AHFS*LIST	ICD-9-CM Diagnosis Code
28:16.08	Tranquilizers	969.5
	benzodiazepine-based	969.4
	butyrophenone-based	969.2
	major NEC	969.3
	phenothiazine-based	969.1
28:16.12	Other Psychotherapeutic Agents	969.8
28:20	Respiratory and Cerebral Stimulants	970.9
	analeptics	970.0
	anorexigenic agents	977.0
	psychostimulants	969.7
	specified type NEC	970.8
28:24	Sedatives and Hypnotics	967.9
	barbiturates	967.0
	benzodiazepine-based tranquilizers	969.4
	chloral hydrate group	967.1
	glutethamide group	967.5
	intravenous anesthetics	968.3
	methaqualone	967.4
	paraldehyde	967.2
	phenothiazine-based tranquilizers	969.1
	specified type NEC	967.8
	thiobarbiturates	968.3
	tranquilizer NEC	969.5
36:00	**DIAGNOSTIC AGENTS**	977.8
40:00	**ELECTROLYTE, CALORIC, AND WATER BALANCE AGENTS NEC**	974.5
40:04	Acidifying Agents	963.2
40:08	Alkalinizing Agents	963.3
40:10	Ammonia Detoxicants	974.5
40:12	Replacement Solutions NEC	974.5
	plasma volume expanders	964.8
40:16	Sodium-Removing Resins	974.5
40:18	Potassium-Removing Resins	974.5
40:20	Caloric Agents	974.5
40:24	Salt and Sugar Substitutes	974.5
40:28	Diuretics NEC	974.4
	carbonic acid anhydrase inhibitors	974.2
	mercurials	974.0
	purine derivatives	974.1
	saluretics	974.3
40:36	Irrigating Solutions	974.5
40:40	Uricosuric Agents	974.7
44:00	**ENZYMES NEC**	963.4
	fibrinolysis-affecting agents	964.4
	gastric agents	973.4
48:00	**EXPECTORANTS AND COUGH PREPARATIONS**	
	antihistamine agents	963.0
	antitussives	975.4
	codeine derivatives	965.09
	expectorants	975.5
	narcotic agents NEC	965.09

	AHFS*LIST	ICD-9-CM Diagnosis Code
52:00	**EYE, EAR, NOSE, AND THROAT PREPARATIONS**	
52:04	Anti-Infectives	
	ENT	976.6
	ophthalmic	976.5
52:04.04	Antibiotics	
	ENT	976.6
	ophthalmic	976.5
52:04.06	Antivirals	
	ENT	976.6
	ophthalmic	976.5
52:04.08	Sulfonamides	
	ENT	976.6
	ophthalmic	976.5
52:04.12	Miscellaneous Anti-Infectives	
	ENT	976.6
	ophthalmic	976.5
52:08	Anti-Inflammatory Agents	
	ENT	976.6
	ophthalmic	976.5
52:10	Carbonic Anhydrase Inhibitors	974.2
52:12	Contact Lens Solutions	976.5
52:16	Local Anesthetics	968.5
52:20	Miotics	971.0
52:24	Mydriatics	
	adrenergics	971.2
	anticholinergics	971.1
	antimuscarinics	971.1
	parasympatholytics	971.1
	spasmolytics	971.1
	sympathomimetics	971.2
52:28	Mouth Washes and Gargles	976.6
52:32	Vasoconstrictors	971.2
52:36	Unclassified Agents	
	ENT	976.6
	ophthalmic	976.5
56:00	**GASTROINTESTINAL DRUGS**	
56:04	Antacids and Absorbants	973.0
56:08	Anti-Diarrhea Agents	973.5
56:10	Antiflatulents	973.8
56:12	Cathartics NEC	973.3
	emollients	973.2
	irritants	973.1
56:16	Digestants	973.4
56:20	Emetics and Antiemetics	
	antiemetics	963.0
	emetics	973.6
56:24	Lipotropic Agents	977.1
60:00	**GOLD COMPOUNDS**	965.6
64:00	**HEAVY METAL ANTAGONISTS**	963.8
68:00	**HORMONES AND SYNTHETIC SUBSTITUTES**	
68:04	Adrenals	962.0
68:08	Androgens	962.1

	AHFS*LIST	ICD-9-CM Diagnosis Code
68:12	Contraceptives	962.2
68:16	Estrogens	962.2
68:18	Gonadotropins	962.4
68:20	Insulins and Antidiabetic Agents	962.3
68:20.08	Insulins	962.3
68:24	Parathyroid	962.6
68:28	Pituitary	
	anterior	962.4
	posterior	962.5
68:32	Progestogens	962.2
68:34	Other Corpus Luteum Hormones	962.2
68:36	Thyroid and Antithyroid	
	antithyroid	962.8
	thyroid	962.7
72:00	**LOCAL ANESTHETICS NEC**	968.9
	topical (surface) agents	968.5
	infiltrating agents (intradermal) (subcutaneous) (submucosal)	968.5
	nerve blocking agents (peripheral) (plexus)(regional)	968.6
	spinal	968.7
76:00	**OXYTOCICS**	975.0
78:00	**RADIOACTIVE AGENTS**	990
80:00	**SERUMS, TOXOIDS, AND VACCINES**	
80:04	Serums	979.9
	immune globulin (gamma) (human)	964.6
80:08	Toxoids NEC	978.8
	diphtheria	978.5
	and tetanus	978.9
	with pertussis component	978.6
	tetanus	978.4
	and diphtheria	978.9
	with pertussis component	978.6
80:12	Vaccines NEC	979.9
	bacterial NEC	978.8
	with	
	other bacterial component	978.9
	pertussis component	978.6
	viral and rickettsial component	979.7
	rickettsial NEC	979.6
	with	
	bacterial component	979.7
	pertussis component	978.6
	viral component	979.7
	viral NEC	979.6
	with	
	bacterial component	979.7
	pertussis component	978.6
	rickettsial component	979.7
84:00	**SKIN AND MUCOUS MEMBRANE PREPARATIONS**	
84:04	Anti-Infectives	976.0
84:04.04	Antibiotics	976.0
84:04.08	Fungicides	976.0
84:04.12	Scabicides and Pediculicides	976.0
84:04.16	Miscellaneous Local Anti-Infectives	976.0

	AHFS*LIST	ICD-9-CM Diagnosis Code
84:06	Anti-Inflammatory Agents	976.0
84:08	Antipruritics and Local Anesthetics	
	antipruritics	976.1
	local anesthetics	968.5
84:12	Astringents	976.2
84:16	Cell Stimulants and Proliferants	976.8
84:20	Detergents	976.2
84:24	Emollients, Demulcents, and Protectants	976.3
84:28	Keratolytic Agents	976.4
84:32	Keratoplastic Agents	976.4
84:36	Miscellaneous Agents	976.8
86:00	**SPASMOLYTIC AGENTS**	975.1
	antiasthmatics	975.7
	papaverine	972.5
	theophyllin	974.1
88:00	**VITAMINS**	
88:04	Vitamin A	963.5
88:08	Vitamin B Complex	963.5
	hematopoietic vitamin	964.1
	nicotinic acid derivatives	972.2
88:12	Vitamin C	963.5
88:16	Vitamin D	963.5
88:20	Vitamin E	963.5
88:24	Vitamin K Activity	964.3
88:28	Multivitamin Preparations	963.5
92:00	**UNCLASSIFIED THERAPEUTIC AGENTS**	

APPENDIX D:
CLASSIFICATION OF INDUSTRIAL ACCIDENTS
ACCORDING TO AGENCY

Annex B to the Resolution concerning Statistics of Employment Injuries adopted by the Tenth International Conference of Labor Statisticians on 12 October 1962

1 MACHINES

11 Prime-Movers, except Electrical Motors
111 Steam engines
112 Internal combustion engines
119 Others

12 Transmission Machinery
121 Transmission shafts
122 Transmission belts, cables, pulleys, pinions, chains, gears
129 Others

13 Metalworking Machines
131 Power presses
132 Lathes
133 Milling machines
134 Abrasive wheels
135 Mechanical shears
136 Forging machines
137 Rolling-mills
139 Others

14 Wood and Assimilated Machines
141 Circular saws
142 Other saws
143 Molding machines
144 Overhand planes
149 Others

15 Agricultural Machines
151 Reapers (including combine reapers)
152 Threshers
159 Others

16 Mining Machinery
161 Under-cutters
169 Others

19 Other Machines Not Elsewhere Classified
191 Earth-moving machines, excavating and scraping machines, except means of transport
192 Spinning, weaving and other textile machines
193 Machines for the manufacture of foodstuffs and beverages
194 Machines for the manufacture of paper
195 Printing machines
199 Others

2 MEANS OF TRANSPORT AND LIFTING EQUIPMENT

21 Lifting Machines and Appliances
211 Cranes
212 Lifts and elevators
213 Winches
214 Pulley blocks
219 Others

22 Means of Rail Transport
221 Inter-urban railways
222 Rail transport in mines, tunnels, quarries, industrial establishments, docks, etc.
229 Others

23 Other Wheeled Means of Transport, Excluding Rail Transport
231 Tractors
232 Lorries

2 MEANS OF TRANSPORT AND LIFTING EQUIPMENT *continued*

233 Trucks
234 Motor vehicles, not elsewhere classified
235 Animal-drawn vehicles
236 Hand-drawn vehicles
239 Others

24 Means of Air Transport

25 Means of Water Transport
251 Motorized means of water transport
252 Non-motorized means of water transport

26 Other Means of Transport
261 Cable-cars
262 Mechanical conveyors, except cable-cars
269 Others

3 OTHER EQUIPMENT

31 Pressure Vessels
311 Boilers
312 Pressurized containers
313 Pressurized piping and accessories
314 Gas cylinders
315 Caissons, diving equipment
319 Others

32 Furnaces, Ovens, Kilns
321 Blast furnaces
322 Refining furnaces
323 Other furnaces
324 Kilns
325 Ovens

33 Refrigerating Plants

34 Electrical Installations, Including Electric Motors, but Excluding Electric Hand Tools
341 Rotating machines
342 Conductors
343 Transformers
344 Control apparatus
349 Others

35 Electric Hand Tools

36 Tools, Implements, and Appliances, Except Electric Hand Tools
361 Power-driven hand tools, except electric hand tools
362 Hand tools, not power-driven
369 Others

37 Ladders, Mobile Ramps

38 Scaffolding

39 Other Equipment, Not Elsewhere Classified

4 MATERIALS, SUBSTANCES AND RADIATIONS

41 Explosives

42 Dusts, Gases, Liquids and Chemicals, Excluding Explosives
421 Dusts
422 Gases, vapors, fumes
423 Liquids, not elsewhere classified
424 Chemicals, not elsewhere classified

43 Flying Fragments

44 Radiations
441 Ionizing radiations
449 Others

49 Other Materials and Substances Not Elsewhere Classified

5 WORKING ENVIRONMENT

51 Outdoor

511 Weather
512 Traffic and working surfaces
513 Water
519 Others

52 Indoor

521 Floors
522 Confined quarters
523 Stairs
524 Other traffic and working surfaces
525 Floor openings and wall openings
526 Environmental factors (lighting, ventilation, temperature, noise, etc.)
529 Others

53 Underground

531 Roofs and faces of mine roads and tunnels, etc.
532 Floors of mine roads and tunnels, etc.
533 Working-faces of mines, tunnels, etc.
534 Mine shafts
535 Fire
536 Water
539 Others

6 OTHER AGENCIES, NOT ELSEWHERE CLASSIFIED

61 Animals

611 Live animals
612 Animals products

69 Other Agencies, Not Elsewhere Classified

7 AGENCIES NOT CLASSIFIED FOR LACK OF SUFFICIENT DATA

This page intentionally left blank.

APPENDIX E:
LIST OF THREE-DIGIT CATEGORIES

1. INFECTIOUS AND PARASITIC DISEASES

Intestinal infectious diseases (001-009)
- 001 Cholera
- 002 Typhoid and paratyphoid fevers
- 003 Other salmonella infections
- 004 Shigellosis
- 005 Other food poisoning (bacterial)
- 006 Amebiasis
- 007 Other protozoal intestinal diseases
- 008 Intestinal infections due to other organisms
- 009 Ill-defined intestinal infections

Tuberculosis (010-018)
- 010 Primary tuberculous infection
- 011 Pulmonary tuberculosis
- 012 Other respiratory tuberculosis
- 013 Tuberculosis of meninges and central nervous system
- 014 Tuberculosis of intestines, peritoneum, and mesenteric glands
- 015 Tuberculosis of bones and joints
- 016 Tuberculosis of genitourinary system
- 017 Tuberculosis of other organs
- 018 Miliary tuberculosis

Zoonotic bacterial diseases (020-027)
- 020 Plague
- 021 Tularemia
- 022 Anthrax
- 023 Brucellosis
- 024 Glanders
- 025 Melioidosis
- 026 Rat-bite fever
- 027 Other zoonotic bacterial diseases

Other bacterial diseases (030-041)
- 030 Leprosy
- 031 Diseases due to other mycobacteria
- 032 Diphtheria
- 033 Whooping cough
- 034 Streptococcal sore throat and scarlet fever
- 035 Erysipelas
- 036 Meningococcal infection
- 037 Tetanus
- 038 Septicemia
- 039 Actinomycotic infections
- 040 Other bacterial diseases
- 041 Bacterial infection in conditions classified elsewhere and of unspecified site

Human immunodeficiency virus (HIV) infection (042)
- 042 Human immunodeficiency virus [HIV] disease

Poliomyelitis and other non-arthropod-borne viral diseases of central nervous system (045-049)
- 045 Acute poliomyelitis
- 046 Slow virus infections and prion diseases of central nervous system
- 047 Meningitis due to enterovirus
- 048 Other enterovirus diseases of central nervous system
- 049 Other non-arthropod-borne viral diseases of central nervous system

Viral diseases generally accompanied by exanthem (050-059)
- 050 Smallpox
- 051 Cowpox and paravaccinia
- 052 Chickenpox
- 053 Herpes zoster
- 054 Herpes simplex
- 055 Measles
- 056 Rubella

1. INFECTIOUS AND PARASITIC DISEASES *continued*

057　Other viral exanthemata
058　Other human herpesviruses
059　Other poxvirus infections

Arthropod-borne viral diseases (060-066)
060　Yellow fever
061　Dengue
062　Mosquito-borne viral encephalitis
063　Tick-borne viral encephalitis
064　Viral encephalitis transmitted by other and unspecified arthropods
065　Arthropod-borne hemorrhagic fever
066　Other arthropod-borne viral diseases

Other diseases due to viruses and Chlamydiae (070-079)
070　Viral hepatitis
071　Rabies
072　Mumps
073　Ornithosis
074　Specific diseases due to Coxsackie virus
075　Infectious mononucleosis
076　Trachoma
077　Other diseases of conjunctiva due to viruses and Chlamydiae
078　Other diseases due to viruses and Chlamydiae
079　Viral and Chlamydial infection in conditions classified elsewhere and of unspecified
　　　site

Rickettsioses and other arthropod-borne diseases (080-088)
080　Louse-borne [epidemic] typhus
081　Other typhus
082　Tick-borne rickettsioses
083　Other rickettsioses
084　Malaria
085　Leishmaniasis
086　Trypanosomiasis
087　Relapsing fever
088　Other arthropod-borne diseases

Syphilis and other venereal diseases (090-099)
090　Congenital syphilis
091　Early syphilis, symptomatic
092　Early syphilis, latent
093　Cardiovascular syphilis
094　Neurosyphilis
095　Other forms of late syphilis, with symptoms
096　Late syphilis, latent
097　Other and unspecified syphilis
098　Gonococcal infections
099　Other venereal diseases

Other spirochetal diseases (100-104)
100　Leptospirosis
101　Vincent's angina
102　Yaws
103　Pinta
104　Other spirochetal infection

Mycoses (110-118)
110　Dermatophytosis
111　Dermatomycosis, other and unspecified
112　Candidiasis
114　Coccidioidomycosis
115　Histoplasmosis
116　Blastomycotic infection
117　Other mycoses
118　Opportunistic mycoses

Helminthiases (120-129)
120　Schistosomiasis [bilharziasis]
121　Other trematode infections

1. INFECTIOUS AND PARASITIC DISEASES *continued*

122 Echinococcosis
123 Other cestode infection
124 Trichinosis
125 Filarial infection and dracontiasis
126 Ancylostomiasis and necatoriasis
127 Other intestinal helminthiases
128 Other and unspecified helminthiases
129 Intestinal parasitism, unspecified

Other infectious and parasitic diseases (130-136)

130 Toxoplasmosis
131 Trichomoniasis
132 Pediculosis and phthirus infestation
133 Acariasis
134 Other infestation
135 Sarcoidosis
136 Other and unspecified infectious and parasitic diseases

Late effects of infectious and parasitic diseases (137-139)

137 Late effects of tuberculosis
138 Late effects of acute poliomyelitis
139 Late effects of other infectious and parasitic diseases

2. NEOPLASMS

Malignant neoplasm of lip, oral cavity, and pharynx (140-149)

140 Malignant neoplasm of lip
141 Malignant neoplasm of tongue
142 Malignant neoplasm of major salivary glands
143 Malignant neoplasm of gum
144 Malignant neoplasm of floor of mouth
145 Malignant neoplasm of other and unspecified parts of mouth
146 Malignant neoplasm of oropharynx
147 Malignant neoplasm of nasopharynx
148 Malignant neoplasm of hypopharynx
149 Malignant neoplasm of other and ill-defined sites within the lip, oral cavity, and pharynx

Malignant neoplasm of digestive organs and peritoneum (150-159)

150 Malignant neoplasm of esophagus
151 Malignant neoplasm of stomach
152 Malignant neoplasm of small intestine, including duodenum
153 Malignant neoplasm of colon
154 Malignant neoplasm of rectum, rectosigmoid junction, and anus
155 Malignant neoplasm of liver and intrahepatic bile ducts
156 Malignant neoplasm of gallbladder and extrahepatic bile ducts
157 Malignant neoplasm of pancreas
158 Malignant neoplasm of retroperitoneum and peritoneum
159 Malignant neoplasm of other and ill-defined sites within the digestive organs and peritoneum

Malignant neoplasm of respiratory and intrathoracic organs (160-165)

160 Malignant neoplasm of nasal cavities, middle ear, and accessory sinuses
161 Malignant neoplasm of larynx
162 Malignant neoplasm of trachea, bronchus, and lung
163 Malignant neoplasm of pleura
164 Malignant neoplasm of thymus, heart, and mediastinum
165 Malignant neoplasm of other and ill-defined sites within the respiratory system and intrathoracic organs

Malignant neoplasm of bone, connective tissue, skin, and breast (170-176)

170 Malignant neoplasm of bone and articular cartilage
171 Malignant neoplasm of connective and other soft tissue
172 Malignant melanoma of skin
173 Other and unspecified malignant neoplasm of skin
174 Malignant neoplasm of female breast
175 Malignant neoplasm of male breast
176 Kaposi's sarcoma

2. NEOPLASMS *continued*

Malignant neoplasm of genitourinary organs (179-189)

179 Malignant neoplasm of uterus, part unspecified
180 Malignant neoplasm of cervix uteri
181 Malignant neoplasm of placenta
182 Malignant neoplasm of body of uterus
183 Malignant neoplasm of ovary and other uterine adnexa
184 Malignant neoplasm of other and unspecified female genital organs
185 Malignant neoplasm of prostate
186 Malignant neoplasm of testis
187 Malignant neoplasm of penis and other male genital organs
188 Malignant neoplasm of bladder
189 Malignant neoplasm of kidney and other and unspecified urinary organs

Malignant neoplasm of other and unspecified sites (190-199)

190 Malignant neoplasm of eye
191 Malignant neoplasm of brain
192 Malignant neoplasm of other and unspecified parts of nervous system
193 Malignant neoplasm of thyroid gland
194 Malignant neoplasm of other endocrine glands and related structures
195 Malignant neoplasm of other and ill-defined sites
196 Secondary and unspecified malignant neoplasm of lymph nodes
197 Secondary malignant neoplasm of respiratory and digestive systems
198 Secondary malignant neoplasm of other specified sites
199 Malignant neoplasm without specification of site

Malignant neoplasm of lymphatic and hematopoietic tissue (200-208)

200 Lymphosarcoma and reticulosarcoma and other specified malignant tumors of
       lymphatic tissue
201 Hodgkin's disease
202 Other malignant neoplasm of lymphoid and histiocytic tissue
203 Multiple myeloma and immunoproliferative neoplasms
204 Lymphoid leukemia
205 Myeloid leukemia
206 Monocytic leukemia
207 Other specified leukemia
208 Leukemia of unspecified cell type

Neuroendocrine tumors (209)

209 Neuroendocrine tumors

Benign neoplasms (210-229)

210 Benign neoplasm of lip, oral cavity, and pharynx
211 Benign neoplasm of other parts of digestive system
212 Benign neoplasm of respiratory and intrathoracic organs
213 Benign neoplasm of bone and articular cartilage
214 Lipoma
215 Other benign neoplasm of connective and other soft tissue
216 Benign neoplasm of skin
217 Benign neoplasm of breast
218 Uterine leiomyoma
219 Other benign neoplasm of uterus
220 Benign neoplasm of ovary
221 Benign neoplasm of other female genital organs
222 Benign neoplasm of male genital organs
223 Benign neoplasm of kidney and other urinary organs
224 Benign neoplasm of eye
225 Benign neoplasm of brain and other parts of nervous system
226 Benign neoplasm of thyroid gland
227 Benign neoplasm of other endocrine glands and related structures
228 Hemangioma and lymphangioma, any site
229 Benign neoplasm of other and unspecified sites

Carcinoma in situ (230-234)

230 Carcinoma in situ of digestive organs
231 Carcinoma in situ of respiratory system
232 Carcinoma in situ of skin
233 Carcinoma in situ of breast and genitourinary system
234 Carcinoma in situ of other and unspecified sites

2. NEOPLASMS *continued*

Neoplasms of uncertain behavior (235-238)

235 Neoplasm of uncertain behavior of digestive and respiratory systems
236 Neoplasm of uncertain behavior of genitourinary organs
237 Neoplasm of uncertain behavior of endocrine glands and nervous system
238 Neoplasm of uncertain behavior of other and unspecified sites and tissues

Neoplasm of unspecified nature (239)

239 Neoplasm of unspecified nature

3. ENDOCRINE, NUTRITIONAL AND METABOLIC DISEASES, AND IMMUNITY DISORDERS

Disorders of thyroid gland (240-246)

240 Simple and unspecified goiter
241 Nontoxic nodular goiter
242 Thyrotoxicosis with or without goiter
243 Congenital hypothyroidism
244 Acquired hypothyroidism
245 Thyroiditis
246 Other disorders of thyroid

Diseases of other endocrine glands (249-259)

249 Secondary diabetes mellitus
250 Diabetes mellitus
251 Other disorders of pancreatic internal secretion
252 Disorders of parathyroid gland
253 Disorders of the pituitary gland and its hypothalamic control
254 Diseases of thymus gland
255 Disorders of adrenal glands
256 Ovarian dysfunction
257 Testicular dysfunction
258 Polyglandular dysfunction and related disorders
259 Other endocrine disorders

Nutritional deficiencies (260-269)

260 Kwashiorkor
261 Nutritional marasmus
262 Other severe protein-calorie malnutrition
263 Other and unspecified protein-calorie malnutrition
264 Vitamin A deficiency
265 Thiamine and niacin deficiency states
266 Deficiency of B-complex components
267 Ascorbic acid deficiency
268 Vitamin D deficiency
269 Other nutritional deficiencies

Other metabolic and immunity disorders (270-279)

270 Disorders of amino-acid transport and metabolism
271 Disorders of carbohydrate transport and metabolism
272 Disorders of lipoid metabolism
273 Disorders of plasma protein metabolism
274 Gout
275 Disorders of mineral metabolism
276 Disorders of fluid, electrolyte, and acid-base balance
277 Other and unspecified disorders of metabolism
278 Overweight, obesity and other hyperalimentation
279 Disorders involving the immune mechanism

4. DISEASES OF THE BLOOD AND BLOOD-FORMING ORGANS

Diseases of blood and blood-forming organs (280-289)

280 Iron deficiency anemias
281 Other deficiency anemias
282 Hereditary hemolytic anemias
283 Acquired hemolytic anemias
284 Aplastic anemia and other bone marrow failure syndromes
285 Other and unspecified anemias
286 Coagulation defects
287 Purpura and other hemorrhagic conditions

5. MENTAL DISORDERS

        288   Diseases of white blood cells
        289   Other diseases of blood and blood-forming organs

Organic psychotic conditions (290-294)
        290   Dementias
        291   Alcohol-induced mental disorders
        292   Drug-induced mental disorders
        293   Transient mental disorders due to conditions classified elsewhere
        294   Persistent mental disorders due to conditions classified elsewhere

Other psychoses (295-299)
        295   Schizophrenic disorders
        296   Episodic mood disorders
        297   Delusional disorders
        298   Other nonorganic psychoses
        299   Pervasive developmental disorders

Neurotic disorders, personality disorders, and other nonpsychotic mental disorders (300-316)
        300   Anxiety, dissociative and somatoform disorders
        301   Personality disorders
        302   Sexual and gender identity disorders
        303   Alcohol dependence syndrome
        304   Drug dependence
        305   Nondependent abuse of drugs
        306   Physiological malfunction arising from mental factors
        307   Special symptoms or syndromes, not elsewhere classified
        308   Acute reaction to stress
        309   Adjustment reaction
        310   Specific nonpsychotic mental disorders due to brain damage
        311   Depressive disorder, not elsewhere classified
        312   Disturbance of conduct, not elsewhere classified
        313   Disturbance of emotions specific to childhood and adolescence
        314   Hyperkinetic syndrome of childhood
        315   Specific delays in development
        316   Psychic factors associated with diseases classified elsewhere

Mental retardation (317-319)
        317   Mild intellectual disabilities
        318   Other specified intellectual disabilities
        319   Unspecified intellectual disabilities

6. DISEASES OF THE NERVOUS SYSTEM AND SENSE ORGANS

Inflammatory diseases of the central nervous system (320-326)
        320   Bacterial meningitis
        321   Meningitis due to other organisms
        322   Meningitis of unspecified cause
        323   Encephalitis, myelitis, and encephalomyelitis
        324   Intracranial and intraspinal abscess
        325   Phlebitis and thrombophlebitis of intracranial venous sinuses
        326   Late effects of intracranial abscess or pyogenic infection

Organic sleep disorders (327)
        327   Organic sleep disorders

Hereditary and degenerative diseases of the central nervous system (330-337)
        330   Cerebral degenerations usually manifest in childhood
        331   Other cerebral degenerations
        332   Parkinson's disease
        333   Other extrapyramidal disease and abnormal movement disorders
        334   Spinocerebellar disease
        335   Anterior horn cell disease
        336   Other diseases of spinal cord
        337   Disorders of the autonomic nervous system

Pain (338)
        338   Pain, not elsewhere classified

Other headache syndromes (339)
        339   Other headache syndromes

6. DISEASES OF THE NERVOUS SYSTEM AND SENSE ORGANS *continued*

Other disorders of the central nervous system (340-349)

- 340 Multiple sclerosis
- 341 Other demyelinating diseases of central nervous system
- 342 Hemiplegia and hemiparesis
- 343 Infantile cerebral palsy
- 344 Other paralytic syndromes
- 345 Epilepsy and recurrent seizures
- 346 Migraine
- 347 Cataplexy and narcolepsy
- 348 Other conditions of brain
- 349 Other and unspecified disorders of the nervous system

Disorders of the peripheral nervous system (350-359)

- 350 Trigeminal nerve disorders
- 351 Facial nerve disorders
- 352 Disorders of other cranial nerves
- 353 Nerve root and plexus disorders
- 354 Mononeuritis of upper limb and mononeuritis multiplex
- 355 Mononeuritis of lower limb and unspecified site
- 356 Hereditary and idiopathic peripheral neuropathy
- 357 Inflammatory and toxic neuropathy
- 358 Myoneural disorders
- 359 Muscular dystrophies and other myopathies

Disorders of the eye and adnexa (360-379)

- 360 Disorders of the globe
- 361 Retinal detachments and defects
- 362 Other retinal disorders
- 363 Chorioretinal inflammations, scars and other disorders of choroid
- 364 Disorders of iris and ciliary body
- 365 Glaucoma
- 366 Cataract
- 367 Disorders of refraction and accommodation
- 368 Visual disturbances
- 369 Blindness and low vision
- 370 Keratitis
- 371 Corneal opacity and other disorders of cornea
- 372 Disorders of conjunctiva
- 373 Inflammation of eyelids
- 374 Other disorders of eyelids
- 375 Disorders of lacrimal system
- 376 Disorders of the orbit
- 377 Disorders of optic nerve and visual pathways
- 378 Strabismus and other disorders of binocular eye movements
- 379 Other disorders of eye

Diseases of the ear and mastoid process (380-389)

- 380 Disorders of external ear
- 381 Nonsuppurative otitis media and Eustachian tube disorders
- 382 Suppurative and unspecified otitis media
- 383 Mastoiditis and related conditions
- 384 Other disorders of tympanic membrane
- 385 Other disorders of middle ear and mastoid
- 386 Vertiginous syndromes and other disorders of vestibular system
- 387 Otosclerosis
- 388 Other disorders of ear
- 389 Hearing loss

7. DISEASES OF THE CIRCULATORY SYSTEM

Acute rheumatic fever (390-392)

- 390 Rheumatic fever without mention of heart involvement
- 391 Rheumatic fever with heart involvement
- 392 Rheumatic chorea

Chronic rheumatic heart disease (393-398)

- 393 Chronic rheumatic pericarditis
- 394 Diseases of mitral valve

7. DISEASES OF THE CIRCULATORY SYSTEM *continued*

    395   Diseases of aortic valve
    396   Diseases of mitral and aortic valves
    397   Diseases of other endocardial structures
    398   Other rheumatic heart disease

Hypertensive disease (401-405)
    401   Essential hypertension
    402   Hypertensive heart disease
    403   Hypertensive chronic kidney disease
    404   Hypertensive heart and chronic kidney disease
    405   Secondary hypertension

Ischemic heart disease (410-414)
    410   Acute myocardial infarction
    411   Other acute and subacute form of ischemic heart disease
    412   Old myocardial infarction
    413   Angina pectoris
    414   Other forms of chronic ischemic heart disease

Diseases of pulmonary circulation (415-417)
    415   Acute pulmonary heart disease
    416   Chronic pulmonary heart disease
    417   Other diseases of pulmonary circulation

Other forms of heart disease (420-429)
    420   Acute pericarditis
    421   Acute and subacute endocarditis
    422   Acute myocarditis
    423   Other diseases of pericardium
    424   Other diseases of endocardium
    425   Cardiomyopathy
    426   Conduction disorders
    427   Cardiac dysrhythmias
    428   Heart failure
    429   Ill-defined descriptions and complications of heart disease

Cerebrovascular disease (430-438)
    430   Subarachnoid hemorrhage
    431   Intracerebral hemorrhage
    432   Other and unspecified intracranial hemorrhage
    433   Occlusion and stenosis of precerebral arteries
    434   Occlusion of cerebral arteries
    435   Transient cerebral ischemia
    436   Acute but ill-defined cerebrovascular disease
    437   Other and ill-defined cerebrovascular disease
    438   Late effects of cerebrovascular disease

Diseases of arteries, arterioles, and capillaries (440-449)
    440   Atherosclerosis
    441   Aortic aneurysm and dissection
    442   Other aneurysm
    443   Other peripheral vascular disease
    444   Arterial embolism and thrombosis
    445   Atheroembolism
    446   Polyarteritis nodosa and allied conditions
    447   Other disorders of arteries and arterioles
    448   Diseases of capillaries
    449   Septic arterial embolism

Diseases of veins and lymphatics, and other diseases of circulatory system (451-459)
    451   Phlebitis and thrombophlebitis
    452   Portal vein thrombosis
    453   Other venous embolism and thrombosis
    454   Varicose veins of lower extremities
    455   Hemorrhoids
    456   Varicose veins of other sites
    457   Noninfective disorders of lymphatic channels
    458   Hypotension
    459   Other disorders of circulatory system

8. DISEASES OF THE RESPIRATORY SYSTEM

Acute respiratory infections (460-466)
- 460 Acute nasopharyngitis [common cold]
- 461 Acute sinusitis
- 462 Acute pharyngitis
- 463 Acute tonsillitis
- 464 Acute laryngitis and tracheitis
- 465 Acute upper respiratory infections of multiple or unspecified sites
- 466 Acute bronchitis and bronchiolitis

Other diseases of upper respiratory tract (470-478)
- 470 Deviated nasal septum
- 471 Nasal polyps
- 472 Chronic pharyngitis and nasopharyngitis
- 473 Chronic sinusitis
- 474 Chronic disease of tonsils and adenoids
- 475 Peritonsillar abscess
- 476 Chronic laryngitis and laryngotracheitis
- 477 Allergic rhinitis
- 478 Other diseases of upper respiratory tract

Pneumonia and influenza (480-488)
- 480 Viral pneumonia
- 481 Pneumococcal pneumonia [*Streptococcus pneumoniae* pneumonia]
- 482 Other bacterial pneumonia
- 483 Pneumonia due to other specified organism
- 484 Pneumonia in infectious diseases classified elsewhere
- 485 Bronchopneumonia, organism unspecified
- 486 Pneumonia, organism unspecified
- 487 Influenza
- 488 Influenza due to certain identified influenza viruses

Chronic obstructive pulmonary disease and allied conditions (490-496)
- 490 Bronchitis, not specified as acute or chronic
- 491 Chronic bronchitis
- 492 Emphysema
- 493 Asthma
- 494 Bronchiectasis
- 495 Extrinsic allergic alveolitis
- 496 Chronic airway obstruction, not elsewhere classified

Pneumoconioses and other lung diseases due to external agents (500-508)
- 500 Coal workers' pneumoconiosis
- 501 Asbestosis
- 502 Pneumoconiosis due to other silica or silicates
- 503 Pneumoconiosis due to other inorganic dust
- 504 Pneumopathy due to inhalation of other dust
- 505 Pneumoconiosis, unspecified
- 506 Respiratory conditions due to chemical fumes and vapors
- 507 Pneumonitis due to solids and liquids
- 508 Respiratory conditions due to other and unspecified external agents

Other diseases of respiratory system (510-519)
- 510 Empyema
- 511 Pleurisy
- 512 Pneumothorax and air leak
- 513 Abscess of lung and mediastinum
- 514 Pulmonary congestion and hypostasis
- 515 Postinflammatory pulmonary fibrosis
- 516 Other alveolar and parietoalveolar pneumopathy
- 517 Lung involvement in conditions classified elsewhere
- 518 Other diseases of lung
- 519 Other diseases of respiratory system

9. DISEASES OF THE DIGESTIVE SYSTEM

Diseases of oral cavity, salivary glands, and jaws (520-529)
- 520 Disorders of tooth development and eruption
- 521 Diseases of hard tissues of teeth
- 522 Diseases of pulp and periapical tissues

9. DISEASES OF THE DIGESTIVE SYSTEM *continued*

523 Gingival and periodontal diseases
524 Dentofacial anomalies, including malocclusion
525 Other diseases and conditions of the teeth and supporting structures
526 Diseases of the jaws
527 Diseases of the salivary glands
528 Diseases of the oral soft tissues, excluding lesions specific for gingiva and tongue
529 Diseases and other conditions of the tongue

Diseases of esophagus, stomach, and duodenum (530-538)

530 Diseases of esophagus
531 Gastric ulcer
532 Duodenal ulcer
533 Peptic ulcer, site unspecified
534 Gastrojejunal ulcer
535 Gastritis and duodenitis
536 Disorders of function of stomach
537 Other disorders of stomach and duodenum
538 Gastrointestinal mucositis (ulcerative)
539 Complications of bariatric procedures

Appendicitis (540-543)

540 Acute appendicitis
541 Appendicitis, unqualified
542 Other appendicitis
543 Other diseases of appendix

Hernia of abdominal cavity (550-553)

550 Inguinal hernia
551 Other hernia of abdominal cavity, with gangrene
552 Other hernia of abdominal cavity, with obstruction, but without mention of gangrene
553 Other hernia of abdominal cavity without mention of obstruction or gangrene

Noninfectious enteritis and colitis (555-558)

555 Regional enteritis
556 Ulcerative colitis
557 Vascular insufficiency of intestine
558 Other and unspecified noninfectious gastroenteritis and colitis

Other diseases of intestines and peritoneum (560-569)

560 Intestinal obstruction without mention of hernia
562 Diverticula of intestine
564 Functional digestive disorders, not elsewhere classified
565 Anal fissure and fistula
566 Abscess of anal and rectal regions
567 Peritonitis and retroperitoneal infections
568 Other disorders of peritoneum
569 Other disorders of intestine

Other diseases of digestive system (570-579)

570 Acute and subacute necrosis of liver
571 Chronic liver disease and cirrhosis
572 Liver abscess and sequelae of chronic liver disease
573 Other disorders of liver
574 Cholelithiasis
575 Other disorders of gallbladder
576 Other disorders of biliary tract
577 Diseases of pancreas
578 Gastrointestinal hemorrhage
579 Intestinal malabsorption

10. DISEASES OF THE GENITOURINARY SYSTEM

Nephritis, nephrotic syndrome, and nephrosis (580-589)

580 Acute glomerulonephritis
581 Nephrotic syndrome
582 Chronic glomerulonephritis
583 Nephritis and nephropathy, not specified as acute or chronic
584 Acute kidney failure
585 Chronic kidney disease (CKD)

10. DISEASES OF THE GENITOURINARY SYSTEM *continued*

586 Renal failure, unspecified
587 Renal sclerosis, unspecified
588 Disorders resulting from impaired renal function
589 Small kidney of unknown cause

Other diseases of urinary system (590-599)

590 Infections of kidney
591 Hydronephrosis
592 Calculus of kidney and ureter
593 Other disorders of kidney and ureter
594 Calculus of lower urinary tract
595 Cystitis
596 Other disorders of bladder
597 Urethritis, not sexually transmitted, and urethral syndrome
598 Urethral stricture
599 Other disorders of urethra and urinary tract

Diseases of male genital organs (600-608)

600 Hyperplasia of prostate
601 Inflammatory diseases of prostate
602 Other disorders of prostate
603 Hydrocele
604 Orchitis and epididymitis
605 Redundant prepuce and phimosis
606 Infertility, male
607 Disorders of penis
608 Other disorders of male genital organs

Disorders of breast (610-612)

610 Benign mammary dysplasias
611 Other disorders of breast
612 Deformity and disproportion of reconstructed breast

Inflammatory disease of female pelvic organs (614-616)

614 Inflammatory disease of ovary, fallopian tube, pelvic cellular tissue, and peritoneum
615 Inflammatory diseases of uterus, except cervix
616 Inflammatory disease of cervix, vagina, and vulva

Other disorders of female genital tract (617-629)

617 Endometriosis
618 Genital prolapse
619 Fistula involving female genital tract
620 Noninflammatory disorders of ovary, fallopian tube, and broad ligament
621 Disorders of uterus, not elsewhere classified
622 Noninflammatory disorders of cervix
623 Noninflammatory disorders of vagina
624 Noninflammatory disorders of vulva and perineum
625 Pain and other symptoms associated with female genital organs
626 Disorders of menstruation and other abnormal bleeding from female genital tract
627 Menopausal and postmenopausal disorders
628 Infertility, female
629 Other disorders of female genital organs

11. COMPLICATIONS OF PREGNANCY, CHILDBIRTH AND THE PUERPERIUM

Ectopic and molar pregnancy (630-633)

630 Hydatidiform mole
631 Other abnormal product of conception
632 Missed abortion
633 Ectopic pregnancy

Other pregnancy with abortive outcome (634-639)

634 Abortion
635 Legally induced abortion
636 Illegally induced abortion
637 Unspecified abortion
638 Failed attempted abortion
639 Complications following abortion and ectopic and molar pregnancies

11. COMPLICATIONS OF PREGNANCY, CHILDBIRTH AND THE PUERPERIUM *continued*

Complications mainly related to pregnancy (640-649)

640 Hemorrhage in early pregnancy
641 Antepartum hemorrhage, abruptio placentae, and placenta previa
642 Hypertension complicating pregnancy, childbirth, and the puerperium
643 Excessive vomiting in pregnancy
644 Early or threatened labor
645 Late pregnancy
646 Other complications of pregnancy, not elsewhere classified
647 Infectious and parasitic conditions in the mother classifiable elsewhere but complicating pregnancy, childbirth, and the puerperium
648 Other current conditions in the mother classifiable elsewhere but complicating pregnancy, childbirth, and the puerperium
649 Other conditions or status of the mother complicating pregnancy, childbirth or the puerperium

Normal delivery, and other indications for care in pregnancy, labor, and delivery (650-659)

650 Normal delivery
651 Multiple gestation
652 Malposition and malpresentation of fetus
653 Disproportion
654 Abnormality of organs and soft tissues of pelvis
655 Known or suspected fetal abnormality affecting management of mother
656 Other known or suspected fetal and placental problems affecting management of mother
657 Polyhydramnios
658 Other problems associated with amniotic cavity and membranes
659 Other indications for care or intervention related to labor and delivery and not elsewhere classified

Complications occurring mainly in the course of labor and delivery (660-669)

660 Obstructed labor
661 Abnormality of forces of labor
662 Long labor
663 Umbilical cord complications
664 Trauma to perineum and vulva during delivery
665 Other obstetrical trauma
666 Postpartum hemorrhage
667 Retained placenta or membranes, without hemorrhage
668 Complications of the administration of anesthetic or other sedation in labor and delivery
669 Other complications of labor and delivery, not elsewhere classified

Complications of the puerperium (670-677)

670 Major puerperal infection
671 Venous complications in pregnancy and the puerperium
672 Pyrexia of unknown origin during the puerperium
673 Obstetrical pulmonary embolism
674 Other and unspecified complications of the puerperium, not elsewhere classified
675 Infections of the breast and nipple associated with childbirth
676 Other disorders of the breast associated with childbirth, and disorders of lactation
677 Late effect of complication of pregnancy, childbirth, and the puerperium

Other maternal and fetal complications (678-679)

678 Other fetal conditions
679 Complications of in utero procedures

12. DISEASES OF THE SKIN AND SUBCUTANEOUS TISSUE

Infections of skin and subcutaneous tissue (680-686)

680 Carbuncle and furuncle
681 Cellulitis and abscess of finger and toe
682 Other cellulitis and abscess
683 Acute lymphadenitis
684 Impetigo
685 Pilonidal cyst
686 Other local infections of skin and subcutaneous tissue

Other inflammatory conditions of skin and subcutaneous tissue (690-698)

690 Erythematosquamous dermatosis
691 Atopic dermatitis and related conditions

12. DISEASES OF THE SKIN AND SUBCUTANEOUS TISSUE *continued*

692　Contact dermatitis and other eczema
693　Dermatitis due to substances taken internally
694　Bullous dermatoses
695　Erythematous conditions
696　Psoriasis and similar disorders
697　Lichen
698　Pruritus and related conditions

Other diseases of skin and subcutaneous tissue (700-709)

700　Corns and callosities
701　Other hypertrophic and atrophic conditions of skin
702　Other dermatoses
703　Diseases of nail
704　Diseases of hair and hair follicles
705　Disorders of sweat glands
706　Diseases of sebaceous glands
707　Chronic ulcer of skin
708　Urticaria
709　Other disorders of skin and subcutaneous tissue

13. DISEASES OF THE MUSCULOSKELETAL SYSTEM AND CONNECTIVE TISSUE

Arthropathies and related disorders (710-719)

710　Diffuse diseases of connective tissue
711　Arthropathy associated with infections
712　Crystal arthropathies
713　Arthropathy associated with other disorders classified elsewhere
714　Rheumatoid arthritis and other inflammatory polyarthropathies
715　Osteoarthrosis and allied disorders
716　Other and unspecified arthropathies
717　Internal derangement of knee
718　Other derangement of joint
719　Other and unspecified disorder of joint

Dorsopathies (720-724)

720　Ankylosing spondylitis and other inflammatory spondylopathies
721　Spondylosis and allied disorders
722　Intervertebral disc disorders
723　Other disorders of cervical region
724　Other and unspecified disorders of back

Rheumatism, excluding the back (725-729)

725　Polymyalgia rheumatica
726　Peripheral enthesopathies and allied syndromes
727　Other disorders of synovium, tendon, and bursa
728　Disorders of muscle, ligament, and fascia
729　Other disorders of soft tissues

Osteopathies, chondropathies, and acquired musculoskeletal deformities (730-739)

730　Osteomyelitis, periostitis, and other infections involving bone
731　Osteitis deformans and osteopathies associated with other disorders classified
　　　elsewhere
732　Osteochondropathies
733　Other disorders of bone and cartilage
734　Flat foot
735　Acquired deformities of toe
736　Other acquired deformities of limbs
737　Curvature of spine
738　Other acquired deformity
739　Nonallopathic lesions, not elsewhere classified

14. CONGENITAL ANOMALIES

740　Anencephalus and similar anomalies
741　Spina bifida
742　Other congenital anomalies of nervous system
743　Congenital anomalies of eye
744　Congenital anomalies of ear, face, and neck
745　Bulbus cordis anomalies and anomalies of cardiac septal closure

14. CONGENITAL ANOMALIES *continued*

746 Other congenital anomalies of heart
747 Other congenital anomalies of circulatory system
748 Congenital anomalies of respiratory system
749 Cleft palate and cleft lip
750 Other congenital anomalies of upper alimentary tract
751 Other congenital anomalies of digestive system
752 Congenital anomalies of genital organs
753 Congenital anomalies of urinary system
754 Certain congenital musculoskeletal deformities
755 Other congenital anomalies of limbs
756 Other congenital musculoskeletal anomalies
757 Congenital anomalies of the integument
758 Chromosomal anomalies
759 Other and unspecified congenital anomalies

15. CERTAIN CONDITIONS ORIGINATING IN THE PERINATAL PERIOD

Maternal causes of perinatal morbidity and mortality (760-763)

760 Fetus or newborn affected by maternal conditions which may be unrelated to present pregnancy
761 Fetus or newborn affected by maternal complications of pregnancy
762 Fetus or newborn affected by complications of placenta, cord, and membranes
763 Fetus or newborn affected by other complications of labor and delivery

Other conditions originating in the perinatal period (764-779)

764 Slow fetal growth and fetal malnutrition
765 Disorders relating to short gestation and low birthweight
766 Disorders relating to long gestation and high birthweight
767 Birth trauma
768 Intrauterine hypoxia and birth asphyxia
769 Respiratory distress syndrome
770 Other respiratory conditions of fetus and newborn
771 Infections specific to the perinatal period
772 Fetal and neonatal hemorrhage
773 Hemolytic disease of fetus or newborn, due to isoimmunization
774 Other perinatal jaundice
775 Endocrine and metabolic disturbances specific to the fetus and newborn
776 Hematological disorders of newborn
777 Perinatal disorders of digestive system
778 Conditions involving the integument and temperature regulation of fetus and newborn
779 Other and ill-defined conditions originating in the perinatal period

16. SYMPTOMS, SIGNS, AND ILL-DEFINED CONDITIONS

Symptoms (780-789)

780 General symptoms
781 Symptoms involving nervous and musculoskeletal systems
782 Symptoms involving skin and other integumentary tissue
783 Symptoms concerning nutrition, metabolism, and development
784 Symptoms involving head and neck
785 Symptoms involving cardiovascular system
786 Symptoms involving respiratory system and other chest symptoms
787 Symptoms involving digestive system
788 Symptoms involving urinary system
789 Other symptoms involving abdomen and pelvis

Nonspecific abnormal findings (790-796)

790 Nonspecific findings on examination of blood
791 Nonspecific findings on examination of urine
792 Nonspecific abnormal findings in other body substances
793 Nonspecific (abnormal) findings on radiological and other examination of body structure
794 Nonspecific abnormal results of function studies
795 Other and nonspecific abnormal cytological, histological, immunological and DNA test findings
796 Other nonspecific abnormal findings

Ill-defined and unknown causes of morbidity and mortality (797-799)

797 Senility without mention of psychosis

16. SYMPTOMS, SIGNS, AND ILL-DEFINED CONDITIONS *continued*

798   Sudden death, cause unknown
799   Other ill-defined and unknown causes of morbidity and mortality

17. INJURY AND POISONING

Fracture of skull (800-804)

800   Fracture of vault of skull
801   Fracture of base of skull
802   Fracture of face bones
803   Other and unqualified skull fractures
804   Multiple fractures involving skull or face with other bones

Fracture of neck and trunk (805-809)

805   Fracture of vertebral column without mention of spinal cord injury
806   Fracture of vertebral column with spinal cord injury
807   Fracture of rib(s), sternum, larynx, and trachea
808   Fracture of pelvis
809   Ill-defined fractures of bones of trunk

Fracture of upper limb (810-819)

810   Fracture of clavicle
811   Fracture of scapula
812   Fracture of humerus
813   Fracture of radius and ulna
814   Fracture of carpal bone(s)
815   Fracture of metacarpal bone(s)
816   Fracture of one or more phalanges of hand
817   Multiple fractures of hand bones
818   Ill-defined fractures of upper limb
819   Multiple fractures involving both upper limbs, and upper limb with rib(s) and sternum

Fracture of lower limb (820-829)

820   Fracture of neck of femur
821   Fracture of other and unspecified parts of femur
822   Fracture of patella
823   Fracture of tibia and fibula
824   Fracture of ankle
825   Fracture of one or more tarsal and metatarsal bones
826   Fracture of one or more phalanges of foot
827   Other, multiple, and ill-defined fractures of lower limb
828   Multiple fractures involving both lower limbs, lower with upper limb, and lower
          limb(s) with rib(s) and sternum
829   Fracture of unspecified bones

Dislocation (830-839)

830   Dislocation of jaw
831   Dislocation of shoulder
832   Dislocation of elbow
833   Dislocation of wrist
834   Dislocation of finger
835   Dislocation of hip
836   Dislocation of knee
837   Dislocation of ankle
838   Dislocation of foot
839   Other, multiple, and ill-defined dislocations

Sprains and strains of joints and adjacent muscles (840-848)

840   Sprains and strains of shoulder and upper arm
841   Sprains and strains of elbow and forearm
842   Sprains and strains of wrist and hand
843   Sprains and strains of hip and thigh
844   Sprains and strains of knee and leg
845   Sprains and strains of ankle and foot
846   Sprains and strains of sacroiliac region
847   Sprains and strains of other and unspecified parts of back
848   Other and ill-defined sprains and strains

Intracranial injury, excluding those with skull fracture (850-854)

850   Concussion
851   Cerebral laceration and contusion

17. INJURY AND POISONING *continued*

852 Subarachnoid, subdural, and extradural hemorrhage, following injury
853 Other and unspecified intracranial hemorrhage following injury
854 Intracranial injury of other and unspecified nature

Internal injury of thorax, abdomen, and pelvis (860-869)

860 Traumatic pneumothorax and hemothorax
861 Injury to heart and lung
862 Injury to other and unspecified intrathoracic organs
863 Injury to gastrointestinal tract
864 Injury to liver
865 Injury to spleen
866 Injury to kidney
867 Injury to pelvic organs
868 Injury to other intra-abdominal organs
869 Internal injury to unspecified or ill-defined organs

Open wound of head, neck, and trunk (870-879)

870 Open wound of ocular adnexa
871 Open wound of eyeball
872 Open wound of ear
873 Other open wound of head
874 Open wound of neck
875 Open wound of chest (wall)
876 Open wound of back
877 Open wound of buttock
878 Open wound of genital organs (external), including traumatic amputation
879 Open wound of other and unspecified sites, except limbs

Open wound of upper limb (880-887)

880 Open wound of shoulder and upper arm
881 Open wound of elbow, forearm, and wrist
882 Open wound of hand except finger(s) alone
883 Open wound of finger(s)
884 Multiple and unspecified open wound of upper limb
885 Traumatic amputation of thumb (complete) (partial)
886 Traumatic amputation of other finger(s) (complete) (partial)
887 Traumatic amputation of arm and hand (complete) (partial)

Open wound of lower limb (890-897)

890 Open wound of hip and thigh
891 Open wound of knee, leg [except thigh], and ankle
892 Open wound of foot except toe(s) alone
893 Open wound of toe(s)
894 Multiple and unspecified open wound of lower limb
895 Traumatic amputation of toe(s) (complete) (partial)
896 Traumatic amputation of foot (complete) (partial)
897 Traumatic amputation of leg(s) (complete) (partial)

Injury to blood vessels (900-904)

900 Injury to blood vessels of head and neck
901 Injury to blood vessels of thorax
902 Injury to blood vessels of abdomen and pelvis
903 Injury to blood vessels of upper extremity
904 Injury to blood vessels of lower extremity and unspecified sites

Late effects of injuries, poisonings, toxic effects, and other external causes (905-909)

905 Late effects of musculoskeletal and connective tissue injuries
906 Late effects of injuries to skin and subcutaneous tissues
907 Late effects of injuries to the nervous system
908 Late effects of other and unspecified injuries
909 Late effects of other and unspecified external causes

Superficial injury (910-919)

910 Superficial injury of face, neck, and scalp except eye
911 Superficial injury of trunk
912 Superficial injury of shoulder and upper arm
913 Superficial injury of elbow, forearm, and wrist
914 Superficial injury of hand(s) except finger(s) alone
915 Superficial injury of finger(s)

17. INJURY AND POISONING *continued*

916   Superficial injury of hip, thigh, leg, and ankle
917   Superficial injury of foot and toe(s)
918   Superficial injury of eye and adnexa
919   Superficial injury of other, multiple, and unspecified sites

Contusion with intact skin surface (920-924)

920   Contusion of face, scalp, and neck except eye(s)
921   Contusion of eye and adnexa
922   Contusion of trunk
923   Contusion of upper limb
924   Contusion of lower limb and of other and unspecified sites

Crushing injury (925-929)

925   Crushing injury of face, scalp, and neck
926   Crushing injury of trunk
927   Crushing injury of upper limb
928   Crushing injury of lower limb
929   Crushing injury of multiple and unspecified sites

Effects of foreign body entering through orifice (930-939)

930   Foreign body on external eye
931   Foreign body in ear
932   Foreign body in nose
933   Foreign body in pharynx and larynx
934   Foreign body in trachea, bronchus, and lung
935   Foreign body in mouth, esophagus, and stomach
936   Foreign body in intestine and colon
937   Foreign body in anus and rectum
938   Foreign body in digestive system, unspecified
939   Foreign body in genitourinary tract

Burns (940-949)

940   Burn confined to eye and adnexa
941   Burn of face, head, and neck
942   Burn of trunk
943   Burn of upper limb, except wrist and hand
944   Burn of wrist(s) and hand(s)
945   Burn of lower limb(s)
946   Burns of multiple specified sites
947   Burn of internal organs
948   Burns classified according to extent of body surface involved
949   Burn, unspecified

Injury to nerves and spinal cord (950-957)

950   Injury to optic nerve and pathways
951   Injury to other cranial nerve(s)
952   Spinal cord injury without evidence of spinal bone injury
953   Injury to nerve roots and spinal plexus
954   Injury to other nerve(s) of trunk excluding shoulder and pelvic girdles
955   Injury to peripheral nerve(s) of shoulder girdle and upper limb
956   Injury to peripheral nerve(s) of pelvic girdle and lower limb
957   Injury to other and unspecified nerves

Certain traumatic complications and unspecified injuries (958-959)

958   Certain early complications of trauma
959   Injury, other and unspecified

Poisoning by drugs, medicinal and biological substances (960-979)

960   Poisoning by antibiotics
961   Poisoning by other anti-infectives
962   Poisoning by hormones and synthetic substitutes
963   Poisoning by primarily systemic agents
964   Poisoning by agents primarily affecting blood constituents
965   Poisoning by analgesics, antipyretics, and antirheumatics
966   Poisoning by anticonvulsants and anti-Parkinsonism drugs
967   Poisoning by sedatives and hypnotics
968   Poisoning by other central nervous system depressants and anesthetics
969   Poisoning by psychotropic agents
970   Poisoning by central nervous system stimulants

17. INJURY AND POISONING *continued*

971   Poisoning by drugs primarily affecting the autonomic nervous system
972   Poisoning by agents primarily affecting the cardiovascular system
973   Poisoning by agents primarily affecting the gastrointestinal system
974   Poisoning by water, mineral, and uric acid metabolism drugs
975   Poisoning by agents primarily acting on the smooth and skeletal muscles and respiratory system
976   Poisoning by agents primarily affecting skin and mucous membrane, ophthalmological, otorhinolaryngological, and dental drugs
977   Poisoning by other and unspecified drugs and medicinals
978   Poisoning by bacterial vaccines
979   Poisoning by other vaccines and biological substances

Toxic effects of substances chiefly nonmedicinal as to source (980-989)

980   Toxic effect of alcohol
981   Toxic effect of petroleum products
982   Toxic effect of solvents other than petroleum-based
983   Toxic effect of corrosive aromatics, acids, and caustic alkalis
984   Toxic effect of lead and its compounds (including fumes)
985   Toxic effect of other metals
986   Toxic effect of carbon monoxide
987   Toxic effect of other gases, fumes, or vapors
988   Toxic effect of noxious substances eaten as food
989   Toxic effect of other substances, chiefly nonmedicinal as to source

Other and unspecified effects of external causes (990-995)

990   Effects of radiation, unspecified
991   Effects of reduced temperature
992   Effects of heat and light
993   Effects of air pressure
994   Effects of other external causes
995   Certain adverse effects, not elsewhere classified

Complications of surgical and medical care, not elsewhere classified (996-999)

996   Complications peculiar to certain specified procedures
997   Complications affecting specified body systems, not elsewhere classified
998   Other complications of procedures, not elsewhere classified
999   Complications of medical care, not elsewhere classified

SUPPLEMENTARY CLASSIFICATION OF FACTORS INFLUENCING HEALTH STATUS AND CONTACT WITH HEALTH SERVICES

Persons with potential health hazards related to communicable diseases (V01-V06)

V01   Contact with or exposure to communicable diseases
V02   Carrier or suspected carrier of infectious diseases
V03   Need for prophylactic vaccination and inoculation against bacterial diseases
V04   Need for prophylactic vaccination and inoculation against certain viral diseases
V05   Need for other prophylactic vaccination and inoculation against single diseases
V06   Need for prophylactic vaccination and inoculation against combinations of diseases

Persons with need for isolation, other potential health hazards and prophylactic measures (V07-V09)

V07   Need for isolation and other prophylactic or treatment measures
V08   Asymptomatic human immunodeficiency virus (HIV) infection status
V09   Infection with drug-resistant microorganisms

Persons with potential health hazards related to personal and family history (V10-V19)

V10   Personal history of malignant neoplasm
V11   Personal history of mental disorder
V12   Personal history of certain other diseases
V13   Personal history of other diseases
V14   Personal history of allergy to medicinal agents
V15   Other personal history presenting hazards to health
V16   Family history of malignant neoplasm
V17   Family history of certain chronic disabling diseases
V18   Family history of certain other specific conditions
V19   Family history of other conditions

Persons encountering health services in circumstances related to reproduction and development (V20-V29)

V20   Health supervision of infant or child
V21   Constitutional states in development

SUPPLEMENTARY CLASSIFICATION...HEALTH STATUS/HEALTH SERVICES *continued*

V22 Normal pregnancy
V23 Supervision of high-risk pregnancy
V24 Postpartum care and examination
V25 Encounter for contraceptive management
V26 Procreative management
V27 Outcome of delivery
V28 Encounter for antenatal screening of mother
V29 Observation and evaluation of newborns and infants for suspected condition not found

Liveborn infants according to type of birth (V30-V39)
V30 Single liveborn
V31 Twin, mate liveborn
V32 Twin, mate stillborn
V33 Twin, unspecified
V34 Other multiple, mates all liveborn
V35 Other multiple, mates all stillborn
V36 Other multiple, mates live- and stillborn
V37 Other multiple, unspecified
V39 Unspecified

Persons with a condition influencing their health status (V40-V49)
V40 Mental and behavioral problems
V41 Problems with special senses and other special functions
V42 Organ or tissue replaced by transplant
V43 Organ or tissue replaced by other means
V44 Artificial opening status
V45 Other postprocedural states
V46 Other dependence on machines and devices
V47 Other problems with internal organs
V48 Problems with head, neck, and trunk
V49 Other conditions influencing health status

Persons encountering health services for specific procedures and aftercare (V50-V59)
V50 Elective surgery for purposes other than remedying health states
V51 Aftercare involving the use of plastic surgery
V52 Fitting and adjustment of prosthetic device and implant
V53 Fitting and adjustment of other device
V54 Other orthopedic aftercare
V55 Attention to artificial openings
V56 Encounter for dialysis and dialysis catheter care
V57 Care involving use of rehabilitation procedures
V58 Encounter for other and unspecified procedures and aftercare
V59 Donors

Persons encountering health services in other circumstances (V60-V69)
V60 Housing, household, and economic circumstances
V61 Other family circumstances
V62 Other psychosocial circumstances
V63 Unavailability of other medical facilities for care
V64 Persons encountering health services for specific procedures, not carried out
V65 Other persons seeking consultation
V66 Convalescence and palliative care
V67 Follow-up examination
V68 Encounters for administrative purposes
V69 Problems related to lifestyle

Persons without reported diagnosis encountered during examination and investigation of individuals and populations (V70-V86)
V70 General medical examination
V71 Observation and evaluation for suspected conditions not found
V72 Special investigations and examinations
V73 Special screening examination for viral and chlamydial diseases
V74 Special screening examination for bacterial and spirochetal diseases
V75 Special screening examination for other infectious diseases
V76 Special screening for malignant neoplasms
V77 Special screening for endocrine, nutritional, metabolic, and immunity disorders
V78 Special screening for disorders of blood and blood-forming organs

SUPPLEMENTARY CLASSIFICATION...HEALTH STATUS/HEALTH SERVICES *continued*

V79   Special screening for mental disorders and developmental handicaps
V80   Special screening for neurological, eye, and ear diseases
V81   Special screening for cardiovascular, respiratory, and genitourinary diseases
V82   Special screening for other conditions
V83   Genetic carrier status
V84   Genetic susceptibility to disease
V85   Body mass index
V86   Estrogen receptor status
V87   Other specified personal exposures and history presenting hazards to health
V88   Acquired absence of other organs and tissue
V89   Other suspected conditions not found

Retained Foreign Body (V90)
V90   Retained foreign body

Multiple Gestation Placenta Status (V91)
V91   Multiple gestation placenta status

SUPPLEMENTARY CLASSIFICATION OF EXTERNAL CAUSES OF INJURY AND POISONING

External cause status (E000)
E000   External cause status

Activity (E001-E030)
E001   Activities involving walking and running
E002   Activities involving water and water craft
E003   Activities involving ice and snow
E004   Activities involving climbing, rappelling and jumping off
E005   Activities involving dancing and other rhythmic movement
E006   Activities involving other sports and athletics played individually
E007   Activities involving other sports and athletics played as a team or group
E008   Activities involving other specified sports and athletics
E009   Activities involving other cardiorespiratory exercise
E010   Activities involving other muscle strengthening exercises
E011   Activities involving computer technology and electronic devices
E012   Activities involving arts and handcrafts
E013   Activities involving personal hygiene and household maintenance
E014   Activities involving person providing caregiving
E015   Activities involving food preparation, cooking and grilling
E016   Activities involving property and land maintenance, building and construction
E017   Activities involving roller coasters and other types of external motion
E018   Activities involving playing musical instruments
E019   Activities involving animal care
E029   Other activity
E030   Unspecified activity

Railway accidents (E800-E807)
E800   Railway accident involving collision with rolling stock
E801   Railway accident involving collision with other object
E802   Railway accident involving derailment without antecedent collision
E803   Railway accident involving explosion, fire, or burning
E804   Fall in, on, or from railway train
E805   Hit by rolling stock
E806   Other specified railway accident
E807   Railway accident of unspecified nature

Motor vehicle traffic accidents (E810-E819)
E810   Motor vehicle traffic accident involving collision with train
E811   Motor vehicle traffic accident involving re-entrant collision with another motor vehicle
E812   Other motor vehicle traffic accident involving collision with another motor vehicle
E813   Motor vehicle traffic accident involving collision with other vehicle
E814   Motor vehicle traffic accident involving collision with pedestrian
E815   Other motor vehicle traffic accident involving collision on the highway
E816   Motor vehicle traffic accident due to loss of control, without collision on the highway
E817   Noncollision motor vehicle traffic accident while boarding or alighting
E818   Other noncollision motor vehicle traffic accident
E819   Motor vehicle traffic accident of unspecified nature

SUPPLEMENTARY CLASSIFICATION...INJURY AND POISONING *continued*

Motor vehicle nontraffic accidents (E820-E825)

E820 Nontraffic accident involving motor-driven snow vehicle
E821 Nontraffic accident involving other off-road motor vehicle
E822 Other motor vehicle nontraffic accident involving collision with moving object
E823 Other motor vehicle nontraffic accident involving collision with stationary object
E824 Other motor vehicle nontraffic accident while boarding and alighting
E825 Other motor vehicle nontraffic accident of other and unspecified nature

Other road vehicle accidents (E826-E829)

E826 Pedal cycle accident
E827 Animal-drawn vehicle accident
E828 Accident involving animal being ridden
E829 Other road vehicle accidents

Water transport accidents (E830-E838)

E830 Accident to watercraft causing submersion
E831 Accident to watercraft causing other injury
E832 Other accidental submersion or drowning in water transport accident
E833 Fall on stairs or ladders in water transport
E834 Other fall from one level to another in water transport
E835 Other and unspecified fall in water transport
E836 Machinery accident in water transport
E837 Explosion, fire, or burning in watercraft
E838 Other and unspecified water transport accident

Air and space transport accidents (E840-E845)

E840 Accident to powered aircraft at takeoff or landing
E841 Accident to powered aircraft, other and unspecified
E842 Accident to unpowered aircraft
E843 Fall in, on, or from aircraft
E844 Other specified air transport accidents
E845 Accident involving spacecraft

Vehicle accidents, not elsewhere classifiable (E846-E849)

E846 Accidents involving powered vehicles used solely within the buildings and premises of an industrial or commercial establishment
E847 Accidents involving cable cars not running on rails
E848 Accidents involving other vehicles, not elsewhere classifiable
E849 Place of occurrence

Accidental poisoning by drugs, medicinal substances, and biologicals (E850-E858)

E850 Accidental poisoning by analgesics, antipyretics, and antirheumatics
E851 Accidental poisoning by barbiturates
E852 Accidental poisoning by other sedatives and hypnotics
E853 Accidental poisoning by tranquilizers
E854 Accidental poisoning by other psychotropic agents
E855 Accidental poisoning by other drugs acting on central and autonomic nervous systems
E856 Accidental poisoning by antibiotics
E857 Accidental poisoning by other anti-infectives
E858 Accidental poisoning by other drugs

Accidental poisoning by other solid and liquid substances, gases, and vapors (E860-E869)

E860 Accidental poisoning by alcohol, not elsewhere classified
E861 Accidental poisoning by cleansing and polishing agents, disinfectants, paints, and varnishes
E862 Accidental poisoning by petroleum products, other solvents and their vapors, not elsewhere classified
E863 Accidental poisoning by agricultural and horticultural chemical and pharmaceutical preparations other than plant foods and fertilizers
E864 Accidental poisoning by corrosives and caustics, not elsewhere classified
E865 Accidental poisoning from poisonous foodstuffs and poisonous plants
E866 Accidental poisoning by other and unspecified solid and liquid substances
E867 Accidental poisoning by gas distributed by pipeline
E868 Accidental poisoning by other utility gas and other carbon monoxide
E869 Accidental poisoning by other gases and vapors

Misadventures to patients during surgical and medical care (E870-E876)

E870 Accidental cut, puncture, perforation, or hemorrhage during medical care
E871 Foreign object left in body during procedure
E872 Failure of sterile precautions during procedure

SUPPLEMENTARY CLASSIFICATION...INJURY AND POISONING *continued*

E873 Failure in dosage
E874 Mechanical failure of instrument or apparatus during procedure
E875 Contaminated or infected blood, other fluid, drug, or biological substance
E876 Other and unspecified misadventures during medical care

Surgical and medical procedures as the cause of abnormal reaction of patient or later complication, without mention of misadventure at the time of procedure (E878-E879)

E878 Surgical operation and other surgical procedures as the cause of abnormal reaction of patient, or of later complication, without mention of misadventure at the time of operation
E879 Other procedures, without mention of misadventure at the time of procedure, as the cause of abnormal reaction of patient, or of later complication

Accidental falls (E880-E888)

E880 Fall on or from stairs or steps
E881 Fall on or from ladders or scaffolding
E882 Fall from or out of building or other structure
E883 Fall into hole or other opening in surface
E884 Other fall from one level to another
E885 Fall on same level from slipping, tripping, or stumbling
E886 Fall on same level from collision, pushing or shoving, by or with other person
E887 Fracture, cause unspecified
E888 Other and unspecified fall

Accidents caused by fire and flames (E890-E899)

E890 Conflagration in private dwelling
E891 Conflagration in other and unspecified building or structure
E892 Conflagration not in building or structure
E893 Accident caused by ignition of clothing
E894 Ignition of highly inflammable material
E895 Accident caused by controlled fire in private dwelling
E896 Accident caused by controlled fire in other and unspecified building or structure
E897 Accident caused by controlled fire not in building or structure
E898 Accident caused by other specified fire and flames
E899 Accident caused by unspecified fire

Accidents due to natural and environmental factors (E900-E909)

E900 Excessive heat
E901 Excessive cold
E902 High and low air pressure and changes in air pressure
E903 Travel and motion
E904 Hunger, thirst, exposure, and neglect
E905 Venomous animals and plants as the cause of poisoning and toxic reactions
E906 Other injury caused by animals
E907 Lightning
E908 Cataclysmic storms, and floods resulting from storms
E909 Cataclysmic earth surface movements and eruptions

Accidents caused by submersion, suffocation, and foreign bodies (E910-E915)

E910 Accidental drowning and submersion
E911 Inhalation and ingestion of food causing obstruction of respiratory tract or suffocation
E912 Inhalation and ingestion of other object causing obstruction of respiratory tract or suffocation
E913 Accidental mechanical suffocation
E914 Foreign body accidentally entering eye and adnexa
E915 Foreign body accidentally entering other orifice

Other accidents (E916-E928)

E916 Struck accidentally by falling object
E917 Striking against or struck accidentally by objects or persons
E918 Caught accidentally in or between objects
E919 Accidents caused by machinery
E920 Accidents caused by cutting and piercing instruments or objects
E921 Accident caused by explosion of pressure vessel
E922 Accident caused by firearm and air gun missile
E923 Accident caused by explosive material
E924 Accident caused by hot substance or object, caustic or corrosive material, and steam
E925 Accident caused by electric current
E926 Exposure to radiation

SUPPLEMENTARY CLASSIFICATION...INJURY AND POISONING *continued*

    E927 Overexertion and strenuous and repetitive movements or loads
    E928 Other and unspecified environmental and accidental causes

Late effects of accidental injury (E929)
    E929 Late effects of accidental injury

Drugs, medicinal and biological substances causing adverse effects in therapeutic use (E930-E949)
    E930 Antibiotics
    E931 Other anti-infectives
    E932 Hormones and synthetic substitutes
    E933 Primarily systemic agents
    E934 Agents primarily affecting blood constituents
    E935 Analgesics, antipyretics, and antirheumatics
    E936 Anticonvulsants and anti-Parkinsonism drugs
    E937 Sedatives and hypnotics
    E938 Other central nervous system depressants and anesthetics
    E939 Psychotropic agents
    E940 Central nervous system stimulants
    E941 Drugs primarily affecting the autonomic nervous system
    E942 Agents primarily affecting the cardiovascular system
    E943 Agents primarily affecting gastrointestinal system
    E944 Water, mineral, and uric acid metabolism drugs
    E945 Agents primarily acting on the smooth and skeletal muscles and respiratory system
    E946 Agents primarily affecting skin and mucous membrane, ophthalmological, otorhinolaryngological, and dental drugs
    E947 Other and unspecified drugs and medicinal substances
    E948 Bacterial vaccines
    E949 Other vaccines and biological substances

Suicide and self-inflicted injury (E950-E959)
    E950 Suicide and self-inflicted poisoning by solid or liquid substances
    E951 Suicide and self-inflicted poisoning by gases in domestic use
    E952 Suicide and self-inflicted poisoning by other gases and vapors
    E953 Suicide and self-inflicted injury by hanging, strangulation, and suffocation
    E954 Suicide and self-inflicted injury by submersion [drowning]
    E955 Suicide and self-inflicted injury by firearms, air guns and explosives
    E956 Suicide and self-inflicted injury by cutting and piercing instruments
    E957 Suicide and self-inflicted injuries by jumping from high place
    E958 Suicide and self-inflicted injury by other and unspecified means
    E959 Late effects of self-inflicted injury

Homicide and injury purposely inflicted by other persons (E960-E969)
    E960 Fight, brawl, and rape
    E961 Assault by corrosive or caustic substance, except poisoning
    E962 Assault by poisoning
    E963 Assault by hanging and strangulation
    E964 Assault by submersion [drowning]
    E965 Assault by firearms and explosives
    E966 Assault by cutting and piercing instrument
    E967 Perpetrator of child and adult abuse
    E968 Assault by other and unspecified means
    E969 Late effects of injury purposely inflicted by other person

Legal intervention (E970-E978)
    E970 Injury due to legal intervention by firearms
    E971 Injury due to legal intervention by explosives
    E972 Injury due to legal intervention by gas
    E973 Injury due to legal intervention by blunt object
    E974 Injury due to legal intervention by cutting and piercing instruments
    E975 Injury due to legal intervention by other specified means
    E976 Injury due to legal intervention by unspecified means
    E977 Late effects of injuries due to legal intervention
    E978 Legal execution
    E979 Terrorism

SUPPLEMENTARY CLASSIFICATION...INJURY AND POISONING *continued*

Injury undetermined whether accidentally or purposely inflicted (E980-E989)

E980 Poisoning by solid or liquid substances, undetermined whether accidentally or purposely inflicted

E981 Poisoning by gases in domestic use, undetermined whether accidentally or purposely inflicted

E982 Poisoning by other gases, undetermined whether accidentally or purposely inflicted

E983 Hanging, strangulation, or suffocation, undetermined whether accidentally or purposely inflicted

E984 Submersion [drowning], undetermined whether accidentally or purposely inflicted

E985 Injury by firearms, air guns and explosives, undetermined whether accidentally or purposely inflicted

E986 Injury by cutting and piercing instruments, undetermined whether accidentally or purposely inflicted

E987 Falling from high place, undetermined whether accidentally or purposely inflicted

E988 Injury by other and unspecified means, undetermined whether accidentally or purposely inflicted

E989 Late effects of injury, undetermined whether accidentally or purposely inflicted

Injury resulting from operations of war (E990-E999)

E990 Injury due to war operations by fires and conflagrations

E991 Injury due to war operations by bullets and fragments

E992 Injury due to war operations by explosion of marine weapons

E993 Injury due to war operations by other explosion

E994 Injury due to war operations by destruction of aircraft

E995 Injury due to war operations by other and unspecified forms of conventional warfare

E996 Injury due to war operations by nuclear weapons

E997 Injury due to war operations by other forms of unconventional warfare

E998 Injury due to war operations but occurring after cessation of hostilities

E999 Late effects of injury due to war operations and terrorism

APPENDIX F:
LIST OF THREE-DIGIT ICD-9-CM CATEGORIES MAPPED TO ICD-10-CM

WHAT ARE GENERAL EQUIVALENCE MAPPINGS?

General Equivalence Mappings (GEMs), more commonly referred to as just mapping, are a tool that can be used to convert data from ICD-9-CM to ICD-10-CM and ICD-10-PCS and vice versa. Mapping from ICD-10-CM and ICD-10-PCS codes back to ICD-9-CM codes is referred to as backward mapping. Mapping from ICD-9-CM codes to ICD-10-CM and ICD-10-PCS codes is referred to as forward mapping.

The Centers for Medicare & Medicaid Services (CMS) and the Centers for Disease Control and Prevention (CDC) created the national version of the General Equivalence Mappings (GEM) to ensure that consistency in national data is maintained. They have made a commitment to update the GEMs annually along with the updates to International Classification of Diseases, 10th Edition, Clinical Modification (ICD-10-CM) and Procedure Coding System (PCS) during the transition period prior to ICD-10 implementation. CMS and CDC will maintain the GEMs for at least three years beyond October 1, 2014, which is the compliance date for implementation of ICD-10 for all covered entities.

The following tables list ICD-9-CM three-digit codes mapped to ICD-10-CM three-digit codes. The three-digit mapping table provides a quick reference for reviewing and learning the basic hierarchy of the ICD-10 coding system.

ICD-9-CM Code and Description	ICD-10-CM Code and Description

1. INFECTIOUS AND PARASITIC DISEASES
Intestinal infectious diseases (001-009)

001	Cholera	A00	Cholera
002	Typhoid and paratyphoid fevers	A01	Typhoid and paratyphoid fevers
003	Other salmonella infections	A02	Other salmonella infections
004	Shigellosis	A03	Shigellosis
005	Other food poisoning (bacterial)	A05	Other bacterial foodborne intoxications, not elsewhere classified
006	Amebiasis	A06	Amebiasis
007	Other protozoal intestinal diseases	A07	Other protozoal intestinal diseases
008	Intestinal infections due to other organisms	A04	Other bacterial intestinal infections
		A08	Viral and other specified intestinal infections
009	Ill-defined intestinal infections	A09	Infectious gastroenteritis and colitis unspecified
010	Primary tuberculous infection	A18	Tuberculosis of other organs
011	Pulmonary tuberculosis	A15	Respiratory tuberculosis
012	Other respiratory tuberculosis	A15	Respiratory tuberculosis
013	Tuberculosis of meninges and central nervous system	A17	Tuberculosis of nervous system
014	Tuberculosis of intestines, peritoneum, and mesenteric glands	A18	Tuberculosis of other organs
015	Tuberculosis of bones and joints	A18	Tuberculosis of other organs
018	Miliary tuberculosis	A19	Miliary tuberculosis

ICD-9-CM Code and Description	ICD-10-CM Code and Description

Zoonotic bacterial diseases (020-027)

020	Plague	A20	Plague
021	Tularemia	A21	Tularemia
022	Anthrax	A22	Anthrax
023	Brucellosis	A23	Brucellosis
024	Glanders	A24	Glanders and melioidosis
026	Rat-bite fever	A25	Rat-bite fever
027	Other zoonotic bacterial diseases	A26	Erysipeloid
		A28	Other zoonotic bacterial diseases, not elsewhere classified
		A32	Listeriosis

Other bacterial diseases (030-041)

030	Leprosy	A30	Leprosy (Hansen's disease)
031	Diseases due to other mycobacteria	A31	Infection due to other mycobacteria
032	Diphtheria	A36	Diphtheria
033	Whooping cough	A37	Whooping cough
034	Streptococcal sore throat and scarlet fever	A38	Scarlet fever
		J02	Acute nasopharyngitis [common cold]
		J03	Acute tonsillitis
035	Erysipelas	A46	Erysipelas
036	Meningococcal infection	A39	Meningococcal infection
037	Tetanus	A35	Other tetanus
038	Septicemia	A40	Streptococcal sepsis
		A41	Other sepsis
039	Actinomycotic infections	A42	Actinomycosis
		A43	Nocardiosis
040	Other bacterial diseases	A48	Other bacterial diseases, NEC
041	Bacterial infection in conditions classified elsewhere and of unspecified site	A49	Staphylococcal infection of unspecified site
		B95	Streptococcus, Staphylococcus, and Enterococcus as the cause of diseases classified elsewhere
		J20	Acute bronchitis

Human immunodeficiency virus (HIV) infection (042)

042	Human immunodeficiency virus [hiv] disease	B20	Human immunodeficiency virus [HIV] disease

Poliomyelitis and other non-arthropod-borne viral diseases of central nervous system (045-049)

045	Acute poliomyelitis	A80	Acute poliomyelitis
046	Slow virus infections and prion diseases of central nervous system	A81	Atypical virus infections of central nervous system
047	Meningitis due to enterovirus	A87	Viral meningitis
047	Meningitis due to enterovirus	B01	Varicella [chickenpox]

ICD-9-CM Code and Description	ICD-10-CM Code and Description
048 Other enterovirus diseases of central nervous system	A88 Other viral infections of central nervous system, not elsewhere classified
049 Other non-arthropod-borne viral diseases of central nervous system	A85 Other viral encephalitis, not elsewhere classified
	A86 Unspecified viral encephalitis
	A89 Unspecified viral infection of central nervous system

Viral diseases generally accompanied by exanthem (050-059)

050 Smallpox	B03 Smallpox
051 Cowpox and paravaccinia	B08 Cowpox
053 Herpes zoster	B02 Zoster [herpes zoster]
054 Herpes simplex	A60 Anogenital herpesviral [herpes simplex] infections
054 Herpes simplex	B00 Herpesviral [herpes simplex] infections
055 Measles	B05 Measles
056 Rubella	B06 Rubella [German measles]
057 Other viral exanthemata	B09 Other human herpesviruses
058 Other human herpesviruses	B10 Other human herpesviruses
059 Other poxvirus infections	B04 Monkeypox

Arthropod-borne viral diseases (060-066)

060 Yellow fever	A95 Yellow fever
061 Dengue	A90 Dengue fever [classical dengue]
062 Mosquito-borne viral encephalitis	A83 Mosquito-borne viral encephalitis
063 Tick-borne viral encephalitis	A84 Tick-borne viral encephalitis
064 Viral encephalitis transmitted by other and unspecified arthropods	A85 Other viral encephalitis, not elsewhere classified
065 Arthropod-borne hemorrhagic fever	A91 Dengue hemorrhagic fever
	A92 Other mosquito-borne viral fevers
	A98 Other viral hemorrhagic fevers, not elsewhere classified
	A99 Unspecified viral hemorrhagic fever
066 Other arthropod-borne viral diseases	A93 Other arthropod-borne viral fevers, not elsewhere classified
	A94 Unspecified arthropod-borne viral fever

Other diseases due to viruses and Chlamydiae (070-079)

070 Viral hepatitis	B15 Acute hepatitis A
	B16 Acute hepatitis B
	B17 Other acute viral hepatitis
	B18 Chronic viral hepatitis
	B19 Unspecified viral hepatitis
071 Rabies	A82 Rabies
072 Mumps	B26 Mumps
073 Ornithosis	A70 Chlamydia psittaci infections
074 Specific diseases due to coxsackie virus	B33 Other viral diseases, not elsewhere classified
075 Infectious mononucleosis	B27 Infectious mononucleosis
076 Trachoma	A71 Trachoma

ICD-9-CM Code and Description		ICD-10-CM Code and Description	
077	Other diseases of conjunctiva due to viruses and chlamydiae	A74	Other diseases caused by chlamydiae
		B30	Viral conjunctivitis
078	Other diseases due to viruses and chlamydiae	A63	Other predominantly sexually transmitted diseases, not elsewhere classified
		A96	Arenaviral hemorrhagic fever
		B07	Viral warts
		B25	Cytomegaloviral disease
079	Viral and chlamydial infection in conditions classified elsewhere and of unspecified	B34	Viral infection of unspecified site
		B97	Viral agents as the cause of diseases classified elsewhere

Rickettsioses and other arthropod-borne diseases (080-088)

080	Louse-borne [epidemic] typhus	A75	Typhus fever
081	Other typhus	A77	Spotted fever [tick-borne rickettsioses]
082	Tick-borne rickettsioses	A75	Typhus fever
083	Other rickettsioses	A78	Q fever
083	Other rickettsioses	A79	Other rickettsioses
084	Malaria	B50	Plasmodium falciparum malaria
		B51	Plasmodium vivax malaria
		B52	Plasmodium malariae malaria
		B53	Other specified malaria
		B54	Unspecified malaria
085	Leishmaniasis	B55	Leishmaniasis
086	Trypanosomiasis	B56	African trypanosomiasis
		B57	Chagas' disease
087	Relapsing fever	A68	Relapsing fevers
088	Other arthropod-borne diseases	A44	Bartonellosis
		B60	Other protozoal diseases, not elsewhere classified
		B64	Unspecified protozoal disease

Syphilis and other venereal diseases (090-099)

090	Congenital syphilis	A50	Congenital syphilis
091	Early syphilis, symptomatic	A51	Early syphilis
092	Early syphilis, latent	A51	Early syphilis
093	Cardiovascular syphilis	A52	Late syphilis
094	Neurosyphilis	A50	Congenital syphilis
		A52	Late syphilis
095	Other forms of late syphilis, with symptoms	A52	Late syphilis
097	Other and unspecified syphilis	A53	Other and unspecified syphilis
098	Gonococcal infections	A54	Gonococcal infection
099	Other venereal diseases	A55	Chlamydial lymphogranuloma (venereum)
		A56	Other sexually transmitted chlamydial diseases
		A57	Chancroid

ICD-9-CM Code and Description	ICD-10-CM Code and Description
	A58 Granuloma inguinale
	A64 Unspecified sexually transmitted disease

Other spirochetal diseases (100-104)

100 Leptospirosis	A27 Leptospirosis
101 Vincent's angina	A69 Other spirochetal infections
102 Yaws	A66 Yaws
103 Pinta	A67 Pinta [carate]
104 Other spirochetal infection	A65 Nonvenereal syphilis

Mycoses (110-118)

110 Dermatophytosis	B35 Dermatophytosis
111 Dermatomycosis, other and unspecified	B36 Other superficial mycoses
112 Candidiasis	B37 Candidiasis
114 Coccidioidomycosis	B38 Coccidioidomycosis
115 Histoplasmosis	B39 Histoplasmosis
116 Blastomycotic infection	B40 Blastomycosis
	B41 Paracoccidioidomycosis
	B48 Other mycoses, not elsewhere classified
117 Other mycoses	B42 Sporotrichosis
	B43 Chromomycosis and pheomycotic abscess
	B44 Aspergillosis
	B45 Cryptococcosis
	B46 Zygomycosis
	B47 Mycetoma
	B49 Unspecified mycosis
118 Opportunistic mycoses	B48 Other mycoses, not elsewhere classified

Helminthiases (120-129)

120 Schistosomiasis [bilharziasis]	B65 Schistosomiasis [bilharziasis]
121 Other trematode infections	B66 Other fluke infections
122 Echinococcosis	B67 Echinococcosis
123 Other cestode infection	B68 Taeniasis
	B69 Cysticercosis
	B70 Diphyllobothriasis and sparganosis
	B71 Other cestode infections
124 Trichinosis	B75 Trichinellosis
125 Filarial infection and dracontiasis	B72 Dracunculiasis
	B73 Onchocerciasis
	B74 Filariasis
126 Ancylostomiasis and necatoriasis	B76 Hookworm diseases
127 Other intestinal helminthiases	B77 Ascariasis
	B78 Strongyloidiasis
	B79 Trichuriasis
	B80 Enterobiasis
	B81 Other intestinal helminthiases, not elsewhere classified

ICD-9-CM Code and Description		ICD-10-CM Code and Description	
		B82	Unspecified intestinal parasitism
128	Other and unspecified helminthiases	B83	Other helminthiases
129	Intestinal parasitism, unspecified	B82	Unspecified intestinal parasitism

Other infectious and parasitic diseases (130-136)

130	Toxoplasmosis	B58	Toxoplasmosis
131	Trichomoniasis	A59	Trichomoniasis
132	Pediculosis and Phthirus infestation	B85	Pediculosis and phthiriasis
133	Acariasis	B86	Scabies
		B88	Other infestations
134	Other infestation	B87	Myiasis
135	Sarcoidosis	D86	Sarcoidosis
136	Other and unspecified infectious and parasitic diseases	B59	Pneumocystosis
		B89	Unspecified parasitic disease
		B99	Other and unspecified infectious diseases

Late effects of infectious and parasitic diseases (137-139)

137	Late effects of tuberculosis	B90	Sequelae of tuberculosis
138	Late effects of acute poliomyelitis	B91	Sequelae of poliomyelitis
		G14	Postpolio syndrome
139	Late effects of other infectious and parasitic diseases	B92	Sequelae of leprosy
		B94	Sequelae of other and unspecified infectious and parasitic diseases

2. NEOPLASMS

Malignant neoplasm of lip, oral cavity, and pharynx (140-149)

140	Malignant neoplasm of lip	C00	Malignant neoplasm of lip
141	Malignant neoplasm of tongue	C01	Malignant neoplasm of base of tongue
		C02	Malignant neoplasm of other and unspecified parts of tongue
142	Malignant neoplasm of major salivary glands	C07	Malignant neoplasm of parotid gland
		C08	Malignant neoplasm of other and unspecified major salivary glands
143	Malignant neoplasm of gum	C03	Malignant neoplasm of gum
144	Malignant neoplasm of floor of mouth	C04	Malignant neoplasm of floor of mouth
145	Malignant neoplasm of other and unspecified parts of mouth	C05	Malignant neoplasm of palate
		C06	Malignant neoplasm of other and unspecified parts of mouth
146	Malignant neoplasm of oropharynx	C09	Malignant neoplasm of tonsil
		C10	Malignant neoplasm of oropharynx
147	Malignant neoplasm of nasopharynx	C11	Malignant neoplasm of nasopharynx
148	Malignant neoplasm of hypopharynx	C12	Malignant neoplasm of pyriform sinus
		C13	Malignant neoplasm of hypopharynx
149	Malignant neoplasm of other and ill-defined sites within the lip, oral cavity, and	C14	Malignant neoplasm of other and ill-defined sites in the lip, oral cavity and pharynx

ICD-9-CM Code and Description	ICD-10-CM Code and Description

Malignant neoplasm of digestive organs and peritoneum (150-159)

150	Malignant neoplasm of esophagus	C15	Malignant neoplasm of esophagus
151	Malignant neoplasm of stomach	C16	Malignant neoplasm of stomach
152	Malignant neoplasm of small intestine, including duodenum	C17	Malignant neoplasm of small intestine
153	Malignant neoplasm of colon	C18	Malignant neoplasm of colon
154	Malignant neoplasm of rectum, rectosigmoid junction, and anus	C19	Malignant neoplasm of rectosigmoid junction
		C20	Malignant neoplasm of rectum
		C21	Malignant neoplasm of anus and anal canal
155	Malignant neoplasm of liver and intrahepatic bile ducts	C22	Malignant neoplasm of liver and intrahepatic bile ducts
156	Malignant neoplasm of gallbladder and extrahepatic bile ducts	C23	Malignant neoplasm of gallbladder
		C24	Malignant neoplasm of other and unspecified parts of biliary tract
157	Malignant neoplasm of pancreas	C25	Malignant neoplasm of pancreas
158	Malignant neoplasm of retroperitoneum and peritoneum	C48	Malignant neoplasm of retroperitoneum and peritoneum
159	Malignant neoplasm of other and ill-defined sites within the digestive organs and	C26	Malignant neoplasm of other and ill-defined digestive organs

Malignant neoplasm of respiratory and intrathoracic organs (160-165)

160	Malignant neoplasm of nasal cavities, middle ear, and accessory sinuses	C30	Malignant neoplasm of nasal cavity and middle ear
		C31	Malignant neoplasm of accessory sinuses
161	Malignant neoplasm of larynx	C32	Malignant neoplasm of larynx
162	Malignant neoplasm of trachea, bronchus, and lung	C33	Malignant neoplasm of trachea
		C34	Malignant neoplasm of bronchus and lung
163	Malignant neoplasm of pleura	C45	Mesothelioma
164	Malignant neoplasm of thymus, heart, and mediastinum	C37	Malignant neoplasm of thymus
		C38	Malignant neoplasm of heart, mediastinum and pleura
165	Malignant neoplasm of other and ill-defined sites within the respiratory system and	C39	Malignant neoplasm of other and ill-defined sites in the respiratory system and intrathoracic organs

Malignant neoplasm of bone, connective tissue, skin, and breast (170-176)

170	Malignant neoplasm of bone and articular cartilage	C40	Malignant neoplasm of bone and articular cartilage of limbs
		C41	Malignant neoplasm of bone and articular cartilage of other and unspecified sites

ICD-9-CM Code and Description		ICD-10-CM Code and Description	
171	Malignant neoplasm of connective and other soft tissue	C47	Malignant neoplasm of peripheral nerves and autonomic nervous system
		C49	Malignant neoplasm of other connective and soft tissue
172	Malignant melanoma of skin	C43	Malignant melanoma of skin
		D03	Melanoma in situ
173	Other malignant neoplasm of skin	C44	Other and unspecified malignant neoplasm of skin
174	Malignant neoplasm of female breast	C50	Malignant neoplasm of breast
176	Kaposi's sarcoma	C46	Kaposi's sarcoma

Malignant neoplasm of genitourinary organs (179-189)

179	Malignant neoplasm of uterus, part unspecified	C55	Malignant neoplasm of uterus, part unspecified
180	Malignant neoplasm of cervix uteri	C53	Malignant neoplasm of cervix uteri
181	Malignant neoplasm of placenta	C58	Malignant neoplasm of placenta
182	Malignant neoplasm of body of uterus	C54	Malignant neoplasm of corpus uteri
183	Malignant neoplasm of ovary and other uterine adnexa	C56	Malignant neoplasm of ovary
		C57	Malignant neoplasm of other and unspecified female genital organs
184	Malignant neoplasm of other and unspecified female genital organs	C57	Malignant neoplasm of other and unspecified female genital organs
		C52	Malignant neoplasm of vagina
185	Malignant neoplasm of prostate	C61	Malignant neoplasm of prostate
186	Malignant neoplasm of testis	C62	Malignant neoplasm of testis
187	Malignant neoplasm of penis and other male genital organs	C60	Malignant neoplasm of penis
		C63	Malignant neoplasm of other and unspecified male genital organs
188	Malignant neoplasm of bladder	C67	Malignant neoplasm of bladder
189	Malignant neoplasm of kidney and other and unspecified urinary organs	C64	Malignant neoplasm of kidney, except renal pelvis
		C65	Malignant neoplasm of renal pelvis
		C66	Malignant neoplasm of ureter
		C68	Malignant neoplasm of other and unspecified urinary organs

Malignant neoplasm of other and unspecified sites (190-199)

190	Malignant neoplasm of eye	C69	Malignant neoplasm of eye and adnexa
191	Malignant neoplasm of brain	C71	Malignant neoplasm of brain
192	Malignant neoplasm of other and unspecified parts of nervous system	C70	Malignant neoplasm of meninges
		C72	Malignant neoplasm of spinal cord, cranial nerves and other parts of central nervous system
193	Malignant neoplasm of thyroid gland	C73	Malignant neoplasm of thyroid gland
194	Malignant neoplasm of other endocrine glands and related structures	C74	Malignant neoplasm of adrenal gland
		C75	Malignant neoplasm of other endocrine glands and related structures
195	Malignant neoplasm of other and ill-defined sites	C76	Malignant neoplasm of other and ill-defined sites

ICD-9-CM Code and Description | **ICD-10-CM Code and Description**

196	Secondary and unspecified malignant neoplasm of lymph nodes	C77	Secondary and unspecified malignant neoplasm of lymph nodes
197	Secondary malignant neoplasm of respiratory and digestive systems	C78	Secondary malignant neoplasm of respiratory and digestive organs
198	Secondary malignant neoplasm of other specified sites	C79	Secondary malignant neoplasm of other and unspecified sites
199	Malignant neoplasm without specification of site	C80	Malignant neoplasm without specification of site
		G73	Malignant neoplasm of thyroid gland

Malignant neoplasm of lymphatic and hematopoietic tissue (200-208)

200	Lymphosarcoma and reticulosarcoma and other specified malignant tumors of	C83	Non-follicular lymphoma
201	Hodgkin's disease	C81	Hodgkin lymphoma
202	Other malignant neoplasm of lymphoid and histiocytic tissue	C82	Follicular lymphoma
		C84	Mature T/NK-cell lymphomas
		C85	Other specified and unspecified types of non-Hodgkin lymphoma
		C86	Other specified types of T/NK-cell lymphoma
		C96	Other and unspecified malignant neoplasms of lymphoid, hematopoietic and related tissue
203	Multiple myeloma and immunoproliferative neoplasms	C90	Multiple myeloma and malignant plasma cell neoplasms
204	Lymphoid leukemia	C91	Lymphoid leukemia
205	Myeloid leukemia	C92	Myeloid leukemia
206	Monocytic leukemia	C93	Monocytic leukemia
207	Other specified leukemia	C94	Other leukemias of specified cell type
207	Other specified leukemia	D45	Polycythemia vera
208	Leukemia of unspecified cell type	C95	Leukemia of unspecified cell type

Neuroendocrine tumors (209)

209	Neuroendocrine tumors	C4A	Merkel cell carcinoma
		C7A	Malignant neuroendocrine tumors
		C7B	Secondary neuroendocrine tumors
		D3A	Benign carcinoid tumor of unspecified site

Benign neoplasms (210-229)

210	Benign neoplasm of lip, oral cavity, and pharynx	D10	Benign neoplasm of mouth and pharynx
		D11	Benign neoplasm of major salivary glands
211	Benign neoplasm of other parts of digestive system	D12	Benign neoplasm of colon, rectum, anus and anal canal
		D13	Benign neoplasm of other and ill-defined parts of digestive system
		D20	Benign neoplasm of soft tissue of retroperitoneum and peritoneum

ICD-9-CM Code and Description	ICD-10-CM Code and Description
212 Benign neoplasm of respiratory and intrathoracic organs	D14 Benign neoplasm of middle ear and respiratory system
	D15 Benign neoplasm of other and unspecified intrathoracic organs
	D19 Benign neoplasm of mesothelial tissue
213 Benign neoplasm of bone and articular cartilage	D16 Benign neoplasm of bone and articular cartilage
214 Lipoma	D17 Benign lipomatous neoplasm
215 Other benign neoplasm of connective and other soft tissue	D21 Other benign neoplasms of connective and other soft tissue
216 Benign neoplasm of skin	D22 Melanocytic nevi
	D23 Other benign neoplasms of skin
217 Benign neoplasm of breast	D24 Benign neoplasm of breast
218 Uterine leiomyoma	D25 Leiomyoma of uterus
219 Other benign neoplasm of uterus	D26 Other benign neoplasms of uterus
220 Benign neoplasm of ovary	D27 Benign neoplasm of ovary
221 Benign neoplasm of other female genital organs	D28 Benign neoplasm of other and unspecified female genital organs
222 Benign neoplasm of male genital organs	D29 Benign neoplasm of male genital organs
223 Benign neoplasm of kidney and other urinary organs	D30 Benign neoplasm of urinary organs
224 Benign neoplasm of eye	D31 Benign neoplasm of eye and adnexa
225 Benign neoplasm of brain and other parts of nervous system	D32 Benign neoplasm of meninges
	D33 Benign neoplasm of brain and other parts of central nervous system
226 Benign neoplasm of thyroid gland	D34 Benign neoplasm of thyroid gland
227 Benign neoplasm of other endocrine glands and related structures	D35 Benign neoplasm of other and unspecified endocrine glands
228 Hemangioma and lymphangioma, any site	D18 Hemangioma and lymphangioma, any site
229 Benign neoplasm of other and unspecified sites	D36 Benign neoplasm of other and unspecified sites

Carcinoma in situ (230-234)

230 Carcinoma in situ of digestive organs	D00 Carcinoma in situ of oral cavity, esophagus and stomach
230 Carcinoma in situ of digestive organs	D01 Carcinoma in situ of other and unspecified digestive organs
231 Carcinoma in situ of respiratory system	D02 Carcinoma in situ of middle ear and respiratory system
232 Carcinoma in situ of skin	D04 Carcinoma in situ of skin
233 Carcinoma in situ of breast and genitourinary system	D05 Carcinoma in situ of breast
	D06 Carcinoma in situ of cervix uteri
	D07 Carcinoma in situ of other and unspecified genital organs
	D09 Carcinoma in situ of other and unspecified sites
234 Carcinoma in situ of other and unspecified sites	D09 Carcinoma in situ of other and unspecified sites

ICD-9-CM Code and Description   **ICD-10-CM Code and Description**

Neoplasms of uncertain behavior (235-238)

235	Neoplasm of uncertain behavior of digestive and respiratory systems	D37	Neoplasm of uncertain behavior of oral cavity and digestive organs
		D38	Neoplasm of uncertain behavior of middle ear and respiratory and intrathoracic organs
236	Neoplasm of uncertain behavior of genitourinary organs	D39	Neoplasm of uncertain behavior of female genital organs
		D40	Neoplasm of uncertain behavior of male genital organs
		D41	Neoplasm of uncertain behavior of urinary organs
237	Neoplasm of uncertain behavior of endocrine glands and nervous system	D42	Neoplasm of uncertain behavior of meninges
		D43	Neoplasm of uncertain behavior of brain and central nervous system
		D44	Neoplasm of uncertain behavior of endocrine glands
		Q85	Phakomatoses, not elsewhere classified
238	Neoplasm of uncertain behavior of other and unspecified sites and tissues	D46	Myelodysplastic syndromes
		D47	Other neoplasms of uncertain behavior of lymphoid, hematopoietic and related tissue
		D48	Neoplasm of uncertain behavior of other and unspecified sites

Neoplasm of unspecified nature (239)

239	Neoplasm of unspecified nature	D49	Neoplasms of unspecified behavior

3. ENDOCRINE, NUTRITIONAL AND METABOLIC DISEASES, AND IMMUNITY DISORDERS

Disorders of thyroid gland (240-246)

240	Simple and unspecified goiter	E01	Iodine-deficiency related thyroid disorders and allied conditions
		E04	Other nontoxic goiter
241	Nontoxic nodular goiter	E04	Other nontoxic goiter
242	Thyrotoxicosis with or without goiter	E05	Thyrotoxicosis [hyperthyroidism]
243	Congenital hypothyroidism	E00	Congenital iodine-deficiency syndrome
		E03	Other hypothyroidism
244	Acquired hypothyroidism	E02	Subclinical iodine-deficiency hypothyroidism
		E89	Postprocedural endocrine and metabolic complications and disorders, not elsewhere classified
245	Thyroiditis	E06	Thyroiditis
246	Other disorders of thyroid	E07	Other disorders of thyroid
		E35	Disorders of endocrine glands in diseases classified elsewhere

Diseases of other endocrine glands (249-259)

249	Secondary diabetes mellitus	E09	Drug or chemical induced diabetes mellitus

ICD-9-CM Code and Description	ICD-10-CM Code and Description

250	Diabetes mellitus	E10	Type 1 diabetes mellitus
		E11	Type 2 diabetes mellitus
		E13	Other specified diabetes mellitus
251	Other disorders of pancreatic internal secretion	E08	Diabetes mellitus due to underlying condition
		E15	Nondiabetic hypoglycemic coma
		E16	Other disorders of pancreatic internal secretion
252	Disorders of parathyroid gland	E20	Hypoparathyroidism
		E21	Hyperparathyroidism and other disorders of parathyroid gland
253	Disorders of the pituitary gland and its hypothalamic control	E22	Hyperfunction of pituitary gland
		E23	Hypofunction and other disorders of the pituitary gland
254	Diseases of thymus gland	E32	Diseases of thymus
255	Disorders of adrenal glands	E24	Cushing's syndrome
		E25	Adrenogenital disorders
		E26	Hyperaldosteronism
		E27	Other disorders of adrenal gland
256	Ovarian dysfunction	E28	Ovarian dysfunction
257	Testicular dysfunction	E29	Testicular dysfunction
258	Polyglandular dysfunction and related disorders	E31	Polyglandular dysfunction
259	Other endocrine disorders	E30	Disorders of puberty, not elsewhere classified
		E34	Other endocrine disorders

Nutritional deficiencies (260-269)

260	Kwashiorkor	E40	Kwashiorkor
		E42	Marasmic kwashiorkor
261	Nutritional marasmus	E41	Nutritional marasmus
262	Other severe protein-calorie malnutrition	E43	Unspecified severe protein-calorie malnutrition
263	Other and unspecified protein-calorie malnutrition	E44	Protein-calorie malnutrition of moderate and mild degree
		E45	Retarded development following protein-calorie malnutrition
		E46	Unspecified protein-calorie malnutrition
		E64	Sequelae of malnutrition and other nutritional deficiencies
264	Vitamin a deficiency	E50	Vitamin A deficiency
265	Thiamine and niacin deficiency states	E51	Thiamine deficiency
		E52	Niacin deficiency [pellagra]
266	Deficiency of b-complex components	E53	Deficiency of other B group vitamins
267	Ascorbic acid deficiency	E54	Ascorbic acid deficiency
268	Vitamin d deficiency	E55	Vitamin D deficiency
		M83	Puerperal osteomalacia
269	Other nutritional deficiencies	E56	Other vitamin deficiencies
		E58	Dietary calcium deficiency

ICD-9-CM Code and Description		ICD-10-CM Code and Description	
		E59	Dietary selenium deficiency
		E60	Dietary zinc deficiency
		E61	Deficiency of other nutrient elements
		E63	Other nutritional deficiencies

Other metabolic and immunity disorders (270-279)

270	Disorders of amino-acid transport and metabolism	E70	Disorders of aromatic amino-acid metabolism
		E71	Disorders of branched-chain amino-acid metabolism and fatty-acid metabolism
		E72	Other disorders of amino-acid metabolism
271	Disorders of carbohydrate transport and metabolism	E73	Lactose intolerance
		E74	Other disorders of carbohydrate metabolism
272	Disorders of lipoid metabolism	E77	Disorders of glycoprotein metabolism
		E78	Disorders of lipoprotein metabolism and other lipidemias
273	Disorders of plasma protein metabolism	C88	Malignant immunoproliferative diseases and certain other B-cell lymphomas
		D89	Other disorders involving the immune mechanism, not elsewhere classified
		E88	Other and unspecified metabolic disorders
274	Gout	M10	Idiopathic gout unspecified site
		M1A	Idiopathic chronic gout unspecified site without tophus (tophi)
275	Disorders of mineral metabolism	E83	Disorders of mineral metabolism
276	Disorders of fluid, electrolyte, and acid-base balance	E86	Volume depletion
		E87	Other disorders of fluid, electrolyte and acid-base balance
277	Other and unspecified disorders of metabolism	E76	Disorders of glycosaminoglycan metabolism
		E80	Disorders of porphyrin and bilirubin metabolism
		E84	Cystic fibrosis
		E85	Amyloidosis
278	Overweight, obesity and other hyperalimentation	E65	Localized adiposity
		E66	Overweight and obesity
		E67	Other hyperalimentation
		E68	Sequelae of hyperalimentation
279	Disorders involving the immune mechanism	D80	Immunodeficiency with predominantly antibody defects
		D81	Combined immunodeficiencies
		D82	Immunodeficiency associated with other major defects
		D83	Common variable immunodeficiency
		D84	Other immunodeficiencies

ICD-9-CM Code and Description	ICD-10-CM Code and Description

4. DISEASES OF THE BLOOD AND BLOOD-FORMING ORGANS

Diseases of blood and blood-forming organs (280-289)

ICD-9-CM		ICD-10-CM	
280	Iron deficiency anemias	D50	Iron deficiency anemia
281	Other deficiency anemias	D51	Vitamin B12 deficiency anemia
		D52	Folate deficiency anemia
		D53	Other nutritional anemias
282	Hereditary hemolytic anemias	D55	Anemia due to enzyme disorders
		D56	Thalassemia
		D57	Sickle-cell disorders
		D58	Other hereditary hemolytic anemias
283	Acquired hemolytic anemias	D59	Acquired hemolytic anemia
284	Aplastic anemia and other bone marrow failure syndromes	D60	Acquired pure red cell aplasia [erythroblastopenia]
		D61	Other aplastic anemias and other bone marrow failure syndromes
285	Other and unspecified anemias	D62	Acute posthemorrhagic anemia
		D63	Anemia in chronic diseases classified elsewhere
		D64	Other anemias
286	Coagulation defects	D65	Disseminated intravascular coagulation [defibrination syndrome]
		D66	Hereditary factor VIII deficiency
		D67	Hereditary factor IX deficiency
		D68	Other coagulation defects
287	Purpura and other hemorrhagic conditions	D69	Purpura and other hemorrhagic conditions
288	Diseases of white blood cells	D70	Neutropenia
		D71	Functional disorders of polymorphonuclear neutrophils
		D72	Other disorders of white blood cells
		D76	Other specified diseases with participation of lymphoreticular and reticulohistiocytic tissue
289	Other diseases of blood and blood-forming organs	D73	Diseases of spleen
		D74	Methemoglobinemia
		D75	Other and unspecified diseases of blood and blood-forming organs
		D77	Other disorders of blood and blood-forming organs in diseases classified elsewhere
		I88	Nonspecific lymphadenitis

5. MENTAL DISORDERS

Organic psychotic conditions (290-294)

ICD-9-CM		ICD-10-CM	
290	Dementias	F01	Vascular dementia
		F03	Unspecified dementia
291	Alcohol-induced mental disorders	F10	Alcohol related disorders

ICD-9-CM Code and Description	ICD-10-CM Code and Description
292 Drug induced mental disorders	F19 Other psychoactive substance related disorders
293 Transient mental disorders due to conditions classified elsewhere	F05 Delirium due to known physiological condition
	F06 Unspecified dementia
294 Persistent mental disorders due to conditions classified elsewhere	F02 Dementia in other diseases classified elsewhere
	F04 Amnestic disorder due to known physiological condition

Other psychoses (295-299)

295 Schizophrenic disorders	F25 Schizoaffective disorders
296 Episodic mood disorders	F30 Manic episode
	F31 Bipolar disorder
	F32 Major depressive disorder, single episode
	F33 Major depressive disorder, recurrent
	F39 Unspecified mood [affective] disorder
297 Delusional disorders	F22 Delusional disorders
	F24 Shared psychotic disorder
298 Other nonorganic psychoses	F23 Brief psychotic disorder
	F28 Other psychotic disorder not due to a substance or known physiological condition
	F29 Unspecified psychosis not due to a substance or known physiological condition
299 Pervasive developmental disorders	F84 Pervasive developmental disorders

Neurotic disorders, personality disorders, and other nonpsychotic mental disorders (300-316)

300 Anxiety, dissociative and somatoform disorders	F40 Phobic anxiety disorders
	F41 Other anxiety disorders
	F42 Obsessive-compulsive disorder
	F44 Dissociative and conversion disorders
	F45 Somatoform disorders
	F48 Other nonpsychotic mental disorders
	F99 Mental disorder not otherwise specified
301 Personality disorders	F21 Schizotypal disorder
	F34 Persistent mood [affective] disorders
	F60 Specific personality disorders
	F68 Other disorders of adult personality and behavior
	F69 Unspecified disorder of adult personality and behavior
302 Sexual and gender identity disorders	F52 Sexual dysfunction not due to a substance or known physiological condition
	F64 Gender identity disorders
	F65 Paraphilias

ICD-9-CM Code and Description		ICD-10-CM Code and Description	
		F66	Other sexual disorders
		R37	Sexual dysfunction, unspecified
303	Alcohol dependence syndrome	F10	Alcohol related disorders
304	Drug dependence	F14	Cocaine related disorders
305	Nondependent abuse of drugs	F10	Alcohol related disorders
		F11	Opioid related disorders
		F12	Cannabis related disorders
		F13	Sedative, hypnotic, or anxiolytic related disorders
		F14	Cocaine related disorders
		F15	Other stimulant related disorders
		F16	Hallucinogen related disorders
		F17	Nicotine dependence
		F18	Inhalant related disorders
		F19	Other psychoactive substance related disorders
		F55	Abuse of non-psychoactive substances
306	Physiological malfunction arising from mental factors	F59	Unspecified behavioral syndromes associated with physiological disturbances and physical factors
307	Special symptoms or syndromes, not elsewhere classified	F50	Eating disorders
		F95	Tic disorder
		F98	Other behavioral and emotional disorders with onset usually occurring in childhood and adolescence
308	Acute reaction to stress	F43	Reaction to severe stress, and adjustment disorders
309	Adjustment reaction	F93	Emotional disorders with onset specific to childhood
310	Specific nonpsychotic mental disorders due to brain damage	F07	Other mental disorders due to known physiological condition
		F09	Personality and behavioral disorders due to known physiological condition
311	Depressive disorder, not elsewhere classified	F32	Major depressive disorder, single episode
312	Disturbance of conduct, not elsewhere classified	F63	Impulse disorders
		F91	Conduct disorders
313	Disturbance of emotions specific to childhood and adolescence	F94	Disorders of social functioning with onset specific to childhood and adolescence
314	Hyperkinetic syndrome of childhood	F90	Attention-deficit hyperactivity disorders
315	Specific delays in development	F80	Specific developmental disorders of speech and language
		F81	Specific developmental disorders of scholastic skills
		F82	Specific developmental disorder of motor function
		F88	Other disorders of psychological development
		F89	Unspecified disorder of psychological development
		R48	Dyslexia and other symbolic dysfunctions, not elsewhere classified

ICD-9-CM Code and Description		ICD-10-CM Code and Description	
316	Psychic factors associated with diseases classified elsewhere	F54	Psychological and behavioral factors associated with disorders or diseases classified elsewhere

Mental retardation (317-319)

317	Mild mental retardation	F70	Mild intellectual disabilities
318	Other specified mental retardation	F71	Moderate mental retardation
		F72	Severe intellectual disabilities
		F73	Profound intellectual disabilities
319	Unspecified mental retardation	F78	Other intellectual disabilities
		F79	Unspecified intellectual disabilities

6. DISEASES OF THE NERVOUS SYSTEM AND SENSE ORGANS
Inflammatory diseases of the central nervous system (320-326)

320	Bacterial meningitis	G00	Bacterial meningitis, not elsewhere classified
		G01	Meningitis in bacterial diseases classified elsewhere
321	Meningitis due to other organisms	G02	Meningitis in other infectious and parasitic diseases classified elsewhere
322	Meningitis of unspecified cause	G03	Meningitis due to other and unspecified causes
323	Encephalitis, myelitis, and encephalomyelitis	G04	Encephalitis, myelitis and encephalomyelitis
		G05	Encephalitis, myelitis and encephalomyelitis in diseases classified elsewhere
		G92	Toxic encephalopathy
324	Intracranial and intraspinal abscess	G06	Intracranial and intraspinal abscess and granuloma
		G07	Intracranial and intraspinal abscess and granuloma in diseases classified elsewhere
325	Phlebitis and thrombophlebitis of intracranial venous sinuses	G08	Intracranial and intraspinal phlebitis and thrombophlebitis
326	Late effects of intracranial abscess or pyogenic infection	G09	Sequelae of inflammatory diseases of central nervous system

Organic sleep disorders (327)

327	Organic sleep disorders	F51	Sleep disorders not due to a substance or known physiological condition

Hereditary and degenerative diseases of the central nervous system (330-337)

330	Cerebral degenerations usually manifest in childhood	E75	Disorders of sphingolipid metabolism and other lipid storage disorders
331	Other cerebral degenerations	G30	Alzheimer's disease
		G31	Other degenerative diseases of nervous system, not elsewhere classified
		G91	Hydrocephalus
		G94	Other disorders of brain in diseases classified elsewhere
332	Parkinson's disease	G20	Parkinson's disease

ICD-9-CM Code and Description	ICD-10-CM Code and Description
333 Other extrapyramidal disease and abnormal movement disorders	G10 Huntington's disease
	G21 Secondary parkinsonism
	G23 Other degenerative diseases of basal ganglia
	G24 Dystonia
	G25 Other extrapyramidal and movement disorders
	G26 Extrapyramidal and movement disorders in diseases classified elsewhere
334 Spinocerebellar disease	G11 Hereditary ataxia
335 Anterior horn cell disease	G12 Spinal muscular atrophy and related syndromes
336 Other diseases of spinal cord	G32 Other degenerative disorders of nervous system in diseases classified elsewhere
	G95 Other and unspecified diseases of spinal cord
337 Disorders of the autonomic nervous system	G90 Disorders of autonomic nervous system
	G99 Other disorders of nervous system in diseases classified elsewhere

Pain (338)

338 Pain, not elsewhere classified	G89 Pain, not elsewhere classified
	R52 Pain, unspecified

Other headache syndromes (339)

339 Other headache syndromes	G44 Other headache syndromes

Other disorders of the central nervous system (340-349)

340 Multiple sclerosis	G35 Multiple sclerosis
341 Other demyelinating diseases of central nervous system	G36 Other acute disseminated demyelination
	G37 Other demyelinating diseases of central nervous system
342 Hemiplegia and hemiparesis	G81 Hemiplegia and hemiparesis
343 Infantile cerebral palsy	G80 Cerebral palsy
344 Other paralytic syndromes	G82 Paraplegia (paraparesis) and quadriplegia (quadriparesis)
	G83 Other paralytic syndromes
345 Epilepsy and recurrent seizures	G40 Epilepsy and recurrent seizures
346 Migraine	G43 Migraine
348 Other conditions of brain	G93 Other disorders of brain
349 Other and unspecified disorders of the nervous system	G96 Other disorders of central nervous system
	G98 Other disorders of nervous system not elsewhere classified

ICD-9-CM Code and Description	ICD-10-CM Code and Description

Disorders of the peripheral nervous system (350-359)

350	Trigeminal nerve disorders	G50	Disorders of trigeminal nerve
351	Facial nerve disorders	G51	Facial nerve disorders
352	Disorders of other cranial nerves	G52	Disorders of other cranial nerves
		G53	Cranial nerve disorders in diseases classified elsewhere
353	Nerve root and plexus disorders	G54	Nerve root and plexus disorders
		G55	Mononeuropathies of upper limb
354	Mononeuritis of upper limb and mononeuritis multiplex	G56	Mononeuropathies of lower limb
		G58	Other mononeuropathies
355	Mononeuritis of lower limb and unspecified site	G57	Mononeuropathy in diseases classified elsewhere
		G59	Hereditary and idiopathic neuropathy
356	Hereditary and idiopathic peripheral neuropathy	G60	Disorders of trigeminal nerve
357	Inflammatory and toxic neuropathy	G13	Systemic atrophies primarily affecting central nervous system in diseases classified elsewhere
		G61	Inflammatory polyneuropathy
		G62	Other and unspecified polyneuropathies
		G63	Polyneuropathy in diseases classified elsewhere
		G64	Other disorders of peripheral nervous system
		G65	Sequelae of inflammatory and toxic polyneuropathies
358	Myoneural disorders	G70	Myasthenia gravis and other myoneural disorders
359	Muscular dystrophies and other myopathies	G71	Primary disorders of muscles
		G72	Other and unspecified myopathies

Disorders of the eye and adnexa (360-379)

360	Disorders of the globe	H44	Disorders of globe
361	Retinal detachments and defects	H33	Retinal detachments and breaks
362	Other retinal disorders	H34	Retinal vascular occlusions
		H35	Other retinal disorders
		H36	Retinal disorders in diseases classified elsewhere
363	Chorioretinal inflammations, scars and other disorders of choroid	H30	Chorioretinal inflammation
		H31	Other disorders of choroid
		H32	Chorioretinal disorders in diseases classified elsewhere
364	Disorders of iris and ciliary body	H20	Iridocyclitis
		H21	Other disorders of iris and ciliary body
		H22	Disorders of iris and ciliary body in diseases classified elsewhere
365	Glaucoma	H40	Glaucoma
		H42	Glaucoma in diseases classified elsewhere

ICD-9-CM Code and Description		ICD-10-CM Code and Description	
366	Cataract	H25	Age-related cataract
		H26	Other cataract
		H28	Cataract in diseases classified elsewhere
367	Disorders of refraction and accommodation	H52	Disorders of refraction and accommodation
368	Visual disturbances	H53	Visual disturbances
369	Blindness and low vision	H54	Blindness and low vision
370	Keratitis	H16	Keratitis
371	Corneal opacity and other disorders of cornea	H17	Corneal scars and opacities
		H18	Other disorders of cornea
372	Disorders of conjunctiva	H10	Conjunctivitis
		H11	Other disorders of conjunctiva
373	Inflammation of eyelids	H00	Hordeolum and chalazion
		H01	Other inflammation of eyelid
374	Other disorders of eyelids	H02	Other disorders of eyelid
375	Disorders of lacrimal system	H04	Disorders of lacrimal system
376	Disorders of the orbit	H05	Disorders of orbit
377	Disorders of optic nerve and visual pathways	H46	Optic neuritis
		H47	Other disorders of optic [2nd] nerve and visual pathways
378	Strabismus and other disorders of binocular eye movements	H49	Paralytic strabismus
		H50	Other strabismus
		H51	Other disorders of binocular movement
379	Other disorders of eye	H15	Disorders of sclera
		H27	Other disorders of lens
		H43	Disorders of vitreous body
		H55	Nystagmus and other irregular eye movements
		H57	Other disorders of eye and adnexa

Diseases of the ear and mastoid process (380-389)

380	Disorders of external ear	H60	Otitis externa
		H61	Other disorders of external ear
		H62	Disorders of external ear in diseases classified elsewhere
381	Nonsuppurative otitis media and eustachian tube disorders	H65	Nonsuppurative otitis media
		H68	Eustachian salpingitis and obstruction
		H69	Other and unspecified disorders of Eustachian tube
382	Suppurative and unspecified otitis media	H66	Suppurative and unspecified otitis media
		H67	Otitis media in diseases classified elsewhere
383	Mastoiditis and related conditions	H70	Mastoiditis and related conditions
		H75	Other disorders of middle ear and mastoid in diseases classified elsewhere

ICD-9-CM Code and Description		ICD-10-CM Code and Description	
		H95	Intraoperative and postprocedural complications and disorders of ear and mastoid process, not elsewhere classified
384	Other disorders of tympanic membrane	H72	Perforation of tympanic membrane
		H73	Other disorders of tympanic membrane
385	Other disorders of middle ear and mastoid	H71	Cholesteatoma of middle ear
		H74	Other disorders of middle ear mastoid
386	Vertiginous syndromes and other disorders of vestibular system	H81	Disorders of vestibular function
		H82	Vertiginous syndromes in diseases classified elsewhere
		H83	Other diseases of inner ear
387	Otosclerosis	H80	Otosclerosis
388	Other disorders of ear	H92	Otalgia and effusion of ear
		H93	Other disorders of ear, not elsewhere classified
		H94	Other disorders of ear in diseases classified elsewhere
389	Hearing loss	H90	Conductive and sensorineural hearing loss
		H91	Other and unspecified hearing loss

7. DISEASES OF THE CIRCULATORY SYSTEM

Acute rheumatic fever (390-392)

390	Rheumatic fever without mention of heart involvement	I00	Rheumatic fever without heart involvement
391	Rheumatic fever with heart involvement	I01	Rheumatic fever with heart involvement
392	Rheumatic chorea	I02	Rheumatic chorea

Chronic rheumatic heart disease (393-398)

393	Chronic rheumatic pericarditis	I09	Other rheumatic heart diseases
394	Diseases of mitral valve	I05	Rheumatic mitral valve diseases
395	Diseases of aortic valve	I06	Rheumatic aortic valve diseases
396	Diseases of mitral and aortic valves	I08	Multiple valve diseases
397	Diseases of other endocardial structures	I07	Rheumatic tricuspid valve diseases
398	Other rheumatic heart disease	I09	Other rheumatic heart diseases

Hypertensive disease (401-405)

401	Essential hypertension	I10	Essential (primary) hypertension
402	Hypertensive heart disease	I11	Hypertensive heart disease
403	Hypertensive chronic kidney disease	I12	Hypertensive chronic kidney disease
404	Hypertensive heart and chronic kidney disease	I13	Hypertensive heart and chronic kidney disease
405	Secondary hypertension	I15	Secondary hypertension

ICD-9-CM Code and Description	ICD-10-CM Code and Description

Ischemic heart disease (410-414)

410	Acute myocardial infarction	I21	ST elevation (STEMI) and non-ST elevation (NSTEMI) myocardial infarction
		I22	Subsequent ST elevation (STEMI) and non-ST elevation (NSTEMI) myocardial infarction
411	Other acute and subacute form of ischemic heart disease	I20	Angina pectoris
		I24	Other acute ischemic heart diseases
412	Old myocardial infarction	I25	Chronic ischemic heart disease
414	Other forms of chronic ischemic heart disease	I25	Chronic ischemic heart disease

Diseases of pulmonary circulation (415-417)

415	Acute pulmonary heart disease	I26	Pulmonary embolism
416	Chronic pulmonary heart disease	I27	Other pulmonary heart diseases
417	Other diseases of pulmonary circulation	I28	Other diseases of pulmonary vessels

Other forms of heart disease (420-429)

420	Acute pericarditis	I30	Acute pericarditis
		I32	Pericarditis in diseases classified elsewhere
421	Acute and subacute endocarditis	I33	Acute and subacute endocarditis
		I39	Endocarditis and heart valve disorders in diseases classified elsewhere
422	Acute myocarditis	I40	Acute myocarditis
		I41	Myocarditis in diseases classified elsewhere
423	Other diseases of pericardium	I31	Other diseases of pericardium
424	Other diseases of endocardium	I34	Nonrheumatic mitral valve disorders
		I35	Nonrheumatic aortic valve disorders
		I36	Nonrheumatic tricuspid valve disorders
		I37	Nonrheumatic pulmonary valve disorders
		I38	Endocarditis, valve unspecified
425	Cardiomyopathy	I42	Cardiomyopathy
		I43	Cardiomyopathy in diseases classified elsewhere
426	Conduction disorders	I44	Atrioventricular and left bundle-branch block
		I45	Other conduction disorders
427	Cardiac dysrhythmias	I46	Cardiac arrest
		I47	Paroxysmal tachycardia
		I48	Atrial fibrillation and flutter
		I49	Other cardiac arrhythmias
428	Heart failure	I50	Heart failure
429	Ill-defined descriptions and complications of heart disease	I23	Certain current complications following ST elevation (STEMI) and non-ST elevation (NSTEMI) myocardial infarction (within the 28 day period)

ICD-9-CM Code and Description	ICD-10-CM Code and Description

429	Ill-defined descriptions and complications of heart disease	I51	Complications and ill-defined descriptions of heart disease
		I52	Other heart disorders in diseases classified elsewhere
		I97	Intraoperative and postprocedural complications and disorders of circulatory system, not elsewhere classified

Cerebrovascular disease (430-438)

430	Subarachnoid hemorrhage	I60	Nontraumatic subarachnoid hemorrhage
431	Intracerebral hemorrhage	I61	Nontraumatic intracerebral hemorrhage
432	Other and unspecified intracranial hemorrhage	I62	Other and unspecified nontraumatic intracranial hemorrhage
433	Occlusion and stenosis of precerebral arteries	I63	Cerebral infarction
		I65	Occlusion and stenosis of precerebral arteries, not resulting in cerebral infarction
434	Occlusion of cerebral arteries	I66	Occlusion and stenosis of cerebral arteries, not resulting in cerebral infarction
435	Transient cerebral ischemia	G45	Transient cerebral ischemic attacks and related syndromes
		G46	Vascular syndromes of brain in cerebrovascular diseases
437	Other and ill-defined cerebrovascular disease	I67	Other cerebrovascular diseases
		I68	Cerebrovascular disorders in diseases classified elsewhere
438	Late effects of cerebrovascular disease	I69	Sequelae of cerebrovascular disease

Diseases of arteries, arterioles, and capillaries (440-449)

440	Atherosclerosis	I70	Atherosclerosis
441	Aortic aneurysm and dissection	I71	Aortic aneurysm and dissection
		I79	Disorders of arteries, arterioles and capillaries in diseases classified elsewhere
442	Other aneurysm	I72	Other aneurysm
443	Other peripheral vascular disease	I73	Other peripheral vascular diseases
444	Arterial embolism and thrombosis	I74	Arterial embolism and thrombosis
445	Atheroembolism	I75	Atheroembolism
446	Polyarteritis nodosa and allied conditions	M30	Polyarteritis nodosa and related conditions
		M31	Other necrotizing vasculopathies
447	Other disorders of arteries and arterioles	I77	Diseases of capillaries
448	Diseases of capillaries	I78	Disorders of arteries, arterioles and capillaries in diseases classified elsewhere
449	Septic arterial embolism	I76	Other disorders of arteries and arterioles

Diseases of veins and lymphatics, and other diseases of circulatory system (451-459)

451	Phlebitis and thrombophlebitis	I80	Phlebitis and thrombophlebitis
452	Portal vein thrombosis	I81	Portal vein thrombosis

ICD-9-CM Code and Description		ICD-10-CM Code and Description	
453	Other venous embolism and thrombosis	I82	Other venous embolism and thrombosis
454	Varicose veins of lower extremities	I83	Varicose veins of lower extremities
455	Hemorrhoids	I84	Unspecified thrombosed hemorrhoids
456	Varicose veins of other sites	I85	Esophageal varices
		I86	Varicose veins of other sites
457	Noninfective disorders of lymphatic channels	I89	Other noninfective disorders of lymphatic vessels and lymph nodes
458	Hypotension	I95	Hypotension
459	Other disorders of circulatory system	I87	Other disorders of veins
459	Other disorders of circulatory system	I99	Other and unspecified disorders of circulatory system
		R58	Hemorrhage not elsewhere classified

8. DISEASES OF THE RESPIRATORY SYSTEM

Acute respiratory infections (460-466)

460	Acute nasopharyngitis [common cold]	J00	Acute nasopharyngitis [common cold]
461	Acute sinusitis	J01	Acute sinusitis
464	Acute laryngitis and tracheitis	J04	Acute laryngitis and tracheitis
		J05	Acute obstructive laryngitis [croup] and epiglottitis
465	Acute upper respiratory infections of multiple or unspecified sites	J06	Acute upper respiratory infections of multiple and unspecified sites
466	Acute bronchitis and bronchiolitis	J21	Acute bronchiolitis

Other diseases of upper respiratory tract (470-478)

470	Deviated nasal septum	J34	Other and unspecified disorders of nose and nasal sinuses
471	Nasal polyps	J33	Nasal polyp
472	Chronic pharyngitis and nasopharyngitis	J31	Chronic rhinitis, nasopharyngitis and pharyngitis
473	Chronic sinusitis	J32	Chronic sinusitis
474	Chronic disease of tonsils and adenoids	J35	Chronic diseases of tonsils and adenoids
475	Peritonsillar abscess	J36	Peritonsillar abscess
476	Chronic laryngitis and laryngotracheitis	J37	Chronic laryngitis and laryngotracheitis
477	Allergic rhinitis	J30	Vasomotor and allergic rhinitis
478	Other diseases of upper respiratory tract	J34	Other and unspecified disorders of nose and nasal sinuses
		J38	Diseases of vocal cords and larynx, not elsewhere classified
		J39	Other diseases of upper respiratory tract

Pneumonia and influenza (480-488)

480	Viral pneumonia	J12	Viral pneumonia, not elsewhere classified
481	Pneumococcal pneumonia [streptococcus pneumoniae pneumonia]	J13	Pneumonia due to Streptococcus pneumoniae

ICD-9-CM Code and Description		ICD-10-CM Code and Description	
482	Other bacterial pneumonia	J14	Pneumonia due to Hemophilus influenzae
		J15	Bacterial pneumonia, not elsewhere classified
483	Pneumonia due to other specified organism	J16	Pneumonia due to other infectious organisms, not elsewhere classified
484	Pneumonia in infectious diseases classified elsewhere	J17	Pneumonia in diseases classified elsewhere
485	Bronchopneumonia, organism unspecified	J18	Pneumonia, unspecified organism
486	Pneumonia, organism unspecified	J18	Pneumonia, unspecified organism
487	Influenza	J10	Influenza due to other identified influenza virus
488	Influenza due to certain identified influenza viruses	J09	Influenza due to certain identified influenza viruses

Chronic obstructive pulmonary disease and allied conditions (490-496)

490	Bronchitis, not specified as acute or chronic	J40	Bronchitis, not specified as acute or chronic
491	Chronic bronchitis	J41	Simple and mucopurulent chronic bronchitis
		J42	Unspecified chronic bronchitis
		J44	Other chronic obstructive pulmonary disease
492	Emphysema	J43	Emphysema
493	Asthma	J45	Asthma
494	Bronchiectasis	J47	Bronchiectasis
495	Extrinsic allergic alveolitis	J67	Hypersensitivity pneumonitis due to organic dust
496	Chronic airway obstruction, not elsewhere classified	J44	Other chronic obstructive pulmonary disease

Pneumoconioses and other lung diseases due to external agents (500-508)

500	Coal workers' pneumoconiosis	J60	Coalworker's pneumoconiosis
501	Asbestosis	J61	Pneumoconiosis due to asbestos and other mineral fibers
502	Pneumoconiosis due to other silica or silicates	J62	Pneumoconiosis due to dust containing silica
503	Pneumoconiosis due to other inorganic dust	J63	Pneumoconiosis due to other inorganic dusts
504	Pneumopathy due to inhalation of other dust	J66	Airway disease due to specific organic dust
505	Pneumoconiosis, unspecified	J64	Unspecified pneumoconiosis
		J65	Pneumoconiosis associated with tuberculosis
506	Respiratory conditions due to chemical fumes and vapors	J68	Respiratory conditions due to inhalation of chemicals, gases, fumes and vapors
507	Pneumonitis due to solids and liquids	J69	Pneumonitis due to solids and liquids
508	Respiratory conditions due to other and unspecified external agents	J70	Respiratory conditions due to other external agents

ICD-9-CM Code and Description	ICD-10-CM Code and Description

Other diseases of respiratory system (510-519)

510	Empyema	J86	Pyothorax
511	Pleurisy	J90	Pleural effusion, not elsewhere classified
		J91	Pleural effusion in conditions classified elsewhere
		J92	Pleural plaque
		J94	Other pleural conditions
512	Pneumothorax	J93	Pneumothorax and air leak
513	Abscess of lung and mediastinum	J85	Abscess of lung and mediastinum
514	Pulmonary congestion and hypostasis	J18	Pneumonia, unspecified organism
		J81	Pulmonary edema
515	Postinflammatory pulmonary fibrosis		
516	Other alveolar and parietoalveolar pneumopathy	J84	Other interstitial pulmonary diseases
517	Lung involvement in conditions classified elsewhere	J99	Respiratory disorders in diseases classified elsewhere
518	Other diseases of lung	J80	Acute respiratory distress syndrome
		J81	Pulmonary edema
		J82	Pulmonary eosinophilia, not elsewhere classified
		J96	Respiratory failure, not elsewhere classified
519	Other diseases of respiratory system	J22	Unspecified acute lower respiratory infection
		J95	Intraoperative and postprocedural complications and disorders of respiratory system, not elsewhere classified
		J98	Other respiratory disorders

9. DISEASES OF THE DIGESTIVE SYSTEM

Diseases of oral cavity, salivary glands, and jaws (520-529)

520	Disorders of tooth development and eruption	K00	Disorders of tooth development and eruption
		K01	Embedded and impacted teeth
521	Diseases of hard tissues of teeth	K02	Dental caries
		K03	Other diseases of hard tissues of teeth
522	Diseases of pulp and periapical tissues	K04	Diseases of pulp and periapical tissues
523	Gingival and periodontal diseases	K05	Gingivitis and periodontal diseases
		K06	Other disorders of gingiva and edentulous alveolar ridge
524	Dentofacial anomalies, including malocclusion	M26	Dentofacial anomalies [including malocclusion]
525	Other diseases and conditions of the teeth and supporting structures	K08	Other disorders of teeth and supporting structures
526	Diseases of the jaws	K09	Cysts of oral region, not elsewhere classified
		M27	Other diseases of jaws
527	Diseases of the salivary glands	K11	Diseases of salivary glands

ICD-9-CM Code and Description	ICD-10-CM Code and Description
528 Diseases of the oral soft tissues, excluding lesions specific for gingiva and tongue	A69 Other spirochetal infections
	K12 Stomatitis and related lesions
	K13 Other diseases of lip and oral mucosa
529 Diseases and other conditions of the tongue	K14 Diseases of tongue

Diseases of esophagus, stomach, and duodenum (530-539)

530 Diseases of esophagus	K20 Esophagitis
	K21 Gastro-esophageal reflux disease
	K22 Other diseases of esophagus
	K23 Disorders of esophagus in diseases classified elsewhere
531 Gastric ulcer	K25 Gastric ulcer
532 Duodenal ulcer	K26 Duodenal ulcer
533 Peptic ulcer, site unspecified	K27 Peptic ulcer, site unspecified
534 Gastrojejunal ulcer	K28 Gastrojejunal ulcer
535 Gastritis and duodenitis	K29 Gastritis and duodenitis
536 Disorders of function of stomach	K30 Functional dyspepsia
	K31 Other diseases of stomach and duodenum
537 Other disorders of stomach and duodenum	K31 Other diseases of stomach and duodenum
538 Gastrointestinal mucositis (ulcerative)	K92 Other diseases of digestive system
539 Complications of bariatric procedures	K95 Complications of bariatric procedures

Appendicitis (540-543)

540 Acute appendicitis	K35 Acute appendicitis
541 Appendicitis, unqualified	K37 Unspecified appendicitis
542 Other appendicitis	K36 Other appendicitis
543 Other diseases of appendix	K38 Other diseases of appendix

Hernia of abdominal cavity (550-553)

550 Inguinal hernia	K40 Inguinal hernia
552 Other hernia of abdominal cavity, with obstruction, but without mention of gangrene	K41 Femoral hernia
	K42 Umbilical hernia
	K43 Ventral hernia
	K44 Diaphragmatic hernia
	K45 Other abdominal hernia
	K46 Unspecified abdominal hernia
553 Other hernia of abdominal cavity without mention of obstruction or gangrene	K41 Femoral hernia

Noninfectious enteritis and colitis (555-558)

555 Regional enteritis	K50 Crohn's disease [regional enteritis]
556 Ulcerative colitis	K51 Ulcerative colitis
557 Vascular insufficiency of intestine	K55 Vascular disorders of intestine

ICD-9-CM Code and Description	ICD-10-CM Code and Description
558 Other and unspecified noninfectious gastroenteritis and colitis	K52 Other and unspecified noninfective gastroenteritis and colitis

Other diseases of intestines and peritoneum (560-569)

ICD-9-CM	ICD-10-CM
560 Intestinal obstruction without mention of hernia	K56 Paralytic ileus and intestinal obstruction without hernia
562 Diverticula of intestine	K57 Diverticular disease of intestine
564 Functional digestive disorders, not elsewhere classified	K58 Irritable bowel syndrome
	K59 Fissure and fistula of anal and rectal regions
	K91 Intraoperative and postprocedural complications and disorders of digestive system, not elsewhere classified
565 Anal fissure and fistula	K60 Abscess of anal and rectal regions
566 Abscess of anal and rectal regions	K61 Other diseases of anus and rectum
567 Peritonitis and retroperitoneal infections	K65 Peritonitis
	K67 Disorders of peritoneum in infectious diseases classified elsewhere
	K68 Disorders of retroperitoneum
568 Other disorders of peritoneum	K66 Other disorders of peritoneum
569 Other disorders of intestine	K62 Other diseases of intestine
	K63 Hemorrhoids and perianal venous thrombosis
	K94 Complications of artificial openings of the digestive system

Other diseases of digestive system (570-579)

ICD-9-CM	ICD-10-CM
570 Acute and subacute necrosis of liver	K72 Hepatic failure, not elsewhere classified
571 Chronic liver disease and cirrhosis	K70 Alcoholic liver disease
	K73 Chronic hepatitis, not elsewhere classified
	K74 Fibrosis and cirrhosis of liver
	K76 Other diseases of liver
572 Liver abscess and sequelae of chronic liver disease	K75 Other inflammatory liver diseases
573 Other disorders of liver	K71 Toxic liver disease
	K77 Liver disorders in diseases classified elsewhere
574 Cholelithiasis	K80 Cholelithiasis
575 Other disorders of gallbladder	K81 Cholecystitis
	K82 Other diseases of gallbladder
576 Other disorders of biliary tract	K83 Other diseases of biliary tract
	K87 Disorders of gallbladder biliary tract and pancreas in diseases classified elsewhere
577 Diseases of pancreas	K85 Acute pancreatitis
	K86 Other diseases of pancreas
578 Gastrointestinal hemorrhage	K92 Other diseases of digestive system
579 Intestinal malabsorption	K90 Intestinal malabsorption

ICD-9-CM Code and Description	ICD-10-CM Code and Description

10. DISEASES OF THE GENITOURINARY SYSTEM
Nephritis, nephrotic syndrome, and nephrosis (580-589)

580	Acute glomerulonephritis	N00	Acute nephritic syndrome
		N01	Rapidly progressive nephritic syndrome
581	Nephrotic syndrome	N02	Recurrent and persistent hematuria
		N04	Nephrotic syndrome
582	Chronic glomerulonephritis	N03	Chronic nephritic syndrome
583	Nephritis and nephropathy, not specified as acute or chronic	N05	Unspecified nephritic syndrome
		N06	Isolated proteinuria with specified morphological lesion
		N07	Hereditary nephropathy, not elsewhere classified
		N08	Glomerular disorders in diseases classified elsewhere
		N14	Drug- and heavy-metal-induced tubulointerstitial and tubular conditions
		N15	Other renal tubulointerstitial diseases
		N16	Renal tubulointerstitial disorders in diseases classified elsewhere
584	Acute kidney failure	N17	Acute kidney failure
585	Chronic kidney disease (ckd)	N18	Chronic kidney disease (CKD)
586	Renal failure, unspecified	N19	Unspecified kidney failure
587	Renal sclerosis, unspecified	N26	Unspecified contracted kidney
588	Disorders resulting from impaired renal function	N25	Disorders resulting from impaired renal tubular function
589	Small kidney of unknown cause	N27	Small kidney of unknown cause

Other diseases of urinary system (590-599)

590	Infections of kidney	N10	Acute tubulointerstitial nephritis
		N11	Chronic tubulointerstitial nephritis
		N12	Tubulo-interstitial nephritis not specified as acute or chronic
591	Hydronephrosis	N13	Obstructive and reflux uropathy
592	Calculus of kidney and ureter	N20	Calculus of kidney and ureter
		N22	Calculus of urinary tract in diseases classified elsewhere
593	Other disorders of kidney and ureter	N28	Other disorders of kidney and ureter, not elsewhere classified
		N29	Other disorders of kidney and ureter in diseases classified elsewhere
594	Calculus of lower urinary tract	N21	Calculus of lower urinary tract
595	Cystitis	N30	Cystitis
596	Other disorders of bladder	N31	Neuromuscular dysfunction of bladder, not elsewhere classified
		N32	Other disorders of bladder
		N34	Urethritis and urethral syndrome
597	Urethritis, not sexually transmitted, and urethral syndrome	N35	Urethral stricture
598	Urethral stricture	N30	Cystitis
		N37	Urethral disorders in diseases classified elsewhere

ICD-9-CM Code and Description	ICD-10-CM Code and Description
599 Other disorders of urethra and urinary tract	N36 Other disorders of urethra
	N39 Other disorders of urinary system
	R31 Hematuria

Diseases of male genital organs (600-608)

600 Hyperplasia of prostate	N40 Enlarged prostate
601 Inflammatory diseases of prostate	N41 Inflammatory diseases of prostate
602 Other disorders of prostate	N42 Other and unspecified disorders of prostate
603 Hydrocele	N43 Hydrocele and spermatocele
604 Orchitis and epididymitis	N45 Orchitis and epididymitis
605 Redundant prepuce and phimosis	N47 Disorders of prepuce
606 Infertility, male	N46 Male infertility
607 Disorders of penis	N48 Other disorders of penis
	N52 Male erectile dysfunction
608 Other disorders of male genital organs	N44 Noninflammatory disorders of testis
	N49 Inflammatory disorders of male genital organs, not elsewhere classified
	N50 Other and unspecified disorders of male genital organs
	N51 Disorders of male genital organs in diseases classified elsewhere
	N53 Other male sexual dysfunction

Disorders of breast (610-612)

610 Benign mammary dysplasias	N60 Benign mammary dysplasia
611 Other disorders of breast	N61 Inflammatory disorders of breast
	N62 Hypertrophy of breast
	N63 Unspecified lump in breast
	N64 Other disorders of breast
612 Deformity and disproportion of reconstructed breast	N65 Deformity and disproportion of reconstructed breast

Inflammatory disease of female pelvic organs (614-616)

614 Inflammatory disease of ovary, fallopian tube, pelvic cellular tissue, and peritoneum	N70 Salpingitis and oophoritis
	N73 Other female pelvic inflammatory diseases
	N74 Female pelvic inflammatory disorders in diseases classified elsewhere
615 Inflammatory diseases of uterus, except cervix	N71 Acute inflammatory disease of uterus
616 Inflammatory disease of cervix, vagina, and vulva	N72 Inflammatory disease of cervix uteri
	N75 Diseases of Bartholin's gland
	N76 Other inflammation of vagina and vulva
	N77 Vulvovaginal ulceration and inflammation in diseases classified elsewhere

ICD-9-CM Code and Description		ICD-10-CM Code and Description	

Other disorders of female genital tract (617-629)

617	Endometriosis	N80	Endometriosis
618	Genital prolapse	N81	Female genital prolapse
619	Fistula involving female genital tract	N82	Fistulae involving female genital tract
620	Noninflammatory disorders of ovary, fallopian tube, and broad ligament	N83	Noninflammatory disorders of ovary, fallopian tube and broad ligament
621	Disorders of uterus, not elsewhere classified	N84	Polyp of female genital tract
		N85	Other noninflammatory disorders of uterus, except cervix
622	Noninflammatory disorders of cervix	N86	Erosion and ectropion of cervix uteri
		N87	Dysplasia of cervix uteri
		N88	Other noninflammatory disorders of cervix uteri
623	Noninflammatory disorders of vagina	N89	Other noninflammatory disorders of vagina
624	Noninflammatory disorders of vulva and perineum	N90	Other noninflammatory disorders of vulva and perineum
625	Pain and other symptoms associated with female genital organs	N94	Pain and other conditions associated with female genital organs and menstrual cycle
626	Disorders of menstruation and other abnormal bleeding from female genital tract	N91	Absent, scanty and rare menstruation
		N92	Excessive, frequent and irregular menstruation
		N93	Other abnormal uterine and vaginal bleeding
627	Menopausal and postmenopausal disorders	N95	Menopausal and other perimenopausal disorders
628	Infertility, female	N97	Female infertility
629	Other disorders of female genital organs	N96	Recurrent pregnancy loss

11. COMPLICATIONS OF PREGNANCY, CHILDBIRTH AND THE PUERPERIUM

Ectopic and molar pregnancy (630-633)

630	Hydatidiform mole	O01	Hydatidiform mole
631	Other abnormal product of conception	O02	Other abnormal products of conception
633	Ectopic pregnancy	O00	Ectopic pregnancy

Other pregnancy with abortive outcome (634-639)

634	Abortion	O03	Spontaneous abortion
635	Legally induced abortion	O04	Complications following (induced) termination of pregnancy
638	Failed attempted abortion	O07	Failed attempted termination of pregnancy
639	Complications following abortion and ectopic and molar pregnancies	A34	Obstetrical tetanus
		O08	Complications following ectopic and molar pregnancy

ICD-9-CM Code and Description	ICD-10-CM Code and Description

Complications mainly related to pregnancy (640-649)

641	Antepartum hemorrhage, abruptio placentae, and placenta previa	O44	Placenta previa
		O45	Premature separation of placenta [abruptio placentae]
		O46	Antepartum hemorrhage, not elsewhere classified
		O67	Labor and delivery complicated by intrapartum hemorrhage, not elsewhere classified
642	Hypertension complicating pregnancy, childbirth, and the puerperium	O10	Pre-existing hypertension complicating pregnancy, childbirth and the puerperium
		O11	Pre-existing hypertension with pre-eclampsia
		O13	Gestational [pregnancy-induced] hypertension without significant proteinuria
		O14	Pre-eclampsia
		O15	Eclampsia
		O16	Unspecified maternal hypertension
643	Excessive vomiting in pregnancy	O21	Excessive vomiting in pregnancy
644	Early or threatened labor	O47	False labor
		O60	Preterm labor
645	Late pregnancy	O48	Late pregnancy
646	Other complications of pregnancy, not elsewhere classified	O12	Gestational [pregnancy-induced] edema and proteinuria without hypertension
		O23	Infections of genitourinary tract in pregnancy
		O26	Maternal care for other conditions predominantly related to pregnancy
		O29	Complications of anesthesia during pregnancy
		O31	Complications specific to multiple gestation
647	Infectious and parasitic conditions in the mother classifiable elsewhere but	O98	Maternal infectious and parasitic diseases classifiable elsewhere but complicating pregnancy, childbirth and the puerperium
648	Other current conditions in the mother classifiable elsewhere but complicating	F53	Puerperal psychosis
		O24	Diabetes mellitus in pregnancy, childbirth, and the puerperium
		O25	Malnutrition in pregnancy, childbirth and the puerperium
		O33	Maternal care for disproportion
		O99	Other maternal diseases classifiable elsewhere but complicating pregnancy, childbirth and the puerperium
		O9A	Maternal malignant neoplasms, traumatic injuries and abuse classifiable elsewhere but complicating pregnancy, childbirth and the puerperium
649	Other conditions or status of the mother complicating pregnancy, childbirth, or the puerperium	O99	Other maternal diseases classifiable elsewhere but complicating pregnancy, childbirth and the puerperium

ICD-9-CM Code and Description		ICD-10-CM Code and Description	

Normal delivery, and other indications for care in pregnancy, labor, and delivery (650-659)

650	Normal delivery	O80	Encounter for full-term uncomplicated delivery
651	Multiple gestation	O30	Multiple gestation
652	Malposition and malpresentation of fetus	O32	Maternal care for malpresentation of fetus
653	Disproportion	O65	Obstructed labor due to maternal pelvic abnormality
654	Abnormality of organs and soft tissues of pelvis	O34	Maternal care for abnormality of pelvic organs
655	Known or suspected fetal abnormality affecting management of mother	O35	Maternal care for known or suspected fetal abnormality and damage
656	Other known or suspected fetal and placental problems affecting management of	O36	Maternal care for other fetal problems
		O43	Placental disorders
		O68	Labor and delivery complicated by abnormality of fetal acid-base balance
		O77	Other fetal stress complicating labor and delivery
657	Polyhydramnios	O40	Polyhydramnios
658	Other problems associated with amniotic cavity and membranes	O41	Other disorders of amniotic fluid and membranes
		O42	Premature rupture of membranes
659	Other indications for care or intervention related to labor and delivery and not	O61	Failed induction of labor
		O76	Abnormality in fetal heart rate and rhythm complicating labor and delivery

Complications occurring mainly in the course of labor and delivery (660-669)

660	Obstructed labor	O64	Obstructed labor due to malposition and malpresentation of fetus
		O66	Other obstructed labor
661	Abnormality of forces of labor	O62	Abnormalities of forces of labor
662	Long labor	O63	Long labor
663	Umbilical cord complications	O69	Labor and delivery complicated by umbilical cord complications
664	Trauma to perineum and vulva during delivery	O70	Perineal laceration during delivery
665	Other obstetrical trauma	O71	Other obstetric trauma
666	Postpartum hemorrhage	O72	Postpartum hemorrhage
667	Retained placenta or membranes, without hemorrhage	O73	Retained placenta and membranes, without hemorrhage
668	Complications of the administration of anesthetic or other sedation in labor and	O74	Complications of anesthesia during labor and delivery
		O89	Complications of anesthesia during the puerperium
669	Other complications of labor and delivery, not elsewhere classified	O75	Other complications of labor and delivery, not elsewhere classified
		O82	Encounter for cesarean delivery without indication

ICD-9-CM Code and Description	ICD-10-CM Code and Description

Complications of the puerperium (670-677)

670	Major puerperal infection	O85	Puerperal sepsis
671	Venous complications in pregnancy and the puerperium	O22	Venous complications and hemorrhoids in pregnancy
		O87	Venous complications and hemorrhoids in the puerperium
672	Pyrexia of unknown origin during the puerperium		
673	Obstetrical pulmonary embolism	O88	Obstetric embolism
674	Other and unspecified complications of the puerperium, not elsewhere classified	O86	Other puerperal infections
		O90	Complications of the puerperium, not elsewhere classified
675	Infections of the breast and nipple associated with childbirth	O91	Infections of breast associated with pregnancy, the puerperium and lactation
676	Other disorders of the breast associated with childbirth, and disorders of lactation	O92	Other disorders of breast and disorders of lactation associated with pregnancy and the puerperium
677	Late effect of complication of pregnancy, childbirth, and the puerperium	O94	Sequelae of complication of pregnancy, childbirth, and the puerperium

Other maternal and fetal complications (678-679)

678	Other fetal conditions	O35	Maternal care for known or suspected fetal abnormality and damage
		O36	Maternal care for other fetal problems
		O30	Multiple gestation
679	Complications of in utero procedures	O26	Maternal care for other conditions predominantly related to pregnancy
		O75	Other complications of labor and delivery, not elsewhere classified
		O90	Complications of the puerperium, not elsewhere classified
		O35	Maternal care for known or suspected fetal abnormality and damage

12. DISEASES OF THE SKIN AND SUBCUTANEOUS TISSUE

Infections of skin and subcutaneous tissue (680-686)

680	Carbuncle and furuncle	L02	Cutaneous abscess, furuncle and carbuncle
681	Cellulitis and abscess of finger and toe	L03	Cellulitis and acute lymphangitis
682	Other cellulitis and abscess	L02	Cutaneous abscess, furuncle and carbuncle
683	Acute lymphadenitis	L04	Acute lymphadenitis
684	Impetigo	L01	Impetigo
685	Pilonidal cyst	L05	Pilonidal cyst and sinus
686	Other local infections of skin and subcutaneous tissue	L08	Other local infections of skin and subcutaneous tissue
		L88	Pyoderma gangrenosum
		L98	Other disorders of skin and subcutaneous tissue, not elsewhere classified

ICD-9-CM Code and Description		ICD-10-CM Code and Description	

Other inflammatory conditions of skin and subcutaneous tissue (690-698)

690	Erythematosquamous dermatosis	L21	Seborrheic dermatitis
691	Atopic dermatitis and related conditions	L20	Atopic dermatitis
		L22	Diaper dermatitis
692	Contact dermatitis and other eczema	L23	Allergic contact dermatitis
		L24	Irritant contact dermatitis
		L25	Unspecified contact dermatitis
		L30	Other and unspecified dermatitis
		L55	Sunburn
		L56	Other acute skin changes due to ultraviolet radiation
		L58	Radiodermatitis
		L59	Other disorders of skin and subcutaneous tissue related to radiation
693	Dermatitis due to substances taken internally	L27	Dermatitis due to substances taken internally
694	Bullous dermatoses	L10	Pemphigus
		L12	Pemphigoid
		L13	Other bullous disorders
		L14	Bullous disorders in diseases classified elsewhere
695	Erythematous conditions	L00	Staphylococcal scalded skin syndrome
		L26	Exfoliative dermatitis
		L49	Exfoliation due to erythematous conditions according to extent of body surface involved
		L51	Erythema multiforme
		L52	Erythema nodosum
		L53	Other erythematous conditions
		L54	Erythema in diseases classified elsewhere
		L71	Rosacea
		L92	Granulomatous disorders of skin and subcutaneous tissue
		L93	Lupus erythematosus
696	Psoriasis and similar disorders	L40	Psoriasis
696	Psoriasis and similar disorders	L41	Parapsoriasis
		L42	Pityriasis rosea
		L44	Other papulosquamous disorders
		L45	Papulosquamous disorders in diseases classified elsewhere
697	Lichen	L43	Lichen planus
698	Pruritus and related conditions	L28	Lichen simplex chronicus and prurigo
		L29	Pruritus

Other diseases of skin and subcutaneous tissue (700-709)

700	Corns and callosities	L84	Corns and callosities
701	Other hypertrophic and atrophic conditions of skin	L11	Other acantholytic disorders
		L83	Acanthosis nigricans

ICD-9-CM Code and Description		ICD-10-CM Code and Description	
		L85	Other epidermal thickening
		L86	Keratoderma in diseases classified elsewhere
		L87	Transepidermal elimination disorders
		L90	Atrophic disorders of skin
		L91	Hypertrophic disorders of skin
		L94	Other localized connective tissue disorders
		L99	Other disorders of skin and subcutaneous tissue in diseases classified elsewhere
702	Other dermatoses	L57	Skin changes due to chronic exposure to nonionizing radiation
		L82	Seborrheic keratosis
703	Diseases of nail	L60	Nail disorders
		L62	Nail disorders in diseases classified elsewhere
704	Diseases of hair and hair follicles	L63	Alopecia areata
		L64	Androgenic alopecia
		L65	Other nonscarring hair loss
		L66	Cicatricial alopecia [scarring hair loss]
		L67	Hair color and hair shaft abnormalities
		L68	Hypertrichosis
705	Disorders of sweat glands	L74	Eccrine sweat disorders
		L75	Apocrine sweat disorders
706	Diseases of sebaceous glands	L70	Acne
		L72	Follicular cysts of skin and subcutaneous tissue
		L73	Other follicular disorders
707	Chronic ulcer of skin	L89	Pressure ulcer
		L97	Non-pressure chronic ulcer of lower limb, not elsewhere classified
708	Urticaria	L50	Urticaria
709	Other disorders of skin and subcutaneous tissue	L80	Vitiligo
		L81	Other disorders of pigmentation
		L95	Vasculitis limited to skin, not elsewhere classified

13. DISEASES OF THE MUSCULOSKELETAL SYSTEM AND CONNECTIVE TISSUE

Arthropathies and related disorders (710-719)

710	Diffuse diseases of connective tissue	M32	Systemic lupus erythematosus (SLE)
		M33	Dermatopolymyositis
		M34	Systemic sclerosis [scleroderma]
		M35	Other systemic involvement of connective tissue
		M36	Systemic disorders of connective tissue in diseases classified elsewhere
711	Arthropathy associated with infections	M00	Pyogenic arthritis
		M01	Direct infections of joint in infectious and parasitic diseases classified elsewhere
712	Crystal arthropathies	M11	Other crystal arthropathies

ICD-9-CM Code and Description		ICD-10-CM Code and Description	
713	Arthropathy associated with other disorders classified elsewhere	M02	Postinfective and reactive arthropathies
		M07	Enteropathic arthropathies
		M14	Arthropathies in other diseases classified elsewhere
714	Rheumatoid arthritis and other inflammatory polyarthropathies	M05	Rheumatoid arthritis with rheumatoid factor
		M06	Other rheumatoid arthritis
		M08	Juvenile arthritis
		M12	Other and unspecified arthropathy
715	Osteoarthrosis and allied disorders	M15	Polyosteoarthritis
		M16	Osteoarthritis of hip
		M17	Osteoarthritis of knee
		M18	Osteoarthritis of first carpometacarpal joint
		M19	Other and unspecified osteoarthritis
716	Other and unspecified arthropathies	M13	Other arthritis
717	Internal derangement of knee	M23	Internal derangement of knee
718	Other derangement of joint	M22	Disorder of patella
		M24	Other specific joint derangements
719	Other and unspecified disorder of joint	M25	Other joint disorder, not elsewhere classified

Dorsopathies (720-724)

720	Ankylosing spondylitis and other inflammatory spondylopathies	M45	Ankylosing spondylitis
		M46	Other inflammatory spondylopathies
		M49	Spondylopathies in diseases classified elsewhere
721	Spondylosis and allied disorders	M47	Spondylosis
722	Intervertebral disc disorders	M50	Cervical disc disorders
		M51	Thoracic, thoracolumbar, and lumbosacral intervertebral disc disorders
723	Other disorders of cervical region	M53	Other and unspecified dorsopathies, not elsewhere classified
		M54	Dorsalgia
724	Other and unspecified disorders of back	M48	Other spondylopathies

Rheumatism, excluding the back (725-729)

725	Polymyalgia rheumatica	M35	Other systemic involvement of connective tissue
726	Peripheral enthesopathies and allied syndromes	M75	Shoulder lesions
		M76	Enthesopathies, lower limb, excluding foot
		M77	Other enthesopathies
727	Other disorders of synovium, tendon, and bursa	M65	Synovitis and tenosynovitis
		M66	Spontaneous rupture of synovium and tendon
		M67	Other disorders of synovium and tendon

ICD-9-CM Code and Description	ICD-10-CM Code and Description
	M70 Soft tissue disorders related to use, overuse and pressure
	M71 Other bursopathies
728 Disorders of muscle, ligament, and fascia	M60 Myositis
	M61 Calcification and ossification of muscle
	M62 Other disorders of muscle
	M63 Disorders of muscle in diseases classified elsewhere
	M72 Fibroblastic disorders
729 Other disorders of soft tissues	M79 Other and unspecified soft tissue disorders, not elsewhere classified

Osteopathies, chondropathies, and acquired musculoskeletal deformities (730-739)

730 Osteomyelitis, periostitis, and other infections involving bone	M86 Osteomyelitis
731 Osteitis deformans and osteopathies associated with other disorders classified	M88 Osteitis deformans [Paget's disease of bone]
	M90 Osteopathies in diseases classified elsewhere
732 Osteochondropathies	M42 Spinal osteochondrosis
	M91 Juvenile osteochondrosis of hip and pelvis
	M92 Other juvenile osteochondrosis
	M93 Other osteochondropathies
733 Other disorders of bone and cartilage	M80 Osteoporosis with current pathological fracture
	M81 Osteoporosis without current pathological fracture
	M84 Disorder of continuity of bone
	M85 Other disorders of bone density and structure
	M87 Osteonecrosis
	M89 Other disorders of bone
	M94 Other disorders of cartilage
734 Flat foot	M21 Other acquired deformities of limbs
735 Acquired deformities of toe	M20 Acquired deformities of fingers and toes
736 Other acquired deformities of limbs	M20 Acquired deformities of fingers and toes
	M21 Other acquired deformities of limbs
737 Curvature of spine	M40 Kyphosis and lordosis
	M41 Scoliosis
738 Other acquired deformity	M43 Other deforming dorsopathies
	M95 Other acquired deformities of musculoskeletal system and connective tissue
739 Nonallopathic lesions, not elsewhere classified	M99 Biomechanical lesions, not elsewhere classified

14. CONGENITAL ANOMALIES

740 Anencephalus and similar anomalies	O00 Anencephaly and similar malformations
741 Spina bifida	Q05 Spina bifida

ICD-9-CM Code and Description		ICD-10-CM Code and Description	
		O07	Other congenital malformations of nervous system
742	Other congenital anomalies of nervous system	Q01	Encephalocele
		Q02	Microcephaly
		Q03	Congenital hydrocephalus
		Q04	Other congenital malformations of brain
		Q06	Other congenital malformations of spinal cord
743	Congenital anomalies of eye	Q10	Congenital malformations of eyelid, lacrimal apparatus and orbit
		Q11	Anophthalmos, microphthalmos and macrophthalmos
		Q12	Congenital lens malformations
		Q13	Congenital malformations of anterior segment of eye
		Q14	Congenital malformations of posterior segment of eye
		Q15	Other congenital malformations of eye
744	Congenital anomalies of ear, face, and neck	Q16	Congenital malformations of ear causing impairment of hearing
		Q17	Other congenital malformations of ear
		Q18	Other congenital malformations of face and neck
745	Bulbus cordis anomalies and anomalies of cardiac septal closure	Q20	Congenital malformations of cardiac chambers and connections
		Q21	Congenital malformations of cardiac septa
746	Other congenital anomalies of heart	Q22	Congenital malformations of pulmonary and tricuspid valves
		Q23	Congenital malformations of aortic and mitral valves
		Q24	Other congenital malformations of heart
747	Other congenital anomalies of circulatory system	Q25	Congenital malformations of great arteries
		Q26	Congenital malformations of great veins
		Q27	Other congenital malformations of peripheral vascular system
		Q28	Other congenital malformations of circulatory system
748	Congenital anomalies of respiratory system	Q30	Congenital malformations of nose
		Q31	Congenital malformations of larynx
		Q32	Congenital malformations of trachea and bronchus
		Q33	Congenital malformations of lung
		Q34	Other congenital malformations of respiratory system
749	Cleft palate and cleft lip	Q35	Cleft palate
		Q36	Cleft lip
		Q37	Cleft palate with cleft lip
750	Other congenital anomalies of upper alimentary tract	Q38	Other congenital malformations of tongue, mouth and pharynx

ICD-9-CM Code and Description		ICD-10-CM Code and Description	
		Q39	Congenital malformations of esophagus
		Q40	Other congenital malformations of upper alimentary tract
751	Other congenital anomalies of digestive system	Q41	Congenital absence, atresia and stenosis of small intestine
		Q42	Congenital absence, atresia and stenosis of large intestine
		Q43	Other congenital malformations of intestine
		Q44	Congenital malformations of gallbladder, bile ducts and liver
		Q45	Other congenital malformations of digestive system
752	Congenital anomalies of genital organs	Q50	Congenital malformations of ovaries, fallopian tubes and broad ligaments
		Q51	Congenital malformations of uterus and cervix
		Q52	Other congenital malformations of female genitalia
		Q53	Undescended and ectopic testicle
		Q54	Hypospadias
		Q55	Other congenital malformations of male genital organs
		Q56	Indeterminate sex and pseudohermaphroditism
		Q64	Other congenital malformations of urinary system
753	Congenital anomalies of urinary system	Q60	Renal agenesis and other reduction defects of kidney
		Q61	Cystic kidney disease
		Q62	Congenital obstructive defects of renal pelvis and congenital malformations of ureter
		Q63	Other congenital malformations of kidney
754	Certain congenital musculoskeletal deformities	Q65	Congenital deformities of hip
		Q66	Congenital deformities of feet
		Q67	Congenital musculoskeletal deformities of head, face, spine and chest
		Q68	Other congenital musculoskeletal deformities
755	Other congenital anomalies of limbs	Q69	Polydactyly
		Q70	Syndactyly
		Q71	Reduction defects of upper limb
		Q72	Reduction defects of lower limb
		Q73	Reduction defects of unspecified limb
		Q74	Other congenital malformations of limb(s)
		Q87	Other specified congenital malformation syndromes affecting multiple systems
756	Other congenital musculoskeletal anomalies	Q75	Other congenital malformations of skull and face bones
		Q76	Congenital malformations of spine and bony thorax
		Q77	Osteochondrodysplasia with defects of growth of tubular bones and spine

ICD-9-CM Code and Description	ICD-10-CM Code and Description
	Q78 Other osteochondrodysplasias
	Q79 Congenital malformations of musculoskeletal system, not elsewhere classified
757 Congenital anomalies of the integument	Q80 Congenital ichthyosis
	Q81 Epidermolysis bullosa
	Q82 Other congenital malformations of skin
	Q83 Congenital malformations of breast
	Q84 Other congenital malformations of integument
758 Chromosomal anomalies	Q90 Down syndrome
	Q91 Trisomy 18 and Trisomy 13
	Q92 Other trisomies and partial trisomies of the autosomes, not elsewhere classified
	Q93 Monosomies and deletions from the autosomes, not elsewhere classified
	Q95 Balanced rearrangements and structural markers, not elsewhere classified
	Q96 Turner's syndrome
	Q97 Other sex chromosome abnormalities, female phenotype, not elsewhere classified
	Q98 Other sex chromosome abnormalities, male phenotype, not elsewhere classified
	Q99 Other chromosome abnormalities, not elsewhere classified
759 Other and unspecified congenital anomalies	Q89 Other congenital malformations, not elsewhere classified

15. CERTAIN CONDITIONS ORIGINATING IN THE PERINATAL PERIOD

Maternal causes of perinatal morbidity and mortality (760-763)

760 Fetus or newborn affected by maternal conditions which may be unrelated to present	P00 Newborn (suspected to be) affected by maternal conditions that may be unrelated to present pregnancy
	Q86 Congenital malformation syndromes due to known exogenous causes, not elsewhere classified
761 Fetus or newborn affected by maternal complications of pregnancy	P01 Newborn (suspected to be) affected by maternal complications of pregnancy
762 Fetus or newborn affected by complications of placenta, cord, and membranes	P02 Newborn (suspected to be) affected by complications of placenta, cord and membranes
763 Fetus or newborn affected by other complications of labor and delivery	P03 Newborn (suspected to be) affected by other complications of labor and delivery
	P04 Newborn (suspected to be) affected by noxious substances transmitted via placenta or breast milk

Other conditions originating in the perinatal period (764-779)

764 Slow fetal growth and fetal malnutrition	P05 Disorders of newborn related to slow fetal growth and fetal malnutrition
765 Disorders relating to short gestation and low birthweight	P07 Disorders of newborn related to short gestation and low birth weight, not elsewhere classified

ICD-9-CM Code and Description		ICD-10-CM Code and Description	
766	Disorders relating to long gestation and high birthweight	P08	Disorders of newborn related to long gestation and high birth weight
767	Birth trauma	P10	Intracranial laceration and hemorrhage due to birth injury
		P11	Other birth injuries to central nervous system
		P12	Birth injury to scalp
		P13	Birth injury to skeleton
		P14	Birth injury to peripheral nervous system
		P15	Other birth injuries
768	Intrauterine hypoxia and birth asphyxia	P19	Metabolic acidemia in newborn
		P84	Other problems with newborn
769	Respiratory distress syndrome	P22	Respiratory distress of newborn
770	Other respiratory conditions of fetus and newborn	P23	Congenital pneumonia
		P24	Neonatal aspiration
		P25	Interstitial emphysema and related conditions originating in the perinatal period
		P26	Pulmonary hemorrhage originating in the perinatal period
		P27	Chronic respiratory disease originating in the perinatal period
		P28	Other respiratory conditions originating in the perinatal period
771	Infections specific to the perinatal period	A33	Tetanus neonatorum
		P35	Congenital viral diseases
		P36	Bacterial sepsis of newborn
		P37	Other congenital infectious and parasitic diseases
		P38	Omphalitis of newborn
		P39	Other infections specific to the perinatal period
772	Fetal and neonatal hemorrhage	P50	Newborn affected by intrauterine (fetal) blood loss
		P51	Umbilical hemorrhage of newborn
		P52	Intracranial nontraumatic hemorrhage of newborn
		P54	Other neonatal hemorrhages
773	Hemolytic disease of fetus or newborn, due to isoimmunization	P55	Hemolytic disease of newborn
		P56	Hydrops fetalis due to hemolytic disease
		P57	Kernicterus
774	Other perinatal jaundice	P58	Neonatal jaundice due to other excessive hemolysis
		P59	Neonatal jaundice from other and unspecified causes
775	Endocrine and metabolic disturbances specific to the fetus and newborn	P70	Transitory disorders of carbohydrate metabolism specific to newborn
		P71	Transitory neonatal disorders of calcium and magnesium metabolism

ICD-9-CM Code and Description		ICD-10-CM Code and Description	
		P72	Other transitory neonatal endocrine disorders
		P74	Other transitory neonatal electrolyte and metabolic disturbances
		P94	Disorders of muscle tone of newborn
776	Hematological disorders of newborn	P53	Hemorrhagic disease of newborn
		P60	Disseminated intravascular coagulation of newborn
		P61	Other perinatal hematological disorders
777	Perinatal disorders of digestive system	P76	Other intestinal obstruction of newborn
		P77	Necrotizing enterocolitis of newborn
		P78	Other perinatal digestive system disorders
778	Conditions involving the integument and temperature regulation of fetus and newborn	P80	Hypothermia of newborn
		P81	Other disturbances of temperature regulation of newborn
		P83	Other conditions of integument specific to newborn
779	Other and ill-defined conditions originating in the perinatal period	P29	Cardiovascular disorders originating in the perinatal period
		P90	Convulsions of newborn
		P91	Other disturbances of cerebral status of newborn
		P92	Feeding problems of newborn
		P93	Reactions and intoxications due to drugs administered to newborn
		P95	Stillbirth
		P96	Other conditions originating in the perinatal period

16. SYMPTOMS, SIGNS, AND ILL-DEFINED CONDITIONS

Symptoms (780-789)

780	General symptoms	G47	Sleep disorders
		R40	Somnolence, stupor and coma
		R41	Other symptoms and signs involving cognitive functions and awareness
		R42	Dizziness and giddiness
		R44	Other symptoms and signs involving general sensations and perceptions
		R50	Fever of other and unknown origin
		R53	Malaise and fatigue
		R55	Syncope and collapse
		R56	Convulsions, not elsewhere classified
		R61	Generalized hyperhidrosis
		R68	Other general symptoms and signs
781	Symptoms involving nervous and musculoskeletal systems	R25	Abnormal involuntary movements
		R26	Abnormalities of gait and mobility
		R27	Other lack of coordination
		R29	Other symptoms and signs involving the nervous and musculoskeletal systems

ICD-9-CM Code and Description		ICD-10-CM Code and Description	
		R43	Disturbances of smell and taste
782	Symptoms involving skin and other integumentary tissue	R17	Unspecified jaundice
		R20	Disturbances of skin sensation
		R21	Rash and other nonspecific skin eruption
		R22	Localized swelling, mass and lump of skin and subcutaneous tissue
		R23	Other skin changes
		R60	Edema, not elsewhere classified
783	Symptoms concerning nutrition, metabolism, and development	R62	Lack of expected normal physiological development in childhood and adults
		R63	Symptoms and signs concerning food and fluid intake
784	Symptoms involving head and neck	R04	Hemorrhage from respiratory passages
		R07	Pain in throat and chest
		R47	Speech disturbances, not elsewhere classified
		R49	Voice and resonance disorders
		R51	Headache
		R90	Abnormal findings on diagnostic imaging of central nervous system
785	Symptoms involving cardiovascular system	I96	Gangrene, not elsewhere classified
		R00	Abnormalities of heart beat
		R01	Cardiac murmurs and other cardiac sounds
		R57	Shock, not elsewhere classified
		R59	Enlarged lymph nodes
786	Symptoms involving respiratory system and other chest symptoms	R05	Cough
		R06	Abnormalities of breathing
787	Symptoms involving digestive system	R11	Nausea and vomiting
		R12	Heartburn
		R13	Aphagia and dysphagia
		R14	Flatulence and related conditions
		R15	Fecal incontinence
788	Symptoms involving urinary system	N23	Unspecified renal colic
		R30	Pain associated with micturition
		R32	Unspecified urinary incontinence
		R33	Retention of urine
		R34	Polyuria
		R35	Polyuria
		R36	Urethral discharge
		R39	Other and unspecified symptoms and signs involving the genitourinary system
789	Other symptoms involving abdomen and pelvis	R10	Abdominal and pelvic pain
		R16	Hepatomegaly and splenomegaly, not elsewhere classified
		R18	Ascites
		R19	Other symptoms and signs involving the digestive system and abdomen

ICD-9-CM Code and Description	ICD-10-CM Code and Description

Nonspecific abnormal findings (790-796)

790	Nonspecific findings on examination of blood	E79	Disorders of purine and pyrimidine metabolism
		R70	Elevated erythrocyte sedimentation rate and abnormality of plasma viscosity
		R71	Abnormality of red blood cells
		R73	Elevated blood glucose level
		R74	Abnormal serum enzyme levels
		R77	Other abnormalities of plasma proteins
		R78	Findings of drugs and other substances, not normally found in blood
		R79	Other abnormal findings of blood chemistry
791	Nonspecific findings on examination of urine	R80	Proteinuria
		R81	Glycosuria
		R82	Other and unspecified abnormal findings in urine
792	Nonspecific abnormal findings in other body substances	O28	Abnormal findings on antenatal screening of mother
		R83	Abnormal findings in cerebrospinal fluid
		R84	Abnormal findings in specimens from respiratory organs and thorax
		R85	Abnormal findings in specimens from digestive organs and abdominal cavity
		R86	Abnormal findings in specimens from male genital organs
		R87	Abnormal findings in specimens from female genital organs
		R88	Abnormal findings in other body fluids and substances
		R89	Abnormal findings in specimens from other organs, systems and tissues
793	Nonspecific (abnormal) findings on radiological and other examination of body	R91	Abnormal findings on diagnostic imaging of lung
		R92	Abnormal and inconclusive findings on diagnostic imaging of breast
		R93	Abnormal findings on diagnostic imaging of other body structures
794	Nonspecific abnormal results of function studies	R94	Abnormal results of function studies
795	Other and nonspecific abnormal cytological, histological, immunological and DNA	R75	Inconclusive laboratory evidence of human immunodeficiency virus [HIV]
		R76	Other abnormal immunological findings in serum
		R97	Abnormal tumor markers
796	Other nonspecific abnormal findings	P09	Abnormal findings on neonatal screening
		R03	Abnormal blood-pressure reading, without diagnosis

ICD-9-CM Code and Description	ICD-10-CM Code and Description

Ill-defined and unknown causes of morbidity and mortality (797-799)

797	Senility without mention of psychosis	R54	Age-related physical debility
798	Sudden death, cause unknown	R99	Ill-defined and unknown cause of mortality
799	Other ill-defined and unknown causes of morbidity and mortality	R09	Other symptoms and signs involving the circulatory and respiratory system
		R45	Symptoms and signs involving emotional state
		R46	Symptoms and signs involving appearance and behavior
		R64	Cachexia
		R65	Symptoms and signs specifically associated with systemic inflammation and infection

17. INJURY AND POISONING

Fracture of skull (800-804)

800	Fracture of vault of skull	S02	Fracture of skull and facial bones
801	Fracture of base of skull	S02	Fracture of skull and facial bones
		S06	Intracranial injury
802	Fracture of face bones	S02	Fracture of skull and facial bones
803	Other and unqualified skull fractures	S02	Fracture of skull and facial bones
		S06	Intracranial injury
804	Multiple fractures involving skull or face with other bones	S02	Fracture of skull and facial bones
		S06	Intracranial injury

Fracture of neck and trunk (805-809)

805	Fracture of vertebral column without mention of spinal cord injury	S12	Fracture of cervical vertebra and other parts of neck
		S22	Fracture of rib(s), sternum and thoracic spine
		S32	Fracture of lumbar spine and pelvis
806	Fracture of vertebral column with spinal cord injury	S12	Fracture of cervical vertebra and other parts of neck
		S14	Injury of nerves and spinal cord at neck level
807	Fracture of rib(s), sternum, larynx, and trachea	S22	Fracture of rib(s), sternum and thoracic spine
808	Fracture of pelvis	S32	Fracture of lumbar spine and pelvis
809	Ill-defined fractures of bones of trunk	S22	Fracture of rib(s), sternum and thoracic spine

Fracture of upper limb (810-819)

810	Fracture of clavicle	S42	Fracture of shoulder and upper arm
811	Fracture of scapula		
812	Fracture of humerus	S49	Other and unspecified injuries of shoulder and upper arm

ICD-9-CM Code and Description		ICD-10-CM Code and Description	
813	Fracture of radius and ulna	S52	Fracture of forearm
		S59	Other and unspecified injuries of elbow and forearm
814	Fracture of carpal bone(s)	S62	Fracture at wrist and hand level
815	Fracture of metacarpal bone(s)	S62	Fracture at wrist and hand level
816	Fracture of one or more phalanges of hand	S62	Fracture at wrist and hand level
817	Multiple fractures of hand bones	S62	Fracture at wrist and hand level
818	Ill-defined fractures of upper limb	S62	Fracture at wrist and hand level
819	Multiple fractures involving both upper limbs, and upper limb with rib(s) and sternum	S22	Fracture of rib(s), sternum and thoracic spine

Fracture of lower limb (820-829)

820	Fracture of neck of femur	S72	Fracture of femur
		S79	Other and unspecified injuries of hip and thigh
821	Fracture of other and unspecified parts of femur	S72	Fracture of femur
822	Fracture of patella	S82	Fracture of lower leg, including ankle
823	Fracture of tibia and fibula	S89	Other and unspecified injuries of lower leg
824	Fracture of ankle	S82	Fracture of lower leg, including ankle
825	Fracture of one or more tarsal and metatarsal bones	S92	Fracture of foot and toe, except ankle
826	Fracture of one or more phalanges of foot	S92	Fracture of foot and toe, except ankle
827	Other, multiple, and ill-defined fractures of lower limb	T14	Injury of unspecified body region
828	Multiple fractures involving both lower limbs, lower with upper limb, and lower limb(s) with rib(s) and sternum	T07	Unspecified multiple injuries
829	Fracture of unspecified bones	T14	Injury of unspecified body region

Dislocation (830-839)

830	Dislocation of jaw	S03	Dislocation and sprain of joints and ligaments of head
831	Dislocation of shoulder	S43	Dislocation and sprain of joints and ligaments of shoulder girdle
832	Dislocation of elbow	S53	Dislocation and sprain of joints and ligaments of elbow
833	Dislocation of wrist	S63	Dislocation and sprain of joints and ligaments at wrist and hand level
834	Dislocation of finger		
835	Dislocation of hip	S73	Dislocation and sprain of joint and ligaments of hip
836	Dislocation of knee	S83	Dislocation and sprain of joints and ligaments of knee
837	Dislocation of ankle	S93	Dislocation and sprain of joints and ligaments at ankle, foot and toe level

ICD-9-CM Code and Description		ICD-10-CM Code and Description	
839	Other, multiple, and ill-defined dislocations	S13	Dislocation and sprain of joints and ligaments at neck level
		S23	Dislocation and sprain of joints and ligaments of thorax
		S33	Dislocation and sprain of joints and ligaments of lumbar spine and pelvis

Sprains and strains of joints and adjacent muscles (840-848)

840	Sprains and strains of shoulder and upper arm	S43	Dislocation and sprain of joints and ligaments of shoulder girdle
		S46	Injury of muscle, fascia and tendon at shoulder and upper arm level
841	Sprains and strains of elbow and forearm	S53	Dislocation and sprain of joints and ligaments of elbow
842	Sprains and strains of wrist and hand	S63	Dislocation and sprain of joints and ligaments at wrist and hand level
843	Sprains and strains of hip and thigh	S73	Dislocation and sprain of joint and ligaments of hip
844	Sprains and strains of knee and leg	S83	Dislocation and sprain of joints and ligaments of knee
845	Sprains and strains of ankle and foot	S93	Dislocation and sprain of joints and ligaments at ankle, foot and toe level
846	Sprains and strains of sacroiliac region	S33	Dislocation and sprain of joints and ligaments of lumbar spine and pelvis
847	Sprains and strains of other and unspecified parts of back	S16	Injury of muscle, fascia and tendon at neck level
848	Other and ill-defined sprains and strains	S03	Dislocation and sprain of joints and ligaments of head

Intracranial injury, excluding those with skull fracture (850-854)

850	Concussion	S06	Intracranial injury
851	Cerebral laceration and contusion	S06	Intracranial injury
852	Subarachnoid, subdural, and extradural hemorrhage, following injury	S06	Intracranial injury
853	Other and unspecified intracranial hemorrhage following injury	S06	Intracranial injury
854	Intracranial injury of other and unspecified nature	S06	Intracranial injury

Internal injury of thorax, abdomen, and pelvis (860-869)

860	Traumatic pneumothorax and hemothorax	S27	Injury of other and unspecified intrathoracic organs
861	Injury to heart and lung	S26	Injury of heart
862	Injury to other and unspecified intrathoracic organs	S27	Injury of other and unspecified intrathoracic organs
863	Injury to gastrointestinal tract	S36	Injury of intra-abdominal organs
864	Injury to liver	S36	Injury of intra-abdominal organs
865	Injury to spleen	S36	Injury of intra-abdominal organs
866	Injury to kidney	S37	Injury of urinary and pelvic organs
867	Injury to pelvic organs	S37	Injury of urinary and pelvic organs
868	Injury to other intra-abdominal organs	S36	Injury of intra-abdominal organs

ICD-9-CM Code and Description		ICD-10-CM Code and Description	
869	Internal injury to unspecified or ill-defined organs	S36	Injury of intra-abdominal organs
		S37	Injury of urinary and pelvic organs

Open wound of head, neck, and trunk (870-879)

870	Open wound of ocular adnexa	S01	Open wound of head
871	Open wound of eyeball	S05	Injury of eye and orbit
872	Open wound of ear	S01	Open wound of head
873	Other open wound of head	S01	Open wound of head
		S08	Avulsion and traumatic amputation of part of head
874	Open wound of neck	S11	Open wound of neck
875	Open wound of chest (wall)	S21	Open wound of thorax
876	Open wound of back	S31	Open wound of abdomen, lower back, pelvis and external genitals
877	Open wound of genital organs (external), including traumatic amputation	S31	Open wound of abdomen, lower back, pelvis and external genitals
878	Open wound of genital organs (external), including traumatic amputation	S31	Open wound of abdomen, lower back, pelvis and external genitals
879	Open wound of other and unspecified sites, except limbs	S21	Open wound of thorax

Open wound of upper limb (880-887)

880	Open wound of shoulder and upper arm	S41	Open wound of shoulder and upper arm
881	Open wound of elbow, forearm, and wrist	S51	Open wound of elbow and forearm
882	Open wound of hand except finger(s) alone	S66	Injury of muscle, fascia and tendon at wrist and hand level
883	Open wound of finger(s)	S61	Open wound of wrist, hand and fingers
884	Multiple and unspecified open wound of upper limb		
885	Traumatic amputation of thumb (complete) (partial)	S68	Traumatic amputation of wrist, hand and fingers
886	Traumatic amputation of other finger(s) (complete) (partial)	S68	Traumatic amputation of wrist, hand and fingers
887	Traumatic amputation of arm and hand (complete) (partial)	S48	Traumatic amputation of shoulder and upper arm
		S58	Traumatic amputation of elbow and forearm

Open wound of lower limb (890-897)

890	Open wound of hip and thigh	S71	Open wound of hip and thigh
891	Open wound of knee, leg [except thigh], and ankle	S81	Open wound of knee and lower leg
		S91	Open wound of ankle, foot and toes
892	Open wound of foot except toe(s) alone	S91	Open wound of ankle, foot and toes
893	Open wound of toe(s)	S91	Open wound of ankle, foot and toes

ICD-9-CM Code and Description	ICD-10-CM Code and Description
894 Multiple and unspecified open wound of lower limb	S71 Open wound of hip and thigh
895 Traumatic amputation of toe(s) (complete) (partial)	S98 Traumatic amputation of ankle and foot
896 Traumatic amputation of foot (complete) (partial)	S98 Traumatic amputation of ankle and foot
897 Traumatic amputation of leg(s) (complete) (partial)	S78 Traumatic amputation of hip and thigh
	S88 Traumatic amputation of lower leg

Injury to blood vessels (900-904)

900 Injury to blood vessels of head and neck	S09 Other and unspecified injuries of head
	S15 Injury of blood vessels at neck level
901 Injury to blood vessels of thorax	S25 Injury of blood vessels of thorax
902 Injury to blood vessels of abdomen and pelvis	S35 Injury of blood vessels at abdomen, lower back and pelvis level
903 Injury to blood vessels of upper extremity	S45 Injury of blood vessels at shoulder and upper arm level
	S55 Injury of blood vessels at forearm level
	S65 Injury of blood vessels at wrist and hand level
904 Injury to blood vessels of lower extremity and unspecified sites	S75 Injury of blood vessels at hip and thigh level
	S85 Injury of blood vessels at lower leg level
	S95 Injury of blood vessels at ankle and foot level

Late effects of injuries, poisonings, toxic effects, and other external causes (905-909)

905 Late effects of musculoskeletal and connective tissue injuries	M67 Other disorders of synovium and tendon
	M84 Disorder of continuity of bone
	S02 Fracture of skull and facial bones
	S03 Dislocation and sprain of joints and ligaments of head
	S12 Fracture of cervical vertebra and other parts of neck
	S13 Dislocation and sprain of joints and ligaments at neck level
	S22 Fracture of rib(s), sternum and thoracic spine
	S23 Dislocation and sprain of joints and ligaments of thorax
	S32 Fracture of lumbar spine and pelvis
	S33 Dislocation and sprain of joints and ligaments of lumbar spine and pelvis
	S42 Fracture of shoulder and upper arm
	S43 Dislocation and sprain of joints and ligaments of shoulder girdle
	S46 Injury of muscle, fascia and tendon at shoulder and upper arm level

ICD-9-CM Code and Description	ICD-10-CM Code and Description
	S48 Traumatic amputation of shoulder and upper arm
	S52 Fracture of forearm
	S53 Dislocation and sprain of joints and ligaments of elbow
	S56 Injury of muscle, fascia and tendon at forearm level
	S58 Traumatic amputation of elbow and forearm
	S62 Fracture at wrist and hand level
	S63 Dislocation and sprain of joints and ligaments at wrist and hand level
	S66 Injury of muscle, fascia and tendon at wrist and hand level
	S68 Traumatic amputation of wrist, hand and fingers
	S72 Fracture of femur
	S73 Dislocation and sprain of joint and ligaments of hip
	S76 Injury of muscle, fascia and tendon at hip and thigh level
	S78 Traumatic amputation of hip and thigh
	S79 Other and unspecified injuries of hip and thigh
	S82 Fracture of lower leg, including ankle
	S83 Dislocation and sprain of joints and ligaments of knee
	S88 Traumatic amputation of lower leg
	S92 Fracture of foot and toe, except ankle
	S93 Dislocation and sprain of joints and ligaments at ankle, foot and toe
	S96 Injury of muscle and tendon at ankle and foot level
906 Late effects of injuries to skin and subcutaneous tissues	S00 Superficial injury of head
	S01 Open wound of head
	S07 Crushing injury of head
	S10 Superficial injury of neck
	S11 Open wound of neck
	S17 Crushing injury of neck
	S20 Superficial injury of thorax
	S21 Open wound of thorax
	S28 Crushing injury of thorax, and traumatic amputation of part of thorax
	S30 Superficial injury of abdomen, lower back, pelvis and external genitals
	S31 Open wound of abdomen, lower back, pelvis and external genitals
	S38 Crushing injury and traumatic amputation of abdomen, lower back, pelvis and external genitals

ICD-9-CM Code and Description	ICD-10-CM Code and Description	
	S40	Superficial injury of shoulder and upper arm
	S41	Open wound of shoulder and upper arm
	S47	Crushing injury of shoulder and upper arm
	S50	Superficial injury of elbow and forearm
	S51	Open wound of elbow and forearm
	S57	Crushing injury of elbow and forearm
	S60	Superficial injury of wrist, hand and fingers
	S61	Open wound of wrist, hand and fingers
	S67	Crushing injury of wrist, hand and fingers
	S70	Superficial injury of hip and thigh
	S71	Open wound of hip and thigh
	S77	Crushing injury of hip and thigh
	S80	Superficial injury of knee and lower leg
	S81	Open wound of knee and lower leg
	S87	Crushing injury of lower leg
	S90	Superficial injury of ankle, foot and toes
	S91	Open wound of ankle, foot and toes
	S97	Crushing injury of ankle and foot
	T20	Burn and corrosion of head, face, and neck
	T21	Burn and corrosion of trunk
	T22	Burn and corrosion of shoulder and upper limb, except wrist and hand
	T23	Burn and corrosion of wrist and hand
	T24	Burn and corrosion of lower limb, except ankle and foot
	T28	Burn and corrosion of other internal organs
907 Late effects of injuries to the nervous system	S04	Injury of cranial nerve
	S06	Intracranial injury
	S14	Injury of nerves and spinal cord at neck level
	S24	Injury of nerves and spinal cord at thorax level
	S34	Injury of lumbar and sacral spinal cord and nerves at abdomen, lower back and pelvis level
	S44	Injury of nerves at shoulder and upper arm level
	S54	Injury of nerves at forearm level
	S64	Injury of nerves at wrist and hand level
	S74	Injury of nerves at hip and thigh level
	S84	Injury of nerves at lower leg level
	S94	Injury of nerves at ankle and foot level

ICD-9-CM Code and Description	ICD-10-CM Code and Description
908 Late effects of other and unspecified injuries	S09 Other and unspecified injuries of head
	S15 Injury of blood vessels at neck level
	S16 Injury of muscle, fascia and tendon at neck level
	S25 Injury of blood vessels of thorax
	S26 Injury of heart
	S27 Injury of other and unspecified intrathoracic organs
	S29 Other and unspecified injuries of thorax
	S35 Injury of blood vessels at abdomen, lower back and pelvis level
	S36 Injury of intra-abdominal organs
	S37 Injury of urinary and pelvic organs
	S39 Other and unspecified injuries of abdomen, lower back, pelvis and external genitals
	S45 Injury of blood vessels at shoulder and upper arm level
	S49 Other and unspecified injuries of shoulder and upper arm
	S55 Injury of blood vessels at forearm level
	S59 Other and unspecified injuries of elbow and forearm
	S65 Injury of blood vessels at wrist and hand level
	S69 Other and unspecified injuries of wrist, hand and finger(s)
	S75 Injury of blood vessels at hip and thigh level
	S79 Other and unspecified injuries of hip and thigh
	S85 Injury of blood vessels at lower leg level
	S89 Other and unspecified injuries of lower leg
	S95 Injury of blood vessels at ankle and foot level
	S99 Other and unspecified injuries of ankle and foot
	T15 Foreign body on external eye
	T16 Foreign body in ear
	T17 Foreign body in respiratory tract
	T18 Foreign body in alimentary tract
	T19 Foreign body in genitourinary tract
	T79 Certain early complications of trauma, not elsewhere classified

ICD-9-CM Code and Description	ICD-10-CM Code and Description
909 Late effects of other and unspecified external causes	L59 Other disorders of skin and subcutaneous tissue related to radiation
	T50 Poisoning by, adverse effect of and underdosing of diuretics and other and unspecified drugs, medicaments and biological substances
	T65 Toxic effect of other and unspecified substances
	T75 Other and unspecified effects of other external causes
	T78 Adverse effects, not elsewhere classified
	T88 Other complications of surgical and medical care, not elsewhere classified

Superficial injury (910-919)

910 Superficial injury of face, neck, and scalp except eye	L08 Other specified local infections of the skin and subcutaneous tissue
	S00 Insect bite (nonvenomous) of scalp, initial encounter
	S10 Abrasion of unspecified part of neck, initial encounter
911 Superficial injury of trunk	L08 Other specified local infections of the skin and subcutaneous tissue
	S20 Abrasion of unspecified parts of thorax, initial encounter
	S30 Blister (nonthermal) of lower back and pelvis, initial encounter
912 Superficial injury of shoulder and upper arm	L08 Other local infections of skin and subcutaneous tissue
913 Superficial injury of elbow, forearm, and wrist	L08 Other local infections of skin and subcutaneous tissue
	S50 Superficial injury of elbow and forearm
	S60 Superficial injury of wrist, hand and fingers
914 Superficial injury of hand(s) except finger(s) alone	L08 Other local infections of skin and subcutaneous tissue
	S60 Superficial injury of wrist, hand and fingers
915 Superficial injury of finger(s)	L08 Other local infections of skin and subcutaneous tissue
	S60 Superficial injury of wrist, hand and fingers
916 Superficial injury of hip, thigh, leg, and ankle	L08 Other local infections of skin and subcutaneous tissue
	S70 Superficial injury of hip and thigh
	S80 Superficial injury of knee and lower leg
	S90 Superficial injury of ankle, foot and toes
917 Superficial injury of foot and toe(s)	L08 Other local infections of skin and subcutaneous tissue
	S90 Superficial injury of ankle, foot and toes
918 Superficial injury of eye and adnexa	S00 Superficial injury of head
	S05 Injury of eye and orbit

ICD-9-CM Code and Description	ICD-10-CM Code and Description

919	Superficial injury of other, multiple, and unspecified sites	L08	Other local infections of skin and subcutaneous tissue
		T07	Unspecified multiple injuries

Contusion with intact skin surface (920-924)

920	Contusion of face, scalp, and neck except eye(s)	S10	Superficial injury of neck
922	Contusion of trunk	S20	Superficial injury of thorax
		S30	Superficial injury of abdomen, lower back, pelvis and external genitals
923	Contusion of upper limb	S40	Superficial injury of shoulder and upper arm
		S50	Superficial injury of elbow and forearm
		S60	Superficial injury of wrist, hand and fingers
924	Contusion of lower limb and of other and unspecified sites	S70	Superficial injury of hip and thigh
		S80	Superficial injury of knee and lower leg
		S90	Superficial injury of ankle, foot and toes

Crushing injury (925-929)

925	Crushing injury of face, scalp, and neck	S07	Crushing injury of head
		S17	Crushing injury of neck
926	Crushing injury of trunk	S28	Crushing injury of thorax, and traumatic amputation of part of thorax
		S38	Crushing injury and traumatic amputation of abdomen, lower back, pelvis and external genitals
927	Crushing injury of upper limb	S47	Crushing injury of shoulder and upper arm
		S57	Crushing injury of elbow and forearm
		S67	Crushing injury of wrist, hand and fingers
928	Crushing injury of lower limb	S77	Crushing injury of hip and thigh
		S87	Crushing injury of lower leg
		S97	Crushing injury of ankle and foot
929	Crushing injury of multiple and unspecified sites		

Effects of foreign body entering through orifice (930-939)

930	Foreign body on external eye	T15	Foreign body on external eye
931	Foreign body in ear	T16	Foreign body in ear
932	Foreign body in nose	T17	Foreign body in respiratory tract
933	Foreign body in pharynx and larynx	T17	Foreign body in respiratory tract
934	Foreign body in trachea, bronchus, and lung	T17	Foreign body in respiratory tract
935	Foreign body in mouth, esophagus, and stomach	T18	Foreign body in alimentary tract
936	Foreign body in intestine and colon	T18	Foreign body in alimentary tract
937	Foreign body in anus and rectum	T18	Foreign body in alimentary tract

ICD-9-CM Code and Description	ICD-10-CM Code and Description
938 Foreign body in digestive system, unspecified	T18 Foreign body in alimentary tract
939 Foreign body in genitourinary tract	T19 Foreign body in genitourinary tract

Burns (940-949)

940 Burn confined to eye and adnexa	T26 Burn and corrosion confined to eye and adnexa
941 Burn of face, head, and neck	T20 Burn and corrosion of head, face, and neck
942 Burn of trunk	T21 Burn and corrosion of trunk
943 Burn of upper limb, except wrist and hand	T22 Burn and corrosion of shoulder and upper limb, except wrist and hand
944 Burn of wrist(s) and hand(s)	T23 Burn and corrosion of wrist and hand
945 Burn of lower limb(s)	T24 Burn and corrosion of lower limb, except ankle and foot
	T25 Burn and corrosion of ankle and foot
946 Burns of multiple specified sites	
947 Burn of internal organs	T27 Burn and corrosion of respiratory tract
	T28 Burn and corrosion of other internal organs
948 Burns classified according to extent of body surface involved	T31 Burns classified according to extent of body surface involved
	T32 Corrosions classified according to extent of body surface involved
949 Burn, unspecified	T30 Burn and corrosion, body region unspecified

Injury to nerves and spinal cord (950-957)

950 Injury to optic nerve and pathways	S04 Injury of cranial nerve
951 Injury to other cranial nerve(s)	
952 Spinal cord injury without evidence of spinal bone injury	S14 Injury of nerves and spinal cord at neck level
	S24 Injury of nerves and spinal cord at thorax level
	S34 Injury of lumbar and sacral spinal cord and nerves at abdomen, lower back and pelvis level
953 Injury to nerve roots and spinal plexus	
954 Injury to other nerve(s) of trunk excluding shoulder and pelvic girdles	
955 Injury to peripheral nerve(s) of shoulder girdle and upper limb	S44 Injury of nerves at shoulder and upper arm level
	S54 Injury of nerves at forearm level
	S64 Injury of nerves at wrist and hand level
956 Injury to peripheral nerve(s) of pelvic girdle and lower limb	S74 Injury of nerves at hip and thigh level
	S84 Injury of nerves at lower leg level
	S94 Injury of nerves at ankle and foot level
957 Injury to other and unspecified nerves	

Certain traumatic complications and unspecified injuries (958-959)

958 Certain early complications of trauma	T79 Certain early complications of trauma, not elsewhere classified

ICD-9-CM Code and Description		ICD-10-CM Code and Description	
959	Injury, other and unspecified	S19	Other specified and unspecified injuries of neck
		S29	Other and unspecified injuries of thorax
		S39	Other and unspecified injuries of abdomen, lower back, pelvis and external genitals
		S46	Injury of muscle, fascia and tendon at shoulder and upper arm level
		S56	Injury of muscle, fascia and tendon at forearm level
		S66	Injury of muscle, fascia and tendon at wrist and hand level
		S69	Other and unspecified injuries of wrist, hand and finger(s)
		S76	Injury of muscle, fascia and tendon at hip and thigh level
		S86	Injury of muscle, fascia and tendon at lower leg level
		S96	Injury of muscle and tendon at ankle and foot level
		S99	Other and unspecified injuries of ankle and foot
		T07	Unspecified multiple injuries
		T14	Injury of unspecified body region

Poisoning by drugs, medicinal and biological substances (960-979)

960	Poisoning by antibiotics	T36	Poisoning by, adverse effect of and underdosing of systemic antibiotics
961	Poisoning by other anti-infectives	T37	Poisoning by, adverse effect of and underdosing of other systemic anti-infectives and antiparasitics
962	Poisoning by hormones and synthetic substitutes	T38	Poisoning by, adverse effect of and underdosing of hormones and their synthetic substitutes and antagonists, not elsewhere classified
		T50	Poisoning by, adverse effect of and underdosing of diuretics and other and unspecified drugs, medicaments and biological substances
963	Poisoning by primarily systemic agents	T45	Poisoning by, adverse effect of and underdosing of primarily systemic and hematological agents, not elsewhere classified
964	Poisoning by agents primarily affecting blood constituents	T45	Poisoning by, adverse effect of and underdosing of primarily systemic and hematological agents, not elsewhere classified
965	Poisoning by agents primarily affecting blood constituents	T39	Poisoning by, adverse effect of and underdosing of nonopioid analgesics, antipyretics and antirheumatics
		T40	Poisoning by, adverse effect of and underdosing of narcotics and psychodysleptics [hallucinogens]
966	Poisoning by anticonvulsants and anti-parkinsonism drugs	T42	Poisoning by, adverse effect of and underdosing of antiepileptic, sedative-hypnotic and antiparkinsonism drugs
967	Poisoning by sedatives and hypnotics	T42	Poisoning by, adverse effect of and underdosing of antiepileptic, sedative-hypnotic and antiparkinsonism drugs

ICD-9-CM Code and Description	ICD-10-CM Code and Description
968 Poisoning by other central nervous system depressants and anesthetics	T41 Poisoning by, adverse effect of and underdosing of anesthetics and therapeutic gases
969 Poisoning by psychotropic agents	T43 Poisoning by, adverse effect of and underdosing of psychotropic drugs, not elsewhere classified
970 Poisoning by central nervous system stimulants	T50 Poisoning by, adverse effect of and underdosing of diuretics and other and unspecified drugs, medicaments and biological substances
971 Poisoning by drugs primarily affecting the autonomic nervous system	T44 Poisoning by, adverse effect of and underdosing of drugs primarily affecting the autonomic nervous system
972 Poisoning by agents primarily affecting the cardiovascular system	T46 Poisoning by, adverse effect of and underdosing of agents primarily affecting the cardiovascular system
973 Poisoning by agents primarily affecting the gastrointestinal system	T47 Poisoning by, adverse effect of and underdosing of agents primarily affecting the gastrointestinal system
974 Poisoning by water, mineral, and uric acid metabolism drugs	T48 Poisoning by, adverse effect of and underdosing of agents primarily acting on smooth and skeletal muscles and the respiratory system
975 Poisoning by agents primarily acting on the smooth and skeletal muscles and	T49 Poisoning by, adverse effect of and underdosing of topical agents primarily affecting skin and mucous membrane and by ophthalmological, otorhinolaryngological and dental drugs
976 Poisoning by agents primarily affecting skin and mucous membrane,	T46 Poisoning by, adverse effect of and underdosing of agents primarily affecting the cardiovascular system
977 Poisoning by other and unspecified drugs and medicinals	T50 Poisoning by, adverse effect of and underdosing of diuretics and other and unspecified drugs, medicaments and biological substances
978 Poisoning by bacterial vaccines	T50 Poisoning by, adverse effect of and underdosing of diuretics and other and unspecified drugs, medicaments and biological substances
979 Poisoning by other vaccines and biological substances	T50 Poisoning by, adverse effect of and underdosing of diuretics and other and unspecified drugs, medicaments and biological substances

Toxic effects of substances chiefly nonmedicinal as to source (980-989)

980	Toxic effect of alcohol	T51	Toxic effect of alcohol
981	Toxic effect of petroleum products	T52	Toxic effect of organic solvents
982	Toxic effect of solvents other than petroleum-based	T53	Toxic effect of halogen derivatives of aliphatic and aromatic hydrocarbons
983	Toxic effect of corrosive aromatics, acids, and caustic alkalis	T54	Toxic effect of corrosive substances
984	Toxic effect of lead and its compounds (including fumes)	T56	Toxic effect of metals
985	Toxic effect of other metals	T57	Toxic effect of other inorganic substances
986	Toxic effect of carbon monoxide	T58	Toxic effect of carbon monoxide
987	Toxic effect of other gases, fumes, or vapors	T59	Toxic effect of other gases, fumes and vapors

ICD-9-CM Code and Description		ICD-10-CM Code and Description	
988	Toxic effect of noxious substances eaten as food	T61	Toxic effect of noxious substances eaten as seafood
988	Toxic effect of noxious substances eaten as food	T62	Toxic effect of other noxious substances eaten as food
tbl9 89	Toxic effect of other substances, chiefly nonmedicinal as to source	T55	Toxic effect of soaps and detergents
		T60	Toxic effect of pesticides
		T63	Toxic effect of contact with venomous animals and plants
		T64	Toxic effect of aflatoxin and other mycotoxin food contaminants
		T65	Toxic effect of other and unspecified substances

Other and unspecified effects of external causes (990-995)

990	Effects of radiation, unspecified	T66	Radiation sickness, unspecified
991	Effects of reduced temperature	T33	Superficial frostbite
		T34	Frostbite with tissue necrosis
		T68	Hypothermia
		T69	Other effects of reduced temperature
992	Effects of heat and light	T67	Effects of heat and light
993	Effects of air pressure	T70	Effects of air pressure and water pressure
994	Effects of other external causes	T71	Asphyxiation
		T73	Effects of other deprivation
		T75	Other and unspecified effects of other external causes
995	Certain adverse effects, not elsewhere classified	R65	Symptoms and signs specifically associated with systemic inflammation and infection
		T74	Adult and child abuse, neglect and other maltreatment, confirmed
		T76	Adult and child abuse, neglect and other maltreatment, suspected
		T78	Adverse effects, not elsewhere classified

Complications of surgical and medical care, not elsewhere classified (996-999)

996	Complications peculiar to certain specified procedures	T82	Complications of cardiac and vascular prosthetic devices, implants and grafts
		T83	Complications of genitourinary prosthetic devices, implants and grafts
		T84	Complications of internal orthopedic prosthetic devices, implants and grafts
		T85	Complications of other internal prosthetic devices, implants and grafts
		T86	Complications of transplanted organs and tissue
		T87	Complications peculiar to reattachment and amputation
997	Complications affecting specified body systems, not elsewhere classified	G97	Intraoperative and postprocedural complications and disorders of nervous system, not elsewhere classified
		H59	Intraoperative and postprocedural complications and disorders of eye and adnexa, not elsewhere classified

ICD-9-CM Code and Description		ICD-10-CM Code and Description	
		N99	Intraoperative and postprocedural complications and disorders of genitourinary system, not elsewhere classified
998	Other complications of procedures, not elsewhere classified	D78	Intraoperative and postprocedural complications of the spleen
		E36	Intraoperative complications of endocrine system
		L76	Intraoperative and postprocedural complications of skin and subcutaneous tissue
		T81	Complications of procedures, not elsewhere classified
999	Complications of medical care, not elsewhere classified	N98	Complications associated with artificial fertilization
		T80	Complications following infusion, transfusion and therapeutic injection
		T88	Other complications of surgical and medical care, not elsewhere classified
		B96	Other bacterial agents as the cause of diseases classified elsewhere

SUPPLEMENTARY CLASSIFICATION OF FACTORS INFLUENCING HEALTH STATUS AND CONTACT WITH HEALTH SERVICES

Persons with potential health hazards related to communicable diseases (V01-V06)

V01	Contact with or exposure to communicable diseases	Z20	Contact with and (suspected) exposure to communicable diseases
V02	Carrier or suspected carrier of infectious diseases	Z22	Encounter for immunization
V03	Need for prophylactic vaccination and inoculation against bacterial diseases	Z23	Immunization not carried out and underimmunization status
V04	Need for prophylactic vaccination and inoculation against certain viral diseases	Z23	Immunization not carried out and underimmunization status
V05	Need for other prophylactic vaccination and inoculation against single diseases	Z23	Immunization not carried out and underimmunization status
V06	Need for prophylactic vaccination and inoculation against combinations of diseases	Z23	Immunization not carried out and underimmunization status

Persons with need for isolation, other potential health hazards and prophylactic measures (V07-V09)

V08	Asymptomatic human immunodeficiency virus [hiv] infection status	Z21	Asymptomatic human immunodeficiency virus [HIV] infection status
V09	Infection with drug-resistant microorganisms	Z16	Resistance to antimicrobial drugs

Persons with potential health hazards related to personal and family history (V10-V19)

V10	Personal history of malignant neoplasm	Z85	Personal history of malignant neoplasm
V10	Personal history of malignant neoplasm	Z86	Personal history of certain other diseases
V11	Personal history of mental disorder	Z65	Problems related to other psychosocial services

ICD-9-CM Code and Description		ICD-10-CM Code and Description	
V12	Personal history of certain other diseases	Z87	Personal history of other diseases and conditions
V14	Personal history of allergy to medicinal agents	Z88	Allergy status to drugs, medicaments and biological substances
V15	Other personal history presenting hazards to health	Z91	Personal risk factors, not elsewhere classified
		Z92	Personal history of medical treatment
V16	Family history of malignant neoplasm	Z80	Family history of primary malignant neoplasm
V17	Family history of certain chronic disabling diseases	Z82	Family history of certain disabilities and chronic diseases (leading to disablement)
V18	Family history of certain other specific conditions	Z81	Family history of mental and behavioral disorders
V19	Family history of other conditions	Z83	Family history of other specific disorders
		Z84	Family history of other conditions

Persons encountering health services in circumstances related to reproduction and development (V20-V29)

V20	Health supervision of infant or child	Z00	Encounter for general examination without complaint, suspected or reported diagnosis
V21	Constitutional states in development	P07	Disorders of newborn related to short gestation and low birth weight, not elsewhere classified
V22	Normal pregnancy	Z33	Pregnant state
		Z34	Encounter for supervision of normal pregnancy
V23	Supervision of high-risk pregnancy	O09	Supervision of high risk pregnancy
V24	Postpartum care and examination	Z39	Encounter for maternal postpartum care and examination
V25	Encounter for contraceptive management	Z30	Encounter for contraceptive management
V26	Procreative management	Z31	Encounter for procreative management
V27	Outcome of delivery	Z37	Outcome of delivery
V28	Encounter for antenatal screening of mother	Z36	Encounter for antenatal screening of mother
V29	Observation and evaluation of newborns and infants for suspected condition not found	P00	Newborn (suspected to be) affected by maternal conditions that may be unrelated to present pregnancy

Liveborn infants according to type of birth (V30-V39)

V30	Single liveborn	Z38	Liveborn infants according to place of birth and type of delivery
V31	Twin, mate liveborn	Z38	Liveborn infants according to place of birth and type of delivery
V32	Twin, mate stillborn	Z38	Liveborn infants according to place of birth and type of delivery
V33	Twin, unspecified	Z38	Liveborn infants according to place of birth and type of delivery
V34	Other multiple, mates all liveborn	Z38	Liveborn infants according to place of birth and type of delivery

ICD-9-CM Code and Description		ICD-10-CM Code and Description	
V35	Other multiple, mates all stillborn	Z38	Liveborn infants according to place of birth and type of delivery
V36	Other multiple, mates live- and stillborn	Z38	Liveborn infants according to place of birth and type of delivery
V37	Other multiple, unspecified	Z38	Liveborn infants according to place of birth and type of delivery
V39	Unspecified	Z38	Liveborn infants according to place of birth and type of delivery

Persons with a condition influencing their health status (V40-V49)

V40	Mental and behavioral problems	F81	Specific developmental disorders of scholastic skills
		Z86	Personal history of certain other diseases
		F48	Other nonpsychotic mental disorders
V41	Problems with special senses and other special functions	Z97	Presence of other devices
V42	Organ or tissue replaced by transplant	Z94	Transplanted organ and tissue status
V43	Organ or tissue replaced by other means	Z96	Presence of other functional implants
		Z97	Presence of other devices
V44	Artificial opening status	Z93	Artificial opening status
V45	Other postprocedural states	M96	Intraoperative and postprocedural complications and disorders of musculoskeletal system, not elsewhere classified
		Z90	Acquired absence of organs, not elsewhere classified
		Z95	Presence of cardiac and vascular implants and grafts
		Z98	Other postprocedural states
V46	Other dependence on machines and devices	Z99	Dependence on enabling machines and devices, not elsewhere classified
V47	Other problems with internal organs	R68	Other general symptoms and signs
V48	Problems with head, neck, and trunk	R68	Other general symptoms and signs
V49	Other conditions influencing health status	Z74	Problems related to care provider dependency
		Z78	Other specified health status
		Z89	Acquired absence of limb

Persons encountering health services for specific procedures and aftercare (V50-V59)

V50	Elective surgery for purposes other than remedying health states	Z40	Encounter for prophylactic surgery
		Z41	Encounter for procedures for purposes other than remedying health state
V51	Carrier or suspected carrier of infectious diseases	Z42	Encounter for plastic and reconstructive surgery following medical procedure
V52	Need for prophylactic vaccination and inoculation against bacterial diseases	Z44	Encounter for fitting and adjustment of external prosthetic device
V53	Infection with drug-resistant microorganisms	Z45	Encounter for adjustment and management of implanted device

ICD-9-CM Code and Description		ICD-10-CM Code and Description	
		Z46	Encounter for fitting and adjustment of other devices
V54	Personal history of malignant neoplasm	Z47	Orthopedic aftercare
V55	Personal history of malignant neoplasm	Z43	Encounter for attention to artificial openings
V57	Care involving use of rehabilitation procedures	Z51	Encounter for other aftercare
V56	Personal history of certain other diseases	Z49	Encounter for attention to artificial openings
V58	Personal history of allergy to medicinal agents	Z48	Encounter for other postprocedural aftercare
		Z51	Encounter for other aftercare
		Z79	Long term (current) drug therapy
V59	Family history of malignant neoplasm	Z52	Donors of organs and tissues

Persons encountering health services in other circumstances (V60-V69)

V60	Family history of certain chronic disabling diseases	Z59	Problems related to housing and economic circumstances
V61	Family history of certain other specific conditions	Z62	Problems related to upbringing
		Z63	Other problems related to primary support group, including family circumstances
		Z64	Problems related to certain psychosocial circumstances
		Z69	Encounter for mental health services for victim and perpetrator of abuse
V62	Normal pregnancy	Z55	Problems related to education and literacy
		Z56	Problems related to employment and unemployment
		Z57	Occupational exposure to risk factors
		Z60	Problems related to social environment
		Z65	Problems related to other psychosocial circumstances
V63	Outcome of delivery	Z75	Problems related to medical facilities and other health care
V64	Encounter for antenatal screening of mother	Z28	Immunization not carried out and underimmunization status
		Z53	Persons encountering health services for specific procedures and treatment, not carried out
V65	Organ or tissue replaced by transplant	Z70	Counseling related to sexual attitude, behavior and orientation
		Z71	Persons encountering health services for other counseling and medical advice, not elsewhere classified
V67	Artificial opening status	Z08	Encounter for follow-up examination after completed treatment for malignant neoplasm

ICD-9-CM Code and Description		ICD-10-CM Code and Description	
		Z09	Encounter for follow-up examination after completed treatment for conditions other than malignant neoplasm
V68	Other postprocedural states	Z76	Persons encountering health services in other circumstances
V69	Other postprocedural states	Z72	Problems related to lifestyle
		Z73	Problems related to life management difficulty

Persons without reported diagnosis encountered during examination and investigation of individuals and populations (V70-V86)

V70	Other postprocedural states	Z00	Encounter for general examination without complaint, suspected or reported diagnosis
		Z02	Encounter for administrative examination
V71	Other conditions influencing health status	Z03	Encounter for medical observation for suspected diseases and conditions ruled out
		Z04	Encounter for examination and observation for other reasons
V72	Other conditions influencing health status	Z01	Encounter for other special examination without complaint, suspected or reported diagnosis
		Z32	Encounter for pregnancy test and childbirth and childcare instruction
V73	Special screening examination for viral and chlamydial diseases	Z11	Encounter for screening for infectious and parasitic diseases
V74	Elective surgery for purposes other than remedying health states	Z11	Encounter for screening for infectious and parasitic diseases
V75	Special screening examination for other infectious diseases	Z11	Encounter for screening for infectious and parasitic diseases
V76	Aftercare involving the use of plastic surgery	Z12	Encounter for screening for malignant neoplasms
V77	Special screening for endocrine, nutritional, metabolic, and immunity disorders	Z13	Encounter for screening for other diseases and disorders
V78	Fitting and adjustment of prosthetic device and implant	Z13	Encounter for screening for other diseases and disorders
V79	Special screening for mental disorders and developmental handicaps	Z13	Encounter for screening for other diseases and disorders
V80	Special screening for neurological, eye, and ear diseases	Z13	Encounter for screening for other diseases and disorders
V81	Special screening for cardiovascular, respiratory, and genitourinary diseases	Z13	Encounter for screening for other diseases and disorders
V82	Special screening for other conditions	Z13	Encounter for screening for other diseases and disorders
V83	Fitting and adjustment of other device	Z14	Genetic carrier
V84	Fitting and adjustment of other device	Z15	Genetic susceptibility to disease
V85	Other orthopedic aftercare	Z68	Body mass index [BMI]
V86	Attention to artificial openings	Z17	Estrogen receptor status
V87	Other specified personal exposures and history presenting hazards to health	Z77	Other contact with and (suspected) exposures hazardous to health

ICD-9-CM Code and Description		ICD-10-CM Code and Description	
V88	Acquired absence of other organs and tissue	Z90	Acquired absence of organs, not elsewhere classified
V89	Other suspected conditions not found	Z03	Encounter for medical observation for suspected diseases and conditions ruled out

Retained Foreign Body (V90)

V90	Retained foreign body	Z18	Retained foreign body fragments

Multiple Gestation Placenta Status (V91)

V91	Multiple gestation placenta status	O30	Multiple gestation

SUPPLEMENTARY CLASSIFICATION OF EXTERNAL CAUSES OF INJURY AND POISONING

External cause status (E000)

E000	External cause status	Y99	External cause status

Activity (E001-E030)

E001	Activities involving walking and running	Y93	Activity codes
E002	Activities involving water and water craft	Y93	Activity codes
E003	Activities involving snow and ice	Y93	Activity codes
E004	Activities involving climbing, rappelling and jumping off	Y93	Activity codes
E005	Activities involving dancing and other rhythmic movement	Y93	Activity codes
E006	Activities involving other sports and athletics played individually	Y93	Activity codes
E007	Activities involving other sports and athletics played as a group	Y93	Activity codes
E008	Activities involving other specified sports and athletics	Y93	Activity codes
E009	Activity involving other cardiorespiratory exercise	Y93	Activity codes
E010	Activity involving other muscle strengthening exercises	Y93	Activity codes
E011	Activities involving computer technology and electronic devices	Y93	Activity codes
E012	Activities involving arts and handcrafts	Y93	Activity codes
lpar E013	Activities involving personal hygiene and household maintenance	Y93	Activity codes
E014	Activities involving person providing caregiving	Y93	Activity codes
E015	Activities involving food preparation, cooking and grilling	Y93	Activity codes
E016	Activities involving property and land maintenance, building and construction	Y93	Activity codes
E017	Activities involving roller coasters and other types of external motion	Y93	Activity codes
E018	Activities involving playing musical instrument	Y93	Activity codes

ICD-9-CM Code and Description	ICD-10-CM Code and Description
E019 Activities involving animal care	Y93 Activity codes
E029 Other activity	Y93 Activity codes
E030 Unspecified activity	Y93 Activity codes

Railway accidents (E800-E807)

E800 Railway accident involving collision with rolling stock	V15 Pedal cycle rider injured in collision with railway train or railway vehicle
	V81 Occupant of railway train or railway vehicle injured in transport accident
E801 Railway accident involving collision with other object	V15 Pedal cycle rider injured in collision with railway train or railway vehicle
	V81 Occupant of railway train or railway vehicle injured in transport accident
	V82 Occupant of powered streetcar injured in transport accident
E802 Railway accident involving derailment without antecedent collision	V15 Pedal cycle rider injured in collision with railway train or railway vehicle
	V81 Occupant of railway train or railway vehicle injured in transport accident
E803 Railway accident involving explosion fire or burning	V15 Pedal cycle rider injured in collision with railway train or railway vehicle
	V81 Occupant of railway train or railway vehicle injured in transport accident
E804 Fall in on or from railway train	V15 Pedal cycle rider injured in collision with railway train or railway vehicle
	V81 Occupant of railway train or railway vehicle injured in transport accident
E805 Hit by rolling stock	V05 Pedestrian injured in collision with railway train or railway vehicle
	V15 Pedal cycle rider injured in collision with railway train or railway vehicle
	V81 Occupant of railway train or railway vehicle injured in transport accident
E806 Other specified railway accident	V15 Pedal cycle rider injured in collision with railway train or railway vehicle
	V81 Occupant of railway train or railway vehicle injured in transport accident
E807 Railway accident of unspecified nature	V05 Pedestrian injured in collision with railway train or railway vehicle
	V15 Pedal cycle rider injured in collision with railway train or railway vehicle
	V81 Occupant of railway train or railway vehicle injured in transport accident

Motor vehicle traffic accidents (E810-E819)

E810 Motor vehicle traffic accident involving collision with train	V05 Pedestrian injured in collision with railway train or railway vehicle
	V15 Pedal cycle rider injured in collision with railway train or railway vehicle
	V25 Motorcycle rider injured in collision with railway train or railway vehicle
	V45 Car occupant injured in collision with railway train or railway vehicle
	V80 Animal-rider or occupant of animal-drawn vehicle injured in transport accident
	V82 Occupant of powered streetcar injured in transport accident
E811 Motor vehicle traffic accident involving re-entrant collision with another motor vehicle	V03 Pedestrian injured in collision with car, pick-up truck or van

ICD-9-CM Code and Description		ICD-10-CM Code and Description	
		V13	Pedal cycle rider injured in collision with car, pick-up truck or van
		V29	Motorcycle rider injured in other and unspecified transport accidents
		V49	Car occupant injured in other and unspecified transport accidents
		V80	Animal-rider or occupant of animal-drawn vehicle injured in transport accident
		V82	Occupant of powered streetcar injured in transport accident
E812	Other motor vehicle traffic accident involving collision with motor vehicle	V03	Pedestrian injured in collision with car, pick-up truck or van
		V13	Pedal cycle rider injured in collision with car, pick-up truck or van
		V29	Motorcycle rider injured in other and unspecified transport accidents
		V43	Car occupant injured in collision with car, pick-up truck or van
		V49	Car occupant injured in other and unspecified transport accidents
		V80	Animal-rider or occupant of animal-drawn vehicle injured in transport accident
		V82	Occupant of powered streetcar injured in transport accident
		V87	Traffic accident of specified type but victim's mode of transport unknown
E813	Motor vehicle traffic accident involving collision with other vehicle	V03	Pedestrian injured in collision with car, pick-up truck or van
		V19	Pedal cycle rider injured in other and unspecified transport accidents
		V21	Motorcycle rider injured in collision with pedal cycle
		V26	Motorcycle rider injured in collision with other nonmotor vehicle
		V46	Car occupant injured in collision with other nonmotor vehicle
		V80	Animal-rider or occupant of animal-drawn vehicle injured in transport accident
		V82	Occupant of powered streetcar injured in transport accident
		V87	Traffic accident of specified type but victim's mode of transport unknown
E814	Motor vehicle traffic accident involving collision with pedestrian	V03	Pedestrian injured in collision with car, pick-up truck or van
		V13	Pedal cycle rider injured in collision with car, pick-up truck or van
		V20	Motorcycle rider injured in collision with pedestrian or animal
		V40	Car occupant injured in collision with pedestrian or animal
		V80	Animal-rider or occupant of animal-drawn vehicle injured in transport accident
		V82	Occupant of powered streetcar injured in transport accident
E815	Other motor vehicle traffic accident involving collision on the highway	V03	Pedestrian injured in collision with car, pick-up truck or van
		V13	Pedal cycle rider injured in collision with car, pick-up truck or van
		V27	Motorcycle rider injured in collision with fixed or stationary object

ICD-9-CM Code and Description	ICD-10-CM Code and Description
	V29 Motorcycle rider injured in other and unspecified transport accidents
	V80 Animal-rider or occupant of animal-drawn vehicle injured in transport accident
	V82 Occupant of powered streetcar injured in transport accident
	V86 Occupant of special all-terrain or other off-road motor vehicle, injured in transport accident
E816 Motor vehicle traffic accident due to loss of control without collision on the highway	V09 Pedestrian injured in other and unspecified transport accidents
	V19 Pedal cycle rider injured in other and unspecified transport accidents
	V28 Motorcycle rider injured in noncollision transport accident
	V48 Car occupant injured in noncollision transport accident
	V80 Animal-rider or occupant of animal-drawn vehicle injured in transport accident
	V82 Occupant of powered streetcar injured in transport accident
E817 Noncollision motor vehicle traffic accident while boarding or alighting	V09 Pedestrian injured in other and unspecified transport accidents
	V18 Pedal cycle rider injured in noncollision transport accident
	V28 Motorcycle rider injured in noncollision transport accident
	V48 Car occupant injured in noncollision transport accident
	V80 Animal-rider or occupant of animal-drawn vehicle injured in transport accident
	V82 Occupant of powered streetcar injured in transport accident
	V87 Traffic accident of specified type but victim's mode of transport unknown
E818 Other noncollision motor vehicle traffic accident	V09 Pedestrian injured in other and unspecified transport accidents
	V18 Pedal cycle rider injured in noncollision transport accident
	V28 Motorcycle rider injured in noncollision transport accident
	V48 Car occupant injured in noncollision transport accident
	V78 Bus occupant injured in noncollision transport accident
	V80 Animal-rider or occupant of animal-drawn vehicle injured in transport accident
	V82 Occupant of powered streetcar injured in transport accident
	V87 Traffic accident of specified type but victim's mode of transport unknown
E819 Motor vehicle traffic accident of unspecified nature	V09 Pedestrian injured in other and unspecified transport accidents
	V19 Pedal cycle rider injured in other and unspecified transport accidents
	V29 Motorcycle rider injured in other and unspecified transport accidents
	V49 Car occupant injured in other and unspecified transport accidents

ICD-9-CM Code and Description	ICD-10-CM Code and Description
	V59 Occupant of pick-up truck or van injured in other and unspecified transport accidents
	V69 Occupant of heavy transport vehicle injured in other and unspecified transport accidents
	V80 Animal-rider or occupant of animal-drawn vehicle injured in transport accident
	V82 Occupant of powered streetcar injured in transport accident
	V89 Motor- or nonmotor-vehicle accident, type of vehicle unspecified

Motor vehicle nontraffic accidents (E820-E825)

E820 Nontraffic accident involving motor-driven snow vehicle	V86 Occupant of special all-terrain or other off-road motor vehicle, injured in transport accident
	V86 Occupant of special all-terrain or other off-road motor vehicle, injured in transport accident
	V88 Nontraffic accident of specified type but victim's mode of transport unknown
E821 Nontraffic accident involving other off-road motor vehicle	V86 Occupant of special all-terrain or other off-road motor vehicle, injured in transport accident
	V88 Nontraffic accident of specified type but victim's mode of transport unknown
E822 Other motor vehicle nontraffic accident involving collision with moving object	V03 Pedestrian injured in collision with car, pick-up truck or van
	V19 Pedal cycle rider injured in other and unspecified transport accidents
	V20 Motorcycle rider injured in collision with pedestrian or animal
	V40 Car occupant injured in collision with pedestrian or animal
	V80 Animal-rider or occupant of animal-drawn vehicle injured in transport accident
E822 Other motor vehicle nontraffic accident involving collision with moving object	V82 Occupant of powered streetcar injured in transport accident
E823 Other motor vehicle nontraffic accident involving collision with stationary object	V09 Pedestrian injured in other and unspecified transport accidents
	V17 Pedal cycle rider injured in collision with fixed or stationary object
	V27 Motorcycle rider injured in collision with fixed or stationary object
	V47 Car occupant injured in collision with fixed or stationary object
	V57 Occupant of pick-up truck or van injured in collision with fixed or stationary object
	V80 Animal-rider or occupant of animal-drawn vehicle injured in transport accident
	V82 Occupant of powered streetcar injured in transport accident
E824 Other motor vehicle nontraffic accident while boarding and alighting	V09 Pedestrian injured in other and unspecified transport accidents
	V18 Pedal cycle rider injured in noncollision transport accident

ICD-9-CM Code and Description	ICD-10-CM Code and Description
	V23 Motorcycle rider injured in collision with car, pick-up truck or van
	V43 Car occupant injured in collision with car, pick-up truck or van
	V80 Animal-rider or occupant of animal-drawn vehicle injured in transport accident
	V82 Occupant of powered streetcar injured in transport accident
	V88 Nontraffic accident of specified type but victim's mode of transport unknown
E825 Other motor vehicle nontraffic accident of other and unspecified nature	V09 Pedestrian injured in other and unspecified transport accidents
	V19 Pedal cycle rider injured in other and unspecified transport accidents
	V28 Motorcycle rider injured in noncollision transport accident
	V29 Motorcycle rider injured in other and unspecified transport accidents
	V49 Car occupant injured in other and unspecified transport accidents
	V58 Occupant of pick-up truck or van injured in noncollision transport accident
	V80 Animal-rider or occupant of animal-drawn vehicle injured in transport accident
	V82 Occupant of powered streetcar injured in transport accident
	V89 Motor- or nonmotor-vehicle accident, type of vehicle unspecified

Other road vehicle accidents (E826-E829)

ICD-9-CM Code and Description	ICD-10-CM Code and Description
E826 Pedal cycle accident	V01 Pedestrian injured in collision with pedal cycle
	V10 Pedal cycle rider injured in collision with pedestrian or animal
	V18 Pedal cycle rider injured in noncollision transport accident
	V80 Animal-rider or occupant of animal-drawn vehicle injured in transport accident
	V80 Animal-rider or occupant of animal-drawn vehicle injured in transport accident
	V82 Occupant of powered streetcar injured in transport accident
E827 Animal-drawn vehicle accident	V09 Pedestrian injured in other and unspecified transport accidents
	V80 Animal-rider or occupant of animal-drawn vehicle injured in transport accident
	V82 Occupant of powered streetcar injured in transport accident
	V88 Nontraffic accident of specified type but victim's mode of transport unknown
E828 Accident involving animal being ridden	V09 Pedestrian injured in other and unspecified transport accidents
	V80 Animal-rider or occupant of animal-drawn vehicle injured in transport accident
	V82 Occupant of powered streetcar injured in transport accident
	V88 Nontraffic accident of specified type but victim's mode of transport unknown

ICD-9-CM Code and Description	ICD-10-CM Code and Description
E829 Other road vehicle accidents	V06 Pedestrian injured in collision with other nonmotor vehicle
	V82 Occupant of powered streetcar injured in transport accident
	V88 Nontraffic accident of specified type but victim's mode of transport unknown
	V89 Motor- or nonmotor-vehicle accident, type of vehicle unspecified

Water transport accidents (E830-E838)

E830 Accident to watercraft causing submersion	V90 Drowning and submersion due to accident to watercraft
E831 Accident to watercraft causing other injury	V91 Other injury due to accident to watercraft
E832 Other accidental submersion or drowning in water transport accident	V92 Drowning and submersion due to accident on board watercraft, without accident to watercraft
E833 Fall on stairs or ladders in water transport	V93 Other injury due to accident on board watercraft, without accident to watercraft
E834 Other fall from one level to another in water transport	V93 Other injury due to accident on board watercraft, without accident to watercraft
E835 Other and unspecified fall in water transport	V93 Other injury due to accident on board watercraft, without accident to watercraft
E836 Machinery accident in water transport	V93 Other injury due to accident on board watercraft, without accident to watercraft
E837 Explosion fire or burning in watercraft	V93 Other injury due to accident on board watercraft, without accident to watercraft
E838 Other and unspecified water transport accident	V94 Other and unspecified water transport accidents

Air and space transport accidents (E840-E845)

E840 Accident to powered aircraft at takeoff or landing	V95 Accident to powered aircraft causing injury to occupant
	V97 Other specified air transport accidents
E841 Accident to powered aircraft other and unspecified	V95 Accident to powered aircraft causing injury to occupant
	V97 Other specified air transport accidents
E842 Accident to unpowered aircraft	V96 Accident to nonpowered aircraft causing injury to occupant
E842 Accident to unpowered aircraft	V97 Other specified air transport accidents
E843 Fall in on or from aircraft	V97 Other specified air transport accidents
E844 Other specified air transport accidents	V97 Other specified air transport accidents
E845 Accident involving spacecraft	V83 Occupant of special vehicle mainly used on industrial premises injured in transport accident
	V95 Accident to powered aircraft causing injury to occupant
	V95 Accident to powered aircraft causing injury to occupant
	V97 Other specified air transport accidents

Vehicle accidents, not elsewhere classifiable (E846-E849)

E847 Accidents involving cable cars not running on rails	V98 Other specified transport accidents
E848 Accidents involving other vehicles not elsewhere classifiable	V98 Other specified transport accidents
E849 Place of occurrence	Y92 Place of occurrence of the external cause

ICD-9-CM Code and Description	ICD-10-CM Code and Description

Accidental poisoning by drugs, medicinal substances, and biologicals (E850-E858)

E850	Accidental poisoning by analgesics, antipyretics, and antirheumatics	—	No ICD-10 equivalent
E851	Accidental poisoning by barbiturates	—	No ICD-10 equivalent
E852	Accidental poisoning by other sedatives and hypnotics	—	No ICD-10 equivalent
E853	Accidental poisoning by tranquilizers	—	No ICD-10 equivalent
E854	Accidental poisoning by other psychotropic agents	—	No ICD-10 equivalent
E855	Accidental poisoning by other drugs acting on central and autonomic nervous systems	—	No ICD-10 equivalent
E856	Accidental poisoning by antibiotics	—	No ICD-10 equivalent
E857	Accidental poisoning by other anti-infectives	—	No ICD-10 equivalent
E858	Accidental poisoning by other drugs	—	No ICD-10 equivalent

Accidental poisoning by other solid and liquid substances, gases, and vapors (E860-E869)

E860	Accidental poisoning by alcohol, not elsewhere classified	—	No ICD-10 equivalent
E861	Accidental poisoning by cleansing and polishing agents, disinfectants, paints, and Varnishes	—	No ICD-10 equivalent
E862	Accidental poisoning by petroleum products, other solvents and their vapors, not elsewhere classified	—	No ICD-10 equivalent
E863	Accidental poisoning by agricultural and horticultural chemical and pharmaceutical preparations other than plant foods and fertilizers	—	No ICD-10 equivalent
E864	Accidental poisoning by corrosives and caustics, not elsewhere classified	—	No ICD-10 equivalent
E865	Accidental poisoning from poisonous foodstuffs and poisonous plants	—	No ICD-10 equivalent
E866	Accidental poisoning by other and unspecified solid and liquid substances	—	No ICD-10 equivalent
E867	Accidental poisoning by gas distributed by pipeline	—	No ICD-10 equivalent
E868	Accidental poisoning by other utility gas and other carbon monoxide	—	No ICD-10 equivalent
E869	Accidental poisoning by other gases and vapors	—	No ICD-10 equivalent

Misadventures to patients during surgical and medical care (E870-E876)

E870	Accidental cut, puncture, perforation, or hemorrhage during medical care	—	No ICD-10 equivalent
E871	Foreign object left in body during procedure	—	No ICD-10 equivalent
E872	Failure of sterile precautions during procedure	Y62	Failure of sterile precautions during surgical and medical care

ICD-9-CM Code and Description		ICD-10-CM Code and Description	
E873	Failure in dosage	Y63	Failure in dosage during surgical and medical care
E874	Mechanical failure of instrument or apparatus during procedure	Y65	Other misadventures during surgical and medical care
E875	Contaminated or infected blood other fluid drug or biological substance	Y64	Contaminated medical or biological substances
E876	Other and unspecified misadventures during medical care	Y65	Other misadventures during surgical and medical care
		Y69	Unspecified misadventure during surgical and medical care

Surgical and medical procedures as the cause of abnormal reaction of patient or later complication, without mention of misadventure at the time of procedure (E878-E879)

E878	Surgical operation and other surgical procedures as the cause of abnormal reaction of patient or of later complication without mention of misadventure at the time of operation	Y83	Surgical operation and other surgical procedures as the cause of abnormal reaction of the patient, or of later
E879	Other procedures without mention of misadventure at the time of procedure as the cause of abnormal reaction of patient or of later complication	Y84	Other medical procedures as the cause of abnormal reaction of the patient, or of later complication, without

Accidental falls (E880-E888)

E880	Accidental fall on or from stairs or steps	W10	Fall on and from stairs and steps
E880	Accidental fall on or from stairs or steps	W10	Fall on and from stairs and steps
		W11	Fall on and from ladder
		W12	Fall on and from scaffolding
E881	Accidental fall on or from ladders or scaffolding	W16	Fall, jump or diving into water
E882	Accidental fall from or out of building or other structure	W13	Fall from, out of or through building or structure
		W16	Fall, jump or diving into water
		W17	Other fall from one level to another
E883	Accidental fall into hole or other opening in surface	W17	Other fall from one level to another
E884	Other accidental falls from one level to another	W05	Fall from non-moving wheelchair, nonmotorized scooter and motorized mobility scooter
		W06	Fall from bed
		W07	Fall from chair
		W08	Fall from other furniture
		W09	Fall on and from playground equipment
		W14	Fall from tree
		W15	Fall from cliff
		W17	Other fall from one level to another
		W18	Other slipping, tripping and stumbling and falls
E885	Accidental fall on same level from slipping tripping or stumbling	V00	Pedestrian conveyance accident
		W18	Other slipping, tripping and stumbling and falls

ICD-9-CM Code and Description		ICD-10-CM Code and Description	
E886	Accidental fall on same level from collision pushing or shoving by or with other person	V00	Pedestrian conveyance accident
		W03	Other fall on same level due to collision with another person
E887	Fracture cause unspecified	W19	Unspecified fall
E888	Other and unspecified fall	W01	Fall on same level from slipping, tripping and stumbling
		W18	Other slipping, tripping and stumbling and falls
		W19	Unspecified fall

Accidents caused by fire and flames (E890-E899)

E890	Conflagration in private dwelling	X00	Exposure to uncontrolled fire in building or structure
		X08	Exposure to other specified smoke, fire and flames
E891	Conflagration in other and unspecified building or structure	X00	Exposure to uncontrolled fire in building or structure
		X08	Exposure to other specified smoke, fire and flames
E892	Conflagration not in building or structure	X01	Exposure to uncontrolled fire, not in building or structure
E893	Accident caused by ignition of clothing	X02	Exposure to controlled fire in building or structure
		X03	Exposure to controlled fire, not in building or structure
		X05	Exposure to ignition or melting of nightwear
		X06	Exposure to ignition or melting of other clothing and apparel
		X08	Exposure to other specified smoke, fire and flames
E894	Ignition of highly inflammable material	X04	Exposure to ignition of highly flammable material
E895	Accident caused by controlled fire in private dwelling	X02	Exposure to controlled fire in building or structure
E896	Accident caused by controlled fire in other and unspecified building or structure	X02	Exposure to controlled fire in building or structure
E897	Accident caused by controlled fire not in building or structure	X03	Exposure to controlled fire, not in building or structure
E898	Accident caused by other specified fire and flames	X08	Exposure to other specified smoke, fire and flames
		X08	Exposure to other specified smoke, fire and flames
E899	Accident caused by unspecified fire	X08	Exposure to other specified smoke, fire and flames

Accidents due to natural and environmental factors (E900-E909)

E900	Accident caused by excessive heat	W92	Exposure to excessive heat of man-made origin
		X30	Exposure to excessive natural heat
E901	Accidents due to excessive cold	W93	Exposure to excessive cold of man-made origin
		X31	Exposure to excessive natural cold
E902	Accident due to high and low air pressure and changes in air pressure	W94	Exposure to high and low air pressure and changes in air pressure
		W99	Exposure to other man-made environmental factors

ICD-9-CM Code and Description		ICD-10-CM Code and Description	
E903	Accident due to travel and motion	—	No ICD-10 equivalent
E904	Accident due to hunger, thirst, exposure, and neglect	—	No ICD-10 equivalent
E905	Accident due to venomous animals and plants as the cause of poisoning and toxic reactions	—	No ICD-10 equivalent
E906	Other injury caused by animals	W53	Contact with rodent
		W54	Contact with dog
		W55	Contact with other mammals
		W57	Bitten or stung by nonvenomous insect and other nonvenomous arthropods
		W59	Contact with other nonvenomous reptiles
		W64	Exposure to other animate mechanical forces
E907	Accident due to lightning	X39	Exposure to other forces of nature
E908	Accident due to cataclysmic storms and floods resulting from storms	X37	Cataclysmic storm
		X38	Flood
E909	Accident due to cataclysmic earth surface movements and eruptions	X34	Earthquake
		X35	Volcanic eruption
		X36	Avalanche, landslide and other earth movements
		X37	Cataclysmic storm
		X39	Exposure to other forces of nature

Accidents caused by submersion, suffocation, and foreign bodies (E910-E915)

E910	Accidental drowning and submersion	W65	Accidental drowning and submersion while in bath-tub
		W67	Accidental drowning and submersion while in swimming-pool
		W69	Accidental drowning and submersion while in natural water
		W74	Unspecified cause of accidental drowning and submersion
E911	Inhalation and ingestion of food causing obstruction of respiratory tract or suffocation	—	No ICD-10 equivalent
E912	Inhalation and ingestion of other object causing obstruction of respiratory tract or suffocation	—	No ICD-10 equivalent
E913	Accidental mechanical suffocation	—	No ICD-10 equivalent
E914	Foreign body accidentally entering eye and adnexa	—	No ICD-10 equivalent
E915	Foreign body accidentally entering other orifice	—	No ICD-10 equivalent

Other accidents (E916-E928)

E916	Struck accidentally by falling object	W20	Struck by thrown, projected or falling object
E917	Striking against or struck accidentally by objects or persons	W18	Other slipping, tripping and stumbling and falls
		W18	Other slipping, tripping and stumbling and falls
		W20	Struck by thrown, projected or falling object

ICD-9-CM Code and Description	ICD-10-CM Code and Description
	W21 Striking against or struck by sports equipment
	W22 Striking against or struck by other objects
	W50 Accidental hit, strike, kick, twist, bite or scratch by another person
	W51 Accidental striking against or bumped into by another person
	W52 Crushed, pushed or stepped on by crowd or human stampede
E918 Caught accidentally in or between objects	W23 Caught, crushed, jammed or pinched in or between objects
E919 Accidents caused by machinery	W24 Contact with lifting and transmission devices, not elsewhere classified
	W24 Contact with lifting and transmission devices, not elsewhere classified
	W30 Contact with agricultural machinery
	W31 Contact with other and unspecified machinery
E920 Accidents caused by cutting and piercing instruments or objects	W26 Contact with knife, sword or dagger
	W27 Contact with nonpowered hand tool
	W28 Contact with powered lawn mower
	W29 Contact with other powered hand tools and household machinery
	W45 Foreign body or object entering through skin
	W46 Contact with hypodermic needle
E921 Accident caused by explosion of pressure vessel	W35 Explosion and rupture of boiler
	W36 Explosion and rupture of gas cylinder
	W38 Explosion and rupture of other specified pressurized devices
E922 Accident caused by firearm and air gun missile	W32 Accidental handgun discharge and malfunction
	W33 Accidental rifle, shotgun and larger firearm discharge and malfunction
	W34 Accidental discharge and malfunction from other and unspecified firearms and guns
E923 Accident caused by explosive material	W39 Discharge of firework
	W40 Explosion of other materials
E924 Accident caused by hot substance or object caustic or corrosive material and steam	X11 Contact with hot tap-water
	X12 Contact with other hot fluids
	X19 Contact with other heat and hot substances
E925 Accident caused by electric current	W85 Exposure to electric transmission lines
	W86 Exposure to other specified electric current
E926 Exposure to radiation	W88 Exposure to ionizing radiation
	W89 Exposure to man-made visible and ultraviolet light
	W90 Exposure to other nonionizing radiation
E927 Overexertion and strenuous and repetitive movements or loads	—— No ICD-10 equivalent
E928 Other and unspecified environmental and accidental causes	W42 Exposure to noise

ICD-9-CM Code and Description

ICD-10-CM Code and Description

W49	Exposure to other inanimate mechanical forces
W50	Accidental hit, strike, kick, twist, bite or scratch by another person
X52	Prolonged stay in weightless environment
X58	Exposure to other specified factors

Late effects of accidental injury (E929)

E929 Late effects of accidental injury	

V87	Traffic accident of specified type but victim's mode of transport unknown
V88	Nontraffic accident of specified type but victim's mode of transport unknown
V89	Motor- or nonmotor-vehicle accident, type of vehicle unspecified
V97	Other specified air transport accidents
V98	Other specified transport accidents
V99	Unspecified transport accident
W17	Other fall from one level to another
W18	Other slipping, tripping and stumbling and falls
W19	Unspecified fall
W92	Exposure to excessive heat of man-made origin
W99	Exposure to other man-made environmental factors
X39	Exposure to other forces of nature
X58	Exposure to other specified factors
Y33	Other specified events, undetermined intent

Drugs, medicinal and biological substances causing adverse effects in therapeutic use (E930-E949)

E930	Antibiotics	—	No ICD-10 equivalent
E931	Other anti-infectives	—	No ICD-10 equivalent
E932	Hormones and synthetic substitutes	—	No ICD-10 equivalent
E933	Primarily systemic agents	—	No ICD-10 equivalent
E934	Agents primarily affecting blood constituents	—	No ICD-10 equivalent
E935	Analgesics, antipyretics, and antirheumatics	—	No ICD-10 equivalent
E936	Anticonvulsants and anti-Parkinsonism drugs	—	No ICD-10 equivalent
E937	Sedatives and hypnotics	—	No ICD-10 equivalent
E938	Other central nervous system depressants and anesthetics	—	No ICD-10 equivalent
E939	Psychotropic agents	—	No ICD-10 equivalent
E940	Central nervous system stimulants	—	No ICD-10 equivalent
E941	Drugs primarily affecting the autonomic nervous system	—	No ICD-10 equivalent

ICD-9-CM Code and Description	ICD-10-CM Code and Description
E942 Agents primarily affecting the cardiovascular system	— No ICD-10 equivalent
E943 Agents primarily affecting gastrointestinal system	— No ICD-10 equivalent
E944 Water, mineral, and uric acid metabolism drugs	— No ICD-10 equivalent
E945 Agents primarily acting on the smooth and skeletal muscles and respiratory system	— No ICD-10 equivalent
lpha E946 Agents primarily affecting skin and mucous membrane, ophthalmological, otorhinolaryngological, and dental drugs	— No ICD-10 equivalent
E947 Other and unspecified drugs and medicinal substances	— No ICD-10 equivalent
E948 Bacterial vaccines	— No ICD-10 equivalent
E949 Other vaccines and biological substances	— No ICD-10 equivalent

Suicide and self-inflicted injury (E950-E959)

E950 Suicide and self-inflicted poisoning by solid or liquid substances	— No ICD-10 equivalent
E951 Suicide and self-inflicted poisoning by gases in domestic use	— No ICD-10 equivalent
E952 Suicide and self-inflicted poisoning by other gases and vapors	— No ICD-10 equivalent
E953 Suicide and self-inflicted injury by hanging, strangulation, and suffocation	— No ICD-10 equivalent
E954 Suicide and self-inflicted injury by submersion (drowning)	X71 Intentional self-harm by drowning and submersion
E955 Suicide and self-inflicted injury by firearms air guns and explosives	X72 Intentional self-harm by handgun discharge
	X73 Intentional self-harm by rifle, shotgun and larger firearm discharge
	X74 Intentional self-harm by other and unspecified firearm and gun discharge
	X75 Intentional self-harm by explosive material
E956 Suicide and self-inflicted injury by cutting and piercing instrument	X78 Intentional self-harm by sharp object
E957 Suicide and self-inflicted injuries by jumping from high place	X80 Intentional self-harm by jumping from a high place
	Y92 Place of occurrence of the external cause
E958 Suicide and self-inflicted injury by other and unspecified means	X76 Intentional self-harm by smoke, fire and flames
	X77 Intentional self-harm by steam, hot vapors and hot objects
	X81 Intentional self-harm by jumping or lying in front of moving object
	X82 Intentional self-harm by crashing of motor vehicle
	X83 Intentional self-harm by other specified means
E959 Late effects of self-inflicted injury	X71 Intentional self-harm by drowning and submersion

ICD-9-CM Code and Description		ICD-10-CM Code and Description	
		X72	Intentional self-harm by handgun discharge
		X73	Intentional self-harm by rifle, shotgun and larger firearm discharge
		X74	Intentional self-harm by other and unspecified firearm and gun discharge
		X75	Intentional self-harm by explosive material
		X76	Intentional self-harm by smoke, fire and flames
		X77	Intentional self-harm by steam, hot vapors and hot objects
		X78	Intentional self-harm by sharp object
		X81	Intentional self-harm by jumping or lying in front of moving object
		X82	Intentional self-harm by crashing of motor vehicle
		X83	Intentional self-harm by other specified means

Homicide and injury purposely inflicted by other persons (E960-E969)

E960	Fight brawl rape	Y04	Assault by bodily force
E961	Assault by corrosive or caustic substance, except poisoning	—	No ICD-10 equivalent
E962	Assault by poisoning	—	No ICD-10 equivalent
E963	Assault by hanging and strangulation	—	No ICD-10 equivalent
E964	Assault by submersion (drowning)	X92	Assault by drowning and submersion
E965	Assault by firearms and explosives	X93	Assault by handgun discharge
		X94	Assault by rifle, shotgun and larger firearm discharge
		X95	Assault by other and unspecified firearm and gun discharge
		X96	Assault by explosive material
E966	Assault by cutting and piercing instrument	X99	Assault by sharp object
E967	Perpetrator of child and adult abuse	Y07	Perpetrator of assault, maltreatment and neglect
E968	Assault by other and unspecified means	X95	Assault by other and unspecified firearm and gun discharge
		X97	Assault by smoke, fire and flames
		X98	Assault by steam, hot vapors and hot objects
		Y00	Assault by blunt object
		Y01	Assault by pushing from high place
		Y03	Assault by crashing of motor vehicle
		Y04	Assault by bodily force
		Y07	Perpetrator of assault, maltreatment and neglect
		Y08	Assault by other specified means
E969	Late effects of injury purposely inflicted by other person	X92	Assault by drowning and submersion
		X95	Assault by other and unspecified firearm and gun discharge
		X96	Assault by explosive material
		X98	Assault by steam, hot vapors and hot objects
		X99	Assault by sharp object
		Y00	Assault by blunt object

ICD-9-CM Code and Description	ICD-10-CM Code and Description
	Y01 Assault by pushing from high place
	Y03 Assault by crashing of motor vehicle
	Y04 Assault by bodily force
	Y08 Assault by other specified means

Legal intervention (E970-E978)

E970 Injury due to legal intervention by firearms	Y35 Legal intervention
E971 Injury due to legal intervention by explosives	Y35 Legal intervention
E972 Injury due to legal intervention by gas	Y35 Legal intervention
E973 Injury due to legal intervention by blunt object	Y35 Legal intervention
E974 Injury due to legal intervention by cutting and piercing instruments	Y35 Legal intervention
E975 Injury due to legal intervention by other specified means	Y35 Legal intervention
E976 Injury due to legal intervention by unspecified means	Y35 Legal intervention
E977 Late effects of injuries due to legal intervention	Y35 Legal intervention
E978 Legal execution	— No ICD-10 equivalent
E979 Terrorism	Y38 Terrorism

Injury undetermined whether accidentally or purposely inflicted (E980-E989)

E980 Poisoning by solid or liquid substances, undetermined whether accidentally or purposely inflicted	— No ICD-10 equivalent
E981 Poisoning by gases in domestic use, undetermined whether accidentally or purposely inflicted	— No ICD-10 equivalent
E982 Poisoning by other gases, undetermined whether accidentally or purposely inflicted	— No ICD-10 equivalent
E983 Hanging, strangulation, or suffocation, undetermined whether accidentally or purposely inflicted	— No ICD-10 equivalent
E984 Submersion [drowning], undetermined whether accidentally or purposely inflicted	— No ICD-10 equivalent
E985 Injury by firearms air guns and explosives undetermined whether accidentally or purposely inflicted	Y22 Handgun discharge, undetermined intent
	Y23 Rifle, shotgun and larger firearm discharge, undetermined intent
	Y24 Other and unspecified firearm discharge, undetermined intent
	Y25 Contact with explosive material, undetermined intent
E986 Injury by cutting and piercing instruments undetermined whether accidentally or purposely inflicted	Y28 Contact with sharp object, undetermined intent

ICD-9-CM Code and Description	ICD-10-CM Code and Description
E987 Falling from high place undetermined whether accidentally or purposely inflicted	Y30 Falling, jumping or pushed from a high place, undetermined intent
E988 Injury by other and unspecified means undetermined whether accidentally or purposely inflicted	Y26 Exposure to smoke, fire and flames, undetermined intent
	Y27 Contact with steam, hot vapors and hot objects, undetermined intent
	Y31 Falling, lying or running before or into moving object, undetermined intent
	Y32 Crashing of motor vehicle, undetermined intent
	Y33 Other specified events, undetermined intent

Injury resulting from operations of war (E990-E999)

E990	Injury due to war operations by fires and conflagrations	Y36	Operations of war
E991	Injury due to war operations by bullets and fragments	Y36	Operations of war
E992	Injury due to war operations by explosion of marine weapons	Y36	Operations of war
E993	Injury due to war operations by other explosion	Y36	Operations of war
E994	Injury due to war operations by destruction of aircraft	Y36	Operations of war
E995	Injury due to war operations by other and unspecified forms of conventional warfare	Y36	Operations of war
E996	Injury due to war operations by nuclear weapons	Y36	Operations of war
E997	Injury due to war operations by other forms of unconventional warfare	Y36	Operations of war
E998	Injury due to war operations but occurring after cessation of hostilities	Y36	Operations of war
E999	Late effect of injury due to war operations and terrorism	Y36	Operations of war

DISEASES: ALPHABETIC INDEX

VOLUME 2

A

AAT (alpha-1 antitrypsin) deficiency 273.4
AAV (disease) (illness) (infection)—*see* Human
   immunodeficiency virus (disease) (illness)
   (infection)
Abactio —*see* Abortion, induced
Abactus venter —*see* Abortion, induced
Abarognosis 781.99
Abasia (-astasia) 307.9
   atactica 781.3
   choreic 781.3
   hysterical 300.11
   paroxysmal trepidant 781.3
   spastic 781.3
   trembling 781.3
   trepidans 781.3
Abderhalden-Kaufmann-Lignac syndrome
   (cystinosis) 270.0
Abdomen, abdominal —*see also* condition
   accordion 306.4
   acute 789.0
   angina 557.1
   burst 868.00
   convulsive equivalent (*see also* Epilepsy) 345.5
   heart 746.87
   muscle deficiency syndrome 756.79
   obstipum 756.79
Abdominalgia 789.0
   periodic 277.31
Abduction contracture, hip or other joint —*see*
   Contraction, joint
Abercrombie's syndrome (amyloid
   degeneration) 277.39
Aberrant (congenital)—*see also* Malposition,
   congenital
   adrenal gland 759.1
   blood vessel NEC 747.60
      arteriovenous NEC 747.60
      cerebrovascular 747.81
      gastrointestinal 747.61
      lower limb 747.64
      renal 747.62
      spinal 747.82
      upper limb 747.63
   breast 757.6
   endocrine gland NEC 759.2
   gastrointestinal vessel (peripheral) 747.61
   hepatic duct 751.69
   lower limb vessel (peripheral) 747.64
   pancreas 751.7
   parathyroid gland 759.2
   peripheral vascular vessel NEC 747.60
   pituitary gland (pharyngeal) 759.2
   renal blood vessel 747.62
   sebaceous glands, mucous membrane, mouth
      750.26
   spinal vessel 747.82
   spleen 759.0
   testis (descent) 752.51
   thymus gland 759.2
   thyroid gland 759.2
   upper limb vessel (peripheral) 747.63
Aberratio
   lactis 757.6
   testis 752.51
Aberration —*see also* Anomaly
   chromosome—*see* Anomaly, chromosome(s)
   distantial 368.9

Aberration—*continued*
   mental (*see also* Disorder, mental,
      nonpsychotic) 300.9
Abetalipoproteinemia 272.5
Abionarce 780.79
Abiotrophy 799.89
Ablatio
   placentae—*see* Placenta, ablatio
   retinae (*see also* Detachment, retina) 361.9
Ablation
   pituitary (gland) (with hypofunction) 253.7
   placenta—*see* Placenta, ablatio
   uterus 621.8
Ablepharia, ablepharon, ablephary 743.62
Ablepsia —*see* Blindness
Ablepsy —*see* Blindness
Ablutomania 300.3
Abnormal, abnormality, abnormalities —*see*
   also Anomaly
   acid-base balance 276.4
      fetus or newborn—*see* Distress, fetal
   adaptation curve, dark 368.63
   alveolar ridge 525.9
   amnion 658.9
      affecting fetus or newborn 762.9
   anatomical relationship NEC 759.9
   apertures, congenital, diaphragm 756.6
   auditory perception NEC 388.40
   autosomes NEC 758.5
      13 758.1
      18 758.2
      21 or 22 758.0
      D₁ 758.1
      E₃ 758.2
      G 758.0
   ballistocardiogram 794.39
   basal metabolic rate (BMR) 794.7
   biosynthesis, testicular androgen 257.2
   blood level (of)
      cobalt 790.6
      copper 790.6
      iron 790.6
      lead 790.6
      lithium 790.6
      magnesium 790.6
      mineral 790.6
      zinc 790.6
   blood pressure
      elevated (without diagnosis of hypertension)
         796.2
      low (*see also* Hypotension) 458.9
         reading (incidental) (isolated) (nonspecific)
            796.3
   blood sugar 790.29
   bowel sounds 787.5
   breathing behavior—*see* Respiration
   caloric test 794.19
   cervix (acquired) NEC 622.9
      congenital 752.40
      in pregnancy or childbirth 654.6
         causing obstructed labor 660.2
            affecting fetus or newborn 763.1
   chemistry, blood NEC 790.6
   chest sounds 786.7
   chorion 658.9
      affecting fetus or newborn 762.9
   chromosomal NEC 758.89

Abnormal, abnormality—*continued*
  analysis, nonspecific result 795.2
  autosomes (*see also* Abnormal, autosomes
    NEC) 758.5
  fetal, (suspected) affecting management of
    pregnancy 655.1
    sex 758.81
  clinical findings NEC 796.4
  communication—*see* Fistula
  configuration of pupils 379.49
  coronary
    artery 746.85
    vein 746.9
  cortisol-binding globulin 255.8
  course, Eustachian tube 744.24
  creatinine clearance 794.4
  dentofacial NEC 524.9
    functional 524.50
    specified type NEC 524.89
  development, developmental NEC 759.9
    bone 756.9
    central nervous system 742.9
  direction, teeth 524.30
  Dynia (*see also* Defect, coagulation) 286.9
  Ebstein 746.2
  echocardiogram 793.2
  echoencephalogram 794.01
  echogram NEC—*see* Findings, abnormal,
    structure
  electrocardiogram (ECG) (EKG) 794.31
  electroencephalogram (EEG) 794.02
  electromyogram (EMG) 794.17
    ocular 794.14
  electro-oculogram (EOG) 794.12
  electroretinogram (ERG) 794.11
  erythrocytes 289.9
    congenital, with perinatal jaundice 282.9
     [774.0]
  Eustachian valve 746.9
  excitability under minor stress 301.9
  fat distribution 782.9
  feces 787.7
  fetal heart rate—*see* Distress, fetal
  fetus NEC
    affecting management of pregnancy—*see*
     Pregnancy, management affected by, fetal
    causing disproportion 653.7
     affecting fetus or newborn 763.1
     causing obstructed labor 660.1
      affecting fetus or newborn 763.1
  findings without manifest disease—*see*
    Findings, abnormal
  fluid
    amniotic 792.3
    cerebrospinal 792.0
    peritoneal 792.9
    pleural 792.9
    synovial 792.9
    vaginal 792.9
  forces of labor NEC 661.9
    affecting fetus or newborn 763.7
  form, teeth 520.2
  function studies
    auditory 794.15
    bladder 794.9
    brain 794.00
    cardiovascular 794.30
    endocrine NEC 794.6
    kidney 794.4
    liver 794.8
    nervous system
     central 794.00

Abnormal, abnormality—*continued*
    peripheral 794.19
    oculomotor 794.14
    pancreas 794.9
    placenta 794.9
    pulmonary 794.2
    retina 794.11
    special senses 794.19
    spleen 794.9
    thyroid 794.5
    vestibular 794.16
  gait 781.2
    hysterical 300.11
  gastrin secretion 251.5
  globulin
    cortisol-binding 255.8
    thyroid-binding 246.8
  glucagon secretion 251.4
  glucose 790.29
    in pregnancy, childbirth, or puerperium 648.8
     fetus or newborn 775.0
    non-fasting 790.29
  gravitational (G) forces or states 994.9
  hair NEC 704.2
  hard tissue formation in pulp 522.3
  head movement 781.0
  heart
    rate
     fetus, affecting liveborn infant
      before the onset of labor 763.81
      during labor 763.82
      unspecified as to time of onset 763.83
     intrauterine
      before the onset of labor 763.81
      during labor 763.82
      unspecified as to time of onset 763.83
     newborn
      before the onset of labor 763.81
      during labor 763.82
      unspecified as to time of onset 763.83
    shadow 793.2
    sounds NEC 785.3
  hemoglobin (*see also* Disease, hemoglobin)
    282.7
    trait—*see* Trait, hemoglobin, abnormal
  hemorrhage, uterus—*see* Hemorrhage, uterus
  histology NEC 795.4
  increase in
    appetite 783.6
    development 783.9
  involuntary movement 781.0
  jaw closure 524.51
  karyotype 795.2
  knee jerk 796.1
  labor NEC 661.9
    affecting fetus or newborn 763.7
  laboratory findings—*see* Findings, abnormal
  length, organ or site, congenital—*see* Distortion
  liver function test 790.6
  loss of height 781.91
  loss of weight 783.21
  lung shadow 793.19
  mammogram 793.80
    calcification 793.89
    calculus 793.89
    microcalcification 793.81
  Mantoux test 795.51
  membranes (fetal)
    affecting fetus or newborn 762.9
    complicating pregnancy 658.8
  menstruation—*see* Menstruation

Abnormal, abnormality —*continued*
metabolism (*see also* condition) 783.9
movement 781.0
  disorder, NEC 333.90
    sleep related, unspecified 780.58
    specified, NEC 333.99
  head 781.0
  involuntary 781.0
  specified type NEC 333.99
muscle contraction, localized 728.85
myoglobin (Aberdeen) (Annapolis) 289.9
narrowness, eyelid 743.62
optokinetic response 379.57
organs or tissues of pelvis NEC
  in pregnancy or childbirth 654.9
    affecting fetus or newborn 763.89
    causing obstructed labor 660.2
      affecting fetus or newborn 763.1
origin—*see* Malposition, congenital
palmar creases 757.2
Papanicolaou (smear)
  anus 796.70
    with
      atypical squamous cells
        cannot exclude high grade squamous
          intraepithelial lesion (ASC-H)
          796.72
        of undetermined significance (ASC-US)
          796.71
      cytologic evidence of malignancy 796.76
      high grade squamous intraepithelial lesion
        (HGSIL) 796.74
      low grade squamous intraepithelial lesion
        (LGSIL) 796.73
    glandular 796.70
    specified finding NEC 796.79
  cervix 795.00
    with
      atypical squamous cell
        cannot exclude high grade squamous
          intraepithelial lesion (ASC-H)
          795.02
        of undetermined significance (ASC-US)
          795.01
      cytologic evidence of malignancy 795.06
      favor benign (ASCUS favor benign)
        795.01
      favor dysplasia (ASCUS favor dysplasia)
        795.02
      high grade squamous intraepithelial lesion
        (HGSIL) 795.04
      low grade squamous intraepithelial lesion
        (LGSIL) 795.03
    nonspecific finding NEC 795.09
  other site 796.9
  vagina 795.10
    with
      atypical squamous cells
        cannot exclude high grade squamous
          intraepithelial lesion (ASC-H)
          795.12
        of undetermined significance (ASC-US)
          795.11
      cytologic evidence of malignancy 795.16
      high grade squamous intraepithelial lesion
        (HGSIL) 795.14
      low grade squamous intraepithelial lesion
        (LGSIL) 795.13
    glandular 795.10
    specified finding NEC 795.19

Abnormal, abnormality —*continued*
parturition
  affecting fetus or newborn 763.9
  mother—*see* Delivery, complicated
pelvis (bony)—*see* Deformity, pelvis
percussion, chest 786.7
periods (grossly) (*see also* Menstruation) 626.9
phonocardiogram 794.39
placenta—*see* Placenta, abnormal
plantar reflex 796.1
plasma protein—*see* Deficiency, plasma, protein
pleural folds 748.8
position—*see also* Malposition
  gravid uterus 654.4
    causing obstructed labor 660.2
      affecting fetus or newborn 763.1
posture NEC 781.92
presentation (fetus)—*see* Presentation, fetus,
  abnormal
product of conception NEC 631.8
puberty—*see* Puberty
pulmonary
  artery 747.39
  function, newborn 770.89
  test results 794.2
  ventilation, newborn 770.89
    hyperventilation 786.01
pulsations in neck 785.1
pupil reflexes 379.40
quality of milk 676.8
radiological examination 793.99
  abdomen NEC 793.6
  biliary tract 793.3
  breast 793.89
    mammogram NOS 793.80
    mammographic
      calcification 793.89
      calculus 793.89
      microcalcification 793.81
  gastrointestinal tract 793.4
  genitourinary organs 793.5
  head 793.0
  image test inconclusive due to excess body fat
    793.91
  intrathoracic organ NEC 793.2
  lung (field) 793.19
  musculoskeletal system 793.7
  retroperitoneum 793.6
  skin and subcutaneous tissue 793.99
  skull 793.0
red blood cells 790.09
  morphology 790.09
  volume 790.09
reflex NEC 796.1
renal function test 794.4
respiration signs—*see* Respiration
response to nerve stimulation 794.10
retinal correspondence 368.34
rhythm, heart—*see also* Arrhythmia fetus—*see*
  Distress, fetal
saliva 792.4
scan
  brain 794.09
  kidney 794.4
  liver 794.8
  lung 794.2
  thyroid 794.5
secretion
  gastrin 251.5
  glucagon 251.4
semen 792.2

Abnormal, abnormality —*continued*
serum level (of)
    acid phosphatase 790.5
    alkaline phosphatase 790.5
    amylase 790.5
    enzymes NEC 790.5
    lipase 790.5
shape
    cornea 743.41
    gallbladder 751.69
    gravid uterus 654.4
        affecting fetus or newborn 763.89
        causing obstructed labor 660.2
            affecting fetus or newborn 763.1
    head (*see also* Anomaly, skull) 756.0
    organ or site, congenital NEC—*see* Distortion
    sinus venosus 747.40
size
    fetus, complicating delivery 653.5
        causing obstructed labor 660.1
    gallbladder 751.69
    head (*see also* Anomaly, skull) 756.0
    organ or site, congenital NEC—*see* Distortion
    teeth 520.2
skin and appendages, congenital NEC 757.9
soft parts of pelvis—*see* Abnormal, organs or
    tissues of pelvis
spermatozoa 792.2
sputum (amount) (color) (excessive) (odor)
    (purulent) 786.4
stool NEC 787.7
    bloody 578.1
        occult 792.1
    bulky 787.7
    color (dark) (light) 792.1
    content (fat) (mucus) (pus) 792.1
    occult blood 792.1
synchondrosis 756.9
test results without manifest disease—*see*
    Findings, abnormal
thebesian valve 746.9
thermography—*see* Findings, abnormal,
    structure
threshold, cones or rods (eye) 368.63
thyroid-binding globulin 246.8
thyroid product 246.8
toxicology (findings) NEC 796.0
tracheal cartilage (congenital) 748.3
transport protein 273.8
ultrasound results—*see* Findings, abnormal,
    structure
umbilical cord
    affecting fetus or newborn 762.6
    complicating delivery 663.9
    specified NEC 663.8
union
    cricoid cartilage and thyroid cartilage 748.3
    larynx and trachea 748.3
    thyroid cartilage and hyoid bone 748.3
urination NEC 788.69
    psychogenic 306.53
    stream
        intermittent 788.61
        slowing 788.62
        splitting 788.61
        weak 788.62
    urgency 788.63
urine (constituents) NEC 791.9

Abnormal, abnormality —*continued*
uterine hemorrhage (*see also* Hemorrhage,
    uterus) 626.9
    climacteric 627.0
    postmenopausal 627.1
vagina (acquired) (congenital)
    in pregnancy or childbirth 654.7
        affecting fetus or newborn 763.89
        causing obstructed labor 660.2
            affecting fetus or newborn 763.1
vascular sounds 785.9
vectorcardiogram 794.39
visually evoked potential (VEP) 794.13
vulva (acquired) (congenital)
    in pregnancy or childbirth 654.8
        affecting fetus or newborn 763.89
        causing obstructed labor 660.2
            affecting fetus or newborn 763.1
weight
    gain 783.1
        of pregnancy 646.1
            with hypertension—*see* Toxemia, of
                pregnancy
    loss 783.21
x-ray examination—*see* Abnormal, radiological
    examination
Abnormally formed uterus —*see* Anomaly,
uterus
Abnormity (any organ or part)—*see* Anomaly
ABO
hemolytic disease 773.1
incompatibility (due to transfusion of blood or
    blood products)
    with hemolytic transfusion reaction (HTR)
        (not specified as acute or delayed) 999.61
        24 hours or more after transfusion 999.63
        acute 999.62
        delayed 999.63
        less than 24 hours after transfusion 999.62
        unspecified time after transfusion 999.61
    reaction 999.60
        specified NEC 999.69
Abocclusion 524.20
Abolition, language 784.69
Aborter, habitual or recurrent NEC
without current pregnancy 629.81
current abortion (*see also* Abortion,
    spontaneous) 634.9
    affecting fetus or newborn 761.8
observation in current pregnancy 646.3
Abortion (complete) (incomplete) (inevitable)
    (with retained products of conception) 637.9

*Note—Use the following fifth-digit
subclassification with categories 634-637:*

0   unspecified
1   incomplete
2   complete

with
    complication(s) (any) following previous
        abortion—*see* category 639
    damage to pelvic organ (laceration) (rupture)
        (tear) 637.2
    embolism (air) (amniotic fluid) (blood clot)
        (pulmonary) (pyemic) (septic) (soap)
        637.6
    genital tract and pelvic infection 637.0
    hemorrhage, delayed or excessive 637.1
    metabolic disorder 637.4
    renal failure (acute) 637.3

Abortion—*continued*

sepsis (genital tract) (pelvic organ) 637.0
    urinary tract 637.7
shock (postoperative) (septic) 637.5
specified complication NEC 637.7
toxemia 637.3
unspecified complication(s) 637.8
urinary tract infection 637.7
accidental—*see* Abortion, spontaneous
artificial—*see* Abortion, induced
attempted (failed)—*see* Abortion, failed
criminal—*see* Abortion, illegal
early—*see* Abortion, spontaneous
elective—*see* Abortion, legal
failed (legal) 638.9
with
    damage to pelvic organ (laceration) (rupture)
        (tear) 638.2
    embolism (air) (amniotic fluid) (blood clot)
        (pulmonary) (pyemic) (septic) (soap)
        638.6
    genital tract and pelvic infection 638.0
    hemorrhage, delayed or excessive 638.1
    metabolic disorder 638.4
    renal failure (acute) 638.3
    sepsis (genital tract) (pelvic organ) 638.0
        urinary tract 638.7
    shock (postoperative) (septic) 638.5
    specified complication NEC 638.7
    toxemia 638.3
    unspecified complication(s) 638.8
    urinary tract infection 638.7
fetal indication—*see* Abortion, legal
fetus 779.6
following threatened abortion—*see* Abortion, by
    type
habitual or recurrent (care during pregnancy)
    646.3
with current abortion (*see also* Abortion,
    spontaneous) 634.9
    affecting fetus or newborn 761.8
without current pregnancy 629.81
homicidal—*see* Abortion, illegal
illegal 636.9
with
    damage to pelvic organ (laceration) (rupture)
        (tear) 636.2
    embolism (air) (amniotic fluid) (blood clot)
        (pulmonary) (pyemic) (septic) (soap)
        636.6
    genital tract and pelvic infection 636.0
    hemorrhage, delayed or excessive 636.1
    metabolic disorder 636.4
    renal failure 636.3
    sepsis (genital tract) (pelvic organ) 636.0
        urinary tract 636.7
    shock (postoperative) (septic) 636.5
    specified complication NEC 636.7
    toxemia 636.3
    unspecified complication(s) 636.8
    urinary tract infection 636.7
fetus 779.6
induced 637.9
    illegal—*see* Abortion, illegal
    legal indications—*see* Abortion, legal
    medical indications—*see* Abortion, legal
    therapeutic—*see* Abortion, legal
late—*see* Abortion, spontaneous

Abortion—*continued*

legal (legal indication) (medical indication)
    (under medical supervision) 635.9
with
    damage to pelvic organ (laceration) (rupture)
        (tear) 635.2
    embolism (air) (amniotic fluid) (blood clot)
        (pulmonary) (pyemic) (septic) (soap) 635.6
    genital tract and pelvic infection 635.0
    hemorrhage, delayed or excessive 635.1
    metabolic disorder 635.4
    renal failure (acute) 635.3
    sepsis (genital tract) (pelvic organ) 635.0
        urinary tract 635.7
    shock (postoperative) (septic) 635.5
    specified complication NEC 635.7
    toxemia 635.3
    unspecified complication(s) 635.8
    urinary tract infection 635.7
fetus 779.6
medical indication—*see* Abortion, legal
mental hygiene problem—*see* Abortion, legal
missed 632
operative—*see* Abortion, legal
psychiatric indication—*see* Abortion, legal
recurrent—*see* Abortion, spontaneous
self-induced—*see* Abortion, illegal
septic—*see* Abortion, by type, with sepsis
spontaneous 634.9
with
    damage to pelvic organ (laceration) (rupture)
        (tear) 634.2
    embolism (air) (amniotic fluid) (blood clot)
        (pulmonary) (pyemic) (septic) (soap)
        634.6
    genital tract and pelvic infection 634.0
    hemorrhage, delayed or excessive 634.1
    metabolic disorder 634.4
    renal failure 634.3
    sepsis (genital tract) (pelvic organ) 634.0
        urinary tract 634.7
    shock (postoperative) (septic) 634.5
    specified complication NEC 634.7
    toxemia 634.3
    unspecified complication(s) 634.8
    urinary tract infection 634.7
fetus 761.8
threatened 640.0
    affecting fetus or newborn 762.1
surgical—*see* Abortion, legal
therapeutic—*see* Abortion, legal
threatened 640.0
    affecting fetus or newborn 762.1
tubal—*see* Pregnancy, tubal
voluntary—*see* Abortion, legal
Abortus fever 023.9
Aboulomania 301.6
Abrachia 755.20
Abrachiatism 755.20
Abrachiocephalia 759.89
Abrachiocephalus 759.89
Abrami's disease (acquired hemolytic jaundice)
    283.9
Abramov-Fiedler myocarditis (acute isolated
    myocarditis) 422.91
Abrasion —*see also* Injury, superficial, by site
    cornea 918.1

Abrasion—*continued*
  dental 521.20
    extending into
      dentine 521.22
      pulp 521.23
    generalized 521.25
    limited to enamel 521.21
    localized 521.24
  teeth, tooth (dentifrice) (habitual) (hard tissues)
    (occupational) (ritual) (traditional) (wedge
    defect) (*see also* Abrasion, dental) 521.20
Abrikossov's tumor (M9580/0)—*see also*
  Neoplasm, connective tissue, benign
  malignant (M9580/3)—*see* Neoplasm,
  connective tissue, malignant
Abrism 988.8
Abruption, placenta —*see* Placenta, abruptio
Abruptio placentae —*see* Placenta, abruptio
Abscess (acute) (chronic) (infectional)
  (lymphangitic) (metastatic) (multiple)
  (pyogenic) (septic) (with lymphangitis) (*see
  also* Cellulitis) 682.9
  abdomen, abdominal
    cavity 567.22
    wall 682.2
  abdominopelvic 567.22
  accessory sinus (chronic) (*see also* Sinusitis)
    473.9
  adrenal (capsule) (gland) 255.8
  alveolar 522.5
    with sinus 522.7
  amebic 006.3
    bladder 006.8
    brain (with liver or lung abscess) 006.5
    liver (without mention of brain or lung
      abscess) 006.3
      with
        brain abscess (and lung abscess) 006.5
        lung abscess 006.4
    lung (with liver abscess) 006.4
      with brain abscess 006.5
    seminal vesicle 006.8
    specified site NEC 006.8
    spleen 006.8
  anaerobic 040.0
  ankle 682.6
  anorectal 566
  antecubital space 682.3
  antrum (chronic) (Highmore) (*see also* Sinusitis,
    maxillary) 473.0
  anus 566
  apical (tooth) 522.5
    with sinus (alveolar) 522.7
  appendix 540.1
  areola (acute) (chronic) (nonpuerperal) 611.0
    puerperal, postpartum 675.1
  arm (any part, above wrist) 682.3
  artery (wall) 447.2
  atheromatous 447.2
  auditory canal (external) 380.10
  auricle (ear) (staphylococcal) (streptococcal)
    380.10
  axilla, axillary (region) 682.3
    lymph gland or node 683
  back (any part) 682.2

Abscess—*continued*
  Bartholin's gland 616.3
    with
      abortion—*see* Abortion, by type, with sepsis
      ectopic pregnancy (*see also* categories
        633.0-633.9) 639.0
      molar pregnancy (*see also* categories
        630-632) 639.0
    complicating pregnancy or puerperium 646.6
    following
      abortion 639.0
      ectopic or molar pregnancy 639.0
  bartholinian 616.3
  Bezold's 383.01
  bile, biliary, duct or tract (*see also* Cholecystitis)
    576.8
  bilharziasis 120.1
  bladder (wall) 595.89
    amebic 006.8
  bone (subperiosteal) (*see also* Osteomyelitis)
    730.0
    accessory sinus (chronic) (*see also* Sinusitis)
      473.9
    acute 730.0
    chronic or old 730.1
    jaw (lower) (upper) 526.4
    mastoid—*see* Mastoiditis, acute
    petrous (*see also* Petrositis) 383.20
    spinal (tuberculous) (*see also* Tuberculosis)
      015.0 *[730.88]*
      nontuberculous 730.08
  bowel 569.5
  brain (any part) 324.0
    amebic (with liver or lung abscess) 006.5
    cystic 324.0
    late effect—*see* category 326
    otogenic 324.0
    tuberculous (*see also* Tuberculosis) 013.3
  breast (acute) (chronic) (nonpuerperal) 611.0
    newborn 771.5
    puerperal, postpartum 675.1
    tuberculous (*see also* Tuberculosis) 017.9
  broad ligament (chronic) (*see also* Disease,
    pelvis, inflammatory) 614.4
    acute 614.3
  Brodie's (chronic) (localized) (*see also*
    Osteomyelitis) 730.1
  bronchus 519.19
  buccal cavity 528.3
  bulbourethral gland 597.0
  bursa 727.89
    pharyngeal 478.29
  buttock 682.5
  canaliculus, breast 611.0
  canthus 372.20
  cartilage 733.99
  cecum 569.5
    with appendicitis 540.1
  cerebellum, cerebellar 324.0
    late effect—*see* category 326
  cerebral (embolic) 324.0
    late effect—*see* category 326
  cervical (neck region) 682.1
    lymph gland or node 683
    stump (*see also* Cervicitis) 616.0
  cervix (stump) (uteri) (*see also* Cervicitis) 616.0
  cheek, external 682.0
    inner 528.3
  chest 510.9
    with fistula 510.0
    wall 682.2

Abscess—*continued*
chin 682.0
choroid 363.00
ciliary body 364.3
circumtonsillar 475
cold (tuberculous)—*see also* Tuberculosis,
    abscess
    articular—*see* Tuberculosis, joint
colon (wall) 569.5
colostomy or enterostomy 569.6
conjunctiva 372.00
connective tissue NEC 682.9
cornea 370.55
    with ulcer 370.00
corpus
    cavernosum 607.2
    luteum (*see also* Salpingo-oophoritis) 614.2
Cowper's gland 597.0
cranium 324.0
cul-de-sac (Douglas') (posterior) (*see also*
    Disease, pelvis, inflammatory) 614.4
    acute 614.3
dental 522.5
    with sinus (alveolar) 522.7
dentoalveolar 522.5
    with sinus (alveolar) 522.7
diaphragm, diaphragmatic 567.22
digit NEC 681.9
Douglas' cul-de-sac or pouch (*see also* Disease,
    pelvis, inflammatory) 614.4
    acute 614.3
Dubois' 090.5
ductless gland 259.8
ear
    acute 382.00
    external 380.10
    inner 386.30
    middle—*see* Otitis media
elbow 682.3
endamebic—*see* Abscess, amebic
entamebic—*see* Abscess, amebic
enterostomy 569.6
epididymis 604.0
epidural 324.9
    brain 324.0
    late effect—*see* category 326
    spinal cord 324.1
epiglottis 478.79
epiploon, epiploic 567.22
erysipelatous (*see also* Erysipelas) 035
esophagostomy 530.86
esophagus 530.19
ethmoid (bone) (chronic) (sinus) (*see also*
    Sinusitis, ethmoidal) 473.2
external auditory canal 380.10
extradural 324.9
    brain 324.0
    late effect—*see* category 326
    spinal cord 324.1
extraperitoneal—*see* Abscess, peritoneum
eye 360.00
eyelid 373.13
face (any part, except eye) 682.0
fallopian tube (*see also* Salpingo-oophoritis)
    614.2
fascia 728.89
fauces 478.29
fecal 569.5
femoral (region) 682.6
filaria, filarial (*see also* Infestation, filarial)
    125.9

Abscess—*continued*
finger (any) (intrathecal) (periosteal)
    (subcutaneous) (subcuticular) 681.00
fistulous NEC 682.9
flank 682.2
foot (except toe) 682.7
forearm 682.3
forehead 682.0
frontal (sinus) (chronic) (*see also* Sinusitis,
    frontal) 473.1
gallbladder (*see also* Cholecystitis, acute) 575.0
gastric 535.0
genital organ or tract NEC
    female 616.9
        with
            abortion—*see* Abortion, by type, with
                sepsis
            ectopic pregnancy (*see also* categories
                633.0-633.9) 639.0
            molar pregnancy (*see also* categories
                630-632) 639.0
        following
            abortion 639.0
            ectopic or molar pregnancy 639.0
        puerperal, postpartum, childbirth 670.8
    male 608.4
genitourinary system, tuberculous (*see also*
    Tuberculosis) 016.9
gingival 523.30
gland, glandular (lymph) (acute) NEC 683
glottis 478.79
gluteal (region) 682.5
gonorrheal NEC (*see also* Gonococcus) 098.0
groin 682.2
gum 523.30
hand (except finger or thumb) 682.4
head (except face) 682.8
heart 429.89
heel 682.7
helminthic (*see also* Infestation, by specific
    parasite) 128.9
hepatic 572.0
    amebic (*see also* Abscess, liver, amebic) 006.3
    duct 576.8
hip 682.6
    tuberculous (active) (*see also* Tuberculosis)
        015.1
ileocecal 540.1
ileostomy (bud) 569.6
iliac (region) 682.2
    fossa 540.1
iliopsoas 567.31
    tuberculous (see also Tuberculosis) 015.0
        [730.88]
infraclavicular (fossa) 682.3
inguinal (region) 682.2
    lymph gland or node 683
intersphincteric (anus) 566
intestine, intestinal 569.5
    rectal 566
intra-abdominal (*see also* Abscess, peritoneum)
    567.22
    postoperative 998.59
intracranial 324.0
    late effect—*see* category 326
intramammary—*see* Abscess, breast
intramastoid (*see also* Mastoiditis, acute) 383.00
intraorbital 376.01
intraperitoneal 567.22
intraspinal 324.1
    late effect—*see* category 326

Abscess—*continued*
  intratonsillar 475
  iris 364.3
  ischiorectal 566
  jaw (bone) (lower) (upper) 526.4
    skin 682.0
  joint (*see also* Arthritis, pyogenic) 711.0
    vertebral (tuberculous) (*see also* Tuberculosis)
      015.0 *[730.88]*
      nontuberculous 724.8
  kidney 590.2
    with
      abortion—*see* Abortion, by type, with
        urinary tract infection
      calculus 592.0
      ectopic pregnancy (*see also* categories
        633.0-633.9) 639.8
      molar pregnancy (*see also* categories
        630-632) 639.8
    complicating pregnancy or puerperium 646.6
      affecting fetus or newborn 760.1
    following
      abortion 639.8
      ectopic or molar pregnancy 639.8
  knee 682.6
    joint 711.06
    tuberculous (active) (*see also* Tuberculosis)
      015.2
  labium (majus) (minus) 616.4
    complicating pregnancy, childbirth, or
      puerperium 646.6
  lacrimal (passages) (sac) (*see also*
      Dacryocystitis) 375.30
    caruncle 375.30
    gland (*see also* Dacryoadenitis) 375.00
  lacunar 597.0
  larynx 478.79
  lateral (alveolar) 522.5
    with sinus 522.7
  leg, except foot 682.6
  lens 360.00
  lid 373.13
  lingual 529.0
    tonsil 475
  lip 528.5
  Littre's gland 597.0
  liver 572.0
    amebic 006.3
      with
        brain abscess (and lung abscess) 006.5
        lung abscess 006.4
      due to Entamoeba histolytica 006.3
      dysenteric (*see also* Abscess, liver, amebic)
        006.3
      pyogenic 572.0
      tropical (*see also* Abscess, liver, amebic)
        006.3
  loin (region) 682.2
  lumbar (tuberculous) (*see also* Tuberculosis)
      015.0 *[730.88]*
    nontuberculous 682.2
  lung (miliary) (putrid) 513.0
    amebic (with liver abscess) 006.4
      with brain abscess 006.5
  lymph, lymphatic, gland or node (acute) 683
    any site, except mesenteric 683
    mesentery 289.2
  lymphangitic, acute—*see* Cellulitis
  malar 526.4
  mammary gland—*see* Abscess, breast
  marginal (anus) 566

Abscess—*continued*
  mastoid (process) (*see also* Mastoiditis, acute)
      383.00
    subperiosteal 383.01
  maxilla, maxillary 526.4
    molar (tooth) 522.5
      with sinus 522.7
    premolar 522.5
    sinus (chronic) (*see also* Sinusitis, maxillary)
      473.0
  mediastinum 513.1
  meibomian gland 373.12
  meninges (*see also* Meningitis) 320.9
  mesentery, mesenteric 567.22
  mesosalpinx (*see also* Salpingo-oophoritis)
      614.2
  milk 675.1
  Monro's (psoriasis) 696.1
  mons pubis 682.2
  mouth (floor) 528.3
  multiple sites NEC 682.9
  mural 682.2
  muscle 728.89
    psoas 567.31
  myocardium 422.92
  nabothian (follicle) (*see also* Cervicitis) 616.0
  nail (chronic) (with lymphangitis) 681.9
    finger 681.02
    toe 681.11
  nasal (fossa) (septum) 478.19
    sinus (chronic) (*see also* Sinusitis) 473.9
  nasopharyngeal 478.29
  nates 682.5
  navel 682.2
    newborn NEC 771.4
  neck (region) 682.1
    lymph gland or node 683
  nephritic (*see also* Abscess, kidney) 590.2
  nipple 611.0
    puerperal, postpartum 675.0
  nose (septum) 478.19
    external 682.0
  omentum 567.22
  operative wound 998.59
  orbit, orbital 376.01
  ossifluent—*see* Abscess, bone
  ovary, ovarian (corpus luteum) (*see also*
      Salpingo-oophoritis) 614.2
  oviduct (*see also* Salpingo-oophoritis) 614.2
  palate (soft) 528.3
    hard 526.4
  palmar (space) 682.4
  pancreas (duct) 577.0
  paradontal 523.30
  parafrenal 607.2
  parametric, parametrium (chronic) (*see also*
      Disease, pelvis, inflammatory) 614.4
    acute 614.3
  paranephric 590.2
  parapancreatic 577.0
  parapharyngeal 478.22
  pararectal 566
  parasinus (*see also* Sinusitis) 473.9
  parauterine (*see also* Disease, pelvis,
      inflammatory) 614.4
    acute 614.3
  paravaginal (*see also* Vaginitis) 616.10
  parietal region 682.8
  parodontal 523.30
  parotid (duct) (gland) 527.3
    region 528.3

Abscess—*continued*
parumbilical 682.2
  newborn 771.4
pectoral (region) 682.2
pelvirectal 567.22
pelvis, pelvic
  female (chronic) (*see also* Disease, pelvis,
    inflammatory) 614.4
    acute 614.3
  male, peritoneal (cellular tissue)—*see*
    Abscess, peritoneum
  tuberculous (*see also* Tuberculosis) 016.9
penis 607.2
  gonococcal (acute) 098.0
    chronic or duration of 2 months or over
      098.2
perianal 566
periapical 522.5
  with sinus (alveolar) 522.7
periappendiceal 540.1
pericardial 420.99
pericecal 540.1
pericemental 523.30
pericholecystic (*see also* Cholecystitis, acute)
  575.0
pericoronal 523.30
peridental 523.30
perigastric 535.0
perimetric (*see also* Disease, pelvis,
  inflammatory) 614.4
  acute 614.3
perinephric, perinephritic (*see also* Abscess,
  kidney) 590.2
perineum, perineal (superficial) 682.2
  deep (with urethral involvement) 597.0
  urethra 597.0
periodontal (parietal) 523.31
  apical 522.5
periosteum, periosteal (*see also* Periostitis)
  730.3
  with osteomyelitis (*see also* Osteomyelitis)
    730.2
    acute or subacute 730.0
    chronic or old 730.1
peripleuritic 510.9
  with fistula 510.0
periproctic 566
periprostatic 601.2
perirectal (staphylococcal) 566
perirenal (tissue) (*see also* Abscess, kidney)
  590.2
perisinuous (nose) (*see also* Sinusitis) 473.9
peritoneum, peritoneal (perforated) (ruptured)
  567.22
  with
    abortion—*see* Abortion, by type, with sepsis
    appendicitis 540.1
    ectopic pregnancy (*see also* categories
      633.0-633.9) 639.0
    molar pregnancy (*see also* categories
      630-632) 639.0
  following
    abortion 639.0
    ectopic or molar pregnancy 639.0
  pelvic, female (*see also* Disease, pelvis,
    inflammatory) 614.4
    acute 614.3
  postoperative 998.59
  puerperal, postpartum, childbirth 670.8
  tuberculous (*see also* Tuberculosis) 014.0
peritonsillar 475

Abscess—*continued*
perityphlic 540.1
periureteral 593.89
periurethral 597.0
  gonococcal (acute) 098.0
    chronic or duration of 2 months or over
      098.2
periuterine (*see also* Disease, pelvis,
  inflammatory) 614.4
  acute 614.3
perivesical 595.89
pernicious NEC 682.9
petrous bone—*see* Petrositis
phagedenic NEC 682.9
  chancroid 099.0
pharynx, pharyngeal (lateral) 478.29
phlegmonous NEC 682.9
pilonidal 685.0
pituitary (gland) 253.8
pleura 510.9
  with fistula 510.0
popliteal 682.6
postanal 566
postcecal 540.1
postlaryngeal 478.79
postnasal 478.19
postpharyngeal 478.24
posttonsillar 475
posttyphoid 002.0
Pott's (*see also* Tuberculosis) 015.0 *[730.88]*
pouch of Douglas (chronic) (*see also* Disease,
  pelvis, inflammatory) 614.4
premammary—*see* Abscess, breast
prepatellar 682.6
prostate (*see also* Prostatitis) 601.2
  gonococcal (acute) 098.12
    chronic or duration of 2 months or over 098.32
psoas 567.31
  tuberculous (*see also* Tuberculosis) 015.0
    [730.88]
pterygopalatine fossa 682.8
pubis 682.2
puerperal—Puerperal, abscess, by site
pulmonary—*see* Abscess, lung
pulp, pulpal (dental) 522.0
  finger 681.01
  toe 681.10
pyemic—*see* Septicemia
pyloric valve 535.0
rectovaginal septum 569.5
rectovesical 595.89
rectum 566
regional NEC 682.9
renal (*see also* Abscess, kidney) 590.2
retina 363.00
retrobulbar 376.01
retrocecal 567.22
retrolaryngeal 478.79
retromammary—*see* Abscess, breast
retroperineal 682.2
retroperitoneal 567.38
  postprocedural 998.59
retropharyngeal 478.24
  tuberculous (*see also* Tuberculosis) 012.8
retrorectal 566
retrouterine (*see also* Disease, pelvis,
  inflammatory) 614.4
  acute 614.3
retrovesical 595.89
root, tooth 522.5
  with sinus (alveolar) 522.7

Abscess—*continued*
round ligament (*see also* Disease, pelvis,
  inflammatory) 614.4
  acute 614.3
rupture (spontaneous) NEC 682.9
sacrum (tuberculous) (*see also* Tuberculosis)
  015.0 *[730.88]*
  nontuberculous 730.08
salivary duct or gland 527.3
scalp (any part) 682.8
scapular 730.01
sclera 379.09
scrofulous (*see also* Tuberculosis) 017.2
scrotum 608.4
seminal vesicle 608.0
  amebic 006.8
septal, dental 522.5
  with sinus (alveolar) 522.7
septum (nasal) 478.19
serous (*see also* Periostitis) 730.3
shoulder 682.3
side 682.2
sigmoid 569.5
sinus (accessory) (chronic) (nasal) (*see also*
  Sinusitis) 473.9
  intracranial venous (any) 324.0
  late effect—*see* category 326
Skene's duct or gland 597.0
skin NEC 682.9
  tuberculous (primary) (*see also* Tuberculosis)
    017.0
sloughing NEC 682.9
specified site NEC 682.8
  amebic 006.8
spermatic cord 608.4
sphenoidal (sinus) (*see also* Sinusitis,
  sphenoidal) 473.3
spinal
  cord (any part) (staphylococcal) 324.1
    tuberculous (*see also* Tuberculosis) 013.5
  epidural 324.1
spine (column) (tuberculous) (*see also*
  Tuberculosis) 015.0 *[730.88]*
  nontuberculous 730.08
spleen 289.59
  amebic 006.8
staphylococcal NEC 682.9
stitch 998.59
stomach (wall) 535.0
strumous (tuberculous) (*see also* Tuberculosis)
  017.2
subarachnoid 324.9
  brain 324.0
  cerebral 324.0
  late effect—*see* category 326
  spinal cord 324.1
subareolar—*see also* Abscess, breast
  puerperal, postpartum 675.1
subcecal 540.1
subcutaneous NEC 682.9
subdiaphragmatic 567.22
subdorsal 682.2
subdural 324.9
  brain 324.0
  late effect—*see* category 326
  spinal cord 324.1
subgaleal 682.8
subhepatic 567.22
sublingual 528.3
  gland 527.3
submammary—*see* Abscess, breast

Abscess—*continued*
submandibular (region) (space) (triangle) 682.0
  gland 527.3
submaxillary (region) 682.0
  gland 527.3
submental (pyogenic) 682.0
  gland 527.3
subpectoral 682.2
subperiosteal—*see* Abscess, bone
subperitoneal 567.22
subphrenic—*see also* Abscess, peritoneum
  567.22
  postoperative 998.59
subscapular 682.2
subungual 681.9
suburethral 597.0
sudoriparous 705.89
suppurative NEC 682.9
supraclavicular (fossa) 682.3
suprahepatic 567.22
suprapelvic (*see also* Disease, pelvis,
  inflammatory) 614.4
  acute 614.3
suprapubic 682.2
suprarenal (capsule) (gland) 255.8
sweat gland 705.89
syphilitic 095.8
teeth, tooth (root) 522.5
  with sinus (alveolar) 522.7
  supporting structures NEC 523.30
temple 682.0
temporal region 682.0
temporosphenoidal 324.0
  late effect—*see* category 326
tendon (sheath) 727.89
testicle—*see* Orchitis
thecal 728.89
thigh (acquired) 682.6
thorax 510.9
  with fistula 510.0
throat 478.29
thumb (intrathecal) (periosteal) (subcutaneous)
  (subcuticular) 681.00
thymus (gland) 254.1
thyroid (gland) 245.0
toe (any) (intrathecal) (periosteal)
  (subcutaneous) (subcuticular) 681.10
tongue (staphylococcal) 529.0
tonsil(s) (lingual) 475
tonsillopharyngeal 475
tooth, teeth (root) 522.5
  with sinus (alveolar) 522.7
  supporting structure NEC 523.30
trachea 478.9
trunk 682.2
tubal (*see also* Salpingo-oophoritis) 614.2
tuberculous—*see* Tuberculosis, abscess
tubo-ovarian (*see also* Salpingo-oophoritis)
  614.2
tunica vaginalis 608.4
umbilicus NEC 682.2
  newborn 771.4
upper arm 682.3
upper respiratory 478.9
urachus 682.2
urethra (gland) 597.0
urinary 597.0

Abscess—*continued*
uterus, uterine (wall) (*see also* Endometritis)
   615.9
   ligament (*see also* Disease, pelvis,
      inflammatory) 614.4
      acute 614.3
   neck (*see also* Cervicitis) 616.0
uvula 528.3
vagina (wall) (*see also* Vaginitis) 616.10
vaginorectal (*see also* Vaginitis) 616.10
vas deferens 608.4
vermiform appendix 540.1
vertebra (column) (tuberculous) (*see also*
   Tuberculosis) 015.0 *[730.88]*
   nontuberculous 730.0
vesical 595.89
vesicouterine pouch (*see also* Disease, pelvis,
   inflammatory) 614.4
vitreous (humor) (pneumococcal) 360.04
vocal cord 478.5
von Bezold's 383.01
vulva 616.4
   complicating pregnancy, childbirth, or
      puerperium 646.6
vulvovaginal gland (*see also* Vaginitis) 616.3
web-space 682.4
wrist 682.4
Absence (organ or part) (complete or partial)
acoustic nerve 742.8
adrenal (gland) (congenital) 759.1
   acquired V45.79
albumin (blood) 273.8
alimentary tract (complete) (congenital) (partial)
   751.8
   lower 751.5
   upper 750.8
alpha-fucosidase 271.8
alveolar process (acquired) 525.8
   congenital 750.26
anus, anal (canal) (congenital) 751.2
aorta (congenital) 747.22
aortic valve (congenital) 746.89
appendix, congenital 751.2
arm (acquired) V49.60
   above elbow V49.66
   below elbow V49.65
   congenital (*see also* Deformity, reduction,
      upper limb) 755.20
      lower—*see* Absence, forearm, congenital
      upper (complete) (partial) (with absence of
         distal elements, incomplete) 755.24
         with
            complete absence of distal elements
               755.21
            forearm (incomplete) 755.23
artery (congenital) (peripheral) NEC (*see also*
   Anomaly, peripheral vascular system)
   747.60
   brain 747.81
   cerebral 747.81
   coronary 746.85
   pulmonary 747.31
   umbilical 747.5
atrial septum 745.69
auditory canal (congenital) (external) 744.01
auricle (ear) (with stenosis or atresia of auditory
   canal), congenital 744.01
bile, biliary duct (common) or passage
   (congenital) 751.61
   bladder (acquired) V45.74
      congenital 753.8

Absence—*continued*
bone (congenital) NEC 756.9
   marrow 284.9
      acquired (secondary) 284.89
      congenital 284.09
      hereditary 284.09
      idiopathic 284.9
   skull 756.0
bowel sounds 787.5
brain 740.0
   specified part 742.2
breast(s) (acquired) V45.71
   congenital 757.6
broad ligament (congenital) 752.19
bronchus (congenital) 748.3
calvarium, calvaria (skull) 756.0
canaliculus lacrimalis, congenital 743.65
carpal(s) (congenital) (complete) (partial) (with
      absence of distal elements, incomplete) (*see
      also* Deformity, reduction, upper limb)
   755.28
   with complete absence of distal elements
      755.21
cartilage 756.9
caudal spine 756.13
cecum (acquired) (postoperative)
      (posttraumatic) V45.72
   congenital 751.2
cementum 520.4
cerebellum (congenital) (vermis) 742.2
cervix (acquired) (uteri) V88.01
   with remaining uterus V88.03
   and uterus V88.01
   congenital 752.43
chin, congenital 744.89
cilia (congenital) 743.63
   acquired 374.89
circulatory system, part NEC 747.89
clavicle 755.51
clitoris (congenital) 752.49
coccyx, congenital 756.13
cold sense (*see also* Disturbance, sensation)
   782.0
colon (acquired) (postoperative) V45.72
   congenital 751.2
congenital
   lumen—*see* Atresia
   organ or site NEC—*see* Agenesis
   septum—*see* Imperfect, closure
corpus callosum (congenital) 742.2
cricoid cartilage 748.3
diaphragm (congenital) (with hernia) 756.6
   with obstruction 756.6
digestive organ(s) or tract, congenital (complete)
      (partial) 751.8
   acquired V45.79
   lower 751.5
   upper 750.8
ductus arteriosus 747.89
duodenum (acquired) (postoperative) V45.72
   congenital 751.1
ear, congenital 744.09
   acquired V45.79
   auricle 744.01
   external 744.01
   inner 744.05
   lobe, lobule 744.21
   middle, except ossicles 744.03
      ossicles 744.04
   ossicles 744.04
ejaculatory duct (congenital) 752.89

Absence—*continued*

  endocrine gland NEC (congenital) 759.2
  epididymis (congenital) 752.89
    acquired V45.77
  epiglottis, congenital 748.3
  epileptic (atonic) (typical) (*see also* Epilepsy)
    345.0
  erythrocyte 284.9
  erythropoiesis 284.9
    congenital 284.01
  esophagus (congenital) 750.3
  Eustachian tube (congenital) 744.24
  extremity (acquired)
    congenital (*see also* Deformity, reduction)
      755.4
    lower V49.70
    upper V49.60
  extrinsic muscle, eye 743.69
  eye (acquired) V45.78
    adnexa (congenital) 743.69
    congenital 743.00
    muscle (congenital) 743.69
  eyelid (fold), congenital 743.62
    acquired 374.89
  face
    bones NEC 756.0
    specified part NEC 744.89
  fallopian tube(s) (acquired) V45.77
    congenital 752.19
  femur, congenital (complete) (partial) (with
      absence of distal elements, incomplete) (*see
      also* Deformity, reduction, lower limb)
      755.34
    with
      complete absence of distal elements 755.31
      tibia and fibula (incomplete) 755.33
  fibrin 790.92
    fibrinogen (congenital) 286.3
      acquired 286.6
  fibula, congenital (complete) (partial) (with
      absence of distal elements, incomplete) (*see
      also* Deformity, reduction, lower limb)
      755.37
    with
      complete absence of distal elements 755.31
      tibia 755.35
        with
          complete absence of distal elements
            755.31
          femur (incomplete) 755.33
            with complete absence of distal
              elements 755.31
  finger (acquired) V49.62
    congenital (complete) (partial) (*see also*
      Deformity, reduction, upper limb) 755.29
      meaning all fingers (complete) (partial)
        755.21
      transverse 755.21
  fissures of lungs (congenital) 748.5
  foot (acquired) V49.73
    congenital (complete) 755.31
  forearm (acquired) V49.65
    congenital (complete) (partial) (with absence
      of distal elements, incomplete) (*see also*
      Deformity, reduction, upper limb) 755.25
    with
      complete absence of distal elements (hand
        and fingers) 755.21
      humerus (incomplete) 755.23
  fovea centralis 743.55

Absence—*continued*

  fucosidase 271.8
    gallbladder (acquired) V45.79
    congenital 751.69
  gamma globulin (blood) 279.00
  genital organs
    acquired V45.77
    congenital
      female 752.89
        external 752.49
        internal NEC 752.89
      male 752.89
        penis 752.69
  genitourinary organs, congenital NEC 752.89
  glottis 748.3
  gonadal, congenital NEC 758.6
  hair (congenital) 757.4
    acquired—*see* Alopecia
  hand (acquired) V49.63
    congenital (complete) (*see also* Deformity,
      reduction, upper limb) 755.21
  heart (congenital) 759.89
    acquired—*see* Status, organ replacement
  heat sense (*see also* Disturbance, sensation)
    782.0
  humerus, congenital (complete) (partial) (with
      absence of distal elements, incomplete) (*see
      also* Deformity, reduction, upper limb)
      755.24
    with
      complete absence of distal elements 755.21
      radius and ulna (incomplete) 755.23
  hymen (congenital) 752.49
  ileum (acquired) (postoperative) (posttraumatic)
      V45.72
    congenital 751.1
  immunoglobulin, isolated NEC 279.03
    IgA 279.01
    IgG 279.03
    IgM 279.02
  incus (acquired) 385.24
    congenital 744.04
  internal ear (congenital) 744.05
  intestine (acquired) (small) V45.72
    congenital 751.1
    large 751.2
    large V45.72
      congenital 751.2
  iris (congenital) 743.45
  jaw—*see* Absence, mandible
  jejunum (acquired) V45.72
    congenital 751.1
  joint (acquired) (following prior explantation of
      joint prosthesis) (with or without presence of
      antibiotic-impregnated cement spacer) NEC
      V88.29
    congenital NEC 755.8
    hip V88.21
    knee V88.22
  kidney(s) (acquired) V45.73
    congenital 753.0
  labium (congenital) (majus) (minus) 752.49
  labyrinth, membranous 744.05
  lacrimal apparatus (congenital) 743.65
  larynx (congenital) 748.3
  leg (acquired) V49.70
    above knee V49.76
    below knee V49.75

Absence—*continued*
  congenital (partial) (unilateral) (*see also*
    Deformity, reduction, lower limb) 755.31
  lower (complete) (partial) (with absence of
    distal elements, incomplete) 755.35
    with
      complete absence of distal elements
        (foot and toes) 755.31
      thigh (incomplete) 755.33
        with complete absence of distal
          elements 755.31
    upper—*see* Absence, femur
  lens (congenital) 743.35
    acquired 379.31
  ligament, broad (congenital) 752.19
  limb (acquired)
    congenital (complete) (partial) (*see also*
      Deformity, reduction) 755.4
    lower 755.30
      complete 755.31
      incomplete 755.32
      longitudinal—*see* Deficiency, lower limb,
        longitudinal
      transverse 755.31
    upper 755.20
      complete 755.21
      incomplete 755.22
      longitudinal—*see* Deficiency, upper limb,
        longitudinal
      transverse 755.21
    lower NEC V49.70
    upper NEC V49.60
  lip 750.26
  liver (congenital) (lobe) 751.69
  lumbar (congenital) (vertebra) 756.13
    isthmus 756.11
    pars articularis 756.11
  lumen—*see* Atresia
  lung (bilateral) (congenital) (fissure) (lobe)
    (unilateral) 748.5
    acquired (any part) V45.76
  mandible (congenital) 524.09
  maxilla (congenital) 524.09
  menstruation 626.0
  metacarpal(s), congenital (complete) (partial)
    (with absence of distal elements,
    incomplete) (*see also* Deformity, reduction,
    upper limb) 755.28
    with all fingers, complete 755.21
  metatarsal(s), congenital (complete) (partial)
    (with absence of distal elements,
    incomplete) (*see also* Deformity, reduction,
    lower limb) 755.38
    with complete absence of distal elements
      755.31
  muscle (congenital) (pectoral) 756.81
    ocular 743.69
  musculoskeletal system (congenital) NEC 756.9
  nail(s) (congenital) 757.5
  neck, part 744.89
  nerve 742.8
  nervous system, part NEC 742.8
  neutrophil 288.00
  nipple (congenital) 757.6
    acquired V45.71
  nose (congenital) 748.1
    acquired 738.0
  nuclear 742.8
  ocular muscle (congenital) 743.69

Absence—*continued*
  organ
    of Corti (congenital) 744.05
    or site
      acquired V45.79
      congenital NEC 759.89
  osseous meatus (ear) 744.03
  ovary (acquired) V45.77
    congenital 752.0
  oviduct (acquired) V45.77
    congenital 752.19
  pancreas (congenital) 751.7
    acquired (postoperative) (posttraumatic)
      V88.11
    partial V88.12
    total V88.11
  parathyroid gland (congenital) 759.2
  parotid gland(s) (congenital) 750.21
  patella, congenital 755.64
  pelvic girdle (congenital) 755.69
  penis (congenital) 752.69
    acquired V45.77
  pericardium (congenital) 746.89
  perineal body (congenital) 756.81
  phalange(s), congenital 755.4
    lower limb (complete) (intercalary) (partial)
      (terminal) (*see also* Deformity, reduction,
      lower limb) 755.39
      meaning all toes (complete) (partial) 755.31
      transverse 755.31
    upper limb (complete) (intercalary) (partial)
      (terminal) (*see also* Deformity, reduction,
      upper limb) 755.29
      meaning all digits (complete) (partial)
        755.21
      transverse 755.21
  pituitary gland (congenital) 759.2
  postoperative—*see* Absence, by site, acquired
  prostate (congenital) 752.89
    acquired V45.77
  pulmonary
    artery 747.31
    trunk 747.31
    valve (congenital) 746.01
    vein 747.49
  punctum lacrimale (congenital) 743.65
  radius, congenital (complete) (partial) (with
    absence of distal elements, incomplete)
    755.26
    with
      complete absence of distal elements 755.21
      ulna 755.25
      with
        complete absence of distal elements
          755.21
        humerus (incomplete) 755.23
  ray, congenital 755.4
    lower limb (complete) (partial) (*see also*
      Deformity, reduction, lower limb) 755.38
      meaning all rays 755.31
      transverse 755.31
    upper limb (complete) (partial) (*see also*
      Deformity, reduction, upper limb) 755.28
      meaning all rays 755.21
      transverse 755.21
  rectum (congenital) 751.2
    acquired V45.79
  red cell 284.9
    acquired (secondary) 284.81
    congenital 284.01
    hereditary 284.01
    idiopathic 284.9

Absence—*continued*
respiratory organ (congenital) NEC 748.9
rib (acquired) 738.3
  congenital 756.3
roof of orbit (congenital) 742.0
round ligament (congenital) 752.89
sacrum, congenital 756.13
salivary gland(s) (congenital) 750.21
scapula 755.59
scrotum, congenital 752.89
seminal tract or duct (congenital) 752.89
  acquired V45.77
septum (congenital)—*see also* Imperfect,
  closure, septum
  atrial 745.69
  and ventricular 745.7
  between aorta and pulmonary artery 745.0
  ventricular 745.3
  and atrial 745.7
sex chromosomes 758.81
shoulder girdle, congenital (complete) (partial)
  755.59
skin (congenital) 757.39
skull bone 756.0
  with
    anencephalus 740.0
    encephalocele 742.0
    hydrocephalus 742.3
      with spina bifida (*see also* Spina bifida)
      741.0
    microcephalus 742.1
spermatic cord (congenital) 752.89
spinal cord 742.59
spine, congenital 756.13
spleen (congenital) 759.0
  acquired V45.79
sternum, congenital 756.3
stomach (acquired) (partial) (postoperative)
  V45.75
  congenital 750.7
  with postgastric surgery syndrome 564.2
submaxillary gland(s) (congenital) 750.21
superior vena cava (congenital) 747.49
tarsal(s), congenital (complete) (partial) (with
  absence of distal elements, incomplete) (*see
  also* Deformity, reduction, lower limb)
  755.38
teeth, tooth (congenital) 520.0
  with abnormal spacing 524.30
  acquired 525.10
    due to
      caries 525.13
      extraction 525.10
      periodontal disease 525.12
      trauma 525.11
    with malocclusion 524.30
tendon (congenital) 756.81
testis (congenital) 752.89
  acquired V45.77
thigh (acquired) 736.89
thumb (acquired) V49.61
  congenital 755.29
thymus gland (congenital) 759.2
thyroid (gland) (surgical) 246.8
  with hypothyroidism 244.0
  cartilage, congenital 748.3
  congenital 243

Absence—*continued*
tibia, congenital (complete) (partial) (with absence
  of distal elements, incomplete) (*see also*
  Deformity, reduction, lower limb) 755.36
  with
    complete absence of distal elements 755.31
    fibula 755.35
      with
        complete absence of distal elements
        755.31
        femur (incomplete) 755.33
          with complete absence of distal
          elements 755.31
toe (acquired) V49.72
  congenital (complete) (partial) 755.39
    meaning all toes 755.31
    transverse 755.31
  great V49.71
tongue (congenital) 750.11
tooth, teeth, (congenital) 520.0
  with abnormal spacing 524.30
  acquired 525.10
    due to
      caries 525.13
      extraction 525.10
      periodontal disease 525.12
      trauma 525.11
    with malocclusion 524.30
trachea (cartilage) (congenital) (rings) 748.3
transverse aortic arch (congenital) 747.21
tricuspid valve 746.1
ulna, congenital (complete) (partial) (with
  absence of distal elements, incomplete) (*see
  also* Deformity, reduction, upper limb)
  755.27
  with
    complete absence of distal elements 755.21
    radius 755.25
      with
        complete absence of distal elements
        755.21
      humerus (incomplete) 755.23
umbilical artery (congenital) 747.5
ureter (congenital) 753.4
  acquired V45.74
urethra, congenital 753.8
  acquired V45.74
urinary system, part NEC, congenital 753.8
  acquired V45.74
uterus (acquired) V88.01
  with remaining cervical stump V88.02
  and cervix V88.01
  congenital 752.31
uvula (congenital) 750.26
vagina, congenital 752.45
  acquired V45.77
vas deferens (congenital) 752.89
  acquired V45.77
vein (congenital) (peripheral) NEC (*see also*
  Anomaly, peripheral vascular system)
  747.60
  brain 747.81
  great 747.49
  portal 747.49
  pulmonary 747.49
vena cava (congenital) (inferior) (superior)
  747.49
ventral horn cell 742.59
ventricular septum 745.3
vermis of cerebellum 742.2
vertebra, congenital 756.13
vulva, congenital 752.49

Absentia epileptica (*see also* Epilepsy) 345.0
Absinthemia (*see also* Dependence) 304.6
Absinthism (*see also* Dependence) 304.6
Absorbent system disease 459.89
Absorption
  alcohol, through placenta or breast milk 760.71
  antibiotics, through placenta or breast milk
    760.74
  anticonvulsants, through placenta or breast milk
    760.77
  antifungals, through placenta or breast milk
    760.74
  anti-infective, through placenta or breast milk
    760.74
  antimetabolics, through placenta or breast milk
    760.78
  chemical NEC 989.9
    specified chemical or substance—*see* Table of
      drugs and chemicals
    through placenta or breast milk (fetus or
      newborn) 760.70
      alcohol 760.71
      anticonvulsants 760.77
      antifungals 760.74
      anti-infective agents 760.74
      antimetabolics 760.78
      cocaine 760.75
      "crack" 760.75
      diethylstilbestrol *[DES]* 760.76
      hallucinogenic agents 760.73
      medicinal agents NEC 760.79
      narcotics 760.72
      obstetric anesthetic or analgesic drug 763.5
      specified agent NEC 760.79
      suspected, affecting management of
        pregnancy 655.5
  cocaine, through placenta or breast milk 760.75
  drug NEC (*see also* Reaction, drug)
    through placenta or breast milk (fetus or
      newborn) 760.70
      alcohol 760.71
      anticonvulsants 760.77
      antifungals 760.74
      anti-infective agents 760.74
      antimetabolics 760.78
      cocaine 760.75
      "crack" 760.75
      diethylstilbestrol (DES) 760.76
      hallucinogenic agents 760.73
      medicinal agents NEC 760.79
      narcotics 760.72
      obstetric anesthetic or analgesic drug 763.5
      specified agent NEC 760.79
      suspected, affecting management of
        pregnancy 655.5
  fat, disturbance 579.8
  hallucinogenic agents, through placenta or
    breast milk 760.73
  immune sera, through placenta or breast milk
    760.79
  lactose defect 271.3
  medicinal agents NEC, through placenta or
    breast milk 760.79
  narcotics, through placenta or breast milk
    760.72
  noxious substance,—*see* Absorption, chemical
  protein, disturbance 579.8
  pus or septic, general—*see* Septicemia
  quinine, through placenta or breast milk 760.74
  toxic substance—*see* Absorption, chemical
  uremic—*see* Uremia

Abstinence symptoms or syndrome
  alcohol 291.81
  drug 292.0
  neonatal 779.5
Abt-Letterer-Siwe syndrome (acute
    histiocytosis X) (M9722/3) 202.5
Abulia 799.89
Abulomania 301.6
Abuse
  adult 995.80
    emotional 995.82
    multiple forms 995.85
    neglect (nutritional) 995.84
    physical 995.81
    psychological 995.82
    sexual 995.83
  alcohol (*see also* Alcoholism) 305.0
    dependent 303.9
    non-dependent 305.0
  child 995.50
    counseling
      perpetrator
        non-parent V62.83
        parent V61.22
      victim V61.21
    emotional 995.51
    multiple forms 995.59
    neglect (nutritional) 995.52
    physical 995.54
      shaken infant syndrome 995.55
    psychological 995.51
    sexual 995.53
  drugs, nondependent 305.9

> *Note—Use the following fifth-digit
> subclassification with the following codes:
> 305.0, 305.2-305.9:*
>
> *0 unspecifidd*
> *1 continuous*
> *2 episodic*
> *3 in remission*

    amphetamine type 305.7
    antidepressants 305.8
    anxiolytic 305.4
    barbiturates 305.4
    caffeine 305.9
    cannabis 305.2
    cocaine type 305.6
    hallucinogens 305.3
    hashish 305.2
    hypnotic 305.4
    inhalant 305.9
    LSD 305.3
    marijuana 305.2
    mixed 305.9
    morphine type 305.5
    opioid type 305.5
    phencyclidine (PCP) 305.9
    sedative 305.4
    specified NEC 305.9
    tranquilizers 305.4
  spouse 995.80
  tobacco 305.1
Acalcerosis 275.40
Acalcicosis 275.40
Acalculia 784.69
  developmental 315.1
Acanthocheilonemiasis 125.4
Acanthocytosis 272.5
Acanthokeratodermia 701.1

Acantholysis 701.8
bullosa 757.39
Acanthoma (benign) (M8070/0)—*see also*
Neoplasm, by site, benign
malignant (M8070/3)—*see* Neoplasm, by site,
malignant
Acanthosis (acquired) (nigricans) 701.2
adult 701.2
benign (congenital) 757.39
congenital 757.39
glycogenic
esophagus 530.8
juvenile 701.2
tongue 529.8
Acanthrocytosis 272.5
Acapnia 276.3
Acarbia 276.2
Acardia 759.89
Acardiacus amorphus 759.89
Acardiotrophia 429.1
Acardius 759.89
Acariasis 133.9
sarcoptic 133.0
Acaridiasis 133.9
Acarinosis 133.9
Acariosis 133.9
Acarodermatitis 133.9
urticarioides 133.9
Acarophobia 300.29
Acatalasemia 277.89
Acatalasia 277.89
Acatamathesia 784.69
Acataphasia 784.59
Acathisia 781.0
due to drugs 333.99
Acceleration, accelerated
atrioventricular conduction 426.7
idioventricular rhythm 427.89
Accessory (congenital)
adrenal gland 759.1
anus 751.5
appendix 751.5
atrioventricular conduction 426.7
auditory ossicles 744.04
auricle (ear) 744.1
autosome(s) NEC 758.5
21 or 22 758.0
biliary duct or passage 751.69
bladder 753.8
blood vessels (peripheral) (congenital) NEC (*see
also* Anomaly, peripheral vascular system)
747.60
cerebral 747.81
coronary 746.85
bone NEC 756.9
foot 755.67
breast tissue, axilla 757.6
carpal bones 755.56
cecum 751.5
cervix 752.44
chromosome(s) NEC 758.5
13-15 758.1
16-18 758.2
21 or 22 758.0
autosome(s) NEC 758.5
D₁ 758.1
E₃ 758.2
G 758.0
sex 758.81
coronary artery 746.85

Accessory—*continued*
cusp(s), heart valve NEC 746.89
pulmonary 746.09
cystic duct 751.69
digits 755.00
ear (auricle) (lobe) 744.1
endocrine gland NEC 759.2
external os 752.44
eyelid 743.62
eye muscle 743.69
face bone(s) 756.0
fallopian tube (fimbria) (ostium) 752.19
fingers 755.01
foreskin 605
frontonasal process 756.0
gallbladder 751.69
genital organ(s)
female 752.89
external 752.49
internal NEC 752.89
male NEC 752.89
penis 752.69
genitourinary organs NEC 752.89
heart 746.89
valve NEC 746.89
pulmonary 746.09
hepatic ducts 751.69
hymen 752.49
intestine (large) (small) 751.5
kidney 753.3
lacrimal canal 743.65
leaflet, heart valve NEC 746.89
pulmonary 746.09
ligament, broad 752.19
liver (duct) 751.69
lobule (ear) 744.1
lung (lobe) 748.69
muscle 756.82
navicular of carpus 755.56
nervous system, part NEC 742.8
nipple 757.6
nose 748.1
organ or site NEC—*see* Anomaly, specified type NEC
ovary 752.0
oviduct 752.19
pancreas 751.7
parathyroid gland 759.2
parotid gland (and duct) 750.22
pituitary gland 759.2
placental lobe—*see* Placenta, abnormal
preauricular appendage 744.1
prepuce 605
renal arteries (multiple) 747.62
rib 756.3
cervical 756.2
roots (teeth) 520.2
salivary gland 750.22
sesamoids 755.8
sinus—*see* condition
skin tags 757.39
spleen 759.0
sternum 756.3
submaxillary gland 750.22
tarsal bones 755.67
teeth, tooth 520.1
causing crowding 524.31
tendon 756.89
thumb 755.01
thymus gland 759.2
thyroid gland 759.2
toes 755.02

Accessory—*continued*
  tongue 750.13
  tragus 744.1
  ureter 753.4
  urethra 753.8
  urinary organ or tract NEC 753.8
  uterus 752.2
  vagina 752.49
  valve, heart NEC 746.89
    pulmonary 746.09
  vertebra 756.19
  vocal cords 748.3
  vulva 752.49
Accident, accidental —*see also* condition
  birth NEC 767.9
  cardiovascular (*see also* Disease,
    cardiovascular) 429.2
  cerebral (*see also* Disease, cerebrovascular,
    acute) 434.91
  cerebrovascular (current) (CVA) (*see also*
    Disease, cerebrovascular, acute) 434.91
    aborted 434.91
    embolic 434.11
    healed or old V12.54
    hemorrhagic—*see* Hemorrhage, brain
    impending 435.9
    ischemic 434.91
    late effect—*see* Late effect(s) (of)
      cerebrovascular disease
    postoperative 997.02
    thrombotic 434.01
  coronary (*see also* Infarct, myocardium) 410.9
  craniovascular (*see also* Disease,
    cerebrovascular, acute) 436
  during pregnancy, to mother
    affecting fetus or newborn 760.5
  heart, cardiac (*see also* Infarct, myocardium)
    410.9
  intrauterine 779.89
  vascular—*see* Disease, cerebrovascular, acute
Accommodation
  disorder of 367.51
    drug-induced 367.89
    toxic 367.89
  insufficiency of 367.4
  paralysis of 367.51
    hysterical 300.11
  spasm of 367.53
Accouchement —*see* Delivery
Accreta placenta (without hemorrhage) 667.0
  with hemorrhage 666.0
Accretio cordis (nonrheumatic) 423.1
Accretions on teeth 523.6
Accumulation secretion, prostate 602.8
Acephalia, acephalism, acephaly 740.0
Acephalic monster 740.0
Acephalobrachia monster 759.89
Acephalocardia 759.89
Acephalocardius 759.89
Acephalochiria 759.89
Acephalochirus monster 759.89
Acephalogaster 759.89
Acephalostomus monster 759.89
Acephalothorax 759.89
Acephalus 740.0
Acetonemia 790.6
  diabetic 250.1
  due to secondary diabetes 249.1
Acetonglycosuria 982.8
Acetonuria 791.6

Achalasia 530.0
  cardia 530.0
  digestive organs congenital NEC 751.8
  esophagus 530.0
  pelvirectal 751.3
  psychogenic 306.4
  pylorus 750.5
  sphincteral NEC 564.89
Achard-Thiers syndrome (adrenogenital) 255.2
Ache (s)—*see* Pain
Acheilia 750.26
Acheiria 755.21
Achillobursitis 726.71
Achillodynia 726.71
Achlorhydria, achlorhydric 536.0
  anemia 280.9
  diarrhea 536.0
  neurogenic 536.0
  postvagotomy 564.2
  psychogenic 306.4
  secondary to vagotomy 564.2
Achloroblepsia 368.52
Achloropsia 368.52
Acholia 575.8
Acholuric jaundice (familial) (splenomegalic)
  (*see also* Spherocytosis) 282.0
  acquired 283.9
Achondroplasia 756.4
Achrestic anemia 281.8
Achroacytosis, lacrimal gland 375.00
  tuberculous (*see also* Tuberculosis) 017.3
Achroma, cutis 709.00
Achromate (congenital) 368.54
Achromatopia 368.54
Achromatopsia (congenital) 368.54
Achromia
  congenital 270.2
  parasitica 111.0
  unguium 703.8
Achylia
  gastrica 536.8
    neurogenic 536.3
    psychogenic 306.4
  pancreatica 577.1
Achylosis 536.8
Acid
  burn—*see also* Burn, by site
    from swallowing acid—*see* Burn, internal
      organs
  deficiency
    amide nicotinic 265.2
    amino 270.9
    ascorbic 267
    folic 266.2
    nicotinic (amide) 265.2
    pantothenic 266.2
  intoxication 276.2
  peptic disease 536.8
  stomach 536.8
    psychogenic 306.4
Acidemia 276.2
  arginosuccinic 270.6
  fetal
    affecting management of pregnancy 656.3
    before onset of labor, in liveborn infant 768.2
    during labor and delivery, in liveborn infant
      768.3
    intrauterine—*see* Distress, fetal 656.3
    unspecified as to time of onset, in liveborn
      infant 768.4

Acidemia—*continued*
　newborn 775.81
　pipecolic 270.7
Acidity, gastric (high) (low) 536.8
　psychogenic 306.4
Acidocytopenia 288.59
Acidocytosis 288.3
Acidopenia 288.59
Acidosis 276.2
　diabetic 250.1
　　due to secondary diabetes 249.1
　fetal, affecting management of pregnancy 656.8
　fetal, affecting newborn 775.81
　kidney tubular 588.89
　lactic 276.2
　metabolic NEC 276.2
　　with respiratory acidosis 276.4
　　　of newborn 775.81
　　late, of newborn 775.7
　newborn 775.81
　renal
　　hyperchloremic 588.89
　　tubular (distal) (proximal) 588.89
　respiratory 276.2
　　complicated by
　　　metabolic acidosis 276.4
　　　　of newborn 775.81
　　　metabolic alkalosis 276.4
Aciduria 791.9
　arginosuccinic 270.6
　beta-aminoisobutyric (BAIB) 277.2
　glutaric
　　type I 270.7
　　type II (type IIA, IIB, IIC) 277.85
　　type III 277.86
　glycolic 271.8
　methylmalonic 270.3
　　with glycinemia 270.7
　organic 270.9
　orotic (congenital) (hereditary) (pyrimidine
　　deficiency) 281.4
Acladiosis 111.8
　skin 111.8
Aclasis
　diaphyseal 756.4
　tarsoepiphyseal 756.59
Acleistocardia 745.5
Aclusion 524.4
Acmesthesia 782.0
Acne (pustular) (vulgaris) 706.1
　agminata (*see also* Tuberculosis) 017.0
　artificialis 706.1
　atrophica 706.0
　cachecticorum (Hebra) 706.1
　conglobata 706.1
　conjunctiva 706.1
　cystic 706.1
　decalvans 704.09
　erythematosa 695.3
　eyelid 706.1
　frontalis 706.0
　indurata 706.1
　keloid 706.1
　lupoid 706.0
　necrotic, necrotica 706.0
　　miliaris 704.8
　neonatal 706.1
　nodular 706.1
　occupational 706.1
　papulosa 706.1
　rodens 706.0

Acne—*continued*
　rosacea 695.3
　scorbutica 267
　scrofulosorum (Bazin) (*see also* Tuberculosis)
　　017.0
　summer 692.72
　tropical 706.1
　varioliformis 706.0
Acneiform drug eruptions 692.3
Acnitis (primary) (*see also* Tuberculosis) 017.0
Acomia 704.00
Acontractile bladder 344.61
Aconuresis (*see also* Incontinence) 788.30
Acosta's disease 993.2
Acousma 780.1
Acoustic —*see* condition
Acousticophobia 300.29
Acquired —*see* condition
Acquired immunodeficiency syndrome —*see*
　　Human immunodeficiency virus (disease)
　　(illness) (infection)
Acragnosis 781.99
Acrania (monster) 740.0
Acroagnosis 781.99
Acroangiodermatitis 448.9
Acroasphyxia, chronic 443.89
Acrobrachycephaly 756.0
Acrobystiolith 608.89
Acrobystitis 607.2
Acrocephalopolysyndactyly 755.55
Acrocephalosyndactyly 755.55
Acrocephaly 756.0
Acrochondrohyperplasia 759.82
Acrocyanosis 443.89
　newborn 770.83
Acrodermatitis 686.8
　atrophicans (chronica) 701.8
　continua (Hallopeau) 696.1
　enteropathica 686.8
　Hallopeau's 696.1
　perstans 696.1
　pustulosa continua 696.1
　recalcitrant pustular 696.1
Acrodynia 985.0
Acrodysplasia 755.55
Acrohyperhidrosis (*see also* Hyperhidrosis)
　　780.8
Acrokeratosis verruciformis 757.39
Acromastitis 611.0
Acromegaly, acromegalia (skin) 253.0
Acromelalgia 443.82
Acromicria, acromikria 756.59
Acronyx 703.0
Acropachy, thyroid (*see also* Thyrotoxicosis)
　　242.9
Acropachyderma 757.39
Acroparesthesia 443.89
　simple (Schultz's type) 443.89
　vasomotor (Nothnagel's type) 443.89
Acropathy thyroid (*see also* Thyrotoxicosis) 242.9
Acrophobia 300.29
Acroposthitis 607.2
Acroscleriasis (*see also* Scleroderma) 710.1
Acroscleroderma (*see also* Scleroderma) 710.1
Acrosclerosis (*see also* Scleroderma) 710.1
Acrosphacelus 785.4
Acrosphenosyndactylia 755.55
Acrospiroma, eccrine (M8402/0)—*see*
　　Neoplasm, skin, benign
Acrostealgia 732.9

Acrosyndactyly (*see also* Syndactylism) 755.10
Acrotrophodynia 991.4
Actinic —*see also* condition
  cheilitis (due to sun) 692.72
    chronic NEC 692.74
    due to radiation, except from sun 692.82
  conjunctivitis 370.24
  dermatitis (due to sun) (*see also* Dermatitis,
    actinic) 692.70
    due to
      roentgen rays or radioactive substance
        692.82
      ultraviolet radiation, except from sun 692.82
      sun NEC 692.70
  elastosis solare 692.74
  granuloma 692.73
  keratitis 370.24
  ophthalmia 370.24
  reticuloid 692.73
Actinobacillosis, general 027.8
Actinobacillus
  lignieresii 027.8
  mallei 024
  muris 026.1
Actinocutitis NEC (*see also* Dermatitis, actinic)
  692.70
Actinodermatitis NEC (*see also* Dermatitis,
  actinic) 692.70
Actinomyces
  israelii (infection)—*see* Actinomycosis
  muris-ratti (infection) 026.1
Actinomycosis actinomycotic 039.9
  with
    pneumonia 039.1
  abdominal 039.2
  cervicofacial 039.3
  cutaneous 039.0
  pulmonary 039.1
  specified site NEC 039.8
  thoracic 039.1
Actinoneuritis 357.89
Action, heart
  disorder 427.9
    postoperative 997.1
  irregular 427.9
    postoperative 997.1
    psychogenic 306.2
Active —*see* condition
Activity decrease, functional 780.99
Acute —*see also* condition
  abdomen NEC 789.0
  gallbladder (*see also* Cholecystitis, acute) 575.0
Acyanoblepsia 368.53
Acyanopsia 368.53
Acystia 753.8
Acystinervia —*see* Neurogenic, bladder
Acystineuria —*see* Neurogenic, bladder
Adactylia, adactyly (congenital) 755.4
  lower limb (complete) (intercalary) (partial)
    (terminal) (*see also* Deformity, reduction,
    lower limb) 755.39
    meaning all digits (complete) (partial) 755.31
    transverse (complete) (partial) 755.31
  upper limb (complete) (intercalary) (partial)
    (terminal) (*see also* Deformity, reduction,
    upper limb) 755.29
    meaning all digits (complete) (partial) 755.21
    transverse (complete) (partial) 755.21
Adair-Dighton syndrome (brittle bones and blue
  sclera, deafness) 756.51

Adamantinoblastoma (M9310/0)—*see*
  Ameloblastoma
Adamantinoma (M9310/0)—*see* Ameloblastoma
Adamantoblastoma (M9310/0)—*see*
  Ameloblastoma
Adams-Stokes (-Morgagni) disease or syndrome
  (syncope with heart block) 426.9
Adaptation reaction (*see also* Reaction,
  adjustment) 309.9
Addiction —*see also* Dependence
  absinthe 304.6
  alcoholic (ethyl) (methyl) (wood) 303.9
    complicating pregnancy, childbirth, or
      puerperium 648.4
    affecting fetus or newborn 760.71
    suspected damage to fetus affecting
      management of pregnancy 655.4
  drug (*see also* Dependence) 304.9
  ethyl alcohol 303.9
  heroin 304.0
  hospital 301.51
  methyl alcohol 303.9
  methylated spirit 303.9
  morphine (-like substances) 304.0
  nicotine 305.1
  opium 304.0
  tobacco 305.1
  wine 303.9
Addison's
  anemia (pernicious) 281.0
  disease (bronze) (primary adrenal insufficiency)
    255.41
    tuberculous (*see also* Tuberculosis) 017.6
  keloid (morphea) 701.0
  melanoderma (adrenal cortical hypofunction)
    255.41
Addison-Biermer anemia (pernicious) 281.0
Addison-Gull disease —*see* Xanthoma
Addisonian crisis or melanosis (acute
  adrenocortical insufficiency) 255.41
Additional —*see also* Accessory
  chromosome(s) 758.5
    13-15 758.1
    16-18 758.2
    21 758.0
    autosome(s) NEC 758.5
    sex 758.81
Adduction contracture, hip or other joint —*see*
  Contraction, joint
**ADEM (acute disseminated encephalomyelitis)
  (postinfectious)** 136.9 *[323.61]*
  infectious 136.9 *[323.61]*
  noninfectious 323.81
Adenasthenia gastrica 536.0
Aden fever 061
Adenitis (*see also* Lymphadenitis) 289.3
  acute, unspecified site 683
    epidemic infectious 075
  axillary 289.3
    acute 683
    chronic or subacute 289.1
  Bartholin's gland 616.89
  bulbourethral gland (*see also* Urethritis) 597.89
  cervical 289.3
    acute 683
    chronic or subacute 289.1
  chancroid (Ducrey's bacillus) 099.0
  chronic (any lymph node, except mesenteric)
    289.1
    mesenteric 289.2
  Cowper's gland (*see also* Urethritis) 597.89

Adenitis——*continued*
epidemic, acute 075
gangrenous 683
gonorrheal NEC 098.89
groin 289.3
  acute 683
  chronic or subacute 289.1
infectious 075
inguinal (region) 289.3
  acute 683
  chronic or subacute 289.1
lymph gland or node, except mesenteric 289.3
  acute 683
  chronic or subacute 289.1
  mesenteric (acute) (chronic) (nonspecific)
    (subacute) 289.2
  mesenteric (acute) (chronic) (nonspecific)
    (subacute) 289.2
  due to Pasteurella multocida (P. septica) 027.2
parotid gland (suppurative) 527.2
phlegmonous 683
salivary duct or gland (any) (recurring)
  (suppurative) 527.2
scrofulous (*see also* Tuberculosis) 017.2
septic 289.3
Skene's duct or gland (*see also* Urethritis)
  597.89
strumous, tuberculous (*see also* Tuberculosis)
  017.2
subacute, unspecified site 289.1
sublingual gland (suppurative) 527.2
submandibular gland (suppurative) 527.2
submaxillary gland (suppurative) 527.2
suppurative 683
tuberculous—*see* Tuberculosis, lymph gland
urethral gland (*see also* Urethritis) 597.89
venereal NEC 099.8
Wharton's duct (suppurative) 527.2
Adenoacanthoma (M8570/3)—*see* Neoplasm, by
site, malignant
Adenoameloblastoma (M9300/0) 213.1
upper jaw (bone) 213.0
Adenocarcinoma (M8140/3)—*see also*
Neoplasm, by site, malignant

> *Note—The list of adjectival modifiers below is
> not exhaustive. A description of
> adenocarcinoma that does not appear in this list
> should be coded in the same manner as
> carcinoma with that description. Thus, "mixed
> acidophil-basophil adenocarcinoma," should be
> coded in the same manner as "mixed
> acidophil-basophil carcinoma," which appears
> in the list under "Carcinoma."*
>
> *Except where otherwise indicated, the
> morphological varieties of adenocarcinoma in
> the list below should be coded by site as for
> "Neoplasm, malignant."*

with
  apocrine metaplasia (M8573/3)
  cartilaginous (and osseous) metaplasia
    (M8571/3)
  osseous (and cartilaginous) metaplasia
    (M8571/3)
  spindle cell metaplasia (M8572/3)
  squamous metaplasia (M8570/3)
acidophil (M8280/3)
  specified site—*see* Neoplasm, by site,
    malignant
  unspecified site 194.3

Adenocarcinoma—*continued*
acinar (M8550/3)
acinic cell (M8550/3)
adrenal cortical (M8370/3) 194.0
alveolar (M8251/3)
and
  epidermoid carcinoma, mixed (M8560/3)
  squamous cell carcinoma, mixed (M8560/3)
apocrine (M8401/3)
  breast—*see* Neoplasm, breast, malignant
  specified site NEC—*see* Neoplasm, skin,
    malignant
  unspecified site 173.99
basophil (M8300/3)
  specified site—*see* Neoplasm, by site,
    malignant
  unspecified site 194.3
  bile duct type (M8160/3)
  sliver 155.1
  specified site NEC—*see* Neoplasm, by site,
    malignant
  unspecified site 155.1
bronchiolar (M8250/3)—*see* Neoplasm, lung,
  malignant
ceruminous (M8420/3) 173.29
chromophobe (M8270/3)
  specified site—*see* Neoplasm, by site,
    malignant
  unspecified site 194.3
clear cell (mesonephroid type) (M8310/3)
colloid (M8480/3)
cylindroid type (M8200/3)
diffuse type (M8145/3)
  pecified site—*see* Neoplasm, by site,
    malignant
  unspecified site 151.9
duct (infiltrating) (M8500/3)
  with Paget's disease (M8541/3)—*see*
    Neoplasm, breast, malignant
  specified site—*see* Neoplasm, by site,
    malignant
  unspecified site 174.9
embryonal (M9070/3)
endometrioid (M8380/3)—*see* Neoplasm, by
  site, malignant
eosinophil (M8280/3)
  specified site—*see* Neoplasm, by site,
    malignant
  unspecified site 194.3
follicular (M8330/3)
  and papillary (M8340/3) 193
  moderately differentiated type (M8332/3) 193
  pure follicle type (M8331/3) 193
  specified site—*see* Neoplasm, by site,
    malignant
  trabecular type (M8332/3) 193
  unspecified type 193
  well differentiated type (M8331/3) 193
gelatinous (M8480/3)
granular cell (M8320/3)
Hürthle cell (M8290/3) 193
in
  adenomatous
    polyp (M8210/3)
    polyposis coli (M8220/3) 153.9
    polypoid adenoma (M8210/3)
    tubular adenoma (M8210/3)
    villous adenoma (M8261/3)
  infiltrating duct (M8500/3)
    with Paget's disease (M8541/3)—*see*
      Neoplasm, breast, malignant

Adenocarcinoma—*continued*
    specified site—*see* Neoplasm, by site,
        malignant
    unspecified site 174.9
    inflammatory (M8530/3)
    specified site—*see* Neoplasm, by site,
        malignant
    unspecified site 174.9
    in situ (M8140/2)—*see* Neoplasm, by site, in
        situ
    intestinal type (M8144/3)
    specified site—*see* Neoplasm, by site,
        malignant
    unspecified site 151.9
    intraductal (noninfiltrating) (M8500/2)
        papillary (M8503/2)
            specified site—*see* Neoplasm, by site, in situ
            unspecified site 233.0
        specified site—*see* Neoplasm, by site, in situ
        unspecified site 233.0
    islet cell (M8150/3)
        and exocrine, mixed (M8154/3)
            specified site—*see* Neoplasm, by site,
                malignant
            unspecified site 157.9
        pancreas 157.4
        specified site NEC—*see* Neoplasm, by site,
            malignant
        unspecified site 157.4
    lobular (M8520/3)
        specified site—*see* Neoplasm, by site,
            malignant
        unspecified site 174.9
    medullary (M8510/3)
    mesonephric (M9110/3)
    mixed cell (M8323/3)
    mucinous (M8480/3)
    mucin-producing (M8481/3)
    mucoid (M8480/3)—*see also* Neoplasm, by site,
        malignant
        cell (M8300/3)
            specified site—*see* Neoplasm, by site,
                malignant
            unspecified site 194.3
    nonencapsulated sclerosing (M8350/3) 193
    oncocytic (M8290/3)
    oxyphilic (M8290/3)
    papillary (M8260/3)
        and follicular (M8340/3) 193
        intraductal (noninfiltrating) (M8503/2)
            specified site—*see* Neoplasm, by site, in situ
            unspecified site 233.0
        serous (M8460/3)
            specified site—*see* Neoplasm, by site,
                malignant
            unspecified site 183.0
    papillocystic (M8450/3)
        specified site—*see* Neoplasm, by site,
            malignant
        unspecified site 183.0
    pseudomucinous (M8470/3)
        specified site—*see* Neoplasm, by site,
            malignant
        unspecified site 183.0
    renal cell (M8312/3) 189.0
    sebaceous (M8410/3)
    serous (M8441/3)—*see also* Neoplasm, by site,
        malignant
        papillary
            specified site—*see* Neoplasm, by site,
                malignant
            unspecified site 183.0

Adenocarcinoma—*continued*
    signet ring cell (M8490/3)
    superficial spreading (M8143/3)
    sweat gland (M8400/3)—*see* Neoplasm, skin,
        malignant
    trabecular (M8190/3)
    tubular (M8211/3)
    villous (M8262/3)
    water-clear cell (M8322/3) 194.1
Adenofibroma (M9013/0)
    clear cell (M8313/0)—*see* Neoplasm, by site,
        benign
    endometrioid (M8381/0) 220
        borderline malignancy (M8381/1) 236.2
        malignant (M8381/3) 183.0
    mucinous (M9015/0)
        specified site—*see* Neoplasm, by site, benign
        unspecified site 220
    prostate 600.20
        with other lower urinary tract symptoms
            (LUTS) 600.21
        with urinary
            obstruction 600.21
            retention 600.21
    serous (M9014/0)
        specified site—*see* Neoplasm, by site, benign
        unspecified site 220
    specified site—*see* Neoplasm, by site, benign
    unspecified site 220
Adenofibrosis
    breast 610.2
    endometrioid 617.0
Adenoiditis 474.01
    acute 463
    chronic 474.01
        with chronic tonsillitis 474.02
Adenoids (congenital) (of nasal fossa) 474.9
    hypertrophy 474.12
    vegetations 474.2
Adenolipomatosis (symmetrical) 272.8
Adenolymphoma (M8561/0)
    specified site—*see* Neoplasm, by site, benign
    unspecified site 210.2
Adenoma (sessile) (M8140/0)—*see also*
    Neoplasm, by site, benign

> *Note—Except where otherwise indicated, the*
> *morphological varieties of adenoma in the list*
> *below should be coded by site as for*
> *"Neoplasm, benign."*

    acidophil (M8280/0)
        specified site—*see* Neoplasm, by site, benign
        unspecified site 227.3
    acinar (cell) (M8550/0)
    acinic cell (M8550/0)
    adrenal (cortex) (cortical) (functioning)
        (M8370/0) 227.0
        clear cell type (M8373/0) 227.0
        compact cell type (M8371/0) 227.0
        glomerulosa cell type (M8374/0) 227.0
        heavily pigmented variant (M8372/0) 227.0
        mixed cell type (M8375/0) 227.0
    alpha cell (M8152/0)
        pancreas 211.7
        specified site NEC—*see* Neoplasm, by site,
            benign
        unspecified site 211.7
    alveolar (M8251/0)
    apocrine (M8401/0)
        breast 217

Adenoma—*continued*
  specified site NEC—*see* Neoplasm, skin,
    benign
  unspecified site 216.9
basal cell (M8147/0)
basophil (M8300/0)
  specified site—*see* Neoplasm, by site, benign
  unspecified site 227.3
beta cell (M8151/0)
  pancreas 211.7
  specified site NEC—*see* Neoplasm, by site,
    benign
  unspecified site 211.7
bile duct (M8160/0) 211.5
black (M8372/0) 227.0
bronchial (M8140/1) 235.7
  carcinoid type (M8240/3)—*see* Neoplasm,
    lung, malignant
  cylindroid type (M8200/3)—*see* Neoplasm,
    lung, malignant
ceruminous (M8420/0) 216.2
chief cell (M8321/0) 227.1
  chromophobe (M8270/0)
  (specified site—*see* Neoplasm, by site, benign
  unspecified site 227.3
clear cell (M8310/0)
colloid (M8334/0)
  specified site—*see* Neoplasm, by site, benign
  unspecified site 226
cylindroid type, bronchus (M8200/3)—*see*
    Neoplasm, lung, malignant
duct (M8503/0)
embryonal (M8191/0)
endocrine, multiple (M8360/1)
  single specified site—*see* Neoplasm, by site,
    uncertain behavior
  two or more specified sites 237.4
  unspecified site 237.4
endometrioid (M8380/0)—*see also* Neoplasm,
  by site, benign
  borderline malignancy (M8380/1)—*see*
    Neoplasm, by site, uncertain behavior
eosinophil (M8280/0)
  specified site—*see* Neoplasm, by site, benign
  unspecified site 227.3
fetal (M8333/0)
  specified site—*see* Neoplasm, by site, benign
  unspecified site 226
follicular (M8330/0)
  specified site—*see* Neoplasm, by site, benign
  unspecified site 226
hepatocellular (M8170/0) 211.5
Hürthle cell (M8290/0) 226
intracystic papillary (M8504/0)
islet cell (functioning) (M8150/0)
  pancreas 211.7
  specified site NEC—*see* Neoplasm, by site,
    benign
  unspecified site 211.7
liver cell (M8170/0) 211.5
macrofollicular (M8334/0)
  specified site NEC—*see* Neoplasm, by site,
    benign
  unspecified site 226
malignant, malignum (M8140/3)—*see*
    Neoplasm, by site, malignant
mesonephric (M9110/0)
microfollicular (M8333/0)
  specified site—*see* Neoplasm, by site, benign
  unspecified site 226
mixed cell (M8323/0)

Adenoma—*continued*
monomorphic (M8146/0)
mucinous (M8480/0)
mucoid cell (M8300/0)
  specified site—*see* Neoplasm, by site, benign
  unspecified site 227.3
multiple endocrine (M8360/1)
  single specified site—*see* Neoplasm, by site,
    uncertain behavior
  two or more specified sites 237.4
  unspecified site 237.4
nipple (M8506/0) 217
oncocytic (M8290/0)
oxyphilic (M8290/0)
papillary (M8260/0)—*see also* Neoplasm, by
  site, benign
  intracystic (M8504/0)
papillotubular (M8263/0)
Pick's tubular (M8640/0)
  specified site—*see* Neoplasm, by site, benign
  unspecified site
    female 220
    male 222.0
pleomorphic (M8940/0)
polypoid (M8210/0)
prostate (benign) 600.20
  with
    other lower urinary tract symptoms (LUTS)
      600.21
    urinary
      obstruction 600.21
      retention 600.21
rete cell 222.0
sebaceous, sebaceum (gland) (senile)
    (M8410/0)—*see also* Neoplasm, skin,
    benign
  disseminata 759.5
Sertoli cell (M8640/0)
  specified site—*see* Neoplasm, by site, benign
  unspecified site
    female 220
    male 222.0
skin appendage (M8390/0)—*see* Neoplasm,
  skin, benign
sudoriferous gland (M8400/0)—*see* Neoplasm,
  skin, benign
sweat gland or duct (M8400/0)—*see* Neoplasm,
  skin, benign
testicular (M8640/0)
  specified site—*see* Neoplasm, by site, benign
  unspecified site
    female 220
    male 222.0
thyroid 226
trabecular (M8190/0)
tubular (M8211/0)—*see also* Neoplasm, by site,
  benign
  papillary (M8460/3)
  Pick's (M8640/0)
    specified site—*see* Neoplasm, by site, benign
    unspecified site
      female 220
      male 222.0
tubulovillous (M8263/0)
villoglandular (M8263/0)
villous (M8261/1)—*see* Neoplasm, by site,
  uncertain behavior
water-clear cell (M8322/0) 227.1
wolffian duct (M9110/0)

Adenomatosis (M8220/0)
  endocrine (multiple) (M8360/1)
    single specified site—*see* Neoplasm, by site, uncertain behavior
    two or more specified sites 237.4
    unspecified site 237.4
  erosive of nipple (M8506/0) 217
  pluriendocrine—*see* Adenomatosis, endocrine
  pulmonary (M8250/1) 235.7
    malignant (M8250/3)—*see* Neoplasm, lung, malignant
    specified site—*see* Neoplasm, by site, benign
    unspecified site 211.3
Adenomatous
  cyst, thyroid (gland)—*see* Goiter, nodular
  goiter (nontoxic) (*see also* Goiter, nodular) 241.9
    toxic or with hyperthyroidism 242.3
Adenomyoma (M8932/0)—*see also* Neoplasm, by site, benign
  prostate 600.20
    with
      other lower urinary tract symptoms (LUTS) 600.21
      urinary
        obstruction 600.21
        retention 600.21
Adenomyometritis 617.0
Adenomyosis (uterus) (internal) 617.0
Adenopathy (lymph gland) 785.6
  inguinal 785.6
  mediastinal 785.6
  mesentery 785.6
  syphilitic (secondary) 091.4
    tracheobronchial 785.6
  tuberculous (*see also* Tuberculosis) 012.1
    primary, progressive 010.8
  tuberculous (*see also* Tuberculosis, lymph gland) 017.2
    primary, progressive 010.8
    tracheobronchial 012.1
    primary, progressive 010.8
Adenopharyngitis 462
Adenophlegmon 683
Adenosalpingitis 614.1
Adenosarcoma (M8960/3) 189.0
Adenosclerosis 289.3
Adenosis
  breast (sclerosing) 610.2
  vagina, congenital 752.49
Adentia (complete) (partial) (*see also* Absence, teeth) 520.0
Adherent
  labium (minus) 624.4
  pericardium (nonrheumatic) 423.1
    rheumatic 393
  placenta 667.0
    with hemorrhage 666.0
  prepuce 605
  scar (skin) NEC 709.2
  tendon in scar 709.2
Adhesion(s), adhesive (postinfectional)(postoperative)
  abdominal (wall) (*see also* Adhesions, peritoneum) 568.0
  amnion to fetus 658.8
    affecting fetus or newborn 762.8
  appendix 543.9
  arachnoiditis—*see* Meningitis
  auditory tube (Eustachian) 381.89
  bands—*see also* Adhesions, peritoneum
    cervix 622.3
    uterus 621.5

Adhesion(s)—*continued*
  bile duct (any) 576.8
  bladder (sphincter) 596.89
  bowel (*see also* Adhesions, peritoneum) 568.0
  cardiac 423.1
    rheumatic 398.99
  cecum (*see also* Adhesions, peritoneum) 568.0
  cervicovaginal 622.3
    congenital 752.49
    postpartal 674.8
    old 622.3
  cervix 622.3
  clitoris 624.4
  colon (*see also* Adhesions, peritoneum) 568.0
  common duct 576.8
  congenital—*see also* Anomaly, specified type NEC
    fingers (*see also* Syndactylism, fingers) 755.11
    labium (majus) (minus) 752.49
    omental, anomalous 751.4
    ovary 752.0
    peritoneal 751.4
    toes (*see also* Syndactylism, toes) 755.13
    tongue (to gum or roof of mouth) 750.12
  conjunctiva (acquired) (localized) 372.62
    congenital 743.63
    extensive 372.63
  cornea—*see* Opacity, cornea
  cystic duct 575.8
  diaphragm (*see also* Adhesions, peritoneum) 568.0
  due to foreign body—*see* Foreign body
  duodenum (*see also* Adhesions, peritoneum) 568.0
    with obstruction 537.3
  ear, middle—*see* Adhesions, middle ear
  epididymis 608.89
  epidural—*see* Adhesions, meninges
  epiglottis 478.79
  Eustachian tube 381.89
  eyelid 374.46
    postoperative 997.99
    surgically created V45.69
  gallbladder (*see also* Disease, gallbladder) 575.8
  globe 360.89
  heart 423.1
    rheumatic 398.99
  ileocecal (coil) (*see also* Adhesions, peritoneum) 568.0
  ileum (*see also* Adhesions, peritoneum) 568.0
  intestine (postoperative) (*see also* Adhesions, peritoneum) 568.0
    with obstruction 560.81
      with hernia—*see also* Hernia, by site, with obstruction
        gangrenous—*see* Hernia, by site, with gangrene
  intra-abdominal (*see also* Adhesions, peritoneum) 568.0
  iris 364.70
    to corneal graft 996.79
  joint (*see also* Ankylosis) 718.5
  kidney 593.89
  labium (majus) (minus), congenital 752.49
  liver 572.8
  lung 511.0
  mediastinum 519.3
  meninges 349.2
    cerebral (any) 349.2
      congenital 742.4
    congenital 742.8

Admission—*continued*
for —*continued*
  antineoplastic
    chemotherapy (oral) (intravenous) V58.11
    immunotherapy V58.12
  assisted reproductive fertility procedure cycle
    V26.81
  artificial insemination V26.1
  attention to artificial opening (of) V55.9
    artificial vagina V55.7
    colostomy V55.3
    cystostomy V55.5
    enterostomy V55.4
    gastrostomy V55.1
    ileostomy V55.2
    jejunostomy V55.4
    nephrostomy V55.6
    specified site NEC V55.8
      intestinal tract V55.4
      urinary tract V55.6
    tracheostomy V55.0
    ureterostomy V55.6
    urethrostomy V55.6
  battery replacement
    cardiac pacemaker V53.31
  blood typing V72.86
    Rh typing V72.86
  boarding V65.0
  breast
    augmentation or reduction V50.1
    implant exchange (different material)
      (different size) V52.4
    reconstruction following mastectomy V51.0
    removal
      prophylactic V50.41
      tissue expander without synchronous
        insertion of permanent implant V52.4
  change of
    cardiac pacemaker (battery) V53.31
    carotid sinus pacemaker V53.39
    catheter in artificial opening—*see* Attention
      to, artificial, opening
    drains V58.49
    dressing
      wound V58.30
        nonsurgical V58.30
        surgical V58.31
    fixation device
      external V54.89
      internal V54.01
    Kirschner wire V54.89
    neuropacemaker device (brain) (peripheral
      nerve) (spinal cord) V53.02
    nonsurgical wound dressing V58.30
    pacemaker device
      brain V53.02
      cardiac V53.31
      carotid sinus V53.39
      nervous system V53.02
    plaster cast V54.89
    splint, external V54.89
    Steinmann pin V54.89
    surgical wound dressing V58.31
    traction device V54.89
    wound packing V58.30
      nonsurgical V58.30
      surgical V58.31
  checkup only V70.0
  chemotherapy, (oral) (intravenous)
    antineoplastic V58.11
  circumcision, ritual or routine (in absence of
    medical indication) V50.2

Admission—*continued*
for —*continued*
  clinical research investigation (control)
    (normal comparison) (participant) V70.7
  closure of artificial opening—*see* Attention to,
    artificial, opening
  contraceptive
    counseling V25.09
      emergency V25.03
      postcoital V25.03
    management V25.9
      specified type NEC V25.8
  convalescence following V66.9
    chemotherapy V66.2
    psychotherapy V66.3
    radiotherapy V66.1
    surgery V66.0
    treatment (for) V66.5
      combined V66.6
      fracture V66.4
      mental disorder NEC V66.3
      specified condition NEC V66.5
  cosmetic surgery NEC V50.1
    breast reconstruction following mastectomy
      V51.0
    following healed injury or operation V51.8
  counseling (*see also* Counseling) V65.40
    without complaint or sickness V65.49
    contraceptive management V25.09
      emergency V25.03
      postcoital V25.03
    dietary V65.3
    exercise V65.41
    fertility preservation (prior to cancer
      therapy) (prior to surgical removal of
      gonads) V26.42
    for
      nonattending third party V65.19
      pediatric
        pre-adoption visit for adoptive parent(s)
          V65.11
        pre-birth visit for expectant parent(s)
          V65.11
      victim of abuse
        child V61.21
        partner or spouse V61.11
    genetic V26.33
    gonorrhea V65.45
    HIV V65.44
    human immunodeficiency virus V65.44
    injury prevention V65.43
    insulin pump training V65.46
    natural family planning
      procreative V26.41
      to avoid pregnancy V25.04
    procreative management V26.49
      using natural family planning V26.41
    sexually transmitted disease NEC V65.45
      HIV V65.44
    specified reason NEC V65.49
    substance use and abuse V65.42
    syphilis V65.45
    victim of abuse
      child V61.21
      partner or spouse V61.11
  desensitization to allergens V07.1
  dialysis V56.0
    catheter
      fitting and adjustment
        extracorporeal V56.1
        peritoneal V56.2

Admission—*continued*
  for —*continued*
    dialysis—*continued*
      removal or replacement
        extracorporeal V56.1
        peritoneal V56.2
      extracorporeal (renal) V56.0
      peritoneal V56.8
      renal V56.0
    dietary surveillance and counseling V65.3
    drug monitoring, therapeutic V58.83
    ear piercing V50.3
    elective surgery V50.9
      breast
        augmentation or reduction V50.1
        removal, prophylactic V50.41
        reconstruction following mastectomy
          V51.0
      circumcision, ritual or routine (in absence of
        medical indication) V50.2
      cosmetic NEC V50.1
        breast reconstruction following mastecomy
          V51.0
        following healed injury or operation V51.8
      ear piercing V50.3
      face-lift V50.1
      hair transplant V50.0
      plastic
        breast reconstruction following mastecomy
          V51.0
        cosmetic NEC V50.1
        following healed injury or operation V51.8
      prophylactic organ removal V50.49
        breast V50.41
        ovary V50.42
      repair of scarred tissue (following healed
        injury or operation) V51.8
      specified type NEC V50.8
    end-of-life care V66.7
    examination (*see also* Examination) V70.9
      administrative purpose NEC V70.3
      adoption V70.3
      allergy V72.7
      antibody response V72.61
      at health care facility V70.0
      athletic team V70.3
      camp V70.3
      cardiovascular, preoperative V72.81
      clinical research investigation (control)
        (participant) V70.7
      dental V72.2
      developmental testing (child) (infant) V20.2
      donor (potential) V70.8
      driver's license V70.3
      ear V72.19
      employment V70.5
      eye V72.0
      follow-up (routine)—*see* Examination,
        follow-up
      for admission to
        old age home V70.3
        school V70.3
      general V70.9
        specified reason NEC V70.8
      gynecological V72.31
      health supervision
        child (over 28 days old) V20.2
        infant (over 28 days old) V20.2
        newborn
          8 to 28 days old V20.32
          under 8 days old V20.31

Admission—*continued*
  for —*continued*
    examination—*continued*
      hearing V72.19
        following failed hearing screening V72.11
      immigration V70.3
      infant
        8 to 28 days old V20.32
        over 28 days old, routine V20.2
        under 8 days old V20.31
      insurance certification V70.3
      laboratory V72.60
        ordered as part of a routine general
          medical examination V72.62
        pre-operative V72.63
        pre-procedural V72.63
        specified NEC V72.69
      marriage license V70.3
      medical (general) (*see also* Examination,
        medical) V70.9
      medicolegal reasons V70.4
      naturalization V70.3
      pelvic (annual) (periodic) V72.31
      postpartum checkup V24.2
      pregnancy (possible) (unconfirmed) V72.40
        negative result V72.41
        positive result V72.42
      preoperative V72.84
        cardiovascular V72.81
        respiratory V72.82
        specified NEC V72.83
      preprocedural V72.84
        cardiovascular V72.81
        general physical V72.83
        respiratory V72.82
        specified NEC V72.83
      prior to chemotherapy V72.83
      prison V70.3
      psychiatric (general) V70.2
        requested by authority V70.1
      radiological NEC V72.5
      respiratory, preoperative V72.82
      school V70.3
      screening—*see* Screening
      skin hypersensitivity V72.7
      specified type NEC V72.85
      sport competition V70.3
      vision V72.0
      well baby and child care V20.2
    exercise therapy V57.1
    face-lift, cosmetic reason V50.1
    fertility preservation (prior to cancer therapy)
      (prior to surgical removal of gonads)
      V26.82
    fitting (of)
      artificial
        arm (complete) (partial) V52.0
        eye V52.2
        leg (complete) (partial) V52.1
      biliary drainage tube V58.82
      brain neuropacemaker V53.02
      breast V52.4
        implant V50.1
        prosthesis V52.4
      cardiac pacemaker V53.31
      catheter
        non-vascular V58.82
        vascular V58.81
      cerebral ventricle (communicating) shunt
        V53.01
      chest tube V58.82

Admission—*continued*
  for —*continued*
    fitting (of)—*continued*
      colostomy belt V53.5
      contact lenses V53.1
      cystostomy device V53.6
      dental prosthesis V52.3
      device, unspecified type V53.90
        abdominal V53.59
        cerebral ventricle (communicating) shunt
          V53.01
        gastrointestinal NEC V53.59
        insulin pump V53.91
        intestinal V53.50
        intrauterine contraceptive
          insertion V25.11
          removal V25.12
            and reinsertion V25.13
          replacement V25.13
        nervous system V53.09
        orthodontic V53.4
        other device V53.99
        prosthetic V52.9
          breast V52.4
          dental V52.3
          eye V52.2
        special senses V53.09
        substitution
          auditory V53.09
          nervous system V53.09
          visual V53.09
      diaphragm (contraceptive) V25.02
      fistula (sinus tract) drainage tube V58.82
      gastric lap band V53.51
      gastrointestinal appliance and device NEC
        V53.59
      growth rod V54.02
      hearing aid V53.2
      ileostomy device V53.5
      intestinal appliance and device V53.50
      intrauterine contraceptive device
        insertion V25.11
        removal V25.12
          and reinsertion V25.13
        replacement V25.13
      neuropacemaker (brain) (peripheral nerve)
        (spinal cord) V53.02
      orthodontic device V53.4
      orthopedic (device) V53.7
        brace V53.7
        cast V53.7
        shoes V53.7
      pacemaker
        brain V53.02
        cardiac V53.31
        carotid sinus V53.39
        spinal cord V53.02
      pleural drainage tube V58.82
      portacath V58.81
      prosthesis V52.9
        arm (complete) (partial) V52.0
        breast V52.4
        dental V52.3
        eye V52.2
        leg (complete) (partial) V52.1
        specified type NEC V52.8
      spectacles V53.1
      wheelchair V53.8
    follow-up examination (routine) (following)
      V67.9
      cancer chemotherapy V67.2
      chemotherapy V67.2

Admission—*continued*
  for —*continued*
    follow-up examination—*continued*
      high-risk medication NEC V67.51
      injury NEC V67.59
      psychiatric V67.3
      psychotherapy V67.3
      radiotherapy V67.1
      specified surgery NEC V67.09
        surgery V67.00
      treatment (for) V67.9
        combined V67.6
        fracture V67.4
        involving high-risk medication NEC
          V67.51
        mental disorder V67.3
        specified NEC V67.59
      vaginal pap smear V67.01
    hair transplant, for cosmetic reason V50.0
    health advice, education, or instruction V65.4
    hearing conservation and treatment V72.12
    hormone replacement therapy
      (postmenopausal) V07.4
    hospice care V66.7
    immunizations (childhood) appropriate for age
      V20.2
    immunotherapy, antineoplastic V58.12
    in vitro fertilization cycle V26.81
    insertion (of)
      intrauterine contraceptive device V25.11
      subdermal implantable contraceptive V25.5
    insulin pump titration V53.91
    insulin pump training V65.46
    intrauterine device
      insertion V25.11
      removal V25.12
        and reinsertion V25.13
      management V25.42
      replacement V25.13
    investigation to determine further disposition
      V63.8
    isolation V07.0
    issue of
      disability examination certificate V68.01
      medical certificate NEC V68.09
      repeat prescription NEC V68.1
        contraceptive device NEC V25.49
    kidney dialysis V56.0
    lengthening of growth rod V54.02
    mental health evaluation V70.2
      requested by authority V70.1
    natural family planning counseling and advice
      procreative V26.41
      to avoid pregnancy V25.04
    nonmedical reason NEC V68.89
    nursing care evaluation V63.8
    observation (without need for further medical
      care) (*see also* Observation) V71.9
      accident V71.4
      alleged rape or seduction V71.5
      criminal assault V71.6
      following accident V71.4
        at work V71.3
      foreign body ingestion V71.89
      growth and development variations,
        childhood V21.0
      inflicted injury NEC V71.6
      ingestion of deleterious agent or foreign
        body V71.89
      injury V71.6
      malignant neoplasm V71.1
      mental disorder V71.09

Admission—*continued*
　for —*continued*
　　observation—*continued*
　　　newborn—*see* Observation, suspected
　　　　condition, newborn
　　　rape V71.5
　　　specified NEC V71.89
　　　suspected
　　　　abuse V71.81
　　　　accident V71.4
　　　　　at work V71.3
　　　　benign neoplasm V71.89
　　　　cardiovascular V71.7
　　　　disorder V71.9
　　　　exposure
　　　　　anthrax V71.82
　　　　　biological agent NEC V71.83
　　　　　SARS V71.83
　　　　heart V71.7
　　　　inflicted injury NEC V71.6
　　　　malignant neoplasm V71.1
　　　　maternal and fetal problem not found
　　　　　amniotic cavity and membrane V89.01
　　　　　cervical shortening V89.05
　　　　　fetal anomaly V89.03
　　　　　fetal growth V89.04
　　　　　oligohydramnios V89.01
　　　　　other specified NEC V89.09
　　　　　placenta V89.02
　　　　　polyhydramnios V89.01
　　　　mental NEC V71.09
　　　　neglect V71.81
　　　　specified condition NEC V71.89
　　　　tuberculosis V71.2
　　　　tuberculosis V71.2
　　occupational therapy V57.21
　　organ transplant, donor—*see* Donor
　　ovary, ovarian removal, prophylactic V50.42
　　palliative care V66.7
　　Papanicolaou smear
　　　cervix V76.2
　　　　for suspected malignant neoplasm V76.2
　　　　　no disease found V71.1
　　　　routine, as part of gynecological
　　　　　examination V72.31
　　　　to confirm findings of recent normal smear
　　　　　following initial abnormal smear
　　　　　V72.32
　　　vaginal V76.47
　　　　following hysterectomy for malignant
　　　　　condition V67.01
　　passage of sounds or bougie in artificial
　　　opening—*see* Attention to, artificial, opening
　　paternity testing V70.4
　　peritoneal dialysis V56.8
　　physical therapy NEC V57.1
　　plastic surgery
　　　breast reconstruction following mastectomy
　　　　V51.0
　　　cosmetic NEC V50.1
　　　following healed injury or operation V51.8
　　postmenopausal hormone replacement therapy
　　　V07.4
　　postpartum observation
　　　immediately after delivery V24.0
　　　routine follow-up V24.2
　　poststerilization (for restoration) V26.0
　　procreative management V26.9
　　　assisted reproductive fertility procedure
　　　　cycle V26.81
　　　in vitro fertilization cycle V26.81
　　　specified type NEC V26.89

Admission—*continued*
　for —*continued*
　　prophylactic
　　　administration of
　　　　antibiotics, long-term V58.62
　　　　　short term use—*omit code*
　　　　antitoxin, any V07.2
　　　　antivenin V07.2
　　　　chemotherapeutic agent NEC V07.39
　　　　chemotherapy NEC V07.39
　　　　diphtheria antitoxin V07.2
　　　　fluoride V07.31
　　　　gamma globulin V07.2
　　　　immune sera (gamma globulin) V07.2
　　　　RhoGAM V07.2
　　　　tetanus antitoxin V07.2
　　　breathing exercises V57.0
　　　chemotherapy NEC V07.39
　　　fluoride V07.31
　　　measure V07.9
　　　　specified type NEC V07.8
　　　organ removal V50.49
　　　　breast V50.41
　　　　ovary V50.42
　　psychiatric examination (general) V70.2
　　　requested by authority V70.1
　　radiation management V58.0
　　radiotherapy V58.0
　　reconstruction following mastectomy V51.0
　　reforming of artificial opening—*see* Attention
　　　to, artificial, opening
　　rehabilitation V57.9
　　　multiple types V57.89
　　　occupational V57.21
　　　orthoptic V57.4
　　　orthotic V57.81
　　　physical NEC V57.1
　　　specified type NEC V57.89
　　　speech (-language) V57.3
　　　vocational V57.22
　　removal of
　　　breast tissue expander without synchronous
　　　　insertion of permanent implant V52.4
　　　cardiac pacemaker V53.31
　　　cast (plaster) V54.89
　　　catheter from artificial opening—*see*
　　　　Attention to, artificial, opening
　　　cerebral ventricle (communicating) shunt
　　　　V53.01
　　　cystostomy catheter V55.5
　　　device
　　　　cerebral ventricle (communicating) shunt
　　　　　V53.01
　　　　fixation
　　　　　external V54.89
　　　　　internal V54.01
　　　　intrauterine contraceptive V25.12
　　　　traction, external V54.89
　　　drains V58.49
　　　dressing
　　　　wound V58.30
　　　　　nonsurgical V58.30
　　　　　surgical V58.31
　　　fixation device
　　　　external V54.89
　　　　internal V54.01
　　　intrauterine contraceptive device V25.12
　　　Kirschner wire V54.89
　　　neuropacemaker (brain) (peripheral nerve)
　　　　(spinal cord) V53.02
　　　nonsurgical wound dressing V58.30

Admission—*continued*
  for —*continued*
    removal of—*continued*
      orthopedic fixation device
        external V54.89
        internal V54.01
      pacemaker device
        brain V53.02
        cardiac V53.31
        carotid sinus V53.39
        nervous system V53.02
      plaster cast V54.89
      plate (fracture) V54.01
      rod V54.01
      screw (fracture) V54.01
      splint, traction V54.89
      staples V58.32
      Steinmann pin V54.89
      subdermal implantable contraceptive V25.43
      surgical wound dressing V58.31
      sutures V58.32
      traction device, external V54.89
      ureteral stent V53.6
      wound packing V58.30
        nonsurgical V58.30
        surgical V58.31
    repair of scarred tissue (following healed
      injury or operation) V51.8
    replacement of intrauterine contraceptive
      device V25.13
    reprogramming of cardiac pacemaker V53.31
    respirator (ventilator) dependence
      during
        mechanical failure V46.14
        power failure V46.12
      for weaning V46.13
    restoration of organ continuity
      (poststerilization) (tuboplasty) (vasoplasty)
      V26.0
    Rh typing V72.86
    routine infant and child vision and hearing
      testing V20.2
    sensitivity test—*see also* Test, skin
      allergy NEC V72.7
      bacterial disease NEC V74.9
      Dick V74.8
      Kveim V82.89
      Mantoux V74.1
      mycotic infection NEC V75.4
      parasitic disease NEC V75.8
      Schick V74.3
      Schultz-Charlton V74.8
    social service (agency) referral or evaluation
      V63.8
    speech(-language) therapy V57.3
    sterilization V25.2
    suspected disorder (ruled out) (without need
      for further care)—*see* Observation
    terminal care V66.7
    tests only—*see* Test
    therapeutic drug monitoring V58.83
    therapy
      blood transfusion, without reported
        diagnosis V58.2
      breathing exercises V57.0
      chemotherapy, antineoplastic V58.11
        prophylactic NEC V07.39
          fluoride V07.31

Admission—*continued*
  for —*continued*
    therapy—*continued*
      dialysis (intermittent) (treatment)
        extracorporeal V56.0
        peritoneal V56.8
        renal V56.0
        specified type NEC V56.8
      exercise (remedial) NEC V57.1
        breathing V57.0
      immunotherapy, antineoplastic V58.12
      long-term (current) (prophylactic) drug use
        NEC V58.69
        antibiotics V58.62
          short-term use—*omit code*
        anticoagulants V58.61
        anti-inflammatories, non-steroidal
          (NSAID) V58.64
        antiplatelets V58.63
        antithrombotics V58.63
        aspirin V58.66
        bisphosphonates V58.68
        high-risk medications NEC V58.69
        insulin V58.67
        methadone for pain control V58.69
        opiate analgesic V58.69
        steroids V58.65
      occupational V57.21
      orthoptic V57.4
      physical NEC V57.1
      radiation V58.0
      speech(-language) V57.3
      vocational V57.22
    toilet or cleaning
      of artificial opening — *see* Attention to,
        artificial, opening
      of non-vascular catheter V58.82
      of vascular catheter V58.81
    treatment
      measure V07.9
        specified type NEC V07.8
    tubal ligation V25.2
    tuboplasty for previous sterilization V26.0
    ultrasound, routine fetal V28.3
    vaccination, prophylactic (against)
      arthropod-borne virus, viral NEC V05.1
        disease NEC V05.1
        encephalitis V05.0
      Bacille Calmette Guérin (BCG) V03.2
      BCG V03.2
      chickenpox V05.4
      cholera alone V03.0
        with typhoid-paratyphoid (cholera + TAB)
          V06.0
      common cold V04.7
      dengue V05.1
      diphtheria alone V03.5
      diphtheria-tetanus-pertussis (DTP) (DTaP)
        V06.1
        with
          poliomyelitis (DTP + polio) V06.3
          typhoid-paratyphoid (DTP + TAB)
            V06.2
      diphtheria-tetanus [Td] [DT] without
        pertussis V06.5
      disease (single) NEC V05.9
        bacterial NEC V03.9
          specified type NEC V03.89
        combinations NEC V06.9
          specified type NEC V06.8
        specified type NEC V05.8
        viral NEC V04.89

Admission—*continued*

for —*continued*

vaccination—*continued*

encephalitis, viral, arthropod-borne V05.0

Hemophilus influenzae, type B [Hib] V03.81

hepatitis, viral V05.3

human papillomavirus (HPV) V04.89

immune sera (gamma globulin) V07.2

influenza V04.81

with

Streptococcus pneumoniae [pneumococcus] V06.6

Leishmaniasis V05.2

measles alone V04.2

measles-mumps-rubella (MMR) V06.4

mumps alone V04.6

with measles and rubella (MMR) V06.4

not done because of contraindication V64.09

pertussis alone V03.6

plague V03.3

pneumonia V03.82

poliomyelitis V04.0

with diphtheria-tetanus-pertussis (DTP + polio) V06.3

rabies V04.5

respiratory syncytial virus (RSV) V04.82

rubella alone V04.3

with measles and mumps (MMR) V06.4

smallpox V04.1

specified type NEC V05.8

Streptococcus pneumoniae [pneumococcus] V03.82

with

influenza V06.6

tetanus toxoid alone V03.7

with diphtheria [Td] [DT] V06.5

and pertussis (DTP) (DTaP) V06.1

tuberculosis (BCG) V03.2

tularemia V03.4

typhoid alone V03.1

with diphtheria-tetanus-pertussis (TAB + DTP) V06.2

typhoid-paratyphoid alone (TAB) V03.1

typhus V05.8

varicella V05.4

viral encephalitis, arthropod-borne V05.0

viral hepatitis V05.3

yellow fever V04.4

vasectomy V25.2

vasoplasty for previous sterilization V26.0

vision examination V72.0

vocational therapy V57.22

waiting period for admission to other facility V63.2

undergoing social agency investigation V63.8

well baby and child care V20.2

x-ray of chest

for suspected tuberculosis V71.2

routine V72.5

Adnexitis (suppurative) (*see also* Salpingo-oophoritis) 614.2

Adolescence NEC V21.2

Adoption

agency referral V68.89

examination V70.3

held for V68.89

Adrenal gland —*see* condition

Adrenalism 255.9

tuberculous (*see also* Tuberculosis) 017.6

Adrenalitis, adrenitis 255.8

meningococcal hemorrhagic 036.3

Adrenarche, precocious 259.1

Adrenocortical syndrome 255.2

Adrenogenital syndrome (acquired) (congenital) 255.2

iatrogenic, fetus or newborn 760.79

Adrenoleukodystrophy 277.86

neonatal 277.86

x-linked 277.86

Adrenomyeloneuropathy 277.86

Adventitious bursa —*see* Bursitis

Adynamia (episodica) (hereditary) (periodic) 359.3

Adynamic

ileus or intestine (*see also* ileus) 560.1

ureter 753.22

Aeration lung imperfect, newborn 770.5

Aerobullosis 993.3

Aerocele —*see* Embolism, air

Aerodermectasia

subcutaneous (traumatic) 958.7

surgical 998.81

surgical 998.81

Aerodontalgia 993.2

Aeroembolism 993.3

Aerogenes capsulatus infection (*see also* Gangrene, gas) 040.0

Aero-otitis media 993.0

Aerophagy, aerophagia 306.4

psychogenic 306.4

Aerosinusitis 993.1

Aerotitis 993.0

Affection, affections —*see also* Disease

sacroiliac (joint), old 724.6

shoulder region NEC 726.2

Afibrinogenemia 286.3

acquired 286.6

congenital 286.3

postpartum 666.3

African

sleeping sickness 086.5

tick fever 087.1

trypanosomiasis 086.5

Gambian 086.3

Rhodesian 086.4

Aftercare V58.9

amputation stump V54.89

artificial openings—*see* Attention to, artificial, opening

blood transfusion without reported diagnosis V58.2

breathing exercise V57.0

cardiac device V53.39

defibrillator, automatic implantable (with synchronous cardiac pacemaker) V53.32

pacemaker V53.31

carotid sinus V53.39

carotid sinus pacemaker V53.39

cerebral ventricle (communicating) shunt V53.01

chemotherapy (oral) (intravenous) session (adjunctive) (maintenance) V58.11

defibrillator, automatic implantable cardiac (with synchronous cardiac pacemaker) V53.32

exercise (remedial) (therapeutic) V57.1

breathing V57.0

extracorporeal dialysis (intermittent) (treatment) V56.0

Aftercare—*continued*
  following surgery NEC V58.49
    wound closure, planned V58.41
    for
      injury V58.43
      neoplasm V58.42
      organ transplant V58.44
      trauma V58.43
    joint
      explantation of prosthesis (staged procedure)
        V54.82
      replacement V54.81
    of
      circulatory system V58.73
      digestive system V58.75
      genital organs V58.76
      genitourinary system V58.76
      musculoskeletal system V58.78
      nervous system V58.72
      oral cavity V58.75
      respiratory system V58.74
      sense organs V58.71
      skin V58.77
      subcutaneous tissue V58.77
      teeth V58.75
      urinary system V58.76
    spinal —*see* Aftercare, following surgery, of,
      specified body system
  fracture V54.9
    healing V54.89
      pathologic
        ankle V54.29
        arm V54.20
          lower V54.22
          upper V54.21
        finger V54.29
        foot V54.29
        hand V54.29
        hip V54.23
        leg V54.24
          lower V54.26
          upper V54.25
        pelvis V54.29
        specified site NEC V54.29
        toe(s) V54.29
        vertebrae V54.27
        wrist V54.29
      traumatic
        ankle V54.19
        arm V54.10
          lower V54.12
          upper V54.11
        finger V54.19
        foot V54.19
        hand V54.19
        hip V54.13
        leg V54.14
          lower V54.16
          upper V54.15
        pelvis V54.19
        specified site NEC V54.19
        toe(s) V54.19
        vertebrae V54.17
        wrist V54.19
    removal of
      external fixation device V54.89
      internal fixation device V54.01
    specified care NEC V54.89
  gait training V57.1
    for use of artificial limb(s) V57.81
  internal fixation device V54.09

Aftercare—*continued*
  involving
    dialysis (intermittent) (treatment)
      extracorporeal V56.0
      peritoneal V56.8
      renal V56.0
    gait training V57.1
      for use of artificial limb(s) V57.81
    growth rod
      adjustment V54.02
      lengthening V54.02
    internal fixation device V54.09
    orthoptic training V57.4
    orthotic training V57.81
    radiotherapy session V58.0
    removal of
      drains V58.49
      dressings
        wound V58.30
          nonsurgical V58.30
          surgical V58.31
      fixation device
        external V54.89
        internal V54.01
      fracture plate V54.01
      nonsurgical wound dressing V58.30
      pins V54.01
      plaster cast V54.89
      rods V54.01
      screws V54.01
      staples V58.32
      surgical wound dressings V58.31
      sutures V58.32
      traction device, external V54.89
      wound packing V58.30
        nonsurgical V58.30
        surgical V58.31
  neuropacemaker (brain) (peripheral nerve)
    (spinal cord) V53.02
  occupational therapy V57.21
  orthodontic V58.5
  orthopedic V54.9
    change of external fixation or traction device
      V54.8
    following joint
      explantation of prosthesis (staged procedure)
        V54.82
      replacement V54.81
    internal fixation device V54.09
    removal of fixation device
      external V54.89
      internal V54.01
    specified care NEC V54.89
  orthoptic training V57.4
  orthotic training V57.81
  pacemaker
    brain V53.02
    cardiac V53.31
    carotid sinus V53.39
    peripheral nerve V53.02
    spinal cord V53.02
  peritoneal dialysis (intermittent) (treatment)
    V56.8
  physical therapy NEC V57.1
    breathing exercises V57.0
  radiotherapy session V58.0
  rehabilitation procedure V57.9
    breathing exercises V57.0
    multiple types V57.89
    occupational V57.21
    orthoptic V57.4

Aftercare—*continued*
rehabilitation procedure—*continued*
orthotic V57.81
physical therapy NEC V57.1
remedial exercises V57.1
specified type NEC V57.89
speech(-language) V57.3
therapeutic exercises V57.1
vocational V57.22
renal dialysis (intermittent) (treatment) V56.0
specified type NEC V58.89
removal of non-vascular catheter V58.82
removal of vascular catheter V58.81
speech(-language) therapy V57.3
stump, amputation V54.89
vocational rehabilitation V57.22
After-cataract 366.50
obscuring vision 366.53
specified type, not obscuring vision 366.52
Agalactia 676.4
Agammaglobulinemia 279.00
with lymphopenia 279.2
acquired (primary) (secondary) 279.06
Bruton's X-linked 279.04
infantile sex-linked (Bruton's) (congenital)
279.04
Swiss-type 279.2
Aganglionosis (bowel) (colon) 751.3
Age (old) (*see also* Senile) 797
Agenesis —*see also* Absence, by site, congenital
acoustic nerve 742.8
adrenal (gland) 759.1
alimentary tract (complete) (partial) NEC 751.8
lower 751.2
upper 750.8
anus, anal (canal) 751.2
aorta 747.22
appendix 751.2
arm (complete) (partial) (*see also* Deformity,
reduction, upper limb) 755.20
artery (peripheral) NEC (*see also* Anomaly,
peripheral vascular system) 747.60
brain 747.81
coronary 746.85
pulmonary 747.31
umbilical 747.5
auditory (canal) (external) 744.01
auricle (ear) 744.01
bile, biliary duct or passage 751.61
bone NEC 756.9
brain 740.0
specified part 742.2
breast 757.6
bronchus 748.3
canaliculus lacrimalis 743.65
carpus NEC (*see also* Deformity, reduction,
upper limb) 755.28
cartilage 756.9
cecum 751.2
cerebellum 742.2
cervix 752.43
chin 744.89
cilia 743.63
circulatory system, part NEC 747.89
clavicle 755.51
clitoris 752.49
coccyx 756.13
colon 751.2
corpus callosum 742.2
diaphragm (with hernia) 756.6

Agenesis—*continued*
digestive organ(s) or tract (complete) (partial)
NEC 751.8
lower 751.2
upper 750.8
ductus arteriosus 747.89
duodenum 751.1
ear NEC 744.09
auricle 744.01
lobe 744.21
ejaculatory duct 752.89
endocrine (gland) NEC 759.2
epiglottis 748.3
esophagus 750.3
Eustachian tube 744.24
extrinsic muscle, eye 743.69
eye 743.00
adnexa 743.69
eyelid (fold) 743.62
face
bones NEC 756.0
specified part NEC 744.89
fallopian tube 752.19
femur NEC (*see also* Absence, femur,
congenital) 755.34
fibula NEC (*see also* Absence, fibula,
congenital) 755.37
finger NEC (*see also* Absence, finger,
congenital) 755.29
foot (complete) (*see also* Deformity, reduction,
lower limb) 755.31
gallbladder 751.69
gastric 750.8
genitalia, genital (organ)
female 752.89
external 752.49
internal NEC 752.89
male 752.89
penis 752.69
glottis 748.3
gonadal 758.6
hair 757.4
hand (complete) (*see also* Deformity, reduction,
upper limb) 755.21
heart 746.89
valve NEC 746.89
aortic 746.89
mitral 746.89
pulmonary 746.01
hepatic 751.69
humerus NEC (*see also* Absence, humerus,
congenital) 755.24
hymen 752.49
ileum 751.1
incus 744.04
intestine (small) 751.1
large 751.2
iris (dilator fibers) 743.45
jaw 524.09
jejunum 751.1
kidney(s) (partial) (unilateral) 753.0
labium (majus) (minus) 752.49
labyrinth, membranous 744.05
lacrimal apparatus (congenital) 743.65
larynx 748.3
leg NEC (*see also* Deformity, reduction, lower
limb) 755.30
lens 743.35
limb (complete) (partial) (*see also* Deformity,
reduction) 755.4
lower NEC 755.30
upper 755.20

Agranulocytosis (see also Neutropenia) 288.09
  chronic 288.09
  cyclical 288.02
  due to infection 288.04
  genetic 288.01
  infantile 288.01
  periodic 288.02
  pernicious 288.09
Agraphia (absolute) 784.69
  with alexia 784.61
  developmental 315.39
Agrypnia (*see also* Insomnia) 780.52
Ague (*see also* Malaria) 084.6
  brass-founders' 985.8
  dumb 084.6
  tertian 084.1
Agyria 742.2
AHTR (acute hemolytic transfusion reaction)
  —*see* Complications, transfusion
Ahumada-del Castillo syndrome (nonpuerperal
  galactorrhea and amenorrhea) 253.1
AIDS 042
AIDS-associated retrovirus (disease) (illness) 042
  infection—*see* Human immunodeficiency virus,
    infection
AIDS-associated virus (disease) (illness) 042
  infection—*see* Human immunodeficiency virus,
    infection
AIDS-like disease (illness) (syndrome) 042
AIDS-related complex 042
AIDS-related conditions 042
AIDS-related virus (disease) (illness) 042
  infection—*see* Human immunodeficiency virus,
    infection
AIDS virus (disease) (illness) 042
  infection—*see* Human immunodeficiency virus,
    infection
Ailment, heart —*see* Disease, heart
Ailurophobia 300.29
AIN I (anal intraepithelial neoplasia I)
  (histologically confirmed) 569.44
AIN II (anal intraepithelial neoplasia II)
  (histologically confirmed) 569.44
AIN III (anal intraepithelial neoplasia III)
  230.6
  anal canal 230.5
Ainhum (disease) 136.0
AIPHI (acute idiopathic pulmonary hemorrhage
  in infants (over 28 days old)) 786.31
Air
  anterior mediastinum 518.1
  compressed, disease 993.3
  embolism (any site) (artery) (cerebral) 958.0
    with
      abortion—*see* Abortion, by type, with
        embolism
      ectopic pregnancy (*see also* categories
        633.0-633.9) 639.6
      molar pregnancy (*see also* categories
        630-632) 639.6
    due to implanted device—*see* Complications,
      due to (presence of) any device, implant,
      or graft classified to 996.0-996.5 NEC
    following
      abortion 639.6
      ectopic or molar pregnancy 639.6
    infusion, perfusion, or transfusion 999.1
    in pregnancy, childbirth, or puerperium 673.0
    traumatic 958.0
  hunger 786.09
    psychogenic 306.1

Air —*continued*
  leak (lung) (pulmonary) (thorax) 512.84
    iatrogenic 512.1
    persistant 512.84
    postoperative 512.2
  rarefied, effects of—*see* Effect, adverse, high altitude
  sickness 994.6
Airplane sickness 994.6
Akathisia, acathisia 781.0
  due to drugs 333.99
  neuroleptic-induced acute 333.99
Akinesia algeria 352.6
Akiyami 100.89
Akureyri disease (epidemic neuromyasthenia) 049.8
Alacrima (congenital) 743.65
Alactasia (hereditary) 271.3
Alagille syndrome 759.89
Alalia 784.3
  developmental 315.31
    receptive-expressive 315.32
  secondary to organic lesion 784.3
Alaninemia 270.8
Alastrim 050.1
Albarrán's disease (colibacilluria) 791.9
Albers-Schönberg's disease (marble bones)
  756.52
Albert's disease 726.71
Albinism, albino (choroid) (cutaneous) (eye)
  (generalized) (isolated) (ocular)
  (oculocutaneous) (partial) 270.2
Albinismus 270.2
Albright (-Martin) (-Bantam) disease
  (pseudohypoparathyroidism) 275.49
Albright (-McCune) (-Sternberg) syndrome
  (osteitis fibrosa disseminata) 756.59
Albuminous —*see* condition
Albuminuria, albuminuric (acute) (chronic)
  (subacute) 791.0
  Bence-Jones 791.0
  cardiac 785.9
  complicating pregnancy, childbirth, or
    puerperium 646.2
    with hypertension—*see* Toxemia, of
      pregnancy
    affecting fetus or newborn 760.1
  cyclic 593.6
  gestational 646.2
  gravidarum 646.2
    with hypertension—*see* Toxemia, of
      pregnancy
    affecting fetus or newborn 760.1
  heart 785.9
  idiopathic 593.6
  orthostatic 593.6
  postural 593.6
  pre-eclamptic (mild) 642.4
    affecting fetus or newborn 760.0
    severe 642.5
      affecting fetus or newborn 760.0
  recurrent physiologic 593.6
  scarlatinal 034.1
Albumosuria 791.0
  Bence-Jones 791.0
  myelopathic (M9730/3) 203.0
Alcaptonuria 270.2
Alcohol, alcoholic
  abstinence 291.81
  acute intoxication 305.0
    with dependence 303.0

Alcohol, alcoholic—*continued*
　addiction (*see also* Alcoholism) 303.9
　　maternal
　　　with suspected fetal damage affecting
　　　　management of pregnancy 655.4
　　　affecting fetus or newborn 760.71
　amnestic disorder, persisting 291.1
　anxiety 291.89
　brain syndrome, chronic 291.2
　cardiopathy 425.5
　chronic (*see also* Alcoholism) 303.9
　cirrhosis (liver) 571.2
　delirium 291.0
　　acute 291.0
　　chronic 291.1
　　tremens 291.0
　　withdrawal 291.0
　dementia NEC 291.2
　deterioration 291.2
　drunkenness (simple) 305.0
　hallucinosis (acute) 291.3
　induced
　　circadian rhythm sleep disorder 291.82
　　hypersomnia 291.82
　　insomnia 291.82
　　mental disorder 291.9
　　　anxiety 291.89
　　　mood 291.89
　　　sexual 291.89
　　　sleep 291.82
　　　specified type 291.89
　　parasomnia 291.82
　　persisting
　　　amnestic disorder 291.1
　　　dementia 291.2
　　psychotic disorder
　　　with
　　　　delusions 291.5
　　　　hallucinations 291.3
　　sleep disorder 291.82
　insanity 291.9
　intoxication (acute) 305.0
　　with dependence 303.0
　　pathological 291.4
　jealousy 291.5
　Korsakoff's, Korsakov's, Korsakow's 291.1
　liver NEC 571.3
　　acute 571.1
　　chronic 571.2
　mania (acute) (chronic) 291.9
　mood 291.89
　paranoia 291.5
　paranoid (type) psychosis 291.5
　pellagra 265.2
　poisoning, accidental (acute) NEC 980.9
　　specified type of alcohol—*see* Table of drugs
　　　and chemicals
　psychosis (*see also* Psychosis, alcoholic) 291.9
　　Korsakoff's, Korsakov's, Korsakow's 291.1
　　polyneuritic 291.1
　　with
　　　delusions 291.5
　　　hallucinations 291.3
　related disorder 291.9
　withdrawal symptoms, syndrome NEC 291.81
　　delirium 291.0
　　hallucinosis 291.3

Alcoholism 303.9

> *Note*—*Use the following fifth-digit*
> *subclassification with category 303:*
>
> *0　unspecifhed*
> *1　continuous*
> *2　episodic*
> *3　in remission*

　with psychosis (*see also* Psychosis, alcoholic)
　　291.9
　acute 303.0
　chronic 303.9
　　with psychosis 291.9
　complicating pregnancy, childbirth, or
　　puerperium 648.4
　　affecting fetus or newborn 760.71
　history V11.3
　Korsakoff's, Korsakov's, Korsakow's 291.1
　suspected damage to fetus affecting
　　management of pregnancy 655.4
Alder's anomaly or syndrome (leukocyte
　granulation anomaly) 288.2
Alder-Reilly anomaly (leukocyte granulation) 288.2
Aldosteronism (primary) 255.10
　congenital 255.10
　familial type I 255.11
　glucocorticoid-remediable 255.11
　secondary 255.14
Aldosteronoma (M8370/1) 237.2
Aldrich (-Wiskott) syndrome
　(eczema-thrombocytopenia) 279.12
Aleppo boil 085.1
Aleukemic —*see* condition
Aleukia
　congenital 288.09
　hemorrhagica 284.9
　　acquired (secondary) 284.89
　　congenital 284.09
　　idiopathic 284.9
　splenica 289.4
Alexia (congenital) (developmental) 315.01
　secondary to organic lesion 784.61
Algoneurodystrophy 733.7
Algophobia 300.29
Alibert's disease (mycosis fungoides) (M9700/3)
　202.1
Alibert-Bazin disease (M9700/3) 202.1
Alice in Wonderland syndrome 293.89
Alienation, mental (*see also* Psychosis) 298.9
Alkalemia 276.3
Alkalosis 276.3
　metabolic 276.3
　　with respiratory acidosis 276.4
　respiratory 276.3
Alkaptonuria 270.2
Allen-Masters syndrome 620.6
Allergic bronchopulmonary aspergillosis 518.6
Allergy, allergic (reaction) 995.3
　air-borne substance (*see also* Fever, hay) 477.9
　　specified allergen NEC 477.8
　alveolitis (extrinsic) 495.9
　　due to
　　　Aspergillus clavatus 495.4
　　　cryptostroma corticale 495.6
　　　organisms (fungal, thermophilic
　　　　actinomycete, other) growing in
　　　　ventilation (air conditioning systems)
　　　　495.7
　　　specified type NEC 495.8

Allergy, allergic—*continued*
  anaphylactic reaction or shock 995.0
    due to
      food—*see* Anaphylactic reaction or shock,
        due to, food
  angioedema 995.1
  angioneurotic edema 995.1
  animal (cat) (dog) (epidermal) 477.8
    dander 477.2
    hair 477.2
  arthritis (*see also* Arthritis, allergic) 716.2
  asthma—*see* Asthma
  bee sting (anaphylactic shock) 989.5
  biological—*see* Allergy, drug
  bronchial asthma—*see* Asthma
  conjunctivitis (eczematous) 372.14
  dander, animal (cat) (dog) 477.2
  dandruff 477.8
  dermatitis (venenata)—*see* Dermatitis
  diathesis V15.09
  drug, medicinal substance, and biological (any)
    (correct medicinal substance properly
    administered) (external) (internal) 995.27
    wrong substance given or taken NEC 977.9
      specified drug or substance—*see* Table of
        drugs and chemicals
  dust (house) (stock) 477.8
  eczema—*see* Eczema
  endophthalmitis 360.19
  epidermal (animal) 477.8
  existing dental restorative material 525.66
  feathers 477.8
  food (any) (ingested) 693.1
    atopic 691.8
    in contact with skin 692.5
  gastritis 535.4
  gastroenteritis 558.3
  gastrointestinal 558.3
  grain 477.0
  grass (pollen) 477.0
    asthma (*see also* Asthma) 493.0
    hay fever 477.0
  hair, animal (cat) (dog) 477.2
  hay fever (grass) (pollen) (ragweed) (tree) (*see*
    also Fever, hay) 477.9
  history (of) V15.09
    to
      arachnid bite V15.06
      eggs V15.03
      food additives V15.05
      insect bite V15.06
      latex V15.07
      milk products V15.02
      nuts V15.05
        peanuts V15.01
      radiographic dye V15.08
      seafood V15.04
      specified food NEC V15.05
      spider bite V15.06
  horse serum—*see* Allergy, serum
  inhalant 477.9
    dust 477.8
    pollen 477.0
    specified allergen other than pollen 477.8
  kapok 477.8
  medicine—*see* Allergy, drug
  migraine 339.00
  milk protein 558.3
  pannus 370.62
  pneumonia 518.3

Allergy, allergic—*continued*
  pollen (any) (hay fever) 477.0
    asthma (*see also* Asthma) 493.0
  primrose 477.0
  primula 477.0
  purpura 287.2
  ragweed (pollen) (Senecio jacobae) 477.0
    asthma (*see also* Asthma) 493.0
    hay fever 477.0
  respiratory (*see also* Allergy, inhalant) 477.9
    due to
      drug—*see* Allergy, drug
      food—*see* Allergy, food
  rhinitis (*see also* Fever, hay) 477.9
    due to food 477.1
  rose 477.0
  Senecio jacobae 477.0
  serum (prophylactic) (therapeutic) 999.59
    anaphylactic reaction or shock 999.49
  shock (anaphylactic)
    due to
      adverse effect of correct medicinal substance
        properly administered 995.0
      food—*see* Anaphylactic reaction or shock,
        due to, food
    from
      administration of blood products 999.41
      immunization 999.42
      serum NEC 999.49
  sinusitis (*see also* Fever, hay) 477.9
  skin reaction 692.9
    specified substance—*see* Dermatitis, due to
  tree (any) (hay fever) (pollen) 477.0
    asthma (*see also* Asthma) 493.0
  upper respiratory (*see also* Fever, hay) 477.9
  urethritis 597.89
  urticaria 708.0
  vaccine—*see* Allergy, serum
Allescheriosis 117.6
Alligator skin disease (ichthyosis congenita) 757.1
  acquired 701.1
Allocheiria, allochiria (*see also* Disturbance,
  sensation) 782.0
Almeida's disease (Brazilian blastomycosis) 116.1
Alopecia (atrophicans) (pregnancy) (premature)
  (senile) 704.00
  adnata 757.4
  areata 704.01
  celsi 704.01
  cicatrisata 704.09
  circumscripta 704.01
  congenital, congenitalis 757.4
  disseminata 704.01
  effluvium (telogen) 704.02
  febrile 704.09
  generalisata 704.09
  hereditaria 704.09
  marginalis 704.01
  mucinosa 704.09
  postinfectional 704.09
  seborrheica 704.09
  specific 091.82
  syphilitic (secondary) 091.82
  telogen effluvium 704.02
  totalis 704.09
  toxica 704.09
  universalis 704.09
  x-ray 704.09
Alper's disease 330.8
Alpha-lipoproteinemia 272.4
Alpha thalassemia 282.43
Alphos 696.1

Alpine sickness 993.2
Alport's syndrome (hereditary
hematuria-nephropathy-deafness) 759.89
**ALPS (autoimmune lymphoproliferative
syndrome)** 279.41
ALTE (apparent life threatening event) in
newborn and infant 799.82
Alteration (of), altered
awareness 780.09
transient 780.02
consciousness 780.09
persistent vegetative state 780.03
transient 780.02
mental status 780.97
amnesia (retrograde) 780.93
memory loss 780.93
Alternaria (infection) 118
Alternating —*see* condition
Altitude, high (effects)—*see* Effect, adverse,
high altitude
Aluminosis (of lung) 503
Alvarez syndrome (transient cerebral ischemia) 435.9
Alveolar capillary block syndrome 516.64
Alveolitis
allergic (extrinsic) 495.9
due to organisms (fungal, thermophilic
actinomycete, other) growing in ventilation
(air conditioning systems) 495.7
specified type NEC 495.8
due to
Aspergillus clavatus 495.4
Cryptostroma corticale 495.6
fibrosing (chronic) (cryptogenic) (lung) 516.31
idiopathic 516.30
rheumatoid 714.81
jaw 526.5
sicca dolorosa 526.5
Alveolus, alveolar —*see* condition
Alymphocytosis (pure) 279.2
Alymphoplasia, thymic 279.2
Alzheimer's
dementia (senile)
with behavioral disturbance 331.0 *[294.11]*
without behavioral disturbance 331.0 *[294.10]*
disease or sclerosis 331.0
with dementia—*see* Alzheimer's, dementia
Amastia (*see also* Absence, breast) 611.89
Amaurosis (acquired) (congenital) (*see also*
Blindness) 369.00
fugax 362.34
hysterical 300.11
Leber's (congenital) 362.76
tobacco 377.34
uremic—*see* Uremia
Amaurotic familial idiocy (infantile) (juvenile)
(late) 330.1
Ambisexual 752.7
Amblyopia (acquired) (congenital) (partial) 368.00
color 368.59
acquired 368.55
deprivation 368.02
ex anopsia 368.00
hysterical 300.11
nocturnal 368.60
vitamin A deficiency 264.5
refractive 368.03
strabismic 368.01
suppression 368.01
tobacco 377.34
toxic NEC 377.34
uremic—*see* Uremia

Ameba, amebic (histolytica)–*see also* Amebiasis
abscess 006.3
bladder 006.8
brain (with liver and lung abscess) 006.5
liver 006.3
with brain abscess (and lung abscess) 006.5
with lung abscess 006.4
lung (with liver abscess) 006.4
with brain abscess 006.5
seminal vesicle 006.8
spleen 006.8
carrier (suspected of) V02.2
meningoencephalitis
due to Naegleria (gruberi) 136.29
primary 136.29
Amebiasis NEC 006.9
with
brain abscess (with liver or lung abscess) 006.5
liver abscess (without mention of brain or lung
abscess) 006.3
lung abscess (with liver abscess) 006.4
with brain abscess 006.5
acute 006.0
bladder 006.8
chronic 006.1
cutaneous 006.6
cutis 006.6
due to organism other than Entamoeba
histolytica 007.8
hepatic (*see also* Abscess, liver, amebic) 006.3
nondysenteric 006.2
seminal vesicle 006.8
specified
organism NEC 007.8
site NEC 006.8
Ameboma 006.8
Amelia 755.4
lower limb 755.31
upper limb 755.21
Ameloblastoma (M9310/0) 213.1
jaw (bone) (lower) 213.1
upper 213.0
long bones (M9261/3)—*see* Neoplasm, bone,
malignant
malignant (M9310/3) 170.1
jaw (bone) (lower) 170.1
upper 170.0
mandible 213.1
tibial (M9261/3) 170.7
Amelogenesis imperfecta 520.5
nonhereditaria (segmentalis) 520.4
Amenorrhea (primary) (secondary) 626.0
due to ovarian dysfunction 256.8
hyperhormonal 256.8
Amentia (*see also* Disability, intellectual) 319
Meynert's (nonalcoholic) 294.0
alcoholic 291.1
nevoid 759.6
American
leishmaniasis 085.5
mountain tick fever 066.1
trypanosomiasis—*see* Trypanosomiasis,
American
Ametropia (*see also* Disorder, accommodation) 367.9
Amianthosis 501
Amimia 784.69
Amino acid
deficiency 270.9
anemia 281.4
metabolic disorder (*see also* Disorder, amino
acid) 270.9

Aminoaciduria 270.9
  imidazole 270.5
Amnesia (retrograde) 780.93
  auditory 784.69
    developmental 315.31
    secondary to organic lesion 784.69
  dissociative 300.12
  hysterical or dissociative type 300.12
  psychogenic 300.12
  transient global 437.7
Amnestic (confabulatory) syndrome 294.0
  alcohol-induced persisting 291.1
  drug-induced persisting 292.83
  posttraumatic 294.0
Amniocentesis screening (for) V28.2
  alphafetoprotein level, raised V28.1
  chromosomal anomalies V28.0
Amnion, amniotic —*see also* condition
  nodosum 658.8
Amnionitis (complicating pregnancy) 658.4
  affecting fetus or newborn 762.7
Amoral trends 301.7
Amotio retinae (*see also* Detachment, retina) 361.9
Ampulla
  lower esophagus 530.89
  phrenic 530.89
Amputation
  any part of fetus, to facilitate delivery 763.89
  cervix (supravaginal) (uteri) 622.8
    in pregnancy or childbirth 654.6
      affecting fetus or newborn 763.89
  clitoris—*see* Wound, open, clitoris
  congenital
    lower limb 755.31
    upper limb 755.21
  neuroma (traumatic)—*see also* Injury, nerve, by
    site
  surgical complications (late) 997.61
  penis—*see* Amputation, traumatic, penis
  status (without complication)—*see* Absence, by
    site, acquired
  stump (surgical)(posttraumatic)
    abnormal, painful, or with complication (late)
      997.60
    healed or old NEC —*see also* Absence, by
      site, acquired
      lower V49.70
      upper V49.60
  traumatic (complete) (partial)

Note—*"Complicated" includes traumatic
amputation with delayed healing, delayed
treatment, foreign body, or infection.*

  arm 887.4
    at or above elbow 887.2
      complicated 887.3
    below elbow 887.0
      complicated 887.1
    both (bilateral) (any level(s)) 887.6
      complicated 887.7
    complicated 887.5
    finger(s) (one or both hands) 886.0
      with thumb(s) 885.0
        complicated 885.1
      complicated 886.1
    foot (except toe(s) only) 896.0
      and other leg 897.6
        complicated 897.7
      both (bilateral) 896.2
        complicated 896.3
      complicated 896.1

Amputation—*continued*
    toe(s) only (one or both feet) 895.0
      complicated 895.1
    genital organ(s) (external) NEC 878.8
      complicated 878.9
    hand (except finger(s) only) 887.0
      and other arm 887.6
        complicated 887.7
      both (bilateral) 887.6
        complicated 887.7
      complicated 887.1
    finger(s) (one or both hands) 886.0
      with thumb(s) 885.0
        complicated 885.1
      complicated 886.1
    thumb(s) (with fingers of either hand) 885.0
      complicated 885.1
    head 874.9
    late effect—*see* Late, effects (of), amputation
    leg 897.4
      and other foot 897.6
        complicated 897.7
      at or above knee 897.2
        complicated 897.3
      below knee 897.0
        complicated 897.1
      both (bilateral) 897.6
        complicated 897.7
      complicated 897.5
    lower limb(s) except toe(s)—*see* Amputation,
      traumatic, leg
    nose—*see* Wound, open, nose
    penis 878.0
      complicated 878.1
    sites other than limbs—*see* Wound, open, by site
    thumb(s) (with finger(s) of either hand) 885.0
      complicated 885.1
    toe(s) (one or both feet) 895.0
      complicated 895.1
    upper limb(s)—*see* Amputation, traumatic, arm
Amputee (bilateral) (old) —*see also* Absence, by
  site, acquired V49.70
Amusia 784.69
  developmental 315.39
  secondary to organic lesion 784.69
Amyelencephalus 740.0
Amyelia 742.59
Amygdalitis— *see* Tonsillitis
Amygdalolith 474.8
Amyloid disease or degeneration 277.30
  heart 277.39 [425.7]
Amyloidosis (familial) (general) (generalized)
  (genetic) (primary) 277.30
  with lung involvement 277.39 [517.8]
  cardiac, hereditary 277.39
  heart 277.39 [425.7]
  nephropathic 277.39 [583.81]
  neuropathic (Portuguese) (Swiss) 277.39
    [357.4]
  pulmonary 277.39 [517.8]
  secondary 277.39
  systemic, inherited 277.39
Amylopectinosis (brancher enzyme deficiency)
  271.0
Amylophagia 307.52
Amyoplasia, congenita 756.89
Amyotonia 728.2
  congenita 358.8

Amyotrophia, amyotrophy, amyotrophic 728.2
congenita 756.89
diabetic 250.6 *[353.5]*
due to secondary diabetes 249.6 *[353.5]*
lateral sclerosis (syndrome) 335.20
neuralgic 353.5
sclerosis (lateral) 335.20
spinal progressive 335.21
Anacidity
gastric 536.0
psychogenic 306.4
Anaerosis of newborn 770.88
Analbuminemia 273.8
Analgesia (*see also* Anesthesia) 782.0
Analphalipoproteinemia 272.5
Anaphylactic reaction or shock (correct
substance properly administered) 995.0
due to
administration of blood and blood products
999.41
chemical - *see* Table of Drugs and Chemicals
correct medicinal substance properly
administered 995.0
drug or medicinal substance
correct substance properly administered
995.0
overdose or wrong substance given or taken
977.9
specified drug - *see* Table of Drugs and
Chemicals
following sting(s) 989.5
food 995.60
additives 995.66
crustaceans 995.62
eggs 995.68
fish 995.65
fruits 995.63
milk products 995.67
nuts (tree) 995.64
peanuts 995.61
*see*ds 995.64
specified NEC 995.69
tree nuts 995.64
vegetables 995.63
immunization 999.42
overdose or wrong substance given or taken
977.9
specified drug—*see* Table of drugs and
chemicals
serum NEC 999.49
following sting(s) 989.5
purpura 287.0
serum NEC 999.49
Anaphylactoid reaction or shock —*see*
Anaphylactic reaction or shock
Anaphylaxis —*see* Anaphylactic reaction or
shock
Anaplasia, cervix 622.10
Anaplasmosis, human 082.49
Anarthria 784.51
Anarthritic rheumatoid disease 446.5
Anasarca 782.3
cardiac (*see also* Failure, heart) 428.0
fetus or newborn 778.0
lung 514
nutritional 262
pulmonary 514
renal (*see also* Nephrosis) 581.9
Anaspadias 752.62

Anastomosis
aneurysmal—*see* Aneurysm
arteriovenous, congenital NEC (*see also*
Anomaly, arteriovenous) 747.60
ruptured, of brain (*see also* Hemorrhage,
subarachnoid) 430
intestinal 569.89
complicated NEC 997.49
involving urinary tract 997.5
retinal and choroidal vessels 743.58
acquired 362.17
Anatomical narrow angle (glaucoma) 365.02
Ancylostoma (infection) (infestation) 126.9
americanus 126.1
braziliense 126.2
caninum 126.8
ceylanicum 126.3
duodenale 126.0
Necator americanus 126.1
Ancylostomiasis (intestinal) 126.9
Ancylostoma
americanus 126.1
caninum 126.8
ceylanicum 126.3
duodenale 126.0
braziliense 126.2
Necator americanus 126.1
Anders' disease or syndrome (adiposis tuberosa
simplex) 272.8
Andersen's glycogen storage disease 271.0
Anderson's disease 272.7
Andes disease 993.2
Andrews' disease (bacterid) 686.8
Androblastoma (M8630/1)
benign (M8630/0)
specified site—*see* Neoplasm, by site, benign
unspecified site
female 220
male 222.0
malignant (M8630/3)
specified site—*see* Neoplasm, by site,
malignant
unspecified site
female 183.0
male 186.9
specified site—*see* Neoplasm, by site, uncertain
behavior
tubular (M8640/0)
with lipid storage (M8641/0)
specified site—*see* Neoplasm, by site,
benign
unspecified site
female 220
male 222.0
specified site—*see* Neoplasm, by site, benign
unspecified site
female 220
male 222.0
unspecified site
female 236.2
male 236.4
Android pelvis 755.69
with disproportion (fetopelvic) 653.3
affecting fetus or newborn 763.1
causing obstructed labor 660.1
affecting fetus or newborn 763.1
Anectasis, pulmonary (newborn or fetus) 770.5

Anemia 285.9
in
  chronic illness NEC 285.29
  chronic kidney disease 285.21
  end-stage renal disease 285.21
  neoplastic disease 285.22
with
  disorder of
    anaerobic glycolysis 282.3
    pentose phosphate pathway 282.2
  koilonychia 280.9
6-phosphogluconic dehydrogenase deficiency
  282.2
achlorhydric 280.9
achrestic 281.8
Addison's (pernicious) 281.0
Addison-Biermer (pernicious) 281.0
agranulocytic 288.09
amino acid deficiency 281.4
antineoplastic chemotherapy induced 285.3
aplastic 284.9
  acquired (secondary) 284.89
  congenital 284.01
  constitutional 284.01
  due to
    antineoplastic chemotherapy 284.89
    chronic systemic disease 284.89
    drugs 284.89
    infection 284.89
    radiation 284.89
  idiopathic 284.9
  myxedema 244.9
  of or complicating pregnancy 648.2
  red cell (acquired) (adult) (with thymoma)
    284.81
    congenital 284.01
    pure 284.01
  specified type NEC 284.89
  toxic (paralytic) 284.89
aregenerative 284.9
  congenital 284.01
asiderotic 280.9
atypical (primary) 285.9
autohemolysis of Selwyn and Dacie (type I)
  282.2
autoimmune hemolytic 283.0
Baghdad Spring 282.2
Balantidium coli 007.0
Biermer's (pernicious) 281.0
blood loss (chronic) 280.0
  acute 285.1
bothriocephalus 123.4
brickmakers' (*see also* Ancylostomiasis) 126.9
cerebral 437.8
childhood 282.9
chlorotic 280.9
chronica congenita aregenerativa 284.01
chronic 285.9
  blood loss 280.0
  hemolytic 282.9
    idiopathic 283.9
  simple 281.9
combined system disease NEC 281.0 *[336.2]*
  due to dietary deficiency 281.1 *[336.2]*
complicating pregnancy or childbirth 648.2
congenital (following fetal blood loss) 776.5
  aplastic 284.01
  due to isoimmunization NEC 773.2
  Heinz-body 282.7
  hereditary hemolytic NEC 282.9

Anemia—*continued*
congenital—*continued*
  nonspherocytic
    Type I 282.2
    Type II 282.3
  pernicious 281.0
  spherocytic (*see also* Spherocytosis) 282.0
Cooley's (erythroblastic) 282.44
crescent—*see* Disease, sickle-cell
cytogenic 281.0
Dacie's (nonspherocytic)
  Type I 282.2
  Type II 282.3
Davidson's (refractory) 284.9
deficiency 281.9
  2, 3 diphosphoglycurate mutase 282.3
  2, 3 PG 282.3
  6-PGD 282.2
  6-phosphogluronic dehydrogenase 282.2
  amino acid 281.4
  combined B_{12} and folate 281.3
  enzyme, drug-induced (hemolytic) 282.2
  erythrocytic glutathione 282.2
  folate 281.2
    dietary 281.2
    drug-induced 281.2
  folic acid 281.2
    dietary 281.2
    drug-induced 281.2
  G-6-PD 282.2
  GGS-R 282.2
  glucose-6-phosphate dehydrogenase (G-6-PD)
    282.2
  glucose-phosphate isomerase 282.3
  glutathione peroxidase 282.2
  glutathione reductase 282.2
  glyceraldehyde phosphate dehydrogenase
    282.3
  GPI 282.3
  G SH 282.2
  hexokinase 282.3
  iron (Fe) 280.9
    specified NEC 280.8
  nutritional 281.9
    with
      poor iron absorption 280.9
      specified deficiency NEC 281.8
    due to inadequate dietary iron intake 280.1
    specified type NEC 281.8
  of or complicating pregnancy 648.2
  pentose phosphate pathway 282.2
  PFK 282.3
  phosphofructo-aldolase 282.3
  phosphofructokinase 282.3
  phosphoglycerate kinase 282.3
  PK 282.3
  protein 281.4
  pyruvate kinase (PK) 282.3
    TPI 282.3
    triosephosphate isomerase 282.3
    vitamin B_{12} NEC 281.1
      dietary 281.1
      pernicious 281.0
Diamond-Blackfan (congenital hypoplastic)
  284.01
dibothriocephalus 123.4
dimorphic 281.9
diphasic 281.8
diphtheritic 032.89
Diphyllobothrium 123.4

Anemia—*continued*
  hemolytic—*continued*
    type II 282.3
    type I 282.2
    type II 282.3
    of or complicating pregnancy 648.2
    resulting from presence of shunt or other
        internal prosthetic device 283.19
    secondary 283.19
      autoimmune 283.0
    sickle-cell—*see* Disease, sickle-cell
    Stransky-Regala type (Hb-E) (*see also*
        Disease, hemoglobin) 282.7
    symptomatic 283.19
      autoimmune 283.0
    toxic (acquired) 283.19
    uremic (adult) (child) 283.11
    warm type (secondary) (symptomatic) 283.0
  hemorrhagic (chronic) 280.0
    acute 285.1
  HEMPAS 285.8
  hereditary erythroblast multinuclearity- positive
      acidified serum test 285.8
  Herrick's (hemoglobin S disease) 282.61
  hexokinase deficiency 282.3
  high A$_2$ 282.46
  hookworm (*see also* Ancylostomiasis) 126.9
  hypochromic (idiopathic) (microcytic)
      (normoblastic) 280.9
    with iron loading 285.0
    due to blood loss (chronic) 280.0
      acute 285.1
    familial sex linked 285.0
    pyridoxine-responsive 285.0
  hypoplasia, red blood cells 284.81
    congenital or familial 284.01
  hypoplastic (idiopathic) 284.9
    congenital 284.01
    familial 284.01
    of childhood 284.09
  idiopathic 285.9
    hemolytic, chronic 283.9
  infantile 285.9
  infective, infectional 285.9
  intertropical (*see also* Ancylostomiasis) 126.9
  iron (Fe) deficiency 280.9
    due to blood loss (chronic) 280.0
      acute 285.1
    of or complicating pregnancy 648.2
    specified NEC 280.8
  Jaksch's (pseudoleukemia infantum) 285.8
  Joseph-Diamond-Blackfan (congenital
      hypoplastic) 284.01
  labyrinth 386.50
  Lederer's (acquired infectious hemolytic
      anemia) 283.19
  leptocytosis (hereditary) 282.40
  leukoerythroblastic 284.2
  macrocytic 281.9
    nutritional 281.2
    of or complicating pregnancy 648.2
    tropical 281.2
  malabsorption (familial), selective B$_{12}$ with
      proteinuria 281.1
  malarial (*see also* Malaria) 084.6
  malignant (progressive) 281.0
  malnutrition 281.9
  marsh (*see also* Malaria) 084.6
  Mediterranean 282.40
    with hemoglobinopathy 282.49

Anemia—*continued*
  megaloblastic 281.9
    combined B$_{12}$ and folate deficiency 281.3
    nutritional (of infancy) 281.2
    of infancy 281.2
    of or complicating pregnancy 648.2
    refractory 281.3
    specified NEC 281.3
  megalocytic 281.9
  microangiopathic hemolytic 283.19
  microcytic (hypochromic) 280.9
    due to blood loss (chronic) 280.0
      acute 285.1
    familial 282.49
    hypochromic 280.9
  microdrepanocytosis 282.41
  miners' (*see also* Ancylostomiasis) 126.9
  myelopathic 285.8
  myelophthisic (normocytic) 284.2
  newborn (*see also* Disease, hemolytic) 773.2
    due to isoimmunization (*see also* Disease,
        hemolytic) 773.2
    late, due to isoimmunization 773.5
    posthemorrhagic 776.5
  nonregenerative 284.9
  nonspherocytic hemolytic—*see* Anemia,
      hemolytic, nonspherocytic
  normocytic (infectional) (not due to blood loss)
      285.9
    due to blood loss (chronic) 280.0
      acute 285.1
    myelophthisic 284.2
  nutritional (deficiency) 281.9
    with
      poor iron absorption 280.9
      specified deficiency NEC 281.8
    due to inadequate dietary iron intake 280.1
    megaloblastic (of infancy) 281.2
  of childhood 282.9
  of chronic
    disease NEC 285.29
    illness NEC 285.29
  of or complicating pregnancy 648.2
    affecting fetus or newborn 760.8
  of prematurity 776.6
  orotic aciduric (congenital) (hereditary) 281.4
  osteosclerotic 289.89
  ovalocytosis (hereditary) (*see also*
      Elliptocytosis) 282.1
  paludal (*see also* Malaria) 084.6
  pentose phosphate pathway deficiency 282.2
  pernicious (combined system disease)
      (congenital) (dorsolateral spinal
      degeneration) (juvenile) (myelopathy)
      (neuropathy) (posterior sclerosis) (primary)
      (progressive) (spleen) 281.0
    of or complicating pregnancy 648.2
  pleochromic 285.9
    of sprue 281.8
  portal 285.8
  posthemorrhagic (chronic) 280.0
    acute 285.1
    newborn 776.5
  postoperative
    due to (acute) blood loss 285.1
      chronic blood loss 280.0
    other 285.9
  postpartum 648.2
  pressure 285.9
  primary 285.9
  profound 285.9

Anemia—*continued*
progressive 285.9
  malignant 281.0
  pernicious 281.0
protein-deficiency 281.4
pseudoleukemica infantum 285.8
puerperal 648.2
pure red cell 284.81
  congenital 284.01
pyridoxine-responsive (hypochromic) 285.0
pyruvate kinase (PK) deficiency 282.3
refractoria sideroblastica 238.72
refractory (primary) 238.72
  with
    excess
      blasts-1 (RAEB-1) 238.72
      blasts-2 (RAEB-2) 238.73
    hemochromatosis 238.72
    ringed sideroblasts (RARS) 238.72
  due to
    drug 285.0
    myelodysplastic syndrome 238.72
    toxin 285.0
  hereditary 285.0
  idiopathic 238.72
  megaloblastic 281.3
  sideroblastic 238.72
    hereditary 285.0
  sideropenic 280.9
Rietti-Greppi-Micheli (thalassemia minor) 282.46
scorbutic 281.8
secondary (to) 285.9
  blood loss (chronic) 280.0
    acute 285.1
  hemorrhage 280.0
    acute 285.1
  inadequate dietary iron intake 280.1
semiplastic 284.9
septic 285.9
sickle-cell (*see also* Disease, sickle-cell) 282.60
sideroachrestic 285.0
sideroblastic (acquired) (any type) (congenital)
    (drug-induced) (due to disease) (hereditary)
    (primary) (secondary) (sex-linked
    hypochromic) (vitamin B$_6$ responsive) 285.0
  refractory 238.72
    congenital 285.0
    drug-induced 285.0
    hereditary 285.0
    sex-linked hypochromic 285.0
    vitamin B$_6$-responsive 285.0
  sideropenic (refractory) 280.9
    due to blood loss (chronic) 280.0
      acute 285.1
simple chronic 281.9
specified type NEC 285.8
spherocytic (hereditary) (*see also* Spherocytosis) 282.0
splenic 285.8
  familial (Gaucher's) 272.7
splenomegalic 285.8
stomatocytosis 282.8
syphilitic 095.8
target cell (oval) 285.8
  with thalassemia —*see* Thalassemia
thalassemia 282.40
thrombocytopenic (*see also* Thrombocytopenia) 287.5
toxic 284.89
triosephosphate isomerase deficiency 282.3

Anemia—*continued*
tropical, macrocytic 281.2
tuberculous (*see also* Tuberculosis) 017.9
vegan's 281.1
vitamin
  B$_6$-responsive 285.0
  B$_{12}$ deficiency (dietary) 281.1
    pernicious 281.0
von Jaksch's (pseudoleukemia infantum) 285.8
Witts' (achlorhydric anemia) 280.9
Zuelzer (-Ogden) (nutritional megaloblastic anemia) 281.2
Anencephalus, anencephaly 740.0
fetal, affecting management of pregnancy 655.0
Anergasia (*see also* Psychosis, organic) 294.9
senile 290.0
Anesthesia, anesthetic 782.0
complication or reaction NEC 995.22
  due to
    correct substance properly administered 995.22
    overdose or wrong substance given 968.4
      specified anesthetic—*see* Table of drugs and chemicals
  cornea 371.81
  death from
    correct substance properly administered 995.4
    during delivery 668.9
    overdose or wrong substance given 968.4
      specified anesthetic—*see* Table of drugs and chemicals
  eye 371.81
  functional 300.11
  hyperesthetic, thalamic 338.0
  hysterical 300.11
  local skin lesion 782.0
  olfactory 781.1
  sexual (psychogenic) 302.72
  shock
    due to
      correct substance properly administered 995.4
      overdose or wrong substance given 968.4
      specified anesthetic—*see* Table of drugs and chemicals
  skin 782.0
  tactile 782.0
  testicular 608.9
  thermal 782.0
Anetoderma (maculosum) 701.3
Aneuploidy NEC 758.5
Aneurin deficiency 265.1
Aneurysm (anastomotic) (artery) (cirsoid)
    (diffuse) (false) (fusiform) (multiple)
    (ruptured) (saccular) (varicose) 442.9
abdominal (aorta) 441.4
  ruptured 441.3
  syphilitic 093.0
aorta, aortic (nonsyphilitic) 441.9
  abdominal 441.4
    dissecting 441.02
    ruptured 441.3
    syphilitic 093.0
  arch 441.2
    ruptured 441.1
  arteriosclerotic NEC 441.9
    ruptured 441.5
  ascending 441.2
    ruptured 441.1
  congenital 747.29

Aneurysm—*continued*
aorta—*continued*
  descending 441.9
    abdominal 441.4
      ruptured 441.3
      ruptured 441.5
    thoracic 441.2
      ruptured 441.1
    dissecting 441.00
      abdominal 441.02
      thoracic 441.01
      thoracoabdominal 441.03
    due to coarctation (aorta) 747.10
    ruptured 441.5
    sinus, right 747.29
    syphilitic 093.0
    thoracoabdominal 441.7
      ruptured 441.6
    thorax, thoracic (arch) (nonsyphilitic) 441.2
      dissecting 441.01
      ruptured 441.1
      syphilitic 093.0
    transverse 441.2
      ruptured 441.1
    valve (heart) (*see also* Endocarditis, aortic)
        424.1
  arteriosclerotic NEC 442.9
    cerebral 437.3
      ruptured (*see also* Hemorrhage,
        subarachnoid) 430
  arteriovenous (congenital) (peripheral) NEC
      (*see also* Anomaly, arteriovenous) 747.32
    acquired NEC 447.0
      brain 437.3
        ruptured (*see also* Hemorrhage,
          subarachnoid) 430
      coronary 414.11
      pulmonary 417.0
    brain (cerebral) 747.81
      ruptured (*see also* Hemorrhage,
        subarachnoid) 430
    coronary 746.85
    pulmonary 747.3
    retina 743.58
    specified site NEC 747.89
      acquired 447.0
    traumatic (*see also* Injury, blood vessel, by
      site) 904.9
  basal—*see* Aneurysm, brain
  berry (congenital) (ruptured) (*see also*
      Hemorrhage, subarachnoid) 430
    nonruptured 437.3
  brain 437.3
    arteriosclerotic 437.3
      ruptured (*see also* Hemorrhage,
        subarachnoid) 430
    arteriovenous 747.81
      acquired 437.3
        ruptured (*see also* Hemorrhage,
          subarachnoid) 430
      ruptured (*see also* Hemorrhage,
        subarachnoid) 430
    berry (congenital) (ruptured) (*see also*
        Hemorrhage, subarachnoid) 430
      nonruptured 437.3
    congenital 747.81
      ruptured (*see also* Hemorrhage,
        subarachnoid) 430
    meninges 437.3
      ruptured (*see also* Hemorrhage,
        subarachnoid) 430

Aneurysm—*continued*
brain—*continued*
  miliary (congenital) (ruptured) (*see also*
      Hemorrhage, subarachnoid) 430
  mycotic 421.0
    ruptured (*see also* Hemorrhage,
      subarachnoid) 430
  nonruptured 437.3
  ruptured (*see also* Hemorrhage, subarachnoid)
      430
    syphilitic 094.87
  syphilitic (hemorrhage) 094.87
  traumatic—*see* Injury, intracranial
cardiac (false) (*see also* Aneurysm, heart)
    414.10
carotid artery (common) (external) 442.81
  internal (intracranial portion) 437.3
    extracranial portion 442.81
    ruptured into brain (*see also* Hemorrhage,
      subarachnoid) 430
  syphilitic 093.89
  intracranial 094.87
cavernous sinus (*see also* Aneurysm, brain)
    437.3
  arteriovenous 747.81
    ruptured (*see also* Hemorrhage,
      subarachnoid) 430
  congenital 747.81
    ruptured (*see also* Hemorrhage,
      subarachnoid) 430
celiac 442.84
central nervous system, syphilitic 094.89
cerebral—*see* Aneurysm, brain
chest—*see* Aneurysm, thorax
circle of Willis (*see also* Aneurysm, brain)
    437.3
  congenital 747.81
    ruptured (*see also* Hemorrhage,
      subarachnoid) 430
  ruptured (*see also* Hemorrhage, subarachnoid)
      430
common iliac artery 442.2
congenital (peripheral) NEC 747.60
  brain 747.81
    ruptured (*see also* Hemorrhage,
      subarachnoid) 430
  cerebral—*see* Aneurysm, brain, congenital
  coronary 746.85
  gastrointestinal 747.61
  lower limb 747.64
  pulmonary 747.32
  renal 747.62
  retina 743.58
  specified site NEC 747.89
  spinal 747.82
  upper limb 747.63
conjunctiva 372.74
conus arteriosus (*see also* Aneurysm, heart) 414.10
coronary (arteriosclerotic) (artery) (vein) (*see
    also* Aneurysm, heart) 414.11
  arteriovenous 746.85
  congenital 746.85
  syphilitic 093.89
cylindrical 441.9
  ruptured 441.5
  syphilitic 093.9
dissecting 442.9
  aorta 441.00
    abdominal 441.02
    thoracic 441.01
    thoracoabdominal 441.03
  syphilitic 093.9

Aneurysm—*continued*
ductus arteriosus 747.0
embolic—*see* Embolism, artery
endocardial, infective (any valve) 421.0
femoral 442.3
gastroduodenal 442.84
gastroepiploic 442.84
heart (chronic or with a stated duration of over 8 weeks) (infectional) (wall) 414.10
  acute or with a stated duration of 8 weeks or less (*see also* Infarct, myocardium) 410.9
  congenital 746.89
  valve—*see* Endocarditis
hepatic 442.84
iliac (common) 442.2
infective (any valve) 421.0
innominate (nonsyphilitic) 442.89
  syphilitic 093.89
interauricular septum (*see also* Aneurysm, heart) 414.10
interventricular septum (*see also* Aneurysm, heart) 414.10
intracranial—*see* Aneurysm, brain
intrathoracic (nonsyphilitic) 441.2
  ruptured 441.1
  syphilitic 093.0
jugular vein (acute) 453.89
  chronic 453.76
lower extremity 442.3
lung (pulmonary artery) 417.1
malignant 093.9
mediastinal (nonsyphilitic) 442.89
  syphilitic 093.89
miliary (congenital) (ruptured) (*see also* Hemorrhage, subarachnoid) 430
mitral (heart) (valve) 424.0
mural (arteriovenous) (heart) (*see also* Aneurysm, heart) 414.10
mycotic, any site 421.0
  ruptured, brain (*see also* Hemorrhage, subarachnoid) 430
  without endocarditis —*see* Aneurysm, by site
myocardium (*see also* Aneurysm, heart) 414.10
neck 442.81
pancreaticoduodenal 442.84
patent ductus arteriosus 747.0
peripheral NEC 442.89
  congenital NEC (*see also* Aneurysm, congenital) 747.60
popliteal 442.3
pulmonary 417.1
  arteriovenous 747.32
    acquired 417.0
  syphilitic 093.89
  valve (heart) (*see also* Endocarditis, pulmonary) 424.3
racemose 442.9
  congenital (peripheral) NEC 747.60
radial 442.0
Rasmussen's (*see also* Tuberculosis) 011.2
renal 442.1
retinal (acquired) 362.17
  congenital 743.58
  diabetic 250.5 *[362.01]*
    due to secondary diabetes 249.5 *[362.01]*
sinus, aortic (of Valsalva) 747.29
specified site NEC 442.89
spinal (cord) 442.89
  congenital 747.82
  syphilitic (hemorrhage) 094.89
spleen, splenic 442.83

Aneurysm—*continued*
subclavian 442.82
  syphilitic 093.89
superior mesenteric 442.84
syphilitic 093.9
  aorta 093.0
  central nervous system 094.89
  congenital 090.5
  spine, spinal 094.89
thoracoabdominal 441.7
  ruptured 441.6
thorax, thoracic (arch) (nonsyphilitic) 441.2
  dissecting 441.01
  ruptured 441.1
  syphilitic 093.0
traumatic (complication) (early)—*see* Injury, blood vessel, by site
tricuspid (heart) (valve)—*see* Endocarditis, tricuspid
ulnar 442.0
upper extremity 442.0
valve, valvular—*see* Endocarditis
venous 456.8
  congenital NEC (*see also* Aneurysm, congenital) 747.60
ventricle (arteriovenous) (*see also* Aneurysm, heart) 414.10
visceral artery NEC 442.84
Angiectasis 459.89
Angiectopia 459.9
Angiitis 447.6
allergic granulomatous 446.4
hypersensitivity 446.20
  Goodpasture's syndrome 446.21
  specified NEC 446.29
necrotizing 446.0
Wegener's (necrotizing respiratory granulomatosis) 446.4
Angina (attack) (cardiac) (chest) (effort) (heart) (pectoris) (syndrome) (vasomotor) 413.9
abdominal 557.1
accelerated 411.1
agranulocytic 288.03
aphthous 074.0
catarrhal 462
crescendo 411.1
croupous 464.4
cruris 443.9
  due to atherosclerosis NEC (*see also* Arteriosclerosis, extremities) 440.20
decubitus 413.0
diphtheritic (membranous) 032.0
equivalent 413.9
erysipelatous 034.0
erythematous 462
exudative, chronic 476.0
faucium 478.29
gangrenous 462
  diphtheritic 032.0
infectious 462
initial 411.1
intestinal 557.1
ludovici 528.3
Ludwig's 528.3
malignant 462
  diphtheritic 032.0
membranous 464.4
  diphtheritic 032.0
mesenteric 557.1
monocytic 075
nocturnal 413.0

Angina—*continued*
  phlegmonous 475
    diphtheritic 032.0
  preinfarctional 411.1
  Prinzmetal's 413.1
  progressive 411.1
  pseudomembranous 101
  psychogenic 306.2
  pultaceous, diphtheritic 032.0
  scarlatinal 034.1
  septic 034.0
  simple 462
  stable NEC 413.9
  staphylococcal 462
  streptococcal 034.0
  stridulous, diphtheritic 032.3
  syphilitic 093.9
    congenital 090.5
  tonsil 475
  trachealis 464.4
  unstable 411.1
  variant 413.1
  Vincent's 101
Angioblastoma (M9161/1)—*see* Neoplasm,
  connective tissue, uncertain behavior
Angiocholecystitis (*see also* Cholecystitis, acute)
  575.0
Angiocholitis (*see also* Cholecystitis, acute) 576.1
Angiodysgensis spinalis 336.1
Angiodysplasia (intestinalis) (intestine) 569.84
  with hemorrhage 569.85
  duodenum 537.82
    with hemorrhage 537.83
  stomach 537.82
    with hemorrhage 537.83
Angioedema (allergic) (any site) (with urticaria)
  995.1
  hereditary 277.6
Angioendothelioma (M9130/1)—*see also*
  Neoplasm, by site, uncertain behavior
  benign (M9130/0) (*see also* Hemangioma, by
    site) 228.00
  bone (M9260/3)—*see* Neoplasm, bone, malignant
  Ewing's (M9260/3)—*see* Neoplasm, bone,
    malignant
  nervous system (M9130/0) 228.09
Angiofibroma (M9160/0)—*see also* Neoplasm,
  by site, benign
  juvenile (M9160/0) 210.7
    specified site—*see* Neoplasm, by site, benign
    unspecified site 210.7
Angiohemophilia (A) (B) 286.4
Angioid streaks (choroid) (retina) 363.43
Angiokeratoma (M9141/0)—*see also* Neoplasm,
  skin, benign
  corporis diffusum 272.7
Angiokeratosis
  diffuse 272.7
Angioleiomyoma (M8894/0)—*see* Neoplasm,
  connective tissue, benign
Angioleucitis 683
Angiolipoma (M8861/0) (*see also* Lipoma, by
  site) 214.9
  infiltrating (M8861/1)—*see* Neoplasm,
    connective tissue, uncertain behavior
Angioma (M9120/0) (*see also* Hemangioma, by
  site) 228.00
  capillary 448.1
  hemorrhagicum hereditaria 448.0
  malignant (M9120/3)—*see* Neoplasm,
    connective tissue, malignant

Angioma—*continued*
  pigmentosum et atrophicum 757.33
  placenta—*see* Placenta, abnormal
  plexiform (M9131/0)—*see* Hemangioma, by site
  senile 448.1
  serpiginosum 709.1
  spider 448.1
  stellate 448.1
Angiomatosis 757.32
  bacillary 083.8
  corporis diffusum universale 272.7
  cutaneocerebral 759.6
  encephalocutaneous 759.6
  encephalofacial 759.6
  encephalotrigeminal 759.6
  hemorrhagic familial 448.0
  hereditary familial 448.0
  heredofamilial 448.0
  meningo-oculofacial 759.6
  multiple sites 228.09
  neuro-oculocutaneous 759.6
  retina (Hippel's disease) 759.6
  retinocerebellosa 759.6
  retinocerebral 759.6
  systemic 228.09
Angiomyolipoma (M8860/0)
  specified site—*see* Neoplasm, connective tissue, benign
  unspecified site 223.0
Angiomyoliposarcoma (M8860/3)—*see*
  Neoplasm, connective tissue, malignant
Angiomyoma (M8894/0)—*see* Neoplasm,
  connective tissue, benign
Angiomyosarcoma (M8894/3)—*see* Neoplasm,
  connective tissue, malignant
Angioneurosis 306.2
Angioneurotic edema (allergic) (any site) (with
  urticaria) 995.1
  hereditary 277.6
Angiopathia, angiopathy 459.9
  diabetic (peripheral) 250.7 *[443.81]*
    due to secondary diabetes 249.7 [443.81]
  peripheral 443.9
    diabetic 250.7 *[443.81]*
      due to secondary diabetes 249.7 [443.81]
    specified type NEC 443.89
  retinae syphilitica 093.89
  retinalis (juvenilis) 362.18
    background 362.10
    diabetic 250.5 *[362.01]*
      due to secondary diabetes 249.5 [362.01]
    proliferative 362.29
    tuberculous (*see also* Tuberculosis) 017.3 *[362.18]*
Angiosarcoma (M9120/3)—*see* Neoplasm,
  connective tissue, malignant
Angiosclerosis —*see* Arteriosclerosis
Angioscotoma, enlarged 368.42
Angiospasm 443.9
  brachial plexus 353.0
  cerebral 435.9
  cervical plexus 353.2
  nerve
    arm 354.9
      axillary 353.0
      median 354.1
      ulnar 354.2
    autonomic (*see also* Neuropathy, peripheral,
      autonomic) 337.9
    axillary 353.0
    leg 355.8
      plantar 355.6
    lower extremity—*see* Angiospasm, nerve, leg

Angiospasm—*continued*
  median 354.1
  peripheral NEC 355.9
  spinal NEC 355.9
  sympathetic (*see also* Neuropathy, peripheral,
    autonomic) 337.9
  ulnar 354.2
  upper extremity—*see* Angiospasm, nerve, arm
  peripheral NEC 443.9
  traumatic 443.9
    foot 443.9
    leg 443.9
    vessel 443.9
Angiospastic disease or edema 443.9
Angle's
  class I 524.21
  class II 524.22
  class III 524.23
Anguillulosis 127.2
Angulation
  cecum (*see also* Obstruction, intestine) 560.9
  coccyx (acquired) 738.6
    congenital 756.19
  femur (acquired) 736.39
    congenital 755.69
  intestine (large) (small) (*see also* Obstruction,
    intestine) 560.9
  sacrum (acquired) 738.5
    congenital 756.19
  sigmoid (flexure) (*see also* Obstruction,
    intestine) 560.9
  spine (*see also* Curvature, spine) 737.9
  tibia (acquired) 736.89
    congenital 755.69
  ureter 593.3
  wrist (acquired) 736.09
    congenital 755.59
Angulus infectiosus 686.8
Anhedonia 780.99
Anhidrosis (lid) (neurogenic) (thermogenic)
  705.0
Anhydration 276.51
  with
    hypernatremia 276.0
    hyponatremia 276.1
Anhydremia 276.52
  with
    hypernatremia 276.0
    hyponatremia 276.1
Anidrosis 705.0
Aniridia (congenital) 743.45
Anisakiasis (infection) (infestation) 127.1
Anisakis larva infestation 127.1
Aniseikonia 367.32
Anisocoria (pupil) 379.41
  congenital 743.46
Anisocytosis 790.09
Anisometropia (congenital) 367.31
Ankle —*see* condition
Ankyloblepharon (acquired) (eyelid) 374.46
  filiforme (adnatum) (congenital) 743.62
  total 743.62
Ankylodactly (*see also* Syndactylism) 755.10
Ankyloglossia 750.0
Ankylosis (fibrous) (osseous) 718.50
  ankle 718.57
  any joint, produced by surgical fusion V45.4
  cricoarytenoid (cartilage) (joint) (larynx) 478.79
  dental 521.6
  ear ossicle NEC 385.22
    malleus 385.21

Ankylosis—*continued*
  elbow 718.52
  finger 718.54
  hip 718.55
  incostapedial joint (infectional) 385.22
  joint, produced by surgical fusion NEC V45.4
  knee 718.56
  lumbosacral (joint) 724.6
  malleus 385.21
  multiple sites 718.59
  postoperative (status) V45.4
  sacroiliac (joint) 724.6
  shoulder 718.51
  specified site NEC 718.58
  spine NEC 724.9
  surgical V45.4
  teeth, tooth (hard tissues) 521.6
  temporomandibular joint 524.61
  wrist 718.53
Ankylostoma —*see* Ancylostoma
Ankylostomiasis (intestinal)—*see*
  Ancylostomiasis
Ankylurethria (*see also* Stricture, urethra) 598.9
Annular —*see also* condition
  detachment, cervix 622.8
  organ or site, congenital NEC—*see* Distortion
  pancreas (congenital) 751.7
Anodontia (complete) (partial) (vera) 520.0
  with abnormal spacing 524.30
  acquired 525.10
    causing malocclusion 524.30
    due to
      caries 525.13
      extraction 525.10
      periodontal disease 525.12
      trauma 525.11
Anomaly, anomalous (congenital) (unspecified
  type) 759.9
  abdomen 759.9
  abdominal wall 756.70
  acoustic nerve 742.9
  adrenal (gland) 759.1
  Alder (-Reilly) (leukocyte granulation) 288.2
  alimentary tract 751.9
    lower 751.5
    specified type NEC 751.8
    upper (any part, except tongue) 750.9
      tongue 750.10
        specified type NEC 750.19
  alveolar 524.70
    ridge (process) 525.8
    specified NEC 524.79
  ankle (joint) 755.69
  anus, anal (canal) 751.5
  aorta, aortic 747.20
    arch 747.21
    coarctation (postductal) (preductal) 747.10
    cusp or valve NEC 746.9
    septum 745.0
    specified type NEC 747.29
  aorticopulmonary septum 745.0
  apertures, diaphragm 756.6
  appendix 751.5
  aqueduct of Sylvius 742.3
    with spina bifida (*see also* Spina bifida) 741.0
  arm 755.50
    reduction (*see also* Deformity, reduction,
      upper limb) 755.20

Anomaly, anomalous—*continued*
arteriovenous (congenital) (peripheral) NEC
747.60
brain 747.81
cerebral 747.81
coronary 746.85
gastrointestinal 747.61
acquired—*see* Angiodysplasia
lower limb 747.64
renal 747.62
specified site NEC 747.69
spinal 747.82
upper limb 747.63
artery (*see also* Anomaly, peripheral vascular
system) NEC 747.60
brain 747.81
cerebral 747.81
coronary 746.85
eye 743.9
pulmonary 747.39
renal 747.62
retina 743.9
umbilical 747.5
arytenoepiglottic folds 748.3
atrial
bands 746.9
folds 746.9
septa 745.5
atrioventricular
canal 745.69
common 745.69
conduction 426.7
excitation 426.7
septum 745.4
atrium—*see* Anomaly, atrial
auditory canal 744.3
specified type NEC 744.29
with hearing impairment 744.02
auricle
ear 744.3
causing impairment of hearing 744.02
heart 746.9
septum 745.5
autosomes, autosomal NEC 758.5
Axenfeld's 743.44
back 759.9
band
atrial 746.9
heart 746.9
ventricular 746.9
Bartholin's duct 750.9
biliary duct or passage 751.60
atresia 751.61
bladder (neck) (sphincter) (trigone) 753.9
specified type NEC 753.8
blood vessel 747.9
artery—*see* Anomly, artery
peripheral vascular—*see* Anomaly, peripheral
vascular system
vein—*see* Anomaly, vein
bone NEC 756.9
ankle 755.69
arm 755.50
chest 756.3
cranium 756.0
face 756.0
finger 755.50
foot 755.67
forearm 755.50
frontal 756.0
head 756.0

Anomaly, anomalous—*continued*
bone—*continued*
hip 755.63
leg 755.60
lumbosacral 756.10
nose 748.1
pelvic girdle 755.60
rachitic 756.4
rib 756.3
shoulder girdle 755.50
skull 756.0
with
anencephalus 740.0
encephalocele 742.0
hydrocephalus 742.3
with spina bifida (*see also* Spina bifida)
741.0
microcephalus 742.1
toe 755.66
brain 742.9
multiple 742.4
reduction 742.2
specified type NEC 742.4
vessel 747.81
branchial cleft NEC 744.49
cyst 744.42
fistula 744.41
persistent 744.41
sinus (external) (internal) 744.41
breast 757.6
broad ligament 752.10
specified type NEC 752.19
bronchus 748.3
bulbar septum 745.0
bulbus cordis 745.9
persistent (in left ventricle) 745.8
bursa 756.9
canal of Nuck 752.9
canthus 743.9
capillary NEC (*see also* Anomaly, peripheral
vascular system) 747.60
cardiac 746.9
septal closure 745.9
acquired 429.71
valve NEC 746.9
pulmonary 746.00
specified type NEC 746.89
cardiovascular system 746.9
complicating pregnancy, childbirth, or
puerperium 648.5
carpus 755.50
cartilage, trachea 748.3
cartilaginous 756.9
caruncle, lacrimal, lachrymal 743.9
cascade stomach 750.7
cauda equina 742.59
cecum 751.5
cerebral—*see also* Anomaly, brain
vessels 747.81
cerebrovascular system 747.81
cervix (uterus) 752.40
with doubling of vagina and uterus 752.2
in pregnancy or childbirth 654.6
affecting fetus or newborn 763.89
causing obstructed labor 660.2
affecting fetus or newborn 763.1
Chédiak-Higashi (-Steinbrinck) (congenital
gigantism of peroxidase granules) 288.2
cheek 744.9
chest (wall) 756.3

Anomaly, anomalous—*continued*
  chin 744.9
    specified type NEC 744.89
  chordae tendineae 746.9
  choroid 743.9
    plexus 742.9
  chromosomes, chromosomal 758.9
    13 (13-15) 758.1
    18 (16-18) 758.2
    21 or 22 758.0
    autosomes NEC (*see also* Abnormality,
        autosomes) 758.5
      deletion 758.39
    Christchurch 758.39
    D₁ 758.1
    E₃ 758.2
    G 758.0
    mitochondrial 758.9
    mosaics 758.89
    sex 758.81
      complement, XO 758.6
      complement, XXX 758.81
      complement, XYY 758.81
      gonadal dysgenesis 758.6
      Klinefelter's 758.7
      Turner's 758.6
    trisomy 21 758.0
  cilia 743.9
  circulatory system 747.9
    specified type NEC 747.89
  clavicle 755.51
  clitoris 752.40
  coccyx 756.10
  colon 751.5
  common duct 751.60
  communication
    coronary artery 746.85
    left ventricle with right atrium 745.4
  concha (ear) 744.3
  connection
    renal vessels with kidney 747.62
    total pulmonary venous 747.41
  connective tissue 756.9
    specified type NEC 756.89
  cornea 743.9
    shape 743.41
    size 743.41
    specified type NEC 743.49
  coronary
    artery 746.85
    vein 746.89
  cranium—*see* Anomaly, skull
  cricoid cartilage 748.3
  cushion, endocardial 745.60
    specified type NEC 745.69
  cystic duct 751.60
  dental arch 524.20
    specified NEC 524.29
  dental arch relationship 524.20
    angle's class I 524.21
    angle's class II 524.22
    angle's class III 524.23
    articulation
      anterior 524.27
      posterior 524.27
      reverse 524.27
    disto-occlusion 524.22
      division I 524.22
      division II 524.22
    excessive horizontal overlap 524.26
    interarch distance (excessive) (inadequate)
        524.28

Anomaly, anomalous—*continued*
  dental arch relationship—*continued*
    mesio-occlusion 524.23
    neutro-occlusion 524.21
    open
      anterior occlusal relationship 524.24
      posterior occlusal relationship 524.25
    specified NEC 524.29
  dentition 520.6
  dentofacial NEC 524.9
    functional 524.50
    specified type NEC 524.89
  dermatoglyphic 757.2
  Descemet's membrane 743.9
    specified type NEC 743.49
  development
    cervix 752.40
    vagina 752.40
    vulva 752.40
  diaphragm, diaphragmatic (apertures) NEC
      756.6
  digestive organ(s) or system 751.9
    lower 751.5
    specified type NEC 751.8
    upper 750.9
  distribution, coronary artery 746.85
  ductus
    arteriosus 747.0
    Botalli 747.0
  duodenum 751.5
  dura 742.9
    brain 742.4
    spinal cord 742.59
  ear 744.3
    causing impairment of hearing 744.00
      specified type NEC 744.09
    external 744.3
      causing impairment of hearing 744.02
      specified type NEC 744.29
    inner (causing impairment of hearing) 744.05
    middle, except ossicles (causing impairment
        of hearing) 744.03
      ossicles 744.04
    ossicles 744.04
    prominent auricle 744.29
    specified type NEC 744.29
      with hearing impairment 744.09
  Ebstein's (heart) 746.2
    tricuspid valve 746.2
  ectodermal 757.9
  Eisenmenger's (ventricular septal defect) 745.4
  ejaculatory duct 752.9
    specified type NEC 752.89
  elbow (joint) 755.50
  endocardial cushion 745.60
    specified type NEC 745.69
  endocrine gland NEC 759.2
  epididymis 752.9
  epiglottis 748.3
  esophagus 750.9
    specified type NEC 750.4
  Eustachian tube 744.3
    specified type NEC 744.24
  eye (any part) 743.9
    adnexa 743.9
      specified type NEC 743.69
    anophthalmos 743.00
    anterior
      chamber and related structures 743.9
        angle 743.9
          specified type NEC 743.44
        specified type NEC 743.44

Anomaly, anomalous—*continued*
  eye—*continued*
    segment 743.9
      combined 743.48
      multiple 743.48
      specified type NEC 743.49
    cataract (*see also* Cataract) 743.30
    glaucoma (*see also* Buphthalmia) 743.20
    lid 743.9
      specified type NEC 743.63
    microphthalmos (*see also* Microphthalmos) 743.10
    posterior segment 743.9
      specified type NEC 743.59
      vascular 743.58
      vitreous 743.9
        specified type NEC 743.51
    ptosis (eyelid) 743.61
    retina 743.9
      specified type NEC 743.59
    sclera 743.9
      specified type NEC 743.47
    specified type NEC 743.8
  eyebrow 744.89
  eyelid 743.9
    specified type NEC 743.63
  face (any part) 744.9
    bone(s) 756.0
    specified type NEC 744.89
  fallopian tube 752.10
    specified type NEC 752.19
  fascia 756.9
    specified type NEC 756.89
  femur 755.60
  fibula 755.60
  finger 755.50
    supernumerary 755.01
    webbed (*see also* Syndactylism, fingers) 755.11
  fixation, intestine 751.4
  flexion (joint) 755.9
    hip or thigh (*see also* Dislocation, hip,
      congenital) 754.30
  folds, heart 746.9
  foot 755.67
  foramen
    Botalli 745.5
    ovale 745.5
  forearm 755.50
  forehead (*see also* Anomaly, skull) 756.0
  form, teeth 520.2
  fovea centralis 743.9
  frontal bone (*see also* Anomaly, skull) 756.0
  gallbladder 751.60
  Gartner's duct 752.41
  gastrointestinal tract 751.9
    specified type NEC 751.8
    vessel 747.61
  genitalia, genital organ(s) or system
    female 752.9
      external 752.40
        specified type NEC 752.49
      internal NEC 752.9
    male (external and internal) 752.9
      epispadias 752.62
      hidden penis 752.65
      hydrocele, congenital 778.6
      hypospadias 752.61
      micropenis 752.64
      testis, undescended 752.51
        retractile 752.52
    specified type NEC 752.89
  genitourinary NEC 752.9

Anomaly, anomalous—*continued*
  Gerbode 745.4
  globe (eye) 743.9
  glottis 748.3
  granulation or granulocyte, genetic 288.2
    constitutional 288.2
    leukocyte 288.2
  gum 750.9
  gyri 742.9
  hair 757.9
    specified type NEC 757.4
  hand 755.50
  hard tissue formation in pulp 522.3
  head (*see also* Anomaly, skull) 756.0
  heart 746.9
    auricle 746.9
    bands 746.9
    fibroelastosis cordis 425.3
    folds 746.9
    malposition 746.87
    maternal, affecting fetus or newborn 760.3
    obstructive NEC 746.84
    patent ductus arteriosus (Botalli) 747.0
    septum 745.9
      acquired 429.71
      aortic 745.0
      aorticopulmonary 745.0
      atrial 745.5
      auricular 745.5
      between aorta and pulmonary artery 745.0
      endocardial cushion type 745.60
        specified type NEC 745.69
      interatrial 745.5
      interventricular 745.4
        with pulmonary stenosis or atresia,
          dextraposition of aorta, and
          hypertrophy of right ventricle 745.2
        acquired 429.71
      specified type NEC 745.8
      ventricular 745.4
        with pulmonary stenosis or atresia,
          dextraposition of aorta, and
          hypertrophy of right ventricle 745.2
        acquired 429.71
    specified type NEC 746.89
    tetralogy of Fallot 745.2
    valve NEC 746.9
      aortic 746.9
        atresia 746.89
        bicuspid valve 746.4
        insufficiency 746.4
        specified type NEC 746.89
        stenosis 746.3
          subaortic 746.81
          supravalvular 747.22
      mitral 746.9
        atresia 746.89
        insufficiency 746.6
        specified type NEC 746.89
        stenosis 746.5
      pulmonary 746.00
        atresia 746.01
        insufficiency 746.09
        stenosis 746.02
          infundibular 746.83
          subvalvular 746.83
      tricuspid 746.9
        atresia 746.1
        stenosis 746.1
    ventricle 746.9
  heel 755.67

Anomaly, anomalous—*continued*
　nerve 742.9
　　acoustic 742.9
　　　specified type NEC 742.8
　　optic 742.9
　　　specified type NEC 742.8
　　specified type NEC 742.8
　nervous system NEC 742.9
　　brain 742.9
　　　specified type NEC 742.4
　　specified type NEC 742.8
　neurological 742.9
　nipple 757.6
　nonteratogenic NEC 754.89
　nose, nasal (bone) (cartilage) (septum) (sinus)
　　　748.1
　ocular muscle 743.9
　omphalomesenteric duct 751.0
　opening, pulmonary veins 747.49
　optic
　　disc 743.9
　　　specified type NEC 743.57
　　nerve 742.9
　opticociliary vessels 743.9
　orbit (eye) 743.9
　　specified type NEC 743.66
　organ
　　of Corti (causing impairment of hearing)
　　　744.05
　　or site 759.9
　　　specified type NEC 759.89
　origin
　　both great arteries from same ventricle 745.11
　　coronary artery 746.85
　　innominate artery 747.69
　　left coronary artery from pulmonary artery
　　　746.85
　　pulmonary artery 747.39
　　renal vessels 747.62
　　subclavian artery (left) (right) 747.21
　osseous meatus (ear) 744.03
　ovary 752.0
　oviduct 752.10
　palate (hard) (soft) 750.9
　　cleft (*see also* Cleft, palate) 749.00
　pancreas (duct) 751.7
　papillary muscles 746.9
　parathyroid gland 759.2
　paraurethral ducts 753.9
　parotid (gland) 750.9
　patella 755.64
　Pelger-Huët (hereditary hyposegmentation)
　　　288.2
　pelvic girdle 755.60
　　specified type NEC 755.69
　pelvis (bony) 755.60
　　complicating delivery 653.0
　　rachitic 268.1
　　　fetal 756.4
　penis (glans) 752.69
　pericardium 746.89
　peripheral vascular system NEC 747.60
　　gastrointestinal 747.61
　　lower limb 747.64
　　renal 747.62
　　specified site NEC 747.69
　　spinal 747.82
　　upper limb 747.63
　Peter's 743.44
　pharynx 750.9
　　branchial cleft 744.41
　　specified type NEC 750.29

Anomaly, anomalous—*continued*
　Pierre Robin 756.0
　pigmentation NEC 709.00
　　congenital 757.33
　pituitary (gland) 759.2
　pleural folds 748.8
　portal vein 747.40
　position tooth, teeth 524.30
　　crowding 524.31
　　displacement 524.30
　　　horizontal 524.33
　　　vertical 524.34
　　distance
　　　interocclusal
　　　　excessive 524.37
　　　　insufficient 524.36
　　excessive spacing 524.32
　　rotation 524.35
　　specified NEC 524.39
　preauricular sinus 744.46
　prepuce 752.9
　prostate 752.9
　pulmonary 748.60
　　artery 747.39
　　circulation 747.39
　　specified type NEC 748.69
　　valve 746.00
　　　atresia 746.01
　　　insufficiency 746.09
　　　specified type NEC 746.09
　　　stenosis 746.02
　　　　infundibular 746.83
　　　　subvalvular 746.83
　　vein 747.40
　　venous
　　　connection 747.49
　　　　partial 747.42
　　　　total 747.41
　　　return 747.49
　　　　partial 747.42
　　　　total (TAPVR) (complete)
　　　　　(subdiaphragmatic)
　　　　　(supradiaphragmatic) 747.41
　pupil 743.9
　pylorus 750.9
　　hypertrophy 750.5
　　stenosis 750.5
　rachitic, fetal 756.4
　radius 755.50
　rectovaginal (septum) 752.40
　rectum 751.5
　refraction 367.9
　renal 753.9
　　vessel 747.62
　respiratory system 748.9
　　specified type NEC 748.8
　rib 756.3
　　cervical 756.2
　Rieger's 743.44
　rings, trachea 748.3
　rotation—*see also* Malrotation
　　hip or thigh (*see also* Subluxation, congenital,
　　　hip) 754.32
　round ligament 752.9
　sacroiliac (joint) 755.69
　sacrum 756.10
　saddle
　　back 754.2
　　nose 754.0
　　　syphilitic 090.5
　salivary gland or duct 750.9
　　specified type NEC 750.26

Anomaly, anomalous—*continued*
scapula 755.50
sclera 743.9
  specified type NEC 743.47
scrotum 752.9
sebaceous gland 757.9
seminal duct or tract 752.9
sense organs 742.9
  specified type NEC 742.8
septum
  heart—*see* Anomaly, heart, septum
  nasal 748.1
sex chromosomes NEC (*see also* Anomaly,
    chromosomes) 758.81
shoulder (girdle) (joint) 755.50
  specified type NEC 755.59
sigmoid (flexure) 751.5
sinus of Valsalva 747.29
site NEC 759.9
skeleton generalized NEC 756.50
skin (appendage) 757.9
  specified type NEC 757.39
skull (bone) 756.0
  with
    anencephalus 740.0
    encephalocele 742.0
    hydrocephalus 742.3
      with spina bifida (*see also* Spina bifida)
        741.0
    microcephalus 742.1
specified type NEC
  adrenal (gland) 759.1
  alimentary tract (complete) (partial) 751.8
    lower 751.5
    upper 750.8
  ankle 755.69
  anus, anal (canal) 751.5
  aorta, aortic 747.29
    arch 747.21
  appendix 751.5
  arm 755.59
  artery (peripheral) NEC (*see also* Anomaly,
    peripheral vascular system) 747.60
    brain 747.81
    coronary 746.85
    eye 743.58
    pulmonary 747.39
    retinal 743.58
    umbilical 747.5
  auditory canal 744.29
    causing impairment of hearing 744.02
  bile duct or passage 751.69
  bladder 753.8
    neck 753.8
  bone(s) 756.9
    arm 755.59
    face 756.0
    leg 755.69
    pelvic girdle 755.69
    shoulder girdle 755.59
    skull 756.0
      with
        anencephalus 740.0
        encephalocele 742.0
        hydrocephalus 742.3
          with spina bifida (*see also* Spina
            bifida) 741.0
        microcephalus 742.1
  brain 742.4
  breast 757.6
  broad ligament 752.19
  bronchus 748.3

Anomaly, anomalous—*continued*
specified type NEC—*continued*
  canal of Nuck 752.89
  cardiac septal closure 745.8
  carpus 755.59
  cartilaginous 756.9
  cecum 751.5
  cervix 752.49
  chest (wall) 756.3
  chin 744.89
  ciliary body 743.46
  circulatory system 747.89
  clavicle 755.51
  clitoris 752.49
  coccyx 756.19
  colon 751.5
  common duct 751.69
  connective tissue 756.89
  cricoid cartilage 748.3
  cystic duct 751.69
  diaphragm 756.6
  digestive organ(s) or tract 751.8
    lower 751.5
    upper 750.8
  duodenum 751.5
  ear 744.29
    auricle 744.29
      causing impairment of hearing 744.02
    causing impairment of hearing 744.09
    inner (causing impairment of hearing)
      744.05
    middle, except ossicles 744.03
      ossicles 744.04
  ejaculatory duct 752.89
  endocrine 759.2
  epiglottis 748.3
  esophagus 750.4
  Eustachian tube 744.24
  eye 743.8
    lid 743.63
    muscle 743.69
  face 744.89
    bone(s) 756.0
  fallopian tube 752.19
  fascia 756.89
  femur 755.69
  fibula 755.69
  finger 755.59
  foot 755.67
  fovea centralis 743.55
  gallbladder 751.69
  Gartner's duct 752.89
  gastrointestinal tract 751.8
  genitalia, genital organ(s)
    female 752.89
      external 752.49
      internal NEC 752.89
    male 752.89
      penis 752.69
      scrotal transposition 752.81
  genitourinary tract NEC 752.89
  glottis 748.3
  hair 757.4
  hand 755.59
  heart 746.89
    valve NEC 746.89
      pulmonary 746.09
  hepatic duct 751.69
  hydatid of Morgagni 752.89
  hymen 752.49
  integument 757.8

Anomaly, anomalous—*continued*
specified type NEC—*continued*
  intestine (large) (small) 751.5
    fixational type 751.4
  iris 743.46
  jejunum 751.5
  joint 755.8
  kidney 753.3
  knee 755.64
  labium (majus) (minus) 752.49
  labyrinth, membranous 744.05
  larynx 748.3
  leg 755.69
  lens 743.39
  limb, except reduction deformity 755.8
    lower 755.69
      reduction deformity (*see also* Deformity,
        reduction, lower limb) 755.30
    upper 755.59
      reduction deformity (*see also* Deformity,
        reduction, upper limb) 755.20
  lip 750.26
  liver 751.69
  lung (fissure) (lobe) 748.69
  meatus urinarius 753.8
  metacarpus 755.59
  mouth 750.26
  Müllerian
    cervix 752.49
    uterus 752.39
    vagina 752.49
  muscle 756.89
    eye 743.69
  musculoskeletal system, except limbs 756.9
  nail 757.5
  neck 744.89
  nerve 742.8
    acoustic 742.8
    optic 742.8
  nervous system 742.8
  nipple 757.6
  nose 748.1
  organ NEC 759.89
    of Corti 744.05
  osseous meatus (ear) 744.03
  ovary 752.0
  oviduct 752.19
  pancreas 751.7
  parathyroid 759.2
  patella 755.64
  pelvic girdle 755.69
  penis 752.69
  pericardium 746.89
  peripheral vascular system NEC (*see also*
    Anomaly, peripheral vascular system)
    747.60
  pharynx 750.29
  pituitary 759.2
  prostate 752.89
  radius 755.59
  rectum 751.5
  respiratory system 748.8
  rib 756.3
  round ligament 752.89
  sacrum 756.19
  salivary duct or gland 750.26
  scapula 755.59
  sclera 743.47
  scrotum 752.89
    transposition 752.81
  seminal duct or tract 752.89

Anomaly, anomalous—*continued*
specified type NEC—*continued*
  shoulder girdle 755.59
  site NEC 759.89
  skin 757.39
  skull (bone(s)) 756.0
    with
      anencephalus 740.0
      encephalocele 742.0
      hydrocephalus 742.3
        with spina bifida (*see also* Spina bifida)
          741.0
      microcephalus 742.1
  specified organ or site NEC 759.89
  spermatic cord 752.89
  spinal cord 742.59
  spine 756.19
  spleen 759.0
  sternum 756.3
  stomach 750.7
  tarsus 755.67
  tendon 756.89
  testis 752.89
  thorax (wall) 756.3
  thymus 759.2
  thyroid (gland) 759.2
    cartilage 748.3
  tibia 755.69
  toe 755.66
  tongue 750.19
  trachea (cartilage) 748.3
  ulna 755.59
  urachus 753.7
  ureter 753.4
    obstructive 753.29
  urethra 753.8
    obstructive 753.6
  urinary tract 753.8
  uterus (Müllerian) 752.39
  uvula 750.26
  vagina 752.49
  vascular NEC (*see also* Anomaly, peripheral
    vascular system) 747.60
    brain 747.81
  vas deferens 752.89
  vein(s) (peripheral) NEC (*see also* Anomaly,
    peripheral vascular system) 747.60
    brain 747.81
    great 747.49
    portal 747.49
    pulmonary 747.49
  vena cava (inferior) (superior) 747.49
  vertebra 756.19
  vulva 752.49
spermatic cord 752.9
spine, spinal 756.10
  column 756.10
  cord 742.9
    meningocele (*see also* Spina bifida) 741.9
    specified type NEC 742.59
    spina bifida (*see also* Spina bifida) 741.9
    vessel 747.82
  meninges 742.59
  nerve root 742.9
spleen 759.0
Sprengel's 755.52
sternum 756.3
stomach 750.9
  specified type NEC 750.7
submaxillary gland 750.9
superior vena cava 747.40

Anomaly, anomalous—*continued*
 talipes—*see* Talipes
 tarsus 755.67
  with complete absence of distal elements
   755.31
 teeth, tooth NEC 520.9
  position 524.30
   crowding 524.31
   displacement 524.30
    horizontal 524.33
    vertical 524.34
   distance
    interocclusal
     excessive 524.37
     insufficient 524.36
   excessive spacing 524.32
   rotation 524.35
   specified NEC 524.39
   spacing 524.30
 tendon 756.9
  specified type NEC 756.89
 termination
  coronary artery 746.85
 testis 752.9
 thebesian valve 746.9
 thigh 755.60
  flexion (*see also* Subluxation, congenital, hip)
   754.32
 thorax (wall) 756.3
 throat 750.9
 thumb 755.50
  supernumerary 755.01
 thymus gland 759.2
 thyroid (gland) 759.2
  cartilage 748.3
 tibia 755.60
  saber 090.5
 toe 755.66
  supernumerary 755.02
  webbed (*see also* Syndactylism, toes) 755.13
 tongue 750.10
  specified type NEC 750.19
 trachea, tracheal 748.3
  cartilage 748.3
  rings 748.3
 tragus 744.3
 transverse aortic arch 747.21
 trichromata 368.59
 trichromatopsia 368.59
 tricuspid (leaflet) (valve) 746.9
  atresia 746.1
  Ebstein's 746.2
  specified type NEC 746.89
  stenosis 746.1
 trunk 759.9
 Uhl's (hypoplasia of myocardium, right
  ventricle) 746.84
 ulna 755.50
 umbilicus 759.9
  artery 747.5
 union, trachea with larynx 748.3
 unspecified site 759.9
 upper extremity 755.50
  vessel 747.63
 urachus 753.7
  specified type NEC 753.7
 ureter 753.9
  obstructive 753.20
  specified type NEC 753.4
   obstructive 753.29

Anomaly, anomalous—*continued*
 urethra (valve) 753.9
  obstructive 753.6
  specified type NEC 753.8
 urinary tract or system (any part, except
  urachus) 753.9
  specified type NEC 753.8
  urachus 753.7
 uterus 752.39
  with only one functioning horn 752.33
  in pregnancy or childbirth 654.0
   affecting fetus or newborn 763.89
   causing obstructed labor 660.2
    affecting fetus or newborn 763.1
 uvula 750.9
 vagina 752.40
 valleculae 748.3
 valve (heart) NEC 746.9
  formation, ureter 753.29
  pulmonary 746.00
  specified type NEC 746.89
 vascular NEC (*see also* Anomaly, peripheral
  vascular system) 747.60
  ring 747.21
 vas deferens 752.9
 vein(s) (peripheral) NEC (*see also* Anomaly,
  peripheral vascular system) 747.60
  brain 747.81
  cerebral 747.81
  coronary 746.89
  great 747.40
   specified type NEC 747.49
  portal 747.40
  pulmonary 747.40
  retina 743.9
 vena cava (inferior) (superior) 747.40
 venous—*see* Anomaly, vein
 venous return (pulmonary) 747.49
  partial 747.42
  total 747.41
 ventricle, ventricular (heart) 746.9
  bands 746.9
  folds 746.9
  septa 745.4
 vertebra 756.10
 vesicourethral orifice 753.9
 vessels NEC (*see also* Anomaly, peripheral
  vascular system) 747.60
  optic papilla 743.9
 vitelline duct 751.0
 vitreous humor 743.9
  specified type NEC 743.51
 vulva 752.40
 wrist (joint) 755.50
Anomia 784.69
Anonychia 757.5
 acquired 703.8
Anophthalmos, anophthalmus (clinical)
 (congenital) (globe) 743.00
 acquired V45.78
Anopsia (altitudinal) (quadrant) 368.46
Anorchia 752.89
Anorchism, anorchidism 752.89
Anorexia 783.0
 hysterical 300.11
 nervosa 307.1
Anosmia (*see also* Disturbance, sensation) 781.1
 hysterical 300.11
 postinfectional 478.9
 psychogenic 306.7
 traumatic 951.8
Anosognosia 780.99

Anosphrasia 781.1
Anosteoplasia 756.50
Anotia 744.09
Anovulatory cycle 628.0
Anoxemia 799.02
  newborn 770.88
Anoxia 799.02
  altitude 993.2
  cerebral 348.1
    with
      abortion—*see* Abortion, by type,
        with specified complication NEC
      ectopic pregnancy (*see also* categories
        633.0-633.9) 639.8
      molar pregnancy (*see also* categories
        630-632) 639.8
    complicating
      delivery (cesarean) (instrumental) 669.4
      ectopic or molar pregnancy 639.8
      obstetric anesthesia or sedation 668.2
    during or resulting from a procedure 997.01
    following
      abortion 639.8
      ectopic or molar pregnancy 639.8
    newborn (*see also* Distress, fetal, liveborn
      infant) 770.88
  due to drowning 994.1
  fetal, affecting newborn 770.88
  heart—*see* Insufficiency, coronary
  high altitude 993.2
  intrauterine
    fetal death (before onset of labor) 768.0
      during labor 768.1
    liveborn infant—*see* Distress, fetal, liveborn
      infant
  myocardial—*see* Insufficiency, coronary
  newborn 768.9
    mild or moderate 768.6
    severe 768.5
  pathological 799.02
Anteflexion —*see* Anteversion
Antenatal
  care, normal pregnancy V22.1
    first V22.0
  sampling
    chorionic villus V28.89
  screening of mother (for) V28.9
    based on amniocentesis NEC V28.2
      chromosomal anomalies V28.0
      raised alphafetoprotein levels V28.1
    chromosomal anomalies V28.0
    fetal growth retardation using ultrasonics
      V28.4
    genomic V28.89
    isoimmunization V28.5
    malformations using ultrasonics V28.3
    proteomic V28.89
    raised alphafetoprotein levels in amniotic fluid
      V28.1
    risk
      pre-term labor V28.82
    specified condition NEC V28.89
    Streptococcus B V28.6
    survey
      fetal anatomic V28.81
    testing
      nuchal translucency V28.89
Antepartum —*see* condition
Anterior —*see also* condition
  spinal artery compression syndrome 721.1
Antero-occlusion 524.24

Anteversion
  cervix (—*see* Anteversion, uterus)
  femur (neck), congenital 755.63
  uterus, uterine (cervix) (postinfectional)
    (postpartal, old) 621.6
    congenital 752.39
    in pregnancy or childbirth 654.4
      affecting fetus or newborn 763.89
      causing obstructed labor 660.2
        affecting fetus or newborn 763.1
Anthracosilicosis (occupational) 500
Anthracosis (lung) (occupational) 500
  lingua 529.3
Anthrax 022.9
  with pneumonia 022.1 *[484.5]*
  colitis 022.2
  cutaneous 022.0
  gastrointestinal 022.2
  intestinal 022.2
  pulmonary 022.1
  respiratory 022.1
  septicemia 022.3
  specified manifestation NEC 022.8
Anthropoid pelvis 755.69
  with disproportion (fetopelvic) 653.2
    affecting fetus or newborn 763.1
    causing obstructed labor 660.1
      affecting fetus or newborn 763.1
Anthropophobia 300.29
Antibioma, breast 611.0
Antibodies
  maternal (blood group) (*see also*
    Incompatibility) 656.2
    anti-D, cord blood 656.1
      fetus or newborn 773.0
Antibody
  anticardiolipin 795.79
    with
      hemorrhagic disorder 286.53
      hypercoagulable state 289.81
  antiphosphatidylglycerol 795.79
    with
      hemorrhagic disorder 286.53
      hypercoagulable state 289.81
  antiphosphatidylinositol 795.79
    with
      hemorrhagic disorder 286.53
      hypercoagulable state 289.81
  antiphosphatidylserine 795.79
    with
      hemorrhagic disorder 286.53
      hypercoagulable state 289.81
  antiphospholipid 795.79
    with
      hemorrhagic disorder 286.53
      hypercoagulable state 289.81
  deficiency syndrome
    agammaglobulinemic 279.00
    congenital 279.04
    hypogammaglobulinemic 279.00
Anticoagulant
  intrinsic, circulating, causing hemorrhagic
    disorder (see also Circulating,
    anticoagulants) 286.59
  lupus (LAC) 795.79
    with
      hemorrhagic disorder 286.53
      hypercoagulable state 289.81
Antimongolism syndrome 758.39
Antimonial cholera 985.4
Antisocial personality 301.7

Antithrombinemia (*see also* Circulating anticoagulants) 286.59
Antithromboplastinemia (*see also* Circulating anticoagulants) 286.59
Antithromboplastinogenemia (*see also* Circulating anticoagulants) 286.59
Antitoxin complication or reaction —*see* Complications, vaccination
Anton (-Babinski) syndrome (hemiasomatognosia) 307.9
Antritis (chronic) 473.0
 maxilla 473.0
 acute 461.0
 stomach 535.4
Antrum, antral —*see* condition
Anuria 788.5
 with
  abortion—*see* Abortion, by type, with renal failure
  ectopic pregnancy (*see also* categories 633.0-633.9) 639.3
  molar pregnancy (*see also* categories 630-632) 639.3
 calculus (impacted) (recurrent) 592.9
  kidney 592.0
  ureter 592.1
 congenital 753.3
 due to a procedure 997.5
 following
  abortion 639.3
  ectopic or molar pregnancy 639.3
 newborn 753.3
 postrenal 593.4
 puerperal, postpartum, childbirth 669.3
 specified as due to a procedure 997.5
 sulfonamide
  correct substance properly administered 788.5
  overdose or wrong substance given or taken 961.0
 traumatic (following crushing) 958.5
Anus, anal —*see also* condition
 high risk human papillomavirus (HPV) DNA test positive 796.75
 low risk human papillomavirus (HPV) DNA test positive 796.79
Anusitis 569.49
Anxiety (neurosis) (reaction) (state) 300.00
 alcohol-induced 291.89
 depression 300.4
 drug-induced 292.89
 due to or associated with physical condition 293.84
 generalized 300.02
 hysteria 300.20
 in
  acute stress reaction 308.0
  transient adjustment reaction 309.24
 panic type 300.01
 separation, abnormal 309.21
 syndrome (organic) (transient) 293.84
Aorta, aortic —*see* condition
Aortectasia (*see also* Ectasia, aortic) 447.70
 with aneurysm 441.9
Aortitis (nonsyphilitic) 447.6
 arteriosclerotic 440.0
 calcific 447.6
 Döhle-Heller 093.1
 luetic 093.1
 rheumatic (*see also* Endocarditis, acute, rheumatic) 391.1
 rheumatoid—*see* Arthritis, rheumatoid
 specific 093.1
 syphilitic 093.1
  congenital 090.5

Apathetic 799.25
 thyroid storm (*see also* Thyrotoxicosis) 242.9
Apathy 799.25
Apepsia 536.8
 achlorhydric 536.0
 psychogenic 306.4
Aperistalsis, esophagus 530.0
Apert's syndrome (acrocephalosyndactyly) 755.55
Apert-Gallais syndrome (adrenogenital) 255.2
Apertognathia 524.20
Aphagia 787.20
 psychogenic 307.1
Aphakia (acquired) (bilateral) (postoperative) (unilateral) 379.31
 congenital 743.35
Aphalangia (congenital) 755.4
 lower limb (complete) (intercalary) (partial) (terminal) 755.39
  meaning all digits (complete) (partial) 755.31
  transverse 755.31
 upper limb (complete) (intercalary) (partial) (terminal) 755.29
  meaning all digits (complete) (partial) 755.21
  transverse 755.21
Aphasia (amnestic) (ataxic) (auditory) (Broca's) (choreatic) (classic) (expressive) (global) (ideational) (ideokinetic) (ideomotor) (jargon) (motor) (nominal) (receptive) (semantic) (sensory) (syntactic) (verbal) (visual) (Wernicke's) 784.3
 developmental 315.31
 syphilis, tertiary 094.89
 uremic—*see* Uremia
Aphemia 784.3
 uremic—*see* Uremia
Aphonia 784.41
 clericorum 784.49
 hysterical 300.11
 organic 784.41
 psychogenic 306.1
Aphthae, aphthous —*see also* condition
 Bednar's 528.2
 cachectic 529.0
 epizootic 078.4
 fever 078.4
 oral 528.2
 stomatitis 528.2
 thrush 112.0
 ulcer (oral) (recurrent) 528.2
  genital organ(s) NEC
   female 616.50
   male 608.89
  larynx 478.79
Apical —*see* condition
Apical ballooning syndrome 429.83
Aplasia —*see also* Agenesis
 alveolar process (acquired) 525.8
  congenital 750.26
 aorta (congenital) 747.22
 aortic valve (congenital) 746.89
 axialis extracorticalis (congenital) 330.0
 bone marrow (myeloid) 284.9
  acquired (secondary) 284.89
  congenital 284.01
  idiopathic 284.9
 brain 740.0
  specified part 742.2
 breast 757.6
 bronchus 748.3
 cementum 520.4

Aplasia—*continued*
cerebellar 742.2
congenital (pure) red cell 284.01
corpus callosum 742.2
erythrocyte 284.81
   congenital 284.01
extracortical axial 330.0
eye (congenital) 743.00
fovea centralis (congenital) 743.55
germinal (cell) 606.0
iris 743.45
labyrinth, membranous 744.05
limb (congenital) 755.4
   lower NEC 755.30
   upper NEC 755.20
lung (bilateral) (congenital) (unilateral) 748.5
nervous system NEC 742.8
nuclear 742.8
ovary 752.0
Pelizaeus-Merzbacher 330.0
prostate (congenital) 752.89
red cell (with thymoma) 284.81
   acquired (secondary) 284.81
      due to drugs 284.81
   adult 284.81
   congenital 284.01
   hereditary 284.01
   of infants 284.01
   primary 284.01
   pure 284.01
      due to drugs 284.81
round ligament (congenital) 752.89
salivary gland 750.21
skin (congenital) 757.39
spinal cord 742.59
spleen 759.0
testis (congenital) 752.89
thymic, with immunodeficiency 279.2
thyroid 243
uterus 752.39
ventral horn cell 742.59
Apleuria 756.3
Apnea, apneic (spells) 786.03
newborn, neonatorum 770.81
   essential 770.81
   obstructive 770.82
   primary 770.81
   sleep 770.81
   specified NEC 770.82
psychogenic 306.1
sleep, unspecified 780.57
   with
      hypersomnia, unspecified 780.53
      hyposomnia, unspecified 780.51
      insomnia, unspecified 780.51
      sleep disturbance 780.57
   central, in conditions classified elsewhere
      327.27
   obstructive (adult) (pediatric) 327.23
   organic 327.20
   other 327.29
   primary central 327.21
Apneumatosis newborn 770.4
Apodia 755.31
Apophysitis (bone) (*see also* Osteochondrosis)
   732.9
calcaneus 732.5
juvenile 732.6
Apoplectiform convulsions (*see also* Disease,
   cerebrovascular, acute) 436

Apoplexia, apoplexy, apoplectic (*see also*
   Disease, cerebrovascular, acute) 436
abdominal 569.89
adrenal 036.3
attack 436
basilar (*see also* Disease, cerebrovascular,
   acute) 436
brain (*see also* Disease, cerebrovascular, acute) 436
bulbar (*see also* Disease, cerebrovascular, acute) 436
capillary (*see also* Disease, cerebrovascular,
   acute) 436
cardiac (*see also* Infarct, myocardium) 410.9
cerebral (*see also* Disease, cerebrovascular,
   acute) 436
chorea (*see also* Disease, cerebrovascular,
   acute) 436
congestive (*see also* Disease, cerebrovascular,
   acute) 436
   newborn 767.4
embolic (*see also* Embolism, brain) 434.1
fetus 767.0
fit (*see also* Disease, cerebrovascular, acute) 436
healed or old V12.54
heart (auricle) (ventricle) (*see also* Infarct,
   myocardium) 410.9
heat 992.0
hemiplegia (*see also* Disease, cerebrovascular,
   acute) 436
hemorrhagic (stroke) (*see also* Hemorrhage,
   brain) 432.9
ingravescent (*see also* Disease, cerebrovascular,
   acute) 436
late effect—*see* Late effect(s) (of)
   cerebrovascular disease
lung—*see* Embolism, pulmonary
meninges, hemorrhagic (*see also* Hemorrhage,
   subarachnoid) 430
neonatorum 767.0
newborn 767.0
pancreatitis 577.0
placenta 641.2
progressive (*see also* Disease, cerebrovascular,
   acute) 436
pulmonary (artery) (vein)—*see* Embolism,
   pulmonary
sanguineous (*see also* Disease, cerebrovascular,
   acute) 436
seizure (*see also* Disease, cerebrovascular,
   acute) 436
serous (*see also* Disease, cerebrovascular, acute)
   436
spleen 289.59
stroke (*see also* Disease, cerebrovascular, acute)
   436
thrombotic (*see also* Thrombosis, brain) 434.0
uremic—*see* Uremia
uteroplacental 641.2
Appendage
fallopian tube (cyst of Morgagni) 752.11
intestine (epiploic) 751.5
preauricular 744.1
testicular (organ of Morgagni) 752.89
Appendicitis 541
with
   perforation, peritonitis (generalized), or
      rupture 540.0
      with peritoneal abscess 540.1
   peritoneal abscess 540.1

Apendicitis—*continued*
acute (catarrhal) (fulminating) (gangrenous)
   (inflammatory) (obstructive) (retrocecal)
   (suppurative) 540.9
   with
      perforation, peritonitis, or rupture 540.0
         with peritoneal abscess 540.1
      peritoneal abscess 540.1
amebic 006.8
chronic (recurrent) 542
exacerbation—*see* Appendicitis, acute
fulminating—*see* Appendicitis, acute
gangrenous—*see* Appendicitis, acute
healed (obliterative) 542
interval 542
neurogenic 542
obstructive 542
pneumococcal 541
recurrent 542
relapsing 542
retrocecal 541
subacute (adhesive) 542
subsiding 542
suppurative—*see* Appendicitis, acute
tuberculous (*see also* Tuberculosis) 014.8
Appendiclausis 543.9
Appendicolithiasis 543.9
Appendicopathia oxyurica 127.4
Appendix, appendicular —*see also* condition
Morgagni (male) 752.89
   fallopian tube 752.11
Appetite
depraved 307.52
excessive 783.6
   psychogenic 307.51
lack or loss (*see also* Anorexia) 783.0
   nonorganic origin 307.59
perverted 307.52
   hysterical 300.11
Apprehension, apprehensiveness (abnormal)
   (state) 300.00
specified type NEC 300.09
Approximal wear 521.10
Apraxia (classic) (ideational) (ideokinetic)
   (ideomotor) (motor) 784.69
oculomotor, congenital 379.51
verbal 784.69
Aptyalism 527.7
Aqueous misdirection 365.83
Arabicum elephantiasis (*see also* Infestation,
   filarial) 125.9
Arachnidism 989.5
Arachnitis —*see* Meningitis
Arachnodactyly 759.82
Arachnoidism 989.5
Arachnoiditis (acute) (adhesive) (basic) (brain)
   (cerebrospinal) (chiasmal) (chronic) (spinal)
   (*see also* Meningitis) 322.9
meningococcal (chronic) 036.0
syphilitic 094.2
tuberculous (*see also* Tuberculosis, meninges)
   013.0
Araneism 989.5
Arboencephalitis, Australian 062.4
Arborization block (heart) 426.6
Arbor virus, arbovirus (infection) NEC 066.9
ARC 042
Arches —*see* condition
Arcuate uterus 752.36
Arcuatus uterus 752.36

Arcus (cornea)
juvenilis 743.43
   interfering with vision 743.42
senilis 371.41
Arc-welders' lung 503
Arc-welders' syndrome (photokeratitis) 370.24
Areflexia 796.1
Areola —*see* condition
Argentaffinoma (M8241/1)—*see also* Neoplasm,
   by site, uncertain behavior
benign (M8241/0)—*see* Neoplasm, by site,
   benign
malignant (M8241/3)—*see* Neoplasm, by site,
   malignant
syndrome 259.2
Argentinian hemorrhagic fever 078.7
Arginosuccinicaciduria 270.6
Argonz-Del Castillo syndrome (nonpuerperal
   galactorrhea and amenorrhea) 253.1
**Argyll-Robertson phenomenon pupil, or
   syndrome** (syphilitic) 094.89
atypical 379.45
nonluetic 379.45
nonsyphilitic 379.45
reversed 379.45
Argyria, argyriasis NEC 985.8
conjunctiva 372.55
cornea 371.16
from drug or medicinal agent
   correct substance properly administered 709.09
   overdose or wrong substance given or taken 961.2
Arhinencephaly 742.2
Arias-Stella phenomenon 621.30
Ariboflavinosis 266.0
Arizona enteritis 008.1
Arm —*see* condition
Armenian disease 277.31
Arnold-Chiari obstruction or syndrome (*see
   also* Spina bifida) 741.0
type I 348.4
type II (*see also* Spina bifida) 741.0
type III 742.0
type IV 742.2
Arousals
confusional 327.41
Arrest, arrested
active phase of labor 661.1
   affecting fetus or newborn 763.7
any plane in pelvis
   complicating delivery 660.1
      affecting fetus or newborn 763.1
bone marrow (*see also* Anemia, aplastic) 284.9
cardiac 427.5
   with
      abortion—*see* Abortion, by type, with
         specified complication NEC
      ectopic pregnancy (*see also* categories
         633.0-633.9) 639.8
      molar pregnancy (*see also* categories
         630-632) 639.8
   complicating
      anesthesia
         correct substance properly administered 427.5
         obstetric 668.1
         overdose or wrong substance given 968.4
            specified anesthetic—*see* Table of drugs
               and chemicals
      delivery (cesarean) (instrumental) 669.4
      ectopic or molar pregnancy 639.8
      surgery (nontherapeutic) (therapeutic) 997.1
   fetus or newborn 779.85

Arrest, arrested—*continued*
  cardiac—*continued*
    following
      abortion 639.8
      ectopic or molar pregnancy 639.8
    personal history, successfully rescucitated
      V12.53
    postoperative (immediate) 997.1
      long-term effect of cardiac surgery 429.4
  cardiorespiratory (*see also* Arrest, cardiac) 427.5
  deep transverse 660.3
    affecting fetus or newborn 763.1
  development or growth
    bone 733.91
    child 783.40
    fetus 764.9
      affecting management of pregnancy 656.5
    tracheal rings 748.3
  epiphyseal 733.91
  granulopoiesis 288.09
  heart—*see* Arrest, cardiac
  respiratory 799.1
    newborn 770.87
  sinus 426.6
  transverse (deep) 660.3
    affecting fetus or newborn 763.1
Arrhenoblastoma (M8630.1)
  benign (M8630/0)
    specified site—*see* Neoplasm, by site, benign
    unspecified site
      female 220
      male 222.0
  malignant (M8630/3)
    specified site— *see* Neoplasm, by site,
      malignant
    unspecified site
      female 183.0
      male 186.9
  specified site—*see* Neoplasm, by site, uncertain
    behavior
  unspecified site
    female 236.2
    male 236.4
Arrhinencephaly 742.2
  due to
    trisomy 13 (13-15) 758.1
    trisomy 18 (16-l8) 758.2
Arrhythmia (auricle) (cardiac) (cordis) (gallop
  rhythm) (juvenile) (nodal) (reflex) (sinus)
  (supraventricular) (transitory) (ventricle) 427.9
  bigeminal rhythm 427.89
  block 426.9
  bradycardia 427.89
  contractions, premature 427.60
  coronary sinus 427.89
  ectopic 427.89
  extrasystolic 427.60
  postoperative 997.1
  psychogenic 306.2
  vagal 780.2
Arrillaga-Ayerza syndrome (pulmonary artery
  sclerosis with pulmonary hypertension) 416.0
Arsenical
  dermatitis 692.4
  keratosis 692.4
  pigmentation 985.1
    from drug or medicinal agent
      correct substance properly administered
        709.09
      overdose or wrong substance given or taken
        961.1

Arsenism 985.1
  from drug or medicinal agent
    correct substance properly administered 692.4
    overdose or wrong substance given or taken
      961.1
Arterial —*see* condition
Arteriectasis 447.8
Arteriofibrosis —*see* Arteriosclerosis
Arteriolar sclerosis —*see* Arteriosclerosis
Arteriolith —*see* Arteriosclerosis
Arteriolitis 447.6
  necrotizing, kidney 447.5
  renal—*see* Hypertension, kidney
Arteriolosclerosis —*see* Arteriosclerosis
Arterionephrosclerosis (*see also* Hypertension,
  kidney) 403.90
Arteriopathy 447.9
Arteriosclerosis, arteriosclerotic (artery)
  (deformans) (diffuse) (disease) (endarteritis)
  (general) (obliterans) (obliterative) (occlusive)
  (senile) (with calcification) 440.9
  with
    gangrene 440.24
    psychosis (*see also* Psychosis, arteriosclerotic)
      290.40
    ulceration 440.23
  aorta 440.0
  arteries of extremities NEC — *see*
    Arteriosclerosis, extremities
  basilar (artery) (*see also* Occlusion, artery,
    basilar) 433.0
  brain 437.0
  bypass graft
    coronary artery 414.05
      autologous artery (gastroepiploic) (internal
        mammary) 414.04
      autologous vein 414.02
      nonautologous biological 414.03
      of transplanted heart 414.07
    extremity 440.30
      autologous vein 440.31
      nonautologous biological 440.32
  cardiac — *see* Arteriosclerosis, coronary
  cardiopathy — *see* Arteriosclerosis, coronary
  cardiorenal (*see also* Hypertension, cardiorenal)
    404.90
  cardiovascular (*see also* Disease,
    cardiovascular) 429.2
  carotid (artery) (common) (internal) (*see also*
    Occlusion, artery, carotid) 433.1
  central nervous system 437.0
  cerebral 437.0
    late effect—*see* Late effect(s) (of)
      cerebrovascular disease
  cerebrospinal 437.0
  cerebrovascular 437.0
  coronary (artery) 414.00
    due to
      calcified coronary lesion (severely) 414.4
      lipid rich plaque 414.3
    graft—*see* Arteriosclerosis, bypass graft
    native artery 414.01
      of transplanted heart 414.06
    of transplanted heart 414.06
  extremities (native artery) 440.20
    bypass graft 440.30
      autologous vein 440.31
      nonautologous biological 440.32

Arteriosclerosis, arteriosclerotic—*continued*
  extremities—*continued*
    claudication (intermittent) 440.21
    and
      gangrene 440.24
      rest pain 440.22
      and
        gangrene 440.24
        ulceration 440.23
          and gangrene 440.24
      ulceration 440.23
        and gangrene 440.24
    gangrene 440.24
    rest pain 440.22
      and gangrene 440.24
      and ulceration 440.23
        and gangrene 440.24
    specified site NEC 440.29
    ulceration 440.23
      and gangrene 440.24
  heart (disease) — *see also* Arteriosclerosis, coronary
    valve 424.99
      aortic 424.1
      mitral 424.0
      pulmonary 424.3
      tricuspid 424.2
  iliac 440.8
  kidney (*see also* Hypertension, kidney) 403.90
  labyrinth, labyrinthine 388.00
  medial NEC 440.20
  mesentery (artery) 557.1
  Mönckeberg's 440.20
  myocarditis 429.0
  nephrosclerosis (*see also* Hypertension, kidney)
    403.90
  peripheral (of extremities) *see* Arteriosclerosis,
    extremities
  precerebral 433.9
    specified artery NEC 433.8
  pulmonary (idiopathic) 416.0
  renal (*see also* Hypertension, kidney) 403.90
    arterioles (*see also* Hypertension, kidney)
      403.90
    artery 440.1
  retinal (vascular) 440.8 *[362.13]*
  specified artery NEC 440.8
    with gangrene 440.8 *[785.4]*
  spinal (cord) 437.0
  vertebral (artery) (*see also* Occlusion, artery,
    vertebral) 433.2
Arteriospasm 443.9
Arteriovenous —*see* condition
Arteritis 447.6
  allergic (*see also* Angiitis, hypersensitivity)
    446.20
  aorta (nonsyphilitic) 447.6
    syphilitic 093.1
  aortic arch 446.7
  brachiocephalica 446.7
  brain 437.4
    syphilitic 094.89
  branchial 446.7
  cerebral 437.4
    late effect—*see* Late effect(s) (of)
      cerebrovascular disease
    syphilitic 094.89
  coronary (artery) —*see also* Arteriosclerosis,
    coronary
    rheumatic 391.9
      chronic 398.99
    syphilitic 093.89

Arteritis—*continued*
  cranial (left) (right) 446.5
  deformans—*see* Arteriosclerosis
  giant cell 446.5
  necrosing or necrotizing 446.0
  nodosa 446.0
  obliterans—*see also* Arteriosclerosis
    subclaviocarotica 446.7
  pulmonary 417.8
  retina 362.18
  rheumatic—*see* Fever, rheumatic
  senile—*see* Arteriosclerosis
  suppurative 447.2
  syphilitic (general) 093.89
    brain 094.89
    coronary 093.89
    spinal 094.89
  temporal 446.5
  young female, syndrome 446.7
Artery, arterial —*see* condition
Arthralgia (*see also* Pain, joint) 719.4
  allergic (*see also* Pain, joint) 719.4
  in caisson disease 993.3
  psychogenic 307.89
  rubella 056.71
  Salmonella 003.23
  temporomandibular joint 524.62
Arthritis, arthritic (acute) (chronic) (subacute)
  716.9

---

*Note—Use the following fifth-digit
subclassification with categories 711-712,
715-716:*

0 site unspecified
1 shoulder region
2 upper arm
3 forearm
4 hand
5 pelvic region and thigh
6 lower leg
7 ankle and foot
8 other specified sites
9 multiple sites

---

  allergic 716.2
  ankylosing (crippling) (spine) 720.0
    sites other than spine 716.9
  atrophic 714.0
    spine 720.9
  back (*see also* Arthritis, spine) 721.90
  Bechterew's (ankylosing spondylitis) 720.0
  blennorrhagic 098.50
  cervical, cervicodorsal (*see also* Spondylosis,
    cervical) 721.0
  Charcot's 094.0 *[713.5]*
    diabetic 250.6 *[713.5]*
      due to secondary diabetes 249.6 *[713.5]*
    syringomyelic 336.0 *[713.5]*
    tabetic 094.0 *[713.5]*
  chylous (*see also* Filariasis) 125.9 *[711.7]*
  climacteric NEC 716.3
  coccyx 721.8
  cricoarytenoid 478.79
  crystal (-induced)—*see* Arthritis, due to crystals
  deformans (*see also* Osteoarthrosis) 715.9
    spine 721.90
      with myelopathy 721.91
  degenerative (*see also* Osteoarthrosis) 715.9
    idiopathic 715.09
    polyarticular 715.09
    spine 721.90
      with myelopathy 721.91

Arthritis, arthritic— *continued*
dermatoarthritis, lipoid 272.8 *[713.0]*
due to or associated with
  acromegaly 253.0 *[713.0]*
  actinomycosis 039.8 *[711.4]*
  amyloidosis 277.39 *[713.7]*
  bacterial disease NEC 040.89 *[711.4]*
  Behçet's syndrome 136.1 *[711.2]*
  blastomycosis 116.0 *[711.6]*
  brucellosis (*see also* Brucellosis) 023.9
    [711.4]
  caisson disease 993.3
  coccidioidomycosis 114.3 *[711.6]*
  coliform (Escherichia coli) 711.0
  colitis, ulcerative (*see also* Colitis, ulcerative)
    556.9 *[713.1]*
  cowpox 051.01 *[711.5]*
  crystals (*see also* Gout)
    dicalcium phosphate 275.49 *[712.1]*
    pyrophosphate 275.49 *[712.2]*
    specified NEC 275.49 *[712.8]*
  dermatoarthritis, lipoid 272.8 *[713.0]*
  dermatological disorder NEC 709.9 *[713.3]*
  diabetes 250.6 *[713.5]*
    due to secondary diabetes 249.6 *[713.5]*
  diphtheria 032.89 *[711.4]*
  dracontiasis 125.7 *[711.7]*
  dysentery 009.0 *[711.3]*
  endocrine disorder NEC 259.9 *[713.0]*
  enteritis NEC 009.1 *[711.3]*
    infectious (*see also* Enteritis, infectious)
      009.0 *[711.3]*
      specified organism NEC 008.8 *[711.3]*
    regional (*see also* Enteritis, regional) 555.9
      [713.1]
    specified organism NEC 008.8 *[711.3]*
  epiphyseal slip, nontraumatic (old) 716.8
  erysipelas 035 *[711.4]*
  erythema
    epidemic 026.1
    multiforme 695.10 *[713.3]*
    nodosum 695.2 *[713.3]*
  Escherichia coli 711.0
  filariasis NEC 125.9 *[711.7]*
  gastrointestinal condition NEC 569.9 *[713.1]*
  glanders 024 *[711.4]*
  Gonococcus 098.50
  gout 274.00
  H. influenzae 711.0
  helminthiasis NEC 128.9 *[711.7]*
  hematological disorder NEC 289.9 *[713.2]*
  hemochromatosis 275.03 *[713.0]*
  hemoglobinopathy NEC (*see also* Disease,
    hemoglobin) 282.7 *[713.2]*
  hemophilia (*see also* Hemophilia) 286.0
    [713.2]
  Hemophilus influenzae (H. influenzae) 711.0
  Henoch (-Schönlein) purpura 287.0 *[713.6]*
  histoplasmosis NEC (*see also* Histoplasmosis)
    115.99 *[711.6]*
  human parvovirus 079.83 *[711.5]*
  hyperparathyroidism 252.00 *[713.0]*
  hypersensitivity reaction NEC 995.3 *[713.6]*
  hypogammaglobulinemia (*see also*
    Hypogammaglobulinemia) 279.00 *[713.0]*
  hypothyroidism NEC 244.9 *[713.0]*
  infection (*see also* Arthritis, infectious) 711.9
  infectious disease NEC 136.9 *[711.8]*
  leprosy (*see also* Leprosy) 030.9 *[711.4]*
  leukemia NEC (M9800/3) 208.9 *[713.2]*
  lipoid dermatoarthritis 272.8 *[713.0]*

Arthritis, arthritic— *continued*
due to or associated with— *continued*
  Lyme disease 088.81 *[711.8]*
  meaning Osteoarthritis—*see* Osteoarthrosis
  Mediterranean fever, familial 277.31 *[713.7]*
  meningococcal infection 036.82
  metabolic disorder NEC 277.9 *[713.0]*
  multiple myelomatosis (M9730/3) 203.0
    [713.2]
  mumps 072.79 *[711.5]*
  mycobacteria 031.8 *[711.4]*
  mycosis NEC 117.9 *[711.6]*
  neurological disorder NEC 349.9 *[713.5]*
  ochronosis 270.2 *[713.0]*
  O'Nyong Nyong 066.3 *[711.5]*
  parasitic disease NEC 136.9 *[711.8]*
  paratyphoid fever (*see also* Fever,
    paratyphoid) 002.9 *[711.3]*
  parvovirus B19 079.83 *[711.5]*
  Pneumococcus 711.0
  poliomyelitis (*see also* Poliomyelitis) 045.9
    [711.5]
  Pseudomonas 711.0
  psoriasis 696.0
  pyogenic organism (E. coli) (H. influenzae)
    (Pseudomonas) (Streptococcus) 711.0
  rat-bite fever 026.1 *[711.4]*
  regional enteritis (*see also* Enteritis, regional)
    555.9 *[713.1]*
  Reiter's disease 099.3 *[711.1]*
  respiratory disorder NEC 519.9 *[713.4]*
  reticulosis, malignant (M9720/3) 202.3
    [713.2]
  rubella 056.71
  salmonellosis 003.23
  sarcoidosis 135 *[713.7]*
  serum sickness 999.59 *[713.6]*
  Staphylococcus 711.0
  Streptococcus 711.0
  syphilis (*see also* Syphilis) 094.0 *[711.4]*
  syringomyelia 336.0 *[713.5]*
  thalassemia (*see also* Thalassemia) 282.40
    [713.2]
  tuberculosis (*see also* Tuberculosis, arthritis)
    015.9 *[711.4]*
  typhoid fever 002.0 *[711.3]*
  ulcerative colitis (*see also* Colitis, ulcerative)
    556.9 *[713.1]*
  urethritis
    nongonococcal (*see also* Urethritis,
      nongonococcal) 099.40 *[711.1]*
    nonspecific (*see also* Urethritis,
      nongonococcal) 099.40 *[711.1]*
    Reiter's 099.3 *[711.1]*
  viral disease NEC 079.99 *[711.5]*
erythema epidemic 026.1
gonococcal 098.50
gouty 274.00
  acute 274.01
hypertrophic (*see also* Osteoarthrosis) 715.9
  spine 721.90
    with myelopathy 721.91
idiopathic, blennorrheal 099.3
in caisson disease 993.3 *[713.8]*
infectious or infective (acute) (chronic)
  (subacute) NEC 711.9
  nonpyogenic 711.9
  spine 720.9
inflammatory NEC 714.9

Arthritis, arthritic—*continued*
  juvenile rheumatoid (chronic) (polyarticular)
    714.30
    acute 714.31
    monoarticular 714.33
    pauciarticular 714.32
  lumbar (*see also* Spondylosis, lumbar) 721.3
  meningococcal 036.82
  menopausal NEC 716.3
  migratory—*see* Fever, rheumatic
  neuropathic (Charcot's) 094.0 *[713.5]*
    diabetic 250.6 *[713.5]*
      due to secondary diabetes 249.6 *[713.5]*
    nonsyphilitic NEC 349.9 *[713.5]*
    syringomyelic 336.0 *[713.5]*
    tabetic 094.0 *[713.5]*
  nodosa (*see also* Osteoarthrosis) 715.9
    spine 721.90
      with myelopathy 721.91
  nonpyogenic NEC 716.9
    spine 721.90
      with myelopathy 721.91
  ochronotic 270.2 *[713.0]*
  palindromic (*see also* Rheumatism,
    palindromic) 719.3
  pneumococcal 711.0
  postdysenteric 009.0 *[711.3]*
  postrheumatic, chronic (Jaccoud's) 714.4
  primary progressive 714.0
    spine 720.9
  proliferative 714.0
    spine 720.0
  psoriatic 696.0
  purulent 711.0
  pyogenic or pyemic 711.0
  reactive 099.3
  rheumatic 714.0
    acute or subacute—*see* Fever, rheumatic
    chronic 714.0
    spine 720.9
  rheumatoid (nodular) 714.0
    with
      splenoadenomegaly and leukopenia 714.1
      visceral or systemic involvement 714.2
    aortitis 714.89
    carditis 714.2
    heart disease 714.2
    juvenile (chronic) (polyarticular) 714.30
      acute 714.31
      monoarticular 714.33
      pauciarticular 714.32
    spine 720.0
  rubella 056.71
  sacral, sacroiliac, sacrococcygeal (*see also*
    Spondylosis, sacral) 721.3
  scorbutic 267
  senile or senescent (*see also* Osteoarthrosis)
    715.9
    spine 721.90
      with myelopathy 721.91
  septic 711.0
  serum (nontherapeutic) (therapeutic) 999.59
    [713.6]
  specified form NEC 716.8
  spine 721.90
    with myelopathy 721.91
    atrophic 720.9
    degenerative 721.90
      with myelopathy 721.91
    hypertrophic (with deformity) 721.90
      with myelopathy 721.91

Arthritis, arthritic— *continued*
  spine—*continued*
    infectious or infective NEC 720.9
    Marie-Strümpell 720.0
    nonpyogenic 721.90
      with myelopathy 721.91
    pyogenic 720.9
    rheumatoid 720.0
    traumatic (old) 721.7
    tuberculous (*see also* Tuberculosis) 015.0
      [720.81]
  staphylococcal 711.0
  streptococcal 711.0
  suppurative 711.0
  syphilitic 094.0 *[713.5]*
    congenital 090.49 *[713.5]*
  syphilitica deformans (Charcot) 094.0 *[713.5]*
  temporomandibular joint 524.69
  thoracic (*see also* Spondylosis, thoracic) 721.2
  toxic of menopause 716.3
  transient 716.4
  traumatic (chronic) (old) (post) 716.1
    current injury—*see* nature of injury
  tuberculous (*see also* Tuberculosis, arthritis)
    015.9 *[711.4]*
  urethritica 099.3 *[711.1]*
  urica, uratic 274.00
  venereal 099.3 *[711.1]*
  vertebral (*see also* Arthritis, spine) 721.90
  villous 716.8
  von Bechterew's 720.0
Arthrocele (*see also* Effusion, joint) 719.0
Arthrochondritis —*see* Arthritis
Arthrodesis status V45.4
Arthrodynia (*see also* Pain, joint) 719.4
  psychogenic 307.89
Arthrodysplasia 755.9
Arthrofibrosis, joint (*see also* Ankylosis) 718.5
Arthrogryposis 728.3
  multiplex, congenita 754.89
Arthrokatadysis 715.35
Arthrolithiasis 274.00
Arthro-onychodysplasia 756.89
Arthro-osteo-onychodysplasia 756.89
Arthropathy (*see also* Arthritis) 716.9

---

*Note—Use the following fifth-digit
subclassification with categories 711-712, 716:*

0 site unspecified
1 shoulder region
2 upper arm
3 forearm
4 hand
5 pelvic region and thigh
6 lower leg
7 ankle and foot
8 other specified sites
9 multiple sites

  Behçet's 136.1 *[711.2]*
  Charcot's 094.0 *[713.5]*
    diabetic 250.6 *[713.5]*
      due to secondary diabetes 249.6 *[713.5]*
    syringomyelic 336.0 *[713.5]*
    tabetic 094.0 *[713.5]*
  crystal (-induced)—*see* Arthritis, due to crystals

Arthropathy—*continued*
  gouty 274.00
    acute 274.01
    chronic (without mention of tophus (tophi))
      274.02
      with tophus (tophi) 274.03
  neurogenic, neuropathic (Charcot's) (tabetic)
    094.0 *[713.5]*
    diabetic 250.6 *[713.5]*
      due to secondary diabetes 249.6 *[713.5]*
    nonsyphilitic NEC 349.9 *[713.5]*
    syringomyelic 336.0 *[713.5]*
  postdysenteric NEC 009.0 *[711.3]*
  postrheumatic, chronic (Jaccoud's) 714.4
  psoriatic 696.0
  pulmonary 731.2
  specified NEC 716.8
  syringomyelia 336.0 *[713.5]*
  tabes dorsalis 094.0 *[713.5]*
  tabetic 094.0 *[713.5]*
  transient 716.4
  traumatic 716.1
  uric acid 274.00
Arthrophyte (*see also* Loose, body, joint) 718.1
Arthrophytis 719.80
  ankle 719.87
  elbow 719.82
  foot 719.87
  hand 719.84
  hip 719.85
  knee 719.86
  multiple sites 719.89
  pelvic region 719.85
  shoulder (region) 719.81
  specified site NEC 719.88
  wrist 719.83
Arthropyosis (*see also* Arthritis, pyogenic) 711.0
Arthroscopic surgical procedure converted to
  open procedure V64.43
Arthrosis (deformans) (degenerative) (*see also*
  Osteoarthrosis) 715.9
  Charcot's 094.0 *[713.5]*
  polyarticular 715.09
  spine (*see also* Spondylosis) 721.90
Arthus' phenomenon 995.21
  due to
    correct substance properly administered 995.21
    overdose or wrong substance given or taken
      977.9
      specified drug—*see* Table of drugs and
        chemicals
  serum 999.59
Articular —*see also* condition
  disc disorder (reducing or non-reducing) 524.63
  spondylolisthesis 756.12
Articulation
  anterior 524.27
  posterior 524.27
  reverse 524.27
Artificial
  device (prosthetic)—*see* Fitting, device
  insemination V26.1
  menopause (states) (symptoms) (syndrome)
    627.4
  opening status (functioning) (without
    complication) V44.9
    anus (colostomy) V44.3
    colostomy V44.3
    cystostomy V44.50
      appendico-vesicostomy V44.52
      cutaneous-vesicostomy V44.51
      specified type NEC V44.59

Artificial—*continued*
  opening status—*continued*
    enterostomy V44.4
    gastrostomy V44.1
    ileostomy V44.2
    intestinal tract NEC V44.4
    jejunostomy V44.4
    nephrostomy V44.6
    specified site NEC V44.8
    tracheostomy V44.0
    ureterostomy V44.6
    urethrostomy V44.6
    urinary tract NEC V44.6
    vagina V44.7
  vagina status V44.7
ARV (disease) (illness) (infection)—*see* Human
  immunodeficiency virus (disease) (illness)
  (infection)
Arytenoid —*see* condition
Asbestosis (occupational) 501
Asboe-Hansen's disease (incontinentia pigmenti)
  757.33
Ascariasis (intestinal) (lung) 127.0
Ascaridiasis 127.0
Ascaridosis 127.0
Ascaris 127.0
  lumbricoides (infestation) 127.0
  pneumonia 127.0
Ascending —*see* condition
ASC-H (atypical squamous cells cannot exclude
  high grade squamous intraepithelial lesion)
  anus 796.72
  cervix 795.02
  vagina 795.12
Aschoff's bodies (*see also* Myocarditis,
  rheumatic) 398.0
Ascites 789.59
  abdominal NEC 789.59
  cancerous (M8000/6) 789.51
  cardiac 428.0
  chylous (nonfilarial) 457.8
    filarial (*see also* Infestation, filarial) 125.9
  congenital 778.0
  due to S. japonicum 120.2
  fetal, causing fetopelvic disproportion 653.7
  heart 428.0
  joint (*see also* Effusion, joint) 719.0
  malignant (M8000/6) 789.51
  pseudochylous 789.59
  syphilitic 095.2
  tuberculous (*see also* Tuberculosis) 014.0
Ascorbic acid (vitamin C) deficiency (scurvy)
  267
ASC-US (atypical squamous cells of
  undetermined significance)
  anus 796.71
  cervix 795.01
  vagina 795.11
ASCVD (arteriosclerotic cardiovascular disease)
  429.2
Aseptic —*see* condition
Asherman's syndrome 621.5
Asialia 527.7
Asiatic cholera (*see also* Cholera) 001.9
Asocial personality or trends 301.7
Asomatognosia 781.8
Aspergillosis 117.3
  with pneumonia 117.3 *[484.6]*
  allergic bronchopulmonary 518.6
  nonsyphilitic NEC 117.3

Aspergillus (flavus) (fumigatus) (infection)
  (terreus) 117.3
Aspermatogenesis 606.0
Aspermia (testis) 606.0
Asphyxia, asphyxiation (by) 799.01
  antenatal—*see* Distress, fetal
  bedclothes 994.7
  birth (*see also* Asphyxia, newborn) 768.9
  bunny bag 994.7
  carbon monoxide 986
  caul (*see also* Asphyxia, newborn) 768.9
  cave-in 994.7
    crushing—*see* Injury, internal, intrathoracic
      organs
  constriction 994.7
  crushing—*see* Injury, internal, intrathoracic
    organs
  drowning 994.1
  fetal, affecting newborn 768.9
  food or foreign body (in larynx) 933.1
    bronchioles 934.8
    bronchus (main) 934.1
    lung 934.8
    nasopharynx 933.0
    nose, nasal passages 932
    pharynx 933.0
    respiratory tract 934.9
      specified part NEC 934.8
    throat 933.0
    trachea 934.0
  gas, fumes, or vapor NEC 987.9
    specified—*see* Table of drugs and chemicals
  gravitational changes 994.7
  hanging 994.7
  inhalation—*see* Inhalation
  intrauterine
    fetal death (before onset of labor) 768.0
      during labor 768.1
    liveborn infant—*see* Distress, fetal, liveborn
      infant
  local 443.0
  mechanical 994.7
    during birth (*see also* Distress, fetal) 768.9
  mucus 933.1
    bronchus (main) 934.1
    larynx 933.1
    lung 934.8
    nasal passages 932
    newborn 770.18
    pharynx 933.0
    respiratory tract 934.9
      specified part NEC 934.8
    throat 933.0
    trachea 934.0
    vaginal (fetus or newborn) 770.18
  newborn 768.9
    blue 768.6
    livida 768.6
    mild or moderate 768.6
    pallida 768.5
    severe 768.5
    white 768.5
    with neurologic involvement 768.5
  pathological 799.01
  plastic bag 994.7
  postnatal (*see also* Asphyxia, newborn) 768.9
    mechanical 994.7
  pressure 994.7
  reticularis 782.61
  strangulation 994.7
  submersion 994.1

Asphyxia, asphyxiation—*continued*
  traumatic NEC—*see* Injury, internal,
    intrathoracic organs
  vomiting, vomitus—*see* Asphyxia, food or
    foreign body
Aspiration
  acid pulmonary (syndrome) 997.39
    obstetric 668.0
  amniotic fluid 770.13
    with respiratory symptoms 770.14
  bronchitis 507.0
  clear amniotic fluid 770.13
    with
      pneumonia 770.14
      pneumonitis 770.14
      respiratory symptoms 770.14
  contents of birth canal 770.17
    with respiratory symptoms 770.18
  fetal 770.10
    blood 770.15
      with
        pneumonia 770.16
        pneumonitis 770.16
      pneumonitis 770.18
  food, foreign body, or gasoline (with
    asphyxiation)—*see* Asphyxia, food or
    foreign body
  meconium 770.11
    with
      pneumonia 770.12
      pneumonitis 770.12
      respiratory symptoms 770.12
    below vocal cords 770.11
      with respiratory symptoms 770.12
  mucus 933.1
    into
      bronchus (main) 934.1
      lung 934.8
      respiratory tract 934.9
        specified part NEC 934.8
      trachea 934.0
    newborn 770.17
    vaginal (fetus or newborn) 770.17
  newborn 770.10
    with respiratory symptoms 770.18
    blood 770.15
      with
        pneumonia 770.16
        pneumonitis 770.16
        respiratory symptoms 770.16
  pneumonia 507.0
    fetus or newborn 770.18
      meconium 770.12
  pneumonitis 507.0
    fetus or newborn 770.18
      meconium 770.12
    obstetric 668.0
  postnatal stomach contents 770.85
    with
      pneumonia 770.86
      pneumonitis 770.86
      respiratory symptoms 770.86
  syndrome of newborn (massive) 770.18
    meconium 770.12
  vernix caseosa 770.17
Asplenia 759.0
  with mesocardia 746.87
Assam fever 085.0

Assimilation, pelvis
  with disproportion 653.2
    affecting fetus or newborn 763.1
    causing obstructed labor 660.1
      affecting fetus or newborn 763.1
Assmann's focus (*see also* Tuberculosis) 011.0
Astasia (-abasia) 307.9
  hysterical 300.11
Asteatosis 706.8
  cutis 706.8
Astereognosis 780.99
Asterixis 781.3
  in liver disease 572.8
Asteroid hyalitis 379.22
Asthenia, asthenic 780.79
  cardiac (*see also* Failure, heart) 428.9
    psychogenic 306.2
  cardiovascular (*see also* Failure, heart) 428.9
    psychogenic 306.2
  heart (*see also* Failure, heart) 428.9
    psychogenic 306.2
  hysterical 300.11
  myocardial (*see also* Failure, heart) 428.9
    psychogenic 306.2
  nervous 300.5
  neurocirculatory 306.2
  neurotic 300.5
  psychogenic 300.5
  psychoneurotic 300.5
  psychophysiologic 300.5
  reaction, psychoneurotic 300.5
  senile 797
  Stiller's 780.79
  tropical anhidrotic 705.1
Asthenopia 368.13
  accommodative 367.4
  hysterical (muscular) 300.11
  psychogenic 306.7
Asthenospermia 792.2
Asthma, asthmatic (bronchial) (catarrh)
  (spasmodic) 493.9

Note—The following fifth digit
subclassification is for use with codes
493.0-493.2, 493.9:

0 unspecified
1 with status asthmaticus
2 with (acute) exacerbation

---

with
  chronic obstructive pulmonary disease
    (COPD) 493.2
  hay fever 493.0
  rhinitis, allergic 493.0
allergic 493.9
  stated cause (external allergen) 493.0
atopic 493.0
cardiac (*see also* Failure, ventricular, left) 428.1
cardiobronchial (*see also* Failure, ventricular,
    left) 428.1
cardiorenal (*see also* Hypertension, cardiorenal)
    404.90
childhood 493.0
colliers' 500
cough variant 493.82
croup 493.9
detergent 507.8
due to
  detergent 507.8
  inhalation of fumes 506.3
  internal immunological process 493.0

Asthma, asthmatic—*continued*
  endogenous (intrinsic) 493.1
  eosinophilic 518.3
  exercise induced bronchospasm 493.81
  exogenous (cosmetics) (dander or dust) (drugs)
    (dust) (feathers) (food) (hay) (platinum)
    (pollen) 493.0
  extrinsic 493.0
  grinders' 502
  hay 493.0
  heart (*see also* Failure, ventricular, left) 428.1
  IgE 493.0
  infective 493.1
  intrinsic 493.1
  Kopp's 254.8
  late-onset 493.1
  meat-wrappers' 506.9
  Millar's (laryngismus stridulus) 478.75
  millstone makers' 502
  miners' 500
  Monday morning 504
  New Orleans (epidemic) 493.0
  platinum 493.0
  pneumoconiotic (occupational) NEC 505
  potters' 502
  psychogenic 316 *[493.9]*
  pulmonary eosinophilic 518.3
  red cedar 495.8
  Rostan's (*see also* Failure, ventricular, left) 428.1
  sandblasters' 502
  sequoiosis 495.8
  stonemasons' 502
  thymic 254.8
  tuberculous (*see also* Tuberculosis, pulmonary) 011.9
  Wichmann's (laryngismus stridulus) 478.75
  wood 495.8
Astigmatism (compound) (congenital) 367.20
  irregular 367.22
  regular 367.21
Astroblastoma (M9430/3)
  nose 748.1
  specified site—*see* Neoplasm, by site,
    malignant
  unspecified site 191.9
Astrocytoma (cystic) (M9400/3)
  anaplastic type (M9401/3)
    specified site—*see* Neoplasm, by site,
      malignant
    unspecified site 191.9
  fibrillary (M9420/3)
    specified site—*see* Neoplasm, by site,
      malignant
    unspecified site 191.9
  fibrous (M9420/3)
    specified site—*see* Neoplasm, by site,
      malignant
    unspecified site 191.9
  gemistocytic (M9411/3)
    specified site—*see* Neoplasm, by site,
      malignant
    unspecified site 191.9
  juvenile (M9421/3)
    specified site—*see* Neoplasm, by site,
      malignant
    unspecified site 191.9
  nose 748.1
  pilocytic (M9421/3)
    specified site—*see* Neoplasm, by site,
      malignant
    unspecified site 191.9

Atonia, atony, atonic
abdominal wall 728.2
bladder (sphincter) 596.4
neurogenic NEC 596.54
with cauda equina syndrome 344.61
capillary 448.9
cecum 564.89
psychogenic 306.4
colon 564.89
psychogenic 306.4
congenital 779.89
dyspepsia 536.3
psychogenic 306.4
intestine 564.89
psychogenic 306.4
stomach 536.3
neurotic or psychogenic 306.4
psychogenic 306.4
uterus 661.2
affecting fetus or newborn 763.7
with hemorrhage (postpartum) 666.1
without hemorrhage
intrapartum 661.2
postpartum 669.8
vesical 596.4
Atopy NEC V15.09
Atransferrinemia, congenital 273.8
Atresia, atretic (congenital) 759.89
alimentary organ or tract NEC 751.8
lower 751.2
upper 750.8
ani, anus, anal (canal) 751.2
aorta 747.22
with hypoplasia of ascending aorta and
defective development of left ventricle
(with mitral valve atresia) 746.7
arch 747.11
ring 747.21
aortic (orifice) (valve) 746.89
arch 747.11
aqueduct of Sylvius 742.3
with spina bifida (*see also* Spina bifida) 741.0
artery NEC (*see also* Atresia, blood vessel)
747.60
cerebral 747.81
coronary 746.85
eye 743.58
pulmonary 747.31
umbilical 747.5
auditory canal (external) 744.02
bile, biliary duct (common) or passage 751.61
acquired (*see also* Obstruction, biliary) 576.2
bladder (neck) 753.6
blood vessel (peripheral) NEC 747.60
cerebral 747.81
gastrointestinal 747.61
lower limb 747.64
pulmonary (artery) 747.31
renal 747.62
spinal 747.82
upper limb 747.63
bronchus 748.3
canal, ear 744.02
cardiac
valve 746.89
aortic 746.89
mitral 746.89
pulmonary 746.01
tricuspid 746.1
cecum 751.2

Atresia, atretic—*continued*
cervix (acquired) 622.4
congenital 752.43
in pregnancy or childbirth 654.6
affecting fetus or newborn 763.89
causing obstructed labor 660.2
affecting fetus or newborn 763.1
choana 748.0
colon 751.2
cystic duct 751.61
acquired 575.8
with obstruction (*see also* Obstruction,
gallbladder) 575.2
digestive organs NEC 751.8
duodenum 751.1
ear canal 744.02
ejaculatory duct 752.89
epiglottis 748.3
esophagus 750.3
Eustachian tube 744.24
fallopian tube (acquired) 628.2
congenital 752.19
follicular cyst 620.0
foramen of
Luschka 742.3
with spina bifida (*see also* Spina bifida) 741.0
Magendie 742.3
with spina bifida (*see also* Spina bifida)
741.0
gallbladder 751.69
genital organ
external
female 752.49
male NEC 752.89
penis 752.69
internal
female 752.89
male 752.89
glottis 748.3
gullet 750.3
heart
valve NEC 746.89
aortic 746.89
mitral 746.89
pulmonary 746.01
tricuspid 746.1
hymen 752.42
acquired 623.3
postinfective 623.3
ileum 751.1
intestine (small) 751.1
large 751.2
iris, filtration angle (*see also* Buphthalmia)
743.20
jejunum 751.1
kidney 753.3
lacrimal, apparatus 743.65
acquired—*see* Stenosis, lacrimal
larynx 748.3
ligament, broad 752.19
lung 748.5
meatus urinarius 753.6
mitral valve 746.89
with atresia or hypoplasia of aortic orifice or
valve, with hypoplasia of ascending aorta
and defective development of left ventricle
746.7
nares (anterior) (posterior) 748.0
nasolacrimal duct 743.65
nasopharynx 748.8

Atresia, atretic—*continued*
  nose, nostril 748.0
    acquired 738.0
  organ or site NEC—*see* Anomaly, specified
      type NEC
  osseous meatus (ear) 744.03
  oviduct (acquired) 628.2
    congenital 752.19
  parotid duct 750.23
    acquired 527.8
  pulmonary (artery) 747.31
    valve 746.01
    vein 747.49
  pulmonic 746.01
  pupil 743.46
  rectum 751.2
  salivary duct or gland 750.23
    acquired 527.8
  sublingual duct 750.23
    acquired 527.8
  submaxillary duct or gland 750.23
    acquired 527.8
  trachea 748.3
  tricuspid valve 746.1
  ureter 753.29
  ureteropelvic junction 753.21
  ureterovesical orifice 753.22
  urethra (valvular) 753.6
  urinary tract NEC 753.29
  uterus 752.31
    acquired 621.8
  vagina (acquired) 623.2
    congenital (total) (partial) 752.45
    postgonococcal (old) 098.2
    postinfectional 623.2
    senile 623.2
  vascular NEC (*see also* Atresia, blood vessel)
      747.60
    cerebral 747.81
  vas deferens 752.89
  vein NEC (*see also* Atresia, blood vessel)
      747.60
    cardiac 746.89
    great 747.49
    portal 747.49
    pulmonary 747.49
  vena cava (inferior) (superior) 747.49
  vesicourethral orifice 753.6
  vulva 752.49
    acquired 624.8
Atrichia, atrichosis 704.00
  congenital (universal) 757.4
Atrioventricularis commune 745.69
Atrophia —*see also* Atrophy
  alba 709.09
  cutis 701.8
    idiopathica progressiva 701.8
    senilis 701.8
  dermatological, diffuse (idiopathic) 701.8
  flava hepatis (acuta) (subacuta) (*see also*
      Necrosis, liver) 570
  gyrata of choroid and retina (central) 363.54
    generalized 363.57
  senilis 797
    dermatological 701.8
  unguium 703.8
    congenita 757.5

Atrophoderma, atrophodermia 701.9
  diffusum (idiopathic) 701.8
  maculatum 701.3
    et striatum 701.3
      due to syphilis 095.8
    syphilitic 091.3
  neuriticum 701.8
  pigmentosum 757.33
  reticulatum symmetricum faciei 701.8
  senile 701.8
  symmetrical 701.8
  vermiculata 701.8
Atrophy, atrophic
  adrenal (autoimmune) (capsule) (cortex) (gland) 255.41
    with hypofunction 255.41
  alveolar process or ridge (edentulous) 525.20
    mandible 525.20
      minimal 525.21
      moderate 525.22
      severe 525.23
    maxilla 525.20
      minimal 525.24
      moderate 525.25
      severe 525.26
  appendix 543.9
  Aran-Duchenne muscular 335.21
  arm 728.2
  arteriosclerotic—*see* Arteriosclerosis
  arthritis 714.0
    spine 720.9
  bile duct (any) 576.8
  bladder 596.89
  blanche (of Milian) 701.3
  bone (senile) 733.99
    due to
      disuse 733.7
      infection 733.99
      tabes dorsalis (neurogenic) 094.0
    posttraumatic 733.99
  brain (cortex) (progressive) 331.9
    with dementia 290.10
    Alzheimer's 331.0
      with dementia—*see* Alzheimer's dementia
    circumscribed (Pick's) 331.11
      with dementia
        with behavioral disturbance 331.11
          [294.11]
        without behavioral disturbance 331.11
          [294.10]
    congenital 742.4
    hereditary 331.9
    senile 331.2
  breast 611.4
    puerperal, postpartum 676.3
  buccal cavity 528.9
  cardiac (brown) (senile) (*see also* Degeneration,
      myocardial) 429.1
  cartilage (infectional) (joint) 733.99
  cast, plaster of Paris 728.2
  cerebellar—*see* Atrophy, brain
  cerebral—*see* Atrophy, brain
  cervix (endometrium) (mucosa) (myometrium)
      (senile) (uteri) 622.8
    menopausal 627.8
  Charcot-Marie-Tooth 356.1

Atrophy, atrophic—*continued*
choroid 363.40
  diffuse secondary 363.42
  hereditary (*see also* Dystrophy, choroid)
    363.50
    gyrate
      central 363.54
      diffuse 363.57
      generalized 363.57
    senile 363.41
ciliary body 364.57
colloid, degenerative 701.3
conjunctiva (senile) 372.89
corpus cavernosum 607.89
cortical (*see also* Atrophy, brain) 331.9
Cruveilhier's 335.21
cystic duct 576.8
dacryosialadenopathy 710.2
degenerative
  colloid 701.3
  senile 701.3
Déjérine-Thomas 333.0
diffuse idiopathic, dermatological 701.8
disuse
  bone 733.7
  muscle 728.2
  pelvic muscles and anal sphincter 618.83
Duchenne-Aran 335.21
ear 388.9
edentulous alveolar ridge 525.20
  mandible 525.20
    minimal 525.21
    moderate 525.22
    severe 525.23
  maxilla 525.20
    minimal 525.24
    moderate 525.25
    severe 525.26
emphysema, lung 492.8
endometrium (senile) 621.8
  cervix 622.8
enteric 569.89
epididymis 608.3
eyeball, cause unknown 360.41
eyelid (senile) 374.50
facial (skin) 701.9
facioscapulohumeral (Landouzy-Déjérine) 359.1
fallopian tube (senile), acquired 620.3
fatty, thymus (gland) 254.8
gallbladder 575.8
gastric 537.89
gastritis (chronic) 535.1
gastrointestinal 569.89
genital organ, male 608.89
glandular 289.3
globe (phthisis bulbi) 360.41
gum (*see also* Recession, gingival) 523.20
hair 704.2
heart (brown) (senile) (*see also* Degeneration,
  myocardial) 429.1
hemifacial 754.0
  Romberg 349.89
hydronephrosis 591
infantile 261
  paralysis, acute (*see also* Poliomyelitis, with
    paralysis) 045.1
intestine 569.89
iris (generalized) (postinfectional) (sector
  shaped) 364.59
  essential 364.51
  progressive 364.51
  sphincter 364.54

Atrophy, atrophic—*continued*
kidney (senile) (*see also* Sclerosis, renal) 587
  with hypertension (*see also* Hypertension,
    kidney) 403.90
  congenital 753.0
  hydronephrotic 591
  infantile 753.0
lacrimal apparatus (primary) 375.13
  secondary 375.14
Landouzy-Déjérine 359.1
laryngitis, infection 476.0
larynx 478.79
Leber's optic 377.16
lip 528.5
liver (acute) (subacute) (*see also* Necrosis, liver)
  570
  chronic (yellow) 571.8
  yellow (congenital) 570
    with
      abortion—*see* Abortion, by type, with
        specified complication NEC
      ectopic pregnancy (*see also* categories
        633.0-633.9) 639.8
      molar pregnancy (*see also* categories
        630-632) 639.8
    chronic 571.8
    complicating pregnancy 646.7
    following
      abortion 639.8
      ectopic or molar pregnancy 639.8
    from injection, inoculation or transfusion
      (onset within 8 months after
      administration)—*see* Hepatitis, viral
    healed 571.5
    obstetric 646.7
    postabortal 639.8
    postimmunization—*see* Hepatitis, viral
    posttransfusion—*see* Hepatitis, viral
    puerperal, postpartum 674.8
lung (senile) 518.89
  congenital 748.69
macular (dermatological) 701.3
  syphilitic, skin 091.3
    striated 095.8
muscle, muscular 728.2
  disuse 728.2
  Duchenne-Aran 335.21
  extremity (lower) (upper) 728.2
  familial spinal 335.11
  general 728.2
  idiopathic 728.2
  infantile spinal 335.0
  myelopathic (progressive) 335.10
  myotonic 359.21
  neuritic 356.1
  neuropathic (peroneal) (progressive) 356.1
  peroneal 356.1
  primary (idiopathic) 728.2
  progressive (familial) (hereditary) (pure)
    335.21
    adult (spinal) 335.19
    infantile (spinal) 335.0
    juvenile (spinal) 335.11
    spinal 335.10
      adult 335.19
      hereditary or familial 335.11
      infantile 335.0
  pseudohypertrophic 359.1
    spinal (progressive) 335.10
    adult 335.19
    Aran-Duchenne 335.21
    familial 335.11

Atrophy, atrophic—*continued*
tunica vaginalis 608.89
turbinate 733.99
tympanic membrane (nonflaccid) 384.82
flaccid 384.81
ulcer (*see also* Ulcer, skin) 707.9
upper respiratory tract 478.9
uterus, uterine (acquired) (senile) 621.8
cervix 622.8
due to radiation (intended effect) 621.8
vagina (senile) 627.3
vascular 459.89
vas deferens 608.89
vertebra (senile) 733.99
vulva (primary) (senile) 624.1
Werdnig-Hoffmann 335.0
yellow (acute) (congenital) (liver) (subacute)
(*see also* Necrosis, liver) 570
chronic 571.8
resulting from administration of blood,
plasma, serum, or other biological
substance (within 8 months of
administration)—*see* Hepatitis, viral
Attack
akinetic (*see also* Epilepsy) 345.0
angina—*see* Angina
apoplectic (*see also* Disease, cerebrovascular,
acute) 436
benign shuddering 333.93
bilious—*see* Vomiting
cataleptic 300.11
cerebral (*see also* Disease, cerebrovascular,
acute) 436
coronary (*see also* Infarct, myocardium) 410.9
cyanotic, newborn 770.83
epileptic (*see also* Epilepsy) 345.9
epileptiform 780.39
heart (*see also* Infarct, myocardium) 410.9
hemiplegia (*see also* Disease, cerebrovascular,
acute) 436
hysterical 300.11
jacksonian (*see also* Epilepsy) 345.5
myocardium, myocardial (*see also* Infarct,
myocardium) 410.9
myoclonic (*see also* Epilepsy) 345.1
panic 300.01
paralysis (*see also* Disease, cerebrovascular,
acute) 436
paroxysmal 780.39
psychomotor (*see also* Epilepsy) 345.4
salaam (*see also* Epilepsy) 345.6
schizophreniform (*see also* Schizophrenia)
295.4
sensory and motor 780.39
syncope 780.2
toxic, cerebral 780.39
transient ischemic (TIA) 435.9
unconsciousness 780.2
hysterical 300.11
vasomotor 780.2
vasovagal (idiopathic) (paroxysmal) 780.2
Attention to
artificial
opening (of) V55.9
digestive tract NEC V55.4
specified site NEC V55.8
urinary tract NEC V55.6
vagina V55.7
colostomy V55.3
cystostomy V55.5

Attention to— *continued*
dressing
wound V58.30
nonsurgical V58.30
surgical V58.31
gastrostomy V55.1
ileostomy V55.2
jejunostomy V55.4
nephrostomy V55.6
surgical dressings V58.31
sutures V58.32
tracheostomy V55.0
ureterostomy V55.6
urethrostomy V55.6
Attrition
gum (*see also* Recession, gingival) 523.20
teeth (hard tissues) 521.10
excessive 521.10
extending into
dentine 521.12
pulp 521.13
generalized 521.15
limited to enamel 521.11
localized 521.14
Atypical —*see also* condition
cells
endocervical 795.00
endometrial 795.00
glandular
anus 796.70
cervical 795.00
vaginal 795.10
distribution, vessel (congenital) (peripheral)
NEC 747.60
endometrium 621.9
kidney 593.89
Atypism, cervix 622.10
Audible tinnitus (*see also* Tinnitus) 388.30
Auditory —*see* condition
Audry's syndrome (acropachyderma) 757.39
Aujeszky's disease 078.89
Aura
jacksonian (*see also* Epilepsy) 345.5
persistent migraine 346.5
with cerebral infarction 346.6
without cerebral infarction 346.5
Aurantiasis, cutis 278.3
Auricle, auricular —*see* condition
Auriculotemporal syndrome 350.8
Australian
Q fever 083.0
X disease 062.4
Autism, autistic (child) (infantile) 299.0
Autodigestion 799.89
Autoerythrocyte sensitization 287.2
Autographism 708.3
Autoimmune
cold sensitivity 283.0
disease NEC 279.49
hemolytic anemia 283.0
inhibitors to clotting factors 286.52
lymphoproliferative syndrome (ALPS) 279.41
thyroiditis 245.2
Autoinfection, septic —*see* Septicemia
Autointoxication 799.89
Automatism 348.89
epileptic (*see also* Epilepsy) 345.4
paroxysmal, idiopathic (*see also* Epilepsy) 345.4
with temporal sclerosis 348.81

Autonomic, autonomous
bladder 596.54
  neurogenic 596.54
    with cauda equine 344.61
dysreflexia 337.3
faciocephalalgia (*see also* Neuropathy,
  peripheral, autonomic) 337.9
hysterical seizure 300.11
imbalance (*see also* Neuropathy, peripheral,
  autonomic) 337.9
Autophony 388.40
Autosensitivity, erythrocyte 287.2
Autotopagnosia 780.99
Autotoxemia 799.89
Autumn —*see* condition
Avellis' syndrome 344.89
Aversion
oral 783.3
  newborn 779.31
  nonorganic origin 307.59
Aviators
disease or sickness (*see also* Effect, adverse,
  high altitude) 993.2
ear 993.0
effort syndrome 306.2
Avitaminosis (multiple NEC) (*see also*
  Deficiency, vitamin) 269.2
A 264.9
B 266.9
  with
    beriberi 265.0
    pellagra 265.2
B_1 265.1
B_2 266.0
B_6 266.1
B_{12} 266.2
C (with scurvy) 267
D 268.9
  with
    osteomalacia 268.2
    rickets 268.0
E 269.1
G 266.0
H 269.1
K 269.0
multiple 269.2
nicotinic acid 265.2
P 269.1
Avulsion (traumatic) 879.8
blood vessel—*see* Injury, blood vessel, by site
cartilage—*see also* Dislocation, by site
  knee, current (*see also* Tear, meniscus) 836.2
  symphyseal (inner), complicating delivery 665.6
complicated 879.9
diaphragm—*see* Injury, internal, diaphragm
ear—*see* Wound, open, ear
epiphysis of bone—*see* Fracture, by site
external site other than limb—*see* Wound, open,
  by site
eye 871.3
fingernail—*see* Wound, open, finger
fracture—*see* Fracture, by site
genital organs, external—*see* Wound, open,
  genital organs
head (intracranial) NEC—*see also* Injury,
  intracranial, with open intracranial wound
  complete 874.9
  external site NEC 873.8
    complicated 873.9
internal organ or site—*see* Injury, internal, by site

Avulsion—*continued*
joint—*see also* Dislocation, by site
  capsule—*see* Sprain, by site
ligament—*see* Sprain, by site
limb—*see also* Amputation, traumatic, by site
  skin and subcutaneous tissue—*see* Wound,
    open, by site
muscle—*see* Sprain, by site
nerve (root)—*see* Injury, nerve, by site
scalp—*see* Wound, open, scalp
skin and subcutaneous tissue—*see* Wound,
  open, by site
symphyseal cartilage (inner), complicating
  delivery 665.6
tendon—*see also* Sprain, by site
  with open wound—*see* Wound, open, by site
toenail—*see* Wound, open, toe(s)
tooth 873.63
  complicated 873.73
Awaiting organ transplant status V49.83
Awareness of heart beat 785.1
Axe grinders' disease 502
Axenfeld's anomaly or syndrome 743.44
Axilla, axillary —*see also* condition
breast 757.6
Axonotmesis —*see* Injury, nerve, by site
Ayala's disease 756.89
Ayerza's disease or syndrome (pulmonary
  artery sclerosis with pulmonary hypertension)
  416.0
Azoospermia 606.0
Azorean disease (of the nervous system) 334.8
Azotemia 790.6
meaning uremia (*see also* Uremia) 586
Aztec ear 744.29
Azygos lobe, lung (fissure) 748.69

B

Baader's syndrome (erythema multiforme exudativum) 695.19
Baastrup's syndrome 721.5
Babesiasis 088.82
Babesiosis 088.82
Babington's disease (familial hemorrhagic telangiectasia) 448.0
Babinski's syndrome (cardiovascular syphilis) 093.89
Babinski-Fröhlich syndrome (adiposogenital dystrophy) 253.8
Babinski-Nageotte syndrome 344.89
Bacillary —*see* condition
Bacilluria 791.9
  asymptomatic, in pregnancy or puerperium 646.5
  tuberculous (*see also* Tuberculosis) 016.9
Bacillus —*see also* Infection, bacillus
  abortus infection 023.1
  anthracis infection 022.9
  coli
    infection 041.49
     generalized 038.42
     intestinal 008.00
     pyemia 038.42
     septicemia 038.42
  Flexner's 004.1
  fusiformis infestation 101
  mallei infection 024
  Shiga's 004.0
  suipestifer infection (*see also* Infection, Salmonella) 003.9
Back —*see* condition
Backache (postural) 724.5
  psychogenic 307.89
  sacroiliac 724.6
Backflow (pyelovenous) (*see also* Disease, renal) 593.9
Backknee (*see also* Genu, recurvatum) 736.5
Bacteremia (*see also* Infection, bacillus) 790.7
  newborn 771.83
Bacteria
  in blood (*see also* Bacteremia) 790.7
  in urine (*see also* Bacteriuria) 599.0
Bacterial —*see* condition
Bactericholia (*see also* Cholecystitis, acute) 575.0
Bacterid, bacteride (Andrews' pustular) 686.8
Bacteriuria, bacteruria 791.9
  with
    urinary tract infection 599.0
  asymptomatic 791.9
    in pregnancy or puerperium 646.5
     affecting fetus or newborn 760.1
Bad
  breath 784.99
  heart—*see* Disease, heart
  trip (*see also* Abuse, drugs, nondependent) 305.3
Baehr-Schiffrin disease (thrombotic thrombocytopenic purpura) 446.6
Baelz's disease (cheilitis glandularis apostematosa) 528.5
Baerensprung's disease (eczema marginatum) 110.3
Bagassosis (occupational) 495.1
Baghdad boil 085.1

Bagratuni's syndrome (temporal arteritis) 446.5
Baker's
  cyst (knee) 727.51
    tuberculous (*see also* Tuberculosis) 015.2
  itch 692.89
Bakwin-Krida syndrome (craniometaphyseal dysplasia) 756.89
Balanitis (circinata) (gangraenosa) (infectious) (vulgaris) 607.1
  amebic 006.8
  candidal 112.2
  chlamydial 099.53
  due to Ducrey's bacillus 099.0
  erosiva circinata et gangraenosa 607.1
  gangrenous 607.1
  gonococcal (acute) 098.0
    chronic or duration of 2 months or over 098.2
  nongonococcal 607.1
  phagedenic 607.1
  venereal NEC 099.8
  xerotica obliterans 607.81
Balanoposthitis 607.1
  chlamydial 099.53
  gonococcal (acute) 098.0
    chronic or duration of 2 months or over 098.2
  ulcerative NEC 099.8
Balanorrhagia —*see* Balanitis
Balantidiasis 007.0
Balantidiosis 007.0
Balbuties, balbutio (*see also* Disorder, fluency) 315.35
Bald
  patches on scalp 704.00
  tongue 529.4
Baldness (*see also* Alopecia) 704.00
Balfour's disease (chloroma) 205.3
Balint's syndrome (psychic paralysis of visual fixation) 368.16
Balkan grippe 083.0
Ball
  food 938
  hair 938
Ballantyne (-Runge) syndrome (postmaturity) 766.22
Balloon disease (*see also* Effect, adverse, high altitude) 993.2
Ballooning posterior leaflet syndrome 424.0
Baló's disease or concentric sclerosis 341.1
Bamberger's disease (hypertrophic pulmonary osteoarthropathy) 731.2
Bamberger-Marie disease (hypertrophic pulmonary osteoarthropathy) 731.2
Bamboo spine 720.0
Bancroft's filariasis 125.0
Band(s)
  adhesive (*see also* Adhesions, peritoneum) 568.0
  amniotic 658.8
    affecting fetus or newborn 762.8
  anomalous or congenital—*see also* Anomaly, specified type NEC
    atrial 746.9
    heart 746.9
    intestine 751.4
    omentum 751.4
    ventricular 746.9
  cervix 622.3
  gallbladder (congenital) 751.69

Band(s)—*continued*
  intestinal (adhesive) (*see also* Adhesions,
    peritoneum) 568.0
    congenital 751.4
  obstructive (*see also* Obstruction, intestine)
    560.81
  periappendiceal (congenital) 751.4
  peritoneal (adhesive) (*see also* Adhesions,
    peritoneum) 568.0
    with intestinal obstruction 560.81
    congenital 751.4
  uterus 621.5
  vagina 623.2
Bandemia (without diagnosis of specific
  infection) 288.66
Bandl's ring (contraction)
  complicating delivery 661.4
    affecting fetus or newborn 763.7
Bang's disease (Brucella abortus) 023.1
Bangkok hemorrhagic fever 065.4
Bannister's disease 995.1
Bantam-Albright-Martin disease
  (pseudohypoparathyroidism) 275.49
Banti's disease or syndrome (with cirrhosis)
  (with portal hypertension)—*see* Cirrhosis, liver
Bar
  calcaneocuboid 755.67
  calcaneonavicular 755.67
  cubonavicular 755.67
  prostate 600.90
    with
      other lower urinary tract symptoms (LUTS)
        600.91
      urinary
        obstruction 600.91
        retention 600.91
  talocalcaneal 755.67
Baragnosis 780.99
Barasheh, barashek 266.2
Barcoo disease or rot (*see also* Ulcer, skin) 707.9
Bard-Pic syndrome (carcinoma, head of
  pancreas) 157.0
Bärensprung's disease (eczema marginatum)
  110.3
Baritosis 503
Barium lung disease 503
Barlow's syndrome (meaning mitral valve
  prolapse) 424.0
Barlow (-Möller) disease or syndrome (meaning
  infantile scurvy) 267
Barodontalgia 993.2
Baron Münchausen syndrome 301.51
Barosinusitis 993.1
Barotitis 993.0
Barotrauma 993.2
  odontalgia 993.2
  otitic 993.0
  sinus 993.1
Barraquer's disease or syndrome (progressive
  lipodystrophy) 272.6
Barré-Guillain syndrome 357.0
Barré-Liéou syndrome (posterior cervical
  sympathetic) 723.2
Barrel chest 738.3
Barrett's esophagus 530.85
Barrett's syndrome or ulcer (chronic peptic
  ulcer of esophagus) 530.85
Bársony-Polgár syndrome (corkscrew
  esophagus) 530.5
Bársony-Teschendorf syndrome (corkscrew
  esophagus) 530.5

Barth syndrome 759.89
Bartholin's
  adenitis (*see also* Bartholinitis) 616.89
  gland—*see* condition
Bartholinitis (suppurating) 616.89
  gonococcal (acute) 098.0
    chronic or duration of 2 months or over 098.2
Bartonellosis 088.0
Bartter's syndrome (secondary
  hyperaldosteronism with juxtaglomerular
  hyperplasia) 255.13
Basal—*see* condition
Basan's (hidrotic) ectodermal dysplasia 757.31
Baseball finger 842.13
Basedow's disease or syndrome (exophthalmic
  goiter) 242.0
Basic —*see* condition
Basilar —*see* condition
Bason's (hidrotic) ectodermal dysplasia 757.31
Basopenia 288.59
Basophilia 288.65
Basophilism (corticoadrenal) (Cushing's)
  (pituitary) (thymic) 255.0
Bassen-Kornzweig syndrome
  (abetalipoproteinemia) 272.5
Bat ear 744.29
Bateman's
  disease 078.0
  purpura (senile) 287.2
Bathing cramp 994.1
Bathophobia 300.23
Batten's disease, retina 330.1 *[362.71]*
Batten-Mayou disease 330.1 *[362.71]*
Batten-Steinert syndrome 359.21
Battered
  adult (syndrome) 995.81
  baby or child (syndrome) 995.54
  spouse (syndrome) 995.81
Battey mycobacterium infection 031.0
Battledore placenta —*see* Placenta, abnormal
Battle exhaustion (*see also* Reaction, stress,
  acute) 308.9
Baumgarten-Cruveilhier (cirrhosis) disease, or
  syndrome 571.5
Bauxite
  fibrosis (of lung) 503
  workers' disease 503
Bayle's disease (dementia paralytica) 094.1
Bazin's disease (primary) (*see also* Tuberculosis)
  017.1
Beach ear 380.12
Beaded hair (congenital) 757.4
Beals syndrome 759.82
Beard's disease (neurasthenia) 300.5
Bearn-Kunkel (-Slater) syndrome (lupoid
  hepatitis) 571.49
Beat
  elbow 727.2
  hand 727.2
  knee 727.2
Beats
  ectopic 427.60
  escaped, heart 427.60
    postoperative 997.1
  premature (nodal) 427.60
    atrial 427.61
    auricular 427.61
    postoperative 997.1
    specified type NEC 427.69
    supraventricular 427.61
    ventricular 427.69

Beau's
  disease or syndrome (*see also* Degeneration,
    myocardial) 429.1
  lines (transverse furrows on fingernails) 703.8
Bechterew's disease (ankylosing spondylitis)
  720.0
Bechterew-Strümpell-Marie syndrome
  (ankylosing spondylitis) 720.0
Beck's syndrome (anterior spinal artery
  occlusion) 433.8
Becker's
  disease
    idiopathic mural endomyocardial disease 425.2
    myotonia congenita, recessive form 359.22
  dystrophy 359.22
Beckwith (-Wiedemann) syndrome 759.89
Bedbugs bite(s) —*see* Injury, superfiical, by site
Bed confinement status V49.84
Bedclothes, asphyxiation or suffocation by
  994.7
Bednar's aphthae 528.2
Bedsore (*see also* Ulcer, pressure) 707.00
  with gangrene 707.00 *[785.4]*
Bedwetting (*see also* Enuresis) 788.36
Beer-drinkers' heart (disease) 425.5
Bee sting (with allergic or anaphylactic shock)
  989.5
Begbie's disease (exophthalmic goiter) 242.0
Behavior disorder, disturbance —*see also*
  Disturbance, conduct
  antisocial, without manifest psychiatric disorder
    adolescent V71.02
    adult V71.01
    child V71.02
  dyssocial, without manifest psychiatric disorder
    adolescent V71.02
    adult V71.01
    child V71.02
  high-risk—*see* Problem
Behçet's syndrome 136.1
Behr's disease 362.50
Beigel's disease or morbus (white piedra) 111.2
Bejel 104.0
Bekhterev's disease (ankylosing spondylitis) 720.0
Bekhterev-Strümpell-Marie syndrome
  (ankylosing spondylitis) 720.0
Belching (*see also* Eructation) 787.3
Bell's
  disease (*see also* Psychosis, affective) 296.0
  mania (*see also* Psychosis, affective) 296.0
  palsy, paralysis 351.0
    infant 767.5
    newborn 767.5
    syphilitic 094.89
  spasm 351.0
Bence-Jones albuminuria, albuminosuria, or
  proteinuria 791.0
Bends 993.3
Benedikt's syndrome (paralysis) 344.89
Benign —*see also* condition
  cellular changes, cervix 795.09
  prostate
    hyperplasia 600.20
      with urinary retention 600.21
    neoplasm 222.2
    with
      other lower urinary tract symptoms (LUTS)
        600.21
      urinary
        obstruction 600.21
        retention 600.21

Bennett's
  disease (leukemia) 208.9
  fracture (closed) 815.01
    open 815.11
Benson's disease 379.22
Bent
  back (hysterical) 300.11
  nose 738.0
    congenital 754.0
Bereavement V62.82
  as adjustment reaction 309.0
Berger's paresthesia (lower limb) 782.0
Bergeron's disease (hysteroepilepsy) 300.11
Beriberi (acute) (atrophic) (chronic) (dry)
  (subacute) (wet) 265.0
  with polyneuropathy 265.0 *[357.4]*
  heart (disease) 265.0 *[425.7]*
  leprosy 030.1
  neuritis 265.0 *[357.4]*
Berlin's disease or edema (traumatic) 921.3
Berloque dermatitis 692.72
Bernard-Horner syndrome (*see also*
  Neuropathy, peripheral, autonomic) 337.9
Bernard-Sergent syndrome (acute
  adrenocortical insufficiency) 255.41
Bernard-Soulier disease or thrombopathy 287.1
Bernhardt's disease or paresthesia 355.1
Bernhardt-Roth disease or syndrome
  (paresthesia) 355.1
Bernheim's syndrome (*see also* Failure, heart)
  428.0
Bertielliasis 123.8
Bertolotti's syndrome (sacralization of fifth
  lumbar vertebra) 756.15
Berylliosis (acute) (chronic) (lung) (occupational)
  503
Besnier's
  lupus pernio 135
  prurigo (atopic dermatitis) (infantile eczema)
    691.8
Besnier-Boeck disease or sarcoid 135
Besnier-Boeck-Schaumann disease
  (sarcoidosis) 135
Best's disease 362.76
Bestiality 302.1
Beta-adrenergic hyperdynamic circulatory
  state 429.82
Beta-aminoisobutyric aciduria 277.2
Beta-mercaptolactate-cysteine disulfiduria
  270.0
Beta thalassemia (mixed) 282.46
  major 282.44
  minor 282.46
Beurmann's disease (sporotrichosis) 117.1
Bezoar 938
  intestine 936
  stomach 935.2
Bezold's abscess (*see also* Mastoiditis) 383.01
Bianchi's syndrome (aphasia-apraxia-alexia)
  784.69
Bicornuate or bicornis uterus (complete)
  (partial) 752.34
  in pregnancy or childbirth 654.0
    with obstructed labor 660.2
      affecting fetus or newborn 763.1
    affecting fetus or newborn 763.89
Bicuspid aortic valve 746.4
Biedl-Bardet syndrome 759.89
Bielschowsky's disease 330.1

Bielschowsky-Jansky
  amaurotic familial idiocy 330.1
  disease 330.1
Biemond's syndrome (obesity, polydactyly, and
  intellectual disabilities) 759.89
Biermer's anemia or disease (pernicious
  anemia) 281.0
Biett's disease 695.4
Bifid (congenital)—*see also* Imperfect, closure
  apex, heart 746.89
  clitoris 752.49
  epiglottis 748.3
  kidney 753.3
  nose 748.1
  patella 755.64
  scrotum 752.89
  toe 755.66
  tongue 750.13
  ureter 753.4
  uterus 752.34
  uvula 749.02
    with cleft lip (*see also* Cleft, palate, with cleft
      lip) 749.20
Biforis uterus (suprasimplex) 752.34
Bifurcation (congenital)—*see also* Imperfect,
  closure
  gallbladder 751.69
  kidney pelvis 753.3
  renal pelvis 753.3
  rib 756.3
  tongue 750.13
  trachea 748.3
  ureter 753.4
  urethra 753.8
  uvula 749.02
    with cleft lip (*see also* Cleft, palate, with cleft
      lip) 749.20
  vertebra 756.19
Bigeminal pulse 427.89
Bigeminy 427.89
Big spleen syndrome 289.4
Bilateral —*see* condition
Bile duct —*see* condition
Bile pigments in urine 791.4
Bilharziasis (*see also* Schistosomiasis) 120.9
  chyluria 120.0
  cutaneous 120.3
  galacturia 120.0
  hematochyluria 120.0
  intestinal 120.1
  lipemia 120.9
  lipuria 120.0
  Oriental 120.2
  piarhemia 120.9
  pulmonary 120.2
  tropical hematuria 120.0
  vesical 120.0
Biliary —*see* condition
Bilious (attack)—*see also* Vomiting
  fever, hemoglobinuric 084.8
Bilirubinuria 791.4
Biliuria 791.4
Billroth's disease
  meningocele (*see also* Spina bifida) 741.9
Bilobate placenta —*see* Placenta, abnormal
Bilocular
  heart 745.7
  stomach 536.8
Bing-Horton syndrome (histamine cephalgia)
  339.00

Binswanger's disease or dementia 290.12
Biörck (-Thorson) syndrome (malignant
  carcinoid) 259.2
Biparta, bipartite —*see also* Imperfect, closure
  carpal scaphoid 755.59
  patella 755.64
  placenta—*see* Placenta, abnormal
  vagina 752.49
Bird
  face 756.0
  fanciers' lung or disease 495.2
  flu (*see also* Influenza, avian) 488.02
Bird's disease (oxaluria) 271.8
Birth
  abnormal fetus or newborn 763.9
  accident, fetus or newborn—*see* Birth, injury
  complications in mother—*see* Delivery,
    complicated
  compression during NEC 767.9
  defect—*see* Anomaly
  delayed, fetus 763.9
  difficult NEC, affecting fetus or newborn 763.9
  dry, affecting fetus or newborn 761.1
  forced, NEC, affecting fetus or newborn 763.89
  forceps, affecting fetus or newborn 763.2
  hematoma of sternomastoid 767.8
  immature 765.1
    extremely 765.0
  inattention, after or at 995.52
  induced, affecting fetus or newborn 763.89
  infant—*see* Newborn
  injury NEC 767.9
    adrenal gland 767.8
    basal ganglia 767.0
    brachial plexus (paralysis) 767.6
    brain (compression) (pressure) 767.0
    cerebellum 767.0
    cerebral hemorrhage 767.0
    conjunctiva 767.8
    eye 767.8
    fracture
      bone, any except clavicle or spine 767.3
      clavicle 767.2
      femur 767.3
      humerus 767.3
      long bone 767.3
      radius and ulna 767.3
      skeleton NEC 767.3
      skull 767.3
      spine 767.4
      tibia and fibula 767.3
    hematoma 767.8
      liver (subcapsular) 767.8
      mastoid 767.8
      skull 767.19
      sternomastoid 767.8
      testes 767.8
      vulva 767.8
    intracranial (edema) 767.0
    laceration
      brain 767.0
      by scalpel 767.8
      peripheral nerve 767.7
    liver 767.8
    meninges
      brain 767.0
      spinal cord 767.4
    nerves (cranial, peripheral) 767.7
      brachial plexus 767.6
      facial 767.5

Birth—*continued*
  injury—*continued*
    paralysis 767.7
      brachial plexus 767.6
      Erb (-Duchenne) 767.6
      facial nerve 767.5
      Klumpke (-Déjérine) 767.6
      radial nerve 767.6
      spinal (cord) (hemorrhage) (laceration)
        (rupture) 767.4
    rupture
      intracranial 767.0
      liver 767.8
      spinal cord 767.4
      spleen 767.8
      viscera 767.8
    scalp 767.19
    scalpel wound 767.8
    skeleton NEC 767.3
    specified NEC 767.8
    spinal cord 767.4
    spleen 767.8
    subdural hemorrhage 767.0
    tentorial, tear 767.0
    testes 767.8
    vulva 767.8
  instrumental, NEC, affecting fetus or newborn
    763.2
  lack of care, after or at 995.52
  multiple
    affected by maternal complications of
      pregnancy 761.5
    healthy liveborn—*see* Newborn, multiple
  neglect, after or at 995.52
  newborn—*see* Newborn
  palsy or paralysis NEC 767.7
  precipitate, fetus or newborn 763.6
  premature (infant) 765.1
  prolonged, affecting fetus or newborn 763.9
  retarded, fetus or newborn 763.9
  shock, newborn 779.89
  strangulation or suffocation
    due to aspiration of clear amniotic fluid 770.13
      with respiratory symptoms 770.14
    mechanical 767.8
  trauma NEC 767.9
  triplet
    affected by maternal complications of
      pregnancy 761.5
    healthy liveborn—*see* Newborn, multiple
  twin
    affected by maternal complications of
      pregnancy 761.5
    healthy liveborn—*see* Newborn, twin
  ventouse, affecting fetus or newborn 763.3
Birt-Hogg-Dube syndrome 759.89
Birthmark 757.32
Bisalbuminemia 273.8
Biskra button 085.1
Bite(s)
  with intact skin surface—*see* Contusion
  animal—*see* Wound, open, by site
    intact skin surface—*see* Contusion
  bedbug—*see* Injury, superficial, by site
  centipede 989.5
  chigger 133.8
  fire ant 989.5
  flea—*see* Injury, superficial, by site
  human (open wound)—*see also* Wound, open,
    by site
    intact skin surface—*see* Contusion

Bite(s)—*continued*
  insect
    nonvenomous—*see* Injury, superficial, by site
    venomous 989.5
  mad dog (death from) 071
  open
    anterior 524.24
    posterior 524.25
  poisonous 989.5
  red bug 133.8
  reptile 989.5
    nonvenomous—*see* Wound, open, by site
  snake 989.5
    nonvenomous—*see* Wound, open, by site
  spider (venomous) 989.5
    nonvenomous—*see* Injury, superficial, by site
  venomous 989.5
Biting
  cheek or lip 528.9
  nail 307.9
Black
  death 020.9
  eye NEC 921.0
  hairy tongue 529.3
  heel 924.20
  lung disease 500
  palm 923.20
Blackfan-Diamond anemia or syndrome
  (congenital hypoplastic anemia) 284.01
Blackhead 706.1
Blackout 780.2
Blackwater fever 084.8
Bladder —*see* Condition
Blast
  blindness 921.3
  concussion—*see* Blast, injury
  injury 869.0
    with open wound into cavity 869.1
    abdomen or thorax—*see* Injury, internal, by
      site
    brain (*see also* Concussion, brain) 850.9
      with skull fracture—*see* Fracture, skull
    ear (acoustic nerve trauma) 951.5
      with perforation, tympanic membrane—*see*
        Wound, open, ear, drum
    lung (*see also* Injury, internal, lung) 861.20
    otitic (explosive) 388.11
Blastomycosis, blastomycotic (chronic)
  (cutaneous) (disseminated) (lung) (pulmonary)
  (systemic) 116.0
  Brazilian 116.1
  European 117.5
  keloidal 116.2
  North American 116.0
  primary pulmonary 116.0
  South American 116.1
Bleb(s) 709.8
  emphysematous (bullous) (diffuse) (lung)
    (ruptured) (solitary) 492.0
  filtering, eye (postglaucoma) (status) V45.69
    with complication 997.99
    postcataract extraction (complication) 997.99
  lung (ruptured) 492.0
    congenital 770.5
  subpleural (emphysematous) 492.0
Bleeder (familial) (hereditary) (*see also* Defect,
  coagulation) 286.9
  nonfamilial 286.9

Bleeding (*see also* Hemorrhage) 459.0
  anal 569.3
  anovulatory 628.0
  atonic, following delivery 666.1
  capillary 448.9
  due to subinvolution 621.1
    puerperal 666.2
  ear 388.69
  excessive, associated with menopausal onset
    627.0
  familial (*see also* Defect, coagulation) 286.9
  following intercourse 626.7
  gastrointestinal 578.9
  gums 523.8
  hemorrhoids—*see* Hemorrhoids, bleeding
  intermenstrual
    irregular 626.6
    regular 626.5
  intraoperative 998.11
  irregular NEC 626.4
  menopausal 627.0
  mouth 528.9
  nipple 611.79
  nose 784.7
  ovulation 626.5
  postclimacteric 627.1
  postcoital 626.7
  postmenopausal 627.1
    following induced menopause 627.4
  postoperative 998.11
  preclimacteric 627.0
  puberty 626.3
    excessive, with onset of menstrual periods
    626.3
  rectum, rectal 569.3
  tendencies (*see also* Defect, coagulation) 286.9
  throat 784.8
  umbilical stump 772.3
  umbilicus 789.9
  unrelated to menstrual cycle 626.6
  uterus, uterine 626.9
    climacteric 627.0
    dysfunctional 626.8
    functional 626.8
    unrelated to menstrual cycle 626.6
  vagina, vaginal 623.8
    functional 626.8
  vicarious 625.8
Blennorrhagia, blennorrhagic —*see*
  Blennorrhea
Blennorrhea (acute) 098.0
  adultorum 098.40
  alveolaris 523.40
  chronic or duration of 2 months or over 098.2
  gonococcal (neonatorum) 098.40
  inclusion (neonatal) (newborn) 771.6
  neonatorum 098.40
Blepharelosis (*see also* Entropion) 374.00
Blepharitis (eyelid) 373.00
  angularis 373.01
  ciliaris 373.00
    with ulcer 373.01
  marginal 373.00
    with ulcer 373.01
  scrofulous (*see also* Tuberculosis) 017.3
    [373.00]
  squamous 373.02
  ulcerative 373.01
Blepharochalasis 374.34
  congenital 743.62
Blepharoclonus 333.81

Blepharoconjunctivitis (*see also* Conjunctivitis)
  372.20
  angular 372.21
  contact 372.22
Blepharophimosis (eyelid) 374.46
  congenital 743.62
Blepharoplegia 374.89
Blepharoptosis 374.30
  congenital 743.61
Blepharopyorrhea 098.49
Blepharospasm 333.81
  due to drugs 333.85
Blessig's cyst 362.62
Blighted ovum 631.8
Blind
  bronchus (congenital) 748.3
  eye—*see also* Blindness
    hypertensive 360.42
    hypotensive 360.41
  loop syndrome (postoperative) 579.2
  sac, fallopian tube (congenital) 752.19
  spot, enlarged 368.42
  tract or tube (congenital) NEC—*see* Atresia
Blindness (acquired) (congenital) (both eyes) 369.00
  with deafness V49.85
  blast 921.3
    with nerve injury—*see* Injury, nerve, optic
  Bright's—*see* Uremia
  color (congenital) 368.59
    acquired 368.55
    blue 368.53
    green 368.52
    red 368.51
    total 368.54
  concussion 950.9
  cortical 377.75
  day 368.10
    acquired 368.10
    congenital 368.10
    hereditary 368.10
    specified type NEC 368.10
  due to
    injury NEC 950.9
    refractive error—*see* Error, refractive
  eclipse (total) 363.31
  emotional 300.11
  face 368.16
  hysterical 300.11
  legal (both eyes) (USA definition) 369.4
    with impairment of better (less impaired) eye
      near-total 369.02
      with
        lesser eye impairment 369.02
          near-total 369.04
          total 369.03
      profound 369.05
      with
        lesser eye impairment 369.05
          near-total 369.07
          profound 369.08
          total 369.06
      severe 369.21
      with
        lesser eye impairment 369.21
          blind 369.11
          near-total 369.13
          profound 369.14
          severe 369.22
          total 369.12
      total
        with lesser eye impairment total 369.01

Blindness—*continued*
  mind 784.69
  moderate
    both eyes 369.25
      with impairment of lesser eye (specified as)
        blind, not further specified 369.15
        low vision, not further specified 369.23
        near-total 369.17
        profound 369.18
        severe 369.24
        total 369.16
    one eye 369.74
      with vision of other eye (specified as)
        near-normal 369.75
        normal 369.76
  near-total
    both eyes 369.04
      with impairment of lesser eye (specified as)
        blind, not further specified 369.02
        total 369.03
    one eye 369.64
      with vision of other eye (specified as)
        near-normal 369.65
        normal 369.66
  night 368.60
    acquired 368.62
    congenital (Japanese) 368.61
    hereditary 368.61
    specified type NEC 368.69
    vitamin A deficiency 264.5
  nocturnal—*see* Blindness, night
  one eye 369.60
    with low vision of other eye 369.10
  profound
    both eyes 369.08
      with impairment of lesser eye (specified as)
        blind, not further specified 369.05
        near-total 369.07
        total 369.06
    one eye 369.67
      with vision of other eye (specified as)
        near-normal 369.68
        normal 369.69
  psychic 784.69
  severe
    both eyes 369.22
      with impairment of lesser eye (specified as)
        blind, not further specified 369.11
        low vision, not further specified 369.21
        near-total 369.13
        profound 369.14
        total 369.12
    one eye 369.71
      with vision of other eye (specified as)
        near-normal 369.72
        normal 369.73
  snow 370.24
  sun 363.31
  temporary 368.12
  total
    both eyes 369.01
    one eye 369.61
      with vision of other eye (specified as)
        near-normal 369.62
        normal 369.63
  transient 368.12
  traumatic NEC 950.9
  word (developmental) 315.01
    acquired 784.61
    secondary to organic lesion 784.61

Blister —*see also* Injury, superficial, by site
  beetle dermatitis 692.89
  due to burn—*see* Burn, by site, second degree
  fever 054.9
  fracture—*omit code*
  multiple, skin, nontraumatic 709.8
Bloating 787.3
Bloch-Siemens syndrome (incontinentia
    pigmenti) 757.33
Bloch-Stauffer dyshormonal dermatosis 757.33
Bloch-Sulzberger disease or syndrome
    (incontinentia pigmenti) (melanoblastosis) 757.33
Block
  alveolar capillary 516.8
  arborization (heart) 426.6
  arrhythmic 426.9
  atrioventricular (AV) (incomplete) (partial)
      426.10
    with
      2:1 atrioventricular response block 426.13
      atrioventricular dissociation 426.0
    first degree (incomplete) 426.11
    second degree (Mobitz type I) 426.13
      Mobitz (type) II 426.12
    third degree 426.0
    complete 426.0
      congenital 746.86
    congenital 746.86
    Mobitz (incomplete)
      type I (Wenckebach's) 426.13
      type II 426.12
    partial 426.13
  auriculoventricular (*see also* Block,
      atrioventricular) 426.10
    complete 426.0
      congenital 746.86
    congenital 746.86
  bifascicular (cardiac) 426.53
  bundle branch (complete) (false) (incomplete)
      426.50
    bilateral 426.53
    left (complete) (main stem) 426.3
      with right bundle branch block 426.53
      anterior fascicular 426.2
        with
          posterior fascicular block 426.3
          right bundle branch block 426.52
      hemiblock 426.2
      incomplete 426.2
        with right bundle branch block 426.53
      posterior fascicular 426.2
        with
          anterior fascicular block 426.3
          right bundle branch block 426.51
    right 426.4
      with
        left bundle branch block (incomplete)
          (main stem) 426.53
        left fascicular block 426.53
          anterior 426.52
          posterior 426.51
      Wilson's type 426.4
  cardiac 426.9
  conduction 426.9
    complete 426.0
  Eustachian tube (*see also* Obstruction,
      Eustachian tube) 381.60
  fascicular (left anterior) (left posterior) 426.2

Block—*continued*
foramen Magendie (acquired) 331.3
  congenital 742.3
    with spina bifida (*see also* Spina bifida) 741.0
heart 426.9
  first degree (atrioventricular) 426.11
  second degree (atrioventricular) 426.13
  third degree (atrioventricular) 426.0
  bundle branch (complete) (false) (incomplete)
    426.50
    bilateral 426.53
    left (*see also* Block, bundle branch, left)
      426.3
    right (*see also* Block, bundle branch, right)
      426.4
  complete (atrioventricular) 426.0
  congenital 746.86
  incomplete 426.13
  intra-atrial 426.6
  intraventricular NEC 426.6
  sinoatrial 426.6
  specified type NEC 426.6
hepatic vein 453.0
intraventricular (diffuse) (myofibrillar) 426.6
  bundle branch (complete) (false) (incomplete)
    426.50
    bilateral 426.53
    left (*see also* Block, bundle branch, left)
      426.3
    right (*see also* Block, bundle branch, right)
      426.4
kidney (*see also* Disease, renal) 593.9
  postcystoscopic 997.5
myocardial (*see also* Block, heart) 426.9
nodal 426.10
optic nerve 377.49
organ or site (congenital) NEC—*see* Atresia
parietal 426.6
peri-infarction 426.6
portal (vein) 452
sinoatrial 426.6
sinoauricular 426.6
spinal cord 336.9
trifascicular 426.54
tubal 628.2
vein NEC 453.9
Blocq's disease or syndrome (astasia-abasia)
  307.9
Blood
constituents, abnormal NEC 790.6
disease 289.9
  specified NEC 289.89
donor V59.01
  other blood components V59.09
  stem cells V59.02
  whole blood V59.01
dyscrasia 289.9
  with
    abortion—*see* Abortion, by type, with
      hemorrhage, delayed or excessive
    ectopic pregnancy (*see also* categories
      633.0-633.9) 639.1
    molar pregnancy (*see also* categories
      630-632) 639.1
  following
    abortion 639.1
    ectopic or molar pregnancy 639.1
  newborn NEC 776.9
  puerperal, postpartum 666.3
flukes NEC (*see also* Infestation, Schistosoma)
  120.9

Blood—*continued*
in
  feces (*see also* Melena) 578.1
    occult 792.1
  urine (*see also* Hematuria) 599.70
mole 631.8
occult 792.1
poisoning (*see also* Septicemia) 038.9
pressure
  decreased, due to shock following injury 958.4
  fluctuating 796.4
  high (*see also* Hypertension) 401.9
    borderline 796.2
    incidental reading (isolated) (nonspecific),
      without diagnosis of hypertension 796.2
  low (*see also* Hypotension) 458.9
    incidental reading (isolated) (nonspecific),
      without diagnosis of hypotension 796.3
spitting (*see also* Hemoptysis) 786.30
staining cornea 371.12
transfusion
  without reported diagnosis V58.2
  donor V59.01
    stem cells V59.02
  reaction or complication—*see* Complications,
    transfusion
tumor—*see* Hematoma
vessel rupture—*see* Hemorrhage
vomiting (*see also* Hematemesis) 578.0
Blood-forming organ disease 289.9
Bloodgood's disease 610.1
Bloodshot eye 379.93
Bloom (-Machacek) (-Torre) syndrome 757.39
Blotch, palpebral 372.55
Blount's disease (tibia vara) 732.4
Blount-Barber syndrome (tibia vara) 732.4
Blue
baby 746.9
bloater 491.20
  with acute bronchitis 491.22
  with exacerbation (acute) 491.21
diaper syndrome 270.0
disease 746.9
dome cyst 610.0
drum syndrome 381.02
sclera 743.47
  with fragility of bone and deafness 756.51
toe syndrome 445.02
Blueness (cyanosis) 782.5
Blurred vision 368.8
Blushing (abnormal) (excessive) 782.62
BMI (body mass index)
adult
  25.0-25.9 V85.21
  26.0-26.9 V85.22
  27.0-27.9 V85.23
  28.0-28.9 V85.24
  29.0-29.9 V85.25
  30.0-30.9 V85.30
  31.0-31.9 V85.31
  32.0-32.9 V85.32
  33.0-33.9 V85.33
  34.0-34.9 V85.34
  35.0-35.9 V85.35
  36.0-36.9 V85.36
  37.0-37.9 V85.37
  38.0-38.9 V85.38
  39.0-39.9 V85.39
  40.0-44.9 V85.41
  45.0-49.9 V85.42
  50.0-59.9 V85.43

BMI (body mass index)—*continued*
  60.0-69.9 V85.44
  70 and over V85.45
  between 19-24 V85.1
  less than 19 V85.0
  pediatric
    5th percentile to less than 85th percentile for
      age V85.52
    85th percentile to less than 95th percentile for
      age V85.53
    greater than or equal to 95th percentile for age
      V85.54
    less than 5th percentile for age V85.51
Boarder, hospital V65.0
  infant V65.0
Bockhart's impetigo (superficial folliculitis) 704.8
Bodechtel-Guttmann disease (subacute
  sclerosing panencephalitis) 046.2
Boder-Sedgwick syndrome (ataxia-
  telangiectasia) 334.8
Body, bodies
  Aschoff (*see also* Myocarditis, rheumatic) 398.0
  asteroid, vitreous 379.22
  choroid, colloid (degenerative) 362.57
    hereditary 362.77
  cytoid (retina) 362.82
  drusen (retina) (*see also* Drusen) 362.57
    optic disc 377.21
  fibrin, pleura 511.0
  foreign—*see* Foreign body
  Hassall-Henle 371.41
  loose
    joint (*see also* Loose, body, joint) 718.1
      knee 717.6
    knee 717.6
    sheath, tendon 727.82
  Mallory's 034.1
  mass index (BMI)
    adult
      25.0-25.9 V85.21
      26.0-26.9 V85.22
      27.0-27.9 V85.23
      28.0-28.9 V85.24
      29.0-29.9 V85.25
      30.0-30.9 V85.30
      31.0-31.9 V85.31
      32.0-32.9 V85.32
      33.0-33.9 V85.33
      34.0-34.9 V85.34
      35.0-35.9 V85.35
      36.0-36.9 V85.36
      37.0-37.9 V85.37
      38.0-38.9 V85.38
      39.0-39.9 V85.39
      40.0-44.9 V85.41
      45.0-49.9 V85.42
      50.0-59.9 V85.43
      60.0-69.9 V85.44
      70 and over V85.45
      between 19-24 V85.1
      less than 19 V85.0
    pediatric
      5th percentile to less than 85th percentile for
        age V85.52
      85th percentile to less than 95th percentile
        for age V85.53
      greater than or equal to 95th percentile for
        age V85.54
      less than 5th percentile for age V85.51
  Mooser 081.0
  Negri 071

Body, bodies—*continued*
  rice (joint) (*see also* Loose, body, joint) 718.1
    knee 717.6
  rocking 307.3
Boeck's
  disease (sarcoidosis) 135
  lupoid (miliary) 135
  sarcoid 135
Boerhaave's syndrome (spontaneous esophageal
  rupture) 530.4
Boggy
  cervix 622.8
  uterus 621.8
Boil (*see also* Carbuncle) 680.9
  abdominal wall 680.2
  Aleppo 085.1
  ankle 680.6
  anus 680.5
  arm (any part, above wrist) 680.3
  auditory canal, external 680.0
  axilla 680.3
  back (any part) 680.2
  Baghdad 085.1
  breast 680.2
  buttock 680.5
  chest wall 680.2
  corpus cavernosum 607.2
  Delhi 085.1
  ear (any part) 680.0
  eyelid 373.13
  face (any part, except eye) 680.0
  finger (any) 680.4
  flank 680.2
  foot (any part) 680.7
  forearm 680.3
  Gafsa 085.1
  genital organ, male 608.4
  gluteal (region) 680.5
  groin 680.2
  hand (any part) 680.4
  head (any part, except face) 680.8
  heel 680.7
  hip 680.6
  knee 680.6
  labia 616.4
  lacrimal (*see also* Dacryocystitis) 375.30
    gland (*see also* Dacryoadenitis) 375.00
    passages (duct) (sac) (*see also* Dacryocystitis)
      375.30
  leg, any part except foot 680.6
  multiple sites 680.9
  Natal 085.1
  neck 680.1
  nose (external) (septum) 680.0
  orbit, orbital 376.01
  partes posteriores 680.5
  pectoral region 680.2
  penis 607.2
  perineum 680.2
  pinna 680.0
  scalp (any part) 680.8
  scrotum 608.4
  seminal vesicle 608.0
  shoulder 680.3
  skin NEC 680.9
  specified site NEC 680.8
  spermatic cord 608.4
  temple (region) 680.0
  testis 608.4
  thigh 680.6
  thumb 680.4
  toe (any) 680.7

Boil —*continued*
tropical 085.1
trunk 680.2
tunica vaginalis 608.4
umbilicus 680.2
upper arm 680.3
vas deferens 608.4
vulva 616.4
wrist 680.4
Bold hives (*see also* Urticaria) 708.9
Bolivian hemorrhagic fever 078.7
Bombé, iris 364.74
Bomford-Rhoads anemia (refractory) 238.72
Bone —*see* condition
Bonnevie-Ullrich syndrome 758.6
Bonnier's syndrome 386.19
Bonvale Dam fever 780.79
Bony block of joint 718.80
ankle 718.87
elbow 718.82
foot 718.87
hand 718.84
hip 718.85
knee 718.86
multiple sites 718.89
pelvic region 718.85
shoulder (region) 718.81
specified site NEC 718.88
wrist 718.83
BOOP (bronchiolitis obliterans organized
penumonia) 516.8
Borderline
diabetes mellitus 790.29
hypertension 796.2
intellectual functioning V62.89
osteopenia 733.90
pelvis 653.1
with obstruction during labor 660.1
affecting fetus or newborn 763.1
psychosis (*see also* Schizophrenia) 295.5
of childhood (*see also* Psychosis, childhood)
299.8
schizophrenia (*see also* Schizophrenia) 295.5
Borna disease 062.9
Bornholm disease (epidemic pleurodynia) 074.1
Borrelia vincentii (mouth) (pharynx) (tonsils) 101
Bostock's catarrh (*see also* Fever, hay) 477.9
Boston exanthem 048
Botalli, ductus (patent) (persistent) 747.0
Bothriocephalus latus infestation 123.4
Botulism 005.1
food poisoning 005.1
infant 040.41
non-foodborne 040.42
wound 040.42
Bouba (*see also* Yaws) 102.9
Bouffée délirante 298.3
Bouillaud's disease or syndrome (rheumatic
heart disease) 391.9
Bourneville's disease (tuberous sclerosis) 759.5
Boutonneuse fever 082.1
Boutonniere
deformity (finger) 736.21
hand (intrinsic) 736.21
Bouveret (-Hoffmann) disease or syndrome
(paroxysmal tachycardia) 427.2
Bovine heart —*see* Hypertrophy, cardiac
Bowel —*see* condition
Bowen's
dermatosis (precancerous) (M8081/2)—*see*
Neoplasm, skin, in situ

Bowen's—*continued*
disease (M8081/2)—*see* Neoplasm, skin, in situ
epithelioma (M8081/2)—*see* Neoplasm, skin, in
situ
type
epidermoid carcinoma in situ (M8081/2)—*see*
Neoplasm, skin, in situ
intraepidermal squamous cell carcinoma
(M8081/2)-*see* Neoplasm, skin, in situ
Bowing
femur 736.89
congenital 754.42
fibula 736.89
congenital 754.43
forearm 736.09
away from midline (cubitus valgus) 736.01
toward midline (cubitus varus) 736.02
leg(s), long bones, congenital 754.44
radius 736.09
away from midline (cubitus valgus) 736.01
toward midline (cubitus varus) 736.02
tibia 736.89
congenital 754.43
Bowleg (s) 736.42
congenital 754.44
rachitic 268.1
Boyd's dysentery 004.2
Brachial —*see* condition
Brachman-de Lange syndrome (Amsterdam
dwarf, intellectual disabilities, and
brachycephaly) 759.89
Brachycardia 427.89
Brachycephaly 756.0
Brachymorphism and ectopia lentis 759.89
Bradley's disease (epidemic vomiting) 078.82
Bradycardia 427.89
chronic (sinus) 427.81
newborn 779.81
nodal 427.89
postoperative 997.1
reflex 337.09
sinoatrial 427.89
with paroxysmal tachyarrhythmia or
tachycardia 427.81
chronic 427.81
sinus 427.89
with paroxysmal tachyarrhythmia or
tachycardia 427.81
chronic 427.81
persistent 427.81
severe 427.81
tachycardia syndrome 427.81
vagal 427.89
Bradykinesia 781.0
Bradypnea 786.09
Brailsford's disease 732.3
radial head 732.3
tarsal scaphoid 732.5
Brailsford-Morquio disease or syndrome
(mucopolysaccharidosis IV) 277.5
Brain —*see also* condition
death 348.82
syndrome (acute) (chronic) (nonpsychotic)
(organic) (with neurotic reaction) (with
behavioral reaction) (*see also* Syndrome,
brain) 310.9
with
presenile brain disease 290.10
psychosis, psychotic reaction (*see also*
Psychosis, organic) 294.9
congenital (*see also* Disability, intellectual) 319

Branched-chain amino-acid disease 270.3
Branchial —*see* condition
Brandt's syndrome (acrodermatitis
    enteropathica) 686.8
Brash (water) 787.1
Brass-founders' ague 985.8
Bravais-Jacksonian epilepsy (*see also* Epilepsy)
    345.5
Braxton Hicks contractions 644.1
Braziers' disease 985.8
Brazilian
    blastomycosis 116.1
    leishmaniasis 085.5
BRBPR (bright red blood per rectum) 569.3
Break
    cardiorenal—*see* Hypertension, cardiorenal
    retina (*see also* Defect, retina) 361.30
Breakbone fever 061
Breakdown
    device, implant, or graft—*see* Complications,
      mechanical
    nervous (*see also* Disorder, mental,
      nonpsychotic) 300.9
    perineum 674.2
Breast —*see also* condition
    buds 259.1
      in newborn 779.89
    dense 793.82
    nodule 793.89
Breast feeding difficulties 676.8
Breath
    foul 784.99
    holder, child 312.81
    holding spells 786.9
    shortness 786.05
Breathing
    asymmetrical 786.09
    bronchial 786.09
    exercises V57.0
    labored 786.09
    mouth 784.99
      causing malocclusion 524.59
    periodic 786.09
      high altitude 327.22
    tic 307.20
Breathlessness 786.09
Breda's disease (*see also* Yaws) 102.9
Breech
    delivery, affecting fetus or newborn 763.0
    extraction, affecting fetus or newborn 763.0
    presentation (buttocks) (complete) (frank) 652.2
      with successful version 652.1
      before labor, affecting fetus or newborn 761.7
      during labor, affecting fetus or newborn 763.0
Breisky's disease (kraurosis vulvae) 624.09
Brennemann's syndrome (acute mesenteric
    lymphadenitis) 289.2
Brenner's
    tumor (benign) (M9000/0) 220
      borderline malignancy (M9000/1) 236.2
      malignant (M9000/3) 183.0
      proliferating (M9000/1) 236.2
Bretonneau's disease (diphtheritic malignant
    angina) 032.0
Breus' mole 631.8
Brevicollis 756.16
Bricklayers' itch 692.89
Brickmakers' anemia 126.9
Bridge
    myocardial 746.85

Bright's
    blindness—*see* Uremia
    disease (*see also* Nephritis) 583.9
      arteriosclerotic (*see also* Hypertension,
        kidney) 403.90
Bright red blood per rectum (BRBPR) 569.3
Brill's disease (recrudescent typhus) 081.1
    flea-borne 081.0
    louse-borne 081.1
Brill-Symmers disease (follicular lymphoma)
    (M9690/3) 202.0
Brill-Zinsser disease (recrudescent typhus) 081.1
Brinton's disease (linitis plastica) (M8142/3) 151.9
Brion-Kayser disease (*see also* Fever,
    paratyphoid) 002.9
Briquet's disorder or syndrome 300.81
Brissaud's
    infantilism (infantile myxedema) 244.9
    motor-verbal tic 307.23
Brissaud-Meige syndrome (infantile myxedema)
    244.9
Brittle
    bones (congenital) 756.51
    nails 703.8
      congenital 757.5
Broad —*see also* condition
    beta disease 272.2
    ligament laceration syndrome 620.6
Brock's syndrome (atelectasis due to enlarged
    lymph nodes) 518.0
Brocq's disease 691.8
    atopic (diffuse) neurodermatitis 691.8
    lichen simplex chronicus 698.3
    parakeratosis psoriasiformis 696.2
    parapsoriasis 696.2
Brocq-Duhring disease (dermatitis
    herpetiformis) 694.0
Brodie's
    abscess (localized) (chronic) (*see also*
      Osteomyelitis) 730.1
    disease (joint) (*see also* Osteomyelitis) 730.1
Broken
    arches 734
      congenital 755.67
    back—*see* Fracture, vertebra, by site
    bone—*see* Fracture, by site
    compensation—*see* Disease, heart
    heart syndrome 429.83
    implant or internal device—*see* listing under
      Complications, mechanical
    neck—*see* Fracture, vertebra, cervical
    nose 802.0
      open 802.1
    tooth, teeth 873.63
      complicated 873.73
Bromhidrosis 705.89
Bromidism, bromism
    acute 967.3
      correct substance properly administered 349.82
      overdose or wrong substance given or taken
        967.3
    chronic (*see also* Dependence) 304.1
Bromidrosiphobia 300.23
Bromidrosis 705.89
Bronchi, bronchial —*see* condition
Bronchiectasis (cylindrical) (diffuse) (fusiform)
    (localized) (moniliform) (postinfectious)
    (recurrent) (saccular) 494.0
    with acute exacerbation 494.1
    congenital 748.61
    tuberculosis (*see also* Tuberculosis) 011.5

Bronchiolectasis —*see* Bronchiectasis
Bronchiolitis (acute) (infectious) (subacute)
466.19
with
bronchospasm or obstruction 466.19
influenza, flu, or grippe (*see also* Influenza)
487.1
catarrhal (acute) (subacute) 466.19
chemical 506.0
chronic 506.4
chronic (obliterative) 491.8
due to external agent—*see* Bronchitis, acute,
due to
fibrosa obliterans 491.8
influenzal (*see also* Influenza) 487.1
obliterans 491.8
status post lung transplant 996.84
with organizing pneumonia (BOOP) 516.8
obliterative (chronic) (diffuse) (subacute) 491.8
due to fumes or vapors 506.4
respiratory syncytial virus 466.11
vesicular—*see* Pneumonia, broncho-
Bronchitis (diffuse) (hypostatic) (infectious)
(inflammatory) (simple) 490
with
emphysema—*see* Emphysema
influenza, flu, or grippe(*see also* Influenza)
487.1
obstruction airway, chronic 491.20
with
acute bronchitis 491.22
exacerbation (acute) 491.21
tracheitis 490
acute or subacute 466.0
with bronchospasm or obstruction 466.0
chronic 491.8
acute or subacute 466.0
with
bronchiectasis 494.1
bronchospasm 466.0
obstruction 466.0
tracheitis 466.0
chemical (due to fumes or vapors) 506.0
due to
fumes or vapors 506.0
radiation 508.8
allergic (acute) (*see also* Asthma) 493.9
arachidic 934.1
aspiration 507.0
due to fumes or vapors 506.0
asthmatic (acute) 493.90
with
acute exacerbation 493.92
status asthmaticus 493.91
chronic 493.2
capillary 466.19
with bronchospasm or obstruction 466.19
chronic 491.8
caseous (*see also* Tuberculosis) 011.3
Castellani's 104.8
catarrhal 490
acute—*see* Bronchitis, acute
chronic 491.0
chemical (acute) (subacute) 506.0
chronic 506.4
due to fumes or vapors (acute) (subacute)
506.0
chronic 506.4
chronic 491.9
with
tracheitis (chronic) 491.8
asthmatic 493.2

Bronchitis—*continued*
chronic—*continued*
catarrhal 491.0
chemical (due to fumes and vapors) 506.4
due to
fumes or vapors (chemical) (inhalation) 506.4
radiation 508.8
tobacco smoking 491.0
mucopurulent 491.1
obstructive 491.20
with
acute bronchitis 491.22
exacerbation (acute) 491.21
purulent 491.1
simple 491.0
specified type NEC 491.8
croupous 466.0
with bronchospasm or obstruction 466.0
due to fumes or vapors 506.0
emphysematous 491.20
with
acute bronchitis 491.22
exacerbation (acute) 491.21
exudative 466.0
fetid (chronic) (recurrent) 491.1
fibrinous, acute or subacute 466.0
with bronchospasm or obstruction 466.0
grippal (*see also* Influenza) 487.1
influenzal (*see also* Influenza) 487.1
membranous, acute or subacute 466.0
with bronchospasm or obstruction 466.0
moulders' 502
mucopurulent (chronic) (recurrent) 491.1
acute or subacute 466.0
non-obstructive 491.0
obliterans 491.8
obstructive (chronic) 491.20
with
acute bronchitis 491.22
exacerbation (acute) 491.21
pituitous 491.1
plastic (inflammatory) 466.0
pneumococcal, acute or subacute 466.0
with bronchospasm or obstruction 466.0
pseudomembranous 466.0
purulent (chronic) (recurrent) 491.1
acute or subacute 466.0
with bronchospasm or obstruction 466.0
putrid 491.1
scrofulous (*see also* Tuberculosis) 011.3
senile 491.9
septic, acute or subacute 466.0
with bronchospasm or obstruction 466.0
smokers' 491.0
spirochetal 104.8
suffocative, acute or subacute 466.0
summer (*see also* Asthma) 493.9
suppurative (chronic) 491.1
acute or subacute 466.0
tuberculous (*see also* Tuberculosis) 011.3
ulcerative 491.8
Vincent's 101
Vincent's 101
viral, acute or subacute 466.0
with bronchospasm or obstruction 466.0
Bronchoalveolitis 485
Bronchoaspergillosis 117.3
Bronchocele
meaning
dilatation of bronchus 519.19
goiter 240.9
Bronchogenic carcinoma 162.9

Bronchohemisporosis 117.9
Broncholithiasis 518.89
tuberculous (*see also* Tuberculosis) 011.3
Bronchomalacia 748.3
Bronchomoniliasis 112.89
Bronchomycosis 112.89
Bronchonocardiosis 039.1
Bronchopleuropneumonia —*see* Pneumonia, broncho-
Bronchopneumonia —*see* Pneumonia, broncho-
Bronchopneumonitis —*see* Pneumonia, broncho-
Bronchopulmonary —*see* condition
Bronchopulmonitis —*see* Pneumonia, broncho-
Bronchorrhagia 786.30
newborn 770.3
tuberculous (*see also* Tuberculosis) 011.3
Bronchorrhea (chronic) (purulent) 491.0
acute 466.0
Bronchospasm 519.11
with
asthma—*see* Asthma
bronchiolitis, acute 466.19
due to respiratory syncytial virus 466.11
bronchitis—*see* Bronchitis
chronic obstructive pulmonary disease
(COPD) 496
emphysema—*see* Emphysema
due to external agent—*see* Condition, respiratory, acture, due to
acute 519.11
due to external agent—*see* Condition, respiratory, acute, due to
exercise induced 493.81
Bronchospirochetosis 104.8
Bronchostenosis 519.19
Bronchus —*see* condition
Bronze, bronzed
diabetes 275.01
disease (Addison's) (skin) 255.41
tuberculous (*see also* Tuberculosis) 017.6
Brooke's disease or tumor (M8100/0)—*see* Neoplasm, skin, benign
Brow presentation complicating delivery 652.4
Brown's tendon sheath syndrome 378.61
Brown enamel of teeth (hereditary) 520.5
Brown-Séquard's paralysis (syndrome) 344.89
Brucella, brucellosis (infection) 023.9
abortus 023.1
canis 023.3
dermatitis, skin 023.9
melitensis 023.0
mixed 023.8
suis 023.2
Bruck's disease 733.99
Bruck-de Lange disease or syndrome
(Amsterdam dwarf, intellectual disabilities, and brachycephaly) 759.89
Brugada syndrome 746.89
Brug's filariasis 125.1
Brugsch's syndrome (acropachyderma) 757.39
Bruhl's disease (splenic anemia with fever) 285.8
Bruise (skin surface intact)—*see also* Contusion
with
fracture—*see* Fracture, by site
open wound—*see* Wound, open, by site
internal organ (abdomen, chest, or pelvis)—*see* Injury, internal, by site
umbilical cord 663.6
affecting fetus or newborn 762.6

Bruit 785.9
arterial (abdominal) (carotid) 785.9
supraclavicular 785.9
Brushburn —*see* Injury, superficial, by site
Bruton's X-linked agammaglobulinemia 279.04
Bruxism 306.8
sleep related 327.53
Bubbly lung syndrome 770.7
Bubo 289.3
blennorrhagic 098.89
chancroidal 099.0
climatic 099.1
due to Hemophilus ducreyi 099.0
gonococcal 098.89
indolent NEC 099.8
inguinal NEC 099.8
chancroidal 099.0
climatic 099.1
due to H. ducreyi 099.0
scrofulous (*see also* Tuberculosis) 017.2
soft chancre 099.0
suppurating 683
syphilitic 091.0
congenital 090.0
tropical 099.1
venereal NEC 099.8
virulent 099.0
Bubonic plague 020.0
Bubonocele —*see* Hernia, inguinal
Buccal —*see* condition
Buchanan's disease (juvenile osteochondrosis of iliac crest) 732.1
Buchem's syndrome (hyperostosis corticalis) 733.3
Buchman's disease (osteochondrosis, juvenile) 732.1
Bucket handle fracture (semilunar cartilage) (*see also* Tear, meniscus) 836.2
Budd-Chiari syndrome (hepatic vein thrombosis) 453.0
Budgerigar-fanciers' disease or lung 495.2
Büdinger-Ludloff-Läwen disease 717.89
Buds
breast 259.1
in newborn 779.89
Buerger's disease (thromboangiitis obliterans) 443.1
Bulbar —*see* condition
Bulbus cordis 745.9
persistent (in left ventricle) 745.8
Bulging fontanels (congenital) 756.0
Bulimia 783.6
nervosa 307.51
nonorganic origin 307.51
Bulky uterus 621.2
Bulla(e) 709.8
lung (emphysematous) (solitary) 492.0
Bullet wound —*see also* Wound, open, by site
fracture—*see* Fracture, by site, open
internal organ (abdomen, chest, or pelvis)—*see* Injury, internal, by site, with open wound
intracranial—*see* Laceration, brain, with open wound
Bullis fever 082.8
Bullying (*see also* Disturbance, conduct) 312.0
Bundle
branch block (complete) (false) (incomplete) 426.50
bilateral 426.53
left (*see also* Block, bundle branch, left) 426.3
hemiblock 426.2
right (*see also* Block, bundle branch, right) 426.4

Bundle—*continued*
of His—*see* condition
of Kent syndrome (anomalous atrioventricular excitation) 426.7
Bungpagga 040.81
Bunion 727.1
Bunionette 727.1
Bunyamwera fever 066.3
Buphthalmia, buphthalmos (congenital) 743.20
associated with
keratoglobus, congenital 743.22
megalocornea 743.22
ocular anomalies NEC 743.22
isolated 743.21
simple 743.21
Bürger-Grütz disease or syndrome (essential familial hyperlipemia) 272.3
Buried roots 525.3
Burke's syndrome 577.8
Burkitt's
tumor (M9750/3) 200.2
type malignant, lymphoma, lymphoblastic, or undifferentiated (M9750/3) 200.2
Burn (acid) (cathode ray) (caustic) (chemical) (electric heating appliance) (electricity) (fire) (flame) (hot liquid or object) (irradiation) (lime) (radiation) (steam) (thermal) (x-ray) 949.0

Note—Use the following fifth-digit subclassification with category 948 to indicate the percent of body surface with third degree burn:

0 less than 10% or unspecified
1 10-19%
2 20-29%
3 30-39%
4 40-49%
5 50-59%
6 60-69%
7 70-79%
8 80-89%
9 90% or more of body surface

---

with
blisters—*see* Burn, by site, second degree
erythema—*see* Burn, by site, first degree
skin loss (epidermal)—*see also* Burn, by site, second degree
full thickness—*see also* Burn, by site, third degree
with necrosis of underlying tissues—*see* Burn, by site, third degree, deep
first degree—*see* Burn, by site, first degree
second degree—*see* Burn, by site, second degree
third degree—*see also* Burn, by site, third degree
deep—*see* Burn, by site, third degree, deep
abdomen, abdominal (muscle) (wall) 942.03
with
trunk—*see* Burn, trunk, multiple sites
first degree 942.13
second degree 942.23
third degree 942.33
deep 942.43
with loss of body part 942.53
ankle 945.03
with
lower limb(s)–*see* Burn, leg, multiple sites
first degree 945.13
second degree 945.23

Burn—*continued*
ankle—*continued*
third degree 945.33
deep 945.43
with loss of body part 945.53
anus—*see* Burn, trunk, specified site NEC
arm(s) 943.00
first degree 943.10
second degree 943.20
third degree 943.30
deep 943.40
with loss of body part 943.50
lower—*see* Burn, forearm(s)
multiple sites, except hand(s) or wrist(s) 943.09
first degree 943.19
second degree 943.29
third degree 943.39
deep 943.49
with loss of body part 943.59
upper 943.03
first degree 943.13
second degree 943.23
third degree 943.33
deep 943.43
with loss of body part 943.53
auditory canal (external)—*see* Burn, ear
auricle (ear)—*see* Burn, ear
axilla 943.04
with
upper limb(s) except hand(s) or wrist(s)—*see* Burn, arm(s), multiple sites
first degree 943.14
second degree 943.24
third degree 943.34
deep 943.44
with loss of body part 943.54
back 942.04
with
trunk—*see* Burn, trunk, multiple sites
first degree 942.14
second degree 942.24
third degree 942.34
deep 942.44
with loss of body part 942.54
biceps
brachii—*see* Burn, arm(s), upper
femoris—*see* Burn, thigh
breast(s) 942.01
with
trunk—*see* Burn, trunk, multiple sites
first degree 942.11
second degree 942.21
third degree 942.31
deep 942.41
with loss of body part 942.51
brow—*see* Burn, forehead
buttock(s)—*see* Burn, back
canthus (eye) 940.1
chemical 940.0
cervix (uteri) 947.4
cheek (cutaneous) 941.07
with
face or head—*see* Burn, head, multiple sites
first degree 941.17
second degree 941.27
third degree 941.37
deep 941.47
with loss of body part 941.57

Burn—*continued*
chest wall (anterior) 942.02
with
trunk—*see* Burn, trunk, multiple sites
first degree 942.12
second degree 942.22
third degree 942.32
deep 942.42
with loss of body part 942.52
chin 941.04
with
face or head—*see* Burn, head, multiple sites
first degree 941.14
second degree 941.24
third degree 941.34
deep 941.44
with loss of body part 941.54
clitoris—*see* Burn, genitourinary organs,
external
colon 947.3
conjunctiva (and cornea) 940.4
chemical
acid 940.3
alkaline 940.2
cornea (and conjunctiva) 940.4
chemical
acid 940.3
alkaline 940.2
costal region—*see* Burn, chest wall
due to ingested chemical agent—*see* Burn,
internal organs
ear (auricle) (canal) (drum) (external) 941.01
with
face or head—*see* Burn, head, multiple sites
first degree 941.11
second degree 941.21
third degree 941.31
deep 941.41
with loss of a body part 941.51
elbow 943.02
with
hand(s) and wrist(s)—*see* Burn, multiple
specified sites
upper limb(s) except hand(s) or
wrist(s)—*see also* Burn, arm(s), multiple
sites
first degree 943.12
second degree 943.22
third degree 943.32
deep 943.42
with loss of body part 943.52
electricity, electric current—*see* Burn, by site
entire body—*see* Burn, multiple, specified sites
epididymis—*see* Burn, genitourinary organs,
external
epigastric region—*see* Burn, abdomen
epiglottis 947.1
esophagus 947.2
extent (percent of body surface)
less than 10 percent 948.0
10-19 percent 948.1
20-29 percent 948.2
30-39 percent 948.3
40-49 percent 948.4
50-59 percent 948.5
60-69 percent 948.6
70-79 percent 948.7
80-89 percent 948.8
90 percent or more 948.9

Burn—*continued*
extremity
lower—*see* Burn, leg
upper—*see* Burn, arm(s)
eye(s) (and adnexa) (only) 940.9
with
face, head, or neck 941.02
first degree 941.12
second degree 941.22
third degree 941.32
deep 941.42
with loss of body part 941.52
other sites (classifiable to more than one
category in 940-945)—*see* Burn,
multiple, specified sites
resulting rupture and destruction of eyeball
940.5
specified part—*see* Burn, by site
eyeball—*see also* Burn, eye
with resulting rupture and destruction of
eyeball 940.5
eyelid(s) 940.1
chemical 940.0
face—*see* Burn, head
finger (nail) (subungual) 944.01
with
hand(s)—*see* Burn, hand(s), multiple sites
other sites—*see* Burn, multiple, specified
sites
thumb 944.04
first degree 944.14
second degree 944.24
third degree 944.34
deep 944.44
with loss of body part 944.54
first degree 944.11
second degree 944.21
third degree 944.31
deep 944.41
with loss of body part 944.51
multiple (digits) 944.03
with thumb—*see* Burn, finger, with thumb
first degree 944.13
second degree 944.23
third degree 944.33
deep 944.43
with loss of body part 944.53
flank—*see* Burn, abdomen
foot 945.02
with
lower limb(s)—*see* Burn, leg, multiple sites
first degree 945.12
second degree 945.22
third degree 945.32
deep 945.42
with loss of body part 945.52
forearm(s) 943.01
with
upper limb(s) except hand(s) or
wrist(s)—*see* Burn, arm(s), multiple sites
first degree 943.11
second degree 943.21
third degree 943.31
deep 943.41
with loss of body part 943.51
forehead 941.07
with
face or head—*see* Burn, head, multiple sites
first degree 941.17
second degree 941.27

Burn—*continued*
  forehead—*continued*
    third degree 941.37
      deep 941.47
        with loss of body part 941.57
  fourth degree—*see* Burn, by site, third degree,
      deep
  friction—*see* Injury, superficial, by site
  from swallowing caustic or corrosive substance
      NEC—*see* Burn, internal organs
  full thickness—*see* Burn, by site, third degree
  gastrointestinal tract 947.3
  genitourinary organs
    external 942.05
      with
        trunk—*see* Burn, trunk, multiple sites
      first degree 942.15
      second degree 942.25
      third degree 942.35
        deep 942.45
          with loss of body part 942.55
    internal 947.8
  globe (eye)—*see* Burn, eyeball
  groin—*see* Burn, abdomen
  gum 947.0
  hand(s) (phalanges) (and wrist) 944.00
    first degree 944.10
    second degree 944.20
    third degree 944.30
      deep 944.40
        with loss of body part 944.50
    back (dorsal surface) 944.06
      first degree 944.16
      second degree 944.26
      third degree 944.36
        deep 944.46
          with loss of body part 944.56
    multiple sites 944.08
      first degree 944.18
      second degree 944.28
      third degree 944.38
        deep 944.48
          with loss of body part 944.58
  head (and face) 941.00
    eye(s) only 940.9
      specified part—*see* Burn, by site
    first degree 941.10
    second degree 941.20
    third degree 941.30
      deep 941.40
        with loss of body part 941.50
    multiple sites 941.09
      with eyes—*see* Burn, eyes, with face, head,
          or neck
      first degree 941.19
      second degree 941.29
      third degree 941.39
        deep 941.49
          with loss of body part 941.59
  heel—*see* Burn, foot
  hip—*see* Burn, trunk, specified site NEC
  iliac region—*see* Burn, trunk, specified site
      NEC
  infected 958.3
  inhalation (*see also* Burn, internal organs) 947.9
  internal organs 947.9
    from caustic or corrosive substance
        (swallowing) NEC 947.9
    specified NEC (*see also* Burn, by site) 947.8
  interscapular region—*see* Burn, back
  intestine (large) (small) 947.3

Burn—*continued*
  iris—*see* Burn, eyeball
  knee 945.05
    with
      lower limb(s)—*see* Burn, leg, multiple sites
    first degree 945.15
    second degree 945.25
    third degree 945.35
      deep 945.45
        with loss of body part 945.55
  labium (majus) (minus)—*see* Burn,
      genitourinary organs, external
  lacrimal apparatus, duct, gland, or sac 940.1
    chemical 940.0
  larynx 947.1
  late effect—*see* Late, effects (of), burn
  leg 945.00
    first degree 945.10
    second degree 945.20
    third degree 945.30
      deep 945.40
        with loss of body part 945.50
    lower 945.04
      with other part(s) of lower limb(s)—*see*
          Burn, leg, multiple sites
      first degree 945.14
      second degree 945.24
      third degree 945.34
        deep 945.44
          with loss of body part 945.54
    multiple sites 945.09
      first degree 945.19
      second degree 945.29
      third degree 945.39
        deep 945.49
          with loss of body part 945.59
    upper—*see* Burn, thigh
  lightning—*see* Burn, by site
  limb(s)
    lower (including foot or toe(s))—*see* Burn, leg
    upper (except wrist and hand)—*see* Burn,
        arm(s)
  lip(s) 941.03
    with
      face or head—*see* Burn, head, multiple sites
    first degree 941.13
    second degree 941.23
    third degree 941.33
      deep 941.43
        with loss of body part 941.53
  lumbar region—*see* Burn, back
  lung 947.1
  malar region—*see* Burn, cheek
  mastoid region—*see* Burn, scalp
  membrane, tympanic—*see* Burn, ear
  midthoracic region—*see* Burn, chest wall
  mouth 947.0
  multiple (*see also* Burn, unspecified) 949.0
    specified sites (classifiable to more than one
        category in 940-945) 946.0
      first degree 946.1
      second degree 946.2
      third degree 946.3
        deep 946.4
          with loss of body part 946.5
  muscle, abdominal—*see* Burn, abdomen
  nasal (septum)—*see* Burn, nose
  neck 941.08
    with
      face or head—*see* Burn, head, multiple sites
    first degree 941.18

Burn—*continued*
  neck—*continued*
    second degree 941.28
    third degree 941.38
      deep 941.48
        with loss of body part 941.58
  nose (septum) 941.05
    with
      face or head—*see* Burn, head, multiple sites
    first degree 941.15
    second degree 941.25
    third degree 941.35
      deep 941.45
        with loss of body part 941.55
  occipital region—*see* Burn, scalp
  orbit region 940.1
    chemical 940.0
  oronasopharynx 947.0
  palate 947.0
  palm(s) 944.05
    with
      hand(s) and wrist(s)—*see* Burn, hand(s),
        multiple sites
    first degree 944.15
    second degree 944.25
    third degree 944.35
      deep 944.45
        with loss of a body part 944.55
  parietal region—*see* Burn, scalp
  penis–*see* Burn, genitourinary organs, external
  perineum—*see* Burn, genitourinary organs,
    external
  periocular area 940.1
    chemical 940.0
  pharynx 947.0
  pleura 947.1
  popliteal space—*see* Burn, knee
  prepuce—*see* Burn, genitourinary organs,
    external
  pubic region—*see* Burn, genitourinary organs,
    external
  pudenda—*see* Burn, genitourinary organs,
    external
  rectum 947.3
  sac, lacrimal 940.1
    chemical 940.0
  sacral region—*see* Burn, back
  salivary (ducts) (glands) 947.0
  scalp 941.06
    with
      face or neck—*see* Burn, head, multiple sites
    first degree 941.16
    second degree 941.26
    third degree 941.36
      deep 941.46
        with loss of body part 941.56
  scapular region 943.06
    with
      upper limb(s), except hand(s) or
        wrist(s)—*see* Burn, arm(s), multiple sites
    first degree 943.16
    second degree 943.26
    third degree 943.36
      deep 943.46
        with loss of body part 943.56
  sclera—*see* Burn, eyeball
  scrotum—*see* Burn, genitourinary organs,
    external
  septum, nasal—*see* Burn, nose

Burn—*continued*
  shoulder(s) 943.05
    with
      hand(s) and wrist(s)—*see* Burn, multiple,
        specified sites
      upper limb(s), except hand(s) or
        wrist(s)—*see* Burn, arm(s), multiple sites
    first degree 943.15
    second degree 943.25
    third degree 943.35
      deep 943.45
        with loss of body part 943.55
  skin NEC (*see also* Burn, unspecified) 949.0
  skull—*see* Burn, head
  small intestine 947.3
  sternal region—*see* Burn, chest wall
  stomach 947.3
  subconjunctival—*see* Burn, conjunctiva
  subcutaneous—*see* Burn, by site, third degree
  submaxillary region—*see* Burn, head
  submental region—*see* Burn, chin
  sun—*see* Sunburn
  supraclavicular fossa—*see* Burn, neck
  supraorbital—*see* Burn, forehead
  temple—*see* Burn, scalp
  temporal region—*see* Burn, scalp
  testicle—*see* Burn, genitourinary organs,
    external
  testis—*see* Burn, genitourinary organs, external
  thigh 945.06
    with
      lower limb(s)–*see* Burn, leg, multiple sites
    first degree 945.16
    second degree 945.26
    third degree 945.36
      deep 945.46
        with loss of body part 945.56
  thorax (external)—*see* Burn, chest wall
  throat 947.0
  thumb(s) (nail) (subungual) 944.02
    with
      finger(s)—*see* Burn, finger, with other sites,
        thumb
      hand(s) and wrist(s)—*see* Burn, hand(s),
        multiple sites
    first degree 944.12
    second degree 944.22
    third degree 944.32
      deep 944.42
        with loss of body part 944.52
  toe (nail) (subungual) 945.01
    with
      lower limb(s)—*see* Burn, leg, multiple sites
    first degree 945.11
    second degree 945.21
    third degree 945.31
      deep 945.41
        with loss of body part 945.51
  tongue 947.0
  tonsil 947.0
  trachea 947.1
  trunk 942.00
    first degree 942.10
    second degree 942.20
    third degree 942.30
      deep 942.40
        with loss of body part 942.50

Burn—*continued*
 trunk—*continued*
  multiple sites 942.09
   first degree 942.19
   second degree 942.29
   third degree 942.39
    deep 942.49
     with loss of body part 942.59
  specified site NEC 942.09
   first degree 942.19
   second degree 942.29
   third degree 942.39
    deep 942.49
     with loss of body part 942.59
 tunica vaginalis—*see* Burn, genitourinary
  organs, external
 tympanic membrane—*see* Burn, ear
 tympanum—*see* Burn, ear
 ultraviolet 692.82
 unspecified site (multiple) 949.0
  with extent of body surface involved specified
   less than 10 percent 948.0
    10-19 percent 948.1
    20-29 percent 948.2
    30-39 percent 948.3
    40-49 percent 948.4
    50-59 percent 948.5
    60-69 percent 948.6
    70-79 percent 948.7
    80-89 percent 948.8
    90 percent or more 948.9
  first degree 949.1
  second degree 949.2
  third degree 949.3
   deep 949.4
    with loss of body part 949.5
 uterus 947.4
 uvula 947.0
 vagina 947.4
 vulva—*see* Burn, genitourinary organs, external
 wrist(s) 944.07
  with
   hand(s)—*see* Burn, hand(s), multiple sites
  first degree 944.17
  second degree 944.27
  third degree 944.37
   deep 944.47
    with loss of body part 944.57
Burnett's syndrome (milk-alkali) 275.42
Burnier's syndrome (hypophyseal dwarfism)
 253.3
Burning
 feet syndrome 266.2
 sensation (*see also* Disturbance, sensation)
  782.0
 tongue 529.6
Burns' disease (osteochondrosis, lower ulna)
 732.3
Bursa —*see also* condition
 pharynx 478.29
Bursitis NEC 727.3
 Achilles tendon 726.71
 adhesive 726.90
  shoulder 726.0
 ankle 726.79
 buttock 726.5
 calcaneal 726.79
 collateral ligament
  fibular 726.63
  tibial 726.62
 Duplay's 726.2

Bursitis—*continued*
 elbow 726.33
 finger 726.8
 foot 726.79
 gonococcal 098.52
 hand 726.4
 hip 726.5
 infrapatellar 726.69
 ischiogluteal 726.5
 knee 726.60
 occupational NEC 727.2
 olecranon 726.33
 pes anserinus 726.61
 pharyngeal 478.29
 popliteal 727.51
 prepatellar 726.65
 radiohumeral 727.3
 scapulohumeral 726.19
  adhesive 726.0
 shoulder 726.10
  adhesive 726.0
 subacromial 726.19
  adhesive 726.0
 subcoracoid 726.19
 subdeltoid 726.19
  adhesive 726.0
 subpatellar 726.69
 syphilitic 095.7
 Thornwaldt's, Tornwaldt's (pharyngeal) 478.29
 toe 726.79
 trochanteric area 726.5
 wrist 726.4
Burst stitches or sutures (complication of
  surgery) (external) (*see also* Dehiscence)
  998.32
 internal 998.31
Buruli ulcer 031.1
Bury's disease (erythema elevatum diutinum)
 695.89
Buschke's disease or scleredema (adultorum)
 710.1
Busquet's disease (osteoperiostitis) (*see also*
  Osteomyelitis) 730.1
Busse-Buschke disease (cryptococcosis) 117.5
Buttock —*see* condition
Button
 Biskra 085.1
 Delhi 085.1
 oriental 085.1
Buttonhole hand (intrinsic) 736.21
Bwamba fever (encephalitis) 066.3
Byssinosis (occupational) 504
Bywaters' syndrome 958.5

C

Cacergasia 300.9
Cachexia 799.4
  cancerous —*see also* Neoplasm, by site,
    malignant 799.4
  cardiac—*see* Disease, heart
  dehydration 276.51
  with
    hypernatremia 276.0
    hyponatremia 276.1
  due to malnutrition 799.4
  exophthalmic 242.0
  heart—*see* Disease, heart
  hypophyseal 253.2
  hypopituitary 253.2
  lead 984.9
    specified type of lead—*see* Table of drugs and
      chemicals
  malaria 084.9
  malignant —*see also* Neoplasm, by site,
    malignant 799.4
  marsh 084.9
  nervous 300.5
  old age 797
  pachydermic—*see* Hypothyroidism
  paludal 084.9
  pituitary (postpartum) 253.2
  renal (*see also* Disease, renal) 593.9
  saturnine 984.9
    specified type of lead—*see* Table of drugs and
      chemicals
  senile 797
  Simmonds' (pituitary cachexia) 253.2
  splenica 289.59
  strumipriva (*see also* Hypothyroidism) 244.9
  tuberculous NEC (*see also* Tuberculosis) 011.9
café au lait spots 709.09
Caffey's disease or syndrome (infantile cortical
  hyperostosis) 756.59
Caisson disease 993.3
Caked breast (puerperal, postpartum) 676.2
Cake kidney 753.3
Calabar swelling 125.2
Calcaneal spur 726.73
Calcaneoapophysitis 732.5
Calcaneonavicular bar 755.67
Calcareous —*see* condition
Calcicosis (occupational) 502
Calciferol (vitamin D) deficiency 268.9
  with
    osteomalacia 268.2
    rickets (*see also* Rickets) 268.0
Calcification
  adrenal (capsule) (gland) 255.41
    tuberculous (*see also* Tuberculosis) 017.6
  aorta 440.0
  artery (annular)—*see* Arteriosclerosis
  auricle (ear) 380.89
  bladder 596.98
    due to S. hematobium 120.0
  brain (cortex)—*see* Calcification, cerebral
  bronchus 519.19
  bursa 727.82
  cardiac (*see also* Degeneration, myocardial) 429.1
  cartilage (postinfectional) 733.99
  cerebral (cortex) 348.89
    artery 437.0
  cervix (uteri) 622.8

Calcification—*continued*
  choroid plexus 349.2
  conjunctiva 372.54
  corpora cavernosa (penis) 607.89
  cortex (brain)—*see* Calcification, cerebral
  dental pulp (nodular) 522.2
  dentinal papilla 520.4
  disc, intervertebral 722.90
    cervical, cervicothoracic 722.91
    lumbar, lumbosacral 722.93
    thoracic, thoracolumbar 722.92
  fallopian tube 620.8
  falx cerebri—*see* Calcification, cerebral
  fascia 728.89
  gallbladder 575.8
  general 275.40
  heart (*see also* Degeneration, myocardial) 429.1
    valve—*see* Endocarditis
  intervertebral cartilage or disc (postinfectional)
    722.90
    cervical, cervicothoracic 722.91
    lumbar, lumbosacral 722.93
    thoracic, thoracolumbar 722.92
  intracranial—*see* Calcification, cerebral
  intraspinal ligament 728.89
  joint 719.80
    ankle 719.87
    elbow 719.82
    foot 719.87
    hand 719.84
    hip 719.85
    knee 719.86
    multiple sites 719.89
    pelvic region 719.85
    shoulder (region) 719.81
    specified site NEC 719.88
    wrist 719.83
  kidney 593.89
    tuberculous (*see also* Tuberculosis) 016.0
  larynx (senile) 478.79
  lens 366.8
  ligament 728.89
    intraspinal 728.89
    knee (medial collateral) 717.89
  lung 518.89
    active 518.89
    postinfectional 518.89
    tuberculous (*see also* Tuberculosis,
      pulmonary) 011.9
  lymph gland or node (postinfectional) 289.3
    tuberculous (*see also* Tuberculosis, lymph
      gland) 017.2
  mammographic 793.89
  massive (paraplegic) 728.10
  medial NEC (*see also* Arteriosclerosis,
    extremities) 440.20
  meninges (cerebral) 349.2
  metastatic 275.40
  Mönckeberg's—*see* Arteriosclerosis
  muscle 728.10
    heterotopic, postoperative 728.13
  myocardium, myocardial (*see also*
    Degeneration, myocardial) 429.1
  ovary 620.8
  pancreas 577.8
  penis 607.99
  periarticular 728.89
  pericardium (*see also* Pericarditis) 423.8

Calcification—*continued*
 pineal gland 259.8
 pleura 511.0
  postinfectional 518.89
  tuberculous (*see also* Tuberculosis, pleura)
   012.0
 pulp (dental) (nodular) 522.2
 renal 593.89
 rider's bone 733.99
 sclera 379.16
 semilunar cartilage 717.89
 spleen 289.59
 subcutaneous 709.3
 suprarenal (capsule) (gland) 255.41
 tendon (sheath) 727.82
  with bursitis, synovitis or tenosynovitis 727.82
 trachea 519.19
 ureter 593.89
 uterus 621.8
 vitreous 379.29
Calcified —*see also* Calcification
 hematoma NEC 959.9
Calcinosis (generalized) (interstitial) (tumoral)
  (universalis) 275.49
 circumscripta 709.3
 cutis 709.3
 intervertebralis 275.49 *[722.90]*
 Raynaud's
  phenomenonsclerodactylytelangiectasis
   (CRST) 710.1
Calciphylaxis (*see also* Calcification, by site)
 275.49
Calcium
 blood
  high (*see also* Hypercalcemia) 275.42
  low (*see also* Hypocalcemia) 275.41
 deposits—*see also* Calcification, by site
  in bursa 727.82
  in tendon (sheath) 727.82
   with bursitis, synovitis or tenosynovitis
    727.82
 salts or soaps in vitreous 379.22
Calciuria 791.9
Calculi —*see* Calculus
Calculosis, intrahepatic —*see*
  Choledocholithiasis
Calculus, calculi, calculous 592.9
 ampulla of Vater—*see* Choledocholithiasis
 anuria (impacted) (recurrent) 592.0
 appendix 543.9
 bile duct (any)—*see* Choledocholithiasis
 biliary—*see* Cholelithiasis
 bilirubin, multiple—*see* Cholelithiasis
 bladder (encysted) (impacted) (urinary) 594.1
  diverticulum 594.0
 bronchus 518.89
 calyx (kidney) (renal) 592.0
  congenital 753.3
 cholesterol (pure) (solitary)—*see* Cholelithiasis
 common duct (bile)—*see* Choledocholithiasis
 conjunctiva 372.54
 cystic 594.1
  duct—*see* Cholelithiasis
 dental 523.6
  subgingival 523.6
  supragingival 523.6
 epididymis 608.89

Calculus, calculi, calculous—*continued*
 gallbladder—*see also* Cholelithiasis
  congenital 751.69
 hepatic (duct)—*see* Choledocholithiasis
 intestine (impaction) (obstruction) 560.39
 kidney (impacted) (multiple) (pelvis) (recurrent)
   (staghorn) 592.0
  congenital 753.3
 lacrimal (passages) 375.57
 liver (impacted)—*see* Choledocholithiasis
 lung 518.89
 mammographic 793.89
 nephritic (impacted) (recurrent) 592.0
 nose 478.19
 pancreas (duct) 577.8
 parotid gland 527.5
 pelvis, encysted 592.0
 prostate 602.0
 pulmonary 518.89
 renal (impacted) (recurrent) 592.0
  congenital 753.3
 salivary (duct) (gland) 527.5
 seminal vesicle 608.89
 staghorn 592.0
 Stensen's duct 527.5
 sublingual duct or gland 527.5
  congenital 750.26
 submaxillary duct, gland, or region 527.5
 suburethral 594.8
 tonsil 474.8
 tooth, teeth 523.6
 tunica vaginalis 608.89
 ureter (impacted) (recurrent) 592.1
 urethra (impacted) 594.2
 urinary (duct) (impacted) (passage) (tract) 592.9
  lower tract NEC 594.9
   specified site 594.8
 vagina 623.8
 vesical (impacted) 594.1
 Wharton's duct 527.5
Caliectasis 593.89
California
 disease 114.0
 encephalitis 062.5
Caligo cornea 371.03
Callositas, callosity (infected) 700
Callus (infected) 700
 bone 726.91
 excessive, following fracture—*see also* Late,
   effect (of), fracture
Calvé (-Perthes) disease (osteochondrosis,
   femoral capital) 732.1
Calvities (*see also* Alopecia) 704.00
Cameroon fever (*see also* Malaria) 084.6
Camptocormia 300.11
Camptodactyly (congenital) 755.59
Camurati-Engelmann disease (diaphyseal
   sclerosis) 756.59
Canal —*see* condition
Canaliculitis (lacrimal) (acute) 375.31
 Actinomyces 039.8
 chronic 375.41
Canavan's disease 330.0

Cancer (M8000/3)—*see also* Neoplasm, by site, malignant

Note—The term "cancer" when modified by an adjective or adjectival phrase indicating a morphological type should be coded in the same manner as "carcinoma" with that adjective or phrase. Thus, "squamous-cell cancer" should be coded in the same manner as "squamous-cell carcinoma," which appears in the list under "Carcinoma."

  bile duct type (M8160/3), liver 155.1
  hepatocellular (M8170/3) 155.0
Cancerous (M8000/3)—*see* Neoplasm, by site, malignant
Cancerphobia 300.29
Cancrum oris 528.1
Candidiasis, candidal 112.9
  with pneumonia 112.4
  balanitis 112.2
  congenital 771.7
  disseminated 112.5
  endocarditis 112.81
  esophagus 112.84
  intertrigo 112.3
  intestine 112.85
  lung 112.4
  meningitis 112.83
  mouth 112.0
  nails 112.3
  neonatal 771.7
  onychia 112.3
  otitis externa 112.82
  otomycosis 112.82
  paronychia 112.3
  perionyxis 112.3
  pneumonia 112.4
  pneumonitis 112.4
  skin 112.3
  specified site NEC 112.89
  systemic 112.5
  urogenital site NEC 112.2
  vagina 112.1
  vulva 112.1
  vulvovaginitis 112.1
Candidiosis —*see* Candidiasis
Candiru infection or infestation 136.8
Canities (premature) 704.3
  congenital 757.4
Canker (mouth) (sore) 528.2
  rash 034.1
Cannabinosis 504
Canton fever 081.9
Cap
  cradle 690.11
Capillariasis 127.5
Capillary —*see* condition
Caplan's syndrome 714.81
Caplan-Colinet syndrome 714.81
Capsule —*see* condition
Capsulitis (joint) 726.90
  adhesive (shoulder) 726.0
  hip 726.5
  knee 726.60
  labyrinthine 387.8
  thyroid 245.9
  wrist 726.4
Caput
  crepitus 756.0
  medusae 456.8
  succedaneum 767.19

Carapata disease 087.1
Carate —*see* Pinta
Carbohydrate-deficient glycoprotein syndrome (CDGS) 271.8
Carboxyhemoglobinemia 986
Carbuncle 680.9
  abdominal wall 680.2
  ankle 680.6
  anus 680.5
  arm (any part, above wrist) 680.3
  auditory canal, external 680.0
  axilla 680.3
  back (any part) 680.2
  breast 680.2
  buttock 680.5
  chest wall 680.2
  corpus cavernosum 607.2
  ear (any part) (external) 680.0
  eyelid 373.13
  face (any part, except eye) 680.0
  finger (any) 680.4
  flank 680.2
  foot (any part) 680.7
  forearm 680.3
  genital organ (male) 608.4
  gluteal (region) 680.5
  groin 680.2
  hand (any part) 680.4
  head (any part, except face) 680.8
  heel 680.7
  hip 680.6
  kidney (*see also* Abscess, kidney) 590.2
  knee 680.6
  labia 616.4
  lacrimal
    gland (*see also* Dacryoadenitis) 375.00
    passages (duct) (sac) (*see also* Dacryocystitis) 375.30
  leg, any part except foot 680.6
  lower extremity, any part except foot 680.6
  malignant 022.0
  multiple sites 680.9
  neck 680.1
  nose (external) (septum) 680.0
  orbit, orbital 376.01
  partes posteriores 680.5
  pectoral region 680.2
  penis 607.2
  perineum 680.2
  pinna 680.0
  scalp (any part) 680.8
  scrotum 608.4
  seminal vesicle 608.0
  shoulder 680.3
  skin NEC 680.9
  specified site NEC 680.8
  spermatic cord 608.4
  temple (region) 680.0
  testis 608.4
  thigh 680.6
  thumb 680.4
  toe (any) 680.7
  trunk 680.2
  tunica vaginalis 608.4
  umbilicus 680.2
  upper arm 680.3
  urethra 597.0
  vas deferens 608.4
  vulva 616.4
  wrist 680.4
Carbunculus (*see also* Carbuncle) 680.9

Carcinoid (tumor) (M8240/1)—see Tumor,
  carcinoid
Carcinoidosis 259.2
Carcinoma (M8010/3)—see also Neoplasm, by
  site, malignant

> *Note—Except where otherwise indicated, the*
> *morphological varieties of carcinoma in the list*
> *below should be coded by site as for*
> *"Neoplasm, malignant."*

with
  apocrine metaplasia (M8573/3)
  cartilaginous (and osseous) metaplasia
    (M8571/3)
  osseous (and cartilaginous) metaplasia
    (M8571/3)
  productive fibrosis (M8141/3)
  spindle cell metaplasia (M8572/3)
  squamous metaplasia (M8570/3)
acidophil (M8280/3)
  specified site—see Neoplasm, by site,
    malignant
  unspecified site 194.3
acidophil-basophil, mixed (M8281/3)
  specified site—see Neoplasm, by site,
    malignant
  unspecified site 194.3
acinar (cell) (M8550/3)
acinic cell (M8550/3)
adenocystic (M8200/3)
adenoid
  cystic (M8200/3)
  squamous cell (M8075/3)
adenosquamous (M8560/3)
adnexal (skin) (M8390/3)—see Neoplasm, skin,
  malignant
adrenal cortical (M8370/3) 194.0
alveolar (M8251/3)
  cell (M8250/3)—see Neoplasm, lung,
    malignant
anaplastic type (M8021/3)
apocrine (M8401/3)
  breast—see Neoplasm, breast, malignant
  specified site NEC—see Neoplasm, skin,
    malignant
  unspecified site 173.99
basal cell (pigmented) (M8090/3) (see also
    Neoplasm, skin, malignant) 173.91
  fibro-epithelial type (M8093/3)—see
    Neoplasm, skin, malignant
  morphea type (M8092/3)—see Neoplasm,
    skin, malignant
  multicentric (M8091/3)—see Neoplasm, skin,
    malignant
basaloid (M8123/3)
basal-squamous cell, mixed (M8094/3)—see
  Neoplasm, skin, malignant
basophil (M8300/3)
  specified site—see Neoplasm, by site,
    malignant
  unspecified site 194.3
basophil-acidophil, mixed (M8281/3)
  specified site—see Neoplasm, by site,
    malignant
  unspecified site 194.3
basosquamous (M8094/3)—see Neoplasm, skin,
  malignant

Carcinoma—*continued*
bile duct type (M8160/3)
  and hepatocellular, mixed (M8180/3) 155.0
  liver 155.1
  specified site NEC—see Neoplasm, by site,
    malignant
  unspecified site 155.1
branchial or branchiogenic 146.8
bronchial or bronchogenic—see Neoplasm,
  lung, malignant
bronchiolar (terminal) (M8250/3)—see
  Neoplasm, lung, malignant
bronchiolo-alveolar (M8250/3)—see Neoplasm,
  lung, malignant
bronchogenic (epidermoid) 162.9
C cell (M8510/3)
  specified site—see Neoplasm, by site,
    malignant
  unspecified site 193
ceruminous (M8420/3) 173.29
chorionic (M9100/3)
  specified site—see Neoplasm, by site,
    malignant
  unspecified site
    female 181
    male 186.9
chromophobe (M8270/3)
  specified site—see Neoplasm, by site,
    malignant
  unspecified site 194.3
clear cell (mesonephroid type) (M8310/3)
cloacogenic (M8124/3)
  specified site—see Neoplasm, by site,
    malignant
  unspecified site 154.8
colloid (M8480/3)
cribriform (M8201/3)
cylindroid type (M8200/3)
diffuse type (M8145/3)
  specified site—see Neoplasm, by site,
    malignant
  unspecified site 151.9
duct (cell) (M8500/3)
  with Paget's disease (M8541/3)—see
    Neoplasm, breast, malignant
  infiltrating (M8500/3)
    specified site—see Neoplasm, by site,
      malignant
    unspecified site 174.9
ductal (M8500/3)
ductular, infiltrating (M8521/3)
embryonal (M9070/3)
  and teratoma, mixed (M9081/3)
  combined with choriocarcinoma
    (M9101/3)—see Neoplasm, by site,
    malignant
  infantile type (M9071/3)
  liver 155.0
  polyembryonal type (M9072/3)
endometrioid (M8380/3)
eosinophil (M8280/3)
  specified site—see Neoplasm, by site,
    malignant
  unspecified site 194.3
epidermoid (M8070/3)—see also Carcinoma,
    squamous cell
  and adenocarcinoma, mixed (M8560/3)
  in situ, Bowen's type (M8081/2)—see
    Neoplasm, skin, in situ
  intradermal—see Neoplasm, skin, in situ

Carcinoma—*continued*
  fibroepithelial type basal cell (M8093/3)—*see*
      Neoplasm, skin, malignant
  follicular (M8330/3)
      and papillary (mixed) (M8340/3) 193
      moderately differentiated type (M8332/3) 193
      pure follicle type (M8331/3) 193
      specified site—*see* Neoplasm, by site,
          malignant
      trabecular type (M8332/3) 193
      unspecified site 193
      well differentiated type (M8331/3) 193
  gelatinous (M8480/3)
  giant cell (M8031/3)
      and spindle cell (M8030/3)
  granular cell (M8320/3)
  granulosa cell (M8620/3) 183.0
  hepatic cell (M8170/3) 155.0
  hepatocellular (M8170/3) 155.0
      and bile duct, mixed (M8180/3)
          155.0
  hepatocholangiolitic (M8180/3) 155.0
  Hurthle cell (thyroid) 193
  hypernephroid (M8311/3)
  in
      adenomatous
          polyp (M8210/3)
          polyposis coli (M8220/3) 153.9
      pleomorphic adenoma (M8940/3)
      polypoid adenoma (M8210/3)
      situ (M8010/3)—*see* Carcinoma,
          in situ
      tubular adenoma (M8210/3)
      villous adenoma (M8261/3)
  infiltrating duct (M8500/3)
      with Paget's disease (M8541/3)—*see*
          Neoplasm, breast, malignant
      specified site—*see* Neoplasm, by site,
          malignant
      unspecified site 174.9
  inflammatory (M8530/3)
      specified site—*see* Neoplasm, by site,
          malignant
      unspecified site 174.9
  in situ (M8010/2)—*see also* Neoplasm, by site,
      in situ
      epidermoid (M8070/2)—*see also* Neoplasm,
          by site, in situ
          with questionable stromal invasion
              (M8076/2)
              specified site—*see* Neoplasm, by site, in
                  situ
              unspecified site 233.1
          Bowen's type (M8081/2)—*see* Neoplasm,
              skin, in situ
      intraductal (M8500/2)
          specified site—*see* Neoplasm, by site, in situ
          unspecified site 233.0
      lobular (M8520/2)
          specified site—*see* Neoplasm, by site, in situ
          unspecified site 233.0
      papillary (M8050/2)—*see* Neoplasm, by site,
          in situ
      squamous cell (M8070/2)—*see also*
          Neoplasm, by site, in situ
          with questionable stromal invasion
              (M8076/2)
          specified site—*see* Neoplasm, by site, in situ
          unspecified site 233.1
      transitional cell (M8120/2)—*see* Neoplasm,
          by site, in situ

Carcinoma—*continued*
  intestinal type (M8144/3)
      specified site—*see* Neoplasm, by site,
          malignant
      unspecified site 151.9
  intraductal (noninfiltrating) (M8500/2)
      papillary (M8503/2)
          specified site—*see* Neoplasm, by site, in situ
          unspecified site 233.0
      specified site—*see* Neoplasm, by site, in situ
      unspecified site 233.0
  intraepidermal (M8070/2)—*see also* Neoplasm,
      skin, in situ
      squamous cell, Bowen's type (M8081/2)—*see*
          Neoplasm, skin, in situ
  intraepithelial (M8010/2)—*see also* Neoplasm,
      by site, in situ
      squamous cell (M8072/2)—*see* Neoplasm, by
          site, in situ
  intraosseous (M9270/3) 170.1
      upper jaw (bone) 170.0
  islet cell (M8150/3)
      and exocrine, mixed (M8154/3)
          specified site—*see* Neoplasm, by site,
              malignant
          unspecified site 157.9
      pancreas 157.4
      specified site NEC—*see* Neoplasm, by site,
          malignant
      unspecified site 157.4
  juvenile, breast (M8502/3)—*see* Neoplasm,
      breast, malignant
  Kulchitsky's cell (carcinoid tumor of intestine)
      259.2
  large cell (M8012/3)
      squamous cell, nonkeratinizing type
          (M8072/3)
  Leydig cell (testis) (M8650/3)
      specified site—*see* Neoplasm, by site,
          malignant
      unspecified site 186.9
          female 183.0
          male 186.9
  liver cell (M8170/3) 155.0
  lobular (infiltrating) (M8520/3)
      non-infiltrating (M8520/3)
          specified site—*see* Neoplasm, by site, in situ
          unspecified site 233.0
      specified site—*see* Neoplasm, by site,
          malignant
      unspecified site 174.9
  lymphoepithelial (M8082/3)
  medullary (M8510/3)
      with
          amyloid stroma (M8511/3)
              specified site—*see* Neoplasm, by site,
                  malignant
              unspecified site 193
          lymphoid stroma (M8512/3)
              specified site—*see* Neoplasm, by site,
                  malignant
              unspecified site 174.9

Carcinoma—*continued*
  Merkel cell 209.36
    buttock 209.36
    ear 209.31
    eyelid, including canthus 209.31
    face 209.31
    genitals 209.36
    lip 209.31
    lower limb 209.34
    neck 209.32
    nodal presentation 209.75
    scalp 209.32
    secondary (any site) 209.75
    specified site NEC 209.36
    trunk 209.35
    unknown primary site 209.75
    upper limb 209.33
    visceral metastatic presentation 209.75
  mesometanephric (M9110/3)
  mesonephric (M9110/3)
  metastatic (M8010/6)—*see* Metastasis, cancer
  metatypical (M8095/3)—*see* Neoplasm, skin, malignant
  morphea type basal cell (M8092/3)—*see* Neoplasm, skin, malignant
  mucinous (M8480/3)
  mucin-producing (M8481/3)
  mucin-secreting (M8481/3)
  mucoepidermoid (M8430/3)
  mucoid (M8480/3)
    cell (M8300/3)
      specified site—*see* Neoplasm, by site, malignant
      unspecified site 194.3
  mucous (M8480/3)
  neuroendocrine
    high grade (M8240/3) 209.30
    malignant poorly differentiated (M8240/3) 209.30
  nonencapsulated sclerosing (M8350/3) 193
  noninfiltrating
    intracystic (M8504/2)—*see* Neoplasm, by site, in situ
    intraductal (M8500/2)
      papillary (M8503/2)
        specified site—*see* Neoplasm, by site, in situ
        unspecified site 233.0
      specified site—*see* Neoplasm, by site, in situ
      unspecified site 233.0
    lobular (M8520/2)
      specified site—*see* Neoplasm, by site, in situ
      unspecified site 233.0
  oat cell (M8042/3)
    specified site—*see* Neoplasm, by site, malignant
    unspecified site 162.9
  odontogenic (M9270/3) 170.1
    upper jaw (bone) 170.0
  onocytic (M8290/3)
  oxyphilic (M8290/3)
  papillary (M8050/3)
    and follicular (mixed) (M8340/3) 193
    epidermoid (M8052/3)
    intraductal (noninfiltrating) (M8503/2)
      specified site—*see* Neoplasm, by site, in situ
      unspecified site 233.0

Carcinoma—*continued*
  papillary—*continued*
    serous (M8460/3)
      specified site—*see* Neoplasm, by site, malignant
      surface (M8461/3)
        specified site—*see* Neoplasm, by site, malignant
        unspecified site 183.0
      unspecified site 183.0
    squamous cell (M8052/3)
    transitional cell (M8130/3)
  papillocystic (M8450/3)
    specified site—*see* Neoplasm, by site, malignant
    unspecified site 183.0
  parafollicular cell (M8510/3)
    specified site—*see* Neoplasm, by site, malignant
    unspecified site 193
  pleomorphic (M8022/3)
  polygonal cell (M8034/3)
  prickle cell (M8070/3)
  pseudoglandular, squamous cell (M8075/3)
  pseudomucinous (M8470/3)
    specified site—*see* Neoplasm, by site, malignant
    unspecified site 183.0
  pseudosarcomatous (M8033/3)
  regaud type (M8082/3)—*see* Neoplasm, nasopharynx, malignant
  renal cell (M8312/3) 189.0
  reserve cell (M8041/3)
  round cell (M8041/3)
  Schmincke (M8082/3)—*see* Neoplasm, nasopharynx, malignant
  Schneiderian (M8121/3)
    specified site—*see* Neoplasm, by site, malignant
    unspecified site 160.0
  scirrhous (M8141/3)
  sebaceous (M8410/3)—*see* Neoplasm, skin, malignant
  secondary (M8010/6)—*see* Neoplasm, by site, malignant, secondary
  secretory, breast (M8502/3)—*see* Neoplasm, breast, malignant
  serous (M8441/3)
    papillary (M8460/3)
      specified site—*see* Neoplasm, by site, malignant
      unspecified site 183.0
    surface, papillary (M8461/3)
      specified site—*see* Neoplasm, by site, malignant
      unspecified site 183.0
  Sertoli cell (M8640/3)
    specified site—*see* Neoplasm, by site, malignant
    unspecified site 186.9
  signet ring cell (M8490/3)
    metastatic (M8490/6)—*see* Neoplasm, by site, secondary
  simplex (M8231/3)
  skin appendage (M8390/3)—*see* Neoplasm, skin, malignant
  small cell (M8041/3)
    fusiform cell type (M8043/3)
    squamous cell, non-keratinizing type (M8073/3)

Carcinoma—*continued*
　solid (M8230/3)
　　with amyloid stroma (M8511/3)
　　　specified site—*see* Neoplasm, by site,
　　　　malignant
　　　unspecified site 193
　spheroidal cell (M8035/3)
　spindle cell (M8032/3)
　　and giant cell (M8030/3)
　spinous cell (M8070/3)
　squamous (cell) (M8070/3)
　　adenoid type (M8075/3)
　　and adenocarcinoma, mixed (M8560/3)
　　intraepidermal, Bowen's type—*see* Neoplasm,
　　　skin, in situ
　　keratinizing type (large cell) (M8071/3)
　　large cell, non-keratinizing type (M8072/3)
　　microinvasive (M8076/3)
　　　specified site—*see* Neoplasm, by site,
　　　　malignant
　　　unspecified site 180.9
　　non-keratinizing type (M8072/3)
　　papillary (M8052/3)
　　pseudoglandular (M8075/3)
　　skin (see also Neoplasm, skin, malignant) 173.92
　　small cell, non-keratinizing type (M8073/3)
　　spindle cell type (M8074/3)
　　verrucous (M8051/3)
　superficial spreading (M8143/3)
　sweat gland (M8400/3)—*see* Neoplasm, skin,
　　malignant
　theca cell (M8600/3) 183.0
　thymic (M8580/3) 164.0
　trabecular (M8190/3)
　transitional (cell) (M8120/3)
　　papillary (M8130/3)
　　spindle cell type (M8122/3)
　tubular (M8211/3)
　undifferentiated type (M8020/3)
　urothelial (M8120/3)
　ventriculi 151.9
　verrucous (epidermoid) (squamous cell)
　　(M8051/3)
　villous (M8262/3)
　water-clear cell (M8322/3) 194.1
　wolffian duct (M9110/3)
Carcinomaphobia 300.29
Carcinomatosis
　peritonei (M8010/6) 197.6
　specified site NEC (M8010/3)—*see* Neoplasm,
　　by site, malignant
　unspecified site (M8010/6) 199.0
Carcinosarcoma (M8980/3)—*see also*
　Neoplasm, by site, malignant
　embryonal type (M8981/3)—*see* Neoplasm, by
　　site, malignant
Cardia, cardial —*see* condition
Cardiac —*see also* condition
　death—*see* Disease, heart
　device
　　defibrillator, automatic implantable (with
　　　synchronous cardiac pacemaker) V45.02
　　in situ NEC V45.00
　　pacemaker
　　　cardiac
　　　　fitting or adjustment V53.3
　　　　in situ V45.01
　　　carotid sinus
　　　　fitting or adjustment V53.3
　　　　in situ V45.09
　pacemaker—*see* Cardiac, device, pacemaker
　tamponade 423.3

Cardialgia (*see also* Pain, precordial) 786.51
Cardiectasis —*see* Hypertrophy, cardiac
Cardiochalasia 530.81
Cardiomalacia (*see also* Degeneration,
　myocardial) 429.1
Cardiomegalia glycogenica diffusa 271.0
Cardiomegaly (*see also* Hypertrophy, cardiac)
　429.3
　congenital 746.89
　glycogen 271.0
　hypertensive (*see also* Hypertension, heart)
　　402.90
　idiopathic 429.3
Cardiomyoliposis (*see also* Degeneration,
　myocardial) 429.1
Cardiomyopathy (congestive) (constrictive)
　(familial) (infiltrative) (obstructive)
　(restrictive) (sporadic) 425.4
　alcoholic 425.5
　amyloid 277.39 *[425.7]*
　beriberi 265.0 *[425.7]*
　cobalt-beer 425.5
　congenital 425.3
　due to
　　amyloidosis 277.39 *[425.7]*
　　beriberi 265.0 *[425.7]*
　　cardiac glycogenesis 271.0 *[425.7]*
　　Chagas' disease 086.0
　　Friedreich's ataxia 334.0 *[425.8]*
　　mucopolysaccharidosis 277.5 *[425.7]*
　　myotonia atrophica 359.21 *[425.8]*
　　progressive muscular dystrophy 359.1 *[425.8]*
　　sarcoidosis 135 *[425.8]*
　glycogen storage 271.0 *[425.7]*
　hypertensive—*see* Hypertension, with, heart
　　involvement
　hypertrophic 425.18
　　nonobstructive 425.18
　　obstructive 425.11
　　　congenital 746.84
　idiopathic (concentric) 425.4
　in
　　Chagas' disease 086.0
　　sarcoidosis 135 *[425.8]*
　ischemic 414.8
　metabolic NEC 277.9 *[425.7]*
　　amyloid 277.39 *[425.7]*
　　thyrotoxic (*see also* Thyrotoxicosis) 242.9
　　　[425.7]
　　thyrotoxicosis (*see also* Thyrotoxicosis) 242.9
　　　[425.7]
　newborn 425.4
　　congenital 425.3
　nutritional 269.9 *[425.7]*
　　beriberi 265.0 *[425.7]*
　obscure of Africa 425.2
　peripartum 674.5
　postpartum 674.5
　primary 425.4
　secondary 425.9
　stress induced 429.83
　takotsubo 429.83
　thyrotoxic (*see also* Thyrotoxicosis) 242.9 *[425.7]*
　toxic NEC 425.9
　tuberculous (*see also* Tuberculosis) 017.9 *[425.8]*
Cardionephritis —*see* Hypertension, cardiorenal
Cardionephropathy —*see* Hypertension,
　cardiorenal
Cardionephrosis —*see* Hypertension,
　cardiorenal
Cardioneurosis 306.2
Cardiopathia nigra 416.0

Cardiopathy (*see also* Disease, heart) 429.9
  hypertensive (*see also* Hypertension, heart) 402.90
  idiopathic 425.4
  mucopolysaccharidosis 277.5 *[425.7]*
Cardiopericarditis (*see also* Pericarditis) 423.9
Cardiophobia 300.29
Cardioptosis 746.87
Cardiorenal —*see* condition
Cardiorrhexis (*see also* Infarct, myocardium)
  410.9
Cardiosclerosis —*see* Arteriosclerosis, coronary
Cardiosis —*see* Disease, heart
Cardiospasm (esophagus) (reflex) (stomach)
  530.0
  congenital 750.7
Cardiostenosis —*see* Disease, heart
Cardiosymphysis 423.1
Cardiothyrotoxicosis —*see* Hyperthyroidism
Cardiovascular —*see* condition
Carditis (acute) (bacterial) (chronic) (subacute)
  429.89
  Coxsackie 074.20
  hypertensive (*see also* Hypertension, heart)
    402.90
  meningococcal 036.40
  rheumatic—*see* Disease, heart, rheumatic
  rheumatoid 714.2
Care (of)
  child (routine) V20.1
  convalescent following V66.9
    chemotherapy V66.2
    medical NEC V66.5
    psychotherapy V66.3
    radiotherapy V66.1
    surgery V66.0
    surgical NEC V66.0
    treatment (for) V66.5
      combined V66.6
      fracture V66.4
      mental disorder NEC V66.3
      specified type NEC V66.5
  end-of-life care V66.7
  family member (handicapped) (sick)
    creating problem for family V61.49
    provided away from home for holiday relief
      V60.5
    unavailable, due to
      absence (person rendering care) (sufferer)
        V60.4
      inability (any reason) of person rendering
        care V60.4
  holiday relief V60.5
  hospice V66.7
  lack of (at or after birth) (infant) (child) 995.52
    adult 995.84
  lactation of mother V24.1
  palliative V66.7
  postpartum
    immediately after delivery V24.0
    routine follow-up V24.2
  prenatal V22.1
    first pregnancy V22.0
    high risk pregnancy V23.9
      inconclusive fetal viability V23.87
      specified problem NEC V23.8
  terminal V66.7
  unavailable, due to
    absence of person rendering care V60.4
    inability (any reason) of person rendering care
      V60.4
  well baby V20.1

Caries (bone) (*see also* Tuberculosis, bone) 015.9
  [730.8]
  arrested 521.04
  cementum 521.03
  cerebrospinal (tuberculous) 015.0 *[730.88]*
  dental (acute) (chronic) (incipient) (infected)
    521.00
    with pulp exposure 521.03
    extending to
      dentine 521.02
      pulp 521.03
    other specified NEC 521.09
    pit and fissure 521.06
    primary
      pit and fissure origin 521.06
      root surface 521.08
      smooth surface origin 521.07
    root surface 521.08
    smooth surface 521.07
  dentin (acute) (chronic) 521.02
  enamel (acute) (chronic) (incipient) 521.01
  external meatus 380.89
  hip (*see also* Tuberculosis) 015.1 *[730.85]*
  initial 521.01
  knee 015.2 *[730.86]*
  labyrinth 386.8
  limb NEC 015.7 *[730.88]*
  mastoid (chronic) (process) 383.1
  middle ear 385.89
  nose 015.7 *[730.88]*
  orbit 015.7 *[730.88]*
  ossicle 385.24
  petrous bone 383.20
  sacrum (tuberculous) 015.0 *[730.88]*
  spine, spinal (column) (tuberculous) 015.0
    [730.88]
  syphilitic 095.5
    congenital 090.0 *[730.8]*
  teeth (internal) 521.00
    initial 521.01
  vertebra (column) (tuberculous) 015.0 *[730.88]*
Carini's syndrome (ichthyosis congenita) 757.1
Carious teeth 521.00
Carneous mole 631.8
Carnosinemia 270.5
Carotid body or sinus syndrome 337.01
Carotidynia 337.01
Carotinemia (dietary) 278.3
Carotinosis (cutis) (skin) 278.3
Carpal tunnel syndrome 354.0
Carpenter's syndrome 759.89
Carpopedal spasm (*see also* Tetany) 781.7
Carpoptosis 736.05
Carrier (suspected) of
  amebiasis V02.2
  bacterial disease (meningococcal,
    staphylococcal, streptococcal) NEC V02.59
  cholera V02.0
  cystic fibrosis gene V83.81
  defective gene V83.89
  diphtheria V02.4
  dysentery (bacillary) V02.3
    amebic V02.2
  Endamoeba histolytica V02.2
  gastrointestinal pathogens NEC V02.3
  genetic defect V83.89
  gonorrhea V02.7
  group B streptococcus V02.51
  HAA (hepatitis Australian-antigen) V02.61
  hemophilia A (asymptomatic) V83.01
    symptomatic V83.02

Carrier—*continued*
  hepatitis V02.60
    Australian-antigen (HAA) V02.61
    B V02.61
    C V02.62
    serum V02.61
    specified type NEC V02.69
    viral V02.60
  infective organism NEC V02.9
  malaria V02.9
  paratyphoid V02.3
  Salmonella V02.3
    typhosa V02.1
  serum hepatitis V02.61
  Shigella V02.3
  Staphylococcus NEC V02.59
    methicillin
      resistant Staphylococcus aureus V02.54
      susceptible Staphylococcus aureus V02.53
  Streptococcus NEC V02.52
    group B V02.51
  typhoid V02.1
  venereal disease NEC V02.8
Carrión's disease (Bartonellosis) 088.0
Car sickness 994.6
Carter's
  relapsing fever (Asiatic) 087.0
Cartilage —*see* condition
Caruncle (inflamed)
  abscess, lacrimal (*see also* Dacryocystitis) 375.30
  conjunctiva 372.00
    acute 372.00
  eyelid 373.00
  labium (majus) (minus) 616.89
  lacrimal 375.30
  urethra (benign) 599.3
  vagina (wall) 616.89
Cascade stomach 537.6
Caseation lymphatic gland (*see also*
    Tuberculosis) 017.2
Caseous
  bronchitis—*see* Tuberculosis, pulmonary
  meningitis 013.0
  pneumonia—*see* Tuberculosis, pulmonary
Cassidy (-Scholte) syndrome (malignant
    carcinoid) 259.2
Castellani's bronchitis 104.8
Castleman's tumor or lymphoma (mediastinal
    lymph node hyperplasia) 785.6
Castration, traumatic 878.2
  complicated 878.3
Casts in urine 791.7
Cat's ear 744.29
Catalepsy 300.11
  catatonic (acute) (*see also* Schizophrenia) 295.2
  hysterical 300.11
  schizophrenic (*see also* Schizophrenia) 295.2
Cataphasia (*see also* Disorder, fluency) 315.35
Cataplexy (idiopathic) *see also* Narcolepsy
Cataract (anterior cortical) (anterior polar)
    (black) (capsular) (central) (cortical)
    (hypermature) (immature) (incipient) (mature)
    366.9
  anterior
    and posterior axial embryonal 743.33
    pyramidal 743.31
    subcapsular polar
      infantile, juvenile, or presenile 366.01
      senile 366.13

Cataract—*continued*
  associated with
    calcinosis 275.40 *[366.42]*
    craniofacial dysostosis 756.0 *[366.44]*
    galactosemia 271.1 *[366.44]*
    hypoparathyroidism 252.1 *[366.42]*
    myotonic disorders 359.21 *[366.43]*
    neovascularization 366.33
  blue dot 743.39
  cerulean 743.39
  complicated NEC 366.30
  congenital 743.30
    capsular or subcapsular 743.31
    cortical 743.32
    nuclear 743.33
    specified type NEC 743.39
    total or subtotal 743.34
    zonular 743.32
  coronary (congenital) 743.39
    acquired 366.12
  cupuliform 366.14
  diabetic 250.5 *[366.41]*
    due to secondary diabetes 249.5 *[366.41]*
  drug-induced 366.45
  due to
    chalcosis 360.24 *[366.34]*
    chronic choroiditis (*see also* Choroiditis)
        363.20 *[366.32]*
    degenerative myopia 360.21 *[366.34]*
    glaucoma (*see also* Glaucoma) 365.9 *[366.31]*
    infection, intraocular NEC 366.32
    inflammatory ocular disorder NEC 366.32
    iridocyclitis, chronic 364.10 *[366.33]*
    pigmentary retinal dystrophy 362.74 *[366.34]*
    radiation 366.46
  electric 366.46
  glassblowers' 366.46
  heat ray 366.46
  heterochromic 366.33
  in eye disease NEC 366.30
  infantile (*see also* Cataract, juvenile) 366.00
  intumescent 366.12
  irradiational 366.46
  juvenile 366.00
    anterior subcapsular polar 366.01
    combined forms 366.09
    cortical 366.03
    lamellar 366.03
    nuclear 366.04
    posterior subcapsular polar 366.02
    specified NEC 366.09
    zonular 366.03
  lamellar 743.32
    infantile, juvenile, or presenile 366.03
  morgagnian 366.18
  myotonic 359.21 *[366.43]*
  myxedema 244.9 *[366.44]*
  nuclear 366.16
  posterior, polar (capsular) 743.31
    infantile, juvenile, or presenile 366.02
    senile 366.14
  presenile (*see also* Cataract, juvenile) 366.00
  punctate
    acquired 366.12
    congenital 743.39
  secondary (membrane) 366.50
    obscuring vision 366.53
    specified type, not obscuring vision 366.52

Cataract—*continued*
  senile 366.10
    anterior subcapsular polar 366.13
    combined forms 366.19
    cortical 366.15
    hypermature 366.18
    immature 366.12
    incipient 366.12
    mature 366.17
    nuclear 366.16
    posterior subcapsular polar 366.14
    specified NEC 366.19
    total or subtotal 366.17
  snowflake 250.5 *[366.41]*
    due to secondary diabetes 249.5 *[366.41]*
  specified NEC 366.8
  subtotal (senile) 366.17
    congenital 743.34
  sunflower 360.24 *[366.34]*
  tetanic NEC 252.1 *[366.42]*
  total (mature) (senile) 366.17
    congenital 743.34
    localized 366.21
    traumatic 366.22
  toxic 366.45
  traumatic 366.20
    partially resolved 366.23
    total 366.22
  zonular (perinuclear) 743.32
    infantile, juvenile, or presenile 366.03
Cataracta 366.10
  brunescens 366.16
  cerulea 743.39
  complicata 366.30
  congenita 743.30
  coralliformis 743.39
  coronaria (congenital) 743.39
    acquired 366.12
  diabetic 250.5 *[366.41]*
    due to secondary diabetes 249.5 *[366.41]*
  floriformis 360.24 *[366.34]*
  membranacea
    accreta 366.50
    congenita 743.39
  nigra 366.16
Catarrh, catarrhal (inflammation) (*see also*
    condition) 460
  acute 460
  asthma, asthmatic (*see also* Asthma) 493.9
  Bostock's (*see also* Fever, hay) 477.9
  bowel—*see* Enteritis
  bronchial 490
    acute 466.0
    chronic 491.0
    subacute 466.0
  cervix, cervical (canal) (uteri)—*see* Cervicitis
  chest (*see also* Bronchitis) 490
  chronic 472.0
  congestion 472.0
  conjunctivitis 372.03
  due to syphilis 095.9
    congenital 090.0
  enteric—*see* Enteritis
  epidemic (*see also* Influenza) 487.1
  Eustachian 381.50
  eye (acute) (vernal) 372.03
  fauces (*see also* Pharyngitis) 462
  febrile 460
  fibrinous acute 466.0
  gastroenteric—*see* Enteritis
  gastrointestinal—*see* Enteritis

Catarrh, catarrhal—*continued*
  gingivitis 523.00
  hay (*see also* Fever, hay) 477.9
  infectious 460
  intestinal—*see* Enteritis
  larynx (*see also* Laryngitis, chronic) 476.0
  liver 070.1
    with hepatic coma 070.0
  lung (*see also* Bronchitis) 490
    acute 466.0
    chronic 491.0
  middle ear (chronic)—*see* Otitis media, chronic
  mouth 528.00
  nasal (chronic) (*see also* Rhinitis) 472.0
    acute 460
  nasobronchial 472.2
  nasopharyngeal (chronic) 472.2
    acute 460
  nose—*see* Catarrh, nasal
  ophthalmia 372.03
  pneumococcal, acute 466.0
  pulmonary (*see also* Bronchitis) 490
    acute 466.0
    chronic 491.0
  spring (eye) 372.13
  suffocating (*see also* Asthma) 493.9
  summer (hay) (*see also* Fever, hay) 477.9
  throat 472.1
  tracheitis 464.10
    with obstruction 464.11
  tubotympanal 381.4
    acute (*see also* Otitis media, acute,
        nonsuppurative) 381.00
    chronic 381.10
  vasomotor (*see also* Fever, hay) 477.9
  vesical (bladder)—*see* Cystitis
Catarrhus aestivus (*see also* Fever, hay) 477.9
Catastrophe, cerebral (*see also* Disease,
    cerebrovascular, acute) 436
Catatonia, catatonic (acute) 781.99
  agitation 295.2
  dementia (praecox) 295.2
  due to or associated with physical condition 293.89
  excitation 295.2
  excited type 295.2
  in conditions classified elsewhere 293.89
  schizophrenia 295.2
  stupor 295.2
  with
    affective psychosis —*see* Psychosis, affective
Cat-scratch —*see also* Injury, superficial
  disease or fever 078.3
Cauda equina —*see also* condition syndrome
    344.60
Cauliflower ear 738.7
Caul over face 768.9
Causalgia 355.9
  lower limb 355.71
  upper limb 354.4
Cause
  external, general effects NEC 994.9
  not stated 799.9
  unknown 799.9
Caustic burn —*see also* Burn, by site
  from swallowing caustic or corrosive
      substance—*see* Burn, internal organs
Cavare's disease (familial periodic paralysis) 359.3
Cave-in, injury
  crushing (severe) (*see also* Crush, by site) 869.1
  suffocation 994.7
Cavernitis (penis) 607.2
  lymph vessel—*see* Lymphangioma

Cavernositis 607.2
Cavernous —*see* condition
Cavitation of lung (*see also* Tuberculosis) 011.2
  nontuberculous 518.89
  primary, progressive 010.8
Cavity
  lung—*see* Cavitation of lung
  optic papilla 743.57
  pulmonary—*see* Cavitation of lung
  teeth 521.00
  vitreous (humor) 379.21
Cavovarus foot, congenital 754.59
Cavus foot (congenital) 754.71
  acquired 736.73
Cazenave's
  disease (pemphigus) NEC 694.4
  lupus (erythematosus) 695.4
CDGS (carbohydrate-deficient glycoprotein syndrome) 271.8
Cecitis —*see* Appendicitis
Cecocele —*see* Hernia
Cecum —*see* condition
Celiac
  artery compression syndrome 447.4
  disease 579.0
  infantilism 579.0
Cell, cellular —*see also* condition
  anterior chamber (eye) (positive aqueous ray) 364.04
Cellulitis (diffuse) (with lymphangitis) (*see also* Abscess) 682.9
  abdominal wall 682.2
  anaerobic (*see also* Gas gangrene) 040.0
  ankle 682.6
  anus 566
  areola 611.0
  arm (any part, above wrist) 682.3
  auditory canal (external) 380.10
  axilla 682.3
  back (any part) 682.2
  breast 611.0
    postpartum 675.1
  broad ligament (*see also* Disease, pelvis, inflammatory) 614.4
    acute 614.3
  buttock 682.5
  cervical (neck region) 682.1
  cervix (uteri) (*see also* Cervicitis) 616.0
  cheek, external 682.0
    internal 528.3
  chest wall 682.2
  chronic NEC 682.9
  colostomy 569.61
  corpus cavernosum 607.2
  digit 681.9
  Douglas' cul-de-sac or pouch (chronic) (*see also* Disease, pelvis, inflammatory) 614.4
    acute 614.3
  drainage site (following operation) 998.59
  ear, external 380.10
  enterostomy 569.61
  erysipelar (*see also* Erysipelas) 035
  esophagostomy 530.86
  eyelid 373.13
  face (any part, except eye) 682.0
  finger (intrathecal) (periosteal) (subcutaneous) (subcuticular) 681.00
  flank 682.2
  foot (except toe) 682.7
  forearm 682.3
  gangrenous (*see also* Gangrene) 785.4

Cellulitis—*continued*
  genital organ NEC
    female—*see* Abscess, genital organ, female
    male 608.4
  glottis 478.71
  gluteal (region) 682.5
  gonococcal NEC 098.0
  groin 682.2
  hand (except finger or thumb) 682.4
  head (except face) NEC 682.8
  heel 682.7
  hip 682.6
  jaw (region) 682.0
  knee 682.6
  labium (majus) (minus) (*see also* Vulvitis) 616.10
  larynx 478.71
  leg, except foot 682.6
  lip 528.5
  mammary gland 611.0
  mouth (floor) 528.3
  multiple sites NEC 682.9
  nasopharynx 478.21
  navel 682.2
    newborn NEC 771.4
  neck (region) 682.1
  nipple 611.0
  nose 478.19
    external 682.0
  orbit, orbital 376.01
  palate (soft) 528.3
  pectoral (region) 682.2
  pelvis, pelvic
    with
      abortion—*see* Abortion, by type, with sepsis
      ectopic pregnancy (*see also* categories 633.0-633.9) 639.0
      molar pregnancy (*see also* categories 630-632) 639.0
    female (*see also* Disease, pelvis, inflammatory) 614.4
      acute 614.3
    following
      abortion 639.0
      ectopic or molar pregnancy 639.0
    male 567.21
  puerperal, postpartum, childbirth 670.8
  penis 607.2
  perineal, perineum 682.2
  perirectal 566
  peritonsillar 475
  periurethral 597.0
  periuterine (*see also* Disease, pelvis, inflammatory) 614.4
    acute 614.3
  pharynx 478.21
  phlegmonous NEC 682.9
  rectum 566
  retromammary 611.0
  retroperitoneal (*see also* Peritonitis) 567.238
  round ligament (*see also* Disease, pelvis, inflammatory) 614.4
    acute 614.3
  scalp (any part) 682.8
    dissecting 704.8
  scrotum 608.4
  seminal vesicle 608.0
  septic NEC 682.9
  shoulder 682.3
  specified sites NEC 682.8
  spermatic cord 608.4

Cellulitis—*continued*
  submandibular (region) (space) (triangle) 682.0
    gland 527.3
  submaxillary 528.3
    gland 527.3
  submental (pyogenic) 682.0
    gland 527.3
  suppurative NEC 682.9
  testis 608.4
  thigh 682.6
  thumb (intrathecal) (periosteal) (subcutaneous)
    (subcuticular) 681.00
  toe (intrathecal) (periosteal) (subcutaneous)
    (subcuticular) 681.10
  tonsil 475
  trunk 682.2
  tuberculous (primary) (*see also* Tuberculosis) 017.0
  tunica vaginalis 608.4
  umbilical 682.2
    newborn NEC 771.4
  vaccinal 999.39
  vagina—*see* Vaginitis
  vas deferens 608.4
  vocal cords 478.5
  vulva (*see also* Vulvitis) 616.10
  wrist 682.4
Cementoblastoma, benign (M9273/0) 213.1
  upper jaw (bone) 213.0
Cementoma (M9273/0) 213.1
  gigantiform (M9275/0) 213.1
    upper jaw (bone) 213.0
  upper jaw (bone) 213.0
Cementoperiostitis 523.40
  acute 523.33
  apical 523.40
Cephalgia, cephalalgia (*see also* Headache) 784.0
  histamine 339.00
  nonorganic origin 307.81
  other trigeminal autonomic (TACS) 339.09
  psychogenic 307.81
  tension 307.81
Cephalhematocele, cephalematocele
  due to birth injury 767.19
  fetus or newborn 767.19
  traumatic (*see also* Contusion, head) 920
Cephalhematoma, cephalematoma (calcified)
  due to birth injury 767.19
  fetus or newborn 767.19
  traumatic (*see also* Contusion, head) 920
Cephalic —*see* condition
Cephalitis —*see* Encephalitis
Cephalocele 742.0
Cephaloma —*see* Neoplasm, by site,
  malignant
Cephalomenia 625.8
Cephalopelvic —*see* condition
Cercomoniasis 007.3
Cerebellitis —*see* Encephalitis
Cerebellum (cerebellar)—*see* condition
Cerebral —*see* condition
Cerebritis —*see* Encephalitis
Cerebrohepatorenal syndrome 759.89
Cerebromacular degeneration 330.1
Cerebromalacia (*see also* Softening, brain) 348.89
  due to cerebrovascular accident 438.89
Cerebrosidosis 272.7
Cerebrospasticity —*see* Palsy, cerebral
Cerebrospinal —*see* condition
Cerebrum —*see* condition
Ceroid storage disease 272.7
Cerumen (accumulation) (impacted) 380.4

Cervical —*see also* condition
  auricle 744.43
  high risk human papillomavirus (HPV) DNA
    test positive 795.05
  intraepithelial glandular neoplasia 233.1
  low rish human papillomavirus (Hpv) DNA test
    positive 795.09
  rib 756.2
  shortening —*see* Short, cervical
Cervicalgia 723.1
Cervicitis (acute) (chronic) (nonvenereal)
    (subacute) (with erosion or ectropion) 616.0
  with
    abortion—*see* Abortion, by type, with sepsis
    ectopic pregnancy (*see also* categories
      633.0-633.9) 639.0
    molar pregnancy (*see also* categories 630-632)
      639.0
    ulceration 616.0
  chlamydial 099.53
  complicating pregnancy or puerperium 646.6
    affecting fetus or newborn 760.8
  following
    abortion 639.0
    ectopic or molar pregnancy 639.0
  gonococcal (acute) 098.15
    chronic or duration of 2 months or more 098.35
  senile (atrophic) 616.0
  syphilitic 095.8
  trichomonal 131.09
  tuberculous (*see also* Tuberculosis) 016.7
Cervicoaural fistula 744.49
Cervicocolpitis (emphysematosa) (*see also*
  Cervicitis) 616.0
Cervix —*see* condition
Cesarean delivery, operation or section NEC
    669.7
  affecting fetus or newborn 763.4
  (planned) occurring after 37 completed weeks of
    gestation but before 39 completed weeks
    gestation due to (spontaneous) onset of labor
    649.8
  post mortem, affecting fetus or newborn 761.6
  previous, affecting management of pregnancy
    654.2
Céstan's syndrome 344.89
Céstan-Chenais paralysis 344.89
Céstan-Raymond syndrome 433.8
Cestode infestation NEC 123.9
  specified type NEC 123.8
Cestodiasis 123.9
CGF (congenital generalized fibromatosis) 759.89
Chaberts' disease 022.9
Chacaleh 266.2
Chafing 709.8
Chagas' disease (*see also* Trypanosomiasis,
  American) 086.2
  with heart involvement 086.0
Chagres fever 084.0
Chalasia (cardiac sphincter) 530.81
Chalazion 373.2
Chalazoderma 757.39
Chalcosis 360.24
  cornea 371.15
  crystalline lens 360.24 *[366.34]*
  retina 360.24
Chalicosis (occupational) (pulmonum) 502
Chancre (any genital site) (hard) (indurated)
    (infecting) (primary) (recurrent) 091.0
  congenital 090.0
  conjunctiva 091.2

Chancre—*continued*
 Ducrey's 099.0
 extragenital 091.2
 eyelid 091.2
 Hunterian 091.0
 lip (syphilis) 091.2
 mixed 099.8
 nipple 091.2
 Nisbet's 099.0
 of
  carate 103.0
  pinta 103.0
  yaws 102.0
 palate, soft 091.2
 phagedenic 099.0
 Ricord's 091.0
 Rollet's (syphilitic) 091.0
 seronegative 091.0
 seropositive 091.0
 simple 099.0
 soft 099.0
  bubo 099.0
 urethra 091.0
 yaws 102.0
Chancriform syndrome 114.1
Chancroid 099.0
 anus 099.0
 penis (Ducrey's bacillus) 099.0
 perineum 099.0
 rectum 099.0
 scrotum 099.0
 urethra 099.0
 vulva 099.0
Chandipura fever 066.8
Chandler's disease (osteochondritis dissecans, hip) 732.7
Change(s) (of)—*see also* Removal of
 arteriosclerotic—*see* Arteriosclerosis
 battery
  cardiac pacemaker V53.31
 bone 733.90
  diabetic 250.8 *[731.8]*
   due to secondary diabetes 249.8 [731.8]
  in disease, unknown cause 733.90
 bowel habits 787.99
 cardiorenal (vascular) (*see also* Hypertension, cardiorenal) 404.90
 cardiovascular—*see* Disease, cardiovascular
 circulatory 459.9
 cognitive or personality change of other type, nonpsychotic 310.1
 color, teeth, tooth
  during formation 520.8
  extrinsic 523.6
  intrinsic posteruptive 521.7
 contraceptive device V25.42
 cornea, corneal
  degenerative NEC 371.40
  membrane NEC 371.30
  senile 371.41
 coronary (*see also* Ischemia, heart) 414.9
 degenerative
  chamber angle (anterior) (iris) 364.56
  ciliary body 364.57
  spine or vertebra (*see also* Spondylosis) 721.90
 dental pulp, regressive 522.2
 drains V58.49
 dressing
  wound V58.30
   nonsurgical V58.30
   surgical V58.31

Change(s) (of)—*continued*
 fixation device V54.89
  external V54.89
  internal V54.01
 heart—*see also* Disease, heart
 hip joint 718.95
 hyperplastic larynx 478.79
 hypertrophic
  nasal sinus (*see also* Sinusitis) 473.9
  turbinate, nasal 478.0
  upper respiratory tract 478.9
 inflammatory—*see* Inflammation
 joint (*see also* Derangement, joint) 718.90
  sacroiliac 724.6
 Kirschner wire V54.89
 knee 717.9
 macular, congenital 743.55
 malignant (M——/3)—*see also* Neoplasm, by site, malignant

> *Note—for malignant change occurring in a neoplasm, use the appropriate M code with behavior digit /3 e.g., malignant change in uterine fibroid—M8890/3. For malignant change occurring in a nonneoplastic condition (e.g., gastric ulcer) use the M code M8000/3.*

 mental (status) NEC 780.97
  due to or associated with physical condition—*see* Syndrome, brain
 myocardium, myocardial—*see* Degeneration, myocardial
 of life (*see also* Menopause) 627.2
 pacemaker battery (cardiac) V53.31
 peripheral nerve 355.9
 personality (nonpsychotic) NEC 310.1
 plaster cast V54.89
 refractive, transient 367.81
 regressive, dental pulp 522.2
 retina 362.9
  myopic (degenerative) (malignant) 360.21
  vascular appearance 362.13
 sacroiliac joint 724.6
 scleral 379.19
  degenerative 379.16
 senile (*see also* Senility) 797
 sensory (*see also* Disturbance, sensation) 782.0
 skin texture 782.8
 spinal cord 336.9
 splint, external V54.89
 subdermal implantable contraceptive V25.5
 suture V58.32
 traction device V54.89
 trophic 355.9
  arm NEC 354.9
  leg NEC 355.8
  lower extremity NEC 355.8
  upper extremity NEC 354.9
 vascular 459.9
 vasomotor 443.9
 voice 784.49
  psychogenic 306.1
 wound packing V58.30
  nonsurgical V58.30
  surgical V58.31
Changing sleep-work schedule, affecting sleep 327.36
Changuinola fever 066.0
Chapping skin 709.8
Character
 depressive 301.12
Charcot's
 arthropathy 094.0 *[713.5]*
 cirrhosis—*see* Cirrhosis, biliary

Charcot's—*continued*
  disease 094.0
    spinal cord 094.0
    fever (biliary) (hepatic) (intermittent)—*see*
      Choledocholithiasis
    joint (disease) 094.0 *[713.5]*
      diabetic 250.6 *[713.5]*
        due to secondary diabetes 249.6 [713.5]
      syringomyelic 336.0 *[713.5]*
    syndrome (intermittent claudication) 443.9
      due to atherosclerosis 440.21
Charcot-Marie-Tooth disease paralysis, or
  syndrome 356.1
CHARGE association (syndrome) 759.89
Charleyhorse (quadriceps) 843.8
  muscle, except quadriceps—*see* Sprain, by site
Charlouis' disease (*see also* Yaws) 102.9
Chauffeur's fracture —*see* Fracture, ulna, lower
  end
Cheadle (-Möller) (-Barlow) disease or syndrome
  (infantile scurvy) 267
Checking (of)
  contraceptive device (intrauterine) V25.42
  device
    fixation V54.89
      external V54.89
      internal V54.09
      traction V54.89
    Kirschner wire V54.89
    plaster cast V54.89
    splint, external V54.89
Checkup
  following treatment—*see* Examination
  health V70.0
  infant (over 28 days old) (not sick) V20.2
  newborn, routine
    8 to 28 days old V20.32
    over 28 days old, routine V20.2
    under 8 days old V20.31
    weight V20.32
  pregnancy (normal) V22.1
    first V22.0
    high risk pregnancy V23.9
      inconclusive fetal viability V23.87
      specified problem NEC V23.8
Chédiak-Higashi (-Steinbrinck) anomaly,
  disease, or syndrome (congenital gigantism of
  peroxidase granules) 288.2
Cheek —*see also* condition
  biting 528.9
Cheese itch 133.8
Cheese washers' lung 495.8
Cheilitis 528.5
  actinic (due to sun) 692.72
    chronic NEC 692.74
      due to radiation, except from sun 692.82
    due to radiation, except from sun 692.82
  acute 528.5
  angular 528.5
  catarrhal 528.5
  chronic 528.5
  exfoliative 528.5
  gangrenous 528.5
  glandularis apostematosa 528.5
  granulomatosa 351.8
  infectional 528.5
  membranous 528.5
  Miescher's 351.8
  suppurative 528.5
  ulcerative 528.5
  vesicular 528.5
Cheilodynia 528.5

Cheilopalatoschisis (*see also* Cleft, palate, with
  cleft lip) 749.20
Cheilophagia 528.9
Cheiloschisis (*see also* Cleft, lip) 749.10
Cheilosis 528.5
  with pellagra 265.2
  angular 528.5
  due to
    dietary deficiency 266.0
    vitamin deficiency 266.0
Cheiromegaly 729.89
Cheiropompholyx 705.81
Cheloid (*see also* Keloid) 701.4
Chemical burn —*see also* Burn, by site
  from swallowing chemical—*see* Burn, internal
    organs
Chemodectoma (M8693/1)—*see* Paraganglioma,
  nonchromaffin
Chemoprophylaxis NEC V07.39
Chemosis, conjunctiva 372.73
Chemotherapy
  convalescence V66.2
  encounter (for) (oral) (intravenous) V58.11
  maintenance (oral) (intravenous) V58.11
  prophylactic NEC V07.39
    fluoride V07.31
Cherubism 526.89
Chest —*see* condition
Cheyne-Stokes respiration (periodic) 786.04
Chiari's
  disease or syndrome (hepatic vein thrombosis)
    453.0
  malformation
    type I 348.4
    type II (*see also* Spina bifida) 741.0
    type III 742.0
    type IV 742.2
  network 746.89
Chiari-Frommel syndrome 676.6
Chicago disease (North American blastomycosis)
  116.0
Chickenpox (*see also* Varicella) 052.9
  exposure to V01.71
  vaccination and inoculation (prophylactic) V05.4
Chiclero ulcer 085.4
Chiggers 133.8
Chignon 111.2
  fetus or newborn (from vacuum extraction)
    767.19
Chigoe disease 134.1
Chikungunya fever 066.3
Chilaiditi's syndrome (subphrenic displacement,
  colon) 751.4
Chilblains 991.5
  lupus 991.5
Child
  behavior causing concern V61.20
    adopted child V61.24
    biological child V61.23
    foster child V61.25
Childbed fever 670.8
Childbirth —*see also* Delivery
  puerperal complications—*see* Puerperal
Childhood, period of rapid growth V21.0
Chill (s) 780.64
  with fever 780.60
  without fever 780.64
  congestive 780.99
    in malarial regions 084.6
  septic—*see* Septicemia
  urethral 599.84

Chilomastigiasis 007.8
Chin —*see* condition
Chinese dysentery 004.9
Chiropractic dislocation (*see also* Lesion,
    nonallopathic, by site) 739.9
Chitral fever 066.0
Chlamydia, chlamydial -*see* **condition**
Chloasma 709.09
  cachecticorum 709.09
  eyelid 374.52
    congenital 757.33
    hyperthyroid 242.0
  gravidarum 646.8
  idiopathic 709.09
  skin 709.09
  symptomatic 709.09
Chloroma (M9930/3) 205.3
Chlorosis 280.9
  Egyptian (*see also* Ancylostomiasis) 126.9
  miners' (*see also* Ancylostomiasis) 126.9
Chlorotic anemia 280.9
Chocolate cyst (ovary) 617.1
Choked
  disk or disc—*see* Papilledema
  on food, phlegm, or vomitus NEC (*see also*
      Asphyxia, food) 933.1
  phlegm 933.1
  while vomiting NEC (*see also* Asphyxia, food) 933.1
Chokes (resulting from bends) 993.3
Choking sensation 784.99
Cholangiectasis (*see also* Disease, gallbladder)
    575.8
Cholangiocarcinoma (M8160/3)
  and hepatocellular carcinoma, combined
      (M8180/3) 155.0
  liver 155.1
  specified site NEC—*see* Neoplasm, by site, malignant
  unspecified site 155.1
Cholangiohepatitis 575.8
  due to fluke infestation 121.1
Cholangiohepatoma (M8180/3) 155.0
Cholangiolitis (acute) (chronic) (extrahepatic)
    (gangrenous) 576.1
  intrahepatic 575.8
  paratyphoidal (*see also* Fever, paratyphoid) 002.9
  typhoidal 002.0
Cholangioma (M8160/0) 211.5
  malignant—*see* Cholangiocarcinoma
Cholangitis (acute) (ascending) (catarrhal)
    (chronic) (infective) (malignant) (primary)
    (recurrent) (sclerosing) (secondary)
    (stenosing) (suppurative) 576.1
  chronic nonsuppurative destructive 571.6
  nonsuppurative destructive (chronic) 571.6
Cholecystdocholithiasis —*see* Choledocholithiasis
Cholecystitis 575.10
  with
    calculus, stones in
      bile duct (common) (hepatic)—*see*
          Choledocholithiasis
      gallbladder—*see* Cholelithiasis
  acute 575.0
  acute and chronic 575.12
  chronic 575.11
  emphysematous (acute) (*see also* Cholecystitis,
      acute) 575.0
  gangrenous (*see also* Cholecystitis, acute) 575.0
  paratyphoidal, current (*see also* Fever,
      paratyphoid) 002.9
  suppurative (*see also* Cholecystitis, acute) 575.0
  typhoidal 002.0

Choledochitis (suppurative) 576.1
Choledocholith —*see* Choledocholithiasis
Choledocholithiasis 574.5

> *Note—Use the following fifth-digit*
> *subclassification with category 574:*
>
> *0 without mention of obstruction*
> *1 with obstruction*

  with
    cholecystitis 574.4
      acute 574.3
      chronic 574.4
    cholelithiasis 574.9
      with
        cholecystitis 574.7
          acute 574.6
            and chronic 574.8
          chronic 574.7
Cholelithiasis (impacted) (multiple) 574.2

> *Note—Use the following fifth-digit*
> *subclassification with category 574:*
>
> *0 without mention of obstruction*
> *1 with obstruction*

  with
    cholecystitis 574.1
      acute 574.0
      chronic 574.1
    choledocholithiasis 574.9
      with
        cholecystitis 574.7
          acute 574.6
            and chronic 574.8
          chronic cholecystitis 574.7
Cholemia (*see also* Jaundice) 782.4
  familial 277.4
  Gilbert's (familial nonhemolytic) 277.4
Cholemic gallstone —*see* Cholelithiasis
Choleperitoneum, choleperitonitis (*see also*
    Disease, gallbladder) 567.81
Cholera (algid) (Asiatic) (asphyctic) (epidemic)
    (gravis) (Indian) (malignant) (morbus)
    (pestilential) (spasmodic) 001.9
  antimonial 985.4
  carrier (suspected) of V02.0
  classical 001.0
  contact V01.0
  due to
    Vibrio
      cholerae (Inaba, Ogawa, Hikojima
          serotypes) 001.0
      El Tor 001.1
  El Tor 001.1
  exposure to V01.0
  vaccination, prophylactic (against) V03.0
Cholerine (*see also* Cholera) 001.9
Cholestasis 576.8
  due to total parenteral nutrition (TPN) 573.8
Cholesteatoma (ear) 385.30
  attic (primary) 385.31
  diffuse 385.35
  external ear (canal) 380.21
  marginal (middle ear) 385.32
    with involvement of mastoid cavity 385.33
    secondary (with middle ear involvement) 385.33
  mastoid cavity 385.30

Cholesteatoma—*continued*
middle ear (secondary) 385.32
  with involvement of mastoid cavity 385.33
postmastoidectomy cavity (recurrent) 383.32
primary 385.31
recurrent, postmastoidectomy cavity 383.32
secondary (middle ear) 385.32
  with involvement of mastoid cavity 385.33
Cholesteatosis (middle ear) (*see also*
  Cholesteatoma) 385.30
diffuse 385.35
Cholesteremia 272.0
Cholesterin
granuloma, middle ear 385.82
in vitreous 379.22
Cholesterol
deposit
  retina 362.82
  vitreous 379.22
elevated (high) 272.0
  with elevated (high) triglycerides 272.2
imbibition of gallbladder (*see also* Disease,
  gallbladder) 575.6
Cholesterolemia 272.0
essential 272.0
familial 272.0
hereditary 272.0
Cholesterosis, cholesterolosis (gallbladder) 575.6
middle ear (*see also* Cholesteatoma) 385.30
with
  cholecystitis—*see* Cholecystitis
  cholelithiasis—*see* Cholelithiasis
Cholocolic fistula (*see also* Fistula, gallbladder)
  575.5
Choluria 791.4
Chondritis (purulent) 733.99
auricle 380.03
costal 733.6
  Tietze's 733.6
patella, posttraumatic 717.7
pinna 380.03
posttraumatica patellae 717.7
tuberculous (active) (*see also* Tuberculosis) 015.9
  intervertebral 015.0 *[730.88]*
Chondroangiopathia calcarea seu punctate
  756.59
Chondroblastoma (M9230/0)—*see also*
  Neoplasm, bone, benign
malignant (M9230/3)—*see* Neoplasm, bone,
  malignant
Chondrocalcinosis (articular) (crystal deposition)
  (dihydrate) (*see also* Arthritis, due to, crystals)
  275.49 *[712.3]*
due to
  calcium pyrophosphate 275.49 *[712.2]*
  dicalcium phosphate crystals 275.49 *[712.1]*
  pyrophosphate crystals 275.4 *[712.2]*
Chondrodermatitis nodularis helicis 380.00
Chondrodysplasia 756.4
angiomatose 756.4
calcificans congenita 756.59
epiphysialis punctata 756.59
hereditary deforming 756.4
rhizomelic punctata 277.86
Chondrodystrophia (fetalis) 756.4
calcarea 756.4
calcificans congenita 756.59
fetalis hypoplastica 756.59
hypoplastica calcinosa 756.59
punctata 756.59
tarda 277.5

Chondrodystrophy (familial) (hypoplastic) 756.4
myotonic (congenital) 359.23
Chondroectodermal dysplasia 756.55
Chondrolysis 733.99
Chondroma (M9220/0)—*see also* Neoplasm
  cartilage, benign
juxtacortical (M9221/0)—*see* Neoplasm, bone,
  benign
periosteal (M9221/0)—*see* Neoplasm, bone,
  benign
Chondromalacia 733.92
epiglottis (congenital) 748.3
generalized 733.92
knee 717.7
larynx (congenital) 748.3
localized, except patella 733.92
patella, patellae 717.7
systemic 733.92
tibial plateau 733.92
trachea (congenital) 748.3
Chondromatosis (M9220/1)—*see* Neoplasm,
  cartilage, uncertain behavior
Chondromyxosarcoma (M9220/3)—*see*
  Neoplasm, cartilage, malignant
Chondro-osteodysplasia (Morquio-Brailsford
  type) 277.5
Chondro-osteodystrophy 277.5
Chondro-osteodystrophy 277.5
Chondro-osteoma (M9210/0)—*see* Neoplasm,
  bone, benign
Chondropathia tuberosa 733.6
Chondrosarcoma (M9220/3)—*see also*
  Neoplasm, cartilage, malignant
juxtacortical (M9221/3)—*see* Neoplasm, bone,
  malignant
mesenchymal (M9240/3)—*see* Neoplasm,
  connective tissue, malignant
Chordae tendineae rupture (chronic) 429.5
Chordee (nonvenereal) 607.89
congenital 752.63
gonococcal 098.2
Chorditis (fibrinous) (nodosa) (tuberosa) 478.5
Chordoma (M9370/3)—*see* Neoplasm, by site,
  malignant
Chorea (gravis) (minor) (spasmodic) 333.5
with
  heart involvement—*see* Chorea with
    rheumatic heart disease
  rheumatic heart disease (chronic, inactive, or
    quiescent) (conditions classifiable to
    393-398)—*see also* Rheumatic heart
    condition involved
    active or acute (conditions classifiable to
      391) 392.0
acute—*see* Chorea, Sydenham's
apoplectic (*see also* Disease, cerebrovascular,
  acute) 436
chronic 333.4
electric 049.8
gravidarum—*see* Eclampsia, pregnancy
habit 307.22
hereditary 333.4
Huntington's 333.4
posthemiplegic 344.89
pregnancy—*see* Eclampsia, pregnancy
progressive 333.4
  chronic 333.4
  hereditary 333.4
rheumatic (chronic) 392.9
  with heart disease or involvement—*see*
    Chorea, with rheumatic heart disease

Chorea—*continued*
  senile 333.5
  Sydenham's 392.9
    with heart involvement—*see* Chorea, with
      rheumatic heart disease
    nonrheumatic 333.5
  variabilis 307.23
Choreoathetosis (paroxysmal) 333.5
Chorioadenoma (destruens) (M9100/1) 236.1
Chorioamnionitis 658.4
  affecting fetus or newborn 762.7
Chorioangioma (M9120/0) 219.8
Choriocarcinoma (M9100/3)
  combined with
    embryonal carcinoma (M9101/3)—*see*
      Neoplasm, by site, malignant
    teratoma (M9101/3)—*see* Neoplasm, by site,
      malignant
  specified site—*see* Neoplasm, by site, malignant
  unspecified site
    female 181
    male 186.9
Chorioencephalitis, lymphocytic (acute)
  (serous) 049.0
Chorioepithelioma (M9100/3)—*see*
  Choriocarcinoma
Choriomeningitis (acute) (benign) (lymphocytic)
  (serous) 049.0
Chorionepithelioma (M9100/3)—*see*
  Choriocarcinoma
Chorionitis (*see also* Scleroderma) 710.1
Chorioretinitis 363.20
  disseminated 363.10
    generalized 363.13
    in
      neurosyphilis 094.83
      secondary syphilis 091.51
    peripheral 363.12
    posterior pole 363.11
    tuberculous (*see also* Tuberculosis) 017.3
      [363.13]
  due to
    histoplasmosis (*see also* Histoplasmosis) 115.92
    toxoplasmosis (acquired) 130.2
      congenital (active) 771.2
  focal 363.00
    juxtapapillary 363.01
    peripheral 363.04
    posterior pole NEC 363.03
  juxtapapillaris, juxtapapillary 363.01
  progressive myopia (degeneration) 360.21
  syphilitic (secondary) 091.51
    congenital (early) 090.0 *[363.13]*
      late 090.5 *[363.13]*
    late 095.8 *[363.13]*
  tuberculous (*see also* Tuberculosis) 017.3 *[363.13]*
Choristoma —*see* Neoplasm, by site, benign
Choroid —*see* condition
Choroideremia, choroidermia (initial stage)
  (late stage) (partial or total atrophy) 363.55
Choroiditis (*see also* Chorioretinitis) 363.20
  leprous 030.9 *[363.13]*
  senile guttate 363.41
  sympathetic 360.11
  syphilitic (secondary) 091.51
    congenital (early) 090.0 *[363.13]*
      late 090.5 *[363.13]*
    late 095.8 *[363.13]*
  Tay's 363.41
  tuberculous (*see also* Tuberculosis) 017.3
    [363.13]

Choroidopathy NEC 363.9
  degenerative (*see also* Degeneration, choroid)
    363.40
  hereditary (*see also* Dystrophy, choroid) 363.50
  specified type NEC 363.8
Choroidoretinitis —*see* Chorioretinitis
Choroidosis, central serous 362.41
Choroidretinopathy, serous 362.41
Christian's syndrome (chronic histiocytosis X)
  277.89
Christian-Weber disease (nodular
  nonsuppurative panniculitis) 729.30
Christmas disease 286.1
Chromaffinoma (M8700/0)—*see also*
  Neoplasm, by site, benign
  malignant (M8700/3)—*see* Neoplasm, by site,
    malignant
Chromatopsia 368.59
Chromhidrosis, chromidrosis 705.89
Chromoblastomycosis 117.2
Chromomycosis 117.2
Chromophytosis 111.0
Chromotrichomycosis 111.8
Chronic —*see* condition
Churg-Strauss syndrome 446.4
Chyle cyst, mesentery 457.8
Chylocele (nonfilarial) 457.8
  filarial (*see also* Infestation, filarial) 125.9
  tunica vaginalis (nonfilarial) 608.84
    filarial (*see also* Infestation, filarial) 125.9
Chylomicronemia (fasting) (with
  hyperprebetalipoproteinemia) 272.3
Chylopericardium (acute) 420.90
Chylothorax (nonfilarial) 457.8
  filarial (*see also* Infestation, filarial) 125.9
Chylous
  ascites 457.8
  cyst of peritoneum 457.8
  hydrocele 603.9
  hydrothorax (nonfilarial) 457.8
    filarial (*see also* Infestation, filarial) 125.9
Chyluria 791.1
  bilharziasis 120.0
  due to
    Brugia (malayi) 125.1
    Wuchereria (bancrofti) 125.0
      malayi 125.1
  filarial (*see also* Infestation, filarial) 125.9
  filariasis (*see also* Infestation, filarial) 125.9
  nonfilarial 791.1
Cicatricial (deformity)—*see* Cicatrix
Cicatrix (adherent) (contracted) (painful)
  (vicious) 709.2
  adenoid 474.8
  alveolar process 525.8
  anus 569.49
  auricle 380.89
  bile duct (*see also* Disease, biliary) 576.8
  bladder 596.89
  bone 733.99
  brain 348.89
  cervix (postoperative) (postpartal) 622.3
    in pregnancy or childbirth 654.6
      causing obstructed labor 660.2
  chorioretinal 363.30
    disseminated 363.35
    macular 363.32
    peripheral 363.34
    posterior pole NEC 363.33
  choroid—*see* Cicatrix, chorioretinal

Cicatrix—*continued*
  common duct (*see also* Disease, biliary) 576.8
  congenital 757.39
  conjunctiva 372.64
  cornea 371.00
    tuberculous (*see also* Tuberculosis) 017.3 *[371.05]*
  duodenum (bulb) 537.3
  esophagus 530.3
  eyelid 374.46
    with
      ectropion—*see* Ectropion
      entropion—*see* Entropion
  hypopharynx 478.29
  knee, semilunar cartilage 717.5
  lacrimal
    canaliculi 375.53
    duct
      acquired 375.56
      neonatal 375.55
    punctum 375.52
    sac 375.54
  larynx 478.79
  limbus (cystoid) 372.64
  lung 518.89
  macular 363.32
    disseminated 363.35
    peripheral 363.34
  middle ear 385.89
  mouth 528.9
  muscle 728.89
  nasolacrimal duct
    acquired 375.56
    neonatal 375.55
  nasopharynx 478.29
  palate (soft) 528.9
  penis 607.89
  prostate 602.8
  rectum 569.49
  retina 363.30
    disseminated 363.35
    macular 363.32
    peripheral 363.34
    posterior pole NEC 363.33
  semilunar cartilage—*see* Derangement,
    meniscus
  seminal vesicle 608.89
  skin 709.2
    infected 686.8
    postinfectional 709.2
    tuberculous (*see also* Tuberculosis) 017.0
  specified site NEC 709.2
  throat 478.29
  tongue 529.8
  tonsil (and adenoid) 474.8
  trachea 478.9
  tuberculous NEC (*see also* Tuberculosis) 011.9
  ureter 593.89
  urethra 599.84
  uterus 621.8
  vagina 623.4
    in pregnancy or childbirth 654.7
      causing obstructed labor 660.2
  vocal cord 478.5
  wrist, constricting (annular) 709.2
CIDP (chronic inflammatory demyelinating
  polyneuropathy) 357.81
CIN I (cervical intraepithelial neoplasia I) 622.11
CIN II (cervical intraepithelial neoplasia II) 622.12
CIN III (cervical intraepithelial neoplasia III) 233.1

Cinchonism
  correct substance properly administered 386.9
  overdose or wrong substance given or taken
    961.4
Circine herpes 110.5
Circle of Willis —*see* condition
Circular —*see also* condition
  hymen 752.49
Circulating anticoagulants, antibodies or
  inhibitors (*see also* Anticoagulants) 286.59
  extrinsic 287.8
  following childbirth 666.3
  intrinsic, causing hemorrhagic disorder 286.59
    with
      acquired hemophilia 286.52
      antiphospholipid antibody 286.53
  postpartum 666.3
Circulation
  collateral (venous), any site 459.89
  defective 459.9
    congenital 747.9
    lower extremity 459.89
  embryonic 747.9
  failure 799.89
    fetus or newborn 779.89
    peripheral 785.59
  fetal, persistent 747.83
  heart, incomplete 747.9
Circulatory system —*see* condition
Circulus senilis 371.41
Circumcision
  in absence of medical indication V50.2
  ritual V50.2
  routine V50.2
Circumscribed —*see* condition
Circumvallata placenta —*see* Placenta,
  abnormal
Cirrhosis, cirrhotic 571.5
  with alcoholism 571.2
  alcoholic (liver) 571.2
  atrophic (of liver)—*see* Cirrhosis, portal
  Baumgarten-Cruveilhier 571.5
  biliary (cholangiolitic) (cholangitic)
    (cholestatic) (extrahepatic) (hypertrophic)
    (intrahepatic) (nonobstructive) (obstructive)
    (pericholangiolitic) (posthepatic) (primary)
    (secondary) (xanthomatous) 571.6
    due to
      clonorchiasis 121.1
      flukes 121.3
  brain 331.9
  capsular—*see* Cirrhosis, portal
  cardiac 571.5
    alcoholic 571.2
  central (liver)—*see* Cirrhosis, liver
  Charcot's 571.6
  cholangiolitic—*see* Cirrhosis, biliary
  cholangitic—*see* Cirrhosis, biliary
  cholestatic—*see* Cirrhosis, biliary
  clitoris (hypertrophic) 624.2
  coarsely nodular 571.5
  congestive (liver)—*see* Cirrhosis, cardiac
  Cruveilhier-Baumgarten 571.5
  cryptogenic (of liver) 571.5
    alcoholic 571.2
  dietary (*see also* Cirrhosis, portal) 571.5
  due to
    bronzed diabetes 275.01
    congestive hepatomegaly—*see* Cirrhosis, cardiac
    cystic fibrosis 277.00

Cirrhosis, cirrhotic—*continued*
due to—*continued*
hemochromatosis (*see also* Hemochromatosis) 275.03
hepatolenticular degeneration 275.1
passive congestion (chronic)—*see* Cirrhosis, cardiac
Wilson's disease 275.1
xanthomatosis 272.2
extrahepatic (obstructive)—*see* Cirrhosis, biliary
fatty 571.8
alcoholic 571.0
florid 571.2
Glisson's—*see* Cirrhosis, portal
Hanot's (hypertrophic)—*see* Cirrhosis, biliary
hepatic—*see* Cirrhosis, liver
hepatolienal—*see* Cirrhosis, liver
hobnail—*see* Cirrhosis, portal
hypertrophic—*see also* Cirrhosis, liver
biliary—*see* Cirrhosis, biliary
Hanot's—*see* Cirrhosis, biliary
infectious NEC—*see* Cirrhosis, portal
insular—*see* Cirrhosis, portal
intrahepatic (obstructive) (primary)
(secondary)—*see* Cirrhosis, biliary
juvenile (*see also* Cirrhosis, portal) 571.5
kidney (*see also* Sclerosis, renal) 587
Laennec's (of liver) 571.2
nonalcoholic 571.5
liver (chronic) (hepatolienal) (hypertrophic)
(nodular) (splenomegalic) (unilobar) 571.5
with alcoholism 571.2
alcoholic 571.2
congenital (due to failure of obliteration of
umbilical vein) 777.8
cryptogenic 571.5
alcoholic 571.2
fatty 571.8
alcoholic 571.0
macronodular 571.5
alcoholic 571.2
micronodular 571.5
alcoholic 571.2
nodular, diffuse 571.5
alcoholic 571.2
pigmentary 275.01
portal 571.5
alcoholic 571.2
postnecrotic 571.5
alcoholic 571.2
syphilitic 095.3
lung (chronic) (*see also* Fibrosis, lung) 515
macronodular (of liver) 571.5
alcoholic 571.2
malarial 084.9
metabolic NEC 571.5
micronodular (of liver) 571.5
alcoholic 571.2
monolobular—*see* Cirrhosis, portal
multilobular—*see* Cirrhosis, portal
nephritis (*see also* Sclerosis, renal) 587
nodular—*see* Cirrhosis, liver
nutritional (fatty) 571.5
obstructive (biliary) (extrahepatic)
(intrahepatic)—*see* Cirrhosis, biliary
ovarian 620.8
paludal 084.9
pancreas (duct) 577.8
pericholangiolitic—*see* Cirrhosis, biliary
periportal—*see* Cirrhosis, portal
pigment, pigmentary (of liver) 275.01

Cirrhosis, cirrhotic— *continued*
portal (of liver) 571.5
alcoholic 571.2
posthepatitic (*see also* Cirrhosis, postnecrotic) 571.5
postnecrotic (of liver) 571.5
alcoholic 571.2
primary (intrahepatic)—*see* Cirrhosis, biliary
pulmonary (*see also* Fibrosis, lung) 515
renal (*see also* Sclerosis, renal) 587
septal (*see also* Cirrhosis, postnecrotic) 571.5
spleen 289.51
splenomegalic (of liver)—*see* Cirrhosis, liver
stasis (liver)—*see* Cirrhosis, liver
stomach 535.4
Todd's (*see also* Cirrhosis, biliary) 571.6
toxic (nodular)—*see* Cirrhosis, postnecrotic
trabecular—*see* Cirrhosis, postnecrotic
unilobar—*see* Cirrhosis, liver
vascular (of liver)—*see* Cirrhosis, liver
xanthomatous (biliary) (*see also* Cirrhosis,
biliary) 571.6
due to xanthomatosis (familial) (metabolic)
(primary) 272.2
Cistern, subarachnoid 793.0
Citrullinemia 270.6
Citrullinuria 270.6
Ciuffini-Pancoast tumor (M8010/3) (carcinoma,
pulmonary apex) 162.3
Civatte's disease or poikiloderma 709.09
CJD (Creutzfeldt-Jakob disease) 046.19
variant (vCJD) 046.11
**CLABSI (central line-associated bloodstream
infection)** 999.32
Clam diggers' itch 120.3
Clap —*see* Gonorrhea
Clark's paralysis 343.9
Clarke-Hadfield syndrome (pancreatic
infantilism) 577.8
Clastothrix 704.2
Claude's syndrome 352.6
Claude Bernard-Horner syndrome (*see also*
Neuropathy, peripheral, autonomic) 337.9
Claudication, intermittent 443.9
cerebral (artery) (*see also* Ischemia, cerebral,
transient) 435.9
due to atherosclerosis 440.21
spinal cord (arteriosclerotic) 435.1
syphilitic 094.89
spinalis 435.1
venous (axillary) 453.89
Claudicatio venosa intermittens 453.89
Claustrophobia 300.29
Clavus (infected) 700
Claw foot (congenital) 754.71
acquired 736.74
Claw hand (acquired) 736.06
congenital 755.59
Clawtoe (congenital) 754.71
acquired 735.5
Clay eating 307.52
Clay shovelers' fracture —*see* Fracture,
vertebra, cervical
Cleansing of artificial opening (*see also*
Attention to artificial opening) V55.9
Cleft (congenital)—*see also* Imperfect, closure
alveolar process 525.8
branchial (persistent) 744.41
cyst 744.42
clitoris 752.49
cricoid cartilage, posterior 748.3
facial (*see also* Cleft, lip) 749.10

Cleft—*continued*
lip 749.10
  with cleft palate 749.20
    bilateral (lip and palate) 749.24
      with unilateral lip or palate 749.25
      complete 749.23
      incomplete 749.24
    unilateral (lip and palate) 749.22
      with bilateral lip or palate 749.25
      complete 749.21
      incomplete 749.22
    bilateral 749.14
      with cleft palate, unilateral 749.25
      complete 749.13
      incomplete 749.14
    unilateral 749.12
      with cleft palate, bilateral 749.25
      complete 749.11
      incomplete 749.12
  nose 748.1
palate 749.00
  with cleft lip 749.20
    bilateral (lip and palate) 749.24
      with unilateral lip or palate 749.25
      complete 749.23
      incomplete 749.24
    unilateral (lip and palate) 749.22
      with bilateral lip or palate 749.25
      complete 749.21
      incomplete 749.22
    bilateral 749.04
      with cleft lip, unilateral 749.25
      complete 749.03
      incomplete 749.04
    unilateral 749.02
      with cleft lip, bilateral 749.25
      complete 749.01
      incomplete 749.02
  penis 752.69
  posterior, cricoid cartilage 748.3
  scrotum 752.89
  sternum (congenital) 756.3
  thyroid cartilage (congenital) 748.3
  tongue 750.13
  uvula 749.02
    with cleft lip (*see also* Cleft, lip, with cleft
      palate) 749.20
  water 366.12
Cleft hand (congenital) 755.58
Cleidocranial dysostosis 755.59
Cleidotomy, fetal 763.89
Cleptomania 312.32
Clérambault's syndrome 297.8
  erotomania 302.89
Clergyman's sore throat 784.49
Click, clicking
  systolic syndrome 785.2
Clifford's syndrome (postmaturity) 766.22
Climacteric (*see also* Menopause) 627.2
  arthritis NEC (*see also* Arthritis, climacteric)
    716.3
  depression (*see also* Psychosis, affective) 296.2
  disease 627.2
    recurrent episode 296.3
    single episode 296.2
  female (symptoms) 627.2
  male (symptoms) (syndrome) 608.89
  melancholia (*see also* Psychosis, affective) 296.2
    recurrent episode 296.3
    single episode 296.2
  paranoid state 297.2

Climacteric—*continued*
  paraphrenia 297.2
  polyarthritis NEC 716.39
    male 608.89
  symptoms (female) 627.2
Clinical research investigation (control)
  (participant) V70.7
Clinodactyly 755.59
Clitoris —*see* condition
Cloaca, persistent 751.5
Clonorchiasis 121.1
Clonorchiosis 121.1
Clonorchis infection, liver 121.1
Clonus 781.0
Closed bite 524.20
Closed surgical procedure converted to open
    procedure
  arthroscopic V64.43
  laparoscopic V64.41
  thoracoscopic V64.42
Closure
  artificial opening (*see also* Attention to artificial
    opening) V55.9
  congenital, nose 748.0
  cranial sutures, premature 756.0
  defective or imperfect NEC—*see* Imperfect,
    closure
  fistula, delayed—*see* Fistula
  fontanelle, delayed 756.0
  foramen ovale, imperfect 745.5
  hymen 623.3
  interauricular septum, defective 745.5
  interventricular septum, defective 745.4
  lacrimal duct 375.56
    congenital 743.65
    neonatal 375.55
  nose (congenital) 748.0
    acquired 738.0
  primary angle without glaucoma damage 365.06
  vagina 623.2
  valve—*see* Endocarditis
  vulva 624.8
Clot (blood)
  artery (obstruction) (occlusion) (*see also*
    Embolism) 444.9
  atrial appendage 429.89
  bladder 596.7
  brain (extradural or intradural) (*see also*
    Thrombosis, brain) 434.0
    late effect—*see* Late effect(s) (of)
      cerebrovascular disease
  circulation 444.9
  heart (*see also* Infarct, myocardium) 410.9
    without myocardial infarction 429.89
  vein (*see also* Thrombosis) 453.9
Clotting defect NEC (*see also* Defect,
    coagulation) 286.9
Clouded state 780.09
  epileptic (*see also* Epilepsy) 345.9
  paroxysmal (idiopathic) (*see also* Epilepsy) 345.9
Clouding
  corneal graft 996.51
Cloudy
  antrum, antra 473.0
  dialysis effluent 792.5
Clouston's (hidrotic) ectodermal dysplasia 757.31
Clubbing of fingers 781.5
Clubfinger 736.29
  acquired 736.29
  congenital 754.89

Clubfoot (congenital) 754.70
  acquired 736.71
  equinovarus 754.51
  paralytic 736.71
Club hand (congenital) 754.89
  acquired 736.07
Clubnail (acquired) 703.8
  congenital 757.5
Clump kidney 753.3
Clumsiness 781.3
  syndrome 315.4
Cluttering (see also Disorder, fluency) 315.35
Clutton's joints 090.5
Coagulation, intravascular (diffuse)
  (disseminated) (see also Fibrinolysis) 286.6
  newborn 776.2
Coagulopathy (see also Defect, coagulation) 286.9
  consumption 286.6
  intravascular (disseminated) NEC 286.6
    newborn 776.2
Coalition
  calcaneoscaphoid 755.67
  calcaneus 755.67
  tarsal 755.67
Coal miners'
  elbow 727.2
  lung 500
Coal workers' lung or pneumoconiosis 500
Coarctation
  aorta (postductal) (preductal) 747.10
  pulmonary artery 747.31
Coated tongue 529.3
Coats' disease 362.12
Cocainism (see also Dependence) 304.2
Coccidioidal granuloma 114.3
Coccidioidomycosis 114.9
  with pneumonia 114.0
  cutaneous (primary) 114.1
  disseminated 114.3
  extrapulmonary (primary) 114.1
  lung 114.5
    acute 114.0
    chronic 114.4
    primary 114.0
  meninges 114.2
  primary (pulmonary) 114.0
    acute 114.0
  prostate 114.3
  pulmonary 114.5
    acute 114.0
    chronic 114.4
    primary 114.0
  specified site NEC 114.3
Coccidioidosis 114.9
  lung 114.5
    acute 114.0
    chronic 114.4
    primary 114.0
  meninges 114.2
Coccidiosis (colitis) (diarrhea) (dysentery) 007.2
Cocciuria 791.9
Coccus in urine 791.9
Coccydynia 724.79
Coccygodynia 724.79
Coccyx —see condition
Cochin-China
  diarrhea 579.1
    anguilluliasis 127.2
  ulcer 085.1
Cock's peculiar tumor 706.2
Cockayne's disease or syndrome (microcephaly
  and dwarfism) 759.89

Cockayne-Weber syndrome (epidermolysis
  bullosa) 757.39
Cocked-up toe 735.2
Codman's tumor (benign chondroblastoma)
  (M9230/0)—see Neoplasm, bone, benign
Coenurosis 123.8
Coffee workers' lung 495.8
Cogan's syndrome 370.52
  congenital oculomotor apraxia 379.51
  nonsyphilitic interstitial keratitis 370.52
Coiling, umbilical cord —see Complications,
  umbilical cord
Coitus, painful (female) 625.0
  male 608.89
  psychogenic 302.76
Cold 460
  with influenza, flu, or grippe (see also
    Influenza) 487.1
  abscess—see also Tuberculosis, abscess
    articular—see Tuberculosis, joint
  agglutinin
    disease (chronic) or syndrome 283.0
    hemoglobinuria 283.0
      paroxysmal (cold) (nocturnal) 283.2
  allergic (see also Fever, hay) 477.9
  bronchus or chest—see Bronchitis
    with grippe or influenza (see also Influenza)
      487.1
  common (head) 460
    vaccination, prophylactic (against) V04.7
  deep 464.10
  effects of 991.9
    specified effect NEC 991.8
  excessive 991.9
    specified effect NEC 991.8
  exhaustion from 991.8
  exposure to 991.9
    specified effect NEC 991.8
  grippy (see also Influenza) 487.1
  head 460
  injury syndrome (newborn) 778.2
  intolerance 780.99
  on lung—see Bronchitis
  rose 477.0
  sensitivity, autoimmune 283.0
  virus 460
Coldsore (see also Herpes, simplex) 054.9
Colibacillosis 041.49
  generalized 038.42
Colibacilluria 791.9
Colic (recurrent) 789.7
  abdomen 789.7
    (recurrent)psychogenic 307.89
  appendicular 543.9
  appendix 543.9
  bile duct—see Choledocholithiasis
  biliary—see Cholelithiasis
  bilious—see Cholelithiasis
  common duct—see Choledocholithiasis
  Devonshire NEC 984.9
    specified type of lead—see Table of drugs and
      chemicals
  flatulent 787.3
  gallbladder or gallstone—see Cholelithiasis
  gastric 536.8
  hepatic (duct)—see Choledocholithiasis
  hysterical 300.11
  in
    adult 789.0
    child over 12 months old 789.0
    infant 789.7

Colic—*continued*
  infantile 789.7
  intestinal 789.7
  kidney 788.0
  lead NEC 984.9
    specified type of lead—*see* Table of drugs and
      chemicals
  liver (duct)—*see* Choledocholithiasis
  mucous 564.9
    psychogenic 316 *[564.9]*
  nephritic 788.0
  painter's NEC 984.9
  pancreas 577.8
  psychogenic 306.4
  renal 788.0
  saturnine NEC 984.9
    specified type of lead—*see* Table of drugs and
      chemicals
  spasmodic 789.7
  ureter 788.0
  urethral 599.84
    due to calculus 594.2
  uterus 625.8
    menstrual 625.3
  vermicular 543.9
  virus 460
  worm NEC 128.9
Colicystitis (*see also* Cystitis) 595.9
Colitis (acute) (catarrhal) (croupous) (cystica
    superficialis) (exudative) (hemorrhagic)
    (noninfectious) (phlegmonous) (presumed
    noninfectious) 558.9
  adaptive 564.9
  allergic 558.3
  amebic (*see also* Amebiasis) 006.9
    nondysenteric 006.2
  anthrax 022.2
  bacillary (*see also* Infection, Shigella) 004.9
  balantidial 007.0
  chronic 558.9
    ulcerative (*see also* Colitis, ulcerative) 556.9
  coccidial 007.2
  dietetic 558.9
  due to radiation 558.1
  eosinophilic 558.42
  functional 558.9
  gangrenous 009.0
  giardial 007.1
  granulomatous 555.1
  gravis (*see also* Colitis, ulcerative) 556.9
  infectious (*see also* Enteritis, due to, specific
      organism) 009.0
    presumed 009.1
  ischemic 557.9
    acute 557.0
    chronic 557.1
    due to mesenteric artery insufficiency 557.1
  membranous 564.9
    psychogenic 316 *[564.9]*
  mucous 564.9
    psychogenic 316 *[564.9]*
  necrotic 009.0
  polyposa (*see also* Colitis, ulcerative) 556.9
  protozoal NEC 007.9
  pseudomembranous 008.45
  pseudomucinous 564.9
  regional 555.1
  segmental 555.1
  septic (*see also* Enteritis, due to, specific
      organism) 009.0
  spastic 564.9
    psychogenic 316 *[564.9]*

Colitis—*continued*
  staphylococcus 008.41
    food 005.0
  thromboulcerative 557.0
  toxic 558.2
  transmural 555.1
  trichomonal 007.3
  tuberculous (ulcerative) 014.8
  ulcerative (chronic) (idiopathic) (nonspecific)
      556.9
    entero- 556.0
    fulminant 557.0
    ileo- 556.1
    left-sided 556.5
    procto- 556.2
    proctosigmoid 556.3
    psychogenic 316 *[556]*
    specified NEC 556.8
    universal 556.6
Collagen disease NEC 710.9
  nonvascular 710.9
  vascular (allergic) (*see also* Angiitis,
      hypersensitivity) 446.20
Collagenosis (*see also* Collagen disease) 710.9
  cardiovascular 425.4
  mediastinal 519.3
Collapse 780.2
  adrenal 255.8
  cardiorenal (*see also* Hypertension, cardiorenal)
      404.90
  cardiorespiratory 785.51
    fetus or newborn 779.85
  cardiovascular (*see also* Disease, heart) 785.51
    fetus or newborn 779.85
  circulatory (peripheral) 785.59
    with
      abortion—*see* Abortion, by type, with shock
      ectopic pregnancy (*see also* categories
          633.0-633.9) 639.5
      molar pregnancy (*see also* categories
          630-632) 639.5
    during or after labor and delivery 669.1
    fetus or newborn 779.85
    following
      abortion 639.5
      ectopic or molar pregnancy 639.5
    during or after labor and delivery 669.1
    fetus or newborn 779.89
  during or resulting from a surgical procedure
      998.00
  external ear canal 380.50
    secondary to
      inflammation 380.53
      surgery 380.52
      trauma 380.51
  general 780.2
  heart—*see* Disease, heart
  heat 992.1
  hysterical 300.11
  labyrinth, membranous (congenital) 744.05
  lung (massive) (*see also* Atelectasis) 518.0
    pressure, during labor 668.0
  myocardial—*see* Disease, heart
  nervous (*see also* Disorder, mental,
      nonpsychotic) 300.9
  neurocirculatory 306.2
  nose 738.0
  postoperative (cardiovascular) 998.09
  pulmonary (*see also* Atelectasis) 518.0
    fetus or newborn 770.5
      partial 770.5
      primary 770.4

Collapse—*continued*
thorax 512.89
iatrogenic 512.1
postoperative 512.1
trachea 519.19
valvular—*see* Endocarditis
vascular (peripheral) 785.59
with
abortion—*see* Abortion, by type, with shock
ectopic pregnancy (*see also* categories 633.0-633.9) 639.5
molar pregnancy (*see also* categories 630-632) 639.5
cerebral (*see also* Disease, cerebrovascular, acute) 436
during or after labor and delivery 669.1
fetus or newborn 779.89
following
abortion 639.5
ectopic or molar pregnancy 639.5
vasomotor 785.59
vertebra 733.13
Collateral —*see also* condition
circulation (venous) 459.89
dilation, veins 459.89
Colles' fracture (closed) (reversed) (separation) 813.41
open 813.51
Collet's syndrome 352.6
Collet-Sicard syndrome 352.6
Colliculitis urethralis (*see also* Urethritis) 597.89
Colliers'
asthma 500
lung 500
phthisis (*see also* Tuberculosis) 011.4
Collodion baby (ichthyosis congenita) 757.1
Colloid milium 709.3
Coloboma NEC 743.49
choroid 743.59
fundus 743.52
iris 743.46
lens 743.36
lids 743.62
optic disc (congenital) 743.57
acquired 377.23
retina 743.56
sclera 743.47
Coloenteritis —*see* Enteritis
Colon —*see* condition
Colonization
MRSA (methicillin resistant Staphylococcus aureus) V02.54
MSSA (methicillin susceptible Staphylococcus aureus) V02.53
Coloptosis 569.89
Color
amblyopia NEC 368.59
acquired 368.55
blindness NEC (congenital) 368.59
acquired 368.55
Colostomy
attention to V55.3
fitting or adjustment V53.5
malfunctioning 569.62
status V44.3
Colpitis (*see also* Vaginitis) 616.10
Colpocele 618.6
Colpocystitis (*see also* Vaginitis) 616.10
Colporrhexis 665.4
Colpospasm 625.1
Column, spinal, vertebral —*see* condition

Coma 780.01
apoplectic (*see also* Disease, cerebrovascular, acute) 436
diabetic (with ketoacidosis) 250.3
due to secondary diabetes 249.3
hyperosmolar 250.2
due to secondary diabetes 249.2
eclamptic (*see also* Eclampsia) 780.39
epileptic 345.3
hepatic 572.2
hyperglycemic 250.2
due to secondary diabetes 249.2
hyperosmolar (diabetic) (nonketotic) 250.2
due to secondary diabetes 249.2
hypoglycemic 251.0
diabetic 250.3
due to secondary diabetes 249.3
insulin 250.3
due to secondary diabetes 249.3
hyperosmolar 250.2
due to secondary diabetes 249.2
non-diabetic 251.0
organic hyperinsulinism 251.0
Kussmaul's (diabetic) 250.3
due to secondary diabetes 249.3
liver 572.2
newborn 779.2
prediabetic 250.2
due to secondary diabetes 249.2
uremic—*see* Uremia
Combat fatigue (*see also* Reaction, stress, acute) 308.9
Combined —*see* condition
Comedo 706.1
Comedocarcinoma (M8501/3)—*see also* Neoplasm, breast, malignant
noninfiltrating (M8501/2)
specified site—*see* Neoplasm, by site, in situ
unspecified site 233.0
Comedomastitis 610.4
Comedones 706.1
lanugo 757.4
Comma bacillus, carrier (suspected) of V02.3
Comminuted fracture —*see* Fracture, by site
Common
aortopulmonary trunk 745.0
atrioventricular canal (defect) 745.69
atrium 745.69
cold (head) 460
vaccination, prophylactic (against) V04.7
truncus (arteriosus) 745.0
ventricle 745.3
Commotio (current)
cerebri (*see also* Concussion, brain) 850.9
with skull fracture—*see* Fracture, skull, by site
retinae 921.3
spinalis—*see* Injury, spinal, by site
Commotion (current)
brain (without skull fracture) (*see also* Concussion, brain) 850.9
with skull fracture—*see* Fracture, skull, by site
spinal cord—*see* Injury, spinal, by site
Communication
abnormal—*see also* Fistula
between
base of aorta and pulmonary artery 745.0
left ventricle and right atrium 745.4
pericardial sac and pleural sac 748.8
pulmonary artery and pulmonary vein 747.39

Communication—*continued*

congenital, between uterus and
  anterior abdominal wall 752.39
    bladder 752.39
    intestine 752.39
    rectum 752.39
  left ventricular-right atrial 745.4
  pulmonary artery-pulmonary vein 747.39
Compartment syndrome —*see* Syndrome,
  compartment
Compensation
  broken—*see* Failure, heart
  failure—*see* Failure, heart
  neurosis, psychoneurosis 300.11
Complaint —*see also* Disease
  bowel, functional 564.9
    psychogenic 306.4
  intestine, functional 564.9
    psychogenic 306.4
  kidney (*see also* Disease, renal) 593.9
  liver 573.9
  miners' 500
Complete —*see* condition
Complex
  cardiorenal (*see also* Hypertension, cardiorenal)
    404.90
  castration 300.9
  Costen's 524.60
  ego-dystonic homosexuality 302.0
  Eisenmenger's (ventricular septal defect) 745.4
  homosexual, ego-dystonic 302.0
  hypersexual 302.89
  inferiority 301.9
  jumped process
    spine—*see* Dislocation, vertebra
  primary, tuberculosis (*see also* Tuberculosis) 010.0
  regional pain syndrome 355.9
    type I 337.20
      lower limb 337.22
      specified site NEC 337.29
      upper limb 337.21
    type II
      lower limb 355.71
      upper limb 354.4
  Taussig-Bing (transposition, aorta and
    overriding pulmonary artery) 745.11
Complications
  abortion NEC—*see* categories 634-639
  accidental puncture or laceration during a
    procedure 998.2
  amniocentesis, fetal 679.1
  amputation stump (late) (surgical) 997.60
    traumatic—*see* Amputation, traumatic
  anastomosis (and bypass)—*see also*
    Complications, due to (presence of) any
    device, implant, or graft classified to
    996.0-996.5 NEC
    hemorrhage NEC 998.11
    intestinal (internal) NEC 997.49
      involving urinary tract 997.5
    mechanical—*see* Complications, mechanical,
      graft
    urinary tract (involving intestinal tract) 997.5
  anesthesia, anesthetic NEC (*see also* Anesthesia,
    complication) 995.22
    in labor and delivery 668.9
      affecting fetus or newborn 763.5
      cardiac 668.1
      central nervous system 668.2
      pulmonary 668.0
      specified type NEC 668.8

Complications—*continued*

aortocoronary (bypass) graft 996.03
  atherosclerosis —*see* Arteriosclerosis,
    coronary
  embolism 996.72
  occlusion NEC 996.72
  thrombus 996.72
arthroplasty (*see also* Complications, prosthetic
  joint) 996.49
artificial opening
  cecostomy 569.60
  colostomy 569.6
  cystostomy 596.83
    infection 596.81
    mechanical 596.82
    specified complication NEC 596.83
  enterostomy 569.60
  esophagostomy 530.87
    infection 530.86
    mechanical 530.87
  gastrostomy 536.40
  ileostomy 569.60
  jejunostomy 569.60
  nephrostomy 997.5
  tracheostomy 519.00
  ureterostomy 997.5
  urethrostomy 997.5
bariatric surgery
  gastric band procedure 539.09
    infection 539.01
  specified procedure NEC 539.89
    infection 539.81
bile duct implant (prosthetic) NEC 996.79
  infection or inflammation 996.69
  mechanical 996.59
bleeding (intraoperative) (postoperative) 998.11
blood vessel graft 996.1
  aortocoronary 996.03
    atherosclerosis —*see* Arteriosclerosis,
      coronary
    embolism 996.72
    occlusion NEC 996.72
    thrombus 996.72
  atherosclerosis —*see* Arteriosclerosis,
    extremities
  embolism 996.74
  occlusion NEC 996.74
  thrombus 996.74
bone growth stimulator NEC 996.78
  infection or inflammation 996.67
bone marrow transplant 996.85
breast implant (prosthetic) NEC 996.79
  infection or inflammation 996.69
  mechanical 996.54
bypass—*see also* Complications, anastomosis
  aortocoronary 996.03
    atherosclerosis —*see* Arteriosclerosis,
      coronary
    embolism 996.72
    occlusion NEC 996.72
    thrombus 996.72
  carotid artery 996.1
    atherosclerosis —*see* Arteriosclerosis,
      extremities
    embolism 996.74
    occlusion NEC 996.74
    thrombus 996.74
cardiac (*see also* Disease, heart) 429.9
  device, implant, or graft NEC 996.72
    infection or inflammation 996.61
    long-term effect 429.4

Complications—*continued*
  cardiac—*continued*
    device—*continued*
      mechanical (*see also* Complications,
        mechanical, by type) 996.00
      valve prosthesis 996.71
        infection or inflammation 996.61
    postoperative NEC 997.1
      long-term effect 429.4
  cardiorenal (*see also* Hypertension, cardiorenal)
    404.90
  carotid artery bypass graft 996.1
    atherosclerosis —*see* Arteriosclerosis,
      extremities
    embolism 996.74
    occlusion NEC 996.74
    thrombus 996.74
  cataract fragments in eye 998.82
  catheter device—*see also* Complications, due to
    (presence of) any device, implant, or graft
    classified to 996.0-996.5 NEC
    mechanical—*see* Complications, mechanical,
      catheter
  cecostomy 569.60
  cesarean section wound 674.3
  chemotherapy (antineoplastic) 995.29
  chin implant (prosthetic) NEC 996.79
    infection or inflammation 996.69
    mechanical 996.59
  colostomy (enterostomy) 569.60
    specified type NEC 569.69
  contraceptive device, intrauterine NEC 996.76
    infection 996.65
    inflammation 996.65
    mechanical 996.32
  cord (umbilical)—*see* Complications, umbilical cord
  cornea
    due to contact lens 371.82
  coronary (artery) bypass (graft) NEC 996.03
    atherosclerosis —*see* Arteriosclerosis, coronary
    embolism 996.72
    infection or inflammation 996.61
    mechanical 996.03
    occlusion NEC 996.72
    specified type NEC 996.72
    thrombus 996.72
  cystostomy 596.83
    infection 596.81
    mechanical 596.82
    specified complication NEC 596.83
  delivery 669.9
    procedure (instrumental) (manual) (surgical) 669.4
    specified type NEC 669.8
  dialysis (hemodialysis) (peritoneal) (renal) NEC
    999.9
    catheter NEC—*see also* Complications, due to
      (presence of) any device, implant or graft
      classified to 996.0-996.5 NEC
      infection or inflammation 996.62
        peritoneal 996.68
      mechanical 996.1
        peritoneal 996.56
  drug NEC 995.29
  due to (presence of) any device, implant, or graft
    classified to 996.0-996.5 NEC 996.70
    with infection or inflammation—*see*
      Complications, infection or inflammation,
      due to (presence of) any device, implant,
      or graft classified to 996.0-996.5 NEC

Complications—*continued*
  due to—*continued*
    arterial NEC 996.74
      coronary NEC 996.03
        atherosclerosis —*see* Arteriosclerosis,
          coronary
        embolism 996.72
        occlusion NEC 996.72
        specified type NEC 996.72
        thrombus 996.72
      renal dialysis 996.73
    arteriovenous fistula or shunt NEC 996.74
    bone growth stimulator 996.78
    breast NEC 996.79
    cardiac NEC 996.72
      defibrillator 996.72
      pacemaker 996.72
      valve prosthesis 996.71
    catheter NEC 996.79
      spinal 996.75
      urinary, indwelling 996.76
      vascular NEC 996.74
        renal dialysis 996.73
      ventricular shunt 996.75
    coronary (artery) bypass (graft) NEC 996.03
      atherosclerosis —*see* Arteriosclerosis,
        coronary
      embolism 996.72
      occlusion NEC 996.72
      thrombus 996.72
    electrodes
      brain 996.75
      heart 996.72
    esophagostomy 530.87
    gastrointestinal NEC 996.79
    genitourinary NEC 996.76
    heart valve prosthesis NEC 996.71
    infusion pump 996.74
    insulin pump 996.57
    internal
      joint prosthesis 996.77
      orthopedic NEC 996.78
      specified type NEC 996.79
    intrauterine contraceptive device NEC 996.76
    joint prosthesis, internal NEC 996.77
    mechanical—*see* Complications, mechanical
    nervous system NEC 996.75
    ocular lens NEC 996.79
    orbital NEC 996.79
    orthopedic NEC 996.78
      joint, internal 996.77
    renal dialysis 996.73
    specified type NEC 996.79
    urinary catheter, indwelling 996.76
    vascular NEC 996.74
    ventricular shunt 996.75
    during dialysis NEC 999.9
    ectopic or molar pregnancy NEC 639.9
    electroshock therapy NEC 999.9
    enterostomy 569.60
      specified type NEC 569.69
    esophagostomy 530.87
      infection 530.86
      mechanical 530.87
    external (fixation) device with internal
      component(s) NEC 996.78
      infection or inflammation 996.67
      mechanical 996.49
    extracorporeal circulation NEC 999.9

Complications—*continued*
inhalation therapy NEC 999.9
injection (procedure) 999.9
  drug reaction (*see also* Reaction, drug) 995.27
  infection NEC 999.39
  sepsis NEC 999.39
  serum (prophylactic) (therapeutic)—*see*
    Complications, vaccination
  vaccine (any)—*see* Complications,
    vaccination
inoculation (any)—*see* Complications, vaccination
insulin pump 996.57
internal device (catheter) (electronic) (fixation)
    (prosthetic) NEC—*see also* Complications,
    due to (presence of) any device, implant, or
    graft classified to 996.0-996.5 NEC
  mechanical—*see* Complications, mechanical
intestinal pouch, specified NEC 569.79
intestinal transplant (immune or nonimmune
    cause) 996.87
intraoperative bleeding or hemorrhage 998.11
intrauterine contraceptive device (*see also*
    Complications, contraceptive device) 996.76
  infection or inflammation 996.65
  with fetal damage affecting management of
    pregnancy 655.8
in utero procedure
  fetal 679.1
  maternal 679.0
jejunostomy 569.60
kidney transplant (immune or nonimmune
    cause) 996.81
labor 669.9
  specified condition NEC 669.8
liver transplant (immune or nonimmune cause)
    996.82
lumbar puncture 349.0
mechanical
  anastomosis—*see* Complications, mechanical,
    graft
  artificial heart 996.09
  bypass—*see* Complications, mechanical, graft
  catheter NEC 996.59
    cardiac 996.09
    cystostomy 596.82
    dialysis (hemodialysis) 996.1
      peritoneal 996.56
    during a procedure 998.2
    urethral, indwelling 996.31
  colostomy 569.62
  device NEC 996.59
    balloon (counterpulsation), intra-aortic 996.1
    cardiac 996.00
      automatic implantable defibrillator 996.04
      long-term effect 429.4
      specified NEC 996.09
    contraceptive, intrauterine 996.32
    counterpulsation, intra-aortic 996.1
    fixation, external, with internal components
      996.49
    fixation, internal (nail, rod, plate) 996.40
    genitourinary 996.30
      specified NEC 996.39
    insulin pump 996.57
    nervous system 996.2
    orthopedic, internal 996.40
      prosthetic joint (*see also* Complications,
        mechanical device, orthopedic,
        prosthetic, joint) 996.47

Complications—*continued*
mechanical—*continued*
  device—*continued*
    prosthetic NEC 996.59
      joint 996.47
        articular bearing surface wear 996.46
        aseptic loosening 996.41
        breakage 996.43
        dislocation 996.42
        failure 996.47
        fracture 996.43
          around prosthetic 996.44
          peri-prosthetic 996.44
        instability 996.42
        loosening 996.41
        peri-prosthetic osteolysis 996.45
        subluxation 996.42
        wear 996.46
      umbrella, vena cava 996.1
      vascular 996.1
  dorsal column stimulator 996.2
  electrode NEC 996.59
    brain 996.2
    cardiac 996.01
    spinal column 996.2
  enterostomy 569.62
  esophagostomy 530.87
  fistula, arteriovenous, surgically created 996.1
  gastrostomy 536.42
  graft NEC 996.52
    aortic (bifurcation) 996.1
    aortocoronary bypass 996.03
    blood vessel NEC 996.1
    bone 996.49
    cardiac 996.00
    carotid artery bypass 996.1
    cartilage 996.49
    corneal 996.51
    coronary bypass 996.03
    decellularized allodermis 996.55
    genitourinary 996.30
      specified NEC 996.39
    muscle 996.49
    nervous system 996.2
    organ (immune or nonimmune cause) 996.80
      heart 996.83
      intestines 996.87
      kidney 996.81
      liver 996.82
      lung 996.84
      pancreas 996.86
      specified NEC 996.89
    orthopedic, internal 996.49
    peripheral nerve 996.2
    prosthetic NEC 996.59
    skin 996.52
      artificial 996.55
    specified NEC 996.59
    tendon 996.49
    tissue NEC 996.52
    tooth 996.59
    ureter, without mention of resection 996.39
    vascular 996.1
  heart valve prosthesis 996.02
    long-term effect 429.4
  implant NEC 996.59
    cardiac 996.00
      automatic implantable defibrillator 996.04
      long-term effect 429.4
      specified NEC 996.09

Complications—*continued*
  respiratory—*continued*
    distress syndrome, adult, following trauma and surgery 518.52
    insufficiency, acute, postoperative 518.52
    postoperative NEC 997.39
    therapy NEC 999.9
  sedation during labor and delivery 668.9
    affecting fetus or newborn 763.5
    cardiac 668.1
    central nervous system 668.2
    pulmonary 668.0
    specified type NEC 668.8
  seroma (intraoperative) (postoperative) (noninfected) 998.13
    infected 998.51
  shunt—*see also* Complications, due to (presence of) any device, implant, or graft classified to 996.0-996.5 NEC
    mechanical—*see* Complications, mechanical, shunt
  specified body system NEC
    device, implant, or graft—*see* Complications, due to (presence of) any device, implant, or graft classified to 996.0-996.5 NEC
    postoperative NEC 997.99
  spinal puncture or tap 349.0
  stoma, external
    gastrointestinal tract
      colostomy 569.60
      enterostomy 569.60
      esophagostomy 530.87
        infection 530.86
        mechanical 530.87
      gastrostomy 536.40
    urinary tract 997.5
  stomach banding 539.09
  stomach stapling 539.89
  surgical procedures 998.9
    accidental puncture or laceration 998.2
    amputation stump (late) 997.60
    anastomosis—*see* Complications, anastomosis
    burst stitches or sutures (external) (*see also* Dehiscence) 998.32
      internal 998.31
    cardiac 997.1
      long-term effect following cardiac surgery 429.4
    cataract fragments in eye 998.82
    catheter device—*see* Complications, catheter device
    cecostomy malfunction 569.62
    colostomy malfunction 569.62
    cystostomy malfunction 596.82
      infection 596.81
      mechanical 596.82
      specified complication NEC 596.83
    dehiscence (of incision) (external) (*see also* Dehiscence) 998.32
      internal 998.31
    dialysis NEC (*see also* Complications, dialysis) 999.9
    disruption (*see also* Dehiscence)
      anastomosis (internal)—*see* Complications, mechanical, graft
      internal suture (line) 998.31
      wound (external) 998.32
        internal 998.31
    dumping syndrome (postgastrectomy) 564.2
    elephantiasis or lymphedema 997.99
      postmastectomy 457.0

Complications—*continued*
  surgical procedures—*continued*
    emphysema (surgical) 998.81
    enterostomy malfunction 569.62
    esophagostomy malfunction 530.87
    evisceration 998.32
    fistula (persistent postoperative) 998.6
    foreign body inadvertently left in wound (sponge) (suture) (swab) 998.4
    from nonabsorbable surgical material (Dacron) (mesh) (permanent suture) (reinforcing) (Teflon)—*see* Complications, due to (presence of) any device, implant, or graft classified to 996.0-996.5 NEC
    gastrointestinal NEC 997.49
    gastrostomy malfunction 536.42
    hematoma 998.12
    hemorrhage 998.11
    ileostomy malfunction 569.62
    internal prosthetic device NEC (*see also* Complications, internal device) 996.70
      hemolytic anemia 283.19
      infection or inflammation 996.60
      malfunction—*see* Complications, mechanical
      mechanical complication—*see* Complications, mechanical
      thrombus 996.70
    jejunostomy malfunction 569.62
    nervous system NEC 997.00
    obstruction, internal anastomosis—*see* Complications, mechanical, graft
    other body system NEC 997.99
    peripheral vascular NEC 997.2
    postcardiotomy syndrome 429.4
    postcholecystectomy syndrome 576.0
    postcommissurotomy syndrome 429.4
    postgastrectomy dumping syndrome 564.2
    postmastectomy lymphedema syndrome 457.0
    postmastoidectomy 383.30
      cholesteatoma, recurrent 383.32
      cyst, mucosal 383.31
      granulation 383.33
      inflammation, chronic 383.33
    postvagotomy syndrome 564.2
    postvalvulotomy syndrome 429.4
    reattached extremity (infection) (rejection) (*see also* Complications, reattached, extremity) 996.90
    respiratory NEC 997.39
    seroma 998.13
    shock (endotoxic) (septic) 998.02
      hypovolemic 998.09
    shunt, prosthetic (thrombus)—*see also* Complications, due to (presence of) any device, implant, or graft classified to 996.0-996.5 NEC
      hemolytic anemia 283.19
    specified complication NEC 998.89
    stitch abscess 998.59
    transplant—*see* Complications, graft
    ureterostomy malfunction 997.5
    urethrostomy malfunction 997.5
    urinary NEC 997.5
    vascular
      mesenteric artery 997.71
      other vessels 997.79
      peripheral vessels 997.2
      renal artery 997.72
    wound infection 998.59

Compression—*continued*
  bronchus 519.19
  by cicatrix—*see* Cicatrix
  cardiac 423.9
  cauda equina 344.60
    with neurogenic bladder 344.61
  celiac (artery) (axis) 447.4
  cerebral—*see* Compression, brain
  cervical plexus 353.2
  cord (umbilical)—*see* Compression, umbilical
      cord
  cranial nerve 352.9
    second 377.49
    third (partial) 378.51
      total 378.52
    fourth 378.53
    fifth 350.8
    sixth 378.54
    seventh 351.8
  divers' squeeze 993.3
  duodenum (external) (*see also* Obstruction,
      duodenum) 537.3
  during birth 767.9
  esophagus 530.3
    congenital, external 750.3
  Eustachian tube 381.63
  facies (congenital) 754.0
  fracture—*see* Fracture, by site
  heart—*see* Disease, heart
  intestine (*see also* Obstruction, intestine) 560.9
    with hernia—*see* Hernia, by site, with
      obstruction
  laryngeal nerve, recurrent 478.79
  leg NEC 355.8
  lower extremity NEC 355.8
  lumbosacral plexus 353.1
  lung 518.89
  lymphatic vessel 457.1
  medulla—*see* Compression, brain
  nerve NEC—*see also* Disorder, nerve
    arm NEC 354.9
    autonomic nervous system (*see also*
      Neuropathy, peripheral, autonomic) 337.9
    axillary 353.0
    cranial NEC 352.9
    due to displacement of intervertebral disc
      722.2
      with myelopathy 722.70
    cervical 722.0
      with myelopathy 722.71
    lumbar, lumbosacral 722.10
      with myelopathy 722.73
    thoracic, thoracolumbar 722.11
      with myelopathy 722.72
    iliohypogastric 355.79
    ilioinguinal 355.79
    leg NEC 355.8
    lower extremity NEC 355.8
    median (in carpal tunnel) 354.0
    obturator 355.79
    optic 377.49
    plantar 355.6
    posterior tibial (in tarsal tunnel) 355.5
    root (by scar tissue) NEC 724.9
      cervical NEC 723.4
      lumbar NEC 724.4
      lumbosacral 724.4
      thoracic 724.4
    saphenous 355.79
    sciatic (acute) 355.0
    sympathetic 337.9

Compression—*continued*
  nerve—*continued*
    traumatic—*see* Injury, nerve
    ulnar 354.2
    upper extremity NEC 354.9
  peripheral—*see* Compression, nerve
  spinal (cord) (old or nontraumatic) 336.9
    by displacement of intervertebral disc—*see*
      Displacement, intervertebral disc
    nerve
      root NEC 724.9
        postoperative 722.80
          cervical region 722.81
          lumbar region 722.83
          thoracic region 722.82
        traumatic—*see* Injury, nerve, spinal
      traumatic—*see* Injury, nerve, spinal
    spondylogenic 721.91
      cervical 721.1
      lumbar, lumbosacral 721.42
      thoracic 721.41
    traumatic—*see also* Injury, spinal, by site
      with fracture, vertebra—*see* Fracture,
        vertebra, by site, with spinal cord injury
    spondylogenic—*see* Compression, spinal cord,
      spondylogenic
  subcostal nerve (syndrome) 354.8
  sympathetic nerve NEC 337.9
  syndrome 958.5
  thorax 512.89
    iatrogenic 512.1
    postoperative 512.1
  trachea 519.19
    congenital 748.3
  ulnar nerve (by scar tissue) 354.2
  umbilical cord
    affecting fetus or newborn 762.5
      cord prolapsed 762.4
    complicating delivery 663.2
      cord around neck 663.1
      cord prolapsed 663.0
  upper extremity NEC 354.9
  ureter 593.3
  urethra—*see* Stricture, urethra
  vein 459.2
  vena cava (inferior) (superior) 459.2
  vertebral NEC—*see* Compression, spinal (cord)
Compulsion, compulsive
  eating 307.51
  neurosis (obsessive) 300.3
  personality 301.4
  states (mixed) 300.3
  swearing 300.3
    in Gilles de la Tourette's syndrome 307.23
  tics and spasms 307.22
  water drinking NEC (syndrome) 307.9
Concato's disease (pericardial polyserositis) 423.2
  peritoneal 568.82
  pleural—*see* Pleurisy
Concavity, chest wall 738.3
Concealed
  hemorrhage NEC 459.0
  penis 752.65
Concentric fading 368.12
Concern (normal) about sick person in family
    V61.49
Concrescence (teeth) 520.2
Concretio cordis 423.1
  rheumatic 393

Concretion —*see also* Calculus
  appendicular 543.9
  canaliculus 375.57
  clitoris 624.8
  conjunctiva 372.54
  eyelid 374.56
  intestine (impaction) (obstruction) 560.39
  lacrimal (passages) 375.57
  prepuce (male) 605
    female (clitoris) 624.8
  salivary gland (any) 527.5
  seminal vesicle 608.89
  stomach 537.89
  tonsil 474.8
Concussion (current) 850.9
  with
    loss of consciousness 850.5
      brief (less than one hour)
        30 minutes or less 850.11
        31-59 minutes 850.12
      moderate (1-24 hours) 850.2
      prolonged (more than 24 hours) (with
        complete recovery) (with return to
        pre-existing conscious level) 850.3
        without return to pre-existing conscious
          level 850.4
    mental confusion or disorientation (without
      loss of consciousness) 850.0
      with loss of consciousness—*see* Concussion,
        with, loss of consciousness
    without loss of consciousness 850.0
  blast (air) (hydraulic) (immersion) (underwater)
    869.0
    with open wound into cavity 869.1
  abdomen or thorax—*see* Injury, internal, by site
  brain—*see* Concussion, brain
  ear (acoustic nerve trauma) 951.5
    with perforation, tympanic membrane—*see*
      Wound, open, ear drum
  thorax—*see* Injury, internal, intrathoracic
    organs NEC
  brain or cerebral (without skull fracture) 850.9
    with
      loss of consciousness 850.5
        brief (less than one hour)
          30 minutes or less 850.11
          31-59 minutes 850.12
        moderate (1-24 hours) 850.2
        prolonged (more than 24 hours) (with
          complete recovery) (with return to
          pre-existing conscious level) 850.3
          without return to pre-existing conscious
            level 850.4
      mental confusion or disorientation (without
        loss of consciousness) 850.0
        with loss of consciousness—*see*
          Concussion, brain, with, loss of
          consciousness
    skull fracture—*see* Fracture, skull, by site
    without loss of consciousness 850.0
  cauda equina 952.4
  cerebral—*see* Concussion, brain
  conus medullaris (spine) 952.4
  hydraulic—*see* Concussion, blast
  internal organs—*see* Injury, internal, by site
  labyrinth—*see* Injury, intracranial
  ocular 921.3
  osseous labyrinth—*see* Injury, intracranial

Concussion—*continued*
  spinal (cord)—*see also* Injury, spinal, by site
    due to
      broken
        back—*see* Fracture, vertebra, by site, with
          spinal cord injury
        neck—*see* Fracture, vertebra, cervical,
          with spinal cord injury
      fracture, fracture dislocation, or compression
        fracture of spine or vertebra—*see*
        Fracture, vertebra, by site, with spinal
        cord injury
    syndrome 310.2
  underwater blast—*see* Concussion, blast
Condition —*see also* Disease
  fetal hematologic 678.0
  psychiatric 298.9
  respiratory NEC 519.9
    acute or subacute NEC 519.9
      due to
        external agent 508.9
          specified type NEC 508.8
        fumes or vapors (chemical) (inhalation) 506.3
        radiation 508.0
        smoke inhalation 508.2
    chronic NEC 519.9
      due to
        external agent 508.9
          specified type NEC 508.8
        fumes or vapors (chemical) (inhalation) 506.4
        radiation 508.1
    due to
      external agent 508.9
        specified type NEC 508.8
      fumes or vapors (chemical) (inhalation)
        506.9
Conduct disturbance (*see also* Disturbance,
    conduct) 312.9
  adjustment reaction 309.3
  hyperkinetic 314.2
Condyloma NEC 078.11
  acuminatum 078.11
  gonorrheal 098.0
  latum 091.3
  syphilitic 091.3
    congenital 090.0
  venereal, syphilitic 091.3
Confinement —*see* Delivery
Conflagration —*see also* Burn, by site
  asphyxia (by inhalation of gases, fumes, or
    vapors) 987.9
  specified agent—*see* Table of drugs and
    chemicals
Conflict
  family V61.9
    specified circumstance NEC V61.8
  interpersonal NEC V62.81
  marital V61.10
    involving
      divorce V61.03
      estrangement V61.09
  parent(guardian)-child V61.20
    adopted child V61.24
    biological child V61.23
    foster child V61.25
  partner V61.10
Confluent —*see* condition
Confusion, confused (mental) (state) (*see also*
    State, confusional) 298.9
  acute 293.0
  epileptic 293.0

Confusion, confused—*continued*
  postoperative 293.9
  psychogenic 298.2
  reactive (from emotional stress, psychological
    trauma) 298.2
  subacute 293.1
Confusional arousals 327.41
Congelation 991.9
Congenital —*see also* condition
  aortic septum 747.29
  generalized fibromatosis (CGF) 759.89
  intrinsic factor deficiency 281.0
  malformation—*see* Anomaly
Congestion, congestive
  asphyxia, newborn 768.9
  bladder 596.89
  bowel 569.89
  brain (*see also* Disease, cerebrovascular NEC)
    437.8
    malarial 084.9
  breast 611.79
  bronchi 519.19
  bronchial tube 519.19
  catarrhal 472.0
  cerebral—*see* Congestion, brain
  cerebrospinal—*see* Congestion, brain
  chest 786.9
  chill 780.99
    malarial (*see also* Malaria) 084.6
  circulatory NEC 459.9
  conjunctiva 372.71
  due to disturbance of circulation 459.9
  duodenum 537.3
  enteritis—*see* Enteritis
  eye 372.71
  fibrosis syndrome (pelvic) 625.5
  gastroenteritis—*see* Enteritis
  general 799.89
  glottis 476.0
  heart (*see also* Failure, heart) 428.0
  hepatic 573.0
  hypostatic (lung) 514
  intestine 569.89
  intracranial—*see* Congestion, brain
  kidney 593.89
  labyrinth 386.50
  larynx 476.0
  liver 573.0
  lung 786.9
    active or acute (*see also* Pneumonia) 486
      congenital 770.0
    chronic 514
    hypostatic 514
    idiopathic, acute 518.52
    passive 514
  malaria, malarial (brain) (fever) (*see also*
    Malaria) 084.6
  medulla—*see* Congestion, brain
  nasal 478.19
  nose 478.19
  orbit, orbital 376.33
    inflammatory (chronic) 376.10
      acute 376.00
  ovary 620.8
  pancreas 577.8
  pelvic, female 625.5
  pleural 511.0
  prostate (active) 602.1
  pulmonary—*see* Congestion, lung
  renal 593.89
  retina 362.89

Congestion, congestive—*continued*
  seminal vesicle 608.89
  spinal cord 336.1
  spleen 289.51
    chronic 289.51
  stomach 537.89
  trachea 464.11
  urethra 599.84
  uterus 625.5
    with subinvolution 621.1
  viscera 799.89
Congestive —*see* Congestion
Conical
  cervix 622.6
  cornea 371.60
  teeth 520.2
Conjoined twins 759.4
  causing disproportion (fetopelvic) 678.1
  fetal 678.1
Conjugal maladjustment V61.10
  involving
    divorce V61.03
    estrangement V61.09
Conjunctiva —*see* condition
Conjunctivitis (exposure) (infectious)
    (nondiphtheritic) (pneumococcal) (pustular)
    (staphylococcal) (streptococcal) NEC 372.30
  actinic 370.24
  acute 372.00
    atopic 372.05
    chemical 372.06
    contagious 372.03
    follicular 372.02
    hemorrhagic (viral) 077.4
    toxic 372.06
  adenoviral (acute) 077.3
  allergic (chronic) 372.14
    with hay fever 372.05
  anaphylactic 372.05
  angular 372.03
  Apollo (viral) 077.4
  atopic 372.05
  blennorrhagic (neonatorum) 098.40
  catarrhal 372.03
  chemical 372.06
    allergic 372.05
    meaning corrosion, *see* Burn, conjunctiva
  chlamydial 077.98
    due to
      Chlamydial trachomatis—*see* Trachoma
      paratrachoma 077.0
  chronic 372.10
    allergic 372.14
    follicular 372.12
    simple 372.11
    specified type NEC 372.14
    vernal 372.13
  diphtheritic 032.81
  due to
    dust 372.05
    enterovirus type 70 077.4
    erythema multiforme 695.10 *[372.33]*
    filariasis (*see also* Filariasis) 125.9 *[372.15]*
    mucocutaneous
      disease NEC 372.33
      leishmaniasis 085.5 *[372.15]*
    Reiter's disease 099.3 *[372.33]*
    syphilis 095.8 *[372.10]*
    toxoplasmosis (acquired) 130.1
      congenital (active) 771.2
    trachoma—*see* Trachoma

Conjunctivitis—*continued*
  dust 372.05
  eczematous 370.31
  epidemic 077.1
    hemorrhagic 077.4
  follicular (acute) 372.02
    adenoviral (acute) 077.3
    chronic 372.12
  glare 370.24
  gonococcal (neonatorum) 098.40
  granular (trachomatous) 076.1
    late effect 139.1
  hemorrhagic (acute) (epidemic) 077.4
  herpetic (simplex) 054.43
    zoster 053.21
  inclusion 077.0
  infantile 771.6
  influenzal 372.03
  Koch-Weeks 372.03
  light 372.05
  medicamentosa 372.05
  membranous 372.04
  meningococcic 036.89
  Morax-Axenfeld 372.02
  mucopurulent NEC 372.03
  neonatal 771.6
    gonococcal 098.40
  Newcastle's 077.8
  nodosa 360.14
  of Beal 077.3
  parasitic 372.15
    filariasis (*see also* Filariasis) 125.9 *[372.15]*
    mucocutaneous leishmaniasis 085.5 *[372.15]*
  Parinaud's 372.02
  petrificans 372.39
  phlyctenular 370.31
  pseudomembranous 372.04
    diphtheritic 032.81
  purulent 372.03
  Reiter's 099.3 *[372.33]*
  rosacea 695.3 *[372.31]*
  serous 372.01
    viral 077.99
  simple chronic 372.11
  specified NEC 372.39
  sunlamp 372.04
  swimming pool 077.0
  toxic 372.06
  trachomatous (follicular) 076.1
    acute 076.0
    late effect 139.1
  traumatic NEC 372.39
  tuberculous (*see also* Tuberculosis) 017.3 *[370.31]*
  tularemic 021.3
  tularensis 021.3
  vernal 372.13
    limbar 372.13 *[370.32]*
  viral 077.99
    acute hemorrhagic 077.4
    specified NEC 077.8
Conjunctivochalasis 372.81
Conjunctoblepharitis —*see* Conjunctivitis
Conn (-Louis) syndrome (primary aldosteronism) 255.12
Connective tissue —*see* condition
Conradi (-Hünermann) syndrome or disease (chondrodysplasia calcificans congenita) 756.59
Consanguinity V19.7
Consecutive —*see* condition
Consolidated lung (base)—*see* Pneumonia, lobar

Constipation 564.00
  atonic 564.09
  drug induced
    correct substance properly administered 564.09
    overdose or wrong substance given or taken 977.9
      specified drug—*see* Table of drugs and chemicals
  neurogenic 564.09
  other specified NEC 564.09
  outlet dysfunction 564.02
  psychogenic 306.4
  simple 564.00
  slow transit 564.01
  spastic 564.09
Constitutional —*see also* condition
  arterial hypotension (*see also* Hypotension) 458.9
  obesity 278.00
    morbid 278.01
  psychopathic state 301.9
  short stature in childhood 783.43
  state, developmental V21.9
    specified development NEC V21.8
  substandard 301.6
Constitutionally substandard 301.6
Constriction
  anomalous, meningeal bands or folds 742.8
  aortic arch (congenital) 747.10
  asphyxiation or suffocation by 994.7
  bronchus 519.19
  canal, ear (*see also* Stricture, ear canal, acquired) 380.50
  duodenum 537.3
  gallbladder (*see also* Obstruction, gallbladder) 575.2
    congenital 751.69
  intestine (*see also* Obstruction, intestine) 560.9
  larynx 478.74
    congenital 748.3
  meningeal bands or folds, anomalous 742.8
  organ or site, congenital NEC—*see* Atresia
  prepuce (congenital) 605
  pylorus 537.0
    adult hypertrophic 537.0
    congenital or infantile 750.5
    newborn 750.5
  ring (uterus) 661.4
    affecting fetus or newborn 763.7
  spastic—*see also* Spasm
    ureter 593.3
    urethra—*see* Stricture, urethra
  stomach 537.89
  ureter 593.3
  urethra—*see* Stricture, urethra
  visual field (functional) (peripheral) 368.45
Constrictive —*see* condition
Consultation V65.9
  medical—*see also* Counseling, medical
  specified reason NEC V65.8
  without complaint or sickness V65.9
    feared complaint unfounded V65.5
    specified reason NEC V65.8
Consumption —*see* Tuberculosis
Contact —see also Exposure (suspected)
  with
    AIDS virus V01.79
    anthrax V01.81
    asbestos V15.84
    cholera V01.0
    communicable disease V01.9
      specified type NEC V01.89
      viral NEC V01.79
    Escherichia coli (E. coli) V01.83

Contact—*continued*
  with—*continued*
    German measles V01.4
    gonorrhea V01.6
    HIV V01.79
    human immunodeficiency virus V01.79
    lead V15.86
    meningococcus V01.84
    parasitic disease NEC V01.89
    poliomyelitis V01.2
    potentially hazardous body fluids V15.85
    rabies V01.5
    rubella V01.4
    SARS-associated coronavirus V01.82
    smallpox V01.3
    syphilis V01.6
    tuberculosis V01.1
    varicella V01.71
    venereal disease V01.6
    viral disease NEC V01.79
  dermatitis—*see* Dermatitis
Contamination, food (*see also* Poisoning, food) 005.9
Contraception, contraceptive
  advice NEC V25.09
    family planning V25.09
    fitting of diaphragm V25.02
    prescribing or use of
      oral contraceptive agent V25.01
      specified agent NEC V25.02
  counseling NEC V25.09
    emergency V25.03
    family planning V25.09
    fitting of diaphragm V25.02
    prescribing or use of
      oral contraceptive agent V25.01
        emergency V25.03
        postcoital V25.03
      specified agent NEC V25.02
  device (in situ) V45.59
    causing menorrhagia 996.76
    checking V25.42
    complications 996.32
    insertion V25.11
    intrauterine V45.51
    reinsertion V25.13
    removal V25.12
      and reinsertion V25.13
    replacement V25.13
    subdermal V45.52
  fitting of diaphragm V25.02
  insertion
    intrauterine contraceptive device V25.11
    subdermal implantable V25.5
  maintenance V25.40
    examination V25.40
      intrauterine device V25.42
      oral contraceptive V25.41
      specified method NEC V25.49
      subdermal implantable V25.43
    intrauterine device V25.42
    oral contraceptive V25.41
    specified method NEC V25.49
    subdermal implantable V25.43
  management NEC V25.49
  prescription
    oral contraceptive agent V25.01
      emergency V25.03
      postcoital V25.03
      repeat V25.41
    specified agent NEC V25.02
      repeat V25.49

Contraception, contraceptive—*continued*
  sterilization V25.2
  surveillance V25.40
    intrauterine device V25.42
    oral contraceptive agent V25.41
    specified method NEC V25.49
    subdermal implantable V25.43
Contraction, contracture, contracted
  Achilles tendon (*see also* Short, tendon,
    Achilles) 727.81
  anus 564.89
  axilla 729.90
  bile duct (*see also* Disease, biliary) 576.8
  bladder 596.89
    neck or sphincter 596.0
  bowel (*see also* Obstruction, intestine) 560.9
  Braxton Hicks 644.1
  breast implant, capsular 611.83
  bronchus 519.19
  burn (old)—*see* Cicatrix
  capsular, of breast implant 611.83
  cecum (*see also* Obstruction, intestine) 560.9
  cervix (*see also* Stricture, cervix) 622.4
    congenital 752.49
  cicatricial—*see* Cicatrix
  colon (*see also* Obstruction, intestine) 560.9
  conjunctiva trachomatous, active 076.1
    late effect 139.1
  Dupuytren's 728.6
  eyelid 374.41
  eye socket (after enucleation) 372.64
  face 729.90
  fascia (lata) (postural) 728.89
    Dupuytren's 728.6
    palmar 728.6
    plantar 728.71
  finger NEC 736.29
    congenital 755.59
    joint (*see also* Contraction, joint) 718.44
  flaccid, paralytic
    joint (*see also* Contraction, joint) 718.4
    muscle 728.85
      ocular 378.50
  gallbladder (*see also* Obstruction, gallbladder)
    575.2
  hamstring 728.89
    tendon 727.81
  heart valve—*see* Endocarditis
  Hicks' 644.1
  hip (*see also* Contraction, joint) 718.4
  hourglass
    bladder 596.89
      congenital 753.8
    gallbladder (*see also* Obstruction, gallbladder)
      575.2
      congenital 751.69
    stomach 536.8
      congenital 750.7
      psychogenic 306.4
    uterus 661.4
      affecting fetus or newborn 763.7
  hysterical 300.11
  infantile (*see also* Epilepsy) 345.6
  internal os (*see also* Stricture, cervix) 622.4
  intestine (*see also* Obstruction, intestine) 560.9
  joint (abduction) (acquired) (adduction)
    (flexion) (rotation) 718.40
    ankle 718.47
    congenital NEC 755.8
      generalized or multiple 754.89
        lower limb joints 754.89

Contraction—*continued*
    hip (*see also* Subluxation, congenital, hip)
      754.32
    lower limb (including pelvic girdle) not
      involving hip 754.89
    upper limb (including shoulder girdle)
      755.59
    elbow 718.42
    foot 718.47
    hand 718.44
    hip 718.45
    hysterical 300.11
    knee 718.46
    multiple sites 718.49
    pelvic region 718.45
    shoulder (region) 718.41
    specified site NEC 718.48
    wrist 718.43
  kidney (granular) (secondary) (*see also*
    Sclerosis, renal) 587
    congenital 753.3
    hydronephritic 591
    pyelonephritic (*see also* Pyelitis, chronic)
      590.00
    tuberculous (*see also* Tuberculosis) 016.0
  ligament 728.89
    congenital 756.89
  liver—*see* Cirrhosis, liver
  muscle (postinfectional) (postural) NEC 728.85
    congenital 756.89
      sternocleidomastoid 754.1
    extraocular 378.60
    eye (extrinsic) (*see also* Strabismus) 378.9
      paralytic (*see also* Strabismus, paralytic)
        378.50
    flaccid 728.85
    hysterical 300.11
    ischemic (Volkmann's) 958.6
    paralytic 728.85
    posttraumatic 958.6
    psychogenic 306.0
      specified as conversion reaction 300.11
  myotonic 728.85
  neck (*see also* Torticollis) 723.5
    congenital 754.1
    psychogenic 306.0
  ocular muscle (*see also* Strabismus) 378.9
    paralytic (*see also* Strabismus, paralytic) 378.50
  organ or site, congenital NEC—*see* Atresia
  outlet (pelvis)—*see* Contraction, pelvis
  palmar fascia 728.6
  paralytic
    joint (*see also* Contraction, joint) 718.4
    muscle 728.85
    ocular (*see also* Strabismus, paralytic) 378.50
  pelvis (acquired) (general) 738.6
    affecting fetus or newborn 763.1
    complicating delivery 653.1
      causing obstructed labor 660.1
      generally contracted 653.1
        causing obstructed labor 660.1
      inlet 653.2
        causing obstructed labor 660.1
      midpelvic 653.8
        causing obstructed labor 660.1
      midplane 653.8
        causing obstructed labor 660.1
      outlet 653.3
        causing obstructed labor 660.1
  plantar fascia 728.71

Contraction—*continued*
  premature
    atrial 427.61
    auricular 427.61
    auriculoventricular 427.61
    heart (junctional) (nodal) 427.60
    supraventricular 427.61
    ventricular 427.69
  prostate 602.8
  pylorus (*see also* Pylorospasm) 537.81
  rectosigmoid (*see also* Obstruction, intestine) 560.9
  rectum, rectal (sphincter) 564.89
    psychogenic 306.4
  ring (Bandl's) 661.4
    affecting fetus or newborn 763.7
  scar—*see* Cicatrix
  sigmoid (*see also* Obstruction, intestine) 560.9
  socket, eye 372.64
  spine (*see also* Curvature, spine) 737.9
  stomach 536.8
    hourglass 536.8
      congenital 750.7
      psychogenic 306.4
    psychogenic 306.4
  tendon (sheath) (*see also* Short, tendon) 727.81
  toe 735.8
  ureterovesical orifice (postinfectional) 593.3
  urethra 599.84
  uterus 621.8
    abnormal 661.9
      affecting fetus or newborn 763.7
    clonic, hourglass or tetanic 661.4
      affecting fetus or newborn 763.7
    dyscoordinate 661.4
      affecting fetus or newborn 763.7
    hourglass 661.4
      affecting fetus or newborn 763.7
    hypotonic NEC 661.2
      affecting fetus or newborn 763.7
    incoordinate 661.4
      affecting fetus or newborn 763.7
    inefficient or poor 661.2
      affecting fetus or newborn 763.7
    irregular 661.2
      affecting fetus or newborn 763.7
    tetanic 661.4
      affecting fetus or newborn 763.7
  vagina (outlet) 623.2
  vesical 596.89
    neck or urethral orifice 596.0
  visual field, generalized 368.45
  Volkmann's (ischemic) 958.6
Contusion (skin surface intact) 924.9
  with
    crush injury—*see* Crush
    dislocation—*see* Dislocation, by site
    fracture—*see* Fracture, by site
    internal injury—*see also* Injury, internal, by
      site
      heart—*see* Contusion, cardiac
      kidney—*see* Contusion, kidney
      liver—*see* Contusion, liver
      lung—*see* Contusion, lung
      spleen—*see* Contusion, spleen
    intracranial injury—*see* Injury, intracranial
    nerve injury—*see* Injury, nerve
    open wound—*see* Wound, open, by site
  abdomen, abdominal (muscle) (wall) 922.2
    organ(s) NEC 868.00
  adnexa, eye NEC 921.9

Contusion—*continued*

ankle 924.21
  with other parts of foot 924.20
arm 923.9
  lower (with elbow) 923.10
  upper 923.03
    with shoulder or axillary region 923.09
auditory canal (external) (meatus) (and other
  part(s) of neck, scalp, or face, except eye)
  920
auricle, ear (and other part(s) of neck, scalp, or
  face except eye) 920
axilla 923.02
  with shoulder or upper arm 923.09
back 922.31
bone NEC 924.9
brain (cerebral) (membrane) (with hemorrhage)
  851.8

Note—Use the following fifth-digit
subclassification with categories 851-854:

0 unspecified state of consciousness
1 with no loss of consciousness
2 with brief [less than one hour] loss
  of consciousness
3 with moderate [1-24 hours] loss of
  consciousness
4 with prolonged [more than 24 hours] loss of
  consciousness and return to pre-existing
  conscious level
5 with prolonged [more than 24 hours] loss of
  consciousness, without return to pre-existing
  conscious level
Use fifth-digit 5 to designate when a patient is
unconscious and dies before regaining
conciousness, regardless of the duration of the
loss of conciousness
6 with loss of consciousness of unspecified
  duration
9 with concussion, unspecified

---

with
  open intracranial wound 851.9
  skull fracture—*see* Fracture, skull, by site
  cerebellum 851.4
    with open intracranial wound 851.5
  cortex 851.0
    with open intracranial wound 851.1
  occipital lobe 851.4
    with open intracranial wound 851.5
  stem 851.4
    with open intracranial wound 851.5
breast 922.0
brow (and other part(s) of neck, scalp, or face,
  except eye) 920
buttock 922.32
canthus 921.1
cardiac 861.01
  with open wound into thorax 861.11
cauda equina (spine) 952.4
cerebellum—*see* Contusion, brain, cerebellum
cerebral—*see* Contusion, brain
cheek(s) (and other part(s) of neck, scalp, or
  face, except eye) 920
chest (wall) 922.1
chin (and other part(s) of neck, scalp, or face,
  except eye) 920
clitoris 922.4
conjunctiva 921.1
conus medullaris (spine) 952.4
cornea 921.3

Contusion—*continued*

corpus cavernosum 922.4
cortex (brain) (cerebral)—*see* Contusion, brain,
  cortex
costal region 922.1
ear (and other part(s) of neck, scalp, or face
  except eye) 920
elbow 923.11
  with forearm 923.10
epididymis 922.4
epigastric region 922.2
eye NEC 921.9
eyeball 921.3
eyelid(s) (and periocular area) 921.1
face (and neck, or scalp any part, except eye)
  920
femoral triangle 922.2
fetus or newborn 772.6
finger(s) (nail) (subungual) 923.3
flank 922.2
foot (with ankle) (excluding toe(s)) 924.20
forearm (and elbow) 923.10
forehead (and other part(s) of neck, scalp, or
  face, except eye) 920
genital organs, external 922.4
globe (eye) 921.3
groin 922.2
gum(s) (and other part(s) of neck, scalp, or face,
  except eye) 920
hand(s) (except fingers alone) 923.20
head (any part, except eye) (and face) (and neck)
  920
heart—*see* Contusion, cardiac
heel 924.20
hip 924.01
  with thigh 924.00
iliac region 922.2
inguinal region 922.2
internal organs (abdomen, chest, or pelvis)
  NEC—*see* Injury, internal, by site
interscapular region 922.33
iris (eye) 921.3
kidney 866.01
  with open wound into cavity 866.11
knee 924.11
  with lower leg 924.10
labium (majus) (minus) 922.4
lacrimal apparatus, gland, or sac 921.1
larynx (and other part(s) of neck, scalp, or face,
  except eye) 920
late effect—*see* Late, effects (of), contusion
leg 924.5
  lower (with knee) 924.10
lens 921.3
lingual (and other part(s) of neck, scalp, or face,
  except eye) 920
lip(s) (and other part(s) of neck, scalp, or face,
  except eye) 920
liver 864.01
  with
    laceration—*see* Laceration, liver
    open wound into cavity 864.11
lower extremity 924.5
  multiple sites 924.4
lumbar region 922.31
lung 861.21
  with open wound into thorax 861.31
malar region (and other part(s) of neck, scalp, or
  face, except eye) 920
mandibular joint (and other part(s) of neck,
  scalp, or face, except eye) 920

Contusion—*continued*
  mastoid region (and other part(s) of neck, scalp, or face, except eye) 920
  membrane, brain—*see* Contusion, brain
  midthoracic region 922.1
  mouth (and other part(s) of neck, scalp, or face, except eye) 920
  multiple sites (not classifiable to same three-digit category) 924.8
    lower limb 924.4
    trunk 922.8
    upper limb 923.8
  muscle NEC 924.9
  myocardium—*see* Contusion, cardiac
  nasal (septum) (and other part(s) of neck, scalp, or face, except eye) 920
  neck (and scalp, or face any part, except eye) 920
  nerve—*see* Injury, nerve, by site
  nose (and other part(s) of neck, scalp, or face, except eye) 920
  occipital region (scalp) (and neck or face, except eye) 920
    lobe—*see* Contusion, brain, occipital lobe
  orbit (region) (tissues) 921.2
  palate (soft) (and other part(s) of neck, scalp, or face, except eye) 920
  parietal region (scalp) (and neck, or face, except eye) 920
    lobe—*see* Contusion, brain
  penis 922.4
  pericardium—*see* Contusion, cardiac
  perineum 922.4
  periocular area 921.1
  pharynx (and other part(s) of neck, scalp, or face, except eye) 920
  popliteal space (*see also* Contusion, knee) 924.11
  prepuce 922.4
  pubic region 922.4
  pudenda 922.4
  pulmonary—*see* Contusion, lung
  quadriceps femoralis 924.00
  rib cage 922.1
  sacral region 922.32
  salivary ducts or glands (and other part(s) of neck, scalp, or face, except eye) 920
  scalp (and neck, or face any part, except eye) 920
  scapular region 923.01
    with shoulder or upper arm 923.09
  sclera (eye) 921.3
  scrotum 922.4
  shoulder 923.00
    with upper arm or axillar regions 923.09
  skin NEC 924.9
  skull 920
  spermatic cord 922.4
  spinal cord—*see also* Injury, spinal, by site
    cauda equina 952.4
    conus medullaris 952.4
  spleen 865.01
    with open wound into cavity 865.11
  sternal region 922.1
  stomach—*see* Injury, internal, stomach
  subconjunctival 921.1
  subcutaneous NEC 924.9
  submaxillary region (and other part(s) of neck, scalp, or face, except eye) 920
  submental region (and other part(s) of neck, scalp, or face, except eye) 920

Contusion—*continued*
  subperiosteal NEC 924.9
  supraclavicular fossa (and other part(s) of neck, scalp, or face, except eye) 920
  supraorbital (and other part(s) of neck, scalp, or face, except eye) 920
  temple (region) (and other part(s) of neck, scalp, or face, except eye) 920
  testis 922.4
  thigh (and hip) 924.00
  thorax 922.1
    organ—*see* Injury, internal, intrathoracic
  throat (and other part(s) of neck, scalp, or face, except eye) 920
  thumb(s) (nail) (subungual) 923.3
  toe(s) (nail) (subungual) 924.3
  tongue (and other part(s) of neck, scalp, or face, except eye) 920
  trunk 922.9
    multiple sites 922.8
    specified site—*see* Contusion, by site
  tunica vaginalis 922.4
  tympanum (membrane) (and other part(s) of neck, scalp, or face, except eye) 920
  upper extremity 923.9
    multiple sites 923.8
  uvula (and other part(s) of neck, scalp, or face, except eye) 920
  vagina 922.4
  vocal cord(s) (and other part(s) of neck, scalp, or face, except eye) 920
  vulva 922.4
  wrist 923.21
    with hand(s), except finger(s) alone 923.20
Conus (any type) (congenital) 743.57
  acquired 371.60
  medullaris syndrome 336.8
Convalescence (following) V66.9
  chemotherapy V66.2
  medical NEC V66.5
  psychotherapy V66.3
  radiotherapy V66.1
  surgery NEC V66.0
  treatment (for) NEC V66.5
    combined V66.6
    fracture V66.4
    mental disorder NEC V66.3
    specified disorder NEC V66.5
Conversion
  closed surgical procedure to open procedure
    arthroscopic V64.43
    laparoscopic V64.41
    thoracoscopic V64.42
  hysteria, hysterical, any type 300.11
  neurosis, any 300.11
  reaction, any 300.11
Converter, tuberculosis (test reaction) 795.51
Convulsions (idiopathic) 780.39
  apoplectiform (*see also* Disease, cerebrovascular, acute) 436
  brain 780.39
  cerebral 780.39
  cerebrospinal 780.39
  due to trauma NEC—*see* Injury, intracranial
  eclamptic (*see also* Eclampsia) 780.39
  epileptic (*see also* Epilepsy) 345.9
  epileptiform (*see also* Seizure, epileptiform) 780.39
  epileptoid (*see also* Seizure, epileptiform) 780.39

Convulsions—*continued*
ether
anesthetic
correct substance properly administered 780.39
overdose or wrong substance given 968.2
other specified type—*see* Table of drugs and chemicals
febrile (simple) 780.31
complex 780.32
generalized 780.39
hysterical 300.11
infantile 780.39
epilepsy—*see* Epilepsy
internal 780.39
jacksonian (*see also* Epilepsy) 345.5
myoclonic 333.2
newborn 779.0
paretic 094.1
pregnancy (nephritic) (uremic)—*see* Eclampsia, pregnancy
psychomotor (*see also* Epilepsy) 345.4
puerperal, postpartum—*see* Eclampsia, pregnancy
recurrent 780.39
epileptic—*see* Epilepsy
reflex 781.0
repetitive 780.39
epileptic—*see* Epilepsy
salaam (*see also* Epilepsy) 345.6
scarlatinal 034.1
spasmodic 780.39
tetanus, tetanic (*see also* Tetanus) 037
thymic 254.8
uncinate 780.39
uremic 586
Convulsive —*see also* Convulsions
disorder or state 780.39
epileptic—*see* Epilepsy
equivalent, abdominal (*see also* Epilepsy) 345.5
Cooke-Apert-Gallais syndrome (adrenogenital) 255.2
Cooley's anemia (erythroblastic) 282.44
Coolie itch 126.9
Cooper's
disease 610.1
hernia—*see* Hernia, Cooper's
Coordination disturbance 781.3
Copper wire arteries, retina 362.13
Copra itch 133.8
Coprolith 560.39
Coprophilia 302.89
Coproporphyria, hereditary 277.1
Coprostasis 560.32
with hernia—*see also* Hernia, by site, with obstruction
gangrenous—*see* Hernia, by site, with gangrene
Cor
biloculare 745.7
bovinum—*see* Hypertrophy, cardiac
bovis—*see also* Hypertrophy, cardiac
pulmonale (chronic) 416.9
acute 415.0
triatriatum, triatrium 746.82
triloculare 745.8
biatriatum 745.3
biventriculare 745.69
Corbus' disease 607.1

Cord —*see also* condition
around neck (tightly) (with compression)
affecting fetus or newborn 762.5
complicating delivery 663.1
without compression 663.3
affecting fetus or newborn 762.6
bladder NEC 344.61
tabetic 094.0
prolapse
affecting fetus or newborn 762.4
complicating delivery 663.0
Cord's angiopathy (*see also* Tuberculosis) 017.3
[362.18]
Cordis ectopia 746.87
Corditis (spermatic) 608.4
Corectopia 743.46
Cori type glycogen storage disease —*see* Disease, glycogen storage
Cork-handlers' disease or lung 495.3
Corkscrew esophagus 530.5
Corlett's pyosis (impetigo) 684
Corn (infected) 700
Cornea—*see also* condition
donor V59.5
guttata (dystrophy) 371.57
plana 743.41
Cornelia de Lange's syndrome (Amsterdam dwarf, intellectual disabilities, and brachycephaly) 759.89
Cornual gestation or pregnancy —*see* Pregnancy, cornual
Cornu cutaneum 702.8
Coronary (artery)—*see also* condition
arising from aorta or pulmonary trunk 746.85
Corpora —*see also* condition
amylacea (prostate) 602.8
cavernosa—*see* condition
Corpulence (*see also* Obesity) 278.0
Corpus —*see* condition
Corrigan's disease —*see* Insufficiency, aortic
Corrosive burn —*see* Burn, by site
Corsican fever (*see also* Malaria) 084.6
Cortical —*see also* condition
blindness 377.75
necrosis, kidney (bilateral) 583.6
Corticoadrenal —*see* condition
Corticosexual syndrome 255.2
Coryza (acute) 460
with grippe or influenza (*see also* Influenza) 487.1
syphilitic 095.8
congenital (chronic) 090.0
Costen's syndrome or complex 524.60
Costiveness (*see also* Constipation) 564.00
Costochondritis 733.6
Cotard's syndrome (paranoia) 297.1
Cot death 798.0
Cotia virus 059.8
Cotungo's disease 724.3
Cough 786.2
with hemorrhage (*see also* Hemoptysis) 786.39
affected 786.2
bronchial 786.2
with grippe or influenza (*see also* Influenza) 487.1
chronic 786.2
epidemic 786.2
functional 306.1
hemorrhagic 786.39

Cough—*continued*
hysterical 300.11
laryngeal, spasmodic 786.2
nervous 786.2
psychogenic 306.1
smokers' 491.0
tea tasters' 112.89
Counseling NEC V65.40
without complaint or sickness V65.49
abuse victim NEC V62.89
child V61.21
partner V61.11
spouse V61.11
child abuse, maltreatment, or neglect V61.21
contraceptive NEC V25.09
device (intrauterine) V25.02
maintenance V25.40
intrauterine contraceptive device V25.42
oral contraceptive (pill) V25.41
specified type NEC V25.49
subdermal implantable V25.43
management NEC V25.9
oral contraceptive (pill) V25.01
emergency V25.03
postcoital V25.03
prescription NEC V25.02
oral contraceptive (pill) V25.01
emergency V25.03
postcoital V25.03
repeat prescription V25.41
repeat prescription V25.40
subdermal implantable V25.43
surveillance V25.40
dietary V65.3
exercise V65.41
expectant parents(s)
pediatric pre-adoption visit V65.11
pediatric pre-birth visit V65.11
explanation of
investigation finding NEC V65.49
medication NEC V65.49
family planning V25.09
natural
procreative V26.41
to avoid pregnancy V25.04
for nonattending third party V65.19
genetic V26.33
gonorrhea V65.45
health (advice) (education) (instruction) NEC
V65.49
HIV V65.44
human immunodeficiency virus V65.44
injury prevention V65.43
insulin pump training V65.46
marital V61.10
medical (for) V65.9
boarding school resident V60.6
condition not demonstrated V65.5
feared complaint and no disease found V65.5
institutional resident V60.6
on behalf of another V65.19
person living alone V60.3
natural family planning
procreative V26.41
to avoid pregnancy V25.04
parent(guardian)-child conflict V61.20
adopted child V61.24
biological child V61.23
foster child V61.25
specified problem NEC V61.29

Counseling—*continued*
partner abuse
perpetrator V61.12
victim V61.11
pediatric
pre-adoption visit for adoptive parent(s)
V65.11
pre-birth visit for expectant parent(s) V65.11
perpetrator of
child abuse V62.83
parental V61.22
partner abuse V61.12
spouse abuse V61.12
procreative V65.49
sex NEC V65.49
transmitted disease NEC V65.45
HIV V65.44
specified reason NEC V65.49
spousal abuse
perpetrator V61.12
victim V61.11
substance use and abuse V65.42
syphilis V65.45
victim (of)
abuse NEC V62.89
child abuse V61.21
partner abuse V61.11
spousal abuse V61.11
Coupled rhythm 427.89
Couvelaire uterus (complicating delivery)—*see*
Placenta, separation
Cowper's gland —*see* condition
Cowperitis (*see also* Urethritis) 597.89
gonorrheal (acute) 098.0
chronic or duration of 2 months or over 098.2
Cowpox (abortive) 051.01
due to vaccination 999.0
eyelid 051.01 *[373.5]*
postvaccination 999.0 *[373.5]*
Coxa
plana 732.1
valga (acquired) 736.31
congenital 755.61
late effect of rickets 268.1
vara (acquired) 736.32
congenital 755.62
late effect of rickets 268.1
Coxae malum senilis 715.25
Coxalgia (nontuberculous) 719.45
tuberculous (*see also* Tuberculosis) 015.1 *[730.85]*
Coxalgic pelvis 736.30
Coxitis 716.65
Coxsackie (infection) (virus) 079.2
central nervous system NEC 048
endocarditis 074.22
enteritis 008.67
meningitis (aseptic) 047.0
myocarditis 074.23
pericarditis 074.21
pharyngitis 074.0
pleurodynia 074.1
specific disease NEC 074.8
Crabs, meaning pubic lice 132.2
Crack baby 760.75
Cracked
nipple 611.2
puerperal, postpartum 676.1
puerperal, postpartum 676.1
tooth 521.81
Cradle cap 690.11
Craft neurosis 300.89

Craigiasis 007.8
Cramp(s) 729.82
　abdominal 789.0
　bathing 994.1
　colic 789.7
　　infantile 789.7
　　psychogenic 306.4
　due to immersion 994.1
　extremity (lower) (upper) NEC 729.82
　fireman 992.2
　heat 992.2
　hysterical 300.11
　immersion 994.1
　intestinal 789.0
　　psychogenic 306.4
　linotypist's 300.89
　　organic 333.84
　muscle (extremity) (general) 729.82
　　due to immersion 994.1
　　hysterical 300.11
　occupational (hand) 300.89
　　organic 333.84
　psychogenic 307.89
　salt depletion 276.1
　sleep related leg 327.52
　stoker 992.2
　stomach 789.0
　telegraphers' 300.89
　　organic 333.84
　typists' 300.89
　　organic 333.84
　uterus 625.8
　　menstrual 625.3
　writers' 333.84
　　organic 333.84
　　psychogenic 300.89
Cranial —*see* condition
Cranioclasis, fetal 763.89
Craniocleidodysostosis 755.59
Craniofenestria (skull) 756.0
Craniolacunia (skull) 756.0
Craniopagus 759.4
Craniopathy, metabolic 733.3
Craniopharyngeal —*see* condition
Craniopharyngioma (M9350/1) 237.0
Craniorachischisis (totalis) 740.1
Cranioschisis 756.0
Craniostenosis 756.0
Craniosynostosis 756.0
Craniotabes (cause unknown) 733.3
　rachitic 268.1
　syphilitic 090.5
Craniotomy, fetal 763.89
Cranium —*see* condition
Craw-craw 125.3
CRBSI (catheter-related bloodstream infection) 999.31
Creaking joint 719.60
　ankle 719.67
　elbow 719.62
　foot 719.67
　hand 719.64
　hip 719.65
　knee 719.66
　multiple sites 719.69
　pelvic region 719.65
　shoulder (region) 719.61
　specified site NEC 719.68
　wrist 719.63

Creeping
　eruption 126.9
　palsy 335.21
　paralysis 335.21
Crenated tongue 529.8
Creotoxism 005.9
Crepitus
　caput 756.0
　joint 719.60
　　ankle 719.67
　　elbow 719.62
　　foot 719.67
　　hand 719.64
　　hip 719.65
　　knee 719.66
　　multiple sites 719.69
　　pelvic region 719.65
　　shoulder (region) 719.61
　　specified site NEC 719.68
　　wrist 719.63
Crescent or conus choroid, congenital 743.57
Cretin, cretinism (athyrotic) (congenital) (endemic) (metabolic) (nongoitrous) (sporadic) 243
　goitrous (sporadic) 246.1
　pelvis (dwarf type) (male type) 243
　　with disproportion (fetopelvic) 653.1
　　　affecting fetus or newborn 763.1
　　　causing obstructed labor 660.1
　　　　affecting fetus or newborn 763.1
　pituitary 253.3
Cretinoid degeneration 243
Creutzfeldt-Jakob disease (CJD) (syndrome) 046.19
　with dementia
　　with behavioral disturbance 046.19 *[294.11]*
　　without behavioral disturbance 046.19 *[294.10]*
　familial 046.19
　iatrogenic 046.19
　specified NEC 046.19
　sporadic 046.19
　variant (vCJD) 046.11
　　with dementia
　　　with behavioral disturbance 046.11 *[294.11]*
　　　without behavioral disturbance 046.11 *[294.10]*
Crib death 798.0
Cribriform hymen 752.49
Cri-du-chat syndrome 758.31
Crigler-Najjar disease or syndrome (congenital hyperbilirubinemia) 277.4
Crimean hemorrhagic fever 065.0
Criminalism 301.7
Crisis
　abdomen 789.0
　addisonian (acute adrenocortical insufficiency) 255.41
　adrenal (cortical) 255.41
　asthmatic—*see* Asthma
　brain, cerebral (*see also* Disease, cerebrovascular, acute) 436
　celiac 579.0
　Dietl's 593.4
　emotional NEC 309.29
　　acute reaction to stress 308.0
　　adjustment reaction 309.9
　　specific to childhood or adolescence 313.9
　gastric (tabetic) 094.0
　glaucomatocyclitic 364.22
　heart (*see also* Failure, heart) 428.9

Crisis—*continued*
  hypertensive—*see* Hypertension
  nitritoid
    correct substance properly administered
      458.29
    overdose or wrong substance given or taken
      961.1
  oculogyric 378.87
    psychogenic 306.7
  Pel's 094.0
  psychosexual identity 302.6
  rectum 094.0
  renal 593.81
  sickle cell 282.62
  stomach (tabetic) 094.0
  tabetic 094.0
  thyroid (*see also* Thyrotoxicosis) 242.9
  thyrotoxic (*see also* Thyrotoxicosis) 242.9
  vascular—*see* Disease, cerebrovascular, acute
Crocq's disease (acrocyanosis) 443.89
Crohn's disease (*see also* Enteritis, regional) 555.9
Cronkhite-Canada syndrome 211.3
Crooked septum, nasal 470
Cross
  birth (of fetus) complicating delivery 652.3
    with successful version 652.1
    causing obstructed labor 660.0
  bite, anterior or posterior 524.27
  eye (*see also* Esotropia) 378.00
Crossed ectopia of kidney 753.3
Crossfoot 754.50
Croup, croupous (acute) (angina) (catarrhal)
    (infective) (inflammatory) (laryngeal)
    (membranous) (nondiphtheritic)
    (pseudomembranous) 464.4
  asthmatic (*see also* Asthma) 493.9
  bronchial 466.0
  diphtheritic (membranous) 032.3
  false 478.75
  spasmodic 478.75
    diphtheritic 032.3
  stridulous 478.75
    diphtheritic 032.3
Crouzon's disease (craniofacial dysostosis)
  756.0
Crowding, teeth 524.31
CRST syndrome (cutaneous systemic sclerosis)
  710.1
Cruchet's disease (encephalitis lethargica) 049.8
Cruelty in children (*see also* Disturbance,
  conduct) 312.9
Crural ulcer (*see also* Ulcer, lower extremity)
  707.10
Crush, crushed, crushing (injury) 929.9
  abdomen 926.19
    internal—*see* Injury, internal, abdomen
  ankle 928.21
    with other parts of foot 928.20
  arm 927.9
    lower (and elbow) 927.10
    upper 927.03
      with shoulder or axillary region 927.09
  axilla 927.02
    with shoulder or upper arm 927.09
  back 926.11
  breast 926.19
  buttock 926.12
  cheek 925.1
  chest—*see* Injury, internal, chest
  ear 925.1

Crush, crushed, crushing—*continued*
  elbow 927.11
    with forearm 927.10
  face 925.1
  finger(s) 927.3
    with hand(s) 927.20
      and wrist(s) 927.21
  flank 926.19
  foot, excluding toe(s) alone (with ankle) 928.20
  forearm (and elbow) 927.10
  genitalia, external (female) 926.0
    internal—*see* Injury, internal, genital organ NEC
  hand, except finger(s) alone (and wrist) 927.20
  head—*see* Fracture, skull, by site
  heel 928.20
  hip 928.01
    with thigh 928.00
  internal organ (abdomen, chest, or pelvis)—*see*
    Injury, internal, by site
  knee 928.11
    with leg, lower 928.10
  labium (majus) (minus) 926.0
  larynx 925.2
  late effect—*see* Late, effects (of), crushing
  leg 928.9
    lower 928.10
      and knee 928.11
    upper 928.00
  limb
    lower 928.9
      multiple sites 928.8
    upper 927.9
      multiple sites 927.8
  multiple sites NEC 929.0
  neck 925.2
  nerve—*see* Injury, nerve, by site
  nose 802.0
    open 802.1
  penis 926.0
  pharynx 925.2
  scalp 925.2
  scapular region 927.01
    with shoulder or upper arm 927.09
  scrotum 926.0
  shoulder 927.00
    with upper arm or axillary region 927.09
  skull or cranium—*see* Fracture, skull, by site
  spinal cord—*see* Injury, spinal, by site
  syndrome (complication of trauma) 958.5
  testis 926.0
  thigh (with hip) 928.00
  throat 925.2
  thumb(s) (and fingers) 927.3
  toe(s) 928.3
    with foot 928.20
      and ankle 928.21
  tonsil 925.2
  trunk 926.9
    chest—*see* Injury, internal, intrathoracic
      organs NEC
    internal organ—*see* Injury, internal, by site
    multiple sites 926.8
    specified site NEC 926.19
  vulva 926.0
  wrist 927.21
    with hand(s), except fingers alone 927.20
Crusta lactea 690.11
Crusts 782.8
Crutch paralysis 953.4
Cruveilhier's disease 335.21
Cruveilhier-Baumgarten cirrhosis, disease, or
  syndrome 571.5

Cruz-Chagas disease (*see also* Trypanosomiasis) 086.2
Crying
constant, continuous
adolescent 780.95
adult 780.95
baby 780.92
child 780.95
infant 780.92
newborn 780.92
excessive
adolescent 780.95
adult 780.95
baby 780.92
child 780.95
infant 780.92
newborn 780.92
Cryofibrinogenemia 273.2
Cryoglobulinemia (mixed) 273.2
Crypt (anal) (rectal) 569.49
Cryptitis (anal) (rectal) 569.49
Cryptococcosis (European) (pulmonary) (systemic) 117.5
Cryptococcus 117.5
epidermicus 117.5
neoformans, infection by 117.5
Cryptopapillitis (anus) 569.49
Cryptophthalmos (eyelid) 743.06
Cryptorchid, cryptorchism, cryptorchidism 752.51
Cryptosporidiosis 007.4
hepatobiliary 136.8
respiratory 136.8
Cryptotia 744.29
Crystallopathy
calcium pyrophosphate (*see also* Arthritis) 275.49 *[712.2]*
dicalcium phosphate (*see also* Arthritis) 275.49 *[712.1]*
gouty 274.00
pyrophosphate NEC (*see also* Arthritis) 275.49 *[712.2]*
uric acid 274.00
Crystalluria 791.9
Csillag's disease (lichen sclerosus et atrophicus) 701.0
Cuban itch 050.1
Cubitus
valgus (acquired) 736.01
congenital 755.59
late effect of rickets 268.1
varus (acquired) 736.02
congenital 755.59
late effect of rickets 268.1
Cultural deprivation V62.4
Cupping of optic disc 377.14
Curling's ulcer —*see* Ulcer, duodenum
Curling esophagus 530.5
Curschmann (-Batten) (-Steinert) disease or syndrome 359.21
Curvature
organ or site, congenital NEC—*see* Distortion
penis (lateral) 752.69
Pott's (spinal) (*see also* Tuberculosis) 015.0 *[737.43]*
radius, idiopathic, progressive (congenital) 755.54

Curvature—*continued*
spine (acquired) (angular) (idiopathic) (incorrect) (postural) 737.9
congenital 754.2
due to or associated with
Charcot-Marie-Tooth disease 356.1 *[737.40]*
mucopolysaccharidosis 277.5 *[737.40]*
neurofibromatosis 237.71 *[737.40]*
osteitis
deformans 731.0 *[737.40]*
fibrosa cystica 252.01 *[737.40]*
osteoporosis (*see also* Osteoporosis) 733.00 *[737.40]*
poliomyelitis (*see also* Poliomyelitis) 138 *[737.40]*
tuberculosis (Pott's curvature) (*see also* Tuberculosis) 015.0 *[737.43]*
kyphoscoliotic (*see also* Kyphoscoliosis) 737.30
kyphotic (*see also* Kyphosis) 737.10
late effect of rickets 268.1 *[737.40]*
Pott's 015.0 *[737.40]*
scoliotic (*see also* Scoliosis) 737.30
specified NEC 737.8
tuberculous 015.0 *[737.40]*
Cushing's
basophilism, disease, or syndrome (iatrogenic) (idiopathic) (pituitary basophilism) (pituitary dependent) 255.0
ulcer—*see* Ulcer, peptic
Cushingoid due to steroid therapy
correct substance properly administered 255.0
overdose or wrong substance given or taken 962.0
Cut (external)—*see* Wound, open, by site
Cutaneous —*see also* condition
hemorrhage 782.7
horn (cheek) (eyelid) (mouth) 702.8
larva migrans 126.9
Cutis —*see also* condition
hyperelastic 756.83
acquired 701.8
laxa 756.83
senilis 701.8
marmorata 782.61
osteosis 709.3
pendula 756.83
acquired 701.8
rhomboidalis nuchae 701.8
verticis gyrata 757.39
acquired 701.8
Cyanopathy, newborn 770.83
Cyanosis 782.5
autotoxic 289.7
common atrioventricular canal 745.69
congenital 770.83
conjunctiva 372.71
due to
endocardial cushion defect 745.60
nonclosure, foramen botalli 745.5
patent foramen botalli 745.5
persistent foramen ovale 745.5
enterogenous 289.7
fetus or newborn 770.83
ostium primum defect 745.61
paroxysmal digital 443.0
retina, retinal 362.10
Cycle
anovulatory 628.0
menstrual, irregular 626.4
Cyclencephaly 759.89

Cyclical vomiting 536.2
   associated with migraine 346.2
   psychogenic 306.4
Cyclitic membrane 364.74
Cyclitis (*see also* Iridocyclitis) 364.3
   acute 364.00
      primary 364.01
      recurrent 364.02
   chronic 364.10
      in
         sarcoidosis 135 *[364.11]*
         tuberculosis (*see also* Tuberculosis) 017.3
            [364.11]
   Fuchs' heterochromic 364.21
   granulomatous 364.10
   lens induced 364.23
   nongranulomatous 364.00
   posterior 363.21
   primary 364.01
   recurrent 364.02
   secondary (noninfectious) 364.04
      infectious 364.03
   subacute 364.00
      primary 364.01
      recurrent 364.02
Cyclokeratitis —*see* Keratitis
Cyclophoria 378.44
Cyclopia, cyclops 759.89
Cycloplegia 367.51
Cyclospasm 367.53
Cyclosporiasis 007.5
Cyclothymia 301.13
Cyclothymic personality 301.13
Cyclotropia 378.33
Cyesis —*see* Pregnancy
Cylindroma (M8200/3)—*see also* Neoplasm, by
   site, malignant
   eccrine dermal (M8200/0)—*see* Neoplasm, skin, benign
   skin (M8200/0)—*see* Neoplasm, skin, benign
Cylindruria 791.7
Cyllosoma 759.89
Cynanche
   diphtheritic 032.3
   tonsillaris 475
Cynorexia 783.6
Cyphosis —*see* Kyphosis
Cyprus fever (*see also* Brucellosis) 023.9
Cyriax's syndrome (slipping rib) 733.99
Cyst (mucus) (retention) (serous) (simple)

---

*Note—In general, cysts are not neoplastic and
are classified to the appropriate category for
disease of the specified anatomical site. This
generalization does not apply to certain types of
cysts which are neoplastic in nature, for
example, dermoid, nor does it apply to cysts of
certain structures, for example, branchial cleft,
which are classified as developmental
anomalies. The following listing includes some
of the most frequently reported sites of cysts as
well as qualifiers which indicate the type of cyst.
The latter qualifiers usually are not repeated
under the anatomical sites. Since the code
assignment for a given site may vary depending
upon the type of cyst, the coder should refer to
the listings under the specified type of cyst
before consideration is given to the site.*

---

   accessory, fallopian tube 752.11
   adenoid (infected) 474.8
   adrenal gland 255.8
      congenital 759.1

Cyst —*continued*
   air, lung 518.89
   allantoic 753.7
   alveolar process (jaw bone) 526.2
   amnion, amniotic 658.8
   anterior chamber (eye) 364.60
      exudative 364.62
      implantation (surgical) (traumatic) 364.61
      parasitic 360.13
   anterior nasopalatine 526.1
   antrum 478.19
   anus 569.49
   apical (periodontal) (tooth) 522.8
   appendix 543.9
   arachnoid, brain 348.0
   arytenoid 478.79
   auricle 706.2
   Baker's (knee) 727.51
      tuberculous (*see also* Tuberculosis) 015.2
   Bartholin's gland or duct 616.2
   bile duct (*see also* Disease, biliary) 576.8
   bladder (multiple) (trigone) 596.89
   Blessig's 362.62
   blood, endocardial (*see also* Endocarditis)
      424.90
   blue dome 610.0
   bone (local) 733.20
      aneurysmal 733.22
      jaw 526.2
         developmental (odontogenic) 526.0
         fissural 526.1
         latent 526.89
      solitary 733.21
      unicameral 733.21
   brain 348.0
      congenital 742.4
      hydatid (*see also* Echinococcus) 122.9
      third ventricle (colloid) 742.4
   branchial (cleft) 744.42
   branchiogenic 744.42
   breast (benign) (blue dome) (pedunculated)
      (solitary) (traumatic) 610.0
      involution 610.4
      sebaceous 610.8
   broad ligament (benign) 620.8
      embryonic 752.11
   bronchogenic (mediastinal) (sequestration)
      518.89
      congenital 748.4
   buccal 528.4
   bulbourethral gland (Cowper's) 599.89
   bursa, bursal 727.49
      pharyngeal 478.26
   calcifying odontogenic (M9301/0) 213.1
      upper jaw (bone) 213.0
   canal of Nuck (acquired) (serous) 629.1
      congenital 752.41
   canthus 372.75
   carcinomatous (M8010/3)—*see* Neoplasm, by
      site, malignant
   cartilage (joint)—*see* Derangement, joint
   cauda equina 336.8
   cavum septi pellucidi NEC 348.0
   celomic (pericardium) 746.89
   cerebellopontine (angle)—*see* Cyst, brain
   cerebellum—*see* Cyst, brain
   cerebral—*see* Cyst, brain
   cervical lateral 744.42
   cervix 622.8
      embryonal 752.41
      nabothian (gland) 616.0

Cyst —*continued*
  chamber, anterior (eye) 364.60
    exudative 364.62
    implantation (surgical) (traumatic) 364.61
    parasitic 360.13
  chiasmal, optic NEC (*see also* Lesion, chiasmal)
      377.54
  chocolate (ovary) 617.1
  choledochal (congenital) 751.69
    acquired 576.8
  choledochus 751.69
  chorion 658.8
  choroid plexus 348.0
  chyle, mesentery 457.8
  ciliary body 364.60
    exudative 364.64
    implantation 364.61
    primary 364.63
  clitoris 624.8
  coccyx (*see also* Cyst, bone) 733.20
  colloid
    third ventricle (brain) 742.4
    thyroid gland—*see* Goiter
  colon 569.89
  common (bile) duct (*see also* Disease, biliary)
      576.8
  congenital NEC 759.89
    adrenal glands 759.1
    epiglottis 748.3
    esophagus 750.4
    fallopian tube 752.11
    kidney 753.10
      multiple 753.19
      single 753.11
    larynx 748.3
    liver 751.62
    lung 748.4
    mediastinum 748.8
    ovary 752.0
    oviduct 752.11
    pancreas 751.7
    periurethral (tissue) 753.8
    prepuce NEC 752.69
      penis 752.69
    sublingual 750.26
    submaxillary gland 750.26
    thymus (gland) 759.2
    tongue 750.19
    ureterovesical orifice 753.4
    vulva 752.41
  conjunctiva 372.75
  cornea 371.23
  corpora quadrigemina 348.0
  corpus
    albicans (ovary) 620.2
    luteum (ruptured) 620.1
  Cowper's gland (benign) (infected) 599.89
  cranial meninges 348.0
  craniobuccal pouch 253.8
  craniopharyngeal pouch 253.8
  cystic duct (*see also* Disease, gallbladder) 575.8
  Cysticercus (any site) 123.1
  Dandy-Walker 742.3
    with spina bifida (*see also* Spina bifida) 741.0
  dental 522.8
    developmental 526.0
    eruption 526.0
    lateral periodontal 526.0
    primordial (keratocyst) 526.0
    root 522.8

Cyst —*continued*
  dentigerous 526.0
    mandible 526.0
    maxilla 526.0
  dermoid (M9084/0)—*see also* Neoplasm, by
      site, benign
    with malignant transformation (M9084/3)
        183.0
    implantation
      external area or site (skin) NEC 709.8
      iris 364.61
      skin 709.8
      vagina 623.8
      vulva 624.8
    mouth 528.4
    oral soft tissue 528.4
    sacrococcygeal 685.1
      with abscess 685.0
  developmental of ovary, ovarian 752.0
  dura (cerebral) 348.0
    spinal 349.2
  ear (external) 706.2
  echinococcal (*see also* Echinococcus) 122.9
  embryonal
    cervix uteri 752.41
    genitalia, female external 752.41
    uterus 752.39
    vagina 752.41
  endometrial 621.8
    ectopic 617.9
  endometrium (uterus) 621.8
    ectopic—*see* Endometriosis
  enteric 751.5
  enterogenous 751.5
  epidermal (inclusion) (*see also* Cyst, skin) 706.2
  epidermoid (inclusion) (*see also* Cyst, skin)
      706.2
    mouth 528.4
    not of skin—*see* Cyst, by site
    oral soft tissue 528.4
  epididymis 608.89
  epiglottis 478.79
  epiphysis cerebri 259.8
  epithelial (inclusion) (*see also* Cyst, skin) 706.2
  epoophoron 752.11
  eruption 526.0
  esophagus 530.89
  ethmoid sinus 478.19
  eye (retention) 379.8
    congenital 743.03
    posterior segment, congenital 743.54
  eyebrow 706.2
  eyelid (sebaceous) 374.84
    infected 373.13
    sweat glands or ducts 374.84
  falciform ligament (inflammatory) 573.8
  fallopian tube 620.8
    congenital 752.11
  female genital organs NEC 629.89
  fimbrial (congenital) 752.11
  fissural (oral region) 526.1
  follicle (atretic) (graafian) (ovarian) 620.0
    nabothian (gland) 616.0
  follicular (atretic) (ovarian) 620.0
    dentigerous 526.0
  frontal sinus 478.19
  gallbladder or duct 575.8
  ganglion 727.43
  Gartner's duct 752.41
  gas, of mesentery 568.89
  gingiva 523.8

Cyst —*continued*
  gland of moll 374.84
  globulomaxillary 526.1
  graafian follicle 620.0
  granulosal lutein 620.2
  hemangiomatous (M9121/0) (*see also*
      Hemangioma) 228.00
  hydatid (*see also* Echinococcus) 122.9
    fallopian tube (Morgagni) 752.11
    liver NEC 122.8
    lung NEC 122.9
    Morgagni 752.89
      fallopian tube 752.11
    specified site NEC 122.9
  hymen 623.8
    embryonal 752.41
  hypopharynx 478.26
  hypophysis, hypophyseal (duct) (recurrent)
      253.8
    cerebri 253.8
  implantation (dermoid)
    anterior chamber (eye) 364.61
    external area or site (skin) NEC 709.8
    iris 364.61
    vagina 623.8
    vulva 624.8
  incisor, incisive canal 526.1
  inclusion (epidermal) (epithelial) (epidermoid)
      (mucous) (squamous) (*see also* Cyst, skin)
      706.2
    not of skin—*see* Neoplasm, by site, benign
  intestine (large) (small) 569.89
  intracranial—*see* Cyst, brain
  intraligamentous 728.89
    knee 717.89
  intrasellar 253.8
  iris (idiopathic) 364.60
    exudative 364.62
    implantation (surgical) (traumatic) 364.61
    miotic pupillary 364.55
    parasitic 360.13
  Iwanoff's 362.62
  jaw (bone) (aneurysmal) (extravasation)
      (hemorrhagic) (traumatic) 526.2
    developmental (odontogenic) 526.0
    fissural 526.1
  keratin 706.2
  kidney (congenital) 753.10
    acquired 593.2
    calyceal (*see also* Hydronephrosis) 591
    multiple 753.19
    pyelogenic (*see also* Hydronephrosis) 591
    simple 593.2
    single 753.11
    solitary (not congenital) 593.2
  labium (majus) (minus) 624.8
    sebaceous 624.8
  lacrimal
    apparatus 375.43
    gland or sac 375.12
  larynx 478.79
  lens 379.39
    congenital 743.39
  lip (gland) 528.5
  liver 573.8
    congenital 751.62
    hydatid (*see also* Echinococcus) 122.8
      granulosis 122.0
      multilocularis 122.5

Cyst —*continued*
  lung 518.89
    congenital 748.4
    giant bullous 492.0
  lutein 620.1
  lymphangiomatous (M9173/0) 228.1
  lymphoepithelial
    mouth 528.4
    oral soft tissue 528.4
  macula 362.54
  malignant (M8000/3)—*see* Neoplasm, by site,
      malignant
  mammary gland (sweat gland) (*see also* Cyst,
      breast) 610.0
  mandible 526.2
    dentigerous 526.0
    radicular 522.8
  maxilla 526.2
    dentigerous 526.0
    radicular 522.8
  median
    anterior maxillary 526.1
    palatal 526.1
  mediastinum (congenital) 748.8
  meibomian (gland) (retention) 373.2
    infected 373.12
  membrane, brain 348.0
  meninges (cerebral) 348.0
    spinal 349.2
  meniscus knee 717.5
  mesentery, mesenteric (gas) 568.89
    chyle 457.8
    gas 568.89
  mesonephric duct 752.89
  mesothelial
    peritoneum 568.89
    pleura (peritoneal) 568.89
  milk 611.5
  miotic pupillary (iris) 364.55
  Morgagni (hydatid) 752.89
    fallopian tube 752.11
  mouth 528.4
  Müllerian duct 752.89
    appendix testis 608.89
    cervix (embryonal) 752.41
    fallopian tube 752.11
    prostatic utricle 599.89
    vagina (embryonal) 752.41
  multilocular (ovary) (M8000/1) 239.5
  myometrium 621.8
  nabothian (follicle) (ruptured) 616.0
  nasal sinus 478.19
  nasoalveolar 528.4
  nasolabial 528.4
  nasopalatine (duct) 526.1
    anterior 526.1
  nasopharynx 478.26
  neoplastic (M8000/1)—*see also* Neoplasm, by
      site, unspecified nature
    benign (M8000/0)—*see* Neoplasm, by site, benign
      uterus 621.8
  nervous system—*see* Cyst, brain
  neuroenteric 742.59
  neuroepithelial ventricle 348.0
  nipple 610.0
  nose 478.19
    skin of 706.2
  odontogenic, developmental 526.0
  omentum (lesser) 568.89
    congenital 751.8

Cyst —*continued*
  oral soft tissue (dermoid) (epidermoid)
      (lymphoepithelial) 528.4
  ora serrata 361.19
  orbit 376.81
  ovary, ovarian (twisted) 620.2
    adherent 620.2
    chocolate 617.1
    corpus
      albicans 620.2
      luteum 620.1
    dermoid (M9084/0) 220
    developmental 752.0
    due to failure of involution NEC 620.2
    endometrial 617.1
    follicular (atretic) (graafian) (hemorrhagic)
        620.0
    hemorrhagic 620.2
    in pregnancy or childbirth 654.4
      affecting fetus or newborn 763.89
      causing obstructed labor 660.2
        affecting fetus or newborn 763.1
    multilocular (M8000/1) 239.5
    pseudomucinous (M8470/0) 220
    retention 620.2
    serous 620.2
    theca lutein 620.2
    tuberculous (*see also* Tuberculosis) 016.6
    unspecified 620.2
  oviduct 620.8
  palatal papilla (jaw) 526.1
  palate 526.1
    fissural 526.1
    median (fissural) 526.1
  palatine, of papilla 526.1
  pancreas, pancreatic 577.2
    congenital 751.7
    false 577.2
    hemorrhagic 577.2
    true 577.2
  paralabral
    hip 718.85
    shoulder 840.7
  paramesonephric duct - see Cyst, Müllerian duct
  paranephric 593.2
  para ovarian 752.11
  paraphysis, cerebri 742.4
  parasitic NEC 136.9
  parathyroid (gland) 252.8
  paratubal (fallopian) 620.8
  paraurethral duct 599.89
  paroophoron 752.11
  parotid gland 527.6
    mucous extravasation or retention 527.6
  parovarian 752.11
  pars planus 364.60
    exudative 364.64
    primary 364.63
  pelvis, female
    in pregnancy or childbirth 654.4
      affecting fetus or newborn 763.89
      causing obstructed labor 660.2
        affecting fetus or newborn 763.1
  penis (sebaceous) 607.89
  periapical 522.8
  pericardial (congenital) 746.89
    acquired (secondary) 423.8
  pericoronal 526.0
  perineural (Tarlov's) 355.9
  periodontal 522.8
    lateral 526.0

Cyst —*continued*
  peripancreatic 577.2
  peripelvic (lymphatic) 593.2
  peritoneum 568.89
    chylous 457.8
  pharynx (wall) 478.26
  pilar 704.41
  pilonidal (infected) (rectum) 685.1
    with abscess 685.0
    malignant (M9084/3) 173.59
  pituitary (duct) (gland) 253.8
  placenta (amniotic)—*see* Placenta, abnormal
  pleura 519.8
  popliteal 727.51
  porencephalic 742.4
    acquired 348.0
  postanal (infected) 685.1
    with abscess 685.0
  posterior segment of eye, congenital 743.54
  postmastoidectomy cavity 383.31
  preauricular 744.47
  prepuce 607.89
    congenital 752.69
  primordial (jaw) 526.0
  prostate 600.3
  pseudomucinous (ovary) (M8470/0) 220
  pudenda (sweat glands) 624.8
  pupillary, miotic 364.55
    sebaceous 624.8
  radicular (residual) 522.8
  radiculodental 522.8
  ranular 527.6
  Rathke's pouch 253.8
  rectum (epithelium) (mucous) 569.49
  renal—*see* Cyst, kidney
  residual (radicular) 522.8
  retention (ovary) 620.2
  retina 361.19
    macular 362.54
    parasitic 360.13
    primary 361.13
    secondary 361.14
  retroperitoneal 568.89
  sacrococcygeal (dermoid) 685.1
    with abscess 685.0
  salivary gland or duct 527.6
    mucous extravasation or retention 527.6
  Sampson's 617.1
  sclera 379.19
  scrotum (sebaceous) 706.2
    sweat glands 706.2
  sebaceous (duct) (gland) 706.2
    breast 610.8
    eyelid 374.84
    genital organ NEC
      female 629.89
      male 608.89
    scrotum 706.2
  semilunar cartilage (knee) (multiple) 717.5
  seminal vesicle 608.89
  serous (ovary) 620.2
  sinus (antral) (ethmoidal) (frontal) (maxillary)
      (nasal) (sphenoidal) 478.19
  Skene's gland 599.89
  skin (epidermal) (epidermoid, inclusion)
      (epithelial) (inclusion) (retention)
      (sebaceous) 706.2
    breast 610.8
    eyelid 374.84
    genital organ NEC
      female 629.89
      male 608.89

Cystadenoma (M8440/0)—*see also* Neoplasm,
  by site, benign
 bile duct (M8161/0) 211.5
 endometrioid (M8380/0)—*see also* Neoplasm,
  by site, benign
  borderline malignancy (M8380/1)—*see*
   Neoplasm, by site, uncertain behavior
 malignant (M8440/3)—*see* Neoplasm, by site,
  malignant
 mucinous (M8470/0)
  borderline malignancy (M8470/1)
   specified site—*see* Neoplasm, uncertain
    behavior
   unspecified site 236.2
  papillary (M8471/0)
   borderline malignancy (M8471/1)
    specified site—*see* Neoplasm, by site,
     uncertain behavior
    unspecified site 236.2
   specified site—*see* Neoplasm, by site,
    benign
   unspecified site 220
  specified site—*see* Neoplasm, by site, benign
  unspecified site 220
 papillary (M8450/0)
  borderline malignancy (M8450/1)
   specified site—*see* Neoplasm, by site,
    uncertain behavior
   unspecified site 236.2
  lymphomatosum (M8561/0) 210.2
  mucinous (M8471/0)
   borderline malignancy (M8471/1)
    specified site—*see* Neoplasm, by site,
     uncertain behavior
    unspecified site 236.2
   specified site—*see* Neoplasm, by site,
    benign
   unspecified site 220
  pseudomucinous (M8471/0)
   borderline malignancy (M8471/1)
    specified site—*see* Neoplasm, by site,
     uncertain behavior
    unspecified site 236.2
   specified site—*see* Neoplasm, by site,
    benign
   unspecified site 220
  serous (M8460/0)
   borderline malignancy (M8460/1)
    specified site—*see* Neoplasm, by site,
     uncertain behavior
    unspecified site 236.2
   specified site—*see* Neoplasm, by site,
    benign
   unspecified site 220
  specified site—*see* Neoplasm, by site, benign
  unspecified site 220
 pseudomucinous (M8470/0)
  borderline malignancy (M8470/1)
   specified site—*see* Neoplasm, by site,
    uncertain behavior
   unspecified site 236.2
  papillary (M8471/0)
   borderline malignancy (M8471/1)
    specified site—*see* Neoplasm, by site,
     uncertain behavior
    unspecified site 236.2
   specified site—*see* Neoplasm, by site,
    benign
   unspecified site 220
  specified site—*see* Neoplasm, by site, benign
  unspecified site 220

Cystadenoma—*continued*
 serous (M8441/0)
  borderline malignancy (M8441/1)
   specified site—*see* Neoplasm, by site,
    uncertain behavior
   unspecified site 236.2
  papillary (M8460/0)
   borderline malignancy (M8460/1)
    specified site—*see* Neoplasm, by site,
     uncertain behavior
    unspecified site 236.2
   specified site—*see* Neoplasm, by site,
    benign
   unspecified site 220
  specified site—*see* Neoplasm, by site, benign
  unspecified site 220
 thyroid 226
Cystathioninemia 270.4
Cystathioninuria 270.4
Cystic —*see also* condition
 breast, chronic 610.1
 corpora lutea 620.1
 degeneration, congenital
  brain 742.4
  kidney (*see also* Cystic, disease, kidney)
   753.10
 disease
  breast, chronic 610.1
  kidney, congenital 753.10
   medullary 753.16
   multiple 753.19
   polycystic—*see* Polycystic, kidney
   single 753.11
   specified NEC 753.19
  liver, congenital 751.62
  lung 518.89
   congenital 748.4
  pancreas, congenital 751.7
  semilunar cartilage 717.5
 duct—*see* condition
 eyeball, congenital 743.03
 fibrosis (pancreas) 277.00
  with
   manifestations
    gastrointestinal 277.03
    pulmonary 277.02
    specified NEC 277.09
   meconium ileus 277.01
   pulmonary exacerbation 277.02
 hygroma (M9173/0) 228.1
 kidney, congenital 753.10
  medullary 753.16
  multiple 753.19
  polycystic—*see* Polycystic, kidney
  single 753.11
  specified NEC 753.19
 liver, congenital 751.62
 lung 518.89
  congenital 748.4
 mass—*see* Cyst
 mastitis, chronic 610.1
 ovary 620.2
 pancreas, congenital 751.7
Cysticerciasis 123.1
Cysticercosis (mammary) (subretinal) 123.1
Cysticercus 123.1
 cellulosae infestation 123.1
Cystinosis (malignant) 270.0
Cystinuria 270.0

Cystitis (bacillary) (colli) (diffuse) (exudative)
    (hemorrhagic) (purulent) (recurrent) (septic)
    (suppurative) (ulcerative) 595.9
  with
    abortion—*see* Abortion, by type, with urinary
        tract infection
    ectopic pregnancy (*see also* categories
        633.0-633.9) 639.8
    fibrosis 595.1
    leukoplakia 595.1
    malakoplakia 595.1
    metaplasia 595.1
    molar pregnancy (*see also* categories 630-632)
        639.8
  actinomycotic 039.8 *[595.4]*
  acute 595.0
    of trigone 595.3
  allergic 595.89
  amebic 006.8 *[595.4]*
  bilharzial 120.9 *[595.4]*
  blennorrhagic (acute) 098.11
    chronic or duration of 2 months or more
        098.31
  bullous 595.89
  calculous 594.1
  chlamydial 099.53
  chronic 595.2
    interstitial 595.1
    of trigone 595.3
  complicating pregnancy, childbirth, or
      puerperium 646.6
    affecting fetus or newborn 760.1
  cystic(a) 595.81
  diphtheritic 032.84
  echinococcal
    granulosus 122.3 *[595.4]*
    multilocularis 122.6 *[595.4]*
  emphysematous 595.89
  encysted 595.81
  follicular 595.3
  following
    abortion 639.8
    ectopic or molar pregnancy 639.8
  gangrenous 595.89
  glandularis 595.89
  gonococcal (acute) 098.11
    chronic or duration of 2 months or more
        098.31
  incrusted 595.89
  interstitial 595.1
  irradiation 595.82
  irritation 595.89
  malignant 595.89
  monilial 112.2
  of trigone 595.3
  panmural 595.1
  polyposa 595.89
  prostatic 601.3
  radiation 595.82
  Reiter's (abacterial) 099.3
  specified NEC 595.89
  subacute 595.2
  submucous 595.1
  syphilitic 095.8
  trichomoniasis 131.09
  tuberculous (*see also* Tuberculosis) 016.1
  ulcerative 595.1

Cystocele
  female (without uterine prolapse) 618.01
    with uterine prolapse 618.4
      complete 618.3
      incomplete 618.2
    lateral 618.02
    midline 618.01
    paravaginal 618.02
  in pregnancy or childbirth 654.4
    affecting fetus or newborn 763.89
    causing obstructed labor 660.2
      affecting fetus or newborn 763.1
  male 596.89
Cystoid
  cicatrix limbus 372.64
  degeneration macula 362.53
Cystolithiasis 594.1
Cystoma (M8440/0)—*see also* Neoplasm, by
    site, benign
  endometrial, ovary 617.1
  mucinous (M8470/0)
    specified site—*see* Neoplasm, by site, benign
    unspecified site 220
  serous (M8441/0)
    specified site—*see* Neoplasm, by site, benign
    unspecified site 220
  simple (ovary) 620.2
Cystoplegia 596.53
Cystoptosis 596.89
Cystopyelitis (*see also* Pyelitis) 590.80
Cystorrhagia 596.89
Cystosarcoma phyllodes (M9020/1) 238.3
  benign (M9020/0) 217
  malignant (M9020/3)—*see* Neoplasm, breast,
    malignant
Cystostomy status V44.50
  appendico-vesicostomy V44.52
  cutaneous-vesicostomy V44.51
  specified type NEC V44.59
  with complication 596.83
    infection 596.81
    mechanical 596.82
    specified complication NEC 596.83
Cystourethritis (*see also* Urethritis) 597.89
Cystourethrocele (*see also* Cystocele)
  female (without uterine prolapse) 618.09
    with uterine prolapse 618.4
      complete 618.3
      incomplete 618.2
  male 596.89
Cytomegalic inclusion disease 078.5
  congenital 771.1
Cytomycosis, reticuloendothelial (*see also*
    Histoplasmosis, American) 115.00
Cytopenia 289.9
  refractory
    with
      multilineage dysplasia (RCMD) 238.72
        and ringed sideroblasts (RCMD-RS)
          238.72

D

Daae (-Finsen) disease (epidemic pleurodynia) 074.1
Dabney's grip 074.1
Da Costa's syndrome (neurocirculatory asthenia) 306.2
Dacryoadenitis, dacryadenitis 375.00
  acute 375.01
  chronic 375.02
Dacryocystitis 375.30
  acute 375.32
  chronic 375.42
  neonatal 771.6
  phlegmonous 375.33
  syphilitic 095.8
    congenital 090.0
  trachomatous, active 076.1
    late effect 139.1
  tuberculous (*see also* Tuberculosis) 017.3
Dacryocystoblennorrhea 375.42
Dacryocystocele 375.43
Dacryolith, dacryolithiasis 375.57
Dacryoma 375.43
Dacryopericystitis (acute) (subacute) 375.32
  chronic 375.42
Dacryops 375.11
Dacryosialadenopathy, atrophic 710.2
Dacryostenosis 375.56
  congenital 743.65
Dactylitis
  bone (*see also* Osteomyelitis) 730.2
  sickle-cell 282.62
    Hb-C 282.64
    Hb-SS 282.62
    specified NEC 282.69
  syphilitic 095.5
  tuberculous (*see also* Tuberculosis) 015.5
Dactylolysis spontanea 136.0
Dactylosymphysis (*see also* Syndactylism) 755.10
Damage
  arteriosclerotic—*see* Arteriosclerosis
  brain 348.9
    anoxic, hypoxic 348.1
      during or resulting from a procedure 997.01
      ischemic, in newborn 768.70
        mild 768.71
        moderate 768.72
        severe 768.73
    child NEC 343.9
    due to birth injury 767.0
    minimal (child) (*see also* Hyperkinesia) 314.9
    newborn 767.0
  cardiac—*see also* Disease, heart
  cardiorenal (vascular) (*see also* Hypertension, cardiorenal) 404.90
  central nervous system—*see* Damage, brain
  cerebral NEC—*see* Damage, brain
  coccyx, complicating delivery 665.6
  coronary (*see also* Ischemia, heart) 414.9
  eye, birth injury 767.8
  heart—*see also* Disease, heart
    valve—*see* Endocarditis
  hypothalamus NEC 348.9
  liver 571.9
    alcoholic 571.3
  medication 995.20

Damage—*continued*
  myocardium (*see also* Degeneration, myocardial) 429.1
  pelvic
    joint or ligament, during delivery 665.6
    organ NEC
      with
        abortion—*see* Abortion, by type, with damage to pelvic organs
        ectopic pregnancy (*see also* categories 633.0-633.9) 639.2
        molar pregnancy (*see also* categories 630-632) 639.2
      during delivery 665.5
      following
        abortion 639.2
        ectopic or molar pregnancy 639.2
  renal (*see also* Disease, renal) 593.9
  skin, solar 692.79
    acute 692.72
    chronic 692.74
  subendocardium, subendocardial (*see also* Degeneration, myocardial) 429.1
  vascular 459.9
Dameshek's syndrome (erythroblastic anemia) 282.49
Dana-Putnam syndrome (subacute combined sclerosis with pernicious anemia) 281.0
  [336.2]
Danbolt (-Closs) syndrome (acrodermatitis enteropathica) 686.8
Dandruff 690.18
Dandy fever 061
Dandy-Walker deformity or syndrome (atresia, foramen of Magendie) 742.3
  with spina bifida (*see also* Spina bifida) 741.0
Dangle foot 736.79
Danielssen's disease (anesthetic leprosy) 030.1
Danlos' syndrome 756.83
Darier's disease (congenital) (keratosis follicularis) 757.39
  due to vitamin A deficiency 264.8
  meaning erythema annulare centrifugum 695.0
Darier-Roussy sarcoid 135
Dark area on retina 239.81
Darling's
  disease (*see also* Histoplasmosis, American) 115.00
  histoplasmosis (*see also* Histoplasmosis, American) 115.00
Dartre 054.9
Darwin's tubercle 744.29
Davidson's anemia (refractory) 284.9
Davies' disease 425.0
Davies-Colley syndrome (slipping rib) 733.99
Dawson's encephalitis 046.2
Day blindness (*see also* Blindness, day) 368.60
Dead
  fetus
    retained (in utero) 656.4
      early pregnancy (death before 22 completed weeks gestation) 632
      late (death after 22 completed weeks gestation) 656.4
    syndrome 641.3
  labyrinth 386.50
  ovum, retained 631.8

Deaf and dumb NEC 389.7
Deaf mutism (acquired) (congenital) NEC 389.7
  endemic 243
  hysterical 300.11
  syphilitic, congenital 090.0
Deafness (acquired) (complete) (congenital)
  (hereditary) (middle ear) (partial) 389.9
  with
    blindness V49.85
    blue sclera and fragility of bone 756.51
  auditory fatigue 389.9
  aviation 993.0
    nerve injury 951.5
  boilermakers' 951.5
  central 389.14
    with conductive hearing loss 389.20
      bilateral 389.22
      unilateral 389.21
  conductive (air) 389.00
    with sensorineural hearing loss 389.20
      bilateral 389.22
      unilateral 389.21
    bilateral 389.06
    combined types 389.08
    external ear 389.01
    inner ear 389.04
    middle ear 389.03
    multiple types 389.08
    tympanic membrane 389.02
    unilateral 389.05
  emotional (complete) 300.11
  functional (complete) 300.11
  high frequency 389.8
  hysterical (complete) 300.11
  injury 951.5
  low frequency 389.8
  mental 784.69
  mixed conductive and sensorineural 389.20
    bilateral 389.22
    unilateral 389.21
  nerve
    with conductive hearing loss 389.20
      bilateral 389.22
      unilateral 389.21
    bilateral 389.12
    unilateral 389.13
  neural
    with conductive hearing loss 389.20
      bilateral 389.22
      unilateral 389.21
    bilateral 389.12
    unilateral 389.13
  noise-induced 388.12
    nerve injury 951.5
  nonspeaking 389.7
  perceptive 389.10
    with conductive hearing loss 389.20
      bilateral 389.22
      unilateral 389.21
    central 389.14
    neural
      bilateral 389.12
      unilateral 389.13
    sensorineural 389.10
      asymmetrical 389.16
      bilateral 389.18
      unilateral 389.15
    sensory
      bilateral 389.11
      unilateral 389.17
  psychogenic (complete) 306.7

Deafness—*continued*
  sensorineural (*see also* Deafness, perceptive)
    389.10
    asymmetrical 389.16
    bilateral 389.18
    unilateral 389.15
  sensory
    with conductive hearing loss 389.20
      bilateral 389.22
      unilateral 389.21
    bilateral 389.11
    unilateral 389.17
  specified type NEC 389.8
  sudden NEC 388.2
  syphilitic 094.89
  transient ischemic 388.02
  transmission—*see* Deafness, conductive
  traumatic 951.5
  word (secondary to organic lesion) 784.69
    developmental 315.31
Death
  after delivery (cause not stated) (sudden) 674.9
  anesthetic
    due to
      correct substance properly administered
        995.4
      overdose or wrong substance given 968.4
        specified anesthetic—*see* Table of drugs
          and chemicals
    during delivery 668.9
  brain 348.82
  cardiac (sudden) (SCD)—code to underlying
    condition
    family history of V17.41
    personal history of, successfully resuscitated
      V12.53
  cause unknown 798.2
  cot (infant) 798.0
  crib (infant) 798.0
  fetus, fetal (cause not stated) (intrauterine) 779.9
    early, with retention (before 22 completed
      weeks gestation) 632
    from asphyxia or anoxia (before labor) 768.0
      during labor 768.1
    late, affecting management of pregnancy (after
      22 completed weeks gestation) 656.4
  from pregnancy NEC 646.9
  instantaneous 798.1
  intrauterine (*see also* Death, fetus) 779.9
    complicating pregnancy 656.4
  maternal, affecting fetus or newborn 761.6
  neonatal NEC 779.9
  sudden (cause unknown) 798.1
    cardiac (SCD)
      family history of V17.41
      personal history of, successfully resuscitated
        V12.53
    during delivery 669.9
      under anesthesia NEC 668.9
    infant, syndrome (SIDS) 798.0
    puerperal, during puerperium 674.9
  unattended (cause unknown) 798.9
  under anesthesia NEC
    due to
      correct substance properly administered
        995.4
      overdose or wrong substance given 968.4
        specified anesthetic—*see* Table of drugs
          and chemicals
    during delivery 668.9
  violent 798.1

de Beurmann-Gougerot disease (sporotrichosis) 117.1

Debility (general) (infantile) (postinfectional) 799.3
  with nutritional difficulty 269.9
  congenital or neonatal NEC 779.9
  nervous 300.5
  old age 797
  senile 797

Débove's disease (splenomegaly) 789.2

Decalcification
  bone (see also Osteoporosis) 733.00
  teeth 521.89

Decapitation 874.9
  fetal (to facilitate delivery) 763.89

Decapsulation, kidney 593.89

Decay
  dental 521.00
  senile 797
  tooth, teeth 521.00

Decensus, uterus —see Prolapse, uterus

Deciduitis (acute)
  with
    abortion—see Abortion, by type, with sepsis
    ectopic pregnancy (see also categories 633.0-633.9) 639.0
    molar pregnancy (see also categories 630-632) 639.0
  affecting fetus or newborn 760.8
  following
    abortion 639.0
    ectopic or molar pregnancy 639.0
  in pregnancy 646.6
  puerperal, postpartum 670.1

Deciduoma malignum (M9100/3) 181

Deciduous tooth (retained) 520.6

Decline (general) (see also Debility) 799.3

Decompensation
  cardiac (acute) (chronic) (see also Disease, heart) 429.9
    failure—see Failure, heart
  cardiorenal (see also Hypertension, cardiorenal) 404.90
  cardiovascular (see also Disease, cardiovascular) 429.2
  heart (see also Disease, heart) 429.9
    failure—see Failure, heart
  hepatic 572.2
  myocardial (acute) (chronic) (see also Disease, heart) 429.9
    failure—see Failure, heart
  respiratory 519.9

Decompression sickness 993.3

Decrease, decreased
  blood
    platelets (see also Thrombocytopenia) 287.5
    pressure 796.3
      due to shock following
        injury 958.4
        operation 998.00
    white cell count 288.50
      specified NEC 288.59
  cardiac reserve—see Disease, heart
  estrogen 256.39
    postablative 256.2
  fetal movements 655.7
  fragility of erythrocytes 289.89
  function
    adrenal (cortex) 255.41
      medulla 255.5
    ovary in hypopituitarism 253.4

Decrease, decreased—continued
  parenchyma of pancreas 577.8
  pituitary (gland) (lobe) (anterior) 253.2
    posterior (lobe) 253.8
  functional activity 780.99
  glucose 790.29
  haptoglobin (serum) NEC 273.8
  leukocytes 288.50
  libido 799.81
  lymphocytes 288.51
  platelets (see also Thrombocytopenia) 287.5
  pulse pressure 785.9
  respiration due to shock following injury 958.4
  sexual desire 799.81
  tear secretion NEC 375.15
  tolerance
    fat 579.8
    salt and water 276.9
  vision NEC 369.9
  white blood cell count 288.50

Decubital gangrene (see also Ulcer, pressure) 707.00 [785.4]

Decubiti (see also Ulcer, pressure) 707.00

Decubitus (ulcer) (see also Ulcer, pressure) 707.00
  with gangrene 707.00 [785.4]
  ankle 707.06
  back
    lower 707.03
    upper 707.02
  buttock 707.05
  coccyx 707.03
  elbow 707.01
  head 707.09
  heel 707.07
  hip 707.04
  other site 707.09
  sacrum 707.03
  shoulder blades 707.02

Deepening acetabulum 718.85

Defect, defective 759.9
  3-beta-hydroxysteroid dehydrogenase 255.2
  11-hydroxylase 255.2
  21-hydroxylase 255.2
  abdominal wall, congenital 756.70
  aorticopulmonary septum 745.0
  aortic septal 745.0
  atrial septal (ostium secundum type) 745.5
    acquired 429.71
    ostium primum type 745.61
    sinus venosus 745.8
  atrioventricular
    canal 745.69
    septum 745.4
      acquired 429.71
  atrium secundum 745.5
    acquired 429.71
  auricular septal 745.5
    acquired 429.71
  bilirubin excretion 277.4
  biosynthesis, testicular androgen 257.2
  bridge 525.60
  bulbar septum 745.0
  butanol-insoluble iodide 246.1
  chromosome—see Anomaly, chromosome
  circulation (acquired) 459.9
    congenital 747.9
    newborn 747.9
  clotting NEC (see also Defect, coagulation) 286.9

Defect, defective—*continued*
coagulation (factor) (*see also* Deficiency,
    coagulation factor) 286.9
  with
    abortion—*see* Abortion, by type, with
      hemorrhage
    ectopic pregnancy (*see also* categories
      634-638) 639.1
    molar pregnancy (*see also* categories
      630-632) 639.1
  acquired (any) 286.7
  antepartum or intrapartum 641.3
    affecting fetus or newborn 762.1
  causing hemorrhage of pregnancy or delivery
    641.3
  complicating pregnancy, childbirth, or the
    puerperium 649.3
  due to
    liver disease 286.7
    vitamin K deficiency 286.7
  newborn, transient 776.3
  postpartum 666.3
  specified type NEC 286.9
conduction (heart) 426.9
  bone (*see also* Deafness, conductive) 389.00
congenital, organ or site NEC—*see also*
  Anomaly
circulation 747.9
Descemet's membrane 743.9
  specified type NEC 743.49
diaphragm 756.6
ectodermal 757.9
esophagus 750.9
pulmonic cusps—*see* Anomaly, heart valve
respiratory system 748.9
  specified type NEC 748.8
crown 525.60
cushion endocardial 745.60
dental restoration 525.60
dentin (hereditary) 520.5
Descemet's membrane (congenital) 743.9
  acquired 371.30
  specific type NEC 743.49
deutan 368.52
developmental—*see also* Anomaly, by site
  cauda equina 742.59
  left ventricle 746.9
    with atresia or hypoplasia of aortic orifice or
      valve, with hypoplasia of ascending
      aorta 746.7
    in hypoplastic left heart syndrome 746.7
  testis 752.9
  vessel 747.9
diaphragm
  with elevation, eventration, or hernia—*see*
    Hernia, diaphragm
  congenital 756.6
    with elevation, eventration, or hernia 756.6
    gross (with elevation, eventration, or hernia)
      756.6
ectodermal, congenital 757.9
Eisenmenger's (ventricular septal defect) 745.4
endocardial cushion 745.60
  specified type NEC 745.69
esophagus, congenital 750.9
extensor retinaculum 728.9
fibrin polymerization (*see also* Defect,
  coagulation) 286.3

Defect, defective—*continued*
filling
  biliary tract 793.3
  bladder 793.5
  dental 525.60
  gallbladder 793.3
  kidney 793.5
  stomach 793.4
  ureter 793.5
fossa ovalis 745.5
gene, carrier (suspected) of V83.89
Gerbode 745.4
glaucomatous, without elevated tension 365.89
Hageman (factor) (*see also* Defect, coagulation)
  286.3
hearing (*see also* Deafness) 389.9
high grade 317
homogentisic acid 270.2
interatrial septal 745.5
  acquired 429.71
interauricular septal 745.5
  acquired 429.71
interventricular septal 745.4
  with pulmonary stenosis or atresia,
    dextroposition of aorta, and hypertrophy of
    right ventricle 745.2
  acquired 429.71
  in tetralogy of Fallot 745.2
iodide trapping 246.1
iodotyrosine dehalogenase 246.1
kynureninase 270.2
learning, specific 315.2
major osseous 731.3
mental (*see also* Disability, intellectual) 319
osseous, major 731.3
osteochondral NEC 738.8
ostium
  primum 745.61
  secundum 745.5
pericardium 746.89
peroxidase-binding 246.1
placental blood supply—*see* Placenta,
  insufficiency
platelet (qualitative) 287.1
  constitutional 286.4
postural, spine 737.9
protan 368.51
pulmonic cusps, congenital 746.00
renal pelvis 753.9
  obstructive 753.29
  specified type NEC 753.3
respiratory system, congenital 748.9
  specified type NEC 748.8
retina, retinal 361.30
  with detachment (*see also* Detachment, retina,
    with retinal defect) 361.00
  multiple 361.33
    with detachment 361.02
  nerve fiber bundle 362.85
  single 361.30
    with detachment 361.01
septal (closure) (heart) NEC 745.9
  acquired 429.71
  atrial 745.5
  specified type NEC 745.8
speech NEC 784.59
  developmental 315.39
  late effect of cerebrovascular disease — *see*
    Late effect(s) (of) cerebrovascular disease,
    speech and language deficit
  secondary to organic lesion 784.59

Defect, defective—*continued*
Taussig-Bing (transposition, aorta and overriding pulmonary artery) 745.11
teeth, wedge 521.20
thyroid hormone synthesis 246.1
tritan 368.53
ureter 753.9
  obstructive 753.29
vascular (acquired) (local) 459.9
  congenital (peripheral) NEC 747.60
    gastrointestinal 747.61
    lower limb 747.64
    renal 747.62
    specified NEC 747.69
    spinal 747.82
    upper limb 747.63
ventricular septal 745.4
  with pulmonary stenosis or atresia, dextraposition of aorta, and hypertrophy of right ventricle 745.2
  acquired 429.71
  atrioventricular canal type 745.69
  between infundibulum and anterior portion 745.4
  in tetralogy of Fallot 745.2
  isolated anterior 745.4
vision NEC 369.9
visual field 368.40
  arcuate 368.43
  heteronymous, bilateral 368.47
  homonymous, bilateral 368.46
  localized NEC 368.44
  nasal step 368.44
  peripheral 368.44
  sector 368.43
voice and resonance 784.40
wedge, teeth (abrasion) 521.20
Defeminization syndrome 255.2
Deferentitis 608.4
  gonorrheal (acute) 098.14
  chronic or duration of 2 months or over 098.34
Defibrination syndrome (*see also* Fibrinolysis) 286.6
Deficiency, deficient
3-beta-hydroxysteroid dehydrogenase 255.2
6-phosphogluconic dehydrogenase (anemia) 282.2
11-beta-hydroxylase 255.2
17-alpha-hydroxylase 255.2
18-hydroxysteroid dehydrogenase 255.2
20-alpha-hydroxylase 255.2
21-hydroxylase 255.2
AAT (alpha-1 antitrypsin) 273.4
abdominal muscle syndrome 756.79
accelerator globulin (Ac G) (blood) (*see also* Defect, coagulation) 286.3
AC globulin (congenital) (*see also* Defect, coagulation) 286.3
  acquired 286.7
activating factor (blood) (*see also* Defect, coagulation) 286.3
adenohypophyseal 253.2
adenosine deaminase 277.2
aldolase (hereditary) 271.2
alpha-1-antitrypsin 273.4
alpha-1-trypsin inhibitor 273.4
alpha-fucosidase 271.8
alpha-lipoprotein 272.5
alpha-mannosidase 271.8
amino acid 270.9
anemia—*see* Anemia, deficiency

Deficiency, deficient—*continued*
aneurin 265.1
  with beriberi 265.0
antibody NEC 279.00
antidiuretic hormone 253.5
antihemophilic
  factor (A) 286.0
    B 286.1
    C 286.2
  globulin (AHG) NEC 286.0
antithrombin III 289.81
antitrypsin 273.4
argininosuccinate synthetase or lyase 270.6
ascorbic acid (with scurvy) 267
autoprothrombin
  I (*see also* Defect, coagulation) 286.3
  II 286.1
  C (*see also* Defect, coagulation) 286.3
bile salt 579.8
biotin 266.2
biotinidase 277.6
bradykinase-1 277.6
brancher enzyme (amylopectinosis) 271.0
calciferol 268.9
  with
    osteomalacia 268.2
    rickets (*see also* Rickets) 268.0
calcium 275.40
  dietary 269.3
calorie, severe 261
carbamyl phosphate synthetase 270.6
cardiac (*see also* Insufficiency, myocardial) 428.0
carnitine 277.81
  due to
    hemodialysis 277.83
    inborn errors of metabolism 277.82
    valproic acid therapy 277.83
  iatrogenic 277.83
  palmitoyltransferase (CPT1, CPT2) 277.85
  palmityl transferase (CPT1, CPT2) 277.85
  primary 277.81
  secondary 277.84
carotene 264.9
Carr factor (*see also* Defect, coagulation) 286.9
central nervous system 349.9
ceruloplasmin 275.1
cevitamic acid (with scurvy) 267
choline 266.2
Christmas factor 286.1
chromium 269.3
citrin 269.1
clotting (blood) (*see also* Defect, coagulation) 286.9
coagulation factor NEC 286.9
  with
    abortion—*see* Abortion, by type, with hemorrhage
    ectopic pregnancy (*see also* categories 634-638) 639.1
    molar pregnancy (*see also* categories 630-632) 639.1
  acquired (any) 286.7
  antepartum or intrapartum 641.3
    affecting fetus or newborn 762.1
  complicating pregnancy, childbirth, or the puerperium 649.3
  due to
    liver disease 286.7
    vitamin K deficiency 286.7
  newborn, transient 776.3

Deficiency, deficient—*continued*
  coagulation factor —*continued*
    postpartum 666.3
    specified type NEC 286.3
  color vision (congenital) 368.59
    acquired 368.55
  combined glucocorticoid and mineralocorticoid
    255.41
  combined, two or more coagulation factors (*see
    also* Defect, coagulation) 286.9
  complement factor NEC 279.8
  contact factor (*see also* Defect, coagulation)
    286.3
  copper NEC 275.1
  corticoadrenal 255.41
  craniofacial axis 756.0
  cyanocobalamin (vitamin B$_{12}$) 266.2
  debrancher enzyme (limit dextrinosis) 271.0
  desmolase 255.2
  diet 269.9
  dihydrofolate reductase 281.2
  dihydropteridine reductase 270.1
  dihydropyrimidine dehydrogenase (DPD) 277.6
  disaccharidase (intestinal) 271.3
  disease NEC 269.9
  ear(s) V48.8
  edema 262
  endocrine 259.9
  enzymes, circulating NEC (*see also* Deficiency,
    by specific enzyme) 277.6
  ergosterol 268.9
    with
      osteomalacia 268.2
      rickets (*see also* Rickets) 268.0
  erythrocytic glutathione (anemia) 282.2
  eyelid(s) V48.8
  factor (*see also* Defect, coagulation) 286.9
    I (congenital) (fibrinogen) 286.3
      antepartum or intrapartum 641.3
        affecting fetus or newborn 762.1
      newborn, transient 776.3
      postpartum 666.3
    II (congenital) (prothrombin) 286.3
    V (congenital) (labile) 286.3
    VII (congenital) (stable) 286.3
    VIII (congenital) (functional) 286.0
      with
        functional defect 286.0
        vascular defect 286.4
    IX (Christmas) (congenital) (functional) 286.1
    X (congenital) (Stuart-Prower) 286.3
    XI (congenital) (plasma thromboplastin
      antecedent) 286.2
    XII (congenital) (Hageman) 286.3
    XIII (congenital) (fibrin stabilizing) 286.3
    Hageman 286.3
    multiple (congenital) 286.9
      acquired 286.7
  fibrinase (*see also* Defect, coagulation) 286.3
  fibrinogen (congenital) (*see also* Defect,
    coagulation) 286.3
    acquired 286.6
  fibrin stabilizing factor (congenital) (*see also*
    Defect, coagulation) 286.3
    acquired 286.7
  finger—*see* Absence, finger
  Fletcher factor (*see also* Defect, coagulation)
    286.9
  fluorine 269.3
  folate, anemia 281.2
  folic acid (vitamin B$_c$) 266.2
    anemia 281.2

Deficiency, deficient—*continued*
  follicle-stimulating hormone (FSH) 253.4
  fructokinase 271.2
  fructose-1, 6-diphosphate 271.2
  fructose-1-phosphate aldolase 271.2
  FSH (follicle-stimulating hormone) 253.4
  fucosidase 271.8
  galactokinase 271.1
  galactose-1-phosphate uridyl transferase 271.1
  gamma globulin in blood 279.00
  glass factor (*see also* Defect, coagulation) 286.3
  glucocorticoid 255.41
  glucose-6-phosphatase 271.0
  glucose-6-phosphate dehydrogenase anemia 282.2
  glucuronyl transferase 277.4
  glutathione-reductase (anemia) 282.2
  glycogen synthetase 271.0
  growth hormone 253.3
  Hageman factor (congenital) (*see also* Defect,
    coagulation) 286.3
  head V48.0
  hemoglobin (*see also* Anemia) 285.9
  hepatophosphorylase 271.0
  hexose monophosphate (HMP) shunt 282.2
  HGH (human growth hormone) 253.3
  HG-PRT 277.2
  homogentisic acid oxidase 270.2
  hormone—*see also* Deficiency, by specific
      hormone
    anterior pituitary (isolated) (partial) NEC
      253.4
      growth (human) 253.3
    follicle-stimulating 253.4
    growth (human) (isolated) 253.3
    human growth 253.3
    interstitial cell-stimulating 253.4
    luteinizing 253.4
    melanocyte-stimulating 253.4
    testicular 257.2
  human growth hormone 253.3
  humoral 279.00
    with
      hyper-IgM 279.05
        autosomal recessive 279.05
        X-linked 279.05
      increased IgM 279.05
    congenital hypogammaglobulinemia 279.04
      non-sex-linked 279.06
    selective immunoglobulin NEC 279.03
      IgA 279.01
      IgG 279.03
      IgM 279.02
        increased 279.05
    specified NEC 279.09
  hydroxylase 255.2
  hypoxanthine-guanine
      phosphoribosyltransferase (HG-PRT) 277.2
  ICSH (interstitial cell-stimulating hormone)
      253.4
  immunity NEC 279.3
    cell-mediated 279.10
      with
        hyperimmunoglobulinemia 279.2
        thrombocytopenia and eczema 279.12
      specified NEC 279.19
    combined (severe) 279.2
      syndrome 279.2
    common variable 279.06
    humoral NEC 279.00
      IgA (secretory) 279.01
      IgG 279.03
      IgM 279.02

Deficiency, deficient—*continued*
immunoglobulin, selective NEC 279.03
 IgA 279.01
 IgG 279.03
 IgM 279.02
inositol (B complex) 266.2
interferon 279.49
internal organ V47.0
interstitial cell-stimulating hormone (ICSH)
 253.4
intrinsic (urethral) sphincter (ISD) 599.82
intrinsic factor (Castle's) (congenital) 281.0
invertase 271.3
iodine 269.3
iron, anemia 280.9
labile factor (congenital) (*see also* Defect,
 coagulation) 286.3
 acquired 286.7
lacrimal fluid (acquired) 375.15
 congenital 743.64
lactase 271.3
Laki-Lorand factor (*see also* Defect,
 coagulation) 286.3
lecithin-cholesterol acyltranferase 272.5
LH (luteinizing hormone) 253.4
limb V49.0
 lower V49.0
  congenital (*see also* Deficiency, lower limb,
   congenital) 755.30
 upper V49.0
  congenital (*see also* Deficiency, upper limb,
   congenital) 755.20
lipocaic 577.8
lipoid (high-density) 272.5
lipoprotein (familial) (high density) 272.5
liver phosphorylase 271.0
long chain 3-hydroxyacyl CoA dehydrogenase
 (LCHAD) 277.85
long chain/very long chain acyl CoA
 dehydrogenase (LCAD, VLCAD) 277.85
lower limb V49.0
 congenital 755.30
  with complete absence of distal elements
   755.31
  longitudinal (complete) (partial) (with distal
   deficiencies, incomplete) 755.32
   with complete absence of distal elements
    755.31
   combined femoral, tibial, fibular
    (incomplete) 755.33
   femoral 755.34
   fibular 755.37
   metatarsal(s) 755.38
   phalange(s) 755.39
    meaning all digits 755.31
   tarsal(s) 755.38
   tibia 755.36
   tibiofibular 755.35
  transverse 755.31
luteinizing hormone (LH) 253.4
lysosomal alpha-1, 4 glucosidase 271.0
magnesium 275.2
mannosidase 271.8
medium chain acyl CoA dehydrogenase
 (MCAD) 277.85
melanocyte-stimulating hormone (MSH) 253.4
menadione (vitamin K) 269.0
 newborn 776.0
mental (familial) (hereditary) (*see also*
 Disability, intellectual) 319

Deficiency, deficient—*continued*
methylenetetrahydrofolate reductase (MTHFR)
 270.4
mineral NEC 269.3
mineralocorticoid 255.42
molybdenum 269.3
moral 301.7
multiple, syndrome 260
myocardial (*see also* Insufficiency myocardial)
 428.0
myophosphorylase 271.0
NADH (DPNH) -methemoglobin-reductase
 (congenital) 289.7
NADH diaphorase or reductase (congenital)
 289.7
neck V48.1
niacin (amide) (-tryptophan) 265.2
nicotinamide 265.2
nicotinic acid (amide) 265.2
nose V48.8
number of teeth (*see also* Anodontia) 520.0
nutrition, nutritional 269.9
 specified NEC 269.8
ornithine transcarbamylase 270.6
ovarian 256.39
oxygen (*see also* Anoxia) 799.02
pantothenic acid 266.2
parathyroid (gland) 252.1
phenylalanine hydroxylase 270.1
phosphoenolpyruvate carboxykinase 271.8
phosphofructokinase 271.2
phosphoglucomutase 271.0
phosphohexosisomerase 271.0
phosphomannomutase 271.8
phosphomannose isomerase 271.8
phosphomannosyl mutase 271.8
phosphorylase kinase, liver 271.0
pituitary (anterior) 253.2
 posterior 253.5
placenta—*see* Placenta, insufficiency
plasma
 cell 279.00
 protein (paraproteinemia) (pyroglobulinemia)
  273.8
  gamma globulin 279.00
 thromboplastin
  antecedent (PTA) 286.2
  component (PTC) 286.1
platelet NEC 287.1
 constitutional 286.4
polyglandular 258.9
potassium (K) 276.8
proaccelerin (congenital) (*see also* Defect,
 congenital) 286.3
 acquired 286.7
proconvertin factor (congenital) (*see also*
 Defect, coagulation) 286.3
 acquired 286.7
prolactin 253.4
protein 260
 anemia 281.4
 C 289.81
 plasma—*see* Deficiency, plasma, protein
 S 289.81
prothrombin (congenital) (*see also* Defect,
 coagulation) 286.3
 acquired 286.7
Prower factor (*see also* Defect, coagulation)
 286.3
PRT 277.2
pseudocholinesterase 289.89

Deficiency, deficient—*continued*
psychobiological 301.6
PTA 286.2
PTC 286.1
purine nucleoside phosphorylase 277.2
pyracin (alpha) (beta) 266.1
pyridoxal 266.1
pyridoxamine 266.1
pyridoxine (derivatives) 266.1
pyruvate carboxylase 271.8
pyruvate dehydrogenase 271.8
pyruvate kinase (PK) 282.3
riboflavin (vitamin B_2) 266.0
saccadic eye movements 379.57
salivation 527.7
salt 276.1
secretion
  ovary 256.39
  salivary gland (any) 527.7
  urine 788.5
selenium 269.3
serum
  antitrypsin, familial 273.4
  protein (congenital) 273.8
short chain acyl CoA dehydrogenase (SCAD) 277.85
short stature homeobox gene (SHOX)
with
  dyschondrosteosis 756.89
  short stature (idiopathic) 783.43
  Turner's syndrome 758.6
smooth pursuit movements (eye) 379.58
sodium (Na) 276.1
SPCA (*see also* Defect, coagulation) 286.3
specified NEC 269.8
stable factor (congenital) (*see also* Defect, coagulation) 286.3
  acquired 286.7
Stuart (-Prower) factor (*see also* Defect, coagulation) 286.3
sucrase 271.3
sucrase-isomaltase 271.3
sulfite oxidase 270.0
syndrome, multiple 260
thiamine, thiaminic (chloride) 265.1
thrombokinase (*see also* Defect, coagulation) 286.3
  newborn 776.0
thrombopoieten 287.39
thymolymphatic 279.2
thyroid (gland) 244.9
tocopherol 269.1
toe—*see* Absence, toe
tooth bud (*see also* Anodontia) 520.0
trunk V48.1
UDPG-glycogen transferase 271.0
upper limb V49.0
  congenital 755.20
    with complete absence of distal elements 755.21
    longitudinal (complete) (partial) (with distal deficiencies, incomplete) 755.22
      carpal(s) 755.28
      combined humeral, radial, ulnar (incomplete) 755.23
      humeral 755.24
      metacarpal(s) 755.28
      phalange(s) 755.29
        meaning all digits 755.21
      radial 755.26
      radioulnar 755.25
      ulnar 755.27
    transverse (complete) (partial) 755.21

Deficiency, deficient—*continued*
vascular 459.9
vasopressin 253.5
viosterol (*see also* Deficiency, calciferol) 268.9
vitamin (multiple) NEC 269.2
  A 264.9
  with
    Bitôt's spot 264.1
      corneal 264.2
        with corneal ulceration 264.3
    keratomalacia 264.4
    keratosis, follicular 264.8
    night blindness 264.5
    scar of cornea, xerophthalmic 264.6
    specified manifestation NEC 264.8
      ocular 264.7
    xeroderma 264.8
    xerophthalmia 264.7
    xerosis
      conjunctival 264.0
        with Bitôt's spot 264.1
      corneal 264.2
        with corneal ulceration 264.3
  B (complex) NEC 266.9
  with
    beriberi 265.0
    pellagra 265.2
    specified type NEC 266.2
  B_1 NEC 265.1
    beriberi 265.0
  B_2 266.0
  B_6 266.1
  B_{12} 266.2
  B_c (folic acid) 266.2
  C (ascorbic acid) (with scurvy) 267
  D (calciferol) (ergosterol) 268.9
  with
    osteomalacia 268.2
    rickets (*see also* Rickets) 268.0
  E 269.1
  folic acid 266.2
  G 266.0
  H 266.2
  K 269.0
    of newborn 776.0
  nicotinic acid 265.2
  P 269.1
  PP 265.2
  specified NEC 269.1
  zinc 269.3
Deficient —*see also* Deficiency
blink reflex 374.45
craniofacial axis 756.0
number of teeth (*see also* Anodontia) 520.0
secretion of urine 788.5
Deficit
attention 799.51
cognitive communication 799.52
concentration 799.51
executive function 799.55
frontal lobe 799.55
neurologic NEC 781.99
  due to
    cerebrovascular lesion (*see also* Disease, cerebrovascular, acute) 436
    late effect—*see* Late effect(s) (of) cerebrovascular disease
    transient ischemic attack 435.9

Deficit—*continued*
  neurologic—*continued*
    ischemic
      reversible (RIND) 434.91
        history of (personal) V12.54
      prolonged (PRIND) 434.91
        history of (personal) V12.54
    oxygen 799.02
    psychomotor 799.54
    visuospatial 799.53
Deflection
  radius 736.09
  septum (acquired) (nasal) (nose) 470
  spine—*see* Curvature, spine
  turbinate (nose) 470
Defluvium
  capillorum (*see also* Alopecia) 704.00
  ciliorum 374.55
  unguium 703.8
Deformity 738.9
  abdomen, congenital 759.9
  abdominal wall
    acquired 738.8
    congenital 756.70
    muscle deficiency syndrome 756.79
  acquired (unspecified site) 738.9
    specified site NEC 738.8
  adrenal gland (congenital) 759.1
  alimentary tract, congenital 751.9
    lower 751.5
      specified type NEC 751.8
    upper (any part, except tongue) 750.9
      specified type NEC 750.8
      tongue 750.10
        specified type NEC 750.19
  ankle (joint) (acquired) 736.70
    abduction 718.47
    congenital 755.69
    contraction 718.47
    specified NEC 736.79
  anus (congenital) 751.5
    acquired 569.49
  aorta (congenital) 747.20
    acquired 447.8
    arch 747.21
      acquired 447.8
    coarctation 747.10
  aortic
    arch 747.21
      acquired 447.8
    cusp or valve (congenital) 746.9
      acquired (*see also* Endocarditis, aortic)
        424.1
    ring 747.21
  appendix 751.5
  arm (acquired) 736.89
    congenital 755.50
  arteriovenous (congenital) (peripheral) NEC
      747.60
    gastrointestinal 747.61
    lower limb 747.64
    renal 747.62
    specified NEC 747.69
    spinal 747.82
    upper limb 747.63
  artery (congenital) (peripheral) NEC (*see also*
      Deformity, vascular) 747.60
    acquired 447.8
    cerebral 747.81
    coronary (congenital) 746.85
      acquired (*see also* Ischemia, heart) 414.9

Deformity—*continued*
  artery—*continued*
    retinal 743.9
    umbilical 747.5
  atrial septal (congenital) (heart) 745.5
  auditory canal (congenital) (external) (*see also*
      Deformity, ear) 744.3
    acquired 380.50
  auricle
    ear (congenital) (*see also* Deformity, ear)
        744.3
      acquired 380.32
    heart (congenital) 746.9
  back (acquired)—*see* Deformity, spine
  Bartholin's duct (congenital) 750.9
  bile duct (congenital) 751.60
    acquired 576.8
      with calculus, choledocholithiasis, or
        stones—*see* Choledocholithiasis
  biliary duct or passage (congenital) 751.60
    acquired 576.8
      with calculus, choledocholithiasis, or
        stones—*see* Choledocholithiasis
  bladder (neck) (sphincter) (trigone) (acquired)
      596.89
    congenital 753.9
  bone (acquired) NEC 738.9
    congenital 756.9
    turbinate 738.0
  boutonniere (finger) 736.21
  brain (congenital) 742.9
    acquired 348.89
    multiple 742.4
    reduction 742.2
    vessel (congenital) 747.81
  breast (acquired) 611.89
    congenital 757.6
    reconstructed 612.0
  bronchus (congenital) 748.3
    acquired 519.19
  bursa, congenital 756.9
  canal of Nuck 752.9
  canthus (congenital) 743.9
    acquired 374.89
  capillary (acquired) 448.9
    congenital NEC (*see also* Deformity, vascular)
        747.60
  cardiac—*see* Deformity, heart
  cardiovascular system (congenital) 746.9
  caruncle, lacrimal (congenital) 743.9
    acquired 375.69
  cascade, stomach 537.6
  cecum (congenital) 751.5
    acquired 569.89
  cerebral (congenital) 742.9
    acquired 348.89
  cervix (acquired) (uterus) 622.8
    congenital 752.40
  cheek (acquired) 738.19
    congenital 744.9
  chest (wall) (acquired) 738.3
    congenital 754.89
    late effect of rickets 268.1
  chin (acquired) 738.19
    congenital 744.9
  choroid (congenital) 743.9
    acquired 363.8
    plexus (congenital) 742.9
      acquired 349.2
  cicatricial—*see* Cicatrix

Deformity—*continued*
  cilia (congenital) 743.9
    acquired 374.89
  circulatory system (congenital) 747.9
  clavicle (acquired) 738.8
    congenital 755.51
  clitoris (congenital) 752.40
    acquired 624.8
  clubfoot—*see* Clubfoot
  coccyx (acquired) 738.6
    congenital 756.10
  colon (congenital) 751.5
    acquired 569.89
  concha (ear) (congenital) (*see also* Deformity,
      ear) 744.3
    acquired 380.32
  congenital, organ or site not listed (*see also*
      Anomaly) 759.9
  cornea (congenital) 743.9
    acquired 371.70
  coronary artery (congenital) 746.85
    acquired (*see also* Ischemia, heart) 414.9
  cranium (acquired) 738.19
    congenital (*see also* Deformity, skull,
        congenital) 756.0
  cricoid cartilage (congenital) 748.3
    acquired 478.79
  cystic duct (congenital) 751.60
    acquired 575.8
  Dandy-Walker 742.3
    with spina bifida (*see also* Spina bifida) 741.0
  diaphragm (congenital) 756.6
    acquired 738.8
  digestive organ(s) or system (congenital) NEC
      751.9
    specified type NEC 751.8
  ductus arteriosus 747.0
  duodenal bulb 537.89
  duodenum (congenital) 751.5
    acquired 537.89
  dura (congenital) 742.9
    brain 742.4
      acquired 349.2
    spinal 742.59
      acquired 349.2
  ear (congenital) 744.3
    acquired 380.32
    auricle 744.3
      causing impairment of hearing 744.02
    causing impairment of hearing 744.00
    external 744.3
      causing impairment of hearing 744.02
    internal 744.05
    lobule 744.3
    middle 744.03
      ossicles 744.04
    ossicles 744.04
  ectodermal (congenital) NEC 757.9
    specified type NEC 757.8
  ejaculatory duct (congenital) 752.9
    acquired 608.89
  elbow (joint) (acquired) 736.00
    congenital 755.50
    contraction 718.42
  endocrine gland NEC 759.2
  epididymis (congenital) 752.9
    acquired 608.89
    torsion 608.24
  epiglottis (congenital) 748.3
    acquired 478.79
  esophagus (congenital) 750.9
    acquired 530.89

Deformity—*continued*
  Eustachian tube (congenital) NEC 744.3
    specified type NEC 744.24
  extremity (acquired) 736.9
    congenital, except reduction deformity 755.9
      lower 755.60
      upper 755.50
    reduction—*see* Deformity, reduction
  eye (congenital) 743.9
    acquired 379.8
    muscle 743.9
  eyebrow (congenital) 744.89
  eyelid (congenital) 743.9
    acquired 374.89
    specified type NEC 743.62
  face (acquired) 738.19
    congenital (any part) 744.9
    due to intrauterine malposition and pressure 754.0
  fallopian tube (congenital) 752.10
    acquired 620.8
  femur (acquired) 736.89
    congenital 755.60
  fetal
    with fetopelvic disproportion 653.7
      affecting fetus or newborn 763.1
    causing obstructed labor 660.1
      affecting fetus or newborn 763.1
    known or suspected, affecting management of
        pregnancy 655.9
  finger (acquired) 736.20
    boutonniere type 736.21
    congenital 755.50
    flexion contracture 718.44
    swan neck 736.22
  flexion (joint) (acquired) 736.9
    congenital NEC 755.9
    hip or thigh (acquired) 736.39
      congenital (*see also* Subluxation, congenital,
          hip) 754.32
  foot (acquired) 736.70
    cavovarus 736.75
      congenital 754.59
    congenital NEC 754.70
      specified type NEC 754.79
    valgus (acquired) 736.79
      congenital 754.60
        specified type NEC 754.69
    varus (acquired) 736.79
      congenital 754.50
        specified type NEC 754.59
  forearm (acquired) 736.00
    congenital 755.50
  forehead (acquired) 738.19
    congenital (*see also* Deformity, skull,
        congenital) 756.0
  frontal bone (acquired) 738.19
    congenital (*see also* Deformity, skull,
        congenital) 756.0
  gallbladder (congenital) 751.60
    acquired 575.8
  gastrointestinal tract (congenital) NEC 751.9
    acquired 569.89
    specified type NEC 751.8
  genitalia, genital organ(s) or system NEC
    congenital 752.9
    female (congenital) 752.9
      acquired 629.89
      external 752.40
      internal 752.9
    male (congenital) 752.9
      acquired 608.89

Deformity—*continued*
  globe (eye) (congenital) 743.9
    acquired 360.89
  gum (congenital) 750.9
    acquired 523.9
  gunstock 736.02
  hand (acquired) 736.00
    claw 736.06
    congenital 755.50
    minus (and plus) (intrinsic) 736.09
    pill roller (intrinsic) 736.09
    plus (and minus) (intrinsic) 736.09
    swan neck (intrinsic) 736.09
  head (acquired) 738.10
    congenital (*see also* Deformity, skull,
      congenital) 756.0
    specified NEC 738.19
  heart (congenital) 746.9
    auricle (congenital) 746.9
    septum 745.9
      auricular 745.5
      specified type NEC 745.8
      ventricular 745.4
    valve (congenital) NEC 746.9
      acquired—*see* Endocarditis
      pulmonary (congenital) 746.00
      specified type NEC 746.89
    ventricle (congenital) 746.9
  heel (acquired) 736.76
    congenital 755.67
  hepatic duct (congenital) 751.60
    acquired 576.8
    with calculus, choledocholithiasis, or
      stones—*see* Choledocholithiasis
  hip (joint) (acquired) 736.30
    congenital NEC 755.63
    flexion 718.45
      congenital (*see also* Subluxation, congenital,
      hip) 754.32
  hourglass—*see* Contraction, hourglass
  humerus (acquired) 736.89
    congenital 755.50
  hymen (congenital) 752.40
  hypophyseal (congenital) 759.2
  ileocecal (coil) (valve) (congenital) 751.5
    acquired 569.89
  ileum (intestine) (congenital) 751.5
    acquired 569.89
  ilium (acquired) 738.6
    congenital 755.60
  integument (congenital) 757.9
  intervertebral cartilage or disc (acquired)—*see*
    also Displacement, intervertebral disc
    congenital 756.10
  intestine (large) (small) (congenital) 751.5
    acquired 569.89
  iris (acquired) 364.75
    congenital 743.9
    prolapse 364.89
  ischium (acquired) 738.6
    congenital 755.60
  jaw (acquired) (congenital) NEC 524.9
    due to intrauterine malposition and pressure
      754.0
  joint (acquired) NEC 738.8
    congenital 755.9
    contraction (abduction) (adduction) (extension)
      (flexion)—*see* Contraction, joint
  kidney(s) (calyx) (pelvis) (congenital) 753.9
    acquired 593.89
    vessel 747.62
      acquired 459.9

Deformity—*continued*
  Klippel-Feil (brevicollis) 756.16
  knee (acquired) NEC 736.6
    congenital 755.64
  labium (majus) (minus) (congenital) 752.40
    acquired 624.8
  lacrimal apparatus or duct (congenital) 743.9
    acquired 375.69
  larynx (muscle) (congenital) 748.3
    acquired 478.79
    web (glottic) (subglottic) 748.2
  leg (lower) (upper) (acquired) NEC 736.89
    congenital 755.60
    reduction—*see* Deformity, reduction, lower limb
  lens (congenital) 743.9
    acquired 379.39
  lid (fold) (congenital) 743.9
    acquired 374.89
  ligament (acquired) 728.9
    congenital 756.9
  limb (acquired) 736.9
    congenital, except reduction deformity 755.9
      lower 755.60
        reduction (*see also* Deformity, reduction,
          lower limb) 755.30
      upper 755.50
        reduction (*see also* Deformity, reduction,
          lower limb) 755.20
    specified NEC 736.89
  lip (congenital) NEC 750.9
    acquired 528.5
    specified type NEC 750.26
  liver (congenital) 751.60
    acquired 573.8
    duct (congenital) 751.60
      acquired 576.8
      with calculus, choledocholithiasis, or
        stones—*see* Choledocholithiasis
  lower extremity—*see* Deformity, leg
  lumbosacral (joint) (region) (congenital) 756.10
    acquired 738.5
  lung (congenital) 748.60
    acquired 518.89
    specified type NEC 748.69
  lymphatic system, congenital 759.9
  Madelung's (radius) 755.54
  maxilla (acquired) (congenital) 524.9
  meninges or membrane (congenital) 742.9
    brain 742.4
      acquired 349.2
    spinal (cord) 742.59
      acquired 349.2
  mesentery (congenital) 751.9
    acquired 568.89
  metacarpus (acquired) 736.00
    congenital 755.50
  metatarsus (acquired) 736.70
    congenital 754.70
  middle ear, except ossicles (congenital) 744.03
    ossicles 744.04
  mitral (leaflets) (valve) (congenital) 746.9
    acquired—*see* Endocarditis, mitral
    Ebstein's 746.89
    parachute 746.5
    specified type NEC 746.89
    stenosis, congenital 746.5
  mouth (acquired) 528.9
    congenital NEC 750.9
      specified type NEC 750.26
  multiple, congenital NEC 759.7
    specified type NEC 759.89

Deformity—*continued*
 rotation (joint) (acquired) 736.9
  congenital 755.9
  hip or thigh 736.39
   congenital (*see also* Subluxation, congenital, hip) 754.32
 sacroiliac joint (congenital) 755.69
  acquired 738.5
 sacrum (acquired) 738.5
  congenital 756.10
 saddle
  back 737.8
  nose 738.0
   syphilitic 090.5
 salivary gland or duct (congenital) 750.9
  acquired 527.8
 scapula (acquired) 736.89
  congenital 755.50
 scrotum (congenital) 752.9
  acquired 608.89
 sebaceous gland, acquired 706.8
 seminal tract or duct (congenital) 752.9
  acquired 608.89
 septum (nasal) (acquired) 470
  congenital 748.1
 shoulder (joint) (acquired) 736.89
  congenital 755.50
   specified type NEC 755.59
  contraction 718.41
 sigmoid (flexure) (congenital) 751.5
  acquired 569.89
 sinus of Valsalva 747.29
 skin (congenital) 757.9
  acquired NEC 709.8
 skull (acquired) 738.19
  congenital 756.0
   with
    anencephalus 740.0
    encephalocele 742.0
    hydrocephalus 742.3
     with spina bifida (*see also* Spina bifida) 741.0
    microcephalus 742.1
    due to intrauterine malposition and pressure 754.0
 soft parts, organs or tissues (of pelvis)
  in pregnancy or childbirth NEC 654.9
   affecting fetus or newborn 763.89
   causing obstructed labor 660.2
    affecting fetus or newborn 763.1
 spermatic cord (congenital) 752.9
  acquired 608.89
  torsion 608.22
   extravaginal 608.21
   intravaginal 608.22
 spinal
  column—*see* Deformity, spine
  cord (congenital) 742.9
   acquired 336.8
   vessel (congenital) 747.82
  nerve root (congenital) 742.9
   acquired 724.9
  vessel 747.82
 spine (acquired) NEC 738.5
  congenital 756.10
   due to intrauterine malposition and pressure 754.2
  kyphoscoliotic (*see also* Kyphoscoliosis) 737.30
  kyphotic (*see also* Kyphosis) 737.10
  lordotic (*see also* Lordosis) 737.20
  rachitic 268.1
  scoliotic (*see also* Scoliosis) 737.30

Deformity—*continued*
 spleen
  acquired 289.59
  congenital 759.0
 Sprengel's (congenital) 755.52
 sternum (acquired) 738.3
  congenital 756.3
 stomach (congenital) 750.9
  acquired 537.89
 submaxillary gland (congenital) 750.9
  acquired 527.8
 swan neck (acquired)
  finger 736.22
  hand 736.09
 talipes—*see* Talipes
 teeth, tooth NEC 520.9
 testis (congenital) 752.9
  acquired 608.89
  torsion 608.20
 thigh (acquired) 736.89
  congenital 755.60
 thorax (acquired) (wall) 738.3
  congenital 754.89
  late effect of rickets 268.1
 thumb (acquired) 736.20
  congenital 755.50
 thymus (tissue) (congenital) 759.2
 thyroid (gland) (congenital) 759.2
  cartilage 748.3
   acquired 478.79
 tibia (acquired) 736.89
  congenital 755.60
  saber 090.5
 toe (acquired) 735.9
  congenital 755.66
  specified NEC 735.8
 tongue (congenital) 750.10
  acquired 529.8
 tooth, teeth NEC 520.9
 trachea (rings) (congenital) 748.3
  acquired 519.19
 transverse aortic arch (congenital) 747.21
 tricuspid (leaflets) (valve) (congenital) 746.9
  acquired—*see* Endocarditis, tricuspid
  atresia or stenosis 746.1
  specified type NEC 746.89
 trunk (acquired) 738.3
  congenital 759.9
 ulna (acquired) 736.00
  congenital 755.50
 upper extremity—*see* Deformity, arm
 urachus (congenital) 753.7
 ureter (opening) (congenital) 753.9
  acquired 593.89
 urethra (valve) (congenital) 753.9
  acquired 599.84
 urinary tract or system (congenital) 753.9
  urachus 753.7
 uterus (congenital) 752.39
  acquired 621.8
 uvula (congenital) 750.9
  acquired 528.9
 vagina (congenital) 752.40
  acquired 623.8
 valve, valvular (heart) (congenital) 746.9
  acquired—*see* Endocarditis
  pulmonary 746.00
  specified type NEC 746.89
 vascular (congenital) (peripheral) NEC 747.60
  acquired 459.9
  gastrointestinal 747.61
  lower limb 747.64

Deformity—*continued*
  vascular—*continued*
    renal 747.62
    specified site NEC 747.69
    spinal 747.82
    upper limb 747.63
  vas deferens (congenital) 752.9
    acquired 608.89
  vein (congenital) NEC (*see also* Deformity,
      vascular) 747.60
    brain 747.81
    coronary 746.9
    great 747.40
  vena cava (inferior) (superior) (congenital)
      747.40
  vertebra—*see* Deformity, spine
  vesicourethral orifice (acquired) 596.89
    congenital NEC 753.9
      specified type NEC 753.8
  vessels of optic papilla (congenital) 743.9
  visual field (contraction) 368.45
  vitreous humor (congenital) 743.9
    acquired 379.29
  vulva (congenital) 752.40
    acquired 624.8
  wrist (joint) (acquired) 736.00
    congenital 755.50
    contraction 718.43
    valgus 736.03
      congenital 755.59
    varus 736.04
      congenital 755.59

Degeneration, degenerative
  adrenal (capsule) (gland) 255.8
    with hypofunction 255.41
    fatty 255.8
    hyaline 255.8
    infectional 255.8
    lardaceous 277.39
  amyloid (any site) (general) 277.39
  anterior cornua, spinal cord 336.8
  anterior labral 840.8
  aorta, aortic 440.0
    fatty 447.8
    valve (heart) (*see also* Endocarditis, aortic)
        424.1
  arteriovascular—*see* Arteriosclerosis
  artery, arterial (atheromatous) (calcareous)—*see
      also* Arteriosclerosis
    amyloid 277.39
    lardaceous 277.39
    medial NEC (*see also* Arteriosclerosis,
        extremities) 440.20
  articular cartilage NEC (*see also* Disorder,
      cartilage, articular) 718.0
    elbow 718.02
    knee 717.5
    patella 717.7
    shoulder 718.01
    spine (*see also* Spondylosis) 721.90
  atheromatous—*see* Arteriosclerosis
  bacony (any site) 277.39
  basal nuclei or ganglia NEC 333.0
  bone 733.90
  brachial plexus 353.0
  brain (cortical) (progressive) 331.9
    arteriosclerotic 437.0
    childhood 330.9
      specified type NEC 330.8
    congenital 742.4

Degeneration, degenerative—*continued*
  brain—*continued*
    cystic 348.0
      congenital 742.4
    familial NEC 331.89
    grey matter 330.8
    heredofamilial NEC 331.89
    in
      alcoholism 303.9 *[331.7]*
      beriberi 265.0 *[331.7]*
      cerebrovascular disease 437.9 *[331.7]*
      congenital hydrocephalus 742.3 *[331.7]*
        with spina bifida (*see also* Spina bifida)
            741.0 *[331.7]*
      Fabry's disease 272.7 *[330.2]*
      Gaucher's disease 272.7 *[330.2]*
      Hunter's disease or syndrome 277.5 *[330.3]*
      lipidosis
        cerebral 330.1
        generalized 272.7 *[330.2]*
      mucopolysaccharidosis 277.5 *[330.3]*
      myxedema (*see also* Myxedema) 244.9
          [331.7]
      neoplastic disease NEC (M8000/1) 239.9
          [331.7]
      Niemann-Pick disease 272.7 *[330.2]*
      sphingolipidosis 272.7 *[330.2]*
      vitamin B₁₂ deficiency 266.2 *[331.7]*
    motor centers 331.89
    senile 331.2
    specified type NEC 331.89
  breast—*see* Disease, breast
  Bruch's membrane 363.40
  bundle of His 426.50
    left 426.3
    right 426.4
  calcareous NEC 275.49
  capillaries 448.9
    amyloid 277.39
    fatty 448.9
    lardaceous 277.39
  cardiac (brown) (calcareous) (fatty) (fibrous)
      (hyaline) (mural) (muscular) (pigmentary)
      (senile) (with arteriosclerosis) (*see also*
      Degeneration, myocardial) 429.1
    valve, valvular—*see* Endocarditis
  cardiorenal (*see also* Hypertension, cardiorenal)
      404.90
  cardiovascular (*see also* Disease, cardiovascular)
      429.2
    renal (*see also* Hypertension, cardiorenal) 404.90
  cartilage (joint)—*see* Derangement, joint
  cerebellar NEC 334.9
    primary (hereditary) (sporadic) 334.2
  cerebral—*see* Degeneration, brain
  cerebromacular 330.1
  cerebrovascular 437.1
    due to hypertension 437.2
    late effect—*see* Late effect(s) (of)
        cerebrovascular disease
  cervical plexus 353.2
  cervix 622.8
    due to radiation (intended effect) 622.8
      adverse effect or misadventure 622.8
  changes, spine or vertebra (*see also*
      Spondylosis) 721.90
  chitinous 277.39
  chorioretinal 363.40
    congenital 743.53
    hereditary 363.50

Degeneration, degenerative—*continued*
  choroid (colloid) (drusen) 363.40
    hereditary 363.50
    senile 363.41
      diffuse secondary 363.42
  cochlear 386.8
  collateral ligament (knee) (medial) 717.82
    lateral 717.81
  combined (spinal cord) (subacute) 266.2 *[336.2]*
    with anemia (pernicious) 281.0 *[336.2]*
    due to dietary deficiency 281.1 *[336.2]*
    due to vitamin B$_{12}$ deficiency anemia (dietary)
      281.1 *[336.2]*
  conjunctiva 372.50
    amyloid 277.39 *[372.50]*
  cornea 371.40
    calcerous 371.44
    familial (hereditary) (*see also* Dystrophy,
      cornea) 371.50
      macular 371.55
      reticular 371.54
    hyaline (of old scars) 371.41
    marginal (Terrien's) 371.48
    mosaic (shagreen) 371.41
    nodular 371.46
    peripheral 371.48
    senile 371.41
  cortical (cerebellar) (parenchymatous) 334.2
    alcoholic 303.9 *[334.4]*
    diffuse, due to arteriopathy 437.0
  corticobasal 331.6
  corticostriatal-spinal 334.8
  cretinoid 243
  cruciate ligament (knee) (posterior) 717.84
    anterior 717.83
  cutis 709.3
    amyloid 277.39
  dental pulp 522.2
  disc disease—*see* Degeneration, intervertebral
    disc
  dorsolateral (spinal cord)—*see* Degeneration,
    combined
  endocardial 424.90
  extrapyramidal NEC 333.90
  eye NEC 360.40
    macular (*see also* Degeneration, macula) 362.50
      congenital 362.75
      hereditary 362.76
  fatty (diffuse) (general) 272.8
    liver 571.8
      alcoholic 571.0
    localized site—*see* Degeneration, by site, fatty
    placenta—*see* Placenta, abnormal
  globe (eye) NEC 360.40
    macular—*see* Degeneration, macula
  grey matter 330.8
  heart (brown) (calcareous) (fatty) (fibrous)
    (hyaline) (mural) (muscular) (pigmentary)
    (senile) (with arteriosclerosis) (*see also*
    Degeneration, myocardial) 429.1
    amyloid 277.39 *[425.7]*
    atheromatous —*see* Arteriosclerosis, coronary
    gouty 274.82
    hypertensive (*see also* Hypertension, heart)
      402.90
    ischemic 414.9
    valve, valvular—*see* Endocarditis
  hepatolenticular (Wilson's) 275.1
  hepatorenal 572.4
  heredofamilial
    brain NEC 331.89
    spinal cord NEC 336.8

Degeneration, degenerative—*continued*
  hyaline (diffuse) (generalized) 728.9
    localized—*see also* Degeneration, by site
      cornea 371.41
      keratitis 371.41
  hypertensive vascular—*see* Hypertension
  infrapatellar fat pad 729.31
  internal semilunar cartilage 717.3
  intervertebral disc 722.6
    with myelopathy 722.70
    cervical, cervicothoracic 722.4
      with myelopathy 722.71
    lumbar, lumbosacral 722.52
      with myelopathy 722.73
    thoracic, thoracolumbar 722.51
      with myelopathy 722.72
  intestine 569.89
    amyloid 277.39
    lardaceous 277.39
  iris (generalized) (*see also* Atrophy, iris) 364.59
    pigmentary 364.53
    pupillary margin 364.54
  ischemic—*see* Ischemia
  joint disease (*see also* Osteoarthrosis) 715.9
    multiple sites 715.09
    spine (*see also* Spondylosis) 721.90
  kidney (*see also* Sclerosis, renal) 587
    amyloid 277.39 *[583.81]*
    cyst, cystic (multiple) (solitary) 593.2
      congenital (*see also* Cystic, disease, kidney)
        753.10
    fatty 593.89
    fibrocystic (congenital) 753.19
    lardaceous 277.39 *[583.81]*
    polycystic (congenital) 753.12
      adult type (APKD) 753.13
      autosomal dominant 753.13
      autosomal recessive 753.14
      childhood type (CPKD) 753.14
      infantile type 753.14
    waxy 277.39 *[583.81]*
  Kuhnt-Junius (retina) 362.52
  labyrinth, osseous 386.8
  lacrimal passages, cystic 375.12
  lardaceous (any site) 277.39
  lateral column (posterior), spinal cord (*see also*
    Degeneration, combined) 266.2 *[336.2]*
  lattice 362.63
  lens 366.9
    infantile, juvenile, or presenile 366.00
    senile 366.10
  lenticular (familial) (progressive) (Wilson's)
    (with cirrhosis of liver) 275.1
    striate artery 437.0
  lethal ball, prosthetic heart valve 996.02
  ligament
    collateral (knee) (medial) 717.82
      lateral 717.81
    cruciate (knee) (posterior) 717.84
      anterior 717.83
  liver (diffuse) 572.8
    amyloid 277.39
    congenital (cystic) 751.62
    cystic 572.8
      congenital 751.62
    fatty 571.8
      alcoholic 571.0
    hypertrophic 572.8
    lardaceous 277.39
    parenchymatous, acute or subacute (*see also*
      Necrosis, liver) 570

Degeneration, degenerative—*continued*
  liver—*continued*
    pigmentary 572.8
    toxic (acute) 573.8
    waxy 277.39
  lung 518.8
  lymph gland 289.3
    hyaline 289.3
    lardaceous 277.39
  macula (acquired) (senile) 362.50
    atrophic 362.51
    Best's 362.76
    congenital 362.75
    cystic 362.54
    cystoid 362.53
    disciform 362.52
    dry 362.51
    exudative 362.52
    familial pseudoinflammatory 362.77
    hereditary 362.76
    hole 362.54
    juvenile (Stargardt's) 362.75
    nonexudative 362.51
    pseudohole 362.54
    wet 362.52
  medullary—*see* Degeneration, brain
  membranous labyrinth, congenital (causing
      impairment of hearing) 744.05
  meniscus—*see* Derangement, joint
  microcystoid 362.62
  mitral—*see* Insufficiency, mitral
  Mönckeberg's (*see also* Arteriosclerosis,
      extremities) 440.20
  moral 301.7
  motor centers, senile 331.2
  mural (*see also* Degeneration, myocardial) 429.1
    heart, cardiac (*see also* Degeneration,
        myocardial) 429.1
    myocardium, myocardial (*see also*
        Degeneration, myocardial) 429.1
  muscle 728.9
    fatty 728.9
    fibrous 728.9
    heart (*see also* Degeneration, myocardial)
        429.1
    hyaline 728.9
  muscular progressive 728.2
  myelin, central nervous system NEC 341.9
  myocardium, myocardial (brown) (calcareous)
      (fatty) (fibrous) (hyaline) (mural) (muscular)
      (pigmentary) (senile) (with arteriosclerosis)
      429.1
    with rheumatic fever (conditions classifiable
        to 390) 398.0
      active, acute, or subacute 391.2
        with chorea 392.0
      inactive or quiescent (with chorea) 398.0
    amyloid 277.39 *[425.7]*
    congenital 746.89
    fetus or newborn 779.89
    gouty 274.82
    hypertensive (*see also* Hypertension, heart)
        402.90
    ischemic 414.8
    rheumatic (*see also* Degeneration,
        myocardium, with rheumatic fever) 398.0
    syphilitic 093.82
  nasal sinus (mucosa) (*see also* Sinusitis) 473.9
    frontal 473.1
    maxillary 473.0
  nerve—*see* Disorder, nerve

Degeneration, degenerative—*continued*
  nervous system 349.89
    amyloid 277.39 *[357.4]*
    autonomic (*see also* Neuropathy, peripheral,
        autonomic) 337.9
    fatty 349.89
    peripheral autonomic NEC (*see also*
        Neuropathy, peripheral, autonomic) 337.9
  nipple 611.9
  nose 478.19
  oculoacousticocerebral, congenital (progressive)
      743.8
  olivopontocerebellar (familial) (hereditary) 333.0
  osseous labyrinth 386.8
  ovary 620.8
    cystic 620.2
    microcystic 620.2
  pallidal, pigmentary (progressive) 333.0
  pancreas 577.8
    tuberculous (*see also* Tuberculosis) 017.9
  papillary muscle 429.81
  paving stone 362.61
  penis 607.89
  peritoneum 568.89
  pigmentary (diffuse) (general)
    localized—*see* Degeneration, by site
    pallidal (progressive) 333.0
    secondary 362.65
  pineal gland 259.8
  pituitary (gland) 253.8
  placenta (fatty) (fibrinoid) (fibroid)—*see*
      Placenta, abnormal
  popliteal fat pad 729.31
  posterolateral (spinal cord) (*see also*
      Degeneration, combined) 266.2 *[336.2]*
  pulmonary valve (heart) (*see also* Endocarditis,
      pulmonary) 424.3
  pulp (tooth) 522.2
  pupillary margin 364.54
  renal (*see also* Sclerosis, renal) 587
    fibrocystic 753.19
    polycystic 753.12
      adult type (APKD) 753.13
      autosomal dominant 753.13
      autosomal recessive 753.14
      childhood type (CPKD) 753.14
      infantile type 753.14
  reticuloendothelial system 289.89
  retina (peripheral) 362.60
    with retinal defect (*see also* Detachment,
        retina, with retinal defect) 361.00
    cystic (senile) 362.50
    cystoid 362.53
    hereditary (*see also* Dystrophy, retina) 362.70
      cerebroretinal 362.71
      congenital 362.75
      juvenile (Stargardt's) 362.75
      macula 362.76
    Kuhnt-Junius 362.52
    lattice 362.63
    macular (*see also* Degeneration, macula) 362.50
    microcystoid 362.62
    palisade 362.63
    paving stone 362.61
    pigmentary (primary) 362.74
      secondary 362.65
    posterior pole (*see also* Degeneration, macula)
        362.50
    secondary 362.66
    senile 362.60
      cystic 362.53
      reticular 362.64

Degeneration, degenerative—*continued*
saccule, congenital (causing impairment of hearing) 744.05
sacculocochlear 386.8
senile 797
  brain 331.2
  cardiac, heart, or myocardium (*see also* Degeneration, myocardial) 429.1
  motor centers 331.2
  reticule 362.64
  retina, cystic 362.50
  vascular—*see* Arteriosclerosis
silicone rubber poppet (prosthetic valve) 996.02
sinus (cystic) (*see also* Sinusitis) 473.9
  polypoid 471.1
skin 709.3
  amyloid 277.39
  colloid 709.3
spinal (cord) 336.8
  amyloid 277.39
  column 733.90
  combined (subacute) (*see also* Degeneration, combined) 266.2 *[336.2]*
    with anemia (pernicious) 281.0 *[336.2]*
  dorsolateral (*see also* Degeneration, combined) 266.2 *[336.2]*
  familial NEC 336.8
  fatty 336.8
  funicular (*see also* Degeneration, combined) 266.2 *[336.2]*
  heredofamilial NEC 336.8
  posterolateral (*see also* Degeneration, combined) 266.2 *[336.2]*
  subacute combined—*see* Degeneration, combined
  tuberculous (*see also* Tuberculosis) 013.8
spine 733.90
spleen 289.59
  amyloid 277.39
  lardaceous 277.39
stomach 537.89
  lardaceous 277.39
strionigral 333.0
sudoriparous (cystic) 705.89
suprarenal (capsule) (gland) 255.8
  with hypofunction 255.41
sweat gland 705.89
synovial membrane (pulpy) 727.9
tapetoretinal 362.74
  adult or presenile form 362.50
testis (postinfectional) 608.89
thymus (gland) 254.8
  fatty 254.8
  lardaceous 277.39
thyroid (gland) 246.8
tricuspid (heart) (valve)—*see* Endocarditis, tricuspid
tuberculous NEC (*see also* Tuberculosis) 011.9
turbinate 733.90
uterus 621.8
  cystic 621.8
vascular (senile)—*see also* Arteriosclerosis
  hypertensive—*see* Hypertension
vitreoretinal (primary) 362.73
  secondary 362.66
vitreous humor (with infiltration) 379.21
wallerian NEC—*see* Disorder, nerve
waxy (any site) 277.39
Wilson's hepatolenticular 275.1

Deglutition
paralysis 784.99
  hysterical 300.11
pneumonia 507.0
Degos' disease or syndrome 447.8
Degradation disorder, branched-chain amino-acid 270.3
Dehiscence
anastomosis—*see* Complications, anastomosis
cesarean wound 674.1
closure of
  cornea 998.32
  fascia, superficial or muscular 998.31
  internal organ 998.31
  mucosa 998.32
  muscle or muscle flap 998.31
  ribs or rib cage 998.31
  skin 998.32
  skull or craniotomy 998.31
  sternum or sternotomy 998.31
  subcutaneous tissue 998.32
  tendon or ligament 998.31
  traumatic laceration (external) (internal) 998.33
episiotomy 674.2
operation wound 998.32
  deep 998.31
  external 998.32
  internal 998.31
  superficial 998.32
perineal wound (postpartum) 674.2
postoperative 998.32
  abdomen 998.32
    internal 998.31
  internal 998.31
traumatic injury wound repair 998.33
uterine wound 674.1
Dehydration (cachexia) 276.51
newborn 775.5
with
  hypernatremia 276.0
  hyponatremia 276.1
Deiters' nucleus syndrome 386.19
Déjérine's disease 356.0
Déjérine-Klumpke paralysis 767.6
Déjérine-Roussy syndrome 338.0
Déjérine-Sottas disease or neuropathy (hypertrophic) 356.0
Déjérine-Thomas atrophy or syndrome 333.0
de Lange's syndrome (Amsterdam dwarf, intellectual disabilities, and brachycephaly) 759.89
Delay, delayed
adaptation, cones or rods 368.63
any plane in pelvis
  affecting fetus or newborn 763.1
  complicating delivery 660.1
birth or delivery NEC 662.1
  affecting fetus or newborn 763.9
  second twin, triplet, or multiple mate 662.3
closure—*see also* Fistula
  cranial suture 756.0
  fontanel 756.0
coagulation NEC 790.92
conduction (cardiac) (ventricular) 426.9
delivery NEC 662.1
  second twin, triplet, etc. 662.3
    affecting fetus or newborn 763.89
development
  in childhood 783.40
    physiological 783.40
  intellectual NEC 315.9
  learning NEC 315.2

Delay, delayed—*continued*
development—*continued*
reading 315.00
sexual 259.0
speech 315.39
and language due to hearing loss 315.34
associated with hyperkinesis 314.1
spelling 315.09
gastric emptying 536.8
menarche 256.39
due to pituitary hypofunction 253.4
menstruation (cause unknown) 626.8
milestone in childhood 783.42
motility—*see* Hypomotility
passage of meconium (newborn) 777.1
primary respiration 768.9
puberty 259.0
separation of umbilical cord 779.83
sexual maturation, female 259.0
vaccination V64.00
Del Castillo's syndrome (germinal aplasia) 606.0
Deleage's disease 359.89
Deletion syndrome
5p 758.31
22q11.2 758.32
autosomal NEC 758.39
constitutional 5q deletion 758.39
Delhi (boil) (button) (sore) 085.1
Delinquency (juvenile) 312.9
group (*see also* Disturbance, conduct) 312.2
neurotic 312.4
Delirium, delirious 780.09
acute 780.09
due to conditions classified elsewhere 293.0
alcoholic 291.0
acute 291.0
chronic 291.1
alcoholicum 291.0
chronic (*see also* Psychosis) 293.89
due to or associated with physical
condition—*see* Psychosis, organic
due to conditions classified elsewhere 293.0
drug-induced 292.81
eclamptic (*see also* Eclampsia) 780.39
exhaustion (*see also* Reaction, stress, acute)
308.9
hysterical 300.11
in
presenile dementia 290.11
senile dementia 290.3
induced by drug 292.81
manic, maniacal (acute) (*see also* Psychosis,
affective) 296.0
recurrent episode 296.1
single episode 296.0
puerperal 293.9
senile 290.3
subacute (psychotic) 293.1
thyroid (*see also* Thyrotoxicosis) 242.9
traumatic—*see also* Injury, intracranial
with
lesion, spinal cord—*see* Injury, spinal, by
site
shock, spinal—*see* Injury, spinal, by site
tremens (impending) 291.0
uremic—*see* Uremia
withdrawal
alcoholic (acute) 291.0
chronic 291.1
drug 292.0

Delivery

*Note—Use the following fifth-digit
subclassification with categories
640-649, 651-676:*

0 unspecified as to episode of care
1 delivered, with or without mention of
   antepartum condition
2 delivered, with mention of
   postpartum complication
3 antepartum condition or complication
4 postpartum condition or
   complication

breech (assisted) (spontaneous) 652.2
affecting fetus or newborn 763.0
extraction NEC 669.6
cesarean (for) 669.7
abnormal
cervix 654.6
pelvic organs or tissues 654.9
pelvis (bony) (major) NEC 653.0
presentation or position 652.9
in multiple gestation 652.6
size, fetus 653.5
soft parts (of pelvis) 654.9
uterus, congenital 654.0
vagina 654.7
vulva 654.8
abruptio placentae 641.2
acromion presentation 652.8
affecting fetus or newborn 763.4
anteversion, cervix or uterus 654.4
atony, uterus 661.2
with hemorrhage 666.1
bicornis or bicornuate uterus 654.0
breech presentation 652.2
brow presentation 652.4
cephalopelvic disproportion (normally formed
fetus) 653.4
chin presentation 652.4
cicatrix of cervix 654.6
contracted pelvis (general) 653.1
inlet 653.2
outlet 653.3
cord presentation or prolapse 663.0
cystocele 654.4
deformity (acquired) (congenital)
pelvic organs or tissues NEC 654.9
pelvis (bony) NEC 653.0
displacement, uterus NEC 654.4
disproportion NEC 653.9
distress
fetal 656.8
maternal 669.0
eclampsia 642.6
face presentation 652.4
failed
forceps 660.7
trial of labor NEC 660.6
vacuum extraction 660.7
ventouse 660.7
fetal deformity 653.7
fetal-maternal hemorrhage 656.0
fetus, fetal
distress 656.8
prematurity 656.8
fibroid (tumor) (uterus) 654.1
footling 652.8
with successful version 652.1

Delivery—*continued*

cesarean—*continued*

hemorrhage (antepartum) (intrapartum) NEC 641.9

hydrocephalic fetus 653.6

incarceration of uterus 654.3

incoordinate uterine action 661.4

inertia, uterus 661.2

 primary 661.0

 secondary 661.1

lateroversion, uterus or cervix 654.4

mal lie 652.9

malposition

 fetus 652.9

  in multiple gestation 652.6

 pelvic organs or tissues NEC 654.9

 uterus NEC or cervix 654.4

malpresentation NEC 652.9

 in multiple gestation 652.6

maternal

 diabetes mellitus (conditions classifiable to 249 and 250) 648.0

 heart disease NEC 648.6

meconium in liquor 656.8

 staining only 792.3

oblique presentation 652.3

oversize fetus 653.5

pelvic tumor NEC 654.9

placental insufficiency 656.5

placenta previa 641.0

 with hemorrhage 641.1

(planned) occurring after 37 completed weeks of gestation but before 39 completed weeks gestation due to (spontaneous) onset of labor 649.8

poor dilation, cervix 661.0

pre-eclampsia 642.4

 severe 642.5

previous

 cesarean delivery 654.2

 surgery (to)

  cervix 654.6

  gynecological NEC 654.9

  rectum 654.8

  uterus NEC 654.9

   from previous cesarean delivery 654.2

  vagina 654.7

prolapse

 arm or hand 652.7

 uterus 654.4

prolonged labor 662.1

rectocele 654.4

retroversion, uterus or cervix 654.3

rigid

 cervix 654.6

 pelvic floor 654.4

 perineum 654.8

 vagina 654.7

 vulva 654.8

sacculation, pregnant uterus 654.4

scar(s)

 cervix 654.6

 cesarean delivery 654.2

 uterus NEC 654.9

  due to previous cesarean delivery 654.2

Shirodkar suture in situ 654.5

shoulder presentation 652.8

stenosis or stricture, cervix 654.6

transverse presentation or lie 652.3

tumor, pelvic organs or tissues NEC 654.4

umbilical cord presentation or prolapse 663.0

Delivery—*continued*

completely normal case—*see* category 650

complicated (by) NEC 669.9

abdominal tumor, fetal 653.7

 causing obstructed labor 660.1

abnormal, abnormality of

 cervix 654.6

  causing obstructed labor 660.2

 forces of labor 661.9

 formation of uterus 654.0

 pelvic organs or tissues 654.9

  causing obstructed labor 660.2

 pelvis (bony) (major) NEC 653.0

  causing obstructed labor 660.1

 presentation or position NEC 652.9

  causing obstructed labor 660.0

 size, fetus 653.5

  causing obstructed labor 660.1

 soft parts (of pelvis) 654.9

  causing obstructed labor 660.2

 uterine contractions NEC 661.9

 uterus (formation) 654.0

  causing obstructed labor 660.2

 vagina 654.7

  causing obstructed labor 660.2

abnormally formed uterus (any type) (congenital) 654.0

 causing obstructed labor 660.2

acromion presentation 652.8

 causing obstructed labor 660.0

adherent placenta 667.0

 with hemorrhage 666.0

adhesions, uterus (to abdominal wall) 654.4

advanced maternal age NEC 659.6

 multigravida 659.6

 primigravida 659.5

air embolism 673.0

amnionitis 658.4

amniotic fluid embolism 673.1

anesthetic death 668.9

annular detachment, cervix 665.3

antepartum hemorrhage—*see* Delivery, complicated, hemorrhage

anteversion, cervix or uterus 654.4

 causing obstructed labor 660.2

apoplexy 674.0

 placenta 641.2

arrested active phase 661.1

asymmetrical pelvis bone 653.0

 causing obstructed labor 660.1

atony, uterus with hemorrhage (hypotonic) (inertia) 666.1

 hypertonic 661.4

Bandl's ring 661.4

battledore placenta—*see* Placenta, abnormal

bicornis or bicornuate uterus 654.0

 causing obstructed labor 660.2

birth injury to mother NEC 665.9

bleeding (*see also* Delivery, complicated, hemorrhage) 641.9

breech presentation (assisted) (buttocks) (complete) (frank) (spontaneous) 652.2

 with successful version 652.1

brow presentation 652.4

cephalopelvic disproportion (normally formed fetus) 653.4

 causing obstructed labor 660.1

cerebral hemorrhage 674.0

cervical dystocia 661.2

chin presentation 652.4

 causing obstructed labor 660.0

Delivery—*continued*
  complicated by—*continued*
    cicatrix
      cervix 654.6
        causing obstructed labor 660.2
      vagina 654.7
        causing obstructed labor 660.2
    coagulation defect 649.3
    colporrhexis 665.4
      with perineal laceration 664.0
    compound presentation 652.8
      causing obstructed labor 660.0
    compression of cord (umbilical) 663.2
      around neck 663.1
      cord prolapsed 663.0
    contraction, contracted pelvis 653.1
      causing obstructed labor 660.1
      general 653.1
        causing obstructed labor 660.1
      inlet 653.2
        causing obstructed labor 660.1
      midpelvic 653.8
        causing obstructed labor 660.1
      midplane 653.8
        causing obstructed labor 660.1
      outlet 653.3
        causing obstructed labor 660.1
    contraction ring 661.4
    cord (umbilical) 663.9
      around neck, tightly or with compression 663.1
        without compression 663.3
      bruising 663.6
      complication NEC 663.9
        specified type NEC 663.8
      compression NEC 663.2
      entanglement NEC 663.3
        with compression 663.2
      forelying 663.0
      hematoma 663.6
      marginal attachment 663.8
      presentation 663.0
      prolapse (complete) (occult) (partial) 663.0
      short 663.4
      specified complication NEC 663.8
      thrombosis (vessels) 663.6
      vascular lesion 663.6
      velamentous insertion 663.8
    Couvelaire uterus 641.2
    cretin pelvis (dwarf type) (male type) 653.1
      causing obstructed labor 660.1
    crossbirth 652.3
      with successful version 652.1
      causing obstructed labor 660.0
    cyst (Gartner's duct) 654.7
    cystocele 654.4
      causing obstructed labor 660.2
    death of fetus (near term) 656.4
      early (before 22 completed weeks'
        gestation) 632
    deformity (acquired) (congenital)
      fetus 653.7
        causing obstructed labor 660.1
      pelvic organs or tissues NEC 654.9
        causing obstructed labor 660.2
      pelvis (bony) NEC 653.0
        causing obstructed labor 660.1
    delay, delayed
      delivery in multiple pregnancy 662.3
        due to locked mates 660.5
      following rupture of membranes
        (spontaneous) 658.2
        artificial 658.3

Delivery—*continued*
  complicated by—*continued*
    depressed fetal heart tones 659.7
    diastasis recti 665.8
    dilatation
      bladder 654.4
        causing obstructed labor 660.2
      cervix, incomplete, poor or slow 661.0
    diseased placenta 656.7
    displacement uterus NEC 654.4
      causing obstructed labor 660.2
    disproportion NEC 653.9
      causing obstructed labor 660.1
    disruptio uteri—*see* Delivery, complicated,
      rupture, uterus
    distress
      fetal 656.8
      maternal 669.0
    double uterus (congenital) 654.0
      causing obstructed labor 660.2
    dropsy amnion 657
    dysfunction, uterus 661.9
      hypertonic 661.4
      hypotonic 661.2
        primary 661.0
        secondary 661.1
      incoordinate 661.4
    dystocia
      cervical 661.2
      fetal—*see* Delivery, complicated, abnormal,
        presentation
      maternal—*see* Delivery, complicated,
        prolonged labor
      pelvic—*see* Delivery, complicated,
        contraction pelvis
      positional 652.8
      shoulder girdle 660.4
    eclampsia 642.6
    ectopic kidney 654.4
      causing obstructed labor 660.2
    edema, cervix 654.6
      causing obstructed labor 660.2
    effusion, amniotic fluid 658.1
    elderly multigravida 659.6
    elderly primigravida 659.5
    embolism (pulmonary) 673.2
      air 673.0
      amniotic fluid 673.1
      blood-clot 673.2
      cerebral 674.0
      fat 673.8
      pyemic 673.3
      septic 673.3
    entanglement, umbilical cord 663.3
      with compression 663.2
      around neck (with compression) 663.1
    eversion, cervix or uterus 665.2
    excessive
      fetal growth 653.5
        causing obstructed labor 660.1
      size of fetus 653.5
        causing obstructed labor 660.1
    face presentation 652.4
      causing obstructed labor 660.0
      to pubes 660.3
    failure, fetal head to enter pelvic brim 652.5
      causing obstructed labor 660.0
    female genital mutilation 660.8

Delivery—*continued*
  complicated by—*continued*
    fetal
      acid-base balance 656.8
      death (near term) NEC 656.4
        early (before 22 completed weeks'
          gestation) 632
      deformity 653.7
        causing obstructed labor 660.1
      distress 656.8
      heart rate or rhythm 659.7
      reduction of multiple fetuses reduced to
        single fetus 651.7
    fetopelvic disproportion 653.4
      causing obstructed labor 660.1
    fever during labor 659.2
    fibroid (tumor) (uterus) 654.1
      causing obstructed labor 660.2
    fibromyomata 654.1
      causing obstructed labor 660.2
    forelying umbilical cord 663.0
    fracture of coccyx 665.6
    hematoma 664.5
      broad ligament 665.7
      ischial spine 665.7
      pelvic 665.7
      perineum 664.5
      soft tissues 665.7
      subdural 674.0
      umbilical cord 663.6
      vagina 665.7
      vulva or perineum 664.5
    hemorrhage (uterine) (antepartum)
      (intrapartum) (pregnancy) 641.9
      accidental 641.2
      associated with
        afibrinogenemia 641.3
        coagulation defect 641.3
          hyperfibrinolysis 641.3
          hypofibrinogenemia 641.3
      cerebral 674.0
      due to
        low-lying placenta 641.1
        placenta previa 641.1
        premature separation of placenta (normally
          implanted) 641.2
        retained placenta 666.0
        trauma 641.8
        uterine leiomyoma 641.8
      marginal sinus rupture 641.2
      placenta NEC 641.9
      postpartum (atonic) (immediate) (within 24
        hours) 666.1
        with retained or trapped placenta 666.0
        third stage 666.0
        delayed 666.2
        secondary 666.2
    hourglass contraction, uterus 661.4
    hydramnios 657
    hydrocephalic fetus 653.6
      causing obstructed labor 660.1
    hydrops fetalis 653.7
      causing obstructed labor 660.1
    hypertension—*see* Hypertension, complicating
      pregnancy
    hypertonic uterine dysfunction 661.4
    hypotonic uterine dysfunction 661.2
    impacted shoulders 660.4
    incarceration, uterus 654.3
      causing obstructed labor 660.2
    incomplete dilation (cervix) 661.0
    incoordinate uterus 661.4

Delivery—*continued*
  complicated by—*continued*
    indication NEC 659.9
      specified type NEC 659.8
    inertia, uterus 661.2
      hypertonic 661.4
      hypotonic 661.2
      primary 661.0
      secondary 661.1
    infantile
      genitalia 654.4
        causing obstructed labor 660.2
      uterus (os) 654.4
        causing obstructed labor 660.2
    injury (to mother) NEC 665.9
    intrauterine fetal death (near term) NEC 656.4
      early (before 22 completed weeks'
        gestation) 632
    inversion, uterus 665.2
    kidney, ectopic 654.4
      causing obstructed labor 660.2
    knot (true), umbilical cord 663.2
    labor
      onset (spontaneous) after 37 completed
        weeks of gestation but before 39
        completed weeks gestation with delivery
        by (planned) cesarean section 649.8
      premature (before 37 completed weeks
        gestation) 644.2
    laceration 664.9
      anus (sphincter) (healed) (old) 654.8
        not associated with third-degree perineal
          laceration 664.6
        with mucosa 664.3
      bladder (urinary) 665.5
      bowel 665.5
      central 664.4
      cervix (uteri) 665.3
      fourchette 664.0
      hymen 664.0
      labia (majora) (minora) 664.0
      pelvic
        floor 664.1
        organ NEC 665.5
      perineum, perineal 664.4
        first degree 664.0
        second degree 664.1
        third degree 664.2
        fourth degree 664.3
        central 664.4
        extensive NEC 664.4
        muscles 664.1
        skin 664.0
        slight 664.0
      peritoneum (pelvic) 665.5
      periurethral tissue 664.8
      rectovaginal (septum) (without perineal
        laceration) 665.4
        with perineum 664.2
          with anal or rectal mucosa 664.3
      skin (perineum) 664.0
      specified site or type NEC 664.8
      sphincter ani (healed) (old) 654.8
        not associated with third-degree perineal
          laceration 664.6
        with mucosa 664.3
      urethra 665.5
      uterus 665.1
        before labor 665.0

Delivery—*continued*
  complicated by—*continued*
    laceration—*continued*
      vagina, vaginal (deep) (high) (sulcus) (wall)
          (without perineal laceration) 665.4
        with perineum 664.0
        muscles, with perineum 664.1
        vulva 664.0
      lateroversion, uterus or cervix 654.4
        causing obstructed labor 660.2
      locked mates 660.5
      low implantation of placenta—*see* Delivery,
          complicated, placenta, previa
      mal lie 652.9
      malposition
        fetus NEC 652.9
          causing obstructed labor 660.0
        pelvic organs or tissues NEC 654.9
          causing obstructed labor 660.2
        placenta 641.1
          without hemorrhage 641.0
        uterus NEC or cervix 654.4
          causing obstructed labor 660.2
      malpresentation 652.9
        causing obstructed labor 660.0
      marginal sinus (bleeding) (rupture) 641.2
      maternal hypotension syndrome 669.2
      meconium in liquor 656.8
      membranes, retained—*see* Delivery,
          complicated, placenta, retained
      mentum presentation 652.4
        causing obstructed labor 660.0
      metrorrhagia (myopathia)—*see* Delivery,
          complicated, hemorrhage
      metrorrhexis—*see* Delivery, complicated,
          rupture, uterus
      multiparity (grand) 659.4
      myelomeningocele, fetus 653.7
        causing obstructed labor 660.1
      Nägele's pelvis 653.0
        causing obstructed labor 660.1
      nonengagement, fetal head 652.5
        causing obstructed labor 660.0
      oblique presentation 652.3
        causing obstructed labor 660.0
      obstetric
        shock 669.1
        trauma NEC 665.9
      obstructed labor 660.9
        due to
          abnormality pelvic organs or tissues
              (conditions classifiable to 654.0-654.9)
              660.2
          deep transverse arrest 660.3
          impacted shoulders 660.4
          locked twins 660.5
          malposition and malpresentation of fetus
              (conditions classifiable to 652.0-652.9)
              660.0
          persistent occipitoposterior 660.3
          shoulder dystocia 660.4
      occult prolapse of umbilical cord 663.0
      oversize fetus 653.5
        causing obstructed labor 660.1
      pathological retraction ring, uterus 661.4
      pelvic
        arrest (deep) (high) (of fetal head)
            (transverse) 660.3
        deformity (bone)—*see also* Deformity,
            pelvis, with disproportion
          soft tissue 654.9
            causing obstructed labor 660.2

Delivery—*continued*
  complicated by—*continued*
    pelvic—*continued*
      tumor NEC 654.9
        causing obstructed labor 660.2
      penetration, pregnant uterus by instrument 665.1
      perforation—*see* Delivery, complicated,
          laceration
      persistent
        hymen 654.8
          causing obstructed labor 660.2
        occipitoposterior 660.3
      placenta, placental
        ablatio 641.2
        abnormality 656.7
          with hemorrhage 641.2
        abruptio 641.2
        accreta 667.0
          with hemorrhage 666.0
        adherent (without hemorrhage) 667.0
          with hemorrhage 666.0
        apoplexy 641.2
        battledore 663.8
        detachment (premature) 641.2
        disease 656.7
        hemorrhage NEC 641.9
        increta (without hemorrhage) 667.0
          with hemorrhage 666.0
        low (implantation) 641.1
          without hemorrhage 641.0
        malformation 656.7
          with hemorrhage 641.2
        malposition 641.1
          without hemorrhage 641.0
        marginal sinus rupture 641.2
        percreta 667.0
          with hemorrhage 666.0
        premature separation 641.2
        previa (central) (lateral) (marginal) (partial)
            641.1
          without hemorrhage 641.0
        retained (with hemorrhage) 666.0
          without hemorrhage 667.0
        rupture of marginal sinus 641.2
        separation (premature) 641.2
        trapped 666.0
          without hemorrhage 667.0
        vicious insertion 641.1
      polyhydramnios 657
      polyp, cervix 654.6
        causing obstructed labor 660.2
      precipitate labor 661.3
      premature
        labor (before 37 completed weeks gestation)
            644.2
        rupture, membranes 658.1
          delayed delivery following 658.2
      presenting umbilical cord 663.0
      previous
        cesarean delivery 654.2
        surgery
          cervix 654.6
            causing obstructed labor 660.2
          gynecological NEC 654.9
            causing obstructed labor 660.2
          perineum 654.8
          rectum 654.8
          uterus NEC 654.9
            due to previous cesarean delivery 654.2
          vagina 654.7
            causing obstructed labor 660.2
          vulva 654.8

Delivery—*continued*
  complicated by—*continued*
    primary uterine inertia 661.0
    primipara, elderly or old 659.5
    prolapse
      arm or hand 652.7
        causing obstructed labor 660.0
      cord (umbilical) 663.0
      fetal extremity 652.8
      foot or leg 652.8
        causing obstructed labor 660.0
      umbilical cord (complete) (occult) (partial)
        663.0
      uterus 654.4
        causing obstructed labor 660.2
    prolonged labor 662.1
      active phase 661.2
      due to
        cervical dystocia 661.2
        contraction ring 661.4
        tetanic uterus 661.4
        uterine inertia 661.2
          primary 661.0
          secondary 661.1
      first stage 662.0
      latent phase 661.0
      second stage 662.2
    pyrexia during labor 659.2
    rachitic pelvis 653.2
      causing obstructed labor 660.1
    rectocele 654.4
      causing obstructed labor 660.2
    retained membranes or portions of placenta
      666.2
      without hemorrhage 667.1
    retarded (prolonged) birth 662.1
    retention secundines (with hemorrhage) 666.2
      without hemorrhage 667.1
    retroversion, uterus or cervix 654.3
      causing obstructed labor 660.2
    rigid
      cervix 654.6
        causing obstructed labor 660.2
      pelvic floor 654.4
        causing obstructed labor 660.2
      perineum or vulva 654.8
        causing obstructed labor 660.2
      vagina 654.7
        causing obstructed labor 660.2
    Robert's pelvis 653.0
      causing obstructed labor 660.1
    rupture—*see also* Delivery, complicated,
        laceration
      bladder (urinary) 665.5
      cervix 665.3
      marginal sinus 641.2
      membranes, premature 658.1
      pelvic organ NEC 665.5
      perineum (without mention of other
          laceration)—*see* Delivery, complicated,
          laceration, perineum
      peritoneum (pelvic) 665.5
      urethra 665.5
      uterus (during labor) 665.1
        before labor 665.0
    sacculation, pregnant uterus 654.4
    sacral teratomas, fetal 653.7
      causing obstructed labor 660.1

Delivery—*continued*
  complicated by—*continued*
    scar(s)
      cervix 654.6
        causing obstructed labor 660.2
      cesarean delivery 654.2
        causing obstructed labor 660.2
      perineum 654.8
        causing obstructed labor 660.2
      uterus NEC 654.9
        causing obstructed labor 660.2
        due to previous cesarean delivery 654.2
      vagina 654.7
        causing obstructed labor 660.2
      vulva 654.8
        causing obstructed labor 660.2
    scoliotic pelvis 653.0
      causing obstructed labor 660.1
    secondary uterine inertia 661.1
    secundines, retained—*see* Delivery,
        complicated, placenta, retained
    separation
      placenta (premature) 641.2
      pubic bone 665.6
      symphysis pubis 665.6
    septate vagina 654.7
      causing obstructed labor 660.2
    shock (birth) (obstetric) (puerperal) 669.1
    short cord syndrome 663.4
    shoulder
      girdle dystocia 660.4
      presentation 652.8
        causing obstructed labor 660.0
    Siamese twins 678.1
    slow slope active phase 661.2
    spasm
      cervix 661.4
      uterus 661.4
    spondylolisthesis, pelvis 653.3
      causing obstructed labor 660.1
    spondylolysis (lumbosacral) 653.3
      causing obstructed labor 660.1
    spondylosis 653.0
      causing obstructed labor 660.1
    stenosis or stricture
      cervix 654.6
        causing obstructed labor 660.2
      vagina 654.7
        causing obstructed labor 660.2
    sudden death, unknown cause 669.9
    tear (pelvic organ) (*see also* Delivery,
        complicated, laceration) 664.9
      anal sphincter (healed) (old) 654.8
        not associated with third-degree perineal
          laceration 664.6
    teratomas, sacral, fetal 653.7
      causing obstructed labor 660.1
    tetanic uterus 661.4
    tipping pelvis 653.0
      causing obstructed labor 660.1
    transverse
      arrest (deep) 660.3
      presentation or lie 652.3
        with successful version 652.1
        causing obstructed labor 660.0
    trauma (obstetrical) NEC 665.9
      periurethral 664.8

Delivery—*continued*
  complicated by—*continued*
    tumor
      abdominal, fetal 653.7
        causing obstructed labor 660.1
      pelvic organs or tissues NEC 654.9
        causing obstructed labor 660.2
    umbilical cord (*see also* Delivery,
        complicated, cord) 663.9
      around neck tightly, or with compression
        663.1
      entanglement NEC 663.3
        with compression 663.2
      prolapse (complete) (occult) (partial) 663.0
    unstable lie 652.0
      causing obstructed labor 660.0
    uterine
      inertia (*see also* Delivery, complicated,
        inertia, uterus) 661.2
      spasm 661.4
    vasa previa 663.5
    velamentous insertion of cord 663.8
    young maternal age 659.8
  delayed NEC 662.1
    following rupture of membranes (spontaneous)
        658.2
      artificial 658.3
    second twin, triplet, etc. 662.3
  difficult NEC 669.9
    previous, affecting management of pregnancy
        or childbirth V23.49
    specified type NEC 669.8
  early onset (spontaneous) 644.2
  forceps NEC 669.5
    affecting fetus or newborn 763.2
  footling 652.8
    with successful version 652.1
  missed (at or near term) 656.4
  multiple gestation NEC 651.9
    with fetal loss and retention of one or more
        fetus(es) 651.6
    following (elective) fetal reduction 651.7
    specified type NEC 651.8
      with fetal loss and retention of one or more
        fetus(es) 651.6
      following (elective) fetal reduction 651.7
  nonviable infant 656.4
  normal—*see* category 650
  precipitate 661.3
    affecting fetus or newborn 763.6
  premature NEC (before 37 completed weeks
      gestation) 644.2
    previous, affecting management of pregnancy
        V23.41
  quadruplet NEC 651.2
    with fetal loss and retention of one or more
        fetus(es) 651.5
    following (elective) fetal reduction 651.7
  quintuplet NEC 651.8
    with fetal loss and retention of one or more
        fetus(es) 651.6
    following (elective) fetal reduction 651.7
  sextuplet NEC 651.8
    with fetal loss and retention of one or more
        fetus(es) 651.6
    following (elective) fetal reduction 651.7
  specified complication NEC 669.8
  stillbirth (near term) NEC 656.4
    early (before 22 completed weeks' gestation)
        632

Delivery—*continued*
  term pregnancy (live birth) NEC—*see* category
      650
    stillbirth NEC 656.4
  threatened premature 644.2
  triplets NEC 651.1
    with fetal loss and retention of one or more
        fetus(es) 651.4
    delayed delivery (one or more mates) 662.3
    following (elective) fetal reduction 651.7
    locked mates 660.5
  twins NEC 651.0
    with fetal loss and retention of one or more
        fetus(es) 651.3
    delayed delivery (one or more mates) 662.3
    following (elective) fetal reduction 651.7
    locked mates 660.5
  uncomplicated—*see* category 650
  vacuum extractor NEC 669.5
    affecting fetus or newborn 763.3
  ventouse NEC 669.5
    affecting fetus or newborn 763.3
Dellen, cornea 371.41
Delusions (paranoid) 297.9
  grandiose 297.1
  parasitosis 300.29
  systematized 297.1
Dementia 294.20
  with behavioral disturbance (aggressive)
      (combative) (violent) 294.21
  alcohol-induced persisting (*see also* Psychosis,
      alcoholic) 291.2
  Alzheimer's—*see* Alzheimer's dementia
  arteriosclerotic (simple type) (uncomplicated)
      290.40
    with
      acute confusional state 290.41
      delirium 290.41
      delusions 290.42
      depressed mood 290.43
    depressed type 290.43
    paranoid type 290.42
  Binswanger's 290.12
  catatonic (acute) (*see also* Schizophrenia) 295.2
  congenital (*see also* Disability, intellectual) 319
  degenerative 290.9
    presenile-onset—*see* Dementia, presenile
    senile-onset—*see* Dementia, senile
  developmental (*see also* Schizophrenia) 295.9
  dialysis 294.8
    transient 293.9
  drug-induced persisting (*see also* Psychosis,
      drug) 292.82
  due to or associated with condition(s) classified
      elsewhere
    Alzheimer's
      with behavioral disturbance 331.0 *[294.11]*
      without behavioral disturbance 331.0
        [294.10]
    cerebral lipidoses
      with behavioral disturbance 330.1 *[294.11]*
      without behavioral disturbance 330.1
        [294.10]
    epilepsy
      with behavioral disturbance 345.9 *[294.11]*
      without behavioral disturbance 345.9
        [294.10]
    hepatolenticular degeneration
      with behavioral disturbance 275.1 *[294.11]*
      without behavioral disturbance 275.1
        [294.10]

Dementia—*continued*
  due to or associated with—*continued*
    HIV
      with behavioral disturbance 042 *[294.11]*
      without behavioral disturbance 042 *[294.10]*
    Huntington's chorea
      with behavioral disturbance 333.4 *[294.11]*
      without behavioral disturbance 333.4
        [294.10]
    Jakob-Creutzfeldt disease (CJD)
      with behavioral disturbance 046.19 *[294.11]*
      without behavioral disturbance 046.19
        [294.10]
      variant (vCJD) 046.11
        with dementia
          with behavioral disturbance 046.11
            [294.11]
          without behavioral disturbance 046.11
            [294.10]
    Lewy bodies
      with behavioral disturbance 331.82 *[294.11]*
      without behavioral disturbance 331.82
        [294.10]
    multiple sclerosis
      with behavioral disturbance 340 *[294.11]*
      without behavioral disturbance 340 *[294.10]*
    neurosyphilis
      with behavioral disturbance 094.9 *[294.11]*
      without behavioral disturbance 094.9
        [294.10]
    Parkinsonism
      with behavioral disturbance 331.82 *[294.11]*
      without behavioral disturbance 331.82
        [294.10]
    Parkinson's disease
      with behavioral disturbance 332.0 *[294.11]*
      without behavioral disturbance 332.0
        [294.10]
    Pelizaeus-Merzbacher disease
      with behavioral disturbance 333.0 *[294.11]*
      without behavioral disturbance 333.0
        [294.10]
    Pick's disease
      with behavioral disturbance 331.11 *[294.11]*
      without behavioral disturbance 331.11
        [294.10]
    polyarteritis nodosa
      with behavioral disturbance 446.0 *[294.11]*
      without behavioral disturbance 446.0
        [294.10]
    syphilis
      with behavioral disturbance 094.1 *[294.11]*
      without behavioral disturbance 094.1
        [294.10]
    Wilson's disease
      with behavioral disturbance 275.1 *[294.11]*
      without behavioral disturbance 275.1
        [294.10]
  frontal 331.19
    with behavioral disturbance 331.19 *[294.11]*
    without behavioral disturbance 331.19
      [294.10]
  frontotemporal 331.19
    with behavioral disturbance 331.19 *[294.11]*
    without behavioral disturbance 331.19
      [294.10]
  hebephrenic (acute) 295.1
  Heller's (infantile psychosis) (*see also*
    Psychosis, childhood) 299.1
  idiopathic 290.9
    presenile-onset—*see* Dementia, presenile
    senile-onset—*see* Dementia, senile

Dementia—*continued*
  in
    arteriosclerotic brain disease 290.40
    senility 290.0
  induced by drug 292.82
  infantile, infantilia (*see also* Psychosis,
    childhood) 299.0
  Lewy body 331.82
    with behavioral disturbance 331.82 *[294.11]*
    without behavioral disturbance 331.82 *[294.10]*
  multi-infarct (cerebrovascular) (*see also*
    Dementia, arteriosclerotic) 290.40
  old age 290.0
  paralytica, paralytic 094.1
    juvenilis 090.40
    syphilitic 094.1
      congenital 090.40
    tabetic form 094.1
  paranoid (*see also* Schizophrenia) 295.3
  paraphrenic (*see also* Schizophrenia) 295.3
  paretic 094.1
  praecox (*see also* Schizophrenia) 295.9
  presenile 290.10
    with
      acute confusional state 290.11
      delirium 290.11
      delusional features 290.12
      depressive features 290.13
    depressed type 290.13
    paranoid type 290.12
    simple type 290.10
    uncomplicated 290.10
  primary (acute) (*see also* Schizophrenia) 295.0
  progressive, syphilitic 094.1
  puerperal—*see* Psychosis, puerperal
  schizophrenic (*see also* Schizophrenia) 295.9
  senile 290.0
    with
      acute confusional state 290.3
      delirium 290.3
      delusional features 290.20
      depressive features 290.21
    depressed type 290.21
    exhaustion 290.0
    paranoid type 290.20
  simple type (acute) (*see also* Schizophrenia) 295.0
  simplex (acute) (*see also* Schizophrenia) 295.0
  syphilitic 094.1
  uremic—*see* Uremia
  vascular 290.40
    with
      delirium 290.41
      delusions 290.42
      depressed mood 290.43
Demerol dependence (*see also* Dependence)
  304.0
Demineralization, ankle (*see also* Osteoporosis)
  733.00
Demodex folliculorum (infestation) 133.8
Demoralization 799.25
de Morgan's spots (senile angiomas) 448.1
Demyelinating
  polyneuritis, chronic inflammatory 357.81
Demyelination, demyelinization
  central nervous system 341.9
    specified NEC 341.8
  corpus callosum (central) 341.8
  global 340
Dengue (fever) 061
  sandfly 061
  vaccination, prophylactic (against) V05.1
  virus hemorrhagic fever 065.4

Dens
evaginatus 520.2
in dente 520.2
invaginatus 520.2
Dense breast(s) 793.82
Density
increased, bone (disseminated) (generalized)
(spotted) 733.99
lung (nodular) 518.89
Dental —*see also* condition
examination only V72.2
Dentia praecox 520.6
Denticles (in pulp) 522.2
Dentigerous cyst 526.0
Dentin
irregular (in pulp) 522.3
opalescent 520.5
secondary (in pulp) 522.3
sensitive 521.89
Dentinogenesis imperfecta 520.5
Dentinoma (M9271/0) 213.1
upper jaw (bone) 213.0
Dentition 520.7
abnormal 520.6
anomaly 520.6
delayed 520.6
difficult 520.7
disorder of 520.6
precocious 520.6
retarded 520.6
Denture sore (mouth) 528.9
Dependence

---

*Note—Use the following fifth-digit
subclassification with category 304:*

0 unspecified
1 continuous
2 episodic
3 in remission

---

with
withdrawal symptoms
alcohol 291.81
drug 292.0
14-hydroxy-dihydromorphinone 304.0
absinthe 304.6
acemorphan 304.0
acetanilid(e) 304.6
acetophenetidin 304.6
acetorphine 304.0
acetyldihydrocodeine 304.0
acetyldihydrocodeinone 304.0
Adalin 304.1
Afghanistan black 304.3
agrypnal 304.1
alcohol, alcoholic (ethyl) (methyl) (wood) 303.9
maternal, with suspected fetal damage
affecting management of pregnancy 655.4
allobarbitone 304.1
allonal 304.1
allylisopropylacetylurea 304.1
alphaprodine (hydrochloride) 304.0
Alurate 304.1
Alvodine 304.0
amethocaine 304.6
amidone 304.0
amidopyrine 304.6
aminopyrine 304.6
amobarbital 304.1
amphetamine(s) (type) (drugs classifiable to
969.7) 304.4

Dependence—*continued*
amylene hydrate 304.6
amylobarbitone 304.1
amylocaine 304.6
Amytal (sodium) 304.1
analgesic (drug) NEC 304.6
synthetic with morphine-like effect 304.0
anesthetic (agent) (drug) (gas) (general) (local)
NEC 304.6
Angel dust 304.6
anileridine 304.0
antipyrine 304.6
anxiolytic 304.1
aprobarbital 304.1
aprobarbitone 304.1
atropine 304.6
Avertin (bromide) 304.6
barbenyl 304.1
barbital(s) 304.1
barbitone 304.1
barbiturate(s) (compounds) (drugs classifiable to
967.0) 304.1
barbituric acid (and compounds) 304.1
benzedrine 304.4
benzylmorphine 304.0
Beta-chlor 304.1
bhang 304.3
blue velvet 304.0
Brevital 304.1
bromal (hydrate) 304.1
bromide(s) NEC 304.1
bromine compounds NEC 304.1
bromisovalum 304.1
bromoform 304.1
Bromo-seltzer 304.1
bromural 304.1
butabarbital (sodium) 304.1
butabarpal 304.1
butallylonal 304.1
butethal 304.1
buthalitone (sodium) 304.1
Butisol 304.1
butobarbitone 304.1
butyl chloral (hydrate) 304.1
caffeine 304.4
cannabis (indica) (sativa) (resin) (derivatives)
(type) 304.3
carbamazepine 304.6
Carbrital 304.1
carbromal 304.1
carisoprodol 304.6
Catha (edulis) 304.4
chloral (betaine) (hydrate) 304.1
chloralamide 304.1
chloralformamide 304.1
chloralose 304.1
chlordiazepoxide 304.1
Chloretone 304.1
chlorobutanol 304.1
chlorodyne 304.1
chloroform 304.6
Cliradon 304.0
coca (leaf) and derivatives 304.2
cocaine 304.2
hydrochloride 304.2
salt (any) 304.2
codeine 304.0
combination of drugs (excluding morphine or
opioid type drug) NEC 304.8
morphine or opioid type drug with any other
drug 304.7

Dependence—*continued*
croton-chloral 304.1
cyclobarbital 304.1
cyclobarbitone 304.1
dagga 304.3
Delvinal 304.1
Demerol 304.0
desocodeine 304.0
desomorphine 304.0
desoxyephedrine 304.4
DET 304.5
dexamphetamine 304.4
dexedrine 304.4
dextromethorphan 304.0
dextromoramide 304.0
dextronorpseudoephedrine 304.4
dextrorphan 304.0
diacetylmorphine 304.0
Dial 304.1
diallylbarbituric acid 304.1
diamorphine 304.0
diazepam 304.1
dibucaine 304.6
dichloroethane 304.6
diethyl barbituric acid 304.1
diethylsulfone-diethylmethane 304.1
difencloxazine 304.0
dihydrocodeine 304.0
dihydrocodeinone 304.0
dihydrohydroxycodeinone 304.0
dihydroisocodeine 304.0
dihydromorphine 304.0
dihydromorphinone 304.0
dihydroxcodeinone 304.0
Dilaudid 304.0
dimenhydrinate 304.6
dimethylmeperidine 304.0
dimethyltriptamine 304.5
Dionin 304.0
diphenoxylate 304.6
dipipanone 304.0
d-lysergic acid diethylamide 304.5
DMT 304.5
Dolophine 304.0
DOM 304.2
Doriden 304.1
dormiral 304.1
Dormison 304.1
Dromoran 304.0
drug NEC 304.9
    analgesic NEC 304.6
    combination (excluding morphine or opioid
        type drug) NEC 304.8
        morphine or opioid type drug with any other
            drug 304.7
    complicating pregnancy, childbirth, or
        puerperium 648.3
        affecting fetus or newborn 779.5
    hallucinogenic 304.5
    hypnotic NEC 304.1
    narcotic NEC 304.9
    psychostimulant NEC 304.4
    sedative 304.1
    soporific NEC 304.1
    specified type NEC 304.6
    suspected damage to fetus affecting
        management of pregnancy 655.5
    synthetic, with morphine-like effect 304.0
    tranquilizing 304.1
duboisine 304.6

Dependence—*continued*
ectylurea 304.1
Endocaine 304.6
Equanil 304.1
Eskabarb 304.1
ethchlorvynol 304.1
ether (ethyl) (liquid) (vapor) (vinyl) 304.6
ethidene 304.6
ethinamate 304.1
ethoheptazine 304.6
ethyl
    alcohol 303.9
    bromide 304.6
    carbamate 304.6
    chloride 304.6
    morphine 304.0
ethylene (gas) 304.6
    dichloride 304.6
ethylidene chloride 304.6
etilfen 304.1
etorphine 304.0
etoval 304.1
eucodal 304.0
euneryl 304.1
Evipal 304.1
Evipan 304.1
fentanyl 304.0
ganja 304.3
gardenal 304.1
gardenpanyl 304.1
gelsemine 304.6
Gelsemium 304.6
Gemonil 304.1
glucochloral 304.1
glue (airplane) (sniffing) 304.6
glutethimide 304.1
hallucinogenics 304.5
hashish 304.3
headache powder NEC 304.6
Heavenly Blue 304.5
hedonal 304.1
hemp 304.3
heptabarbital 304.1
Heptalgin 304.0
heptobarbitone 304.1
heroin 304.0
    salt (any) 304.0
hexethal (sodium) 304.1
hexobarbital 304.1
Hycodan 304.0
hydrocodone 304.0
hydromorphinol 304.0
hydromorphinone 304.0
hydromorphone 304.0
hydroxycodeine 304.0
hypnotic NEC 304.1
Indian hemp 304.3
inhalant 304.6
intranarcon 304.1
Kemithal 304.1
ketobemidone 304.0
khat 304.4
kif 304.3
Lactuca (virosa) extract 304.1
lactucarium 304.1
laudanum 304.0
Lebanese red 304.3
Leritine 304.0

Dependence—*continued*
lettuce opium 304.1
Levanil 304.1
Levo-Dromoran 304.0
levo-iso-methadone 304.0
levorphanol 304.0
Librium 304.1
Lomotil 304.6
Lotusate 304.1
LSD (-25) (and derivatives) 304.5
Luminal 304.1
lysergic acid 304.5
  amide 304.5
maconha 304.3
magic mushroom 304.5
marijuana 304.3
MDA (methylene dioxyamphetamine) 304.4
Mebaral 304.1
Medinal 304.1
Medomin 304.1
megahallucinogenics 304.5
meperidine 304.0
mephobarbital 304.1
meprobamate 304.1
mescaline 304.5
methadone 304.0
methamphetamine(s) 304.4
methaqualone 304.1
metharbital 304.1
methitural 304.1
methobarbitone 304.1
methohexital 304.1
methopholine 304.6
methyl
  alcohol 303.9
  bromide 304.6
  morphine 304.0
  sulfonal 304.1
methylated spirit 303.9
methylbutinol 304.6
methyldihydromorphinone 304.0
methylene
  chloride 304.6
  dichloride 304.6
  dioxyamphetamine (MDA) 304.4
methylparafynol 304.1
methylphenidate 304.4
methyprylone 304.1
metopon 304.0
Miltown 304.1
morning glory *see*ds 304.5
morphinan(s) 304.0
morphine (sulfate) (sulfite) (type) (drugs
  classifiable to 965.00-965.09) 304.0
morphine or opioid type drug (drugs classifiable
  to 965.00-965.09) with any other drug 304.7
morphinol(s) 304.0
morphinon 304.0
morpholinylethylmorphine 304.0
mylomide 304.1
myristicin 304.5
narcotic (drug) NEC 304.9
nealbarbital 304.1
nealbarbitone 304.1
Nembutal 304.1
Neonal 304.1
Neraval 304.1
Neravan 304.1
neurobarb 304.1
nicotine 305.1
Nisentil 304.0

Dependence—*continued*
nitrous oxide 304.6
Noctec 304.1
Noludar 304.1
nonbarbiturate sedatives and tranquilizers with
  similar effect 304.1
noptil 304.1
normorphine 304.0
noscapine 304.0
Novocaine 304.6
Numorphan 304.0
nunol 304.1
Nupercaine 304.6
Oblivon 304.1
on
  aspirator V46.0
  hemodialysis V45.11
  hyperbaric chamber V46.8
  iron lung V46.11
  machine (enabling) V46.9
    specified type NEC V46.8
  peritoneal dialysis V45.11
  Possum (Patient-Operated-Selector-
    Mechanism) V46.8
  renal dialysis machine V45.11
  respirator (ventilator) V46.11
    encounter
      during
        mechanical failure V46.14
        power failure V46.12
      for weaning V46.13
  supplemental oxygen V46.2
  wheelchair V46.3
opiate 304.0
opioids 304.0
opioid type drug 304.0
  with any other drug 304.7
opium (alkaloids) (derivatives) (tincture) 304.0
ortal 304.1
Oxazepam 304.1
oxycodone 304.0
oxymorphone 304.0
Palfium 304.0
Panadol 304.6
pantopium 304.0
pantopon 304.0
papaverine 304.0
paracetamol 304.6
paracodin 304.0
paraldehyde 304.1
paregoric 304.0
Parzone 304.0
PCP (phencyclidine) 304.6
Pearly Gates 304.5
pentazocine 304.0
pentobarbital 304.1
pentobarbitone (sodium) 304.1
Pentothal 304.1
Percaine 304.6
Percodan 304.0
Perichlor 304.1
Pernocton 304.1
Pernoston 304.1
peronine 304.0
pethidine (hydrochloride) 304.0
petrichloral 304.1
peyote 304.5
Phanodorn 304.1
phenacetin 304.6
phenadoxone 304.0
phenaglycodol 304.1
phenazocine 304.0

Dependence—*continued*
  phencyclidine 304.6
  phenmetrazine 304.4
  phenobal 304.1
  phenobarbital 304.1
  phenobarbitone 304.1
  phenomorphan 304.0
  phenonyl 304.1
  phenoperidine 304.0
  pholcodine 304.0
  piminodine 304.0
  Pipadone 304.0
  Pitkin's solution 304.6
  Placidyl 304.1
  polysubstance 304.8
  Pontocaine 304.6
  pot 304.3
  potassium bromide 304.1
  Preludin 304.4
  Prinadol 304.0
  probarbital 304.1
  procaine 304.6
  propanal 304.1
  propoxyphene 304.6
  psilocibin 304.5
  psilocin 304.5
  psilocybin 304.5
  psilocyline 304.5
  psilocyn 304.5
  psychedelic agents 304.5
  psychostimulant NEC 304.4
  psychotomimetic agents 304.5
  pyrahexyl 304.3
  Pyramidon 304.6
  quinalbarbitone 304.1
  racemoramide 304.0
  racemorphan 304.0
  Rela 304.6
  scopolamine 304.6
  secobarbital 304.1
  Seconal 304.1
  sedative NEC 304.1
    nonbarbiturate with barbiturate effect 304.1
  Sedormid 304.1
  sernyl 304.1
  sodium bromide 304.1
  Soma 304.6
  Somnal 304.1
  Somnos 304.1
  Soneryl 304.1
  soporific (drug) NEC 304.1
  specified drug NEC 304.6
  speed 304.4
  spinocaine 304.6
  Stovaine 304.6
  STP 304.5
  stramonium 304.6
  Sulfonal 304.1
  sulfonethylmethane 304.1
  sulfonmethane 304.1
  Surital 304.1
  synthetic drug with morphine-like effect 304.0
  talbutal 304.1
  tetracaine 304.6
  tetrahydrocannabinol 304.3
  tetronal 304.1
  THC 304.3
  thebacon 304.0
  thebaine 304.0
  thiamil 304.1
  thiamylal 304.1

Dependence—*continued*
  thiopental 304.1
  tobacco 305.1
  toluene, toluol 304.6
  tranquilizer NEC 304.1
    nonbarbiturate with barbiturate effect 304.1
  tribromacetaldehyde 304.6
  tribromethanol 304.6
  tribromomethane 304.6
  trichloroethanol 304.6
  trichoroethyl phosphate 304.1
  triclofos 304.1
  Trional 304.1
  Tuinal 304.1
  Turkish Green 304.3
  urethan(e) 304.6
  Valium 304.1
  Valmid 304.1
  veganin 304.0
  veramon 304.1
  Veronal 304.1
  versidyne 304.6
  vinbarbital 304.1
  vinbarbitone 304.1
  vinyl bitone 304.1
  vitamin B$_6$ 266.1
  wine 303.9
  Zactane 304.6
Dependency
  passive 301.6
  reactions 301.6
Depersonalization (episode, in neurotic state)
    (neurotic) (syndrome) 300.6
Depletion
  carbohydrates 271.9
  complement factor 279.8
  extracellular fluid 276.52
  plasma 276.52
  potassium 276.8
    nephropathy 588.89
  salt or sodium 276.1
    causing heat exhaustion or prostration 992.4
    nephropathy 593.9
  volume 276.50
    extracellular fluid 276.52
    plasma 276.52
Deployment (military)
  personal history of V62.22
  returned from V62.22
  status V62.21
Deposit
  argentous, cornea 371.16
  bone, in Boeck's sarcoid 135
  calcareous, calcium—*see* Calcification
  cholesterol
    retina 362.82
    skin 709.3
    vitreous (humor) 379.22
  conjunctival 372.56
  cornea, corneal NEC 371.10
    argentous 371.16
    in
      cystinosis 270.0 *[371.15]*
      mucopolysaccharidosis 277.5 *[371.15]*
  crystalline, vitreous (humor) 379.22
  hemosiderin, in old scars of cornea 371.11
  metallic, in lens 366.45
  skin 709.3
  teeth, tooth (betel) (black) (green) (materia alba)
      (orange) (soft) (tobacco) 523.6
  urate, in kidney (*see also* Disease, renal) 593.9
Depraved appetite 307.52

Depression 311
acute (*see also* Psychosis, affective) 296.2
  recurrent episode 296.3
  single episode 296.2
agitated (*see also* Psychosis, affective) 296.2
  recurrent episode 296.3
  single episode 296.2
anaclitic 309.21
anxiety 300.4
arches 734
  congenital 754.61
autogenous (*see also* Psychosis, affective) 296.2
  recurrent episode 296.3
  single episode 296.2
basal metabolic rate (BMR) 794.7
bone marrow 289.9
central nervous system 799.1
  newborn 779.2
cerebral 331.9
  newborn 779.2
cerebrovascular 437.8
  newborn 779.2
chest wall 738.3
endogenous (*see also* Psychosis, affective) 296.2
  recurrent episode 296.3
  single episode 296.2
functional activity 780.99
hysterical 300.11
involutional, climacteric, or menopausal (*see also* Psychosis, affective) 296.2
  recurrent episode 296.3
  single episode 296.2
major 296.2
  recurrent episode 296.3
  single episode 296.2
manic (*see also* Psychosis, affective) 296.80
medullary 348.89
  newborn 779.2
mental 300.4
metatarsal heads—*see* Depression, arches
metatarsus—*see* Depression, arches
monopolar (*see also* Psychosis, affective) 296.2
  recurrent episode 296.3
  single episode 296.2
nervous 300.4
neurotic 300.4
nose 738.0
postpartum 648.4
psychogenic 300.4
  reactive 298.0
psychoneurotic 300.4
psychotic (*see also* Psychosis, affective) 296.2
  reactive 298.0
  recurrent episode 296.3
  single episode 296.2
reactive 300.4
  neurotic 300.4
  psychogenic 298.0
  psychoneurotic 300.4
  psychotic 298.0
recurrent 296.3
respiratory center 348.89
  newborn 770.89
scapula 736.89
senile 290.21
situational (acute) (brief) 309.0
  prolonged 309.1
skull 754.0
sternum 738.3
visual field 368.40

Depressive reaction —*see also* Reaction, depressive
acute (transient) 309.0
  with anxiety 309.28
prolonged 309.1
situational (acute) 309.0
  prolonged 309.1
Deprivation
cultural V62.4
emotional V62.89
  affecting
    adult 995.82
    infant or child 995.51
food 994.2
  specific substance NEC 269.8
protein (familial) (kwashiorkor) 260
sleep V69.4
social V62.4
  affecting
    adult 995.82
    infant or child 995.51
symptoms, syndrome
  alcohol 291.81
  drug 292.0
vitamins (*see also* Deficiency, vitamin) 269.2
water 994.3
de Quervain's
disease (tendon sheath) 727.04
thyroiditis (subacute granulomatous thyroiditis) 245.1
syndrome 259.51
Derangement
ankle (internal) 718.97
  current injury (*see also* Dislocation, ankle) 837.0
  recurrent 718.37
cartilage (articular) NEC (*see also* Disorder, cartilage, articular) 718.0
  knee 717.9
    recurrent 718.36
  recurrent 718.3
collateral ligament (knee) (medial) (tibial) 717.82
  current injury 844.1
    lateral (fibular) 844.0
  lateral (fibular) 717.81
    current injury 844.0
cruciate ligament (knee) (posterior) 717.84
  anterior 717.83
    current injury 844.2
  current injury 844.2
elbow (internal) 718.92
  current injury (*see also* Dislocation, elbow) 832.00
  recurrent 718.32
gastrointestinal 536.9
heart—*see* Disease, heart
hip (joint) (internal) (old) 718.95
  current injury (*see also* Dislocation, hip) 835.00
  recurrent 718.35
intervertebral disc—*see* Displacement, intervertebral disc
joint (internal) 718.90
  ankle 718.97
  current injury—*see also* Dislocation, by site
    knee, meniscus or cartilage (*see also* Tear, meniscus) 836.2
  elbow 718.92
  foot 718.97
  hand 718.94
  hip 718.95

Derangement—*continued*
 joint—*continued*
  knee 717.9
  multiple sites 718.99
  pelvic region 718.95
  recurrent 718.30
   ankle 718.37
   elbow 718.32
   foot 718.37
   hand 718.34
   hip 718.35
   knee 718.36
   multiple sites 718.39
   pelvic region 718.35
   shoulder (region) 718.31
   specified site NEC 718.38
   temporomandibular (old) 524.69
   wrist 718.33
  shoulder (region) 718.91
  specified site NEC 718.98
  spine NEC 724.9
  temporomandibular 524.69
  wrist 718.93
 knee (cartilage) (internal) 717.9
  current injury (*see also* Tear, meniscus) 836.2
 ligament 717.89
  capsular 717.85
  collateral—*see* Derangement, collateral
   ligament
  cruciate—*see* Derangement, cruciate
   ligament
  specified NEC 717.85
  recurrent 718.36
 low back NEC 724.9
 meniscus NEC (knee) 717.5
  current injury (*see also* Tear, meniscus) 836.2
  lateral 717.40
   anterior horn 717.42
   posterior horn 717.43
   specified NEC 717.49
  medial 717.3
   anterior horn 717.1
   posterior horn 717.2
  recurrent 718.3
  site other than knee—*see* Disorder, cartilage,
   articular
 mental (*see also* Psychosis) 298.9
 rotator cuff (recurrent) (tear) 726.10
  current 840.4
 sacroiliac (old) 724.6
  current—*see* Dislocation, sacroiliac
 semilunar cartilage (knee) 717.5
  current injury 836.2
   lateral 836.1
   medial 836.0
  recurrent 718.3
 shoulder (internal) 718.91
  current injury (*see also* Dislocation, shoulder)
   831.00
  recurrent 718.31
 spine (recurrent) NEC 724.9
  current—*see* Dislocation, spine
 temporomandibular (internal) (joint) (old)
  524.69
  current—*see* Dislocation, jaw
Dercum's disease or syndrome (adiposis
 dolorosa) 272.8
Derealization (neurotic) 300.6
Dermal —*see* condition
Dermaphytid —*see* Dermatophytosis
Dermatergosis —*see* Dermatitis

Dermatitis (allergic) (contact) (occupational)
 (venenata) 692.9
 ab igne 692.82
 acneiform 692.9
 actinic (due to sun) 692.70
  acute 692.72
  chronic NEC 692.74
  other than from sun NEC 692.82
 ambustionis
  due to
   burn or scald—*see* Burn, by site
   sunburn (*see also* Sunburn) 692.71
 amebic 006.6
 ammonia 691.0
 anaphylactoid NEC 692.9
 arsenical 692.4
 artefacta 698.4
  psychogenic 316 *[698.4]*
 asthmatic 691.8
 atopic (allergic) (intrinsic) 691.8
  psychogenic 316 *[691.8]*
 atrophicans 701.8
  diffusa 701.8
  maculosa 701.3
 autoimmune progesterone 279.49
 berlock, berloque 692.72
 blastomycetic 116.0
 blister beetle 692.89
 Brucella NEC 023.9
 bullosa 694.9
  striata pratensis 692.6
 bullous 694.9
  mucosynechial, atrophic 694.60
   with ocular involvement 694.61
  seasonal 694.8
 calorica
  due to
   burn or scald—*see* Burn, by site
   cold 692.89
   sunburn (*see also* Sunburn) 692.71
 caterpillar 692.89
 cercarial 120.3
 combustionis
  due to
   burn or scald—*see* Burn, by site
   sunburn (*see also* Sunburn) 692.71
 congelationis 991.5
 contusiformis 695.2
 diabetic 250.8
 diaper 691.0
 diphtheritica 032.85
 due to
  acetone 692.2
  acids 692.4
  adhesive plaster 692.4
  alcohol (skin contact) (substances classifiable
   to 980.0-980.9) 692.4
   taken internally 693.8
  alkalis 692.4
  allergy NEC 692.9
  ammonia (household) (liquid) 692.4
  animal
   dander (cat) (dog) 692.84
   hair (cat) (dog) 692.84
  arnica 692.3
  arsenic 692.4
   taken internally 693.8
  blister beetle 692.89
  cantharides 692.3
  carbon disulphide 692.2
  caterpillar 692.89

Dermatitis—*continued*
  due to—*continued*
    caustics 692.4
    cereal (ingested) 693.1
      contact with skin 692.5
    chemical(s) NEC 692.4
      internal 693.8
      irritant NEC 692.4
      taken internally 693.8
    chlorocompounds 692.2
    coffee (ingested) 693.1
      contact with skin 692.5
    cold weather 692.89
    cosmetics 692.81
    cyclohexanes 692.2
    dander, animal (cat) (dog) 692.84
    deodorant 692.81
    detergents 692.0
    dichromate 692.4
    drugs and medicinals (correct substance
      properly administered) (internal use) 693.0
      external (in contact with skin) 692.3
        wrong substance given or taken 976.9
          specified substance—*see* Table of drugs
            and chemicals
      wrong substance given or taken 977.9
        specified substance—*see* Table of drugs
          and chemicals
    dyes 692.89
      hair 692.89
    epidermophytosis—*see* Dermatophytosis
    esters 692.2
    external irritant NEC 692.9
      specified agent NEC 692.89
    eye shadow 692.81
    fish (ingested) 693.1
      contact with skin 692.5
    flour (ingested) 693.1
      contact with skin 692.5
    food (ingested) 693.1
      in contact with skin 692.5
    fruit (ingested) 693.1
      contact with skin 692.5
    fungicides 692.3
    furs 692.84
    glycols 692.2
    greases NEC 692.1
    hair, animal (cat) (dog) 692.84
    hair dyes 692.89
    hot
      objects and materials—*see* Burn, by site
      weather or places 692.89
    hydrocarbons 692.2
    infrared rays, except from sun 692.82
      solar NEC (*see also* Dermatitis, due to, sun)
        692.70
    ingested substance 693.9
      drugs and medicinals (*see also* Dermatitis,
        due to, drugs and medicinals) 693.0
      food 693.1
      specified substance NEC 693.8
    ingestion or injection of
      chemical 693.8
      drug (correct substance properly
        administered) 693.0
        wrong substance given or taken 977.9
          specified substance—*see* Table of drugs
            and chemicals
    insecticides 692.4

Dermatitis—*continued*
  due to—*continued*
    internal agent 693.9
      drugs and medicinals (*see also* Dermatitis,
        due to, drugs and medicinals) 693.0
      food (ingested) 693.1
        in contact with skin 692.5
      specified agent NEC 693.8
    iodine 692.3
    iodoform 692.3
    irradiation 692.82
    jewelry 692.83
    keratolytics 692.3
    ketones 692.2
    lacquer tree (Rhus verniciflua) 692.6
    light (sun) NEC (*see also* Dermatitis, due to,
      sun) 692.70
      other 692.82
    low temperature 692.89
    mascara 692.81
    meat (ingested) 693.1
      contact with skin 692.5
    mercury, mercurials 692.3
    metals 692.83
    milk (ingested) 693.1
      contact with skin 692.5
    Neomycin 692.3
    nylon 692.4
    oils NEC 692.1
    paint solvent 692.2
    pediculocides 692.3
    petroleum products (substances classifiable to
      981) 692.4
    phenol 692.3
    photosensitiveness, photosensitivity (sun)
      692.72
      other light 692.82
    plants NEC 692.6
    plasters, medicated (any) 692.3
    plastic 692.4
    poison
      ivy (Rhus toxicodendron) 692.6
      oak (Rhus diversiloba) 692.6
      plant or vine 692.6
      sumac (Rhus venenata) 692.6
      vine (Rhus radicans) 692.6
    preservatives 692.89
    primrose (primula) 692.6
    primula 692.6
    radiation 692.82
      sun NEC (*see also* Dermatitis, due to, sun)
        692.70
      tanning bed 692.82
    radioactive substance 692.82
    radium 692.82
    ragweed (Senecio jacobae) 692.6
    Rhus (diversiloba) (radicans) (toxicodendron)
      (venenata) (verniciflua) 692.6
    rubber 692.4
    scabicides 692.3
    Senecio jacobae 692.6
    solar radiation—*see* Dermatitis, due to, sun
    solvents (any) (substances classifiable to
      982.0-982.8) 692.2
      chlorocompound group 692.2
      cyclohexane group 692.2
      ester group 692.2
      glycol group 692.2
      hydrocarbon group 692.2
      ketone group 692.2
      paint 692.2

Dermatitis—*continued*
  due to—*continued*
    specified agent NEC 692.89
    sun 692.70
      acute 692.72
      chronic NEC 692.74
      specified NEC 692.79
    sunburn (*see also* Sunburn) 692.71
    sunshine NEC (*see also* Dermatitis, due to,
        sun) 692.70
    tanning bed 692.82
    tetrachlorethylene 692.2
    toluene 692.2
    topical medications 692.3
    turpentine 692.2
    ultraviolet rays, except from sun 692.82
      sun NEC (*see also* Dermatitis, due to, sun)
          692.70
    vaccine or vaccination (correct substance
        properly administered) 693.0
      wrong substance given or taken
        bacterial vaccine 978.8
          specified—*see* Table of drugs and
              chemicals
        other vaccines NEC 979.9
          specified—*see* Table of drugs and
              chemicals
    varicose veins (*see also* Varicose, vein,
        inflamed or infected) 454.1
    x-rays 692.82
  dyshydrotic 705.81
  dysmenorrheica 625.8
  eczematoid NEC 692.9
    infectious 690.8
  eczematous NEC 692.9
  epidemica 695.89
  erysipelatosa 695.81
  escharotica—*see* Burn, by site
  exfoliativa, exfoliative 695.89
    generalized 695.89
    infantum 695.81
    neonatorum 695.81
  eyelid 373.31
    allergic 373.32
    contact 373.32
    eczematous 373.31
    herpes (zoster) 053.20
      simplex 054.41
    infective 373.5
      due to
        actinomycosis 039.3 *[373.5]*
        herpes
          simplex 054.41
          zoster 053.20
        impetigo 684 *[373.5]*
        leprosy (*see also* Leprosy) 030.0 *[373.4]*
        lupus vulgaris (tuberculous) (*see also*
            Tuberculosis) 017.0 *[373.4]*
        mycotic dermatitis (*see also*
            Dermatomycosis) 111.9 *[373.5]*
        vaccinia 051.02 *[373.5]*
          postvaccination 999.0 *[373.5]*
        yaws (*see also* Yaws) 102.9 *[373.4]*
  facta, factitia 698.4
    psychogenic 316 *[698.4]*
  ficta 698.4
    psychogenic 316 *[698.4]*
  flexural 691.8
  follicularis 704.8
  friction 709.8

Dermatitis—*continued*
  fungus 111.9
    specified type NEC 111.8
  gangrenosa, gangrenous (infantum) (*see also*
      Gangrene) 785.4
  gestationis 646.8
  gonococcal 098.89
  gouty 274.89
  harvest mite 133.8
  heat 692.89
  herpetiformis (bullous) (erythematous)
      (pustular) (vesicular) 694.0
    juvenile 694.2
    senile 694.5
  hiemalis 692.89
  hypostatic, hypostatica 454.1
    with ulcer 454.2
  impetiginous 684
  infantile (acute) (chronic) (intertriginous)
      (intrinsic) (seborrheic) 690.12
  infectiosa eczematoides 690.8
  infectious (staphylococcal) (streptococcal) 686.9
    eczematoid 690.8
  infective eczematoid 690.8
  Jacquet's (diaper dermatitis) 691.0
  leptus 133.8
  lichenified NEC 692.9
  lichenoid, chronic 701.0
  lichenoides purpurica pigmentosa 709.1
  meadow 692.6
  medicamentosa (correct substance properly
      administered) (internal use) (*see also*
      Dermatitis, due to, drugs or medicinals)
      693.0
    due to contact with skin 692.3
  mite 133.8
  multiformis 694.0
    juvenile 694.2
    senile 694.5
  napkin 691.0
  neuro 698.3
  neurotica 694.0
  nummular NEC 692.9
  osteatosis, osteatotic 706.8
  papillaris capillitii 706.1
  pellagrous 265.2
  perioral 695.3
  perstans 696.1
  photosensitivity (sun) 692.72
    other light 692.82
  pigmented purpuric lichenoid 709.1
  polymorpha dolorosa 694.0
  primary irritant 692.9
  pruriginosa 694.0
  pruritic NEC 692.9
  psoriasiform nodularis 696.2
  psychogenic 316
  purulent 686.00
  pustular contagious 051.2
  pyococcal 686.00
  pyocyaneus 686.09
  pyogenica 686.00
  radiation 692.82
  repens 696.1
  Ritter's (exfoliativa) 695.81
  Schamberg's (progressive pigmentary
      dermatosis) 709.09
  schistosome 120.3
  seasonal bullous 694.8
  seborrheic 690.10
    infantile 690.12

Dermatitis—*continued*
  sensitization NEC 692.9
  septic (*see also* Septicemia) 686.00
    gonococcal 098.89
  solar, solare NEC (*see also* Dermatitis, due to,
    sun) 692.70
  stasis 454.1
    due to
      postphlebitic syndrome 459.12
        with ulcer 459.13
      varicose veins—*see* Varicose
    ulcerated or with ulcer (varicose) 454.2
  sunburn (*see also* Sunburn) 692.71
  suppurative 686.00
  traumatic NEC 709.8
  trophoneurotica 694.0
  ultraviolet, except from sun 692.82
    due to sun NEC (*see also* Dermatitis, due to,
      sun) 692.70
  varicose 454.1
    with ulcer 454.2
  vegetans 686.8
  verrucosa 117.2
  xerotic 706.8
Dermatoarthritis, lipoid 272.8 *[713.0]*
Dermatochalasia, dermatochalasis 374.87
Dermatofibroma (lenticulare) (M8832/0)—*see
  also* Neoplasm, skin, benign
  protuberans (M8832/1)—*see* Neoplasm, skin,
    uncertain behavior
Dermatofibrosarcoma (protuberans) (M8832/3)
  see Neoplasm, skin, malignant
Dermatographia 708.3
Dermatolysis (congenital) (exfoliativa) 757.39
  acquired 701.8
  eyelids 374.34
  palpebrarum 374.34
  senile 701.8
Dermatomegaly NEC 701.8
Dermatomucomyositis 710.3
Dermatomycosis 111.9
  furfuracea 111.0
  specified type NEC 111.8
Dermatomyositis (acute) (chronic) 710.3
Dermatoneuritis of children 985.0
Dermatophiliasis 134.1
Dermatophytide —*see* Dermatophytosis
Dermatophytosis (Epidermophyton) (infection)
  (microsporum) (tinea) (Trichophyton) 110.9
  beard 110.0
  body 110.5
  deep seated 110.6
  fingernails 110.1
  foot 110.4
  groin 110.3
  hand 110.2
  nail 110.1
  perianal (area) 110.3
  scalp 110.0
  scrotal 110.8
  specified site NEC 110.8
  toenails 110.1
  vulva 110.8
Dermatopolyneuritis 985.0
Dermatorrhexis 756.83
  acquired 701.8
Dermatosclerosis (*see also* Scleroderma) 710.1
  localized 701.0
Dermatosis 709.9
  Andrews' 686.8
  atopic 691.8

Dermatosis—*continued*
  Bowen's (M8081/2)—*see* Neoplasm, skin, in situ
  bullous 694.9
    specified type NEC 694.8
  erythematosquamous 690.8
  exfoliativa 695.89
  factitial 698.4
  gonococcal 098.89
  herpetiformis 694.0
    juvenile 694.2
    senile 694.5
  hysterical 300.11
  linear IgA 694.8
  menstrual NEC 709.8
  neutrophilic, acute febrile 695.89
  occupational (*see also* Dermatitis) 692.9
  papulosa nigra 709.8
  pigmentary NEC 709.00
    progressive 709.09
    Schamberg's 709.09
    Siemens-Bloch 757.33
  progressive pigmentary 709.09
  psychogenic 316
  pustular subcorneal 694.1
  Schamberg's (progressive pigmentary) 709.09
  senile NEC 709.3
  Unna's (seborrheic dermatitis) 690.10
Dermographia 708.3
Dermographism 708.3
Dermoid (cyst) (M9084/0)—*see also* Neoplasm,
  by site, benign
  with malignant transformation (M9084/3) 183.0
Dermopathy
  infiltrative, with thyrotoxicosis 242.0
  nephrogenic fibrosing 701.8
  senile NEC 709.3
Dermophytosis —*see* Dermatophytosis
Descemet's membrane —*see* condition
Descemetocele 371.72
Descending —*see* condition
Descensus uteri (complete) (incomplete) (partial)
  (without vaginal wall prolapse) 618.1
  with mention of vaginal wall prolapse—*see*
    Prolapse, uterovaginal
Desensitization to allergens V07.1
Desert
  rheumatism 114.0
  sore (*see also* Ulcer, skin) 707.9
Desertion (child) (newborn) 995.52
  adult 995.84
Desmoid (extra-abdominal) (tumor) (M8821/1)—*see
  also* Neoplasm, connective tissue, uncertain behavior
  abdominal (M8822/1)—*see* Neoplasm,
    connective tissue, uncertain behavior
Despondency 300.4
Desquamative dermatitis NEC 695.89
Destruction
  articular facet (*see also* Derangement, joint) 718.9
    vertebra 724.9
  bone 733.90
    syphilitic 095.5
  joint (*see also* Derangement, joint) 718.9
    sacroiliac 724.6
  kidney 593.89
  live fetus to facilitate birth NEC 763.89
  ossicles (ear) 385.24
  rectal sphincter 569.49
  septum (nasal) 478.19
  tuberculous NEC (*see also* Tuberculosis) 011.9
  tympanic membrane 384.82
  tympanum 385.89
  vertebral disc—*see* Degeneration, intervertebral disc

Destructiveness (*see also* Disturbance, conduct)
312.9
adjustment reaction 309.3
Detachment
cartilage—*see also* Sprain, by site
knee—*see* Tear, meniscus
cervix, annular 622.8
complicating delivery 665.3
choroid (old) (postinfectional) (simple)
(spontaneous) 363.70
hemorrhagic 363.72
serous 363.71
knee, medial meniscus (old) 717.3
current injury 836.0
ligament—*see* Sprain, by site
placenta (premature)—*see* Placenta, separation
retina (recent) 361.9
with retinal defect (rhegmatogenous) 361.00
giant tear 361.03
multiple 361.02
partial
with
giant tear 361.03
multiple defects 361.02
retinal dialysis (juvenile) 361.04
single defect 361.01
retinal dialysis (juvenile) 361.04
single 361.01
subtotal 361.05
total 361.05
delimited (old) (partial) 361.06
old
delimited 361.06
partial 361.06
total or subtotal 361.07
pigment epithelium (RPE) (serous) 362.42
exudative 362.42
hemorrhagic 362.43
rhegmatogenous (*see also* Detachment, retina,
with retinal defect) 361.00
serous (without retinal defect) 361.2
specified type NEC 361.89
traction (with vitreoretinal organization)
361.81
vitreous humor 379.21
Detergent asthma 507.8
Deterioration
epileptic
with behavioral disturbance 345.9 *[294.11]*
without behavioral disturbance 345.9 *[294.10]*
heart, cardiac (*see also* Degeneration,
myocardial) 429.1
mental (*see also* Psychosis) 298.9
myocardium, myocardial (*see also*
Degeneration, myocardial) 429.1
senile (simple) 797
transplanted organ—*see* Complications,
transplant, organ, by site
de Toni-Fanconi syndrome (cystinosis) 270.0
Deuteranomaly 368.52
Deuteranopia (anomalous trichromat) (complete)
(incomplete) 368.52
Deutschländer's disease —*see* Fracture, foot
Development
abnormal, bone 756.9
arrested 783.40
bone 733.91
child 783.40
due to malnutrition (protein-calorie) 263.2
fetus or newborn 764.9
tracheal rings (congenital) 748.3

Development—*continued*
defective, congenital—*see also* Anomaly
cauda equina 742.59
left ventricle 746.9
with atresia or hypoplasia of aortic orifice or
valve with hypoplasia of ascending aorta
746.7
in hypoplastic left heart syndrome 746.7
delayed (*see also* Delay, development) 783.40
arithmetical skills 315.1
language (skills) 315.31
and speech due to hearing loss 315.34
expressive 315.31
mixed receptive-expressive 315.32
learning skill, specified NEC 315.2
mixed skills 315.5
motor coordination 315.4
reading 315.00
specified
learning skill NEC 315.2
type NEC, except learning 315.8
speech 315.39
and language due to hearing loss 315.34
associated with hyperkinesia 314.1
phonological 315.39
spelling 315.09
written expression 315.2
imperfect, congenital—*see also* Anomaly
heart 746.9
lungs 748.60
improper (fetus or newborn) 764.9
incomplete (fetus or newborn) 764.9
affecting management of pregnancy 656.5
bronchial tree 748.3
organ or site not listed—*see* Hypoplasia
respiratory system 748.9
sexual, precocious NEC 259.1
tardy, mental (*see also* Disability, intellectual) 319
Developmental —*see* condition
Devergie's disease (pityriasis rubra pilaris) 696.4
Deviation
conjugate (eye) 378.87
palsy 378.81
spasm, spastic 378.82
esophagus 530.89
eye, skew 378.87
mandible, opening and closing 524.53
midline (jaw) (teeth) 524.29
specified site NEC—*see* Malposition
occlusal plane 524.76
organ or site, congenital NEC—*see* Malposition,
congenital
septum (acquired) (nasal) 470
congenital 754.0
sexual 302.9
bestiality 302.1
coprophilia 302.89
ego-dystonic
homosexuality 302.0
lesbianism 302.0
erotomania 302.89
Clérambault's 297.8
exhibitionism (sexual) 302.4
fetishism 302.81
transvestic 302.3
frotteurism 302.89
homosexuality, ego-dystonic 302.0
pedophilic 302.2
lesbianism, ego-dystonic 302.0
masochism 302.83
narcissism 302.89
necrophilia 302.89

Deviation—*continued*
    sexual—*continued*
        nymphomania 302.89
        pederosis 302.2
        pedophilia 302.2
        sadism 302.84
        sadomasochism 302.84
        satyriasis 302.89
        specified type NEC 302.89
        transvestic fetishism 302.3
        transvestism 302.3
        voyeurism 302.82
        zoophilia (erotica) 302.1
    teeth, midline 524.29
    trachea 519.19
    ureter (congenital) 753.4
Devic's disease 341.0
Device
    cerebral ventricle (communicating) in situ V45.2
    contraceptive—*see* Contraceptive, device
    drainage, cerebrospinal fluid V45.2
Devil's
    grip 074.1
    pinches (purpura simplex) 287.2
Devitalized tooth 522.9
Devonshire colic 984.9
    specified type of lead—*see* Table of drugs and
        chemicals
Dextraposition, aorta 747.21
    with ventricular septal defect, pulmonary
        stenosis or atresia, and hypertrophy of right
        ventricle 745.2
    in tetralogy of Fallot 745.2
Dextratransposition, aorta 745.11
Dextrinosis, limit (debrancher enzyme
        deficiency) 271.0
Dextrocardia (corrected) (false) (isolated)
        (secondary) (true) 746.87
    with
        complete transposition of viscera 759.3
        situs inversus 759.3
Dextroversion, kidney (left) 753.3
Dhobie itch 110.3
DHTR (delayed hemolytic transfusion reaction) -
        see Complications, transfusion
Diabetes, diabetic (brittle) (congenital) (familial)
        (mellitus) (severe) (slight) (without
        complication) 250.0

> *Note—Use the following fifth-digit*
> *subclassification with category 250:*
>
> 0 *type II or unspecified type, not stated as*
>   *uncontrolled*
>   *Fifth-digit 0 is for use for type II patients,*
>   *even if the patient requires insulin*
> 1 *type I [juvenile type], not stated as*
>   *uncontrolled*
> 2 *type II or unspecified type, uncontrolled*
>   *Fifth-digit 2 is for use for type II patients,*
>   *even if the paiten requires insulin*
> 3 *type I [juvenile type], uncontrolled*

    with
        coma (with ketoacidosis) 250.3
            due to secondary diabetes 249.3
            hyperosmolar (nonketotic) 250.2
                due to secondary diabetes 249.2
        complication NEC 250.9
            due to secondary diabetes 249.9
            specified NEC 250.8
                due to secondary diabetes 249.8

Diabetes, diabetic—*continued*
    with—*continued*
        gangrene 250.7 *[785.4]*
            due to secondary diabetes 249.7 *[785.4]*
        hyperglycemia — code to Diabetes, by type,
            with 5th digit for not stated as uncontrolled
        hyperosmolarity 250.2
            due to secondary diabetes 249.2
        ketosis, ketoacidosis 250.1
            due to secondary diabetes 249.1
        loss of protective sensation (LOPS) - *see*
            Diabetes, neuropathy
        osteomyelitis 250.8 *[731.8]*
            due to secondary diabetes 249.8 *[731.8]*
        specified manifestations NEC 250.8
            due to secondary diabetes 249.8
    acetonemia 250.1
        due to secondary diabetes 249.1
    acidosis 250.1
        due to secondary diabetes 249.1
    amyotrophy 250.6 *[353.5]*
        due to secondary diabetes 249.6 *[353.5]*
    angiopathy, peripheral 250.7 *[443.81]*
        due to secondary diabetes 249.7 *[443.81]*
    asymptomatic 790.29
    autonomic neuropathy (peripheral) 250.6 *[337.1]*
        due to secondary diabetes 249.6 *[337.1]*
    bone change 250.8 *[731.8]*
        due to secondary diabetes 249.8 *[731.8]*
    borderline 790.29
    bronze, bronzed 275.01
    cataract 250.5 *[366.41]*
        due to secondary diabetes 249.5 *[366.41]*
    chemical induced—see Diabetes, secondary
    complicating pregnancy, childbirth, or
        puerperium 648.0
    coma (with ketoacidosis) 250.3
        due to secondary diabetes 249.3
        hyperglycemic 250.3
            due to secondary diabetes 249.3
        hyperosmolar (nonketotic) 250.2
            due to secondary diabetes 249.2
        hypoglycemic 250.3
            due to secondary diabetes 249.3
        insulin 250.3
            due to secondary diabetes 249.3
    complicating pregnancy, childbirth, or
        puerperium (maternal) (conditions
        classifiable to 249 and 250) 648.0
        affecting fetus or newborn 775.0
    complication NEC 250.9
        due to secondary diabetes 249.9
        specified NEC 250.8
            due to secondary diabetes 249.8
    dorsal sclerosis 250.6 *[340]*
        due to secondary diabetes 249.6 *[340]*
    drug induced—*see also* Diabetes, secondary
        overdose or wrong substance given or taken
            — *see* Table of Drugs and Chemicals
    due to
        cystic fibrosis — *see* Diabetes, secondary
        infection — *see* Diabetes, secondary
    dwarfism-obesity syndrome 258.1
    gangrene 250.7 *[785.4]*
        due to secondary diabetes 249.7 *[785.4]*
    gastroparesis 250.6 *[536.3]*
        due to secondary diabetes 249.6 *[536.3]*
    gestational 648.8
        complicating pregnancy, childbirth, or
            puerperium 648.8
    glaucoma 250.5 *[365.44]*
        due to secondary diabetes 249.5 *[365.44]*

Diabetes, diabetic—*continued*
  glomerulosclerosis (intercapillary) 250.4 *[581.81]*
    due to secondary diabetes 249.4 *[581.81]*
  glycogenosis, secondary 250.8 *[259.8]*
    due to secondary diabetes 249.8 *[259.8]*
  hemochromatosis (*see also* Hemochromatosis)
    275.03
  hyperosmolar coma 250.2
    due to secondary diabetes 249.2
  hyperosmolarity 250.2
    due to secondary diabetes 249.2
  hypertension-nephrosis syndrome 250.4 *[581.81]*
    due to secondary diabetes 249.4 *[581.81]*
  hypoglycemia 250.8
    due to secondary diabetes 249.8
  hypoglycemic shock 250.8
    due to secondary diabetes 249.8
  inadequately controlled—code to Diabetes, by
    type, with 5th digit for not stated as
    uncontrolled
  insipidus 253.5
    nephrogenic 588.1
    pituitary 253.5
    vasopressin-resistant 588.1
  intercapillary glomerulosclerosis 250.4 *[581.81]*
    due to secondary diabetes 249.4 *[581.81]*
  iritis 250.5 *[364.42]*
    due to secondary diabetes 249.5 *[364.42]*
  ketosis, ketoacidosis 250.1
    due to secondary diabetes 249.1
  Kimmelstiel (-Wilson) disease or syndrome
    (intercapillary glomerulosclerosis) 250.4
    [581.81]
    due to secondary diabetes 249.4 *[581.81]*
  Lancereaux's (diabetes mellitus with marked
    emaciation) 250.8 *[261]*
    due to secondary diabetes 249.8 *[261]*
  latent (chemical)—*see* Diabetes, secondary
    complicating pregnancy, childbirth, or
    puerperium 648.0
  lipoidosis 250.8 *[272.7]*
    due to secondary diabetes 249.8 *[272.7]*
  macular edema 250.5 *[362.07]*
    due to secondary diabetes 249.5 *[362.07]*
  maternal
    with manifest disease in the infant 775.1
    affecting fetus or newborn 775.0
  microaneurysms, retinal 250.5 *[362.01]*
    due to secondary diabetes 249.5 *[362.01]*
  mononeuropathy 250.6 *[355.9]*
    due to secondary diabetes 249.6 *[355.9]*
  neonatal, transient 775.1
  nephropathy 250.4 *[583.81]*
    due to secondary diabetes 249.4 *[583.81]*
  nephrosis (syndrome) 250.4 *[581.81]*
    due to secondary diabetes 249.4 *[581.81]*
  neuralgia 250.6 *[357.2]*
    due to secondary diabetes 249.6 *[357.2]*
  neuritis 250.6 *[357.2]*
    due to secondary diabetes 249.6 *[357.2]*
  neurogenic arthropathy 250.6 *[713.5]*
    due to secondary diabetes 249.6 *[713.5]*
  neuropathy 250.6 *[357.2]*
    autonomic (peripheral) 250.6 *[337.1]*
      due to secondary diabetes 249.6 *[337.1]*
    due to secondary diabetes 249.6 *[357.2]*
  nonclinical 790.29
  osteomyelitis 250.8 *[731.8]*
    due to secondary diabetes 249.8 *[731.8]*
  out of control—code to Diabetes, by type, with
    5th digit for uncontrolled

Diabetes, diabetic—*continued*
  peripheral autonomic neuropathy 250.6 *[337.1]*
    due to secondary diabetes 249.6 *[337.1]*
  phosphate 275.3
  polyneuropathy 250.6 *[357.2]*
    due to secondary diabetes 249.6 *[357.2]*
  poorly controlled—code to Diabetes, by type,
    with 5th digit for not stated as uncontrolled
  renal (true) 271.4
  retinal
    edema 250.5 *[362.07]*
      due to secondary diabetes 249.5 *[362.07]*
    hemorrhage 250.5 *[362.01]*
      due to secondary diabetes 249.5 *[362.01]*
    microaneurysms 250.5 *[362.01]*
      due to secondary diabetes 249.5 *[362.01]*
  retinitis 250.5 *[362.01]*
    due to secondary diabetes 249.5 *[362.01]*
  retinopathy 250.5 *[362.01]*
    due to secondary diabetes 249.5 *[362.01]*
    background 250.5 *[362.01]*
      due to secondary diabetes 249.5 *[362.01]*
    nonproliferative 250.5 *[362.03]*
      due to secondary diabetes 249.5 *[362.03]*
    mild 250.5 *[362.04]*
      due to secondary diabetes 249.5 *[362.04]*
    moderate 250.5 *[362.05]*
      due to secondary diabetes 249.5 *[362.05]*
    severe 250.5 *[362.06]*
      due to secondary diabetes 249.5 *[362.06]*
    proliferative 250.5 *[362.02]*
      due to secondary diabetes 249.5 *[362.02]*
  secondary (chemical-induced) (due to chronic
    condition) (due to infection) (drug-induced)
    249.0
    with
      coma (with ketoacidosis) 249.3
        hyperosmolar (nonketotic) 249.2
      complication NEC 249.9
        specified NEC 249.8
      gangrene 249.7 *[785.4]*
      hyperosmolarity 249.2
      ketosis, ketoacidosis 249.1
      osteomyelitis 249.8 *[731.8]*
      specified manifestations NEC 249.8
    acetonemia 249.1
    acidosis 249.1
    amyotrophy 249.6 *[353.5]*
    angiopathy, peripheral 249.7 *[443.81]*
    autonomic neuropathy (peripheral) 249.6 *[337.1]*
    bone change 249.8 *[731.8]*
    cataract 249.5 *[366.41]*
    coma (with ketoacidosis) 249.3
      hyperglycemic 249.3
      hyperosmolar (nonketotic) 249.2
      hypoglycemic 249.3
      insulin 249.3
    complicating pregnancy, childbirth, or
      puerperium (maternal) 648.0
      affecting fetus or newborn 775.0
    complication NEC 249.9
      specified NEC 249.8
    dorsal sclerosis 249.6 *[340]*
    due to overdose or wrong substance given or
      taken — *see* Table of Drugs and
      Chemicals
    gangrene 249.7 *[785.4]*
    gastroparesis 249.6 *[536.3]*
    glaucoma 249.5 *[365.44]*
    glomerulosclerosis (intercapillary) 249.4 *[581.81]*
    glycogenosis, secondary 249.8 *[259.8]*
    hyperosmolar coma 249.2

Diarrhea, diarrheal—*continued*
due to
achylia gastrica 536.8
Aerobacter aerogenes 008.2
Bacillus coli—*see* Enteritis, E. coli
bacteria NEC 008.5
bile salts 579.8
Capillaria
hepatica 128.8
philippinensis 127.5
Clostridium perfringens (C) (F) 008.46
Enterobacter aerogenes 008.2
enterococci 008.49
Escherichia coli—*see* Enteritis, E. coli
Giardia lamblia 007.1
Heterophyes heterophyes 121.6
irritating foods 787.91
Metagonimus yokogawai 121.5
Necator americanus 126.1
Paracolobactrum arizonae 008.1
Paracolon bacillus NEC 008.47
Arizona 008.1
Proteus (bacillus) (mirabilis) (Morganii) 008.3
Pseudomonas aeruginosa 008.42
S. japonicum 120.2
specified organism NEC 008.8
bacterial 008.49
viral NEC 008.69
Staphylococcus 008.41
Streptococcus 008.49
anaerobic 008.46
Strongyloides stercoralis 127.2
Trichuris trichiuria 127.3
virus NEC (*see also* Enteritis, viral) 008.69
dysenteric 009.2
due to specified organism NEC 008.8
dyspeptic 787.91
endemic 009.3
epidemic 009.3
fermentative 787.91
flagellate 007.9
Flexner's (ulcerative) 004.1
functional 564.5
following gastrointestinal surgery 564.4
psychogenic 306.4
giardial 007.1
Giardia lamblia 007.1
hill 579.1
hyperperistalsis (nervous) 306.4
infectious 009.2
presumed 009.3
inflammatory 787.91
due to specified organism NEC 008.8
malarial (*see also* Malaria) 084.6
mite 133.8
mycotic 117.9
nervous 306.4
neurogenic 564.5
parenteral NEC 009.2
postgastrectomy 564.4
postvagotomy 564.4
prostaglandin induced 579.8
protozoal NEC 007.9
psychogenic 306.4
septic 009.2
due to specified organism NEC 008.8
specified organism NEC 008.8
bacterial 008.49
viral NEC 008.69
Staphylococcus 008.41

Diarrhea, diarrheal—*continued*
Streptococcus 008.49
anaerobic 088.46
toxic 558.2
travelers' 009.2
due to specified organism NEC 008.8
trichomonal 007.3
tropical 579.1
tuberculous 014.8
ulcerative (chronic) (*see also* Colitis, ulcerative)
556.9
viral (*see also* Enteritis, viral) 008.8
zymotic NEC 009.2
Diastasis
cranial bones 733.99
congenital 756.0
joint (traumatic)—*see* Dislocation, by site
muscle 728.84
congenital 756.89
recti (abdomen) 728.84
complicating delivery 665.8
congenital 756.79
Diastema, teeth, tooth 524.30
Diastematomyelia 742.51
Diataxia, cerebral, infantile 343.0
Diathesis
allergic V15.09
bleeding (familial) 287.9
cystine (familial) 270.0
gouty 274.9
hemorrhagic (familial) 287.9
newborn NEC 776.0
oxalic 271.8
scrofulous (*see also* Tuberculosis) 017.2
spasmophilic (*see also* Tetany) 781.7
ulcer 536.9
uric acid 274.9
Diaz's disease or osteochondrosis 732.5
Dibothriocephaliasis 123.4
larval 123.5
Dibothriocephalus (infection) (infestation)
(latus) 123.4
larval 123.5
Dicephalus 759.4
Dichotomy, teeth 520.2
Dichromat, dichromata (congenital) 368.59
Dichromatopsia (congenital) 368.59
Dichuchwa 104.0
Dicroceliasis 121.8
Didelphys, didelphic (*see also* Double uterus)
752.2
Didymitis (*see also* Epididymitis) 604.90
Died —*see also* Death
without
medical attention (cause unknown) 798.9
sign of disease 798.2
Dientamoeba diarrhea 007.8
Dietary
inadequacy or deficiency 269.9
surveillance and counseling V65.3
Dietl's crisis 593.4
Dieulafoy lesion (hemorrhagic) of
duodenum 537.84
esophagus 530.82
intestine 569.86
stomach 537.84
Dieulafoy's ulcer —*see* Ulcer, stomach
Difficult
birth, affecting fetus or newborn 763.9
delivery NEC 669.9

Difficulty
  feeding 783.3
    adult 783.3
    breast 676.8
    child 783.3
    elderly 783.3
    infant 783.3
    newborn 779.31
    nonorganic (infant) NEC 307.59
  mechanical, gastroduodenal stoma 537.89
  reading 315.00
  specific, spelling 315.09
  swallowing (*see also* Dysphagia) 787.20
  walking 719.7
Diffuse —*see* condition
Diffused ganglion 727.42
DiGeorge's syndrome (thymic hypoplasia)
  279.11
Digestive —*see* condition
Di Guglielmo's disease or syndrome (M9841/3)
  207.0
Dihydropyrimidine dehydrogenase disease
  (DPD) 277.6
Diktyoma (M9051/3)—*see* Neoplasm, by site,
  malignant
Dilaceration, tooth 520.4
Dilatation
  anus 564.89
    venule—*see* Hemorrhoids
  aorta (focal) (general) (*see also* Ectasia, aortic)
    447.70
    with aneurysm 441.9
    congenital 747.29
    infectional 093.0
    ruptured 441.5
    syphilitic 093.0
  appendix (cystic) 543.9
  artery 447.8
  bile duct (common) (congenital) 751.69
    acquired 576.8
  bladder (sphincter) 596.89
    congenital 753.8
    in pregnancy or childbirth 654.4
      causing obstructed labor 660.2
        affecting fetus or newborn 763.1
  blood vessel 459.89
  bronchus, bronchi 494.0
    with acute exacerbation 494.1
  calyx (due to obstruction) 593.89
  capillaries 448.9
  cardiac (acute) (chronic) (*see also* Hypertrophy,
    cardiac) 429.3
    congenital 746.89
      valve NEC 746.89
        pulmonary 746.09
    hypertensive (*see also* Hypertension, heart)
      402.90
  cavum septi pellucidi 742.4
  cecum 564.89
    psychogenic 306.4
  cervix (uteri)—*see also* Incompetency, cervix
    incomplete, poor, slow
      affecting fetus or newborn 763.7
      complicating delivery 661.0
        affecting fetus or newborn 763.7
  colon 564.7
    congenital 751.3
    due to mechanical obstruction 560.89
    psychogenic 306.4

Dilatation—*continued*
  common bile duct (congenital) 751.69
    acquired 576.8
      with calculus, choledocholithiasis, or
        stones—*see* Choledocholithiasis
  cystic duct 751.69
    acquired (any bile duct) 575.8
  duct, mammary 610.4
  duodenum 564.89
  esophagus 530.89
    congenital 750.4
    due to
      achalasia 530.0
      cardiospasm 530.0
  Eustachian tube, congenital 744.24
  fontanel 756.0
  gallbladder 575.8
    congenital 751.69
  gastric 536.8
    acute 536.1
    psychogenic 306.4
  heart (acute) (chronic) (*see also* Hypertrophy,
    cardiac) 429.3
    congenital 746.89
    hypertensive (*see also* Hypertension, heart)
      402.90
    valve—*see also* Endocarditis
      congenital 746.89
  ileum 564.89
    psychogenic 306.4
  inguinal rings—*see* Hernia, inguinal
  jejunum 564.89
    psychogenic 306.4
  kidney (calyx) (collecting structures) (cystic)
    (parenchyma) (pelvis) 593.89
  lacrimal passages 375.69
  lymphatic vessel 457.1
  mammary duct 610.4
  Meckel's diverticulum (congenital) 751.0
  meningeal vessels, congenital 742.8
  myocardium (acute) (chronic) (*see also*
    Hypertrophy, cardiac) 429.3
  organ or site, congenital NEC—*see* Distortion
  pancreatic duct 577.8
  pelvis, kidney 593.89
  pericardium—*see* Pericarditis
  pharynx 478.29
  prostate 602.8
  pulmonary
    artery (idiopathic) 417.8
      congenital 747.39
    valve, congenital 746.09
  pupil 379.43
  rectum 564.89
  renal 593.89
  saccule vestibularis, congenital 744.05
  salivary gland (duct) 527.8
  sphincter ani 564.89
  stomach 536.8
    acute 536.1
    psychogenic 306.4
  submaxillary duct 527.8
  trachea, congenital 748.3
  ureter (idiopathic) 593.89
    congenital 753.20
    due to obstruction 593.5
  urethra (acquired) 599.84
  vasomotor 443.9
  vein 459.89

Dilatation—*continued*
  ventricular, ventricle (acute) (chronic) (*see also*
      Hypertrophy, cardiac) 429.3
    cerebral, congenital 742.4
    hypertensive (*see also* Hypertension, heart) 402.90
  venule 459.89
    anus—*see* Hemorrhoids
  vesical orifice 596.89
Dilated, dilation —*see* Dilatation
Diminished
  hearing (acuity) (*see also* Deafness) 389.9
  pulse pressure 785.9
  vision NEC 369.9
  vital capacity 794.2
Diminuta taenia 123.6
Diminution, sense or sensation (cold) (heat)
    (tactile) (vibratory) (*see also* Disturbance,
    sensation) 782.0
Dimitri-Sturge-Weber disease
    (encephalocutaneous angiomatosis) 759.6
Dimple
  parasacral 685.1
    with abscess 685.0
  pilonidal 685.1
    with abscess 685.0
  postanal 685.1
    with abscess 685.0
Dioctophyma renale (infection) (infestation) 128.8
Dipetalonemiasis 125.4
Diphallus 752.69
Diphtheria, diphtheritic (gangrenous)
    (hemorrhagic) 032.9
  carrier (suspected) of V02.4
  cutaneous 032.85
  cystitis 032.84
  faucial 032.0
  infection of wound 032.85
  inoculation (anti) (not sick) V03.5
  laryngeal 032.3
  myocarditis 032.82
  nasal anterior 032.2
  nasopharyngeal 032.1
  neurological complication 032.89
  peritonitis 032.83
  specified site NEC 032.89
Diphyllobothriasis (intestine) 123.4
  larval 123.5
Diplacusis 388.41
Diplegia (upper limbs) 344.2
  brain or cerebral 437.8
  congenital 343.0
  facial 351.0
    congenital 352.6
  infantile or congenital (cerebral) (spastic)
      (spinal) 343.0
  lower limbs 344.1
  syphilitic, congenital 090.49
Diplococcus, diplococcal —*see* condition
Diplomyelia 742.59
Diplopia 368.2
  refractive 368.15
Dipsomania (*see also* Alcoholism) 303.9
  with psychosis (*see also* Psychosis, alcoholic) 291.9
Dipylidiasis 123.8
  intestine 123.8
Direction, teeth, abnormal 524.30
Dirt-eating child 307.52

Disability, disabilities
  heart—*see* Disease, heart
  intellectual 319
    borderline V62.89
    mild, IQ 50-70 317
    moderate, IQ 35-49 318.0
    profound, IQ under 20 318.2
    severe, IQ 20-34 318.1
  learning NEC 315.2
  special spelling 315.09
Disarticulation (*see also* Derangement, joint) 718.9
  meaning
    amputation
      status—*see* Absence, by site
      traumatic —*see* Amputation, traumatic
    dislocation, traumatic or congenital—*see*
        Dislocation
Disaster, cerebrovascular (*see also* Disease,
    cerebrovascular, acute) 436
Discharge
  anal NEC 787.99
  breast (female) (male) 611.79
  conjunctiva 372.89
  continued locomotor idiopathic (*see also*
      Epilepsy) 345.5
  diencephalic autonomic idiopathic (*see also*
      Epilepsy) 345.5
  ear 388.60
    blood 388.69
    cerebrospinal fluid 388.61
  excessive urine 788.42
  eye 379.93
  nasal 478.19
  nipple 611.79
  patterned motor idiopathic (*see also* Epilepsy) 345.5
  penile 788.7
  postnasal—*see* Sinusitis
  sinus, from mediastinum 510.0
  umbilicus 789.9
  urethral 788.7
    bloody 599.84
  vaginal 623.5
Discitis 722.90
  cervical, cervicothoracic 722.91
  lumbar, lumbosacral 722.93
  thoracic, thoracolumbar 722.92
Discogenic syndrome —*see* Displacement,
    intervertebral disc
Discoid
  kidney 753.3
  meniscus, congenital 717.5
  semilunar cartilage 717.5
Discoloration
  mouth 528.9
  nails 703.8
  teeth 521.7
    due to
      drugs 521.7
      metals (copper) (silver) 521.7
      pulpal bleeding 521.7
    during formation 520.8
    extrinsic 523.6
    intrinsic posteruptive 521.7
Discomfort
  chest 786.59
  visual 368.13
Discomycosis —*see* Actinomycosis
Discontinuity, ossicles, ossicular chain 385.23

Discrepancy
centric occlusion
  maximum intercuspation 524.55
  of teeth 524.55
leg length (acquired) 736.81
  congenital 755.30
uterine size-date 649.6
Discrimination
political V62.4
racial V62.4
religious V62.4
sex V62.4
Disease, diseased —*see also* Syndrome
Abrami's (acquired hemolytic jaundice) 283.9
absorbent system 459.89
accumulation—*see* Thesaurismosis
acid-peptic 536.8
Acosta's 993.2
Adams-Stokes (-Morgagni) (syncope with heart
  block) 426.9
Addison's (bronze) (primary adrenal
  insufficiency) 255.41
  anemia (pernicious) 281.0
  tuberculous (*see also* Tuberculosis) 017.6
Addison-Gull—*see* Xanthoma
adenoids (and tonsils) (chronic) 474.9
adrenal (gland) (capsule) (cortex) 255.9
  hyperfunction 255.3
  hypofunction 255.41
  specified type NEC 255.8
ainhum (dactylolysis spontanea) 136.0
akamushi (scrub typhus) 081.2
Akureyri (epidemic neuromyasthenia) 049.8
Albarrán's (colibacilluria) 791.9
Albers-Schönberg's (marble bones) 756.52
Albert's 726.71
Albright (-Martin) (-Bantam) 275.49
Alibert's (mycosis fungoides) (M9700/3) 202.1
Alibert-Bazin (M9700/3) 202.1
alimentary canal 569.9
alligator skin (ichthyosis congenital) 757.1
  acquired 701.1
Almeida's (Brazilian blastomycosis) 116.1
Alpers' 330.8
alpine 993.2
altitude 993.2
alveoli, teeth 525.9
Alzheimer's—*see* Alzheimer's
amyloid (any site) 277.30
anarthritic rheumatoid 446.5
Anders' (adiposis tuberosa simplex) 272.8
Andersen's (glycogenosis IV) 271.0
Anderson's (angiokeratoma corporis diffusum)
  272.7
Andes 993.2
Andrews' (bacterid) 686.8
angiospastic, angiospasmodic 443.9
  cerebral 435.9
    with transient neurologic deficit 435.9
  vein 459.89
anterior
  chamber 364.9
  horn cell 335.9
    specified type NEC 335.8
antral (chronic) 473.0
  acute 461.0
anus NEC 569.49
aorta (nonsyphilitic) 447.9
  syphilitic NEC 093.89
aortic (heart) (valve) (*see also* Endocarditis,
  aortic) 424.1

Disease, diseased—*continued*
apollo 077.4
aponeurosis 726.90
appendix 543.9
aqueous (chamber) 364.9
arc-welders' lung 503
Armenian 277.31
Arnold-Chiari (*see also* Spina bifida) 741.0
arterial 447.9
  occlusive (*see also* Occlusion, by site) 444.22
    with embolus or thrombus—*see* Occlusion,
      by site
  due to stricture or stenosis 447.1
  specified type NEC 447.8
arteriocardiorenal (*see also* Hypertension,
  cardiorenal) 404.90
arteriolar (generalized) (obliterative) 447.9
  specified type NEC 447.8
arteriorenal—*see* Hypertension, kidney
arteriosclerotic—*see also* Arteriosclerosis
  cardiovascular 429.2
  coronary —*see* Arteriosclerosis, coronary
  heart —*see* Arteriosclerosis, coronary
artery 447.9
  cerebral 437.9
  coronary —*see* Arteriosclerosis, coronary
  specified type NEC 447.8
arthropod-borne NEC 088.9
  specified type NEC 088.89
Asboe-Hansen's (incontinentia pigmenti) 757.33
atticoantral, chronic (with posterior or superior
  marginal perforation of ear drum) 382.2
auditory canal, ear 380.9
Aujeszky's 078.89
auricle, ear NEC 380.30
Australian X 062.4
autoimmune NEC 279.49
  hemolytic (cold type) (warm type) 283.0
  parathyroid 252.1
  thyroid 245.2
aviators' (*see also* Effect, adverse, high altitude)
  993.2
ax(e)-grinders' 502
Ayala's 756.89
Ayerza's (pulmonary artery sclerosis with
  pulmonary hypertension) 416.0
Azorean (of the nervous system) 334.8
Babington's (familial hemorrhagic
  telangiectasia) 448.0
back bone NEC 733.90
bacterial NEC 040.89
  zoonotic NEC 027.9
    specified type NEC 027.8
Baehr-Schiffrin (thrombotic thrombocytopenic
  purpura) 446.6
Baelz's (cheilitis glandularis apostematosa)
  528.5
Baerensprung's (eczema marginatum) 110.3
Balfour's (chloroma) 205.3
balloon (*see also* Effect, adverse, high altitude)
  993.2
Baló's 341.1
Bamberger (-Marie) (hypertrophic pulmonary
  osteoarthropathy) 731.2
Bang's (Brucella abortus) 023.1
Bannister's 995.1
Banti's (with cirrhosis) (with portal
  hypertension)—*see* Cirrhosis, liver
Barcoo (*see also* Ulcer, skin) 707.9
barium lung 503
Barlow (-Möller) (infantile scurvy) 267

Disease, diseased—*continued*
  barometer makers' 985.0
  Barraquer (-Simons) (progressive lipodystrophy)
      272.6
  basal ganglia 333.90
    degenerative NEC 333.0
    specified NEC 333.89
  Basedow's (exophthalmic goiter) 242.0
  basement membrane NEC 583.89
    with
      pulmonary hemorrhage (Goodpasture's
          syndrome) 446.21 *[583.81]*
  Bateman's 078.0
    purpura (senile) 287.2
  Batten's 330.1 *[362.71]*
  Batten-Mayou (retina) 330.1 *[362.71]*
  Batten-Steinert 359.21
  Battey 031.0
  Baumgarten-Cruveilhier (cirrhosis of liver) 571.5
  bauxite-workers' 503
  Bayle's (dementia paralytica) 094.1
  Bazin's (primary) (*see also* Tuberculosis) 017.1
  Beard's (neurasthenia) 300.5
  Beau's (*see also* Degeneration, myocardial) 429.1
  Bechterew's (ankylosing spondylitis) 720.0
  Becker's
    idiopathic mural endomyocardial disease 425.2
    myotonia congenita, recessive form 359.22
  Begbie's (exophthalmic goiter) 242.0
  Behr's 362.50
  Beigel's (white piedra) 111.2
  Bekhterev's (ankylosing spondylitis) 720.0
  Bell's (*see also* Psychosis, affective) 296.0
  Bennett's (leukemia) 208.9
  Benson's 379.22
  Bergeron's (hysteroepilepsy) 300.11
  Berlin's 921.3
  Bernard-Soulier (thrombopathy) 287.1
  Bernhardt (-Roth) 355.1
  beryllium 503
  Besnier-Boeck (-Schaumann) (sarcoidosis) 135
  Best's 362.76
  Beurmann's (sporotrichosis) 117.1
  Bielschowsky (-Jansky) 330.1
  Biermer's (pernicious anemia) 281.0
  Biett's (discoid lupus erythematosus) 695.4
  bile duct (*see also* Disease, biliary) 576.9
  biliary (duct) (tract) 576.9
    with calculus, choledocholithiasis, or
        stones—*see* Choledocholithiasis
  Billroth's (meningocele) (*see also* Spina bifida)
      741.9
  Binswanger's 290.12
  Bird's (oxaluria) 271.8
  bird fanciers' 495.2
  black lung 500
  bladder 596.9
    specified NEC 596.89
  bleeder's 286.0
  Bloch-Sulzberger (incontinentia pigmenti) 757.33
  Blocq's (astasia-abasia) 307.9
  blood (-forming organs) 289.9
    specified NEC 289.89
    vessel 459.9
  Bloodgood's 610.1
  Blount's (tibia vara) 732.4
  blue 746.9
  Bodechtel-Guttmann (subacute sclerosing
      panencephalitis) 046.2
  Boeck's (sarcoidosis) 135

Disease, diseased—*continued*
  bone 733.90
    fibrocystic NEC 733.29
      jaw 526.2
    marrow 289.9
    Paget's (osteitis deformans) 731.0
    specified type NEC 733.99
    von Recklinghausen's (osteitis fibrosa cystica)
        252.01
  Bonfils'—*see* Disease, Hodgkin's
  Borna 062.9
  Bornholm (epidemic pleurodynia) 074.1
  Bostock's (*see also* Fever, hay) 477.9
  Bouchard's (myopathic dilatation of the
      stomach) 536.1
  Bouillaud's (rheumatic heart disease) 391.9
  Bourneville (-Brissaud) (tuberous sclerosis) 759.5
  Bouveret (-Hoffmann) (paroxysmal tachycardia)
      427.2
  bowel 569.9
    functional 564.9
    psychogenic 306.4
  Bowen's (M8081/2)—*see* Neoplasm, skin, in situ
  Bozzolo's (multiple myeloma) (M9730/3) 203.0
  Bradley's (epidemic vomiting) 078.82
  Brailsford's 732.3
    radius, head 732.3
    tarsal, scaphoid 732.5
  Brailsford-Morquio (mucopolysaccharidosis IV)
      277.5
  brain 348.9
    Alzheimer's 331.0
      with dementia—*see* Alzheimer's, dementia
    arterial, artery 437.9
    arteriosclerotic 437.0
    congenital 742.9
    degenerative—*see* Degeneration, brain
    inflammatory—*see also* Encephalitis
    late effect—*see* category 326
    organic 348.9
      arteriosclerotic 437.0
    parasitic NEC 123.9
    Pick's 331.11
      with dementia
        with behavioral disturbance 331.11
            [294.11]
        without behavioral disturbance 331.11
            [294.10]
    senile 331.2
  braziers' 985.8
  breast 611.9
    cystic (chronic) 610.1
    fibrocystic 610.1
    inflammatory 611.0
    Paget's (M8540/3) 174.0
    puerperal, postpartum NEC 676.3
    specified NEC 611.89
  Breda's (*see also* Yaws) 102.9
  Breisky's (kraurosis vulvae) 624.09
  Bretonneau's (diphtheritic malignant angina)
      032.0
  Bright's (*see also* Nephritis) 583.9
    arteriosclerotic (*see also* Hypertension,
        kidney) 403.90
  Brill's (recrudescent typhus) 081.1
    flea-borne 081.0
    louse-borne 081.1
  Brill-Symmers (follicular lymphoma)
      (M9690/3) 202.0
  Brill-Zinsser (recrudescent typhus) 081.1

Disease, diseased—*continued*

Brinton's (leather bottle stomach) (M8142/3)
151.9
Brion-Kayser (*see also* Fever, paratyphoid)
002.9
broad
beta 272.2
ligament, noninflammatory 620.9
specified NEC 620.8
Brocq's 691.8
meaning
atopic (diffuse) neurodermatitis 691.8
dermatitis herpetiformis 694.0
lichen simplex chronicus 698.3
parapsoriasis 696.2
prurigo 698.2
Brocq-Duhring (dermatitis herpetiformis) 694.0
Brodie's (joint) (*see also* Osteomyelitis) 730.1
bronchi 519.19
bronchopulmonary 519.19
bronze (Addison's) 255.41
tuberculous (*see also* Tuberculosis) 017.6
Brown-Séquard 344.89
Bruck's 733.99
Bruck-de Lange (Amsterdam dwarf, intellectual
disabilities, and brachycephaly) 759.89
Bruhl's (splenic anemia with fever) 285.8
Bruton's (X-linked agammaglobulinemia)
279.04
buccal cavity 528.9
Buchanan's (juvenile osteochondrosis, iliac
crest) 732.1
Buchman's (osteochondrosis juvenile) 732.1
Budgerigar-fanciers' 495.2
Büdinger-Ludloff-Läwen 717.89
Buerger's (thromboangiitis obliterans) 443.1
Bürger-Grütz (essential familial hyperlipemia)
272.3
Burns' (lower ulna) 732.3
bursa 727.9
Bury's (erythema elevatum diutinum) 695.89
Buschke's 710.1
Busquet's (*see also* Osteomyelitis) 730.1
Busse-Buschke (cryptococcosis) 117.5
C₂ (*see also* Alcoholism) 303.9
Caffey's (infantile cortical hyperostosis) 756.59
caisson 993.3
calculous 592.9
California 114.0
Calvé (-Perthes) (osteochondrosis, femoral
capital) 732.1
Camurati-Engelmann (diaphyseal sclerosis)
756.59
Canavan's 330.0
capillaries 448.9
Carapata 087.1
cardiac-*see* Disease, heart
cardiopulmonary, chronic 416.9
cardiorenal (arteriosclerotic) (hepatic)
(hypertensive) (vascular) (*see also*
Hypertension, cardiorenal) 404.90
cardiovascular (arteriosclerotic) 429.2
congenital 746.9
hypertensive (*see also* Hypertension, heart)
402.90
benign 402.10
malignant 402.00
renal (*see also* Hypertension, cardiorenal)
404.90
syphilitic (asymptomatic) 093.9
carotid gland 259.8

Disease, diseased—*continued*

Carrión's (Bartonellosis) 088.0
cartilage NEC 733.90
specified NEC 733.99
Castellani's 104.8
cat-scratch 078.3
Cavare's (familial periodic paralysis) 359.3
Cazenave's (pemphigus) 694.4
cecum 569.9
celiac (adult) 579.0
infantile 579.0
cellular tissue NEC 709.9
central core 359.0
cerebellar, cerebellum—*see* Disease, brain
cerebral (*see also* Disease, brain) 348.9
arterial, artery 437.9
degenerative—*see* Degeneration, brain
cerebrospinal 349.9
cerebrovascular NEC 437.9
acute 436
embolic—*see* Embolism, brain
late effect—*see* Late effect(s) (of)
cerebrovascular disease
puerperal, postpartum, childbirth 674.0
thrombotic—*see* Thrombosis, brain
arteriosclerotic 437.0
embolic—*see* Embolism, brain
ischemic, generalized NEC 437.1
late effect—*see* Late effect(s) (of)
cerebrovascular disease
occlusive 437.1
puerperal, postpartum, childbirth 674.0
specified type NEC 437.8
thrombotic—*see* Thrombosis, brain
ceroid storage 272.7
cervix (uteri)
inflammatory 616.0
noninflammatory 622.9
specified NEC 622.8
Chabert's 022.9
Chagas' (*see also* Trypanosomiasis, American)
086.2
Chandler's (osteochondritis dissecans, hip)
732.7
Charcot's (joint) 094.0 *[713.5]*
spinal cord 094.0
Charcot-Marie-Tooth 356.1
Charlouis' (*see also* Yaws) 102.9
Cheadle (-Möller) (-Barlow) (infantile scurvy)
267
Chédiak-Steinbrinck (-Higashi) (congenital
gigantism of peroxidase granules) 288.2
cheek, inner 528.9
chest 519.9
Chiari's (hepatic vein thrombosis) 453.0
Chicago (North American blastomycosis) 116.0
chignon (white piedra) 111.2
chigoe, chigo (jigger) 134.1
childhood granulomatous 288.1
Chinese liver fluke 121.1
chlamydial NEC 078.88
cholecystic (*see also* Disease, gallbladder) 575.9
choroid 363.9
degenerative (*see also* Degeneration, choroid)
363.40
hereditary (*see also* Dystrophy, choroid)
363.50
specified type NEC 363.8
Christian's (chronic histiocytosis X) 277.89
Christian-Weber (nodular nonsuppurative
panniculitis) 729.30

Disease, diseased—*continued*
Christmas 286.1
ciliary body 364.9
   specified NEC 364.89
circulatory (system) NEC 459.9
   chronic, maternal, affecting fetus or newborn
      760.3
   specified NEC 459.89
   syphilitic 093.9
      congenital 090.5
Civatte's (poikiloderma) 709.09
climacteric 627.2
   male 608.89
coagulation factor deficiency (congenital) (*see
   also* Defect, coagulation) 286.9
Coats' 362.12
coccidioidal pulmonary 114.5
   acute 114.0
   chronic 114.4
   primary 114.0
   residual 114.4
Cockayne's (microcephaly and dwarfism)
   759.89
Cogan's 370.52
cold
   agglutinin 283.0
      or hemoglobinuria 283.0
         paroxysmal (cold) (nocturnal) 283.2
   hemagglutinin (chronic) 283.0
collagen NEC 710.9
   nonvascular 710.9
   specified NEC 710.8
   vascular (allergic) (*see also* Angiitis,
      hypersensitivity) 446.20
colon 569.9
   functional 564.9
      congenital 751.3
   ischemic 557.0
combined system (of spinal cord) 266.2 *[336.2]*
   with anemia (pernicious) 281.0 *[336.2]*
compressed air 993.3
Concato's (pericardial polyserositis) 423.2
   peritoneal 568.82
   pleural—*see* Pleurisy
congenital NEC 799.89
conjunctiva 372.9
   chlamydial 077.98
      specified NEC 077.8
   specified type NEC 372.89
   viral 077.99
      specified NEC 077.8
connective tissue, diffuse (*see also* Disease,
   collagen) 710.9
Conor and Bruch's (boutonneuse fever) 082.1
Conradi (-Hünermann) 756.59
Cooley's (erythroblastic anemia) 282.44
Cooper's 610.1
Corbus' 607.1
cork-handlers' 495.3
cornea (*see also* Keratopathy) 371.9
coronary (*see also* Ischemia, heart) 414.9
   congenital 746.85
   ostial, syphilitic 093.20
      aortic 093.22
      mitral 093.21
      pulmonary 093.24
      tricuspid 093.23
Corrigan's—*see* Insufficiency, aortic
Cotugno's 724.3
Coxsackie (virus) NEC 074.8
cranial nerve NEC 352.9

Disease, diseased—*continued*
Creutzfeldt-Jakob (CJD) 046.19
   with dementia
      with behavioral disturbance 046.19 *[294.11]*
      without behavioral disturbance 046.19
         [294.10]
   familial 046.19
   iatrogenic 046.19
   specified NEC 046.19
   sporadic 046.19
   variant (vCJD) 046.11
      with dementia
         with behavioral disturbance 046.11
            [294.11]
         without behavioral disturbance 046.11
            [294.10]
Crigler-Najjar (congenital hyperbilirubinemia)
   277.4
Crocq's (acrocyanosis) 443.89
Crohn's (intestine) (*see also* Enteritis, regional)
   555.9
Crouzon's (craniofacial dysostosis) 756.0
Cruchet's (encephalitis lethargica) 049.8
Cruveilhier's 335.21
Cruz-Chagas (*see also* Trypanosomiasis,
   American) 086.2
crystal deposition (*see also* Arthritis, due to,
   crystals) 712.9
Csillag's (lichen sclerosus et atrophicus) 701.0
Curschmann's 359.21
Cushing's (pituitary basophilism) 255.0
cystic
   breast (chronic) 610.1
   kidney, congenital (*see also* Cystic, disease,
      kidney) 753.10
   liver, congenital 751.62
   lung 518.89
      congenital 748.4
   pancreas 577.2
      congenital 751.7
   renal, congenital (*see also* Cystic, disease,
      kidney) 753.10
   semilunar cartilage 717.5
cysticercus 123.1
cystine storage (with renal sclerosis) 270.0
cytomegalic inclusion (generalized) 078.5
   with
      pneumonia 078.5 *[484.1]*
   congenital 771.1
Daae (-Finsen) (epidemic pleurodynia) 074.1
dancing 297.8
Danielssen's (anesthetic leprosy) 030.1
Darier's (congenital) (keratosis follicularis)
   757.39
   erythema annulare centrifugum 695.0
   vitamin A deficiency 264.8
Darling's (histoplasmosis) (*see also*
   Histoplasmosis, American) 115.00
Davies' 425.0
de Beurmann-Gougerot (sporotrichosis) 117.1
Débove's (splenomegaly) 789.2
deer fly (*see also* Tularemia) 021.9
deficiency 269.9
degenerative—*see also* Degeneration
   disc—*see* Degeneration, intervertebral disc
Degos' 447.8
Déjérine (-Sottas) 356.0
Deleage's 359.89
demyelinating, demyelinizating (brain stem)
   (central nervous system) 341.9
   multiple sclerosis 340
   specified NEC 341.8

Disease, diseased—*continued*
de Quervain's (tendon sheath) 727.04
 thyroid (subacute granulomatous thyroiditis)
  245.1
Dercum's (adiposis dolorosa) 272.8
Deutschländer's—*see* Fracture, foot
Devergie's (pityriasis rubra pilaris) 696.4
Devic's 341.0
diaphorase deficiency 289.7
diaphragm 519.4
diarrheal, infectious 009.2
diatomaceous earth 502
Diaz's (osteochondrosis astragalus) 732.5
digestive system 569.9
Di Guglielmo's (erythemic myelosis) (M9841/3)
  207.0
Dimitri-Sturge-Weber (encephalocutaneous
  angiomatosis) 759.6
disc, degenerative—*see* Degeneration,
  intervertebral disc
discogenic (*see also* Disease, intervertebral disc)
  722.90
diverticular—*see* Diverticula
Down's (mongolism) 758.0
Dubini's (electric chorea) 049.8
Dubois' (thymus gland) 090.5
Duchenne's 094.0
 locomotor ataxia 094.0
 muscular dystrophy 359.1
 paralysis 335.22
 pseudohypertrophy, muscles 359.1
Duchenne-Griesinger 359.1
ductless glands 259.9
Duhring's (dermatitis herpetiformis) 694.0
Dukes (-Filatov) 057.8
duodenum NEC 537.9
 specified NEC 537.89
Duplay's 726.2
Dupré's (meningism) 781.6
Dupuytren's (muscle contracture) 728.6
Durand-Nicolas-Favre (climatic bubo) 099.1
Duroziez's (congenital mitral stenosis) 746.5
Dutton's (trypanosomiasis) 086.9
Eales' 362.18
ear (chronic) (inner) NEC 388.9
 middle 385.9
  adhesive (*see also* Adhesions, middle ear)
   385.10
  specified NEC 385.89
Eberth's (typhoid fever) 002.0
Ebstein's
 heart 746.2
 meaning diabetes 250.4 *[581.81]*
  due to secondary diabetes 249.4 *[581.81]*
Echinococcus (*see also* Echinococcus) 122.9
ECHO virus NEC 078.89
Economo's (encephalitis lethargica) 049.8
Eddowes' (brittle bones and blue sclera) 756.51
Edsall's 992.2
Eichstedt's (pityriasis versicolor) 111.0
Ellis-van Creveld (chondroectodermal
  dysplasia) 756.55
endocardium—*see* Endocarditis
endocrine glands or system NEC 259.9
 specified NEC 259.8
endomyocardial, idiopathic mural 425.2
Engel-von Recklinghausen (osteitis fibrosa
  cystica) 252.01
Engelmann's (diaphyseal sclerosis) 756.59
English (rickets) 268.0
Engman's (infectious eczematoid dermatitis)
  690.8

Disease, diseased—*continued*
enteroviral, enterovirus NEC 078.89
 central nervous system NEC 048
 epidemic NEC 136.9
epididymis 608.9
epigastric, functional 536.9
 psychogenic 306.4
Erb (-Landouzy) 359.1
Erb-Goldflam 358.00
Erdheim-Chester (ECD) 277.89
Erichsen's (railway spine) 300.16
esophagus 530.9
 functional 530.5
 psychogenic 306.4
Eulenburg's (congenital paramyotonia) 359.29
Eustachian tube 381.9
Evans' (thrombocytopenic purpura) 287.32
external auditory canal 380.9
extrapyramidal NEC 333.90
eye 379.90
 anterior chamber 364.9
 inflammatory NEC 364.3
 muscle 378.9
eyeball 360.9
eyelid 374.9
eyeworm of Africa 125.2
Fabry's (angiokeratoma corporis diffusum)
  272.7
facial nerve (seventh) 351.9
 newborn 767.5
Fahr-Volhard (malignant nephrosclerosis)
  403.00
fallopian tube, noninflammatory 620.9
 specified NEC 620.8
familial periodic 277.31
 paralysis 359.3
Fanconi's (congenital pancytopenia) 284.09
Farber's (disseminated lipogranulomatosis)
  272.8
fascia 728.9
 inflammatory 728.9
Fauchard's (periodontitis) 523.40
Favre-Durand-Nicolas (climatic bubo) 099.1
Favre-Racouchot (elastoidosis cutanea
  nodularis) 701.8
Fede's 529.0
Feer's 985.0
Felix's (juvenile osteochondrosis, hip) 732.1
Fenwick's (gastric atrophy) 537.89
Fernels' (aortic aneurysm) 441.9
fibrocaseous, of lung (*see also* Tuberculosis,
  pulmonary) 011.9
fibrocystic—*see also* Fibrocystic, disease
 newborn 277.01
Fiedler's (leptospiral jaundice) 100.0
fifth 057.0
Filatoff's (infectious mononucleosis) 075
Filatov's (infectious mononucleosis) 075
file-cutters' 984.9
 specified type of lead—*see* Table of drugs and
  chemicals
filterable virus NEC 078.89
fish skin 757.1
 acquired 701.1
Flajani (-Basedow) (exophthalmic goiter) 242.0
Flatau-Schilder 341.1
flax-dressers' 504
Fleischner's 732.3
flint 502
fluke—*see* Infestation, fluke
Følling's (phenylketonuria) 270.1
foot and mouth 078.4

Disease, diseased—*continued*
foot process 581.3
Forbes' (glycogenosis III) 271.0
Fordyce's (ectopic sebaceous glands) (mouth) 750.26
Fordyce-Fox (apocrine miliaria) 705.82
Fothergill's
meaning scarlatina anginosa 034.1
neuralgia (*see also* Neuralgia, trigeminal) 350.1
Fournier's 608.83
female 616.89
fourth 057.8
Fox (-Fordyce) (apocrine miliaria) 705.82
Francis' (*see also* Tularemia) 021.9
Franklin's (heavy chain) 273.2
Frei's (climatic bubo) 099.1
Freiberg's (flattening metatarsal) 732.5
Friedländer's (endarteritis obliterans)—*see* Arteriosclerosis
Friedreich's
combined systemic or ataxia 334.0
facial hemihypertrophy 756.0
myoclonia 333.2
Fröhlich's (adiposogenital dystrophy) 253.8
Frommel's 676.6
frontal sinus (chronic) 473.1
acute 461.1
Fuller's earth 502
fungus, fungous NEC 117.9
Gaisböck's (polycythemia hypertonica) 289.0
gallbladder 575.9
congenital 751.60
Gamna's (siderotic splenomegaly) 289.51
Gamstorp's (adynamia episodica hereditaria) 359.3
Gandy-Nanta (siderotic splenomegaly) 289.51
gannister (occupational) 502
Garré's (*see also* Osteomyelitis) 730.1
gastric (*see also* Disease, stomach) 537.9
gastroesophageal reflux (GERD) 530.81
gastrointestinal (tract) 569.9
amyloid 277.39
functional 536.9
psychogenic 306.4
Gaucher's (adult) (cerebroside lipidosis) (infantile) 272.7
Gayet's (superior hemorrhagic polioencephalitis) 265.1
Gee (-Herter) (-Heubner) (-Thaysen) (nontropical sprue) 579.0
generalized neoplastic (M8000/6) 199.0
genital organs NEC
female 629.9
specified NEC 629.89
male 608.9
Gerhardt's (erythromelalgia) 443.82
Gerlier's (epidemic vertigo) 078.81
Gibert's (pityriasis rosea) 696.3
Gibney's (perispondylitis) 720.9
Gierke's (glycogenosis I) 271.0
Gilbert's (familial nonhemolytic jaundice) 277.4
Gilchrist's (North American blastomycosis) 116.0
Gilford (-Hutchinson) (progeria) 259.8
Gilles de la Tourette's (motor-verbal tic) 307.23
Giovannini's 117.9
gland (lymph) 289.9
Glanzmann's (hereditary hemorrhagic thrombasthenia) 287.1
glassblowers' 527.1

Disease, diseased—*continued*
Glénard's (enteroptosis) 569.89
Glisson's (*see also* Rickets) 268.0
glomerular
membranous, idiopathic 581.1
minimal change 581.3
glycogen storage (Andersen's) (Cori types 1-7) (Forbes') (McArdle-Schmid-Pearson) (Pompe's) (types I-VII) 271.0
cardiac 271.0 *[425.7]*
generalized 271.0
glucose-6-phosphatase deficiency 271.0
heart 271.0 *[425.7]*
hepatorenal 271.0
liver and kidneys 271.0
myocardium 271.0 *[425.7]*
von Gierke's (glycogenosis I) 271.0
Goldflam-Erb 358.00
Goldscheider's (epidermolysis bullosa) 757.39
Goldstein's (familial hemorrhagic telangiectasia) 448.0
gonococcal NEC 098.0
Goodall's (epidemic vomiting) 078.82
Gordon's (exudative enteropathy) 579.8
Gougerot's (trisymptomatic) 709.1
Gougerot-Carteaud (confluent reticulate papillomatosis) 701.8
Gougerot-Hailey-Hailey (benign familial chronic pemphigus) 757.39
graft-versus-host 279.50
acute 279.51
on chronic 279.53
chronic 279.52
grain-handlers' 495.8
Grancher's (splenopneumonia)—*see* Pneumonia
granulomatous (childhood) (chronic) 288.1
graphite lung 503
Graves' (exophthalmic goiter) 242.0
Greenfield's 330.0
green monkey 078.89
Griesinger's (*see also* Ancylostomiasis) 126.9
grinders' 502
Grisel's 723.5
Gruby's (tinea tonsurans) 110.0
Guertin's (electric chorea) 049.8
Guillain-Barré 357.0
Guinon's (motor-verbal tic) 307.23
Gull's (thyroid atrophy with myxedema) 244.8
Gull and Sutton's—*see* Hypertension, kidney
gum NEC 523.9
Günther's (congenital erythropoietic porphyria) 277.1
gynecological 629.9
specified NEC 629.89
H 270.0
Haas' 732.3
Habermann's (acute parapsoriasis varioliformis) 696.2
Haff 985.1
Hageman (congenital factor XII deficiency) (*see also* Defect, congenital) 286.3
Haglund's (osteochondrosis os tibiale externum) 732.5
Hagner's (hypertrophic pulmonary osteoarthropathy) 731.2
Hailey-Hailey (benign familial chronic pemphigus) 757.39
hair (follicles) NEC 704.9
specified type NEC 704.8
Hallervorden-Spatz 333.0

Disease, diseased—*continued*
 Hallopeau's (lichen sclerosus et atrophicus) 701.0
 Hamman's (spontaneous mediastinal emphysema) 518.1
 hand, foot, and mouth 074.3
 Hand-Schüller-Christian (chronic histiocytosis X) 277.89
 Hanot's—*see* Cirrhosis, biliary
 Hansen's (leprosy) 030.9
  benign form 030.1
  malignant form 030.0
 Harada's 363.22
 Harley's (intermittent hemoglobinuria) 283.2
 Hart's (pellagra-cerebellar ataxia renal aminoaciduria) 270.0
 Hartnup (pellagra-cerebellar ataxia-renal aminoaciduria) 270.0
 Hashimoto's (struma lymphomatosa) 245.2
 Hb—*see* Disease, hemoglobin
 heart (organic) 429.9
  with
   acute pulmonary edema (*see also* Failure, ventricular, left) 428.1
    hypertensive 402.91
     with renal failure 404.92
     benign 402.11
      with renal failure 404.12
     malignant 402.01
      with renal failure 404.02
   kidney disease—*see* Hypertension, cardiorenal
   rheumatic fever (conditions classifiable to 390)
    active 391.9
     with chorea 392.0
    inactive or quiescent (with chorea) 398.90
  amyloid 277.39 *[425.7]*
  aortic (valve) (*see also* Endocarditis, aortic) 424.1
  arteriosclerotic or sclerotic (minimal) (senile)—*see* Arteriosclerosis, coronary
  artery, arterial —*see* Arteriosclerosis, coronary
  atherosclerotic —*see* Arteriosclerosis, coronary
  beer drinkers' 425.5
  beriberi 265.0 *[425.7]*
  black 416.0
  congenital NEC 746.9
   cyanotic 746.9
   maternal, affecting fetus or newborn 760.3
   specified type NEC 746.89
  congestive (*see also* Failure, heart) 428.0
  coronary 414.9
  cryptogenic 429.9
  due to
   amyloidosis 277.39 *[425.7]*
   beriberi 265.0 *[425.7]*
   cardiac glycogenosis 271.0 *[425.7]*
   Friedreich's ataxia 334.0 *[425.8]*
   gout 274.82
   mucopolysaccharidosis 277.5 *[425.7]*
   myotonia atrophica 359.21 *[425.8]*
   progressive muscular dystrophy 359.1 *[425.8]*
   sarcoidosis 135 *[425.8]*
  fetal 746.9
   inflammatory 746.89
  fibroid (*see also* Myocarditis) 429.0

Disease, diseased—*continued*
 heart—*continued*
  functional 427.9
   postoperative 997.1
   psychogenic 306.2
  glycogen storage 271.0 *[425.7]*
  gonococcal NEC 098.85
  gouty 274.82
  hypertensive (*see also* Hypertension, heart) 402.90
   benign 402.10
   malignant 402.00
  hyperthyroid (*see also* Hyperthyroidism) 242.9 *[425.7]*
  incompletely diagnosed—*see* Disease, heart
  ischemic (chronic) (*see also* Ischemia, heart) 414.9
   acute (*see also* Infarct, myocardium) 410.9
    without myocardial infarction 411.89
     with coronary (artery) occlusion 411.81
   asymptomatic 412
   diagnosed on ECG or other special investigation but currently presenting no symptoms 412
  kyphoscoliotic 416.1
  mitral (*see also* Endocarditis, mitral) 394.9
  muscular (*see also* Degeneration, myocardial) 429.1
  postpartum 674.8
  psychogenic (functional) 306.2
  pulmonary (chronic) 416.9
   acute 415.0
   specified NEC 416.8
  rheumatic (chronic) (inactive) (old) (quiescent) (with chorea) 398.90
   active or acute 391.9
    with chorea (active) (rheumatic) (Sydenham's) 392.0
   specified type NEC 391.8
   maternal, affecting fetus or newborn 760.3
  rheumatoid—*see* Arthritis, rheumatoid
  sclerotic —*see* Arteriosclerosis, coronary
  senile (*see also* Myocarditis) 429.0
  specified type NEC 429.89
  syphilitic 093.89
   aortic 093.1
    aneurysm 093.0
   asymptomatic 093.89
   congenital 090.5
  thyroid (gland) (*see also* Hyperthyroidism) 242.9 *[425.7]*
  thyrotoxic (*see also* Thyrotoxicosis) 242.9 *[425.7]*
  tuberculous (*see also* Tuberculosis) 017.9 *[425.8]*
  valve, valvular (obstructive) (regurgitant)—*see also* Endocarditis
   congenital NEC (*see also* Anomaly, heart, valve) 746.9
   pulmonary 746.00
   specified type NEC 746.89
  vascular—*see* Disease, cardiovascular
 heavy-chain (gamma G) 273.2
 Heberden's 715.04
 Hebra's
  dermatitis exfoliativa 695.89
  erythema multiforme exudativum 695.19
  pityriasis
   maculata et circinata 696.3
   rubra 695.89
    pilaris 696.4
  prurigo 698.2

Disease, diseased—*continued*
 Heerfordt's (uveoparotitis) 135
 Heidenhain's 290.10
  with dementia 290.10
 Heilmeyer-Schöner (M9842/3) 207.1
 Heine-Medin (*see also* Poliomyelitis) 045.9
 Heller's (*see also* Psychosis, childhood) 299.1
 Heller-Döhle (syphilitic aortitis) 093.1
 hematopoietic organs 289.9
 hemoglobin (Hb) 282.7
  with thalassemia 282.49
  abnormal (mixed) NEC 282.7
   with thalassemia 282.49
  AS genotype 282.5
  Bart's 282.43
  C (Hb-C) 282.7
   with other abnormal hemoglobin NEC 282.7
   elliptocytosis 282.7
   Hb-S (without crisis) 282.63
    with
     crisis 282.64
      vaso-occlusive pain 282.64
    sickle-cell (without crisis) 282.63
     with
      crisis 282.64
       vaso-occlusive pain 282.64
    thalassemia 282.49
  constant spring 282.7
  D (Hb-D) 282.7
   with other abnormal hemoglobin NEC 282.7
   Hb-S (without crisis) 282.68
    with crisis 282.69
   sickle-cell (without crisis) 282.68
    with crisis 282.69
   thalassemia 282.49
  E (Hb-E) 282.7
   with other abnormal hemoglobin NEC 282.7
   Hb-S (without crisis) 282.68
    with crisis 282.69
   sickle-cell (without crisis) 282.68
    with crisis 282.69
   thalassemia 282.47
  elliptocytosis 282.7
  F (Hb-F) 282.7
  G (Hb-G) 282.7
  H (Hb-H) 282.43
  hereditary persistence, fetal (HPFH) ("Swiss
   variety") 282.7
  high fetal gene 282.7
  I thalassemia 282.49
  M 289.7
  S—*see also* Disease, sickle-cell, Hb-S
   thalassemia (without crisis) 282.41
    with
     crisis 282.42
      vaso-occlusive pain 282.42
  spherocytosis 282.7
  unstable, hemolytic 282.7
  Zurich (Hb-Zurich) 282.7
 hemolytic (fetus) (newborn) 773.2
  autoimmune (cold type) (warm type) 283.0
  due to or with
   incompatibility
    ABO (blood group) 773.1
    blood (group) (Duffy) (Kell) (Kidd)
     (Lewis) (M) (S) NEC 773.2
    Rh (blood group) (factor) 773.0
   Rh negative mother 773.0
  unstable hemoglobin 282.7
 hemorrhagic 287.9
  newborn 776.0

Disease, diseased—*continued*
 Henoch (-Schönlein) (purpura nervosa) 287.0
 hepatic—*see* Disease, liver
 hepatolenticular 275.1
 heredodegenerative NEC
  brain 331.89
  spinal cord 336.8
 Hers' (glycogenosis VI) 271.0
 Herter (-Gee) (-Heubner) (nontropical sprue) 579.0
 Herxheimer's (diffuse idiopathic cutaneous
  atrophy) 701.8
 Heubner's 094.89
 Heubner-Herter (nontropical sprue) 579.0
 high fetal gene or hemoglobin thalassemia (*see
  also* Thalassemia) 282.40
 Hildenbrand's (typhus) 081.9
 hip (joint) NEC 719.95
  congenital 755.63
  suppurative 711.05
  tuberculous (*see also* Tuberculosis) 015.1
   [730.85]
 Hippel's (retinocerebral angiomatosis) 759.6
 Hirschfeld's (acute diabetes mellitus) (*see also*
  Diabetes) 250.0
  due to secondary diabetes 249.0
 Hirschsprung's (congenital megacolon) 751.3
 His (-Werner) (trench fever) 083.1
 HIV 042
 Hodgkin's (M9650/3) 201.9

---

*Note—Use the following fifth-digit
subclassification with categories 201:*

0 *unspecified site*
1 *lymph nodes of head, face, and neck*
2 *intrathoracic lymph nodes*
3 *intra-abdominal lymph nodes*
4 *lymph nodes of axilla and upper limb*
5 *lymph nodes of inguinal region and
   lower limb*
6 *intrapelvic lymph nodes*
7 *spleen*
8 *lymph nodes of multiple sites*

---

  lymphocytic
   depletion (M9653/3) 201.7
    diffuse fibrosis (M9654/3) 201.7
    reticular type (M9655/3) 201.7
   predominance (M9651/3) 201.4
  lymphocytic-histiocytic predominance
   (M9651/3) 201.4
  mixed cellularity (M9652/3) 201.6
  nodular sclerosis (M9656/3) 201.5
   cellular phase (M9657/3) 201.5
 Hodgson's 441.9
  ruptured 441.5
 Hoffa (-Kastert) (liposynovitis prepatellaris)
  272.8
 Holla (*see also* Spherocytosis) 282.0
 homozygous-Hb-S 282.61
 hoof and mouth 078.4
 hookworm (*see also* Ancylostomiasis) 126.9
 Horton's (temporal arteritis) 446.5
 host-versus-graft (immune or nonimmune cause)
  279.50
 HPFH (hereditary persistence of fetal
  hemoglobin) ("Swiss variety") 282.7
 Huchard's (continued arterial hypertension)
  401.9
 Huguier's (uterine fibroma) 218.9
 human immunodeficiency (virus) 042
 hunger 251.1

Disease, diseased—*continued*
  Hunt's
    dyssynergia cerebellaris myoclonica 334.2
    herpetic geniculate ganglionitis 053.11
  Huntington's 333.4
  Huppert's (multiple myeloma) (M9730/3) 203.0
  Hurler's (mucopolysaccharidosis I) 277.5
  Hutchinson's, meaning
    angioma serpiginosum 709.1
    cheiropompholyx 705.81
    prurigo estivalis 692.72
  Hutchinson-Boeck (sarcoidosis) 135
  Hutchinson-Gilford (progeria) 259.8
  hyaline (diffuse) (generalized) 728.9
    membrane (lung) (newborn) 769
  hydatid (*see also* Echinococcus) 122.9
  Hyde's (prurigo nodularis) 698.3
  hyperkinetic (*see also* Hyperkinesia) 314.9
    heart 429.82
  hypertensive (*see also* Hypertension) 401.9
  hypophysis 253.9
    hyperfunction 253.1
    hypofunction 253.2
  Iceland (epidemic neuromyasthenia) 049.8
  I cell 272.7
  ill-defined 799.89
  immunologic NEC 279.9
  immunoproliferative 203.8
  inclusion 078.5
    salivary gland 078.5
  infancy, early NEC 779.9
  infective NEC 136.9
  inguinal gland 289.9
  internal semilunar cartilage, cystic 717.5
  intervertebral disc 722.90
    with myelopathy 722.70
    cervical, cervicothoracic 722.91
      with myelopathy 722.71
    lumbar, lumbosacral 722.93
      with myelopathy 722.73
    thoracic, thoracolumbar 722.92
      with myelopathy 722.72
  intestine 569.9
    functional 564.9
      congenital 751.3
      psychogenic 306.4
    lardaceous 277.39
    organic 569.9
    protozoal NEC 007.9
  iris 364.9
    specified NEC 364.89
  iron
    metabolism (*see also* Hemochromatosis) 275.09
    storage (*see also* Hemochromatosis) 275.03
  Isambert's (*see also* Tuberculosis, larynx) 012.3
  Iselin's (osteochondrosis, fifth metatarsal) 732.5
  Island (scrub typhus) 081.2
  itai-itai 985.5
  Jadassohn's (maculopapular erythroderma) 696.2
  Jadassohn-Pellizari's (anetoderma) 701.3
  Jakob-Creutzfeldt (CJD) 046.19
    with dementia
      with behavioral disturbance 046.19 *[294.11]*
      without behavioral disturbance 046.19
        [294.10]
    familial 046.19
    iatrogenic 046.19
    specified NEC 046.19
    sporadic 046.19

Disease, diseased—*continued*
  variant (vCJD) 046.11
    with dementia
      with behavioral disturbance 046.11 *[294.11]*
      without behavioral disturbance 046.11
        [294.10]
  Jaksch (-Luzet) (pseudoleukemia infantum) 285.8
  Janet's 300.89
  Jansky-Bielschowsky 330.1
  jaw NEC 526.9
    fibrocystic 526.2
  Jensen's 363.05
  Jeune's (asphyxiating thoracic dystrophy) 756.4
  jigger 134.1
  Johnson-Stevens (erythema multiforme
      exudativum) 695.13
  joint NEC 719.9
    ankle 719.97
    Charcot 094.0 *[713.5]*
    degenerative (*see also* Osteoarthrosis) 715.9
      multiple 715.09
      spine (*see also* Spondylosis) 721.90
    elbow 719.92
    foot 719.97
    hand 719.94
    hip 719.95
    hypertrophic (chronic) (degenerative) (*see also*
        Osteoarthrosis) 715.9
      spine (*see also* Spondylosis) 721.90
    knee 719.96
    Luschka 721.90
    multiple sites 719.99
    pelvic region 719.95
    sacroiliac 724.6
    shoulder (region) 719.91
    specified site NEC 719.98
    spine NEC 724.9
      pseudarthrosis following fusion 733.82
      sacroiliac 724.6
    wrist 719.93
  Jourdain's (acute gingivitis) 523.00
  Jüngling's (sarcoidosis) 135
  Kahler (-Bozzolo) (multiple myeloma)
      (M9730/3) 203.0
  Kalischer's 759.6
  Kaposi's 757.33
    lichen ruber 697.8
      acuminatus 696.4
      moniliformis 697.8
    xeroderma pigmentosum 757.33
  Kaschin-Beck (endemic polyarthritis) 716.00
    ankle 716.07
    arm 716.02
      lower (and wrist) 716.03
      upper (and elbow) 716.02
    foot (and ankle) 716.07
    forearm (and wrist) 716.03
    hand 716.04
    leg 716.06
      lower 716.06
      upper 716.05
    multiple sites 716.09
    pelvic region (hip) (thigh) 716.05
    shoulder region 716.01
    specified site NEC 716.08
  Katayama 120.2
  Kawasaki 446.1
  Kedani (scrub typhus) 081.2

Disease, diseased—*continued*
kidney (functional) (pelvis) (*see also* Disease,
renal) 593.9
chronic 585.9
requiring chronic dialysis 585.6
stage
I 585.1
II (mild) 585.2
III (moderate) 585.3
IV (severe) 585.4
V 585.5
cystic (congenital) 753.10
multiple 753.19
single 753.11
specified NEC 753.19
fibrocystic (congenital) 753.19
in gout 274.10
polycystic (congenital) 753.12
adult type (APKD) 753.13
autosomal dominant 753.13
autosomal recessive 753.14
childhood type (CPKD) 753.14
infantile type 753.14
Kienböck's (carpal lunate) (wrist) 732.3
Kimmelstiel (-Wilson) (intercapillary
glomerulosclerosis) 250.4 *[581.81]*
due to secondary diabetes 249.4 *[581.81]*
Kinnier Wilson's (hepatolenticular
degeneration) 275.1
kissing 075
Kleb's (*see also* Nephritis) 583.9
Klinger's 446.4
Klippel's 723.8
Klippel-Feil (brevicollis) 756.16
knight's 911.1
Köbner's (epidermolysis bullosa) 757.39
Koenig-Wichmann (pemphigus) 694.4
Köhler's
first (osteoarthrosis juvenilis) 732.5
second (Freiberg's infraction, metatarsal head)
732.5
patellar 732.4
tarsal navicular (bone) (osteoarthrosis
juvenilis) 732.5
Köhler-Freiberg (infraction, metatarsal head) 732.5
Köhler-Mouchet (osteoarthrosis juvenilis) 732.5
Köhler-Pellegrini-Stieda (calcification, knee
joint) 726.62
Kok 759.89
König's (osteochondritis dissecans) 732.7
Korsakoff's (nonalcoholic) 294.0
alcoholic 291.1
Kostmann's (infantile genetic agranulocytosis)
288.01
Krabbe's 330.0
Kraepelin-Morel (*see also* Schizophrenia) 295.9
Kraft-Weber-Dimitri 759.6
Kufs' 330.1
Kugelberg-Welander 335.11
Kuhnt-Junius 362.52
Kümmell's (-Verneuil) (spondylitis) 721.7
Kundrat's (lymphosarcoma) 200.1
kuru 046.0
Kussmaul (-Meier) (polyarteritis nodosa) 446.0
Kyasanur Forest 065.2
Kyrle's (hyperkeratosis follicularis in cutem
penetrans) 701.1
labia
inflammatory 616.10
noninflammatory 624.9
specified NEC 624.8

Disease, diseased—*continued*
labyrinth, ear 386.8
lacrimal system (apparatus) (passages) 375.9
gland 375.00
specified NEC 375.89
Lafora's 333.2
Lagleyze-von Hippel (retinocerebral
angiomatosis) 759.6
Lancereaux-Mathieu (leptospiral jaundice) 100.0
Landry's 357.0
Lane's 569.89
lardaceous (any site) 277.39
Larrey-Weil (leptospiral jaundice) 100.0
Larsen (-Johansson) (juvenile osteopathia
patellae) 732.4
larynx 478.70
Lasègue's (persecution mania) 297.9
Leber's 377.16
Lederer's (acquired infectious hemolytic
anemia) 283.19
Legg's (capital femoral osteochondrosis) 732.1
Legg-Calvé-Perthes (capital femoral
osteochondrosis) 732.1
Legg-Calvé-Waldenström (femoral capital
osteochondrosis) 732.1
Legg-Perthes (femoral capital osteochondrosis)
732.1
Legionnaires' 482.84
Leigh's 330.8
Leiner's (exfoliative dermatitis) 695.89
Leloir's (lupus erythematosus) 695.4
Lenegre's 426.0
lens (eye) 379.39
Leriche's (osteoporosis, posttraumatic) 733.7
Letterer-Siwe (acute histiocytosis X) (M9722/3)
202.5
Lev's (acquired complete heart block) 426.0
Lewandowski's (*see also* Tuberculosis) 017.0
Lewandowski-Lutz (epidermodysplasia
verruciformis) 078.19
Lewy body 331.82
with dementia
with behavioral disturbance 331.82 *[294.11]*
without behavioral disturbance 331.82
[294.10]
Leyden's (periodic vomiting) 536.2
Libman-Sacks (verrucous endocarditis) 710.0
[424.91]
Lichtheim's (subacute combined sclerosis with
pernicious anemia) 281.0 *[336.2]*
ligament 728.9
light chain 203.0
Lightwood's (renal tubular acidosis) 588.89
Lignac's (cystinosis) 270.0
Lindau's (retinocerebral angiomatosis) 759.6
Lindau-von Hippel (angiomatosis
retinocerebellosa) 759.6
lip NEC 528.5
lipidosis 272.7
lipoid storage NEC 272.7
Lipschütz's 616.50
Little's—*see* Palsy, cerebral
liver 573.9
alcoholic 571.3
acute 571.1
chronic 571.3
chronic 571.9
alcoholic 571.3
cystic, congenital 751.62
drug-induced 573.3

Disease, diseased—*continued*
  liver—*continued*
    due to
      chemicals 573.3
      fluorinated agents 573.3
      hypersensitivity drugs 573.3
      isoniazids 573.3
    end stage NEC 572.8
      due to hepatitis —*see* Hepatitis
    fibrocystic (congenital) 751.62
    glycogen storage 271.0
    organic 573.9
    polycystic (congenital) 751.62
  Lobo's (keloid blastomycosis) 116.2
  Lobstein's (brittle bones and blue sclera) 756.61
  locomotor system 334.9
  Lorain's (pituitary dwarfism) 253.3
  Lou Gehrig's 335.20
  Lucas-Championnière (fibrinous bronchitis) 466.0
  Ludwig's (submaxillary cellulitis) 528.3
  luetic—*see* Syphilis
  lumbosacral region 724.6
  lung NEC 518.89
    black 500
    congenital 748.60
    cystic 518.89
      congenital 748.4
    fibroid (chronic) (*see also* Fibrosis, lung) 515
    fluke 121.2
      Oriental 121.2
    in
      amyloidosis 277.39 *[517.8]*
      polymyositis 710.4 *[517.8]*
      sarcoidosis 135 *[517.8]*
      Sjögren's syndrome 710.2 *[517.8]*
      syphilis 095.1
      systemic lupus erythematosus 710.0 *[517.8]*
      systemic sclerosis 710.1 *[517.2]*
    interstitial (chronic) 515
      acute 136.3
      respiratory bronchiolitis 516.34
    nonspecific, chronic 496
    obstructive (chronic) (COPD) 496
      with
        acute
          bronchitis 491.22
          exacerbation NEC 491.21
        alveolitis, allergic (*see also* Alveolitis,
          allergic) 495.9
        asthma (chronic) (obstructive) 493.2
        bronchiectasis 494.0
          with exacerbation (acute) 494.1
        bronchitis (chronic) 491.20
          with
            acute bronchitis 491.22
            exacerbation (acute) 491.21
        decompensated 491.21
          with exacerbation 491.21
        emphysema NEC 492.8
      diffuse (with fibrosis) 496
    of childhood, specified NEC 516.69
    polycystic 518.89
      asthma (chronic) (obstructive) 493.2
      congenital 748.4
    purulent (cavitary) 513.0
    restrictive 518.89
    rheumatoid 714.81
      diffuse interstitial 714.81
    specified NEC 518.89
  Lutembacher's (atrial septal defect with mitral
    stenosis) 745.5

Disease, diseased—*continued*
  Lutz-Miescher (elastosis perforans serpiginosa)
    701.1
  Lutz-Splendore-de Almeida (Brazilian
    blastomycosis) 116.1
  Lyell's (toxic epidermal necrolysis) 695.15
    due to drug
      correct substance properly administered
        695.15
      overdose or wrong substance given or taken
        977.9
        specific drug—*see* Table of drugs and
          chemicals
  Lyme 088.81
  lymphatic (gland) (system) 289.9
    channel (noninfective) 457.9
    vessel (noninfective) 457.9
    specified NEC 457.8
  lymphoproliferative (chronic) (M9970/1) 238.79
    X linked 759.89
  Machado-Joseph 334.8
  Madelung's (lipomatosis) 272.8
  Madura (actinomycotic) 039.9
    mycotic 117.4
  Magitot's 526.4
  Majocchi's (purpura annularis telangiectodes)
    709.1
  malarial (*see also* Malaria) 084.6
  Malassez's (cystic) 608.89
  Malibu 919.8
    infected 919.9
  malignant (M8000/3)—*see also* Neoplasm, by
    site, malignant
    previous, affecting management of pregnancy
      V23.8
  Manson's 120.1
  maple bark 495.6
  maple syrup (urine) 270.3
  Marburg (virus) 078.89
  Marchiafava (-Bignami) 341.8
  Marfan's 090.49
    congenital syphilis 090.49
    meaning Marfan's syndrome 759.82
  Marie-Bamberger (hypertrophic pulmonary
    osteoarthropathy) (secondary) 731.2
    primary or idiopathic (acropachyderma)
      757.39
    pulmonary (hypertrophic osteoarthropathy)
      731.2
  Marie-Strümpell (ankylosing spondylitis) 720.0
  Marion's (bladder neck obstruction) 596.0
  Marsh's (exophthalmic goiter) 242.0
  Martin's 715.27
  mast cell 757.33
    systemic (M9741/3) 202.6
  mastoid (*see also* Mastoiditis) 383.9
    process 385.9
  maternal, unrelated to pregnancy NEC, affecting
    fetus or newborn 760.9
  Mathieu's (leptospiral jaundice) 100.0
  Mauclaire's 732.3
  Mauriac's (erythema nodosum syphiliticum)
    091.3
  Maxcy's 081.0
  McArdle (-Schmid-Pearson) (glycogenosis V)
    271.0
  mediastinum NEC 519.3
  Medin's (*see also* Poliomyelitis) 045.9
  Mediterranean 282.40
    with hemoglobinopathy 282.49
  medullary center (idiopathic) (respiratory) 348.89

Disease, diseased—*continued*
Meige's (chronic hereditary edema) 757.0
Meleda 757.39
Ménétrier's (hypertrophic gastritis) 535.2
Ménière's (active) 386.00
  cochlear 386.02
  cochleovestibular 386.01
  inactive 386.04
  in remission 386.04
  vestibular 386.03
meningeal—*see* Meningitis
mental (*see also* Psychosis) 298.9
Merzbacher-Pelizaeus 330.0
mesenchymal 710.9
mesenteric embolic 557.0
metabolic NEC 277.9
metal polishers' 502
metastatic—*see* Metastasis
Mibelli's 757.39
microdrepanocytic 282.41
microvascular —*code to condition*
microvillus
  atrophy 751.5
  inclusion (MVD) 751.5
Miescher's 709.3
Mikulicz's (dryness of mouth, absent or
  decreased lacrimation) 527.1
Milkman (-Looser) (osteomalacia with
  pseudofractures) 268.2
Miller's (osteomalacia) 268.2
Mills' 335.29
Milroy's (chronic hereditary edema) 757.0
Minamata 985.0
Minor's 336.1
Minot's (hemorrhagic disease, newborn) 776.0
Minot-von Willebrand-Jürgens
  (angiohemophilia) 286.4
Mitchell's (erythromelalgia) 443.82
mitral—*see* Endocarditis, mitral
Mljet (mal de Meleda) 757.39
Möbius', Moebius' 346.2
Moeller's 267
Möller (-Barlow) (infantile scurvy) 267
Mönckeberg's (*see also* arteriosclerosis,
  extremities) 440.20
Mondor's (thrombophlebitis of breast) 451.89
Monge's 993.2
Morel-Kraepelin (*see also* Schizophrenia) 295.9
Morgagni's (syndrome) (hyperostosis frontalis
  interna) 733.3
Morgagni-Adams-Stokes (syncope with heart
  block) 426.9
Morquio (-Brailsford) (-Ullrich)
  (mucopolysaccharidosis IV) 277.5
Morton's (with metatarsalgia) 355.6
Morvan's 336.0
motor neuron (bulbar) (mixed type) 335.20
Mouchet's (juvenile osteochondrosis, foot)
  732.5
mouth 528.9
Moyamoya 437.5
Mucha's (acute parapsoriasis varioliformis)
  696.2
mu-chain 273.2
mucolipidosis (I) (II) (III) 272.7
Münchmeyer's (exostosis luxurians) 728.11
Murri's (intermittent hemoglobinuria) 283.2
muscle 359.9
  inflammatory 728.9
  ocular 378.9
musculoskeletal system 729.90

Disease, diseased—*continued*
mushroom workers' 495.5
Myà's (congenital dilation, colon) 751.3
mycotic 117.9
myeloproliferative (chronic) (M9960/1) 238.79
myocardium, myocardial (*see also*
  Degeneration, myocardial) 429.1
  hypertensive (*see also* Hypertension, heart)
    402.90
  primary (idiopathic) 425.4
myoneural 358.9
Naegeli's 287.1
nail 703.9
  specified type NEC 703.8
Nairobi sheep 066.1
nasal 478.19
  cavity NEC 478.19
  sinus (chronic)—*see* Sinusitis
navel (newborn) NEC 779.89
  delayed separation of umbilical cord 779.83
nemaline body 359.0
neoplastic, generalized (M8000/6) 199.0
nerve—*see* Disorder, nerve
nervous system (central) 349.9
  autonomic, peripheral (*see also* Neuropathy,
    peripheral, autonomic) 337.9
  congenital 742.9
  inflammatory—*see* Encephalitis
  parasympathetic (*see also* Neuropathy,
    peripheral, autonomic) 337.9
  peripheral NEC 355.9
  prion NEC 046.79
  specified NEC 349.89
  sympathetic (*see also* Neuropathy, peripheral,
    autonomic) 337.9
  vegetative (*see also* Neuropathy, peripheral,
    autonomic) 337.9
Nettleship's (urticaria pigmentosa) 757.33
Neumann's (pemphigus vegetans) 694.4
neurologic (central) NEC (*see also* Disease,
  nervous system) 349.9
  peripheral NEC 355.9
neuromuscular system NEC 358.9
Newcastle 077.8
Nicolas (-Durand) -Favre (climatic bubo) 099.1
Niemann-Pick (lipid histiocytosis) 272.7
nipple 611.9
  Paget's (M8540/3) 174.0
Nishimoto (-Takeuchi) 437.5
nonarthropod-borne NEC 078.89
  central nervous system NEC 049.9
  enterovirus NEC 078.89
non-autoimmune hemolytic NEC 283.10
Nonne-Milroy-Meige (chronic hereditary
  edema) 757.0
Norrie's (congenital progressive
  oculoacousticocerebral degeneration) 743.8
nose 478.19
nucleus pulposus—*see* Disease, intervertebral
  disc
nutritional 269.9
  maternal, affecting fetus or newborn 760.4
oasthouse, urine 270.2
obliterative vascular 447.1
Odelberg's (juvenile osteochondrosis) 732.1
Oguchi's (retina) 368.61
Ohara's (*see also* Tularemia) 021.9
Ollier's (chondrodysplasia) 756.4
Opitz's (congestive splenomegaly) 289.51
Oppenheim's 358.8

Disease, diseased—*continued*
 Oppenheim-Urbach (necrobiosis lipoidica
  diabeticorum) 250.8 *[709.3]*
  due to secondary diabetes 249.8 *[709.3]*
 optic nerve NEC 377.49
 orbit 376.9
  specified NEC 376.89
 Oriental liver fluke 121.1
 Oriental lung fluke 121.2
 Ormond's 593.4
 Osgood's tibia (tubercle) 732.4
 Osgood-Schlatter 732.4
 Osler (-Vaquez) (polycythemia vera) (M9950/1)
  238.4
 Osler-Rendu (familial hemorrhagic
  telangiectasia) 448.0
 osteofibrocystic 252.01
 Otto's 715.35
 outer ear 380.9
 ovary (noninflammatory) NEC 620.9
  cystic 620.2
  polycystic 256.4
  specified NEC 620.8
 Owren's (congenital) (*see also* Defect,
  coagulation) 286.3
 Paas' 756.59
 Paget's (osteitis deformans) 731.0
  with infiltrating duct carcinoma of the breast
   (M8541/3)—*see* Neoplasm, breast, malignant
  bone 731.0
   osteosarcoma in (M9184/3)—*see* Neoplasm,
    bone, malignant
  breast (M8540/3) 174.0
  extramammary (M8542/3)—*see also*
   Neoplasm, skin, malignant
   anus 154.3
    skin 173.59
  malignant (M8540/3)
   breast 174.0
   specified site NEC (M8542/3)—*see*
    Neoplasm, skin, malignant
   unspecified site 174.0
  mammary (M8540/3) 174.0
  nipple (M8540/3) 174.0
 palate (soft) 528.9
 Paltauf-Sternberg 201.9
 pancreas 577.9
  cystic 577.2
   congenital 751.7
  fibrocystic 277.00
 Panner's 732.3
  capitellum humeri 732.3
  head of humerus 732.3
  tarsal navicular (bone) (osteochondrosis) 732.5
 panvalvular—*see* Endocarditis, mitral
 parametrium 629.9
 parasitic NEC 136.9
  cerebral NEC 123.9
  intestinal NEC 129
  mouth 112.0
  skin NEC 134.9
  specified type—*see* Infestation
  tongue 112.0
 parathyroid (gland) 252.9
  specified NEC 252.8
 Parkinson's 332.0
 parodontal 523.9
 Parrot's (syphilitic osteochondritis) 090.0
 Parry's (exophthalmic goiter) 242.0
 Parson's (exophthalmic goiter) 242.0
 Pavy's 593.6

Disease, diseased—*continued*
 Paxton's (white piedra) 111.2
 Payr's (splenic flexure syndrome) 569.89
 pearl-workers' (chronic osteomyelitis) (*see also*
  Osteomyelitis) 730.1
 Pel-Ebstein—*see* Disease, Hodgkin's
 Pelizaeus-Merzbacher 330.0
  with dementia
   with behavioral disturbance 330.0 *[294.11]*
   without behavioral disturbance 330.0
    [294.10]
 Pellegrini-Stieda (calcification, knee joint) 726.62
 pelvis, pelvic
  female NEC 629.9
   specified NEC 629.89
  gonococcal (acute) 098.19
   chronic or duration of 2 months or over 098.39
  infection (*see also* Disease, pelvis, inflammatory)
   614.9
  inflammatory (female) (PID) 614.9
   with
    abortion—*see* Abortion, by type, with sepsis
    ectopic pregnancy (*see also* categories
     633.0-633.9) 639.0
    molar pregnancy (*see also* categories
     630-632) 639.0
   acute 614.3
   chronic 614.4
   complicating pregnancy 646.6
    affecting fetus or newborn 760.8
   following
    abortion 639.0
    ectopic or molar pregnancy 639.0
   peritonitis (acute) 614.5
    chronic NEC 614.7
   puerperal, postpartum, childbirth 670.8
   specified NEC 614.8
  organ, female NEC 629.9
   specified NEC 629.89
  peritoneum, female NEC 629.9
   specified NEC 629.89
 penis 607.9
  inflammatory 607.2
 peptic NEC 536.9
  acid 536.8
 periapical tissues NEC 522.9
 pericardium 423.9
  specified type NEC 423.8
 perineum
  female
   inflammatory 616.9
    specified NEC 616.89
   noninflammatory 624.9
    specified NEC 624.8
  male (inflammatory) 682.2
 periodic (familial) (Reimann's) NEC 277.31
  paralysis 359.3
 periodontal NEC 523.9
  specified NEC 523.8
 periosteum 733.90
 peripheral
  arterial 443.9
  autonomic nervous system (*see also*
   Neuropathy, autonomic) 337.9
  nerve NEC (*see also* Neuropathy) 356.9
   multiple—*see* Polyneuropathy
  vascular 443.9
   specified type NEC 443.89
 peritoneum 568.9
  pelvic, female 629.9
   specified NEC 629.89

Disease, diseased—*continued*
Perrin-Ferraton (snapping hip) 719.65
persistent mucosal (middle ear) (with posterior
 or superior marginal perforation of ear
 drum) 382.2
Perthes' (capital femoral osteochondrosis) 732.1
Petit's (*see also* Hernia, lumbar) 553.8
Peutz-Jeghers 759.6
Peyronie's 607.85
Pfeiffer's (infectious mononucleosis) 075
pharynx 478.20
Phocas' 610.1
photochromogenic (acid-fast bacilli)
 (pulmonary) 031.0
 nonpulmonary 031.9
Pick's
 brain 331.11
 with dementia
 with behavioral disturbance 331.11
 [294.11]
 without behavioral disturbance 331.11
 [294.10]
 cerebral atrophy 331.11
 with dementia
 with behavioral disturbance 331.11
 [294.11]
 without behavioral disturbance 331.11
 [294.10]
 lipid histiocytosis 272.7
 liver (pericardial pseudocirrhosis of liver) 423.2
 pericardium (pericardial pseudocirrhosis of
 liver) 423.2
 polyserositis (pericardial pseudocirrhosis of
 liver) 423.2
Pierson's (osteochondrosis) 732.1
pigeon fancier's or breeders' 495.2
pineal gland 259.8
pink 985.0
Pinkus' (lichen nitidus) 697.1
pinworm 127.4
pituitary (gland) 253.9
 hyperfunction 253.1
 hypofunction 253.2
pituitary snuff-takers' 495.8
placenta
 affecting fetus or newborn 762.2
 complicating pregnancy or childbirth 656.7
pleura (cavity) (*see also* Pleurisy) 511.0
Plummer's (toxic nodular goiter) 242.3
pneumatic
 drill 994.9
 hammer 994.9
policeman's 729.2
Pollitzer's (hidradenitis suppurativa) 705.83
polycystic (congenital) 759.89
 kidney or renal 753.12
 adult type (APKD) 753.13
 autosomal dominant 753.13
 autosomal recessive 753.14
 childhood type (CPKD) 753.14
 infantile type 753.14
 liver or hepatic 751.62
 lung or pulmonary 518.89
 congenital 748.4
 ovary, ovaries 256.4
 spleen 759.0
polyethylene 996.45
Pompe's (glycogenosis II) 271.0
Poncet's (tuberculous rheumatism) (*see also*
 Tuberculosis) 015.9
Posada-Wernicke 114.9

Disease, diseased—*continued*
Potain's (pulmonary edema) 514
Pott's (*see also* Tuberculosis) 015.0 *[730.88]*
 osteomyelitis 015.0 *[730.88]*
 paraplegia 015.0 *[730.88]*
 spinal curvature 015.0 *[737.43]*
 spondylitis 015.0 *[720.81]*
Potter's 753.0
Poulet's 714.2
pregnancy NEC (*see also* Pregnancy) 646.9
Preiser's (osteoporosis) 733.09
Pringle's (tuberous sclerosis) 759.5
Profichet's 729.90
prostate 602.9
 specified type NEC 602.8
protozoal NEC 136.8
 intestine, intestinal NEC 007.9
pseudo-Hurler's (mucolipidosis III) 272.7
psychiatric (*see also* Psychosis) 298.9
psychotic (*see also* Psychosis) 298.9
Puente's (simple glandular cheilitis) 528.5
puerperal NEC (*see also* Puerperal) 674.9
pulmonary—*see also* Disease, lung
 amyloid 277.39 *[517.8]*
 artery 417.9
 circulation, circulatory 417.9
 specified NEC 417.8
 diffuse obstructive (chronic) 496
 with
 acute bronchitis 491.22
 asthma (chronic) (obstructive) 493.2
 bronchitis (chronic) 491.20
 with exacerbation (acute) 491.21
 exacerbation NEC (acute) 491.21
 heart (chronic) 416.9
 specified NEC 416.8
 hypertensive (vascular) 416.0
 cardiovascular 416.0
 obstructive diffuse (chronic) 496
 decompensated 491.21
 with exacerbation 491.21
 with
 acute bronchitis 491.22
 asthma (chronic) (obstructive) 493.2
 bronchitis (chronic) 491.20
 with
 exacerbation (acute) 491.21
 acute 491.22
 exacerbation NEC (acute) 491.21
 valve (*see also* Endocarditis, pulmonary) 424.3
 pulp (dental) NEC 522.9
 pulseless 446.7
Putnam's (subacute combined sclerosis with
 pernicious anemia) 281.0 *[336.2]*
Pyle (-Cohn) (craniometaphyseal dysplasia) 756.89
pyramidal tract 333.90
Quervain's
 tendon sheath 727.04
 thyroid (subacute granulomatous thyroiditis)
 245.1
Quincke's—*see* Edema, angioneurotic
Quinquaud (acne decalvans) 704.09
rag sorters' 022.1
Raynaud's (Paroxysmal digital cyanosis) 443.0
reactive airway—*see* Asthma
Recklinghausen's (M9540/1) 237.71
 bone (osteitis fibrosa cystica) 252.01
Recklinghausen-Applebaum (hemochromatosis)
 (*see also* Hemochromatosis) 275.03
Reclus' (cystic) 610.1

Disease, diseased—*continued*
rectum NEC 569.49
Refsum's (heredopathia atactica
  polyneuritiformis) 356.3
Reichmann's (gastrosuccorrhea) 536.8
Reimann's (periodic) 277.31
Reiter's 099.3
renal (functional) (pelvis) (*see also* Disease,
  kidney) 593.9
with
  edema (*see also* Nephrosis) 581.9
  exudative nephritis 583.89
  lesion of interstitial nephritis 583.89
  stated generalized cause—*see* Nephritis
acute 593.9
basement membrane NEC 583.89
  with
    pulmonary hemorrhage (Goodpasture's
      syndrome) 446.21 *[583.81]*
chronic (*see also* Disease, kidney, chronic)
  585.9
complicating pregnancy or puerperium NEC
  646.2
  with hypertension—*see* Toxemia, of
    pregnancy
  affecting fetus or newborn 760.1
cystic, congenital (*see also* Cystic, disease,
  kidney) 753.10
diabetic 250.4 *[583.81]*
  due to secondary diabetes 249.4 *[581.81]*
due to
  amyloidosis 277.39 *[583.81]*
  diabetes mellitus 250.4 *[583.81]*
    due to secondary diabetes 249.4 *[581.81]*
  systemic lupus erythematosis 710.0 *[583.81]*
end-stage 585.6
exudative 583.89
fibrocystic (congenital) 753.19
gonococcal 098.19 *[583.81]*
gouty 274.10
hypertensive (*see also* Hypertension, kidney)
  403.90
immune complex NEC 583.89
interstitial (diffuse) (focal) 583.89
lupus 710.0 *[583.81]*
maternal, affecting fetus or newborn 760.1
  hypertensive 760.0
phosphate-losing (tubular) 588.0
polycystic (congenital) 753.12
  adult type (APKD) 753.13
  autosomal dominant 753.13
  autosomal recessive 753.14
  childhood type (CPKD) 753.14
  infantile type 753.14
specified lesion or cause NEC (*see also*
  Glomerulonephritis) 583.89
subacute 581.9
syphilitic 095.4
tuberculous (*see also* Tuberculosis) 016.0
  [583.81]
tubular (*see also* Nephrosis, tubular) 584.5
Rendu-Olser-Weber (familial hemorrhagic
  telangiectasia) 448.0
renovascular (arteriosclerotic) (*see also*
  Hypertension, kidney) 403.90
respiratory (tract) 519.9
  acute or subacute (upper) NEC 465.9
    due to fumes or vapors 506.3
    multiple sites NEC 465.8
    noninfectious 478.9
    streptococcal 034.0

Disease, diseased—*continued*
respiratory (tract)—*continued*
chronic 519.9
  arising in the perinatal period 770.7
  due to fumes or vapors 506.4
due to
  aspiration of liquids or solids 508.9
  external agents NEC 508.9
    specified NEC 508.8
  fumes or vapors 506.9
    acute or subacute NEC 506.3
    chronic 506.4
fetus or newborn NEC 770.9
obstructive 496
smoke inhalation 508.2
specified type NEC 519.8
upper (acute) (infectious) NEC 465.9
  multiple sites NEC 465.8
  noninfectious NEC 478.9
  streptococcal 034.0
retina, retinal NEC 362.9
  Batten's or Batten-Mayou 330.1 *[362.71]*
  degeneration 362.89
  vascular lesion 362.17
rheumatic (*see also* Arthritis) 716.8
  heart—*see* Disease, heart, rheumatic
rheumatoid (heart)—*see* Arthritis, rheumatoid
rickettsial NEC 083.9
  specified type NEC 083.8
Riedel's (ligneous thyroiditis) 245.3
Riga (-Fede) (cachectic aphthae) 529.0
Riggs' (compound periodontitis) 523.40
Ritter's 695.81
Rivalta's (cervicofacial actinomycosis) 039.3
Robles' (onchocerciasis) 125.3 *[360.13]*
Roger's (congenital interventricular septal
  defect) 745.4
Rokitansky's (*see also* Necrosis, liver) 570
Romberg's 349.89
Rosenthal's (factor XI deficiency) 286.2
Rossbach's (hyperchlorhydria) 536.8
  psychogenic 306.4
Roth (-Bernhardt) 355.1
Runeberg's (progressive pernicious anemia)
  281.0
Rust's (tuberculous spondylitis) (*see also*
  Tuberculosis) 015.0 *[720.81]*
Rustitskii's (multiple myeloma) (M9730/3)
  203.0
Ruysch's (Hirschsprung's disease) 751.3
Sachs (-Tay) 330.1
sacroiliac NEC 724.6
salivary gland or duct NEC 527.9
  inclusion 078.5
    streptococcal 034.0
  virus 078.5
Sander's (paranoia) 297.1
Sandhoff's 330.1
sandworm 126.9
Savill's (epidemic exfoliative dermatitis) 695.89
Schamberg's (progressive pigmentary
  dermatosis) 709.09
Schaumann's (sarcoidosis) 135
Schenck's (sporotrichosis) 117.1
Scheuermann's (osteochondrosis) 732.0
Schilder (-Flatau) 341.1
Schimmelbusch's 610.1
Schlatter's tibia (tubercle) 732.4
Schlatter-Osgood 732.4

Disease, diseased—*continued*
Stuttgart 100.89
Sudeck's 733.7
supporting structures of teeth NEC 525.9
suprarenal (gland) (capsule) 255.9
  hyperfunction 255.3
  hypofunction 255.41
Sutton's 709.09
Sutton and Gull's—*see* Hypertension, kidney
sweat glands NEC 705.9
  specified type NEC 705.89
sweating 078.2
Sweeley-Klionsky 272.7
Swift (-Feer) 985.0
swimming pool (bacillus) 031.1
swineherd's 100.89
Sylvest's (epidemic pleurodynia) 074.1
Symmers (follicular lymphoma) (M9690/3)
  202.0
sympathetic nervous system (*see also*
  Neuropathy, peripheral, autonomic) 337.9
synovium 727.9
syphilitic—*see* Syphilis
systemic tissue mast cell (M9741/3) 202.6
Taenzer's 757.4
Takayasu's (pulseless) 446.7
Talma's 728.85
Tangier (familial high-density lipoprotein
  deficiency) 272.5
Tarral-Besnier (pityriasis rubra pilaris) 696.4
Tay-Sachs 330.1
Taylor's 701.8
tear duct 375.69
teeth, tooth 525.9
  hard tissues 521.9
    specified NEC 521.89
  pulp NEC 522.9
tendon 727.9
  inflammatory NEC 727.9
terminal vessel 443.9
testis 608.9
Thaysen-Gee (nontropical sprue) 579.0
Thomsen's 359.22
Thomson's (congenital poikiloderma) 757.33
Thornwaldt's, Tornwaldt's (pharyngeal bursitis)
  478.29
throat 478.20
  septic 034.0
thromboembolic (*see also* Embolism) 444.9
thymus (gland) 254.9
  specified NEC 254.8
thyroid (gland) NEC 246.9
  heart (*see also* Hyperthyroidism) 242.9
    [425.7]
  lardaceous 277.39
  specified NEC 246.8
Tietze's 733.6
Tommaselli's
  correct substance properly administered
    599.70
  overdose or wrong substance given or taken
    961.4
tongue 529.9
tonsils, tonsillar (and adenoids) (chronic) 474.9
  specified NEC 474.8
tooth, teeth 525.9
  hard tissues 521.9
    specified NEC 521.89
  pulp NEC 522.9
Tornwaldt's (pharyngeal bursitis) 478.29
Tourette's 307.23

Disease, diseased—*continued*
trachea 519.19
tricuspid—*see* Endocarditis, tricuspid
triglyceride-storage, type I, II, III 272.7
triple vessel (coronary arteries) —*see*
  Arteriosclerosis, coronary
trisymptomatic, Gougerot's 709.1
trophoblastic (*see also* Hydatidiform mole) 630
  previous, affecting management of pregnancy
    V23.1
tsutsugamushi (scrub typhus) 081.2
tube (fallopian), noninflammatory 620.9
  specified NEC 620.8
tuberculous NEC (*see also* Tuberculosis) 011.9
tubo-ovarian
  inflammatory (*see also* Salpingo-oophoritis)
    614.2
  noninflammatory 620.9
    specified NEC 620.8
tubotympanic, chronic (with anterior perforation
  of ear drum) 382.1
tympanum 385.9
Uhl's 746.84
umbilicus (newborn) NEC 779.89
  delayed separation 779.83
Underwood's (sclerema neonatorum) 778.1
undiagnosed 799.9
Unna's (seborrheic dermatitis) 690.18
unstable hemoglobin hemolytic 282.7
Unverricht (-Lundborg) 345.1
Urbach-Oppenheim (necrobiosis lipoidica
  diabeticorum) 250.8 *[709.3]*
  due to secondary diabetes 249.8 *[709.3]*
Urbach-Wiethe (lipoid proteinosis) 272.8
ureter 593.9
urethra 599.9
  specified type NEC 599.84
urinary (tract) 599.9
  bladder 596.9
    specified NEC 596.89
  maternal, affecting fetus or newborn 760.1
Usher-Senear (pemphigus erythematosus) 694.4
uterus (organic) 621.9
  infective (*see also* Endometritis) 615.9
  inflammatory (*see also* Endometritis) 615.9
  noninflammatory 621.9
    specified type NEC 621.8
uveal tract
  anterior 364.9
  posterior 363.9
vagabonds' 132.1
vagina, vaginal
  inflammation 616.10
  noninflammatory 623.9
    specified NEC 623.8
Valsuani's (progressive pernicious anemia,
  puerperal) 648.2
  complicating pregnancy or puerperium 648.2
valve, valvular—*see also* Endocarditis
  congenital NEC (*see also* Anomaly, heart,
    valve) 746.9
  pulmonary 746.00
    specified type NEC 746.89
van Bogaert-Nijssen (-Peiffer) 330.0
van Creveld-von Gierke (glycogenosis I) 271.0
van den Bergh's (enterogenous cyanosis) 289.7
van Neck's (juvenile osteochondrosis) 732.1
Vaquez (-Osler) (polycythemia vera) (M9950/1)
  238.4

Disease, diseased—*continued*
  vascular 459.9
    arteriosclerotic—*see* Arteriosclerosis
    hypertensive—*see* Hypertension
    obliterative 447.1
      peripheral 443.9
    occlusive 459.9
    peripheral (occlusive) 443.9
      in (due to) (with) diabetes mellitus 250.7
        [443.81]
      in (due to) (with) secondary diabetes 249.7
        [443.81]
      specified type NEC 443.89
  vas deferens 608.9
  vasomotor 443.9
  vasospastic 443.9
  vein 459.9
  venereal 099.9
    fifth 099.1
    sixth 099.1
    chlamydial NEC 099.50
      anus 099.52
      bladder 099.53
      cervix 099.53
      epididymis 099.54
      genitourinary NEC 099.55
        lower 099.53
        specified NEC 099.54
      pelvic inflammatory disease 099.54
      perihepatic 099.56
      peritoneum 099.56
      pharynx 099.51
      rectum 099.52
      specified site NEC 099.59
      testis 099.54
      vagina 099.53
      vulva 099.53
    complicating pregnancy, childbirth, or
        puerperium 647.2
    specified nature or type NEC 099.8
      chlamydial—*see* Disease, venereal,
        chlamydial
  Verneuil's (syphilitic bursitis) 095.7
  Verse's (calcinosis intervertebralis) 275.49
    [722.90]
  vertebra, vertebral NEC 733.90
    disc—*see* Disease, Intervertebral disc
  vibration NEC 994.9
  Vidal's (lichen simplex chronicus) 698.3
  Vincent's (trench mouth) 101
  Virchow's 733.99
  virus (filterable) NEC 078.89
    arbovirus NEC 066.9
    arthropod-borne NEC 066.9
    central nervous system NEC 049.9
      specified type NEC 049.8
    complicating pregnancy, childbirth, or
        puerperium 647.6
    contact (with) V01.79
      varicella V01.71
    exposure to V01.79
      varicella V01.71
    Marburg 078.89
    maternal
      with fetal damage affecting management of
        pregnancy 655.3
    nonarthropod-borne NEC 078.89
      central nervous system NEC 049.9
        specified NEC 049.8
    vaccination, prophylactic (against) V04.89
  vitreous 379.29

Disease, diseased—*continued*
  vocal cords NEC 478.5
  Vogt's (Cecile) 333.71
  Vogt-Spielmeyer 330.1
  Volhard-Fahr (malignant nephrosclerosis)
    403.00
  Volkmann's
    acquired 958.6
  von Bechterew's (ankylosing spondylitis) 720.0
  von Economo's (encephalitis lethargica) 049.8
  von Eulenburg's (congenital paramyotonia)
    359.29
  von Gierke's (glycogenosis I) 271.0
  von Graefe's 378.72
  von Hippel's (retinocerebral angiomatosis)
    759.6
  von Hippel-Lindau (angiomatosis
    retinocerebellosa) 759.6
  von Jaksch's (pseudoleukemia infantum) 285.8
  von Recklinghausen's (M9540/1) 237.71
    bone (osteitis fibrosa cystica) 252.01
  von Recklinghausen-Applebaum (hemochromatosis)
    (*see also* Hemochromatosis) 275.03
  von Willebrand (-Jürgens) (angiohemophilia)
    286.4
  von Zambusch's (lichen sclerosus et atrophicus)
    701.0
  Voorhoeve's (dyschondroplasia) 756.4
  Vrolik's (osteogenesis imperfecta) 756.51
  vulva
    inflammatory 616.10
    noninflammatory 624.9
      specified NEC 624.8
  Wagner's (colloid milium) 709.3
  Waldenström's (osteochondrosis capital
    femoral) 732.1
  Wallgren's (obstruction of splenic vein with
    collateral circulation) 459.89
  Wardrop's (with lymphangitis) 681.9
    finger 681.02
    toe 681.11
  Wassilieff's (leptospiral jaundice) 100.0
  wasting NEC 799.4
    due to malnutrition 261
    paralysis 335.21
  Waterhouse-Friderichsen 036.3
  waxy (any site) 277.39
  Weber-Christian (nodular nonsuppurative
    panniculitis) 729.30
  Wegner's (syphilitic osteochondritis) 090.0
  Weil's (leptospiral jaundice) 100.0
    of lung 100.0
  Weir Mitchell's (erythromelalgia) 443.82
  Werdnig-Hoffmann 335.0
  Werlhof's (*see also* Purpura, thrombocytopenic)
    287.39
  Werner's 258.01
  Werner's (progeria adultorum) 259.8
  Werner-His (trench fever) 083.1
  Werner-Schultz (agranulocytosis) 288.09
  Wernicke's (superior hemorrhagic
    polioencephalitis) 265.1
  Wernicke-Posadas 114.9
  Whipple's (intestinal lipodystrophy) 040.2
  whipworm 127.3
  white
    blood cell 288.9
      specified NEC 288.8
    spot 701.0
  White's (congenital) (keratosis follicularis)
    757.39

Disease, diseased—*continued*
  Whitmore's (melioidosis) 025
  Widal-Abrami (acquired hemolytic jaundice)
    283.9
  Wilkie's 557.1
  Wilkinson-Sneddon (subcorneal pustular
    dermatosis) 694.1
  Willis' (diabetes mellitus) (*see also* Diabetes)
    250.0
    due to secondary diabetes 249.0
  Wilson's (hepatolenticular degeneration) 275.1
  Wilson-Brocq (dermatitis exfoliativa) 695.89
  winter vomiting 078.82
  Wise's 696.2
  Wohlfart-Kugelberg-Welander 335.11
  Woillez's (acute idiopathic pulmonary
    congestion) 518.52
  Wolman's (primary familial xanthomatosis)
    272.7
  wool-sorters' 022.1
  Zagari's (xerostomia) 527.7
  Zahorsky's (exanthem subitum) 058.10
  Ziehen-Oppenheim 333.6
  zoonotic, bacterial NEC 027.9
    specified type NEC 027.8
Disfigurement (due to scar) 709.2
  head V48.6
  limb V49.4
  neck V48.7
  trunk V48.7
Disgerminoma —*see* Dysgerminoma
Disinsertion, retina 361.04
Disintegration, complete, of the body 799.89
  traumatic 869.1
Disk kidney 753.3
Dislocatable hip, congenita l (*see also*
  Dislocation, hip, congenital) 754.30
Dislocation (articulation) (closed) (displacement)
  (simple) (subluxation) 839.8

> *Note—"Closed" includes simple, complete,*
> *partial, uncomplicated, and unspecified*
> *dislocation. "Open" includes dislocation*
> *specified as infected or compound and*
> *dislocation with foreign body. "Chronic,"*
> *"habitual," "old," or "recurrent" dislocations*
> *should be coded as indicated under the entry*
> *"Dislocation, recurrent"; and "pathological"*
> *as indicated under the entry "Dislocation,*
> *pathological." For late effect of dislocation see*
> *Late, effect, dislocation.*

  with fracture—*see* Fracture, by site
  acromioclavicular (joint) (closed) 831.04
    open 831.14
  anatomical site (closed)
    specified NEC 839.69
      open 839.79
    unspecified or ill-defined 839.8
      open 839.9
  ankle (scaphoid bone) (closed) 837.0
    open 837.1
  arm (closed) 839.8
    open 839.9
  astragalus (closed) 837.0
    open 837.1
  atlanto-axial (closed) 839.01
    open 839.11
  atlas (closed) 839.01
    open 839.11
  axis (closed) 839.02
    open 839.12

Dislocation—*continued*
  back (closed) 839.8
    open 839.9
  Bell-Daly 723.8
  breast bone (closed) 839.61
    open 839.71
  capsule, joint—*see* Dislocation, by site
  carpal (bone)—*see* Dislocation, wrist
  carpometacarpal (joint) (closed) 833.04
    open 833.14
  cartilage (joint)—*see also* Dislocation, by site
    knee—*see* Tear, meniscus
  cervical, cervicodorsal, or cervicothoracic
    (spine) (vertebra)—*see* Dislocation,
    vertebra, cervical
  chiropractic (*see also* Lesion, nonallopathic)
    739.9
  chondrocostal—*see* Dislocation, costochondral
  chronic—*see* Dislocation, recurrent
  clavicle (closed) 831.04
    open 831.14
  coccyx (closed) 839.41
    open 839.51
  collar bone (closed) 831.04
    open 831.14
  compound (open) NEC 839.9
  congenital NEC 755.8
    hip (*see also* Dislocation, hip, congenital)
      754.30
    lens 743.37
    rib 756.3
    sacroiliac 755.69
    spine NEC 756.19
    vertebra 756.19
  coracoid (closed) 831.09
    open 831.19
  costal cartilage (closed) 839.69
    open 839.79
  costochondral (closed) 839.69
    open 839.79
  cricoarytenoid articulation (closed) 839.69
    open 839.79
  cricothyroid (cartilage) articulation (closed)
    839.69
    open 839.79
  dorsal vertebrae (closed) 839.21
    open 839.31
  ear ossicle 385.23
  elbow (closed) 832.00
    anterior (closed) 832.01
      open 832.11
    congenital 754.89
    divergent (closed) 832.09
      open 832.19
    lateral (closed) 832.04
      open 832.14
    medial (closed) 832.03
      open 832.13
    open 832.10
    posterior (closed) 832.02
      open 832.12
    recurrent 718.32
    specified type NEC 832.09
      open 832.19
  eye 360.81
    lateral 376.36
  eyeball 360.81
    lateral 376.36

Dislocation—*continued*

femur
  distal end (closed) 836.50
    anterior 836.52
      open 836.62
    lateral 836.54
      open 836.64
    medial 836.53
      open 836.63
    open 836.60
    posterior 836.51
      open 836.61
  proximal end (closed) 835.00
    anterior (pubic) 835.03
      open 835.13
    obturator 835.02
      open 835.12
    open 835.10
    posterior 835.01
      open 835.11
fibula
  distal end (closed) 837.0
    open 837.1
  proximal end (closed) 836.59
    open 836.69
finger(s) (phalanx) (thumb) (closed) 834.00
  interphalangeal (joint) 834.02
    open 834.12
  metacarpal (bone), distal end 834.01
    open 834.11
  metacarpophalangeal (joint) 834.01
    open 834.11
  open 834.10
  recurrent 718.34
foot (closed) 838.00
  open 838.10
  recurrent 718.37
forearm (closed) 839.8
  open 839.9
fracture—*see* Fracture, by site
glenoid (closed) 831.09
  open 831.19
habitual—*see* Dislocation, recurrent
hand (closed) 839.8
  open 839.9
hip (closed) 835.00
  anterior 835.03
    obturator 835.02
      open 835.12
    open 835.13
  congenital (unilateral) 754.30
    with subluxation of other hip 754.35
    bilateral 754.31
  developmental 718.75
  open 835.10
  posterior 835.01
    open 835.11
  recurrent 718.35
humerus (closed) 831.00
  distal end (*see also* Dislocation, elbow) 832.00
  open 831.10
  proximal end (closed) 831.00
    anterior (subclavicular) (subcoracoid)
      (subglenoid) (closed) 831.01
      open 831.11
    inferior (closed) 831.03
      open 831.13
    open 831.10
    posterior (closed) 831.02
      open 831.12
implant—*see* Complications, mechanical

Dislocation—*continued*

incus 385.23
infracoracoid (closed) 831.01
  open 831.11
innominate (pubic junction) (sacral junction)
    (closed) 839.69
  acetabulum (*see also* Dislocation, hip) 835.00
  open 839.79
interphalangeal (joint)
  finger or hand (closed) 834.02
    open 834.12
  foot or toe (closed) 838.06
    open 838.16
jaw (cartilage) (meniscus) (closed) 830.0
  open 830.1
  recurrent 524.69
joint NEC (closed) 839.8
  developmental 718.7
  open 839.9
  pathological—*see* Dislocation, pathological
  recurrent—*see* Dislocation, recurrent
knee (closed) 836.50
  anterior 836.51
    open 836.61
  congenital (with genu recurvatum) 754.41
  habitual 718.36
  lateral 836.54
    open 836.64
  medial 836.53
    open 836.63
  old 718.36
  open 836.60
  posterior 836.52
    open 836.62
  recurrent 718.36
  rotatory 836.59
    open 836.69
lacrimal gland 375.16
leg (closed) 839.8
  open 839.9
lens (crystalline) (complete) (partial) 379.32
  anterior 379.33
  congenital 743.37
  ocular implant 996.53
  posterior 379.34
  traumatic 921.3
ligament—*see* Dislocation, by site
lumbar (vertebrae) (closed) 839.20
  open 839.30
lumbosacral (vertebrae) (closed) 839.20
  congenital 756.19
  open 839.30
mandible (closed) 830.0
  open 830.1
maxilla (inferior) (closed) 830.0
  open 830.1
meniscus (knee)—*see also* Tear, meniscus
  other sites—*see* Dislocation, by site
metacarpal (bone)
  distal end (closed) 834.01
    open 834.11
  proximal end (closed) 833.05
    open 833.15
metacarpophalangeal (joint) (closed) 834.01
  open 834.11
metatarsal (bone) (closed) 838.04
  open 838.14
metatarsophalangeal (joint) (closed) 838.05
  open 838.15
midcarpal (joint) (closed) 833.03
  open 833.13

Dislocation—*continued*
  midtarsal (joint) (closed) 838.02
    open 838.12
  Monteggia's—*see* Dislocation, hip
  multiple locations (except fingers only or toes
    only) (closed) 839.8
    open 839.9
  navicular (bone) foot (closed) 837.0
    open 837.1
  neck (*see also* Dislocation, vertebra, cervical)
    839.00
  Nélaton's—*see* Dislocation, ankle
  nontraumatic (joint)—*see* Dislocation,
    pathological
  nose (closed) 839.69
    open 839.79
  not recurrent, not current injury—*see*
    Dislocation, pathological
  occiput from atlas (closed) 839.01
    open 839.11
  old—*see* Dislocation, recurrent
  open (compound) NEC 839.9
  ossicle, ear 385.23
  paralytic (flaccid) (spastic)—*see* Dislocation,
    pathological
  patella (closed) 836.3
    congenital 755.64
    open 836.4
  pathological NEC 718.20
    ankle 718.27
    elbow 718.22
    foot 718.27
    hand 718.24
    hip 718.25
    knee 718.26
    lumbosacral joint 724.6
    multiple sites 718.29
    pelvic region 718.25
    sacroiliac 724.6
    shoulder (region) 718.21
    specified site NEC 718.28
    spine 724.8
      sacroiliac 724.6
    wrist 718.23
  pelvis (closed) 839.69
    acetabulum (*see also* Dislocation, hip) 835.00
    open 839.79
  phalanx
    foot or toe (closed) 838.09
      open 838.19
    hand or finger (*see also* Dislocation, finger)
      834.00
  postpoliomyelitic—*see* Dislocation,
    pathological
  prosthesis, internal—*see* Complications,
    mechanical
  radiocarpal (joint) (closed) 833.02
    open 833.12
  radioulnar (joint)
    distal end (closed) 833.01
      open 833.11
    proximal end (*see also* Dislocation, elbow)
      832.00
  radius
    distal end (closed) 833.00
      open 833.10
    proximal end (closed) 832.01
      open 832.11

Dislocation—*continued*
  recurrent (*see also* Derangement, joint,
    recurrent) 718.3
    elbow 718.32
    hip 718.35
    joint NEC 718.38
    knee 718.36
    lumbosacral (joint) 724.6
    patella 718.36
    sacroiliac 724.6
    shoulder 718.31
    temporomandibular 524.69
  rib (cartilage) (closed) 839.69
    congenital 756.3
    open 839.79
  sacrococcygeal (closed) 839.42
    open 839.52
  sacroiliac (joint) (ligament) (closed) 839.42
    congenital 755.69
    open 839.52
    recurrent 724.6
  sacrum (closed) 839.42
    open 839.52
  scaphoid (bone)
    ankle or foot (closed) 837.0
      open 837.1
    wrist (closed) (*see also* Dislocation, wrist)
      833.00
      open 833.10
  scapula (closed) 831.09
    open 831.19
  semilunar cartilage, knee—*see* Tear, meniscus
  septal cartilage (nose) (closed) 839.69
    open 839.79
  septum (nasal) (old) 470
  sesamoid bone—*see* Dislocation, by site
  shoulder (blade) (ligament) (closed) 831.00
    anterior (subclavicular) (subcoracoid)
      (subglenoid) (closed) 831.01
      open 831.11
    chronic 718.31
    inferior 831.03
      open 831.13
    open 831.10
    posterior (closed) 831.02
      open 831.12
    recurrent 718.31
  skull—*see* Injury, intracranial
  Smith's—*see* Dislocation, foot
  spine (articular process) (*see also* Dislocation,
    vertebra) (closed) 839.40
    atlanto-axial (closed) 839.01
      open 839.11
      recurrent 723.8
    cervical, cervicodorsal, cervicothoracic
      (closed) (*see also* Dislocation, vertebrae,
      cervical) 839.00
      open 839.10
      recurrent 723.8
    coccyx 839.41
      open 839.51
    congenital 756.19
    due to birth trauma 767.4
    open 839.50
    recurrent 724.9
    sacroiliac 839.42
      recurrent 724.6
    sacrum (sacrococcygeal) (sacroiliac) 839.42
      open 839.52
  spontaneous—*see* Dislocation, pathological

Dislocation—*continued*
 sternoclavicular (joint) (closed) 839.61
  open 839.71
 sternum (closed) 839.61
  open 839.71
 subastragalar—*see* Dislocation, foot
 subglenoid (closed) 831.01
  open 831.11
 symphysis
  jaw (closed) 830.0
   open 830.1
  mandibular (closed) 830.0
   open 830.1
 pubis (closed) 839.69
  open 839.79
 tarsal (bone) (joint) 838.01
  open 838.11
 tarsometatarsal (joint) 838.03
  open 838.13
 temporomandibular (joint) (closed) 830.0
  open 830.1
  recurrent 524.69
 thigh
  distal end (*see also* Dislocation, femur, distal
   end) 836.50
  proximal end (*see also* Dislocation, hip) 835.00
 thoracic (vertebrae) (closed) 839.21
  open 839.31
 thumb(s) (*see also* Dislocation, finger) 834.00
 thyroid cartilage (closed) 839.69
  open 839.79
 tibia
  distal end (closed) 837.0
   open 837.1
  proximal end (closed) 836.50
   anterior 836.51
    open 836.61
   lateral 836.54
    open 836.64
   medial 836.53
    open 836.63
   open 836.60
   posterior 836.52
    open 836.62
   rotatory 836.59
    open 836.69
 tibiofibular
  distal (closed) 837.0
   open 837.1
  superior (closed) 836.59
   open 836.69
 toe(s) (closed) 838.09
  open 838.19
 trachea (closed) 839.69
  open 839.79
 ulna
  distal end (closed) 833.09
   open 833.19
  proximal end—*see* Dislocation, elbow
 vertebra (articular process) (body) (closed)
   (traumatic) 839.40
  cervical, cervicodorsal or cervicothoracic
   (closed) 839.00
   first (atlas) 839.01
    open 839.11
   second (axis) 839.02
    open 839.12
   third 839.03
    open 839.13
   fourth 839.04
    open 839.14

Dislocation—*continued*
 vertebra—*continued*
  cervical—*continued*
   fifth 839.05
    open 839.15
   sixth 839.06
    open 839.16
   seventh 839.07
    open 839.17
   congenital 756.19
   multiple sites 839.08
    open 839.18
   open 839.10
  congenital 756.19
  dorsal 839.21
   open 839.31
   recurrent 724.9
  lumbar, lumbosacral 839.20
   open 839.30
  non-traumatic —*see* Displacement,
   intervertebral disc
  open NEC 839.50
  recurrent 724.9
  specified region NEC 839.49
   open 839.59
  thoracic 839.21
   open 839.31
 wrist (carpal bone) (scaphoid) (semilunar)
   (closed) 833.00
  carpometacarpal (joint) 833.04
   open 833.14
  metacarpal bone, proximal end 833.05
   open 833.15
  midcarpal (joint) 833.03
   open 833.13
  open 833.10
  radiocarpal (joint) 833.02
   open 833.12
  radioulnar (joint) 833.01
   open 833.11
  recurrent 718.33
  specified site NEC 833.09
   open 833.19
 xiphoid cartilage (closed) 839.61
  open 839.71
Dislodgement
 artificial skin graft 996.55
 decellularized allodermis graft 996.55
Disobedience, hostile (covert) (overt) (*see also*
  Disturbance, conduct) 312.0
Disorder —*see also* Disease
 academic underachievement, childhood and
  adolescence 313.83
 accommodation 367.51
  drug-induced 367.89
  toxic 367.89
 adjustment (*see also* Reaction, adjustment) 309.9
  with
   anxiety 309.24
   anxiety and depressed mood 309.28
   depressed mood 309.0
   disturbance of conduct 309.3
   disturbance of emotions and conduct 309.4
 adrenal (capsule) (cortex) (gland) 255.9
  specified type NEC 255.8
 adrenogenital 255.2
 affective (*see also* Psychosis, affective) 296.90
  atypical 296.81
 aggressive, unsocialized (*see also* Disturbance,
  conduct) 312.0

Disorder—*continued*
  cervical root (nerve) NEC 353.2
  character NEC (*see also* Disorder, personality)
    301.9
  ciliary body 364.9
    specified NEC 364.89
  coagulation (factor) (*see also* Defect,
    coagulation) 286.9
    factor VIII (congenital) (functional) 286.0
    factor IX (congenital) (functional) 286.1
    neonatal, transitory 776.3
  coccyx 724.70
    specified NEC 724.79
  cognitive 294.9
  colon 569.9
    functional 564.9
      congenital 751.3
  communication 307.9
  conduct (*see also* Disturbance, conduct) 312.9
    adjustment reaction 309.3
    adolescent onset type 312.82
    childhood onset type 312.81
    compulsive 312.30
      specified type NEC 312.39
    hyperkinetic 314.2
    onset unspecified 312.89
    socialized (type) 312.20
      aggressive 312.23
      unaggressive 312.21
    specified NEC 312.89
  conduction, heart 426.9
    specified NEC 426.89
  conflict
    sexual orientation 302.0
  congenital
    glycosylation (CDG) 271.8
  convulsive (secondary) (*see also* Convulsions)
    780.39
    due to injury at birth 767.0
    idiopathic 780.39
  coordination 781.3
  cornea NEC 371.89
    due to contact lens 371.82
  corticosteroid metabolism NEC 255.2
  cranial nerve—*see* Disorder, nerve, cranial
  cyclothymic 301.13
  degradation, branched-chain amino acid 270.3
  delusional 297.1
  dentition 520.6
  depersonalization 300.6
  depressive NEC 311
    atypical 296.82
    major (*see also* Psychosis, affective) 296.2
      recurrent episode 296.3
      single episode 296.2
  development, specific 315.9
    associated with hyperkinesia 314.1
    coordination 315.4
    language 315.31
      and speech due to hearing loss 315.34
    learning 315.2
      arithmetical 315.1
      reading 315.00
    mixed 315.5
    motor coordination 315.4
    specified type NEC 315.8
    speech 315.39
      and language due to hearing loss 315.34
  diaphragm 519.4

Disorder—*continued*
  digestive 536.9
    fetus or newborn 777.9
      specified NEC 777.8
    psychogenic 306.4
  disintegrative, childhood 299.1
  dissociative 300.15
    identity 300.14
    nocturnal 307.47
  drug-related 292.9
  dysmorphic body 300.7
  dysthymic 300.4
  ear 388.9
    degenerative NEC 388.00
    external 380.9
      specified 380.89
    pinna 380.30
    specified type NEC 388.8
    vascular NEC 388.00
  eating NEC 307.50
  electrolyte NEC 276.9
    with
      abortion—*see* Abortion, by type, with
        metabolic disorder
      ectopic pregnancy (*see also* categories
        633.0-633.9) 639.4
      molar pregnancy (*see also* categories
        630-632) 639.4
    acidosis 276.2
      metabolic 276.2
      respiratory 276.2
    alkalosis 276.3
      metabolic 276.3
      respiratory 276.3
    following
      abortion 639.4
      ectopic or molar pregnancy 639.4
    neonatal, transitory NEC 775.5
  emancipation as adjustment reaction 309.22
  emotional (*see also* Disorder, mental,
    nonpsychotic) V40.9
  endocrine 259.9
    specified type NEC 259.8
  esophagus 530.9
    functional 530.5
    psychogenic 306.4
  explosive
    intermittent 312.34
    isolated 312.35
  expressive language 315.31
  eye 379.90
    globe—*see* Disorder, globe
    ill-defined NEC 379.99
    limited duction NEC 378.63
    specified NEC 379.8
  eyelid 374.9
    degenerative 374.50
    sensory 374.44
    specified type NEC 374.89
    vascular 374.85
  factitious (with combined psychological and
    physical signs and symptoms) (with
    predominantly physical signs and
    symptoms) 300.19
    with predominantly psychological signs and
      symptoms 300.16
  factor, coagulation (*see also* Defect, coagulation)
    286.9
    VIII (congenital) (functional) 286.0
    IX (congenital) (functional) 286.1
  fascia 728.9

Disorder—*continued*
  fatty acid oxidation 277.85
  feeding —*see* Feeding
  female sexual arousal 302.72
  fluency 315.35
    adult onset 307.0
    childhood onset 315.35
    due to late effect of cerebrovascular accident 438.14
    in conditions classified elsewhere 784.52
  fluid NEC 276.9
  gastric (functional) 536.9
    motility 536.8
    psychogenic 306.4
    secretion 536.8
  gastrointestinal (functional) NEC 536.9
    newborn (neonatal) 777.9
      specified NEC 777.8
    psychogenic 306.4
  gender (child) 302.6
    adult 302.85
  gender identity (childhood) 302.6
    adolescents 302.85
    adults (-life) 302.85
  genitourinary system, psychogenic 306.50
  globe 360.9
    degenerative 360.20
      specified NEC 360.29
    specified type NEC 360.89
  hearing—*see also* Deafness
    conductive type (air) (*see also* Deafness, conductive) 389.00
    mixed conductive and sensorineural 389.20
      bilateral 389.22
      unilateral 389.21
    nerve
      bilateral 389.12
      unilateral 389.13
    perceptive (*see also* Deafness, perceptive) 389.10
    sensorineural type NEC (*see also* Deafness, sensorineural) 389.10
  heart action 427.9
    postoperative 997.1
  hematological, transient neonatal 776.9
    specified type NEC 776.8
  hematopoietic organs 289.9
  hemorrhagic NEC 287.9
    due to intrinsic circulating anticoagulants, antibodies or inhibitors 286.59
      with
        acquired hemophilia 286.52
        antiphospholipid antibody 286.53
    specified type NEC 287.8
  hemostasis (*see also* Defect, coagulation) 286.9
  homosexual conflict 302.0
  hypomanic (chronic) 301.11
  identity
    childhood and adolescence 313.82
      gender 302.6
    gender 302.6
  immune mechanism (immunity) 279.9
    single complement (C_1-C_9) 279.8
    specified type NEC 279.8
  impulse control (*see also* Disturbance, conduct, compulsive) 312.30
  infant sialic acid storage 271.8
  integument, fetus or newborn 778.9
    specified type NEC 778.8
  interactional psychotic (childhood) (*see also* Psychosis, childhood) 299.1

Disorder—*continued*
  intermittent explosive 312.34
  intervertebral disc 722.90
    cervical, cervicothoracic 722.91
    lumbar, lumbosacral 722.93
    thoracic, thoracolumbar 722.92
  intestinal 569.9
    functional NEC 564.9
      congenital 751.3
      postoperative 564.4
    psychogenic 306.4
  introverted, of childhood and adolescence 313.22
  involuntary emotional expression (IEED) 310.81
  iris 364.9
    specified NEC 364.89
  iron, metabolism 275.09
    specified type NEC 275.09
  isolated explosive 312.35
  joint NEC 719.90
    ankle 719.97
    elbow 719.92
    foot 719.97
    hand 719.94
    hip 719.95
    knee 719.96
    multiple sites 719.99
    pelvic region 719.95
    psychogenic 306.0
    shoulder (region) 719.91
    specified site NEC 719.98
    temporomandibular 524.60
      sounds on opening or closing 524.64
      specified NEC 524.69
    wrist 719.93
  kidney 593.9
    functional 588.9
      specified NEC 588.89
  labyrinth, labyrinthine 386.9
    specified type NEC 386.8
  lactation 676.9
  language (developmental) (expressive) 315.31
    mixed receptive-expressive 315.32
  learning 315.9
  ligament 728.9
  ligamentous attachments, peripheral—*see also* Enthesopathy
    spine 720.1
  limb NEC 729.90
    psychogenic 306.0
  lipid
    metabolism, congenital 272.9
    storage 272.7
  lipoprotein deficiency (familial) 272.5
  low back NEC 724.9
    psychogenic 306.0
  lumbosacral
    plexus 353.1
    root (nerve) NEC 353.4
  lymphoproliferative (chronic) NEC (M9970/1) 238.79
    post-transplant (PTLD) 238.77
  major depressive (*see also* Psychosis, affective) 296.2
    recurrent episode 296.3
    single episode 296.2
  male erectile 607.84
    nonorganic origin 302.72
  manic (*see also* Psychosis, affective) 296.0
    atypical 296.81
  mathematics 315.1

Disorder—*continued*
  meniscus NEC (*see also* Disorder, cartilage,
      articular) 718.0
  menopausal 627.9
    specified NEC 627.8
  menstrual 626.9
    psychogenic 306.52
    specified NEC 626.8
  mental (nonpsychotic) 300.9
    affecting management of pregnancy,
        childbirth, or puerperium 648.4
    drug-induced 292.9
      hallucinogen persistent perception 292.89
      specified type NEC 292.89
    due to or associated with
      alcoholism 291.9
      drug consumption NEC 292.9
        specified type NEC 292.89
      physical condition NEC 293.9
    induced by drug 292.9
      specified type NEC 292.89
    neurotic (*see also* Neurosis) 300.9
    of infancy, childhood or adolescence 313.9
    persistent
      other
        due to conditions classified elsewhere 294.8
      unspecified
        due to conditions classified elsewhere 294.9
    presenile 310.1
      psychotic NEC 290.10
    previous, affecting management of pregnancy
        V23.8
    psychoneurotic (*see also* Neurosis) 300.9
    psychotic (*see also* Psychosis) 298.9
      brief 298.8
      senile 290.20
    specific, following organic brain damage 310.9
      cognitive or personality change of other type
          310.1
      frontal lobe syndrome 310.0
      postconcussional syndrome 310.2
      specified type NEC 310.89
    transient
      in conditions classified elsewhere 293.9
  metabolism NEC 277.9
    with
      abortion—*see* Abortion, by type, with
          metabolic disorder
      ectopic pregnancy (*see also* categories
          633.0-633.9) 639.4
      molar pregnancy (*see also* categories
          630-632) 639.4
    alkaptonuria 270.2
    amino acid (*see also* Disorder, amino acid)
        270.9
      specified type NEC 270.8
    ammonia 270.6
    arginine 270.6
    argininosuccinic acid 270.6
    basal 794.7
    bilirubin 277.4
    calcium 275.40
    carbohydrate 271.9
      specified type NEC 271.8
    cholesterol 272.9
    citrulline 270.6
    copper 275.1
    corticosteroid 255.2
    cystine storage 270.0
    cystinuria 270.0
    fat 272.9
    fatty acid oxidation 277.85

Disorder—*continued*
  metabolism—*continued*
    following
      abortion 639.4
      ectopic or molar pregnancy 639.4
    fructosemia 271.2
    fructosuria 271.2
    fucosidosis 271.8
    due to conditions classified elsewhere 294.8
    galactose-1-phosphate uridyl transferase 271.1
    glutamine 270.7
    glycine 270.7
    glycogen storage NEC 271.0
      hepatorenal 271.0
    hemochromatosis (*see also* Hemochromatosis)
        275.03
    in labor and delivery 669.0
    iron 275.09
    lactose 271.3
    lipid 272.9
      specified type NEC 272.8
      storage 272.7
    lipoprotein—*see also* Hyperlipemia deficiency
        (familial) 272.5
    lysine 270.7
    magnesium 275.2
    mannosidosis 271.8
    mineral 275.9
      specified type NEC 275.8
    mitochondrial 277.87
    mucopolysaccharide 277.5
    nitrogen 270.9
    ornithine 270.6
    oxalosis 271.8
    pentosuria 271.8
    phenylketonuria 270.1
    phosphate 275.3
    phosphorus 275.3
    plasma protein 273.9
      specified type NEC 273.8
    porphyrin 277.1
    purine 277.2
    pyrimidine 277.2
    serine 270.7
    sodium 276.9
    specified type NEC 277.89
    steroid 255.2
    threonine 270.7
    urea cycle 270.6
    xylose 271.8
  micturition NEC 788.69
    psychogenic 306.53
  misery and unhappiness, of childhood and
      adolescence 313.1
  mitochondrial metabolism 277.87
  mitral valve 424.0
  mood (*see also* Disorder, bipolar) 296.90
    alcohol-induced 291.89
    episodic 296.90
      specified NEC 296.99
    in conditions classified elsewhere 293.83
  motor tic 307.20
    chronic 307.22
    transient (childhood) 307.21
  movement NEC 333.90
    hysterical 300.11
    medication-induced 333.90
    periodic limb 327.51
    sleep related, unspecified 780.58
      other organic 327.59
    specified type NEC 333.99
    stereotypic 307.3

Disorder—*continued*
 mucopolysaccharide 277.5
 muscle 728.9
  psychogenic 306.0
  specified type NEC 728.3
 muscular attachments, peripheral—*see also*
   Enthesopathy
  spine 720.1
 musculoskeletal system NEC 729.90
  psychogenic 306.0
 myeloproliferative (chronic) NEC (M9960/1)
   238.79
 myoneural 358.9
  due to lead 358.2
  specified type NEC 358.8
  toxic 358.2
 myotonic 359.29
 neck region NEC 723.9
 nerve 349.9
  abducens NEC 378.54
  accessory 352.4
  acoustic 388.5
  auditory 388.5
  auriculotemporal 350.8
  axillary 353.0
  cerebral—*see* Disorder, nerve, cranial
  cranial 352.9
   first 352.0
   second 377.49
   third
    partial 378.51
    total 378.52
   fourth 378.53
   fifth 350.9
   sixth 378.54
   seventh NEC 351.9
   eighth 388.5
   ninth 352.2
   tenth 352.3
   eleventh 352.4
   twelfth 352.5
   multiple 352.6
  entrapment—*see* Neuropathy, entrapment
  facial 351.9
   specified NEC 351.8
  femoral 355.2
  glossopharyngeal NEC 352.2
  hypoglossal 352.5
  iliohypogastric 355.79
  ilioinguinal 355.79
  intercostal 353.8
  lateral
   cutaneous of thigh 355.1
   popliteal 355.3
  lower limb NEC 355.8
  medial, popliteal 355.4
  median NEC 354.1
  obturator 355.79
  oculomotor
   partial 378.51
   total 378.52
  olfactory 352.0
  optic 377.49
   hypoplasia 377.43
   ischemic 377.41
   nutritional 377.33
   toxic 377.34
  peroneal 355.3
  phrenic 354.8
  plantar 355.6
  pneumogastric 352.3

Disorder—*continued*
 nerve—*continued*
  posterior tibial 355.5
  radial 354.3
  recurrent laryngeal 352.3
  root 353.9
   specified NEC 353.8
  saphenous 355.79
  sciatic NEC 355.0
  specified NEC 355.9
   lower limb 355.79
   upper limb 354.8
  spinal 355.9
  sympathetic NEC 337.9
  trigeminal 350.9
   specified NEC 350.8
  trochlear 378.53
  ulnar 354.2
  upper limb NEC 354.9
  vagus 352.3
 nervous system NEC 349.9
  autonomic (peripheral) (*see also* Neuropathy,
    peripheral, autonomic) 337.9
  cranial 352.9
  parasympathetic (*see also* Neuropathy,
    peripheral, autonomic) 337.9
  specified type NEC 349.89
  sympathetic (*see also* Neuropathy, peripheral,
    autonomic) 337.9
  vegetative (*see also* Neuropathy, peripheral,
    autonomic) 337.9
 neurohypophysis NEC 253.6
 neurological NEC 781.99
  peripheral NEC 355.9
 neuromuscular NEC 358.9
  hereditary NEC 359.1
  specified NEC 358.8
  toxic 358.2
 neurotic 300.9
  specified type NEC 300.89
 neutrophil, polymorphonuclear (functional) 288.1
 nightmare 307.47
 night terror 307.46
 obsessive-compulsive 300.3
 oppositional defiant, childhood and adolescence
   313.81
 optic
  chiasm 377.54
   associated with
    inflammatory disorders 377.54
    neoplasm NEC 377.52
     pituitary 377.51
    pituitary disorders 377.51
    vascular disorders 377.53
  nerve 377.49
  radiations 377.63
  tracts 377.63
 orbit 376.9
  specified NEC 376.89
 orgasmic
  female 302.73
  male 302.74
 overanxious, of childhood and adolescence
   313.0
 oxidation, fatty acid 277.85
 pancreas, internal secretion (other than diabetes
   mellitus) 251.9
  specified type NEC 251.8
 panic 300.01
  with agoraphobia 300.21
 papillary muscle NEC 429.81

Disorder—*continued*
  paranoid 297.9
    induced 297.3
    shared 297.3
  parathyroid 252.9
    specified type NEC 252.8
  paroxysmal, mixed 780.39
  pentose phosphate pathway with anemia 282.2
  periodic limb movement 327.51
  peroxisomal 277.86
  personality 301.9
    affective 301.10
    aggressive 301.3
    amoral 301.7
    anancastic, anankastic 301.4
    antisocial 301.7
    asocial 301.7
    asthenic 301.6
    avoidant 301.82
    borderline 301.83
    compulsive 301.4
    cyclothymic 301.13
    dependent-passive 301.6
    dyssocial 301.7
    emotional instability 301.59
    epileptoid 301.3
    explosive 301.3
    following organic brain damage 310.1
    histrionic 301.50
    hyperthymic 301.11
    hypomanic (chronic) 301.11
    hypothymic 301.12
    hysterical 301.50
    immature 301.89
    inadequate 301.6
    introverted 301.21
    labile 301.59
    moral deficiency 301.7
    narcissistic 301.81
    obsessional 301.4
    obsessive-compulsive 301.4
    overconscientious 301.4
    paranoid 301.0
    passive (-dependent) 301.6
    passive-aggressive 301.84
    pathological NEC 301.9
    pseudosocial 301.7
    psychopathic 301.9
    schizoid 301.20
      introverted 301.21
      schizotypal 301.22
    schizotypal 301.22
    seductive 301.59
    type A 301.4
    unstable 301.59
  pervasive developmental 299.9
    childhood-onset 299.8
    specified NEC 299.8
  phonological 315.39
  pigmentation, choroid (congenital) 743.53
  pinna 380.30
    specified type NEC 380.39
  pituitary, thalamic 253.9
    anterior NEC 253.4
    iatrogenic 253.7
    postablative 253.7
    specified NEC 253.8
  pityriasis-like NEC 696.8
  platelets (blood) 287.1
  polymorphonuclear neutrophils (functional) 288.1
  porphyrin metabolism 277.1

Disorder—*continued*
  postmenopausal 627.9
    specified type NEC 627.8
  post-transplant lymphoproliferative (PTLD) 238.77
  post-traumatic stress (PTSD) 309.81
    acute 309.81
    brief 309.81
    chronic 309.81
  premenstrual dysphoric (PMDD) 625.4
  psoriatic-like NEC 696.8
  psychic, with diseases classified elsewhere 316
  psychogenic NEC (*see also* condition) 300.9
    allergic NEC
      respiratory 306.1
    anxiety 300.00
      atypical 300.00
      generalized 300.02
    appetite 307.59
    articulation, joint 306.0
    asthenic 300.5
    blood 306.8
    cardiovascular (system) 306.2
    compulsive 300.3
    cutaneous 306.3
    depressive 300.4
    digestive (system) 306.4
    dysmenorrheic 306.52
    dyspneic 306.1
    eczematous 306.3
    endocrine (system) 306.6
    eye 306.7
    feeding 307.59
    functional NEC 306.9
    gastric 306.4
    gastrointestinal (system) 306.4
    genitourinary (system) 306.50
    heart (function) (rhythm) 306.2
    hemic 306.8
    hyperventilatory 306.1
    hypochondriacal 300.7
    hysterical 300.10
    intestinal 306.4
    joint 306.0
    learning 315.2
    limb 306.0
    lymphatic (system) 306.8
    menstrual 306.52
    micturition 306.53
    monoplegic NEC 306.0
    motor 307.9
    muscle 306.0
    musculoskeletal 306.0
    neurocirculatory 306.2
    obsessive 300.3
    occupational 300.89
    organ or part of body NEC 306.9
    organs of special sense 306.7
    paralytic NEC 306.0
    phobic 300.20
    physical NEC 306.9
    pruritic 306.3
    rectal 306.4
    respiratory (system) 306.1
    rheumatic 306.0
    sexual (function) 302.70
      specified type NEC 302.79
    sexual orientation conflict 302.0
    skin (allergic) (eczematous) (pruritic) 306.3

Disorder—*continued*
somatization 300.81
somatoform (atypical) (undifferentiated) 300.82
   severe 300.81
   specified type NEC 300.89
speech NEC 784.59
   nonorganic origin 307.9
spine NEC 724.9
   ligamentous or muscular attachments,
      peripheral 720.1
steroid metabolism NEC 255.2
stomach (functional) (*see also* Disorder, gastric) 536.9
   psychogenic 306.4
storage, iron 275.09
stress (*see also* Reaction, stress, acute) 308.3
   posttraumatic
      acute 309.81
      brief 309.81
      chronic 309.81
substitution 300.11
suspected—*see* Observation
synovium 727.9
temperature regulation, fetus or newborn 778.4
temporomandibular joint NEC 524.60
   sounds on opening or closing 524.64
   specified NEC 524.69
tendon 727.9
   shoulder region 726.10
thoracic root (nerve) NEC 353.3
thyrocalcitonin secretion 246.0
thyroid (gland) NEC 246.9
   specified type NEC 246.8
tic 307.20
   chronic (motor or vocal) 307.22
   motor-verbal 307.23
   organic origin 333.1
   transient (of childhood) 307.21
tooth NEC 525.9
   development NEC 520.9
      specified type NEC 520.8
   eruption 520.6
   specified type NEC 525.8
Tourette's 307.23
transport, carbohydrate 271.9
   specified type NEC 271.8
tubular, phosphate-losing 588.0
tympanic membrane 384.9
unaggressive, unsocialized (*see also*
   Disturbance, conduct) 312.1
undersocialized, unsocialized—*see also*
   Disturbance, conduct
   aggressive (type) 312.0
   unaggressive (type) 312.1
vision, visual NEC 368.9
   binocular NEC 368.30
   cortex 377.73
      associated with
         inflammatory disorders 377.73
         neoplasms 377.71
         vascular disorders 377.72
   pathway NEC 377.63
      associated with
         inflammatory disorders 377.63
         neoplasms 377.61
         vascular disorders 377.62
vocal tic
   chronic 307.22
wakefulness (*see also* Hypersomnia) 780.54
   nonorganic origin (transient) 307.43
   persistent 307.44
written expression 315.2

Disorganized globe 360.29
Displacement, displaced

> *Note—For acquired displacement of bones,
> cartilage, joints, tendons, due to injury, see also
> Dislocation. Displacements at ages under one
> year should be considered congenital, provided
> there is no indication the condition was
> acquired after birth.*

acquired traumatic of bond, cartilage, joint,
   tendon NEC (without fracture) (*see also*
   Dislocation) 839.8
   with fracture—*see* Fracture, by site
adrenal gland (congenital) 759.1
alveolus and teeth, vertical 524.75
appendix, retrocecal (congenital) 751.5
auricle (congenital) 744.29
bladder (acquired) 596.89
   congenital 753.8
brachial plexus (congenital) 742.8
brain stem, caudal 742.4
canaliculus lacrimalis 743.65
cardia, through esophageal hiatus 750.6
cerebellum, caudal 742.4
cervix —*see* Displacement, uterus
colon (congenital) 751.4
device, implant, or graft—*see* Complications,
   mechanical
epithelium
   columnar of cervix 622.10
   cuboidal, beyond limits of external os (uterus)
      752.49
esophageal mucosa into cardia of stomach,
   congenital 750.4
esophagus (acquired) 530.89
   congenital 750.4
eyeball (acquired) (old) 376.36
   congenital 743.8
   current injury 871.3
   lateral 376.36
fallopian tube (acquired) 620.4
   congenital 752.19
   opening (congenital) 752.19
gallbladder (congenital) 751.69
gastric mucosa 750.7
   into
      duodenum 750.7
      esophagus 750.7
      Meckel's diverticulum, congenital 750.7
globe (acquired) (lateral) (old) 376.36
   current injury 871.3
graft
   artificial skin graft 996.55
   decellularized allodermis graft 996.55
heart (congenital) 746.87
   acquired 429.89
hymen (congenital) (upward) 752.49
internal prosthesis NEC—*see* Complications,
   mechanical
intervertebral disc (with neuritis, radiculitis,
   sciatica, or other pain) 722.2
   with myelopathy 722.70
   cervical, cervicodorsal, cervicothoracic 722.0
      with myelopathy 722.71
      due to major trauma—*see* Dislocation,
         vertebra, cervical
   due to trauma—*see* Dislocation, vertebra
   lumbar, lumbosacral 722.10
      with myelopathy 722.73
      due to major trauma—*see* Dislocation,
         vertebra, lumbar

Displacement, displaced—*continued*
 intervertebral disc—*continued*
  thoracic, thoracolumbar 722.11
   with myelopathy 722.72
   due to major trauma—*see* Dislocation,
     vertebra, thoracic
 intrauterine device 996.32
 kidney (acquired) 593.0
  congenital 753.3
 lacrimal apparatus or duct (congenital) 743.65
 macula (congenital) 743.55
 Meckel's diverticulum (congenital) 751.0
 nail (congenital) 757.5
  acquired 703.8
 opening of Wharton's duct in mouth 750.26
 organ or site, congenital NEC—*see* Malposition,
   congenital
 ovary (acquired) 620.4
  congenital 752.0
  free in peritoneal cavity (congenital) 752.0
  into hernial sac 620.4
 oviduct (acquired) 620.4
  congenital 752.19
 parathyroid (gland) 252.8
 parotid gland (congenital) 750.26
 punctum lacrimale (congenital) 743.65
 sacroiliac (congenital) (joint) 755.69
  current injury—*see* Dislocation, sacroiliac
  old 724.6
 spine (congenital) 756.19
 spleen, congenital 759.0
 stomach (congenital) 750.7
  acquired 537.89
 subglenoid (closed) 831.01
 sublingual duct (congenital) 750.26
 teeth, tooth 524.30
  horizontal 524.33
  vertical 524.34
 tongue (congenital) (downward) 750.19
 trachea (congenital) 748.3
 ureter or ureteric opening or orifice (congenital)
   753.4
 uterine opening of oviducts or fallopian tubes
   752.19
 uterus, uterine (*see also* Malposition, uterus) 621.6
  congenital 752.39
 ventricular septum 746.89
  with rudimentary ventricle 746.89
 xyphoid bone (process) 738.3
Disproportion 653.9
 affecting fetus or newborn 763.1
 breast, reconstructed 612.1
  between native and reconstructed 612.1
 caused by
  conjoined twins 678.1
  contraction, pelvis (general) 653.1
   inlet 653.2
   midpelvic 653.8
   midplane 653.8
   outlet 653.3
  fetal
   ascites 653.7
   hydrocephalus 653.6
   hydrops 653.7
   meningomyelocele 653.7
   sacral teratoma 653.7
   tumor 653.7
  hydrocephalic fetus 653.6
  pelvis, pelvic, abnormality (bony) NEC 653.0
  unusually large fetus 653.5
 causing obstructed labor 660.1

Disproportion—*continued*
 cephalopelvic, normally formed fetus 653.4
  causing obstructed labor 660.1
 fetal NEC 653.5
  causing obstructed labor 660.1
 fetopelvic, normally formed fetus 653.4
  causing obstructed labor 660.1
 mixed maternal and fetal origin, normally
   formed fetus 653.4
 pelvis, pelvic (bony) NEC 653.1
  causing obstructed labor 660.1
 specified type NEC 653.8
Disruption
 cesarean wound 674.1
 family V61.09
  due to
   child in
    care of non-parental family member
      V61.06
    foster care V61.06
    welfare custody V61.05
   death of family member V61.07
   divorce V61.03
   estrangement V61.09
    parent-child V61.04
   extended absence of family member NEC
     V61.08
   family member
    on military deployment V61.01
    return from military deployment V61.02
   legal separation V61.03
 gastrointestinal anastomosis 997.49
 ligament(s)—*see also* Sprain
  knee
   current injury—*see* Dislocation, knee
   old 717.89
    capsular 717.85
    collateral (medial) 717.82
     lateral 717.81
    cruciate (posterior) 717.84
     anterior 717.83
    specified site NEC 717.85
 marital V61.10
  involving
   divorce V61.03
   estrangement V61.09
 operation wound (external) (*see also*
   Dehiscence) 998.32
  internal 998.31
 organ transplant, anastomosis site—*see*
   Complications, transplant, organ, by site
 ossicles, ossicular chain 385.23
  traumatic—*see* Fracture, skull, base
 parenchyma
  liver (hepatic)—*see* Laceration, liver, major
  spleen—*see* Laceration, spleen, parenchyma,
    massive
 phase-shift, of 24 hour sleep wake cycle,
   unspecified 780.55
  nonorganic origin 307.45
 sleep wake cycle (24 hour), unspecified 780.55
  circadian rhythm 327.33
  nonorganic origin 307.45
 suture line (external) (*see also* Dehiscence)
   998.32
  internal 998.31
 wound 998.30
  cesarean operation 674.1
  episiotomy 674.2
  operation (surgical) 998.32
   cesarean 674.1
   internal 998.31

Disruption—*continued*
  wound—*continued*
    perineal (obstetric) 674.2
    uterine 674.1
Disruptio uteri —*see also* Rupture, uterus
  complicating delivery—*see* Delivery,
    complicated, rupture, uterus
Dissatisfaction with
  employment V62.29
  school environment V62.3
Dissecting —*see* condition
Dissection
  aorta 441.00
    abdominal 441.02
    thoracic 441.01
    thoracoabdominal 441.03
  artery, arterial
    carotid 443.21
    coronary 414.12
    iliac 443.22
    renal 443.23
    specified NEC 443.29
    vertebral 443.24
  vascular 459.9
  wound—*see* Wound, open, by site
Disseminated —*see* condition
Dissociated personality NEC 300.15
Dissociation
  auriculoventricular or atrioventricular (any
    degree) (AV) 426.89
    with heart block 426.0
  interference 426.89
  isorhythmic 426.89
  rhythm
    atrioventricular (AV) 426.89
    interference 426.89
Dissociative
  identity disorder 300.14
  reaction NEC 300.15
Dissolution, vertebra (*see also* Osteoporosis)
  733.00
Distention
  abdomen (gaseous) 787.3
  bladder 596.89
  cecum 569.89
  colon 569.89
  gallbladder 575.8
  gaseous (abdomen) 787.3
  intestine 569.89
  kidney 593.89
  liver 573.9
  seminal vesicle 608.89
  stomach 536.8
    acute 536.1
    psychogenic 306.4
  ureter 593.5
  uterus 621.8
Distichia, distichiasis (eyelid) 743.63
Distoma hepaticum infestation 121.3
Distomiasis 121.9
  bile passages 121.3
    due to Clonorchis sinensis 121.1
  hemic 120.9
  hepatic (liver) 121.3
    due to Clonorchis sinensis (clonorchiasis) 121.1
  intestinal 121.4
  liver 121.3
    due to Clonorchis sinensis 121.1
  lung 121.2
  pulmonary 121.2
Distomolar (fourth molar) 520.1
  causing crowding 524.31

Disto-occlusion (division I) (division II) 524.22
Distortion (congenital)
  adrenal (gland) 759.1
  ankle (joint) 755.69
  anus 751.5
  aorta 747.29
  appendix 751.5
  arm 755.59
  artery (peripheral) NEC (*see also* Distortion,
    peripheral vascular system) 747.60
    cerebral 747.81
    coronary 746.85
    pulmonary 747.39
    retinal 743.58
    umbilical 747.5
  auditory canal 744.29
    causing impairment of hearing 744.02
  bile duct or passage 751.69
  bladder 753.8
  brain 742.4
  bronchus 748.3
  cecum 751.5
  cervix (uteri) 752.49
  chest (wall) 756.3
  clavicle 755.51
  clitoris 752.49
  coccyx 756.19
  colon 751.5
  common duct 751.69
  cornea 743.41
  cricoid cartilage 748.3
  cystic duct 751.69
  duodenum 751.5
  ear 744.29
    auricle 744.29
      causing impairment of hearing 744.02
    causing impairment of hearing 744.09
    external 744.29
      causing impairment of hearing 744.02
    inner 744.05
    middle, except ossicles 744.03
      ossicles 744.04
    ossicles 744.04
  endocrine (gland) NEC 759.2
  epiglottis 748.3
  Eustachian tube 744.24
  eye 743.8
    adnexa 743.69
  face bone(s) 756.0
  fallopian tube 752.19
  femur 755.69
  fibula 755.69
  finger(s) 755.59
  foot 755.67
  gallbladder 751.69
  genitalia, genital organ(s)
    female 752.89
      external 752.49
      internal NEC 752.89
    male 752.89
      penis 752.69
  glottis 748.3
  gyri 742.4
  hand bone(s) 755.59
  heart (auricle) (ventricle) 746.89
    valve (cusp) 746.89
  hepatic duct 751.69
  humerus 755.59
  hymen 752.49
  ileum 751.5

Distortion—*continued*
intestine (large) (small) 751.5
  with anomalous adhesions, fixation or
    malrotation 751.4
jaw NEC 524.89
jejunum 751.5
kidney 753.3
knee (joint) 755.64
labium (majus) (minus) 752.49
larynx 748.3
leg 755.69
lens 743.36
liver 751.69
lumbar spine 756.19
  with disproportion (fetopelvic) 653.0
    affecting fetus or newborn 763.1
    causing obstructed labor 660.1
lumbosacral (joint) (region) 756.19
lung (fissures) (lobe) 748.69
nerve 742.8
nose 748.1
organ
  of Corti 744.05
  or site not listed—*see* Anomaly, specified type NEC
ossicles, ear 744.04
ovary 752.0
oviduct 752.19
pancreas 751.7
parathyroid (gland) 759.2
patella 755.64
peripheral vascular system NEC 747.60
  gastrointestinal 747.61
  lower limb 747.64
  renal 747.62
  spinal 747.82
  upper limb 747.63
pituitary (gland) 759.2
radius 755.59
rectum 751.5
rib 756.3
sacroiliac joint 755.69
sacrum 756.19
scapula 755.59
shoulder girdle 755.59
site not listed—*see* Anomaly, specified type NEC
skull bone(s) 756.0
  with
    anencephalus 740.0
    encephalocele 742.0
    hydrocephalus 742.3
      with spina bifida (*see also* Spina bifida) 741.0
    microcephalus 742.1
spinal cord 742.59
spine 756.19
spleen 759.0
sternum 756.3
thorax (wall) 756.3
thymus (gland) 759.2
thyroid (gland) 759.2
  cartilage 748.3
tibia 755.69
toe(s) 755.66
tongue 750.19
trachea (cartilage) 748.3
ulna 755.59
ureter 753.4
  causing obstruction 753.20
urethra 753.8
  causing obstruction 753.6
uterus 752.39
vagina 752.49

Distortion—*continued*
vein (peripheral) NEC (*see also* Distortion,
  peripheral vascular system) 747.60
  great 747.49
  portal 747.49
  pulmonary 747.49
vena cava (inferior) (superior) 747.49
vertebra 756.19
visual NEC 368.15
  shape or size 368.14
vulva 752.49
wrist (bones) (joint) 755.59
Distress
abdomen 789.0
colon 789.0
emotional V40.9
epigastric 789.0
fetal (syndrome) 768.4
  affecting management of pregnancy or
    childbirth 656.8
  liveborn infant 768.4
    first noted
      before onset of labor 768.2
      during labor and delivery 768.3
    stillborn infant (death before onset of labor)
      768.0
      death during labor 768.1
gastrointestinal (functional) 536.9
  psychogenic 306.4
intestinal (functional) NEC 564.9
  psychogenic 306.4
intrauterine (*see* Distress, fetal)
leg 729.5
maternal 669.0
mental V40.9
respiratory 786.09
  acute (adult) 518.82
  adult syndrome (following trauma and
    surgery) 518.52
    specified NEC 518.82
  fetus or newborn 770.89
  syndrome (idiopathic) (newborn) 769
stomach 536.9
  psychogenic 306.4
Distribution vessel, atypical NEC 747.60
coronary artery 746.85
spinal 747.82
Districhiasis 704.2
Disturbance —*see also* Disease
absorption NEC 579.9
  calcium 269.3
  carbohydrate 579.8
  fat 579.8
  protein 579.8
  specified type NEC 579.8
  vitamin (*see also* Deficiency, vitamin) 269.2
acid-base equilibrium 276.9
activity and attention, simple, with hyperkinesis
  314.01
amino acid (metabolic) (*see also* Disorder,
  amino acid) 270.9
  imidazole 270.5
  maple syrup (urine) disease 270.3
  transport 270.0
assimilation, food 579.9
attention, simple 314.00
  with hyperactivity 314.01
auditory, nerve, except deafness 388.5
behavior (*see also* Disturbance, conduct) 312.9
blood clotting (hypoproteinemia) (mechanism)
  (*see also* Defect, coagulation) 286.9

Disturbance—*continued*
  central nervous system NEC 349.9
  cerebral nerve NEC 352.9
  circulatory 459.9
  conduct 312.9

---

*Note—Use the following fifth-digit
subclassification with categories 312.0-312.2:*

0 *unspecified*
1 *mild*
2 *moderate*
3 *severe*

---

    adjustment reaction 309.3
    adolescent onset type 312.82
    childhood onset type 312.81
    compulsive 312.30
      intermittent explosive disorder 312.34
      isolated explosive disorder 312.35
      kleptomania 312.32
      pathological gambling 312.31
      pyromania 312.33
    hyperkinetic 314.2
    intermittent explosive 312.34
    isolated explosive 312.35
    memory (*see also* Amnesia) 780.99
    mixed with emotions 312.4
    socialized (type) 312.20
      aggressive 312.23
      unaggressive 312.21
    specified type NEC 312.89
    undersocialized, unsocialized
      aggressive (type) 312.0
      unaggressive (type) 312.1
  coordination 781.3
  cranial nerve NEC 352.9
  deep sensibility—*see* Disturbance, sensation
  digestive 536.9
    psychogenic 306.4
  electrolyte—*see* Imbalance, electrolyte
  emotions specific to childhood or adolescence
    313.9
    with
      academic underachievement 313.83
      anxiety and fearfulness 313.0
      elective mutism 313.23
      identity disorder 313.82
      jealousy 313.3
      misery and unhappiness 313.1
      oppositional defiant disorder 313.81
      overanxiousness 313.0
      sensitivity 313.21
      shyness 313.21
      social withdrawal 313.22
      withdrawal reaction 313.22
    involving relationship problems 313.3
    mixed 313.89
    specified type NEC 313.89
  endocrine (gland) 259.9
    neonatal, transitory 775.9
    specified NEC 775.89
  equilibrium 780.4
  feeding (elderly) (infant) 783.3
    newborn 779.31
    nonorganic origin NEC 307.59
    psychogenic NEC 307.59
  fructose metabolism 271.2
  gait 781.2
    hysterical 300.11

Disturbance—*continued*
  gastric (functional) 536.9
    motility 536.8
    psychogenic 306.4
    secretion 536.8
  gastrointestinal (functional) 536.9
    psychogenic 306.4
  habit, child 307.9
  hearing, except deafness 388.40
  heart, functional (conditions classifiable to 426,
    427, 428)
    due to presence of (cardiac) prosthesis 429.4
    postoperative (immediate) 997.1
      long-term effect of cardiac surgery 429.4
    psychogenic 306.2
  hormone 259.9
  innervation uterus, sympathetic,
    parasympathetic 621.8
  keratinization NEC
    gingiva 523.10
    lip 528.5
    oral (mucosa) (soft tissue) 528.79
      residual ridge mucosa
        excessive 528.72
        minimal 528.71
    tongue 528.79
  labyrinth, labyrinthine (vestibule) 386.9
  learning, specific NEC 315.2
  memory (*see also* Amnesia) 780.93
    mild, following organic brain damage 310.89
  mental (*see also* Disorder, mental) 300.9
    associated with diseases classified elsewhere
    316
  metabolism (acquired) (congenital) (*see also*
    Disorder, metabolism) 277.9
    with
      abortion—*see* Abortion, by type, with
        metabolic disorder
      ectopic pregnancy (*see also* categories
        633.0-633.9) 639.4
      molar pregnancy (*see also* categories
        630-632) 639.4
    amino acid (*see also* Disorder, amino acid)
      270.9
      aromatic NEC 270.2
      branched-chain 270.3
      specified type NEC 270.8
      straight-chain NEC 270.7
      sulfur-bearing 270.4
      transport 270.0
    ammonia 270.6
    arginine 270.6
    argininosuccinic acid 270.6
    carbohydrate NEC 271.9
    cholesterol 272.9
    citrulline 270.6
    cystathionine 270.4
    fat 272.9
    following
      abortion 639.4
      ectopic or molar pregnancy 639.4
    general 277.9
      carbohydrate 271.9
      iron 275.09
      phosphate 275.3
      sodium 276.9
    glutamine 270.7
    glycine 270.7
    histidine 270.5
    homocystine 270.4
    in labor or delivery 669.0

Disturbance—*continued*
  metabolism—*continued*
    iron 275.09
    isoleucine 270.3
    leucine 270.3
    lipoid 272.9
      specified type NEC 272.8
    lysine 270.7
    methionine 270.4
    neonatal, transitory 775.9
      specified type NEC 775.89
    nitrogen 788.99
    ornithine 270.6
    phosphate 275.3
    phosphatides 272.7
    serine 270.7
    sodium NEC 276.9
    threonine 270.7
    tryptophan 270.2
    tyrosine 270.2
    urea cycle 270.6
    valine 270.3
  motor 796.1
  nervous functional 799.21
  neuromuscular mechanism (eye) due to syphilis
    094.84
  nutritional 269.9
    nail 703.8
  ocular motion 378.87
    psychogenic 306.7
  oculogyric 378.87
    psychogenic 306.7
  oculomotor NEC 378.87
    psychogenic 306.7
  olfactory nerve 781.1
  optic nerve NEC 377.49
  oral epithelium, including tongue 528.79
    residual ridge mucosa
      excessive 528.72
      minimal 528.71
  personality (pattern) (trait) (*see also* Disorder,
    personality) 301.9
    following organic brain damage 310.1
  polyglandular 258.9
  psychomotor 307.9
  pupillary 379.49
  reflex 796.1
  rhythm, heart 427.9
    postoperative (immediate) 997.1
      long-term effect of cardiac surgery 429.4
    psychogenic 306.2
  salivary secretion 527.7
  sensation (cold) (heat) (localization) (tactile
    discrimination localization) (texture)
    (vibratory) NEC 782.0
    hysterical 300.11
    skin 782.0
    smell 781.1
    taste 781.1
  sensory (*see also* Disturbance, sensation) 782.0
    innervation 782.0
  situational (transient) (*see also* Reaction,
    adjustment) 309.9
    acute 308.3
  sleep 780.50
    initiation or maintenance (*see also* Insomnia)
      780.52
      nonorganic origin 307.41
    nonorganic origin 307.40
      specified type NEC 307.49
    specified NEC 780.59
      nonorganic origin 307.49

Disturbance—*continued*
  sleep—*continued*
    wakefulness (*see also* Hypersomnia) 780.54
      nonorganic origin 307.43
    with apnea—*see* Apnea, sleep
  sociopathic 301.7
  speech NEC 784.59
    developmental 315.39
      associated with hyperkinesis 314.1
    secondary to organic lesion 784.59
  stomach (functional) (*see also* Disturbance,
    gastric) 536.9
  sympathetic (nerve) (*see also* Neuropathy,
    peripheral, autonomic) 337.9
  temperature sense 782.0
    hysterical 300.11
  tooth
    eruption 520.6
    formation 520.4
    structure, hereditary NEC 520.5
  touch (*see also* Disturbance, sensation) 782.0
  vascular 459.9
    arteriosclerotic—*see* Arteriosclerosis
  vasomotor 443.9
  vasospastic 443.9
  vestibular labyrinth 386.9
  vision, visual NEC 368.9
    psychophysical 368.16
    specified NEC 368.8
    subjective 368.10
  voice and resonance784.40
  wakefulness (initiation or maintenance) (*see
    also* Hypersomnia) 780.54
    nonorganic origin 307.43
Disulfiduria, beta-mercaptolactate-cysteine 270.0
Disuse atrophy, bone 733.7
Ditthomska syndrome 307.81
Diuresis 788.42
Divers'
  palsy or paralysis 993.3
  squeeze 993.3
Diverticula, diverticulosis, diverticulum (acute)
  (multiple) (perforated) (ruptured) 562.10
  with diverticulitis 562.11
  aorta (Kommerell's) 747.21
  appendix (noninflammatory) 543.9
  bladder (acquired) (sphincter) 596.3
    congenital 753.8
  broad ligament 620.8
  bronchus (congenital) 748.3
    acquired 494.0
      with acute exacerbation 494.1
  calyx, calyceal (kidney) 593.89
  cardia (stomach) 537.1
  cecum 562.10
    with
      diverticulitis 562.11
        with hemorrhage 562.13
      hemorrhage 562.12
    congenital 751.5
  colon (acquired) 562.10
    with
      diverticulitis 562.11
        with hemorrhage 562.13
      hemorrhage 562.12
    congenital 751.5
  duodenum 562.00
    with
      diverticulitis 562.01
        with hemorrhage 562.03
      hemorrhage 562.02
    congenital 751.5

Diverticula, diverticulosis—*continued*
 epiphrenic (esophagus) 530.6
 esophagus (congenital) 750.4
  acquired 530.6
  epiphrenic 530.6
  pulsion 530.6
  traction 530.6
  Zenker's 530.6
 Eustachian tube 381.89
 fallopian tube 620.8
 gallbladder (congenital) 751.69
 gastric 537.1
 heart (congenital) 746.89
 ileum 562.00
  with
   diverticulitis 562.01
    with hemorrhage 562.03
   hemorrhage 562.02
 intestine (large) 562.10
  with
   diverticulitis 562.11
    with hemorrhage 562.13
   hemorrhage 562.12
  congenital 751.5
  small 562.00
   with
    diverticulitis 562.01
     with hemorrhage 562.03
    hemorrhage 562.02
   congenital 751.5
 jejunum 562.00
  with
   diverticulitis 562.01
    with hemorrhage 562.03
   hemorrhage 562.02
 kidney (calyx) (pelvis) 593.89
  with calculus 592.0
 Kommerell's 747.21
 laryngeal ventricle (congenital) 748.3
 Meckel's (displaced) (hypertrophic) 751.0
 midthoracic 530.6
 organ or site, congenital NEC—*see* Distortion
 pericardium (congenital) (cyst) 746.89
  acquired (true) 423.8
 pharyngoesophageal (pulsion) 530.6
 pharynx (congenital) 750.27
 pulsion (esophagus) 530.6
 rectosigmoid 562.10
  with
   diverticulitis 562.11
    with hemorrhage 562.13
   hemorrhage 562.12
  congenital 751.5
 rectum 562.10
  with
   diverticulitis 562.11
    with hemorrhage 562.13
   hemorrhage 562.12
 renal (calyces) (pelvis) 593.89
  with calculus 592.0
 Rokitansky's 530.6
 seminal vesicle 608.0
 sigmoid 562.10
  with
   diverticulitis 562.11
    with hemorrhage 562.13
   hemorrhage 562.12
  congenital 751.5
 small intestine 562.00
  with
   diverticulitis 562.01
    with hemorrhage 562.03

Diverticula, diverticulosis— *continued*
  hemorrhage 562.02
 stomach (cardia) (juxtacardia) (juxtapyloric)
  (acquired) 537.1
  congenital 750.7
 subdiaphragmatic 530.6
 trachea (congenital) 748.3
  acquired 519.19
 traction (esophagus) 530.6
 ureter (acquired) 593.89
  congenital 753.4
 ureterovesical orifice 593.89
 urethra (acquired) 599.2
  congenital 753.8
 ventricle, left (congenital) 746.89
 vesical (urinary) 596.3
  congenital 753.8
 Zenker's (esophagus) 530.6
Diverticulitis (acute) (*see also* Diverticula) 562.11
 with hemorrhage 562.13
 bladder (urinary) 596.3
 cecum (perforated) 562.11
  with hemorrhage 562.13
 colon (perforated) 562.11
  with hemorrhage 562.13
 duodenum 562.01
  with hemorrhage 562.03
 esophagus 530.6
 ileum (perforated) 562.01
  with hemorrhage 562.03
 intestine (large) (perforated) 562.11
  with hemorrhage 562.13
  small 562.01
   with hemorrhage 562.03
 jejunum (perforated) 562.01
  with hemorrhage 562.03
 Meckel's (perforated) 751.0
 pharyngoesophageal 530.6
 rectosigmoid (perforated) 562.11
  with hemorrhage 562.13
 rectum 562.11
  with hemorrhage 562.13
 sigmoid (old) (perforated) 562.11
  with hemorrhage 562.13
 small intestine (perforated) 562.01
  with hemorrhage 562.03
 vesical (urinary) 596.3
Diverticulosis —*see* Diverticula
Division
 cervix uteri 622.8
  external os into two openings by frenum 752.44
 external (cervical) into two openings by frenum
  752.44
 glans penis 752.69
 hymen 752.49
 labia minora (congenital) 752.49
 ligament (partial or complete) (current)—*see
  also* Sprain, by site
  with open wound—*see* Wound, open, by site
 muscle (partial or complete) (current)—*see also*
  Sprain, by site
  with open wound—*see* Wound, open, by site
 nerve—*see* Injury, nerve, by site
 penis glans 752.69
 spinal cord—*see* Injury, spinal, by site
 vein 459.9
 traumatic—*see* Injury, vascular, by site
Divorce V61.03
Dix-Hallpike neurolabyrinthitis 386.12
Dizziness 780.4
 hysterical 300.11
 psychogenic 306.9

Doan-Wiseman syndrome (primary splenic
   neutropenia) 289.53
Dog bite —*see* Wound, open, by site
Döhle-Heller aortitis 093.1
Döhle body-panmyelopathic syndrome 288.2
Dolichocephaly, dolichocephalus 754.0
Dolichocolon 751.5
Dolichostenomelia 759.82
Donohue's syndrome (leprechaunism) 259.8
Donor
   blood V59.01
      other blood components V59.09
      stem cells V59.02
      whole blood V59.01
   bone V59.2
      marrow V59.3
   cornea V59.5
   egg (oocyte) (ovum) V59.70
      age 35 and over V59.73
         anonymous recipient V59.73
         designated recipient V59.74
      under age 35 V59.71
         anonymous recipient V59.71
         designated recipient V59.72
   heart V59.8
   kidney V59.4
   liver V59.6
   lung V59.8
   lymphocyte V59.8
   organ V59.9
      specified NEC V59.8
   potential, examination of V70.8
   skin V59.1
   specified organ or tissue NEC V59.8
   sperm V59.8
   stem cells V59.02
   tissue V59.9
      specified type NEC V59.8
Donovanosis (granuloma venereum) 099.2
DOPS (diffuse obstructive pulmonary syndrome) 496
Double
   albumin 273.8
   aortic arch 747.21
   auditory canal 744.29
   auricle (heart) 746.82
   bladder 753.8
   external (cervical) os 752.44
   kidney with double pelvis (renal) 753.3
   larynx 748.3
   meatus urinarius 753.8
   organ or site NEC—*see* Accessory
   orifice
      heart valve NEC 746.89
         pulmonary 746.09
   outlet, right ventricle 745.11
   pelvis (renal) with double ureter 753.4
   penis 752.69
   tongue 750.13
   ureter (one or both sides) 753.4
      with double pelvis (renal) 753.4
   urethra 753.8
   urinary meatus 753.8
   uterus (any degree) 752.2
      with doubling of cervix and vagina 752.2
      in pregnancy or childbirth 654.0
         affecting fetus or newborn 763.89
   vagina 752.47
      with doubling of cervix and uterus 752.2
   vision 368.2
   vocal cords 748.3
   vulva 752.49
   whammy (syndrome) 360.81

Douglas' pouch, cul-de-sac —*see* condition
Down's disease or syndrome (mongolism) 758.0
Down-growth, epithelial (anterior chamber) 364.61
DPD (dihydropyrimidine dehydrogenase
   deficiency) 277.6
Dracontiasis 125.7
Dracunculiasis 125.7
Dracunculosis 125.7
Drainage
   abscess (spontaneous)—*see* Abscess
   anomalous pulmonary veins to hepatic veins or
      right atrium 747.41
   stump (amputation) (surgical) 997.62
   suprapubic, bladder 596.89
Dream state, hysterical 300.13
Drepanocytic anemia (*see also* Disease, sickle
   cell) 282.60
Dresbach's syndrome (elliptocytosis) 282.1
Dreschlera (infection) 118
   hawaiiensis 117.8
Dressler's syndrome (postmyocardial infarction)
   411.0
Dribbling (post-void) 788.35
Drift, ulnar 736.09
Drinking (alcohol)—*see also* Alcoholism
   excessive, to excess NEC (*see also* Abuse,
      drugs, nondependent) 305.0
      bouts, periodic 305.0
      continual 303.9
      episodic 305.0
      habitual 303.9
      periodic 305.0
Drip, postnasal (chronic) 784.91
   due to
      allergic rhinitis —*see* Rhinitis, allergic
      common cold 460
      gastroesophageal reflux —*see* Reflux,
         gastroesophageal
      nasopharyngitis —*see* Nasopharyngitis
      other known condition —*code to condition*
      sinusitis —*see* Sinusitis
Drivers' license examination V70.3
Droop
   Cooper's 611.81
   facial 781.94
Drop
   finger 736.29
   foot 736.79
   hematocrit (precipitous) 790.01
   hemoglobin 790.01
   toe 735.8
   wrist 736.05
Dropped
   dead 798.1
   heart beats 426.6
Dropsy, dropsical (*see also* Edema) 782.3
   abdomen 789.59
   amnion (*see also* Hydramnios) 657
   brain—*see* Hydrocephalus
   cardiac (*see also* Failure, heart) 428.0
   cardiorenal (*see also* Hypertension, cardiorenal)
      404.90
   chest 511.9
   fetus or newborn 778.0
      due to isoimmunization 773.3
   gangrenous (*see also* Gangrene) 785.4
   heart (*see also* Failure, heart) 428.0
   hepatic—*see* Cirrhosis, liver
   infantile—*see* Hydrops, fetalis
   kidney (*see also* Nephrosis) 581.9
   liver—*see* Cirrhosis, liver

Dropsy, dropsical—*continued*
  lung 514
  malarial (*see also* Malaria) 084.9
  neonatorum—*see* Hydrops, fetalis
  nephritic 581.9
  newborn—*see* Hydrops, fetalis
  nutritional 269.9
  ovary 620.8
  pericardium (*see also* Pericarditis) 423.9
  renal (*see also* Nephrosis) 581.9
  uremic—*see* Uremia
Drowned, drowning (near) 994.1
  lung 518.52
Drowsiness 780.09
Drug —*see also* condition
  addiction (*see also* listing under Dependence) 304.9
  adverse effect, correct substance properly
    administered 995.20
  allergy 995.27
  dependence (*see also* listing under Dependence) 304.9
  habit (*see also* listing under Dependence) 304.9
  hypersensitivity 995.27
  induced
    circadian rhythm sleep disorder 292.85
    hypersomnia 292.85
    insomnia 292.85
    mental disorder 292.9
      anxiety 292.89
      mood 292.84
      sexual 292.89
      sleep 292.85
      specified type 292.89
    parasomnia 292.85
    persisting
      amnestic disorder 292.83
      dementia 292.82
    psychotic disorder
      with
        delusions 292.11
        hallucinations 292.12
    sleep disorder 292.85
  intoxication 292.89
  overdose—*see* Table of drugs and chemicals
  poisoning—*see* Table of drugs and chemicals
  therapy (maintenance) status NEC
    chemotherapy, antineoplastic V58.11
    immunotherapy, antineoplastic V58.12
    long-term (current) (prophylactic) use V58.69
      antibiotics V58.62
      anticoagulants V58.61
      anti-inflammatories, non-steroidal (NSAID)
        V58.64
      antiplatelets V58.63
      antithrombotics V58.63
      aspirin V58.66
      bisphosphonates V58.68
      high-risk medications NEC V58.69
      insulin V58.67
      methadone for pain control V58.69
      opiate analgesic V58.69
      steroids V58.65
    methadone 304.00
  wrong substance given or taken in error—*see*
    Table of drugs and chemicals
Drunkenness (*see also* Abuse, drugs,
  nondependent) 305.0
  acute in alcoholism (*see also* Alcoholism) 303.0
  chronic (*see also* Alcoholism) 303.9
  pathologic 291.4
  simple (acute) 305.0
    in alcoholism 303.0
  sleep 307.47

Drusen
  optic disc or papilla 377.21
  retina (colloid) (hyaloid degeneration) 362.57
    hereditary 362.77
Drusenfieber 075
Dry, dryness —*see also* condition
  eye 375.15
    syndrome 375.15
  larynx 478.79
  mouth 527.7
  nose 478.19
  skin syndrome 701.1
  socket (teeth) 526.5
  throat 478.29
DSAP (disseminated superficial actinic
  porokeratosis) 692.75
DSTR (delayed serologic transfusion reaction)
  due to or resulting from incompatibility
    ABO 999.69
    non-ABO antigen (minor) (Duffy) (Kell)
      (Kidd) (Lewis) (M) (N) (P) (S) 999.79
    Rh antigen (C) (c) (D) (E) (e) 999.74
Duane's retraction syndrome 378.71
Duane-Stilling-Turk syndrome (ocular
  retraction syndrome) 378.71
Dubin-Johnson disease or syndrome 277.4
Dubini's disease (electric chorea) 049.8
Dubois' abscess or disease 090.5
Duchenne's
  disease 094.0
    locomotor ataxia 094.0
    muscular dystrophy 359.1
    pseudohypertrophy, muscles 359.1
  paralysis 335.22
  syndrome 335.22
Duchenne-Aran myelopathic muscular atrophy
  (nonprogressive) (progressive) 335.21
Duchenne-Griesinger disease 359.1
Ducrey's
  bacillus 099.0
  chancre 099.0
  disease (chancroid) 099.0
Duct, ductus —*see* condition
Duengero 061
Duhring's disease (dermatitis herpetiformis) 694.0
Dukes (-Filatov) disease 057.8
Dullness
  cardiac (decreased) (increased) 785.3
Dumb ague (*see also* Malaria) 084.6
Dumbness (*see also* Aphasia) 784.3
Dumdum fever 085.0
Dumping syndrome (postgastrectomy) 564.2
  nonsurgical 536.8
Duodenitis (nonspecific) (peptic) 535.60
  due to
    Strongyloides stercoralis 127.2
  with hemorrhage 535.61
Duodenocholangitis 575.8
Duodenum, duodenal —*see* condition
Duplay's disease, periarthritis, or syndrome
  726.2
Duplex —*see also* Accessory
  kidney 753.3
  placenta—*see* Placenta, abnormal
  uterus 752.2
Duplication —*see also* Accessory
  anus 751.5
  aortic arch 747.21
  appendix 751.5
  biliary duct (any) 751.69
  bladder 753.8

Duplication—*continued*
  cecum 751.5
    and appendix 751.5
  cervical, cervix 752.44
  clitoris 752.49
  cystic duct 751.69
  digestive organs 751.8
  duodenum 751.5
  esophagus 750.4
  fallopian tube 752.19
  frontonasal process 756.0
  gallbladder 751.69
  ileum 751.5
  intestine (large) (small) 751.5
  jejunum 751.5
  kidney 753.3
  liver 751.69
  nose 748.1
  pancreas 751.7
  penis 752.69
  respiratory organs NEC 748.9
  salivary duct 750.22
  spinal cord (incomplete) 742.51
  stomach 750.7
  ureter 753.4
  vagina 752.47
  vas deferens 752.89
  vocal cords 748.3
Dupré's disease or syndrome (meningism) 781.6
Dupuytren's
  contraction 728.6
  disease (muscle contracture) 728.6
  fracture (closed) 824.4
    ankle (closed) 824.4
      open 824.5
    fibula (closed) 824.4
      open 824.5
    open 824.5
    radius (closed) 813.42
      open 813.52
  muscle contracture 728.6
Durand-Nicolas-Favre disease (climatic bubo) 099.1
Durotomy incidental (inadvertent) (*see also* Tear, dural) 349.31
Duroziez's disease (congenital mitral stenosis) 746.5
Dust
  conjunctivitis 372.05
  reticulation (occupational) 504
Dutton's
  disease (trypanosomiasis) 086.9
  relapsing fever (West African) 087.1
Dwarf, dwarfism 259.4
  with infantilism (hypophyseal) 253.3
  achondroplastic 756.4
  Amsterdam 759.89
  bird-headed 759.89
  congenital 259.4
  constitutional 259.4
  hypophyseal 253.3
  infantile 259.4
  Levi type 253.3
  Lorain-Levi (pituitary) 253.3
  Lorain type (pituitary) 253.3
  metatropic 756.4
  nephrotic-glycosuric, with hypophosphatemic rickets 270.0
  nutritional 263.2
  ovarian 758.6
  pancreatic 577.8
  pituitary 253.3
  polydystrophic 277.5

Dwarf, dwarfism—*continued*
  primordial 253.3
  psychosocial 259.4
  renal 588.0
    with hypertension—*see* Hypertension, kidney
  Russell's (uterine dwarfism and craniofacial dysostosis) 759.89
Dyke-Young anemia or syndrome (acquired macrocytic hemolytic anemia) (secondary) (symptomatic) 283.9
Dynia abnormality (*see also* Defect, coagulation) 286.9
Dysacousis 388.40
Dysadrenocortism 255.9
  hyperfunction 255.3
  hypofunction 255.41
Dysarthria 784.51
  due to late effect of cerebrovascular disease (*see also* Late effect(s) (of) cerebrovascular disease) 438.13
Dysautonomia (*see also* Neuropathy, peripheral, autonomic) 337.9
  familial 742.8
Dysbarism 993.3
Dysbasia 719.7
  angiosclerotica intermittens 443.9
  due to atherosclerosis 440.21
  hysterical 300.11
  lordotica (progressiva) 333.6
  nonorganic origin 307.9
  psychogenic 307.9
Dysbetalipoproteinemia (familial) 272.2
Dyscalculia 315.1
Dyschezia (*see also* Constipation) 564.00
Dyschondroplasia (with hemangiomata) 756.4
  Voorhoeve's 756.4
Dyschondrosteosis 756.59
Dyschromia 709.00
Dyscollagenosis 710.9
Dyscoria 743.41
Dyscraniopyophalangy 759.89
Dyscrasia
  blood 289.9
    with antepartum hemorrhage 641.3
    hemorrhage, subungual 287.8
    puerperal, postpartum 666.3
  ovary 256.8
  plasma cell 273.9
  pluriglandular 258.9
  polyglandular 258.9
Dysdiadochokinesia 781.3
Dysectasia, vesical neck 596.89
Dysendocrinism 259.9
Dysentery, dysenteric (bilious) (catarrhal) (diarrhea) (epidemic) (gangrenous) (hemorrhagic) (infectious) (sporadic) (tropical) (ulcerative) 009.0
  abscess, liver (*see also* Abscess, amebic) 006.3
  amebic (*see also* Amebiasis) 006.9
    with abscess—*see* Abscess, amebic
    acute 006.0
    carrier (suspected) of V02.2
    chronic 006.1
  arthritis (*see also* Arthritis, due to, dysentery) 009.0 *[711.3]*
    bacillary 004.9 *[711.3]*
  asylum 004.9
  bacillary 004.9
    arthritis 004.9 *[711.3]*
    Boyd 004.2
    Flexner 004.1

Dysentery, dysenteric—*continued*
  bacillary—*continued*
    Schmitz (-Stutzer) 004.0
    Shiga 004.0
    Shigella 004.9
      group A 004.0
      group B 004.1
      group C 004.2
      group D 004.3
      specified type NEC 004.8
    Sonne 004.3
    specified type NEC 004.8
  bacterium 004.9
  balantidial 007.0
  Balantidium coli 007.0
  Boyd's 004.2
  Chilomastix 007.8
  Chinese 004.9
  choleriform 001.1
  coccidial 007.2
  Dientamoeba fragilis 007.8
  due to specified organism NEC—*see* Enteritis,
    due to, by organism
  Embadomonas 007.8
  Endolimax nana—*see* Dysentery, amebic
  Entamoba, entamebic—*see* Dysentery, amebic
  Flexner's 004.1
  Flexner-Boyd 004.2
  giardial 007.1
  Giardia lamblia 007.1
  Hiss-Russell 004.1
  lamblia 007.1
  leishmanial 085.0
  malarial (*see also* Malaria) 084.6
  metazoal 127.9
  Monilia 112.89
  protozoal NEC 007.9
  Russell's 004.8
  salmonella 003.0
  schistosomal 120.1
  Schmitz (-Stutzer) 004.0
  Shiga 004.0
  Shigella NEC (*see also* Dysentery, bacillary)
    004.9
    boydii 004.2
    dysenteriae 004.0
      Schmitz 004.0
      Shiga 004.0
    flexneri 004.1
    Group A 004.0
    Group B 004.1
    Group C 004.2
    Group D 004.3
    Schmitz 004.0
    Shiga 004.0
    Sonnei 004.3
  Sonne 004.3
  strongyloidiasis 127.2
  trichomonal 007.3
  tuberculous (*see also* Tuberculosis) 014.8
  viral (*see also* Enteritis, viral) 008.8
Dysequilibrium 780.4
Dysesthesia 782.0
  hysterical 300.11
Dysfibrinogenemia (congenital) (*see also* Defect,
    coagulation) 286.3
Dysfunction
  adrenal (cortical) 255.9
    hyperfunction 255.3
    hypofunction 255.41

Dysfunction—*continued*
  associated with sleep stages or arousal from
    sleep 780.56
    nonorganic origin 307.47
  bladder NEC 596.59
  bleeding, uterus 626.8
  brain, minimal (*see also* Hyperkinesia) 314.9
  cerebral 348.30
  colon 564.9
    psychogenic 306.4
  colostomy or enterostomy 569.62
  cystic duct 575.8
  diastolic 429.9
    with heart failure—*see* Failure, heart
    due to
      cardiomyopathy—*see* Cardiomyopathy
      hypertension—*see* Hypertension, heart
  endocrine NEC 259.9
  endometrium 621.8
  enteric stoma 569.62
  enterostomy 569.62
  erectile 607.84
    nonorganic origin 302.72
  esophagostomy 530.87
  Eustachian tube 381.81
  gallbladder 575.8
  gastrointestinal 536.9
  gland, glandular NEC 259.9
  heart 427.9
    postoperative (immediate) 997.1
      long-term effect of cardiac surgery 429.4
  hemoglobin 289.89
  hepatic 573.9
  hepatocellular NEC 573.9
  hypophysis 253.9
    hyperfunction 253.1
    hypofunction 253.2
    posterior lobe 253.6
      hypofunction 253.5
  kidney (*see also* Disease, renal) 593.9
  labyrinthine 386.50
    specified NEC 386.58
  liver 573.9
    constitutional 277.4
  minimal brain (child) (*see also* Hyperkinesia)
    314.9
  ovary, ovarian 256.9
    hyperfunction 256.1
      estrogen 256.0
    hypofunction 256.39
      postablative 256.2
    postablative 256.2
    specified NEC 256.8
  papillary muscle 429.81
    with myocardial infarction 410.8
  parathyroid 252.8
    hyperfunction 252.00
    hypofunction 252.1
  pineal gland 259.8
  pituitary (gland) 253.9
    hyperfunction 253.1
    hypofunction 253.2
    posterior 253.6
      hypofunction 253.5
  placental—*see* Placenta, insufficiency
  platelets (blood) 287.1
  polyglandular 258.9
    specified NEC 258.8

Dysfunction—*continued*
psychosexual 302.70
  with
    dyspareunia (functional) (psychogenic)
      302.76
    frigidity 302.72
    impotence 302.72
    inhibition
      orgasm
        female 302.73
        male 302.74
      sexual
        desire 302.71
        excitement 302.72
    premature ejaculation 302.75
    sexual aversion 302.79
    specified disorder NEC 302.79
    vaginismus 306.51
pylorus 537.9
rectum 564.9
  psychogenic 306.4
segmental (*see also* Dysfunction, somatic) 739.9
senile 797
sexual 302.70
sinoatrial node 427.81
somatic 739.9
  abdomen 739.9
  acromioclavicular 739.7
  cervical 739.1
  cervicothoracic 739.1
  costochondral 739.8
  costovertebral 739.8
  extremities
    lower 739.6
    upper 739.7
  head 739.0
  hip 739.5
  umbar, lumbosacral 739.3
  occipitocervical 739.0
  pelvic 739.5
  pubic 739.5
  rib cage 739.8
  sacral 739.4
  sacrococcygeal 739.4
  sacroiliac 739.4
  specified site NEC 739.9
  sternochondral 739.8
  sternoclavicular 739.7
  temporomandibular 739.0
  thoracic, thoracolumbar 739.2
stomach 536.9
  psychogenic 306.4
suprarenal 255.9
  hyperfunction 255.3
  hypofunction 255.41
symbolic NEC 784.60
  specified type NEC 784.69
systolic 429.9
  with heart failure—*see* Failure, heart
temporomandibular (joint)
  (joint-pain-syndrome) NEC 524.60
  sounds on opening or closing 524.64
  specified NEC 524.69
testicular 257.9
  hyperfunction 257.0
  hypofunction 257.2
  specified type NEC 257.8
thymus 254.9

Dysfunction—*continued*
thyroid 246.9
  complicating pregnancy, childbirth, or
    puerperium 648.1
  hyperfunction—*see* Hyperthyroidism
  hypofunction—*see* Hypothyroidism
uterus, complicating delivery 661.9
  affecting fetus or newborn 763.7
  hypertonic 661.4
  hypotonic 661.2
    primary 661.0
    secondary 661.1
velopharyngeal (acquired) 528.9
  congenital 750.29
ventricular 429.9
  with congestive heart failure (*see also* Failure,
    heart) 428.0
  due to
    cardiomyopathy—*see* Cardiomyopathy
    hypertension—*see* Hypertension, heart
  left, reversible following sudden emotional
    stress 429.83
vesicourethral NEC 596.59
vestibular 386.50
  specified type NEC 386.58
Dysgammaglobulinemia 279.06
Dysgenesis
gonadal (due to chromosomal anomaly) 758.6
  pure 752.7
kidney(s) 753.0
ovarian 758.6
renal 753.0
reticular 279.2
seminiferous tubules 758.6
tidal platelet 287.31
Dysgerminoma (M9060/3)
specified site—*see* Neoplasm, by site, malignant
unspecified site
  female 183.0
  male 186.9
Dysgeusia 781.1
Dysgraphia 781.3
Dyshidrosis 705.81
Dysidrosis 705.81
Dysinsulinism 251.8
Dyskaryotic cervical smear 795.09
Dyskeratosis (*see also* Keratosis) 701.1
bullosa hereditaria 757.39
cervix 622.10
congenital 757.39
follicularis 757.39
  vitamin A deficiency 264.8
gingiva 523.8
oral soft tissue NEC 528.79
tongue 528.79
uterus NEC 621.8
Dyskinesia 781.3
biliary 575.8
esophagus 530.5
hysterical 300.11
intestinal 564.89
neuroleptic-induced tardive 333.85
nonorganic origin 307.9
orofacial 333.82
  due to drugs 333.85
psychogenic 307.9
subacute, due to drugs 333.85
tardive (oral) 333.85
Dyslalia 784.59
developmental 315.39

Dyslexia 784.61
  developmental 315.02
  secondary to organic lesion 784.61
Dyslipidemia 272.4
Dysmaturity (*see also* Immaturity) 765.1
  lung 770.4
  pulmonary 770.4
Dysmenorrhea (essential) (exfoliative)
    (functional) (intrinsic) (membranous)
    (primary) (secondary) 625.3
  psychogenic 306.52
Dysmetabolic syndrome X 277.7
Dysmetria 781.3
Dysmorodystrophia mesodermalis congenita
    759.82
Dysnomia 784.3
Dysorexia 783.0
  hysterical 300.11
Dysostosis
  cleidocranial, cleidocranialis 755.59
  craniofacial 756.0
  Fairbank's (idiopathic familial generalized
      osteophytosis) 756.50
  mandibularis 756.0
  mandibulofacial, incomplete 756.0
  multiplex 277.5
  orodigitofacial 759.89
Dyspareunia (female) 625.0
  male 608.89
  psychogenic 302.76
Dyspepsia (allergic) (congenital) (fermentative)
    (flatulent) (functional) (gastric) (gastrointestinal)
    (neurogenic) (occupational) (reflex) 536.8
  acid 536.8
  atonic 536.3
    psychogenic 306.4
  diarrhea 787.91
    psychogenic 306.4
  intestinal 564.89
    psychogenic 306.4
  nervous 306.4
  neurotic 306.4
  psychogenic 306.4
Dysphagia 787.20
  cervical 787.29
  functional 300.11
  hysterical 300.11
  nervous 300.11
  neurogenic 787.29
  oral phase 787.21
  oropharyngeal phase 787.22
  pharyngeal phase 787.23
  pharyngoesophageal phase 787.24
  psychogenic 306.4
  sideropenic 280.8
  spastica 530.5
  specified NEC 787.29
Dysphagocytosis, congenital 288.1
Dysphasia 784.59
Dysphonia 784.42
  clericorum 784.49
  functional 300.11
  hysterical 300.11
  psychogenic 306.1
  spastica 478.79
Dyspigmentation —*see also* Pigmentation
  eyelid (acquired) 374.52
Dyspituitarism 253.9
  hyperfunction 253.1
  hypofunction 253.2
  posterior lobe 253.6

Dysplasia —*see also* Anomaly
  alveolar capillary, with vein misalignment
      516.64
  anus 569.44
    intraepithelial neoplasia I (AIN I)
        (histologically confirmed) 569.44
    intraepithelial neoplasia II (AIN II)
        (histologically confirmed) 569.44
    intraepithelial neoplasia III (AIN III) 230.6
      anal canal 230.5
    mild (histologically confirmed) 569.44
    moderate (histologically confirmed) 569.44
    severe 230.6
      anal canal 230.5
  artery
    fibromuscular NEC 447.8
      carotid 447.8
      renal 447.3
  bladder 596.89
  bone (fibrous) NEC 733.29
    diaphyseal, progressive 756.59
    jaw 526.89
    monostotic 733.29
    polyostotic 756.54
    solitary 733.29
  brain 742.9
  bronchopulmonary, fetus or newborn 770.7
  cervix (uteri) 622.10
    cervical intraepithelial neoplasia I (CIN 1)
        622.11
    cervical intraepithelial neoplasia II (CIN II)
        622.12
    cervical intraepithelial neoplasia III (CIN III)
        233.1
    CIN I 622.11
    CIN II 622.12
    CIN III 233.1
    mild 622.11
    moderate 622.12
    severe 233.1
  chondroectodermal 756.55
  chondromatose 756.4
  colon 211.3
  craniocarpotarsal 759.89
  craniometaphyseal 756.89
  dentinal 520.5
  diaphyseal, progressive 756.59
  ectodermal (anhidrotic) (Bason) (Clouston's)
      (congenital) (Feinmesser) (hereditary)
      (hidrotic) (Marshall) (Robinson's) 757.31
  epiphysealis 756.9
    multiplex 756.56
    punctata 756.59
  epiphysis 756.9
    multiple 756.56
  epithelial
    epiglottis 478.79
    uterine cervix 622.10
  erythroid NEC 289.89
  eye (*see also* Microphthalmos) 743.10
  familial metaphyseal 756.89
  fibromuscular, artery NEC 447.8
    carotid 447.8
    renal 447.3
  fibrous
    bone NEC 733.29
    diaphyseal, progressive 756.59
    jaw 526.89
    monostotic 733.29
    polyostotic 756.54
    solitary 733.29

Dysplasia—*continued*
high grade, focal—*see* Neoplasm, by site, benign
hip (congenital) 755.63
with dislocation (*see also* Dislocation, hip,
congenital) 754.30
hypohidrotic ectodermal 757.31
joint 755.8
kidney 753.15
leg 755.69
linguofacialis 759.89
lung 748.5
macular 743.55
mammary (benign) (gland) 610.9
cystic 610.1
specified type NEC 610.8
metaphyseal 756.9
familial 756.89
monostotic fibrous 733.29
muscle 756.89
myeloid NEC 289.89
nervous system (general) 742.9
neuroectodermal 759.6
oculoauriculovertebral 756.0
oculodentodigital 759.89
olfactogenital 253.4
osteo-onycho-arthro (hereditary) 756.89
periosteum 733.99
polyostotic fibrous 756.54
progressive diaphyseal 756.59
prostate 602.3
intraepithelial neoplasia I (PIN I) 602.3
intraepithelial neoplasia II (PIN II) 602.3
intraepithelial neoplasia III (PIN III) 233.4
renal 753.15
renofacialis 753.0
retinal NEC 743.56
retrolental (*see also* Retinopathy of prematurity)
362.21
skin 709.8
spinal cord 742.9
thymic, with immunodeficiency 279.2
vagina 623.0
mild 623.0
moderate 623.0
severe 233.31
vocal cord 478.5
vulva 624.8
intraepithelial neoplasia I (VIN I) 624.01
intraepithelial neoplasia II (VIN II) 624.02
intraepithelial neoplasia III (VIN III) 233.32
mild 624.01
moderate 624.02
severe 233.32
VIN I 624.01
VIN II 624.02
VIN III 233.32
Dyspnea (nocturnal) (paroxysmal) 786.09
asthmatic (bronchial) (*see also* Asthma) 493.9
with bronchitis (*see also* Asthma) 493.9
chronic 493.2
cardiac (*see also* Failure, ventricular, left) 428.1
cardiac (*see also* Failure, ventricular, left) 428.1
functional 300.11
hyperventilation 786.01
hysterical 300.11
Monday morning 504
newborn 770.89
psychogenic 306.1
uremic—*see* Uremia
Dyspraxia 781.3
syndrome 315.4

Dysproteinemia 273.8
transient with copper deficiency 281.4
Dysprothrombinemia (constitutional) (*see also*
Defect, coagulation) 286.3
Dysreflexia, autonomic 337.3
Dysrhythmia
cardiac 427.9
postoperative (immediate) 997.1
long-term effect of cardiac surgery 429.4
specified type NEC 427.89
cerebral or cortical 348.30
Dyssecretosis, mucoserous 710.2
**Dyssocial reaction without manifest psychiatric
disorder**
adolescent V71.02
adult V71.01
child V71.02
Dyssomnia NEC 780.56
nonorganic origin 307.47
Dyssplenism 289.4
Dyssynergia
biliary (*see also* Disease, biliary) 576.8
cerebellaris myoclonica 334.2
detrusor sphincter (bladder) 596.55
ventricular 429.89
Dystasia, hereditary areflexic 334.3
Dysthymia 300.4
Dysthymic disorder 300.4
Dysthyroidism 246.9
Dystocia 660.9
affecting fetus or newborn 763.1
cervical 661.2
affecting fetus or newborn 763.7
contraction ring 661.4
affecting fetus or newborn 763.7
fetal 660.9
abnormal size 653.5
affecting fetus or newborn 763.1
deformity 653.7
maternal 660.9
affecting fetus or newborn 763.1
positional 660.0
affecting fetus or newborn 763.1
shoulder (girdle) 660.4
affecting fetus or newborn 763.1
uterine NEC 661.4
affecting fetus or newborn 763.7
Dystonia
acute
due to drugs 333.72
neuroleptic-induced acute 333.72
deformans progressiva 333.6
lenticularis 333.6
musculorum deformans 333.6
torsion (idiopathic) 333.6
acquired 333.79
fragments (of) 333.89
genetic 333.6
symptomatic 333.79
Dystonic
movements 781.0
Dystopia kidney 753.3
Dystrophy, dystrophia 783.9
adiposogenital 253.8
asphyxiating thoracic 756.4
Becker's type 359.22
brevicollis 756.16
Bruch's membrane 362.77
cervical (sympathetic) NEC 337.09
chondro-osseous with punctate epiphyseal
dysplasia 756.59

Dystrophy, dystrophia—*continued*
  choroid (hereditary) 363.50
    central (areolar) (partial) 363.53
      total (gyrate) 363.54
    circinate 363.53
    circumpapillary (partial) 363.51
      total 363.52
    diffuse
      partial 363.56
      total 363.57
    generalized
      partial 363.56
      total 363.57
    gyrate
      central 363.54
      generalized 363.57
    helicoid 363.52
    peripapillary—*see* Dystrophy, choroid,
      circumpapillary
    serpiginous 363.54
  cornea (hereditary) 371.50
    anterior NEC 371.52
    Cogan's 371.52
    combined 371.57
    crystalline 371.56
    endothelial (Fuchs') 371.57
    epithelial 371.50
      juvenile 371.51
      microscopic cystic 371.52
    granular 371.53
    lattice 371.54
    macular 371.55
    marginal (Terrien's) 371.48
    Meesman's 371.51
    microscopic cystic (epithelial) 371.52
    nodular, Salzmann's 371.46
    polymorphous 371.58
    posterior NEC 371.58
    ring-like 371.52
    Salzmann's nodular 371.46
    stromal NEC 371.56
  dermatochondrocorneal 371.50
  Duchenne's 359.1
  due to malnutrition 263.9
  Erb's 359.1
  familial
    hyperplastic periosteal 756.59
    osseous 277.5
  foveal 362.77
  Fuchs', cornea 371.57
  Gowers' muscular 359.1
  hair 704.2
  hereditary, progressive muscular 359.1
  hypogenital, with diabetic tendency 759.81
  Landouzy-Déjérine 359.1
  Leyden-Möbius 359.1
  mesodermalis congenita 759.82
  muscular 359.1
    congenital (hereditary) 359.0
      myotonic 359.22
    distal 359.1
    Duchenne's 359.1
    Erb's 359.1
    fascioscapulohumeral 359.1
    Gowers' 359.1
    hereditary (progressive) 359.1
    Landouzy-Déjérine 359.1
    limb-girdle 359.1
    myotonic 359.21
    progressive (hereditary) 359.1
      Charcot-Marie-Tooth 356.1
    pseudohypertrophic (infantile) 359.1

Dystrophy, dystrophia—*continued*
  myocardium, myocardial (*see also*
    Degeneration, myocardial) 429.1
  myotonic 359.21
  myotonica 359.21
  nail 703.8
    congenital 757.5
  neurovascular (traumatic) (*see also* Neuropathy,
    peripheral, autonomic) 337.9
  nutritional 263.9
  ocular 359.1
  oculocerebrorenal 270.8
  oculopharyngeal 359.1
  ovarian 620.8
  papillary (and pigmentary) 701.1
  pelvicrural atrophic 359.1
  pigmentary (*see also* Acanthosis) 701.2
  pituitary (gland) 253.8
  polyglandular 258.8
  posttraumatic sympathetic—*see* Dystrophy,
    sympathetic
  progressive ophthalmoplegic 359.1
  reflex neuromuscular—*see* Dystrophy,
    sympathetic
  retina, retinal (hereditary) 362.70
    albipunctate 362.74
    Bruch's membrane 362.77
    cone, progressive 362.75
    hyaline 362.77
    in
      Bassen-Kornzweig syndrome 272.5
        [362.72]
      cerebroretinal lipidosis 330.1 *[362.71]*
      Refsum's disease 356.3 *[362.72]*
      systemic lipidosis 272.7 *[362.71]*
    juvenile (Stargardt's) 362.75
    pigmentary 362.74
    pigment epithelium 362.76
    progressive cone (-rod) 362.75
    pseudoinflammatory foveal 362.77
    rod, progressive 362.75
    sensory 362.75
    vitelliform 362.76
  Salzmann's nodular 371.46
  scapuloperoneal 359.1
  skin NEC 709.9
  sympathetic (posttraumatic) (reflex) 337.20
    lower limb 337.22
    specified NEC 337.29
    upper limb 337.21
  tapetoretinal NEC 362.74
  thoracic asphyxiating 756.4
  unguium 703.8
    congenital 757.5
  vitreoretinal (primary) 362.73
    secondary 362.66
  vulva 624.09
Dysuria 788.1
  psychogenic 306.53

E

Eagle-Barrett syndrome 756.71
Eales' disease (syndrome) 362.18
Ear —*see also* condition
 ache 388.70
  otogenic 388.71
  referred 388.72
 lop 744.29
 piercing V50.3
 swimmers' acute 380.12
 tank 380.12
 tropical 111.8 *[380.15]*
 wax 380.4
Earache 388.70
 otogenic 388.71
 referred 388.72
Early satiety 780.94
Eaton-Lambert syndrome (*see also* Syndrome,
  Lambert-Eaton) 358.30
Eberth's disease (typhoid fever) 002.0
Ebstein's
 anomaly or syndrome (downward displacement,
  tricuspid valve into right ventricle) 746.2
 disease (diabetes) 250.4 *[581.81]*
  due to secondary diabetes 249.4 *[581.81]*
Eccentro-osteochondrodysplasia 277.5
Ecchondroma (M9210/0)—*see* Neoplasm, bone,
  benign
Ecchondrosis (M9210/1) 238.0
Ecchordosis physaliphora 756.0
Ecchymosis (multiple) 459.89
 conjunctiva 372.72
 eye (traumatic) 921.0
 eyelids (traumatic) 921.1
 newborn 772.6
 spontaneous 782.7
 traumatic—*see* Contusion
ECD (Erdheim-Chester disease) 277.89
Echinococciasis —*see* Echinococcus
Echinococcosis —*see* Echinococcus
Echinococcus (infection) 122.9
 granulosus 122.4
  liver 122.0
  lung 122.1
  orbit 122.3 *[376.13]*
  specified site NEC 122.3
  thyroid 122.2
 liver NEC 122.8
  granulosus 122.0
  multilocularis 122.5
 lung NEC 122.9
  granulosus 122.1
  multilocularis 122.6
 multilocularis 122.7
  liver 122.5
  specified site NEC 122.6
 orbit 122.9 *[376.13]*
  granulosus 122.3 *[376.13]*
  multilocularis 122.6 *[376.13]*
 specified site NEC 122.9
  granulosus 122.3
  multilocularis 122.6 *[376.13]*
 thyroid NEC 122.9
  granulosus 122.2
  multilocularis 122.6
Echinorhynchiasis 127.7
Echinostomiasis 121.8
Echolalia 784.69
ECHO virus infection NEC 079.1

Eclampsia, eclamptic (coma) (convulsions)
  (delirium) 780.39
 female, child-bearing age NEC—*see* Eclampsia,
  pregnancy
 gravidarum—*see* Eclampsia, pregnancy
 male 780.39
 not associated with pregnancy or childbirth
  780.39
 pregnancy, childbirth or puerperium 642.6
  with pre-existing hypertension 642.7
  affecting fetus or newborn 760.0
 uremic 586
Eclipse blindness (total) 363.31
Economic circumstance affecting care V60.9
 specified type NEC V60.89
Economo's disease (encephalitis lethargica) 049.8
Ectasia, ectasis
 annuloaortic 424.1
 aorta (*see also* Ectasia, aortic) 447.70
  with aneurysm 441.9
  ruptured 441.5
 aortic 447.70
  with aneurysm 441.9
  abdominal 447.72
  thoracic 447.71
  thoracoabdominal 447.73
 breast 610.4
 capillary 448.9
 cornea (marginal) (postinfectional) 371.71
 duct (mammary) 610.4
 gastric antral vascular (GAVE) 537.82
  with hemorrhage 537.83
  without hemorrhage 537.82
 kidney 593.89
 mammary duct (gland) 610.4
 papillary 448.9
 renal 593.89
 salivary gland (duct) 527.8
 scar, cornea 371.71
 sclera 379.11
Ecthyma 686.8
 contagiosum 051.2
 gangrenosum 686.09
 infectiosum 051.2
Ectocardia 746.87
Ectodermal dysplasia, congenital 757.31
Ectodermosis erosiva pluriorificialis 695.19
Ectopic, ectopia (congenital) 759.89
 abdominal viscera 751.8
  due to defect in anterior abdominal wall
   756.79
 ACTH syndrome 255.0
 adrenal gland 759.1
 anus 751.5
 auricular beats 427.61
 beats 427.60
 bladder 753.5
 bone and cartilage in lung 748.69
 brain 742.4
 breast tissue 757.6
 cardiac 746.87
 cerebral 742.4
 cordis 746.87
 endometrium 617.9
 gallbladder 751.69
 gastric mucosa 750.7
 gestation—*see* Pregnancy, ectopic
 heart 746.87

Ectopic, ectopia—*continued*
  hormone secretion NEC 259.3
  hyperparathyroidism 259.3
  kidney (crossed) (intrathoracic) (pelvis) 753.3
    in pregnancy or childbirth 654.4
      causing obstructed labor 660.2
  lens 743.37
  lentis 743.37
  mole—*see* Pregnancy, ectopic
  organ or site NEC—*see* Malposition, congenital
  ovary 752.0
  pancreas, pancreatic tissue 751.7
  pregnancy—*see* Pregnancy, ectopic
  pupil 364.75
  renal 753.3
  sebaceous glands of mouth 750.26
  secretion
    ACTH 255.0
    adrenal hormone 259.3
    adrenalin 259.3
    adrenocorticotropin 255.0
    antidiuretic hormone (ADH) 259.3
    epinephrine 259.3
    hormone NEC 259.3
    norepinephrine 259.3
    pituitary (posterior) 259.3
  spleen 759.0
  testis 752.51
  thyroid 759.2
  ureter 753.4
  ventricular beats 427.69
  vesicae 753.5
Ectrodactyly 755.4
  finger (*see also* Absence, finger, congenital) 755.29
  toe (*see also* Absence, toe, congenital) 755.39
Ectromelia 755.4
  lower limb 755.30
  upper limb 755.20
Ectropion 374.10
  anus 569.49
  cervix 622.0
    with mention of cervicitis 616.0
  cicatricial 374.14
  congenital 743.62
  eyelid 374.10
    cicatricial 374.14
    congenital 743.62
    mechanical 374.12
    paralytic 374.12
    senile 374.11
    spastic 374.13
  iris (pigment epithelium) 364.54
  lip (congenital) 750.26
    acquired 528.5
  mechanical 374.12
  paralytic 374.12
  rectum 569.49
  senile 374.11
  spastic 374.13
  urethra 599.84
  uvea 364.54
Eczema (acute) (allergic) (chronic)
    (erythematous) (fissum) (occupational)
    (rubrum) (squamous) 692.9
  asteatotic 706.8
  atopic 691.8
  contact NEC 692.9
  dermatitis NEC 692.9
  due to specified cause—*see* Dermatitis, due to
  dyshidrotic 705.81
  external ear 380.22
  flexural 691.8

Eczema—*continued*
  gouty 274.89
  herpeticum 054.0
  hypertrophicum 701.8
  hypostatic—*see* Varicose, vein
  impetiginous 684
  infantile (acute) (chronic) (due to any substance)
    (intertriginous) (seborrheic) 690.12
  intertriginous NEC 692.9
    infantile 690.12
  intrinsic 691.8
  lichenified NEC 692.9
  marginatum 110.3
  nummular 692.9
  pustular 686.8
  seborrheic 690.18
    infantile 690.12
  solare 692.72
  stasis (lower extremity) 454.1
    ulcerated 454.2
  vaccination, vaccinatum 999.0
  varicose (lower extremity)—*see* Varicose, vein
  verrucosum callosum 698.3
Eczematoid, exudative 691.8
Eddowes' syndrome (brittle bones and blue
    sclera) 756.51
Edema, edematous 782.3
  with nephritis (*see also* Nephrosis) 581.9
  allergic 995.1
  angioneurotic (allergic) (any site) (with
    urticaria) 995.1
    hereditary 277.6
  angiospastic 443.9
  Berlin's (traumatic) 921.3
  brain (cytotoxic) (vasogenic) 348.5
    due to birth injury 767.8
    fetus or newborn 767.8
  cardiac (*see also* Failure, heart) 428.0
  cardiovascular (*see also* Failure, heart) 428.0
  cerebral—*see* Edema, brain
  cerebrospinal vessel—*see* Edema, brain
  cervix (acute) (uteri) 622.8
    puerperal, postpartum 674.8
  chronic hereditary 757.0
  circumscribed, acute 995.1
    hereditary 277.6
  complicating pregnancy (gestational) 646.1
    with hypertension—*see* Toxemia, of pregnancy
  conjunctiva 372.73
  connective tissue 782.3
  cornea 371.20
    due to contact lenses 371.24
    idiopathic 371.21
    secondary 371.22
  due to
    lymphatic obstruction—*see* Edema, lymphatic
    salt retention 276.0
  epiglottis—*see* Edema, glottis
  essential, acute 995.1
    hereditary 277.6
  extremities, lower—*see* Edema, legs
  eyelid NEC 374.82
  familial, hereditary (legs) 757.0
  famine 262
  fetus or newborn 778.5
  genital organs
    female 629.89
    male 608.86
  gestational 646.1
    with hypertension—*see* Toxemia, of pregnancy

Edema, edematous—*continued*
glottis, glottic, glottides (obstructive) (passive)
478.6
allergic 995.1
hereditary 277.6
due to external agent—*see* Condition,
respiratory, acute, due to specified agent
heart (*see also* Failure, heart) 428.0
newborn 779.89
heat 992.7
hereditary (legs) 757.0
inanition 262
infectious 782.3
intracranial 348.5
due to injury at birth 767.8
iris 364.89
joint (*see also* Effusion, joint) 719.0
larynx (*see also* Edema, glottis) 478.6
legs 782.3
due to venous obstruction 459.2
hereditary 757.0
localized 782.3
due to venous obstruction 459.2
lower extremity 459.2
lower extremities—*see* Edema, legs
lungs 514
acute 518.4
with heart disease or failure (*see also*
Failure, ventricular, left) 428.1
congestive 428.0
chemical (due to fumes or vapors) 506.1
due to
external agent(s) NEC 508.9
specified NEC 508.8
fumes and vapors (chemical) (inhalation)
506.1
radiation 508.0
chemical (acute) 506.1
chronic 506.4
chronic 514
chemical (due to fumes or vapors) 506.4
due to
external agent(s) NEC 508.9
specified NEC 508.8
fumes or vapors (chemical) (inhalation)
506.4
radiation 508.1
due to
external agent 508.9
specified NEC 508.8
high altitude 993.2
near drowning 994.1
postoperative 518.4
terminal 514
lymphatic 457.1
due to mastectomy operation 457.0
macula 362.83
cystoid 362.53
diabetic 250.5 *[362.07]*
due to secondary diabetes 249.5 *[362.07]*
malignant (*see also* Gangrene, gas) 040.0
Milroy's 757.0
nasopharynx 478.25
neonatorum 778.5
nutritional (newborn) 262
with dyspigmentation, skin and hair 260
optic disc or nerve—*see* Papilledema
orbit 376.33
circulatory 459.89
palate (soft) (hard) 528.9
pancreas 577.8

Edema, edematous—*continued*
penis 607.83
periodic 995.1
hereditary 277.6
pharynx 478.25
pitting 782.3
pulmonary—*see* Edema, lung
Quincke's 995.1
hereditary 277.6
renal (*see also* Nephrosis) 581.9
retina (localized) (macular) (peripheral) 362.83
cystoid 362.53
diabetic 250.5 *[362.07]*
due to secondary diabetes 249.5 *[362.07]*
salt 276.0
scrotum 608.86
seminal vesicle 608.86
spermatic cord 608.86
spinal cord 336.1
starvation 262
stasis (*see also* Hypertension, venous) 459.30
subconjunctival 372.73
subglottic (*see also* Edema, glottis) 478.6
supraglottic (*see also* Edema, glottis) 478.6
testis 608.86
toxic NEC 782.3
traumatic NEC 782.3
tunica vaginalis 608.86
vas deferens 608.86
vocal cord—*see* Edema, glottis
vulva (acute) 624.8
Edentia (complete) (partial) (*see also* Absence,
tooth) 520.0
acquired (*see also* Edentulism) 525.40
due to
caries 525.13
extraction 525.10
periodontal disease 525.12
specified NEC 525.19
trauma 525.11
causing malocclusion 524.30
congenital (deficiency of tooth buds) 520.0
Edentulism 525.40
complete 525.40
class I 525.41
class II 525.42
class III 525.43
class IV 525.44
partial 525.50
class I 525.51
class II 525.52
class III 525.53
class IV 525.54
Edsall's disease 992.2
Educational handicap V62.3
Edwards' syndrome 758.2
Effect, adverse NEC
abnormal gravitational (G) forces or states 994.9
air pressure—*see* Effect, adverse, atmospheric
pressure
altitude (high)—*see* Effect, adverse, high altitude
anesthetic
in labor and delivery NEC 668.9
affecting fetus or newborn 763.5
antitoxin—*see* Complications, vaccination
atmospheric pressure 993.9
due to explosion 993.4
high 993.3
low—*see* Effect, adverse, high altitude
specified effect NEC 993.8

Effect, adverse—*continued*
  biological, correct substance properly
    administered (*see also* Effect, adverse, drug)
    995.20
  blood (derivatives) (serum) (transfusion)—*see*
    Complications, transfusion
  chemical substance NEC 989.9
    specified—*see* Table of drugs and chemicals
  cobalt, radioactive (*see also* Effect, adverse,
    radioactive substance) 990
  cold (temperature) (weather) 991.9
    chilblains 991.5
    frostbite—*see* Frostbite
    specified effect NEC 991.8
  drugs and medicinals 995.20
    correct substance properly administered
      995.20
    overdose or wrong substance given or taken
      977.9
    specified drug—*see* Table of drugs and
      chemicals
  electric current (shock) 994.8
    burn—*see* Burn, by site
  electricity (electrocution) (shock) 994.8
    burn—*see* Burn, by site
  exertion (excessive) 994.5
  exposure 994.9
    exhaustion 994.4
  external cause NEC 994.9
  fallout (radioactive) NEC 990
  fluoroscopy NEC 990
  foodstuffs
    allergic reaction (*see also* Allergy, food) 693.1
    anaphylactic reaction or shock due to food
      NEC—*see* Anaphylactic reaction or shock,
      due to food
    noxious 988.9
      specified type NEC (*see also* Poisoning, by
      name of noxious foodstuff) 988.8
  gases, fumes, or vapors—*see* Table of drugs and
    chemicals
  glue (airplane) sniffing 304.6
  heat—*see* Heat
  high altitude NEC 993.2
    anoxia 993.2
    on
      fears 993.0
      sinuses 993.1
    polycythemia 289.0
  hot weather—*see* Heat
  hunger 994.2
  immersion, foot 991.4
  immunization—*see* Complications, vaccination
  immunological agents—*see* Complications,
    vaccination
  implantation (removable) of isotope or radium
    NEC 990
  infrared (radiation) (rays) NEC 990
    burn—*see* Burn, by site
    dermatitis or eczema 692.82
  infusion—*see* Complications, infusion
  ingestion or injection of isotope (therapeutic)
    NEC 990
  irradiation NEC (*see also* Effect, adverse,
    radiation) 990
  isotope (radioactive) NEC 990
  lack of care (child) (infant) (newborn) 995.52
    adult 995.84
  lightning 994.0
    burn—*see* Burn, by site
  Lirugin—*see* Complications, vaccination

Effect, adverse—*continued*
  medicinal substance, correct, properly
    administered (*see also* Effect, adverse,
    drugs) 995.20
  mesothorium NEC 990
  motion 994.6
  noise, inner ear 388.10
  other drug, medicinal and biological substance
    995.29
  overheated places—*see* Heat
  polonium NEC 990
  psychosocial, of work environment V62.1
  radiation (diagnostic) (fallout) (infrared) (natural
    source) (therapeutic) (tracer) (ultraviolet)
    (x-ray) NEC 990
    with pulmonary manifestations
      acute 508.0
      chronic 508.1
    dermatitis or eczema 692.82
      due to sun NEC (*see also* Dermatitis, due to,
      sun) 692.70
    fibrosis of lungs 508.1
    maternal with suspected damage to fetus
      affecting management of pregnancy 655.6
    pneumonitis 508.0
  radioactive substance NEC 990
    dermatitis or eczema 692.82
  radioactivity NEC 990
  radiotherapy NEC 990
    dermatitis or eczema 692.82
  radium NEC 990
  reduced temperature 991.9
    frostbite—*see* Frostbite
    immersion, foot (hand) 991.4
    specified effect NEC 991.8
  roentgenography NEC 990
  roentgenoscopy NEC 990
  roentgen rays NEC 990
  serum (prophylactic) (therapeutic) NEC 999.59
  specified NEC 995.89
    external cause NEC 994.9
  strangulation 994.7
  submersion 994.1
  teletherapy NEC 990
  thirst 994.3
  transfusion—*see* Complications, transfusion
  ultraviolet (radiation) (rays) NEC 990
    burn—*see also* Burn, by site
      from sun (*see also* Sunburn) 692.71
    dermatitis or eczema 692.82
      due to sun NEC (*see also* Dermatitis, due to,
      sun) 692.70
  uranium NEC 990
  vaccine (any)—*see* Complications, vaccination
  weightlessness 994.9
  whole blood—*see also* Complications,
    transfusion
    overdose or wrong substance given (*see also*
      Table of drugs and chemicals) 964.7
  working environment V62.1
  x-rays NEC 990
    dermatitis or eczema 692.82
Effect, remote
  of cancer —*see* condition
Effects, late —*see* Late, effect (of)
Effluvium, telogen 704.02
Effort
  intolerance 306.2
  syndrome (aviators) (psychogenic) 306.2

Effusion
  Amniotic fluid (*see also* Rupture, membranes,
    premature) 658.1
  brain (serous) 348.5
  bronchial (*see also* Bronchitis) 490
  cerebral 348.5
  cerebrospinal (*see also* Meningitis) 322.9
    vessel 348.5
  chest—*see* Effusion, pleura
  intracranial 348.5
  joint 719.00
    ankle 719.07
    elbow 719.02
    foot 719.07
    hand 719.04
    hip 719.05
    knee 719.06
    multiple sites 719.09
    pelvic region 719.05
    shoulder (region) 719.01
    specified site NEC 719.08
    wrist 719.03
  meninges (*see also* Meningitis) 322.9
  pericardium, pericardial (*see also* Pericarditis) 423.9
    acute 420.90
  peritoneal (chronic) 568.82
  pleura, pleurisy, pleuritic, pleuropericardial 511.9
    bacterial, nontuberculous 511.1
    fetus or newborn 511.9
    malignant 511.81
    nontuberculous 511.9
      bacterial 511.1
    pneumococcal 511.1
    staphylococcal 511.1
    streptococcal 511.1
    tuberculous (*see also* Tuberculosis, pleura) 012.0
      primary progressive 010.1
    traumatic 862.29
      with open wound 862.39
  pulmonary—*see* Effusion, pleura
  spinal (*see also* Meningitis) 322.9
  thorax, thoracic—*see* Effusion, pleura
Egg (oocyte) (ovum)
  donor V59.70
    age 35 and over V59.73
      anonymous recipient V59.73
      designated recipient V59.74
    under age 35 V59.71
      anonymous recipient V59.71
      designated recipient V59.72
Eggshell nails 703.8
  congenital 757.5
Ego-dystonic
  homosexuality 302.0
  lesbianism 302.0
  sexual orientation 302.0
Egyptian splenomegaly 120.1
Ehlers-Danlos syndrome 756.83
Ehrlichiosis 082.40
  chaffeensis 082.41
  specified type NEC 082.49
Eichstedt's disease (pityriasis versicolor) 111.0
EIN (endometrial intraepithelial neoplasia) 621.35
Eisenmenger's complex or syndrome
  (ventricular septal defect) 745.4
Ejaculation, semen
  painful 608.89
    psychogenic 306.59
  premature 302.75
  retrograde 608.87
Ekbom syndrome (restless legs) 333.94

Ekman's syndrome (brittle bones and blue
  sclera) 756.51
Elastic skin 756.83
  acquired 701.8
Elastofibroma (M8820/0)—*see* Neoplasm,
  connective tissue, benign
Elastoidosis
  cutanea nodularis 701.8
  cutis cystica et comedonica 701.8
Elastoma 757.39
  juvenile 757.39
  Miescher's (elastosis perforans serpiginosa) 701.1
Elastomyofibrosis 425.3
Elastosis 701.8
  atrophicans 701.8
  perforans serpiginosa 701.1
  reactive perforating 701.1
  senilis 701.8
  solar (actinic) 692.74
Elbow —*see* condition
Electric
  current, electricity, effects (concussion) (fatal)
    (nonfatal) (shock) 994.8
    burn—*see* Burn, by site
  feet (foot) syndrome 266.2
  shock from electroshock gun (taser) 994.8
Electrocution 994.8
Electrolyte imbalance 276.9
  with
    abortion—*see* Abortion, by type, with
      metabolic disorder
    ectopic pregnancy (*see also* categories
      633.0-633.9) 639.4
    hyperemesis gravidarum (before 22 completed
      weeks gestation) 643.1
    molar pregnancy (*see also* categories 630-632)
      639.4
  following
    abortion 639.4
    ectopic or molar pregnancy 639.4
Elephant man syndrome 237.71
Elephantiasis (nonfilarial) 457.1
  arabicum (*see also* Infestation, filarial) 125.9
  congenita hereditaria 757.0
  congenital (any site) 757.0
  due to
    Brugia (malayi) 125.1
    mastectomy operation 457.0
    Wuchereria (bancrofti) 125.0
      malayi 125.1
  eyelid 374.83
  filarial (*see also* Infestation, filarial) 125.9
  filariensis (*see also* Infestation, filarial) 125.9
  gingival 523.8
  glandular 457.1
  graecorum 030.9
  lymphangiectatic 457.1
  lymphatic vessel 457.1
    due to mastectomy operation 457.0
  neuromatosa 237.71
  postmastectomy 457.0
  scrotum 457.1
  streptococcal 457.1
  surgical 997.99
    postmastectomy 457.0
  telangiectodes 457.1
  vulva (nonfilarial) 624.8
Elevated —*see also* Elevation
  findings on laboratory examination — see
    Findings, abnormal, without diagnosis
    (examination) (laboratory test)

Elevated—*continued*
  GFR (glomerular filtration rate) — see Findings,
    abnormal, without diagnosis (examination)
    (laboratory test)
Elevation
  17-ketosteroids 791.9
  acid phosphatase 790.5
  alkaline phosphatase 790.5
  amylase 790.5
  antibody titers 795.79
  basal metabolic rate (BMR) 794.7
  blood pressure (*see also* Hypertension) 401.9
    reading (incidental) (isolated) (nonspecific),
      no diagnosis of hypertension 796.2
  blood sugar 790.29
  body temperature (of unknown origin) (*see also*
    Pyrexia) 780.60
  C-reactive protein (CRP) 790.95
  cancer antigen 125 [CA 125] 795.82
  carcinoembryonic antigen [CEA] 795.81
  cholesterol 272.0
    with high triglycerides 272.2
  conjugate, eye 378.81
  CRP (C-reactive protein) 790.95
  diaphragm, congenital 756.6
  GFR (glomerular filtration rate) — see Findings,
    abnormal, without diagnosis (examination)
    (laboratory test)
  glucose
    fasting 790.21
    tolerance test 790.22
  immunoglobulin level 795.79
  indolacetic acid 791.9
  lactic acid dehydrogenase (LDH) level 790.4
  leukocytes 288.60
  lipase 790.5
  lipoprotein a level 272.8
  liver function test (LFT) 790.6
    alkaline phosphatase 790.5
    aminotransferase 790.4
    bilirubin 782.4
    hepatic enzyme NEC 790.5
    lactate dehydrogenase 790.4
  lymphocytes 288.61
  prostate specific antigen (PSA) 790.93
  renin 790.99
    in hypertension (*see also* Hypertension,
      renovascular) 405.91
  Rh titer (see also Complications, transfusion)
    999.70
  scapula, congenital 755.52
  sedimentation rate 790.1
  SGOT 790.4
  SGPT 790.4
  transaminase 790.4
  triglycerides 272.1
    with high cholesterol 272.2
  vanillylmandelic acid 791.9
  venous pressure 459.89
  VMA 791.9
  white blood cell count 288.60
    specified NEC 288.69
Elliptocytosis (congenital) (hereditary) 282.1
  Hb-C (disease) 282.7
  hemoglobin disease 282.7
  sickle-cell (disease) 282.60
    trait 282.5
Ellis-van Creveld disease or syndrome
  (chondroectodermal dysplasia) 756.55
Ellison-Zollinger syndrome (gastric
  hypersecretion with pancreatic islet cell
  tumor) 251.5

Elongation, elongated (congenital)—*see also*
  Distortion
  bone 756.9
  cervix (uteri) 752.49
    acquired 622.6
    hypertrophic 622.6
  colon 751.5
  common bile duct 751.69
  cystic duct 751.69
  frenulum, penis 752.69
  labia minora, acquired 624.8
  ligamentum patellae 756.89
  petiolus (epiglottidis) 748.3
  styloid bone (process) 733.99
  tooth, teeth 520.2
  uvula 750.26
    acquired 528.9
Elschnig bodies or pearls 366.51
El Tor cholera 001.1
Emaciation (due to malnutrition) 261
Emancipation disorder 309.22
Embadomoniasis 007.8
Embarrassment heart, cardiac —*see* Disease,
  heart
Embedded
  fragment (status) - *see* Foreign body, retained
  splinter (status) - *see* Foreign body, retained
  tooth, teeth 520.6
    root only 525.3
Embolic —*see* condition
Embolism 444.9
  with
    abortion—*see* Abortion, by type, with
      embolism
    ectopic pregnancy (*see also* categories
      633.0-633.9) 639.6
    molar pregnancy (*see also* categories 630-632)
      639.6
  air (any site) 958.0
    with
      abortion—*see* Abortion, by type, with
        embolism
      ectopic pregnancy (*see also* categories
        633.0-633.9) 639.6
      molar pregnancy (*see also* categories
        630-632) 639.6
    due to implanted device—*see* Complications,
      due to (presence of) any device, implant,
      or graft classified to 996.0-996.5 NEC
    following
      abortion 639.6
      ectopic or molar pregnancy 639.6
      infusion, perfusion, or transfusion 999.1
    in pregnancy, childbirth, or puerperium 673.0
    traumatic 958.0
  amniotic fluid (pulmonary) 673.1
    with
      abortion—*see* Abortion, by type, with
        embolism
      ectopic pregnancy (*see also* categories
        633.0-633.9) 639.6
      molar pregnancy (*see also* categories
        630-632) 639.6
    following
      abortion 639.6
      ectopic or molar pregnancy 639.6
  aorta, aortic 444.1
    abdominal 444.09
      saddle 444.01
    bifurcation 444.09
    saddle 444.01
    thoracic 444.1

Embolism—*continued*
  artery 444.9
    auditory, internal 433.8
    basilar (*see also* Occlusion, artery, basilar)
      433.0
    bladder 444.89
    carotid (common) (internal) (*see also*
      Occlusion, artery, carotid) 433.1
    cerebellar (anterior inferior) (posterior
      inferior) (superior) 433.8
    cerebral (*see also* Embolism, brain) 434.1
    choroidal (anterior) 433.8
    communicating posterior 433.8
    coronary (*see also* Infarct, myocardium) 410.9
      without myocardial infarction 411.81
    extremity 444.22
      lower 444.22
      upper 444.21
    hypophyseal 433.8
    mesenteric (with gangrene) 557.0
    ophthalmic (*see also* Occlusion, retina) 362.30
    peripheral 444.22
    pontine 433.8
    precerebral NEC—*see* Occlusion, artery,
      precerebral
    pulmonary—*see* Embolism, pulmonary
    pyemic 449
      pulmonary 415.12
    renal 593.81
    retinal (*see also* Occlusion, retina) 362.30
    septic 449
      pulmonary 415.12
    specified site NEC 444.89
    vertebral (*see also* Occlusion, artery,
      vertebral) 433.2
  auditory, internal 433.8
  basilar (artery) (*see also* Occlusion, artery,
    basilar) 433.0
  birth, mother—*see* Embolism, obstetrical
  blood-clot
    with
      abortion—*see* Abortion, by type, with embolism
      ectopic pregnancy (*see also* categories
        633.0-633.9) 639.6
      molar pregnancy (*see also* categories
        630-632) 639.6
    following
      abortion 639.6
      ectopic or molar pregnancy 639.6
    in pregnancy, childbirth, or puerperium 673.2
  brain 434.1
    with
      abortion—*see* Abortion, by type, with embolism
      ectopic pregnancy (*see also* categories
        633.0-633.9) 639.6
      molar pregnancy (*see also* categories
        630-632) 639.6
    following
      abortion 639.6
      ectopic or molar pregnancy 639.6
    late effect—*see* Late effect(s) (of)
      cerebrovascular disease
    puerperal, postpartum, childbirth 674.0
  capillary 448.9
  cardiac (*see also* Infarct, myocardium) 410.9
  carotid (artery) (common) (internal) (*see also*
    Occlusion, artery, carotid) 433.1
  cavernous sinus (venous)—*see* Embolism,
    intracranial venous sinus
  cerebral (*see also* Embolism, brain) 434.1
  cholesterol—*see* Atheroembolism
  choroidal (anterior) (artery) 433.8

Embolism—*continued*
  coronary (artery or vein) (systemic) (*see also*
    Infarct, myocardium) 410.9
    without myocardial infarction 411.81
  due to (presence of) any device, implant, or graft
    classifiable to 996.0-996.5 —*see*
    Complications, due to (presence of) any
    device, implant, or graft classified to
    996.0-996.5 NEC
  encephalomalacia (*see also* Embolism, brain) 434.1
  extremities 444.22
    lower 444.22
    upper 444.21
  eye 362.30
  fat (cerebral) (pulmonary) (systemic) 958.1
    with
      abortion—*see* Abortion, by type, with embolism
      ectopic pregnancy (*see also* categories
        633.0-633.9) 639.6
      molar pregnancy (*see also* categories
        630-632) 639.6
    complicating delivery or puerperium 673.8
    following
      abortion 639.6
      ectopic or molar pregnancy 639.6
    in pregnancy, childbirth, or the puerperium 673.8
  femoral (artery) 444.22
    vein 453.6
      deep 453.41
  following
    abortion 639.6
    ectopic or molar pregnancy 639.6
    infusion, perfusion, or transfusion
      air 999.1
      thrombus 999.2
  heart (fatty) (*see also* Infarct, myocardium) 410.9
  hepatic (vein) 453.0
  iliac (artery) 444.81
  iliofemoral 444.81
  in pregnancy, childbirth, or puerperium
    (pulmonary)—*see* Embolism, obstetrical
  intestine (artery) (vein) (with gangrene) 557.0
  intracranial (*see also* Embolism, brain) 434.1
    venous sinus (any) 325
      late effect—*see* category 326
      nonpyogenic 437.6
        in pregnancy or puerperium 671.5
  kidney (artery) 593.81
  lateral sinus (venous)—*see* Embolism,
    intracranial venous sinus
  longitudinal sinus (venous)—*see* Embolism,
    intracranial venous sinus
  lower extremity 444.22
  lung (massive)—*see* Embolism, pulmonary
  meninges (*see also* Embolism, brain) 434.1
  mesenteric (artery) (with gangrene) 557.0
  multiple NEC 444.9
  obstetrical (pulmonary) 673.2
    air 673.0
    amniotic fluid (pulmonary) 673.1
    blood-clot 673.2
    cardiac 674.8
    fat 673.8
    heart 674.8
    pyemic 673.3
    septic 673.3
    specified NEC 674.8
  ophthalmic (*see also* Occlusion, retina) 362.30
  paradoxical NEC 444.9
  penis 607.82

Embolism—*continued*
  peripheral arteries NEC 444.22
    lower 444.22
    upper 444.21
  pituitary 253.8
  popliteal (artery) 444.22
  portal (vein) 452
  postoperative NEC 997.2
    cerebral 997.02
    mesenteric artery 997.71
    other vessels 997.79
    peripheral vascular 997.2
    pulmonary 415.11
      septic 415.11
    renal artery 997.72
  precerebral artery (*see also* Occlusion, artery,
    precerebral) 433.9
  puerperal—*see* Embolism, obstetrical
  pulmonary (acute) (artery) (vein) 415.19
    with
      abortion—*see* Abortion, by type, with
        embolism
      ectopic pregnancy (*see also* categories
        633.0-633.9) 639.6
      molar pregnancy (*see also* categories
        630-632) 639.6
    chronic 416.2
    following
      abortion 639.6
      ectopic or molar pregnancy 639.6
    healed or old V12.55
    iatrogenic 415.11
    in pregnancy, childbirth, or puerperium—*see*
      Embolism, obstetrical
    personal history of V12.55
    postoperative 415.11
    septic 415.12
  pyemic (multiple) (*see also* Septicemia) 415.12
    with
      abortion—*see* Abortion, by type, with embolism
      ectopic pregnancy (*see also* categories
        633.0-633.9) 639.6
      molar pregnancy (*see also* categories
        630-632) 639.6
    Aerobacter aerogenes 415.12
    enteric gram-negative bacilli 415.12
    Enterobacter aerogenes 415.12
    Escherichia coli 415.12
    following
      abortion 639.6
      ectopic or molar pregnancy 639.6
    Hemophilus influenzae 415.12
    pneumococcal 415.12
    Proteus vulgaris 415.12
    Pseudomonas (aeruginosa) 415.12
    puerperal, postpartum, childbirth (any
      organism) 673.3
    Serratia 415.12
    specified organism NEC 415.12
    staphylococcal 415.12
      aureus 415.12
      specified organism NEC 415.12
    streptococcal 415.12
  renal (artery) 593.81
    vein 453.3
  retina, retinal (*see also* Occlusion, retina) 362.30
  saddle
    abdominal aorta 444.01
    pulmonary artery 415.13
  septic 415.12
    arterial 449
  septicemic—*see* Embolism, pyemic

Embolism—*continued*
  sinus—*see* Embolism, intracranial venous sinus
  soap
    with
      abortion—*see* Abortion, by type, with embolism
      ectopic pregnancy (*see also* categories
        633.0-633.9) 639.6
      molar pregnancy (*see also* categories
        630-632) 639.6
    following
      abortion 639.6
      ectopic or molar pregnancy 639.6
  spinal cord (nonpyogenic) 336.1
    in pregnancy or puerperium 671.5
    pyogenic origin 324.1
    late effect—*see* category 326
  spleen, splenic (artery) 444.89
  thrombus (thromboembolism) following
    infusion, perfusion, or transfusion 999.2
  upper extremity 444.21
  vein 453.9
    with inflammation or phlebitis—*see*
      Thrombophlebitis
    antecubital (acute) 453.81
      chronic 453.71
    axillary (acute) 453.84
      chronic 453.74
    basilic (acute) 453.81
      chronic 453.71
    brachial (acute) 453.82
      chronic 453.72
    brachiocephalic (acute) (innominate) 453.87
      chronic 453.77
    cephalic (acute) 453.81
      chronic 453.71
    cerebral (*see also* Embolism, brain) 434.1
    coronary (*see also* Infarct, myocardium) 410.9
      without myocardial infarction 411.81
    hepatic 453.0
    internal jugular (acute) 453.86
      chronic 453.76
    lower extremity (superficial) 453.6
      deep 453.40
        acute 453.40
          calf 453.42
          distal (lower leg) 453.42
          femoral 453.41
          iliac 453.41
          lower leg 453.42
          peroneal 453.42
          popliteal 453.41
          proximal (upper leg) 453.41
          thigh 453.41
          tibial 453.42
        chronic 453.50
          calf 453.52
          distal (lower leg) 453.52
          femoral 453.51
          iliac 453.51
          lower leg 453.52
          peroneal 453.52
          popliteal 453.51
          proximal (upper leg) 453.51
          thigh 453.51
          tibial 453.52
      saphenous (greater) (lesser) 453.6
      superficial 453.6
    mesenteric (with gangrene) 557.0
    portal 452
    pulmonary—*see* Embolism, pulmonary
    radial (acute) 453.82
      chronic 453.72

Embolism—*continued*
  vein—*continued*
    renal 453.3
    saphenous (greater) (lesser) 453.6
    specified NEC (acute) 453.89
      chronic 453.79
      with inflammation or phlebitis—*see*
        Thrombophlebitis
    subclavian (acute) 453.85
      chronic 453.75
    superior vena cava (acute) 453.87
      chronic 453.77
    thoracic (acute) 453.87
      chronic 453.77
    ulnar (acute(453.82
      chronic 453.72
    upper extremity (acute) 453.83
      chronic 453.73
        deep 453.72
        superficial 453.71
      deep 453.82
      superficial 453.81
    vena cava
      inferior 453.2
      superior (acute) 453.87
        chronic 453.77
    vessels of brain (*see also* Embolism, brain)
      434.1
Embolization —*see* Embolism
Embolus —*see* Embolism
Embryoma (M9080/1)—*see also* Neoplasm, by
    site, uncertain behavior
  benign (M9080/0)—*see* Neoplasm, by site, benign
  kidney (M8960/3) 189.0
  liver (M8970/3) 155.0
  malignant (M9080/3)—*see also* Neoplasm, by
    site, malignant
  kidney (M8960/3) 189.0
  liver (M8970/3) 155.0
  testis (M9070/3) 186.9
    undescended 186.0
  testis (M9070/3) 186.9
    undescended 186.0
Embryonic
  circulation 747.9
  heart 747.9
  vas deferens 752.89
Embryopathia NEC 759.9
Embryotomy, fetal 763.89
Embryotoxon 743.43
  interfering with vision 743.42
Emesis —*see also* Vomiting
  bilious 787.04
  gravidarum—*see* Hyperemesis, gravidarum
Emissions, nocturnal (semen) 608.89
Emotional
  crisis—*see* Crisis, emotional
  disorder (*see also* Disorder, mental) 300.9
  instability (excessive) 301.3
  lability 799.24
  overlay—*see* Reaction, adjustment
  upset 300.9
Emotionality, pathological 301.3
Emotogenic disease (*see also* Disorder,
    psychogenic) 306.9

Emphysema (atrophic) (centriacinar)
    (centrilobular) (chronic) (diffuse) (essential)
    (hypertrophic) (interlobular) (lung)
    (obstructive) (panlobular) (paracicatricial)
    (paracinar) (postural) (pulmonary) (senile)
    (subpleural) (traction) (unilateral) (unilobular)
    (vesicular) 492.8
  with bronchitis
    chronic 491.20
      with
        acute bronchitis 491.22
        exacerbation (acute) 491.21
  bullous (giant) 492.0
  cellular tissue 958.7
    surgical 998.81
  compensatory 518.2
  congenital 770.2
  conjunctiva 372.89
  connective tissue 958.7
    surgical 998.81
  due to fumes or vapors 506.4
  eye 376.89
  eyelid 374.85
    surgical 998.81
    traumatic 958.7
  fetus or newborn (interstitial) (mediastinal)
      (unilobular) 770.2
  heart 416.9
  interstitial 518.1
    congenital 770.2
    fetus or newborn 770.2
  laminated tissue 958.7
    surgical 998.81
  mediastinal 518.1
    fetus or newborn 770.2
  newborn (interstitial) (mediastinal) (unilobular)
      770.2
  obstructive diffuse with fibrosis 492.8
  orbit 376.89
  subcutaneous 958.7
    due to trauma 958.7
    nontraumatic 518.1
    surgical 998.81
  surgical 998.81
  thymus (gland) (congenital) 254.8
  traumatic 958.7
  tuberculous (*see also* Tuberculosis, pulmonary)
      011.9
Employment examination (certification) V70.5
Empty sella (turcica) syndrome 253.8
Empyema (chest) (diaphragmatic) (double)
    (encapsulated) (general) (interlobar) (lung)
    (medial) (necessitatis) (perforating chest wall)
    (pleura) (pneumococcal) (residual) (sacculated)
    (streptococcal) (supradiaphragmatic) 510.9
  with fistula 510.0
  accessory sinus (chronic) (*see also* Sinusitis) 473.9
  acute 510.9
    with fistula 510.0
  antrum (chronic) (*see also* Sinusitis, maxillary)
      473.0
  brain (any part) (*see also* Abscess, brain) 324.0
  ethmoidal (sinus) (chronic) (*see also* Sinusitis,
      ethmoidal) 473.2
  extradural (*see also* Abscess, extradural) 324.9
  frontal (sinus) (chronic) (*see also* Sinusitis,
      frontal) 473.1
  gallbladder (*see also* Cholecystitis, acute) 575.0
  mastoid (process) (acute) (*see also* Mastoiditis,
      acute) 383.00

Empyema—*continued*
  maxilla, maxillary 526.4
    sinus (chronic) (*see also* Sinusitis, maxillary)
      473.0
  nasal sinus (chronic) (*see also* Sinusitis) 473.9
  sinus (accessory) (nasal) (*see also* Sinusitis) 473.9
  sphenoidal (chronic) (sinus) (*see also* Sinusitis,
    sphenoidal) 473.3
  subarachnoid (*see also* Abscess, extradural) 324.9
  subdural (*see also* Abscess, extradural) 324.9
  tuberculous (*see also* Tuberculosis, pleura) 012.0
  ureter (*see also* Ureteritis) 593.89
  ventricular (*see also* Abscess, brain) 324.0
Enameloma 520.2
Encephalitis (bacterial) (chronic) (hemorrhagic)
    (idiopathic) (nonepidemic) (spurious)
    (subacute) 323.9
  acute—*see also* Encephalitis, viral
    disseminated (postinfectious) NEC 136.9 *[323.61]*
      postimmunization or postvaccination 323.51
    inclusional 049.8
    inclusion body 049.8
    necrotizing 049.8
  arboviral, arbovirus NEC 064
  arthropod-borne (*see also* Encephalitis, viral,
    arthropod-borne) 064
  Australian X 062.4
  Bwamba fever 066.3
  California (virus) 062.5
  Central European 063.2
  Czechoslovakian 063.2
  Dawson's (inclusion body) 046.2
  diffuse sclerosing 046.2
  due to
    actinomycosis 039.8 *[323.41]*
    cat-scratch disease 078.3 *[323.01]*
    human herpesvirus 6 058.21
    human herpesvirus 7 058.29
    human herpesvirus NEC 058.29
    human immunodeficiency virus [HIV] disease
      042 *[323.01]*
    infectious mononucleosis 075 *[323.01]*
    malaria (*see also* Malaria) 084.6 *[323.2]*
    Negishi virus 064
    ornithosis 073.7 *[323.01]*
    other infection classified elsewhere 136.9
      [323.41]
    prophylactic inoculation against smallpox 323.51
    rickettsiosis (*see also* Rickettsiosis) 083.9
      [323.1]
    rubella 056.01
    toxoplasmosis (acquired) 130.0
      congenital (active) 771.2 *[323.41]*
    typhus (fever) (*see also* Typhus) 081.9 *[323.1]*
    vaccination (smallpox) 323.51
  Eastern equine 062.2
  endemic 049.8
  epidemic 049.8
  equine (acute) (infectious) (viral) 062.9
    Eastern 062.2
    Venezuelan 066.2
    Western 062.1
  Far Eastern 063.0
  following vaccination or other immunization
    procedure 323.51
  herpes 054.3
  human herpesvirus 6 058.21
  human herpesvirus 7 058.29
  human herpesvirus NEC 058.29
  Ilheus (virus) 062.8
  inclusion body 046.2
  infectious (acute) (virus) NEC 049.8

Encephalitis—*continued*
  influenzal (*see also* Influenza) 487.8 *[323.41]*
    lethargic 049.8
  Japanese (B type) 062.0
  La Crosse 062.5
  Langat 063.8
  late effect—*see* Late, effect, encephalitis
  lead 984.9 *[323.71]*
  lethargic (acute) (infectious) (influenzal) 049.8
  lethargica 049.8
  louping ill 063.1
  lupus 710.0 *[323.81]*
  lymphatica 049.0
  Mengo 049.8
  meningococcal 036.1
  mumps 072.2
  Murray Valley 062.4
  myoclonic 049.8
  Negishi virus 064
  otitic NEC 382.4 *[323.41]*
  parasitic NEC 123.9 *[323.41]*
  periaxialis (concentrica) (diffusa) 341.1
  postchickenpox 052.0
  postexanthematous NEC 057.9 *[323.62]*
  postimmunization 323.51
  postinfectious NEC 136.9 *[323.62]*
  postmeasles 055.0
  posttraumatic 323.81
  postvaccinal (smallpox) 323.51
  postvaricella 052.0
  postviral NEC 079.99 *[323.62]*
    postexanthematous 057.9 *[323.62]*
    specified NEC 057.8 *[323.62]*
  Powassan 063.8
  progressive subcortical (Binswanger's) 290.12
  Rasmussen 323.81
  Rio Bravo 049.8
  rubella 056.01
  Russian
    autumnal 062.0
    spring-summer type (taiga) 063.0
  saturnine 984.9 *[323.71]*
  Semliki Forest 062.8
  serous 048
  slow-acting virus NEC 046.8
  specified cause NEC 323.81
  St. Louis type 062.3
  subacute sclerosing 046.2
  subcorticalis chronica 290.12
  summer 062.0
  suppurative 324.0
  syphilitic 094.81
    congenital 090.41
  tick-borne 063.9
  torula, torular 117.5 *[323.41]*
  toxic NEC 989.9 *[323.71]*
  toxoplasmic (acquired) 130.0
    congenital (active) 771.2 *[323.41]*
  trichinosis 124 *[323.41]*
  Trypanosomiasis (*see also* Trypanosomiasis)
    086.9 *[323.2]*
  tuberculous (*see also* Tuberculosis) 013.6
  type B (Japanese) 062.0
  type C 062.3
  van Bogaert's 046.2
  Venezuelan 066.2
  Vienna type 049.8

Encephalitis—*continued*
viral, virus 049.9
  arthropod-borne NEC 064
    mosquito-borne 062.9
      Australian X disease 062.4
      California virus 062.5
      Eastern equine 062.2
      Ilheus virus 062.8
      Japanese (B type) 062.0
      Murray Valley 062.4
      specified type NEC 062.8
      St. Louis 062.3
      type B 062.0
      type C 062.3
      Western equine 062.1
    tick-borne 063.9
      biundulant 063.2
      Central European 063.2
      Czechoslovakian 063.2
      diphasic meningoencephalitis 063.2
      Far Eastern 063.0
      Langat 063.8
      louping ill 063.1
      Powassan 063.8
      Russian spring-summer (taiga) 063.0
      specified type NEC 063.8
    vector unknown 064
  slow acting NEC 046.8
  specified type NEC 049.8
  vaccination, prophylactic (against) V05.0
  von Economo's 049.8
  Western equine 062.1
  West Nile type 066.41
Encephalocele 742.0
  orbit 376.81
Encephalocystocele 742.0
**Encephaloduroarteriomyosynangiosis
  (EDAMS)** 437.5
Encephalomalacia (brain) (cerebellar) (cerebral)
    (cerebrospinal) (*see also* Softening, brain)
    348.89
  due to
    hemorrhage (*see also* Hemorrhage, brain) 431
    recurrent spasm of artery 435.9
  embolic (cerebral) (*see also* Embolism, brain)
    434.1
  subcorticalis chronicus arteriosclerotica 290.12
  thrombotic (*see also* Thrombosis, brain) 434.0
Encephalomeningitis —*see* Meningoencephalitis
Encephalomeningocele 742.0
Encephalomeningomyelitis —*see*
  Meningoencephalitis
Encephalomeningopathy (*see also*
  Meningoencephalitis) 349.9
Encephalomyelitis (chronic) (granulomatous)
    (myalgic, benign) (*see also* Encephalitis)
    323.9
  abortive disseminated 049.8
  acute disseminated (ADEM) (postinfectious)
    136.9 *[323.61]*
    infectious 136.9 *[323.61]*
    noninfectious 323.81
    postimmunization 323.51
  due to
    cat-scratch disease 078.3 *[323.01]*
    infectious mononucleosis 075 *[323.01]*
    ornithosis 073.7 *[323.01]*
    vaccination (any) 323.51
  equine (acute) (infectious) 062.9
    Eastern 062.2
    Venezuelan 066.2
    Western 062.1

Encephalomyelitis—*continued*
  funicularis infectiosa 049.8
  late effect—*see* Late, effect, encephalitis
  Munch-Peterson's 049.8
  postchickenpox 052.0
  postimmunization 323.51
  postmeasles 055.0
  postvaccinal (smallpox) 323.51
  rubella 056.01
  specified cause NEC 323.81
  syphilitic 094.81
  West Nile 066.41
Encephalomyelocele 742.0
Encephalomyelomeningitis —*see*
  Meningoencephalitis
Encephalomyeloneuropathy 349.9
Encephalomyelopathy 349.9
  subacute necrotizing (infantile) 330.8
Encephalomyeloradiculitis (acute) 357.0
Encephalomyeloradiculoneuritis (acute) 357.0
Encephalomyeloradiculopathy 349.9
Encephalomyocarditis 074.23
**Encephalopathia hyperbilirubinemica
  newborn** 774.7
  due to isoimmunization (conditions classifiable
    to 773.0-773.2) 773.4
Encephalopathy (acute) 348.30
  alcoholic 291.2
  anoxic—*see* Damage, brain, anoxic
  arteriosclerotic 437.0
    late effect—*see* Late effect(s) (of)
      cerebrovascular disease
  bilirubin, newborn 774.7
    due to isoimmunization 773.4
  congenital 742.9
  demyelinating (callosal) 341.8
  due to
    birth injury (intracranial) 767.8
    dialysis 294.8
      transient 293.9
    drugs (—*see also* Table of Drugs and
      Chemicals) 349.82
    hyperinsulinism—*see* Hyperinsulinism
    influenza (virus) (*see also* Influenza) 487.8
      identified
        avian 488.09
        (novel) 2009 H1N1 488.19
    lack of vitamin (*see also* Deficiency, vitamin)
      269.2
    nicotinic acid deficiency 291.2
    serum (nontherapeutic) (therapeutic) 999.59
    syphilis 094.81
    trauma (postconcussional) 310.2
      current (*see also* Concussion, brain) 850.9
        with skull fracture—*see* Fracture, skull, by
          site, with intracranial injury
    vaccination 323.51
  hepatic 572.2
  hyperbilirubinemic, newborn 774.7
    due to isoimmunization (conditions
      classifiable to 773.0-773.2) 773.4
  hypertensive 437.2
  hypoglycemic 251.2
  hypoxic—*see also* Damage, brain, anoxic
    ischemic (HIE) 768.70
      mild 768.71
      moderate 768.72
      severe 768.73
  infantile cystic necrotizing (congenital) 341.8
  lead 984.9 *[323.71]*
  leukopolio 330.0

Encephalopathy—*continued*
  metabolic (*see also* Delirium) 348.31
    drug induced 349.82
    toxic 349.82
  necrotizing
    hemorrhagic (acute) 323.61
    subacute 330.8
  other specified type NEC 348.39
  pellagrous 265.2
  portal-systemic 572.2
  postcontusional 310.2
  posttraumatic 310.2
  saturnine 984.9 *[323.71]*
  septic 348.31
  spongioform, subacute (viral) 046.19
  subacute
    necrotizing 330.8
    spongioform 046.19
    viral, spongioform 046.19
  subcortical progressive (Schilder) 341.1
    chronic (Binswanger's) 290.12
  toxic 349.82
    metabolic 349.82
  traumatic (postconcussional) 310.2
    current (*see also* Concussion, brain) 850.9
      with skull fracture—*see* Fracture, skull, by
        site, with intracranial injury
  vitamin B deficiency NEC 266.9
  Wernicke's (superior hemorrhagic
    polioencephalitis) 265.1
Enchephalorrhagia (*see also* Hemorrhage,
  brain) 432.9
  healed or old V12.54
  late effect—*see* Late effect(s) (of)
    cerebrovascular disease
Encephalosis, posttraumatic 310.2
Enchondroma (M9220/0)—*see also* Neoplasm,
  bone, benign
  multiple, congenital 756.4
Enchondromatosis (cartilaginous) (congenital)
  (multiple) 756.4
Enchondroses, multiple (cartilaginous)
  (congenital) 756.4
Encopresis (*see also* Incontinence, feces) 787.60
  nonorganic origin 307.7
Encounter for —*see also* Admission for
  administrative purpose only V68.9
    referral of patient without examination or
      treatment V68.81
    specified purpose NEC V68.89
  chemotherapy, (oral) (intravenous)
    antineoplastic V58.11
  determination of fetal viability of pregnancy
    V23.87
  disability examination V68.01
  end-of-life care V66.7
  hospice care V66.7
  immunizations (childhood) appropriate for age V20.2
  immunotherapy, antineoplastic V58.12
  joint prosthesis insertion following prior
    explantation of joint prosthesis V54.82
  palliative care V66.7
  radiotherapy V58.0
  respirator (ventilator) dependence
    during
      mechanical failure V46.14
      power failure V46.12
    for weaning V46.13
  routine infant and child vision and hearing
    testing V20.2

Encounter for—*continued*
  school examination V70.3
    following surgery V67.09
  screening mammogram NEC V76.12
    for high-risk patient V76.11
  paternity testing V70.4
  terminal care V66.7
  weaning from respirator (ventilator) V46.13
Encystment —*see* Cyst
End-of-life care V66.7
Endamebiasis —*see* Amebiasis
Endamoeba —*see* Amebiasis
Endarteritis (bacterial, subacute) (infective)
  (septic) 447.6
  brain, cerebral or cerebrospinal 437.4
    late effect—*see* Late effect(s) (of)
      cerebrovascular disease
  coronary (artery) —*see* Arteriosclerosis,
    coronary
  deformans—*see* Arteriosclerosis
  embolic (*see also* Embolism) 444.9
  obliterans—*see also* Arteriosclerosis
    pulmonary 417.8
  pulmonary 417.8
  retina 362.18
  senile—*see* Arteriosclerosis
  syphilitic 093.89
    brain or cerebral 094.89
    congenital 090.5
    spinal 094.89
  tuberculous (*see also* Tuberculosis) 017.9
Endemic —*see* condition
Endocarditis (chronic) (indeterminate)
  (interstitial) (marantic) (nonbacterial
  thrombotic) (residual) (sclerotic) (sclerous)
  (senile) (valvular) 424.90
  with
    rheumatic fever (conditions classifiable to
      390)
      active—*see* Endocarditis, acute, rheumatic
      inactive or quiescent (with chorea) 397.9
  acute or subacute 421.9
    rheumatic (aortic) (mitral) (pulmonary)
      (tricuspid) 391.1
      with chorea (acute) (rheumatic)
        (Sydenham's) 392.0
  aortic (heart) (nonrheumatic) (valve) 424.1
    with
      mitral (valve) disease 396.9
        active or acute 391.1
          with chorea (acute) (rheumatic)
            (Sydenham's) 392.0
      rheumatic fever (conditions classifiable to
        390)
        active—*see* Endocarditis, acute, rheumatic
        inactive or quiescent (with chorea) 395.9
          with mitral disease 396.9
    acute or subacute 421.9
    arteriosclerotic 424.1
    congenital 746.89
    hypertensive 424.1
    rheumatic (chronic) (inactive) 395.9
      with mitral (valve) disease 396.9
        active or acute 391.1
          with chorea (acute) (rheumatic)
            (Sydenham's) 392.0
      active or acute 391.1
        with chorea (acute) (rheumatic)
          (Sydenham's) 392.0
    specified cause, except rheumatic 424.1
    syphilitic 093.22

Endocarditis—*continued*
arteriosclerotic or due to arteriosclerosis 424.99
atypical verrucous (Libman-Sacks) 710.0
    [424.91]
bacterial (acute) (any valve) (chronic) (subacute)
    421.0
blastomycotic 116.0 *[421.1]*
candidal 112.81
congenital 425.3
constrictive 421.0
Coxsackie 074.22
due to
    blastomycosis 116.0 *[421.1]*
    candidiasis 112.81
    Coxsackie (virus) 074.22
    disseminated lupus erythematosus 710.0
        [424.91]
    histoplasmosis (*see also* Histoplasmosis) 115.94
    hypertension (benign) 424.99
    moniliasis 112.81
    prosthetic cardiac valve 996.61
    Q fever 083.0 *[421.1]*
    serratia marcescens 421.0
    typhoid (fever) 002.0 *[421.1]*
fetal 425.3
gonococcal 098.84
hypertensive 424.99
infectious or infective (acute) (any valve)
    (chronic) (subacute) 421.0
lenta (acute) (any valve) (chronic) (subacute)
    421.0
Libman-Sacks 710.0 *[424.91]*
Loeffler's (parietal fibroplastic) 421.0
malignant (acute) (any valve) (chronic)
    (subacute) 421.0
meningococcal 036.42
mitral (chronic) (double) (fibroid) (heart)
    (inactive) (valve) (with chorea) 394.9
    with
        aortic (valve) disease 396.9
            active or acute 391.1
                with chorea (acute) (rheumatic)
                    (Sydenham's) 392.0
            rheumatic fever (conditions classifiable to
                390)
                active—*see* Endocarditis, acute, rheumatic
                inactive or quiescent (with chorea) 394.9
                    with aortic valve disease 396.9
    active or acute 391.1
        bacterial 421.0
        with chorea (acute) (rheumatic)
            (Sydenham's) 392.0
    arteriosclerotic 424.0
    congenital 746.89
    hypertensive 424.0
    nonrheumatic 424.0
        acute or subacute 421.9
    syphilitic 093.21
monilial 112.81
mycotic (acute) (any valve) (chronic) (subacute)
    421.0
pneumococcic (acute) (any valve) (chronic)
    (subacute) 421.0
pulmonary (chronic) (heart) (valve) 424.3
    with
        rheumatic fever (conditions classifiable to 390)
            active—*see* Endocarditis, acute, rheumatic
            inactive or quiescent (with chorea) 397.1
    acute or subacute 421.9
        rheumatic 391.1
            with chorea (acute) (rheumatic)
                (Sydenham's) 392.0

Endocarditis—*continued*
pulmonary—*continued*
    arteriosclerotic or due to arteriosclerosis 424.3
    congenital 746.09
    hypertensive or due to hypertension (benign)
        424.3
    rheumatic (chronic) (inactive) (with chorea)
        397.1
        active or acute 391.1
            with chorea (acute) (rheumatic)
                (Sydenham's) 392.0
    syphilitic 093.24
purulent (acute) (any valve) (chronic) (subacute)
    421.0
rheumatic (chronic) (inactive) (with chorea)
    397.9
    active or acute (aortic) (mitral) (pulmonary)
        (tricuspid) 391.1
        with chorea (acute) (rheumatic)
            (Sydenham's) 392.0
septic (acute) (any valve) (chronic) (subacute)
    421.0
specified cause, except rheumatic 424.99
streptococcal (acute) (any valve) (chronic)
    (subacute) 421.0
subacute—*see* Endocarditis, acute
suppurative (any valve) (acute) (chronic)
    (subacute) 421.0
syphilitic NEC 093.20
toxic (*see also* Endocarditis, acute) 421.9
tricuspid (chronic) (heart) (inactive) (rheumatic)
    (valve) (with chorea) 397.0
    with
        rheumatic fever (conditions classifiable to
            390)
            active—*see* Endocarditis, acute, rheumatic
            inactive or quiescent (with chorea) 397.0
    active or acute 391.1
        with chorea (acute) (rheumatic)
            (Sydenham's) 392.0
    arteriosclerotic 424.2
    congenital 746.89
    hypertensive 424.2
    nonrheumatic 424.2
        acute or subacute 421.9
    specified cause, except rheumatic 424.2
    syphilitic 093.23
tuberculous (*see also* Tuberculosis) 017.9
    [424.91]
typhoid 002.0 *[421.1]*
ulcerative (acute) (any valve) (chronic)
    (subacute) 421.0
vegetative (acute) (any valve) (chronic)
    (subacute) 421.0
verrucous (acute) (any valve) (chronic)
    (subacute) NEC 710.0 *[424.91]*
    nonbacterial 710.0 *[424.91]*
    nonrheumatic 710.0 *[424.91]*
Endocardium, endocardial —*see also* condition
cushion defect 745.60
    specified type NEC 745.69
Endocervicitis (*see also* Cervicitis) 616.0
due to
    intrauterine (contraceptive) device 996.65
gonorrheal (acute) 098.15
    chronic or duration of 2 months or over 098.35
hyperplastic 616.0
syphilitic 095.8
trichomonal 131.09
tuberculous (*see also* Tuberculosis) 016.7
Endocrine —*see* condition
Endocrinopathy, pluriglandular 258.9

Endodontitis 522.0
Endomastoiditis (*see also* Mastoiditis) 383.9
Endometrioma 617.9
Endometriosis 617.9
  appendix 617.5
  bladder 617.8
  bowel 617.5
  broad ligament 617.3
  cervix 617.0
  colon 617.5
  cul-de-sac (Douglas') 617.3
  exocervix 617.0
  fallopian tube 617.2
  female genital organ NEC 617.8
  gallbladder 617.8
  in scar of skin 617.6
  internal 617.0
  intestine 617.5
  lung 617.8
  myometrium 617.0
  ovary 617.1
  parametrium 617.3
  pelvic peritoneum 617.3
  peritoneal (pelvic) 617.3
  rectovaginal septum 617.4
  rectum 617.5
  round ligament 617.3
  skin 617.6
  specified site NEC 617.8
  stromal (M8931/1) 236.0
  umbilicus 617.8
  uterus 617.0
    internal 617.0
  vagina 617.4
  vulva 617.8
Endometritis (nonspecific) (purulent) (septic)
  (suppurative) 615.9
  with
    abortion—*see* Abortion, by type, with sepsis
    ectopic pregnancy (*see also* categories
      633.0-633.9) 639.0
    molar pregnancy (*see also* categories 630-632)
      639.0
  acute 615.0
  blennorrhagic 098.16
    acute 098.16
    chronic or duration of 2 months or over 098.36
  cervix, cervical (*see also* Cervicitis) 616.0
    hyperplastic 616.0
  chronic 615.1
  complicating pregnancy 670.1
    affecting fetus or newborn 760.8
    septic 670.2
  decidual 615.9
  following
    abortion 639.0
    ectopic or molar pregnancy 639.0
  gonorrheal (acute) 098.16
    chronic or duration of 2 months or over 098.36
  hyperplastic (*see also* Hyperplasia,
    endometrium) 621.30
    cervix 616.0
  polypoid—*see* Endometritis, hyperplastic
  puerperal, postpartum, childbirth 670.1
    septic 670.2
  senile (atrophic) 615.9
  subacute 615.0
  tuberculous (*see also* Tuberculosis) 016.7
Endometrium —*see* condition
Endomyocardiopathy, South African 425.2

Endomyocarditis —*see* Endocarditis
Endomyofibrosis 425.0
Endomyometritis (*see also* Endometritis) 615.9
Endopericarditis —*see* Endocarditis
Endoperineuritis —*see* Disorder, nerve
Endophlebitis (*see also* Phlebitis) 451.9
  leg 451.2
    deep (vessels) 451.19
    superficial (vessels) 451.0
  portal (vein) 572.1
  retina 362.18
  specified site NEC 451.89
  syphilitic 093.89
Endophthalmia (*see also* Endophthalmitis) 360.00
  gonorrheal 098.42
Endophthalmitis (globe) (infective) (metastatic)
  (purulent) (subacute) 360.00
  acute 360.01
  bleb associated 379.63
  chronic 360.03
  parasitic 360.13
  phacoanaphylactic 360.19
  specified type NEC 360.19
  sympathetic 360.11
Endosalpingioma (M9111/1) 236.2
Endosalpingiosis 629.89
Endosteitis —*see* Osteomyelitis
Endothelioma, bone (M9260/3)—*see* Neoplasm,
  bone, malignant
Endotheliosis 287.8
  hemorrhagic infectional 287.8
Endotoxemia —*code to condition*
Endotoxic shock 785.52
  postoperative 998.02
Endotrachelitis (*see also* Cervicitis) 616.0
Enema rash 692.89
Engel-von Recklinghausen disease or
  syndrome (osteitis fibrosa cystica) 252.01
Engelmann's disease (diaphyseal sclerosis)
  756.59
English disease (*see also* Rickets) 268.0
Engman's disease (infectious eczematoid
  dermatitis) 690.8
Engorgement
  breast 611.79
    newborn 778.7
    puerperal, postpartum 676.2
  liver 573.9
  lung 514
  pulmonary 514
  retina, venous 362.37
  stomach 536.8
  venous, retina 362.37
Enlargement, enlarged —*see also* Hypertrophy
  abdomen 789.3
  adenoids 474.12
    and tonsils 474.10
  alveolar process or ridge 525.8
  apertures of diaphragm (congenital) 756.6
  blind spot, visual field 368.42
  gingival 523.8
  heart, cardiac (*see also* Hypertrophy, cardiac) 429.3
  lacrimal gland, chronic 375.03
  liver (*see also* Hypertrophy, liver) 789.1
  lymph gland or node 785.6
  orbit 376.46
  organ or site, congenital NEC—*see* Anomaly,
    specified type NEC
  parathyroid (gland) 252.01
  pituitary fossa 793.0

Enlargement, enlarged—*continued*
  prostate (simple) (soft) 600.00
    with
      other lower urinary tract symptoms (LUTS)
          600.01
      urinary
        obstruction 600.01
        retention 600.01
  sella turcica 793.0
  spleen (*see also* Splenomegaly) 789.2
    congenital 759.0
  thymus (congenital) (gland) 254.0
  thyroid (gland) (*see also* Goiter) 240.9
  tongue 529.8
  tonsils 474.11
    and adenoids 474.10
  uterus 621.2
Enophthalmos 376.50
  due to
    atrophy of orbital tissue 376.51
    surgery 376.52
    trauma 376.52
Enostosis 526.89
Entamebiasis —*see* Amebiasis
Entamebic —*see* Amebiasis
Entanglement, umbilical cord (s) 663.3
  with compression 663.2
  affecting fetus or newborn 762.5
  around neck with compression 663.1
  twins in monoamniotic sac 663.2
Enteralgia 789.0
Enteric —*see* condition
Enteritis (acute) (catarrhal) (choleraic) (chronic)
    (congestive) (diarrheal) (exudative) (follicular)
    (hemorrhagic) (infantile) (lienteric)
    (noninfectious) (perforative) (phlegmonous)
    (presumed noninfectious)
    (pseudomembranous) 558.9
  adaptive 564.9
  aertrycke infection 003.0
  allergic 558.3
  amebic (*see also* Amebiasis) 006.9
    with abscess—*see* Abscess, amebic
    acute 006.0
      with abscess—*see* Abscess, amebic
      nondysenteric 006.2
    chronic 006.1
      with abscess—*see* Abscess, amebic
      nondysenteric 006.2
    nondysenteric 006.2
  anaerobic (cocci) (gram-negative)
      (gram-positive) (mixed) NEC 008.46
  bacillary NEC 004.9
  bacterial NEC 008.5
    specified NEC 008.49
  Bacteroides (fragilis) (melaninogeniscus)
      (oralis) 008.46
  Butyrivibrio (fibriosolvens) 008.46
  Campylobacter 008.43
  Candida 112.85
  Chilomastix 007.8
  choleriformis 001.1
  chronic 558.9
    ulcerative (*see also* Colitis, ulcerative) 556.9
  cicatrizing (chronic) 555.0
  Clostridium
    botulinum 005.1
    difficile 008.45
    haemolyticum 008.46
    novyi 008.46
    perfringens (C) (F) 008.46
    specified type NEC 008.46

Enteritis—*continued*
  coccidial 007.2
  dietetic 558.9
  due to
    achylia gastrica 536.8
    adenovirus 008.62
    Aerobacter aerogenes 008.2
    anaerobes—*see* Enteritis, anaerobic 008.46
    Arizona (bacillus) 008.1
    astrovirus 008.66
    Bacillus coli—*see* Enteritis, E. coli 008.0
    bacteria NEC 008.5
      specified NEC 008.49
    Bacteroides 008.46
    Butyrivibrio (fibriosolvens) 008.46
    calicivirus 008.65
    Campylobacter 008.43
    Clostridium—*see* Enteritis, Clostridium
    Cockle agent 008.64
    Coxsackie (virus) 008.67
    Ditchling agent 008.64
    ECHO virus 008.67
    Enterobacter aerogenes 008.2
    enterococci 008.49
    enterovirus NEC 008.67
    Escherichia coli—*see* Enteritis, E. coli
    Eubacterium 008.46
    Fusobacterium (nucleatum) 008.46
    gram-negative bacteria NEC 008.47
      anaerobic NEC 008.46
    Hawaii agent 008.63
    irritating foods 558.9
    Klebsiella aerogenes 008.47
    Marin County agent 008.66
    Montgomery County agent 008.63
    norovirus 008.63
    Norwalk-like agent 008.63
    Norwalk virus 008.63
    Otofuke agent 008.63
    Paracolobactrum arizonae 008.1
    paracolon bacillus NEC 008.47
      Arizona 008.1
    Paramatta agent 008.64
    Peptococcus 008.46
    Peptostreptococcus 008.46
    Propionibacterium 008.46
    Proteus (bacillus) (mirabilis) (morganii) 008.3
    Pseudomonas aeruginosa 008.42
    radiation 558.1
    Rotavirus 008.61
    Sapporo agent 008.63
    small round virus (SRV) NEC 008.64
      featureless NEC 008.63
      structured NEC 008.63
    Snow Mountain (SM) agent 008.63
    specified
      bacteria NEC 008.49
      organism, nonbacterial NEC 008.8
      virus NEC 008.69
    Staphylococcus 008.41
    Streptococcus 008.49
      anaerobic 008.46
    Taunton agent 008.63
    Torovirus 008.69
    Treponema 008.46
    Veillonella 008.46
    virus 008.8
      specified type NEC 008.69
    Wollan (W) agent 008.64
    Yersinia enterocolitica 008.44
  dysentery—*see* Dysentery

Enteritis—*continued*
  E. coli 008.00
    enterohemorrhagic 008.04
    enteroinvasive 008.03
    enteropathogenic 008.01
    enterotoxigenic 008.02
    specified type NEC 008.09
  el tor 001.1
  embadomonial 007.8
  eosinophilic 558.41
  epidemic 009.0
  Eubacterium 008.46
  fermentative 558.9
  fulminant 557.0
  Fusobacterium (nucleatum) 008.46
  gangrenous (*see also* Enteritis, due to, by
    organism) 009.0
  giardial 007.1
  gram-negative bacteria NEC 008.47
    anaerobic NEC 008.46
  infectious NEC (*see also* Enteritis, due to, by
    organism) 009.0
    presumed 009.1
  influenzal (*see also* *I*nfluenza) 487.8
  ischemic 557.9
    acute 557.0
    chronic 557.1
    due to mesenteric artery insufficiency 557.1
  membranous 564.9
  mucous 564.9
  myxomembranous 564.9
  necrotic (*see also* Enteritis, due to, by organism) 009.0
  necroticans 005.2
  necrotizing of fetus or newborn (*see also*
    Enterocolitis, necrotizing, newborn) 777.50
  neurogenic 564.9
  newborn 777.8
    necrotizing (*see also* Enterocolitis,
     necrotizing, newborn) 777.50
  parasitic NEC 129
  paratyphoid (fever) (*see also* Fever,
    paratyphoid) 002.9
  Peptococcus 008.46
  Peptostreptococcus 008.46
  Propionibacterium 008.46
  protozoal NEC 007.9
  radiation 558.1
  regional (of) 555.9
    intestine
      large (bowel, colon, or rectum) 555.1
        with small intestine 555.2
      small (duodenum, ileum, or jejunum) 555.0
        with large intestine 555.2
  Salmonella infection 003.0
  salmonellosis 003.0
  segmental (*see also* Enteritis, regional) 555.9
  septic (*see also* Enteritis, due to, by organism)
    009.0
  Shigella 004.9
  simple 558.9
  spasmodic 564.9
  spastic 564.9
  staphylococcal 008.41
    due to food 005.0
  streptococcal 008.49
    anaerobic 008.46
  toxic 558.2
  Treponema (denticola) (macrodentium) 008.46
  trichomonal 007.3
  tuberculous (*see also* Tuberculosis) 014.8
  typhosa 002.0

Enteritis—*continued*
  ulcerative (chronic) (*see also* Colitis, ulcerative)
    556.9
  Veillonella 008.46
  viral 008.8
    adenovirus 008.62
    enterovirus 008.67
    specified virus NEC 008.69
  Yersinia enterocolitica 008.44
  zymotic 009.0
Enteroarticular syndrome 099.3
Enterobiasis 127.4
Enterobius vermicularis 127.4
Enterocele (*see also* Hernia) 553.9
  pelvis, pelvic (acquired) (congenital) 618.6
  vagina, vaginal (acquired) (congenital) 618.6
Enterocolitis —*see also* Enteritis
  fetus or newborn (*see also* Enterocolitis,
    necrotizing, newborn) 777.8
  necrotizing 777.50
  fulminant 557.0
  granulomatous 555.2
  hemorrhagic (acute) 557.0
    chronic 557.1
  necrotizing (acute) (membranous) 557.0
    newborn 777.50
      with
        perforation 777.53
        pneumatosis without perforation 777.52
        pneumatosis and perforation 777.53
      stage I 777.51
      stage II 777.52
      stage III 777.53
      without pneumatosis, without perforation
        777.51
  primary necrotizing (*see also* Enterocolitis,
    necrotizing, newborn) 777.50
  pseudomembranous 008.45
    newborn 008.45
  radiation 558.1
    newborn (*see also* Enterocolitis, necrotizing,
     newborn) 777.50
  ulcerative 556.0
Enterocystoma 751.5
Enterogastritis —*see* Enteritis
Enterogenous cyanosis 289.7
Enterolith, enterolithiasis (impaction) 560.39
  with hernia—*see also* Hernia, by site, with
    obstruction
    gangrenous—*see* Hernia, by site, with
     gangrene
Enteropathy 569.9
  exudative (of Gordon) 579.8
  gluten 579.0
  hemorrhagic, terminal 557.0
  protein-losing 579.8
Enteroperitonitis (*see also* Peritonitis) 567.9
Enteroptosis 569.89
Enterorrhagia 578.9
Enterospasm 564.9
  psychogenic 306.4
Enterostenosis (*see also* Obstruction, intestine)
  560.9
Enterostomy status V44.4
  with complication 569.60
Enthesopathy 726.39
  ankle and tarsus 726.70
  elbow region 726.30
    specified NEC 726.39
  hip 726.5

Enthesopathy—*continued*
  knee 726.60
  peripheral NEC 726.8
  shoulder region 726.10
    adhesive 726.0
  spinal 720.1
  wrist and carpus 726.4
Entrance, air into vein —*see* Embolism, air
Entrapment, nerve —*see* Neuropathy,
  entrapment
Entropion (eyelid) 374.00
  cicatricial 374.04
  congenital 743.62
  late effect of trachoma (healed) 139.1
  mechanical 374.02
  paralytic 374.02
  senile 374.01
  spastic 374.03
Enucleation of eye (current) (traumatic) 871.3
Enuresis 788.30
  habit disturbance 307.6
  nocturnal 788.36
    psychogenic 307.6
  nonorganic origin 307.6
  psychogenic 307.6
Enzymopathy 277.9
Eosinopenia 288.59
Eosinophilia 288.3
  with
    angiolymphoid hyperplasia (ALHE) 228.01
  allergic 288.3
  hereditary 288.3
  idiopathic 288.3
  infiltrative 518.3
  Loeffler's 518.3
  myalgia syndrome 710.5
  pulmonary (tropical) 518.3
  secondary 288.3
  tropical 518.3
Eosinophilic —*see also* condition
  fasciitis 728.89
  granuloma (bone) 277.89
  infiltration lung 518.3
Ependymitis (acute) (cerebral) (chronic)
  (granular) (*see also* Meningitis) 322.9
Ependymoblastoma (M9392/3)
  specified site—*see* Neoplasm, by site, malignant
  unspecified site 191.9
Ependymoma (epithelial) (malignant) (M9391/3)
  anaplastic type (M9392/3)
    specified site—*see* Neoplasm, by site, malignant
    unspecified site 191.9
  benign (M9391/0)
    specified site—*see* Neoplasm, by site, benign
    unspecified site 225.0
  myxopapillary (M9394/1) 237.5
  papillary (M9393/1) 237.5
  specified site—*see* Neoplasm, by site, malignant
  unspecified site 191.9
Ependymopathy 349.2
  spinal cord 349.2
Ephelides, ephelis 709.09
Ephemeral fever (*see also* Pyrexia) 780.60
Epiblepharon (congenital) 743.62
Epicanthus, epicanthic fold (congenital) (eyelid)
  743.63
Epicondylitis (elbow) (lateral) 726.32
  medial 726.31

Epicystitis (*see also* Cystitis) 595.9
Epidemic —*see* condition
Epidermidalization, cervix —*see* condition
Epidermidization, cervix —*see* condition
Epidermis, epidermal —*see* condition
Epidermization, cervix —*see* condition
Epidermodysplasia verruciformis 078.19
Epidermoid
  cholesteatoma—*see* Cholesteatoma
  inclusion (*see also* Cyst, skin) 706.2
Epidermolysis
  acuta (combustiformis) (toxica) 695.15
  bullosa 757.39
  necroticans combustiformis 695.15
    due to drug
      correct substance properly administered 695.15
      overdose or wrong substance given or taken
        977.9
      specified drug—*see* Table of drugs and
        chemicals
Epidermophytid —*see* Dermatophytosis
Epidermophytosis (infected)—*see*
  Dermatophytosis
Epidermosis, ear (middle) (*see also*
  Cholesteatoma) 385.30
Epididymis —*see* condition
Epididymitis (nonvenereal) 604.90
  with abscess 604.0
  acute 604.99
  blennorrhagic (acute) 098.0
    chronic or duration of 2 months or over 098.2
  caseous (*see also* Tuberculosis) 016.4
  chlamydial 099.54
  diphtheritic 032.89 *[604.91]*
  filarial 125.9 *[604.91]*
  gonococcal (acute) 098.0
    chronic or duration of 2 months or over 098.2
  recurrent 604.99
  residual 604.99
  syphilitic 095.8 *[604.91]*
  tuberculous (*see also* Tuberculosis) 016.4
Epididymo-orchitis (*see also* Epididymitis)
  604.90
  with abscess 604.0
  chlamydial 099.54
  gonococcal (acute) 098.13
    chronic or duration of 2 months or over 098.33
Epidural —*see* condition
Epigastritis (*see also* Gastritis) 535.5
Epigastrium, epigastric —*see* condition
Epigastrocele (*see also* Hernia, epigastric) 553.29
Epiglottiditis (acute) 464.30
  with obstruction 464.31
  chronic 476.1
  viral 464.30
    with obstruction 464.31
Epiglottis —*see* condition
Epiglottitis (acute) 464.30
  with obstruction 464.31
  chronic 476.1
  viral 464.30
    with obstruction 464.31
Epignathus 759.4
Epilepsia
  partialis continua (*see also* Epilepsy) 345.7
  procursiva (*see also* Epilepsy) 345.8

Epilepsy, epileptic (idiopathic) 345.9

> *Note—use the following fifth-digit subclassification with categories 345.0, 345.1, 345.4-345.9*
>
> *0 without mention of intractable epilepsy*
> *1 with intractable epilepsy*
> > *pharmacoresistant (pharmacologically resistant)*
> > *poorly controlled*
> > *refractory (medically)*
> > *treatment resistant*

abdominal 345.5
absence (attack) 345.0
akinetic 345.0
  psychomotor 345.4
automatism 345.4
autonomic diencephalic 345.5
brain 345.9
Bravais-Jacksonian 345.5
cerebral 345.9
climacteric 345.9
clonic 345.1
clouded state 345.9
coma 345.3
communicating 345.4
complicating pregnancy, childbirth or the
  puerperium 649.4
congenital 345.9
convulsions 345.9
cortical (focal) (motor) 345.5
cursive (running) 345.8
cysticercosis 123.1
deterioration
  with behavioral disturbance 345.9 *[294.11]*
  without behavioral disturbance 345.9 *[294.10]*
due to syphilis 094.89
equivalent 345.5
fit 345.9
focal (motor) 345.5
gelastic 345.8
generalized 345.9
  convulsive 345.1
  flexion 345.1
  nonconvulsive 345.0
grand mal (idiopathic) 345.1
Jacksonian (motor) (sensory) 345.5
Kojevnikoff's, Kojevnikov's, Kojewnikoff's
  345.7
laryngeal 786.2
limbic system 345.4
localization related (focal) (partial) and epileptic
  syndromes
  with
    complex partial seizures 345.4
    simple partial seizures 345.5
major (motor) 345.1
minor 345.0
mixed (type) 345.9
motor partial 345.5
musicogenic 345.1
myoclonus, myoclonic 345.1
  progressive (familial) 345.1
nonconvulsive, generalized 345.0
parasitic NEC 123.9

Epilepsy, epileptic—*continued*
partial (focalized) 345.5
  with
    impairment of consciousness 345.4
     memory and ideational disturbances 345.4
  abdominal type 345.5
  motor type 345.5
  psychomotor type 345.4
  psychosensory type 345.4
  secondarily generalized 345.4
  sensory type 345.5
  somatomotor type 345.5
  somatosensory type 345.5
  temporal lobe type 345.4
  visceral type 345.5
  visual type 345.5
  without impairment of consciousness 345.5
peripheral 345.9
petit mal 345.0
photokinetic 345.8
progressive myoclonic (familial) 345.1
psychic equivalent 345.5
psychomotor 345.4
psychosensory 345.4
reflex 345.1
seizure 345.9
senile 345.9
sensory-induced 345.5
sleep (*see also* Narcolepsy) 347.00
somatomotor type 345.5
somatosensory 345.5
specified type NEC 345.8
status (grand mal) 345.3
  focal motor 345.7
  petit mal 345.2
  psychomotor 345.7
  temporal lobe 345.7
symptomatic 345.9
temporal lobe 345.4
tonic (-clonic) 345.1
traumatic (injury unspecified) 907.0
  injury specified—*see* Late, effect (of)
    specified injury
twilight 293.0
uncinate (gyrus) 345.4
Unverricht (-Lundborg) (familial myoclonic)
  345.1
visceral 345.5
visual 345.5
Epileptiform
convulsions 780.39
seizure 780.39
Epiloia 759.5
Epimenorrhea 626.2
Epipharyngitis (*see also* Nasopharyngitis) 460
Epiphora 375.20
due to
  excess lacrimation 375.21
  insufficient drainage 375.22
Epiphyseal arrest 733.91
femoral head 732.2
Epiphyseolysis, epiphysiolysis (*see also* Osteochondrosis) 732.9
Epiphysitis (*see also* Osteochondrosis) 732.9
juvenile 732.6
marginal (Scheuermann's) 732.0
os calcis 732.5
syphilitic (congenital) 090.0
vertebral (Scheuermann's) 732.0
Epiplocele (*see also* Hernia) 553.9
Epiploitis (*see also* Peritonitis) 567.9

Epiplosarcomphalocele (*see also* Hernia, umbilicus) 553.1
Episcleritis 379.00
  gouty 274.89 *[379.09]*
  nodular 379.02
  periodica fugax 379.01
    angioneurotic—*see* Edema, angioneurotic
  specified NEC 379.09
  staphylococcal 379.00
  suppurative 379.00
  syphilitic 095.0
  tuberculous (*see also* Tuberculosis) 017.3 *[379.09]*
Episode
  brain (*see also* Disease, cerebrovascular, acute) 436
  cerebral (*see also* Disease, cerebrovascular, acute) 436
  depersonalization (in neurotic state) 300.6
  hyporesponsive 780.09
  psychotic (*see also* Psychosis) 298.9
    organic, transient 293.9
  schizophrenic (acute) NEC (*see also* Schizophrenia) 295.4
Epispadias
  female 753.8
  male 752.62
Episplenitis 289.59
Epistaxis (multiple) 784.7
  hereditary 448.0
  vicarious menstruation 625.8
Epithelioma (malignant) (M8011/3)—*see also* Neoplasm, by site, malignant
  adenoides cysticum (M8100/0)—*see* Neoplasm, skin, benign
  basal cell (M8090/3)—*see* Neoplasm, skin, malignant
  benign (M8011/0)—*see* Neoplasm, by site, benign
  Bowen's (M8081/2)—*see* Neoplasm, skin, in situ
  calcifying (benign) (Malherbe's) (M8110/0)—*see* Neoplasm, skin, benign
  external site—*see* Neoplasm, skin, malignant
  intraepidermal, Jadassohn (M8096/0)—*see* Neoplasm, skin, benign
  squamous cell (M8070/3)—*see* Neoplasm, by site, malignant
Epitheliopathy
  pigment, retina 363.15
  posterior multifocal placoid (acute) 363.15
Epithelium, epithelial —*see* condition
Epituberculosis (allergic) (with atelectasis) (*see also* Tuberculosis) 010.8
Eponychia 757.5
Epstein's
  nephrosis or syndrome (*see also* Nephrosis) 581.9
  pearl (mouth) 528.4
Epstein-Barr infection (viral) 075
  chronic 780.79 *[139.8]*
Epulis (giant cell) (gingiva) 523.8
Equinia 024
Equinovarus (congenital) 754.51
  acquired 736.71
Equivalent
  angina 413.9
  convulsive (abdominal) (*see also* Epilepsy) 345.5
  epileptic (psychic) (*see also* Epilepsy) 345.5

Erb's
  disease 359.1
  palsy, paralysis (birth) (brachial) (newborn) 767.6
    spinal (spastic) syphilitic 094.89
  pseudohypertrophic muscular dystrophy 359.1
Erb (-Duchenne) paralysis (birth injury) (newborn) 767.6
Erb-Goldflam disease or syndrome 358.00
Erdheim-Chester disease (ECD) 277.89
Erdheim's syndrome (acromegalic macrospondylitis) 253.0
Erection, painful (persistent) 607.3
Ergosterol deficiency (vitamin D) 268.9
  with
    osteomalacia 268.2
    rickets (*see also* Rickets) 268.0
Ergotism (ergotized grain) 988.2
  from ergot used as drug (migraine therapy)
    correct substance properly administered 349.82
    overdose or wrong substance given or taken 975.0
Erichsen's disease (railway spine) 300.16
Erlacher-Blount syndrome (tibia vara) 732.4
Erosio interdigitalis blastomycetica 112.3
Erosion
  arteriosclerotic plaque—*see* Arteriosclerosis, by site
  artery NEC 447.2
    without rupture 447.8
  bone 733.99
  bronchus 519.19
  cartilage (joint) 733.99
  cervix (uteri) (acquired) (chronic) (congenital) 622.0
    with mention of cervicitis 616.0
  cornea (recurrent) (*see also* Keratitis) 371.42
    traumatic 918.1
  dental (idiopathic) (occupational) 521.30
    extending into
      dentine 521.32
      pulp 521.33
    generalized 521.35
    limited to enamel 521.31
    localized 521.34
  duodenum, postpyloric—*see* Ulcer, duodenum
  esophagus 530.89
  gastric 535.4
  implanted vaginal mesh
    in, into
      pelvic floor muscles 629.31
      surrounding organ(s) or tissue 629.31
  intestine 569.89
  lymphatic vessel 457.8
  pylorus, pyloric (ulcer) 535.4
  sclera 379.16
  spine, aneurysmal 094.89
  spleen 289.59
  stomach 535.4
  teeth (idiopathic) (occupational) (*see also* Erosion, dental) 521.30
    due to
      medicine 521.30
      persistent vomiting 521.30
  urethra 599.84
  uterus 621.8
  vaginal prosthetic materials NEC
    in, into
      pelvic floor muscles 629.31
      surrounding organ(s) or tissue 629.31
  vertebra 733.99
Erotomania 302.89
  Clérambault's 297.8

Erythredema 985.0
   polyneuritica 985.0
   polyneuropathy 985.0
Erythremia (acute) (M9841/3) 207.0
   chronic (M9842/3) 207.1
   secondary 289.0
Erythroblastopenia (acquired) 284.89
   congenital 284.01
Erythroblastophthisis 284.01
Erythroblastosis (fetalis) (newborn) 773.2
   due to
      ABO
         antibodies 773.1
         incompatibility, maternal/fetal 773.1
         isoimmunization 773.1
      Rh
         antibodies 773.0
         incompatibility, maternal/fetal 773.0
         isoimmunization 773.0
Erythrocyanosis (crurum) 443.89
Erythrocythemia —see Erythremia
Erythrocytopenia 285.9
Erythrocytosis (megalosplenic)
   familial 289.6
   oval, hereditary (see also Elliptocytosis) 282.1
   secondary 289.0
   stress 289.0
Erythroderma (see also Erythema) 695.9
   desquamativa (in infants) 695.89
   exfoliative 695.89
   ichthyosiform, congenital 757.1
   infantum 695.89
   maculopapular 696.2
   neonatorum 778.8
   psoriaticum 696.1
   secondary 695.9
Erythrodysesthesia, palmar plantar (PPE) 693.0
Erythrogenesis imperfecta 284.09
Erythroleukemia (M9840/3) 207.0
Erythromelalgia 443.82
Erythromelia 701.8
Erythropenia 285.9
Erythrophagocytosis 289.9
Erythrophobia 300.23
Erythroplakia
   oral mucosa 528.79
   tongue 528.79
Erythroplasia (Queyrat) (M8080/2)
   specified site—see Neoplasm, skin, in situ
   unspecified site 233.5
Erythropoiesis, idiopathic ineffective 285.0
Escaped beats, heart 427.60
   postoperative 997.1
Escherichia coli (E. coli) —see Infection,
      Escherichia coli
Esoenteritis —see Enteritis
Esophagalgia 530.89
Esophagectasis 530.89
   due to cardiospasm 530.0
Esophagismus 530.5
Esophagitis (alkaline) (chemical) (chronic)
      (infectional) (necrotic) (postoperative) 530.10
   acute 530.12
   candidal 112.84
   eosinophilic 530.13
   reflux 530.11
   specified NEC 530.19
   tuberculous (see also Tuberculosis) 017.8
   ulcerative 530.19
Esophagocele 530.6
Esophagodynia 530.89

Esophagomalacia 530.89
Esophagoptosis 530.89
Esophagospasm 530.5
Esophagostenosis 530.3
Esophagostomiasis 127.7
Esophagostomy
   complication 530.87
      infection 530.86
      malfunctioning 530.87
      mechanical 530.87
Esophagotracheal —see condition
Esophagus —see condition
Esophoria 378.41
   convergence, excess 378.84
   divergence, insufficiency 378.85
Esotropia (nonaccommodative) 378.00
   accommodative 378.35
   alternating 378.05
      with
         A pattern 378.06
         specified noncomitancy NEC 378.08
         V pattern 378.07
         X pattern 378.08
         Y pattern 378.08
      intermittent 378.22
   intermittent 378.20
      alternating 378.22
      monocular 378.21
   monocular 378.01
      with
         A pattern 378.02
         specified noncomitancy NEC 378.04
         V pattern 378.03
         X pattern 378.04
         Y pattern 378.04
      intermittent 378.21
Espundia 085.5
Essential —see condition
Esterapenia 289.89
Esthesioneuroblastoma (M9522/3) 160.0
Esthesioneurocytoma (M9521/3) 160.0
Esthesioneuroepithelioma (M9523/3) 160.0
Esthiomene 099.1
Estivo-autumnal
   fever 084.0
   malaria 084.0
Estrangement V61.09
Estriasis 134.0
Ethanolaminuria 270.8
Ethanolism (see also Alcoholism) 303.9
Ether dependence, dependency (see also
      Dependence) 304.6
Etherism (see also Dependence) 304.6
Ethmoid, ethmoidal —see condition
Ethmoiditis (chronic) (nonpurulent) (purulent)
      (see also Sinusitis, ethmoidal) 473.2
   influenzal (see also Influenza) 487.1
   Woakes' 471.1
Ethylism (see also Alcoholism) 303.9
Eulenburg's disease (congenital paramyotonia)
      359.29
Eunuchism 257.2
Eunuchoidism 257.2
   hypogonadotropic 257.2
European blastomycosis 117.5
Eustachian —see condition
Euthyroid sick syndrome 790.94
Euthyroidism 244.9

Evaluation
fetal lung maturity 659.8
for suspected condition (*see also* Observation) V71.9
  abuse V71.81
  exposure
    antrax V71.82
    biologic agent NEC V71.83
    SARS V71.83
  neglect V71.81
  newborn—*see* Observation, suspected,
    condition, newborn
  specified condition NEC V71.89
mental health V70.2
requested by authority V70.1
nursing care V63.8
social service V63.8
Evans' syndrome (thrombocytopenic purpura) 287.32
**Event, apparent life threatening in newborn
  and infant (ALTE)** 799.82
Eventration
colon into chest—*see* Hernia, diaphragm
diaphragm (congenital) 756.6
Eversion
bladder 596.89
cervix (uteri) 622.0
  with mention of cervicitis 616.0
foot NEC 736.79
  congenital 755.67
lacrimal punctum 375.51
punctum lacrimale (postinfectional) (senile) 375.51
ureter (meatus) 593.89
urethra (meatus) 599.84
uterus 618.1
  complicating delivery 665.2
    affecting fetus or newborn 763.89
  puerperal, postpartum 674.8
Evidence
of malignancy
  cytologic
    without histologic confirmation
      anus 796.76
      cervix 795.06
      vagina 795.16
Evisceration
birth injury 767.8
bowel (congenital)—*see* Hernia, ventral
congenital (*see also* Hernia, ventral) 553.29
operative wound 998.32
traumatic NEC 869.1
  eye 871.3
Evulsion —*see* Avulsion
Ewing's
angioendothelioma (M9260/3)—*see* Neoplasm,
  bone, malignant
sarcoma (M9260/3)—*see* Neoplasm, bone,
  malignant
tumor (M9260/3)—*see* Neoplasm, bone, malignant
Exaggerated lumbosacral angle (with impinging
  spine) 756.12
Examination (general) (routine) (of) (for) V70.9
allergy V72.7
annual V70.0
cardiovascular preoperative V72.81
cervical Papanicolaou smear V76.2
  as a part of routine gynecological examination
    V72.31
  to confirm findings of recent normal smear
    following initial abnormal smear V72.32
child care (routine) V20.2
clinical research investigation (normal control
  patient) (participant) V70.7

Examination—*continued*
dental V72.2
developmental testing (child) (infant) V20.2
donor (potential) V70.8
ear V72.19
eye V72.0
following
  accident (motor vehicle) V71.4
  alleged rape or seduction (victim or culprit) V71.5
  inflicted injury (victim or culprit) NEC V71.6
  rape or seduction, alleged (victim or culprit) V71.5
  treatment (for) V67.9
    combined V67.6
    fracture V67.4
    involving high-risk medication NEC V67.51
    mental disorder V67.3
    specified condition NEC V67.59
follow-up (routine) (following) V67.9
  cancer chemotherapy V67.2
  chemotherapy V67.2
  disease NEC V67.59
  high-risk medication NEC V67.51
  injury NEC V67.59
population survey V70.6
postpartum V24.2
psychiatric V67.3
psychotherapy V67.3
radiotherapy V67.1
specified surgery NEC V67.09
surgery V67.00
  vaginal pap smear V67.01
gynecological V72.31
  for contraceptive maintenance V25.40
    intrauterine device V25.42
    pill V25.41
    specified method NEC V25.49
health (of)
  armed forces personnel V70.5
  checkup V70.0
  child, routine V20.2
  defined subpopulation NEC V70.5
  inhabitants of institutions V70.5
  occupational V70.5
  pre-employment screening V70.5
  preschool children V70.5
    for admission to school V70.3
  prisoners V70.5
    for entrance into prison V70.3
  prostitutes V70.5
  refugees V70.5
  school children V70.5
  students V70.5
hearing V72.19
  following failed hearing screening V72.11
infant
  8 to 28 days old V20.32
  over 28 days old, routine V20.2
  under 8 days old V20.31
laboratory V72.60
  ordered as part of a routine general medical
    examination V72.62
  pre-operative V72.63
  pre-procedural V72.63
  specified NEC V72.69
lactating mother V24.1
medical (for) (of) V70.9
  administrative purpose NEC V70.3
  admission to
    old age home V70.3
    prison V70.3
    school V70.3
  adoption V70.3

Examination—*continued*
  medical (for) (of)—*continued*
    armed forces personnel V70.5
    at health care facility V70.0
    camp V70.3
    child, routine V20.2
    clinical research investigation (control)
        (normal comparison) (participant) V70.7
    defined subpopulation NEC V70.5
    donor (potential) V70.8
    driving license V70.3
    general V70.9
      routine V70.0
      specified reason NEC V70.8
    immigration V70.3
    inhabitants of institutions V70.5
    insurance certification V70.3
    marriage V70.3
    medicolegal reasons V70.4
    naturalization V70.3
    occupational V70.5
    population survey V70.6
    pre-employment V70.5
    preschool children V70.5
      for admission to school V70.3
    prison V70.3
    prisoners V70.5
      for entrance into prison V70.3
    prostitutes V70.5
    refugees V70.5
    school children V70.5
    specified reason NEC V70.8
    sport competition V70.3
    students V70.5
  medicolegal reason V70.4
  pelvic (annual) (periodic) V72.31
  periodic (annual) (routine) V70.0
  postpartum
    immediately after delivery V24.0
    routine follow-up V24.2
  pregnancy (unconfirmed) (possible) V72.40
    negative result V72.41
    positive result V72.42
  prenatal V22.1
    first pregnancy V22.0
    high-risk pregnancy V23.9
      specified problem NEC V23.8
      to determine fetal viability V23.87
  preoperative V72.84
    cardiovascular V72.81
    respiratory V72.82
    specified NEC V72.83
  preprocedural V72.84
    cardiovascular V72.81
    general physical V72.83
    respiratory V72.82
    specified NEC V72.83
  prior to chemotherapy V72.83
  psychiatric V70.2
    follow-up not needing further care V67.3
    requested by authority V70.1
  radiological NEC V72.5
  respiratory preoperative V72.82
  screening—*see* Screening
  sensitization V72.7
  skin V72.7
    hypersensitivity V72.7
  special V72.9
  specified type or reason NEC V72.85
    preoperative V72.83
      specified NEC V72.83

Examination—*continued*
  teeth V72.2
  vaginal Papanicolaou smear V76.47
    following hysterectomy for malignant
        condition V67.01
  victim or culprit following
    alleged rape or seduction V71.5
    inflicted injury NEC V71.6
  vision V72.0
  well baby V20.2
Exanthem, exanthema (*see also* Rash) 782.1
  Boston 048
  epidemic, with meningitis 048
  lichenoid psoriasiform 696.2
  subitum 058.10
    due to
      human herpesvirus 6 058.11
      human herpesvirus 7 058.12
  viral, virus NEC 057.9
    specified type NEC 057.8
Excess, excessive, excessively
  alcohol level in blood 790.3
  carbohydrate tissue, localized 278.1
  carotene (dietary) 278.3
  cold 991.9
    specified effect NEC 991.8
  convergence 378.84
  crying 780.95
    of
      adolescent 780.95
      adult 780.95
      baby 780.92
      child 780.95
      infant (baby) 780.92
      newborn 780.92
  development, breast 611.1
  diaphoresis (*see also* Hyperhidrosis) 780.8
  distance, interarch 524.28
  divergence 378.85
  drinking (alcohol) NEC (*see also* Abuse, drugs,
        nondependent) 305.0
    continual (*see also* Alcoholism) 303.9
    habitual (*see also* Alcoholism) 303.9
  eating 783.6
  eyelid fold (congenital) 743.62
  fat 278.02
    in heart (*see also* Degeneration, myocardial) 429.1
    tissue, localized 278.1
  foreskin 605
  gas 787.3
  gastrin 251.5
  glucagon 251.4
  heat (*see also* Heat) 992.9
  horizontal
    overjet 524.26
    overlap 524.26
  interarch distance 524.28
  intermaxillary vertical dimension 524.37
  interocclusal distance of teeth 524.37
  large
    colon 564.7
      congenital 751.3
    fetus or infant 766.0
      with obstructed labor 660.1
        affecting management of pregnancy 656.6
        causing disproportion 653.5
    newborn (weight of 4500 grams or more) 766.0

Excess, excessive, excessively—*continued*
long
  colon 751.5
  organ or site, congenital NEC—*see* Anomaly,
    specified type NEC
  umbilical cord (entangled)
    affecting fetus or newborn 762.5
    in pregnancy or childbirth 663.3
      with compression 663.2
menstruation 626.2
number of teeth 520.1
  causing crowding 524.31
nutrients (dietary) NEC 783.6
potassium (K) 276.7
salivation (*see also* Ptyalism) 527.7
secretion—*see also* Hypersecretion
  milk 676.6
  sputum 786.4
  sweat (*see also* Hyperhidrosis) 780.8
short
  organ or site, congenital NEC—*see* Anomaly,
    specified type NEC
  umbilical cord
    affecting fetus or newborn 762.6
    in pregnancy or childbirth 663.4
skin NEC 701.9
  eyelid 743.62
    acquired 374.30
sodium (Na) 276.0
spacing of teeth 524.32
sputum 786.4
sweating (*see also* Hyperhidrosis) 780.8
tearing (ducts) (eye) (*see also* Epiphora) 375.20
thirst 783.5
  due to deprivation of water 994.3
tissue in reconstructed breast 612.0
tuberosity 524.07
vitamin
  A (dietary) 278.2
    administered as drug (chronic) (prolonged
      excessive intake) 278.2
    reaction to sudden overdose 963.5
  D (dietary) 278.4
    administered as drug (chronic) (prolonged
      excessive intake) 278.4
    reaction to sudden overdose 963.5
weight 278.02
  gain 783.1
    of pregnancy 646.1
  loss 783.21
Excitability, abnormal, under minor stress
  309.29
Excitation
catatonic (*see also* Schizophrenia) 295.2
psychogenic 298.1
reactive (from emotional stress, psychological
  trauma) 298.1
Excitement
manic (*see also* Psychosis, affective) 296.0
  recurrent episode 296.1
  single episode 296.0
mental, reactive (from emotional stress,
  psychological trauma) 298.1
state, reactive (from emotional stress,
  psychological trauma) 298.1
Excluded pupils 364.76
Excoriation (traumatic) (*see also* Injury,
  superficial, by site) 919.8
neurotic 698.4
Excyclophoria 378.44
Excyclotropia 378.33
Exencephalus, exencephaly 742.0

Exercise
breathing V57.0
remedial NEC V57.1
therapeutic NEC V57.1
Exfoliation
skin
  due to erythematous condition 695.50
    involving (percent of body surface)
      less than 10 percent 695.50
      10-19 percent 695.51
      20-29 percent 695.52
      30-39 percent 695.53
      40-49 percent 695.54
      50-59 percent 695.55
      60-69 percent 695.56
      70-79 percent 695.57
      80-89 percent 695.58
      90 percent or more 695.59
teeth
  due to systemic causes 525.0
Exfoliative —*see also* condition
dermatitis 695.89
Exhaustion, exhaustive (physical NEC) 780.79
battle (*see also* Reaction, stress, acute) 308.9
cardiac (*see also* Failure, heart) 428.9
delirium (*see also* Reaction, stress, acute) 308.9
due to
  cold 991.8
  excessive exertion 994.5
  exposure 994.4
  overexertion 994.5
fetus or newborn 779.89
heart (*see also* Failure, heart) 428.9
heat 992.5
  due to
    salt depletion 992.4
    water depletion 992.3
manic (*see also* Psychosis, affective) 296.0
  recurrent episode 296.1
  single episode 296.0
maternal, complicating delivery 669.8
  affecting fetus or newborn 763.89
mental 300.5
myocardium, myocardial (*see also* Failure,
  heart) 428.9
nervous 300.5
old age 797
postinfectional NEC 780.79
psychogenic 300.5
psychosis (*see also* Reaction, stress, acute)
  308.9
senile 797
  dementia 290.0
Exhibitionism (sexual) 302.4
Exomphalos 756.72
Exophoria 378.42
convergence, insufficiency 378.83
divergence, excess 378.85
Exophthalmic
cachexia 242.0
goiter 242.0
ophthalmoplegia 242.0 *[376.22]*
Exophthalmos 376.30
congenital 743.66
constant 376.31
endocrine NEC 259.9 *[376.22]*
hyperthyroidism 242.0 *[376.21]*
intermittent NEC 376.34
malignant 242.0 *[376.21]*
pulsating 376.35
  endocrine NEC 259.9 *[376.22]*
thyrotoxic 242.0 *[376.21]*

Exostosis 726.91
  cartilaginous (M9210/0)—*see* Neoplasm, bone,
    benign
  congenital 756.4
  ear canal, external 380.81
  gonococcal 098.89
  hip 726.5
  intracranial 733.3
  jaw (bone) 526.81
  luxurians 728.11
  multiple (cancellous) (congenital) (hereditary) 756.4
  nasal bones 726.91
  orbit, orbital 376.42
  osteocartilaginous (M9210/0)—*see* Neoplasm,
    bone, benign
  spine 721.8
    with spondylosis—*see* Spondylosis
  syphilitic 095.5
  wrist 726.4
Exotropia 378.10
  alternating 378.15
    with
      A pattern 378.16
      specified noncomitancy 378.18
      V pattern 378.17
      X pattern 378.18
      Y pattern 378.18
    intermittent 378.24
  intermittent 378.20
    alternating 378.24
    monocular 378.23
  monocular 378.11
    with
      A pattern 378.12
      specified noncomitancy NEC 378.14
      V pattern 378.13
      X pattern 378.14
      Y pattern 378.14
    intermittent 378.23
Explanation of
  investigation finding V65.4
  medication V65.4
Exposure (suspected) 994.9
  algae bloom V87.32
  cold 991.9
    specified effect NEC 991.8
  effects of 994.9
  exhaustion due to 994.4
  implanted vaginal mesh
    into vagina 629.32
    through vaginal wall 629.32
  to
    AIDS virus V01.79
    anthrax V01.81
    aromatic
      amines V87.11
      dyes V87.19
    arsenic V87.01
    asbestos V15.84
    benzene V87.12
    body fluids (hazardous) V15.85
    cholera V01.0
    communicable disease V01.9
      specified type NEC V01.89
    chromium compounds V87.09
    dyes V87.2
      aromatic V87.19
    Escherichia coli (E. coli) V01.83
    German measles V01.4
    gonorrhea V01.6

Exposure—*continued*
  to —*continued*
    hazardous
      aromatic compounds NEC V87.19
      body fluids V15.85
      chemicals NEC V87.2
      metals V87.09
      substances V87.39
    HIV V01.79
    human immunodeficiency virus V01.79
    lead V15.86
    meningococcus V01.84
    mold V87.31
    nickel dust V87.09
    parasitic disease V01.89
    poliomyelitis V01.2
    polycyclic aromatic hydrocarbons V87.19
    potentially hazardous body fluids V15.85
    rabies V01.5
    rubella V01.4
    SARS-associated coronavirus V01.82
    smallpox V01.3
    syphilis V01.6
    tuberculosis V01.1
    uranium V87.02
    varicella V01.71
    venereal disease V01.6
    viral disease NEC V01.79
      varicella V01.71
  vaginal prosthetic materials NEC
    into vagina 629.32
    through vaginal wall 629.32
Exsanguination, fetal 772.0
Exstrophy
  abdominal content 751.8
  bladder (urinary) 753.5
Extensive —*see* condition
Extra —*see also* Accessory
  rib 756.3
    cervical 756.2
Extraction
  with hook 763.89
  breech NEC 669.6
    affecting fetus or newborn 763.0
  cataract postsurgical V45.61
  manual NEC 669.8
    affecting fetus or newborn 763.89
Extrasystole 427.60
  atrial 427.61
  postoperative 997.1
  ventricular 427.69
Extrauterine gestation or pregnancy —*see*
  Pregnancy, ectopic
Extravasation
  blood 459.0
    lower extremity 459.0
  chemotherapy, vesicant 999.81
  chyle into mesentery 457.8
  pelvicalyceal 593.4
  pyelosinus 593.4
  urine 788.8
    from ureter 788.8
  vesicant
    agent NEC 999.82
    chemotherapy 999.81
Extremity —*see* condition
Extrophy —*see* Exstrophy

Extroversion
  bladder 753.5
  uterus 618.1
    complicating delivery 665.2
      affecting fetus or newborn 763.89
    postpartal (old) 618.1
Extruded tooth 524.34
Extrusion
  alveolus and teeth 524.75
  breast implant (prosthetic) 996.54
  device, implant, or graft—*see* Complications,
      mechanical
  eye implant (ball) (globe) 996.59
  intervertebral disc—*see* Displacement,
      intervertebral disc
  lacrimal gland 375.43
  mesh (reinforcing) 996.59
  ocular lens implant 996.53
  prosthetic device NEC—*see* Complications,
      mechanical
  vitreous 379.26
Exudate, pleura —*see* Effusion, pleura
Exudates, retina 362.82
Exudative —*see* condition
Eye, eyeball, eyelid—*see* condition
Eyestrain 368.13
Eyeworm disease of Africa 125.2

F

Faber's anemia or syndrome (achlorhydric anemia) 280.9
Fabry's disease (angiokeratoma corporis diffusum) 272.7
Face, facial —*see* condition
Facet of cornea 371.44
Faciocephalalgia, autonomic (*see also* Neuropathy, peripheral, autonomic) 337.9
Facioscapulohumeral myopathy 359.1
Factitious disorder, illness —*see* Illness, factitious
Factor
  deficiency—*see* Deficiency, factor
  psychic, associated with diseases classified elsewhere 316
  risk—*see* Problem
  V Leiden mutation 289.81
Fahr-Volhard disease (malignant nephrosclerosis) 403.00
Failure, failed
  adenohypophyseal 253.2
  attempted abortion (legal) (*see also* Abortion, failed) 638.9
  bone marrow (anemia) 284.9
    acquired (secondary) 284.89
    congenital 284.09
    idiopathic 284.9
  cardiac (*see also* Failure, heart) 428.9
    newborn 779.89
  cardiorenal (chronic) 428.9
    hypertensive (*see also* Hypertension, cardiorenal) 404.93
  cardiorespiratory 799.1
    specified during or due to a procedure 997.1
    long-term effect of cardiac surgery 429.4
  cardiovascular (chronic) 428.9
  cerebrovascular 437.8
  cervical dilatation in labor 661.0
    affecting fetus or newborn 763.7
  circulation, circulatory 799.89
    fetus or newborn 779.89
    peripheral 785.50
    postoperative 998.00
  compensation—*see* Disease, heart
  conscious sedation, during procedure 995.24
  congestive (*see also* Failure, heart) 428.0
  coronary (*see also* Insufficiency, coronary) 411.89
  dental implant 525.79
    due to
      infection 525.71
      lack of attached gingiva 525.72
      occlusal trauma (caused by poor prosthetic design) 525.72
      parafunctional habits 525.72
      periodontal infection (peri-implantitis) 525.72
      poor oral hygiene 525.72
      unintentional loading 525.71
    endosseous NEC 525.79
    mechanical 525.73
    osseointegration 525.71
      due to
        complications of systemic disease 525.71
        poor bone quality 525.71
        premature loading 525.71
      iatrogenic 525.71
      prior to intentional prosthetic loading 525.71

Failure, failed—*continued*
  dental implant—*continued*
    post-osseointegration
      biological 525.72
      iatrogenic 525.72
      due to complications of systemic disease 525.72
      mechanical 525.73
    pre-integration 525.71
    pre-osseointegration 525.71
  dental prosthesis causing loss of dental implant 525.73
  dental restoration
    marginal integrity 525.61
    periodontal anatomical integrity 525.65
  descent of head (at term) 652.5
    affecting fetus or newborn 763.1
    in labor 660.0
      affecting fetus or newborn 763.1
  device, implant, or graft—*see* Complications, mechanical
  engagement of head NEC 652.5
    in labor 660.0
  extrarenal 788.99
  fetal head to enter pelvic brim 652.5
    affecting fetus or newborn 763.1
    in labor 660.0
      affecting fetus or newborn 763.1
  forceps NEC 660.7
    affecting fetus or newborn 763.1
  fusion (joint) (spinal) 996.49
  growth in childhood 783.43
  heart (acute) (sudden) 428.9
    with
      abortion—*see* Abortion, by type, with specified complication NEC
      acute pulmonary edema (*see also* Failure, ventricular, left) 428.1
        with congestion (*see also* Failure, heart) 428.0
      decompensation (*see also* Failure, heart) 428.0
      dilation—*see* Disease, heart
      ectopic pregnancy (*see also* categories 633.0-633.9) 639.8
      molar pregnancy (*see also* categories 630-632) 639.8
    arteriosclerotic 440.9
    combined left-right sided 428.0
    combined systolic and diastolic 428.40
      acute 428.41
      acute on chronic 428.43
      chronic 428.42
    compensated (*see also* Failure, heart) 428.0
    complicating
      abortion—*see* Abortion, by type, with specified complication NEC
      delivery (cesarean) (instrumental) 669.4
      ectopic pregnancy (*see also* categories 633.0-633.9) 639.8
      molar pregnancy (*see also* categories 630-632) 639.8
      obstetric anesthesia or sedation 668.1
      surgery 997.1
    congestive (compensated) (decompensated) (*see also* Failure, heart) 428.0
      with rheumatic fever (conditions classifiable to 390)
        active 391.8
        inactive or quiescent (with chorea) 398.91

Failure, failed—*continued*
　heart—*continued*
　　congestive—*continued*
　　　fetus or newborn 779.89
　　　hypertensive (*see also* Hypertension, heart)
　　　　402.91
　　　　with renal disease (*see also* Hypertension,
　　　　　cardiorenal) 404.91
　　　　　with renal failure 404.93
　　　　benign 402.11
　　　　malignant 402.01
　　　rheumatic (chronic) (inactive) (with chorea)
　　　　398.91
　　　　active or acute 391.8
　　　　　with chorea (Sydenham's) 392.0
　　　decompensated (*see also* Failure, heart) 428.0
　　　degenerative (*see also* Degeneration,
　　　　myocardial) 429.1
　　　diastolic 428.30
　　　　acute 428.31
　　　　acute or chronic 428.33
　　　　chronic 428.32
　　　due to presence of (cardiac) prosthesis 429.4
　　　fetus or newborn 779.89
　　　following
　　　　abortion 639.8
　　　　cardiac surgery 429.4
　　　　ectopic or molar pregnancy 639.8
　　　high output NEC 428.9
　　　hypertensive (*see also* Hypertension, heart) 402.91
　　　　with renal disease (*see also* Hypertension,
　　　　　cardiorenal) 404.91
　　　　　with renal failure 404.93
　　　　benign 402.11
　　　　malignant 402.01
　　　left (ventricular) (*see also* Failure, ventricular,
　　　　left) 428.1
　　　　with right-sided failure (*see also* Failure,
　　　　　heart) 428.0
　　　low output (syndrome) NEC 428.9
　　　organic—*see* Disease, heart
　　　postoperative (immediate) 997.1
　　　　long term effect of cardiac surgery 429.4
　　　rheumatic (chronic) (congestive) (inactive) 398.91
　　　right (secondary to left heart failure,
　　　　conditions classifiable to 428.1)
　　　　(ventricular) (*see also* Failure, heart) 428.0
　　　senile 797
　　　specified during or due to a procedure 997.1
　　　　long-term effect of cardiac surgery 429.4
　　　systolic 428.20
　　　　acute 428.21
　　　　acute on chronic 428.23
　　　　chronic 428.22
　　　thyrotoxic (*see also* Thyrotoxicosis) 242.9 *[425.7]*
　　　valvular—*see* Endocarditis
　　hepatic 572.8
　　　acute 570
　　　due to a procedure 997.49
　　hepatorenal 572.4
　　hypertensive heart (*see also* Hypertension,
　　　heart) 402.91
　　　benign 402.11
　　　malignant 402.01
　　induction (of labor) 659.1
　　　abortion (legal) (*see also* Abortion, failed)
　　　　638.9
　　　affecting fetus or newborn 763.89
　　　by oxytocic drugs 659.1
　　　instrumental 659.0
　　　mechanical 659.0

Failure, failed—*continued*
　induction (of labor)—*continued*
　　medical 659.1
　　surgical 659.0
　initial alveolar expansion, newborn 770.4
　involution, thymus (gland) 254.8
　kidney—*see* Failure, renal
　lactation 676.4
　Leydig's cell, adult 257.2
　liver 572.8
　　acute 570
　medullary 799.89
　mitral—*see* Endocarditis, mitral
　moderate sedation, during procedure 995.24
　myocardium, myocardial (*see also* Failure,
　　heart) 428.9
　　chronic (*see also* Failure, heart) 428.0
　　congestive (*see also* Failure, heart) 428.0
　ovarian (primary) 256.39
　　iatrogenic 256.2
　　postablative 256.2
　　postirradiation 256.2
　　postsurgical 256.2
　ovulation 628.0
　prerenal 788.99
　renal (kidney) 586
　　with
　　　abortion—*see* Abortion, by type, with renal
　　　　failure
　　　ectopic pregnancy (*see also* categories
　　　　633.0-633.9) 639.3
　　　edema (*see also* Nephrosis) 581.9
　　　hypertension (*see also* Hypertension,
　　　　kidney) 403.91
　　　hypertensive heart disease (conditions
　　　　classifiable to 402) 404.92
　　　　with heart failure 404.93
　　　　benign 404.12
　　　　　with heart failure 404.13
　　　　malignant 404.02
　　　　　with heart failure 404.03
　　　molar pregnancy (*see also* categories
　　　　630-632) 639.3
　　　tubular necrosis (acute) 584.5
　　acute 584.9
　　　with lesion of
　　　　necrosis
　　　　　cortical (renal) 584.6
　　　　　medullary (renal) (papillary) 584.7
　　　　　tubular 584.5
　　　　specified pathology NEC 584.8
　　chronic 585.9
　　　hypertensive or with hypertension (*see also*
　　　　Hypertension, kidney) 403.91
　　due to a procedure 997.5
　　following
　　　abortion 639.3
　　　crushing 958.5
　　　ectopic or molar pregnancy 639.3
　　　labor and delivery (acute) 669.3
　　　hypertensive (*see also* Hypertension, kidney)
　　　　403.91
　　puerperal, postpartum 669.3
　　respiration, respiratory 518.81
　　　acute 518.81
　　　　following trauma and surgery 518.51
　　　acute and chronic 518.84
　　　　following trauma and surgery 518.53
　　　center 348.89
　　　　newborn 770.84
　　　chronic 518.83

Failure, failed—*continued*
respiration, respiratory—*continued*
following trauma and surgery or shock 518.51
newborn 770.84
rotation
cecum 751.4
colon 751.4
intestine 751.4
kidney 753.3
sedation, during procedure
conscious 995.24
moderate 995.24
segmentation—*see also* Fusion
fingers (*see also* Syndactylism, fingers) 755.11
toes (*see also* Syndactylism, toes) 755.13
seminiferous tubule, adult 257.2
senile (general) 797
with psychosis 290.20
testis, primary (seminal) 257.2
to progress 661.2
to thrive
adult 783.7
child 783.41
newborn 779.34
transplant 996.80
bone marrow 996.85
organ (immune or nonimmune cause) 996.80
bone marrow 996.85
heart 996.83
intestines 996.87
kidney 996.81
liver 996.82
lung 996.84
pancreas 996.86
specified NEC 996.89
skin 996.52
artificial 996.55
decellularized allodermis 996.55
temporary allograft or pigskin graft—*omit code*
stem cell(s) 996.88
from
peripheral blood 996.88
umbilical blood 996.88
trial of labor NEC 660.6
affecting fetus or newborn 763.1
tubal ligation 998.89
urinary 586
vacuum extraction
abortion—*see* Abortion, failed
delivery NEC 660.7
affecting fetus or newborn 763.1
vasectomy 998.89
ventouse NEC 660.7
affecting fetus or newborn 763.1
ventricular (*see also* Failure, heart) 428.9
left 428.1
with rheumatic fever (conditions classifiable
to 390)
active 391.8
with chorea 392.0
inactive or quiescent (with chorea) 398.91
hypertensive (*see also* Hypertension, heart)
402.91
benign 402.11
malignant 402.01
rheumatic (chronic) (inactive) (with chorea)
398.91
active or acute 391.8
with chorea 392.0
right (*see also* Failure, heart) 428.0
vital centers, fetus or newborn 779.8
weight gain in childhood 783.41

Fainting (fit) (spell) 780.2
Falciform hymen 752.49
Fall, maternal, affecting fetus or newborn 760.5
Fallen arches 734
Falling, any organ or part —*see* Prolapse
Fallopian
insufflation
fertility testing V26.21
following sterilization reversal V26.22
tube—*see* condition
Fallot's
pentalogy 745.2
tetrad or tetralogy 745.2
triad or trilogy 746.09
Fallout, radioactive (adverse effect) NEC 990
False —*see also* condition
bundle branch block 426.50
bursa 727.89
croup 478.75
joint 733.82
labor (pains) 644.1
opening, urinary, male 752.69
passage, urethra (prostatic) 599.4
positive
serological test for syphilis 795.6
Wassermann reaction 795.6
pregnancy 300.11
Family, familial —*see also* condition
affected by
family member
currently on deployment (military) V61.01
returned from deployment (military) (current
or past conflict) V61.02
disruption (*see also* Disruption, family) V61.09
estrangement V61.09
hemophagocytic
lymphohistiocytosis 288.4
reticulosis 288.4
Li-fraumeni (syndrome) V84.01
planning advice V25.09
natural
procreative V26.41
to avoid pregnancy V25.04
problem V61.9
specified circumstance NEC V61.8
retinoblastoma (syndrome) 190.5
Famine 994.2
edema 262
Fanconi's anemia (congenital pancytopenia) 284.09
Fanconi (-de Toni) (-Debré) syndrome
(cystinosis) 270.0
Farber (-Uzman) syndrome or disease
(disseminated lipogranulomatosis) 272.8
Farcin 024
Farcy 024
Farmers'
lung 495.0
skin 692.74
Farsightedness 367.0
Fascia —*see* condition
Fasciculation 781.0
Fasciculitis optica 377.32
Fasciitis 729.4
eosinophilic 728.89
necrotizing 728.86
nodular 728.79
perirenal 593.4
plantar 728.71
pseudosarcomatous 728.79
traumatic (old) NEC 728.79
current—*see* Sprain, by site

Fasciola hepatica infestation 121.3
Fascioliasis 121.3
Fasciolopsiasis (small intestine) 121.4
Fasciolopsis (small intestine) 121.4
Fast pulse 785.0
Fat
  embolism (cerebral) (pulmonary) (systemic)
    958.1
    with
      abortion—*see* Abortion, by type, with
        embolism
      ectopic pregnancy (*see also* categories
        633.0-633.9) 639.6
      molar pregnancy (*see also* categories
        630-632) 639.6
    complicating delivery or puerperium 673.8
    following
      abortion 639.6
      ectopic or molar pregnancy 639.6
    in pregnancy, childbirth, or the puerperium
      673.8
  excessive 278.02
    in heart (*see also* Degeneration, myocardial)
      429.1
  general 278.02
  hernia, herniation 729.30
    eyelid 374.34
    knee 729.31
    orbit 374.34
    retro-orbital 374.34
    retropatellar 729.31
    specified site NEC 729.39
  indigestion 579.8
  in stool 792.1
  localized (pad) 278.1
    heart (*see also* Degeneration, myocardial) 429.1
    knee 729.31
    retropatellar 729.31
  necrosis—*see also* Fatty, degeneration
    breast (aseptic) (segmental) 611.3
    mesentery 567.82
    omentum 567.82
    peritoneum 567.82
  pad 278.1
Fatal familial insomnia (FFI) 046.72
Fatal syncope 798.1
Fatigue 780.79
  auditory deafness (*see also* Deafness) 389.9
  chronic, syndrome 780.71
  combat (*see also* Reaction, stress, acute) 308.9
  during pregnancy 646.8
  general 780.79
    psychogenic 300.5
  heat (transient) 992.6
  muscle 729.89
  myocardium (*see also* Failure, heart) 428.9
  nervous 300.5
  neurosis 300.5
  operational 300.89
  postural 729.89
  posture 729.89
  psychogenic (general) 300.5
  senile 797
  syndrome NEC 300.5
    chronic 780.71
  undue 780.79
  voice 784.49
Fatness 278.02

Fatty —*see also* condition
  apron 278.1
  degeneration (diffuse) (general) NEC 272.8
    localized—*see* Degeneration, by site, fatty
    placenta—*see* Placenta, abnormal
    heart (enlarged) (*see also* Degeneration,
      myocardial) 429.1
  infiltration (diffuse) (general) (*see also*
    Degeneration, by site, fatty) 272.8
    heart (enlarged) (*see also* Degeneration,
      myocardial) 429.1
  liver 571.8
    alcoholic 571.0
    necrosis—*see* Degeneration, fatty
  phanerosis 272.8
Fauces —*see* condition
Fauchard's disease (periodontitis) 523.40
Faucitis 478.29
Faulty —*see also* condition
  position of teeth 524.30
Favism (anemia) 282.2
Favre-Racouchot disease (elastoidosis cutanea
  nodularis) 701.8
Favus 110.9
  beard 110.0
  capitis 110.0
  corporis 110.5
  eyelid 110.8
  foot 110.4
  hand 110.2
  scalp 110.0
  specified site NEC 110.8
Fear, fearfulness (complex) (reaction) 300.20
  child 313.0
  of
    animals 300.29
    closed spaces 300.29
    crowds 300.29
    eating in public 300.23
    heights 300.29
    open spaces 300.22
      with panic attacks 300.21
    public speaking 300.23
    streets 300.22
      with panic attacks 300.21
    travel 300.22
      with panic attacks 300.21
    washing in public 300.23
  transient 308.0
Feared complaint unfounded V65.5
Febricula (continued) (simple) (*see also* Pyrexia)
  780.60
Febrile (*see also* Pyrexia) 780.60
  convulsion (simple) 780.31
    complex 780.32
  nonhemolytic transfusion reaction (FNHTR)
    780.66
  seizure (simple) 780.31
    atypical 780.32
    complex 780.32
    complicated 780.32
Febris (*see also* Fever) 780.60
  aestiva (*see also* Fever, hay) 477.9
  flava (*see also* Fever, yellow) 060.9
  melitensis 023.0
  pestis (*see also* Plague) 020.9
  puerperalis 672
  recurrens (*see also* Fever, relapsing) 087.9
    pediculo vestimenti 087.0
  rubra 034.1
  typhoidea 002.0
  typhosa 002.0

Fecal —*see* condition
Fecalith (impaction) 560.32
  with hernia—*see also* Hernia, by site, with
    obstruction
  gangrenous—*see* Hernia, by site, with gangrene
    appendix 543.9
    congenital 777.1
Fede's disease 529.0
Feeble-minded 317
Feeble rapid pulse due to shock following
    injury 958.4
Feeding
  faulty (elderly) (infant) 783.3
    newborn 779.31
  formula check V20.2
  improper (elderly) (infant) 783.3
    newborn 779.31
  problem (elderly) (infant) 783.3
    newborn 779.31
    nonorganic origin 307.59
Feeling of foreign body in throat 784.99
Feer's disease 985.0
Feet —*see* condition
Feigned illness V65.2
Feil-Klippel syndrome (brevicollis) 756.16
Feinmesser's (hidrotic) ectodermal dysplasia
    757.31
Felix's disease (juvenile osteochondrosis, hip)
    732.1
Felon (any digit) (with lymphangitis) 681.01
  herpetic 054.6
Felty's syndrome (rheumatoid arthritis with
    splenomegaly and leukopenia) 714.1
Feminism in boys 302.6
Feminization, testicular 259.51
  with pseudohermaphroditism, male 259.51
Femoral hernia —*see* Hernia, femoral
Femora vara 736.32
Femur, femoral —*see* condition
Fenestrata placenta —*see* Placenta, abnormal
Fenestration, fenestrated —*see also* Imperfect,
    closure
  aorta-pulmonary 745.0
  aorticopulmonary 745.0
  aortopulmonary 745.0
  cusps, heart valve NEC 746.89
    pulmonary 746.09
  hymen 752.49
  pulmonic cusps 746.09
Fenwick's disease 537.89
Fermentation (gastric) (gastrointestinal)
    (stomach) 536.8
  intestine 564.89
    psychogenic 306.4
  psychogenic 306.4
Fernell's disease (aortic aneurysm) 441.9
Fertile eunuch syndrome 257.2
Fertility, meaning multiparity—*see* Multiparity
Fetal
  alcohol syndrome 760.71
  anemia 678.0
  thrombocytopenia 678.0
  twin to twin transfusion 678.0
Fetalis uterus 752.39
Fetid
  breath 784.99
  sweat 705.89
Fetishism 302.81
  transvestic 302.3

Fetomaternal hemorrhage
  affecting management of pregnancy 656.0
  fetus or newborn 772.0
Fetus, fetal —*see also* condition
  papyraceous 779.89
  type lung tissue 770.4
Fever 780.60
  with chills 780.60
    in malarial regions (*see also* Malaria) 084.6
  abortus NEC 023.9
  Aden 061
  African tick-borne 087.1
  American
    mountain tick 066.1
    spotted 082.0
  and ague (*see also* Malaria) 084.6
  aphthous 078.4
  arbovirus hemorrhagic 065.9
  Assam 085.0
  Australian A or Q 083.0
  Bangkok hemorrhagic 065.4
  biliary, Charcot's intermittent—*see*
    Choledocholithiasis
  bilious, hemoglobinuric 084.8
  blackwater 084.8
  blister 054.9
  Bonvale Dam 780.79
  boutonneuse 082.1
  brain 323.9
    late effect—*see* category 326
  breakbone 061
  Bullis 082.8
  Bunyamwera 066.3
  Burdwan 085.0
  Bwamba (encephalitis) 066.3
  Cameroon (*see also* Malaria) 084.6
  Canton 081.9
  catarrhal (acute) 460
    chronic 472.0
  cat-scratch 078.3
  cerebral 323.9
    late effect—*see* category 326
  cerebrospinal (meningococcal) (*see also*
    Meningitis, cerebrospinal) 036.0
  Chagres 084.0
  Chandipura 066.8
  changuinola 066.0
  Charcot's (biliary) (hepatic) (intermittent)—*see*
    Choledocholithiasis
  Chikungunya (viral) 066.3
    hemorrhagic 065.4
  childbed 670.8
  Chitral 066.0
  Colombo (*see also* Fever, paratyphoid) 002.9
  Colorado tick (virus) 066.1
  congestive
    malarial (*see also* Malaria) 084.6
    remittent (*see also* Malaria) 084.6
  Congo virus 065.0
  continued 780.60
    malarial 084.0
  Corsican (*see also* Malaria) 084.6
  Crimean hemorrhagic 065.0
  Cyprus (*see also* Brucellosis) 023.9
  dandy 061
  deer fly (*see also* Tularemia) 021.9
  dehydration, newborn 778.4
  dengue (virus) 061
    hemorrhagic 065.4
  desert 114.0
  due to heat 992.0
  Dumdum 085.0

Fever—*continued*
enteric 002.0
ephemeral (of unknown origin) (*see also*
   Pyrexia) 780.60
epidemic, hemorrhagic of the Far East 065.0
erysipelatous (*see also* Erysipelas) 035
estivo-autumnal (malarial) 084.0
etiocholanolone 277.31
famine—*see also* Fever, relapsing
   meaning typhus—*see* Typhus
Far Eastern hemorrhagic 065.0
five day 083.1
Fort Bragg 100.89
gastroenteric 002.0
gastromalarial (*see also* Malaria) 084.6
Gibraltar (*see also* Brucellosis) 023.9
glandular 075
Guama (viral) 066.3
Haverhill 026.1
hay (allergic) (with rhinitis) 477.9
   with
      asthma (bronchial) (*see also* Asthma) 493.0
   due to
      dander, animal (cat) (dog) 477.2
      dust 477.8
      fowl 477.8
      hair, animal (cat) (dog) 477.2
      pollen, any plant or tree 477.0
      specified allergen other than pollen 477.8
heat (effects) 992.0
hematuric, bilious 084.8
hemoglobinuric (malarial) 084.8
   bilious 084.8
hemorrhagic (arthropod-borne) NEC 065.9
   with renal syndrome 078.6
   arenaviral 078.7
   Argentine 078.7
   Bangkok 065.4
   Bolivian 078.7
   Central Asian 065.0
   chikungunya 065.4
   Crimean 065.0
   dengue (virus) 065.4
   Ebola 065.8
   epidemic 078.6
      of Far East 065.0
   Far Eastern 065.0
   Junin virus 078.7
   Korean 078.6
   Kyasanur forest 065.2
   Machupo virus 078.7
   mite-borne NEC 065.8
   mosquito-borne 065.4
   Omsk 065.1
   Philippine 065.4
   Russian (Yaroslav) 078.6
   Singapore 065.4
   Southeast Asia 065.4
   Thailand 065.4
   tick-borne NEC 065.3
hepatic (*see also* Cholecystitis) 575.8
   intermittent (Charcot's)—*see*
      Choledocholithiasis
herpetic (*see also* Herpes) 054.9
Hyalomma tick 065.0
icterohemorrhagic 100.0
inanition 780.60
   newborn 778.4
in conditions classified elsewhere 780.61
infective NEC 136.9

Fever—*continued*
intermittent (bilious) (*see also* Malaria) 084.6
   hepatic (Charcot)—*see* Choledocholithiasis
   of unknown origin (*see also* Pyrexia) 780.60
pernicious 084.0
iodide
   correct substance properly administered
      780.60
   overdose or wrong substance given or taken
      975.5
Japanese river 081.2
jungle yellow 060.0
Junin virus, hemorrhagic 078.7
Katayama 120.2
Kedani 081.2
Kenya 082.1
Korean hemorrhagic 078.6
Lassa 078.89
Lone Star 082.8
lung—*see* Pneumonia
Machupo virus, hemorrhagic 078.7
malaria, malarial (*see also* Malaria) 084.6
Malta (*see also* Brucellosis) 023.9
Marseilles 082.1
marsh (*see also* Malaria) 084.6
Mayaro (viral) 066.3
Mediterranean (*see also* Brucellosis) 023.9
   familial 277.31
   tick 082.1
meningeal—*see* Meningitis
metal fumes NEC 985.8
Meuse 083.1
Mexican—*see* Typhus, Mexican
Mianeh 087.1
miasmatic (*see also* Malaria) 084.6
miliary 078.2
milk, female 672
mill 504
mite-borne hemorrhagic 065.8
Monday 504
mosquito-borne NEC 066.3
   hemorrhagic NEC 065.4
mountain 066.1
   meaning
      Rocky Mountain spotted 082.0
      undulant fever (*see also* Brucellosis) 023.9
   tick (American) 066.1
Mucambo (viral) 066.3
mud 100.89
Neapolitan (*see also* Brucellosis) 023.9
neutropenic 288.00
newborn (environmentally induced) 778.4
nine-mile 083.0
nonexanthematous tick 066.1
North Asian tick-borne typhus 082.2
Omsk hemorrhagic 065.1
O'nyong-nyong (viral) 066.3
Oropouche (viral) 066.3
Oroya 088.0
paludal (*see also* Malaria) 084.6
Panama 084.0
pappataci 066.0
paratyphoid 002.9
   A 002.1
   B (Schottmüller's) 002.2
   C (Hirschfeld) 002.3
parrot 073.9
periodic 277.31
pernicious, acute 084.0
persistent (of unknown origin) (*see also*
      Pyrexia) 780.60

Fever—*continued*
  petechial 036.0
  pharyngoconjunctival 077.2
    adenoviral type 3 077.2
  Philippine hemorrhagic 065.4
  phlebotomus 066.0
  Piry 066.8
  Pixuna (viral) 066.3
  Plasmodium ovale 084.3
  pleural (*see also* Pleurisy) 511.0
  pneumonic—*see* Pneumonia
  polymer fume 987.8
  postimmunization 780.63
  postoperative 780.62
    due to infection 998.59
  posttransfusion 780.66
  postvaccination 780.63
  pretibial 100.89
  puerperal, postpartum 672
  putrid—*see* Septicemia
  pyemic—*see* Septicemia
  Q 083.0
    with pneumonia 083.0 *[484.8]*
  quadrilateral 083.0
  quartan (malaria) 084.2
  Queensland (coastal) 083.0
    seven-day 100.89
  Quintan (A) 083.1
  quotidian 084.0
  rabbit (*see also* Tularemia) 021.9
  rat-bite 026.9
    due to
      Spirillum minor or minus 026.0
      Spirochaeta morsus muris 026.0
      Streptobacillus moniliformis 026.1
  recurrent—*see* Fever, relapsing
  relapsing 087.9
    Carter's (Asiatic) 087.0
    Dutton's (West African) 087.1
    Koch's 087.9
    louse-borne (epidemic) 087.0
    Novy's (American) 087.1
    Obermeyer's (European) 087.0
    spirillum NEC 087.9
    tick-borne (endemic) 087.1
  remittent (bilious) (congestive) (gastric) (*see also* Malaria) 084.6
  rheumatic (active) (acute) (chronic) (subacute) 390
    with heart involvement 391.9
      carditis 391.9
      endocarditis (aortic) (mitral) (pulmonary) (tricuspid) 391.1
      multiple sites 391.8
      myocarditis 391.2
      pancarditis, acute 391.8
      pericarditis 391.0
      specified type NEC 391.8
      valvulitis 391.1
    inactive or quiescent with cardiac hypertrophy 398.99
      carditis 398.90
      endocarditis 397.9
        aortic (valve) 395.9
          with mitral (valve) disease 396.9
        mitral (valve) 394.9
          with aortic (valve) disease 396.9
        pulmonary (valve) 397.1
        tricuspid (valve) 397.0
      heart conditions (classifiable to 429.3, 429.6, 429.9) 398.99
      failure (congestive) (conditions classifiable to 428.0, 428.9) 398.91

Fever—*continued*
  rheumatic—*continued*
    inactive—*continued*
      left ventricular failure (conditions classifiable to 428.1) 398.91
      myocardial degeneration (conditions classifiable to 429.1) 398.0
      myocarditis (conditions classifiable to 429.0) 398.0
      pancarditis 398.99
      pericarditis 393
  Rift Valley (viral) 066.3
  Rocky Mountain spotted 082.0
  rose 477.0
  Ross river (viral) 066.3
  Russian hemorrhagic 078.6
  sandfly 066.0
  San Joaquin (valley) 114.0
  São Paulo 082.0
  scarlet 034.1
  septic—*see* Septicemia
  seven-day 061
    Japan 100.89
    Queensland 100.89
  shin bone 083.1
  Singapore hemorrhagic 065.4
  solar 061
  sore 054.9
  South African tick-bite 087.1
  Southeast Asia hemorrhagic 065.4
  spinal—*see* Meningitis
  spirillary 026.0
  splenic (*see also* Anthrax) 022.9
  spotted (Rocky Mountain) 082.0
    American 082.0
    Brazilian 082.0
    Colombian 082.0
    meaning
      cerebrospinal meningitis 036.0
      typhus 082.9
  spring 309.23
  steroid
    correct substance properly administered 780.60
    overdose or wrong substance given or taken 962.0
  streptobacillary 026.1
  subtertian 084.0
  Sumatran mite 081.2
  sun 061
  swamp 100.89
  sweating 078.2
  swine 003.8
  sylvatic yellow 060.0
  Tahyna 062.5
  tertian—*see* Malaria, tertian
  Thailand hemorrhagic 065.4
  thermic 992.0
  three day 066.0
    with Coxsackie exanthem 074.8
  tick
    American mountain 066.1
    Colorado 066.1
    Kemerovo 066.1
    Mediterranean 082.1
    mountain 066.1
    nonexanthematous 066.1
    Quaranfil 066.1
  tick-bite NEC 066.1
  tick-borne NEC 066.1
    hemorrhagic NEC 065.3
  transitory of newborn 778.4

Fever—*continued*
  trench 083.1
  tsutsugamushi 081.2
  typhogastric 002.0
  typhoid (abortive) (ambulant) (any site)
      (hemorrhagic) (infection) (intermittent)
      (malignant) (rheumatic) 002.0
  typhomalarial (*see also* Malaria) 084.6
  typhus—*see* Typhus
  undulant (*see also* Brucellosis) 023.9
  unknown origin (*see also* Pyrexia) 780.60
  uremic—*see* Uremia
  uveoparotid 135
  valley (Coccidioidomycosis) 114.0
  Venezuelan equine 066.2
  Volhynian 083.1
  Wesselsbron (viral) 066.3
  West
    African 084.8
    Nile (viral) 066.40
      with
        cranial nerve disorders 066.42
        encephalitis 066.41
        optic neuritis 066.42
        other complications 066.49
        other neurologic manifestations 066.42
        polyradiculitis 066.42
  Whitmore's 025
  Wolhynian 083.1
  worm 128.9
  Yaroslav hemorrhagic 078.6
  yellow 060.9
    jungle 060.0
    sylvatic 060.0
    urban 060.1
    vaccination, prophylactic (against) V04.4
  Zika (viral) 066.3
Fibrillation
  atrial (established) (paroxysmal) 427.31
  auricular (atrial) (established) 427.31
  cardiac (ventricular) 427.41
  coronary (*see also* Infarct, myocardium) 410.9
  heart (ventricular) 427.41
  muscular 728.9
  postoperative 997.1
  ventricular 427.41
Fibrin
  ball or bodies, pleural (sac) 511.0
  chamber, anterior (eye) (gelatinous exudate)
      364.04
Fibrinogenolysis (hemorrhagic)—*see*
    Fibrinolysis
Fibrinogenopenia (congenital) (hereditary) (*see
    also* Defect, coagulation) 286.3
  acquired 286.6
Fibrinolysis (acquired) (hemorrhagic)
    (pathologic) 286.6
  with
    abortion—*see* Abortion, by type, with
        hemorrhage, delayed or excessive
    ectopic pregnancy (*see also* categories
        633.0-633.9) 639.1
    molar pregnancy (*see also* categories 630-632)
        639.1
  antepartum or intrapartum 641.3
    affecting fetus or newborn 762.1
  following
    abortion 639.1
    ectopic or molar pregnancy 639.1
  newborn, transient 776.2
  postpartum 666.3

Fibrinopenia (hereditary) (*see also* Defect,
    coagulation) 286.3
  acquired 286.6
Fibrinopurulent —*see* condition
Fibrinous —*see* condition
Fibroadenoma (M9010/0)
  cellular intracanalicular (M9020/0) 217
  giant (intracanalicular) (M9020/0) 217
  intracanalicular (M9011/0)
    cellular (M9020/0) 217
    giant (M9020/0) 217
    specified site—*see* Neoplasm, by site, benign
    unspecified site 217
  juvenile (M9030/0) 217
  pericanalicular (M9012/0)
    specified site—*see* Neoplasm, by site, benign
    unspecified site 217
  phyllodes (M9020/0) 217
  prostate 600.20
    with
      other lower urinary tract symptoms (LUTS)
          600.21
      urinary
        obstruction 600.21
        retention 600.21
  specified site—*see* Neoplasm, by site, benign
  unspecified site 217
Fibroadenosis, breast (chronic) (cystic) (diffuse)
    (periodic) (segmental) 610.2
Fibroangioma (M9160/0)—*see also* Neoplasm,
    by site, benign
  juvenile (M9160/0)
    specified site—*see* Neoplasm, by site, benign
    unspecified site 210.7
Fibrocellulitis progressiva ossificans 728.11
Fibrochondrosarcoma (M9220/3)—*see*
    Neoplasm, cartilage, malignant
Fibrocystic
  disease 277.00
    bone NEC 733.29
    breast 610.1
    jaw 526.2
    kidney (congenital) 753.19
    liver 751.62
    lung 518.89
      congenital 748.4
    pancreas 277.00
  kidney (congenital) 753.19
Fibrodysplasia ossificans multiplex
    (progressiva) 728.11
Fibroelastosis (cordis) (endocardial)
    (endomyocardial) 425.3
Fibroid (tumor) (M8890/0)—*see also* Neoplasm,
    connective tissue, benign
  disease, lung (chronic) (*see also* Fibrosis, lung)
      515
  heart (disease) (*see also* Myocarditis) 429.0
  induration, lung (chronic) (*see also* Fibrosis,
      lung) 515
  in pregnancy or childbirth 654.1
    affecting fetus or newborn 763.89
    causing obstructed labor 660.2
      affecting fetus or newborn 763.1
  liver—*see* Cirrhosis, liver
  lung (*see also* Fibrosis, lung) 515
  pneumonia (chronic) (*see also* Fibrosis, lung)
      515
  uterus (M8890/0) (*see also* Leiomyoma, uterus)
      218.9
Fibrolipoma (M8851/0) (*see also* Lipoma, by
    site) 214.9

Fibroliposarcoma (M8850/3)—*see* Neoplasm, connective tissue, malignant
Fibroma (M8810/0)—*see also* Neoplasm, connective tissue, benign
  ameloblastic (M9330/0) 213.1
    upper jaw (bone) 213.0
  bone (nonossifying) 733.99
    ossifying (M9262/0)—*see* Neoplasm, bone, benign
    cementifying (M9274/0)—*see* Neoplasm, bone, benign
    chondromyxoid (M9241/0)—*see* Neoplasm, bone, benign
    desmoplastic (M8823/1)—*see* Neoplasm, connective tissue, uncertain behavior
    facial (M8813/0)—*see* Neoplasm, connective tissue, benign
    invasive (M8821/1)—*see* Neoplasm, connective tissue, uncertain behavior
    molle (M8851/0) (*see also* Lipoma, by site) 214.9
    myxoid (M8811/0)—*see* Neoplasm, connective tissue, benign
    nasopharynx, nasopharyngeal (juvenile) (M9160/0) 210.7
    nonosteogenic (nonossifying)—*see* Dysplasia, fibrous
    odontogenic (M9321/0) 213.1
      upper jaw (bone) 213.0
    ossifying (M9262/0)—*see* Neoplasm, bone, benign
    periosteal (M8812/0)—*see* Neoplasm, bone, benign
    prostate 600.20
      with
        other lower urinary tract symptoms (LUTS) 600.21
        urinary
          obstruction 600.21
          retention 600.21
    soft (M8851/0) (*see also* Lipoma, by site) 214.9
Fibromatosis 728.79
  abdominal (M8822/1)—*see* Neoplasm, connective tissue, uncertain behavior
  aggressive (M8821/1)—*see* Neoplasm, connective tissue, uncertain behavior
  congenital generalized (CGF) 759.89
  Dupuytren's 728.6
  gingival 523.8
  plantar fascia 728.71
  proliferative 728.79
  pseudosarcomatous (proliferative) (subcutaneous) 728.79
  subcutaneous pseudosarcomatous (proliferative) 728.79
Fibromyalgia 729.1
Fibromyoma (M8890/0)—*see also* Neoplasm, connective tissue, benign
  uterus (corpus) (*see also* Leiomyoma, uterus) 218.9
    in pregnancy or childbirth 654.1
      affecting fetus or newborn 763.89
      causing obstructed labor 660.2
        affecting fetus or newborn 763.1
Fibromyositis (*see also* Myositis) 729.1
  scapulohumeral 726.2
Fibromyxolipoma (M8852/0) (*see also* Lipoma, by site) 214.9
Fibromyxoma (M8811/0)—*see* Neoplasm, connective tissue, benign
Fibromyxosarcoma (M8811/3)—*see* Neoplasm, connective tissue, malignant
Fibro-odontoma, ameloblastic (M9290/0) 213.1
  upper jaw (bone) 213.0

Fibro-osteoma (M9262/0)—*see* Neoplasm, bone, benign
Fibroplasia, retrolental (*see also* Retinopathy of prematurity) 362.21
Fibropurulent —*see* condition
Fibrosarcoma (M8810/3)—*see also* Neoplasm, connective tissue, malignant
  ameloblastic (M9330/3) 170.1
    upper jaw (bone) 170.0
  congenital (M8814/3)—*see* Neoplasm, connective tissue, malignant
  fascial (M8813/3)—*see* Neoplasm, connective tissue, malignant
  infantile (M8814/3)—*see* Neoplasm, connective tissue, malignant
  odontogenic (M9330/3) 170.1
    upper jaw (bone) 170.0
  periosteal (M8812/3)—*see* Neoplasm, bone, malignant
Fibrosclerosis
  breast 610.3
  corpora cavernosa (penis) 607.89
  familial multifocal NEC 710.8
  multifocal (idiopathic) NEC 710.8
  penis (corpora cavernosa) 607.89
Fibrosis, fibrotic
  adrenal (gland) 255.8
  alveolar (diffuse) 516.31
  amnion 658.8
  anal papillae 569.49
  anus 569.49
  appendix, appendiceal, noninflammatory 543.9
  arteriocapillary—*see* Arteriosclerosis
  bauxite (of lung) 503
  biliary 576.8
    due to Clonorchis sinensis 121.1
  bladder 596.89
    interstitial 595.1
    localized submucosal 595.1
    panmural 595.1
  bone, diffuse 756.59
  breast 610.3
  capillary—*see also* Arteriosclerosis
    lung (chronic) (*see also* Fibrosis, lung) 515
  cardiac (*see also* Myocarditis) 429.0
  cervix 622.8
  chorion 658.8
  corpus cavernosum 607.89
  cystic (of pancreas) 277.00
    with
      manifestations
        gastrointestinal 277.03
        pulmonary 277.02
        specified NEC 277.09
      meconium ileus 277.01
      pulmonary exacerbation 277.02
  due to (presence of) any device, implant, or graft—*see* Complications, due to (presence of) any device, implant, or graft classified to 996.0-996.5 NEC
  ejaculatory duct 608.89
  endocardium (*see also* Endocarditis) 424.90
  endomyocardial (African) 425.0
  epididymis 608.89
  eye muscle 378.62
  graphite (of lung) 503
  heart (*see also* Myocarditis) 429.0
  hepatic—*see also* Cirrhosis, liver
    due to Clonorchis sinensis 121.1
  hepatolienal—*see* Cirrhosis, liver
  hepatosplenic—*see* Cirrhosis, liver

Fibrosis, fibrotic—*continued*
infrapatellar fat pad 729.31
interstitial pulmonary, newborn 770.7
intrascrotal 608.89
kidney (*see also* Sclerosis, renal) 587
liver—*see* Cirrhosis, liver
lung (atrophic) (capillary) (chronic) (confluent)
    (massive) (perialveolar) (peribronchial) 515
  with
    anthracosilicosis (occupational) 500
    anthracosis (occupational) 500
    asbestosis (occupational) 501
    bagassosis (occupational) 495.1
    bauxite 503
    berylliosis (occupational) 503
    byssinosis (occupational) 504
    calcicosis (occupational) 502
    chalicosis (occupational) 502
    dust reticulation (occupational) 504
    farmers' lung 495.0
    gannister disease (occupational) 502
    graphite 503
    pneumonoconiosis (occupational) 505
    pneumosiderosis (occupational) 503
    siderosis (occupational) 503
    silicosis (occupational) 502
  tuberculosis (*see also* Tuberculosis) 011.4
  diffuse (idiopathic) (interstitial) 516.31
  due to
    bauxite 503
    fumes or vapors (chemical) (inhalation) 506.4
    graphite 503
  following radiation 508.1
  postinflammatory 515
  silicotic (massive) (occupational) 502
  tuberculous (*see also* Tuberculosis) 011.4
lymphatic gland 289.3
median bar 600.90
  with
    other lower urinary tract symptoms (LUTS)
        600.91
    urinary
      obstruction 600.91
      retention 600.91
mediastinum (idiopathic) 519.3
meninges 349.2
muscle NEC 728.2
  iatrogenic (from injection) 999.9
myocardium, myocardial (*see also* Myocarditis)
    429.0
oral submucous 528.8
ovary 620.8
oviduct 620.8
pancreas 577.8
  cystic 277.00
    with
      manifestations
        gastrointestinal 277.03
        pulmonary 277.02
        specified NEC 277.09
      meconium ileus 277.01
      pulmonary exacerbation 277.02
penis 607.89
periappendiceal 543.9
periarticular (*see also* Ankylosis) 718.5
pericardium 423.1
perineum, in pregnancy or childbirth 654.8
  affecting fetus or newborn 763.89
  causing obstructed labor 660.2
    affecting fetus or newborn 763.1

Fibrosis, fibrotic—*continued*
perineural NEC 355.9
  foot 355.6
periureteral 593.89
placenta—*see* Placenta, abnormal
pleura 511.0
popliteal fat pad 729.31
preretinal 362.56
prostate (chronic) 600.90
  with
    other lower urinary tract symptoms (LUTS)
        600.91
    urinary
      obstruction 600.91
      retention 600.91
pulmonary (chronic) (*see also* Fibrosis, lung)
    515
  alveolar capillary block 516.8
  idiopathic 516.31
  interstitial
    diffuse (idiopathic) 516.31
    newborn 770.7
radiation—*see* Effect, adverse, radiation
rectal sphincter 569.49
retroperitoneal, idiopathic 593.4
sclerosing mesenteric (idiopathic) 567.82
scrotum 608.89
seminal vesicle 608.89
senile 797
skin NEC 709.2
spermatic cord 608.89
spleen 289.59
  bilharzial (*see also* Schistosomiasis) 120.9
subepidermal nodular (M8832/0)—*see*
    Neoplasm, skin, benign
submucous NEC 709.2
  oral 528.8
  tongue 528.8
syncytium—*see* Placenta, abnormal
testis 608.89
  chronic, due to syphilis 095.8
thymus (gland) 254.8
tunica vaginalis 608.89
ureter 593.89
urethra 599.84
uterus (nonneoplastic) 621.8
  bilharzial (*see also* Schistosomiasis) 120.9
  neoplastic (*see also* Leiomyoma, uterus) 218.9
vagina 623.8
valve, heart (*see also* Endocarditis) 424.90
vas deferens 608.89
vein 459.89
  lower extremities 459.89
vesical 595.1
Fibrositis (periarticular) (rheumatoid) 729.0
  humeroscapular region 726.2
  nodular, chronic
    Jaccoud's 714.4
    rheumatoid 714.4
  ossificans 728.11
  scapulohumeral 726.2
Fibrothorax 511.0
Fibrotic —*see* Fibrosis
Fibrous —*see* condition
Fibroxanthoma (M8831/0)—*see also* Neoplasm,
    connective tissue, benign
  atypical (M8831/1)—*see* Neoplasm, connective
    tissue, uncertain behavior
  malignant (M8831/3)—*see* Neoplasm,
    connective tissue, malignant
Fibroxanthosarcoma (M8831/3)—*see*
    Neoplasm, connective tissue, malignant

Fiedler's
disease (leptospiral jaundice) 100.0
myocarditis or syndrome (acute isolated
myocarditis) 422.91
Fiessinger-Leroy (-Reiter) syndrome 099.3
Fiessinger-Rendu syndrome (erythema
muliforme exudativum) 695.19
Fifth disease (eruptive) 057.0
venereal 099.1
Filaria, filarial —*see* Infestation, filarial
Filariasis (*see also* Infestation, filarial) 125.9
bancroftian 125.0
Brug's 125.1
due to
bancrofti 125.0
Brugia (Wuchereria) (malayi) 125.1
Loa loa 125.2
malayi 125.1
organism NEC 125.6
Wuchereria (bancrofti) 125.0
malayi 125.1
Malayan 125.1
ozzardi 125.5
specified type NEC 125.6
Filatoff's, Filatov's, Filatow's disease
(infectious mononucleosis) 075
File-cutters' disease 984.9
specified type of lead—*see* Table of drugs and
chemicals
Filling defect
biliary tract 793.3
bladder 793.5
duodenum 793.4
gallbladder 793.3
gastrointestinal tract 793.4
intestine 793.4
kidney 793.5
stomach 793.4
ureter 793.5
Filtering bleb, eye (postglaucoma) (status)
V45.69
with complication or rupture 997.99
postcataract extraction (complication) 997.99
Fimbrial cyst (congenital) 752.11
Fimbriated hymen 752.49
Financial problem affecting care V60.2
Findings (abnormal), without diagnosis
(examination) (laboratory test) 796.4
17-ketosteroids, elevated 791.9
acetonuria 791.6
acid phosphatase 790.5
albumin-globulin ratio 790.99
albuminuria 791.0
alcohol in blood 790.3
alkaline phosphatase 790.5
amniotic fluid 792.3
amylase 790.5
anisocytosis 790.09
antenatal screening 796.5
anthrax positive 795.31
antibody titers, elevated 795.79
anticardiolipin antibody 795.79
antigen-antibody reaction 795.79
antiphosphatidylglycerol antibody 795.79
antiphosphatidylinositol antibody 795.79
antiphosphatidylserine antibody 795.79
antiphospholipid antibody 795.79
bacteriuria 791.9
ballistocardiogram 794.39
bicarbonate 276.9
bile in urine 791.4

Findings —*continued*
bilirubin 277.4
bleeding time (prolonged) 790.92
blood culture, positive 790.7
blood gas level 790.91
blood sugar level 790.29
high 790.29
fasting glucose 790.21
glucose tolerance test 790.22
low 251.2
C-reactive protein (CRP) 790.95
calcium 275.40
cancer antigen 125 [CA 125] 795.82
carbonate 276.9
carcinoembryonic antigen [CEA] 795.81
casts, urine 791.7
catecholamines 791.9
cells, urine 791.7
cerebrospinal fluid (color) (content) (pressure)
792.0
cervical
high risk human papillomavirus (HPV) DNA
test positive 795.05
low risk human papillomavirus (HPV) DNA
test positive 795.09
non-atypical endometrial cells 795.09
chloride 276.9
cholesterol 272.9
high 272.0
with high triglycerides 272.2
chromosome analysis 795.2
chyluria 791.1
circulation time 794.39
cloudy dialysis effluent 792.5
cloudy urine 791.9
coagulation study 790.92
cobalt, blood 790.6
color of urine (unusual) NEC 791.9
copper, blood 790.6
creatinine clearance 794.4
crystals, urine 791.9
culture, positive NEC 795.39
blood 790.7
HIV V08
human immunodeficiency virus V08
nose 795.39
Staphylococcus — *see* Carrier (suspected)
of, Staphylococcus
skin lesion NEC 795.39
spinal fluid 792.0
sputum 795.39
stool 792.1
throat 795.39
urine 791.9
viral
human immunodeficiency V08
wound 795.39
cytology specified site NEC 796.9
echocardiogram 793.2
echoencephalogram 794.01
echogram NEC—*see* Findings, abnormal,
structure
electrocardiogram (ECG) (EKG) 794.31
electroencephalogram (EEG) 794.02
electrolyte level, urinary 791.9
electromyogram (EMG) 794.17
ocular 794.14
electro-oculogram (EOG) 794.12
electroretinogram (ERG) 794.11
enzymes, serum NEC 790.5
fibrinogen titer coagulation study 790.92

Findings—*continued*
  filling defect—*see* Filling defect
  function study NEC 794.9
    auditory 794.15
    bladder 794.9
    brain 794.00
    cardiac 794.30
    endocrine NEC 794.6
      thyroid 794.5
    kidney 794.4
    liver 794.8
    nervous system
      central 794.00
      peripheral 794.19
    oculomotor 794.14
    pancreas 794.9
    placenta 794.9
    pulmonary 794.2
    retina 794.11
    special senses 794.19
    spleen 794.9
    vestibular 794.16
  gallbladder, nonvisualization 793.3
  glucose 790.29
    elevated
      fasting 790.21
      tolerance test 790.22
  glycosuria 791.5
  heart
    shadow 793.2
    sounds 785.3
  hematinuria 791.2
  hematocrit
    drop (precipitous) 790.01
    elevated 282.7
    low 285.9
  hematologic NEC 790.99
  hematuria 599.70
  hemoglobin
    drop 790.01
    elevated 282.7
    low 285.9
  hemoglobinuria 791.2
  histological NEC 795.4
  hormones 259.9
  immunoglobulins, elevated 795.79
  indolacetic acid, elevated 791.9
  iron 790.6
  karyotype 795.2
  ketonuria 791.6
  lactic acid dehydrogenase (LDH) 790.4
  lead 790.6
  lipase 790.5
  lipids NEC 272.9
  lithium, blood 790.6
  liver function test 790.6
  lung field (shadow) 793.19
    coin lesion 793.11
  magnesium, blood 790.6
  mammogram 793.80
    calcification 793.89
    caclulus 793.89
    dense breasts 793.82
    inconclusive 793.82
      due to dense breasts 793.82
    microcalcification 793.81
  mediastinal shift 793.2
  melanin, urine 791.9
  microbiologic NEC 795.39
  mineral, blood NEC 790.6
  myoglobinuria 791.3
  nasal swab, anthrax 795.31

Findings—*continued*
  neonatal screening 796.6
  nitrogen derivatives, blood 790.6
  nonvisualization of gallbladder 793.3
  nose culture, positive 795.39
  odor of urine (unusual) NEC 791.9
  oxygen saturation 790.91
  Papanicolaou (smear) 796.9
    anus 796.70
      with
        atypical squamous cells
          cannot exclude high grade squamous
            intraepithelial lesion (ASC-H)
            796.72
          of undetermined significance (ASC-US)
            796.71
        cytologic evidence of malignancy 796.76
        high grade squamous intraepithelial lesion
          (HGSIL) 796.74
        low grade squamous intraepithelial lesion
          (LGSIL) 796.73
      glandular 796.70
      specified finding NEC 796.79
    cervix 795.00
      with
        atypical squamous cells
          cannot exclude high grade squamous
            intrepithelial lesion (ASC-H) 795.02
          of undetermined significance (ASC-US)
            795.01
        cytologic evidence of malignancy 795.06
        high grade squamous intraepithelial lesion
          (HGSIL) 795.04
        low grade squamous intraepithelial lesion
          (LGSIL) 795.03
        non-atypical endometrial cells 795.09
      dyskaryotic 795.09
      non-atypical endometrial cells 795.09
      nonspecific finding NEC 795.09
    other site 796.9
    vagina 795.10
      with
        atypical squamous cells
          cannot exclude high grade squamous
            intraepithelial lesion (ASC-H)
            795.12
          of undetermined significance (ASC-US)
            795.11
        cytologic evidence of malignancy 795.16
        high grade squamous intraepithelial lesion
          (HGSIL) 795.14
        low grade squamous intraepithelial lesion
          (LGSIL) 795.13
      glandular 795.10
      specified NEC 795.19
  peritoneal fluid 792.9
  phonocardiogram 794.39
  phosphorus 275.3
  pleural fluid 792.9
  pneumoencephalogram 793.0
  PO_2-oxygen ratio 790.91
  poikilocytosis 790.09
  potassium
    deficiency 276.8
    excess 276.7
  PPD 795.51
  prostate specific antigen (PSA) 790.93
  protein, serum NEC 790.99
  proteinuria 791.0
  prothrombin time (partial) (prolonged) (PT)
    (PTT) 790.92
  pyuria 791.9

Findings —*continued*
  radiologic (x-ray) 793.99
    abdomen 793.6
    biliary tract 793.3
    breast 793.89
      abnormal mammogram NOS 793.80
      mammographic
        calcification 793.89
        calculus 793.89
        microcalcification 793.81
    gastrointestinal tract 793.4
    genitourinary organs 793.5
    head 793.0
    image test inconclusive due to excess body fat
      793.91
    intrathoracic organs NEC 793.2
    lung 793.19
    musculoskeletal 793.7
    placenta 793.99
    retroperitoneum 793.6
    skin 793.99
    skull 793.0
    subcutaneous tissue 793.99
  red blood cell 790.09
    count 790.09
    morphology 790.09
    sickling 790.09
    volume 790.09
  saliva 792.4
  scan NEC 794.9
    bladder 794.9
    bone 794.9
    brain 794.09
    kidney 794.4
    liver 794.8
    lung 794.2
    pancreas 794.9
    placental 794.9
    spleen 794.9
    thyroid 794.5
  sedimentation rate, elevated 790.1
  semen 792.2
  serological (for)
    human immunodeficiency virus (HIV)
      inconclusive 795.71
      positive V08
    syphilis—*see* Findings, serology for syphilis
  serology for syphilis
    false positive 795.6
    positive 097.1
      false 795.6
      follow-up of latent syphilis—*see* Syphilis,
        latent
      only finding—*see* Syphilis, latent
  serum 790.99
    blood NEC 790.99
    enzymes NEC 790.5
    proteins 790.99
  SGOT 790.4
  SGPT 790.4
  sickling of red blood cells 790.09
  skin test, positive 795.79
    tuberculin (without active tuberculosis) 795.51
  sodium 790.6
    deficiency 276.1
    excess 276.0
  specified NEC 796.9
  spermatozoa 792.2
  spinal fluid 792.0
    culture, positive 792.0
  sputum culture, positive 795.39

Findings —*continued*
  for acid-fast bacilli 795.39
  stool NEC 792.1
    bloody 578.1
      occult 792.1
    color 792.1
    culture, positive 792.1
    occult blood 792.1
  stress test 794.39
  structure, body (echogram) (thermogram)
    (ultrasound) (x-ray) NEC 793.99
    abdomen 793.6
    breast 793.89
      abnormal mammogram 793.80
      mammographic
        calcification 793.89
        calculus 793.89
        microcalcification 793.81
    gastrointestinal tract 793.4
    genitourinary organs 793.5
    head 793.0
      echogram (ultrasound) 794.01
    intrathoracic organs NEC 793.2
    lung 793.19
    musculoskeletal 793.7
    placenta 793.99
    retroperitoneum 793.6
    skin 793.99
    subcutaneous tissue NEC 793.99
  synovial fluid 792.9
  thermogram—*see* Finding, abnormal, structure
  throat culture, positive 795.39
  thyroid (function) 794.5
    metabolism (rate) 794.5
    scan 794.5
    uptake 794.5
  total proteins 790.99
  toxicology (drugs) (heavy metals) 796.0
  transaminase (level) 790.4
  triglycerides 272.9
    high 272.1
      with high cholesterol 272.2
  tuberculin skin test (without active tuberculosis)
    795.51
  tumor markers NEC 795.89
  ultrasound—*see also* Finding, abnormal,
    structure
    cardiogram 793.2
  uric acid, blood 790.6
  urine, urinary constituents 791.9
    acetone 791.6
    albumin 791.0
    bacteria 791.9
    bile 791.4
    blood 599.70
    casts or cells 791.7
    chyle 791.1
    culture, positive 791.9
    glucose 791.5
    hemoglobin 791.2
    ketone 791.6
    protein 791.0
    pus 791.9
    sugar 791.5
  vaginal
    fluid 792.9
    high risk human papillomavirus (HPV) DNA
      test positive 795.15
    low risk human papillomavirus (HPV) DNA
      test positive 795.19
  vanillylmandelic acid, elevated 791.9

Fistula—*continued*
  carotid-cavernous
    congenital 747.81
      with hemorrhage 430
    traumatic 900.82
      with hemorrhage (*see also* Hemorrhage,
        brain, traumatic) 853.0
      late effect 908.3
  cecosigmoidal 569.81
  cecum 569.81
  cerebrospinal (fluid) 349.81
  cervical, lateral (congenital) 744.41
  cervicoaural (congenital) 744.49
  cervicosigmoidal 619.1
  cervicovesical 619.0
  cervix 619.8
  chest (wall) 510.0
  cholecystocolic (*see also* Fistula, gallbladder)
    575.5
  cholecystocolonic (*see also* Fistula, gallbladder)
    575.5
  cholecystoduodenal (*see also* Fistula,
    gallbladder) 575.5
  cholecystoenteric (*see also* Fistula, gallbladder)
    575.5
  cholecystogastric (*see also* Fistula, gallbladder)
    575.5
  cholecystointestinal (*see also* Fistula,
    gallbladder) 575.5
  choledochoduodenal 576.4
  cholocolic (*see also* Fistula, gallbladder) 575.5
  coccyx 685.1
    with abscess 685.0
  colon 569.81
  colostomy 569.69
  colovaginal (acquired) 619.1
  common duct (bile duct) 576.4
  congenital, NEC—*see* Anomaly, specified type
    NEC
  cornea, causing hypotony 360.32
  coronary, arteriovenous 414.19
    congenital 746.85
  costal region 510.0
  cul-de-sac, Douglas' 619.8
  cutaneous 686.9
  cystic duct (*see also* Fistula, gallbladder) 575.5
    congenital 751.69
  cystostomy 596.83
  dental 522.7
  diaphragm 510.0
    bronchovisceral 510.0
    pleuroperitoneal 510.0
    pulmonoperitoneal 510.0
  duodenum 537.4
  ear (canal) (external) 380.89
  enterocolic 569.81
  enterocutaneous 569.81
  enteroenteric 569.81
  entero-uterine 619.1
    congenital 752.39
  enterovaginal 619.1
    congenital 752.49
  enterovesical 596.1
  epididymis 608.89
    tuberculous (*see also* Tuberculosis) 016.4
  esophagobronchial 530.89
    congenital 750.3
  esophagocutaneous 530.89
  esophagopleurocutaneous 530.89
  esophagotracheal 530.84
    congenital 750.3

Fistula—*continued*
  esophagus 530.89
    congenital 750.4
  ethmoid (*see also* Sinusitis, ethmoidal) 473.2
  eyeball (cornea) (sclera) 360.32
  eyelid 373.11
  fallopian tube (external) 619.2
  fecal 569.81
    congenital 751.5
  from periapical lesion 522.7
  frontal sinus (*see also* Sinusitis, frontal) 473.1
  gallbladder 575.5
    with calculus, cholelithiasis, stones (*see also*
      Cholelithiasis) 574.2
    congenital 751.69
  gastric 537.4
  gastrocolic 537.4
    congenital 750.7
    tuberculous (*see also* Tuberculosis) 014.8
  gastroenterocolic 537.4
  gastroesophageal 537.4
  gastrojejunal 537.4
  gastrojejunocolic 537.4
  genital
    organs
      female 619.9
        specified site NEC 619.8
      male 608.89
    tract-skin (female) 619.2
  hepatopleural 510.0
  hepatopulmonary 510.0
  horseshoe 565.1
  ileorectal 569.81
  ileosigmoidal 569.81
  ileostomy 569.69
  ileovesical 596.1
  ileum 569.81
  in ano 565.1
    tuberculous (*see also* Tuberculosis) 014.8
  inner ear (*see also* Fistula, labyrinth) 386.40
  intestine 569.81
  intestinocolonic (abdominal) 569.81
  intestinoureteral 593.82
  intestinouterine 619.1
  intestinovaginal 619.1
    congenital 752.49
  intestinovesical 596.1
  involving female genital tract 619.9
    digestive-genital 619.1
    genital tract-skin 619.2
    specified site NEC 619.8
    urinary-genital 619.0
  ischiorectal (fossa) 566
  jejunostomy 569.69
  jejunum 569.81
  joint 719.80
    ankle 719.87
    elbow 719.82
    foot 719.87
    hand 719.84
    hip 719.85
    knee 719.86
    multiple sites 719.89
    pelvic region 719.85
    shoulder (region) 719.81
    specified site NEC 719.88
    tuberculous—*see* Tuberculosis, joint
    wrist 719.83
  kidney 593.89
  labium (majus) (minus) 619.8

Fistula—*continued*
  labyrinth, labyrinthine NEC 386.40
    combined sites 386.48
    multiple sites 386.48
    oval window 386.42
    round window 386.41
  semicircular canal 386.43
  lacrimal, lachrymal (duct) (gland) (sac) 375.61
  lacrimonasal duct 375.61
  laryngotracheal 748.3
  larynx 478.79
  lip 528.5
    congenital 750.25
  lumbar, tuberculous (*see also* Tuberculosis)
    015.0 *[730.8]*
  lung 510.0
  lymphatic (node) (vessel) 457.8
  mamillary 611.0
  mammary (gland) 611.0
    puerperal, postpartum 675.1
  mastoid (process) (region) 383.1
  maxillary (*see also* Sinusitis, maxillary) 473.0
  mediastinal 510.0
  mediastinobronchial 510.0
  mediastinocutaneous 510.0
  middle ear 385.89
  mouth 528.3
  nasal 478.19
    sinus (*see also* Sinusitis) 473.9
  nasopharynx 478.29
  nipple—*see* Fistula, breast
  nose 478.19
  oral (cutaneous) 528.3
    maxillary (*see also* Sinusitis, maxillary) 473.0
    nasal (with cleft palate) (*see also* Cleft, palate)
      749.00
  orbit, orbital 376.10
  oro-antral (*see also* Sinusitis, maxillary) 473.0
  oval window (internal ear) 386.42
  oviduct (external) 619.2
  palate (hard) 526.89
    soft 528.9
  pancreatic 577.8
  pancreaticoduodenal 577.8
  parotid (gland) 527.4
    region 528.3
  pelvoabdominointestinal 569.81
  penis 607.89
  perianal 565.1
  pericardium (pleura) (sac) (*see also* Pericarditis)
    423.8
  pericecal 569.81
  perineal—*see* Fistula, perineum
  perineorectal 569.81
  perineosigmoidal 569.81
  perineo-urethroscrotal 608.89
  perineum, perineal (with urethral involvement)
    NEC 599.1
    tuberculous (*see also* Tuberculosis) 017.9
    ureter 593.82
  perirectal 565.1
    tuberculous (*see also* Tuberculosis) 014.8
  peritoneum (*see also* Peritonitis) 567.22
  periurethral 599.1
  pharyngo-esophageal 478.29
  pharynx 478.29
    branchial cleft (congenital) 744.41
  pilonidal (infected) (rectum) 685.1
    with abscess 685.0

Fistula—*continued*
  pleura, pleural, pleurocutaneous,
    pleuroperitoneal 510.0
    stomach 510.0
    tuberculous (*see also* Tuberculosis) 012.0
  pleuropericardial 423.8
  postauricular 383.81
  postoperative, persistent 998.6
  preauricular (congenital) 744.46
  prostate 602.8
  pulmonary 510.0
    arteriovenous 417.0
      congenital 747.39
    tuberculous (*see also* Tuberculosis,
      pulmonary) 011.9
  pulmonoperitoneal 510.0
  rectolabial 619.1
  rectosigmoid (intercommunicating) 569.81
  rectoureteral 593.82
  rectourethral 599.1
    congenital 753.8
  rectouterine 619.1
    congenital 752.39
  rectovaginal 619.1
    congenital 752.49
    old, postpartal 619.1
    tuberculous (*see also* Tuberculosis) 014.8
  rectovesical 596.1
    congenital 753.8
  rectovesicovaginal 619.1
  rectovulvar 619.1
    congenital 752.49
  rectum (to skin) 565.1
    tuberculous (*see also* Tuberculosis) 014.8
  renal 593.89
  retroauricular 383.81
  round window (internal ear) 386.41
  salivary duct or gland 527.4
    congenital 750.24
  sclera 360.32
  scrotum (urinary) 608.89
    tuberculous (*see also* Tuberculosis) 016.5
  semicircular canals (internal ear) 386.43
  sigmoid 569.81
    vesicoabdominal 596.1
  sigmoidovaginal 619.1
    congenital 752.49
  skin 686.9
    ureter 593.82
    vagina 619.2
  sphenoidal sinus (*see also* Sinusitis, sphenoidal)
    473.3
  splenocolic 289.59
  stercoral 569.81
  stomach 537.4
  sublingual gland 527.4
    congenital 750.24
  submaxillary
    gland 527.4
      congenital 750.24
    region 528.3
  thoracic 510.0
    duct 457.8
  thoracicoabdominal 510.0
  thoracicogastric 510.0
  thoracicointestinal 510.0
  thoracoabdominal 510.0
  thoracogastric 510.0
  thorax 510.0
  thyroglossal duct 759.2
  thyroid 246.8
  trachea (congenital) (external) (internal) 748.3

Fistula—*continued*
tracheoesophageal 530.84
  congenital 750.3
  following tracheostomy 519.09
traumatic
  arteriovenous (*see also* Injury, blood vessel,
    by site) 904.9
  brain—*see* Injury, intracranial
tuberculous—*see* Tuberculosis, by site
typhoid 002.0
umbilical 759.89
umbilico-urinary 753.8
urachal, urachus 753.7
ureter (persistent) 593.82
ureteroabdominal 593.82
ureterocervical 593.82
ureterorectal 593.82
ureterosigmoido-abdominal 593.82
ureterovaginal 619.0
ureterovesical 596.2
urethra 599.1
  congenital 753.8
  tuberculous (*see also* Tuberculosis) 016.3
urethroperineal 599.1
urethroperineovesical 596.2
urethrorectal 599.1
  congenital 753.8
urethroscrotal 608.89
urethrovaginal 619.0
urethrovesical 596.2
urethrovesicovaginal 619.0
urinary (persistent) (recurrent) 599.1
uteroabdominal (anterior wall) 619.2
  congenital 752.39
uteroenteric 619.1
uterofecal 619.1
uterointestinal 619.1
  congenital 752.39
uterorectal 619.1
  congenital 752.39
uteroureteric 619.0
uterovaginal 619.8
uterovesical 619.0
  congenital 752.39
uterus 619.8
vagina (wall) 619.8
  postpartal, old 619.8
vaginocutaneous (postpartal) 619.2
vaginoileal (acquired) 619.1
vaginoperineal 619.2
vesical NEC 596.2
vesicoabdominal 596.2
vesicocervicovaginal 619.0
vesicocolic 596.1
vesicocutaneous 596.2
vesicoenteric 596.1
vesicointestinal 596.1
vesicometrorectal 619.1
vesicoperineal 596.2
vesicorectal 596.1
  congenital 753.8
vesicosigmoidal 596.1
vesicosigmoidovaginal 619.1
vesicoureteral 596.2
vesicoureterovaginal 619.0
vesicourethral 596.2
vesicourethrorectal 596.1
vesicouterine 619.0
  congenital 752.39
vesicovaginal 619.0
vulvorectal 619.1
  congenital 752.49

Fit 780.39
apoplectic (*see also* Disease, cerebrovascular,
  acute) 436
late effect—*see* Late effect(s) (of)
  cerebrovascular disease
epileptic (*see also* Epilepsy) 345.9
fainting 780.2
hysterical 300.11
newborn 779.0
Fitting (of)
artificial
  arm (complete) (partial) V52.0
  breast V52.4
    implant exchange (different material)
      (different size) V52.4
  eye(s) V52.2
  leg(s) (complete) (partial) V52.1
brain neuropacemaker V53.02
cardiac pacemaker V53.31
carotid sinus pacemaker V53.39
cerebral ventricle (communicating) shunt V53.01
colostomy belt V53.5
contact lenses V53.1
cystostomy device V53.6
defibrillator, automatic implantable (with
  synchronous cardiac pacemaker) V53.32
dentures V52.3
device, unspecified type V53.90
  abdominal V53.59
  cardiac
    defibrillator, automatic implantable (with
      synchronous cardiac pacemaker) V53.32
    pacemaker V53.31
    specified NEC V53.39
  cerebral ventricle (communicating) shunt
    V53.01
  gastrointestinal NEC V53.59
  insulin pump V53.91
  intestinal V53.50
  intrauterine contraceptive
    insertion V25.11
    removal V25.12
      and reinsertion V25.13
    replacement V25.13
  nervous system V53.09
  orthodontic V53.4
  orthoptic V53.1
  other device V53.99
  prosthetic V52.9
    breast V52.4
    dental V52.3
    eye V52.2
    specified type NEC V52.8
  special senses V53.09
  substitution
    auditory V53.09
    nervous system V53.09
    visual V53.09
  urinary V53.6
diaphragm (contraceptive) V25.02
gastric lap band V53.51
gastrointestinal appliance and device NEC V53.59
glasses (reading) V53.1
growth rod V54.02
hearing aid V53.2
ileostomy device V53.5
intestinal appliance and device V53.50
intrauterine contraceptive device
  insertion V25.11
  removal V25.12
    and reinsertion V25.13
  replacement V25.13

Fitting—*continued*
  neuropacemaker (brain) (peripheral nerve)
      (spinal cord) V53.02
  orthodontic device V53.4
  orthopedic (device) V53.7
    brace V53.7
    cast V53.7
    corset V53.7
    shoes V53.7
  pacemaker (cardiac) V53.31
    brain V53.02
    carotid sinus V53.39
    peripheral nerve V53.02
    spinal cord V53.02
  prosthesis V52.9
    arm (complete) (partial) V52.0
    breast V52.4
      implant exchange (different material)
          (different size) V52.4
    dental V52.3
    eye V52.2
    leg (complete) (partial) V52.1
    specified type NEC V52.8
  spectacles V53.1
  wheelchair V53.8
Fitz's syndrome (acute hemorrhagic pancreatitis)
    577.0
Fitz-Hugh and Curtis syndrome 098.86
  due to
    Chlamydia trachomatis 099.56
    Neisseria gonorrhoeae (gonococcal peritonitis)
        098.86
Fixation
  joint—*see* Ankylosis
  larynx 478.79
  pupil 364.76
  stapes 385.22
    deafness (*see also* Deafness, conductive) 389.04
  uterus (acquired)—*see* Malposition, uterus
  vocal cord 478.5
Flaccid —*see* condition
  foot 736.79
  forearm 736.09
  palate, congenital 750.26
Flail
  chest 807.4
    newborn 767.3
  joint (paralytic) 718.80
    ankle 718.87
    elbow 718.82
    foot 718.87
    hand 718.84
    hip 718.85
    knee 718.86
    multiple sites 718.89
    pelvic region 718.85
    shoulder (region) 718.81
    specified site NEC 718.88
    wrist 718.83
Flajani (-Basedow) syndrome or disease
    (exophthalmic goiter) 242.0
Flap, liver 572.8
Flare, anterior chamber (aqueous) (eye) 364.04
Flashback phenomena (drug) (hallucinogenic) 292.89
Flat
  chamber (anterior) (eye) 360.34
  chest, congenital 754.89
  electroencephalogram (EEG) 348.89

Flat —*continued*
  foot (acquired) (fixed type) (painful) (postural)
      (spastic) 734
    congenital 754.61
      rocker bottom 754.61
      vertical talus 754.61
    rachitic 268.1
    rocker bottom (congenital) 754.61
    vertical talus, congenital 754.61
  organ or site, congenital NEC—*see* Anomaly,
      specified type NEC
  pelvis 738.6
    with disproportion (fetopelvic) 653.2
      affecting fetus or newborn 763.1
      causing obstructed labor 660.1
        affecting fetus or newborn 763.1
    congenital 755.69
Flatau-Schilder disease 341.1
Flattening
  head, femur 736.39
  hip 736.39
  lip (congenital) 744.89
  nose (congenital) 754.0
    acquired 738.0
Flatulence 787.3
Flatus 787.3
  vaginalis 629.89
Flax dressers' disease 504
Flea bite —*see* Injury, superficial, by site
Fleischer (-Kayser) ring (corneal pigmentation)
    275.1 *[371.14]*
Fleischner's disease 732.3
Fleshy mole 631.8
Flexibilitas cerea (*see also* Catalepsy) 300.11
Flexion
  cervix —*see* Flexion, uterus
  contracture, joint (*see also* Contraction, joint) 718.4
  deformity, joint (*see also* Contraction, joint) 736.9
    hip, congenital (*see also* Subluxation,
        congenital, hip) 754.32
  uterus (*see also* Malposition, uterus) 621.6
Flexner's
  bacillus 004.1
  diarrhea (ulcerative) 004.1
  dysentery 004.1
Flexner-Boyd dysentery 004.2
Flexure —*see* condition
Floater, vitreous 379.24
Floating
  cartilage (joint) (*see also* Disorder, cartilage,
      articular) 718.0
    knee 717.6
  gallbladder (congenital) 751.69
  kidney 593.0
    congenital 753.3
  liver (congenital) 751.69
  rib 756.3
  spleen 289.59
Flooding 626.2
Floor —*see* condition
Floppy
  infant NEC 781.99
  iris syndrome 364.81
  valve syndrome (mitral) 424.0
Flu —*see also* Influenza
  bird (*see also* Influenza, avian) 488.02
  gastric NEC 008.8
  swine —*see* Influenza, (novel) 2009 H1N1
Fluctuating blood pressure 796.4

Fluid
abdomen 789.59
chest (see also Pleurisy, with effusion) 511.9
heart (see also Failure, heart) 428.0
joint (see also Effusion, joint) 719.0
loss (acute) 276.50
with
hypernatremia 276.0
hyponatremia 276.1
lung—see also Edema, lung
encysted 511.89
peritoneal cavity 789.59
malignant 789.51
pleural cavity (see also Pleurisy, with effusion) 511.9
retention 276.69
Flukes NEC (see also Infestation, fluke) 121.9
blood NEC (see also Infestation, Schistosoma) 120.9
liver 121.3
Fluor (albus) (vaginalis) 623.5
trichomonal (Trichomonas vaginalis) 131.00
Fluorosis (dental) (chronic) 520.3
Flushing 782.62
menopausal 627.2
Flush syndrome 259.2
Flutter
atrial or auricular 427.32
heart (ventricular) 427.42
atrial 427.32
impure 427.32
postoperative 997.1
ventricular 427.42
Flux (bloody) (serosanguineous) 009.0
FNHTR (febrile hemolytic transfusion reaction) 780.66
Focal —see condition
Fochier's abscess —see Abscess, by site
Focus, Assmann's (see also Tuberculosis) 011.0
Fogo selvagem 694.4
Foix-Alajouanine syndrome 336.1
Folds, anomalous —see also Anomaly, specified type NEC
Bowman's membrane 371.31
Descemet's membrane 371.32
epicanthic 743.63
heart 746.89
posterior segment of eye, congenital 743.54
Folie à deux 297.3
Follicle
cervix (nabothian) (ruptured) 616.0
graafian, ruptured, with hemorrhage 620.0
nabothian 616.0
Folliclis (primary) (see also Tuberculosis) 017.0
Follicular —see also condition
cyst (atretic) 620.0
Folliculitis 704.8
abscedens et suffodiens 704.8
decalvans 704.09
gonorrheal (acute) 098.0
chronic or duration of 2 months or more 098.2
keloid, keloidalis 706.1
pustular 704.8
ulerythematosa reticulata 701.8
Folliculosis, conjunctival 372.02
Folling's disease (phenylketonuria) 270.1
Follow-up (examination) (routine) (following) V67.9
cancer chemotherapy V67.2
chemotherapy V67.2
fracture V67.4
high-risk medication V67.51

Follow-up—continued
injury NEC V67.59
postpartum
immediately after delivery V24.0
routine V24.2
psychiatric V67.3
psychotherapy V67.3
radiotherapy V67.1
specified condition NEC V67.59
specified surgery NEC V67.09
surgery V67.00
vaginal pap smear V67.01
treatment V67.9
combined NEC V67.6
fracture V67.4
involving high-risk medication NEC V67.51
mental disorder V67.3
specified NEC V67.59
Fong's syndrome (hereditary osteoonychodysplasia) 756.89
Food
allergy 693.1
anaphylactic shock—see Anaphylactic reaction or shock, due to, food
asphyxia (from aspiration or inhalation) (see also Asphyxia, food) 933.1
choked on (see also Asphyxia, food) 933.1
deprivation 994.2
specified kind of food NEC 269.8
intoxication (see also Poisoning, food) 005.9
lack of 994.2
poisoning (see also Poisoning, food) 005.9
refusal or rejection NEC 307.59
strangulation or suffocation (see also Asphyxia, food) 933.1
toxemia (see also Poisoning, food) 005.9
Foot —see also condition
and mouth disease 078.4
process disease 581.3
Foramen ovale (nonclosure) (patent) (persistent) 745.5
Forbes' (glycogen storage) disease 271.0
Forbes-Albright syndrome (nonpuerperal amenorrhea and lactation associated with pituitary tumor) 253.1
Forced birth or delivery NEC 669.8
affecting fetus or newborn NEC 763.89
Forceps
delivery NEC 669.5
affecting fetus or newborn 763.2
Fordyce's disease (ectopic sebaceous glands) (mouth) 750.26
Fordyce-Fox disease (apocrine miliaria) 705.82
Forearm —see condition
Foreign body

> Note—For foreign body with open wound or other injury, see Wound, open, or the type of injury specified.

accidentally left during a procedure 998.4
anterior chamber (eye) 871.6
magnetic 871.5
retained or old 360.51
retained or old 360.61
ciliary body (eye) 871.6
magnetic 871.5
retained or old 360.52
retained or old 360.62

Foreign body—*continued*
  entering through orifice (current) (old)
    accessory sinus 932
    air passage (upper) 933.0
      lower 934.8
    alimentary canal 938
    alveolar process 935.0
    antrum (Highmore) 932
    anus 937
    appendix 936
    asphyxia due to (*see also* Asphyxia, food)
      933.1
    auditory canal 931
    auricle 931
    bladder 939.0
    bronchioles 934.8
    bronchus (main) 934.1
    buccal cavity 935.0
    canthus (inner) 930.1
    cecum 936
    cervix (canal) uterine 939.1
    coil, ileocecal 936
    colon 936
    conjunctiva 930.1
    conjunctival sac 930.1
    cornea 930.0
    digestive organ or tract NEC 938
    duodenum 936
    ear (external) 931
    esophagus 935.1
    eye (external) 930.9
      combined sites 930.8
      intraocular—*see* Foreign body, by site
      specified site NEC 930.8
    eyeball 930.8
      intraocular—*see* Foreign body, intraocular
    eyelid 930.1
      retained or old 374.86
    frontal sinus 932
    gastrointestinal tract 938
    genitourinary tract 939.9
    globe 930.8
      penetrating 871.6
        magnetic 871.5
          retained or old 360.50
        retained or old 360.60
    gum 935.0
    Highmore's antrum 932
    hypopharynx 933.0
    ileocecal coil 936
    ileum 936
    inspiration (of) 933.1
    intestine (large) (small) 936
    lacrimal apparatus, duct, gland, or sac 930.2
    larynx 933.1
    lung 934.8
    maxillary sinus 932
    mouth 935.0
    nasal sinus 932
    nasopharynx 933.0
    nose (passage) 932
    nostril 932
    oral cavity 935.0
    palate 935.0
    penis 939.3
    pharynx 933.0
    pyriform sinus 933.0
    rectosigmoid 937
      junction 937
    rectum 937

Foreign body—*continued*
  entering through—*continued*
    respiratory tract 934.9
      specified part NEC 934.8
    sclera 930.1
    sinus 932
      accessory 932
      frontal 932
      maxillary 932
      nasal 932
      pyriform 933.0
    small intestine 936
    stomach (hairball) 935.2
    suffocation by (*see also* Asphyxia, food) 933.1
    swallowed 938
      tongue 933.0
    tear ducts or glands 930.2
    throat 933.0
    tongue 935.0
      swallowed 933.0
    tonsil, tonsillar 933.0
      fossa 933.0
    trachea 934.0
    ureter 939.0
    urethra 939.0
    uterus (any part) 939.1
    vagina 939.2
    vulva 939.2
    wind pipe 934.0
  feeling of, in throat 784.99
  granuloma (old) 728.82
    bone 733.99
    in operative wound (inadvertently left) 998.4
      due to surgical material intentionally
        left—*see* Complications, due to
        (presence of) any device, implant, or
        graft classified to 996.0-996.5 NEC
    muscle 728.82
    skin 709.4
    soft tissue 709.1
    subcutaneous tissue 709.4
  in
    bone (residual) 733.99
    open wound—*see* Wound, open, by site
      complicated
    soft tissue (residual) 729.6
  inadvertently left in operation wound (causing
    adhesions, obstruction, or perforation) 998.4
  ingestion, ingested NEC 938
  inhalation or inspiration (*see also* Asphyxia,
    food) 933.1
  internal organ, not entering through an
    orifice—*see* Injury, internal, by site, with
    open wound
  intraocular (nonmagnetic) 871.6
    combined sites 871.6
      magnetic 871.5
        retained or old 360.59
      retained or old 360.69
    magnetic 871.5
      retained or old 360.50
    retained or old 360.60
    specified site NEC 871.6
      magnetic 871.5
        retained or old 360.59
      retained or old 360.69
  iris (nonmagnetic) 871.6
    magnetic 871.5
      retained or old 360.52
    retained or old 360.62

Foreign body—*continued*
 lens (nonmagnetic) 871.6
   magnetic 871.5
     retained or old 360.53
   retained or old 360.63
 lid, eye 930.1
 ocular muscle 870.4
   retained or old 376.6
 old or residual
   bone 733.99
   eyelid 374.86
   middle ear 385.83
   muscle 729.6
     ocular 376.6
   retrobulbar 376.6
   skin 729.6
     with granuloma 709.4
   soft tissue 729.6
     with granuloma 709.4
   subcutaneous tissue 729.6
     with granuloma 709.4
 operation wound, left accidentally 998.4
 orbit 870.4
   retained or old 376.6
 posterior wall, eye 871.6
   magnetic 871.5
     retained or old 360.55
   retained or old 360.65
 respiratory tree 934.9
   specified site NEC 934.8
 retained (old) (nonmagnetic) (in) V90.9
   anterior chamber (eye) 360.61
     magnetic 360.51
   ciliary body 360.62
     magnetic 360.52
   eyelid 374.86
   fragment(s)
     acrylics V90.2
     animal quills V90.31
     animal spines V90.31
     cement V90.83
     concrete V90.83
     crystalline V90.83
     depleted
       isotope V90.09
       uranium V90.01
     diethylhexylphthalates V90.2
     glass V90.81
     isocyanate V90.2
     metal V90.10
       magnetic V90.11
       nonmagnetic V90.12
     organic NEC V90.39
     plastic V90.2
     radioactive
       nontherapeutic V90.09
       specified NEC V90.09
     stone V90.83
     tooth V90.32
     wood V90.33
   globe 360.60
     magnetic 360.50
   intraocular 360.60
     magnetic 360.50
     specified site NEC 360.69
       magnetic 360.59
   iris 360.62
     magnetic 360.52
   lens 360.63
     magnetic 360.53
   muscle 729.6

Foreign body—*continued*
 retained—*continued*
   orbit 376.6
   posterior wall of globe 360.65
     magnetic 360.55
   retina 360.65
     magnetic 360.55
   retrobulbar 376.6
   skin 729.6
     with granuloma 709.4
   soft tissue 729.6
     with granuloma 709.4
   specified NEC V90.89
   subcutaneous tissue 729.6
     with granuloma 709.4
   vitreous 360.64
     magnetic 360.54
 retina 871.6
   magnetic 871.5
     retained or old 360.55
   retained or old 360.65
 superficial, without major open wound (*see also* Injury, superficial, by site) 919.6
 swallowed NEC 938
 throat, feeling of 784.99
 vitreous (humor) 871.6
   magnetic 871.5
     retained or old 360.54
   retained or old 360.64
Forking, aqueduct of Sylvius 742.3
 with spina bifida (*see also* Spina bifida) 741.0
Formation
 bone in scar tissue (skin) 709.3
 connective tissue in vitreous 379.25
 Elschnig pearls (postcataract extraction) 366.51
 hyaline in cornea 371.49
 sequestrum in bone (due to infection) (*see also* Osteomyelitis) 730.1
 valve
   colon, congenital 751.5
   ureter (congenital) 753.29
Formication 782.0
Fort Bragg fever 100.89
Fossa —*see also* condition
 pyriform—*see* condition
Foster care (status) V60.81
Foster-Kennedy syndrome 377.04
Fothergill's
 disease, meaning scarlatina anginosa 034.1
 neuralgia (*see also* Neuralgia, trigeminal) 350.1
Foul breath 784.99
Found dead (cause unknown) 798.9
Foundling V20.0
Fournier's disease (idiopathic gangrene) 608.83
 female 616.89
Fourth
 cranial nerve—*see* condition
 disease 057.8
 molar 520.1
Foville's syndrome 344.89
Fox's
 disease (apocrine miliaria) 705.82
 impetigo (contagiosa) 684
Fox-Fordyce disease (apocrine miliaria) 705.82

Fracture—*continued*
cricoid cartilage (closed) 807.5
  open 807.6
cuboid (ankle) (closed) 825.23
  open 825.33
cuneiform
  foot (closed) 825.24
    open 825.34
  wrist (closed) 814.03
    open 814.13
dental implant 525.73
dental restorative material
  with loss of material 525.64
  without loss of material 525.63
due to
  birth injury—*see* Birth injury, fracture
  gunshot—*see* Fracture, by site, open
  neoplasm—*see* Fracture, pathologic
  osteoporosis—*see* Fracture, pathologic
Dupuytren's (ankle) (fibula) (closed) 824.4
  open 824.5
  radius 813.42
    open 813.52
Duverney's—*see* Fracture, ilium
elbow—*see also* Fracture, humerus, lower end
  olecranon (process) (closed) 813.01
    open 813.11
  supracondylar (closed) 812.41
    open 812.51
ethmoid (bone) (sinus)—*see* Fracture, skull, base
face bone(s) (closed) NEC 802.8
  with
    other bone(s)—*see also* Fracture, multiple, skull
    skull—*see also* Fracture, skull
      involving other bones—*see* Fracture,
        multiple, skull
  open 802.9
fatigue—*see* Fracture, march
femur, femoral (closed) 821.00
  cervicotrochanteric 820.03
    open 820.13
  condyles, epicondyles 821.21
    open 821.31
  distal end—*see* Fracture, femur, lower end
  epiphysis (separation)
    capital 820.01
      open 820.11
    head 820.01
      open 820.11
    lower 821.22
      open 821.32
    trochanteric 820.01
      open 820.11
    upper 820.01
      open 820.11
  head 820.09
    open 820.19
  lower end or extremity (distal end) (closed)
    821.20
    condyles, epicondyles 821.21
      open 821.31
    epiphysis (separation) 821.22
      open 821.32
    multiple sites 821.29
      open 821.39
    open 821.30
    specified site NEC 821.29
      open 821.39
    supracondylar 821.23
      open 821.33
    T-shaped 821.21
      open 821.31

Fracture—*continued*
femur—*continued*
  neck (closed) 820.8
    base (cervicotrochanteric) 820.03
      open 820.13
    extracapsular 820.20
      open 820.30
    intertrochanteric (section) 820.21
      open 820.31
    intracapsular 820.00
      open 820.10
    intratrochanteric 820.21
      open 821.31
    midcervical 820.02
      open 820.12
    open 820.9
    pathologic 733.14
      specified part NEC 733.15
    specified site NEC 820.09
      open 820.19
    stress 733.96
    transcervical 820.02
      open 820.12
    transtrochanteric 820.20
      open 820.30
  open 821.10
  pathologic 733.14
    specified part NEC 733.15
  peritrochanteric (section) 820.20
    open 820.30
  shaft (lower third) (middle third) (upper third)
    821.01
    open 821.11
    stress 733.97
  subcapital 820.09
    open 820.19
  subtrochanteric (region) (section) 820.22
    open 820.32
  supracondylar 821.23
    open 821.33
  transepiphyseal 820.01
    open 820.11
  trochanter (greater) (lesser) (*see also* Fracture,
    femur, neck, by site) 820.20
    open 820.30
  T-shaped, into knee joint 821.21
    open 821.31
  upper end 820.8
    open 820.9
fibula (closed) 823.81
  with tibia 823.82
    open 823.92
  distal end 824.8
    open 824.9
  epiphysis
    lower 824.8
      open 824.9
    upper—*see* Fracture, fibula, upper end
  head—*see* Fracture, fibula, upper end
  involving ankle 824.2
    open 824.3
  lower end or extremity 824.8
    open 824.9
  malleolus (external) (lateral) 824.2
    open 824.3
  open NEC 823.91
  pathologic 733.16
  proximal end—*see* Fracture, fibula, upper end
  shaft 823.21
    with tibia 823.22
      open 823.32
    open 823.31

Fracture—*continued*
fibula—*continued*
stress 733.93
torus 853.41
with tibia 823.42
upper end or extremity (epiphysis) (head)
(proximal end) (styloid) 823.01
with tibia 823.02
open 823.12
open 823.11
finger(s), of one hand (closed) (*see also*
Fracture, phalanx, hand) 816.00
with
metacarpal bone(s), of same hand 817.0
open 817.1
thumb of same hand 816.03
open 816.13
open 816.10
foot, except toe(s) alone (closed) 825.20
open 825.30
forearm (closed) NEC 813.80
lower end (distal end) (lower epiphysis)
813.40
open 813.50
open 813.90
shaft 813.20
open 813.30
upper end (proximal end) (upper epiphysis)
813.00
open 813.10
fossa, anterior, middle, or posterior—*see*
Fracture, skull, base
frontal (bone)—*see also* Fracture, skull, vault
sinus—*see* Fracture, skull base
Galeazzi's—*see* Fracture, radius, lower end
glenoid (cavity) (fossa) (scapula) (closed)
811.03
open 811.13
Gosselin's—*see* Fracture, ankle
greenstick—*see* Fracture, by site
grenade-throwers'—*see* Fracture, humerus,
shaft
gutter—*see* Fracture, skull, vault
hamate (closed) 814.08
open 814.18
hand, one (closed) 815.00
carpals 814.00
open 814.10
specified site NEC 814.09
open 814.19
metacarpals 815.00
open 815.10
multiple, bones of one hand 817.0
open 817.1
open 815.10
phalanges (*see also* Fracture, phalanx, hand)
816.00
open 816.10
healing
aftercare (*see also* Aftercare, fracture) V54.89
change of cast V54.89
complications—*see* condition
convalescence V66.4
removal of
cast V54.89
fixation device
external V54.89
internal V54.01
heel bone (closed) 825.0
open 825.1
Hill-Sachs 812.09

Fracture—*continued*
hip (closed) (*see also* Fracture, femur, neck)
820.8
open 820.9
pathologic 733.14
humerus (closed) 812.20
anatomical neck 812.02
open 812.12
articular process (*see also* Fracture, humerus,
condyle(s) 812.44
open 812.54
capitellum 812.49
open 812.59
condyle(s) 812.44
lateral (external) 812.42
open 812.52
medial (internal epicondyle) 812.43
open 812.53
open 812.54
distal end—*see* Fracture, humerus, lower end
epiphysis
lower (*see also* Fracture, humerus,
condyle(s)) 812.44
open 812.54
upper 812.09
open 812.19
external condyle 812.42
open 812.52
great tuberosity 812.03
open 812.13
head 812.09
open 812.19
internal epicondyle 812.43
open 812.53
lesser tuberosity 812.09
open 812.19
lower end or extremity (distal end) (*see also*
Fracture, humerus, by site) 812.40
multiple sites NEC 812.49
open 812.59
open 812.50
specified site NEC 812.49
open 812.59
neck 812.01
open 812.11
open 812.30
pathologic 733.11
proximal end—*see* Fracture, humerus, upper
end
shaft 812.21
open 812.31
supracondylar 812.41
open 812.51
surgical neck 812.01
open 812.11
trochlea 812.49
open 812.59
T-shaped 812.44
open 812.54
tuberosity—*see* Fracture, humerus, upper end
upper end or extremity (proximal end) (*see
also* Fracture, humerus, by site) 812.00
open 812.10
specified site NEC 812.09
open 812.19
hyoid bone (closed) 807.5
open 807.6
hyperextension—*see* Fracture, radius, lower end
ilium (with visceral injury) (closed) 808.41
open 808.51
impaction, impacted—*see* Fracture, by site
incus—*see* Fracture, skull, base

Fracture—*continued*
  innominate bone (with visceral injury) (closed)
      808.49
    open 808.59
  instep, of one foot (closed) 825.20
    with toe(s) of same foot 827.0
      open 827.1
    open 825.30
  insufficiency—*see* Fracture, pathologic, by site
  internal
    ear—*see* Fracture, skull, base
    semilunar cartilage, knee—*see* Tear,
        meniscus, medial
  intertrochanteric—*see* Fracture, femur, neck,
      intertrochanteric
  ischium (with visceral injury) (closed) 808.42
    open 808.52
  jaw (bone) (lower) (closed) (*see also* Fracture,
      mandible) 802.20
    angle 802.25
      open 802.35
    open 802.30
    upper—*see* Fracture, maxilla
  knee
    cap (closed) 822.0
      open 822.1
    cartilage (semilunar)—*see* Tear, meniscus
  labyrinth (osseous)—*see* Fracture, skull, base
  larynx (closed) 807.5
    open 807.6
  late effect—*see* Late, effects (of), fracture
  Le Fort's—*see* Fracture, maxilla
  leg (closed) 827.0
    with rib(s) or sternum 828.0
      open 828.1
    both (any bones) 828.0
      open 828.1
    lower—*see* Fracture, tibia
    open 827.1
    upper—*see* Fracture, femur
  limb
    lower (multiple) (closed) NEC 827.0
      open 827.1
    upper (multiple) (closed) NEC 818.0
      open 818.1
  long bones, due to birth trauma—*see* Birth
      injury, fracture
  lumbar—*see* Fracture, vertebra, lumbar
  lunate bone (closed) 814.02
    open 814.12
  malar bone (closed) 802.4
    open 802.5
  Malgaigne's (closed) 808.43
    open 808.53
  malleolus (closed)0 824.8
    bimalleolar 824.4
      open 824.5
    lateral 824.2
      and medial—*see also* Fracture, malleolus,
          bimalleolar
        with lip of tibia—*see* Fracture, malleolus,
            trimalleolar
      open 824.3
    medial (closed) 824.0
      and lateral—*see also* Fracture, malleolus,
          bimalleolar
        with lip of tibia—*see* Fracture, malleolus,
            trimalleolar
      open 824.1
    open 824.9
    trimalleolar (closed) 824.6
      open 824.7

Fracture—*continued*
  malleus—*see* Fracture, skull, base
  malunion 733.81
  mandible (closed) 802.20
    angle 802.25
      open 802.35
    body 802.28
      alveolar border 802.27
        open 802.37
      open 802.38
      symphysis 802.26
        open 802.36
    condylar process 802.21
      open 802.31
    coronoid process 802.23
      open 802.33
    multiple sites 802.29
      open 802.39
    open 802.30
    ramus NEC 802.24
      open 802.34
    subcondylar 802.22
      open 802.32
  manubrium—*see* Fracture, sternum
  march 733.95
    femoral neck 733.96
    fibula 733.93
    metatarsals 733.94
    pelvis 733.98
    shaft of femur 733.97
    tibia 733.93
  maxilla, maxillary (superior) (upper jaw)
      (closed) 802.4
    inferior—*see* Fracture, mandible
    open 802.5
  meniscus, knee—*see* Tear, meniscus
  metacarpus, metacarpal (bone(s)), of one hand
      (closed) 815.00
    with phalanx, phalanges, hand (finger(s))
        (thumb) of same hand 817.0
      open 817.1
    base 815.02
      first metacarpal 815.01
        open 815.11
      open 815.12
      thumb 815.01
        open 815.11
    multiple sites 815.09
      open 815.19
    neck 815.04
      open 815.14
    open 815.10
    shaft 815.03
      open 815.13
  metatarsus, metatarsal (bone(s)), of one foot
      (closed) 825.25
    with tarsal bone(s) 825.29
      open 825.39
    open 825.35
  Monteggia's (closed) 813.03
    open 813.13
  Moore's—*see* Fracture, radius, lower end
  multangular bone (closed)
    larger 814.05
      open 814.15
    smaller 814.06
      open 814.16

Fracture—*continued*
  multiple (closed) 829.0

> *Note—Multiple fractures of sites classifiable to the same three- or four-digit category are coded to that category, except for sites classifiable to 810-818 or 820-827 in different limbs.*
>
> *Multiple fractures of sites classifiable to different fourth-digit subdivisions within the same three-digit category should be dealt with according to coding rules.*
>
> *Multiple fractures of sites classifiable to different three-digit categories (identifiable from the listing under "Fracture"), and of sites classifiable to 810-818 or 820-827 in different limbs should be coded according to the following list, which should be referred to in the following priority order: skull or face bones, pelvis or vertebral column, legs, arms.*

      arm (multiple bones in same arm except in hand alone) (sites classifiable to 810-817 with sites classifiable to a different three-digit category in 810-817 in same arm) (closed) 818.0
        open 818.1
      arms, both or arm(s) with rib(s) or sternum (sites classifiable to 810-818 with sites classifiable to same range of categories in other limb or to 807) (closed) 819.0
        open 819.1
      bones of trunk NEC (closed) 809.0
        open 809.1
      hand, metacarpal bone(s) with phalanx or phalanges of same hand (sites classifiable to 815 with sites classifiable to 816 in same hand) (closed) 817.0
        open 817.1
      leg (multiple bones in same leg) (sites classifiable to 820-826 with sites classifiable to a different three-digit category in that range in same leg) (closed) 827.0
        open 827.1
      legs, both or leg(s) with arm(s), rib(s), or sternum (sites classifiable to 820-827 with sites classifiable to same range of categories in other leg or to 807 or 810-819) (closed) 828.0
        open 828.1
      open 829.1
      pelvis with other bones except skull or face bones (sites classifiable to 808 with sites classifiable to 805-807 or 810-829) (closed) 809.0
        open 809.1
      skull, specified or unspecified bones, or face bone(s) with any other bone(s) (sites classifiable to 800-803 with sites classifiable to 805-829) (closed) 804.0

Fracture—*continued*
  multiple—*continued*

> *Note—Use the following fifth-digit subclassification with categories 800, 801, 803, and 804:*
>
> 0 *unspecified state of consciousness*
> 1 *with no loss of consciousness*
> 2 *with brief [less than one hour] loss of consciousness*
> 3 *with moderate [1-24 hours] loss of consciousness*
> 4 *with prolonged [more than 24 hours] loss of consciousness and return to pre-existing conscious level*
> 5 *with prolonged [more than 24 hours] loss of consciousness, without return to pre-existing conscious level*
> *Use fifth-digit 5 to designate when a patient is unconcious and dies before regaining conciousness, regardless of the duration of the loss of conciousness*
> 6 *with loss of consciousness of unspecified duration*
> 9 *with concussion, unspecified*

      with
        contusion, cerebral 804.1
        epidural hemorrhage 804.2
        extradural hemorrhage 804.2
        hemorrhage (intracranial) NEC 804.3
        intracranial injury NEC 804.4
        laceration, cerebral 804.1
        subarachnoid hemorrhage 804.2
        subdural hemorrhage 804.2
      open 804.5
        with
          contusion, cerebral 804.6
          epidural hemorrhage 804.7
          extradural hemorrhage 804.7
          hemorrhage (intracranial) NEC 804.8
          intracranial injury NEC 804.9
          laceration, cerebral 804.6
          subarachnoid hemorrhage 804.7
          subdural hemorrhage 804.7
      vertebral column with other bones, except skull or face bones (sites classifiable to 805 or 806 with sites classifiable to 807-808 or 810-829) (closed) 809.0
        open 809.1
  nasal (bone(s)) (closed) 802.0
    open 802.1
  sinus—Fracture, skull, base
  navicular
    carpal (wrist) (closed) 814.01
      open 814.11
    tarsal (ankle) (closed) 825.22
      open 825.32
  neck—*see* Fracture, vertebra, cervical
  neural arch—*see* Fracture, vertebra, by site
  nonunion 733.82
  nose, nasal (bone) (septum) (closed) 802.0
    open 802.1
  occiput—*see* Fracture, skull, base
  odontoid process—*see* Fracture, vertebra, cervical

Fracture—*continued*
olecranon (process) (ulna) (closed) 813.01
  open 813.11
  open 829.1
orbit, orbital (bone) (region) (closed) 802.8
  floor (blow-out) 802.6
  open 802.7
  open 802.9
  roof—*see* Fracture, skull, base
  specified part NEC 802.8
  open 802.9
os
  calcis (closed) 825.0
  open 825.1
  magnum (closed) 814.07
  open 814.17
  pubis (with visceral injury) (closed) 808.2
  open 808.3
  triquetrum (closed) 814.03
  open 814.13
osseous
  auditory meatus—*see* Fracture, skull, base
  labyrinth—*see* Fracture, skull, base
  ossicles, auditory (incus) (malleus)
    (stapes)—*see* Fracture, skull, base
osteoporotic—*see* Fracture, pathologic
palate (closed) 802.8
  open 802.9
paratrooper—*see* Fracture, tibia, lower end
parietal bone—*see* Fracture, skull, vault
parry—*see* Fracture, Monteggia's
patella (closed) 822.0
  open 822.1
pathologic (cause unknown) 733.10
  ankle 733.16
  femur (neck) 733.14
    specified NEC 733.15
  fibula 733.16
  hip 733.14
  humerus 733.11
  radius 733.12
  specified site NEC 733.19
  tibia 733.16
  ulna 733.12
  vertebrae (collapse) 733.13
  wrist 733.12
pedicle (of vertebral arch)—*see* Fracture,
    vertebra, by site
pelvis, pelvic (bone(s)) (with visceral injury)
    (closed) 808.8
  multiple
    with
      disruption of pelvic circle 808.43
        open 808.53
      disruption of pelvic ring 808.43
        open 808.53
    without
      disruption of pelvic circle 808.44
        open 808.54
      disruption of pelvic ring 808.44
        open 808.54
  open 808.9
  rim (closed) 808.49
    open 808.59
  stress 733.98
peritrochanteric (closed) 820.20
  open 820.30
phalanx, phalanges, of one
  foot (closed) 826.0
    with bone(s) of same lower limb 827.0
      open 827.1
    open 826.1

Fracture—*continued*
phalanx, phalanges—*continued*
  hand (closed) 816.00
    with metacarpal bone(s) of same hand 817.0
      open 817.1
    distal 816.02
      open 816.12
    middle 816.01
      open 816.11
    multiple sites NEC 816.03
      open 816.13
    open 816.10
    proximal 816.01
      open 816.11
pisiform (closed) 814.04
  open 814.14
pond—Fracture, skull, vault
Pott's (closed) 824.4
  open 824.5
prosthetic device, internal—*see* Complications,
    mechanical
pubis (with visceral injury) (closed) 808.2
  open 808.3
Quervain's (closed) 814.01
  open 814.11
radius (alone) (closed) 813.81
  with ulna NEC 813.83
    open 813.93
  distal end—*see* Fracture, radius, lower end
  epiphysis
    lower—*see* Fracture, radius, lower end
    upper—*see* Fracture, radius, upper end
  head—*see* Fracture, radius, upper end
  lower end or extremity (distal end) (lower
      epiphysis) 813.42
    with ulna (lower end) 813.44
      open 813.54
    open 813.52
    torus 813.45
      with ulna 813.47
  neck—*see* Fracture, radius, upper end
  open NEC 813.91
  pathologic 733.12
  proximal end—*see* Fracture, radius, upper end
  shaft (closed) 813.21
    with ulna (shaft) 813.23
      open 813.33
    open 813.31
  upper end 813.07
    with ulna (upper end) 813.08
      open 813.18
    epiphysis 813.05
      open 813.15
    head 813.05
      open 813.15
    multiple sites 813.07
      open 813.17
    neck 813.06
      open 813.16
    open 813.17
    specified site NEC 813.07
      open 813.17
ramus
  inferior or superior (with visceral injury)
      (closed) 808.2
    open 808.3
  ischium—*see* Fracture, ischium
  mandible 802.24
    open 802.34

Fracture—*continued*
  rib(s) (closed) 807.0

---

*Note—Use the following fifth-digit
subclassification with categories 807.0-807.1:*

0 rib(s), unspecified
1 one rib
2 two ribs
3 three ribs
4 four ribs
5 five ribs
6 six ribs
7 seven ribs
8 eight or more ribs
9 multiple ribs, unspecified

---

  with flail chest (open) 807.4
  open 807.1
 root, tooth 873.63
  complicated 873.73
 sacrum—*see* Fracture, vertebra, sacrum
 scaphoid
  ankle (closed) 825.22
   open 825.32
  wrist (closed) 814.01
   open 814.11
 scapula (closed) 811.00
  acromial, acromion (process) 811.01
   open 811.11
  body 811.09
   open 811.19
  coracoid process 811.02
   open 811.12
  glenoid (cavity) (fossa) 811.03
   open 811.13
  neck 811.03
   open 811.13
  open 811.10
 semilunar
  bone, wrist (closed) 814.02
   open 814.12
  cartilage (interior) (knee)—*see* Tear, meniscus
 sesamoid bone—*see* Fracture, by site
 Shepherd's (closed) 825.21
  open 825.31
 shoulder—*see also* Fracture, humerus, upper
   end
  blade—*see* Fracture, scapula
 silverfork—*see* Fracture, radius, lower end
 sinus (ethmoid) (frontal) (maxillary) (nasal)
  (sphenoidal)—*see* Fracture, skull, base
  maxillary—*see* Fracture, maxilla
 Skillern's—*see* Fracture, radius, shaft

Fracture—*continued*
  skull (multiple NEC) (with face bones) (closed)
   803.0

---

*Note—Use the following fifth-digit
subclassification with categories 800, 801, 803,
and 804:*

0 unspecified state of consciousness
1 with no loss of consciousness
*2 with brief [less than one hour] loss of
   consciousness*
*3 with moderate [1-24 hours] loss of
   consciousness*
*4 with prolonged [more than 24 hours] loss of
   consciousness and return to pre-existing
   conscious level*
*5 with prolonged [more than 24 hours] loss of
   consciousness, without return to pre-existing
   conscious level*
*Use fifth-digit 5 to designate when a patient is
unconscious and dies before regaining
consciousness, regardless of the duration of the
loss of consciousness*
*6 with loss of consciousness of unspecified
   duration*
9 with concussion, unspecified

---

  with
   contusion, cerebral 803.1
   epidural hemorrhage 803.2
   extradural hemorrhage 803.2
   hemorrhage (intracranial) NEC 803.3
   intracranial injury NEC 803.4
   laceration, cerebral 803.1
   other bones—*see* Fracture, multiple, skull
   subarachnoid hemorrhage 803.2
   subdural hemorrhage 803.2
  base (antrum) (ethmoid bone) (fossa) (internal
   ear) (nasal sinus) (occiput) (sphenoid)
   (temporal bone) (closed) 801.0
   with
    contusion, cerebral 801.1
    epidural hemorrhage 801.2
    extradural hemorrhage 801.2
    hemorrhage (intracranial) NEC 801.3
    intracranial injury NEC 801.4
    laceration, cerebral 801.1
    subarachnoid hemorrhage 801.2
    subdural hemorrhage 801.2
   open 801.5
    with
     contusion, cerebral 801.6
     epidural hemorrhage 801.7
     extradural hemorrhage 801.7
     hemorrhage (intracranial) NEC 801.8
     intracranial injury NEC 801.9
     laceration, cerebral 801.6
     subarachnoid hemorrhage 801.7
     subdural hemorrhage 801.7
  birth injury 767.3
  face bones—*see* Fracture, face bones
  open 803.5
   with
    contusion, cerebral 803.6
    epidural hemorrhage 803.7
    extradural hemorrhage 803.7
    hemorrhage (intracranial) NEC 803.8
    intracranial injury NEC 803.9
    laceration, cerebral 803.6
    subarachnoid hemorrhage 803.7
    subdural hemorrhage 803.7

Fracture—*continued*
skull—*continued*
vault (frontal bone) (parietal bone) (vertex) (closed) 800.0
with
contusion, cerebral 800.1
epidural hemorrhage 800.2
extradural hemorrhage 800.2
hemorrhage (intracranial) NEC 800.3
intracranial injury NEC 800.4
laceration, cerebral 800.1
subarachnoid hemorrhage 800.2
subdural hemorrhage 800.2
open 800.5
with
contusion, cerebral 800.6
epidural hemorrhage 800.7
extradural hemorrhage 800.7
hemorrhage (intracranial) NEC 800.8
intracranial injury NEC 800.9
laceration, cerebral 800.6
subarachnoid hemorrhage 800.7
subdural hemorrhage 800.7
Smith's 813.41
open 813.51
sphenoid (bone) (sinus)—*see* Fracture, skull, base
spine—*see also* Fracture, vertebra, by site
due to birth trauma 767.4
spinous process—*see* Fracture, vertebra, by site
spontaneous—*see* Fracture, pathologic
sprinters'—*see* Fracture, ilium
stapes—*see* Fracture, skull, base
stave—*see also* Fracture, metacarpus, metacarpal bone(s)
spine—*see* Fracture, tibia, upper end
sternum (closed) 807.2
with flail chest (open) 807.4
open 807.3
Stieda's—*see* Fracture, femur, lower end
stress 733.95
femoral neck 733.96
fibula 733.93
metatarsals 733.94
pelvis 733.98
shaft of femur 733.97
specified site NEC 733.95
tibia 733.93
styloid process
metacarpal (closed) 815.02
open 815.12
radius—*see* Fracture, radius, lower end
temporal bone—*see* Fracture, skull, base
ulna—*see* Fracture, ulna, lower end
supracondylar, elbow 812.41
open 812.51
symphysis pubis (with visceral injury) (closed) 808.2
open 808.3
talus (ankle bone) (closed) 825.21
open 825.31
tarsus, tarsal bone(s) (with metatarsus) of one foot (closed) NEC 825.29
open 825.39
temporal bone (styloid)—*see* Fracture, skull, base
tendon—*see* Sprain, by site
thigh—*see* Fracture, femur, shaft
thumb (and finger(s)) of one hand (closed) (*see also* Fracture, phalanx, hand) 816.00
with metacarpal bone(s) of same hand 817.0
open 817.1

Fracture—*continued*
thumb—*continued*
metacarpal(s)—*see* Fracture, metacarpus
open 816.10
thyroid cartilage (closed) 807.5
open 807.6
tibia (closed) 823.80
with fibula 823.82
open 823.92
condyles—*see* Fracture, tibia, upper end
distal end 824.8
open 824.9
epiphysis
lower 824.8
open 824.9
upper—*see* Fracture, tibia, upper end
head (involving knee joint)—*see* Fracture, tibia, upper end
intercondyloid eminence—*see* Fracture, tibia, upper end
involving ankle 824.0
open 824.1
lower end or extremity (anterior lip) (posterior lip) 824.8
open 824.9
malleolus (internal) (medial) 824.0
open 824.1
open NEC 823.90
pathologic 733.16
proximal end—*see* Fracture, tibia, upper end
shaft 823.20
with fibula 823.22
open 823.32
open 823.30
spine—*see* Fracture, tibia, upper end
stress 733.93
torus 823.40
with tibia 823.42
tuberosity—*see* Fracture, tibia, upper end
upper end or extremity (condyle) (epiphysis) (head) (spine) (proximal end) (tuberosity) 823.00
with fibula 823.02
open 823.12
open 823.10
toe(s), of one foot (closed) 826.0
with bone(s) of same lower limb 827.0
open 827.1
open 826.1
tooth (root) 873.63
complicated 873.73
torus
fibula 823.41
with tibia 823.42
humerus 812.49
radius (alone) 813.45
with ulna 813.47
tibia 823.40
with fibula 823.42
ulna (alone) 813.46
with radius 813.47
trachea (closed) 807.5
open 807.6
transverse process—*see* Fracture, vertebra, by site
trapezium (closed) 814.05
open 814.15
trapezoid bone (closed) 814.06
open 814.16
trimalleolar (closed) 824.6
open 824.7

Fracture—*continued*
triquetral (bone) (closed) 814.03
  open 814.13
trochanter (greater) (lesser) (closed) (*see also*
  Fracture, femur, neck, by site) 820.20
  open 820.30
trunk (bones) (closed) 809.0
  open 809.1
tuberosity (external)—*see* Fracture, by site
ulna (alone) (closed) 813.82
  with radius NEC 813.83
    open 813.93
  coronoid process (closed) 813.02
    open 813.12
  distal end—*see* Fracture, ulna, lower end
  epiphysis
    lower—*see* Fracture, ulna, lower end
    upper—*see* Fracture, ulna, upper, end
  head—*see* Fracture, ulna, lower end
  lower end (distal end) (head) (lower epiphysis)
    (styloid process) 813.43
    with radius (lower end) 813.44
      open 813.54
    open 813.53
  olecranon process (closed) 813.01
    open 813.11
  open NEC 813.92
  pathologic 733.12
  proximal end—*see* Fracture, ulna, upper end
  shaft 813.22
    with radius (shaft) 813.23
      open 813.33
    open 813.32
  styloid process—*see* Fracture, ulna, lower end
  torus 813.46
    with radius 813.47
  transverse—*see* Fracture, ulna, by site
  upper end (epiphysis) 813.04
    with radius (upper end) 813.08
      open 813.18
    multiple sites 813.04
      open 813.14
    open 813.14
    specified site NEC 813.04
      open 813.14
unciform (closed) 814.08
  open 814.18
vertebra, vertebral (back) (body) (column)
  (neural arch) (pedicle) (spine) (spinous
  process) (transverse process) (closed) 805.8
  with
    hematomyelia—*see* Fracture, vertebra, by
      site, with spinal cord injury
    injury to
      cauda equina—*see* Fracture, vertebra,
        sacrum, with spinal cord injury
      nerve—*see* Fracture, vertebra, by site, with
        spinal cord injury
      paralysis—*see* Fracture, vertebra, by site,
        with spinal cord injury
      paraplegia—*see* Fracture, vertebra, by site,
        with spinal cord injury
      quadriplegia—*see* Fracture, vertebra, by site,
        with spinal cord injury
      spinal concussion—*see* Fracture, vertebra,
        by site, with spinal cord injury

Fracture—*continued*
  vertebra—*continued*
    with—*continued*
      spinal cord injury (closed) NEC 806.8

Note—Use the following fifth-digit
subclassification with categories 806.0-806.3:

C_1-C_4 *or unspecified level and* D_1-D_6 (T_1-T_6) *or*
unspecified level with:

0 *unspecified spinal cord injury*
1 *complete lesion of cord*
2 *anterior cord syndrome*
3 *central cord syndrome*
4 *specified injury NEC*

C_5-C_7 *level and* D_7-D_{12} *level with:*

5 *unspecified spinal cord injury*
6 *complete lesion of cord*
7 *anterior cord syndrome*
8 *central cord syndrome*
9 *specified injury NEC*

---

      cervical 806.0
        open 806.1
      dorsal, dorsolumbar 806.2
        open 806.3
      open 806.9
      thoracic, thoracolumbar 806.2
        open 806.3
    atlanto-axial—*see* Fracture, vertebra, cervical
    cervical (hangman) (teardrop) (closed) 805.00
      with spinal cord injury—*see* Fracture,
        vertebra, with spinal cord injury, cervical
      first (atlas) 805.01
        open 805.11
      second (axis) 805.02
        open 805.12
      third 805.03
        open 805.13
      fourth 805.04
        open 805.14
      fifth 805.05
        open 805.15
      sixth 805.06
        open 805.16
      seventh 805.07
        open 805.17
      multiple sites 805.08
        open 805.18
      open 805.10
    chronic 733.13
    coccyx (closed) 805.6
      with spinal cord injury (closed) 806.60
        cauda equina injury 806.62
          complete lesion 806.61
            open 806.71
          open 806.72
        open 806.70
        specified type NEC 806.69
          open 806.79
      open 805.7
    collapsed 733.13
    compression, not due to trauma 733.13
    dorsal (closed) 805.2
      with spinal cord injury—*see* Fracture,
        vertebra, with spinal cord injury, dorsal
      open 805.3

Fracture—*continued*
vertebra—*continued*
dorsolumbar (closed) 805.2
with spinal cord injury—*see* Fracture,
vertebra, with spinal cord injury, dorsal
open 805.3
due to osteoporosis 733.13
fetus or newborn 767.4
lumbar (closed) 805.4
with spinal cord injury (closed) 806.4
open 806.5
open 805.5
nontraumatic 733.13
open NEC 805.9
pathologic 733.13
sacrum (closed) 805.6
with spinal cord injury 806.60
cauda equina injury 806.62
complete lesion 806.61
open 806.71
open 806.72
open 806.70
specified type NEC 806.69
open 806.79
open 805.7
site unspecified (closed) 805.8
with spinal cord injury (closed) 806.8
open 806.9
open 805.9
stress (any site) 733.95
thoracic (closed) 805.2
with spinal cord injury—*see* Fracture,
vertebra, with spinal cord injury,
thoracic
open 805.3
vertex—*see* Fracture, skull, vault
vomer (bone) 802.0
open 802.1
Wagstaffe's—*see* Fracture, ankle
wrist (closed) 814.00
open 814.10
pathologic 733.12
xiphoid (process)—*see* Fracture, sternum
zygoma (zygomatic arch) (closed) 802.4
open 802.5
Fragile X syndrome 759.83
Fragilitas
crinium 704.2
hair 704.2
ossium 756.51
with blue sclera 756.51
unguium 703.8
congenital 757.5
Fragility
bone 756.51
with deafness and blue sclera 756.51
capillary (hereditary) 287.8
hair 704.2
nails 703.8
Fragmentation —*see* Fracture, by site
Frailty 797
Frambesia, frambesial (tropica) (*see also* Yaws)
102.9
initial lesion or ulcer 102.0
primary 102.0
Frambeside
gummatous 102.4
of early yaws 102.2
Frambesioma 102.1
Franceschetti's syndrome (mandibulofacial
dysostosis) 756.0
Francis' disease (*see also* Tularemia) 021.9

Frank's essential thrombocytopenia (*see also*
Purpura, thrombocytopenic) 287.39
Franklin's disease (heavy chain) 273.2
Fraser's syndrome 759.89
Freckle 709.09
malignant melanoma in (M8742/3)—*see*
Melanoma
melanotic (of Hutchinson) (M8742/2)—*see*
Neoplasm, skin, in situ
retinal 239.81
Freeman-Sheldon syndrome 759.89
Freezing 991.9
specified effect NEC 991.8
Frei's disease (climatic bubo) 099.1
Freiberg's
disease (osteochondrosis, second metatarsal) 732.5
infraction of metatarsal head 732.5
osteochondrosis 732.5
Fremitus, friction, cardiac 785.3
Frenulum lingua 750.0
Frenum
external os 752.44
tongue 750.0
Frequency (urinary) NEC 788.41
micturition 788.41
nocturnal 788.43
psychogenic 306.53
Frey's syndrome (auriculotemporal syndrome)
705.22
Friction
burn (*see also* Injury, superficial, by site) 919.0
fremitus, cardiac 785.3
precordial 785.3
sounds, chest 786.7
Friderichsen-Waterhouse syndrome or disease
036.3
Friedländer's
B (bacillus) NEC (*see also* condition) 041.3
sepsis or septicemia 038.49
disease (endarteritis obliterans)—*see*
Arteriosclerosis
Friedreich's
ataxia 334.0
combined systemic disease 334.0
disease 333.2
combined systemic 334.0
myoclonia 333.2
sclerosis (spinal cord) 334.0
Friedrich-Erb-Arnold syndrome
(acropachyderma) 757.39
Frigidity 302.72
psychic or psychogenic 302.72
Fröhlich's disease or syndrome (adiposogenital
dystrophy) 253.8
Froin's syndrome 336.8
Frommel's disease 676.6
Frommel-Chiari syndrome 676.6
Frontal —*see also* condition
lobe syndrome 310.0
Frostbite 991.3
face 991.0
foot 991.2
hand 991.1
specified site NEC 991.3
Frotteurism 302.89
Frozen 991.9
pelvis 620.8
shoulder 726.0
Fructosemia 271.2
Fructosuria (benign) (essential) 271.2

Fuchs'
black spot (myopic) 360.21
corneal dystrophy (endothelial) 371.57
heterochromic cyclitis 364.21
Fucosidosis 271.8
Fugue 780.99
dissociative 300.13
hysterical (dissociative) 300.13
reaction to exceptional stress (transient) 308.1
Fukuhara syndrome 277.87
Fuller Albright's syndrome (osteitis fibrosa
disseminata) 756.59
Fuller's earth disease 502
Fulminant, fulminating —*see* condition
Functional —*see* condition
Functioning
borderline intellectual V62.89
Fundus —*see also* condition
flavimaculatus 362.76
Fungemia 117.9
Fungus, fungous
cerebral 348.89
disease NEC 117.9
infection—*see* Infection, fungus
testis (*see also* Tuberculosis) 016.5 *[608.81]*
Funiculitis (acute) 608.4
chronic 608.4
endemic 608.4
gonococcal (acute) 098.14
chronic or duration of 2 months or over 098.34
tuberculous (*see also* Tuberculosis) 016.5
FUO (fever of unknown origin) (*see also* Pyrexia)
780.60
Funnel
breast (acquired) 738.3
congenital 754.81
late effect of rickets 268.1
chest (acquired) 738.3
congenital 754.81
late effect of rickets 268.1
pelvis (acquired) 738.6
with disproportion (fetopelvic) 653.3
affecting fetus or newborn 763.1
causing obstructed labor 660.1
affecting fetus or newborn 763.1
congenital 755.69
tuberculous (*see also* Tuberculosis) 016.9
Furfur 690.18
microsporon 111.0
Furor, paroxysmal (idiopathic) (*see also*
Epilepsy) 345.8
Furriers' lung 495.8
Furrowed tongue 529.5
congenital 750.13
Furrowing nail (s) (transverse) 703.8
congenital 757.5
Furuncle 680.9
abdominal wall 680.2
ankle 680.6
anus 680.5
arm (any part, above wrist) 680.3
auditory canal, external 680.0
axilla 680.3
back (any part) 680.2
breast 680.2
buttock 680.5
chest wall 680.2
corpus cavernosum 607.2
ear (any part) 680.0
eyelid 373.13

Furuncle—*continued*
face (any part, except eye) 680.0
finger (any) 680.4
flank 680.2
foot (any part) 680.7
forearm 680.3
gluteal (region) 680.5
groin 680.2
hand (any part) 680.4
head (any part, except face) 680.8
heel 680.7
hip 680.6
kidney (*see also* Abscess, kidney) 590.2
knee 680.6
labium (majus) (minus) 616.4
lacrimal
gland (*see also* Dacryoadenitis) 375.00
passages (duct) (sac) (*see also* Dacryocystitis)
375.30
leg, any part except foot 680.6
malignant 022.0
multiple sites 680.9
neck 680.1
nose (external) (septum) 680.0
orbit 376.01
partes posteriores 680.5
pectoral region 680.2
penis 607.2
perineum 680.2
pinna 680.0
scalp (any part) 680.8
scrotum 608.4
seminal vesicle 608.0
shoulder 680.3
skin NEC 680.9
specified site NEC 680.8
spermatic cord 608.4
temple (region) 680.0
testis 604.90
thigh 680.6
thumb 680.4
toe (any) 680.7
trunk 680.2
tunica vaginalis 608.4
umbilicus 680.2
upper arm 680.3
vas deferens 608.4
vulva 616.4
wrist 680.4
Furunculosis (*see also* Furuncle) 680.9
external auditory meatus 680.0 *[380.13]*
Fusarium (infection) 118
Fusion, fused (congenital)
anal (with urogenital canal) 751.5
aorta and pulmonary artery 745.0
astragaloscaphoid 755.67
atria 745.5
atrium and ventricle 745.69
auditory canal 744.02
auricles, heart 745.5
binocular, with defective stereopsis 368.33
bone 756.9
cervical spine—*see* Fusion, spine
choanal 748.0
commissure, mitral valve 746.5
cranial sutures, premature 756.0
cusps, heart valve NEC 746.89
mitral 746.5
tricuspid 746.89
ear ossicles 744.04
fingers (*see also* Syndactylism, fingers) 755.11

Fusion, fused—*continued*
  hymen 752.42
  hymeno-urethral 599.89
    causing obstructed labor 660.1
      affecting fetus or newborn 763.1
  joint (acquired)—*see also* Ankylosis
    congenital 755.8
  kidneys (incomplete) 753.3
  labium (majus) (minus) 752.49
  larynx and trachea 748.3
  limb 755.8
    lower 755.69
    upper 755.59
  lobe, lung 748.5
  lumbosacral (acquired) 724.6
    congenital 756.15
    surgical V45.4
  nares (anterior) (posterior) 748.0
  nose, nasal 748.0
  nostril(s) 748.0
  organ or site NEC—*see* Anomaly, specified
    type NEC
  ossicles 756.9
    auditory 744.04
  pulmonary valve segment 746.02
  pulmonic cusps 746.02
  ribs 756.3
  sacroiliac (acquired) (joint) 724.6
    congenital 755.69
    surgical V45.4
  skull, imperfect 756.0
  spine (acquired) 724.9
    arthrodesis status V45.4
    congenital (vertebra) 756.15
    postoperative status V45.4
  sublingual duct with submaxillary duct at
    opening in mouth 750.26
  talonavicular (bar) 755.67
  teeth, tooth 520.2
  testes 752.89
  toes (*see also* Syndactylism, toes) 755.13
  trachea and esophagus 750.3
  twins 759.4
  urethral-hymenal 599.89
  vagina 752.49
  valve cusps—*see* Fusion, cusps, heart valve
  ventricles, heart 745.4
  vertebra (arch)—*see* Fusion, spine
  vulva 752.49
Fusospirillosis (mouth) (tongue) (tonsil) 101
Fussy infant (baby) 780.91

G

Gafsa boil 085.1
Gain, weight (abnormal) (excessive) (see also
  Weight, gain) 783.1
Gaisböck's disease or syndrome (polycythemia
  hypertonica) 289.0
Gait
  abnormality 781.2
    hysterical 300.11
  ataxic 781.2
    hysterical 300.11
  disturbance 781.2
    hysterical 300.11
  paralytic 781.2
  scissor 781.2
  spastic 781.2
  staggering 781.2
    hysterical 300.11
Galactocele (breast) (infected) 611.5
  puerperal, postpartum 676.8
Galactophoritis 611.0
  puerperal, postpartum 675.2
Galactorrhea 676.6
  not associated with childbirth 611.6
Galactosemia (classic) (congenital) 271.1
Galactosuria 271.1
Galacturia 791.1
  bilharziasis 120.0
Galen's vein —see condition
Gallbladder —see also condition
  acute (see also Disease, gallbladder) 575.0
Gall duct —see condition
Gallop rhythm 427.89
Gallstone (cholemic) (colic) (impacted)—see
  also Cholelithiasis
  causing intestinal obstruction 560.31
Gambling, pathological 312.31
Gammaloidosis 277.39
Gammopathy 273.9
  macroglobulinemia 273.3
  monoclonal (benign) (essential) (idiopathic)
    (with lymphoplasmacytic dyscrasia) 273.1
Gamna's disease (siderotic splenomegaly)
  289.51
Gampsodactylia (congenital) 754.71
Gamstorp's disease (adynamia episodica
  hereditaria) 359.3
Gandy-Nanta disease (siderotic splenomegaly)
  289.51
Gang activity without manifest psychiatric
  disorder V71.09
  adolescent V71.02
  adult V71.01
  child V71.02
Gangliocytoma (M9490/0)—see Neoplasm,
  connective tissue, benign
Ganglioglioma (M9505/1)—see Neoplasm, by
  site, uncertain behavior
Ganglion 727.43
  joint 727.41
  of yaws (early) (late) 102.6
  periosteal (see also Periostitis) 730.3
  tendon sheath (compound) (diffuse) 727.42
  tuberculous (see also Tuberculosis) 015.9
Ganglioneuroblastoma (M9490/3)—see
  Neoplasm, connective tissue, malignant
Ganglioneuroma (M9490/0)—see also
  Neoplasm, connective tissue, benign

Ganglioneuroma—continued
  malignant (M9490/3)—see Neoplasm,
    connective tissue, malignant
Ganglioneuromatosis (M9491/0)—see
  Neoplasm, connective tissue, benign
Ganglionitis
  fifth nerve (see also Neuralgia, trigeminal)
    350.1
  gasserian 350.1
  geniculate 351.1
    herpetic 053.11
    newborn 767.5
  herpes zoster 053.11
  herpetic geniculate (Hunt's syndrome) 053.11
Gangliosidosis 330.1
Gangosa 102.5
Gangrene, gangrenous (anemia) (artery)
    (cellulitis) (dermatitis) (dry) (infective)
    (moist) (pemphigus) (septic) (skin) (stasis)
    (ulcer) 785.4
  with
    arteriosclerosis (native artery) 440.24
      bypass graft 440.30
        autologous vein 440.31
        nonautologous biological 440.32
    diabetes (mellitus) 250.7 [785.4]
      due to secondary diabetes 249.7 [785.4]
  abdomen (wall) 785.4
  adenitis 683
  alveolar 526.5
  angina 462
    diphtheritic 032.0
  anus 569.49
  appendices epiploicae—see Gangrene,
    mesentery
  appendix—see Appendicitis, acute
  arteriosclerotic —see Arteriosclerosis, with,
    gangrene
  auricle 785.4
  Bacillus welchii (see also Gangrene, gas) 040.0
  bile duct (see also Cholangitis) 576.8
  bladder 595.89
  bowel—see Gangrene, intestine
  cecum—see Gangrene, intestine
  Clostridium perfringens or welchii (see also
    Gangrene, gas) 040.0
  colon—see Gangrene, intestine
  connective tissue 785.4
  cornea 371.40
  corpora cavernosa (infective) 607.2
    noninfective 607.89
  cutaneous, spreading 785.4
  decubital (see also Ulcer, pressure) 707.00
    [785.4]
  diabetic (any site) 250.7 [785.4]
    due to secondary diabetes 249.7 [785.4]
  dropsical 785.4
  emphysematous (see also Gangrene, gas) 040.0
  epidemic (ergotized grain) 988.2
  epididymis (infectional) (see also Epididymitis)
    604.99
  erysipelas (see also Erysipelas) 035
  extremity (lower) (upper) 785.4
  gallbladder or duct (see also Cholecystitis,
    acute) 575.0

Gangrene, gangrenous—*continued*
gas (bacillus) 040.0
 with
  abortion—*see* Abortion, by type, with sepsis
  ectopic pregnancy (*see also* categories
   633.0-633.9) 639.0
  molar pregnancy (*see also* categories
   630-632) 639.0
 following
  abortion 639.0
  ectopic or molar pregnancy 639.0
 puerperal, postpartum, childbirth 670.8
glossitis 529.0
gum 523.8
hernia—*see* Hernia, by site, with gangrene
hospital noma 528.1
intestine, intestinal (acute) (hemorrhagic)
  (massive) 557.0
 with
  hernia—*see* Hernia, by site, with gangrene
  mesenteric embolism or infarction 557.0
  obstruction (*see also* Obstruction, intestine)
   560.9
laryngitis 464.00
 with obstruction 464.01
liver 573.8
lung 513.0
 spirochetal 104.8
lymphangitis 457.2
Meleney's (cutaneous) 686.09
mesentery 557.0
 with
  embolism or infarction 557.0
  intestinal obstruction (*see also* Obstruction,
   intestine) 560.9
mouth 528.1
noma 528.1
orchitis 604.90
ovary (*see also* Salpingo-oophoritis) 614.2
pancreas 577.0
penis (infectional) 607.2
 noninfective 607.89
perineum 785.4
pharynx 462
 septic 034.0
pneumonia 513.0
Pott's 440.24
presenile 443.1
pulmonary 513.0
pulp, tooth 522.1
quinsy 475
Raynaud's (symmetric gangrene) 443.0 *[785.4]*
rectum 569.49
retropharyngeal 478.24
rupture—*see* Hernia, by site, with gangrene
scrotum 608.4
 noninfective 608.83
senile 440.24
sore throat 462
spermatic cord 608.4
 noninfective 608.89
spine 785.4
spirochetal NEC 104.8
spreading cutaneous 785.4
stomach 537.89
stomatitis 528.1
symmetrical 443.0 *[785.4]*
testis (infectional) (*see also* Orchitis) 604.99
 noninfective 608.89
throat 462
 diphtheritic 032.0

Gangrene, gangrenous— *continued*
thyroid (gland) 246.8
tonsillitis (acute) 463
tooth (pulp) 522.1
tuberculous NEC (*see also* Tuberculosis) 011.9
tunica vaginalis 608.4
 noninfective 608.89
umbilicus 785.4
uterus (*see also* Endometritis) 615.9
uvulitis 528.3
vas deferens 608.4
 noninfective 608.89
vulva (*see also* Vulvitis) 616.10
Gannister disease (occupational) 502
 with tuberculosis—*see* Tuberculosis, pulmonary
Ganser's syndrome, hysterical 300.16
Gardner-Diamond syndrome (autoerythrocyte
  sensitization) 287.2
Gargoylism 277.5
Garré's
 disease (*see also* Osteomyelitis) 730.1
 osteitis (sclerosing) (*see also* Osteomyelitis)
  730.1
 osteomyelitis (*see also* Osteomyelitis) 730.1
Garrod's pads, knuckle 728.79
Gartner's duct
 cyst 752.41
 persistent 752.41
Gas 787.3
 asphyxia, asphyxiation, inhalation, poisoning,
  suffocation NEC 987.9
  specified gas—*see* Table of drugs and
   chemicals
 bacillus gangrene or infection—*see* Gas,
  gangrene
 cyst, mesentery 568.89
 excessive 787.3
 gangrene 040.0
  with
   abortion—*see* Abortion, by type, with sepsis
   ectopic pregnancy (*see also* categories
    633.0-633.9) 639.0
   molar pregnancy (*see also* categories
    630-632) 639.0
  following
   abortion 639.0
   ectopic or molar pregnancy 639.0
  puerperal, postpartum, childbirth 670.8
 on stomach 787.3
 pains 787.3
Gastradenitis 535.0
Gastralgia 536.8
 psychogenic 307.89
Gastrectasis, gastrectasia 536.1
 psychogenic 306.4
Gastric —*see* condition
Gastrinoma (M8153/1)
 malignant (M8153/3)
  pancreas 157.4
  specified site NEC—*see* Neoplasm, by site,
   malignant
  unspecified site 157.4
 specified site—*see* Neoplasm, by site,
  uncertain behavior
 unspecified site 235.5

Gastritis 535.5

> *Note—Use the following fifth-digit*
> *subclassification for category 535:*
>
> 0 *without mention of hemorrhage*
> 1 *with hemorrhage*

acute 535.0
alcoholic 535.3
allergic 535.4
antral 535.4
atrophic 535.1
atrophic-hyperplastic 535.1
bile-induced 535.4
catarrhal 535.0
chronic (atrophic) 535.1
cirrhotic 535.4
corrosive (acute) 535.4
dietetic 535.4
due to diet deficiency 269.9 *[535.4]*
eosinophilic 535.7
erosive 535.4
follicular 535.4
   chronic 535.1
giant hypertrophic 535.2
glandular 535.4
   chronic 535.1
hypertrophic (mucosa) 535.2
   chronic giant 211.1
irritant 535.4
nervous 306.4
phlegmonous 535.0
psychogenic 306.4
sclerotic 535.4
spastic 536.8
subacute 535.0
superficial 535.4
suppurative 535.0
toxic 535.4
tuberculous (*see also* Tuberculosis) 017.9
Gastrocarcinoma (M8010/3) 151.9
Gastrocolic —*see* condition
Gastrocolitis —*see* Enteritis
Gastrodisciasis 121.8
Gastroduodenitis (*see also* Gastritis) 535.5
catarrhal 535.0
infectional 535.0
virus, viral 008.8
   specified type NEC 008.69
Gastrodynia 536.8
Gastroenteritis (acute) (catarrhal) (congestive)
   (hemorrhagic) (noninfectious) (*see also*
   Enteritis) 558.9
aertrycke infection 003.0
allergic 558.3
chronic 558.9
   ulcerative (*see also* Colitis, ulcerative) 556.9
dietetic 558.9
due to
   antineoplastic chemotherapy 558.9
   food poisoning (*see also* Poisoning, food) 005.9
   radiation 558.1
eosinophilic 558.41
epidemic 009.0
functional 558.9
infectious (*see also* Enteritis, due to, by
   organism) 009.0
   presumed 009.1
salmonella 003.0
septic (*see also* Enteritis, due to, by organism)
   009.0

Gastroenteritis—*continued*
toxic 558.2
tuberculous (*see also* Tuberculosis) 014.8
ulcerative (*see also* Colitis, ulcerative) 556.9
viral NEC 008.8
   specified type NEC 008.69
zymotic 009.0
Gastroenterocolitis —*see* Enteritis
Gastroenteropathy, protein-losing 579.8
Gastroenteroptosis 569.89
Gastroesophageal laceration-hemorrhage
   syndrome 530.7
Gastroesophagitis 530.19
Gastrohepatitis (*see also* Gastritis) 535.5
Gastrointestinal —*see* condition
Gastrojejunal —*see* condition
Gastrojejunitis (*see also* Gastritis) 535.5
Gastrojejunocolic —*see* condition
Gastroliths 537.89
Gastromalacia 537.89
Gastroparalysis 536.3
diabetic 250.6 *[536.3]*
   due to secondary diabetes 249.6 *[536.3]*
Gastroparesis 536.3
diabetic 250.6 *[536.3]*
   due to secondary diabetes 249.6 *[536.3]*
Gastropathy 537.9
congestive portal 537.89
erythematous 535.5
exudative 579.8
portal hypertension 537.89
Gastroptosis 537.5
Gastrorrhagia 578.0
Gastrorrhea 536.8
psychogenic 306.4
Gastroschisis (congenital) 756.73
acquired 569.89
Gastrospasm (neurogenic) (reflex) 536.8
neurotic 306.4
psychogenic 306.4
Gastrostaxis 578.0
Gastrostenosis 537.89
Gastrostomy
attention to V55.1
complication 536.40
   specified type 536.49
infection 536.41
malfunctioning 536.42
status V44.1
Gastrosuccorrhea (continuous) (intermittent) 536.8
neurotic 306.4
psychogenic 306.4
Gaucher's
disease (adult) (cerebroside lipidosis) (infantile)
   272.7
hepatomegaly 272.7
splenomegaly (cerebroside lipidosis) 272.7
GAVE (gastric antral vascular ectasia) 537.82
with hemorrhage 537.83
without hemorrhage 537.82
Gayet's disease (superior hemorrhagic
   polioencephalitis) 265.1
Gayet-Wernicke's syndrome (superior
   hemorrhagic polioencephalitis) 265.1
Gee (-Herter) (-Heubner) (-Thaysen) disease or
   syndrome (nontropical sprue) 579.0
Gélineau's syndrome (*see also* Narcolepsy) 347.00
Gemination, teeth 520.2
Gemistocytoma (M9411/3)
specified site—*see* Neoplasm, by site, malignant
unspecified site 191.9

General, generalized —*see* condition
Genetic
 susceptibility to
  MEN (multiple endocrine neoplasia) V84.81
  neoplasia
   multiple endocrine (MEN) V84.81
  neoplasm
   malignant, of
    breast V84.01
    endometrium V84.04
    other V84.09
    ovary V84.02
    prostate V84.03
   specified disease NEC V84.89
Genital —*see* condition
 warts 078.11
Genito-anorectal syndrome 099.1
Genitourinary system —*see* condition
Genu
 congenital 755.64
 extrorsum (acquired) 736.42
  congenital 755.64
  late effects of rickets 268.1
 introrsum (acquired) 736.41
  congenital 755.64
  late effects of rickets 268.1
 rachitic (old) 268.1
 recurvatum (acquired) 736.5
  congenital 754.40
   with dislocation of knee 754.41
  late effects of rickets 268.1
 valgum (acquired) (knock-knee) 736.41
  congenital 755.64
  late effects of rickets 268.1
 varum (acquired) (bowleg) 736.42
  congenital 755.64
  late effects of rickets 268.1
Geographic tongue 529.1
Geophagia 307.52
Geotrichosis 117.9
 intestine 117.9
 lung 117.9
 mouth 117.9
Gephyrophobia 300.29
Gerbode defect 745.4
GERD (gastroesophageal reflux disease) 530.81
Gerhardt's
 disease (erythromelalgia) 443.82
 syndrome (vocal cord paralysis) 478.30
Gerlier's disease (epidemic vertigo) 078.81
German measles 056.9
 exposure to V01.4
Germinoblastoma (diffuse) (M9614/3) 202.8
 follicular (M9692/3) 202.0
Germinoma (M9064/3)—*see* Neoplasm, by site,
 malignant
Gerontoxon 371.41
Gerstmann's syndrome (finger agnosia) 784.69
Gerstmann-Sträussler-Scheinker syndrome
 (GSS) 046.71
Gestation (period)—*see also* Pregnancy
 ectopic NEC (*see also* Pregnancy, ectopic) 633.90
  with intrauterine pregnancy 633.91

Gestation (period)—*continued*
 multiple
  placenta status
   quadruplet
    two or more monoamniotic fetuses V91.22
    two or more monochorionic fetuses
     V91.21
    unable to determine number of placenta
     and number of amniotic sacs V91.29
    unspecified number of placenta and
     unspecified number of amniotic sacs
     V91.20
   specified (greater than quadruplets) NEC
    two or more monoamniotic fetuses V91.92
    two or more monochorionic fetuses
     V91.91
    unable to determine number of placenta
     and number of amniotic sacs V91.99
    unspecified number of placenta and
     unspecified number of amniotic sacs
     V91.90
   triplet
    two or more monoamniotic fetuses V91.12
    two or more monochorionic fetuses
     V91.11
    unable to determine number of placenta
     and number of amniotic sacs V91.19
    unspecified number of placenta,
     unspecified number of amniotic sacs
     V91.10
   twin
    dichorionic/diamniotic (two placentae, two
     amniotic sacs) V91.03
    monochorionic/diamniotic (one placenta,
     two amniotic sacs) V91.02
    monochorionic/monoamniotic (one
     placenta, one amniotic sac) V91.01
    unable to determine number of placenta
     and number of amniotic sacs V91.09
    unspecified number of placenta,
     unspecified number of amniotic sacs
     V91.00
Gestational proteinuria 646.2
 with hypertension—*see* Toxemia, of pregnancy
Ghon tubercle primary infection (*see also*
 Tuberculosis) 010.0
Ghost
 teeth 520.4
 vessels, cornea 370.64
Ghoul hand 102.3
Gianotti Crosti syndrome 057.8
 due to known virus—*see* Infection, virus
 due to unknown virus 057.8
Giant
 cell
  epulis 523.8
   peripheral (gingiva) 523.8
  tumor, tendon sheath 727.02
 colon (congenital) 751.3
 esophagus (congenital) 750.4
 kidney 753.3
 urticaria 995.1
  hereditary 277.6
Giardia lamblia infestation 007.1
Giardiasis 007.1
Gibert's disease (pityriasis rosea) 696.3
Gibraltar fever —*see* Brucellosis
Giddiness 780.4
 hysterical 300.11
 psychogenic 306.9
Gierke's disease (glycogenosis I) 271.0

Gigantism (cerebral) (hypophyseal) (pituitary) 253.0
Gilbert's disease or cholemia (familial nonhemolytic jaundice) 277.4
Gilchrist's disease (North American blastomycosis) 116.0
Gilford (-Hutchinson) disease or syndrome (progeria) 259.8
Gilles de la Tourette's disease (motor-verbal tic) 307.23
Gillespie's syndrome (dysplasia oculodentodigitalis) 759.89
Gingivitis 523.10
  acute 523.00
    necrotizing 101
    non-plaque induced 523.01
    plaque induced 523.00
  catarrhal 523.00
  chronic 523.10
    non-plaque induced 523.11
  desquamative 523.10
  expulsiva 523.40
  hyperplastic 523.10
  marginal, simple 523.10
  necrotizing, acute 101
  non-plaque induced 523.11
  pellagrous 265.2
  plaque induced 523.10
  ulcerative 523.10
    acute necrotizing 101
  Vincent's 101
Gingivoglossitis 529.0
Gingivopericementitis 523.40
Gingivosis 523.10
Gingivostomatitis 523.10
  herpetic 054.2
Giovannini's disease 117.9
GISA (glycopeptide intermediate staphylococcus aureus) V09.8
Gland, glandular —see condition
Glanders 024
Glanzmann (-Naegeli) disease or thrombasthenia 287.1
Glassblowers' disease 527.1
Glaucoma (capsular) (inflammatory) (noninflammatory) (primary) 365.9
  with increased episcleral venous pressure 365.82
  absolute 360.42
  acute 365.22
    narrow angle 365.22
    secondary 365.60
  angle closure 365.20
    acute 365.22
    attack 365.22
    chronic 365.23
    crisis 365.22
    intermittent 365.21
    interval 365.21
    primary 365.20
      chronic 365.23
    residual stage 365.24
    subacute 365.21
  angle recession 365.65
  border line 365.00
  chronic 365.11
    noncongestive 365.11
    open angle 365.11
    simple 365.11
  closed angle—see Glaucoma, angle closure

Glaucoma—*continued*
  congenital 743.20
    associated with other eye anomalies 743.22
    simple 743.21
  congestive—*see* Glaucoma, narrow angle
  corticosteroid-induced (glaucomatous stage) 365.31
    residual stage 365.32
  exfoliation 365.52
  hemorrhagic 365.60
  hypersecretion 365.81
  in or with
    aniridia 365.42
    Axenfeld's anomaly 365.41
    congenital syndromes NEC 759.89 *[365.44]*
    disorder of lens NEC 365.59
    inflammation, ocular 365.62
    iris
      anomalies NEC 365.42
      atrophy, essential 365.42
      bombé 365.61
    microcornea 365.43
    neurofibromatosis 237.71 *[365.44]*
    ocular
      cysts NEC 365.64
      disorders NEC 365.60
      trauma 365.65
      tumors NEC 365.64
    pupillary block or seclusion 365.61
    Rieger's anomaly or syndrome 365.41
    seclusion of pupil 365.61
    Sturge-Weber (-Dimitri) syndrome 759.6 *[365.44]*
    systemic syndrome NEC 365.44
    tumor of globe 365.64
    vascular disorders NEC 365.63
  infantile 365.14
    congenital 743.20
      associated with other eye anomalies 743.22
      simple 743.21
  inflammatory 365.62
  juvenile 365.14
  low tension 365.12
  malignant 365.83
  narrow angle (primary) 365.20
    acute 365.22
    chronic 365.23
    intermittent 365.21
    interval 365.21
    residual stage 365.24
    subacute 365.21
  neovascular 365.63
  newborn 743.20
    associated with other eye anomalies 743.22
    simple 743.21
  noncongestive (chronic) 365.11
  nonobstructive (chronic) 365.11
  normal tension 365.12
  obstructive 365.60
    due to lens changes 365.59
  open angle 365.10
    with
      abnormal optic disc appearance or asymmetry 365.01
      borderline findings
        high risk 365.05
        intraocular pressure 365.01
        low risk 365.01
      cupping of optic discs 365.01
      thin central corneal thickness (pachymetry) 365.01

Glaucoma—*continued*
  open angle—*continued*
    high risk 365.05
    low risk 365.01
    primary 365.11
    residual stage 365.15
  phacoanaphylactic 365.59
  phacolytic 365.51
  phacomorphic
    acute 365.22
    borderline 365.06
  pigment dispersion 365.13
  pigmentary 365.13
  postinfectious 365.60
  pseudoexfoliation 365.52
  secondary NEC 365.60
    due to
      steroids 365.31
      surgery 365.60
  simple (chronic) 365.11
  simplex 365.11
  stage
    advanced 365.73
    early 365.71
    end-stage 365.73
    indeterminate 365.74
    mild 365.71
    moderate 365.72
    severe 365.73
    unspecified 365.70
  steroid
    induced 365.31
    responders 365.03
  suspect 365.00
    primary angle closure 365.02
  syphilitic 095.8
  traumatic NEC 365.65
    newborn 767.8
  uveitic 365.62
  wide angle (*see also* Glaucoma, open angle)
    365.10
Glaucomatous flecks (subcapsular) 366.31
Glazed tongue 529.4
Gleet 098.2
Glénard's disease or syndrome (enteroptosis)
  569.89
Glinski-Simmonds syndrome (pituitary
  cachexia) 253.2
Glioblastoma (multiforme) (M9440/3)
  with sarcomatous component (M9442/3)
    specified site—*see* Neoplasm, by site,
      malignant
    unspecified site 191.9
  giant cell (M9441/3)
    specified site—*see* Neoplasm, by site, malignant
    unspecified site 191.9
  specified site—*see* Neoplasm, by site, malignant
  unspecified site 191.9
Glioma (malignant) (M9380/3)
  astrocytic (M9400/3)
    specified site—*see* Neoplasm, by site,
      malignant
    unspecified site 191.9
  mixed (M9382/3)
    specified site—*see* Neoplasm, by site,
      malignant
    unspecified site 191.9
  nose 748.1
  specified site NEC—*see* Neoplasm, by site,
    malignant
  subependymal (M9383/1) 237.5
  unspecified site 191.9

Gliomatosis cerebri (M9381/3) 191.0
Glioneuroma (M9505/1)—*see* Neoplasm, by
  site, uncertain behavior
Gliosarcoma (M9380/3)
  specified site—*see* Neoplasm, by site, malignant
  unspecified site 191.9
Gliosis (cerebral) 349.89
  spinal 336.0
Glisson's
  cirrhosis—*see* Cirrhosis, portal
  disease (*see also* Rickets) 268.0
Glissonitis 573.3
Globinuria 791.2
Globus 306.4
  hystericus 300.11
Glomangioma (M8712/0) (*see also*
  Hemangioma) 228.00
Glomangiosarcoma (M8710/3)—*see* Neoplasm,
  connective tissue, malignant
Glomerular nephritis (*see also* Nephritis) 583.9
Glomerulitis (*see also* Nephritis) 583.9
Glomerulonephritis (*see also* Nephritis) 583.9
  with
    edema (*see also* Nephrosis) 581.9
    lesion of
      exudative nephritis 583.89
      interstitial nephritis (diffuse) (focal) 583.89
      necrotizing glomerulitis 583.4
        acute 580.4
        chronic 582.4
      renal necrosis 583.9
        cortical 583.6
        medullary 583.7
      specified pathology NEC 583.89
        acute 580.89
        chronic 582.89
    necrosis, renal 583.9
      cortical 583.6
      medullary (papillary) 583.7
    specified pathology or lesion NEC 583.89
  acute 580.9
    with
      exudative nephritis 580.89
      interstitial nephritis (diffuse) (focal) 580.89
      necrotizing glomerulitis 580.4
    extracapillary with epithelial crescents 580.4
    poststreptococcal 580.0
    proliferative (diffuse) 580.0
    rapidly progressive 580.4
    specified pathology NEC 580.89
  arteriolar (*see also* Hypertension, kidney) 403.90
  arteriosclerotic (*see also* Hypertension, kidney)
    403.90
  ascending (*see also* Pyelitis) 590.80
  basement membrane NEC 583.89
    with
      pulmonary hemorrhage (Goodpasture's
        syndrome) 446.21 *[583.81]*
  chronic 582.9
    with
      exudative nephritis 582.89
      interstitial nephritis (diffuse) (focal) 582.89
      necrotizing glomerulitis 582.4
      specified pathology or lesion NEC 582.89
    endothelial 582.2
    extracapillary with epithelial crescents 582.4
    hypocomplementemic persistent 582.2
    lobular 582.2
    membranoproliferative 582.2
    membranous 582.1
      and proliferative (mixed) 582.2
      sclerosing 582.1

Glomerulonephritis—*continued*
  chronic—*continued*
    mesangiocapillary 582.2
    mixed membranous and proliferative 582.2
    proliferative (diffuse) 582.0
    rapidly progressive 582.4
    sclerosing 582.1
  cirrhotic—*see* Sclerosis, renal
  desquamative—*see* Nephrosis
  due to or associated with
    amyloidosis 277.39 *[583.81]*
      with nephrotic syndrome 277.39 *[581.81]*
      chronic 277.39 *[582.81]*
    diabetes mellitus 250.4 *[583.81]*
      due to secondary diabetes 249.4 *[581.81]*
      with nephrotic syndrome 250.4 *[581.81]*
        due to secondary diabetes 249.4 *[581.81]*
    diphtheria 032.89 *[580.81]*
    gonococcal infection (acute) 098.19 *[583.81]*
      chronic or duration or 2 months or over
        098.39 *[583.81]*
    infectious hepatitis 070.9 *[580.81]*
    malaria (with nephrotic syndrome) 084.9
      [581.81]
    mumps 072.79 *[580.81]*
    polyarteritis (nodosa) (with nephrotic
      syndrome) 446.0 *[581.81]*
    specified pathology NEC 583.89
      acute 580.89
      chronic 582.89
    streptotrichosis 039.8 *[583.81]*
    subacute bacterial endocarditis 421.0 *[580.81]*
    syphilis (late) 095.4
      congenital 090.5 *[583.81]*
      early 091.69 *[583.81]*
    systemic lupus erythematosus 710.0 *[583.81]*
      with nephrotic syndrome 710.0 *[581.81]*
      chronic 710.0 *[582.81]*
    tuberculosis (*see also* Tuberculosis) 016.0
      [583.81]
    typhoid fever 002.0 *[580.81]*
  extracapillary with epithelial crescents 583.4
    acute 580.4
    chronic 582.4
  exudative 583.89
    acute 580.89
    chronic 582.89
  focal (*see also* Nephritis) 583.9
    embolic 580.4
  granular 582.89
  granulomatous 582.89
  hydremic (*see also* Nephrosis) 581.9
  hypocomplementemic persistent 583.2
    with nephrotic syndrome 581.2
    chronic 582.2
  immune complex NEC 583.89
  infective (*see also* Pyelitis) 590.80
  interstitial (diffuse) (focal) 583.89
    with nephrotic syndrome 581.89
    acute 580.89
    chronic 582.89
  latent or quiescent 582.9
  lobular 583.2
    with nephrotic syndrome 581.2
    chronic 582.2
  membranoproliferative 583.2
    with nephrotic syndrome 581.2
    chronic 582.2

Glomerulonephritis—*continued*
  membranous 583.1
    with nephrotic syndrome 581.1
    and proliferative (mixed) 583.2
      with nephrotic syndrome 581.2
      chronic 582.2
    chronic 582.1
    sclerosing 582.1
      with nephrotic syndrome 581.1
    mesangiocapillary 583.2
      with nephrotic syndrome 581.2
      chronic 582.2
    minimal change 581.3
    mixed membranous and proliferative 583.2
      with nephrotic syndrome 581.2
      chronic 582.2
    necrotizing 583.4
      acute 580.4
      chronic 582.4
    nephrotic (*see also* Nephrosis) 581.9
    old—*see* Glomerulonephritis, chronic
    parenchymatous 581.89
    poststreptococcal 580.0
    proliferative (diffuse) 583.0
      with nephrotic syndrome 581.0
      acute 580.0
      chronic 582.0
    purulent (*see also* Pyelitis) 590.80
    quiescent—*see* Nephritis, chronic
    rapidly progressive 583.4
      acute 580.4
      chronic 582.4
    sclerosing membranous (chronic) 582.1
      with nephrotic syndrome 581.1
    septic (*see also* Pyelitis) 590.80
    specified pathology or lesion NEC 583.89
      with nephrotic syndrome 581.89
      acute 580.89
      chronic 582.89
    suppurative (acute) (disseminated) (*see also*
      Pyelitis) 590.80
    toxic—*see* Nephritis, acute
    tubal, tubular—*see* Nephrosis, tubular
    type II (Ellis)—*see* Nephrosis
    vascular—*see* Hypertension, kidney
Glomerulosclerosis (*see also* Sclerosis, renal) 587
  focal 582.1
    with nephrotic syndrome 581.1
  intercapillary (nodular) (with diabetes) 250.4
    [581.81]
    due to secondary diabetes 249.4 *[581.81]*
Glossagra 529.6
Glossalgia 529.6
Glossitis 529.0
  areata exfoliativa 529.1
  atrophic 529.4
  benign migratory 529.1
  gangrenous 529.0
  Hunter's 529.4
  median rhomboid 529.2
  Moeller's 529.4
  pellagrous 265.2
Glossocele 529.8
Glossodynia 529.6
  exfoliativa 529.4
Glossoncus 529.8
Glossophytia 529.3
Glossoplegia 529.8
Glossoptosis 529.8
Glossopyrosis 529.6

Glossotrichia 529.3
Glossy skin 701.9
Glottis —*see* condition
Glottitis —*see* Glossitis
Glucagonoma (M8152/0)
  malignant (M8152/3)
    pancreas 157.4
    specified site NEC—*see* Neoplasm, by site,
      malignant
    unspecified site 157.4
    pancreas 211.7
    specified site NEC—*see* Neoplasm, by site, benign
    unspecified site 211.7
Glucoglycinuria 270.7
Glue ear syndrome 381.20
Glue sniffing (airplane glue) (*see also*
  Dependence) 304.6
Glycinemia (with methylmalonic acidemia) 270.7
Glycinuria (renal) (with ketosis) 270.0
Glycogen
  infiltration (*see also* Disease, glycogen storage)
    271.0
  storage disease (*see also* Disease, glycogen
    storage) 271.0
Glycogenosis (*see also* Disease, glycogen
  storage) 271.0
  cardiac 271.0 *[425.7]*
  Cori, types I-VII 271.0
  diabetic, secondary 250.8 *[259.8]*
    due to secondary diabetes 249.8 *[259.8]*
  diffuse (with hepatic cirrhosis) 271.0
  generalized 271.0
  glucose-6-phosphatase deficiency 271.0
  hepatophosphorylase deficiency 271.0
  hepatorenal 271.0
  myophosphorylase deficiency 271.0
  pulmonary interstitial 516.62
Glycopenia 251.2
Glycopeptide
  intermediate staphylococcus aureus (GISA) V09.8
  resistant
    enterococcus V09.8
    staphylococcus aureus (GRSA) V09.8
Glycoprolinuria 270.8
Glycosuria 791.5
  renal 271.4
Gnathostoma (spinigerum) (infection)
  (infestation) 128.1
  wandering swellings from 128.1
Gnathostomiasis 128.1
Goiter (adolescent) (colloid) (diffuse) (dipping)
  (due to iodine deficiency) (endemic)
  (euthyroid) (heart) (hyperplastic) (internal)
  (intrathoracic) (juvenile) (mixed type)
  (nonendemic) (parenchymatous) (plunging)
  (sporadic) (subclavicular) (substernal) 240.9
  with
    hyperthyroidism (recurrent) (*see also* Goiter,
      toxic) 242.0
    thyrotoxicosis (*see also* Goiter, toxic) 242.0
  adenomatous (*see also* Goiter, nodular) 241.9
  cancerous (M8000/3) 193
  complicating pregnancy, childbirth, or
    puerperium 648.1
  congenital 246.1
  cystic (*see also* Goiter, nodular) 241.9
  due to enzyme defect in synthesis of thyroid
    hormone (butane-insoluble iodine)
    (coupling) (deiodinase) (iodide trapping or
    organification) (iodotyrosine dehalogenase)
    (peroxidase) 246.1

Goiter—*continued*
  dyshormonogenic 246.1
  exophthalmic (*see also* Goiter, toxic) 242.0
  familial (with deaf-mutism) 243
  fibrous 245.3
  lingual 759.2
  lymphadenoid 245.2
  malignant (M8000/3) 193
  multinodular (nontoxic) 241.1
    toxic or with hyperthyroidism (*see also* Goiter,
      toxic) 242.2
  nodular (nontoxic) 241.9
    with
      hyperthyroidism (*see also* Goiter, toxic)
        242.3
      thyrotoxicosis (*see also* Goiter, toxic) 242.3
    endemic 241.9
    exophthalmic (diffuse) (*see also* Goiter, toxic)
      242.0
    multinodular (nontoxic) 241.1
    sporadic 241.9
    toxic (*see also* Goiter, toxic) 242.3
    uninodular (nontoxic) 241.0
  nontoxic (nodular) 241.9
    multinodular 241.1
    uninodular 241.0
  pulsating (*see also* Goiter, toxic) 242.0
  simple 240.0
  toxic 242.0

> *Note—Use the following fifth-digit*
> *subclassification with category 242:*
>
> *0 without mention of thyrotoxic crisis*
> *or storm*
> *1 with mention of thyrotoxic crisis or storm*

    adenomatous 242.3
      multinodular 242.2
      uninodular 242.1
    multinodular 242.2
    nodular 242.3
      multinodular 242.2
      uninodular 242.1
    uninodular 242.1
  uninodular (nontoxic) 241.0
    toxic or with hyperthyroidism (*see also* Goiter,
      toxic) 242.1
Goldberg (-Maxwell) (-Morris) syndrome
  (testicular feminization) 259.51
Goldblatt's
  hypertension 440.1
  kidney 440.1
Goldenhar's syndrome (oculoauriculovertebral
  dysplasia) 756.0
Goldflam-Erb disease or syndrome 358.00
Goldscheider's disease (epidermolysis bullosa)
  757.39
Goldstein's disease (familial hemorrhagic
  telangiectasia) 448.0
Golfer's elbow 726.32
Goltz-Gorlin syndrome (dermal hypoplasia)
  757.39
Gonadoblastoma (M9073/1)
  specified site—*see* Neoplasm, by site uncertain
    behavior
  unspecified site
    female 236.2
    male 236.4
Gonecystitis (*see also* Vesiculitis) 608.0
Gongylonemiasis 125.6
  mouth 125.6

Goniosynechiae 364.73
Gonococcemia 098.89
Gonococcus, gonococcal (disease) (infection)
    (*see also* condition) 098.0
    anus 098.7
    bursa 098.52
    chronic NEC 098.2
    complicating pregnancy, childbirth, or
        puerperium 647.1
        affecting fetus or newborn 760.2
    conjunctiva, conjunctivitis (neonatorum) 098.40
    dermatosis 098.89
    endocardium 098.84
    epididymo-orchitis 098.13
        chronic or duration of 2 months or over 098.33
    eye (newborn) 098.40
    fallopian tube (chronic) 098.37
        acute 098.17
    genitourinary (acute) (organ) (system) (tract)
        (*see also* Gonorrhea) 098.0
        lower 098.0
            chronic 098.2
        upper 098.10
            chronic 098.30
    heart NEC 098.85
    joint 098.50
    keratoderma 098.81
    keratosis (blennorrhagica) 098.81
    lymphatic (gland) (node) 098.89
    meninges 098.82
    orchitis (acute) 098.13
        chronic or duration of 2 months or over 098.33
    pelvis (acute) 098.19
        chronic or duration of 2 months or over 098.39
    pericarditis 098.83
    peritonitis 098.86
    pharyngitis 098.6
    pharynx 098.6
    proctitis 098.7
    pyosalpinx (chronic) 098.37
        acute 098.17
    rectum 098.7
    septicemia 098.89
    skin 098.89
    specified site NEC 098.89
    synovitis 098.51
    tendon sheath 098.51
    throat 098.6
    urethra (acute) 098.0
        chronic or duration of 2 months or over 098.2
    vulva (acute) 098.0
        chronic or duration of 2 months or over 098.2
Gonocytoma (M9073/1)
    specified site—*see* Neoplasm, by site, uncertain
        behavior
    unspecified site
        female 236.2
        male 236.4
Gonorrhea 098.0
    acute 098.0
    Bartholin's gland (acute) 098.0
        chronic or duration of 2 months or over 098.2
    bladder (acute) 098.11
        chronic or duration of 2 months or over 098.31
    carrier (suspected of) V02.7
    cervix (acute) 098.15
        chronic or duration of 2 months or over 098.35
    chronic 098.2
    complicating pregnancy, childbirth, or
        puerperium 647.1
        affecting fetus or newborn 760.2

Gonorrhea—*continued*
    conjunctiva, conjunctivitis (neonatorum) 098.40
    contact V01.6
    Cowper's gland (acute) 098.0
        chronic or duration of 2 months or over 098.2
    duration of two months or over 098.2
    exposure to V01.6
    fallopian tube (chronic) 098.37
        acute 098.17
    genitourinary (acute) (organ) (system) (tract)
        098.0
        chronic 098.2
        duration of two months or over 098.2
    kidney (acute) 098.19
        chronic or duration of 2 months or over 098.39
    ovary (acute) 098.19
        chronic or duration of 2 months or over 098.39
    pelvis (acute) 098.19
        chronic or duration of 2 months or over 098.39
    penis (acute) 098.0
        chronic or duration of 2 months or over 098.2
    prostate (acute) 098.12
        chronic or duration of 2 months or over 098.32
    seminal vesicle (acute) 098.14
        chronic or duration of 2 months or over 098.34
    specified site NEC—*see* Gonococcus
    spermatic cord (acute) 098.14
        chronic or duration of 2 months or over 098.34
    urethra (acute) 098.0
        chronic or duration of 2 months or over 098.2
    vagina (acute) 098.0
        chronic or duration of 2 months or over 098.2
    vas deferens (acute) 098.14
        chronic or duration of 2 months or over 098.34
    vulva (acute) 098.0
        chronic or duration of 2 months or over 098.2
Goodpasture's syndrome (pneumorenal) 446.21
Good's syndrome 279.06
Gopalan's syndrome (burning feet) 266.2
Gordon's disease (exudative enteropathy) 579.8
Gorlin-Chaudhry-Moss syndrome 759.89
Gougerot's syndrome (trisymptomatic) 709.1
Gougerot-Blum syndrome (pigmented purpuric
    lichenoid dermatitis) 709.1
Gougerot-Carteaud disease or syndrome
    (confluent reticulate papillomatosis) 701.8
Gougerot-Hailey-Hailey disease (benign familial
    chronic pemphigus) 757.39
Gougerot (-Houwer) -Sjögren syndrome
    (keratoconjunctivitis sicca) 710.2
Gouley's syndrome (constrictive pericarditis)
    423.2
Goundou 102.6
Gout, gouty 274.9
    with
        specified manifestations NEC 274.89
        tophi (tophus) 274.03
    acute 274.01
    arthritis 274.00
        acute 274.01
    arthropathy 274.00
        acute 274.01
        chronic (without mention of tophus (tophi))
            274.02
            with tophus (tophi) 274.03
    attack 274.01
    chronic 274.02
        tophaceous 274.03
    degeneration, heart 274.82
    diathesis 274.9
    eczema 274.89

Gout, gouty—*continued*
episcleritis 274.89 *[379.09]*
external ear (tophus) 274.81
flare 274.01
glomerulonephritis 274.10
iritis 274.89 *[364.11]*
joint 274.00
kidney 274.10
lead 984.9
  specified type of lead—*see* Table of drugs and
    chemicals
nephritis 274.10
neuritis 274.89 *[357.4]*
phlebitis 274.89 *[451.9]*
rheumatic 714.0
saturnine 984.9
  specified type of lead—*see* Table of drugs and
    chemicals
spondylitis 274.00
synovitis 274.00
syphilitic 095.8
tophi 274.03
  ear 274.81
  heart 274.82
  specified site NEC 274.82
Gowers'
muscular dystrophy 359.1
syndrome (vasovagal attack) 780.2
Gowers-Paton-Kennedy syndrome 377.04
Gradenigo's syndrome 383.02
Graft-versus-host disease 279.50
due to organ transplant NEC—*see*
  Complications, transplant, organ
Graham Steell's murmur (pulmonic
  regurgitation) (*see also* Endocarditis,
  pulmonary) 424.3
Grain-handlers' disease or lung 495.8
Grain mite (itch) 133.8
Grand
mal (idiopathic) (*see also* Epilepsy) 345.1
  hysteria of Charcot 300.11
  nonrecurrent or isolated 780.39
multipara
  affecting management of labor and delivery
    659.4
  status only (not pregnant) V61.5
Granite workers' lung 502
Granular —*see also* condition
inflammation, pharynx 472.1
kidney (contracting) (*see also* Sclerosis, renal) 587
liver—*see* Cirrhosis, liver
nephritis—*see* Nephritis
Granulation tissue, abnormal —*see also*
  Granuloma
abnormal or excessive 701.5
postmastoidectomy cavity 383.33
postoperative 701.5
skin 701.5
Granulocytopenia, granulocytopenic (primary)
  288.00
malignant 288.09
Granuloma NEC 686.1
abdomen (wall) 568.89
  skin (pyogenicum) 686.1
    from residual foreign body 709.4
annulare 695.89
anus 569.49
apical 522.6
appendix 543.9
aural 380.23

Granuloma—*continued*
beryllium (skin) 709.4
  lung 503
bone (*see also* Osteomyelitis) 730.1
  eosinophilic 277.89
  from residual foreign body 733.99
canaliculus lacrimalis 375.81
cerebral 348.89
cholesterin, middle ear 385.82
coccidioidal (progressive) 114.3
  lung 114.4
  meninges 114.2
  primary (lung) 114.0
colon 569.89
conjunctiva 372.61
dental 522.6
ear, middle (cholesterin) 385.82
  with otitis media—*see* Otitis media
eosinophilic 277.89
  bone 277.89
  lung 277.89
  oral mucosa 528.9
exuberant 701.5
eyelid 374.89
facial
  lethal midline 446.3
  malignant 446.3
faciale 701.8
fissuratum (gum) 523.8
foot NEC 686.1
foreign body (in soft tissue) NEC 728.82
  bone 733.99
  in operative wound 998.4
  muscle 728.82
  skin 709.4
  subcutaneous tissue 709.4
fungoides 202.1
gangraenescens 446.3
giant cell (central) (jaw) (reparative) 526.3
  gingiva 523.8
  peripheral (gingiva) 523.8
gland (lymph) 289.3
Hodgkin's (M9661/3) 201.1
ileum 569.89
infectious NEC 136.9
inguinale (Donovan) 099.2
  venereal 099.2
intestine 569.89
iridocyclitis 364.10
jaw (bone) 526.3
  reparative giant cell 526.3
kidney (*see also* Infection, kidney) 590.9
lacrimal sac 375.81
larynx 478.79
lethal midline 446.3
lipid 277.89
lipoid 277.89
liver 572.8
lung (infectious) (*see also* Fibrosis, lung) 515
  coccidioidal 114.4
  eosinophilic 277.89
lymph gland 289.3
Majocchi's 110.6
malignant, face 446.3
mandible 526.3
mediastinum 519.3
midline 446.3
monilial 112.3
muscle 728.82
  from residual foreign body 728.82
nasal sinus (*see also* Sinusitis) 473.9

Granuloma—*continued*
  operation wound 998.59
    foreign body 998.4
    stitch (external) 998.89
      internal organ 998.89
    talc 998.7
  oral mucosa, eosinophilic or pyogenic 528.9
  orbit, orbital 376.11
  paracoccidioidal 116.1
  penis, venereal 099.2
  periapical 522.6
  peritoneum 568.89
    due to ova of helminths NEC (*see also*
      Helminthiasis) 128.9
  postmastoidectomy cavity 383.33
  postoperative–*see* Granuloma, operation wound
  prostate 601.8
  pudendi (ulcerating) 099.2
  pudendorum (ulcerative) 099.2
  pulp, internal (tooth) 521.49
  pyogenic, pyogenicum (skin) 686.1
    maxillary alveolar ridge 522.6
    oral mucosa 528.9
  rectum 569.49
  reticulohistiocytic 277.89
  rubrum nasi 705.89
  sarcoid 135
  Schistosoma 120.9
  septic (skin) 686.1
  silica (skin) 709.4
  sinus (accessory) (infectional) (nasal) (*see also*
    Sinusitis) 473.9
  skin (pyogenicum) 686.1
    from foreign body or material 709.4
  sperm 608.89
  spine
    syphilitic (epidural) 094.89
    tuberculous (*see also* Tuberculosis) 015.0
      [730.88]
  stitch (postoperative) 998.89
    internal wound 998.89
  suppurative (skin) 686.1
  suture (postoperative) 998.89
    internal wound 998.89
  swimming pool 031.1
  talc 728.82
    in operation wound 998.7
  telangiectaticum (skin) 686.1
  tracheostomy 519.09
  trichophyticum 110.6
  tropicum 102.4
  umbilicus 686.1
    newborn 771.4
  urethra 599.84
  uveitis 364.10
  vagina 099.2
  venereum 099.2
  vocal cords 478.5
  Wegener's (necrotizing respiratory
    granulomatosis) 446.4
Granulomatosis NEC 686.1
  disciformis chronica et progressiva 709.3
  infantiseptica 771.2
  lipoid 277.89
  lipophagic, intestinal 040.2
  miliary 027.0
  necrotizing, respiratory 446.4
  progressive, septic 288.1
  Wegener's (necrotizing respiratory) 446.4
Granulomatous tissue —*see* Granuloma
Granulosis rubra nasi 705.89
Graphite fibrosis (of lung) 503

Graphospasm 300.89
  organic 333.84
Grating scapula 733.99
Gravel (urinary) (*see also* Calculus) 592.9
Graves' disease (exophthalmic goiter) (*see also*
  Goiter, toxic) 242.0
Gravis —*see* condition
Grawitz's tumor (hypernephroma) (M8312/3)
  189.0
Grayness, hair (premature) 704.3
  congenital 757.4
Gray or grey syndrome (chloramphenicol)
  (newborn) 779.4
Greenfield's disease 330.0
Green sickness 280.9
Greenstick fracture —*see* Fracture, by site
Greig's syndrome (hypertelorism) 756.0
Grief 309.0
Griesinger's disease (*see also* Ancylostomiasis)
  126.9
Grinder's
  asthma 502
  lung 502
  phthisis (*see also* Tuberculosis) 011.4
Grinding, teeth 306.8
Grip
  Dabney's 074.1
  devil's 074.1
Grippe, grippal —*see also* Influenza
  Balkan 083.0
  intestinal (*see also* Influenza) 487.8
  summer 074.8
Grippy cold (*see also* Influenza) 487.1
Grisel's disease 723.5
Groin —*see* condition
Grooved
  nails (transverse) 703.8
  tongue 529.5
    congenital 750.13
Ground itch 126.9
Growing pains, children 781.99
Growth (fungoid) (neoplastic) (new)
  (M8000/1)—*see also* Neoplasm, by site,
  unspecified nature
  adenoid (vegetative) 474.12
  benign (M8000/0)—*see* Neoplasm, by site,
    benign
  fetal, poor 764.9
    affecting management of pregnancy 656.5
  malignant (M8000/3)—*see* Neoplasm, by site
    malignant
  rapid, childhood V21.0
  secondary (M8000/6)—*see* Neoplasm, by site,
    malignant, secondary
GRSA (glycopeptide resistant staphylococcus
  aureus) V09.8
Gruber's hernia —*see* Hernia, Gruber's
Gruby's disease (tinea tonsurans) 110.0
GSS (Gerstmann-Straussler-Scheinker syndrome)
  046.71
G-trisomy 758.0
Guama fever 066.3
Gubler (-Millard) paralysis or syndrome 344.89
Guérin-Stern syndrome (arthrogryposis
  multiplex congenita) 754.89
Guertin's disease (electric chorea) 049.8
Guillain-Barré disease or syndrome 357.0
Guinea worms (infection) (infestation) 125.7
Guinon's disease (motor-verbal tic) 307.23
Gull's disease (thyroid atrophy with myxedema)
  244.8

Gull and Sutton's disease —*see* Hypertension, kidney
Gum —*see* condition
Gumboil 522.7
Gumma (syphilitic) 095.9
  artery 093.89
    cerebral or spinal 094.89
  bone 095.5
    of yaws (late) 102.6
  brain 094.89
  cauda equina 094.89
  central nervous system NEC 094.9
  ciliary body 095.8 *[364.11]*
  congenital 090.5
    testis 090.5
  eyelid 095.8 *[373.5]*
  heart 093.89
  intracranial 094.89
  iris 095.8 *[364.11]*
  kidney 095.4
  larynx 095.8
  leptomeninges 094.2
  liver 095.3
  meninges 094.2
  myocardium 093.82
  nasopharynx 095.8
  neurosyphilitic 094.9
  nose 095.8
  orbit 095.8
  palate (soft) 095.8
  penis 095.8
  pericardium 093.81
  pharynx 095.8
  pituitary 095.8
  scrofulous (*see also* Tuberculosis) 017.0
  skin 095.8
  specified site NEC 095.8
  spinal cord 094.89
  tongue 095.8
  tonsil 095.8
  trachea 095.8
  tuberculous (*see also* Tuberculosis) 017.0
  ulcerative due to yaws 102.4
  ureter 095.8
  yaws 102.4
    bone 102.6
Gunn's syndrome (jaw-winking syndrome) 742.8
Gunshot wound —*see also* Wound, open, by site
  fracture—*see* Fracture, by site, open
  internal organs (abdomen, chest, or pelvis)—*see* Injury, internal, by site, with open wound
  intracranial—*see* Laceration, brain, with open intracranial wound
Günther's disease or syndrome (congenital erythropoietic porphyria) 277.1
Gustatory hallucination 780.1
Gynandrism 752.7
Gynandroblastoma (M8632/1)
  specified site—*see* Neoplasm, by site, uncertain behavior
  unspecified site
    female 236.2
    male 236.4
Gynandromorphism 752.7
Gynatresia (congenital) 752.49
Gynecoid pelvis, male 738.6
Gynecological examination V72.31
  for contraceptive maintenance V25.40
Gynecomastia 611.1
Gynephobia 300.29

Gyrate scalp 757.39

H

Haas' disease (osteochondrosis head of humerus) 732.3
Habermann's disease (acute parapsoriasis varioliformis) 696.2
Habit, habituation
chorea 307.22
disturbance, child 307.9
drug (*see also* Dependence) 304.9
laxative (*see also* Abuse, drugs, nondependent) 305.9
spasm 307.20
chronic 307.22
transient (of childhood) 307.21
tic 307.20
chronic 307.22
transient (of childhood) 307.21
use of
nonprescribed drugs (*see also* Abuse, drugs, nondependent) 305.9
patent medicines (*see also* Abuse, drugs, nondependent) 305.9
vomiting 536.2
Hadfield-Clarke syndrome (pancreatic infantilism) 577.8
Haff disease 985.1
Hageman factor defect, deficiency, or disease (*see also Defect, coagulation*) 286.3
Haglund's disease (osteochondrosis os tibiale externum) 732.5
Haglund-Läwen-Fründ syndrome 717.89
Hagner's disease (hypertrophic pulmonary osteoarthropathy) 731.2
Hag teeth, tooth 524.39
Hailey-Hailey disease (benign familial chronic pemphigus) 757.39
Hair —*see also* condition
plucking 307.9
Hairball in stomach 935.2
Hairy black tongue 529.3
Half vertebra 756.14
Halitosis 784.99
Hallermann-Streiff syndrome 756.0
Hallervorden-Spatz disease or syndrome 333.0
Hallopeau's
acrodermatitis (continua) 696.1
disease (lichen sclerosis et atrophicus) 701.0
Hallucination (auditory) (gustatory) (olfactory) (tactile) 780.1
alcohol-induced 291.3
drug-induced 292.12
visual 368.16
Hallucinosis 298.9
alcohol-induced (acute) 291.3
drug-induced 292.12
Hallus —*see* Hallux
Hallux 735.9
limitus 735.8
malleus (acquired) 735.3
rigidus (acquired) 735.2
congenital 755.66
late effects of rickets 268.1
valgus (acquired) 735.0
congenital 755.66
varus (acquired) 735.1
congenital 755.66
Halo, visual 368.15
Hamartoblastoma 759.6

Hamartoma 759.6
epithelial (gingival), odontogenic, central, or peripheral (M9321/0) 213.1
upper jaw (bone) 213.0
vascular 757.32
Hamartosis, hamartoses NEC 759.6
Hamman's disease or syndrome (spontaneous mediastinal emphysema) 518.1
Hamman-Rich syndrome (diffuse interstitial pulmonary fibrosis) 516.33
Hammer toe (acquired) 735.4
congenital 755.66
late effects of rickets 268.1
Hand —*see* condition
Hand-Schüller-Christian disease or syndrome (chronic histiocytosis x) 277.89
Hand-foot syndrome 693.0
Hanging (asphyxia) (strangulation) (suffocation) 994.7
Hangnail (finger) (with lymphangitis) 681.02
Hangover (alcohol) (*see also* Abuse, drugs, nondependent) 305.0
Hanot's cirrhosis or disease —*see* Cirrhosis, biliary
Hanot-Chauffard (-Troisier) syndrome (bronze diabetes) 275.01
Hansen's disease (leprosy) 030.9
benign form 030.1
malignant form 030.0
Harada's disease or syndrome 363.22
Hard chancre 091.0
Hard firm prostate 600.10
with
urinary
obstruction 600.11
retention 600.11
Hardening
artery—*see* Arteriosclerosis
brain 348.89
liver 571.8
Hare's syndrome (M8010/3) (carcinoma, pulmonary apex) 162.3
Harelip (*see also* Cleft, lip) 749.10
Harkavy's syndrome 446.0
Harlequin (fetus) 757.1
color change syndrome 779.89
Harley's disease (intermittent hemoglobinuria) 283.2
Harris'
lines 733.91
syndrome (organic hyperinsulinism) 251.1
Hart's disease or syndrome (pellagra-cerebellar ataxia-renal aminoaciduria) 270.0
Hartmann's pouch (abnormal sacculation of gallbladder neck) 575.8
of intestine V44.3
attention to V55.3
Hartnup disease (pellagra-cerebellar ataxia-renal aminoaciduria) 270.0
Harvester lung 495.0
Hashimoto's disease or struma (struma lymphomatosa) 245.2
Hassall-Henle bodies (corneal warts) 371.41
Haut mal (*see also* Epilepsy) 345.1
Haverhill fever 026.1
Hawaiian wood rose dependence 304.5
Hawkins' keloid 701.4

Hay
  asthma (*see also* Asthma) 493.0
    fever (allergic) (with rhinitis) 477.9with
        asthma (bronchial) (*see also* Asthma) 493.0
    allergic, due to grass, pollen, ragweed, or tree
        477.0
    conjunctivitis 372.05
    due to
      dander, animal (cat) (dog) 477.2
      dust 477.8
      fowl 477.8
      hair, animal (cat) (dog) 477.2
      pollen 477.0
      specified allergen other than pollen 477.8
Hayem-Faber syndrome (achlorhydric anemia)
    280.9
Hayem-Widal syndrome (acquired hemolytic
    jaundice) 283.9
Haygarth's nodosities 715.04
Hazard-Crile tumor (M8350/3) 193
Hb (abnormal)
    disease—*see* Disease, hemoglobin
    trait—*see* Trait
H disease 270.0
Head —*see also* condition
    banging 307.3
Headache 784.0
  allergic 339.00
  associated with sexual activity 339.82
  cluster 339.00
    chronic 339.02
    episodic 339.01
  daily
    chronic 784.0
    new persistent (NPDH) 339.42
  drug induced 339.3
  due to
    loss, spinal fluid 349.0
    lumbar puncture 349.0
    saddle block 349.0
  emotional 307.81
  histamine 339.00
  hypnic 339.81
  lumbar puncture 349.0
  medication overuse 339.3
  menopausal 627.2
  menstrual 346.4
  migraine 346.9
  nasal septum 784.0
  nonorganic origin 307.81
  orgasmic 339.82
  postspinal 349.0
  post-traumatic 339.20
    acute 339.21
    chronic 339.22
  premenstrual 346.4
  preorgasmic 339.82
  primary
    cough 339.83
    exertional 339.84
    stabbing 339.85
    thunderclap 339.43
  psychogenic 307.81
  psychophysiologic 307.81
  rebound 339.3
  short lasting unilateral neuralgiform with
      conjunctival injection and tearing (SUNCT)
      339.05
  sick 346.9

Headache—*continued*
  spinal 349.0
    complicating labor and delivery 668.8
    postpartum 668.8
  spinal fluid loss 349.0
  syndrome
    cluster 339.00
    complicated NEC 339.44
    periodic in child or adolescent 346.2
    specified NEC 339.89
  tension 307.81
    type 339.10
      chronic 339.12
      episodic 339.11
  vascular 784.0
    migraine type 346.9
  vasomotor 346.9
Health
  advice V65.4
  audit V70.0
  checkup V70.0
  education V65.4
  hazard (*see also* History of) V15.9
    falling V15.88
    specified cause NEC V15.89
  instruction V65.4
  services provided because (of)
    boarding school residence V60.6
    holiday relief for person providing home care
        V60.5
    inadequate
      housing V60.1
      resources V60.2
    lack of housing V60.0
    no care available in home V60.4
    person living alone V60.3
    poverty V60.3
    residence in institution V60.6
    specified cause NEC V60.89
    vacation relief for person providing home care
        V60.5
Healthy
  donor (*see also* Donor) V59.9
  infant or child
    accompanying sick mother V65.0
    receiving care V20.1
  person
    accompanying sick relative V65.0
    admitted for sterilization V25.2
    receiving prophylactic inoculation or
        vaccination (*see also* Vaccination,
        prophylactic) V05.9
Hearing
  conservation and treatment V72.12
  examination V72.19
    following failed hearing screening V72.11
Heart —*see* condition
Heartburn 787.1
  psychogenic 306.4
Heat (effects) 992.9
  apoplexy 992.0
  burn—*see also* Burn, by site
    from sun (*see also* Sunburn) 692.71
  collapse 992.1
  cramps 992.2
  dermatitis or eczema 692.89
  edema 992.7
  erythema—*see* Burn, by site
  excessive 992.9
    specified effect NEC 992.8

Heat —*continued*
  exhaustion 992.5
    anhydrotic 992.3
    due to
      salt (and water) depletion 992.4
      water depletion 992.3
  fatigue (transient) 992.6
  fever 992.0
  hyperpyrexia 992.0
  prickly 705.1
  prostration—*see* Heat, exhaustion
  pyrexia 992.0
  rash 705.1
  specified effect NEC 992.8
  stroke 992.0
  sunburn (*see also* Sunburn) 692.71
  syncope 992.1
Heavy-chain disease 273.2
Heavy-for-dates (fetus or infant) 766.1
  4500 grams or more 766.0
  exceptionally 766.0
Hebephrenia, hebephrenic (acute) (*see also*
    Schizophrenia) 295.1
  dementia (praecox) (*see also* Schizophrenia)
    295.1
  schizophrenia (*see also* Schizophrenia) 295.1
Heberden's
  disease or nodes 715.04
  syndrome (angina pectoris) 413.9
Hebra's disease
  dermatitis exfoliativa 695.89
  erythema multiforme exudativum 695.19
  pityriasis 695.89
    maculata et circinata 696.3
    rubra 695.89
      pilaris 696.4
  prurigo 698.2
Hebra, nose 040.1
Hedinger's syndrome (malignant carcinoid)
    259.2
Heel —*see* condition
Heerfordt's disease or syndrome (uveoparotitis)
    135
Hegglin's anomaly or syndrome 288.2
Heidenhain's disease 290.10
  with dementia 290.10
Heilmeyer-Schöner disease (M9842/3) 207.1
Heine-Medin disease (*see also* Poliomyelitis)
    045.9
Heinz-body anemia, congenital 282.7
Heller's disease or syndrome (infantile
    psychosis) (*see also* Psychosis, childhood) 299.1
H.E.L.L.P. 642.5
Helminthiasis (*see also* Infestation, by specific
    parasite) 128.9
  Ancylostoma (*see also* Ancylostoma) 126.9
  intestinal 127.9
    mixed types (types classifiable to more than
      one of the titles 120.0-127.7) 127.8
    specified type 127.7
  mixed types (intestinal) (types classifiable to
    more than one of the titles 120.0-127.7) 127.8
  Necator americanus 126.1
  specified type NEC 128.8
  Trichinella 124
Heloma 700
Hemangioblastoma (M9161/1)—*see also*
    Neoplasm, connective tissue, uncertain
    behavior
  malignant (M9161//3)—*see* Neoplasm,
    connective tissue, malignant

Hemangioblastomatosis, cerebelloretinal 759.6
Hemangioendothelioma (M9130/1)—*see also*
    Neoplasm, by site, uncertain behavior
  benign (M9130/0) 228.00
  bone (diffuse) (M9130/3)—*see* Neoplasm, bone,
    malignant
  malignant (M9130/3)—*see* Neoplasm,
    connective tissue, malignant
  nervous system (M9130/0) 228.09
Hemangioendotheliosarcoma (M9130/3)—*see*
    Neoplasm, connective tissue, malignant
Hemangiofibroma (M9160/0)—*see* Neoplasm,
    by site, benign
Hemangiolipoma (M8861/0)—*see* Lipoma
Hemangioma (M9120/0) 228.00
  arteriovenous (M9123/0)—*see* Hemangioma, by
    site
  brain 228.02
  capillary (M9131/0)—*see* Hemangioma, by site
  cavernous (M9121/0)—*see* Hemangioma, by
    site
  central nervous system NEC 228.09
  choroid 228.09
  heart 228.09
  infantile (M9131/0)—*see* Hemangioma, by site
  intra-abdominal structures 228.04
  intracranial structures 228.02
  intramuscular (M9132/0)—*see* Hemangioma, by site
  iris 228.09
  juvenile (M9131/0)—*see* Hemangioma, by site
  malignant (M9120/3)—*see* Neoplasm,
    connective tissue, malignant
  meninges 228.09
    brain 228.02
    spinal cord 228.09
  peritoneum 228.04
  placenta—*see* Placenta, abnormal
  plexiform (M9131/0)—*see* Hemangioma, by
    site
  racemose (M9123/0)—*see* Hemangioma, by site
  retina 228.03
  retroperitoneal tissue 228.04
  sclerosing (M8832/0)—*see* Neoplasm, skin,
    benign
  simplex (M9131/0)—*see* Hemangioma, by site
  skin and subcutaneous tissue 228.01
  specified site NEC 228.09
  spinal cord 228.09
  venous (M9122/0)—*see* Hemangioma, by site
  verrucous keratotic (M9142/0)—*see*
    Hemangioma, by site
Hemangiomatosis (systemic) 757.32
  involving single site—*see* Hemangioma
Hemangiopericytoma (M9150/1)—*see also*
    Neoplasm, connective tissue, uncertain
    behavior
  benign (M9150/0)—*see* Neoplasm, connective
    tissue, benign
  malignant (M9150/3)—*see* Neoplasm,
    connective tissue, malignant
Hemangiosarcoma (M9120/3)—*see* Neoplasm,
    connective tissue, malignant
Hemarthrosis (nontraumatic) 719.0
  ankle 719.17
  elbow 719.12
  foot 719.17
  hand 719.14
  hip 719.15
  knee 719.16
  multiple sites 719.19
  pelvic region 719.15
  shoulder (region) 719.11

Hemarthrosis—*continued*
  specified site NEC 719.18
  traumatic—*see* Sprain, by site
  wrist 719.13
Hematemesis 578.0
  with ulcer—*see* Ulcer, by site, with hemorrhage
  due to S. japonicum 120.2
  Goldstein's (familial hemorrhagic
    telangiectasia) 448.0
  newborn 772.4
    due to swallowed maternal blood 777.3
Hematidrosis 705.89
Hematinuria (*see also* Hemoglobinuria) 791.2
  malarial 084.8
  paroxysmal 283.2
Hematite miners' lung 503
Hematobilia 576.8
Hematocele (congenital) (diffuse) (idiopathic)
  608.83
  broad ligament 620.7
  canal of Nuck 629.0
  cord, male 608.83
  fallopian tube 620.8
  female NEC 629.0
  ischiorectal 569.89
  male NEC 608.83
  ovary 629.0
  pelvis, pelvic
    female 629.0
      with ectopic pregnancy (*see also* Pregnancy,
        ectopic) 633.90
        with intrauterine pregnancy 633.91
    male 608.83
  periuterine 629.0
  retrouterine 629.0
  scrotum 608.83
  spermatic cord (diffuse) 608.83
  testis 608.84
  traumatic—*see* Injury, internal, pelvis
  tunica vaginalis 608.83
  uterine ligament 629.0
  uterus 621.4
  vagina 623.6
  vulva 624.5
Hematocephalus 742.4
Hematochezia (*see also* Melena) 578.1
Hematochyluria (*see also* Infestation, filarial)
  125.9
Hematocolpos 626.8
Hematocornea 371.12
Hematogenous —*see* condition
Hematoma (skin surface intact) (traumatic)—*see*
  also Contusion

*Note—Hematomas are coded according to
origin and the nature and site of the hematoma
or the accompanying injury. Hematomas of
unspecified origin are coded as injuries of the
sites involved, except:*
(a) *hematomas of genital organs which are
coded as diseases of the organ involved
unless they complicate pregnancy or
delivery*
(b) *hematomas of the eye which are coded as
diseases of the eye.*

*For late effect of hematoma classifiable to
920-924 see Late, effect, contusion*

Hematoma—*continued*
  with
    crush injury—*see* Crush
    fracture—*see* Fracture, by site
    injury of internal organs—*see also* Injury,
      internal, by site
      kidney—*see* Hematoma, kidney, traumatic
      liver—*see* Hematoma, liver, traumatic
      spleen—*see* Hematoma, spleen
    nerve injury—*see* Injury, nerve
    open wound—*see* Wound, open, by site
    skin surface intact—*see* Contusion
  abdomen (wall)—*see* Contusion, abdomen
  amnion 658.8
  aorta, dissecting 441.00
    abdominal 441.02
    thoracic 441.01
    thoracoabdominal 441.03
  aortic intramural—*see* Dissection, aorta
  arterial (complicating trauma) 904.9
    specified site—*see* Injury, blood vessel, by site
  auricle (ear) 380.31
  birth injury 767.8
    skull 767.19
  brain (traumatic) 853.0

*Note—Use the following fifth-digit
subclassification with categories 851-854:*

0 *unspecified state of consciousness*
1 *with no loss of consciousness*
2 *with brief [less than one hour] loss of
   consciousness*
3 *with moderate [1-24 hours] loss of
   consciousness*
4 *with prolonged [more than 24 hours] loss of
   consciousness and return to pre-existing
   conscious level*
5 *with prolonged [more than 24 hours] loss of
   consciousness, without return to pre-existing
   conscious level*
*Use fifth-digit 5 to designate when a patient is
unconscious and dies before regaining
consciousness, regardless of the duration of the
loss of consciousness*
6 *with loss of consciousness of unspecified
   duration*
9 *with concussion, unspecified*

  with
    cerebral
      contusion—*see* Contusion, brain
      laceration—*see* Laceration, brain
    open intracranial wound 853.1
    skull fracture—*see* Fracture, skull, by site
  extradural or epidural 852.4
    with open intracranial wound 852.5
    fetus or newborn 767.0
    nontraumatic 432.0
  fetus or newborn NEC 767.0
  nontraumatic (*see also* Hemorrhage, brain) 431
    epidural or extradural 432.0
    newborn NEC 772.8
    subarachnoid, arachnoid, or meningeal (*see
      also* Hemorrhage, subarachnoid) 430
    subdural (*see also* Hemorrhage, subdural)
      432.1
  subarachnoid, arachnoid, or meningeal 852.0
    with open intracranial wound 852.1
    fetus or newborn 772.2
    nontraumatic (*see also* Hemorrhage,
      subarachnoid) 430

Hematoma—*continued*
 brain—*continued*
  subdural 852.2
   with open intracranial wound 852.3
   fetus or newborn (localized) 767.0
   nontraumatic (*see also* Hemorrhage,
    subdural) 432.1
 breast (nontraumatic) 611.89
 broad ligament (nontraumatic) 620.7
  complicating delivery 665.7
  traumatic—*see* Injury, internal, broad
   ligament
 calcified NEC 959.9
 capitis 920
  due to birth injury 767.19
  newborn 767.19
 cerebral—*see* Hematoma, brain
 cesarean section wound 674.3
 chorion—*see* Placenta, abnormal
 complicating delivery (perineum) (vulva) 664.5
  pelvic 665.7
  vagina 665.7
 corpus
  cavernosum (nontraumatic) 607.82
  luteum (nontraumatic) (ruptured) 620.1
 dura (mater)—*see* Hematoma, brain, subdural
 epididymis (nontraumatic) 608.83
 epidural (traumatic)—*see also* Hematoma,
  brain, extradural
  spinal—*see* Injury, spinal, by site
 episiotomy 674.3
 external ear 380.31
 extradural—*see also* Hematoma, brain,
  extradural
  fetus or newborn 767.0
  nontraumatic 432.0
   fetus or newborn 767.0
 fallopian tube 620.8
 genital organ (nontraumatic)
  female NEC 629.89
  male NEC 608.83
  traumatic (external site) 922.4
   internal—*see* Injury, internal, genital organ
 graafian follicle (ruptured) 620.0
 internal organs (abdomen, chest, or pelvis)—*see*
  also Injury, internal, by site
  kidney—*see* Hematoma, kidney, traumatic
  liver—*see* Hematoma, liver, traumatic
  spleen—*see* Hematoma, spleen
 intracranial—*see* Hematoma, brain
 kidney, cystic 593.81
  traumatic 866.01
   with open wound into cavity 866.11
 labia (nontraumatic) 624.5
 lingual (and other parts of neck, scalp, or face,
  except eye) 920
 liver (subcapsular) 573.8
  birth injury 767.8
  fetus or newborn 767.8
  traumatic NEC 864.01
   with
    laceration—*see* Laceration, liver
    open wound into cavity 864.11
 mediastinum—*see* Injury, internal, mediastinum
 meninges, meningeal (brain)—*see also*
  Hematoma, brain, subarachnoid
  spinal—*see* Injury, spinal, by site
 mesosalpinx (nontraumatic) 620.8
  traumatic—*see* Injury, internal, pelvis
 muscle (traumatic)—*see* Contusion, by site
  nontraumatic 729.92

Hematoma—*continued*
 nasal (septum) (and other part(s) of neck, scalp,
  or face, except eye) 920
 obstetrical surgical wound 674.3
 orbit, orbital (nontraumatic) 376.32
  traumatic 921.2
 ovary (corpus luteum) (nontraumatic) 620.1
  traumatic—*see* Injury, internal, ovary
 pelvis (female) (nontraumatic) 629.89
  complicating delivery 665.7
  male 608.83
  traumatic—*see also* Injury, internal, pelvis
   specified organ NEC (*see also* Injury,
    internal, pelvis) 867.6
 penis (nontraumatic) 607.82
 pericranial (and neck, or face any part, except
  eye) 920
  due to injury at birth 767.19
 perineal wound (obstetrical) 674.3
  complicating delivery 664.5
 perirenal, cystic 593.81
 pinna 380.31
 placenta—*see* Placenta, abnormal
 postoperative 998.12
 retroperitoneal (nontraumatic) 568.81
  traumatic—*see* Injury, internal,
   retroperitoneum
 retropubic, male 568.81
 scalp (and neck, or face any part, except eye)
  920
  fetus or newborn 767.19
 scrotum (nontraumatic) 608.83
  traumatic 922.4
 seminal vesicle (nontraumatic) 608.83
  traumatic—*see* Injury, internal, seminal
   vesicle
 soft tissue 729.92
 spermatic cord—*see also* Injury, internal,
  spermatic cord
  nontraumatic 608.83
 spinal (cord) (meninges)—*see also* Injury,
  spinal, by site
  fetus or newborn 767.4
  nontraumatic 336.1
 spleen 865.01
  with
   laceration—*see* Laceration, spleen
   open wound into cavity 865.11
 sternocleidomastoid, birth injury 767.8
 sternomastoid, birth injury 767.8
 subarachnoid—*see also* Hematoma, brain,
  subarachnoid
  fetus or newborn 772.2
  nontraumatic (*see also* Hemorrhage,
   subarachnoid) 430
  newborn 772.2
 subdural—*see also* Hematoma, brain, subdural
  fetus or newborn (localized) 767.0
  nontraumatic (*see also* Hemorrhage, subdural)
   432.1
 subperiosteal (syndrome) 267
  traumatic—*see* Hematoma, by site
 superficial, fetus or newborn 772.6
 syncytium—*see* Placenta, abnormal
 testis (nontraumatic) 608.83
  birth injury 767.8
  traumatic 922.4
 tunica vaginalis (nontraumatic) 608.83
 umbilical cord 663.6
  affecting fetus or newborn 762.6
 uterine ligament (nontraumatic) 620.7
  traumatic—*see* Injury, internal, pelvis

Hematoma—*continued*
uterus 621.4
traumatic—*see* Injury, internal, pelvis
vagina (nontraumatic) (ruptured) 623.6
complicating delivery 665.7
traumatic 922.4
vas deferens (nontraumatic) 608.83
traumatic—*see* Injury, internal, vas deferens
vitreous 379.23
vocal cord 920
vulva (nontraumatic) 624.5
complicating delivery 664.5
fetus or newborn 767.8
traumatic 922.4
Hematometra 621.4
Hematomyelia 336.1
with fracture of vertebra (*see also* Fracture,
vertebra, by site, with spinal cord injury)
806.8
fetus or newborn 767.4
Hematomyelitis 323.9
late effect—*see* category 326
Hematoperitoneum (*see also* Hemoperitoneum)
568.81
Hematopneumothorax (*see also* Hemothorax)
511.89
Hematopoiesis, cyclic 288.02
Hematoporphyria (acquired) (congenital) 277.1
Hematoporphyrinuria (acquired) (congenital)
277.1
Hematorachis, hematorrhachis 336.1
fetus or newborn 767.4
Hematosalpinx 620.8
with
ectopic pregnancy (*see also* categories
633.0-633.9) 639.2
molar pregnancy (*see also* categories 630-632)
639.2
infectional (*see also* Salpingo-oophoritis) 614.2
Hematospermia 608.82
Hematothorax (*see also* Hemothorax) 511.89
Hematotympanum 381.03
Hematuria (benign) (essential) (idiopathic)
599.70
due to S. hematobium 120.0
endemic 120.0
gross 599.71
intermittent 599.70
malarial 084.8
microscopic 599.72
paroxysmal 599.70
sulfonamide
correct substance properly administered
599.70
overdose or wrong substance given or taken
961.0
tropical (bilharziasis) 120.0
tuberculous (*see also* Tuberculosis) 016.9
Hematuric bilious fever 084.8
Hemeralopia 368.10
acquired 286.5
Hemiabiotrophy 799.89
Hemi-akinesia 781.8
Hemianalgesia (*see also* Disturbance, sensation)
782.0
Hemianencephaly 740.0
Hemianesthesia (*see also* Disturbance, sensation)
782.0

Hemianopia, hemianopsia (altitudinal)
(homonymous) 368.46
binasal 368.47
bitemporal 368.47
heteronymous 368.47
syphilitic 095.8
Hemiasomatognosia 307.9
Hemiathetosis 781.0
Hemiatrophy 799.89
cerebellar 334.8
face 349.89
progressive 349.89
fascia 728.9
leg 728.2
tongue 529.8
Hemiballism (us) 333.5
Hemiblock (cardiac) (heart) (left) 426.2
Hemicardia 746.89
Hemicephalus, hemicephaly 740.0
Hemichorea 333.5
Hemicrania 346.9
congenital malformation 740.0
continua 339.41
paroxysmal 339.03
chronic 339.04
episodic 339.03
Hemidystrophy —*see* Hemiatrophy
Hemiectromelia 755.4
Hemihypalgesia (*see also* Disturbance,
sensation) 782.0
Hemihypertrophy (congenital) 759.89
cranial 756.0
Hemihypesthesia (*see also* Disturbance,
sensation) 782.0
Hemi-inattention 781.8
Hemimelia 755.4
lower limb 755.30
paraxial (complete) (incomplete) (intercalary)
(terminal) 755.32
fibula 755.37
tibia 755.36
transverse (complete) (partial) 755.31
upper limb 755.20
paraxial (complete) (incomplete) (intercalary)
(terminal) 755.22
radial 755.26
ulnar 755.27
transverse (complete) (partial) 755.21
Hemiparalysis (*see also* Hemiplegia) 342.9
Hemiparesis (*see also* Hemiplegia) 342.9
Hemiparesthesia (*see also* Disturbance,
sensation) 782.0
Hemiplegia 342.9
acute (*see also* Disease, cerebrovascular, acute)
436
alternans facialis 344.89
apoplectic (*see also* Disease, cerebrovascular,
acute) 436
late effect or residual
affecting
dominant side 438.21
nondominant side 438.22
unspecified side 438.20
arteriosclerotic 437.0
late effect or residual
affecting
dominant side 438.21
nondominant side 438.22
unspecified side 438.20
ascending (spinal) NEC 344.89

Hemiplegia—*continued*
attack (*see also* Disease, cerebrovascular, acute)
436
brain, cerebral (current episode) 437.8
congenital 343.1
cerebral—*see* Hemiplegia, brain
congenital (cerebral) (spastic) (spinal) 343.1
conversion neurosis (hysterical) 300.11
cortical—*see* Hemiplegia, brain
due to
arteriosclerosis 437.0
late effect or residual
affecting
dominant side 438.21
nondominant side 438.22
unspecified side 438.20
cerebrovascular lesion (*see also* Disease,
cerebrovascular, acute) 436
late effect
affecting
dominant side 438.21
nondominant side 438.22
unspecified side 438.20
embolic (current) (*see also* Embolism, brain)
434.1
late effect
affecting
dominant side 438.21
nondominant side 438.22
unspecified side 438.20
flaccid 342.0
hypertensive (current episode) 437.8
infantile (postnatal) 343.4
late effect
birth injury, intracranial or spinal 343.4
cerebrovascular lesion—*see* Late effect(s) (of)
cerebrovascular disease
viral encephalitis 139.0
middle alternating NEC 344.89
newborn NEC 767.0
seizure (current episode) (*see also* Disease,
cerebrovascular, acute) 436
spastic 342.1
congenital or infantile 343.1
specified NEC 342.8
thrombotic (current) (*see also* Thrombosis,
brain) 434.0
late effect—*see* late effect(s) (of)
cerebrovascular disease
Hemisection, spinal cord —*see* Fracture,
vertebra, by site, with spinal cord injury
Hemispasm 781.0
facial 781.0
Hemispatial neglect 781.8
Hemisporosis 117.9
Hemitremor 781.0
Hemivertebra 756.14
Hemobilia 576.8
Hemocholecyst 575.8
Hemochromatosis (acquired) (liver)
(myocardium) (secondary) 275.03
diabetic 275.03
due to repeated red blood cell transfusions
275.02
hereditary 275.01
primary idiopathic 275.01
specified NEC 275.03
transfusion associated (red blood cell) 275.02
with refractory anemia 238.72
Hemodialysis V56.0

Hemoglobin —*see also* condition
abnormal (disease)—*see* Disease, hemoglobin
AS genotype 282.5
fetal, hereditary persistence 282.7
H Constant Spring 282.43
H disease 282.43
high-oxygen-affinity 289.0
low NEC 285.9
S (Hb-S), heterozygous 282.5
Hemoglobinemia 283.2
due to blood transfusion NEC 999.89
bone marrow 996.85
paroxysmal 283.2
Hemoglobinopathy (mixed) (*see also* Disease,
hemoglobin) 282.7
with thalassemia 282.49
sickle-cell 282.60
with thalassemia (without crisis) 282.41
with
crisis 282.42
vaso-occlusive pain 282.42
Hemoglobinuria, hemoglobinuric 791.2
with anemia, hemolytic, acquired (chronic) NEC
283.2
cold (agglutinin) (paroxysmal) (with Raynaud's
syndrome) 283.2
due to
exertion 283.2
hemolysis (from external causes) NEC 283.2
exercise 283.2
fever (malaria) 084.8
infantile 791.2
intermittent 283.2
malarial 084.8
march 283.2
nocturnal (paroxysmal) 283.2
paroxysmal (cold) (nocturnal) 283.2
Hemolymphangioma (M9175/0) 228.1
Hemolysis
fetal—*see* Jaundice, fetus or newborn
intravascular (disseminated) NEC 286.6
with
abortion—*see* Abortion, by type, with
hemorrhage, delayed or excessive
ectopic pregnancy (*see also* categories
633.0-633.9) 639.1
hemorrhage of pregnancy 641.3
affecting fetus or newborn 762.1
molar pregnancy (*see also* categories
630-632) 639.1
acute 283.2
following
abortion 639.1
ectopic or molar pregnancy 639.1
neonatal—*see* Jaundice, fetus or newborn
transfusion NEC 999.89
bone marrow 996.85
Hemolytic —*see also* condition
anemia—*see* Anemia, hemolytic
uremic syndrome 283.11
Hemometra 621.4
Hemopericardium (with effusion) 423.0
newborn 772.8
traumatic (*see also* Hemothorax, traumatic) 860.2
with open wound into thorax 860.3
Hemoperitoneum 568.81
infectional (*see also* Peritonitis) 567.29
traumatic—*see* Injury, internal, peritoneum
Hemophagocytic syndrome 288.4
infection-associated 288.4

Hemophilia (familial) (hereditary) 286.0
A 286.0
  carrier (asymptomatic) V83.01
    symptomatic V83.02
acquired 286.52
autoimmune 286.52
B (Leyden) 286.1
C 286.2
calcipriva (*see also* Fibrinolysis) 286.7
classical 286.0
nonfamilial 286.7
secondary 286.52
vascular 286.4
Hemophilus influenzae NEC 041.5
arachnoiditis (basic) (brain) (spinal) 320.0
  late effect—*see* category 326
bronchopneumonia 482.2
cerebral ventriculitis 320.0
  late effect—*see* category 326
cerebrospinal inflammation 320.0
  late effect—*see* category 326
infection NEC 041.5
leptomeningitis 320.0
  late effect—*see* category 326
meningitis (cerebral) (cerebrospinal) (spinal)
  320.0
  late effect—*see* category 326
meningomyelitis 320.0
  late effect—*see* category 326
pachymeningitis (adhesive) (fibrous)
  (hemorrhagic) (hypertrophic) (spinal) 320.0
  late effect—*see* category 326
pneumonia (broncho-) 482.2
Hemophthalmos 360.43
Hemopneumothorax (*see also* Hemothorax)
  511.89
traumatic 860.4
  with open wound into thorax 860.5
Hemoptysis 786.30
due to Paragonimus (westermani) 121.2
newborn 770.3
specified NEC 786.39
tuberculous (*see also* Tuberculosis, pulmonary)
  011.9
Hemorrhage, hemorrhagic (nontraumatic) 459.0
abdomen 459.0
accidental (antepartum) 641.2
  affecting fetus or newborn 762.1
adenoid 474.8
adrenal (capsule) (gland) (medulla) 255.41
  newborn 772.5
after labor—*see* Hemorrhage, postpartum
alveolar
  lung, newborn 770.3
  process 525.8
alveolus 525.8
amputation stump (surgical) 998.11
  secondary, delayed 997.69
anemia (chronic) 280.0
  acute 285.1
antepartum—*see* Hemorrhage, pregnancy
anus (sphincter) 569.3
apoplexy (stroke) 432.9
arachnoid—*see* Hemorrhage, subarachnoid
artery NEC 459.0
  brain (*see also* Hemorrhage, brain) 431
  middle meningeal—*see* Hemorrhage,
    subarachnoid
basilar (ganglion) (*see also* Hemorrhage, brain)
  431
bladder 596.89
blood dyscrasia 289.9

Hemorrhage, hemorrhagic—*continued*
bowel 578.9
  newborn 772.4
brain (miliary) (nontraumatic) 431
  with
    birth injury 767.0
  arachnoid—*see* Hemorrhage, subarachnoid
  due to
    birth injury 767.0
    rupture of aneurysm (congenital) (*see also*
      Hemorrhage, subarachnoid) 430
    mycotic 431
    syphilis 094.89
  epidural or extradural—*see* Hemorrhage,
    extradural
  fetus or newborn (anoxic) (hypoxic) (due to
    birth trauma) (nontraumatic) 767.0
  intraventricular 772.10
    grade I 772.11
    grade II 772.12
    grade III 772.13
    grade IV 772.14
  iatrogenic 997.02
  postoperative 997.02
  puerperal, postpartum, childbirth 674.0
  stem 431
  subarachnoid, arachnoid or meningeal—*see*
    Hemorrhage, subarachnoid
  subdural—*see* Hemorrhage, subdural
  traumatic NEC 853.0

---

*Note—Use the following fifth-digit
subclassification with categories 851-854:*

0 unspecified state of consciousness
1 with no loss of consciousness
*2 with brief [less than one hour] loss of
consciousness*
*3 with moderate [1-24 hours] loss of
consciousness*
*4 with prolonged [more than 24 hours] loss of
consciousness and return to pre-existing
conscious level*
*5 with prolonged [more than 24 hours] loss of
consciousness, without return to pre-existing
conscious level
Use fifth-digit 5 to designate when a patient is
unconscious and dies before regaining
consciousness, regardless of the duration of the
loss of consciousness*
*6 with loss of consciousness of unspecified
duration*
9 with concussion, unspecified

---

  with
    cerebral
      contusion—*see* Contusion, brain
      laceration—*see* Laceration, brain
      open intracranial wound 853.1
      skull fracture—*see* Fracture, skull, by site
    extradural or epidural 852.4
      with open intracranial wound 852.5
    subarachnoid 852.0
      with open intracranial wound 852.1
    subdural 852.2
      with open intracranial wound 852.3
breast 611.79
bronchial tube—*see* Hemorrhage, lung
bronchopulmonary—*see* Hemorrhage, lung
bronchus (cause unknown) (*see also*
  Hemorrhage, lung) 786.30
bulbar (*see also* Hemorrhage, brain) 431

Hemorrhage, hemorrhagic—*continued*
  bursa 727.89
  capillary 448.9
    primary 287.8
  capsular—*see* Hemorrhage, brain
  cardiovascular 429.89
  cecum 578.9
  cephalic (*see also* Hemorrhage, brain) 431
  cerebellar (*see also* Hemorrhage, brain) 431
  cerebellum (*see also* Hemorrhage, brain) 431
  cerebral (*see also* Hemorrhage, brain) 431
    fetus or newborn (anoxic) (traumatic) 767.0
  cerebromeningeal (*see also* Hemorrhage, brain)
    431
  cerebrospinal (*see also* Hemorrhage, brain) 431
  cerebrovascular accident—*see* Hemorrhage,
    brain
  cerebrum (*see also* Hemorrhage, brain) 431
  cervix (stump) (uteri) 622.8
  cesarean section wound 674.3
  chamber, anterior (eye) 364.41
  childbirth—*see* Hemorrhage, complicating,
    delivery
  choroid 363.61
    expulsive 363.62
  ciliary body 364.41
  cochlea 386.8
  colon—*see* Hemorrhage, intestine
  complicating
    delivery 641.9
      affecting fetus or newborn 762.1
      associated with
        afibrinogenemia 641.3
          affecting fetus or newborn 763.89
        coagulation defect 641.3
          affecting fetus or newborn 763.89
        hyperfibrinolysis 641.3
          affecting fetus or newborn 763.89
        hypofibrinogenemia 641.3
          affecting fetus or newborn 763.89
      due to
        low-lying placenta 641.1
          affecting fetus or newborn 762.0
        placenta previa 641.1
          affecting fetus or newborn 762.0
        premature separation of placenta 641.2
          affecting fetus or newborn 762.1
        retained
          placenta 666.0
          secundines 666.2
        trauma 641.8
          affecting fetus or newborn 763.89
        uterine leiomyoma 641.8
          affecting fetus or newborn 763.89
    surgical procedure 998.11
  complication(s)
    of dental implant placement 525.71
  concealed NEC 459.0
  congenital 772.9
  conjunctiva 372.72
    newborn 772.8
  cord, newborn 772.0
    slipped ligature 772.3
    stump 772.3
  corpus luteum (ruptured) 620.1
  cortical (*see also* Hemorrhage, brain) 431
  cranial 432.9
  cutaneous 782.7
    newborn 772.6

Hemorrhage, hemorrhagic—*continued*
  cyst, pancreas 577.2
  cystitis—*see* Cystitis
  delayed
    with
      abortion—*see* Abortion, by type, with
        hemorrhage, delayed or excessive
      ectopic pregnancy (*see also* categories
        633.0-633.9) 639.1
      molar pregnancy (*see also* categories
        630-632) 639.1
    following
      abortion 639.1
      ectopic or molar pregnancy 639.1
    postpartum 666.2
  diathesis (familial) 287.9
    newborn 776.0
  disease 287.9
    newborn 776.0
    specified type NEC 287.8
  disorder 287.9
    due to intrinsic circulating anticoagulants,
      antibodies, or inhibitors 286.59
      with
        acquired hemophilia 286.52
        antiphospholipid antibody 286.53
    specified type NEC 287.8
  due to
    any device, implant, or graft (presence of)
      classifiable to 996.0-996.5—*see*
      Complications, due to (presence of) any
      device, implant, or graft classified to
      996.0—996.5 NEC
    intrinsic circulating anticoagulant, antibodies,
      or inhibitors 286.59
      with
        acquired hemophilia 286.52
        antiphospholipid antibody 286.53
  duodenum, duodenal 537.89
    ulcer—*see* Ulcer, duodenum, with hemorrhage
  dura mater—*see* Hemorrhage, subdural
  endotracheal—*see* Hemorrhage, lung
  epicranial subaponeurotic (massive) 767.11
  epidural—*see* Hemorrhage, extradural
  episiotomy 674.3
  esophagus 530.82
    varix (*see also* Varix, esophagus, bleeding) 456.0
  excessive
    with
      abortion—*see* Abortion, by type, with
        hemorrhage, delayed or excessive
      ectopic pregnancy (*see also* categories
        633.0-633.9) 639.1
      molar pregnancy (*see also* categories
        630-632) 639.1
    following
      abortion 639.1
      ectopic or molar pregnancy 639.1
  external 459.0
  extradural (traumatic)—*see also* Hemorrhage,
    brain, traumatic, extradural
    birth injury 767.0
    fetus or newborn (anoxic) (traumatic) 767.0
    nontraumatic 432.0
  eye 360.43
    chamber (anterior) (aqueous) 364.41
    fundus 362.81
  eyelid 374.81
  fallopian tube 620.8

Hemorrhage, hemorrhagic—*continued*
fetomaternal 772.0
  affecting management of pregnancy or
    puerperium 656.0
fetus, fetal, affecting newborn 772.0
  from
    cut end of co-twin's cord 772.0
    placenta 772.0
    ruptured cord 772.0
    vasa previa 772.0
  into
    co-twin 772.0
    mother's circulation 772.0
      affecting management of pregnancy or
        puerperium 656.0
fever (*see also* Fever, hemorrhagic) 065.9
  with renal syndrome 078.6
  arthropod-borne NEC 065.9
  Bangkok 065.4
  Crimean 065.0
  dengue virus 065.4
  epidemic 078.6
  Junin virus 078.7
  Korean 078.6
  Machupo virus 078.7
  mite-borne 065.8
  mosquito-borne 065.4
  Philippine 065.4
  Russian (Yaroslav) 078.6
  Singapore 065.4
  southeast Asia 065.4
  Thailand 065.4
  tick-borne NEC 065.3
fibrinogenolysis (*see also* Fibrinolysis) 286.6
fibrinolytic (acquired) (*see also* Fibrinolysis)
  286.6
fontanel 767.19
from tracheostomy stoma 519.09
fundus, eye 362.81
funis
  affecting fetus or newborn 772.0
  complicating delivery 663.8
gastric (*see also* Hemorrhage, stomach) 578.9
gastroenteric 578.9
  newborn 772.4
gastrointestinal (tract) 578.9
  newborn 772.4
genitourinary (tract) NEC 599.89
gingiva 523.8
globe 360.43
gravidarum—*see* Hemorrhage, pregnancy
gum 523.8
heart 429.89
hypopharyngeal (throat) 784.8
intermenstrual 626.6
  irregular 626.6
  regular 626.5
internal (organs) 459.0
  capsule (*see also* Hemorrhage, brain) 431
  ear 386.8
  newborn 772.8
intestine 578.9
  congenital 772.4
  newborn 772.4
  into
    bladder wall 596.7
    bursa 727.89
    corpus luysii (*see also* Hemorrhage, brain) 431
intra-abdominal 459.0
  during or following surgery 998.11
intra-alveolar, newborn (lung) 770.3
intracerebral (*see also* Hemorrhage, brain) 431

Hemorrhage, hemorrhagic—*continued*
intracranial NEC 432.9
  puerperal, postpartum, childbirth 674.0
  traumatic—*see* Hemorrhage, brain, traumatic
intramedullary NEC 336.1
intraocular 360.43
intraoperative 998.11
intrapartum—*see* Hemorrhage, complicating,
  delivery
intrapelvic
  female 629.89
  male 459.0
intraperitoneal 459.0
intrapontine (*see also* Hemorrhage, brain) 431
intrauterine 621.4
  complicating delivery—*see* Hemorrhage,
    complicating, delivery
  in pregnancy or childbirth—*see* Hemorrhage,
    pregnancy
  postpartum (*see also* Hemorrhage,
    postpartum) 666.1
intraventricular (*see also* Hemorrhage, brain) 431
  fetus or newborn (anoxic) (traumatic) 772.10
    grade I 772.11
    grade II 772.12
    grade III 772.13
    grade IV 772.14
intravesical 596.7
iris (postinfectional) (postinflammatory) (toxic)
  364.41
joint (nontraumatic) 719.10
  ankle 719.17
  elbow 719.12
  foot 719.17
  forearm 719.13
  hand 719.14
  hip 719.15
  knee 719.16
  lower leg 719.16
  multiple sites 719.19
  pelvic region 719.15
  shoulder (region) 719.11
  specified site NEC 719.18
  thigh 719.15
  upper arm 719.12
  wrist 719.13
kidney 593.81
knee (joint) 719.16
labyrinth 386.8
leg NEC 459.0
lenticular striate artery (*see also* Hemorrhage,
  brain) 431
ligature, vessel 998.11
liver 573.8
lower extremity NEC 459.0
lung 786.30
  newborn 770.3
  tuberculous (*see also* Tuberculosis,
    pulmonary) 011.9
malaria 084.8
marginal sinus 641.2
massive subaponeurotic, birth injury 767.11
maternal, affecting fetus or newborn 762.1
mediastinum 786.30
medulla (*see also* Hemorrhage, brain) 431
membrane (brain) (*see also* Hemorrhage,
  subarachnoid) 430
  spinal cord—*see* Hemorrhage, spinal cord
meninges, meningeal (brain) (middle) (*see also*
  Hemorrhage, subarachnoid) 430
  spinal cord—*see* Hemorrhage, spinal cord
mesentery 568.81

Hemorrhage, hemorrhagic—*continued*
  metritis 626.8
  midbrain (*see also* Hemorrhage, brain) 431
  mole 631.8
  mouth 528.9
  mucous membrane NEC 459.0
    newborn 772.8
  muscle 728.89
  nail (subungual) 703.8
  nasal turbinate 784.7
    newborn 772.8
  nasopharynx 478.29
  navel, newborn 772.3
  newborn 772.9
    adrenal 772.5
    alveolar (lung) 770.3
    brain (anoxic) (hypoxic) (due to birth trauma) 767.0
    cerebral (anoxic) (hypoxic) (due to birth
        trauma) 767.0
    conjunctiva 772.8
    cutaneous 772.6
    diathesis 776.0
    due to vitamin K deficiency 776.0
    epicranial subaponeurotic (massive) 767.11
    gastrointestinal 772.4
    internal (organs) 772.8
    intestines 772.4
    intra-alveolar (lung) 770.3
    intracranial (from any perinatal cause) 767.0
    intraventricular (from any perinatal cause) 772.10
      grade I 772.11
      grade II 772.12
      grade III 772.13
      grade IV 772.14
    lung 770.3
    pulmonary (massive) 770.3
    spinal cord, traumatic 767.4
    stomach 772.4
    subaponeurotic (massive) 767.11
    subarachnoid (from any perinatal cause) 772.2
    subconjunctival 772.8
    subgaleal 767.11
    umbilicus 772.0
      slipped ligature 772.3
      vasa previa 772.0
  nipple 611.79
  nose 784.7
    newborn 772.8
  obstetrical surgical wound 674.3
  omentum 568.89
    newborn 772.4
  optic nerve (sheath) 377.42
  orbit 376.32
  ovary 620.1
  oviduct 620.8
  pancreas 577.8
  parathyroid (gland) (spontaneous) 252.8
  parturition—*see* Hemorrhage, complicating,
      delivery
  penis 607.82
  pericardium, pericarditis 423.0
  perineal wound (obstetrical) 674.3
  peritoneum, peritoneal 459.0
  peritonsillar tissue 474.8
    after operation on tonsils 998.11
    due to infection 475
  petechial 782.7
  pituitary (gland) 253.8
  placenta NEC 641.9
    affecting fetus or newborn 762.1
    from surgical or instrumental damage 641.8
      affecting fetus or newborn 762.1

Hemorrhage, hemorrhagic—*continued*
  placenta previa 641.1
    affecting fetus or newborn 762.0
  pleura—*see* Hemorrhage, lung
  polioencephalitis, superior 265.1
  polymyositis—*see* Polymyositis
  pons (*see also* Hemorrhage, brain) 431
  pontine (*see also* Hemorrhage, brain) 431
  popliteal 459.0
  postcoital 626.7
  postextraction (dental) 998.11
  postmenopausal 627.1
  postnasal 784.7
  postoperative 998.11
  postpartum (atonic) (following delivery of
      placenta) 666.1
    delayed or secondary (after 24 hours) 666.2
    retained placenta 666.0
    third stage 666.0
  pregnancy (concealed) 641.9
    accidental 641.2
      affecting fetus or newborn 762.1
    affecting fetus or newborn 762.1
    before 22 completed weeks gestation 640.9
      affecting fetus or newborn 762.1
    due to
      abruptio placenta 641.2
        affecting fetus or newborn 762.1
      afibrinogenemia or other coagulation defect
          (conditions classifiable to 286.0-286.9)
          641.3
        affecting fetus or newborn 762.1
      coagulation defect 641.3
        affecting fetus or newborn 762.1
      hyperfibrinolysis 641.3
        affecting fetus or newborn 762.1
      hypofibrinogenemia 641.3
        affecting fetus or newborn 762.1
      leiomyoma, uterus 641.8
        affecting fetus or newborn 762.1
      low-lying placenta 641.1
        affecting fetus or newborn 762.1
      marginal sinus (rupture) 641.2
        affecting fetus or newborn 762.1
      placenta previa 641.1
        affecting fetus or newborn 762.0
      premature separation of placenta (normally
          implanted) 641.2
        affecting fetus or newborn 762.1
      threatened abortion 640.0
        affecting fetus or newborn 762.1
      trauma 641.8
        affecting fetus or newborn 762.1
    early (before 22 completed weeks gestation)
        640.9
      affecting fetus or newborn 762.1
    previous, affecting management of pregnancy
        or childbirth V23.49
    unavoidable—*see* Hemorrhage, pregnancy,
        due to placenta previa
  prepartum (mother)—*see* Hemorrhage,
      pregnancy
  preretinal, cause unspecified 362.81
  prostate 602.1
  puerperal (*see also* Hemorrhage, postpartum)
      666.1
  pulmonary (*see also* Hemorrhage, lung) 786.30
    acute idiopathic in infants (AIPHI) (over 28
        days old) 786.31
    newborn (massive) 770.3
    renal syndrome 446.21

Hemorrhage, hemorrhagic—*continued*
 purpura (primary) (*see also* Purpura,
  thrombocytopenic) 287.39
 rectum (sphincter) 569.3
 recurring, following initial hemorrhage at time
  of injury 958.2
 renal 593.81
  pulmonary syndrome 446.21
 respiratory tract (*see also* Hemorrhage, lung)
  786.30
 retina, retinal (deep) (superficial) (vessels) 362.81
  diabetic 250.5 *[362.01]*
   due to secondary diabetes 249.5 *[362.01]*
  due to birth injury 772.8
 retrobulbar 376.89
 retroperitoneal 459.0
 retroplacental (*see also* Placenta, separation) 641.2
 scalp 459.0
  due to injury at birth 767.19
 scrotum 608.83
 secondary (nontraumatic) 459.0
  following initial hemorrhage at time of injury
   958.2
 seminal vesicle 608.83
 skin 782.7
  newborn 772.6
 spermatic cord 608.83
 spinal (cord) 336.1
  aneurysm (ruptured) 336.1
   syphilitic 094.89
  due to birth injury 767.4
  fetus or newborn 767.4
 spleen 289.59
 spontaneous NEC 459.0
  petechial 782.7
 stomach 578.9
  newborn 772.4
  ulcer—*see* Ulcer, stomach, with hemorrhage
 subaponeurotic, newborn 767.11
  massive (birth injury) 767.11
 subarachnoid (nontraumatic) 430
  fetus or newborn (anoxic) (traumatic) 772.2
  puerperal, postpartum, childbirth 674.0
  traumatic—*see* Hemorrhage, brain, traumatic,
   subarachnoid
 subconjunctival 372.72
  due to birth injury 772.8
  newborn 772.8
 subcortical (*see also* Hemorrhage, brain) 431
 subcutaneous 782.7
 subdiaphragmatic 459.0
 subdural (nontraumatic) 432.1
  due to birth injury 767.0
  fetus or newborn (anoxic) (hypoxic) (due to
   birth trauma) 767.0
  puerperal, postpartum, childbirth 674.0
  spinal 336.1
  traumatic—*see* Hemorrhage, brain, traumatic,
   subdural
 subgaleal 767.11
 subhyaloid 362.81
 subperiosteal 733.99
 subretinal 362.81
 subtentorial (*see also* Hemorrhage, subdural) 432.1
 subungual 703.8
  due to blood dyscrasia 287.8
 suprarenal (capsule) (gland) 255.41
  fetus or newborn 772.5
 tentorium (traumatic)—*see also* Hemorrhage,
  brain, traumatic
  fetus or newborn 767.0
  nontraumatic—*see* Hemorrhage, subdural

Hemorrhage, hemorrhagic—*continued*
 testis 608.83
 thigh 459.0
 third stage 666.0
 thorax—*see* Hemorrhage, lung
 throat 784.8
 thrombocythemia 238.71
 thymus (gland) 254.8
 thyroid (gland) 246.3
  cyst 246.3
 tongue 529.8
 tonsil 474.8
  postoperative 998.11
 tooth socket (postextraction) 998.11
 trachea—*see* Hemorrhage, lung
 traumatic—*see also* nature of injury
  brain—*see* Hemorrhage, brain, traumatic
  recurring or secondary (following initial
   hemorrhage at time of injury) 958.2
 tuberculous NEC (*see also* Tuberculosis,
  pulmonary) 011.9
 tunica vaginalis 608.83
 ulcer—*see* Ulcer, by site, with hemorrhage
 umbilicus, umbilical cord 772.0
  after birth, newborn 772.3
  complicating delivery 663.8
   affecting fetus or newborn 772.0
  slipped ligature 772.3
  stump 772.3
 unavoidable (due to placenta previa) 641.1
  affecting fetus or newborn 762.0
 upper extremity 459.0
 urethra (idiopathic) 599.84
 uterus, uterine (abnormal) 626.9
  climacteric 627.0
  complicating delivery—*see* Hemorrhage,
   complicating, delivery
  due to
   intrauterine contraceptive device 996.76
   perforating uterus 996.32
  functional or dysfunctional 626.8
  in pregnancy—*see* Hemorrhage, pregnancy
  intermenstrual 626.6
   irregular 626.6
   regular 626.5
  postmenopausal 627.1
  postpartum (*see also* Hemorrhage,
   postpartum) 666.1
  prepubertal 626.8
  pubertal 626.3
  puerperal (immediate) 666.1
 vagina 623.8
 vasa previa 663.5
  affecting fetus or newborn 772.0
 vas deferens 608.83
 ventricular (*see also* Hemorrhage, brain) 431
 vesical 596.89
 viscera 459.0
  newborn 772.8
 vitreous (humor) (intraocular) 379.23
 vocal cord 478.5
 vulva 624.8
Hemorrhoids (anus) (rectum) (without
  complication) 455.6
 bleeding, prolapsed, strangulated, or ulcerated
  NEC 455.8
  external 455.5
  internal 455.2
 complicated NEC 455.8
 complicating pregnancy and puerperium 671.8

Hemorrhoids—*continued*
external 455.3
  with complication NEC 455.5
  bleeding, prolapsed, strangulated, or ulcerated 455.5
  thrombosed 455.4
internal 455.0
  with complication NEC 455.2
  bleeding, prolapsed, strangulated, or ulcerated 455.2
  thrombosed 455.1
residual skin tag 455.9
sentinel pile 455.9
thrombosed NEC 455.7
  external 455.4
  internal 455.1
Hemosalpinx 620.8
Hemosiderosis 275.09
dietary 275.09
pulmonary (idiopathic) 275.09 *[516.1]*
transfusion NEC 275.02
  bone marrow 996.85
Hemospermia 608.82
Hemothorax 511.89
bacterial, nontuberculous 511.1
newborn 772.8
nontuberculous 511.89
  bacterial 511.1
pneumococcal 511.1
postoperative 998.11
staphylococcal 511.1
streptococcal 511.1
traumatic 860.2
  with
    open wound into thorax 860.3
    pneumothorax 860.4
      with open wound into thorax 860.5
tuberculous (*see also* Tuberculosis, pleura) 012.0
Hemotympanum 385.89
Hench-Rosenberg syndrome (palindromic arthritis) (*see also* Rheumatism, palindromic) 719.3
Henle's warts 371.41
Henoch (-Schönlein)
disease or syndrome (allergic purpura) 287.0
purpura (allergic) 287.0
Henpue, henpuye 102.6
Heparitinuria 277.5
Hepar lobatum 095.3
Heparin-induced thrombocytopenia (HIT) 289.84
Hepatalgia 573.8
Hepatic —*see also* condition
flexure syndrome 569.89
Hepatitis 573.3
acute (*see also* Necrosis, liver) 570
  alcoholic 571.1
  infective 070.1
    with hepatic coma 070.0
alcoholic 571.1
amebic—*see* Abscess, liver, amebic
anicteric (acute)—*see* Hepatitis, viral
antigen-associated (HAA) *see* Hepatitis, viral, type B
Australian antigen (positive) *see* Hepatitis, viral, type B
autoimmune 571.42

Hepatitis—*continued*
catarrhal (acute) 070.1
  with hepatic coma 070.0
  chronic 571.40
  newborn 070.1
    with hepatic coma 070.0
chemical 573.3
cholangiolitic 573.8
cholestatic 573.8
chronic 571.40
  active 571.49
    viral—*see* Hepatitis, viral
  aggressive 571.49
  persistent 571.41
  viral—*see* Hepatitis, viral
cytomegalic inclusion virus 078.5 *[573.1]*
diffuse 573.3
"dirty needle"—*see* Hepatitis, viral
  with hepatic coma 070.2
drug-induced 573.3
due to
  Coxsackie 074.8 *[573.1]*
  cytomegalic inclusion virus 078.5 *[573.1]*
  infectious mononucleosis 075 *[573.1]*
  malaria 084.9 *[573.2]*
  mumps 072.71
  secondary syphilis 091.62
  toxoplasmosis (acquired) 130.5
    congenital (active) 771.2
epidemic—*see* Hepatitis, viral, type A
fetus or newborn 774.4
fibrous (chronic) 571.49
  acute 570
from injection, inoculation, or transfusion (blood) (other substance) (plasma) (serum) (onset within 8 months after administration) *see* Hepatitis, viral
fulminant (viral) (*see also* Hepatitis, viral) 070.9
  with hepatic coma 070.6
  type A 070.1
    with hepatic coma 070.0
  type B—*see* Hepatitis, viral, Type B
giant cell (neonatal) 774.4
hemorrhagic 573.8
history of
  B V12.09
  C V12.09
homologous serum—*see* Hepatitis, viral
hypertrophic (chronic) 571.49
  acute 570
nfectious, infective (acute) (chronic) (subacute) 070.1
  with hepatic coma 070.0
inoculation—*see* Hepatitis, viral
interstitial (chronic) 571.49
  acute 570
lupoid 571.49
malarial 084.9 *[573.2]*
malignant (*see also* Necrosis, liver) 570
neonatal (toxic) 774.4
newborn 774.4
parenchymatous (acute) (*see also* Necrosis, liver) 570
peliosis 573.3
persistent, chronic 571.41
plasma cell 571.49
postimmunization—*see* Hepatitis, viral
postnecrotic 571.49
posttransfusion—*see* Hepatitis, viral
recurrent 571.49

Hepatitis—*continued*
  septic 573.3
  serum—*see* Hepatitis, viral
    carrier (suspected) of V02.61
  subacute (*see also* Necrosis, liver) 570
  suppurative (diffuse) 572.0
  syphilitic (late) 095.3
    congenital (early) 090.0 *[573.2]*
      late 090.5 *[573.2]*
    secondary 091.62
  toxic (noninfectious) 573.3
    fetus or newborn 774.4
  tuberculous (*see also* Tuberculosis) 017.9
  viral (acute) (anicteric) (cholangiolitic)
    (cholestatic) (chronic) (subacute) 070.9
    with hepatic coma 070.6
    AU-SH type virus—*see* Hepatitis, viral, type
      B
    Australian antigen—*see* Hepatitis, viral, type
      B
    B-antigen—*see* Hepatitis, viral, type B
    Coxsackie 074.8 *[573.1]*
    cytomegalic inclusion 078.5 *[573.1]*
    IH (virus)—*see* Hepatitis, viral, type A
    infectious hepatitis virus—*see* Hepatitis, viral,
      type A
    serum hepatitis virus—*see* Hepatitis, viral,
      type B
    SH—*see* Hepatitis, viral, type B
    specified type NEC 070.59
      with hepatic coma 070.49
    type A 070.1
      with hepatic coma 070.0
    type B (acute) 070.30
      with
        hepatic coma 070.20
          with hepatitis delta 070.21
        hepatitis delta 070.31
          with hepatic coma 070.21
      carrier status V02.61
      chronic 070.32
      with
        hepatic coma 070.22
          with hepatitis delta 070.23
        hepatitis delta 070.33
          with hepatic coma 070.23
    type C
      with hepatic coma 070.41
      acute 070.51
        with hepatic coma 070.41
      carrier status V02.62
      chronic 070.54
        with hepatic coma 070.44
      in remission 070.54
      unspecified 070.70
        with hepatic coma 070.71
    type delta (with hepatitis B carrier state)
      070.52
      with
        active hepatitis B disease—*see* Hepatitis,
          viral, type B
        hepatic coma 070.42
    type E 070.53
      with hepatic coma 070.43
    vaccination and inoculation (prophylactic)
      V05.3
  Waldenström's (lupoid hepatitis) 571.49
Hepatization, lung (acute)—*see also* Pneumonia,
  lobar
  chronic (*see also* Fibrosis, lung) 515
Hepatoblastoma (M8970/3) 155.0
Hepatocarcinoma (M8170/3) 155.0

Hepatocholangiocarcinoma (M8180/3) 155.0
Hepatocholangioma, benign (M8180/0) 211.5
Hepatocholangitis 573.8
Hepatocystitis (*see also* Cholecystitis) 575.10
Hepatodystrophy 570
Hepatolenticular degeneration 275.1
Hepatolithiasis —*see* Choledocholithiasis
Hepatoma (malignant) (M8170/3) 155.0
  benign (M8170/0) 211.5
  congenital (M8970/3) 155.0
  embryonal (M8970/3) 155.0
Hepatomegalia glycogenica diffusa 271.0
Hepatomegaly (*see also* Hypertrophy, liver)
  789.1
  congenital 751.69
    syphilitic 090.0
  due to Clonorchis sinensis 121.1
  Gaucher's 272.7
  syphilitic (congenital) 090.0
Hepatoptosis 573.8
Hepatorrhexis 573.8
Hepatosis, toxic 573.8
Hepatosplenomegaly 571.8
  due to S. japonicum 120.2
  hyperlipemic (Burger-Grutz type) 272.3
Herald patch 696.3
Hereditary —*see* condition
Heredodegeneration 330.9
  macular 362.70
Heredopathia atactica polyneuritiformis 356.3
Heredosyphilis (*see also* Syphilis, congenital)
  090.9
Hermaphroditism (true) 752.7
  with specified chromosomal anomaly—*see*
    Anomaly, chromosomes, sex
Hernia, hernial (acquired) (recurrent) 553.9
  with
    gangrene (obstructed) NEC 551.9
    obstruction NEC 552.9
      and gangrene 551.9
  abdomen (wall)—*see* Hernia, ventral
  abdominal, specified site NEC 553.8
    with
      gangrene (obstructed) 551.8
      obstruction 552.8
        and gangrene 551.8
  appendix 553.8
    with
      gangrene (obstructed) 551.8
      obstruction 552.8
        and gangrene 551.8
  bilateral (inguinal)—*see* Hernia, inguinal
  bladder (sphincter)
    congenital (female) (male) 756.71
    female (*see also* Cystocele, female) 618.01
    male 596.89
  brain 348.4
    congenital 742.0
  broad ligament 553.8
  cartilage, vertebral—*see* Displacement,
    intervertebral disc
  cerebral 348.4
    congenital 742.0
    endaural 742.0
  ciliary body 364.89
    traumatic 871.1
  colic 553.9
    with
      gangrene (obstructed) 551.9
      obstruction 552.9
        and gangrene 551.9

Hernia, hernial—*continued*
  colon 553.9
    with
      gangrene (obstructed) 551.9
      obstruction 552.9
        and gangrene 551.9
  colostomy (stoma) 569.69
  Cooper's (retroperitoneal) 553.8
    with
      gangrene (obstructed) 551.8
      obstruction 552.8
        and gangrene 551.8
  crural—*see* Hernia, femoral
  cystostomy 596.83
  diaphragm, diaphragmatic 553.3
    with
      gangrene (obstructed) 551.3
      obstruction 552.3
        and gangrene 551.3
    congenital 756.6
    due to gross defect of diaphragm 756.6
    traumatic 862.0
      with open wound into cavity 862.1
  direct (inguinal)—*see* Hernia, inguinal
  disc, intervertebral—*see* Displacement,
    intervertebral disc
  diverticulum, intestine 553.9
    with
      gangrene (obstructed) 551.9
      obstruction 552.9
        and gangrene 551.9
  double (inguinal)—*see* Hernia, inguinal
  due to adhesion with obstruction 552.9
  duodenojejunal 553.8
    with
      gangrene (obstructed) 551.8
      obstruction 552.8
        and gangrene 551.8
  en glissade—*see* Hernia, inguinal
  enterostomy (stoma) 569.69
  epigastric 553.29
    with
      gangrene (obstruction) 551.29
      obstruction 552.29
        and gangrene 551.29
    recurrent 553.21
      with
        gangrene (obstructed) 551.21
        obstruction 552.21
          and gangrene 551.21
  esophageal hiatus (sliding) 553.3
    with
      gangrene (obstructed) 551.3
      obstruction 552.3
        and gangrene 551.3
    congenital 750.6
  external (inguinal)—*see* Hernia, inguinal
  fallopian tube 620.4
  fascia 728.89
  fat 729.30
    eyelid 374.34
    orbital 374.34
    pad 729.30
      eye, eyelid 374.34
      knee 729.31
      orbit 374.34
      popliteal (space) 729.31
      specified site NEC 729.39

Hernia, hernial—*continued*
  femoral (unilateral) 553.00
    with
      gangrene (obstructed) 551.00
      obstruction 552.00
        with gangrene 551.00
    bilateral 553.02
      gangrenous (obstructed) 551.02
      obstructed 552.02
        with gangrene 551.02
    recurrent 553.03
      gangrenous (obstructed) 551.03
      obstructed 552.03
        with gangrene 551.03
    recurrent (unilateral) 553.01
      bilateral 553.03
        gangrenous (obstructed) 551.03
        obstructed 552.03
          with gangrene 551.03
      gangrenous (obstructed) 551.01
      obstructed 552.01
        with gangrene 551.01
  foramen
    Bochdalek 553.3
      with
        gangrene (obstructed) 551.3
        obstruction 552.3
          and gangrene 551.3
      congenital 756.6
    magnum 348.4
    Morgagni, morgagnian 553.3
      with
        gangrene 551.3
        obstruction 552.3
          and gangrene 551.3
      congenital 756.6
  funicular (umbilical) 553.1
    with
      gangrene (obstructed) 551.1
      obstruction 552.1
        and gangrene 551.1
    spermatic cord—*see* Hernia, inguinal
  gangrenous—*see* Hernia, by site, with gangrene
  gastrointestinal tract 553.9
    with
      gangrene (obstructed) 551.9
      obstruction 552.9
        and gangrene 551.9
  gluteal—*see* Hernia, femoral
  Gruber's (internal mesogastric) 553.8
    with
      gangrene (obstructed) 551.8
      obstruction 552.8
        and gangrene 551.8
  Hesselbach's 553.8
    with
      gangrene (obstructed) 551.8
      obstruction 552.8
        and gangrene 551.8
  hiatal (esophageal) (sliding) 553.3
    with
      gangrene (obstructed) 551.3
      obstruction 552.3
        and gangrene 551.3
    congenital 750.6
  incarcerated (*see also* Hernia, by site, with
      obstruction) 552.9
    gangrenous (*see also* Hernia, by site, with
        gangrene) 551.9

Hernia, hernial—*continued*
  incisional 553.21
    with
      gangrene (obstructed) 551.21
      obstruction 552.21
        and gangrene 551.21
  lumbar—*see* Hernia, lumbar
  recurrent 553.21
    with
      gangrene (obstructed) 551.21
      obstruction 552.21
        and gangrene 551.21
  indirect (inguinal)—*see* Hernia, inguinal
  infantile—*see* Hernia, inguinal
  infrapatellar fat pad 729.31
  inguinal (direct) (double) (encysted) (external)
    (funicular) (indirect) (infantile) (internal)
    (interstitial) (oblique) (scrotal) (sliding)
    550.9

> *Note—Use the following fifth-digit*
> *subclassification with category 550:*
>
> *0 unilateral or unspecified (not specified as*
>   *recurrent)*
> *1 unilateral or unspecified, recurrent*
> *2 bilateral (not specified as recurrent)*
> *3 bilateral, recurrent*

    with
      gangrene (obstructed) 550.0
      obstruction 550.1
        and gangrene 550.0
  internal 553.8
    with
      gangrene (obstructed) 551.8
      obstruction 552.8
        and gangrene 551.8
    inguinal—*see* Hernia, inguinal
  interstitial 553.9
    with
      gangrene (obstructed) 551.9
      obstruction 552.9
        and gangrene 551.9
    inguinal—*see* Hernia, inguinal
  intervertebral cartilage or disc—*see*
    Displacement, intervertebral disc
  intestine, intestinal 553.9
    with
      gangrene (obstructed) 551.9
      obstruction 552.9
        and gangrene 551.9
  intra-abdominal 553.9
    with
      gangrene (obstructed) 551.9
      obstruction 552.9
        and gangrene 551.9
  intraparietal 553.9
    with
      gangrene (obstructed) 551.9
      obstruction 552.9
        and gangrene 551.9
  iris 364.89
    traumatic 871.1
  irreducible (*see also* Hernia, by site, with
    obstruction) 552.9
    gangrenous (with obstruction) (*see also*
      Hernia, by site, with gangrene) 551.9
  ischiatic 553.8
    with
      gangrene (obstructed) 551.8
      obstruction 552.8
        and gangrene 551.8

Hernia, hernial—*continued*
  ischiorectal 553.8
    with
      gangrene (obstructed) 551.8
      obstruction 552.8
        and gangrene 551.8
  lens 379.32
    traumatic 871.1
  linea
    alba—*see* Hernia, epigastric
    semilunaris—*see* Hernia, spigelian
  Littre's (diverticular) 553.9
    with
      gangrene (obstructed) 551.9
      obstruction 552.9
        and gangrene 551.9
  lumbar 553.8
    with
      gangrene (obstructed) 551.8
      obstruction 552.8
        and gangrene 551.8
    intervertebral disc 722.10
  lung (subcutaneous) 518.89
    congenital 748.69
  mediastinum 519.3
  mesenteric (internal) 553.8
    with
      gangrene (obstructed) 551.8
      obstruction 552.8
        and gangrene 551.8
  mesocolon 553.8
    with
      gangrene (obstructed) 551.8
      obstruction 552.8
        and gangrene 551.8
  muscle (sheath) 728.89
  nucleus pulposus—*see* Displacement,
    intervertebral disc
  oblique (inguinal)—*see* Hernia, inguinal
  obstructive (*see also* Hernia, by site, with
    obstruction) 552.9
    gangrenous (with obstruction) (*see also*
      Hernia, by site, with gangrene) 551.9
  obturator 553.8
    with
      gangrene (obstructed) 551.8
      obstruction 552.8
        and gangrene 551.8
  omental 553.8
    with
      gangrene (obstructed) 551.8
      obstruction 552.8
        and gangrene 551.8
  orbital fat (pad) 374.34
  ovary 620.4
  oviduct 620.4
  paracolostomy (stoma) 569.69
  paraduodenal 553.8
    with
      gangrene (obstructed) 551.8
      obstruction 552.8
        and gangrene 551.8
  paraesophageal 553.3
    with
      gangrene (obstructed) 551.3
      obstruction 552.3
        and gangrene 551.3
    congenital 750.6

Hernia, hernial—*continued*
  parahiatal 553.3
    with
      gangrene (obstructed) 551.3
      obstruction 552.3
        and gangrene 551.3
  paraumbilical 553.1
    with
      gangrene (obstructed) 551.1
      obstruction 552.1
        and gangrene 551.1
  parietal 553.9
    with
      gangrene (obstructed) 551.9
      obstruction 552.9
        and gangrene 551.9
  perineal 553.8
    with
      gangrene (obstructed) 551.8
      obstruction 552.8
        and gangrene 551.8
  peritoneal sac, lesser 553.8
    with
      gangrene (obstructed) 551.8
      obstruction 552.8
        and gangrene 551.8
  popliteal fat pad 729.31
  postoperative 553.21
    with
      gangrene (obstructed) 551.21
      obstruction 552.21
        and gangrene 551.21
  pregnant uterus 654.4
  prevesical 596.89
  properitoneal 553.8
    with
      gangrene (obstructed) 551.8
      obstruction 552.8
        and gangrene 551.8
  pudendal 553.8
    with
      gangrene (obstructed) 551.8
      obstruction 552.8
        and gangrene 551.8
  rectovaginal 618.6
  retroperitoneal 553.8
    with
      gangrene (obstructed) 551.8
      obstruction 552.8
        and gangrene 551.8
  Richter's (parietal) 553.9
    with
      gangrene (obstructed) 551.9
      obstruction 552.9
        and gangrene 551.9
  Rieux's, Riex's (retrocecal) 553.8
    with
      gangrene (obstructed) 551.8
      obstruction 552.8
        and gangrene 551.8
  sciatic 553.8
    with
      gangrene (obstructed) 551.8
      obstruction 552.8
        and gangrene 551.8
  scrotum, scrotal—*see* Hernia, inguinal
  sliding (inguinal)—*see also* Hernia, inguinal
    hiatus—*see* Hernia, hiatal

Hernia, hernial—*continued*
  spigelian 553.29
    with
      gangrene (obstructed) 551.29
      obstruction 552.29
        and gangrene 551.29
  spinal (*see also* Spina bifida) 741.9
    with hydrocephalus 741.0
  strangulated (*see also* Hernia, by site, with
      obstruction) 552.9
  gangrenous (with obstruction) (*see also*
      Hernia, by site, with gangrene) 551.9
  supraumbilicus (linea alba)—*see* Hernia,
      epigastric
  tendon 727.9
  testis (nontraumatic) 550.9
    meaning
      scrotal hernia 550.9
      symptomatic late syphilis 095.8
  Treitz's (fossa) 553.8
    with
      gangrene (obstructed) 551.8
      obstruction 552.8
        and gangrene 551.8
  tunica
    albuginea 608.89
    vaginalis 752.89
  umbilicus, umbilical 553.1
    with
      gangrene (obstructed) 551.1
      obstruction 552.1
        and gangrene 551.1
  ureter 593.89
    with obstruction 593.4
  uterus 621.8
    pregnant 654.4
  vaginal (posterior) 618.6
  Velpeau's (femoral) (*see also* Hernia, femoral)
      553.00
  ventral 553.20
    with
      gangrene (obstructed) 551.20
      obstruction 552.20
        and gangrene 551.20
    recurrent 553.21
      with
        gangrene (obstructed) 551.21
        obstruction 552.21
          and gangrene 551.21
  vesical
    congenital (female) (male) 756.71
    female (*see also* Cystocele, female) 618.01
    male 596.89
  vitreous (into anterior chamber) 379.21
    traumatic 871.1
Herniation —*see also* Hernia
  brain (stem) 348.4
  cerebral 348.4
  gastric mucosa (into duodenal bulb) 537.89
  mediastinum 519.3
  nucleus pulposus—*see* Displacement,
      intervertebral disc
Herpangina 074.0
Herpes, herpetic 054.9
  auricularis (zoster) 053.71
    simplex 054.73
  blepharitis (zoster) 053.20
    simplex 054.41
  circinate 110.5
  circinatus 110.5
    bullous 694.5

Hiccup (*see also* Hiccough) 786.8
Hicks (-Braxton) contractures 644.1
Hidden penis 752.65
Hidradenitis (axillaris) (suppurative) 705.83
Hidradenoma (nodular) (M8400/0)—*see also*
  Neoplasm, skin, benign
  clear cell (M8402/0)—*see* Neoplasm, skin,
    benign
  papillary (M8405/0)—*see* Neoplasm, skin,
    benign
Hidrocystoma (M8404/0)—*see* Neoplasm, skin,
  benign
HIE (hypoxic-ischemic encephalopathy) 768.70
  mild 768.71
  moderate 768.72
  severe 768.73
High
  A$_2$ anemia 282.46
  altitude effects 993.2
    anoxia 993.2
    on
      ears 993.0
      sinuses 993.1
    polycythemia 289.0
  arch
    foot 755.67
    palate 750.26
  artery (arterial) tension (*see also* Hypertension)
    401.9
    without diagnosis of hypertension 796.2
  basal metabolic rate (BMR) 794.7
  blood pressure (*see also* Hypertension) 401.9
    borderline 796.2
    incidental reading (isolated) (nonspecific), no
      diagnosis of hypertension 796.2
  cholesterol 272.0
    with high triglycerides 272.2
  compliance bladder 596.4
  diaphragm (congenital) 756.6
  frequency deafness (congenital) (regional) 389.8
  head at term 652.5
  output failure (cardiac) (*see also* Failure, heart)
    428.9
  oxygen-affinity hemoglobin 289.0
  palate 750.26
  risk
    behavior —*see* Problem
    family situation V61.9
      specified circumstance NEC V61.8
    human papillomavirus (HPV) DNA test
      positive
      anal 796.75
      cervical 795.05
      vaginal 795.15
    individual NEC V62.89
    infant NEC V20.1
    patient taking drugs (prescribed) V67.51
      nonprescribed (*see also* Abuse, drugs,
        nondependent) 305.9
    pregnancy V23.9
      inadequate prenatal care V23.7
      inconclusive fetal viability V23.87
      specified problem NEC V23.8
  temperature (of unknown origin) (*see also*
    Pyrexia) 780.60
  thoracic rib 756.3
  triglycerides 272.1
    with high cholesterol 272.2
Hildenbrand's disease (typhus) 081.9
Hilger's syndrome 337.09

Hill diarrhea 579.1
Hilliard's lupus (*see also* Tuberculosis) 017.0
Hilum —*see* condition
Hip —*see* condition
Hippel's disease (retinocerebral angiomatosis) 759.6
Hippus 379.49
Hirschfeld's disease (acute diabetes mellitus) (*see*
  also Diabetes) 250.0
  due to secondary diabetes 249.0
Hirschsprung's disease or megacolon
  (congenital) 751.3
Hirsuties (*see also* Hypertrichosis) 704.1
Hirsutism (*see also* Hypertrichosis) 704.1
Hirudiniasis (external) (internal) 134.2
His-Werner disease (trench fever) 083.1
Hiss-Russell dysentery 004.1
Histamine cephalgia 339.00
Histidinemia 270.5
Histidinuria 270.5
Histiocytic syndromes 288.4
Histiocytoma (M8832/0)—*see also* Neoplasm,
  skin, benign
  fibrous (M8830/0)—*see also* Neoplasm, skin,
    benign
    atypical (M8830/1)—*see* Neoplasm,
      connective tissue, uncertain behavior
    malignant (M8830/0)—*see* Neoplasm,
      connective tissue, malignant
Histiocytosis (acute) (chronic) (subacute) 277.89
  acute differentiated progressive (M9722/3) 202.5
  adult pulmonary Langerhans cell (PLCH) 516.5
  cholesterol 277.89
  essential 277.89
  lipid, lipoid (essential) 272.7
  lipochrome (familial) 288.1
  malignant (M9720/3) 202.3
  non-Langerhans cell 277.89
  polyostotic sclerosing 277.89
  X (chronic) 277.89
    acute (progressive) (M9722/3) 202.5
Histoplasmosis 115.90
  with
    endocarditis 115.94
    meningitis 115.91
    pericarditis 115.93
    pneumonia 115.95
    retinitis 115.92
    specified manifestation NEC 115.99
  African (due to Histoplasma duboisii) 115.10
    with
      endocarditis 115.14
      meningitis 115.11
      pericarditis 115.13
      pneumonia 115.15
      retinitis 115.12
      specified manifestation NEC 115.19
  American (due to Histoplasma capsulatum) 115.00
    with
      endocarditis 115.04
      meningitis 115.01
      pericarditis 115.03
      pneumonia 115.05
      retinitis 115.02
      specified manifestation NEC 115.09
  Darling's—*see* Histoplasmosis, American
  large form (*see also* Histoplasmosis, African) 115.10
  lung 115.05
  small form (*see also* Histoplasmosis, American)
    115.00

History (personal) of
abuse
  emotional V15.42
  neglect V15.42
  physical V15.41
  sexual V15.41
affective psychosis V11.1
alcoholism V11.3
  specified as drinking problem (*see also* Abuse, drugs, nondependent) 305.0
allergy (to) V15.09
  analgesic agent NEC V14.6
  anesthetic NEC V14.4
  antibiotic agent NEC V14.1
    penicillin V14.0
  anti-infective agent NEC V14.3
  arachnid bite V15.06
  diathesis V15.09
  drug V14.9
    specified type NEC V14.8
  eggs V15.03
  food additives V15.05
  insect bite V15.06
  latex V15.07
  medicinal agents V14.9
    specified type NEC V14.8
  milk products V15.02
  narcotic agent NEC V14.5
  nuts V15.05
    peanuts V15.01
  penicillin V14.0
  radiographic dye V15.08
  seafood V15.04
  serum V14.7
  specified food NEC V15.05
  specified nonmedicinal agents NEC V15.09
  spider bite V15.06
  sulfa V14.2
  sulfonamides V14.2
  therapeutic agent NEC V15.09
  vaccine V14.7
anaphylactic reaction or shock V13.81
anaphylaxis V13.81
anemia V12.3
arrest, sudden cardiac V12.53
arthritis V13.4
attack, transient ischemic (TIA) V12.54
benign neoplasm of brain V12.41
blood disease V12.3
calculi, urinary V13.01
cardiovascular disease V12.50
  myocardial infarction 412
chemotherapy, antineoplastic V87.41
child abuse V15.41
cigarette smoking V15.82
circulatory system disease V12.50
  myocardial infarction 412
cleft lip and palate, corrected V13.64
combat and operational stress reaction V11.4
congenital malformation (corrected)
  circulatory system V13.65
  digestive system V13.67
  ear V13.64
  eye V13.64
  face V13.64
  genitourinary system V13.62
  heart V13.65
  integument V13.68
  limbs V13.68
  musculoskeletal V13.68
  neck V13.64

History—*continued*
congenital malformation—*continued*
  nervous system V13.63
  respiratory system V13.66
  specified type NEC V13.69
contraception V15.7
death, sudden, successfully resuscitated V12.53
deficit
  prolonged reversible ischemic neurologic (PRIND) V12.54
  reversible ischemic neurologic (RIND) V12.54
diathesis, allergic V15.09
digestive system disease V12.70
  peptic ulcer V12.71
  polyps, colonic V12.72
  specified NEC V12.79
disease (of) V13.9
  blood V12.3
  blood-forming organs V12.3
  cardiovascular system V12.50
  circulatory system V12.50
    specified NEC V12.59
  digestive system V12.70
    peptic ulcer V12.71
    polyps, colonic V12.72
    specified NEC V12.79
  infectious V12.00
    malaria V12.03
    methicillin resistant Staphylococcus aureus (MRSA) V12.04
    MRSA (methicillin resistant Staphylococcus aureus) V12.04
    poliomyelitis V12.02
    specified NEC V12.09
    tuberculosis V12.01
  parasitic V12.00
    specified NEC V12.09
  respiratory system V12.60
    pneumonia V12.61
    specified NEC V12.69
  skin V13.3
  specified site NEC V13.89
  subcutaneous tissue V13.3
  trophoblastic V13.1
    affecting management of pregnancy V23.1
disorder (of) V13.9
  endocrine V12.29
    gestational diabetes V12.21
  genital system V13.29
  hematological V12.3
  immunity V12.29
  mental V11.9
    affective type V11.1
    manic-depressive V11.1
    neurosis V11.2
    schizophrenia V11.0
    specified type NEC V11.8
  metabolic V12.29
  musculoskeletal NEC V13.59
  nervous system V12.40
    specified type NEC V12.49
  obstetric V13.29
    affecting management of current pregnancy V23.49
      ectopic pregnancy V23.42
      pre-term labor V13.21
  sense organs V12.40
    specified type NEC V12.49
  specified site NEC V13.89

History—*continued*
  malignant neoplasm—*continued*
    mediastinum V10.29
    melanoma (of skin) V10.82
    middle ear V10.22
    mouth V10.02
      specified part NEC V10.02
    nasal cavities V10.22
    nasopharynx V10.02
    nervous system NEC V10.86
    nose V10.22
    oropharynx V10.02
    ovary V10.43
    pancreas V10.09
    parathyroid V10.88
    penis V10.49
    pharynx V10.02
    pineal V10.88
    pituitary V10.88
    placenta V10.44
    pleura V10.29
    prostate V10.46
    rectosigmoid junction V10.06
    rectum V10.06
    renal pelvis V10.53
    respiratory organs NEC V10.20
    salivary gland V10.02
    skin V10.83
      melanoma V10.82
    small intestine NEC V10.09
    soft tissue NEC V10.89
    specified site NEC V10.89
    stomach V10.04
    testis V10.47
    thymus V10.29
    thyroid V10.87
    tongue V10.01
    trachea V10.12
    ureter V10.59
    urethra V10.59
    urinary organ V10.50
    uterine adnexa V10.44
    uterus V10.42
    vagina V10.44
    vulva V10.44
  manic-depressive psychosis V11.1
  meningitis V12.42
  mental disorder V11.9
    affective type V11.1
    manic-depressive V11.1
    neurosis V11.2
    schizophrenia V11.0
    specified type NEC V11.8
  Merkel cell carcinoma V10.91
  metabolic disorder V12.29
  methicillin resistant Staphylococcus aureus
    (MRSA) V12.04
  MRSA (methicillin resistant Staphylococcus
    aureus) V12.04
  musculoskeletal disorder NEC V13.59
  myocardial infarction 412
  neglect (emotional) V15.42
  nephrotic syndrome V13.03
  nervous system disorder V12.40
    specified type NEC V12.49
  neurosis V11.2
  noncompliance with medical treatment V15.81
  nutritional deficiency V12.1

History—*continued*
  obstetric disorder V13.29
    affecting management of current pregnancy
      V23.49
    ectopic pregnancy 23.42
    pre-term labor V23.41
  pre-term labor V13.41
  parasitic disease V12.00
    specified NEC V12.09
  perinatal problems V13.7
    low birth weight (*see also* Status, low birth
      weight) V21.30
  physical abuse V15.41
  poisoning V15.6
  poliomyelitis V12.02
  polyps, colonic V12.72
  poor obstetric V23.49
    affecting management of current pregnancy
      V23.49
    ectopic pregnancy 23.42
    pre-term labor V23.41
  pre-term labor V13.41
  prolonged reversible ischemic neurologic
    deficits (PRIND) V12.54
  psychiatric disorder V11.9
    affective type V11.1
    manic-depressive V11.1
    neurosis V11.2
    schizophrenia V11.0
    specified type NEC V11.8
  psychological trauma V15.49
    emotional abuse V15.42
    neglect V15.42
    physical abuse V15.41
    rape V15.41
  psychoneurosis V11.2
  radiation therapy V15.3
  rape V15.41
  respiratory system disease V12.60
    pneumonia V12.61
    specified NEC V12.69
  reticulosarcoma V10.71
  return from military deployment V62.22
  reversible ischemic neurologic deficit (RIND)
    V12.54
  schizophrenia V11.0
  skin disease V13.3
  smoking (tobacco) V15.82
  steroid therapy V87.45
    inhaled V87.44
    systemic V87.45
  stroke without residual deficits V12.54
  subcutaneous tissue disease V13.3
  sudden
    cardiac
      arrest V12.53
      death (successfully resuscitated) V12.53
  surgery (to)
    great vessels V15.1
    heart V15.1
    in utero
      during pregnancy V15.21
      while a fetus V15.22
    organs NEC V15.29
  syndrome, nephrotic V13.03
  therapy
    antineoplastic drug V87.41
    drug NEC V87.49
    estrogen V87.43
    immunosuppression V87.46
    monoclonal drug V87.42

History—*continued*
  therapy—*continued*
    steroid V87.45
      inhaled V87.44
      systemic V87.45
    thrombophlebitis V12.52
    thrombosis V12.51
      pulmonary V12.55
    tobacco use V15.82
    trophoblastic disease V13.1
      affecting management of pregnancy V23.1
    tuberculosis V12.01
    ulcer, peptic V12.71
    urinary system disorder V13.00
      calculi V13.01
      infection V13.02
      nephrotic syndrome V13.03
      specified NEC V13.09
HIT (heparin-induced thrombocytopenia) 289.84
HIV infection (disease) (illness)—*see* Human
  immunodeficiency virus (disease) (illness)
  (infection)
Hives (bold) (*see also* Urticaria) 708.9
Hoarseness 784.42
Hobnail liver —*see* Cirrhosis, portal
Hobo, hoboism V60.0
Hodgkin's
  disease (M9650/3) 201.9
    lymphocytic
      depletion (M9653/3) 201.7
        diffuse fibrosis (M9654/3) 201.7
        reticular type (M9655/3) 201.7
      predominance (M9651/3) 201.4
    lymphocytic-histiocytic predominance
      (M9651/3) 201.4
    mixed cellularity (M9652/3) 201.6
    nodular sclerosis (M9656/3) 201.5
      cellular phase (M9657/3) 201.5
    granuloma (M9661/3) 201.1
    lymphogranulomatosis (M9650/3) 201.9
    lymphoma (M9650/3) 201.9
    lymphosarcoma (M9650/3) 201.9
    paragranuloma (M9660/3) 201.0
    sarcoma (M9662/3) 201.2
Hodgson's disease (aneurysmal dilatation of
  aorta) 441.9
  ruptured 441.5
Hodi-potsy 111.0
Hoffa -(Kastert) disease or syndrome
  (liposynovitis prepatellaris) 272.8
Hoffmann's syndrome 244.9 *[359.5]*
Hoffmann-Bouveret syndrome (paroxysmal
  tachycardia) 427.2
Hole
  macula 362.54
  optic disc, crater-like 377.22
  retina (macula) 362.54
    round 361.31
      with detachment 361.01
Holla disease (*see also* Spherocytosis) 282.0
Holländer-Simons syndrome (progressive
  lipodystrophy) 272.6
Hollow foot (congenital) 754.71
  acquired 736.73
Holmes' syndrome (visual disorientation) 368.16
Holoprosencephaly 742.2
  due to
    trisomy 13 758.1
    trisomy 18 758.2

Holthouse's hernia —*see* Hernia, inguinal
Homesickness 309.89
Homicidal ideation V62.85
Homocystinemia 270.4
Homocystinuria 270.4
Homologous serum jaundice (prophylactic)
  (therapeutic)—*see* Hepatitis, viral
Homosexuality —*omit code*
  ego-dystonic 302.0
  pedophilic 302.2
  problems with 302.0
Homozygous Hb-S disease 282.61
Honeycomb lung 518.89
  congenital 748.4
Hong Kong ear 117.3
HOOD (hereditary osteo-onychodysplasia) 756.89
Hooded
  clitoris 752.49
  penis 752.69
Hookworm (anemia) (disease) (infestation)—*see*
  Ancylostomiasis
Hoppe-Goldflam syndrome 358.00
Hordeolum (external) (eyelid) 373.11
  internal 373.12
Horn
  cutaneous 702.8
    cheek 702.8
    eyelid 702.8
    penis 702.8
  iliac 756.89
  nail 703.8
    congenital 757.5
  papillary 700
Horner's
  syndrome (*see also* Neuropathy, peripheral,
    autonomic) 337.9
    traumatic 954.0
  teeth 520.4
Horseshoe kidney (congenital) 753.3
Horton's
  disease (temporal arteritis) 446.5
  headache or neuralgia 339.00
Hospice care V66.7
Hospitalism (in children) NEC 309.83
Hourglass contraction, contracture
  bladder 596.89
  gallbladder 575.2
    congenital 751.69
  stomach 536.8
    congenital 750.7
    psychogenic 306.4
  uterus 661.4
    affecting fetus or newborn 763.7
Household circumstance affecting care V60.9
  specified type NEC V60.89
Housemaid's knee 727.2
Housing circumstance affecting care V60.9
  specified type NEC V60.89
HTLV-I infection 079.51
HTLV-II infection 079.52
HTLV-III (disease) (illness) (infection)—*see*
  Human immunodeficiency virus (disease)
  (illness) (infection)
HTLV-III/LAV
  (disease) (illness) (infection)—*see* Human
    immunodeficiency virus (disease) (illness)
    (infection)

HTR (hemolytic transfusion reaction)
due to or resulting from
 incompatibility
  ABO 999.61
   acute 999.62
   delayed 999.63
  non-ABO antigen (minor) (Duffy) (Kell)
   (Kidd) (Lewis) (M) (N) (P) (S) 999.76
   acute 999.77
   delayed 999.78
  Rh antigen (C) (c) (D) (E) (e) 999.71
   acture 999.72
   delayed 999.73
Huchard's disease (continued arterial
 hypertension) 401.9
Hudson-Stähli lines 371.11
Huguier's disease (uterine fibroma) 218.9
Hum, venous —omit code
Human bite (open wound)—see also Wound,
 open, by site
 intact skin surface—see Contusion
Human immunodeficiency virus (disease)
 (illness) 042
 infection V08
  with symptoms, symptomatic 042
Human immunodeficiency virus-2 infection
 079.53
Human immunovirus (disease) (illness)
 (infection)—see Human immunodeficiency
 virus (disease) (illness) (infection)
Human papillomavirus 079.4
 high risk, DNA test positive
  anal 796.75
  cervical 795.05
  vaginal 795.15
 low risk, DNA test positive
  anal 796.79
  cervical 795.09
  vaginal 795.19
Human parovirus 079.83
Human T-cell lymphotrophic virus I infection
 079.51
Human T-cell lymphotrophic virus II infection
 079.52
Human T-cell lymphotropic virus-III (disease)
 (illness) (infection)—see Human
 immunodeficiency virus (disease) (illness)
 (infection)
Hungry bone syndrome 275.5
Humpback (acquired) 737.9
 congenital 756.19
Hunchback (acquired) 737.9
 congenital 756.19
Hunger 994.2
 air, psychogenic 306.1
 disease 251.1
Hunner's ulcer (see also Cystitis) 595.1
Hunt's
 neuralgia 053.11
 syndrome (herpetic geniculate ganglionitis)
  053.11
 dyssynergia cerebellaris myoclonica 334.2
Hunter's glossitis 529.4
Hunter (-Hurler) syndrome
 (mucopolysaccharidosis II) 277.5
Hunterian chancre 091.0
Huntington's
 chorea 333.4
 disease 333.4
Huppert's disease (multiple myeloma)
 (M9730/3) 203.0

Hurler (-Hunter) disease or syndrome
 (mucopolysaccharidosis II) 277.5
Hürthle cell
 adenocarcinoma (M8290/3) 193
 adenoma (M8290/0) 226
 carcinoma (M8290/3) 193
 tumor (M8290/0) 226
Hutchinson's
 disease meaning
  angioma serpiginosum 709.1
  cheiropompholyx 705.81
  prurigo estivalis 692.72
  summer eruption, or summer prurigo 692.72
 incisors 090.5
 melanotic freckle (M8742/2)—see also
  Neoplasm, skin, in situ
 malignant melanoma in (M8742/3)—see
  Melanoma
 teeth or incisors (congenital syphilis) 090.5
Hutchinson-Boeck disease or syndrome
 (sarcoidosis) 135
Hutchinson-Gilford disease or syndrome
 (progeria) 259.8
Hyaline
 degeneration (diffuse) (generalized) 728.9
  localized—see Degeneration, by site
 membrane (disease) (lung) (newborn) 769
Hyalinosis cutis et mucosae 272.8
Hyalin plaque, sclera, senile 379.16
Hyalitis (asteroid) 379.22
 syphilitic 095.8
Hydatid
 cyst or tumor—see also Echinococcus
  fallopian tube 752.11
 mole—see Hydatidiform mole
 Morgagni (congenital) 752.89
  fallopian tube 752.11
Hydatidiform mole (benign) (complicating
 pregnancy) (delivered) (undelivered) 630
 invasive (M9100/1) 236.1
 malignant (M9100/1) 236.1
 previous, affecting management of pregnancy
  V23.1
Hydatidosis —see Echinococcus
Hyde's disease (prurigo nodularis) 698.3
Hydradenitis 705.83
Hydradenoma (M8400/0)—see Hidradenoma
Hydralazine lupus or syndrome
 correct substance properly administered 695.4
 overdose or wrong substance given or taken
  972.6
Hydramnios 657
 affecting fetus or newborn 761.3
Hydrancephaly 742.3
 with spina bifida (see also Spina bifida) 741.0
Hydranencephaly 742.3
 with spina bifida (see also Spina bifida) 741.0
Hydrargyrism NEC 985.0
Hydrarthrosis (see also Effusion, joint) 719.0
 gonococcal 098.50
 intermittent (see also Rheumatism, palindromic)
  719.3
 of yaws (early) (late) 102.6
 syphilitic 095.8
  congenital 090.5
Hydremia 285.9
Hydrencephalocele (congenital) 742.0
Hydrencephalomeningocele (congenital) 742.0

Hydroa 694.0
  aestivale 692.72
  gestationis 646.8
  herpetiformis 694.0
  pruriginosa 694.0
  vacciniforme 692.72
Hydroadenitis 705.83
Hydrocalycosis (*see also* Hydronephrosis) 591
  congenital 753.29
Hydrocalyx (*see also* Hydronephrosis) 591
Hydrocele (calcified) (chylous) (idiopathic)
    (infantile) (inguinal canal) (recurrent) (senile)
    (spermatic cord) (testis) (tunica vaginalis) 603.9
  canal of Nuck (female) 629.1
    male 603.9
  congenital 778.6
  encysted 603.0
    congenital 778.6
  female NEC 629.89
  infected 603.1
  round ligament 629.89
  specified type NEC 603.8
    congenital 778.6
  spinalis (*see also* Spina bifida) 741.9
  vulva 624.8
Hydrocephalic fetus
  affecting management of pregnancy 655.0
  causing disproportion 653.6
    with obstructed labor 660.1
      affecting fetus or newborn 763.1
Hydrocephalus (acquired) (external) (internal)
    (malignant) (noncommunicating) (obstructive)
    (recurrent) 331.4
  aqueduct of Sylvius stricture 742.3
    with spina bifida (*see also* Spina bifida) 741.0
  chronic 742.3
    with spina bifida (*see also* Spina bifida) 741.0
  communicating 331.3
  congenital (external) (internal) 742.3
    with spina bifida (*see also* Spina bifida) 741.0
  due to
    stricture of aqueduct of Sylvius 742.3
      with spina bifida (*see also* Spina bifida)
        741.0
    toxoplasmosis (congenital) 771.2
  fetal affecting management of pregnancy 655.0
  foramen Magendie block (acquired) 331.3
    congenital 742.3
      with spina bifida (*see also* Spina bifida)
        741.0
  newborn 742.3
    with spina bifida (*see also* Spina bifida) 741.0
  normal pressure 331.5
    idiopathic (INPH) 331.5
    secondary 331.3
  otitic 348.2
  syphilitic, congenital 090.49
  tuberculous (*see also* Tuberculosis) 013.8
Hydrocolpos (congenital) 623.8
Hydrocystoma (M8404/0)—*see* Neoplasm, skin,
    benign
Hydroencephalocele (congenital) 742.0
Hydroencephalomeningocele (congenital) 742.0
Hydrohematopneumothorax (*see also*
    Hemothorax) 511.89
Hydromeningitis —*see* Meningitis
Hydromeningocele (spinal) (*see also* Spina
    bifida) 741.9
  cranial 742.0
Hydrometra 621.8
Hydrometrocolpos 623.8

Hydromicrocephaly 742.1
Hydromphalus (congenital) (since birth) 757.39
Hydromyelia 742.53
Hydromyelocele (*see also* Spina bifida) 741.9
Hydronephrosis 591
  atrophic 591
  congenital 753.29
  due to S. hematobium 120.0
  early 591
  functionless (infected) 591
  infected 591
  intermittent 591
  primary 591
  secondary 591
  tuberculous (*see also* Tuberculosis) 016.0
Hydropericarditis (*see also* Pericarditis) 423.9
Hydropericardium (*see also* Pericarditis) 423.9
Hydroperitoneum 789.59
Hydrophobia 071
Hydrophthalmos (*see also* Buphthalmia) 743.20
Hydropneumohemothorax (*see also*
    Hemothorax) 511.89
Hydropneumopericarditis (*see also* Pericarditis)
    423.9
Hydropneumopericardium (*see also*
    Pericarditis) 423.9
Hydropneumothorax 511.89
  nontuberculous 511.89
    bacterial 511.1
  pneumococcal 511.1
  staphylococcal 511.1
  streptococcal 511.1
  traumatic 860.0
    with open wound into thorax 860.1
  tuberculous (*see also* Tuberculosis, pleural) 012.0
Hydrops 782.3
  abdominis 789.59
  amnii (complicating pregnancy) (*see also*
    Hydramnios) 657
  articulorum intermittens (*see also* Rheumatism,
    palindromic) 719.3
  cardiac (*see also* Failure, heart) 428.0
  congenital—*see* Hydrops, fetalis
  endolymphatic (*see also* Disease, Ménière's)
    386.00
  fetal, fetalis or newborn 778.0
    due to
      alpha thalassemia 282.43
      isoimmunization 773.3
    not due to isoimmunization 778.0
  gallbladder 575.3
  idiopathic (fetus or newborn) 778.0
  joint (*see also* Effusion, joint) 719.0
  labyrinth (*see also* Disease, Ménière's) 386.00
  meningeal NEC 331.4
  nutritional 262
  pericardium—*see* Pericarditis
  pleura (*see also* Hydrothorax) 511.89
  renal (*see also* Nephrosis) 581.9
  spermatic cord (*see also* Hydrocele) 603.9
Hydropyonephrosis (*see also* Pyelitis) 590.80
  chronic 590.00
Hydrorachis 742.53
Hydrorrhea (nasal) 478.19
  gravidarum 658.1
  pregnancy 658.1
Hydrosadenitis 705.83
Hydrosalpinx (fallopian tube) (follicularis) 614.1

Hydrothorax (double) (pleural) 511.89
  chylous (nonfilarial) 457.8
    filaria (*see also* Infestation, filarial) 125.9
  nontuberculous 511.89
    bacterial 511.1
  pneumococcal 511.1
  staphylococcal 511.1
  streptococcal 511.1
  traumatic 862.29
    with open wound into thorax 862.39
  tuberculous (*see also* Tuberculosis, pleura) 012.0
Hydroureter 593.5
  congenital 753.22
Hydroureteronephrosis (*see also*
  Hydronephrosis) 591
Hydrourethra 599.84
Hydroxykynureninuria 270.2
Hydroxyprolinemia 270.8
Hydroxyprolinuria 270.8
Hygroma (congenital) (cystic) (M9173/0) 228.1
  prepatellar 727.3
  subdural—*see* Hematoma, subdural
Hymen —*see* condition
Hymenolepiasis (diminuta) (infection)
  (infestation) (nana) 123.6
Hymenolepis (diminuta) (infection) (infestation)
  (nana) 123.6
Hypalgesia (*see also* Disturbance, sensation)
  782.0
Hyperabduction syndrome 447.8
Hyperacidity, gastric 536.8
  psychogenic 306.4
Hyperactive, hyperactivity 314.01
  basal cell, uterine cervix 622.10
  bladder 596.51
  bowel (syndrome) 564.9
    sounds 787.5
  cervix epithelial (basal) 622.10
  child 314.01
  colon 564.9
  gastrointestinal 536.8
    psychogenic 306.4
  intestine 564.9
  labyrinth (unilateral) 386.51
    with loss of labyrinthine reactivity 386.58
    bilateral 386.52
  nasal mucous membrane 478.19
  stomach 536.8
  thyroid (gland) (*see also* Thyrotoxicosis) 242.9
Hyperacusis 388.42
Hyperadrenalism (cortical) 255.3
  medullary 255.6
Hyperadrenocorticism 255.3
  congenital 255.2
  iatrogenic
    correct substance properly administered 255.3
    overdose or wrong substance given or taken 962.0
Hyperaffectivity 301.11
Hyperaldosteronism (atypical) (hyperplastic)
  (normoaldosteronal) (normotensive) (primary)
  255.10
  secondary 255.14
Hyperalgesia (*see also* Disturbance, sensation)
  782.0
Hyperalimentation 783.6
  carotene 278.3
  specified NEC 278.8
  vitamin A 278.2
  vitamin D 278.4

Hyperaminoaciduria 270.9
  arginine 270.6
  citrulline 270.6
  cystine 270.0
  glycine 270.0
  lysine 270.7
  ornithine 270.6
  renal (types I, II, III) 270.0
Hyperammonemia (congenital) 270.6
Hyperamnesia 780.99
Hyperamylasemia 790.5
Hyperaphia 782.0
Hyperazotemia 791.9
Hyperbetalipoproteinemia (acquired) (essential)
  (familial) (hereditary) (primary) (secondary)
  272.0
  with pre-betalipoproteinemia 272.2
Hyperbilirubinemia 782.4
  congenital 277.4
  constitutional 277.4
  neonatal (transient) (*see also* Jaundice, fetus or
    newborn) 774.6
  of prematurity 774.2
Hyperbilirubinemica encephalopathia,
  newborn 774.7
  due to isoimmunization 773.4
Hypercalcemia, hypercalcemic (idiopathic) 275.42
  nephropathy 588.89
Hypercalcinuria 275.40
Hypercapnia 786.09
  with mixed acid-base disorder 276.4
  fetal, affecting newborn 770.89
Hypercarotinemia 278.3
Hypercementosis 521.5
Hyperchloremia 276.9
Hyperchlorhydria 536.8
  neurotic 306.4
  psychogenic 306.4
Hypercholesterinemia —*see*
  Hypercholesterolemia
Hypercholesterolemia 272.0
  with hyperglyceridemia, endogenous 272.2
  essential 272.0
  familial 272.0
  hereditary 272.0
  primary 272.0
  pure 272.0
Hypercholesterolosis 272.0
Hyperchylia gastricsa 536.8
  psychogenic 306.4
Hyperchylomicronemia (familial) (with
  hyperbetalipoproteinemia) 272.3
Hypercoagulation syndrome (primary) 289.81
  secondary 289.82
Hypercorticosteronism
  correct substance properly administered 255.3
  overdose or wrong substance given or taken
    962.0
Hypercortisonism
  correct substance properly administered 255.3
  overdose or wrong substance given or taken
    962.0
Hyperdynamic beta-adrenergic state or
  syndrome (circulatory) 429.82
Hyperekplexia 759.89
Hyperelectrolytemia 276.9

Hyperemesis 536.2
arising during pregnancy—*see* Hyperemesis, gravidarum
gravidarum (mild) (before 22 completed weeks gestation) 643.0
with
carbohydrate depletion 643.1
dehydration 643.1
electrolyte imbalance 643.1
metabolic disturbance 643.1
affecting fetus or newborn 761.8
severe (with metabolic disturbance) 643.1
psychogenic 306.4
Hyperemia (acute) 780.99
anal mucosa 569.49
bladder 596.7
cerebral 437.8
conjunctiva 372.71
ear, internal, acute 386.30
enteric 564.89
eye 372.71
eyelid (active) (passive) 374.82
intestine 564.89
iris 364.41
kidney 593.81
labyrinth 386.30
liver (active) (passive) 573.8
lung 514
ovary 620.8
passive 780.99
pulmonary 514
renal 593.81
retina 362.89
spleen 289.59
stomach 537.89
Hyperesthesia (body surface) (*see also* Disturbance, sensation) 782.0
larynx (reflex) 478.79
hysterical 300.11
pharynx (reflex) 478.29
Hyperestrinism 256.0
Hyperestrogenism 256.0
Hyperestrogenosis 256.0
Hyperexplexia 759.89
Hyperextension, joint 718.80
ankle 718.87
elbow 718.82
foot 718.87
hand 718.84
hip 718.85
knee 718.86
multiple sites 718.89
pelvic region 718.85
shoulder (region) 718.81
specified site NEC 718.88
wrist 718.83
Hyperfibrinolysis —*see* Fibrinolysis
Hyperfolliculinism 256.0
Hyperfructosemia 271.2
Hyperfunction
adrenal (cortex) 255.3
androgenic, acquired benign 255.3
medulla 255.6
virilism 255.2
corticoadrenal NEC 255.3
labyrinth—*see* Hyperactive, labyrinth
medulloadrenal 255.6
ovary 256.1
estrogen 256.0
pancreas 577.8
parathyroid (gland) 252.00

Hyperfunction—*continued*
pituitary (anterior) (gland) (lobe) 253.1
testicular 257.0
Hypergammaglobulinemia 289.89
monoclonal, benign (BMH) 273.1
polyclonal 273.0
Waldenström's 273.0
Hyperglobulinemia 273.8
Hyperglycemia 790.29
maternal
affecting fetus or newborn 775.0
manifest diabetes in infant 775.1
postpancreatectomy (complete) (partial) 251.3
Hyperglyceridemia 272.1
endogenous 272.1
essential 272.1
familial 272.1
hereditary 272.1
mixed 272.3
pure 272.1
Hyperglycinemia 270.7
Hypergonadism
ovarian 256.1
testicular (infantile) (primary) 257.0
Hyperheparinemia (*see also* Circulating, intrinsic anticoagulants) 287.5
Hyperhidrosis, hyperidrosis 705.21
axilla 705.21
face 705.21
focal (localized) 705.21
primary 705.21
axilla 705.21
face 705.21
palms 705.21
soles 705.21
secondary 705.22
axilla 705.22
face 705.22
palms 705.22
soles 705.22
generalized 780.8
palms 705.21
psychogenic 306.3
secondary 780.8
soles 705.21
Hyperhistidinemia 270.5
Hyperinsulinism (ectopic) (functional) (organic) NEC 251.1
iatrogenic 251.0
reactive 251.2
spontaneous 251.2
therapeutic misadventure (from administration of insulin) 962.3
Hyperiodemia 276.9
Hyperirritability (cerebral), in newborn 779.1
Hyperkalemia 276.7
Hyperkeratosis (*see also* Keratosis) 701.1
cervix 622.2
congenital 757.39
cornea 371.89
due to yaws (early) (late) (palmar or plantar) 102.3
eccentrica 757.39
figurata centrifuga atrophica 757.39
follicularis 757.39
in cutem penetrans 701.1
limbic (cornea) 371.89
palmoplantaris climacterica 701.1
pinta (carate) 103.1
senile (with pruritus) 702.0
tongue 528.79
universalis congenita 757.1

Hyperkeratosis—*continued*
vagina 623.1
vocal cord 478.5
vulva 624.09
Hyperkinesia, hyperkinetic (disease) (reaction)
   (syndrome) 314.9
with
   attention deficit —*see* Disorder, attention deficit
   conduct disorder 314.2
   developmental delay 314.1
   simple disturbance of activity and attention
      314.01
   specified manifestation NEC 314.8
heart (disease) 429.82
of childhood or adolescence NEC 314.9
Hyperlacrimation (*see also* Epiphora) 375.20
Hyperlipemia (*see also* Hyperlipidemia) 272.4
Hyperlipidemia 272.4
carbohydrate-induced 272.1
combined 272.2
endogenous 272.1
exogenous 272.3
fat-induced 272.3
group
   A 272.0
   B 272.1
   C 272.2
   D 272.3
mixed 272.2
specified type NEC 272.4
Hyperlipidosis 272.7
hereditary 272.7
Hyperlipoproteinemia (acquired) (essential)
   (familial) (hereditary) (primary) (secondary)
   272.4
Fredrickson type
   I 272.3
   IIa 272.0
   IIb 272.2
   III 272.2
   IV 272.1
   V 272.3
low-density-lipoid-type (LDL) 272.0
very-low-density-lipoid-type [VLDL] 272.1
Hyperlucent lung, unilateral 492.8
Hyperluteinization 256.1
Hyperlysinemia 270.7
Hypermagnesemia 275.2
neonatal 775.5
Hypermaturity (fetus or newborn)
post-term infant 766.21
prolonged gestation infant 766.22
Hypermenorrhea 626.2
Hypermetabolism 794.7
Hypermethioninemia 270.4
Hypermetropia (congenital) 367.0
Hypermobility
cecum 564.9
coccyx 724.71
colon 564.9
   psychogenic 306.4
ileum 564.89
joint (acquired) 718.80
   ankle 718.87
   elbow 718.82
   foot 718.87
   hand 718.84
   hip 718.85
   knee 718.86
   multiple sites 718.89

Hypermobility—*continued*
pelvic region 718.85
shoulder (region) 718.81
specified site NEC 718.88
wrist 718.83
kidney, congenital 753.3
meniscus (knee) 717.5
scapula 718.81
stomach 536.8
   psychogenic 306.4
syndrome 728.5
testis, congenital 752.52
urethral 599.81
Hypermotility
gastrointestinal 536.8
intestine 564.9
   psychogenic 306.4
stomach 536.8
Hypernasality 784.43
Hypernatremia 276.0
with water depletion 276.0
Hypernephroma (M8312/3) 189.0
Hyperopia 367.0
Hyperorexia 783.6
Hyperornithinemia 270.6
Hyperosmia (*see also* Disturbance, sensation)
   781.1
Hyperosmolality 276.0
Hyperosteogenesis 733.99
Hyperostosis 733.99
calvarial 733.3
cortical 733.3
   infantile 756.59
frontal, internal of skull 733.3
interna frontalis 733.3
monomelic 733.99
skull 733.3
   congenital 756.0
vertebral 721.8
   with spondylosis—*see* Spondylosis
   ankylosing 721.6
Hyperovarianism 256.1
Hyperovarism, hyperovaria 256.1
Hyperoxaluria (primary) 271.8
Hyperoxia 987.8
Hyperparathyroidism 252.00
ectopic 259.3
other 252.08
primary 252.01
secondary (of renal origin) 588.81
   non-renal 252.02
tertiary 252.08
Hyperpathia (*see also* Disturbance, sensation)
   782.0
psychogenic 307.80
Hyperperistalsis 787.4
psychogenic 306.4
Hyperpermeability, capillary 448.9
Hyperphagia 783.6
Hyperphenylalaninemia 270.1
Hyperphoria 378.40
alternating 378.45
Hyperphosphatemia 275.3
Hyperpiesia (*see also* Hypertension) 401.9
Hyperpiesis (*see also* Hypertension) 401.9
Hyperpigmentation —*see* Pigmentation
Hyperpinealism 259.8
Hyperpipecolatemia 270.7
Hyperpituitarism 253.1

Hyperplasia, hyperplastic
adenoids (lymphoid tissue) 474.12
  and tonsils 474.10
adrenal (capsule) (cortex) (gland) 255.8
  with
    sexual precocity (male) 255.2
    virilism, adrenal 255.2
    virilization (female) 255.2
  congenital 255.2
  due to excess ACTH (ectopic) (pituitary) 255.0
  medulla 255.8
alpha cells (pancreatic)
  with
    gastrin excess 251.5
    glucagon excess 251.4
angiolymphoid, with eosinophilia (ALHE)
    228.01
appendix (lymphoid) 543.0
artery, fibromuscular NEC 447.8
  carotid 447.8
  renal 447.3
bone 733.99
  marrow 289.9
breast (*see also* Hypertrophy, breast) 611.1
  ductal 610.8
    atypical 610.8
carotid artery 447.8
cementation, cementum (teeth) (tooth) 521.5
cervical gland 785.6
cervix (uteri) 622.10
  basal cell 622.10
  congenital 752.49
  endometrium 622.10
  polypoid 622.10
chin 524.05
clitoris, congenital 752.49
dentin 521.5
endocervicitis 616.0
endometrium, endometrial (adenomatous)
    (atypical) (cystic) (glandular) (polypoid)
    (uterus) 621.30
  with atypia 621.33
  without atypia
    complex 621.32
    simple 621.31
  benign 621.34
  cervix 622.10
epithelial 709.8
  focal, oral, including tongue 528.79
  mouth (focal) 528.79
  nipple 611.89
  skin 709.8
  tongue (focal) 528.79
  vaginal wall 623.0
erythroid 289.9
fascialis ossificans (progressiva) 728.11
fibromuscular, artery NEC 447.8
  carotid 447.8
  renal 447.3
genital
  female 629.89
  male 608.89
gingiva 523.8
glandularis
  cystica uteri 621.30
  endometrium (uterus) 621.30
  interstitialis uteri 621.30
granulocytic 288.69
gum 523.8
hymen, congenital 752.49
islands of Langerhans 251.1

Hyperplasia, hyperplastic—*continued*
islet cell (pancreatic) 251.9
  alpha cells
    with excess
      gastrin 251.5
      glucagon 251.4
  beta cells 251.1
juxtaglomerular (complex) (kidney) 593.89
kidney (congenital) 753.3
liver (congenital) 751.69
lymph node (gland) 785.6
lymphoid (diffuse) (nodular) 785.6
  appendix 543.0
  intestine 569.89
mandibular 524.02
  alveolar 524.72
  unilateral condylar 526.89
Marchand multiple nodular (liver)—*see*
    Cirrhosis, postnecrotic
maxillary 524.01
  alveolar 524.71
medulla, adrenal 255.8
myometrium, myometrial 621.2
neuroendocrine cell, of infancy 516.61
nose (lymphoid) (polypoid) 478.19
oral soft tissue (inflammatory) (irritative)
    (mucosa) NEC 528.9
  gingiva 523.8
  tongue 529.8
organ or site, congenital NEC—*see* Anomaly,
    specified type NEC
ovary 620.8
palate, papillary 528.9
pancreatic islet cells 251.9
  alpha
    with excess
      gastrin 251.5
      glucagon 251.4
  beta 251.1
parathyroid (gland) 252.01
persistent, vitreous (primary) 743.51
pharynx (lymphoid) 478.29
prostate 600.90
  with
    other lower urinary tract symptoms (LUTS)
      600.91
    urinary
      obstruction 600.91
      retention 600.91
  adenofibromatous 600.20
    with
      other lower urinary tract symptoms
        (LUTS) 600.21
      urinary
        obstruction 600.21
        retention 600.21
  nodular 600.10
    with
      urinary
        obstruction 600.11
        retention 600.11
renal artery (fibromuscular) 447.3
reticuloendothelial (cell) 289.9
salivary gland (any) 527.1
Schimmelbusch's 610.1
suprarenal (capsule) (gland) 255.8
thymus (gland) (persistent) 254.0
thyroid (*see also* Goiter) 240.9
  primary 242.0
  secondary 242.2

Hyperplasia, hyperplastic—*continued*
  tonsil (lymphoid tissue) 474.11
    and adenoids 474.10
  urethrovaginal 599.89
  uterus, uterine (myometrium) 621.2
    endometrium (*see also* Hyperplasia,
      endometrium) 621.30
  vitreous (humor), primary persistent 743.51
  vulva 624.3
  zygoma 738.11
Hyperpnea (*see also* Hyperventilation) 786.01
Hyperpotassemia 276.7
Hyperprebetalipoproteinemia 272.1
  with chylomicronemia 272.3
  familial 272.1
Hyperprolactinemia 253.1
Hyperprolinemia 270.8
Hyperproteinemia 273.8
Hyperprothrombinemia 289.89
Hyperpselaphesia 782.0
Hyperpyrexia 780.60
  heat (effects of) 992.0
  malarial (*see also* Malaria) 084.6
  malignant, due to anesthetic 995.86
  rheumatic—*see* Fever, rheumatic
  unknown origin (*see also* Pyrexia) 780.60
Hyperreactor, vascular 780.2
Hyperreflexia 796.1
  bladder, autonomic 596.54
    with cauda equina 344.61
  detrusor 344.61
Hypersalivation (*see also* Ptyalism) 527.7
Hypersarcosinemia 270.8
Hypersecretion
  ACTH 255.3
  androgens (ovarian) 256.1
  calcitonin 246.0
  corticoadrenal 255.3
  cortisol 255.0
  estrogen 256.0
  gastric 536.8
    psychogenic 306.4
  gastrin 251.5
  glucagon 251.4
  hormone
    ACTH 255.3
    anterior pituitary 253.1
    growth NEC 253.0
    ovarian androgen 256.1
    testicular 257.0
    thyroid stimulating 242.8
  insulin—*see* Hyperinsulinism
  lacrimal glands (*see also* Epiphora) 375.20
  medulloadrenal 255.6
  milk 676.6
  ovarian androgens 256.1
  pituitary (anterior) 253.1
  salivary gland (any) 527.7
  testicular hormones 257.0
  thyrocalcitonin 246.0
  upper respiratory 478.9
Hypersegmentation, hereditary 288.2
  eosinophils 288.2
  neutrophil nuclei 288.2
Hypersensitive, hypersensitiveness,
  hypersensitivity —*see also* Allergy
  angiitis 446.20
    specified NEC 446.29
  carotid sinus 337.01
  colon 564.9
    psychogenic 306.4

Hypersensitive, hypersensitivity—*continued*
  DNA (deoxyribonucleic acid) NEC 287.2
  drug (*see also* Allergy, drug) 995.27
    due to correct medicinal substance properly
      administered 995.27
  esophagus 530.89
  insect bites—*see* Injury, superficial, by site
  labyrinth 386.58
  pain (*see also* Disturbance, sensation) 782.0
  pneumonitis NEC 495.9
  reaction (*see also* Allergy) 995.3
    upper respiratory tract NEC 478.8
  stomach (allergic) (nonallergic) 536.8
    psychogenic 306.4
Hypersomatotropism (classic) 253.0
Hypersomnia, unspecified 780.54
  with sleep apnea, unspecified 780.53
  alcohol induced 291.82
  drug induced 291.85
  due to
    medical condition classified elsewhere 327.14
    mental disorder 327.15
  idiopathic
    with long sleep time 327.11
    without long sleep time 327.12
  menstrual related 327.13
  nonorganic origin 307.43
    persistent (primary) 307.44
    transient 307.43
  organic 327.10
  other 327.19
  primary 307.44
  recurrent 327.13
Hypersplenia 289.4
Hypersplenism 289.4
Hypersteatosis 706.3
Hyperstimulation, ovarian 256.1
Hypersuprarenalism 255.3
Hypersusceptibility —*see* Allergy
Hyper-TBG-nemia 246.8
Hypertelorism 756.0
  orbit, orbital 376.41

       "H" listing resumes after
       Hypertension table...

Hypertension, hypertensive

	Malignant	Benign	Unspecified
(arterial) (arteriolar) (crisis) (degeneration) (disease) (essential) (fluctuating) (idiopathic) (intermittent) (labile) (low renin) (orthostatic) (paroxysmal) (primary) (systemic) (uncontrolled) (vascular)	401.0	401.1	401.9
with			
chronic kidney disease			
stage I through stage IV, or unspecified	403.00	403.10	403.90
stage V or end stage renal disease	403.01	403.11	403.91
heart involvement (conditions classifiable to 429.0-429.3, 429.8, 429.9 due to hypertension) (*see also* Hypertension, heart)	402.00	402.10	402.90
with kidney involvement—*see* Hypertension, cardiorenal			
renal (kidney) involvement (only conditions classifiable to 585, 587) (excludes conditions classifiable to 584) (*see also* Hypertension, kidney)	403.00	403.10	403.90
with heart involvement—*see* Hypertension, cardiorenal			
failure (and sclerosis) (*see also* Hypertension, kidney) . .	403.01	403.11	403.91
sclerosis without failure (*see also* Hypertension, kidney) .	403.00	403.10	403.90
accelerated (*see also* Hypertension, by type, malignant)	401.0	—	—
antepartum—*see* Hypertension complicating pregnancy, childbirth, or the puerperium			
borderline	—	—	796.2
cardiorenal (disease)	404.00	404.10	404.90
with			
chronic kidney disease			
stage I through stage IV, or unspecified	404.00	404.10	404.90
and heart failure	404.01	404.11	404.91
stage V or end stage renal disease	404.02	404.12	404.92
and heart failure	404.03	404.13	404.93
heart failure.	404.01	404.11	404.91
and chronic kidney disease.	404.01	404.11	404.91
stage I through stage IV or unspecified	404.01	404.11	404.91
stage V or end stage renal disease.	404.03	404.13	404.93
cardiovascular disease (arteriosclerotic) (sclerotic)	402.00	402.10	402.90
with			
heart failure	402.01	402.11	402.91
renal involvement (conditions classifiable to 403) (*see also* Hypertension, cardiorenal)	404.00	404.10	404.90
cardiovascular renal (disease) (sclerosis) (*see also* Hypertension cardiorenal)	404.00	404.10	404.90
cerebrovascular disease NEC	437.2	437.2	437.2
complicating pregnancy, childbirth, or the puerperium	642.2	642.0	642.9
with			
albuminuria (and edema) (mild)	—	—	642.4
severe	—	—	642.5
chronic kidney disease	642.2	642.2	642.2
and heart disease	642.2	642.2	642.2
edema (mild)	—	—	642.4
severe	—	—	642.5
heart disease	642.2	642.2	642.2
and chronic kidney disease.	642.2	642.2	642.2
renal disease	642.2	642.2	642.2
and heart disease	642.2	642.2	642.2
chronic	642.2	642.0	642.0
with pre-eclampsia or eclampsia	642.7	642.7	642.7
fetus or newborn	760.0	760.0	760.0
essential.	—	642.0	642.0
with pre-eclampsia or eclampsia	—	642.7	642.7
fetus or newborn	760.0	760.0	760.0
fetus or newborn	760.0	760.0	760.0
gestational	—	—	642.3
pre-existing	642.2	642.0	642.0
with pre-eclampsia or eclampsia	642.7	642.7	642.7
fetus or newborn	760.0	760.0	760.0
secondary to renal disease	642.1	642.1	642.1
with pre-eclampsia or eclampsia	642.7	642.7	642.7
fetus or newborn	760.0	760.0	760.0
transient.	—	—	642.3
due to			
aldosteronism, primary	405.09	405.19	405.99
brain tumor.	405.09	405.19	405.99
bulbar poliomyelitis	405.09	405.19	405.99
calculus			
kidney	405.09	405.19	405.99
ureter.	405.09	405.19	405.99
coarctation, aorta	405.09	405.19	405.99
Cushing's disease	405.09	405.19	405.99

	Malignant	Benign	Unspecified
glomerulosclerosis (*see also* Hypertension, kidney)	403.00	403.10	403.90
periarteritis nodosa	405.09	405.19	405.99
pheochromocytoma	405.09	405.19	405.99
polycystic kidney(s)	405.09	405.19	405.99
polycythemia	405.09	405.19	405.99
porphyria	405.09	405.19	405.99
pyelonephritis	405.09	405.19	405.99
renal (artery)			
aneurysm	405.01	405.11	405.91
anomaly	405.01	405.11	405.91
embolism	405.01	405.11	405.91
fibromuscular hyperplasia	405.01	405.11	405.91
occlusion	405.01	405.11	405.91
stenosis	405.01	405.11	405.91
thrombosis	405.01	405.11	405.91
encephalopathy	437.2	437.2	437.2
gestational (transient) NEC	—	—	642.3
Goldblatt's	440.1	440.1	440.1
heart (disease) (conditions classifiable to 429.0-429.3, 429.8,			
429.9 due to hypertension)	402.00	402.10	402.90
with			
heart failure	402.01	402.11	402.91
hypertensive kidney disease (conditions classifiable to 403) (*see*			
also Hypertension, cardiorenal)	404.00	404.10	404.90
renal sclerosis (*see also* Hypertension, cardiorenal)	404.00	404.10	404.90
intracranial, benign	—	348.2	—
intraocular	—	—	365.04
kidney	403.00	403.10	403.90
with			
chronic kidney disease			
stage I through stage IV, or unspecified	403.00	403.10	403.90
stage V or end stage renal disease	403.01	403.11	403.91
heart involvement (conditions classifiable to 429.0-429.3,			
429.8, 429.9 due to hypertension) (*see also*			
Hypertension cardiorenal)	404.00	404.10	404.90
hypertensive heart (disease) (conditions classifiable to 402)			
(*see also* Hypertension, cardiorenal)	404.00	404.10	404.90
lesser circulation	—	—	416.0
necrotizing	401.0	—	—
ocular	—	—	365.04
pancreatic duct—code to underlying condition			
with chronic pancreatitis	—	—	577.1
portal (due to chronic liver disease)	—	—	572.3
postoperative	—	—	997.91
psychogenic	—	—	306.2
puerperal, postpartum—*see* Hypertension, complicating			
pregnancy, childbirth, or the puerperium			
pulmonary (artery) (secondary)	—	—	416.8
idiopathic	—	—	416.0
primary	—	—	416.0
of newborn	—	—	747.83
with			
cor pulmonale (chronic)	—	—	416.8
acute	—	—	415.0
right heart ventricular strain/failure	—	—	416.8
acute	—	—	415.0
secondary	—	—	416.8
renal (disease) (*see also* Hypertension, kidney)	403.00	403.10	403.90
renovascular NEC	405.01	405.11	405.91
secondary NEC	405.09	405.19	405.99
due to			
aldosteronism, primary	405.09	405.19	405.99
brain tumor	405.09	405.19	405.99
bulbar poliomyelitis	405.09	405.19	405.99
calculus			
kidney	405.09	405.19	405.99
ureter	405.09	405.19	405.99
coarctation, aorta	405.09	405.19	405.99
Cushing's disease	405.09	405.19	405.99
glomerulosclerosis (*see also* Hypertension, kidney)	403.00	403.10	403.90
periarteritis nodosa	405.09	405.19	405.99
pheochromocytoma	405.09	405.19	405.99
polycystic kidney(s)	405.09	405.19	405.99
polycythemia	405.09	405.19	405.99
porphyria	405.09	405.19	405.99
pyelonephritis	405.09	405.19	405.99
renal (artery)			
aneurysm	405.01	405.11	405.91
anomaly	405.01	405.11	405.91

	Malignant	Benign	Unspecified
embolism.	405.01	405.11	405.91
fibromuscular hyperplasia	405.01	405.11	405.91
occlusion	405.01	405.11	405.91
stenosis.	405.01	405.11	405.91
thrombosis	405.01	405.11	405.91
transient	—	—	796.2
of pregnancy	—	—	642.3
venous, chronic (asymptomatic) (idiopathic)	—	—	459.30
with			
complication, NEC	—	—	459.39
due to			
deep vein thrombosis (*see also* Syndrome, postphlebetic) .	—	—	459.10
inflammation	—	—	459.32
with ulcer.	—	—	459.33
ulcer.	—	—	459.31
with inflammation	—	—	459.33

Hypertensive urgency —*see* Hypertension
Hyperthecosis, ovary 256.8
Hyperthermia (of unknown origin) (*see also* Pyrexia) 780.60
  malignant (due to anesthesia) 995.86
  newborn 778.4
Hyperthymergasia (*see also* Psychosis, affective) 296.0
  reactive (from emotional stress, psychological trauma) 298.1
  recurrent episode 296.1
  single episode 296.0
Hyperthymism 254.8
Hyperthyroid (recurrent)—*see* Hyperthyroidism
Hyperthyroidism (latent) (preadult) (recurrent) (without goiter) 242.9

> *Note—Use the following fifth-digit subclassification with category 242:*
>
> *0 without mention of thyrotoxic crisis or storm*
> *1 with mention of thyrotoxic crisis or storm*

  with
    goiter (diffuse) 242.0
      adenomatous 242.3
        multinodular 242.2
        uninodular 242.1
      nodular 242.3
        multinodular 242.2
        uninodular 242.1
      thyroid nodule 242.1
    complicating pregnancy, childbirth, or puerperium 648.1
    neonatal (transient) 775.3
Hypertonia —Hypertonicity
Hypertonicity
  bladder 596.51
  fetus or newborn 779.89
  gastrointestinal (tract) 536.8
  infancy 779.89
    due to electrolyte imbalance 779.89
  muscle 728.85
  stomach 536.8
    psychogenic 306.4
  uterus, uterine (contractions) 661.4
    affecting fetus or newborn 763.7
Hypertony —*see* Hypertonicity
Hypertransaminemia 790.4
Hypertrichosis 704.1
  congenital 757.4
  eyelid 374.54
  lanuginosa 757.4
    acquired 704.1
Hypertriglyceridemia, essential 272.1
Hypertrophy, hypertrophic
  adenoids (infectional) 474.12
    and tonsils (faucial) (infective) (lingual) (lymphoid) 474.10
  adrenal 255.8
  alveolar process or ridge 525.8
  anal papillae 569.49
  apocrine gland 705.82
  artery NEC 447.8
    carotid 447.8
    congenital (peripheral) NEC 747.60
    gastrointestinal 747.61
    lower limb 747.64
    renal 747.62
    specified NEC 747.69
    spinal 747.82

Hypertrophy, hypertrophic—*continued*
  arthritis (chronic) (*see also* Osteoarthrosis) 715.9
    spine (*see also* Spondylosis) 721.90
  arytenoid 478.79
  asymmetrical (heart) 429.9
  auricular—*see* Hypertrophy, cardiac
  Bartholin's gland 624.8
  bile duct 576.8
  bladder (sphincter) (trigone) 596.89
  blind spot, visual field 368.42
  bone 733.99
  brain 348.89
  breast 611.1
    cystic 610.1
    fetus or newborn 778.7
    fibrocystic 610.1
    massive pubertal 611.1
    puerperal, postpartum 676.3
    senile (parenchymatous) 611.1
  cardiac (chronic) (idiopathic) 429.3
    with
      rheumatic fever (conditions classifiable to 390)
        active 391.8
          with chorea 392.0
        inactive or quiescent (with chorea) 398.99
    congenital NEC 746.89
    fatty (*see also* Degeneration, myocardial) 429.1
    hypertensive (*see also* Hypertension, heart) 402.90
    rheumatic (with chorea) 398.99
      active or acute 391.8
        with chorea 392.0
    valve (*see also* Endocarditis) 424.90
      congenital NEC 746.89
  cartilage 733.99
  cecum 569.89
  cervix (uteri) 622.6
    congenital 752.49
    elongation 622.6
  clitoris (cirrhotic) 624.2
    congenital 752.49
  colon 569.89
    congenital 751.3
  conjunctiva, lymphoid 372.73
  cornea 371.89
  corpora cavernosa 607.89
  duodenum 537.89
  endometrium (uterus) (*see also* Hyperplasia, endometrium) 621.30
    cervix 622.6
  epididymis 608.89
  esophageal hiatus (congenital) 756.6
    with hernia—*see* Hernia, diaphragm
  eyelid 374.30
  falx, skull 733.99
  fat pad 729.30
    infrapatellar 729.31
    knee 729.31
    orbital 374.34
    popliteal 729.31
    prepatellar 729.31
    retropatellar 729.31
    specified site NEC 729.39
  foot (congenital) 755.67
  frenum, frenulum (tongue) 529.8
    linguae 529.8
    lip 528.5
  gallbladder or cystic duct 575.8
  gastric mucosa 535.2

Hypertrophy, hypertrophic—*continued*
gingiva 523.8
gland, glandular (general) NEC 785.6
gum (mucous membrane) 523.8
heart (idiopathic)—*see also* Hypertrophy,
  cardiac
  valve—*see also* Endocarditis
  congenital NEC 746.89
hemifacial 754.0
hepatic—*see* Hypertrophy, liver
hiatus (esophageal) 756.6
hilus gland 785.6
hymen, congenital 752.49
ileum 569.89
infrapatellar fat pad 729.31
intestine 569.89
jejunum 569.89
kidney (compensatory) 593.1
  congenital 753.3
labial frenulum 528.5
labium (majus) (minus) 624.3
lacrimal gland, chronic 375.03
ligament 728.9
  spinal 724.8
linguae frenulum 529.8
lingual tonsil (infectional) 474.11
lip (frenum) 528.5
  congenital 744.81
liver 789.1
  acute 573.8
  cirrhotic—*see* Cirrhosis, liver
  congenital 751.69
  fatty—*see* Fatty, liver
lymph gland 785.6
  tuberculous—*see* Tuberculosis, lymph gland
mammary gland—*see* Hypertrophy, breast
maxillary frenulum 528.5
Meckel's diverticulum (congenital) 751.0
medial meniscus, acquired 717.3
median bar 600.90
  with
    other lower urinary tract symptoms (LUTS)
      600.91
    urinary
      obstruction 600.91
      retention 600.91
mediastinum 519.3
meibomian gland 373.2
meniscus, knee, congenital 755.64
metatarsal head 733.99
metatarsus 733.99
mouth 528.9
mucous membrane
  alveolar process 523.8
  nose 478.19
  turbinate (nasal) 478.0
muscle 728.9
muscular coat, artery NEC 447.8
  carotid 447.8
  renal 447.3
myocardium (*see also* Hypertrophy, cardiac)
  429.3
  idiopathic 425.18
myometrium 621.2
nail 703.8
  congenital 757.5
nasal 478.19
  alae 478.19
  bone 738.0
  cartilage 478.19
  mucous membrane (septum) 478.19
  sinus (*see also* Sinusitis) 473.9

Hypertrophy, hypertrophic—*continued*
nasal—*continued*
  turbinate 478.0
nasopharynx, lymphoid (infectional) (tissue)
  (wall) 478.29
neck, uterus 622.6
nipple 611.1
normal aperture diaphragm (congenital) 756.6
nose (*see also* Hypertrophy, nasal) 478.19
orbit 376.46
organ or site, congenital NEC—*see* Anomaly,
  specified type NEC
osteoarthropathy (pulmonary) 731.2
ovary 620.8
palate (hard) 526.89
  soft 528.9
pancreas (congenital) 751.7
papillae
  anal 569.49
  tongue 529.3
parathyroid (gland) 252.01
parotid gland 527.1
penis 607.89
phallus 607.89
  female (clitoris) 624.2
pharyngeal tonsil 474.12
pharyngitis 472.1
pharynx 478.29
  lymphoid (infectional) (tissue) (wall) 478.29
pituitary (fossa) (gland) 253.8
popliteal fat pad 729.31
preauricular (lymph) gland (Hampstead) 785.6
prepuce (congenital) 605
  female 624.2
prostate (asymptomatic) (early) (recurrent) 600.90
  with
    other lower urinary tract symptoms (LUTS)
      600.91
    urinary
      obstruction 600.91
      retention 600.91
  adenofibromatous 600.20
    with
      other lower urinary tract symptoms
        (LUTS) 600.21
      urinary
        obstruction 600.21
        retention 600.21
  benign 600.00
    with
      other lower urinary tract symptoms
        (LUTS) 600.01
      urinary
        obstruction 600.01
        retention 600.01
  congenital 752.89
psuedoedematous hypodermal 757.0
pseudomuscular 359.1
pylorus (muscle) (sphincter) 537.0
  congenital 750.5
  infantile 750.5
rectal sphincter 569.49
rectum 569.49
renal 593.1
rhinitis (turbinate) 472.0
salivary duct or gland 527.1
  congenital 750.26
scaphoid (tarsal) 733.99
scar 701.4
scrotum 608.89
sella turcica 253.8

Hypertrophy, hypertrophic—*continued*
  seminal vesicle 608.89
  sigmoid 569.89
  skin condition NEC 701.9
  spermatic cord 608.89
  spinal ligament 724.8
  spleen—*see* Splenomegaly
  spondylitis (spine) (*see also* Spondylosis) 721.90
  stomach 537.89
  subaortic stenosis (idiopathic) 425.11
  sublingual gland 527.1
    congenital 750.26
  submaxillary gland 527.1
  suprarenal (gland) 255.8
  tendon 727.9
  testis 608.89
    congenital 752.89
  thymic, thymus (congenital) (gland) 254.0
  thyroid (gland) (*see also* Goiter) 240.9
    primary 242.0
    secondary 242.2
  toe (congenital) 755.65
    acquired 735.8
  tongue 529.8
    congenital 750.15
    frenum 529.8
    papillae (foliate) 529.3
  tonsil (faucial) (infective) (lingual) (lymphoid) 474.11
    and adenoids 474.10
    with
      adenoiditis 474.01
      tonsillitis 474.00
        and adenoiditis 474.02
  tunica vaginalis 608.89
  turbinate (mucous membrane) 478.0
  ureter 593.89
  urethra 599.84
  uterus 621.2
    puerperal, postpartum 674.8
  uvula 528.9
  vagina 623.8
  vas deferens 608.89
  vein 459.89
  ventricle, ventricular (heart) (left) (right)—*see also* Hypertrophy, cardiac
    congenital 746.89
    due to hypertension (left) (right) (*see also* Hypertension, heart) 402.90
      benign 402.10
      malignant 402.00
    right with ventricular septal defect, pulmonary stenosis or atresia, and dextraposition of aorta 745.2
  verumontanum 599.89
  vesical 596.89
  vocal cord 478.5
  vulva 624.3
    stasis (nonfilarial) 624.3
Hypertropia (intermittent) (periodic) 378.31
Hypertyrosinemia 270.2
Hyperuricemia 790.6
Hypervalinemia 270.3
Hyperventilation (tetany) 786.01
  hysterical 300.11
  psychogenic 306.1
  syndrome 306.1
Hyperviscidosis 277.00
Hyperviscosity (of serum) (syndrome) NEC 273.3
  polycythemic 289.0
  sclerocythemic 282.8

Hypervitaminosis (dietary) NEC 278.8
  A (dietary) 278.2
  D (dietary) 278.4
  from excessive administration or use of vitamin preparations (chronic) 278.8
  reaction to sudden overdose 963.5
  vitamin A 278.2
    reaction to sudden overdose 963.5
  vitamin D 278.4
    reaction to sudden overdose 963.5
  vitamin K
    correct substance properly administered 278.8
    overdose or wrong substance given or taken 964.3
Hypervolemia 276.69
Hypesthesia (*see also* Disturbance, sensation) 782.0
  cornea 371.81
Hyphema (anterior chamber) (ciliary body) (iris) 364.41
  traumatic 921.3
Hyphemia —*see* Hyphema
Hypoacidity, gastric 536.8
  psychogenic 306.4
Hypoactive labyrinth (function)—*see* Hypofunction, labyrinth
Hypoadrenalism 255.41
  tuberculous (*see also* Tuberculosis) 017.6
Hypoadrenocorticism 255.41
  pituitary 253.4
Hypoalbuminemia 273.8
Hypoaldosteronism 255.42
Hypoalphalipoproteinemia 272.5
Hypobarism 993.2
Hypobaropathy 993.2
Hypobetalipoproteinemia (familial) 272.5
Hypocalcemia 275.41
  cow's milk 775.4
  dietary 269.3
  neonatal 775.4
  phosphate-loading 775.4
Hypocalcification, teeth 520.4
Hypochloremia 276.9
Hypochlorhydria 536.8
  neurotic 306.4
  psychogenic 306.4
Hypocholesteremia 272.5
Hypochondria (reaction) 300.7
Hypochondriac 300.7
Hypochondriasis 300.7
Hypochromasia blood cells 280.9
Hypochromic anemia 280.9
  due to blood loss (chronic) 280.0
    acute 285.1
  microcytic 280.9
Hypocoagulability (*see also* Defect, coagulation) 286.9
Hypocomplementemia 279.8
Hypocythemia (progressive) 284.9
Hypodontia (*see also* Anodontia) 520.0
Hypoeosinophilia 288.59
Hypoesthesia (*see also* Disturbance, sensation) 782.0
  cornea 371.81
  tactile 782.0
Hypoestrinism 256.39
Hypoestrogenism 256.39
Hypoferremia 280.9
  due to blood loss (chronic) 280.0

Hypoplasia, hypoplasis—*continued*
  artery (congenital) (peripheral) NEC 747.60
    brain 747.81
    cerebral 747.81
    coronary 746.85
    gastrointestinal 747.61
    lower limb 747.64
    pulmonary 747.31
    renal 747.62
    retinal 743.58
    specified NEC 747.69
    spinal 747.82
    umbilical 747.5
    upper limb 747.63
  auditory canal 744.29
    causing impairment of hearing 744.02
  biliary duct (common) or passage 751.61
  bladder 753.8
  bone NEC 756.9
    face 756.0
    malar 756.0
    mandible 524.04
      alveolar 524.74
    marrow 284.9
      acquired (secondary) 284.89
      congenital 284.09
      idiopathic 284.9
    maxilla 524.03
      alveolar 524.73
    skull (*see also* Hypoplasia, skull) 756.0
  brain 742.1
    gyri 742.2
    specified part 742.2
  breast (areola) 611.82
  bronchus (tree) 748.3
  cardiac 746.89
    valve—*see* Hypoplasia, heart, valve
    vein 746.89
  carpus (*see also* Absence, carpal, congenital)
    755.28
  cartilaginous 756.9
  cecum 751.2
  cementum 520.4
    hereditary 520.5
  cephalic 742.1
  cerebellum 742.2
  cervix (uteri) 752.43
  chin 524.06
  clavicle 755.51
  coccyx 756.19
  colon 751.2
  corpus callosum 742.2
  cricoid cartilage 748.3
  dermal, focal (Goltz) 757.39
  digestive organ(s) or tract NEC 751.8
    lower 751.2
    upper 750.8
  ear 744.29
    auricle 744.23
    lobe 744.29
    middle, except ossicles 744.03
      ossicles 744.04
    ossicles 744.04
  enamel of teeth (neonatal) (postnatal) (prenatal)
    520.4
    hereditary 520.5
  endocrine (gland) NEC 759.2
  endometrium 621.8
  epididymis 752.89
  epiglottis 748.3
  erythroid, congenital 284.01

Hypoplasia, hypoplasis—*continued*
  erythropoietic, chronic acquired 284.81
  esophagus 750.3
  Eustachian tube 744.24
  eye (*see also* Microphthalmos) 743.10
    lid 743.62
  face 744.89
    bone(s) 756.0
  fallopian tube 752.19
  femur (*see also* Absence, femur, congenital)
    755.34
  fibula (*see also* Absence, fibula, congenital)
    755.37
  finger (*see also* Absence, finger, congenital)
    755.29
  focal dermal 757.39
  foot 755.31
  gallbladder 751.69
  genitalia, genital organ(s)
    female 752.89
      external 752.49
      internal NEC 752.89
    in adiposogenital dystrophy 253.8
    male 752.89
      penis 752.69
  glottis 748.3
  hair 757.4
  hand 755.21
  heart 746.89
    left (complex) (syndrome) 746.7
    valve NEC 746.89
      pulmonary 746.01
  humerus (*see also* Absence, humerus,
    congenital) 755.24
  hymen 752.49
  intestine (small) 751.1
    large 751.2
  iris 743.46
  jaw 524.09
  kidney(s) 753.0
  labium (majus) (minus) 752.49
  labyrinth, membranous 744.05
  lacrimal duct (apparatus) 743.65
  larynx 748.3
  leg (*see also* Absence, limb, congenital, lower)
    755.30
  limb 755.4
    lower (*see also* Absence, limb, congenital,
      lower) 755.30
    upper (*see also* Absence, limb, congenital,
      upper) 755.20
  liver 751.69
  lung (lobe) 748.5
  mammary (areolar) 611.82
  mandibular 524.04
    alveolar 524.74
    unilateral condylar 526.89
  maxillary 524.03
    alveolar 524.73
  medullary 284.9
  megakaryocytic 287.30
  metacarpus (*see also* Absence, metacarpal,
    congenital) 755.28
  metatarsus (*see also* Absence, metatarsal,
    congenital) 755.38
  muscle 756.89
    eye 743.69
  myocardium (congenital) (Uhl's anomaly)
    746.84
  nail(s) 757.5
  nasolacrimal duct 743.65

Hypoplasia, hypoplasis—*continued*
nervous system NEC 742.8
neural 742.8
nose, nasal 748.1
ophthalmic (*see also* Microphthalmos) 743.10
optic nerve 377.43
organ
of Corti 744.05
or site NEC—*see* Anomaly, by site
osseous meatus (ear) 744.03
ovary 752.0
oviduct 752.19
pancreas 751.7
parathyroid (gland) 759.2
parotid gland 750.26
patella 755.64
pelvis, pelvic girdle 755.69
penis 752.69
peripheral vascular system (congenital) NEC 747.60
gastrointestinal 747.61
lower limb 747.64
renal 747.62
specified NEC 747.69
spinal 747.82
upper limb 747.63
pituitary (gland) 759.2
pulmonary 748.5
arteriovenous 747.32
artery 747.31
valve 746.01
punctum lacrimale 743.65
radioulnar (*see also* Absence, radius, congenital, with ulna) 755.25
radius (*see also* Absence, radius, congenital) 755.26
rectum 751.2
respiratory system NEC 748.9
rib 756.3
sacrum 756.19
scapula 755.59
shoulder girdle 755.59
skin 757.39
skull (bone) 756.0
with
anencephalus 740.0
encephalocele 742.0
hydrocephalus 742.3
with spina bifida (*see also* Spina bifida) 741.0
microcephalus 742.1
spinal (cord) (ventral horn cell) 742.59
vessel 747.82
spine 756.19
spleen 759.0
sternum 756.3
tarsus (*see also* Absence, tarsal, congenital) 755.38
testis, testicle 752.89
thymus (gland) 279.11
thyroid (gland) 243
cartilage 748.3
tibiofibular (*see also* Absence, tibia, congenital, with fibula) 755.35
toe (*see also* Absence, toe, congenital) 755.39
tongue 750.16
trachea (cartilage) (rings) 748.3
Turner's (tooth) 520.4
ulna (*see also* Absence, ulna, congenital) 755.27
umbilical artery 747.5
ureter 753.29
uterus 752.32
vagina 752.45
vascular (peripheral) NEC (*see also* Hypoplasia, peripheral vascular system) 747.60
brain 747.81

Hypoplasia, hypoplasis—*continued*
vein(s) (peripheral) NEC (*see also* Hypoplasia, peripheral vascular system 747.60
brain 747.81
cardiac 746.89
great 747.49
portal 747.49
pulmonary 747.49
vena cava (inferior) (superior) 747.49
vertebra 756.19
vulva 752.49
zonule (ciliary) 743.39
zygoma 738.12
Hypopotassemia 276.8
Hypoproaccelerinemia (*see also* Defect, coagulation) 286.3
Hypoproconvertinemia (congenital) (*see also* Defect, coagulation) 286.3
Hypoproteinemia (essential) (hypermetabolic) (idiopathic) 273.8
Hypoproteinosis 260
Hypoprothrombinemia (congenital) (hereditary) (idiopathic) (*see also* Defect, coagulation) 286.3
acquired 286.7
newborn 776.3
Hypopselaphesia 782.0
Hypopyon (anterior chamber) (eye) 364.05
iritis 364.05
ulcer (cornea) 370.04
Hypopyrexia 780.99
Hyporeflex 796.1
Hyporeninemia, extreme 790.99
in primary aldosteronism 255.10
Hyporesponsive episode 780.09
Hyposecretion
ACTH 253.4
ovary 256.39
postablative 256.2
salivary gland (any) 527.7
Hyposegmentation of neutrophils, hereditary 288.2
Hyposiderinemia 280.9
Hyposmolality 276.1
syndrome 276.1
Hyposomatotropism 253.3
Hyposomnia, unspecified (*see also* Insomnia) 780.52
with sleep apnea, unspecified 780.51
Hypospadias (male) 752.61
female 753.8
Hypospermatogenesis 606.1
Hyposphagma 372.72
Hyposplenism 289.59
Hypostasis, pulmonary 514
Hypostatic —*see* condition
Hyposthenuria 593.89
Hyposuprarenalism 255.41
Hypo-TBG-nemia 246.8
Hypotension (arterial) (constitutional) 458.9
chronic 458.1
iatrogenic 458.29
maternal, syndrome (following labor and delivery) 669.2
of hemodialysis 458.21
orthostatic (chronic) 458.0
dysautonomic-dyskinetic syndrome 333.0
permanent idiopathic 458.1
postoperative 458.29

Hypotension—*continued*
  postural 458.0
  specified type NEC 458.8
  transient 796.3
Hypothermia (accidental) 991.6
  anesthetic 995.89
  associated with low environmental temperature
    991.6
  newborn NEC 778.3
  not associated with low environmental
    temperature 780.65
Hypothymergasia (*see also* Psychosis, affective)
    296.2
  recurrent episode 296.3
  single episode 296.2
Hypothyroidism (acquired) 244.9
  complicating pregnancy, childbirth, or
    puerperium 648.1
  congenital 243
  due to
    ablation 244.1
      radioactive iodine 244.1
      surgical 244.0
    iodine (administration) (ingestion) 244.2
      radioactive 244.1
    irradiation therapy 244.1
    p-aminosalicylic acid (PAS) 244.3
    phenylbutazone 244.3
    resorcinol 244.3
    specified cause NEC 244.8
    surgery 244.0
  goitrous (sporadic) 246.1
  iatrogenic NEC 244.3
  iodine 244.2
  pituitary 244.8
  postablative NEC 244.1
  postsurgical 244.0
  primary 244.9
  secondary NEC 244.8
  specified cause NEC 244.8
  sporadic goitrous 246.1
Hypotonia, hypotonicity, hypotony 781.3
  benign congenital 358.8
  bladder 596.4
  congenital 779.89
    benign 358.8
  eye 360.30
    due to
      fistula 360.32
      ocular disorder NEC 360.33
    following loss of aqueous or vitreous 360.33
    primary 360.31
  infantile muscular (benign) 359.0
  muscle 728.9
  uterus, uterine (contractions)—*see* Inertia,
    uterus
Hypotrichosis 704.09
  congenital 757.4
  lid (congenital) 757.4
    acquired 374.55
  postinfectional NEC 704.09
Hypotropia 378.32
Hypoventilation 786.09
  congenital central alveolar syndrome 327.25
  idiopathic sleep related nonobstructive alveolar
    327.24
  obesity 278.03
  sleep related, in conditions classifiable
    elsewhere 327.26
Hypovitaminosis (*see also* Deficiency, vitamin)
    269.2

Hypovolemia 276.52
  surgical shock 998.09
  traumatic (shock) 958.4
Hypoxemia (*see also* Anoxia) 799.02
  sleep related, in conditions classifiable
    elsewhere 327.26
Hypoxia (*see also* Anoxia) 799.02
  cerebral 348.1
    during or resulting from a procedure 997.01
    newborn 770.88
      mild or moderate 768.6
      severe 768.5
  fetal, affecting newborn 770.88
  intrauterine—*see* Distress, fetal
  myocardial (*see also* Insufficiency, coronary)
    411.89
    arteriosclerotic —*see* Arteriosclerosis,
      coronary
  newborn 770.88
  sleep related 327.24
Hypoxic-ischemic encephalopathy (HIE) 768.70
  mild 768.71
  moderate 768.72
  severe 768.73
Hypsarrhythmia (*see also* Epilepsy) 345.6
Hysteralgia, pregnant uterus 646.8
Hysteria, hysterical 300.10
  anxiety 300.20
  Charcot's gland 300.11
  conversion (any manifestation) 300.11
  dissociative type NEC 300.15
  psychosis, acute 298.1
Hysteroepilepsy 300.11
Hysterotomy, affecting fetus or newborn
    763.89

I

Iatrogenic syndrome of excess cortisol 255.0
IBM (inclusion body myositis) 359.71
Iceland disease (epidemic neuromyasthenia) 049.8
Ichthyosis (congenita) 757.1
  acquired 701.1
  fetalis gravior 757.1
  follicularis 757.1
  hystrix 757.39
  lamellar 757.1
  lingual 528.6
  palmaris and plantaris 757.39
  simplex 757.1
  vera 757.1
  vulgaris 757.1
Ichthyotoxism 988.0
  bacterial (*see also* Poisoning, food) 005.9
Icteroanemia, hemolytic (acquired) 283.9
  congenital (*see also* Spherocytosis) 282.0
Icterus (*see also* Jaundice) 782.4
  catarrhal—*see* Icterus, infectious
  conjunctiva 782.4
    newborn 774.6
  epidemic—*see* Icterus, infectious
  febrilis—*see* Icterus, infectious
  fetus or newborn—*see* Jaundice, fetus or newborn
  gravis (*see also* Necrosis, liver) 570
    complicating pregnancy 646.7
      affecting fetus or newborn 760.8
    fetus or newborn NEC 773.0
    obstetrical 646.7
      affecting fetus or newborn 760.8
  hematogenous (acquired) 283.9
  hemolytic (acquired) 283.9
    congenital (*see also* Spherocytosis) 282.0
  hemorrhagic (acute) 100.0
    leptospiral 100.0
    newborn 776.0
    spirochetal 100.0
  infectious 070.1
    with hepatic coma 070.0
    leptospiral 100.0
    spirochetal 100.0
  intermittens juvenilis 277.4
  malignant (*see also* Necrosis, liver) 570
  neonatorum (*see also* Jaundice, fetus or
    newborn) 774.6
  pernicious (*see also* Necrosis, liver) 570
  spirochetal 100.0
Ictus solaris, solis 992.0
Ideation
  homicidal V62.85
  suicidal V62.84
Identity disorder 313.82
  dissociative 300.14
  gender role (child) 302.6
    adult 302.85
  psychosexual (child) 302.6
    adult 302.85
Idioglossia 307.9
Idiopathic —*see* condition
Idiosyncrasy (*see also* Allergy) 995.3
  drug, medicinal substance, and biological—*see*
    Allergy, drug

Idiot, idiocy (congenital) 318.2
  amaurotic (Bielschowsky) (-Jansky) (family)
    (infantile (late)) (juvenile (late))
    (Vogt-Spielmeyer) 330.1
  microcephalic 742.1
  Mongolian 758.0
  oxycephalic 756.0
Id reaction (due to bacteria) 692.89
**IEED (involuntary emotional expression
  disorder)** 310.81
IFIS (intraoperative floppy iris syndrome)
  364.81
IgE asthma 493.0
Ileitis (chronic) (*see also* Enteritis) 558.9
  infectious 009.0
  noninfectious 558.9
  regional (ulcerative) 555.0
    with large intestine 555.2
  segmental 555.0
    with large intestine 555.2
  terminal (ulcerative) 555.0
    with large intestine 555.2
Ileocolitis (*see also* Enteritis) 558.9
  infectious 009.0
  regional 555.2
  ulcerative 556.1
Ileostomy status V44.2
  with complication 569.60
Ileotyphus 002.0
Ileum —*see* condition
Ileus (adynamic) (bowel) (colon) (inhibitory)
  (intestine) (neurogenic) (paralytic) 560.1
  arteriomesenteric duodenal 537.2
  due to gallstone (in intestine) 560.31
  duodenal, chronic 537.2
  following gastrointestinal surgery 997.49
  gallstone 560.31
  mechanical (*see also* Obstruction, intestine) 560.9
  meconium 777.1
    due to cystic fibrosis 277.01
  myxedema 564.89
  postoperative 997.49
  transitory, newborn 777.4
Iliac —*see* condition
Iliotibial band friction syndrome 728.89
Ill, louping 063.1
Illegitimacy V61.6
Illness —*see also* Disease
  factitious 300.19
    with
      combined psychological and physical signs
        and symptoms 300.19
      physical symptoms 300.19
      predominantly
        physical signs and symptoms 300.19
        psychological symptoms 300.16
    chronic (with physical symptoms) 301.51
  heart—*see* Disease, heart
  manic-depressive (*see also* Psychosis, affective)
    296.80
  mental (*see also* Disorder, mental) 300.9
Imbalance 781.2
  autonomic (*see also* Neuropathy, peripheral,
    autonomic) 337.9

Imbalance—*continued*
electrolyte 276.9
  with
    abortion—*see* Abortion, by type, with
      metabolic disorder
    ectopic pregnancy (*see also* categories
      633.0-633.9) 639.4
    hyperemesis gravidarum (before 22
      completed weeks gestation) 643.1
    molar pregnancy (*see also* categories
      630-632) 639.4
    following
      abortion 639.4
      ectopic or molar pregnancy 639.4
    neonatal, transitory NEC 775.5
  endocrine 259.9
  eye muscle NEC 378.9
  heterophoria—*see* Heterophoria
  glomerulotubular NEC 593.89
  hormone 259.9
  hysterical (*see also* Hysteria) 300.10
  labyrinth NEC 386.50
  posture 729.90
  sympathetic (*see also* Neuropathy, peripheral,
    autonomic) 337.9
Imbecile, imbecility 318.0
  moral 301.7
  old age 290.9
  senile 290.9
  specified IQ—*see* IQ
  unspecified IQ 318.0
Imbedding, intrauterine device 996.32
Imbibition, cholesterol (gallbladder) 575.6
Imerslund (-Gräsbeck) syndrome (anemia due to
  familial selective vitamin B$_{12}$ malabsorption)
  281.1
Iminoacidopathy 270.8
Iminoglycinuria, familial 270.8
Immature —*see also* Immaturity
  personality 301.89
Immaturity 765.1
  extreme 765.0
  fetus or infant light-for-dates—*see*
    Light-for-dates
  lung, fetus or newborn 770.4
  organ or site NEC—*see* Hypoplasia
  pulmonary, fetus or newborn 770.4
  reaction 301.89
  sexual (female) (male) 259.0
Immersion 994.1
  foot 991.4
  hand 991.4
Immobile, immobility
  complete
    due to severe physical disability or frality
      780.72
  intestine 564.89
  joint—*see* Ankylosis
  syndrome (paraplegic) 728.3
Immunization
  ABO
    affecting management of pregnancy 656.2
      fetus or newborn 773.1
    complication—*see* Complications, vaccination
  Rh factor
    affecting management of pregnancy 656.1
      fetus or newborn 773.0
    from transfusion (*see also* Complications,
      transfusion) 999.70

Immunodeficiency 279.3
  with
    adenosine-deaminase deficiency 279.2
    defect, predominant
      B-cell 279.00
      T-cell 279.10
    hyperimmunoglobulinemia 279.2
    lymphopenia, hereditary 279.2
    thrombocytopenia and eczema 279.12
    thymic
      aplasia 279.2
      dysplasia 279.2
  autosomal recessive, Swiss-type 279.2
  common variable 279.06
  severe combined (SCID) 279.2
  to Rh factor
    affecting management of pregnancy 656.1
    fetus or newborn 773.0
  X-linked, with increased IgM 279.05
Immunotherapy, prophylactic V07.2
  antineoplastic V58.12
Impaction, impacted
  bowel, colon, rectum 560.30
    with hernia—*see also* Hernia, by site, with
      obstruction
      gangrenous—*see* Hernia, by site, with
        gangrene
    by
      calculus 560.32
      gallstone 560.31
    fecal 560.32
    specified type NEC 560.32
  calculus—*see* Calculus
  cerumen (ear) (external) 380.4
  cuspid 520.6
  dental 520.6
  fecal, feces 560.32
    with hernia—*see also* Hernia, by site, with
      obstruction
      gangrenous—*see* Hernia, by site, with
        gangrene
  fracture—*see* Fracture, by site
  gallbladder—*see* Cholelithiasis
  gallstone(s)—*see* Cholelithiasis
    in intestine (any part) 560.31
  intestine(s) 560.30
    with hernia—*see also* Hernia, by site, with
      obstruction
      gangrenous—*see* Hernia, by site, with
        gangrene
    by
      calculus 560.32
      gallstone 560.31
    fecal 560.32
    specified type NEC 560.32
  intrauterine device (IUD) 996.32
  molar 520.6
  shoulder 660.4
    affecting fetus or newborn 763.1
  tooth, teeth 520.6
  turbinate 733.99
Impaired, impairment (function)
  arm V49.1
    movement, involving
      musculoskeletal system V49.1
      nervous system V49.2
  auditory discrimination 388.43
  back V48.3
  body (entire) V49.89
  cognitive, mild, so stated 331.83
  combined visual hearing V49.85

Impaired, impairment—*continued*
dual sensory V49.85
glucose
  fasting 790.21
  tolerance test (oral) 790.22
hearing (*see also* Deafness) 389.9
  combined with visual impairment V49.85
heart—*see* Disease, heart
kidney (*see also* Disease, renal) 593.9
  disorder resulting from 588.9
    specified NEC 588.89
leg V49.1
  movement, involving
    musculoskeletal system V49.1
    nervous system V49.2
limb V49.1
  movement, involving
    musculoskeletal system V49.1
    nervous system V49.2
liver 573.8
mastication 524.9
mild cognitive, so stated 331.83
mobility
  ear ossicles NEC 385.22
  incostapedial joint 385.22
  malleus 385.21
myocardium, myocardial (*see also*
    Insufficiency, myocardial) 428.0
neuromusculoskeletal NEC V49.89
  back V48.3
  head V48.2
  limb V49.2
  neck V48.3
  spine V48.3
  trunk V48.3
rectal sphincter 787.99
renal (*see also* Disease, renal) 593.9
  disorder resulting from 588.9
    specified NEC 588.89
spine V48.3
vision NEC 369.9
  both eyes NEC 369.3
  combined with hearing impairment V49.85
  moderate 369.74
    both eyes 369.25
      with impairment of lesser eye (specified
        as)
        blind, not further specified 369.15
        low vision, not further specified 369.23
        near-total 369.17
        profound 369.18
        severe 369.24
        total 369.16
    one eye 369.74
      with vision of other eye (specified as)
        near-normal 369.75
        normal 369.76
  near-total 369.64
    both eyes 369.04
      with impairment of lesser eye (specified
        as)
        blind, not further specified 369.02
        total 369.03
    one eye 369.64
      with vision of other eye (specified as)
        near-normal 369.65
        normal 369.66
  one eye 369.60
    with low vision of other eye 369.10

Impaired, impairment—*continued*
vision—*continued*
  profound 369.67
    both eyes 369.08
      with impairment of lesser eye (specified
        as)
        blind, not further specified 369.05
        near-total 369.07
        total 369.06
    one eye 369.67
      with vision of other eye (specified as)
        near-normal 369.68
        normal 369.69
  severe 369.71
    both eyes 369.22
      with impairment of lesser eye (specified as)
        blind, not further specified 369.11
        low vision, not further specified 369.21
        near-total 369.13
        profound 369.14
        total 369.12
    one eye 369.71
      with vision of other eye (specified as)
        near-normal 369.72
        normal 369.73
  total
    both eyes 369.01
    one eye 369.61
      with vision of other eye (specified as)
        near-normal 369.62
        normal 369.63
Impaludism —*see* Malaria
Impediment, speech NEC 784.59
  psychogenic 307.9
  secondary to organic lesion 784.59
Impending
  cerebrovascular accident or attack 435.9
  coronary syndrome 411.1
  delirium tremens 291.0
  myocardial infarction 411.1
Imperception, auditory (acquired) (congenital)
    389.9
Imperfect
  aeration, lung (newborn) 770.5
  closure (congenital)
    alimentary tract NEC 751.8
      lower 751.5
      upper 750.8
    atrioventricular ostium 745.69
    atrium (secundum) 745.5
      primum 745.61
    branchial cleft or sinus 744.41
    choroid 743.59
    cricoid cartilage 748.3
    cusps, heart valve NEC 746.89
      pulmonary 746.09
    ductus
      arteriosus 747.0
      Botalli 747.0
    ear drum 744.29
      causing impairment of hearing 744.03
    endocardial cushion 745.60
    epiglottis 748.3
    esophagus with communication to bronchus or
        trachea 750.3
    Eustachian valve 746.89
    eyelid 743.62
    face, facial (*see also* Cleft, lip) 749.10
    foramen
      Botalli 745.5
      ovale 745.5

Imperfect—*continued*
　closure (congenital)—*continued*
　　genitalia, genital organ(s) or system
　　　female 752.89
　　　　external 752.49
　　　　internal NEC 752.89
　　　　uterus 752.39
　　　male 752.89
　　　　penis 752.69
　　glottis 748.3
　　heart valve (cusps) NEC 746.89
　　interatrial ostium or septum 745.5
　　interauricular ostium or septum 745.5
　　interventricular ostium or septum 745.4
　　iris 743.46
　　kidney 753.3
　　larynx 748.3
　　lens 743.36
　　lip (*see also* Cleft, lip) 749.10
　　nasal septum or sinus 748.1
　　nose 748.1
　　omphalomesenteric duct 751.0
　　optic nerve entry 743.57
　　organ or site NEC—*see* Anomaly, specified
　　　type, by site
　　ostium
　　　interatrial 745.5
　　　interauricular 745.5
　　　interventricular 745.4
　　palate (*see also* Cleft, palate) 749.00
　　preauricular sinus 744.46
　　retina 743.56
　　roof of orbit 742.0
　　sclera 743.47
　　septum
　　　aortic 745.0
　　　aorticopulmonary 745.0
　　　atrial (secundum) 745.5
　　　　primum 745.61
　　　between aorta and pulmonary artery 745.0
　　　heart 745.9
　　　interatrial (secundum) 745.5
　　　　primum 745.61
　　　interauricular (secundum) 745.5
　　　　primum 745.61
　　　interventricular 745.4
　　　　with pulmonary stenosis or atresia,
　　　　　dextraposition of aorta, and
　　　　　hypertrophy of right ventricle 745.2
　　　　in tetralogy of Fallot 745.2
　　　nasal 748.1
　　　ventricular 745.4
　　　　with pulmonary stenosis or atresia,
　　　　　dextraposition of aorta, and
　　　　　hypertrophy of right ventricle 745.2
　　　　in tetralogy of Fallot 745.2
　　skull 756.0
　　　with
　　　　anencephalus 740.0
　　　　encephalocele 742.0
　　　　hydrocephalus 742.3
　　　　　with spina bifida (*see also* Spina bifida)
　　　　　　741.0
　　　　microcephalus 742.1
　　　spine (with meningocele) (*see also* Spina
　　　　bifida) 741.90
　　thyroid cartilage 748.3
　　trachea 748.3
　　tympanic membrane 744.29
　　　causing impairment of hearing 744.03
　　uterus (with communication to bladder,
　　　intestine, or rectum) 752.39

Imperfect—*continued*
　closure (congenital)—*continued*
　　uvula 749.02
　　　with cleft lip (*see also* Cleft, palate, with
　　　　cleft lip) 749.20
　　vitelline duct 751.0
　development—*see* Anomaly, by site
　erection 607.84
　fusion—*see* Imperfect, closure
　inflation lung (newborn) 770.5
　intestinal canal 751.5
　poise 729.90
　rotation—*see* Malrotation
　septum, ventricular 745.4
Imperfectly descended testis 752.51
Imperforate (congenital)—*see also* Atresia
　anus 751.2
　bile duct 751.61
　cervix (uteri) 752.49
　esophagus 750.3
　hymen 752.42
　intestine (small) 751.1
　　large 751.2
　jejunum 751.1
　pharynx 750.29
　rectum 751.2
　salivary duct 750.23
　urethra 753.6
　urinary meatus 753.6
　vagina 752.49
Impervious (congenital)—*see also* Atresia
　anus 751.2
　bile duct 751.61
　esophagus 750.3
　intestine (small) 751.1
　　large 751.5
　rectum 751.2
　urethra 753.6
Impetiginization of other dermatoses 684
Impetigo (any organism) (any site) (bullous)
　　(circinate) (contagiosa) (neonatorum)
　　(simplex) 684
　Bockhart's (superficial folliculitis) 704.8
　external ear 684 [*380.13*]
　eyelid 684 [*373.5*]
　Fox's (contagiosa) 684
　furfuracea 696.5
　herpetiformis 694.3
　　nonobstetrical 694.3
　staphylococcal infection 684
　ulcerative 686.8
　vulgaris 684
Impingement, soft tissue between teeth 524.89
　anterior 524.81
　posterior 524.82
Implant, endometrial 617.9
Implantation
　anomalous—*see also* Anomaly, specified type,
　　by site
　　ureter 753.4
　cyst
　　external area or site (skin) NEC 709.8
　　iris 364.61
　　vagina 623.8
　　vulva 624.8
　dermoid (cyst)
　　external area or site (skin) NEC 709.8
　　iris 364.61
　　vagina 623.8
　　vulva 624.8
　placenta, low or marginal—*see* Placenta previa

Impotence (sexual) 607.84
  organic origin NEC 607.84
  psychogenic 302.72
Impoverished blood 285.9
Impression, basilar 756.0
Imprisonment V62.5
Improper
  development, infant 764.9
Improperly tied umbilical cord (causing
  hemorrhage) 772.3
Impulses, obsessional 300.3
Impulsive 799.23
  neurosis 300.3
Impulsiveness 799.23
Inaction, kidney (*see also* Disease, renal) 593.9
Inactive —*see* condition
Inadequate, inadequacy
  aesthetics of dental restoration 525.67
  biologic 301.6
  cardiac and renal—*see* Hypertension, cardiorenal
  constitutional 301.6
  development
    child 783.40
    fetus 764.9
      affecting management of pregnancy 656.5
    genitalia
      after puberty NEC 259.0
      congenital—*see* Hypoplasia, genitalia
    lungs 748.5
    organ or site NEC—*see* Hypoplasia, by site
  dietary 269.9
  distance, interarch 524.28
  education V62.3
  environment
    economic problem V60.2
    household condition NEC V60.1
    poverty V60.2
    unemployment V62.0
  functional 301.6
  household care, due to
    family member
      handicapped or ill V60.4
      temporarily away from home V60.4
        on vacation V60.5
    technical defects in home V60.1
    temporary absence from home of person
      rendering care V60.4
  housing (heating) (space) V60.1
  interarch distance 524.28
  material resources V60.2
  mental (*see also* Disability, intellectual) 319
  nervous system 799.29
  personality 301.6
  prenatal care in current pregnancy V23.7
  pulmonary
    function 786.09
      newborn 770.89
    ventilation, newborn 770.89
  respiration 786.09
    newborn 770.89
  sample
    cytology
      anal 796.78
      cervical 795.08
      vaginal 795.18
  social 301.6
Inanition 263.9
  with edema 262
  due to
    deprivation of food 994.2
    malnutrition 263.9
  fever 780.60

Inappropriate
  change in quantitative human chorionic
    gonadotropin (hCG) in early pregnancy
    631.0
  level of quantitative human chorionic
    gonadotropin (hCG) for gestational age in
    early pregnancy 631.0
  secretion
    ACTH 255.0
    antidiuretic hormone (ADH) (excessive) 253.6
    deficiency 253.5
    ectopic hormone NEC 259.3
    pituitary (posterior) 253.6
Inattention after or at birth 995.52
Inborn errors of metabolism —*see* Disorder,
  metabolism
Incarceration, incarcerated
  bubonocele—*see also* Hernia, inguinal, with
    obstruction
    gangrenous—*see* Hernia, inguinal, with
      gangrene
  colon (by hernia)—*see also* Hernia, by site, with
    obstruction
    gangrenous—*see* Hernia, by site, with
      gangrene
  enterocele 552.9
    gangrenous 551.9
  epigastrocele 552.29
    gangrenous 551.29
  epiplocele 552.9
    gangrenous 551.9
  exomphalos 552.1
    gangrenous 551.1
  fallopian tube 620.8
  hernia—*see also* Hernia, by site, with
    obstruction
    gangrenous—*see* Hernia, by site, with
      gangrene
  iris, in wound 871.1
  lens, in wound 871.1
  merocele (*see also* Hernia, femoral, with
    obstruction) 552.00
  Omentum (by hernia)—*see also* Hernia, by site,
    with obstruction
    gangrenous—*see* Hernia, by site, with
      gangrene
  omphalocele 756.72
  rupture (meaning hernia) (*see also* Hernia, by
    site, with obstruction) 552.9
    gangrenous (*see also* Hernia, by site, with
      gangrene) 551.9
  sarcoepiplocele 552.9
    gangrenous 551.9
  sarcoepiplomphalocele 552.1
    with gangrene 551.1
  uterus 621.8
    gravid 654.3
      causing obstructed labor 660.2
        affecting fetus or newborn 763.1
Incident, cerebrovascular (*see also* Disease,
  cerebrovascular, acute) 436
Incineration (entire body) (from fire,
  conflagration, electricity, or lightning)—*see*
  Burn, multiple, specified sites
Incised wound
  external—*see* Wound, open, by site
  internal organs (abdomen, chest, or pelvis)—*see*
    Injury, internal, by site, with open wound
Incision, incisional
  hernia—*see* Hernia, incisional
  surgical, complication—*see* Complications,
    surgical procedures

Increase, increased—*continued*
  cold sense (*see also* Disturbance, sensation)
    782.0
  estrogen 256.0
  function
    adrenal (cortex) 255.3
      medulla 255.6
    pituitary (anterior) (gland) (lobe) 253.1
      posterior 253.6
  heat sense (*see also* Disturbance, sensation) 782.0
  intracranial pressure 781.99
    injury at birth 767.8
  light reflex of retina 362.13
  permeability, capillary 448.9
  pressure
    intracranial 781.99
      injury at birth 767.8
    intraocular 365.00
  pulsations 785.9
  pulse pressure 785.9
  sphericity, lens 743.36
  splenic activity 289.4
  venous pressure 459.89
    portal 572.3
Incrustation, cornea, lead or zinc 930.0
Incyclophoria 378.44
Incyclotropia 378.33
Indeterminate sex 752.7
India rubber skin 756.83
Indicanuria 270.2
Indigestion (bilious) (functional) 536.8
  acid 536.8
  catarrhal 536.8
  due to decomposed food NEC 005.9
  fat 579.8
  nervous 306.4
  psychogenic 306.4
Indirect —*see* condition
Indolent bubo NEC 099.8
Induced
  abortion—*see* Abortion, induced
  birth, affecting fetus or newborn 763.89
  delivery—*see* Delivery
  labor—*see* Delivery
Induration, indurated
  brain 348.89
  breast (fibrous) 611.79
    puerperal, postpartum 676.3
  broad ligament 620.8
  chancre 091.0
    anus 091.1
    congenital 090.0
    extragenital NEC 091.2
  corpora cavernosa (penis) (plastic) 607.89
  liver (chronic) 573.8
    acute 573.8
  lung (black) (brown) (chronic) (fibroid) (*see
    also* Fibrosis, lung) 515
    essential brown 275.09 *[516.1]*
  penile 607.89
  phlebitic—*see* Phlebitis
  skin 782.8
  stomach 537.89
Induratio penis plastica 607.89
Industrial —*see* condition
Inebriety (*see also* Abuse, drugs, nondependent)
  305.0
Inefficiency
  kidney (*see also* Disease, renal) 593.9
  thyroid (acquired) (gland) 244.9

Inelasticity, skin 782.8
Inequality, leg (acquired) (length) 736.81
  congenital 755.30
Inertia
  bladder 596.4
    neurogenic 596.54
      with cauda equina syndrome 344.61
  stomach 536.8
    psychogenic 306.4
  uterus, uterine 661.2
    affecting fetus or newborn 763.7
    primary 661.0
    secondary 661.1
  vesical 596.4
    neurogenic 596.54
      with cauda equina 344.61
Infant —*see also* condition
  excessive crying of 780.92
  fussy (baby) 780.91
  held for adoption V68.89
  newborn—*see* Newborn
  post-term (gestation period over 40 completed
    weeks to 42 completed weeks) 766.21
  prolonged gestation of (period over 42
    completed weeks) 766.22
  syndrome of diabetic mother 775.0
"Infant Hercules" syndrome 255.2
Infantile —*see also* condition
  genitalia, genitals 259.0
    in pregnancy or childbirth NEC 654.4
      affecting fetus or newborn 763.89
      causing obstructed labor 660.2
        affecting fetus or newborn 763.1
  heart 746.9
  kidney 753.3
  lack of care 995.52
  macula degeneration 362.75
  melanodontia 521.05
  os, uterus (*see also* Infantile, genitalia) 259.0
  pelvis 738.6
    with disproportion (fetopelvic) 653.1
      affecting fetus or newborn 763.1
      causing obstructed labor 660.1
        affecting fetus or newborn 763.1
  penis 259.0
  testis 257.2
  uterus (*see also* Infantile, genitalia) 259.0
  vulva 752.49
Infantilism 259.9
  with dwarfism (hypophyseal) 253.3
  Brissaud's (infantile myxedema) 244.9
  celiac 579.0
  Herter's (nontropical sprue) 579.0
  hypophyseal 253.3
  hypothalamic (with obesity) 253.8
  idiopathic 259.9
  intestinal 579.0
  pancreatic 577.8
  pituitary 253.3
  renal 588.0
  sexual (with obesity) 259.0
Infants, healthy liveborn —*see* Newborn
Infarct, infarction
  adrenal (capsule) (gland) 255.41
  amnion 658.8
  anterior (with contiguous portion of
    intraventricular septum) NEC (*see also*
    Infarct, myocardium) 410.1
  appendices epiploicae 557.0
  bowel 557.0

Infarct, infarction—*continued*
placenta (complicating pregnancy) 656.7
  affecting fetus or newborn 762.2
pontine—*see* Infarct, brain
posterior NEC (*see also* Infarct, myocardium)
  410.6
prostate 602.8
pulmonary (artery) (hemorrhagic) (vein) 415.19
  with
    abortion—*see* Abortion, by type, with
      embolism
    ectopic pregnancy (*see also* categories
      633.0-633.9) 639.6
    molar pregnancy (*see also* categories
      630-632) 639.6
  following
    abortion 639.6
    ectopic or molar pregnancy 639.6
  iatrogenic 415.11
  in pregnancy, childbirth, or puerperium—*see*
    Embolism, obstetrical
  postoperative 415.11
  septic 415.12
renal 593.81
  embolic or thrombotic 593.81
retina, retinal 362.84
  with occlusion—*see* Occlusion, retina
spinal (acute) (cord) (embolic) (nonembolic) 336.1
spleen 289.59
  embolic or thrombotic 444.89
subchorionic—*see* Infarct, placenta
subendocardial (*see also* Infarct, myocardium)
  410.7
suprarenal (capsule) (gland) 255.41
syncytium—*see* Infarct, placenta
testis 608.83
thrombotic (*see also* Thrombosis) 453.9
  artery, arterial—*see* Embolism
thyroid (gland) 246.3
ventricle (heart) (*see also* Infarct, myocardium)
  410.9
Infecting —*see* condition
Infection, infected, infective (opportunistic) 136.9
  with
    influenza viruses occurring in pigs or other
      animals - *see* Influenza, due to identified,
      novel influenza A virus
    lymphangitis - *see* Lymphangitis
  abortion—*see* Abortion, by type, with sepsis
  abscess (skin)—*see* Abscess, by site
  Absidia 117.7
  Acanthocheilonema (perstans) 125.4
    streptocerca 125.6
  acanthamoeba 136.21
  accessory sinus (chronic) (*see also* Sinusitis)
    473.9
  Achorion—*see* Dermatophytosis
  Acremonium falciforme 117.4
  acromioclavicular (joint) 711.91
  actinobacillus
    lignieresii 027.8
    mallei 024
    muris 026.1
  actinomadura—*see* Actinomycosis
  Actinomyces (israelii)—*see also* Actinomycosis
    muris-ratti 026.1
  Actinomycetales (actinomadura) (Actinomyces)
    (Nocardia) (Streptomyces)—*see*
    Actinomycosis
  actinomycotic NEC (*see also* Actinomycosis)
    039.9

Infection, infected, infective—*continued*
adenoid (chronic) 474.01
  acute 463
  and tonsil (chronic) 474.02
    acute or subacute 463
adenovirus NEC 079.0
  in diseases classified elsewhere—*see* category 079
  unspecified nature or site 079.0
Aerobacter aerogenes NEC 041.85
  enteritis 008.2
aerogenes capsulatus (*see also* Gangrene, gas) 040.0
aertrycke (*see also* Infection, Salmonella) 003.9
ajellomyces dermatitidis 116.0
alimentary canal NEC (*see also* Enteritis, due to,
  by organism) 009.0
Allescheria boydii 117.6
Alternaria 118
alveolus, alveolar (process) (pulpal origin) 522.4
ameba, amebic (histolytica) (*see also*
  Amebiasis) 006.9
  acute 006.0
  chronic 006.1
  free-living 136.29
  hartmanni 007.8
  specified
    site NEC 006.8
    type NEC 007.8
amniotic fluid or cavity 658.4
  affecting fetus or newborn 762.7
anaerobes (cocci) (gram-negative) (gram
  positive) (mixed) NEC 041.84
anal canal 569.49
Ancylostoma braziliense 126.2
Angiostrongylus cantonensis 128.8
anisakiasis 127.1
Anisakis larva 127.1
anthrax (*see also* Anthrax) 022.9
antrum (chronic) (*see also* Sinusitis, maxillary)
  473.0
anus (papillae) (sphincter) 569.49
arbor virus NEC 066.9
arbovirus NEC 066.9
argentophil-rod 027.0
Ascaris lumbricoides 127.0
ascomycetes 117.4
Aspergillus (flavus) (fumigatus) (terreus) 117.3
atypical
  acid-fast (bacilli) (*see also* Mycobacterium,
    atypical) 031.9
  mycobacteria (*see also* Mycobacterium,
    atypical) 031.9
auditory meatus (circumscribed) (diffuse)
  (external) (*see also* Otitis, externa) 380.10
auricle (ear) (*see also* Otitis, externa) 380.10
axillary gland 683
Babesiasis 088.82
Babesiosis 088.82
Bacillus NEC 041.89
  abortus 023.1
  anthracis (*see also* Anthrax) 022.9
  cereus (food poisoning) 005.89
  coli—*see* Infection, Escherichia coli
  coliform NEC 041.85
  Ducrey's (any location) 099.0
  Flexner's 004.1
  Friedländer's NEC 041.3
  fusiformis 101
  gas (gangrene) (*see also* Gangrene, gas) 040.0
  mallei 024
  melitensis 023.0

Infection, infected, infective—*continued*
Bacillus—*continued*
paratyphoid, paratyphosus 002.9
A 002.1
B 002.2
C 002.3
Schmorl's 040.3
Shiga 004.0
suipestifer (*see also* Infection, Salmonella) 003.9
swimming pool 031.1
typhosa 002.0
welchii (*see also* Gangrene, gas) 040.0
Whitmore's 025
bacterial NEC 041.9
specified NEC 041.89
anaerobic NEC 041.84
gram-negative NEC 041.85
anaerobic NEC 041.84
Bacterium
paratyphosum 002.9
A 002.1
B 002.2
C 002.3
typhosum 002.0
Bacteroides (fragilis) (melaninogenicus) (oralis) NEC 041.82
balantidium coli 007.0
Bartholin's gland 616.89
Basidiobolus 117.7
Bedsonia 079.98
specified NEC 079.88
bile duct 576.1
bladder (*see also* Cystitis) 595.9
Blastomyces, blastomycotic 116.0
brasiliensis 116.1
dermatitidis 116.0
European 117.5
Loboi 116.2
North American 116.0
South American 116.1
bleb
postprocedural 379.60
stage 1 379.61
stage 2 379.62
stage 3 379.63
blood stream—*see also* Septicemia
catheter-related (CRBSI) 999.31
central line-associated (CLABSI) 999.32
due to central venous catheter 999.32
bone 730.9
specified—*see* Osteomyelitis
Bordetella 033.9
bronchiseptica 033.8
parapertussis 033.1
pertussis 033.0
Borrelia
bergdorfi 088.81
vincentii (mouth) (pharynx) (tonsil) 101
bovine stomatitis 059.11
brain (*see also* Encephalitis) 323.9
late effect—*see* category 326
membranes—(*see also* Meningitis) 322.9
septic 324.0
late effect—*see* category 326
meninges (*see also* Meningitis) 320.9
branchial cyst 744.42

Infection, infected, infective—*continued*
breast 611.0
puerperal, postpartum 675.2
with nipple 675.9
specified type NEC 675.8
nonpurulent 675.2
purulent 675.1
bronchus (*see also* Bronchitis) 490
fungus NEC 117.9
Brucella 023.9
abortus 023.1
canis 023.3
melitensis 023.0
mixed 023.8
suis 023.2
Brugia (Wuchereria) malayi 125.1
bursa—*see* Bursitis
buttocks (skin) 686.9
Candida (albicans) (tropicalis) (*see also* Candidiasis) 112.9
congenital 771.7
Candiru 136.8
Capillaria
hepatica 128.8
philippinensis 127.5
cartilage 733.99
cat liver fluke 121.0
catheter-related bloodstream (CRBSI) 999.31
cellulitis—*see* Cellulitis, by site
central line-associated 999.31
bloodstream 999.32
Cephalosporum falciforme 117.4
Cercomonas hominis (intestinal) 007.3
cerebrospinal (*see also* Meningitis) 322.9
late effect—*see* category 326
cervical gland 683
cervix (*see also* Cervicitis) 616.0
cesarean section wound 674.3
Chilomastix (intestinal) 007.8
Chlamydia 079.98
specified NEC 079.88
Cholera (*see also* Cholera) 001.9
chorionic plate 658.8
Cladosporium
bantianum 117.8
carrionii 117.2
mansoni 111.1
trichoides 117.8
wernecki 111.1
Clonorchis (sinensis) (liver) 121.1
Clostridium (haemolyticum) (novyi) NEC 041.84
botulinum 005.1
histolyticum (*see also* Gangrene, gas) 040.0
oedematiens (*see also* Gangrene, gas) 040.0
perfringens 041.83
due to food 005.2
septicum (*see also* Gangrene, gas) 040.0
sordelii (*see also* Gangrene, gas) 040.0
welchii (*see also* Gangrene, gas) 040.0
due to food 005.2
Coccidioides (immitis) (*see also* Coccidioidomycosis) 114.9
coccus NEC 041.89
colon (*see also* Enteritis, due to, by organism) 009.0
bacillus—*see* Infection, Escherichia coli
colostomy or enterostomy 569.61
common duct 576.1
complicating pregnancy, childbirth, or puerperium NEC 647.9
affecting fetus or newborn 760.2

Infection, infected, infective—*continued*
  Condiobolus 117.7
  congenital NEC 771.89
    Candida albicans 771.7
    chronic 771.2
    Cytomegalovirus 771.1
    hepatitis, viral 771.2
    Herpes simplex 771.2
    listeriosis 771.2
    malaria 771.2
    poliomyelitis 535.6
    rubella 771.0
    toxoplasmosis 771.2
    tuberculosis 771.2
    urinary (tract) 771.82
    vaccinia 771.2
  coronavirus 079.89
    SARS-associated 079.82
  corpus luteum (*see also* Salpingo-oophoritis) 614.2
  Corynebacterium diphtheriae—*see* Diphtheria
  cotia virus 059.8
  Coxsackie (*see also* Coxsackie) 079.2
    endocardium 074.22
    heart NEC 074.20
    in diseases classified elsewhere—*see* category 079
    meninges 047.0
    myocardium 074.23
    pericardium 074.21
    pharynx 074.0
    specified disease NEC 074.8
    unspecified nature or site 079.2
  Cryptococcus neoformans 117.5
  Cryptosporidia 007.4
  Cunninghamella 117.7
  cyst—*see* Cyst
  Cysticercus cellulosae 123.1
  cystostomy 596.83
  cytomegalovirus 078.5
    congenital 771.1
  dental (pulpal origin) 522.4
  deuteromycetes 117.4
  Dicrocoelium dendriticum 121.8
  Dipetalonema (perstans) 125.4
    streptocerca 125.6
  diphtherial—*see* Diphtheria
  Diphyllobothrium (adult) (latum) (pacificum) 123.4
    larval 123.5
  Diplogonoporus (grandis) 123.8
  Dipylidium (caninum) 123.8
  Dirofilaria 125.6
  dog tapeworm 123.8
  Dracunculus medinensis 125.7
  Dreschlera 118
    hawaiiensis 117.8
  Ducrey's bacillus (any site) 099.0
  due to or resulting from
    central venous catheter (*see also*
      Complications, due to, catheter, central
      venous) 999.31
      bloodstream 999.32
      localized 999.33
    device, implant, or graft (any) (presence
      of)—*see* Complications, infection and
      inflammation, due to (presence of) any
      device, implant, or graft classified to
      996.0-996.5 NEC

Infection, infected, infective—*continued*
  due to or resulting from—*continued*
    injection, inoculation, infusion, transfusion, or
      vaccination (prophylactic) (therapeutic)
      999.39
      blood and blood products
        acute 999.34
    injury NEC—*see* Wound, open, by site,
      complicated
    surgery 998.59
  duodenum 535.6
  ear—*see also* Otitis
    external (*see also* Otitis, externa) 380.10
    inner (*see also* Labyrinthitis) 386.30
    middle —*see* Otitis, media
  Eaton's agent NEC 041.81
  Eberthella typhosa 002.0
  Ebola 078.89
  echinococcosis 122.9
  Echinococcus (*see also* Echinococcus) 122.9
  Echinostoma 121.8
  ECHO virus 079.1
    in diseases classified elsewhere—*see* category
      079
    unspecified nature or site 079.1
  Ehrlichiosis 082.40
    chaffeensis 082.41
    specified type NEC 082.49
  Endamoeba—*see* Infection, ameba
  endocardium (*see also* Endocarditis) 421.0
  endocervix (*see also* Cervicitis) 616.0
  Entamoeba—*see* Infection, ameba
  enteric (*see also* Enteritis, due to, by organism) 009.0
  Enterobacter aerogenes NEC 041.85
  Enterobacter sakazakii 041.85
  Enterobius vermicularis 127.4
  enterococcus NEC 041.04
  enterovirus NEC 079.89
    central nervous system NEC 048
    enteritis 008.67
    meningitis 047.9
  Entomophthora 117.7
  Epidermophyton—*see* Dermatophytosis
  epidermophytosis—*see* Dermatophytosis
  episiotomy 674.3
  Epstein-Barr virus 075
    chronic 780.79 *[139.8]*
  erysipeloid 027.1
  Erysipelothrix (insidiosa) (rhusiopathiae) 027.1
  erythema infectiosum 057.0
  Escherichia coli (E. coli) 041.49
    enteritis—*see* Enteritis, E. coli
    generalized 038.42
    intestinal—*see* Enteritis, E. coli
    non-Shiga toxin-producing 041.49
    Shiga toxin-producing (STEC) 041.43
      with
        unspecified O group 041.43
      non-O157 (with known O group) 041.42
      O157 (with confirmation of Shiga toxin
        when H antigen is unknown, or is not
        H7) 041.41
      O157:H- (nonmotile) with confirmation of
        Shiga toxin 041.41
      O157:H7 with or without confirmation of
        Shiga toxin-production 041.41
      specified NEC 041.42
  esophagostomy 530.86
  ethmoidal (chronic) (sinus) (*see also* Sinusitis,
    ethmoidal) 473.2

Infection, infected, infective—*continued*
  Eubacterium 041.84
  Eustachian tube (ear) 381.50
    acute 381.51
    chronic 381.52
  exanthema subitum (*see also* Exanthem
    subitum) 058.10
  exit site 999.33
  external auditory canal (meatus) (*see also* Otitis,
    externa) 380.10
  eye NEC 360.00
  eyelid 373.9
    specified NEC 373.8
  fallopian tube (*see also* Salpingo-oophoritis)
    614.2
  fascia 728.89
  Fasciola
    gigantica 121.3
    hepatica 121.3
  Fasciolopsis (buski) 121.4
  fetus (intra-amniotic)—*see* Infection, congenital
  filarial—*see* Infestation, filarial
  finger (skin) 686.9
    abscess (with lymphangitis) 681.00
      pulp 681.01
    cellulitis (with lymphangitis) 681.00
    distal closed space (with lymphangitis) 681.00
    nail 681.02
      fungus 110.1
  fish tapeworm 123.4
    larval 123.5
  flagellate, intestinal 007.9
  fluke—*see* Infestation, fluke
  focal
    teeth (pulpal origin) 522.4
    tonsils 474.00
      and adenoids 474.02
  Fonsecaea
    compactum 117.2
    pedrosoi 117.2
  food (*see also* Poisoning, food) 005.9
  foot (skin) 686.9
    fungus 110.4
  Francisella tularensis (*see also* Tularemia) 021.9
  frontal sinus (chronic) (*see also* Sinusitis,
    frontal) 473.1
  fungus NEC 117.9
    beard 110.0
    body 110.5
    dermatiacious NEC 117.8
    foot 110.4
    groin 110.3
    hand 110.2
    nail 110.1
    pathogenic to compromised host only 118
    perianal (area) 110.3
    scalp 110.0
    scrotum 110.8
    skin 111.9
      foot 110.4
      hand 110.2
    toenails 110.1
    trachea 117.9
  Fusarium 118
  Fusobacterium 041.84
  gallbladder (*see also* Cholecystitis, acute) 575.0
  Gardnerella vaginalis 041.89
  gas bacillus (*see also* Gas, gangrene) 040.0
  gastric (*see also* Gastritis) 535.5
  Gastrodiscoides hominis 121.8
  gastroenteric (*see also* Enteritis, due to, by
    organism) 009.0

Infection, infected, infective—*continued*
  gastrointestinal (*see also* Enteritis, due to, by
    organism) 009.0
  gastrostomy 536.41
  generalized NEC (*see also* Septicemia) 038.9
  genital organ or tract NEC
    female 614.9
      with
        abortion—*see* Abortion, by type, with sepsis
        ectopic pregnancy (*see also* categories
          633.0-633.9) 639.0
        molar pregnancy (*see also* categories
          630-632) 639.0
      complicating pregnancy 646.6
        affecting fetus or newborn 760.8
      following
        abortion 639.0
        ectopic or molar pregnancy 639.0
      puerperal, postpartum, childbirth 670.8
        minor or localized 646.6
          affecting fetus or newborn 760.8
    male 608.4
  genitourinary tract NEC 599.0
  Ghon tubercle, primary (*see also* Tuberculosis)
    010.0
  Giardia lamblia 007.1
  gingival (chronic) 523.10
    acute 523.00
    Vincent's 101
  glanders 024
  Glenosporopsis amazonica 116.2
  Gnathostoma spinigerum 128.1
  Gongylonema 125.6
  gonococcal NEC (*see also* Gonococcus) 098.0
  gram-negative bacilli NEC 041.85
    anaerobic 041.84
  guinea worm 125.7
  gum (*see also* Infection, gingival) 523.10
  Hantavirus 079.81
  heart 429.89
  Helicobacter pylori [*H. pylori*] 041.86
  helminths NEC 128.9
    intestinal 127.9
      mixed (types classifiable to more than one
        category in 120.0-127.7) 127.8
      specified type NEC 127.7
    specified type NEC 128.8
  Hemophilus influenzae NEC 041.5
    generalized 038.41
  Herpes (simplex) (*see also* Herpes, simplex)
    054.9
    congenital 771.2
    zoster (*see also* Herpes, zoster) 053.9
      eye NEC 053.29
  Heterophyes heterophyes 121.6
  Histoplasma (*see also* Histoplasmosis) 115.90
    capsulatum (*see also* Histoplasmosis,
      American) 115.00
    duboisii (*see also* Histoplasmosis, African)
      115.10
  HIV V08
    with symptoms, symptomatic 042
  hookworm (*see also* Ancylostomiasis) 126.9
  human herpesvirus 6 058.81
  human herpesvirus 7 058.82
  human herpesvirus 8 058.89
  human herpesvirus NEC 058.89
  human immunodeficiency virus V08
    with symptoms, symptomatic 042
  human papillomavirus 079.4
  hydrocele 603.1
  hydronephrosis 591

Infection, infected, infective—*continued*
Hymenolepis 123.6
hypopharynx 478.29
inguinal glands 683
  due to soft chancre 099.0
insertion site 999.33
intestine, intestinal (*see also* Enteritis, due to, by
  organism) 009.0
intrauterine (*see also* Endometritis) 615.9
  complicating delivery 646.6
isospora belli or hominis 007.2
Japanese B encephalitis 062.0
jaw (bone) (acute) (chronic) (lower) (subacute)
  (upper) 526.4
joint—*see* Arthritis, infectious or infective
Kaposi's sarcoma-associated herpesvirus 058.89
kidney (cortex) (hematogenous) 590.9
  with
    abortion—*see* Abortion, by type, with
      urinary tract infection
    calculus 592.0
    ectopic pregnancy (*see also* categories
      633.0-633.9) 639.8
    molar pregnancy (*see also* categories
      630-632) 639.8
  complicating pregnancy or puerperium 646.6
    affecting fetus or newborn 760.1
  following
    abortion 639.8
    ectopic or molar pregnancy 639.8
  pelvis and ureter 590.3
Klebsiella pneumoniae NEC 041.3
knee (skin) NEC 686.9
  joint—*see* Arthritis, infectious
Koch's (*see also* Tuberculosis, pulmonary) 011.9
labia (majora) (minora) (*see also* Vulvitis)
  616.10
lacrimal
  gland (*see also* Dacryoadenitis) 375.00
  passages (duct) (sac) (*see also* Dacryocystitis)
    375.30
larynx NEC 478.79
leg (skin) NEC 686.9
Leishmania (*see also* Leishmaniasis) 085.9
  braziliensis 085.5
  donovani 085.0
  Ethiopica 085.3
  furunculosa 085.1
  infantum 085.0
  mexicana 085.4
  tropica (minor) 085.1
    major 085.2
Leptosphaeria senegalensis 117.4
leptospira (*see also* Leptospirosis) 100.9
  Australis 100.89
  Bataviae 100.89
  pyrogenes 100.89
  specified type NEC 100.89
leptospirochetal NEC (*see also* Leptospirosis)
  100.9
Leptothrix—*see* Actinomycosis
Listeria monocytogenes (listeriosis) 027.0
  congenital 771.2
liver fluke—*see* Infestation, fluke, liver
Loa loa 125.2
  eyelid 125.2 *[373.6]*
Loboa loboi 116.2
local, skin (staphylococcal) (streptococcal) NEC
  686.9
  abscess—*see* Abscess, by site
  cellulitis—*see* Cellulitis, by site
  ulcer (*see also* Ulcer, skin) 707.9

Infection, infected, infective—*continued*
Loefflerella
  mallei 024
  whitmori 025
lung 518.89
  atypical Mycobacterium 031.0
  tuberculous (*see also* Tuberculosis,
    pulmonary) 011.9
  basilar 518.89
  chronic 518.89
  fungus NEC 117.9
  spirochetal 104.8
  virus—*see* Pneumonia, virus
lymph gland (axillary) (cervical) (inguinal) 683
  mesenteric 289.2
lymphoid tissue, base of tongue or posterior
  pharynx, NEC 474.00
madurella
  grisea 117.4
  mycetomii 117.4
major
  with
    abortion—*see* Abortion, by type, with sepsis
    ectopic pregnancy (*see also* categories
      633.0-633.9) 639.0
    molar pregnancy (*see also* categories
      630-632) 639.0
  following
    abortion 639.0
    ectopic or molar pregnancy 639.0
  puerperal, postpartum, childbirth 670.0
malarial—*see* Malaria
Malassezia furfur 111.0
Malleomyces
  mallei 024
  pseudomallei 025
mammary gland 611.0
  puerperal, postpartum 675.2
Mansonella (ozzardi) 125.5
mastoid (suppurative)—*see* Mastoiditis
maxilla, maxillary 526.4
  sinus (chronic) (*see also* Sinusitis, maxillary)
    473.0
mediastinum 519.2
medina 125.7
meibomian
  cyst 373.12
  gland 373.12
melioidosis 025
meninges (*see also* Meningitis) 320.9
meningococcal (*see also* condition) 036.9
  brain 036.1
  cerebrospinal 036.0
  endocardium 036.42
  generalized 036.2
  meninges 036.0
  meningococcemia 036.2
  specified site NEC 036.89
mesenteric lymph nodes or glands NEC 289.2
Metagonimus 121.5
metatarsophalangeal 711.97
methicillin
  resistant Staphylococcus aureus (MRSA) 041.12
  susceptible Staphylococcus aureus (MSSA)
    041.11
microorganism resistant to drugs—*see*
  Resistance (to), drugs by microorganisms
Microsporidia 136.8
microsporum, microsporic—*see*
  Dermatophytosis
Mima polymorpha NEC 041.85
mixed flora NEC 041.89

Infection, infected, infective—*continued*
  Monilia (*see also* Candidiasis) 112.9
    neonatal 771.7
  monkeypox 059.01
  Monosporium apiospermum 117.6
  mouth (focus) NEC 528.9
    parasitic 112.0
  MRSA (methicillin resistant Staphylococcus
      aureus) 041.12
  MSSA (methicillin susceptible Staphylococcus
      aureus) 041.11
  Mucor 117.7
  muscle NEC 728.89
  mycelium NEC 117.9
  mycetoma
    actinomycotic NEC (*see also* Actinomycosis) 039.9
    mycotic NEC 117.4
  Mycobacterium, mycobacterial (*see also*
      Mycobacterium) 031.9
  mycoplasma NEC 041.81
  mycotic NEC 117.9
    pathogenic to compromised host only 118
    skin NEC 111.9
    systemic 117.9
  myocardium NEC 422.90
  nail (chronic) (with lymphangitis) 681.9
    finger 681.02
      fungus 110.1
    ingrowing 703.0
    toe 681.11
      fungus 110.1
  nasal sinus (chronic) (*see also* Sinusitis) 473.9
  nasopharynx (chronic) 478.29
    acute 460
  navel 686.9
    newborn 771.4
  Neisserian—*see* Gonococcus
  Neotestudina rosatii 117.4
  newborn, generalized 771.89
  nipple 611.0
    puerperal, postpartum 675.0
      with breast 675.9
        specified type NEC 675.8
  Nocardia—*see* Actinomycosis
  nose 478.19
  nostril 478.19
  obstetrical surgical wound 674.3
  Oesophagostomum (apiostomum) 127.7
  Oestrus ovis 134.0
  Oidium albicans (*see also* Candidiasis) 112.9
  Onchocerca (volvulus) 125.3
    eye 125.3 [360.13]
    eyelid 125.3 [373.6]
  operation wound 998.59
  Opisthorchis (felineus) (tenuicollis) (viverrini)
      121.0
  orbit 376.00
    chronic 376.10
  orthopoxvirus 059.00
    specified NEC 059.09
  ovary (*see also* Salpingo-oophoritis) 614.2
  Oxyuris vermicularis 127.4
  pancreas 577.0
  Paracoccidioides brasiliensis 116.1
  Paragonimus (westermani) 121.2
  parainfluenza virus 079.89
  parameningococcus NEC 036.9
    with meningitis 036.0
  parapoxvirus 059.10
    specified NEC 059.19
  parasitic NEC 136.9

Infection, infected, infective—*continued*
  paratyphoid 002.9
    Type A 002.1
    Type B 002.2
    Type C 002.3
  paraurethral ducts 597.89
  parotid gland 527.2
  Pasteurella NEC 027.2
    multocida (cat-bite) (dog-bite) 027.2
    pestis (*see also* Plague) 020.9
    pseudotuberculosis 027.2
    septica (cat-bite) (dog-bite) 027.2
    tularensis (*see also* Tularemia) 021.9
  pelvic, female (*see also* Disease, pelvis,
      inflammatory) 614.9
  penis (glans) (retention) NEC 607.2
    herpetic 054.13
  Peptococcus 041.84
  Peptostreptococcus 041.84
  periapical (pulpal origin) 522.4
  peridental 523.30
  perineal wound (obstetrical) 674.3
  periodontal 523.31
  periorbital 376.00
    chronic 376.10
  perirectal 569.49
  perirenal (*see also* Infection, kidney) 590.9
  peritoneal (*see also* Peritonitis) 567.9
  periureteral 593.89
  periurethral 597.89
  Petriellidium boydii 117.6
  pharynx 478.29
    Coxsackie virus 074.0
    phlegmonous 462
    posterior, lymphoid 474.00
  Phialophora
    gougerotii 117.8
    jeanselmei 117.8
    verrucosa 117.2
  Piedraia hortai 111.3
  pinna, acute 380.11
  pinta 103.9
    intermediate 103.1
    late 103.2
    mixed 103.3
    primary 103.0
  pinworm 127.4
  pityrosporum furfur 111.0
  pleuropneumonia-like organisms NEC (PPLO)
      041.81
  pneumococcal NEC 041.2
    generalized (purulent) 038.2
  Pneumococcus NEC 041.2
  port 999.33
  postoperative wound 998.59
  posttraumatic NEC 958.3
  postvaccinal 999.39
  poxvirus 059.9
    specified NEC 059.8
  prepuce 607.1
  Propionibacterium 041.84
  prostate (capsule) (*see also* Prostatitis) 601.9
  Proteus (mirabilis) (morganii) (vulgaris) NEC
      041.6
    enteritis 008.3
  protozoal NEC 136.8
    intestinal NEC 007.9
  Pseudomonas NEC 041.7
    mallei 024
    pneumonia 482.1
    pseudomallei 025

Infection, infected, infective—*continued*
  psittacosis 073.9
  puerperal, postpartum (major) 670.0
    minor 646.6
  pulmonary—*see* Infection, lung
  purulent—*see* Abscess
  putrid, generalized—*see* Septicemia
  pyemic—*see* Septicemia
  Pyrenochaeta romeroi 117.4
  Q fever 083.0
  rabies 071
  rectum (sphincter) 569.49
  renal (*see also* Infection, kidney) 590.9
    pelvis and ureter 590.3
  reservoir 999.33
  resistant to drugs—*see* Resistance (to), drugs by
    microorganisms
  respiratory 519.8
    chronic 519.8
    influenzal (acute) (upper) (*see also* Influenza)
      487.1
    lung 518.89
    rhinovirus 460
    syncytial virus 079.6
    upper (acute) (infectious) NEC 465.9
      with flu, grippe, or influenza (*see also*
        Influenza) 487.1
      influenzal (*see also* Influenza) 487.1
      multiple sites NEC 465.8
      streptococcal 034.0
      viral NEC 465.9
  respiratory syncytial virus (RSV) 079.6
  resulting from presence of shunt or other
    internal prosthetic device—*see*
    Complications, infection and inflammation,
    due to (presence of) any device, implant, or
    graft classified to 996.0-996.5 NEC
  retroperitoneal 567.39
  retrovirus 079.50
    human immunodeficiency virus type 2
      (HIV-2) 079.53
    human T-cell lymphotrophic virus type I
      (HTLV-I) 079.51
    human T-cell lymphotrophic virus type II
      (HTLV-II) 079.52
    specified NEC 079.59
  Rhinocladium 117.1
  Rhinosporidium (*see*beri) 117.0
  rhinovirus
    in diseases classified elsewhere—*see* category
      079
    unspecified nature or site 079.3
  Rhizopus 117.7
  rickettsial 083.9
  rickettsialpox 083.2
  rubella (*see also* Rubella) 056.9
    congenital 771.0
  Saccharomyces (*see also* Candidiasis) 112.9
  Saksenaea 117.7
  salivary duct or gland (any) 527.2
  Salmonella (aertrycke) (callinarum)
    (choleraesuis) (enteritidis) (suipestifer)
    (typhimurium) 003.9
    with
      arthritis 003.23
      gastroenteritis 003.0
      localized infection 003.20
        specified type NEC 003.29
      meningitis 003.21
      osteomyelitis 003.24
      pneumonia 003.22

Infection, infected, infective—*continued*
  septicemia 003.1
    specified manifestation NEC 003.8
  due to food (poisoning) (any serotype) (*see
    also* Poisoning, food, due to, Salmonella)
  hirschfeldii 002.3
  localized 003.20
    specified type NEC 003.29
  paratyphi 002.9
    A 002.1
    B 002.2
    C 002.3
  schottmuelleri 002.2
  specified type NEC 003.8
  typhi 002.0
  typhosa 002.0
  saprophytic 136.8
  Sarcocystis, lindemanni 136.5
  SARS-associated coronavirus 079.82
  scabies 133.0
  Schistosoma—*see* Infestation, Schistosoma
  Schmorl's bacillus 040.3
  scratch or other superficial injury—*see* Injury,
    superficial, by site
  scrotum (acute) NEC 608.4
  sealpox 059.12
  secondary, burn or open wound (dislocation)
    (fracture) 958.3
  seminal vesicle (*see also* Vesiculitis) 608.0
  septic
    generalized—*see* Septicemia
    localized, skin (*see also* Abscess) 682.9
  septicemic—*see* Septicemia
  seroma 998.51
  Serratia (marcescens) 041.85
    generalized 038.44
  sheep liver fluke 121.3
  Shigella 004.9
    boydii 004.2
    dysenteriae 004.0
    Flexneri 004.1
    group
      A 004.0
      B 004.1
      C 004.2
      D 004.3
    Schmitz (-Stutzer) 004.0
    Schmitzii 004.0
    Shiga 004.0
    Sonnei 004.3
    specified type NEC 004.8
  Sin Nombre virus 079.81
  sinus (*see also* Sinusitis) 473.9
    pilonidal 685.1
      with abscess 685.0
    skin NEC 686.9
  Skene's duct or gland (*see also* Urethritis) 597.89
  skin (local) (staphylococcal) (streptococcal)
    NEC 686.9
    abscess—*see* Abscess, by site
    cellulitis—*see* Cellulitis, by site
    due to fungus 111.9
      specified type NEC 111.8
    mycotic 111.9
      specified type NEC 111.8
    ulcer (*see also* Ulcer, skin) 707.9
  slow virus 046.9
    specified condition NEC 046.8
  Sparganum (mansoni) (proliferum) 123.5
  spermatic cord NEC 608.4

Infection, infected, infective—*continued*
  sphenoidal (chronic) (sinus) (*see also* Sinusitis, sphenoidal) 473.3
  Spherophorus necrophorus 040.3
  spinal cord NEC (*see also* Encephalitis) 323.9
    abscess 324.1
      late effect—*see* category 326
    late effect—*see* category 326
    meninges—*see* Meningitis
    streptococcal 320.2
  Spirillum
    minus or minor 026.0
    morsus muris 026.0
    obermeieri 087.0
  spirochetal NEC 104.9
    lung 104.8
    specified nature or site NEC 104.8
  spleen 289.59
  Sporothrix schenckii 117.1
  Sporotrichum (schenckii) 117.1
  Sporozoa 136.8
  staphylococcal NEC 041.10
    aureus 041.11
      methicillin
        resistant (MRSA) 041.12
        susceptible MSSA) 041.11
    food poisoning 005.0
    generalized (purulent) 038.10
      aureus 038.11
        methicillin
          resistant 038.12
          susceptible 038.11
      specified organism NEC 038.19
    pneumonia 482.40
      aureus 482.41
        methicillin
          resistant (MRSA) 482.42
          susceptible (MSSA) 482.41
      MRSA (methicillin resistant staphylococcus aureus) 482.42
      MSSA (methicillin susceptible staphylococcus aureus) 482.41
      specified type NEC 482.49
    septicemia 038.10
      aureus 038.11
        methicillin
          resistant (MRSA) 038.12
          susceptible (MSSA) 038.11
      MRSA (methicillin resistant staphylococcus aureus) 038.12
      MSSA (methicillin susceptible staphylococcus aureus) 038.11
      specified organism NEC 038.19
    specified NEC 041.19
  steatoma 706.2
  Stellantchasmus falcatus 121.6
  Streptobacillus moniliformis 026.1
  streptococcal NEC 041.00
    generalized (purulent) 038.0
    group
      A 041.01
      B 041.02
      C 041.03
      D [enterococcus] 041.04
      G 041.05
    pneumonia—*see* Pneumonia, streptococcal 482.3
    septicemia 038.0
    sore throat 034.0
    specified NEC 041.09
  Streptomyces—*see* Actinomycosis

Infection, infected, infective—*continued*
  streptotrichosis—*see* Actinomycosis
  Strongyloides (stercoralis) 127.2
  stump (amputation) (posttraumatic) (surgical) 997.62
    traumatic—*see* Amputation, traumatic, by site, complicated
  subcutaneous tissue, local NEC 686.9
  submaxillary region 528.9
  suipestifer (*see also* Infection, Salmonella) 003.9
  swimming pool bacillus 031.1
  syphilitic—*see* Syphilis
  systemic—*see* Septicemia
  Taenia—*see* Infestation, Taenia
  Taeniarhynchus saginatus 123.2
  tanapox 059.21
  tapeworm—*see* Infestation, tapeworm
  tendon (sheath) 727.89
  Ternidens diminutus 127.7
  testis (*see also* Orchitis) 604.90
  thigh (skin) 686.9
  threadworm 127.4
  throat 478.29
    pneumococcal 462
    staphylococcal 462
    streptococcal 034.0
    viral NEC (*see also* Pharyngitis) 462
  thumb (skin) 686.9
    abscess (with lymphangitis) 681.00
      pulp 681.01
    cellulitis (with lymphangitis) 681.00
    nail 681.02
  thyroglossal duct 529.8
  toe (skin) 686.9
    abscess (with lymphangitis) 681.10
    cellulitis (with lymphangitis) 681.10
    nail 681.11
      fungus 110.1
  tongue NEC 529.0
    parasitic 112.0
  tonsil (faucial) (lingual) (pharyngeal) 474.00
    acute or subacute 463
    and adenoid 474.02
    tag 474.00
  tooth, teeth 522.4
    periapical (pulpal origin) 522.4
    peridental 523.30
    periodontal 523.31
    pulp 522.0
    socket 526.5
  TORCH - see Infection, congenital NEC
    without active infection 760.2
  Torula histolytica 117.5
  Toxocara (cani) (cati) (felis) 128.0
  Toxoplasma gondii (*see also* Toxoplasmosis) 130.9
  trachea, chronic 491.8
    fungus 117.9
  traumatic NEC 958.3
  trematode NEC 121.9
  trench fever 083.1
  Treponema
    denticola 041.84
    macrodenticum 041.84
    pallidum (*see also* Syphilis) 097.9
  Trichinella (spiralis) 124
  Trichomonas 131.9
    bladder 131.09
    cervix 131.09
    hominis 007.3
    intestine 007.3
    prostate 131.03
    specified site NEC 131.8

Infection, infected, infective—*continued*
   urethra 131.02
   urogenitalis 131.00
   vagina 131.01
   vulva 131.01
Trichophyton, trichophytid—*see*
   Dermatophytosis
Trichosporon (beigelii) cutaneum 111.2
Trichostrongylus 127.6
Trichuris (trichiuria) 127.3
Trombicula (irritans) 133.8
Trypanosoma (*see also* Trypanosomiasis) 086.9
   cruzi 086.2
tubal (*see also* Salpingo-oophoritis) 614.2
tuberculous NEC (*see also* Tuberculosis) 011.9
tubo-ovarian (*see also* Salpingo-oophoritis)
   614.2
tunica vaginalis 608.4
tunnel 999.33
tympanic membrane—*see* Myringitis
typhoid (abortive) (ambulant) (bacillus) 002.0
typhus 081.9
   flea-borne (endemic) 081.0
   louse-borne (epidemic) 080
   mite-borne 081.2
   recrudescent 081.1
   tick-borne 082.9
     African 082.1
     North Asian 082.2
umbilicus (septic) 686.9
   newborn NEC 771.4
ureter 593.89
urethra (*see also* Urethritis) 597.80
urinary (tract) NEC 599.0
   with
     abortion—*see* Abortion, by type, with
       urinary tract infection
     ectopic pregnancy (*see also* categories
       633.0-633.9) 639.8
     molar pregnancy (*see also* categories
       630-632) 639.8
   candidal 112.2
   complicating pregnancy, childbirth, or
     puerperium 646.6
     affecting fetus or newborn 760.1
     asymptomatic 646.5
     affecting fetus or newborn 760.1
   diplococcal (acute) 098.0
     chronic 098.2
   due to Trichomonas (vaginalis) 131.00
   following
     abortion 639.8
     ectopic or molar pregnancy 639.8
   gonococcal (acute) 098.0
     chronic or duration of 2 months or over
       098.2
   newborn 771.82
   trichomonal 131.00
   tuberculous (*see also* Tuberculosis) 016.3
uterus, uterine (*see also* Endometritis) 615.9
utriculus masculinus NEC 597.89
vaccination 999.39
vagina (granulation tissue) (wall) (*see also*
   Vaginitis) 616.10
varicella 052.9
varicose veins—*see* Varicose, veins
variola 050.9
   major 050.0
   minor 050.1
vas deferens NEC 608.4
Veillonella 041.84

Infection, infected, infective—*continued*
   verumontanum 597.89
   vesical (*see also* Cystitis) 595.9
   Vibrio
     cholerae 001.0
     El Tor 001.1
     parahaemolyticus (food poisoning) 005.4
     vulnificus 041.85
   Vincent's (gums) (mouth) (tonsil) 101
   virus, viral 079.99
     adenovirus
       in diseases classified elsewhere—*see*
         category 079
       unspecified nature or site 079.0
     central nervous system NEC 049.9
       enterovirus 048
         meningitis 047.9
         specified type NEC 047.8
       slow virus 046.9
         specified condition NEC 046.8
     chest 519.8
     conjunctivitis 077.99
       specified type NEC 077.8
     coronavirus 079.89
       SARS-associated 079.82
     Coxsackie (*see also* Infection, Coxsackie) 079.2
     Ebola 065.8
     ECHO
       in diseases classified elsewhere—*see*
         category 079
       unspecified nature or site 079.1
     encephalitis 049.9
       arthropod-borne NEC 064
       tick-borne 063.9
         specified type NEC 063.8
     enteritis NEC (*see also* Enteritis, viral) 008.8
     exanthem NEC 057.9
     Hantavirus 079.81
     human papilloma 079.4
     in diseases classified elsewhere—*see* category 079
     intestine (*see also* Enteritis, viral) 008.8
     lung—*see* Pneumonia, viral
     respiratory syncytial virus (RSV) 079.6
     rhinovirus
       in diseases classified elsewhere—*see*
         category 079
       unspecified nature or site 079.3
     salivary gland disease 078.5
     slow 046.9
       specified condition NEC 046.8
     specified type NEC 079.89
       in diseases classified elsewhere—*see*
         category 079
       unspecified nature or site 079.99
     warts 078.10
       specified NEC 078.19
     yaba monkey tumor 059.22
   vulva (*see also* Vulvitis) 616.10
   whipworm 127.3
   Whitmore's bacillus 025
   wound (local) (posttraumatic) NEC 958.3
     with
       dislocation—*see* Dislocation, by site, open
       fracture—*see* Fracture, by site, open
       open wound—*see* Wound, open, by site,
         complicated
     postoperative 998.59
     surgical 998.59
   Wuchereria 125.0
     bancrofti 125.0
     malayi 125.1

Infection, infected, infective—*continued*
  yaba monkey tumor virus 059.22
  yatapoxvirus 059.20
  yaws—*see* Yaws
  yeast (*see also* Candidiasis) 112.9
  yellow fever (*see also* Fever, yellow) 060.9
  Yersinia pestis (*see also* Plague) 020.9
  Zeis' gland 373.12
  zoonotic bacterial NEC 027.9
  Zopfia senegalensis 117.4
Infective, infectious —*see* condition
Inferiority complex 301.9
  constitutional psychopathic 301.9
Infertility
  female 628.9
   age related 628.8
   associated with
    adhesions, peritubal 614.6 *[628.2]*
    anomaly
     cervical mucus 628.4
     congenital
      cervix 628.4
      fallopian tube 628.2
      uterus 628.3
      vagina 628.4
    anovulation 628.0
    dysmucorrhea 628.4
    endometritis, tuberculous (*see also*
     Tuberculosis) 016.7 *[628.3]*
    Stein-Leventhal syndrome 256.4 *[628.0]*
   due to
    adiposogenital dystrophy 253.8 *[628.1]*
    anterior pituitary disorder NEC 253.4
     [628.1]
     hyperfunction 253.1 *[628.1]*
    cervical anomaly 628.4
    fallopian tube anomaly 628.2
    ovarian failure 256.39 *[628.0]*
    Stein-Leventhal syndrome 256.4 *[628.0]*
    uterine anomaly 628.3
    vaginal anomaly 628.4
   nonimplantation 628.3
   origin
    cervical 628.4
    pituitary-hypothalamus NEC 253.8 *[628.1]*
     anterior pituitary NEC 253.4 *[628.1]*
      hyperfunction NEC 253.1 *[628.1]*
     dwarfism 253.3 *[628.1]*
     panhypopituitarism 253.2 *[628.1]*
    specified NEC 628.8
    tubal (block) (occlusion) (stenosis) 628.2
     adhesions 614.6 *[628.2]*
    uterine 628.3
    vaginal 628.4
   previous, requiring supervision of pregnancy
    V23.0
  male 606.9
   absolute 606.0
   due to
    azoospermia 606.0
    drug therapy 606.8
    extratesticular cause NEC 606.8
    germinal cell
     aplasia 606.0
     desquamation 606.1
    hypospermatogenesis 606.1
    infection 606.8
    obstruction, afferent ducts 606.8
    oligospermia 606.1
    radiation 606.8

Infertility—*continued*
  male—*continued*
    spermatogenic arrest (complete) 606.0
     incomplete 606.1
    systemic disease 606.8
Infestation 134.9
  Acanthocheilonema (perstans) 125.4
   streptocerca 125.6
  Acariasis 133.9
   demodex folliculorum 133.8
   Sarcoptes scabiei 133.0
   trombiculae 133.8
  Agamofilaria streptocerca 125.6
  Ancylostoma, Ankylostoma 126.9
   americanum 126.1
   braziliense 126.2
   canium 126.8
   ceylanicum 126.3
   duodenale 126.0
   new world 126.1
   old world 126.0
  Angiostrongylus cantonensis 128.8
  anisakiasis 127.1
  Anisakis larva 127.1
  arthropod NEC 134.1
  Ascaris lumbricoides 127.0
  Bacillus fusiformis 101
  Balantidium coli 007.0
  beef tapeworm 123.2
  Bothriocephalus (latus) 123.4
   larval 123.5
  broad tapeworm 123.4
   larval 123.5
  Brugia malayi 125.1
  Candiru 136.8
  Capillaria
   hepatica 128.8
   philippinensis 127.5
  cat liver fluke 121.0
  Cercomonas hominis (intestinal) 007.3
  cestodes 123.9
   specified type NEC 123.8
  chigger 133.8
  chigoe 134.1
  Chilomastix 007.8
  Clonorchis (sinensis) (liver) 121.1
  coccidia 007.2
  complicating pregnancy, childbirth, or
   puerperium 647.9
   affecting fetus or newborn 760.8
  Cysticercus cellulosae 123.1
  Demodex folliculorum 133.8
  Dermatobia (hominis) 134.0
  Dibothriocephalus (latus) 123.4
   larval 123.5
  Dicrocoelium dendriticum 121.8
  Diphyllobothrium (adult) (intestinal) (latum)
   (pacificum) 123.4
   larval 123.5
  Diplogonoporus (grandis) 123.8
  Dipylidium (caninum) 123.8
  Distoma hepaticum 121.3
  dog tapeworm 123.8
  Dracunculus medinensis 125.7
  dragon worm 125.7
  dwarf tapeworm 123.6
  Echinococcus (*see also* Echinococcus) 122.9
  Echinostoma ilocanum 121.8
  Embadomonas 007.8
  Endamoeba (histolytica)—*see* Infection, ameba
  Entamoeba (histolytica)—*see* Infection, ameba

Infestation—*continued*
  Enterobius vermicularis 127.4
  Epidermophyton—*see* Dermatophytosis
  eyeworm 125.2
  Fasciola
    gigantica 121.3
    hepatica 121.3
  Fasciolopsis (buski) (small intestine) 121.4
  filarial 125.9
    due to
      Acanthocheilonema (perstans) 125.4
        streptocerca 125.6
      Brugia (Wuchereria) malayi 125.1
      Dracunculus medinensis 125.7
      guinea worms 125.7
      Mansonella (ozzardi) 125.5
      Onchocerca volvulus 125.3
        eye 125.3 *[360.13]*
        eyelid 125.3 *[373.6]*
      Wuchereria (bancrofti) 125.0
        malayi 125.1
    specified type NEC 125.6
  fish tapeworm 123.4
    larval 123.5
  fluke 121.9
    blood NEC (*see also* Schistosomiasis) 120.9
    cat liver 121.0
    intestinal (giant) 121.4
    liver (sheep) 121.3
      cat 121.0
      Chinese 121.1
      clonorchiasis 121.1
      fascioliasis 121.3
      Oriental 121.1
    lung (oriental) 121.2
    sheep liver 121.3
  fly larva 134.0
  Gasterophilus (intestinalis) 134.0
  Gastrodiscoides hominis 121.8
  Giardia lamblia 007.1
  Gnathostoma (spinigerum) 128.1
  Gongylonema 125.6
  guinea worm 125.7
  helminth NEC 128.9
    intestinal 127.9
      mixed (types classifiable to more than one
        category in 120.0-127.7) 127.8
      specified type NEC 127.7
    specified type NEC 128.8
  Heterophyes heterophyes (small intestine) 121.6
  hookworm (*see also* Infestation, ancylostoma)
    126.9
  Hymenolepis (diminuta) (nana) 123.6
  intestinal NEC 129
  leeches (aquatic) (land) 134.2
  Leishmania—*see* Leishmaniasis
  lice (*see also* infestation, pediculus) 132.9
  Linguatulidae, linguatula (pentastoma) (serrata)
    134.1
  Loa loa 125.2
    eyelid 125.2 *[373.6]*
  louse (*see also* Infestation, pediculus) 132.9
    body 132.1
    head 132.0
    pubic 132.2
  maggots 134.0
  Mansonella (ozzardi) 125.5
  medina 125.7
  Metagonimus yokogawai (small intestine) 121.5
  Microfilaria streptocerca 125.3
    eye 125.3 *[360.13]*
    eyelid 125.3 *[373.6]*

Infestation—*continued*
  Microsporon furfur 111.0
  microsporum—*see* Dermatophytosis
  mites 133.9
    scabic 133.0
    specified type NEC 133.8
  Monilia (albicans) (*see also* Candidiasis) 112.9
    vagina 112.1
    vulva 112.1
  mouth 112.0
  Necator americanus 126.1
  nematode (intestinal) 127.9
    Ancylostoma (*see also* Ancylostoma) 126.9
    Ascaris lumbricoides 127.0
    conjunctiva NEC 128.9
    Dioctophyma 128.8
    Enterobius vermicularis 127.4
    Gnathostoma spinigerum 128.1
    Oesophagostomum (apiostomum) 127.7
    Physaloptera 127.4
    specified type NEC 127.7
    Strongyloides stercoralis 127.2
    Ternidens diminutus 127.7
    Trichinella spiralis 124
    Trichostrongylus 127.6
    Trichuris (trichiuria) 127.3
  Oesophagostomum (apiostomum) 127.7
  Oestrus ovis 134.0
  Onchocerca (volvulus) 125.3
    eye 125.3 *[360.13]*
    eyelid 125.3 *[373.6]*
  Opisthorchis (felineus) (tenuicollis) (viverrini)
    121.0
  Oxyuris vermicularis 127.4
  Paragonimus (westermani) 121.2
  parasite, parasitic NEC 136.9
    eyelid 134.9 *[373.6]*
    intestinal 129
    mouth 112.0
    orbit 376.13
    skin 134.9
    tongue 112.0
  pediculus 132.9
    capitis (humanus) (any site) 132.0
    corporis (humanus) (any site) 132.1
    eyelid 132.0 *[373.6]*
    mixed (classifiable to more than one category
      in 132.0-132.2) 132.3
    pubis (any site) 132.2
  phthirus (pubis) (any site) 132.2
    with any infestation classifiable to 132.0 and
      132.1 132.3
  pinworm 127.4
  pork tapeworm (adult) 123.0
  protozoal NEC 136.8
  pubic louse 132.2
  rat tapeworm 123.6
  red bug 133.8
  roundworm (large) NEC 127.0
  sand flea 134.1
  saprophytic NEC 136.8
  Sarcoptes scabiei 133.0
  scabies 133.0
  Schistosoma 120.9
    bovis 120.8
    cercariae 120.3
    hematobium 120.0
    intercalatum 120.8
    japonicum 120.2
    mansoni 120.1
    mattheii 120.8

Infestation—*continued*
Schistosoma —*continued*
specified
site—*see* Schistosomiasis
type NEC 120.8
spindale 120.8
screw worms 134.0
skin NEC 134.9
Sparganum (mansoni) (proliferum) 123.5
larval 123.5
specified type NEC 134.8
Spirometra larvae 123.5
Sporozoa NEC 136.8
Stellantchasmus falcatus 121.6
Strongyloides 127.2
Strongylus (gibsoni) 127.7
Taenia 123.3
diminuta 123.6
Echinococcus (*see also* Echinococcus) 122.9
mediocanellata 123.2
nana 123.6
saginata (mediocanellata) 123.2
solium (intestinal form) 123.0
larval form 123.1
Taeniarhynchus saginatus 123.2
tapeworm 123.9
beef 123.2
broad 123.4
larval 123.5
dog 123.8
dwarf 123.6
fish 123.4
larval 123.5
pork 123.0
rat 123.6
Ternidens diminutus 127.7
Tetranychus molestissimus 133.8
threadworm 127.4
tongue 112.0
Toxocara (cani) (cati) (felis) 128.0
trematode(s) NEC 121.9
Trichina spiralis 124
Trichinella spiralis 124
Trichocephalus 127.3
Trichomonas 131.9
bladder 131.09
cervix 131.09
intestine 007.3
prostate 131.03
specified site NEC 131.8
urethra (female) (male) 131.02
urogenital 131.00
vagina 131.01
vulva 131.01
Trichophyton—*see* Dermatophytosis
Trichostrongylus instabilis 127.6
Trichuris (trichiuria) 127.3
Trombicula (irritans) 133.8
Trypanosoma—*see* Trypanosomiasis
Tunga penetrans 134.1
Uncinaria americana 126.1
whipworm 127.3
worms NEC 128.9
intestinal 127.9
Wuchereria 125.0
bancrofti 125.0
malayi 125.1
Infiltrate, infiltration
with an iron compound 275.09
amyloid (any site) (generalized) 277.39
calcareous (muscle) NEC 275.49
localized—*see* Degeneration, by site

Infiltrate, infiltration—*continued*
calcium salt (muscle) 275.49
chemotherapy, vesicant 999.81
corneal (*see also* Edema, cornea) 371.20
eyelid 373.9
fatty (diffuse) (generalized) 272.8
localized—*see* Degeneration, by site, fatty
glycogen, glycogenic (*see also* Disease,
glycogen storage) 271.10
heart, cardiac
fatty (*see also* Degeneration, myocardial)
429.1
glycogenic 271.0 *[425.7]*
inflammatory in vitreous 379.29
kidney (*see also* Disease, renal) 593.9
leukemic (M9800/3)—*see* Leukemia
liver 573.8
fatty—*see* Fatty, liver
glycogen (*see also* Disease, glycogen storage)
271.0
lung (*see also* Infiltrate, pulmonary) 793.19
eosinophilic 518.3
x-ray finding only 793.19
lymphatic (*see also* Leukemia, lymphatic) 204.9
gland, pigmentary 289.3
muscle, fatty 728.9
myelogenous (*see also* Leukemia, myeloid)
205.9
myocardium, myocardial
fatty (*see also* Degeneration, myocardial)
429.1
glycogenic 271.0 *[425.7]*
pulmonary 793.19
with
eosinophilia 518.3
pneumonia—*see* Pneumonia, by type
x-ray finding only 793.19
Ranke's primary (*see also* Tuberculosis) 010.0
skin, lymphocyctic (benign) 709.8
thymus (gland) (fatty) 254.8
urine 788.8
vesicant
agent NEC 999.82
chemotherapy 999.81
vitreous humor 379.29
Infirmity 799.89
senile 797
Inflammation, inflamed, inflammatory (with
exudation)
abducens (nerve) 378.54
accessory sinus (chronic) (*see also* Sinusitis)
473.9
adrenal (gland) 255.8
alimentary canal—*see* Enteritis
alveoli (teeth) 526.5
scorbutic 267
amnion—*see* Amnionitis
anal canal 569.49
antrum (chronic) (*see also* Sinusitis, maxillary)
473.0
anus 569.49
appendix (*see also* Appendicitis) 541
arachnoid—*see* Meningitis
areola 611.0
puerperal, postpartum 675.0
areolar tissue NEC 686.9
artery—*see* Arteritis
auditory meatus (external) (*see also* Otitis,
externa) 380.10
Bartholin's gland 616.89
bile duct or passage 576.1
bladder (*see also* Cystitis) 595.9

Inflammation—*continued*
bleb
    postprocedural 379.60
      stage 1 379.61
      stage 2 379.62
      stage 3 379.63
bone—*see* Osteomyelitis
bowel (*see also* Enteritis) 558.9
brain (*see also* Encephalitis) 323.9
    late effect—*see* category 326
    membrane—*see* Meningitis
breast 611.0
    puerperal, postpartum 675.2
broad ligament (*see also* Disease, pelvis,
    inflammatory) 614.4
    acute 614.3
bronchus—*see* Bronchitis
bursa—*see* Bursitis
capsule
    liver 573.3
    spleen 289.59
catarrhal (*see also* Catarrh) 460
    vagina 616.10
cecum (*see also* Appendicitis) 541
cerebral (*see also* Encephalitis) 323.9
    late effect—*see* category 326
    membrane—*see* Meningitis
cerebrospinal (*see also* Meningitis) 322.9
    late effect—*see* category 326
    meningococcal 036.0
    tuberculous (*see also* Tuberculosis) 013.6
cervix (uteri) (*see also* Cervicitis) 616.0
chest 519.9
choroid NEC (*see also* Choroiditis) 363.20
cicatrix (tissue)—*see* Cicatrix
colon (*see also* Enteritis) 558.9
    granulomatous 555.1
    newborn 558.9
connective tissue (diffuse) NEC 728.9
cornea (*see also* Keratitis) 370.9
    with ulcer (*see also* Ulcer, cornea) 370.00
corpora cavernosa (penis) 607.2
cranial nerve—*see* Disorder, nerve, cranial
diarrhea—*see* Diarrhea
disc (intervertebral) (space) 722.90
    cervical, cervicothoracic 722.91
    lumbar, lumbosacral 722.93
    thoracic, thoracolumbar 722.93
Douglas' cul-de-sac or pouch (chronic) (*see also*
    Disease, pelvis, inflammatory) 614.4
    acute 614.3
due to (presence of) any device, implant, or graft
    classifiable to 996.0-996.5—*see*
    Complications, infection and inflammation,
    due to (presence of) any device, implant, or
    graft classified to 996.0-996.5 NEC
duodenum 535.6
dura mater—*see* Meningitis
ear—*see also* Otitis
    external (*see also* Otitis, externa) 380.10
    inner (*see also* Labyrinthitis) 386.30
    middle—*see* Otitis media
esophagus 530.10
ethmoidal (chronic) (sinus) (*see also* Sinusitis,
    ethmoidal) 473.2
Eustachian tube (catarrhal) 381.50
    acute 381.51
    chronic 381.52
extrarectal 569.49
eye 379.99
eyelid 373.9
    specified NEC 373.8

Inflammation—*continued*
fallopian tube (*see also* Salpingo-oophoritis)
    614.2
fascia 728.9
fetal membranes (acute) 658.4
    affecting fetus or newborn 762.7
follicular, pharynx 472.1
frontal (chronic) (sinus) (*see also* Sinusitis,
    frontal) 473.1
gallbladder (*see also* Cholecystitis, acute) 575.0
gall duct (*see also* Cholecystitis) 575.10
gastrointestinal (*see also* Enteritis) 558.9
genital organ (diffuse) (internal)
    female 614.9
      with
        abortion—*see* Abortion, by type, with
          sepsis
        ectopic pregnancy (*see also* categories
          633.0-633.9) 639.0
        molar pregnancy (*see also* categories
          630-632) 639.0
      complicating pregnancy, childbirth, or
        puerperium 646.6
        affecting fetus or newborn 760.8
      following
        abortion 639.0
        ectopic or molar pregnancy 639.0
    male 608.4
gland (lymph) (*see also* Lymphadenitis) 289.3
glottis (*see also* Laryngitis) 464.00
    with obstruction 464.01
granular, pharynx 472.1
gum 523.10
heart (*see also* Carditis) 429.89
hepatic duct 576.8
hernial sac—*see* Hernia, by site
ileum (*see also* Enteritis) 558.9
    terminal or regional 555.0
    with large intestine 555.2
intervertebral disc 722.90
    cervical, cervicothoracic 722.91
    lumbar, lumbosacral 722.93
    thoracic, thoracolumbar 722.92
intestine (*see also* Enteritis) 558.9
jaw (acute) (bone) (chronic) (lower)
    (suppurative) (upper) 526.4
jejunum—*see* Enteritis
joint NEC (*see also* Arthritis) 716.9
    sacroiliac 720.2
kidney (*see also* Nephritis) 583.9
knee (joint) 716.66
    tuberculous (active) (*see also* Tuberculosis)
      015.2
labium (majus) (minus) (*see also* Vulvitis) 616.10
lacrimal
    gland (*see also* Dacryoadenitis) 375.00
    passages (duct) (sac) (*see also* Dacryocystitis)
      375.30
larynx (*see also* Laryngitis) 464.00
    with obstruction 464.01
    diphtheritic 032.3
leg NEC 686.9
lip 528.5
liver (capsule) (*see also* Hepatitis) 573.3
    acute 570
    chronic 571.40
    suppurative 572.0
lung (acute) (*see also* Pneumonia) 486
    chronic (interstitial) 518.89
lymphatic vessel (*see also* Lymphangitis) 457.2
lymph node or gland (*see also* Lymphadenitis)
    289.3

Inflammation—*continued*
  mammary gland 611.0
    puerperal, postpartum 675.2
  maxilla, maxillary 526.4
    sinus (chronic) (*see also* Sinusitis, maxillary)
      473.0
  membranes of brain or spinal cord—*see*
    Meningitis
  meninges—*see* Meningitis
  mouth 528.00
  muscle 728.9
  myocardium (*see also* Myocarditis) 429.0
  nasal sinus (chronic) (*see also* Sinusitis) 473.9
  nasopharynx—*see* Nasopharyngitis
  navel 686.9
    newborn NEC 771.4
  nerve NEC 729.2
  nipple 611.0
    puerperal, postpartum 675.0
  nose 478.19
    suppurative 472.0
  oculomotor nerve 378.51
  optic nerve 377.30
  orbit (chronic) 376.10
    acute 376.00
    chronic 376.10
  ovary (*see also* Salpingo-oophoritis) 614.2
  oviduct (*see also* Salpingo-oophoritis) 614.2
  pancreas—*see* Pancreatitis
  parametrium (chronic) (*see also* Disease, pelvis,
    inflammatory) 614.4
    acute 614.3
  parotid region 686.9
    gland 527.2
  pelvis, female (*see also* Disease, pelvis,
    inflammatory) 614.9
  penis (corpora cavernosa) 607.2
  perianal 569.49
  pericardium (*see also* Pericarditis) 423.9
  perineum (female) (male) 686.9
  perirectal 569.49
  peritoneum (*see also* Peritonitis) 567.9
  periuterine (*see also* Disease, pelvis,
    inflammatory) 614.9
  perivesical (*see also* Cystitis) 595.9
  petrous bone (*see also* Petrositis) 383.20
  pharynx (*see also* Pharyngitis) 462
    follicular 472.1
    granular 472.1
  pia mater—*see* Meningitis
  pleura—*see* Pleurisy
  postmastoidectomy cavity 383.30
    chronic 383.33
  pouch, internal ileoanal 569.71
  prostate (*see also* Prostatitis) 601.9
  rectosigmoid—*see* Rectosigmoiditis
  rectum (*see also* Proctitis) 569.49
  respiratory, upper (*see also* Infection,
    respiratory, upper) 465.9
    chronic, due to external agent—*see* Condition,
      respiratory, chronic, due to, external agent
    due to
      fumes or vapors (chemical) (inhalation)
        506.2
      radiation 508.1
  retina (*see also* Retinitis) 363.20
  retrocecal (*see also* Appendicitis) 541
  retroperitoneal (*see also* Peritonitis) 567.9
  salivary duct or gland (any) (suppurative) 527.2
  scorbutic, alveoli, teeth 267
  scrotum 608.4
  sigmoid—*see* Enteritis

Inflammation—*continued*
  sinus (*see also* Sinusitis) 473.9
  Skene's duct or gland (*see also* Urethritis)
    597.89
  skin 686.9
  spermatic cord 608.4
  sphenoidal (sinus) (*see also* Sinusitis,
    sphenoidal) 473.3
  spinal
    cord (*see also* Encephalitis) 323.9
      late effect—*see* category 326
    membrane—*see* Meningitis
    nerve—*see* Disorder, nerve
  spine (*see also* Spondylitis) 720.9
  spleen (capsule) 289.59
  stomach—*see* Gastritis
  stricture, rectum 569.49
  subcutaneous tissue NEC 686.9
  suprarenal (gland) 255.8
  synovial (fringe) (membrane)—*see* Bursitis
  tendon (sheath) NEC 726.90
  testis (*see also* Orchitis) 604.90
  thigh 686.9
  throat (*see also* Sore throat) 462
  thymus (gland) 254.8
  thyroid (gland) (*see also* Thyroiditis) 245.9
  tongue 529.0
  tonsil—*see* Tonsillitis
  trachea—*see* Tracheitis
  trochlear nerve 378.53
  tubal (*see also* Salpingo-oophoritis) 614.2
  tuberculous NEC (*see also* Tuberculosis) 011.9
  tubo-ovarian (*see also* Salpingo-oophoritis)
    614.2
  tunica vaginalis 608.4
  tympanic membrane—*see* Myringitis
  umbilicus, umbilical 686.9
    newborn NEC 771.4
  uterine ligament (*see also* Disease, pelvis,
    inflammatory) 614.4
    acute 614.3
  uterus (catarrhal) (*see also* Endometritis) 615.9
  uveal tract (anterior) (*see also* Iridocyclitis)
    364.3
    posterior—*see* Chorioretinitis
    sympathetic 360.11
  vagina (*see also* Vaginitis) 616.10
  vas deferens 608.4
  vein (*see also* Phlebitis) 451.9
    thrombotic 451.9
      cerebral (*see also* Thrombosis, brain) 434.0
      leg 451.2
        deep (vessels) NEC 451.19
        superficial (vessels) 451.0
      lower extremity 451.2
        deep (vessels) NEC 451.19
        superficial (vessels) 451.0
  vocal cord 478.5
  vulva (*see also* Vulvitis) 616.10
Inflation, lung imperfect (newborn) 770.5
Influenza, influenzal 487.1
  with
    bronchitis 487.1
    bronchopneumonia 487.0
    cold (any type) 487.1
    digestive manifestations 487.8
    hemoptysis 487.1
    involvement of
      gastrointestinal tract 487.8
      nervous system 487.8
    laryngitis 487.1

Influenza—*continued*
with—*continued*
manifestations NEC 487.8
respiratory 487.1
pneumonia 487.0
pharyngitis 487.1
pneumonia (any form classifiable to 480-483, 485-486) 487.0
respiratory manifestations NEC 487.1
sinusitis 487.1
sore throat 487.1
tonsillitis 487.1
tracheitis 487.1
upper respiratory infection (acute) 487.1
A/H5N1 see also Influenza, avian) 488.02
abdominal 487.8
Asian 487.1
avian 488.02
with involvement of gastrointestinal tract 488.09
bronchopneumonia 488.01
laryngitis 488.02
manifestations NEC 488.09
respiratory 488.02
pharyngitis 488.02
pneumonia (any form classifiable to 480-483, 485-486) 488.01
respiratory infection (acute) (upper) 488.02
bronchial 487.1
bronchopneumonia 487.0
catarrhal 487.1
due to identified
animal origin influenza virus - see Influenza, due to identified, novel influenza A virus
avian influenza virus 488.02
with
manifestations NEC 488.09
respiratory 488.02
pneumonia (any form classifiable to 480-483, 485-486) 488.01
(novel) 2009 H1N1 influenza virus 488.12
with
manifestations NEC 488.19
respiratory 488.12
pneumonia 488.11
novel influenza A virus 488.82
with
encephalopathy 488.89
involvement of gastrointestinal tract 488.89
laryngitis 488.82
manifestations NEC 488.89
respiratory (acute) (upper) 488.82
pharyngitis 488.82
pneumonia 488.81
epidemic 487.1
gastric 487.8
intestinal 487.8
laryngitis 487.1
maternal affecting fetus or newborn 760.2
manifest influenza in infant 771.2
(novel) 2009 H1N1 488.12
with involvement of gastrointestinal tract 488.19
bronchopneumonia 488.11
laryngitis 488.12
manifestations NEC 488.19
respiratory 488.12
pharyngitis 488.12
pneumonia (any form classifiable to 480-483, 485-486) 488.11
respiratory infection (acute) (upper) 488.12

Influenza—*continued*
novel A/H1N1 (*see also* Influenza, (novel) 2009 H1N1) 488.12
novel influenza A viruses not previously found in humans — *see* Influenza, due to identified, novel influenza A virus
pharyngitis 487.1
pneumonia (any form) 487.0
respiratory (upper) 487.1
specified NEC 487.1
stomach 487.8
vaccination, prophylactic (against) V04.81
Influenza-like disease (*see also* Influenza) 487.1
Infraction, Freiberg's (metatarsal head) 732.5
Infraeruption, teeth 524.34
Infusion complication, misadventure or reaction —*see* Complication, infusion
Ingestion
chemical—*see* Table of drugs and chemicals
drug or medicinal substance
overdose or wrong substance given or taken 977.9
specified drug—*see* Table of drugs and chemicals
foreign body NEC (*see also* Foreign body) 938
Ingrowing
hair 704.8
nail (finger) (toe) (infected) 703.0
Inguinal —*see also* condition
testis 752.51
Inhalation
carbon monoxide 986
flame
mouth 947.0
lung 947.1
food or foreign body (*see also* Asphyxia, food or foreign body) 933.1
gas, fumes, or vapor (noxious) 987.9
specified agent—*see* Table of drugs and chemicals
liquid or vomitus (*see also* Asphyxia, food or foreign body) 933.1
lower respiratory tract NEC 934.9
meconium (fetus or newborn) 770.11
with respiratory symptoms 770.12
mucus (*see also* Asphyxia, mucus) 933.1
oil (causing suffocation) (*see also* Asphyxia, food or foreign body) 933.1
pneumonia—*see* Pneumonia, aspiration
smoke 508.2
steam 987.9
stomach contents or secretions (*see also* Asphyxia, food or foreign body) 933.1
in labor and deliver 668.0
Inhibition, inhibited
academic as adjustment reaction 309.23
orgasm
female 302.73
male 302.74
sexual
desire 302.71
excitement 302.72
work as adjustment reaction 309.23
Inhibitor
autoimmune, to clotting factors 286.52
systemic lupus erythematosus (presence of) 795.79
with
hemorrhagic disorder 286.53
hypercoagulable state 289.81
Iniencephalus, iniencephaly 740.2

Injected eye 372.74
Injury 959.9

> *Note—For abrasion, insect bite (nonvenomous),*
> *blister, or scratch, see Injury, superficial. For*
> *laceration, traumatic rupture, tear, or*
> *penetrating wound of internal organs, such as*
> *heart, lung, liver, kidney, pelvic organs, whether*
> *or not accompanied by open wound in the same*
> *region, see Injury, internal. For nerve injury,*
> *see Injury, nerve. For late effect of injuries*
> *classifiable to 850-854, 860-869, 900-919,*
> *950-959, see Late, effect, injury, by type.*

abdomen, abdominal (viscera)—*see also* Injury,
   internal, abdomen
   muscle or wall 959.12
acoustic, resulting in deafness 951.5
adenoid 959.09
adrenal (gland)—*see* Injury, internal, adrenal
alveolar (process) 959.09
ankle (and foot) (and knee) (and leg, except
   thigh) 959.7
anterior chamber, eye 921.3
anus 959.19
aorta (thoracic) 901.0
   abdominal 902.0
appendix—*see* Injury, internal, appendix
arm, upper (and shoulder) 959.2
artery (complicating trauma) (*see also* Injury,
   blood vessel, by site) 904.9
   cerebral or meningeal (*see also* Hemorrhage,
      brain, traumatic, subarachnoid) 852.0
auditory canal (external) (meatus) 959.09
auricle, auris, ear 959.09
axilla 959.2
back 959.19
bile duct—*see* Injury, internal, bile duct
birth—*see also* Birth, injury
   canal NEC, complicating delivery 665.9
bladder (sphincter)—*see* Injury, internal,
   bladder
blast (air) (hydraulic) (immersion) (underwater)
   NEC 869.0
   with open wound into cavity NEC 869.1
   abdomen or thorax—*see* Injury, internal, by
      site
brain—*see* Concussion, brain
ear (acoustic nerve trauma) 951.5
   with perforation of tympanic
      membrane—*see* Wound, open, ear, drum
blood vessel NEC 904.9
   abdomen 902.9
      multiple 902.87
      specified NEC 902.89
   aorta (thoracic) 901.0
      abdominal 902.0
   arm NEC 903.9
   axillary 903.00
      artery 903.01
      vein 903.02
   azygos vein 901.89
   basilic vein 903.1
   brachial (artery) (vein) 903.1
   bronchial 901.89
   carotid artery 900.00
      common 900.01
      external 900.02
      internal 900.03
   celiac artery 902.20
      specified branch NEC 902.24
   cephalic vein (arm) 903.1
   colica dextra 902.26

Injury—*continued*
   blood vessel—*continued*
      cystic
         artery 902.24
         vein 902.39
      deep plantar 904.6
      digital (artery) (vein) 903.5
      due to accidental puncture or laceration during
         procedure 998.2
      extremity
         lower 904.8
            multiple 904.7
            specified NEC 904.7
         upper 903.9
            multiple 903.8
            specified NEC 903.8
      femoral
         artery (superficial) 904.1
            above profunda origin 904.0
            common 904.0
         vein 904.2
      gastric
         artery 902.21
         vein 902.39
      head 900.9
         intracranial—*see* Injury, intracranial
         multiple 900.82
         specified NEC 900.89
      hemiazygos vein 901.89
      hepatic
         artery 902.22
         vein 902.11
      hypogastric 902.59
         artery 902.51
         vein 902.52
      ileocolic
         artery 902.26
         vein 902.31
      iliac 902.50
         artery 902.53
         specified branch NEC 902.59
         vein 902.54
      innominate
         artery 901.1
         vein 901.3
      intercostal (artery) (vein) 901.81
      jugular vein (external) 900.81
         internal 900.1
      leg NEC 904.8
      mammary (artery) (vein) 901.82
      mesenteric
         artery 902.20
            inferior 902.27
            specified branch NEC 902.29
            superior (trunk) 902.25
               branches, primary 902.26
         vein 902.39
            inferior 902.32
            superior (and primary subdivisions) 902.31
      neck 900.9
         multiple 900.82
         specified NEC 900.89
      ovarian 902.89
         artery 902.81
         vein 902.82
      palmar artery 903.4
      pelvis 902.9
         multiple 902.87
         specified NEC 902.89
      plantar (deep) (artery) (vein) 904.6

Injury—*continued*
  blood vessel—*continued*
    popliteal 904.40
      artery 904.41
      vein 904.42
    portal 902.33
    pulmonary 901.40
      artery 901.41
      vein 901.42
    radial (artery) (vein) 903.2
    renal 902.40
      artery 902.41
      specified NEC 902.49
      vein 902.42
    saphenous
      artery 904.7
      vein (greater) (lesser) 904.3
    splenic
      artery 902.23
      vein 902.34
    subclavian
      artery 901.1
      vein 901.3
    suprarenal 902.49
    thoracic 901.9
      multiple 901.83
      specified NEC 901.89
    tibial 904.50
      artery 904.50
        anterior 904.51
        posterior 904.53
      vein 904.50
        anterior 904.52
        posterior 904.54
    ulnar (artery) (vein) 903.3
    uterine 902.59
      artery 902.55
      vein 902.56
    vena cava
      inferior 902.10
        specified branches NEC 902.19
      superior 901.2
  brachial plexus 953.4
    newborn 767.6
  brain (traumatic) NEC (*see also* Injury, intracranial) 854.0
    due to fracture of skull—see Fracture, skull, by site
  breast 959.19
  broad ligament—*see* Injury, internal, broad ligament
  bronchus, bronchi—*see* Injury, internal, bronchus
  brow 959.09
  buttock 959.19
  canthus, eye 921.1
  cathode ray 990
  cauda equina 952.4
    with fracture, vertebra—*see* Fracture, vertebra, sacrum
  cavernous sinus (*see also* Injury, intracranial) 854.0
  cecum—*see* Injury, internal, cecum
  celiac ganglion or plexus 954.1
  cerebellum (*see also* Injury, intracranial) 854.0
  cervix (uteri)—*see* Injury, internal, cervix
  cheek 959.09
  chest—*see* Injury, internal, chest
    wall 959.11
  childbirth—*see also* Birth, injury
    maternal NEC 665.9
  chin 959.09

Injury—*continued*
  choroid (eye) 921.3
  clitoris 959.14
  coccyx 959.19
    complicating delivery 665.6
  colon—*see* Injury, internal, colon
  common duct—*see* Injury, internal, common duct
  conjunctiva 921.1
    superficial 918.2
  cord
    spermatic—*see* Injury, internal, spermatic cord
    spinal—*see* Injury, spinal, by site
  cornea 921.3
    abrasion 918.1
    due to contact lens 371.82
    penetrating—*see* Injury, eyeball, penetrating
    superficial 918.1
      due to contact lens 371.82
  cortex (cerebral) (*see also* Injury, intracranial) 854.0
    visual 950.3
  costal region 959.11
  costochondral 959.11
  cranial
    bones—*see* Fracture, skull, by site
    cavity (*see also* Injury, intracranial) 854.0
    nerve—*see* Injury, nerve, cranial
  crushing—*see* Crush
  cutaneous sensory nerve
    lower limb 956.4
    upper limb 955.5
  deep tissue—*see* Contusion, by site
    meaning pressure ulcer 707.25
  delivery—*see also* Birth, injury
    maternal NEC 665.9
  Descemet's membrane—*see* Injury, eyeball, penetrating
  diaphragm—*see* Injury, internal, diaphragm
  diffuse axonal—*see* Injury, intracranial
  duodenum—*see* Injury, internal, duodenum
  ear (auricle) (canal) (drum) (external) 959.09
  elbow (and forearm) (and wrist) 959.3
  epididymis 959.14
  epigastric region 959.12
  epiglottis 959.09
  epiphyseal, current—*see* Fracture, by site
  esophagus—*see* Injury, internal, esophagus
  Eustachian tube 959.09
  extremity (lower) (upper) NEC 959.8
  eye 921.9
    penetrating eyeball—*see* Injury, eyeball, penetrating
    superficial 918.9
  eyeball 921.3
    penetrating 871.7
      with
        partial loss (of intraocular tissue) 871.12
        prolapse or exposure (of intraocular tissue) 871.1
      without prolapse 871.0
      foreign body (nonmagnetic) 871.6
        magnetic 871.5
    superficial 918.9
  eyebrow 959.09
  eyelid(s) 921.1
    laceration—*see* Laceration, eyelid
    superficial 918.0
  face (and neck) 959.09
  fallopian tube—*see* Injury, internal, fallopian tube

Injury—*continued*
  finger(s) (nail) 959.5
  flank 959.19
  foot (and ankle) (and knee) (and leg except
    thigh) 959.7
  forceps NEC 767.9
    scalp 767.19
  forearm (and elbow) (and wrist) 959.3
  forehead 959.09
  gallbladder—*see* Injury, internal, gallbladder
  gasserian ganglion 951.2
  gastrointestinal tract—*see* Injury, internal,
    gastrointestinal tract
  genital organ(s)
    with
      abortion—*see* Abortion, by type, with,
        damage to pelvic organs
      ectopic pregnancy (*see also* categories
        633.0-633.9) 639.2
      molar pregnancy (*see also* categories
        630-632) 639.2
    external 959.14
      fracture of corpus cavernosum penis 959.13
    following
      abortion 639.2
      ectopic or molar pregnancy 639.2
    internal—*see* Injury, internal, genital organs
    obstetrical trauma NEC 665.9
      affecting fetus or newborn 763.89
  gland
    lacrimal 921.1
      laceration 870.8
    parathyroid 959.09
    salivary 959.09
    thyroid 959.09
  globe (eye) (*see also* Injury, eyeball) 921.3
  grease gun—*see* Wound, open, by site,
    complicated
  groin 959.19
  gum 959.09
  hand(s) (except fingers) 959.4
  head NEC 959.01
    with
      loss of consciousness 850.5
      skull fracture—*see* Fracture, skull, by site
  heart—*see* Injury, internal, heart
  heel 959.7
  hip (and thigh) 959.6
  hymen 959.14
  hyperextension (cervical) (vertebra) 847.0
  ileum—*see* Injury, internal, ileum
  iliac region 959.19
  infrared rays NEC 990
  instrumental (during surgery) 998.2
    birth injury—*see* Birth, injury
    nonsurgical (*see also* Injury, by site) 959.9
    obstetrical 665.9
      affecting fetus or newborn 763.89
      bladder 665.5
      cervix 665.3
      high vaginal 665.4
      perineal NEC 664.9
      urethra 665.5
      uterus 665.5

Injury—*continued*
  internal 869.0

> *Note—For injury of internal organ(s) by foreign
> body entering through a natural orifice (e.g.,
> inhaled, ingested, or swallowed)—see Foreign
> body, entering through orifice.*
>
> *For internal injury of any of the following sites
> with internal injury of any other of the sites—
> see Injury, internal, multiple.*

  with
    fracture
      pelvis—*see* Fracture, pelvis
      specified site, except pelvis—*see* Injury,
        internal, by site
    open wound into cavity 869.1
  abdomen, abdominal (viscera) NEC 868.00
    with
      fracture, pelvis—*see* Fracture, pelvis
      open wound into cavity 868.10
    specified site NEC 868.09
      with open wound into cavity 868.19
  adrenal (gland) 868.01
    with open wound into cavity 868.11
  aorta (thoracic) 901.0
    abdominal 902.0
  appendix 863.85
    with open wound into cavity 863.95
  bile duct 868.02
    with open wound into cavity 868.12
  bladder (sphincter) 867.0
    with
      abortion—*see* Abortion, by type, with,
        damage to pelvic organs
      ectopic pregnancy (*see also* categories
        633.0-633.9) 639.2
      molar pregnancy (*see also* categories
        630-632) 639.2
      open wound into cavity 867.1
    following
      abortion 639.2
      ectopic or molar pregnancy 639.2
    obstetrical trauma 665.5
      affecting fetus or newborn 763.89
  blood vessel—*see* Injury, blood vessel, by site
  broad ligament 867.6
    with open wound into cavity 867.7
  bronchus, bronchi 862.21
    with open wound into cavity 862.31
  cecum 863.89
    with open wound into cavity 863.99
  cervix (uteri) 867.4
    with
      abortion—*see* Abortion, by type, with
        damage to pelvic organs
      ectopic pregnancy (*see also* categories
        633.0-633.9) 639.2
      molar pregnancy (*see also* categories
        630-632) 639.2
      open wound into cavity 867.5
    following
      abortion 639.2
      ectopic or molar pregnancy 639.2
    obstetrical trauma 665.3
      affecting fetus or newborn 763.89
  chest (*see also* Injury, internal, intrathoracic
    organs) 862.8
    with open wound into cavity 862.9

Injury—*continued*
  internal—*continued*
    colon 863.40
      with
        open wound into cavity 863.50
        rectum 863.46
          with open wound into cavity 863.56
      ascending (right) 863.41
        with open wound into cavity 863.51
      descending (left) 863.43
        with open wound into cavity 863.53
      multiple sites 863.46
        with open wound into cavity 863.56
      sigmoid 863.44
        with open wound into cavity 863.54
      specified site NEC 863.49
        with open wound into cavity 863.59
      transverse 863.42
        with open wound into cavity 863.52
    common duct 868.02
      with open wound into cavity 868.12
    complicating delivery 665.9
      affecting fetus or newborn 763.89
    diaphragm 862.0
      with open wound into cavity 862.1
    duodenum 863.21
      with open wound into cavity 863.31
    esophagus (intrathoracic) 862.22
      with open wound into cavity 862.32
      cervical region 874.4
        complicated 874.5
    fallopian tube 867.6
      with open wound into cavity 867.7
    gallbladder 868.02
      with open wound into cavity 868.12
    gastrointestinal tract NEC 863.80
      with open wound into cavity 863.90
    genital organ NEC 867.6
      with open wound into cavity 867.7
    heart 861.00
      with open wound into thorax 861.10
    ileum 863.29
      with open wound into cavity 863.39
    intestine NEC 863.89
      with open wound into cavity 863.99
      large NEC 863.40
        with open wound into cavity 863.50
      small NEC 863.20
        with open wound into cavity 863.30
    intra-abdominal (organ) 868.00
      with open wound into cavity 868.10
      multiple sites 868.09
        with open wound into cavity 868.19
      specified site NEC 868.09
        with open wound into cavity 868.19
    intrathoracic organs (multiple) 862.8
      with open wound into cavity 862.9
      diaphragm (only)—*see* Injury, internal,
        diaphragm
      heart (only)—*see* Injury, internal, heart
      lung (only)—*see* Injury, internal, lung
      specified site NEC 862.29
        with open wound into cavity 862.39
    intrauterine (*see also* Injury, internal, uterus)
      867.4
      with open wound into cavity 867.5
    jejunum 863.29
      with open wound into cavity 863.39

Injury—*continued*
  internal—*continued*
    kidney (subcapsular) 866.00
      with
        disruption of parenchyma (complete)
          866.03
          with open wound into cavity 866.13
        hematoma (without rupture of capsule)
          866.01
          with open wound into cavity 866.11
        laceration 866.02
          with open wound into cavity 866.12
        open wound into cavity 866.10
    liver 864.00
      with
        contusion 864.01
          with open wound into cavity 864.11
        hematoma 864.01
          with open wound into cavity 864.11
        laceration 864.05
          with open wound into cavity 864.15
          major (disruption of hepatic
            parenchyma) 864.04
            with open wound into cavity 864.14
          minor (capsule only) 864.02
            with open wound into cavity 864.12
          moderate (involving parenchyma) 864.03
            with open wound into cavity 864.13
          multiple 864.04
          stellate 864.04
            with open wound in cavity 864.14
      open wound into cavity 864.10
    lung 861.20
      with open wound into thorax 861.30
      aspiration 507.0
      hemopneumothorax—*see*
        Hemopneumothorax, traumatic
      hemothorax—*see* Hemothorax, traumatic
      pneumohemothorax—*see*
        Pneumohemothorax, traumatic
      pneumothorax—*see* Pneumothorax,
        traumatic
      transfusion related, acute (TRALI) 518.7
    mediastinum 862.29
      with open wound into cavity 862.39
    mesentery 863.89
      with open wound into cavity 863.99
    mesosalpinx 867.6
      with open wound into cavity 867.7
    multiple 869.0

> *Note*—*Multiple internal injuries of sites
> classifiable to the same three- or four-digit
> category should be classified to that category.
> Multiple injuries classifiable to different
> fourth-digit subdivisions of 861 (heart and lung
> injuries) should be dealt with according to
> coding rules.*

      with open wound into cavity 869.1
      intra-abdominal organ (sites classifiable to
        863-868)
        with
          intrathoracic organ(s) (sites classifiable
            to 861-862) 869.0
            with open wound into cavity 869.1
          other intra-abdominal organ(s) (sites
            classifiable to 863-868, except where
            classifiable to the same three-digit
            category) 868.09
            with open wound into cavity 868.19

Injury—*continued*
  internal—*continued*
    multiple—*continued*
      intrathoracic organ (sites classifiable to
          861-862)
        with
          intra-abdominal organ(s) (sites
              classifiable to 863-868) 869.0
            with open wound into cavity 869.1
          other intrathoracic organ(s) (sites
              classifiable to 861-862, except where
              classifiable to the same three-digit
              category) 862.8
            with open wound into cavity 862.9
    myocardium—*see* Injury, internal, heart
    ovary 867.6
      with open wound into cavity 867.7
    pancreas (multiple sites) 863.84
      with open wound into cavity 863.94
      body 863.82
        with open wound into cavity 863.92
      head 863.81
        with open wound into cavity 863.91
      tail 863.83
        with open wound into cavity 863.93
    pelvis, pelvic (organs) (viscera) 867.8
      with
        fracture, pelvis—*see* Fracture, pelvis
        open wound into cavity 867.9
      specified site NEC 867.6
        with open wound into cavity 867.7
    peritoneum 868.03
      with open wound into cavity 868.13
    pleura 862.29
      with open wound into cavity 862.39
    prostate 867.6
      with open wound into cavity 867.7
    rectum 863.45
      with
        colon 863.46
          with open wound into cavity 863.56
        open wound into cavity 863.55
    retroperitoneum 868.04
      with open wound into cavity 868.14
    round ligament 867.6
      with open wound into cavity 867.7
    seminal vesicle 867.6
      with open wound into cavity 867.7
    spermatic cord 867.6
      with open wound into cavity 867.7
    scrotal—*see* Wound, open, spermatic cord
    spleen 865.00
      with
        disruption of parenchyma (massive)
            865.04
          with open wound into cavity 865.14
        hematoma (without rupture of capsule)
            865.01
          with open wound into cavity 865.11
        open wound into cavity 865.10
        tear, capsular 865.02
          with open wound into cavity 865.12
          extending into parenchyma 865.03
            with open wound into cavity 865.13
    stomach 863.0
      with open wound into cavity 863.1

Injury—*continued*
  internal—*continued*
    suprarenal gland (multiple) 868.01
      with open wound into cavity 868.11
    thorax, thoracic (cavity) (organs) (multiple)
        (*see also* Injury, internal, intrathoracic
        organs) 862.8
      with open wound into cavity 862.9
    thymus (gland) 862.29
      with open wound into cavity 862.39
    trachea (intrathoracic) 862.29
      with open wound into cavity 862.39
      cervical region (*see also* Wound, open,
          trachea) 874.02
    ureter 867.2
      with open wound into cavity 867.3
    urethra (sphincter) 867.0
      with
        abortion—*see* Abortion, by type, with,
            damage to pelvic organs
        ectopic pregnancy (*see also* categories
            633.0-633.9) 639.2
        molar pregnancy (*see also* categories
            630-632) 639.2
        open wound into cavity 867.1
      following
        abortion 639.2
        ectopic or molar pregnancy 639.2
      obstetrical trauma 665.5
        affecting fetus or newborn 763.89
    uterus 867.4
      with
        abortion—*see* Abortion, by type, with,
            damage to pelvic organs
        ectopic pregnancy (*see also* categories
            633.0-633.9) 639.2
        molar pregnancy (*see also* categories
            630-632) 639.2
        open wound into cavity 867.5
      following
        abortion 639.2
        ectopic or molar pregnancy 639.2
      obstetrical trauma NEC 665.5
        affecting fetus or newborn 763.89
    vas deferens 867.6
      with open wound into cavity 867.7
    vesical (sphincter) 867.0
      with open wound into cavity 867.1
    viscera (abdominal) (*see also* Injury, internal,
        multiple) 868.00
      with
        fracture, pelvis—*see* Fracture, pelvis
        open wound into cavity 868.10
      thoracic NEC (*see also* Injury, internal,
          intrathoracic organs) 862.8
        with open wound into cavity 862.9
  interscapular region 959.19
  intervertebral disc 959.19
  intestine—*see* Injury, internal, intestine
  intra-abdominal (organs) NEC—*see* Injury,
      internal, intra-abdominal

Injury—*continued*
  intracranial (traumatic) 854.0

Note—*Use the following fifth-digit*
subclassification with categories 851-854:

0 *unspecifidd state of consciousness*
1 *with no loss of consciousness*
2 *with brief [less than one hour] loss of*
   consciousness
3 *with moderate [1-24 hours] loss of*
   consciousness
4 *with prolonged [more than 24 hours] loss of*
   consciousness and return to pre-existing
   conscious level
5 *with prolonged [more than 24 hours] loss of*
   consciousness, without return to pre-existing
   conscious level
Use fifth-digit 5 to designate when a patient is
unconscious and dies before regaining
consciousness, regardless of the duration of the
loss of consciousness
6 *with loss of consciousness of unspecified*
   duration
9 *with concussion, unspecified*

---

  with
    open intracranial wound 854.1
    skull fracture—*see* Fracture, skull, by site
  contusion 851.8
    with open intracranial wound 851.9
    brain stem 851.4
      with open intracranial wound 851.5
    cerebellum 851.4
      with open intracranial wound 851.5
    cortex (cerebral) 851.0
      with open intracranial wound 851.2
  hematoma—*see* Injury, intracranial,
      hemorrhage
  hemorrhage 853.0
    with
      laceration—*see* Injury, intracranial,
          laceration
      open intracranial wound 853.1
    extradural 852.4
      with open intracranial wound 852.5
    subarachnoid 852.0
      with open intracranial wound 852.1
    subdural 852.2
      with open intracranial wound 852.3
  laceration 851.8
    with open intracranial wound 851.9
    brain stem 851.6
      with open intracranial wound 851.7
    cerebellum 851.6
      with open intracranial wound 851.7
    cortex (cerebral) 851.2
      with open intracranial wound 851.3
  intraocular—*see* Injury, eyeball, penetrating
  intrathoracic organs (multiple)—*see* Injury,
      internal, intrathoracic organs
  intrauterine—*see* Injury, internal, intrauterine
  iris 921.3
    penetrating—*see* Injury, eyeball, penetrating
  jaw 959.09
  jejunum—*see* Injury, internal, jejunum

Injury—*continued*
  joint NEC 959.9
    old or residual 718.80
      ankle 718.87
      elbow 718.82
      foot 718.87
      hand 718.84
      hip 718.85
      knee 718.86
      multiple sites 718.89
      pelvic region 718.85
      shoulder (region) 718.81
      specified site NEC 718.88
      wrist 718.83
  kidney—*see* Injury, internal, kidney
    acute (nontraumatic) 584.9
  knee (and ankle) (and foot) (and leg, except
      thigh) 959.7
  labium (majus) (minus) 959.14
  labyrinth, ear 959.09
  lacrimal apparatus, gland, or sac 921.1
    laceration 870.8
  larynx 959.09
  late effect—*see* Late, effects (of), injury
  leg except thigh (and ankle) (and foot) (and
      knee) 959.7
    upper or thigh 959.6
  lens, eye 921.3
    penetrating—*see* Injury, eyeball, penetrating
  lid, eye—*see* Injury, eyelid
  lip 959.09
  liver—*see* Injury, internal, liver
  lobe, parietal—*see* Injury, intracranial
  lumbar (region) 959.19
    plexus 953.5
  lumbosacral (region) 959.19
    plexus 953.5
  lung—*see* Injury, internal, lung
  malar region 959.09
  mastoid region 959.09
  maternal, during pregnancy, affecting fetus or
      newborn 760.5
  maxilla 959.09
  mediastinum—*see* Injury, internal, mediastinum
  membrane
    brain (*see also* Injury, intracranial) 854.0
    tympanic 959.09
  meningeal artery—*see* Hemorrhage, brain,
      traumatic, subarachnoid
  meninges (cerebral)—*see* Injury, intracranial
  mesenteric
    artery—*see* Injury, blood vessel, mesenteric,
        artery
    plexus, inferior 954.1
    vein—*see* Injury, blood vessel, mesenteric,
        vein
  mesentery—*see* Injury, internal, mesentery
  mesosalpinx—*see* Injury, internal, mesosalpinx
  middle ear 959.09
  midthoracic region 959.11
  mouth 959.09
  multiple (sites not classifiable to the same
      four-digit category in 959.0-959.7) 959.8
    internal 869.0
      with open wound into cavity 869.1
  musculocutaneous nerve 955.4
  nail
    finger 959.5
    toe 959.7

Injury—*continued*
  nasal (septum) (sinus) 959.09
  nasopharynx 959.09
  neck (and face) 959.09
  nerve 957.9
    abducens 951.3
    abducent 951.3
    accessory 951.6
    acoustic 951.5
    ankle and foot 956.9
    anterior crural, femoral 956.1
    arm (*see also* Injury, nerve, upper limb) 955.9
    auditory 951.5
    axillary 955.0
    brachial plexus 953.4
    cervical sympathetic 954.0
    cranial 951.9
      first or olfactory 951.8
      second or optic 950.0
      third or oculomotor 951.0
      fourth or trochlear 951.1
      fifth or trigeminal 951.2
      sixth or abducens 951.3
      seventh or facial 951.4
      eighth, acoustic, or auditory 951.5
      ninth or glossopharyngeal 951.8
      tenth, pneumogastric, or vagus 951.8
      eleventh or accessory 951.6
      twelfth or hypoglossal 951.7
      newborn 767.7
    cutaneous sensory
      lower limb 956.4
      upper limb 955.5
    digital (finger) 955.6
      toe 956.5
    facial 951.4
      newborn 767.5
    femoral 956.1
    finger 955.9
    foot and ankle 956.9
    forearm 955.9
    glossopharyngeal 951.8
    hand and wrist 955.9
    head and neck, superficial 957.0
    hypoglossal 951.7
    involving several parts of body 957.8
    leg (*see also* Injury, nerve, lower limb) 956.9
    lower limb 956.9
      multiple 956.8
      specified site NEC 956.5
    lumbar plexus 953.5
    lumbosacral plexus 953.5
    median 955.1
      forearm 955.1
      wrist and hand 955.1
    multiple (in several parts of body) (sites not
        classifiable to the same three-digit
        category) 957.8
    musculocutaneous 955.4
    musculospiral 955.3
      upper arm 955.3
    oculomotor 951.0
    olfactory 951.8
    optic 950.0
    pelvic girdle 956.9
      multiple sites 956.8
      specified site NEC 956.5
    peripheral 957.9
      multiple (in several regions) (sites not
          classifiable to the same three-digit
          category) 957.8
      specified site NEC 957.1

Injury—*continued*
  nerve—*continued*
    peroneal 956.3
      ankle and foot 956.3
      lower leg 956.3
    plantar 956.5
    plexus 957.9
      celiac 954.1
      mesenteric, inferior 954.1
      spinal 953.9
        brachial 953.4
        lumbosacral 953.5
        multiple sites 953.8
      sympathetic NEC 954.1
    pneumogastric 951.8
    radial 955.3
      wrist and hand 955.3
    sacral plexus 953.5
    sciatic 956.0
      thigh 956.0
    shoulder girdle 955.9
      multiple 955.8
      specified site NEC 955.7
    specified site NEC 957.1
    spinal 953.9
      plexus—*see* Injury, nerve, plexus, spinal
      root 953.9
        cervical 953.0
        dorsal 953.1
        lumbar 953.2
        multiple sites 953.8
        sacral 953.3
    splanchnic 954.1
    sympathetic NEC 954.1
      cervical 954.0
    thigh 956.9
    tibial 956.5
      ankle and foot 956.2
      lower leg 956.5
      posterior 956.2
    toe 956.9
    trigeminal 951.2
    trochlear 951.1
    trunk, excluding shoulder and pelvic girdles
        954.9
      specified site NEC 954.8
      sympathetic NEC 954.1
    ulnar 955.2
      forearm 955.2
      wrist (and hand) 955.2
    upper limb 955.9
      multiple 955.8
      specified site NEC 955.7
    vagus 951.8
    wrist and hand 955.9
  nervous system, diffuse 957.8
  nose (septum) 959.09
  obstetrical NEC 665.9
    affecting fetus or newborn 763.89
  occipital (region) (scalp) 959.09
    lobe (*see also* Injury, intracranial) 854.0
  optic 950.9
    chiasm 950.1
    cortex 950.3
    nerve 950.0
    pathways 950.2
  orbit, orbital (region) 921.2
    penetrating 870.3
      with foreign body 870.4
  ovary—*see* Injury, internal, ovary
  paint-gun—*see* Wound, open, by site,
      complicated

Injury—*continued*
  palate (soft) 959.09
  pancreas—*see* Injury, internal, pancreas
  parathyroid (gland) 959.09
  parietal (region) (scalp) 959.09
    lobe—*see* Injury, intracranial
  pelvic
    floor 959.19
      complicating delivery 664.1
        affecting fetus or newborn 763.89
      joint or ligament, complicating delivery 665.6
        affecting fetus or newborn 763.89
      organs—*see also* Injury, internal, pelvis
        with
          abortion—*see* Abortion, by type, with
            damage to pelvic organs
          ectopic pregnancy (*see also* categories
            633.0-633.9) 639.2
          molar pregnancy (*see also* categories
            633.0-633.9) 639.2
        following
          abortion 639.2
          ectopic or molar pregnancy 639.2
        obstetrical trauma 665.5
          affecting fetus or newborn 763.89
  pelvis 959.19
  penis 959.14
    fracture of corpus cavernosum 959.13
  perineum 959.14
  peritoneum—*see* Injury, internal, peritoneum
  periurethral tissue
    with
      abortion—*see* Abortion, by type, with
        damage to pelvic organs
      ectopic pregnancy (*see also* categories
        633.0-633.9) 639.2
      molar pregnancy (*see also* categories
        630-632) 639.2
    complicating delivery 664.8
      affecting fetus or newborn 763.89
    following
      abortion 639.2
      ectopic or molar pregnancy 639.2
  phalanges
    foot 959.7
    hand 959.5
  pharynx 959.09
  pleura—*see* Injury, internal, pleura
  popliteal space 959.7
  post-cardiac surgery (syndrome) 429.4
  prepuce 959.14
  prostate—*see* Injury, internal, prostate
  pubic region 959.19
  pudenda 959.14
  radiation NEC 990
  radioactive substance or radium NEC 990
  rectovaginal septum 959.14
  rectum—*see* Injury, internal, rectum
  retina 921.3
    penetrating—*see* Injury, eyeball, penetrating
  retroperitoneal—*see* Injury, internal,
    retroperitoneum
  roentgen rays NEC 990
  round ligament—*see* Injury, internal, round
    ligament
  sacral (region) 959.19
    plexus 953.5
  sacroiliac ligament NEC 959.19
  sacrum 959.19
  salivary ducts or glands 959.09

Injury—*continued*
  scalp 959.09
    due to birth trauma 767.19
    fetus or newborn 767.19
  scapular region 959.2
  sclera 921.3
    penetrating—*see* Injury, eyeball, penetrating
    superficial 918.2
  scrotum 959.14
  seminal vesicle—*see* Injury, internal, seminal
    vesicle
  shoulder (and upper arm) 959.2
  sinus
    cavernous (*see also* Injury, intracranial) 854.0
    nasal 959.09
  skeleton NEC, birth injury 767.3
  skin NEC 959.9
  skull—*see* Fracture, skull, by site
  soft tissue (of external sites) (severe)—*see*
    Wound, open, by site
  specified site NEC 959.8
  spermatic cord—*see* Injury, internal, spermatic
    cord
  spinal (cord) 952.9
    with fracture, vertebra—*see* Fracture, vertebra,
      by site, with spinal cord injury
    cervical (C_1-C_4) 952.00
      with
        anterior cord syndrome 952.02
        central cord syndrome 952.03
        complete lesion of cord 952.01
        incomplete lesion NEC 952.04
        posterior cord syndrome 952.04
      C_5-C_7 level 952.05
        with
          anterior cord syndrome 952.07
          central cord syndrome 952.08
          complete lesion of cord 952.06
          incomplete lesion NEC 952.09
          posterior cord syndrome 952.09
        specified type NEC 952.09
      specified type NEC 952.04
    dorsal (D_1-D_6) (T_1-T_6) (thoracic) 952.10
      with
        anterior cord syndrome 952.12
        central cord syndrome 952.13
        complete lesion of cord 952.11
        incomplete lesion NEC 952.14
        posterior cord syndrome 952.14
      D_7-D_{12} level (T_7-T_{12}) 952.15
        with
          anterior cord syndrome 952.17
          central cord syndrome 952.18
          complete lesion of cord 952.16
          incomplete lesion NEC 952.19
          posterior cord syndrome 952.19
        specified type NEC 952.19
      specified type NEC 952.14
    lumbar 952.2
    multiple sites 952.8
    nerve (root) NEC—*see* Injury, nerve, spinal,
      root
    plexus 953.9
      brachial 953.4
      lumbosacral 953.5
      multiple sites 953.8
    sacral 952.3
    thoracic (*see also* Injury, spinal, dorsal)
      952.10
  spleen—*see* Injury, internal, spleen
  stellate ganglion 954.1

Injury—*continued*
  sternal region 959.11
  stomach—*see* Injury, internal, stomach
  subconjunctival 921.1
  subcutaneous 959.9
  subdural—*see* Injury, intracranial
  submaxillary region 959.09
  submental region 959.09
  subungual
    fingers 959.5
    toes 959.7
  superficial 919

Note—Use the following fourth-digit subdivisions with categories 910-919:

.0 *Abrasion or friction burn without mention of infection*
.1 *Abrasion or friction burn, infected*
.2 *Blister without mention of infection*
.3 *Blister, infected*
.4 *Insect bite, nonvenomous, without mention of infection*
.5 *Insect bite, nonvenomous, infected*
.6 *Superficial foreign body (splinter) without major open wound and without mention of infection*
.7 *Superficial foreign body (splinter) without major open wound, infected*
.8 *Other and unspecified superficial injury without mention of infection*
.9 *Other and unspecified superficial injury, infected*

For late effects of superficial injury, see category 906.2.

---

  abdomen, abdominal (muscle) (wall) (and other part(s) of trunk) 911
  ankle (and hip, knee, leg, or thigh) 916
  anus (and other part(s) of trunk) 911
  arm 913
    upper (and shoulder) 912
  auditory canal (external) (meatus) (and other part(s) of face, neck, or scalp, except eye) 910
  axilla (and upper arm) 912
  back (and other part(s) of trunk) 911
  breast (and other part(s) of trunk) 911
  brow (and other part(s) of face, neck or scalp, except eye) 910
  buttock (and other part(s) of trunk) 911
  canthus, eye 918.0
  cheek(s) (and other part(s) of face, neck, or scalp, except eye) 910
  chest wall (and other part(s) of trunk) 911
  chin (and other part(s) of face, neck, or scalp, except eye) 910
  clitoris (and other part(s) of trunk) 911
  conjunctiva 918.2
  cornea 918.1
    due to contact lens 371.82
  costal region (and other part(s) of trunk) 911
  ear(s) (auricle) (canal) (drum) (external) (and other part(s) of face, neck, or scalp, except eye) 910
  elbow (and forearm) (and wrist) 913
  epididymis (and other part(s) of trunk) 911
  epigastric region (and other part(s) of trunk) 911
  epiglottis (and other part(s) of face, neck, or scalp, except eye) 910

Injury—*continued*
  superficial—*continued*
    eye(s) (and adnexa) NEC 918.9
    eyelid(s) (and periocular area) 918.0
    face (any part(s), except eye) (and neck or scalp) 910
    finger(s) (nail) (any) 915
    flank (and other part(s) of trunk) 911
    foot (phalanges) (and toe(s)) 917
    forearm (and elbow) (and wrist) 913
    forehead (and other part(s) of face, neck, or scalp, except eye) 910
    globe (eye) 918.9
    groin (and other part(s) of trunk) 911
    gum(s) (and other part(s) of face, neck, or scalp, except eye) 910
    hand(s) (except fingers alone) 914
    head (and other part(s) of face, neck, or scalp, except eye) 910
    heel (and foot or toe) 917
    hip (and ankle, knee, leg, or thigh) 916
    iliac region (and other part(s) of trunk) 911
    interscapular region (and other part(s) of trunk) 911
    iris 918.9
    knee (and ankle, hip, leg, or thigh) 916
    labium (majus) (minus) (and other part(s) of trunk) 911
    lacrimal (apparatus) (gland) (sac) 918.0
    leg (lower) (upper) (and ankle, hip, knee, or thigh) 916
    lip(s) (and other part(s) of face, neck, or scalp, except eye) 910
    lower extremity (except foot) 916
    lumbar region (and other part(s) of trunk) 911
    malar region (and other part(s) of face, neck, or scalp, except eye) 910
    mastoid region (and other part(s) of face, neck, or scalp, except eye) 910
    midthoracic region (and other part(s) of trunk) 911
    mouth (and other part(s) of face, neck, or scalp, except eye) 910
    multiple sites (not classifiable to the same three-digit category) 919
    nasal (septum) (and other part(s) of face, neck, or scalp, except eye) 910
    neck (and face or scalp, any part(s), except eye) 910
    nose (septum) (and other part(s) of face, neck, or scalp, except eye) 910
    occipital region (and other part(s) of face, neck, or scalp, except eye) 910
    orbital region 918.0
    palate (soft) (and other part(s) of face, neck, or scalp, except eye) 910
    parietal region (and other part(s) of face, neck, or scalp, except eye) 910
    penis (and other part(s) of trunk) 911
    perineum (and other part(s) of trunk) 911
    periocular area 918.0
    pharynx (and other part(s) of face, neck, or scalp, except eye) 910
    popliteal space (and ankle, hip, leg, or thigh) 916
    prepuce (and other part(s) of trunk) 911
    pubic region (and other part(s) of trunk) 911
    pudenda (and other part(s) of trunk) 911
    sacral region (and other part(s) of trunk) 911
    salivary (ducts) (glands) (and other part(s) of face, neck, or scalp, except eye) 910

Injury—*continued*
  superficial—*continued*
    scalp (and other part(s) of face or neck, except eye) 910
    scapular region (and upper arm) 912
    sclera 918.2
    scrotum (and other part(s) of trunk) 911
    shoulder (and upper arm) 912
    skin NEC 919
    specified site(s) NEC 919
    sternal region (and other part(s) of trunk) 911
    subconjunctival 918.2
    subcutaneous NEC 919
    submaxillary region (and other part(s) of face, neck, or scalp, except eye) 910
    submental region (and other part(s) of face, neck, or scalp, except eye) 910
    supraclavicular fossa (and other part(s) of face, neck or scalp, except eye) 910
    supraorbital 918.0
    temple (and other part(s) of face, neck, or scalp, except eye) 910
    temporal region (and other part(s) of face, neck, or scalp, except eye) 910
    testis (and other part(s) of trunk) 911
    thigh (and ankle, hip, knee, or leg) 916
    thorax, thoracic (external) (and other part(s) of trunk) 911
    throat (and other part(s) of face, neck, or scalp, except eye) 910
    thumb(s) (nail) 915
    toe(s) (nail) (subungual) (and foot) 917
    tongue (and other part(s) of face, neck, or scalp, except eye) 910
    tooth, teeth (*see also* Abrasion, dental) 521.20
    trunk (any part(s)) 911
    tunica vaginalis (and other part(s) of trunk) 911
    tympanum, tympanic membrane (and other part(s) of face, neck, or scalp, except eye) 910
    upper extremity NEC 913
    uvula (and other part(s) of face, neck, or scalp, except eye) 910
    vagina (and other part(s) of trunk) 911
    vulva (and other part(s) of trunk) 911
    wrist (and elbow) (and forearm) 913
  supraclavicular fossa 959.19
  supraorbital 959.09
  surgical complication (external or internal site) 998.2
  symphysis pubis 959.19
    complicating delivery 665.6
      affecting fetus or newborn 763.89
  temple 959.09
  temporal region 959.09
  testis 959.14
  thigh (and hip) 959.6
  thorax, thoracic (external) 959.11
    cavity—*see* Injury, internal, thorax
    internal—*see* Injury, internal, intrathoracic organs
  throat 959.09
  thumb(s) (nail) 959.5
  thymus—*see* Injury, internal, thymus
  thyroid (gland) 959.09
  toe (nail) (any) 959.7
  tongue 959.09
  tonsil 959.09
  tooth NEC 873.63
    complicated 873.73

Injury—*continued*
  trachea—*see* Injury, internal, trachea
  trunk 959.19
  tunica vaginalis 959.14
  tympanum, tympanic membrane 959.09
  ultraviolet rays NEC 990
  ureter—*see* Injury, internal, ureter
  urethra (sphincter)—*see* Injury, internal, urethra
  uterus—*see* Injury, internal, uterus
  uvula 959.09
  vagina 959.14
  vascular—*see* Injury, blood vessel
  vas deferens—*see* Injury, internal, vas deferens
  vein (*see also* Injury, blood vessel, by site) 904.9
  vena cava
    inferior 902.10
    superior 901.2
  vesical (sphincter)—*see* Injury, internal, vesical
  viscera (abdominal)—*see* Injury, internal, viscera
    with fracture, pelvis—*see* Fracture, pelvis
  visual 950.9
    cortex 950.3
  vitreous (humor) 871.2
  vulva 959.14
  whiplash (cervical spine) 847.0
  wringer—*see* Crush, by site
  wrist (and elbow) (and forearm) 959.3
  x-ray NEC 990
Inoculation —*see also* Vaccination
  complication or reaction—*see* Complication, vaccination
INPH (idiopathic normal pressure hydrocephalus) 331.5
Insanity, insane (*see also* Psychosis) 298.9
  adolescent (*see also* Schizophrenia) 295.9
  alternating (*see also* Psychosis, affective, circular) 296.7
  confusional 298.9
    acute 293.0
    subacute 293.1
  delusional 298.9
  paralysis, general 094.1
    progressive 094.1
  paresis, general 094.1
  senile 290.20
Insect
  bite—*see* Injury, superficial, by site
  venomous, poisoning by 989.5
Insemination, artificial V26.1
Insensitivity
  adrenocorticotropin hormone (ACTH) 255.41
  androgen 259.50
    complete 259.51
    partial 259.52
Insertion
  cord (umbilical) lateral or velamentous 663.8
    affecting fetus or newborn 762.6
  intrauterine contraceptive device V25.11
  placenta, vicious—*see* Placenta, previa
  subdermal implantable contraceptive V25.5
  velamentous, umbilical cord 663.8
    affecting fetus or newborn 762.6
Insolation 992.0
  meaning sunstroke 992.0
Insomnia, unspecified 780.52
  with sleep apnea, unspecified 780.51
  adjustment 307.41
  alcohol induced 291.82
  behavioral, of childhood V69.5

Insufficiency, insufficient—*continued*
mesenteric 557.1
mitral (valve) 424.0
  with
    aortic (valve) disease 396.3
      insufficiency, incompetence, or
        regurgitation 396.3
      stenosis or obstruction 396.2
    obstruction or stenosis 394.2
      with aortic valve disease 396.8
    congenital 746.6
    rheumatic 394.1
      with
        aortic (valve) disease 396.3
          insufficiency, incompetence, or
            regurgitation 396.3
          stenosis or obstruction 396.2
        obstruction or stenosis 394.2
          with aortic valve disease 396.8
        active or acute 391.1
          with chorea, rheumatic (Sydenham's)
            392.0
    specified cause, except rheumatic 424.0
muscle
  heart—*see* Insufficiency, myocardial
  ocular (*see also* Strabismus) 378.9
myocardial, myocardium (with arteriosclerosis)
    428.0
  with rheumatic fever (conditions classifiable
      to 390)
    active, acute, or subacute 391.2
      with chorea 392.0
    inactive or quiescent (with chorea) 398.0
  congenital 746.89
  due to presence of (cardiac) prosthesis 429.4
  fetus or newborn 779.89
  following cardiac surgery 429.4
  hypertensive (*see also* Hypertension, heart)
    402.91
    benign 402.11
    malignant 402.01
  postoperative 997.1
    long-term effect of cardiac surgery 429.4
  rheumatic 398.0
    active, acute, or subacute 391.2
      with chorea (Sydenham's) 392.0
  syphilitic 093.82
nourishment 994.2
organic 799.89
ovary 256.39
  postablative 256.2
pancreatic 577.8
parathyroid (gland) 252.1
peripheral vascular (arterial) 443.9
pituitary (anterior) 253.2
  posterior 253.5
placental—*see* Placenta, insufficiency
platelets 287.5
prenatal care in current pregnancy V23.7
progressive pluriglandular 258.9
pseudocholinesterase 289.89
pulmonary (acute) 518.82
  following
    shock 518.52
    surgery 518.52
    trauma 518.52
  newborn 770.89
  valve (*see also* Endocarditis, pulmonary)
    424.3
    congenital 746.09
pyloric 537.0

Insufficiency, insufficient—*continued*
renal 593.9
  acute 593.9
  chronic 585.9
  due to a procedure 997.5
respiratory 786.09
  acute 518.82
    following trauma and surgery 518.52
  newborn 770.89
rotation—*see* Malrotation
suprarenal 255.41
  medulla 255.5
tarso-orbital fascia, congenital 743.66
tear film 375.15
testis 257.2
thyroid (gland) (acquired)—*see also*
    Hypothyroidism
  congenital 243
tricuspid (*see also* Endocarditis, tricuspid) 397.0
  congenital 746.89
  syphilitic 093.23
urethral sphincter 599.84
valve, valvular (heart) (*see also* Endocarditis)
    424.90
vascular 459.9
  intestine NEC 557.9
  mesenteric 557.1
  peripheral 443.9
  renal (*see also* Hypertension, kidney) 403.90
velopharyngeal
  acquired 528.9
  congenital 750.29
venous (peripheral) 459.81
ventricular—*see* Insufficiency, myocardial
vertebral artery 435.1
vertibrobasilar artery 435.3
weight gain during pregnancy 646.8
zinc 269.3
Insufflation
fallopian
  fertility testing V26.21
  following sterilization reversal V26.22
meconium 770.11
  with respiratory symptoms 770.12
Insular —*see* condition
Insulinoma (M8151/0)
malignant (M8151/3)
  pancreas 157.4
  specified site—*see* Neoplasm, by site,
    malignant
  unspecified site 157.4
pancreas 211.7
specified site—*see* Neoplasm, by site, benign
unspecified site 211.7
Insuloma —*see* Insulinoma
Insult
brain 437.9
  acute 436
cerebral 437.9
  acute 436
cerebrovascular 437.9
  acute 436
vascular NEC 437.9
  acute 436
Insurance examination (certification) V70.3
Intemperance (*see also* Alcoholism) 303.9
Interception of pregnancy (menstrual
    extraction) V25.3
Interference
balancing side 524.56
non-working side 524.56

Intermenstrual
bleeding 626.6
irregular 626.6
regular 626.5
hemorrhage 626.6
irregular 626.6
regular 626.5
ain(s) 625.2
Intermittent— *see* condition
Internal —*see* condition
Interproximal wear 521.10
Interrogation
cardiac defibrillator (automatic) (implantable)
V53.32
cardiac pacemaker V53.31
cardiac (event) (loop) recorder V53.39
infusion pump (implanted) (intrathecal) V53.09
neurostimulator V53.02
Interruption
aortic arch 747.11
bundle of His 426.50
fallopian tube (for sterilization) V25.2
phase-shift, sleep cycle 307.45
repeated REM-sleep 307.48
sleep
due to perceived environmental disturbances
307.48
phase-shift, of 24-hour sleep-wake cycle
307.45
repeated REM-sleep type 307.48
vas deferens (for sterilization) V25.2
Intersexuality 752.7
Interstitial —*see* condition
Intertrigo 695.89
labialis 528.5
Intervertebral disc —*see* condition
Intestine, intestinal —*see also* condition
flu 487.8
Intolerance
carbohydrate NEC 579.8
cardiovascular exercise, with pain (at rest) (with
less than ordinary activity) (with ordinary
activity) V47.2
cold 780.99
disaccharide (hereditary) 271.3
drug
correct substance properly administered 995.27
wrong substance given or taken in error 977.9
specified drug—*see* Table of drugs and
chemicals
effort 306.2
fat NEC 579.8
foods NEC 579.8
fructose (hereditary) 271.2
glucose (-galactose) (congenital) 271.3
gluten 579.0
lactose (hereditary) (infantile) 271.3
lysine (congenital) 270.7
milk NEC 579.8
protein (familial) 270.7
starch NEC 579.8
sucrose (-isomaltose) (congenital) 271.3
Intoxicated NEC (*see also* Alcoholism) 305.0
Intoxication
acid 276.2
acute
alcoholic 305.0
with alcoholism 303.0
hangover effects 305.0
caffeine 305.9
hallucinogenic (*see also* Abuse, drugs,
nondependent) 305.3

Intoxication—*continued*
alcohol (acute) 305.0
with alcoholism 303.0
hangover effects 305.0
idiosyncratic 291.4
pathological 291.4
alimentary canal 558.2
ammonia (hepatic) 572.2
caffeine 305.9
chemical—*see also* Table of drugs and chemicals
via placenta or breast milk 760.70
alcohol 760.71
anticonvulsants 760.77
antifungals 760.74
anti-infective agents 760.74
antimetabolics 760.78
cocaine 760.75
"crack" 760.75
hallucinogenic agents NEC 760.73
medicinal agents NEC 760.79
narcotics 760.72
obstetric anesthetic or analgesic drug 763.5
specified agent NEC 760.79
suspected, affecting management of
pregnancy 655.5
cocaine, through placenta or breast milk 760.75
delirium
alcohol 291.0
drug 292.81
drug 292.89
with delirium 292.81
correct substance properly administered (*see
also* Allergy, drug) 995.27
newborn 779.4
obstetric anesthetic or sedation 668.9
affecting fetus or newborn 763.5
overdose or wrong substance given or
taken—*see* Table of drugs and chemicals
pathologic 292.2
specific to newborn 779.4
via placenta or breast milk 760.70
alcohol 760.71
anticonvulsants 760.77
antifungals 760.74
anti-infective agents 760.74
antimetabolics 760.78
cocaine 760.75
"crack" 760.75
hallucinogenic agents 760.73
medicinal agents NEC 760.79
narcotics 760.72
obstetric anesthetic or analgesic drug 763.5
specified agent NEC 760.79
suspected, affecting management of
pregnancy 655.5
enteric—*see* Intoxication, intestinal
fetus or newborn, via placenta or breast milk
760.70
alcohol 760.71
anticonvulsants 760.77
antifungals 760.74
anti-infective agents 760.74
antimetabolics 760.78
cocaine 760.75
"crack" 760.75
hallucinogenic agents 760.73
medicinal agents NEC 760.79
narcotics 760.72
obstetric anesthetic or analgesic drug 763.5
specified agent NEC 760.79
suspected, affecting management of pregnancy
655.5

Intoxication—*continued*
  food—*see* Poisoning, food
  gastrointestinal 558.2
  hallucinogenic (acute) 305.3
  hepatocerebral 572.2
  idiosyncratic alcohol 291.4
  intestinal 569.89
    due to putrefaction of food 005.9
  methyl alcohol (*see also* Alcoholism) 305.0
    with alcoholism 303.0
  non-foodborne due to toxins of Clostridium
    botulinum [*C. botulinum*] —*see* Botulism
  pathologic 291.4
    drug 292.2
  potassium (K) 276.7
  septic
    with
      abortion—*see* Abortion, by type, with sepsis
      ectopic pregnancy (*see also* categories
        633.0-633.9) 639.0
      molar pregnancy (*see also* categories
        630-632) 639.0
    during labor 659.3
    following
      abortion 639.0
      ectopic or molar pregnancy 639.0
    generalized—*see* Septicemia
    puerperal, postpartum, childbirth 670.2
  serum (prophylactic) (therapeutic) 999.59
  uremic—*see* Uremia
  water 276.69
Intracranial —*see* condition
Intrahepatic gallbladder 751.69
Intraligamentous —*see also* condition
  pregnancy—*see* Pregnancy, cornual
Intraocular —*see also* condition
  sepsis 360.00
Intrathoracic —*see also* condition
  kidney 753.3
  stomach—*see* Hernia, diaphragm
Intrauterine contraceptive device
  checking V25.42
  insertion V25.11
  in situ V45.51
  management V25.42
  prescription V25.02
    repeat V25.42
  reinsertion V25.13
  removal V25.12
    and reinsertion V25.13
  replacement V25.13
Intraventricular —*see* condition
Intrinsic deformity —*see* Deformity
Intruded tooth 524.34
Intrusion, repetitive, of sleep (due to
  environmental disturbances) (with atypical
  polysomnographic features) 307.48
Intumescent, lens (eye) NEC 366.9
  senile 366.12
Intussusception (colon) (enteric) (intestine)
  (rectum) 560.0
  appendix 543.9
  congenital 751.5
  fallopian tube 620.8
  ileocecal 560.0
  ileocolic 560.0
  ureter (with obstruction) 593.4
Invagination
  basilar 756.0
  colon or intestine 560.0
Invalid (since birth) 799.89
Invalidism (chronic) 799.89

Inversion
  albumin-globulin (A-G) ratio 273.8
  bladder 596.89
  cecum (*see also* Intussusception) 560.0
  cervix 622.8
  nipple 611.79
    congenital 757.6
    puerperal, postpartum 676.3
  optic papilla 743.57
  organ or site, congenital NEC—*see* Anomaly,
    specified type NEC
  sleep rhythm 327.39
    nonorganic origin 307.45
  testis (congenital) 752.51
  uterus (postinfectional) (postpartal, old) 621.7
    chronic 621.7
    complicating delivery 665.2
      affecting fetus or newborn 763.89
  vagina—*see* Prolapse, vagina
Investigation
  allergens V72.7
  clinical research (control) (normal comparison)
    (participant) V70.7
Inviability —*see* Immaturity
Involuntary movement, abnormal 781.0
Involution, involutional —*see also* condition
  breast, cystic or fibrocystic 610.1
  depression (*see also* Psychosis, affective) 296.2
    recurrent episode 296.3
    single episode 296.2
  melancholia (*see also* Psychosis, affective) 296.2
    recurrent episode 296.3
    single episode 296.2
  ovary, senile 620.3
  paranoid state (reaction) 297.2
  paraphrenia (climacteric) (menopause) 297.2
  psychosis 298.8
  thymus failure 254.8
IQ
  under 20 318.2
  20-34 318.1
  35-49 318.0
  50-70 317
IRDS 769
Irideremia 743.45
Iridis rubeosis 364.42
  diabetic 250.5 *[364.42]*
    due to secondary diabetes 249.5 *[364.42]*
Iridochoroiditis (panuveitis) 360.12
Iridocyclitis NEC 364.3
  acute 364.00
    primary 364.01
    recurrent 364.02
  chronic 364.10
    in
      lepromatous leprosy 030.0 *[364.11]*
      sarcoidosis 135 *[364.11]*
      tuberculosis (*see also* Tuberculosis) 017.3
        [364.11]
  due to allergy 364.04
  endogenous 364.01
  gonococcal 098.41
  granulomatous 364.10
  herpetic (simplex) 054.44
    zoster 053.22
  hypopyon 364.05
  lens induced 364.23
  nongranulomatous 364.00
  primary 364.01
  recurrent 364.02
  rheumatic 364.10

Iridocyclitis—*continued*
  secondary 364.04
    infectious 364.03
    noninfectious 364.04
  subacute 364.00
    primary 364.01
    recurrent 364.02
  sympathetic 360.11
  syphilitic (secondary) 091.52
  tuberculous (chronic) (*see also* Tuberculosis)
    017.3 *[364.11]*
Iridocyclochoroiditis (panuveitis) 360.12
Iridodialysis 364.76
Iridodonesis 364.89
Iridoplegia (complete) (partial) (reflex) 379.49
Iridoschisis 364.52
**IRIS (Immune Reconstitution Inflammatory
    Syndrome)** 995.90
Iris —*see* condition
Iritis 364.3
  acute 364.00
    primary 364.01
    recurrent 364.02
  chronic 364.10
    in
      sarcoidosis 135 *[364.11]*
      tuberculosis (*see also* Tuberculosis) 017.3
        [364.11]
  diabetic 250.5 *[364.42]*
    due to secondary diabetes 249.5 *[364.42]*
  due to
    allergy 364.04
    herpes simplex 054.44
    leprosy 030.0 *[364.11]*
  endogenous 364.01
  gonococcal 098.41
  gouty 274.89 *[364.11]*
  granulomatous 364.10
  hypopyon 364.05
  lens induced 364.23
  nongranulomatous 364.00
  papulosa 095.8 *[364.11]*
  primary 364.01
  recurrent 364.02
  rheumatic 364.10
  secondary 364.04
    infectious 364.03
    noninfectious 364.04
  subacute 364.00
    primary 364.01
    recurrent 364.02
  sympathetic 360.11
  syphilitic (secondary) 091.52
    congenital 090.0 *[364.11]*
    late 095.8 *[364.11]*
  tuberculous (*see also* Tuberculosis) 017.3 *[364.11]*
  uratic 274.89 *[364.11]*
Iron
  deficiency anemia 280.9
  metabolism disease 275.09
  storage disease 275.09
Iron-miners' lung 503
Irradiated enamel (tooth, teeth) 521.89
Irradiation
  burn—*see* Burn, by site
  effects, adverse 990
Irreducible, irreducibility —*see* condition
Irregular, irregularity
  action, heart 427.9
  alveolar process 525.8
  bleeding NEC 626.4

Irregular, irregularity—*continued*
  breathing 786.09
  colon 569.89
  contour
    of cornea 743.41
      acquired 371.70
    reconstructed breast 612.0
  dentin in pulp 522.3
  eye movements NEC 379.59
  menstruation (cause unknown) 626.4
  periods 626.4
  prostate 602.9
  pupil 364.75
  respiratory 786.09
  septum (nasal) 470
  shape, organ or site, congenital NEC—*see*
    Distortion
  sleep-wake rhythm (non-24-hour) 327.39
    nonorganic origin 307.45
  vertebra 733.99
Irritability 799.22
  bladder 596.89
    neurogenic 596.54
      with cauda equina syndrome 344.61
  bowel (syndrome) 564.1
  bronchial (*see also* Bronchitis) 490
  cerebral, newborn 779.1
  colon 564.1
    psychogenic 306.4
  duodenum 564.89
  heart (psychogenic) 306.2
  ileum 564.89
  jejunum 564.89
  myocardium 306.2
  nervousness 799.21
  rectum 564.89
  stomach 536.9
    psychogenic 306.4
  sympathetic (nervous system) (*see also*
    Neuropathy, peripheral, autonomic) 337.9
  urethra 599.84
  ventricular (heart) (psychogenic) 306.2
Irritable —(*see also* Irritability) 799.22
Irritation
  anus 569.49
  axillary nerve 353.0
  bladder 596.89
  brachial plexus 353.0
  brain (traumatic) (*see also* Injury, intracranial)
    854.0
    nontraumatic—*see* Encephalitis
  bronchial (*see also* Bronchitis) 490
  cerebral (traumatic) (*see also* Injury,
    intracranial) 854.0
    nontraumatic—*see* Encephalitis
  cervical plexus 353.2
  cervix (*see also* Cervicitis) 616.0
  choroid, sympathetic 360.11
  cranial nerve—*see* Disorder, nerve, cranial
  digestive tract 536.9
    psychogenic 306.4
  gastric 536.9
    psychogenic 306.4
  gastrointestinal (tract) 536.9
    functional 536.9
    psychogenic 306.4
  globe, sympathetic 360.11
  intestinal (bowel) 564.9
  labyrinth 386.50
  lumbosacral plexus 353.1

Irritation—*continued*
  meninges (traumatic) (*see also* Injury,
    intracranial) 854.0
    nontraumatic—*see* Meningitis
  myocardium 306.2
  nerve—*see* Disorder, nerve
  nervous 799.21
  nose 478.19
  penis 607.89
  perineum 709.9
  peripheral
    autonomic nervous system (*see also*
      Neuropathy, peripheral, autonomic) 337.9
    nerve—*see* Disorder, nerve
  peritoneum (*see also* Peritonitis) 567.9
  pharynx 478.29
  plantar nerve 355.6
  spinal (cord) (traumatic)—*see also* Injury,
    spinal, by site
    nerve—*see also* Disorder, nerve
      root NEC 724.9
      traumatic—*see* Injury, nerve, spinal
    nontraumatic—*see* Myelitis
  stomach 536.9
    psychogenic 306.4
  sympathetic nerve NEC (*see also* Neuropathy,
    peripheral, autonomic) 337.9
  ulnar nerve 354.2
  vagina 623.9
Isambert's disease 012.3
Ischemia, ischemic 459.9
  basilar artery (with transient neurologic deficit)
    435.0
  bone NEC 733.40
  bowel (transient) 557.9
    acute 557.0
    chronic 557.1
    due to mesenteric artery insufficiency 557.1
  brain—*see also* Ischemia, cerebral
    recurrent focal 435.9
  cardiac (*see also* Ischemia, heart) 414.9
  cardiomyopathy 414.8
  carotid artery (with transient neurologic deficit)
    435.8
  cerebral (chronic) (generalized) 437.1
    arteriosclerotic 437.0
    intermittent (with transient neurologic deficit)
      435.9
    newborn 779.2
    puerperal, postpartum, childbirth 674.0
    recurrent focal (with transient neurologic
      deficit) 435.9
    transient (with transient neurologic deficit)
      435.9
  colon 557.9
    acute 557.0
    chronic 557.1
    due to mesenteric artery insufficiency 557.1
  coronary (chronic) (*see also* Ischemia, heart)
    414.9
  demand 411.89
  heart (chronic or with a stated duration of over 8
    weeks) 414.9
    acute or with a stated duration of 8 weeks or
      less (*see also* Infarct, myocardium) 410.9
      without myocardial infarction 411.89
        with coronary (artery) occlusion 411.81
    subacute 411.89
  intestine (transient) 557.9
    acute 557.0
    chronic 557.1
    due to mesenteric artery insufficiency 557.1

Ischemia, ischemic— *continued*
  kidney 593.81
  labyrinth 386.50
  muscles, leg 728.89
  myocardium, myocardial (chronic or with a
    stated duration of over 8 weeks) 414.8
    acute (*see also* Infarct, myocardium) 410.9
      without myocardial infarction 411.89
        with coronary (artery) occlusion 411.81
  renal 593.81
  retina, retinal 362.84
  small bowel 557.9
    acute 557.0
    chronic 557.1
    due to mesenteric artery insufficiency 557.1
  spinal cord 336.1
  subendocardial (*see also* Insufficiency,
    coronary) 411.89
  supply (*see also* Angina) 414.9
  vertebral artery (with transient neurologic
    deficit) 435.1
Ischialgia (*see also* Sciatica) 724.3
Ischiopagus 759.4
Ischium, ischial —*see* condition
Ischomenia 626.8
Ischuria 788.5
Iselin's disease or osteochondrosis 732.5
Islands of
  parotid tissue in
    lymph nodes 750.26
    neck structures 750.26
  submaxillary glands in
    fascia 750.26
    lymph nodes 750.26
    neck muscles 750.26
Islet cell tumor, pancreas (M8150/0) 211.7
Isoimmunization NEC (*see also* Incompatibility)
  656.2
  anti-E 656.2
  fetus or newborn 773.2
    ABO blood groups 773.1
    Rhesus (Rh) factor 773.0
Isolation V07.0
  social V62.4
Isosporosis 007.2
Issue
  medical certificate NEC V68.09
    cause of death V68.09
    disability examination V68.01
    fitness V68.09
    incapacity V68.09
  repeat prescription NEC V68.1
    appliance V68.1
    contraceptive V25.40
      device NEC V25.49
        intrauterine V25.42
        specified type NEC V25.49
      pill V25.41
    glasses V68.1
    medicinal substance V68.1
Itch (*see also* Pruritus) 698.9
  bakers' 692.89
  barbers' 110.0
  bricklayers' 692.89
  cheese 133.8
  clam diggers' 120.3
  coolie 126.9
  copra 133.8
  Cuban 050.1
  dew 126.9
  dhobie 110.3

Itch —*continued*
  eye 379.99
  filarial (*see also* Infestation, filarial) 125.9
  grain 133.8
  grocers' 133.8
  ground 126.9
  harvest 133.8
  jock 110.3
  Malabar 110.9
    beard 110.0
    foot 110.4
    scalp 110.0
  meaning scabies 133.0
  Norwegian 133.0
  perianal 698.0
  poultrymen's 133.8
  sarcoptic 133.0
  scrub 134.1
  seven year V61.10
    meaning scabies 133.0
  straw 133.8
  swimmers' 120.3
  washerwoman's 692.4
  water 120.3
  winter 698.8
Itsenko-Cushing syndrome (pituitary
    basophilism) 255.0
Ivemark's syndrome (asplenia with congenital
    heart disease) 759.0
Ivory bones 756.52
Ixodes 134.8
Ixodiasis 134.8

J

Jaccoud's nodular fibrositis, chronic (Jaccoud's syndrome) 714.4
Jackson's
  membrane 751.4
  paralysis or syndrome 344.89
  veil 751.4
Jacksonian
  epilepsy (*see also* Epilepsy) 345.5
  seizures (focal) (*see also* Epilepsy) 345.5
Jacob's ulcer (M8090/3)—*see* Neoplasm, skin, malignant, by site
Jacquet's dermatitis (diaper dermatitis) 691.0
Jadassohn's
  blue nevus (M8780/0)—*see* Neoplasm, skin, benign
  disease (maculopapular erythroderma) 696.2
  intraepidermal epithelioma (M8096/0)—*see* Neoplasm, skin, benign
Jadassohn-Lewandowski syndrome (pachyonychia congenita) 757.5
Jadassohn-Pellizari's disease (anetoderma) 701.3
Jadassohn-Tièche nevus (M8780/0)—*see* Neoplasm, skin, benign
Jaffe-Lichtenstein (-Uehlinger) syndrome 252.01
Jahnke's syndrome (encephalocutaneous angiomatosis) 759.6
Jakob-Creutzfeldt disease (CJD) (syndrome) 046.19
  with dementia
    with behavioral disturbance 046.19 *[294.11]*
    without behavioral disturbance 046.19 *[294.10]*
  familial 046.19
  iatrogenic 046.19
  specified NEC 046.19
  sporadic 046.19
  variant (vCJD) 046.11
    with dementia
      with behavioral disturbance 046.11 *[294.11]*
      without behavioral disturbance 046.11 *[294.10]*
Jaksch (-Luzet) disease or syndrome (pseudoleukemia infantum) 285.8
Jamaican
  neuropathy 349.82
  paraplegic tropical ataxic-spastic syndrome 349.82
Janet's disease (psychasthenia) 300.89
Janiceps 759.4
Jansky-Bielschowsky amaurotic familial idiocy 330.1
Japanese
  B type encephalitis 062.0
  river fever 081.2
  seven-day fever 100.89
Jaundice (yellow) 782.4
  acholuric (familial) (splenomegalic) (*see also* Spherocytosis) 282.0
    acquired 283.9
  breast milk 774.39
  catarrhal (acute) 070.1
    with hepatic coma 070.0
    chronic 571.9
    epidemic—*see* Jaundice, epidemic
  cholestatic (benign) 782.4
  chronic idiopathic 277.4
  epidemic (catarrhal) 070.1

Jaundice—*continued*
  with hepatic coma 070.0
    leptospiral 100.0
    spirochetal 100.0
  febrile (acute) 070.1
    with hepatic coma 070.0
    leptospiral 100.0
    spirochetal 100.0
  fetus or newborn 774.6
    due to or associated with
      ABO
        antibodies 773.1
        incompatibility, maternal/fetal 773.1
        isoimmunization 773.1
      absence or deficiency of enzyme system for bilirubin conjugation (congenital) 774.39
      blood group incompatibility NEC 773.2
      breast milk inhibitors to conjugation 774.39
        associated with preterm delivery 774.2
      bruising 774.1
      Crigler-Najjar syndrome 277.4 *[774.31]*
      delayed conjugation 774.30
        associated with preterm delivery 774.2
      development 774.39
      drugs or toxins transmitted from mother 774.1
      G-6-PD deficiency 282.2 *[774.0]*
      galactosemia 271.1 *[774.5]*
      Gilbert's syndrome 277.4 *[774.31]*
      hepatocellular damage 774.4
      hereditary hemolytic anemia (*see also* Anemia, hemolytic) 282.9 *[774.0]*
      hypothyroidism, congenital 243 *[774.31]*
      incompatibility, maternal/fetal NEC 773.2
      infection 774.1
      inspissated bile syndrome 774.4
      isoimmunization NEC 773.2
      mucoviscidosis 277.01 *[774.5]*
      obliteration of bile duct, congenital 751.61 *[774.5]*
      polycythemia 774.1
      preterm delivery 774.2
      red cell defect 282.9 *[774.0]*
      Rh
        antibodies 773.0
        incompatibility, maternal/fetal 773.0
        isoimmunization 773.0
      spherocytosis (congenital) 282.0 *[774.0]*
      swallowed maternal blood 774.1
    physiological NEC 774.6
  from injection, inoculation, infusion, or transfusion (blood) (plasma) (serum) (other substance) (onset within 8 months after administration)—*see* Hepatitis, viral
  Gilbert's (familial nonhemolytic) 277.4
  hematogenous 283.9
  hemolytic (acquired) 283.9
    congenital (*see also* Spherocytosis) 282.0
  hemorrhagic (acute) 100.0
    leptospiral 100.0
    newborn 776.0
    spirochetal 100.0
  hepatocellular 573.8
  homologous (serum)—*see* Hepatitis, viral
  idiopathic, chronic 277.4
  infectious (acute) (subacute) 070.1
    with hepatic coma 070.0
    leptospiral 100.0
    spirochetal 100.0

Jaundice—*continued*
  leptospiral 100.0
  malignant (*see also* Necrosis, liver) 570
  newborn (physiological) (*see also* Jaundice,
    fetus or newborn) 774.6
  nonhemolytic, congenital familial (Gilbert's)
    277.4
  nuclear, newborn (*see also* Kernicterus of
    newborn) 774.7
  obstructive NEC (*see also* Obstruction, biliary)
    576.8
  postimmunization—*see* Hepatitis, viral
  posttransfusion—*see* Hepatitis, viral
  regurgitation (*see also* Obstruction, biliary)
    576.8
  serum (homologous) (prophylactic)
    (therapeutic)—*see* Hepatitis, viral
  spirochetal (hemorrhagic) 100.0
  symptomatic 782.4
    newborn 774.6
Jaw —*see* condition
Jaw-blinking 374.43
  congenital 742.8
Jaw-winking phenomenon or syndrome 742.8
Jealousy
  alcoholic 291.5
  childhood 313.3
  sibling 313.3
Jejunitis (*see also* Enteritis) 558.9
Jejunostomy status V44.4
Jejunum, jejunal —*see* condition
Jensen's disease 363.05
Jericho boil 085.1
Jerks, myoclonic 333.2
Jervell-Lange-Nielsen syndrome 426.82
Jeune's disease or syndrome (asphyxiating
    thoracic dystrophy) 756.4
Jigger disease 134.1
Job's syndrome (chronic granulomatous disease)
    288.1
Jod-Basedow phenomenon 242.8
Johnson-Stevens disease (erythema multiforme
    exudativum) 695.13
Joint —*see also* condition
  Charcot's 094.0 *[713.5]*
  false 733.82
  flail—*see* Flail, joint
  mice—*see* Loose, body, joint, by site
  sinus to bone 730.9
  von Gies' 095.8
Jordan's anomaly or syndrome 288.2
Josephs-Diamond-Blackfan anemia (congenital
    hypoplastic) 284.01
Joubert syndrome 759.89
Jumpers' knee 727.2
Jungle yellow fever 060.0
Jüngling's disease (sarcoidosis) 135
Junin virus hemorrhagic fever 078.7
Juvenile —*see also* condition
  delinquent 312.9
    group (*see also* Disturbance, conduct) 312.2
    neurotic 312.4

K

Kabuki syndrome 759.89
Kahler (-Bozzolo) disease (multiple myeloma)
(M9730/3) 203.0
Kakergasia 300.9
Kakke 265.0
Kala-azar (Indian) (infantile) (Mediterranean)
(Sudanese) 085.0
Kalischer's syndrome (encephalocutaneous
angiomatosis) 759.6
Kallmann's syndrome (hypogonadotropic
hypogonadism with anosmia) 253.4
Kanner's syndrome (autism) (*see also*
Psychosis, childhood) 299.0
Kaolinosis 502
Kaposi's
disease 757.33
lichen ruber 696.4
acuminatus 696.4
moniliformis 697.8
xeroderma pigmentosum 757.33
sarcoma (M9140/3) 176.9
adipose tissue 176.1
aponeurosis 176.1
artery 176.1
associated herpesvirus infection 058.89
blood vessel 176.1
bursa 176.1
connective tissue 176.1
external genitalia 176.8
fascia 176.1
fatty tissue 176.1
fibrous tissue 176.1
gastrointestinal tract NEC 176.3
ligament 176.1
lung 176.4
lymph
gland(s) 176.5
node(s) 176.5
lymphatic(s) NEC 176.1
muscle (skeletal) 176.1
oral cavity NEC 176.8
palate 176.2
scrotum 176.8
skin 176.0
soft tissue 176.1
specified site NEC 176.8
subcutaneous tissue 176.1
synovia 176.1
tendon (sheath) 176.1
vein 176.1
vessel 176.1
viscera NEC 176.9
vulva 176.8
varicelliform eruption 054.0
vaccinia 999.0
Kartagener's syndrome or triad (sinusitis,
bronchiectasis, situs inversus) 759.3
Kasabach-Merritt syndrome (capillary
hemangioma associated with
thrombocytopenic purpura) 287.39
Kaschin-Beck disease (endemic
polyarthritis)—*see* Disease, Kaschin-Beck
Kast's syndrome (dyschondroplasia with
hemangiomas) 756.4
Katatonia (*see also* Schizophrenia) 295.2
Katayama disease or fever 120.2
Kathisophobia 781.0
Kawasaki disease 446.1

Kayser-Fleischer ring (cornea) (pseudosclerosis)
275.1 *[371.14]*
Kaznelson's syndrome (congenital hypoplastic
anemia) 284.01
Kearns-Sayre syndrome 277.87
Kedani fever 081.2
Kelis 701.4
Kelly (-Patterson) syndrome (sideropenic
dysphagia) 280.8
Keloid, cheloid 701.4
Addison's (morphea) 701.0
cornea 371.00
Hawkins' 701.4
scar 701.4
Keloma 701.4
Kenya fever 082.1
Keratectasia 371.71
congenital 743.41
Keratinization NEC
alveolar ridge mucosa
excessive 528.72
minimal 528.71
Keratitis (nodular) (nonulcerative) (simple)
(zonular) NEC 370.9
with ulceration (*see also* Ulcer, cornea) 370.00
actinic 370.24
arborescens 054.42
areolar 370.22
bullosa 370.8
deep—*see* Keratitis, interstitial
dendritic(a) 054.42
desiccation 370.34
diffuse interstitial 370.52
disciform(is) 054.43
varicella 052.7 *[370.44]*
epithelialis vernalis 372.13 *[370.32]*
exposure 370.34
filamentary 370.23
gonococcal (congenital) (prenatal) 098.43
herpes, herpetic (simplex) NEC 054.43
zoster 053.21
hypopyon 370.04
in
chickenpox 052.7 *[370.44]*
exanthema (*see also* Exanthem) 057.9
[370.44]
paravaccinia (*see also* Paravaccinia) 051.9
[370.44]
smallpox (*see also* Smallpox) 050.9 *[370.44]*
vernal conjunctivitis 372.13 *[370.32]*
interstitial (nonsyphilitic) 370.50
with ulcer (*see also* Ulcer, cornea) 370.00
diffuse 370.52
herpes, herpetic (simplex) 054.43
zoster 053.21
syphilitic (congenital) (hereditary) 090.3
tuberculous (*see also* Tuberculosis) 017.3
[370.59]
lagophthalmic 370.34
macular 370.22
neuroparalytic 370.35
neurotrophic 370.35
nummular 370.22
oyster-shuckers' 370.8
parenchymatous—*see* Keratitis, interstitial
petrificans 370.8
phlyctenular 370.31

Keraunoparalysis 994.0
Kerion (celsi) 110.0
Kernicterus of newborn (not due to
   isoimmunization) 774.7
   due to isoimmunization (conditions classifiable
      to 773.0-773.2) 773.4
Ketoacidosis 276.2
   diabetic 250.1
   due to secondary diabetes 249.1
Ketonuria 791.6
   branched-chain, intermittent 270.3
Ketosis 276.2
   diabetic 250.1
   due to secondary diabetes 249.1
Kidney —*see* condition
Kienböck's
   disease 732.3
   adult 732.8
   osteochondrosis 732.3
Kimmelstiel (-Wilson) disease or syndrome
   (intercapillary glomerulosclerosis) 250.4
   [581.81]
   due to secondary diabetes 249.4 *[581.81]*
Kink, kinking
   appendix 543.9
   artery 447.1
   cystic duct, congenital 751.61
   hair (acquired) 704.2
   ileum or intestine (*see also* Obstruction,
      intestine) 560.9
   Lane's (*see also* Obstruction, intestine) 560.9
   organ or site, congenital NEC—*see* Anomaly,
      specified type NEC, by site
   ureter (pelvic junction) 593.3
      congenital 753.20
   vein(s) 459.2
      caval 459.2
      peripheral 459.2
Kinnier Wilson's disease (hepatolenticular
   degeneration) 275.1
Kissing
   osteophytes 721.5
   spine 721.5
   vertebra 721.5
Klauder's syndrome (erythema multiforme
   exudativum) 695.19
Kleb's disease (*see also* Nephritis) 583.9
Klein-Waardenburg syndrome
   (ptosisepicanthus) 270.2
Kleine-Levin syndrome 327.13
Kleptomania 312.32
Klinefelter's syndrome 758.7
Klinger's disease 446.4
Klippel's disease 723.8
Klippel-Feil disease or syndrome (brevicollis)
   756.16
Klippel-Trenaunay syndrome 759.89
Klumpke (-Déjérine) palsy, paralysis (birth)
   (newborn) 767.6
Klüver-Bucy (-Terzian) syndrome 310.0
Knee —*see* condition
Knifegrinders' rot (*see also* Tuberculosis) 011.4
Knock-knee (acquired) 736.41
   congenital 755.64
Knot
   intestinal, syndrome (volvulus) 560.2
   umbilical cord (true) 663.2
      affecting fetus or newborn 762.5
Knots, surfer 919.8
   infected 919.9

Knotting (of)
   hair 704.2
   intestine 560.2
Knuckle pads (Garrod's) 728.79
Köbner's disease (epidermolysis bullosa) 757.39
Koch's
   infection (*see also* Tuberculosis, pulmonary)
      011.9
   relapsing fever 087.9
Koch-Weeks conjunctivitis 372.03
Koenig-Wichman disease (pemphigus) 694.4
Köhler's disease (osteochondrosis) 732.5
   first (osteochondrosis juvenilis) 732.5
   second (Freiburg's infarction, metatarsal head)
      732.5
   patellar 732.4
   tarsal navicular (bone) (osteoarthosis juvenilis)
      732.5
Köhler-Mouchet disease (osteoarthrosis
   juvenilis) 732.5
Köhler-Pellegrini-Stieda disease or syndrome
   (calcification, knee joint) 726.62
Koilonychia 703.8
   congenital 757.5
Kojevnikov's, Kojewnikoff's epilepsy (*see also*
   Epilepsy) 345.7
König's
   disease (osteochondritis dissecans) 732.7
   syndrome 564.89
Koniophthisis (*see also* Tuberculosis) 011.4
Koplik's spots 055.9
Kopp's asthma 254.8
Korean hemorrhagic fever 078.6
Korsakoff (-Wernicke) disease, psychosis, or
   syndrome (nonalcoholic) 294.0
   alcoholic 291.1
Korsakov's disease —*see* Korsakoff's disease
Korsakow's disease —*see* Korsakoff's disease
Kostmann's disease or syndrome (infantile
   genetic agranulocytosis) 288.01
Krabbe's
   disease (leukodystrophy) 330.0
   syndrome
      congenital muscle hypoplasia 756.89
      cutaneocerebral angioma 759.6
Kraepelin-Morel disease (*see also*
   Schizophrenia) 295.9
Kraft-Weber-Dimitri disease 759.6
Kraurosis
   ani 569.49
   penis 607.0
   vagina 623.8
   vulva 624.09
Kreotoxism 005.9
Krukenberg's
   spindle 371.13
   tumor (M8490/6) 198.6
Kufs' disease 330.1
Kugelberg-Welander disease 335.11
Kuhnt-Junius degeneration or disease 362.52
Kulchitsky's cell carcinoma (carcinoid tumor of
   intestine) 259.2
Kümmell's disease or spondylitis 721.7
Kundrat's disease (lymphosarcoma) 200.1
Kunekune —*see* Dermatophytosis
Kunkel syndrome (lupoid hepatitis) 571.49
Kupffer cell sarcoma (M9124/3) 155.0
Kuru 046.0

Kussmaul's
  coma (diabetic) 250.3
    due to secondary diabetes 249.3
  disease (polyarteritis nodosa) 446.0
  respiration (air hunger) 786.09
Kwashiorkor (marasmus type) 260
Kyasanur Forest disease 065.2
Kyphoscoliosis, kyphoscoliotic (acquired) (*see*
    also Scoliosis) 737.30
  congenital 756.19
  due to radiation 737.33
  heart (disease) 416.1
  idiopathic 737.30
    infantile
      progressive 737.32
      resolving 737.31
  late effect of rickets 268.1 *[737.43]*
  specified NEC 737.39
  thoracogenic 737.34
  tuberculous (*see also* Tuberculosis) 015.0
    [737.43]
Kyphosis, kyphotic (acquired) (postural) 737.10
  adolescent postural 737.0
  congenital 756.19
  dorsalis juvenilis 732.0
  due to or associated with
    Charcot-Marie-Tooth disease 356.1 *[737.41]*
    mucopolysaccharidosis 277.5 *[737.41]*
    neurofibromatosis 237.71 *[737.41]*
    osteitis
      deformans 731.0 *[737.41]*
      fibrosa cystica 252.01 *[737.41]*
    osteoporosis (*see also* Osteoporosis) 733.0
      [737.41]
    poliomyelitis (*see also* Poliomyelitis) 138
      [737.41]
    radiation 737.11
    tuberculosis (*see also* Tuberculosis) 015.0
      [737.41]
  Kümmell's 721.7
  late effect of rickets 268.1 *[737.41]*
  Morquio-Brailsford type (spinal) 277.5 *[737.41]*
  pelvis 738.6
  postlaminectomy 737.12
  specified cause NEC 737.19
  syphilitic, congenital 090.5 *[737.41]*
  tuberculous (*see also* Tuberculosis) 015.0
    [737.41]
Kyrle's disease (hyperkeratosis follicularis in
    cutem penetrans) 701.1

L

Labia, labium —*see* condition
Labiated hymen 752.49
Labile
blood pressure 796.2
emotions, emotionality 301.3
vasomotor system 443.9
Lability, emotional 799.24
Labioglossal paralysis 335.22
Labium leporinum (*see also* Cleft, lip) 749.10
Labor (*see also* Delivery)
with complications—*see* Delivery, complicated
abnormal NEC 661.9
affecting fetus or newborn 763.7
arrested active phase 661.1
affecting fetus or newborn 763.7
desultory 661.2
affecting fetus or newborn 763.7
dyscoordinate 661.4
affecting fetus or newborn 763.7
early onset (22-36 weeks gestation) 644.2
failed
induction 659.1
mechanical 659.0
medical 659.1
surgical 659.0
trial (vaginal delivery) 660.6
false 644.1
forced or induced, affecting fetus or newborn
763.89
hypertonic 661.4
affecting fetus or newborn 763.7
hypotonic 661.2
affecting fetus or newborn 763.7
primary 661.0
affecting fetus or newborn 763.7
secondary 661.1
affecting fetus or newborn 763.7
incoordinate 661.4
affecting fetus or newborn 763.7
irregular 661.2
affecting fetus or newborn 763.7
long—*see* Labor, prolonged
missed (at or near term) 656.4
obstructed NEC 660.9
affecting fetus or newborn 763.1
due to female genital mutilation 660.8
specified cause NEC 660.8
affecting fetus or newborn 763.1
pains, spurious 644.1
precipitate 661.3
affecting fetus or newborn 763.6
premature 644.2
threatened 644.0
prolonged or protracted 662.1
affecting fetus or newborn 763.89
first stage 662.0
affecting fetus or newborn 763.89
second stage 662.2
affecting fetus or newborn 763.89
threatened NEC 644.1
undelivered 644.1
Labored breathing (*see also* Hyperventilation)
786.09

Labyrinthitis (inner ear) (destructive) (latent)
386.30
circumscribed 386.32
diffuse 386.31
focal 386.32
purulent 386.33
serous 386.31
suppurative 386.33
syphilitic 095.8
toxic 386.34
viral 386.35
Laceration —*see also* Wound, open, by site
accidental, complicating surgery 998.2
Achilles tendon 845.09
with open wound 892.2
anus (sphincter) 879.6
with
abortion—*see* Abortion, by type, with
damage to pelvic organs
ectopic pregnancy (*see also* categories
633.0-633.9) 639.2
molar pregnancy (*see also* categories
630-632) 639.2
complicated 879.7
complicating delivery (healed) (old) 654.8
with laceration of anal or rectal mucosa
664.3
not associated with third-degree perineal
laceration 664.6
following
abortion 639.2
ectopic or molar pregnancy 639.2
nontraumatic, nonpuerperal (healed) (old)
569.43
bladder (urinary)
with
abortion—*see* Abortion, by type, with
damage to pelvic organs
ectopic pregnancy (*see also* categories
633.0-633.9) 639.2
molar pregnancy (*see also* categories
630-632) 639.2
following
abortion 639.2
ectopic or molar pregnancy 639.2
obstetrical trauma 665.5
blood vessel—*see* Injury, blood vessel, by site
bowel
with
abortion—*see* Abortion, by type, with
damage to pelvic organs
ectopic pregnancy (*see also* categories
633.0-633.9) 639.2
molar pregnancy (*see also* categories
630-632) 639.2
following
abortion 639.2
ectopic or molar pregnancy 639.2
obstetrical trauma 665.5
brain (with hemorrhage) (cerebral) (membrane)
851.8

Laceration— *continued*

Note—Use the following fifth-digit subclassification with categories 851-854: 0 *unspecified state of consciousness* 1 *with no loss of consciousness* 2 *with brief [less than one hour] loss of consciousness* 3 *with moderate [1-24 hours] loss of consciousness* 4 *with prolonged [more than 24 hours] loss of consciousness and return to pre-existing conscious level* 5 *with prolonged [more than 24 hours] loss of consciousness, without return to pre-existing conscious level* *Use fifth-digit 5 to designate when a patient is unconscious and dies before regaining consciousness, regardless of the duration of the loss of consciousness* 6 *with loss of consciousness of unspecified duration* 9 *with concussion, unspecified*

with
   open intracranial wound 851.9
   skull fracture—*see* Fracture, skull, by site
  cerebellum 851.6
   with open intracranial wound 851.7
  cortex 851.2
   with open intracranial wound 851.3
  during birth 767.0
  stem 851.6
   with open intracranial wound 851.7
broad ligament
  with
    abortion—*see* Abortion, by type, with damage to pelvic organs
    ectopic pregnancy (*see also* categories 633.0-633.9) 639.2
    molar pregnancy (*see also* categories 630-632) 639.2
  following
    abortion 639.2
    ectopic or molar pregnancy 639.2
  nontraumatic 620.6
  obstetrical trauma 665.6
  syndrome (nontraumatic) 620.6
capsule, joint—*see* Sprain, by site
cardiac—*see* Laceration, heart
causing eversion of cervix uteri (old) 622.0
central, complicating delivery 664.4
cerebellum—*see* Laceration, brain, cerebellum
cerebral—*see also* Laceration, brain
  during birth 767.0
cervix (uteri)
  with
    abortion—*see* Abortion, by type, with damage to pelvic organs
    ectopic pregnancy (*see also* categories 633.0-633.9) 639.2
    molar pregnancy (*see also* categories 630-632) 639.2
  following
    abortion 639.2
    ectopic or molar pregnancy 639.2
  nonpuerperal, nontraumatic 622.3
  obstetrical trauma (current) 665.3
  old (postpartal) 622.3
  traumatic—*see* Injury, internal, cervix
chordae heart 429.5

Laceration— *continued*
complicated 879.9
cornea—*see* Laceration, eyeball
  superficial 918.1
cortex (cerebral)—*see* Laceration, brain, cortex
esophagus 530.89
eye(s)—*see* Laceration, ocular
eyeball NEC 871.4
  with prolapse or exposure of intraocular tissue 871.1
  penetrating—*see* Penetrating wound, eyeball
  specified as without prolapse of intraocular tissue 871.0
eyelid NEC 870.8
  full thickness 870.1
   involving lacrimal passages 870.2
  skin (and periocular area) 870.0
  penetrating—*see* Penetrating wound, orbit
fourchette
  with
    abortion—*see* Abortion, by type, with damage to pelvic organs
    ectopic pregnancy (*see also* categories 633.0-633.9) 639.2
    molar pregnancy (*see also* categories 630-632) 639.2
  complicating delivery 664.0
  following
    abortion 639.2
    ectopic or molar pregnancy 639.2
heart (without penetration of heart chambers) 861.02
  with
    open wound into thorax 861.12
    penetration of heart chambers 861.03
     with open wound into thorax 861.13
hernial sac—*see* Hernia, by site
internal organ (abdomen) (chest) (pelvis)
  NEC—*see* Injury, internal, by site
kidney (parenchyma) 866.02
  with
    complete disruption of parenchyma (rupture) 866.03
     with open wound into cavity 866.13
    open wound into cavity 866.12
labia
  complicating delivery 664.0
ligament—*see also* Sprain, by site
  with open wound—*see* Wound, open, by site
liver 864.05
  with open wound into cavity 864.15
  major (disruption of hepatic parenchyma) 864.04
   with open wound into cavity 864.14
  minor (capsule only) 864.02
   with open wound into cavity 864.12
  moderate (involving parenchyma without major disruption) 864.03
   with open wound into cavity 864.13
  multiple 864.04
   with open wound into cavity 864.14
  stellate 864.04
   with open wound into cavity 864.14
lung 861.22
  with open wound into thorax 861.32
meninges—*see* Laceration, brain
meniscus (knee) (*see also* Tear, meniscus) 836.2
  old 717.5
  site other than knee—*see also* Sprain, by site
   old NEC (*see also* Disorder, cartilage, articular) 718.0

Laceration—*continued*
muscle—*see also* Sprain, by site
  with open wound—*see* Wound, open, by site
myocardium—*see* Laceration, heart
nerve—*see* Injury, nerve, by site
ocular NEC (*see also* Laceration, eyeball) 871.4
  adnexa NEC 870.8
    penetrating 870.3
      with foreign body 870.4
  orbit (eye) 870.8
    penetrating 870.3
      with foreign body 870.4
pelvic
  floor (muscles)
    with
      abortion—*see* Abortion, by type, with
        damage to pelvic organs
      ectopic pregnancy (*see also* categories
        633.0-633.9) 639.2
      molar pregnancy (*see also* categories
        630-632) 639.2
    complicating delivery 664.1
    following
      abortion 639.2
      ectopic or molar pregnancy 639.2
    nonpuerperal 618.7
    old (postpartal) 618.7
  organ NEC
    with
      abortion—*see* Abortion, by type, with
        damage to pelvic organs
      ectopic pregnancy (*see also* categories
        633.0-633.9) 639.2
      molar pregnancy (*see also* categories
        630-632) 639.2
    complicating delivery 665.5
      affecting fetus or newborn 763.89
    following
      abortion 639.2
      ectopic or molar pregnancy 639.2
    obstetrical trauma 665.5
perineum, perineal (old) (postpartal) 618.7
  with
    abortion—*see* Abortion, by type, with
      damage to pelvic floor
    ectopic pregnancy (*see also* categories
      633.0-633.9) 639.2
    molar pregnancy (*see also* categories
      630-632) 639.2
  complicating delivery 664.4
    first degree 664.0
    second degree 664.1
    third degree 664.2
    fourth degree 664.3
    central 664.4
    involving
      anal sphincter (healed) (old) 654.8
        not associated with third-degree perineal
          laceration 664.6
      fourchette 664.0
      hymen 664.0
      labia 664.0
      pelvic floor 664.1
      perineal muscles 664.1
      rectovaginal septum 664.2
        with anal mucosa 664.3
      skin 664.0
      sphincter (anal) (healed) (old) 654.8
        not associated with third-degree perineal
          laceration 664.6
        with anal mucosa 664.3

Laceration—*continued*
  vagina 664.0
  vaginal muscles 664.1
  vulva 664.0
  secondary 674.2
  following
    abortion 639.2
    ectopic or molar pregnancy 639.2
  male 879.6
    complicated 879.7
  muscles, complicating delivery 664.1
  nonpuerperal, current injury 879.6
    complicated 879.7
  secondary (postpartal) 674.2
peritoneum
  with
    abortion—*see* Abortion, by type, with
      damage to pelvic organs
    ectopic pregnancy (*see also* categories
      633.0-633.9) 639.2
    molar pregnancy (*see also* categories
      630-632) 639.2
  following
    abortion 639.2
    ectopic or molar pregnancy 639.2
  obstetrical trauma 665.5
periurethral tissue
  with
    abortion—*see* Abortion, by type, with
      damage to pelvic organs
    ectopic pregnancy (*see also* categories
      633.0-633.9) 639.2
    molar pregnancy (*see also* categories
      630-632) 639.2
  following
    abortion 639.2
    ectopic or molar pregnancy 639.2
  obstetrical trauma 664.8
rectovaginal (septum)
  with
    abortion—*see* Abortion, by type, with
      damage to pelvic organs
    ectopic pregnancy (*see also* categories
      633.0-633.9) 639.2
    molar pregnancy (*see also* categories
      630-632) 639.2
  complicating delivery 665.4
    with perineum 664.2
      involving anal or rectal mucosa 664.3
  following
    abortion 639.2
    ectopic or molar pregnancy 639.2
  nonpuerperal 623.4
  old (postpartal) 623.4
spinal cord (meninges)—*see also* Injury, spinal,
  by site
  due to injury at birth 767.4
  fetus or newborn 767.4
spleen 865.09
  with
    disruption of parenchyma (massive) 865.04
      with open wound into cavity 865.14
    open wound into cavity 865.19
  capsule (without disruption of parenchyma)
    865.02
    with open wound into cavity 865.12
  parenchyma 865.03
    with open wound into cavity 865.13
    massive disruption (rupture) 865.04
      with open wound into cavity 865.14

Laceration—*continued*
tendon 848.9
  with open wound–*see* Wound, open, by site
  Achilles 845.09
    with open wound 892.2
  lower limb NEC 844.9
    with open wound NEC 894.2
  upper limb NEC 840.9
    with open wound NEC 884.2
tentorium cerebelli—*see* Laceration, brain,
    cerebellum
tongue 873.64
  complicated 873.74
urethra
  with
    abortion—*see* Abortion, by type, with
        damage to pelvic organs
    ectopic pregnancy (*see also* categories
        633.0- 633.9) 639.2
    molar pregnancy (*see also* categories
        630-632) 639.2
  following
    abortion 639.2
    ectopic or molar pregnancy 639.2
  nonpuerperal, nontraumatic 599.84
  obstetrical trauma 665.5
uterus
  with
    abortion—*see* Abortion, by type, with
        damage to pelvic organs
    ectopic pregnancy (*see also* categories
        633.0-633.9) 639.2
    molar pregnancy (*see also* categories
        630-632) 639.2
  following
    abortion 639.2
    ectopic or molar pregnancy 639.2
  nonpuerperal, nontraumatic 621.8
  obstetrical trauma NEC 665.5
  old (postpartal) 621.8
vagina
  with
    abortion—*see* Abortion, by type, with
        damage to pelvic organs
    ectopic pregnancy (*see also* categories
        633.0-633.9) 639.2
    molar pregnancy (*see also* categories
        630-632) 639.2
    perineal involvement, complicating delivery
        664.0
  complicating delivery 665.4
    first degree 664.0
    second degree 664.1
    third degree 664.2
    fourth degree 664.3
    high 665.4
    muscles 664.1
    sulcus 665.4
    wall 665.4
  following
    abortion 639.2
    ectopic or molar pregnancy 639.2
  nonpuerperal, nontraumatic 623.4
  old (postpartal) 623.4
valve, heart—*see* Endocarditis
vulva
  with
    abortion—*see* Abortion, by type, with
        damage to pelvic organs
    ectopic pregnancy (*see also* categories
        633.0-633.9) 639.2

Laceration—*continued*
  molar pregnancy (*see also* categories
      630-632) 639.2
  complicating delivery 664.0
  following
    abortion 639.2
    ectopic or molar pregnancy 639.2
  nonpuerperal, nontraumatic 624.4
  old (postpartal) 624.4
Lachrymal —*see* condition
Lachrymonasal duct —*see* condition
Lack of
  adequate intermaxillary vertical dimension 524.36
  appetite (*see also* Anorexia) 783.0
  care
    in home V60.4
    of adult 995.84
    of infant (at or after birth) 995.52
  coordination 781.3
  development—*see also* Hypoplasia
    physiological in childhood 783.40
  education V62.3
  energy 780.79
  financial resources V60.2
  food 994.2
    in environment V60.89
  growth in childhood 783.43
  heating V60.1
  housing (permanent) (temporary) V60.0
    adequate V60.1
  material resources V60.2
  medical attention 799.89
  memory (*see also* Amnesia) 780.93
    mild, following organic brain damage 310.89
  ovulation 628.0
  person able to render necessary care V60.4
  physical exercise V69.0
  physiologic development in childhood 783.40
  posterior occlusal support 524.57
  prenatal care in current pregnancy V23.7
  shelter V60.0
  sleep V69.4
  water 994.3
Lacrimal —*see* condition
Lacrimation, abnormal (*see also* Epiphora) 375.20
Lacrimonasal duct —*see* condition
Lactation, lactating (breast) (puerperal)
    (postpartum)
  defective 676.4
  disorder 676.9
    specified type NEC 676.8
  excessive 676.6
  failed 676.4
  mastitis NEC 675.2
  mother (care and/or examination) V24.1
  nonpuerperal 611.6
  suppressed 676.5
Lacticemia 271.3
  excessive 276.2
Lactosuria 271.3
Lacunar skull 756.0
Laennec's cirrhosis (alcoholic) 571.2
  nonalcoholic 571.5
Lafora's disease 333.2
Lag, lid (nervous) 374.41
Lagleyze-von Hippel disease (retinocerebral
    angiomatosis) 759.6

Lagophthalmos (eyelid) (nervous) 374.20
  cicatricial 374.23
  keratitis (*see also* Keratitis) 370.34
  mechanical 374.22
  paralytic 374.21
La grippe —*see* Influenza
Lahore sore 085.1
Lakes, venous (cerebral) 437.8
Laki-Lorand factor deficiency (*see also* Defect,
  coagulation) 286.3
Lalling 307.9
Lambliasis 007.1
Lame back 724.5
Lancereaux's diabetes (diabetes mellitus with
  marked emaciation) 250.8 *[261]*
  due to secondary diabetes 249.8 *[261]*
Landau-Kleffner syndrome 345.8
Landouzy-Déjérine dystrophy
  (fascioscapulohumeral atrophy) 359.1
Landry's disease or paralysis 357.0
Landry-Guillain-Barré syndrome 357.0
Lane's
  band 751.4
  disease 569.89
  kink (*see also* Obstruction, intestine) 560.9
Langdon Down's syndrome (mongolism) 758.0
Language abolition 784.69
Lanugo (persistent) 757.4
Laparoscopic surgical procedure converted to
  open procedure V64.41
Lardaceous
  degeneration (any site) 277.39
  disease 277.39
  kidney 277.39 *[583.81]*
  liver 277.39
Large
  baby (regardless of gestational age) 766.1
    exceptionally (weight of 4500 grams or more)
     766.0
    of diabetic mother 775.0
  ear 744.22
  fetus—*see also* Oversize, fetus
    causing disproportion 653.5
     with obstructed labor 660.1
  for dates
    fetus or newborn (regardless of gestational
     age) 766.1
     affecting management of pregnancy 656.6
     exceptionally (weight of 4500 grams or
      more) 766.0
  physiological cup 743.57
  stature 783.9
  waxy liver 277.39
  white kidney—*see* Nephrosis
Larsen's syndrome (flattened facies and multiple
  congenital dislocations) 755.8
Larsen-Johansson disease (juvenile osteopathia
  patellae) 732.4
Larva migrans
  cutaneous NEC 126.9
    ancylostoma 126.9
  of Diptera in vitreous 128.0
  visceral NEC 128.0
Laryngeal —*see also* condition
  syncope 786.2
Laryngismus (acute) (infectious) (stridulous)
  478.75
  congenital 748.3
  diphtheritic 032.3

Laryngitis (acute) (edematous) (fibrinous)
  (gangrenous) (infective) (infiltrative)
  (malignant) (membranous) (phlegmonous)
  (pneumococcal) (pseudomembranous) (septic)
  (subglottic) (suppurative) (ulcerative) (viral)
  464.00
  with
    influenza, flu, or grippe (*see also* Influenza)
     487.1
    obstruction 464.01
    tracheitis (*see also* Laryngotracheitis) 464.20
     with obstruction 464.21
     acute 464.20
      with obstruction 464.21
     chronic 476.1
  atrophic 476.0
  Borrelia vincentii 101
  catarrhal 476.0
  chronic 476.0
    with tracheitis (chronic) 476.1
    due to external agent—*see* Condition,
     respiratory, chronic, due to
  diphtheritic (membranous) 032.3
  due to external agent—*see* Inflammation,
    respiratory, upper, due to
  H. influenzae 464.00
    with obstruction 464.01
  Hemophilus influenzae 464.00
    with obstruction 464.01
  hypertrophic 476.0
  influenzal (*see also* Influenza) 487.1
  pachydermic 478.79
  sicca 476.0
  spasmodic 478.75
    acute 464.00
     with obstruction 464.01
  streptococcal 034.0
  stridulous 478.75
  syphilitic 095.8
    congenital 090.5
  tuberculous (*see also* Tuberculosis, larynx)
    012.3
  Vincent's 101
Laryngocele (congenital) (ventricular) 748.3
Laryngofissure 478.79
  congenital 748.3
Laryngomalacia (congenital) 748.3
Laryngopharyngitis (acute) 465.0
  chronic 478.9
    due to external agent—*see* Condition,
     respiratory, chronic, due to
  due to external agent—*see* Inflammation,
    respiratory, upper, due to
  septic 034.0
Laryngoplegia (*see also* Paralysis, vocal cord)
  478.30
Laryngoptosis 478.79
Laryngospasm 478.75
  due to external agent—*see* Condition,
    respiratory, acute, due to
Laryngostenosis 478.74
  congenital 748.3
Laryngotracheitis (acute) (infectional) (viral)
  (*see also* Laryngitis) 464.20
  with obstruction 464.21
  atrophic 476.1
  Borrelia vincentii 101
  catarrhal 476.1
  chronic 476.1
    due to external agent—*see* Condition,
     respiratory, chronic, due to

Laryngotracheitis—*continued*
   diphtheritic (membranous) 032.3
   due to external agent—*see* Inflammation,
      respiratory, upper, due to
   H. influenzae 464.20
      with obstruction 464.21
   hypertrophic 476.1
   influenzal (*see also* Influenza) 487.1
   pachydermic 478.75
   sicca 476.1
   spasmodic 478.75
      acute 464.20
         with obstruction 464.21
   streptococcal 034.0
   stridulous 478.75
   syphilitic 095.8
      congenital 090.5
   tuberculous (*see also* Tuberculosis, larynx)
      012.3
   Vincent's 101
Laryngotracheobronchitis (*see also* Bronchitis)
      490
   acute 466.0
   chronic 491.8
   viral 466.0
Laryngotracheobronchopneumonitis —*see*
      Pneumonia, broncho-
Larynx, laryngeal —*see* condition
Lasègue's disease (persecution mania) 297.9
Lassa fever 078.89
Lassitude (*see also* Weakness) 780.79
Late —*see also* condition
   infant
      post-term (gestation period over 40
         completed weeks to 42 completed
         weeks) 766.21
      prolonged gestation (period over 42
         completed weeks) 766.22
Late effect(s) (of) —*see also* condition
   abscess
      intracranial or intraspinal (conditions
         classifiable to 324)–*see* category 326
   adverse effect of drug, medicinal or biological
      substance 909.5
   allergic reaction 909.9
   amputation
      postoperative (late) 997.60
      traumatic (injury classifiable to 885-887 and
         895-897) 905.9
   burn (injury classifiable to 948-949) 906.9
      extremities NEC (injury classifiable to 943 or
         945) 906.7
         hand or wrist (injury classifiable to 944)
            906.6
      eye (injury classifiable to 940) 906.5
      face, head, and neck (injury classifiable to
         941) 906.5
      specified site NEC (injury classifiable to 942
         and 946-947) 906.8
   cerebrovascular disease (conditions classifiable
      to 430-437) 438.9
      with
         alterations of sensations 438.6
         aphasia 438.11
         apraxia 438.81
         ataxia 438.84
         cognitive deficits 438.0
         disturbances of vision 438.7
         dysarthria 438.13
         dysphagia 438.82
         dysphasia 438.12
         facial droop 438.83

Late effect(s) (of)—*continued*
   cerebrovascular disease—*continued*
      with—*continued*
         facial weakness 438.83
         fluency disorder 438.14
         hemiplegia/hemiparesis
            affecting
               dominant side 438.21
               nondominant side 438.22
               unspecified side 438.20
         monoplegia of lower limb
            affecting
               dominant side 438.41
               nondominant side 438.42
               unspecified side 438.40
         monoplegia of upper limb
            affecting
               dominant side 438.31
               nondominant side 438.32
               unspecified side 438.30
         paralytic syndrome NEC
            affecting
               bilateral 438.53
               dominant side 438.51
               nondominant side 438.52
               unspecified side 438.50
         speech and language deficit 438.10
            specified type NEC 438.19
         stuttering 438.14
         vertigo 438.85
      specified type NEC 438.89
   childbirth complication(s) 677
   complication(s) of
      childbirth 677
      delivery 677
      pregnancy 677
      puerperium 677
      surgical and medical care (conditions
         classifiable to 996-999) 909.3
      trauma (conditions classifiable to 958) 908.6
   contusion (injury classifiable to 920-924) 906.3
   crushing (injury classifiable to 925-929) 906.4
   delivery complication(s) 677
   dislocation (injury classifiable to 830-839) 905.6
   encephalitis or encephalomyelitis (conditions
      classifiable to 323)—*see* category 326
      in infectious diseases 139.8
         viral (conditions classifiable to 049.8, 049.9,
            062-064) 139.0
   external cause NEC (conditions classifiable to
      995) 909.9
      certain conditions classifiable to categories
         991-994 909.4
   foreign body in orifice (injury classifiable to
      930-939) 908.5
   fracture (multiple) (injury classifiable to
      828-829) 905.5
      extremity
         lower (injury classifiable to 821-827) 905.4
            neck of femur (injury classifiable to 820)
               905.3
         upper (injury classifiable to 810-819) 905.2
      face and skull (injury classifiable to 800-804)
         905.0
      skull and face (injury classifiable to 800-804)
         905.0
      spine and trunk (injury classifiable to 805 and
         807-809) 905.1
         with spinal cord lesion (injury classifiable to
            806) 907.2

Late effect(s) (of)—*continued*
infection
pyogenic, intracranial—*see* category 326
infectious diseases (conditions classifiable to
001-136) NEC 139.8
injury (injury classifiable to 959) 908.9
blood vessel 908.3
abdomen and pelvis (injury classifiable to
902) 908.4
extremity (injury classifiable to 903-904)
908.3
head and neck (injury classifiable to 900)
908.3
intracranial (injury classifiable to 850-854)
907.0
with skull fracture 905.0
thorax (injury classifiable to 901) 908.4
internal organ NEC (injury classifiable to 867
and 869) 908.2
abdomen (injury classifiable to 863-866 and
868) 908.1
thorax (injury classifiable to 860-862) 908.0
intracranial (injury classifiable to 850-854)
907.0
with skull fracture (injury classifiable to
800-801 and 803-804) 905.0
nerve NEC (injury classifiable to 957) 907.9
cranial (injury classifiable to 950-951) 907.1
peripheral NEC (injury classifiable to 957)
907.9
lower limb and pelvic girdle (injury
classifiable to 956) 907.5
upper limb and shoulder girdle (injury
classifiable to 955) 907.4
roots and plexus(es), spinal (injury
classifiable to 953) 907.3
trunk (injury classifiable to 954) 907.3
pregnancy complication(s) 677
puerperal complication(s) 677
spinal
cord (injury classifiable to 806 and 952)
907.2
nerve root(s) and plexus(es) (injury
classifiable to 953) 907.3
superficial (injury classifiable to 910-919)
906.2
tendon (tendon injury classifiable to 840-848,
880-884 with .2, and 890-894 with .2)
905.8
meningitis
bacterial (conditions classifiable to 320)—*see*
category 326
unspecified cause (conditions classifiable to
322)—*see* category 326
myelitis (*see also* Late, effect(s) (of),
encephalitis)—*see* category 326
parasitic diseases (conditions classifiable to
001-136 NEC) 139.8
phlebitis or thrombophlebitis of intracranial
venous sinuses (conditions classifiable to
325)—*see* category 326
poisoning due to drug, medicinal or biological
substance (conditions classifiable to
960-979) 909.0
poliomyelitis, acute (conditions classifiable to
045) 138
radiation (conditions classifiable to 990) 909.2
rickets 268.1
sprain and strain without mention of tendon
injury (injury classifiable to 840-848, except
tendon injury) 905.7
tendon involvement 905.8

Late effect(s) (of)—*continued*
toxic effect of
drug, medicinal or biological substance
(conditions classifiable to 960-979) 909.0
nonmedical substance (conditions classifiable
to 980-989) 909.1
trachoma (conditions classifiable to 076) 139.1
tuberculosis 137.0
bones and joints (conditions classifiable to
015) 137.3
central nervous system (conditions classifiable
to 013) 137.1
genitourinary (conditions classifiable to 016)
137.2
pulmonary (conditions classifiable to 010-012)
137.0
specified organs NEC (conditions classifiable
to 014, 017-018) 137.4
viral encephalitis (conditions classifiable to
049.8, 049.9, 062-064) 139.0
wound, open
extremity (injury classifiable to 880-884 and
890-894, except .2) 906.1
tendon (injury classifiable to 880-884 with
.2 and 890-894 with .2) 905.8
head, neck, and trunk (injury classifiable to
870-879) 906.0
Latent —*see* condition
Lateral —*see* condition
Laterocession —*see* Lateroversion
Lateroflexion —*see* Lateroversion
Lateroversion
cervix—*see* Lateroversion, uterus
uterus, uterine (cervix) (postinfectional)
(postpartal, old) 621.6
congenital 752.39
in pregnancy or childbirth 654.4
affecting fetus or newborn 763.89
Lathyrism 988.2
Launois' syndrome (pituitary gigantism) 253.0
Launois-Bensaude's lipomatosis 272.8
Launois-Cléret syndrome (adiposogenital
dystrophy) 253.8
Laurence-Moon-Biedl syndrome (obesity,
polydactyly, and intellectual disabilities)
759.89
LAV (disease) (illness) (infection)—*see* Human
immunodeficiency virus (disease) (illness)
(infection)
LAV/HTLV-III (disease) (illness)
(infection)—*see* Human immunodeficiency
virus (disease) (illness) (infection)
Lawford's syndrome (encephalocutaneous
angiomatosis) 759.6
Lax, laxity —*see also* Relaxation
ligament 728.4
skin (acquired) 701.8
congenital 756.83
Laxative habit (*see also* Abuse, drugs,
nondependent) 305.9
Lazy leukocyte syndrome 288.09
LCAD (long chain/very long chain acyl CoA
dehydrogenase deficiency, VLCAD) 277.85
LCHAD (long chain 3-hydroxyacyl CoA
dehydrogenase deficiency) 277.85
Lead —*see also* condition
exposure (suspected) to V15.86
incrustation of cornea 371.15
poisoning 984.9
specified type of lead—*see* Table of drugs and
chemicals

Lead miner's lung 503
Leakage
amniotic fluid 658.1
with delayed delivery 658.2
affecting fetus or newborn 761.1
bile from drainage tube (T tube) 997.49
blood (microscopic), fetal, into maternal
circulation 656.0
affecting management of pregnancy or
puerperium 656.0
device, implant, or graft—*see* Complications,
mechanical
spinal fluid at lumbar puncture site 997.09
urine, continuous 788.37
Leaky heart —*see* Endocarditis
Learning defect, specific NEC
(strephosymbolia) 315.2
Leather bottle stomach (M8142/3) 151.9
Leber's
congenital amaurosis 362.76
optic atrophy (hereditary) 377.16
Lederer's anemia or disease (acquired
infectious hemolytic anemia) 283.19
Lederer-Brill syndrome (acquired infectious
hemolytic anemia) 283.19
Leeches (aquatic) (land) 134.2
Left-sided neglect 781.8
Leg —*see* condition
Legal investigation V62.5
Legg (-Calvé) -Perthes disease or syndrome
(osteochondrosis, femoral capital) 732.1
Legionnaires' disease 482.84
Leigh's disease 330.8
Leiner's disease (exfoliative dermatitis) 695.89
Leiofibromyoma (M8890/0)—*see also*
Leiomyoma
uterus (cervix) (corpus) (*see also* Leiomyoma,
uterus) 218.9
Leiomyoblastoma (M8891/1)—*see* Neoplasm,
connective tissue, uncertain behavior
Leiomyofibroma (M8890/0)—*see also*
Neoplasm, connective tissue, benign
uterus (cervix) (corpus) (*see also* Leiomyoma,
uterus) 218.9
Leiomyoma (M8890/0)—*see also* Neoplasm,
connective tissue, benign
bizarre (M8893/0)—*see* Neoplasm, connective
tissue, benign
cellular (M8892/1)—*see* Neoplasm, connective
tissue, uncertain behavior
epithelioid (M8891/1)—*see* Neoplasm,
connective tissue, uncertain behavior
prostate (polypoid) 600.20
with
other lower urinary tract symptoms (LUTS)
600.21
urinary
obstruction 600.21
retention 600.21
uterus (cervix) (corpus) 218.9
interstitial 218.1
intramural 218.1
submucous 218.0
subperitoneal 218.2
subserous 218.2
vascular (M8894/0)—*see* Neoplasm,
connective tissue, benign
Leiomyomatosis (intravascular) (M8890/1)—*see*
Neoplasm, connective tissue, uncertain
behavior

Leiomyosarcoma (M8890/3)—*see also*
Neoplasm, connective tissue, malignant
epithelioid (M8891/3)—*see* Neoplasm,
connective tissue, malignant
Leishmaniasis 085.9
American 085.5
cutaneous 085.4
mucocutaneous 085.5
Asian desert 085.2
Brazilian 085.5
cutaneous 085.9
acute necrotizing 085.2
American 085.4
Asian desert 085.2
diffuse 085.3
dry form 085.1
Ethiopian 085.3
eyelid 085.5 *[373.6]*
late 085.1
lepromatous 085.3
recurrent 085.1
rural 085.2
ulcerating 085.1
urban 085.1
wet form 085.2
zoonotic form 085.2
dermal—*see also* Leishmaniasis, cutaneous
post kala-azar 085.0
eyelid 085.5 *[373.6]*
infantile 085.0
Mediterranean 085.0
mucocutaneous (American) 085.5
naso-oral 085.5
nasopharyngeal 085.5
Old World 085.1
tegumentaria diffusa 085.4
vaccination, prophylactic (against) V05.2
visceral (Indian) 085.0
Leishmanoid, dermal —*see also* Leishmaniasis,
cutaneous
post kala-azar 085.0
Leloir's disease 695.4
Lemiere syndrome 451.89
Lenegre's disease 426.0
Lengthening, leg 736.81
Lennox-Gastaut syndrome 345.0
with tonic seizures 345.1
Lennox's syndrome (*see also* Epilepsy) 345.0
Lens —*see* condition
Lenticonus (anterior) (posterior) (congenital)
743.36
Lenticular degeneration, progressive 275.1
Lentiglobus (posterior) (congenital) 743.36
Lentigo (congenital) 709.09
juvenile 709.09
Maligna (M8742/2)—*see also* Neoplasm, skin,
in situ
melanoma (M8742/3)—*see* Melanoma
senile 709.09
Leonine leprosy 030.0
Leontiasis
ossium 733.3
syphilitic 095.8
congenital 090.5
Léopold-Lévi's syndrome (paroxysmal thyroid
instability) 242.9
Lepore hemoglobin syndrome 282.45
Lepothrix 039.0
Lepra 030.9
Willan's 696.1
Leprechaunism 259.8

Lepromatous leprosy 030.0
Leprosy 030.9
  anesthetic 030.1
  beriberi 030.1
  borderline (group B) (infiltrated) (neuritic) 030.3
  cornea (*see also* Leprosy, by type) 030.9
    [371.89]
  dimorphous (group B) (infiltrated)
    (lepromatous) (neuritic) (tuberculoid) 030.3
  eyelid 030.0 *[373.4]*
  indeterminate (group I) (macular) (neuritic)
    (uncharacteristic) 030.2
  leonine 030.0
  lepromatous (diffuse) (infiltrated) (macular)
    (neuritic) (nodular) (type L) 030.0
  macular (early) (neuritic) (simple) 030.2
  maculoanesthetic 030.1
  mixed 030.0
  neuro 030.1
  nodular 030.0
  primary neuritic 030.3
  specified type or group NEC 030.8
  tubercular 030.1
  tuberculoid (macular) (maculoanesthetic)
    (major) (minor) (neuritic) (type T) 030.1
Leptocytosis, hereditary 282.40
Leptomeningitis (chronic) (circumscribed)
    (hemorrhagic) (nonsuppurative) (*see also*
    Meningitis) 322.9
  aseptic 047.9
    adenovirus 049.1
    Coxsackie virus 047.0
    ECHO virus 047.1
    enterovirus 047.9
    lymphocytic choriomeningitis 049.0
  epidemic 036.0
  late effect—*see* category 326
  meningococcal 036.0
  pneumococcal 320.1
  syphilitic 094.2
  tuberculous (*see also* Tuberculosis, meninges)
    013.0
Leptomeningopathy (*see also* Meningitis) 322.9
Leptospiral —*see* condition
Leptospirochetal —*see* condition
Leptospirosis 100.9
  autumnalis 100.89
  canicula 100.89
  grippotyphosa 100.89
  hebdomidis 100.89
  icterohemorrhagica 100.0
  nanukayami 100.89
  pomona 100.89
  Weil's disease 100.0
Leptothricosis —*see* Actinomycosis
Leptothrix infestation —*see* Actinomycosis
Leptotricosis —*see* Actinomycosis
Leptus dermatitis 133.8
Léri's pleonosteosis 756.89
Léri-Weill syndrome 756.59
Leriche syndrome (aortic bifurcation occlusion)
    444.09
Lermoyez's syndrome (*see also* Disease,
    Ménière's) 386.00
Lesbianism —*omit code*
  egodystonic 302.0
  problems with 302.0
Lesch-Nyhan syndrome (hypoxanthine-guanine-
    phosphoribosyltransferase deficiency) 277.2

Lesion(s)
  abducens nerve 378.54
  alveolar process 525.8
  anorectal 569.49
  aortic (valve)—*see* Endocarditis, aortic
  auditory nerve 388.5
  basal ganglion 333.90
  bile duct (*see also* Disease, biliary) 576.8
  bladder 596.9
  bone 733.90
  brachial plexus 353.0
  brain 348.89
    congenital 742.9
    vascular (*see also* Lesion, cerebrovascular)
      437.9
      degenerative 437.1
      healed or old without residuals V12.54
      hypertensive 437.2
      late effect—*see* Late effect(s) (of)
        cerebrovascular disease
  buccal 528.9
  calcified—*see* Calcification
  canthus 373.9
  carate—*see* Pinta, lesions
  cardia 537.89
  cardiac—*see also* Disease, heart congenital 746.9
    valvular—*see* Endocarditis
  cauda equina 344.60
    with neurogenic bladder 344.61
  cecum 569.89
  cerebral—*see* Lesion, brain
  cerebrovascular (*see also* Disease,
      cerebrovascular NEC) 437.9
    degenerative 437.1
    healed or old without residuals V12.54
    hypertensive 437.2
    specified type NEC 437.8
  cervical root (nerve) NEC 353.2
  chiasmal 377.54
    associated with
      inflammatory disorders 377.54
      neoplasm NEC 377.52
      pituitary 377.51
      pituitary disorders 377.51
      vascular disorders 377.53
  chorda tympani 351.8
  coin, lung 793.11
  colon 569.89
  congenital—*see* Anomaly
  conjunctiva 372.9
  coronary artery (*see also* Ischemia, heart) 414.9
  cranial nerve 352.9
    first 352.0
    second 377.49
    third
      partial 378.51
      total 378.52
    fourth 378.53
    fifth 350.9
    sixth 378.54
    seventh 351.9
    eighth 388.5
    ninth 352.2
    tenth 352.3
    eleventh 352.4
    twelfth 352.5
  cystic—*see* Cyst
  degenerative—*see* Degeneration
  dermal (skin) 709.9

Lesion(s)—*continued*
  Dieulafoy (hemorrhagic)
    of
      duodenum 537.84
      intestine 569.86
      stomach 537.84
    duodenum 537.89
      with obstruction 537.3
  eyelid 373.9
  gasserian ganglion 350.8
  gastric 537.89
  gastroduodenal 537.89
  gastrointestinal 569.89
  glossopharyngeal nerve 352.2
  heart (organic)—*see also* Disease, heart
    vascular—*see* Disease, cardiovascular
  helix (ear) 709.9
  high grade myelodysplastic syndrome 238.73
  hyperchromic, due to pinta (carate) 103.1
  hyperkeratotic (*see also* Hyperkeratosis) 701.1
  hypoglossal nerve 352.5
  hypopharynx 478.29
  hypothalamic 253.9
  ileocecal coil 569.89
  ileum 569.89
  iliohypogastric nerve 355.79
  ilioinguinal nerve 355.79
  in continuity—*see* Injury, nerve, by site
  inflammatory—*see* Inflammation
  intestine 569.89
  intracerebral—*see* Lesion, brain
  intrachiasmal (optic) (*see also* Lesion, chiasmal)
    377.54
  intracranial, space-occupying NEC 784.2
  joint 719.90
    ankle 719.97
    elbow 719.92
    foot 719.97
    hand 719.94
    hip 719.95
    knee 719.96
    multiple sites 719.99
    pelvic region 719.95
    sacroiliac (old) 724.6
    shoulder (region) 719.91
    specified site NEC 719.98
    wrist 719.93
  keratotic (*see also* Keratosis) 701.1
  kidney (*see also* Disease, renal) 593.9
  laryngeal nerve (recurrent) 352.3
  leonine 030.0
  lip 528.5
  liver 573.8
  low grade myelodysplastic syndrome 238.72
  lumbosacral
    plexus 353.1
    root (nerve) NEC 353.4
  lung 518.89
    coin 793.11
  maxillary sinus 473.0
  mitral—*see* Endocarditis, mitral
  Morel Lavallée — see Hematoma, by site
  motor cortex 348.89
  nerve (*see also* Disorder, nerve) 355.9
  nervous system 349.9
    congenital 742.9

Lesion(s)—*continued*
  nonallopathic NEC 739.9
    in region (of)
      abdomen 739.9
      acromioclavicular 739.7
      cervical, cervicothoracic 739.1
      costochondral 739.8
      costovertebral 739.8
      extremity
        lower 739.6
        upper 739.7
      head 739.0
      hip 739.5
      lower extremity 739.6
      lumbar, lumbosacral 739.3
      occipitocervical 739.0
      pelvic 739.5
      pubic 739.5
      rib cage 739.8
      sacral, sacrococcygeal, sacroiliac 739.4
      sternochondral 739.8
      sternoclavicular 739.7
      thoracic, thoracolumbar 739.2
      upper extremity 739.7
  nose (internal) 478.19
  obstructive—*see* Obstruction
  obturator nerve 355.79
  occlusive
    artery—*see* Embolism, artery
  organ or site NEC—*see* Disease, by site
  osteolytic 733.90
  paramacular, of retina 363.32
  peptic 537.89
  periodontal, due to traumatic occlusion 523.8
  perirectal 569.49
  peritoneum (granulomatous) 568.89
  pigmented (skin) 709.00
  pinta—*see* Pinta, lesions
  polypoid—*see* Polyp
  prechiasmal (optic) (*see also* Lesion, chiasmal)
    377.54
  primary—*see also* Syphilis, primary
    carate 103.0
    pinta 103.0
    yaws 102.0
  pulmonary 518.89
    valve (*see also* Endocarditis, pulmonary)
      424.3
  pylorus 537.89
  radiation NEC 990
  radium NEC 990
  rectosigmoid 569.89
  retina, retinal—*see also* Retinopathy
    vascular 362.17
  retroperitoneal 568.89
  romanus 720.1
  sacroiliac (joint) 724.6
  salivary gland 527.8
    benign lymphoepithelial 527.8
  saphenous nerve 355.79
  secondary—*see* Syphilis, secondary
  sigmoid 569.89
  sinus (accessory) (nasal) (*see also* Sinusitis)
    473.9
  skin 709.9
    suppurative 686.00
  SLAP (superior glenoid labrum) 840.7
  space-occupying, intracranial NEC 784.2

Lesion(s)—*continued*
  spinal cord 336.9
    congenital 742.9
    traumatic (complete) (incomplete)
      (transverse)—*see also* Injury, spinal, by
      site
      with
        broken
          back—*see* Fracture, vertebra, by site,
            with spinal cord injury
          neck—*see* Fracture, vertebra, cervical,
            with spinal cord injury
        fracture, vertebra—*see* Fracture, vertebra,
          by site, with spinal cord injury
  spleen 289.50
  stomach 537.89
  superior glenoid labrum (SLAP) 840.7
  syphilitic—*see* Syphilis
  tertiary—*see* Syphilis, tertiary
  thoracic root (nerve) 353.3
  tonsillar fossa 474.9
  tooth, teeth 525.8
    white spot 521.01
  traumatic NEC (*see also* nature and site of
    injury) 959.9
  tricuspid (valve)—*see* Endocarditis, tricuspid
  trigeminal nerve 350.9
  ulcerated or ulcerative—*see* Ulcer
  uterus NEC 621.9
  vagina 623.8
  vagus nerve 352.3
  valvular—*see* Endocarditis
  vascular 459.9
    affecting central nervous system (*see also*
      Lesion, cerebrovascular) 437.9
    following trauma (*see also* Injury, blood
      vessel, by site) 904.9
    retina 362.17
    traumatic—*see* Injury, blood vessel, by site
    umbilical cord 663.6
      affecting fetus or newborn 762.6
  visual
    cortex NEC (*see also* Disorder, visual, cortex)
      377.73
    pathway NEC (*see also* Disorder, visual,
      pathway) 377.63
  warty—*see* Verruca
  white spot, on teeth 521.01
  x-ray NEC 990
Lethargic —*see* condition
Lethargy 780.79
Letterer-Siwe disease (acute histiocytosis X)
  (M9722/3) 202.5
Leucinosis 270.3
Leucocoria 360.44
Leucosarcoma (M9850/3) 207.8
Leukasmus 270.2
Leukemia, leukemic (congenital) (M9800/3) 208.9

*Note—Use the following fifth-digit
subclassification for categories 203-208:*

*0 without mention of having achieved
   remission, failed remission*
1 in remission
2 in relapse

  acute NEC (M9801/3) 208.0
  aleukemic NEC (M9804/3) 208.8
    granulocytic (M9864/3) 205.8
  basophilic (M9870/3) 205.1
  blast (cell) (M9801/3) 208.0

Leukemia, leukemic—*continued*
  blastic (M9801/3) 208.0
    granulocytic (M9861/3) 205.0
  chronic NEC (M9803/3) 208.1
  compound (M9810/3) 207.8
  eosinophilic (M9880/3) 205.1
  giant cell (M9910/3) 207.2
  granulocytic (M9860/3) 205.9
    acute (M9861/3) 205.0
    aleukemic (M9864/3) 205.8
    blastic (M9861/3) 205.0
    chronic (M9863/3) 205.1
    subacute (M9862/3) 205.2
    subleukemic (M9864/3) 205.8
  hairy cell (M9940/3) 202.4
  hemoblastic (M9801/3) 208.0
  histiocytic (M9890/3) 206.9
  lymphatic (M9820/3) 204.9
    acute (M9821/3) 204.0
    aleukemic (M9824/3) 204.8
    chronic (M9823/3) 204.1
    subacute (M9822/3) 204.2
    subleukemic (M9824/3) 204.8
  lymphoblastic (M9821/3) 204.0
  lymphocytic (M9820/3) 204.9
    acute (M9821/3) 204.0
    aleukemic (M9824/3) 204.8
    chronic (M9823/3) 204.1
    granular
      large T-cell 204.8
    subacute (M9822/3) 204.2
    subleukemic (M9824/3) 204.8
  lymphogenous (M9820/3)—*see* Leukemia,
    lymphoid
  lymphoid (M9820/3) 204.9
    acute (M9821/3) 204.0
    aleukemic (M9824/3) 204.8
    blastic (M9821/3) 204.0
    chronic (M9823/3) 204.1
    subacute (M9822/3) 204.2
    subleukemic (M9824/3) 204.8
  lymphosarcoma cell (M9850/3) 207.8
  mast cell (M9900/3) 207.8
  megakaryocytic (M9910/3) 207.2
  megakaryocytoid (M9910/3) 207.2
  mixed (cell) (M9810/3) 207.8
  monoblastic (M9891/3) 206.0
  monocytic (Schilling-type) (M9890/3) 206.9
    acute (M9891/3) 206.0
    aleukemic (M9894/3) 206.8
    chronic (M9893/3) 206.1
    Naegeli-type (M9863/3) 205.1
    subacute (M9892/3) 206.2
    subleukemic (M9894/3) 206.8
  monocytoid (M9890/3) 206.9
    acute (M9891/3) 206.0
    aleukemic (M9894/3) 206.8
    chronic (M9893/3) 206.1
    myelogenous (M9863/3) 205.1
    subacute (M9892/3) 206.2
    subleukemic (M9894/3) 206.8
  monomyelocytic (M9860/3)—*see* Leukemia,
    myelomonocytic
  myeloblastic (M9861/3) 205.0
  myelocytic (M9863/3) 205.1
    acute (M9861/3) 205.0
  myelogenous (M9860/3) 205.9
    acute (M9861/3) 205.0
    aleukemic (M9864/3) 205.8
    chronic (M9863/3) 205.1
    monocytoid (M9863/3) 205.1

Leukemia, leukemic—*continued*
 myelogenous—*continued*
  subacute (M9862/3) 205.2
  subleukemic (M9864) 205.8
 myeloid (M9860/3) 205.9
  acute (M9861/3) 205.0
  aleukemic (M9864/3) 205.8
  chronic (M9863/3) 205.1
  subacute (M9862/3) 205.2
  subleukemic (M9864/3) 205.8
 myelomonocytic (M9860/3) 205.9
  acute (M9861/3) 205.0
  chronic (M9863/3) 205.1
 Naegeli-type monocytic (M9863/3) 205.1
 neutrophilic (M9865/3) 205.1
 plasma cell (M9830/3) 203.1
 plasmacytic (M9830/3) 203.1
 prolymphocytic (M9825/3)—*see* Leukemia,
  lymphoid
 promyelocytic, acute (M9866/3) 205.0
 Schilling-type monocytic (M9890/3)—*see*
  Leukemia, monocytic
 stem cell (M9801/3) 208.0
 subacute NEC (M9802/3) 208.2
 subleukemic NEC (M9804/3) 208.8
 thrombocytic (M9910/3) 207.2
 undifferentiated (M9801/3) 208.0
Leukemoid reaction (basophilic) (lymphocytic)
  (monocytic) (myelocytic) (neutrophilic) 288.62
Leukoaraiosis (hypertensive) 437.1
Leukoariosis —*see* Leukoaraiosis
Leukoclastic vasculitis 446.29
Leukocoria 360.44
Leukocythemia —*see* Leukemia
Leukocytopenia 288.50
Leukocytosis 288.60
 basophilic 288.8
 eosinophilic 288.3
 lymphocytic 288.8
 monocytic 288.8
 neutrophilic 288.8
Leukoderma 709.09
 syphilitic 091.3
  late 095.8
Leukodermia (*see also* Leukoderma) 709.09
Leukodystrophy (cerebral) (globoid cell)
  (metachromatic) (progressive) (sudanophilic)
  330.0
Leukoedema, mouth or tongue 528.79
Leukoencephalitis
 acute hemorrhagic (postinfectious) NEC 136.9
  [323.61]
  postimmunization or postvaccinal 323.51
 subacute sclerosing 046.2
  van Bogaert's 046.2
 van Bogaert's (sclerosing) 046.2
Leukoencephalopathy (*see also* Encephalitis) 323.9
 acute necrotizing hemorrhagic (postinfectious)
  136.9 *[323.61]*
  postimmunization or postvaccinal 323.51
 arteriosclerotic 437.0
 Binswanger's 290.12
 metachromatic 330.0
 multifocal (progressive) 046.3
 progressive multifocal 046.3
 reversible, posterior 348.5
Leukoerythroblastosis 289.9
Leukoerythrosis 289.0

Leukokeratosis (*see also* Leukoplakia) 702.8
 mouth 528.6
 nicotina palati 528.79
 tongue 528.6
Leukokoria 360.44
Leukokraurosis vulva, vulvae 624.09
Leukolymphosarcoma (M9850/3) 207.8
Leukoma (cornea) (interfering with central
  vision) 371.03
 adherent 371.04
Leukomalacia, periventricular 779.7
Leukomelanopathy, hereditary 288.2
Leukonychia (punctata) (striata) 703.8
 congenital 757.5
Leukopathia
 unguium 703.8
  congenital 757.5
Leukopenia 288.50
 basophilic 288.59
 cyclic 288.02
 eosinophilic 288.59
 familial 288.59
 malignant (see also Agranulocytosis) 288.09
 periodic 288.02
 transitory neonatal 776.7
Leukopenic —*see* condition
Leukoplakia 702.8
 anus 569.49
 bladder (postinfectional) 596.89
 buccal 528.6
 cervix (uteri) 622.2
 esophagus 530.83
 gingiva 528.6
 kidney (pelvis) 593.89
 larynx 478.79
 lip 528.6
 mouth 528.6
 oral soft tissue (including tongue) (mucosa) 528.6
 palate 528.6
 pelvis (kidney) 593.89
 penis (infectional) 607.0
 rectum 569.49
 syphilitic 095.8
 tongue 528.6
 tonsil 478.29
 ureter (postinfectional) 593.89
 urethra (postinfectional) 599.84
 uterus 621.8
 vagina 623.1
 vesical 596.89
 vocal cords 478.5
 vulva 624.09
Leukopolioencephalopathy 330.0
Leukorrhea (vagina) 623.5
 due to trichomonas (vaginalis) 131.00
 trichomonal (Trichomonas vaginalis) 131.00
Leukosarcoma (M9850/3) 207.8
Leukosis (M9800/3)—*see* Leukemia
Lev's disease or syndrome (acquired complete
  heart block) 426.0
Levi's syndrome (pituitary dwarfism) 253.3
Levocardia (isolated) 746.87
 with situs inversus 759.3
Levulosuria 271.2
Lewandowski's disease (primary) (*see also*
  Tuberculosis) 017.0
Lewandowski-Lutz disease (epidermodysplasia
  verruciformis) 078.19
Lewy body dementia 331.82
Lewy body disease 331.82
Leyden's disease (periodic vomiting) 536.2
Leyden's-Möbius dystrophy 359.1

Leydig cell
carcinoma (M8650/3)
  specified site—*see* Neoplasm, by site, malignant
  unspecified site
    female 183.0
    male 186.9
tumor (M8650/1)
  benign (M8650/0)
    specified site—*see* Neoplasm, by site, benign
    unspecified site
      female 220
      male 222.0
  malignant (M8650/3)
    specified site—*see* Neoplasm, by site, malignant
    unspecified site
      female 183.0
      male 186.9
  specified site—*see* Neoplasm, by site, uncertain behavior
  unspecified site
    female 236.2
    male 236.4
Leydig-Sertoli cell tumor (M8631/0)
  specified site—*see* Neoplasm, by site, benign
  unspecified site
    female 220
    male 222.0
LGSIL (low grade squamous intraepithelial lesion)
  anus 796.73
  cervix 795.03
  vagina 795.13
Liar, pathologic 301.7
Libman-Sacks disease or syndrome 710.0 [424.91]
Lice (infestation) 132.9
  body (pediculus corporis) 132.1
  crab 132.2
  head (pediculus capitis) 132.0
  mixed (classifiable to more than one of the categories 132.0-132.2) 132.3
  pubic (pediculus pubis) 132.2
Lichen 697.9
  albus 701.0
  annularis 695.89
  atrophicus 701.0
  corneus obtusus 698.3
  myxedematous 701.8
  nitidus 697.1
  pilaris 757.39
    acquired 701.1
  planopilaris 697.0
  planus (acute) (chronicus) (hypertrophic) (verrucous) 697.0
    morphoeicus 701.0
    sclerosus (et atrophicus) 701.0
  ruber 696.4
    acuminatus 696.4
    moniliformis 697.8
    obtusus corneus 698.3
    of Wilson 697.0
    planus 697.0
  sclerosus (et atrophicus) 701.0
  scrofulosus (primary) (*see also* Tuberculosis) 017.0
  simplex (Vidal's) 698.3
    chronicus 698.3
    circumscriptus 698.3
  spinulosus 757.39
    mycotic 117.9
  striata 697.8
  urticatus 698.2

Lichenification 698.3
  nodular 698.3
Lichenoides tuberculosis (primary) (*see also* Tuberculosis) 017.0
Lichtheim's disease or syndrome (subacute combined sclerosis with pernicious anemia) 281.0 [336.2]
Lien migrans 289.59
Lientery (*see also* Diarrhea) 787.91
  infectious 009.2
Life circumstance problem NEC V62.89
Li-Fraumeni cancer syndrome V84.01
Ligament —*see* condition
Light-for-dates (infant) 764.0
  with signs of fetal malnutrition 764.1
  affecting management of pregnancy 656.5
Light-headedness 780.4
Lightning (effects) (shock) (stroke) (struck by) 994.0
  burn—*see* Burn, by site
  foot 266.2
Lightwood's disease or syndrome (renal tubular acidosis) 588.89
Lignac's disease (cystinosis) 270.0
Lignac (-de Toni) (-Fanconi) (-Debré) syndrome (cystinosis) 270.0
Lignac (-Fanconi) syndrome (cystinosis) 270.0
Ligneous thyroiditis 245.3
Likoff's syndrome (angina in menopausal women) 413.9
Limb —*see* condition
Limitation of joint motion (*see also* Stiffness, joint) 719.5
  sacroiliac 724.6
Limit dextrinosis 271.0
Limited
  cardiac reserve—*see* Disease, heart
  duction, eye NEC 378.63
  mandibular range of motion 524.52
Lindau's disease (retinocerebral angiomatosis) 759.6
Lindau (-von Hippel) disease (angiomatosis retinocerebellosa) 759.6
Linea corneae senilis 371.41
Lines
  Beau's (transverse furrows on fingernails) 703.8
  Harris' 733.91
  Hudson-Stähli 371.11
  Stähli's 371.11
Lingua
  geographical 529.1
  nigra (villosa) 529.3
  plicata 529.5
    congenital 750.13
  tylosis 528.6
Lingual (tongue)—*see also* condition
  thyroid 759.2
Linitis (gastric) 535.4
  plastica (M8142/3) 151.9
Lioderma essentialis (cum melanosis et telangiectasia) 757.33
Lip —*see also* condition
  biting 528.9
Lipalgia 272.8
Lipedema —*see* Edema
Lipemia (*see also* Hyperlipidemia) 272.4
  retina, retinalis 272.3
Lipidosis 272.7
  cephalin 272.7
  cerebral (infantile) (juvenile) (late) 330.1
  cerebroretinal 330.1 [362.71]
  cerebroside 272.7

Lipidosis—*continued*
  cerebrospinal 272.7
  chemically-induced 272.7
  cholesterol 272.7
  diabetic 250.8 *[272.7]*
    due to secondary diabetes 249.8 *[272.7]*
  dystopic (hereditary) 272.7
  glycolipid 272.7
  hepatosplenomegalic 272.3
  hereditary, dystopic 272.7
  sulfatide 330.0
Lipoadenoma (M8324/0)—*see* Neoplasm, by
  site, benign
Lipoblastoma (M8881/0)—*see* Lipoma, by site
Lipoblastomatosis (M8881/0)—*see* Lipoma, by
  site
Lipochondrodystrophy 277.5
Lipochrome histiocytosis (familial) 288.1
Lipodermatosclerosis 729.39
Lipodystrophia progressiva 272.6
Lipodystrophy (progressive) 272.6
  insulin 272.6
  intestinal 040.2
  mesenteric 567.82
Lipofibroma (M8851/0)—*see* Lipoma, by site
Lipoglycoproteinosis 272.8
Lipogranuloma, sclerosing 709.8
Lipogranulomatosis (disseminated) 272.8
  kidney 272.8
Lipoid —*see* condition
  histiocytosis 272.7
    essential 272.7
  nephrosis (*see also* Nephrosis) 581.3
  proteinosis of Urbach 272.8
Lipoidemia (*see also* Hyperlipidemia) 272.4
Lipoidosis (*see also* Lipidosis) 272.7
Lipoma (M8850/0) 214.9
  breast (skin) 214.1
  face 214.0
  fetal (M8881/0)—*see also* Lipoma, by site
    fat cell (M8880/0)—*see* Lipoma, by site
  infiltrating (M8856/0)—*see* Lipoma, by site
  intra-abdominal 214.3
  intramuscular (M8856/0)—*see* Lipoma, by site
  intrathoracic 214.2
  kidney 214.3
  mediastinum 214.2
  muscle 214.8
  peritoneum 214.3
  retroperitoneum 214.3
  skin 214.1
    face 214.0
  spermatic cord 214.4
  spindle cell (M8857/0)—*see* Lipoma, by site
  stomach 214.3
  subcutaneous tissue 214.1
    face 214.0
  thymus 214.2
  thyroid gland 214.2
Lipomatosis (dolorosa) 272.8
  epidural 214.8
  fetal (M8881/0)—*see* Lipoma, by site
  Launois-Bensaude's 272.8
Lipomyohemangioma (M8860/0)
  specified site—*see* Neoplasm, connective tissue,
    benign
  unspecified site 223.0
Lipomyoma (M8860/0)
  specified site—*see* Neoplasm, connective tissue,
    benign
  unspecified site 223.0

Lipomyxoma (M8852/0)—*see* Lipoma, by site
Lipomyxosarcoma (M8852/3)—*see* Neoplasm,
  connective tissue, malignant
Lipophagocytosis 289.89
Lipoproteinemia (alpha) 272.4
  broad-beta 272.2
  floating-beta 272.2
  hyper-pre-beta 272.1
Lipoproteinosis (Rössle-Urbach-Wiethe) 272.8
Liposarcoma (M8850/3)—*see also* Neoplasm,
  connective tissue, malignant
  differentiated type (M8851/3)—*see* Neoplasm,
    connective tissue, malignant
  embryonal (M8852/3)—*see* Neoplasm,
    connective tissue, malignant
  mixed type (M8855/3)—*see* Neoplasm,
    connective tissue, malignant
  myxoid (M8852/3)—*see* Neoplasm, connective
    tissue, malignant
  pleomorphic (M8854/3)—*see* Neoplasm,
    connective tissue, malignant
  round cell (M8853/3)—*see* Neoplasm,
    connective tissue, malignant
  well differentiated type (M8851/3)—*see*
    Neoplasm, connective tissue, malignant
Liposynovitis prepatellaris 272.8
Lipping
  cervix 622.0
  spine (*see also* Spondylosis) 721.90
  vertebra (*see also* Spondylosis) 721.90
Lip pits (mucus), congenital 750.25
Lipschütz disease or ulcer 616.50
Lipuria 791.1
  bilharziasis 120.0
Liquefaction, vitreous humor 379.21
Lisping 307.9
Lissauer's paralysis 094.1
Lissencephalia, lissencephaly 742.2
Listerellose 027.0
Listeriose 027.0
Listeriosis 027.0
  congenital 771.2
  fetal 771.2
  suspected fetal damage affecting management of
    pregnancy 655.4
Listlessness 780.79
Lithemia 790.6
Lithiasis —*see also* Calculus
  hepatic (duct)—*see* Choledocholithiasis
  urinary 592.9
Lithopedion 779.9
  affecting management of pregnancy 656.8
Lithosis (occupational) 502
  with tuberculosis—*see* Tuberculosis, pulmonary
Lithuria 791.9
Litigation V62.5
Little
  league elbow 718.82
  stroke syndrome 435.9
Little's disease —*see* Palsy, cerebral
Littre's
  gland—*see* condition
  hernia—*see* Hernia, Littre's
Littritis (*see also* Urethritis) 597.89
Livedo 782.61
  annularis 782.61
  racemose 782.61
  reticularis 782.61
Live flesh 781.0
Liver —*see also* condition
  donor V59.6

Livida, asphyxia
    newborn 768.6
Living
    alone V60.3
        with handicapped person V60.4
Lloyd's syndrome 258.1
Loa loa 125.2
Loasis 125.2
Lobe, lobar —*see* condition
Lobo's disease or blastomycosis 116.2
Lobomycosis 116.2
Lobotomy syndrome 310.0
Lobstein's disease (brittle bones and blue sclera)
    756.51
Lobster-claw hand 755.58
Lobulation (congenital)—*see also* Anomaly,
        specified type NEC, by site
    kidney, fetal 753.3
    liver, abnormal 751.69
    spleen 759.0
Lobule, lobular —*see* condition
Local, localized —*see* condition
Locked bowel or intestine (*see also* Obstruction,
        intestine) 560.9
Locked twins 660.5
    affecting fetus or newborn 763.1
Locked-in state 344.81
Locking
    joint (*see also* Derangement, joint) 718.90
    knee 717.9
Lockjaw (*see also* Tetanus) 037
Locomotor ataxia (progressive) 094.0
Löffler's
    endocarditis 421.0
    eosinophilia or syndrome 518.3
    pneumonia 518.3
    syndrome (eosinophilic pneumonitis) 518.3
Löfgren's syndrome (sarcoidosis) 135
Loiasis 125.2
    eyelid 125.2 *[373.6]*
Loneliness V62.89
Lone star fever 082.8
Long labor 662.1
    affecting fetus or newborn 763.89
    first stage 662.0
    second stage 662.2
Long-term (current) (prophylactic) drug use
    V58.69
    antibiotics V58.62
    anticoagulants V58.61
    anti-inflammatories, non-steroidal (NSAID) V58.64
    antiplatelets/antithrombotics V58.63
    aspirin V58.66
    bisphosphonates V58.68
    high-risk medications NEC V58.69
    insulin V58.67
    methadone for pain control V58.69
    opiate analgesic V58.69
    pain killers V58.69
        anti-inflammatory non-steroidal (NSAID)
            V58.64
        aspirin V58.66
    steroids V58.65
    tamoxifen V07.51
Longitudinal stripes or grooves, nails 703.8
    congenital 757.5
Loop
    intestine (*see also* Volvulus) 560.2
    intrascleral nerve 379.29
    vascular on papilla (optic) 743.57

Loose —*see also* condition
    body
        in tendon sheath 727.82
        joint 718.10
            ankle 718.17
            elbow 718.12
            foot 718.17
            hand 718.14
            hip 718.15
            knee 717.6
            multiple sites 718.19
            pelvic region 718.15
            prosthetic implant—*see* Complications,
                mechanical
            shoulder (region) 718.11
            specified site NEC 718.18
            wrist 718.13
        cartilage (joint) (*see also* Loose, body, joint)
            718.1
            knee 717.6
        facet (vertebral) 724.9
        prosthetic implant—*see* Complications,
            mechanical
        sesamoid, joint (*see also* Loose, body, joint)
            718.1
        tooth, teeth 525.8
Loosening epiphysis 732.9
Looser (-Debray) -Milkman syndrome
    (osteomalacia with pseudofractures) 268.2
Lop ear (deformity) 744.29
Lorain's disease or syndrome (pituitary
    dwarfism) 253.3
Lorain-Levi syndrome (pituitary dwarfism)
    253.3
Lordosis (acquired) (postural) 737.20
    congenital 754.2
    due to or associated with
        Charcot-Marie-Tooth disease 356.1 *[737.42]*
        mucopolysaccharidosis 277.5 *[737.42]*
        neurofibromatosis 237.71 *[737.42]*
        osteitis
            deformans 731.0 *[737.42]*
            fibrosa cystica 252.01 *[737.42]*
        osteoporosis (*see also* Osteoporosis) 733.00
            [737.42]
        poliomyelitis (*see also* Poliomyelitis) 138
            [737.42]
        tuberculosis (*see also* Tuberculosis) 015.0
            [737.42]
    late effect of rickets 268.1 *[737.42]*
    postlaminectomy 737.21
    postsurgical NEC 737.22
    rachitic 268.1 *[737.42]*
    specified NEC 737.29
    tuberculous (*see also* Tuberculosis) 015.0 *[737.42]*
Loss
    appetite 783.0
        hysterical 300.11
        nonorganic origin 307.59
        psychogenic 307.59
    blood—*see* Hemorrhage
    central vision 368.41
    consciousness 780.09
        transient 780.2
    control, sphincter, rectum 787.60
        nonorganic origin 307.7
    ear ossicle, partial 385.24
    elasticity, skin 782.8
    extremity or member, traumatic, current—*see*
        Amputation, traumatic

Loss —*continued*
fluid (acute) 276.50
  with
    hypernatremia 276.0
    hyponatremia 276.1
    fetus or newborn 775.5
hair 704.00
hearing—*see also* Deafness
  central 389.14
  conductive (air) 389.00
    with sensorineural hearing loss 389.20
      bilateral 389.22
      unilateral 389.21
    bilateral 389.06
    combined types 389.08
    external ear 389.01
    inner ear 389.04
    middle ear 389.03
    multiple types 389.08
    tympanic membrane 389.02
    unilateral 389.05
  mixed conductive and sensorineural 389.20
    bilateral 389.22
    unilateral 389.21
  mixed type 389.20
    bilateral 389.22
    unilateral 389.21
  nerve
    bilateral 389.12
    unilateral 389.13
  neural
    bilateral 389.12
    unilateral 389.13
  noise-induced 388.12
  perceptive NEC (*see also* Loss, hearing,
    sensorineural) 389.10
  sensorineural 389.10
    with conductive hearing loss 389.20
      bilateral 389.22
      unilateral 389.21
    asymmetrical 389.16
    bilateral 389.18
    central 389.14
    neural
      bilateral 389.12
      unilateral 389.13
    sensory
      bilateral 389.11
      unilateral 389.17
    unilateral 389.15
  sensory
    bilateral 389.11
    unilateral 389.17
  specified type NEC 389.8
  sudden NEC 388.2
height 781.91
labyrinthine reactivity (unilateral) 386.55
  bilateral 386.56
memory (*see also* Amnesia) 780.93
  mild, following organic brain damage 310.89
mind (*see also* Psychosis) 298.9
occusal vertical dimension 524.37
organ or part—*see* Absence, by site, acquired
recurrent pregnancy—*see* Pregnancy,
  management affected by, abortion, habitual
sensation 782.0
sense of
  smell (*see also* Disturbance, sensation) 781.1
  taste (*see also* Disturbance, sensation) 781.1
  touch (*see also* Disturbance, sensation) 781.1
sight (acquired) (complete) (congenital)—*see*
  Blindness

Loss —*continued*
spinal fluid
  headache 349.0
substance of
  bone (*see also* Osteoporosis) 733.00
  cartilage 733.99
  ear 380.32
  vitreous (humor) 379.26
tooth, teeth
  acquired 525.10
    due to
      caries 525.13
      extraction 525.10
      periodontal disease 525.12
      specified NEC 525.19
      trauma 525.11
vision, visual (*see also* Blindness) 369.9
  both eyes (*see also* Blindness, both eyes)
    369.3
  complete (*see also* Blindness, both eyes) 369.00
  one eye 369.8
  sudden 368.11
  transient 368.12
vitreous 379.26
voice (*see also* Aphonia) 784.41
weight (cause unknown) 783.21
Lou Gehrig's disease 335.20
Louis-Bar syndrome (ataxia-telangiectasia) 334.8
Louping ill 063.1
Lousiness —*see* Lice
Low
back syndrome 724.2
basal metabolic rate (BMR) 794.7
birthweight 765.1
  extreme (less than 1000 grams) 765.0
  for gestational age 764.0
  status (*see also* Status, low birth weight)
    V21.30
bladder compliance 596.52
blood pressure (*see also* Hypotension) 458.9
  reading (incidental) (isolated) (nonspecific)
    796.3
cardiac reserve—*see* Disease, heart
compliance bladder 596.52
frequency deafness—*see* Disorder, hearing
function—*see also* Hypofunction
  kidney (*see also* Disease, renal) 593.9
  liver 573.9
hemoglobin 285.9
implantation, placenta—*see* Placenta, previa
insertion, placenta—*see* Placenta, previa
lying
  kidney 593.0
  organ or site, congenital—*see* Malposition,
    congenital
  placenta—*see* Placenta, previa
output syndrome (cardiac) (*see also* Failure,
  heart) 428.9
platelets (blood) (*see also* Thrombocytopenia)
  287.5
reserve, kidney (*see also* Disease, renal) 593.9
risk
  human papillomavirus (HPV) DNA test
    positive
      anal 796.79
      cervical 795.09
      vaginal 795.19
salt syndrome 593.9
tension glaucoma 365.12
vision 369.9
  both eyes 369.20
  one eye 369.70

Lowe (-Terrey-MacLachlan) syndrome (oculocerebrorenal dystrophy) 270.8
Lower extremity —*see* condition
Lown (-Ganong)-Levine syndrome (short P-R interval, normal QRS complex, and paroxysmal supraventricular tachycardia) 426.81
LSD reaction (*see also* Abuse, drugs, nondependent) 305.3
L-shaped kidney 753.3
Lucas-Championnière disease (fibrinous bronchitis) 466.0
Lucey-Driscoll syndrome (jaundice due to delayed conjugation) 774.30
Ludwig's
    angina 528.3
    disease (submaxillary cellulitis) 528.3
Lues (venerea), luetic—*see* Syphilis
Luetscher's syndrome (dehydration) 276.51
Lumbago 724.2
    due to displacement, intervertebral disc 722.10
Lumbalgia 724.2
    due to displacement, intervertebral disc 722.10
Lumbar —*see* condition
Lumbarization, vertebra 756.15
Lumbermen's itch 133.8
Lump —*see also* Mass
    abdominal 789.3
    breast 611.72
    chest 786.6
    epigastric 789.3
    head 784.2
    kidney 753.3
    liver 789.1
    lung 786.6
    mediastinal 786.6
    neck 784.2
    nose or sinus 784.2
    pelvic 789.3
    skin 782.2
    substernal 786.6
    throat 784.2
    umbilicus 789.3
Lunacy (*see also* Psychosis) 298.9
Lunatomalacia 732.3
Lung —*see also* condition
    donor V59.8
    drug addict's 417.8
    mainliners' 417.8
    vanishing 492.0
Lupoid (miliary) of Boeck 135
Lupus 710.0
    anticoagulant 795.79
        with
            hemorrhagic disorder 286.53
            hypercoagulable state 289.81
    Cazenave's (erythematosus) 695.4
    discoid (local) 695.4
    disseminated 710.0
    erythematodes (discoid) (local) 695.4
    erythematosus (discoid) (local) 695.4
        disseminated 710.0
        eyelid 373.34
        systemic 710.0
            with
                encephalitis 710.0 *[323.81]*
                lung involvement 710.0 *[517.8]*
            inhibitor (presence of) 795.79
                with hypercoagulable state 289.81
    exedens 017.0

Lupus—*continued*
    eyelid (*see also* Tuberculosis) 017.0 *[373.4]*
    Hilliard's 017.0
    hydralazine
        correct substance properly administered 695.4
        overdose or wrong substance given or taken 972.6
    miliaris disseminatus faciei 017.0
    nephritis 710.0 *[583.81]*
        acute 710.0 *[580.81]*
        chronic 710.0 *[582.81]*
    nontuberculous, not disseminated 695.4
    pernio (Besnier) 135
    tuberculous (*see also* Tuberculosis) 017.0
        eyelid (*see also* Tuberculosis) 017.0 *[373.4]*
    vulgaris 017.0
Luschka's joint disease 721.90
Luteinoma (M8610/0) 220
Lutembacher's disease or syndrome (atrial septal defect with mitral stenosis) 745.5
Luteoma (M8610/0) 220
Lutz-Miescher disease (elastosis perforans serpiginosa) 701.1
Lutz-Splendore-de Almeida disease (Brazilian blastomycosis) 116.1
Luxatio
    bulbi due to birth injury 767.8
    coxae congenita (*see also* Dislocation, hip, congenital) 754.30
    erecta—*see* Dislocation, shoulder
    imperfecta—*see* Sprain, by site
    perinealis—*see* Dislocation, hip
Luxation —*see also* Dislocation, by site
    eyeball 360.81
        due to birth injury 767.8
        lateral 376.36
    genital organs (external) NEC—*see* Wound, open, genital organs
    globe (eye) 360.81
        lateral 376.36
    lacrimal gland (postinfectional) 375.16
    lens (old) (partial) 379.32
        congenital 743.37
            syphilitic 090.49 *[379.32]*
        Marfan's disease 090.49
        spontaneous 379.32
    penis—*see* Wound, open, penis
    scrotum—*see* Wound, open, scrotum
    testis—*see* Wound, open, testis
L-xyloketosuria 271.8
Lycanthropy (*see also* Psychosis) 298.9
Lyell's disease or syndrome (toxic epidermal necrolysis) 695.15
    due to drug
        correct substance properly administered 695.15
        overdose or wrong substance given or taken 977.9
        specified drug—*see* Table of drugs and chemicals
Lyme disease 088.81
Lymph
    gland or node—*see* condition
    scrotum (*see also* Infestation, filarial) 125.9
Lymphadenitis 289.3
    with
        abortion—*see* Abortion, by type, with sepsis
        ectopic pregnancy (*see also* categories 633.0-633.9) 639.0
        molar pregnancy (*see also* categories 630-632) 639.0

Lymphadenitis—*continued*
  acute 683
    mesenteric 289.2
  any site, except mesenteric 289.3
    acute 683
    chronic 289.1
    mesenteric (acute) (chronic) (nonspecific)
        (subacute) 289.2
    subacute 289.1
      mesenteric 289.2
  breast, puerperal, postpartum 675.2
  chancroidal (congenital) 099.0
  chronic 289.1
    mesenteric 289.2
  dermatopathic 695.89
  due to
    anthracosis (occupational) 500
    Brugia (Wuchereria) malayi 125.1
    diphtheria (toxin) 032.89
    lymphogranuloma venereum 099.1
    Wuchereria bancrofti 125.0
  following
    abortion 639.0
    ectopic or molar pregnancy 639.0
  generalized 289.3
  gonorrheal 098.89
  granulomatous 289.1
  infectional 683
  mesenteric (acute) (chronic) (nonspecific)
      (subacute) 289.2
    due to Bacillus typhi 002.0
    tuberculous (*see also* Tuberculosis) 014.8
  mycobacterial 031.8
  purulent 683
  pyogenic 683
  regional 078.3
  septic 683
  streptococcal 683
  subacute, unspecified site 289.1
  suppurative 683
  syphilitic (early) (secondary) 091.4
    late 095.8
  tuberculous—*see* Tuberculosis, lymph gland
  venereal 099.1
Lymphadenoid goiter 245.2
Lymphadenopathy (general) 785.6
  due to toxoplasmosis (acquired) 130.7
  congenital (active) 771.2
Lymphadenopathy-associated virus (disease)
    (illness) (infection)—*see* Human Immuno-
    deficiency virus (disease) (illness) (infection)
Lymphadenosis 785.6
  acute 075
Lymphangiectasis 457.1
  conjunctiva 372.89
  postinfectional 457.1
  scrotum 457.1
Lymphangiectatic elephantiasis , nonfilarial
    457.1
Lymphangioendothelioma (M9170/0) 228.1
  malignant (M9170/3)—*see* Neoplasm,
    connective tissue, malignant
Lymphangioleiomyomatosis 516.4
Lymphangioma (M9170/0) 228.1
  capillary (M9171/0) 228.1
  cavernous (M9172/0) 228.1
  cystic (M9173/0) 228.1
  malignant (M9170/3)—*see* Neoplasm,
    connective tissue, malignant
Lymphangiomyoma (M9174/0) 228.1
Lymphangiomyomatosis 516.4

Lymphangiosarcoma (M9170/3)—*see*
    Neoplasm, connective tissue, malignant
Lymphangitis 457.2
  with
    abortion—*see* Abortion, by type, with sepsis
    abscess—*see* Abscess, by site
    cellulitis—*see* Abscess, by site
    ectopic pregnancy (*see also* categories
        633.0-633.9) 639.0
    molar pregnancy (*see also* categories 630-632)
        639.0
  acute (with abscess or cellulitis) 682.9
    specified site—*see* Abscess, by site
  breast, puerperal, postpartum 675.2
  chancroidal 099.0
  chronic (any site) 457.2
  due to
    Brugia (Wuchereria) malayi 125.1
    Wuchereria bancrofti 125.0
  following
    abortion 639.0
    ectopic or molar pregnancy 639.0
  gangrenous 457.2
  penis
    acute 607.2
    gonococcal (acute) 098.0
      chronic or duration of 2 months or more 098.2
  puerperal, postpartum, childbirth 670.8
  strumous, tuberculous (*see also* Tuberculosis)
      017.2
  subacute (any site) 457.2
  tuberculous—*see* Tuberculosis, lymph gland
Lymphatic (vessel)—*see* condition
Lymphatism 254.8
  scrofulous (*see also* Tuberculosis) 017.2
Lymphectasia 457.1
Lymphedema (*see also* Elephantiasis) 457.1
  acquired (chronic) 457.1
  chronic hereditary 757.0
  congenital 757.0
  idiopathic hereditary 757.0
  praecox 457.1
  secondary 457.1
  surgical NEC 997.99
    postmastectomy (syndrome) 457.0
Lymph-hemangioma (M9120/0)—*see*
    Hemangioma, by site
Lymphoblastic —*see* condition
Lymphoblastoma (diffuse) (M9630/3) 200.1
  giant follicular (M9690/3) 202.0
  macrofollicular (M9690/3) 202.0
Lymphoblastosis, acute benign 075
Lymphocele 457.8
Lymphocythemia 288.51
Lymphocytic —*see also* condition
  chorioencephalitis (acute) (serous) 049.0
  choriomeningitis (acute) (serous) 049.0
Lymphocytoma (diffuse) (malignant) (M9620/3)
    200.1
Lymphocytomatosis (M9620/3) 200.1
Lymphocytopenia 288.51
Lymphocytosis (symptomatic) 288.61
  infectious (acute) 078.89
Lymphoepithelioma (M8082/3)—*see* Neoplasm,
    by site, malignant
Lymphogranuloma (malignant) (M9650/3) 201.9
  inguinale 099.1
  venereal (any site) 099.1
    with stricture of rectum 099.1
  venereum 099.1

Lymphogranulomatosis (malignant) (M9650/3)
    201.9
    benign (Boeck's sarcoid) (Schaumann's) 135
    Hodgkin's (M9650/3) 201.9
Lymphohistiocytosis, familial hemophagocytic
    288.4
Lymphoid —*see* condition
Lympholeukoblastoma (M9850/3) 207.8
Lympholeukosarcoma (M9850/3) 207.8
Lymphoma (malignant) (M9590/3) 202.8

> *Note—Use the following fifth-digit
> subclassification with categories 200-202:*
>
> *0 unspecifidd site*
> *1 lymph nodes of head, face and neck*
> *2 intrathoracic lymph nodes*
> *3 intra-abdominal lymph nodes*
> *4 lymph nodes of axilla and upper limb*
> *5 lymph nodes of inguinal region and
>   lower limb*
> *6 intrapelvic lymph nodes*
> *7 spleen*
> *8 lymph nodes of multiple sites*

    wenign (M9580/0)—*see* Neoplasm, by site, benign
    Burkitt's type (lymphoblastic) (undifferentiated)
        (M9750/3) 200.2
    Castleman's (mediastinal lymph node hyperplasia)
        785.6
    centroblastic-centrocytic
        diffuse (M9614/3) 202.8
        follicular (M9692/3) 202.0
    centroblastic type (diffuse) (M9632/3) 202.8
        follicular (M9697/3) 202.0
    centrocytic (M9622/3) 202.8
    compound (M9613/3) 200.8
    convoluted cell type (lymphoblastic) (M9602/3)
        202.8
    diffuse NEC (M9590/3) 202.8
        large B cell 202.8
    follicular (giant) (M9690/3) 202.0
        center cell (diffuse) (M9615/3) 202.8
            cleaved (diffuse) (M9623/3) 202.8
                follicular (M9695/3) 202.0
            non-cleaved (diffuse) (M9633/3) 202.8
                follicular (M9698/3) 202.0
        centroblastic-centrocytic (M9692/3) 202.0
        centroblastic type (M9697/3) 202.0
        large cell 202.0
        lymphocytic
            intermediate differentiation (M9694/3) 202.0
            poorly differentiated (M9696/3) 202.0
        mixed (cell type) (lymphocytic-histiocytic)
            (small cell and large cell) (M9691/3) 202.0
    germinocytic (M9622/3) 202.8
    giant, follicular or follicle (M9690/3) 202.0
    histiocytic (diffuse) (M9640/3) 200.0
        nodular (M9642/3) 200.0
        pleomorphic cell type (M9641/3) 200.0
    Hodgkin's (M9650/3) (*see also* Disease,
        Hodgkin's) 201.9
    immunoblastic (type) (M9612/3) 200.8
    large cell (M9640/3) 200.7
        anaplastic 200.6
        nodular (M9642/3) 202.0
        pleomorphic cell type (M9641/3) 200.0
    lymphoblastic (diffuse) (M9630/3) 200.1
        Burkitt's type (M9750/3) 200.2
        convoluted cell type (M9602/3) 202.8

Lymphoma—*continued*
    lymphocytic (cell type) (diffuse) (M9620/3) 200.1
        with plasmacytoid differentiation, diffuse
            (M9611/3) 200.8
        intermediate differentiation (diffuse)
            (M9621/3) 200.1
            follicular (M9694/3) 202.0
            nodular (M9694/3) 202.0
        nodular (M9690/3) 202.0
        poorly differentiated (diffuse) (M9630/3) 200.1
            follicular (M9696/3) 202.0
            nodular (M9696/3) 202.0
        well differentiated (diffuse) (M9620/3) 200.1
            follicular (M9693/3) 202.0
            nodular (M9693/3) 202.0
    lymphocytic-histiocytic, mixed (diffuse)
        (M9613/3) 200.8
        follicular (M9691/3) 202.0
        nodular (M9691/3) 202.0
    lymphoplasmacytoid type (M9611/3) 200.8
    lymphosarcoma type (M9610/3) 200.1
    macrofollicular (M9690/3) 202.0
    mantle cell 200.4
    marginal zone 200.3
        extranodal B-cell 200.3
        nodal B-cell 200.3
        splenic B-cell 200.3
    mixed cell type (diffuse) (M9613/3) 200.8
        follicular (M9691/3) 202.0
        nodular (M9691/3) 202.0
    nodular (M9690/3) 202.0
        histiocytic (M9642/3) 200.0
        lymphocytic (M9690.3) 202.0
            intermediate differentiation (M9694/3) 202.0
            poorly differentiated (M9696/3) 202.0
        mixed (cell type) (lymphocytic-histiocytic)
            (small cell and large cell) (M9691/3) 202.0
    non-Hodgkin's type NEC (M9591/3) 202.8
    peripheral T-cell 202.7
    primary central nervous system 200.5
    reticulum cell (type) (M9640/3) 200.0
    small cell and large cell, mixed (diffuse)
        (M9613/3) 200.8
        follicular (M9691/3) 202.0
        nodular (M9691/3) 202.0
    stem cell (type) (M9601/3) 202.8
    T-cell 202.1
        peripheral 202.7
    undifferentiated (cell type) (non-Burkitt's)
        (M9600/3) 202.8
        Burkitt's type (M9750/3) 200.2
Lymphomatosis (M9590/3)—*see also*
    Lymphoma
    granulomatous 099.1
Lymphopathia
    venereum 099.1
    veneris 099.1
Lymphopenia 288.51
    familial 279.2
Lymphoreticulosis, benign (of inoculation)
    078.3
Lymphorrhea 457.8
Lymphosarcoma (M9610/3) 200.1
    diffuse (M9610/3) 200.1
        with plasmacytoid differentiation (M9611/3)
            200.8
        lymphoplasmacytic (M9611/3) 200.8
    follicular (giant) (M9690/3) 202.0
        lymphoblastic (M9696/3) 202.0
        lymphocytic, intermediate differentiation
            (M9694/3) 202.0
        mixed cell type (M9691/3) 202.0

Lymphosarcoma—*continued*
  giant follicular (M9690/3) 202.0
  Hodgkin's (M9650/3) 201.9
  immunoblastic (M9612/3) 200.8
  lymphoblastic (diffuse) (M9630/3) 200.1
    follicular (M9696/3) 202.0
    nodular (M9696/3) 202.0
  lymphocytic (diffuse) (M9620/3) 200.1
    intermediate differentiation (diffuse)
      (M9621/3) 200.1
      follicular (M9694/3) 202.0
      nodular (M9694/3) 202.0
  mixed cell type (diffuse) (M9613/3) 200.8
    follicular (M9691/3) 202.0
    nodular (M9691/3) 202.0
  nodular (M9690/3) 202.0
    lymphoblastic (M9696/3) 202.0
    lymphocytic, intermediate differentiation
      (M9694/3) 202.0
    mixed cell type (M9691/3) 202.0
  prolymphocytic (M9631/3) 200.1
  reticulum cell (M9640/3) 200.0
Lymphostasis 457.8
Lypemania (*see also* Melancholia) 296.2
Lyssa 071

M

Macacus ear 744.29
Maceration
  fetus (cause not stated) 779.9
  wet feet, tropical (syndrome) 991.4
Machado-Joseph disease 334.8
Machupo virus hemorrhagic fever 078.7
Macleod's syndrome (abnormal transradiancy, one lung) 492.8
Macrocephalia, macrocephaly 756.0
Macrocheilia (congenital) 744.81
Macrochilia (congenital) 744.81
Macrocolon (congenital) 751.3
Macrocornea 743.41
  associated with buphthalmos 743.22
Macrocytic —see condition
Macrocytosis 289.89
Macrodactylia, macrodactylism (fingers) (thumbs) 755.57
  toes 755.65
Macrodontia 520.2
Macroencephaly 742.4
Macrogenia 524.05
Macrogenitosomia (female) (male) (praecox) 255.2
Macrogingivae 523.8
Macroglobulinemia (essential) (idiopathic) (monoclonal) (primary) (syndrome) (Waldenström's) 273.3
Macroglossia (congenital) 750.15
  acquired 529.8
Macrognathia, macrognathism (congenital) 524.00
  mandibular 524.02
    alveolar 524.72
  maxillary 524.01
    alveolar 524.71
Macrogyria (congenital) 742.4
Macrohydrocephalus (see also Hydrocephalus) 331.4
Macromastia (see also Hypertrophy, breast) 611.1
Macrophage activation syndrome 288.4
Macropsia 368.14
Macrosigmoid 564.7
  congenital 751.3
Macrospondylitis, acromegalic 253.0
Macrostomia (congenital) 744.83
Macrotia (external ear) (congenital) 744.22
Macula
  cornea, corneal
    congenital 743.43
      interfering with vision 743.42
    interfering with central vision 371.03
    not interfering with central vision 371.02
  degeneration (see also Degeneration, macula) 362.50
  hereditary (see also Dystrophy, retina) 362.70
  edema, cystoid 362.53
Maculae ceruleae 132.1
Macules and papules 709.8
Maculopathy, toxic 362.55
Madarosis 374.55
Madelung's
  deformity (radius) 755.54
  disease (lipomatosis) 272.8
  lipomatosis 272.8

Madness (see also Psychosis) 298.9
  myxedema (acute) 293.0
    subacute 293.1
Madura
  disease (actinomycotic) 039.9
    mycotic 117.4
  foot (actinomycotic) 039.4
    mycotic 117.4
Maduromycosis (actinomycotic) 039.9
  mycotic 117.4
Maffucci's syndrome (dyschondroplasia with hemangiomas) 756.4
Magenblase syndrome 306.4
Main en griffe (acquired) 736.06
  congenital 755.59
Maintenance
  chemotherapy regimen or treatment V58.11
  dialysis regimen or treatment
    extracorporeal (renal) V56.0
    peritoneal V56.8
    renal V56.0
  drug therapy or regimen
    chemotherapy, antineoplastic V58.11
    immunotherapy, antineoplastic V58.12
  external fixation NEC V54.89
  methadone 304.00
  radiotherapy V58.0
  traction NEC V54.89
Majocchi's
  disease (purpura annularis telangiectodes) 709.1
  granuloma 110.6
Major —see condition
Mal
  cerebral (idiopathic) (see also Epilepsy) 345.9
  comital (see also Epilepsy) 345.9
  de los pintos (see also Pinta) 103.9
  de Meleda 757.39
  de mer 994.6
  lie—see Presentation, fetal
  perforant (see also Ulcer, lower extremity) 707.15
Malabar itch 110.9
  beard 110.0
  foot 110.4
  scalp 110.0
Malabsorption 579.9
  calcium 579.8
  carbohydrate 579.8
  disaccharide 271.3
  drug-induced 579.8
  due to bacterial overgrowth 579.8
  fat 579.8
  folate, congenital 281.2
  galactose 271.1
  glucose-galactose (congenital) 271.3
  intestinal 579.9
  isomaltose 271.3
  lactose (hereditary) 271.3
  methionine 270.4
  monosaccharide 271.8
  postgastrectomy 579.3
  postsurgical 579.3
  protein 579.8
  sucrose (-isomaltose) (congenital) 271.3
  syndrome 579.9
    postgastrectomy 579.3
    postsurgical 579.3

MNO

Malformation—*continued*
pelvic organs or tissues
in pregnancy or childbirth 654.9
affecting fetus or newborn 763.89
causing obstructed labor 660.2
affecting fetus or newborn 763.1
placenta (*see also* Placenta, abnormal) 656.7
respiratory organs 748.9
specified type NEC 748.8
Rieger's 743.44
sense organs NEC 742.9
specified type NEC 742.8
skin 757.9
specified type NEC 757.8
spinal cord 742.9
teeth, tooth NEC 520.9
tendon 756.9
throat 750.9
umbilical cord (complicating delivery) 663.9
affecting fetus or newborn 762.6
umbilicus 759.9
urinary system NEC 753.9
specified type NEC 753.8
venous —*see* Anomaly, vein
Malfunction —*see also* Dysfunction
arterial graft 996.1
cardiac pacemaker 996.01
catheter device—*see* Complications,
mechanical, catheter
colostomy 569.62
valve 569.62
cystostomy 596.82
infection 596.81
mechanical 596.82
specified complication NEC 596.83
device, implant, or graft NEC—*see*
Complications, mechanical
enteric stoma 569.62
enterostomy 569.62
esophagostomy 530.87
gastroenteric 536.8
gastrostomy 536.42
ileostomy
valve 569.62
nephrostomy 997.5
pacemaker—*see* Complications, mechanical,
pacemaker
prosthetic device, internal—*see* Complications,
mechanical
tracheostomy 519.02
valve
colostomy 569.62
ileostomy 569.62
vascular graft or shunt 996.1
Malgaigne's fracture (closed) 808.43
open 808.53
Malherbe's
calcifying epithelioma (M8110/0)—*see*
Neoplasm, skin, benign
tumor (M8110/0)—*see* Neoplasm, skin, benign
Malibu disease 919.8
infected 919.9
Malignancy (M8000/3)—*see* Neoplasm, by site,
malignant
Malignant —*see* condition
Malingerer, malingering V65.2
Mallet, finger (acquired) 736.1
congenital 755.59
late effect of rickets 268.1
Malleus 024
Mallory's bodies 034.1
Mallory-Weiss syndrome 530.7

Malnutrition (calorie) 263.9
complicating pregnancy 648.9
degree
first 263.1
second 263.0
third 262
mild (protein) 263.1
moderate (protein) 263.0
severe 261
protein-calorie 262
fetus 764.2
"light-for-dates" 764.1
following gastrointestinal surgery 579.3
intrauterine or fetal 764.2
fetus or infant "light-for-dates" 764.1
lack of care, or neglect (child) (infant) 995.52
adult 995.84
malignant 260
mild (protein) 263.1
moderate (protein) 263.0
protein 260
protein-calorie 263.9
mild 263.1
moderate 263.0
severe 262
specified type NEC 263.8
severe 261
protein-calorie NEC 262
Malocclusion (teeth) 524.4
angle's class I 524.21
angle's class II 524.22
angle's class III 524.23
due to
abnormal swallowing 524.59
accessory teeth (causing crowding) 524.31
dentofacial abnormality NEC 524.89
impacted teeth (causing crowding) 520.6
missing teeth 524.30
mouth breathing 524.59
sleep posture 524.59
supernumerary teeth (causing crowding)
524.31
thumb sucking 524.59
tongue, lip, or finger habits 524.59
temporomandibular (joint) 524.69
Malposition
cardiac apex (congenital) 746.87
cervix—*see* Malposition, uterus
congenital
adrenal (gland) 759.1
alimentary tract 751.8
lower 751.5
upper 750.8
aorta 747.21
appendix 751.5
arterial trunk 747.29
artery (peripheral) NEC (*see also* Malposition,
congenital, peripheral vascular system)
747.60
coronary 746.85
pulmonary 747.39
auditory canal 744.29
causing impairment of hearing 744.02
auricle (ear) 744.29
causing impairment of hearing 744.02
cervical 744.43
biliary duct or passage 751.69
bladder (mucosa) 753.8
exteriorized or extroverted 753.5
brachial plexus 742.8
brain tissue 742.4

Malposition—*continued*
  congenital—*continued*
  breast 757.6
  bronchus 748.3
  cardiac apex 746.87
  cecum 751.5
  clavicle 755.51
  colon 751.5
  digestive organ or tract NEC 751.8
    lower 751.5
    upper 750.8
  ear (auricle) (external) 744.29
    ossicles 744.04
  endocrine (gland) NEC 759.2
  epiglottis 748.3
  Eustachian tube 744.24
  eye 743.8
  facial features 744.89
  fallopian tube 752.19
  finger(s) 755.59
    supernumerary 755.01
  foot 755.67
  gallbladder 751.69
  gastrointestinal tract 751.8
  genitalia, genital organ(s) or tract
    female 752.89
      external 752.49
      internal NEC 752.89
    male 752.89
      penis 752.69
      scrotal transposition 752.81
  glottis 748.3
  hand 755.59
  heart 746.87
    dextrocardia 746.87
      with complete transposition of viscera
        759.3
  hepatic duct 751.69
  hip (joint) (*see also* Dislocation, hip,
    congenital) 754.30
  intestine (large) (small) 751.5
    with anomalous adhesions, fixation, or
      malrotation 751.4
  joint NEC 755.8
  kidney 753.3
  larynx 748.3
  limb 755.8
    lower 755.69
    upper 755.59
  liver 751.69
  lung (lobe) 748.69
  nail(s) 757.5
  nerve 742.8
  nervous system NEC 742.8
  nose, nasal (septum) 748.1
  organ or site NEC—*see* Anomaly, specified
    type NEC, by site
  ovary 752.0
  pancreas 751.7
  parathyroid (gland) 759.2
  patella 755.64
  peripheral vascular system 747.60
    gastrointestinal 747.61
    lower limb 747.64
    renal 747.62
    specified NEC 747.69
    spinal 747.82
    upper limb 747.63
  pituitary (gland) 759.2
  respiratory organ or system NEC 748.9

Malposition—*continued*
  congenital—*continued*
  rib (cage) 756.3
    supernumerary in cervical region 756.2
  scapula 755.59
  shoulder 755.59
  spinal cord 742.59
  spine 756.19
  spleen 759.0
  sternum 756.3
  stomach 750.7
  symphysis pubis 755.69
  testis (undescended) 752.51
  thymus (gland) 759.2
  thyroid (gland) (tissue) 759.2
    cartilage 748.3
  toe(s) 755.66
    supernumerary 755.02
  tongue 750.19
  trachea 748.3
  uterus 752.39
  vein(s) (peripheral) NEC (*see also*
    Malposition, congenital, peripheral
    vascular system) 747.60
    great 747.49
    portal 747.49
    pulmonary 747.49
  vena cava (inferior) (superior) 747.49
  device, implant, or graft—*see* Complications,
    mechanical
  fetus NEC (*see also* Presentation, fetal) 652.9
    with successful version 652.1
    affecting fetus or newborn 763.1
    before labor, affecting fetus or newborn 761.7
    causing obstructed labor 660.0
    in multiple gestation (one fetus or more) 652.6
      with locking 660.5
      causing obstructed labor 660.0
  gallbladder (*see also* Disease, gallbladder) 575.8
  gastrointestinal tract 569.89
    congenital 751.8
  heart (*see also* Malposition, congenital, heart) 746.87
  intestine 569.89
    congenital 751.5
  pelvic organs or tissues
    in pregnancy or childbirth 654.4
      affecting fetus or newborn 763.89
      causing obstructed labor 660.2
        affecting fetus or newborn 763.1
  placenta—*see* Placenta, previa
  stomach 537.89
    congenital 750.7
  tooth, teeth 524.30
    with impaction 520.6
  uterus (acquired) (acute) (adherent) (any degree)
    (asymptomatic) (postinfectional) (postpartal,
    old) 621.6
    anteflexion or anteversion (*see also*
      Anteversion, uterus) 621.6
    congenital 752.39
    flexion 621.6
      lateral (*see also* Lateroversion, uterus) 621.6
    in pregnancy or childbirth 654.4
      affecting fetus or newborn 763.89
      causing obstructed labor 660.2
        affecting fetus or newborn 763.1
    inversion 621.6
    lateral (flexion) (version) (*see also*
      Lateroversion, uterus) 621.6
    lateroflexion (*see also* Lateroversion, uterus)
      621.6

Malposition—*continued*
  uterus—*continued*
    lateroversion (*see also* Lateroversion, uterus)
      621.6
    retroflexion or retroversion (*see also*
      Retroversion, uterus) 621.6
Malposture 729.90
Malpresentation, fetus (*see also* Presentation,
  fetal) 652.9
Malrotation
  cecum 751.4
  colon 751.4
  intestine 751.4
  kidney 753.3
MALT (mucosa associated lymphoid tissue) 200.3
Malt workers' lung 495.4
Malta fever (*see also* Brucellosis) 023.9
Maltosuria 271.3
Maltreatment (of)
  adult 995.80
    emotional 995.82
    multiple forms 995.85
    neglect (nutritional) 995.84
    physical 995.81
    psychological 995.82
    sexual 995.83
  child 995.50
    emotional 995.51
    multiple forms 995.59
    neglect (nutritional) 995.52
    psychological 995.51
    physical 995.54
      shaken infant syndrome 995.55
    sexual 995.53
  spouse (*see also* Maltreatment, adult) 995.80
Malum coxae senilis 715.25
Malunion, fracture 733.81
Mammillitis (*see also* Mastitis) 611.0
  puerperal, postpartum 675.2
Mammitis (*see also* Mastitis) 611.0
  puerperal, postpartum 675.2
Mammographic
  calcification 793.89
  calculus 793.89
  microcalcification 793.81
Mammoplasia 611.1
Management
  contraceptive V25.9
    specified type NEC V25.8
  procreative V26.9
    specified type NEC V26.89
Mangled NEC (*see also* nature and site of injury)
  959.9
Mania (monopolar) (*see also* Psychosis,
  affective) 296.0
  alcoholic (acute) (chronic) 291.9
  Bell's—*see* Mania, chronic
  chronic 296.0
    recurrent episode 296.1
    single episode 296.0
  compulsive 300.3
  delirious (acute) 296.0
    recurrent episode 296.1
    single episode 296.0
  epileptic (*see also* Epilepsy) 345.4
  hysterical 300.10
  inhibited 296.89
  puerperal (after delivery) 296.0
    recurrent episode 296.1
    single episode 296.0

Mania—*continued*
  recurrent episode 296.1
  senile 290.8
  single episode 296.0
  stupor 296.89
  stuporous 296.89
  unproductive 296.89
Manic-depressive insanity, psychosis reaction, or
  syndrome (*see also* Psychosis, affective) 296.80
  circular (alternating) 296.7
    currently
      depressed 296.5
      episode unspecified 296.7
      hypomanic, previously depressed 296.4
      manic 296.4
      mixed 296.6
  depressed (type), depressive 296.2
    atypical 296.82
    recurrent episode 296.3
    single episode 296.2
  hypomanic 296.0
    recurrent episode 296.1
    single episode 296.0
  manic 296.0
    atypical 296.81
    recurrent episode 296.1
    single episode 296.0
  mixed NEC 296.89
  perplexed 296.89
  stuporous 296.89
Manifestations, rheumatoid
  lungs 714.81
  pannus—*see* Arthritis, rheumatoid
  subcutaneous nodules—*see* Arthritis, rheumatoid
Mankowsky's syndrome (familial dysplastic
  osteopathy) 731.2
Mannoheptulosuria 271.8
Mannosidosis 271.8
Manson's
  disease (schistosomiasis) 120.1
  pyosis (pemphigus contagiosus) 684
  schistosomiasis 120.1
Mansonellosis 125.5
Manual —*see* condition
Maple bark disease 495.6
Maple bark-strippers' lung 495.6
Maple syrup (urine) disease or syndrome 270.3
Marable's syndrome (celiac artery compression)
  447.4
Marasmus 261
  brain 331.9
  due to malnutrition 261
  intestinal 569.89
  nutritional 261
  senile 797
  tuberculous NEC (*see also* Tuberculosis) 011.9
Marble
  bones 756.52
  skin 782.61
Marburg disease (virus) 078.89
March
  foot 733.94
  hemoglobinuria 283.2
Marchand multiple nodular hyperplasia (liver)
  571.5
Marchesani (-Weill) syndrome
  (brachymorphism and ectopia lentis) 759.89
Marchiafava (-Bignami) disease or syndrome 341.8
Marchiafava-Micheli syndrome (paroxysmal
  nocturnal hemoglobinuria) 283.2

Marcus Gunn's syndrome (jaw-winking syndrome) 742.8

Marfan's
  congenital syphilis 090.49
  disease 090.49
  syndrome (arachnodactyly) 759.82
    meaning congenital syphilis 090.49
      with luxation of lens 090.49 *[379.32]*

Marginal
  implantation, placenta—*see* Placenta, previa
  placenta—*see* Placenta, previa
  sinus (hemorrhage) (rupture) 641.2
    affecting fetus or newborn 762.1

Marie's
  cerebellar ataxia 334.2
  syndrome (acromegaly) 253.0

Marie-Bamberger disease or syndrome
  (hypertrophic) (pulmonary) (secondary) 731.2
  idiopathic (acropachyderma) 757.39
  primary (acropachyderma) 757.39

Marie-Charcot-Tooth neuropathic atrophy, muscle 356.1

Marie-Strümpell arthritis or disease
  (ankylosing spondylitis) 720.0

Marihuana, marijuana
  abuse (*see also* Abuse, drugs, nondependent) 305.2
  dependence (*see also* Dependence) 304.3

Marion's disease (bladder neck obstruction) 596.0

Marital conflict V61.10

Mark
  port wine 757.32
  raspberry 757.32
  strawberry 757.32
  stretch 701.3
  tattoo 709.09

Maroteaux-Lamy syndrome
  (mucopolysaccharidosis VI) 277.5

Marriage license examination V70.3

Marrow (bone)
  arrest 284.9
  megakaryocytic 287.30
  poor function 289.9

Marseilles fever 082.1

Marsh's disease (exophthalmic goiter) 242.0

Marshall's (hidrotic) ectodermal dysplasia 757.31

Marsh fever (*see also* Malaria) 084.6

Martin's disease 715.27

Martin-Albright syndrome
  (pseudohypoparathyroidism) 275.49

Martorell-Fabre syndrome (pulseless disease) 446.7

Masculinization, female with adrenal hyperplasia 255.2

Masculinovoblastoma (M8670/0) 220

Masochism 302.83

Masons' lung 502

Mass
  abdominal 789.3
  anus 787.99
  bone 733.90
  breast 611.72
  cheek 784.2
  chest 786.6
  cystic—*see* Cyst
  ear 388.8
  epigastric 789.3
  eye 379.92
  female genital organ 625.8
  gum 784.2
  head 784.2

Mass—*continued*
  intracranial 784.2
  joint 719.60
    ankle 719.67
    elbow 719.62
    foot 719.67
    hand 719.64
    hip 719.65
    knee 719.66
    multiple sites 719.69
    pelvic region 719.65
    shoulder (region) 719.61
    specified site NEC 719.68
    wrist 719.63
  kidney (*see also* Disease, kidney) 593.9
  lung 786.6
  lymph node 785.6
  malignant (M8000/3)—*see* Neoplasm, by site, malignant
  mediastinal 786.6
  mouth 784.2
  muscle (limb) 729.89
  neck 784.2
  nose or sinus 784.2
  palate 784.2
  pelvis, pelvic 789.3
  penis 607.89
  perineum 625.8
  rectum 787.99
  scrotum 608.89
  skin 782.2
  specified organ NEC—*see* Disease of specified organ or site
  splenic 789.2
  substernal 786.6
    thyroid (*see also* Goiter) 240.9
  superficial (localized) 782.2
  testes 608.89
  throat 784.2
  tongue 784.2
  umbilicus 789.3
  uterus 625.8
  vagina 625.8
  vulva 625.8

Massive —*see* condition

Mastalgia 611.71
  psychogenic 307.89

Mast cell
  disease 757.33
    systemic (M9741/3) 202.6
  leukemia (M9900/3) 207.8
  sarcoma (M9740/3) 202.6
  tumor (M9740/1) 238.5
    malignant (M9740/3) 202.6

Masters-Allen syndrome 620.6

Mastitis (acute) (adolescent) (diffuse)
    (interstitial) (lobular) (nonpuerperal)
    (nonsuppurative) (parenchymatous)
    (phlegmonous) (simple) (subacute)
    (suppurative) 611.0
  chronic (cystic) (fibrocystic) 610.1
  cystic 610.1
    Schimmelbusch's type 610.1
  fibrocystic 610.1
  infective 611.0
  lactational 675.2
  lymphangitis 611.0
  neonatal (noninfective) 778.7
    infective 771.5
  periductal 610.4
  plasma cell 610.4

Mastitis—*continued*
puerperal, postpartum, (interstitial)
  (nonpurulent) (parenchymatous) 675.2
  purulent 675.1
  stagnation 676.2
puerperalis 675.2
retromammary 611.0
  puerperal, postpartum 675.1
submammary 611.0
  puerperal, postpartum 675.1
Mastocytoma (M9740/1) 238.5
malignant (M9740/3) 202.6
Mastocytosis 757.33
malignant (M9741/3) 202.6
systemic (M9741/3) 202.6
Mastodynia 611.71
psychogenic 307.89
Mastoid —*see* condition
Mastoidalgia (*see also* Otalgia) 388.70
Mastoiditis (coalescent) (hemorrhagic)
  (pneumococcal) (streptococcal) (suppurative)
  383.9
acute or subacute 383.00
  with
    Gradenigo's syndrome 383.02
    petrositis 383.02
    specified complication NEC 383.02
    subperiosteal abscess 383.01
chronic (necrotic) (recurrent) 383.1
tuberculous (*see also* Tuberculosis) 015.6
Mastopathy, mastopathia 611.9
chronica cystica 610.1
diffuse cystic 610.1
estrogenic 611.89
ovarian origin 611.89
Mastoplasia 611.1
Masturbation 307.9
Maternal condition, affecting fetus or newborn
acute yellow atrophy of liver 760.8
albuminuria 760.1
anesthesia or analgesia 763.5
blood loss 762.1
chorioamnionitis 762.7
circulatory disease, chronic (conditions
  classifiable to 390-459, 745-747) 760.3
congenital heart disease (conditions classifiable
  to 745-746) 760.3
cortical necrosis of kidney 760.1
death 761.6
diabetes mellitus 775.0
  manifest diabetes in the infant 775.1
disease NEC 760.9
  circulatory system, chronic (conditions
    classifiable to 390-459, 745-747) 760.3
  genitourinary system (conditions classifiable
    to 580-599) 760.1
  respiratory (conditions classifiable to 490-519,
    748) 760.3
eclampsia 760.0
hemorrhage NEC 762.1
hepatitis acute, malignant, or subacute 760.8
hyperemesis (gravidarum) 761.8
hypertension (arising during pregnancy)
  (conditions classifiable to 642) 760.0
infection
  disease classifiable to 001-136 760.2
  genital tract NEC 760.8
  urinary tract 760.1
influenza 760.2
  manifest influenza in the infant 771.2

Maternal condition—*continued*
injury (conditions classifiable to 800-996) 760.5
malaria 760.2
  manifest malaria in infant or fetus 771.2
malnutrition 760.4
necrosis of liver 760.8
nephritis (conditions classifiable to 580-583)
  760.1
nephrosis (conditions classifiable to 581) 760.1
noxious substance transmitted via breast milk or
  placenta 760.70
  alcohol 760.71
  anticonvulsants 760.77
  antifungals 760.74
  anti-infective agents 760.74
  antimetabolics 760.78
  cocaine 760.75
  "crack" 760.75
  diethylstilbestrol [DES] 760.76
  hallucinogenic agents 760.73
  medicinal agents NEC 760.79
  narcotics 760.72
  obstetric anesthetic or analgesic drug 760.72
  specified agent NEC 760.79
nutritional disorder (conditions classifiable to
  260-269) 760.4
operation unrelated to current delivery (*see also*
  Newborn, affected by) 760.64
pre-eclampsia 760.04
pyelitis or pyelonephritis, arising during
  pregnancy (conditions classifiable to 590)
  760.1
renal disease or failure 760.1
respiratory disease, chronic (conditions
  classifiable to 490-519, 748) 760.3
rheumatic heart disease (chronic) (conditions
  classifiable to 393-398) 760.3
rubella (conditions classifiable to 056) 760.2
  manifest rubella in the infant or fetus 771.0
surgery unrelated to current delivery (*see also*
  Newborn, affected by) 760.6
  to uterus or pelvic organs 760.64
syphilis (conditions classifiable to 090-097)
  760.2
  manifest syphilis in the infant or fetus 090.0
thrombophlebitis 760.3
toxemia (of pregnancy) 760.0
  pre-eclamptic 760.0
toxoplasmosis (conditions classifiable to 130)
  760.2
  manifest toxoplasmosis in the infant or fetus
    771.2
transmission of chemical substance through the
  placenta 760.70
  alcohol 760.71
  anticonvulsants 760.77
  antifungals 760.74
  anti-infective agents 760.74
  antimetabolics 760.78
  cocaine 760.75
  "crack" 760.75
  diethylstilbestrol [DES] 760.76
  hallucinogenic agents 760.73
  narcotics 760.72
  specified substance NEC 760.79
uremia 760.1
urinary tract conditions (conditions classifiable
  to 580-599) 760.1
vomiting (pernicious) (persistent) (vicious) 761.8
Maternity —*see* Delivery
Matheiu's disease (leptospiral jaundice) 100.0
Mauclaire's disease or osteochondrosis 732.3

Maxcy's disease 081.0
Maxilla, maxillary —*see* condition
May (-Hegglin) anomaly or syndrome 288.2
Mayaro fever 066.3
Mazoplasia 610.8
MBD (minimal brain dysfunction), child (*see also* Hyperkinesia) 314.9
MCAD (medium chain acyl CoA dehydrogenase deficiency) 277.85
McArdle (-Schmid-Pearson) disease or syndrome (glycogenosis V) 271.0
McCune-Albright syndrome (osteitis fibrosa disseminata) 756.59
MCLS (mucocutaneous lymph node syndrome) 446.1
McQuarrie's syndrome (idiopathic familial hypoglycemia) 251.2
Measles (black) (hemorrhagic) (suppressed) 055.9
　with
　　encephalitis 055.0
　　keratitis 055.71
　　keratoconjunctivitis 055.71
　　otitis media 055.2
　　pneumonia 055.1
　complication 055.8
　　specified type NEC 055.79
　encephalitis 055.0
　French 056.9
　German 056.9
　keratitis 055.71
　keratoconjunctivitis 055.71
　liberty 056.9
　otitis media 055.2
　pneumonia 055.1
　specified complications NEC 055.79
　vaccination, prophylactic (against) V04.2
Meatitis, urethral (*see also* Urethritis) 597.89
Meat poisoning —*see* Poisoning, food
Meatus, meatal —*see* condition
Meat-wrappers' asthma 506.9
Meckel's
　diverticulitis 751.0
　diverticulum (displaced) (hypertrophic) 751.0
Meconium
　aspiration 770.11
　　with
　　　pneumonia 770.12
　　　pneumonitis 770.12
　　　respiratory symptoms 770.12
　　below vocal cords 770.11
　　　with respiratory symptoms 770.12
　　syndrome 770.12
　delayed passage in newborn 777.1
　ileus 777.1
　　due to cystic fibrosis 277.01
　in liquor 792.3
　　noted during delivery 656.8
　insufflation 770.11
　　with respiratory symptoms 770.12
　obstruction
　　fetus or newborn 777.1
　　　in mucoviscidosis 277.01
　passage of 792.3
　　noted during delivery 763.84
　peritonitis 777.6
　plug syndrome (newborn) NEC 777.1
　staining 779.84

Median —*see also* condition
　arcuate ligament syndrome 447.4
　bar (prostate) 600.90
　　with
　　　other lower urinary tract symptoms (LUTS) 600.91
　　　urinary
　　　　obstruction 600.91
　　　　retention 600.91
　vesical orifice 600.90
　　with
　　　other lower urinary tract symptoms (LUTS) 600.91
　　　urinary
　　　　obstruction 600.91
　　　　retention 600.91
　rhomboid glossitis 529.2
Mediastinal shift 793.2
Mediastinitis (acute) (chronic) 519.2
　actinomycotic 039.8
　syphilitic 095.8
　tuberculous (*see also* Tuberculosis) 012.8
Mediastinopericarditis (*see also* Pericarditis) 423.9
　acute 420.90
　chronic 423.8
　　rheumatic 393
　rheumatic, chronic 393
Mediastinum, mediastinal —*see* condition
Medical services provided for —*see* Health, services provided because (of)
Medicine poisoning (by overdose) (wrong substance given or taken in error) 977.9
　specified drug or substance—*see* Table of drugs and chemicals
Medin's disease (poliomyelitis) 045.9
Mediterranean
　anemia 282.40
　　with other hemoglobinopathy 282.49
　disease or syndrome (hemopathic) 282.40
　　with other hemoglobinopathy 282.49
　fever (*see also* Brucellosis) 023.9
　　familial 277.31
　kala-azar 085.0
　leishmaniasis 085.0
　tick fever 082.1
Medulla —*see* condition
Medullary
　cystic kidney 753.16
　sponge kidney 753.17
Medullated fibers
　optic (nerve) 743.57
　retina 362.85
Medulloblastoma (M9470/3)
　desmoplastic (M9471/3) 191.6
　specified site—*see* Neoplasm, by site, malignant
　unspecified site 191.6
Medulloepithelioma (M9501/3)—*see also* Neoplasm, by site, malignant
　teratoid (M9502/3)—*see* Neoplasm, by site, malignant
Medullomyoblastoma (M9472/3)
　specified site—*see* Neoplasm, by site, malignant
　unspecified site 191.6
Meekeren-Ehlers-Danlos syndrome 756.83
Megacaryocytic —*see* condition
Megacolon (acquired) (functional) (not Hirschsprung's disease) 564.7
　aganglionic 751.3
　congenital, congenitum 751.3
　Hirschsprung's (disease) 751.3

Megacolon—*continued*
  psychogenic 306.4
  toxic (*see also* Colitis, ulcerative) 556.9
Megaduodenum 537.3
Megaesophagus (functional) 530.0
  congenital 750.4
Megakaryocytic —*see* condition
Megalencephaly 742.4
Megalerythema (epidermicum) (infectiosum)
  057.0
Megalia, cutis et ossium 757.39
Megaloappendix 751.5
Megalocephalus, megalocephaly NEC 756.0
Megalocornea 743.41
  associated with buphthalmos 743.22
Megalocytic anemia 281.9
Megalodactylia (fingers) (thumbs) 755.57
  toes 755.65
Megaloduodenum 751.5
Megaloesophagus (functional) 530.0
  congenital 750.4
Megalogastria (congenital) 750.7
Megalomania 307.9
Megalophthalmos 743.8
Megalopsia 368.14
Megalosplenia (*see also* Splenomegaly) 789.2
Megaloureter 593.89
  congenital 753.22
Megarectum 569.49
Megasigmoid 564.7
  congenital 751.3
Megaureter 593.89
  congenital 753.22
Megrim 346.9
Meibomian
  cyst 373.2
    infected 373.12
  gland—*see* condition
  infarct (eyelid) 374.85
  stye 373.11
Meibomitis 373.12
Meige
  Milroy disease (chronic hereditary edema) 757.0
  syndrome (blepharospasm-oromandibular
    dystonia) 333.82
Melalgia, nutritional 266.2
Melancholia (*see also* Psychosis, affective)
  296.90
  climacteric 296.2
    recurrent episode 296.3
    single episode 296.2
  hypochondriac 300.7
  intermittent 296.2
    recurrent episode 296.3
    single episode 296.2
  involutional 296.2
    recurrent episode 296.3
    single episode 296.2
  menopausal 296.2
    recurrent episode 296.3
    single episode 296.2
  puerperal 296.2
  reactive (from emotional stress, psychological
    trauma) 298.0
  recurrent 296.3
  senile 290.21
  stuporous 296.2
    recurrent episode 296.3
    single episode 296.2
Melanemia 275.0

Melanoameloblastoma (M9363/0)—*see*
  Neoplasm, bone, benign
Melanoblastoma (M8720/3)—*see* Melanoma
Melanoblastosis
  Block-Sulzberger 757.33
  cutis linearis sive systematisata 757.33
Melanocarcinoma (M8720/3)—*see* Melanoma
Melanocytoma, eyeball (M8726/0) 224.0
Melanocytosis, neurocutaneous 757.33
Melanoderma, melanodermia 709.09
  Addison's (primary adrenal insufficiency) 255.41
Melanodontia, infantile 521.05
Melanodontoclasia 521.05
Melanoepithelioma (M8720/3)—*see* Melanoma
Melanoma (malignant) (M8720/3) 172.9

*Note—Except where otherwise indicated, the
morphological varieties of melanoma in the list
below should be coded by site as for
"Melanoma (malignant)." Internal sites should
be coded to malignant neoplasm of those sites.*

  abdominal wall 172.5
  ala nasi 172.3
  amelanotic (M8730/3)—*see* Melanoma, by site
  ankle 172.7
  anus, anal 154.3
    canal 154.2
  arm 172.6
  auditory canal (external) 172.2
  auricle (ear) 172.2
  auricular canal (external) 172.2
  axilla 172.5
  axillary fold 172.5
  back 172.5
  balloon cell (M8722/3)—*see* Melanoma, by site
  benign (M8720/0)—*see* Neoplasm, skin, benign
  breast (female) (male) 172.5
  brow 172.3
  buttock 172.5
  canthus (eye) 172.1
  cheek (external) 172.3
  chest wall 172.5
  chin 172.3
  choroid 190.6
  conjunctiva 190.3
  ear (external) 172.2
  epithelioid cell (M8771/3)—*see also* Melanoma,
    by site
    and spindle cell, mixed (M8775/3)—*see*
      Melanoma, by site
  external meatus (ear) 172.2
  eye 190.9
  eyebrow 172.3
  eyelid (lower) (upper) 172.1
  face NEC 172.3
  female genital organ (external) NEC 184.4
  finger 172.6
  flank 172.5
  foot 172.7
  forearm 172.6
  forehead 172.3
  foreskin 187.1
  gluteal region 172.5
  groin 172.5
  hand 172.6
  heel 172.7
  helix 172.2
  hip 172.7

Melanoma—*continued*
in
  giant pigmented nevus (M8761/3)—*see*
    Melanoma, by site
  Hutchinson's melanotic freckle
    (M8742/3)—*see* Melanoma, by site
  junctional nevus (M8740/3)—*see* Melanoma,
    by site
  precancerous melanosis (M8741/3)—*see*
    Melanoma, by site
in situ—*see* Melanoma, by site
  skin 172.9
interscapular region 172.5
iris 190.0
jaw 172.3
juvenile (M8770/0)—*see* Neoplasm, skin, benign
knee 172.7
labium
  majus 184.1
  minus 184.2
lacrimal gland 190.2
leg 172.7
lip (lower) (upper) 172.0
liver 197.7
lower limb NEC 172.7
male genital organ (external) NEC 187.9
meatus, acoustic (external) 172.2
meibomian gland 172.1
metastatic
  of or from specified site—*see* Melanoma, by site
  site not of skin—*see* Neoplasm, by site,
    malignant, secondary
  to specified site—*see* Neoplasm, by site,
    malignant, secondary
  unspecified site 172.9
nail 172.9
  finger 172.6
  toe 172.7
neck 172.4
nodular (M8721/3)—*see* Melanoma, by site
nose, external 172.3
orbit 190.1
penis 187.4
perianal skin 172.5
perineum 172.5
pinna 172.2
popliteal (fossa) (space) 172.7
prepuce 187.1
pubes 172.5
pudendum 184.4
retina 190.5
scalp 172.4
scrotum 187.7
septum nasal (skin) 172.3
shoulder 172.6
skin NEC 172.8
  in situ 172.9
spindle cell (M8772/3)—*see also* Melanoma, by
  site
  type A (M8773/3) 190.0
  type B (M8774/3) 190.0
submammary fold 172.5
superficial spreading (M8743/3)—*see*
  Melanoma, by site
temple 172.3
thigh 172.7
toe 172.7
trunk NEC 172.5
umbilicus 172.5
upper limb NEC 172.6
vagina vault 184.0
vulva 184.4

Melanoplakia 528.9
Melanosarcoma (M8720/3)—*see also* Melanoma
  epithelioid cell (M8771/3)—*see* Melanoma
Melanosis 709.09
  addisonian (primary adrenal insufficiency)
    255.41
  tuberculous (*see also* Tuberculosis) 017.6
  adrenal 255.41
  colon 569.89
  conjunctiva 372.55
    congenital 743.49
  corii degenerativa 757.33
  cornea (presenile) (senile) 371.12
    congenital 743.43
      interfering with vision 743.42
    prenatal 743.43
      interfering with vision 743.42
  eye 372.55
    congenital 743.49
  jute spinners' 709.09
  lenticularis progressiva 757.33
  liver 573.8
  precancerous (M8741/2)—*see also* Neoplasm,
    skin, in situ
    malignant melanoma in (M8741/3)—*see* Melanoma
  Riehl's 709.09
  sclera 379.19
    congenital 743.47
  suprarenal 255.41
  tar 709.09
  toxic 709.09
Melanuria 791.9
MELAS syndrome (mitochondrial
  encephalopathy, lactic acidosis and stroke-like
  episodes) 277.87
Melasma 709.09
  adrenal (gland) 255.41
  suprarenal (gland) 255.41
Melena 578.1
  due to
    swallowed maternal blood 777.3
    ulcer—*see* Ulcer, by site, with hemorrhage
  newborn 772.4
    due to swallowed maternal blood 777.3
Meleney's
  gangrene (cutaneous) 686.09
  ulcer (chronic undermining) 686.09
Melioidosis 025
Melitensis, febris 023.0
Melitococcosis 023.0
Melkersson (-Rosenthal) syndrome 351.8
Mellitus, diabetes —*see* Diabetes
Melorheostosis (bone) (leri) 733.99
Meloschisis 744.83
Melotia 744.29
Membrana
  capsularis lentis posterior 743.39
  epipapillaris 743.57
Membranacea placenta —*see* Placenta,
  abnormal
Membranaceous uterus 621.8
Membrane, membranous —*see also* condition
  folds, congenital—*see* Web
  Jackson's 751.4
  over face (causing asphyxia), fetus or newborn
    768.9
  premature rupture—*see* Rupture, membranes,
    premature
  pupillary 364.74
    persistent 743.46

Membrane, membranous—*continued*
retained (complicating delivery) (with
hemorrhage) 666.2
without hemorrhage 667.1
secondary (eye) 366.50
unruptured (causing asphyxia) 768.9
vitreous humor 379.25
Membranitis, fetal 658.4
affecting fetus or newborn 762.7
Memory disturbance, loss or lack (*see also*
Amnesia) 780.93
mild, following organic brain damage 310.89
MEN (multiple endocrine neoplasia) syndrome
type 1 258.01
type IIA 258.02
type IIB 258.03
Menadione (vitamin K) deficiency 269.0
Menarche, precocious 259.1
Mendacity, pathologic 301.7
Mende's syndrome (ptosis-epicanthus) 270.2
Mendelson's syndrome (resulting from a
procedure) 997.32
obstetric 668.0
Ménétrier's disease or syndrome (hypertrophic
gastritis) 535.2
Ménière's disease, syndrome, or vertigo 386.00
cochlear 386.02
cochleovestibular 386.01
inactive 386.04
in remission 386.04
vestibular 386.03
Meninges, meningeal —*see* condition
Meningioma (M9530/0)—*see also* Neoplasm,
meninges, benign
angioblastic (M9535/0)—*see* Neoplasm,
meninges, benign
angiomatous (M9534/0)—*see* Neoplasm,
meninges, benign
endotheliomatous (M9531/0)—*see* Neoplasm,
meninges, benign
fibroblastic (M9532/0)—*see* Neoplasm,
meninges, benign
fibrous (M9532/0)—*see* Neoplasm, meninges,
benign
hemangioblastic (M9535/0)—*see* Neoplasm,
meninges, benign
hemangiopericytic (M9536/0)—*see* Neoplasm,
meninges, benign
malignant (M9530/3)—*see* Neoplasm,
meninges, malignant
meningiothelial (M9531/0)—*see* Neoplasm,
meninges, benign
meningotheliomatous (M9531/0)—*see*
Neoplasm, meninges, benign
mixed (M9537/0)—*see* Neoplasm, meninges,
benign
multiple (M9530/1) 237.6
papillary (M9538/1) 237.6
psammomatous (M9533/0)—*see* Neoplasm,
meninges, benign
syncytial (M9531/0)—*see* Neoplasm, meninges,
benign
transitional (M9537/0)—*see* Neoplasm,
meninges, benign
Meningiomatosis (diffuse) (M9530/1) 237.6
Meningism (*see also* Meningismus) 781.6
Meningismus (infectional) (pneumococcal) 781.6
due to serum or vaccine 997.09 *[321.8]*
influenzal NEC (*see also* Influenza) 487.8

Meningitis (basal) (basic) (basilar) (brain) (cerebral)
(cervical) (congestive) (diffuse) (hemorrhagic)
(infantile) (membranous) (metastatic)
(nonspecific) (pontine) (progressive) (simple)
(spinal) (subacute) (sympathetica) (toxic) 322.9
abacterial NEC (*see also* Meningitis, aseptic) 047.9
actinomycotic 039.8 *[320.7]*
adenoviral 049.1
Aerobacter aerogenes 320.82
anaerobes (cocci) (gram-negative)
(gram-positive) (mixed) (NEC) 320.81
arbovirus NEC 066.9 *[321.2]*
specified type NEC 066.8 *[321.2]*
aseptic (acute) NEC 047.9
adenovirus 049.1
Coxsackie virus 047.0
due to
adenovirus 049.1
Coxsackie virus 047.0
ECHO virus 047.1
enterovirus 047.9
mumps 072.1
poliovirus (*see also* Poliomyelitis) 045.2 *[321.2]*
ECHO virus 047.1
herpes (simplex) virus 054.72
zoster 053.0
leptospiral 100.81
lymphocytic choriomeningitis 049.0
noninfective 322.0
Bacillus pyocyaneus 320.89
bacterial NEC 320.9
anaerobic 320.81
gram-negative 320.82
anaerobic 320.81
Bacteroides (fragilis) (oralis) (melaninogenicus)
320.81
cancerous (M8000/6) 198.4
candidal 112.83
carcinomatous (M8010/6) 198.4
caseous (*see also* Tuberculosis, meninges) 013.0
cerebrospinal (acute) (chronic) (diplococcal)
(endemic) (epidemic) (fulminant) (infectious)
(malignant) (meningococcal) (sporadic) 036.0
carrier (suspected) of V02.59
chronic NEC 322.2
clear cerebrospinal fluid NEC 322.0
Clostridium (haemolyticum) (novyi) NEC 320.81
coccidioidomycosis 114.2
Coxsackie virus 047.0
cryptococcal 117.5 *[321.0]*
diplococcal 036.0
gram-negative 036.0
gram-positive 320.1
Diplococcus pneumoniae 320.1
due to
actinomycosis 039.8 *[320.7]*
adenovirus 049.1
coccidiomycosis 114.2
enterovirus 047.9
specified NEC 047.8
histoplasmosis (*see also* Histoplasmosis) 115.91
Listerosis 027.0 *[320.7]*
Lyme disease 088.81 *[320.7]*
moniliasis 112.83
mumps 072.1
neurosyphilis 094.2
nonbacterial organisms NEC 321.8
oidiomycosis 112.83
poliovirus (*see also* Poliomyelitis) 045.2
[321.2]

Meningitis—*continued*
  due to—*continued*
    preventive immunization, inoculation, or
        vaccination 997.09 *[321.8]*
    sarcoidosis 135 *[321.4]*
    sporotrichosis 117.1 *[321.1]*
    syphilis 094.2
      acute 091.81
      congenital 090.42
      secondary 091.81
    trypanosomiasis (*see also* Trypanosomiasis)
        086.9 *[321.3]*
    whooping cough 033.9 *[320.7]*
  E. coli 320.82
  ECHO virus 047.1
  endothelial-leukocytic, benign, recurrent 047.9
  Enterobacter aerogenes 320.82
  enteroviral 047.9
    specified type NEC 047.8
  enterovirus 047.9
    specified NEC 047.8
  eosinophilic 322.1
  epidemic NEC 036.0
  Escherichia coli (E. coli) 320.82
  Eubacterium 320.81
  fibrinopurulent NEC 320.9
    specified type NEC 320.89
  Friedländer (bacillus) 320.82
  fungal NEC 117.9 *[321.1]*
  Fusobacterium 320.81
  gonococcal 098.82
  gram-negative bacteria NEC 320.82
    anaerobic 320.81
    cocci 036.0
      specified NEC 320.82
  gram-negative cocci NEC 036.0
    specified NEC 320.82
  gram-positive cocci NEC 320.9
  H. influenzae 320.0
  herpes (simplex) virus 054.72
    zoster 053.0
  infectious NEC 320.9
  influenzal 320.0
  Klebsiella pneumoniae 320.82
  late effect—*see* Late, effect, meningitis
  leptospiral (aseptic) 100.81
  Listerella (monocytogenes) 027.0 *[320.7]*
  Listeria monocytogenes 027.0 *[320.7]*
  lymphocytic (acute) (benign) (serous) 049.0
    choriomeningitis virus 049.0
  meningococcal (chronic) 036.0
  Mima polymorpha 320.82
  Mollaret's 047.9
  monilial 112.83
  mumps (virus) 072.1
  mycotic NEC 117.9 *[321.1]*
  Neisseria 036.0
  neurosyphilis 094.2
  nonbacterial NEC (*see also* Meningitis, aseptic) 047.9
  nonpyogenic NEC 322.0
  oidiomycosis 112.83
  ossificans 349.2
  Peptococcus 320.81
  Peptostreptococcus 320.81
  pneumococcal 320.1
  poliovirus (*see also* Poliomyelitis) 045.2 *[321.2]*
  Proprionibacterium 320.81
  Proteus morganii 320.82
  Pseudomonas (aeruginosa) (pyocyaneus) 320.82
  purulent NEC 320.9
    specified organism NEC 320.89

Meningitis—*continued*
  pyogenic NEC 320.9
    specified organism NEC 320.89
  Salmonella 003.21
  septic NEC 320.9
    specified organism NEC 320.89
  serosa circumscripta NEC 322.0
  serous NEC (*see also* Meningitis, aseptic) 047.9
    lymphocytic 049.0
    syndrome 348.2
  Serratia (marcescens) 320.82
  specified organism NEC 320.89
  sporadic cerebrospinal 036.0
  sporotrichosis 117.1 *[321.1]*
  staphylococcal 320.3
  sterile 997.09
  streptococcal (acute) 320.2
  suppurative 320.9
    specified organism NEC 320.89
  syphilitic 094.2
    acute 091.81
    congenital 090.42
    secondary 091.81
  torula 117.5 *[321.0]*
  traumatic (complication of injury) 958.8
  Treponema (denticola) (macrodenticum) 320.81
  trypanosomiasis 086.1 *[321.3]*
  tuberculous (*see also* Tuberculosis, meninges) 013.0
  typhoid 002.0 *[320.7]*
  Veillonella 320.81
  Vibrio vulnificus 320.82
  viral, virus NEC (*see also* Meningitis, aseptic)
      047.9
  Wallgren's (*see also* Meningitis, aseptic) 047.9
Meningocele (congenital) (spinal) (*see also* Spina
      bifida) 741.9
  acquired (traumatic) 349.2
  cerebral 742.0
  cranial 742.0
Meningocerebritis —*see* Meningoencephalitis
Meningococcemia (acute) (chronic) 036.2
Meningococcus, meningococcal (*see also*
      condition) 036.9
  adrenalitis, hemorrhagic 036.3
  carditis 036.40
  carrier (suspected) of V02.59
  cerebrospinal fever 036.0
  encephalitis 036.1
  endocarditis 036.42
  exposure to V01.84
  infection NEC 036.9
  meningitis (cerebrospinal) 036.0
  myocarditis 036.43
  optic neuritis 036.81
  pericarditis 036.41
  septicemia (chronic) 036.2
Meningoencephalitis (*see also* Encephalitis)
      323.9
  acute NEC 048
  bacterial, purulent, pyogenic, or septic—*see*
      Meningitis
  chronic NEC 094.1
  diffuse NEC 094.1
  diphasic 063.2
  due to
    actinomycosis 039.8 *[320.7]*
    blastomycosis NEC (*see also* Blastomycosis)
        116.0 *[323.41]*
    free-living amebae 136.29
    Listeria monocytogenes 027.0 *[320.7]*
    Lyme disease 088.81 *[320.7]*

Meningoencephalitis—*continued*
  due to—*continued*
    mumps 072.2
    Naegleria (amebae) (gruberi) (organisms)
      136.29
    rubella 056.01
    sporotrichosis 117.1 *[321.1]*
    toxoplasmosis (acquired) 130.0
      congenital (active) 771.2 *[323.41]*
    Trypanosoma 086.1 *[323.2]*
  epidemic 036.0
  herpes 054.3
  herpetic 054.3
  H. influenzae 320.0
  infectious (acute) 048
  influenzal 320.0
  late effect—*see* category 326
  Listeria monocytogenes 027.0 *[320.7]*
  lymphocytic (serous) 049.0
  mumps 072.2
  parasitic NEC 123.9 *[323.41]*
  pneumococcal 320.1
  primary amebic 136.29
  rubella 056.01
  serous 048
    lymphocytic 049.0
  specific 094.2
  staphylococcal 320.3
  streptococcal 320.2
  syphilitic 094.2
  toxic NEC 989.9 *[323.71]*
    due to
      carbon tetrachloride (vapor) 987.8 *[323.71]*
      hydroxyquinoline derivatives poisoning
        961.3 *[323.71]*
      lead 984.9 *[323.71]*
      mercury 985.0 *[323.71]*
      thallium 985.8 *[323.71]*
  toxoplasmosis (acquired) 130.0
  trypanosomic 086.1 *[323.2]*
  tuberculous (*see also* Tuberculosis, meninges)
    013.0
  virus NEC 048
Meningoencephalocele 742.0
  syphilitic 094.89
    congenital 090.49
Meningoencephalomyelitis (*see also*
  Meningoencephalitis) 323.9
  acute NEC 048
    disseminated (postinfectious) 136.9 *[323.61]*
      postimmunization or postvaccination 323.51
  due to
    actinomycosis 039.8 *[320.7]*
    torula 117.5 *[323.41]*
    toxoplasma or toxoplasmosis (acquired) 130.0
      congenital (active) 771.2 *[323.41]*
  late effect—*see* category 326
Meningoencephalomyelopathy (*see also*
  Meningoencephalomyelitis) 349.9
Meningoencephalopathy (*see also*
  Meningoencephalitis) 348.39
Meningoencephalopoliomyelitis (*see also*
  Poliomyelitis, bulbar) 045.0
  late effect 138
Meningomyelitis (*see also* Meningoencephalitis)
  323.9
  blastomycotic NEC (*see also* Blastomycosis)
    116.0 *[323.41]*

Meningomyelitis—*continued*
  due to
    actinomycosis 039.8 *[320.7]*
    blastomycosis (*see also* Blastomycosis) 116.0
      [323.41]
    Meningococcus 036.0
    sporotrichosis 117.1 *[323.41]*
    torula 117.5 *[323.41]*
  late effect—*see* category 326
  lethargic 049.8
  meningococcal 036.0
  syphilitic 094.2
  tuberculous (*see Tuberculosis, meninges*) 013.0
Meningomyelocele (*see also* Spina bifida) 741.9
  syphilitic 094.89
Meningomyeloneuritis —*see*
  Meningoencephalitis
Meningoradiculitis —*see* Meningitis
Meningovascular —*see* condition
Meniscocytosis 282.60
Menkes' syndrome —*see* Syndrome, Menkes'
Menolipsis 626.0
Menometrorrhagia 626.2
Menopause, menopausal (symptoms)
  (syndrome) 627.2
  arthritis (any site) NEC 716.3
  artificial 627.4
  bleeding 627.0
  crisis 627.2
  depression (*see also* Psychosis, affective) 296.2
    agitated 296.2
      recurrent episode 296.3
      single episode 296.2
    psychotic 296.2
      recurrent episode 296.3
      single episode 296.2
    recurrent episode 296.3
    single episode 296.2
  melancholia (*see also* Psychosis, affective) 296.2
    recurrent episode 296.3
    single episode 296.2
  paranoid state 297.2
  paraphrenia 297.2
  postsurgical 627.4
  premature 256.31
    postirradiation 256.2
    postsurgical 256.2
  psychoneurosis 627.2
  psychosis NEC 298.8
  surgical 627.4
  toxic polyarthritis NEC 716.39
Menorrhagia (primary) 626.2
  climacteric 627.0
  menopausal 627.0
  postclimacteric 627.1
  postmenopausal 627.1
  preclimacteric 627.0
  premenopausal 627.0
  puberty (menses retained) 626.3
Menorrhalgia 625.3
Menoschesis 626.8
Menostaxis 626.2
Menses, retention 626.8
Menstrual —*see* Menstruation
  cycle, irregular 626.4
  disorders NEC 626.9
  extraction V25.3
  fluid, retained 626.8
  molimen 625.4
  period, normal V65.5
  regulation V25.3

Menstruation
absent 626.0
anovulatory 628.0
delayed 626.8
difficult 625.3
disorder 626.9
psychogenic 306.52
specified NEC 626.8
during pregnancy 640.8
excessive 626.2
frequent 626.2
infrequent 626.1
irregular 626.4
latent 626.8
membranous 626.8
painful (primary) (secondary) 625.3
psychogenic 306.52
passage of clots 626.2
precocious 259.1
protracted 626.8
retained 626.8
retrograde 626.8
scanty 626.1
suppression 626.8
vicarious (nasal) 625.8
Mentagra (*see also* Sycosis) 704.8
Mental —*see also* condition
deficiency (*see also* Disability, intellectual) 319
deterioration (*see also* Psychosis) 298.9
disorder (*see also* Disorder, mental) 300.9
exhaustion 300.5
insufficiency (congenital) (*see also* Disability, intellectual) 319
observation without need for further medical care NEC V71.09
retardation —*see* Disability, intellectual
subnormality (*see also* Disability, intellectual) 319
mild 317
moderate 318.0
profound 318.2
severe 318.1
upset (*see also* Disorder, mental) 300.9
Meralgia paresthetica 355.1
Mercurial —*see* condition
Mercurialism NEC 985.0
Merergasia 300.9
Merkel cell tumor —*see* Carcinoma, Merkel cell
Merocele (*see also* Hernia, femoral) 553.00
Meromelia 755.4
lower limb 755.30
intercalary 755.32
femur 755.34
tibiofibular (complete) (incomplete) 755.33
fibula 755.37
metatarsal(s) 755.38
tibia 755.36
tibiofibular 755.35
terminal (complete) (partial) (transverse) 755.31
longitudinal 755.32
metatarsal(s) 755.38
phalange(s) 755.39
tarsal(s) 755.38
transverse 755.31

Meromelia—*continued*
upper limb 755.20
intercalary 755.22
carpal(s) 755.28
humeral 755.24
radioulnar (complete) (incomplete) 755.23
metacarpal(s) 755.28
phalange(s) 755.29
radial 755.26
radioulnar 755.25
ulnar 755.27
terminal (complete) (partial) (transverse) 755.21
longitudinal 755.22
carpal(s) 755.28
metacarpal(s) 755.28
phalange(s) 755.29
transverse 755.21
Merosmia 781.1
MERRF syndrome (myoclonus with epilepsy and with ragged red fibers) 277.87
Merycism (*see also* Rumination)—*see also* Vomiting
psychogenic 307.53
Merzbacher-Pelizaeus disease 330.0
Mesaortitis —*see* Aortitis
Mesarteritis —*see* Arteritis
Mesencephalitis (*see also* Encephalitis) 323.9
late effect—*see* category 326
Mesenchymoma (M8990/1)—*see also* Neoplasm, connective tissue, uncertain behavior
benign (M8990/0)—*see* Neoplasm, connective tissue, benign
malignant (M8990/3)—*see* Neoplasm, connective tissue, malignant
Mesenteritis
retractile 567.82
sclerosing 567.82
Mesentery, mesenteric —*see* condition
Mesiodens, mesiodentes 520.1
causing crowding 524.31
Mesio-occlusion 524.23
Mesocardia (with asplenia) 746.87
Mesocolon —*see* condition
Mesonephroma (malignant) (M9110/3)—*see also* Neoplasm, by site, malignant
benign (M9110/0)—*see* Neoplasm, by site, benign
Mesophlebitis —*see* Phlebitis
Mesostromal dysgenesis 743.51
Mesothelioma (malignant) (M9050/3)—*see also* Neoplasm, by site, malignant
benign (M9050/0)—*see* Neoplasm, by site, benign
biphasic type (M9053/3)—*see also* Neoplasm, by site, malignant
benign (M9053/0)—*see* Neoplasm, by site, benign
epithelioid (M9052/3)—*see also* Neoplasm, by site, malignant
benign (M9052/0)—*see* Neoplasm, by site, benign
fibrous (M9051/3)—*see also* Neoplasm, by site, malignant
benign (M9051/0)—*see* Neoplasm, by site, benign
Metabolic syndrome 277.7
Metabolism disorder 277.9
specified type NEC 277.89
Metagonimiasis 121.5
Metagonimus infestation (small intestine) 121.5

Metal
  pigmentation (skin) 709.00
  polishers' disease 502
Metalliferous miners' lung 503
Metamorphopsia 368.14
Metaplasia
  bone, in skin 709.3
  breast 611.89
  cervix—*omit code*
  endometrium (squamous) 621.8
  esophagus 530.85
  intestinal, of gastric mucosa 537.89
  kidney (pelvis) (squamous) (*see also* Disease,
    renal) 593.89
  myelogenous 289.89
  myeloid 289.89
    agnogenic 238.76
    megakaryocytic 238.76
  spleen 289.59
  squamous cell
    amnion 658.8
    bladder 596.89
    cervix—*see* condition
    trachea 519.19
    tracheobronchial tree 519.19
    uterus 621.8
      cervix—*see* condition
Metastasis, metastatic
  abscess—*see* Abscess
  calcification 275.40
  cancer, neoplasm, or disease
    from specified site (M8000/3)—*see*
      Neoplasm, by site, malignant
    to specified site (M8000/6)—*see* Neoplasm,
      by site, secondary
  deposits (in) (M8000/6)—*see* Neoplasm, by site,
    secondary
  mesentery, of neuroendocrine tumor 209.74
  pneumonia 038.8 *[484.8]*
  spread (to) (M8000/6)—*see* Neoplasm, by site,
    secondary
Metatarsalgia 726.70
  anterior 355.6
  due to Freiberg's disease 732.5
  Morton's 355.6
Metatarsus, metatarsal —*see also* condition
  adductus varus (congenital) 754.53
  abductus valgus (congenital) 764.60
  primus varus 754.52
  valgus (adductus) (congenital) 754.60
  varus (abductus) (congenital) 754.53
    primus 754.52
Methadone use 304.00
Methemoglobinemia 289.7
  acquired (with sulfhemoglobinemia) 289.7
  congenital 289.7
  enzymatic 289.7
  Hb-M disease 289.7
  hereditary 289.7
  toxic 289.7
Methemoglobinuria (*see also* Hemoglobinuria)
  791.2
Methicillin
  resistant staphylococcus aureus (MRSA) 041.12
    colonization V02.54
    personal history of V12.04
  susceptible staphylococcus aureus (MSSA)
    041.11
    colonization V02.53
Methioninemia 270.4

Metritis (catarrhal) (septic) (suppurative) (*see
    also* Endometritis) 615.9
  blennorrhagic 098.16
    chronic or duration of 2 months or over 098.36
  cervical (*see also* Cervicitis) 616.0
  gonococcal 098.16
    chronic or duration of 2 months or over 098.36
  hemorrhagic 626.8
  puerperal, postpartum, childbirth 670.1
    septic 670.2
  tuberculous (*see also* Tuberculosis) 016.7
Metropathia hemorrhagica 626.8
Metroperitonitis (*see also* Peritonitis, pelvic,
    female) 614.5
Metrorrhagia 626.6
  arising during pregnancy—*see* Hemorrhage,
    pregnancy
  postpartum NEC 666.2
  primary 626.6
  psychogenic 306.59
  puerperal 666.2
Metrorrhexis —*see* Rupture, uterus
Metrosalpingitis (*see also* Salpingo-oophoritis)
  614.2
Metrostaxis 626.6
Metrovaginitis (*see also* Endometritis) 615.9
  gonococcal (acute) 098.16
    chronic or duration of 2 months or over 098.36
Mexican fever —*see* Typhus, Mexican
Meyenburg-Altherr-Uehlinger syndrome
  733.99
Meyer-Schwickerath and Weyers syndrome
  (dysplasia oculodentodigitalis) 759.89
Meynert's amentia (nonalcoholic) 294.0
  alcoholic 291.1
Mibelli's disease 757.39
Mice, joint (*see also* Loose, body, joint) 718.1
  knee 717.6
Micheli-Rietti syndrome (thalassemia minor)
  282.46
Michotte's syndrome 721.5
Micrencephalon, micrencephaly 742.1
Microalbuminuria 791.0
Microaneurysm, retina 362.14
  diabetic 250.5 *[362.01]*
    due to secondary diabetes 249.5 *[362.01]*
Microangiopathy 443.9
  diabetic (peripheral) 250.7 *[443.81]*
    due to secondary diabetes 249.7 *[443.81]*
    retinal 250.5 *[362.01]*
      due to secondary diabetes 249.5 *[362.01]*
  peripheral 443.9
    diabetic 250.7 *[443.81]*
      due to secondary diabetes 249.7 *[443.81]*
  retinal 362.18
    diabetic 250.5 *[362.01]*
      due to secondary diabetes 249.5 *[362.01]*
  thrombotic 446.6
    Moschcowitz's (thrombotic thrombocytopenic
      purpura) 446.6
Microcalcification, mammographic 793.81
Microcephalus, microcephalic, microcephaly
  742.1
  due to toxoplasmosis (congenital) 771.2
Microcheilia 744.82
Microcolon (congenital) 751.5
Microcornea (congenital) 743.41
Microcytic —*see* condition
Microdeletions NEC 758.33
Microdontia 520.2

Microdrepanocytosis (thalassemia-Hb-S disease) 282.41
　with sickle cell crisis 282.42
Microembolism
　atherothrombotic—*see also* Atheroembolism
　retina 362.33
Microencephalon 742.1
Microfilaria streptocerca infestation 125.3
Microgastria (congenital) 750.7
Microgenia 524.06
Microgenitalia (congenital) 752.89
　penis 752.64
Microglioma (M9710/3)
　specified site—*see* Neoplasm, by site, malignant
　unspecified site 191.9
Microglossia (congenital) 750.16
Micrognathia, micrognathism (congenital) 524.00
　mandibular 524.04
　　alveolar 524.74
　maxillary 524.03
　　alveolar 524.73
Microgyria (congenital) 742.2
Microinfarct, heart (*see also* Insufficiency, coronary) 411.89
Microlithiasis, alveolar, pulmonary 516.2
Micromastia 611.82
Micromyelia (congenital) 742.59
Micropenis 752.64
Microphakia (congenital) 743.36
Microphthalmia (congenital) (*see also* Microphthalmos) 743.10
Microphthalmos (congenital) 743.10
　associated with eye and adnexal anomalies NEC 743.12
　due to toxoplasmosis (congenital) 771.2
　isolated 743.11
　simple 743.11
　syndrome 759.89
Micropsia 368.14
Microsporidiosis 136.8
Microsporon furfur infestation 111.0
Microsporosis (*see also* Dermatophytosis) 110.9
　nigra 111.1
Microstomia (congenital) 744.84
Microthelia 757.6
Microthromboembolism —*see* Embolism
Microtia (congenital) (external ear) 744.23
Microtropia 378.34
Microvillus inclusion disease (MVD) 751.5
Micturition
　disorder NEC 788.69
　　psychogenic 306.53
　frequency 788.41
　　psychogenic 306.53
　nocturnal 788.43
　painful 788.1
　　psychogenic 306.53
Middle
　ear—*see* condition
　lobe (right) syndrome 518.0
Midplane —*see* condition
Miescher's disease 709.3
　cheilitis 351.8
　granulomatosis disciformis 709.3
Miescher-Leder syndrome or granulomatosis 709.3
Mieten's syndrome 759.89

Migraine (idiopathic) 346.9

Note: The following fifth digit subclassification is for use with category 346

0　*without mention of intractable migraine*
　　without mention of status migrainosus
　　　without mention of refractory migraine
　　　without mention of status migrainosus
1　*with intractable migraine, so stated, without mention of status migrainosus*
　　with refractory migraine, so stated, without mention of status migrainosus
2　*without mention of intractable migraine with status migrainosus*
　　without mention of refractory migraine with status migrainosus
3　*with intractable migraine, so stated, with status migrainosus*
　　with refractory migraine, so stated, with status migrainosus

---

　with aura (acute-onset) (without headache) (prolonged) (typical) 346.0
　without aura 346.1
　　chronic 346.7
　　transformed 346.7
　abdominal (syndrome) 346.2
　allergic (histamine) 346.2
　atypical 346.8
　basilar 346.0
　chronic without aura 346.7
　classic(al) 346.0
　common 346.1
　comlicated 346.0
　hemiplegic 346.3
　　familial 346.3
　　sporadic 346.3
　lower-half 339.00
　menstrual 346.4
　menstrually related 346.4
　ophthalmic 346.8
　ophthalmoplegic 346.2
　premenstrual 346.4
　pure menstrual 346.4
　retinal 346.0
　specified form NEC 346.8
　transformed without aura 346.7
　variant 346.2
Migrant, social V60.0
Migratory, migrating —*see also* condition
　person V60.0
　testis, congenital 752.52
Mikulicz's disease or syndrome (dryness of mouth, absent or decreased lacrimation) 527.1
Milian atrophia blanche 701.3
Miliaria (crystallina) (rubra) (tropicalis) 705.1
　apocrine 705.82
Miliary —*see* condition
Milium (*see also* Cyst, sebaceous) 706.2
　colloid 709.3
　eyelid 374.84
Milk
　crust 690.11
　excess secretion 676.6
　fever, female 672
　poisoning 988.8
　retention 676.2
　sickness 988.8
　spots 423.1
Milkers' nodes 051.1

Milk-leg (deep vessels) 671.4
  complicating pregnancy 671.3
  nonpuerperal 451.19
  puerperal, postpartum, childbirth 671.4
Milkman (-Looser) disease or syndrome
  (osteomalacia with pseudofractures) 268.2
Milky urine (*see also* Chyluria) 791.1
Millar's asthma (laryngismus stridulus) 478.75
Millard-Gubler paralysis or syndrome 344.89
Millard-Gubler-Foville paralysis 344.89
Miller-Dieker syndrome 758.33
Miller's disease (osteomalacia) 268.2
Miller Fisher's syndrome 357.0
Milles' syndrome (encephalocutaneous
  angiomatosis) 759.6
Mills' disease 335.29
Millstone makers' asthma or lung 502
Milroy's disease (chronic hereditary edema) 757.0
Miners' —*see also* condition
  asthma 500
  elbow 727.2
  knee 727.2
  lung 500
  nystagmus 300.89
  phthisis (*see also* Tuberculosis) 011.4
  tuberculosis (*see also* Tuberculosis) 011.4
Minkowski-Chauffard syndrome (*see also*
  Spherocytosis) 282.0
Minor —*see* condition
Minor's disease 336.1
Minot's disease (hemorrhagic disease, newborn)
  776.0
Minot-von Willebrand (-Jürgens) disease or
  syndrome (angiohemophilia) 286.4
Minus (and plus) hand (intrinsic) 736.09
Miosis (persistent) (pupil) 379.42
Mirizzi's syndrome (hepatic duct stenosis) (*see
  also* Obstruction, biliary) 576.2
  with calculus, cholelithiasis, or stones—*see*
    Choledocholithiasis
Mirror writing 315.09
  secondary to organic lesion 784.69
Misadventure (prophylactic) (therapeutic) (*see
  also* Complications) 999.9
  administration of insulin 962.3
  infusion—*see* Complications, infusion
  local applications (of fomentations, plasters,
    etc.) 999.9
    burn or scald—*see* Burn, by site
  medical care (early) (late) NEC 999.9
    adverse effect of drugs or chemicals—*see*
      Table of drugs and chemicals
    burn or scald—*see* Burn, by site
  radiation NEC 990
  radiotherapy NEC 990
  surgical procedure (early) (late)—*see*
    Complications, surgical procedure
  transfusion—*see* Complications, transfusion
  vaccination or other immunological
    procedure—*see* Complications, vaccination
Misanthropy 301.7
Miscarriage —*see* Abortion, spontaneous
Mischief, malicious, child (*see also* Disturbance,
  conduct) 312.0
Misdirection
  aqueous 365.83
Mismanagement, feeding 783.3

Misplaced, misplacement
  kidney (*see also* Disease, renal) 593.0
    congenital 753.3
  organ or site, congenital NEC—*see* Malposition,
    congenital
Missed
  abortion 632
  delivery (at or near term) 656.4
  labor (at or near term) 656.4
Misshapen reconstructed breast 612.0
Missing —*see also* Absence
  teeth (acquired) 525.10
    congenital (*see also* Anodontia) 520.0
    due to
      caries 525.13
      extraction 525.10
      periodontal disease 525.12
      trauma 525.11
      specified NEC 525.19
  vertebrae (congenital) 756.13
Misuse of drugs NEC (*see also* Abuse, drug,
  nondependent) 305.9
Mitchell's disease (erythromelalgia) 443.82
Mite (s)
  diarrhea 133.8
  grain (itch) 133.8
  hair follicle (itch) 133.8
  in sputum 133.8
**Mitochondrial encephalopathy, lactic acidosis
  and stroke-like episodes** (MELAS
  syndrome) 277.87
**Mitochondrial neurogastrointestinal
  encephalopathy syndrome (MNGIE)** 277.87
Mitral —*see* condition
Mittelschmerz 625.2
Mixed —*see* condition
Mljet disease (mal de Meleda) 757.39
Mobile, mobility
  cecum 751.4
  coccyx 733.99
  excessive—*see* Hypermobility
  gallbladder 751.69
  kidney 593.0
    congenital 753.3
  organ or site, congenital NEC—*see* Malposition,
    congenital
  spleen 289.59
Mobitz heart block (atrioventricular) 426.10
  type I (Wenckebach's) 426.13
  type II 426.12
Möbius'
  disease 346.2
  syndrome
    congenital oculofacial paralysis 352.6
    ophthalmoplegic migraine 346.2
Moeller (-Barlow) disease (infantile scurvy) 267
  glossitis 529.4
Mohr's syndrome (Types I and II) 759.89
Mola destruens (M9100/1) 236.1
Molarization, premolars 520.2
Molar pregnancy 631.8
  hydatidiform (delivered) (undelivered) 630
Mold (s) in vitreous 117.9
Molding, head (during birth)—*omit code*
Mole (pigmented) (M8720/0)—*see also*
  Neoplasm, skin, benign
  blood 631.8
  Breus' 631.8
  cancerous (M8720/3)—*see* Melanoma
  carneous 631.8
  destructive (M9100/1) 236.1

Mole—*continued*
ectopic—*see* Pregnancy, ectopic
fleshy 631.8
hemorrhagic 631.8
hydatid, hydatidiform (benign) (complicating
    pregnancy) (delivered) (undelivered) (*see
    also* Hydatidiform mole) 630
    invasive (M9100/1) 236.1
    malignant (M9100/1) 236.1
    previous, affecting management of pregnancy
        V23.1
invasive (hydatidiform) (M9100/1) 236.1
malignant
    meaning
        malignant hydatidiform mole (M9100/1) 236.1
        melanoma (M8720/3)—*see* Melanoma
    nonpigmented (M8730/0)—*see* Neoplasm, skin,
        benign
pregnancy NEC 631.8
skin (M8720/0)—*see* Neoplasm, skin, benign
stone 631.8
tubal—*see* Pregnancy, tubal
vesicular (*see also* Hydatidiform mole) 630
Molimen, molimina (menstrual) 625.4
Mollaret's meningitis 047.9
Mollities (cerebellar) (cerebral) 437.8
ossium 268.2
Molluscum
contagiosum 078.0
epitheliale 078.0
fibrosum (M8851/0)—*see* Lipoma, by site
pendulum (M8851/0)—*see* Lipoma, by site
**Mönckeberg's arteriosclerosis, degeneration
    disease, or sclerosis** (*see also*
    Arteriosclerosis, extremities) 440.20
Monday fever 504
Monday morning dyspnea or asthma 504
Mondini's malformation (cochlea) 744.05
Mondor's disease (thrombophlebitis of breast)
    451.89
**Mongolian, mongolianism, mongolism
    mongoloid** 758.0
spot 757.33
Monilethrix (congenital) 757.4
Monilia infestation —*see* Candidiasis
Moniliasis —*see also* Candidiasis
neonatal 771.7
vulvovaginitis 112.1
Monkeypox 059.01
Monoarthritis 716.60
ankle 716.67
arm 716.62
    lower (and wrist) 716.63
    upper (and elbow) 716.62
foot (and ankle) 716.67
forearm (and wrist) 716.63
hand 716.64
leg 716.66
    lower 716.66
    upper 716.65
pelvic region (hip) (thigh) 716.65
shoulder (region) 716.61
specified site NEC 716.68
Monoblastic —*see* condition
Monochromatism (cone) (rod) 368.54
Monocytic —*see* condition
Monocytopenia 288.59
Monocytosis (symptomatic) 288.63
Monofixation syndrome 378.34
Monomania (*see also* Psychosis) 298.9

Mononeuritis 355.9
cranial nerve—*see* Disorder, nerve, cranial
femoral nerve 355.2
lateral
    cutaneous nerve of thigh 355.1
    popliteal nerve 355.3
lower limb 355.8
    specified nerve NEC 355.79
medial popliteal nerve 355.4
median nerve 354.1
multiplex 354.5
plantar nerve 355.6
posterior tibial nerve 355.5
radial nerve 354.3
sciatic nerve 355.0
ulnar nerve 354.2
upper limb 354.9
    specified nerve NEC 354.8
vestibular 388.5
Mononeuropathy (*see also* Mononeuritis) 355.9
diabetic NEC 250.6 *[355.9]*
    due to secondary diabetes 249.6 *[355.9]*
    lower limb 250.6 *[355.8]*
        due to secondary diabetes 249.6 *[355.8]*
    upper limb 250.6 *[354.9]*
        due to secondary diabetes 249.6 *[354.9]*
iliohypogastric nerve 355.79
ilioinguinal nerve 355.79
obturator nerve 355.79
saphenous nerve 355.79
Mononucleosis, infectious 075
with hepatitis 075 *[573.1]*
Monoplegia 344.5
brain (current episode) (*see also* Paralysis,
    brain) 437.8
fetus or newborn 767.8
cerebral (current episode) (*see also* Paralysis,
    brain) 437.8
congenital or infantile (cerebral) (spastic)
    (spinal) 343.3
embolic (current) (*see also* Embolism, brain)
    434.1
    late effect—*see* Late effect(s) (of)
        cerebrovascular disease
infantile (cerebral) (spastic) (spinal) 343.3
lower limb 344.30
    affecting
        dominant side 344.31
        nondominant side 344.32
    due to late effect of cerebrovascular accident
        —*see* Late effect(s) (of) cerebrovascular
        accident
newborn 767.8
psychogenic 306.0
    specified as conversion reaction 300.11
thrombotic (current) (*see also* Thrombosis,
    brain) 434.0
    late effect—*see* Late effect(s) (of)
        cerebrovascular disease
transient 781.4
upper limb 344.40
    affecting
        dominant side 344.41
        nondominant side 344.42
    due to late effect of cerebrovascular accident
        —*see* Late effect(s) (of) cerebrovascular
        accident
Monorchism, monorchidism 752.89
Monteggia's fracture (closed) 813.03
open 813.13

Mood swings
brief compensatory 296.99
rebound 296.99
Moore's syndrome (*see also* Epilepsy) 345.5
Mooren's ulcer (cornea) 370.07
Mooser-Neill reaction 081.0
Mooser bodies 081.0
Moral
deficiency 301.7
imbecility 301.7
Morax-Axenfeld conjunctivitis 372.03
Morbilli (*see also* Measles) 055.9
Morbus
anglicus, anglorum 268.0
Beigel 111.2
caducus (*see also* Epilepsy) 345.9
caeruleus 746.89
celiacus 579.0
comitialis (*see also* Epilepsy) 345.9
cordis—*see also* Disease, heart
valvulorum—*see* Endocarditis
coxae 719.95
tuberculous (*see also* Tuberculosis) 015.1
hemorrhagicus neonatorum 776.0
maculosus neonatorum 772.6
renum 593.0
senilis (*see also* Osteoarthrosis) 715.9
Morel-Kraepelin disease (*see also* Schizophrenia) 295.9
Morel-Moore syndrome (hyperostosis frontalis interna) 733.3
Morel-Morgagni syndrome (hyperostosis frontalis interna) 733.3
Morgagni
cyst, organ, hydatid, or appendage 752.89
fallopian tube 752.11
disease or syndrome (hyperostosis frontalis interna) 733.3
Morgagni-Adams-Stokes syndrome (syncope with heart block) 426.9
Morgagni-Stewart-Morel syndrome (hyperostosis frontalis interna) 733.3
Moria (*see also* Psychosis) 298.9
Morning sickness 643.0
Moron 317
Morphea (guttate) (linear) 701.0
Morphine dependence (*see also* Dependence) 304.0
Morphinism (*see also* Dependence) 304.0
Morphinomania (*see also* Dependence) 304.0
Morphoea 701.0
Morquio (-Brailsford) (-Ullrich) disease or syndrome (mucopolysaccharidosis IV) 277.5
kyphosis 277.5
Morris syndrome (testicular feminization) 259.51
Morsus humanus (open wound)—*see also* Wound, open, by site
skin surface intact—*see* Contusion
Mortification (dry) (moist) (*see also* Gangrene) 785.4
Morton's
disease 355.6
foot 355.6
metatarsalgia (syndrome) 355.6
neuralgia 355.6
neuroma 355.6
syndrome (metatarsalgia) (neuralgia) 355.6
toe 355.6
Morvan's disease 336.0

Mosaicism, mosaic (chromosomal) 758.9
autosomal 758.5
sex 758.81
Moschcowitz's syndrome (thrombotic thrombocytopenic purpura) 446.6
Mother yaw 102.0
Motion sickness (from travel, any vehicle) (from roundabouts or swings) 994.6
Mottled teeth (enamel) (endemic) (nonendemic) 520.3
Mottling enamel (endemic) (nonendemic) (teeth) 520.3
Mouchet's disease 732.5
Mould (s) (in vitreous) 117.9
Moulders'
bronchitis 502
tuberculosis (*see also* Tuberculosis) 011.4
Mounier-Kuhn syndrome 748.3
with
acute exacerbation 494.1
bronchiectasis 494.0
with (acute) exacerbation 494.1
acquired 519.19
with bronchiectasis 494.0
with (acute) exacerbation 494.1
Mountain
fever—*see* Fever, mountain
sickness 993.2
with polycythemia, acquired 289.0
acute 289.0
tick fever 066.1
Mouse, joint (*see also* Loose, body, joint) 718.1
knee 717.6
Mouth —*see* condition
Movable
coccyx 724.71
kidney (*see also* Disease, renal) 593.0
congenital 753.3
organ or site, congenital NEC—*see* Malposition, congenital
spleen 289.59
Movement
abnormal (dystonic) (involuntary) 781.0
decreased fetal 655.7
paradoxical facial 374.43
Moya Moya disease 437.5
Mozart's ear 744.29
MRSA (methicillin resistant staphylococcus aureus) 041.12
colonization V02.54
personal history of V12.04
MSSA (methicillin susceptible staphylococcus aureus) 041.11
colonization V02.53
Mucha's disease (acute parapsoriasis varioliformis) 696.2
Mucha-Haberman syndrome (acute parapsoriasis varioliformis) 696.2
Mu-chain disease 273.2
Mucinosis (cutaneous) (papular) 701.8
Mucocele
appendix 543.9
buccal cavity 528.9
gallbladder (*see also* Disease, gallbladder) 575.3
lacrimal sac 375.43
orbit (eye) 376.81
salivary gland (any) 527.6
sinus (accessory) (nasal) 478.19
turbinate (bone) (middle) (nasal) 478.19
uterus 621.8

Mucocutaneous lymph node syndrome (acute) (febrile) (infantile) 446.1
Mucoenteritis 564.9
Mucolipidosis I, II, III 272.7
Mucopolysaccharidosis (types 1-6) 277.5
  cardiopathy 277.5 *[425.7]*
Mucormycosis (lung) 117.7
Mucosa associated lymphoid tissue (MALT) 200.3
Mucositis —*see also* Inflammation, by site 528.00
  cervix (ulcerative) 616.81
  due to
    antineoplastic therapy (ulcerative) 528.01
    other drugs (ulcerative) 528.02
    specified NEC 528.09
  gastrointestinal (ulcerative) 538
  nasal (ulcerative) 478.11
  necroticans agranulocytica (*see also*
    Agranulocytosis) 288.09
  ulcerative 528.00
  vagina (ulcerative) 616.81
  vulva (ulcerative) 616.81
Mucous —*see also* condition
  patches (syphilitic) 091.3
    congenital 090.0
Mucoviscidosis 277.00
  with meconium obstruction 277.01
Mucus
  asphyxia or suffocation (*see also* Asphyxia,
    mucus) 933.1
    newborn 770.18
  in stool 792.1
  plug (*see also* Asphyxia, mucus) 933.1
    aspiration, of newborn 770.17
    tracheobronchial 519.19
    newborn 770.18
Muguet 112.0
Mulberry molars 090.5
Müllerian mixed tumor (M8950/3)—*see*
  Neoplasm, by site, malignant
Multicystic kidney 753.19
Multilobed placenta —*see* Placenta, abnormal
Multinodular prostate 600.10
  with
    urinary
      obstruction 600.11
      retention 600.11
Multiparity V61.5
  affecting
    fetus or newborn 763.89
  management of
    labor and delivery 659.4
    pregnancy V23.3
  requiring contraceptive management (*see also*
    Contraception) V25.9
Multipartita placenta —*see* Placenta, abnormal
Multiple, multiplex —*see also* condition
  birth
    affecting fetus or newborn 761.5
    healthy liveborn—*see* Newborn, multiple
  digits (congenital) 755.00
    fingers 755.01
    toes 755.02
  organ or site NEC—*see* Accessory
  personality 300.14
  renal arteries 747.62
Mumps 072.9
  with complication 072.8
    specified type NEC 072.79
  encephalitis 072.2
  hepatitis 072.71

Mumps—*continued*
  meningitis (aseptic) 072.1
  meningoencephalitis 072.2
  oophoritis 072.79
  orchitis 072.0
  pancreatitis 072.3
  polyneuropathy 072.72
  vaccination, prophylactic (against) V04.6
Mumu (*see also* Infestation, filarial) 125.9
Münchausen syndrome 301.51
Münchmeyer's disease or syndrome (exostosis luxurians) 728.11
Mural —*see* condition
Murmur (cardiac) (heart) (nonorganic) (organic) 785.2
  abdominal 787.5
  aortic (valve) (*see also* Endocarditis, aortic) 424.1
  benign—*omit code*
  cardiorespiratory 785.2
  diastolic—*see* condition
  Flint (*see also* Endocarditis, aortic) 424.1
  functional—*omit code*
  Graham Steell (pulmonic regurgitation) (*see also* Endocarditis, pulmonary) 424.3
  innocent—*omit code*
  insignificant—*omit code*
  midsystolic 785.2
  mitral (valve)—*see* stenosis, mitral
  physiologic—*see* condition
  presystolic, mitral—*see* Insufficiency, mitral
  pulmonic (valve) (*see also* Endocarditis, pulmonary) 424.3
  Still's (vibratory)—*omit code*
  systolic (valvular)—*see* condition
  tricuspid (valve)—*see* Endocarditis, tricuspid
  valvular—*see* condition
  vibratory—*omit code*
  undiagnosed 785.2
Murri's disease (intermittent hemoglobinuria) 283.2
Muscae volitantes 379.24
Muscle, muscular —*see* condition
Musculoneuralgia 729.1
Mushrooming hip 718.95
Mushroom workers' (pickers') lung 495.5
Mutation(s)
  factor V Leiden 289.81
  prothrombin gene 289.81
  surfactant, of lung 516.63
Mutism (*see also* Aphasia) 784.3
  akinetic 784.3
  deaf (acquired) (congenital) 389.7
  hysterical 300.11
  selective (elective) 313.23
    adjustment reaction 309.83
MVD (microvillus inclusion disease) 751.5
MVID (microvillus inclusion disease) 751.5
Myà's disease (congenital dilation, colon) 751.3
Myalgia (intercostal) 729.1
  eosinophilia syndrome 710.5
  epidemic 074.1
    cervical 078.89
  psychogenic 307.89
  traumatic NEC 959.9
Myasthenia 358.00
  cordis—*see* Failure, heart
  gravis 358.00
    with exacerbation (acute) 358.01
    in crisis 358.01
    neonatal 775.2
    pseudoparalytica 358.00

Myasthenia—*continued*
  stomach 536.8
    psychogenic 306.4
  syndrome in
    botulism 005.1 *[358.1]*
    diabetes mellitus 250.6 *[358.1]*
      due to secondary diabetes 249.6 *[358.1]*
    hypothyroidism (*see also* Hypothyroidism)
      244.9 *[358.1]*
    malignant neoplasm NEC 199.1 *[358.1]*
    pernicious anemia 281.0 *[358.1]*
    thyrotoxicosis (*see also* Thyrotoxicosis) 242.9
      [358.1]
Myasthenic 728.87
Mycelium infection NEC 117.9
Mycetismus 988.1
Mycetoma (actinomycotic) 039.9
  bone 039.8
    mycotic 117.4
  foot 039.4
    mycotic 117.4
  madurae 039.9
    mycotic 117.4
  maduromycotic 039.9
    mycotic 117.4
  mycotic 117.4
  nocardial 039.9
Mycobacteriosis —*see* Mycobacterium
Mycobacterium, mycobacterial (infection) 031.9
  acid-fast (bacilli) 031.9
  anonymous (*see also* Mycobacterium, atypical)
    031.9
  atypical (acid-fast bacilli) 031.9
    cutaneous 031.1
    pulmonary 031.0
      tuberculous (*see also* Tuberculosis,
        pulmonary) 011.9
    specified site NEC 031.8
  avium 031.0
    intracellulare complex bacteremia (MAC) 031.2
  balnei 031.1
  Battey 031.0
  cutaneous 031.1
  disseminated 031.2
    avium-intracellulare complex (DMAC) 031.2
  fortuitum 031.0
  intracellulare (battey bacillus) 031.0
  kakerifu 031.8
  kansasii 031.0
  kasongo 031.8
  leprae—*see* Leprosy
  luciflavum 031.0
  marinum 031.1
  pulmonary 031.0
    tuberculous (*see also* Tuberculosis,
      pulmonary) 011.9
  scrofulaceum 031.1
  tuberculosis (human, bovine)—*see also* Tuberculosis
    avian type 031.0
  ulcerans 031.1
  xenopi 031.0
Mycosis, mycotic 117.9
  cutaneous NEC 111.9
  ear 111.8 *[380.15]*
  fungoides (M9700/3) 202.1
  mouth 112.0
  pharynx 117.9
  skin NEC 111.9
  stomatitis 112.0
  systemic NEC 117.9
  tonsil 117.9
  vagina, vaginitis 112.1

Mydriasis (persistent) (pupil) 379.43
Myelatelia 742.59
Myelinoclasis, perivascular, acute
    (postinfectious) NEC 136.9 *[323.61]*
  postimmunization or postvaccinal 323.51
Myelinosis, central pontine 341.8
Myelitis (ascending) (cerebellar) (childhood)
    (chronic) (descending) (diffuse) (disseminated)
    (pressure) (progressive) (spinal cord) (subacute)
    (*see also* Encephalitis) 323.9
  acute (transverse) 341.20
    idiopathic 341.22
    in conditions classified elsewhere 341.21
  due to
    other infection classified elsewhere 136.9
      [323.42]
    specified cause NEC 323.82
    vaccination (any) 323.52
    viral diseases classified elsewhere 323.02
  herpes simplex 054.74
  herpes zoster 053.14
  late effect—*see* category 326
  optic neuritis in 341.0
  postchickenpox 052.2
  postimmunization 323.52
  postinfectious 136.9 *[323.63]*
  postvaccinal 323.52
  postvaricella 052.2
  syphilitic (transverse) 094.89
  toxic 989.9 *[323.72]*
  transverse 323.82
    acute 341.20
      idiopathic 341.22
      in conditions classified elsewhere 341.21
    idiopathic 341.22
  tuberculous (*see also* Tuberculosis) 013.6
  virus 049.9
Myeloblastic —*see* condition
Myelocele (*see also* Spina bifida) 741.9
  with hydrocephalus 741.0
Myelocystocele (*see also* Spina bifida) 741.9
Myelocytic —*see* condition
Myelocytoma 205.1
Myelodysplasia (spinal cord) 742.59
  meaning myelodysplastic syndrome—*see*
    Syndrome, myelodysplastic
Myeloencephalitis —*see* Encephalitis
Myelofibrosis 289.83
  with myeloid metaplasia 238.76
  idiopathic (chronic) 238.76
  megakaryocytic 238.79
  primary 238.76
  secondary 289.83
Myelogenous —*see* condition
Myeloid —*see* condition
Myelokathexis 288.09
Myeloleukodystrophy 330.0
Myelolipoma (M8870/0)—*see* Neoplasm, by site,
    benign
Myeloma (multiple) (plasma cell) (plasmacytic)
    (M9730/3) 203.0
  monostotic (M9731/1) 238.6
  solitary (M9731/1) 238.6
Myelomalacia 336.8
Myelomata, multiple (M9730/3) 203.0
Myelomatosis (M9730/3) 203.0
Myelomeningitis —*see* Meningoencephalitis
Myelomeningocele (spinal cord) (*see also* Spina
    bifida) 741.9
  fetal, causing fetopelvic disproportion 653.7

Myelo-osteo-musculodysplasia hereditaria
  756.89
Myelopathic —*see* condition
Myelopathy (spinal cord) 336.9
  cervical 721.1
  diabetic 250.6 *[336.3]*
    due to secondary diabetes 249.6 *[336.3]*
  drug-induced 336.8
  due to or with
    carbon tetrachloride 987.8 *[323.72]*
    degeneration or displacement, intervertebral
      disc 722.70
      cervical, cervicothoracic 722.71
      lumbar, lumbosacral 722.73
      thoracic, thoracolumbar 722.72
    hydroxyquinoline derivatives 961.3 *[323.72]*
    infection—*see* Encephalitis
    intervertebral disc disorder 722.70
      cervical, cervicothoracic 722.71
      lumbar, lumbosacral 722.73
      thoracic, thoracolumbar 722.72
    lead 984.9 *[323.72]*
    mercury 985.0 *[323.72]*
    neoplastic disease (*see also* Neoplasm, by site)
      239.9 *[336.3]*
    pernicious anemia 281.0 *[336.3]*
    spondylosis 721.91
      cervical 721.1
      lumbar, lumbosacral 721.42
      thoracic 721.41
    thallium 985.8 *[323.72]*
  lumbar, lumbosacral 721.42
  necrotic (subacute) 336.1
  radiation-induced 336.8
  spondylogenic NEC 721.91
    cervical 721.1
    lumbar, lumbosacral 721.42
    thoracic 721.41
  thoracic 721.41
  toxic NEC 989.9 *[323.72]*
  transverse (*see also* Myelitis) 323.82
  vascular 336.1
Myelophthisis 284.2
Myeloproliferative disease (M9960/1) 238.79
Myeloradiculitis (*see also* Polyneuropathy) 357.0
Myeloradiculodysplasia (spinal) 742.59
Myelosarcoma (M9930/3) 205.3
Myelosclerosis 289.89
  with myeloid metaplasia (M9961/1) 238.76
  disseminated, of nervous system 340
  megakaryocytic (M9961/1) 238.79
Myelosis (M9860/3) (*see also* Leukemia,
  myeloid) 205.9
  acute (M9861/3) 205.0
  aleukemic (M9864/3) 205.8
  chronic (M9863/3) 205.1
  erythremic (M9840/3) 207.0
    acute (M9841/3) 207.0
  megakaryocytic (M9920/3) 207.2
  nonleukemic (chronic) 288.8
  subacute (M9862/3) 205.2
Myesthenia —*see* Myasthenia
Myiasis (cavernous) 134.0
  orbit 134.0 *[376.13]*
Myoadenoma, prostate 600.20
  with
    other lower urinary tract symptoms (LUTS)
      600.21
    urinary
      obstruction 600.21
      retention 600.21

Myoblastoma
  granular cell (M9580/0)—*see also* Neoplasm,
    connective tissue, benign
  malignant (M9580/3)—*see* Neoplasm,
    connective tissue, malignant
  tongue (M9580/0) 210.1
Myocardial —*see* condition
Myocardiopathy (congestive) (constrictive)
  (familial) (idiopathic) (infiltrative)
  (obstructive) (primary) (restrictive) (sporadic)
  425.4
  alcoholic 425.5
  amyloid 277.39 *[425.7]*
  beriberi 265.0 *[425.7]*
  cobalt-beer 425.5
  due to
    amyloidosis 277.39 *[425.7]*
    beriberi 265.0 *[425.7]*
    cardiac glycogenosis 271.0 *[425.7]*
    Chagas' disease 086.0
    Friedreich's ataxia 334.0 *[425.8]*
    influenza (*see also* Influenza) 487.8 *[425.8]*
    mucopolysaccharidosis 277.5 *[425.7]*
    myotonia atrophica 359.21 *[425.8]*
    progressive muscular dystrophy 359.1 *[425.8]*
    sarcoidosis 135 *[425.8]*
  glycogen storage 271.0 *[425.7]*
  hypertrophic 425.18
    nonobstructive 425.18
    obstructive 425.11
  metabolic NEC 277.9 *[425.7]*
  nutritional 269.9 *[425.7]*
  obscure (African) 425.2
  peripartum 674.5
  postpartum 674.5
  secondary 425.9
  thyrotoxic (*see also* Thyrotoxicosis) 242.9
    [425.7]
  toxic NEC 425.9
Myocarditis (fibroid) (interstitial) (old)
  (progressive) (senile) (with arteriosclerosis)
  429.0
  with
    rheumatic fever (conditions classifiable to
      390) 398.0
      active (*see also* Myocarditis, acute,
        rheumatic) 391.2
      inactive or quiescent (with chorea) 398.0
  active (nonrheumatic) 422.90
    rheumatic 391.2
      with chorea (acute) (rheumatic)
        (Sydenham's) 392.0
  acute or subacute (interstitial) 422.90
    due to Streptococcus (beta-hemolytic) 391.2
    idiopathic 422.91
    rheumatic 391.2
      with chorea (acute) (rheumatic)
        (Sydenham's) 392.0
    specified type NEC 422.99
  aseptic of newborn 074.23
  bacterial (acute) 422.92
  chagasic 086.0
  chronic (interstitial) 429.0
  congenital 746.89
  constrictive 425.4
  Coxsackie (virus) 074.23
  diphtheritic 032.82

Myocarditis—*continued*
  due to or in
    Coxsackie (virus) 074.23
    diphtheria 032.82
    epidemic louse-borne typhus 080 *[422.0]*
    influenza (*see also* Influenza) 487.8 *[422.0]*
    Lyme disease 088.81 *[422.0]*
    scarlet fever 034.1 *[422.0]*
    toxoplasmosis (acquired) 130.3
    tuberculosis (*see also* Tuberculosis) 017.9
      [422.0]
    typhoid 002.0 *[422.0]*
    typhus NEC 081.9 *[422.0]*
  eosinophilic 422.91
  epidemic of newborn 074.23
  Fiedler's (acute) (isolated) (subacute) 422.91
  giant cell (acute) (subacute) 422.91
  gonococcal 098.85
  granulomatous (idiopathic) (isolated)
    (nonspecific) 422.91
  hypertensive (*see also* Hypertension, heart)
    402.90
  idiopathic 422.91
    granulomatous 422.91
  infective 422.92
  influenzal (*see also* Influenza) 487.8 *[422.0]*
  isolated (diffuse) (granulomatous) 422.91
  malignant 422.99
  meningococcal 036.43
  nonrheumatic, active 422.90
  parenchymatous 422.90
  pneumococcal (acute) (subacute) 422.92
  rheumatic (chronic) (inactive) (with chorea)
    398.0
    active or acute 391.2
      with chorea (acute) (rheumatic)
        (Sydenham's) 392.0
  septic 422.92
  specific (giant cell) (productive) 422.91
  staphylococcal (acute) (subacute) 422.92
  suppurative 422.92
  syphilitic (chronic) 093.82
  toxic 422.93
    rheumatic (*see also* Myocarditis, acute
      rheumatic) 391.2
  tuberculous (*see also* Tuberculosis) 017.9
    [422.0]
  typhoid 002.0 *[422.0]*
  valvular—*see* Endocarditis
  viral, except Coxsackie 422.91
    Coxsackie 074.23
    of newborn (Coxsackie) 074.23
Myocardium, myocardial —*see* condition
Myocardosis (*see also* Cardiomyopathy) 425.4
Myoclonia (essential) 333.2
  epileptica 345.1
  Friedrich's 333.2
  massive 333.2
Myoclonic
  epilepsy, familial (progressive) 345.1
  jerks 333.2
Myoclonus (familial essential) (multifocal)
  (simplex) 333.2
  with epilepsy and with ragged red fibers
    (MERRF syndrome) 277.87
  facial 351.8
  massive (infantile) 333.2
  palatal 333.2
  pharyngeal 333.2

Myocytolysis 429.1
Myodiastasis 728.84
Myoendocarditis —*see also* Endocarditis
  acute or subacute 421.9
Myoepithelioma (M8982/0)—*see* Neoplasm, by
  site, benign
Myofascitis (acute) 729.1
  low back 724.2
Myofibroma (M8890/0)—*see also* Neoplasm,
  connective tissue, benign
  uterus (cervix) (corpus) (*see also* Leiomyoma)
    218.9
Myofibromatosis
  infantile 759.89
Myofibrosis 728.2
  heart (*see also* Myocarditis) 429.0
  humeroscapular region 726.2
  scapulohumeral 726.2
Myofibrositis (*see also* Myositis) 729.1
  scapulohumeral 726.2
Myogelosis (occupational) 728.89
Myoglobinuria 791.3
Myoglobulinuria, primary 791.3
Myokymia —*see also* Myoclonus
  facial 351.8
Myolipoma (M8860/0)
  specified site—*see* Neoplasm, connective tissue,
    benign
  unspecified site 223.0
Myoma (M8895/0)—*see also* Neoplasm,
  connective tissue, benign
  cervix (stump) (uterus) (*see also* Leiomyoma)
    218.9
  malignant (M8895/3)—*see* Neoplasm,
    connective tissue, malignant
  prostate 600.20
    with
      other lower urinary tract symptoms (LUTS)
        600.21
      urinary
        obstruction 600.21
        retention 600.21
  uterus (cervix) (corpus) (*see also* Leiomyoma)
    218.9
    in pregnancy or childbirth 654.1
      affecting fetus or newborn 763.89
      causing obstructed labor 660.2
        affecting fetus or newborn 763.1
Myomalacia 728.9
  cordis, heart (*see also* Degeneration,
    myocardial) 429.1
Myometritis (*see also* Endometritis) 615.9
Myometrium —*see* condition
Myonecrosis, clostridial 040.0
Myopathy 359.9
  alcoholic 359.4
  amyloid 277.39 *[359.6]*
  benign congenital 359.0
  central core 359.0
  centronuclear 359.0
  congenital (benign) 359.0
  critical illness 359.81
  distal 359.1
  due to drugs 359.4
  endocrine 259.9 *[359.5]*
    specified type NEC 259.8 *[359.5]*
  extraocular muscles 376.82
  facioscapulohumeral 359.1

Myopathy—*continued*
  in
    Addison's disease 255.41 *[359.5]*
    amyloidosis 277.39 *[359.6]*
    cretinism 243 *[359.5]*
    Cushing's syndrome 255.0 *[359.5]*
    disseminated lupus erythematosus 710.0 *[359.6]*
    giant cell arteritis 446.5 *[359.6]*
    hyperadrenocorticism NEC 255.3 *[359.5]*
    hyperparathyroidism 252.01 *[359.5]*
    hypopituitarism 253.2 *[359.5]*
    hypothyroidism (*see also* Hypothyroidism)
      244.9 *[359.5]*
    malignant neoplasm NEC (M8000/3) 199.1
      [359.6]
    myxedema (*see also* Myxedema) 244.9 *[359.5]*
    polyarteritis nodosa 446.0 *[359.6]*
    rheumatoid arthritis 714.0 *[359.6]*
    sarcoidosis 135 *[359.6]*
    scleroderma 710.1 *[359.6]*
    Sjögren's disease 710.2 *[359.6]*
    thyrotoxicosis (*see also* Thyrotoxicosis) 242.9
      [359.5]
  inflammatory 359.79
    immune NEC 359.79
    specified NEC 359.79
  intensive care (ICU) 359.81
  limb-girdle 359.1
  myotubular 359.0
  necrotizing, acute 359.81
  nemaline 359.0
  ocular 359.1
  oculopharyngeal 359.1
  of critical illness 359.81
  primary 359.89
  progressive NEC 359.89
  proximal myotonic (PROMM) 359.21
  quadriplegic, acute 359.81
  rod body 359.0
  scapulohumeral 359.1
  specified type NEC 359.89
  toxic 359.4
Myopericarditis (*see also* Pericarditis) 423.9
Myopia (axial) (congenital) (increased curvature
    or refraction, nucleus of lens) 367.1
  degenerative, malignant 360.21
  malignant 360.21
  progressive high (degenerative) 360.21
Myosarcoma (M8895/3)—*see* Neoplasm,
    connective tissue, malignant
Myosis (persistent) 379.42
  stromal (endolymphatic) (M8931/1) 236.0
Myositis 729.1
  clostridial 040.0
  due to posture 729.1
  epidemic 074.1
  fibrosa or fibrous (chronic) 728.2
    Volkmann's (complicating trauma) 958.6
  inclusion body (IBM) 359.71
  infective 728.0
  interstitial 728.81
  multiple—*see* Polymyositis
  occupational 729.1
  orbital, chronic 376.12
  ossificans 728.12
    circumscribed 728.12
    progressive 728.11
    traumatic 728.12
  progressive fibrosing 728.11

Mpurulent 728.0
  rheumatic 729.1
  rheumatoid 729.1
  suppurative 728.0
  syphilitic 095.6
  traumatic (old) 729.1
Myospasia impulsiva 307.23
Myotonia (acquisita) (intermittens) 728.85
  atrophica 359.21
  congenita 359.22
    acetazolamide responsive 359.22
    dominant form 359.22
    recessive form 359.22
  drug-induced 359.24
  dystrophica 359.21
  fluctuans 359.29
  levior 359.22
  permanens 359.29
Myotonic pupil 379.46
Myriapodiasis 134.1
Myringitis
  with otitis media—*see* Otitis media
  acute 384.00
    specified type NEC 384.09
  bullosa hemorrhagica 384.01
  bullous 384.01
  chronic 384.1
Mysophobia 300.29
Mytilotoxism 988.0
Myxadenitis labialis 528.5
Myxedema (adult) (idiocy) (infantile) (juvenile)
    (thyroid gland) (*see also* Hypothyroidism)
    244.9
  circumscribed 242.9
  congenital 243
  cutis 701.8
  localized (pretibial) 242.9
  madness (acute) 293.0
    subacute 293.1
  papular 701.8
  pituitary 244.8
  postpartum 674.8
  pretibial 242.9
  primary 244.9
Myxochondrosarcoma (M9220/3)—*see*
    Neoplasm, cartilage, malignant
Myxofibroma (M8811/0)—*see also* Neoplasm,
    connective tissue, benign
  odontogenic (M9320/0) 213.1
    upper jaw (bone) 213.0
Myxofibrosarcoma (M8811/3)—*see* Neoplasm,
    connective tissue, malignant
Myxolipoma (M8852/0) (*see also* Lipoma, by
    site) 214.9
Myxoliposarcoma (M8852/3)—*see* Neoplasm,
    connective tissue, malignant
Myxoma (M8840/0)—*see also* Neoplasm,
    connective tissue, benign
  odontogenic (M9320/0) 213.1
    upper jaw (bone) 213.0
Myxosarcoma (M8840/3)—*see* Neoplasm,
    connective tissue, malignant

N

Naegeli's
disease (hereditary hemorrhagic
thrombasthenia) 287.1
leukemia, monocytic (M9863/3) 205.1
syndrome (incontinentia pigmenti) 757.33
Naffziger's syndrome 353.0
Naga sore (*see also* Ulcer, skin) 707.9
Nägele's pelvis 738.6
with disproportion (fetopelvic) 653.0
affecting fetus or newborn 763.1
causing obstructed labor 660.1
affecting fetus or newborn 763.1
Nager-de Reynier syndrome (dysostosis
mandibularis) 756.0
Nail —*see also* condition
biting 307.9
patella syndrome (hereditary
osteo-onychodysplasia) 756.89
Nanism, nanosomia (*see also* Dwarfism) 259.4
hypophyseal 253.3
pituitary 253.3
renis, renalis 588.0
Nanukayami 100.89
Napkin rash 691.0
Narcissism 301.81
Narcolepsy 347.00
with cataplexy 347.01
in conditions classified elsewhere 347.10
with cataplexy 347.11
Narcosis
carbon dioxide (respiratory) 786.09
due to drug
correct substance properly administered 780.09
overdose or wrong substance given or taken
977.9
specified drug—*see* Table of drugs and
chemicals
Narcotism (chronic) (*see also* listing under
Dependence) 304.9
acute
correct substance properly administered 349.82
overdose or wrong substance given or taken
967.8
specified drug—*see* Table of drugs and
chemicals
NARP syndrome (Neuropathy, ataxia and
retinitis pigmentosa) 277.87
Narrow
anterior chamber angle 365.02
pelvis (inlet) (outlet)—*see* Contraction, pelvis
Narrowing
artery NEC 447.1
auditory, internal 433.8
basilar 433.0
with other precerebral artery 433.3
bilateral 433.3
carotid 433.1
with other precerebral artery 433.3
bilateral 433.3
cerebellar 433.8
choroidal 433.8
communicating posterior 433.8
coronary —*see also* Arteriosclerosis, coronary
congenital 746.85
due to syphilis 090.5
hypophyseal 433.8
pontine 433.8

Narrowing—*continued*
precerebral NEC 433.9
multiple or bilateral 433.3
specified NEC 433.8
vertebral 433.2
with other precerebral artery 433.3
bilateral 433.3
auditory canal (external) (*see also* Stricture, ear
canal, acquired) 380.50
cerebral arteries 437.0
cicatricial—*see* Cicatrix
congenital—*see* Anomaly, congenital
coronary artery—*see* Narrowing, artery,
coronary
ear, middle 385.22
Eustachian tube (*see also* Obstruction,
Eustachian tube) 381.60
eyelid 374.46
congenital 743.62
intervertebral disc or space NEC—*see*
Degeneration, intervertebral disc
joint space, hip 719.85
larynx 478.74
lids 374.46
congenital 743.62
mesenteric artery (with gangrene) 557.0
palate 524.89
palpebral fissure 374.46
retinal artery 362.13
ureter 593.3
urethra (*see also* Stricture, urethra) 598.9
Narrowness, abnormal, eyelid 743.62
Nasal —*see* condition
Nasolacrimal —*see* condition
Nasopharyngeal —*see also* condition
bursa 478.29
pituitary gland 759.2
torticollis 723.5
Nasopharyngitis (acute) (infective) (subacute) 460
chronic 472.2
due to external agent—*see* Condition,
respiratory, chronic, due to
due to external agent—*see* Condition,
respiratory, due to
septic 034.0
streptococcal 034.0
suppurative (chronic) 472.2
ulcerative (chronic) 472.2
Nasopharynx, nasopharyngeal —*see* condition
Natal tooth, teeth 520.6
Nausea (*see also* Vomiting) 787.02
epidemic 078.82
gravidarum—*see* Hyperemesis, gravidarum
marina 994.6
with vomiting 787.01
Naval —*see* condition
Neapolitan fever (*see also* Brucellosis) 023.9
Near drowning 994.1
Nearsightedness 367.1
Near-syncope 780.2
Nebécourt's syndrome 253.3
Nebula, cornea (eye) 371.01
congenital 743.43
interfering with vision 743.42
Necator americanus infestation 126.1
Necatoriasis 126.1
Neck —*see* condition
Necrencephalus (*see also* Softening, brain) 437.8

Necrobacillosis 040.3
Necrobiosis 799.89
  brain or cerebral (*see also* Softening, brain) 437.8
  lipoidica 709.3
    diabeticorum 250.8 *[709.3]*
    due to secondary diabetes 249.8 *[709.3]*
Necrodermolysis 695.15
Necrolysis, toxic epidermal 695.15
  due to drug
    correct substance properly administered 695.15
    overdose or wrong substance given or taken
      977.9
      specified drug—*see* Table of drugs and
        chemicals
  Stevens-Johnson syndrome overlap (SJS-TEN
    overlap syndrome) 695.14
Necrophilia 302.89
Necrosis, necrotic
  adrenal (capsule) (gland) 255.8
  antrum, nasal sinus 478.19
  aorta (hyaline) (*see also* Aneurysm, aorta) 441.9
    cystic medial 441.00
      abdominal 441.02
      thoracic 441.01
      thoracoabdominal 441.03
    ruptured 441.5
  arteritis 446.0
  artery 447.5
  aseptic, bone 733.40
    femur (head) (neck) 733.42
      medial condyle 733.43
    humoral head 733.41
    jaw 733.45
    medial femoral condyle 733.43
    specified site NEC 733.49
    talus 733.44
  avascular, bone NEC (*see also* Necrosis, aseptic,
    bone) 733.40
  bladder (aseptic) (sphincter) 596.89
  bone (*see also* Osteomyelitis) 730.1
    acute 730.0
    aseptic or avascular 733.40
      femur (head) (neck) 733.42
        medial condyle 733.43
      humoral head 733.41
      jaw 733.45
      medial femoral condyle 733.43
      specified site NEC 733.49
      talus 733.44
    ethmoid 478.19
    ischemic 733.40
    jaw 526.4
      aseptic 733.45
    marrow 289.89
    Paget's (osteitis deformans) 731.0
    tuberculous—*see* Tuberculosis, bone
  brain (softening) (*see also* Softening, brain) 437.8
  breast (aseptic) (fat) (segmental) 611.3
  bronchus, bronchi 519.19
  central nervous system NEC (*see also*
    Softening, brain) 437.8
  cerebellar (*see also* Softening, brain) 437.8
  cerebral (softening) (*see also* Softening, brain) 437.8
  cerebrospinal (softening) (*see also* Softening,
    brain) 437.8
  colon 557.0
  cornea (*see also* Keratitis) 371.40
  cortical, kidney 583.6
  cystic medial (aorta) 441.00
    abdominal 441.02
    thoracic 441.01
    thoracoabdominal 441.03

Necrosis, necrotic—*continued*
  dental 521.09
    pulp 522.1
  due to swallowing corrosive substance—*see*
    Burn, by site
  ear (ossicle) 385.24
  esophagus 530.89
  ethmoid (bone) 478.19
  eyelid 374.50
  fat, fatty (generalized) (*see also* Degeneration,
    fatty) 272.8
    abdominal wall 567.82
    breast (aseptic) (segmental) 611.3
    intestine 569.89
    localized—*see* Degeneration, by site, fatty
    mesentery 567.82
    omentum 567.82
    pancreas 577.8
    peritoneum 567.82
    skin (subcutaneous) 709.3
      newborn 778.1
  femur (aseptic) (avascular) 733.42
    head 733.42
    medial condyle 733.43
    neck 733.42
  gallbladder (*see also* Cholecystitis, acute) 575.0
  gangrenous 785.4
  gastric 537.89
  glottis 478.79
  heart (myocardium)—*see* Infarct, myocardium
  hepatic (*see also* Necrosis, liver) 570
  hip (aseptic) (avascular) 733.42
  intestine (acute) (hemorrhagic) (massive) 557.0
  ischemic 785.4
  jaw 526.4
    aseptic 733.45
  kidney (bilateral) 583.9
    acute 584.9
    cortical 583.6
      acute 584.6
        with
          abortion—*see* Abortion, by type, with
            renal failure
          ectopic pregnancy (*see also* categories
            633.0-633.9) 639.3
          molar pregnancy (*see also* categories
            630-632) 639.3
        complicating pregnancy 646.2
          affecting fetus or newborn 760.1
        following labor and delivery 669.3
    medullary (papillary) (*see also* Pyelitis) 590.80
      in
        acute renal failure 584.7
        nephritis, nephropathy 583.7
    papillary (*see also* Pyelitis) 590.80
      in
        acute renal failure 584.7
        nephritis, nephropathy 583.7
    tubular 584.5
      with
        abortion—*see* Abortion, by type, with
          renal failure
        ectopic pregnancy (*see also* categories
          633.0-633.9) 639.3
        molar pregnancy (*see also* categories
          630-632) 639.3
      complicating
        abortion 639.3
        ectopic or molar pregnancy 639.3
        pregnancy 646.2
          affecting fetus or newborn 760.1

Necrosis, necrotic—*continued*
kidney—*continued*
tubular—*continued*
following labor and delivery 669.3
traumatic 958.5
larynx 478.79
liver (acute) (congenital) (diffuse) (massive) (subacute) 570
with
abortion—*see* Abortion, by type, with specified complication NEC
ectopic pregnancy (*see also* categories 633.0-633.9) 639.8
molar pregnancy (*see also* categories 630-632) 639.8
complicating pregnancy 646.7
affecting fetus or newborn 760.8
following
abortion 639.8
ectopic or molar pregnancy 639.8
obstetrical 646.7
postabortal 639.8
puerperal, postpartum 674.8
toxic 573.3
lung 513.0
lymphatic gland 683
mammary gland 611.3
mastoid (chronic) 383.1
mesentery 557.0
fat 567.82
mitral valve—*see* Insufficiency, mitral
myocardium, myocardial—*see* Infarct, myocardium
nose (septum) 478.19
omentum 557.0
with mesenteric infarction 557.0
fat 567.82
orbit, orbital 376.10
ossicles, ear (aseptic) 385.24
ovary (*see also* Salpingo-oophoritis) 614.2
pancreas (aseptic) (duct) (fat) 577.8
acute 577.0
infective 577.0
papillary, kidney (*see also* Pyelitis) 590.80
perineum 624.8
peritoneum 557.0
with mesenteric infarction 557.0
fat 567.82
pharynx 462
in granulocytopenia 288.09
phosphorus 983.9
pituitary (gland) (postpartum) (Sheehan) 253.2
placenta (*see also* Placenta, abnormal) 656.7
pneumonia 513.0
pulmonary 513.0
pulp (dental) 522.1
pylorus 537.89
radiation—*see* Necrosis, by site
radium—*see* Necrosis, by site
renal—*see* Necrosis, kidney
sclera 379.19
scrotum 608.89
skin or subcutaneous tissue 709.8
due to burn—*see* Burn, by site
gangrenous 785.4
spine, spinal (column) 730.18
acute 730.18
cord 336.1
spleen 289.59
stomach 537.89
stomatitis 528.1

Necrosis, necrotic—*continued*
subcutaneous fat 709.3
fetus or newborn 778.1
subendocardial—*see* Infarct, myocardium
suprarenal (capsule) (gland) 255.8
teeth, tooth 521.09
testis 608.89
thymus (gland) 254.8
tonsil 474.8
trachea 519.19
tuberculous NEC—*see* Tuberculosis
tubular (acute) (anoxic) (toxic) 584.5
due to a procedure 997.5
umbilical cord, affecting fetus or newborn 762.6
vagina 623.8
vertebra (lumbar) 730.18
acute 730.18
tuberculous (*see also* Tuberculosis) 015.0 *[730.8]*
vesical (aseptic) (bladder) 596.89
vulva 624.8
x-ray—*see* Necrosis, by site
Necrospermia 606.0
Necrotizing angiitis 446.0
Negativism 301.7
Neglect (child) (newborn) NEC 995.52
adult 995.84
after or at birth 995.52
hemispatial 781.8
left-sided 781.8
sensory 781.8
visuospatial 781.8
Negri bodies 071
Neill-Dingwall syndrome (microcephaly and dwarfism) 759.89
Neisserian infection NEC—*see* Gonococcus
Nematodiasis NEC (*see also* Infestation, Nematode) 127.9
ancylostoma (*see also* Ancylostomiasis) 126.9
Neoformans cryptococcus infection 117.5
Neonatal —*see also* condition
abstinence syndrome 779.5
adrenoleukodystrophy 277.86
teeth, tooth 520.6
Neonatorum —*see* condition
Neoplasia
anal intraepithelial I (AIN I) (histologically confirmed) 569.44
anal intraepithelial II (AIN II) (histologically confirmed) 569.44
anal intraepithelial III (AIN III) 230.6
anal canal 230.5
endometrial intraepithelial (EIN) 621.35
multiple endocine (MEN)
type I 258.01
type II A 258.02
type II B 258.03
vaginal intraepithelial I (VAIN I) 623.0
vaginal intraepithelial II (VAIN II) 623.0
vaginal intraepithelial III (VAIN III) 233.31
vulvar intraepithelial I (VIN I) 624.01
vulvar intraepithelial II (VIN II) 624.02
vulvar intraepithelial III (VIN III) 233.32

"N" listing resumes after
"Neoplasm, neoplastic" table…

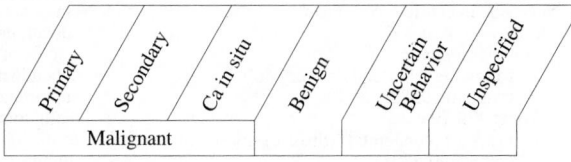

	Malignant					
	Primary	Secondary	Ca in situ	Benign	Uncertain Behavior	Unspecified
Neoplasm, neoplastic	199.1	199.1	234.9	229.9	238.9	239.9

> *Note—1. The list below gives the code numbers for neoplasms by anatomical site. For each site there are six possible code numbers according to whether the neoplasm in question is malignant, benign, in situ, of uncertain behavior, or of unspecified nature. The description of the neoplasm will often indicate which of the six columns is appropriate; e.g., malignant melanoma of skin, benign fibroadenoma of breast, carcinoma in situ of cervix uteri.*
>
> *Where such descriptors are not present, the remainder of the Index should be consulted where guidance is given to the appropriate column for each morphological (histological) variety listed; e.g., Mesonephroma—see Neoplasm, malignant; Embryoma—see also Neoplasm, uncertain behavior; Disease, Bowen's—see Neoplasm, skin, in situ. However, the guidance in the Index can be overridden if one of the descriptors mentioned above is present; e.g., malignant adenoma of colon is coded to 153.9 and not to 211.3 as the adjective "malignant" overrides the Index entry "Adenoma—see also Neoplasm, benign."*
>
> *Note—2. Sites marked with the sign * (e.g., face NEC*) should be classified to malignant neoplasm of skin of these sites if the variety of neoplasm is a squamous cell carcinoma or an epidermoid carcinoma and to benign neoplasm of skin of these sites if the variety of neoplasm is a papilloma (any type).*

	Primary	Secondary	Ca in situ	Benign	Uncertain Behavior	Unspecified
abdomen, abdominal	195.2	198.89	234.8	229.8	238.8	239.89
cavity	195.2	198.89	234.8	229.8	238.8	239.89
organ	195.2	198.89	234.8	229.8	238.8	239.89
viscera	195.2	198.89	234.8	229.8	238.8	239.89
wall	173.50	198.2	232.5	216.5	238.2	239.2
basal cell carcinoma	173.51	—	—	—	—	—
connective tissue	171.5	198.89	—	215.5	238.1	239.2
specified type NEC	173.59	—	—	—	—	—
squamous cell carcinoma	173.52	—	—	—	—	—
abdominopelvic	195.8	198.89	234.8	229.8	238.8	239.89
accessory sinus—*see* Neoplasm, sinus						
acoustic nerve	192.0	198.4	—	225.1	237.9	239.7
acromion (process)	170.4	198.5	—	213.4	238.0	239.2
adenoid (pharynx) (tissue)	147.1	198.89	230.0	210.7	235.1	239.0
adipose tissue (*see also* Neoplasm, connective tissue)	171.9	198.89	—	215.9	238.1	239.2
adnexa (uterine)	183.9	198.82	233.39	221.8	236.3	239.5
adrenal (cortex) (gland) (medulla)	194.0	198.7	234.8	227.0	237.2	239.7
ala nasi (external)	173.30	198.2	232.3	216.3	238.2	239.2
alimentary canal or tract NEC	159.9	197.8	230.9	211.9	235.5	239.0
alveolar	143.9	198.89	230.0	210.4	235.1	239.0
mucosa	143.9	198.89	230.0	210.4	235.1	239.0
lower	143.1	198.89	230.0	210.4	235.1	239.0
upper	143.0	198.89	230.0	210.4	235.1	239.0
ridge or process	170.1	198.5	—	213.1	238.0	239.2
carcinoma	143.9	—	—	—	—	—
lower	143.1	—	—	—	—	—
upper	143.0	—	—	—	—	—
lower	170.1	198.5	—	213.1	238.0	239.2
mucosa	143.9	198.89	230.0	210.4	235.1	239.0
lower	143.1	198.89	230.0	210.4	235.1	239.0
upper	143.0	198.89	230.0	210.4	235.1	239.0
upper	170.0	198.5	—	213.0	238.0	239.2
sulcus	145.1	198.89	230.0	210.4	235.1	239.0
alveolus	143.9	198.89	230.0	210.4	235.1	239.0
lower	143.1	198.89	230.0	210.4	235.1	239.0
upper	143.0	198.89	230.0	210.4	235.1	239.0
ampulla of Vater	156.2	197.8	230.8	211.5	235.3	239.0
ankle NEC*	195.5	198.89	232.7	229.8	238.8	239.89
anorectum, anorectal (junction)	154.8	197.5	230.7	211.4	235.2	239.0

| | Malignant | | | | | |
	Primary	Secondary	Ca in situ	Benign	Uncertain Behavior	Unspecified
antecubital fossa or space*.	195.4	198.89	232.6	229.8	238.8	239.89
antrum (Highmore)						
(maxillary)	160.2	197.3	231.8	212.0	235.9	239.1
pyloric	151.2	197.8	230.2	211.1	235.2	239.0
tympanicum	160.1	197.3	231.8	212.0	235.9	239.1
anus, anal.	154.3	197.5	230.6	211.4	235.5	239.0
canal	154.2	197.5	230.5	211.4	235.5	239.0
contiguous sites with rectosigmoid						
junction or rectum	154.8	—	—	—	—	—
margin (see also Neoplasm, anus,						
skin)	173.50	198.2	232.5	216.5	238.2	239.2
skin	173.50	198.2	232.5	216.5	238.2	239.2
basal cell carcinoma	173.51	—	—	—	—	—
specified type NEC.	173.59	—	—	—	—	—
squamous cell carcinoma	173.52	—	—	—	—	—
sphincter	154.2	197.5	230.5	211.4	235.5	239.0
aorta (thoracic)	171.4	198.89	—	215.4	238.1	239.2
abdominal	171.5	198.89	—	215.5	238.1	239.2
aortic body	194.6	198.89	—	227.6	237.3	239.7
aponeurosis.	171.9	198.89	—	215.9	238.1	239.2
palmar	171.2	198.89	—	215.2	238.1	239.2
plantar	171.3	198.89	—	215.3	238.1	239.2
appendix	153.5	197.5	230.3	211.3	235.2	239.0
arachnoid (cerebral)	192.1	198.4	—	225.2	237.6	239.7
spinal	192.3	198.4	—	225.4	237.6	239.7
areola (female)	174.0	198.81	233.0	217	238.3	239.3
male	175.0	198.81	233.0	217	238.3	239.3
arm NEC*	195.4	198.89	232.6	229.8	238.8	239.89
artery—see Neoplasm, connective tissue						
aryepiglottic fold	148.2	198.89	230.0	210.8	235.1	239.0
hypopharyngeal aspect	148.2	198.89	230.0	210.8	235.1	239.0
laryngeal aspect	161.1	197.3	231.0	212.1	235.6	239.1
marginal zone	148.2	198.89	230.0	210.8	235.1	239.0
arytenoid (cartilage)	161.3	197.3	231.0	212.1	235.6	239.1
fold—see Neoplasm, aryepiglottic						
associated with transplanted organ. .	199.2	—	—	—	—	—
atlas.	170.2	198.5	—	213.2	238.0	239.2
atrium, cardiac	164.1	198.89	—	212.7	238.8	239.89
auditory						
canal (external) (skin) (see also						
Neoplasm, skin, ear)	173.20	198.2	232.2	216.2	238.2	239.2
internal	160.1	197.3	231.8	212.0	235.9	239.1
nerve	192.0	198.4	—	225.1	237.9	239.7
tube.	160.1	197.3	231.8	212.0	235.9	239.1
opening.	147.2	198.89	230.0	210.7	235.1	239.0
auricle, ear (see also Neoplasm,						
skin, ear)	173.20	198.2	232.2	216.2	238.2	239.2
cartilage	171.0	198.89	—	215.0	238.1	239.2
auricular canal (external) (see also						
Neoplasm, skin, ear)	173.20	198.2	232.2	216.2	238.2	239.2
internal	160.1	197.3	231.8	212.0	235.9	239.1
autonomic nerve or nervous						
system NEC.	171.9	198.89	—	215.9	238.1	239.2
axilla, axillary	195.1	198.89	234.8	229.8	238.8	239.89
fold (see also Neoplasm, skin,						
trunk).	173.50	198.2	232.5	216.5	238.2	239.2
back NEC*	195.8	198.89	232.5	229.8	238.8	239.89
Bartholin's gland.	184.1	198.82	233.32	221.2	236.3	239.5
basal ganglia	191.0	198.3	—	225.0	237.5	239.6
basis pedunculi	191.7	198.3	—	225.0	237.5	239.6
bile or biliary (tract)	156.9	197.8	230.8	211.5	235.3	239.0
canaliculi (biliferi)						
(intrahepatic)	155.1	197.8	230.8	211.5	235.3	239.0

	Primary	Secondary	Ca in situ	Benign	Uncertain Behavior	Unspecified
	Malignant					
canals, interlobular	155.1	197.8	230.8	211.5	235.3	239.0
contiguous sites	156.8	—	—	—	—	—
duct or passage (common) (cyst)						
(extrahepatic).	156.1	197.8	230.8	211.5	235.3	239.0
contiguous sites with						
gallbladder	156.8	—	—	—	—	—
interlobular	155.1	197.8	230.8	211.5	235.3	239.0
intrahepatic	155.1	197.8	230.8	211.5	235.3	239.0
and extrahepatic	156.9	197.8	230.8	211.5	235.3	239.0
bladder (urinary)	188.9	198.1	233.7	223.3	236.7	239.4
contiguous sites	188.8	—	—	—	—	—
dome	188.1	198.1	233.7	223.3	236.7	239.4
neck	188.5	198.1	233.7	223.3	236.7	239.4
orifice.	188.9	198.1	233.7	223.3	236.7	239.4
ureteric	188.6	198.1	233.7	223.3	236.7	239.4
urethral	188.5	198.1	233.7	223.3	236.7	239.4
sphincter	188.8	198.1	233.7	223.3	236.7	239.4
trigone	188.0	198.1	233.7	223.3	236.7	239.4
urachus	188.7	—	233.7	223.3	236.7	239.4
wall	188.9	198.1	233.7	223.3	236.7	239.4
anterior	188.3	198.1	233.7	223.3	236.7	239.4
lateral	188.2	198.1	233.7	223.3	236.7	239.4
posterior	188.4	198.1	233.7	223.3	236.7	239.4
blood vessel—*see* Neoplasm, connective tissue						
bone (periosteum)	170.9	198.5	—	213.9	238.0	239.2

Note—Carcinomas and adenocarcinomas, of any type other than intraosseous or odontogenic, of the sites listed under "Neoplasm, bone" should be considered as constituting metastatic spread from an unspecified primary site and coded to 198.5 for morbidity coding .

	Primary	Secondary	Ca in situ	Benign	Uncertain Behavior	Unspecified
acetabulum	170.6	198.5	—	213.6	238.0	239.2
acromion (process)	170.4	198.5	—	213.4	238.0	239.2
ankle	170.8	198.5	—	213.8	238.0	239.2
arm NEC	170.4	198.5	—	213.4	238.0	239.2
astragalus	170.8	198.5	—	213.8	238.0	239.2
atlas	170.2	198.5	—	213.2	238.0	239.2
axis	170.2	198.5	—	213.2	238.0	239.2
back NEC	170.2	198.5	—	213.2	238.0	239.2
calcaneus	170.8	198.5	—	213.8	238.0	239.2
calvarium	170.0	198.5	—	213.0	238.0	239.2
carpus (any)	170.5	198.5	—	213.5	238.0	239.2
cartilage NEC	170.9	198.5	—	213.9	238.0	239.2
clavicle	170.3	198.5	—	213.3	238.0	239.2
clivus	170.0	198.5	—	213.0	238.0	239.2
coccygeal vertebra	170.6	198.5	—	213.6	238.0	239.2
coccyx	170.6	198.5	—	213.6	238.0	239.2
costal cartilage	170.3	198.5	—	213.3	238.0	239.2
costovertebral joint	170.3	198.5	—	213.3	238.0	239.2
cranial	170.0	198.5	—	213.0	238.0	239.2
cuboid	170.8	198.5	—	213.8	238.0	239.2
cuneiform	170.9	198.5	—	213.9	238.0	239.2
ankle	170.8	198.5	—	213.8	238.0	239.2
wrist	170.5	198.5	—	213.5	238.0	239.2
digital	170.9	198.5	—	213.9	238.0	239.2
finger	170.5	198.5	—	213.5	238.0	239.2
toe	170.8	198.5	—	213.8	238.0	239.2
elbow	170.4	198.5	—	213.4	238.0	239.2
ethmoid (labyrinth).	170.0	198.5	—	213.0	238.0	239.2
face	170.0	198.5	—	213.0	238.0	239.2
lower jaw	170.1	198.5	—	213.1	238.0	239.2
femur (any part)	170.7	198.5	—	213.7	238.0	239.2
fibula (any part)	170.7	198.5	—	213.7	238.0	239.2
finger (any)	170.5	198.5	—	213.5	238.0	239.2
foot	170.8	198.5	—	213.8	238.0	239.2

	Malignant			Benign	Uncertain Behavior	Unspecified
	Primary	Secondary	Ca in situ			
forearm	170.4	198.5	—	213.4	238.0	239.2
frontal	170.0	198.5	—	213.0	238.0	239.2
hand	170.5	198.5	—	213.5	238.0	239.2
heel	170.8	198.5	—	213.8	238.0	239.2
hip	170.6	198.5	—	213.6	238.0	239.2
humerus (any part)	170.4	198.5	—	213.4	238.0	239.2
hyoid	170.0	198.5	—	213.0	238.0	239.2
ilium	170.6	198.5	—	213.6	238.0	239.2
innominate	170.6	198.5	—	213.6	238.0	239.2
intervertebral cartilage or						
disc.	170.2	198.5	—	213.2	238.0	239.2
ischium	170.6	198.5	—	213.6	238.0	239.2
jaw (lower)	170.1	198.5	—	213.1	238.0	239.2
upper	170.0	198.5	—	213.0	238.0	239.2
knee	170.7	198.5	—	213.7	238.0	239.2
leg NEC	170.7	198.5	—	213.7	238.0	239.2
limb NEC.	170.9	198.5	—	213.9	238.0	239.2
lower (long bones)	170.7	198.5	—	213.7	238.0	239.2
short bones	170.8	198.5	—	213.8	238.0	239.2
upper (long bones)	170.4	198.5	—	213.4	238.0	239.2
short bones	170.5	198.5	—	213.5	238.0	239.2
long.	170.9	198.5	—	213.9	238.0	239.2
lower limbs NEC.	170.7	198.5	—	213.7	238.0	239.2
upper limbs NEC.	170.4	198.5	—	213.4	238.0	239.2
malar	170.0	198.5	—	213.0	238.0	239.2
mandible	170.1	198.5	—	213.1	238.0	239.2
marrow NEC	202.9	198.5	—	—	—	238.79
mastoid	170.0	198.5	—	213.0	238.0	239.2
maxilla, maxillary						
(superior)	170.0	198.5	—	213.0	238.0	239.2
inferior	170.1	198.5	—	213.1	238.0	239.2
metacarpus (any)	170.5	198.5	—	213.5	238.0	239.2
metatarsus (any)	170.8	198.5	—	213.8	238.0	239.2
navicular (ankle)	170.8	198.5	—	213.8	238.0	239.2
hand	170.5	198.5	—	213.5	238.0	239.2
nose, nasal	170.0	198.5	—	213.0	238.0	239.2
occipital	170.0	198.5	—	213.0	238.0	239.2
orbit	170.0	198.5	—	213.0	238.0	239.2
parietal	170.0	198.5	—	213.0	238.0	239.2
patella	170.8	198.5	—	213.8	238.0	239.2
pelvic	170.6	198.5	—	213.6	238.0	239.2
phalanges	170.9	198.5	—	213.9	238.0	239.2
foot	170.8	198.5	—	213.8	238.0	239.2
hand	170.5	198.5	—	213.5	238.0	239.2
pubic	170.6	198.5	—	213.6	238.0	239.2
radius (any part)	170.4	198.5	—	213.4	238.0	239.2
rib.	170.3	198.5	—	213.3	238.0	239.2
sacral vertebra	170.6	198.5	—	213.6	238.0	239.2
sacrum	170.6	198.5	—	213.6	238.0	239.2
scaphoid (of hand)	170.5	198.5	—	213.5	238.0	239.2
of ankle.	170.8	198.5	—	213.8	238.0	239.2
scapula (any part)	170.4	198.5	—	213.4	238.0	239.2
sella turcica.	170.0	198.5	—	213.0	238.0	239.2
short	170.9	198.5	—	213.9	238.0	239.2
lower limb	170.8	198.5	—	213.8	238.0	239.2
upper limb	170.5	198.5	—	213.5	238.0	239.2
shoulder	170.4	198.5	—	213.4	238.0	239.2
skeleton, skeletal NEC	170.9	198.5	—	213.9	238.0	239.2
skull	170.0	198.5	—	213.0	238.0	239.2
sphenoid	170.0	198.5	—	213.0	238.0	239.2
spine, spinal (column)	170.2	198.5	—	213.2	238.0	239.2
coccyx	170.6	198.5	—	213.6	238.0	239.2
sacrum	170.6	198.5	—	213.6	238.0	239.2

	Malignant			Benign	Uncertain Behavior	Unspecified
	Primary	Secondary	Ca in situ			
sternum	170.3	198.5	—	213.3	238.0	239.2
tarsus (any)	170.8	198.5	—	213.8	238.0	239.2
temporal	170.0	198.5	—	213.0	238.0	239.2
thumb	170.5	198.5	—	213.5	238.0	239.2
tibia (any part)	170.7	198.5	—	213.7	238.0	239.2
toe (any)	170.8	198.5	—	213.8	238.0	239.2
trapezium	170.5	198.5	—	213.5	238.0	239.2
trapezoid	170.5	198.5	—	213.5	238.0	239.2
turbinate	170.0	198.5	—	213.0	238.0	239.2
ulna (any part)	170.4	198.5	—	213.4	238.0	239.2
unciform	170.5	198.5	—	213.5	238.0	239.2
vertebra (column)	170.2	198.5	—	213.2	238.0	239.2
coccyx	170.6	198.5	—	213.6	238.0	239.2
sacrum	170.6	198.5	—	213.6	238.0	239.2
vomer	170.0	198.5	—	213.0	238.0	239.2
wrist	170.5	198.5	—	213.5	238.0	239.2
xiphoid process	170.3	198.5	—	213.3	238.0	239.2
zygomatic	170.0	198.5	—	213.0	238.0	239.2
book-leaf (mouth)	145.8	198.89	230.0	210.4	235.1	239.0
bowel—see Neoplasm, intestine						
brachial plexus	171.2	198.89	—	215.2	238.1	239.2
brain NEC	191.9	198.3	—	225.0	237.5	239.6
basal ganglia	191.0	198.3	—	225.0	237.5	239.6
cerebellopontine angle	191.6	198.3	—	225.0	237.5	239.6
cerebellum NOS	191.6	198.3	—	225.0	237.5	239.6
cerebrum	191.0	198.3	—	225.0	237.5	239.6
choroid plexus	191.5	198.3	—	225.0	237.5	239.6
contiguous sites	191.8	—	—	—	—	—
corpus callosum	191.8	198.3	—	225.0	237.5	239.6
corpus striatum	191.0	198.3	—	225.0	237.5	239.6
cortex (cerebral)	191.0	198.3	—	225.0	237.5	239.6
frontal lobe	191.1	198.3	—	225.0	237.5	239.6
globus pallidus	191.0	198.3	—	225.0	237.5	239.6
hippocampus	191.2	198.3	—	225.0	237.5	239.6
hypothalamus	191.0	198.3	—	225.0	237.5	239.6
internal capsule	191.0	198.3	—	225.0	237.5	239.6
medulla oblongata	191.7	198.3	—	225.0	237.5	239.6
meninges	192.1	198.4	—	225.2	237.6	239.7
midbrain	191.7	198.3	—	225.0	237.5	239.6
occipital lobe	191.4	198.3	—	225.0	237.5	239.6
parietal lobe	191.3	198.3	—	225.0	237.5	239.6
peduncle	191.7	198.3	—	225.0	237.5	239.6
pons	191.7	198.3	—	225.0	237.5	239.6
stem	191.7	198.3	—	225.0	237.5	239.6
tapetum	191.8	198.3	—	225.0	237.5	239.6
temporal lobe	191.2	198.3	—	225.0	237.5	239.6
thalamus	191.0	198.3	—	225.0	237.5	239.6
uncus	191.2	198.3	—	225.0	237.5	239.6
ventricle (floor)	191.5	198.3	—	225.0	237.5	239.6
branchial (cleft) (vestiges)	146.8	198.89	230.0	210.6	235.1	239.0
breast (connective tissue) (female) (glandular tissue) (soft parts)	174.9	198.81	233.0	217	238.3	239.3
areola	174.0	198.81	233.0	217	238.3	239.3
male	175.0	198.81	233.0	217	238.3	239.3
axillary tail	174.6	198.81	233.0	217	238.3	239.3
central portion	174.1	198.81	233.0	217	238.3	239.3
contiguous sites	174.8	—	—	—	—	—
ectopic sites	174.8	198.81	233.0	217	238.3	239.3
inner	174.8	198.81	233.0	217	238.3	239.3
lower	174.8	198.81	233.0	217	238.3	239.3
lower-inner quadrant	174.3	198.81	233.0	217	238.3	239.3
lower-outer quadrant	174.5	198.81	233.0	217	238.3	239.3

	Malignant					
	Primary	Secondary	Ca in situ	Benign	Uncertain Behavior	Unspecified
male	175.9	198.81	233.0	217	238.3	239.3
areola	175.0	198.81	233.0	217	238.3	239.3
ectopic tissue	175.9	198.81	233.0	217	238.3	239.3
nipple	175.0	198.81	233.0	217	238.3	239.3
mastectomy site (skin) (*see also* Neoplasm, mastectomy site)	173.50	198.2	—	—	—	—
specified as breast tissue	174.8	198.81	—	—	—	—
midline	174.8	198.81	233.0	217	238.3	239.3
nipple	174.0	198.81	233.0	217	238.3	239.3
male	175.0	198.81	233.0	217	238.3	239.3
outer	174.8	198.81	233.0	217	238.3	239.3
skin (*see also* Neoplasm, mastectomy site)	173.50	198.2	232.5	216.5	238.2	239.2
tail (axillary)	174.6	198.81	233.0	217	238.3	239.3
upper	174.8	198.81	233.0	217	238.3	239.3
upper-inner quadrant	174.2	198.81	233.0	217	238.3	239.3
upper-outer quadrant	174.4	198.81	233.0	217	238.3	239.3
broad ligament	183.3	198.82	233.39	221.0	236.3	239.5
bronchiogenic, bronchogenic (lung)	162.9	197.0	231.2	212.3	235.7	239.1
bronchiole	162.9	197.0	231.2	212.3	235.7	239.1
bronchus	162.9	197.0	231.2	212.3	235.7	239.1
carina	162.2	197.0	231.2	212.3	235.7	239.1
contiguous sites with lung or trachea	162.8	—	—	—	—	—
lower lobe of lung	162.5	197.0	231.2	212.3	235.7	239.1
main	162.2	197.0	231.2	212.3	235.7	239.1
middle lobe of lung	162.4	197.0	231.2	212.3	235.7	239.1
upper lobe of lung	162.3	197.0	231.2	212.3	235.7	239.1
brow	173.30	198.2	232.3	216.3	238.2	239.2
basal cell carcinoma	173.31	—	—	—	—	—
specified type NEC	173.39	—	—	—	—	—
squamous cell carcinoma	173.32	—	—	—	—	—
buccal (cavity)	145.9	198.89	230.0	210.4	235.1	239.0
commissure	145.0	198.89	230.0	210.4	235.1	239.0
groove (lower) (upper)	145.1	198.89	230.0	210.4	235.1	239.0
mucosa	145.0	198.89	230.0	210.4	235.1	239.0
sulcus (lower) (upper)	145.1	198.89	230.0	210.4	235.1	239.0
bulbourethral gland	189.3	198.1	233.9	223.81	236.99	239.5
bursa—*see* Neoplasm, connective tissue						
buttock NEC*	195.3	198.89	232.5	229.8	238.8	239.89
calf*	195.5	198.89	232.7	229.8	238.8	239.89
calvarium	170.0	198.5	—	213.0	238.0	239.2
calyx, renal	189.1	198.0	233.9	223.1	236.91	239.5
canal						
anal	154.2	197.5	230.5	211.4	235.5	239.0
auditory (external) (*see also* Neoplasm, skin, ear)	173.20	198.2	232.2	216.2	238.2	239.2
auricular (external) (*see also* Neoplasm, skin, ear)	173.20	198.2	232.2	216.2	238.2	239.2
canaliculi, biliary (biliferi) (intrahepatic)	155.1	197.8	230.8	211.5	235.3	239.0
canthus (eye) (inner) (outer)	173.10	198.2	232.1	216.1	238.2	239.2
basal cell carcinoma	173.11	—	—	—	—	—
specified type NEC	173.19	—	—	—	—	—
squamous cell carcinoma	173.12	—	—	—	—	—
capillary—*see* Neoplasm, connective tissue						
caput coli	153.4	197.5	230.3	211.3	235.2	239.0
cardia (gastric)	151.0	197.8	230.2	211.1	235.2	239.0
cardiac orifice (stomach)	151.0	197.8	230.2	211.1	235.2	239.0
cardio-esophageal junction	151.0	197.8	230.2	211.1	235.2	239.0

	Malignant			Benign	Uncertain Behavior	Unspecified
	Primary	Secondary	Ca in situ			
cardio-esophagus	151.0	197.8	230.2	211.1	235.2	239.0
carina (bronchus)	162.2	197.0	231.2	212.3	235.7	239.1
carotid (artery)	171.0	198.89	—	215.0	238.1	239.2
body	194.5	198.89	—	227.5	237.3	239.7
carpus (any bone)	170.5	198.5	—	213.5	238.0	239.2
cartilage (articular) (joint) NEC—*see also*						
Neoplasm, bone	170.9	198.5	—	213.9	238.0	239.2
arytenoid	161.3	197.3	231.0	212.1	235.6	239.1
auricular	171.0	198.89	—	215.0	238.1	239.2
bronchi	162.2	197.3	—	212.3	235.7	239.1
connective tissue—*see* Neoplasm, connective tissue						
costal	170.3	198.5	—	213.3	238.0	239.2
cricoid	161.3	197.3	231.0	212.1	235.6	239.1
cuneiform	161.3	197.3	231.0	212.1	235.6	239.1
ear (external)	171.0	198.89	—	215.0	238.1	239.2
ensiform	170.3	198.5	—	213.3	238.0	239.2
epiglottis	161.1	197.3	231.0	212.1	235.6	239.1
anterior surface	146.4	198.89	230.0	210.6	235.1	239.0
eyelid	171.0	198.89	—	215.0	238.1	239.2
intervertebral	170.2	198.5	—	213.2	238.0	239.2
larynx, laryngeal	161.3	197.3	231.0	212.1	235.6	239.1
nose, nasal	160.0	197.3	231.8	212.0	235.9	239.1
pinna	171.0	198.89	—	215.0	238.1	239.2
rib	170.3	198.5	—	213.3	238.0	239.2
semilunar (knee)	170.7	198.5	—	213.7	238.0	239.2
thyroid	161.3	197.3	231.0	212.1	235.6	239.1
trachea	162.0	197.3	231.1	212.2	235.7	239.1
cauda equina	192.2	198.3	—	225.3	237.5	239.7
cavity						
buccal	145.9	198.89	230.0	210.4	235.1	239.0
nasal	160.0	197.3	231.8	212.0	235.9	239.1
oral	145.9	198.89	230.0	210.4	235.1	239.0
peritoneal	158.9	197.6	—	211.8	235.4	239.0
tympanic	160.1	197.3	231.8	212.0	235.9	239.1
cecum	153.4	197.5	230.3	211.3	235.2	239.0
central						
nervous system—*see* Neoplasm, nervous system						
white matter	191.0	198.3	—	225.0	237.5	239.6
cerebellopontine (angle)	191.6	198.3	—	225.0	237.5	239.6
cerebellum, cerebellar	191.6	198.3	—	225.0	237.5	239.6
cerebrum, cerebral (cortex) (hemisphere)						
(white matter)	191.0	198.3	—	225.0	237.5	239.6
meninges	192.1	198.4	—	225.2	237.6	239.7
peduncle	191.7	198.3	—	225.0	237.5	239.6
ventricle (any)	191.5	198.3	—	225.0	237.5	239.6
cervical region	195.0	198.89	234.8	229.8	238.8	239.89
cervix (cervical) (uteri)						
(uterus)	180.9	198.82	233.1	219.0	236.0	239.5
canal	180.0	198.82	233.1	219.0	236.0	239.5
contiguous sites	180.8	—	—	—	—	—
endocervix (canal) (gland)	180.0	198.82	233.1	219.0	236.0	239.5
exocervix	180.1	198.82	233.1	219.0	236.0	239.5
external os	180.1	198.82	233.1	219.0	236.0	239.5
internal os	180.0	198.82	233.1	219.0	236.0	239.5
nabothian gland	180.0	198.82	233.1	219.0	236.0	239.5
squamocolumnar junction	180.8	198.82	233.1	219.0	236.0	239.5
stump	180.8	198.82	233.1	219.0	236.0	239.5
cheek	195.0	198.89	234.8	229.8	238.8	239.89
external	173.30	198.2	232.3	216.3	238.2	239.2
basal cell carcinoma	173.31	—	—	—	—	—

	Malignant			Benign	Uncertain Behavior	Unspecified
	Primary	Secondary	Ca in situ			
specified type NEC.	173.39	—	—	—	—	—
squamous cell carcinoma	173.32	—	—	—	—	—
inner aspect.	145.0	198.89	230.0	210.4	235.1	239.0
internal	145.0	198.89	230.0	210.4	235.1	239.0
mucosa	145.0	198.89	230.0	210.4	235.1	239.0
chest (wall) NEC.	195.1	198.89	234.8	229.8	238.8	239.89
chiasma opticum	192.0	198.4	—	225.1	237.9	239.7
chin.	173.30	198.2	232.3	216.3	238.2	239.2
basal cell carcinoma	173.31	—	—	—	—	—
specified type NEC.	173.39	—	—	—	—	—
squamous cell carcinoma	173.32	—	—	—	—	—
choana	147.3	198.89	230.0	210.7	235.1	239.0
cholangiole	155.1	197.8	230.8	211.5	235.3	239.0
choledochal duct	156.1	197.8	230.8	211.5	235.3	239.0
choroid	190.6	198.4	234.0	224.6	238.8	239.81
plexus.	191.5	198.3	—	225.0	237.5	239.6
ciliary body.	190.0	198.4	234.0	224.0	238.8	239.89
clavicle	170.3	198.5	—	213.3	238.0	239.2
clitoris	184.3	198.82	233.32	221.2	236.3	239.5
clivus	170.0	198.5	—	213.0	238.0	239.2
cloacogenic zone	154.8	197.5	230.7	211.4	235.5	239.0
coccygeal						
body or glomus.	194.6	198.89	—	227.6	237.3	239.7
vertebra.	170.6	198.5	—	213.6	238.0	239.2
coccyx	170.6	198.5	—	213.6	238.0	239.2
colon—*see also* Neoplasm,						
intestine, large	153.9	197.5	230.3	211.3	235.2	239.0
with rectum.	154.0	197.5	230.4	211.4	235.2	239.0
column, spinal—*see* Neoplasm, spine						
columnella (*see also* Neoplasm,						
skin, face)	173.30	198.2	232.3	216.3	238.2	239.2
commissure						
labial, lip	140.6	198.89	230.0	210.4	235.1	239.0
laryngeal	161.0	197.3	231.0	212.1	235.6	239.1
common (bile) duct	156.1	197.8	230.8	211.5	235.3	239.0
concha (*see also* Neoplasm, skin,						
ear)	173.20	198.2	232.2	216.2	238.2	239.2
nose	160.0	197.3	231.8	212.0	235.9	239.1
conjunctiva	190.3	198.4	234.0	224.3	238.8	239.89
connective tissue NEC	171.9	198.89	—	215.9	238.1	239.2

Note—For neoplasms of connective tissue (blood vessel, bursa, fasica, ligament, muscle, peripheral nerves, sympathetic and parasympathetic nerves, and ganglia, synovia, tendon, etc.) or of morphological types that indicate connective tissue, code according to the list under "Neoplasm, connective tissue;" for sites that do not appear in this list, code to neoplasm of that site; e.g.: liposarcoma, shoulder 171.2; leiomyosarcoma, stomach 151.9; neurofibroma, chest wall 215.4.

Morphological types that indicate connective tissue appear in their proper palce in the alphabetic index with the instruction "see Neoplasm, connective tissue..."

	Malignant			Benign	Uncertain Behavior	Unspecified
abdomen	171.5	198.89	—	215.5	238.1	239.2
abdominal wall	171.5	198.89	—	215.5	238.1	239.2
ankle	171.3	198.89	—	215.3	238.1	239.2
antecubital fossa or space	171.2	198.89	—	215.2	238.1	239.2
arm	171.2	198.89	—	215.2	238.1	239.2
auricle (ear).	171.0	198.89	—	215.0	238.1	239.2
axilla	171.4	198.89	—	215.4	238.1	239.2
back	171.7	198.89	—	215.7	238.1	239.2
breast (female) (*see also*						
Neoplasm, breast).	174.9	198.81	233.0	217	238.3	239.3
male	175.9	198.81	233.0	217	238.3	239.3
buttock	171.6	198.89	—	215.6	238.1	239.2
calf	171.3	198.89	—	215.3	238.1	239.2
cervical region	171.0	198.89	—	215.0	238.1	239.2
cheek	171.0	198.89	—	215.0	238.1	239.2

	Malignant			Benign	Uncertain Behavior	Unspecified
	Primary	Secondary	Ca in situ			
chest (wall)	171.4	198.89	—	215.4	238.1	239.2
chin	171.0	198.89	—	215.0	238.1	239.2
contiguous sites	171.8	—	—	—	—	—
diaphragm	171.4	198.89	—	215.4	238.1	239.2
ear (external)	171.0	198.89	—	215.0	238.1	239.2
elbow	171.2	198.89	—	215.2	238.1	239.2
extrarectal	171.6	198.89	—	215.6	238.1	239.2
extremity	171.8	198.89	—	215.8	238.1	239.2
lower	171.3	198.89	—	215.3	238.1	239.2
upper	171.2	198.89	—	215.2	238.1	239.2
eyelid	171.0	198.89	—	215.0	238.1	239.2
face	171.0	198.89	—	215.0	238.1	239.2
finger	171.2	198.89	—	215.2	238.1	239.2
flank	171.7	198.89	—	215.7	238.1	239.2
foot	171.3	198.89	—	215.3	238.1	239.2
forearm	171.2	198.89	—	215.2	238.1	239.2
forehead	171.0	198.89	—	215.0	238.1	239.2
gastric	171.5	198.89	—	215.5	238.1	—
gastrointestinal	171.5	198.89	—	215.5	238.1	—
gluteal region	171.6	198.89	—	215.6	238.1	239.2
great vessels NEC	171.4	198.89	—	215.4	238.1	239.2
groin	171.6	198.89	—	215.6	238.1	239.2
hand	171.2	198.89	—	215.2	238.1	239.2
head	171.0	198.89	—	215.0	238.1	239.2
heel	171.3	198.89	—	215.3	238.1	239.2
hip	171.3	198.89	—	215.3	238.1	239.2
hypochondrium	171.5	198.89	—	215.5	238.1	239.2
iliopsoas muscle	171.6	198.89	—	215.5	238.1	239.2
infraclavicular region	171.4	198.89	—	215.4	238.1	239.2
inguinal (canal) (region)	171.6	198.89	—	215.6	238.1	239.2
intestine	171.5	198.89	—	215.5	238.1	—
intrathoracic	171.4	198.89	—	215.4	238.1	239.2
ischorectal fossa	171.6	198.89	—	215.6	238.1	239.2
jaw	143.9	198.89	230.0	210.4	235.1	239.0
knee	171.3	198.89	—	215.3	238.1	239.2
leg	171.3	198.89	—	215.3	238.1	239.2
limb NEC	171.9	198.89	—	215.8	238.1	239.2
lower	171.3	198.89	—	215.3	238.1	239.2
upper	171.2	198.89	—	215.2	238.1	239.2
nates	171.6	198.89	—	215.6	238.1	239.2
neck	171.0	198.89	—	215.0	238.1	239.2
orbit	190.1	198.4	234.0	224.1	238.8	239.89
pararectal	171.6	198.89	—	215.6	238.1	239.2
para-urethral	171.6	198.89	—	215.6	238.1	239.2
paravaginal	171.6	198.89	—	215.6	238.1	239.2
pelvis (floor)	171.6	198.89	—	215.6	238.1	239.2
pelvo-abdominal	171.8	198.89	—	215.8	238.1	239.2
perineum	171.6	198.89	—	215.6	238.1	239.2
perirectal (tissue)	171.6	198.89	—	215.6	238.1	239.2
periurethral (tissue)	171.6	198.89	—	215.6	238.1	239.2
popliteal fossa or space	171.3	198.89	—	215.3	238.1	239.2
presacral	171.6	198.89	—	215.6	238.1	239.2
psoas muscle	171.5	198.89	—	215.5	238.1	239.2
pterygoid fossa	171.0	198.89	—	215.0	238.1	239.2
rectovaginal septum or wall	171.6	198.89	—	215.6	238.1	239.2
rectovesical	171.6	198.89	—	215.6	238.1	239.2
retroperitoneum	158.0	197.6	—	211.8	235.4	239.0
sacrococcygeal region	171.6	198.89	—	215.6	238.1	239.2
scalp	171.0	198.89	—	215.0	238.1	239.2
scapular region	171.4	198.89	—	215.4	238.1	239.2
shoulder	171.2	198.89	—	215.2	238.1	239.2
skin (dermis) NEC	173.90	198.2	232.9	216.9	238.2	239.2

Primary	**Secondary**	**Ca in situ**	**Benign**	**Uncertain Behavior**	**Unspecified**
	Malignant				

	Primary	Secondary	Ca in situ	Benign	Uncertain Behavior	Unspecified
stomach.	171.5	198.89	—	215.5	238.1	—
submental.	171.0	198.89	—	215.0	238.1	239.2
supraclavicular region	171.0	198.89	—	215.0	238.1	239.2
temple	171.0	198.89	—	215.0	238.1	239.2
temporal region.	171.0	198.89	—	215.0	238.1	239.2
thigh	171.3	198.89	—	215.3	238.1	239.2
thoracic (duct) (wall).	171.4	198.89	—	215.4	238.1	239.2
thorax.	171.4	198.89	—	215.4	238.1	239.2
thumb.	171.2	198.89	—	215.2	238.1	239.2
toe	171.3	198.89	—	215.3	238.1	239.2
trunk	171.7	198.89	—	215.7	238.1	239.2
umbilicus	171.5	198.89	—	215.5	238.1	239.2
vesicorectal.	171.6	198.89	—	215.6	238.1	239.2
wrist	171.2	198.89	—	215.2	238.1	239.2
conus medullaris	192.2	198.3	—	225.3	237.5	239.7
cord (true) (vocal)	161.0	197.3	231.0	212.1	235.6	239.1
false	161.1	197.3	231.0	212.1	235.6	239.1
spermatic	187.6	198.82	233.6	222.8	236.6	239.5
spinal (cervical) (lumbar)						
(thoracic)	192.2	198.3	—	225.3	237.5	239.7
cornea (limbus).	190.4	198.4	234.0	224.4	238.8	239.89
corpus						
albicans.	183.0	198.6	233.39	220	236.2	239.5
callosum, brain	191.8	198.3	—	225.0	237.5	239.6
cavernosum.	187.3	198.82	233.5	222.1	236.6	239.5
gastric	151.4	197.8	230.2	211.1	235.2	239.0
penis	187.3	198.82	233.5	222.1	236.6	239.5
striatum, cerebrum	191.0	198.3	—	225.0	237.5	239.6
uteri.	182.0	198.82	233.2	219.1	236.0	239.5
isthmus	182.1	198.82	233.2	219.1	236.0	239.5
cortex						
adrenal	194.0	198.7	234.8	227.0	237.2	239.7
cerebral.	191.0	198.3	—	225.0	237.5	239.6
costal cartilage	170.3	198.5	—	213.3	238.0	239.2
costovertebral joint.	170.3	198.5	—	213.3	238.0	239.2
Cowper's gland.	189.3	198.1	233.9	223.81	236.99	239.5
cranial (fossa, any)	191.9	198.3	—	225.0	237.5	239.6
meninges	192.1	198.4	—	225.2	237.6	239.7
nerve (any)	192.0	198.4	—	225.1	237.9	239.7
craniobuccal pouch.	194.3	198.89	234.8	227.3	237.0	239.7
craniopharyngeal (duct)						
(pouch)	194.3	198.89	234.8	227.3	237.0	239.7
cricoid	148.0	198.89	230.0	210.8	235.1	239.0
cartilage	161.3	197.3	231.0	212.1	235.6	239.1
cricopharynx	148.0	198.89	230.0	210.8	235.1	239.0
crypt of Morgagni	154.8	197.5	230.7	211.4	235.2	239.0
crystalline lens	190.0	198.4	234.0	224.0	238.8	239.89
cul-de-sac (Douglas')	158.8	197.6	—	211.8	235.4	239.0
cuneiform cartilage.	161.3	197.3	231.0	212.1	235.6	239.1
cutaneous—*see* Neoplasm, skin						
cutis—*see* Neoplasm, skin						
cystic (bile) duct (common)	156.1	197.8	230.8	211.5	235.3	239.0
dermis—*see* Neoplasm, skin						
diaphragm	171.4	198.89	—	215.4	238.1	239.2
digestive organs, system,						
tube, tract NEC	159.9	197.8	230.9	211.9	235.5	239.0
contiguous sites with						
peritoneum.	159.8	—	—	—	—	—
disc, intervertebral	170.2	198.5	—	213.2	238.0	239.2
disease, generalized	199.0	199.0	234.9	229.9	238.9	199.0
disseminated	199.0	199.0	234.9	229.9	238.9	199.0
Douglas' cul-de-sac or pouch	158.8	197.6	—	211.8	235.4	239.0
duodenojejunal junction	152.8	197.4	230.7	211.2	235.2	239.0

	Primary	Secondary	Ca in situ	Benign	Uncertain Behavior	Unspecified
		Malignant				
duodenum	152.0	197.4	230.7	211.2	235.2	239.0
dura (cranial) (mater)	192.1	198.4	—	225.2	237.6	239.7
cerebral	192.1	198.4	—	225.2	237.6	239.7
spinal	192.3	198.4	—	225.4	237.6	239.7
ear (external) (see also Neoplasm, ear, skin)	173.20	198.2	232.2	216.2	238.2	239.2
auricle or auris (see also Neoplasm, ear, skin)	173.20	198.2	232.2	216.2	238.2	239.2
canal, external (see also Neoplasm, ear, skin)	173.20	198.2	232.2	216.2	238.2	239.2
cartilage	171.0	198.89	—	215.0	238.1	239.2
external meatus (see also Neoplasm, ear, skin)	173.20	198.2	232.2	216.2	238.2	239.2
inner	160.1	197.3	231.8	212.0	235.9	239.89
lobule (see also Neoplasm, ear, skin)	173.20	198.2	232.2	216.2	238.2	239.2
middle	160.1	197.3	231.8	212.0	235.9	239.89
contiguous sites with accessory sinuses or nasal cavities	160.8	—	—	—	—	—
skin	173.20	198.2	232.2	216.2	238.2	239.2
basal cell carcinoma	173.21	—	—	—	—	—
specified type NEC	173.29	—	—	—	—	—
squamous cell carcinoma	173.22	—	—	—	—	—
earlobe	173.20	198.2	232.2	216.2	238.2	239.2
basal cell carcinoma	173.21	—	—	—	—	—
specified type NEC	173.29	—	—	—	—	—
squamous cell carcinoma	173.22	—	—	—	—	—
ejaculatory duct	187.8	198.82	233.6	222.8	236.6	239.5
elbow NEC*	195.4	198.89	232.6	229.8	238.8	239.89
endocardium	164.1	198.89	—	212.7	238.8	239.89
endocervix (canal) (gland)	180.0	198.82	233.1	219.0	236.0	239.5
endocrine gland NEC	194.9	198.89	—	227.9	237.4	239.7
pluriglandular NEC	194.8	198.89	234.8	227.8	237.4	239.7
endometrium (gland) (stroma)	182.0	198.82	233.2	219.1	236.0	239.5
ensiform cartilage	170.3	198.5	—	213.3	238.0	239.2
enteric—*see* Neoplasm, intestine						
ependyma (brain)	191.5	198.3	—	225.0	237.5	239.6
epicardium	164.1	198.89	—	212.7	238.8	239.89
epididymis	187.5	198.82	233.6	222.3	236.6	239.5
epidural	192.9	198.4	—	225.9	237.9	239.7
epiglottis	161.1	197.3	231.0	212.1	235.6	239.1
anterior aspect or surface	146.4	198.89	230.0	210.6	235.1	239.0
cartilage	161.3	197.3	231.0	212.1	235.6	239.1
free border (margin)	146.4	198.89	230.0	210.6	235.1	239.0
junctional region	146.5	198.89	230.0	210.6	235.1	239.0
posterior (laryngeal) surface	161.1	197.3	231.0	212.1	235.6	239.1
suprahyoid portion	161.1	197.3	231.0	212.1	235.6	239.1
esophagogastric junction	151.0	197.8	230.2	211.1	235.2	239.0
esophagus	150.9	197.8	230.1	211.0	235.5	239.0
abdominal	150.2	197.8	230.1	211.0	235.5	239.0
cervical	150.0	197.8	230.1	211.0	235.5	239.0
contiguous sites	150.8	—	—	—	—	—
distal (third)	150.5	197.8	230.1	211.0	235.5	239.0
lower (third)	150.5	197.8	230.1	211.0	235.5	239.0
middle (third)	150.4	197.8	230.1	211.0	235.5	239.0
proximal (third)	150.3	197.8	230.1	211.0	235.5	239.0
specified part NEC	150.8	197.8	230.1	211.0	235.5	239.0
thoracic	150.1	197.8	230.1	211.0	235.5	239.0
upper (third)	150.3	197.8	230.1	211.0	235.5	239.0
ethmoid (sinus)	160.3	197.3	231.8	212.0	235.9	239.1

	Malignant			Benign	Uncertain Behavior	Unspecified
	Primary	Secondary	Ca in situ			
bone or labyrinth	170.0	198.5	—	213.0	238.0	239.2
Eustachian tube.	160.1	197.3	231.8	212.0	235.9	239.1
exocervix.	180.1	198.82	233.1	219.0	236.0	239.5
external						
meatus (ear) (see also Neoplasm,						
skin, ear)	173.20	198.2	232.2	216.2	238.2	239.2
os, cervix uteri	180.1	198.82	233.1	219.0	236.0	239.5
extradural.	192.9	198.4	—	225.9	237.9	239.7
extrahepatic (bile) duct.	156.1	197.8	230.8	211.5	235.3	239.0
contiguous sites with						
gallbladder.	156.8	—	—	—	—	—
extraocular muscle	190.1	198.4	234.0	224.1	238.8	239.89
extrarectal	195.3	198.89	234.8	229.8	238.8	239.89
extremity*	195.8	198.89	232.8	229.8	238.8	239.89
lower*	195.5	198.89	232.7	229.8	238.8	239.89
upper*	195.4	198.89	232.6	229.8	238.8	239.89
eye NEC	190.9	198.4	234.0	224.9	238.8	239.89
contiguous sites	190.8	—	—	—	—	—
specified sites NEC	190.8	198.4	234.0	224.8	238.8	239.89
eyeball	190.0	198.4	234.0	224.0	238.8	239.89
eyebrow	173.30	198.2	232.3	216.3	238.2	239.2
basal cell carcinoma	173.31	—	—	—	—	—
specified type NEC.	173.39	—	—	—	—	—
squamous cell carcinoma	173.32	—	—	—	—	—
eyelid (lower) (skin) (upper)	173.10	198.2	232.1	216.1	238.2	239.2
basal cell carcinoma	173.11	—	—	—	—	—
cartilage	171.0	198.89	—	215.0	238.1	239.2
specified type NEC.	173.19	—	—	—	—	—
squamous cell carcinoma	173.12	—	—	—	—	—
face NEC*	195.0	198.89	232.3	229.8	238.8	239.89
fallopian tube (accessory)	183.2	198.82	233.39	221.0	236.3	239.5
falx (cerebelli) (cerebri)	192.1	198.4	—	225.2	237.6	239.7
fascia—see also Neoplasm, connective tissue						
palmar	171.2	198.89	—	215.2	238.1	239.2
plantar	171.3	198.89	—	215.3	238.1	239.2
fatty tissue—see Neoplasm, connective tissue						
fauces, faucial NEC	146.9	198.89	230.0	210.6	235.1	239.0
pillars.	146.2	198.89	230.0	210.6	235.1	239.0
tonsil	146.0	198.89	230.0	210.5	235.1	239.0
femur (any part)	170.7	198.5	—	213.7	238.0	239.2
fetal membrane	181	198.82	233.2	219.8	236.1	239.5
fibrous tissue—see Neoplasm, connective tissue						
fibula (any part)	170.7	198.5	—	213.7	238.0	239.2
filum terminale	192.2	198.3	—	225.3	237.5	239.7
finger NEC*	195.4	198.89	232.6	229.8	238.8	239.89
flank NEC*.	195.8	198.89	232.5	229.8	238.8	239.89
follicle, nabothian	180.0	198.82	233.1	219.0	236.0	239.5
foot NEC*	195.5	198.89	232.7	229.8	238.8	239.89
forearm NEC*	195.4	198.89	232.6	229.8	238.8	239.89
forehead (skin)	173.30	198.2	232.3	216.3	238.2	239.2
basal cell carcinoma	173.31	—	—	—	—	—
specified type NEC.	173.39	—	—	—	—	—
squamous cell carcinoma	173.32	—	—	—	—	—
foreskin.	187.1	198.82	233.5	222.1	236.6	239.5
fornix						
pharyngeal	147.3	198.89	230.0	210.7	235.1	239.0
vagina	184.0	198.82	233.31	221.1	236.3	239.5
fossa (of)						
anterior (cranial)	191.9	198.3	—	225.0	237.5	239.6
cranial	191.9	198.3	—	225.0	237.5	239.6
ischiorectal	195.3	198.89	234.8	229.8	238.8	239.89
middle (cranial)	191.9	198.3	—	225.0	237.5	239.6
pituitary	194.3	198.89	234.8	227.3	237.0	239.7

	Malignant			Benign	Uncertain Behavior	Unspecified
	Primary	Secondary	Ca in situ			
posterior (cranial)	191.9	198.3	—	225.0	237.5	239.6
pterygoid	171.0	198.89	—	215.0	238.1	239.2
pyriform	148.1	198.89	230.0	210.8	235.1	239.0
Rosenmüller	147.2	198.89	230.0	210.7	235.1	239.0
tonsillar	146.1	198.89	230.0	210.6	235.1	239.0
fourchette	184.4	198.82	233.32	221.2	236.3	239.5
frenulum						
labii—*see* Neoplasm, lip, internal						
linguae	141.3	198.89	230.0	210.1	235.1	239.0
frontal						
bone	170.0	198.5	—	213.0	238.0	239.2
lobe, brain	191.1	198.3	—	225.0	237.5	239.6
meninges	192.1	198.4	—	225.2	237.6	239.7
pole	191.1	198.3	—	225.0	237.5	239.6
sinus	160.4	197.3	231.8	212.0	235.9	239.1
fundus						
stomach	151.3	197.8	230.2	211.1	235.2	239.0
uterus	182.0	198.82	233.2	219.1	236.0	239.5
gall duct (extrahepatic)	156.1	197.8	230.8	211.5	235.3	239.0
intrahepatic	155.1	197.8	230.8	211.5	235.3	239.0
gallbladder	156.0	197.8	230.8	211.5	235.3	239.0
contiguous sites with						
extrahepatic bile ducts	156.8	—	—	—	—	—
ganglia (*see also* Neoplasm,						
connective tissue)	171.9	198.89	—	215.9	238.1	239.2
basal	191.0	198.3	—	225.0	237.5	239.6
ganglion (*see also* Neoplasm,						
connective tissue)	171.9	198.89	—	215.9	238.1	239.2
cranial nerve	192.0	198.4	—	225.1	237.9	239.7
Gartner's duct	184.0	198.82	233.31	221.1	236.3	239.5
gastric—*see* Neoplasm, stomach						
gastrocolic	159.8	197.8	230.9	211.9	235.5	239.0
gastroesophageal junction	151.0	197.8	230.2	211.1	235.2	239.0
gastrointestinal (tract) NEC	159.9	197.8	230.9	211.9	235.5	239.0
generalized	199.0	199.0	234.9	229.9	238.9	199.0
genital organ or tract						
female NEC	184.9	198.82	233.39	221.9	236.3	239.5
contiguous sites	184.8	—	—	—	—	—
specified site NEC	184.8	198.82	233.39	221.8	236.3	239.5
male NEC	187.9	198.82	233.6	222.9	236.6	239.5
contiguous sites	187.8	—	—	—	—	—
specified site NEC	187.8	198.82	233.6	222.8	236.6	239.5
genitourinary tract						
female	184.9	198.82	233.39	221.9	236.3	239.5
male	187.9	198.82	233.6	222.9	236.6	239.5
gingiva (alveolar) (marginal)	143.9	198.89	230.0	210.4	235.1	239.0
lower	143.1	198.89	230.0	210.4	235.1	239.0
mandibular	143.1	198.89	230.0	210.4	235.1	239.0
maxillary	143.0	198.89	230.0	210.4	235.1	239.0
upper	143.0	198.89	230.0	210.4	235.1	239.0
gland, glandular (lymphatic)						
(system)—*see also* Neoplasm,						
lymph gland						
endocrine NEC	194.9	198.89	—	227.9	237.4	239.7
salivary—*see* Neoplasm,						
salivary, gland						
glans penis	187.2	198.82	233.5	222.1	236.6	239.5
globus pallidus	191.0	198.3	—	225.0	237.5	239.6
glomus						
coccygeal	194.6	198.89	—	227.6	237.3	239.7
jugularis	194.6	198.89	—	227.6	237.3	239.7
glosso-epiglottic fold(s)	146.4	198.89	230.0	210.6	235.1	239.0
glossopalatine fold	146.2	198.89	230.0	210.6	235.1	239.0

	Malignant			Benign	Uncertain Behavior	Unspecified
	Primary	Secondary	Ca in situ			
glossopharyngeal sulcus	146.1	198.89	230.0	210.6	235.1	239.0
glottis.	161.0	197.3	231.0	212.1	235.6	239.1
gluteal region*	195.3	198.89	232.5	229.8	238.8	239.89
great vessels NEC	171.4	198.89	—	215.4	238.1	239.2
groin NEC*	195.3	198.89	232.5	229.8	238.8	239.89
gum.	143.9	198.89	230.0	210.4	235.1	239.0
contiguous sites	143.8	—	—	—	—	—
lower	143.1	198.89	230.0	210.4	235.1	239.0
upper	143.0	198.89	230.0	210.4	235.1	239.0
hand NEC*	195.4	198.89	232.6	229.8	238.8	239.89
head NEC*	195.0	198.89	232.4	229.8	238.8	239.89
heart	164.1	198.89	—	212.7	238.8	239.89
contiguous sites with mediastinum or thymus	164.8	—	—	—	—	—
heel NEC*	195.5	198.89	232.7	229.8	238.8	239.89
helix (*see also* Neoplasm, skin, ear) .	173.20	198.2	232.2	216.2	238.2	239.2
hematopoietic, hemopoietic tissue NEC	202.8	198.89	—	—	—	238.79
hemisphere, cerebral	191.0	198.3	—	225.0	237.5	239.6
hemorrhoidal zone	154.2	197.5	230.5	211.4	235.5	239.0
hepatic	155.2	197.7	230.8	211.5	235.3	239.0
duct (bile)	156.1	197.8	230.8	211.5	235.3	239.0
flexure (colon)	153.0	197.5	230.3	211.3	235.2	239.0
primary	155.0	—	—	—	—	—
hilus of lung	162.2	197.0	231.2	212.3	235.7	239.1
hip NEC*	195.5	198.89	232.7	229.8	238.8	239.89
hippocampus, brain	191.2	198.3	—	225.0	237.5	239.6
humerus (any part)	170.4	198.5	—	213.4	238.0	239.2
hymen	184.0	198.82	233.31	221.1	236.3	239.5
hypopharynx, hypopharyngeal NEC	148.9	198.89	230.0	210.8	235.1	239.0
contiguous sites	148.8	—	—	—	—	—
postcricoid region	148.0	198.89	230.0	210.8	235.1	239.0
posterior wall.	148.3	198.89	230.0	210.8	235.1	239.0
pyriform fossa (sinus)	148.1	198.89	230.0	210.8	235.1	239.0
specified site NEC	148.8	198.89	230.0	210.8	235.1	239.0
wall	148.9	198.89	230.0	210.8	235.1	239.0
posterior	148.3	198.89	230.0	210.8	235.1	239.0
hypophysis	194.3	198.89	234.8	227.3	237.0	239.7
hypothalamus.	191.0	198.3	—	225.0	237.5	239.6
ileocecum, ileocecal (coil, junction, valve)	153.4	197.5	230.3	211.3	235.2	239.0
ileum	152.2	197.4	230.7	211.2	235.2	239.0
ilium	170.6	198.5	—	213.6	238.0	239.2
immunoproliferative NEC	203.8	—	—	—	—	—
infraclavicular (region)*	195.1	198.89	232.5	229.8	238.8	239.89
inguinal (region)*	195.3	198.89	232.5	229.8	238.8	239.89
insula	191.0	198.3	—	225.0	237.5	239.6
insular tissue (pancreas)	157.4	197.8	230.9	211.7	235.5	239.0
brain	191.0	198.3	—	225.0	237.5	239.6
interarytenoid fold	148.2	198.89	230.0	210.8	235.1	239.0
hypopharyngeal aspect.	148.2	198.89	230.0	210.8	235.1	239.0
laryngeal aspect	161.1	197.3	231.0	212.1	235.6	239.1
marginal zone	148.2	198.89	230.0	210.8	235.1	239.0
interdental papillae.	143.9	198.89	230.0	210.4	235.1	239.0
lower	143.1	198.89	230.0	210.4	235.1	239.0
upper	143.0	198.89	230.0	210.4	235.1	239.0
internal capsule	191.0	198.3	—	225.0	237.5	239.6
os (cervix)	180.0	198.82	233.1	219.0	236.0	239.5
intervertebral cartilage or disc	170.2	198.5	—	213.2	238.0	239.2

| | Malignant | | | | | |
	Primary	Secondary	Ca in situ	Benign	Uncertain Behavior	Unspecified
intestine, intestinal	159.0	197.8	230.7	211.9	235.2	239.0
large	153.9	197.5	230.3	211.3	235.2	239.0
appendix	153.5	197.5	230.3	211.3	235.2	239.0
caput coli	153.4	197.5	230.3	211.3	235.2	239.0
cecum	153.4	197.5	230.3	211.3	235.2	239.0
colon	153.9	197.5	230.3	211.3	235.2	239.0
and rectum	154.0	197.5	230.4	211.4	235.2	239.0
ascending	153.6	197.5	230.3	211.3	235.2	239.0
caput	153.4	197.5	230.3	211.3	235.2	239.0
contiguous sites	153.8	—	—	—	—	—
descending	153.2	197.5	230.3	211.3	235.2	239.0
distal	153.2	197.5	230.3	211.3	235.2	239.0
left	153.2	197.5	230.3	211.3	235.2	239.0
pelvic	153.3	197.5	230.3	211.3	235.2	239.0
right	153.6	197.5	230.3	211.3	235.2	239.0
sigmoid (flexure)	153.3	197.5	230.3	211.3	235.2	239.0
transverse	153.1	197.5	230.3	211.3	235.2	239.0
contiguous sites	153.8	—	—	—	—	—
hepatic flexure	153.0	197.5	230.3	211.3	235.2	239.0
ileocecum,ileocecal						
(coil, valve)	153.4	197.5	230.3	211.3	235.2	239.0
sigmoid flexure (lower)						
(upper)	153.3	197.5	230.3	211.3	235.2	239.0
splenic flexure	153.7	197.5	230.3	211.3	235.2	239.0
small	152.9	197.4	230.7	211.2	235.2	239.0
contiguous sites	152.8	—	—	—	—	—
duodenum	152.0	197.4	230.7	211.2	235.2	239.0
ileum	152.2	197.4	230.7	211.2	235.2	239.0
jejunum	152.1	197.4	230.7	211.2	235.2	239.0
tract NEC	159.0	197.8	230.7	211.9	235.2	239.0
intra-abdominal	195.2	198.89	234.8	229.8	238.8	239.89
intracranial NEC	191.9	198.3	—	225.0	237.5	239.6
intrahepatic (bile) duct	155.1	197.8	230.8	211.5	235.3	239.0
intraocular	190.0	198.4	234.0	224.0	238.8	239.89
intraorbital	190.1	198.4	234.0	224.1	238.8	239.89
intrasellar	194.3	198.89	234.8	227.3	237.0	239.7
intrathoracic (cavity)						
(organs NEC)	195.1	198.89	234.8	229.8	238.8	239.89
contiguous sites with respiratory						
organs	165.8	—	—	—	—	—
iris	190.0	198.4	234.0	224.0	238.8	239.89
ischiorectal (fossa)	195.3	198.89	234.8	229.8	238.8	239.89
ischium	170.6	198.5	—	213.6	238.0	239.2
island of Reil	191.0	198.3	—	225.0	237.5	239.6
islands or islets of Langerhans	157.4	197.8	230.9	211.7	235.5	239.0
isthmus uteri	182.1	198.82	233.2	219.1	236.0	239.5
jaw	195.0	198.89	234.8	229.8	238.8	239.89
bone	170.1	198.5	—	213.1	238.0	239.2
carcinoma	143.9	—	—	—	—	—
lower	143.1	—	—	—	—	—
upper	143.0	—	—	—	—	—
lower	170.1	198.5	—	213.1	238.0	239.2
upper	170.0	198.5	—	213.0	238.0	239.2
carcinoma (any type)						
(lower) (upper)	195.0	—	—	—	—	—
skin (*see also* Neoplasm, skin						
face)	173.30	198.2	232.3	216.3	238.2	239.2
soft tissues	143.9	198.89	230.0	210.4	235.1	239.0
lower	143.1	198.89	230.0	210.4	235.1	239.0
upper	143.0	198.89	230.0	210.4	235.1	239.0
jejunum	152.1	197.4	230.7	211.2	235.2	239.0
joint NEC (*see also*						
Neoplasm, bone)	170.9	198.5	—	213.9	238.0	239.2

	Malignant			Benign	Uncertain Behavior	Unspecified
	Primary	Secondary	Ca in situ			
acromioclavicular	170.4	198.5	—	213.4	238.0	239.2
bursa or synovial membrane—*see* Neoplasm, connective tissue						
costovertebral	170.3	198.5	—	213.3	238.0	239.2
sternocostal	170.3	198.5	—	213.3	238.0	239.2
temporomandibular	170.1	198.5	—	213.1	238.0	239.2
junction						
anorectal	154.8	197.5	230.7	211.4	235.5	239.0
cardioesophageal	151.0	197.8	230.2	211.1	235.2	239.0
esophagogastric	151.0	197.8	230.2	211.1	235.2	239.0
gastroesophageal	151.0	197.8	230.2	211.1	235.2	239.0
hard and soft palate	145.5	198.89	230.0	210.4	235.1	239.0
ileocecal	153.4	197.5	230.3	211.3	235.2	239.0
pelvirectal	154.0	197.5	230.4	211.4	235.2	239.0
pelviureteric	189.1	198.0	233.9	223.1	236.91	239.5
rectosigmoid	154.0	197.5	230.4	211.4	235.2	239.0
squamocolumnar, of cervix	180.8	198.82	233.1	219.0	236.0	239.5
kidney (parenchyma)	189.0	198.0	233.9	223.0	236.91	239.5
calyx	189.1	198.0	233.9	223.1	236.91	239.5
hilus	189.1	198.0	233.9	223.1	236.91	239.5
pelvis	189.1	198.0	233.9	223.1	236.91	239.5
knee NEC*	195.5	198.89	232.7	229.8	238.8	239.89
labia (skin)	184.4	198.82	233.32	221.2	236.3	239.5
majora	184.1	198.82	233.32	221.2	236.3	239.5
minora	184.2	198.82	233.32	221.2	236.3	239.5
labial—*see also* Neoplasm, lip						
sulcus (lower) (upper)	145.1	198.89	230.0	210.4	235.1	239.0
labium (skin)	184.4	198.82	233.32	221.2	236.3	239.5
majus	184.1	198.82	233.32	221.2	236.3	239.5
minus	184.2	198.82	233.32	221.2	236.3	239.5
lacrimal						
canaliculi	190.7	198.4	234.0	224.7	238.8	239.89
duct (nasal)	190.7	198.4	234.0	224.7	238.8	239.89
gland	190.2	198.4	234.0	224.2	238.8	239.89
punctum	190.7	198.4	234.0	224.7	238.8	239.89
sac	190.7	198.4	234.0	224.7	238.8	239.89
Langerhans, islands or islets	157.4	197.8	230.9	211.7	235.5	239.0
laryngopharynx	148.9	198.89	230.0	210.8	235.1	239.0
larynx, laryngeal NEC	161.9	197.3	231.0	212.1	235.6	239.1
aryepiglottic fold	161.1	197.3	231.0	212.1	235.6	239.1
cartilage (arytenoid) (cricoid) (cuneiform) (thyroid)	161.3	197.3	231.0	212.1	235.6	239.1
commissure (anterior) (posterior)	161.0	197.3	231.0	212.1	235.6	239.1
contiguous sites	161.8	—	—	—	—	—
extrinsic NEC	161.1	197.3	231.0	212.1	235.6	239.1
meaning hypopharynx	148.9	198.89	230.0	210.8	235.1	239.0
interarytenoid fold	161.1	197.3	231.0	212.1	235.6	239.1
intrinsic	161.0	197.3	231.0	212.1	235.6	239.1
ventricular band	161.1	197.3	231.0	212.1	235.6	239.1
leg NEC*	195.5	198.89	232.7	229.8	238.8	239.89
lens, crystalline	190.0	198.4	234.0	224.0	238.8	239.89
lid (lower) (upper)	173.10	198.2	232.1	216.1	238.2	239.2
basal cell carcinoma	173.11	—	—	—	—	—
specified type NEC	173.19	—	—	—	—	—
squamous cell carcinoma	173.12	—	—	—	—	—
ligament—*see also* Neoplasm, connective tissue						
broad	183.3	198.82	233.39	221.0	236.3	239.5
Mackenrodt's	183.8	198.82	233.39	221.8	236.3	239.5
non-uterine—*see* Neoplasm, connective tissue						

	Malignant					
	Primary	Secondary	Ca in situ	Benign	Uncertain Behavior	Unspecified
round	183.5	198.82	—	221.0	236.3	239.5
sacro-uterine	183.4	198.82	—	221.0	236.3	239.5
uterine	183.4	198.82	—	221.0	236.3	239.5
utero-ovarian	183.8	198.82	233.39	221.8	236.3	239.5
uterosacral	183.4	198.82	—	221.0	236.3	239.5
limb*	195.8	198.89	232.8	229.8	238.8	239.89
lower*	195.5	198.89	232.7	229.8	238.8	239.89
upper*	195.4	198.89	232.6	229.8	238.8	239.89
limbus of cornea	190.4	198.4	234.0	224.4	238.8	239.89
lingual NEC (*see also* Neoplasm, tongue)	141.9	198.89	230.0	210.1	235.1	239.0
lingula, lung	162.3	197.0	231.2	212.3	235.7	239.1
lip (external) (lipstick area) (vermillion border)	140.9	198.89	230.0	210.0	235.1	239.0
buccal aspect—*see* Neoplasm, lip, internal						
commissure.	140.6	198.89	230.0	210.4	235.1	239.0
contiguous sites	140.8	—	—	—	—	—
with oral cavity or pharynx	149.8	—	—	—	—	—
frenulum—*see* Neoplasm, lip, internal						
inner aspect—*see* Neoplasm, lip, internal						
internal (buccal) (frenulum) (mucosa) (oral)	140.5	198.89	230.0	210.0	235.1	239.0
lower	140.4	198.89	230.0	210.0	235.1	239.0
upper	140.3	198.89	230.0	210.0	235.1	239.0
lower	140.1	198.89	230.0	210.0	235.1	239.0
internal (buccal) (frenulum) (mucosa) (oral).	140.4	198.89	230.0	210.0	235.1	239.0
mucosa—*see* Neoplasm, lip, internal						
oral aspect—*see* Neoplasm, lip, internal						
skin (commissure) (lower)(upper) .	173.00	198.2	232.0	216.0	238.2	239.2
basal cell carcinoma	173.01	—	—	—	—	—
specified type NEC.	173.09	—	—	—	—	—
squamous cell carcinoma	173.02	—	—	—	—	—
upper	140.0	198.89	230.0	210.0	235.1	239.0
internal (buccal) (frenulum) (mucosa) (oral).	140.3	198.89	230.0	210.0	235.1	239.0
liver.	155.2	197.7	230.8	211.5	235.3	239.0
primary	155.0	—	—	—	—	—
lobe						
azygos	162.3	197.0	231.2	212.3	235.7	239.1
frontal	191.1	198.3	—	225.0	237.5	239.6
lower	162.5	197.0	231.2	212.3	235.7	239.1
middle	162.4	197.0	231.2	212.3	235.7	239.1
occipital	191.4	198.3	—	225.0	237.5	239.6
parietal	191.3	198.3	—	225.0	237.5	239.6
temporal	191.2	198.3	—	225.0	237.5	239.6
upper	162.3	197.0	231.2	212.3	235.7	239.1
lumbosacral plexus.	171.6	198.4	—	215.6	238.1	239.2
lung.	162.9	197.0	231.2	212.3	235.7	239.1
azygos lobe.	162.3	197.0	231.2	212.3	235.7	239.1
carina.	162.2	197.0	231.2	212.3	235.7	239.1
contiguous sites with bronchus or trachea	162.8	—	—	—	—	—
hilus	162.2	197.0	231.2	212.3	235.7	239.1
lingula	162.3	197.0	231.2	212.3	235.7	239.1
lobe NEC.	162.9	197.0	231.2	212.3	235.7	239.1
lower lobe	162.5	197.0	231.2	212.3	235.7	239.1
main bronchus	162.2	197.0	231.2	212.3	235.7	239.1
middle lobe.	162.4	197.0	231.2	212.3	235.7	239.1
upper lobe	162.3	197.0	231.2	212.3	235.7	239.1
lymph, lymphatic						

	Malignant			Benign	Uncertain Behavior	Unspecified
	Primary	Secondary	Ca in situ			
channel NEC (*see also* Neoplasm, connective tissue)	171.9	198.89	—	215.9	238.1	239.2
gland (secondary)	—	196.9	—	229.0	238.8	239.89
abdominal	—	196.2	—	229.0	238.8	239.89
aortic	—	196.2	—	229.0	238.8	239.89
arm	—	196.3	—	229.0	238.8	239.89
auricular (anterior) (posterior)	—	196.0	—	229.0	238.8	239.89
axilla, axillary	—	196.3	—	229.0	238.8	239.89
brachial	—	196.3	—	229.0	238.8	239.89
bronchial	—	196.1	—	229.0	238.8	239.89
bronchopulmonary	—	196.1	—	229.0	238.8	239.89
celiac	—	196.2	—	229.0	238.8	239.89
cervical	—	196.0	—	229.0	238.8	239.89
cervicofacial	—	196.0	—	229.0	238.8	239.89
Cloquet	—	196.5	—	229.0	238.8	239.89
colic	—	196.2	—	229.0	238.8	239.89
common duct	—	196.2	—	229.0	238.8	239.89
cubital	—	196.3	—	229.0	238.8	239.89
diaphragmatic	—	196.1	—	229.0	238.8	239.89
epigastric, inferior	—	196.6	—	229.0	238.8	239.89
epitrochlear	—	196.3	—	229.0	238.8	239.89
esophageal	—	196.1	—	229.0	238.8	239.89
face	—	196.0	—	229.0	238.8	239.89
femoral	—	196.5	—	229.0	238.8	239.89
gastric	—	196.2	—	229.0	238.8	239.89
groin	—	196.5	—	229.0	238.8	239.89
head	—	196.0	—	229.0	238.8	239.89
hepatic	—	196.2	—	229.0	238.8	239.89
hilar (pulmonary)	—	196.1	—	229.0	238.8	239.89
splenic	—	196.2	—	229.0	238.8	239.89
hypogastric	—	196.6	—	229.0	238.8	239.89
ileocolic	—	196.2	—	229.0	238.8	239.89
iliac	—	196.6	—	229.0	238.8	239.89
infraclavicular	—	196.3	—	229.0	238.8	239.89
inguina, inguinal	—	196.5	—	229.0	238.8	239.89
innominate	—	196.1	—	229.0	238.8	239.89
intercostal	—	196.1	—	229.0	238.8	239.89
intestinal	—	196.2	—	229.0	238.8	239.89
intrabdominal	—	196.2	—	229.0	238.8	239.89
intrapelvic	—	196.6	—	229.0	238.8	239.89
intrathoracic	—	196.1	—	229.0	238.8	239.9
jugular	—	196.0	—	229.0	238.8	239.89
leg	—	196.5	—	229.0	238.8	239.89
limb						
lower	—	196.5	—	229.0	238.8	239.9
upper	—	196.3	—	229.0	238.8	239.89
lower limb	—	196.5	—	229.0	238.8	238.9
lumbar	—	196.2	—	229.0	238.8	239.89
mandibular	—	196.0	—	229.0	238.8	239.89
mediastinal	—	196.1	—	229.0	238.8	239.89
mesenteric (inferior) (superior)	—	196.2	—	229.0	238.8	239.89
midcolic	—	196.2	—	229.0	238.8	239.89
multiple sites in categories 196.0-196.6	—	196.8	—	229.0	238.8	239.89
neck	—	196.0	—	229.0	238.8	239.89
obturator	—	196.6	—	229.0	238.8	239.89
occipital	—	196.0	—	229.0	238.8	239.89
pancreatic	—	196.2	—	229.0	238.8	239.89
para-aortic	—	196.2	—	229.0	238.8	239.89
paracervical	—	196.6	—	229.0	238.8	239.89
parametrial	—	196.6	—	229.0	238.8	239.89

	Malignant			Benign	Uncertain Behavior	Unspecified
	Primary	Secondary	Ca in situ			
parasternal	—	196.1	—	229.0	238.8	239.89
parotid	—	196.0	—	229.0	238.8	239.89
pectoral	—	196.3	—	229.0	238.8	239.89
pelvic	—	196.6	—	229.0	238.8	239.89
peri-aortic	—	196.2	—	229.0	238.8	239.89
peripancreatic	—	196.2	—	229.0	238.8	239.89
popliteal	—	196.5	—	229.0	238.8	239.89
porta hepatis	—	196.2	—	229.0	238.8	239.89
portal	—	196.2	—	229.0	238.8	239.89
preauricular	—	196.0	—	229.0	238.8	239.89
prelaryngeal	—	196.0	—	229.0	238.8	239.89
presymphysial	—	196.6	—	229.0	238.8	239.89
pretracheal	—	196.0	—	229.0	238.8	239.89
primary (any site) NEC	202.9	—	—	—	—	—
pulmonary (hiler)	—	196.1	—	229.0	238.8	239.89
pyloric	—	196.2	—	229.0	238.8	239.89
retroperitoneal	—	196.2	—	229.0	238.8	239.89
retropharyngeal	—	196.0	—	229.0	238.8	239.89
Rosenmüller's	—	196.5	—	229.0	238.8	239.89
sacral	—	196.6	—	229.0	238.8	239.89
scalene	—	196.0	—	229.0	238.8	239.89
site NEC	—	196.9	—	229.0	238.8	239.89
splenic (hilar)	—	196.2	—	229.0	238.8	239.89
subclavicular	—	196.3	—	229.0	238.8	239.89
subinguinal	—	196.5	—	229.0	238.8	239.89
sublingual	—	196.0	—	229.0	238.8	239.89
submandibular	—	196.0	—	229.0	238.8	239.89
submaxillary	—	196.0	—	229.0	238.8	239.89
submental	—	196.0	—	229.0	238.8	239.89
subscapular	—	196.3	—	229.0	238.8	239.89
supraclavicular	—	196.0	—	229.0	238.8	239.89
thoracic	—	196.1	—	229.0	238.8	239.89
tibial	—	196.5	—	229.0	238.8	239.89
tracheal	—	196.1	—	229.0	238.8	239.89
tracheobronchial	—	196.1	—	229.0	238.8	239.89
upper limb	—	196.3	—	229.0	238.8	239.89
Virchow's	—	196.0	—	229.0	238.8	239.89
node—*see also* Neoplasm, lymph gland						
primary NEC	202.9	—	—	—	—	—
vessel (*see also* Neoplasm, connective tissue)	171.9	198.89	—	215.9	238.1	239.2
Mackenrodt's ligament	183.8	198.82	233.39	221.8	236.3	239.5
malar	170.0	198.5	—	213.0	238.0	239.2
region—*see* Neoplasm, cheek						
mammary gland—*see* Neoplasm, breast						
mandible	170.1	198.5	—	213.1	238.0	239.2
alveolar						
mucosa	143.1	198.89	230.0	210.4	235.1	239.0
ridge or process	170.1	198.5	—	213.1	238.0	239.2
carcinoma	143.1	—	—	—	—	—
carcinoma	143.1	—	—	—	—	—
marrow (bone) NEC	202.9	198.5	—	—	—	238.79
mastectomy site (skin)	173.50	198.2	—	—	—	—
basal cell carcinoma	173.51	—	—	—	—	—
specified as breast tissue	174.8	198.81	—	—	—	—
specified type NEC	173.59	—	—	—	—	—
squamous cell carcinoma	173.52	—	—	—	—	—
mastoid (air cells) (antrum) (cavity)	160.1	197.3	231.8	212.0	235.9	239.1
bone or process	170.0	198.5	—	213.0	238.0	239.2
maxilla, maxillary (superior)	170.0	198.5	—	213.0	238.0	239.2

	Malignant			Benign	Uncertain Behavior	Unspecified
	Primary	Secondary	Ca in situ			
alveolar						
mucosa	143.0	198.89	230.0	210.4	235.1	239.0
ridge or process	170.0	198.5	—	213.0	238.0	239.2
carcinoma	143.0	—	—	—	—	—
antrum	160.2	197.3	231.8	212.0	235.9	239.1
carcinoma	143.0	—	—	—	—	—
inferior—*see* Neoplasm, mandible						
sinus	160.2	197.3	231.8	212.0	235.9	239.1
meatus						
external (ear) (*see also* Neoplasm,						
skin, ear)	173.20	198.2	232.2	216.2	238.2	239.2
Meckel's diverticulum	152.3	197.4	230.7	211.2	235.2	239.0
mediastinum, mediastinal	164.9	197.1	—	212.5	235.8	239.89
anterior	164.2	197.1	—	212.5	235.8	239.89
contiguous sites with heart						
and thymus	164.8	—	—	—	—	—
posterior	164.3	197.1	—	212.5	235.8	239.89
medulla						
adrenal	194.0	198.7	234.8	227.0	237.2	239.7
oblongata	191.7	198.3	—	225.0	237.5	239.6
meibomian gland	173.10	198.2	232.1	216.1	238.2	239.2
basal cell carcinoma	173.11					
specified type NEC	173.19	—	—	—	—	—
squamous cell carcinoma	173.12	—	—	—	—	—
melanoma —*see* Melanoma						
meninges (brain) (cerebral)						
(cranial) (intracranial)	192.1	198.4	—	225.2	237.6	239.7
spinal (cord)	192.3	198.4	—	225.4	237.6	239.7
meniscus, knee joint						
(lateral) (medial)	170.7	198.5	—	213.7	238.0	239.2
mesentery, mesenteric	158.8	197.6	—	211.8	235.4	239.0
mesoappendix	158.8	197.6	—	211.8	235.4	239.0
mesocolon	158.8	197.6	—	211.8	235.4	239.0
mesopharynx—*see* Neoplasm, oropharynx						
mesosalpinx	183.3	198.82	233.39	221.0	236.3	239.5
mesovarium	183.3	198.82	233.39	221.0	236.3	239.5
metacarpus (any bone)	170.5	198.5	—	213.5	238.0	239.2
metastatic NEC—*see also* Neoplasm,						
by site, secondary	—	199.1	—	—	—	—
metatarsus (any bone)	170.8	198.5	—	213.8	238.0	239.2
midbrain	191.7	198.3	—	225.0	237.5	239.6
milk duct—*see* Neoplasm, breast						
mons						
pubis	184.4	198.82	233.32	221.2	236.3	239.5
veneris	184.4	198.82	233.32	221.2	236.3	239.5
motor tract	192.9	198.4	—	225.9	237.9	239.7
brain	191.9	198.3	—	225.0	237.5	239.6
spinal	192.2	198.3	—	225.3	237.5	239.7
mouth	145.9	198.89	230.0	210.4	235.1	239.0
contiguous sites	145.8	—	—	—	—	—
floor	144.9	198.89	230.0	210.3	235.1	239.0
anterior portion	144.0	198.89	230.0	210.3	235.1	239.0
contiguous sites	144.8	—	—	—	—	—
lateral portion	144.1	198.89	230.0	210.3	235.1	239.0
roof	145.5	198.89	230.0	210.4	235.1	239.0
specified part NEC	145.8	198.89	230.0	210.4	235.1	239.0
vestibule	145.1	198.89	230.0	210.4	235.1	239.0
mucosa						
alveolar (ridge or process)	143.9	198.89	230.0	210.4	235.1	239.0
lower	143.1	198.89	230.0	210.4	235.1	239.0
upper	143.0	198.89	230.0	210.4	235.1	239.0
buccal	145.0	198.89	230.0	210.4	235.1	239.0
cheek	145.0	198.89	230.0	210.4	235.1	239.0

	Malignant			Benign	Uncertain Behavior	Unspecified
	Primary	Secondary	Ca in situ			
lip—*see* Neoplasm, lip, internal						
nasal	160.0	197.3	231.8	212.0	235.9	239.1
oral	145.0	198.89	230.0	210.4	235.1	239.0
Müllerian duct						
female	184.8	198.82	233.39	221.8	236.3	239.5
male	187.8	198.82	233.6	222.8	236.6	239.5
multiple sites NEC	199.0	199.0	234.9	229.9	238.9	199.0
muscle—*see also* Neoplasm, connective tissue						
extraocular	190.1	198.4	234.0	224.1	238.8	239.89
myocardium	164.1	198.89	—	212.7	238.8	239.89
myometrium	182.0	198.82	233.2	219.1	236.0	239.5
myopericardium	164.1	198.89	—	212.7	238.8	239.89
nabothian gland (follicle)	180.0	198.82	233.1	219.0	236.0	239.5
nail	173.90	198.2	232.9	216.9	238.2	239.2
finger (see also Neoplasm, skin, limb, upper)	173.60	198.2	232.6	216.6	238.2	239.2
toe (see also Neoplasm, skin, limb, lower)	173.70	198.2	232.7	216.7	238.2	239.2
nares, naris (anterior) (posterior)	160.0	197.3	231.8	212.0	235.9	239.1
nasal—*see* Neoplasm, nose						
nasolabial groove (*see also* Neoplasm, skin, face)	173.30	198.2	232.3	216.3	238.2	239.2
nasolacrimal duct	190.7	198.4	234.0	224.7	238.8	239.89
nasopharynx, nasopharyngeal	147.9	198.89	230.0	210.7	235.1	239.0
contiguous sites	147.8	—	—	—	—	—
floor	147.3	198.89	230.0	210.7	235.1	239.0
roof	147.0	198.89	230.0	210.7	235.1	239.0
specified site NEC	147.8	198.89	230.0	210.7	235.1	239.0
wall	147.9	198.89	230.0	210.7	235.1	239.0
anterior	147.3	198.89	230.0	210.7	235.1	239.0
lateral	147.2	198.89	230.0	210.7	235.1	239.0
posterior	147.1	198.89	230.0	210.7	235.1	239.0
superior	147.0	198.89	230.0	210.7	235.1	239.0
nates (*see also* Neoplasm, skin, trunk)	173.50	198.2	232.5	216.5	238.2	239.2
neck NEC*	195.0	198.89	234.8	229.8	238.8	239.89
skin	173.40	198.2	232.4	216.4	238.2	239.2
basal cell carcinoma	173.41	—	—	—	—	—
specified type NEC	173.49	—	—	—	—	—
squamous cell carcinoma	173.42	—	—	—	—	—
nerve (autonomic) (ganglion) (parasympathetic) (peripheral) (sympathetic)—*see also* Neoplasm, connective tissue						
abducens	192.0	198.4	—	225.1	237.9	239.7
accessory (spinal)	192.0	198.4	—	225.1	237.9	239.7
acoustic	192.0	198.4	—	225.1	237.9	239.7
auditory	192.0	198.4	—	225.1	237.9	239.7
brachial	171.2	198.89	—	215.2	238.1	239.2
cranial (any)	192.0	198.4	—	225.1	237.9	239.7
facial	192.0	198.4	—	225.1	237.9	239.7
femoral	171.3	198.89	—	215.3	238.1	239.2
glossopharyngeal	192.0	198.4	—	225.1	237.9	239.7
hypoglossal	192.0	198.4	—	225.1	237.9	239.7
intercostal	171.4	198.89	—	215.4	238.1	239.2
lumbar	171.7	198.89	—	215.7	238.1	239.2
median	171.2	198.89	—	215.2	238.1	239.2
obturator	171.3	198.89	—	215.3	238.1	239.2
oculomotor	192.0	198.4	—	225.1	237.9	239.7
olfactory	192.0	198.4	—	225.1	237.9	239.7
optic	192.0	198.4	—	225.1	237.9	239.7

	Malignant					
	Primary	Secondary	Ca in situ	Benign	Uncertain Behavior	Unspecified
peripheral NEC.	171.9	198.89	—	215.9	238.1	239.2
radial	171.2	198.89	—	215.2	238.1	239.2
sacral	171.6	198.89	—	215.6	238.1	239.2
sciatic.	171.3	198.89	—	215.3	238.1	239.2
spinal NEC	171.9	198.89	—	215.9	238.1	239.2
trigeminal.	192.0	198.4	—	225.1	237.9	239.7
trochlear	192.0	198.4	—	225.1	237.9	239.7
ulnar	171.2	198.89	—	215.2	238.1	239.2
vagus	192.0	198.4	—	225.1	237.9	239.7
nervous system (central)						
NEC.	192.9	198.4	—	225.9	237.9	239.7
autonomic NEC	171.9	198.89	—	215.9	238.1	239.2
brain—*see also* Neoplasm, brain						
membrane or meninges	192.1	198.4	—	225.2	237.6	239.7
contiguous sites	192.8	—	—	—	—	—
parasympathetic NEC	171.9	198.89	—	215.9	238.1	239.2
sympathetic NEC.	171.9	198.89	—	215.9	238.1	239.2
nipple (female).	174.0	198.81	233.0	217	238.3	239.3
male	175.0	198.81	233.0	217	238.3	239.3
nose, nasal	195.0	198.89	234.8	229.8	238.8	239.89
ala (external) (*see also* Neoplasm,						
nose, skin)	173.30	198.2	232.3	216.3	238.2	239.2
bone	170.0	198.5	—	213.0	238.0	239.2
cartilage	160.0	197.3	231.8	212.0	235.9	239.1
cavity.	160.0	197.3	231.8	212.0	235.9	239.1
contiguous sites with accessory						
sinuses or middle ear	160.8	—	—	—	—	—
choana	147.3	198.89	230.0	210.7	235.1	239.0
external (skin) (*see also* Neoplasm,						
nose, skin)	173.30	198.2	232.3	216.3	238.2	239.2
fossa	160.0	197.3	231.8	212.0	235.9	239.1
internal	160.0	197.3	231.8	212.0	235.9	239.1
mucosa	160.0	197.3	231.8	212.0	235.9	239.1
septum	160.0	197.3	231.8	212.0	235.9	239.1
posterior margin	147.3	198.89	230.0	210.7	235.1	239.0
sinus—*see* Neoplasm, sinus						
skin.	173.30	198.2	232.3	216.3	238.2	239.2
basal cell carcinoma	173.31	—	—	—	—	—
specified type NEC.	173.39	—	—	—	—	—
squamous cell carcinoma	173.32	—	—	—	—	—
turbinate (mucosa)	160.0	197.3	231.8	212.0	235.9	239.1
bone	170.0	198.5	—	213.0	238.0	239.2
vestibule	160.0	197.3	231.8	212.0	235.9	239.1
nostril.	160.0	197.3	231.8	212.0	235.9	239.1
nucleus pulposus	170.2	198.5	—	213.2	238.0	239.2
occipital						
bone	170.0	198.5	—	213.0	238.0	239.2
lobe or pole, brain	191.4	198.3	—	225.0	237.5	239.6
odontogenic—*see* Neoplasm,						
jaw bone						
oesophagus—*see* Neoplasm,						
esophagus						
olfactory nerve or bulb	192.0	198.4	—	225.1	237.9	239.7
olive (brain)	191.7	198.3	—	225.0	237.5	239.6
omentum	158.8	197.6	—	211.8	235.4	239.0
operculum (brain)	191.0	198.3	—	225.0	237.5	239.6
optic nerve, chiasm, or tract	192.0	198.4	—	225.1	237.9	239.7
oral (cavity)	145.9	198.89	230.0	210.4	235.1	239.0
contiguous sites with lip						
or pharynx	149.8	—	—	—	—	—
ill-defined	149.9	198.89	230.0	210.4	235.1	239.0
mucosa	145.9	198.89	230.0	210.4	235.1	239.0
orbit.	190.1	198.4	234.0	224.1	238.8	239.89

| | Malignant | | | Benign | Uncertain Behavior | Unspecified |
	Primary	Secondary	Ca in situ			
bone	170.0	198.5	—	213.0	238.0	239.2
eye	190.1	198.4	234.0	224.1	238.8	239.89
soft parts	190.1	198.4	234.0	224.1	238.8	239.89
organ of Zuckerkandl	194.6	198.89	—	227.6	237.3	239.7
oropharynx	146.9	198.89	230.0	210.6	235.1	239.0
branchial cleft (vestige)	146.8	198.89	230.0	210.6	235.1	239.0
contiguous sites	146.8	—	—	—	—	—
junctional region	146.5	198.89	230.0	210.6	235.1	239.0
lateral wall	146.6	198.89	230.0	210.6	235.1	239.0
pillars of fauces	146.2	198.89	230.0	210.6	235.1	239.0
posterior wall	146.7	198.89	230.0	210.6	235.1	239.0
specified part NEC	146.8	198.89	230.0	210.6	235.1	239.0
vallecula	146.3	198.89	230.0	210.6	235.1	239.0
os						
external	180.1	198.82	233.1	219.0	236.0	239.5
internal	180.0	198.82	233.1	219.0	236.0	239.5
ovary	183.0	198.6	233.39	220	236.2	239.5
oviduct	183.2	198.82	233.39	221.0	236.3	239.5
palate	145.5	198.89	230.0	210.4	235.1	239.0
hard	145.2	198.89	230.0	210.4	235.1	239.0
junction of hard and soft						
palate	145.5	198.89	230.0	210.4	235.1	239.0
soft	145.3	198.89	230.0	210.4	235.1	239.0
nasopharyngeal surface	147.3	198.89	230.0	210.7	235.1	239.0
posterior surface	147.3	198.89	230.0	210.7	235.1	239.0
superior surface	147.3	198.89	230.0	210.7	235.1	239.0
palatoglossal arch	146.2	198.89	230.0	210.6	235.1	239.0
palatopharyngeal arch	146.2	198.89	230.0	210.6	235.1	239.0
pallium	191.0	198.3	—	225.0	237.5	239.6
palpebra	173.10	198.2	232.1	216.1	238.2	239.2
basal cell carcinoma	173.11	—	—	—	—	—
specified type NEC	173.19	—	—	—	—	—
squamous cell carcinoma	173.12	—	—	—	—	—
pancreas	157.9	197.8	230.9	211.6	235.5	239.0
body	157.1	197.8	230.9	211.6	235.5	239.0
contiguous sites	157.8	—	—	—	—	—
duct (of Santorini) (of						
Wirsung)	157.3	197.8	230.9	211.6	235.5	239.0
ectopic tissue	157.8	197.8	230.9	211.6	235.5	239.0
head	157.0	197.8	230.9	211.6	235.5	239.0
islet cells	157.4	197.8	230.9	211.7	235.5	239.0
neck	157.8	197.8	230.9	211.6	235.5	239.0
tail	157.2	197.8	230.9	211.6	235.5	239.0
para-aortic body	194.6	198.89	—	227.6	237.3	239.7
paraganglion NEC	194.6	198.89	—	227.6	237.3	239.7
parametrium	183.4	198.82	—	221.0	236.3	239.5
paranephric	158.0	197.6	—	211.8	235.4	239.0
pararectal	195.3	198.89	—	229.8	238.8	239.89
parasagittal (region)	195.0	198.89	234.8	229.8	238.8	239.89
parasellar	192.9	198.4	—	225.9	237.9	239.7
parathyroid (gland)	194.1	198.89	234.8	227.1	237.4	239.7
paraurethral	195.3	198.89	—	229.8	238.8	239.89
gland	189.4	198.1	233.9	223.89	236.99	239.5
paravaginal	195.3	198.89	—	229.8	238.8	239.89
parenchyma, kidney	189.0	198.0	233.9	223.0	236.91	239.5
parietal						
bone	170.0	198.5	—	213.0	238.0	239.2
lobe, brain	191.3	198.3	—	225.0	237.5	239.6
paroophoron	183.3	198.82	233.39	221.0	236.3	239.5
parotid (duct) (gland)	142.0	198.89	230.0	210.2	235.0	239.0
parovarium	183.3	198.82	233.39	221.0	236.3	239.5
patella	170.8	198.5	—	213.8	238.0	239.2
peduncle, cerebral	191.7	198.3	—	225.0	237.5	239.6

	Malignant			Benign	Uncertain Behavior	Unspecified
	Primary	Secondary	Ca in situ			
pelvirectal junction	154.0	197.5	230.4	211.4	235.2	239.0
pelvis, pelvic	195.3	198.89	234.8	229.8	238.8	239.89
bone	170.6	198.5	—	213.6	238.0	239.2
floor	195.3	198.89	234.8	229.8	238.8	239.89
renal	189.1	198.0	233.9	223.1	236.91	239.5
viscera	195.3	198.89	234.8	229.8	238.8	239.89
wall	195.3	198.89	234.8	229.8	238.8	239.89
pelvo-abdominal	195.8	198.89	234.8	229.8	238.8	239.89
penis	187.4	198.82	233.5	222.1	236.6	239.5
body	187.3	198.82	233.5	222.1	236.6	239.5
corpus (cavernosum)	187.3	198.82	233.5	222.1	236.6	239.5
glans	187.2	198.82	233.5	222.1	236.6	239.5
skin NEC	187.4	198.82	233.5	222.1	236.6	239.5
periadrenal (tissue)	158.0	197.6	—	211.8	235.4	239.0
perianal (skin) (*see also* Neoplasm, skin, anus)	173.50	198.2	232.5	216.5	238.2	239.2
pericardium	164.1	198.89	—	212.7	238.8	239.89
perinephric	158.0	197.6	—	211.8	235.4	239.0
perineum	195.3	198.89	234.8	229.8	238.8	239.89
periodontal tissue NEC	143.9	198.89	230.0	210.4	235.1	239.0
periosteum—*see* Neoplasm, bone						
peripancreatic	158.0	197.6	—	211.8	235.4	239.0
peripheral nerve NEC	171.9	198.89	—	215.9	238.1	239.2
perirectal (tissue)	195.3	198.89	—	229.8	238.8	239.89
perirenal (tissue)	158.0	197.6	—	211.8	235.4	239.0
peritoneum, peritoneal (cavity)	158.9	197.6	—	211.8	235.4	239.0
contiguous sites	158.8	—	—	—	—	—
with digestive organs	159.8	—	—	—	—	—
parietal	158.8	197.6	—	211.8	235.4	239.0
pelvic	158.8	197.6	—	211.8	235.4	239.0
specified part NEC	158.8	197.6	—	211.8	235.4	239.0
peritonsillar (tissue)	195.0	198.89	234.8	229.8	238.8	239.89
periurethral tissue	195.3	198.89	—	229.8	238.8	239.89
phalanges	170.9	198.5	—	213.9	238.0	239.2
foot	170.8	198.5	—	213.8	238.0	239.2
hand	170.5	198.5	—	213.5	238.0	239.2
pharynx, pharyngeal	149.0	198.89	230.0	210.9	235.1	239.0
bursa	147.1	198.89	230.0	210.7	235.1	239.0
fornix	147.3	198.89	230.0	210.7	235.1	239.0
recess	147.2	198.89	230.0	210.7	235.1	239.0
region	149.0	198.89	230.0	210.9	235.1	239.0
tonsil	147.1	198.89	230.0	210.7	235.1	239.0
wall (lateral) (posterior)	149.0	198.89	230.0	210.9	235.1	239.0
pia mater (cerebral) (cranial)	192.1	198.4	—	225.2	237.6	239.7
spinal	192.3	198.4	—	225.4	237.6	239.7
pillars of fauces	146.2	198.89	230.0	210.6	235.1	239.0
pineal (body) (gland)	194.4	198.89	234.8	227.4	237.1	239.7
pinna (ear) NEC (*see also* Neoplasm, skin, ear)	173.20	198.2	232.2	216.2	238.2	239.2
cartilage	171.0	198.89	—	215.0	238.1	239.2
piriform fossa or sinus	148.1	198.89	230.0	210.8	235.1	239.0
pituitary (body) (fossa) (gland) (lobe)	194.3	198.89	234.8	227.3	237.0	239.7
placenta	181	198.82	233.2	219.8	236.1	239.5
pleura, pleural (cavity)	163.9	197.2	—	212.4	235.8	239.1
contiguous sites	163.8	—	—	—	—	—
parietal	163.0	197.2	—	212.4	235.8	239.1
visceral	163.1	197.2	—	212.4	235.8	239.1
plexus						
brachial	171.2	198.89	—	215.2	238.1	239.2
cervical	171.0	198.89	—	215.0	238.1	239.2
choroid	191.5	198.3	—	225.0	237.5	239.6

	Malignant					
	Primary	Secondary	Ca in situ	Benign	Uncertain Behavior	Unspecified
lumbosacral	171.6	198.89	—	215.6	238.1	239.2
sacral	171.6	198.89	—	215.6	238.1	239.2
pluri-endocrine	194.8	198.89	234.8	227.8	237.4	239.7
pole						
frontal	191.1	198.3	—	225.0	237.5	239.6
occipital	191.4	198.3	—	225.0	237.5	239.6
pons (varolii)	191.7	198.3	—	225.0	237.5	239.6
popliteal fossa or space*	195.5	198.89	234.8	229.8	238.8	239.89
postcricoid (region)	148.0	198.89	230.0	210.8	235.1	239.0
posterior fossa (cranial)	191.9	198.3	—	225.0	237.5	239.6
postnasal space	147.9	198.89	230.0	210.7	235.1	239.0
prepuce	187.1	198.82	233.5	222.1	236.6	239.5
prepylorus	151.1	197.8	230.2	211.1	235.2	239.0
presacral (region)	195.3	198.89	—	229.8	238.8	239.89
prostate (gland)	185	198.82	233.4	222.2	236.5	239.5
utricle	189.3	198.1	233.9	223.81	236.99	239.5
pterygoid fossa	171.0	198.89	—	215.0	238.1	239.2
pubic bone	170.6	198.5	—	213.6	238.0	239.2
pudenda, pudendum (female)	184.4	198.82	233.32	221.2	236.3	239.5
pulmonary	162.9	197.0	231.2	212.3	235.7	239.1
putamen	191.0	198.3	—	225.0	237.5	239.6
pyloric						
antrum	151.2	197.8	230.2	211.1	235.2	239.0
canal	151.1	197.8	230.2	211.1	235.2	239.0
pylorus	151.1	197.8	230.2	211.1	235.2	239.0
pyramid (brain)	191.7	198.3	—	225.0	237.5	239.6
pyriform fossa or sinus	148.1	198.89	230.0	210.8	235.1	239.0
radius (any part)	170.4	198.5	—	213.4	238.0	239.2
Rathke's pouch	194.3	198.89	234.8	227.3	237.0	239.7
rectosigmoid (colon) (junction)	154.0	197.5	230.4	211.4	235.2	239.0
contiguous sites with anus or rectum	154.8	—	—	—	—	—
rectouterine pouch	158.8	197.6	—	211.8	235.4	239.0
rectovaginal septum or wall	195.3	198.89	234.8	229.8	238.8	239.89
rectovesical septum	195.3	198.89	234.8	229.8	238.8	239.89
rectum (ampulla)	154.1	197.5	230.4	211.4	235.2	239.0
and colon	154.0	197.5	230.4	211.4	235.2	239.0
contiguous sites with anus or rectosigmoid junction	154.8	—	—	—	—	—
renal	189.0	198.0	233.9	223.0	236.91	239.5
calyx	189.1	198.0	233.9	223.1	236.91	239.5
hilus	189.1	198.0	233.9	223.1	236.91	239.5
parenchyma	189.0	198.0	233.9	223.0	236.91	239.5
pelvis	189.1	198.0	233.9	223.1	236.91	239.5
respiratory						
organs or system NEC	165.9	197.3	231.9	212.9	235.9	239.1
contiguous sites with intrathoracic organs	165.8	—	—	—	—	—
specified sites NEC	165.8	197.3	231.8	212.8	235.9	239.1
tract NEC	165.9	197.3	231.9	212.9	235.9	239.1
upper	165.0	197.3	231.9	212.9	235.9	239.1
retina	190.5	198.4	234.0	224.5	238.8	239.81
retrobulbar	190.1	198.4	—	224.1	238.8	239.89
retrocecal	158.0	197.6	—	211.8	235.4	239.0
retromolar (area) (triangle) (trigone)	145.6	198.89	230.0	210.4	235.1	239.0
retro-orbital	195.0	198.89	234.8	229.8	238.8	239.89
retroperitoneal (space) (tissue)	158.0	197.6	—	211.8	235.4	239.0
contiguous sites	158.8	—	—	—	—	—
retroperitoneum	158.0	197.6	—	211.8	235.4	239.0
contiguous sites	158.8	—	—	—	—	—

	Malignant					
	Primary	Secondary	Ca in situ	Benign	Uncertain Behavior	Unspecified
retropharyngeal	149.0	198.89	230.0	210.9	235.1	239.0
retrovesical (septum)	195.3	198.89	234.8	229.8	238.8	239.89
rhinencephalon	191.0	198.3	—	225.0	237.5	239.6
rib	170.3	198.5	—	213.3	238.0	239.2
Rosenmüller's fossa	147.2	198.89	230.0	210.7	235.1	239.0
round ligament	183.5	198.82	—	221.0	236.3	239.5
sacrococcyx, sacrococcygeal	170.6	198.5	—	213.6	238.0	239.2
region	195.3	198.89	234.8	229.8	238.8	239.89
sacrouterine ligament	183.4	198.82	—	221.0	236.3	239.5
sacrum, sacral (vertebra)	170.6	198.5	—	213.6	238.0	239.2
salivary gland or duct						
(major)	142.9	198.89	230.0	210.2	235.0	239.0
contiguous sites	142.8	—	—	—	—	—
minor NEC	145.9	198.89	230.0	210.4	235.1	239.0
parotid	142.0	198.89	230.0	210.2	235.0	239.0
pluriglandular	142.8	198.89	230.0	210.2	235.0	239.0
sublingual	142.2	198.89	230.0	210.2	235.0	239.0
submandibular	142.1	198.89	230.0	210.2	235.0	239.0
submaxillary	142.1	198.89	230.0	210.2	235.0	239.0
salpinx (uterine)	183.2	198.82	233.39	221.0	236.3	239.5
Santorini's duct	157.3	197.8	230.9	211.6	235.5	239.0
scalp	173.40	198.2	232.4	216.4	238.2	239.2
basal cell carcinoma	173.41	—	—	—	—	—
specified type NEC	173.49	—	—	—	—	—
squamous cell carcinoma	173.42	—	—	—	—	—
scapula (any part)	170.4	198.5	—	213.4	238.0	239.2
scapular region	195.1	198.89	234.8	229.8	238.8	239.89
scar NEC (see also						
Neoplasm, skin)	173.90	198.2	232.9	216.9	238.2	239.2
sciatic nerve	171.3	198.89	—	215.3	238.1	239.2
sclera	190.0	198.4	234.0	224.0	238.8	239.89
scrotum (skin)	187.7	198.82	233.6	222.4	236.6	239.5
sebaceous gland—see Neoplasm, skin						
sella turcica	194.3	198.89	234.8	227.3	237.0	239.7
bone	170.0	198.5	—	213.0	238.0	239.2
semilunar cartilage (knee)	170.7	198.5	—	213.7	238.0	239.2
seminal vesicle	187.8	198.82	233.6	222.8	236.6	239.5
septum						
nasal	160.0	197.3	231.8	212.0	235.9	239.1
posterior margin	147.3	198.89	230.0	210.7	235.1	239.0
rectovaginal	195.3	198.89	234.8	229.8	238.8	239.89
rectovesical	195.3	198.89	234.8	229.8	238.8	239.89
urethrovaginal	184.9	198.82	233.39	221.9	236.3	239.5
vesicovaginal	184.9	198.82	233.39	221.9	236.3	239.5
shoulder NEC*	195.4	198.89	232.6	229.8	238.8	239.89
sigmoid flexure (lower)						
(upper)	153.3	197.5	230.3	211.3	235.2	239.0
sinus (accessory)	160.9	197.3	231.8	212.0	235.9	239.1
bone (any)	170.0	198.5	—	213.0	238.0	239.2
contiguous sites with middle ear or						
nasal cavities	160.8	—	—	—	—	—
ethmoidal	160.3	197.3	231.8	212.0	235.9	239.1
frontal	160.4	197.3	231.8	212.0	235.9	239.1
maxillary	160.2	197.3	231.8	212.0	235.9	239.1
nasal, paranasal NEC	160.9	197.3	231.8	212.0	235.9	239.1
pyriform	148.1	198.89	230.0	210.8	235.1	239.0
sphenoidal	160.5	197.3	231.8	212.0	235.9	239.1
skeleton, skeletal NEC	170.9	198.5	—	213.9	238.0	239.2
Skene's gland	189.4	198.1	233.9	223.89	236.99	239.5
skin NOS	173.90	198.2	232.9	216.9	238.2	239.2
abdominal wall	173.50	198.2	232.5	216.5	238.2	239.2
basal cell carcinoma	173.51	—	—	—	—	—
specified type NEC	173.59	—	—	—	—	—

	Malignant			Benign	Uncertain Behavior	Unspecified
	Primary	Secondary	Ca in situ			
squamous cell carcinoma 173.52	—	—	—	—	—	
ala nasi (*see also* Neoplasm, skin, face) 173.30	198.2	232.3	216.3	238.2	239.2	
ankle (*see also* Neoplasm, skin, limb, lower) 173.70	198.2	232.7	216.7	238.2	239.2	
antecubital space (*see also* Neoplasm skin, limb, upper). 173.60	198.2	232.6	216.6	238.2	239.2	
anus. 173.50	198.2	232.5	216.5	238.2	239.2	
basal cell carcinoma 173.51	—	—	—	—	—	
specified type NEC. 173.59	—	—	—	—	—	
squamous cell carcinoma 173.52	—	—	—	—	—	
arm (see also Neoplasm, skin limb, upper) 173.60	198.2	232.6	216.6	238.2	239.2	
auditory canal (external) (*see also* Neoplasm, skin, ear) 173.20	198.2	232.2	216.2	238.2	239.2	
auricle (ear) (*see also*Neoplasm, skin, ear). 173.20	198.2	232.2	216.2	238.2	239.2	
auricular canal (external) (*see also* Neoplasm, skin, ear) 173.20	198.2	232.2	216.2	238.2	239.2	
axilla, axillary fold (*see also* Neoplasm, skin, trunk). 173.50	198.2	232.5	216.5	238.2	239.2	
back 173.50	198.2	232.5	216.5	238.2	239.2	
basal cell carcinoma 173.51	—	—	—	—	—	
specified type NEC. 173.59	—	—	—	—	—	
squamous cell carcinoma 173.52	—	—	—	—	—	
basal cell carcinoma, unspecified site. 173.91	—	—	—	—	—	
breast (*see also* Neoplasm, skin, trunk) 173.50	198.2	232.5	216.5	238.2	239.2	
brow (*see also* Neoplasm, skin, face) 173.30	198.2	232.3	216.3	238.2	239.2	
buttock (*see also* Neoplasm, skin, trunk). 173.50	198.2	232.5	216.5	238.2	239.2	
calf (*see also* Neoplasm, skin, limb, lower) 173.70	198.2	232.7	216.7	238.2	239.2	
canthus (eye) (inner)(outer) 173.10	198.2	232.1	216.1	238.2	239.2	
basal cell carcinoma 173.11	—	—	—	—	—	
specified type NEC. 173.19	—	—	—	—	—	
squamous cell carcinoma 173.12	—	—	—	—	—	
cervical region (*see also* Neoplasm, skin, neck) 173.40	198.2	232.4	216.4	238.2	239.2	
cheek (external) (*see also* Neoplasm, skin, face) 173.30	198.2	232.3	216.3	238.2	239.2	
chest (wall) (*see also* Neoplasm, skin, trunk). 173.50	198.2	232.5	216.5	238.2	239.2	
chin (*see also* Neoplasm, skin, face) 173.30	198.2	232.3	216.3	238.2	239.2	
clavicular area (*see also* Neoplasm, skin, trunk). 173.50	198.2	232.5	216.5	238.2	239.2	
clitoris 184.3	198.82	233.32	221.2	236.3	239.5	
columnella (*see also* Neoplasm, skin, face) 173.30	198.2	232.3	216.3	238.2	239.2	
concha (*see also* Neoplasm, skin ear) 173.20	198.2	232.2	216.2	238.2	239.2	
contiguous sites 173.80	—	—	—	—	—	
basal cell carcinoma 173.81	—	—	—	—	—	
specified type NEC. 173.89	—	—	—	—	—	
squamous cell carcinoma 173.82	—	—	—	—	—	
ear (external) 173.20	198.2	232.2	216.2	238.2	239.2	
basal cell carcinoma 173.21	—	—	—	—	—	
specified type NEC. 173.29	—	—	—	—	—	
squamous cell carcinoma 173.22	—	—	—	—	—	

	Malignant			Benign	Uncertain Behavior	Unspecified
	Primary	Secondary	Ca in situ			
elbow (*see also* Neoplasm, skin, limb, upper)	173.60	198.2	232.6	216.6	238.2	239.2
eyebrow (*see also* Neoplasm, skin, face)	173.30	198.2	232.3	216.3	238.2	239.2
eyelid	173.10	198.2	232.1	216.1	238.2	239.2
basal cell carcinoma	173.11	—	—	—	—	—
specified type NEC	173.19	—	—	—	—	—
squamous cell carcinoma	173.12	—	—	—	—	—
face NEC	173.30	198.2	232.3	216.3	238.2	239.2
basal cell carcinoma	173.31	—	—	—	—	—
specified type NEC	173.39	—	—	—	—	—
squamous cell carcinoma	173.32	—	—	—	—	—
female genital organs (external)	184.4	198.82	233.30	221.2	236.3	239.5
clitoris	184.3	198.82	233.32	221.2	236.3	239.5
labium NEC	184.4	198.82	233.32	221.2	236.3	239.5
majus	184.1	198.82	233.32	221.2	236.3	239.5
minus	184.2	198.82	233.32	221.2	236.3	239.5
pudendum	184.4	198.82	233.32	221.2	236.3	239.5
vulva	184.4	198.82	233.32	221.2	236.3	239.5
finger (*see also* Neoplasm, skin, limb, upper)	173.60	198.2	232.6	216.6	238.2	239.2
flank (*see also* Neoplasm, skin, trunk)	173.50	198.2	232.5	216.5	238.2	239.2
foot(*see also* Neoplasm, skin, limb, lower)	173.70	198.2	232.7	216.7	238.2	239.2
forearm (*see also* Neoplasm, skin, limb, upper)	173.60	198.2	232.6	216.6	238.2	239.2
forehead (*see also* Neoplasm, skin, face)	173.30	198.2	232.3	216.3	238.2	239.2
glabella (*see also* Neoplasm, skin, face)	173.30	198.2	232.3	216.3	238.2	239.2
gluteal region (*see also* Neoplasm, skin, trunk)	173.50	198.2	232.5	216.5	238.2	239.2
groin (*see also* Neoplasm, skin, trunk)	173.50	198.2	232.5	216.5	238.2	239.2
hand (*see also* Neoplasm, skin, limb, upper)	173.60	198.2	232.6	216.6	238.2	239.2
head NEC (*see also* Neoplasm, skin, scalp)	173.40	198.2	232.4	216.4	238.2	239.2
heel (*see also* Neoplasm, skin, limb, lower)	173.70	198.2	232.7	216.7	238.2	239.2
helix (*see also* Neoplasm, skin, ear)	173.20	198.2	232.2	216.2	238.2	239.2
hip	173.70	198.2	232.7	216.7	238.2	239.2
basal cell carcinoma	173.71	—	—	—	—	—
specified type NEC	173.79	—	—	—	—	—
squamous cell carcinoma	173.72	—	—	—	—	—
infraclavicular region (*see also* Neoplasm, skin, trunk)	173.50	198.2	232.5	216.5	238.2	239.2
inguinal region (*see also* Neoplasm, skin, trunk)	173.50	198.2	232.5	216.5	238.2	239.2
jaw (*see also* Neoplasm, skin, face)	173.30	198.2	232.3	216.3	238.2	239.2
knee (*see also* Neoplasm, skin, limb, lower)	173.70	198.2	232.7	216.7	238.2	239.2
labia						
majora	184.1	198.82	233.32	221.2	236.3	239.5
minora	184.2	198.82	233.32	221.2	236.3	239.5
leg (*see also* Neoplasm, skin, limb, lower)	173.70	198.2	232.7	216.7	238.2	239.2
lid (lower) (upper)	173.10	198.2	232.1	216.1	238.2	239.2
basal cell carcinoma	173.11	—	—	—	—	—
specified type NEC	173.19	—	—	—	—	—

| | Malignant | | | | | |
	Primary	Secondary	Ca in situ	Benign	Uncertain Behavior	Unspecified
squamous cell carcinoma	173.12	—	—	—	—	—
limb NEC.	173.90	198.2	232.9	216.9	238.2	239.5
lower	173.70	198.2	232.7	216.7	238.2	239.2
basal cell carcinoma	173.71	—	—	—	—	—
specified type NEC.	173.79	—	—	—	—	—
squamous cell carcinoma	173.72	—	—	—	—	—
upper	173.60	198.2	232.6	216.6	238.2	239.2
basal cell carcinoma	173.61	—	—	—	—	—
specified type NEC.	173.69	—	—	—	—	—
squamous cell carcinoma	173.62	—	—	—	—	—
lip (lower) (upper)	173.00	198.2	232.0	216.0	238.2	239.2
basal cell carcinoma	173.01	—	—	—	—	—
specified type NEC.	173.09	—	—	—	—	—
squamous cell carcinoma	173.02	—	—	—	—	—
male genital organs.	187.9	198.82	233.6	222.9	236.6	239.5
penis	187.4	198.82	233.5	222.1	236.6	239.5
prepuce	187.1	198.82	233.5	222.1	236.6	239.5
scrotum	187.7	198.82	233.6	222.4	236.6	239.5
mastectomy site (*see also* Neoplasm, skin, trunk)	173.50	198.2	—	—	—	—
specified as breast tissue	174.8	198.81	—	—	—	—
meatus, acoustic (external) (*see also* Neoplasm, skin, ear)	173.20	198.2	232.2	216.2	238.2	239.2
melanoma —*see* Melanoma						
nates (*see also* Neoplasm, skin, trunk)	173.50	198.2	232.5	216.5	238.2	239.2
neck	173.40	198.2	232.4	216.4	238.2	239.2
basal cell carcinoma	173.41	—	—	—	—	—
specified type NEC.	173.49	—	—	—	—	—
squamous cell carcinoma	173.42	—	—	—	—	—
nose (external) (*see also* Neoplasm, skin, face)	173.30	198.2	232.3	216.3	238.2	239.2
palm (*see also* Neoplasm, skin, limb, upper)	173.60	198.2	232.6	216.6	238.2	239.2
palpebra	173.10	198.2	232.1	216.1	238.2	239.2
basal cell carcinoma	173.11	—	—	—	—	—
specified type NEC.	173.19	—	—	—	—	—
squamous cell carcinoma	173.12	—	—	—	—	—
penis NEC	187.4	198.82	233.5	222.1	236.6	239.5
perianal (*see also* Neoplasm, skin, anus)	173.50	198.2	232.5	216.5	238.2	239.2
perineum (*see also* Neoplasm, skin, anus)	173.50	198.2	232.5	216.5	238.2	239.2
pinna (*see also* Neoplasm, skin, ear)	173.20	198.2	232.2	216.2	238.2	239.2
plantar (*see also* Neoplasm, skin, limb, lower)	173.70	198.2	232.7	216.7	238.2	239.2
popliteal fossa or space (*see also* Neoplasm, skin, limb, lower)	173.70	198.2	232.7	216.7	238.2	239.2
prepuce	187.1	198.82	233.5	222.1	236.6	239.5
pubes (*see also* Neoplasm, skin, trunk)	173.50	198.2	232.5	216.5	238.2	239.2
sacrococcygeal region (*see also* Neoplasm, skin, trunk)	173.50	198.2	232.5	216.5	238.2	239.2
scalp	173.40	198.2	232.4	216.4	238.2	239.2
basal cell carcinoma	173.41	—	—	—	—	—
specified type NEC.	173.49	—	—	—	—	—
squamous cell carcinoma	173.42	—	—	—	—	—
scapular region (*see also* Neoplasm, skin, trunk)	173.50	198.2	232.5	216.5	238.2	239.2
scrotum	187.7	198.82	233.6	222.4	236.6	239.5
shoulder	173.60	198.2	232.6	216.6	238.2	239.2
basal cell carcinoma	173.61	—	—	—	—	—
specified type NEC.	173.69	—	—	—	—	—

	Malignant			Benign	Uncertain Behavior	Unspecified
	Primary	Secondary	Ca in situ			
squamous cell carcinoma	173.62	—	—	—	—	—
sole (foot) (see also Neoplasm, skin, limb, lower)	173.70	198.2	232.7	216.7	238.2	239.2
specified sites NEC	173.80	198.2	232.8	216.8	232.8	239.2
basal cell carcinoma	173.81	—	—	—	—	—
specified type NEC.	173.89	—	—	—	—	—
squamous cell carcinoma	173.82	—	—	—	—	—
specified type NEC, unspecified site	173.99	—	—	—	—	—
squamous cell carcinoma, unspecified site	173.92	—	—	—	—	—
submammary fold (see also Neoplasm, skin, turnk)	173.50	198.2	232.5	216.5	238.2	239.2
supraclavicular region (see also Neoplasm, skin, neck)	173.40	198.2	232.4	216.4	238.2	239.2
temple (see also Neoplasm, skin, face)	173.30	198.2	232.3	216.3	238.2	239.2
thigh (see also Neoplasm, skin, limb, lower)	173.70	198.2	232.7	216.7	238.2	239.2
thoracic wall (see also Neoplasm, skin, trunk)	173.50	198.2	232.5	216.5	238.2	239.2
thumb (see also Neoplasm, skin, limb, upper)	173.60	198.2	232.6	216.6	238.2	239.2
toe (see also Neoplasm, skin, limb, lower)	173.70	198.2	232.7	216.7	238.2	239.2
tragus (see also Neoplasm, skin, ear)	173.20	198.2	232.2	216.2	238.2	239.2
trunk	173.50	198.2	232.5	216.5	238.2	239.2
basal cell carcinoma	173.51	—	—	—	—	—
specified type NEC.	173.59	—	—	—	—	—
squamous cell carcinoma	173.52	—	—	—	—	—
umbilicus (see also Neoplasm, skin, trunk)	173.50	198.2	232.5	216.5	238.2	239.2
vulva	184.4	198.82	233.32	221.2	236.3	239.5
wrist (see also Neoplasm, skin, limb, upper)	173.60	198.2	232.6	216.6	238.2	239.2
skull	170.0	198.5	—	213.0	238.0	239.2
soft parts or tissues—see Neoplasm, connective tissue						
specified site NEC	195.8	198.89	234.8	229.8	238.8	239.89
spermatic cord	187.6	198.82	233.6	222.8	236.6	239.5
sphenoid	160.5	197.3	231.8	212.0	235.9	239.1
bone	170.0	198.5	—	213.0	238.0	239.2
sinus	160.5	197.3	231.8	212.0	235.9	239.1
sphincter						
anal	154.2	197.5	230.5	211.4	235.5	239.0
of Oddi	156.1	197.8	230.8	211.5	235.3	239.0
spine, spinal (column)	170.2	198.5	—	213.2	238.0	239.2
bulb	191.7	198.3	—	225.0	237.5	239.6
coccyx	170.6	198.5	—	213.6	238.0	239.2
cord (cervical) (lumbar) (sacral) (thoracic)	192.2	198.3	—	225.3	237.5	239.7
dura mater	192.3	198.4	—	225.4	237.6	239.7
lumbosacral	170.2	198.5	—	213.2	238.0	239.2
membrane	192.3	198.4	—	225.4	237.6	239.7
meninges	192.3	198.4	—	225.4	237.6	239.7
nerve (root)	171.9	198.89	—	215.9	238.1	239.2
pia mater	192.3	198.4	—	225.4	237.6	239.7
root	171.9	198.89	—	215.9	238.1	239.2
sacrum	170.6	198.5	—	213.6	238.0	239.2
spleen, splenic NEC	159.1	197.8	230.9	211.9	235.5	239.0
flexure (colon)	153.7	197.5	230.3	211.3	235.2	239.0
stem, brain	191.7	198.3	—	225.0	237.5	239.6

	Malignant			Benign	Uncertain Behavior	Unspecified
	Primary	Secondary	Ca in situ			
Stensen's duct	142.0	198.89	230.0	210.2	235.0	239.0
sternum	170.3	198.5	—	213.3	238.0	239.2
stomach	151.9	197.8	230.2	211.1	235.2	239.0
antrum (pyloric)	151.2	197.8	230.2	211.1	235.2	239.0
body	151.4	197.8	230.2	211.1	235.2	239.0
cardia	151.0	197.8	230.2	211.1	235.2	239.0
cardiac orifice	151.0	197.8	230.2	211.1	235.2	239.0
contiguous sites	151.8	—	—	—	—	—
corpus	151.4	197.8	230.2	211.1	235.2	239.0
fundus	151.3	197.8	230.2	211.1	235.2	239.0
greater curvature NEC	151.6	197.8	230.2	211.1	235.2	239.0
lesser curvature NEC	151.5	197.8	230.2	211.1	235.2	239.0
prepylorus	151.1	197.8	230.2	211.1	235.2	239.0
pylorus	151.1	197.8	230.2	211.1	235.2	239.0
wall NEC	151.9	197.8	230.2	211.1	235.2	239.0
anterior NEC	151.8	197.8	230.2	211.1	235.2	239.0
posterior NEC	151.8	197.8	230.2	211.1	235.2	239.0
stroma, endometrial	182.0	198.82	233.2	219.1	236.0	239.5
stump, cervical	180.8	198.82	233.1	219.0	236.0	239.5
subcutaneous (nodule) (tissue) NEC—*see* Neoplasm, connective tissue						
subdural	192.1	198.4	—	225.2	237.6	239.7
subglottis, subglottic	161.2	197.3	231.0	212.1	235.6	239.1
sublingual	144.9	198.89	230.0	210.3	235.1	239.0
gland or duct	142.2	198.89	230.0	210.2	235.0	239.0
submandibular gland	142.1	198.89	230.0	210.2	235.0	239.0
submaxillary gland or duct	142.1	198.89	230.0	210.2	235.0	239.0
submental	195.0	198.89	234.8	229.8	238.8	239.89
subpleural	162.9	197.0	—	212.3	235.7	239.1
substernal	164.2	197.1	—	212.5	235.8	239.89
sudoriferous, sudoriparous gland, site unspecified	173.90	198.2	232.9	216.9	238.2	239.2
specified site—*see* Neoplasm, skin						
supraclavicular region	195.0	198.89	234.8	229.8	238.8	239.89
supraglottis	161.1	197.3	231.0	212.1	235.6	239.1
suprarenal (capsule) (cortex) (gland) (medulla)	194.0	198.7	234.8	227.0	237.2	239.7
suprasellar (region)	191.9	198.3	—	225.0	237.5	239.6
sweat gland (apocrine) (eccrine), site unspecified	173.90	198.2	232.9	216.9	238.2	239.2
specified site—*see* Neoplasm, skin						
sympathetic nerve or nervous system NEC	171.9	198.89	—	215.9	238.1	239.2
symphysis pubis	170.6	198.5	—	213.6	238.0	239.2
synovial membrane—*see* Neoplasm, connective tissue						
tapetum, brain	191.8	198.3	—	225.0	237.5	239.6
tarsus (any bone)	170.8	198.5	—	213.8	238.0	239.2
temple (skin) (*see also* Neoplasm, skin, face)	173.30	198.2	232.3	216.3	238.2	239.2
temporal						
bone	170.0	198.5	—	213.0	238.0	239.2
lobe or pole	191.2	198.3	—	225.0	237.5	239.6
region	195.0	198.89	234.8	229.8	238.8	239.89
skin (see also Neoplasm, skin, face)	173.30	198.2	232.3	216.3	238.2	239.2
tendon (sheath)—*see* Neoplasm, connective tissue						
tentorium (cerebelli)	192.1	198.4	—	225.2	237.6	239.7
testis, testes (descended) (scrotal)	186.9	198.82	233.6	222.0	236.4	239.5
ectopic	186.0	198.82	233.6	222.0	236.4	239.5

	Malignant					
	Primary	Secondary	Ca in situ	Benign	Uncertain Behavior	Unspecified
retained.	186.0	198.82	233.6	222.0	236.4	239.5
undescended	186.0	198.82	233.6	222.0	236.4	239.5
thalamus	191.0	198.3	—	225.0	237.5	239.6
thigh NEC*.	195.5	198.89	234.8	229.8	238.8	239.89
thorax, thoracic (cavity)						
(organs NEC)	195.1	198.89	234.8	229.8	238.8	239.89
duct.	171.4	198.89	—	215.4	238.1	239.2
wall NEC.	195.1	198.89	234.8	229.8	238.8	239.89
throat	149.0	198.89	230.0	210.9	235.1	239.0
thumb NEC*	195.4	198.89	232.6	229.8	238.8	239.89
thymus (gland)	164.0	198.89	—	212.6	235.8	239.89
contiguous sites with heart and						
mediastinum	164.8	—	—	—	—	—
thyroglossal duct	193	198.89	234.8	226	237.4	239.7
thyroid (gland)	193	198.89	234.8	226	237.4	239.7
cartilage	161.3	197.3	231.0	212.1	235.6	239.1
tibia (any part)	170.7	198.5	—	213.7	238.0	239.2
toe NEC*.	195.5	198.89	232.7	229.8	238.8	239.89
tongue	141.9	198.89	230.0	210.1	235.1	239.0
anterior (two-thirds) NEC	141.4	198.89	230.0	210.1	235.1	239.0
dorsal surface.	141.1	198.89	230.0	210.1	235.1	239.0
ventral surface	141.3	198.89	230.0	210.1	235.1	239.0
base (dorsal surface)	141.0	198.89	230.0	210.1	235.1	239.0
border (lateral)	141.2	198.89	230.0	210.1	235.1	239.0
contiguous sites	141.8	—	—	—	—	—
dorsal surface NEC.	141.1	198.89	230.0	210.1	235.1	239.0
fixed part NEC	141.0	198.89	230.0	210.1	235.1	239.0
foramen cecum	141.1	198.89	230.0	210.1	235.1	239.0
frenulum linguae	141.3	198.89	230.0	210.1	235.1	239.0
junctional zone	141.5	198.89	230.0	210.1	235.1	239.0
margin (lateral).	141.2	198.89	230.0	210.1	235.1	239.0
midline NEC	141.1	198.89	230.0	210.1	235.1	239.0
mobile part NEC	141.4	198.89	230.0	210.1	235.1	239.0
posterior (third).	141.0	198.89	230.0	210.1	235.1	239.0
root	141.0	198.89	230.0	210.1	235.1	239.0
surface (dorsal).	141.1	198.89	230.0	210.1	235.1	239.0
base.	141.0	198.89	230.0	210.1	235.1	239.0
ventral	141.3	198.89	230.0	210.1	235.1	239.0
tip	141.2	198.89	230.0	210.1	235.1	239.0
tonsil	141.6	198.89	230.0	210.1	235.1	239.0
tonsil	146.0	198.89	230.0	210.5	235.1	239.0
fauces, faucial	146.0	198.89	230.0	210.5	235.1	239.0
lingual	141.6	198.89	230.0	210.1	235.1	239.0
palatine.	146.0	198.89	230.0	210.5	235.1	239.0
pharyngeal	147.1	198.89	230.0	210.7	235.1	239.0
pillar (anterior) (posterior)	146.2	198.89	230.0	210.6	235.1	239.0
tonsillar fossa.	146.1	198.89	230.0	210.6	235.1	239.0
tooth socket NEC	143.9	198.89	230.0	210.4	235.1	239.0
trachea (cartilage) (mucosa)	162.0	197.3	231.1	212.2	235.7	239.1
contiguous sites with						
bronchus or lung	162.8	—	—	—	—	—
tracheobronchial	162.8	197.3	231.1	212.2	235.7	239.1
contiguous sites with lung	162.8	—	—	—	—	—
tragus (see also Neoplasm, skin, ear)	173.20	198.2	232.2	216.2	238.2	239.2
trunk NEC*.	195.8	198.89	232.5	229.8	238.8	239.89
tubo-ovarian	183.8	198.82	233.39	221.8	236.3	239.5
tunica vaginalis.	187.8	198.82	233.6	222.8	236.6	239.5
turbinate (bone)	170.0	198.5	—	213.0	238.0	239.2
nasal	160.0	197.3	231.8	212.0	235.9	239.1
tympanic cavity	160.1	197.3	231.8	212.0	235.9	239.1
ulna (any part)	170.4	198.5	—	213.4	238.0	239.2
umbilicus, umbilical (see also						
Neoplasm, skin, trunk)	173.50	198.2	232.5	216.5	238.2	239.2

	Malignant				
	Primary	Secondary	Ca in situ	Benign	Uncertain Behavior	Unspecified
---	---	---	---	---	---	---
uncus, brain	191.2	198.3	—	225.0	237.5	239.6
unknown site or unspecified	199.1	199.1	234.9	229.9	238.9	239.9
urachus	188.7	198.1	233.7	223.3	236.7	239.4
ureter, ureteral	189.2	198.1	233.9	223.2	236.91	239.5
orifice (bladder)	188.6	198.1	233.7	223.3	236.7	239.4
ureter-bladder (junction)	188.6	198.1	233.7	223.3	236.7	239.4
urethra, urethral (gland)	189.3	198.1	233.9	223.81	236.99	239.5
orifice, internal	188.5	198.1	233.7	223.3	236.7	239.4
urethrovaginal (septum)	184.9	198.82	233.39	221.9	236.3	239.5
urinary organ or system NEC	189.9	198.1	233.9	223.9	236.99	239.5
bladder—*see* Neoplasm, bladder						
contiguous sites	189.8	—	—	—	—	—
specified sites NEC	189.8	198.1	233.9	223.89	236.99	239.5
utero-ovarian	183.8	198.82	233.39	221.8	236.3	239.5
ligament	183.3	198.82	—	221.0	236.3	239.5
uterosacral ligament	183.4	198.82	—	221.0	236.3	239.5
uterus, uteri, uterine	179	198.82	233.2	219.9	236.0	239.5
adnexa NEC	183.9	198.82	233.39	221.8	236.3	239.5
contiguous sites	183.8	—	—	—	—	—
body	182.0	198.82	233.2	219.1	236.0	239.5
contiguous sites	182.8	—	—	—	—	—
cervix	180.9	198.82	233.1	219.0	236.0	239.5
cornu	182.0	198.82	233.2	219.1	236.0	239.5
corpus	182.0	198.82	233.2	219.1	236.0	239.5
endocervix (canal) (gland)	180.0	198.82	233.1	219.0	236.0	239.5
endometrium	182.0	198.82	233.2	219.1	236.0	239.5
exocervix	180.1	198.82	233.1	219.0	236.0	239.5
external os	180.1	198.82	233.1	219.0	236.0	239.5
fundus	182.0	198.82	233.2	219.1	236.0	239.5
internal os	180.0	198.82	233.1	219.0	236.0	239.5
isthmus	182.1	198.82	233.2	219.1	236.0	239.5
ligament	183.4	198.82	—	221.0	236.3	239.5
broad	183.3	198.82	233.39	221.0	236.3	239.5
round	183.5	198.82	—	221.0	236.3	239.5
lower segment	182.1	198.82	233.2	219.1	236.0	239.5
myometrium	182.0	198.82	233.2	219.1	236.0	239.5
squamocolumnar junction	180.8	198.82	233.1	219.0	236.0	239.5
tube	183.2	198.82	233.39	221.0	236.3	239.5
utricle, prostatic	189.3	198.1	233.9	223.81	236.99	239.5
uveal tract	190.0	198.4	234.0	224.0	238.8	239.89
uvula	145.4	198.89	230.0	210.4	235.1	239.0
vagina, vaginal (fornix) (vault) (wall)	184.0	198.82	233.31	221.1	236.3	239.5
vaginovesical	184.9	198.82	233.39	221.9	236.3	239.5
septum	184.9	198.82	233.39	221.9	236.3	239.5
vallecula (epiglottis)	146.3	198.89	230.0	210.6	235.1	239.0
vascular—*see* Neoplasm, connective tissue						
vas deferens	187.6	198.82	233.6	222.8	236.6	239.5
Vater's ampulla	156.2	197.8	230.8	211.5	235.3	239.0
vein, venous—*see* Neoplasm, connective tissue						
vena cava (abdominal) (inferior)	171.5	198.89	—	215.5	238.1	239.2
superior	171.4	198.89	—	215.4	238.1	239.2
ventricle (cerebral) (floor) (fourth) (lateral) (third)	191.5	198.3	—	225.0	237.5	239.6
cardiac (left) (right)	164.1	198.89	—	212.7	238.8	239.89
ventricular band of larynx	161.1	197.3	231.0	212.1	235.6	239.1
ventriculus—*see* Neoplasm, stomach						
vermillion border—*see* Neoplasm, lip						

	Primary	Secondary	Ca in situ	Benign	Uncertain Behavior	Unspecified
	Malignant					
vermis, cerebellum	191.6	198.3	—	225.0	237.5	239.6
vertebra (column)	170.2	198.5	—	213.2	238.0	239.2
coccyx	170.6	198.5	—	213.6	238.0	239.2
sacrum	170.6	198.5	—	213.6	238.0	239.2
vesical—see Neoplasm, bladder						
vesicle, seminal	187.8	198.82	233.6	222.8	236.6	239.5
vesicocervical tissue	184.9	198.82	233.39	221.9	236.3	239.5
vesicorectal.	195.3	198.89	234.8	229.8	238.8	239.89
vesicovaginal.	184.9	198.82	233.39	221.9	236.3	239.5
septum	184.9	198.82	233.39	221.9	236.3	239.5
vessel (blood)—see Neoplasm, connective tissue						
vestibular gland, greater	184.1	198.82	233.32	221.2	236.3	239.5
vestibule						
mouth.	145.1	198.89	230.0	210.4	235.1	239.0
nose.	160.0	197.3	231.8	212.0	235.9	239.1
Virchow's gland	—	196.0	—	229.0	238.8	239.89
viscera NEC	195.8	198.89	234.8	229.8	238.8	239.89
vocal cords (true).	161.0	197.3	231.0	212.1	235.6	239.1
false	161.1	197.3	231.0	212.1	235.6	239.1
vomer.	170.0	198.5	—	213.0	238.0	239.2
vulva	184.4	198.82	233.32	221.2	236.3	239.5
vulvovaginal gland	184.4	198.82	233.32	221.2	236.3	239.5
Waldeyer's ring	149.1	198.89	230.0	210.9	235.1	239.0
Wharton's duct	142.1	198.89	230.0	210.2	235.0	239.0
white matter (central)						
(cerebral)	191.0	198.3	—	225.0	237.5	239.6
windpipe	162.0	197.3	231.1	212.2	235.7	239.1
Wirsung's duct	157.3	197.8	230.9	211.6	235.5	239.0
wolffian (body) (duct)						
female	184.8	198.82	233.39	221.8	236.3	239.5
male	187.8	198.82	233.6	222.8	236.6	239.5
womb—see Neoplasm, uterus						
wrist NEC*	195.4	198.89	232.6	229.8	238.8	239.89
xiphoid process	170.3	198.5	—	213.3	238.0	239.2
Zuckerkandl's organ	194.6	198.89	—	227.6	237.3	239.7

Nephrosis, nephrotic (Epstein's) (syndrome) 581.9
  with
    lesion of
      focal glomerulosclerosis 581.1
      glomerulonephritis
        endothelial 581.2
        hypocomplementemic persistent 581.2
        lobular 581.2
        membranoproliferative 581.2
        membranous 581.1
        mesangiocapillary 581.2
        minimal change 581.3
        mixed membranous and proliferative 581.2
        proliferative 581.0
      segmental hyalinosis 581.1
      specified pathology NEC 581.89
  acute—*see* Nephrosis, tubular
  anoxic—*see* Nephrosis, tubular
  arteriosclerotic (*see also* Hypertension, kidney)
      403.90
  chemical—*see* Nephrosis, tubular
  cholemic 572.4
  complicating pregnancy, childbirth, or
      puerperium—*see* Nephritis, complicating
      pregnancy
  diabetic 250.4 *[581.81]*
    due to secondary diabetes 249.4 *[581.81]*
  Finnish type (congenital) 759.89
  hemoglobinuric—*see* Nephrosis, tubular
  in
    amyloidosis 277.39 *[581.81]*
    diabetes mellitus 250.4 *[581.81]*
      due to secondary diabetes 249.4 *[581.81]*
    epidemic hemorrhagic fever 078.6
    malaria 084.9 *[581.81]*
    polyarteritis 446.0 *[581.81]*
    systemic lupus erythematosus 710.0 *[581.81]*
  ischemic—*see* Nephrosis, tubular
  lipoid 581.3
  lower nephron—*see* Nephrosis, tubular
  lupoid 710.0 *[581.81]*
  lupus 710.0 *[581.81]*
  malarial 084.9 *[581.81]*
  minimal change 581.3
  necrotizing—*see* Nephrosis, tubular
  osmotic (sucrose) 588.89
  polyarteritic 446.0 *[581.81]*
  radiation 581.9
  specified lesion or cause NEC 581.89
  syphilitic 095.4
  toxic—*see* Nephrosis, tubular
  tubular (acute) 584.5
    due to a procedure 997.5
    radiation 581.9
Nephrosonephritis hemorrhagic (endemic)
    078.6
Nephrostomy status V44.6
  with complication 997.5
Nerve —*see* condition
Nerves 799.21
Nervous (*see also* condition) 799.21
  breakdown 300.9
  heart 306.2
  stomach 306.4
  tension 799.21
Nervousness 799.21
Nesidioblastoma (M8150/0)
  pancreas 211.7
  specified site NEC—*see* Neoplasm, by site, benign
  unspecified site 211.7
Netherton's syndrome (ichthyosiform
    erythroderma) 757.1

Nettle rash 708.8
Nettleship's disease (urticaria pigmentosa) 757.33
Neumann's disease (pemphigus vegetans) 694.4
Neuralgia, neuralgic (acute) (*see also* Neuritis)
    729.2
  accessory (nerve) 352.4
  acoustic (nerve) 388.5
  ankle 355.8
  anterior crural 355.8
  anus 787.99
  arm 723.4
  auditory (nerve) 388.5
  axilla 353.0
  bladder 788.1
  brachial 723.4
  brain—*see* Disorder, nerve, cranial
  broad ligament 625.9
  cerebral—*see* Disorder, nerve, cranial
  ciliary 339.00
  cranial nerve—*see also* Disorder, nerve, cranial
    fifth or trigeminal (*see also* Neuralgia,
        trigeminal) 350.1
  ear 388.71
    middle 352.1
  facial 351.8
  finger 354.9
  flank 355.8
  foot 355.8
  forearm 354.9
  Fothergill's (*see also* Neuralgia, trigeminal)
      350.1
    postherpetic 053.12
  glossopharyngeal (nerve) 352.1
  groin 355.8
  hand 354.9
  heel 355.8
  Horton's 339.00
  Hunt's 053.11
  hypoglossal (nerve) 352.5
  iliac region 355.8
  infraorbital (*see also* Neuralgia, trigeminal)
      350.1
  inguinal 355.8
  intercostal (nerve) 353.8
    postherpetic 053.19
  jaw 352.1
  kidney 788.0
  knee 355.8
  loin 355.8
  malarial (*see also* Malaria) 084.6
  mastoid 385.89
  maxilla 352.1
  median thenar 354.1
  metatarsal 355.6
  middle ear 352.1
  migrainous 339.00
  Morton's 355.6
  nerve, cranial—*see* Disorder, nerve, cranial
  nose 352.0
  occipital 723.8
  olfactory (nerve) 352.0
  ophthalmic 377.30
    postherpetic 053.19
  optic (nerve) 377.30
  penis 607.9
  perineum 355.8
  pleura 511.0
  postherpetic NEC 053.19
    geniculate ganglion 053.11
    ophthalmic 053.19
    trifacial 053.12
    trigeminal 053.12

Neuralgia, neuralgic—*continued*
  pubic region 355.8
  radial (nerve) 723.4
  rectum 787.99
  sacroiliac joint 724.3
  sciatic (nerve) 724.3
  scrotum 608.9
  seminal vesicle 608.9
  shoulder 354.9
  Sluder's 337.09
  specified nerve NEC—*see* Disorder, nerve
  spermatic cord 608.9
  sphenopalatine (ganglion) 337.09
  subscapular (nerve) 723.4
  suprascapular (nerve) 723.4
  testis 608.89
  thenar (median) 354.1
  thigh 355.8
  tongue 352.5
  trifacial (nerve) (*see also* Neuralgia, trigeminal)
    350.1
  trigeminal (nerve) 350.1
    postherpetic 053.12
  tympanic plexus 388.71
  ulnar (nerve) 723.4
  vagus (nerve) 352.3
  wrist 354.9
  writers' 300.89
    organic 333.84
Neurapraxia —*see* Injury, nerve
Neurasthenia 300.5
  cardiac 306.2
  gastric 306.4
  heart 306.2
  postfebrile 780.79
  postviral 780.79
Neurilemmoma (M9560/0)—*see also* Neoplasm,
  connective tissue, benign
  acoustic (nerve) 225.1
  malignant (M9560/3)—*see also* Neoplasm,
    connective tissue, malignant
    acoustic (nerve) 192.0
Neurilemmosarcoma (M9560/3)—*see*
  Neoplasm, connective tissue, malignant
Neurilemoma —*see* Neurilemmoma
Neurinoma (M9560/0)—*see* Neurilemmoma
Neurinomatosis (M9560/1)—*see also* Neoplasm,
  connective tissue, uncertain behavior
  centralis 759.5
Neuritis (*see also* Neuralgia) 729.2
  abducens (nerve) 378.54
  accessory (nerve) 352.4
  acoustic (nerve) 388.5
    syphilitic 094.86
  alcoholic 357.5
    with psychosis 291.1
  amyloid, any site 277.39 *[357.4]*
  anterior crural 355.8
  arising during pregnancy 646.4
  arm 723.4
  ascending 355.2
  auditory (nerve) 388.5
  brachial (nerve) NEC 723.4
    due to displacement, intervertebral disc 722.0
  cervical 723.4
  chest (wall) 353.8
  costal region 353.8
  cranial nerve—*see also* Disorder, nerve, cranial
    first or olfactory 352.0
    second or optic 377.30
    third or oculomotor 378.52
    fourth or trochlear 378.53

Neuritis—*continued*
  cranial nerve—*continued*
    fifth or trigeminal (*see also* Neuralgia,
      trigeminal) 350.1
    sixth or abducens 378.54
    seventh or facial 351.8
      newborn 767.5
    eighth or acoustic 388.5
    ninth or glossopharyngeal 352.1
    tenth or vagus 352.3
    eleventh or accessory 352.4
    twelfth or hypoglossal 352.5
  Déjérine-Sottas 356.0
  diabetic 250.6 *[357.2]*
    due to secondary diabetes 249.6 *[357.2]*
  diphtheritic 032.89 *[357.4]*
  due to
    beriberi 265.0 *[357.4]*
    displacement, prolapse, protrusion, or rupture
      of intervertebral disc 722.2
      cervical 722.0
      lumbar, lumbosacral 722.10
      thoracic, thoracolumbar 722.11
    herniation, nucleus pulposus 722.2
      cervical 722.0
      lumbar, lumbosacral 722.10
      thoracic, thoracolumbar 722.11
  endemic 265.0 *[357.4]*
  facial (nerve) 351.8
    newborn 767.5
  general—*see* Polyneuropathy
  geniculate ganglion 351.1
    due to herpes 053.11
  glossopharyngeal (nerve) 352.1
  gouty 274.89 *[357.4]*
  hypoglossal (nerve) 352.5
  ilioinguinal (nerve) 355.8
  in diseases classified elsewhere—*see*
    Polyneuropathy, in
  infectious (multiple) 357.0
  intercostal (nerve) 353.8
  interstitial hypertrophic progressive NEC 356.9
  leg 355.8
  lumbosacral NEC 724.4
  median (nerve) 354.1
    thenar 354.1
  multiple (acute) (infective) 356.9
    endemic 265.0 *[357.4]*
  multiplex endemica 265.0 *[357.4]*
  nerve root (*see also* Radiculitis) 729.2
  oculomotor (nerve) 378.52
  olfactory (nerve) 352.0
  optic (nerve) 377.30
    in myelitis 341.0
    meningococcal 036.81
  pelvic 355.8
  peripheral (nerve)—*see also* Neuropathy,
    peripheral
    complicating pregnancy or puerperium 646.4
    specified nerve NEC—*see* Mononeuritis
  pneumogastric (nerve) 352.3
  postchickenpox 052.7
  postherpetic 053.19
  progressive hypertrophic interstitial NEC 356.9
  puerperal, postpartum 646.4
  radial (nerve) 723.4
  retrobulbar 377.32
    syphilitic 094.85
  rheumatic (chronic) 729.2
  sacral region 355.8
  sciatic (nerve) 724.3
    due to displacement of intervertebral disc 722.10

Neuritis—*continued*
  serum 999.59
  specified nerve NEC—*see* Disorder, nerve
  spinal (nerve) 355.9
    root (*see also* Radiculitis) 729.2
  subscapular (nerve) 723.4
  suprascapular (nerve) 723.4
  syphilitic 095.8
  thenar (median) 354.1
  thoracic NEC 724.4
  toxic NEC 357.7
  trochlear (nerve) 378.53
  ulnar (nerve) 723.4
  vagus (nerve) 352.3
Neuroangiomatosis, encephalofacial 759.6
Neuroastrocytoma (M9505/1)—*see* Neoplasm,
  by site, uncertain behavior
Neuro-avitaminosis 269.2
Neuroblastoma (M9500/3)
  olfactory (M9522/3) 160.0
  specified site—*see* Neoplasm, by site, malignant
  unspecified site 194.0
Neurochorioretinitis (*see also* Chorioretinitis)
  363.20
Neurocirculatory asthenia 306.2
Neurocytoma (M9506/0)—*see* Neoplasm, by
  site, benign
Neurodermatitis (circumscribed) (circumscripta)
  (local) 698.3
  atopic 691.8
  diffuse (Brocq) 691.8
  disseminated 691.8
  nodulosa 698.3
Neuroencephalomyelopathy, optic 341.0
Neuroendocrine tumor —see Tumor,
  neuroendocrine
Neuroepithelioma (M9503/3)—*see also*
  Neoplasm, by site, malignant
  olfactory (M9521/3) 160.0
Neurofibroma (M9540/0)—*see also* Neoplasm,
  connective tissue, benign
  melanotic (M9541/0)—*see* Neoplasm,
    connective tissue, benign
  multiple (M9540/1) 237.70
    Type 1 237.71
    Type 2 237.72
  plexiform (M9550/0)—*see* Neoplasm,
    connective tissue, benign
Neurofibromatosis (multiple) (M9540/1) 237.70
  acoustic 237.72
  malignant (M9540/3)—*see* Neoplasm,
    connective tissue, malignant
  Schwannomatosis 237.73
  specified type NEC 237.79
  Type 1 237.71
  Type 2 237.72
  von Recklinghausen's 237.71
Neurofibrosarcoma (M9540/3)—*see* Neoplasm,
  connective tissue, malignant
Neurogenic —*see also* condition
  bladder (atonic) (automatic) (autonomic)
    (flaccid) (hypertonic) (hypotonic) (inertia)
    (infranuclear) (irritable) (motor) (nonreflex)
    (nuclear) (paralysis) (reflex) (sensory)
    (spastic) (supranuclear) (uninhibited) 596.54
  with cauda equina syndrome 344.61
    bowel 564.81
    heart 306.2
Neuroglioma (M9505/1)—*see* Neoplasm, by site,
  uncertain behavior
Neurolabyrinthitis (of Dix and Hallpike) 386.12

Neurolathyrism 988.2
Neuroleprosy 030.1
Neuroleptic malignant syndrome 333.92
Neurolipomatosis 272.8
Neuroma (M9570/0)—*see also* Neoplasm,
  connective tissue, benign
  acoustic (nerve) (M9560/0) 225.1
  amputation (traumatic)—*see also* Injury, nerve,
    by site
    surgical complication (late) 997.61
  appendix 211.3
  auditory nerve 225.1
  digital 355.6
    toe 355.6
  interdigital (toe) 355.6
  intermetatarsal 355.6
  Morton's 355.6
  multiple 237.70
    Type 1 237.71
    Type 2 237.72
  nonneoplastic 355.9
    arm NEC 354.9
    leg NEC 355.8
    lower extremity NEC 355.8
    specified site NEC—*see* Mononeuritis, by site
    upper extremity NEC 354.9
  optic (nerve) 225.1
  plantar 355.6
  plexiform (M9550/0)—*see* Neoplasm,
    connective tissue, benign
  surgical (nonneoplastic) 355.9
    arm NEC 354.9
    leg NEC 355.8
    lower extremity NEC 355.8
    upper extremity NEC 354.9
  traumatic—*see also* Injury, nerve, by site
    old—*see* Neuroma, nonneoplastic
Neuromyalgia 729.1
Neuromyasthenia (epidemic) 049.8
Neuromyelitis 341.8
  ascending 357.0
  optica 341.0
Neuromyopathy NEC 358.9
Neuromyositis 729.1
Neuronevus (M8725/0)—*see* Neoplasm, skin,
  benign
Neuronitis 357.0
  ascending (acute) 355.2
  vestibular 386.12
Neuroparalytic —*see* condition
Neuropathy, axtaxia and retinitis pigmentosa
  (NARP syndrome) 277.87
Neuropathy, neuropathic (*see also* Disorder,
  nerve) 355.9
  acute motor 357.82
  alcoholic 357.5
    with psychosis 291.1
  arm NEC 354.9
  ataxia and retinitis pigmentosa (NARP
    syndrome) 277.87
  autonomic (peripheral)—*see* Neuropathy,
    peripheral, autonomic
  axillary nerve 353.0
  brachial plexus 353.0
  cervical plexus 353.2
  chronic
    progressive segmentally demyelinating 357.89
    relapsing demyelinating 357.89
  congenital sensory 356.2
  Déjérine-Sottas 356.0

Neuropathy, neuropathic—*continued*
diabetic 250.6 *[357.2]*
  autonomic (peripheral) 250.6 *[337.1]*
  due to secondary diabetes 249.6 *[357.2]*
    autonomic (peripheral) 249.6 *[337.1]*
entrapment 355.9
  iliohypogastric nerve 355.79
  ilioinguinal nerve 355.79
  lateral cutaneous nerve of thigh 355.1
  median nerve 354.0
  obturator nerve 355.79
  peroneal nerve 355.3
  posterior tibial nerve 355.5
  saphenous nerve 355.79
  ulnar nerve 354.2
facial nerve 351.9
hereditary 356.9
  peripheral 356.0
  sensory (radicular) 356.2
hypertrophic
  Charcot-Marie-Tooth 356.1
  Déjérine-Sottas 356.0
  interstitial 356.9
  Refsum 356.3
intercostal nerve 354.8
ischemic—*see* Disorder, nerve
Jamaican (ginger) 357.7
leg NEC 355.8
lower extremity NEC 355.8
lumbar plexus 353.1
median nerve 354.1
motor
  acute 357.82
multiple (acute) (chronic) (*see also*
  Polyneuropathy) 356.9
optic 377.39
  ischemic 377.41
  nutritional 377.33
  toxic 377.34
peripheral (nerve) (*see also* Polyneuropathy) 356.9
  arm NEC 354.9
  autonomic 337.9
    amyloid 277.39 *[337.1]*
    idiopathic 337.00
    in
      amyloidosis 277.39 *[337.1]*
      diabetes (mellitus) 250.6 *[337.1]*
        due to secondary diabetes 249.6 *[337.1]*
      diseases classified elsewhere 337.1
      gout 274.89 *[337.1]*
      hyperthyroidism 242.9 *[337.1]*
  due to
    antitetanus serum 357.6
    arsenic 357.7
    drugs 357.6
    lead 357.7
    organophosphate compounds 357.7
    toxic agent NEC 357.7
  hereditary 356.0
  idiopathic 356.9
    progressive 356.4
    specified type NEC 356.8
  in diseases classified elsewhere—*see*
    Polyneuropathy, in
  leg NEC 355.8
  lower extremity NEC 355.8
  upper extremity NEC 354.9
plantar nerves 355.6
progressive
  hypertrophic interstitial 356.9
  inflammatory 357.89

Neuropathy, neuropathic—*continued*
radicular NEC 729.2
  brachial 723.4
  cervical NEC 723.4
  hereditary sensory 356.2
  lumbar 724.4
  lumbosacral 724.4
  thoracic NEC 724.4
sacral plexus 353.1
sciatic 355.0
spinal nerve NEC 355.9
  root (*see also* Radiculitis) 729.2
toxic 357.7
trigeminal sensory 350.8
ulnar nerve 354.2
upper extremity NEC 354.9
uremic 585.9 *[357.4]*
vitamin B$_{12}$ 266.2 *[357.4]*
  with anemia (pernicious) 281.0 *[357.4]*
    due to dietary deficiency 281.1 *[357.4]*
Neurophthisis —*see also* Disorder, nerve
peripheral 356.9
  diabetic 250.6 *[357.2]*
    due to secondary diabetes 249.6 *[357.2]*
Neuropraxia —*see* Injury,nerve
Neuroretinitis 363.05
syphilitic 094.85
Neurosarcoma 9M9540/3)—sde Neoplasm,
connective tissue, malignant
Neurosclerosis —*see* Disorder, nerve
Neurosis, neurotic 300.9
accident 300.16
anancastic, anankastic 300.3
anxiety (state) 300.00
  generalized 300.02
  panic type 300.01
asthenic 300.5
bladder 306.53
cardiac (reflex) 306.2
cardiovascular 306.2
climacteric, unspecified type 627.2
colon 306.4
compensation 300.16
compulsive, compulsion 300.3
conversion 300.11
craft 300.89
cutaneous 306.3
depersonalization 300.6
depressive (reaction) (type) 300.4
endocrine 306.6
environmental 300.89
fatigue 300.5
functional (*see also* Disorder, psychosomatic)
  306.9
gastric 306.4
gastrointestinal 306.4
genitourinary 306.50
heart 306.2
hypochondriacal 300.7
hysterical 300.10
  conversion type 300.11
  dissociative type 300.15
impulsive 300.3
incoordination 306.0
  larynx 306.1
  vocal cord 306.1
intestine 306.4
larynx 306.1
  hysterical 300.11
  sensory 306.1
menopause, unspecified type 627.2

Neurosis, neurotic—*continued*
  mixed NEC 300.89
  musculoskeletal 306.0
  obsessional 300.3
    phobia 300.3
  obsessive-compulsive 300.3
  occupational 300.89
  ocular 306.7
  oral (*see also* Disorder, fluency) 315.35
  organ (*see also* Disorder, psychosomatic) 306.9
  pharynx 306.1
  phobic 300.20
  posttraumatic (acute) (situational) 309.81
    chronic 309.81
  psychasthenic (type) 300.89
  railroad 300.16
  rectum 306.4
  respiratory 306.1
  rumination 306.4
  senile 300.89
  sexual 302.70
  situational 300.89
  specified type NEC 300.89
  state 300.9
    with depersonalization episode 300.6
  stomach 306.4
  vasomotor 306.2
  visceral 306.4
  war 300.16
Neurospongioblastosis diffusa 759.5
Neurosyphilis (arrested) (early) (inactive) (late)
    (latent) (recurrent) 094.9
  with ataxia (cerebellar) (locomotor) (spastic)
    (spinal) 094.0
  acute meningitis 094.2
  aneurysm 094.89
  arachnoid (adhesive) 094.2
  arteritis (any artery) 094.89
  asymptomatic 094.3
  congenital 090.40
  dura (mater) 094.89
  general paresis 094.1
  gumma 094.9
  hemorrhagic 094.9
  juvenile (asymptomatic) (meningeal) 090.40
  leptomeninges (aseptic) 094.2
  meningeal 094.2
  meninges (adhesive) 094.2
  meningovascular (diffuse) 094.2
  optic atrophy 094.84
  parenchymatous (degenerative) 094.1
  paresis (*see also* Paresis, general) 094.1
  paretic (*see also* Paresis, general) 094.1
  relapse 094.9
  remission in (sustained) 094.9
  serological 094.3
  specified nature or site NEC 094.89
  tabes (dorsalis) 094.0
    juvenile 090.40
  tabetic 094.0
    juvenile 090.40
  taboparesis 094.1
    juvenile 090.40
  thrombosis 094.89
  vascular 094.89
Neurotic (*see also* Neurosis) 300.9
  excoriation 698.4
    psychogenic 306.3
Neurotmesis —*see* Injury, nerve, by site
Neurotoxemia —*see* Toxemia
Neutro-oclusion 524.21

Neutropenia, neutropenic (idiopathic)
    (pernicious) (primary) 288.00
  chronic 288.09
    hypoplastic 288.09
  congenital (nontransient) 288.01
  cyclic 288.02
  drug induced 288.03
  due to infection 288.04
  fever 288.00
  genetic 288.01
  immune 288.09
  infantile 288.01
  malignant 288.09
  neonatal, transitory (isoimmune) (maternal
    transfer) 776.7
  periodic 288.02
  splenic 289.53
  splenomegaly 289.53
  toxic 288.09
Neutrophilia, hereditary giant 288.2
Nevocarcinoma (M8720/3)—*see* Melanoma
Nevus (M8720/0)—*see also* Neoplasm, skin,
    benign

> *Note*—*Except where otherwise indicated, the
> varieties of nevus in the list below that are
> followed by a morphology code number (M‑‑‑‑
> ‑/0) should be coded by site as for "Neoplasm,
> skin, benign."*

  acanthotic 702.8
  achromic (M8730/0)
  amelanotic (M8730/0)
  anemic, anemicus 709.09
  angiomatous (M9120/0) (*see also* Hemangioma)
    228.00
  araneus 448.1
  avasculosus 709.09
  balloon cell (M8722/0)
  bathing trunk (M8761/1) 238.2
  blue (M8780/0)
    cellular (M8790/0)
    giant (M8790/0)
    Jadassohn's (M8780/0)
    malignant (M8780/3)—*see* Melanoma
  capillary (M9131/0) (*see also* Hemangioma)
    228.00
  cavernous (M9121/0) (*see also* Hemangioma)
    228.00
  cellular (M8720/0)
    blue (M8790/0)
  comedonicus 757.33
  compound (M8760/0)
  conjunctiva (M8720/0) 224.3
  dermal (M8750/0)
    and epidermal (M8760/0)
  epithelioid cell (and spindle cell) (M8770/0)
  flammeus 757.32
    osteohypertrophic 759.89
  hairy (M8720/0)
  halo (M8723/0)
  hemangiomatous (M9120/0) (*see also*
    Hemangioma) 228.00
  intradermal (M8750/0)
  intraepidermal (M8740/0)
  involuting (M8724/0)
  Jadassohn's (blue) (M8780/0)
  junction, junctional (M8740/0)
    malignant melanoma in (M8740/3)—*see*
    Melanoma
  juvenile (M8770/0)
  lymphatic (M9170/0) 228.1

Nevus—*continued*
  magnocellular (M8726/0)
    specified site—*see* Neoplasm, by site, benign
    unspecified site 224.0
  malignant (M8720/3)—*see* Melanoma
  meaning hemangioma (M9120/0) (*see also*
    Hemangioma) 228.00
  melanotic (pigmented) (M8720/0)
  multiplex 759.5
  nonneoplastic 448.1
  nonpigmented (M8730/0)
  nonvascular (M8720/0)
  oral mucosa, white sponge 750.26
  osteohypertrophic, flammeus 759.89
  papillaris (M8720/0)
  papillomatosus (M8720/0)
  pigmented (M8720/0)
    giant (M8761/1)—*see also* Neoplasm, skin,
      uncertain behavior
      malignant melanoma in (M8761/3)—*see*
        Melanoma
  systematicus 757.33
  pilosus (M8720/0)
  port wine 757.32
  sanguineous 757.32
  sebaceous (senile) 702.8
  senile 448.1
  spider 448.1
  spindle cell (and epithelioid cell) (M8770/0)
  stellar 448.1
  strawberry 757.32
  syringocystadenomatous papilliferous
    (M8406/0)
  unius lateris 757.33
  Unna's 757.32
  vascular 757.32
  verrucous 757.33
  white sponge (oral mucosa) 750.26
Newborn (infant) (liveborn)
  abstinence syndrome 779.5
  affected by
    amniocentesis 760.61
    maternal abuse of drugs (gestational) (via
      placenta) (via breast milk) (see also
      Noxious, substances transmitted through
      placenta or breast milk (affecting fetus or
      newborn)) 760.70
      methamphetamine(s) 760.72
    procedure
      amniocentesis 760.61
      in utero NEC 760.62
      surgical on mother
        during pregnancy NEC 760.63
        previous not associated with pregnancy
          760.64
  apnea 770.81
    obstructive 770.82
    specified NEC 770.82
  breast buds 779.89
  cardiomyopathy 425.4
    congenital 425.3
  convulsion 779.0
  electrolyte imbalance NEC (transitory) 775.5
  fever (environmentally-induced) 778.4
  gestation
    24 completed weeks 765.22
    25-26 completed weeks 765.23
    27-28 completed weeks 765.24
    29-30 completed weeks 765.25
    31-32 completed weeks 765.26
    33-34 completed weeks 765.27

Newborn—*continued*
  gestation—*continued*
    35-36 completed weeks 765.28
    37 or more completed weeks 765.29
    less than 24 completed weeks 765.21
    unspecified completed weeks 765.20
  infection 771.89
    candida 771.7
    mastitis 771.5
    specified NEC 771.89
    urinary tract 771.82
  mastitis 771.5
  multiple NEC
    born in hospital (without mention of cesarean
      delivery or section) V37.00
      with cesarean delivery or section V37.01
    born outside hospital
      hospitalized V37.1
      not hospitalized V37.2
    mates all liveborn
      born in hospital (without mention of
        cesarean delivery or section) V34.00
      with cesarean delivery or section V34.01
      born outside hospital
        hospitalized V34.1
        not hospitalized V34.2
    mates all stillborn
      born in hospital (without mention of
        cesarean delivery or section) V35.00
      with cesarean delivery or section V35.01
      born outside hospital
        hospitalized V35.1
        not hospitalized V35.2
    mates liveborn and stillborn
      born in hospital (without mention of
        cesarean delivery or section) V36.00
      with cesarean delivery or section V36.01
      born outside hospital
        hospitalized V36.1
        not hospitalized V36.2
  omphalitis 771.4
  seizure 779.0
  sepsis 771.81
  single
    born in hospital (without mention of cesarean
      delivery or section) V30.00
      with cesarean delivery or section V30.01
    born outside hospital
      hospitalized V30.1
      not hospitalized V30.2
  specified condition NEC 779.89
  twin NEC
    born in hospital (without mention of cesarean
      delivery or section) V33.00
      with cesarean delivery or section V33.01
    born outside hospital
      hospitalized V33.1
      not hospitalized V33.2
    mate liveborn
      born in hospital V31.0
      born outside hospital
        hospitalized V31.1
        not hospitalized V31.2
    mate stillborn
      born in hospital V32.0
      born outside hospital
        hospitalized V32.1
        not hospitalized V32.2

Newborn—*continued*
  unspecified as to single or multiple birth
    born in hospital (without mention of cesarean
      delivery or section) V39.00
      with cesarean delivery or section V39.01
    born outside hospital
      hospitalized V39.1
      not hospitalized V39.2
  weight check V20.32
Newcastle's conjunctivitis or disease 077.8
Nezelof's syndrome (pure alymphocytosis) 279.13
Niacin (amide) deficiency 265.2
Nicolas-Durand-Favre disease (climatic bubo)
  099.1
Nicolas-Favre disease (climatic bubo) 099.1
Nicotinic acid (amide) deficiency 265.2
Niemann-Pick disease (lipid histiocytosis)
  (splenomegaly) 272.7
Night
  blindness (*see also* Blindness, night) 368.60
    congenital 368.61
      vitamin A deficiency 264.5
  cramps 729.82
  sweats 780.8
  terrors, child 307.46
Nightmare 307.47
  REM-sleep type 307.47
Nipple —*see* condition
Nisbet's chancre 099.0
Nishimoto (-Takeuchi) disease 437.5
Nitritoid crisis or reaction —*see* Crisis, nitritoid
Nitrogen retention, extrarenal 788.99
Nitrosohemoglobinemia 289.89
Njovera 104.0
No
  diagnosis 799.9
  disease (found) V71.9
  room at the inn V65.0
Nocardiasis —*see* Nocardiosis
Nocardiosis 039.9
  with pneumonia 039.1
  lung 039.1
  specified type NEC 039.8
Nocturia 788.43
  psychogenic 306.53
Nocturnal —*see also* condition
  dyspnea (paroxysmal) 786.09
  emissions 608.89
  enuresis 788.36
    psychogenic 307.6
  frequency (micturition) 788.43
    psychogenic 306.53
Nodal rhythm disorder 427.89
Nodding of head 781.0
Node (s)—*see also* Nodule
  Heberden's 715.04
  larynx 478.79
  lymph—*see* condition
  milkers' 051.1
  Osler's 421.0
  rheumatic 729.89
  Schmorl's 722.30
    lumbar, lumbosacral 722.32
    specified region NEC 722.39
    thoracic, thoracolumbar 722.31
  singers' 478.5
  skin NEC 782.2
  tuberculous—*see* Tuberculosis, lymph gland
  vocal cords 478.5
Nodosities, Haygarth's 715.04

Nodule(s), nodular
  actinomycotic (*see also* Actinomycosis) 039.9
  arthritic—*see* Arthritis, nodosa
  breast 793.89
  cutaneous 782.2
  Haygarth's 715.04
  inflammatory—*see* Inflammation
  juxta-articular 102.7
    syphilitic 095.7
    yaws 102.7
  larynx 478.79
  lung
    emphysematous 492.8
    solitary 793.11
  milkers' 051.1
  prostate 600.10
    with
      urinary
        obstruction 600.11
        retention 600.11
  pulmonary, solitary (subsegmental branch of the
    bronchial tree) 793.11
    multiple 793.19
  retrocardiac 785.9
  rheumatic 729.89
  rheumatoid—*see* Arthritis rheumatoid
  scrotum (inflammatory) 608.4
  singers' 478.5
  skin NEC 782.2
  solitary, lung 518.89
    emphysematous 492.8
  subcutaneous 782.2
  thyroid (gland) (nontoxic) (uninodular) 241.0
    with
      hyperthyroidism 242.1
      thyrotoxicosis 242.1
    toxic or with hyperthyroidism 242.1
  vocal cords 478.5
Noma (gangrenous) (hospital) (infective) 528.1
  auricle (*see also* Gangrene) 785.4
  mouth 528.1
  pudendi (*see also* Vulvitis) 616.10
  vulvae (*see also* Vulvitis) 616.10
Nomadism V60.0
Non-adherence
  artificial skin graft 996.55
  decellularized allodermis graft 996.55
Non-autoimmune hemolytic anemia NEC 283.10
Nonclosure —*see also* Imperfect, closure
  ductus
    arteriosus 747.0
    Botalli 747.0
  Eustachian valve 746.89
  foramen
    Botalli 745.5
    ovale 745.5
Noncompliance with medical treatment V15.81
  renal dialysis V45.12
Nondescent (congenital)—*see also* Malposition,
  congenital
  cecum 751.4
  colon 751.4
  testis 752.51
Nondevelopment
  brain 742.1
    specified part 742.2
  heart 746.89
  organ or site, congenital NEC—*see* Hypoplasia
Nonengagement
  head NEC 652.5
    in labor 660.1
      affecting fetus or newborn 763.1

Nonexanthematous tick fever 066.1
Nonexpansion, lung (newborn) NEC 770.4
Nonfunctioning
　cystic duct (*see also* Disease, gallbladder) 575.8
　gallbladder (*see also* Disease, gallbladder) 575.8
　kidney (*see also* Disease, renal) 593.9
　labyrinth 386.58
Nonhealing
　stump (surgical) 997.60
　wound, surgical 998.83
Nonimplantation of ovum, causing infertility 628.3
Noninsufflation, fallopian tube 628.2
Nonne-Milroy-Meige syndrome (chronic hereditary edema) 757.0
Nonovulation 628.0
Nonpatent fallopian tube 628.2
Nonpneumatization, lung NEC 770.4
Nonreflex bladder 596.54
　with cauda equina 344.61
Nonretention of food —*see also* Vomiting
Nonrotation —*see* Malrotation
Nonsecretion, urine (*see also* Anuria) 788.5
　newborn 753.3
Nonunion
　fracture 733.82
　organ or site, congenital NEC—*see* Imperfect, closure
　symphysis pubis, congenital 755.69
　top sacrum, congenital 756.19
Nonviability 765.0
Nonvisualization, gallbladder 793.3
Nonvitalized tooth 522.9
Non-working side interference 524.56
Normal
　delivery—*see* category 650
　menses V65.5
　state (feared complaint unfounded) V65.5
Normoblastosis 289.89
Normocytic anemia (infectional) 285.9
　due to blood loss (chronic) 280.0
　　acute 285.1
Norrie's disease (congenital) (progressive oculoacousticocerebral degeneration) 743.8
North American blastomycosis 116.0
Norwegian itch 133.0
Nose, nasal —*see* condition
Nosebleed 784.7
Nosomania 298.9
Nosophobia 300.29
Nostalgia 309.89
Notch of iris 743.46
Notched lip, congenital (*see also* Cleft, lip) 749.10
Notching nose, congenital (tip) 748.1
Nothnagel's
　syndrome 378.52
　vasomotor acroparesthesia 443.89
Novy's relapsing fever (American) 087.1
Noxious
　foodstuffs, poisoning by
　　fish 988.0
　　fungi 988.1
　　mushrooms 988.1
　　plants (food) 988.2
　　shellfish 988.0
　　specified type NEC 988.8
　　toadstool 988.1

Noxious—*continued*
　substances transmitted through placenta or breast milk (affecting fetus or newborn) 760.70
　acetretin 760.78
　alcohol 760.71
　aminopterin 760.78
　antiandrogens 760.79
　anticonvulsant 760.77
　antifungal 760.74
　anti-infective agents 760.74
　antimetabolic 760.78
　atorvastatin 760.78
　carbamazepine 760.77
　cocaine 760.75
　"crack" 760.75
　diethylstilbestrol (DES) 760.76
　divalproex sodium 760.77
　endocrine disrupting chemicals 760.79
　estrogens 760.79
　etretinate 760.78
　fluconazole 760.74
　fluvastatin 760.78
　hallucinogenic agents NEC 760.73
　hormones 760.79
　lithium 760.79
　lovastatin 760.78
　medicinal agents NEC 760.79
　methotrexate 760.78
　misoprostil 760.79
　narcotics 760.72
　obstetric anesthetic or analgesic 763.5
　phenobarbital 760.77
　phenytoin 760.77
　pravastatin 760.78
　progestins 760.79
　retinoic acid 760.78
　simvastatin 760.78
　solvents 760.79
　specified agent NEC 760.79
　statins 760.78
　suspected, affecting management of pregnancy 655.5
　tetracycline 760.74
　thalidomide 760.79
　trimethadione 760.77
　valproate 760.77
　valproic acid 760.77
　vitamin A 760.78
NPDH (new persistent daily headache) 339.42
Nuchal hitch (arm) 652.8
Nucleus pulposus —*see* condition
Numbness 782.0
Nuns' knee 727.2
Nursemaid's
　elbow 832.2
　shoulder 831.0
Nutmeg liver 573.8
Nutrition, deficient or insufficient (particular kind of food) 269.9
　due to
　　insufficient food 994.2
　　lack of
　　　care (child) (infant) 995.52
　　　　adult 995.84
　　　food 994.2
Nyctalopia (*see also* Blindness, night) 368.60
　vitamin A deficiency 264.5

Nycturia 788.43
  psychogenic 306.53
Nymphomania 302.89
Nystagmus 379.50
  associated with vestibular system disorders
      379.54
  benign paroxysmal positional 386.11
  central positional 386.2
  congenital 379.51
  deprivation 379.53
  dissociated 379.55
  latent 379.52
  miners' 300.89
  positional
    benign paroxysmal 386.11
    central 386.2
  specified NEC 379.56
  vestibular 379.54
  visual deprivation 379.53

O

Oasthouse urine disease 270.2
Obermeyer's relapsing fever (European) 087.0
Obesity (constitutional) (exogenous) (familial)
    (nutritional) (simple) 278.00
  adrenal 255.8
  complicating pregnancy, childbirth, or the
    puerperium 649.1
  due to hyperalimentation 278.00
  endocrine NEC 259.9
  endogenous 259.9
  Fröhlich's (adiposogenital dystrophy) 253.8
  glandular NEC 259.9
  hypothyroid (*see also* Hypothyroidism) 244.9
  hypoventilation syndrome 278.03
  morbid 278.01
  of pregnancy 649.1
  pituitary 253.8
  severe 278.01
  thyroid (*see also* Hypothyroidism) 244.9
Oblique —*see also* condition
  lie before labor, affecting fetus or newborn 761.7
Obliquity, pelvis 738.6
Obliteration
  abdominal aorta 446.7
  appendix (lumen) 543.9
  artery 447.1
  ascending aorta 446.7
  bile ducts 576.8
    with calculus, choledocholithiasis, or
      stones—*see* Choledocholithiasis
    congenital 751.61
      jaundice from 751.61 *[774.5]*
  common duct 576.8
    with calculus, choledocholithiasis, or
      stones—*see* Choledocholithiasis
    congenital 751.61
  cystic duct 575.8
    with calculus, choledocholithiasis, or
      stones—*see* Choledocholithiasis
  disease, arteriolar 447.1
  endometrium 621.8
  eye, anterior chamber 360.34
  fallopian tube 628.2
  lymphatic vessel 457.1
    postmastectomy 457.0
  organ or site, congenital NEC—*see* Atresia
  placental blood vessels—*see* Placenta, abnormal
  supra-aortic branches 446.7
  ureter 593.89
  urethra 599.84
  vein 459.9
  vestibule (oral) 525.8
Observation (for) V71.9
  without need for further medical care V71.9
  accident NEC V71.4
    at work V71.3
  criminal assault V71.6
  deleterious agent ingestion V71.89
  disease V71.9
    cardiovascular V71.7
    heart V71.7
    mental V71.09
    specified condition NEC V71.89
  foreign body ingestion V71.89
  growth and development variations V21.8
  injuries (accidental) V71.4
    inflicted NEC V71.6
      during alleged rape or seduction V71.5

Observation—*continued*
  malignant neoplasm, suspected V71.1
  postpartum
    immediately after delivery V24.0
    routine follow-up V24.2
  pregnancy
    high-risk V23.9
      inconclusive fetal viability V23.87
      specified problem NEC V23.8
    normal (without complication) V22.1
      with nonobstetric complication V22.2
      first V22.0
  rape or seduction, alleged V71.5
    injury during V71.5
  suicide attempt, alleged V71.89
  suspected (undiagnosed) (unproven)
    abuse V71.81
    cardiovascular disease V71.7
    child or wife battering victim V71.6
    concussion (cerebral) V71.6
    condition NEC V71.89
      infant—*see* Observation, suspected,
        condition, newborn
      maternal and fetal
        amniotic cavity and membrane problem
          V89.01
        cervical shortening V89.05
        fetal anomaly V89.03
        fetal growth problem V89.04
        oligohydramnios V89.01
        other specified problem NEC V89.09
        placental problem V89.02
        polyhydramnios V89.01
      newborn V29.9
        cardiovascular disease V29.8
        congenital anomaly V29.8
        genetic V29.3
        infectious V29.0
        ingestion foreign object V29.8
        injury V29.8
        metabolic V29.3
        neoplasm V29.8
        neurological V29.1
        poison, poisoning V29.8
        respiratory V29.2
        specified NEC V29.8
    exposure
      anthrax V71.82
      biological agent NEC V71.83
      SARS V71.83
    infectious disease not requiring isolation V71.89
    malignant neoplasm V71.1
    mental disorder V71.09
    neglect V71.81
    neoplasm
      benign V71.89
      malignant V71.1
    specified condition NEC V71.89
    tuberculosis V71.2
  tuberculosis, suspected V71.2
Obsession, obsessional 300.3
  ideas and mental images 300.3
  impulses 300.3
  neurosis 300.3
  phobia 300.3
  psychasthenia 300.3
  ruminations 300.3
  state 300.3
  syndrome 300.3

Obstruction, obstructed—*continued*
foramen of Monro (congenital) 742.3
  with spina bifida (*see also* Spina bifida) 741.0
foreign body—*see* Foreign body
gallbladder 575.2
  with calculus, cholelithiasis, or stones 574.21
    with cholecystitis (chronic) 574.11
      acute 574.01
  congenital 751.69
    jaundice from 751.69 *[774.5]*
gastric outlet 537.0
gastrointestinal (*see also* Obstruction, intestine)
  560.9
glottis 478.79
hepatic 573.8
  duct (*see also* Obstruction, biliary) 576.2
    congenital 751.61
  icterus (*see also* Obstruction, biliary) 576.8
    congenital 751.61
ileocecal coil (*see also* Obstruction, intestine)
  560.9
ileum (*see also* Obstruction, intestine) 560.9
iliofemoral (artery) 444.81
internal anastomosis—*see* Complications,
  mechanical, graft
intestine (mechanical) (neurogenic)
  (paroxysmal) (postinfectional) (reflex) 560.9
  with
    adhesions (intestinal) (peritoneal) 560.81
    hernia—*see also* Hernia, by site, with
      obstruction
    gangrenous—*see* Hernia, by site, with
      gangrene
  adynamic (*see also* Ileus) 560.1
  by gallstone 560.31
  congenital or infantile (small) 751.1
    large 751.2
  due to
    Ascaris lumbricoides 127.0
    mural thickening 560.89
    procedure 997.49
      involving urinary tract 997.5
  impaction 560.32
  infantile—*see* Obstruction, intestine,
    congenital
  newborn
    due to
      fecaliths 777.1
      inspissated milk 777.2
      meconium (plug) 777.1
        in mucoviscidosis 277.01
      transitory 777.4
    specified cause NEC 560.89
    transitory, newborn 777.4
    volvulus 560.2
intracardiac ball valve prosthesis 996.02
jaundice (*see also* Obstruction, biliary) 576.8
  congenital 751.61
jejunum (*see also* Obstruction, intestine) 560.9
kidney 593.89
labor 660.9
  affecting fetus or newborn 763.1
  by
    bony pelvis (conditions classifiable to
      653.0-653.9) 660.1
    deep transverse arrest 660.3
    impacted shoulder 660.4
    locked twins 660.5
    malposition (fetus) (conditions classifiable
      to 652.0-652.9) 660.0
      head during labor 660.3

Obstruction, obstructed—*continued*
  persistent occipitoposterior position 660.3
  soft tissue, pelvic (conditions classifiable to
    654.0-654.9) 660.2
lacrimal
  canaliculi 375.53
  congenital 743.65
  punctum 375.52
  sac 375.54
lacrimonasal duct 375.56
  congenital 743.65
  neonatal 375.55
lacteal, with steatorrhea 579.2
laryngitis (*see also* Laryngitis) 464.01
larynx 478.79
  congenital 748.3
liver 573.8
  cirrhotic (*see also* Cirrhosis, liver) 571.5
lung 518.89
  with
    asthma—*see* Asthma
    bronchitis (chronic) 491.20
    emphysema NEC 492.8
  airway, chronic 496
  chronic NEC 496
    with
      asthma (chronic) (obstructive) 493.2
    disease, chronic 496
      with
        asthma (chronic) (obstructive) 493.2
    emphysematous 492.8
lymphatic 457.1
meconium
  fetus or newborn 777.1
    in mucoviscidosis 277.01
  newborn due to fecaliths 777.1
mediastinum 519.3
mitral (rheumatic)—*see* Stenosis, mitral
nasal 478.19
  duct 375.56
    neonatal 375.55
  sinus—*see* Sinusitis
nasolacrimal duct 375.56
  congenital 743.65
  neonatal 375.55
nasopharynx 478.29
nose 478.19
organ or site, congenital NEC—*see* Atresia
pancreatic duct 577.8
parotid gland 527.8
pelviureteral junction (*see also* Obstruction,
  ureter) 593.4
pharynx 478.29
portal (circulation) (vein) 452
prostate 600.90
  with
    other lower urinary tract symptoms (LUTS)
      600.91
    urinary
      obstruction 600.91
      retention 600.91
  valve (urinary) 596.0
pulmonary
  valve (heart) (*see also* Endocarditis,
    pulmonary) 424.3
  vein, isolated 747.49
pyemic—*see* Septicemia
pylorus (acquired) 537.0
  congenital 750.5
  infantile 750.5
rectosigmoid (*see also* Obstruction, intestine) 560.9

Obstruction, obstructed—*continued*
  rectum 569.49
  renal 593.89
  respiratory 519.8
    chronic 496
  retinal (artery) (vein) (central) (*see also*
      Occlusion, retina) 362.30
  salivary duct (any) 527.8
    with calculus 527.5
  sigmoid (*see also* Obstruction, intestine) 560.9
  sinus (accessory) (nasal) (*see also* Sinusitis)
      473.9
  Stensen's duct 527.8
  stomach 537.89
    acute 536.1
    congenital 750.7
  submaxillary gland 527.8
    with calculus 527.5
  thoracic duct 457.1
  thrombotic—*see* Thrombosis
  tooth eruption 520.6
  trachea 519.19
  tracheostomy airway 519.09
  tricuspid—*see* Endocarditis, tricuspid
  upper respiratory, congenital 748.8
  ureter (functional) 593.4
    congenital 753.20
    due to calculus 592.1
  ureteropelvic junction, congenital 753.21
  ureterovesical junction, congenital 753.22
  urethra 599.60
    congenital 753.6
  urinary (moderate) 599.60
    organ or tract (lower) 599.60
      due to
        benign prostatic hypertrophy (BPH)—*see*
            category 600
        specified NEC 599.69
          due to
            benign prostatic hypertrophy
                (BPH)—*see* category 600
    prostatic valve 596.0
    specified NEC 599.69
      due to
        benign prostatic hypertrophy (BPH)—*see*
            category 600
  uropathy 599.60
  uterus 621.8
  vagina 623.2
  valvular—*see* Endocarditis
  vascular graft or shunt 996.1
    atherosclerosis —*see* Arteriosclerosis,
        coronary
    embolism 996.74
    occlusion NEC 996.74
    thrombus 996.74
  vein, venous 459.2
    caval (inferior) (superior) 459.2
    thrombotic—*see* Thrombosis
  vena cava (inferior) (superior) 459.2
  ventricular shunt 996.2
  vesical 596.0
  vesicourethral orifice 596.0
  vessel NEC 459.9
Obturator —*see* condition
Occlusal
  plane deviation 524.76
  wear, teeth 521.10

Occlusion
  anus 569.49
    congenital 751.2
    infantile 751.2
  aortoiliac (chronic) 444.09
  aqueduct of Sylvius 331.4
    congenital 742.3
      with spina bifida (*see also* Spina bifida) 741.0
  arteries of extremities, lower 444.22
    without thrombus or embolus (*see also*
        Arteriosclerosis, extremities) 440.20
    due to stricture or stenosis 447.1
    upper 444.21
      without thrombus or embolus (*see also*
          Arteriosclerosis, extremities) 440.20
      due to stricture or stenosis 447.1
  artery NEC (*see also* Embolism, artery) 444.9
    auditory, internal 433.8
    basilar 433.0
      with other precerebral artery 433.3
      bilateral 433.3
    brain or cerebral (*see also* Infarct, brain) 434.9
    carotid 433.1
      with other precerebral artery 433.3
      bilateral 433.3
    cerebellar (anterior inferior) (posterior
        inferior) (superior) 433.8
    cerebral (*see also* Infarct, brain) 434.9
    choroidal (anterior) 433.8
    chronic total
      coronary 414.2
      extremity(ies) 440.4
    complete
      coronary 414.2
      extremity(ies) 440.4
    communicating posterior 433.8
    coronary (thrombotic) (*see also* Infarct,
        myocardium) 410.9
      acute 410.9
        without myocardial infarction 411.81
      chronic total 414.2
      complete 414.2
      healed or old 412
      total 414.2
    extremity(ies)
      chronic total 440.4
      complete 440.4
      total 440.4
    hypophyseal 433.8
    iliac 444.81
    mesenteric (embolic) (thrombotic) (with
        gangrene) 557.0
    pontine 433.8
    precerebral NEC 433.9
      late effect—*see* Late effect(s) (of)
          cerebrovascular disease
      multiple or bilateral 433.3
      puerperal, postpartum, childbirth 674.0
      specified NEC 433.8
    renal 593.81
    retinal—*see* Occlusion, retina, artery
    spinal 433.8
    vertebral 433.2
      with other precerebral artery 433.3
      bilateral 433.3
  basilar (artery)—*see* Occlusion, artery, basilar
  bile duct (any) (*see also* Obstruction, biliary)
      576.2
  bowel (*see also* Obstruction, intestine) 560.9
  brain (artery) (vascular) (*see also* Infarct, brain)
      434.9

Occlusion—*continued*
breast (duct) 611.89
carotid (artery) (common) (internal)—*see*
Occlusion, artery, carotid
cerebellar (anterior inferior) (artery) (posterior
inferior) (superior) 433.8
cerebral (artery) (*see also* Infarct, brain) 434.9
cerebrovascular (*see also* Infarct, brain) 434.9
diffuse 437.0
cervical canal (*see also* Stricture, cervix) 622.4
by falciparum malaria 084.0
cervix (uteri) (*see also* Stricture, cervix) 622.4
choanal 748.0
choroidal (artery) 433.8
colon (*see also* Obstruction, intestine) 560.9
communicating posterior artery 433.8
coronary (artery) (thrombotic) (*see also* Infarct,
myocardium) 410.9
acute 410.9
without myocardial infarction 411.81
healed or old 412
without myocardial infarction 411.81
cystic duct (*see also* Obstruction, gallbladder)
575.2
congenital 751.69
disto
division I 524.22
division II 524.22
embolic—*see* Embolism
fallopian tube 628.2
congenital 752.19
gallbladder (*see also* Obstruction, gallbladder)
575.2
congenital 751.69
jaundice from 751.69 *[774.5]*
gingiva, traumatic 523.8
hymen 623.3
congenital 752.42
hypophyseal (artery) 433.8
iliac artery 444.81
intestine (*see also* Obstruction, intestine) 560.9
kidney 593.89
lacrimal apparatus—*see* Stenosis, lacrimal
lung 518.89
lymph or lymphatic channel 457.1
mammary duct 611.89
mesenteric artery (embolic) (thrombotic) (with
gangrene) 557.0
nose 478.1
congenital 748.0
organ or site, congenital NEC—*see* Atresia
oviduct 628.2
congenital 752.19
periodontal, traumatic 523.8
peripheral arteries (lower extremity) 444.22
without thrombus or embolus (*see also*
Arteriosclerosis, extremities) 440.20
due to stricture or stenosis 447.1
upper extremity 444.21
without thrombus or embolus (*see also*
Arteriosclerosis, extremities) 440.20
due to stricture or stenosis 447.1
pontine (artery) 433.8
posterior lingual, of mandibular teeth 524.29
precerebral artery—*see* Occlusion, artery,
precerebral NEC
puncta lacrimalia 375.52
pupil 364.74
pylorus (*see also* Stricture, pylorus) 537.0
renal artery 593.81

Occlusion—*continued*
retina, retinal (vascular) 362.30
artery, arterial 362.30
branch 362.32
central (total) 362.31
partial 362.33
transient 362.34
tributary 362.32
vein 362.30
branch 362.36
central (total) 362.35
incipient 362.37
partial 362.37
tributary 362.36
spinal artery 433.8
stent
coronary 996.72
teeth (mandibular) (posterior lingual) 524.29
thoracic duct 457.1
tubal 628.2
ureter (complete) (partial) 593.4
congenital 753.29
urethra (*see also* Stricture, urethra) 598.9
congenital 753.6
uterus 621.8
vagina 623.2
vascular NEC 459.9
vein—*see* Thrombosis
vena cava
inferior 453.2
superior (acute) 453.87
chronic 453.77
ventricle (brain) NEC 331.4
vertebral (artery)—*see* Occlusion, artery,
vertebral
vessel (blood) NEC 459.9
vulva 624.8
Occlusio pupillae 364.74
Occupational
problems NEC V62.29
therapy V57.21
Ochlophobia 300.29
Ochronosis (alkaptonuric) (congenital)
(endogenous) 270.2
with chloasma of eyelid 270.2
Ocular muscle —*see also* condition
myopathy 359.1
torticollis 781.93
Oculoauriculovertebral dysplasia 756.0
Oculogyric
crisis or disturbance 378.87
psychogenic 306.7
Oculomotor syndrome 378.81
Oddi's sphincter spasm 576.5
Odelberg's disease (juvenile osteochondrosis)
732.1
Odontalgia 525.9
Odontoameloblastoma (M9311/0) 213.1
upper jaw (bone) 213.0
Odontoclasia 521.05
Odontoclasis 873.63
complicated 873.73
Odontodysplasia, regional 520.4
Odontogenesis imperfecta 520.5
Odontoma (M9280/0) 213.1
ameloblastic (M9311/0) 213.1
upper jaw (bone) 213.0
calcified (M9280/0) 213.1
upper jaw (bone) 213.0

Odontoma—*continued*
  complex (M9282/0) 213.1
    upper jaw (bone) 213.0
  compound (M9281/0) 213.1
    upper jaw (bone) 213.0
  fibroameloblastic (M9290/0) 213.1
    upper jaw (bone) 213.0
  follicular 526.0
    upper jaw (bone) 213.0
Odontomyelitis (closed) (open) 522.0
Odontonecrosis 521.09
Odontorrhagia 525.8
Odontosarcoma, ameloblastic (M9290/3) 170.1
  upper jaw (bone) 170.0
Odynophagia 787.20
Oesophagostomiasis 127.7
Oesophagostomum infestation 127.7
Oestriasis 134.0
Ogilvie's syndrome (sympathicotonic colon
  obstruction) 560.89
Oguchi's disease (retina) 368.61
Ohara's disease (*see also* Tularemia) 021.9
Oidiomycosis (*see also* Candidiasis) 112.9
Oidiomycotic meningitis 112.83
Oidium albicans infection (*see also* Candidiasis)
  112.9
Old age 797
  dementia (of) 290.0
Olfactory —*see* condition
Oligemia 285.9
Oligergasia (*see also* Disability, intellectual) 319
Oligoamnios 658.0
  affecting fetus or newborn 761.2
Oligoastrocytoma, mixed (M9382/3)
  specified site—*see* Neoplasm, by site, malignant
  unspecified site 191.9
Oligocythemia 285.9
Oligodendroblastoma (M9460/3)
  specified site—*see* Neoplasm, by site, malignant
  unspecified site 191.9
Oligodendroglioma (M9450/3)
  anaplastic type (M9451/3)
    specified site—*see* Neoplasm, by site, malignant
    unspecified site 191.9
  specified site—*see* Neoplasm, by site, malignant
  unspecified site 191.9
Oligodendroma —*see* Oligodendroglioma
Oligodontia (*see also* Anodontia) 520.0
Oligoencephalon 742.1
Oligohydramnios 658.0
  affecting fetus or newborn 761.2
  due to premature rupture of membranes 658.1
    affecting fetus or newborn 761.2
Oligohydrosis 705.0
Oligomenorrhea 626.1
Oligophrenia (*see also* Disability, intellectual)
  319
  phenylpyruvic 270.1
Oligospermia 606.1
Oligotrichia 704.09
  congenita 757.4
Oliguria 788.5
  with
    abortion—*see* Abortion, by type, with renal failure
    ectopic pregnancy (*see also* categories
      633.0-633.9) 639.3
    molar pregnancy (*see also* categories 630-632)
      639.3

Oliguria—*continued*
  complicating
    abortion 639.3
    ectopic or molar pregnancy 639.3
    pregnancy 646.2
      with hypertension—*see* Toxemia, of
        pregnancy
  due to a procedure 997.5
  following labor and delivery 669.3
  heart or cardiac—*see* Failure, heart
  puerperal, postpartum 669.3
  specified due to a procedure 997.5
Ollier's disease (chondrodysplasia) 756.4
Omentitis (*see also* Peritonitis) 567.9
Omentocele (*see also* Hernia, omental) 553.8
Omentum, omental —*see* condition
Omphalitis (congenital) (newborn) 771.4
  not of newborn 686.9
  tetanus 771.3
Omphalocele 756.72
Omphalomesenteric duct, persistent 751.0
Omphalorrhagia, newborn 772.3
Omsk hemorrhagic fever 065.1
Onanism 307.9
Onchocerciasis 125.3
  eye 125.3 *[360.13]*
Onchocercosis 125.3
Oncocytoma (M8290/0)—*see* Neoplasm, by site,
  benign
Ondine's curse 348.89
Oneirophrenia (*see also* Schizophrenia) 295.4
Onychauxis 703.8
  congenital 757.5
Onychia (with lymphangitis) 681.9
  dermatophytic 110.1
  finger 681.02
  toe 681.11
Onychitis (with lymphangitis) 681.9
  finger 681.02
  toe 681.11
Onychocryptosis 703.0
Onychodystrophy 703.8
  congenital 757.5
Onychogryphosis 703.8
Onychogryposis 703.8
Onycholysis 703.8
Onychomadesis 703.8
Onychomalacia 703.8
Onychomycosis 110.1
  finger 110.1
  toe 110.1
Onycho-osteodysplasia 756.89
Onychophagy 307.9
Onychoptosis 703.8
Onychorrhexis 703.8
  congenital 757.5
Onychoschizia 703.8
Onychotrophia (*see also* Atrophy, nail) 703.8
O'nyong-nyong fever 066.3
Onyxis (finger) (toe) 703.0
Onyxitis (with lymphangitis) 681.9
  finger 681.02
  toe 681.11
Oocyte (egg) (ovum)
  donor V59.70
    age 35 and over V59.73
      anonymous recipient V59.73
      designated recipient V59.74
    under age 35 V59.71
      anonymous recipient V59.71
      designated recipient V59.72

Oophoritis (cystic) (infectional) (interstitial) (*see also* Salpingo-oophoritis) 614.2
  complicating pregnancy 646.6
  fetal (acute) 752.0
  gonococcal (acute) 098.19
    chronic or duration of 2 months or over 098.39
  tuberculous (*see also* Tuberculosis) 016.6
Opacity, opacities
  cornea 371.00
    central 371.03
    congenital 743.43
      interfering with vision 743.42
    degenerative (*see also* Degeneration, cornea) 371.40
    hereditary (*see also* Dystrophy, cornea) 371.50
    inflammatory (*see also* Keratitis) 370.9
    late effect of trachoma (healed) 139.1
    minor 371.01
    peripheral 371.02
  enamel (fluoride) (nonfluoride) (teeth) 520.3
  lens (*see also* Cataract) 366.9
  snowball 379.22
  vitreous (humor) 379.24
    congenital 743.51
Opalescent dentin (hereditary) 520.5
Open, opening
  abnormal, organ or site, congenital—*see* Imperfect, closure
  angle
    with
      borderline findings
        high risk 365.05
        intraocular pressure 365.01
        low risk 365.01
      cupping of discs 365.01
    high risk 365.05
    low risk 365.01
  bite
    anterior 524.24
    posterior 524.25
  false—*see* Imperfect, closure
  margin on tooth restoration 525.61
  restoration margins 525.61
  wound—*see* Wound, open, by site
Operation
  causing mutilation of fetus 763.89
  destructive, on live fetus, to facilitate birth 763.89
  for delivery, fetus or newborn 763.89
  maternal, unrelated to current delivery, affecting fetus or newborn (*see also* Newborn, affected by) 760.64
Operational fatigue 300.89
Operative —*see* condition
Operculitis (chronic) 523.40
  acute 523.30
Operculum, retina 361.32
  with detachment 361.01
Ophiasis 704.01
Ophthalmia (*see also* Conjunctivitis) 372.30
  actinic rays 370.24
  allergic (acute) 372.05
    chronic 372.14
  blennorrhagic (neonatorum) 098.40
  catarrhal 372.03
  diphtheritic 032.81
  Egyptian 076.1
  electric, electrica 370.24
  gonococcal (neonatorum) 098.40
  metastatic 360.11
  migraine 346.8

Ophthalmia—*continued*
  neonatorum, newborn 771.6
    gonococcal 098.40
  nodosa 360.14
  phlyctenular 370.31
    with ulcer (*see also* Ulcer, cornea) 370.00
  sympathetic 360.11
Ophthalmitis —*see* Ophthalmia
Ophthalmocele (congenital) 743.66
Ophthalmoneuromyelitis 341.0
Ophthalmopathy, infiltrative with thyrotoxicosis 242.0
Ophthalmoplegia (*see also* Strabismus) 378.9
  anterior internuclear 378.86
  ataxia-areflexia syndrome 357.0
  bilateral 378.9
  diabetic 250.5 *[378.86]*
    due to secondary diabetes 249.5 *[378.86]*
  exophthalmic 242.0 *[376.22]*
  external 378.55
    progressive 378.72
    total 378.56
  interna(l) (complete) (total) 367.52
  internuclear 378.86
  migraine 346.2
  painful 378.55
  Parinaud's 378.81
  progressive external 378.72
  supranuclear, progressive 333.0
  total (external) 378.56
    internal 367.52
  unilateral 378.9
Opisthognathism 524.00
Opisthorchiasis (felineus) (tenuicollis) (viverrini) 121.0
Opisthotonos, opisthotonus 781.0
Opitz's disease (congestive splenomegaly) 289.51
Opiumism (*see also* Dependence) 304.0
Oppenheim's disease 358.8
Oppenheim-Urbach disease or syndrome (necrobiosis lipoidica diabeticorum) 250.8 *[709.3]*
  due to secondary diabetes 249.8 *[709.3]*
Opsoclonia 379.59
Optic nerve —*see* condition
Orbit —*see* condition
Orchioblastoma (M9071/3) 186.9
Orchitis (nonspecific) (septic) 604.90
  with abscess 604.0
  blennorrhagic (acute) 098.13
    chronic or duration of 2 months or over 098.33
  diphtheritic 032.89 *[604.91]*
  filarial 125.9 *[604.91]*
  gangrenous 604.99
  gonococcal (acute) 098.13
    chronic or duration of 2 months or over 098.33
  mumps 072.0
  parotidea 072.0
  suppurative 604.99
  syphilitic 095.8 *[604.91]*
  tuberculous (*see also* Tuberculosis) 016.5 *[608.81]*
Orf 051.2
Organic —*see also* condition
  heart—*see* Disease, heart
  insufficiency 799.89
Oriental
  bilharziasis 120.2
  schistosomiasis 120.2
  sore 085.1
Orientation
  ego-dystonic sexual 302.0

Orifice —*see* condition
Origin, both great vessels from right ventricle 745.11
Ormond's disease or syndrome 593.4
Ornithosis 073.9
  with
    complication 073.8
      specified NEC 073.7
    pneumonia 073.0
    pneumonitis (lobular) 073.0
Orodigitofacial dysostosis 759.89
Oropouche fever 066.3
Orotaciduria, oroticaciduria (congenital)
    (hereditary) (pyrimidine deficiency) 281.4
Oroya fever 088.0
Orthodontics V58.5
  adjustment V53.4
  aftercare V58.5
  fitting V53.4
Orthopnea 786.02
Orthoptic training V57.4
Os, uterus —*see* condition
Osgood-Schlatter
  disease 732.4
  osteochondrosis 732.4
Osler's
  disease (M9950/1) (polycythemia vera) 238.4
  nodes 421.0
Osler-Rendu disease (familial hemorrhagic
    telangiectasia) 448.0
Osler-Vaquez disease (M9950/1) (polycythemia
    vera) 238.4
Osler-Weber-Rendu syndrome (familial
    hemorrhagic telangiectasia) 448.0
Osmidrosis 705.89
Osseous —*see* condition
Ossification
  artery—*see* Arteriosclerosis
  auricle (ear) 380.39
  bronchus 519.19
  cardiac (*see also* Degeneration, myocardial) 429.1
  cartilage (senile) 733.99
  coronary —*see* Arteriosclerosis, coronary
  diaphragm 728.10
  ear 380.39
    middle (*see also* Otosclerosis) 387.9
  falx cerebri 349.2
  fascia 728.10
  fontanel
    defective or delayed 756.0
    premature 756.0
  heart (*see also* Degeneration, myocardial) 429.1
    valve—*see* Endocarditis
  larynx 478.79
  ligament
    posterior longitudinal 724.8
      cervical 723.7
  meninges (cerebral) 349.2
    spinal 336.8
  multiple, eccentric centers 733.99
  muscle 728.10
    heterotopic, postoperative 728.13
  myocardium, myocardial (*see also*
    Degeneration, myocardial) 429.1
  penis 607.81
  periarticular 728.89
  sclera 379.16
  tendon 727.82
  trachea 519.19
  tympanic membrane (*see also*
    Tympanosclerosis) 385.00
  vitreous (humor) 360.44

Osteitis (*see also* Osteomyelitis) 730.2
  acute 730.0
  alveolar 526.5
  chronic 730.1
  condensans (ilii) 733.5
  deformans (Paget's) 731.0
    due to or associated with malignant neoplasm
      (*see also* Neoplasm, bone, malignant)
      170.9 *[731.1]*
  due to yaws 102.6
  fibrosa NEC 733.29
    cystica (generalisata) 252.01
    disseminata 756.59
    osteoplastica 252.01
  fragilitans 756.51
  Garré's (sclerosing) 730.1
  infectious (acute) (subacute) 730.0
    chronic or old 730.1
  jaw (acute) (chronic) (lower) (neonatal)
    (suppurative) (upper) 526.4
  parathyroid 252.01
  petrous bone (*see also* Petrositis) 383.20
  pubis 733.5
  sclerotic, nonsuppurative 730.1
  syphilitic 095.5
  tuberculosa
    cystica (of Jüngling) 135
    multiplex cystoides 135
Osteoarthritica spondylitis (spine) (*see also*
    Spondylosis) 721.90
Osteoarthritis (*see also* Osteoarthrosis) 715.9
  distal interphalangeal 715.9
  hyperplastic 731.2
  interspinalis (*see also* Spondylosis) 721.90
  spine, spinal NEC (*see also* Spondylosis) 721.90
Osteoarthropathy (*see also* Osteoarthrosis) 715.9
  chronic idiopathic hypertrophic 757.39
  familial idiopathic 757.39
  hypertrophic pulmonary 731.2
    secondary 731.2
  idiopathic hypertrophic 757.39
  primary hypertrophic 731.2
  pulmonary hypertrophic 731.2
  secondary hypertrophic 731.2
Osteoarthrosis (degenerative) (hypertrophic)
    (rheumatoid) 715.9

Note—Use the following fifth-digit
subclassification with category 715:

0 site unspecified
1 shoulder region
2 upper arm
3 forearm
4 hand
5 pelvic region and thigh
6 lower leg
7 ankle and foot
8 other specified sites except spine
9 multiple sites

  deformans alkaptonurica 270.2
  generalized 715.09
  juvenilis (Köhler's) 732.5
  localized 715.3
    idiopathic 715.1
    primary 715.1
    secondary 715.2
  multiple sites, not specified as generalized 715.89
  polyarticular 715.09
  spine (*see also* Spondylosis) 721.90
  temperomandibular joint 524.69

Osteoblastoma (M9200/0)—*see* Neoplasm, bone, benign
Osteochondritis (*see also* Osteochondrosis) 732.9
  dissecans 732.7
    hip 732.7
  ischiopubica 732.1
  multiple 756.59
  syphilitic (congenital) 090.0
Osteochondrodermodysplasia 756.59
Osteochondrodystrophy 277.5
  deformans 277.5
  familial 277.5
  fetalis 756.4
Osteochondrolysis 732.7
Osteochondroma (M9210/0)—*see also*
  Neoplasm, bone, benign
  multiple, congenital 756.4
Osteochondromatosis (M9210/1) 238.0
  synovial 727.82
Osteochondromyxosarcoma (M9180/3)—*see*
  Neoplasm, bone, malignant
Osteochondropathy NEC 732.9
Osteochondrosarcoma (M9180/3)—*see*
  Neoplasm, bone, malignant
Osteochondrosis 732.9
  acetabulum 732.1
  adult spine 732.8
  astragalus 732.5
  Blount's 732.4
  Buchanan's (juvenile osteochondrosis of iliac crest) 732.1
  Buchman's (juvenile osteochondrosis) 732.1
  Burns' 732.3
  calcaneus 732.5
  capitular epiphysis (femur) 732.1
  carpal
    lunate (wrist) 732.3
    scaphoid 732.3
  coxae juvenilis 732.1
  deformans juvenilis (coxae) (hip) 732.1
    Scheuermann's 732.0
    spine 732.0
    tibia 732.4
    vertebra 732.0
  Diaz's (astragalus) 732.5
  dissecans (knee) (shoulder) 732.7
  femoral capital epiphysis 732.1
  femur (head) (juvenile) 732.1
  foot (juvenile) 732.5
  Freiberg's (disease) (second metatarsal) 732.5
  Haas' 732.3
  Haglund's (os tibiale externum) 732.5
  hand (juvenile) 732.3
  head of
    femur 732.1
    humerus (juvenile) 732.3
  hip (juvenile) 732.1
  humerus (juvenile) 732.3
  iliac crest (juvenile) 732.1
  ilium (juvenile) 732.1
  ischiopubic synchondrosis 732.1
  Iselin's (osteochondrosis fifth metatarsal) 732.5
  juvenile, juvenilis 732.6
    arm 732.3
    capital femoral epiphysis 732.1
    capitellum humeri 732.3
    capitular epiphysis 732.1
    carpal scaphoid 732.3
    clavicle, sternal epiphysis 732.6
    coxae 732.1
    deformans 732.1

Osteochondrosis—*continued*
  juvenile—*continued*
    foot 732.5
    hand 732.3
    hip and pelvis 732.1
    lower extremity, except foot 732.4
    lunate, wrist 732.3
    medial cuneiform bone 732.5
    metatarsal (head) 732.5
    metatarsophalangeal 732.5
    navicular, ankle 732.5
    patella 732.4
    primary patellar center (of Köhler) 732.4
    specified site NEC 732.6
    spine 732.0
    tarsal scaphoid 732.5
    tibia (epiphysis) (tuberosity) 732.4
    upper extremity 732.3
    vertebra (body) (Calvé) 732.0
      epiphyseal plates (of Scheuermann) 732.0
  Kienböck's (disease) 732.3
  Köhler's (disease) (navicular, ankle) 732.5
    patellar 732.4
    tarsal navicular 732.5
  Legg-Calvé-Perthes (disease) 732.1
  lower extremity (juvenile) 732.4
  lunate bone 732.3
  Mauclaire's 732.3
  metacarpal heads (of Mauclaire) 732.3
  metatarsal (fifth) (head) (second) 732.5
  navicular, ankle 732.5
  os calcis 732.5
  Osgood-Schlatter 732.4
  os tibiale externum 732.5
  Panner's 732.3
  patella (juvenile) 732.4
  patellar center
    primary (of Köhler) 732.4
    secondary (of Sinding-Larsen) 732.4
  pelvis (juvenile) 732.1
  Pierson's 732.1
  radial head (juvenile) 732.3
  Scheuermann's 732.0
  Sever's (calcaneum) 732.5
  Sinding-Larsen (secondary patellar center) 732.4
  spine (juvenile) 732.0
    adult 732.8
  symphysis pubis (of Pierson) (juvenile) 732.1
  syphilitic (congenital) 090.0
  tarsal (navicular) (scaphoid) 732.5
  tibia (proximal) (tubercle) 732.4
  tuberculous—*see* Tuberculosis, bone
  ulna 732.3
  upper extremity (juvenile) 732.3
  van Neck's (juvenile osteochondrosis) 732.1
  vertebral (juvenile) 732.0
    adult 732.8
Osteoclastoma (M9250/1) 238.0
  malignant (M9250/3)—*see* Neoplasm, bone, malignant
Osteocopic pain 733.90
Osteodynia 733.90
Osteodystrophy
  azotemic 588.0
  chronica deformans hypertrophica 731.0
  congenital 756.50
    specified type NEC 756.59
  deformans 731.0
  fibrosa localisata 731.0
  parathyroid 252.01
  renal 588.0

Osteofibroma (M9262/0)—*see* Neoplasm, bone, benign
Osteofibrosarcoma (M9182/3)—*see* Neoplasm, bone, malignant
Osteogenesis imperfecta 756.51
Osteogenic —*see* condition
Osteoma (M9180/0)—*see also* Neoplasm, bone, benign
   osteoid (M9191/0)—*see also* Neoplasm, bone, benign
   giant (M9200/0)—*see* Neoplasm, bone, benign
Osteomalacia 268.2
   chronica deformans hypertrophica 731.0
   due to vitamin D deficiency 268.2
   infantile (*see also* Rickets) 268.0
   juvenile (*see also* Rickets) 268.0
   oncogenic 275.8
   pelvis 268.2
   vitamin D-resistant 275.3
Osteomalacic bone 268.2
Osteomalacosis 268.2
Osteomyelitis (general) (infective) (localized) (neonatal) (purulent) (pyogenic) (septic) (staphylococcal) (streptococcal) (suppurative) (with periostitis) 730.2

Note—Use the following fifth-digit subclassification with category 730:

0 *site unspecified*
1 *shoulder region*
2 *upper arm*
3 *forearm*
4 *hand*
5 *pelvic region and thigh*
6 *lower leg*
7 *ankle and foot*
8 *other specified sites*
9 *multiple sites*

---

   acute or subacute 730.0
   chronic or old 730.1
   due to or associated with
      diabetes mellitus 250.8 *[731.8]*
         due to secondary diabetes 249.8 *[731.8]*
      tuberculosis (*see also* Tuberculosis, bone) 015.9 *[730.8]*
         limb bones 015.5 *[730.8]*
         specified bones NEC 015.7 *[730.8]*
         spine 015.0 *[730.8]*
         typhoid 002.0 *[730.8]*
   Garré's 730.1
   jaw (acute) (chronic) (lower) (neonatal) (suppurative) (upper) 526.4
   nonsuppurating 730.1
   orbital 376.03
   petrous bone (*see also* Petrositis) 383.20
   Salmonella 003.24
   sclerosing, nonsuppurative 730.1
   sicca 730.1
   syphilitic 095.5
      congenital 090.0 *[730.8]*
   tuberculous—*see* Tuberculosis, bone
   typhoid 002.0 *[730.8]*
Osteomyelofibrosis 289.89
Osteomyelosclerosis 289.89
Osteonecrosis 733.40
   meaning osteomyelitis 730.1
Osteo-onycho-arthro dysplasia 756.89
Osteo-onychodysplasia, hereditary 756.89

Osteopathia
   condensans disseminata 756.53
   hyperostotica multiplex infantilis 756.59
   hypertrophica toxica 731.2
   striata 756.4
Osteopathy resulting from poliomyelitis (*see also* Poliomyelitis) 045.9 *[730.7]*
   familial dysplastic 731.2
Osteopecilia 756.53
Osteopenia 733.90
   borderline 733.90
Osteoperiostitis (*see also* Osteomyelitis) 730.2
   ossificans toxica 731.2
   toxica ossificans 731.2
Osteopetrosis (familial) 756.52
Osteophyte —*see* Exostosis
Osteophytosis —*see* Exostosis
Osteopoikilosis 756.53
Osteoporosis (generalized) 733.00
   circumscripta 731.0
   disuse 733.03
   drug-induced 733.09
   idiopathic 733.02
   postmenopausal 733.01
   posttraumatic 733.7
   screening V82.81
   senile 733.01
   specified type NEC 733.09
Osteoporosis-osteomalacia syndrome 268.2
Osteopsathyrosis 756.51
Osteoradionecrosis, jaw 526.89
Osteosarcoma (M9180/3)—*see also* Neoplasm, bone, malignant
   chondroblastic (M9181/3)—*see* Neoplasm, bone, malignant
   fibroblastic (M9182/3)—*see* Neoplasm, bone, malignant
   in Paget's disease of bone (M9184/3)—*see* Neoplasm, bone, malignant
   juxtacortical (M9190/3)—*see* Neoplasm, bone, malignant
   parosteal (M9190/3)—*see* Neoplasm, bone, malignant
   telangiectatic (M9183/3)—*see* Neoplasm, bone, malignant
Osteosclerosis 756.52
   fragilis (generalisata) 756.52
Osteosclerotic anemia 289.89
Osteosis
   acromegaloid 757.39
   cutis 709.3
   parathyroid 252.01
   renal fibrocystic 588.0
Österreicher-Turner syndrome 756.89
Ostium
   atrioventriculare commune 745.69
   primum (arteriosum) (defect) (persistent) 745.61
   secundum (arteriosum) (defect) (patent) (persistent) 745.5
Ostrum-Furst syndrome 756.59
Otalgia 388.70
   otogenic 388.71
   referred 388.72
Othematoma 380.31
Otitic hydrocephalus 348.2
Otitis 382.9
   with effusion 381.4
      purulent 382.4
      secretory 381.4
      serous 381.4
      suppurative 382.4

Otitis—*continued*
  acute 382.9
  adhesive (*see also* Adhesions, middle ear)
    385.10
  chronic 382.9
    with effusion 381.3
    mucoid, mucous (simple) 381.20
    purulent 382.3
    secretory 381.3
    serous 381.10
    suppurative 382.3
  diffuse parasitic 136.8
  externa (acute) (diffuse) (hemorrhagica) 380.10
    actinic 380.22
    candidal 112.82
    chemical 380.22
    chronic 380.23
      mycotic—*see* Otitis, externa, mycotic
      specified type NEC 380.23
    circumscribed 380.10
    contact 380.22
    due to
      erysipelas 035 *[380.13]*
      impetigo 684 *[380.13]*
      seborrheic dermatitis 690.10 *[380.13]*
    eczematoid 380.22
    furuncular 680.0 *[380.13]*
    infective 380.10
      chronic 380.16
    malignant 380.14
    mycotic (chronic) 380.15
      due to
        aspergillosis 117.3 *[380.15]*
        moniliasis 112.82
        otomycosis 111.8 *[380.15]*
    reactive 380.22
    specified type NEC 380.22
    tropical 111.8 *[380.15]*
  insidiosa (*see also* Otosclerosis) 387.9
  interna (*see also* Labyrinthitis) 386.30
  media (hemorrhagic) (staphylococcal)
    (streptococcal) 382.9
    acute 382.9
      with effusion 381.00
      allergic 381.04
        mucoid 381.05
        sanguineous 381.06
        serous 381.04
      catarrhal 381.00
      exudative 381.00
      mucoid 381.02
        allergic 381.05
      necrotizing 382.00
        with spontaneous rupture of ear drum
          382.01
        in
          influenza (*see also* Influenza) 487.8
            [382.02]
          measles 055.2
          scarlet fever 034.1 *[382.02]*
      nonsuppurative 381.00
      purulent 382.00
        with spontaneous rupture of ear drum
          382.01
      sanguineous 381.03
        allergic 381.06
      secretory 381.01
      seromucinous 381.02
      serous 381.01
        allergic 381.04

Otitis—*continued*
  media—*continued*
    acute—*continued*
      suppurative 382.00
        with spontaneous rupture of ear drum
          382.01
        due to
          influenza (*see also* Influenza) 487.8
            [382.02]
          scarlet fever 034.1 *[382.02]*
      transudative 381.00
    adhesive (*see also* Adhesions, middle ear) 385.10
    allergic 381.4
      acute 381.04
        mucoid 381.05
        sanguineous 381.06
        serous 381.04
      chronic 381.3
    catarrhal 381.4
      acute 381.00
      chronic (simple) 381.10
    chronic 382.9
      with effusion 381.3
      adhesive (*see also* Adhesions, middle ear)
        385.10
      allergic 381.3
      atticoantral, suppurative (with posterior or
        superior marginal perforation of ear
        drum) 382.2
      benign suppurative (with anterior perforation
        of ear drum) 382.1
      catarrhal 381.10
      exudative 381.3
      mucinous 381.20
      mucoid, mucous (simple) 381.20
      mucosanguineous 381.29
      nonsuppurative 381.3
      purulent 382.3
      secretory 381.3
      seromucinous 381.3
      serosanguineous 381.19
      serous (simple) 381.10
      suppurative 382.3
        atticoantral (with posterior or superior
          marginal perforation of ear drum)
          382.2
        benign (with anterior perforation of ear
          drum) 382.1
        tuberculous (*see also* Tuberculosis) 017.4
        tubotympanic 382.1
      transudative 381.3
    exudative 381.4
      acute 381.00
      chronic 381.3
    fibrotic (*see also* Adhesions, middle ear)
      385.10
    mucoid, mucous 381.4
      acute 381.02
      chronic (simple) 381.20
    mucosanguineous, chronic 381.29
    nonsuppurative 381.4
      acute 381.00
      chronic 381.3
    postmeasles 055.2
    purulent 382.4
      acute 382.00
        with spontaneous rupture of ear drum
          382.01
      chronic 382.3
    sanguineous, acute 381.03
      allergic 381.06

Otitis—*continued*
  media—*continued*
    secretory 381.4
      acute or subacute 381.01
      chronic 381.3
    seromucinous 381.4
      acute or subacute 381.02
      chronic 381.3
    serosanguineous, chronic 381.19
    serous 381.4
      acute or subacute 381.01
      chronic (simple) 381.10
    subacute—*see* Otitis, media, acute
    suppurative 382.4
      acute 382.00
        with spontaneous rupture of ear drum 382.01
      chronic 382.3
        atticoantral 382.2
        benign 382.1
        tuberculous (*see also* Tuberculosis) 017.4
        tubotympanic 382.1
    transudative 381.4
      acute 381.00
      chronic 381.3
    tuberculous (*see also* Tuberculosis) 017.4
    postmeasles 055.2
Otoconia 386.8
Otolith syndrome 386.19
Otomycosis 111.8 *[380.15]*
  in
    aspergillosis 117.3 *[380.15]*
    moniliasis 112.82
Otopathy 388.9
Otoporosis (*see also* Otosclerosis) 387.9
Otorrhagia 388.69
  traumatic—*see* nature of injury
Otorrhea 388.60
  blood 388.69
  cerebrospinal (fluid) 388.61
Otosclerosis (general) 387.9
  cochlear (endosteal) 387.2
  involving
    otic capsule 387.2
    oval window
      nonobliterative 387.0
      obliterative 387.1
    round window 387.2
  nonobliterative 387.0
  obliterative 387.1
  specified type NEC 387.8
Otospongiosis (*see also* Otosclerosis) 387.9
Otto's disease or pelvis 715.35
Outburst, aggressive (*see also* Disturbance, conduct) 312.0
  in children or adolescents 313.9
Outcome of delivery
  multiple birth NEC V27.9
    all liveborn V27.5
    all stillborn V27.7
    some liveborn V27.6
    unspecified V27.9
  single V27.9
    liveborn V27.0
    stillborn V27.1
  twins V27.9
    both liveborn V27.2
    both stillborn V27.4
    one liveborn, one stillborn V27.3
Outlet —*see also* condition
  syndrome (thoracic) 353.0
Outstanding ears (bilateral) 744.29

Ovalocytosis (congenital) (hereditary) (*see also* Elliptocytosis) 282.1
Ovarian —*see also* condition
  pregnancy—*see* Pregnancy, ovarian
  remnant syndrome 620.8
  vein syndrome 593.4
Ovaritis (cystic) (*see also* Salpingo-oophoritis) 614.2
Ovary, ovarian —*see* condition
Overactive —*see also* Hyperfunction
  bladder 596.51
  eye muscle (*see also* Strabismus) 378.9
  hypothalamus 253.8
  thyroid (*see also* Thyrotoxicosis) 242.9
Overactivity, child 314.01
Overbite (deep) (excessive) (horizontal) (vertical) 524.29
Overbreathing (*see also* Hyperventilation) 786.01
Overconscientious personality 301.4
Overdevelopment —*see also* Hypertrophy
  breast (female) (male) 611.1
  nasal bones 738.0
  prostate, congenital 752.89
Overdistention —*see* Distention
Overdose overdosage (drug) 977.9
  specified drug or substance—*see* Table of drugs and chemicals
Overeating 783.6
  with obesity 278.0
  nonorganic origin 307.51
Overexertion (effects) (exhaustion) 994.5
Overexposure (effects) 994.9
  exhaustion 994.4
Overfeeding (*see also* Overeating) 783.6
Overfill, endodontic 526.62
Overgrowth, bone NEC 733.99
Overhanging
  tooth restoration 525.62
  unrepairable, dental restorative materials 525.62
Overheated (effects) (places)—*see* Heat
Overinhibited child 313.0
Overjet 524.29
  excessive horizontal 524.26
Overlaid, overlying (suffocation) 994.7
Overlap
  excessive horizontal 524.26
Overlapping toe (acquired) 735.8
  congenital (fifth toe) 755.66
Overload
  fluid 276.69
    due to transfusion (blood) (blood components) 276.61
  iron, due to repeated red blood cell transfusions 275.02
  potassium (K) 276.7
  sodium (Na) 276.0
  transfusion associated circulatory (TACO) 276.61
Overnutrition (*see also* Hyperalimentation) 783.6
Overproduction —*see also* Hypersecretion
  ACTH 255.3
  cortisol 255.0
  growth hormone 253.0
  thyroid-stimulating hormone (TSH) 242.8
Overriding
  aorta 747.21
  finger (acquired) 736.29
    congenital 755.59
  toe (acquired) 735.8
    congenital 755.66

Oversize
  fetus (weight of 4500 grams or more) 766.0
    affecting management of pregnancy 656.6
    causing disproportion 653.5
      with obstructed labor 660.1
      affecting fetus or newborn 763.1
Overstimulation, ovarian 256.1
Overstrained 780.79
  heart—*see* Hypertrophy, cardiac
Overweight (*see also* Obesity) 278.02
Overwork 780.79
Oviduct —*see* condition
Ovotestis 752.7
Ovulation (cycle)
  failure or lack of 628.0
  pain 625.2
Ovum
  blighted 631.8
  donor V59.70
    age 35 and over V59.73
      anonymous recipient V59.73
      designated recipient V59.74
    under age 35 V59.71
      anonymous recipient V59.71
      designated recipient V59.72
  dropsical 631.8
  pathologic 631.8
Owren's disease or syndrome (parahemophilia)
  (*see also* Defect, coagulation) 286.3
Oxalosis 271.8
Oxaluria 271.8
Ox heart —*see* Hypertrophy, cardiac
OX syndrome 758.6
Oxycephaly, oxycephalic 756.0
  syphilitic, congenital 090.0
Oxyuriasis 127.4
Oxyuris vermicularis (infestation) 127.4
Ozena 472.0

P

Pacemaker syndrome 429.4
Pachyderma, pachydermia 701.8
  laryngis 478.5
  laryngitis 478.79
  larynx (verrucosa) 478.79
Pachydermatitis 701.8
Pachydermatocele (congenital) 757.39
  acquired 701.8
Pachydermatosis 701.8
Pachydermoperiostitis
  secondary 731.2
Pachydermoperiostosis
  primary idiopathic 757.39
  secondary 731.2
Pachymeningitis (adhesive) (basal) (brain)
  (cerebral) (cervical) (chronic) (circumscribed)
  (external) (fibrous) (hemorrhagic)
  (hypertrophic) (internal) (purulent) (spinal)
  (suppurative) (*see also* Meningitis) 322.9
  gonococcal 098.82
Pachyonychia (congenital) 757.5
  acquired 703.8
Pachyperiosteodermia
  primary or idiopathic 757.39
  secondary 731.2
Pachyperiostosis
  primary or idiopathic 757.39
  secondary 731.2
Pacinian tumor (M9507/0)—*see* Neoplasm,
  skin, benign
Pads, knuckle or Garrod's 728.79
Paget's disease (osteitis deformans) 731.0
  with infiltrating duct carcinoma of the breast
    (M8541/3)—*see* Neoplasm, breast,
    malignant
  bone 731.0
    osteosarcoma in (M9184/3)—*see* Neoplasm,
     bone, malignant
  breast (M8540/3) 174.0
  extramammary (M8542/3)—*see also* Neoplasm,
    skin, malignant
    anus 154.3
    skin 173.59
  malignant (M8540/3)
    breast 174.0
    specified site NEC (M8542/3)—*see*
     Neoplasm, skin, malignant
    unspecified site 174.0
  mammary (M8540/3) 174.0
  necrosis of bone 731.0
  nipple (M8540/3) 174.0
  osteitis deformans 731.0
Paget-Schroetter syndrome (intermittent venous
  claudication) 453.89
Pain(s) (*see also* Painful) 780.96
  abdominal 789.0
  acute 338.19
    due to trauma 338.11
    postoperative 338.18
     post-thoracotomy 338.12
  adnexa (uteri) 625.9
  alimentary, due to vascular insufficiency 557.9
  anginoid (*see also* Pain, precordial) 786.51
  anus 569.42
  arch 729.5
  arm 729.5
  axillary 729.5

Pain(s)—*continued*
  back (postural) 724.5
    low 724.2
    psychogenic 307.89
  bile duct 576.9
  bladder 788.99
  bone 733.90
  breast 611.71
    psychogenic 307.89
  broad ligament 625.9
  cancer associated 338.3
  cartilage NEC 733.90
  cecum 789.0
  cervicobrachial 723.3
  chest (central) 786.50
    atypical 786.59
    midsternal 786.51
    musculoskeletal 786.59
    noncardiac 786.59
    substernal 786.51
    wall (anterior) 786.52
  chronic 338.29
    associated with significant psychosocial
     dysfunction 338.4
    due to trauma 338.21
    postoperative 338.28
     post-thoracotomy 338.22
    syndrome 338.4
  coccyx 724.79
  colon 789.0
  common duct 576.9
  coronary—*see* Angina
  costochondral 786.52
  diaphragm 786.52
  due to (presence of) any device, implant, or graft
    classifiable to 996.0-996.5—*see*
    Complications, due to (presence of) any
    device, implant, or graft classified to
    996.0-996.5 NEC
  malignancy (primary) (secondary) 338.3
  ear (*see also* Otalgia) 388.70
  epigastric, epigastrium 789.0
  extremity (lower) (upper) 729.5
  eye 379.91
  face, facial 784.0
    atypical 350.2
    nerve 351.8
  false (labor) 644.1
  female genital organ NEC 625.9
    psychogenic 307.89
  finger 729.5
  flank 789.0
  foot 729.5
  gallbladder 575.9
  gas (intestinal) 787.3
  gastric 536.8
  generalized 780.96
  genital organ
    female 625.9
    male 608.9
    psychogenic 307.89
  groin 789.0
  growing 781.99
  hand 729.5
  head (*see also* Headache) 784.0
  heart (*see also* Pain, precordial) 786.51
  infraorbital (*see also* Neuralgia, trigeminal)
    350.1

PQR

Pain(s)—*continued*
  intermenstrual 625.2
  jaw 784.92
  joint 719.40
    ankle 719.47
    elbow 719.42
    foot 719.47
    hand 719.44
    hip 719.45
    knee 719.46
    multiple sites 719.49
    pelvic region 719.45
    psychogenic 307.89
    shoulder (region) 719.41
    specified site NEC 719.48
    wrist 719.43
  kidney 788.0
  labor, false or spurious 644.1
  laryngeal 784.1
  leg 729.5
  limb 729.5
  low back 724.2
  lumbar region 724.2
  mandible, mandibular 784.92
  mastoid (*see also* Otalgia) 388.70
  maxilla 784.92
  menstrual 625.3
  metacarpophalangeal (joint) 719.44
  metatarsophalangeal (joint) 719.47
  mouth 528.9
  muscle 729.1
    intercostal 786.59
  musculoskeletal (*see also* Pain, by site) 729.1
  nasal 478.19
  nasopharynx 478.29
  neck NEC 723.1
    psychogenic 307.89
  neoplasm related (acute) (chronic) 338.3
  nerve NEC 729.2
  neuromuscular 729.1
  nose 478.19
  ocular 379.91
  ophthalmic 379.91
  orbital region 379.91
  osteocopic 733.90
  ovary 625.9
    psychogenic 307.89
  over heart (*see also* Pain, precordial) 786.51
  ovulation 625.2
  pelvic (female) 625.9
    male NEC 789.0
      psychogenic 307.89
    psychogenic 307.89
  penis 607.9
    psychogenic 307.89
  pericardial (*see also* Pain, precordial) 786.51
  perineum
    female 625.9
    male 608.9
  pharynx 478.29
  pleura, pleural, pleuritic 786.52
  post-operative 338.18
    acute 338.18
    chronic 338.28
  post-thoracotomy 338.12
    acute 338.12
    chronic 338.22
  preauricular 388.70
  precordial (region) 786.51
    psychogenic 307.89
  premenstrual 625.4
  psychogenic 307.80

Pain(s)—*continued*
  cardiovascular system 307.89
  gastrointestinal system 307.89
  genitourinary system 307.89
  heart 307.89
  musculoskeletal system 307.89
  respiratory system 307.89
  skin 306.3
  radicular (spinal) (*see also* Radiculitis) 729.2
  rectum 569.42
  respiration 786.52
  retrosternal 786.51
  rheumatic NEC 729.0
    muscular 729.1
  rib 786.50
  root (spinal) (*see also* Radiculitis) 729.2
  round ligament (stretch) 625.9
  sacroiliac 724.6
  sciatic 724.3
  scrotum 608.9
    psychogenic 307.89
  seminal vesicle 608.9
  sinus 478.19
  skin 782.0
  spermatic cord 608.9
  spinal root (*see also* Radiculitis) 729.2
  stomach 536.8
    psychogenic 307.89
  substernal 786.51
  temporomandibular (joint) 524.62
  testis 608.9
    psychogenic 307.89
  thoracic spine 724.1
    with radicular and visceral pain 724.4
  throat 784.1
  tibia 733.90
  toe 729.5
  tongue 529.6
  tooth 525.9
  total hip replacement 996.77
  total knee replacement 996.77
  trigeminal (*see also* Neuralgia, trigeminal) 350.1
  tumor associated 338.3
  umbilicus 789.0
  ureter 788.0
  urinary (organ) (system) 788.0
  uterus 625.9
    psychogenic 307.89
  vagina 625.9
  vertebrogenic (syndrome) 724.5
  vesical 788.99
  vulva 625.9
  xiphoid 733.90
Painful —*see also* Pain
  arc syndrome 726.19
  coitus
    female 625.0
    male 608.89
      psychogenic 302.76
  ejaculation (semen) 608.89
    psychogenic 302.79
  erection 607.3
  feet syndrome 266.2
  menstruation 625.3
    psychogenic 306.52
  micturition 788.1
  ophthalmoplegia 378.55
  respiration 786.52
  scar NEC 709.2
  urination 788.1
  wire sutures 998.89

Painters' colic 984.9
  specified type of lead—*see* Table of drugs and
    chemicals
Palate —*see* condition
Palatoplegia 528.9
Palatoschisis (*see also* Cleft, palate) 749.00
Palilalia 784.69
Palindromic arthritis (*see also* Rheumatism,
    palindromic) 719.3
Palliative care V66.7
Pallor 782.61
  temporal, optic disc 377.15
Palmar —*see also* condition
  fascia—*see* condition
Palpable
  cecum 569.89
  kidney 593.89
  liver 573.9
  lymph nodes 785.6
  ovary 620.8
  prostate 602.9
  spleen (*see also* Splenomegaly) 789.2
  uterus 625.8
Palpitation (heart) 785.1
  psychogenic 306.2
Palsy (*see also* Paralysis) 344.9
  atrophic diffuse 335.20
  Bell's 351.0
    newborn 767.5
  birth 767.7
  brachial plexus 353.0
    fetus or newborn 767.6
  brain—*see also* Palsy, cerebral
    noncongenital or noninfantile 344.89
      due to vascular lesion—*see* category 438
      late effect—*see* Late effect(s) (of)
        cerebrovascular disease
    syphilitic 094.89
      congenital 090.49
  bulbar (chronic) (progressive) 335.22
    pseudo NEC 335.23
    supranuclear NEC 344.89
  cerebral (congenital) (infantile) (spastic) 343.9
    athetoid 333.71
    diplegic 343.0
      mue to prevhous vascular lesion—*see*
        category 438
      late effect—*see* Late effect(s) (of)
        cerebrovascular disease
    hemiplegic 343.1
    monoplegic 343.3
    noncongenital or noninfantile 437.8
      mue to prevhous vascular lesion—*see*
        category 438
      late effect—*see* Late effect(s) (of)
        cerebrovascular disease
    paraplegic 343.0
    quadriplegic 343.2
    spastic, not congenital or infantile 344.89
    syphilitic 094.89
      congenital 090.49
    tetraplegic 343.2
  cranial nerve—*see also* Disorder, nerve, cranial
    multiple 352.6
  creeping 335.21
  divers' 993.3
  Erb's (birth injury) 767.6
  facial 351.0
    newborn 767.5
  glossopharyngeal 352.2
  Klumpke (-Déjérine) 767.6

Palsy—*continued*
  lead 984.9
    specified type of lead—*see* Table of drugs and
      chemicals
  median nerve (tardy) 354.0
  peroneal nerve (acute) (tardy) 355.3
  progressive supranuclear 333.0
  pseudobulbar NEC 335.23
  radial nerve (acute) 354.3
  seventh nerve 351.0
    newborn 767.5
  shaking (*see also* Parkinsonism) 332.0
  spastic (cerebral) (spinal) 343.9
    hemiplegic 343.1
  specified nerve NEC—*see* Disorder, nerve
  supranuclear NEC 356.8
    progressive 333.0
  ulnar nerve (tardy) 354.2
  wasting 335.21
Paltauf-Sternberg disease 201.9
Paludism —*see* Malaria
Panama fever 084.0
Panaris (with lymphangitis) 681.9
  finger 681.02
  toe 681.11
Panaritium (with lymphangitis) 681.9
  finger 681.02
  toe 681.11
Panarteritis (nodosa) 446.0
  brain or cerebral 437.4
Pancake heart 793.2
  with cor pulmonale (chronic) 416.9
Pancarditis (acute) (chronic) 429.89
  with
    rheumatic fever (active) (acute) (chronic)
      (subacute) 391.8
      inactive or quiescent 398.99
    rheumatic, acute 391.8
    chronic or inactive 398.99
Pancoast's syndrome or tumor (carcinoma,
    pulmonary apex) (M8010/3) 162.3
Pancoast-Tobias syndrome (M8010/3)
    (carcinoma, pulmonary apex) 162.3
Pancolitis 556.6
Pancreas, pancreatic —*see* condition
Pancreatitis 577.0
  acute (edematous) (hemorrhagic) (recurrent) 577.0
  annular 577.0
  apoplectic 577.0
  calcereous 577.0
  chronic (infectious) 577.1
    recurrent 577.1
  cystic 577.2
  fibrous 577.8
  gangrenous 577.0
  hemorrhagic (acute) 577.0
  interstitial (chronic) 577.1
    acute 577.0
  malignant 577.0
  mumps 072.3
  painless 577.1
  recurrent 577.1
  relapsing 577.1
  subacute 577.0
  suppurative 577.0
  syphilitic 095.8
Pancreatolithiasis 577.8
Pancytolysis 289.9

Pancytopenia (acquired) 284.19
  with
    malformations 284.09
    myelodysplastic syndrome — *see* Syndrome,
      myelodysplastic
  congenital 284.09
  due to
    antineoplastic chemotherapy 284.11
    drug, specified NEC 284.12
  specified NEC 284.19
Panencephalitis —*see also* Encephalitis
  subacute, sclerosing 046.2
Panhematopenia 284.81
  congenital 284.09
  constitutional 284.09
  splenic, primary 289.4
Panhemocytopenia 284.81
  congenital 284.09
  constitutional 284.09
Panhypogonadism 257.2
Panhypopituitarism 253.2
  prepubertal 253.3
Panic (attack) (state) 300.01
  reaction to exceptional stress (transient) 308.0
Panmyelopathy, familial constitutional 284.09
Panmyelophthisis 284.2
  acquired (secondary) 284.81
  congenital 284.2
  idiopathic 284.9
Panmyelosis (acute) (M9951/1) 238.79
Panner's disease 732.3
  capitellum humeri 732.3
  head of humerus 732.3
  tarsal navicular (bone) (osteochondrosis) 732.5
Panneuritis endemica 265.0 *[357.4]*
Panniculitis 729.30
  back 724.8
  knee 729.31
  mesenteric 567.82
  neck 723.6
  nodular, nonsuppurative 729.30
  sacral 724.8
  specified site NEC 729.39
Panniculus adiposus (abdominal) 278.1
Pannus (corneal) 370.62
  abdominal (symptomatic) 278.1
  allergic eczematous 370.62
  degenerativus 370.62
  keratic 370.62
  rheumatoid—*see* Arthritis, rheumatoid
  trachomatosus, trachomatous (active) 076.1
    [370.62]
  late effect 139.1
Panophthalmitis 360.02
Panotitis —*see* Otitis media
Pansinusitis (chronic) (hyperplastic)
  (nonpurulent) (purulent) 473.8
  acute 461.8
  due to fungus NEC 117.9
  tuberculous (*see also* Tuberculosis) 012.8
Panuveitis 360.12
  sympathetic 360.11
Panvalvular disease —*see* Endocarditis, mitral
Papageienkrankheit 073.9

Papanicolaou smear
  anus 796.70
    with
      atypical squamous cells
        cannot exclude high grade squamous
          intraepithelial lesion (ASC-H) 796.72
        of undetermined significance (ASC-US)
          796.71
      cytologic evidence of malignancy 796.76
      high grade squamous intraepithelial lesion
        (HGSIL) 796.74
      low grade squamous intraepithelial lesion
        (LGSIL) 796.73
    glandular 796.70
    specified finding NEC 796.79
    unsatisfactory cytology 796.78
  cervix (screening test) V76.2
    as part of gynecological examination V72.31
    for suspected malignant neoplasm V76.2
      no disease found V71.1
    inadequate cytology sample 795.08
    nonspecific abnormal finding 795.00
      with
        atypical squamous cells—changes of
          undetermined significance
          cannot exclude high grade squamous
            intraepithelial lesion (ASC-H)
            795.02
          of undetermined significance (ASC-US)
            795.01
        cytologic evidence of malignancy 795.06
        high grade squamous intraepithelial lesion
          (HGSIL) 795.04
        low grade squamous intraepithelial lesion
          (LGSIL) 795.03
      nonspecific finding NEC 795.09
      satisfactory smear but lacking
        transformation zone 795.07
    to confirm findings of recent normal smear
      following initial abnormal smear V72.32
    unsatisfactory cervical cytology 795.08
  other specified site—*see also* Screening,
    malignant neoplasm
    for suspected malignant neoplasm—*see also*
      Screening, malignant neoplasm
    no disease found V71.1
    nonspecific abnormal finding 796.9
  vagina V76.47
    with
      atypical squamous cells
        cannot exclude high grade squamous
          intraepithelial lesion (ASC-H) 795.12
        of undetermined significance (ASC-US)
          795.11
      cytologic evidence of malignancy 795.16
      high grade squamous intraepithelial lesion
        (HGSIL) 795.14
      low grade squamous intraepithelial lesion
        (LGSIL) 795.13
    abnormal NEC 795.19
    following hysterectomy for malignant
      condition V67.01
    inadequate cytology sample 795.18
    unsatisfactory cytology 795.18
Papilledema 377.00
  associated with
    decreased ocular pressure 377.02
    increased intracranial pressure 377.01
    retinal disorder 377.03
  choked disc 377.00
  infectional 377.00

Papillitis 377.31
  anus 569.49
  chronic lingual 529.4
  necrotizing, kidney 584.7
  optic 377.31
  rectum 569.49
  renal, necrotizing 584.7
  tongue 529.0
Papilloma (M8050/0)—*see also* Neoplasm, by
  site, benign

> *Note—Except where otherwise indicated, the*
> *morphological varieties of papilloma in the list*
> *below should be coded by site as for*
> *"Neoplasm, benign."*

  acuminatum (female) (male) 078.11
  bladder (urinary) (transitional cell) (M8120/1)
    236.7
    benign (M8120/0) 223.3
  choroid plexus (M9390/0) 225.0
    anaplastic type (M9390/3) 191.5
    malignant (M9390/3) 191.5
  ductal (M8503/0)
  dyskeratotic (M8052/0)
  epidermoid (M8052/0)
  hyperkeratotic (M8052/0)
  intracystic (M8504/0)
  intraductal (M8503/0)
  inverted (M8053/0)
  keratotic (M8052/0)
  parakeratotic (M8052/0)
  pinta (primary) 103.0
  renal pelvis (transitional cell) (M8120/1) 236.99
    benign (M8120/0) 223.1
  Schneiderian (M8121/0)
    specified site—*see* Neoplasm, by site, benign
    unspecified site 212.0
  serous surface (M8461/0)
    borderline malignancy (M8461/1)
      specified site—*see* Neoplasm, by site,
        uncertain behavior
      unspecified site 236.2
    specified site—*see* Neoplasm, by site, benign
    unspecified site 220
  squamous (cell) (M8052/0)
  transitional (cell) (M8120/0)
    bladder (urinary) (M8120/1) 236.7
    inverted type (M8121/1)—*see* Neoplasm, by
      site, uncertain behavior
    renal pelvis (M8120/1) 236.91
    ureter (M8120/1) 236.91
  ureter (transitional cell) (M8120/1) 236.91
    benign (M8120/0) 223.2
  urothelial (M8120/1)—*see* Neoplasm, by site,
    uncertain behavior
  verrucous (M8051/0)
  villous (M8261/1)—*see* Neoplasm, by site,
    uncertain behavior
  yaws, plantar or palmar 102.1
Papillomata, multiple, of yaws 102.1
Papillomatosis (M8060/0)—*see also* Neoplasm,
  by site, benign
  confluent and reticulate 701.8
  cutaneous 701.8
  ductal, breast 610.1
  Gougerot-Carteaud (confluent reticulate) 701.8
  intraductal (diffuse) (M8505/0)—*see* Neoplasm,
    by site, benign
  subareolar duct (M8506/0) 217
Papillon-Léage and Psaume syndrome
  (orodigitofacial dysostosis) 759.89

Papule 709.8
  carate (primary) 103.0
  fibrous, of nose (M8724/0) 216.3
  pinta (primary) 103.0
Papulosis
  lymphomatoid 709.8
  malignant 447.8
Papyraceous fetus 779.89
  complicating pregnancy 646.0
Paracephalus 759.7
Parachute mitral valve 746.5
Paracoccidioidomycosis 116.1
  mucocutaneous-lymphangitic 116.1
  pulmonary 116.1
  visceral 116.1
Paracoccidiomycosis —*see*
  Paracoccidioidomycosis
Paracusis 388.40
Paradentosis 523.5
Paradoxical facial movements 374.43
Paraffinoma 999.9
Paraganglioma (M8680/1)
  adrenal (M8700/0) 227.0
    malignant (M8700/3) 194.0
  aortic body (M8691/1) 237.3
    malignant (M8691/3) 194.6
  carotid body (M8692/1) 237.3
    malignant (M8692/3) 194.5
  chromaffin (M8700/0)—*see also* Neoplasm, by
    site, benign
    malignant (M8700/3)—*see* Neoplasm, by site,
      malignant
  extra-adrenal (M8693/1)
    malignant (M8693/3)
      specified site—*see* Neoplasm, by site,
        malignant
      unspecified site 194.6
    specified site—*see* Neoplasm, by site,
      uncertain behavior
    unspecified site 237.3
  glomus jugulare (M8690/1) 237.3
    malignant (M8690/3) 194.6
  jugular (M8690/1) 237.3
    malignant (M8680/3)
      specified site—*see* Neoplasm, by site,
        malignant
    unspecified site 194.6
  nonchromaffin (M8693/1)
    malignant (M8693/3)
      specified site—*see* Neoplasm, by site,
        malignant
      unspecified site 194.6
    specified site—*see* Neoplasm, by site,
      uncertain behavior
    unspecified site 237.3
  parasympathetic (M8682/1)
    specified site—*see* Neoplasm, by site,
      uncertain behavior
    unspecified site 237.3
  specified site—*see* Neoplasm, by site, uncertain
    behavior
  sympathetic (M8681/1)
    specified site—*see* Neoplasm, by site,
      uncertain behavior
    unspecified site 237.3
  unspecified site 237.3
Parageusia 781.1
  psychogenic 306.7
Paragonimiasis 121.2
Paragranuloma, Hodgkin's (M9660/3) 201.0

Parahemophilia (*see also* Defect, coagulation) 286.3
Parakeratosis 690.8
  psoriasiformis 696.2
  variegata 696.2
Paralysis, paralytic (complete) (incomplete) 344.9
  with
    broken
      back—*see* Fracture, vertebra, by site, with spinal cord injury
      neck—*see* Fracture, vertebra, cervical, with spinal cord injury
    fracture, vertebra—*see* Fracture, vertebra, by site, with spinal cord injury
    syphilis 094.89
  abdomen and back muscles 355.9
  abdominal muscles 355.9
  abducens (nerve) 378.54
  abductor 355.9
    lower extremity 355.8
    upper extremity 354.9
  accessory nerve 352.4
  accommodation 367.51
    hysterical 300.11
  acoustic nerve 388.5
  agitans 332.0
    arteriosclerotic 332.0
  alternating 344.89
    oculomotor 344.89
  amyotrophic 335.20
  ankle 355.8
  anterior serratus 355.9
  anus (sphincter) 569.49
  apoplectic (current episode) (*see also* Disease, cerebrovascular, acute) 436
    late effect—*see* Late effect(s) (of) cerebrovascular disease
    category 438
  arm 344.40
    affecting
      dominant side 344.41
      nondominant side 344.42
    both 344.2
    due to old CVA—*see* Category 438
    hysterical 300.11
    late effect—*see* Late effect(s) (of) cerebrovascular disease
    psychogenic 306.0
    transient 781.4
      traumatic NDC (*see also* Injury, nerve, upper limb) 955.9
  arteriosclerotic (current episode) 437.0
    late effect—*see* Late effect(s) (of) cerebrovascular disease
  ascending (spinal), acute 357.0
  associated, nuclear 344.89
  asthenic bulbar 358.00
  ataxic NEC 334.9
    general 094.1
  athetoid 333.71
  atrophic 356.9
    infantile, acute (*see also* Poliomyelitis, with paralysis) 045.1
    muscle NEC 355.9
    progressive 335.21
    spinal (acute) (*see also* Poliomyelitis, with paralysis) 045.1
  attack (*see also* Disease, cerebrovascular, acute) 436
  axillary 353.0
  Babinski-Nageotte's 344.89

Paralysis, paralytic—*continued*
  Bell's 351.0
    newborn 767.5
  Benedikt's 344.89
  birth (injury) 767.7
    brain 767.0
    intracranial 767.0
    spinal cord 767.4
  bladder (sphincter) 596.53
    neurogenic 596.54
      with cauda equina syndrome 344.61
    puerperal, postpartum, childbirth 665.5
    sensory 596.54
      with cauda equina 344.61
    spastic 596.54
      with cauda equina 344.61
  bowel, colon, or intestine (*see also* Ileus) 560.1
  brachial plexus 353.0
    due to birth injury 767.6
    newborn 767.6
  brain
    congenital—*see* Palsy, cerebral
    current episode 437.8
    diplegia 344.2
    due to previous vascular lesion—*see* category 438
    hemiplegia 342.9
      due to previous vascular lesion—*see* category 438
      late effect—*see* Late effect(s) (of) cerebrovascular disease
    infantile—*see* Palsy, cerebral
    late effect—*see* Late effect(s) (of) cerebrovascular disease
    monoplegia—*see also* Monoplegia
      due to previous vascular lesion—*see* category 438
      late effect—*see* Late effect(s) (of) cerebrovascular disease
    paraplegia 344.1
    quadriplegia —*see* Quadriplegia
    syphilitic, congenital 090.49
    triplegia 344.89
  bronchi 519.19
  Brown-Séquard's 344.89
  bulbar (chronic) (progressive) 335.22
    infantile (*see also* Poliomyelitis, bulbar) 045.0
    poliomyelitic (*see also* Poliomyelitis, bulbar) 045.0
    pseudo 335.23
    supranuclear 344.89
  bulbospinal 358.00
  cardiac (*see also* Failure, heart) 428.9
  cerebral
    current episode 437.8
    spastic, infantile—*see* Palsy, cerebral
  cerebrocerebellar 437.8
    diplegic infantile 343.0
  cervical
    plexus 353.2
    sympathetic NEC 337.09
  Céstan-Chenais 344.89
  Charcot-Marie-Tooth type 356.1
  childhood—*see* Palsy, cerebral
  Clark's 343.9
  colon (*see also* Ileus) 560.1
  compressed air 993.3
  compression
    arm NEC 354.9
    cerebral—*see* Paralysis, brain
    leg NEC 355.8
    lower extremity NEC 355.8
    upper extremity NEC 354.9

Paralysis, paralytic—*continued*
  congenital (cerebral) (spastic) (spinal)—*see*
    Palsy, cerebral
  conjugate movement (of eye) 378.81
    cortical (nuclear) (supranuclear) 378.81
  convergence 378.83
  cordis (*see also* Failure, heart) 428.9
  cortical (*see also* Paralysis, brain) 437.8
  cranial or cerebral nerve (*see also* Disorder,
    nerve, cranial) 352.9
  creeping 335.21
  crossed leg 344.89
  crutch 953.4
  deglutition 784.99
    hysterical 300.11
  dementia 094.1
  descending (spinal) NEC 335.9
  diaphragm (flaccid) 519.4
    due to accidental section of phrenic nerve
      during procedure 998.2
  digestive organs NEC 564.89
  diplegic—*see* Diplegia
  divergence (nuclear) 378.85
  divers' 993.3
  Duchenne's 335.22
  due to intracranial or spinal birth injury—*see*
    Palsy, cerebral
  embolic (current episode) (*see also* Embolism,
    brain) 434.1
    late effect —*see* Late effect(s) (of)
      cerebrovascular disease
  enteric (*see also* Ileus) 560.1
    with hernia—*see* Hernia, by site, with
      obstruction
  Erb's syphilitic spastic spinal 094.89
  Erb (-Duchenne) (birth) (newborn) 767.6
  esophagus 530.89
  essential, infancy (*see also* Poliomyelitis) 045.9
  extremity
    lower —*see* Paralysis, leg
    spastic (hereditary) 343.3
      noncongenital or noninfantile 344.1
    transient (cause unknown) 781.4
    upper —*see* Paralysis, arm
  eye muscle (extrinsic) 378.55
    intrinsic 367.51
  facial (nerve) 351.0
    birth injury 767.5
    congenital 767.5
    following operation NEC 998.2
    newborn 767.5
  familial 359.3
    periodic 359.3
    spastic 334.1
  fauces 478.29
  finger NEC 354.9
  foot NEC 355.8
  gait 781.2
  gastric nerve 352.3
  gaze 378.81
  general 094.1
    ataxic 094.1
    insane 094.1
    juvenile 090.40
    progressive 094.1
    tabetic 094.1
  glossopharyngeal (nerve) 352.2
  glottis (*see also* Paralysis, vocal cord) 478.30
  gluteal 353.4
  Gubler (-Millard) 344.89

Paralysis, paralytic—*continued*
  hand 354.9
    hysterical 300.11
    psychogenic 306.0
  heart (*see also* Failure, heart) 428.9
  hemifacial, progressive 349.89
  hemiplegic—*see* Hemiplegia
  hyperkalemic periodic (familial) 359.3
  hypertensive (current episode) 437.8
  hypoglossal (nerve) 352.5
  hypokalemic periodic 359.3
  Hyrtl's sphincter (rectum) 569.49
  hysterical 300.11
  ileus (*see also* Ileus) 560.1
  infantile (*see also* Poliomyelitis) 045.9
    atrophic acute 045.1
    bulbar 045.0
    cerebral—*see* Palsy, cerebral
    paralytic 045.1
    progressive acute 045.9
    spastic—*see* Palsy, cerebral
    spinal 045.9
  infective (*see also* Poliomyelitis) 045.9
  inferior nuclear 344.9
  insane, general or progressive 094.1
  internuclear 378.86
  interosseous 355.9
  intestine (*see also* Ileus) 560.1
  intracranial (current episode) (*see also* Paralysis,
    brain) 437.8
    due to birth injury 767.0
  iris 379.49
    due to diphtheria (toxin) 032.81 *[379.49]*
  ischemic, Volkmann's (complicating trauma)
    958.6
  isolated sleep, recurrent 327.43
  Jackson's 344.89
  jake 357.7
  Jamaica ginger (jake) 357.7
  juvenile general 090.40
  Klumpke (-Déjérine) (birth) (newborn) 767.6
  labioglossal (laryngeal) (pharyngeal) 335.22
  Landry's 357.0
  laryngeal nerve (recurrent) (superior) (*see also*
    Paralysis, vocal cord) 478.30
  larynx (*see also* Paralysis, vocal cord) 478.30
    due to diphtheria (toxin) 032.3
  late effect
    due to
      birth injury, brain or spinal (cord)—*see*
        Palsy, cerebral
      edema, brain or cerebral—*see* Paralysis,
        brain
      lesion
        cerebrovascular—*see* category 438
        late effect—*see* Late effect(s) (of)
          cerebrovascular disease
        spinal (cord)—*see* Paralysis, spinal
  lateral 335.24
  lead 984.9
    specified type of lead—*see* Table of drugs and
      chemicals
  left side—*see* Hemiplegia
  leg 344.30
    affecting
      dominant side 344.31
      nondominant side 344.32
    both (*see also* Paraplegia) 344.1
    crossed 344.89
    hysterical 300.11
    psychogenic 306.0
    transient or transitory 781.4

Paralysis, paralytic—*continued*
  leg —*continued*
    traumatic NEC (*see also* Injury, nerve, lower
      limb) 956.9
  levator palpebrae superioris 374.31
  limb NEC 344.5
    all four—*see* Quadriplegia
    quadriplegia—*see* Quadriplegia
  lip 528.5
  Lissauer's 094.1
  local 355.9
  lower limb—*see also* Paralysis, leg
    both (*see also* Paraplegia) 344.1
  lung 518.89
    newborn 770.89
  median nerve 354.1
  medullary (tegmental) 344.89
  mesencephalic NEC 344.89
    tegmental 344.89
  middle alternating 344.89
  Millard-Gubler-Foville 344.89
  monoplegic—*see* Monoplegia
  motor NEC 344.9
    cerebral—*see* Paralysis, brain
    spinal—*see* Paralysis, spinal
  multiple
    cerebral—*see* Paralysis, brain
    spinal—*see* Paralysis, spinal
  muscle (flaccid) 359.9
    due to nerve lesion NEC 355.9
    eye (extrinsic) 378.55
      intrinsic 367.51
      oblique 378.51
    iris sphincter 364.89
    ischemic (complicating trauma) (Volkmann's)
      958.6
    pseudohypertrophic 359.1
  muscular (atrophic) 359.9
    progressive 335.21
  musculocutaneous nerve 354.9
  musculospiral 354.9
  nerve—*see also* Disorder, nerve
    third or oculomotor (partial) 378.51
      total 378.52
    fourth or trochlear 378.53
    sixth or abducens 378.54
    seventh or facial 351.0
      birth injury 767.5
      due to
        injection NEC 999.9
        operation NEC 997.09
      newborn 767.5
    accessory 352.4
    auditory 388.5
    birth injury 767.7
    cranial or cerebral (*see also* Disorder, nerve,
      cranial) 352.9
    facial 351.0
      birth injury 767.5
      newborn 767.5
    laryngeal (*see also* Paralysis, vocal cord) 478.30
      newborn 767.7
    phrenic 354.8
      newborn 767.7
    radial 354.3
      birth injury 767.6
      newborn 767.6
    syphilitic 094.89
    traumatic NEC (*see also* Injury, nerve, by site)
      957.9
    trigeminal 350.9
    ulnar 354.2

Paralysis, paralytic—*continued*
  newborn NEC 767.0
  normokalemic periodic 359.3
  obstetrical, newborn 767.7
  ocular 378.9
  oculofacial, congenital 352.6
  oculomotor (nerve) (partial) 378.51
    alternating 344.89
    external bilateral 378.55
    total 378.52
  olfactory nerve 352.0
  palate 528.9
  palatopharyngolaryngeal 352.6
  paratrigeminal 350.9
  periodic (familial) (hyperkalemic) (hypokalemic)
    (normokalemic) (potassium sensitive)
    (secondary) 359.3
  peripheral
    autonomic nervous system—*see* Neuropathy,
      peripheral, autonomic
    nerve NEC 355.9
  peroneal (nerve) 355.3
  pharynx 478.29
  phrenic nerve 354.8
  plantar nerves 355.6
  pneumogastric nerve 352.3
  poliomyelitis (current) (*see also* Poliomyelitis,
    with paralysis) 045.1
    bulbar 045.0
  popliteal nerve 355.3
  pressure (*see also* Neuropathy, entrapment)
    355.9
  progressive 335.21
    atrophic 335.21
    bulbar 335.22
    general 094.1
    hemifacial 349.89
    infantile, acute (*see also* Poliomyelitis) 045.9
    multiple 335.20
  pseudobulbar 335.23
  pseudohypertrophic 359.1
    muscle 359.1
  psychogenic 306.0
  pupil, pupillary 379.49
  quadriceps 355.8
  quadriplegic (*see also* Quadriplegia) 344.0
  radial nerve 354.3
    birth injury 767.6
  rectum (sphincter) 569.49
  rectus muscle (eye) 378.55
  recurrent
    isolated sleep 327.43
    laryngeal nerve (*see also* Paralysis, vocal
      cord) 478.30
  respiratory (muscle) (system) (tract) 786.09
    center NEC 344.89
      fetus or newborn 770.87
    congenital 768.9
    newborn 768.9
  right side—*see* Hemiplegia
  Saturday night 354.3
  saturnine 984.9
    specified type of lead—*see* Table of drugs and
      chemicals
  sciatic nerve 355.0
  secondary—*see* Paralysis, late effect
  seizure (cerebral) (current episode) (*see also*
    Disease, cerebrovascular, acute) 436
    late effect—*see* Late effect(s) (of)
      cerebrovascular disease
  senile NEC 344.9

Paralysis, paralytic—*continued*
 serratus magnus 355.9
 shaking (*see also* Parkinsonism) 332.0
 shock (*see also* Disease, cerebrovascular, acute)
   436
  late effect—*see* Late effect(s) (of)
    cerebrovascular disease
 shoulder 354.9
 soft palate 528.9
 spasmodic—*see* Paralysis, spastic
 spastic 344.9
  cerebral infantile—*see* Palsy, cerebral
  congenital (cerebral)—*see* Palsy, cerebral
  familial 334.1
  hereditary 334.1
  infantile 343.9
  noncongenital or noninfantile, cerebral 344.9
  syphilitic 094.0
   spinal 094.89
 sphincter, bladder (*see also* Paralysis, bladder)
   596.53
 spinal (cord) NEC 344.1
  accessory nerve 352.4
  acute (*see also* Poliomyelitis) 045.9
  ascending acute 357.0
  atrophic (acute) (*see also* Poliomyelitis, with
    paralysis) 045.1
   spastic, syphilitic 094.89
  congenital NEC 343.9
  hemiplegic —*see* Hemiplegia
  hereditary 336.8
  infantile (*see also* Poliomyelitis) 045.9
  late effect NEC 344.89
  monoplegic—*see* Monoplegia
  nerve 355.9
  progressive 335.10
  quadriplegic —*see* Quadriplegia
  spastic NEC 343.9
  traumatic—*see* Injury, spinal, by site
 sternomastoid 352.4
 stomach 536.3
  diabetic 250.6 *[536.3]*
   due to secondary diabetes 249.6 *[536.3]*
  nerve (nondiabetic) 352.3
 stroke (current episode) *see* Infarct, brain
  late effect—*see* Late effect(s) (of)
    cerebrovascular disease
 subscapularis 354.8
 superior nuclear NEC 334.9
 supranuclear 356.8
 sympathetic
  cervical NEC 337.09
  nerve NEC (*see also* Neuropathy, peripheral,
    autonomic) 337.9
  nervous system—*see* Neuropathy, peripheral,
    autonomic
 syndrome 344.9
  specified NEC 344.89
 syphilitic spastic spinal (Erb's) 094.89
 tabetic general 094.1
 thigh 355.8
 throat 478.29
  diphtheritic 032.0
  muscle 478.29
 thrombotic (current episode) (*see also*
    Thrombosis, brain) 434.0
  late effect—*see* Late effect(s) (of)
    cerebrovascular disease
 thumb NEC 354.9
 tick (-bite) 989.5

Paralysis, paralytic—*continued*
 Todd's (postepileptic transitory paralysis)
   344.89
 toe 355.6
 tongue 529.8
 transient
  arm or leg NEC 781.4
  traumatic NEC (*see also* Injury, nerve, by site)
    957.9
 trapezius 352.4
 traumatic, transient NEC (*see also* Injury, nerve,
    by site) 957.9
 trembling (*see also* Parkinsonism) 332.0
 triceps brachii 354.9
 trigeminal nerve 350.9
 trochlear nerve 378.53
 ulnar nerve 354.2
 upper limb —*see also* Paralysis, arm
  both (*see also* Diplegia) 344.2
 uremic—*see* Uremia
 uveoparotitic 135
 uvula 528.9
  hysterical 300.11
  postdiphtheritic 032.0
 vagus nerve 352.3
 vasomotor NEC 337.9
 velum palati 528.9
 vesical (*see also* Paralysis, bladder) 596.53
 vestibular nerve 388.5
 visual field, psychic 368.16
 vocal cord 478.30
  bilateral (partial) 478.33
   complete 478.34
  complete (bilateral) 478.34
  unilateral (partial) 478.31
   complete 478.32
 Volkmann's (complicating trauma) 958.6
 wasting 335.21
 Weber's 344.89
 wrist NEC 354.9
Paramedial orifice, urethrovesical 753.8
Paramenia 626.9
Parametritis (chronic) (*see also* Disease, pelvis,
   inflammatory) 614.4
 acute 614.3
 puerperal, postpartum, childbirth 670.8
Parametrium, parametric —*see* condition
Paramnesia (*see also* Amnesia) 780.93
Paramolar 520.1
 causing crowding 524.31
Paramyloidosis 277.30
Paramyoclonus multiplex 333.2
Paramyotonia 359.29
 congenita (of von Eulenburg) 359.29
Paraneoplastic syndrome —*see* condition
Parangi (*see also* Yaws) 102.9
Paranoia 297.1
 alcoholic 291.5
 querulans 297.8
 senile 290.20
Paranoid
 dementia (*see also* Schizophrenia) 295.3
  praecox (acute) 295.3
  senile 290.20
 personality 301.0
 psychosis 297.9
  alcoholic 291.5
  climacteric 297.2
  drug-induced 292.11
  involutional 297.2

Paranoid—*continued*
  psychosis—*continued*
    menopausal 297.2
    protracted reactive 298.4
    psychogenic 298.4
      acute 298.3
      senile 290.20
    reaction (chronic) 297.9
      acute 298.3
    schizophrenia (acute) (*see also* Schizophrenia)
      295.3
    state 297.9
      alcohol-induced 291.5
      climacteric 297.2
      drug-induced 292.11
      due to or associated with
        arteriosclerosis (cerebrovascular) 290.42
        presenile brain disease 290.12
        senile brain disease 290.20
      involutional 297.2
      menopausal 297.2
      senile 290.20
      simple 297.0
      specified type NEC 297.8
    tendencies 301.0
    traits 301.0
    trends 301.0
    type, psychopathic personality 301.0
Paraparesis (*see also* Paraplegia) 344.1
Paraphasia 784.3
Paraphilia (*see also* Deviation, sexual) 302.9
Paraphimosis (congenital) 605
  chancroidal 099.0
Paraphrenia, paraphrenic (late) 297.2
  climacteric 297.2
  dementia (*see also* Schizophrenia) 295.3
  involutional 297.2
  menopausal 297.2
  schizophrenia (acute) (*see also* Schizophrenia)
    295.3
Paraplegia 344.1
  with
    broken back—*see* Fracture, vertebra, by site,
      with spinal cord injury
    fracture, vertebra—*see* Fracture, vertebra, by
      site, with spinal cord injury
    ataxic—*see* Degeneration, combined, spinal
      cord
    brain (current episode) (*see also* Paralysis,
      brain) 437.8
    cerebral (current episode) (*see also* Paralysis,
      brain) 437.8
    congenital or infantile (cerebral) (spastic)
      (spinal) 343.0
    cortical—*see* Paralysis, brain
    familial spastic 334.1
    functional (hysterical) 300.11
    hysterical 300.11
    infantile 343.0
    late effect 344.1
    Pott's (*see also* Tuberculosis) 015.0 *[730.88]*
    psychogenic 306.0
    spastic
      Erb's spinal 094.89
      hereditary 334.1
      not infantile or congenital 344.1
    spinal (cord)
      traumatic NEC—*see* Injury, spinal, by site
    syphilitic (spastic) 094.89
    traumatic NEC—*see* Injury, spinal, by site

Paraproteinemia 273.2
  benign (familial) 273.1
  monoclonal 273.1
  secondary to malignant or inflammatory disease
    273.1
Parapsoriasis 696.2
  en plaques 696.2
  guttata 696.2
  lichenoides chronica 696.2
  retiformis 696.2
  varioliformis (acuta) 696.2
Parascarlatina 057.8
Parasitic —*see also* condition
  disease NEC (*see also* Infestation, parasitic)
    136.9
    contact V01.89
    exposure to V01.89
    intestinal NEC 129
    skin NEC 134.9
  stomatitis 112.0
  sycosis 110.0
    beard 110.0
    scalp 110.0
  twin 759.4
Parasitism NEC 136.9
  intestinal NEC 129
  skin NEC 134.9
  specified—*see* Infestation
Parasitophobia 300.29
Parasomnia 307.47
  alcohol induced 291.82
  drug induced 292.85
  nonorganic origin 307.47
  organic 327.40
    in conditions classified elsewhere 327.44
    other 327.49
Paraspadias 752.69
Paraspasm facialis 351.8
Parathyroid gland —*see* condition
Parathyroiditis (autoimmune) 252.1
Parathyroprival tetany 252.1
Paratrachoma 077.0
Paratyphilitis (*see also* Appendicitis) 541
Paratyphoid (fever)—*see* Fever, paratyphoid
Paratyphus —*see* Fever, paratyphoid
Paraurethral duct 753.8
Para-urethritis 597.89
  gonococcal (acute) 098.0
  chronic or duration of 2 months or over 098.2
Paravaccinia NEC 051.9
  milkers' node 051.1
Paravaginitis (*see also* Vaginitis) 616.10
Parencephalitis (*see also* Encephalitis) 323.9
  late effect—*see* category 326
Parergasia 298.9
Paresis (*see also* Paralysis) 344.9
  accommodation 367.51
  bladder (spastic) (sphincter) (*see also* Paralysis,
    bladder) 596.53
    tabetic 094.0
  bowel, colon, or intestine (*see also* Ileus) 560.1
  brain or cerebral—*see* Paralysis, brain
  extrinsic muscle, eye 378.55
  general 094.1
    arrested 094.1
    brain 094.1
    cerebral 094.1
    insane 094.1
    juvenile 090.40
      remission 090.49

Paresis—*continued*
  general—*continued*
    progressive 094.1
    remission (sustained) 094.1
    tabetic 094.1
  heart (*see also* Failure, heart) 428.9
  infantile (*see also* Poliomyelitis) 045.9
  insane 094.1
  juvenile 090.40
  late effect—*see* Paralysis, late effect
  luetic (general) 094.1
  peripheral progressive 356.9
  pseudohypertrophic 359.1
  senile NEC 344.9
  stomach 536.3
    diabetic 250.6 *[536.3]*
      due to secondary diabetes 249.6 *[536.3]*
  syphilitic (general) 094.1
    congenital 090.40
  transient, limb 781.4
  vesical (sphincter) NEC 596.53
Paresthesia (*see also* Disturbance, sensation) 782.0
  Berger's (paresthesia of lower limb) 782.0
  Bernhardt 355.1
  Magnan's 782.0
Paretic —*see* condition
Parinaud's
  conjunctivitis 372.02
  oculoglandular syndrome 372.02
  ophthalmoplegia 378.81
  syndrome (paralysis of conjugate upward gaze) 378.81
Parkes Weber and Dimitri syndrome (encephalocutaneous angiomatosis) 759.6
Parkinson's disease, syndrome, or tremor —*see* Parkinsonism
Parkinsonism (arteriosclerotic) (idiopathic) (primary) 332.0
  associated with orthostatic hypotension (idiopathic) (symptomatic) 333.0
  due to drugs 332.1
  neuroleptic-induced 332.1
  secondary 332.1
  syphilitic 094.82
Parodontitis 523.40
Parodontosis 523.5
Paronychia (with lymphangitis) 681.9
  candidal (chronic) 112.3
  chronic 681.9
    candidal 112.3
    finger 681.02
    toe 681.11
  finger 681.02
  toe 681.11
  tuberculous (primary) (*see also* Tuberculosis) 017.0
Parorexia NEC 307.52
  hysterical 300.11
Parosmia 781.1
  psychogenic 306.7
Parotid gland —*see* condition
Parotiditis (*see also* Parotitis) 527.2
  epidemic 072.9
  infectious 072.9
Parotitis 527.2
  allergic 527.2
  chronic 527.2
  epidemic (*see also* Mumps) 072.9
  infectious (*see also* Mumps) 072.9
  noninfectious 527.2

Parotitis—*continued*
  nonspecific toxic 527.2
  not mumps 527.2
  postoperative 527.2
  purulent 527.2
  septic 527.2
  suppurative (acute) 527.2
  surgical 527.2
  toxic 527.2
Paroxysmal —*see also* condition
  dyspnea (nocturnal) 786.09
Parrot's disease (syphilitic osteochondritis) 090.0
Parrot fever 073.9
Parry's disease or syndrome (exophthalmic goiter) 242.0
Parry-Romberg syndrome 349.89
Parson's disease (exophthalmic goiter) 242.0
Parsonage-Aldren-Turner syndrome 353.5
Parsonage-Turner syndrome 353.5
Pars planitis 363.21
Particolored infant 757.39
Parturition —*see* Delivery
Parvovirus 079.83
  B19 079.83
  human 079.83
Passage
  false, urethra 599.4
  meconium noted during delivery 763.84
  of sounds or bougies (*see also* Attention to artificial opening) V55.9
Passive —*see* condition
Pasteurella septica 027.2
Pasteurellosis (*see also* Infection, Pasteurella) 027.2
PAT (paroxysmal atrial tachycardia) 427.0
Patau's syndrome (trisomy D₁) 758.1
Patch
  herald 696.3
Patches
  mucous (syphilitic) 091.3
    congenital 090.0
  smokers' (mouth) 528.6
Patellar —*see* condition
Patellofemoral syndrome 719.46
Patent —*see also* Imperfect closure
  atrioventricular ostium 745.69
  canal of Nuck 752.41
  cervix 622.5
    complicating pregnancy 654.5
      affecting fetus or newborn 761.0
  ductus arteriosus or Botalli 747.0
  Eustachian
    tube 381.7
    valve 746.89
  foramen
    Botalli 745.5
    ovale 745.5
  interauricular septum 745.5
  interventricular septum 745.4
  omphalomesenteric duct 751.0
  os (uteri)—*see* Patent, cervix
  ostium secundum 745.5
  urachus 753.7
  vitelline duct 751.0
Paternity testing V70.4
Paterson's syndrome (sideropenic dysphagia) 280.8
Paterson (-Brown) (-Kelly) syndrome (sideropenic dysphagia) 280.8

Paterson-Kelly syndrome or web (sideropenic dysphagia) 280.8
Pathologic, pathological —*see also* condition
asphyxia 799.01
drunkenness 291.4
emotionality 301.3
liar 301.7
personality 301.9
resorption, tooth 521.40
external 521.42
internal 521.41
specified NEC 521.49
sexuality (*see also* Deviation, sexual) 302.9
Pathology (of)—*see also* Disease
periradicular, associated with previous endodontic treatment 526.69
Patterned motor discharges, idiopathic (*see also* Epilepsy) 345.5
Patulous —*see also* Patent
anus 569.49
Eustachian tube 381.7
Pause, sinoatrial 427.81
Pavor nocturnus 307.46
Pavy's disease 593.6
Paxton's disease (white piedra) 111.2
Payr's disease or syndrome (splenic flexure syndrome) 569.89
PBA (pseudobulbar affect) 310.81
Pearls
Elschnig 366.51
enamel 520.2
Pearl-workers' disease (chronic osteomyelitis) (*see also* Osteomyelitis) 730.1
Pectenitis 569.49
Pectenosis 569.49
Pectoral —*see* condition
Pectus
carinatum (congenital) 754.82
acquired 738.3
rachitic (*see also* Rickets) 268.0
excavatum (congenital) 754.81
acquired 738.3
rachitic (*see also* Rickets) 268.0
recurvatum (congenital) 754.81
acquired 738.3
Pedatrophia 261
Pederosis 302.2
Pediculosis (infestation) 132.9
capitis (head louse) (any site) 132.0
corporis (body louse) (any site) 132.1
eyelid 132.0 *[373.6]*
mixed (classifiable to more than one category in 132.0-132.2) 132.3
pubis (pubic louse) (any site) 132.2
vestimenti 132.1
vulvae 132.2
Pediculus (infestation)—*see* Pediculosis
Pedophilia 302.2
Peg-shaped teeth 520.2
Pel's crisis 094.0
Pel-Ebstein disease —*see* Disease, Hodgkin's
Pelade 704.01
Pelger-Huët anomaly or syndrome (hereditary hyposegmentation) 288.2
Peliosis (rheumatica) 287.0
Pelizaeus-Merzbacher
disease 330.0
sclerosis, diffuse cerebral 330.0
Pellagra (alcoholic or with alcoholism) 265.2
with polyneuropathy 265.2 *[357.4]*

Pellagra-cerebellar-ataxia-renal aminoaciduria syndrome 270.0
Pellegrini's disease (calcification, knee joint) 726.62
Pellegrini (-Stieda) disease or syndrome (calcification, knee joint) 726.62
Pellizzi's syndrome (pineal) 259.8
Pelvic —*see also* condition
congestion-fibrosis syndrome 625.5
kidney 753.3
Pelvioectasis 591
Pelviolithiasis 592.0
Pelviperitonitis
female (*see also* Peritonitis, pelvic, female) 614.5
male (*see also* Peritonitis) 567.21
Pelvis, pelvic —*see also* condition or type
infantile 738.6
Nägele's 738.6
obliquity 738.6
Robert's 755.69
Pemphigoid 694.5
benign, mucous membrane 694.60
with ocular involvement 694.61
bullous 694.5
cicatricial 694.60
with ocular involvement 694.61
juvenile 694.2
Pemphigus 694.4
benign 694.5
chronic familial 757.39
Brazilian 694.4
circinatus 694.0
congenital, traumatic 757.39
conjunctiva 694.61
contagiosus 684
erythematodes 694.4
erythematosus 694.4
foliaceus 694.4
frambesiodes 694.4
gangrenous (*see also* Gangrene) 785.4
malignant 694.4
neonatorum, newborn 684
ocular 694.61
papillaris 694.4
seborrheic 694.4
South American 694.4
syphilitic (congenital) 090.0
vegetans 694.4
vulgaris 694.4
wildfire 694.4
Pendred's syndrome (familial goiter with deaf-mutism) 243
Pendulous
abdomen 701.9
in pregnancy or childbirth 654.4
affecting fetus or newborn 763.89
breast 611.89
Penetrating wound —*see also* Wound, open, by site
with internal injury—*see* Injury, internal, by site, with open wound
eyeball 871.7
with foreign body (nonmagnetic) 871.6
magnetic 871.5
ocular (*see also* Penetrating wound, eyeball) 871.7
adnexa 870.3
with foreign body 870.4
orbit 870.3
with foreign body 870.4

Penetration, pregnant uterus by instrument
  with
    abortion—*see* Abortion, by type, with damage
      to pelvic organs
    ectopic pregnancy (*see also* categories
      633.0-633.9) 639.2
    molar pregnancy (*see also* categories 630-632)
      639.2
  complication of delivery 665.1
    affecting fetus or newborn 763.89
  following
    abortion 639.2
    ectopic or molar pregnancy 639.2
Penfield's syndrome (*see also* Epilepsy) 345.5
Penicilliosis of lung 117.3
Penis —*see* condition
Penitis 607.2
Penta X syndrome 758.81
Pentalogy (of Fallot) 745.2
Pentosuria (benign) (essential) 271.8
Peptic acid disease 536.8
Peregrinating patient V65.2
Perforated —*see* Perforation
Perforation, perforative (nontraumatic)
  antrum (*see also* Sinusitis, maxillary) 473.0
  appendix 540.0
    with peritoneal abscess 540.1
  atrial septum, multiple 745.5
  attic, ear 384.22
    healed 384.81
  bile duct, except cystic (*see also* Disease,
    biliary) 576.3
    cystic 575.4
  bladder (urinary) 596.6
    with
      abortion—*see* Abortion, by type, with
        damage to pelvic organs
      ectopic pregnancy (*see also* categories
        633.0-633.9) 639.2
      molar pregnancy (*see also* categories
        630-632) 639.2
    following
      abortion 639.2
      ectopic or molar pregnancy 639.2
    obstetrical trauma 665.5
  bowel 569.83
    with
      abortion—*see* Abortion, by type, with
        damage to pelvic organs
      ectopic pregnancy (*see also* categories
        633.0-633.9) 639.2
      molar pregnancy (*see also* categories
        630-632) 639.2
    fetus or newborn 777.6
    following
      abortion 639.2
      ectopic or molar pregnancy 639.2
    obstetrical trauma 665.5
  broad ligament
    with
      abortion—*see* Abortion, by type, with
        damage to pelvic organs
      ectopic pregnancy (*see also* categories
        633.0-633.9) 639.2
      molar pregnancy (*see also* categories
        630-632) 639.2
    following
      abortion 639.2
      ectopic or molar pregnancy 639.2
    obstetrical trauma 665.6

Perforation, perforative—*continued*
  by
    device, implant, or graft—*see* Complications,
      mechanical
    foreign body left accidentally in operation
      wound 998.4
    instrument (any) during a procedure,
      accidental 998.2
  cecum 540.0
    with peritoneal abscess 540.1
  cervix (uteri)—*see also* Injury, internal, cervix
    with
      abortion—*see* Abortion, by type, with
        damage to pelvic organs
      ectopic pregnancy (*see also* categories
        633.0-633.9) 639.2
      molar pregnancy (*see also* categories
        630-632) 639.2
    following
      abortion 639.2
      ectopic or molar pregnancy 639.2
    obstetrical trauma 665.3
  colon 569.83
  common duct (bile) 576.3
  cornea (*see also* Ulcer, cornea) 370.00
    due to ulceration 370.06
  cystic duct 575.4
  diverticulum (*see also* Diverticula) 562.10
    small intestine 562.00
  duodenum, duodenal (ulcer)—*see* Ulcer,
    duodenum, with perforation
  ear drum—*see* Perforation, tympanum
  enteritis—*see* Enteritis
  esophagus 530.4
  ethmoidal sinus (*see also* Sinusitis, ethmoidal)
    473.2
  foreign body (external site)—*see also* Wound,
    open, by site, complicated
    internal site, by ingested object—*see* Foreign
      body
  frontal sinus (*see also* Sinusitis, frontal) 473.1
  gallbladder or duct (*see also* Disease,
    gallbladder) 575.4
  gastric (ulcer)—*see* Ulcer, stomach, with
    perforation
  heart valve—*see* Endocarditis
  ileum (*see also* Perforation, intestine) 569.83
  instrumental
    external—*see* Wound, open, by site
    pregnant uterus, complicating delivery 665.9
    surgical (accidental) (blood vessel) (nerve)
      (organ) 998.2
  intestine 569.83
    with
      abortion—*see* Abortion, by type, with
        damage to pelvic organs
      ectopic pregnancy (*see also* categories
        633.0-633.9) 639.2
      molar pregnancy (*see also* categories
        630-632) 639.2
    fetus or newborn 777.6
    obstetrical trauma 665.5
    ulcerative NEC 569.83
  jejunum, jejunal 569.83
    ulcer—*see* Ulcer, gastrojejunal, with
      perforation
  mastoid (antrum) (cell) 383.89
  maxillary sinus (*see also* Sinusitis, maxillary)
    473.0
  membrana tympani—*see* Perforation, tympanum

Perforation, perforative—*continued*
nasal
  septum 478.19
    congenital 748.1
    syphilitic 095.8
  sinus (*see also* Sinusitis) 473.9
    congenital 748.1
palate (hard) 526.89
  soft 528.9
    syphilitic 095.8
  syphilitic 095.8
palatine vault 526.89
  syphilitic 095.8
    congenital 090.5
pelvic
  floor
    with
      abortion—*see* Abortion, by type, with
        damage to pelvic organs
      ectopic pregnancy (*see also* categories
        633.0-633.9) 639.2
      molar pregnancy (*see also* categories
        630-632) 639.2
      obstetrical trauma 664.1
  organ
    with
      abortion—*see* Abortion, by type, with
        damage to pelvic organs
      ectopic pregnancy (*see also* categories
        633.0-633.9) 639.2
      molar pregnancy (*see also* categories
        630-632) 639.2
    following
      abortion 639.2
      ectopic or molar pregnancy 639.2
      obstetrical trauma 665.5
perineum—*see* Laceration, perineum
periurethral tissue
  with
    abortion—*see* Abortion, by type, with
      damage to pelvic organs
    ectopic pregnancy (*see also* categories
      630-632) 639.2
    molar pregnancy (*see also* categories
      630-632) 639.2
pharynx 478.29
pylorus, pyloric (ulcer)—*see* Ulcer, stomach,
  with perforation
rectum 569.49
root canal space 526.61
sigmoid 569.83
sinus (accessory) (chronic) (nasal) (*see also*
  Sinusitis) 473.9
sphenoidal sinus (*see also* Sinusitis, sphenoidal)
  473.3
stomach (due to ulcer)—*see* Ulcer, stomach,
  with perforation
surgical (accidental) (by instrument) (blood
  vessel) (nerve) (organ) 998.2
traumatic
  external—*see* Wound, open, by site
  eye (*see also* Penetrating wound, ocular) 871.7
  internal organ—*see* Injury, internal, by site
tympanum (membrane) (persistent
  posttraumatic) (postinflammatory) 384.20
  with
    otitis media—*see* Otitis media
  attic 384.22
  central 384.21
  healed 384.81
  marginal NEC 384.23

Perforation, perforative—*continued*
tympanum—*continued*
  multiple 384.24
  pars flaccida 384.22
  total 384.25
  traumatic—*see* Wound, open, ear, drum
typhoid, gastrointestinal 002.0
ulcer—*see* Ulcer, by site, with perforation
ureter 593.89
urethra
  with
    abortion—*see* Abortion, by type, with
      damage to pelvic organs
    ectopic pregnancy (*see also* categories
      633.0-633.9) 639.2
    molar pregnancy (*see also* categories
      630-632) 639.2
  following
    abortion 639.2
    ectopic or molar pregnancy 639.2
    obstetrical trauma 665.5
uterus—*see also* Injury, internal, uterus
  with
    abortion—*see* Abortion, by type, with
      damage to pelvic organs
    ectopic pregnancy (*see also* categories
      633.0-633.9) 639.2
    molar pregnancy (*see also* categories
      630-632) 639.2
    by intrauterine contraceptive device 996.32
  following
    abortion 639.2
    ectopic or molar pregnancy 639.2
    obstetrical trauma—*see* Injury, internal,
      uterus, obstetrical trauma
uvula 528.9
  syphilitic 095.8
vagina—*see* Laceration, vagina
viscus NEC 799.89
  traumatic 868.00
    with open wound into cavity 868.10
Periadenitis mucosa necrotica recurrens 528.2
Periangiitis 446.0
Periantritis 535.4
Periappendicitis (acute) (*see also* Appendicitis)
  541
Periarteritis (disseminated) (infectious)
  (necrotizing) (nodosa) 446.0
Periarthritis (joint) 726.90
  Duplay's 726.2
  gonococcal 098.50
  humeroscapularis 726.2
  scapulohumeral 726.2
  shoulder 726.2
  wrist 726.4
Periarthrosis (angioneural)—*see* Periarthritis
Peribronchitis 491.9
  tuberculous (*see also* Tuberculosis) 011.3
Pericapsulitis, adhesive (shoulder) 726.0
Pericarditis (granular) (with decompensation)
  (with effusion) 423.9
  with
    rheumatic fever (conditions classifiable to
      390)
      active (*see also* Pericarditis, rheumatic)
        391.0
      inactive or quiescent 393
  actinomycotic 039.8 *[420.0]*

Pericarditis—*continued*
  acute (nonrheumatic) 420.90
    with chorea (acute) (rheumatic) (Sydenham's)
      392.0
    bacterial 420.99
    benign 420.91
    hemorrhagic 420.90
    idiopathic 420.91
    infective 420.90
    nonspecific 420.91
    rheumatic 391.0
      with chorea (acute) (rheumatic)
        (Sydenham's) 392.0
    sicca 420.90
    viral 420.91
  adhesive or adherent (external) (internal) 423.1
    acute—*see* Pericarditis, acute
    rheumatic (external) (internal) 393
  amebic 006.8 *[420.0]*
  bacterial (acute) (subacute) (with serous or
    seropurulent effusion) 420.99
  calcareous 423.2
  cholesterol (chronic) 423.8
    acute 420.90
  chronic (nonrheumatic) 423.8
    rheumatic 393
  constrictive 423.2
  Coxsackie 074.21
  due to
    actinomycosis 039.8 *[420.0]*
    amebiasis 006.8 *[420.0]*
    Coxsackie (virus) 074.21
    histoplasmosis (*see also* Histoplasmosis) 115.93
    nocardiosis 039.8 *[420.0]*
    tuberculosis (*see also* Tuberculosis) 017.9
      [420.0]
  fibrinocaseous (*see also* Tuberculosis) 017.9
    [420.0]
  fibrinopurulent 420.99
  fibrinous—*see* Pericarditis, rheumatic
  fibropurulent 420.99
  fibrous 423.1
  gonococcal 098.83
  hemorrhagic 423.0
  idiopathic (acute) 420.91
  infective (acute) 420.90
  meningococcal 036.41
  neoplastic (chronic) 423.8
    acute 420.90
  nonspecific 420.91
  obliterans, obliterating 423.1
  plastic 423.1
  pneumococcal (acute) 420.99
  postinfarction 411.0
  purulent (acute) 420.99
  rheumatic (active) (acute) (with effusion) (with
    pneumonia) 391.0
    with chorea (acute) (rheumatic) (Sydenham's)
      392.0
    chronic or inactive (with chorea) 393
  septic (acute) 420.99
  serofibrinous—*see* Pericarditis, rheumatic
  staphylococcal (acute) 420.99
  streptococcal (acute) 420.99
  suppurative (acute) 420.99
  syphilitic 093.81
  tuberculous (acute) (chronic) (*see also*
    Tuberculosis) 017.9 *[420.0]*
  uremic 585.9 *[420.0]*
  viral (acute) 420.91
Pericardium, pericardial —*see* condition
Pericellulitis (*see also* Cellulitis) 682.9

Pericementitis 523.40
  acute 523.30
  chronic (suppurative) 523.40
Pericholecystitis (*see also* Cholecystitis) 575.10
Perichondritis
  auricle 380.00
    acute 380.01
    chronic 380.02
  bronchus 491.9
  ear (external) 380.00
    acute 380.01
    chronic 380.02
  larynx 478.71
    syphilitic 095.8
    typhoid 002.0 *[478.71]*
  nose 478.19
  pinna 380.00
    acute 380.01
    chronic 380.02
  trachea 478.9
Periclasia 523.5
Pericolitis 569.89
Pericoronitis (chronic) 523.40
  acute 523.33
Pericystitis (*see also* Cystitis) 595.9
Pericytoma (M9150/1)—*see also* Neoplasm,
    connective tissue, uncertain behavior
  benign (M9150/0)—*see* Neoplasm, connective
    tissue, benign
  malignant (M9150/3)—*see* Neoplasm,
    connective tissue, malignant
Peridacryocystitis, acute 375.32
Peridiverticulitis (*see also* Diverticulitis) 562.11
Periduodenitis 535.6
Periendocarditis (*see also* Endocarditis) 424.90
  acute or subacute 421.9
Periepididymitis (*see also* Epididymitis) 604.90
Perifolliculitis (abscedens) 704.8
  capitis, abscedens et suffodiens 704.8
  dissecting, scalp 704.8
  scalp 704.8
  superficial pustular 704.8
Perigastritis (acute) 535.0
Perigastrojejunitis (acute) 535.0
Perihepatitis (acute) 573.3
  chlamydial 099.56
  gonococcal 098.86
Peri-ileitis (subacute) 569.89
Perilabyrinthitis (acute)—*see* Labyrinthitis
Perimeningitis —*see* Meningitis
Perimetritis (*see also* Endometritis) 615.9
Perimetrosalpingitis (*see also*
    Salpingo-oophoritis) 614.2
Perineocele 618.05
Perinephric —*see* condition
Perinephritic —*see* condition
Perinephritis (*see also* Infection, kidney) 590.9
  purulent (*see also* Abscess, kidney) 590.2
Perineum, perineal —*see* condition
Perineuritis NEC 729.2
Periodic —*see also* condition
  disease (familial) 277.31
  edema 995.1
    hereditary 277.6
  fever 277.31
  headache syndrome in child or adolescent 346.2
  limb movement disorder 327.51
  paralysis (familial) 359.3
  peritonitis 277.31
  polyserositis 277.31
  somnolence (*see also* Narcolepsy) 347.00

Periodontal
  cyst 522.8
  pocket 523.8
Periodontitis (chronic) (complex) (compound)
    (simplex) 523.40
  acute 523.33
  aggressive 523.30
    generalized 523.32
    localized 523.31
  apical 522.6
    acute (pulpal origin) 522.4
  generalized 523.42
  localized 523.41
Periodontoclasia 523.5
Periodontosis 523.5
Periods —*see also* Menstruation
  heavy 626.2
  irregular 626.4
Perionychia (with lymphangitis) 681.9
  finger 681.02
  toe 681.11
Perioophoritis (*see also* Salpingo-oophoritis) 614.2
Periorchitis (*see also* Orchitis) 604.90
Periosteum, periosteal —*see* condition
Periostitis (circumscribed) (diffuse) (infective) 730.3

Note—Use the following fifth-digit
subclassification with category 730:
0 site unspdcified
1 shoulder region
2 upper arm
3 forearm
4 hand
5 pelvic region and thigh
6 lower leg
7 ankle and foot
8 other specified sites
9 multiple sites

  with osteomyelitis (*see also* Osteomyelitis) 730.2
    acute or subacute 730.0
    chronic or old 730.1
  albuminosa, albuminosus 730.3
  alveolar 526.5
  alveolodental 526.5
  dental 526.5
  gonorrheal 098.89
  hyperplastica, generalized 731.2
  jaw (lower) (upper) 526.4
  monomelic 733.99
  orbital 376.02
  syphilitic 095.5
    congenital 090.0 *[730.8]*
    secondary 091.61
  tuberculous (*see also* Tuberculosis, bone) 015.9
    [730.8]
  yaws (early) (hypertrophic) (late) 102.6
Periostosis (*see also* Periostitis) 730.3
  with osteomyelitis (*see also* Osteomyelitis) 730.2
    acute or subacute 730.0
    chronic or old 730.1
  hyperplastic 756.59
Peripartum cardiomyopathy 674.5
Periphlebitis (*see also* Phlebitis) 451.9
  lower extremity 451.2
    deep (vessels) 451.19
    superficial (vessels) 451.0
  portal 572.1
  retina 362.18
    superficial (vessels) 451.0
  tuberculous (*see also* Tuberculosis) 017.9
    retina 017.3 *[362.18]*

Peripneumonia —*see* Pneumonia
Periproctitis 569.49
Periprostatitis (*see also* Prostatitis) 601.9
Perirectal —*see* condition
Perirenal —*see* condition
Perisalpingitis (*see also* Salpingo-oophoritis)
    614.2
Perisigmoiditis 569.89
Perisplenitis (infectional) 289.59
Perispondylitis —*see* Spondylitis
Peristalsis reversed or visible 787.4
Peritendinitis (*see also* Tenosynovitis) 726.90
  adhesive (shoulder) 726.0
Perithelioma (M9150/1)—*see* Pericytoma
Peritoneum, peritoneal —*see also* condition
  equilibration test V56.32
Peritonitis (acute) (adhesive) (fibrinous)
    (hemorrhagic) (idiopathic) (localized)
    (perforative) (primary) (with adhesions) (with
    effusion) 567.9
  with or following
    abortion—*see* Abortion, by type, with sepsis
    abscess 567.21
    appendicitis 540.0
      with peritoneal abscess 540.1
    ectopic pregnancy (*see also* categories
        633.0-633.9) 639.0
    molar pregnancy (*see also* categories 630-632)
        639.0
  aseptic 998.7
  bacterial 567.29
    spontaneous 567.23
  bile, biliary 567.81
  chemical 998.7
  chlamydial 099.56
  chronic proliferative 567.89
  congenital NEC 777.6
  diaphragmatic 567.22
  diffuse NEC 567.29
  diphtheritic 032.83
  disseminated NEC 567.29
  due to
    bile 567.81
    foreign
      body or object accidentally left during a
          procedure (instrument) (sponge) (swab)
          998.4
      substance accidentally left during a procedure
          (chemical) (powder) (talc) 998.7
    talc 998.7
    urine 567.89
  fibrinopurulent 567.29
  fibrinous 567.29
  fibrocaseous (*see also* Tuberculosis) 014.0
  fibropurulent 567.29
  general, generalized (acute) 567.21
  gonococcal 098.86
  in infective disease NEC 136.9 *[567.0]*
  meconium (newborn) 777.6
  pancreatic 577.8
  paroxysmal, benign 277.31
  pelvic
    female (acute) 614.5
      chronic NEC 614.7
        with adhesions 614.6
      puerperal, postpartum, childbirth 670.8
    male (acute) 567.21
  periodic (familial) 277.31
  phlegmonous 567.29
  pneumococcal 567.1
  postabortal 639.0

Peritonitis—*continued*
  proliferative, chronic 567.89
  puerperal, postpartum, childbirth 670.8
  purulent 567.29
  septic 567.29
  spontaneous bacterial 567.23
  staphylococcal 567.29
  streptococcal 567.29
  subdiaphragmatic 567.29
  subphrenic 567.29
  suppurative 567.29
  syphilitic 095.2
    congenital 090.0 *[567.0]*
  talc 998.7
  tuberculous (*see also* Tuberculosis) 014.0
  urine 567.89
Peritonsillar —*see* condition
Peritonsillitis 475
Perityphlitis (*see also* Appendicitis) 541
Periureteritis 593.89
Periurethral —*see* condition
Periurethritis (gangrenous) 597.89
Periuterine —*see* condition
Perivaginitis (*see also* Vaginitis) 616.10
Perivasculitis, retinal 362.18
Perivasitis (chronic) 608.4
Periventricular leukomalacia 779.7
Perivesiculitis (seminal) (*see also* Vesiculitis)
    608.0
Perlèche 686.8
  due to
    moniliasis 112.0
    riboflavin deficiency 266.0
Pernicious —*see* condition
Pernio, perniosis 991.5
Persecution
  delusion 297.9
  social V62.4
Perseveration (tonic) 784.69
Persistence, persistent (congenital) 759.89
  anal membrane 751.2
  arteria stapedia 744.04
  atrioventricular canal 745.69
  bloody ejaculate 792.2
  branchial cleft 744.41
  bulbus cordis in left ventricle 745.8
  canal of Cloquet 743.51
  capsule (opaque) 743.51
  cilioretinal artery or vein 743.51
  cloaca 751.5
  communication—*see* Fistula, congenital
  convolutions
    aortic arch 747.21
    fallopian tube 752.19
    oviduct 752.19
    uterine tube 752.19
  double aortic arch 747.21
  ductus
    arteriosus 747.0
    Botalli 747.0
  fetal
    circulation 747.83
    form of cervix (uteri) 752.49
    hemoglobin (hereditary) ("Swiss variety")
      282.7
    pulmonary hypertension 747.83
  foramen
    Botalli 745.5
    ovale 745.5
  Gartner's duct 752.41

Persistence, persistent—*continued*
  hemoglobin, fetal (hereditary) (HPFH) 282.7
  hyaloid
    artery (generally incomplete) 743.51
    system 743.51
  hymen (tag)
    in pregnancy or childbirth 654.8
      causing obstructed labor 660.2
  lanugo 757.4
  left
    posterior cardinal vein 747.49
    root with right arch of aorta 747.21
    superior vena cava 747.49
  Meckel's diverticulum 751.0
  mesonephric duct 752.89
    fallopian tube 752.11
  mucosal disease (middle ear) (with posterior or
    superior marginal perforation of ear drum)
    382.2
  nail(s), anomalous 757.5
  occiput, anterior or posterior 660.3
    fetus or newborn 763.1
  omphalomesenteric duct 751.0
  organ or site NEC—*see* Anomaly, specified
    type NEC
  ostium
    atrioventriculare commune 745.69
    primum 745.61
    secundum 745.5
  ovarian rests in fallopian tube 752.19
  pancreatic tissue in intestinal tract 751.5
  primary (deciduous)
    teeth 520.6
    vitreous hyperplasia 743.51
  pulmonary hypertension 747.83
  pupillary membrane 743.46
    iris 743.46
  Rhesus (Rh) titer (*see also* Complications,
    transfusion) 999.70
  right aortic arch 747.21
  sinus
    urogenitalis 752.89
    venosus with imperfect incorporation in right
      auricle 747.49
  thymus (gland) 254.8
    hyperplasia 254.0
  thyroglossal duct 759.2
  thyrolingual duct 759.2
  truncus arteriosus or communis 745.0
  tunica vasculosa lentis 743.39
  umbilical sinus 753.7
  urachus 753.7
  vegetative state 780.03
  vitelline duct 751.0
  wolffian duct 752.89
Person (with)
  admitted for clinical research, as participant or
    control subject V70.7
  affected by
    family member
      currently on deployment (military) V61.01
      returned from deployment (military) (current
        or past conflict) V61.02
  awaiting admission to adequate facility
    elsewhere V63.2
    undergoing social agency investigation V63.8
  concern (normal) about sick person in family
    V61.49

Person—*continued*
  consulting on behalf of another V65.19
    pediatric
      pre-adoption visit for adoptive parents V65.11
      pre-birth visit for expectant parents V65.11
  currently deployed in theater or in support of
    military war, peacekeeping and
    humanitarian operations V62.21
  feared
    complaint in whom no diagnosis was made
      V65.5
    condition not demonstrated V65.5
  feigning illness V65.2
  healthy, accompanying sick person V65.0
  history of military war, peacekeeping and
    humanitarian deployment (current or past
    conflict) V62.22
  living (in)
    alone V60.3
    boarding school V60.6
    residence remote from hospital or medical
      care facility V63.0
    residential institution V60.6
    without
      adequate
        financial resources V60.2
        housing (heating) (space) V60.1
        housing (permanent) (temporary) V60.0
        material resources V60.2
        person able to render necessary care V60.4
        shelter V60.0
  medical services in home not available V63.1
  on waiting list V63.2
    undergoing social agency investigation V63.8
  sick or handicapped in family V61.49
  "worried well" V65.5
Personality
  affective 301.10
  aggressive 301.3
  amoral 301.7
  anancastic, anankastic 301.4
  antisocial 301.7
  asocial 301.7
  asthenic 301.6
  avoidant 301.82
  borderline 301.83
  change 310.1
  compulsive 301.4
  cycloid 301.13
  cyclothymic 301.13
  dependent 301.6
  depressive (chronic) 301.12
  disorder, disturbance NEC 301.9
    with
      antisocial disturbance 301.7
      pattern disturbance NEC 301.9
      sociopathic disturbance 301.7
      trait disturbance 301.9
  dual 300.14
  dyssocial 301.7
  eccentric 301.89
    "haltlose" type 301.89
  emotionally unstable 301.59
  epileptoid 301.3
  explosive 301.3
  fanatic 301.0
  histrionic 301.50
  hyperthymic 301.11
  hypomanic 301.11
  hypothymic 301.12
  hysterical 301.50

Personality—*continued*
  immature 301.89
  inadequate 301.6
  labile 301.59
  masochistic 301.89
  morally defective 301.7
  multiple 300.14
  narcissistic 301.81
  obsessional 301.4
  obsessive-compulsive 301.4
  overconscientious 301.4
  paranoid 301.0
  passive (-dependent) 301.6
  passive-aggressive 301.84
  pathologic NEC 301.9
  pattern defect or disturbance 301.9
  pseudosocial 301.7
  psychoinfantile 301.59
  psychoneurotic NEC 301.89
  psychopathic 301.9
    with
      amoral trend 301.7
      antisocial trend 301.7
      asocial trend 301.7
      pathologic sexuality (*see also* Deviation,
        sexual) 302.9
      mixed types 301.9
  schizoid 301.20
    introverted 301.21
    schizotypal 301.22
  type A 301.4
  unstable (emotional) 301.59
Perthes' disease (capital femoral
  osteochondrosis) 732.1
Pertussis (*see also* Whooping cough) 033.9
  vaccination, prophylactic (against) V03.6
Peruvian wart 088.0
Perversion, perverted
  appetite 307.52
    hysterical 300.11
  function
    pineal gland 259.8
    pituitary gland 253.9
      anterior lobe
        deficient 253.2
        excessive 253.1
      posterior lobe 253.6
    placenta—*see* Placenta, abnormal
  sense of smell or taste 781.1
    psychogenic 306.7
  sexual (*see also* Deviation, sexual) 302.9
Pervious, congenital —*see also* Imperfect,
  closure
  ductus arteriosus 747.0
Pes (congenital) (*see also* Talipes) 754.70
  abductus (congenital) 754.60
    acquired 736.79
  acquired NEC 736.79
    planus 734
  adductus (congenital) 754.79
    acquired 736.79
  cavus 754.71
    acquired 736.73
  planovalgus (congenital) 754.69
    acquired 736.79
  planus (acquired) (any degree) 734
    congenital 754.61
    rachitic 268.1
  valgus (congenital) 754.61
    acquired 736.79
  varus (congenital) 754.50
    acquired 736.79

Pest (*see also* Plague) 020.9
Pestis (*see also* Plague) 020.9
  bubonica 020.0
  fulminans 020.0
  minor 020.8
  pneumonica—*see* Plague, pneumonic
Petechia, petechiae 782.7
  fetus or newborn 772.6
Petechial
  fever 036.0
  typhus 081.9
Petges-Cléjat or Petges-Clégat syndrome
  (poikilodermatomyositis) 710.3
Petit's
  disease (*see also* Hernia, lumbar) 553.8
Petit mal (idiopathic) (*see also* Epilepsy) 345.0
  status 345.2
Petrellidosis 117.6
Petrositis 383.20
  acute 383.21
  chronic 383.22
Peutz-Jeghers disease or syndrome 759.6
Peyronie's disease 607.85
Pfeiffer's disease 075
Phacentocele 379.32
  traumatic 921.3
Phacoanaphylaxis 360.19
Phacocele (old) 379.32
  traumatic 921.3
Phaehyphomycosis 117.8
Phagedena (dry) (moist) (*see also* Gangrene)
  785.4
  arteriosclerotic 440.24
  geometric 686.09
  penis 607.89
  senile 440.24
  sloughing 785.4
  tropical (*see also* Ulcer, skin) 707.9
  vulva 616.50
Phagedenic —*see also* condition
  abscess—*see also* Abscess
  chancroid 099.0
  bubo NEC 099.8
  chancre 099.0
  ulcer (tropical) (*see also* Ulcer, skin) 707.9
Phagomania 307.52
Phakoma 362.89
Phantom limb (syndrome) 353.6
Pharyngeal —*see also* condition
  arch remnant 744.41
  pouch syndrome 279.11
Pharyngitis (acute) (catarrhal) (gangrenous)
  (infective) (malignant) (membranous)
  (phlegmonous) (pneumococcal)
  (pseudomembranous) (simple)
  (staphylococcal) (subacute) (suppurative)
  (ulcerative) (viral) 462
  with influenza, flu, or grippe (*see also*
    Influenza) 487.1
  aphthous 074.0
  atrophic 472.1
  chlamydial 099.51
  chronic 472.1
  Coxsackie virus 074.0
  diphtheritic (membranous) 032.0
  follicular 472.1
  fusospirochetal 101
  gonococcal 098.6
  granular (chronic) 472.1
  herpetic 054.79

Pharyngitis—*continued*
  hypertrophic 472.1
  infectional, chronic 472.1
  influenzal (*see also* Influenza) 487.1
  lymphonodular, acute 074.8
  septic 034.0
  streptococcal 034.0
  tuberculous (*see also* Tuberculosis) 012.8
  vesicular 074.0
Pharyngoconjunctival fever 077.2
Pharyngoconjunctivitis, viral 077.2
Pharyngolaryngitis (acute) 465.0
  chronic 478.9
  septic 034.0
Pharyngoplegia 478.29
Pharyngotonsillitis 465.8
  tuberculous 012.8
Pharyngotracheitis (acute) 465.8
  chronic 478.9
Pharynx, pharyngeal —*see* condition
Phase of life problem NEC V62.89
Phenomenon
  Arthus' 995.21
  flashback (drug) 292.89
  jaw-winking 742.8
  Jod-Basedow 242.8
  L. E. cell 710.0
  lupus erythematosus cell 710.0
  Pelger-Huët (hereditary hyposegmentation) 288.2
  Raynaud's (paroxysmal digital cyanosis)
    (secondary) 443.0
  Reilly's (*see also* Neuropathy, peripheral,
    autonomic) 337.9
  vasomotor 780.2
  vasospastic 443.9
  vasovagal 780.2
  Wenckebach's, heart block (second degree) 426.13
Phenylketonuria (PKU) 270.1
Phenylpyruvicaciduria 270.1
Pheochromoblastoma (M8700/3)
  specified site—*see* Neoplasm, by site, malignant
  unspecified site 194.0
Pheochromocytoma (M8700/0)
  malignant (M8700/3)
    specified site—*see* Neoplasm, by site,
      malignant
    unspecified site 194.0
  specified site—*see* Neoplasm, by site, benign
  unspecified site 227.0
Phimosis (congenital) 605
  chancroidal 099.0
  due to infection 605
Phlebectasia (*see also* Varicose, vein) 454.9
  congenital NEC 747.60
  esophagus (*see also* Varix, esophagus) 456.1
    with hemorrhage (*see also* Varix, esophagus,
      bleeding) 456.0
Phlebitis (infective) (pyemic) (septic)
  (suppurative) 451.9
  antecubital vein 451.82
  arm NEC 451.84
    axillary vein 451.89
    basilic vein 451.82
    deep 451.83
    superficial 451.82
  basilic vein 451.82
  blue 451.19
  brachial vein 451.83
  breast, superficial 451.89

Phlebitis—*continued*
  cavernous (venous) sinus—*see* Phlebitis,
    intracranial sinus
  cephalic vein 451.82
  cerebral (venous) sinus—*see* Phlebitis,
    intracranial sinus
  chest wall, superficial 451.89
  complicating pregnancy or puerperium 671.2
    affecting fetus or newborn 760.3
  cranial (venous) sinus—*see* Phlebitis,
    intracranial sinus
  deep (vessels) 451.19
    femoral vein 451.11
    specified vessel NEC 451.19
  due to implanted device—*see* Complications,
    due to (presence of) any device, implant, or
    graft classified to 996.0-996.5 NEC
  during or resulting from a procedure 997.2
  femoral vein (deep) (superficial) 451.11
  femoropopliteal 451.19
  following infusion, perfusion, or transfusion
    999.2
  gouty 274.89 *[451.9]*
  hepatic veins 451.89
  iliac vein 451.81
  iliofemoral 451.11
  intracranial sinus (any) (venous) 325
    late effect—*see* category 326
    nonpyogenic 437.6
      in pregnancy or puerperium 671.5
  jugular vein 451.89
  lateral (venous) sinus—*see* Phlebitis,
    intracranial sinus
  leg 451.2
    deep (vessels) 451.19
      femoral vein 451.11
      specified vessel NEC 451.19
    superficial (vessels) 451.0
      femoral vein 451.11
  longitudinal sinus—*see* Phlebitis, intracranial
    sinus
  lower extremity 451.2
    deep (vessels) 451.19
      femoral vein 451.11
      specified vessel NEC 451.19
    superficial (vessels) 451.0
      femoral vein 451.11
  migrans, migrating (superficial) 453.1
  pelvic
    with
      abortion—*see* Abortion, by type, with sepsis
      ectopic pregnancy (*see also* categories
        633.0-633.9) 639.0
      molar pregnancy (*see also* categories
        630-632) 639.0
    following
      abortion 639.0
      ectopic or molar pregnancy 639.0
    puerperal, postpartum 671.4
  popliteal vein 451.19
  portal (vein) 572.1
  postoperative 997.2
  pregnancy 671.2
    deep 671.3
    specified type NEC 671.5
    superficial 671.2
  puerperal, postpartum, childbirth 671.2
    deep 671.4
    lower extremities 671.2
    pelvis 671.4
    specified site NEC 671.5
    superficial 671.2

Phlebitis—*continued*
  radial vein 451.83
  retina 362.18
  saphenous (great) (long) 451.0
    accessory or small 451.0
  sinus (meninges)—*see* Phlebitis, intracranial
    sinus
  specified site NEC 451.89
  subclavian vein 451.89
  syphilitic 093.89
  tibial vein 451.19
  ulcer, ulcerative 451.9
    leg 451.2
      deep (vessels) 451.19
        femoral vein 451.11
        specified vessel NEC 451.19
      superficial (vessels) 451.0
        femoral vein 451.11
    lower extremity 451.2
      deep (vessels) 451.19
        femoral vein 451.11
        specified vessel NEC 451.19
      superficial (vessels) 451.0
  ulnar vein 451.83
  umbilicus 451.89
  upper extremity—*see* Phlebitis, arm
  uterus (septic) (*see also* Endometritis) 615.9
  varicose (leg) (lower extremity) (*see also*
    Varicose, vein) 454.1
Phlebofibrosis 459.89
Pheboliths 459.89
Phlebosclerosis 459.89
Phlebothrombosis —*see* Thrombosis
Phlebotomus fever 066.0
Phlegm, choked on 933.1
Phlegmasia
  alba dolens (deep vessels) 451.19
    complicating pregnancy 671.3
    nonpuerperal 451.19
    puerperal, postpartum, childbirth 671.4
  cerulea dolens 451.19
Phlegmon (*see also* Abscess) 682.9
  erysipelatous (*see also* Erysipelas) 035
  iliac 682.2
    fossa 540.1
  throat 478.29
Phlegmonous —*see* condition
Phlyctenulosis (allergic) (keratoconjunctivitis)
    (nontuberculous) 370.31
  cornea 370.31
    with ulcer (*see also* Ulcer, cornea) 370.00
  tuberculous (*see also* Tuberculosis) 017.3
    [370.31]
Phobia, phobic (reaction) 300.20
  animal 300.29
  isolated NEC 300.29
  obsessional 300.3
  simple NEC 300.29
  social 300.23
  specified NEC 300.29
  state 300.20
Phocas' disease 610.1
Phocomelia 755.4
  lower limb 755.32
    complete 755.33
    distal 755.35
    proximal 755.34
  upper limb 755.22
    complete 755.23
    distal 755.25
    proximal 755.24
Phoria (*see also* Heterophoria) 378.40

Phosphate-losing tubular disorder 588.0
Phosphatemia 275.3
Phosphaturia 275.3
Photoallergic response 692.72
Photocoproporphyria 277.1
Photodermatitis (sun) 692.72
  light other than sun 692.82
Photokeratitis 370.24
Photo-ophthalmia 370.24
Photophobia 368.13
Photopsia 368.15
Photoretinitis 363.31
Photoretinopathy 363.31
Photosensitiveness (sun) 692.72
  light other than sun 692.82
Photosensitization (sun) skin 692.72
  light other than sun 692.82
Phototoxic response 692.72
Phrenitis 323.9
Phrynoderma 264.8
Phthiriasis (pubis) (any site) 132.2
  with any infestation classifiable to 132.0
    and 132.1 132.3
Phthirus infestation —*see* Phthiriasis
Phthisis (*see also* Tuberculosis) 011.9
  bulbi (infectional) 360.41
  colliers' 011.4
  cornea 371.05
  eyeball (due to infection) 360.41
  millstone makers' 011.4
  miners' 011.4
  potters' 011.4
  sandblasters' 011.4
  stonemasons' 011.4
Phycomycosis 117.7
Physalopteriasis 127.7
Physical therapy NEC V57.1
  breathing exercises V57.0
Physiological cup, optic papilla
  borderline, glaucoma suspect 365.00
  enlarged 377.14
  glaucomatous 377.14
Phytobezoar 938
  intestine 936
  stomach 935.2
Pian (*see also* Yaws) 102.9
Pianoma 102.1
Piarhemia, piarrhemia (*see also* Hyperlipemia)
  272.4
  bilharziasis 120.9
Pica 307.52
  hysterical 300.11
Pick's
  cerebral atrophy 331.11
    with dementia
      with behavioral disturbance 331.11 *[294.11]*
      without behavioral disturbance 331.11
        [294.10]
  disease
    brain 331.11
      dementia in
        with behavioral disturbance 331.11
          [294.11]
        without behavioral disturbance 331.11
          [294.10]
    lipid histiocytosis 272.7
    liver (pericardial pseudocirrhosis of liver)
      423.2
    pericardium (pericardial pseudocirrhosis of
      liver) 423.2

Pick's—*continued*
  polyserositis (pericardial pseudocirrhosis of
    liver) 423.2
  syndrome
    heart (pericardial pseudocirrhosis of liver)
      423.2
    liver (pericardial pseudocirrhosis of liver)
      423.2
  tubular adenoma (M8640/0)
    specified site—*see* Neoplasm, by site, benign
    unspecified site
      female 220
      male 222.0
Pick-Herxheimer syndrome (diffuse idiopathic
  cutaneous atrophy) 701.8
Pick-Niemann disease (lipid histiocytosis) 272.7
Pickwickian syndrome (cardiopulmonary
  obesity) 278.03
Piebaldism, classic 709.09
Piedra 111.2
  beard 111.2
    black 111.3
    white 111.2
  black 111.3
  scalp 111.3
    black 111.3
    white 111.2
  white 111.2
Pierre Marie's syndrome (pulmonary
  hypertrophic osteoarthropathy) 731.2
Pierre Marie-Bamberger syndrome
  (hypertrophic pulmonary osteoarthropathy)
  731.2
Pierre Mauriac's syndrome
  (diabetes-dwarfism-obesity) 258.1
Pierre Robin deformity or syndrome
  (congenital) 756.0
Pierson's disease or osteochondrosis 732.1
Pigeon
  breast or chest (acquired) 738.3
    congenital 754.82
    rachitic (*see also* Rickets) 268.0
  breeders' disease or lung 495.2
  fanciers' disease or lung 495.2
  toe 735.8
Pigmentation (abnormal) 709.00
  anomaly 709.00
    congenital 757.33
    specified NEC 709.09
  conjunctiva 372.55
  cornea 371.10
    anterior 371.11
    posterior 371.13
    stromal 371.12
  lids (congenital) 757.33
    acquired 374.52
  limbus corneae 371.10
  metals 709.00
  optic papilla, congenital 743.57
  retina (congenital) (grouped) (nevoid) 743.53
    acquired 362.74
  scrotum, congenital 757.33
Piles —*see* Hemorrhoids
Pili
  annulati or torti (congenital) 757.4
  incarnati 704.8
Pill roller hand (intrinsic) 736.09
Pilomatrixoma (M8110/0)—*see* Neoplasm, skin,
  benign
Pilonidal —*see* condition
Pimple 709.8

PIN I (prostatic intraepithelial neoplasia I)
   602.3
PIN II (prostatic intraepithelial neoplasia II)
   602.3
PIN III (prostatic intraepithelial neoplasia III)
   233.4
Pinched nerve —*see* Neuropathy, entrapment
Pineal body or gland —*see* condition
Pinealoblastoma (M9362/3) 194.4
Pinealoma (M9360/1) 237.1
   malignant (M9360/3) 194.4
Pineoblastoma (M9362/3) 194.4
Pineocytoma (M9361/1) 237.1
Pinguecula 372.51
Pingueculitis 372.34
Pinhole meatus (*see also* Stricture, urethra) 598.9
Pink
   disease 985.0
   eye 372.03
   puffer 492.8
Pinkus' disease (lichen nitidus) 697.1
Pinpoint
   meatus (*see also* Stricture, urethra) 598.9
   os (uteri) (*see also* Stricture, cervix) 622.4
Pinselhaare (congenital) 757.4
Pinta 103.9
   cardiovascular lesions 103.2
   chancre (primary) 103.0
   erythematous plaques 103.1
   hyperchromic lesions 103.1
   hyperkeratosis 103.1
   lesions 103.9
      cardiovascular 103.2
      hyperchromic 103.1
      intermediate 103.1
      late 103.2
      mixed 103.3
      primary 103.0
      skin (achromic) (cicatricial) (dyschromic)
         103.2
         hyperchromic 103.1
         mixed (achromic and hyperchromic) 103.3
   papule (primary) 103.0
   skin lesions (achromic) (cicatricial)
      (dyschromic) 103.2
      hyperchromic 103.1
      mixed (achromic and hyperchromic) 103.3
   vitiligo 103.2
Pintid 103.0
Pinworms (disease) (infection) (infestation)
   127.4
Piry fever 066.8
Pistol wound —*see* Gunshot wound
Pit, lip (mucus), congenital 750.25
Pitchers' elbow 718.82
Pithecoid pelvis 755.69
   with disproportion (fetopelvic) 653.2
      affecting fetus or newborn 763.1
      causing obstructed labor 660.1
Pithiatism 300.11
Pitted —*see also* Pitting
   teeth 520.4
Pitting (edema) (*see also* Edema) 782.3
   lip 782.3
   nail 703.8
      congenital 757.5
Pituitary gland —*see* condition
Pituitary snuff-takers' disease 495.8

Pityriasis 696.5
   alba 696.5
   capitis 690.11
   circinata (et maculata) 696.3
   Hebra's (exfoliative dermatitis) 695.89
   lichenoides et varioliformis 696.2
   maculata (et circinata) 696.3
   nigra 111.1
   pilaris 757.39
      acquired 701.1
      Hebra's 696.4
   rosea 696.3
   rotunda 696.3
   rubra (Hebra) 695.89
      pilaris 696.4
   sicca 690.18
   simplex 690.18
   specified type NEC 696.5
   streptogenes 696.5
   versicolor 111.0
      scrotal 111.0
Placenta, placental
   ablatio 641.2
      affecting fetus or newborn 762.1
   abnormal, abnormality 656.7
      with hemorrhage 641.8
         affecting fetus or newborn 762.1
      affecting fetus or newborn 762.2
   abruptio 641.2
      affecting fetus or newborn 762.1
   accessory lobe—*see* Placenta, abnormal
   accreta (without hemorrhage) 667.0
      with hemorrhage 666.0
   adherent (without hemorrhage) 667.0
      with hemorrhage 666.0
   apoplexy—*see* Placenta, separation
   battledore—*see* Placenta, abnormal
   bilobate—*see* Placenta, abnormal
   bipartita—*see* Placenta, abnormal
   carneous mole 631.8
   centralis—*see* Placenta, previa
   circumvallata—*see* Placenta, abnormal
   cyst (amniotic)—*see* Placenta, abnormal
   deficiency—*see* Placenta insufficiency
   degeneration—*see* Placenta, insufficiency
   detachment (partial) (premature) (with
         hemorrhage) 641.2
      affecting fetus or newborn 762.1
   dimidiata—*see* Placenta, abnormal
   disease 656.7
      affecting fetus or newborn 762.2
   duplex—*see* Placenta, abnormal
   dysfunction—*see* Placenta, insufficiency
   fenestrata—*see* Placenta, abnormal
   fibrosis—*see* Placenta, abnormal
   fleshy mole 631.8
   hematoma—*see* Placenta, abnormal
   hemorrhage NEC—*see* Placenta, separation
   hormone disturbance or malfunction—*see*
         Placenta, abnormal
   hyperplasia—*see* Placenta, abnormal
   increta (without hemorrhage) 667.0
      with hemorrhage 666.0
   infarction 656.7
      affecting fetus or newborn 762.2
   insertion, vicious—*see* Placenta, previa
   insufficiency
      affecting
         fetus or newborn 762.2
         management of pregnancy 656.5
   lateral—*see* Placenta, previa

Placenta, placental—*continued*
low implantation or insertion—*see* Placenta, previa
low-lying—*see* Placenta, previa
malformation—*see* Placenta, abnormal
malposition—*see* Placenta, previa
marginalis, marginata—*see* Placenta, previa
marginal sinus (hemorrhage) (rupture) 641.2
  affecting fetus or newborn 762.1
membranacea—*see* Placenta, abnormal
multilobed—*see* Placenta, abnormal
multipartita—*see* Placenta, abnormal
necrosis—*see* Placenta, abnormal
percreta (without hemorrhage) 667.0
  with hemorrhage 666.0
polyp 674.4
previa (central) (centralis) (complete) (lateral) (marginal) (marginalis) (partial) (partialis) (total) (with hemorrhage) 641.1
  affecting fetus or newborn 762.0
  noted
    before labor, without hemorrhage (with cesarean delivery) 641.0
    during pregnancy (without hemorrhage) 641.0
  without hemorrhage (before labor and delivery) (during pregnancy) 641.0
retention (with hemorrhage) 666.0
  fragments, complicating puerperium (delayed hemorrhage) 666.2
    without hemorrhage 667.1
  postpartum, puerperal 666.2
    without hemorrhage 667.0
separation (normally implanted) (partial) (premature) (with hemorrhage) 641.2
  affecting fetus or newborn 762.1
septuplex—*see* Placenta, abnormal
small—*see* Placenta, insufficiency
softening (premature)—*see* Placenta, abnormal
spuria—*see* Placenta, abnormal
succenturiata—*see* Placenta, abnormal
syphilitic 095.8
transfusion syndromes 762.3
transmission of chemical substance—*see* Absorption, chemical, through placenta
trapped (with hemorrhage) 666.0
  without hemorrhage 667.0
trilobate—*see* Placenta, abnormal
tripartita—*see* Placenta, abnormal
triplex—*see* Placenta, abnormal
varicose vessel—*see* Placenta, abnormal
vicious insertion—*see* Placenta, previa
Placentitis
affecting fetus or newborn 762.7
complicating pregnancy 658.4
Plagiocephaly (skull) 754.0
Plague 020.9
abortive 020.8
ambulatory 020.8
bubonic 020.0
cellulocutaneous 020.1
lymphatic gland 020.0
pneumonic 020.5
  primary 020.3
  secondary 020.4
pulmonary—*see* Plague, pneumonic
pulmonic—*see* Plague, pneumonic
septicemic 020.2
tonsillar 020.9
  septicemic 020.2
vaccination, prophylactic (against) V03.3

Planning, family V25.09
contraception V25.9
natural
  procreative V26.41
  to avoid pregnancy V25.04
procreation V26.49
  natural V26.41
Plaque
artery, arterial—*see* Arteriosclerosis
calcareous—*see* Calcification
Hollenhorst's (retinal) 362.33
tongue 528.6
Plasma cell myeloma 203.0
Plasmacytoma, plasmocytoma (solitary) (M9731/1) 238.6
benign (M9731/0)—*see* Neoplasm, by site, benign
malignant (M9731/3) 203.8
Plasmacytopenia 288.59
Plasmacytosis 288.64
Plaster ulcer (*see also* Ulcer, pressure) 707.00
Plateau iris syndrome (without glaucoma) 364.82
with glaucoma 365.23
Platybasia 756.0
Platyonychia (congenital) 757.5
acquired 703.8
Platypelloid pelvis 738.6
with disproportion (fetopelvic) 653.2
  affecting fetus or newborn 763.1
  causing obstructed labor 660.1
    affecting fetus or newborn 763.1
congenital 755.69
Platyspondylia 756.19
Plethora 782.62
newborn 776.4
Pleura, pleural —*see* condition
Pleuralgia 786.52
Pleurisy (acute) (adhesive) (chronic) (costal) (diaphragmatic) (double) (dry) (fetid) (fibrinous) (fibrous) (interlobar) (latent) (lung) (old) (plastic) (primary) (residual) (sicca) (sterile) (subacute) (unresolved) (with adherent pleura) 511.0
with
  effusion (without mention of cause) 511.9
    bacterial, nontuberculous 511.1
    nontuberculous NEC 511.9
      bacterial 511.1
    pneumococcal 511.1
    specified type NEC 511.89
    staphylococcal 511.1
    streptococcal 511.1
    tuberculous (*see also* Tuberculosis, pleura) 012.0
      primary, progressive 010.1
  influenza, flu, or grippe (*see also* Influenza) 487.1
  tuberculosis—*see* Pleurisy, tuberculous
encysted 511.89
exudative (*see also* Pleurisy, with effusion) 511.9
  bacterial, nontuberculous 511.1
fibrinopurulent 510.9
  with fistula 510.0
fibropurulent 510.9
  with fistula 510.0
hemorrhagic 511.89
influenzal (*see also* Influenza) 487.1
pneumococcal 511.0
  with effusion 511.1

Pleurisy—*continued*
  purulent 510.9
    with fistula 510.0
  septic 510.9
    with fistula 510.0
  serofibrinous (*see also* Pleurisy, with effusion) 511.9
    bacterial, nontuberculous 511.1
  seropurulent 510.9
    with fistula 510.0
  serous (*see also* Pleurisy, with effusion) 511.9
    bacterial, nontuberculous 511.1
  staphylococcal 511.0
    with effusion 511.1
  streptococcal 511.0
    with effusion 511.1
  suppurative 510.9
    with fistula 510.0
  traumatic (post) (current) 862.29
    with open wound into cavity 862.39
  tuberculous (with effusion) (*see also*
      Tuberculosis, pleura) 012.0
    primary, progressive 010.1
Pleuritis sicca —*see* Pleurisy
Pleurobronchopneumonia (*see also* Pneumonia,
    broncho-) 485
Pleurodynia 786.52
  epidemic 074.1
  viral 074.1
Pleurohepatitis 573.8
Pleuropericarditis (*see also* Pericarditis) 423.9
  acute 420.90
Pleuropneumonia (acute) (bilateral) (double)
    (septic) (*see also* Pneumonia) 486
  chronic (*see also* Fibrosis, lung) 515
Pleurorrhea (*see also* Hydrothorax) 511.89
Plexitis, brachial 353.0
Plica
  knee 727.83
  polonica 132.0
  tonsil 474.8
Plicae dysphonia ventricularis 784.49
Plicated tongue 529.5
  congenital 750.13
Plug
  bronchus NEC 519.19
  meconium (newborn) NEC 777.1
  mucus—*see* Mucus, plug
Plumbism 984.9
  specified type of lead—*see* Table of drugs and
    chemicals
Plummer's disease (toxic nodular goiter) 242.3
Plummer-Vinson syndrome (sideropenic
    dysphagia) 280.8
Pluricarential syndrome of infancy 260
Plurideficiency syndrome of infancy 260
Plus (and minus) hand (intrinsic) 736.09
PMDD (premenstrual dysphoric disorder)
    625.4
PMS 625.4
Pneumathemia —*see* Air, embolism, by type
Pneumatic drill or hammer disease 994.9
Pneumatocele (lung) 518.89
  intracranial 348.89
  tension 492.0
Pneumatosis
  cystoides intestinalis 569.89
  peritonei 568.89
  pulmonum 492.8
Pneumaturia 599.84
Pneumoblastoma (M8981/3)—*see* Neoplasm,
    lung, malignant

Pneumocephalus 348.89
Pneumococcemia 038.2
Pneumococcus, pneumococcal —*see* condition
Pneumoconiosis (due to) (inhalation of) 505
  aluminum 503
  asbestos 501
  bagasse 495.1
  bauxite 503
  beryllium 503
  carbon electrode makers' 503
  coal
    miners' (simple) 500
    workers' (simple) 500
  cotton dust 504
  diatomite fibrosis 502
  dust NEC 504
    inorganic 503
    lime 502
    marble 502
    organic NEC 504
  fumes or vapors (from silo) 506.9
  graphite 503
  hard metal 503
  mica 502
  moldy hay 495.0
  rheumatoid 714.81
  silica NEC 502
    and carbon 500
  silicate NEC 502
  talc 502
Pneumocystis carinii pneumonia 136.3
Pneumocystis jiroveci pneumonia 136.3
Pneumocystosis 136.3
  with pneumonia 136.3
Pneumoenteritis 025
Pneumohemopericardium (*see also* Pericarditis)
    423.9
Pneumohemothorax (*see also* Hemothorax)
    511.89
  traumatic 860.4
    with open wound into thorax 860.5
Pneumohydropericardium (*see also*
    Pericarditis) 423.9
Pneumohydrothorax (*see also* Hydrothorax)
    511.89
Pneumomediastinum 518.1
  congenital 770.2
  fetus or newborn 770.2
Pneumomycosis 117.9
Pneumonia (acute) (Alpenstich) (benign)
    (bilateral) (brain) (cerebral) (circumscribed)
    (congestive) (creeping) (delayed resolution)
    (double) (epidemic) (fever) (flash) (fulminant)
    (fungoid) (granulomatous) (hemorrhagic)
    (incipient) (infantile) (infectious) (infiltration)
    (insular) (intermittent) (latent) (lobe)
    (migratory) (newborn) (organized)
    (overwhelming) (primary) (progressive)
    (pseudolobar) (purulent) (resolved)
    (secondary) (senile) (septic) (suppurative)
    (terminal) (true) (unresolved) (vesicular) 486
  with influenza, flu, or grippe 487.0
    due to
      identified (virus)
        avian 488.01
        (novel) 2009 H1N1 488.11
        novel influenza A 488.81
  adenoviral 480.0
  adynamic 514
  alba 090.0
  allergic 518.3

Pneumonia—*continued*
  alveolar—*see* Pneumonia, lobar
  anaerobes 482.81
  anthrax 022.1 *[484.5]*
  apex, apical—*see* Pneumonia, lobar
  ascaris 127.0 *[484.8]*
  aspiration 507.0
    due to
      aspiration of microorganisms
        bacterial 482.9
          specified type NEC 482.89
          specified organism NEC 483.8
            bacterial NEC 482.89
          viral 480.9
            specified type NEC 480.8
      food (regurgitated) 507.0
      gastric secretions 507.0
      milk 507.0
      oils, essences 507.1
      solids, liquids NEC 507.8
      vomitus 507.0
    fetal 770.18
      due to
        blood 770.16
        clear amniotic fluid 770.14
        meconium 770.12
        postnatal stomach contents 770.86
      newborn 770.18
        due to
          blood 770.16
          clear amniotic fluid 770.14
          meconium 770.12
          postnatal stomach contents 770.86
  asthenic 514
  atypical (disseminated, focal) (primary) 486
    with influenza (*see also* Influenza) 487.0
  bacillus 482.9
    specified type NEC 482.89
  bacterial 482.9
    specified type NEC 482.89
  Bacteroides (fragilis) (oralis) (melaninogenicus)
    482.81
  basal, basic, basilar—*see* Pneumonia, by type
  bronchiolitis obliterans organized (BOOP) 516.8
  broncho-, bronchial (confluent) (croupous)
    (diffuse) (disseminated) (hemorrhagic)
    (involving lobes) (lobar) (terminal) 485
    with influenza 487.0
      due to
        identified (virus)
          avian 488.01
          (novel) 2009 H1N1 488.11
          novel influenza A 488.81
    allergic 518.3
    aspiration (*see also* Pneumonia, aspiration)
      507.0
    bacterial 482.9
      specified type NEC 482.89
    capillary 466.19
      with bronchospasm or obstruction 466.19
    chronic (*see also* Fibrosis, lung) 515
    congenital (infective) 770.0
    diplococcal 481
    Eaton's agent 483.0
    Escherichia coli (E. coli) 482.82
    Friedländer's bacillus 482.0
    Hemophilus influenzae 482.2
    hiberno-vernal 083.0 *[484.8]*
    hypostatic 514
    influenzal (*see also* Influenza) 487.0
    inhalation (*see also* Pneumonia, aspiration) 507.0
      due to fumes or vapors (chemical) 506.0

Pneumonia—*continued*
  broncho, bronchial—*continued*
    Klebsiella 482.0
    lipid 507.1
      endogenous 516.8
    Mycoplasma (pneumoniae) 483.0
    ornithosis 073.0
    pleuropneumonia-like organisms (PPLO) 483.0
    pneumococcal 481
    Proteus 482.83
    pseudomonas 482.1
    specified organism NEC 483.8
      bacterial NEC 482.89
    staphylococcal 482.40
      aureus 482.41
        methicillin
          resistant (MRSA) 482.42
          susceptible (MSSA) 482.41
        specified type NEC 482.49
    streptococcal—*see* Pneumonia, streptococcal
    typhoid 002.0 *[484.8]*
    viral, virus (*see also* Pneumonia, viral) 480.9
  Butyrivibrio (fibriosolvens) 482.81
  Candida 112.4
  capillary 466.19
    with bronchospasm or obstruction 466.19
  caseous (*see also* Tuberculosis) 011.6
  catarrhal—*see* Pneumonia, broncho-
  central—*see* Pneumonia, lobar
  Chlamydia, chlamydial 483.1
    pneumoniae 483.1
    psittaci 073.0
    specified type NEC 483.1
    trachomatis 483.1
  cholesterol 516.8
  chronic (*see also* Fibrosis, lung) 515
  cirrhotic (chronic) (*see also* Fibrosis, lung) 515
  Clostridium (haemolyticum) (novyi) NEC
    482.81
  confluent—*see* Pneumonia, broncho-
  congenital (infective) 770.0
    aspiration 770.18
  croupous—*see* Pneumonia, lobar
  cryptogenic organizing 516.36
  cytomegalic inclusion 078.5 *[484.1]*
  deglutition (*see also* Pneumonia, aspiration)
    507.0
  desquamative interstitial 516.37
  diffuse—*see* Pneumonia, broncho-
  diplococcal, diplococcus (broncho-) (lobar) 481
  disseminated (focal)—*see* Pneumonia, broncho-
  due to
    adenovirus 480.0
    Bacterium anitratum 482.83
    Chlamydia, chlamydial 483.1
      pneumoniae 483.1
      psittaci 073.0
      specified type NEC 483.1
      trachomatis 483.1
    coccidioidomycosis 114.0
    Diplococcus (pneumoniae) 481
    Eaton's agent 483.0
    Escherichia coli (E. coli) 482.82
    Friedländer's bacillus 482.0
    fumes or vapors (chemical) (inhalation) 506.0
    fungus NEC 117.9 *[484.7]*
      coccidioidomycosis 114.0
    Hemophilus influenzae (H. influenzae) 482.2
    Herellea 482.83
    influenza (*see also* Influenza) 487.0
    Klebsiella pneumoniae 482.0
    Mycoplasma (pneumoniae) 483.0

Pneumonia—*continued*
due to—*continued*
parainfluenza virus 480.2
pleuropneumonia-like organism (PPLO) 483.0
Pneumococcus 481
Pneumocystis carinii 136.3
Pneumocystis jiroveci 136.3
Proteus 482.83
pseudomonas 482.1
respiratory syncytial virus 480.1
rickettsia 083.9 *[484.8]*
SARS-associated coronavirus 480.3
specified
bacteria NEC 482.89
organism NEC 483.8
virus NEC 480.8
Staphylococcus 482.40
aureus 482.41
methicillin
resistant (MRSA) 482.42
susceptible (MSSA) 482.41
specified type NEC 482.49
Streptococcus—*see also* Pneumonia,
streptococcal
pneumoniae 481
virus (*see also* Pneumonia, viral) 480.9
Eaton's agent 483.0
embolic, embolism (*see also* Embolism,
pulmonary) 415.1
eosinophilic 518.3
Escherichia coli (E. coli) 482.82
Eubacterium 482.81
fibrinous—*see* Pneumonia, lobar
fibroid (chronic) (*see also* Fibrosis, lung) 515
fibrous (*see also* Fibrosis, lung) 515
Friedländer's bacillus 482.0
Fusobacterium (nucleatum) 482.81
gangrenous 513.0
giant cell (*see also* Pneumonia, viral) 480.9
gram-negative bacteria NEC 482.83
anaerobic 482.81
grippal (*see also* Influenza) 487.0
Hemophilus influenzae (bronchial) (lobar) 482.2
hypostatic (broncho-) (lobar) 514
in
actinomycosis 039.1
anthrax 022.1 *[484.5]*
aspergillosis 117.3 *[484.6]*
candidiasis 112.4
coccidioidomycosis 114.0
cytomegalic inclusion disease 078.5 *[484.1]*
histoplasmosis (*see also* Histoplasmosis)
115.95
infectious disease NEC 136.9 *[484.8]*
measles 055.1
mycosis, systemic NEC 117.9 *[484.7]*
nocardiasis, nocardiosis 039.1
ornithosis 073.0
pneumocystosis 136.3
psittacosis 073.0
Q fever 083.0 *[484.8]*
salmonellosis 003.22
toxoplasmosis 130.4
tularemia 021.2
typhoid (fever) 002.0 *[484.8]*
varicella 052.1
whooping cough (*see also* Whooping cough)
033.9 *[484.3]*
infective, acquired prenatally 770.0
influenzal (broncho) (lobar) (virus) (*see also*
Influenza) 487.0

Pneumonia—*continued*
inhalation (*see also* Pneumonia, aspiration) 507.0
fumes or vapors (chemical) 506.0
interstitial 516.8
with influenzal (*see also* Influenza) 487.0
acute
due to Pneumocystis (carinii) (jiroveci)
136.3
meaning:
acute interstitial pneumonitis 516.33
atypical pneumonia—*see* Pneumonia,
atypical
bacterial pneumonia—*see* Pneumonia,
bacterial
chronic (*see also* Fibrosis, lung) 515
desquamative 516.37
hypostatic 514
idiopathic 516.30
lymphoid 516.35
lipoid 507.1
lymphoid (due to known underlying cause) 516.8
non-specific (due to known underlying cause)
516.8
organizing (due to known underlying cause)
516.8
plasma cell 136.3
pseudomonas 482.1
intrauterine (infective) 770.0
aspiration 770.18
blood 770.16
clear amniotic fluid 770.14
meconium 770.12
postnatal stomach contents 770.86
Klebsiella pneumoniae 482.0
Legionnaires' 482.84
lipid, lipoid (exogenous) (interstitial) 507.1
endogenous 516.8
lobar (diplococcal) (disseminated) (double)
(interstitial) (pneumococcal, any type) 481
with influenza (*see also* Influenza) 487.0
bacterial 482.9
specified type NEC 482.89
chronic (*see also* Fibrosis, lung) 515
Escherichia coli (E. coli) 482.82
Friedländer's bacillus 482.0
Hemophilus influenzae (H. influenzae) 482.2
hypostatic 514
influenzal (*see also* Influenza) 487.0
Klebsiella 482.0
ornithosis 073.0
Proteus 482.83
pseudomonas 482.1
psittacosis 073.0
specified organism NEC 483.8
bacterial NEC 482.89
staphylococcal 482.40
aureus 482.41
methicillin
resistant (MRSA) 482.42
susceptible (MSSA) 482.41
specified type NEC 482.49
streptococcal—*see* Pneumonia, streptococcal
viral, virus (*see also* Pneumonia, viral) 480.9
lobular (confluent)—*see* Pneumonia, broncho-
Löffler's 518.3
massive—*see* Pneumonia, lobar
meconium aspiration 770.12
metastatic NEC 038.8 *[484.8]*
methicillin resistant Staphylococcus aureus
(MRSA) 482.42
methicillin susceptible Staphylococcus aureus
(MSSA) 482.41

Pneumonia—*continued*
- MRSA (methicillin resistant Staphylococcus aureus) 482.42
- MSSA (methicillin susceptible Staphylococcus aureus) 482.41
- multilobar —*see* Pneumonia, by type
- Mycoplasma (pneumoniae) 483.0
- necrotic 513.0
- nitrogen dioxide 506.9
- orthostatic 514
- parainfluenza virus 480.2
- parenchymatous (*see also* Fibrosis, lung) 515
- passive 514
- patchy—*see* Pneumonia, broncho
- Peptococcus 482.81
- Peptostreptococcus 482.81
- plasma cell 136.3
- pleurolobar—*see* Pneumonia, lobar
- pleuropneumonia-like organism (PPLO) 483.0
- pneumococcal (broncho) (lobar) 481
- Pneumocystis (carinii) (jiroveci) 136.3
- postinfectional NEC 136.9 *[484.8]*
- postmeasles 055.1
- postoperative 997.39
  - aspiration 997.32
- primary atypical 486
- Proprionibacterium 482.81
- Proteus 482.83
- pseudomonas 482.1
- psittacosis 073.0
- radiation 508.0
- respiratory syncytial virus 480.1
- resulting from a procedure 997.39
  - aspiration 997.32
- rheumatic 390 *[517.1]*
- Salmonella 003.22
- SARS-associated coronavirus 480.3
- segmented, segmental—*see* Pneumonia, broncho-
- Serratia (marcescens) 482.83
- specified
  - bacteria NEC 482.89
  - organism NEC 483.8
  - virus NEC 480.8
- spirochetal 104.8 *[484.8]*
- staphylococcal (broncho) (lobar) 482.40
  - aureus 482.41
    - methicillin
      - resistant (MRSA) 482.42
      - susceptible (MSSA) 482.41
  - specified type NEC 482.49
- static, stasis 514
- streptococcal (broncho) (lobar) NEC 482.30
  - Group
    - A 482.31
    - B 482.32
    - specified NEC 482.39
  - pneumoniae 481
  - specified type NEC 482.39
- Streptococcus pneumoniae 481
- traumatic (complication) (early) (secondary) 958.8
- tuberculous (any) (*see also* Tuberculosis) 011.6
- tularemic 021.2
- TWAR agent 483.1
- varicella 052.1
- Veillonella 482.81
- ventilator associated 997.31

Pneumonia—*continued*
- viral, virus (broncho) (interstitial) (lobar) 480.9
  - with influenza, flu, or grippe (*see also* Influenza) 487.0
  - adenoviral 480.0
  - parainfluenza 480.2
  - respiratory syncytial 480.1
  - SARS-associated coronavirus 480.3
  - specified type NEC 480.8
- white (congenital) 090.0

Pneumonic —*see* condition

Pneumonitis (acute) (primary) (*see also* Pneumonia) 486
- allergic 495.9
  - specified type NEC 495.8
- aspiration 507.0
  - due to fumes or gases 506.0
  - fetal 770.18
    - due to
      - blood 770.16
      - clear amniotic fluid 770.14
      - meconium 770.12
      - postnatal stomach contents 770.86
  - newborn 770.18
    - due to
      - blood 770.16
      - clear amniotic fluid 770.14
      - meconium 770.12
      - postnatal stomach contents 770.86
  - obstetric 668.0
- chemical 506.0
  - due to fumes or gases 506.0
  - resulting from a procedure 997.32
- cholesterol 516.8
- chronic (*see also* Fibrosis, lung) 515
- congenital rubella 771.0
- crack 506.0
- due to
  - crack (cocaine) 506.0
  - fumes or vapors 506.0
  - inhalation
    - food (regurgitated), milk, vomitus 507.0
    - oils, essences 507.1
    - saliva 507.0
    - solids, liquids NEC 507.8
  - toxoplasmosis (acquired) 130.4
    - congenital (active) 771.2 *[484.8]*
- eosinophilic 518.3
- fetal aspiration 770.18
  - due to
    - blood 770.16
    - clear amniotic fluid 770.14
    - meconium 770.12
    - postnatal stomach contents 770.86
- hypersensitivity 495.9
- interstitial (chronic) (*see also* Fibrosis, lung) 515
  - acute 516.33
  - idiopathic
    - lymphocytic 516.35
    - non-specific 516.32
  - lymphoid 516.8
- lymphoid, interstitial 516.8
- meconium aspiration 770.12
- postanesthetic
  - correct substance properly administered 507.0
  - obstetric 668.0
  - overdose or wrong substance given 968.4
    - specified anesthetic—*see* Table of drugs and chemicals
- postoperative 997.3
  - aspiration 997.32
  - obstetric 668.0

Pneumonitis—*continued*
  radiation 508.0
  rubella, congenital 771.0
  "ventilation" 495.7
  ventilator associated 997.31
  wood-dust 495.8
Pneumonoconiosis —*see* Pneumoconiosis
Pneumoparotid 527.8
Pneumopathy NEC 518.89
  alveolar 516.9
    specified NEC 516.8
  due to dust NEC 504
  parietoalveolar 516.9
    specified condition NEC 516.8
Pneumopericarditis (*see also* Pericarditis) 423.9
  acute 420.90
Pneumopericardium —*see also* Pericarditis
  congenital 770.2
  fetus or newborn 770.2
  traumatic (post) (*see also* Pneumothorax,
    traumatic) 860.0
    with open wound into thorax 860.1
Pneumoperitoneum 568.89
  fetus or newborn 770.2
Pneumophagia (psychogenic) 306.4
Pneumopleurisy, pneumopleuritis (*see also*
  Pneumonia) 486
Pneumopyopericardium 420.99
Pneumopyothorax (*see also* Pyopneumothorax)
  510.9
  with fistula 510.0
Pneumorrhagia 786.30
  newborn 770.3
  tuberculous (*see also* Tuberculosis, pulmonary)
    011.9
Pneumosiderosis (occupational) 503
Pneumothorax 512.89
  acute 512.89
  chronic 512.83
  congenital 770.2
  due to operative injury of chest wall or lung 512.1
    accidental puncture or laceration 512.1
  fetus or newborn 770.2
  iatrogenic 512.1
  postoperative 512.1
  specified type NEC 512.89
  spontaneous 512.89
    fetus or newborn 770.2
    primary 512.81
    secondary 512.82
    tension 512.0
  sucking 512.89
    iatrogenic 512.1
    postoperative 512.1
  tense valvular, infectional 512.0
  tension 512.0
    iatrogenic 512.1
    postoperative 512.1
    spontaneous 512.0
  traumatic 860.0
    with
      hemothorax 860.4
        with open wound into thorax 860.5
      open wound into thorax 860.1
  tuberculous (*see also* Tuberculosis) 011.7
Pocket(s)
  endocardial (*see also* Endocarditis) 424.90
  periodontal 523.8
Podagra 274.01
Podencephalus 759.89
Poikilocytosis 790.09

Poikiloderma 709.09
  Civatte's 709.09
  congenital 757.33
  vasculare atrophicans 696.2
Poikilodermatomyositis 710.3
Pointed ear 744.29
Poise imperfect 729.90
Poisoned —*see* Poisoning
Poisoning (acute)—*see also* Table of Drugs and
  Chemicals
  Bacillus, B.
    aertrycke (*see also* Infection, Salmonella) 003.9
    botulinus 005.1
    cholerae (suis) (*see also* Infection,
      Salmonella) 003.9
    paratyphosus (*see also* Infection, Salmonella)
      003.9
    suipestifer (*see also* Infection, Salmonella) 003.9
  bacterial toxins NEC 005.9
  berries, noxious 988.2
  blood (general)—*see* Septicemia
  botulism 005.1
  bread, moldy, mouldy—*see* Poisoning, food
  Ciguatera 988.0
  damaged meat—*see* Poisoning, food
  death-cap (Amanita phalloides) (Amanita verna)
    988.1
  decomposed food—*see* Poisoning, food
  diseased food—*see* Poisoning, food
  drug—*see* Table of drugs and chemicals
  epidemic, fish, meat, or other food—*see*
    Poisoning, food
  fava bean 282.2
  fish (bacterial)—*see also* Poisoning, food
    noxious 988.0
  food (acute) (bacterial) (diseased) (infected)
    NEC 005.9
    due to
      Bacillus
        aertrycke (*see also* Poisoning, food, due to
          Salmonella) 003.9
        botulinus 005.1
        cereus 005.89
        choleraesuis (*see also* Poisoning, food, due
          to Salmonella) 003.9
        paratyphosus (*see also* Poisoning, food,
          due to Salmonella) 003.9
        suipestifer (*see also* Poisoning, food, due
          to Salmonella) 003.9
      Clostridium 005.3
        botulinum 005.1
        perfringens 005.2
        welchii 005.2
      Salmonella (aertrycke) (callinarum)
        (choleraesuis) (enteritidis) (paratyphi)
        (suipestifer) 003.9
        with
          gastroenteritis 003.0
          localized infection(s) (*see also* Infection,
            Salmonella) 003.20
          septicemia 003.1
          specified manifestation NEC 003.8
      specified bacterium NEC 005.89
      Staphylococcus 005.0
      Streptococcus 005.8
      Vibrio parahaemolyticus 005.4
      Vibrio vulnificus 005.81
    noxious or naturally toxic 988.0
      berries 988.2
      fish 988.0
      mushroom 988.1
      plants NEC 988.2

Poisoning—*continued*
  ice cream—*see* Poisoning, food
  ichthyotoxism (bacterial) 005.9
  kreotoxism, food 005.9
  malarial—*see* Malaria
  meat—*see* Poisoning, food
  mushroom (noxious) 988.1
  mussel—*see also* Poisoning, food
    noxious 988.0
  noxious foodstuffs (*see also* Poisoning, food,
    noxious) 988.9
    specified type NEC 988.8
  plants, noxious 988.2
  pork—*see also* Poisoning, food
    specified NEC 988.8
    Trichinosis 124
  ptomaine—*see* Poisoning, food
  putrefaction, food—*see* Poisoning, food
  radiation 508.0
  Salmonella (*see also* Infection, Salmonella) 003.9
  sausage—*see also* Poisoning, food
    Trichinosis 124
  saxitoxin 988.0
  shellfish—*see also* Poisoning, food
    noxious (amnesic) (azaspiracid) (diarrheic)
      (neurotoxic) (paralytic) 988.0
  Staphylococcus, food 005.0
  toxic, from disease NEC 799.89
  truffles—*see* Poisoning, food
  uremic—*see* Uremia
  uric acid 274.9
  water 276.69
Poison ivy, oak, sumac or other plant
  dermatitis 692.6
Poker spine 720.0
Policeman's disease 729.2
Polioencephalitis (acute) (bulbar) (*see also*
  Poliomyelitis, bulbar) 045.0
  inferior 335.22
  influenzal (*see also* Influenza) 487.8
  superior hemorrhagic (acute) (Wernicke's)
    265.1
  Wernicke's (superior hemorrhagic) 265.1
Polioencephalomyelitis (acute) (anterior)
  (bulbar) (*see also* Polioencephalitis) 045.0
Polioencephalopathy, superior hemorrhagic
  265.1
  with
    beriberi 265.0
    pellagra 265.2
Poliomeningoencephalitis —*see*
  Meningoencephalitis
Poliomyelitis (acute) (anterior) (epidemic) 045.9

Note—Use the following fifth-digit
subclassification with category 045:

0 poliovirus, unspecified type
1 poliovirus, type I
2 poliovirus, type II
3 poliovirus, type III

  with
    paralysis 045.1
      bulbar 045.0
  abortive 045.2
  ascending 045.9
    progressive 045.9
  bulbar 045.0
  cerebral 045.0
  chronic 335.21

Poliomyelitis— *continued*
  congenital 771.2
  contact V01.2
  deformities 138
  exposure to V01.2
  late effect 138
  nonepidemic 045.9
  nonparalytic 045.2
  old with deformity 138
  posterior, acute 053.19
  residual 138
  sequelae 138
  spinal, acute 045.9
  syphilitic (chronic) 094.89
  vaccination, prophylactic (against) V04.0
Poliosis (eyebrow) (eyelashes) 704.3
  circumscripta (congenital) 757.4
    acquired 704.3
  congenital 757.4
Pollakiuria 788.41
  psychogenic 306.53
Pollinosis 477.0
Pollitzer's disease (hidradenitis suppurativa)
  705.83
Polyadenitis (*see also* Adenitis) 289.3
  malignant 020.0
Polyalgia 729.99
Polyangiitis (essential) 446.0
Polyarteritis (nodosa) (renal) 446.0
Polyarthralgia 719.49
  psychogenic 306.0
Polyarthritis, polyarthropathy NEC 716.59
  due to or associated with other specified
    conditions—*see* Arthritis, due to or
    associated with
  endemic (*see also* Disease, Kaschin-Beck) 716.0
  inflammatory 714.9
    specified type NEC 714.89
  juvenile (chronic) 714.30
    acute 714.31
  migratory—*see* Fever, rheumatic
  rheumatic 714.0
    fever (acute)—*see* Fever, rheumatic
Polycarential syndrome of infancy 260
Polychondritis (atrophic) (chronic) (relapsing)
  733.99
Polycoria 743.46
Polycystic (congenital) (disease) 759.89
  degeneration, kidney—*see* Polycystic, kidney
  kidney (congenital) 753.12
    adult type (APKD) 753.13
    autosomal dominant 753.13
    autosomal recessive 753.14
    childhood type (CPKD) 753.14
    infantile type 753.14
  liver 751.62
  lung 518.89
    congenital 748.4
  ovary, ovaries 256.4
  spleen 759.0
Polycythemia (primary) (rubra) (vera) (M9950/1)
  238.4
  acquired 289.0
  benign 289.0
    familial 289.6
  due to
    donor twin 776.4
    fall in plasma volume 289.0
    high altitude 289.0
    maternal-fetal transfusion 776.4
    stress 289.0

Polycythemia—*continued*
  emotional 289.0
  erythropoietin 289.0
  familial (benign) 289.6
  Gaisböck's (hypertonica) 289.0
  high altitude 289.0
  hypertonica 289.0
  hypoxemic 289.0
  neonatorum 776.4
  nephrogenous 289.0
  relative 289.0
  secondary 289.0
  spurious 289.0
  stress 289.0
Polycytosis cryptogenica 289.0
Polydactylism, polydactyly 755.00
  fingers 755.01
  toes 755.02
Polydipsia 783.5
Polydystrophic oligophrenia 277.5
Polyembryoma (M9072/3)—*see* Neoplasm, by
    site, malignant
Polygalactia 676.6
Polyglandular
  deficiency 258.9
  dyscrasia 258.9
  dysfunction 258.9
  syndrome 258.8
Polyhydramnios (*see also* Hydramnios) 657
Polymastia 757.6
Polymenorrhea 626.2
Polymicrogyria 742.2
Polymyalgia 725
  arteritica 446.5
  rheumatica 725
Polymyositis (acute) (chronic) (hemorrhagic) 710.4
  with involvement of
    lung 710.4 *[517.8]*
    skin 710.3
  ossificans (generalisata) (progressiva) 728.19
  Wagner's (dermatomyositis) 710.3
Polyneuritis, polyneuritic (*see also*
    Polyneuropathy) 356.9
  alcoholic 357.5
    with psychosis 291.1
  cranialis 352.6
  demyelinating, chronic inflammatory (CIDP)
    357.81
  diabetic 250.6 *[357.2]*
    due to secondary diabetes 249.6 *[357.2]*
  due to lack of vitamin NEC 269.2 *[357.4]*
  endemic 265.0 *[357.4]*
  erythredema 985.0
  febrile 357.0
  hereditary ataxic 356.3
  idiopathic, acute 357.0
  infective (acute) 357.0
  nutritional 269.9 *[357.4]*
  postinfectious 357.0
Polyneuropathy (peripheral) 356.9
  alcoholic 357.5
  amyloid 277.39 *[357.4]*
  arsenical 357.7
  critical illness 357.82
  demyelinating, chronic inflammatory (CIDP)
    357.81
  diabetic 250.6 *[357.2]*
    due to secondary diabetes 249.6 *[357.2]*

Polyneuropathy—*continued*
  due to
    antitetanus serum 357.6
    arsenic 357.7
    drug or medicinal substance 357.6
      correct substance properly administered 357.6
      overdose or wrong substance given or taken
        977.9
      specified drug—*see* Table of drugs and
        chemicals
    lack of vitamin NEC 269.2 *[357.4]*
    lead 357.7
    organophosphate compounds 357.7
    pellagra 265.2 *[357.4]*
    porphyria 277.1 *[357.4]*
    serum 357.6
    toxic agent NEC 357.7
  hereditary 356.0
  idiopathic 356.9
    progressive 356.4
  in
    amyloidosis 277.39 *[357.4]*
    avitaminosis 269.2 *[357.4]*
      specified NEC 269.1 *[357.4]*
    beriberi 265.0 *[357.4]*
    collagen vascular disease NEC 710.9 *[357.1]*
    deficiency
      B-complex NEC 266.2 *[357.4]*
      vitamin B 266.9 *[357.4]*
      vitamin B_6 266.1 *[357.4]*
    diabetes 250.6 *[357.2]*
      due to secondary diabetes 249.6 *[357.2]*
    diphtheria (*see also* Diphtheria) 032.89 *[357.4]*
    disseminated lupus erythematosus 710.0 *[357.1]*
    herpes zoster 053.13
    hypoglycemia 251.2 *[357.4]*
    malignant neoplasm (M8000/3) NEC 199.1
      [357.3]
    mumps 072.72
    pellagra 265.2 *[357.4]*
    polyarteritis nodosa 446.0 *[357.1]*
    porphyria 277.1 *[357.4]*
    rheumatoid arthritis 714.0 *[357.1]*
    sarcoidosis 135 *[357.4]*
    uremia 585.9 *[357.4]*
  lead 357.7
  nutritional 269.9 *[357.4]*
    specified NEC 269.8 *[357.4]*
  postherpetic 053.13
  progressive 356.4
  sensory (hereditary) 356.2
  specified NEC 356.8
Polyonychia 757.5
Polyopia 368.2
  refractive 368.15
Polyorchism, polyorchidism (three testes)
    752.89
Polyorrhymenitis (peritoneal) (*see also*
    Polyserositis) 568.82
  pericardial 423.2
Polyostotic fibrous dysplasia 756.54
Polyotia 744.1
Polyp, polypus

Note—*Polyps of organs or sites that do not
appear in the list below should be coded to the
residual category for diseases of the organ or
site concerned.*

  accessory sinus 471.8
  adenoid tissue 471.0

Polyp, polypus—*continued*
  adenomatous (M8210/0)—*see also* Neoplasm,
      by site, benign
    adenocarcinoma in (M8210/3)—*see*
        Neoplasm, by site, malignant
    carcinoma in (M8210/3)—*see* Neoplasm, by
        site, malignant
    multiple (M8221/0)—*see* Neoplasm, by site,
        benign
  antrum 471.8
  anus, anal (canal) (nonadenomatous) 569.0
    adenomatous 211.4
  Bartholin's gland 624.6
  bladder (M8120/1) 236.7
  broad ligament 620.8
  cervix (uteri) 622.7
    adenomatous 219.0
    in pregnancy or childbirth 654.6
      affecting fetus or newborn 763.89
      causing obstructed labor 660.2
    mucous 622.7
    nonneoplastic 622.7
  choanal 471.0
  cholesterol 575.6
  clitoris 624.6
  colon (M8210/0) (*see also* Polyp, adenomatous)
      211.3
  corpus uteri 621.0
  dental 522.0
  ear (middle) 385.30
  endometrium 621.0
  ethmoidal (sinus) 471.8
  fallopian tube 620.8
  female genital organs NEC 624.8
  frontal (sinus) 471.8
  gallbladder 575.6
  gingiva 523.8
  gum 523.8
  labia 624.6
  larynx (mucous) 478.4
  malignant (M8000/3)—*see* Neoplasm, by site,
      malignant
  maxillary (sinus) 471.8
  middle ear 385.30
  myometrium 621.0
  nares
    anterior 471.9
    posterior 471.0
  nasal (mucous) 471.9
    cavity 471.0
    septum 471.9
  nasopharyngeal 471.0
  neoplastic (M8210/0)—*see* Neoplasm, by site,
      benign
  nose (mucous) 471.9
  oviduct 620.8
  paratubal 620.8
  pharynx 478.29
    congenital 750.29
  placenta, placental 674.4
  prostate 600.20
    with
      other lower urinary tract symptoms (LUTS)
          600.21
      urinary
        obstruction 600.21
        retention 600.21
  pudenda 624.6
  pulp (dental) 522.0
  rectosigmoid 211.4

Polyp, polypus—*continued*
  rectum (nonadenomatous) 569.0
    adenomatous 211.4
  septum (nasal) 471.9
  sinus (accessory) (ethmoidal) (frontal)
      (maxillary) (sphenoidal) 471.8
  sphenoidal (sinus) 471.8
  stomach (M8210/0) 211.1
  tube, fallopian 620.8
  turbinate, mucous membrane 471.8
  ureter 593.89
  urethra 599.3
  uterine
    ligament 620.8
    tube 620.8
  uterus (body) (corpus) (mucous) 621.0
    in pregnancy or childbirth 654.1
      affecting fetus or newborn 763.89
      causing obstructed labor 660.2
  vagina 623.7
  vocal cord (mucous) 478.4
  vulva 624.6
Polyphagia 783.6
Polypoid —*see* condition
Polyposis —*see also* Polyp
  coli (adenomatous) (M8220/0) 211.3
    adenocarcinoma in (M8220/3) 153.9
    carcinoma in (M8220/3) 153.9
  familial (M8220/0) 211.3
  intestinal (adenomatous) (M8220/0) 211.3
  multiple (M8221/0)—*see* Neoplasm, by site,
      benign
Polyradiculitis (acute) 357.0
Polyradiculoneuropathy (acute) (segmentally
    demyelinating) 357.0
Polysarcia 278.00
Polyserositis (peritoneal) 568.82
  due to pericarditis 423.2
  paroxysmal (familial) 277.31
  pericardial 423.2
  periodic (familial) 277.31
  pleural—*see* Pleurisy
  recurrent 277.31
  tuberculous (*see also* Tuberculosis,
      polyserositis) 018.9
Polysialia 527.7
Polysplenia syndrome 759.0
Polythelia 757.6
Polytrichia (*see also* Hypertrichosis) 704.1
Polyunguia (congenital) 757.5
  acquired 703.8
Polyuria 788.42
Pompe's disease (glycogenosis II) 271.0
Pompholyx 705.81
Poncet's disease (tuberculous rheumatism) (*see
    also* Tuberculosis) 015.9
Pond fracture —*see* Fracture, skull, vault
Ponos 085.0
Pons, pontine —*see* condition
Poor
  aesthetics of existing restoration of tooth 525.67
  contractions, labor 661.2
    affecting fetus or newborn 763.7
  fetal growth NEC 764.9
    affecting management of pregnancy 656.5
  incorporation
    artificial skin graft 996.55
    decellularized allodermis graft 996.55

Poor —*continued*
  obstetrical history V13.49
    affecting management of current pregnancy V23.49
      ectopic pregnancy V23.42
      pre-term labor V23.41
    pre-term labor V13.41
  sucking reflex (newborn) 796.1
  vision NEC 369.9
Poradenitis, nostras 099.1
Porencephaly (congenital) (development) (true)
    742.4
  acquired 348.0
  nondevelopmental 348.0
  traumatic (post) 310.2
Porocephaliasis 134.1
Porokeratosis 757.39
  disseminated superficial actinic (DSAP) 692.75
Poroma, eccrine (M8402/0)—*see* Neoplasm,
    skin, benign
Porphyria (acute) (congenital) (constitutional)
    (erythropoietic) (familial) (hepatica)
    (idiopathic) (idiosyncratic) (intermittent)
    (latent) (mixed hepatic) (photosensitive)
    (South African genetic) (Swedish) 277.1
  acquired 277.1
  cutaneatarda
    hereditaria 277.1
    symptomatica 277.1
  due to drugs
    correct substance properly administered 277.1
    overdose or wrong substance given or taken 977.9
      specified drug—*see* Table of drugs and
        chemicals
  secondary 277.1
  toxic NEC 277.1
  variegata 277.1
Porphyrinuria (acquired) (congenital)
    (secondary) 277.1
Porphyruria (acquired) (congenital) 277.1
Portal —*see* condition
Port wine nevus or mark 757.32
Posadas-Wernicke disease 114.9
Position
  fetus, abnormal (*see also* Presentation, fetal) 652.9
  teeth, faulty (*see also* Anomaly, position tooth)
    524.30
Positive
  culture (nonspecific) 795.39
    AIDS virus V08
    blood 790.7
    HIV V08
    human immunodeficiency virus V08
    nose 795.39
      Staphylococcus — *see* Carrier (suspected)
        of, Staphylococcus
    skin lesion NEC 795.39
    spinal fluid 792.0
    sputum 795.39
    stool 792.1
    throat 795.39
    urine 791.9
    wound 795.39
  findings, anthrax 795.31
  HIV V08
  human immunodeficiency virus (HIV) V08
  PPD 795.51
  serology
    AIDS virus V08
      inconclusive 795.71

Positive— *continued*
  serology—*continued*
    HIV V08
      inconclusive 795.71
    human immunodeficiency virus V08
      inconclusive 795.71
    syphilis 097.1
      with signs or symptoms—*see* Syphilis, by
        site and stage
      false 795.6
    skin test 795.7
    tuberculin (without active tuberculosis) 795.51
    VDRL 097.1
      with signs or symptoms—*see* Syphilis, by site
        and stage
      false 795.6
    Wassermann reaction 097.1
      false 795.6
Postcardiotomy syndrome 429.4
Postcaval ureter 753.4
Postcholecystectomy syndrome 576.0
Postclimacteric bleeding 627.1
Postcommissurotomy syndrome 429.4
Postconcussional syndrome 310.2
Postcontusional syndrome 310.2
Postcricoid region —*see* condition
Post-dates (pregnancy) —*see* Pregnancy
Postencephalitic —*see also* condition
  syndrome 310.89
Posterior —*see* condition
Posterolateral sclerosis (spinal cord)—*see*
  Degeneration, combined
Postexanthematous —*see* condition
Postfebrile —*see* condition
Postgastrectomy dumping syndrome 564.2
Posthemiplegic chorea 344.89
Posthemorrhagic anemia (chronic) 280.0
  acute 285.1
  newborn 776.5
Posthepatitis syndrome 780.79
Postherpetic neuralgia (intercostal) (syndrome)
    (zoster) 053.19
  geniculate ganglion 053.11
  ophthalmica 053.19
  trigeminal 053.12
Posthitis 607.1
Postimmunization complication or reaction
    —*see* Complications, vaccination
Postinfectious —*see* condition
Postinfluenzal syndrome 780.79
Postlaminectomy syndrome 722.80
  cervical, cervicothoracic 722.81
  kyphosis 737.12
  lumbar, lumbosacral 722.83
  thoracic, thoracolumbar 722.82
Postleukotomy syndrome 310.0
Postlobectomy syndrome 310.0
Postmastectomy lymphedema (syndrome) 457.0
Postmaturity, postmature (fetus or newborn)
    (gestation period over 42 completed weeks)
    766.22
  affecting management of pregnancy
    post-term pregnancy 645.1
    prolonged pregnancy 645.2
  syndrome 766.22
Postmeasles —*see also* condition
  complication 055.8
    specified NEC 055.79

Postmenopausal
  endometrium (atrophic) 627.8
    suppurative (*see also* Endometritis) 615.9
  hormone replacement therapy V07.4
  status (age related) (natural) V49.81
Postnasal drip 784.91
Postnatal —*see* condition
Postoperative —*see also* condition
  confusion state 293.9
  psychosis 293.9
  status NEC (*see also* Status (post)) V45.89
Postpancreatectomy hyperglycemia 251.3
Postpartum —*see also* condition
  anemia 648.2
  cardiomyopathy 674.5
  observation
    immediately after delivery V24.0
    routine follow-up V24.2
Postperfusion syndrome NEC 999.89
  bone marrow 996.85
Postpoliomyelitic —*see* condition
Postsurgery status NEC (*see also* Status (post))
  V45.89
Post-term (pregnancy) 645.1
  infant (gestation period over 40 completed
    weeks to 42 completed weeks) 766.21
Post-transplant lymphoproliferative disorder
  (PTLD) 238.77
Posttraumatic —*see* condition
Posttraumatic brain syndrome, nonpsychotic
  310.2
Post-Traumatic Stress Disorder (PTSD) 309.81
Post-typhoid abscess 002.0
Postures, hysterical 300.11
Postvaccinal reaction or complication —*see*
  Complications, vaccination
Postvagotomy syndrome 564.2
Postvalvulotomy syndrome 429.4
Postvasectomy sperm count V25.8
Potain's disease (pulmonary edema) 514
Potain's syndrome (gastrectasis with dyspepsia)
  536.1
Pott's
  curvature (spinal) (*see also* Tuberculosis) 015.0
    [737.43]
  disease or paraplegia (*see also* Tuberculosis)
    015.0 *[730.88]*
  fracture (closed) 824.4
    open 824.5
  gangrene 440.24
  osteomyelitis (*see also* Tuberculosis) 015.0 *[730.88]*
  spinal curvature (*see also* Tuberculosis) 015.0
    [737.43]
  tumor, puffy (*see also* Osteomyelitis) 730.2
Potter's
  asthma 502
  disease 753.0
  facies 754.0
  lung 502
  syndrome (with renal agenesis) 753.0
Pouch
  bronchus 748.3
  Douglas'—*see* condition
  esophagus, esophageal (congenital) 750.4
    acquired 530.6
  gastric 537.1
  Hartmann's (abnormal sacculation of
    gallbladder neck) 575.8
    of intestine V44.3
      attention to V55.3
  pharynx, pharyngeal (congenital) 750.27

Pouchitis 569.71
Poulet's disease 714.2
Poultrymen's itch 133.8
Poverty V60.2
PPE (plamar plantar erythrodysesthesia) 693.0
Prader-Labhart-Willi-Fanconi syndrome
  (hypogenital dystrophy with diabetic
  tendency) 759.81
Prader-Willi syndrome (hypogenital dystrophy
  with diabetic tendency) 759.81
Preachers' voice 784.49
Pre-AIDS —*see* Human immunodeficiency virus
  (disease) (illness) (infection)
Preauricular appendage 744.1
Prebetalipoproteinemia (acquired) (essential)
  (familial) (hereditary) (primary) (secondary)
  272.1
  with chylomicronemia 272.3
Precipitate labor 661.3
  affecting fetus or newborn 763.6
Preclimacteric bleeding 627.0
  menorrhagia 627.0
Precocious
  adrenarche 259.1
  menarche 259.1
  menstruation 259.1
  pubarche 259.1
  puberty NEC 259.1
  sexual development NEC 259.1
  thelarche 259.1
Precocity, sexual (constitutional) (cryptogenic)
  (female) (idiopathic) (male) NEC 259.1
  with adrenal hyperplasia 255.2
Precordial pain 786.51
  psychogenic 307.89
Predeciduous teeth 520.2
Prediabetes, prediabetic 790.29
  complicating pregnancy, childbirth, or
    puerperium 648.8
  fetus or newborn 775.89
Predislocation status of hip, at birth (*see also*
  Subluxation, congenital, hip) 754.32
Pre-eclampsia (mild) 642.4
  with pre-existing hypertension 642.7
  affecting fetus or newborn 760.0
  severe 642.5
  superimposed on pre-existing hypertensive
    disease 642.7
Preeruptive color change, teeth, tooth 520.8
Preexcitation 426.7
  atrioventricular conduction 426.7
  ventricular 426.7
Preglaucoma 365.00
Pregnancy (single) (uterine) (without sickness)
  V22.2

---

*Note—Use the following fifth-digit
subclassification with categories 640-649,
651-679:*

0 unspecified as to episode of care
*1 delivered, with or without mention of
    antepartum condition*
*2 delivered, with mention of postpartum
    complication*
3 antepartum condition or complication
4 postpartum condition or complication

---

  abdominal (ectopic) 633.00
    affecting fetus or newborn 761.4
    with intrauterine pregnancy 633.01

Pregnancy—*continued*
abnormal NEC 646.9
ampullar—*see* Pregnancy, tubal
biochemical 631.0
broad ligament—*see* Pregnancy, cornual
cervical—*see* Pregnancy, cornual
chemical 631.0
combined (extrauterine and intrauterine)—*see*
Pregnancy, cornual
complicated (by) 646.9
abnormal, abnormality NEC 646.9
cervix 654.6
cord (umbilical) 663.9
glucose tolerance (conditions classifiable to
790.21-790.29) 648.8
pelvic organs or tissues NEC 654.9
pelvis (bony) 653.0
perineum or vulva 654.8
placenta, placental (vessel) 656.7
position
cervix 654.4
placenta 641.1
without hemorrhage 641.0
uterus 654.4
size, fetus 653.5
uterus (congenital) 654.0
abscess or cellulitis
bladder 646.6
genitourinary tract (conditions classifiable to
590, 595, 597, 599.0, 614.0-614.5,
614.7-614.9, 615) 646.6
kidney 646.6
urinary tract NEC 646.6
adhesion, pelvic peritoneal 648.9
air embolism 673.0
albuminuria 646.2
with hypertension—*see* Toxemia, of
pregnancy
amnionitis 658.4
amniotic fluid embolism 673.1
anemia (conditions classifiable to 280-285)
648.2
appendicitis 648.9
atrophy, yellow (acute) (liver) (subacute) 646.7
bacilluria, asymptomatic 646.5
bacteriuria, asymptomatic 646.5
bariatric surgery status 649.2
bicornis or bicornuate uterus 654.0
biliary problems 646.8
bone and joint disorders (conditions
classifiable to 720-724 or conditions
affecting lower limbs classifiable to
711-719, 725-738) 648.7
breech presentation 652.2
with successful version 652.1
cardiovascular disease (conditions classifiable
to 390-398, 410-429) 648.6
congenital (conditions classifiable to
745-747) 648.5
cerebrovascular disorders conditions
(classifiable to 430-434, 436-437) 674.0
cervicitis (conditions classifiable to 616.0)
646.6
chloasma (gravidarum) 646.8
cholelithiasis 646.8
cholestasis 646.7
chorea (gravidarum)—*see* Eclampsia,
pregnancy
coagulation defect 649.3
conjoined twins 678.1

Pregnancy—*continued*
complicated by—*continued*
contraction, pelvis (general) 653.1
inlet 653.2
outlet 653.3
convulsions (eclamptic) (uremic) 642.6
with pre-existing hypertension 642.7
current disease or condition (nonobstetric)
abnormal glucose tolerance 648.8
anemia 648.2
biliary tract 646.7
bone and joint (lower limb) 648.7
cardiovascular 648.6
congenital 648.5
cerebrovascular 674.0
diabetes (conditions classifiable to 249 and
250) 648.0
drug dependence 648.3
female genital mutilation 648.9
genital organ or tract 646.6
gonorrheal 647.1
hypertensive 642.2
chronic kidney 642.2
renal 642.1
infectious 647.9
specified type NEC 647.8
liver 646.7
malarial 647.4
nutritional deficiency 648.9
parasitic NEC 647.8
periodontal disease 648.9
renal 646.2
hypertensive 642.1
rubella 647.5
specified condition NEC 648.9
syphilitic 647.0
thyroid 648.1
tuberculous 647.3
urinary 646.6
venereal 647.2
viral NEC 647.6
cystitis 646.6
cystocele 654.4
death of fetus (near term) 656.4
early pregnancy (before 22 completed weeks
gestation) 632
deciduitis 646.6
decreased fetal movements 655.7
diabetes (mellitus) (conditions classifiable to
249 and 250) 648.0
disorders of liver and biliary tract 646.7
displacement, uterus NEC 654.4
disproportion—*see* Disproportion
double uterus 654.0
drug dependence (conditions classifiable to
304) 648.3
dysplasia, cervix 654.6
early onset of delivery (spontaneous) 644.2
eclampsia, eclamptic (coma) (convulsions)
(delirium) (nephritis) (uremia) 642.6
with pre-existing hypertension 642.7
edema 646.1
with hypertension—*see* Toxemia, of
pregnancy
effusion, amniotic fluid 658.1
delayed delivery following 658.2
embolism
air 673.0
amniotic fluid 673.1
blood-clot 673.2
cerebral 674.0

Pregnancy—*continued*
  complicated by—*continued*
    embolism—*continued*
      pulmonary NEC 673.2
      pyemic 673.3
      septic 673.3
    emesis (gravidarum)—*see* Pregnancy,
      complicated, vomiting
    endometritis (conditions classifiable to
      615.0-615.9) 670.1
      decidual 646.6
    epilepsy 649.4
    excessive weight gain NEC 646.1
    face presentation 652.4
    failure, fetal head to enter pelvic brim 652.5
    false labor (pains) 644.1
    fatigue 646.8
    fatty metamorphosis of liver 646.7
    female genital mutilation 648.9
    fetal
      anemia 678.0
      complications from in utero procedure 679.1
      conjoined twins 678.1
      death (near term) 656.4
        early (before 22 completed weeks
          gestation) 632
      deformity 653.7
      distress 656.8
      hematologic conditions 678.0
      reduction of multiple fetuses reduced to
        single fetus 651.7
      thrombocytopenia 678.0
      twin to twin transfusion 678.0
    fibroid (tumor) (uterus) 654.1
    footling presentation 652.8
      with successful version 652.1
    gallbladder disease 646.8
    gastric banding status 649.2
    gastric bypass status for obesity 649.2
    genital herpes (asymptomatic) (history of)
      (inactive) 647.6
    goiter 648.1
    gonococcal infection (conditions classifiable
      to 098) 647.1
    gonorrhea (conditions classifiable to 098)
      647.1
    hemorrhage 641.9
      accidental 641.2
      before 22 completed weeks gestation NEC
        640.9
      cerebrovascular 674.0
      due to
        afibrinogenemia or other coagulation
          defect (conditions classifiable to
          286.0-286.9) 641.3
        leiomyoma, uterine 641.8
        marginal sinus (rupture) 641.2
        premature separation, placenta 641.2
        trauma 641.8
      early (before 22 completed weeks gestation)
        640.9
      threatened abortion 640.0
      unavoidable 641.1
    hepatitis (acute) (malignant) (subacute) 646.7
      viral 647.6
    herniation of uterus 654.4
    high head at term 652.5
    hydatidiform mole (delivered) (undelivered)
      630
    hydramnios 657
    hydrocephalic fetus 653.6

Pregnancy—*continued*
  complicated by—*continued*
    hydrops amnii 657
    hydrorrhea 658.1
    hyperemesis (gravidarum)—*see* Hyperemesis,
      gravidarum
    hypertension—*see* Hypertension, complicating
      pregnancy
    hypertensive heart and chronic kidney disease
      642.2
    hypertensive
      chronic kidney disease 642.2
      heart and chronic kidney disease 642.2
      heart and renal disease 642.2
      heart disease 642.2
      renal disease 642.2
    hyperthyroidism 648.1
    hypothyroidism 648.1
    hysteralgia 646.8
    icterus gravis 646.7
    incarceration, uterus 654.3
    incompetent cervix (os) 654.5
    infection 647.9
      amniotic fluid 658.4
      bladder 646.6
      genital organ (conditions classifiable to
        614.0-614.5, 614.7-614.9, 615) 646.6
      kidney (conditions classifiable to
        590.0-590.9) 646.6
      urinary (tract) 646.6
        asymptomatic 646.5
    infective and parasitic diseases NEC 647.8
    inflammation
      bladder 646.6
      genital organ (conditions classifiable to
        614.0-614.5, 614.7-614.9, 615) 646.6
      urinary tract NEC 646.6
    injury 648.9
      obstetrical NEC 665.9
    insufficient weight gain 646.8
    insulin resistance 648.8
    intrauterine fetal death (near term) NEC 656.4
      early (before 22 completed weeks'
        gestation) 632
    malaria (conditions classifiable to 084) 647.4
    malformation, uterus (congenital) 654.0
    malnutrition (conditions classifiable to
      260-269) 648.9
    malposition
      fetus—*see* Pregnancy, complicated,
        malpresentation
      uterus or cervix 654.4
    malpresentation 652.9
      with successful version 652.1
      in multiple gestation 652.6
      specified type NEC 652.8
    marginal sinus hemorrhage or rupture 641.2
    maternal complications from in utero
      procedure 679.0
    maternal drug abuse 648.4
    maternal obesity syndrome 646.1
    menstruation 640.8
    mental disorders (conditions classifiable to
      290-303, 305.0, 305.2-305.9, 306-316,
      317-319) 648.4
    mentum presentation 652.4
    missed
      abortion 632
      delivery (at or near term) 656.4
      labor (at or near term) 656.4

Pregnancy—*continued*
  complicated by—*continued*
    necrosis
      genital organ or tract (conditions classifiable
        to 614.0-614.5, 614.7-614.9, 615) 646.6
      liver (conditions classifiable to 570) 646.7
      renal, cortical 646.2
    nephritis or nephrosis (conditions classifiable
      to 580-589) 646.2
      with hypertension 642.1
    nephropathy NEC 646.2
    neuritis (peripheral) 646.4
    nutritional deficiency (conditions classifiable
      to 260-269) 648.9
    obesity 649.1
      surgery status 649.2
    oblique lie or presentation 652.3
      with successful version 652.1
    obstetrical trauma NEC 665.9
    oligohydramnios NEC 658.0
    onset of contractions before 37 weeks 644.0
    oversize fetus 653.5
    papyraceous fetus 646.0
    patent cervix 654.5
    pelvic inflammatory disease (conditions
      classifiable to 614.0-614.5, 614.7-614.9,
      615) 646.6
    pelvic peritoneal adhesion 648.9
    placenta, placental
      abnormality 656.7
      abruptio or ablatio 641.2
      detachment 641.2
      disease 656.7
      infarct 656.7
      low implantation 641.1
        without hemorrhage 641.0
      malformation 656.7
      malposition 641.1
        without hemorrhage 641.0
      marginal sinus hemorrhage 641.2
      previa 641.1
        without hemorrhage 641.0
      separation (premature) (undelivered) 641.2
    placentitis 658.4
    pneumonia 648.9
    polyhydramnios 657
    postmaturity
      post-term 645.1
      prolonged 645.2
    prediabetes 648.8
    pre-eclampsia (mild) 642.4
      severe 642.5
      superimposed on pre-existing hypertensive
        disease 642.7
    premature rupture of membranes 658.1
      with delayed delivery 658.2
    previous
      ectopic pregnancy V23.42
      infertility V23.0
      in utero procedure during previous
        pregnancy V23.86
      nonobstetric condition V23.8
      poor obstetrical history V23.49
      premature delivery V23.41
      trophoblastic disease (conditions classifiable
        to 630) V23.1
    prolapse, uterus 654.4
    proteinuria (gestational) 646.2
      with hypertension—*see* Toxemia, of
        pregnancy
    pruritus (neurogenic) 646.8

Pregnancy—*continued*
  complicated by—*continued*
    psychosis or psychoneurosis 648.4
    ptyalism 646.8
    pyelitis (conditions classifiable to
      590.0-590.9) 646.6
    renal disease or failure NEC 646.2
      with secondary hypertension 642.1
      hypertensive 642.2
    retention, retained dead ovum 631.8
    retroversion, uterus 654.3
    Rh immunization, incompatibility, or
      sensitization 656.1
    rubella (conditions classifiable to 056) 647.5
    rupture
      amnion (premature) 658.1
        with delayed delivery 658.2
      marginal sinus (hemorrhage) 641.2
      membranes (premature) 658.1
        with delayed delivery 658.2
      uterus (before onset of labor) 665.0
    salivation (excessive) 646.8
    salpingo-oophoritis (conditions classifiable to
      614.0-614.2) 646.6
    septicemia (conditions classifiable to
      038.0-038.9) 647.8
      postpartum 670.2
      puerperal 670.2
    smoking 649.0
    spasms, uterus (abnormal) 646.8
    specified condition NEC 646.8
    spotting 649.5
    spurious labor pains 644.1
    status post
      bariatric surgery 649.2
      gastric banding 649.2
      gastric bypass for obesity 649.2
      obesity surgery 649.2
    superfecundation 651.9
    superfetation 651.9
    syphilis (conditions classifiable to 090-097)
      647.0
    threatened
      abortion 640.0
      premature delivery 644.2
      premature labor 644.0
    thrombophlebitis (superficial) 671.2
      deep 671.3
      septic 670.3
    thrombosis 671.2
      venous (superficial) 671.2
      deep 671.3
    thyroid dysfunction (conditions classifiable to
      240-246) 648.1
    thyroiditis 648.1
    thyrotoxicosis 648.1
    tobacco use disorder 649.0
    torsion of uterus 654.4
    toxemia—*see* Toxemia, of pregnancy
    transverse lie or presentation 652.3
      with successful version 652.1
    trauma 648.9
      obstetrical 665.9
    tuberculosis (conditions classifiable to
      010-018) 647.3
    tumor
      cervix 654.6
      ovary 654.4
      pelvic organs or tissue NEC 654.4
      uterus (body) 654.1
        cervix 654.6

Pregnancy—*continued*
complicated by—*continued*
tumor—*continued*
vagina 654.7
vulva 654.8
unstable lie 652.0
uremia—*see* Pregnancy, complicated, renal disease
urethritis 646.6
vaginitis or vulvitis (conditions classifiable to 616.1) 646.6
varicose
placental vessels 656.7
veins (legs) 671.0
perineum 671.1
vulva 671.1
varicosity, labia or vulva 671.1
venereal disease NEC (conditions classifiable to 099) 647.2
venous complication 671.9
viral disease NEC (conditions classifiable to 042, 050-055, 057-079, 795.05, 795.15, 796.75) 647.6
vomiting (incoercible) (pernicious) (persistent) (uncontrollable) (vicious) 643.9
due to organic disease or other cause 643.8
early—*see* Hyperemesis, gravidarum
late (after 22 completed weeks gestation) 643.2
young maternal age 659.8
complications NEC 646.9
cornual 633.80
affecting fetus or newborn 761.4
with intrauterine pregnancy 633.81
death, maternal NEC 646.9
delivered—*see* Delivery
ectopic (ruptured) NEC 633.90
with intrauterine pregnancy 633.91
abdominal—*see* Pregnancy, abdominal
affecting fetus or newborn 761.4
combined (extrauterine and intrauterine)—*see* Pregnancy, cornual
ovarian—*see* Pregnancy, ovarian
specified type NEC 633.80
affecting fetus or newborn 761.4
with intrauterine pregnancy 633.81
tubal—*see* Pregnancy, tubal
examination, pregnancy
negative result V72.41
not confirmed V72.40
positive result V72.42
extrauterine—*see* Pregnancy, ectopic
fallopian—*see* Pregnancy, tubal
false 300.11
labor (pains) 644.1
fatigue 646.8
illegitimate V61.6
incidental finding V22.2
in double uterus 654.0
interstitial—*see* Pregnancy, cornual
intraligamentous—*see* Pregnancy, cornual
intramural—*see* Pregnancy, cornual
intraperitoneal—*see* Pregnancy, abdominal
isthmian—*see* Pregnancy, tubal
management affected by
abnormal, abnormality
fetus (suspected) 655.9
specified NEC 655.8
placenta 656.7
advanced maternal age NEC 659.6
multigravida 659.6
primigravida 659.5

Pregnancy—*continued*
management affected by—*continued*
antibodies (maternal)
anti-c 656.1
anti-d 656.1
anti-e 656.1
blood group (ABO) 656.2
Rh(esus) 656.1
appendicitis 648.9
bariatric surgery status 649.2
coagulation defect 649.3
elderly multigravida 659.6
elderly primigravida 659.5
epilepsy 649.4
fetal (suspected)
abnormality 655.9
abdominal 655.8
acid-base balance 656.8
cardiovascular 655.8
facial 655.8
gastrointestinal 655.8
genitourinary 655.8
heart rate or rhythm 659.7
limb 655.8
specified NEC 655.8
acidemia 656.3
anencephaly 655.0
aneuploidy 655.1
bradycardia 659.7
central nervous system malformation 655.0
chromosomal abnormalities (conditions classifiable to 758.0-758.9) 655.1
damage from
drugs 655.5
obstetric, anesthetic, or sedative 655.5
environmental toxins 655.8
intrauterine contraceptive device 655.8
maternal
alcohol addiction 655.4
disease NEC 655.4
drug use 655.5
listeriosis 655.4
rubella 655.3
toxoplasmosis 655.4
viral infection 655.3
radiation 655.6
death (near term) 656.4
early (before 22 completed weeks gestation) 632
distress 656.8
excessive growth 656.6
growth retardation 656.5
hereditary disease 655.2
hydrocephalus 655.0
intrauterine death 656.4
poor growth 656.5
spina bifida (with myelomeningocele) 655.0
fetal-maternal hemorrhage 656.0
gastric banding status 649.2
gastric bypass status for obesity 649.2
hereditary disease in family (possibly) affecting fetus 655.2
incompatibility, blood groups (ABO) 656.2
rh(esus) 656.1
insufficient prenatal care V23.7
insulin resistance 648.8
intrauterine death 656.4
isoimmunization (ABO) 656.2
rh(esus) 656.1
large-for-dates fetus 656.6
light-for-dates fetus 656.5

Pregnancy—*continued*
  management affected by—*continued*
    meconium in liquor 656.8
    mental disorder (conditions classifiable to
      290-303, 305.0, 305.2-305.9, 306-316,
      317-319) 648.4
    multiparity (grand) 659.4
    obesity 649.1
      surgery status 649.2
    poor obstetric history V23.49
      pre-term labor V23.41
    postmaturity
      post-term 645.1
      prolonged 645.2
    post-term pregnancy 645.1
    previous
      abortion V23.2
        habitual 646.3
      cesarean delivery 654.2
      difficult delivery V23.49
      ectopic pregnancy V23.42
      forceps delivery V23.49
      habitual abortions 646.3
      hemorrhage, antepartum or postpartum
        V23.49
      hydatidiform mole V23.1
      infertility V23.0
      in utero procedure during previous
        pregnancy V23.86
      malignancy NEC V23.8
      nonobstetrical conditions V23.8
      premature delivery V23.41
      recurrent pregnancy loss 646.3
      trophoblastic disease (conditions in 630)
        V23.1
      vesicular mole V23.1
    prolonged pregnancy 645.2
    recurrent pregnancy loss 646.3
    small-for-dates fetus 656.5
    smoking 649.0
    spotting 649.5
    suspected conditions not found
      amniotic cavity and membrane problem
        V89.01
      cervical shortening V89.05
      fetal anomaly V89.03
      fetal growth problem V89.04
      oligohydramnios V89.01
      other specified problem NEC V89.09
      placental problem V89.02
      polyhydramnios V89.01
    tobacco use disorder 649.0
    venous complication 671.9
    young maternal age 659.8
  maternal death NEC 646.9
  mesometric (mural)—*see* Pregnancy, cornual
  molar 631.8
    hydatidiform (*see also* Hydatidiform mole)
      630
      previous, affecting management of
        pregnancy V23.1
    previous, affecting management of pregnancy
      V23.49
  multiple NEC 651.9
    with fetal loss and retention of one or more
      fetus(es) 651.6
    affecting fetus or newborn 761.5
    following (elective) fetal reduction 651.7
    specified type NEC 651.8
      with fetal loss and retention of one or more
        fetus(es) 651.6
      following (elective) fetal reduction 651.7

Pregnancy—*continued*
  mural—*see* Pregnancy, cornual
  observation NEC V22.1
    first pregnancy V22.0
    high-risk V23.9
      inconclusive fetal viability V23.87
      specified problem NEC V23.8
  ovarian 633.20
    affecting fetus or newborn 761.4
    with intrauterine pregnancy 633.21
  possible, not (yet) confirmed V72.40
  postmature
    post-term 645.1
    prolonged 645.2
  post-term 645.1
  prenatal care only V22.1
    first pregnancy V22.0
    high-risk V23.9
      inconclusive fetal viability V23.87
      specified problem NEC V23.8
  prolonged 645.2
  resulting from
    assisted reproductive technology V23.85
    in vitro fertilization V23.85
  quadruplet NEC 651.2
    with fetal loss and retention of one or more
      fetus(es) 651.5
    affecting fetus or newborn 761.5
    following (elective) fetal reduction 651.7
  quintuplet NEC 651.8
    with fetal loss and retention of one or more
      fetus(es) 651.6
    affecting fetus or newborn 761.5
    following (elective) fetal reduction 651.7
  sextuplet NEC 651.8
    with fetal loss and retention of one or more
      fetus(es) 651.6
    affecting fetus or newborn 761.5
    following (elective) fetal reduction 651.7
  spurious 300.11
  superfecundation NEC 651.9
    with fetal loss and retention of one or more
      fetus(es) 651.6
    following (elective) fetal reduction 651.7
  superfetation NEC 651.9
    with fetal loss and retention of one or more
      fetus(es) 651.6
    following (elective) fetal reduction 651.7
  supervision (of) (for)—*see also* Pregnancy,
    management affected by
    elderly
      multigravida V23.82
      primigravida V23.81
    high-risk V23.9
      inconclusive fetal viability V23.87
      insufficient prenatal care V23.7
      specified problem NEC V23.8
    inconclusive fetal viability V23.87
    multiparity V23.3
    normal NEC V22.1
      first V22.0
    poor
      obstetric history V23.49
        ectopic pregnancy V23.42
        pre-term labor V23.41
      reproductive history V23.5
    previous
      abortion V23.2
      hydatidiform mole V23.1
      infertility V23.0
      neonatal death V23.5
      stillbirth V23.5

Pregnancy—*continued*
  supervision—*continued*
    trophoblastic disease V23.1
      vesicular mole V23.1
    specified problem NEC V23.8
    young
      multigravida V23.84
      primigravida V23.83
  triplet NEC 651.1
    with fetal loss and retention of one or more
        fetus(es) 651.4
    affecting fetus or newborn 761.5
    following (elective) fetal reduction 651.7
  tubal (with rupture) 633.10
    affecting fetus or newborn 761.4
    with intrauterine pregnancy 633.11
  twin NEC 651.0
    with fetal loss and retention of one or more
        fetus(es) 651.3
    affecting fetus or newborn 761.5
    conjoined 678.1
    following (elective) fetal reduction 651.7
  unconfirmed V72.40
  undelivered (no other diagnosis) V22.2
    with false labor 644.1
    high-risk V23.9
      specified problem NEC V23.8
  unwanted NEC V61.7
Pregnant uterus —*see* condition
Preiser's disease (osteoporosis) 733.09
Prekwashiorkor 260
Preleukemia 238.75
Preluxation of hip, congenital (*see also*
  Subluxation, congenital, hip) 754.32
Premature —*see also* condition
  beats (nodal) 427.60
    atrial 427.61
    auricular 427.61
    postoperative 997.1
    specified type NEC 427.69
    supraventricular 427.61
    ventricular 427.69
  birth NEC 765.1
  closure
    cranial suture 756.0
    fontanel 756.0
    foramen ovale 745.8
  contractions 427.60
    atrial 427.61
    auricular 427.61
    auriculoventricular 427.61
    heart (extrasystole) 427.60
    junctional 427.60
    nodal 427.60
    postoperative 997.1
    ventricular 427.69
  ejaculation 302.75
  infant NEC 765.1
    excessive 765.0
    light-for-dates—*see* Light-for-dates
  labor 644.2
    threatened 644.0
  lungs 770.4
  menopause 256.31
  puberty 259.1
  rupture of membranes or amnion 658.1
    affecting fetus or newborn 761.1
    delayed delivery following 658.2
  senility (syndrome) 259.8
  separation, placenta (partial)—*see* Placenta,
      separation
  ventricular systole 427.69

Prematurity NEC 765.1
  extreme 765.0
Premenstrual syndrome 625.4
Premenstrual tension 625.4
Premolarization, cuspids 520.2
Premyeloma 273.1
Prenatal
  care, normal pregnancy V22.1
    first V22.0
  death, cause unknown—*see* Death, fetus
  screening—*see* Antenatal, screening
  teeth 520.6
Prepartum —*see* condition
Preponderance, left or right ventricular 429.3
Prepuce —*see* condition
PRES (posterior reversible encephalopathy
  syndrome) 348.39
Presbycardia 797
  hypertensive (*see also* Hypertension, heart) 402.90
Presbycusis 388.01
Presbyesophagus 530.89
Presbyophrenia 310.1
Presbyopia 367.4
Prescription of contraceptives NEC V25.02
  diaphragm V25.02
  oral (pill) V25.01
    emergency V25.03
    postcoital V25.03
    repeat V25.41
  repeat V25.40
    oral (pill) V25.41
Presenile —*see also* condition
  aging 259.8
  dementia (*see also* Dementia, presenile) 290.10
Presenility 259.8
Presentation, fetal
  abnormal 652.9
    with successful version 652.1
    before labor, affecting fetus or newborn 761.7
    causing obstructed labor 660.0
      affecting fetus or newborn, any, except
          breech 763.1
    in multiple gestation (one or more) 652.6
    specified NEC 652.8
  arm 652.7
    causing obstructed labor 660.0
  breech (buttocks) (complete) (frank) 652.2
    with successful version 652.1
    before labor, affecting fetus or newborn
        761.7
    before labor, affecting fetus or newborn 761.7
  brow 652.4
    causing obstructed labor 660.0
  buttocks 652.2
  chin 652.4
  complete 652.2
  compound 652.8
  cord 663.0
  extended head 652.4
  face 652.4
    to pubes 652.8
  footling 652.8
  frank 652.2
  hand, leg, or foot NEC 652.8
  incomplete 652.8
  mentum 652.4
  multiple gestation (one fetus or more) 652.6
  oblique 652.3
    with successful version 652.1
  shoulder 652.8
    affecting fetus or newborn 763.1

Presentation, fetal—*continued*
  transverse 652.3
    with successful version 652.1
  umbilical cord 663.0
  unstable 652.0
Prespondylolisthesis (congenital) (lumbosacral)
  756.11
Pressure
  area, skin ulcer (*see also* Ulcer, pressure) 707.00
  atrophy, spine 733.99
  birth, fetus or newborn NEC 767.9
  brachial plexus 353.0
  brain 348.4
    injury at birth 767.0
  cerebral—*see* Pressure, brain
  chest 786.59
  cone, tentorial 348.4
    injury at birth 767.0
  funis—*see* Compression, umbilical cord
  hyposystolic (*see also* Hypotension) 458.9
  increased
    intracranial 781.99
      due to
        benign intracranial hypertension 348.2
        hydrocephalus—*see* hydrocephalus
        injury at birth 767.8
      intraocular 365.00
  lumbosacral plexus 353.1
  mediastinum 519.3
  necrosis (chronic) (skin) (*see also* Decubitus)
    707.00
  nerve—*see* Compression, nerve
  paralysis (*see also* Neuropathy, entrapment) 355.9
  pre-ulcer skin changes limited to persistent focal
    erythema (*see also* Ulcer, pressure) 707.21
  sore (chronic) (*see also* Ulcer, pressure) 707.00
  spinal cord 336.9
  ulcer (chronic) (*see also* Ulcer, pressure) 707.00
  umbilical cord—*see* Compression, umbilical cord
  venous, increased 459.89
Pre-syncope 780.2
Preterm infant NEC 765.1
  extreme 765.0
Priapism (penis) 607.3
Prickling sensation (*see also* Disturbance,
  sensation) 782.0
Prickly heat 705.1
Primary —*see also* condition
  angle closure suspect 365.02
Primigravida, elderly
  affecting
    fetus or newborn 763.89
    management of pregnancy, labor, and delivery
      659.5
Primipara, old
  affecting
    fetus or newborn 763.89
    management of pregnancy, labor, and delivery
      659.5
Primula dermatitis 692.6
Primus varus (bilateral) (metatarsus) 754.52
**PRIND (prolonged reversible ischemic
  neurologic deficit)** 434.91
  history of personal V12.54
Pringle's disease (tuberous sclerosis) 759.5
Prinzmetal's angina 413.1
Prinzmetal-Massumi syndrome (anterior chest
  wall) 786.52
Prizefighter ear 738.7

Problem (with) V49.9
  academic V62.3
  acculturation V62.4
  adopted child V61.24
  aged
    in-law V61.3
    parent V61.3
    person NEC V61.8
  alcoholism in family V61.41
  anger reaction (*see also* Disturbance, conduct)
    312.0
  behavior, child 312.9
  behavioral V40.9
    specified NEC V40.39
  betting V69.3
  biological child V61.23
  cardiorespiratory NEC V47.2
  care of sick or handicapped person in family or
    household V61.49
  career choice V62.29
  communication V40.1
  conscience regarding medical care V62.6
  delinquency (juvenile) 312.9
  diet, inappropriate V69.1
  digestive NEC V47.3
  ear NEC V41.3
  eating habits, inappropriate V69.1
  economic V60.2
    affecting care V60.9
      specified type NEC V60.89
  educational V62.3
  enuresis, child 307.6
  exercise, lack of V69.0
  eye NEC V41.1
  family V61.9
    specified circumstance NEC V61.8
  fear reaction, child 313.0
  feeding (elderly) (infant) 783.3
    newborn 779.31
    nonorganic 307.59
  fetal, affecting management of pregnancy 656.9
    specified type NEC 656.8
  financial V60.2
  foster child V61.25
  functional V41.9
    specified type NEC V41.8
  gambling V69.3
  genital NEC V47.5
  head V48.9
    deficiency V48.0
    disfigurement V48.6
    mechanical V48.2
    motor V48.2
    movement of V48.2
    sensory V48.4
    specified condition NEC V48.8
  hearing V41.2
  high-risk sexual behavior V69.2
  identity 313.82
  influencing health status NEC V49.89
  internal organ NEC V47.9
    deficiency V47.0
    mechanical or motor V47.1
  interpersonal NEC V62.81
  jealousy, child 313.3
  learning V40.0
  legal V62.5
  life circumstance NEC V62.89
  lifestyle V69.9
    specified NEC V69.8

Problem—*continued*
limb V49.9
  deficiency V49.0
  disfigurement V49.4
  mechanical V49.1
  motor V49.2
  movement, involving
    musculoskeletal system V49.1
    nervous system V49.2
  sensory V49.3
  specified condition NEC V49.5
litigation V62.5
living alone V60.3
loneliness NEC V62.89
marital V61.10
  involving
    divorce V61.03
    estrangement V61.09
    psychosexual disorder 302.9
    sexual function V41.7
  relationship V61.10
mastication V41.6
medical care, within family V61.49
mental V40.9
  specified NEC V40.2
mental hygiene, adult V40.9
multiparity V61.5
nail biting, child 307.9
neck V48.9
  deficiency V48.1
  disfigurement V48.7
  mechanical V48.3
  motor V48.3
  movement V48.3
  sensory V48.5
  specified condition NEC V48.8
neurological NEC 781.99
none (feared complaint unfounded) V65.5
occupational V62.29
parent-child V61.20
  adopted child V61.24
  biological child V61.23
  foster child V61.25
  relationship V61.20
partner V61.10
  relationship V61.10
personal NEC V62.89
  interpersonal conflict NEC V62.81
personality (*see also* Disorder, personality)
  301.9
phase of life V62.89
placenta, affecting management of pregnancy
  656.9
  specified type NEC 656.8
poverty V60.2
presence of sick or handicapped person in
  family or household V61.49
psychiatric 300.9
psychosocial V62.9
  specified type NEC V62.89
relational NEC V62.81
relationship, childhood 313.3
religious or spiritual belief
  other than medical care V62.89
  regarding medical care V62.6
self-damaging behavior V69.8
sexual
  behavior, high-risk V69.2
  function NEC V41.7

Problem—*continued*
sibling
  relational V61.8
  relationship V61.8
sight V41.0
sleep disorder, child 307.40
sleep, lack of V69.4
smell V41.5
speech V40.1
spite reaction, child (*see also* Disturbance,
  conduct) 312.0
spoiled child reaction (*see also* Disturbance,
  conduct) 312.1
substance abuse in family V61.42
swallowing V41.6
tantrum, child (*see also* Disturbance, conduct)
  312.1
taste V41.5
thumb sucking, child 307.9
tic (child) 307.21
trunk V48.9
  deficiency V48.1
  disfigurement V48.7
  mechanical V48.3
  motor V48.3
  movement V48.3
  sensory V48.5
  specified condition NEC V48.8
unemployment V62.0
urinary NEC V47.4
voice production V41.4
Procedure (surgical) not done NEC V64.3
because of
  contraindication V64.1
  patient's decision V64.2
    for reasons of conscience or religion V62.6
  specified reason NEC V64.3
Procidentia
anus (sphincter) 569.1
rectum (sphincter) 569.1
stomach 537.89
uteri 618.1
Proctalgia 569.42
fugax 564.6
spasmodic 564.6
  psychogenic 307.89
Proctitis 569.49
amebic 006.8
chlamydial 099.52
gonococcal 098.7
granulomatous 555.1
idiopathic 556.2
  with ulcerative sigmoiditis 556.3
tuberculous (*see also* Tuberculosis) 014.8
ulcerative (chronic) (nonspecific) 556.2
  with ulcerative sigmoiditis 556.3
Proctocele
female (without uterine prolapse) 618.04
  with uterine prolapse 618.4
    complete 618.3
    incomplete 618.2
male 569.49
Proctocolitis, idiopathic 556.2
with ulcerative sigmoiditis 556.3
Proctoptosis 569.1
Proctosigmoiditis 569.89
ulcerative (chronic) 556.3
Proctospasm 564.6
psychogenic 306.4
Prodromal-AIDS —*see* Human
  immunodeficiency virus (disease) (illness)
  (infection)

Profichet's disease or syndrome 729.90
Progeria (adultorum) (syndrome) 259.8
Prognathism (mandibular) (maxillary) 524.10
Progonoma (melanotic) (M9363/0)—*see*
   Neoplasm, by site, benign
Progressive —*see* condition
Prolapse, prolapsed
   anus, anal (canal) (sphincter) 569.1
   arm or hand, complicating delivery 652.7
      causing obstructed labor 660.0
         affecting fetus or newborn 763.1
      fetus or newborn 763.1
   bladder (acquired) (mucosa) (sphincter)
      congenital (female) (male) 756.71
      female (*see also* Cystocele, female) 618.01
      male 596.89
   breast implant (prosthetic) 996.54
   cecostomy 569.69
   cecum 569.89
   cervix, cervical (hypertrophied) 618.1
      anterior lip, obstructing labor 660.2
         affecting fetus or newborn 763.1
      congenital 752.49
      postpartal (old) 618.1
      stump 618.84
   ciliary body 871.1
   colon (pedunculated) 569.89
   colostomy 569.69
   conjunctiva 372.73
   cord—*see* Prolapse, umbilical cord
   cystostomy 596.83
   disc (intervertebral)—*see* Displacement,
      intervertebral disc
   duodenum 537.89
   eye implant (orbital) 996.59
      lens (ocular) 996.53
   fallopian tube 620.4
   fetal extremity, complicating delivery 652.8
      causing obstructed labor 660.0
      fetus or newborn 763.1
   funis—*see* Prolapse, umbilical cord
   gastric (mucosa) 537.89
   genital, female 618.9
      specified NEC 618.89
   globe 360 81
   ileostomy bud 569.69
   intervertebral disc—*see* Displacement,
      intervertebral disc
   intestine (small) 569.89
   iris 364.89
      traumatic 871.1
   kidney (*see also* Disease, renal) 593.0
      congenital 753.3
   laryngeal muscles or ventricle 478.79
   leg, complicating delivery 652.8
      causing obstructed labor 660.0
      fetus or newborn 763.1
   liver 573.8
   meatus urinarius 599.5
   mitral valve 424.0
   ocular lens implant 996.53
   organ or site, congenital NEC—*see* Malposition,
      congenital
   ovary 620.4
   pelvic (floor), female 618.89
   perineum, female 618.89
   pregnant uterus 654.4
   rectum (mucosa) (sphincter) 569.1
      due to Trichuris trichiuria 127.3
   spleen 289.59
   stomach 537.89

Prolapse, prolapsed—*continued*
   umbilical cord
      affecting fetus or newborn 762.4
      complicating delivery 663.0
   ureter 593.89
      with obstruction 593.4
   ureterovesical orifice 593.89
   urethra (acquired) (infected) (mucosa) 599.5
      congenital 753.8
   uterovaginal 618.4
      complete 618.3
      incomplete 618.2
      specified NEC 618.89
   uterus (first degree) (second degree) (third
         degree) (complete) (without vaginal wall
         prolapse) 618.1
      with mention of vaginal wall prolapse—*see*
         Prolapse, uterovaginal
      congenital 752.39
      in pregnancy or childbirth 654.4
         affecting fetus or newborn 763.1
         causing obstructed labor 660.2
            affecting fetus or newborn 763.1
      postpartal (old) 618.1
   uveal 871.1
   vagina (anterior) (posterior) (vault) (wall)
         (without uterine prolapse) 618.00
      with uterine prolapse 618.4
         complete 618.3
         incomplete 618.2
      paravaginal 618.02
      posthysterectomy 618.5
      specified NEC 618.09
   vitreous (humor) 379.26
      traumatic 871.1
   womb—*see* Prolapse, uterus
Prolapsus, female 618.9
Proliferative —*see* condition
Prolinemia 270.8
Prolinuria 270.8
Prolonged, prolongation
   bleeding time (*see also* Defect, coagulation) 790.92
      "idiopathic" (in von Willebrand's disease) 286.4
   coagulation time (*see also* Defect, coagulation)
         790.92
   gestation syndrome 766.22
   labor 662.1
      affecting fetus or newborn 763.89
      first stage 662.0
      second stage 662.2
   PR interval 426.11
   pregnancy 645.2
   prothrombin time (*see also* Defect, coagulation)
         790.92
   QT interval 794.31
      syndrome 426.82
   rupture of membranes (24 hours or more prior to
         onset of labor) 658.2
   uterine contractions in labor 661.4
      affecting fetus or newborn 763.7
Prominauris 744.29
Prominence
   auricle (ear) (congenital) 744.29
      acquired 380.32
   ischial spine or sacral promontory
      with disproportion (fetopelvic) 653.3
         affecting fetus or newborn 763.1
         causing obstructed labor 660.1
            affecting fetus or newborn 763.1
   nose (congenital) 748.1
      acquired 738.0
PROMM (proximal myotonic myotonia) 359.21

Pronation
ankle 736.79
foot 736.79
congenital 755.67
Prophylactic
administration of
antibiotics, long-term V58.62
short-term—omit code
antitoxin, any V07.2
antivenin V07.2
chemotherapeutic agent NEC V07.39
fluoride V07.31
diphtheria antitoxin V07.2
drug V07.39
gamma globulin V07.2
immune sera (gamma globulin) V07.2
RhoGAM V07.2
tetanus antitoxin V07.2
chemotherapy NEC V07.39
fluoride V07.31
hormone replacement (postmenopausal) V07.4
immunotherapy V07.2
measure V07.9
specified type NEC V07.8
medication V07.39
postmenopausal hormone replacement V07.4
sterilization V25.2
Proptosis (ocular) (*see also* Exophthalmos)
376.30
thyroid 242.0
Propulsion
eyeball 360.81
Prosecution, anxiety concerning V62.5
Prosopagnosia 368.16
Prostate, prostatic —*see* condition
Prostatism 600.90
with
other lower urinary tract symptoms (LUTS) 600.91
urinary
obstruction 600.91
retention 600.91
Prostatitis (congestive) (suppurative) 601.9
acute 601.0
cavitary 601.8
chlamydial 099.54
chronic 601.1
diverticular 601.8
due to Trichomonas (vaginalis) 131.03
fibrous 600.90
with
other lower urinary tract symptoms (LUTS)
600.91
urinary
obstruction 600.91
retention 600.91
gonococcal (acute) 098.12
chronic or duration of 2 months or over 098.32
granulomatous 601.8
hypertrophic 600.00
with
other lower urinary tract symptoms (LUTS)
600.01
urinary
obstruction 600.01
retention 600.01
specified type NEC 601.8
subacute 601.1
trichomonal 131.03
tuberculous (*see also* Tuberculosis) 016.5 *[601.4]*
Prostatocystitis 601.3
Prostatorrhea 602.8
Prostatoseminovesiculitis, trichomonal 131.03

Prostration 780.79
heat 992.5
anhydrotic 992.3
due to
salt (and water) depletion 992.4
water depletion 992.3
nervous 300.5
newborn 779.89
senile 797
Protanomaly 368.51
Protanopia (anomalous trichromat) (complete)
(incomplete) 368.51
Protection (against) (from) —*see* Prophylactic
Protein
deficiency 260
malnutrition 260
sickness (prophylactic) (therapeutic) 999.59
Proteinemia 790.99
Proteinosis
alveolar, lung or pulmonary 516.0
lipid 272.8
Proteinosis
lipoid (of Urbach) 272.8
Proteinuria (*see also* Albuminuria) 791.0
Bence-Jones NEC 791.0
gestational 646.2
with hypertension—*see* Toxemia, of
pregnancy
orthostatic 593.6
postural 593.6
Proteolysis, pathologic 286.6
Protocoproporphyria 277.1
Protoporphyria (erythrohepatic) (erythropoietic)
277.1
Protrusio acetabuli 718.65
Protrusion
acetabulum (into pelvis) 718.65
device, implant, or graft—*see* Complications,
mechanical
ear, congenital 744.29
intervertebral disc—*see* Displacement,
intervertebral disc
nucleus pulposus—*see* Displacement,
intervertebral disc
Proud flesh 701.5
Prune belly (syndrome) 756.71
Prurigo (ferox) (gravis) (Hebra's) (hebrae)
(mitis) (simplex) 698.2
agria 698.3
asthma syndrome 691.8
Besnier's (atopic dermatitis) (infantile eczema)
691.8
eczematodes allergicum 691.8
estivalis (Hutchinson's) 692.72
Hutchinson's 692.72
nodularis 698.3
psychogenic 306.3
Pruritus, pruritic 698.9
ani 698.0
psychogenic 306.3
conditions NEC 698.9
psychogenic 306.3
due to Onchocerca volvulus 125.3
ear 698.9
essential 698.9
genital organ(s) 698.1
psychogenic 306.3
gravidarum 646.8
hiemalis 698.8
neurogenic (any site) 306.3
perianal 698.0

Pruritus, pruritic—*continued*
  psychogenic (any site) 306.3
  scrotum 698.1
    psychogenic 306.3
  senile, senilis 698.8
  Trichomonas 131.9
  vulva, vulvae 698.1
    psychogenic 306.3
Psammocarcinoma (M8140/3)—*see* Neoplasm,
  by site, malignant
Pseudarthrosis, pseudoarthrosis (bone) 733.82
  joint following fusion V45.4
Pseudoacanthosis
  nigricans 701.8
Pseudoaneurysm —*see* Aneurysm
Pseudoangina (pectoris)—*see* Angina
Pseudoangioma 452
Pseudo-Argyll-Robertson pupil 379.45
Pseudoarteriosus 747.89
Pseudoarthrosis —*see* Pseudarthrosis
Pseudoataxia 799.89
Pseudobulbar affect (PBA) 310.81
Pseudobursa 727.89
Pseudocholera 025
Pseudochromidrosis 705.89
Pseudocirrhosis, liver, pericardial 423.2
Pseudocoarctation 747.21
Pseudocowpox 051.1
Pseudocoxalgia 732.1
Pseudocroup 478.75
Pseudocyesis 300.11
Pseudocyst
  lung 518.89
  pancreas 577.2
  retina 361.19
Pseudodementia 300.16
Pseudoelephantiasis neuroarthritica 757.0
Pseudoemphysema 518.89
Pseudoencephalitis
  superior (acute) hemorrhagic 265.1
Pseudoerosion cervix, congenital 752.49
Pseudoexfoliation, lens capsule 366.11
Pseudofracture (idiopathic) (multiple)
  (spontaneous) (symmetrical) 268.2
Pseudoglanders 025
Pseudoglioma 360.44
Pseudogout —*see* Chondrocalcinosis
Pseudohallucination 780.1
Pseudohemianesthesia 782.0
Pseudohemophilia (Bernuth's) (hereditary) (type
  B) 286.4
  type A 287.8
  vascular 287.8
Pseudohermaphroditism 752.7
  with chromosomal anomaly—*see* Anomaly,
    chromosomal
  adrenal 255.2
  female (without adrenocortical disorder) 752.7
    with adrenocortical disorder 255.2
    adrenal 255.2
  male (without gonadal disorder) 752.7
    with
      adrenocortical disorder 255.2
      cleft scrotum 752.7
      feminizing testis 259.51
      gonadal disorder 257.9
      adrenal 255.2
Pseudohole, macula 362.54
Pseudo-Hurler's disease (mucolipidosis III)
  272.7
Pseudohydrocephalus 348.2

Pseudohypertrophic muscular dystrophy
  (Erb's) 359.1
Pseudohypertrophy, muscle 359.1
Pseudohypoparathyroidism 275.49
Psuedopseudohypoparathyroidism 275.49
Pseudoinfluenza (*see also* Influenza) 487.1
Pseudoinsomnia 307.49
Pseudoleukemia 288.8
  infantile 285.8
Pseudomembranous —*see* condition
Pseudomeningocele (cerebral) (infective) 349.2
  postprocedural 997.01
  spinal 349.2
Pseudomenstruation 626.8
Pseudomucinous
  cyst (ovary) (M8470/0) 220
  peritoneum 568.89
Pseudomyeloma 273.1
Pseudomyxoma peritonei (M8480/6) 197.6
Pseudoneuritis optic (nerve) 377.24
  papilla 377.24
  congenital 743.57
Pseudoneuroma —*see* Injury, nerve, by site
Pseudo-obstruction
  intestine (chronic) (idiopathic) (intermittent
    secondary) (primary) 564.89
  acute 560.89
Pseudopapilledema 377.24
Pseudoparalysis
  arm or leg 781.4
  atonic, congenital 358.8
Pseudopelade 704.09
Pseudophakia V43.1
Pseudopolycythemia 289.0
Pseudopolyposis, colon 556.4
Pseudoporencephaly 348.0
Pseudopseudohypoparathyroidism 275.49
Pseudopsychosis 300.16
Pseudopterygium 372.52
Pseudoptosis (eyelid) 374.34
Pseudorabies 078.89
Pseudoretinitis, pigmentosa 362.65
Pseudorickets 588.0
  senile (Pozzi's) 731.0
Pseudorubella 057.8
Pseudoscarlatina 057.8
Pseudosclerema 778.1
Pseudosclerosis (brain)
  Jakob's 046.19
  of Westphal (-Strümpell) (hepatolenticular
    degeneration) 275.1
  spastic 046.19
    with dementia
      with behavioral disturbance 046.19 *[294.11]*
      without behavioral disturbance 046.19
      [294.10]
Pseudoseizure 780.39
  non-psychiatric 780.39
  psychiatric 300.11
Pseudotabes 799.89
  diabetic 250.6 *[337.1]*
  due to secondary diabetes 249.6 *[337.1]*
Pseudotetanus (*see also* Convulsions) 780.39
Pseudotetany 781.7
  hysterical 300.11
Pseudothalassemia 285.0
Pseudotrichinosis 710.3
Pseudotruncus arteriosus 747.29
Pseudotuberculosis, pasteurella (infection) 027.2

Pseudotumor
  cerebri 348.2
  orbit (inflammatory) 376.11
Pseudo-Turner's syndrome 759.89
Pseudoxanthoma elasticum 757.39
Psilosis (sprue) (tropical) 579.1
  Monilia 112.89
  nontropical 579.0
  not sprue 704.00
Psittacosis 073.9
Psoitis 728.89
Psora NEC 696.1
Psoriasis 696.1
  any type, except arthropathic 696.1
  arthritic, arthropathic 696.0
  buccal 528.6
  flexural 696.1
  follicularis 696.1
  guttate 696.1
  inverse 696.1
  mouth 528.6
  nummularis 696.1
  psychogenic 316 *[696.1]*
  punctata 696.1
  pustular 696.1
  rupioides 696.1
  vulgaris 696.1
Psorospermiasis 136.4
Psorospermosis 136.4
  follicularis (vegetans) 757.39
Psychalgia 307.80
Psychasthenia 300.89
  compulsive 300.3
  mixed compulsive states 300.3
  obsession 300.3
Psychiatric disorder or problem NEC 300.9
Psychogenic —*see also* condition
  factors associated with physical conditions 316
Psychoneurosis, psychoneurotic (*see also*
  Neurosis) 300.9
  anxiety (state) 300.00
  climacteric 627.2
  compensation 300.16
  compulsion 300.3
  conversion hysteria 300.11
  depersonalization 300.6
  depressive type 300.4
  dissociative hysteria 300.15
  hypochondriacal 300.7
  hysteria 300.10
    conversion type 300.11
    dissociative type 300.15
  mixed NEC 300.89
  neurasthenic 300.5
  obsessional 300.3
  obsessive-compulsive 300.3
  occupational 300.89
  personality NEC 301.89
  phobia 300.20
  senile NEC 300.89
Psychopathic —*see also* condition
  constitution, posttraumatic 310.2
    with psychosis 293.9
  personality 301.9
    amoral trends 301.7
    antisocial trends 301.7
    asocial trends 301.7
    mixed types 301.7
  state 301.9
Psychopathy, sexual (*see also* Deviation, sexual)
  302.9

Psychophysiologic, psychophysiological
  condition—*see* Reaction, psychophysiologic
Psychose passionelle 297.8
Psychosexual identity disorder 302.6
  adult-life 302.85
  childhood 302.6
Psychosis 298.9
  acute hysterical 298.1
  affecting management of pregnancy, childbirth,
    or puerperium 648.4
  affective (*see also* Disorder, mood) 296.90
    drug induced 292.84
    due to or associated with physical condition
      293.83

> *Note—Use the following fifth-digit*
> *subclassification with categories 296.0-296.6:*
>
> *0 unspecified*
> *1 mild*
> *2 moderate*
> *3 severe, without mention of psychotic*
> *   behavior*
> *4 severe, specified as with psychotic behavior*
> *5 in partial or unspecified remission*
> *6 in full remission*

  involutional 296.2
    recurrent episode 296.3
    single episode 296.2
  manic-depressive 296.80
    circular (alternating) 296.7
      currently depressed 296.5
      currently manic 296.4
    depressed type 296.2
      atypical 296.82
      recurrent episode 296.3
      single episode 296.2
    manic 296.0
      atypical 296.81
      recurrent episode 296.1
      single episode 296.0
    mixed type NEC 296.89
    specified type NEC 296.89
  senile 290.21
  specified type NEC 296.99
  alcoholic 291.9
    with
      anxiety 291.89
      delirium tremens 291.0
      delusions 291.5
      dementia 291.2
      hallucinosis 291.3
      jealousy 291.5
      mood disturbance 291.89
      paranoia 291.5
      persisting amnesia 291.1
      sexual dysfunction 291.89
      sleep disturbance 291.89
    amnestic confabulatory 291.1
    delirium tremens 291.0
    hallucinosis 291.3
    Korsakoff's, Korsakov's, Korsakow's 291.1
    paranoid type 291.5
    pathological intoxication 291.4
    polyneuritic 291.1
    specified type NEC 291.89
  alternating (*see also* Psychosis,
    manic-depressive, circular) 296.7
  anergastic (*see also* Psychosis, organic) 294.9

Psychosis—*continued*
arteriosclerotic 290.40
  with
    acute confusional state 290.41
    delirium 290.41
    delusions 290.42
    depressed mood 290.43
    depressed type 290.43
    paranoid type 290.42
    simple type 290.40
    uncomplicated 290.40
  atypical 298.9
    depressive 296.82
    manic 296.81
  borderline (schizophrenia) (*see also*
      Schizophrenia) 295.5
    of childhood (*see also* Psychosis, childhood)
      299.8
    prepubertal 299.8
  brief reactive 298.8
  childhood, with origin specific to 299.9

> *Note—Use the following fifth-digit
> subclassification with category 299:*
>
> *0 current or active state*
> *1 residual state*

  atypical 299.8
  specified type NEC 299.8
  circular (*see also* Psychosis, manic-depressive,
      circular) 296.7
  climacteric (*see also* Psychosis, involutional)
      298.8
  confusional 298.9
    acute 293.0
    reactive 298.2
    subacute 293.1
  depressive (*see also* Psychosis, affective) 296.2
    atypical 296.82
    involutional 296.2
      recurrent episode 296.3
      single episode 296.2
    psychogenic 298.0
    reactive (emotional stress) (psychological
        trauma) 298.0
    recurrent episode 296.3
      with hypomania (bipolar II) 296.89
    single episode 296.2
  disintegrative, childhood (*see also* Psychosis,
      childhood) 299.1
  drug 292.9
    with
      affective syndrome 292.84
      amnestic syndrome 292.83
      anxiety 292.89
      delirium 292.81
        withdrawal 292.0
      delusions 292.11
      dementia 292.82
      depressive state 292.84
      hallucinations 292.12
      hallucinosis 292.12
      mood disorder 292.84
      mood disturbance 292.84
      organic personality syndrome NEC 292.89
      sexual dysfunction 292.89
      sleep disturbance 292.89
      withdrawal syndrome (and delirium) 292.0
    affective syndrome 292.84
    delusions 292.11
    hallucinatory state 292.12

Psychosis—*continued*
  drug—*continued*
    hallucinosis 292.12
    paranoid state 292.11
    specified type NEC 292.89
    withdrawal syndrome (and delirium) 292.0
  due to or associated with physical condition (*see
      also* Psychosis, organic) 293.9
  epileptic NEC 294.8
  excitation (psychogenic) (reactive) 298.1
  exhaustive (*see also* Reaction, stress, acute) 308.9
  hypomanic (*see also* Psychosis, affective) 296.0
    recurrent episode 296.1
    single episode 296.0
  hysterical 298.8
    acute 298.1
  incipient 298.8
    schizophrenic (*see also* Schizophrenia) 295.5
  induced 297.3
  infantile (*see also* Psychosis, childhood) 299.0
  infective 293.9
    acute 293.0
    subacute 293.1
  in
    conditions classified elsewhere
      with
        delusions 293.81
        hallucinations 293.82
    pregnancy, childbirth, or puerperium 648.4
  interactional (childhood) (*see also* Psychosis,
      childhood) 299.1
  involutional 298.8
    depressive (*see also* Psychosis, affective)
        296.2
      recurrent episode 296.3
      single episode 296.2
    melancholic 296.2
      recurrent episode 296.3
      single episode 296.2
    paranoid state 297.2
    paraphrenia 297.2
  Korsakoff's, Korakov's, Korsakow's
      (nonalcoholic) 294.0
    alcoholic 291.1
  mania (phase) (*see also* Psychosis, affective)
      296.0
    recurrent episode 296.1
    single episode 296.0
  manic (*see also* Psychosis, affective) 296.0
    atypical 296.81
    recurrent episode 296.1
    single episode 296.0
  manic-depressive 296.80
    circular 296.7
      currently
        depressed 296.5
        manic 296.4
      mixed 296.6
    depressive 296.2
      recurrent episode 296.3
        with hypomania (bipolar II) 296.89
      single episode 296.2
    hypomanic 296.0
      recurrent episode 296.1
      single episode 296.0
    manic 296.0
      atypical 296.81
      recurrent episode 296.1
      single episode 296.0
    mixed NEC 296.89
    perplexed 296.89
    stuporous 296.89

Psychosis—*continued*
menopausal (*see also* Psychosis, involutional)
  298.8
mixed schizophrenic and affective (*see also*
  Schizophrenia) 295.7
multi-infarct (cerebrovascular) (*see also*
  Psychosis, arteriosclerotic) 290.40
organic NEC 294.9
  due to or associated with
    addiction
      alcohol (*see also* Psychosis, alcoholic)
        291.9
      drug (*see also* Psychosis, drug) 292.9
    alcohol intoxication, acute (*see also*
      Psychosis, alcoholic) 291.9
    alcoholism (*see also* Psychosis, alcoholic)
      291.9
    arteriosclerosis (cerebral) (*see also*
      Psychosis, arteriosclerotic) 290.40
    cerebrovascular disease
      acute (psychosis) 293.0
      arteriosclerotic (*see also* Psychosis,
        arteriosclerotic) 290.40
    childbirth—*see* Psychosis, puerperal
    dependence
      alcohol (*see also* Psychosis, alcoholic)
        291.9
      drug 292.9
    disease
      alcoholic liver (*see also* Psychosis,
        alcoholic) 291.9
      brain
        arteriosclerotic (*see also* Psychosis,
          arteriosclerotic) 290.40
        cerebrovascular
          acute (psychosis) 293.0
          arteriosclerotic (*see also* Psychosis,
            arteriosclerotic) 290.40
      endocrine or metabolic 293.9
        acute (psychosis) 293.0
        subacute (psychosis) 293.1
      Jakob-Creutzfeldt 046.19
        with behavioral disturbance 046.19
          [294.11]
        without behavioral disturbance 046.19
          [294.10]
        familial 046.19
        iatrogenic 046.19
        specified NEC 046.19
        sporadic 046.19
        variant 046.11
          with dementia
            with behavioral disturbance 046.11
              [294.11]
            without behavioral disturbance
              046.11 *[294.10]*
      liver, alcoholic (*see also* Psychosis,
        alcoholic) 291.9
    disorder
      cerebrovascular
        acute (psychosis) 293.0
      endocrine or metabolic 293.9
        acute (psychosis) 293.0
        subacute (psychosis) 293.1
    epilepsy
      with behavioral disturbance 345.9
        [294.11]
      without behavioral disturbance 345.9
        [294.10]
      transient (acute) 293.0

Psychosis—*continued*
organic—*continued*
  due to—*continued*
    Huntington's chorea
      with behavioral disturbance 333.4
        [294.11]
      without behavioral disturbance 333.4
        [294.10]
    infection
      brain 293.9
        acute (psychosis) 293.0
        chronic 294.8
        subacute (psychosis) 293.1
      intracranial NEC 293.9
        acute (psychosis) 293.0
        chronic 294.8
        subacute (psychosis) 293.1
    intoxication
      alcoholic (acute) (*see also* Psychosis,
        alcoholic) 291.9
      pathological 291.4
      drug (*see also* Psychosis, drug) 292.9
    ischemia
      cerebrovascular (generalized) (*see also*
        Psychosis, arteriosclerotic) 290.40
    Jakob-Creutzfeldt disease (syndrome)
      046.19
      with behavioral disturbance 046.19
        [294.11]
      without behavioral disturbance 046.19
        [294.10]
      variant 046.11
        with dementia
          with behavioral disturbance 046.11
            [294.11]
          without behavioral disturbance 046.11
            [294.10]
    multiple sclerosis
      with behavioral disturbance 340 *[294.11]*
      without behavioral disturbance 340
        [294.10]
    physical condition NEC 293.9
      with
        delusions 293.81
        hallucinations 293.82
    presenility 290.10
    puerperium—*see* Psychosis, puerperal
    sclerosis, multiple
      with behavioral disturbance 340 *[294.11]*
      without behavioral disturbance 340
        [294.10]
    senility 290.20
    status epilepticus
      with behavioral disturbance 345.3
        [294.11]
      without behavioral disturbance 345.3
        [294.10]
    trauma
      brain (birth) (from electrical current)
        (surgical) 293.9
        acute (psychosis) 293.0
        chronic 294.8
        subacute (psychosis) 293.1
    unspecified physical condition 293.9
      with
        delusions 293.81
        hallucinations 293.82
infective 293.9
  acute (psychosis) 293.0
  subacute 293.1

Psychosis—*continued*
  organic—*continued*
    posttraumatic 293.9
      acute 293.0
      subacute 293.1
    specified type NEC 294.8
    transient 293.9
      with
        anxiety 293.84
        delusions 293.81
        depression 293.83
        hallucinations 293.82
      depressive type 293.83
      hallucinatory type 293.82
      paranoid type 293.81
      specified type NEC 293.89
  paranoic 297.1
  paranoid (chronic) 297.9
    alcoholic 291.5
    chronic 297.1
    climacteric 297.2
    involutional 297.2
    menopausal 297.2
    protracted reactive 298.4
    psychogenic 298.4
      acute 298.3
    schizophrenic (*see also* Schizophrenia) 295.3
    senile 290.20
  paroxysmal 298.9
    senile 290.20
  polyneuritic, alcoholic 291.1
  postoperative 293.9
  postpartum—*see* Psychosis, puerperal
  prepsychotic (*see also* Schizophrenia) 295.5
  presbyophrenic (type) 290.8
  presenile (*see also* Dementia, presenile) 290.10
  prison 300.16
  psychogenic 298.8
    depressive 298.0
    paranoid 298.4
      acute 298.3
  puerperal
    specified type—*see* categories 295-298
    unspecified type 293.89
      acute 293.0
      chronic 293.89
      subacute 293.1
  reactive (emotional stress) (psychological
    trauma) 298.8
    brief 298.8
    confusion 298.2
    depressive 298.0
    excitation 298.1
  schizo-affective (depressed) (excited) (*see also*
    Schizophrenia) 295.7
  schizophrenia, schizophrenic (*see also*
    Schizophrenia) 295.9
    borderline type 295.5
    of childhood (*see also* Psychosis, childhood)
      299.8
    catatonic (excited) (withdrawn) 295.2
    childhood type (*see also* Psychosis, childhood)
      299.9
    hebephrenic 295.1
    incipient 295.5
    latent 295.5
    paranoid 295.3
    prepsychotic 295.5
    prodromal 295.5
    pseudoneurotic 295.5
    pseudopsychopathic 295.5

Psychosis—*continued*
  schizophrenic—*continued*
    schizophreniform 295.4
    simple 295.0
    undifferentiated type 295.9
  schizophreniform 295.4
  senile NEC 290.20
    with
      delusional features 290.20
      depressive features 290.21
    depressed type 290.21
    paranoid type 290.20
    simple deterioration 290.20
    specified type—*see* categories 295-298
  shared 297.3
  situational (reactive) 298.8
  symbiotic (childhood) (*see also* Psychosis,
    childhood) 299.1
  toxic (acute) 293.9
Psychotic (*see also* condition) 298.9
  episode 298.9
  due to or associated with physical conditions
    (*see also* Psychosis, organic) 293.9
Pterygium (eye) 372.40
  central 372.43
  colli 744.5
  double 372.44
  peripheral (stationary) 372.41
    progressive 372.42
  recurrent 372.45
Ptilosis 374.55
PTLD (post-transplant lymphoproliferative
  disorder) 238.77
Ptomaine (poisoning) (*see also* Poisoning, food)
  005.9
Ptosis (adiposa) 374.30
  breast 611.81
  cecum 569.89
  colon 569.89
  congenital (eyelid) 743.61
    specified site NEC—*see* Anomaly, specified
      type NEC
  epicanthus syndrome 270.2
  eyelid 374.30
    congenital 743.61
    mechanical 374.33
    myogenic 374.32
    paralytic 374.31
  gastric 537.5
  intestine 569.89
  kidney (*see also* Disease, renal) 593.0
    congenital 753.3
  liver 573.8
  renal (*see also* Disease, renal) 593.0
    congenital 753.3
  splanchnic 569.89
  spleen 289.59
  stomach 537.5
  viscera 569.89
PTP (posttransfusion purpura) 287.41
PTSD (Post-Traumatic Stress Disorder) 309.81
Ptyalism 527.7
  hysterical 300.11
  periodic 527.2
  pregnancy 646.8
  psychogenic 306.4
Ptyalolithiasis 527.5
Pubalgia 848.8
Pubarche, precocious 259.1
Pubertas praecox 259.1

Puberty V21.1
abnormal 259.9
bleeding 626.3
delayed 259.0
precocious (constitutional) (cryptogenic)
(idiopathic) NEC 259.1
due to
adrenal
cortical hyperfunction 255.2
hyperplasia 255.2
cortical hyperfunction 255.2
ovarian hyperfunction 256.1
estrogen 256.0
pineal tumor 259.8
testicular hyperfunction 257.0
premature 259.1
due to
adrenal cortical hyperfunction 255.2
pineal tumor 259.8
pituitary (anterior) hyperfunction 253.1
Puckering, macula 362.56
Pudenda, pudendum —*see* condition
Puente's disease (simple glandular cheilitis)
528.5
Puerperal
abscess
areola 675.1
Bartholin's gland 646.6
breast 675.1
cervix (uteri) 670.8
fallopian tube 670.8
genital organ 670.8
kidney 646.6
mammary 675.1
mesosalpinx 670.8
nabothian 646.6
nipple 675.0
ovary, ovarian 670.8
oviduct 670.8
parametric 670.8
para-uterine 670.8
pelvic 670.8
perimetric 670
periuterine 670.8
retro-uterine 670.8
subareolar 675.1
suprapelvic 670.8
tubal (ruptured) 670.8
tubo-ovarian 670.8
urinary tract NEC 646.6
uterine, uterus 670.8
vagina (wall) 646.6
vaginorectal 646.6
vulvovaginal gland 646.6
accident 674.9
adnexitis 670.8
afibrinogenemia, or other coagulation defect
666.3
albuminuria (acute) (subacute) 646.2
pre-eclamptic 642.4
anemia (conditions classifiable to 280-285)
648.2
anuria 669.3
apoplexy 674.0
asymptomatic bacteriuria 646.5
atrophy, breast 676.3
blood dyscrasia 666.3
caked breast 676.2
cardiomyopathy 674.5
cellulitis—*see* Puerperal, abscess

Puerperal—*continued*
cerebrovascular disorder (conditions classifiable
to 430-434, 436-437) 674.0
cervicitis (conditions classifiable to 616.0) 646.6
coagulopathy (any) 666.3
complications 674.9
specified type NEC 674.8
convulsions (eclamptic) (uremic) 642.6
with pre-existing hypertension 642.7
cracked nipple 676.1
cystitis 646.6
cystopyelitis 646.6
deciduitis (acute) 670.8
delirium NEC 293.9
diabetes (mellitus) (conditions classifiable to
249 and 250) 648.0
disease 674.9
breast NEC 676.3
cerebrovascular (acute) 674.0
nonobstetric NEC (*see also* Pregnancy,
complicated, current disease or condition)
648.9
pelvis inflammatory 670.8
renal NEC 646.2
tubo-ovarian 670.8
Valsuani's (progressive pernicious anemia) 648.2
disorder
lactation 676.9
specified type NEC 676.8
nonobstetric NEC (*see also* Pregnancy,
complicated, current disease or condition)
648.9
disruption
cesarean wound 674.1
episiotomy wound 674.2
perineal laceration wound 674.2
drug dependence (conditions classifiable to 304)
648.3
eclampsia 642.6
with pre-existing hypertension 642.7
embolism (pulmonary) 673.2
air 673.0
amniotic fluid 673.1
blood-clot 673.2
brain or cerebral 674.0
cardiac 674.8
fat 673.8
intracranial sinus (venous) 671.5
pyemic 673.3
septic 673.3
spinal cord 671.5
endometritis (conditions classifiable to
615.0-615.9) 670.1
endophlebitis—*see* Puerperal, phlebitis
endotrachelitis 646.6
engorgement, breasts 676.2
erysipelas 670.8
failure
lactation 676.4
renal, acute 669.3
fever 672
meaning pyrexia (of unknown origin) 672
meaning sepsis 670.2
fissure, nipple 676.1
fistula
breast 675.1
mammary gland 675.1
nipple 675.0
galactophoritis 675.2
galactorrhea 676.6

Puerperal—*continued*
  gangrene
    gas 670.8
      with sepsis 670.2
    uterus 670.8
  gonorrhea (conditions classifiable to 098) 647.1
  hematoma, subdural 674.0
  hematosalpinx, infectional 670.8
  hemiplegia, cerebral 674.0
  hemorrhage 666.1
    brain 674.0
    bulbar 674.0
    cerebellar 674.0
    cerebral 674.0
    cortical 674.0
    delayed (after 24 hours) (uterine) 666.2
    extradural 674.0
    internal capsule 674.0
    intracranial 674.0
    intrapontine 674.0
    meningeal 674.0
    pontine 674.0
    subarachnoid 674.0
    subcortical 674.0
    subdural 674.0
    uterine, delayed 666.2
    ventricular 674.0
  hemorrhoids 671.8
  hepatorenal syndrome 674.8
  hypertrophy
    breast 676.3
    mammary gland 676.3
  induration breast (fibrous) 676.3
  infarction
    lung—*see* Puerperal, embolism
    pulmonary—*see* Puerperal, embolism
  infection
    Bartholin's gland 646.6
    breast 675.2
      with nipple 675.9
        specified type NEC 675.8
    cervix 646.6
    endocervix 646.6
    fallopian tube 670.8
    generalized 670.0
    genital tract (major) 670.0
      minor or localized 646.6
    kidney (bacillus coli) 646.6
    mammary gland 675.2
      with nipple 675.9
        specified type NEC 675.8
    nipple 675.0
      with breast 675.9
        specified type NEC 675.8
    ovary 670.8
    pelvic 670.8
    peritoneum 670.8
    renal 646.6
    tubo-ovarian 670.8
    urinary (tract) NEC 646.6
      asymptomatic 646.5
    uterus, uterine 670.8
    vagina 646.6
  inflammation—*see also* Puerperal, infection
    areola 675.1
    Bartholin's gland 646.6
    breast 675.2
    broad ligament 670.8
    cervix (uteri) 646.6
    fallopian tube 670.8

Puerperal—*continued*
  inflammation—*continued*
    genital organs 670.8
      localized 646.6
    mammary gland 675.2
    nipple 675.0
    ovary 670.8
    oviduct 670.8
    pelvis 670.8
    periuterine 670.8
    tubal 670.8
    vagina 646.6
    vein—*see* Puerperal, phlebitis
  inversion, nipple 676.3
  ischemia, cerebral 674.0
  lymphangitis 670.8
    breast 675.2
  malaria (conditions classifiable to 084) 647.4
  malnutrition 648.9
  mammillitis 675.0
  mammitis 675.2
  mania 296.0
    recurrent episode 296.1
    single episode 296.0
  mastitis 675.2
    purulent 675.1
    retromammary 675.1
    submammary 675.1
  melancholia 296.2
    recurrent episode 296.3
    single episode 296.2
  mental disorder (conditions classifiable to
    290-303, 305.0, 305.2-305.9, 306-316,
    317-319) 648.4
  metritis (suppurative) 670.1
    septic 670.2
  metroperitonitis 670.8
  metrorrhagia 666.2
  metrosalpingitis 670.8
  metrovaginitis 670.8
  milk leg 671.4
  monoplegia, cerebral 674.0
  necrosis
    kidney, tubular 669.3
    liver (acute) (subacute) (conditions classifiable
      to 570) 674.8
    ovary 670.8
    renal cortex 669.3
  nephritis or nephrosis (conditions classifiable to
    580-589) 646.2
    with hypertension 642.1
  nutritional deficiency (conditions classifiable to
    260-269) 648.9
  occlusion, precerebral artery 674.0
  oliguria 669.3
  oophoritis 670.8
  ovaritis 670.8
  paralysis
    bladder (sphincter) 665.5
    cerebral 674.0
  paralytic stroke 674.0
  parametritis 670.8
  paravaginitis 646.6
  pelviperitonitis 670.8
  perimetritis 670.8
  perimetrosalpingitis 670.8
  perinephritis 646.6
  perioophoritis 670.8
  periphlebitis—*see* Puerperal, phlebitis
  perisalpingitis 670.8
  peritoneal infection 670.8

Puerperal—*continued*
  peritonitis (pelvic) 670.8
  perivaginitis 646.6
  phlebitis 671.2
    deep 671.4
    intracranial sinus (venous) 671.5
    pelvic 671.4
    specified site NEC 671.5
    superficial 671.2
  phlegmasia alba dolens 671.4
  placental polyp 674.4
  pneumonia, embolic—*see* Puerperal, embolism
  prediabetes 648.8
  pre-eclampsia (mild) 642.4
    with pre-existing hypertension 642.7
    severe 642.5
  psychosis, unspecified (*see also* Psychosis,
    puerperal) 293.89
  pyelitis 646.6
  pyelocystitis 646.6
  pyelohydronephrosis 646.6
  pyelonephritis 646.6
  pyelonephrosis 646.6
  pyemia 670.2
  pyocystitis 646.6
  pyohemia 670.2
  pyometra 670.8
  pyonephritis 646.6
  pyonephrosis 646.6
  pyo-oophoritis 670.8
  pyosalpingitis 670.8
  pyosalpinx 670.8
  pyrexia (of unknown origin) 672
  renal
    disease NEC 646.2
    failure, acute 669.3
  retention
    decidua (fragments) (with delayed
      hemorrhage) 666.2
      without hemorrhage 667.1
    placenta (fragments) (with delayed
      hemorrhage) 666.2
      without hemorrhage 667.1
    secundines (fragments) (with delayed
      hemorrhage) 666.2
      without hemorrhage 667.1
  retracted nipple 676.0
  rubella (conditions classifiable to 056) 647.5
  salpingitis 670.8
  salpingo-oophoritis 670.8
  salpingo-ovaritis 670.8
  salpingoperitonitis 670.8
  sapremia 670.2
  secondary perineal tear 674.2
  sepsis (pelvic) 670.2
  septicemia 670.2
  subinvolution (uterus) 674.8
  sudden death (cause unknown) 674.9
  suppuration—*see* Puerperal, abscess
  syphilis (conditions classifiable to 090-097)
    647.0
  tetanus 670.8
  thelitis 675.0
  thrombocytopenia 666.3
  thrombophlebitis (superficial) 671.2
    deep 671.4
    pelvic 671.4
    septic 670.3
    specified site NEC 671.5
  thrombosis (venous)—*see* Thrombosis,
    puerperal

Puerperal—*continued*
  thyroid dysfunction (conditions classifiable to
    240-246) 648.1
  toxemia (*see also* Toxemia, of pregnancy) 642.4
    eclamptic 642.6
      with pre-existing hypertension 642.7
    pre-eclamptic (mild) 642.4
      with
        convulsions 642.6
        pre-existing hypertension 642.7
      severe 642.5
  tuberculosis (conditions classifiable to 010-018)
    647.3
  uremia 669.3
  vaginitis (conditions classifiable to 616.1) 646.6
  varicose veins (legs) 671.0
    vulva or perineum 671.1
  venous complication 671.9
  vulvitis (conditions classifiable to 616.1) 646.6
  vulvovaginitis (conditions classifiable to 616.1)
    646.6
  white leg 671.4
Pulled muscle —*see* Sprain, by site
Pulmolithiasis 518.89
Pulmonary —*see* condition
Pulmonitis (unknown etiology) 486
Pulpitis (acute) (anachoretic) (chronic)
    (hyperplastic) (putrescent) (suppurative)
    (ulcerative) 522.0
Pulpless tooth 522.9
Pulse
  alternating 427.89
    psychogenic 306.2
  bigeminal 427.89
  fast 785.0
  feeble, rapid, due to shock following injury
    958.4
  rapid 785.0
  slow 427.89
  strong 785.9
  trigeminal 427.89
  water-hammer (*see also* Insufficiency, aortic)
    424.1
  weak 785.9
Pulseless disease 446.7
Pulsus
  alternans or trigeminy 427.89
    psychogenic 306.2
Punch drunk 310.2
Puncta lacrimalia occlusion 375.52
Punctiform hymen 752.49
Puncture (traumatic)—*see also* Wound, open, by
    site
  accidental, complicating surgery 998.2
  bladder, nontraumatic 596.6
  by
    device, implant, or graft—*see* Complications,
      mechanical
    foreign body
      internal organs—*see also* Injury, internal, by
        site
        by ingested object—*see* Foreign body
      left accidentally in operation wound 998.4
    instrument (any) during a procedure,
      accidental 998.2
  internal organs, abdomen, chest, or pelvis—*see*
    Injury, internal, by site
  kidney, nontraumatic 593.89
Pupil —*see* condition
Pupillary membrane 364.74
  persistent 743.46

Pupillotonia 379.46
  pseudotabetic 379.46
Purpura 287.2
  abdominal 287.0
  allergic 287.0
  anaphylactoid 287.0
  annularis telangiectodes 709.1
  arthritic 287.0
  autoerythrocyte sensitization 287.2
  autoimmune 287.0
  bacterial 287.0
  Bateman's (senile) 287.2
  capillary fragility (hereditary) (idiopathic) 287.8
  cryoglobulinemic 273.2
  devil's pinches 287.2
  fibrinolytic (*see also* Fibrinolysis) 286.6
  fulminans, fulminous 286.6
  gangrenous 287.0
  hemorrhagic (*see also* Purpura,
    thrombocytopenic) 287.39
    nodular 272.7
    nonthrombocytopenic 287.0
    thrombocytopenic 287.39
  Henoch's (purpura nervosa) 287.0
  Henoch-Schönlein (allergic) 287.0
  hypergammaglobulinemic (benign primary)
    (Waldenström's) 273.0
  idiopathic 287.31
    nonthrombocytopenic 287.0
    thrombocytopenic 287.31
  immune thrombocytopenic 287.31
  infectious 287.0
  malignant 287.0
  neonatorum 772.6
  nervosa 287.0
  newborn NEC 772.6
  nonthrombocytopenic 287.2
    hemorrhagic 287.0
    idiopathic 287.0
  nonthrombopenic 287.2
  peliosis rheumatica 287.0
  pigmentaria, progressiva 709.09
  posttransfusion (PTP) 287.41
    from whole blood (fresh) or blood products
      287.41
  primary 287.0
  primitive 287.0
  red cell membrane sensitivity 287.2
  rheumatica 287.0
  Schönlein (-Henoch) (allergic) 287.0
  scorbutic 267
  senile 287.2
  simplex 287.2
  symptomatica 287.0
  telangiectasia annularis 709.1
  thrombocytopenic (*see also* Thrombocytopenia)
    287.30
    congenital 287.33
    essential 287.30
    hereditary 287.31
    idiopathic 287.31
    immune 287.31
    neonatal, transitory (*see also*
      Thrombocytopenia, neonatal transitory)
      776.1
    primary 287.30
    puerperal, postpartum 666.3
    thrombotic 446.6
  thrombohemolytic (*see also* Fibrinolysis) 286.6

Purpura—*continued*
  thrombopenic (*see also* Thrombocytopenia)
    287.30
    congenital 287.33
    essential 287.30
  thrombotic 446.6
    thrombocytic 446.6
    thrombocytopenic 446.6
  toxic 287.0
  variolosa 050.0
  vascular 287.0
  visceral symptoms 287.0
  Werlhof's (*see also* Purpura, thrombocytopenic)
    287.39
Purpuric spots 782.7
Purulent —*see* condition
Pus
  absorption, general—*see* Septicemia
  in
    stool 792.1
    urine 791.9
  tube (rupture) (*see also* Salpingo-oophoritis)
    614.2
Pustular rash 782.1
Pustule 686.9
  malignant 022.0
  nonmalignant 686.9
Putnam's disease (subacute combined sclerosis
  with pernicious anemia) 281.0 *[336.2]*
Putnam-Dana syndrome (subacute combined
  sclerosis with pernicious anemia) 281.0
  [336.2]
Putrefaction, intestinal 569.89
Putrescent pulp (dental) 522.1
Pyarthritis —*see* Pyarthrosis
Pyarthrosis (*see also* Arthritis, pyogenic) 711.0
  tuberculous—*see* Tuberculosis, joint
Pycnoepilepsy, pycnolepsy (idiopathic) (*see also*
  Epilepsy) 345.0
Pyelectasia 593.89
Pyelectasis 593.89
Pyelitis (congenital) (uremic) 590.80
  with
    abortion—*see* Abortion, by type, with
      specified complication NEC
    contracted kidney 590.00
    ectopic pregnancy (*see also* categories
      633.0-633.9) 639.8
    molar pregnancy (*see also* categories 630-632)
      639.8
  acute 590.10
    with renal medullary necrosis 590.11
  chronic 590.00
    with
      renal medullary necrosis 590.01
  complicating pregnancy, childbirth, or
    puerperium 646.6
    affecting fetus or newborn 760.1
  cystica 590.3
  following
    abortion 639.8
    ectopic or molar pregnancy 639.8
  gonococcal 098.19
    chronic or duration of 2 months or over 098.39
  tuberculous (*see also* Tuberculosis) 016.0 *[590.81]*
Pyelocaliectasis 593.89
Pyelocystitis (*see also* Pyelitis) 590.80
Pyelohydronephrosis 591

Pyelonephritis (*see also* Pyelitis) 590.80
  acute 590.10
    with renal medullary necrosis 590.11
  chronic 590.00
  syphilitic (late) 095.4
  tuberculous (*see also* Tuberculosis) 016.0
    [590.81]
Pyelonephrosis (*see also* Pyelitis) 590.80
  chronic 590.00
Pyelophlebitis 451.89
Pyelo-ureteritis cystica 590.3
Pyemia, pyemic (purulent) (*see also* Septicemia)
  038.9
  abscess—*see* Abscess
  arthritis (*see also* Arthritis, pyogenic) 711.0
  Bacillus coli 038.42
  embolism—(*see also* Septicemia) 415.12
  fever 038.9
  infection 038.9
  joint (*see also* Arthritis, pyogenic) 711.0
  liver 572.1
  meningococcal 036.2
  newborn 771.81
  phlebitis—*see* Phlebitis
  pneumococcal 038.2
  portal 572.1
  postvaccinal 999.39
  puerperal 670.2
  specified organism NEC 038.8
  staphylococcal 038.10
    aureus 038.11
      methicillin
        resistant 038.12
        susceptible 038.11
    specified organism NEC 038.19
  streptococcal 038.0
  tuberculous—*see* Tuberculosis, miliary
Pygopagus 759.4
Pykno-epilepsy, pyknolepsy (idiopathic) (*see*
  also Epilepsy) 345.0
Pyle (-Cohn) disease (craniometaphyseal
  dysplasia) 756.89
Pylephlebitis (suppurative) 572.1
Pylethrombophlebitis 572.1
Pylethrombosis 572.1
Pyloritis (*see also* Gastritis) 535.5
Pylorospasm (reflex) 537.81
  congenital or infantile 750.5
  neurotic 306.4
  newborn 750.5
  psychogenic 306.4
Pylorus, pyloric —*see* condition
Pyoarthrosis —*see* Pyarthrosis
Pyocele
  mastoid 383.00
  sinus (accessory) (nasal) (*see also* Sinusitis)
    473.9
  turbinate (bone) 473.9
  urethra (*see also* Urethritis) 597.0
Pyococcal dermatitis 686.00
Pyococcide, skin 686.00
Pyocolpos (*see also* Vaginitis) 616.10
Pyocyaneus dermatitis 686.09
Pyocystitis (*see also* Cystitis) 595.9
Pyoderma, pyodermia NEC 686.00
  gangrenosum 686.01
  specified type NEC 686.09
  vegetans 686.8
Pyodermatitis 686.00
  vegetans 686.8
Pyogenic —*see* condition

Pyohemia —*see* Septicemia
Pyohydronephrosis (*see also* Pyelitis) 590.80
Pyometra 615.9
Pyometritis (*see also* Endometritis) 615.9
Pyometrium (*see also* Endometritis) 615.9
Pyomyositis 728.0
  ossificans 728.19
  tropical (bungpagga) 040.81
Pyonephritis (*see also* Pyelitis) 590.80
  chronic 590.00
Pyonephrosis (congenital) (*see also* Pyelitis)
  590.80
  acute 590.10
Pyo-oophoritis (*see also* Salpingo-oophoritis)
  614.2
Pyo-ovarium (*see also* Salpingo-oophoritis)
  614.2
Pyopericarditis 420.99
Pyopericardium 420.99
Pyophlebitis —*see* Phlebitis
Pyopneumopericardium 420.99
Pyopneumothorax (infectional) 510.9
  with fistula 510.0
  subdiaphragmatic (*see also* Peritonitis) 567.29
  subphrenic (*see also* Peritonitis) 567.29
  tuberculous (*see also* Tuberculosis, pleura) 012.0
Pyorrhea (alveolar) (alveolaris) 523.40
  degenerative 523.5
Pyosalpingitis (*see also* Salpingo-oophoritis) 614.2
Pyosalpinx (*see also* Salpingo-oophoritis) 614.2
Pyosepticemia —*see* Septicemia
Pyosis
  Corlett's (impetigo) 684
  Manson's (pemphigus contagiosus) 684
Pyothorax 510.9
  with fistula 510.0
  tuberculous (*see also* Tuberculosis, pleura)
    012.0
Pyoureter 593.89
  tuberculous (*see also* Tuberculosis) 016.2
Pyramidopallidonigral syndrome 332.0
Pyrexia (of unknown origin) (P.U.O.) 780.60
  atmospheric 992.0
  during labor 659.2
  environmentally-induced
    newborn 778.4
  heat 992.0
  newborn, environmentally-induced 778.4
  puerperal 672
Pyroglobulinemia 273.8
Pyromania 312.33
Pyrosis 787.1
Pyrroloporphyria 277.1
Pyuria (bacterial) 791.9

Q

Q fever 083.0
  with pneumonia 083.0 *[484.8]*
Quadricuspid aortic valve 746.89
Quadrilateral fever 083.0
Quadriparesis —*see* Quadriplegia
  meaning muscle weakness 728.87
Quadriplegia 344.00
  with fracture, vertebra (process)—*see* Fracture,
    vertebra, cervical, with spinal cord injury
  brain (current episode) 437.8
  cerebral (current episode) 437.8
  C1-C4
    complete 344.01
    incomplete 344.02
  C5-C7
    complete 344.03
    incomplete 344.04
  congenital or infantile (cerebral) (spastic)
    (spinal) 343.2
  cortical 437.8
  embolic (current episode) (*see also* Embolism,
    brain) 434.1
  functional 780.72
  infantile (cerebral) (spastic) (spinal) 343.2
  newborn NEC 767.0
  specified NEC 344.09
  thrombotic (current episode) (*see also*
    Thrombosis, brain) 434.0
  traumatic—*see* Injury, spinal, cervical
Quadruplet
  affected by maternal complications of pregnancy
    761.5
  healthy liveborn—*see* Newborn, multiple
  pregnancy (complicating delivery) NEC 651.8
    with fetal loss and retention of one or more
      fetus(es) 651.5
    following (elective) fetal reduction 651.7
Quarrelsomeness 301.3
Quartan
  fever 084.2
  malaria (fever) 084.2
Queensland fever 083.0
  coastal 083.0
  seven-day 100.89
Quervain's disease 727.04
  thyroid (subacute granulomatous thyroiditis)
    245.1
Queyrat's erythroplasia (M8080/2)
  specified site—*see* Neoplasm, skin, in situ
  unspecified site 233.5
Quincke's disease or edema —*see* Edema,
  angioneurotic
Quinquaud's disease (acne decalvans) 704.09
Quinsy (gangrenous) 475
Quintan fever 083.1
Quintuplet
  affected by maternal complications of pregnancy
    761.5
  healthy liveborn—*see* Newborn, multiple
  pregnancy (complicating delivery) NEC 651.2
    with fetal loss and retention of one or more
      fetus(es) 651.6
    following (elective) fetal reduction 651.7
Quotidian
  fever 084.0
  malaria (fever) 084.0

R

Rabbia 071
Rabbit fever (*see also* Tularemia) 021.9
Rabies 071
  contact V01.5
  exposure to V01.5
  inoculation V04.5
    reaction—*see* Complications, vaccination
  vaccination, prophylactic (against) V04.5
Rachischisis (*see also* Spina bifida) 741.9
Rachitic —*see also* condition
  deformities of spine 268.1
  pelvis 268.1
    with disproportion (fetopelvic) 653.2
      affecting fetus or newborn 763.1
      causing obstructed labor 660.1
        affecting fetus or newborn 763.1
Rachitis, rachitism —*see also* Rickets
  acute 268.0
  fetalis 756.4
  renalis 588.0
  tarda 268.0
Racket nail 757.5
Radial nerve —*see* condition
Radiation effects or sickness —*see also* Effect,
  adverse, radiation
  cataract 366.46
  dermatitis 692.82
  sunburn (*see also* Sunburn) 692.71
Radiculitis (pressure) (vertebrogenic) 729.2
  accessory nerve 723.4
  anterior crural 724.4
  arm 723.4
  brachial 723.4
  cervical NEC 723.4
  due to displacement of intervertebral disc—*see*
    Neuritis, due to, displacement intervertebral
    disc
  leg 724.4
  lumbar NEC 724.4
  lumbosacral 724.4
  rheumatic 729.2
  syphilitic 094.89
  thoracic (with visceral pain) 724.4
Radiculomyelitis 357.0
  toxic, due to
    Clostridium tetani 037
    Corynebacterium diphtheriae 032.89
Radiculopathy (*see also* Radiculitis) 729.2
Radioactive substances, adverse effect —*see*
  Effect, adverse, radioactive substance
Radiodermal burns (acute) (chronic)
  (occupational)—*see* Burn, by site
Radiodermatitis 692.82
Radionecrosis —*see* Effect, adverse, radiation
Radiotherapy session V58.0
Radium, adverse effect —*see* Effect, adverse,
  radioactive substance
Raeder-Harbitz syndrome (pulseless disease) 446.7
Rage (*see also* Disturbance, conduct) 312.0
  meaning rabies 071
Rag sorters' disease 022.1
Raillietiniasis 123.8
Railroad neurosis 300.16
Railway spine 300.16
Raised —*see* Elevation
Raiva 071
Rake teeth, tooth 524.39
Rales 786.7

Ramifying renal pelvis 753.3
Ramsay Hunt syndrome (herpetic geniculate
    ganglionitis) 053.11
    meaning dyssynergia cerebellaris myoclonica 334.2
Ranke's primary infiltration (*see also*
    Tuberculosis) 010.0
Ranula 527.6
    congenital 750.26
Rape
    adult 995.83
    alleged, observation or examination V71.5
    child 995.53
Rapid
    feeble pulse, due to shock, following injury 958.4
    heart (beat) 785.0
        psychogenic 306.2
    respiration 786.06
        psychogenic 306.1
    second stage (delivery) 661.3
        affecting fetus or newborn 763.6
    time-zone change syndrome 327.35
Rarefaction, bone 733.99
Rash 782.1
    canker 034.1
    diaper 691.0
    drug (internal use) 693.0
        contact 692.3
    ECHO 9 virus 078.89
    enema 692.89
    food (*see also* Allergy, food) 693.1
    heat 705.1
    napkin 691.0
    nettle 708.8
    pustular 782.1
    rose 782.1
        epidemic 056.9
        of infants 057.8
    scarlet 034.1
    serum (prophylactic) (therapeutic) 999.59
    toxic 782.1
    wandering tongue 529.1
Rasmussen's aneurysm (*see also* Tuberculosis)
    011.2
Rat-bite fever 026.9
    due to Streptobacillus moniliformis 026.1
    spirochetal (morsus muris) 026.0
Rathke's pouch tumor (M9350/1) 237.0
Raymond (-Céstan) syndrome 433.8
Raynaud's
    disease or syndrome (paroxysmal digital
        cyanosis) 443.0
    gangrene (symmetric) 443.0 *[785.4]*
    phenomenon (paroxysmal digital cyanosis)
        (secondary) 443.0
RDS 769
Reaction
    acute situational maladjustment (*see also*
        Reaction, adjustment) 309.9
    adaptation (*see also* Reaction, adjustment) 309.9
    adjustment 309.9
        with
            anxious mood 309.24
                with depressed mood 309.28
            conduct disturbance 309.3
                combined with disturbance of emotions 309.4
            depressed mood 309.0
                brief 309.0
                    with anxious mood 309.28
                prolonged 309.1
            elective mutism 309.83
            mixed emotions and conduct 309.4

Reaction—*continued*
    adjustment—*continued*
        with—*continued*
            mutism, elective 309.83
            physical symptoms 309.82
            predominant disturbance (of)
                conduct 309.3
                emotions NEC 309.29
                    mixed 309.28
                mixed, emotions and conduct 309.4
                specified type NEC 309.89
            specific academic or work inhibition 309.23
            withdrawal 309.83
        depressive 309.0
            with conduct disturbance 309.4
            brief 309.0
            prolonged 309.1
        specified type NEC 309.89
    adverse food NEC 995.7
    affective (*see also* Psychosis, affective) 296.90
        specified type NEC 296.99
    aggressive 301.3
        unsocialized (*see also* Disturbance, conduct)
            312.0
    allergic (*see also* Allergy) 995.3
        drug, medicinal substance, and
            biological—*see* Allergy, drug
        due to correct medical substance properly
            administered 995.27
        food—*see* Allergy, food
        serum 999.59
    anaphylactic—*see* Anaphylactic reaction
    anesthesia—*see* Anesthesia, complication
    anger 312.0
    antisocial 301.7
    antitoxin (prophylactic) (therapeutic)—*see*
        Complications, vaccination
    anxiety 300.00
    Arthus 995.21
    asthenic 300.5
    compulsive 300.3
    conversion (anesthetic) (autonomic)
        (hyperkinetic) (mixed paralytic)
        (paresthetic) 300.11
    deoxyribonuclease (DNA) (DNase)
        hypersensitivity NEC 287.2
    depressive 300.4
        acute 309.0
        affective (*see also* Psychosis, affective) 296.2
            recurrent episode 296.3
            single episode 296.2
        brief 309.0
        manic (*see also* Psychosis, affective) 296.80
        neurotic 300.4
        psychoneurotic 300.4
        psychotic 298.0
    dissociative 300.15
    drug NEC (*see also* Table of Drugs and
        Chemicals) 995.20
        allergic—*see also* Allergy, drug 995.27
        correct substance properly administered 995.20
        obstetric anesthetic or analgesic NEC 668.9
            affecting fetus or newborn 763.5
            specified drug—*see* Table of drugs and
                chemicals
        overdose or poisoning 977.9
            specified drug—*see* Table of drugs and
                chemicals
        specific to newborn 779.4
        transmitted via placenta or breast milk—*see*
            Absorption, drug, through placenta

Reaction—*continued*
  drug—*continued*
    withdrawal NEC 292.0
      infant of dependent mother 779.5
      wrong substance given or taken in error 977.9
      specified drug—*see* Table of drugs and
        chemicals
  dyssocial 301.7
  dystonic, acute, due to drugs 333.72
  erysipeloid 027.1
  fear 300.20
    child 313.0
  fluid loss, cerebrospinal 349.0
  food—*see also* Allergy, food
    adverse NEC 995.7
      anaphylactic shock—*see* Anaphylactic
        reaction or shock, due to food
  foreign
    body NEC 728.82
      in operative wound (inadvertently left) 998.4
      due to surgical material intentionally
        left—*see* Complications, due to
        (presence of) any device, implant, or
        graft classified to 996.0-996.5 NEC
    substance accidentally left during a procedure
      (chemical) (powder) (talc) 998.7
      body or object (instrument) (sponge) (swab)
        998.4
  graft-versus-host (GVH) 279.50
  grief (acute) (brief) 309.0
    prolonged 309.1
  gross stress (*see also* Reaction, stress, acute)
    308.9
  group delinquent (*see also* Disturbance,
    conduct) 312.2
  Herxheimer's 995.91
  hyperkinetic (*see also* Hyperkinesia) 314.9
  hypochondriacal 300.7
  hypoglycemic, due to insulin 251.0
    therapeutic misadventure 962.3
  hypomanic (*see also* Psychosis, affective) 296.0
    recurrent episode 296.1
    single episode 296.0
  hysterical 300.10
    conversion type 300.11
    dissociative 300.15
  id (bacterial cause) 692.89
  immaturity NEC 301.89
    aggressive 301.3
    emotional instability 301.59
  immunization—*see* Complications, vaccination
  incompatibility
    blood group (*see also* Complications,
      transfusion) 999.80
    ABO (due to transfusion of blood or blood
      products) (*see also* Complications,
      transfusion) 999.60
    minor blood group 999.89
    non-ABO (*see also* Complications,
      transfusion) 999.75
    Rh antigen (C) (c) (D) (E) (e) (factor)
      (infusion) (transfusion) (*see also*
      Complications, transfusion) 999.70
  inflammatory—*see* Infection
  infusion—*see* Complications, infusion
  inoculation (immune serum)—*see*
    Complications, vaccination
  insulin 995.23

Reaction—*continued*
  involutional
    paranoid 297.2
    psychotic (*see also* Psychosis, affective,
      depressive) 296.2
  leukemoid (basophilic) (lymphocytic)
    (monocytic) (myelocytic) (neutrophilic)
    288.62
  LSD (*see also* Abuse, drugs, nondependent) 305.3
  lumbar puncture 349.0
  manic-depressive (*see also* Psychosis, affective)
    296.80
    depressed 296.2
      recurrent episode 296.3
      single episode 296.2
    hypomanic 296.0
  neurasthenic 300.5
  neurogenic (*see also* Neurosis) 300.9
  neurotic NEC 300.9
  neurotic-depressive 300.4
  nitritoid—*see* Crisis, nitritoid
  nonspecific
    to
      cell mediated immunity measurement of
        gamma interferon antigen response
        without active tuberculosis 795.52
      QuantiFERON-TB test (QFT) without active
        tuberculosis 795.52
      tuberculin test (*see also* Reaction, tuberculin
        skin test) 795.51
  obsessive-compulsive 300.3
  organic 293.9
    acute 293.0
    subacute 293.1
  overanxious, child or adolescent 313.0
  paranoid (chronic) 297.9
    acute 298.3
    climacteric 297.2
    involutional 297.2
    menopausal 297.2
    senile 290.20
    simple 297.0
  passive
    aggressive 301.84
    dependency 301.6
  personality (*see also* Disorder, personality)
    301.9
  phobic 300.20
  postradiation—*see* Effect, adverse, radiation
  psychogenic NEC 300.9
  psychoneurotic (*see also* Neurosis) 300.9
    anxiety 300.00
    compulsive 300.3
    conversion 300.11
    depersonalization 300.6
    depressive 300.4
    dissociative 300.15
    hypochondriacal 300.7
    hysterical 300.10
      conversion type 300.11
      dissociative type 300.15
    neurasthenic 300.5
    obsessive 300.3
    obsessive-compulsive 300.3
    phobic 300.20
    tension state 300.9
  psychophysiologic NEC (*see also* Disorder,
    psychosomatic) 306.9
    cardiovascular 306.2
    digestive 306.4
    endocrine 306.6

Reaction—*continued*
 psychophysiologic —*continued*
  gastrointestinal 306.4
  genitourinary 306.50
  heart 306.2
  hemic 306.8
  intestinal (large) (small) 306.4
  laryngeal 306.1
  lymphatic 306.8
  musculoskeletal 306.0
  pharyngeal 306.1
  respiratory 306.1
  skin 306.3
  special sense organs 306.7
 psychosomatic (*see also* Disorder,
   psychosomatic) 306.9
 psychotic (*see also* Psychosis) 298.9
  depressive 298.0
  due to or associated with physical condition
    (*see also* Psychosis, organic) 293.9
  involutional (*see also* Psychosis, affective)
    296.2
   recurrent episode 296.3
   single episode 296.2
 pupillary (myotonic) (tonic) 379.46
 radiation—*see* Effect, adverse, radiation
 runaway—*see also* Disturbance, conduct
  socialized 312.2
  undersocialized, unsocialized 312.1
 scarlet fever toxin—*see* Complications,
   vaccination
 schizophrenic (*see also* Schizophrenia) 295.9
  latent 295.5
 serological for syphilis—*see* Serology for
   syphilis
 serum (prophylactic) (therapeutic) 999.59
  anaphylactic 999.49
  due to
   administration of blood and blood products
     999.51
    anaphylactic 999.41
   vaccination 999.52
    anaphylactic 999.41
   immediate 999.49
 situational (*see also* Reaction, adjustment) 309.9
  acute, to stress 308.3
 adjustment (*see also* Reaction, adjustment) 309.9
 somatization (*see also* Disorder, psychosomatic)
   306.9
 spinal puncture 349.0
 spite, child (*see also* Disturbance, conduct) 312.0
 stress, acute 308.9
  bone or cartilage —*see* Fracture, stress
  with predominant disturbance (of)
   consciousness 308.1
   emotions 308.0
   mixed 308.4
   psychomotor 308.2
   specified type NEC 308.3
 surgical procedure—*see* Complications, surgical
   procedure
 tetanus antitoxin—*see* Complications,
   vaccination
 toxin-antitoxin—*see* Complications, vaccination
 transfusion (blood) (bone marrow)
   (lymphocytes) (allergic) (see also
   Complications, transfusion) 999.80
 tuberculin skin test, nonspecific (without active
   tuberculosis) 795.51
  positive (without active tuberculosis) 795.51

Reaction— *continued*
 ultraviolet—*see* Effect, adverse, ultraviolet
 undersocialized, unsocialized—*see also*
   Disturbance, conduct
  aggressive (type) 312.0
  unaggressive (type) 312.1
 vaccination (any)—*see* Complications,
   vaccination
 white graft (skin) 996.52
 withdrawing, child or adolescent 313.22
 x-ray—*see* Effect, adverse, x-rays
Reactive depression (*see also* Reaction,
   depressive) 300.4
 neurotic 300.4
 psychoneurotic 300.4
 psychotic 298.0
Rebound tenderness 789.6
Recalcitrant patient V15.81
Recanalization, thrombus —*see* Thrombosis
Recession, receding
 chamber angle (eye) 364.77
 chin 524.06
 gingival (postinfective) (postoperative) 523.20
  generalized 523.25
  localized 523.24
  minimal 523.21
  moderate 523.22
  servere 523.23
Recklinghausen's disease (M9540/1) 237.71
 bones (osteitis fibrosa cystica) 252.01
Recklinghausen-Applebaum disease
   (hemochromatosis) 275.03
Reclus' disease (cystic) 610.1
Recrudescent typhus (fever) 081.1
Recruitment, auditory 388.44
Rectalgia 569.42
Rectitis 569.49
Rectocele
 female (without uterine prolapse) 618.04
  with uterine prolapse 618.4
   complete 618.3
   incomplete 618.2
 in pregnancy or childbirth 654.4
  causing obstructed labor 660.2
   affecting fetus or newborn 763.1
 male 569.49
 vagina, vaginal (outlet) 618.04
Rectosigmoiditis 569.89
 ulcerative (chronic) 556.3
Rectosigmoid junction —*see* condition
Rectourethral —*see* condition
Rectovaginal —*see* condition
Rectovesical —*see* condition
Rectum, rectal —*see* condition
Recurrent —*see* condition
 pregnancy loss - *see* Pregnancy, management
   affected by, abortion, habitual
Red bugs 133.8
Red cedar asthma 495.8
Redness
 conjunctiva 379.93
 eye 379.93
 nose 478.19
Reduced ventilatory or vital capacity 794.2
Reduction
 function
  kidney (*see also* Disease, renal) 593.9
  liver 573.8
 ventilatory capacity 794.2
 vital capacity 794.2

Redundant, redundancy
abdomen 701.9
anus 751.5
cardia 537.89
clitoris 624.2
colon (congenital) 751.5
foreskin (congenital) 605
intestine 751.5
labia 624.3
organ or site, congenital NEC—*see* Accessory
panniculus (abdominal) 278.1
prepuce (congenital) 605
pylorus 537.89
rectum 751.5
scrotum 608.89
sigmoid 751.5
skin (of face) 701.9
eyelids 374.30
stomach 537.89
uvula 528.9
vagina 623.8
Reduplication —*see* Duplication
Referral
adoption (agency) V68.89
nursing care V63.8
patient without examination or treatment V68.81
social services V63.8
Reflex —*see also* condition
blink, deficient 374.45
hyperactive gag 478.29
neurogenic bladder NEC 596.54
atonic 596.54
with cauda equina syndrome 344.61
vasoconstriction 443.9
Reflux 530.81
acid 530.81
esophageal 530.81
esophagitis 530.11
gastroesophageal 530.81
mitral—*see* Insufficiency, mitral
ureteral —*see* Reflux, vesicoureteral
vasovagal 780.2
vesicoureteral 593.70
with
reflux nephropathy 593.73
bilateral 593.72
unilateral 593.71
Reformed gallbladder 576.0
Reforming, artificial openings (*see also*
Attention to, artificial, opening) V55.9
Refractive error (*see also* Error, refractive) 367.9
Refsum's disease or syndrome (heredopathia
atactica polyneuritiformis) 356.3
Refusal of
food 307.59
hysterical 300.11
treatment because of, due to
patient's decision NEC V64.2
reason of conscience or religion V62.6
Regaud
tumor (M8082/3)—*see* Neoplasm, nasopharynx,
malignant
type carcinoma (M8082/3)—*see* Neoplasm,
nasopharynx, malignant
Regional —*see* condition
Regulation feeding (elderly) (infant) 783.3
newborn 779.31
Regurgitated
food, choked on 933.1
stomach contents, choked on 933.1

Regurgitation 787.03
aortic (valve) (*see also* Insufficiency, aortic) 424.1
congenital 746.4
syphilitic 093.22
food—*see also* Vomiting
with reswallowing—*see* Rumination
newborn 779.33
gastric contents—*see* Vomiting
heart—*see* Endocarditis
mitral (valve)—*see also* Insufficiency, mitral
congenital 746.6
myocardial—*see* Endocarditis
pulmonary (heart) (valve) (*see also*
Endocarditis, pulmonary) 424.3
stomach—*see* Vomiting
tricuspid—*see* Endocarditis, tricuspid
valve, valvular—*see* Endocarditis
vesicoureteral —*see* Reflux, vesicoureteral
Rehabilitation V57.9
multiple types V57.89
occupational V57.21
specified type NEC V57.89
speech(-language) V57.3
vocational V57.22
Reichmann's disease or syndrome
(gastrosuccorrhea) 536.8
Reifenstein's syndrome (hereditary familial
hypogonadism, male) 259.52
Reilly's syndrome or phenomenon (*see also*
Neuropathy, peripheral, autonomic) 337.9
Reimann's periodic disease 277.31
Reinsertion, contraceptive device V25.42
intrauterine V25.13
Reiter's disease, syndrome, or urethritis 099.3
[711.1]
Rejection
food, hysterical 300.11
transplant 996.80
bone marrow 996.85
corneal 996.51
organ (immune or nonimmune cause) 996.80
bone marrow 996.85
heart 996.83
intestines 996.87
kidney 996.81
liver 996.82
lung 996.84
pancreas 996.86
specified NEC 996.89
skin 996.52
artificial 996.55
decellularized allodermis 996.55
stem cell(s) 996.88
from
peripheral blood 996.88
umbilical cord 996.88
Relapsing fever 087.9
Carter's (Asiatic) 087.0
Dutton's (West African) 087.1
Koch's 087.9
louse-borne (epidemic) 087.0
Novy's (American) 087.1
Obermeyer's (European) 087.0
Spirillum 087.9
tick-borne (endemic) 087.1
Relaxation
anus (sphincter) 569.49
due to hysteria 300.11
arch (foot) 734
congenital 754.61
back ligaments 728.4

Relaxation—*continued*
  bladder (sphincter) 596.59
  cardio-esophageal 530.89
  cervix (*see also* Incompetency, cervix) 622.5
  diaphragm 519.4
  inguinal rings—*see* Hernia, inguinal
  joint (capsule) (ligament) (paralytic) (*see also*
      Derangement, joint) 718.90
    congenital 755.8
  lumbosacral joint 724.6
  pelvic floor 618.89
  pelvis 618.89
  perineum 618.89
  posture 729.90
  rectum (sphincter) 569.49
  sacroiliac (joint) 724.6
  scrotum 608.89
  urethra (sphincter) 599.84
  uterus (outlet) 618.89
  vagina (outlet) 618.89
  vesical 596.59
Remains
  canal of Cloquet 743.51
  capsule (opaque) 743.51
Remittent fever (malarial) 084.6
Remnant
  canal of Cloquet 743.51
  capsule (opaque) 743.51
  cervix, cervical stump (acquired) (postoperative)
      622.8
  cystic duct, postcholecystectomy 576.0
  fingernail 703.8
    congenital 757.5
  meniscus, knee 717.5
  thyroglossal duct 759.2
  tonsil 474.8
    infected 474.00
  urachus 753.7
Remote effect of cancer —*see* Condition
Removal (of)
  catheter (urinary) (indwelling) V53.6
    from artificial opening—*see* Attention to,
        artificial, opening
    non-vascular V58.82
    vascular V58.81
  cerebral ventricle (communicating) shunt V53.01
  device—*see also* Fitting (of)
    contraceptive V25.12
      with reinsertion V25.13
    fixation
      external V54.89
      internal V54.01
      traction V54.89
  drains V58.49
  dressing
    wound V58.30
      nonsurgical V58.30
      surgical V58.31
  ileostomy V55.2
  Kirschner wire V54.89
  non-vascular catheter V58.82
  pin V54.01
  plaster cast V54.89
  plate (fracture) V54.01
  rod V54.01
  screw V54.01
  splint, external V54.89
  subdermal implantable contraceptive V25.43
  staples V58.32
  sutures V58.32
  traction device, external V54.89

Removal (of)—*continued*
  vascular catheter V58.81
  wound packing V58.30
    nonsurgical V58.30
    surgical V58.31
Ren
  arcuatus 753.3
  mobile, mobilis (*see also* Disease, renal) 593.0
    congenital 753.3
  unguliformis 753.3
Renal —*see also* condition
  glomerulohyalinosis-diabetic syndrome 250.4
      [581.81]
    due to secondary diabetes 249.4 *[581.81]*
Rendu-Osler-Weber disease or syndrome
    (familial hemorrhagic telangiectasia) 448.0
Reninoma (M8361/1) 236.91
Rénon-Delille syndrome 253.8
Repair
  pelvic floor, previous, in pregnancy or childbirth
      654.4
    affecting fetus or newborn 763.89
  scarred tissue V51.8
Replacement by artificial or mechanical device
    or prosthesis of (*see also* Fitting (of))
  artificial skin V43.83
  bladder V43.5
  blood vessel V43.4
  breast V43.82
  eye globe V43.0
  heart
    with
      assist device V43.21
      fully implantable artificial heart V43.22
    valve V43.3
  intestine V43.89
  joint V43.60
    ankle 43.66
    elbow V43.62
    finger V43.69
    hip (partial) (total) V43.64
    knee V43.65
    shoulder V43.61
    specified NEC V43.69
    wrist V43.63
  kidney V43.89
  larynx V43.81
  lens V43.1
  limb(s) V43.7
  liver V43.89
  lung V43.89
  organ NEC V43.89
  pancreas V43.89
  skin (artificial) V43.83
  tissue NEC V43.89
Reprogramming
  cardiac pacemaker V53.31
Request for expert evidence V68.2
Reserve, decreased or low
  cardiac—*see* Disease, heart
  kidney (*see also* Disease, renal) 593.9
Residual —*see also* condition
  bladder 596.89
  foreign body—*see* Retention, foreign body
  state, schizophrenic (*see also* Schizophrenia)
      295.6
  urine 788.69

Resistance, resistant (to)

Note—Use the following subclassification for categories V09.5, V09.7, V09.8, V09.9.:

0 *without mention of resistance to multiple drugs*
1 *with resistance to multiple drugs*

V09.5 *quinolones and fluoroquinolones*
V09.7 *antimycobacterial agents*
V09.8 *specified drugs NEC*
V09.9 *unspecified drugs*

9 *multiple sites*

activated protein C 289.81
drugs by microorganisms V09.90
 Amikacin V09.4
 aminoglycosides V09.4
 Amodiaquine V09.5
 Amoxicillin V09.0
 Ampicillin V09.0
 antimycobacterial agents V09.7
 Azithromycin V09.2
 Azlocillin V09.0
 Aztreonam V09.1
 B-lactam antibiotics V09.1
 Bacampicillin V09.0
 Bacitracin V09.8
 Benznidazole V09.8
 Capreomycin V09.7
 Carbenicillin V09.0
 Cefaclor V09.1
 Cefadroxil V09.1
 Cefamandole V09.1
 Cefatetan V09.1
 Cefazolin V09.1
 Cefixime V09.1
 Cefonicid V09.1
 Cefoperazone V09.1
 Ceforanide V09.1
 Cefotaxime V09.1
 Cefoxitin V09.1
 Ceftazidine V09.1
 Ceftizoxime V09.1
 Ceftriaxone V09.1
 Cefuroxime V09.1
 Cephalexin V09.1
 Cephaloglycin V09.1
 Cephaloridine V09.1
 cephalosporins V09.1
 Cephalothin V09.1
 Cephapirin V09.1
 Cephradine V09.1
 Chloramphenicol V09.8
 Chloraquine V09.5
 Chlorguanide V09.8
 Chlorproguanil V09.8
 Chlortetracycline V09.3
 Cinoxacin V09.5
 Ciprofloxacin V09.5
 Clarithromycin V09.2
 Clindamycin V09.8
 Clioquinol V09.5
 Clofazimine V09.7
 Cloxacillin V09.0
 Cyclacillin V09.0
 Cycloserine V09.7
 Dapsone [DZ] V09.7
 Demeclocycline V09.3
 Dicloxacillin V09.0

Resistance, resistant (to)—*continued*
 drugs by microorganisms—*continued*
 Doxycycline V09.3
 Enoxacin V09.5
 Erythromycin V09.2
 Ethambutol [EMB] V09.7
 Ethionamide [ETA] V09.7
 fluoroquinolones NEC V09.5
 Gentamicin V09.4
 Halofantrine V09.8
 ImipenemV09.1
 Iodoquinol V09.5
 Isoniazid [INH] V09.7
 Kanamycin V09.4
 macrolides V09.2
 Mafenide V09.6
 MDRO (multiple drug resistant organisms)
  NOS V09.91
 Mefloquine V09.8
 Melassoprol V09.8
 Methacycline V09.3
 Methenamine V09.8
 Methicillin—*see* Infection, methicillin
 Metronidazole V09.8
 Mezlocillin V09.0
 Minocycline V09.3
 multiple drug resistant organisms NOS V09.91
 Nafcillin V09.0
 Nalidixic Acid V09.5
 Natamycin V09.2
 Neomycin V09.4
 Netilmicin V09.4
 Nimorazole V09.8
 Nitrofurantoin V09.8
 Nitrofurtimox V09.8
 Norfloxacin V09.5
 Nystatin V09.2
 Ofloxacin V09.5
 Oleandomycin V09.2
 Oxacillin V09.0
 Oxytetracycline V09.3
 Para-amino salicylic acid [PAS] V09.7
 Paromomycin V09.4
 Penicillin (G)(V)(VK) V09.0
 penicillins V09.0
 Pentamidine V09.8
 Piperacillin V09.0
 Primaquine V09.5
 Proguanil V09.8
 Pyrazinamide [PZA] V09.7
 Pyrimethamine/Sulfalene V09.8
 Pyrimethamine/Sulfodoxine V09.8
 Quinacrine V09.5
 Quinidine V09.8
 Quinine V09.8
 quinolones V09.5
 Rifabutin V09.7
 Rifampin [RIF] V09.7
 Rifamycin V09.7
 Rolitetracycline V09.3
 specified drugs NEC V09.8
 Spectinomycin V09.8
 Spiramycin V09.2
 Streptomycin [SM] V09.4
 Sulfacetamide V09.6
 Sulfacytine V90.6
 Sulfadiazine V09.6
 Sulfadoxine V09.6
 Sulfamethoxazole V09.6
 Sulfapyridine V09.6
 Sulfasalizine V09.6

Retention, retained—*continued*
  decidua (following delivery) (fragments) (with
      hemorrhage) 666.2
    without hemorrhage 667.1
  deciduous tooth 520.6
  dental root 525.3
  fecal (*see also* Constipation) 564.00
  fluid 276.69
  foreign body—*see also* Foreign body, retained
    bone 733.99
    current trauma—*see* Foreign body, by site or type
    middle ear 385.83
    muscle 729.6
    soft tissue NEC 729.6
  gallstones, following cholecystectomy 997.41
  gastric 536.8
  membranes (following delivery) (with
      hemorrhage) 666.2
    with abortion—*see* Abortion, by type
    without hemorrhage 667.1
  menses 626.8
  milk (puerperal) 676.2
  nitrogen, extrarenal 788.99
  placenta (total) (with hemorrhage) 666.0
    with abortion—*see* Abortion, by type
    portions or fragments 666.2
      without hemorrhage 667.1
    without hemorrhage 667.0
  products of conception
    early pregnancy (fetal death before 22
        completed weeks gestation) 632
    following
      abortion—*see* Abortion, by type
      delivery 666.2
        with hemorrhage 666.2
        without hemorrhage 667.1
  secundines (following delivery) (with
      hemorrhage) 666.2
    with abortion—*see* Abortion, by type
    complicating puerperium (delayed
        hemorrhage) 666.2
    without hemorrhage 667.1
  smegma, clitoris 624.8
  urine NEC 788.20
    bladder, incomplete emptying 788.21
    due to benign prostatic hypertrophy
        (BPH)—*see* category 600
    due to benign prostatic hypertrophy
        (BPH)—*see* category 600
    psychogenic 306.53
    specified NEC 788.29
  water (in tissue) (*see also* Edema) 782.3
Reticulation, dust (occupational) 504
Reticulocytosis NEC 790.99
Reticuloendotheliosis
  acute infantile (M9722/3) 202.5
  leukemic (M9940/3) 202.4
  malignant (M9720/3) 202.3
  nonlipid (M9722/3) 202.5
Reticulohistiocytoma (giant cell) 277.89
Reticulohistiocytosis, multicentric 272.8
Reticulolymphosarcoma (diffuse) (M9613/3)
    200.8
  follicular (M9691/3) 202.0
  nodular (M9691/3) 202.0
Reticulosarcoma (M9640/3) 200.0
  odular (M9642/3) 200.0
  pleomorphic cell type (M9641/3) 200.0

Reticulosis (skin)
  acute of infancy (M9722/3) 202.5
  familial hemophagocytic 288.4
  histiocytic medullary (M9721/3) 202.3
  lipomelanotic 695.89
  malignant (M9720/3) 202.3
  Sézary's (M9701/3) 202.2
Retina, retinal —*see* condition
Retinitis (*see also* Chorioretinitis) 363.20
  albuminurica 585.9 *[363.10]*
  arteriosclerotic 440.8 *[362.13]*
  central angiospastic 362.41
  Coat's 362.12
  diabetic 250.5 *[362.01]*
    due to secondary diabetes 249.5 *[362.01]*
  disciformis 362.52
  disseminated 363.10
    metastatic 363.14
    neurosyphilitic 094.83
    pigment epitheliopathy 363.15
  exudative 362.12
  focal 363.00
    in histoplasmosis 115.92
      capsulatum 115.02
      duboisii 115.12
    juxtapapillary 363.05
    macular 363.06
    paramacular 363.06
    peripheral 363.08
    posterior pole NEC 363.07
  gravidarum 646.8
  hemorrhagica externa 362.12
  juxtapapillary (Jensen's) 363.05
  luetic—*see* Retinitis, syphilitic
  metastatic 363.14
  pigmentosa 362.74
  proliferans 362.29
  proliferating 362.29
  punctata albescens 362.76
  renal 585.9 *[363.13]*
  syphilitic (secondary) 091.51
    congenital 090.0 *[363.13]*
    early 091.51
    late 095.8 *[363.13]*
  syphilitica, central, recurrent 095.8 *[363.13]*
  tuberculous (*see also* Tuberculous) 017.3 *[363.13]*
Retinoblastoma (M9510/3) 190.5
  differentiated type (M9511/3) 190.5
  undifferentiated type (M9512/3) 190.5
Retinochoroiditis (*see also* Chorioretinitis) 363.20
  central angiospastic 362.41
  disseminated 363.10
    metastatic 363.14
    neurosyphilitic 094.83
    pigment epitheliopathy 363.15
    syphilitic 094.83
  due to toxoplasmosis (acquired) (focal) 130.2
  focal 363.00
    in histoplasmosis 115.92
      capsulatum 115.02
      duboisii 115.12
    juxtapapillary (Jensen's) 363.05
    macular 363.06
    paramacular 363.06
    peripheral 363.08
    posterior pole NEC 363.07
  juxtapapillaris 363.05
  syphilitic (disseminated) 094.83

Retinopathy (background) 362.10
  arteriosclerotic 440.8 *[362.13]*
  atherosclerotic 440.8 *[362.13]*
  central serous 362.41
  circinate 362.10
  Coat's 362.12
  diabetic 250.5 *[362.01]*
    due to secondary diabetes 249.5 *[362.01]*
    nonproliferative 250.5 *[362.03]*
      due to secondary diabetes 249.5 *[362.03]*
      mild 250.5 *[362.04]*
        due to secondary diabetes 249.5 *[362.04]*
      moderate 250.5 *[362.05]*
        due to secondary diabetes 249.5 *[362.05]*
      severe 250.5 *[362.06]*
        due to secondary diabetes 249.5 *[362.06]*
    proliferative 250.5 *[362.02]*
      due to secondary diabetes 249.5 *[362.02]*
  exudative 362.12
  hypertensive 362.11
  of prematurity 362.20
    cicatricial 362.21
    stage
      0 362.22
      1 362.23
      2 362.24
      3 362.25
      4 362.26
      5 362.27
  nonproliferative
    diabetic 250.5 *[362.03]*
      due to secondary diabetes 249.5 *[362.03]*
      mild 250.5 *[362.04]*
        due to secondary diabetes 249.5 *[362.04]*
      moderate 250.5 *[362.05]*
        due to secondary diabetes 249.5 *[362.05]*
      severe 250.5 *[362.06]*
        due to secondary diabetes 249.5 *[362.06]*
  pigmentary, congenital 362.74
  proliferative 362.29
    diabetic 250.5 *[362.02]*
      due to secondary diabetes 249.5 *[362.02]*
    sickle-cell 282.60 *[362.29]*
  solar 363.31
Retinoschisis 361.10
  bullous 361.12
  congenital 743.56
  flat 361.11
  juvenile 362.73
Retractile testis 752.52
Retraction
  cervix *see* Retraction, uterus
  drum (membrane) 384.82
  eyelid 374.41
  finger 736.29
  head 781.0
  lid 374.41
  lung 518.89
  mediastinum 519.3
  nipple 611.79
    congenital 757.6
    puerperal, postpartum 676.0
  palmar fascia 728.6
  pleura (*see also* Pleurisy) 511.0
  ring, uterus (Bandl's) (pathological) 661.4
    affecting fetus or newborn 763.7
  sternum (congenital) 756.3
    acquired 738.3
    during respiration 786.9
  substernal 738.3
  supraclavicular 738.8

Retraction—*continued*
  syndrome (Duane's) 378.71
  uterus 621.6
  valve (heart)—*see* Endocarditis
Retrobulbar —*see* condition
Retrocaval ureter 753.4
Retrocecal —*see also* condition
  appendix (congenital) 751.5
Retrocession —*see* Retroversion
Retrodisplacement —*see* Retroversion
Retroflection, retroflexion —*see* Retroversion
Retrognathia, retrognathism (mandibular)
  (maxillary) 524.06
Retrograde
  ejaculation 608.87
  menstruation 626.8
Retroiliac ureter 753.4
Retroperineal —*see* condition
Retroperitoneal —*see* condition
Retroperitonitis 567.39
Retropharyngeal —*see* condition
Retroplacental —*see* condition
Retroposition —*see* Retroversion
Retroprosthetic membrane 996.51
Retrosternal thyroid (congenital) 759.2
Retroversion, retroverted
  cervix *see* Retroversion, uterus
  female NEC (*see also* Retroversion, uterus) 621.6
  iris 364.70
  testis (congenital) 752.51
  uterus, uterine (acquired) (acute) (adherent) (any
    degree) (asymptomatic) (cervix)
    (postinfectional) (postpartal, old) 621.6
    congenital 752.39
    in pregnancy or childbirth 654.3
      affecting fetus or newborn 763.89
      causing obstructed labor 660.2
        affecting fetus or newborn 763.1
Retrusion, premaxilla (developmental) 524.04
Rett's syndrome 330.8
Reverse, reversed
  peristalsis 787.4
Reye's syndrome 331.81
Reye-Sheehan syndrome (postpartum pituitary
  necrosis) 253.2
Rh antigen (C) (c) (D) (E) (e) (factor)
  hemolytic disease 773.0
  incompatibility, immunization, or sensitization
    affecting management of pregnancy 656.1
    fetus or newborn 773.0
      transfusion reaction (*see also* Complications,
        transfusion) 999.70
    negative mother, affecting fetus or newborn
      773.0
    titer elevated (*see also* Complications,
      transfusion) 999.70
    transfusion reaction (*see also* Complications,
      transfusion) 999.70
Rhabdomyolysis (idiopathic) 728.88
Rhabdomyoma (M8900/0)—*see also* Neoplasm,
  connective tissue, benign
  adult (M8904/0)—*see* Neoplasm, connective
    tissue, benign
  fetal (M8903/0)—*see* Neoplasm, connective
    tissue, benign
  glycogenic (M8904/0)—*see* Neoplasm,
    connective tissue, benign

Rhabdomyosarcoma (M8900/3)—*see also*
  Neoplasm connective tissue, malignant
  alveolar (M8920/3)—*see* Neoplasm, connective
    tissue, malignant
  embryonal (M8910/3)—*see* Neoplasm,
    connective tissue malignant
  mixed type (M8902/3)—*see* Neoplasm,
    connective tissue, malignant
  pleomorphic (M8901/3)—*see* Neoplasm,
    connective tissue, malignant
Rhabdosarcoma (M8900/3)—*see*
  Rhabdomyosarcoma
Rhesus (factor) (Rh) incompatibility—*see* Rh,
  incompatibility
Rheumaticosis —*see* Rheumatism
Rheumatism, rheumatic (acute NEC) 729.0
  adherent pericardium 393
  arthritis
    acute or subacute—*see* Fever, rheumatic
    chronic 714.0
      spine 720.0
  articular (chronic) NEC (*see also* Arthritis)
    716.9
    acute or subacute—*see* Fever, rheumatic
  back 724.9
  blennorrhagic 098.59
  carditis—*see* Disease, heart, rheumatic
  cerebral—*see* Fever, rheumatic
  chorea (acute)—*see* Chorea, rheumatic
  chronic NEC 729.0
  coronary arteritis 391.9
    chronic 398.99
  degeneration, myocardium (*see also*
    Degeneration, myocardium, with rheumatic
    fever) 398.0
  desert 114.0
  febrile—*see* Fever, rheumatic
  fever—*see* Fever, rheumatic
  gonococcal 098.59
  gout 714.00
  heart
    disease (*see also* Disease, heart, rheumatic)
      398.90
    failure (chronic) (congestive) (inactive) 398.91
  hemopericardium—*see* Rheumatic, pericarditis
  hydropericardium—*see* Rheumatic, pericarditis
  inflammatory (acute) (chronic) (subacute)—*see*
    Fever, rheumatic
  intercostal 729.0
    meaning Tietze's disease 733.6
  joint (chronic) NEC (*see also* Arthritis) 716.9
    acute—*see* Fever, rheumatic
  mediastinopericarditis—*see* Rheumatic,
    pericarditis
  muscular 729.0
  myocardial degeneration (*see also*
    Degeneration, myocardium, with rheumatic
    fever) 398.0
  myocarditis (chronic) (inactive) (with chorea)
    398.0
    active or acute 391.2
      with chorea (acute) (rheumatic)
        (Sydenham's) 392.0
  myositis 729.1
  neck 724.9
  neuralgic 729.0
  neuritis (acute) (chronic) 729.2
  neuromuscular 729.0
  nodose—*see* Arthritis, nodosa
  nonarticular 729.0

Rheumatism, rheumatic— *continued*
  palindromic 719.30
    ankle 719.37
    elbow 719.32
    foot 719.37
    hand 719.34
    hip 719.35
    knee 719.36
    multiple sites 719.39
    pelvic region 719.35
    shoulder (region) 719.31
    specified site NEC 719.38
    wrist 719.33
  pancarditis, acute 391.8
    with chorea (acute) (rheumatic) (Sydenham's)
      392.0
    chronic or inactive 398.99
  pericarditis (active) (acute) (with effusion) (with
    pneumonia) 391.0
    with chorea (acute) (rheumatic) (Sydenham's)
      392.0
    chronic or inactive 393
  pericardium—*see* Rheumatic, pericarditis
  pleuropericarditis—*see* Rheumatic, pericarditis
  pneumonia 390 *[517.1]*
  pneumonitis 390 *[517.1]*
  pneumopericarditis—*see* Rheumatic,
    pericarditis
  polyarthritis
    acute or subacute—*see* Fever, rheumatic
    chronic 714.0
  polyarticular NEC (*see also* Arthritis) 716.9
  psychogenic 306.0
  radiculitis 729.2
  sciatic 724.3
  septic—*see* Fever, rheumatic
  spine 724.9
  subacute NEC 729.0
  torticollis 723.5
  tuberculous NEC (*see also* Tuberculosis) 015.9
  typhoid fever 002.0
Rheumatoid —*see also* condition
  lungs 714.81
Rhinitis (atrophic) (catarrhal) (chronic)
    (croupous) (fibrinous) (hyperplastic)
    (hypertrophic) (membranous) (purulent)
    (suppurative) (ulcerative) 472.0
  with
    hay fever (*see also* Fever, hay) 477.9
      with asthma (bronchial) 493.0
    sore throat—*see* Nasopharyngitis
  acute 460
  allergic (nonseasonal) (seasonal) (*see also*
    Fever, hay) 477.9
    due to food 477.1
    with asthma (*see also* Asthma) 493.0
  granulomatous 472.0
  infective 460
  obstructive 472.0
  pneumococcal 460
  syphilitic 095.8
    congenital 090.0
  tuberculous (*see also* Tuberculosis) 012.8
  vasomotor (*see also* Fever, hay) 477.9
Rhinoantritis (chronic) 473.0
  acute 461.0
Rhinodacryolith 375.57
Rhinolalia (aperta) (clausa) (open) 784.43
Rhinolith 478.19
  nasal sinus (*see also* Sinusitis) 473.9
Rhinomegaly 478.19

Rhinopharyngitis (acute) (subacute) (*see also* Nasopharyngitis) 460
  chronic 472.2
  destructive ulcerating 102.5
  mutilans 102.5
Rhinophyma 695.3
Rhinorrhea 478.19
  cerebrospinal (fluid) 349.81
  paroxysmal (*see also* Fever, hay) 477.9
  spasmodic (*see also* Fever, hay) 477.9
Rhinosalpingitis 381.50
  acute 381.51
  chronic 381.52
Rhinoscleroma 040.1
Rhinosporidiosis 117.0
Rhinovirus infection 079.3
Rhizomelic chrondrodysplasia punctata 277.86
Rhizomelique, pseudopolyarthritic 446.5
Rhoads and Bomford anemia (refractory) 238.72
Rhus
  diversiloba dermatitis 692.6
  radicans dermatitis 692.6
  toxicodendron dermatitis 692.6
  venenata dermatitis 692.6
  verniciflua dermatitis 692.6
Rhythm
  atrioventricular nodal 427.89
  disorder 427.9
    coronary sinus 427.89
    ectopic 427.89
    nodal 427.89
  escape 427.89
  heart, abnormal 427.9
    fetus or newborn—*see* Abnormal, heart rate
  idioventricular 426.89
    accelerated 427.89
  nodal 427.89
  sleep, inversion 327.39
    nonorganic origin 307.45
Rhytidosis facialis 701.8
Rib —*see also* condition
  cervical 756.2
Riboflavin deficiency 266.0
Rice bodies (*see also* Loose, body, joint) 718.1
  knee 717.6
Richter's hernia —*see* Hernia, Richter's
Ricinism 988.2
Rickets (active) (acute) (adolescent) (adult) (chest wall) (congenital) (current) (infantile) (intestinal) 268.0
  celiac 579.0
  fetal 756.4
  hemorrhagic 267
  hypophosphatemic with nephrotic-glycosuric dwarfism 270.0
  kidney 588.0
  late effect 268.1
  renal 588.0
  scurvy 267
  vitamin D-resistant 275.3
Rickettsial disease 083.9
  specified type NEC 083.8
Rickettsialpox 083.2
Rickettsiosis NEC 083.9
  specified type NEC 083.8
  tick-borne 082.9
    specified type NEC 082.8
  vesicular 083.2
Ricord's chancre 091.0
Riddoch's syndrome (visual disorientation) 368.16

Rider's
  bone 733.99
  chancre 091.0
Ridge, alveolus —*see also* condition
  edentulous
    atrophy 525.20
      mandible 525.20
        minimal 525.21
        moderate 525.22
        severe 525.23
      maxilla 525.20
        minimal 525.24
        moderate 525.25
        severe 525.26
    flabby 525.20
Ridged ear 744.29
Riedel's
  disease (ligneous thyroiditis) 245.3
  lobe, liver 751.69
  struma (ligneous thyroiditis) 245.3
  thyroiditis (ligneous) 245.3
Rieger's anomaly or syndrome (mesodermal dysgenesis, anterior ocular segment) 743.44
Riehl's melanosis 709.09
Rietti-Greppi-Micheli anemia or syndrome 282.46
Rieux's hernia —*see* Hernia, Rieux's
Rift Valley fever 066.3
Riga's disease (cachectic aphthae) 529.0
Riga-Fede disease (cachectic aphthae) 529.0
Riggs' disease (compound periodontitis) 523.40
Right middle lobe syndrome 518.0
Rigid, rigidity —*see also* condition
  abdominal 789.4
  articular, multiple congenital 754.89
  back 724.8
  cervix uteri
    in pregnancy or childbirth 654.6
      affecting fetus or newborn 763.89
      causing obstructed labor 660.2
        affecting fetus or newborn 763.1
  hymen (acquired) (congenital) 623.3
  nuchal 781.6
  pelvic floor
    in pregnancy or childbirth 654.4
      affecting fetus or newborn 763.89
      causing obstructed labor 660.2
        affecting fetus or newborn 763.1
  perineum or vulva
    in pregnancy or childbirth 654.8
      affecting fetus or newborn 763.89
      causing obstructed labor 660.2
        affecting fetus or newborn 763.1
  spine 724.8
  vagina
    in pregnancy or childbirth 654.7
      affecting fetus or newborn 763.89
      causing obstructed labor 660.2
        affecting fetus or newborn 763.1
Rigors 780.99
Riley-Day syndrome (familial dysautonomia) 742.8
RIND (reversible ischemic neurological deficit) 434.91
  history of personal V12.54
Ring(s)
  aorta 747.21
  Bandl's, complicating delivery 661.4
    affecting fetus or newborn 763.7
  contraction, complicating delivery 661.4
    affecting fetus or newborn 763.7
  esophageal (congenital) 750.3

Ring(s)—*continued*
  Fleischer (-Kayser) (cornea) 275.1 *[371.14]*
  hymenal, tight (acquired) (congenital) 623.3
  Kayser-Fleischer (cornea) 275.1 *[371.14]*
  retraction, uterus, pathological 661.4
    affecting fetus or newborn 763.7
  Schatzki's (esophagus) (congenital) (lower) 750.3
    acquired 530.3
  Soemmering's 366.51
  trachea, abnormal 748.3
  vascular (congenital) 747.21
  Vossius' 921.3
    late effect 366.21
Ringed hair (congenital) 757.4
Ringing in the ear (*see also* Tinnitus) 388.30
Ringworm 110.9
  beard 110.0
  body 110.5
  Burmese 110.9
  corporeal 110.5
  foot 110.4
  groin 110.3
  hand 110.2
  honeycomb 110.0
  nails 110.1
  perianal (area) 110.3
  scalp 110.0
  specified site NEC 110.8
  Tokelau 110.5
Rise, venous pressure 459.89
Risk
  factor —*see* Problem
  falling V15.88
  suicidal 300.9
Ritter's disease (dermatitis exfoliativa
    neonatorum) 695.81
Rivalry, sibling 313.3
Rivalta's disease (cervicofacial actinomycosis)
    039.3
River blindness 125.3 *[360.13]*
Robert's pelvis 755.69
  with disproportion (fetopelvic) 653.0
    affecting fetus or newborn 763.1
    causing obstructed labor 660.1
      affecting fetus or newborn 763.1
Robin's syndrome 756.0
Robinson's (hidrotic) ectodermal dysplasia 757.31
Robles' disease (onchocerciasis) 125.3 *[360.13]*
Rochalimea —*see* Rickettsial disease
Rocky Mountain fever (spotted) 082.0
Rodent ulcer 9M8090/3)—*see also* Neoplasm,
    skin, malignant
  cornea 370.07
Roentgen ray, adverse effect —*see* Effect,
    adverse, x-ray
Roetheln 056.9
Roger's disease (congenital interventricular
    septal defect) 745.4
Rokitansky's
  disease (*see also* Necrosis, liver) 570
  tumor 620.2
Rokitansky-Aschoff sinuses (mucosal
    outpouching of gallbladder) (*see also* Disease,
    gallbladder) 575.8
Rokitansky-Kuster-Hauser syndrome
    (congenital absence vagina) 752.45
Rollet's chancre (syphilitic) 091.0
Rolling of head 781.0

Romano-Ward syndrome (prolonged QT
    interval syndrome) 426.82
Romanus lesion 720.1
Romberg's disease or syndrome 349.89
Roof, mouth —*see* condition
Rosacea 695.3
  acne 695.3
  keratitis 695.3 *[370.49]*
Rosary, rachitic 268.0
Rose
  cold 477.0
  fever 477.0
  rash 782.1
    epidemic 056.9
    of infants 057.8
Rosen-Castleman-Liebow syndrome
    (pulmonary proteinosis) 516.0
Rosenbach's erysipelatoid or erysipeloid 027.1
Rosenthal's disease (factor XI deficiency) 286.2
Roseola 057.8
  infantum, infantilis (*see also* Exanthem subitum)
    058.10
Rossbach's disease (hyperchlorhydria) 536.8
  psychogenic 306.4
Rössle-Urbach-Wiethe lipoproteinosis 272.8
Ross river fever 066.3
Rostan's asthma (cardiac) (*see also* Failure,
    ventricular, left) 428.1
Rot
  Barcoo (*see also* Ulcer, skin) 707.9
  knife-grinders' (*see also* Tuberculosis) 011.4
Rot-Bernhardt disease 355.1
Rotation
  anomalous, incomplete or insufficient—*see*
    Malrotation
  cecum (congenital) 751.4
  colon (congenital) 751.4
  manual, affecting fetus or newborn 763.89
  spine, incomplete or insufficient 737.8
  tooth, teeth 524.35
  vertebra, incomplete or insufficient 737.8
Röteln 056.9
Roth's disease or meralgia 355.1
Roth-Bernhardt disease or syndrome 355.1
Rothmund (-Thomson) syndrome 757.33
Rotor's disease or syndrome (idiopathic
    hyperbilirubinemia) 277.4
Rotundum ulcus —*see* Ulcer, stomach
Round
  back (with wedging of vertebrae) 737.10
    late effect of rickets 268.1
  hole, retina 361.31
    with detachment 361.01
  ulcer (stomach)—*see* Ulcer, stomach
  worms (infestation) (large) NEC 127.0
Roussy-Lévy syndrome 334.3
Routine postpartum follow-up V24.2
Roy (-Jutras) syndrome (acropachyderma) 757.39
Rubella (German measles) 056.9
  complicating pregnancy, childbirth, or
    puerperium 647.5
  complication 056.8
    neurological 056.00
      encephalomyelitis 056.01
      specified type NEC 056.09
    specified type NEC 056.79
  congenital 771.0
  contact V01.4
  exposure to V01.4

Rubella—*continued*
  maternal
    with suspected fetal damage affecting
        management of pregnancy 655.3
    affecting fetus or newborn 760.2
      manifest rubella in infant 771.0
    specified complications NEC 056.79
  vaccination, prophylactic (against) V04.3
Rubeola (measles) (*see also* Measles) 055.9
  complicated 055.8
  meaning rubella (*see also* Rubella) 056.9
  scarlatinosis 057.8
Rubeosis iridis 364.42
  diabetica 250.5 *[364.42]*
    due to secondary diabetes 249.5 *[364.42]*
Rubinstein-Taybi's syndrome (brachydactylia,
    short stature and intellectual disabilities)
    759.89
Rud's syndrome (mental deficiency, epilepsy,
    and infantilism) 759.89
Rudimentary (congenital)—*see also* Agenesis
  arm 755.22
  bone 756.9
  cervix uteri 752.43
  eye (*see also* Microphthalmos) 743.10
  fallopian tube 752.19
  leg 755.32
  lobule of ear 744.21
  patella 755.64
  respiratory organs in thoracopagus 759.4
  tracheal bronchus 748.3
  uterine horn 752.39
  uterus 752.39
    in male 752.7
    solid or with cavity 752.39
  vagina 752.45
Ruiter-Pompen (-Wyers) syndrome
    (angiokeratoma corporis diffusum) 272.7
Ruled out condition (*see also* Observation,
    suspected) V71.9
Rumination —*see also* Vomiting
  disorder 307.53
  neurotic 300.3
  obsessional 300.3
  psychogenic 307.53
Runaway reaction —*see also* Disturbance,
    conduct
  socialized 312.2
  undersocialized, unsocialized 312.1
Runeberg's disease (progressive pernicious
    anemia) 281.0
Runge's syndrome (postmaturity) 766.22
Runny nose 784.99
Rupia 091.3
  congenital 090.0
  tertiary 095.9
Rupture, ruptured 553.9
  abdominal viscera NEC 799.89
    obstetrical trauma 665.5
  abscess (spontaneous)—*see* Abscess, by site
  amnion—*see* Rupture, membranes
  aneurysm—*see* Aneurysm
  anus (sphincter)—*see* Laceration, anus
  aorta, aortic 441.5
    abdominal 441.3
    arch 441.1
    ascending 441.1
    descending 441.5
      abdominal 441.3
      thoracic 441.1

Rupture, ruptured—*continued*
  aorta, aortic—*continued*
    syphilitic 093.0
    thoracoabdominal 441.6
    thorax, thoracic 441.1
    transverse 441.1
    traumatic (thoracic) 901.0
      abdominal 902.0
    valve or cusp (*see also* Endocarditis, aortic) 424.1
  appendix (with peritonitis) 540.0
    traumatic—*see* Injury, internal,
        gastrointestinal tract
    with peritoneal abscess 540.1
  arteriovenous fistula, brain (congenital) 430
  artery 447.2
    brain (*see also* Hemorrhage, brain) 431
    coronary (*see also* Infarct, myocardium) 410.9
    heart (*see also* Infarct, myocardium) 410.9
    pulmonary 417.8
    traumatic (complication) (*see also* Injury,
        blood vessel, by site) 904.9
  bile duct, except cystic (*see also* Disease,
      biliary) 576.3
    cystic 575.4
    traumatic—*see* Injury, internal,
        intra-abdominal
  bladder (sphincter) 596.6
    with
      abortion—*see* Abortion, by type, with
          damage to pelvic organs
      ectopic pregnancy (*see also* categories
          633.0-633.9) 639.2
      molar pregnancy (*see also* categories
          630-632) 639.2
    following
      abortion 639.2
      ectopic or molar pregnancy 639.2
    nontraumatic 596.6
    obstetrical trauma 665.5
    spontaneous 596.6
    traumatic—*see* Injury, internal, bladder
  blood vessel (*see also* Hemorrhage) 459.0
    brain (*see also* Hemorrhage, brain) 431
    heart (*see also* Infarct, myocardium) 410.9
    traumatic (complication) (*see also* Injury,
        blood vessel, by site) 904.9
  bone—*see* Fracture, by site
  bowel 569.89
    traumatic—*see* Injury, internal, intestine
  Bowman's membrane 371.31
  brain
    aneurysm (congenital) (*see also* Hemorrhage,
        subarachnoid) 430
      late effect—*see* Late effect(s) (of)
          cerebrovascular disease
      syphilitic 094.87
    hemorrhagic (*see also* Hemorrhage, brain) 431
    injury at birth 767.0
    syphilitic 094.89
  capillaries 448.9
  cardiac (*see also* Infarct, myocardium) 410.9
  cartilage (articular) (current)—*see also* Sprain,
      by site
    knee—*see* Tear, meniscus
    semilunar—*see* Tear, meniscus
  cecum (with peritonitis) 540.0
    traumatic 863.89
      with open wound into cavity 863.99
    with peritoneal abscess 540.1

Rupture, ruptured—*continued*
  cerebral aneurysm (congenital) (*see also*
      Hemorrhage, subarachnoid) 430
    late effect—*see* Late effect(s) (of)
        cerebrovascular disease
  cervix (uteri)
    with
      abortion—*see* Abortion, by type, with
          damage to pelvic organs
      ectopic pregnancy (*see also* categories
          633.0-633.9) 639.2
      molar pregnancy (*see also* categories
          630-632) 639.2
    following
      abortion 639.2
      ectopic or molar pregnancy 639.2
    obstetrical trauma 665.3
    traumatic—*see* Injury, internal, cervix
  chordae tendineae 429.5
  choroid (direct) (indirect) (traumatic) 363.63
  circle of Willis (*see also* Hemorrhage,
      subarachnoid) 430
    late effect—*see* Late effect(s) (of)
        cerebrovascular disease
  colon 569.89
    traumatic—*see* Injury, internal, colon
  cornea (traumatic)—*see also* Rupture, eye
    due to ulcer 370.00
  coronary (artery) (thrombotic) (*see also* Infarct,
      myocardium) 410.9
  corpus luteum (infected) (ovary) 620.1
  cyst—*see* Cyst
  cystic duct (*see also* Disease, gallbladder) 575.4
  Descemet's membrane 371.33
    traumatic—*see* Rupture, eye
  diaphragm—*see also* Hernia, diaphragm
    traumatic—*see* Injury, internal, diaphragm
  diverticulum
    bladder 596.3
    intestine (large) (*see also* Diverticula) 562.10
      small 562.00
  duodenal stump 537.89
  duodenum (ulcer)—*see* Ulcer, duodenum, with
      perforation
  ear drum (*see also* Perforation, tympanum) 384.20
    with otitis media—*see* Otitis media
    traumatic—*see* Wound, open, ear
  esophagus 530.4
    traumatic 862.22
      with open wound into cavity 862.32
      cervical region—*see* Wound, open,
          esophagus
  eye (without prolapse of intraocular tissue) 871.0
    with
      exposure of intraocular tissue 871.1
      partial loss of intraocular tissue 871.2
      prolapse of intraocular tissue 871.1
    due to burn 940.5
  fallopian tube 620.8
    due to pregnancy—*see* Pregnancy, tubal
    traumatic—*see* Injury, internal, fallopian tube
  fontanel 767.3
  free wall (ventricle) (*see also* Infarct,
      myocardium) 410.9
  gallbladder or duct (*see also* Disease,
      gallbladder) 575.4
    traumatic—*see* Injury, internal, gallbladder
  gastric (*see also* Rupture, stomach) 537.89
    vessel 459.0
  globe (eye) (traumatic)—*see* Rupture, eye

Rupture, ruptured—*continued*
  graafian follicle (hematoma) 620.0
  heart (auricle) (ventricle) (*see also* Infarct,
      myocardium) 410.9
    infectional 422.90
    traumatic—*see* Rupture, myocardium,
        traumatic
  hymen 623.8
  internal
    organ, traumatic—*see also* Injury, internal, by
        site
      heart—*see* Rupture, myocardium, traumatic
      kidney—*see* Rupture, kidney
      liver—*see* Rupture, liver
      spleen—*see* Rupture, spleen, traumatic
      semilunar cartilage—*see* Tear, meniscus
    intervertebral disc—*see* Displacement,
        intervertebral disc
    traumatic (current)—*see* Dislocation, vertebra
  intestine 569.89
    traumatic—*see* Injury, internal, intestine
  intracranial, birth injury 767.0
  iris 364.76
    traumatic—*see* Rupture, eye
  joint capsule—*see* Sprain, by site
  kidney (traumatic) 866.03
    with open wound into cavity 866.13
    due to birth injury 767.8
    nontraumatic 593.89
  lacrimal apparatus (traumatic) 870.2
  lens (traumatic) 366.20
  ligament—*see also* Sprain, by site
    with open wound—*see* Wound, open, by site
    old (*see also* Disorder, cartilage, articular)
        718.0
  liver (traumatic) 864.04
    with open wound into cavity 864.14
    due to birth injury 767.8
    nontraumatic 573.8
  lymphatic (node) (vessel) 457.8
  marginal sinus (placental) (with hemorrhage) 641.2
    affecting fetus or newborn 762.1
  meaning hernia—*see* Hernia
  membrana tympani (*see also* Perforation,
      tympanum) 384.20
    with otitis media—*see* Otitis media
    traumatic—*see* Wound, open, ear
  membranes (spontaneous)
    artificial
      delayed delivery following 658.3
        affecting fetus or newborn 761.1
      fetus or newborn 761.1
    delayed delivery following 658.2
      affecting fetus or newborn 761.1
    premature (less than 24 hours prior to onset of
        labor) 658.1
      affecting fetus or newborn 761.1
      delayed delivery following 658.2
        affecting fetus or newborn 761.1
  meningeal artery (*see also* Hemorrhage,
      subarachnoid) 430
    late effect—*see* Late effect(s) (of)
        cerebrovascular disease
  meniscus (knee)—*see also* Tear, meniscus
    old (*see also* Derangement, meniscus) 717.5
      site other than knee—*see* Disorder, cartilage,
          articular
    site other than knee—*see* Sprain, by site
  mesentery 568.89
    traumatic—*see* Injury, internal, mesentery
  mitral—*see* Insufficiency, mitral

Rupture, ruptured—*continued*
traumatic—*continued*
external site—*see* Wound, open, by site
eye 871.2
globe (eye)—*see* Wound, open, eyeball
internal organ (abdomen, chest, or
pelvis)—*see also* Injury, internal, by site
heart—*see* Rupture, myocardium, traumatic
kidney—*see* Rupture, kidney
liver—*see* Rupture, liver
spleen—*see* Rupture, spleen, traumatic
ligament, muscle, or tendon—*see also* Sprain,
by site
with open wound—*see* Wound, open, by site
meaning hernia—*see* Hernia
tricuspid (heart) (valve)—*see* Endocarditis,
tricuspid
tube, tubal 620.8
abscess (*see also* Salpingo-oophoritis) 614.2
due to pregnancy—*see* Pregnancy, tubal
tympanum, tympanic (membrane) (*see also*
Perforation, tympanum) 384.20
with otitis media—*see* Otitis media
traumatic—*see* Wound, open, ear, drum
umbilical cord 663.8
fetus or newborn 772.0
ureter (traumatic) (*see also* Injury, internal,
ureter) 867.2
nontraumatic 593.89
urethra 599.84
with
abortion—*see* Abortion, by type, with
damage to pelvic organs
ectopic pregnancy (*see also* categories
633.0-633.9) 639.2
molar pregnancy (*see also* categories
630-632) 639.2
following
abortion 639.2
ectopic or molar pregnancy 639.2
obstetrical trauma 665.5
traumatic—*see* Injury, internal urethra
uterosacral ligament 620.8
uterus (traumatic)—*see also* Injury, internal
uterus
affecting fetus or newborn 763.89
during labor 665.1
nonpuerperal, nontraumatic 621.8
nontraumatic 621.8
pregnant (during labor) 665.1
before labor 665.0
vaginal 878.6
complicated 878.7
complicating delivery—*see* Laceration,
vagina, complicating delivery
valve, valvular (heart)—*see* Endocarditis
varicose vein—*see* Varicose, vein
varix—*see* Varix
vena cava 459.0
ventricle (free wall) (left) (*see also* Infarct,
myocardium) 410.9
vesical (urinary) 596.6
traumatic—*see* Injury, internal, bladder
vessel (blood) 459.0
pulmonary 417.8
viscus 799.89
vulva 878.4
complicated 878.5
complicating delivery 664.0
Russell's dwarf (uterine dwarfism and
craniofacial dysostosis) 759.89
Russell's dysentery 004.8

Russell (-Silver) syndrome (congenital
hemihypertrophy and short stature) 759.89
Russian spring-summer type encephalitis 063.0
Rust's disease (tuberculous spondylitis) 015.0
[720.81]
Rustitskii's disease (multiple myeloma)
(M9730/3) 203.0
Ruysch's disease (Hirschsprung's disease) 751.3
Rytand-Lipsitch syndrome (complete
atrioventricular block) 426.0

S

Saber
  shin 090.5
  tibia 090.5
Sac, lacrimal —*see* condition
Saccharomyces infection (*see also* Candidiasis) 112.9
Saccharopinuria 270.7
Saccular —*see* condition
Sacculation
  aorta (nonsyphilitic) (*see also* Aneurysm, aorta) 441.9
    ruptured 441.5
    syphilitic 093.0
  bladder 596.3
  colon 569.89
  intralaryngeal (congenital) (ventricular) 748.3
  larynx (congenital) (ventricular) 748.3
  organ or site, congenital—*see* Distortion
  pregnant uterus, complicating delivery 654.4
    affecting fetus or newborn 763.1
      causing obstructed labor 660.2
        affecting fetus or newborn 763.1
  rectosigmoid 569.89
  sigmoid 569.89
  ureter 593.89
  urethra 599.2
  vesical 596.3
Sachs (-Tay) disease (amaurotic familial idiocy) 330.1
Sacks-Libman disease 710.0 *[424.91]*
Sacralgia 724.6
Sacralization
  fifth lumbar vertebra 756.15
  incomplete (vertebra) 756.15
Sacrodynia 724.6
Sacroiliac joint —*see* condition
Sacroiliitis NEC 720.2
Sacrum —*see* condition
Saddle
  back 737.8
  embolus
    abdominal aorta 444.01
    pulmonary artery 415.13
  injury—code to condition
  nose 738.0
    congenital 754.0
    due to syphilis 090.5
Sadism (sexual) 302.84
Saemisch's ulcer 370.04
Saenger's syndrome 379.46
Sago spleen 277.39
Sailors' skin 692.74
Saint
  Anthony's fire (*see also* Erysipelas) 035
  Guy's dance—*see* Chorea
  Louis-type encephalitis 062.3
  triad (*see also* Hernia, diaphragm) 553.3
  Vitus' dance—*see* Chorea
Salicylism
  correct substance properly administered 535.4
  overdose or wrong substance given or taken 965.1
Salivary duct or gland —*see also* condition
  virus disease 078.5
Salivation (excessive) (*see also* Ptyalism) 527.7

Salmonella (aertrycke) (choleraesuis) (enteritidis) (gallinarum) (suipestifer) (typhimurium) (*see also* Infection, Salmonella) 003.9
  arthritis 003.23
  carrier (suspected) of V02.3
  meningitis 003.21
  osteomyelitis 003.24
  pneumonia 003.22
  septicemia 003.1
  typhosa 002.0
    carrier (suspected) of V02.1
Salmonellosis 003.0
  with pneumonia 003.22
Salpingitis (catarrhal) (fallopian tube) (nodular) (pseudofollicular) (purulent) (septic) (*see also* Salpingo-oophoritis) 614.2
  ear 381.50
    acute 381.51
    chronic 381.52
  Eustachian (tube) 381.50
    acute 381.51
    chronic 381.52
  follicularis 614.1
  gonococcal (chronic) 098.37
    acute 098.17
  interstitial, chronic 614.1
  isthmica nodosa 614.1
  old—*see* Salpingo-oophoritis, chronic
  puerperal, postpartum, childbirth 670.8
  specific (chronic) 098.37
    acute 098.17
  tuberculous (acute) (chronic) (*see also* Tuberculosis) 016.6
  venereal (chronic) 098.37
    acute 098.17
Salpingocele 620.4
Salpingo-oophoritis (catarrhal) (purulent) (ruptured) (septic) (suppurative) 614.2
  acute 614.0
    with
      abortion—*see* Abortion, by type, with sepsis
      ectopic pregnancy (*see also* categories 633.0-633.9) 639.0
      molar pregnancy (*see also* categories 630-632) 639.0
    following
      abortion 639.0
      ectopic or molar pregnancy 639.0
    gonococcal 098.17
    puerperal, postpartum, childbirth 670.8
    tuberculous (*see also* Tuberculosis) 016.6
  chronic 614.1
    gonococcal 098.37
    tuberculous (*see also* Tuberculosis) 016.6
  complicating pregnancy 646.6
    affecting fetus or newborn 760.8
  gonococcal (chronic) 098.37
    acute 098.17
  old—*see* Salpingo-oophoritis, chronic
  puerperal 670.8
  specific—*see* Salpingo-oophoritis, gonococcal
  subacute (*see also* Salpingo-oophoritis, acute) 614.0
  tuberculous (acute) (chronic) (*see also* Tuberculosis) 016.6
  venereal—*see* Salpingo-oophoritis, gonococcal
Salpingo-ovaritis (*see also* Salpingo-oophoritis) 614.2

Salpingoperitonitis (*see also*
Salpingo-oophoritis) 614.2
Salt-losing
nephritis (*see also* Disease, renal) 593.9
syndrome (*see also* Disease, renal) 593.9
Salt-rheum (*see also* Eczema) 692.9
Salzmann's nodular dystrophy 371.46
Sampling chorionic villus V28.89
Sampson's cyst or tumor 617.1
Sandblasters'
asthma 502
lung 502
Sander's disease (paranoia) 297.1
Sandfly fever 066.0
Sandhoff's disease 330.1
Sanfilippo's syndrome (mucopolysaccharidosis
III) 277.5
Sanger-Brown's ataxia 334.2
San Joaquin Valley fever 114.0
São Paulo fever or typhus 082.0
Saponification, mesenteric 567.89
Sapremia —*see* Septicemia
Sarcocele (benign)
syphilitic 095.8
congenital 090.5
Sarcoepiplocele (*see also* Hernia) 553.9
Sarcoepiplomphalocele (*see also* Hernia,
umbilicus) 553.1
Sarcoid (any site) 135
with lung involvement 135 *[517.8]*
Boeck's 135
Darier-Roussy 135
Spiegler-Fendt 686.8
Sarcoidosis 135
cardiac 135 *[425.8]*
lung 135 *[517.8]*
Sarcoma (M8800/3)—*see also* Neoplasm,
connective tissue, malignant
alveolar soft part (M9581/3)—*see* Neoplasm,
connective tissue, malignant
ameloblastic (M9330/3) 170.1
upper jaw (bone) 170.0
botryoid (M8910/3)—*see* Neoplasm, connective
tissue, malignant
botryoides (M8910/3)—*see* Neoplasm,
connective tissue, malignant
cerebellar (M9480/3) 191.6
circumscribed (arachnoidal) (M9471/3) 191.6
circumscribed (arachnoidal) cerebellar
(M9471/3) 191.6
clear cell, of tendons and aponeuroses
(M9044/3)—*see* Neoplasm, connective
tissue, malignant
embryonal (M8991/3)—*see* Neoplasm,
connective tissue, malignant
endometrial (stromal) (M8930/3) 182.0
isthmus 182.1
endothelial (M9130/3)—*see also* Neoplasm,
connective tissue, malignant
bone (M9260/3)—*see* Neoplasm, bone,
malignant
epithelioid cell (M8804/3)—*see* Neoplasm,
connective tissue, malignant
Ewing's (M9260/3)—*see* Neoplasm, bone,
malignant
follicular dendritic cell 202.9
germinoblastic (diffuse) (M9632/3) 202.8
follicular (M9697/3) 202.0

Sarcoma—*continued*
giant cell (M8802/3)—*see also* Neoplasm,
connective tissue, malignant
bone (M9250/3)—*see* Neoplasm, bone,
malignant
glomoid (M8710/3)—*see* Neoplasm, connective
tissue, malignant
granulocytic (M9930/3) 205.3
hemangioendothelial (M9130/3)—*see*
Neoplasm, connective tissue, malignant
hemorrhagic, multiple (M9140/3)—*see*
Kaposi's, sarcoma
Hodgkin's (M9662/3) 201.2
immunoblastic (M9612/3) 200.8
interdigitating dendritic cell 202.9
Kaposi's (M9140/3)—*see* Kaposi's, sarcoma
Kupffer cell (M9124/3) 155.0
Langerhans cell 202.9
leptomeningeal (M9530/3)—*see* Neoplasm,
meninges, malignant
lymphangioendothelial (M9170/3)—*see*
Neoplasm, connective tissue, malignant
lymphoblastic (M9630/3) 200.1
lymphocytic (M9620/3) 200.1
mast cell (M9740/3) 202.6
melanotic (M8720/3)—*see* Melanoma
meningeal (M9530/3)—*see* Neoplasm,
meninges, malignant
meningothelial (M9530/3)—*see* Neoplasm,
meninges, malignant
mesenchymal (M8800/3)—*see also* Neoplasm,
connective tissue, malignant
mixed (M8990/3)—*see* Neoplasm, connective
tissue, malignant
mesothelial (M9050/3)—*see* Neoplasm, by site,
malignant
monstrocellular (M9481/3)
specified site—*see* Neoplasm, by site, malignant
unspecified site 191.9
myeloid (M9930/3) 205.3
neurogenic (M9540/3)—*see* Neoplasm,
connective tissue, malignant
odontogenic (M9270/3) 170.1
upper jaw (bone) 170.0
osteoblastic (M9180/3)—*see* Neoplasm, bone,
malignant
osteogenic (M9180/3)—*see also* Neoplasm,
bone, malignant
juxtacortical (M9190/3)—*see* Neoplasm,
bone, malignant
periosteal (M9190/3)—*see* Neoplasm, bone,
malignant
periosteal (M8812/3)—*see also* Neoplasm,
bone, malignant
osteogenic (M9190/3)—*see* Neoplasm, bone,
malignant
plasma cell (M9731/3) 203.8
pleomorphic cell (M8802/3)—*see* Neoplasm,
connective tissue, malignant
reticuloendothelial (M9720/3) 202.3
reticulum cell (M9640/3) 200.0
nodular (M9642/3) 200.0
pleomorphic cell type (M9641/3) 200.0
round cell (M8803/3)—*see* Neoplasm,
connective tissue, malignant
small cell (M8803/3)—*see* Neoplasm,
connective tissue, malignant
spindle cell (M8801/3)—*see* Neoplasm,
connective tissue, malignant

Sarcoma—*continued*
  stromal (endometrial) (M8930/3) 182.0
    isthmus 182.1
  synovial (M9040/3)—*see also* Neoplasm,
      connective tissue, malignant
    biphasic type (M9043/3)—*see* Neoplasm,
      connective tissue, malignant
    epithelioid cell type (M9042/3)—*see*
      Neoplasm, connective tissue, malignant
    spindle cell type (M9041/3)—*see* Neoplasm,
      connective tissue, malignant
Sarcomatosis
  meningeal (M9539/3)—*see* Neoplasm,
      meninges, malignant
  specified site NEC (M8800/3)—*see* Neoplasm,
      connective tissue, malignant
  unspecified site (M8800/6) 171.9
Sarcosinemia 270.8
Sarcosporidiosis 136.5
Satiety, early 780.94
Satisfactory smear but lacking transformation
    zone
  anal 796.77
  cervical 795.07
Saturnine —*see* condition
Saturnism 984.9
  specified type of lead—*see* Table of drugs and
    chemicals
Satyriasis 302.89
Sauriasis —*see* Ichthyosis
Sauriderma 757.39
Sauriosis —*see* Ichthyosis
Savill's disease (epidemic exfoliative dermatitis)
    695.89
SBE (subacute bacterial endocarditis) 421.0
Scabies (any site) 133.0
Scabs 782.8
Scaglietti-Dagnini syndrome (acromegalic
    macrospondylitis) 253.0
Scald, scalded —*see also* Burn, by site
  skin syndrome 695.81
Scalenus anticus (anterior) syndrome 353.0
Scales 782.8
Scalp —*see* condition
Scaphocephaly 756.0
Scaphoiditis, tarsal 732.5
Scapulalgia 733.90
Scapulohumeral myopathy 359.1
Scar, scarring (*see also* Cicatrix) 709.2
  adherent 709.2
  atrophic 709.2
  cervix
    in pregnancy or childbirth 654.6
      affecting fetus or newborn 763.89
      causing obstructed labor 660.2
        affecting fetus or newborn 763.1
  cheloid 701.4
  chorioretinal 363.30
    disseminated 363.35
    macular 363.32
    peripheral 363.34
    posterior pole NEC 363.33
  choroid (*see also* Scar, chorioretinal) 363.30
  compression, pericardial 423.9
  congenital 757.39
  conjunctiva 372.64
  cornea 371.00
    xerophthalmic 264.6

Scar, scarring—*continued*
  due to previous cesarean delivery, complicating
      pregnancy or childbirth 654.2
    affecting fetus or newborn 763.89
  duodenal (bulb) (cap) 537.3
  hypertrophic 701.4
  keloid 701.4
  labia 624.4
  lung (base) 518.89
  macula 363.32
    disseminated 363.35
    peripheral 363.34
  muscle 728.89
  myocardium, myocardial 412
  painful 709.2
  papillary muscle 429.81
  posterior pole NEC 363.33
    macular—*see* Scar, macula
  postnecrotic (hepatic) (liver) 571.9
  psychic V15.49
  retina (*see also* Scar, chorioretinal) 363.30
  trachea 478.9
  uterus 621.8
    in pregnancy or childbirth NEC 654.9
      affecting fetus or newborn 763.89
      due to previous cesarean delivery 654.2
  vulva 624.4
Scarabiasis 134.1
Scarlatina 034.1
  anginosa 034.1
  maligna 034.1
  myocarditis, acute 034.1 *[422.0]*
    old (*see also* Myocarditis) 429.0
  otitis media 034.1 *[382.02]*
  ulcerosa 034.1
Scarlatinella 057.8
Scarlet fever (albuminuria) (angina)
    (convulsions) (lesions of lid) (rash) 034.1
Schamberg's disease, dermatitis, or dermatosis
    (progressive pigmentary dermatosis) 709.09
Schatzki's ring (esophagus) (lower) (congenital)
    750.3
  acquired 530.3
Schaufenster krankheit 413.9
Schaumann's
  benign lymphogranulomatosis 135
  disease (sarcoidosis) 135
  syndrome (sarcoidosis) 135
Scheie's syndrome (mucopolysaccharidosis IS)
    277.5
Schenck's disease (sporotrichosis) 117.1
Scheuermann's disease or osteochondrosis
    732.0
Scheuthauer-Marie-Sainton syndrome
    (cleidocranialis dysostosis) 755.59
Schilder (-Flatau) disease 341.1
Schilling-type monocytic leukemia (M9890/3)
    206.9
Schimmelbusch's disease, cystic mastitis, or
    hyperplasia 610.1
Schirmer's syndrome (encephalocutaneous
    angiomatosis) 759.6
Schistocelia 756.79
Schistoglossia 750.13
Schistosoma infestation —*see* Infestation,
    Schistosoma
Schistosomiasis 120.9
  Asiatic 120.2
  bladder 120.0
  chestermani 120.8

Schistosomiasis—*continued*
  colon 120.1
  cutaneous 120.3
  due to
    S. hematobium 120.0
    S. japonicum 120.2
    S. mansoni 120.1
    S. mattheii 120.8
  eastern 120.2
  genitourinary tract 120.0
  intestinal 120.1
  lung 120.2
  Manson's (intestinal) 120.1
  Oriental 120.2
  pulmonary 120.2
  specified type NEC 120.8
  vesical 120.0
Schizencephaly 742.4
Schizo-affective psychosis (*see also*
  Schizophrenia) 295.7
Schizodontia 520.2
Schizoid personality 301.20
  introverted 301.21
  schizotypal 301.22
Schizophrenia, schizophrenic (reaction) 295.9

Note—Use the following fifth-digit
subclassification with category 295:

0 unspecified
1 subchronic
2 chronic
3 subchronic with acute exacerbation
4 chronic with acute exacerbation
5 in remission

---

  acute (attack) NEC 295.8
    episode 295.4
  atypical form 295.8
  borderline 295.5
  catalepsy 295.2
  catatonic (type) (acute) (excited) (withdrawn) 295.2
  childhood (type) (*see also* Psychosis, childhood)
    299.9
  chronic NEC 295.6
  coenesthesiopathic 295.8
  cyclic (type) 295.7
  disorganized (type) 295.1
  flexibilitas cerea 295.2
  hebephrenic (type) (acute) 295.1
  incipient 295.5
  latent 295.5
  paranoid (type) (acute) 295.3
  paraphrenic (acute) 295.3
  prepsychotic 295.5
  primary (acute) 295.0
  prodromal 295.5
  pseudoneurotic 295.5
  pseudopsychopathic 295.5
  reaction 295.9
  residual type (state) 295.6
  restzustand 295.6
  schizo-affective (type) (depressed) (excited)
    295.7
  schizophreniform type 295.4
  simple (type) (acute) 295.0
  simplex (acute) 295.0
  specified type NEC 295.8
  syndrome of childhood NEC (*see also*
    Psychosis, childhood) 299.9
  undifferentiated type 295.9
    acute 295.8
    chronic 295.6

Schizothymia 301.20
  introverted 301.21
  schizotypal 301.22
Schlafkrankheit 086.5
Schlatter's tibia (osteochondrosis) 732.4
Schlatter-Osgood disease (osteochondrosis,
  tibial tubercle) 732.4
Schloffer's tumor (*see also* Peritonitis) 567.29
Schmidt's syndrome
  sphallo-pharyngo-laryngeal hemiplegia 352.6
  thyroid-adrenocortical insufficiency 258.1
  vagoaccessory 352.6
Schmincke
  carcinoma (M8082/3)—*see* Neoplasm,
    nasopharynx, malignant
  tumor (M8082/3)—*see* Neoplasm, nasopharynx,
    malignant
Schmitz (-Stutzer) dysentery 004.0
Schmorl's disease or nodes 722.30
  lumbar, lumbosacral 722.32
  specified region NEC 722.39
  thoracic, thoracolumbar 722.31
Schneider's syndrome 047.9
Schneiderian
  carcinoma (M8121/3)
    specified site—*see* Neoplasm, by site, malignant
    unspecified site 160.0
  papilloma (M8121/0)
    specified site—*see* Neoplasm, by site, benign
    unspecified site 212.0
Schnitzler syndrome 273.1
Schoffer's tumor (*see also* Peritonitis) 567.29
Scholte's syndrome (malignant carcinoid) 259.2
Scholz's disease 330.0
Scholz (-Bielschowsky-Henneberg) syndrome 330.0
Schönlein (-Henoch) disease (primary) (purpura)
  (rheumatic) 287.0
School examination V70.3
  following surgery V67.09
Schottmüller's disease (*see also* Fever,
  paratyphoid) 002.9
Schroeder's syndrome (endocrine-hypertensive) 255.3
Schüller-Christian disease or syndrome
  (chronic histiocytosis X) 277.89
Schultz's disease or syndrome (agranulocytosis)
  288.09
Schultze's acroparesthesia, simple 443.89
Schwalbe-Ziehen-Oppenheimer disease 333.6
Schwannoma (M9560/0)—*see also* Neoplasm,
  connective tissue, benign
  malignant (M9560/3)—*see* Neoplasm,
    connective tissue, malignant
Schwannomatosis 237.73
Schwartz (-Jampel) syndrome 359.23
Schwartz-Bartter syndrome (inappropriate
  secretion of antidiuretic hormone) 253.6
Schweninger-Buzzi disease (macular atrophy) 701.3
Sciatic —*see* condition
Sciatica (infectional) 724.3
  due to
    displacement of intervertebral disc 722.10
    herniation, nucleus pulposus 722.10
  wallet 724.3
Scimitar syndrome (anomalous venous drainage,
  right lung to inferior vena cava) 747.49
Sclera —*see* condition
Sclerectasia 379.11
Scleredema
  adultorum 710.1
  Buschke's 710.1
  newborn 778.1

Sclerema
adiposum (newborn) 778.1
adultorum 710.1
edematosum (newborn) 778.1
neonatorum 778.1
newborn 778.1
Scleriasis —*see* Scleroderma
Scleritis 379.00
with corneal involvement 379.05
anterior (annular) (localized) 379.03
brawny 379.06
granulomatous 379.09
posterior 379.07
specified NEC 379.09
suppurative 379.09
syphilitic 095.0
tuberculous (nodular) (*see also* Tuberculosis)
017.3 *[379.09]*
Sclerochoroiditis (*see also* Scleritis) 379.00
Scleroconjunctivitis (*see also* Scleritis) 379.00
Sclerocystic ovary (syndrome) 256.4
Sclerodactylia 701.0
Scleroderma, sclerodermia (acrosclerotic)
(diffuse) (generalized) (progressive)
(pulmonary) 710.1
circumscribed 701.0
linear 701.0
localized (linear) 701.0
newborn 778.1
Sclerokeratitis 379.05
meaning sclerosing keratitis 370.54
tuberculous (*see also* Tuberculosis) 017.3
[379.09]
Scleroma, trachea 040.1
Scleromalacia
multiple 731.0
perforans 379.04
Scleromyxedema 701.8
Scleroperikeratitis 379.05
Sclerose en plaques 340
Sclerosis, sclerotic
adrenal (gland) 255.8
Alzheimer's 331.0
with dementia—*see* Alzheimer's, dementia
amyotrophic (lateral) 335.20
annularis fibrosi
aortic 424.1
mitral 424.0
aorta, aortic 440.0
valve (*see also* Endocarditis, aortic) 424.1
artery, arterial, arteriolar, arteriovascular—*see*
Arteriosclerosis
ascending multiple 340
Baló's (concentric) 341.1
basilar—*see* Sclerosis, brain
bone (localized) NEC 733.99
brain (general) (lobular) 348.89
Alzheimer's—*see* Alzheimer's dementia
artery, arterial 437.0
atrophic lobar 331.0
with dementia
with behavioral disturbance 331.0
[294.11]
without behavioral disturbance 331.0
[294.10]
diffuse 341.1
familial (chronic) (infantile) 330.0
infantile (chronic) (familial) 330.0
Pelizaeus-Merzbacher type 330.0
disseminated 340
hereditary 334.2

Sclerosis, sclerotic—*continued*
brain—*continued*
hippocampal 348.81
infantile, (degenerative) (diffuse) 330.0
insular 340
Krabbe's 330.0
mesial temporal 348.81
miliary 340
multiple 340
Pelizaeus-Merzbacher 330.0
progressive familial 330.0
senile 437.0
temporal 348.81
mesial 348.81
tuberous 759.5
bulbar, progressive 340
bundle of His 426.50
left 426.3
right 426.4
cardiac —*see* Arteriosclerosis, coronary
cardiorenal (*see also* Hypertension, cardiorenal)
404.90
cardiovascular (*see also* Disease,
cardiovascular) 429.2
renal (*see also* Hypertension, cardiorenal)
404.90
centrolobar, familial 330.0
cerebellar—*see* Sclerosis, brain
cerebral—*see* Sclerosis, brain
cerebrospinal 340
disseminated 340
multiple 340
cerebrovascular 437.0
choroid 363.40
diffuse 363.56
combined (spinal cord)—*see also* Degeneration,
combined
multiple 340
concentric, Baló's 341.1
cornea 370.54
coronary (artery) —*see* Arteriosclerosis,
coronary
corpus cavernosum
female 624.8
male 607.89
Dewitzky's
aortic 424.1
mitral 424.0
diffuse NEC 341.1
disease, heart —*see* Arteriosclerosis, coronary
disseminated 340
dorsal 340
dorsolateral (spinal cord)—*see* Degeneration,
combined
endometrium 621.8
extrapyramidal 333.90
eye, nuclear (senile) 366.16
Friedreich's (spinal cord) 334.0
funicular (spermatic cord) 608.89
gastritis 535.4
general (vascular)—*see* Arteriosclerosis
gland (lymphatic) 457.8
hepatic 571.9
hereditary
cerebellar 334.2
spinal 334.0
hippocampal 348.81
idiopathic cortical (Garré's) (*see also*
Osteomyelitis) 730.1
ilium, piriform 733.5

Sclerosis, sclerotic—*continued*
insular 340
  pancreas 251.8
Islands of Langerhans 251.8
kidney—*see* Sclerosis, renal
larynx 478.79
lateral 335.24
  amyotrophic 335.20
  descending 335.24
  primary 335.24
  spinal 335.24
liver 571.9
lobar, atrophic (of brain) 331.0
  with dementia
    with behavioral disturbance 331.0 *[294.11]*
    without behavioral disturbance 331.0 *[294.10]*
lung (*see also* Fibrosis, lung) 515
mastoid 383.1
mesial temporal 348.81
mitral—*see* Endocarditis, mitral
Mönckeberg's (medial) (*see also*
  Arteriosclerosis, extremities) 440.20
multiple (brain stem) (cerebral) (generalized)
  (spinal cord) 340
myocardium, myocardial —*see*
  Arteriosclerosis, coronary
nuclear (senile), eye 366.16
ovary 620.8
pancreas 577.8
penis 607.89
peripheral arteries NEC (*see also*
  Arteriosclerosis, extremities) 440.20
plaques 340
pluriglandular 258.8
polyglandular 258.8
posterior (spinal cord) (syphilitic) 094.0
posterolateral (spinal cord)—*see* Degeneration,
  combined
prepuce 607.89
primary lateral 335.24
progressive systemic 710.1
pulmonary (*see also* Fibrosis, lung) 515
  artery 416.0
  valve (heart) (*see also* Endocarditis,
    pulmonary) 424.3
renal 587
  with
    cystine storage disease 270.0
    hypertension (*see also* Hypertension,
      kidney) 403.90
    hypertensive heart disease (conditions
      classifiable to 402) (*see also*
      Hypertension, cardiorenal) 404.90
    arteriolar (hyaline) (*see also* Hypertension,
      kidney) 403.90
    hyperplastic (*see also* Hypertension, kidney)
      403.90
retina (senile) (vascular) 362.17
rheumatic
  aortic valve 395.9
  mitral valve 394.9
Schilder's 341.1
senile—*see* Arteriosclerosis
spinal (cord) (general) (progressive) (transverse)
  336.8
  ascending 357.0
  combined—*see also* Degeneration, combined
    multiple 340
    syphilitic 094.89
  disseminated 340
  dorsolateral—*see* Degeneration, combined

Sclerosis, sclerotic—*continued*
hereditary (Friedreich's) (mixed form) 334.0
lateral (amyotrophic) 335.24
multiple 340
posterior (syphilitic) 094.0
stomach 537.89
subendocardial, congenital 425.3
systemic (progressive) 710.1
  with lung involvement 710.1 *[517.2]*
temporal 348.81
  mesial 348.81
tricuspid (heart) (valve)—*see* Endocarditis,
  tricuspid
tuberous (brain) 759.5
tympanic membrane (*see also*
  Tympanosclerosis) 385.00
valve, valvular (heart)—*see* Endocarditis
vascular—*see* Arteriosclerosis
vein 459.89
Sclerotenonitis 379.07
Sclerotitis (*see also* Scleritis) 379.00
  syphilitic 095.0
  tuberculous (*see also* Tuberculosis) 017.3 *[379.09]*
Scoliosis (acquired) (postural) 737.30
  congenital 754.2
  due to or associated with
    Charcot-Marie-Tooth disease 356.1 *[737.43]*
    mucopolysaccharidosis 277.5 *[737.43]*
    neurofibromatosis 237.71 *[737.43]*
    osteitis
      deformans 731.0 *[737.43]*
      fibrosa cystica 252.01 *[737.43]*
    osteoporosis (*see also* Osteoporosis) 733.00
      [737.43]
    poliomyelitis 138 *[737.43]*
    radiation 737.33
    tuberculosis (*see also* Tuberculosis) 015.0
      [737.43]
  idiopathic 737.30
    infantile
      progressive 737.32
      resolving 737.31
  paralytic 737.39
  rachitic 268.1
  sciatic 724.3
  specified NEC 737.39
  thoracogenic 737.34
  tuberculous (*see also* Tuberculosis) 015.0 *[737.43]*
Scoliotic pelvis 738.6
  with disproportion (fetopelvic) 653.0
    affecting fetus or newborn 763.1
    causing obstructed labor 660.1
      affecting fetus or newborn 763.1
Scorbutus, scorbutic 267
  anemia 281.8
Scotoma (ring) 368.44
  arcuate 368.43
  Bjerrum 368.43
  blind spot area 368.42
  central 368.41
  centrocecal 368.41
  paracecal 368.42
  paracentral 368.41
  scintillating 368.12
  Seidel 368.43
Scratch —*see* Injury, superficial, by site
Scratchy throat 784.99
Screening (for) V82.9
  alcoholism V79.1
  anemia, deficiency NEC V78.1
    iron V78.0

Screening (for)—*continued*
  anomaly, congenital V82.89
  antenatal, of mother V28.9
    alphafetoprotein levels, raised V28.1
    based on amniocentesis V28.2
      chromosomal anomalies V28.0
      raised alphafetoprotein levels V28.1
    fetal growth retardation using ultrasonics V28.4
    genomic V28.89
    isoimmunization V28.5
    malformations using ultrasonics V28.3
    proteomic V28.89
    raised alphafetoprotein levels V28.1
    risk
      pre-term labor V28.82
    specified condition NEC V28.89
    Streptococcus B V28.6
  arterial hypertension V81.1
  arthropod-borne viral disease NEC V73.5
  asymptomatic bacteriuria V81.5
  bacterial
    and spirochetal sexually transmitted diseases V74.5
    conjunctivitis V74.4
    disease V74.9
      sexually transmitted V74.5
      specified condition NEC V74.8
  bacteriuria, asymptomatic V81.5
  blood disorder NEC V78.9
    specified type NEC V78.8
  bronchitis, chronic V81.3
  brucellosis V74.8
  cancer—*see* Screening, malignant neoplasm
  cardiovascular disease NEC V81.2
  cataract V80.2
  Chagas' disease V75.3
  chemical poisoning V82.5
  cholera V74.0
  cholesterol level V77.91
  chromosomal
    anomalies
      by amniocentesis, antenatal V28.0
      maternal postnatal V82.4
    athletes V70.3
  colonoscopy V76.51
  condition
    cardiovascular NEC V81.2
    eye NEC V80.2
    genitourinary NEC V81.6
    neurological NEC V80.09
    respiratory NEC V81.4
    skin V82.0
    specified NEC V82.89
  congenital
    anomaly V82.89
      eye V80.2
    dislocation of hip V82.3
    eye condition or disease V80.2
  conjunctivitis, bacterial V74.4
  contamination NEC (*see also* Poisoning) V82.5
  coronary artery disease V81.0
  cystic fibrosis V77.6
  deficiency anemia NEC V78.1
    iron V78.0
  dengue fever V73.5
  depression V79.0
  developmental handicap V79.9
    in early childhood V79.3
    specified type NEC V79.8
  diabetes mellitus V77.1
  diphtheria V74.3

Screening (for)—*continued*
  disease or disorder V82.9
    bacterial V74.9
      specified NEC V74.8
    blood V78.9
      specified type NEC V78.8
    blood-forming organ V78.9
      specified type NEC V78.8
    cardiovascular NEC V81.2
      hypertensive V81.1
      ischemic V81.0
    Chagas' V75.3
    chlamydial V73.98
      specified NEC V73.88
    ear NEC V80.3
    endocrine NEC V77.99
    eye NEC V80.2
    genitourinary NEC V81.6
    heart NEC V81.2
      hypertensive V81.1
      ischemic V81.0
    HPV (human papillomvirus) V73.81
    human papillomavirus (HPV) V73.81
    immunity NEC V77.99
    infectious NEC V75.9
    lipoid NEC V77.91
    mental V79.9
      specified type NEC V79.8
    metabolic NEC V77.99
      inborn NEC V77.7
    neurological NEC V80.09
    nutritional NEC V77.99
    rheumatic NEC V82.2
    rickettsial V75.0
    sexually transmitted V74.5
      bacterial V74.5
      spirochetal V74.5
    sickle-cell V78.2
      trait V78.2
    specified type NEC V82.89
    thyroid V77.0
    vascular NEC V81.2
      ischemic V81.0
    venereal V74.5
    viral V73.99
      arthropod-borne NEC V73.5
      specified type NEC V73.89
  dislocation of hip, congenital V82.3
  drugs in athletes V70.3
  elevated titer V82.9
  emphysema (chronic) V81.3
  encephalitis, viral (mosquito or tick borne) V73.5
  endocrine disorder NEC V77.99
  eye disorder NEC V80.2
    congenital V80.2
  fever
    dengue V73.5
    hemorrhagic V73.5
    yellow V73.4
  filariasis V75.6
  galactosemia V77.4
  genetic V82.79
    disease carrier status V82.71
  genitourinary condition NEC V81.6
  glaucoma V80.1
  gonorrhea V74.5
  gout V77.5
  Hansen's disease V74.2
  heart disease NEC V81.2
    hypertensive V81.1
    ischemic V81.0

Screening (for)—*continued*
  heavy metal poisoning V82.5
  helminthiasis, intestinal V75.7
  hematopoietic malignancy V76.89
  hemoglobinopathies NEC V78.3
  hemorrhagic fever V73.5
  Hodgkin's disease V76.89
  hormones in athletes V70.3
  HPV (human papillomavirus) V73.81
  human papillomavirus (HPV) V73.81
  hypercholesterolemia V77.91
  hyperlipidemia V77.91
  hypertension V81.1
  immunity disorder NEC V77.99
  inborn errors of metabolism NEC V77.7
  infection
    bacterial V74.9
      specified type NEC V74.8
    mycotic V75.4
    parasitic NEC V75.8
  infectious disease V75.9
    specified type NEC V75.8
  ingestion of radioactive substance V82.5
  intellectual disabilities V79.2
  intestinal helminthiasis V75.7
  iron deficiency anemia V78.0
  ischemic heart disease V81.0
  lead poisoning V82.5
  leishmaniasis V75.2
  leprosy V74.2
  leptospirosis V74.8
  leukemia V76.89
  lipoid disorder NEC V77.91
  lymphoma V76.89
  malaria V75.1
  malignant neoplasm (of) V76.9
    bladder V76.3
    blood V76.89
    breast V76.10
      mammogram NEC V76.12
        for high-risk patient V76.11
      specified type NEC V76.19
    cervix V76.2
    colon V76.51
    colorectal V76.51
    hematopoietic system V76.89
    intestine V76.50
      colon V76.51
      small V76.52
    lung V76.0
    lymph (glands) V76.89
    nervous system V76.81
    oral cavity V76.42
    other specified neoplasm NEC V76.89
    ovary V76.46
    prostate V76.44
    rectum V76.41
    respiratory organs V76.0
    skin V76.43
    specified sites NEC V76.49
    testis V76.45
    vagina V76.47
      following hysterectomy for malignant
        condition V67.01
  malnutrition V77.2
  mammogram NEC V76.12
    for high-risk patient V76.11
  maternal postnatal chromosomal anomalies V82.4
  measles V73.2

  mental
    disorder V79.9
      specified type NEC V79.8
    retardation — *see* Screening, intellectual
      disabilities
  metabolic errors, inborn V77.7
  metabolic disorder NEC V77.99
  mucoviscidosis V77.6
  multiphasic V82.6
  mycosis V75.4
  mycotic infection V75.4
  nephropathy V81.5
  neurological condition NEC V80.09
  nutritional disorder V77.99
    obesity V77.8
  obesity V77.8
  osteoporosis V82.81
  parasitic infection NEC V75.8
  phenylketonuria V77.3
  plague V74.8
  poisoning
    chemical NEC V82.5
    contaminated water supply V82.5
    heavy metal V82.5
  poliomyelitis V73.0
  postnatal chromosomal anomalies, maternal V82.4
  prenatal—*see* Screening, antenatal
  pulmonary tuberculosis V74.1
  radiation exposure V82.5
  renal disease V81.5
  respiratory condition NEC V81.4
  rheumatic disorder NEC V82.2
  rheumatoid arthritis V82.1
  rickettsial disease V75.0
  rubella V73.3
  schistosomiasis V75.5
  senile macular lesions of eye V80.2
  sexually transmitted diseases V74.5
    bacterial V74.5
    spirochetal V74.5
  sickle-cell anemia, disease, or trait V78.2
  skin condition V82.0
  sleeping sickness V75.3
  smallpox V73.1
  special V82.9
    specified condition NEC V82.89
  specified type NEC V82.89
  spirochetal disease V74.9
    sexually transmitted V74.5
    specified type NEC V74.8
  stimulants in athletes V70.3
  syphilis V74.5
  tetanus V74.8
  thyroid disorder V77.0
  trachoma V73.6
  traumatic brain injury V80.01
  trypanosomiasis V75.3
  tuberculosis, pulmonary V74.1
  venereal disease V74.5
  viral encephalitis
    mosquito-borne V73.5
    tick-borne V73.5
  whooping cough V74.8
  worms, intestinal V75.7
  yaws V74.8
  yellow fever V73.4
Scrofula (*see also* Tuberculosis) 017.2
Scrofulide (primary) (*see also* Tuberculosis) 017.0
Scrofuloderma, scrofulodermia (any site)
    (primary) (*see also* Tuberculosis) 017.0

Scrofulosis (universal) (*see also* Tuberculosis)
017.2
Scrofulosis lichen (primary) (*see also*
Tuberculosis) 017.0
Scrofulous —*see* condition
Scrotal tongue 529.5
congenital 750.13
Scrotum —*see* condition
Scurvy (gum) (infantile) (rickets) (scorbutic) 267
Sea-blue histiocyte syndrome 272.7
Seabright-Bantam syndrome
(pseudohypoparathyroidism) 275.49
Sealpox 059.12
Seasickness 994.6
Seatworm 127.4
Sebaceous
cyst (*see also* Cyst, sebaceous) 706.2
gland disease NEC 706.9
Sebocystomatosis 706.2
Seborrhea, seborrheic 706.3
adiposa 706.3
capitis 690.11
congestiva 695.4
corporis 706.3
dermatitis 690.10
infantile 690.12
diathesis in infants 695.89
eczema 690.18
infantile 690.12
keratosis 702.19
inflamed 702.11
nigricans 705.89
sicca 690.18
wart 702.19
inflamed 702.11
Seckel's syndrome 759.89
Seclusion pupil 364.74
Seclusiveness, child 313.22
Secondary —*see also* condition
neoplasm—*see* Neoplasm, by site, malignant,
secondary
Secretan's disease or syndrome (posttraumatic
edema) 782.3
Secretion
antidiuretic hormone, inappropriate (syndrome)
253.6
catecholamine, by pheochromocytoma 255.6
hormone
antidiuretic, inappropriate (syndrome) 253.6
by
carcinoid tumor 259.2
pheochromocytoma 255.6
ectopic NEC 259.3
urinary
excessive 788.42
suppression 788.5
Section
cesarean
affecting fetus or newborn 763.4
post mortem, affecting fetus or newborn 761.6
previous, in pregnancy or childbirth 654.2
affecting fetus or newborn 763.89
nerve, traumatic—*see* Injury, nerve, by site
Seeligmann's syndrome (ichthyosis congenita)
757.1
Segmentation, incomplete (congenital)—*see*
also Fusion
bone NEC 756.9
lumbosacral (joint) 756.15
vertebra 756.15
lumbosacral 756.15

Seizure(s) 780.39
akinetic (idiopathic) (*see also* Epilepsy) 345.0
psychomotor 345.4
apoplexy, apoplectic (*see also* Disease,
cerebrovascular, acute) 436
atonic (*see also* Epilepsy) 345.0
autonomic 300.11
brain or cerebral (*see also* Disease,
cerebrovascular, acute) 436
convulsive (*see also* Convulsions) 780.39
cortical (focal) (motor) (*see also* Epilepsy) 345.5
disorder (see also Epilepsy) 345.9
due to stroke 438.89
epilepsy, epileptic (cryptogenic) (*see also*
Epilepsy) 345.9
epileptiform, epileptoid 780.39
focal (*see also* Epilepsy) 345.5
febrile (simple) 780.31
atypical 780.32
complex 780.32
complicated 780.32
with status epilepticus 345.3
heart—*see* Disease, heart
hysterical 300.11
Jacksonian (focal) (*see also* Epilepsy) 345.5
motor type 345.5
sensory type 345.5
migraine triggered 346.0
newborn 779.0
paralysis (*see also* Disease, cerebrovascular,
acute) 436
post traumatic 780.33
recurrent 345.8
epileptic—*see* Epilepsy
repetitive 780.39
epileptic—*see* Epilepsy
salaam (*see also* Epilepsy) 345.6
uncinate (*see also* Epilepsy) 345.4
Self-mutilation 300.9
Semicoma 780.09
Semiconsciousness 780.09
Seminal
vesicle—*see* condition
vesiculitis (*see also* Vesiculitis) 608.0
Seminoma (M9061/3)
anaplastic type (M9062/3)
specified site—*see* Neoplasm, by site,
malignant
unspecified site 186.9
specified site—*see* Neoplasm, by site, malignant
spermatocytic (M9063/3)
specified site—*see* Neoplasm, by site, malignant
unspecified site 186.9
unspecified site 186.9
Semliki Forest encephalitis 062.8
Senear-Usher disease or syndrome (pemphigus
erythematosus) 694.4
Senecio jacobae dermatitis 692.6
Senectus 797
Senescence 797
Senile (*see also* condition) 797
cervix (atrophic) 622.8
degenerative atrophy, skin 701.3
endometrium (atrophic) 621.8
fallopian tube (atrophic) 620.3
heart (failure) 797
lung 492.8
ovary (atrophic) 620.3
syndrome 259.8
vagina, vaginitis (atrophic) 627.3
wart 702.0

Senility 797
  with
    acute confusional state 290.3
    delirium 290.3
    mental changes 290.9
    psychosis NEC (*see also* Psychosis, senile) 290.20
  premature (syndrome) 259.8
Sensation
  burning (*see also* Disturbance, sensation) 782.0
    tongue 529.6
  choking 784.99
  loss of (*see also* Disturbance, sensation) 782.0
  prickling (*see also* Disturbance, sensation) 782.0
  tingling (*see also* Disturbance, sensation) 782.0
Sense loss (touch) (*see also* Disturbance,
    sensation) 782.0
  smell 781.1
  taste 781.1
Sensibility disturbance NEC (cortical) (deep)
    (vibratory) (*see also* Disturbance, sensation)
    782.0
Sensitive dentine 521.89
Sensitiver Beziehungswahn 297.8
Sensitivity, sensitization —*see also* Allergy
  autoerythrocyte 287.2
  carotid sinus 337.01
  child (excessive) 313.21
  cold, autoimmune 283.0
  methemoglobin 289.7
  suxamethonium 289.89
  tuberculin, without clinical or radiological
    symptoms 795.51
Sensory
  extinction 781.8
  neglect 781.8
Separation
  acromioclavicular—see Dislocation, shoulder
  anxiety, abnormal 309.21
  apophysis, traumatic—*see* Fracture, by site
  choroid 363.70
    hemorrhagic 363.72
    serous 363.71
  costochondral (simple) (traumatic)—*see*
    Dislocation, costochondral
  delayed
    umbilical cord 779.83
  epiphysis, epiphyseal
    nontraumatic 732.9
      upper femoral 732.2
    traumatic—*see* Fracture, by site
  fracture—*see* Fracture, by site
  infundibulum cardiac from right ventricle by a
    partition 746.83
  joint (current) (traumatic)—*see* Dislocation, by
    site
  placenta (normally implanted)—*see* Placenta,
    separation
  pubic bone, obstetrical trauma 665.6
  retina, retinal (*see also* Detachment, retina) 361.9
    layers 362.40
      sensory (*see also* Retinoschisis) 361.10
    pigment epithelium (exudative) 362.42
      hemorrhagic 362.43
  sternoclavicular (traumatic)—*see* Dislocation,
    sternoclavicular
  symphysis pubis, obstetrical trauma 665.6
  tracheal ring, incomplete (congenital) 748.3

Sepsis (generalized) 995.91
  with
    abortion—*see* Abortion, by type, with sepsis
    acute organ dysfunction 995.92
    ectopic pregnancy (*see also* categories
      633.0-633.9) 639.0
    molar pregnancy (*see also* categories 630-632)
      639.0
    multiple organ dysfunction (MOD) 995.92
  buccal 528.3
  complicating labor 659.3
  dental (pulpal origin) 522.4
  female genital organ NEC 614.9
  fetus (intrauterine) 771.81
  following
    abortion 639.0
    ectopic or molar pregnancy 639.0
    infusion, perfusion, or transfusion 999.39
  Friedländer's 038.49
  intra-abdominal 567.22
  intraocular 360.00
  localized—code to specific localized infection
    in operation wound 998.59
    skin (*see also* Abscess) 682.9
  malleus 024
  newborn (organism unspecified) NEC 771.81
  oral 528.3
  puerperal, postpartum, childbirth (pelvic) 670.2
  resulting from infusion, injection, transfusion, or
    vaccination 999.39
  severe 995.92
  skin, localized (*see also* Abscess) 682.9
  umbilical (newborn) (organism unspecified)
    771.89
    tetanus 771.3
  urinary 599.0
    meaning sepsis 995.91
    meaning urinary tract infection 599.0
Septate —*see also* Septum
Septic —*see also* condition
  adenoids 474.01
    and tonsils 474.02
  arm (with lymphangitis) 682.3
  embolus—*see* Embolism
  finger (with lymphangitis) 681.00
  foot (with lymphangitis) 682.7
  gallbladder (*see also* Cholecystitis) 575.8
  hand (with lymphangitis) 682.4
  joint (*see also* Arthritis, septic) 711.0
  kidney (*see also* Infection, kidney) 590.9
  leg (with lymphangitis) 682.6
  mouth 528.3
  nail 681.9
    finger 681.02
    toe 681.11
  shock (endotoxic) 785.52
    postoperative 998.02
  sore (*see also* Abscess) 682.9
    throat 034.0
      milk-borne 034.0
      streptococcal 034.0
  spleen (acute) 289.59
  teeth (pulpal origin) 522.4
  throat 034.0
  thrombus—*see* Thrombosis
  toe (with lymphangitis) 681.10
  tonsils 474.00
    and adenoids 474.02
  umbilical cord (newborn) (organism
    unspecified) 771.89
  uterus (*see also* Endometritis) 615.9

Septicemia, septicemic (generalized)
  (suppurative) 038.9
  with
    abortion—*see* Abortion, by type, with sepsis
    ectopic pregnancy (*see also* categories
      633.0-633.9) 639.0
    molar pregnancy (*see also* categories 630-632)
      639.0
  Aerobacter aerogenes 038.49
  anaerobic 038.3
  anthrax 022.3
  Bacillus coli 038.42
  Bacteroides 038.3
  Clostridium 038.3
  complicating labor 659.3
  cryptogenic 038.9
  enteric gram-negative bacilli 038.40
  Enterobacter aerogenes 038.49
  Erysipelothrix (insidiosa) (rhusiopathiae) 027.1
  Escherichia coli 038.42
  following
    abortion 639.0
    ectopic or molar pregnancy 639.0
    infusion, injection, transfusion, or vaccination
      999.39
  Friedländer's (bacillus) 038.49
  gangrenous 038.9
  gonococcal 098.89
  gram-negative (organism) 038.40
    anaerobic 038.3
  Hemophilus influenzae 038.41
  herpes (simplex) 054.5
  herpetic 054.5
  Listeria monocytogenes 027.0
  meningeal—*see* Meningitis
  meningococcal (chronic) (fulminating) 036.2
  methicillin
    resistant Staphylococcus aureus (MRSA) 038.12
    susceptible Staphylococcus aureus (MSSA)
      038.11
  MRSA (methicillin resistant Staphylococcus
    aureus) 038.12
  MSSA (methicillin susceptible Staphylococcus
    aureus) 038.11
  navel, newborn (organism unspecified) 771.89
  newborn (organism unspecified) 771.81
  plague 020.2
  pneumococcal 038.2
  postabortal 639.0
  postoperative 998.59
  Proteus vulgaris 038.49
  Pseudomonas (aeruginosa) 038.43
  puerperal, postpartum 670.2
  Salmonella (aertrycke) (callinarum)
    (choleraesuis) (enteritidis) (suipestifer) 003.1
  Serratia 038.44
  Shigella (*see also* Dysentery, bacillary) 004.9
  specified organism NEC 038.8
  staphylococcal 038.10
    aureus 038.11
      methicillin
        resistant (MRSA) 038.12
        susceptible (MSSA) 038.11
    specified organism NEC 038.19
  streptococcal (anaerobic) 038.0
  suipestifer 003.1
  umbilicus, newborn (organism unspecified) 771.89
  viral 079.99
  Yersinia enterocolitica 038.49

Septum, septate (congenital)—*see also*
  Anomaly, specified type NEC
  anal 751.2
  aqueduct of Sylvius 742.3
    with spina bifida (*see also* Spina bifida) 741.0
  hymen 752.49
  uterus (complete) (partial) 752.35
  vagina
    in pregnancy or childbirth 654.7
      affecting fetus or newborn 763.89
      causing obstructed labor 660.2
        affecting fetus or newborn 763.1
    longitudinal (with or without obstruction) 752.47
    transverse 752.46
Sequestration
  lung (congenital) (extralobar) (intralobar) 748.5
  orbit 376.10
  pulmonary artery (congenital) 747.39
  splenic 289.52
Sequestrum
  bone (*see also* Osteomyelitis) 730.1
    jaw 526.4
  dental 525.8
  jaw bone 526.4
  sinus (accessory) (nasal) (*see also* Sinusitis) 473.9
    maxillary 473.0
Sequoiosis asthma 495.8
Serology for syphilis
  doubtful
    with signs or symptoms—*see* Syphilis, by site
      and stage
    follow-up of latent syphilis—*see* Syphilis, latent
  false positive 795.6
  negative, with signs or symptoms—*see* Syphilis,
    by site and stage
  positive 097.1
    with signs or symptoms—*see* Syphilis, by site
      and stage
    false 795.6
    follow-up of latent syphilis—*see* Syphilis, latent
    only finding—*see* Syphilis, latent
  reactivated 097.1
Seroma (postoperative) (non-infected) 998.13
  infected 998.51
  post-traumatic 729.91
Seropurulent —*see* condition
Serositis, multiple 569.89
  pericardial 423.2
  peritoneal 568.82
  pleural—*see* Pleurisy
Serotonin syndrome 333.99
Serous —*see* condition
Sertoli cell
  adenoma (M8640/0)
    specified site—*see* Neoplasm, by site, benign
    unspecified site
      female 220
      male 222.0
  carcinoma (M8640/3)
    specified site—*see* Neoplasm, by site,
      malignant
    unspecified site 186.9
  syndrome (germinal aplasia) 606.0
  tumor (M8640/0)
    with lipid storage (M8641/0)
      specified site—*see* Neoplasm, by site,
        benign
      unspecified site
        female 220
        male 222.0

Sertoli cell—*continued*
  tumor—*continued*
    specified site—*see* Neoplasm, by site, benign
    unspecified site
      female 220
      male 222.0
Sertoli-Leydig cell tumor (M8631/0)
  specified site—*see* Neoplasm, by site, benign
  unspecified site
    female 220
    male 222.0
Serum
  allergy, allergic reaction 999.59
    shock 999.49
  arthritis 999.59 *[713.6]*
  complication or reaction NEC 999.59
  disease NEC 999.59
  hepatitis 070.3
  intoxication 999.59
  jaundice (homologous) *see* Hepatitis, viral
  neuritis 999.59
  poisoning NEC 999.59
  rash NEC 999.59
  reaction NEC 999.59
  sickness NEC 999.59
Sesamoiditis 733.99
Seven-day fever 061
  of
    Japan 100.89
    Queensland 100.89
Sever's disease or osteochondrosis (calcaneum) 732.5
Sex chromosome mosaics 758.81
Sex reassignment surgery status (*see also*
  Trans-sexualism) 302.50
Sextuplet
  affected by maternal complications of pregnancy
    761.5
  healthy liveborn—*see* Newborn, multiple
  pregnancy (complicating delivery) NEC 651.8
    with fetal loss and retention of one or more
      fetus(es) 651.6
    following (elective) fetal reduction 651.7
Sexual
  anesthesia 302.72
  deviation (*see also* Deviation, sexual) 302.9
  disorder (*see also* Deviation, sexual) 302.9
  frigidity (female) 302.72
  function, disorder of (psychogenic) 302.70
    specified type NEC 302.79
  immaturity (female) (male) 259.0
  impotence 607.84
    organic origin NEC 607.84
    psychogenic 302.72
  precocity (constitutional) (cryptogenic) (female)
    (idiopathic) (male) NEC 259.1
    with adrenal hyperplasia 255.2
  sadism 302.84
Sexuality, pathological (*see also* Deviation,
  sexual) 302.9
Sézary's disease , reticulosis, or syndrome
  (M9701/3) 202.2
Shadow, lung 793.19
Shaken infant syndrome 995.55
Shaking
  head (tremor) 781.0
  palsy or paralysis (*see also* Parkinsonism) 332.0
Shallowness, acetabulum 736.39
Shaver's disease or syndrome (bauxite
  pneumoconiosis) 503
Shearing
  artificial skin graft 996.55
  decellularized allodermis graft 996.55

Sheath (tendon)—*see* condition
Shedding
  nail 703.8
  teeth, premature, primary (deciduous) 520.6
Sheehan's disease or syndrome (postpartum
  pituitary necrosis) 253.2
Shelf, rectal 569.49
Shell
  shock (current) (*see also* Reaction, stress, acute)
    308.9
    lasting state 300.16
  teeth 520.5
Shield kidney 753.3
Shift, mediastinal 793.2
Shifting
  pacemaker 427.89
  sleep-work schedule (affecting sleep) 327.36
Shiga's
  bacillus 004.0
  dysentery 004.0
Shigella (dysentery) (*see also* Dysentery,
  bacillary) 004.9
  carrier (suspected) of V02.3
Shigellosis (*see also* Dysentery, bacillary) 004.9
Shingles (*see also* Herpes, zoster) 053.9
  eye NEC 053.29
Shin splints 844.9
Shipyard eye or disease 077.1
Shirodkar suture, in pregnancy 654.5
Shock 785.50
  with
    abortion—*see* Abortion, by type, with shock
    ectopic pregnancy (*see also* categories
      633.0-633.9) 639.5
    molar pregnancy (*see also* categories 630-632)
      639.5
  allergic—*see* Anaphylactic reaction or shock
  anaclitic 309.21
  anaphylactic—*see also* Anaphylactic reaction or
    shock
    due to administration of blood and blood
      products 999.41
  anaphylactoid—*see* Anaphylactic reaction or
    shock
  anesthetic
    correct substance properly administered 995.4
    overdose or wrong substance given 968.4
      specified anesthetic—*see* Table of drugs and
        chemicals
  birth, fetus or newborn NEC 779.89
  cardiogenic 785.51
  chemical substance—*see* Table of drugs and
    chemicals
  circulatory 785.59
  complicating
    abortion—*see* Abortion, by type, with shock
    ectopic pregnancy (*see also* categories
      633.0-633.9) 639.5
    labor and delivery 669.1
    molar pregnancy (*see also* categories 630-632)
      639.5
  culture 309.29
  due to
    drug 995.0
      correct substance properly administered 995.0
      overdose or wrong substance given or taken
        977.9
      specified drug—*see* Table of drugs and
        chemicals
    food—*see* Anaphylactic shock, due to, food
  during labor and delivery 669.1

Shock—*continued*
 electric 994.8
  from electroshock gun (taser) 994.8
 endotoxic 785.52
  due to surgical procedure 998.02
  postoperative 998.02
 following
  abortion 639.5
  ectopic or molar pregnancy 639.5
  injury (immediate) (delayed) 958.4
  labor and delivery 669.1
 gram-negative 785.52
  postoperative 998.02
 hematogenic 785.59
 hemorrhagic
  due to
   disease 785.59
   surgery (intraoperative) (postoperative)
    998.09
   trauma 958.4
 hypovolemic NEC 785.59
  surgical 998.09
  traumatic 958.4
 insulin 251.0
  therapeutic misadventure 962.3
 kidney 584.5
  traumatic (following crushing) 958.5
 lightning 994.0
 lung 518.82
  related to trauma and surgery 518.52
 nervous (*see also* Reaction, stress, acute) 308.9
 obstetric 669.1
  with
   abortion—*see* Abortion, by type, with shock
   ectopic pregnancy (*see also* categories
    633.0-633.9) 639.5
   molar pregnancy (*see also* categories
    630-632) 639.5
  following
   abortion 639.5
   ectopic or molar pregnancy 639.5
 paralysis, paralytic (*see also* Disease,
  cerebrovascular, acute) 436
 late effect—*see* Late effect(s) (of)
  cerebrovascular disease
 pleural (surgical) 998.09
  due to trauma 958.4
 postoperative 998.00
  with
   abortion—*see* Abortion, by type, with shock
   ectopic pregnancy (*see also* categories
    633.0-633.9) 639.5
   molar pregnancy (*see also* categories
    630-632) 639.5
  cardiogenic 998.01
  following
   abortion 639.5
   ectopic or molar pregnancy 639.5
  hypovolemic 998.09
  specified NEC 998.09
  septic (endotoxic) (gram-negative) 998.02
 psychic (*see also* Reaction, stress, acute) 308.9
  past history (of) V15.49
 psychogenic (*see also* Reaction, stress, acute)
  308.9
 septic 785.52
  with
   abortion—*see* Abortion, by type, with shock
   ectopic pregnancy (*see also* categories
    633.0-633.9) 639.5
   molar pregnancy (*see also* categories
    630-632) 639.5

Shock—*continued*
 septic—*continued*
  due to
   surgical procedure 998.02
   transfusion NEC 999.89
    bone marrow 996.85
  following
   abortion 639.5
   ectopic or molar pregnancy 639.5
   surgical procedure 998.02
   transfusion NEC 999.89
    bone marrow 996.85
  postoperative 998.02
 spinal—*see also* Injury, spinal, by site
  with spinal bone injury—*see* Fracture,
   vertebra, by site, with spinal cord injury
 surgical 998.00
 therapeutic misadventure NEC (*see also*
  Complications) 998.89
 thyroxin 962.7
 toxic 040.82
 transfusion—*see* Complications, transfusion
 traumatic (immediate) (delayed) 958.4
Shoemakers' chest 738.3
Short, shortening, shortness
 Achilles tendon (acquired) 727.81
 arm 736.89
  congenital 755.20
 back 737.9
 bowel syndrome 579.3
 breath 786.05
 cervical, cervix 649.7
  gravid uterus 649.7
  non-gravid uterus 622.5
   acquired 622.5
   congenital 752.49
 chain acyl CoA dehydrogenase deficiency
  (SCAD) 277.85
 common bile duct, congenital 751.69
 cord (umbilical) 663.4
  affecting fetus or newborn 762.6
 cystic duct, congenital 751.69
 esophagus (congenital) 750.4
 femur (acquired) 736.81
  congenital 755.34
 frenulum linguae 750.0
 frenum, lingual 750.0
 hamstrings 727.81
 hip (acquired) 736.39
  congenital 755.63
 leg (acquired) 736.81
  congenital 755.30
 metatarsus (congenital) 754.79
  acquired 736.79
 organ or site, congenital NEC—*see* Distortion
 palate (congenital) 750.26
 P-R interval syndrome 426.81
 radius (acquired) 736.09
  congenital 755.26
 round ligament 629.89
 sleeper 307.49
 stature, constitutional (hereditary) (idiopathic)
  783.43
 tendon 727.81
  Achilles (acquired) 727.81
   congenital 754.79
  congenital 756.89
 thigh (acquired) 736.81
  congenital 755.34
 tibialis anticus 727.81
 umbilical cord 663.4
  affecting fetus or newborn 762.6

Silver wire arteries, retina 362.13
Silvestroni-Bianco syndrome (thalassemia minima) 282.49
Simian crease 757.2
Simmonds' cachexia or disease (pituitary cachexia) 253.2
Simons' disease or syndrome (progressive lipodystrophy) 272.6
Simple, simplex —*see* condition
Sinding-Larsen disease (juvenile osteopathia patellae) 732.4
Singapore hemorrhagic fever 065.4
Singers' node or nodule 478.5
Single
  atrium 745.69
  coronary artery 746.85
  umbilical artery 747.5
  ventricle 745.3
Singultus 786.8
  epidemicus 078.89
Sinus —*see also* Fistula
  abdominal 569.81
  arrest 426.6
  arrhythmia 427.89
  bradycardia 427.89
    chronic 427.81
  branchial cleft (external) (internal) 744.41
  coccygeal (infected) 685.1
    with abscess 685.0
  dental 522.7
  dermal (congenital) 685.1
    with abscess 685.0
  draining—*see* Fistula
  infected, skin NEC 686.9
  marginal, ruptured or bleeding 641.2
    affecting fetus or newborn 762.1
  pause 426.6
  pericranii 742.0
  pilonidal (infected) (rectum) 685.1
    with abscess 685.0
  preauricular 744.46
  rectovaginal 619.1
  sacrococcygeal (dermoid) (infected) 685.1
    with abscess 685.0
  skin
    infected NEC 686.9
    noninfected—*see* Ulcer, skin
  tachycardia 427.89
  tarsi syndrome 726.79
  testis 608.89
  tract (postinfectional)—*see* Fistula
  urachus 753.7
Sinuses, Rokitansky-Aschoff (*see also* Disease, gallbladder) 575.8
Sinusitis (accessory) (nasal) (hyperplastic) (nonpurulent) (purulent) (chronic) 473.9
  with influenza, flu, or grippe (*see also* Influenza) 487.1
  acute 461.9
    ethmoidal 461.2
    frontal 461.1
    maxillary 461.0
    specified type NEC 461.8
    sphenoidal 461.3
  allergic (*see also* Fever, hay) 477.9
  antrum—*see* Sinusitis, maxillary
  due to
    fungus, any sinus 117.9
    high altitude 993.1
  ethmoidal 473.2
    acute 461.2

Sinusitis—*continued*
  frontal 473.1
    acute 461.1
  influenzal (*see also* Influenza) 487.1
  maxillary 473.0
    acute 461.0
  specified site NEC 473.8
  sphenoidal 473.3
    acute 461.3
  syphilitic, any sinus 095.8
  tuberculous, any sinus (*see also* Tuberculosis) 012.8
Sinusitis-bronchiectasis-situs inversus (syndrome) (triad) 759.3
Sipple's syndrome (medullary thyroid carcinoma-pheochromocytoma) 258.02
SIRS (systemic inflammatory response syndrome) 995.90
  due to
    infectious process 995.91
      with acute organ dysfunction 995.92
    non-infectious process 995.93
      with acute organ dysfunction 995.94
Sirenomelia 759.89
Siriasis 992.0
Sirkari's disease 085.0
Siti 104.0
Sitophobia 300.29
Situation, psychiatric 300.9
Situational
  disturbance (transient) (*see also* Reaction, adjustment) 309.9
    acute 308.3
  maladjustment, acute (*see also* Reaction, adjustment) 309.9
  reaction (*see also* Reaction, adjustment) 309.9
    acute 308.3
Situs inversus or transversus 759.3
  abdominalis 759.3
  thoracis 759.3
Sixth disease
  due to
    human herpesvirus 6 058.11
    human herpesvirus 7 058.12
Sjögren (-Gougerot) syndrome or disease (keratoconjunctivitis sicca) 710.2
  with lung involvement 710.2 *[517.8]*
Sjögren-Larsson syndrome (ichthyosis congenita) 757.1
SJS-TEN (Stevens-Johnson syndrome-toxic epidermal necrolysis overlap syndrome) 695.14
Skeletal —*see* condition
Skene's gland —*see* condition
Skenitis (*see also* Urethritis) 597.89
  gonorrheal (acute) 098.0
    chronic or duration of 2 months or over 098.2
Skerljevo 104.0
Skevas-Zerfus disease 989.5
Skin —*see also* condition
  donor V59.1
  hidebound 710.9
SLAP lesion (superior glenoid labrum) 840.7
Slate-dressers' lung 502
Slate-miners' lung 502
Sleep
  deprivation V69.4
  disorder 780.50
    with apnea—*see* Apnea, sleep
    child 307.40
    movement, unspecified 780.58
    nonorganic origin 307.40
      specified type NEC 307.49

Softening
bone 268.2
brain (necrotic) (progressive) 348.89
  arteriosclerotic 437.0
  congenital 742.4
  due to cerebrovascular accident 438.89
  embolic (*see also* Embolism, brain) 434.1
  hemorrhagic (*see also* Hemorrhage, brain) 431
  occlusive 434.9
  thrombotic (*see also* Thrombosis, brain) 434.0
cartilage 733.92
cerebellar—*see* Softening, brain
cerebral—*see* Softening, brain
cerebrospinal—*see* Softening, brain
myocardial, heart (*see also* Degeneration,
  myocardial) 429.1
nails 703.8
spinal cord 336.8
stomach 537.89
Soiling, fecal 787.62
Solar fever 061
Soldier's
heart 306.2
patches 423.1
Solitary
cyst
  bone 733.21
  kidney 593.2
kidney (congenital) 753.0
tubercle, brain (*see also* Tuberculosis, brain) 013.2
ulcer, bladder 596.89
Somatization reaction, somatic reaction (*see*
  also Disorder, psychosomatic) 306.9
disorder 300.81
Somatoform disorder 300.82
atypical 300.82
severe 300.81
undifferentiated 300.82
Somnambulism 307.46
hysterical 300.13
Somnolence 780.09
nonorganic origin 307.43
periodic 349.89
Sonne dysentery 004.3
Soor 112.0
Sore
Delhi 085.1
desert (*see also* Ulcer, skin) 707.9
eye 379.99
Lahore 085.1
mouth 528.9
  canker 528.2
  due to dentures 528.9
muscle 729.1
Naga (*see also* Ulcer, skin) 707.9
oriental 085.1
pressure (*see also* Ulcer, pressure) 707.00
  with gangrene (*see also* Ulcer, pressure)
    707.00 [*785.4*]
skin NEC 709.9
soft 099.0
throat 462
  with influenza, flu, or grippe (*see also*
    Influenza) 487.1
  acute 462
  chronic 472.1
  clergyman's 784.49
  coxsackie (virus) 074.0
  diphtheritic 032.0
  epidemic 034.0
  gangrenous 462

Sore —*continued*
throat—*continued*
  herpetic 054.79
  influenzal (*see also* Influenza) 487.1
  malignant 462
  purulent 462
  putrid 462
  septic 034.0
  streptococcal (ulcerative) 034.0
  ulcerated 462
  viral NEC 462
    Coxsackie 074.0
  tropical (*see also* Ulcer, skin) 707.9
  veldt (*see also* Ulcer, skin) 707.9
Sotos' syndrome (cerebral gigantism) 253.0
Sounds
friction, pleural 786.7
succussion, chest 786.7
temporomandibular joint
  on opening or closing 524.64
South African cardiomyopathy syndrome
  425.2
South American
blastomycosis 116.1
trypanosomiasis—*see* Trypanosomiasis
Southeast Asian hemorrhagic fever 065.4
Spacing, teeth, abnormal 524.30
excessive 524.32
Spade-like hand (congenital) 754.89
Spading nail 703.8
congenital 757.5
Spanemia 285.9
Spanish collar 605
Sparganosis 123.5
Spasm, spastic, spasticity (*see also* condition)
  781.0
accommodation 367.53
ampulla of Vater (*see also* Disease, gallbladder)
  576.8
anus, ani (sphincter) (reflex) 564.6
  psychogenic 306.4
artery NEC 443.9
  basilar 435.0
  carotid 435.8
  cerebral 435.9
    specified artery NEC 435.8
  retinal (*see also* Occlusion, retinal, artery)
    362.30
  vertebral 435.1
  vertebrobasilar 435.3
Bell's 351.0
bladder (sphincter, external or internal) 596.89
bowel 564.9
  psychogenic 306.4
bronchus, bronchiole 519.11
cardia 530.0
cardiac—*see* Angina
carpopedal (*see also* Tetany) 781.7
cecum 564.9
  psychogenic 306.4
cerebral (arteries) (vascular) 435.9
  specified artery NEC 435.8
cerebrovascular 435.9
cervix, complicating delivery 661.4
  affecting fetus or newborn 763.7
ciliary body (of accommodation) 367.53
colon 564.1
  psychogenic 306.4
common duct (*see also* Disease, biliary) 576.8
compulsive 307.22
conjugate 378.82

Spasm, spastic, spasticity—*continued*
  convergence 378.84
  coronary (artery)—*see* Angina
  diaphragm (reflex) 786.8
    psychogenic 306.1
  duodenum, duodenal (bulb) 564.89
  esophagus (diffuse) 530.5
    psychogenic 306.4
  facial 351.8
  fallopian tube 620.8
  gait 781.2
  gastrointestinal (tract) 536.8
    psychogenic 306.4
  glottis 478.75
    hysterical 300.11
    psychogenic 306.1
      specified as conversion reaction 300.11
    reflex through recurrent laryngeal nerve
      478.75
  habit 307.20
    chronic 307.22
    transient (of childhood) 307.21
  heart—*see* Angina
  hourglass—*see* Contraction, hourglass
  hysterical 300.11
  infantile (*see also* Epilepsy) 345.6
  internal oblique, eye 378.51
  intestinal 564.9
    psychogenic 306.4
  larynx, laryngeal 478.75
    hysterical 300.11
    psychogenic 306.1
      specified as conversion reaction 300.11
  levator palpebrae superioris 333.81
  lightning (*see also* Epilepsy) 345.6
  mobile 781.0
  muscle 728.85
    back 724.8
    psychogenic 306.0
  nerve, trigeminal 350.1
  nervous 306.0
  nodding 307.3
    infantile (*see also* Epilepsy) 345.6
  occupational 300.89
  oculogyric 378.87
  ophthalmic artery 362.30
  orbicularis 781.0
  perineal 625.8
  peroneo-extensor (*see also* Flat, foot) 734
  pharynx (reflex) 478.29
    hysterical 300.11
    psychogenic 306.1
      specified as conversion reaction 300.11
  pregnant uterus, complicating delivery 661.4
    psychogenic 306.0
  pylorus 537.81
    adult hypertrophic 537.0
    congenital or infantile 750.5
    psychogenic 306.4
  rectum (sphincter) 564.6
    psychogenic 306.4
  retinal artery NEC (*see also* Occlusion, retina,
    artery) 362.30
  sacroiliac 724.6
  salaam (infantile) (*see also* Epilepsy) 345.6
  saltatory 781.0
  sigmoid 564.9
    psychogenic 306.4
  sphincter of Oddi (*see also* Disease, gallbladder)
    576.5

Spasm, spastic, spasticity—*continued*
  stomach 536.8
    neurotic 306.4
  throat 478.29
    hysterical 300.11
    psychogenic 306.1
      specified as conversion reaction 300.11
  tic 307.20
    chronic 307.22
    transient (of childhood) 307.21
  tongue 529.8
  torsion 333.6
  trigeminal nerve 350.1
    postherpetic 053.12
  ureter 593.89
  urethra (sphincter) 599.84
  uterus 625.8
    complicating labor 661.4
      affecting fetus or newborn 763.7
  vagina 625.1
    psychogenic 306.51
  vascular NEC 443.9
  vasomotor NEC 443.9
  vein NEC 459.89
  vesical (sphincter, external or internal) 596.89
  viscera 789.0
Spasmodic —*see* condition
Spasmophilia (*see also* Tetany) 781.7
Spasmus nutans 307.3
Spastic —*see also* Spasm
  child 343.9
Spasticity —*see also* Spasm
  cerebral, child 343.9
Speakers' throat 784.49
Specific, specified —*see* condition
Speech
  defect, disorder, disturbance, impediment NEC
    784.59
    psychogenic 307.9
  (language) therapy V57.3
Spells 780.39
  breath-holding 786.9
Spencer's disease (epidemic vomiting) 078.82
Spens' syndrome (syncope with heart block)
  426.9
Spermatic cord —*see* condition
Spermatocele 608.1
  congenital 752.89
Spermatocystitis 608.4
Spermatocytoma (M9063/3)
  specified site—*see* Neoplasm, by site, malignant
  unspecified site 186.9
Spermatorrhea 608.89
Sperm counts
  fertility testing V26.21
  following sterilization reversal V26.22
  postvasectomy V25.8
Sphacelus (*see also* Gangrene) 785.4
Sphenoidal —*see* condition
Sphenoiditis (chronic) (*see also* Sinusitis,
  sphenoidal) 473.3
Sphenopalatine ganglion neuralgia 337.09
Sphericity, increased, lens 743.36
Spherocytosis (congenital) (familial) (hereditary)
  282.0
  hemoglobin disease 287.7
  sickle-cell (disease) 282.60
Spherophakia 743.36
Sphincter —*see* condition
Sphincteritis, sphincter of Oddi (*see also*
  Cholecystitis) 576.8

Sphingolipidosis 272.7
Sphingolipodystrophy 272.7
Sphingomyelinosis 272.7
Spicule tooth 520.2
Spider
    finger 755.59
    nevus 448.1
    vascular 448.1
Spiegler-Fendt sarcoid 686.8
Spielmeyer-Stock disease 330.1
Spielmeyer-Vogt disease 330.1
Spina bifida (aperta) 741.9

Note—Use the following fifth-digit
subclassification with category 741:
0 unspecified region
1 cervical region
2 dorsal [thoracic] region
3 lumbar region

    with hydrocephalus 741.0
    fetal (suspected), affecting management of
        pregnancy 655.0
    occulta 756.17
Spindle, Krukenberg's 371.13
Spine, spinal —*see* condition
Spiradenoma (eccrine) (M8403/0)—*see*
    Neoplasm, skin, benign
Spirillosis NEC (*see also* Fever, relapsing) 087.9
Spirillum minus 026.0
Spirillum obermeieri infection 087.0
Spirochetal —*see* condition
Spirochetosis 104.9
    arthritic, arthritica 104.9 *[711.8]*
    bronchopulmonary 104.8
    icterohemorrhagica 100.0
    lung 104.8
Spitting blood (*see also* Hemoptysis) 786.30
Splanchnomegaly 569.89
Splanchnoptosis 569.89
Spleen, splenic —*see also* condition
    agenesis 759.0
    flexure syndrome 569.89
    neutropenia syndrome 289.53
    sequestration syndrome 289.52
Splenectasis (*see also* Splenomegaly) 789.2
Splenitis (interstitial) (malignant) (nonspecific)
    289.59
    malarial (*see also* Malaria) 084.6
    tuberculous (*see also* Tuberculosis) 017.7
Splenocele 289.59
Splenomegalia —*see* Splenomegaly
Splenomegalic —*see* condition
Splenomegaly 789.2
    Bengal 789.2
    cirrhotic 289.51
    congenital 759.0
    congestive, chronic 289.51
    cryptogenic 789.2
    Egyptian 120.1
    Gaucher's (cerebroside lipidosis) 272.7
    idiopathic 789.2
    malarial (*see also* Malaria) 084.6
    neutropenic 289.53
    Niemann-Pick (lipid histiocytosis) 272.7
    siderotic 289.51
    syphilitic 095.8
        congenital 090.0
    tropical (Bengal) (idiopathic) 789.2
Splenopathy 289.50
Splenopneumonia —*see* Pneumonia
Splenoptosis 289.59

Splinter —*see* Injury, superficial, by site
Split, splitting
    heart sounds 427.89
    lip, congenital (*see also* Cleft, lip) 749.10
    nails 703.8
    urinary stream 788.61
Spoiled child reaction (*see also* Disturbance,
    conduct) 312.1
Spondylarthritis (*see also* Spondylosis) 721.90
Spondylarthrosis (*see also* Spondylosis) 721.90
Spondylitis 720.9
    ankylopoietica 720.0
    ankylosing (chronic) 720.0
    atrophic 720.9
        ligamentous 720.9
    chronic (traumatic) (*see also* Spondylosis) 721.90
    deformans (chronic) (*see also* Spondylosis) 721.90
    gonococcal 098.53
    gouty 274.00
    hypertrophic (*see also* Spondylosis) 721.90
    infectious NEC 720.9
    juvenile (adolescent) 720.0
    Kümmell's 721.7
    Marie-Strümpell (ankylosing) 720.0
    muscularis 720.9
    ossificans ligamentosa 721.6
    osteoarthritica (*see also* Spondylosis) 721.90
    posttraumatic 721.7
    proliferative 720.0
    rheumatoid 720.0
    rhizomelica 720.0
    sacroiliac NEC 720.2
    senescent (*see also* Spondylosis) 721.90
    senile (*see also* Spondylosis) 721.90
    static (*see also* Spondylosis) 721.90
    traumatic (chronic) (*see also* Spondylosis) 721.90
    tuberculous (*see also* Tuberculosis) 015.0 *[720.81]*
    typhosa 002.0 *[720.81]*
Spondyloarthrosis (*see also* Spondylosis) 721.90
Spondylolisthesis (congenital) (lumbosacral)
    756.12
    with disproportion (fetopelvic) 653.3
        affecting fetus or newborn 763.1
        causing obstructed labor 660.1
            affecting fetus or newborn 763.1
    acquired 738.4
    degenerative 738.4
    traumatic 738.4
        acute (lumbar)—*see* Fracture, vertebra,
            lumbar
        site other than lumbosacral—*see* Fracture,
            vertebra, by site
Spondylolysis (congenital) 756.11
    acquired 738.4
    cervical 756.19
    lumbosacral region 756.11
        with disproportion (fetopelvic) 653.3
            affecting fetus or newborn 763.1
            causing obstructed labor 660.1
                affecting fetus or newborn 763.1
Spondylopathy
    inflammatory 720.9
        specified type NEC 720.89
    traumatic 721.7
Spondylose rhizomelique 720.0
Spondylosis 721.90
    with
        disproportion 653.3
            affecting fetus or newborn 763.1
            causing obstructed labor 660.1
                affecting fetus or newborn 763.1
        myelopathy NEC 721.91

Spondylosis—*continued*
cervical, cervicodorsal 721.0
  with myelopathy 721.1
  inflammatory 720.9
  lumbar, lumbosacral 721.3
    with myelopathy 721.42
  sacral 721.3
    with myelopathy 721.42
  thoracic 721.2
    with myelopathy 721.41
  traumatic 721.7
Sponge
  divers' disease 989.5
  inadvertently left in operation wound 998.4
  kidney (medullary) 753.17
Spongioblastoma (M9422/3)
  multiforme (M9440/3)
    specified site—*see* Neoplasm, by site, malignant
    unspecified site 191.9
  polare (M9423/3)
    specified site—*see* Neoplasm, by site,
      malignant
    unspecified site 191.9
  primitive polar (M9443/3)
    specified site—*see* Neoplasm, by site,
      malignant
    unspecified site 191.9
  specified site—*see* Neoplasm, by site, malignant
  unspecified site 191.9
Spongiocytoma (M9400/3)
    specified site—*see* Neoplasm, by site, malignant
    unspecified site 191.9
Spongioneuroblastoma (M9504/3)—*see*
  Neoplasm, by site, malignant
Spontaneous —*see also* condition
  fracture—*see* Fracture, pathologic
Spoon nail 703.8
  congenital 757.5
Sporadic —*see* condition
Sporotrichosis (bones) (cutaneous)
  (disseminated) (epidermal) (lymphatic)
  (lymphocutaneous) (mucous membranes)
  (pulmonary) (skeletal) (visceral) 117.1
Sporotrichum schenckii infection 117.1
Spots, spotting
  atrophic (skin) 701.3
  Bitôt's (in the young child) 264.1
  café au lait 709.09
  cayenne pepper 448.1
  complicating pregnancy 649.5
  cotton wool (retina) 362.83
  de Morgan's (senile angiomas) 448.1
  Fúchs' black (myopic) 360.21
  intermenstrual
    irregular 626.6
    regular 626.5
  interpalpebral 372.53
  Koplik's 055.9
  liver 709.09
  Mongolian (pigmented) 757.33
  of pregnancy 649.5
  purpuric 782.7
  ruby 448.1
Spotted fever —*see* Fever, spotted
Sprain, strain (joint) (ligament) (muscle)
  (tendon) 848.9
  abdominal wall (muscle) 848.8
  Achilles tendon 845.09
  acromioclavicular 840.0
  ankle 845.00
    and foot 845.00

Sprain, strain—*continued*
  anterior longitudinal, cervical 847.0
  arm 840.9
    upper 840.9
      and shoulder 840.9
  astragalus 845.00
  atlanto-axial 847.0
  atlanto-occipital 847.0
  atlas 847.0
  axis 847.0
  back (*see also* Sprain, spine) 847.9
  breast bone 848.40
  broad ligament—*see* Injury, internal, broad
    ligament
  calcaneofibular 845.02
  carpal 842.01
  carpometacarpal 842.11
  cartilage
    costal, without mention of injury to sternum
      848.3
      involving sternum 848.42
    ear 848.8
    knee 844.9
      with current tear (*see also* Tear, meniscus)
        836.2
    semilunar (knee) 844.8
      with current tear (*see also* Tear, meniscus)
        836.2
    septal, nose 848.0
    thyroid region 848.2
    xiphoid 848.49
  cervical, cervicodorsal, cervicothoracic 847.0
  chondrocostal, without mention of injury to
    sternum 848.3
    involving sternum 848.42
  chondrosternal 848.42
  chronic (joint)—*see* Derangement, joint
  clavicle 840.9
  coccyx 847.4
  collar bone 840.9
  collateral, knee (medial) (tibial) 844.1
    lateral (fibular) 844.0
    recurrent or old 717.89
      lateral 717.81
      medial 717.82
  coracoacromial 840.8
  coracoclavicular 840.1
  coracohumeral 840.2
  coracoid (process) 840.9
  coronary, knee 844.8
  costal cartilage, without mention of injury to
    sternum 848.3
    involving sternum 848.42
  cricoarytenoid articulation 848.2
  cricothyroid articulation 848.2
  cruciate
    knee 844.2
    old 717.89
      anterior 717.83
      posterior 717.84
  deltoid
    ankle 845.01
    shoulder 840.8
  dorsal (spine) 847.1
  ear cartilage 848.8
  elbow 841.9
    and forearm 841.9
    specified site NEC 841.8
  femur (proximal end) 843.9
    distal end 844.9

Sprain, strain—*continued*
  fibula (proximal end) 844.9
    distal end 845.00
  fibulocalcaneal 845.02
  finger(s) 842.10
  foot 845.10
    and ankle 845.00
  forearm 841.9
    and elbow 841.9
    specified site NEC 841.8
  glenoid (shoulder) (*see also* SLAP lesion) 840.8
  hand 842.10
  hip 843.9
    and thigh 843.9
  humerus (proximal end) 840.9
    distal end 841.9
  iliofemoral 843.0
  infraspinatus 840.3
  innominate
    acetabulum 843.9
    pubic junction 848.5
    sacral junction 846.1
  internal
    collateral, ankle 845.01
    semilunar cartilage 844.8
      with current tear (*see also* Tear, meniscus)
        836.2
      old 717.5
  interphalangeal
    finger 842.13
    toe 845.13
  ischiocapsular 843.1
  jaw (cartilage) (meniscus) 848.1
    old 524.69
  knee 844.9
    and leg 844.9
    old 717.5
      collateral
        lateral 717.81
        medial 717.82
      cruciate
        anterior 717.83
        posterior 717.84
  late effect—*see* Late, effects (of), sprain
  lateral collateral, knee 844.0
    old 717.81
  leg 844.9
    and knee 844.9
  ligamentum teres femoris 843.8
  low back 846.9
  lumbar (spine) 847.2
  lumbosacral 846.0
    chronic or old 724.6
  mandible 848.1
    old 524.69
  maxilla 848.1
  medial collateral, knee 844.1
    old 717.82
  meniscus
    jaw 848.1
      old 524.69
    knee 844.8
      with current tear (*see also* Tear, meniscus)
        836.2
      old 717.5
    mandible 848.1
      old 524.69
    specified site NEC 848.8
  metacarpal 842.10
    distal 842.12
    proximal 842.11

Sprain, strain—*continued*
  metacarpophalangeal 842.12
  metatarsal 845.10
  metatarsophalangeal 845.12
  midcarpal 842.19
  midtarsal 845.19
  multiple sites, except fingers alone or toes alone
    848.8
  neck 847.0
  nose (septal cartilage) 848.0
  occiput from atlas 847.0
  old—*see* Derangement, joint
  orbicular, hip 843.8
  patella(r) 844.8
    old 717.89
  pelvis 848.5
  phalanx
    finger 842.10
    toe 845.10
  radiocarpal 842.02
  radiohumeral 841.2
  radioulnar 841.9
    distal 842.09
  radius, radial (proximal end) 841.9
    and ulna 841.9
      distal 842.09
    collateral 841.0
    distal end 842.00
  recurrent—*see* Sprain, by site
  rib (cage), without mention of injury to sternum
    848.3
    involving sternum 848.42
  rotator cuff (capsule) 840.4
  round ligament—*see also* Injury, internal, round
    ligament
    femur 843.8
  sacral (spine) 847.3
  sacrococcygeal 847.3
  sacroiliac (region) 846.9
    chronic or old 724.6
    ligament 846.1
    specified site NEC 846.8
  sacrospinatus 846.2
  sacrospinous 846.2
  sacrotuberous 846.3
  scaphoid bone, ankle 845.00
  scapula(r) 840.9
  semilunar cartilage (knee) 844.8
    with current tear (*see also* Tear, meniscus)
      836.2
    old 717.5
  septal cartilage (nose) 848.0
  shoulder 840.9
    and arm, upper 840.9
    blade 840.9
    specified site NEC 848.8
  spine 847.9
    cervical 847.0
    coccyx 847.4
    dorsal 847.1
    lumbar 847.2
    lumbosacral 846.0
      chronic or old 724.6
    sacral 847.3
    sacroiliac (*see also* Sprain, sacroiliac) 846.9
      chronic or old 724.6
    thoracic 847.1
  sternoclavicular 848.41
  sternum 848.40
  subglenoid (*see also* SLAP lesion) 840.8
  subscapularis 840.5

Sprain, strain—*continued*
supraspinatus 840.6
symphysis
jaw 848.1
old 524.69
mandibular 848.1
old 524.69
pubis 848.5
talofibular 845.09
tarsal 845.10
tarsometatarsal 845.11
temporomandibular 848.1
old 524.69
teres
ligamentum femoris 843.8
major or minor 840.8
thigh (proximal end) 843.9
and hip 843.9
distal end 844.9
thoracic (spine) 847.1
thorax 848.8
thumb 842.10
thyroid cartilage or region 848.2
tibia (proximal end) 844.9
distal end 845.00
tibiofibular
distal 845.03
superior 844.3
toe(s) 845.10
trachea 848.8
trapezoid 840.8
ulna, ulnar (proximal end) 841.9
collateral 841.1
distal end 842.00
ulnohumeral 841.3
vertebrae (*see also* Sprain, spine) 847.9
cervical, cervicodorsal, cervicothoracic 847.0
wrist (cuneiform) (scaphoid) (semilunar) 842.00
xiphoid cartilage 848.49
Sprengel's deformity (congenital) 755.52
Spring fever 309.23
Sprue 579.1
celiac 579.0
idiopathic 579.0
meaning thrush 112.0
nontropical 579.0
tropical 579.1
Spur —*see also* Exostosis
bone 726.91
calcaneal 726.73
calcaneal 726.73
iliac crest 726.5
nose (septum) 478.19
bone 726.91
septal 478.19
Spuria placenta —*see* Placenta, abnormal
Spurway's syndrome (brittle bones and blue
sclera) 756.51
Sputum, abnormal (amount) (color) (excessive)
(odor) (purulent) 786.4
bloody 786.30
Squamous —*see also* condition
cell metaplasia
bladder 596.89
cervix—*see* condition
epithelium in
cervical canal (congenital) 752.49
uterine mucosa (congenital) 752.39
metaplasia
bladder 596.89
cervix—*see* condition

Squashed nose 738.0
congenital 754.0
Squeeze, divers' 993.3
Squint (*see also* Strabismus) 378.9
accommodative (*see also* Esotropia) 378.00
concomitant (*see also* Heterotropia) 378.30
Stab —*see also* Wound, open, by site
internal organs—*see* Injury, internal, by site,
with open wound
Staggering gait 781.2
hysterical 300.11
Staghorn calculus 592.0
Stähl's
ear 744.29
pigment line (cornea) 371.11
Stähli's pigment lines (cornea) 371.11
Stain, staining
meconium 779.84
port wine 757.32
tooth, teeth (hard tissues) 521.7
due to
accretions 523.6
deposits (betel) (black) (green) (materia
alba) (orange) (tobacco) 523.6
metals (copper) (silver) 521.7
nicotine 523.6
pulpal bleeding 521.7
tobacco 523.6
Stammering (see also Disorder, fluency) 315.35
Standstill
atrial 426.6
auricular 426.6
cardiac (*see also* Arrest, cardiac) 427.5
sinoatrial 426.6
sinus 426.6
ventricular (*see also* Arrest, cardiac) 427.5
Stannosis 503
Stanton's disease (melioidosis) 025
Staphylitis (acute) (catarrhal) (chronic)
(gangrenous) (membranous) (suppurative)
(ulcerative) 528.3
Staphylococcemia 038.10
aureus 038.11
specified organism NEC 038.19
Staphylococcus, staphylococcal —*see* condition
Staphyloderma (skin) 686.00
Staphyloma 379.11
anterior, localized 379.14
ciliary 379.11
cornea 371.73
equatorial 379.13
posterior 379.12
posticum 379.12
ring 379.15
sclera NEC 379.11
Starch eating 307.52
Stargardt's disease 362.75
Starvation (inanition) (due to lack of food) 994.2
edema 262
voluntary NEC 307.1
Stasis
bile (duct) (*see also* Disease, biliary) 576.8
bronchus (*see also* Bronchitis) 490
cardiac (*see also* Failure, heart) 428.0
cecum 564.89
colon 564.89
dermatitis (*see also* Varix, with stasis
dermatitis) 454.1
duodenal 536.8
eczema (*see also* Varix, with stasis dermatitis)
454.1

Stasis—*continued*
edema (*see also* Hypertension, venous) 459.30
foot 991.4
gastric 536.3
ileocecal coil 564.89
ileum 564.89
intestinal 564.89
jejunum 564.89
kidney 586
liver 571.9
  cirrhotic—*see* Cirrhosis, liver
lymphatic 457.8
pneumonia 514
portal 571.9
pulmonary 514
rectal 564.89
renal 586
  tubular 584.5
stomach 536.3
ulcer
  with varicose veins 454.0
  without varicose veins 459.81
urine NEC (*see also* Retention, urine) 788.20
venous 459.81
State
affective and paranoid, mixed, organic psychotic
  294.8
agitated 307.9
  acute reaction to stress 308.2
anxiety (neurotic) (*see also* Anxiety) 300.00
  specified type NEC 300.09
apprehension (*see also* Anxiety) 300.00
  specified type NEC 300.09
climacteric, female 627.2
  following induced menopause 627.4
clouded
  epileptic (*see also* Epilepsy) 345.9
  paroxysmal (idiopathic) (*see also* Epilepsy)
    345.9
compulsive (mixed) (with obsession) 300.3
confusional 298.9
  acute 293.0
    with
      arteriosclerotic dementia 290.41
      presenile brain disease 290.11
      senility 290.3
    alcoholic 291.0
    drug-induced 292.81
  epileptic 293.0
  postoperative 293.9
  reactive (emotional stress) (psychological
    trauma) 298.2
  subacute 293.1
constitutional psychopathic 301.9
convulsive (*see also* Convulsions) 780.39
depressive NEC 311
  induced by drug 292.84
  neurotic 300.4
dissociative 300.15
hallucinatory 780.1
  induced by drug 292.12
hypercoagulable (primary) 289.81
  secondary 289.82
hyperdynamic beta-adrenergic circulatory
  429.82
locked-in 344.81
menopausal 627.2
  artificial 627.4
  following induced menopause 627.4
neurotic NEC 300.9
  with depersonalization episode 300.6

State—*continued*
obsessional 300.3
oneiroid (*see also* Schizophrenia) 295.4
panic 300.01
paranoid 297.9
  alcohol-induced 291.5
  arteriosclerotic 290.42
  climacteric 297.2
  drug-induced 292.11
  in
    presenile brain disease 290.12
    senile brain disease 290.20
  involutional 297.2
  menopausal 297.2
  senile 290.20
  simple 297.0
postleukotomy 310.0
pregnant (*see also* Pregnancy) V22.2
psychogenic, twilight 298.2
psychotic, organic (*see also* Psychosis, organic)
  294.9
  mixed paranoid and affective 294.8
  senile or presenile NEC 290.9
  transient NEC 293.9
    with
      anxiety 293.84
      delusions 293.81
      depression 293.83
      hallucinations 293.82
residual schizophrenic (*see also* Schizophrenia)
  295.6
tension (*see also* Anxiety) 300.9
transient organic psychotic 293.9
  anxiety type 293.84
  depressive type 293.83
  hallucinatory type 293.83
  paranoid type 293.81
  specified type NEC 293.89
twilight
  epileptic 293.0
  psychogenic 298.2
vegetative (persistent) 780.03
Status (post)
absence
  epileptic (*see also* Epilepsy) 345.2
  of organ, acquired (postsurgical)—*see*
    Absence, by site, acquired
administration of tPA (rtPA) in a different
  institution within the last 24 hours prior to
  admission to facility V45.88
anastomosis of intestine (for bypass) V45.3
angioplasty, percutaneous transluminal coronary
  V45.82
anginosus 413.9
ankle prosthesis V43.66
aortocoronary bypass or shunt V45.81
arthrodesis V45.4
artificially induced condition NEC V45.89
artificial opening (of) V44.9
  gastrointestinal tract NEC V44.4
  specified site NEC V44.8
  urinary tract NEC V44.6
  vagina V44.7
aspirator V46.0
asthmaticus (*see also* Asthma) 493.9
awaiting organ transplant V49.83
bariatric surgery V45.86
  complicating pregnancy, childbirth, or the
    puerperium 649.2
bed confinement V49.84

Status—*continued*
  breast
    correction V43.82
    implant removal V45.83
    reconstruction V43.82
  cardiac
    device (in situ) V45.00
      defibrillator, automatic implantable (with synchronous cardiac pacemaker) V45.02
      pacemaker V45.01
        fitting or adjustment V53.3
      carotid sinus V45.09
        fitting or adjustment V53.3
  carotid sinus stimulator V45.09
  cataract extraction V45.61
  chemotherapy V66.2
    current V58.69
  circumcision, female 629.20
  clitorectomy (female genital mutilation type I) 629.21
    with excision of labia minora (female genital mutilation type II) 629.22
  colonization — *see* Carrier (suspected) of
  colostomy V44.3
  contraceptive device V45.59
    intrauterine V45.51
    subdermal V45.52
  convulsivus idiopathicus (*see also* Epilepsy) 345.3
  coronary artery bypass or shunt V45.81
  cutting
    female genital 629.20
      specified NEC 629.29
      type I 629.21
      type II 629.22
      type III 629.23
      type IV 629.29
  cystostomy V44.50
    appendico-vesicostomy V44.52
    cutaneous-vesicostomy V44.51
    specified type NEC V44.59
  defibrillator, automatic implantable cardiac (with synchronous cardiac pacemaker) V45.02
  delinquent immunization V15.83
  dental crowns V45.84
  dental fillings V45.84
  dental restoration V45.84
  dental sealant V49.82
  dialysis (hemo) (peritoneal) V45.11
  do not resuscitate V49.86
  donor V59.9
  drug therapy or regimen V67.59
    high-risk medication NEC V67.51
  elbow prosthesis V43.62
  embedded
    fragment — *see* Foreign body, retained
    splinter — *see* Foreign body, retained
  enterostomy V44.4
  epileptic, epilepticus (absence) (grand mal) (*see also* Epilepsy) 345.3
    focal motor 345.7
    partial 345.7
    petit mal 345.2
    psychomotor 345.7
    temporal lobe 345.7
  estrogen receptor
    negative [ER-] V86.1
    positive [ER+] V86.0
  explantation of joint prosthesis NEC V88.29
    hip V88.21
    knee V88.22

Status—*continued*
  eye (adnexa) surgery V45.69
  female genital
    cutting 629.20
      specified NEC 629.29
      type I 629.21
      type II 629.22
      type III 629.23
      type IV 629.29
    mutilation 629.20
      type IV 629.29
  filtering bleb (eye) (postglaucoma) V45.69
    with rupture or complication 997.99
    postcataract extraction (complication) 997.99
  finger joint prosthesis V43.69
  foster care V60.81
  gastric
    banding V45.86
      complicating pregnancy, childbirth, or the puerperium 649.2
    bypass for obesity V45.86
      complicating pregnancy, childbirth, or the puerperium 649.2
  gastrostomy V44.1
  grand mal 345.3
  heart valve prosthesis V43.3
  hemodialysis V45.11
  hip prosthesis (joint) (partial) (total) V43.64
    explantation V88.21
  hysterectomy V88.01
    partial with remaining cervical stump V88.02
    total V88.01
  ileostomy V44.2
  infibulation (female genital mutilation type III) 629.23
  insulin pump V45.85
  intestinal bypass V45.3
  intrauterine contraceptive device V45.51
  jejunostomy V44.4
  joint prosthesis NEC V43.69
    explantation V88.29
  knee joint prosthesis V43.65
    explantation V88.22
  lacunaris 437.8
  lacunosis 437.8
  lapsed immunization schedule V15.83
  low birth weight V21.30
    less than 500 grams V21.31
    500-999 grams V21.32
    1000-1499 grams V21.33
    1500-1999 grams V21.34
    2000-2500 grams V21.35
  lymphaticus 254.8
  malignant neoplasm, ablated or excised—*see* History, malignant neoplasm
  marmoratus 333.79
  military deployment V62.22
  mutilation, female 629.20
    type I 629.21
    type II 629.22
    type III 629.23
    type IV 629.29
  nephrostomy V44.6
  neuropacemaker NEC V45.89
    brain V45.89
    carotid sinus V45.09
    neurologic NEC V45.89
  obesity surgery V45.86
    complicating pregnancy, childbirth, or the puerperium 649.2

Status—*continued*
  organ replacement
    by artificial or mechanical device or prosthesis of
      artery V43.4
      artificial skin V43.83
      bladder V43.5
      blood vessel V43.4
      breast V43.82
      eye globe V43.0
      heart
        assist device V43.21
        fully implantable artificial heart V43.22
        valve V43.3
      intestine V43.89
      joint V43.60
        ankle V43.66
        elbow V43.62
        finger V43.69
        hip (partial) (total) V43.64
        knee V43.65
        shoulder V43.61
        specified NEC 43.69
        wrist V43.63
      kidney V43.89
      larynx V43.81
      lens V43.1
      limb(s) V43.7
      liver V43.89
      lung V43.89
      organ NEC V43.89
      pancreas V43.89
      skin (artificial) V43.83
      tissue NEC V43.89
      vein V43.4
    by organ transplant (heterologous)
        (homologous)—*see* Status, transplant
  pacemaker
    brain V45.89
    cardiac V45.01
    carotid sinus V45.09
    neurologic NEC V45.89
    specified site NEC V45.89
  percutaneous transluminal coronary angioplasty
      V45.82
  peritoneal dialysis V45.11
  petit mal 345.2
  physical restraints V49.87
  postcommotio cerebri 310.2
  postmenopausal (age related) (natural) V49.81
  postoperative NEC V45.89
  postpartum NEC V24.2
    care immediately following delivery V24.0
    routine follow-up V24.2
  postsurgical NEC V45.89
  renal dialysis V45.11
    noncompliance V45.12
  respirator (ventilator) V46.11
    encounter
      during
        mechanical failure V46.14
        power failure V46.12
      for weaning V46.13
  retained foreign body—*see* Foreign body, retained
  reversed jejunal transposition (for bypass) V45.3
  sex reassignment surgery status (*see also*
      Trans-sexualism) 302.50
  shoulder prosthesis V43.61

Status—*continued*
  shunt
    aortocoronary bypass V45.81
    arteriovenous (for dialysis) V45.11
    cerebrospinal fluid V45.2
    vascular NEC V45.89
      aortocoronary (bypass) V45.81
    ventricular (communicating) (for drainage)
        V45.2
  sterilization
    tubal ligation V26.51
    vasectomy V26.52
  subdermal contraceptive device V45.52
  thymicolymphaticus 254.8
  thymicus 254.8
  thymolymphaticus 254.8
  tooth extraction 525.10
  tracheostomy V44.0
  transplant
    blood vessel V42.89
    bone V42.4
      marrow V42.81
    cornea V42.5
    heart V42.1
      valve V42.2
    intestine V42.84
    kidney V42.0
    liver V42.7
    lung V42.6
    organ V42.9
      removal (due to complication, failure,
          rejection or infection) V45.87
      specified site NEC V42.89
    pancreas V42.83
    peripheral stem cells V42.82
    skin V42.3
    stem cells, peripheral V42.82
    tissue V42.9
      specified type NEC V42.89
    vessel, blood V42.89
  tubal ligation V26.51
  underimmunization V15.83
  ureterostomy V44.6
  urethrostomy V44.6
  vagina, artificial V44.7
  vasectomy V26.52
  vascular shunt NEC V45.89
    aortocoronary (bypass) V45.81
  ventilator (respirator) V46.11
    encounter
      during
        mechanical failure V46.14
        power failure V46.12
      for weaning V46.13
  wheelchair confinement V46.3
  wrist prosthesis V43.63
Stave fracture —*see* Fracture, metacarpus,
    metacarpal bone(s)
Steal
  subclavian artery 435.2
  vertebral artery 435.1
Stealing, solitary, child problem (*see also*
    Disturbance, conduct) 312.1
Steam burn —*see* Burn, by site
Steatocystoma multiplex 706.2
Steatoma (infected) 706.2
  eyelid (cystic) 374.84
    infected 373.13

Steatorrhea (chronic) 579.8
  with lacteal obstruction 579.2
  idiopathic 579.0
    adult 579.0
    infantile 579.0
  pancreatic 579.4
  primary 579.0
  secondary 579.8
  specified cause NEC 579.8
  tropical 579.1
Steatosis 272.8
  heart (*see also* Degeneration, myocardial) 429.1
  kidney 593.89
  liver 571.8
Steele-Richardson (-Olszewski) Syndrome 333.0
Stein's syndrome (polycystic ovary) 256.4
Stein-Leventhal syndrome (polycystic ovary)
  256.4
Steinbrocker's syndrome (*see also* Neuropathy,
  peripheral, autonomic) 337.9
Steinert's disease 359.21
STEMI (ST elevation myocardial infarction) (*see
  also* Infarct, myocardium, ST elevation) 410.9
Stenocardia (*see also* Angina) 413.9
Stenocephaly 756.0
Stenosis (cicatricial)—*see also* Stricture
  ampulla of Vater 576.2
    with calculus, cholelithiasis, or stones—*see*
      Choledocholithiasis
  anus, anal (canal) (sphincter) 569.2
    congenital 751.2
  aorta (ascending) 747.22
    arch 747.10
    arteriosclerotic 440.0
    calcified 440.0
  aortic (valve) 424.1
    with
      mitral (valve)
        insufficiency or incompetence 396.2
        stenosis or obstruction 396.0
    atypical 396.0
    congenital 746.3
    rheumatic 395.0
      with
        insufficiency, incompetency or
          regurgitation 395.2
          with mitral (valve) disease 396.8
        mitral (valve)
          disease (stenosis) 396.0
          insufficiency or incompetence 396.2
          stenosis or obstruction 396.0
    specified cause, except rheumatic 424.1
    syphilitic 093.22
  aqueduct of Sylvius (congenital) 742.3
    with spina bifida (*see also* Spina bifida) 741.0
    acquired 331.4
  artery NEC (*see also* Arteriosclerosis) 447.1
    basilar—*see* Narrowing, artery, basilar
    carotid (common) (internal)—*see* Narrowing,
      artery, carotid
    celiac 447.4
    cerebral 437.0
      due to
        embolism (*see also* Embolism, brain) 434.1
        thrombus (*see also* Thrombosis, brain) 434.0
    extremities 440.20
    precerebral—*see* Narrowing, artery,
      precerebral
    pulmonary (congenital) 747.31
      acquired 417.8
    renal 440.1
    vertebral—*see* Narrowing, artery, vertebral

Stenosis—*continued*
  bile duct or biliary passage (*see also*
    Obstruction, biliary) 576.2
    congenital 751.61
  bladder neck (acquired) 596.0
    congenital 753.6
  brain 348.89
  bronchus 519.19
    syphilitic 095.8
  cardia (stomach) 537.89
    congenital 750.7
  cardiovascular (*see also* Disease,
    cardiovascular) 429.2
  carotid artery—*see* Narrowing, artery, carotid
  cervix, cervical (canal) 622.4
    congenital 752.49
    in pregnancy or childbirth 654.6
      affecting fetus or newborn 763.89
      causing obstructed labor 660.2
        affecting fetus or newborn 763.1
  colon (*see also* Obstruction, intestine) 560.9
    congenital 751.2
  colostomy 569.62
  common bile duct (*see also* Obstruction, biliary)
    576.2
    congenital 751.61
  coronary (artery) —*see* Arteriosclerosis,
    coronary
  cystic duct (*see also* Obstruction, gallbladder)
    575.2
    congenital 751.61
  due to (presence of) any device, implant, or graft
    classifiable to 996.0-996.5—*see*
    Complications, due to (presence of) any
    device, implant, or graft classified to
    996.0-996.5 NEC
  duodenum 537.3
    congenital 751.1
  ejaculatory duct NEC 608.89
  endocervical os—*see* Stenosis, cervix
  enterostomy 569.62
  esophagostomy 530.87
  esophagus 530.3
    congenital 750.3
    syphilitic 095.8
      congenital 090.5
  external ear canal 380.50
    secondary to
      inflammation 380.53
      surgery 380.52
      trauma 380.51
  gallbladder (*see also* Obstruction, gallbladder)
    575.2
  glottis 478.74
  heart valve (acquired)—*see also* Endocarditis
    congenital NEC 746.89
      aortic 746.3
      mitral 746.5
      pulmonary 746.02
      tricuspid 746.1
  hepatic duct (*see also* Obstruction, biliary) 576.2
  hymen 623.3
  hypertrophic subaortic (idiopathic) 425.11
  infundibulum cardiac 746.83
  intestine (*see also* Obstruction, intestine) 560.9
    congenital (small) 751.1
      large 751.2
  lacrimal
    canaliculi 375.53
    duct 375.56
      congenital 743.65

Stenosis—*continued*
  lacrimal—*continued*
    punctum 375.52
      congenital 743.65
    sac 375.54
      congenital 743.65
  lacrimonasal duct 375.56
    congenital 743.65
    neonatal 375.55
  larynx 478.74
    congenital 748.3
    syphilitic 095.8
      congenital 090.5
  mitral (valve) (chronic) (inactive) 394.0
    with
      aortic (valve)
        disease (insufficiency) 396.1
        insufficiency or incompetence 396.1
        stenosis or obstruction 396.0
      incompetency, insufficiency or regurgitation
        394.2
        with aortic valve disease 396.8
    active or acute 391.1
      with chorea (acute) (rheumatic)
        (Sydenham's) 392.0
    congenital 746.5
    specified cause, except rheumatic 424.0
    syphilitic 093.21
  myocardium, myocardial (*see also*
    Degeneration, myocardial) 429.1
    hypertrophic subaortic (idiopathic) 425.11
  nares (anterior) (posterior) 478.19
    congenital 748.0
  nasal duct 375.56
    congenital 743.65
  nasolacrimal duct 375.56
    congenital 743.65
    neonatal 375.55
  organ or site, congenital NEC—*see* Atresia
  papilla of Vater 576.2
    with calculus, cholelithiasis, or stones—*see*
      Choledocholithiasis
  pulmonary (artery) (congenital) 747.31
    with ventricular septal defect, dextraposition
      of aorta and hypertrophy of right ventricle
      745.2
    acquired 417.8
    infundibular 746.83
    in tetralogy of Fallot 745.2
    subvalvular 746.83
    valve (*see also* Endocarditis, pulmonary) 424.3
      congenital 746.02
    vein 747.49
      acquired 417.8
    vessel NEC 417.8
  pulmonic (congenital) 746.02
    infundibular 746.83
    subvalvular 746.83
  pylorus (hypertrophic) 537.0
    adult 537.0
    congenital 750.5
    infantile 750.5
  rectum (sphincter) (*see also* Stricture, rectum) 569.2
  renal artery 440.1
  salivary duct (any) 527.8
  sphincter of Oddi (*see also* Obstruction, biliary) 576.2
  spinal 724.00
    cervical 723.0
    lumbar, lumbosacral (without neurogenic
      claudication) 724.02
      with neurogenic claudication 724.03

Stenosis—*continued*
  spinal—*continued*
    nerve (root) NEC 724.9
      specified region NEC 724.09
    thoracic, thoracolumbar 724.01
  stomach, hourglass 537.6
  subaortic 746.81
    hypertrophic (idiopathic) 425.11
  supra (valvular)-aortic 747.22
  trachea 519.19
    congenital 748.3
    syphilitic 095.8
    tuberculous (*see also* Tuberculosis) 012.8
  tracheostomy 519.02
  tricuspid (valve) (*see also* Endocarditis,
    tricuspid) 397.0
    congenital 746.1
    nonrheumatic 424.2
  tubal 628.2
  ureter (*see also* Stricture, ureter) 593.3
    congenital 753.29
  urethra (*see also* Stricture, urethra) 598.9
  vagina 623.2
    congenital 752.49
    in pregnancy or childbirth 654.7
      affecting fetus or newborn 763.89
      causing obstructed labor 660.2
        affecting fetus or newborn 763.1
  valve (cardiac) (heart) (*see also* Endocarditis) 424.90
    congenital NEC 746.89
      aortic 746.3
      mitral 746.5
      pulmonary 746.02
      tricuspid 746.1
      urethra 753.6
  valvular (*see also* Endocarditis) 424.90
    congenital NEC 746.89
      urethra 753.6
  vascular graft or shunt 996.1
    atherosclerosis —*see* Arteriosclerosis,
      extremities
    embolism 996.74
    occlusion NEC 996.74
    thrombus 996.74
  vena cava (inferior) (superior) 459.2
    congenital 747.49
  ventricular shunt 996.2
  vulva 624.8
Stent jail 996.72
Stercolith (*see also* Fecalith) 560.32
  appendix 543.9
Stercoraceous, stercoral ulcer 569.82
  anus or rectum 569.41
Stereopsis, defective
  with fusion 368.33
  without fusion 368.32
Stereotypies NEC 307.3
Sterility
  female—*see* Infertility, female
  male (*see also* Infertility, male) 606.9
Sterilization, admission for V25.2
  status
    tubal ligation V26.51
    vasectomy V26.52
Sternalgia (*see also* Angina) 413.9
Sternopagus 759.4
Sternum bifidum 756.3
Sternutation 784.99

Steroid
  effects (adverse) (iatrogenic)
    cushingoid
      correct substance properly administered 255.0
      overdose or wrong substance given or taken
        962.0
    diabetes—*see* Diabetes, secondary
      correct substance properly administered 251.8
      overdose or wrong substance given or taken
        962.0
    due to
      correct substance properly administered 255.8
      overdose or wrong substance given or taken
        962.0
    fever
      correct substance properly administered 780.60
      overdose or wrong substance given or taken
        962.0
    withdrawal
      correct substance properly administered 255.41
      overdose or wrong substance given or taken
        962.0
  responder 365.03
Stevens-Johnson disease or syndrome (erythema
    multiforme exudativum) 695.13
  toxic epidermal necrolysis overlap (SJS-TEN
    overlap syndrome) 695.14
Stewart-Morel syndrome (hyperostosis frontalis
    interna) 733.3
Sticker's disease (erythema infectiosum) 057.0
Stickler syndrome 759.89
Sticky eye 372.03
Stieda's disease (calcification, knee joint) 726.62
Stiff
  back 724.8
  neck (*see also* Torticollis) 723.5
Stiff-baby 759.89
Stiff-man syndrome 333.91
Stiffness, joint NEC 719.50
  ankle 719.57
  back 724.8
  elbow 719.52
  finger 719.54
  hip 719.55
  knee 719.56
  multiple sites 719.59
  sacroiliac 724.6
  shoulder 719.51
  specified site NEC 719.58
  spine 724.9
  surgical fusion V45.4
  wrist 719.53
Stigmata, congenital syphilis 090.5
Still's disease or syndrome 714.30
  adult onset 714.2
Still-Felty syndrome (rheumatoid arthritis with
    splenomegaly and leukopenia) 714.1
Stillbirth, stillborn NEC 779.9
Stiller's disease (asthenia) 780.79
Stilling-Türk-Duane syndrome (ocular
    retraction syndrome) 378.71
Stimulation, ovary 256.1
Sting (animal) (bee) (fish) (insect) (jellyfish)
    (Portuguese man-o-war) (wasp) (venomous)
    989.5
  anaphylactic shock or reaction 989.5
  plant 692.6
Stippled epiphyses 756.59

Stitch
  abscess 998.59
  burst (in external operation wound) (*see also*
    Dehiscence) 998.32
    internal 998.31
  in back 724.5
Stojano's (subcostal) syndrome 098.86
Stokes' disease (exophthalmic goiter) 242.0
Stokes-Adams syndrome (syncope with heart
    block) 426.9
Stokvis' (-Talma) disease (enterogenous
    cyanosis) 289.7
Stomach —*see* condition
Stoma malfunction
  colostomy 569.62
  cystostomy 596.82
    infection 596.81
    mechanical 596.82
    specified complication NEC 596.83
  enterostomy 569.62
  esophagostomy 530.87
  gastrostomy 536.42
  ileostomy 569.62
  nephrostomy 997.5
  tracheostomy 519.02
  ureterostomy 997.5
Stomatitis 528.00
  angular 528.5
    due to dietary or vitamin deficiency 266.0
  aphthous 528.2
  bovine 059.11
  candidal 112.0
  catarrhal 528.00
  denture 528.9
  diphtheritic (membranous) 032.0
  due to
    dietary deficiency 266.0
    thrush 112.0
    vitamin deficiency 266.0
  epidemic 078.4
  epizootic 078.4
  follicular 528.00
  gangrenous 528.1
  herpetic 054.2
  herpetiformis 528.2
  malignant 528.00
  membranous acute 528.00
  monilial 112.0
  mycotic 112.0
  necrotic 528.1
    ulcerative 101
  necrotizing ulcerative 101
  parasitic 112.0
  septic 528.00
  specified NEC 528.09
  spirochetal 101
  suppurative (acute) 528.00
  ulcerative 528.00
    necrotizing 101
  ulceromembranous 101
  vesicular 528.00
    with exanthem 074.3
  Vincent's 101
Stomatocytosis 282.8
Stomatomycosis 112.0
Stomatorrhagia 528.9
Stone(s) —*see also* Calculus
  bladder 594.1
    diverticulum 594.0
  cystine 270.0

Stone(s)—*continued*
   heart syndrome (*see also* Failure, ventricular,
      left) 428.1
   kidney 592.0
   prostate 602.0
   pulp (dental) 522.2
   renal 592.0
   salivary duct or gland (any) 527.5
   ureter 592.1
   urethra (impacted) 594.2
   urinary (duct) (impacted) (passage) 592.9
      bladder 594.1
         diverticulum 594.0
      lower tract NEC 594.9
      specified site 594.8
   xanthine 277.2
Stonecutters' lung 502
   tuberculous (*see also* Tuberculosis) 011.4
Stonemasons'
   asthma, disease, or lung 502
   tuberculous (*see also* Tuberculosis) 011.4
   phthisis (*see also* Tuberculosis) 011.4
Stoppage
   bowel (*see also* Obstruction, intestine) 560.9
   heart (*see also* Arrest, cardiac) 427.5
   intestine (*see also* Obstruction, intestine) 560.9
   urine NEC (*see also* Retention, urine) 788.20
Storm, thyroid (apathetic) (*see also*
      Thyrotoxicosis) 242.9
Strabismus (alternating) (congenital)
      (nonparalytic) 378.9
   concomitant (*see also* Heterotropia) 378.30
      convergent (*see also* Esotropia) 378.00
      divergent (*see also* Exotropia) 378.10
   convergent (*see also* Esotropia) 378.00
   divergent (*see also* Exotropia) 378.10
   due to adhesions, scars—*see* Strabismus,
      mechanical
   in neuromuscular disorder NEC 378.73
   intermittent 378.20
      vertical 378.31
   latent 378.40
      convergent (esophoria) 378.41
      divergent (exophoria) 378.42
      vertical 378.43
   mechanical 378.60
      due to
         Brown's tendon sheath syndrome 378.61
         specified musculofascial disorder NEC
            378.62
   paralytic 378.50
      third or oculomotor nerve (partial) 378.51
         total 378.52
      fourth or trochlear nerve 378.53
      sixth or abducens nerve 378.54
   specified type NEC 378.73
   vertical (hypertropia) 378.31
Strain —*see also* Sprain, by site
   eye NEC 368.13
   heart—*see* Disease, heart
   meaning gonorrhea—*see* Gonorrhea
   on urination 788.65
   physical NEC V62.89
   postural 729.90
   psychological NEC V62.89
Strands
   conjunctiva 372.62
   vitreous humor 379.25
Strangulation, strangulated 994.7
   appendix 543.9
   asphyxiation or suffocation by 994.7

Strangulation, strangulated—*continued*
   bladder neck 596.0
   bowel—*see* Strangulation, intestine
   colon—*see* Strangulation, intestine
   cord (umbilical)—*see* Compression, umbilical
      cord
   due to birth injury 767.8
   food or foreign body (*see also* Asphyxia, food)
      933.1
   hemorrhoids 455.8
      external 455.5
      internal 455.2
   hernia—*see also* Hernia, by site, with
      obstruction
      gangrenous—*see* Hernia, by site, with
         gangrene
   intestine (large) (small) 560.2
      with hernia—*see also* Hernia, by site, with
         obstruction
         gangrenous—*see* Hernia, by site, with
            gangrene
      congenital (small) 751.1
         large 751.2
   mesentery 560.2
   mucus (*see also* Asphyxia, mucus) 933.1
      newborn 770.18
   omentum 560.2
   organ or site, congenital NEC—*see* Atresia
   ovary 620.8
      due to hernia 620.4
   penis 607.89
      foreign body 939.3
   rupture (*see also* Hernia, by site, with
      obstruction) 552.9
      gangrenous (*see also* Hernia, by site, with
         gangrene) 551.9
   stomach, due to hernia (*see also* Hernia, by site,
      with obstruction) 552.9
      with gangrene (*see also* Hernia, by site, with
         gangrene) 551.9
   umbilical cord—*see* Compression, umbilical
      cord
   vesicourethral orifice 596.0
Strangury 788.1
Strawberry
   gallbladder (*see also* Disease, gallbladder) 575.6
   mark 757.32
   tongue (red) (white) 529.3
Straw itch 133.8
Streak, ovarian 752.0
Strephosymbolia 315.01
   secondary to organic lesion 784.69
Streptobacillary fever 026.1
Streptobacillus moniliformis 026.1
Streptococcemia 038.0
Streptococcicosis —*see* Infection, streptococcal
Streptococcus, streptococcal —*see* condition
Streptoderma 686.00
Streptomycosis —*see* Actinomycosis
Streptothricosis —*see* Actinomycosis
Streptothrix —*see* Actinomycosis
Streptotrichosis —*see* Actinomycosis
Stress 308.9
   fracture—*see* Fracture, stress
   polycythemia 289.0
   reaction (gross) (*see also* Reaction, stress, acute)
      308.9
Stretching, nerve —*see* Injury, nerve, by site
Striae (albicantes) (atrophicae) (cutis distensae)
      (distensae) 701.3
Striations of nails 703.8

Stricture (*see also* Stenosis) 799.89
  ampulla of Vater 576.2
    with calculus, cholelithiasis, or stones—*see*
      Choledocholithiasis
  anus (sphincter) 569.2
    congenital 751.2
    infantile 751.2
  aorta (ascending) 747.22
    arch 747.10
    arteriosclerotic 440.0
    calcified 440.0
  aortic (valve) (*see also* Stenosis, aortic) 424.1
    congenital 746.3
  aqueduct of Sylvius (congenital) 742.3
    with spina bifida (*see also* Spina bifida) 741.0
    acquired 331.4
  artery 447.1
    basilar—*see* Narrowing, artery, basilar
    carotid (common) (internal)—*see* Narrowing,
      artery, carotid
    celiac 447.4
    cerebral 437.0
      congenital 747.81
      due to
        embolism (*see also* Embolism, brain) 434.1
        thrombus (*see also* Thrombosis, brain)
          434.0
    congenital (peripheral) 747.60
      cerebral 747.81
      coronary 746.85
      gastrointestinal 747.61
      lower limb 747.64
      renal 747.62
      retinal 743.58
      specified NEC 747.69
      spinal 747.82
      umbilical 747.5
      upper limb 747.63
    coronary —*see* Arteriosclerosis, coronary
      congenital 746.85
    precerebral—*see* Narrowing, artery,
      precerebral NEC
    pulmonary (congenital) 747.31
      acquired 417.8
    renal 440.1
    vertebral—*see* Narrowing, artery, vertebral
  auditory canal (congenital) (external) 744.02
    acquired (*see also* Stricture, ear canal,
      acquired) 380.50
  bile duct or passage (any) (postoperative) (*see*
    also Obstruction, biliary) 576.2
    congenital 751.61
  bladder 596.89
    congenital 753.6
    neck 596.0
      congenital 753.6
  bowel (*see also* Obstruction, intestine) 560.9
  brain 348.89
  bronchus 519.19
    syphilitic 095.8
  cardia (stomach) 537.89
    congenital 750.7
  cardiac—*see also* Disease, heart
    orifice (stomach) 537.89
  cardiovascular (*see also* Disease,
    cardiovascular) 429.2
  carotid artery—*see* Narrowing, artery, carotid
  cecum (*see also* Obstruction, intestine) 560.9
  cervix, cervical (canal) 622.4
    congenital 752.49

Stricture—*continued*
  cervix—*continued*
    in pregnancy or childbirth 654.6
      affecting fetus or newborn 763.89
      causing obstructed labor 660.2
        affecting fetus or newborn 763.1
  colon (*see also* Obstruction, intestine) 560.9
    congenital 751.2
  colostomy 569.62
  common bile duct (*see also* Obstruction, biliary)
    576.2
    congenital 751.61
  coronary (artery) —*see* Arteriosclerosis,
    coronary
    congenital 746.85
  cystic duct (*see also* Obstruction, gallbladder)
    575.2
    congenital 751.61
  cystostomy 596.83
  digestive organs NEC, congenital 751.8
  duodenum 537.3
    congenital 751.1
  ear canal (external) (congenital) 744.02
    acquired 380.50
      secondary to
        inflammation 380.53
        surgery 380.52
        trauma 380.51
  ejaculatory duct 608.85
  enterostomy 569.62
  esophagostomy 530.87
  esophagus (corrosive) (peptic) 530.3
    congenital 750.3
    syphilitic 095.8
      congenital 090.5
  Eustachian tube (*see also* Obstruction,
    Eustachian tube) 381.60
    congenital 744.24
  fallopian tube 628.2
    gonococcal (chronic) 098.37
      acute 098.17
    tuberculous (*see also* Tuberculosis) 016.6
  gallbladder (*see also* Obstruction, gallbladder)
    575.2
    congenital 751.69
  glottis 478.74
  heart—*see also* Disease, heart
    congenital NEC 746.89
    valve—*see also* Endocarditis
      congenital NEC 746.89
        aortic 746.3
        mitral 746.5
        pulmonary 746.02
        tricuspid 746.1
  hepatic duct (*see also* Obstruction, biliary) 576.2
  hourglass, of stomach 537.6
  hymen 623.3
  hypopharynx 478.29
  intestine (*see also* Obstruction, intestine) 560.9
    congenital (small) 751.1
      large 751.2
    ischemic 557.1
  lacrimal
    canaliculi 375.53
      congenital 743.65
    punctum 375.52
      congenital 743.65
    sac 375.54
      congenital 743.65
  lacrimonasal duct 375.56
    congenital 743.65
    neonatal 375.55

Stricture—*continued*
  larynx 478.79
    congenital 748.3
    syphilitic 095.8
      congenital 090.5
  lung 518.89
  meatus
    ear (congenital) 744.02
      acquired (*see also* Stricture, ear canal,
        acquired) 380.50
    osseous (congenital) (ear) 744.03
      acquired (*see also* Stricture, ear canal,
        acquired) 380.50
    urinarius (*see also* Stricture, urethra) 598.9
      congenital 753.6
  mitral (valve) (*see also* Stenosis, mitral) 394.0
    congenital 746.5
    specified cause, except rheumatic 424.0
  myocardium, myocardial (*see also*
    Degeneration, myocardial) 429.1
    hypertrophic subaortic (idiopathic) 425.11
  nares (anterior) (posterior) 478.19
    congenital 748.0
  nasal duct 375.56
    congenital 743.65
    neonatal 375.55
  nasolacrimal duct 375.56
    congenital 743.65
    neonatal 375.55
  nasopharynx 478.29
    syphilitic 095.8
  nephrostomy 997.5
  nose 478.19
    congenital 748.0
  nostril (anterior) (posterior) 478.19
    congenital 748.0
  organ or site, congenital NEC—*see* Atresia
  osseous meatus (congenital) (ear) 744.03
    acquired (*see also* Stricture, ear canal,
      acquired) 380.50
  os uteri (*see also* Stricture, cervix) 622.4
  oviduct—*see* Stricture, fallopian tube
  pelviureteric junction 593.3
  pharynx (dilation) 478.29
  prostate 602.8
  pulmonary, pulmonic
    artery (congenital) 747.31
      acquired 417.8
      noncongenital 417.8
    infundibulum (congenital) 746.83
    valve (*see also* Endocarditis, pulmonary)
      424.3
      congenital 746.02
    vein (congenital) 747.49
      acquired 417.8
    vessel NEC 417.8
  punctum lacrimale 375.52
    congenital 743.65
  pylorus (hypertrophic) 537.0
    adult 537.0
    congenital 750.5
    infantile 750.5
  rectosigmoid 569.89
  rectum (sphincter) 569.2
    congenital 751.2
    due to
      chemical burn 947.3
      irradiation 569.2
      lymphogranuloma venereum 099.1
    gonococcal 098.7
    inflammatory 099.1

Stricture—*continued*
  rectum—*continued*
    syphilitic 095.8
    tuberculous (*see also* Tuberculosis) 014.8
  renal artery 440.1
  salivary duct or gland (any) 527.8
  sigmoid (flexure) (*see also* Obstruction,
    intestine) 560.9
  spermatic cord 608.85
  stoma (following) (of)
    colostomy 569.62
    cystostomy 596.83
    enterostomy 569.62
    esophagostomy 530.87
    gastrostomy 536.42
    ileostomy 569.62
    nephrostomy 997.5
    tracheostomy 519.02
    ureterostomy 997.5
  stomach 537.89
    congenital 750.7
    hourglass 537.6
  subaortic 746.81
    hypertrophic (acquired) (idiopathic) 425.11
  subglottic 478.74
  syphilitic NEC 095.8
  tendon (sheath) 727.81
  trachea 519.19
    congenital 748.3
    syphilitic 095.8
    tuberculous (*see also* Tuberculosis) 012.8
  tracheostomy 519.02
  tricuspid (valve) (*see also* Endocarditis,
    tricuspid) 397.0
    congenital 746.1
    nonrheumatic 424.2
  tunica vaginalis 608.85
  ureter (postoperative) 593.3
    congenital 753.29
    tuberculous (*see also* Tuberculosis) 016.2
  ureteropelvic junction 593.3
    congenital 753.21
  ureterovesical orifice 593.3
    congenital 753.22
  urethra (anterior) (meatal) (organic) (posterior)
    (spasmodic) 598.9
    associated with schistosomiasis (*see also*
      Schistosomiasis) 120.9 *[598.01]*
    congenital (valvular) 753.6
    due to
      infection 598.00
        syphilis 095.8 *[598.01]*
      trauma 598.1
    gonococcal 098.2 *[598.01]*
    gonorrheal 098.2 *[598.01]*
    infective 598.00
    late effect of injury 598.1
    postcatheterization 598.2
    postobstetric 598.1
    postoperative 598.2
    specified cause NEC 598.8
    syphilitic 095.8 *[598.01]*
    traumatic 598.1
    valvular, congenital 753.6
  urinary meatus (*see also* Stricture, urethra)
    598.9
    congenital 753.6
  uterus, uterine 621.5
    os (external) (internal)—see Stricture, cervix
  vagina (outlet) 623.2
    congenital 752.49

Stricture—*continued*
  valve (cardiac) (heart) (*see also* Endocarditis) 424.90
    congenital (cardiac) (heart) NEC 746.89
      aortic 746.3
      mitral 746.5
      pulmonary 746.02
      tricuspid 746.1
      urethra 753.6
  valvular (*see also* Endocarditis) 424.90
  vascular graft or shunt 996.1
    atherosclerosis —*see* Arteriosclerosis, extremities
    embolism 996.74
    occlusion NEC 996.74
    thrombus 996.74
  vas deferens 608.85
    congenital 752.89
  vein 459.2
  vena cava (inferior) (superior) NEC 459.2
    congenital 747.49
  ventricular shunt 996.2
  vesicourethral orifice 596.0
    congenital 753.6
  vulva (acquired) 624.8
Stridor 786.1
  congenital (larynx) 748.3
Stridulous —*see* condition
Strippling of nails 703.8
Stroke 434.91
  apoplectic (*see also* Disease, cerebrovascular, acute) 436
  brain—*see* Infarct, brain
  embolic 434.11
  epileptic—*see* Epilepsy
  healed or old V12.54
  heart—*see* Disease, heart
  heat 992.0
  hemorrhagic—*see* Hemorrhage, brain
  iatrogenic 997.02
  in evolution 434.91
  ischemic 434.91
  late effect—*see* Late effect(s) (of) cerebrovascular disease
  lightning 994.0
  paralytic—*see* Infarct, brain
  postoperative 997.02
  progressive 435.9
  thrombotic 434.01
Stromatosis, endometrial (M8931/1) 236.0
Strong pulse 785.9
Strongyloides stercoralis infestation 127.2
Strongyloidiasis 127.2
Strongyloidosis 127.2
Strongylus (gibsoni) infestation 127.7
Strophulus (newborn) 779.89
  pruriginosus 698.2
Struck by lightning 994.0
Struma (*see also* Goiter) 240.9
  fibrosa 245.3
  Hashimoto (struma lymphomatosa) 245.2
  lymphomatosa 245.2
  nodosa (simplex) 241.9
    endemic 241.9
    multinodular 241.1
    sporadic 241.9
    toxic or with hyperthyroidism 242.3
      multinodular 242.2
      uninodular 242.1
    toxicosa 242.3
      multinodular 242.2
      uninodular 242.1

Struma—*continued*
  uninodular 241.0
  ovarii (M9090/0) 220
    and carcinoid (M9091/1) 236.2
    malignant (M9090/3) 183.0
  Riedel's (ligneous thyroiditis) 245.3
  scrofulous (*see also* Tuberculosis) 017.2
  tuberculous (*see also* Tuberculosis) 017.2
    abscess 017.2
    adenitis 017.2
    lymphangitis 017.2
    ulcer 017.2
Strumipriva cachexia (*see also* Hypothyroidism) 244.9
Strümpell-Marie disease or spine (ankylosing spondylitis) 720.0
Strümpell-Westphal pseudosclerosis (hepatolenticular degeneration) 275.1
Stuart's disease (congenital factor X deficiency) (*see also* Defect, coagulation) 286.3
Stuart-Prower factor deficiency (congenital factor X deficiency) (*see also* Defect, coagulation) 286.3
Students' elbow 727.2
Stuffy nose 478.19
Stump —*see also* Amputation
  cervix, cervical (healed) 622.8
Stupor 780.09
  catatonic (*see also* Schizophrenia) 295.2
  circular (*see also* Psychosis, manic-depressive, circular) 296.7
  manic 296.89
  manic-depressive (*see also* Psychosis, affective) 296.89
  mental (anergic) (delusional) 298.9
  psychogenic 298.8
  reaction to exceptional stress (transient) 308.2
  traumatic NEC—*see also* Injury, intracranial
    with spinal (cord)
      lesion—*see* Injury, spinal, by site
      shock—*see* Injury, spinal, by site
Sturge (-Weber) (-Dimitri) disease or syndrome (encephalocutaneous angiomatosis) 759.6
Sturge-Kalischer-Weber syndrome (encephalocutaneous angiomatosis) 759.6
Stuttering 315.35
  adult onset 307.0
  childhood onset 315.35
  due to late effect of cerebrovascular disease (see also Late effect(s) (of) cerebrovascular disease) 438.14
  in conditions classified elsewhere 784.52
Sty, stye 373.11
  external 373.11
  internal 373.12
  meibomian 373.12
Subacidity, gastric 536.8
  psychogenic 306.4
Subacute —*see* condition
Subarachnoid —*see* condition
Subclavian steal syndrome 435.2
Subcortical —*see* condition
Subcostal syndrome 098.86
  nerve compression 354.8
Subcutaneous, subcuticular —*see* condition
Subdelirium 293.1
Subdural —*see* condition
Subendocardium —*see* condition
Subependymoma (M9383/1) 237.5
Suberosis 495.3
Subglossitis —*see* Glossitis

Subhemophilia 286.0
Subinvolution (uterus) 621.1
  breast (postlactational) (postpartum) 611.89
  chronic 621.1
  puerperal, postpartum 674.8
Sublingual —*see* condition
Sublinguitis 527.2
Subluxation —*see also* Dislocation, by site
  congenital NEC—*see also* Malposition,
      congenital
    hip (unilateral) 754.32
      with dislocation of other hip 754.35
      bilateral 754.33
    joint
      lower limb 755.69
      shoulder 755.59
      upper limb 755.59
    lower limb (joint) 755.69
    shoulder (joint) 755.59
    upper limb (joint) 755.59
  lens 379.32
    anterior 379.33
    posterior 379.34
  radial head 832.2
  rotary, cervical region of spine—*see* Fracture,
      vertebra, cervical
Submaxillary —*see* condition
Submersion (fatal) (nonfatal) 994.1
Submissiveness (undue), in child 313.0
Submucous —*see* condition
Subnormal, subnormality
  accommodation (*see also* Disorder,
      accommodation) 367.9
  mental (*see also* Disability, intellectual) 319
    mild 317
    moderate 318.0
    profound 318.2
    severe 318.1
  temperature (accidental) 991.6
    not associated with low environmental
        temperature 780.99
Subphrenic —*see* condition
Subscapular nerve —*see* condition
Subseptus uterus 752.35
Subsiding appendicitis 542
Substance abuse in family V61.42
Substernal thyroid (*see also* Goiter) 240.9
  congenital 759.2
Substitution disorder 300.11
Subtentorial —*see* condition
Subtertian
  fever 084.0
  malaria (fever) 084.0
Subthyroidism (acquired) (*see also*
  Hypothyroidism) 244.9
  congenital 243
Succenturiata placenta —*see* Placenta,
  abnormal
Succussion sounds, chest 786.7
Sucking thumb, child 307.9
Sudamen 705.1
Sudamina 705.1
Sudanese kala-azar 085.0
Sudden
  death, cause unknown (less than 24 hours) 798.1
    cardiac (SCD)
      family history of V17.41
      personal history of, successfully resuscitated
          V12.53
    during childbirth 669.9
    infant 798.0

Sudden—*continued*
  death—*continued*
    puerperal, postpartum 674.9
  hearing loss NEC 388.2
  heart failure (*see also* Failure, heart) 428.9
  infant death syndrome 798.0
Sudeck's atrophy, disease, or syndrome 733.7
SUDS (Sudden unexplained death) 798.2
Suffocation (*see also* Asphyxia) 799.01
  by
    bed clothes 994.7
    bunny bag 994.7
    cave-in 994.7
    constriction 994.7
    drowning 994.1
    inhalation
      food or foreign body (*see also* Asphyxia,
          food or foreign body) 933.1
      oil or gasoline (*see also* Asphyxia, food or
          foreign body) 933.1
    overlying 994.7
    plastic bag 994.7
    pressure 994.7
    strangulation 994.7
  during birth 768.1
  mechanical 994.7
Sugar
  blood
    high 790.29
    low 251.2
  in urine 791.5
Suicide, suicidal (attempted)
  by poisoning—*see* Table of drugs and chemicals
  ideation V62.84
  risk 300.9
  tendencies 300.9
  trauma NEC (*see also* nature and site of injury)
      959.9
Suipestifer infection (*see also* Infection,
  Salmonella) 003.9
Sulfatidosis 330.0
Sulfhemoglobinemia, sulphemoglobinemia
  (acquired) (congenital) 289.7
Sumatran mite fever 081.2
Summer —*see* condition
Sunburn 692.71
  dermatitis 692.71
  due to
    other ultraviolet radiation 692.82
    tanning bed 692.82
  first degree 692.71
  second degree 692.76
  third degree 692.77
SUNCT (Short-lasting Unilateral Neuralgiform
  headache with Conjunctival injection and
  Tearing) 339.05
Sunken
  acetabulum 718.85
  fontanels 756.0
Sunstroke 992.0
Superfecundation 651.9
  with fetal loss and retention of one or more
      fetus(es) 651.6
  following (elective) fetal reduction 651.7
Superfetation 651.9
  with fetal loss and retention of one or more
      fetus(es) 651.6
  following (elective) fetal reduction 651.7
Supernumerary (congenital)
  aortic cusps 746.89
  auditory ossicles 744.04

Supernumerary—*continued*
bone 756.9
breast 757.6
carpal bones 755.56
cusps, heart valve NEC 746.89
mitral 746.5
pulmonary 746.09
digit(s) 755.00
finger 755.01
toe 755.02
ear (lobule) 744.1
fallopian tube 752.19
finger 755.01
hymen 752.49
kidney 753.3
lacrimal glands 743.64
lacrimonasal duct 743.65
lobule (ear) 744.1
mitral cusps 746.5
muscle 756.82
nipples 757.6
organ or site NEC—*see* Accessory
ossicles, auditory 744.04
ovary 752.0
oviduct 752.19
pulmonic cusps 746.09
rib 756.3
cervical or first 756.2
syndrome 756.2
roots (of teeth) 520.2
spinal vertebra 756.19
spleen 759.0
tarsal bones 755.67
teeth 520.1
causing crowding 524.31
testis 752.89
thumb 755.01
toe 755.02
uterus 752.2
vagina 752.49
vertebra 756.19
Supervision (of)
contraceptive method previously prescribed V25.40
intrauterine device V25.42
oral contraceptive (pill) V25.41
specified type NEC V25.49
subdermal implantable contraceptive V25.43
dietary (for) V65.3
allergy (food) V65.3
colitis V65.3
diabetes mellitus V65.3
food allergy intolerance V65.3
gastritis V65.3
hypercholesterolemia V65.3
hypoglycemia V65.3
intolerance (food) V65.3
obesity V65.3
specified NEC V65.3
lactation V24.1
newborn health
8 to 28 days old V20.32
under 8 days old V20.31
pregnancy—*see* Pregnancy, supervision of
Supplemental teeth 520.1
causing crowding 524.31
Suppression
binocular vision 368.31
lactation 676.5
menstruation 626.8
ovarian secretion 256.39
renal 586

Suppression—*continued*
urinary secretion 788.5
urine 788.5
Suppuration, suppurative —*see also* condition
accessory sinus (chronic) (*see also* Sinusitis)
473.9
adrenal gland 255.8
antrum (chronic) (*see also* Sinusitis, maxillary)
473.0
bladder (*see also* Cystitis) 595.89
bowel 569.89
brain 324.0
late effect 326
breast 611.0
puerperal, postpartum 675.1
dental periosteum 526.5
diffuse (skin) 686.00
ear (middle) (*see also* Otitis media) 382.4
external (*see also* Otitis, externa) 380.10
internal 386.33
ethmoidal (sinus) (chronic) (*see also* Sinusitis,
ethmoidal) 473.2
fallopian tube (*see also* Salpingo-oophoritis)
614.2
frontal (sinus) (chronic) (*see also* Sinusitis,
frontal) 473.1
gallbladder (*see also* Cholecystitis, acute) 575.0
gum 523.30
hernial sac—*see* Hernia, by site
intestine 569.89
joint (*see also* Arthritis, suppurative) 711.0
labyrinthine 386.33
lung 513.0
mammary gland 611.0
puerperal, postpartum 675.1
maxilla, maxillary 526.4
sinus (chronic) (*see also* Sinusitis, maxillary)
473.0
muscle 728.0
nasal sinus (chronic) (*see also* Sinusitis) 473.9
pancreas 577.0
parotid gland 527.2
pelvis, pelvic
female (*see also* Disease, pelvis,
inflammatory) 614.4
acute 614.3
male (*see also* Peritonitis) 567.21
pericranial (*see also* Osteomyelitis) 730.2
salivary duct or gland (any) 527.2
sinus (nasal) (*see also* Sinusitis) 473.9
sphenoidal (sinus) (chronic) (*see also* Sinusitis,
sphenoidal) 473.3
thymus (gland) 254.1
thyroid (gland) 245.0
tonsil 474.8
uterus (*see also* Endometritis) 615.9
vagina 616.10
wound—*see also* Wound, open, by site,
complicated
dislocation—*see* Dislocation, by site,
compound
fracture—*see* Fracture, by site, open
scratch or other superficial injury—*see* Injury,
superficial, by site
Supraeruption, teeth 524.34
Supraglottitis 464.50
with obstruction 464.51
Suprapubic drainage 596.89
Suprarenal (gland)—*see* condition

Suprascapular nerve —*see* condition
Suprasellar —*see* condition
Supraspinatus syndrome 726.10
Surfer knots 919.8
   infected 919.9
Surgery
   cosmetic NEC V50.1
      breast reconstruction following mastectomy
         V51.0
      following healed injury or operation V51.8
      hair transplant V50.0
   elective V50.9
      breast
         augmentation or reduction V50.1
         reconstruction following mastectomy V51.0
      circumcision, ritual or routine (in absence of
         medical indication) V50.2
      cosmetic NEC V50.1
      ear piercing V50.3
      face-lift V50.1
      following healed injury or operation V51.8
      hair transplant V50.0
   not done because of
      contraindication V64.1
      patient's decision V64.2
      specified reason NEC V64.3
   plastic
      breast
         augmentation or reduction V50.1
         reconstruction following mastectomy V51.0
      cosmetic V50.1
      face-lift V50.1
      following healed injury or operation V51.8
      repair of scarred tissue (following healed
         injury or operation) V51.8
      specified type NEC V50.8
   previous, in pregnancy or childbirth
      cervix 654.6
         affecting fetus or newborn (*see also*
            Newborn, affected by) 760.63
         causing obstructed labor 660.2
            affecting fetus or newborn 763.1
      pelvic soft tissues NEC 654.9
         affecting fetus or newborn (*see also*
            Newborn, affected by) 760.63
         causing obstructed labor 660.2
            affecting fetus or newborn 763.1
      perineum or vulva 654.8
      uterus NEC 654.9
         affecting fetus or newborn (*see also*
            Newborn, affected by) 760.63
         causing obstructed labor 660.2
            affecting fetus or newborn 763.1
         due to previous cesarean delivery 654.2
      vagina 654.7
Surgical
   abortion—*see* Abortion, legal
   emphysema 998.81
   kidney (*see also* Pyelitis) 590.80
   operation NEC 799.9
   procedures, complication or misadventure—*see*
      Complications, surgical procedure
   shock 998.00
Survey
   fetal anatomic V28.81

Susceptibility
   genetic
      to
         MEN (multiple endocrine neoplasia) V84.81
         neoplasia
            multiple endocrine (MEN) V84.81
         neoplasm
            malignant, of
               breast V84.01
               endometrium V84.04
               other V84.09
               ovary V84.02
               prostate V84.03
               specified disease NEC V84.89
Suspected condition, ruled out (*see also*
      Observation, suspected) V71.9
   specified condition NEC V71.89
Suspended uterus, in pregnancy or childbirth
   654.4
   affecting fetus or newborn 763.89
   causing obstructed labor 660.2
      affecting fetus or newborn 763.1
Sutton's disease 709.09
Sutton and Gull's disease (arteriolar
      nephrosclerosis) (*see also* Hypertension,
      kidney) 403.90
Suture
   burst (in external operation wound) (*see also*
      Dehiscence) 998.32
      internal 998.31
   inadvertently left in operation wound 998.4
   removal V58.32
   Shirodkar, in pregnancy (with or without
      cervical incompetence) 654.5
Swab inadvertently left in operation wound
   998.4
Swallowed, swallowing
   difficulty (*see also* Dysphagia) 787.20
   foreign body NEC (*see also* Foreign body) 938
Swamp fever 100.89
Swan neck hand (intrinsic) 736.09
Sweat (s), sweating
   disease or sickness 078.2
   excessive (*see also* Hyperhidrosis) 780.8
   fetid 705.89
   fever 078.2
   gland disease 705.9
      specified type NEC 705.89
   miliary 078.2
   night 780.8
Sweeley-Klionsky disease (angiokeratoma
      corporis diffusum) 272.7
Sweet's syndrome (acute febrile neutrophilic
      dermatosis) 695.89
Swelling 782.3
   abdominal (not referable to specific organ)
      789.3
   adrenal gland, cloudy 255.8
   ankle 719.07
   anus 787.99
   arm 729.81
   breast 611.72
   Calabar 125.2
   cervical gland 785.6
   cheek 784.2
   chest 786.6
   ear 388.8
   epigastric 789.3
   extremity (lower) (upper) 729.81

Swelling—*continued*
eye 379.92
female genital organ 625.8
finger 729.81
foot 729.81
glands 785.6
gum 784.2
hand 729.81
head 784.2
inflammatory—*see* Inflammation
joint (*see also* Effusion, joint) 719.0
  tuberculous—*see* Tuberculosis, joint
kidney, cloudy 593.89
leg 729.81
limb 729.81
liver 573.8
lung 786.6
lymph nodes 785.6
mediastinal 786.6
mouth 784.2
muscle (limb) 729.81
neck 784.2
nose or sinus 784.2
palate 784.2
pelvis 789.3
penis 607.83
perineum 625.8
rectum 787.99
scrotum 608.86
skin 782.2
splenic (*see also* Splenomegaly) 789.2
substernal 786.6
superficial, localized (skin) 782.2
testicle 608.86
throat 784.2
toe 729.81
tongue 784.2
tubular (*see also* Disease, renal) 593.9
umbilicus 789.3
uterus 625.8
vagina 625.8
vulva 625.8
wandering, due to Gnathostoma (spinigerum)
  128.1
white—*see* Tuberculosis, arthritis
Swift's disease 985.0
Swimmers'
eye (acute) 380.12
itch 120.3
Swimming in the head 780.4
Swollen —*see also* Swelling
glands 785.6
Swyer-James syndrome (unilateral hyperlucent
  lung) 492.8
Swyer's syndrome (XY pure gonadal
  dysgenesis) 752.7
Sycosis 704.8
barbae (not parasitic) 704.8
contagiosa 110.0
lupoid 704.8
mycotic 110.0
parasitic 110.0
vulgaris 704.8
Sydenham's chorea —*see* Chorea, Sydenham's
Sylvatic yellow fever 060.0
Sylvest's disease (epidemic pleurodynia) 074.1
Symblepharon 372.63
congenital 743.62
Symonds' syndrome 348.2
Sympathetic —*see* condition
Sympatheticotonia (*see also* Neuropathy,
  peripheral, autonomic) 337.9

Sympathicoblastoma (M9500/3)
specified site—*see* Neoplasm, by site, malignant
unspecified site 194.0
Sympathicogonioma (M9500/3)—*see*
  Sympathicoblastoma
Sympathoblastoma (M9500/3)—*see*
  Sympathicoblastoma
Sympathogonioma (M9500/3)—*see*
  Sympathicoblastoma
Symphalangy (*see also* Syndactylism) 755.10
Symptoms, specified (general) NEC 780.99
abdomen NEC 789.9
bone NEC 733.90
breast NEC 611.79
cardiac NEC 785.9
cardiovascular NEC 785.9
chest NEC 786.9
cognition 799.59
development NEC 783.9
digestive system NEC 787.99
emotional state NEC 799.29
eye NEC 379.99
gastrointestinal tract NEC 787.99
genital organs NEC
  female 625.9
  male 608.9
head and neck NEC 784.99
heart NEC 785.9
jaw 784.92
joint NEC 719.60
  ankle 719.67
  elbow 719.62
  foot 719.67
  hand 719.64
  hip 719.65
  knee 719.66
  multiple sites 719.69
  pelvic region 719.65
  shoulder (region) 719.61
  specified site NEC 719.68
  temporomandibular 524.69
  wrist 719.63
larynx NEC 784.99
limbs NEC 729.89
lymphatic system NEC 785.9
maxilla 784.92
menopausal 627.2
metabolism NEC 783.9
mouth NEC 528.9
muscle NEC 728.9
musculoskeletal NEC 781.99
  limbs NEC 729.89
nervous system NEC 781.99
neurotic NEC 300.9
nutrition, metabolism, and development NEC 783.9
pelvis NEC 789.9
  female 625.9
peritoneum NEC 789.9
respiratory system NEC 786.9
skin and integument NEC 782.9
subcutaneous tissue NEC 782.9
throat NEC 784.99
tonsil NEC 784.99
urinary system NEC 788.99
vascular NEC 785.9
Sympus 759.89
Synarthrosis 719.80
ankle 719.87
elbow 719.82
foot 719.87
hand 719.84

Synarthrosis—*continued*
  hip 719.85
  knee 719.86
  multiple sites 719.89
  pelvic region 719.85
  shoulder (region) 719.81
  specified site NEC 719.88
  wrist 719.83
Syncephalus 759.4
Synchondrosis 756.9
  abnormal (congenital) 756.9
  ischiopubic (van Neck's) 732.1
Synchysis (senile) (vitreous humor) 379.21
  scintillans 379.22
Syncope (near) (pre-) 780.2
  anginosa 413.9
  bradycardia 427.89
  cardiac 780.2
  carotid sinus 337.01
  complicating delivery 669.2
  due to lumbar puncture 349.0
  fatal 798.1
  heart 780.2
  heat 992.1
  laryngeal 786.2
  tussive 786.2
  vasoconstriction 780.2
  vasodepressor 780.2
  vasomotor 780.2
  vasovagal 780.2
Syncytial infarct —*see* Placenta, abnormal
Syndactylism, syndactyly (multiple sites) 755.10
  fingers (without fusion of bone) 755.11
    with fusion of bone 755.12
  toes (without fusion of bone) 755.13
    with fusion of bone 755.14
Syndrome —*see also* Disease
  5q minus 238.74
  abdominal
    acute 789.0
    migraine 346.2
    muscle deficiency 756.79
  Abercrombie's (amyloid degeneration) 277.39
  abnormal innervation 374.43
  abstinence
    alcohol 291.81
    drug 292.0
    neonatal 779.5
  Abt-Letterer-Siwe (acute histiocytosis X)
    (M9722/3) 202.5
  Achard-Thiers (adrenogenital) 255.2
  acid pulmonary aspiration 997.39
    obstetric (Mendelson's) 668.0
  acquired immune deficiency 042
  acquired immunodeficiency 042
  acrocephalosyndactylism 755.55
  acute abdominal 789.0
  acute chest 517.3
  acute coronary 411.1
  Adair-Dighton (brittle bones and blue sclera,
    deafness) 756.51
  Adams-Stokes (-Morgagni) (syncope with heart
    block) 426.9
  addisonian 255.41
  Adie (-Holmes) (pupil) 379.46
  adiposogenital 253.8
  adrenal
    hemorrhage 036.3
    meningococcic 036.3
  adrenocortical 255.3

Syndrome—*continued*
  adrenogenital (acquired) (congenital) 255.2
    feminizing 255.2
    iatrogenic 760.79
    virilism (acquired) (congenital) 255.2
  affective organic NEC 293.89
    drug-induced 292.84
  afferent loop NEC 537.89
  African macroglobulinemia 273.3
  Ahumada-Del Castillo (nonpuerperal
    galactorrhea and amenorrhea) 253.1
  air blast concussion—*see* Injury, internal, by site
  Alagille 759.89
  Albright (-Martin) (pseudohypoparathyroidism)
    275.49
  Albright-McCune-Sternberg (osteitis fibrosa
    disseminata) 756.59
  alcohol withdrawal 291.81
  Alder's (leukocyte granulation anomaly) 288.2
  Aldrich (-Wiskott) (eczema-thrombocytopenia)
    279.12
  Alibert-Bazin (mycosis, fungoides) (M9700/3)
    202.1
  Alice in Wonderland 293.89
  alien hand 781.8
  Allen-Masters 620.6
  Alligator baby (ichthyosis congenita) 757.1
  Alport's (hereditary hematuria-nephropathy-
    deafness) 759.89
  Alvarez (transient cerebral ischemia) 435.9
  alveolar capillary block 516.8
  Alzheimer's 331.0
    with dementia—*see* Alzheimer's, dementia
  amnestic (confabulatory) 294.0
    alcohol-induced persisting 291.1
    drug-induced 292.83
    posttraumatic 294.0
  amotivational 292.89
  amyostatic 275.1
  amyotrophic lateral sclerosis 335.20
  androgen insensitivity 259.51
    partial 259.52
  Angelman 759.89
  angina (*see also* Angina) 413.9
  ankyloglossia superior 750.0
  anterior
    chest wall 786.52
    compartment (tibial) 958.8
    spinal artery 433.8
      compression 721.1
    tibial (compartment) 958.8
  antibody deficiency 279.00
    agammaglobulinemic 279.00
    congenital 279.04
    hypogammaglobulinemic 279.00
  anticardiolipin antibody 289.81
  antimongolism 758.39
  antiphospholipid antibody 289.81
  Anton (-Babinski) (hemiasomatognosia) 307.9
  anxiety (*see also* Anxiety) 300.00
    organic 293.84
  aortic
    arch 446.7
    bifurcation (occlusion) 444.09
    ring 747.21
  Apert's (acrocephalosyndactyly) 755.55
  Apert-Gallais (adrenogenital) 255.2
  aphasia-apraxia-alexia 784.69
  apical ballooning 429.83
  "approximate answers" 300.16
  arcuate ligament (-celiac axis) 447.4

Syndrome—*continued*

Boder-Sedgwick (ataxia-telangiectasia) 334.8
Boerhaave's (spontaneous esophageal rupture)
530.4
Bonnevie-Ullrich 758.6
Bonnier's 386.19
Borjeson-Forssman-Lehmann 759.89
Bouillaud's (rheumatic heart disease) 391.9
Bourneville (-Pringle) (tuberous sclerosis) 759.5
Bouveret (-Hoffmann) (paroxysmal tachycardia)
427.2
brachial plexus 353.0
Brachman-de Lange (Amsterdam dwarf,
intellectual disabilities, and brachycephaly)
759.89
bradycardia-tachycardia 427.81
Brailsford-Morquio (dystrophy)
(mucopolysaccharidosis IV) 277.5
brain (acute) (chronic) (nonpsychotic) (organic)
(with behavioral reaction) (with neurotic
reaction) 310.9
with
    presenile brain disease (*see also* Dementia,
        presenile) 290.10
    psychosis, psychotic reaction (*see also*
        Psychosis, organic) 294.9
chronic alcoholic 291.2
congenital (*see also* Disability, intellectual)
    319
postcontusional 310.2
posttraumatic
    nonpsychotic 310.2
    psychotic 293.9
        acute 293.0
        chronic (*see also* Psychosis, organic) 294.8
        subacute 293.1
psycho-organic (*see also* Syndrome,
    psycho-organic) 310.9
psychotic (*see also* Psychosis, organic) 294.9
senile (*see also* Dementia, senile) 290.0
branchial arch 744.41
Brandt's (acrodermatitis enteropathica) 686.8
Brennemann's 289.2
Briquet's 300.81
Brissaud-Meige (infantile myxedema) 244.9
broad ligament laceration 620.6
Brock's (atelectasis due to enlarged lymph
nodes) 518.0
broken heart 429.83
Brown's tendon sheath 378.61
Brown-Séquard 344.89
brown spot 756.59
Brugada 746.89
Brugsch's (acropachyderma) 757.39
bubbly lung 770.7
Buchem's (hyperostosis corticalis) 733.3
Budd-Chiari (hepatic vein thrombosis) 453.0
Büdinger-Ludloff-Läwen 717.89
bulbar 335.22
    lateral (*see also* Disease, cerebrovascular,
        acute) 436
Bullis fever 082.8
bundle of Kent (anomalous atrioventricular
excitation) 426.7
Bürger-Grütz (essential familial hyperlipemia)
272.1
Burke's (pancreatic insufficiency and chronic
neutropenia) 577.8
Burnett's (milk-alkali) 275.42
Burnier's (hypophyseal dwarfism) 253.3
burning feet 266.2

Syndrome—*continued*

Bywaters' 958.5
Caffey's (infantile cortical hyperostosis) 756.59
Calvé-Legg-Perthes (osteochondrosis, femoral
capital) 732.1
Caplan (-Colinet) syndrome 714.81
capsular thrombosis (*see also* Thrombosis,
brain) 434.0
carbohydrate-deficient glycoprotein (CDGS) 271.8
carcinogenic thrombophlebitis 453.1
carcinoid 259.2
cardiac asthma (*see also* Failure, ventricular,
left) 428.1
cardiacos negros 416.0
cardiofaciocutaneous 759.89
cardiopulmonary obesity 278.03
cardiorenal (*see also* Hypertension, cardiorenal)
404.90
cardiorespiratory distress (idiopathic), newborn
769
cardiovascular renal (*see also* Hypertension,
cardiorenal) 404.90
cardiovasorenal 272.7
Carini's (ichthyosis congenita) 757.1
carotid
    artery (internal) 435.8
    body or sinus 337.01
carpal tunnel 354.0
Carpenter's 759.89
Cassidy (-Scholte) (malignant carcinoid) 259.2
cat-cry 758.31
cauda equina 344.60
causalgia 355.9
    lower limb 355.71
    upper limb 354.4
cavernous sinus 437.6
celiac 579.0
    artery compression 447.4
    axis 447.4
central pain 338.0
cerebellomedullary malformation (*see also*
Spina bifida) 741.0
cerebral gigantism 253.0
cerebrohepatorenal 759.89
cervical (root) (spine) NEC 723.8
    disc 722.71
    posterior, sympathetic 723.2
    rib 353.0
    sympathetic paralysis 337.09
    traumatic (acute) NEC 847.0
cervicobrachial (diffuse) 723.3
cervicocranial 723.2
cervicodorsal outlet 353.2
Céstan's 344.89
Céstan (-Raymond) 433.8
Céstan-Chenais 344.89
chancriform 114.1
Charcot's (intermittent claudication) 443.9
    angina cruris 443.9
    due to atherosclerosis 440.21
Charcot-Marie-Tooth 356.1
Charcot-Weiss-Baker 337.01
CHARGE association 759.89
Cheadle (-Möller) (-Barlow) (infantile scurvy)
267
Chédiak-Higashi (-Steinbrinck) (congenital
gigantism of peroxidase granules) 288.2
chest wall 786.52
Chiari's (hepatic vein thrombosis) 453.0
Chiari-Frommel 676.6
chiasmatic 368.41

Syndrome—*continued*
cystic duct stump 576.0
Da Costa's (neurocirculatory asthenia) 306.2
Dameshek's (erythroblastic anemia) 282.49
Dana-Putnam (subacute combined sclerosis with
pernicious anemia) 281.0 *[336.2]*
Danbolt (-Closs) (acrodermatitis enteropathica)
686.8
Dandy-Walker (atresia, foramen of Magendie)
742.3
with spina bifida (*see also* Spina bifida) 741.0
Danlos' 756.83
Davies-Colley (slipping rib) 733.99
dead fetus 641.3
defeminization 255.2
defibrination (*see also* Fibrinolysis) 286.6
Degos' 447.8
Deiters' nucleus 386.19
Déjérine-Roussy 338.0
Déjérine-Thomas 333.0
de Lange's (Amsterdam dwarf, intellectual
disabilities, and brachycephaly) (Cornelia)
759.89
Del Castillo's (germinal aplasia) 606.0
deletion chromosomes 758.39
delusional
induced by drug 292.11
dementia-aphonia, of childhood (*see also*
Psychosis, childhood) 299.1
demyelinating NEC 341.9
denial visual hallucination 307.9
depersonalization 300.6
de Quervain's 259.51
Dercum's (adiposis dolorosa) 272.8
de Toni-Fanconi (-Debré) (cystinosis) 270.0
diabetes-dwarfism-obesity (juvenile) 258.1
diabetes mellitus-hypertension-nephrosis 250.4
[581.81]
due to secondary diabetes 249.4 *[581.81]*
diabetes mellitus in newborn infant 775.1
diabetes-nephrosis 250.4 *[581.81]*
due to secondary diabetes 249.4 *[581.81]*
diabetic amyotrophy 250.6 *[353.5]*
due to secondary diabetes 249.6 [353.5]
Diamond-Blackfan (congenital hypoplastic
anemia) 284.01
Diamond-Gardener (autoerythrocyte
sensitization) 287.2
DIC (diffuse or disseminated intravascular
coagulopathy) (*see also* Fibrinolysis) 286.6
diencephalohypophyseal NEC 253.8
diffuse cervicobrachial 723.3
diffuse obstructive pulmonary 496
DiGeorge's (thymic hypoplasia) 279.11
Dighton's 756.51
Di Guglielmo's (erythremic myelosis)
(M9841/3) 207.0
disequilibrium 276.9
disseminated platelet thrombosis 446.6
Ditthomska 307.81
Doan-Wiseman (primary splenic neutropenia)
289.53
Döhle body-panmyelopathic 288.2
Donohue's (leprechaunism) 259.8
dorsolateral medullary (*see also* Disease,
cerebrovascular, acute) 436
double athetosis 333.71
double whammy 360.81
Down's (mongolism) 758.0
Dresbach's (elliptocytosis) 282.1

Syndrome—*continued*
Dressler's (postmyocardial infarction) 411.0
hemoglobinuria 283.2
postcardiotomy 429.4
drug withdrawal, infant, of dependent mother
779.5
dry skin 701.1
eye 375.15
DSAP (disseminated superficial actinic
porokeratosis) 692.75
Duane's (retraction) 378.71
Duane-Stilling-Türk (ocular retraction
syndrome) 378.71
Dubin-Johnson (constitutional
hyperbilirubinemia) 277.4
Dubin-Sprinz (constitutional
hyperbilirubinemia) 277.4
Duchenne's 335.22
due to abnormality
autosomal NEC (*see also* Abnormal,
autosomes NEC) 758.5
13 758.1
18 758.2
21 or 22 758.0
D_1 758.1
E_3 758.2
G 758.0
chromosomal 758.89
sex 758.81
dumping 564.2
nonsurgical 536.8
Duplay's 726.2
Dupré's (meningism) 781.6
Dyke-Young (acquired macrocytic hemolytic
anemia) 283.9
dyspraxia 315.4
dystocia, dystrophia 654.9
Eagle-Barrett 756.71
Eales' 362.18
Eaton-Lambert (*see also* Syndrome,
Lambert-Eaton) 358.30
Ebstein's (downward displacement, tricuspid
valve into right ventricle) 746.2
ectopic ACTH secretion 255.0
eczema-thrombocytopenia 279.12
Eddowes' (brittle bones and blue sclera) 756.51
Edwards' 758.2
efferent loop 537.89
effort (aviators') (psychogenic) 306.2
Ehlers-Danlos 756.83
Eisenmenger's (ventricular septal defect) 745.4
Ekbom's (restless legs) 333.94
Ekman's (brittle bones and blue sclera) 756.51
electric feet 266.2
Elephant man 237.71
Ellison-Zollinger (gastric hypersecretion with
pancreatic islet cell tumor) 251.5
Ellis-van Creveld (chondroectodermal
dysplasia) 756.55
embryonic fixation 270.2
empty sella (turcica) 253.8
endocrine-hypertensive 255.3
Engel-von Recklinghausen (osteitis fibrosa
cystica) 252.01
enteroarticular 099.3
entrapment—*see* Neuropathy, entrapment
eosinophilia myalgia 710.5
epidemic vomiting 078.82
Epstein's—*see* Nephrosis
Erb (-Oppenheim) -Goldflam 358.00
Erdheim-Chester 277.89

Syndrome—*continued*
  Guillain-Barré (-Strohl) 357.0
  Gunn's (jaw-winking syndrome) 742.8
  Günther's (congenital erythropoietic porphyria)
    277.1
  gustatory sweating 350.8
  H3O 759.81
  Hadfield-Clarke (pancreatic infantilism) 577.8
  Haglund-Läwen-Fründ 717.89
  hairless women 257.8
  hair tourniquet—*see also* Injury, superficial, by
    site
    finger 915.8
      infected 915.9
    penis 911.8
      infected 911.9
    toe 917.8
      infected 917.9
  Hallermann-Streiff 756.0
  Hallervorden-Spatz 333.0
  Hamman's (spontaneous mediastinal
    emphysema) 518.1
  Hamman-Rich (diffuse interstitial pulmonary
    fibrosis) 516.33
  Hand-Schüller-Christian (chronic histiocytosis
    X) 277.89
  hand-foot 693.0
  Hanot-Chauffard (-Troisier) (bronze diabetes)
    275.01
  Harada's 363.22
  Hare's (M8010/3) (carcinoma, pulmonary apex)
    162.3
  Harkavy's 446.0
  harlequin color change 779.89
  Harris' (organic hyperinsulinism) 251.1
  Hart's (pellagra-cerebellar ataxia-renal
    aminoaciduria) 270.0
  Hayem-Faber (achlorhydric anemia) 280.9
  Hayem-Widal (acquired hemolytic jaundice) 283.9
  headache — *see* Headache, syndrome
  Heberden's (angina pectoris) 413.9
  Hedinger's (malignant carcinoid) 259.2
  Hegglin's 288.2
  Heller's (infantile psychosis) (*see also*
    Psychosis, childhood) 299.1
  H.E.L.L.P. 642.5
  hemolytic-uremic (adult) (child) 283.11
  hemophagocytic 288.4
    infection-associated 288.4
  Hench-Rosenberg (palindromic arthritis) (*see
    also* Rheumatism, palindromic) 719.3
  Henoch-Schönlein (allergic purpura) 287.0
  hepatic flexure 569.89
  hepatopulmonary 573.5
  hepatorenal 572.4
    due to a procedure 997.49
    following delivery 674.8
  hepatourologic 572.4
  Herrick's (hemoglobin S disease) 282.61
  Herter (-Gee) (nontropical sprue) 579.0
  Heubner-Herter (nontropical sprue) 579.0
  Heyd's (hepatorenal) 572.4
  HHHO 759.81
  high grade myelodysplastic 238.73
    with 5q deletion 238.73
  Hilger's 337.09
  histiocytic 288.4
  Hoffa (-Kastert) (liposynovitis prepatellaris) 272.8
  Hoffmann's 244.9 *[359.5]*
  Hoffmann-Bouveret (paroxysmal tachycardia)
    427.2

Syndrome—*continued*
  Hoffmann-Werdnig 335.0
  Holländer-Simons (progressive lipodystrophy)
    272.6
  Holmes' (visual disorientation) 368.16
  Holmes-Adie 379.46
  Hoppe-Goldflam 358.00
  Yorner's (sde also Neuropathy, peripheral,
    autonomic) 337.9
    traumatic—*see* Injury, nerve, cervical
      sympathetic
  hospital addiction 301.51
  hungry bone 275.5
  Hunt's (herpetic geniculate ganglionitis) 053.11
    dyssynergia cerebellaris myoclonica 334.2
  Hunter (-Hurler) (mucopolysaccharidosis II)
    277.5
  hunterian glossitis 529.4
  Hurler (-Hunter) (mucopolysaccharidosis II)
    277.5
  Hutchinson's incisors or teeth 090.5
  Hutchinson-Boeck (sarcoidosis) 135
  Hutchinson-Gilford (progeria) 259.8
  hydralazine
    correct substance properly administered 695.4
    overdose or wrong substance given or taken
      972.6
  hydraulic concussion (abdomen) (*see also*
    Injury, internal, abdomen) 868.00
  hyperabduction 447.8
  hyperactive bowel 564.9
  hyperaldosteronism with hypokalemic alkalosis
    (Bartter's) 255.13
  hypercalcemic 275.42
  hypercoagulation NEC 289.89
  hypereosinophilic (idiopathic) 288.3
  hyperfusion 997.01
  hyperkalemic 276.7
  hyperkinetic—*see also* Hyperkinesia
    heart 429.82
  hyperlipemia-hemolytic anemia-icterus 571.1
  hypermobility 728.5
  hypernatremia 276.0
  hyperosmolarity 276.0
  hypersomnia-bulimia 349.89
  hypersplenic 289.4
  hypersympathetic (*see also* Neuropathy,
    peripheral, autonomic) 337.9
  hypertransfusion, newborn 776.4
  hyperventilation, psychogenic 306.1
  hyperviscosity (of serum) NEC 273.3
    polycythemic 289.0
    sclerothymic 282.8
  hypoglycemic (familial) (neonatal) 251.2
    functional 251.1
  hypokalemic 276.8
  hypophyseal 253.8
  hypophyseothalamic 253.8
  hypopituitarism 253.2
  hypoplastic left heart 746.7
  hypopotassemia 276.8
  hyposmolality 276.1
  hypotension, maternal 669.2
  hypothenar hammer 443.89
  hypotonia-hypomentia-hypogonadism-obesity
    759.81
  ICF (intravascular coagulation-fibrinolysis) (*see
    also* Fibrinolysis) 286.6
  idiopathic cardiorespiratory distress, newborn 769
  idiopathic nephrotic (infantile) 581.9

Syndrome—*continued*
lateral
  cutaneous nerve of thigh 355.1
  medullary (*see also* Disease, cerebrovascular
    acute) 436
Launois' (pituitary gigantism) 253.0
Launois-Cléret (adiposogenital dystrophy) 253.8
Laurence-Moon (-Bardet) -Biedl (obesity,
  polydactyly, and intellectual disabilities)
  759.8
Lawford's (encephalocutaneous angiomatosis) 759.6
lazy
  leukocyte 288.09
  posture 728.3
Lederer-Brill (acquired infectious hemolytic
  anemia) 283.19
Legg-Calvé-Perthes (osteochondrosis capital
  femoral) 732.1
Lemiere 451.89
Lennox's (*see also* Epilepsy) 345.0
Lennox-Gastaut syndrome 345.0
  with tonic seizures 345.1
lenticular 275.1
Léopold-Lévi's (paroxysmal thyroid instability)
  242.9
Lepore hemoglobin 282.45
Léri-Weill 756.59
Leriche's (aortic bifurcation occlusion) 444.09
Lermoyez's (*see also* Disease, Ménière's)
  386.00
Lesch-Nyhan (hypoxanthine-guanine-
  phosphoribosyltransferase deficiency) 277.2
leukoencephalopathy, reversible, posterior 348.5
Lev's (acquired complete heart block) 426.0
Levi's (pituitary dwarfism) 253.3
Lévy-Roussy 334.3
Lichtheim's (subacute combined sclerosis with
  pernicious anemia) 281.0 *[336.2]*
Li-Fraumeni V84.01
Lightwood's (renal tubular acidosis) 588.89
Lignac (-de Toni) (-Fanconi) (-Debré)
  (cystinosis) 270.0
Likoff's (angina in menopausal women) 413.9
liver-kidney 572.4
Lloyd's 258.1
lobotomy 310.0
Löffler's (eosinophilic pneumonitis) 518.3
Löfgren's (sarcoidosis) 135
long arm 18 or 21 deletion 758.39
Looser (-Debray) -Milkman (osteomalacia with
  pseudofractures) 268.2
Lorain-Levi (pituitary dwarfism) 253.3
Louis-Bar (ataxia-telangiectasia) 334.8
low
  atmospheric pressure 993.2
  back 724.2
    psychogenic 306.0
  output (cardiac) (*see also* Failure, heart) 428.9
Lowe's (oculocerebrorenal dystrophy) 270.8
Lowe-Terrey-MacLachlan (oculocerebrorenal
  dystrophy) 270.8
lower radicular, newborn 767.4
Lown (-Ganong)-Levine (short P-R interval,
  normal QRS complex, and supraventricular
  tachycardia) 426.81
Lucey-Driscoll (jaundice due to delayed
  conjugation) 774.30
Luetscher's (dehydration) 276.51
lumbar vertebral 724.4
Lutembacher's (atrial septal defect with mitral
  stenosis) 745.5

Syndrome—*continued*
Lyell's (toxic epidermal necrolysis) 695.15
  due to drug
    correct substance properly administered
      695.15
    overdose or wrong substance given or taken
      977.9
    specified drug—*see* Table of drugs and
      chemicals
MacLeod's 492.8
macrogenitosomia praecox 259.8
macroglobulinemia 273.3
macrophage activation 288.4
Maffucci's (dyschondroplasia with
  hemangiomas) 756.4
Magenblase 306.4
magnesium-deficiency 781.7
Mal de Debarquement 780.4
malabsorption 579.9
  postsurgical 579.3
  spinal fluid 331.3
malignant carcinoid 259.2
Mallory-Weiss 530.7
mandibulofacial dysostosis 756.0
manic-depressive (*see also* Psychosis, affective)
  296.80
Mankowsky's (familial dysplastic osteopathy)
  731.2
maple syrup (urine) 270.3
Marable's (celiac artery compression) 447.4
Marchesani (-Weill) (brachymorphism and
  ectopia lentis) 759.89
Marchiafava-Bignami 341.8
Marchiafava-Micheli (paroxysmal nocturnal
  hemoglobinuria) 283.2
Marcus Gunn's (jaw-winking syndrome) 742.8
Marfan's (arachnodactyly) 759.82
  meaning congenital syphilis 090.49
  with luxation of lens 090.49 *[379.32]*
Marie's (acromegaly) 253.0
  primary or idiopathic (acropachyderma)
    757.39
  secondary (hypertrophic pulmonary
    osteoarthropathy) 731.2
Markus-Adie 379.46
Maroteaux-Lamy (mucopolysaccharidosis VI)
  277.5
Martin's 715.27
Martin-Albright (pseudohypoparathyroidism)
  275.49
Martorell-Fabré (pulseless disease) 446.7
massive aspiration of newborn 770.18
Masters-Allen 620.6
mastocytosis 757.33
maternal hypotension 669.2
maternal obesity 646.1
May (-Hegglin) 288.2
McArdle (-Schmid) (-Pearson) (glycogenosis V)
  271.0
McCune-Albright (osteitis fibrosa disseminata)
  756.59
McQuarrie's (idiopathic familial hypoglycemia)
  251.2
meconium
  aspiration 770.12
  plug (newborn) NEC 777.1
median arcuate ligament 447.4
mediastinal fibrosis 519.3
Meekeren-Ehlers-Danlos 756.83

Syndrome—*continued*
Noonan's 759.89
Nothnagel's
  ophthalmoplegia-cerebellar ataxia 378.52
  vasomotor acroparesthesia 443.89
nucleus ambiguous-hypoglossal 352.6
OAV (oculoauriculovertebral dysplasia) 756.0
obesity hypoventilation 278.03
obsessional 300.3
oculocutaneous 364.24
oculomotor 378.81
oculourethroarticular 099.3
Ogilvie's (sympathicotonic colon obstruction)
  560.89
ophthalmoplegia-cerebellar ataxia 378.52
Oppenheim-Urbach (necrobiosis lipoidica
  diabeticorum) 250.8 *[709.3]*
  due to secondary diabetes 249.8 *[709.3]*
oral-facial-digital 759.89
organic
  affective NEC 293.83
    drug-induced 292.84
  anxiety 293.84
  delusional 293.81
    alcohol-induced 291.5
    drug-induced 292.11
    due to or associated with
      arteriosclerosis 290.42
      presenile brain disease 290.12
      senility 290.20
  depressive 293.83
    drug-induced 292.84
    due to or associated with
      arteriosclerosis 290.43
      presenile brain disease 290.13
      senile brain disease 290.21
  hallucinosis 293.82
    drug-induced 292.84
  organic affective 293.83
    induced by drug 292.84
  organic personality 310.1
    induced by drug 292.89
Ormond's 593.4
orodigitofacial 759.89
orthostatic hypotensive-dysautonomic-
  dyskinetic 333.0
Osler-Weber-Rendu (familial hemorrhagic
  telangiectasia) 448.0
osteodermopathic hyperostosis 757.39
osteoporosis-osteomalacia 268.2
Österreicher-Turner (hereditary
  osteo-onychodysplasia) 756.89
os trigonum 755.69
Ostrum-Furst 756.59
otolith 386.19
otopalatodigital 759.89
outlet (thoracic) 353.0
ovarian remnant 620.8
Owren's (*see also* Defect, coagulation) 286.3
OX 758.6
pacemaker 429.4
Paget-Schroetter (intermittent venous
  claudication) 453.89
pain—*see also* Pain
  central 338.0
  chronic 338.4

Syndrome—*continued*
pain—*continued*
  complex regional 355.9
    type I 337.20
      lower limb 337.22
      specified site NEC 337.29
      upper limb 337.21
    type II
      lower limb 355.71
      upper limb 354.4
  myelopathic 338.0
  thalamic (hypersthetic) 338.0
painful
  apicocostal vertebral (M8010/3) 162.3
  arc 726.19
  bruising 287.2
  feet 266.2
Pancoast's (carcinoma, pulmonary apex)
  (M8010/3) 162.3
panhypopituitary (postpartum) 253.2
papillary muscle 429.81
  with myocardial infarction 410.8
Papillon-Léage and Psaume (orodigitofacial
  dysostosis) 759.89
parabiotic (transfusion)
  donor (twin) 772.0
  recipient (twin) 776.4
paralysis agitans 332.0
paralytic 344.9
  specified type NEC 344.89
Paraneoplastic —*see* condition
Parinaud's (paralysis of conjugate upward gaze)
  378.81
  oculoglandular 372.02
Parkes Weber and Dimitri (encephalocutaneous
  angiomatosis) 759.6
Parkinson's (*see also* Parkinsonism) 332.0
parkinsonian (*see also* Parkinsonism) 332.0
Parry's (exophthalmic goiter) 242.0
Parry-Romberg 349.89
Parsonage-Aldren-Turner 353.5
Parsonage-Turner 353.5
Patau's (trisomy D_1) 758.1
patella clunk 719.66
patellofemoral 719.46
Paterson (-Brown) (-Kelly) (sideropenic
  dysphagia) 280.8
Payr's (splenic flexure syndrome) 569.89
pectoral girdle 447.8
pectoralis minor 447.8
Pelger-Huët (hereditary hyposegmentation)
  288.2
pellagra-cerebellar ataxia-renal aminoaciduria
  270.0
Pellegrini-Stieda 726.62
pellagroid 265.2
Pellizzi's (pineal) 259.8
pelvic congestion (-fibrosis) 625.5
Pendred's (familial goiter with deaf-mutism)
  243
Penfield's (*see also* Epilepsy) 345.5
Penta X 758.81
peptic ulcer—*see* Ulcer, peptic 533.9
perabduction 447.8
periodic 277.31
periurethral fibrosis 593.4
persistent fetal circulation 747.83
Petges-Cléjat (poikilodermatomyositis) 710.3
Peutz-Jeghers 759.6
Pfeiffer (acrocephalosyndactyly) 755.55

Syndrome—*continued*
pyloroduodenal 537.89
pyramidopallidonigral 332.0
pyriformis 355.0
QT interval prolongation 426.82
radicular NEC 729.2
  lower limbs 724.4
  upper limbs 723.4
    newborn 767.4
Raeder-Harbitz (pulseless disease) 446.7
Ramsay Hunt's
  dyssynergia cerebellaris myoclonica 334.2
  herpetic geniculate ganglionitis 053.11
rapid time-zone change 327.35
Raymond (-Céstan) 433.8
Raynaud's (paroxysmal digital cyanosis) 443.0
RDS (respiratory distress syndrome, newborn)
  769
Refsum's (heredopathia atactica
  polyneuritiformis) 356.3
Reichmann's (gastrosuccorrhea) 536.8
Reifenstein's (hereditary familial
  hypogonadism, male) 259.52
Reilly's (*see also* Neuropathy, peripheral,
  autonomic) 337.9
Reiter's 099.3
renal glomerulohyalinosis-diabetic 250.4
  [581.81]
  due to secondary diabetes 249.4 [581.81]
Rendu-Osler-Weber (familial hemorrhagic
  telangiectasia) 448.0
renofacial (congenital biliary fibroangiomatosis)
  753.0
Rénon-Delille 253.8
respiratory distress (idiopathic) (newborn) 769
  adult (following trauma and surgery) 518.52
    specified NEC 518.82
  type II 770.6
restless legs (RLS) 333.94
retinoblastoma (familial) 190.5
retraction (Duane's) 378.71
retroperitoneal fibrosis 593.4
retroviral seroconversion (acute) V08
Rett's 330.8
Reye's 331.81
Reye-Sheehan (postpartum pituitary necrosis)
  253.2
Riddoch's (visual disorientation) 368.16
Ridley's (*see also* Failure, ventricular, left)
  428.1
Rieger's (mesodermal dysgenesis, anterior
  ocular segment) 743.44
Rietti-Greppi-Micheli (thalassemia minor)
  282.46
right ventricular obstruction—*see* Failure heart
Riley-Day (familial dysautonomia) 742.8
Robin's 756.0
Rokitansky-Kuster-Hauser (congenital absence,
  vagina) 752.45
Romano-Ward (prolonged QT interval
  syndrome) 426.82
Romberg's 349.89
Rosen-Castleman-Liebow (pulmonary
  proteinosis) 516.0
rotator cuff, shoulder 726.10
Roth's 355.1
Rothmund's (congenital poikiloderma) 757.33
Rotor's (idiopathic hyperbilirubinemia) 277.4
Roussy-Lévy 334.3
Roy (-Jutras) (acropachyderma) 757.39

Syndrome—*continued*
rubella (congenital) 771.0
Rubinstein-Taybi's (brachydactylia, short
  stature, and intellectual disabilities) 759.89
Rud's (mental deficiency, epilepsy, and
  infantilism) 759.89
Ruiter-Pompen (-Wyers) (angiokeratoma
  corporis diffusum) 272.7
Runge's (postmaturity) 766.22
Russell (-Silver) (congenital hemihypertrophy
  and short stature) 759.89
Rytand-Lipsitch (complete atrioventricular
  block) 426.0
sacralization-scoliosis-sciatica 756.15
sacroiliac 724.6
Saenger's 379.46
salt
  depletion (*see also* Disease, renal) 593.9
    due to heat NEC 992.8
      causing heat exhaustion or prostration
        992.4
  low (*see also* Disease, renal) 593.9
salt-losing (*see also* Disease, renal) 593.9
Sanfilippo's (mucopolysaccharidosis III) 277.5
Scaglietti-Dagnini (acromegalic
  macrospondylitis) 253.0
scalded skin 695.81
scalenus anticus (anterior) 353.0
scapulocostal 354.8
scapuloperoneal 359.1
scapulovertebral 723.4
Schaumann's (sarcoidosis) 135
Scheie's (mucopolysaccharidosis IS) 277.5
Scheuthauer-Marie-Sainton (cleidocranialis
  dysostosis) 755.59
Schirmer's (encephalocutaneous angiomatosis)
  759.6
schizophrenic, of childhood NEC (*see also*
  Psychosis, childhood) 299.9
Schmidt's
  sphallo-pharyngo-laryngeal hemiplegia 352.6
  thyroid-adrenocortical insufficiency 258.1
  vagoaccessory 352.6
Schneider's 047.9
Schnitzler 273.1
Scholte's (malignant carcinoid) 259.2
Scholz (-Bielschowsky-Henneberg) 330.0
Schroeder's (endocrine-hypertensive) 255.3
Schüller-Christian (chronic histiocytosis X)
  277.89
Schultz's (agranulocytosis) 288.09
Schwachman's—*see* Syndrome, Shwachman's
Schwartz (-Jampel) 359.23
Schwartz-Bartter (inappropriate secretion of
  antidiuretic hormone) 253.6
Scimitar (anomalous venous drainage, right lung
  to inferior vena cave) 747.49
sclerocystic ovary 256.4
sea-blue histiocyte 272.7
Seabright-Bantam (pseudohypoparathyroidism)
  275.49
Seckel's 759.89
Secretan's (posttraumatic edema) 782.3
secretoinhibitor (keratoconjunctivitis sicca)
  710.2
Seeligmann's (ichthyosis congenita) 757.1
Senear-Usher (pemphigus erythematosus) 694.4
senilism 259.8
seroconversion, retroviral (acute) V08
serotonin 333.99

Syndrome—*continued*
serous meningitis 348.2
Sertoli cell (germinal aplasia) 606.0
sex chromosome mosaic 758.81
Sézary's (reticulosis) (M9701/3) 202.2
shaken infant 995.55
Shaver's (bauxite pneumoconiosis) 503
Sheehan's (postpartum pituitary necrosis) 253.2
shock (traumatic) 958.4
  kidney 584.5
    following crush injury 958.5
  lung 518.82
    related to trauma and surgery 518.52
  neurogenic 308.9
  psychic 308.9
Shone's 746.84
short
  bowel 579.3
  P-R interval 426.81
shoulder-arm (*see also* Neuropathy, peripheral,
  autonomic) 337.9
shoulder-girdle 723.4
shoulder-hand (*see also* Neuropathy, peripheral,
  autonomic) 337.9
Shwachman's 288.02
Shy-Drager (orthostatic hypotension with
  multisystem degeneration) 333.0
Sicard's 352.6
sicca (keratoconjunctivitis) 710.2
sick
  cell 276.1
  cilia 759.89
  sinus 427.81
sideropenic 280.8
Siemens'
  ectodermal dysplasia 757.31
  keratosis follicularis spinulosa (decalvans)
    757.39
Silfverskiöld's (osteochondrodystrophy,
  extremities) 756.50
Silver's (congenital hemihypertrophy and short
  stature) 759.89
Silvestroni-Bianco (thalassemia minima) 282.46
Simons' (progressive lipodystrophy) 272.6
sinus tarsi 726.79
sinusitis-bronchiectasis-situs inversus 759.3
Sipple's (medullary thyroid
  carcinoma-pheochromocytoma) 258.02
Sjögren (-Gougerot) (keratoconjunctivitis sicca)
  710.2
  with lung involvement 710.2 *[517.8]*
Sjögren-Larsson (ichthyosis congenita) 757.1
SJS-TEN (Stevens-Johnson syndrome-toxic
  epidermal necrolysis overlap) 695.14
Slocumb's 255.3
Sluder's 337.09
Smith-Lemli-Opitz (cerebrohepatorenal
  syndrome) 759.89
Smith-Magenis 758.33
smokers' 305.1
Sneddon-Wilkinson (subcorneal pustular
  dermatosis) 694.1
Sotos' (cerebral gigantism) 253.0
South African cardiomyopathy 425.2
spasmodic
  upward movement, eyes(s) 378.82
  winking 307.20
Spens' (syncope with heart block) 426.9
spherophakia-brachymorphia 759.89

Syndrome—*continued*
spinal cord injury—*see also* Injury, spinal, by
  site
  with fracture, vertebra—*see* Fracture, vertebra,
    by site, with spinal cord injury
  cervical—*see* Injury, spinal, cervical
  fluid malabsorption (acquired) 331.3
splenic
  agenesis 759.0
  flexure 569.89
  neutropenia 289.53
  sequestration 289.52
Spurway's (brittle bones and blue sclera) 756.51
staphylococcal scalded skin 695.81
Stein's (polycystic ovary) 256.4
Stein-Leventhal (polycystic ovary) 256.4
Steinbrocker's (*see also* Neuropathy, peripheral,
  autonomic) 337.9
Stevens-Johnson (erythema multiforme
  exudativum) 695.13
  toxic epidermal necrolysis overlap (SJS-TEN
    overlap syndrome) 695.14
Stewart-Morel (hyperostosis frontalis interna)
  733.3
Stickler 759.89
stiff-baby 759.89
stiff-man 333.91
Still's (juvenile rheumatoid arthritis) 714.30
Still-Felty (rheumatoid arthritis with
  splenomegaly and leukopenia) 714.1
Stilling-Türk-Duane (ocular retraction
  syndrome) 378.71
Stojano's (subcostal) 098.86
Stokes (-Adams) (syncope with heart block)
  426.9
Stokvis-Talma (enterogenous cyanosis) 289.7
stone heart (*see also* Failure, ventricular, left)
  428.1
straight-back 756.19
stroke (*see also* Disease, cerebrovascular, acute)
  436
  little 435.9
Sturge-Kalischer-Weber (encephalotrigeminal
  angiomatosis) 759.6
Sturge-Weber (-Dimitri) (encephalocutaneous
  angiomatosis) 759.6
subclavian-carotid obstruction (chronic) 446.7
subclavian steal 435.2
subcoracoid-pectoralis minor 447.8
subcostal 098.86
  nerve compression 354.8
subperiosteal hematoma 267
subphrenic interposition 751.4
sudden infant death (SIDS) 798.0
Sudeck's 733.7
Sudeck-Leriche 733.7
superior
  cerebellar artery (*see also* Disease,
    cerebrovascular, acute) 436
  mesenteric artery 557.1
  pulmonary sulcus (tumor) (M8010/3) 162.3
  semi-circular canal dehiscence 386.8
  vena cava 459.2
suprarenal cortical 255.3
supraspinatus 726.10
Susac 348.39
swallowed blood 777.3
sweat retention 705.1
Sweet's (acute febrile neutrophilic dermatosis)
  695.89
Swyer-James (unilateral hyperlucent lung) 492.8

Syndrome—*continued*

Swyer's (XY pure gonadal dysgenesis) 752.7
Symonds' 348.2
sympathetic
    cervical paralysis 337.09
    pelvic 625.5
syndactylic oxycephaly 755.55
syphilitic-cardiovascular 093.89
systemic
    fibrosclerosing 710.8
    inflammatory response (SIRS) 995.90
      due to
        infectious process 995.91
          with acute organ dysfunction 995.92
        non-infectious process 995.93
          with acute organ dysfunction 995.94
systolic click (-murmur) 785.2
Tabagism 305.1
tachycardia-bradycardia 427.81
Takayasu (-Onishi) (pulseless disease) 446.7
Takotsubo 429.83
Tapia's 352.6
tarsal tunnel 355.5
Taussig-Bing (transposition, aorta and
    overriding pulmonary artery) 745.11
Taybi's (otopalatodigital) 759.89
Taylor's 625.5
teething 520.7
tegmental 344.89
telangiectasis-pigmentation-cataract 757.33
temporal 383.02
    lobectomy behavior 310.0
temporomandibular joint-pain-dysfunction
    [TMJ] NEC 524.60
    specified NEC 524.69
Terry's (*see also* Retinopathy of prematurity)
    362.21
testicular feminization 259.51
testis, nonvirilizing 257.8
tethered (spinal) cord 742.59
thalamic 338.0
Thibierge-Weissenbach (cutaneous systemic
    sclerosis) 710.1
Thiele 724.6
thoracic outlet (compression) 353.0
thoracogenous rheumatic (hypertrophic
    pulmonary osteoarthropathy) 731.2
Thorn's (*see also* Disease, renal) 593.9
Thorson-Biörck (malignant carcinoid) 259.2
thrombopenia-hemangioma 287.39
thyroid-adrenocortical insufficiency 258.1
Tietze's 733.6
time-zone (rapid) 327.35
Tobias' (carcinoma, pulmonary apex)
    (M8010/3) 162.3
toilet seat 926.0
Tolosa-Hunt 378.55
Toni-Fanconi (cystinosis) 270.0
Touraine's (hereditary osteo-onychodysplasia)
    756.89
Touraine-Solente-Golé (acropachyderma)
    757.39
toxic
    oil 710.5
    shock 040.82
transfusion
    fetal-maternal 772.0
    twin
      donor (infant) 772.0
      recipient (infant) 776.4
transient left ventricular apical ballooning 429.83

Syndrome—*continued*

Treacher Collins' (incomplete mandibulofacial
    dysostosis) 756.0
trigeminal plate 259.8
triple X female 758.81
trisomy NEC 758.5
    13 or D_1 758.1
    16-18 or E 758.2
    18 or E_3 758.2
    20 758.5
    21 or G (mongolism) 758.0
    22 or G (mongolism) 758.0
    G 758.0
Troisier-Hanot-Chauffard (bronze diabetes) 275.01
tropical wet feet 991.4
Trousseau's (thrombophlebitis migrans visceral
    cancer) 453.1
tumor lysis (following antineoplastic drug
    therapy) (spontaneous) 277.88
Türk's (ocular retraction syndrome) 378.71
Turner's 758.6
Turner-Varny 758.6
Twiddler's (due to)
    automatic implantable defibrillator 996.04
    pacemaker 996.01
twin-to-twin transfusion 762.3
    recipient twin 776.4
Uehlinger's (acropachyderma) 757.39
Ullrich (-Bonnevie) (-Turner) 758.6
Ullrich-Feichtiger 759.89
underwater blast injury (abdominal) (*see also*
    Injury, internal, abdomen) 868.00
universal joint, cervix 620.6
Unverricht (-Lundborg) 345.1
Unverricht-Wagner (dermatomyositis) 710.3
upward gaze 378.81
Urbach-Oppenheim (necrobiosis lipoidica
    diabeticorum) 250.8 *[709.3]*
    due to secondary diabetes 249.8 *[709.3]*
Urbach-Wiethe (lipoid proteinosis) 272.8
uremia, chronic 585.9
urethral 597.81
urethro-oculoarticular 099.3
urethro-oculosynovial 099.3
urohepatic 572.4
uveocutaneous 364.24
uveomeningeal, uveomeningitis 363.22
vagohypoglossal 352.6
vagovagal 780.2
van Buchem's (hyperostosis corticalis) 733.3
van der Hoeve's (brittle bones and blue sclera,
    deafness) 756.51
van der Hoeve-Halbertsma-Waardenburg
    (ptosis-epicanthus) 270.2
van der Hoeve-Waardenburg-Gualdi
    (ptosis-epicanthus) 270.2
van Neck-Odelberg (juvenile osteochondrosis)
    732.1
vanishing twin 651.33
vascular splanchnic 557.0
vasomotor 443.9
vasovagal 780.2
VATER 759.89
Velo-cardio-facial 758.32
vena cava (inferior) (superior) (obstruction)
    459.2
Verbiest's (claudicatio intermittens spinalis)
    435.1
Vernet's 352.6

Synovioma (M9040/3)—*see also* Neoplasm,
    connective tissue, malignant
  benign (M9040/3)—*see* Neoplasm, connective
    tissue, benign
Synoviosarcoma (M9040/3)—*see* Neoplasm,
    connective tissue, malignant
Synovitis (*see also* Tenosynovitis) 727.00
  chronic crepitant, wrist 727.2
  due to crystals—*see* Arthritis, due to crystals
  gonococcal 098.51
  gouty 274.00
  specified NEC 727.09
  syphilitic 095.7
    congenital 090.0
  traumatic, current—*see* Sprain, by site
  tuberculous—*see* Tuberculosis, synovitis
  villonodular 719.20
    ankle 719.27
    elbow 719.22
    foot 719.27
    hand 719.24
    hip 719.25
    knee 719.26
    multiple sites 719.29
    pelvic region 719.25
    shoulder (region) 719.21
    specified site NEC 719.28
    wrist 719.23
Syphilide 091.3
  congenital 090.0
  newborn 090.0
  tubercular 095.8
    congenital 090.0
Syphilis, syphilitic (acquired) 097.9
  with lung involvement 095.1
  abdomen (late) 095.2
  acoustic nerve 094.86
  adenopathy (secondary) 091.4
  adrenal (gland) 095.8
    with cortical hypofunction 095.8
  age under 2 years NEC (*see also* Syphilis,
    congenital) 090.9
    acquired 097.9
  alopecia (secondary) 091.82
  anemia 095.8
  aneurysm (artery) (ruptured) 093.89
    aorta 093.0
    central nervous system 094.89
    congenital 090.5
  anus 095.8
    primary 091.1
    secondary 091.3
  aorta, aortic (arch) (abdominal) (insufficiency)
    (pulmonary) (regurgitation) (stenosis)
    (thoracic) 093.89
    aneurysm 093.0
  arachnoid (adhesive) 094.2
  artery 093.89
    cerebral 094.89
    spinal 094.89
  arthropathy (neurogenic) (tabetic) 094.0 *[713.5]*
  asymptomatic—*see* Syphilis, latent
  ataxia, locomotor (progressive) 094.0
  atrophoderma maculatum 091.3
  auricular fibrillation 093.89
  Bell's palsy 094.89
  bladder 095.8
  bone 095.5
    secondary 091.61
  brain 094.89
  breast 095.8

Syphilis, syphilitic—*continued*
  bronchus 095.8
  bubo 091.0
  bulbar palsy 094.89
  bursa (late) 095.7
  cardiac decompensation 093.89
  cardiovascular (early) (late) (primary)
    (secondary) (tertiary) 093.9
    specified type and site NEC 093.89
    causing death under 2 years of age (*see also*
      Syphilis, congenital) 090.9
      stated to be acquired NEC 097.9
  central nervous system (any site) (early) (late)
    (latent) (primary) (recurrent) (relapse)
    (secondary) (tertiary) 094.9
    with
      ataxia 094.0
      paralysis, general 094.1
        juvenile 090.40
      paresis (general) 094.1
        juvenile 090.40
      tabes (dorsalis) 094.0
        juvenile 090.40
      taboparesis 094.1
        juvenile 090.40
      aneurysm (ruptured) 094.87
    congenital 090.40
    juvenile 090.40
    remission in (sustained) 094.9
    serology doubtful, negative, or positive 094.9
    specified nature or site NEC 094.89
    vascular 094.89
  cerebral 094.89
    meningovascular 094.2
    nerves 094.89
    sclerosis 094.89
    thrombosis 094.89
  cerebrospinal 094.89
    tabetic 094.0
  cerebrovascular 094.89
  cervix 095.8
  chancre (multiple) 091.0
    extragenital 091.2
    Rollet's 091.0
  Charcot's joint 094.0 *[713.5]*
  choked disc 094.89 *[377.00]*
  chorioretinitis 091.51
    congenital 090.0 *[363.13]*
    late 094.83
  choroiditis 091.51
    congenital 090.0 *[363.13]*
    late 094.83
    prenatal 090.0 *[363.13]*
  choroidoretinitis (secondary) 091.51
    congenital 090.0 *[363.13]*
    late 094.83
  ciliary body (secondary) 091.52
    late 095.8 *[364.11]*
  colon (late) 095.8
  combined sclerosis 094.89
  complicating pregnancy, childbirth or
    puerperium 647.0
    affecting fetus or newborn 760.2
  condyloma (latum) 091.3

Syphilis, syphilitic—*continued*
congenital 090.9
  with
    encephalitis 090.41
    paresis (general) 090.40
    tabes (dorsalis) 090.40
    taboparesis 090.40
  chorioretinitis, choroiditis 090.0 *[363.13]*
  early or less than 2 years after birth NEC 090.2
    with manifestations 090.0
    latent (without manifestations) 090.1
      negative spinal fluid test 090.1
      serology, positive 090.1
    symptomatic 090.0
  interstitial keratitis 090.3
  juvenile neurosyphilis 090.40
  late or 2 years or more after birth NEC 090.7
    chorioretinitis, choroiditis 090.5 *[363.13]*
    interstitial keratitis 090.3
    juvenile neurosyphilis NEC 090.40
    latent (without manifestations) 090.6
      negative spinal fluid test 090.6
      serology, positive 090.6
    symptomatic or with manifestations NEC
      090.5
    interstitial keratitis 090.3
conjugal 097.9
  tabes 094.0
conjunctiva 095.8 *[372.10]*
contact V01.6
cord, bladder 094.0
cornea, late 095.8 *[370.59]*
coronary (artery) 093.89
  sclerosis 093.89
coryza 095.8
  congenital 090.0
cranial nerve 094.89
cutaneous—*see* Syphilis, skin
dacryocystitis 095.8
degeneration, spinal cord 094.89
d'emblée 095.8
dementia 094.1
  paralytica 094.1
    juvenilis 090.40
destruction of bone 095.5
dilatation, aorta 093.0
due to blood transfusion 097.9
dura mater 094.89
ear 095.8
  inner 095.8
    nerve (eighth) 094.86
    neurorecurrence 094.86
early NEC 091.0
  cardiovascular 093.9
  central nervous system 094.9
    paresis 094.1
    tabes 094.0
  latent (without manifestations) (less than 2
    years after infection) 092.9
    negative spinal fluid test 092.9
    serological relapse following treatment 092.0
    serology positive 092.9
  paresis 094.1
  relapse (treated, untreated) 091.7
  skin 091.3
  symptomatic NEC 091.89
    extragenital chancre 091.2
    primary, except extragenital chancre 091.0
    secondary (*see also* Syphilis, secondary) 091.3
      relapse (treated, untreated) 091.7
  tabes 094.0
  ulcer 091.3

Syphilis, syphilitic—*continued*
eighth nerve 094.86
endemic, nonvenereal 104.0
endocarditis 093.20
  aortic 093.22
  mitral 093.21
  pulmonary 093.24
  tricuspid 093.23
epididymis (late) 095.8
epiglottis 095.8
epiphysitis (congenital) 090.0
esophagus 095.8
Eustachian tube 095.8
exposure to V01.6
eye 095.8 *[363.13]*
  neuromuscular mechanism 094.85
eyelid 095.8 *[373.5]*
  with gumma 095.8 *[373.5]*
  ptosis 094.89
fallopian tube 095.8
fracture 095.5
gallbladder (late) 095.8
gastric 095.8
  crisis 094.0
  polyposis 095.8
general 097.9
  paralysis 094.1
    juvenile 090.40
genital (primary) 091.0
glaucoma 095.8
gumma (late) NEC 095.9
  cardiovascular system 093.9
  central nervous system 094.9
  congenital 090.5
  heart or artery 093.89
heart 093.89
  block 093.89
  decompensation 093.89
  disease 093.89
  failure 093.89
  valve (*see also* Syphilis, endocarditis) 093.20
hemianesthesia 094.89
hemianopsia 095.8
hemiparesis 094.89
hemiplegia 094.89
hepatic artery 093.89
hepatitis 095.3
hepatomegaly 095.3
  congenital 090.0
hereditaria tarda (*see also* Syphilis, congenital,
  late) 090.7
hereditary (*see also* Syphilis, congenital) 090.9
  interstitial keratitis 090.3
Hutchinson's teeth 090.5
hyalitis 095.8
inactive—*see* Syphilis, latent
infantum NEC (*see also* Syphilis, congenital)
  090.9
inherited—*see* Syphilis, congenital
internal ear 095.8
intestine (late) 095.8
iris, iritis (secondary) 091.52
  late 095.8 *[364.11]*
joint (late) 095.8
keratitis (congenital) (early) (interstitial) (late)
  (parenchymatous) (punctata profunda) 090.3
kidney 095.4
lacrimal apparatus 095.8
laryngeal paralysis 095.8
larynx 095.8

Syphilis, syphilitic—*continued*
late 097.0
  cardiovascular 093.9
  central nervous system 094.9
  latent or 2 years or more after infection
    (without manifestations) 096
    negative spinal fluid test 096
    serology positive 096
  paresis 094.1
  specified site NEC 095.8
  symptomatic or with symptoms 095.9
  tabes 094.0
latent 097.1
  central nervous system 094.9
  date of infection unspecified 097.1
  early or less than 2 years after infection 092.9
  late or 2 years or more after infection 096
  serology
    doubtful
      follow-up of latent syphilis 097.1
        central nervous system 094.9
        date of infection unspecified 097.1
        early or less than 2 years after infection
          092.9
        late or 2 years or more after infection
          096
      positive, only finding 097.1
        date of infection unspecified 097.1
        early or less than 2 years after infection
          097.1
        late or 2 years or more after infection 097.1
lens 095.8
leukoderma 091.3
  late 095.8
lienis 095.8
lip 091.3
  chancre 091.2
  late 095.8
  primary 091.2
Lissauer's paralysis 094.1
liver 095.3
  secondary 091.62
locomotor ataxia 094.0
lung 095.1
lymphadenitis (secondary) 091.4
lymph gland (early) (secondary) 091.4
  late 095.8
macular atrophy of skin 091.3
  striated 095.8
maternal, affecting fetus or newborn 760.2
  manifest syphilis in newborn—*see* Syphilis,
    congenital
mediastinum (late) 095.8
meninges (adhesive) (basilar) (brain) (spinal
    cord) 094.2
meningitis 094.2
  acute 091.81
  congenital 090.42
meningoencephalitis 094.2
meningovascular 094.2
  congenital 090.49
mesarteritis 093.89
  brain 094.89
  spine 094.89
middle ear 095.8
mitral stenosis 093.21
monoplegia 094.89
mouth (secondary) 091.3
  late 095.8
mucocutaneous 091.3
  late 095.8

Syphilis, syphilitic—*continued*
mucous
  membrane 091.3
    late 095.8
  patches 091.3
    congenital 090.0
mulberry molars 090.5
muscle 095.6
myocardium 093.82
myositis 095.6
nasal sinus 095.8
neonatorum NEC (*see also* Syphilis, congenital)
  090.9
nerve palsy (any cranial nerve) 094.89
nervous system, central 094.9
neuritis 095.8
  acoustic nerve 094.86
neurorecidive of retina 094.83
neuroretinitis 094.85
newborn (*see also* Syphilis, congenital) 090.9
nodular superficial 095.8
nonvenereal, endemic 104.0
nose 095.8
  saddle back deformity 090.5
  septum 095.8
    perforated 095.8
occlusive arterial disease 093.89
ophthalmic 095.8 *[363.13]*
ophthalmoplegia 094.89
optic nerve (atrophy) (neuritis) (papilla) 094.84
orbit (late) 095.8
orchitis 095.8
organic 097.9
osseous (late) 095.5
osteochondritis (congenital) 090.0
osteoporosis 095.5
ovary 095.8
oviduct 095.8
palate 095.8
  gumma 095.8
  perforated 090.5
pancreas (late) 095.8
pancreatitis 095.8
paralysis 094.89
  general 094.1
  juvenile 090.40
paraplegia 094.89
paresis (general) 094.1
  juvenile 090.40
paresthesia 094.89
Parkinson's disease or syndrome 094.82
paroxysmal tachycardia 093.89
pemphigus (congenital) 090.0
penis 091.0
  chancre 091.0
  late 095.8
pericardium 093.81
perichondritis, larynx 095.8
periosteum 095.5
  congenital 090.0
  early 091.61
  secondary 091.61
peripheral nerve 095.8
petrous bone (late) 095.5
pharynx 095.8
  secondary 091.3
pituitary (gland) 095.8
placenta 095.8
pleura (late) 095.8
pneumonia, white 090.0
pontine (lesion) 094.89

Syphilis, syphilitic—*continued*
portal vein 093.89
primary NEC 091.2
anal 091.1
and secondary (*see also* Syphilis, secondary) 091.9
cardiovascular 093.9
central nervous system 094.9
extragenital chancre NEC 091.2
fingers 091.2
genital 091.0
lip 091.2
specified site NEC 091.2
tonsils 091.2
prostate 095.8
psychosis (intracranial gumma) 094.89
ptosis (eyelid) 094.89
pulmonary (late) 095.1
artery 093.89
pulmonum 095.1
pyelonephritis 095.4
recently acquired, symptomatic NEC 091.89
rectum 095.8
respiratory tract 095.8
retina
late 094.83
neurorecidive 094.83
retrobulbar neuritis 094.85
salpingitis 095.8
sclera (late) 095.0
sclerosis
cerebral 094.89
coronary 093.89
multiple 094.89
subacute 094.89
scotoma (central) 095.8
scrotum 095.8
secondary (and primary) 091.9
adenopathy 091.4
anus 091.3
bone 091.61
cardiovascular 093.9
central nervous system 094.9
chorioretinitis, choroiditis 091.51
hepatitis 091.62
liver 091.62
lymphadenitis 091.4
meningitis, acute 091.81
mouth 091.3
mucous membranes 091.3
periosteum 091.61
periostitis 091.61
pharynx 091.3
relapse (treated) (untreated) 091.7
skin 091.3
specified form NEC 091.89
tonsil 091.3
ulcer 091.3
viscera 091.69
vulva 091.3
seminal vesicle (late) 095.8
seronegative
with signs or symptoms—*see* Syphilis, by site and stage
seropositive
with signs or symptoms—*see* Syphilis, by site and stage
follow-up of latent syphilis—*see* Syphilis, latent
only finding—*see* Syphilis, latent
seventh nerve (paralysis) 094.89

Syphilis, syphilitic—*continued*
sinus 095.8
sinusitis 095.8
skeletal system 095.5
skin (early) (secondary) (with ulceration) 091.3
late or tertiary 095.8
small intestine 095.8
spastic spinal paralysis 094.0
spermatic cord (late) 095.8
spinal (cord) 094.89
with
paresis 094.1
tabes 094.0
spleen 095.8
splenomegaly 095.8
spondylitis 095.5
staphyloma 095.8
stigmata (congenital) 090.5
stomach 095.8
synovium (late) 095.7
tabes dorsalis (early) (late) 094.0
juvenile 090.40
tabetic type 094.0
juvenile 090.40
taboparesis 094.1
juvenile 090.40
tachycardia 093.89
tendon (late) 095.7
tertiary 097.0
with symptoms 095.8
cardiovascular 093.9
central nervous system 094.9
multiple NEC 095.8
specified site NEC 095.8
testis 095.8
thorax 095.8
throat 095.8
thymus (gland) 095.8
thyroid (late) 095.8
tongue 095.8
tonsil (lingual) 095.8
primary 091.2
secondary 091.3
trachea 095.8
tricuspid valve 093.23
tumor, brain 094.89
tunica vaginalis (late) 095.8
ulcer (any site) (early) (secondary) 091.3
late 095.9
perforating 095.9
foot 094.0
urethra (stricture) 095.8
urogenital 095.8
uterus 095.8
uveal tract (secondary) 091.50
late 095.8 *[363.13]*
uveitis (secondary) 091.50
late 095.8 *[363.13]*
uvula (late) 095.8
perforated 095.8
vagina 091.0
late 095.8
valvulitis NEC 093.20
vascular 093.89
brain or cerebral 094.89
vein 093.89
cerebral 094.89
ventriculi 095.8
vesicae urinariae 095.8
viscera (abdominal) 095.2
secondary 091.69

Syphilis, syphilitic—*continued*
  vitreous (hemorrhage) (opacities) 095.8
  vulva 091.0
    late 095.8
    secondary 091.3
Syphiloma 095.9
  cardiovascular system 093.9
  central nervous system 094.9
  circulatory system 093.9
  congenital 090.5
Syphilophobia 300.29
Syringadenoma (M8400/0)—*see also* Neoplasm,
    skin, benign
  papillary (M8406/0)—*see* Neoplasm, skin,
    benign
Syringobulbia 336.0
Syringocarcinoma (M8400/3)—*see* Neoplasm,
    skin, malignant
Syringocystadenoma (M8400/0)—*see also*
    Neoplasm, skin, benign
  papillary (M8406/0)—*see* Neoplasm, skin,
    benign
Syringocystoma (M8407/0)—*see* Neoplasm,
    skin, benign
Syringoma (M8407/0)—*see also* Neoplasm, skin,
    benign
  chondroid (M8940/0)—*see* Neoplasm, by site,
    benign
Syringomyelia 336.0
Syringomyelitis 323.9
  late effect—*see* category 326
Syringomyelocele (*see also* Spina bifida) 741.9
Syringopontia 336.0
System, systemic —*see also* condition
  disease, combined—*see* Degeneration,
    combined
  fibrosclerosing syndrome 710.8
  inflammatory response syndrome (SIRS) 995.90
    due to
      infectious process 995.91
        with acute organ dysfunction 995.92
      non-infectious process 995.93
        with acute organ dysfunction 995.94
  lupus erythematosus 710.0
    inhibitor 795.79

T

Tab —*see* Tag
Tabacism 989.8
Tabacosis 989.8
Tabardillo 080
  flea-borne 081.0
  louse-borne 080
Tabes, tabetic
  with
    central nervous system syphilis 094.0
    Charcot's joint 094.0 *[713.5]*
    cord bladder 094.0
    crisis, viscera (any) 094.0
    paralysis, general 094.1
    paresis (general) 094.1
    perforating ulcer 094.0
  arthropathy 094.0 *[713.5]*
  bladder 094.0
  bone 094.0
  cerebrospinal 094.0
  congenital 090.40
  conjugal 094.0
  dorsalis 094.0
    neurosyphilis 094.0
  early 094.0
  juvenile 090.40
  latent 094.0
  mesenterica (*see also* Tuberculosis) 014.8
  paralysis insane, general 094.1
  peripheral (nonsyphilitic) 799.89
  spasmodic 094.0
    not dorsal or dorsalis 343.9
  syphilis (cerebrospinal) 094.0
Taboparalysis 094.1
Taboparesis (remission) 094.1
  with
    Charcot's joint 094.1 *[713.5]*
    cord bladder 094.1
    perforating ulcer 094.1
  juvenile 090.40
Tache noir 923.20
Tachyalimentation 579.3
Tachyarrhythmia, tachyrhythmia —*see also*
  Tachycardia
  paroxysmal with sinus bradycardia 427.81
Tachycardia 785.0
  atrial 427.89
  auricular 427.89
  AV nodal re-entry (re-entrant) 427.89
  newborn 779.82
  nodal 427.89
    nonparoxysmal atrioventricular 426.89
  nonparoxysmal atrioventricular (nodal) 426.89
  nonsustained 427.2
  paroxysmal 427.2
    with sinus bradycardia 427.81
    atrial (PAT) 427.0
      psychogenic 316 *[427.0]*
    atrioventricular (AV) 427.0
      psychogenic 316 *[427.0]*
    essential 427.2
    junctional ectopic 427.0
    nodal 427.0
    psychogenic 316 *[427.2]*
      atrial 316 *[427.0]*
      supraventricular 316 *[427.0]*
      ventricular 316 *[427.1]*

Tachycardia—*continued*
  supraventricular 427.0
    psychogenic 316 *[427.0]*
  ventricular 427.1
    psychogenic 316 *[427.1]*
  postoperative 997.1
  psychogenic 306.2
  sick sinus 427.81
  sinoauricular 427.89
  sinus 427.89
  supraventricular 427.89
  sustained 427.2
    supraventricular 427.0
    ventricular 427.1
  ventricular (paroxysmal) 427.1
    psychogenic 316 *[427.1]*
Tachygastria 536.8
Tachypnea 786.06
  hysterical 300.11
  newborn (idiopathic) (transitory) 770.6
  psychogenic 306.1
  transitory, of newborn 770.6
TACO (transfusion associated circulatory
  overload) 276.61
Taenia (infection) (infestation) (*see also*
  Infestation, taenia) 123.3
  diminuta 123.6
  echinococcal infestation (*see also*
    Echinococcus) 122.9
  nana 123.6
  saginata infestation 123.2
  solium (intestinal form) 123.0
    larval form 123.1
Taeniasis (intestine) (*see also* Infestation, Taenia)
  123.3
  saginata 123.2
  solium 123.0
Taenzer's disease 757.4
Tag (hypertrophied skin) (infected) 701.9
  adenoid 474.8
  anus 455.9
  endocardial (*see also* Endocarditis) 424.90
  hemorrhoidal 455.9
  hymen 623.8
  perineal 624.8
  preauricular 744.1
  rectum 455.9
  sentinel 455.9
  skin 701.9
    accessory 757.39
    anus 455.9
    congenital 757.39
    preauricular 744.1
    rectum 455.9
  tonsil 474.8
  urethra, urethral 599.84
  vulva 624.8
Tahyna fever 062.5
Takayasu (-Onishi) disease or syndrome
  (pulseless disease) 446.7
Takotsubo syndrome 429.83
Talc granuloma 728.82
  in operation wound 998.7
Talcosis 502
Talipes (congenital) 754.70
  acquired NEC 736.79
    planus 734

Talipes—*continued*
  asymmetric 754.79
    acquired 736.79
  calcaneovalgus 754.62
    acquired 736.76
  calcaneovarus 754.59
    acquired 736.76
  calcaneus 754.79
    acquired 736.76
  cavovarus 754.59
    acquired 736.75
  cavus 754.71
    acquired 736.73
  equinovalgus 754.69
    acquired 736.72
  equinovarus 754.51
    acquired 736.71
  equinus 754.79
    acquired, NEC 736.72
  percavus 754.71
    acquired 736.73
  planovalgus 754.69
    acquired 736.79
  planus (acquired) (any degree) 734
    congenital 754.61
    due to rickets 268.1
  valgus 754.60
    acquired 736.79
  varus 754.50
    acquired 736.79
Talma's disease 728.85
Talon noir 924.20
  hand 923.20
  heel 924.20
  toe 924.3
Tamponade heart (Rose's) (*see also*
    Pericarditis) 423.3
Tanapox 059.21
Tangier disease (familial high-density
    lipoprotein deficiency) 272.5
Tank ear 380.12
Tantrum (childhood) (*see also* Disturbance,
    conduct) 312.1
Tapeworm (infection) (infestation) (*see also*
    Infestation, tapeworm) 123.9
Tapia's syndrome 352.6
Tarantism 297.8
Target-oval cell anemia 285.8
  with thalassemia—*see* Thalassemia
Tarlov's cyst 355.9
Tarral-Besnier disease (pityriasis rubra pilaris)
    696.4
Tarsalgia 729.2
Tarsal tunnel syndrome 355.5
Tarsitis (eyelid) 373.00
  syphilitic 095.8 *[373.00]*
  tuberculous (*see also* Tuberculosis) 017.0 *[373.4]*
Tartar (teeth) 523.6
Tattoo (mark) 709.09
Taurodontism 520.2
Taussig-Bing defect, heart, or syndrome
    (transposition, aorta and overriding pulmonary
    artery) 745.11
Tay's choroiditis 363.41
Tay-Sachs
  amaurotic familial idiocy 330.1
  disease 330.1
Taybi's syndrome (otopalatodigital) 759.89
Taylor's
  disease (diffuse idiopathic cutaneous atrophy) 701.8
  syndrome 625.5

TBI (traumatic brain injury) (see also Injury,
    intracranial) 854.0
  with skull fracture —see Fracture, skull, by site
Tear, torn (traumatic)—*see also* Wound, open,
    by site
  annular fibrosis 722.51
  anus, anal (sphincter) 863.89
    with open wound in cavity 863.99
    complicating delivery (healed) (old) 654.8
      with mucosa 664.3
      not associated with third-degree perineal
        laceration 664.6
    nontraumatic, nonpuerperal (healed) (old)
      569.43
  articular cartilage, old (*see also* Disorder,
    cartilage, articular) 718.0
  bladder
    with
      abortion—*see* Abortion, by type, with
        damage to pelvic organs
      ectopic pregnancy (*see also* categories
        633.0-633.9) 639.2
      molar pregnancy (*see also* categories
        630-632) 639.2
    following
      abortion 639.2
      ectopic or molar pregnancy 639.2
    obstetrical trauma 665.5
  bowel
    with
      abortion—*see* Abortion, by type, with
        damage to pelvic organs
      ectopic pregnancy (*see also* categories
        633.0-633.9) 639.2
      molar pregnancy (*see also* categories
        630-632) 639.2
    following
      abortion 639.2
      ectopic or molar pregnancy 639.2
    obstetrical trauma 665.5
  broad ligament
    with
      abortion—*see* Abortion, by type, with
        damage to pelvic organs
      ectopic pregnancy (*see also* categories
        633.0-633.9) 639.2
      molar pregnancy (*see also* categories
        630-632) 639.2
    following
      abortion 639.2
      ectopic or molar pregnancy 639.2
    obstetrical trauma 665.6
  bucket handle (knee) (meniscus)—*see* Tear,
    meniscus
  capsule
    joint—*see* Sprain, by site
    spleen—*see* Laceration, spleen, capsule
  cartilage—*see also* Sprain, by site
    articular, old (*see also* Disorder, cartilage,
      articular) 718.0
    knee—*see* Tear, meniscus
    semilunar (knee) (current injury)—*see* Tear,
      meniscus
  cervix
    with
      abortion—*see* Abortion, by type, with
        damage to pelvic organs
      ectopic pregnancy (*see also* categories
        633.0-633.9) 639.2
      molar pregnancy (*see also* categories
        630-632) 639.2

Tear, torn—*continued*
cervix—*continued*
  following
    abortion 639.2
    ectopic or molar pregnancy 639.2
    obstetrical trauma (current) 665.3
  old 622.3
dural 349.31
  accidental puncture or laceration during a
    procedure 349.31
  incidental (inadvertent) 349.31
  nontraumatic NEC 349.39
internal organ (abdomen, chest, or pelvis)—*see*
    Injury, internal, by site
ligament—*see also* Sprain, by site
  with open wound—*see* Wound, open by site
meniscus (knee) (current injury) 836.2
  bucket handle 836.0
    old 717.0
  lateral 836.1
    anterior horn 836.1
      old 717.42
    bucket handle 836.1
      old 717.41
    old 717.40
    posterior horn 836.1
      old 717.43
    specified site NEC 836.1
      old 717.49
  medial 836.0
    anterior horn 836.0
      old 717.1
    bucket handle 836.0
      old 717.0
    old 717.3
    posterior horn 836.0
      old 717.2
  old NEC 717.5
  site other than knee—*see* Sprain, by site
muscle—*see also* Sprain, by site
  with open wound—*see* Wound, open by site
pelvic
  floor, complicating delivery 664.1
  organ NEC
    with
      abortion—*see* Abortion, by type, with
        damage to pelvic organs
      ectopic pregnancy (*see also* categories
        633.0-633.9) 639.2
      molar pregnancy (*see also* categories
        630-632) 639.2
    following
      abortion 639.2
      ectopic or molar pregnancy 639.2
      obstetrical trauma 665.5
perineum—*see also* Laceration, perineum
  obstetrical trauma 665.5
periurethral tissue
  with
    abortion—*see* Abortion, by type, with
      damage to pelvic organs
    ectopic pregnancy (*see also* categories
      633.0-633.9) 639.2
    molar pregnancy (*see also* categories
      630-632) 639.2
  following
    abortion 639.2
    ectopic or molar pregnancy 639.2
    obstetrical trauma 664.8
rectovaginal septum—*see* Laceration,
    rectovaginal septum

Tear, torn—*continued*
retina, retinal (recent) (with detachment) 361.00
  without detachment 361.30
  dialysis (juvenile) (with detachment) 361.04
  giant (with detachment) 361.03
  horseshoe (without detachment) 361.32
  multiple (with detachment) 361.02
    without detachment 361.33
  old
    delimited (partial) 361.06
    partial 361.06
    total or subtotal 361.07
  partial (without detachment)
    giant 361.03
    multiple defects 361.02
    old (delimited) 361.06
    single defect 361.01
  round hole (without detachment) 361.31
  single defect (with detachment) 361.01
  total or subtotal (recent) 361.05
    old 361.07
rotator cuff (traumatic) 840.4
  current injury 840.4
  degenerative 726.10
  nontraumatic (complete) 727.61
    partial 726.13
semilunar cartilage, knee (*see also* Tear,
    meniscus) 836.2
  old 717.5
tendon—*see also* Sprain, by site
  with open wound—*see* Wound, open by site
tentorial, at birth 767.0
umbilical cord
  affecting fetus or newborn 772.0
  complicating delivery 663.8
urethra
  with
    abortion—*see* Abortion, by type, with
      damage to pelvic organs
    ectopic pregnancy (*see also* categories
      633.0-633.9) 639.2
    molar pregnancy (*see also* categories
      630-632) 639.2
  following
    abortion 639.2
    ectopic or molar pregnancy 639.2
    obstetrical trauma 665.5
uterus—*see* Injury, internal, uterus
vagina—*see* Laceration, vagina
vessel, from catheter 998.2
vulva, complicating delivery 664.0
Tear stone 375.57
Teeth, tooth —*see also* condition
  grinding 306.8
  prenatal 520.6
Teething 520.7
  syndrome 520.7
Tegmental syndrome 344.89
Telangiectasia, telangiectasis (verrucous) 448.9
  ataxic (cerebellar) 334.8
  familial 448.0
  hemorrhagic, hereditary (congenital) (senile) 448.0
  hereditary hemorrhagic 448.0
  retina 362.15
  spider 448.1
Telecanthus (congenital) 743.63
Telescoped bowel or intestine (*see also*
    Intussusception) 560.0
Teletherapy, adverse effect NEC 990
Telogen effluvium 704.02

Temperature
  body, high (of unknown origin) (*see also*
    Pyrexia) 780.60
  cold, trauma from 991.9
    newborn 778.2
    specified effect NEC 991.8
  high
    body (of unknown origin) (*see also* Pyrexia)
      780.60
    trauma from—*see* Heat
Temper tantrum (childhood) (*see also*
    Disturbance, conduct) 312.1
Temple —*see* condition
Temporal —*see also* condition
  lobe syndrome 310.0
**Temporomandibular joint-pain-dysfunction
    syndrome** 524.60
Temporosphenoidal —*see* condition
Tendency
  bleeding (*see also* Defect, coagulation) 286.9
  homosexual, ego-dystonic 302.0
  paranoid 301.0
  suicide 300.9
Tenderness
  abdominal (generalized) (localized) 789.6
  rebound 789.6
  skin 782.0
Tendinitis, tendonitis (*see also* Tenosynovitis)
    726.90
  Achilles 726.71
  adhesive 726.90
    shoulder 726.0
  calcific 727.82
    shoulder 726.11
  gluteal 726.5
  patellar 726.64
  peroneal 726.79
  pes anserinus 726.61
  psoas 726.5
  tibialis (anterior) (posterior) 726.72
  trochanteric 726.5
Tendon —*see* condition
Tendosynovitis —*see* Tenosynovitis
Tendovaginitis —*see* Tenosynovitis
Tenesmus 787.99
  rectal 787.99
  vesical 788.99
Tenia —*see* Taenia
Teniasis —*see* Taeniasis
Tennis elbow 726.32
Tenonitis —*see also* Tenosynovitis
  eye (capsule) 376.04
Tenontosynovitis —*see* Tenosynovitis
Tenontothecitis —*see* Tenosynovitis
Tenophyte 727.9
Tenosynovitis (*see also* Synovitis) 727.00
  adhesive 726.90
    shoulder 726.0
  ankle 727.06
  bicipital (calcifying) 726.12
  buttock 727.09
  due to crystals—*see* Arthritis, due to crystals
  elbow 727.09
  finger 727.05
  foot 727.06
  gonococcal 098.51
  hand 727.05
  hip 727.09
  knee 727.09
  radial styloid 727.04

Tenosynovitis—*continued*
  shoulder 726.10
    adhesive 726.0
  specified NEC 727.09
  spine 720.1
  supraspinatus 726.10
  toe 727.06
  tuberculous—*see* Tuberculosis, tenosynovitis
  wrist 727.05
Tenovaginitis —*see* Tenosynovitis
Tension
  arterial, high (*see also* Hypertension) 401.9
    without diagnosis of hypertension 796.2
  headache 307.81
  intraocular (elevated) 365.00
  nervous 799.21
  ocular (elevated) 365.00
  pneumothorax 512.0
    iatrogenic 512.1
    postoperative 512.1
    spontaneous 512.0
  premenstrual 625.4
  state 300.9
Tentorium —*see* condition
Teratencephalus 759.89
Teratism 759.7
Teratoblastoma (malignant) (M9080/3)—*see*
    Neoplasm, by site, malignant
Teratocarcinoma (M9081/3)—*see also*
    Neoplasm, by site, malignant
  liver 155.0
Teratoma (solid) (M9080/1)—*see also*
    Neoplasm, by site, uncertain behavior
  adult (cystic) (M9080/0)—*see* Neoplasm, by
    site, benign
  and embryonal carcinoma, mixed
    (M9081/3)—*see* Neoplasm, by site,
    malignant
  benign (M9080/0)—*see* Neoplasm, by site,
    benign
  combined with choriocarcinoma
    (M9101/3)—*see* Neoplasm, by site,
    malignant
  cystic (adult) (M9080/0)—*see* Neoplasm, by
    site, benign
  differentiated type (M9080/0)—*see* Neoplasm,
    by site, benign
  embryonal (M9080/3)—*see also* Neoplasm, by
    site, malignant
    liver 155.0
  fetal
    sacral, causing fetopelvic disproportion 653.7
  immature (M9080/3)—*see* Neoplasm, by site,
    malignant
  liver (M9080/3) 155.0
    adult, benign, cystic, differentiated type or
      mature (M9080/0) 211.5
  malignant (M9080/3)—*see also* Neoplasm, by
    site, malignant
    anaplastic type (M9082/3)—*see* Neoplasm, by
      site, malignant
    intermediate type (M9083/3)—*see* Neoplasm,
      by site, malignant
    liver (M9080/3) 155.0
    trophoblastic (M9102/3)
      specified site—*see* Neoplasm, by site,
        malignant
      unspecified site 186.9
    undifferentiated type (M9082/3)—*see*
      Neoplasm, by site, malignant

Teratoma—*continued*
  mature (M9080/0)—*see* Neoplasm, by site, benign
    malignant (M9080/3) —see Neoplasm, by site,
      malignant
  ovary (M9080/0) 220
    embryonal, immature, or malignant (M9080/3)
      183.0
  suprasellar (M9080/3)—*see* Neoplasm, by site,
    malignant
  testis (M9080/3) 186.9
    adult, benign, cystic, differentiated type or
      mature (M9080/0) 222.0
    undescended 186.0
Terminal care V66.7
Termination
  anomalous—*see also* Malposition, congenital
    portal vein 747.49
    right pulmonary vein 747.42
  pregnancy (legal) (therapeutic) (*see* Abortion,
    legal) 635.9
    fetus NEC 779.6
    illegal (*see also* Abortion, illegal) 636.9
Ternidens diminutus infestation 127.7
Terrors, night (child) 307.46
Terry's syndrome (*see also* Retinopathy of
  prematurity) 362.21
Tertiary —*see* condition
Tessellated fundus, retina (tigroid) 362.89
Test(s)
  adequacy
    hemodialysis V56.31
    peritoneal dialysis V56.32
  AIDS virus V72.69
  allergen V72.7
  bacterial disease NEC (*see also* Screening, by
    name of disease) V74.9
  basal metabolic rate V72.69
  blood
    alcohol V70.4
    drug V70.4
      for therapeutic drug monitoring V58.83
      for routine general physical examination
        V72.62
      prior to treatment or procedure V72.63
    typing V72.86
      Rh typing V72.86
  developmental, infant or child V20.2
  Dick V74.8
  fertility V26.21
  genetic
    female V26.32
    for genetic disease carrier status
      female V26.31
      male V26.34
    male V26.39
  hearing V72.19
    following failed hearing screening V72.11
    routine, for infant and child V20.2
  HIV V72.69
  human immunodeficiency virus V72.69
  immunity status V72.61
  Kveim V82.89
  laboratory V72.60
    for medicolegal reason V70.4
    ordered as part of a routine general medical
      examination V72.62
    pre-operative V72.63
    pre-procedural V72.63
    specified NEC V72.69
  male partner of female with recurrent pregnancy
    loss V26.35

Test(s)—*continued*
  Mantoux (for tuberculosis) V74.1
  mycotic organism V75.4
  nuchal translucency V28.89
  parasitic agent NEC V75.8
  paternity V70.4
  peritoneal equilibration V56.32
  pregnancy
    negative result V72.41
    positive result V72.42
      first pregnancy V72.42
    unconfirmed V72.40
  preoperative V72.84
    cardiovascular V72.81
    respiratory V72.82
    specified NEC V72.83
  procreative management NEC V26.29
    genetic disease carrier status
      female V26.31
      male V26.34
  Rh typing V72.86
  sarcoidosis V82.89
  Schick V74.3
  Schultz-Charlton V74.8
  skin, diagnostic
    allergy V72.7
    bacterial agent NEC (*see also* Screening, by
      name of disease) V74.9
    Dick V74.8
    hypersensitivity V72.7
    Kveim V82.89
    Mantoux V74.1
    mycotic organism V75.4
    parasitic agent NEC V75.8
    sarcoidosis V82.89
    Schick V74.3
    Schultz-Charlton V74.8
    tuberculin V74.1
  specified type NEC V72.85
  tuberculin V74.1
  vision V72.0
    routine, for infant and child V20.2
  Wassermann
    positive (*see also* Serology for syphilis,
      positive) 097.1
    false 795.6
Testicle, testicular, testis —*see also* condition
  feminization (syndrome) 259.51
Tetanus, tetanic (cephalic) (convulsions) 037
  with
    abortion—*see* Abortion, by type, with sepsis
    ectopic pregnancy (*see also* categories
      633.0-633.9) 639.0
    molar pregnancy (*see* categories 630-632) 639.0
  following
    abortion 639.0
    ectopic or molar pregnancy 639.0
  inoculation V03.7
    reaction (due to serum)—*see* Complications,
      vaccination
  neonatorum 771.3
  puerperal, postpartum, childbirth 670.8
Tetany, tetanic 781.7
  alkalosis 276.3
  associated with rickets 268.0
  convulsions 781.7
    hysterical 300.11
  functional (hysterical) 300.11
  hyperkinetic 781.7
    hysterical 300.11

Tetany, tetanic—*continued*
 hyperpnea 786.01
  hysterical 300.11
  psychogenic 306.1
 hyperventilation 786.01
  hysterical 300.11
  psychogenic 306.1
 hypocalcemic, neonatal 775.4
 hysterical 300.11
 neonatal 775.4
 parathyroid (gland) 252.1
 parathyroprival 252.1
 postoperative 252.1
 postthyroidectomy 252.1
 pseudotetany 781.7
  hysterical 300.11
 psychogenic 306.1
 specified as conversion reaction 300.11
Tetralogy of Fallot 745.2
Tetraplegia —*see* Quadriplegia
Thailand hemorrhagic fever 065.4
Thalassanemia 282.40
Thalassemia (disease) 282.40
 with other hemoglobinopathy 282.49
 alpha (major) (severe) (triple gene defect)
   282.43
  silent carrier 282.46
 beta (homozygous) (major) (severe) 282.44
 delta-beta (homozygous) 282.45
 dominant 282.49
 Hb-S (without crisis) 282.41
  with
   crisis 282.42
   vaso-occlusive pain 282.42
 hemoglobin
  C (Hb-C) 282.49
  D (Hb-D) 282.49
  E (Hb-E) 282.49
  E-beta 282.47
  H (Hb-H) 282.49
  I (Hb-I) 282.49
 high fetal gene (see also Thalassemia) 282.40
 high fetal hemoglobin (see also Thalassemia)
   282.40
 intermedia 282.44
 major 282.44
 minor (alpha) (beta) 282.46
 mixed 282.49
 sickle-cell (without crisis) 282.41
  with
   crisis 282.42
   vaso-occlusive pain 282.42
 specified NEC 282.49
 trait (alpha) (beta) (delta-beta) 282.46
Thalassemic variants 282.49
Thaysen-Gee disease (nontropical sprue) 579.0
Thecoma (M8600/0) 220
 malignant (M8600/3) 183.0
Thelarche, precocious 259.1
Thelitis 611.0
 puerperal, postpartum 675.0
Therapeutic —*see* condition
Therapy V57.9
 blood transfusion, without reported diagnosis
   V58.2
 breathing V57.0
 chemotherapy, antineoplastic V58.11
  fluoride V07.31
  prophylactic NEC V07.39

Therapy—*continued*
 dialysis (intermittent) (treatment)
  extracorporeal V56.0
  peritoneal V56.8
  renal V56.0
  specified type NEC V56.8
 exercise NEC V57.1
  breathing V57.0
 extracorporeal dialysis (renal) V56.0
 fluoride prophylaxis V07.31
 hemodialysis V56.0
 hormone replacement (postmenopausal) V07.4
 immunotherapy, antineoplastic V58.12
 long term oxygen therapy V46.2
 occupational V57.21
 orthoptic V57.4
 orthotic V57.81
 peritoneal dialysis V56.8
 physical NEC V57.1
 postmenopausal hormone replacement V07.4
 radiation V58.0
 speech (-language) V57.3
 vocational V57.22
Thermalgesia 782.0
Thermalgia 782.0
Thermanalgesia 782.0
Thermanesthesia 782.0
Thermic —*see* condition
Thermography (abnormal) 793.99
 breast 793.89
Thermoplegia 992.0
Thesaurismosis
 amyloid 277.39
 bilirubin 277.4
 calcium 275.40
 cystine 270.0
 glycogen (*see also* Disease, glycogen storage)
   271.0
 kerasin 272.7
 lipoid 272.7
 melanin 255.41
 phosphatide 272.7
 urate 274.9
Thiaminic deficiency 265.1
 with beriberi 265.0
Thibierge-Weissenbach syndrome (cutaneous
  systemic sclerosis) 710.1
Thickened endometrium 793.5
Thickening
 bone 733.99
  extremity 733.99
 breast 611.79
 hymen 623.3
 larynx 478.79
 nail 703.8
  congenital 757.5
 periosteal 733.99
 pleura (*see also* Pleurisy) 511.0
 skin 782.8
 subepiglottic 478.79
 tongue 529.8
 valve, heart—*see* Endocarditis
Thiele syndrome 724.6
Thigh —*see* condition
Thinning vertebra (*see also* Osteoporosis) 733.00
Thirst, excessive 783.5
 due to deprivation of water 994.3
Thomsen's disease 359.22
Thomson's disease (congenital poikiloderma) 757.33

Thoracic —*see also* condition
  kidney 753.3
  outlet syndrome 353.0
  stomach—*see* Hernia, diaphragm
Thoracogastroschisis (congenital) 759.89
Thoracopagus 759.4
Thoracoschisis 756.3
Thorax —*see* condition
Thorn's syndrome (*see also* Disease, renal) 593.9
Thornwaldt's, Tornwaldt's
  bursitis (pharyngeal) 478.29
  cyst 478.26
  disease (pharyngeal bursitis) 478.29
Thoracoscopic surgical procedure converted to
  open procedure V64.42
Thorson-Biörck syndrome (malignant
  carcinoid) 259.2
Threadworm (infection) (infestation) 127.4
Threatened
  abortion or miscarriage 640.0
    with subsequent abortion (*see also* Abortion,
      spontaneous) 634.9
    affecting fetus 762.1
  labor 644.1
    affecting fetus or newborn 761.8
    premature 644.0
  miscarriage 640.0
    affecting fetus 762.1
  premature
    delivery 644.2
      affecting fetus or newborn 761.8
    labor 644.0
      before 22 completed weeks gestation 640.0
Three-day fever 066.0
Threshers' lung 495.0
Thrix annulata (congenital) 757.4
Throat —*see* condition
Thrombasthenia (Glanzmann's) (hemorrhagic)
  (hereditary) 287.1
Thromboangiitis 443.1
  obliterans (general) 443.1
    cerebral 437.1
    vessels
      brain 437.1
      spinal cord 437.1
Thromboarteritis —*see* Arteritis
Thromboasthenia (Glanzmann's) (hemorrhagic)
  (hereditary) 287.1
Thrombocytasthenia (Glanzmann's) 287.1
Thrombocythemia (primary) (M9962/1) 238.71
  essential 238.71
  hemorrhagic 238.71
  idiopathic (hemorrhagic) (M9962/1) 238.71
Thrombocytopathy (dystrophic) (granulopenic)
  287.1
Thrombocytopenia, thrombocytopenic 287.5
  with
    absent radii (TAR) syndrome 287.33
    giant hemangioma 287.39
  amegakaryocytic, congenital 287.33
  congenital 287.33
  cyclic 287.39
  dilutional 287.49
  due to
    drugs 287.49
    extracorporeal circulation of blood 287.49
    massive blood transfusion 287.49
    platelet alloimmunization 287.49
  essential 287.30
  fetal 678.0

Thrombocytopenia— *continued*
  heparin-induced (HIT) 289.84
  hereditary 287.33
  Kasabach-Merritt 287.39
  neonatal, transitory 776.1
    due to
      exchange transfusion 776.1
      idiopathic maternal thrombocytopenia 776.1
      isoimmunization 776.1
  primary 287.30
  puerperal, postpartum 666.3
  purpura (*see also* Purpura, thrombocytopenic)
    287.30
    thrombotic 446.6
  secondary NEC 287.49
  sex-linked 287.39
Thrombocytosis 238.71
  essential 238.71
  primary 238.71
Thromboembolism —*see* Embolism
Thrombopathy (Bernard-Soulier) 287.1
  constitutional 286.4
  Willebrand-Jürgens (angiohemophilia) 286.4
Thrombopenia (*see also* Thrombocytopenia) 287.5
Thrombophlebitis 451.9
  antecubital vein 451.82
  antepartum (superficial) 671.2
    affecting fetus or newborn 760.3
    deep 671.3
  arm 451.89
    deep 451.83
    superficial 451.82
  breast, superficial 451.89
  cavernous (venous) sinus—*see*
    Thrombophlebitis, intracranial venous sinus
  cephalic vein 451.82
  cerebral (sinus) (vein) 325
    late effect—*see* category 326
    nonpyogenic 437.6
      in pregnancy or puerperium 671.5
      late effect—*see* Late effect(s) (of)
        cerebrovascular disease
  due to implanted device—*see* Complications,
    due to (presence of) any device, implant, or
    graft classified to 996.0-996.5 NEC
  during or resulting from a procedure NEC 997.2
  femoral 451.11
  femoropopliteal 451.19
  following infusion, perfusion, or transfusion
    999.2
  hepatic (vein) 451.89
  idiopathic, recurrent 453.1
  iliac vein 451.81
  iliofemoral 451.11
  intracranial venous sinus (any) 325
    late effect—*see* category 326
    nonpyogenic 437.6
      in pregnancy or puerperium 671.5
      late effect—*see* Late effect(s) (of)
        cerebrovascular disease
  jugular vein 451.89
  lateral (venous) sinus—*see* Thrombophlebitis,
    intracranial venous sinus
  leg 451.2
    deep (vessels) 451.19
      femoral vein 451.11
      specified vessel NEC 451.19
    superficial (vessels) 451.0
      femoral vein 451.11
  longitudinal (venous) sinus—*see*
    Thrombophlebitis, intracranial venous sinus

Thrombophlebitis—*continued*
  lower extremity 451.2
    deep (vessels) 451.19
      femoral vein 451.11
      specified vessel NEC 451.19
    superficial (vessels) 451.0
  migrans, migrating 453.1
  pelvic
    with
      abortion—*see* Abortion, by type, with sepsis
      ectopic pregnancy (*see also* categories
        633.0-633.9) 639.0
      molar pregnancy (*see also* categories
        630-632) 639.0
    following
      abortion 639.0
      ectopic or molar pregnancy 639.0
    puerperal 671.4
  popliteal vein 451.19
  portal (vein) 572.1
  postoperative 997.2
  pregnancy (superficial) 671.2
    affecting fetus or newborn 760.3
    deep 671.3
  puerperal, postpartum, childbirth (extremities)
    (superficial) 671.2
    deep 671.4
    pelvic 671.4
    septic 670.3
    specified site NEC 671.5
  radial vein 451.83
  saphenous (greater) (lesser) 451.0
  sinus (intracranial)—*see* Thrombophlebitis,
    intracranial venous sinus
  specified site NEC 451.89
  tibial vein 451.19
Thrombosis, thrombotic (marantic) (multiple)
    (progressive) (vein) (vessel) 453.9
  with childbirth or during the puerperium—*see*
    Thrombosis, puerperal, postpartum
  antepartum—*see* Thrombosis, pregnancy
  aorta, aortic 444.1
    abdominal 444.09
      saddle 444.01
    bifurcation 444.09
      saddle 444.01
    terminal 444.09
    thoracic 444.1
    valve—*see* Endocarditis, aortic
  apoplexy (*see also* Thrombosis, brain) 434.0
    late effect—*see* Late effect(s) (of)
      cerebrovascular disease
  appendix, septic—*see* Appendicitis, acute
  arteriolar-capillary platelet, disseminated 446.6
  artery, arteries (postinfectional) 444.9
    auditory, internal 433.8
    basilar (*see also* Occlusion, artery, basilar) 433.0
    carotid (common) (internal) (*see also*
      Occlusion, artery, carotid) 433.1
      with other precerebral artery 433.3
    cerebellar (anterior inferior) (posterior
      inferior) (superior) 433.8
    cerebral (*see also* Thrombosis, brain) 434.0
    choroidal (anterior) 433.8
    communicating posterior 433.8
    coronary (*see also* Infarct, myocardium) 410.9
      due to syphilis 093.89
      healed or specified as old 412
      without myocardial infarction 411.81
    extremities 444.22
      lower 444.22
      upper 444.21

Thrombosis, thrombotic—*continued*
  artery, arteries—*continued*
    femoral 444.22
    hepatic 444.89
    hypophyseal 433.8
    meningeal, anterior or posterior 433.8
    mesenteric (with gangrene) 557.0
    ophthalmic (*see also* Occlusion, retina) 362.30
    pontine 433.8
    popliteal 444.22
    precerebral—*see* Occlusion, artery,
      precerebral NEC
    pulmonary 415.19
      iatrogenic 415.11
      personal history of V12.55
      postoperative 415.11
      septic 415.12
    renal 593.81
    retinal (*see also* Occlusion, retina) 362.30
    specified site NEC 444.89
    spinal, anterior or posterior 433.8
    traumatic (complication) (early) (*see also*
      Injury, blood vessel, by site) 904.9
    vertebral (*see also* Occlusion, artery,
      vertebral) 433.2
      with other precerebral artery 433.3
  atrial (endocardial) 424.90
    due to syphilis 093.89
    without endocarditis 429.89
  auricular (*see also* Infarct, myocardium) 410.9
  axillary (acute) (vein) 453.84
    chronic 453.74
    personal history of V12.51
  basilar (artery) (*see also* Occlusion, artery,
    basilar) 433.0
  bland NEC 453.9
  brain (artery) (stem) 434.0
    due to syphilis 094.89
    iatrogenic 997.02
    late effect—*see* Late effect(s) (of)
      cerebrovascular disease
    postoperative 997.02
    puerperal, postpartum, childbirth 674.0
    sinus (*see also* Thrombosis, intracranial
      venous sinus) 325
  capillary 448.9
    arteriolar, generalized 446.6
  cardiac (*see also* Infarct, myocardium) 410.9
    due to syphilis 093.89
    healed or specified as old 412
    valve—*see* Endocarditis
  carotid (artery) (common) (internal) (*see also*
    Occlusion, artery, carotid) 433.1
    with other precerebral artery 433.3
  cavernous sinus (venous)—*see* Thrombosis,
    intracranial venous sinus
  cerebellar artery (anterior inferior) (posterior
    inferior) (superior) 433.8
    late effect—*see* Late effect(s) (of)
      cerebrovascular disease
  cerebral (arteries) (*see also* Thrombosis, brain)
    434.0
    late effect—*see* Late effect(s) (of)
      cerebrovascular disease
  coronary (artery) (*see also* Infarct, myocardium)
    410.9
    due to syphilis 093.89
    healed or specified as old 412
    without myocardial infarction 411.81
  corpus cavernosum 607.82
  cortical (*see also* Thrombosis, brain) 434.0

Thrombosis, thrombotic—*continued*
  due to (presence of) any device, implant, or graft
    classifiable to 996.0-996.5—*see*
    Complications, due to (presence of) any
    device, implant, or graft classified to
    996.0-996.5 NEC
  effort 453.89
  endocardial—*see* Infarct, myocardium
  eye (*see also* Occlusion, retina) 362.30
  femoral (vein) 453.6
    with inflammation or phlebitis 451.11
    artery 444.22
    deep 453.41
    personal history of V12.51
  genital organ, male 608.83
  heart (chamber) (*see also* Infarct, myocardium)
    410.9
  hepatic (vein) 453.0
    artery 444.89
    infectional or septic 572.1
  iliac (acute) (vein) 453.41
    with inflammation or phlebitis 451.81
    artery (common) (external) (internal) 444.81
    chronic 453.51
    personal history of V12.51
  inflammation, vein—*see* Thrombophlebitis
  internal carotid artery (*see also* Occlusion,
    artery, carotid) 433.1
    with other precerebral artery 433.3
  intestine (with gangrene) 557.0
  intracranial (*see also* Thrombosis, brain) 434.0
    venous sinus (any) 325
      nonpyogenic origin 437.6
      in pregnancy or puerperium 671.5
  intramural (*see also* Infarct, myocardium) 410.9
    without
      cardiac condition 429.89
      coronary artery disease 429.89
      myocardial infarction 429.89
    healed or specified as old 412
  jugular (bulb)
    external (acute) 453.89
      chronic 453.79
    internal (acute) 453.86
      chronic 453.76
  kidney 593.81
    artery 593.81
  lateral sinus (venous)—*see* Thrombosis,
    intracranial venous sinus
  leg (see also Thrombosis, lower extremity)
    453.6
    with inflammation or phlebitis—*see*
      Thrombophlebitis
    deep (vessels) 453.40
      acute 453.40
        lower (distal) 453.42
        upper (proximal) 453.41
      chronic 453.50
        lower (distal) 453.52
        upper (proximal) 453.51
      personal history of V12.51
    superficial (vessels) 453.6
  liver (venous) 453.0
    artery 444.89
    infectional or septic 572.1
    portal vein 452
  longitudinal sinus (venous)—*see* Thrombosis,
    intracranial venous sinus

Thrombosis, thrombotic—*continued*
  lower extremity (superficial) 453.6
    deep vessels 453.40
      acute 453.40
        calf 453.42
        distal (lower leg) 453.42
        femoral 453.41
        iliac 453.41
        lower leg 453.42
        peroneal 453.42
        popliteal 453.41
        proximal (upper leg) 453.41
        thigh 453.41
        tibial 453.42
      chronic 453.50
        calf 453.52
        distal (lower leg) 453.52
        femoral 453.51
        iliac 453.51
        lower leg 453.52
        peroneal 453.52
        popliteal 453.51
        proximal (upper leg) 453.51
        thigh 453.51
        tibial 453.52
    personal history of V12.51
    saphenous (greater) (lesser) 453.6
    superficial 453.6
  lung 415.19
    iatrogenic 415.11
    personal history of V12.55
    postoperative 415.11
    septic 415.12
  marantic, dural sinus 437.6
  meninges (brain) (*see also* Thrombosis, brain)
    434.0
  mesenteric (artery) (with gangrene) 557.0
    vein (inferior) (superior) 557.0
  mitral—*see* Insufficiency, mitral
  mural (heart chamber) (*see also* Infarct,
    myocardium) 410.9
    without
      cardiac condition 429.89
      coronary artery disease 429.89
      myocardial infarction 429.89
    due to syphilis 093.89
    following myocardial infarction 429.79
    healed or specified as old 412
  omentum (with gangrene) 557.0
  ophthalmic (artery) (*see also* Occlusion, retina)
    362.30
  pampiniform plexus (male) 608.83
    female 620.8
  parietal (*see also* Infarct, myocardium) 410.9
  penis, penile 607.82
  peripheral arteries 444.22
    lower 444.22
    upper 444.21
  platelet 446.6
  portal 452
    due to syphilis 093.89
    infectional or septic 572.1
  precerebral artery—*see also* Occlusion, artery,
    precerebral NEC
  pregnancy 671.2
    deep (vein) 671.3
    superficial (vein) 671.2

Thrombosis, thrombotic—*continued*
puerperal, postpartum, childbirth 671.2
  brain (artery) 674.0
    venous 671.5
  cardiac 674.8
  cerebral (artery) 674.0
    venous 671.5
  deep (vein) 671.4
  intracranial sinus (nonpyogenic) (venous)
    671.5
  pelvic 671.4
  pulmonary (artery) 673.2
  specified site NEC 671.5
  superficial 671.2
pulmonary (artery) (vein) 415.19
  iatrogenic 415.11
  personal history of V12.55
  postoperative 415.11
  septic 415.12
radial vein 451.83
renal (artery) 593.81
  vein 453.3
resulting from presence of shunt or other
    internal prosthetic device—*see*
    Complications, due to (presence of) any
    device, implant, or graft classified to
    996.0-996.5 NEC
retina, retinal (artery) 362.30
  arterial branch 362.32
  central 362.31
  partial 362.33
  vein
    central 362.35
    tributary (branch) 362.36
saphenous vein (greater) (lesser) 453.6
scrotum 608.83
seminal vesicle 608.83
sigmoid (venous) sinus (*see* Thrombosis,
    intracranial venous sinus) 325
silent NEC 453.9
sinus, intracranial (venous) (any) (*see also*
    Thrombosis, intracranial venous sinus) 325
softening, brain (*see also* Thrombosis, brain)
    434.0
specified site NEC (acute) 453.89
  chronic 453.79
spermatic cord 608.83
spinal cord 336.1
  due to syphilis 094.89
  in pregnancy or puerperium 671.5
  pyogenic origin 324.1
    late effect—*see* category 326
spleen, splenic 289.59
  artery 444.89
testis 608.83
traumatic (complication) (early) (*see also* Injury,
    blood vessel, by site) 904.9
tricuspid—*see* Endocarditis, tricuspid
tumor—*see* Neoplasm, by site
tunica vaginalis 608.83
umbilical cord (vessels) 663.6
  affecting fetus or newborn 762.6
upper extremity (acute) 453.83
  chronic 453.73
    deep 453.72
    superficial 453.71
  deep 453.82
  superficial 453.81
vas deferens 608.83

Thrombosis, thrombotic—*continued*
vein
  antecubital (acute) 453.81
    chronic 453.71
  axillary (acute) 453.84
    chronic 453.74
  basilic (acute) 453.81
    chronic 453.71
  brachial (acute) 453.82
    chronic 453.72
  brachiocephalic (innominate) (acute) 453.87
    chronic 453.77
  cephalic (acute) 453.81
    chronic 453.71
  deep 453.40
    personal history of V12.51
  internal jugular (acute) 453.86
    chronic 453.76
  lower extremity—*see* Thrombosis, lower
    extremity
  personal history of V12.51
  radial (acute) 453.82
    chronic 453.72
  saphenous (greater) (lesser) 453.6
  specified site NEC (acute) 453.89
    chronic 453.79
  subclavian (acute) 453.85
    chronic 453.75
  superior vena cava (acute) 453.87
    chronic 453.77
  thoracic (acute) 453.87
    chronic 453.77
  ulnar (acute) 453.82
    chronic 453.72
  upper extremity - see Thrombosis, upper
    extremity
vena cava
  inferior 453.2
  personal history of V12.51
  superior (acute) 453.87
    chronic 453.77
Thrombus —*see* Thrombosis
Thrush 112.0
newborn 771.7
Thumb —*see also* condition
gamekeeper's 842.12
sucking (child problem) 307.9
Thygeson's superficial punctate keratitis
  370.21
Thymergasia (*see also* Psychosis, affective)
  296.80
Thymitis 254.8
Thymoma (benign) (M8580/0) 212.6
malignant (M8580/3) 164.0
Thymus, thymic (gland)—*see* condition
Thyrocele (*see also* Goiter) 240.9
Thyroglossal —*see also* condition
cyst 759.2
duct, persistent 759.2
Thyroid (body) (gland)—*see also* condition
hormone resistance 246.8
lingual 759.2
Thyroiditis 245.9
acute (pyogenic) (suppurative) 245.0
  nonsuppurative 245.0
autoimmune 245.2
chronic (nonspecific) (sclerosing) 245.8
  fibrous 245.3
  lymphadenoid 245.2
  lymphocytic 245.2
  lymphoid 245.2

Thyroiditis—*continued*
  complicating pregnancy, childbirth, or
    puerperium 648.1
  de Quervain's (subacute granulomatous) 245.1
  fibrous (chronic) 245.3
  giant (cell) (follicular) 245.1
  granulomatous (de Quervain's) (subacute) 245.1
  Hashimoto's (struma lymphomatosa) 245.2
  iatrogenic 245.4
  invasive (fibrous) 245.3
  ligneous 245.3
  lymphocytic (chronic) 245.2
  lymphoid 245.2
  lymphomatous 245.2
  pseudotuberculous 245.1
  pyogenic 245.0
  radiation 245.4
  Riedel's (ligneous) 245.3
  subacute 245.1
  suppurative 245.0
  tuberculous (*see also* Tuberculosis) 017.5
  viral 245.1
  woody 245.3
Thyrolingual duct, persistent 759.2
Thyromegaly 240.9
Thyrotoxic
  crisis or storm (*see also* Thyrotoxicosis) 242.9
  heart failure (*see also* Thyrotoxicosis) 242.9 *[425.7]*
Thyrotoxicosis 242.9

*Note—Use the following fifth-digit
subclassification with category 242:*

0 without mention of thyrotoxic crisis or storm
1 with mention of thyrotoxic crisis or storm

  with
    goiter (diffuse) 242.0
      adenomatous 242.3
        multinodular 242.2
        uninodular 242.1
      nodular 242.3
        multinodular 242.2
        uninodular 242.1
    infiltrative
      dermopathy 242.0
      ophthalmopathy 242.0
      thyroid acropachy 242.0
  complicating pregnancy, childbirth, or
    puerperium 648.1
  due to
    ectopic thyroid nodule 242.4
    ingestion of (excessive) thyroid material 242.8
    specified cause NEC 242.8
  factitia 242.8
  heart 242.9 *[425.7]*
  neonatal (transient) 775.3
TIA (transient ischemic attack) 435.9
  with transient neurologic deficit 435.9
  late effect—*see* Late effect(s) (of)
    cerebrovascular disease
Tibia vara 732.4
Tic 307.20
  breathing 307.20
  child problem 307.21
  compulsive 307.22
  convulsive 307.20
  degenerative (generalized) (localized) 333.3
    facial 351.8
  douloureux (*see also* Neuralgia, trigeminal)
    350.1
    atypical 350.2

Tic —*continued*
  habit 307.20
    chronic (motor or vocal) 307.22
    transient (of childhood) 307.21
  lid 307.20
    transient (of childhood) 307.21
  motor-verbal 307.23
  occupational 300.89
  orbicularis 307.20
    transient (of childhood) 307.21
  organic origin 333.3
  postchoreic—*see* Chorea
  psychogenic 307.20
    compulsive 307.22
  salaam 781.0
  spasm 307.20
    chronic (motor or vocal) 307.22
    transient (of childhood) 307.21
Tick (-borne) fever NEC 066.1
  American mountain 066.1
  Colorado 066.1
  hemorrhagic NEC 065.3
    Crimean 065.0
    Kyasanur Forest 065.2
    Omsk 065.1
  mountain 066.1
  nonexanthematous 066.1
Tick-bite fever NEC 066.1
  African 087.1
  Colorado (virus) 066.1
  Rocky Mountain 082.0
Tick paralysis 989.5
Tics and spasms, compulsive 307.22
Tietze's disease or syndrome 733.6
Tight, tightness
  anus 564.89
  chest 786.59
  fascia (lata) 728.9
  foreskin (congenital) 605
  hymen 623.3
  introitus (acquired) (congenital) 623.3
  rectal sphincter 564.89
  tendon 727.81
    Achilles (heel) 727.81
  urethral sphincter 598.9
Tilting vertebra 737.9
Timidity, child 313.21
Tinea (intersecta) (tarsi) 110.9
  amiantacea 110.0
  asbestina 110.0
  barbae 110.0
  beard 110.0
  black dot 110.0
  blanca 111.2
  capitis 110.0
  corporis 110.5
  cruris 110.3
  decalvans 704.09
  flava 111.0
  foot 110.4
  furfuracea 111.0
  imbricata (Tokelau) 110.5
  lepothrix 039.0
  manuum 110.2
  microsporic (*see also* Dermatophytosis) 110.9
  nigra 111.1
  nodosa 111.2
  pedis 110.4
  scalp 110.0
  specified site NEC 110.8
  sycosis 110.0

Tortuous
   artery 447.1
   fallopian tube 752.19
   organ or site, congenital NEC—*see* Distortion
   renal vessel, congenital 747.62
   retina vessel (congenital) 743.58
      acquired 362.17
   ureter 593.4
   urethra 599.84
   vein—*see* Varicose, vein
Torula, torular (infection) 117.5
   histolytica 117.5
   lung 117.5
Torulosis 117.5
Torus
   fracture
      fibula 823.41
         with tibia 823.42
      humerus 812.49
      radius (alone) 813.45
         with ulna 813.47
      tibia 823.40
         with fibula 823.42
      ulna (alone) 813.46
         with radius 813.47
   mandibularis 526.81
   palatinus 526.81
Touch, vitreous 997.99
Touraine's syndrome (hereditary
   osteo-onychodysplasia) 756.89
Touraine-Solente-Golé syndrome
   (acropachyderma) 757.39
Tourette's disease (motor-verbal tic) 307.23
Tower skull 756.0
   with exophthalmos 756.0
Toxemia 799.89
   with abortion—*see* Abortion, by type, with toxemia
   bacterial—*see* Septicemia
   biliary (*see also* Disease, biliary) 576.8
   burn—*see* Burn, by site
   congenital NEC 779.89
   eclamptic 642.6
      with pre-existing hypertension 642.7
   erysipelatous (*see also* Erysipelas) 035
   fatigue 799.89
   fetus or newborn NEC 779.89
   food (*see also* Poisoning, food) 005.9
   gastric 537.89
   gastrointestinal 558.2
   intestinal 558.2
   kidney (*see also* Disease, renal) 593.9
   lung 518.89
   malarial NEC (*see also* Malaria) 084.6
   maternal (of pregnancy), affecting fetus or
      newborn 760.0
   myocardial—*see* Myocarditis, toxic
   of pregnancy (mild) (pre-eclamptic) 642.4
      with
         convulsions 642.6
         pre-existing hypertension 642.7
      affecting fetus or newborn 760.0
      severe 642.5
   pre-eclamptic—*see* Toxemia, of pregnancy
   puerperal, postpartum—*see* Toxemia, of
      pregnancy
   pulmonary 518.89
   renal (*see also* Disease, renal) 593.9
   septic (*see also* Septicemia) 038.9
   small intestine 558.2

Toxemia—*continued*
   staphylococcal 038.10
      aureus 038.11
      due to food 005.0
      specified organism NEC 038.19
   stasis 799.89
   stomach 537.89
   uremic (*see also* Uremia) 586
   urinary 586
Toxemica cerebropathia psychica
   (nonalcoholic) 294.0
   alcoholic 291.1
Toxic (poisoning)—*see also* condition
   from drug or poison—*see* Table of drugs and
      chemicals
   oil syndrome 710.5
   shock syndrome 040.82
   thyroid (gland) (*see also* Thyrotoxicosis) 242.9
Toxicemia —*see* Toxemia
Toxicity
   dilantin
      asymptomatic 796.0
      symptomatic—*see* Table of Drugs and Chemicals
   drug
      asymptomatic 796.0
      symptomatic—*see* Table of Drugs and Chemicals
   fava bean 282.2
   from drug or poison
      asymptomatic 796.0
      symptomatic—*see* Table of Drugs and
         Chemicals
Toxicosis (*see also* Toxemia) 799.89
   capillary, hemorrhagic 287.0
Toxinfection 799.89
   gastrointestinal 558.2
Toxocariasis 128.0
Toxoplasma infection, generalized 130.9
Toxoplasmosis (acquired) 130.9
   with pneumonia 130.4
   congenital, active 771.2
   disseminated (multisystemic) 130.8
   maternal
      with suspected damage to fetus affecting
         management of pregnancy 655.4
      affecting fetus or newborn 760.2
         manifest toxoplasmosis in fetus or newborn
            771.2
   multiple sites 130.8
   multisystemic disseminated 130.8
   specified site NEC 130.7
Trabeculation, bladder 596.89
Trachea —*see* condition
Tracheitis (acute)(catarrhal)(infantile)
   (membranous) (plastic) (pneumococcal)
   (septic) (suppurative) (viral) 464.10
   with
      bronchitis 490
         acute or subacute 466.0
         chronic 491.8
         tuberculosis—*see* Tuberculosis, pulmonary
      laryngitis (acute) 464.20
         with obstruction 464.21
         chronic 476.1
         tuberculous (*see also* Tuberculosis, larynx) 012.3
      obstruction 464.11
   chronic 491.8
      with
         bronchitis (chronic) 491.8
         laryngitis (chronic) 476.1
      due to external agent—*see* Condition,
         respiratory, chronic, due to

Tracheitis—*continued*
  diphtheritic (membranous) 032.3
    due to external agent—*see* Inflammation,
      respiratory, upper, due to
  edematous 464.11
  influenzal (*see also* Influenza) 487.1
  streptococcal 034.0
  syphilitic 095.8
  tuberculous (*see also* Tuberculosis) 012.8
Trachelitis (nonvenereal) (*see also* Cervicitis) 616.0
  trichomonal 131.09
Tracheobronchial —*see* condition
Tracheobronchitis (*see also* Bronchitis) 490
  acute or subacute 466.0
    with bronchospasm or obstruction 466.0
  chronic 491.8
  influenzal (*see also* Influenza) 487.1
  senile 491.8
Tracheobronchomegaly (congenital) 748.3
  with bronchiectasis 494.0
    with (acute) exacerbation 494.1
  acquired 519.19
    with bronchiectasis 494.0
      with (acute) exacerbation 494.1
Tracheobronchopneumonitis —*see* Pneumonia,
  broncho
Tracheocele (external) (internal) 519.19
  congenital 748.3
Tracheomalacia 519.19
  congenital 748.3
Tracheopharyngitis (acute) 465.8
  chronic 478.9
    due to external agent—*see* Condition,
      respiratory, chronic, due to
    due to external agent—*see* Inflammation,
      respiratory, upper, due to
Tracheostenosis 519.19
  congenital 748.3
Tracheostomy
  attention to V55.0
  complication 519.00
  granuloma 519.09
  hemorrhage 519.09
  infection 519.01
  malfunctioning 519.02
  obstruction 519.09
  sepsis 519.01
  status V44.0
  stenosis 519.02
Trachoma, trachomatous 076.9
  active (stage) 076.1
  contraction of conjunctiva 076.1
  dubium 076.0
  healed or late effect 139.1
  initial (stage) 076.0
  Türck's (chronic catarrhal laryngitis) 476.0
Trachyphonia 784.49
Traction, vitreomacular 379.27
Training
  insulin pump V65.46
  orthoptic V57.4
  orthotic V57.81
Train sickness 994.6
Trait
  hemoglobin
    abnormal NEC 282.7
      with thalassemia 282.46
    C (*see also* Disease, hemoglobin, C) 282.7
      with elliptocytosis 282.7
    S (Hb-S) 282.5

Trait—*continued*
  Lepore 282.49
    with other abnormal hemoglobin NEC 282.49
  paranoid 301.0
  sickle-cell 282.5
    with
      elliptocytosis 282.5
      spherocytosis 282.5
  thalassemia (alpha) (beta) (delta-beta) 282.46
Traits, paranoid 301.0
Tramp V60.0
Trance 780.09
  hysterical 300.13
Transaminasemia 790.4
Transfusion, blood
  donor V59.01
    stem cells V59.02
  fetal twin to twin 678.0
  incompatible (*see also* Complications,
    transfusion) 999.80
    ABO (*see also* Complications, transfusion)
      999.60
    minor blood group 999.89
    non-ABO (*see also* Complications,
      transfusion) 999.75
    Rh (antigen) (C) (c) (D) (E) (e) (*see also*
      Complications, transfusion) 999.70
  reaction or complication—*see* Complications,
    transfusion
  related acute lung injury (TRALI) 518.7
  syndrome
    fetomaternal 772.0
    twin-to-twin
      blood loss (donor twin) 772.0
      recipient twin 776.4
  twin to twin fetal 678.0
  without reported diagnosis V58.2
Transient —*see also* condition
  alteration of awareness 780.02
  blindness 368.12
  deafness (ischemic) 388.02
  global amnesia 437.7
  hyperglycemia (post-procedural) 790.29
  hypoglycemia (post-procedural) 251.2
  person (homeless) NEC V60.0
Transitional, lumbosacral joint of vertebra
  756.19
Translocation
  autosomes NEC 758.5
    13-15 758.1
    16-18 758.2
    21 or 22 758.0
    balanced in normal individual 758.4
    D_1 758.1
    E_3 758.2
    G 758.0
  balanced autosomal in normal individual 758.4
  chromosomes NEC 758.89
  Down's syndrome 758.0
Translucency, iris 364.53
Transmission of chemical substances through
  the placenta (affecting fetus or newborn)
  760.70
  alcohol 760.71
  anticonvulsants 760.77
  antifungals 760.74
  anti-infective agents 760.74
  antimetabolics 760.78
  cocaine 760.75
  "crack" 760.75
  diethylstilbestrol [DES] 760.76
  hallucinogenic agents 760.73

Tremor—*continued*
  flapping (liver) 572.8
  hereditary 333.1
  hysterical 300.11
  intention 333.1
  medication-induced postural 333.1
  mercurial 985.0
  muscle 728.85
  Parkinson's (*see also* Parkinsonism) 332.0
  psychogenic 306.0
    specified as conversion reaction 300.11
  senilis 797
  specified type NEC 333.1
Trench
  fever 083.1
  foot 991.4
  mouth 101
  nephritis—*see* Nephritis, acute
Treponema pallidum infection (*see also*
    Syphilis) 097.9
Treponematosis 102.9
  due to
    T. pallidum—*see* Syphilis
    T. pertenue (yaws) (*see also* Yaws) 102.9
Triad
  Kartagener's 759.3
  Reiter's (complete) (incomplete) 099.3
  Saint's (*see also* Hernia, diaphragm) 553.3
Trichiasis 704.2
  cicatricial 704.2
  eyelid 374.05
    with entropion (*see also* Entropion) 374.00
Trichinella spiralis (infection) (infestation) 124
Trichinelliasis 124
Trichinellosis 124
Trichiniasis 124
Trichinosis 124
Trichobezoar 938
  intestine 936
  stomach 935.2
Trichocephaliasis 127.3
Trichocephalosis 127.3
Trichocephalus infestation 127.3
Trichoclasis 704.2
Trichoepithelioma (M8100/0)—*see also*
    Neoplasm, skin, benign
  breast 217
  genital organ NEC—*see* Neoplasm, by site,
    benign
  malignant (M8100/3)—*see* Neoplasm, skin,
    malignant
Trichofolliculoma (M8101/0)—*see* Neoplasm,
    skin, benign
Tricholemmoma (M8102/0)—*see* Neoplasm,
    skin, benign
Trichomatosis 704.2
Trichomoniasis 131.9
  bladder 131.09
  cervix 131.09
  intestinal 007.3
  prostate 131.03
  seminal vesicle 131.09
  specified site NEC 131.8
  urethra 131.02
  urogenitalis 131.00
  vagina 131.01
  vulva 131.01
  vulvovaginal 131.01

Trichomycosis 039.0
  axillaris 039.0
  nodosa 111.2
  nodularis 111.2
  rubra 039.0
Trichonocardiosis (axillaris) (palmellina) 039.0
Trichonodosis 704.2
Trichophytid, trichophyton infection (*see also*
    Dermatophytosis) 110.9
Trichophytide —*see* Dermatophytosis
Trichophytobezoar 938
  intestine 936
  stomach 935.2
Trichophytosis —*see* Dermatophytosis
Trichoptilosis 704.2
Trichorrhexis (nodosa) 704.2
Trichosporosis nodosa 111.2
Trichostasis spinulosa (congenital) 757.4
Trichostrongyliasis (small intestine) 127.6
Trichostrongylosis 127.6
Trichostrongylus (instabilis) infection 127.6
Trichotillomania 312.39
Trichromat, anomalous (congenital) 368.59
Trichromatopsia, anomalous (congenital)
    368.59
Trichuriasis 127.3
Trichuris trichiuria (any site) (infection)
    (infestation) 127.3
Tricuspid (valve)—*see* condition
Trifid —*see also* Accessory
  kidney (pelvis) 753.3
  tongue 750.13
Trigeminal neuralgia (*see also* Neuralgia,
    trigeminal) 350.1
Trigeminoencephaloangiomatosis 759.6
Trigeminy 427.89
  postoperative 997.1
Trigger finger (acquired) 727.03
  congenital 756.89
Trigonitis (bladder) (chronic)
    (pseudomembranous) 595.3
  tuberculous (*see also* Tuberculosis) 016.1
Trigonocephaly 756.0
Trihexosidosis 272.7
Trilobate placenta —*see* Placenta, abnormal
Trilocular heart 745.8
Trimethylaminuria 270.8
Tripartita placenta —*see* Placenta, abnormal
Triple —*see also* Accessory
  kidneys 753.3
  uteri 752.2
  X female 758.81
Triplegia 344.89
  congenital or infantile 343.8
Triplet
  affected by maternal complications of pregnancy
    761.5
  healthy liveborn—*see* Newborn, multiple
  pregnancy (complicating delivery) NEC 651.1
    with fetal loss and retention of one or more
      fetus(es) 651.4
    following (elective) fetal reduction 651.7
Triplex placenta —*see* Placenta, abnormal
Triplication —*see* Accessory
Trismus 781.0
  neonatorum 771.3
  newborn 771.3
Trisomy (syndrome) NEC 758.5
  13 (partial) 758.1
  16-18 758.2

Trisomy—*continued*
18 (partial) 758.2
21 (partial) 758.0
22 758.0
autosomes NEC 758.5
D₁ 758.1
E₃ 758.2
G (group) 758.0
group D₁ 758.1
group E 758.2
group G 758.0
Tritanomaly 368.53
Tritanopia 368.53
Troisier-Hanot-Chauffard syndrome (bronze diabetes) 275.01
Trombidiosis 133.8
Trophedema (hereditary) 757.0
congenital 757.0
Trophoblastic disease (*see also* Hydatidiform mole) 630
previous, affecting management of pregnancy V23.1
Tropholymphedema 757.0
Trophoneurosis NEC 356.9
arm NEC 354.9
disseminated 710.1
facial 349.89
leg NEC 355.8
lower extremity NEC 355.8
upper extremity NEC 354.9
Tropical —*see also* condition
maceration feet (syndrome) 991.4
wet foot (syndrome) 991.4
Trouble —*see also* Disease
bowel 569.9
heart—*see* Disease, heart
intestine 569.9
kidney (*see also* Disease, renal) 593.9
nervous 799.21
sinus (*see also* Sinusitis) 473.9
Trousseau's syndrome (thrombophlebitis migrans) 453.1
Truancy, childhood —*see also* Disturbance, conduct
socialized 312.2
undersocialized, unsocialized 312.1
Truncus
arteriosus (persistent) 745.0
common 745.0
communis 745.0
Trunk —*see* condition
Trychophytide —*see* Dermatophytosis
Trypanosoma infestation —*see* Trypanosomiasis
Trypanosomiasis 086.9
with meningoencephalitis 086.9 *[323.2]*
African 086.5
due to Trypanosoma 086.5
gambiense 086.3
rhodesiense 086.4
American 086.2
with
heart involvement 086.0
other organ involvement 086.1
without mention of organ involvement 086.2
Brazilian—*see* Trypanosomiasis, American
Chagas'—*see* Trypanosomiasis, American
due to Trypanosoma
cruzi—*see* Trypanosomiasis, American
gambiense 086.3
rhodesiense 086.4

Trypanosomiasis—*continued*
gambiensis, Gambian 086.3
North American—*see* Trypanosomiasis, American
rhodesiensis, Rhodesian 086.4
South American—*see* Trypanosomiasis, American
T-shaped incisors 520.2
Tsutsugamushi fever 081.2
Tube, tubal, tubular —*see also* condition
ligation, admission for V25.2
Tubercle —*see also* Tuberculosis
brain, solitary 013.2
Darwin's 744.29
epithelioid noncaseating 135
Ghon, primary infection 010.0
Tuberculid, tuberculide (indurating) (lichenoid) (miliary) (papulonecrotic) (primary) (skin) (subcutaneous) (*see also* Tuberculosis) 017.0
Tuberculoma —*see also* Tuberculosis
brain (any part) 013.2
meninges (cerebral) (spinal) 013.1
spinal cord 013.4
Tuberculosis, tubercular, tuberculous (calcification) (calcified) (caseous) (chromogenic acid-fast bacilli) (congenital) (degeneration) (disease) (fibrocaseous) (fistula) (gangrene) (interstitial) (isolated circumscribed lesions) (necrosis) (parenchymatous) (ulcerative) 011.9

> *Note—Use the following fifth-digit subclassification with categories 010-018:*
>
> *0 unspecified*
> *1 bacteriological or histological examination not done*
> *2 bacteriological or histological examination unknown (at present)*
> *3 tubercle bacilli found (in sputum) by microscopy*
> *4 tubercle bacilli not found (in sputum) by microscopy, but found by bacterial culture*
> *5 tubercle bacilli not found by bacteriological examination, but tuberculosis confirmed histologically*
> *6 tubercle bacilli not found by bacteriological or histological examination, but tuberculosis confirmed by other methods [inoculation of animals]*
>
> *For tuberculous conditions specified as late effects or sequelae, see category 137.*

abdomen 014.8
lymph gland 014.8
abscess 011.9
arm 017.9
bone (*see also* Osteomyelitis, due to, tuberculosis) 015.9 *[730.8]*
hip 015.1 *[730.85]*
knee 015.2 *[730.86]*
sacrum 015.0 *[730.88]*
specified site NEC 015.7 *[730.88]*
spinal 015.0 *[730.88]*
vertebra 015.0 *[730.88]*
brain 013.3
breast 017.9
Cowper's gland 016.5
dura (mater) 013.8
brain 013.3
spinal cord 013.5

Tuberculosis, tubercular—*continued*
abscess—*continued*
epidural 013.8
brain 013.3
spinal cord 013.5
frontal sinus—*see* Tuberculosis, sinus
genital organs NEC 016.9
female 016.7
male 016.5
genitourinary NEC 016.9
gland (lymphatic)—*see* Tuberculosis, lymph
gland
hip 015.1
iliopsoas 015.0 *[730.88]*
intestine 014.8
ischiorectal 014.8
joint 015.9
hip 015.1
knee 015.2
specified joint NEC 015.8
vertebral 015.0 *[730.88]*
kidney 016.0 *[590.81]*
knee 015.2
lumbar 015.0 *[730.88]*
lung 011.2
primary, progressive 010.8
meninges (cerebral) (spinal) 013.0
pelvic 016.9
female 016.7
male 016.5
perianal 014.8
fistula 014.8
perinephritic 016.0 *[590.81]*
perineum 017.9
perirectal 014.8
psoas 015.0 *[730.88]*
rectum 014.8
retropharyngeal 012.8
sacrum 015.0 *[730.88]*
scrofulous 017.2
scrotum 016.5
skin 017.0
primary 017.0
spinal cord 013.5
spine or vertebra (column) 015.0 *[730.88]*
strumous 017.2
subdiaphragmatic 014.8
testis 016.5
thigh 017.9
urinary 016.3
kidney 016.0 *[590.81]*
uterus 016.7
accessory sinus—*see* Tuberculosis, sinus
Addison's disease 017.6
adenitis (*see also* Tuberculosis, lymph gland)
017.2
adenoids 012.8
adenopathy (*see also* Tuberculosis, lymph
gland) 017.2
tracheobronchial 012.1
primary progressive 010.8
adherent pericardium 017.9 *[420.0]*
adnexa (uteri) 016.7
adrenal (capsule) (gland) 017.6
air passage NEC 012.8
alimentary canal 014.8
anemia 017.9
ankle (joint) 015.8
bone 015.5 *[730.87]*
anus 014.8
apex (*see also* Tuberculosis, pulmonary) 011.9

Tuberculosis, tubercular— *continued*
apical (*see also* Tuberculosis, pulmonary) 011.9
appendicitis 014.8
appendix 014.8
arachnoid 013.0
artery 017.9
arthritis (chronic) (synovial) 015.9 *[711.40]*
ankle 015.8 *[730.87]*
hip 015.1 *[711.45]*
knee 015.2 *[711.46]*
specified site NEC 015.8 *[711.48]*
spine or vertebra (column) 015.0 *[720.81]*
wrist 015.8 *[730.83]*
articular—*see* Tuberculosis, joint
ascites 014.0
asthma (*see also* Tuberculosis, pulmonary)
011.9
axilla, axillary 017.2
gland 017.2
bilateral (*see also* Tuberculosis, pulmonary)
011.9
bladder 016.1
bone (*see also* Osteomyelitis, due to,
tuberculosis) 015.9 *[730.8]*
hip 015.1 *[730.85]*
knee 015.2 *[730.86]*
limb NEC 015.5 *[730.88]*
sacrum 015.0 *[730.88]*
specified site NEC 015.7 *[730.88]*
spinal or vertebral column 015.0 *[730.88]*
bowel 014.8
miliary 018.9
brain 013.2
breast 017.9
broad ligament 016.7
bronchi, bronchial, bronchus 011.3
ectasia, ectasis 011.5
fistula 011.3
primary, progressive 010.8
gland 012.1
primary, progressive 010.8
isolated 012.2
lymph gland or node 012.1
primary, progressive 010.8
bronchiectasis 011.5
bronchitis 011.3
bronchopleural 012.0
bronchopneumonia, bronchopneumonic 011.6
bronchorrhagia 011.3
bronchotracheal 011.3
isolated 012.2
bronchus—*see* Tuberculosis, bronchi
bronze disease (Addison's) 017.6
buccal cavity 017.9
bulbourethral gland 016.5
bursa (*see also* Tuberculosis, joint) 015.9
cachexia NEC (*see also* Tuberculosis,
pulmonary) 011.9
cardiomyopathy 017.9 *[425.8]*
caries (*see also* Tuberculosis, bone) 015.9
[730.8]
cartilage (*see also* Tuberculosis, bone) 015.9
[730.8]
intervertebral 015.0 *[730.88]*
catarrhal (*see also* Tuberculosis, pulmonary)
011.9
cecum 014.8
cellular tissue (primary) 017.0
cellulitis (primary) 017.0
central nervous system 013.9
specified site NEC 013.8

Tuberculosis, tubercular—*continued*
cerebellum (current) 013.2
cerebral (current) 013.2
  meninges 013.0
cerebrospinal 013.6
  meninges 013.0
cerebrum (current) 013.2
cervical 017.2
  gland 017.2
  lymph nodes 017.2
cervicitis (uteri) 016.7
cervix 016.7
chest (*see also* Tuberculosis, pulmonary) 011.9
childhood type or first infection 010.0
choroid 017.3 *[363.13]*
choroiditis 017.3 *[363.13]*
ciliary body 017.3 *[364.11]*
colitis 014.8
colliers' 011.4
colliquativa (primary) 017.0
colon 014.8
  ulceration 014.8
complex, primary 010.0
complicating pregnancy, childbirth, or
    puerperium 647.3
  affecting fetus or newborn 760.2
congenital 771.2
conjunctiva 017.3 *[370.31]*
connective tissue 017.9
  bone—*see* Tuberculosis, bone
contact V01.1
converter (tuberculin skin test) (without disease)
    795.51
cornea (ulcer) 017.3 *[370.31]*
Cowper's gland 016.5
coxae 015.1 *[730.85]*
coxalgia 015.1 *[730.85]*
cul-de-sac of Douglas 014.8
curvature, spine 015.0 *[737.40]*
cutis (colliquativa) (primary) 017.0
cyst, ovary 016.6
cystitis 016.1
dacryocystitis 017.3 *[375.32]*
dactylitis 015.5
diarrhea 014.8
diffuse (*see also* Tuberculosis, miliary) 018.9
  lung—*see* Tuberculosis, pulmonary
  meninges 013.0
digestive tract 014.8
disseminated (*see also* Tuberculosis, miliary)
    018.9
  meninges 013.0
duodenum 014.8
dura (mater) 013.9
  abscess 013.8
    cerebral 013.3
    spinal 013.5
dysentery 014.8
ear (inner) (middle) 017.4
  bone 015.6
  external (primary) 017.0
  skin (primary) 017.0
elbow 015.8
emphysema—*see* Tuberculosis, pulmonary
empyema 012.0
encephalitis 013.6
endarteritis 017.9
endocarditis (any valve) 017.9 *[424.91]*
endocardium (any valve) 017.9 *[424.91]*
endocrine glands NEC 017.9
endometrium 016.7

Tuberculosis, tubercular—*continued*
enteric, enterica 014.8
enteritis 014.8
enterocolitis 014.8
epididymis 016.4
epididymitis 016.4
epidural abscess 013.8
  brain 013.3
  spinal cord 013.5
epiglottis 012.3
episcleritis 017.3 *[379.00]*
erythema (induratum) (nodosum) (primary) 017.1
esophagus 017.8
Eustachian tube 017.4
exposure to V01.1
exudative 012.0
  primary, progressive 010.1
eye 017.3
eyelid (primary) 017.0
  lupus 017.0 *[373.4]*
fallopian tube 016.6
fascia 017.9
fauces 012.8
finger 017.9
first infection 010.0
fistula, perirectal 014.8
Florida 011.6
foot 017.9
funnel pelvis 137.3
gallbladder 017.9
galloping (*see also* Tuberculosis, pulmonary)
    011.9
ganglionic 015.9
gastritis 017.9
gastrocolic fistula 014.8
gastroenteritis 014.8
gastrointestinal tract 014.8
general, generalized 018.9
  acute 018.0
  chronic 018.8
genital organs NEC 016.9
  female 016.7
  male 016.5
genitourinary NEC 016.9
genu 015.2
glandulae suprarenalis 017.6
glandular, general 017.2
glottis 012.3
grinders' 011.4
groin 017.2
gum 017.9
hand 017.9
heart 017.9 *[425.8]*
hematogenous—*see* Tuberculosis, miliary
hemoptysis (*see also* Tuberculosis, pulmonary)
    011.9
hemorrhage NEC (*see also* Tuberculosis,
    pulmonary) 011.9
hemothorax 012.0
hepatitis 017.9
hilar lymph nodes 012.1
  primary, progressive 010.8
hip (disease) (joint) 015.1
  bone 015.1 *[730.85]*
hydrocephalus 013.8
hydropneumothorax 012.0
hydrothorax 012.0
hypoadrenalism 017.6
hypopharynx 012.8
ileocecal (hyperplastic) 014.8
ileocolitis 014.8

Tuberculosis, tubercular—*continued*
　ileum 014.8
　iliac spine (superior) 015.0 *[730.88]*
　incipient NEC (*see also* Tuberculosis,
　　pulmonary) 011.9
　indurativa (primary) 017.1
　infantile 010.0
　infection NEC 011.9
　　without clinical manifestation 010.0
　infraclavicular gland 017.2
　inguinal gland 017.2
　inguinalis 017.2
　intestine (any part) 014.8
　iris 017.3 *[364.11]*
　iritis 017.3 *[364.11]*
　ischiorectal 014.8
　jaw 015.7 *[730.88]*
　jejunum 014.8
　joint 015.9
　　hip 015.1
　　knee 015.2
　　specified site NEC 015.8
　　vertebral 015.0 *[730.88]*
　keratitis 017.3 *[370.31]*
　　interstitial 017.3 *[370.59]*
　keratoconjunctivitis 017.3 *[370.31]*
　kidney 016.0
　knee (joint) 015.2
　kyphoscoliosis 015.0 *[737.43]*
　kyphosis 015.0 *[737.41]*
　lacrimal apparatus, gland 017.3
　laryngitis 012.3
　larynx 012.3
　latent 795.51
　leptomeninges, leptomeningitis (cerebral)
　　(spinal) 013.0
　lichenoides (primary) 017.0
　linguae 017.9
　lip 017.9
　liver 017.9
　lordosis 015.0 *[737.42]*
　lung—*see* Tuberculosis, pulmonary
　luposa 017.0
　　eyelid 017.0 *[373.4]*
　lymphadenitis—*see* Tuberculosis, lymph gland
　lymphangitis—*see* Tuberculosis, lymph gland
　lymphatic (gland) (vessel)—*see* Tuberculosis,
　　lymph gland
　lymph gland or node (peripheral) 017.2
　　abdomen 014.8
　　bronchial 012.1
　　　primary, progressive 010.8
　　cervical 017.2
　　hilar 012.1
　　　primary, progressive 010.8
　　intrathoracic 012.1
　　　primary, progressive 010.8
　　mediastinal 012.1
　　　primary, progressive 010.8
　　mesenteric 014.8
　　peripheral 017.2
　　retroperitoneal 014.8
　　tracheobronchial 012.1
　　　primary, progressive 010.8
　malignant NEC (*see also* Tuberculosis,
　　pulmonary) 011.9
　mammary gland 017.9
　marasmus NEC (*see also* Tuberculosis,
　　pulmonary) 011.9
　mastoiditis 015.6
　maternal, affecting fetus or newborn 760.2

Tuberculosis, tubercular—*continued*
　mediastinal (lymph) gland or node 012.1
　　primary, progressive 010.8
　mediastinitis 012.8
　　primary, progressive 010.8
　mediastinopericarditis 017.9 *[420.0]*
　mediastinum 012.8
　　primary, progressive 010.8
　medulla 013.9
　　brain 013.2
　　spinal cord 013.4
　melanosis, Addisonian 017.6
　membrane, brain 013.0
　meninges (cerebral) (spinal) 013.0
　meningitis (basilar) (brain) (cerebral)
　　(cerebrospinal) (spinal) 013.0
　meningoencephalitis 013.0
　mesentery, mesenteric 014.8
　　lymph gland or node 014.8
　miliary (any site) 018.9
　　acute 018.0
　　chronic 018.8
　　specified type NEC 018.8
　millstone makers' 011.4
　miners' 011.4
　moulders' 011.4
　mouth 017.9
　multiple 018.9
　　acute 018.0
　　chronic 018.8
　muscle 017.9
　myelitis 013.6
　myocarditis 017.9 *[422.0]*
　myocardium 017.9 *[422.0]*
　nasal (passage) (sinus) 012.8
　nasopharynx 012.8
　neck gland 017.2
　nephritis 016.0 *[583.81]*
　nerve 017.9
　nose (septum) 012.8
　ocular 017.3
　old NEC 137.0
　　without residuals V12.01
　omentum 014.8
　oophoritis (acute) (chronic) 016.6
　optic 017.3 *[377.39]*
　　nerve trunk 017.3 *[377.39]*
　　papilla, papillae 017.3 *[377.39]*
　orbit 017.3
　orchitis 016.5 *[608.81]*
　organ, specified NEC 017.9
　orificialis (primary) 017.0
　osseous (*see also* Tuberculosis, bone) 015.9
　　[730.8]
　osteitis (*see also* Tuberculosis, bone) 015.9
　　[730.8]
　osteomyelitis (*see also* Tuberculosis, bone)
　　015.9 *[730.8]*
　otitis (media) 017.4
　ovaritis (acute) (chronic) 016.6
　ovary (acute) (chronic) 016.6
　oviducts (acute) (chronic) 016.6
　pachymeningitis 013.0
　palate (soft) 017.9
　pancreas 017.9
　papulonecrotic (primary) 017.0
　parathyroid glands 017.9
　paronychia (primary) 017.0
　parotid gland or region 017.9
　pelvic organ NEC 016.9
　　female 016.7
　　male 016.5

Tuberculosis, tubercular—*continued*
pelvis (bony) 015.7 *[730.85]*
penis 016.5
peribronchitis 011.3
pericarditis 017.9 *[420.0]*
pericardium 017.9 *[420.0]*
perichondritis, larynx 012.3
perineum 017.9
periostitis (*see also* Tuberculosis, bone) 015.9
[730.8]
periphlebitis 017.9
eye vessel 017.3 *[362.18]*
retina 017.3 *[362.18]*
perirectal fistula 014.8
peritoneal gland 014.8
peritoneum 014.0
peritonitis 014.0
pernicious NEC (*see also* Tuberculosis,
pulmonary) 011.9
pharyngitis 012.8
pharynx 012.8
phlyctenulosis (conjunctiva) 017.3 *[370.31]*
phthisis NEC (*see also* Tuberculosis,
pulmonary) 011.9
pituitary gland 017.9
placenta 016.7
pleura, pleural, pleurisy, pleuritis (fibrinous)
(obliterative) (purulent) (simple plastic)
(with effusion) 012.0
primary, progressive 010.1
pneumonia, pneumonic 011.6
pneumothorax 011.7
polyserositis 018.9
acute 018.0
chronic 018.8
potters' 011.4
prepuce 016.5
primary 010.9
complex 010.0
complicated 010.8
with pleurisy or effusion 010.1
progressive 010.8
with pleurisy or effusion 010.1
skin 017.0
proctitis 014.8
prostate 016.5 *[601.4]*
prostatitis 016.5 *[601.4]*
pulmonaris (*see also* Tuberculosis, pulmonary)
011.9
pulmonary (artery) (incipient) (malignant)
(multiple round foci) (pernicious)
(reinfection stage) 011.9
cavitated or with cavitation 011.2
primary, progressive 010.8
childhood type or first infection 010.0
chromogenic acid-fast bacilli 795.39
fibrosis or fibrotic 011.4
infiltrative 011.0
primary, progressive 010.9
nodular 011.1
specified NEC 011.8
sputum positive only 795.39
status following surgical collapse of lung NEC
011.9
pyelitis 016.0 *[590.81]*
pyelonephritis 016.0 *[590.81]*
pyemia—*see* Tuberculosis, miliary
pyonephrosis 016.0
pyopneumothorax 012.0
pyothorax 012.0

Tuberculosis, tubercular—*continued*
rectum (with abscess) 014.8
fistula 014.8
reinfection stage (*see also* Tuberculosis,
pulmonary) 011.9
renal 016.0
renis 016.0
reproductive organ 016.7
respiratory NEC (*see also* Tuberculosis,
pulmonary) 011.9
specified site NEC 012.8
retina 017.3 *[363.13]*
retroperitoneal (lymph gland or node) 014.8
gland 014.8
retropharyngeal abscess 012.8
rheumatism 015.9
rhinitis 012.8
sacroiliac (joint) 015.8
sacrum 015.0 *[730.88]*
salivary gland 017.9
salpingitis (acute) (chronic) 016.6
sandblasters' 011.4
sclera 017.3 *[379.09]*
scoliosis 015.0 *[737.43]*
scrofulous 017.2
scrotum 016.5
seminal tract or vesicle 016.5 *[608.81]*
senile NEC (*see also* Tuberculosis, pulmonary)
011.9
septic NEC (*see also* Tuberculosis, miliary)
018.9
shoulder 015.8
blade 015.7 *[730.8]*
sigmoid 014.8
sinus (accessory) (nasal) 012.8
bone 015.7 *[730.88]*
epididymis 016.4
skeletal NEC (*see also* Osteomyelitis, due to
tuberculosis) 015.9 *[730.8]*
skin (any site) (primary) 017.0
small intestine 014.8
soft palate 017.9
spermatic cord 016.5
spinal
column 015.0 *[730.88]*
cord 013.4
disease 015.0 *[730.88]*
medulla 013.4
membrane 013.0
meninges 013.0
spine 015.0 *[730.88]*
spleen 017.7
splenitis 017.7
spondylitis 015.0 *[720.81]*
spontaneous pneumothorax—*see* Tuberculosis,
pulmonary
sternoclavicular joint 015.8
stomach 017.9
stonemasons' 011.4
struma 017.2
subcutaneous tissue (cellular) (primary) 017.0
subcutis (primary) 017.0
subdeltoid bursa 017.9
submaxillary 017.9
region 017.9
supraclavicular gland 017.2
suprarenal (capsule) (gland) 017.6
swelling, joint (*see also* Tuberculosis, joint)
015.9
symphysis pubis 015.7 *[730.88]*

Tuberculosis, tubercular—*continued*
 synovitis 015.9 *[727.01]*
  hip 015.1 *[727.01]*
  knee 015.2 *[727.01]*
  specified site NEC 015.8 *[727.01]*
  spine or vertebra 015.0 *[727.01]*
 systemic—*see* Tuberculosis, miliary
 tarsitis (eyelid) 017.0 *[373.4]*
  ankle (bone) 015.5 *[730.87]*
 tendon (sheath)—*see* Tuberculosis,
   tenosynovitis
 tenosynovitis 015.9 *[727.01]*
  hip 015.1 *[727.01]*
  knee 015.2 *[727.01]*
  specified site NEC 015.8 *[727.01]*
  spine or vertebra 015.0 *[727.01]*
 testis 016.5 *[608.81]*
 throat 012.8
 thymus gland 017.9
 thyroid gland 017.5
 toe 017.9
 tongue 017.9
 tonsil (lingual) 012.8
 tonsillitis 012.8
 trachea, tracheal 012.8
  gland 012.1
   primary, progressive 010.8
   isolated 012.2
  tracheobronchial 011.3
   glandular 012.1
    primary, progressive 010.8
    isolated 012.2
   lymph gland or node 012.1
    primary, progressive 010.8
 tubal 016.6
 tunica vaginalis 016.5
 typhlitis 014.8
 ulcer (primary) (skin) 017.0
  bowel or intestine 014.8
  specified site NEC—*see* Tuberculosis, by site
 unspecified site—*see* Tuberculosis, pulmonary
 ureter 016.2
 urethra, urethral 016.3
 urinary organ or tract 016.3
  kidney 016.0
 uterus 016.7
 uveal tract 017.3 *[363.13]*
 uvula 017.9
 vaccination, prophylactic (against) V03.2
 vagina 016.7
 vas deferens 016.5
 vein 017.9
 verruca (primary) 017.0
 verrucosa (cutis) (primary) 017.0
 vertebra (column) 015.0 *[730.88]*
 vesiculitis 016.5 *[608.81]*
 viscera NEC 014.8
 vulva 016.7 *[616.51]*
 wrist (joint) 015.8
  bone 015.5 *[730.83]*
Tuberculum
 auriculae 744.29
 occlusal 520.2
 paramolare 520.2
Tuberosity
 jaw, excessive 524.07
 maxillary, entire 524.07
Tuberous sclerosis (brain) 759.5
Tubo-ovarian —*see* condition
Tuboplasty, after previous sterilization V26.0
Tubotympanitis 381.10

Tularemia 021.9
 with
  conjunctivitis 021.3
  pneumonia 021.2
 bronchopneumonic 021.2
 conjunctivitis 021.3
 cryptogenic 021.1
 disseminated 021.8
 enteric 021.1
 generalized 021.8
 glandular 021.8
 intestinal 021.1
 oculoglandular 021.3
 ophthalmic 021.3
 pneumonia 021.2
 pulmonary 021.2
 specified NEC 021.8
 typhoidal 021.1
 ulceroglandular 021.0
 vaccination, prophylactic (against) V03.4
Tularensis conjunctivitis 021.3
Tumefaction —*see also* Swelling
 liver (*see also* Hypertrophy, liver) 789.1
Tumor (M8000/1)—*see also* Neoplasm, by site,
   unspecified nature
 Abrikossov's (M9580/0)—*see also* Neoplasm,
   connective tissue, benign
  malignant (M9580/3)—*see* Neoplasm,
   connective tissue, malignant
 acinar cell (M8550/1)—*see* Neoplasm, by site,
   uncertain behavior
 acinic cell (M8550/1)—*see* Neoplasm, by site,
   uncertain behavior
 adenomatoid (M9054/0)—*see also* Neoplasm,
   by site, benign
  odontogenic (M9300/0) 213.1
   upper jaw (bone) 213.0
 adnexal (skin) (M8390/0)—*see* Neoplasm, skin,
   benign
 adrenal
  cortical (benign) (M8370/0) 227.0
   malignant (M8370/3) 194.0
  rest (M8671/0)—*see* Neoplasm, by site, benign
 alpha cell (M8152/0)
  malignant (M8152/3)
   pancreas 157.4
   specified site NEC—*see* Neoplasm, by site,
    malignant
   unspecified site 157.4
  pancreas 211.7
  specified site NEC—*see* Neoplasm, by site,
   benign
  unspecified site 211.7
 aneurysmal (*see also* Aneurysm) 442.9
 aortic body (M8691/1) 237.3
  malignant (M8691/3) 194.6
 argentaffin (M8241/1)—*see* Neoplasm, by site,
   uncertain behavior
 basal cell (M8090/1)—*see also* Neoplasm, skin,
   uncertain behavior
 benign (M8000/0)—*see* Neoplasm, by site, benign
 beta cell (M8151/0)
  malignant (M8151/3)
   pancreas 157.4
   specified site—*see* Neoplasm, by site,
    malignant
   unspecified site 157.4
  pancreas 211.7
  specified site NEC—*see* Neoplasm, by site,
   benign
  unspecified site 211.7
 blood—*see* Hematoma

Tumor—*continued*
  brenner (M9000/0) 220
    borderline malignancy (M9000/1) 236.2
    malignant (M9000/3) 183.0
    proliferating (M9000/1) 236.2
  Brooke's (M8100/0)—*see* Neoplasm, skin, benign
  brown fat (M8880/0)—*see* Lipoma, by site
  Burkitt's (M9750/3) 200.2
  calcifying epithelial odontogenic (M9340/0) 213.1
    upper jaw (bone) 213.0
  carcinoid (M8240/1) 209.60
    benign 209.60
      appendix 209.51
      ascending colon 209.53
      bronchus 209.61
      cecum 209.52
      colon 209.50
      descending colon 209.55
      duodenum 209.41
      foregut 209.65
      hindgut 209.67
      ileum 209.43
      jejunum 209.42
      kidney 209.64
      large intestine 209.50
      lung 209.61
      midgut 209.66
      rectum 209.57
      sigmoid colon 209.56
      small intestine 209.40
      specified NEC 209.69
      stomach 209.63
      thymus 209.62
      transverse colon 209.54
    malignant (of) 209.20
      appendix 209.11
      ascending colon 209.13
      bronchus 209.21
      cecum 209.12
      colon 209.10
      descending colon 209.15
      duodenum 209.01
      foregut 209.25
      hindgut 209.27
      ileum 209.03
      jejunum 209.02
      kidney 209.24
      large intestine 209.10
      lung 209.21
      midgut 209.26
      rectum 209.17
      sigmoid colon 209.16
      small intestine 209.00
      specified NEC 209.29
      stomach 209.23
      thymus 209.22
      transverse colon 209.14
    secondary—see Tumor, neuroendocrine,
      secondary
  carotid body (M8692/1) 237.3
    malignant (M8692/3) 194.5
  Castleman's (mediastinal lymph node
    hyperplasia) 785.6
  cells (M8001/1)—*see also* Neoplasm, by site,
    unspecified nature
    benign (M8001/0)—*see* Neoplasm, by site,
      benign
    malignant (M8001/3)—*see* Neoplasm, by site,
      malignant
    uncertain whether benign or malignant
      (M8001/1)—*see* Neoplasm, by site,
      uncertain nature

Tumor—*continued*
  cervix
    in pregnancy or childbirth 654.6
      affecting fetus or newborn 763.89
      causing obstructed labor 660.2
        affecting fetus or newborn 763.1
  chondromatous giant cell (M9230/0)—*see*
    Neoplasm, bone, benign
  chromaffin (M8700/0)—*see also* Neoplasm, by
    site, benign
    malignant (M8700/3)—*see* Neoplasm, by site,
      malignant
  Cock's peculiar 706.2
  Codman's (benign chondroblastoma)
    (M9230/0)—*see* Neoplasm, bone, benign
  dentigerous, mixed (M9282/0) 213.1
    upper jaw (bone) 213.0
  dermoid (M9084/0)—*see* Neoplasm, by site,
    benign
    with malignant transformation (M9084/3)
      183.0
  desmoid (extra-abdominal) (M8821/1)—*see
    also* Neoplasm, connective tissue, uncertain
    behavior
    abdominal (M8822/1)—*see* Neoplasm,
      connective tissue, uncertain behavior
  embryonal (mixed) (M9080/1)—*see also*
    Neoplasm, by site, uncertain behavior
    liver (M9080/3) 155.0
  endodermal sinus (M9071/3)
    specified site—*see* Neoplasm, by site,
      malignant
    unspecified site
      female 183.0
      male 186.9
  epithelial
    benign (M8010/0)—*see* Neoplasm, by site,
      benign
    malignant (M8010/3)—*see* Neoplasm, by site,
      malignant
  Ewing's (M9260/3)—*see* Neoplasm, bone,
    malignant
  fatty—*see* Lipoma
  fetal, causing disproportion 653.7
    causing obstructed labor 660.1
  fibroid (M8890/0)—*see* Leiomyoma
  G cell (M8153/1)
    malignant (M8153/3)
      pancreas 157.4
      specified site NEC—*see* Neoplasm, by site,
        malignant
      unspecified site 157.4
    specified site—*see* Neoplasm, by site,
      uncertain behavior
    unspecified site 235.5
  giant cell (type) (M8003/1)—*see also*
    Neoplasm, by site, unspecified nature
    bone (M9250/1) 238.0
      malignant (M9250/3)—*see* Neoplasm, bone,
        malignant
    chondromatous (M9230/0)—*see* Neoplasm,
      bone, benign
    malignant (M8003/3)—*see* Neoplasm, by site,
      malignant
    peripheral (gingiva) 523.8
    soft parts (M9251/1)—*see also* Neoplasm,
      connective tissue, uncertain behavior
      malignant (M9251/3)—*see* Neoplasm,
        connective tissue, malignant
    tendon sheath 727.02

Tumor—*continued*

glomus (M8711/0)—*see also* Hemangioma, by site
  jugulare (M8690/1) 237.3
    malignant (M8690/3) 194.6
gonadal stromal (M8590/1)—*see* Neoplasm, by site, uncertain behavior
granular cell (M9580/0)—*see also* Neoplasm, connective tissue, benign
  malignant (M9580/3)—*see* Neoplasm, connective tissue, malignant
granulosa cell (M8620/1) 236.2
  malignant (M8620/3) 183.0
granulosa cell-theca cell (M8621/1) 236.2
  malignant (M8621/3) 183.0
Grawitz's (hypernephroma) (M8312/3) 189.0
hazard-crile (M8350/3) 193
hemorrhoidal—*see* Hemorrhoids
hilar cell (M8660/0) 220
hurthle cell (benign) (M8290/0) 226
  malignant (M8290/3) 193
hydatid (*see also* Echinococcus) 122.9
hypernephroid (M8311/1)—*see also* Neoplasm, by site, uncertain behavior
interstitial cell (M8650/1)—*see also* Neoplasm, by site, uncertain behavior
  benign (M8650/0)—*see* Neoplasm, by site, benign
  malignant (M8650/3)—*see* Neoplasm, by site, malignant
islet cell (M8150/0)
  malignant (M8150/3)
    pancreas 157.4
    specified site—*see* Neoplasm, by site, malignant
    unspecified site 157.4
  pancreas 211.7
  specified site NEC—*see* Neoplasm, by site, benign
  unspecified site 211.7
juxtaglomerular (M8361/1) 236.91
Krukenberg's (M8490/6) 198.6
Leydig cell (M8650/1)
  benign (M8650/0)
    specified site—*see* Neoplasm, by site, benign
    unspecified site
      female 220
      male 220.0
  malignant (M8650/3)
    specified site—*see* Neoplasm, by site, malignant
    unspecified site
      female 183.0
      male 186.9
  specified site—*see* Neoplasm, by site, uncertain behavior
  unspecified site
    female 236.2
    male 236.4
lipid cell, ovary (M8670/0) 220
lipoid cell, ovary (M8670/0) 220
lymphomatous, benign (M9590/0)—*see also* Neoplasm, by site, benign
lysis syndrome (following antineoplastic drug therapy) (spontaneous) 277.88
Malherbe's (M8110/0)—*see* Neoplasm, skin, benign

Tumor—*continued*

malignant (M8000/3)—*see also* Neoplasm, by site, malignant
  fusiform cell (type) (M8004/3)—*see* Neoplasm, by site, malignant
  giant cell (type) (M8003/3)—*see* Neoplasm, by site, malignant
  mixed NEC (M8940/3)—*see* Neoplasm, by site, malignant
  small cell (type) (M8002/3)—*see* Neoplasm, by site, malignant
  spindle cell (type) (M8004/3)—*see* Neoplasm, by site, malignant
mast cell (M9740/1) 238.5
  malignant (M9740/3) 202.6
melanotic, neuroectodermal (M9363/0)—*see* Neoplasm, by site, benign
Merkel cell—*see* Carcinoma, Merkel cell
mesenchymal
  malignant (M8800/3)—*see* Neoplasm, connective tissue, malignant
  mixed (M8990/1)—*see* Neoplasm, connective tissue, uncertain behavior
mesodermal, mixed (M8951/3)—*see also* Neoplasm, by site, malignant
  liver 155.0
mesonephric (M9110/1)—*see also* Neoplasm, by site, uncertain behavior
  malignant (M9110/3)—*see* Neoplasm, by site, malignant
metastatic
  from specified site (M8000/3)—*see* Neoplasm, by site, malignant
  to specified site (M8000/6)—*see* Neoplasm, by site, malignant, secondary
mixed NEC (M8940/0)—*see also* Neoplasm, by site, benign
  malignant (M8940/3)—*see* Neoplasm, by site, malignant
mucocarcinoid, malignant (M8243/3)—*see* Neoplasm, by site, malignant
mucoepidermoid (M8430/1)—*see* Neoplasm, by site, uncertain behavior
Müllerian, mixed (M8950/3)—*see* Neoplasm, by site, malignant
myoepithelial (M8982/0)—*see* Neoplasm, by site, benign
neuroendocrine 209.60
  malignant poorly differentiated 209.30
  secondary 209.70
    bone 209.73
    distant lymph nodes 209.71
    liver 209.72
    peritoneum 209.74
    site specified NEC 209.79
neurogenic olfactory (M9520/3) 160.0
nonencapsulated sclerosing (M8350/3) 193
odontogenic (M9270/1) 238.0
  adenomatoid (M9300/0) 213.1
    upper jaw (bone) 213.0
  benign (M9270/0) 213.1
    upper jaw (bone) 213.0
  calcifying epithelial (M9340/0) 213.1
    upper jaw (bone) 213.0
  malignant (M9270/3) 170.1
    upper jaw (bone) 170.0
  squamous (M9312/0) 213.1
    upper jaw (bone) 213.0
ovarian stromal (M8590/1) 236.2

Tumor—*continued*

ovary

in pregnancy or childbirth 654.4

affecting fetus or newborn 763.89

causing obstructed labor 660.2

affecting fetus or newborn 763.1

pacinian (M9507/0)—*see* Neoplasm, skin, benign

Pancoast's (M8010/3) 162.3

papillary—*see* Papilloma

pelvic, in pregnancy or childbirth 654.9

affecting fetus or newborn 763.89

causing obstructed labor 660.2

affecting fetus or newborn 763.1

phantom 300.11

plasma cell (M9731/1) 238.6

benign (M9731/0)—*see* Neoplasm, by site, benign

malignant (M9731/3) 203.8

polyvesicular vitelline (M9071/3)

specified site—*see* Neoplasm, by site, malignant

unspecified site

female 183.0

male 186.9

Pott's puffy (*see also* Osteomyelitis) 730.2

Rathke's pouch (M9350/1) 237.0

regaud's (M8082/3)—*see* Neoplasm, nasopharynx, malignant

rete cell (M8140/0) 222.0

retinal anlage (M9363/0)—*see* Neoplasm, by site, benign

Rokitansky's 620.2

salivary gland type, mixed (M8940/0)—*see also* Neoplasm, by site, benign

malignant (M8940/3)—*see* Neoplasm, by site, malignant

Sampson's 617.1

Schloffer's (*see also* Peritonitis) 567.29

Schmincke (M8082/3)—*see* Neoplasm, nasopharynx, malignant

sebaceous (*see also* Cyst, sebaceous) 706.2

secondary (M8000/6)—*see* Neoplasm, by site, secondary

carcinoid — *see* Tumor, neuroendocrine, secondary

neuroendocrine — *see* Tumor, neuroendocrine, secondary

Sertoli cell (M8640/0)

with lipid storage (M8641/0)

specified site—*see* Neoplasm, by site, benign

unspecified site

female 220

male 222.0

specified site—*see* Neoplasm, by site, benign

unspecified site

female 220

male 222.0

Sertoli-Leydig cell (M8631/0)

specified site—*see* Neoplasm, by site, benign

unspecified site

female 220

male 222.0

sex cord (-stromal) (M8590/1)—*see* Neoplasm, by site, uncertain behavior

skin appendage (M8390/0)—*see* Neoplasm, skin, benign

Tumor—*continued*

soft tissue

benign (M8800/0)—*see* Neoplasm, connective tissue, benign

malignant (M8800/3)—*see* Neoplasm, connective tissue, malignant

sternomastoid 754.1

stromal

abdomen

benign 215.5

malignant NEC 171.5

uncertain behavior 238.1

digestive system 238.1

benign 215.5

malignant NEC 171.5

uncertain behavior 238.1

endometrium (endometrial) 236.0

gastric 238.1

benign 215.5

malignant NEC 171.5

uncertain behavior 238.1

gastrointestinal 238.1

benign 215.5

malignant NEC 171.5

uncertain behavior 238.1

intestine (small) 238.1

benign 215.5

malignant 152.9

uncertain behavior 238.1

stomach 238.1

benign 215.5

malignant 151.9

uncertain behavior 238.1

superior sulcus (lung) (pulmonary) (syndrome) (M8010/3) 162.3

suprasulcus (M8010/3) 162.3

sweat gland (M8400/1)—*see also* Neoplasm, skin, uncertain behavior

benign (M8400/0)—*see* Neoplasm, skin, benign

malignant (M8400/3)—*see* Neoplasm, skin, malignant

syphilitic brain 094.89

congenital 090.49

testicular stromal (M8590/1) 236.4

theca cell (M8600/0) 220

theca cell-granulosa cell (M8621/1) 236.2

theca-lutein (M8610/0) 220

turban (M8200/0) 216.4

uterus

in pregnancy or childbirth 654.1

affecting fetus or newborn 763.89

causing obstructed labor 660.2

affecting fetus or newborn 763.1

vagina

in pregnancy or childbirth 654.7

affecting fetus or newborn 763.89

causing obstructed labor 660.2

affecting fetus or newborn 763.1

varicose (*see also* Varicose, vein) 454.9

von Recklinghausen's (M9540/1) 237.71

vulva

in pregnancy or childbirth 654.8

affecting fetus or newborn 763.89

causing obstructed labor 660.2

affecting fetus or newborn 763.1

Warthin's (salivary gland) (M8561/0) 210.2

white—*see also* Tuberculosis, arthritis

White-Darier 757.39

Wilms' (nephroblastoma) (M8960/3) 189.0

Tumor—*continued*
  yolk sac (M9071/3)
    specified site—*see* Neoplasm, by site, malignant
    unspecified site
      female 183.0
      male 186.9
Tumorlet (M8040/1)—*see* Neoplasm, by site,
  uncertain behavior
Tungiasis 134.1
Tunica vasculosa lentis 743.39
Tunnel vision 368.45
Turban tumor (M8200/0) 216.4
Türck's trachoma (chronic catarrhal laryngitis)
  476.0
Türk's syndrome (ocular retraction syndrome)
  378.71
Turner's
  hypoplasia (tooth) 520.4
  syndrome 758.6
  tooth 520.4
Turner-Kieser syndrome (hereditary
  osteo-onychodysplasia) 756.89
Turner-Varny syndrome 758.6
Turricephaly 756.0
Tussis convulsiva (*see also* Whooping cough) 033.9
Twiddler's syndrome (due to)
  automatic implantable defibrillator 996.04
  pacemaker 996.01
Twin
  affected by maternal complications of pregnancy
    761.5
  conjoined 759.4
    fetal 678.1
  healthy liveborn—*see* Newborn, twin
  pregnancy (complicating delivery) NEC 651.0
    with fetal loss and retention of one fetus 651.3
    conjoined 678.1
    following (elective) fetal reduction 651.7
Twinning, teeth 520.2
Twist, twisted
  bowel, colon, or intestine 560.2
  hair (congenital) 757.4
  mesentery 560.2
  omentum 560.2
  organ or site, congenital NEC—*see* Anomaly,
    specified type NEC
  ovarian pedicle 620.5
    congenital 752.0
  umbilical cord—*see* Compression, umbilical
    cord
Twitch 781.0
Tylosis 700
  buccalis 528.6
  gingiva 523.8
  linguae 528.6
  palmaris et plantaris 757.39
Tympanism 787.3
Tympanites (abdominal) (intestine) 787.3
Tympanitis —*see* Myringitis
Tympanosclerosis 385.00
  involving
    combined sites NEC 385.09
      with tympanic membrane 385.03
    tympanic membrane 385.01
      with ossicles 385.02
        and middle ear 385.03
Tympanum —*see* condition
Tympany
  abdomen 787.3
  chest 786.7
Typhlitis (*see also* Appendicitis) 541

Typhoenteritis 002.0
Typhogastric fever 002.0
Typhoid (abortive) (ambulant) (any site) (fever)
    (hemorrhagic) (infection) (intermittent)
    (malignant) (rheumatic) 002.0
  with pneumonia 002.0 *[484.8]*
  abdominal 002.0
  carrier (suspected) of V02.1
  cholecystitis (current) 002.0
  clinical (Widal and blood test negative) 002.0
  endocarditis 002.0 *[421.1]*
  inoculation reaction—*see* Complications,
    vaccination
  meningitis 002.0 *[320.7]*
  mesenteric lymph nodes 002.0
  myocarditis 002.0 *[422.0]*
  osteomyelitis (*see also* Osteomyelitis, due to,
    typhoid) 002.0 *[730.8]*
  perichondritis, larynx 002.0 *[478.71]*
  pneumonia 002.0 *[484.8]*
  spine 002.0 *[720.81]*
  ulcer (perforating) 002.0
  vaccination, prophylactic (against) V03.1
  Widal negative 002.0
Typhomalaria (fever) (*see also* Malaria) 084.6
Typhomania 002.0
Typhoperitonitis 002.0
Typhus (fever) 081.9
  abdominal, abdominalis 002.0
  African tick 082.1
  amarillic (*see also* Fever, Yellow) 060.9
  brain 081.9
  cerebral 081.9
  classical 080
  endemic (flea-borne) 081.0
  epidemic (louse-borne) 080
  exanthematic NEC 080
  exanthematicus SAI 080
    brillii SAI 081.1
    Mexicanus SAI 081.0
    pediculo vestimenti causa 080
    typhus murinus 081.0
  flea-borne 081.0
  Indian tick 082.1
  Kenya tick 082.1
  louse-borne 080
  Mexican 081.0
    flea-borne 081.0
    louse-borne 080
    tabardillo 080
  mite-borne 081.2
  murine 081.0
  North Asian tick-borne 082.2
  petechial 081.9
  Queensland tick 082.3
  rat 081.0
  recrudescent 081.1
  recurrent (*see also* Fever, relapsing) 087.9
  São Paulo 082.0
  scrub (China) (India) (Malaya) (New Guinea)
    081.2
  shop (of Malaya) 081.0
  Siberian tick 082.2
  tick-borne NEC 082.9
  tropical 081.2
  vaccination, prophylactic (against) V05.8
Tyrosinemia 270.2
  neonatal 775.89
Tyrosinosis (Medes) (Sakai) 270.2
Tyrosinuria 270.2
Tyrosyluria 270.2

U

Uehlinger's syndrome (acropachyderma) 757.39
Uhl's anomaly or disease (hypoplasia of myocardium, right ventricle) 746.84
Ulcer, ulcerated, ulcerating, ulceration, ulcerative 707.9
  with gangrene 707.9 *[785.4]*
  abdomen (wall) (*see also* Ulcer, skin) 707.8
  ala, nose 478.19
  alveolar process 526.5
  amebic (intestine) 006.9
    skin 006.6
  anastomotic—*see* Ulcer, gastrojejunal
  anorectal 569.41
  antral—*see* Ulcer, stomach
  anus (sphincter) (solitary) 569.41
    varicose—*see* Varicose, ulcer, anus
  aorta —*see* Aneurysm
  aphthous (oral) (recurrent) 528.2
    genital organ(s)
      female 616.50
      male 608.89
    mouth 528.2
  arm (*see also* Ulcer, skin) 707.8
  arteriosclerotic plaque—*see* Arteriosclerosis, by site
  artery NEC 447.2
    without rupture 447.8
  atrophic NEC—*see* Ulcer, skin
  Barrett's (chronic peptic ulcer of esophagus) 530.85
  bile duct 576.8
  bladder (solitary) (sphincter) 596.89
    bilharzial (*see also* Schistosomiasis) 120.9 *[595.4]*
    submucosal (*see also* Cystitis) 595.1
    tuberculous (*see also* Tuberculosis) 016.1
  bleeding NEC—*see* Ulcer, peptic, with hemorrhage
  bone 730.9
  bowel (*see also* Ulcer, intestine) 569.82
  breast 611.0
  bronchitis 491.8
  bronchus 519.19
  buccal (cavity) (traumatic) 528.9
  burn (acute)—*see* Ulcer, duodenum
  Buruli 031.1
  buttock (*see also* Ulcer, skin) 707.8
    decubitus (*see also* Ulcer, pressure) 707.00
  cancerous (M8000/3)—*see* Neoplasm, by site, malignant
  cardia—*see* Ulcer, stomach
  cardio-esophageal (peptic) 530.20
    with bleeding 530.21
  cecum (*see also* Ulcer, intestine) 569.82
  cervix (uteri) (trophic) 622.0
    with mention of cervicitis 616.0
  chancroidal 099.0
  chest (wall) (*see also* Ulcer, skin) 707.8
  Chiclero 085.4
  chin (pyogenic) (*see also* Ulcer, skin) 707.8
  chronic (cause unknown)—*see also* Ulcer, skin
    penis 607.89
  Cochin-China 085.1
  colitis —*see* Colitis, ulcerative
  colon (*see also* Ulcer, intestine) 569.82
  conjunctiva (acute) (postinfectional) 372.00

Ulcer, ulcerated, ulcerating—*continued*
  cornea (infectional) 370.00
    with perforation 370.06
    annular 370.02
    catarrhal 370.01
    central 370.03
    dendritic 054.42
    marginal 370.01
    mycotic 370.05
    phlyctenular, tuberculous (*see also* Tuberculosis) 017.3 *[370.31]*
    ring 370.02
    rodent 370.07
    serpent, serpiginous 370.04
    superficial marginal 370.01
    tuberculous (*see also* Tuberculosis) 017.3 *[370.31]*
  corpus cavernosum (chronic) 607.89
  crural—*see* Ulcer, lower extremity
  Curling's—*see* Ulcer, duodenum
  Cushing's—*see* Ulcer, peptic
  cystitis (interstitial) 595.1
  decubitus (unspecified site) (*see also* Ulcer, pressure) 707.00
    with gangrene 707.00 *[785.4]*
    ankle 707.06
    back
      lower 707.03
      upper 707.02
    buttock 707.05
    coccyx 707.03
    elbow 707.01
    head 707.09
    heel 707.07
    hip 707.04
    other site 707.09
    sacrum 707.03
    shoulder blades 707.02
  dendritic 054.42
  diabetes, diabetic (mellitus) 250.8 *[707.9]*
    due to secondary diabetes 249.8 *[707.9]*
    lower limb 250.8 *[707.10]*
      due to secondary diabetes 249.8 *[707.10]*
      ankle 250.8 *[707.13]*
        due to secondary diabetes 249.8 *[707.13]*
      calf 250.8 *[707.12]*
        due to secondary diabetes 249.8 *[707.12]*
      foot 250.8 *[707.15]*
        due to secondary diabetes 249.8 *[707.15]*
      heel 250.8 *[707.14]*
        due to secondary diabetes 249.8 *[707.14]*
      knee 250.8 *[707.19]*
        due to secondary diabetes 249.8 *[707.19]*
      specified site NEC 250.8 *[707.19]*
        due to secondary diabetes 249.8 *[707.19]*
      thigh 250.8 *[707.11]*
        due to secondary diabetes 249.8 *[707.11]*
      toes 250.8 *[707.15]*
        due to secondary diabetes 249.8 *[707.15]*
    specified site NEC 250.8 *[707.8]*
      due to secondary diabetes 249.8 *[707.8]*
  Dieulafoy—*see* Lesion, Dieulafoy
  due to
    infection NEC—*see* Ulcer, skin
    radiation, radium—*see* Ulcer, by site
    trophic disturbance (any region)—*see* Ulcer, skin
    x-ray—*see* Ulcer, by site

Ulcer, ulcerated, ulcerating—*continued*
  duodenum, duodenal (eroded) (peptic) 532.9

> *Note—Use the following fifth-digit*
> *subclassification with categories 531-534:*
>
> 0 *without mention of obstruction*
> 1 *with obstruction*

  with
    hemorrhage (chronic) 532.4
      and perforation 532.6
    perforation (chronic) 532.5
      and hemorrhage 532.6
  acute 532.3
    with
      hemorrhage 532.0
        and perforation 532.2
      perforation 532.1
        and hemorrhage 532.2
  bleeding (recurrent)—*see* Ulcer, duodenum,
    with hemorrhage
  chronic 532.7
    with
      hemorrhage 532.4
        and perforation 532.6
      perforation 532.5
        and hemorrhage 532.6
  penetrating—*see* Ulcer, duodenum, with
    perforation
  perforating—*see* Ulcer, duodenum, with
    perforation
  dysenteric NEC 009.0
  elusive 595.1
  endocarditis (any valve) (acute) (chronic)
    (subacute) 421.0
  enteritis —*see* Colitis, ulcerative
  enterocolitis 556.0
  epiglottis 478.79
  esophagus (peptic) 530.20
    with bleeding 530.21
    due to ingestion
      aspirin 530.20
      chemicals 530.20
      medicinal agents 530.20
    fungal 530.20
    infectional 530.20
    varicose (*see also* Varix, esophagus) 456.1
      bleeding (*see also* Varix, esophagus,
        bleeding) 456.0
  eye NEC 360.00
    dendritic 054.42
  eyelid (region) 373.01
  face (*see also* Ulcer, skin) 707.8
  fauces 478.29
  Fenwick (-Hunner) (solitary) (*see also* Cystitis)
    595.1
  fistulous NEC—*see* Ulcer, skin
  foot (indolent) (*see also* Ulcer, lower extremity)
    707.15
    perforating 707.15
      leprous 030.1
      syphilitic 094.0
    trophic 707.15
    varicose 454.0
      inflamed or infected 454.2
  frambesial, initial or primary 102.0
  gallbladder or duct 575.8
  gall duct 576.8
  gangrenous (*see also* Gangrene) 785.4
  gastric—*see* Ulcer, stomach
  gastrocolic—*see* Ulcer, gastrojejunal

Ulcer, ulcerated, ulcerating—*continued*
  gastroduodenal—*see* Ulcer, peptic
  gastroesophageal—*see* Ulcer, stomach
  gastrohepatic—*see* Ulcer, stomach
  gastrointestinal—*see* Ulcer, gastrojejunal
  gastrojejunal (eroded) (peptic) 534.9

> *Note—Use the following fifth-digit*
> *subclassification with categories 531-534:*
>
> 0 *without mention of obstruction*
> 1 *with obstruction*

  with
    hemorrhage (chronic) 534.4
      and perforation 534.6
    perforation 534.5
      and hemorrhage 534.6
  acute 534.3
    with
      hemorrhage 534.0
        and perforation 534.2
      perforation 534.1
        and hemorrhage 534.2
  bleeding (recurrent)—*see* Ulcer, gastrojejunal,
    with hemorrhage
  chronic 534.7
    with
      hemorrhage 534.4
        and perforation 534.6
      perforation 534.5
        and hemorrhage 534.6
  penetrating—*see* Ulcer, gastrojejunal, with
    perforation
  perforating—*see* Ulcer, gastrojejunal, with
    perforation
  gastrojejunocolic—*see* Ulcer, gastrojejunal
  genital organ
    female 629.89
    male 608.89
  gingiva 523.8
  gingivitis 523.10
  glottis 478.79
  granuloma of pudenda 099.2
  groin (*see also* Ulcer, skin) 707.8
  gum 523.8
  gumma, due to yaws 102.4
  hand (*see also* Ulcer, skin) 707.8
  hard palate 528.9
  heel (*see also* Ulcer, lower extremity) 707.14
    decubitus (*see also* Ulcer, pressure) 707.07
  hemorrhoids 455.8
    external 455.5
    internal 455.2
  hip (*see also* Ulcer, skin) 707.8
    decubitus (*see also* Ulcer, pressure) 707.04
  Hunner's 595.1
  hypopharynx 478.29
  hypopyon (chronic) (subacute) 370.04
  hypostaticum—*see* Ulcer, varicose
  ileocolitis 556.1
  ileum (*see also* Ulcer, intestine) 569.82
  intestine, intestinal 569.82
    with perforation 569.83
    amebic 006.9
    duodenal—*see* Ulcer, duodenum
    granulocytopenic (with hemorrhage) 288.09
    marginal 569.82
    perforating 569.83
    small, primary 569.82
    stercoraceous 569.82
    stercoral 569.82

Ulcer, ulcerated, ulcerating—*continued*
  tuberculous (*see also* Tuberculosis) 014.8
  typhoid (fever) 002.0
  varicose 456.8
  ischemic 707.9
    lower extremity (*see also* Ulcer, lower
      extremity) 707.10
      ankle 707.13
      calf 707.12
      foot 707.15
      heel 707.14
      knee 707.19
      specified site NEC 707.19
      thigh 707.11
      toes 707.15
  jejunum, jejunal—*see* Ulcer, gastrojejunal
  keratitis (*see also* Ulcer, cornea) 370.00
  knee—*see* Ulcer, lower extremity
  labium (majus) (minus) 616.50
  laryngitis (*see also* Laryngitis) 464.00
    with obstruction 464.01
  larynx (aphthous) (contact) 478.79
    diphtheritic 032.3
  leg—*see* Ulcer, lower extremity
  lip 528.5
  Lipschütz's 616.50
  lower extremity (atrophic) (chronic)
    (neurogenic) (perforating) (pyogenic)
    (trophic) (tropical) 707.10
    with gangrene (*see also* Ulcer, lower
      extremity) 707.10 *[785.4]*
      arteriosclerotic 440.24
    ankle 707.13
    arteriosclerotic 440.23
      with gangrene 440.24
    calf 707.12
    decubitus (*see also* Ulcer, pressure) 707.00
      with gangrene 707.00 *[785.4]*
      ankle 707.06
      buttock 707.05
      heel 707.07
      hip 707.04
    foot 707.15
    heel 707.14
    knee 707.19
    specified site NEC 707.19
    thigh 707.11
    toes 707.15
    varicose 454.0
      inflamed or infected 454.2
  luetic—*see* Ulcer, syphilitic
  lung 518.89
    tuberculous (*see also* Tuberculosis) 011.2
  malignant (M8000/3)—*see* Neoplasm, by site,
    malignant
  marginal NEC—*see* Ulcer, gastrojejunal
  meatus (urinarius) 597.89
  Meckel's diverticulum 751.0
  Meleney's (chronic undermining) 686.09
  Mooren's (cornea) 370.07
  mouth (traumatic) 528.9
  mycobacterial (skin) 031.1
  nasopharynx 478.29
  navel cord (newborn) 771.4
  neck (*see also* Ulcer, skin) 707.8
    uterus 622.0
  neurogenic NEC—*see* Ulcer, skin

Ulcer, ulcerated, ulcerating—*continued*
  nose, nasal (infectional) (passage) 478.19
    septum 478.19
      varicose 456.8
    skin—*see* Ulcer, skin
    spirochetal NEC 104.8
  oral mucosa (traumatic) 528.9
  palate (soft) 528.9
  penetrating NEC—*see* Ulcer, peptic, with
    perforation
  penis (chronic) 607.89
  peptic (site unspecified) 533.9

> *Note—Use the following fifth-digit*
> *subclassification with categories 531-534:*
>
> *0 without mention of obstruction*
> *1 with obstruction*

    with
      hemorrhage 533.4
        and perforation 533.6
      perforation (chronic) 533.5
        and hemorrhage 533.6
    acute 533.3
      with
        hemorrhage 533.0
          and perforation 533.2
        perforation 533.1
          and hemorrhage 533.2
    bleeding (recurrent)—*see* Ulcer, peptic, with
      hemorrhage
    chronic 533.7
      with
        hemorrhage 533.4
          and perforation 533.6
        perforation 533.5
          and hemorrhage 533.6
    penetrating—*see* Ulcer, peptic, with
      perforation
  perforating NEC (*see also* Ulcer, peptic, with
    perforation) 533.5
    skin 707.9
  perineum (*see also* Ulcer, skin) 707.8
  peritonsillar 474.8
  phagedenic (tropical) NEC—*see* Ulcer, skin
  pharynx 478.29
  phlebitis—*see* Phlebitis
  plaster (*see also* Ulcer, pressure) 707.00
  popliteal space—*see* Ulcer, lower extremity
  postpyloric—*see* Ulcer, duodenum
  prepuce 607.89
  prepyloric—*see* Ulcer, stomach
  pressure 707.00
    with
      abrasion, blister, partial thickness skin loss
        involving epidermis and/or dermis
        707.22
      full thickness skin loss involving damage or
        necrosis of subcutaneous tissue 707.23
      gangrene 707.00 [785.4]
      necrosis of soft tissues through to underlying
        muscle, tendon, or bone 707.24
    ankle 707.06
    back
      lower 707.03
      upper 707.02
    buttock 707.05
    coccyx 707.03
    elbow 707.01
    head 707.09
    healed — omit code
    healing — code to Ulcer, pressure, by stage

Ulcer, ulcerated, ulcerating—*continued*
　heel 707.07
　hip 707.04
　other site 707.09
　sacrum 707.03
　shoulder blades 707.02
　stage
　　I (healing) 707.21
　　II (healing) 707.22
　　III (healing) 707.23
　　IV (healing) 707.24
　　unspecified (healing) 707.20
　unstageable 707.25
　primary of intestine 569.82
　　with perforation 569.83
　proctitis 556.2
　　with ulcerative sigmoiditis 556.3
　prostate 601.8
　pseudopeptic—*see* Ulcer, peptic
　pyloric—*see* Ulcer, stomach
　rectosigmoid 569.82
　　with perforation 569.83
　rectum (sphincter) (solitary) 569.41
　　stercoraceous, stercoral 569.41
　　varicose—*see* Varicose, ulcer, anus
　retina (*see also* Chorioretinitis) 363.20
　rodent (M8090/3)—*see also* Neoplasm, skin,
　　malignant
　　cornea 370.07
　round—*see* Ulcer, stomach
　sacrum (region) (*see also* Ulcer, skin) 707.8
　Saemisch's 370.04
　scalp (*see also* Ulcer, skin) 707.8
　sclera 379.09
　scrofulous (*see also* Tuberculosis) 017.2
　scrotum 608.89
　　tuberculous (*see also* Tuberculosis) 016.5
　　varicose 456.4
　seminal vesicle 608.89
　sigmoid 569.82
　　with perforation 569.83
　skin (atrophic) (chronic) (neurogenic)
　　(non-healing) (perforating) (pyogenic)
　　(trophic) 707.9
　　with gangrene 707.9 *[785.4]*
　　amebic 006.6
　　decubitus (*see also* Ulcer, pressure) 707.00
　　　with gangrene 707.00 *[785.4]*
　　in granulocytopenia 288.09
　　lower extremity (*see also* Ulcer, lower
　　　extremity) 707.10
　　　with gangrene 707.10 *[785.4]*
　　　arteriosclerotic 440.24
　　　ankle 707.13
　　　arteriosclerotic 440.23
　　　　with gangrene 440.24
　　　calf 707.12
　　　foot 707.15
　　　heel 707.14
　　　knee 707.19
　　　specified site NEC 707.19
　　　thigh 707.11
　　　toes 707.15
　　mycobacterial 031.1
　　syphilitic (early) (secondary) 091.3
　　tuberculous (primary) (*see also* Tuberculosis)
　　　017.0
　　varicose—*see* Ulcer, varicose
　sloughing NEC—*see* Ulcer, skin
　soft palate 528.9
　solitary, anus or rectum (sphincter) 569.41

Ulcer, ulcerated, ulcerating—*continued*
　sore throat 462
　　streptococcal 034.0
　spermatic cord 608.89
　spine (tuberculous) 015.0 *[730.88]*
　stasis (leg) (venous) 454.0
　　with varicose veins 454.0
　　inflamed or infected 454.2
　　without varicose veins 459.81
　stercoral, stercoraceous 569.82
　　with perforation 569.83
　　anus or rectum 569.41
　stoma, stomal—*see* Ulcer, gastrojejunal
　stomach (eroded) (peptic) (round) 531.9

> *Note—Use the following fifth-digit
> subclassification with categories 531-534:*
>
> *0　without mention of obstruction*
> *1　with obstruction*

　　with
　　　hemorrhage 531.4
　　　　and perforation 531.6
　　　perforation (chronic) 531.5
　　　　and hemorrhage 531.6
　　acute 531.3
　　　with
　　　　hemorrhage 531.0
　　　　　and perforation 531.2
　　　　perforation 531.1
　　　　　and hemorrhage 531.2
　　bleeding (recurrent)—*see* Ulcer, stomach,
　　　with hemorrhage
　　chronic 531.7
　　　with
　　　　hemorrhage 531.4
　　　　　and perforation 531.6
　　　　perforation 531.5
　　　　　and hemorrhage 531.6
　　penetrating—*see* Ulcer, stomach, with
　　　perforation
　　perforating—*see* Ulcer, stomach, with
　　　perforation
　stomatitis 528.00
　stress—*see* Ulcer, peptic
　strumous (tuberculous) (*see also* Tuberculosis)
　　017.2
　submental (*see also* Ulcer, skin) 707.8
　submucosal, bladder 595.1
　syphilitic (any site) (early) (secondary) 091.3
　　late 095.9
　　perforating 095.9
　　　foot 094.0
　testis 608.89
　thigh—*see* Ulcer, lower extremity
　throat 478.29
　　diphtheritic 032.0
　toe—*see* Ulcer, lower extremity
　tongue (traumatic) 529.0
　tonsil 474.8
　　diphtheritic 032.0
　trachea 519.19
　trophic—*see* Ulcer, skin
　tropical NEC (*see also* Ulcer, skin) 707.9
　tuberculous—*see* Tuberculosis, ulcer
　tunica vaginalis 608.89
　turbinate 730.9
　typhoid (fever) 002.0
　　perforating 002.0
　umbilicus (newborn) 771.4
　unspecified site NEC—*see* Ulcer, skin

Ulcer, ulcerated, ulcerating—*continued*
urethra (meatus) (*see also* Urethritis) 597.89
uterus 621.8
  cervix 622.0
    with mention of cervicitis 616.0
  neck 622.0
    with mention of cervicitis 616.0
vagina 616.89
valve, heart 421.0
varicose (lower extremity, any part) 454.0
  anus—*see* Varicose, ulcer, anus
  broad ligament 456.5
  esophagus (*see also* Varix, esophagus) 456.1
    bleeding (*see also* Varix, esophagus,
      bleeding) 456.0
  inflamed or infected 454.2
  nasal septum 456.8
  perineum 456.6
  rectum—*see* Varicose, ulcer, anus
  scrotum 456.4
  specified site NEC 456.8
  sublingual 456.3
  vulva 456.6
vas deferens 608.89
vesical (*see also* Ulcer, bladder) 596.89
vulva (acute) (infectional) 616.50
  Behçet's syndrome 136.1 *[616.51]*
  herpetic 054.12
  tuberculous 016.7 *[616.51]*
vulvobuccal, recurring 616.50
x-ray—*see* Ulcer, by site
yaws 102.4
Ulcerosa scarlatina 034.1
Ulcus —*see also* Ulcer
cutis tuberculosum (*see also* Tuberculosis)
  017.0
duodeni—*see* Ulcer, duodenum
durum 091.0
  extragenital 091.2
gastrojejunale—*see* Ulcer, gastrojejunal
hypostaticum—*see* Ulcer, varicose
molle (cutis) (skin) 099.0
serpens cornea (pneumococcal) 370.04
ventriculi—*see* Ulcer, stomach
Ulegyria 742.4
Ulerythema
acneiforma 701.8
centrifugum 695.4
ophryogenes 757.4
Ullrich (-Bonnevie) (-Turner) syndrome 758.6
Ullrich-Feichtiger syndrome 759.89
Ulnar —*see* condition
Ulorrhagia 523.8
Ulorrhea 523.8
Umbilicus, umbilical —*see also* condition
cord necrosis, affecting fetus or newborn 762.6
Unacceptable
existing dental restoration
  contours 525.65
  morphology 525.65
Unavailability of medical facilities (at) V63.9
due to
  investigation by social service agency V63.8
  lack of services at home V63.1
  remoteness from facility V63.0
  waiting list V63.2
home V63.1
outpatient clinic V63.0
specified reason NEC V63.8
Uncinaria americana infestation 126.1
Uncinariasis (*see also* Ancylostomiasis) 126.9
Unconscious, unconsciousness 780.09

Underdevelopment —*see also* Undeveloped
sexual 259.0
Underfill, endodontic 526.63
Undernourishment 269.9
Undernutrition 269.9
Under observation —*see* Observation
Underweight 783.22
for gestational age—*see* Light-for-dates
Underwood's disease (sclerema neonatorum)
  778.1
Undescended —*see also* Malposition, congenital
cecum 751.4
colon 751.4
testis 752.51
Undetermined diagnosis or cause 799.9
Undeveloped, undevelopment —*see also*
  Hypoplasia
brain (congenital) 742.1
cerebral (congenital) 742.1
fetus or newborn 764.9
heart 746.89
lung 748.5
testis 257.2
uterus 259.0
Undiagnosed (disease) 799.9
Undulant fever (*see also* Brucellosis) 023.9
Unemployment, anxiety concerning V62.0
Unequal leg (acquired) (length) 736.81
congenital 755.30
Unerupted teeth, tooth 520.6
Unextracted dental root 525.3
Unguis incarnatus 703.0
Unicornis uterus 752.33
Unicornuate uterus (with or without a separate
  uterine horn) 752.33
Unicorporeus uterus 752.39
Uniformis uterus 752.39
Unilateral —*see also* condition
development, breast 611.89
organ or site, congenital NEC—*see* Agenesis
vagina 752.49
Unilateralis uterus 752.39
Unilocular heart 745.8
Uninhibited (neurogenic) bladder 596.54
with cauda equina syndrome 344.61
neurogenic—*see* Neurogenic, bladder 596.54
Union, abnormal —*see also* Fusion
divided tendon 727.89
larynx and trachea 748.3
Universal
joint, cervix 620.6
mesentery 751.4
Unknown
cause of death 799.9
diagnosis 799.9
Unna's disease (seborrheic dermatitis) 690.10
Unresponsiveness, adrenocorticotropin
  (ACTH) 255.41
Unsoundness of mind (*see also* Psychosis) 298.9
Unspecified cause of death 799.9
Unsatisfactory
cytology smear
  anal 796.78
  cervical 795.08
  vaginal 795.18
restoration, tooth (existing) 525.60
  specified NEC 525.69
Unstable
back NEC 724.9
colon 569.89
joint—*see* Instability, joint

Unstable—*continued*
lie 652.0
affecting fetus or newborn (before labor) 761.7
causing obstructed labor 660.0
affecting fetus or newborn 763.1
lumbosacral joint (congenital) 756.19
acquired 724.6
sacroiliac 724.6
spine NEC 724.9
Untruthfulness, child problem (*see also*
Disturbance, conduct) 312.0
Unverricht (-Lundborg) disease, syndrome, or
epilepsy 345.1
Unverricht-Wagner syndrome
(dermatomyositis) 710.3
Upper respiratory —*see* condition
Upset
gastric 536.8
psychogenic 306.4
gastrointestinal 536.8
psychogenic 306.4
virus (*see also* Enteritis, viral) 008.8
intestinal (large) (small) 564.9
psychogenic 306.4
menstruation 626.9
mental 300.9
stomach 536.8
psychogenic 306.4
Urachus —*see also* condition
patent 753.7
persistent 753.7
Uratic arthritis 274.00
Urbach's lipoid proteinosis 272.8
Urbach-Oppenheim disease or syndrome
(necrobiosis lipoidica diabeticorum) 250.8
[709.3]
due to secondary diabetes 249.8 *[709.3]*
Urbach-Wiethe disease or syndrome (lipoid
proteinosis) 272.8
Urban yellow fever 060.1
Urea, blood, high —*see* Uremia
Uremia, uremic (absorption) (amaurosis)
(amblyopia) (aphasia) (apoplexy) (coma)
(delirium) (dementia) (dropsy) (dyspnea)
(fever) (intoxication) (mania) (paralysis)
(poisoning) (toxemia) (vomiting) 586
with
abortion—*see* Abortion, by type, with renal
failure
ectopic pregnancy (*see also* categories
633.0-633.9) 639.3
hypertension (*see also* Hypertension, kidney)
403.91
molar pregnancy (*see also* categories 630-632)
639.3
chronic 585.9
complicating
abortion 639.3
ectopic or molar pregnancy 639.3
hypertension (*see also* Hypertension, kidney)
403.91
labor and delivery 669.3
congenital 779.89
extrarenal 788.99
hypertensive (chronic) (*see also* Hypertension,
kidney) 403.91
maternal NEC, affecting fetus or newborn 760.1
neuropathy 585.9 *[357.4]*
pericarditis 585.9 *[420.0]*
prerenal 788.99
pyelitic (*see also* Pyelitis) 590.80

Ureter, ureteral —*see* condition
Ureteralgia 788.0
Ureterectasis 593.89
Ureteritis 593.89
cystica 590.3
due to calculus 592.1
gonococcal (acute) 098.19
chronic or duration of 2 months or over 098.39
nonspecific 593.89
Ureterocele (acquired) 593.89
congenital 753.23
Ureterolith 592.1
Ureterolithiasis 592.1
Ureterostomy status V44.6
with complication 997.5
Urethra, urethral —*see* condition
Urethralgia 788.99
Urethritis (abacterial) (acute) (allergic) (anterior)
(chronic) (nonvenereal) (posterior) (recurrent)
(simple) (subacute) (ulcerative)
(undifferentiated) 597.80
diplococcal (acute) 098.0
chronic or duration of 2 months or over 098.2
due to Trichomonas (vaginalis) 131.02
gonococcal (acute) 098.0
chronic or duration of 2 months or over 098.2
nongonococcal (sexually transmitted) 099.40
Chlamydia trachomatis 099.41
Reiter's 099.3
specified organism NEC 099.49
nonspecific (sexually transmitted) (*see also*
Urethritis, nongonococcal) 099.40
not sexually transmitted 597.80
Reiter's 099.3
trichomonal or due to Trichomonas (vaginalis)
131.02
tuberculous (*see also* Tuberculosis) 016.3
venereal NEC (*see also* Urethritis,
nongonococcal) 099.40
Urethrocele
female 618.03
with uterine prolapse 618.4
complete 618.3
incomplete 618.2
male 599.5
Urethrolithiasis 594.2
Urethro-oculoarticular syndrome 099.3
Urethro-oculosynovial syndrome 099.3
Urethrorectal —*see* condition
Urethrorrhagia 599.84
Urethrorrhea 788.7
Urethrostomy status V44.6
with complication 997.5
Urethrotrigonitis 595.3
Urethrovaginal —*see* condition
Urgency
fecal 787.63
hypertensive—*see* Hypertension
Urhidrosis, uridrosis 705.89
Uric acid
diathesis 274.9
in blood 790.6
Uricacidemia 790.6
Uricemia 790.6
Uricosuria 791.9
Urination
frequent 788.41
painful 788.1
urgency 788.63

Urine, urinary —*see also* condition
abnormality NEC 788.69
blood in (*see also* Hematuria) 599.70
discharge, excessive 788.42
enuresis 788.30
nonorganic origin 307.6
extravasation 788.8
frequency 788.41
hesitancy 788.64
incontinence 788.30
active 788.30
female 788.30
stress 625.6
and urge 788.33
male 788.30
stress 788.32
and urge 788.33
mixed (stress and urge) 788.33
neurogenic 788.39
nonorganic origin 307.6
overflow 788.38
stress (female) 625.6
male NEC 788.32
intermittent stream 788.61
pus in 791.9
retention or stasis NEC 788.20
bladder, incomplete emptying 788.21
psychogenic 306.53
specified NEC 788.29
secretion
deficient 788.5
excessive 788.42
frequency 788.41
strain 788.65
stream
intermittent 788.61
slowing 788.62
splitting 788.61
weak 788.62
urgency 788.63
Urinemia —*see* Uremia
Urinoma NEC 599.9
bladder 596.89
kidney 593.89
renal 593.89
ureter 593.89
urethra 599.84
Uroarthritis, infectious 099.3
Urodialysis 788.5
Urolithiasis 592.9
Uronephrosis 593.89
Uropathy 599.9
obstructive 599.60
Urosepsis 599.0
meaning sepsis 995.91
meaning urinary tract infection 599.0
Urticaria 708.9
with angioneurotic edema 995.1
hereditary 277.6
allergic 708.0
cholinergic 708.5
chronic 708.8
cold, familial 708.2
dermatographic 708.3
due to
cold or heat 708.2
drugs 708.0
food 708.0
inhalants 708.0
plants 708.8
serum 999.59

Uritcaria—*continued*
factitial 708.3
giant 995.1
hereditary 277.6
gigantea 995.1
hereditary 277.6
idiopathic 708.1
larynx 995.1
hereditary 277.6
neonatorum 778.8
nonallergic 708.1
papulosa (Hebra) 698.2
perstans hemorrhagica 757.39
pigmentosa 757.33
recurrent periodic 708.8
serum 999.59
solare 692.72
specified type NEC 708.8
thermal (cold) (heat) 708.2
vibratory 708.4
Urticarioides acarodermatitis 133.9
Use of
agents affecting estrogen receptors and estrogen
levels NEC V07.59
anastrozole (Arimidex) V07.52
aromatase inhibitors V07.52
estrogen receptor downregulators V07.59
exemestane (Aromasin) V07.52
fulvestrant (Faslodex) V07.59
gonadotropin-releasing hormone (GnRH)
agonist V07.59
goserelin acetate (Zoladex) V07.59
letrozole (Femara) V07.52
leuprolide acetate (leuprorelin) (Lupron) V07.59
megestrol acetate (Megace) V07.59
methadone 304.00
nonprescribed drugs (*see also* Abuse, drugs,
nondependent) 305.9
patent medicines (*see also* Abuse, drugs,
nondependent) 305.9
raloxifene (Evista) V07.51
selective estrogen receptor modulators (SERMs)
V07.51
tamoxifen (Nolvadex) V07.51
toremifene (Fareston) V07.51
Usher-Senear disease (pemphigus
erythematosus) 694.4
Uta 085.5
Uterine size-date discrepancy 649.6
Uteromegaly 621.2
Uterovaginal —*see* condition
Uterovesical —*see* condition
Uterus —*see also* condition
with only one functioning horn 752.33
Utriculitis (utriculus prostaticus) 597.89
Uveal —*see* condition
Uveitis (anterior) (*see also* Iridocyclitis) 364.3
acute or subacute 364.00
due to or associated with
gonococcal infection 098.41
herpes (simplex) 054.44
zoster 053.22
primary 364.01
recurrent 364.02
secondary (noninfectious) 364.04
infectious 364.03
allergic 360.11

Uveitis—*continued*
  chronic 364.10
    due to or associated with
      sarcoidosis 135 *[364.11]*
      tuberculosis (*see also* Tuberculosis) 017.3
        [364.11]
    due to
      operation 360.11
      toxoplasmosis (acquired) 130.2
        congenital (active) 771.2
    granulomatous 364.10
    heterochromic 364.21
    lens-induced 364.23
    nongranulomatous 364.00
    posterior 363.20
      disseminated—*see* Chorioretinitis,
        disseminated
      focal—*see* Chorioretinitis, focal
    recurrent 364.02
    sympathetic 360.11
    syphilitic (secondary) 091.50
      congenital 090.0 *[363.13]*
      late 095.8 *[363.13]*
    tuberculous (*see also* Tuberculosis) 017.3
      [364.11]
Uveoencephalitis 363.22
Uveokeratitis (*see also* Iridocyclitis) 364.3
Uveoparotid fever 135
Uveoparotitis 135
Uvula —*see* condition
Uvulitis (acute) (catarrhal) (chronic)
    (gangrenous) (membranous) (suppurative)
    (ulcerative) 528.3

V

Vaccination
complication or reaction—*see* Complications, vaccination
delayed V64.00
not carried out V64.00
  because of
    acute illness V64.01
    allergy to vaccine or component V64.04
    caregiver refusal V64.05
    chronic illness V64.02
    guardian refusal V64.05
    immune compromised state V64.03
    parent refusal V64.05
    patient had disease being vaccinated against V64.08
    patient refusal V64.06
    reason NEC V64.09
    religious reasons V64.07
prophylactic (against) V05.9
  arthropod-borne viral
    disease NEC V05.1
    encephalitis V05.0
  chickenpox V05.4
  cholera (alone) V03.0
    with typhoid-paratyphoid (cholera + TAB) V06.0
  common cold V04.7
  diphtheria (alone) V03.5
    with
      poliomyelitis (DTP + polio) V06.3
      tetanus V06.5
        pertussis combined [DTP] [DTaP] V06.1
      typhoid-paratyphoid (DTP + TAB) V06.2
  disease (single) NEC V05.9
    bacterial NEC V03.9
      specified type NEC V03.89
    combinations NEC V06.9
      specified type NEC V06.8
    specified type NEC V05.8
  encephalitis, viral, arthropod-borne V05.0
  Hemophilus influenzae, type B [Hib] V03.81
  hepatitis, viral V05.3
  influenza V04.81
    with
      Streptococcus pneumoniae [pneumococcus] V06.6
  leishmaniasis V05.2
  measles (alone) V04.2
    with mumps-rubella (MMR) V06.4
  mumps (alone) V04.6
    with measles and rubella (MMR) V06.4
  pertussis alone V03.6
  plague V03.3
  poliomyelitis V04.0
    with diphtheria-tetanus-pertussis (DTP + polio) V06.3
  rabies V04.5
  respiratory syncytial virus (RSV) V04.82
  rubella (alone) V04.3
    with measles and mumps (MMR) V06.4
  smallpox V04.1
  Streptococcus pneumoniae [pneumococcus] V03.82
    with
      influenza V06.6
  tetanus toxoid (alone) V03.7
    with diphtheria [Td] [DT] V06.5
      with
        pertussis [DTP] [DTaP] V06.1

Vaccination—*continued*
    with poliomyelitis (DTP + polio) V06.3
  tuberculosis (BCG) V03.2
  tularemia V03.4
  typhoid-paratyphoid (TAB) (alone) V03.1
    with diphtheria-tetanus-pertussis (TAB + DTP) V06.2
  varicella V05.4
  viral
    disease NEC V04.89
    encephalitis, arthropod-borne V05.0
    hepatitis V05.3
  yellow fever V04.4
Vaccinia (generalized) 999.0
congenital 771.2
conjunctiva 999.39
eyelids 999.0 *[373.5]*
localized 999.39
nose 999.39
not from vaccination 051.02
  eyelid 051.02 *[373.5]*
sine vaccinatione 051.02
without vaccination 051.02
Vacuum
extraction of fetus or newborn 763.3
in sinus (accessory) (nasal) (*see also* Sinusitis) 473.9
Vagabond V60.0
Vagabondage V60.0
Vagabonds' disease 132.1
Vagina, vaginal —*see also* condition
high risk human papillomavirus (HPV) DNA test positive 795.15
low risk human papillomavirus (HPV) DNA test positive 795.19
Vaginalitis (tunica) 608.4
Vaginismus (reflex) 625.1
functional 306.51
hysterical 300.11
psychogenic 306.51
Vaginitis (acute) (chronic) (circumscribed) (diffuse) (emphysematous) (Hemophilus vaginalis) (nonspecific) (nonvenereal) (ulcerative) 616.10
with
  abortion—*see* Abortion, by type, with sepsis
  ectopic pregnancy (*see also* categories 633.0-633.9) 639.0
  molar pregnancy (*see also* categories 630-632) 639.0
adhesive, congenital 752.49
atrophic, postmenopausal 627.3
bacterial 616.10
blennorrhagic (acute) 098.0
  chronic or duration of 2 months or over 098.2
candidal 112.1
chlamydial 099.53
complicating pregnancy or puerperium 646.6
  affecting fetus or newborn 760.8
congenital (adhesive) 752.49
due to
  C. albicans 112.1
  Trichomonas (vaginalis) 131.01
following
  abortion 639.0
  ectopic or molar pregnancy 639.0

Vaginitis—*continued*
gonococcal (acute) 098.0
chronic or duration of 2 months or over 098.2
granuloma 099.2
Monilia 112.1
mycotic 112.1
pinworm 127.4 *[616.11]*
postirradiation 616.10
postmenopausal atrophic 627.3
senile (atrophic) 627.3
syphilitic (early) 091.0
late 095.8
trichomonal 131.01
tuberculous (*see also* Tuberculosis) 016.7
venereal NEC 099.8
Vaginosis —*see* Vaginitis
Vagotonia 352.3
Vagrancy V60.0
VAIN I (vaginal intraepithelial neoplasia I) 623.0
VAIN II (vaginal intraepithelial neoplasia II) 623.0
VAIN III (vaginal intraepithelial neoplasia III) 233.31
Vallecula —*see* condition
Valley fever 114.0
Valsuani's disease (progressive pernicious anemia, puerperal) 648.2
Valve, valvular (formation)—*see also* condition
cerebral ventricle (communicating) in situ V45.2
cervix, internal os 752.49
colon 751.5
congenital NEC—*see* Atresia
formation, congenital NEC—*see* Atresia
heart defect—*see* Anomaly, heart, valve
ureter 753.29
pelvic junction 753.21
vesical orifice 753.22
urethra 753.6
Valvulitis (chronic) (*see also* Endocarditis) 424.90
rheumatic (chronic) (inactive) (with chorea) 397.9
active or acute (aortic) (mitral) (pulmonary) (tricuspid) 391.1
syphilitic NEC 093.20
aortic 093.22
mitral 093.21
pulmonary 093.24
tricuspid 093.23
Valvulopathy —*see* Endocarditis
van Bogaert's leukoencephalitis (sclerosing) (subacute) 046.2
van Bogaert-Nijssen (-Peiffer) disease 330.0
van Buchem's syndrome (hyperostosis corticalis) 733.3
Vancomycin (glycopeptide)
intermediate staphylococcus aureus (VISA/GISA) V09.8
resistant
enterococcus (VRE) V09.8
staphylococcus aureus (VRSA/GRSA) V09.8
van Creveld-von Gierke disease (glycogenosis I) 271.0
van den Bergh's disease (enterogenous cyanosis) 289.7
van der Hoeve's syndrome (brittle bones and blue sclera, deafness) 756.51
van der Hoeve-Halbertsma-Waardenburg syndrome (ptosis-epicanthus) 270.2

van der Hoeve-Waardenburg-Gualdi syndrome (ptosis epicanthus) 270.2
Vanillism 692.89
Vanishing lung 492.0
Vanishing twin 651.33
van Neck (-Odelberg) disease or syndrome (juvenile osteochondrosis) 732.1
Vapor asphyxia or suffocation NEC 987.9
specified agent—*see* Table of drugs and chemicals
Vaquez's disease (M9950/1) 238.4
Vaquez-Osler disease (polycythemia vera) (M9950/1) 238.4
Variance, lethal ball, prosthetic heart valve 996.02
Variants, thalassemic 282.49
Variations in hair color 704.3
Varicella 052.9
with
complication 052.8
specified NEC 052.7
pneumonia 052.1
exposure to V01.71
vaccination and inoculation (prophylactic) V05.4
Varices —*see* Varix
Varicocele (scrotum) (thrombosed) 456.4
ovary 456.5
perineum 456.6
spermatic cord (ulcerated) 456.4
Varicose
aneurysm (ruptured) (*see also* Aneurysm) 442.9
dermatitis (lower extremity)—*see* Varicose, vein, inflamed or infected
eczema—*see* Varicose, vein
phlebitis—*see* Varicose, vein, inflamed or infected
placental vessel—*see* Placenta, abnormal
tumor—*see* Varicose, vein
ulcer (lower extremity, any part) 454.0
anus 455.8
external 455.5
internal 455.2
esophagus (*see also* Varix, esophagus) 456.1
bleeding (*see also* Varix, esophagus, bleeding) 456.0
inflamed or infected 454.2
nasal septum 456.8
perineum 456.6
rectum—*see* Varicose, ulcer, anus
scrotum 456.4
specified site NEC 456.8
vein (lower extremity) (ruptured) (*see also* Varix) 454.9
with
complications NEC 454.8
edema 454.8
inflammation or infection 454.1
ulcerated 454.2
pain 454.8
stasis dermatitis 454.1
with ulcer 454.2
swelling 454.8
ulcer 454.0
inflamed or infected 454.2
anus—*see* Hemorrhoids
broad ligament 456.5
congenital (peripheral) NEC 747.60
gastrointestinal 747.61
lower limb 747.64
renal 747.62

Varicose—*continued*
  specified NEC 747.69
  upper limb 747.63
  esophagus (ulcerated) (*see also* Varix,
    esophagus) 456.1
    bleeding (*see also* Varix, esophagus,
      bleeding) 456.0
  inflamed or infected 454.1
    with ulcer 454.2
  in pregnancy or puerperium 671.0
    vulva or perineum 671.1
  nasal septum (with ulcer) 456.8
  pelvis 456.5
  perineum 456.6
    in pregnancy, childbirth, or puerperium
      671.1
  rectum—*see* Hemorrhoids
  scrotum (ulcerated) 456.4
  specified site NEC 456.8
  sublingual 456.3
  ulcerated 454.0
    inflamed or infected 454.2
  umbilical cord, affecting fetus or newborn
    762.6
  urethra 456.8
  vulva 456.6
    in pregnancy, childbirth, or puerperium
      671.1
  vessel—*see also* Varix
    placenta—*see* Placenta, abnormal
Varicosis, varicosities, varicosity (*see also*
  Varix) 454.9
Variola 050.9
  hemorrhagic (pustular) 050.0
  major 050.0
  minor 050.1
  modified 050.2
Varioloid 050.2
Variolosa, purpura 050.0
Varix (lower extremity) (ruptured) 454.9
  with
    complications NEC 454.8
    edema 454.8
    inflammation or infection 454.1
      with ulcer 454.2
    pain 454.8
    stasis dermatitis 454.1
      with ulcer 454.2
    swelling 454.8
    ulcer 454.0
      with inflammation or infection 454.2
  aneurysmal (*see also* Aneurysm) 442.9
  anus—*see* Hemorrhoids
  arteriovenous (congenital) (peripheral) NEC
    747.60
    gastrointestinal 747.61
    lower limb 747.64
    renal 747.62
    specified NEC 747.69
    spinal 747.82
    upper limb 747.63
  bladder 456.5
  broad ligament 456.5
  congenital (peripheral) NEC 747.60
  esophagus (ulcerated) 456.1
    bleeding 456.0
    in
      cirrhosis of liver 571.5 *[456.20]*
      portal hypertension 572.3 *[456.20]*
    congenital 747.69

Varix—*continued*
  in
    cirrhosis of liver 571.5 *[456.21]*
      with bleeding 571.5 *[456.20]*
    portal hypertension 572.3 *[456.21]*
      with bleeding 572.3 *[456.20]*
  gastric 456.8
  inflamed or infected 454.1
    ulcerated 454.2
  in pregnancy or puerperium 671.0
    perineum 671.1
    vulva 671.1
  labia (majora) 456.6
  orbit 456.8
    congenital 747.69
  ovary 456.5
  papillary 448.1
  pelvis 456.5
  perineum 456.6
    in pregnancy or puerperium 671.1
  pharynx 456.8
  placenta—*see* Placenta, abnormal
  prostate 456.8
  rectum—*see* Hemorrhoids
  renal papilla 456.8
  retina 362.17
  scrotum (ulcerated) 456.4
  sigmoid colon 456.8
  specified site NEC 456.8
  spinal (cord) (vessels) 456.8
  spleen, splenic (vein) (with phlebolith) 456.8
  sublingual 456.3
  ulcerated 454.0
    inflamed or infected 454.2
  umbilical cord, affecting fetus or newborn 762.6
  uterine ligament 456.5
  vocal cord 456.8
  vulva 456.6
    in pregnancy, childbirth, or puerperium 671.1
Vasa previa 663.5
  affecting fetus or newborn 762.6
  hemorrhage from, affecting fetus or newborn 772.0
Vascular —*see also* condition
  loop on papilla (optic) 743.57
  sheathing, retina 362.13
  spasm 443.9
  spider 448.1
Vascularity, pulmonary, congenital 747.39
Vascularization
  choroid 362.16
  cornea 370.60
    deep 370.63
    localized 370.61
  retina 362.16
  subretinal 362.16
Vasculitis 447.6
  allergic 287.0
  cryoglobulinemic 273.2
  disseminated 447.6
  kidney 447.8
  leukocytoclastic 446.29
  nodular 695.2
  retinal 362.18
  rheumatic—*see* Fever, rheumatic
Vasculopathy
  cardiac allograft 996.83
Vas deferens —*see* condition
Vas deferentitis 608.4
Vasectomy, admission for V25.2

Vasitis 608.4
  nodosa 608.4
  scrotum 608.4
  spermatic cord 608.4
  testis 608.4
  tuberculous (*see also* Tuberculosis) 016.5
  tunica vaginalis 608.4
  vas deferens 608.4
Vasodilation 443.9
Vasomotor —*see* condition
Vasoplasty, after previous sterilization V26.0
Vasoplegia, splanchnic (*see also* Neuropathy,
    peripheral, autonomic) 337.9
Vasospasm 443.9
  cerebral (artery) 435.9
    with transient neurologic deficit 435.9
  coronary 413.1
  nerve
    arm NEC 354.9
    autonomic 337.9
    brachial plexus 353.0
    cervical plexus 353.2
    leg NEC 355.8
    lower extremity NEC 355.8
    peripheral NEC 355.9
    spinal NEC 355.9
    sympathetic 337.9
    upper extremity NEC 354.9
  peripheral NEC 443.9
  retina (artery) (*see also* Occlusion, retinal,
    artery) 362.30
Vasospastic —*see* condition
Vasovagal attack (paroxysmal) 780.2
  psychogenic 306.2
Vater's ampulla —*see* condition
VATER syndrome 759.89
vCJD (variant Creutzfeldt-Jakob disease) 046.11
Vegetation, vegetative
  adenoid (nasal fossa) 474.2
  consciousness (persistent) 780.03
  endocarditis (acute) (any valve) (chronic)
    (subacute) 421.0
  heart (mycotic) (valve) 421.0
  state (persistent) 780.03
Veil
  Jackson's 751.4
  over face (causing asphyxia) 768.9
Vein, venous —*see* condition
Veldt sore (*see also* Ulcer, skin) 707.9
Velo-cardio-facial syndrome 758.32
Velpeau's hernia —*see* Hernia, femoral
Venereal
  balanitis NEC 099.8
  bubo 099.1
  disease 099.9
    specified nature or type NEC 099.8
  granuloma inguinale 099.2
  lymphogranuloma (Durand-Nicolas-Favre), any
    site 099.1
  salpingitis 098.37
  urethritis (*see also* Urethritis, nongonococcal)
    099.40
  vaginitis NEC 099.8
  warts 078.11
Vengefulness, in child (*see also* Disturbance,
    conduct) 312.0
Venofibrosis 459.89
Venom, venomous
  bite or sting (animal or insect) 989.5
  poisoning 989.5
Venous —*see* condition

Ventouse delivery NEC 669.5
  affecting fetus or newborn 763.3
Ventral —*see* condition
Ventricle, ventricular —*see also* condition
  escape 427.69
  standstill (*see also* Arrest, cardiac) 427.5
Ventriculitis, cerebral (*see also* Meningitis)
    322.9
Ventriculostomy status V45.2
Verbiest's syndrome (claudicatio intermittens
    spinalis) 435.1
Vernet's syndrome 352.6
Verneuil's disease (syphilitic bursitis) 095.7
Verruca (filiformis) 078.10
  acuminata (any site) 078.11
  necrogenica (primary) (*see also* Tuberculosis)
    017.0
  peruana 088.0
  peruviana 088.0
  plana (juvenilis) 078.19
  plantaris 078.12
  seborrheica 702.19
    inflamed 702.11
  senilis 702.0
  tuberculosa (primary) (*see also* Tuberculosis)
    017.0
  venereal 078.11
  viral 078.10
    specified NEC 078.19
  vulgaris 078.10
Verrucosities (*see also* Verruca) 078.10
Verrucous endocarditis (acute) (any valve)
    (chronic) (subacute) 710.0 *[424.91]*
  nonbacterial 710.0 *[424.91]*
Verruga
  peruana 088.0
  peruviana 088.0
Verse's disease (calcinosis intervertebralis)
    275.49 *[722.90]*
Version
  before labor, affecting fetus or newborn 761.7
  cephalic (correcting previous malposition) 652.1
    affecting fetus or newborn 763.1
  cervix (*see* Version, uterus)
  uterus (postinfectional) (postpartal, old) (*see
    also* Malposition, uterus) 621.6
    forward—*see* Anteversion, uterus
    lateral—*see* Lateroversion, uterus
Vertebra, vertebral —*see* condition
Vertigo 780.4
  auditory 386.19
  aural 386.19
  benign paroxysmal positional 386.11
  central origin 386.2
  cerebral 386.2
  Dix and Hallpike (epidemic) 386.12
  endemic paralytic 078.81
  epidemic 078.81
    Dix and Hallpike 386.12
    Gerlier's 078.81
    Pedersen's 386.12
    vestibular neuronitis 386.12
  epileptic—*see* Epilepsy
  Gerlier's (epidemic) 078.81
  hysterical 300.11
  labyrinthine 386.10
  laryngeal 786.2
  malignant positional 386.2
  Ménière's (*see also* Disease, Ménière's) 386.00
  menopausal 627.2
  otogenic 386.19

Vertigo—*continued*
paralytic 078.81
paroxysmal positional, benign 386.11
Pedersen's (epidemic) 386.12
peripheral 386.10
specified type NEC 386.19
positional
benign paroxysmal 386.11
malignant 386.2
Verumontanitis (chronic) (*see also* Urethritis)
597.89
Vesania (*see also* Psychosis) 298.9
Vesical —*see* condition
Vesicle
cutaneous 709.8
seminal—*see* condition
skin 709.8
Vesicocolic —*see* condition
Vesicoperineal —*see* condition
Vesicorectal —*see* condition
Vesicourethrorectal —*see* condition
Vesicovaginal —*see* condition
Vesicular —*see* condition
Vesiculitis (seminal) 608.0
amebic 006.8
gonorrheal (acute) 098.14
chronic or duration of 2 months or over 098.34
trichomonal 131.09
tuberculous (*see also* Tuberculosis) 016.5
[608.81]
Vestibulitis (ear) (*see also* Labyrinthitis) 386.30
nose (external) 478.19
vulvar 625.71
Vestibulopathy, acute peripheral (recurrent)
386.12
Vestige, vestigial —*see also* Persistence
branchial 744.41
structures in vitreous 743.51
Vibriosis NEC 027.9
Vidal's disease (lichen simplex chronicus) 698.3
Video display tube syndrome 723.8
Vienna type encephalitis 049.8
Villaret's syndrome 352.6
Villous —*see* condition
VIN I (vulvar intraepithelial neoplasia I) 624.01
VIN II (vulvar intraepithelial neoplasia II) 624.02
VIN III (vulvar intraepithelial neoplasia III)
233.32
Vincent's
angina 101
bronchitis 101
disease 101
gingivitis 101
infection (any site) 101
laryngitis 101
stomatitis 101
tonsillitis 101
Vinson-Plummer syndrome (sideropenic
dysphagia) 280.8
Viosterol deficiency (*see also* Deficiency,
calciferol) 268.9
Virchow's disease 733.99
Viremia 790.8
Virilism (adrenal) (female) NEC 255.2
with
3-beta-hydroxysteroid dehydrogenase defect
255.2
11-hydroxylase defect 255.2
21-hydroxylase defect 255.2

Virilism—*continued*
adrenal
hyperplasia 255.2
insufficiency (congenital) 255.2
cortical hyperfunction 255.2
Virilization (female) (suprarenal) (*see also*
Virilism) 255.2
isosexual 256.4
Virulent bubo 099.0
Virus, viral —*see also* condition
infection NEC (*see also* Infection, viral) 079.99
septicemia 079.99
yaba monkey tumor 059.22
VISA (vancomycin intermediate staphylococcus
aureus) V09.8
Viscera, visceral —*see* condition
Visceroptosis 569.89
Visible peristalsis 787.4
Vision, visual
binocular, suppression 368.31
blurred, blurring 368.8
hysterical 300.11
defect, defective (*see also* Impaired, vision)
369.9
disorientation (syndrome) 368.16
disturbance NEC (*see also* Disturbance, vision)
368.9
hysterical 300.11
examination V72.0
field, limitation 368.40
fusion, with defective steropsis 368.33
hallucinations 368.16
halos 368.16
loss 369.9
both eyes (*see also* Blindness, both eyes)
369.3
complete (*see also* Blindness, both eyes)
369.00
one eye 369.8
sudden 368.16
low (both eyes) 369.20
one eye (other eye normal) (*see also* Impaired,
vision) 369.70
blindness, other eye 369.10
perception, simultaneous without fusion 368.32
tunnel 368.45
Vitality, lack or want of 780.79
newborn 779.89
Vitamin deficiency NEC (*see also* Deficiency,
vitamin) 269.2
Vitelline duct, persistent 751.0
Vitiligo 709.01
due to pinta (carate) 103.2
eyelid 374.53
vulva 624.8
Vitium cordis —*see* Disease, heart
Vitreous —*see also* condition
touch syndrome 997.99
VLCAD (long chain/very long chain acyl CoA
dehydrogenase deficiency, LCAD) 277.85
Vocal cord —*see* condition
Vocational rehabilitation V57.22
Vogt's (Cecile) disease or syndrome 333.7
Vogt-Koyanagi syndrome 364.24
Vogt-Spielmeyer disease (amaurotic familial
idiocy) 330.1
Voice
change (*see also* Dysphonia) 784.49
loss (*see also* Aphonia) 784.41
Volhard-Fahr disease (malignant
nephrosclerosis) 403.00

Volhynian fever 083.1
Volkmann's ischemic contracture or paralysis
(complicating trauma) 958.6
Voluntary starvation 307.1
Volvulus (bowel) (colon) (intestine) 560.2
with
hernia—*see also* Hernia, by site, with
obstruction
gangrenous—*see* Hernia, by site, with
gangrene
perforation 560.2
congenital 751.5
duodenum 537.3
fallopian tube 620.5
oviduct 620.5
stomach (due to absence of gastrocolic
ligament) 537.89
Vomiting 787.03
with nausea 787.01
allergic 535.4
asphyxia 933.1
bilious (cause unknown) 787.04
following gastrointestinal surgery 564.3
newborn 779.32
blood (*see also* Hematemesis) 578.0
causing asphyxia, choking, or suffocation (*see
also* Asphyxia, food) 933.1
cyclical 536.2
associated with migraine 346.2
psychogenic 306.4
epidemic 078.82
fecal matter 569.87
following gastrointestinal surgery 564.3
functional 536.8
psychogenic 306.4
habit 536.2
hysterical 300.11
nervous 306.4
neurotic 306.4
newborn 779.33
bilious 779.32
of or complicating pregnancy 643.9
due to
organic disease 643.8
specific cause NEC 643.8
early—*see* Hyperemesis, gravidarum
late (after 22 completed weeks of gestation)
643.2
pernicious or persistent 536.2
complicating pregnancy—*see* Hyperemesis,
gravidarum
psychogenic 306.4
physiological 787.03
bilious 787.04
psychic 306.4
psychogenic 307.54
stercoral 569.89
uncontrollable 536.2
psychogenic 306.4
uremic—*see* Uremia
winter 078.82
von Bechterew (-Strumpell) disease or syndrome
(ankylosing spondylitis) 720.0
von Bezold's abscess 383.01
von Economo's disease (encephalitis lethargica)
049.8
von Eulenburg's disease (congenital
paramyotonia) 359.29
von Gierke's disease (glycogenosis I) 271.0
von Gies' joint 095.8
von Graefe's disease or syndrome 378.72

von Hippel (-Lindau) disease or syndrome
(retinocerebral angiomatosis) 759.6
von Jaksch's anemia or disease
(pseudoleukemia infantum) 285.8
von Recklinghausen's
disease or syndrome (nerves) (skin) (M9540/1)
237.71
bones (osteitis fibrosa cystica) 252.01
tumor (M9540/1) 237.71
von Recklinghausen-Applebaum disease
(hemochromatosis) (*see also*
Hemochromatosis) 275.03
von Schroetter's syndrome (intermittent venous
claudication) 453.89
von Willebrand (-Jürgens) (-Minot) disease or
syndrome (angiohemophilia) 286.4
von Zambusch's disease (lichen sclerosus et
atrophicus) 701.0
Voorhoeve's disease or dyschondroplasia 756.4
Vossius' ring 921.3
late effect 366.21
Voyeurism 302.82
VRE (vancomycin resistant enterococcus) V09.8
Vrolik's disease (osteogenesis imperfecta) 756.51
VRSA (vancomycin resistant staphylococcus
aureus) V09.8
Vulva —*see* condition
Vulvismus 625.1
Vulvitis (acute) (allergic) (chronic) (gangrenous)
(hypertrophic) (intertriginous) 616.10
with
abortion—*see* Abortion, by type, with sepsis
ectopic pregnancy (*see also* categories
633.0-633.9) 639.0
molar pregnancy (*see also* categories 630-632)
639.0
adhesive, congenital 752.49
blennorrhagic (acute) 098.0
chronic or duration of 2 months or over 098.2
chlamydial 099.53
complicating pregnancy or puerperium 646.6
due to Ducrey's bacillus 099.0
following
abortion 639.0
ectopic or molar pregnancy 639.0
gonococcal (acute) 098.0
chronic or duration of 2 months or over 098.2
herpetic 054.11
leukoplakic 624.09
monilial 112.1
puerperal, postpartum, childbirth 646.6
syphilitic (early) 091.0
late 095.8
trichomonal 131.01
Vulvodynia 625.70
specified NEC 625.79
Vulvorectal —*see* condition
Vulvovaginitis (*see also* Vulvitis) 616.10
amebic 006.8
chlamydial 099.53
gonococcal (acute) 098.0
chronic or duration of 2 months or over 098.2
herpetic 054.11
monilial 112.1
trichomonal (Trichomonas vaginalis) 131.01

W

Waardenburg's syndrome 756.89
 meaning ptosis-epicanthus 270.2
Waardenburg-Klein syndrome
 (ptosis-epicanthus) 270.2
Wagner's disease (colloid milium) 709.3
Wagner (-Unverricht) syndrome
 (dermatomyositis) 710.3
Waiting list, person on V63.2
 undergoing social agency investigation V63.8
Wakefulness disorder (see also Hypersomnia)
 780.54
 nonorganic origin 307.43
Waldenström's
 disease (osteochondrosis, capital femoral) 732.1
 hepatitis (lupoid hepatitis) 571.49
 hypergammaglobulinemia 273.0
 macroglobulinemia 273.3
 purpura, hypergammaglobulinemic 273.0
 syndrome (macroglobulinemia) 273.3
Waldenström-Kjellberg syndrome (sideropenic
 dysphagia) 280.8
Walking
 difficulty 719.7
  psychogenic 307.9
 sleep 307.46
  hysterical 300.13
Wall, abdominal —see condition
Wallenberg's syndrome (posterior inferior
 cerebellar artery) (see also Disease,
 cerebrovascular, acute) 436
Wallgren's
 disease (obstruction of splenic vein with
  collateral circulation) 459.89
 meningitis (see also Meningitis, aseptic) 047.9
Wandering
 acetabulum 736.39
 gallbladder 751.69
 in diseases classified elsewhere V40.31
 kidney, congenital 753.3
 organ or site, congenital NEC—see Malposition,
  congenital
 pacemaker (atrial) (heart) 427.89
 spleen 289.59
Wardrop's disease (with lymphangitis) 681.9
 finger 681.02
 toe 681.11
War neurosis 300.16
Wart (digitate) (filiform) (infectious) (juvenile)
 (plantar) (viral) 078.10
 common 078.19
 external genital organs (venereal) 078.11
 fig 078.19
 flat 078.19
 genital 078.11
 Hassall-Henle's (of cornea) 371.41
 Henle's (of cornea) 371.41
 juvenile 078.19
 moist 078.10
 Peruvian 088.0
 plantar 078.12
 prosector (see also Tuberculosis) 017.0
 seborrheic 702.19
  inflamed 702.11
 senile 702.0
 specified NEC 078.19
 syphilitic 091.3
 tuberculous (see also Tuberculosis) 017.0
 venereal (female) (male) 078.11

Warthin's tumor (salivary gland) (M8561/0) 210.2
Washerwoman's itch 692.4
Wassilieff's disease (leptospiral jaundice) 100.0
Wasting
 disease 799.4
  due to malnutrition 261
 extreme (due to malnutrition) 261
 muscular NEC 728.2
 palsy, paralysis 335.21
 pelvic muscle 618.83
Water
 clefts 366.12
 deprivation of 994.3
 in joint (see also Effusion, joint) 719.0
 intoxication 276.69
 itch 120.3
 lack of 994.3
 loading 276.69
 on
  brain—see Hydrocephalus
  chest 511.89
 poisoning 276.69
Waterbrash 787.1
Water-hammer pulse (see also Insufficiency,
 aortic) 424.1
Waterhouse (-Friderichsen) disease or syndrome
 036.3
Water-losing nephritis 588.89
Watermelon stomach 537.82
 with hemorrhage 537.83
 without hemorrhage 537.82
Wax in ear 380.4
Waxy
 degeneration, any site 277.39
 disease 277.39
 kidney 277.39 [583.81]
 liver (large) 277.39
 spleen 277.39
Weak, weakness (generalized) 780.79
 arches (acquired) 734
  congenital 754.61
 bladder sphincter 596.59
 congenital 779.89
 eye muscle—see Strabismus
 facial 781.94
 foot (double)—see Weak, arches
 heart, cardiac (see also Failure, heart) 428.9
  congenital 746.9
 mind 317
 muscle (generalized) 728.87
 myocardium (see also Failure, heart) 428.9
 newborn 779.89
 pelvic fundus
  pubocervical tissue 618.81
  rectovaginal tissue 618.82
 pulse 785.9
 senile 797
 valvular—see Endocarditis
Wear, worn, tooth, teeth (approximal) (hard
 tissues) (interproximal) (occlusal)—see also
 Attrition, teeth 521.10
Weather, weathered
 effects of
  cold NEC 991.9
   specified effect NEC 991.8
  hot (see also Heat) 992.9
 skin 692.74

WXYZ

Web, webbed (congenital)—*see also* Anomaly, specified type NEC
  canthus 743.63
  digits (*see also* Syndactylism) 755.10
  duodenal 751.5
  esophagus 750.3
  fingers (*see also* Syndactylism, fingers) 755.11
  larynx (glottic) (subglottic) 748.2
  neck (pterygium colli) 744.5
  Paterson-Kelly (sideropenic dysphagia) 280.8
  popliteal syndrome 756.89
  toes (*see also* Syndactylism, toes) 755.13
Weber's paralysis or syndrome 344.89
Weber-Christian disease or syndrome (nodular nonsuppurative panniculitis) 729.30
Weber-Cockayne syndrome (epidermolysis bullosa) 757.39
Weber-Dimitri syndrome 759.6
Weber-Gubler syndrome 344.89
Weber-Leyden syndrome 344.89
Weber-Osler syndrome (familial hemorrhagic telangiectasia) 448.0
Wedge-shaped or wedging vertebra (*see also* Osteoporosis) 733.00
Wegener's granulomatosis or syndrome 446.4
Wegner's disease (syphilitic osteochondritis) 090.0
Weight
  gain (abnormal) (excessive) 783.1
    during pregnancy 646.1
      insufficient 646.8
  less than 1000 grams at birth 765.0
  loss (cause unknown) 783.21
Weightlessness 994.9
Weil's disease (leptospiral jaundice) 100.00
Weill-Marchesani syndrome (brachymorphism and ectopia lentis) 759.89
Weingarten's syndrome (tropical eosinophilia) 518.3
Weir Mitchell's disease (erythromelalgia) 443.82
Weiss-Baker syndrome (carotid sinus syncope) 337.01
Weissenbach-Thibierge syndrome (cutaneous systemic sclerosis) 710.1
Wen (*see also* Cyst, sebaceous) 706.2
Wenckebach's phenomenon, heart block (second degree) 426.13
Werdnig-Hoffmann syndrome (muscular atrophy) 335.0
Werlhof's disease (*see also* Purpura, thrombocytopenic) 287.39
Werlhof-Wichmann syndrome (*see also* Purpura, thrombocytopenic) 287.39
Wermer's syndrome or disease (polyendocrine adenomatosis) 258.01
Werner's disease or syndrome (progeria adultorum) 259.8
Werner-His disease (trench fever) 083.1
Werner-Schultz disease (agranulocytosis) 288.09
Wernicke's encephalopathy, disease or syndrome (superior hemorrhagic polioencephalitis) 265.1
Wernicke-Korsakoff syndrome or psychosis (nonalcoholic) 294.0
  alcoholic 291.1
Wernicke-Posadas disease (*see also* Coccidioidomycosis) 114.9
Wesselsbron fever 066.3
West African fever 084.8

West Nile
  encephalitis 066.41
  encephalomyelitis 066.41
  fever 066.40
    with
      cranial nerve disorders 066.42
      encephalitis 066.41
      optic neuritis 066.42
      other complications 066.49
      other neurologic manifestations 066.42
      polyradiculitis 066.42
  virus 066.40
Westphal-Strümpell syndrome (hepatolenticular degeneration) 275.1
Wet
  brain (alcoholic) (*see also* Alcoholism) 303.9
  feet, tropical (syndrome) (maceration) 991.4
  lung (syndrome)
    adult 518.52
    newborn 770.6
Wharton's duct —*see* condition
Wheal 709.8
Wheelchair confinement status V46.3
Wheezing 786.07
Whiplash injury or syndrome 847.0
Whipple's disease or syndrome (intestinal lipodystrophy) 040.2
Whipworm 127.3
"Whistling face" syndrome (craniocarpotarsal dystrophy) 759.89
White —*see also* condition
  kidney
    large—*see* Nephrosis
    small 582.9
  leg, puerperal, postpartum, childbirth 671.4
    nonpuerperal 451.19
  mouth 112.0
  patches of mouth 528.6
  sponge nevus of oral mucosa 750.26
  spot lesions, teeth 521.01
White's disease (congenital) (keratosis follicularis) 757.39
Whitehead 706.2
Whitlow (with lymphangitis) 681.01
  herpetic 054.6
Whitmore's disease or fever (melioidosis) 025
Whooping cough 033.9
  with pneumonia 033.9 *[484.3]*
  due to
    Bordetella
      bronchoseptica 033.8
        with pneumonia 033.8 *[484.3]*
      parapertussis 033.1
        with pneumonia 033.1 *[484.3]*
      pertussis 033.0
        with pneumonia 033.0 *[484.3]*
    specified organism NEC 033.8
      with pneumonia 033.8 *[484.3]*
  vaccination, prophylactic (against) V03.6
Wichmann's asthma (laryngismus stridulus) 478.75
Widal (-Abrami) syndrome (acquired hemolytic jaundice) 283.9
Widening aorta (*see also* Ectasia, aortic) 447.70
  with aneurysm 441.9
  ruptured 441.5
Wilkie's disease or syndrome 557.1
Wilkinson-Sneddon disease or syndrome (subcorneal pustular dermatosis) 694.1
Willan's lepra 696.1
Willan-Plumbe syndrome (psoriasis) 696.1

Willebrand (-Jürgens) syndrome or
thrombopathy (angiohemophilia) 286.4
Willi-Prader syndrome (hypogenital dystrophy
with diabetic tendency) 759.81
Willis' disease (diabetes mellitus) (*see also*
Diabetes) 250.0
due to secondary diabetes 249.0
Wilms' tumor or neoplasm (nephroblastoma)
(M8960/3) 189.0
Wilson's
disease or syndrome (hepatolenticular
degeneration) 275.1
hepatolenticular degeneration 275.1
lichen ruber 697.0
Wilson-Brocq disease (dermatitis exfoliativa)
695.89
Wilson-Mikity syndrome 770.7
Window —*see also* Imperfect, closure
aorticopulmonary 745.0
Winged scapula 736.89
Winter —*see also* condition
vomiting disease 078.82
Wise's disease 696.2
Wiskott-Aldrich syndrome
(eczema-thrombocytopenia) 279.12
Withdrawal symptoms, syndrome
alcohol 291.81
delirium (acute) 291.0
chronic 291.1
newborn 760.71
drug or narcotic 292.0
newborn, infant of dependent mother 779.5
steroid NEC
correct substance properly administered 255.41
overdose or wrong substance given or taken
962.0
Withdrawing reaction, child or adolescent
313.22
Witts' anemia (achlorhydric anemia) 280.9
Witzelsucht 301.9
Woakes' syndrome (ethmoiditis) 471.1
Wohlfart-Kugelberg-Welander disease 335.11
Woillez's disease (acute idiopathic pulmonary
congestion) 518.52
Wolff-Parkinson-White syndrome (anomalous
atrioventricular excitation) 426.7
Wolhynian fever 083.1
Wolman's disease (primary familial
xanthomatosis) 272.7
Wood asthma 495.8
Woolly, wooly hair (congenital) (nevus) 757.4
Wool-sorters' disease 022.1
Word
blindness (congenital) (developmental) 315.01
secondary to organic lesion 784.61
deafness (secondary to organic lesion) 784.69
developmental 315.31
Worm (s) (colic) (fever) (infection) (infestation)
(*see also* Infestation) 128.9
guinea 125.7
in intestine NEC 127.9
Worm-eaten soles 102.3
Worn out (*see also* Exhaustion) 780.79
artificial heart valve 996.02
cardiac defibrillator (with synchronous cardiac
pacemaker) V53.32
cardiac pacemaker lead or battery V53.31
joint prosthesis (see also Complications,
mechanical, device NEC, prosthetic NEC,
joint) 996.46
"Worried well" V65.5

Wound, open (by cutting or piercing instrument)
(by firearms) (cut) (dissection) (incised)
(laceration) (penetration) (perforating)
(puncture) (with initial hemorrhage, not
internal) 879.8

---

*Note—For fracture with open wound, see
Fracture. For laceration, traumatic rupture,
tear or penetrating wound of internal organs,
such as heart, lung, liver, kidney, pelvic organs,
etc., whether or not accompanied by open
wound or fracture in the same region, see
Injury, internal. For contused wound, see
Contusion. For crush injury, see Crush. For
abrasion, insect bite (nonvenomous), blister, or
scratch, see Injury, superficial.*

Complicated includes wounds with:
delayed healing
delayed treatment
foreign body
primary infection

*For late effect of open wound, see Late, effect,
wound, open, by site.*

---

abdomen, abdominal (external) (muscle) 879.2
complicated 879.3
wall (anterior) 879.2
complicated 879.3
lateral 879.4
complicated 879.5
alveolar (process) 873.62
complicated 873.72
ankle 891.0
with tendon involvement 891.2
complicated 891.1
anterior chamber, eye (*see also* Wound, open,
intraocular) 871.9
anus 863.89
arm 884.0
with tendon involvement 884.2
complicated 884.1
forearm 881.00
with tendon involvement 881.20
complicated 881.10
multiple sites—*see* Wound, open, multiple,
upper limb
upper 880.03
with tendon involvement 880.23
complicated 880.13
multiple sites (with axillary or shoulder
regions) 880.09
with tendon involvement 880.29
complicated 880.19
artery—*see* Injury, blood vessel, by site
auditory
canal (external) (meatus) 872.02
complicated 872.12
ossicles (incus) (malleus) (stapes) 872.62
complicated 872.72
auricle, ear 872.01
complicated 872.11
axilla 880.02
with tendon involvement 880.22
complicated 880.12
with tendon involvement 880.29
involving other sites of upper arm 880.09
complicated 880.19
back 876.0
complicated 876.1

Wound, open—*continued*
 heel 892.0
  with tendon involvement 892.2
  complicated 892.1
 high-velocity (grease gun)—*see* Wound, open,
   complicated, by site
 hip 890.0
  with tendon involvement 890.2
  complicated 890.1
 hymen 878.6
  complicated 878.7
 hypochondrium 879.4
  complicated 879.5
 hypogastric region 879.2
  complicated 879.3
 iliac (region) 879.4
  complicated 879.5
 incidental to
  dislocation—*see* Dislocation, open, by site
  fracture—*see* Fracture, open, by site
  intracranial injury—*see* Injury, intracranial,
    with open intracranial wound
  nerve injury—*see* Injury, nerve, by site
 inguinal region 879.4
  complicated 879.5
 instep 892.0
  with tendon involvement 892.2
  complicated 892.1
 interscapular region 876.0
  complicated 876.1
 intracranial—*see* Injury, intracranial, with open
   intracranial wound
 intraocular 871.9
  with
   partial loss (of intraocular tissue) 871.2
   prolapse or exposure (of intraocular tissue)
     871.1
  laceration (*see also* Laceration, eyeball) 871.4
  penetrating 871.7
   with foreign body (nonmagnetic) 871.6
    magnetic 871.5
  without prolapse (of intraocular tissue) 871.0
 iris (*see also* Wound, open, eyeball) 871.9
 jaw (fracture not involved) 873.44
  with fracture—*see* Fracture, jaw
  complicated 873.54
 knee 891.0
  with tendon involvement 891.2
  complicated 891.1
 labium (majus) (minus) 878.4
  complicated 878.5
 lacrimal apparatus, gland, or sac 870.8
  with laceration of eyelid 870.2
 larynx 874.01
  with trachea 874.00
   complicated 874.10
  complicated 874.11
 leg (multiple) 891.0
  with tendon involvement 891.2
  complicated 891.1
  lower 891.0
   with tendon involvement 891.2
   complicated 891.1
  thigh 890.0
   with tendon involvement 890.2
   complicated 890.1
  upper 890.0
   with tendon involvement 890.2
   complicated 890.1
 lens (eye) (alone) (*see also* Cataract, traumatic)
   366.20

Wound, open—*continued*
 with involvement of other eye structures—*see*
   Wound, open, eyeball
 limb
  lower (multiple) NEC 894.0
   with tendon involvement 894.2
   complicated 894.1
  upper (multiple) NEC 884.0
   with tendon involvement 884.2
   complicated 884.1
 lip 873.43
  complicated 873.53
 loin 876.0
  complicated 876.1
 lumbar region 876.0
  complicated 876.1
 malar region 873.41
  complicated 873.51
 mastoid region 873.49
  complicated 873.59
 mediastinum—*see* Injury, internal, mediastinum
 midthoracic region 875.0
  complicated 875.1
 mouth 873.60
  complicated 873.70
  floor 873.64
   complicated 873.74
  multiple sites 873.69
   complicated 873.79
  specified site NEC 873.69
   complicated 873.79
 multiple, unspecified site(s) 879.8

---

*Note—Multiple open wounds of sites
classifiable to the same four-digit category
should be classified to that category unless they
are in different limbs.*

*Multiple open wounds of sites classifiable to
different four-digit categories, or to different
limbs, should be coded separately.*

---

  complicated 879.9
  lower limb(s) (one or both) (sites classifiable
    to more than one three-digit category in
    890 to 893) 894.0
   with tendon involvement 894.2
   complicated 894.1
  upper limb(s) (one or both) (sites classifiable
    to more than one three-digit category in
    880 to 883) 884.0
   with tendon involvement 884.2
   complicated 884.1
 muscle—*see* Sprain, by site
 nail
  finger(s) 883.0
   complicated 883.1
  thumb 883.0
   complicated 883.1
  toe(s) 893.0
   complicated 893.1
 nape (neck) 874.8
  complicated 874.9
  specified part NEC 874.8
   complicated 874.9
 nasal—*see also* Wound, open, nose
  cavity 873.22
   complicated 873.32
  septum 873.21
   complicated 873.31
  sinuses 873.23
   complicated 873.33

Wound, open—*continued*
  complicated 893.1
  tongue 873.64
    complicated 873.74
  tonsil—*see* Wound, open, neck
  trachea (cervical region) 874.02
    with larynx 874.00
      complicated 874.10
    complicated 874.12
    intrathoracic—*see* Injury, internal, trachea
  trunk (multiple) NEC 879.6
    complicated 879.7
    specified site NEC 879.6
      complicated 879.7
  tunica vaginalis 878.2
    complicated 878.3
  tympanic membrane 872.61
    complicated 872.71
  tympanum 872.61
    complicated 872.71
  umbilical region 879.2
    complicated 879.3
  ureter—*see* Injury, internal, ureter
  urethra—*see* Injury, internal, urethra
  uterus—*see* Injury, internal, uterus
  uvula 873.69
    complicated 873.79
  vagina 878.6
    complicated 878.7
  vas deferens—*see* Injury, internal, vas deferens
  vitreous (humor) 871.2
  vulva 878.4
    complicated 878.5
  wrist 881.02
    with tendon involvement 881.22
    complicated 881.12
Wright's syndrome (hyperabduction) 447.8
  pneumonia 390 *[517.1]*
Wringer injury —*see* Crush injury, by site
Wrinkling of skin 701.8
Wrist —*see also* condition
  drop (acquired) 736.05
Wrong drug (given in error) NEC 977.9
  specified drug or substance—*see* Table of drugs
    and chemicals
Wry neck —*see also* Torticollis
  congenital 754.1
Wuchereria infestation 125.0
  bancrofti 125.0
  Brugia malayi 125.1
  malayi 125.1
Wuchereriasis 125.0
Wuchereriosis 125.0
Wuchernde struma langhans (M8332/3) 193

X

Xanthelasma 272.2
  eyelid 272.2 *[374.51]*
  palpebrarum 272.2 *[374.51]*
Xanthelasmatosis (essential) 272.2
Xanthelasmoidea 757.33
Xanthine stones 277.2
Xanthinuria 277.2
Xanthofibroma (M8831/0)—*see* Neoplasm,
  connective tissue, benign
Xanthoma(s), xanthomatosis 272.2
  with
    hyperlipoproteinemia
      type I 272.3
      type III 272.2
      type IV 272.1
      type V 272.3
  bone 272.7
  craniohypophyseal 277.89
  cutaneotendinous 272.7
  diabeticorum 250.8 *[272.2]*
    due to secondary diabetes 249.8 *[272.2]*
  disseminatum 272.7
  eruptive 272.2
  eyelid 272.2 *[374.51]*
  familial 272.7
  hereditary 272.7
  hypercholesterinemic 272.0
  hypercholesterolemic 272.0
  hyperlipemic 272.4
  hyperlipidemic 272.4
  infantile 272.7
  joint 272.7
  juvenile 272.7
  multiple 272.7
  multiplex 272.7
  primary familial 272.7
  tendon (sheath) 272.7
  tuberosum 272.2
  tuberous 272.2
  tubo-eruptive 272.2
Xanthosis 709.09
  surgical 998.81
Xenophobia 300.29
Xeroderma (congenital) 757.39
  acquired 701.1
    eyelid 373.33
  eyelid 373.33
  pigmentosum 757.33
  vitamin A deficiency 264.8
Xerophthalmia 372.53
  vitamin A deficiency 264.7
Xerosis
  conjunctiva 372.53
    with Bitôt's spot 372.53
      vitamin A deficiency 264.1
    vitamin A deficiency 264.0
  cornea 371.40
    with corneal ulceration 370.00
      vitamin A deficiency 264.3
    vitamin A deficiency 264.2
  cutis 706.8
  skin 706.8
Xerostomia 527.7
Xiphodynia 733.90
Xiphoidalgia 733.90
Xiphoiditis 733.99
Xiphopagus 759.4

XO syndrome 758.6
X-ray
  effects, adverse, NEC 990
  of chest
    for suspected tuberculosis V71.2
    routine V72.5
XXX syndrome 758.81
XXXXY syndrome 758.81
XXY syndrome 758.7
Xyloketosuria 271.8
Xylosuria 271.8
Xylulosuria 271.8
XYY syndrome 758.81

Y

Yaba monkey tumor virus 059.22
Yawning 786.09
  psychogenic 306.1
Yaws 102.9
  bone or joint lesions 102.6
  butter 102.1
  chancre 102.0
  cutaneous, less than five years after infection
      102.2
  early (cutaneous) (macular) (maculopapular)
      (micropapular) (papular) 102.2
    frambeside 102.2
    skin lesions NEC 102.2
  eyelid 102.9 *[373.4]*
  ganglion 102.6
  gangosis, gangosa 102.5
  gumma, gummata 102.4
    bone 102.6
  gummatous
    frambeside 102.4
    osteitis 102.6
    periostitis 102.6
  hydrarthrosis 102.6
  hyperkeratosis (early) (late) (palmar) (plantar)
      102.3
  initial lesions 102.0
  joint lesions 102.6
  juxta-articular nodules 102.7
  late nodular (ulcerated) 102.4
  latent (without clinical manifestations) (with
      positive serology) 102.8
  mother 102.0
  mucosal 102.7
  multiple papillomata 102.1
  nodular, late (ulcerated) 102.4
  osteitis 102.6
  papilloma, papillomata (palmar) (plantar) 102.1
  periostitis (hypertrophic) 102.6
  ulcers 102.4
  wet crab 102.1
Yeast infection (*see also* Candidiasis) 112.9
Yellow
  atrophy (liver) 570
    chronic 571.8
    resulting from administration of blood,
        plasma, serum, or other biological
        substance (within 8 months of
        administration)—*see* Hepatitis, viral
  fever—*see* Fever, yellow
  jack (*see also* Fever, yellow) 060.9
  jaundice (*see also* Jaundice) 782.4
Yersinia septica 027.8

Z

Zagari's disease (xerostomia) 527.7
Zahorsky's disease (exanthema subitum) (*see
    also* Exanthem subitum) 058.10
  syndrome (herpangina) 074.0
Zellweger syndrome 277.86
Zenker's diverticulum (esophagus) 530.6
Ziehen-Oppenheim disease 333.6
Zieve's syndrome (jaundice, hyperlipemia, and
    hemolytic anemia) 571.1
Zika fever 066.3
Zollinger-Ellison syndrome (gastric
    hypersecretion with pancreatic islet cell
    tumor) 251.5
Zona (*see also* Herpes, zoster) 053.9
Zoophilia (erotica) 302.1
Zoophobia 300.29
Zoster (herpes) (*see also* Herpes, zoster) 053.9
Zuelzer (-Ogden) anemia or syndrome
    (nutritional megaloblastic anemia) 281.2
Zygodactyly (*see also* Syndactylism) 755.10
Zygomycosis 117.7
Zymotic —*see* condition

SECTION 2

ALPHABETIC INDEX TO POISONING AND EXTERNAL CAUSES OF ADVERSE EFFECTS OF DRUGS AND OTHER CHEMICAL SUBSTANCES

TABLE OF DRUGS AND CHEMICALS

This table contains a classification of drugs and other chemical substances to identify poisoning states and external causes of adverse effects.

Each of the listed substances in the table is assigned a code according to the poisoning classification (960–989). These codes are used when there is a statement of poisoning, overdose, wrong substance given or taken, or intoxication.

The table also contains a listing of external causes of adverse effects. An adverse effect is a pathologic manifestation due to ingestion or exposure to drugs or other chemical substances (e.g., dermatitis, hypersensitivity reaction, aspirin gastritis). The adverse effect is to be identified by the appropriate code found in Section 1, Index to Diseases and Injuries. An external cause code can then be used to identify the circumstances involved. The table headings pertaining to external causes are defined below:

Accidental poisoning (E850–E869)—accidental overdose of drug, wrong substance given or taken, drug taken inadvertently, accidents in the usage of drugs and biologicals in medical and surgical procedures, and to show external causes of poisonings classifiable to 980–989.

Therapeutic use (E930–E949)—a correct substance properly administered in therapeutic or prophylactic dosage as the external cause of adverse effects.

Suicide attempt (E950–E952)—instances in which self–inflicted injuries or poisonings are involved.

Assault (E961–E962)—injury or poisoning inflicted by another person with the intent to injure or kill.

Undetermined (E980–E982)—to be used when the intent of the poisoning or injury cannot be determined whether it was intentional or accidental.

The American Hospital Formulary Service list numbers are included in the table to help classify new drugs not identified in the table by name. The AHFS list numbers are keyed to the continually revised American Hospital Formulary Service (AHFS).* These listings are found in the table under the main term **Drug**.

Excluded from the table are radium and other radioactive substances. The classification of adverse effects and complications pertaining to these substances will be found in Section 1, Index to Diseases and Injuries, and Section 3, Index to External Causes of Injuries.

Although certain substances are indexed with one or more subentries, the majority are listed according to one use or state. It is recognized that many substances may be used in various ways, in medicine and in industry, and may cause adverse effects whatever the state of the agent (solid, liquid, or fumes arising from a liquid). In cases in which the reported data indicates a use or state not in the table, or which is clearly different from the one listed, an attempt should be made to classify the substance in the form which most nearly expresses the reported facts.

*American Hospital Formulary Service, 2 vol. (Washington, DC: American Society of Hospital Pharmacists, 1959)

Substance	Poisoning	Accident	Therapeutic Use	Suicide Attempt	Assault	Undetermined
			External Cause (E-Code)			
1–propanol	980.3	E860.4	—	E950.9	E962.1	E980.9
2–propanol	980.2	E860.3	—	E950.9	E962.1	E980.9
2, 4–D (dichlorophenoxyacetic acid)	989.4	E863.5	—	E950.6	E962.1	E980.7
2, 4–toluene diisocyanate	983.0	E864.0	—	E950.7	E962.1	E980.6
2, 4, 5–T (trichlorophenoxyacetic acid)	989.2	E863.5	—	E950.6	E962.1	E980.7
14–hydroxydihydromorphinone	965.09	E850.2	E935.2	E950.0	E962.0	E980.0
ABOB	961.7	E857	E931.7	E950.4	E962.0	E980.4
Abrus (seed)	988.2	E865.3	—	E950.9	E962.1	E980.9
Absinthe	980.0	E860.1	—	E950.9	E962.1	E980.9
beverage	980.0	E860.0	—	E950.9	E962.1	E980.9
Acenocoumarin, acenocoumarol	964.2	E858.2	E934.2	E950.4	E962.0	E980.4
Acepromazine	969.1	E853.0	E939.1	E950.3	E962.0	E980.3
Acetal	982.8	E862.4	—	E950.9	E962.1	E980.9
Acetaldehyde (vapor)	987.8	E869.8	—	E952.8	E962.2	E982.8
liquid	989.89	E866.8	—	E950.9	E962.1	E980.9
Acetaminophen	965.4	E850.4	E935.4	E950.0	E962.0	E980.0
Acetaminosalol	965.1	E850.3	E935.3	E950.0	E962.0	E980.0
Acetanilid(e)	965.4	E850.4	E935.4	E950.0	E962.0	E980.0
Acetarsol, acetarsone	961.1	E857	E931.1	E950.4	E962.0	E980.4
Acetazolamide	974.2	E858.5	E944.2	E950.4	E962.0	E980.4
Acetic						
acid	983.1	E864.1	—	E950.7	E962.1	E980.6
with sodium acetate (ointment)	976.3	E858.7	E946.3	E950.4	E962.0	E980.4
irrigating solution	974.5	E858.5	E944.5	E950.4	E962.0	E980.4
lotion	976.2	E858.7	E946.2	E950.4	E962.0	E980.4
anhydride	983.1	E864.1	—	E950.7	E962.1	E980.6
ether (vapor)	982.8	E862.4	—	E950.9	E962.1	E980.9
Acetohexamide	962.3	E858.0	E932.3	E950.4	E962.0	E980.4
Acetomenaphthone	964.3	E858.2	E934.3	E950.4	E962.0	E980.4
Acetomorphine	965.01	E850.0	E935.0	E950.0	E962.0	E980.0
Acetone (oils) (vapor)	982.8	E862.4	—	E950.9	E962.1	E980.9
Acetophenazine (maleate)	969.1	E853.0	E939.1	E950.3	E962.0	E980.3
Acetophenetidin	965.4	E850.4	E935.4	E950.0	E962.0	E980.0
Acetophenone	982.0	E862.4	—	E950.9	E962.1	E980.9
Acetorphine	965.09	E850.2	E935.2	E950.0	E962.0	E980.0
Acetosulfone (sodium)	961.8	E857	E931.8	E950.4	E962.0	E980.4
Acetrizoate (sodium)	977.8	E858.8	E947.8	E950.4	E962.0	E980.4
Acetylcarbromal	967.3	E852.2	E937.3	E950.2	E962.0	E980.2
Acetylcholine (chloride)	971.0	E855.3	E941.0	E950.4	E962.0	E980.4
Acetylcysteine	975.5	E858.6	E945.5	E950.4	E962.0	E980.4
Acetyldigitoxin	972.1	E858.3	E942.1	E950.4	E962.0	E980.4
Acetyldihydrocodeine	965.09	E850.2	E935.2	E950.0	E962.0	E980.0
Acetyldihydrocodeinone	965.09	E850.2	E935.2	E950.0	E962.0	E980.0
Acetylene (gas) (industrial)	987.1	E868.1	—	E951.8	E962.2	E981.8
incomplete combustion of — *see* Carbon monoxide, fuel, utility						
tetrachloride (vapor)	982.3	E862.4	—	E950.9	E962.1	E980.9
Acetyliodosalicylic acid	965.1	E850.3	E935.3	E950.0	E962.0	E980.0
Acetylphenylhydrazine	965.8	E850.8	E935.8	E950.0	E962.0	E980.0
Acetylsalicylic acid	965.1	E850.3	E935.3	E950.0	E962.0	E980.0
Achromycin	960.4	E856	E930.4	E950.4	E962.0	E980.4
ophthalmic preparation	976.5	E858.7	E946.5	E950.4	E962.0	E980.4
topical NEC	976.0	E858.7	E946.0	E950.4	E962.0	E980.4
Acidifying agents	963.2	E858.1	E933.2	E950.4	E962.0	E980.4
Acids (corrosive) NEC	983.1	E864.1	—	E950.7	E962.1	E980.6
Aconite (wild)	988.2	E865.4	—	E950.9	E962.1	E980.9
Aconitine (liniment)	976.8	E858.7	E946.8	E950.4	E962.0	E980.4
Aconitum ferox	988.2	E865.4	—	E950.9	E962.1	E980.9
Acridine	983.0	E864.0	—	E950.7	E962.1	E980.6
vapor	987.8	E869.8	—	E952.8	E962.2	E982.8

Substance	Poisoning	Accident	Therapeutic Use	Suicide Attempt	Assault	Undetermined
		External Cause (E-Code)				
Acriflavine	961.9	E857	E931.9	E950.4	E962.0	E980.4
Acrisorcin	976.0	E858.7	E946.0	E950.4	E962.0	E980.4
Acrolein (gas)	987.8	E869.8	—	E952.8	E962.2	E982.8
liquid	989.89	E866.8	—	E950.9	E962.1	E980.9
Actaea spicata	988.2	E865.4	—	E950.9	E962.1	E980.9
Acterol	961.5	E857	E931.5	E950.4	E962.0	E980.4
ACTH	962.4	E858.0	E932.4	E950.4	E962.0	E980.4
Acthar	962.4	E858.0	E932.4	E950.4	E962.0	E980.4
Actinomycin (C) (D)	960.7	E856	E930.7	E950.4	E962.0	E980.4
Adalin (acetyl)	967.3	E852.2	E937.3	E950.2	E962.0	E980.2
Adenosine (phosphate)	977.8	E858.8	E947.8	E950.4	E962.0	E980.4
Adhesives	989.89	E866.6	—	E950.9	E962.1	E980.9
ADH	962.5	E858.0	E932.5	E950.4	E962.0	E980.4
Adicillin	960.0	E856	E930.0	E950.4	E962.0	E980.4
Adiphenine	975.1	E855.6	E945.1	E950.4	E962.0	E980.4
Adjunct, pharmaceutical	977.4	E858.8	E947.4	E950.4	E962.0	E980.4
Adrenal (extract, cortex or medulla) (glucocorticoids) (hormones) (mineralocorticoids)	962.0	E858.0	E932.0	E950.4	E962.0	E980.4
ENT agent	976.6	E858.7	E946.6	E950.4	E962.0	E980.4
ophthalmic preparation	976.5	E858.7	E946.5	E950.4	E962.0	E980.4
topical NEC	976.0	E858.7	E946.0	E950.4	E962.0	E980.4
Adrenalin	971.2	E855.5	E941.2	E950.4	E962.0	E980.4
Adrenergic blocking agents	971.3	E855.6	E941.3	E950.4	E962.0	E980.4
Adrenergics	971.2	E855.5	E941.2	E950.4	E962.0	E980.4
Adrenochrome (derivatives)	972.8	E858.3	E942.8	E950.4	E962.0	E980.4
Adrenocorticotropic hormone	962.4	E858.0	E932.4	E950.4	E962.0	E980.4
Adrenocorticotropin	962.4	E858.0	E932.4	E950.4	E962.0	E980.4
Adriamycin	960.7	E856	E930.7	E950.4	E962.0	E980.4
Aerosol spray — *see* Sprays						
Aerosporin	960.8	E856	E930.8	E950.4	E962.0	E980.4
ENT agent	976.6	E858.7	E946.6	E950.4	E962.0	E980.4
ophthalmic preparation	976.5	E858.7	E946.5	E950.4	E962.0	E980.4
topical NEC	976.0	E858.7	E946.0	E950.4	E962.0	E980.4
Aethusa cynapium	988.2	E865.4	—	E950.9	E962.1	E980.9
Afghanistan black	969.6	E854.1	E939.6	E950.3	E962.0	E980.3
Aflatoxin	989.7	E865.9	—	E950.9	E962.1	E980.9
African boxwood	988.2	E865.4	—	E950.9	E962.1	E980.9
Agar (–agar)	973.3	E858.4	E943.3	E950.4	E962.0	E980.4
Agricultural agent NEC	989.89	E863.9	—	E950.6	E962.1	E980.7
Agrypnal	967.0	E851	E937.0	E950.1	E962.0	E980.1
Air contaminant(s), source or type not specified	987.9	E869.9	—	E952.9	E962.2	E982.9
specified type — *see* specific substance						
Akee	988.2	E865.4	—	E950.9	E962.1	E980.9
Akrinol	976.0	E858.7	E946.0	E950.4	E962.0	E980.4
Alantolactone	961.6	E857	E931.6	E950.4	E962.0	E980.4
Albamycin	960.8	E856	E930.8	E950.4	E962.0	E980.4
Albumin (normal human serum)	964.7	E858.2	E934.7	E950.4	E962.0	E980.4
Albuterol	975.7	E858.6	E945.7	E950.4	E962.0	E980.4
Alcohol	980.9	E860.9	—	E950.9	E962.1	E980.9
absolute	980.0	E860.1	—	E950.9	E962.1	E980.9
beverage	980.0	E860.0	E947.8	E950.9	E962.1	E980.9
amyl	980.3	E860.4	—	E950.9	E962.1	E980.9
antifreeze	980.1	E860.2	—	E950.9	E962.1	E980.9
butyl	980.3	E860.4	—	E950.9	E962.1	E980.9
dehydrated	980.0	E860.1	—	E950.9	E962.1	E980.9
beverage	980.0	E860.0	E947.8	E950.9	E862.1	E980.9
denatured	980.0	E860.1	—	E950.9	E962.1	E980.9
deterrents	977.3	E858.8	E947.3	E950.4	E962.0	E980.4
diagnostic (gastric function)	977.8	E858.8	E947.8	E950.4	E962.0	E980.4

Substance	Poisoning	Accident	Therapeutic Use	Suicide Attempt	Assault	Undetermined
			External Cause (E-Code)			
ethyl	980.0	E860.1	—	E950.9	E962.1	E980.9
beverage	980.0	E860.0	E947.8	E950.9	E962.1	E980.9
grain	980.0	E860.1	—	E950.9	E962.1	E980.9
beverage	980.0	E860.0	E947.8	E950.9	E962.1	E980.9
industrial	980.9	E860.9	—	E950.9	E962.1	E980.9
isopropyl	980.2	E860.3	—	E950.9	E962.1	E980.9
methyl	980.1	E860.2	—	E950.9	E962.1	E980.9
preparation for consumption	980.0	E860.0	E947.8	E950.9	E962.1	E980.9
propyl	980.3	E860.4	—	E950.9	E962.1	E980.9
secondary	980.2	E860.3	—	E950.9	E962.1	E980.9
radiator	980.1	E860.2	—	E950.9	E962.1	E980.9
rubbing	980.2	E860.3	—	E950.9	E962.1	E980.9
specified type NEC	980.8	E860.8	—	E950.9	E962.1	E980.9
surgical	980.9	E860.9	—	E950.9	E962.1	E980.9
vapor (from any type of alcohol)	987.8	E869.8	—	E952.8	E962.2	E982.8
wood	980.1	E860.2	—	E950.9	E962.1	E980.9
Alcuronium chloride	975.2	E858.6	E945.2	E950.4	E962.0	E980.4
Aldactone	974.4	E858.5	E944.4	E950.4	E962.0	E980.4
Aldicarb	989.3	E863.2	—	E950.6	E962.1	E980.7
Aldomet	972.6	E858.3	E942.6	E950.4	E962.0	E980.4
Aldosterone	962.0	E858.0	E932.0	E950.4	E962.0	E980.4
Aldrin (dust)	989.2	E863.0	—	E950.6	E962.1	E980.7
Algeldrate	973.0	E858.4	E943.0	E950.4	E962.0	E980.4
Alidase	963.4	E858.1	E933.4	E950.4	E962.0	E980.4
Aliphatic thiocyanates	989.0	E866.8	—	E950.9	E962.1	E980.9
Alkaline antiseptic solution (aromatic)	976.6	E858.7	E946.6	E950.4	E962.0	E980.4
Alkalinizing agents (medicinal)	963.3	E858.1	E933.3	E950.4	E962.0	E980.4
Alkalis, caustic	983.2	E864.2	—	E950.7	E962.1	E980.6
Alkalizing agents (medicinal)	963.3	E858.1	E933.3	E950.4	E962.0	E980.4
Alka–seltzer	965.1	E850.3	E935.3	E950.0	E962.0	E980.0
Alkavervir	972.6	E858.3	E942.6	E950.4	E962.0	E980.4
Allegron	969.05	E854.0	E939.0	E950.3	E962.0	E980.3
Alleve *see* Naproxen						
Allobarbital, allobarbitone	967.0	E851	E937.0	E950.1	E962.0	E980.1
Allopurinol	974.7	E858.5	E944.7	E950.4	E962.0	E980.4
Allylestrenol	962.2	E858.0	E932.2	E950.4	E962.0	E980.4
Allylisopropylacetylurea	967.8	E852.8	E937.8	E950.2	E962.0	E980.2
Allylisopropylmalonylurea	967.0	E851	E937.0	E950.1	E962.0	E980.1
Allyltribromide	967.3	E852.2	E937.3	E950.2	E962.0	E980.2
Aloe, aloes, aloin	973.1	E858.4	E943.1	E950.4	E962.0	E980.4
Alosetron	973.8	E858.4	E943.8	E950.4	E962.0	E980.4
Aloxidone	966.0	E855.0	E936.0	E950.4	E962.0	E980.4
Aloxiprin	965.1	E850.3	E935.3	E950.0	E962.0	E980.0
Alpha amylase	963.4	E858.1	E933.4	E950.4	E962.0	E980.4
Alpha-1 blockers	971.3	E855.6	E941.3	E950.4	E962.0	E980.4
Alpha tocopherol	963.5	E858.1	E933.5	E950.4	E962.0	E980.4
Alphaprodine (hydrochloride)	965.09	E850.2	E935.2	E950.0	E962.0	E980.0
Alseroxylon	972.6	E858.3	E942.6	E950.4	E962.0	E980.4
Alum (ammonium) (potassium)	983.2	E864.2	—	E950.7	E962.1	E980.6
medicinal (astringent) NEC	976.2	E858.7	E946.2	E950.4	E962.0	E980.4
Aluminium, aluminum (gel) (hydroxide)	973.0	E858.4	E943.0	E950.4	E962.0	E980.4
acetate solution	976.2	E858.7	E946.2	E950.4	E962.0	E980.4
aspirin	965.1	E850.3	E935.3	E950.0	E962.0	E980.0
carbonate	973.0	E858.4	E943.0	E950.4	E962.0	E980.4
glycinate	973.0	E858.4	E943.0	E950.4	E962.0	E980.4
nicotinate	972.2	E858.3	E942.2	E950.4	E962.0	E980.4
ointment (surgical) (topical)	976.3	E858.7	E946.3	E950.4	E962.0	E980.4
phosphate	973.0	E858.4	E943.0	E950.4	E962.0	E980.4
subacetate	976.2	E858.7	E946.2	E950.4	E962.0	E980.4
topical NEC	976.3	E858.7	E946.3	E950.4	E962.0	E980.4

Substance	Poisoning	Accident	Therapeutic Use	Suicide Attempt	Assault	Undetermined
			External Cause (E-Code)			
Alurate	967.0	E851	E937.0	E950.1	E962.0	E980.1
Alverine (citrate)	975.1	E858.6	E945.1	E950.4	E962.0	E980.4
Alvodine	965.09	E850.2	E935.2	E950.0	E962.0	E980.0
Amanita phalloides	988.1	E865.5	—	E950.9	E962.1	E980.9
Amantadine (hydrochloride)	966.4	E855.0	E936.4	E950.4	E962.0	E980.4
Ambazone.	961.9	E857	E931.9	E950.4	E962.0	E980.4
Ambenonium	971.0	E855.3	E941.0	E950.4	E962.0	E980.4
Ambutonium bromide	971.1	E855.4	E941.1	E950.4	E962.0	E980.4
Ametazole.	977.8	E858.8	E947.8	E950.4	E962.0	E980.4
Amethocaine (infiltration) (topical) .	968.5	E855.2	E938.5	E950.4	E962.0	E980.4
nerve block (peripheral) (plexus).	968.6	E855.2	E938.6	E950.4	E962.0	E980.4
spinal.	968.7	E855.2	E938.7	E950.4	E962.0	E980.4
Amethopterin	963.1	E858.1	E933.1	E950.4	E962.0	E980.4
Amfepramone	977.0	E858.8	E947.0	E950.4	E962.0	E980.4
Amidon.	965.02	E850.1	E935.1	E950.0	E962.0	E980.0
Amidopyrine.	965.5	E850.5	E935.5	E950.0	E962.0	E980.0
Aminacrine	976.0	E858.7	E946.0	E950.4	E962.0	E980.4
Aminitrozole.	961.5	E857	E931.5	E950.4	E962.0	E980.4
Aminoacetic acid	974.5	E858.5	E944.5	E950.4	E962.0	E980.4
Amino acids.	974.5	E858.5	E944.5	E950.4	E962.0	E980.4
Aminocaproic acid	964.4	E858.2	E934.4	E950.4	E962.0	E980.4
Aminoethylisothiourium	963.8	E858.1	E933.8	E950.4	E962.0	E980.4
Aminoglutethimide	966.3	E855.0	E936.3	E950.4	E962.0	E980.4
Aminometradine	974.3	E858.5	E944.3	E950.4	E962.0	E980.4
Aminopentamide	971.1	E855.4	E941.1	E950.4	E962.0	E980.4
Aminophenazone	965.5	E850.5	E935.5	E950.0	E962.0	E980.0
Aminophenol	983.0	E864.0	—	E950.7	E962.1	E980.6
Aminophenylpyridone	969.5	E853.8	E939.5	E950.3	E962.0	E980.3
Aminophyllin	975.7	E858.6	E945.7	E950.4	E962.0	E980.4
Aminopterin	963.1	E858.1	E933.1	E950.4	E962.0	E980.4
Aminopyrine.	965.5	E850.5	E935.5	E950.0	E962.0	E980.0
Aminosalicylic acid	961.8	E857	E931.8	E950.4	E962.0	E980.4
Amiphenazole	970.1	E854.3	E940.1	E950.4	E962.0	E980.4
Amiquinsin	972.6	E858.3	E942.6	E950.4	E962.0	E980.4
Amisometradine	974.3	E858.5	E944.3	E950.4	E962.0	E980.4
Amitriptyline	969.05	E854.0	E939.0	E950.3	E962.0	E980.3
Ammonia (fumes) (gas) (vapor)	987.8	E869.8	—	E952.8	E962.2	E982.8
liquid (household) NEC	983.2	E861.4	—	E950.7	E962.1	E980.6
spirit, aromatic	970.89	E854.3	E940.8	E950.4	E962.0	E980.4
Ammoniated mercury	976.0	E858.7	E946.0	E950.4	E962.0	E980.4
Ammonium						
carbonate	983.2	E864.2	—	E950.7	E962.1	E980.6
chloride (acidifying agent)	963.2	E858.1	E933.2	E950.4	E962.0	E980.4
expectorant	975.5	E858.6	E945.5	E950.4	E962.0	E980.4
compounds (household) NEC	983.2	E861.4	—	E950.7	E962.1	E980.6
fumes (any usage)	987.8	E869.8	—	E952.8	E962.2	E982.8
industrial.	983.2	E864.2	—	E950.7	E962.1	E980.6
ichthyosulfonate	976.4	E858.7	E946.4	E950.4	E962.0	E980.4
mandelate	961.9	E857	E931.9	E950.4	E962.0	E980.4
Amobarbital	967.0	E851	E937.0	E950.1	E962.0	E980.1
Amodiaquin(e)	961.4	E857	E931.4	E950.4	E962.0	E980.4
Amopyroquin(e)	961.4	E857	E931.4	E950.4	E962.0	E980.4
Amphenidone	969.5	E853.8	E939.5	E950.3	E962.0	E980.3
Amphetamine	969.72	E854.2	E939.7	E950.3	E962.0	E980.3
Amphomycin	960.8	E856	E930.8	E950.4	E962.0	E980.4
Amphotericin B	960.1	E856	E930.1	E950.4	E962.0	E980.4
topical	976.0	E858.7	E946.0	E950.4	E962.0	E980.4
Ampicillin.	960.0	E856	E930.0	E950.4	E962.0	E980.4
Amprotropine	971.1	E855.4	E941.1	E950.4	E962.0	E980.4
Amygdalin	977.8	E858.8	E947.8	E950.4	E962.0	E980.4
Amyl						

Substance	Poisoning	Accident	Therapeutic Use	Suicide Attempt	Assault	Undetermined
			External Cause (E-Code)			
acetate (vapor)	982.8	E862.4	—	E950.9	E962.1	E980.9
alcohol	980.3	E860.4	—	E950.9	E962.1	E980.9
nitrite (medicinal)	972.4	E858.3	E942.4	E950.4	E962.0	E980.4
Amylase (alpha)	963.4	E858.1	E933.4	E950.4	E962.0	E980.4
Amylene hydrate	980.8	E860.8	—	E950.9	E962.1	E980.9
Amylobarbitone	967.0	E851	E937.0	E950.1	E962.0	E980.1
Amylocaine	968.9	E855.2	E938.9	E950.4	E962.0	E980.4
infiltration (subcutaneous)	968.5	E855.2	E938.5	E950.4	E962.0	E980.4
nerve block (peripheral) (plexus).	968.6	E855.2	E938.6	E950.4	E962.0	E980.4
spinal	968.7	E855.2	E938.7	E950.4	E962.0	E980.4
topical (surface)	968.5	E855.2	E938.5	E950.4	E962.0	E980.4
Amytal (sodium)	967.0	E851	E937.0	E950.1	E962.0	E980.1
Analeptics.	970.0	E854.3	E940.0	E950.4	E962.0	E980.4
Analgesics	965.9	E850.9	E935.9	E950.0	E962.0	E980.0
aromatic NEC	965.4	E850.4	E935.4	E950.0	E962.0	E980.0
non–narcotic NEC.	965.7	E850.7	E935.7	E950.0	E962.0	E980.0
specified NEC	965.8	E850.8	E935.8	E950.0	E962.0	E980.0
Anamirta cocculus	988.2	E865.3	—	E950.9	E962.1	E980.9
Ancillin.	960.0	E856	E930.0	E950.4	E962.0	E980.4
Androgens (anabolic congeners).	962.1	E858.0	E932.1	E950.4	E962.0	E980.4
Androstalone	962.1	E858.0	E932.1	E950.4	E962.0	E980.4
Androsterone	962.1	E858.0	E932.1	E950.4	E962.0	E980.4
Anemone pulsatilla	988.2	E865.4	—	E950.9	E962.1	E980.9
Anesthesia, anesthetic (general) NEC	968.4	E855.1	E938.4	E950.4	E962.0	E980.4
block (nerve) (plexus)	968.6	E855.2	E938.6	E950.4	E962.0	E980.4
gaseous NEC.	968.2	E855.1	E938.2	E950.4	E962.0	E980.4
halogenated hydrocarbon derivatives NEC	968.2	E855.1	E938.2	E950.4	E962.0	E980.4
infiltration (intradermal) (subcutaneous) (submucosal)	968.5	E855.2	E938.5	E950.4	E962.0	E980.4
intravenous.	968.3	E855.1	E938.3	E950.4	E962.0	E980.4
local NEC.	968.9	E855.2	E938.9	E950.4	E962.0	E980.4
nerve blocking (peripheral) (plexus)	968.6	E855.2	E938.6	E950.4	E962.0	E980.4
rectal NEC.	968.3	E855.1	E938.3	E950.4	E962.0	E980.4
spinal	968.7	E855.2	E938.7	E950.4	E962.0	E980.4
surface	968.5	E855.2	E938.5	E950.4	E962.0	E980.4
topical	968.5	E855.2	E938.5	E950.4	E962.0	E980.4
Aneurine	963.5	E858.1	E933.5	E950.4	E962.0	E980.4
Angio–Conray	977.8	E858.8	E947.8	E950.4	E962.0	E980.4
Anginine see Glyceryl trinitrate						
Angiotensin	971.2	E855.5	E941.2	E950.4	E962.0	E980.4
Anhydrohydroxyprogesterone	962.2	E858.0	E932.2	E950.4	E962.0	E980.4
Anhydron	974.3	E858.5	E944.3	E950.4	E962.0	E980.4
Anileridine	965.09	E850.2	E935.2	E950.0	E962.0	E980.0
Aniline (dye) (liquid)	983.0	E864.0	—	E950.7	E962.1	E980.6
analgesic	965.4	E850.4	E935.4	E950.0	E962.0	E980.0
derivatives, therapeutic NEC	965.4	E850.4	E935.4	E950.0	E962.0	E980.0
vapor	987.8	E869.8	—	E952.8	E962.2	E982.8
Anisindione	964.2	E858.2	E934.2	E950.4	E962.0	E980.4
Anisotropine.	971.1	E855.4	E941.1	E950.4	E962.0	E980.4
Anorexic agents	977.0	E858.8	E947.0	E950.4	E962.0	E980.4
Ant (bite) (sting)	989.5	E905.5	—	E950.9	E962.1	E980.9
Antabuse	977.3	E858.8	E947.3	E950.4	E962.0	E980.4
Antacids	973.0	E858.4	E943.0	E950.4	E962.0	E980.4
Antazoline	963.0	E858.1	E933.0	E950.4	E962.0	E980.4
Anthelmintics	961.6	E857	E931.6	E950.4	E962.0	E980.4
Anthralin	976.4	E858.7	E946.4	E950.4	E962.0	E980.4
Anthramycin.	960.7	E856	E930.7	E950.4	E962.0	E980.4
Antiadrenergics.	971.3	E855.6	E941.3	E950.4	E962.0	E980.4
Antiallergic agents	963.0	E858.1	E933.0	E950.4	E962.0	E980.4

Substance	Poisoning	Accident	Therapeutic Use	Suicide Attempt	Assault	Undetermined
		External Cause (E-Code)				
Antianemic agents NEC	964.1	E858.2	E934.1	E950.4	E962.0	E980.4
Antiaris toxicaria	988.2	E865.4	—	E950.9	E962.1	E980.9
Antiarteriosclerotic agents	972.2	E858.3	E942.2	E950.4	E962.0	E980.4
Antiasthmatics	975.7	E858.6	E945.7	E950.4	E962.0	E980.4
Antibiotics	960.9	E856	E930.9	E950.4	E962.0	E980.4
antifungal	960.1	E856	E930.1	E950.4	E962.0	E980.4
antimycobacterial	960.6	E856	E930.6	E950.4	E962.0	E980.4
antineoplastic	960.7	E856	E930.7	E950.4	E962.0	E980.4
cephalosporin (group)	960.5	E856	E930.5	E950.4	E962.0	E980.4
chloramphenicol (group)	960.2	E856	E930.2	E950.4	E962.0	E980.4
macrolides	960.3	E856	E930.3	E950.4	E962.0	E980.4
specified NEC	960.8	E856	E930.8	E950.4	E962.0	E980.4
tetracycline (group)	960.4	E856	E930.4	E950.4	E962.0	E980.4
Anticancer agents NEC	963.1	E858.1	E933.1	E950.4	E962.0	E980.4
antibiotics	960.7	E856	E930.7	E950.4	E962.0	E980.4
Anticholinergics	971.1	E855.4	E941.1	E950.4	E962.0	E980.4
Anticholinesterase (organophosphorus) (reversible)	971.0	E855.3	E941.0	E950.4	E962.0	E980.4
Anticoagulants	964.2	E858.2	E934.2	E950.4	E962.0	E980.4
antagonists	964.5	E858.2	E934.5	E950.4	E962.0	E980.4
Anti–common cold agents NEC	975.6	E858.6	E945.6	E950.4	E962.0	E980.4
Anticonvulsants NEC	966.3	E855.0	E936.3	E950.4	E962.0	E980.4
Antidepressants	969.00	E854.0	E939.0	E950.3	E962.0	E980.3
monoamine oxidase inhibitors (MAOI)	969.01	E854.0	E939.0	E950.3	E962.0	E980.3
specified type NEC	969.09	E854.0	E939.0	E950.3	E962.0	E980.3
SSNRI (selective serotonin and norepinephrine reuptake inhibitors)	969.02	E854.0	E939.0	E950.3	E962.0	E980.3
SSRI (selective serotonin reuptake inhibitors)	969.03	E854.0	E939.0	E950.3	E962.0	E980.3
tetracyclic	969.04	E854.0	E939.0	E950.3	E962.0	E980.3
tricyclic	969.05	E854.0	E939.0	E950.3	E962.0	E980.3
Antidiabetic agents	962.3	E858.0	E932.3	E950.4	E962.0	E980.4
Antidiarrheal agents	973.5	E858.4	E943.5	E950.4	E962.0	E980.4
Antidiuretic hormone	962.5	E858.0	E932.5	E950.4	E962.0	E980.4
Antidotes NEC	977.2	E858.8	E947.2	E950.4	E962.0	E980.4
Antiemetic agents	963.0	E858.1	E933.0	E950.4	E962.0	E980.4
Antiepilepsy agent NEC	966.3	E855.0	E936.3	E950.4	E962.0	E980.4
Antifertility pills	962.2	E858.0	E932.2	E950.4	E962.0	E980.4
Antiflatulents	973.8	E858.4	E943.8	E950.4	E962.0	E980.4
Antifreeze	989.89	E866.8	—	E950.9	E962.1	E980.9
alcohol	980.1	E860.2	—	E950.9	E962.1	E980.9
ethylene glycol	982.8	E862.4	—	E950.9	E962.1	E980.9
Antifungals (nonmedicinal) (sprays)	989.4	E863.6	—	E950.6	E962.1	E980.7
medicinal NEC	961.9	E857	E931.9	E950.4	E962.0	E980.4
antibiotic	960.1	E856	E930.1	E950.4	E962.0	E980.4
topical	976.0	E858.7	E946.0	E950.4	E962.0	E980.4
Antigastric secretion agents	973.0	E858.4	E943.0	E950.4	E962.0	E980.4
Antihelmintics	961.6	E857	E931.6	E950.4	E962.0	E980.4
Antihemophilic factor (human)	964.7	E858.2	E934.7	E950.4	E962.0	E980.4
Antihistamine	963.0	E858.1	E933.0	E950.4	E962.0	E980.4
Antihypertensive agents NEC	972.6	E858.3	E942.6	E950.4	E962.0	E980.4
Anti–infectives NEC	961.9	E857	E931.9	E950.4	E962.0	E980.4
antibiotics	960.9	E856	E930.9	E950.4	E962.0	E980.4
specified NEC	960.8	E856	E930.8	E950.4	E962.0	E980.4
antihelmintic	961.6	E857	E931.6	E950.4	E962.0	E980.4
antimalarial	961.4	E857	E931.4	E950.4	E962.0	E980.4
antimycobacterial NEC	961.8	E857	E931.8	E950.4	E962.0	E980.4
antibiotics	960.6	E856	E930.6	E950.4	E962.0	E980.4
antiprotozoal NEC	961.5	E857	E931.5	E950.4	E962.0	E980.4
blood	961.4	E857	E931.4	E950.4	E962.0	E980.4
antiviral	961.7	E857	E931.7	E950.4	E962.0	E980.4
arsenical	961.1	E857	E931.1	E950.4	E962.0	E980.4

Substance	Poisoning	Accident	Therapeutic Use	Suicide Attempt	Assault	Undetermined
			External Cause (E-Code)			
ENT agents	976.6	E858.7	E946.6	E950.4	E962.0	E980.4
heavy metals NEC	961.2	E857	E931.2	E950.4	E962.0	E980.4
local	976.0	E858.7	E946.0	E950.4	E962.0	E980.4
ophthalmic preparation	976.5	E858.7	E946.5	E950.4	E962.0	E980.4
topical NEC	976.0	E858.7	E946.0	E950.4	E962.0	E980.4
Anti–inflammatory agents (topical)	976.0	E858.7	E946.0	E950.4	E962.0	E980.4
Antiknock (tetraethyl lead)	984.1	E862.1	—	E950.9	E962.1	E980.9
Antilipemics	972.2	E858.3	E942.2	E950.4	E962.0	E980.4
Antimalarials	961.4	E857	E931.4	E950.4	E962.0	E980.4
Antimony (compounds) (vapor) NEC	985.4	E866.2	—	E950.9	E962.1	E980.9
anti–infectives	961.2	E857	E931.2	E950.4	E962.0	E980.4
pesticides (vapor)	985.4	E863.4	—	E950.6	E962.2	E980.7
potassium tartrate	961.2	E857	E931.2	E950.4	E962.0	E980.4
tartrated	961.2	E857	E931.2	E950.4	E962.0	E980.4
Antimuscarinic agents	971.1	E855.4	E941.1	E950.4	E962.0	E980.4
Antimycobacterials NEC	961.8	E857	E931.8	E950.4	E962.0	E980.4
antibiotics	960.6	E856	E930.6	E950.4	E962.0	E980.4
Antineoplastic agents	963.1	E858.1	E933.1	E950.4	E962.0	E980.4
antibiotics	960.7	E856	E930.7	E950.4	E962.0	E980.4
Anti–Parkinsonism agents	966.4	E855.0	E936.4	E950.4	E962.0	E980.4
Antiphlogistics	965.69	E850.6	E935.6	E950.0	E962.0	E980.0
Antiprotozoals NEC	961.5	E857	E931.5	E950.4	E962.0	E980.4
blood	961.4	E857	E931.4	E950.4	E962.0	E980.4
Antipruritics (local)	976.1	E858.7	E946.1	E950.4	E962.0	E980.4
Antipsychotic agents NEC	969.3	E853.8	E939.3	E950.3	E962.0	E980.3
Antipyretics	965.9	E850.9	E935.9	E950.0	E962.0	E980.0
specified NEC	965.8	E850.8	E935.8	E950.0	E962.0	E980.0
Antipyrine	965.5	E850.5	E935.5	E950.0	E962.0	E980.0
Antirabies serum (equine)	979.9	E858.8	E949.9	E950.4	E962.0	E980.4
Antirheumatics	965.69	E850.6	E935.6	E950.0	E962.0	E980.0
Antiseborrheics	976.4	E858.7	E946.4	E950.4	E962.0	E980.4
Antiseptics (external) (medicinal)	976.0	E858.7	E946.0	E950.4	E962.0	E980.4
Antistine	963.0	E858.1	E933.0	E950.4	E962.0	E980.4
Antithyroid agents	962.8	E858.0	E932.8	E950.4	E962.0	E980.4
Antitoxin, any	979.9	E858.8	E949.9	E950.4	E962.0	E980.4
Antituberculars	961.8	E857	E931.8	E950.4	E962.0	E980.4
antibiotics	960.6	E856	E930.6	E950.4	E962.0	E980.4
Antitussives	975.4	E858.6	E945.5	E950.4	E962.0	E980.4
Antivaricose agents (sclerosing)	972.7	E858.3	E942.7	E950.4	E962.0	E980.4
Antivenin (crotaline) (spider–bite)	979.9	E858.8	E949.9	E950.4	E962.0	E980.4
Antivert	963.0	E858.1	E933.0	E950.4	E962.0	E980.4
Antivirals NEC	961.7	E857	E931.7	E950.4	E962.0	E980.4
Ant poisons — *see* Pesticides						
Antrol	989.4	E863.4	—	E950.6	E962.1	E980.7
fungicide	989.4	E863.6	—	E950.6	E962.1	E980.7
Apomorphine hydrochloride (emetic)	973.6	E858.4	E943.6	E950.4	E962.0	E980.4
Appetite depressants, central	977.0	E858.8	E947.0	E950.4	E962.0	E980.4
Apresoline	972.6	E858.3	E942.6	E950.4	E962.0	E980.4
Aprobarbital, aprobarbitone	967.0	E851	E937.0	E950.1	E962.0	E980.1
Apronalide	967.8	E852.8	E937.8	E950.2	E962.0	E980.2
Aqua fortis	983.1	E864.1	—	E950.7	E962.1	E980.6
Arachis oil (topical)	976.3	E858.7	E946.3	E950.4	E962.0	E980.4
cathartic	973.2	E858.4	E943.2	E950.4	E962.0	E980.4
Aralen	961.4	E857	E931.4	E950.4	E962.0	E980.4
Arginine salts	974.5	E858.5	E944.5	E950.4	E962.0	E980.4
Argyrol	976.0	E858.7	E946.0	E950.4	E962.0	E980.4
ENT agent	976.6	E858.7	E946.6	E950.4	E962.0	E980.4
ophthalmic preparation	976.5	E858.7	E946.5	E950.4	E962.0	E980.4
Aristocort	962.0	E858.0	E932.0	E950.4	E962.0	E980.4
ENT agent	976.6	E858.7	E946.6	E950.4	E962.0	E980.4

Substance	Poisoning	Accident	Therapeutic Use	Suicide Attempt	Assault	Undetermined
			External Cause (E-Code)			
ophthalmic preparation	976.5	E858.7	E946.5	E950.4	E962.0	E980.4
topical NEC	976.0	E858.7	E946.0	E950.4	E962.0	E980.4
Aromatics, corrosive	983.0	E864.0	—	E950.7	E962.1	E980.6
disinfectants	983.0	E861.4	—	E950.7	E962.1	E980.6
Arsenate of lead (insecticide)	985.1	E863.4	—	E950.8	E962.1	E980.8
herbicide	985.1	E863.5	—	E950.8	E962.1	E980.8
Arsenic, arsenicals (compounds) (dust)						
(fumes) (vapor) NEC	985.1	E866.3	—	E950.8	E962.1	E980.8
anti–infectives	961.1	E857	E931.1	E950.4	E962.0	E980.4
pesticide (dust) (fumes)	985.1	E863.4	—	E950.8	E962.1	E980.8
Arsine (gas)	985.1	E866.3	—	E950.8	E962.1	E980.8
Arsphenamine (silver)	961.1	E857	E931.1	E950.4	E962.0	E980.4
Arsthinol	961.1	E857	E931.1	E950.4	E962.0	E980.4
Artane	971.1	E855.4	E941.1	E950.4	E962.0	E980.4
Arthropod (venomous) NEC	989.5	E905.5	—	E950.9	E962.1	E980.9
Asbestos	989.81	E866.8	—	E950.9	E962.1	E980.9
Ascaridole	961.6	E857	E931.6	E950.4	E962.0	E980.4
Ascorbic acid	963.5	E858.1	E933.5	E950.4	E962.0	E980.4
Asiaticoside	976.0	E858.7	E946.0	E950.4	E962.0	E980.4
Aspidium (oleoresin)	961.6	E857	E931.6	E950.4	E962.0	E980.4
Aspirin	965.1	E850.3	E935.3	E950.0	E962.0	E980.0
Astringents (local)	976.2	E858.7	E946.2	E950.4	E962.0	E980.4
Atabrine	961.3	E857	E931.3	E950.4	E962.0	E980.4
Ataractics	969.5	E853.8	E939.5	E950.3	E962.0	E980.3
Atonia drug, intestinal	973.3	E858.4	E943.3	E950.4	E962.0	E980.4
Atophan	974.7	E858.5	E944.7	E950.4	E962.0	E980.4
Atropine	971.1	E855.4	E941.1	E950.4	E962.0	E980.4
Attapulgite	973.5	E858.4	E943.5	E950.4	E962.0	E980.4
Attenuvax	979.4	E858.8	E949.4	E950.4	E962.0	E980.4
Aureomycin	960.4	E856	E930.4	E950.4	E962.0	E980.4
ophthalmic preparation	976.5	E858.7	E946.5	E950.4	E962.0	E980.4
topical NEC	976.0	E858.7	E946.0	E950.4	E962.0	E980.4
Aurothioglucose	965.69	E850.6	E935.6	E950.0	E962.0	E980.0
Aurothioglycanide	965.69	E850.6	E935.6	E950.0	E962.0	E980.0
Aurothiomalate	965.69	E850.6	E935.6	E950.0	E962.0	E980.0
Automobile fuel	981	E862.1	—	E950.9	E962.1	E980.9
Autonomic nervous system agents NEC . . .	971.9	E855.9	E941.9	E950.4	E962.0	E980.4
Avlosulfon	961.8	E857	E931.8	E950.4	E962.0	E980.4
Avomine	967.8	E852.8	E937.8	E950.2	E962.0	E980.2
Azacyclonol	969.5	E853.8	E939.5	E950.3	E962.0	E980.3
Azapetine	971.3	E855.6	E941.3	E950.4	E962.0	E980.4
Azaribine	963.1	E858.1	E933.1	E950.4	E962.0	E980.4
Azaserine	960.7	E856	E930.7	E950.4	E962.0	E980.4
Azathioprine	963.1	E858.1	E933.1	E950.4	E962.0	E980.4
Azosulfamide	961.0	E857	E931.0	E950.4	E962.0	E980.4
Azulfidine	961.0	E857	E931.0	E950.4	E962.0	E980.4
Azuresin	977.8	E858.8	E947.8	E950.4	E962.0	E980.4
Bacimycin	976.0	E858.7	E946.0	E950.4	E962.0	E980.4
ophthalmic preparation	976.5	E858.7	E946.5	E950.4	E962.0	E980.4
Bacitracin	960.8	E856	E930.8	E950.4	E962.0	E980.4
ENT agent	976.6	E858.7	E946.6	E950.4	E962.0	E980.4
ophthalmic preparation	976.5	E858.7	E946.5	E950.4	E962.0	E980.4
topical NEC	976.0	E858.7	E946.0	E950.4	E962.0	E980.4
Baking soda	963.3	E858.1	E933.3	E950.4	E962.0	E980.4
BAL	963.8	E858.1	E933.8	E950.4	E962.0	E980.4
Bamethan (sulfate)	972.5	E858.3	E942.5	E950.4	E962.0	E980.4
Bamipine	963.0	E858.1	E933.0	E950.4	E962.0	E980.4
Baneberry	988.2	E865.4	—	E950.9	E962.1	E980.9
Banewort	988.2	E865.4	—	E950.9	E962.1	E980.9
Barbenyl	967.0	E851	E937.0	E950.1	E962.0	E980.1
Barbital, barbitone	967.0	E851	E937.0	E950.1	E962.0	E980.1

Substance	Poisoning	Accident	Therapeutic Use	Suicide Attempt	Assault	Undetermined
			External Cause (E-Code)			
Barbiturates, barbituric acid	967.0	E851	E937.0	E950.1	E962.0	E980.1
anesthetic (intravenous)	968.3	E855.1	E938.3	E950.4	E962.0	E980.4
Barium (carbonate) (chloride) (sulfate)	985.8	E866.4	—	E950.9	E962.1	E980.9
diagnostic agent	977.8	E858.8	E947.8	E950.4	E962.0	E980.4
pesticide	985.8	E863.4	—	E950.6	E962.1	E980.7
rodenticide	985.8	E863.7	—	E950.6	E962.1	E980.7
Barrier cream	976.3	E858.7	E946.3	E950.4	E962.0	E980.4
Battery acid or fluid	983.1	E864.1	—	E950.7	E962.1	E980.6
Bay rum	980.8	E860.8	—	E950.9	E962.1	E980.9
BCG vaccine	978.0	E858.8	E948.0	E950.4	E962.0	E980.4
Bearsfoot	988.2	E865.4	—	E950.9	E962.1	E980.9
Beclamide	966.3	E855.0	E936.3	E950.4	E962.0	E980.4
Bee (sting) (venom)	989.5	E905.3	—	E950.9	E962.1	E980.9
Belladonna (alkaloids)	971.1	E855.4	E941.1	E950.4	E962.0	E980.4
Bemegride	970.0	E854.3	E940.0	E950.4	E962.0	E980.4
Benactyzine	969.8	E855.8	E939.8	E950.3	E962.0	E980.3
Benadryl	963.0	E858.1	E933.0	E950.4	E962.0	E980.4
Bendrofluazide	974.3	E858.5	E944.3	E950.4	E962.0	E980.4
Bendroflumethiazide	974.3	E858.5	E944.3	E950.4	E962.0	E980.4
Benemid	974.7	E858.5	E944.7	E950.4	E962.0	E980.4
Benethamine penicillin G	960.0	E856	E930.0	E950.4	E962.0	E980.4
Benisone	976.0	E858.7	E946.0	E950.4	E962.0	E980.4
Benoquin	976.8	E858.7	E946.8	E950.4	E962.0	E980.4
Benoxinate	968.5	E855.2	E938.5	E950.4	E962.0	E980.4
Bentonite	976.3	E858.7	E946.3	E950.4	E962.0	E980.4
Benzalkonium (chloride)	976.0	E858.7	E946.0	E950.4	E962.0	E980.4
ophthalmic preparation	976.5	E858.7	E946.5	E950.4	E962.0	E980.4
Benzamidosalicylate (calcium)	961.8	E857	E931.8	E950.4	E962.0	E980.4
Benzathine penicillin	960.0	E856	E930.0	E950.4	E962.0	E980.4
Benzcarbimine	963.1	E858.1	E933.1	E950.4	E962.0	E980.4
Benzedrex	971.2	E855.5	E941.2	E950.4	E962.0	E980.4
Benzedrine (amphetamine)	969.72	E854.2	E939.7	E950.3	E962.0	E980.3
Benzene (acetyl) (dimethyl) (methyl) (solvent) (vapor)	982.0	E862.4	—	E950.9	E962.1	E980.9
hexachloride (gamma) (insecticide) (vapor)	989.2	E863.0	—	E950.6	E962.1	E980.7
Benzethonium	976.0	E858.7	E946.0	E950.4	E962.0	E980.4
Benzhexol (chloride)	966.4	E855.0	E936.4	E950.4	E962.0	E980.4
Benzilonium	971.1	E855.4	E941.1	E950.4	E962.0	E980.4
Benzin(e) — see Ligroin						
Benziodarone	972.4	E858.3	E942.4	E950.4	E962.0	E980.4
Benzocaine	968.5	E855.2	E938.5	E950.4	E962.0	E980.4
Benzodiapin	969.4	E853.2	E939.4	E950.3	E962.0	E980.3
Benzodiazepines (tranquilizers) NEC	969.4	E853.2	E939.4	E950.3	E962.0	E980.3
Benzoic acid (with salicylic acid) (anti–infective)	976.0	E858.7	E946.0	E950.4	E962.0	E980.4
Benzoin	976.3	E858.7	E946.3	E950.4	E962.0	E980.4
Benzol (vapor)	982.0	E862.4	—	E950.9	E962.1	E980.9
Benzomorphan	965.09	E850.2	E935.2	E950.0	E962.0	E980.0
Benzonatate	975.4	E858.6	E945.4	E950.4	E962.0	E980.4
Benzothiadiazides	974.3	E858.5	E944.3	E950.4	E962.0	E980.4
Benzoylpas	961.8	E857	E931.8	E950.4	E962.0	E980.4
Benzperidol	969.5	E853.8	E939.5	E950.3	E962.0	E980.3
Benzphetamine	977.0	E858.8	E947.0	E950.4	E962.0	E980.4
Benzpyrinium	971.0	E855.3	E941.0	E950.4	E962.0	E980.4
Benzquinamide	963.0	E858.1	E933.0	E950.4	E962.0	E980.4
Benzthiazide	974.3	E858.5	E944.3	E950.4	E962.0	E980.4
Benztropine	971.1	E855.4	E941.1	E950.4	E962.0	E980.4
Benzyl acetate	982.8	E862.4	—	E950.9	E962.1	E980.9

Substance	Poisoning	Accident	Therapeutic Use	Suicide Attempt	Assault	Undetermined
			External Cause (E-Code)			
benzoate (anti–infective)	976.0	E858.7	E946.0	E950.4	E962.0	E980.4
morphine	965.09	E850.2	E935.2	E950.0	E962.0	E980.0
penicillin	960.0	E856	E930.0	E950.4	E962.0	E980.4
Bephenium hydroxynapthoate	961.6	E857	E931.6	E950.4	E962.0	E980.4
Bergamot oil	989.89	E866.8	—	E950.9	E962.1	E980.9
Berries, poisonous	988.2	E865.3	—	E950.9	E962.1	E980.9
Beryllium (compounds) (fumes)	985.3	E866.4	—	E950.9	E962.1	E980.9
Beta–carotene	976.3	E858.7	E946.3	E950.4	E962.0	E980.4
Beta–Chlor	967.1	E852.0	E937.1	E950.2	E962.0	E980.2
Betamethasone	962.0	E858.0	E932.0	E950.4	E962.0	E980.4
topical	976.0	E858.7	E946.0	E950.4	E962.0	E980.4
Betazole	977.8	E858.8	E947.8	E950.4	E962.0	E980.4
Bethanechol	971.0	E855.3	E941.0	E950.4	E962.0	E980.4
Bethanidine	972.6	E858.3	E942.6	E950.4	E962.0	E980.4
Betula oil	976.3	E858.7	E946.3	E950.4	E962.0	E980.4
Bhang	969.6	E854.1	E939.6	E950.3	E962.0	E980.3
Bialamicol	961.5	E857	E931.5	E950.4	E962.0	E980.4
Bichloride of mercury — *see* Mercury, chloride						
Bichromates (calcium) (crystals) (potassium) (sodium)	983.9	E864.3	—	E950.7	E962.1	E980.6
fumes	987.8	E869.8	—	E952.8	E962.2	E982.8
Biguanide derivatives, oral	962.3	E858.0	E932.3	E950.4	E962.0	E980.4
Biligrafin	977.8	E858.8	E947.8	E950.4	E962.0	E980.4
Bilopaque	977.8	E858.8	E947.8	E950.4	E962.0	E980.4
Bioflavonoids	972.8	E858.3	E942.8	E950.4	E962.0	E980.4
Biological substance NEC	979.9	E858.8	E949.9	E950.4	E962.0	E980.4
Biperiden	966.4	E855.0	E936.4	E950.4	E962.0	E980.4
Bisacodyl	973.1	E858.4	E943.1	E950.4	E962.0	E980.4
Bishydroxycoumarin	964.2	E858.2	E934.2	E950.4	E962.0	E980.4
Bismarsen	961.1	E857	E931.1	E950.4	E962.0	E980.4
Bismuth (compounds) NEC	985.8	E866.4	—	E950.9	E962.1	E980.9
anti–infectives	961.2	E857	E931.2	E950.4	E962.0	E980.4
subcarbonate	973.5	E858.4	E943.5	E950.4	E962.0	E980.4
sulfarsphenamine	961.1	E857	E931.1	E950.4	E962.0	E980.4
Bisphosphonates						
intravenous	963.1	E858.1	E933.7	E950.4	E962.0	E980.4
oral	963.1	E858.1	E933.6	E950.4	E962.0	E980.4
Bithionol	961.6	E857	E931.6	E950.4	E962.0	E980.4
Bitter almond oil	989.0	E866.8	—	E950.9	E962.1	E980.9
Bittersweet	988.2	E865.4	—	E950.9	E962.1	E980.9
Black						
flag	989.4	E863.4	—	E950.6	E962.1	E980.7
henbane	988.2	E865.4	—	E950.9	E962.1	E980.9
leaf (40)	989.4	E863.4	—	E950.6	E962.1	E980.7
widow spider (bite)	989.5	E905.1	—	E950.9	E962.1	E980.9
antivenin	979.9	E858.8	E949.9	E950.4	E962.0	E980.4
Blast furnace gas (carbon monoxide from)	986	E868.8	—	E952.1	E962.2	E982.1
Bleach NEC	983.9	E864.3	—	E950.7	E962.1	E980.6
Bleaching solutions	983.9	E864.3	—	E950.7	E962.1	E980.6
Bleomycin (sulfate)	960.7	E856	E930.7	E950.4	E962.0	E980.4
Blockain	968.9	E855.2	E938.9	E950.4	E962.0	E980.4
infiltration (subcutaneous)	968.5	E855.2	E938.5	E950.4	E962.0	E980.4
nerve block (peripheral) (plexus)	968.6	E855.2	E938.6	E950.4	E962.0	E980.4
topical (surface)	968.5	E855.2	E938.5	E950.4	E962.0	E980.4
Blood (derivatives) (natural) (plasma) (whole)	964.7	E858.2	E934.7	E950.4	E962.0	E980.4
affecting agent	964.9	E858.2	E934.9	E950.4	E962.0	E980.4
specified NEC	964.8	E858.2	E934.8	E950.4	E962.0	E980.4
substitute (macromolecular)	964.8	E858.2	E934.8	E950.4	E962.0	E980.4
Blue velvet	965.09	E850.2	E935.2	E950.0	E962.0	E980.0

Substance	Poisoning	Accident	Therapeutic Use	Suicide Attempt	Assault	Undetermined
			External Cause (E-Code)			
Bone meal	989.89	E866.5	—	E950.9	E962.1	E980.9
Bonine	963.0	E858.1	E933.0	E950.4	E962.0	E980.4
Boracic acid	976.0	E858.7	E946.0	E950.4	E962.0	E980.4
ENT agent	976.6	E858.7	E946.6	E950.4	E962.0	E980.4
ophthalmic preparation	976.5	E858.7	E946.5	E950.4	E962.0	E980.4
Borate (cleanser) (sodium)	989.6	E861.3	—	E950.9	E962.1	E980.9
Borax (cleanser)	989.6	E861.3	—	E950.9	E962.1	E980.9
Boric acid	976.0	E858.7	E946.0	E950.4	E962.0	E980.4
ENT agent	976.6	E858.7	E946.6	E950.4	E962.0	E980.4
ophthalmic preparation	976.5	E858.7	E946.5	E950.4	E962.0	E980.4
Boron hydride NEC	989.89	E866.8	—	E950.9	E962.1	E980.9
fumes or gas	987.8	E869.8	—	E952.8	E962.2	E982.8
Botox	975.3	E858.6	E945.3	E950.4	E962.0	E980.4
Brake fluid vapor	987.8	E869.8	—	E952.8	E962.2	E982.8
Brass (compounds) (fumes)	985.8	E866.4	—	E950.9	E962.1	E980.9
Brasso	981	E861.3	—	E950.9	E962.1	E980.9
Bretylium (tosylate)	972.6	E858.3	E942.6	E950.4	E962.0	E980.4
Brevital (sodium)	968.3	E855.1	E938.3	E950.4	E962.0	E980.4
British antilewisite	963.8	E858.1	E933.8	E950.4	E962.0	E980.4
Bromal (hydrate)	967.3	E852.2	E937.3	E950.2	E962.0	E980.2
Bromelains	963.4	E858.1	E933.4	E950.4	E962.0	E980.4
Bromides NEC	967.3	E852.2	E937.3	E950.2	E962.0	E980.2
Bromine (vapor)	987.8	E869.8	—	E952.8	E962.2	E982.8
compounds (medicinal)	967.3	E852.2	E937.3	E950.2	E962.0	E980.2
Bromisovalum	967.3	E852.2	E937.3	E950.2	E962.0	E980.2
Bromobenzyl cyanide	987.5	E869.3	—	E952.8	E962.2	E982.8
Bromodiphenhydramine	963.0	E858.1	E933.0	E950.4	E962.0	E980.4
Bromoform	967.3	E852.2	E937.3	E950.2	E962.0	E980.2
Bromophenol blue reagent	977.8	E858.8	E947.8	E950.4	E962.0	E980.4
Bromosalicylhydroxamic acid	961.8	E857	E931.8	E950.4	E962.0	E980.4
Bromo–seltzer	965.4	E850.4	E935.4	E950.0	E962.0	E980.0
Brompheniramine	963.0	E858.1	E933.0	E950.4	E962.0	E980.4
Bromural	967.3	E852.2	E937.3	E950.2	E962.0	E980.2
Brown spider (bite) (venom)	989.5	E905.1	—	E950.9	E962.1	E980.9
Brucia	988.2	E865.3	—	E950.9	E962.1	E980.9
Brucine	989.1	E863.7	—	E950.6	E962.1	E980.7
Brunswick green — *see* Copper						
Bruten — *see* Ibuprofen						
Bryonia (alba) (dioica)	988.2	E865.4	—	E950.9	E962.1	E980.9
Buclizine	969.5	E853.8	E939.5	E950.3	E962.0	E980.3
Bufferin	965.1	E850.3	E935.3	E950.0	E962.0	E980.0
Bufotenine	969.6	E854.1	E939.6	E950.3	E962.0	E980.3
Buphenine	971.2	E855.5	E941.2	E950.4	E962.0	E980.4
Bupivacaine	968.9	E855.2	E938.9	E950.4	E962.0	E980.4
infiltration (subcutaneous)	968.5	E855.2	E938.5	E950.4	E962.0	E980.4
nerve block (peripheral) (plexus)	968.6	E855.2	E938.6	E950.4	E962.0	E980.4
Busulfan	963.1	E858.1	E933.1	E950.4	E962.0	E980.4
Butabarbital (sodium)	967.0	E851	E937.0	E950.1	E962.0	E980.1
Butabarbitone	967.0	E851	E937.0	E950.1	E962.0	E980.1
Butabarpal	967.0	E851	E937.0	E950.1	E962.0	E980.1
Butacaine	968.5	E855.2	E938.5	E950.4	E962.0	E980.4
Butallylonal	967.0	E851	E937.0	E950.1	E962.0	E980.1
Butane (distributed in mobile container)	987.0	E868.0	—	E951.1	E962.2	E981.1
distributed through pipes	987.0	E867	—	E951.0	E962.2	E981.0
incomplete combustion of — *see* Carbon monoxide, butane						
Butanol	980.3	E860.4	—	E950.9	E962.1	E980.9
Butanone	982.8	E862.4	—	E950.9	E962.1	E980.9
Butaperazine	969.1	E853.0	E939.1	E950.3	E962.0	E980.3
Butazolidin	965.5	E850.5	E935.5	E950.0	E962.0	E980.0

TABLE OF DRUGS AND CHEMICALS

Substance	Poisoning	Accident	Therapeutic Use	Suicide Attempt	Assault	Undetermined
			External Cause (E-Code)			
Butethal	967.0	E851	E937.0	E950.1	E962.0	E980.1
Butethamate	971.1	E855.4	E941.1	E950.4	E962.0	E980.4
Buthalitone (sodium)	968.3	E855.1	E938.3	E950.4	E962.0	E980.4
Butisol (sodium)	967.0	E851	E937.0	E950.1	E962.0	E980.1
Butobarbital, butobarbitone	967.0	E851	E937.0	E950.1	E962.0	E980.1
Butriptyline	969.05	E854.0	E939.0	E950.3	E962.0	E980.3
Buttercups.	988.2	E865.4	—	E950.9	E962.1	E980.9
Butter of antimony — *see* Antimony						
Butyl						
acetate (secondary)	982.8	E862.4	—	E950.9	E962.1	E980.9
alcohol	980.3	E860.4	—	E950.9	E962.1	E980.9
carbinol	980.8	E860.8	—	E950.9	E962.1	E980.9
carbitol	982.8	E862.4	—	E950.9	E962.1	E980.9
cellosolve	982.8	E862.4	—	E950.9	E962.1	E980.9
chloral (hydrate)	967.1	E852.0	E937.1	E950.2	E962.0	E980.2
formate	982.8	E862.4	—	E950.9	E962.1	E980.9
scopolammonium bromide	971.1	E855.4	E941.1	E950.4	E962.0	E980.4
Butyn	968.5	E855.2	E938.5	E950.4	E962.0	E980.4
Butyrophenone (–based tranquilizers)	969.2	E853.1	E939.2	E950.3	E962.0	E980.3
Cacodyl, cacodylic acid — *see* Arsenic						
Cactinomycin	960.7	E856	E930.7	E950.4	E962.0	E980.4
Cade oil	976.4	E858.7	E946.4	E950.4	E962.0	E980.4
Cadmium (chloride) (compounds) (dust)						
(fumes) (oxide)	985.5	E866.4	—	E950.9	E962.1	E980.9
sulfide (medicinal) NEC	976.4	E858.7	E946.4	E950.4	E962.0	E980.4
Caffeine	969.71	E854.2	E939.7	E950.3	E962.0	E980.3
Calabar bean.	988.2	E865.4	—	E950.9	E962.1	E980.9
Caladium seguinium	988.2	E865.4	—	E950.9	E962.1	E980.9
Calamine (liniment) (lotion)	976.3	E858.7	E946.3	E950.4	E962.0	E980.4
Calciferol	963.5	E858.1	E933.5	E950.4	E962.0	E980.4
Calcium (salts) NEC	974.5	E858.5	E944.5	E950.4	E962.0	E980.4
acetylsalicylate	965.1	E850.3	E935.3	E950.0	E962.0	E980.0
benzamidosalicylate	961.8	E857	E931.8	E950.4	E962.0	E980.4
carbaspirin	965.1	E850.3	E935.3	E950.0	E962.0	E980.0
carbamide (citrated)	977.3	E858.8	E947.3	E950.4	E962.0	E980.4
carbonate (antacid)	973.0	E858.4	E943.0	E950.4	E962.0	E980.4
cyanide (citrated)	977.3	E858.8	E947.3	E950.4	E962.0	E980.4
dioctyl sulfosuccinate	973.2	E858.4	E943.2	E950.4	E962.0	E980.4
disodium edathamil	963.8	E858.1	E933.8	E950.4	E962.0	E980.4
disodium edetate	963.8	E858.1	E933.8	E950.4	E962.0	E980.4
EDTA.	963.8	E858.1	E933.8	E950.4	E962.0	E980.4
hydrate, hydroxide	983.2	E864.2	—	E950.7	E962.1	E980.6
mandelate	961.9	E857	E931.9	E950.4	E962.0	E980.4
oxide	983.2	E864.2	—	E950.7	E962.1	E980.6
Calomel — *see* Mercury, chloride						
Caloric agents NEC.	974.5	E858.5	E944.5	E950.4	E962.0	E980.4
Calusterone	963.1	E858.1	E933.1	E950.4	E962.0	E980.4
Camoquin	961.4	E857	E931.4	E950.4	E962.0	E980.4
Camphor (oil)	976.1	E858.7	E946.1	E950.4	E962.0	E980.4
Candeptin	976.0	E858.7	E946.0	E950.4	E962.0	E980.4
Candicidin	976.0	E858.7	E946.0	E950.4	E962.0	E980.4
Cannabinols	969.6	E854.1	E939.6	E950.3	E962.0	E980.3
Cannabis (derivatives) (indica) (sativa)	969.6	E854.1	E939.6	E950.3	E962.0	E980.3
Canned heat	980.1	E860.2	—	E950.9	E962.1	E980.9
Cantharides, cantharidin, cantharis	976.8	E858.7	E946.8	E950.4	E962.0	E980.4
Capillary agents	972.8	E858.3	E942.8	E950.4	E962.0	E980.4
Capreomycin	960.6	E856	E930.6	E950.4	E962.0	E980.4
Captodiame, captodiamine	969.5	E853.8	E939.5	E950.3	E962.0	E980.3
Caramiphen (hydrochloride)	971.1	E855.4	E941.1	E950.4	E962.0	E980.4
Carbachol	971.0	E855.3	E941.0	E950.4	E962.0	E980.4
Carbacrylamine resins.	974.5	E858.5	E944.5	E950.4	E962.0	E980.4

Substance	Poisoning	Accident	Therapeutic Use	Suicide Attempt	Assault	Undetermined
			External Cause (E-Code)			
Carbamate (sedative)	967.8	E852.8	E937.8	E950.2	E962.0	E980.2
herbicide	989.3	E863.5	—	E950.6	E962.1	E980.7
insecticide	989.3	E863.2	—	E950.6	E962.1	E980.7
Carbamazepine	966.3	E855.0	E936.3	E950.4	E962.0	E980.4
Carbamic esters	967.8	E852.8	E937.8	E950.2	E962.0	E980.2
Carbamide	974.4	E858.5	E944.4	E950.4	E962.0	E980.4
topical	976.8	E858.7	E946.8	E950.4	E962.0	E980.4
Carbamylcholine chloride	971.0	E855.3	E941.0	E950.4	E962.0	E980.4
Carbarsone	961.1	E857	E931.1	E950.4	E962.0	E980.4
Carbaryl	989.3	E863.2	—	E950.6	E962.1	E980.7
Carbaspirin	965.1	E850.3	E935.3	E950.0	E962.0	E980.0
Carbazochrome	972.8	E858.3	E942.8	E950.4	E962.0	E980.4
Carbenicillin	960.0	E856	E930.0	E950.4	E962.0	E980.4
Carbenoxolone	973.8	E858.4	E943.8	E950.4	E962.0	E980.4
Carbetapentane	975.4	E858.6	E945.4	E950.4	E962.0	E980.4
Carbimazole	962.8	E858.0	E932.8	E950.4	E962.0	E980.4
Carbinol	980.1	E860.2	—	E950.9	E962.1	E980.9
Carbinoxamine	963.0	E858.1	E933.0	E950.4	E962.0	E980.4
Carbitol	982.8	E862.4	—	E950.9	E962.1	E980.9
Carbocaine	968.9	E855.2	E938.9	E950.4	E962.0	E980.4
infiltration (subcutaneous)	968.5	E855.2	E938.5	E950.4	E962.0	E980.4
nerve block (peripheral) (plexus)	968.6	E855.2	E938.6	E950.4	E962.0	E980.4
topical (surface)	968.5	E855.2	E938.5	E950.4	E962.0	E980.4
Carbol–fuchsin solution	976.0	E858.7	E946.0	E950.4	E962.0	E980.4
Carbolic acid (*see also* Phenol)	983.0	E864.0	—	E950.7	E962.1	E980.6
Carbomycin	960.8	E856	E930.8	E950.4	E962.0	E980.4
Carbon						
bisulfide (liquid) (vapor)	982.2	E862.4	—	E950.9	E962.1	E980.9
dioxide (gas)	987.8	E869.8	—	E952.8	E962.2	E982.8
disulfide (liquid) (vapor)	982.2	E862.4	—	E950.9	E962.1	E980.9
monoxide (from incomplete combustion of) (in) NEC	986	E868.9	—	E952.1	E962.2	E982.1
blast furnace gas	986	E868.8	—	E952.1	E962.2	E982.1
butane (distributed in mobile container)	986	E868.0	—	E951.1	E962.2	E981.1
distributed through pipes	986	E867	—	E951.0	E962.2	E981.0
charcoal fumes	986	E868.3	—	E952.1	E962.2	E982.1
coal						
gas (piped)	986	E867	—	E951.0	E962.2	E981.0
solid (in domestic stoves, fireplaces)	986	E868.3	—	E952.1	E962.2	E982.1
coke (in domestic stoves, fireplaces)	986	E868.3	—	E952.1	E962.2	E982.1
exhaust gas (motor) not in transit	986	E868.2	—	E952.0	E962.2	E982.0
combustion engine, any not in watercraft	986	E868.2	—	E952.0	E962.2	E982.0
farm tractor, not in transit	986	E868.2	—	E952.0	E962.2	E982.0
gas engine	986	E868.2	—	E952.0	E962.2	E982.0
motor pump	986	E868.2	—	E952.0	E962.2	E982.0
motor vehicle, not in transit	986	E868.2	—	E952.0	E962.2	E982.0
fuel (in domestic use)	986	E868.3	—	E952.1	E962.2	E982.1
gas (piped)	986	E867	—	E951.0	E962.2	E981.0
in mobile container	986	E868.0	—	E951.1	E962.2	E981.1
utility	986	E868.1	—	E951.8	E962.2	E981.1
in mobile container	986	E868.0	—	E951.1	E962.2	E981.1
piped (natural)	986	E867	—	E951.0	E962.2	E981.0
illuminating gas	986	E868.1	—	E951.8	E962.2	E981.8
industrial fuels or gases, any	986	E868.8	—	E952.1	E962.2	E982.1
kerosene (in domestic stoves, fireplaces)	986	E868.3	—	E952.1	E962.2	E982.1
kiln gas or vapor	986	E868.8	—	E952.1	E962.2	E982.1

Substance	Poisoning	Accident	Therapeutic Use	Suicide Attempt	Assault	Undetermined
			External Cause (E-Code)			
motor exhaust gas, not in transit	986	E868.2	—	E952.0	E962.2	E982.0
piped gas (manufactured) (natural)	986	E867	—	E951.0	E962.2	E981.0
producer gas	986	E868.8	—	E952.1	E962.2	E982.1
propane (distributed in mobile container)	986	E868.0	—	E951.1	E962.2	E981.1
distributed through pipes	986	E867	—	E951.0	E962.2	E981.0
specified source NEC	986	E868.8	—	E952.1	E962.2	E982.1
stove gas	986	E868.1	—	E951.8	E962.2	E981.8
piped	986	E867	—	E951.0	E962.2	E981.0
utility gas	986	E868.1	—	E951.8	E962.2	E981.8
piped	986	E867	—	E951.0	E962.2	E981.0
water gas	986	E868.1	—	E951.8	E962.2	E981.8
wood (in domestic stoves, fireplaces)	986	E868.3	—	E952.1	E962.2	E982.1
tetrachloride (vapor) NEC	987.8	E869.8	—	E952.8	E962.2	E982.8
liquid (cleansing agent) NEC	982.1	E861.3	—	E950.9	E962.1	E980.9
solvent	982.1	E862.4	—	E950.9	E962.1	E980.9
Carbonic acid (gas)	987.8	E869.8	—	E952.8	E962.2	E982.8
anhydrase inhibitors	974.2	E858.5	E944.2	E950.4	E962.0	E980.4
Carbowax	976.3	E858.7	E946.3	E950.4	E962.0	E980.4
Carbrital	967.0	E851	E937.0	E950.1	E962.0	E980.1
Carbromal (derivatives)	967.3	E852.2	E937.3	E950.2	E962.0	E980.2
Cardiac						
depressants	972.0	E858.3	E942.0	E950.4	E962.0	E980.4
rhythm regulators	972.0	E858.3	E942.0	E950.4	E962.0	E980.4
Cardiografin	977.8	E858.8	E947.8	E950.4	E962.0	E980.4
Cardio–green	977.8	E858.8	E947.8	E950.4	E962.0	E980.4
Cardiotonic glycosides	972.1	E858.3	E942.1	E950.4	E962.0	E980.4
Cardiovascular agents NEC	972.9	E858.3	E942.9	E950.4	E962.0	E980.4
Cardrase	974.2	E858.5	E944.2	E950.4	E962.0	E980.4
Carfusin	976.0	E858.7	E946.0	E950.4	E962.0	E980.4
Carisoprodol	968.0	E855.1	E938.0	E950.4	E962.0	E980.4
Carmustine	963.1	E858.1	E933.1	E950.4	E962.0	E980.4
Carotene	963.5	E858.1	E933.5	E950.4	E962.0	E980.4
Carphenazine (maleate)	969.1	E853.0	E939.1	E950.3	E962.0	E980.3
Carter's Little Pills	973.1	E858.4	E943.1	E950.4	E962.0	E980.4
Cascara (sagrada)	973.1	E858.4	E943.1	E950.4	E962.0	E980.4
Cassava	988.2	E865.4	—	E950.9	E962.1	E980.9
Castellani's paint	976.0	E858.7	E946.0	E950.4	E962.0	E980.4
Castor						
bean	988.2	E865.3	—	E950.9	E962.1	E980.9
oil	973.1	E858.4	E943.1	E950.4	E962.0	E980.4
Caterpillar (sting)	989.5	E905.5	—	E950.9	E962.1	E980.9
Catha (edulis)	970.89	E854.3	E940.8	E950.4	E962.0	E980.4
Cathartics NEC	973.3	E858.4	E943.3	E950.4	E962.0	E980.4
contact	973.1	E858.4	E943.1	E950.4	E962.0	E980.4
emollient	973.2	E858.4	E943.2	E950.4	E962.0	E980.4
intestinal irritants	973.1	E858.4	E943.1	E950.4	E962.0	E980.4
saline	973.3	E858.4	E943.3	E950.4	E962.0	E980.4
Cathomycin	960.8	E856	E930.8	E950.4	E962.0	E980.4
Caustic(s)	983.9	E864.4	—	E950.7	E962.1	E980.6
alkali	983.2	E864.2	—	E950.7	E962.1	E980.6
hydroxide	983.2	E864.2	—	E950.7	E962.1	E980.6
potash	983.2	E864.2	—	E950.7	E962.1	E980.6
soda	983.2	E864.2	—	E950.7	E962.1	E980.6
specified NEC	983.9	E864.3	—	E950.7	E962.1	E980.6
Ceepryn	976.0	E858.7	E946.0	E950.4	E962.0	E980.4
ENT agent	976.6	E858.7	E946.6	E950.4	E962.0	E980.4
lozenges	976.6	E858.7	E946.6	E950.4	E962.0	E980.4
Celestone	962.0	E858.0	E932.0	E950.4	E962.0	E980.4
topical	976.0	E858.7	E946.0	E950.4	E962.0	E980.4
Cellosolve	982.8	E862.4	—	E950.9	E962.1	E980.9

Substance	Poisoning	Accident	Therapeutic Use	Suicide Attempt	Assault	Undetermined
			External Cause (E-Code)			
Cell stimulants and proliferants	976.8	E858.7	E946.8	E950.4	E962.0	E980.4
Cellulose derivatives, cathartic	973.3	E858.4	E943.3	E950.4	E962.0	E980.4
nitrates (topical)	976.3	E858.7	E946.3	E950.4	E962.0	E980.4
Centipede (bite)	989.5	E905.4	—	E950.9	E962.1	E980.9
Central nervous system						
depressants.	968.4	E855.1	E938.4	E950.4	E962.0	E980.4
anesthetic (general) NEC	968.4	E855.1	E938.4	E950.4	E962.0	E980.4
gases NEC	968.2	E855.1	E938.2	E950.4	E962.0	E980.4
intravenous	968.3	E855.1	E938.3	E950.4	E962.0	E980.4
barbiturates.	967.0	E851	E937.0	E950.1	E962.0	E980.1
bromides.	967.3	E852.2	E937.3	E950.2	E962.0	E980.2
cannabis sativa	969.6	E854.1	E939.6	E950.3	E962.0	E980.3
chloral hydrate	967.1	E852.0	E937.1	E950.2	E962.0	E980.2
hallucinogenics	969.6	E854.1	E939.6	E950.3	E962.0	E980.3
hypnotics	967.9	E852.9	E937.9	E950.2	E962.0	E980.2
specified NEC.	967.8	E852.8	E937.8	E950.2	E962.0	E980.2
muscle relaxants.	968.0	E855.1	E938.0	E950.4	E962.0	E980.4
paraldehyde	967.2	E852.1	E937.2	E950.2	E962.0	E980.2
sedatives.	967.9	E852.9	E937.9	E950.2	E962.0	E980.2
mixed NEC.	967.6	E852.5	E937.6	E950.2	E962.0	E980.2
specified NEC.	967.8	E852.8	E937.8	E950.2	E962.0	E980.2
muscle–tone depressants	968.0	E855.1	E938.0	E950.4	E962.0	E980.4
stimulants	970.9	E854.3	E940.9	E950.4	E962.0	E980.4
amphetamines.	969.72	E854.2	E939.7	E950.3	E962.0	E980.3
analeptics	970.0	E854.3	E940.0	E950.4	E962.0	E980.4
antidepressants	969.00	E854.0	E939.0	E950.3	E962.0	E980.3
opiate antagonists	970.1	E854.3	E940.0	E950.4	E962.0	E980.4
specified NEC	970.89	E854.3	E940.8	E950.4	E962.0	E980.4
Cephalexin	960.5	E856	E930.5	E950.4	E962.0	E980.4
Cephaloglycin	960.5	E856	E930.5	E950.4	E962.0	E980.4
Cephaloridine	960.5	E856	E930.5	E950.4	E962.0	E980.4
Cephalosporins NEC	960.5	E856	E930.5	E950.4	E962.0	E980.4
N (adicillin)	960.0	E856	E930.0	E950.4	E962.0	E980.4
Cephalothin (sodium)	960.5	E856	E930.5	E950.4	E962.0	E980.4
Cerbera (odallam)	988.2	E865.4	—	E950.9	E962.1	E980.9
Cerberin	972.1	E858.3	E942.1	E950.4	E962.0	E980.4
Cerebral stimulants	970.9	E854.3	E940.9	E950.4	E962.0	E980.4
psychotherapeutic	969.79	E854.2	E939.7	E950.3	E962.0	E980.3
specified NEC	970.89	E854.3	E940.8	E950.4	E962.0	E980.4
Cetalkonium (chloride)	976.0	E858.7	E946.0	E950.4	E962.0	E980.4
Cetoxime	963.0	E858.1	E933.0	E950.4	E962.0	E980.4
Cetrimide	976.2	E858.7	E946.2	E950.4	E962.0	E980.4
Cetylpyridinium	976.0	E858.7	E946.0	E950.4	E962.0	E980.4
ENT agent.	976.6	E858.7	E946.6	E950.4	E962.0	E980.4
lozenges.	976.6	E858.7	E946.6	E950.4	E962.0	E980.4
Cevadilla — see Sabadilla						
Cevitamic acid.	963.5	E858.1	E933.5	E950.4	E962.0	E980.4
Chalk, precipitated	973.0	E858.4	E943.0	E950.4	E962.0	E980.4
Charcoal						
fumes (carbon monoxide).	986	E868.3	—	E952.1	E962.2	E982.1
industrial.	986	E868.8	—	E952.1	E962.2	E982.1
medicinal (activated).	973.0	E858.4	E943.0	E950.4	E962.0	E980.4
Chelating agents NEC.	977.2	E858.8	E947.2	E950.4	E962.0	E980.4
Chelidonium majus	988.2	E865.4	—	E950.9	E962.1	E980.9
Chemical substance	989.9	E866.9	—	E950.9	E962.1	E980.9
specified NEC	989.89	E866.8	—	E950.9	E962.1	E980.9
Chemotherapy, antineoplastic	963.1	E858.1	E933.1	E950.4	E962.0	E980.4
Chenopodium (oil)	961.6	E857	E931.6	E950.4	E962.0	E980.4
Cherry laurel	988.2	E865.4	—	E950.9	E962.1	E980.9
Chiniofon.	961.3	E857	E931.3	E950.4	E962.0	E980.4

Substance	Poisoning	Accident	Therapeutic Use	Suicide Attempt	Assault	Undetermined
			External Cause (E-Code)			
Chlophedianol	975.4	E858.6	E945.4	E950.4	E962.0	E980.4
Chloral (betaine) (formamide) (hydrate)	967.1	E852.0	E937.1	E950.2	E962.0	E980.2
Chloralamide	967.1	E852.0	E937.1	E950.2	E962.0	E980.2
Chlorambucil	963.1	E858.1	E933.1	E950.4	E962.0	E980.4
Chloramphenicol	960.2	E856	E930.2	E950.4	E962.0	E980.4
ENT agent	976.6	E858.7	E946.6	E950.4	E962.0	E980.4
ophthalmic preparation	976.5	E858.7	E946.5	E950.4	E962.0	E980.4
topical NEC	976.0	E858.7	E946.0	E950.4	E962.0	E980.4
Chlorate(s) (potassium) (sodium) NEC	983.9	E864.3	—	E950.7	E962.1	E980.6
herbicides	989.4	E863.5	—	E950.6	E962.1	E980.7
Chlorcyclizine	963.0	E858.1	E933.0	E950.4	E962.0	E980.4
Chlordan(e) (dust)	989.2	E863.0	—	E950.6	E962.1	E980.7
Chlordantoin	976.0	E858.7	E946.0	E950.4	E962.0	E980.4
Chlordiazepoxide	969.4	E853.2	E939.4	E950.3	E962.0	E980.3
Chloresium	976.8	E858.7	E946.8	E950.4	E962.0	E980.4
Chlorethiazol	967.1	E852.0	E937.1	E950.2	E962.0	E980.2
Chlorethyl — *see* Ethyl, chloride						
Chloretone	967.1	E852.0	E937.1	E950.2	E962.0	E980.2
Chlorex	982.3	E862.4	—	E950.9	E962.1	E980.9
Chlorhexadol	967.1	E852.0	E937.1	E950.2	E962.0	E980.2
Chlorhexidine (hydrochloride)	976.0	E858.7	E946.0	E950.4	E962.0	E980.4
Chlorhydroxyquinolin	976.0	E858.7	E946.0	E950.4	E962.0	E980.4
Chloride of lime (bleach)	983.9	E864.3	—	E950.7	E962.1	E980.6
Chlorinated						
camphene	989.2	E863.0	—	E950.6	E962.1	E980.7
diphenyl	989.89	E866.8	—	E950.9	E962.1	E980.9
hydrocarbons NEC	989.2	E863.0	—	E950.6	E962.1	E980.7
solvent	982.3	E862.4	—	E950.9	E962.1	E980.9
lime (bleach)	983.9	E864.3	—	E950.7	E962.1	E980.6
naphthalene — *see* Naphthalene						
pesticides NEC	989.2	E863.0	—	E950.6	E962.1	E980.7
soda — *see* Sodium, hypochlorite						
Chlorine (fumes) (gas)	987.6	E869.8	—	E952.8	E962.2	E982.8
bleach	983.9	E864.3	—	E950.7	E962.1	E980.6
compounds NEC	983.9	E864.3	—	E950.7	E962.1	E980.6
disinfectant	983.9	E861.4	—	E950.7	E962.1	E980.6
releasing agents NEC	983.9	E864.3	—	E950.7	E962.1	E980.6
Chlorisondamine	972.3	E858.3	E942.3	E950.4	E962.0	E980.4
Chlormadinone	962.2	E858.0	E932.2	E950.4	E962.0	E980.4
Chlormerodrin	974.0	E858.5	E944.0	E950.4	E962.0	E980.4
Chlormethiazole	967.1	E852.0	E937.1	E950.2	E962.0	E980.2
Chlormethylenecycline	960.4	E856	E930.4	E950.4	E962.0	E980.4
Chlormezanone	969.5	E853.8	E939.5	E950.3	E962.0	E980.3
Chloroacetophenone	987.5	E869.3	—	E952.8	E962.2	E982.8
Chloroaniline	983.0	E864.0	—	E950.7	E962.1	E980.6
Chlorobenzene, chlorobenzol	982.0	E862.4	—	E950.9	E962.1	E980.9
Chlorobutanol	967.1	E852.0	E937.1	E950.2	E962.0	E980.2
Chlorodinitrobenzene	983.0	E864.0	—	E950.7	E962.1	E980.6
dust or vapor	987.8	E869.8	—	E952.8	E962.2	E982.8
Chloroethane — *see* Ethyl, chloride						
Chloroform (fumes) (vapor)	987.8	E869.8	—	E952.8	E962.2	E982.8
anesthetic (gas)	968.2	E855.1	E938.2	E950.4	E962.0	E980.4
liquid NEC	968.4	E855.1	E938.4	E950.4	E962.0	E980.4
solvent	982.3	E862.4	—	E950.9	E962.1	E980.9
Chloroguanide	961.4	E857	E931.4	E950.4	E962.0	E980.4
Chloromycetin	960.2	E856	E930.2	E950.4	E962.0	E980.4
ENT agent	976.6	E858.7	E946.6	E950.4	E962.0	E980.4
ophthalmic preparation	976.5	E858.7	E946.5	E950.4	E962.0	E980.4
otic solution	976.6	E858.7	E946.6	E950.4	E962.0	E980.4
topical NEC	976.0	E858.7	E946.0	E950.4	E962.0	E980.4
Chloronitrobenzene	983.0	E864.0	—	E950.7	E962.1	E980.6

Substance	Poisoning	Accident	Therapeutic Use	Suicide Attempt	Assault	Undetermined
			External Cause (E-Code)			
dust or vapor	987.8	E869.8	—	E952.8	E962.2	E982.8
Chlorophenol	983.0	E864.0	—	E950.7	E962.1	E980.6
Chlorophenothane	989.2	E863.0	—	E950.6	E962.1	E980.7
Chlorophyll (derivatives)	976.8	E858.7	E946.8	E950.4	E962.0	E980.4
Chloropicrin (fumes)	987.8	E869.8	—	E952.8	E962.2	E982.8
fumigant	989.4	E863.8	—	E950.6	E962.1	E980.7
fungicide	989.4	E863.6	—	E950.6	E962.1	E980.7
pesticide (fumes)	989.4	E863.4	—	E950.6	E962.1	E980.7
Chloroprocaine	968.9	E855.2	E938.9	E950.4	E962.0	E980.4
infiltration (subcutaneous)	968.5	E855.2	E938.5	E950.4	E962.0	E980.4
nerve block (peripheral) (plexus)	968.6	E855.2	E938.6	E950.4	E962.0	E980.4
Chloroptic	976.5	E858.7	E946.5	E950.4	E962.0	E980.4
Chloropurine	963.1	E858.1	E933.1	E950.4	E962.0	E980.4
Chloroquine (hydrochloride) (phosphate)	961.4	E857	E931.4	E950.4	E962.0	E980.4
Chlorothen	963.0	E858.1	E933.0	E950.4	E962.0	E980.4
Chlorothiazide	974.3	E858.5	E944.3	E950.4	E962.0	E980.4
Chlorotrianisene	962.2	E858.0	E932.2	E950.4	E962.0	E980.4
Chlorovinyldichloroarsine	985.1	E866.3	—	E950.8	E962.1	E980.8
Chloroxylenol	976.0	E858.7	E946.0	E950.4	E962.0	E980.4
Chlorphenesin (carbamate)	968.0	E855.1	E938.0	E950.4	E962.0	E980.4
topical (antifungal)	976.0	E858.7	E946.0	E950.4	E962.0	E980.4
Chlorpheniramine	963.0	E858.1	E933.0	E950.4	E962.0	E980.4
Chlorophenoxamine	966.4	E855.0	E936.4	E950.4	E962.0	E980.4
Chlorophentermine	977.0	E858.8	E947.0	E950.4	E962.0	E980.4
Chlorproguanil	961.4	E857	E931.4	E950.4	E962.0	E980.4
Chlorpromazine	969.1	E853.0	E939.1	E950.3	E962.0	E980.3
Chlorpropamide	962.3	E858.0	E932.3	E950.4	E962.0	E980.4
Chlorprothixene	969.3	E853.8	E939.3	E950.3	E962.0	E980.3
Chlorquinaldol	976.0	E858.7	E946.0	E950.4	E962.0	E980.4
Chlortetracycline	960.4	E856	E930.4	E950.4	E962.0	E980.4
Chlorthalidone	974.4	E858.5	E944.4	E950.4	E962.0	E980.4
Chlortrianisene	962.2	E858.0	E932.2	E950.4	E962.0	E980.4
Chlor–Trimeton	963.0	E858.1	E933.0	E950.4	E962.0	E980.4
Chlorzoxazone	968.0	E855.1	E938.0	E950.4	E962.0	E980.4
Choke damp	987.8	E869.8	—	E952.8	E962.2	E982.8
Cholebrine	977.8	E858.8	E947.8	E950.4	E962.0	E980.4
Cholera vaccine	978.2	E858.8	E948.2	E950.4	E962.0	E980.4
Cholesterol–lowering agents	972.2	E858.3	E942.2	E950.4	E962.0	E980.4
Cholestyramine (resin)	972.2	E858.3	E942.2	E950.4	E962.0	E980.4
Cholic acid	973.4	E858.4	E943.4	E950.4	E962.0	E980.4
Choline						
dihydrogen citrate	977.1	E858.8	E947.1	E950.4	E962.0	E980.4
salicylate	965.1	E850.3	E935.3	E950.0	E962.0	E980.0
theophyllinate	974.1	E858.5	E944.1	E950.4	E962.0	E980.4
Cholinergics	971.0	E855.3	E941.0	E950.4	E962.0	E980.4
Cholografin	977.8	E858.8	E947.8	E950.4	E962.0	E980.4
Chorionic gonadotropin	962.4	E858.0	E932.4	E950.4	E962.0	E980.4
Chromates	983.9	E864.3	—	E950.7	E962.1	E980.6
dust or mist	987.8	E869.8	—	E952.8	E962.2	E982.8
lead	984.0	E866.0	—	E950.9	E962.1	E980.9
paint	984.0	E861.5	—	E950.9	E962.1	E980.9
Chromic acid	983.9	E864.3	—	E950.7	E962.1	E980.6
dust or mist	987.8	E869.8	—	E952.8	E962.2	E982.8
Chromium	985.6	E866.4	—	E950.9	E962.1	E980.9
compounds — see Chromates						
Chromonar	972.4	E858.3	E942.4	E950.4	E962.0	E980.4
Chromyl chloride	983.9	E864.3	—	E950.7	E962.1	E980.6
Chrysarobin (ointment)	976.4	E858.7	E946.4	E950.4	E962.0	E980.4
Chrysazin	973.1	E858.4	E943.1	E950.4	E962.0	E980.4
Chymar	963.4	E858.1	E933.4	E950.4	E962.0	E980.4

Substance	Poisoning	Accident	Therapeutic Use	Suicide Attempt	Assault	Undetermined
			External Cause (E-Code)			
ophthalmic preparation.	976.5	E858.7	E946.5	E950.4	E962.0	E980.4
Chymotrypsin	963.4	E858.1	E933.4	E950.4	E962.0	E980.4
ophthalmic preparation.	976.5	E858.7	E946.5	E950.4	E962.0	E980.4
Cicuta maculata or virosa	988.2	E865.4	—	E950.9	E962.1	E980.9
Cigarette lighter fluid	981	E862.1	—	E950.9	E962.1	E980.9
Cinchocaine (spinal)	968.7	E855.2	E938.7	E950.4	E962.0	E980.4
topical (surface)	968.5	E855.2	E938.5	E950.4	E962.0	E980.4
Cinchona	961.4	E857	E931.4	E950.4	E962.0	E980.4
Cinchonine alkaloids	961.4	E857	E931.4	E950.4	E962.0	E980.4
Cinchophen	974.7	E858.5	E944.7	E950.4	E962.0	E980.4
Cinnarizine	963.0	E858.1	E933.0	E950.4	E962.0	E980.4
Citanest.	968.9	E855.2	E938.9	E950.4	E962.0	E980.4
infiltration (subcutaneous)	968.5	E855.2	E938.5	E950.4	E962.0	E980.4
nerve block (peripheral) (plexus).	968.6	E855.2	E938.6	E950.4	E962.0	E980.4
Citric acid.	989.89	E866.8	—	E950.9	E962.1	E980.9
Citrovorum factor.	964.1	E858.2	E934.1	E950.4	E962.0	E980.4
Claviceps purpurea	988.2	E865.4	—	E950.9	E962.1	E980.9
Cleaner, cleansing agent type not specified . .	989.89	E861.9	—	E950.9	E962.1	E980.9
of paint or varnish	982.8	E862.9	—	E950.9	E962.1	E980.9
specified type NEC	989.89	E861.3	—	E950.9	E962.1	E980.9
Clematis vitalba	988.2	E865.4	—	E950.9	E962.1	E980.9
Clemizole.	963.0	E858.1	E933.0	E950.4	E962.0	E980.4
penicillin	960.0	E856	E930.0	E950.4	E962.0	E980.4
Clidinium	971.1	E855.4	E941.1	E950.4	E962.0	E980.4
Clindamycin	960.8	E856	E930.8	E950.4	E962.0	E980.4
Cliradon	965.09	E850.2	E935.2	E950.0	E962.0	E980.0
Clocortolone.	962.0	E858.0	E932.0	E950.4	E962.0	E980.4
Clofedanol	975.4	E858.6	E945.4	E950.4	E962.0	E980.4
Clofibrate	972.2	E858.3	E942.2	E950.4	E962.0	E980.4
Clomethiazole	967.1	E852.0	E937.1	E950.2	E962.0	E980.2
Clomiphene	977.8	E858.8	E947.8	E950.4	E962.0	E980.4
Clonazepam	969.4	E853.2	E939.4	E950.3	E962.0	E980.3
Clonidine	972.6	E858.3	E942.6	E950.4	E962.0	E980.4
Clopamide	974.3	E858.5	E944.3	E950.4	E962.0	E980.4
Clorazepate	969.4	E853.2	E939.4	E950.3	E962.0	E980.3
Clorexolone	974.4	E858.5	E944.4	E950.4	E962.0	E980.4
Clorox (bleach)	983.9	E864.3	—	E950.7	E962.1	E980.6
Clortermine	977.0	E858.8	E947.0	E950.4	E962.0	E980.4
Clotrimazole.	976.0	E858.7	E946.0	E950.4	E962.0	E980.4
Cloxacillin	960.0	E856	E930.0	E950.4	E962.0	E980.4
Coagulants NEC	964.5	E858.2	E934.5	E950.4	E962.0	E980.4
Coal (carbon monoxide from) — see also						
Carbon, monoxide, coal						
oil — see Kerosene						
tar NEC.	983.0	E864.0	—	E950.7	E962.1	E980.6
fumes	987.8	E869.8	—	E952.8	E962.2	E982.8
medicinal (ointment)	976.4	E858.7	E946.4	E950.4	E962.0	E980.4
analgesics NEC	965.5	E850.5	E935.5	E950.0	E962.0	E980.0
naphtha (solvent)	981	E862.0	—	E950.9	E962.1	E980.9
Cobalt (fumes) (industrial)	985.8	E866.4	—	E950.9	E962.1	E980.9
Cobra (venom).	989.5	E905.0	—	E950.9	E962.1	E980.9
Coca (leaf)	970.81	E854.3	E940.8	E950.4	E962.0	E980.4
Cocaine (hydrochloride) (salt).	970.81	E854.3	E940.8	E950.4	E962.0	E980.4
topical anesthetic	968.5	E855.2	E938.5	E950.4	E962.0	E980.4
Coccidioidin	977.8	E858.8	E947.8	E950.4	E962.0	E980.4
Cocculus indicus	988.2	E865.3	—	E950.9	E962.1	E980.9
Cochineal	989.89	E866.8	—	E950.9	E962.1	E980.9
medicinal products	977.4	E858.8	E947.4	E950.4	E962.0	E980.4
Codeine.	965.09	E850.2	E935.2	E950.0	E962.0	E980.0
Coffee	989.89	E866.8	—	E950.9	E962.1	E980.9
Cogentin	971.1	E855.4	E941.1	E950.4	E962.0	E980.4

Substance	Poisoning	Accident	Therapeutic Use	Suicide Attempt	Assault	Undetermined
			External Cause (E-Code)			

Substance	Poisoning	Accident	Therapeutic Use	Suicide Attempt	Assault	Undetermined
Coke fumes or gas (carbon monoxide)	986	E868.3	—	E952.1	E962.2	E982.1
industrial use	986	E868.8	—	E952.1	E962.2	E982.1
Colace	973.2	E858.4	E943.2	E950.4	E962.0	E980.4
Colchicine	974.7	E858.5	E944.7	E950.4	E962.0	E980.4
Colchicum	988.2	E865.3	—	E950.9	E962.1	E980.9
Cold cream	976.3	E858.7	E946.3	E950.4	E962.0	E980.4
Colestipol	972.2	E858.3	E942.2	E950.4	E962.0	E980.4
Colistimethate	960.8	E856	E930.8	E950.4	E962.0	E980.4
Colistin	960.8	E856	E930.8	E950.4	E962.0	E980.4
Collagen	977.8	E866.8	E947.8	E950.9	E962.1	E980.9
Collagenase	976.8	E858.7	E946.8	E950.4	E962.0	E980.4
Collodion (flexible)	976.3	E858.7	E946.3	E950.4	E962.0	E980.4
Colocynth	973.1	E858.4	E943.1	E950.4	E962.0	E980.4
Coloring matter — see Dye(s)						
Combustion gas — see Carbon, monoxide						
Compazine	969.1	E853.0	E939.1	E950.3	E962.0	E980.3
Compound						
42 (warfarin)	989.4	E863.7	—	E950.6	E962.1	E980.7
269 (endrin)	989.2	E863.0	—	E950.6	E962.1	E980.7
497 (dieldrin)	989.2	E863.0	—	E950.6	E962.1	E980.7
1080 (sodium fluoroacetate)	989.4	E863.7	—	E950.6	E962.1	E980.7
3422 (parathion)	989.3	E863.1	—	E950.6	E962.1	E980.7
3911 (phorate)	989.3	E863.1	—	E950.6	E962.1	E980.7
3956 (toxaphene)	989.2	E863.0	—	E950.6	E962.1	E980.7
4049 (malathion)	989.3	E863.1	—	E950.6	E962.1	E980.7
4124 (dicapthon)	989.4	E863.4	—	E950.6	E962.1	E980.7
E (cortisone)	962.0	E858.0	E932.0	E950.4	E962.0	E980.4
F (hydrocortisone)	962.0	E858.0	E932.0	E950.4	E962.0	E980.4
Congo red	977.8	E858.8	E947.8	E950.4	E962.0	E980.4
Coniine, conine	965.7	E850.7	E935.7	E950.0	E962.0	E980.0
Conium (maculatum)	988.2	E865.4	—	E950.9	E962.1	E980.9
Conjugated estrogens (equine)	962.2	E858.0	E932.2	E950.4	E962.0	E980.4
Contac	975.6	E858.6	E945.6	E950.4	E962.0	E980.4
Contact lens solution	976.5	E858.7	E946.5	E950.4	E962.0	E980.4
Contraceptives (oral)	962.2	E858.0	E932.2	E950.4	E962.0	E980.4
vaginal	976.8	E858.7	E946.8	E950.4	E962.0	E980.4
Contrast media (roentgenographic)	977.8	E858.8	E947.8	E950.4	E962.0	E980.4
Convallaria majalis	988.2	E865.4	—	E950.9	E962.1	E980.9
Copper (dust) (fumes) (salts) NEC	985.8	E866.4	—	E950.9	E962.1	E980.9
arsenate, arsenite	985.1	E866.3	—	E950.8	E962.1	E980.8
insecticide	985.1	E863.4	—	E950.8	E962.1	E980.8
emetic	973.6	E858.4	E943.6	E950.4	E962.0	E980.4
fungicide	985.8	E863.6	—	E950.6	E962.1	E980.7
insecticide	985.8	E863.4	—	E950.6	E962.1	E980.7
oleate	976.0	E858.7	E946.0	E950.4	E962.0	E980.4
sulfate	983.9	E864.3	—	E950.7	E962.1	E980.6
fungicide	983.9	E863.6	—	E950.7	E962.1	E980.6
cupric	973.6	E858.4	E943.6	E950.4	E962.0	E980.4
cuprous	983.9	E864.3	—	E950.7	E962.1	E980.6
Copperhead snake (bite) (venom)	989.5	E905.0	—	E950.9	E962.1	E980.9
Coral (sting)	989.5	E905.6	—	E950.9	E962.1	E980.9
snake (bite) (venom)	989.5	E905.0	—	E950.9	E962.1	E980.9
Cordran	976.0	E858.7	E946.0	E950.4	E962.0	E980.4
Corn cures	976.4	E858.7	E946.4	E950.4	E962.0	E980.4
Cornhusker's lotion	976.3	E858.7	E946.3	E950.4	E962.0	E980.4
Corn starch	976.3	E858.7	E946.3	E950.4	E962.0	E980.4
Corrosive	983.9	E864.4	—	E950.7	E962.1	E980.6
acids NEC	983.1	E864.1	—	E950.7	E962.1	E980.6
aromatics	983.0	E864.0	—	E950.7	E962.1	E980.6
disinfectant	983.0	E861.4	—	E950.7	E962.1	E980.6

Substance	Poisoning	Accident	Therapeutic Use	Suicide Attempt	Assault	Undetermined
			External Cause (E-Code)			
fumes NEC	987.9	E869.9	—	E952.9	E962.2	E982.9
specified NEC	983.9	E864.3	—	E950.7	E961.1	E980.6
sublimate — *see* Mercury, chloride						
Cortate	962.0	E858.0	E932.0	E950.4	E962.0	E980.4
Cort–Dome	962.0	E858.0	E932.0	E950.4	E962.0	E980.4
ENT agent.	976.6	E858.7	E946.6	E950.4	E962.0	E980.4
ophthalmic preparation	976.5	E858.7	E946.5	E950.4	E962.0	E980.4
topical NEC	976.0	E858.7	E946.0	E950.4	E962.0	E980.4
Cortef	962.0	E858.0	E932.0	E950.4	E962.0	E980.4
ENT agent.	976.6	E858.7	E946.6	E950.4	E962.0	E980.4
ophthalmic preparation	976.5	E858.7	E946.5	E950.4	E962.0	E980.4
topical NEC	976.0	E858.7	E946.0	E950.4	E962.0	E980.4
Corticosteroids (fluorinated)	962.0	E858.0	E932.0	E950.4	E962.0	E980.4
ENT agent.	976.6	E858.7	E946.6	E950.4	E962.0	E980.4
ophthalmic preparation	976.5	E858.7	E946.5	E950.4	E962.0	E980.4
topical NEC	976.0	E858.7	E946.0	E950.4	E962.0	E980.4
Corticotropin	962.4	E858.0	E932.4	E950.4	E962.0	E980.4
Cortisol.	962.0	E858.0	E932.0	E950.4	E962.0	E980.4
ENT agent.	976.6	E858.7	E946.6	E950.4	E962.0	E980.4
ophthalmic preparation	976.5	E858.7	E946.5	E950.4	E962.0	E980.4
topical NEC	976.0	E858.7	E946.0	E950.4	E962.0	E980.4
Cortisone derivatives (acetate)	962.0	E858.0	E932.0	E950.4	E962.0	E980.4
ENT agent.	976.6	E858.7	E946.6	E950.4	E962.0	E980.4
ophthalmic preparation	976.5	E858.7	E946.5	E950.4	E962.0	E980.4
topical NEC	976.0	E858.7	E946.0	E950.4	E962.0	E980.4
Cortogen	962.0	E858.0	E932.0	E950.4	E962.0	E980.4
ENT agent.	976.6	E858.7	E946.6	E950.4	E962.0	E980.4
ophthalmic preparation	976.5	E858.7	E946.5	E950.4	E962.0	E980.4
Cortone.	962.0	E858.0	E932.0	E950.4	E962.0	E980.4
ENT agent.	976.6	E858.7	E946.6	E950.4	E962.0	E980.4
ophthalmic preparation	976.5	E858.7	E946.5	E950.4	E962.0	E980.4
Cortril	962.0	E858.0	E932.0	E950.4	E962.0	E980.4
ENT agent.	976.6	E858.7	E946.6	E950.4	E962.0	E980.4
ophthalmic preparation	976.5	E858.7	E946.5	E950.4	E962.0	E980.4
topical NEC	976.0	E858.7	E946.0	E950.4	E962.0	E980.4
Cosmetics.	989.89	E866.7	—	E950.9	E962.1	E980.9
Cosyntropin	977.8	E858.8	E947.8	E950.4	E962.0	E980.4
Cotarnine	964.5	E858.2	E934.5	E950.4	E962.0	E980.4
Cotton*seed* oil	976.3	E858.7	E946.3	E950.4	E962.0	E980.4
Cough mixtures (antitussives).	975.4	E858.6	E945.4	E950.4	E962.0	E980.4
containing opiates	965.09	E850.2	E935.2	E950.0	E962.0	E980.0
expectorants	975.5	E858.6	E945.5	E950.4	E962.0	E980.4
Coumadin.	964.2	E858.2	E934.2	E950.4	E962.0	E980.4
rodenticide.	989.4	E863.7	—	E950.6	E962.1	E980.7
Coumarin	964.2	E858.2	E934.2	E950.4	E962.0	E980.4
Coumetarol	964.2	E858.2	E934.2	E950.4	E962.0	E980.4
Cowbane	988.2	E865.4	—	E950.9	E962.1	E980.9
Cozyme.	963.5	E858.1	E933.5	E950.4	E962.0	E980.4
Crack.	970.81	E854.3	E940.8	E950.4	E962.0	E980.4
Creolin.	983.0	E864.0	—	E950.7	E962.1	E980.6
disinfectant	983.0	E861.4	—	E950.7	E962.1	E980.6
Creosol (compound).	983.0	E864.0	—	E950.7	E962.1	E980.6
Creosote (beechwood) (coal tar).	983.0	E864.0	—	E950.7	E962.1	E980.6
medicinal (expectorant)	975.5	E858.6	E945.5	E950.4	E962.0	E980.4
syrup	975.5	E858.6	E945.5	E950.4	E962.0	E980.4
Cresol	983.0	E864.0	—	E950.7	E962.1	E980.6
disinfectant	983.0	E861.4	—	E950.7	E962.1	E980.6
Cresylic acid	983.0	E864.0	—	E950.7	E962.1	E980.6
Cropropamide	965.7	E850.7	E935.7	E950.0	E962.0	E980.0
with crotethamide.	970.0	E854.3	E940.0	E950.4	E962.0	E980.4
Crotamiton	976.0	E858.7	E946.0	E950.4	E962.0	E980.4

Substance	Poisoning	Accident	Therapeutic Use	Suicide Attempt	Assault	Undetermined
			External Cause (E-Code)			
Crotethamide 965.7	E850.7	E935.7	E950.0	E962.0	E980.0
with cropropamide 970.0	E854.3	E940.0	E950.4	E962.0	E980.4
Croton (oil) 973.1	E858.4	E943.1	E950.4	E962.0	E980.4
chloral 967.1	E852.0	E937.1	E950.2	E962.0	E980.2
Crude oil 981	E862.1	—	E950.9	E962.1	E980.9
Cryogenine 965.8	E850.8	E935.8	E950.0	E962.0	E980.0
Cryolite (pesticide) 989.4	E863.4	—	E950.6	E962.1	E980.7
Cryptenamine 972.6	E858.3	E942.6	E950.4	E962.0	E980.4
Crystal violet 976.0	E858.7	E946.0	E950.4	E962.0	E980.4
Cuckoopint 988.2	E865.4	—	E950.9	E962.1	E980.9
Cumetharol 964.2	E858.2	E934.2	E950.4	E962.0	E980.4
Cupric sulfate 973.6	E858.4	E943.6	E950.4	E962.0	E980.4
Cuprous sulfate 983.9	E864.3	—	E950.7	E962.1	E980.6
Curare, curarine 975.2	E858.6	E945.2	E950.4	E962.0	E980.4
Cyanic acid — *see* Cyanide(s)					
Cyanide(s) (compounds) (hydrogen)					
(potassium) (sodium) NEC 989.0	E866.8	—	E950.9	E962.1	E980.9
dust or gas (inhalation) NEC 987.7	E869.8	—	E952.8	E962.2	E982.8
fumigant. 989.0	E863.8	—	E950.6	E962.1	E980.7
mercuric — *see* Mercury					
pesticide (dust) (fumes) 989.0	E863.4	—	E950.6	E962.1	E980.7
Cyanocobalamin 964.1	E858.2	E934.1	E950.4	E962.0	E980.4
Cyanogen (chloride) (gas) NEC . . . 987.8	E869.8	—	E952.8	E962.2	E982.8
Cyclaine 968.5	E855.2	E938.5	E950.4	E962.0	E980.4
Cyclamen europaeum 988.2	E865.4	—	E950.9	E962.1	E980.9
Cyclandelate 972.5	E858.3	E942.5	E950.4	E962.0	E980.4
Cyclazocine 965.09	E850.2	E935.2	E950.0	E962.0	E980.0
Cyclizine 963.0	E858.1	E933.0	E950.4	E962.0	E980.4
Cyclobarbital, cyclobarbitone 967.0	E851	E937.0	E950.1	E962.0	E980.1
Cycloguanil 961.4	E857	E931.4	E950.4	E962.0	E980.4
Cyclohexane 982.0	E862.4	—	E950.9	E962.1	E980.9
Cyclohexanol 980.8	E860.8	—	E950.9	E962.1	E980.9
Cyclohexanone 982.8	E862.4	—	E950.9	E962.1	E980.9
Cyclomethycaine 968.5	E855.2	E938.5	E950.4	E962.0	E980.4
Cyclopentamine 971.2	E855.5	E941.2	E950.4	E962.0	E980.4
Cyclopenthiazide 974.3	E858.5	E944.3	E950.4	E962.0	E980.4
Cyclopentolate 971.1	E855.4	E941.1	E950.4	E962.0	E980.4
Cyclophosphamide 963.1	E858.1	E933.1	E950.4	E962.0	E980.4
Cyclopropane 968.2	E855.1	E938.2	E950.4	E962.0	E980.4
Cycloserine 960.6	E856	E930.6	E950.4	E962.0	E980.4
Cyclothiazide 974.3	E858.5	E944.3	E950.4	E962.0	E980.4
Cycrimine 966.4	E855.0	E936.4	E950.4	E962.0	E980.4
Cymarin 972.1	E858.3	E942.1	E950.4	E962.0	E980.4
Cyproheptadine 963.0	E858.1	E933.0	E950.4	E962.0	E980.4
Cyprolidol. 969.09	E854.0	E939.0	E950.3	E962.0	E980.3
Cytarabine 963.1	E858.1	E933.1	E950.4	E962.0	E980.4
Cytisus					
laburnum 988.2	E865.4	—	E950.9	E962.1	E980.9
scoparius 988.2	E865.4	—	E950.9	E962.1	E980.9
Cytomel 962.7	E858.0	E932.7	E950.4	E962.0	E980.4
Cytosine (antineoplastic) 963.1	E858.1	E933.1	E950.4	E962.0	E980.4
Cytoxan 963.1	E858.1	E933.1	E950.4	E962.0	E980.4
Dacarbazine 963.1	E858.1	E933.1	E950.4	E962.0	E980.4
Dactinomycin 960.7	E856	E930.7	E950.4	E962.0	E980.4
DADPS 961.8	E857	E931.8	E950.4	E962.0	E980.4
Dakin's solution (external) 976.0	E858.7	E946.0	E950.4	E962.0	E980.4
Dalmane 969.4	E853.2	E939.4	E950.3	E962.0	E980.3
DAM. 977.2	E858.8	E947.2	E950.4	E962.0	E980.4
Danilone 964.2	E858.2	E934.2	E950.4	E962.0	E980.4
Danthron 973.1	E858.4	E943.1	E950.4	E962.0	E980.4

TABLE OF DRUGS AND CHEMICALS

Substance	Poisoning	Accident	Therapeutic Use	Suicide Attempt	Assault	Undetermined
			External Cause (E-Code)			
Dantrolene	975.2	E858.6	E945.2	E950.4	E962.0	E980.4
Daphne (gnidium) (mezereum)	988.2	E865.4	—	E950.9	E962.1	E980.9
berry	988.2	E865.3	—	E950.9	E962.1	E980.9
Dapsone	961.8	E857	E931.8	E950.4	E962.0	E980.4
Daraprim	961.4	E857	E931.4	E950.4	E962.0	E980.4
Darnel	988.2	E865.3	—	E950.9	E962.1	E980.9
Darvon	965.8	E850.8	E935.8	E950.0	E962.0	E980.0
Daunorubicin	960.7	E856	E930.7	E950.4	E962.0	E980.4
DBI	962.3	E858.0	E932.3	E950.4	E962.0	E980.4
D–Con (rodenticide)	989.4	E863.7	—	E950.6	E962.1	E980.7
DDS	961.8	E857	E931.8	E950.4	E962.0	E980.4
DDT	989.2	E863.0	—	E950.6	E962.1	E980.7
Deadly nightshade	988.2	E865.4	—	E950.9	E962.1	E980.9
berry	988.2	E865.3	—	E950.9	E962.1	E980.9
Deanol	969.79	E854.2	E939.7	E950.3	E962.0	E980.3
Debrisoquine	972.6	E858.3	E942.6	E950.4	E962.0	E980.4
Decaborane	989.89	E866.8	—	E950.9	E962.1	E980.9
fumes	987.8	E869.8	—	E952.8	E962.2	E982.8
Decadron	962.0	E858.0	E932.0	E950.4	E962.0	E980.4
ENT agent	976.6	E858.7	E946.6	E950.4	E962.0	E980.4
ophthalmic preparation	976.5	E858.7	E946.5	E950.4	E962.0	E980.4
topical NEC	976.0	E858.7	E946.0	E950.4	E962.0	E980.4
Decahydronaphthalene	982.0	E862.4	—	E950.9	E962.1	E980.9
Decalin	982.0	E862.4	—	E950.9	E962.1	E980.9
Decamethonium	975.2	E858.6	E945.2	E950.4	E962.0	E980.4
Decholin	973.4	E858.4	E943.4	E950.4	E962.0	E980.4
sodium (diagnostic)	977.8	E858.8	E947.8	E950.4	E962.0	E980.4
Declomycin	960.4	E856	E930.4	E950.4	E962.0	E980.4
Deferoxamine	963.8	E858.1	E933.8	E950.4	E962.0	E980.4
Dehydrocholic acid	973.4	E858.4	E943.4	E950.4	E962.0	E980.4
Dekalin	982.0	E862.4	—	E950.9	E962.1	E980.9
Delalutin	962.2	E858.0	E932.2	E950.4	E962.0	E980.4
Delphinium	988.2	E865.3	—	E950.9	E962.1	E980.9
Deltasone	962.0	E858.0	E932.0	E950.4	E962.0	E980.4
Deltra	962.0	E858.0	E932.0	E950.4	E962.0	E980.4
Delvinal	967.0	E851	E937.0	E950.1	E962.0	E980.1
Demecarium (bromide)	971.0	E855.3	E941.0	E950.4	E962.0	E980.4
Demeclocycline	960.4	E856	E930.4	E950.4	E962.0	E980.4
Demecolcine	963.1	E858.1	E933.1	E950.4	E962.0	E980.4
Demelanizing agents	976.8	E858.7	E946.8	E950.4	E962.0	E980.4
Demerol	965.09	E850.2	E935.2	E950.0	E962.0	E980.0
Demethylchlortetracycline	960.4	E856	E930.4	E950.4	E962.0	E980.4
Demethyltetracycline	960.4	E856	E930.4	E950.4	E962.0	E980.4
Demeton	989.3	E863.1	—	E950.6	E962.1	E980.7
Demulcents	976.3	E858.7	E946.3	E950.4	E962.0	E980.4
Demulen	962.2	E858.0	E932.2	E950.4	E962.0	E980.4
Denatured alcohol	980.0	E860.1	—	E950.9	E962.1	E980.9
Dendrid	976.5	E858.7	E946.5	E950.4	E962.0	E980.4
Dental agents, topical	976.7	E858.7	E946.7	E950.4	E962.0	E980.4
Deodorant spray (feminine hygiene)	976.8	E858.7	E946.8	E950.4	E962.0	E980.4
Deoxyribonuclease	963.4	E858.1	E933.4	E950.4	E962.0	E980.4
Depressants						
appetite, central	977.0	E858.8	E947.0	E950.4	E962.0	E980.4
cardiac	972.0	E858.3	E942.0	E950.4	E962.0	E980.4
central nervous system (anesthetic)	968.4	E855.1	E938.4	E950.4	E962.0	E980.4
psychotherapeutic	969.5	E853.9	E939.5	E950.3	E962.0	E980.3
Dequalinium	976.0	E858.7	E946.0	E950.4	E962.0	E980.4
Dermolate	976.2	E858.7	E946.2	E950.4	E962.0	E980.4
DES	962.2	E858.0	E932.2	E950.4	E962.0	E980.4
Desenex	976.0	E858.7	E946.0	E950.4	E962.0	E980.4
Deserpidine	972.6	E858.3	E942.6	E950.4	E962.0	E980.4

Substance	Poisoning	Accident	Therapeutic Use	Suicide Attempt	Assault	Undetermined
			External Cause (E-Code)			
Desipramine	969.05	E854.0	E939.0	E950.3	E962.0	E980.3
Deslanoside	972.1	E858.3	E942.1	E950.4	E962.0	E980.4
Desocodeine	965.09	E850.2	E935.2	E950.0	E962.0	E980.0
Desomorphine	965.09	E850.2	E935.2	E950.0	E962.0	E980.0
Desonide	976.0	E858.7	E946.0	E950.4	E962.0	E980.4
Desoxycorticosterone derivatives	962.0	E858.0	E932.0	E950.4	E962.0	E980.4
Desoxyephedrine	969.72	E854.2	E939.7	E950.3	E962.0	E980.3
DET	969.6	E854.1	E939.6	E950.3	E962.0	E980.3
Detergents (ingested) (synthetic)	989.6	E861.0	—	E950.9	E962.1	E980.9
external medication	976.2	E858.7	E946.2	E950.4	E962.0	E980.4
Deterrent, alcohol	977.3	E858.8	E947.3	E950.4	E962.0	E980.4
Detrothyronine	962.7	E858.0	E932.7	E950.4	E962.0	E980.4
Dettol (external medication)	976.0	E858.7	E946.0	E950.4	E962.0	E980.4
Dexamethasone	962.0	E858.0	E932.0	E950.4	E962.0	E980.4
ENT agent	976.6	E858.7	E946.6	E950.4	E962.0	E980.4
ophthalmic preparation	976.5	E858.7	E946.5	E950.4	E962.0	E980.4
topical NEC	976.0	E858.7	E946.0	E950.4	E962.0	E980.4
Dexamphetamine	969.72	E854.2	E939.7	E950.3	E962.0	E980.3
Dexedrine	969.72	E854.2	E939.7	E950.3	E962.0	E980.3
Dexpanthenol	963.5	E858.1	E933.5	E950.4	E962.0	E980.4
Dextran	964.8	E858.2	E934.8	E950.4	E962.0	E980.4
Dextriferron	964.0	E858.2	E934.0	E950.4	E962.0	E980.4
Dextroamphetamine	969.72	E854.2	E939.7	E950.3	E962.0	E980.3
Dextro calcium pantothenate	963.5	E858.1	E933.5	E950.4	E962.0	E980.4
Dextromethorphan	975.4	E858.6	E945.4	E950.4	E962.0	E980.4
Dextromoramide	965.09	E850.2	E935.2	E950.0	E962.0	E980.0
Dextro pantothenyl alcohol	963.5	E858.1	E933.5	E950.4	E962.0	E980.4
topical	976.8	E858.7	E946.8	E950.4	E962.0	E980.4
Dextropropoxyphene (hydrochloride)	965.8	E850.8	E935.8	E950.0	E962.0	E980.0
Dextrorphan	965.09	E850.2	E935.2	E950.0	E962.0	E980.0
Dextrose NEC	974.5	E858.5	E944.5	E950.4	E962.0	E980.4
Dextrothyroxin	962.7	E858.0	E932.7	E950.4	E962.0	E980.4
DFP	971.0	E855.3	E941.0	E950.4	E962.0	E980.4
DHE–45	972.9	E858.3	E942.9	E950.4	E962.0	E980.4
Diabinese	962.3	E858.0	E932.3	E950.4	E962.0	E980.4
Diacetyl monoxime	977.2	E858.8	E947.2	E950.4	E962.0	E980.4
Diacetylmorphine	965.01	E850.0	E935.0	E950.0	E962.0	E980.0
Diagnostic agents	977.8	E858.8	E947.8	E950.4	E962.0	E980.4
Dial (soap)	976.2	E858.7	E946.2	E950.4	E962.0	E980.4
sedative	967.0	E851	E937.0	E950.1	E962.0	E980.1
Diallylbarbituric acid	967.0	E851	E937.0	E950.1	E962.0	E980.1
Diaminodiphenylsulfone	961.8	E857	E931.8	E950.4	E962.0	E980.4
Diamorphine	965.01	E850.0	E935.0	E950.0	E962.0	E980.0
Diamox	974.2	E858.5	E944.2	E950.4	E962.0	E980.4
Diamthazole	976.0	E858.7	E946.0	E950.4	E962.0	E980.4
Diaphenylsulfone	961.8	E857	E931.8	E950.4	E962.0	E980.4
Diasone (sodium)	961.8	E857	E931.8	E950.4	E962.0	E980.4
Diazepam	969.4	E853.2	E939.4	E950.3	E962.0	E980.3
Diazinon	989.3	E863.1	—	E950.6	E962.1	E980.7
Diazomethane (gas)	987.8	E869.8	—	E952.8	E962.2	E982.8
Diazoxide	972.5	E858.3	E942.5	E950.4	E962.0	E980.4
Dibenamine	971.3	E855.6	E941.3	E950.4	E962.0	E980.4
Dibenzheptropine	963.0	E858.1	E933.0	E950.4	E962.0	E980.4
Dibenzyline	971.3	E855.6	E941.3	E950.4	E962.0	E980.4
Diborane (gas)	987.8	E869.8	—	E952.8	E962.2	E982.8
Dibromomannitol	963.1	E858.1	E933.1	E950.4	E962.0	E980.4
Dibucaine (spinal)	968.7	E855.2	E938.7	E950.4	E962.0	E980.4
topical (surface)	968.5	E855.2	E938.5	E950.4	E962.0	E980.4
Dibunate sodium	975.4	E858.6	E945.4	E950.4	E962.0	E980.4
Dibutoline	971.1	E855.4	E941.1	E950.4	E962.0	E980.4

Substance	Poisoning	Accident	Therapeutic Use	Suicide Attempt	Assault	Undetermined
			External Cause (E-Code)			
Dicapthon	989.4	E863.4	—	E950.6	E962.1	E980.7
Dichloralphenazone	967.1	E852.0	E937.1	E950.2	E962.0	E980.2
Dichlorodifluoromethane	987.4	E869.2	—	E952.8	E962.2	E982.8
Dichloroethane	982.3	E862.4	—	E950.9	E962.1	E980.9
Dichloroethylene	982.3	E862.4	—	E950.9	E962.1	E980.9
Dichloroethyl sulfide	987.8	E869.8	—	E952.8	E962.2	E982.8
Dichlorohydrin	982.3	E862.4	—	E950.9	E962.1	E980.9
Dichloromethane (solvent) (vapor)	982.3	E862.4	—	E950.9	E962.1	E980.9
Dichlorophen(e)	961.6	E857	E931.6	E950.4	E962.0	E980.4
Dichlorphenamide	974.2	E858.5	E944.2	E950.4	E962.0	E980.4
Dichlorvos	989.3	E863.1	—	E950.6	E962.1	E980.7
Diclofenac sodium	965.69	E850.6	E935.6	E950.0	E962.0	E980.0
Dicoumarin, dicumarol	964.2	E858.2	E934.2	E950.4	E962.0	E980.4
Dicyanogen (gas)	987.8	E869.8	—	E952.8	E962.2	E982.8
Dicyclomine	971.1	E855.4	E941.1	E950.4	E962.0	E980.4
Dieldrin (vapor)	989.2	E863.0	—	E950.6	E962.1	E980.7
Dienestrol	962.2	E858.0	E932.2	E950.4	E962.0	E980.4
Dietetics	977.0	E858.8	E947.0	E950.4	E962.0	E980.4
Diethazine	966.4	E855.0	E936.4	E950.4	E962.0	E980.4
Diethyl						
barbituric acid	967.0	E851	E937.0	E950.1	E962.0	E980.1
carbamazine	961.6	E857	E931.6	E950.4	E962.0	E980.4
carbinol	980.8	E860.8	—	E950.9	E962.1	E980.9
carbonate	982.8	E862.4	—	E950.9	E962.1	E980.9
ether (vapor) — *see* Ether(s)						
propion	977.0	E858.8	E947.0	E950.4	E962.0	E980.4
stilbestrol	962.2	E858.0	E932.2	E950.4	E962.0	E980.4
Diethylene						
dioxide	982.8	E862.4	—	E950.9	E962.1	E980.9
glycol (monoacetate) (monoethyl ether)	982.8	E862.4	—	E950.9	E962.1	E980.9
Diethylsulfone–diethylmethane	967.8	E852.8	E937.8	E950.2	E962.0	E980.2
Difencloxazine	965.09	E850.2	E935.2	E950.0	E962.0	E980.0
Diffusin	963.4	E858.1	E933.4	E950.4	E962.0	E980.4
Diflos	971.0	E855.3	E941.0	E950.4	E962.0	E980.4
Digestants	973.4	E858.4	E943.4	E950.4	E962.0	E980.4
Digitalin(e)	972.1	E858.3	E942.1	E950.4	E962.0	E980.4
Digitalis glycosides	972.1	E858.3	E942.1	E950.4	E962.0	E980.4
Digitoxin	972.1	E858.3	E942.1	E950.4	E962.0	E980.4
Digoxin	972.1	E858.3	E942.1	E950.4	E962.0	E980.4
Dihydrocodeine	965.09	E850.2	E935.2	E950.0	E962.0	E980.0
Dihydrocodeinone	965.09	E850.2	E935.2	E950.0	E962.0	E980.0
Dihydroergocristine	972.9	E858.3	E942.9	E950.4	E962.0	E980.4
Dihydroergotamine	972.9	E858.3	E942.9	E950.4	E962.0	E980.4
Dihydroergotoxine	972.9	E858.3	E942.9	E950.4	E962.0	E980.4
Dihydrohydroxycodeinone	965.09	E850.2	E935.2	E950.0	E962.0	E980.0
Dihydrohydroxymorphinone	965.09	E850.2	E935.2	E950.0	E962.0	E980.0
Dihydroisocodeine	965.09	E850.2	E935.2	E950.0	E962.0	E980.0
Dihydromorphine	965.09	E850.2	E935.2	E950.0	E962.0	E980.0
Dihydromorphinone	965.09	E850.2	E935.2	E950.0	E962.0	E980.0
Dihydrostreptomycin	960.6	E856	E930.6	E950.4	E962.0	E980.4
Dihydrotachysterol	962.6	E858.0	E932.6	E950.4	E962.0	E980.4
Dihydroxyanthraquinone	973.1	E858.4	E943.1	E950.4	E962.0	E980.4
Dihydroxycodeinone	965.09	E850.2	E935.2	E950.0	E962.0	E980.0
Diiodohydroxyquin	961.3	E857	E931.3	E950.4	E962.0	E980.4
topical	976.0	E858.7	E946.0	E950.4	E962.0	E980.4
Diiodohydroxyquinoline	961.3	E857	E931.3	E950.4	E962.0	E980.4
Dilantin	966.1	E855.0	E936.1	E950.4	E962.0	E980.4
Dilaudid	965.09	E850.2	E935.2	E950.0	E962.0	E980.0
Diloxanide	961.5	E857	E931.5	E950.4	E962.0	E980.4
Dimefline	970.0	E854.3	E940.0	E950.4	E962.0	E980.4
Dimenhydrinate	963.0	E858.1	E933.0	E950.4	E962.0	E980.4

Substance	Poisoning	Accident	Therapeutic Use	Suicide Attempt	Assault	Undetermined
			External Cause (E-Code)			
Dimercaprol	963.8	E858.1	E933.8	E950.4	E962.0	E980.4
Dimercaptopropanol.	963.8	E858.1	E933.8	E950.4	E962.0	E980.4
Dimetane	963.0	E858.1	E933.0	E950.4	E962.0	E980.4
Dimethicone.	976.3	E858.7	E946.3	E950.4	E962.0	E980.4
Dimethindene	963.0	E858.1	E933.0	E950.4	E962.0	E980.4
Dimethisoquin	968.5	E855.2	E938.5	E950.4	E962.0	E980.4
Dimethisterone.	962.2	E858.0	E932.2	E950.4	E962.0	E980.4
Dimethoxanate.	975.4	E858.6	E945.4	E950.4	E962.0	E980.4
Dimethyl						
arsine, arsinic acid — *see* Arsenic						
carbinol	980.2	E860.3	—	E950.9	E962.1	E980.9
diguanide	962.3	E858.0	E932.3	E950.4	E962.0	E980.4
ketone	982.8	E862.4	—	E950.9	E962.1	E980.9
vapor	987.8	E869.8	—	E952.8	E962.2	E982.8
meperidine.	965.09	E850.2	E935.2	E950.0	E962.0	E980.0
parathion	989.3	E863.1	—	E950.6	E962.1	E980.7
polysiloxane	973.8	E858.4	E943.8	E950.4	E962.0	E980.4
sulfate (fumes)	987.8	E869.8	—	E952.8	E962.2	E982.8
liquid	983.9	E864.3	—	E950.7	E962.1	E980.6
sulfoxide NEC	982.8	E862.4	—	E950.9	E962.1	E980.9
medicinal	976.4	E858.7	E946.4	E950.4	E962.0	E980.4
triptamine	969.6	E854.1	E939.6	E950.3	E962.0	E980.3
tubocurarine	975.2	E858.6	E945.2	E950.4	E962.0	E980.4
Dindevan	964.2	E858.2	E934.2	E950.4	E962.0	E980.4
Dinitro (–ortho–) cresol (herbicide) (spray) . .	989.4	E863.5	—	E950.6	E962.1	E980.7
insecticide.	989.4	E863.4	—	E950.6	E962.1	E980.7
Dinitrobenzene.	983.0	E864.0	—	E950.7	E962.1	E980.6
vapor	987.8	E869.8	—	E952.8	E962.2	E982.8
Dinitro–orthocresol (herbicide)	989.4	E863.5	—	E950.6	E962.1	E980.7
insecticide.	989.4	E863.4	—	E950.6	E962.1	E980.7
Dinitrophenol (herbicide) (spray)	989.4	E863.5	—	E950.6	E962.1	E980.7
insecticide.	989.4	E863.4	—	E950.6	E962.1	E980.7
Dinoprost	975.0	E858.6	E945.0	E950.4	E962.0	E980.4
Dioctyl sulfosuccinate (calcium) (sodium). . .	973.2	E858.4	E943.2	E950.4	E962.0	E980.4
Diodoquin.	961.3	E857	E931.3	E950.4	E962.0	E980.4
Dione derivatives NEC	966.3	E855.0	E936.3	E950.4	E962.0	E980.4
Dionin	965.09	E850.2	E935.2	E950.0	E962.0	E980.0
Dioxane.	982.8	E862.4	—	E950.9	E962.1	E980.9
Dioxin — *see* herbicide						
Dioxyline	972.5	E858.3	E942.5	E950.4	E962.0	E980.4
Dipentene	982.8	E862.4	—	E950.9	E962.1	E980.9
Diphemanil	971.1	E855.4	E941.1	E950.4	E962.0	E980.4
Diphenadione	964.2	E858.2	E934.2	E950.4	E962.0	E980.4
Diphenhydramine.	963.0	E858.1	E933.0	E950.4	E962.0	E980.4
Diphenidol	963.0	E858.1	E933.0	E950.4	E962.0	E980.4
Diphenoxylate	973.5	E858.4	E943.5	E950.4	E962.0	E980.4
Diphenylchloroarsine	985.1	E866.3	—	E950.8	E962.1	E980.8
Diphenylhydantoin (sodium)	966.1	E855.0	E936.1	E950.4	E962.0	E980.4
Diphenylpyraline	963.0	E858.1	E933.0	E950.4	E962.0	E980.4
Diphtheria						
antitoxin.	979.9	E858.8	E949.9	E950.4	E962.0	E980.4
toxoid.	978.5	E858.8	E948.5	E950.4	E962.0	E980.4
with tetanus toxoid	978.9	E858.8	E948.9	E950.4	E962.0	E980.4
with pertussis component	978.6	E858.8	E948.6	E950.4	E962.0	E980.4
vaccine	978.5	E858.8	E948.5	E950.4	E962.0	E980.4
Dipipanone	965.09	E850.2	E935.2	E950.0	E962.0	E980.0
Diplovax	979.5	E858.8	E949.5	E950.4	E962.0	E980.4
Diprophylline	975.1	E858.6	E945.1	E950.4	E962.0	E980.4
Dipyridamole	972.4	E858.3	E942.4	E950.4	E962.0	E980.4
Dipyrone	965.5	E850.5	E935.5	E950.0	E962.0	E980.0

Substance	Poisoning	Accident	Therapeutic Use	Suicide Attempt	Assault	Undetermined
			External Cause (E-Code)			
Diquat 989.4	E863.5	—	E950.6	E962.1	E980.7
Disinfectant NEC. 983.9	E861.4	—	E950.7	E962.1	E980.6
alkaline 983.2	E861.4	—	E950.7	E962.1	E980.6
aromatic. 983.0	E861.4	—	E950.7	E962.1	E980.6
Disipal 966.4	E855.0	E936.4	E950.4	E962.0	E980.4
Disodium edetate 963.8	E858.1	E933.8	E950.4	E962.0	E980.4
Disulfamide 974.4	E858.5	E944.4	E950.4	E962.0	E980.4
Disulfanilamide 961.0	E857	E931.0	E950.4	E962.0	E980.4
Disulfiram. 977.3	E858.8	E947.3	E950.4	E962.0	E980.4
Dithiazanine 961.6	E857	E931.6	E950.4	E962.0	E980.4
Dithioglycerol 963.8	E858.1	E933.8	E950.4	E962.0	E980.4
Dithranol 976.4	E858.7	E946.4	E950.4	E962.0	E980.4
Diucardin 974.3	E858.5	E944.3	E950.4	E962.0	E980.4
Diupres 974.3	E858.5	E944.3	E950.4	E962.0	E980.4
Diuretics NEC 974.4	E858.5	E944.4	E950.4	E962.0	E980.4
carbonic acid anhydrase inhibitors 974.2	E858.5	E944.2	E950.4	E962.0	E980.4
mercurial 974.0	E858.5	E944.0	E950.4	E962.0	E980.4
osmotic 974.4	E858.5	E944.4	E950.4	E962.0	E980.4
purine derivatives 974.1	E858.5	E944.1	E950.4	E962.0	E980.4
saluretic. 974.3	E858.5	E944.3	E950.4	E962.0	E980.4
Diuril. 974.3	E858.5	E944.3	E950.4	E962.0	E980.4
Divinyl ether 968.2	E855.1	E938.2	E950.4	E962.0	E980.4
D–lysergic acid diethylamide 969.6	E854.1	E939.6	E950.3	E962.0	E980.3
DMCT 960.4	E856	E930.4	E950.4	E962.0	E980.4
DMSO 982.8	E862.4	—	E950.9	E962.1	E980.9
DMT 969.6	E854.1	E939.6	E950.3	E962.0	E980.3
DNOC 989.4	E863.5	—	E950.6	E962.1	E980.7
DOCA 962.0	E858.0	E932.0	E950.4	E962.0	E980.4
Dolophine. 965.02	E850.1	E935.1	E950.0	E962.0	E980.0
Doloxene 965.8	E850.8	E935.8	E950.0	E962.0	E980.0
DOM. 969.6	E854.1	E939.6	E950.3	E962.0	E980.3
Domestic gas — *see* Gas, utility					
Domiphen (bromide) (lozenges) 976.6	E858.7	E946.6	E950.4	E962.0	E980.4
Dopa (levo) 966.4	E855.0	E936.4	E950.4	E962.0	E980.4
Dopamine 971.2	E855.5	E941.2	E950.4	E962.0	E980.4
Doriden 967.5	E852.4	E937.5	E950.2	E962.0	E980.2
Dormiral 967.0	E851	E937.0	E950.1	E962.0	E980.1
Dormison 967.8	E852.8	E937.8	E950.2	E962.0	E980.2
Dornase 963.4	E858.1	E933.4	E950.4	E962.0	E980.4
Dorsacaine 968.5	E855.2	E938.5	E950.4	E962.0	E980.4
Dothiepin hydrochloride 969.05	E854.0	E939.0	E950.3	E962.0	E980.3
Doxapram 970.0	E854.3	E940.0	E950.4	E962.0	E980.4
Doxepin 969.05	E854.0	E939.0	E950.3	E962.0	E980.3
Doxorubicin 960.7	E856	E930.7	E950.4	E962.0	E980.4
Doxycycline 960.4	E856	E930.4	E950.4	E962.0	E980.4
Doxylamine 963.0	E858.1	E933.0	E950.4	E962.0	E980.4
Dramamine 963.0	E858.1	E933.0	E950.4	E962.0	E980.4
Drano (drain cleaner) 983.2	E864.2	—	E950.7	E962.1	E980.6
Dromoran 965.09	E850.2	E935.2	E950.0	E962.0	E980.0
Dromostanolone 962.1	E858.0	E932.1	E950.4	E962.0	E980.4
Droperidol 969.2	E853.1	E939.2	E950.3	E962.0	E980.3
Drotrecogin alfa 964.2	E858.2	E934.2	E950.4	E962.0	E980.4
Drug 977.9	E858.9	E947.9	E950.5	E962.0	E980.5
specified NEC 977.8	E858.8	E947.8	E950.4	E962.0	E980.4
AHFS List					
4:00 antihistamine drugs 963.0	E858.1	E933.0	E950.4	E962.0	E980.4
8:04 amebacides 961.5	E857	E931.5	E950.4	E962.0	E980.4
arsenical anti–infectives. 961.1	E857	E931.1	E950.4	E962.0	E980.4
quinoline derivatives 961.3	E857	E931.3	E950.4	E962.0	E980.4
8:08 anthelmintics. 961.6	E857	E931.6	E950.4	E962.0	E980.4
quinoline derivatives 961.3	E857	E931.3	E950.4	E962.0	E980.4

Substance	Poisoning	Accident	Therapeutic Use	Suicide Attempt	Assault	Undetermined
			External Cause (E-Code)			
8:12.04 antifungal antibiotics	960.1	E856	E930.1	E950.4	E962.0	E980.4
8:12.06 cephalosporins	960.5	E856	E930.5	E950.4	E962.0	E980.4
8:12.08 chloramphenicol	960.2	E856	E930.2	E950.4	E962.0	E980.4
8:12.12 erythromycins	960.3	E856	E930.3	E950.4	E962.0	E980.4
8:12.16 penicillins	960.0	E856	E930.0	E950.4	E962.0	E980.4
8:12.20 streptomycins	960.6	E856	E930.6	E950.4	E962.0	E980.4
8:12.24 tetracyclines	960.4	E856	E930.4	E950.4	E962.0	E980.4
8:12.28 other antibiotics	960.8	E856	E930.8	E950.4	E962.0	E980.4
antimycobacterial	960.6	E856	E930.6	E950.4	E962.0	E980.4
macrolides	960.3	E856	E930.3	E950.4	E962.0	E980.4
8:16 antituberculars	961.8	E857	E931.8	E950.4	E962.0	E980.4
antibiotics	960.6	E856	E930.6	E950.4	E962.0	E980.4
8:18 antivirals	961.7	E857	E931.7	E950.4	E962.0	E980.4
8:20 plasmodicides (antimalarials)	961.4	E857	E931.4	E950.4	E962.0	E980.4
8:24 sulfonamides	961.0	E857	E931.0	E950.4	E962.0	E980.4
8:26 sulfones	961.8	E857	E931.8	E950.4	E962.0	E980.4
8:28 treponemicides	961.2	E857	E931.2	E950.4	E962.0	E980.4
8:32 trichomonacides	961.5	E857	E931.5	E950.4	E962.0	E980.4
quinoline derivatives	961.3	E857	E931.3	E950.4	E962.0	E980.4
nitrofuran derivatives	961.9	E857	E931.9	E950.4	E962.0	E980.4
8:36 urinary germicides	961.9	E857	E931.9	E950.4	E962.0	E980.4
quinoline derivatives	961.3	E857	E931.3	E950.4	E962.0	E980.4
8:40 other anti–infectives	961.9	E857	E931.9	E950.4	E962.0	E980.4
10:00 antineoplastic agents	963.1	E858.1	E933.1	E950.4	E962.0	E980.4
antibiotics	960.7	E856	E930.7	E950.4	E962.0	E980.4
progestogens	962.2	E858.0	E932.2	E950.4	E962.0	E980.4
12:04 parasympathomimetic (cholinergic) agents	971.0	E855.3	E941.0	E950.4	E962.0	E980.4
12:08 parasympatholytic (cholinergic –blocking) agents	971.1	E855.4	E941.1	E950.4	E962.0	E980.4
12:12 Sympathomimetic (adrenergic) agents	971.2	E855.5	E941.2	E950.4	E962.0	E980.4
12:16 sympatholytic (adrenergic– blocking) agents	971.3	E855.6	E941.3	E950.4	E962.0	E980.4
12:20 skeletal muscle relaxants central nervous system muscle-tone depressants	968.0	E855.1	E938.0	E950.4	E962.0	E980.4
myoneural blocking agents	975.2	E858.6	E945.2	E950.4	E962.0	E980.4
16:00 blood derivatives	964.7	E858.2	E934.7	E950.4	E962.0	E980.4
20:04 antianemia drugs	964.1	E858.2	E934.1	E950.4	E962.0	E980.4
20:04.04 iron preparations	964.0	E858.2	E934.0	E950.4	E962.0	E980.4
20:04.08 liver and stomach preparations	964.1	E858.2	E934.1	E950.4	E962.0	E980.4
20:12.04 anticoagulants	964.2	E858.2	E934.2	E950.4	E962.0	E980.4
20:12.08 antiheparin agents	964.5	E858.2	E934.5	E950.4	E962.0	E980.4
20:12.12 coagulants	964.5	E858.2	E934.5	E950.4	E962.0	E980.4
20:12.16 hemostatics NEC	964.5	E858.2	E934.5	E950.4	E962.0	E980.4
capillary active drugs	972.8	E858.3	E942.8	E950.4	E962.0	E980.4
24:04 cardiac drugs	972.9	E858.3	E942.9	E950.4	E962.0	E980.4
cardiotonic agents	972.1	E858.3	E942.1	E950.4	E962.0	E980.4
rhythm regulators	972.0	E858.3	E942.0	E950.4	E962.0	E980.4
24:06 antilipemic agents	972.2	E858.3	E942.2	E950.4	E962.0	E980.4
thyroid derivatives	962.7	E858.0	E932.7	E950.4	E962.0	E980.4
24:08 hypotensive agents	972.6	E858.3	E942.6	E950.4	E962.0	E980.4
adrenergic blocking agents	971.3	E855.6	E941.3	E950.4	E962.0	E980.4
ganglion blocking agents	972.3	E858.3	E942.3	E950.4	E962.0	E980.4
vasodilators	972.5	E858.3	E942.5	E950.4	E962.0	E980.4
24:12 vasodilating agents NEC	972.5	E858.3	E942.5	E950.4	E962.0	E980.4
coronary	972.4	E858.3	E942.4	E950.4	E962.0	E980.4
nicotinic acid derivatives	972.2	E858.3	E942.2	E950.4	E962.0	E980.4
24:16 sclerosing agents	972.7	E858.3	E942.7	E950.4	E962.0	E980.4

Substance	Poisoning	Accident	Therapeutic Use	Suicide Attempt	Assault	Undetermined
			External Cause (E-Code)			
28:04 general anesthetics	968.4	E855.1	E938.4	E950.4	E962.0	E980.4
gaseous anesthetics	968.2	E855.1	E938.2	E950.4	E962.0	E980.4
halothane	968.1	E855.1	E938.1	E950.4	E962.0	E980.4
intravenous anesthetics	968.3	E855.1	E938.3	E950.4	E962.0	E980.4
28:08 analgesics and antipyretics	965.9	E850.9	E935.9	E950.0	E962.0	E980.0
antirheumatics	965.69	E850.6	E935.6	E950.0	E962.0	E980.0
aromatic analgesics	965.4	E850.4	E935.4	E950.0	E962.0	E980.0
non–narcotic NEC	965.7	E850.7	E935.7	E950.0	E962.0	E980.0
opium alkaloids	965.00	E850.2	E935.2	E950.0	E962.0	E980.0
heroin	965.01	E850.0	E935.0	E950.0	E962.0	E980.0
methadone	965.02	E850.1	E935.1	E950.0	E962.0	E980.0
specified type NEC	965.09	E850.2	E935.2	E950.0	E962.0	E980.0
pyrazole derivatives	965.5	E850.5	E935.5	E950.0	E962.0	E980.0
salicylates	965.1	E850.3	E935.3	E950.0	E962.0	E980.0
specified NEC	965.8	E850.8	E935.8	E950.0	E962.0	E980.0
28:10 narcotic antagonists	970.1	E854.3	E940.1	E950.4	E962.0	E980.4
28:12 anticonvulsants	966.3	E855.0	E936.3	E950.4	E962.0	E980.4
barbiturates	967.0	E851	E937.0	E950.1	E962.0	E980.1
benzodiazepine–based tranquilizers	969.4	E853.2	E939.4	E950.3	E962.0	E980.3
bromides	967.3	E852.2	E937.3	E950.2	E962.0	E980.2
hydantoin derivatives	966.1	E855.0	E936.1	E950.4	E962.0	E980.4
oxazolidine (derivatives)	966.0	E855.0	E936.0	E950.4	E962.0	E980.4
succinimides	966.2	E855.0	E936.2	E950.4	E962.0	E980.4
28:16.04 anti-depressants	969.00	E854.0	E939.0	E950.3	E962.0	E980.3
28:16.08 tranquilizers	969.5	E853.9	E939.5	E950.3	E962.0	E980.3
benzodiazepine–based	969.4	E853.2	E939.4	E950.3	E962.0	E980.3
butyrophenone–based	969.2	E853.1	E939.2	E950.3	E962.0	E980.3
major NEC	969.3	E853.8	E939.3	E950.3	E962.0	E980.3
phenothiazine–based	969.1	E853.0	E939.1	E950.3	E962.0	E980.3
28:16.12 other psychotherapeutic agents	969.8	E855.8	E939.8	E950.3	E962.0	E980.3
28:20 respiratory and cerebral stimulants	970.9	E854.3	E940.9	E950.4	E962.0	E980.4
analeptics	970.0	E854.3	E940.0	E950.4	E962.0	E980.4
anorexigenic agents	977.0	E858.8	E947.0	E950.4	E962.0	E980.4
psychostimulants	969.70	E854.2	E939.7	E950.3	E962.0	E980.3
specified NEC	970.89	E854.3	E940.8	E950.4	E962.0	E980.4
28:24 sedatives and hypnotics	967.9	E852.9	E937.9	E950.2	E962.0	E980.2
barbiturates	967.0	E851	E937.0	E950.1	E962.0	E980.1
benzodiazepine–based tranquilizers	969.4	E853.2	E939.4	E950.3	E962.0	E980.3
chloral hydrate (group)	967.1	E852.0	E937.1	E950.2	E962.0	E980.2
glutethamide group	967.5	E852.4	E937.5	E950.2	E962.0	E980.2
intravenous anesthetics	968.3	E855.1	E938.3	E950.4	E962.0	E980.4
methaqualone (compounds)	967.4	E852.3	E937.4	E950.2	E962.0	E980.2
paraldehyde	967.2	E852.1	E937.2	E950.2	E962.0	E980.2
phenothiazine–based tranquilizers	969.1	E853.0	E939.1	E950.3	E962.0	E980.3
specified NEC	967.8	E852.8	E937.8	E950.2	E962.0	E980.2
thiobarbiturates	968.3	E855.1	E938.3	E950.4	E962.0	E980.4
tranquilizer NEC	969.5	E853.9	E939.5	E950.3	E962.0	E980.3
36:04 to 36:88 diagnostic agents	977.8	E858.8	E947.8	E950.4	E962.0	E980.4
40:00 electrolyte, caloric, and water balance agents NEC	974.5	E858.5	E944.5	E950.4	E962.0	E980.4
40:04 acidifying agents	963.2	E858.1	E933.2	E950.4	E962.0	E980.4
40:08 alkalinizing agents	963.3	E858.1	E933.3	E950.4	E962.0	E980.4
40:10 ammonia detoxicants	974.5	E858.5	E944.5	E950.4	E962.0	E980.4
40:12 replacement solutions	974.5	E858.5	E944.5	E950.4	E962.0	E980.4
plasma expanders	964.8	E858.2	E934.8	E950.4	E962.0	E980.4
40:16 sodium–removing resins	974.5	E858.5	E944.5	E950.4	E962.0	E980.4
40:18 potassium–removing resins	974.5	E858.5	E944.5	E950.4	E962.0	E980.4
40:20 caloric agents	974.5	E858.5	E944.5	E950.4	E962.0	E980.4
40:24 salt and sugar substitutes	974.5	E858.5	E944.5	E950.4	E962.0	E980.4
40:28 diuretics NEC	974.4	E858.5	E944.4	E950.4	E962.0	E980.4

Substance	Poisoning	Accident	Therapeutic Use	Suicide Attempt	Assault	Undetermined
			External Cause (E-Code)			
carbonic acid anhydrase inhibitors	974.2	E858.5	E944.2	E950.4	E962.0	E980.4
mercurials	974.0	E858.5	E944.0	E950.4	E962.0	E980.4
purine derivatives	974.1	E858.5	E944.1	E950.4	E962.0	E980.4
saluretics	974.3	E858.5	E944.3	E950.4	E962.0	E980.4
thiazides	974.3	E858.5	E944.3	E950.4	E962.1	E980.4
40:36 irrigating solutions	974.5	E858.5	E944.5	E950.4	E962.0	E980.4
40:40 uricosuric agents	974.7	E858.5	E944.7	E950.4	E962.0	E980.4
44:00 enzymes	963.4	E858.1	E933.4	E950.4	E962.0	E980.4
fibrinolysis–affecting agents	964.4	E858.2	E934.4	E950.4	E962.0	E980.4
gastric agents	973.4	E858.4	E943.4	E950.4	E962.0	E980.4
48:00 expectorants and cough preparations						
antihistamine agents	963.0	E858.1	E933.0	E950.4	E962.0	E980.4
antitussives	975.4	E858.6	E945.4	E950.4	E962.0	E980.4
codeine derivatives	965.09	E850.2	E935.2	E950.0	E962.0	E980.0
expectorants	975.5	E858.6	E945.5	E950.4	E962.0	E980.4
narcotic agents NEC	965.09	E850.2	E935.2	E950.0	E962.0	E980.0
52:04 anti–infectives (EENT)						
ENT agent	976.6	E858.7	E946.6	E950.4	E962.0	E980.4
ophthalmic preparation	976.5	E858.7	E946.5	E950.4	E962.0	E980.4
52:04.04 antibiotics (EENT)						
ENT agent	976.6	E858.7	E946.6	E950.4	E962.0	E980.4
ophthalmic preparation	976.5	E858.7	E946.5	E950.4	E962.0	E980.4
52:04.06 antivirals (EENT)						
ENT agent	976.6	E858.7	E946.6	E950.4	E962.0	E980.4
ophthalmic preparation	976.5	E858.7	E946.5	E950.4	E962.0	E980.4
52:04.08 sulfonamides (EENT)						
ENT agent	976.6	E858.7	E946.6	E950.4	E962.0	E980.4
ophthalmic preparation	976.5	E858.7	E946.5	E950.4	E962.0	E980.4
52:04.12 miscellaneous anti–infectives (EENT)						
ENT agent	976.6	E858.7	E946.6	E950.4	E962.0	E980.4
ophthalmic preparation	976.5	E858.7	E946.5	E950.4	E962.0	E980.4
52:08 anti–inflammatory agents (EENT)						
ENT agent	976.6	E858.7	E946.6	E950.4	E962.0	E980.4
ophthalmic preparation	976.5	E858.7	E946.5	E950.4	E962.0	E980.4
52:10 carbonic anhydrase inhibitors	974.2	E858.5	E944.2	E950.4	E962.0	E980.4
52:12 contact lens solutions	976.5	E858.7	E946.5	E950.4	E962.0	E980.4
52:16 local anesthetics (EENT)	968.5	E855.2	E938.5	E950.4	E962.0	E980.4
52:20 miotics	971.0	E855.3	E941.0	E950.4	E962.0	E980.4
52:24 mydriatics						
adrenergics	971.2	E855.5	E941.2	E950.4	E962.0	E980.4
anticholinergics	971.1	E855.4	E941.1	E950.4	E962.0	E980.4
antimuscarinics	971.1	E855.4	E941.1	E950.4	E962.0	E980.4
parasympatholytics	971.1	E855.4	E941.1	E950.4	E962.0	E980.4
spasmolytics	971.1	E855.4	E941.1	E950.4	E962.0	E980.4
sympathomimetics	971.2	E855.5	E941.2	E950.4	E962.0	E980.4
52:28 mouth washes and gargles	976.6	E858.7	E946.6	E950.4	E962.0	E980.4
52:32 vasoconstrictors (EENT)	971.2	E855.5	E941.2	E950.4	E962.0	E980.4
52:36 unclassified agents (EENT)						
ENT agent	976.6	E858.7	E946.6	E950.4	E962.0	E980.4
ophthalmic preparation	976.5	E858.7	E946.5	E950.4	E962.0	E980.4
56:04 antacids and adsorbents	973.0	E858.4	E943.0	E950.4	E962.0	E980.4
56:08 antidiarrhea agents	973.5	E858.4	E943.5	E950.4	E962.0	E980.4
56:10 antiflatulents	973.8	E858.4	E943.8	E950.4	E962.0	E980.4
56:12 cathartics NEC	973.3	E858.4	E943.3	E950.4	E962.0	E980.4
emollients	973.2	E858.4	E943.2	E950.4	E962.0	E980.4
irritants	973.1	E858.4	E943.1	E950.4	E962.0	E980.4
56:16 digestants	973.4	E858.4	E943.4	E950.4	E962.0	E980.4
56:20 emetics and antiemetics						
antiemetics	963.0	E858.1	E933.0	E950.4	E962.0	E980.4
emetics	973.6	E858.4	E943.6	E950.4	E962.0	E980.4

Substance	Poisoning	Accident	Therapeutic Use	Suicide Attempt	Assault	Undetermined
			External Cause (E-Code)			
56:24 lipotropic agents	977.1	E858.8	E947.1	E950.4	E962.0	E980.4
56:40 miscellaneous G.I. drugs	973.8	E858.4	E943.8	E950.4	E962.0	E980.4
60:00 gold compounds	965.69	E850.6	E935.6	E950.0	E962.0	E980.0
64:00 heavy metal antagonists	963.8	E858.1	E933.8	E950.4	E962.0	E980.4
68:04 adrenals	962.0	E858.0	E932.0	E950.4	E962.0	E980.4
68:08 androgens	962.1	E858.0	E932.1	E950.4	E962.0	E980.4
68:12 contraceptives, oral	962.2	E858.0	E932.2	E950.4	E962.0	E980.4
68:16 estrogens	962.2	E858.0	E932.2	E950.4	E962.0	E980.4
68:18 gonadotropins	962.4	E858.0	E932.4	E950.4	E962.0	E980.4
68:20 insulins and antidiabetic agents	962.3	E858.0	E932.3	E950.4	E962.0	E980.4
68:20.08 insulins	962.3	E858.0	E932.3	E950.4	E962.0	E980.4
68:24 parathyroid	962.6	E858.0	E932.6	E950.4	E962.0	E980.4
68:28 pituitary (posterior)	962.5	E858.0	E932.5	E950.4	E962.0	E980.4
anterior	962.4	E858.0	E932.4	E950.4	E962.0	E980.4
68:32 progestogens	962.2	E858.0	E932.2	E950.4	E962.0	E980.4
68:34 other corpus luteum hormones NEC	962.2	E858.0	E932.2	E950.4	E962.0	E980.4
68:36 thyroid and antithyroid antithyroid	962.8	E858.0	E932.8	E950.4	E962.0	E980.4
thyroid (derivatives)	962.7	E858.0	E932.7	E950.4	E962.0	E980.4
72:00 local anesthetics NEC	968.9	E855.2	E938.9	E950.4	E962.0	E980.4
topical (surface)	968.5	E855.2	E938.5	E950.4	E962.0	E980.4
infiltration (intradermal) (subcutaneous) (submucosal)	968.5	E855.2	E938.5	E950.4	E962.0	E980.4
nerve blocking (peripheral) (plexus) (regional)	968.6	E855.2	E938.6	E950.4	E962.0	E980.4
spinal	968.7	E855.2	E938.7	E950.4	E962.0	E980.4
76:00 oxytocics	975.0	E858.6	E945.0	E950.4	E962.0	E980.4
78:00 radioactive agents	990	—	—	—	—	—
80:04 serums NEC	979.9	E858.8	E949.9	E950.4	E962.0	E980.4
immune gamma globulin (human)	964.6	E858.2	E934.6	E950.4	E962.0	E980.4
80:08 toxoids NEC	978.8	E858.8	E948.8	E950.4	E962.0	E980.4
diphtheria	978.5	E858.8	E948.5	E950.4	E962.0	E980.4
and tetanus	978.9	E858.8	E948.9	E950.4	E962.0	E980.4
with pertussis component	978.6	E858.8	E948.6	E950.4	E962.0	E980.4
tetanus	978.4	E858.8	E948.4	E950.4	E962.0	E980.4
and diphtheria	978.9	E858.8	E948.9	E950.4	E962.0	E980.4
with pertussis component	978.6	E858.8	E948.6	E950.4	E962.0	E980.4
80:12 vaccines	979.9	E858.8	E949.9	E950.4	E962.0	E980.4
bacterial NEC	978.8	E858.8	E948.8	E950.4	E962.0	E980.4
with other bacterial components	978.9	E858.8	E948.9	E950.4	E962.0	E980.4
pertussis component	978.6	E858.8	E948.6	E950.4	E962.0	E980.4
viral and rickettsial components	979.7	E858.8	E949.7	E950.4	E962.0	E980.4
rickettsial NEC	979.6	E858.8	E949.6	E950.4	E962.0	E980.4
with bacterial component	979.7	E858.8	E949.7	E950.4	E962.0	E980.4
pertussis component	978.6	E858.8	E948.6	E950.4	E962.0	E980.4
viral component	979.7	E858.8	E949.7	E950.4	E962.0	E980.4
viral NEC	979.6	E858.8	E949.6	E950.4	E962.0	E980.4
with bacterial component	979.7	E858.8	E949.7	E950.4	E962.0	E980.4
pertussis component	978.6	E858.8	E948.6	E950.4	E962.0	E980.4
rickettsial component	979.7	E858.8	E949.7	E950.4	E962.0	E980.4
84:04.04 antibiotics (skin and mucous membrane)	976.0	E858.7	E946.0	E950.4	E962.0	E980.4
84:04.08 fungicides (skin and mucous membrane)	976.0	E858.7	E946.0	E950.4	E962.0	E980.4
84:04.12 scabicides and pediculicides (skin and mucous membrane)	976.0	E858.7	E946.0	E950.4	E962.0	E980.4

Substance	Poisoning	Accident	Therapeutic Use	Suicide Attempt	Assault	Undetermined
		External Cause (E-Code)				
84:04.16 miscellaneous local anti-infectives (skin and mucous membrane)	976.0	E858.7	E946.0	E950.4	E962.0	E980.4
84:06 anti–inflammatory agents (skin and mucous membrane)	976.0	E858.7	E946.0	E950.4	E962.0	E980.4
84:08 antipruritics and local anesthetics antipruritics	976.1	E858.7	E946.1	E950.4	E962.0	E980.4
local anesthetics	968.5	E855.2	E938.5	E950.4	E962.0	E980.4
84:12 astringents	976.2	E858.7	E946.2	E950.4	E962.0	E980.4
84:16 cell stimulants and proliferants	976.8	E858.7	E946.8	E950.4	E962.0	E980.4
84:20 detergents	976.2	E858.7	E946.2	E950.4	E962.0	E980.4
84:24 emollients, demulcents, and protectants	976.3	E858.7	E946.3	E950.4	E962.0	E980.4
84:28 keratolytic agents	976.4	E858.7	E946.4	E950.4	E962.0	E980.4
84:32 keratoplastic agents	976.4	E858.7	E946.4	E950.4	E962.0	E980.4
84:36 miscellaneous agents (skin and mucous membrane)	976.8	E858.7	E946.8	E950.4	E962.0	E980.4
86:00 spasmolytic agents	975.1	E858.6	E945.1	E950.4	E962.0	E980.4
antiasthmatics	975.7	E858.6	E945.7	E950.4	E962.0	E980.4
papaverine	972.5	E858.3	E942.5	E950.4	E962.0	E980.4
theophylline	974.1	E858.5	E944.1	E950.4	E962.0	E980.4
88:04 vitamin A	963.5	E858.1	E933.5	E950.4	E962.0	E980.4
88:08 vitamin B complex	963.5	E858.1	E933.5	E950.4	E962.0	E980.4
hematopoietic vitamin	964.1	E858.2	E934.1	E950.4	E962.0	E980.4
nicotinic acid derivatives	972.2	E858.3	E942.2	E950.4	E962.0	E980.4
88:12 vitamin C	963.5	E858.1	E933.5	E950.4	E962.0	E980.4
88:16 vitamin D	963.5	E858.1	E933.5	E950.4	E962.0	E980.4
88:20 vitamin E	963.5	E858.1	E933.5	E950.4	E962.0	E980.4
88:24 vitamin K activity	964.3	E858.2	E934.3	E950.4	E962.0	E980.4
88:28 multivitamin preparations	963.5	E858.1	E933.5	E950.4	E962.0	E980.4
92:00 unclassified therapeutic agents	977.8	E858.8	E947.8	E950.4	E962.0	E980.4
Duboisine	971.1	E855.4	E941.1	E950.4	E962.0	E980.4
Dulcolax	973.1	E858.4	E943.1	E950.4	E962.0	E980.4
Duponol (C) (EP)	976.2	E858.7	E946.2	E950.4	E962.0	E980.4
Durabolin	962.1	E858.0	E932.1	E950.4	E962.0	E980.4
Dyclone	968.5	E855.2	E938.5	E950.4	E962.0	E980.4
Dyclonine	968.5	E855.2	E938.5	E950.4	E962.0	E980.4
Dydrogesterone	962.2	E858.0	E932.2	E950.4	E962.0	E980.4
Dyes NEC	989.89	E866.8	—	E950.9	E962.1	E980.9
diagnostic agents	977.8	E858.8	E947.8	E950.4	E962.0	E980.4
pharmaceutical NEC	977.4	E858.8	E947.4	E950.4	E962.0	E980.4
Dyfols	971.0	E855.3	E941.0	E950.4	E962.0	E980.4
Dymelor	962.3	E858.0	E932.3	E950.4	E962.0	E980.4
Dynamite	989.89	E866.8	—	E950.9	E962.1	E980.9
fumes	987.8	E869.8	—	E952.8	E962.2	E982.8
Dyphylline	975.1	E858.6	E945.1	E950.4	E962.0	E980.4
Ear preparations	976.6	E858.7	E946.6	E950.4	E962.0	E980.4
Echothiopate, ecothiopate	971.0	E855.3	E941.0	E950.4	E962.0	E980.4
Ecstasy	969.72	E854.2	E939.7	E950.3	E962.0	E980.3
Ectylurea	967.8	E852.8	E937.8	E950.2	E962.0	E980.2
Edathamil disodium	963.8	E858.1	E933.8	E950.4	E962.0	E980.4
Edecrin	974.4	E858.5	E944.4	E950.4	E962.0	E980.4
Edetate, disodium (calcium)	963.8	E858.1	E933.8	E950.4	E962.0	E980.4
Edrophonium	971.0	E855.3	E941.0	E950.4	E962.0	E980.4
Elase	976.8	E858.7	E946.8	E950.4	E962.0	E980.4
Elaterium	973.1	E858.4	E943.1	E950.4	E962.0	E980.4
Elder	988.2	E865.4	—	E950.9	E962.1	E980.9
berry (unripe)	988.2	E865.3	—	E950.9	E962.1	E980.9
Electrolytes NEC	974.5	E858.5	E944.5	E950.4	E962.0	E980.4
Electrolytic agent NEC	974.5	E858.5	E944.5	E950.4	E962.0	E980.4

Substance	Poisoning	Accident	Therapeutic Use	Suicide Attempt	Assault	Undetermined
			External Cause (E-Code)			
Embramine 963.0	E858.1	E933.0	E950.4	E962.0	E980.4
Emetics. 973.6	E858.4	E943.6	E950.4	E962.0	E980.4
Emetine (hydrochloride) 961.5	E857	E931.5	E950.4	E962.0	E980.4
Emollients. 976.3	E858.7	E946.3	E950.4	E962.0	E980.4
Emylcamate 969.5	E853.8	E939.5	E950.3	E962.0	E980.3
Encyprate 969.09	E854.0	E939.0	E950.3	E962.0	E980.3
Endocaine. 968.5	E855.2	E938.5	E950.4	E962.0	E980.4
Endrin 989.2	E863.0	—	E950.6	E962.1	E980.7
Enflurane 968.2	E855.1	E938.2	E950.4	E962.0	E980.4
Enovid 962.2	E858.0	E932.2	E950.4	E962.0	E980.4
ENT preparations (anti–infectives). 976.6	E858.7	E946.6	E950.4	E962.0	E980.4
Enzodase 963.4	E858.1	E933.4	E950.4	E962.0	E980.4
Enzymes NEC. 963.4	E858.1	E933.4	E950.4	E962.0	E980.4
Epanutin 966.1	E855.0	E936.1	E950.4	E962.0	E980.4
Ephedra (tincture) 971.2	E855.5	E941.2	E950.4	E962.0	E980.4
Ephedrine 971.2	E855.5	E941.2	E950.4	E962.0	E980.4
Epiestriol 962.2	E858.0	E932.2	E950.4	E962.0	E980.4
Epilim — *see* Sodium valproate					
Epinephrine 971.2	E855.5	E941.2	E950.4	E962.0	E980.4
Epsom salt 973.3	E858.4	E943.3	E950.4	E962.0	E980.4
Equanil 969.5	E853.8	E939.5	E950.3	E962.0	E980.3
Equisetum (diuretic) 974.4	E858.5	E944.4	E950.4	E962.0	E980.4
Ergometrine 975.0	E858.6	E945.0	E950.4	E962.0	E980.4
Ergonovine 975.0	E858.6	E945.0	E950.4	E962.0	E980.4
Ergot NEC 988.2	E865.4	—	E950.9	E962.1	E980.9
medicinal (alkaloids). 975.0	E858.6	E945.0	E950.4	E962.0	E980.4
Ergotamine (tartrate) (for migraine) NEC . . . 972.9	E858.3	E942.9	E950.4	E962.0	E980.4
Ergotrate 975.0	E858.6	E945.0	E950.4	E962.0	E980.4
Erythrityl tetranitrate 972.4	E858.3	E942.4	E950.4	E962.0	E980.4
Erythrol tetranitrate 972.4	E858.3	E942.4	E950.4	E962.0	E980.4
Erythromycin 960.3	E856	E930.3	E950.4	E962.0	E980.4
ophthalmic preparation. 976.5	E858.7	E946.5	E950.4	E962.0	E980.4
topical NEC 976.0	E858.7	E946.0	E950.4	E962.0	E980.4
Eserine 971.0	E855.3	E941.0	E950.4	E962.0	E980.4
Eskabarb 967.0	E851	E937.0	E950.1	E962.0	E980.1
Eskalith. 969.8	E855.8	E939.8	E950.3	E962.0	E980.3
Estradiol (cypionate) (dipropionate)					
(valerate). 962.2	E858.0	E932.2	E950.4	E962.0	E980.4
Estriol 962.2	E858.0	E932.2	E950.4	E962.0	E980.4
Estrogens (with progestogens) 962.2	E858.0	E932.2	E950.4	E962.0	E980.4
Estrone 962.2	E858.0	E932.2	E950.4	E962.0	E980.4
Etafedrine 971.2	E855.5	E941.2	E950.4	E962.0	E980.4
Ethacrynate sodium 974.4	E858.5	E944.4	E950.4	E962.0	E980.4
Ethacrynic acid. 974.4	E858.5	E944.4	E950.4	E962.0	E980.4
Ethambutol 961.8	E857	E931.8	E950.4	E962.0	E980.4
Ethamide 974.2	E858.5	E944.2	E950.4	E962.0	E980.4
Ethamivan. 970.0	E854.3	E940.0	E950.4	E962.0	E980.4
Ethamsylate 964.5	E858.2	E934.5	E950.4	E962.0	E980.4
Ethanol 980.0	E860.1	—	E950.9	E962.1	E980.9
beverage. 980.0	E860.0	—	E950.9	E962.1	E980.9
Etchlorvynol 967.8	E852.8	E937.8	E950.2	E962.0	E980.2
Ethebenecid 974.7	E858.5	E944.7	E950.4	E962.0	E980.4
Ether(s) (diethyl) (ethyl) (vapor). 987.8	E869.8	—	E952.8	E962.2	E982.8
anesthetic 968.2	E855.1	E938.2	E950.4	E962.0	E980.4
petroleum — *see* Ligroin					
solvent 982.8	E862.4	—	E950.9	E962.1	E980.9
Ethidine chloride (vapor). 987.8	E869.8	—	E952.8	E962.2	E982.8
liquid (solvent) 982.3	E862.4	—	E950.9	E962.1	E980.9
Ethinamate 967.8	E852.8	E937.8	E950.2	E962.0	E980.2
Ethinylestradiol. 962.2	E858.0	E932.2	E950.4	E962.0	E980.4
Ethionamide 961.8	E857	E931.8	E950.4	E962.0	E980.4

Substance	Poisoning	Accident	Therapeutic Use	Suicide Attempt	Assault	Undetermined
			External Cause (E-Code)			
Ethisterone	962.2	E858.0	E932.2	E950.4	E962.0	E980.4
Ethobral	967.0	E851	E937.0	E950.1	E962.0	E980.1
Ethocaine (infiltration) (topical)	968.5	E855.2	E938.5	E950.4	E962.0	E980.4
nerve block (peripheral) (plexus)	968.6	E855.2	E938.6	E950.4	E962.0	E980.4
spinal	968.7	E855.2	E938.7	E950.4	E962.0	E980.4
Ethoheptazine (citrate)	965.7	E850.7	E935.7	E950.0	E962.0	E980.0
Ethopropazine	966.4	E855.0	E936.4	E950.4	E962.0	E980.4
Ethosuximide	966.2	E855.0	E936.2	E950.4	E962.0	E980.4
Ethotoin	966.1	E855.0	E936.1	E950.4	E962.0	E980.4
Ethoxazene	961.9	E857	E931.9	E950.4	E962.0	E980.4
Ethoxzolamide	974.2	E858.5	E944.2	E950.4	E962.0	E980.4
Ethyl						
acetate (vapor)	982.8	E862.4	—	E950.9	E962.1	E980.9
alcohol	980.0	E860.1	—	E950.9	E962.1	E980.9
beverage	980.0	E860.0	—	E950.9	E962.1	E980.9
aldehyde (vapor)	987.8	E869.8	—	E952.8	E962.2	E982.8
liquid	989.89	E866.8	—	E950.9	E962.1	E980.9
aminobenzoate	968.5	E855.2	E938.5	E950.4	E962.0	E980.4
biscoumacetate	964.2	E858.2	E934.2	E950.4	E962.0	E980.4
bromide (anesthetic)	968.2	E855.1	E938.2	E950.4	E962.0	E980.4
carbamate (antineoplastic)	963.1	E858.1	E933.1	E950.4	E962.0	E980.4
carbinol	980.3	E860.4	—	E950.9	E962.1	E980.9
chaulmoograte	961.8	E857	E931.8	E950.4	E962.0	E980.4
chloride (vapor)	987.8	E869.8	—	E952.8	E962.2	E982.8
anesthetic (local)	968.5	E855.2	E938.5	E950.4	E962.0	E980.4
inhaled	968.2	E855.1	E938.2	E950.4	E962.0	E980.4
solvent	982.3	E862.4	—	E950.9	E962.1	E980.9
estranol	962.1	E858.0	E932.1	E950.4	E962.0	E980.4
ether — see Ether(s)						
formate (solvent) NEC	982.8	E862.4	—	E950.9	E962.1	E980.9
iodoacetate	987.5	E869.3	—	E952.8	E962.2	E982.8
lactate (solvent) NEC	982.8	E862.4	—	E950.9	E962.1	E980.9
methylcarbinol	980.8	E860.8	—	E950.9	E962.1	E980.9
morphine	965.09	E850.2	E935.2	E950.0	E962.0	E980.0
Ethylene (gas)	987.1	E869.8	—	E952.8	E962.2	E982.8
anesthetic (general)	968.2	E855.1	E938.2	E950.4	E962.0	E980.4
chlorohydrin (vapor)	982.3	E862.4	—	E950.9	E962.1	E980.9
dichloride (vapor)	982.3	E862.4	—	E950.9	E962.1	E980.9
glycol(s) (any) (vapor)	982.8	E862.4	—	E950.9	E962.1	E980.9
Ethylidene						
chloride NEC	982.3	E862.4	—	E950.9	E962.1	E980.9
diethyl ether	982.8	E862.4	—	E950.9	E962.1	E980.9
Ethynodiol	962.2	E858.0	E932.2	E950.4	E962.0	E980.4
Etidocaine	968.9	E855.2	E938.9	E950.4	E962.0	E980.4
infiltration (subcutaneous)	968.5	E855.2	E938.5	E950.4	E962.0	E980.4
nerve (peripheral) (plexus)	968.6	E855.2	E938.6	E950.4	E962.0	E980.4
Etilfen	967.0	E851	E937.0	E950.1	E962.0	E980.1
Etomide	965.7	E850.7	E935.7	E950.0	E962.0	E980.0
Etorphine	965.09	E850.2	E935.2	E950.0	E962.0	E980.0
Etoval	967.0	E851	E937.0	E950.1	E962.0	E980.1
Etryptamine	969.01	E854.0	E939.0	E950.3	E962.0	E980.3
Eucaine	968.5	E855.2	E938.5	E950.4	E962.0	E980.4
Eucalyptus (oil) NEC	975.5	E858.6	E945.5	E950.4	E962.0	E980.4
Eucatropine	971.1	E855.4	E941.1	E950.4	E962.0	E980.4
Eucodal	965.09	E850.2	E935.2	E950.0	E962.0	E980.0
Euneryl	967.0	E851	E937.0	E950.1	E962.0	E980.1
Euphthalmine	971.1	E855.4	E941.1	E950.4	E962.0	E980.4
Eurax	976.0	E858.7	E946.0	E950.4	E962.0	E980.4
Euresol	976.4	E858.7	E946.4	E950.4	E962.0	E980.4
Euthroid	962.7	E858.0	E932.7	E950.4	E962.0	E980.4

Substance	Poisoning	Accident	Therapeutic Use	Suicide Attempt	Assault	Undetermined
			External Cause (E-Code)			
Evans blue	977.8	E858.8	E947.8	E950.4	E962.0	E980.4
Evipal	967.0	E851	E937.0	E950.1	E962.0	E980.1
sodium	968.3	E855.1	E938.3	E950.4	E962.0	E980.4
Evipan	967.0	E851	E937.0	E950.1	E962.0	E980.1
sodium	968.3	E855.1	E938.3	E950.4	E962.0	E980.4
Exalgin	965.4	E850.4	E935.4	E950.0	E962.0	E980.0
Excipients, pharmaceutical	977.4	E858.8	E947.4	E950.4	E962.0	E980.4
Exhaust gas — *see* Carbon, monoxide						
Ex–Lax (phenolphthalein)	973.1	E858.4	E943.1	E950.4	E962.0	E980.4
Expectorants	975.5	E858.6	E945.5	E950.4	E962.0	E980.4
External medications (skin) (mucous membrane)	976.9	E858.7	E946.9	E950.4	E962.0	E980.4
dental agent	976.7	E858.7	E946.7	E950.4	E962.0	E980.4
ENT agent	976.6	E858.7	E946.6	E950.4	E962.0	E980.4
ophthalmic preparation	976.5	E858.7	E946.5	E950.4	E962.0	E980.4
specified NEC	976.8	E858.7	E946.8	E950.4	E962.0	E980.4
Eye agents (anti–infective)	976.5	E858.7	E946.5	E950.4	E962.0	E980.4
Factor IX complex (human)	964.5	E858.2	E934.5	E950.4	E962.0	E980.4
Fecal softeners	973.2	E858.4	E943.2	E950.4	E962.0	E980.4
Fenbutrazate	977.0	E858.8	E947.0	E950.4	E962.0	E980.4
Fencamfamin	970.89	E854.3	E940.8	E950.4	E962.0	E980.4
Fenfluramine	977.0	E858.8	E947.0	E950.4	E962.0	E980.4
Fenoprofen	965.61	E850.6	E935.6	E950.0	E962.0	E980.0
Fentanyl	965.09	E850.2	E935.2	E950.0	E962.0	E980.0
Fentazin	969.1	E853.0	E939.1	E950.3	E962.0	E980.3
Fenticlor, fentichlor	976.0	E858.7	E946.0	E950.4	E962.0	E980.4
Fer de lance (bite) (venom)	989.5	E905.0	—	E950.9	E962.1	E980.9
Ferric — *see* Iron						
Ferrocholinate	964.0	E858.2	E934.0	E950.4	E962.0	E980.4
Ferrous fumerate, gluconate, lactate, salt NEC, sulfate (medicinal)	964.0	E858.2	E934.0	E950.4	E962.0	E980.4
Ferrum — *see* Iron						
Fertilizers NEC	989.89	E866.5	—	E950.9	E962.1	E980.4
with herbicide mixture	989.4	E863.5	—	E950.6	E962.1	E980.7
Fibrinogen (human)	964.7	E858.2	E934.7	E950.4	E962.0	E980.4
Fibrinolysin	964.4	E858.2	E934.4	E950.4	E962.0	E980.4
Fibrinolysis–affecting agents	964.4	E858.2	E934.4	E950.4	E962.0	E980.4
Filix mas	961.6	E857	E931.6	E950.4	E962.0	E980.4
Fiorinal	965.1	E850.3	E935.3	E950.0	E962.0	E980.0
Fire damp	987.1	E869.8	—	E952.8	E962.2	E982.8
Fish, nonbacterial or noxious	988.0	E865.2	—	E950.9	E962.1	E980.9
shell	988.0	E865.1	—	E950.9	E962.1	E980.9
Flagyl	961.5	E857	E931.5	E950.4	E962.0	E980.4
Flavoxate	975.1	E858.6	E945.1	E950.4	E962.0	E980.4
Flaxedil	975.2	E858.6	E945.2	E950.4	E962.0	E980.4
Flaxseed (medicinal)	976.3	E858.7	E946.3	E950.4	E962.0	E980.4
Flomax	971.3	E855.6	E941.3	E950.4	E962.0	E980.4
Florantyrone	973.4	E858.4	E943.4	E950.4	E962.0	E980.4
Floraquin	961.3	E857	E931.3	E950.4	E962.0	E980.4
Florinef	962.0	E858.0	E932.0	E950.4	E962.0	E980.4
ENT agent	976.6	E858.7	E946.6	E950.4	E962.0	E980.4
ophthalmic preparation	976.5	E858.7	E946.5	E950.4	E962.0	E980.4
topical NEC	976.0	E858.7	E946.0	E950.4	E962.0	E980.4
Flowers of sulfur	976.4	E858.7	E946.4	E950.4	E962.0	E980.4
Floxuridine	963.1	E858.1	E933.1	E950.4	E962.0	E980.4
Flucytosine	961.9	E857	E931.9	E950.4	E962.0	E980.4
Fludrocortisone	962.0	E858.0	E932.0	E950.4	E962.0	E980.4
ENT agent	976.6	E858.7	E946.6	E950.4	E962.0	E980.4
ophthalmic preparation	976.5	E858.7	E946.5	E950.4	E962.0	E980.4
topical NEC	976.0	E858.7	E946.0	E950.4	E962.0	E980.4
Flumethasone	976.0	E858.7	E946.0	E950.4	E962.0	E980.4

Substance	Poisoning	Accident	Therapeutic Use	Suicide Attempt	Assault	Undetermined
			External Cause (E-Code)			
Flumethiazide	974.3	E858.5	E944.3	E950.4	E962.0	E980.4
Flumidin	961.7	E857	E931.7	E950.4	E962.0	E980.4
Flunitrazepam	969.4	E853.2	E939.4	E950.3	E962.0	E980.3
Fluocinolone	976.0	E858.7	E946.0	E950.4	E962.0	E980.4
Fluocortolone	962.0	E858.0	E932.0	E950.4	E962.0	E980.4
Fluohydrocortisone	962.0	E858.0	E932.0	E950.4	E962.0	E980.4
ENT agent	976.6	E858.7	E946.6	E950.4	E962.0	E980.4
ophthalmic preparation	976.5	E858.7	E946.5	E950.4	E962.0	E980.4
topical NEC	976.0	E858.7	E946.0	E950.4	E962.0	E980.4
Fluonid	976.0	E858.7	E946.0	E950.4	E962.0	E980.4
Fluopromazine	969.1	E853.0	E939.1	E950.3	E962.0	E980.3
Fluoracetate	989.4	E863.7	—	E950.6	E962.1	E980.7
Fluorescein (sodium)	977.8	E858.8	E947.8	E950.4	E962.0	E980.4
Fluoride(s) (pesticides) (sodium) NEC	989.4	E863.4	—	E950.6	E962.1	E980.7
hydrogen — see Hydrofluoric acid						
medicinal	976.7	E858.7	E946.7	E950.4	E962.0	E980.4
not pesticide NEC	983.9	E864.4	—	E950.7	E962.1	E980.6
stannous	976.7	E858.7	E946.7	E950.4	E962.0	E980.4
Fluorinated corticosteroids	962.0	E858.0	E932.0	E950.4	E962.0	E980.4
Fluorine (compounds) (gas)	987.8	E869.8	—	E952.8	E962.2	E982.8
salt — see Fluoride(s)						
Fluoristan	976.7	E858.7	E946.7	E950.4	E962.0	E980.4
Fluoroacetate	989.4	E863.7	—	E950.6	E962.1	E980.7
Fluorodeoxyuridine	963.1	E858.1	E933.1	E950.4	E962.0	E980.4
Fluorometholone (topical) NEC	976.0	E858.7	E946.0	E950.4	E962.0	E980.4
ophthalmic preparation	976.5	E858.7	E946.5	E950.4	E962.0	E980.4
Fluorouracil	963.1	E858.1	E933.1	E950.4	E962.0	E980.4
Fluothane	968.1	E855.1	E938.1	E950.4	E962.0	E980.4
Fluoxetine hydrochloride	969.03	E854.0	E939.0	E950.3	E962.0	E980.3
Fluoxymesterone	962.1	E858.0	E932.1	E950.4	E962.0	E980.4
Fluphenazine	969.1	E853.0	E939.1	E950.3	E962.0	E980.3
Fluprednisolone	962.0	E858.0	E932.0	E950.4	E962.0	E980.4
Flurandrenolide	976.0	E858.7	E946.0	E950.4	E962.0	E980.4
Flurazepam (hydrochloride)	969.4	E853.2	E939.4	E950.3	E962.0	E980.3
Flurbiprofen	965.61	E850.6	E935.6	E950.0	E962.0	E980.0
Flurobate	976.0	E858.7	E946.0	E950.4	E962.0	E980.4
Flurothyl	969.8	E855.8	E939.8	E950.3	E962.0	E980.3
Fluroxene	968.2	E855.1	E938.2	E950.4	E962.0	E980.4
Folacin	964.1	E858.2	E934.1	E950.4	E962.0	E980.4
Folic acid	964.1	E858.2	E934.1	E950.4	E962.0	E980.4
Follicle stimulating hormone	962.4	E858.0	E932.4	E950.4	E962.0	E980.4
Food, foodstuffs, nonbacterial or noxious	988.9	E865.9	—	E950.9	E962.1	E980.9
berries, seeds	988.2	E865.3	—	E950.9	E962.1	E980.9
fish	988.0	E865.2	—	E950.9	E962.1	E980.9
mushrooms	988.1	E865.5	—	E950.9	E962.1	E980.9
plants	988.2	E865.9	—	E950.9	E962.1	E980.9
specified type NEC	988.2	E865.4	—	E950.9	E962.1	E980.9
shellfish	988.0	E865.1	—	E950.9	E962.1	E980.9
specified NEC	988.8	E865.8	—	E950.9	E962.1	E980.9
Fool's parsley	988.2	E865.4	—	E950.9	E962.1	E980.9
Formaldehyde (solution)	989.89	E861.4	—	E950.9	E962.1	E980.9
fungicide	989.4	E863.6	—	E950.6	E962.1	E980.7
gas or vapor	987.8	E869.8	—	E952.8	E962.2	E982.8
Formalin	989.89	E861.4	—	E950.9	E962.1	E980.9
fungicide	989.4	E863.6	—	E950.6	E962.1	E980.7
vapor	987.8	E869.8	—	E952.8	E962.2	E982.8
Formic acid	983.1	E864.1	—	E950.7	E962.1	E980.6
vapor	987.8	E869.8	—	E952.8	E962.2	E982.8
Fowler's solution	985.1	E866.3	—	E950.8	E962.1	E980.8
Foxglove	988.2	E865.4	—	E950.9	E962.1	E980.9

Substance	Poisoning	Accident	Therapeutic Use	Suicide Attempt	Assault	Undetermined
			External Cause (E-Code)			
Fox green	977.8	E858.8	E947.8	E950.4	E962.0	E980.4
Framycetin	960.8	E856	E930.8	E950.4	E962.0	E980.4
Frangula (extract)	973.1	E858.4	E943.1	E950.4	E962.0	E980.4
Frei antigen	977.8	E858.8	E947.8	E950.4	E962.0	E980.4
Freons	987.4	E869.2	—	E952.8	E962.2	E982.8
Fructose	974.5	E858.5	E944.5	E950.4	E962.0	E980.4
Frusemide	974.4	E858.5	E944.4	E950.4	E962.0	E980.4
FSH	962.4	E858.0	E932.4	E950.4	E962.0	E980.4
Fuel						
automobile	981	E862.1	—	E950.9	E962.1	E980.9
exhaust gas, not in transit	986	E868.2	—	E952.0	E962.2	E982.0
vapor NEC	987.1	E869.8	—	E952.8	E962.2	E982.8
gas (domestic use) — see also Carbon, monoxide, fuel						
utility	987.1	E868.1	—	E951.8	E962.2	E981.8
incomplete combustion of — see Carbon, monoxide, fuel, utility						
in mobile container	987.0	E868.0	—	E951.1	E962.2	E981.1
piped (natural)	987.1	E867	—	E951.0	E962.2	E981.0
industrial, incomplete combustion	986	E868.3	—	E952.1	E962.2	E982.1
Fugillin	960.8	E856	E930.8	E950.4	E962.0	E980.4
Fulminate of mercury	985.0	E866.1	—	E950.9	E962.1	E980.9
Fulvicin	960.1	E856	E930.1	E950.4	E962.0	E980.4
Fumadil	960.8	E856	E930.8	E950.4	E962.0	E980.4
Fumagillin	960.8	E856	E930.8	E950.4	E962.0	E980.4
Fumes (from)	987.9	E869.9	—	E952.9	E962.2	E982.9
carbon monoxide — see Carbon, monoxide						
charcoal (domestic use)	986	E868.3	—	E952.1	E962.2	E982.1
chloroform — see Chloroform						
coke (in domestic stoves, fireplaces)	986	E868.3	—	E952.1	E962.2	E982.1
corrosive NEC	987.8	E869.8	—	E952.8	E962.2	E982.8
ether — see Ether(s)						
freons	987.4	E869.2	—	E952.8	E962.2	E982.8
hydrocarbons	987.1	E869.8	—	E952.8	E962.2	E982.8
petroleum (liquefied)	987.0	E868.0	—	E951.1	E962.2	E981.1
distributed through pipes (pure or mixed with air)	987.0	E867	—	E951.0	E962.2	E981.0
lead — see Lead						
metals — see specified metal						
nitrogen dioxide	987.2	E869.0	—	E952.8	E962.2	E982.8
pesticides — see Pesticides						
petroleum (liquefied)	987.0	E868.0	—	E951.1	E962.2	E981.1
distributed through pipes (pure or mixed with air)	987.0	E867	—	E951.0	E962.2	E981.0
polyester	987.8	E869.8	—	E952.8	E962.2	E982.8
specified source, other (see also substance specified)	987.8	E869.8	—	E952.8	E962.2	E982.8
sulfur dioxide	987.3	E869.1	—	E952.8	E962.2	E982.8
Fumigants	989.4	E863.8	—	E950.6	E962.1	E980.7
Fungi, noxious, used as food	988.1	E865.5	—	E950.9	E962.1	E980.9
Fungicides (see also Antifungals)	989.4	E863.6	—	E950.6	E962.1	E980.7
Fungizone	960.1	E856	E930.1	E950.4	E962.0	E980.4
topical	976.0	E858.7	E946.0	E950.4	E962.0	E980.4
Furacin	976.0	E858.7	E946.0	E950.4	E962.0	E980.4
Furadantin	961.9	E857	E931.9	E950.4	E962.0	E980.4
Furazolidone	961.9	E857	E931.9	E950.4	E962.0	E980.4
Furnace (coal burning) (domestic), gas from	986	E868.3	—	E952.1	E962.2	E982.1
industrial	986	E868.8	—	E952.1	E962.2	E982.1
Furniture polish	989.89	E861.2	—	E950.9	E962.1	E980.9
Furosemide	974.4	E858.5	E944.4	E950.4	E962.0	E980.4

Substance	Poisoning	Accident	Therapeutic Use	Suicide Attempt	Assault	Undetermined
		External Cause (E-Code)				
Furoxone 961.9	E857	E931.9	E950.4	E962.0	E980.4
Fusel oil (amyl) (butyl) (propyl). 980.3	E860.4	—	E950.9	E962.1	E980.9
Fusidic acid 960.8	E856	E930.8	E950.4	E962.0	E980.4
Gallamine 975.2	E858.6	E945.2	E950.4	E962.0	E980.4
Gallotannic acid 976.2	E858.7	E946.2	E950.4	E962.0	E980.4
Gamboge 973.1	E858.4	E943.1	E950.4	E962.0	E980.4
Gamimune 964.6	E858.2	E934.6	E950.4	E962.0	E980.4
Gamma–benzene hexachloride (vapor) . . . 989.2	E863.0	—	E950.6	E962.1	E980.7
Gamma globulin 964.6	E858.2	E934.6	E950.4	E962.0	E980.4
Gamma Hydroxy Butyrate (GHB) 968.4	E855.1	E938.4	E950.4	E962.0	E980.4
Gamulin 964.6	E858.2	E934.6	E950.4	E962.0	E980.4
Ganglionic blocking agents. 972.3	E858.3	E942.3	E950.4	E962.0	E980.4
Ganja. 969.6	E854.1	E939.6	E950.3	E962.0	E980.3
Garamycin 960.8	E856	E930.8	E950.4	E962.0	E980.4
ophthalmic preparation 976.5	E858.7	E946.5	E950.4	E962.0	E980.4
topical NEC 976.0	E858.7	E946.0	E950.4	E962.0	E980.4
Gardenal 967.0	E851	E937.0	E950.1	E962.0	E980.1
Gardepanyl 967.0	E851	E937.0	E950.1	E962.0	E980.1
Gas 987.9	E869.9	—	E952.9	E962.2	E982.9
acetylene 987.1	E868.1	—	E951.8	E962.2	E981.8
incomplete combustion of — *see*					
Carbon, monoxide, fuel, utility					
air contaminants, source or type not					
specified 987.9	E869.9	—	E952.9	E962.2	E982.9
anesthetic (general) NEC 968.2	E855.1	E938.2	E950.4	E962.0	E980.4
blast furnace 986	E868.8	—	E952.1	E962.2	E982.1
butane — *see* Butane					
carbon monoxide — *see* Carbon, monoxide					
chlorine 987.6	E869.8	—	E952.8	E962.2	E982.8
coal — *see* Carbon, monoxide, coal					
cyanide 987.7	E869.8	—	E952.8	E962.2	E982.8
dicyanogen. 987.8	E869.8	—	E952.8	E962.2	E982.8
domestic — *see* Gas, utility					
exhaust — *see* Carbon, monoxide, exhaust gas					
from wood– or coal–burning stove or					
fireplace 986	E868.3	—	E952.1	E962.2	E982.1
fuel (domestic use) — *see also* Carbon,					
monoxide, fuel					
industrial use 986	E868.8	—	E952.1	E962.2	E982.1
utility 987.1	E868.1	—	E951.8	E962.2	E981.8
incomplete combustion of — *see*					
Carbon, monoxide, fuel, utility					
in mobile container 987.0	E868.0	—	E951.1	E962.2	E981.1
piped (natural) 987.1	E867	—	E951.0	E962.2	E981.0
garage 986	E868.2	—	E952.0	E962.2	E982.0
hydrocarbon NEC 987.1	E869.8	—	E952.8	E962.2	E982.8
incomplete combustion of — *see*					
Carbon, monoxide, fuel, utility					
liquefied (mobile container) 987.0	E868.0	—	E951.1	E962.2	E981.1
piped 987.0	E867	—	E951.0	E962.2	E981.0
hydrocyanic acid 987.7	E869.8	—	E952.8	E962.2	E982.8
illuminating — *see* Gas, utility					
incomplete combustion, any — *see* Carbon,					
monoxide					
kiln 986	E868.8	—	E952.1	E962.2	E982.1
lacrimogenic 987.5	E869.3	—	E952.8	E962.2	E982.8
marsh. 987.1	E869.8	—	E952.8	E962.2	E982.8
motor exhaust, not in transit 986	E868.8	—	E952.1	E962.2	E982.1
mustard — *see* Mustard, gas					
natural 987.1	E867	—	E951.0	E962.2	E981.0

Substance	Poisoning	Accident	Therapeutic Use	Suicide Attempt	Assault	Undetermined
		External Cause (E-Code)				
nerve (war)	987.9	E869.9	—	E952.9	E962.2	E982.9
oils	981	E862.1	—	E950.9	E962.1	E980.9
petroleum (liquefied) (distributed in mobile containers)	987.0	E868.0	—	E951.1	E962.2	E981.1
piped (pure or mixed with air)	987.0	E867	—	E951.1	E962.2	E981.1
piped (manufactured) (natural) NEC	987.1	E867	—	E951.0	E962.2	E981.0
producer	986	E868.8	—	E952.1	E962.2	E982.1
propane — *see* Propane						
refrigerant (freon)	987.4	E869.2	—	E952.8	E962.2	E982.8
not freon	987.9	E869.9	—	E952.9	E962.2	E982.9
sewer	987.8	E869.8	—	E952.8	E962.2	E982.8
specified source NEC (*see also* substance specified)	987.8	E869.8	—	E952.8	E962.2	E982.8
stove — *see* Gas, utility						
tear	987.5	E869.3	—	E952.8	E962.2	E982.8
utility (for cooking, heating, or lighting) (piped) NEC	987.1	E868.1	—	E951.8	E962.2	E981.8
incomplete combustion of — *see* Carbon, monoxide, fuel, utility						
in mobile container	987.0	E868.0	—	E951.1	E962.2	E981.1
piped (natural)	987.1	E867	—	E951.0	E962.2	E981.0
water	987.1	E868.1	—	E951.8	E962.2	E981.8
incomplete combustion of — *see* Carbon, monoxide, fuel, utility						
Gaseous substance — *see* Gas						
Gasoline, gasolene	981	E862.1	—	E950.9	E962.1	E980.9
vapor	987.1	E869.8	—	E952.8	E962.2	E982.8
Gastric enzymes	973.4	E858.4	E943.4	E950.4	E962.0	E980.4
Gastrografin	977.8	E858.8	E947.8	E950.4	E962.0	E980.4
Gastrointestinal agents	973.9	E858.4	E943.9	E950.4	E962.0	E980.4
specified NEC	973.8	E858.4	E943.8	E950.4	E962.0	E980.4
Gaultheria procumbens	988.2	E865.4	—	E950.9	E962.1	E980.9
Gelatin (intravenous)	964.8	E858.2	E934.8	E950.4	E962.0	E980.4
absorbable (sponge)	964.5	E858.2	E934.5	E950.4	E962.0	E980.4
Gelfilm	976.8	E858.7	E946.8	E950.4	E962.0	E980.4
Gelfoam	964.5	E858.2	E934.5	E950.4	E962.0	E980.4
Gelsemine	970.89	E854.3	E940.8	E950.4	E962.0	E980.4
Gelsemium (sempervirens)	988.2	E865.4	—	E950.9	E962.1	E980.9
Gemonil	967.0	E851	E937.0	E950.1	E962.0	E980.1
Gentamicin	960.8	E856	E930.8	E950.4	E962.0	E980.4
ophthalmic preparation	976.5	E858.7	E946.5	E950.4	E962.0	E980.4
topical NEC	976.0	E858.7	E946.0	E950.4	E962.0	E980.4
Gentian violet	976.0	E858.7	E946.0	E950.4	E962.0	E980.4
Gexane	976.0	E858.7	E946.0	E950.4	E962.0	E980.4
Gila monster (venom)	989.5	E905.0	—	E950.9	E962.1	E980.9
Ginger, Jamaica	989.89	E866.8	—	E950.9	E962.1	E980.9
Gitalin	972.1	E858.3	E942.1	E950.4	E962.0	E980.4
Gitoxin	972.1	E858.3	E942.1	E950.4	E962.0	E980.4
Glandular extract (medicinal) NEC	977.9	E858.9	E947.9	E950.5	E962.0	E980.5
Glaucarubin	961.5	E857	E931.5	E950.4	E962.0	E980.4
Globin zinc insulin	962.3	E858.0	E932.3	E950.4	E962.0	E980.4
Glucagon	962.3	E858.0	E932.3	E950.4	E962.0	E980.4
Glucochloral	967.1	E852.0	E937.1	E950.2	E962.0	E980.2
Glucocorticoids	962.0	E858.0	E932.0	E950.4	E962.0	E980.4
Glucose	974.5	E858.5	E944.5	E950.4	E962.0	E980.4
oxidase reagent	977.8	E858.8	E947.8	E950.4	E962.0	E980.4
Glucosulfone sodium	961.8	E857	E931.8	E950.4	E962.0	E980.4
Glue(s)	989.89	E866.6	—	E950.9	E962.1	E980.9
Glutamic acid (hydrochloride)	973.4	E858.4	E943.4	E950.4	E962.0	E980.4
Glutaraldehyde	989.89	E861.4	—	E950.9	E962.1	E980.9
Glutathione	963.8	E858.1	E933.8	E950.4	E962.0	E980.4

Substance	Poisoning	Accident	Therapeutic Use	Suicide Attempt	Assault	Undetermined
		External Cause (E-Code)				
Glutethimide (group)	967.5	E852.4	E937.5	E950.2	E962.0	E980.2
Glycerin (lotion)	976.3	E858.7	E946.3	E950.4	E962.0	E980.4
Glycerol (topical)	976.3	E858.7	E946.3	E950.4	E962.0	E980.4
Glyceryl						
guaiacolate	975.5	E858.6	E945.5	E950.4	E962.0	E980.4
triacetate (topical)	976.0	E858.7	E946.0	E950.4	E962.0	E980.4
trinitrate	972.4	E858.3	E942.4	E950.4	E962.0	E980.4
Glycine	974.5	E858.5	E944.5	E950.4	E962.0	E980.4
Glycobiarsol	961.1	E857	E931.1	E950.4	E962.0	E980.4
Glycols (ether)	982.8	E862.4	—	E950.9	E962.1	E980.9
Glycopyrrolate	971.1	E855.4	E941.1	E950.4	E962.0	E980.4
Glymidine	962.3	E858.0	E932.3	E950.4	E962.0	E980.4
Gold (compounds) (salts)	965.69	E850.6	E935.6	E950.0	E962.0	E980.0
Golden sulfide of antimony	985.4	E866.2	—	E950.9	E962.1	E980.9
Goldylocks	988.2	E865.4	—	E950.9	E962.1	E980.9
Gonadal tissue extract	962.9	E858.0	E932.9	E950.4	E962.0	E980.4
female	962.2	E858.0	E932.2	E950.4	E962.0	E980.4
male	962.1	E858.0	E932.1	E950.4	E962.0	E980.4
Gonadotropin	962.4	E858.0	E932.4	E950.4	E962.0	E980.4
Grain alcohol	980.0	E860.1	—	E950.9	E962.1	E980.9
beverage	980.0	E860.0	—	E950.9	E962.1	E980.9
Gramicidin	960.8	E856	E930.8	E950.4	E962.0	E980.4
Gratiola officinalis	988.2	E865.4	—	E950.9	E962.1	E980.9
Grease	989.89	E866.8	—	E950.9	E962.1	E980.9
Green hellebore	988.2	E865.4	—	E950.9	E962.1	E980.9
Green soap	976.2	E858.7	E946.2	E950.4	E962.0	E980.4
Grifulvin	960.1	E856	E930.1	E950.4	E962.0	E980.4
Griseofulvin	960.1	E856	E930.1	E950.4	E962.0	E980.4
Growth hormone	962.4	E858.0	E932.4	E950.4	E962.0	E980.4
Guaiacol	975.5	E858.6	E945.5	E950.4	E962.0	E980.4
Guaiac reagent	977.8	E858.8	E947.8	E950.4	E962.0	E980.4
Guaifenesin	975.5	E858.6	E945.5	E950.4	E962.0	E980.4
Guaiphenesin	975.5	E858.6	E945.5	E950.4	E962.0	E980.4
Guanatol	961.4	E857	E931.4	E950.4	E962.0	E980.4
Guanethidine	972.6	E858.3	E942.6	E950.4	E962.0	E980.4
Guano	989.89	E866.5	—	E950.9	E962.1	E980.9
Guanochlor	972.6	E858.3	E942.6	E950.4	E962.0	E980.4
Guanoctine	972.6	E858.3	E942.6	E950.4	E962.0	E980.4
Guanoxan	972.6	E858.3	E942.6	E950.4	E962.0	E980.4
Hair treatment agent NEC	976.4	E858.7	E946.4	E950.4	E962.0	E980.4
Halcinonide	976.0	E858.7	E946.0	E950.4	E962.0	E980.4
Halethazole	976.0	E858.7	E946.0	E950.4	E962.0	E980.4
Hallucinogens	969.6	E854.1	E939.6	E950.3	E962.0	E980.3
Haloperidol	969.2	E853.1	E939.2	E950.3	E962.0	E980.3
Haloprogin	976.0	E858.7	E946.0	E950.4	E962.0	E980.4
Halotex	976.0	E858.7	E946.0	E950.4	E962.0	E980.4
Halothane	968.1	E855.1	E938.1	E950.4	E962.0	E980.4
Halquinols	976.0	E858.7	E946.0	E950.4	E962.0	E980.4
Hand sanitizer	976.0	E858.7	E946.0	E950.4	E962.0	E980.4
Harmonyl	972.6	E858.3	E942.6	E950.4	E962.0	E980.4
Hartmann's solution	974.5	E858.5	E944.5	E950.4	E962.0	E980.4
Hashish	969.6	E854.1	E939.6	E950.3	E962.0	E980.3
Hawaiian wood rose seeds	969.6	E854.1	E939.6	E950.3	E962.0	E980.3
Headache cures, drugs, powders NEC	977.9	E858.9	E947.9	E950.5	E962.0	E980.9
Heavenly Blue (morning glory)	969.6	E854.1	E939.6	E950.3	E962.0	E980.3
Heavy metal						
antagonists	963.8	E858.1	E933.8	E950.4	E962.0	E980.4
anti–infectives	961.2	E857	E931.2	E950.4	E962.0	E980.4
Hedaquinium	976.0	E858.7	E946.0	E950.4	E962.0	E980.4
Hedge hyssop	988.2	E865.4	—	E950.9	E962.1	E980.9

TABLE OF DRUGS AND CHEMICALS

Substance	Poisoning	Accident	Therapeutic Use	Suicide Attempt	Assault	Undetermined
			External Cause (E-Code)			
Heet	976.8	E858.7	E946.8	E950.4	E962.0	E980.4
Helenin	961.6	E857	E931.6	E950.4	E962.0	E980.4
Hellebore (black) (green) (white)	988.2	E865.4	—	E950.9	E962.1	E980.9
Hemlock	988.2	E865.4	—	E950.9	E962.1	E980.9
Hemostatics	964.5	E858.2	E934.5	E950.4	E962.0	E980.4
capillary active drugs	972.8	E858.3	E942.8	E950.4	E962.0	E980.4
Henbane	988.2	E865.4	—	E950.9	E962.1	E980.9
Heparin (sodium)	964.2	E858.2	E934.2	E950.4	E962.0	E980.4
Heptabarbital, heptabarbitone	967.0	E851	E937.0	E950.1	E962.0	E980.1
Heptachlor	989.2	E863.0	—	E950.6	E962.1	E980.7
Heptalgin	965.09	E850.2	E935.2	E950.0	E962.0	E980.0
Herbicides	989.4	E863.5	—	E950.6	E962.1	E980.7
Heroin	965.01	E850.0	E935.0	E950.0	E962.0	E980.0
Herplex	976.5	E858.7	E946.5	E950.4	E962.0	E980.4
HES	964.8	E858.2	E934.8	E950.4	E962.0	E980.4
Hetastarch	964.8	E858.2	E934.8	E950.4	E962.0	E980.4
Hexachlorocyclohexane	989.2	E863.0	—	E950.6	E962.1	E980.7
Hexachlorophene	976.2	E858.7	E946.2	E950.4	E962.0	E980.4
Hexadimethrine (bromide)	964.5	E858.2	E934.5	E950.4	E962.0	E980.4
Hexafluorenium	975.2	E858.6	E945.2	E950.4	E962.0	E980.4
Hexa–germ	976.2	E858.7	E946.2	E950.4	E962.0	E980.4
Hexahydrophenol	980.8	E860.8	—	E950.9	E962.1	E980.9
Hexalin	980.8	E860.8	—	E950.9	E962.1	E980.9
Hexamethonium	972.3	E858.3	E942.3	E950.4	E962.0	E980.4
Hexamethyleneamine	961.9	E857	E931.9	E950.4	E962.0	E980.4
Hexamine	961.9	E857	E931.9	E950.4	E962.0	E980.4
Hexanone	982.8	E862.4	—	E950.9	E962.1	E980.9
Hexapropymate	967.8	E852.8	E937.8	E950.2	E962.0	E980.2
Hexestrol	962.2	E858.0	E932.2	E950.4	E962.0	E980.4
Hexethal (sodium)	967.0	E851	E937.0	E950.1	E962.0	E980.1
Hexetidine	976.0	E858.7	E946.0	E950.4	E962.0	E980.4
Hexobarbital, hexobarbitone	967.0	E851	E937.0	E950.1	E962.0	E980.1
sodium (anesthetic)	968.3	E855.1	E938.3	E950.4	E962.0	E980.4
soluble	968.3	E855.1	E938.3	E950.4	E962.0	E980.4
Hexocyclium	971.1	E855.4	E941.1	E950.4	E962.0	E980.4
Hexoestrol	962.2	E858.0	E932.2	E950.4	E962.0	E980.4
Hexone	982.8	E862.4	—	E950.9	E962.1	E980.9
Hexylcaine	968.5	E855.2	E938.5	E950.4	E962.0	E980.4
Hexylresorcinol	961.6	E857	E931.6	E950.4	E962.0	E980.4
Hinkle's pills	973.1	E858.4	E943.1	E950.4	E962.0	E980.4
Histalog	977.8	E858.8	E947.8	E950.4	E962.0	E980.4
Histamine (phosphate)	972.5	E858.3	E942.5	E950.4	E962.0	E980.4
Histoplasmin	977.8	E858.8	E947.8	E950.4	E962.0	E980.4
Holly berries	988.2	E865.3	—	E950.9	E962.1	E980.9
Homatropine	971.1	E855.4	E941.1	E950.4	E962.0	E980.4
Homo–tet	964.6	E858.2	E934.6	E950.4	E962.0	E980.4
Hormones (synthetic substitute) NEC	962.9	E858.0	E932.9	E950.4	E962.0	E980.4
adrenal cortical steroids	962.0	E858.0	E932.0	E950.4	E962.0	E980.4
antidiabetic agents	962.3	E858.0	E932.3	E950.4	E962.0	E980.4
follicle stimulating	962.4	E858.0	E932.4	E950.4	E962.0	E980.4
gonadotropic	962.4	E858.0	E932.4	E950.4	E962.0	E980.4
growth	962.4	E858.0	E932.4	E950.4	E962.0	E980.4
ovarian (substitutes)	962.2	E858.0	E932.2	E950.4	E962.0	E980.4
parathyroid (derivatives)	962.6	E858.0	E932.6	E950.4	E962.0	E980.4
pituitary (posterior)	962.5	E858.0	E932.5	E950.4	E962.0	E980.4
anterior	962.4	E858.0	E932.4	E950.4	E962.0	E980.4
thyroid (derivative)	962.7	E858.0	E932.7	E950.4	E962.0	E980.4
Hornet (sting)	989.5	E905.3	—	E950.9	E962.1	E980.9
Horticulture agent NEC	989.4	E863.9	—	E950.6	E962.1	E980.7
Hyaluronidase	963.4	E858.1	E933.4	E950.4	E962.0	E980.4
Hyazyme	963.4	E858.1	E933.4	E950.4	E962.0	E980.4

Substance	Poisoning	Accident	Therapeutic Use	Suicide Attempt	Assault	Undetermined
			External Cause (E-Code)			
Hycodan	965.09	E850.2	E935.2	E950.0	E962.0	E980.0
Hydantoin derivatives	966.1	E855.0	E936.1	E950.4	E962.0	E980.4
Hydeltra	962.0	E858.0	E932.0	E950.4	E962.0	E980.4
Hydergine	971.3	E855.6	E941.3	E950.4	E962.0	E980.4
Hydrabamine penicillin	960.0	E856	E930.0	E950.4	E962.0	E980.4
Hydralazine, hydrallazine	972.6	E858.3	E942.6	E950.4	E962.0	E980.4
Hydrargaphen	976.0	E858.7	E946.0	E950.4	E962.0	E980.4
Hydrazine	983.9	E864.3	—	E950.7	E962.1	E980.6
Hydriodic acid	975.5	E858.6	E945.5	E950.4	E962.0	E980.4
Hydrocarbon gas	987.1	E869.8	—	E952.8	E962.2	E982.8
incomplete combustion of — *see* Carbon, monoxide, fuel, utility						
liquefied (mobile container)	987.0	E868.0	—	E951.1	E962.2	E981.1
piped (natural)	987.0	E867	—	E951.0	E962.2	E981.0
Hydrochloric acid (liquid)	983.1	E864.1	—	E950.7	E962.1	E980.6
medicinal	973.4	E858.4	E943.4	E950.4	E962.0	E980.4
vapor	987.8	E869.8	—	E952.8	E962.2	E982.8
Hydrochlorothiazide	974.3	E858.5	E944.3	E950.4	E962.0	E980.4
Hydrocodone	965.09	E850.2	E935.2	E950.0	E962.0	E980.0
Hydrocortisone	962.0	E858.0	E932.0	E950.4	E962.0	E980.4
ENT agent	976.6	E858.7	E946.6	E950.4	E962.0	E980.4
ophthalmic preparation	976.5	E858.7	E946.5	E950.4	E962.0	E980.4
topical NEC	976.0	E858.7	E946.0	E950.4	E962.0	E980.4
Hydrocortone	962.0	E858.0	E932.0	E950.4	E962.0	E980.4
ENT agent	976.6	E858.7	E946.6	E950.4	E962.0	E980.4
ophthalmic preparation	976.5	E858.7	E946.5	E950.4	E962.0	E980.4
topical NEC	976.0	E858.7	E946.0	E950.4	E962.0	E980.4
Hydrocyanic acid — *see* Cyanide(s)						
Hydroflumethiazide	974.3	E858.5	E944.3	E950.4	E962.0	E980.4
Hydrofluoric acid (liquid)	983.1	E864.1	—	E950.7	E962.1	E980.6
vapor	987.8	E869.8	—	E952.8	E962.2	E982.8
Hydrogen	987.8	E869.8	—	E952.8	E962.2	E982.8
arsenide	985.1	E866.3	—	E950.8	E962.1	E980.8
arseniureted	985.1	E866.3	—	E950.8	E962.1	E980.8
cyanide (salts)	989.0	E866.8	—	E950.9	E962.1	E980.9
gas	987.7	E869.8	—	E952.8	E962.2	E982.8
fluoride (liquid)	983.1	E864.1	—	E950.7	E962.1	E980.6
vapor	987.8	E869.8	—	E952.8	E962.2	E982.8
peroxide (solution)	976.6	E858.7	E946.6	E950.4	E962.0	E980.4
phosphureted	987.8	E869.8	—	E952.8	E962.2	E982.8
sulfide (gas)	987.8	E869.8	—	E952.8	E962.2	E982.8
arseniureted	985.1	E866.3	—	E950.8	E962.1	E980.8
sulfureted	987.8	E869.8	—	E952.8	E962.2	E982.8
Hydromorphinol	965.09	E850.2	E935.2	E950.0	E962.0	E980.0
Hydromorphinone	965.09	E850.2	E935.2	E950.0	E962.0	E980.0
Hydromorphone	965.09	E850.2	E935.2	E950.0	E962.0	E980.0
Hydromox	974.3	E858.5	E944.3	E950.4	E962.0	E980.4
Hydrophilic lotion	976.3	E858.7	E946.3	E950.4	E962.0	E980.4
Hydroquinone	983.0	E864.0	—	E950.7	E962.1	E980.6
vapor	987.8	E869.8	—	E952.8	E962.2	E982.8
Hydrosulfuric acid (gas)	987.8	E869.8	—	E952.8	E962.2	E982.8
Hydrous wool fat (lotion)	976.3	E858.7	E946.3	E950.4	E962.0	E980.4
Hydroxide, caustic	983.2	E864.2	—	E950.7	E962.1	E980.6
Hydroxocobalamin	964.1	E858.2	E934.1	E950.4	E962.0	E980.4
Hydroxyamphetamine	971.2	E855.5	E941.2	E950.4	E962.0	E980.4
Hydroxychloroquine	961.4	E857	E931.4	E950.4	E962.0	E980.4
Hydroxydihydrocodeinone	965.09	E850.2	E935.2	E950.0	E962.0	E980.0
Hydroxyethyl starch	964.8	E858.2	E934.8	E950.4	E962.0	E980.4
Hydroxyphenamate	969.5	E853.8	E939.5	E950.3	E962.0	E980.3
Hydroxyphenylbutazone	965.5	E850.5	E935.5	E950.0	E962.0	E980.0

Substance	Poisoning	Accident	Therapeutic Use	Suicide Attempt	Assault	Undetermined
			External Cause (E-Code)			
Hydroxyprogesterone	962.2	E858.0	E932.2	E950.4	E962.0	E980.4
Hydroxyquinoline derivatives	961.3	E857	E931.3	E950.4	E962.0	E980.4
Hydroxystilbamidine	961.5	E857	E931.5	E950.4	E962.0	E980.4
Hydroxyurea	963.1	E858.1	E933.1	E950.4	E962.0	E980.4
Hydroxyzine	969.5	E853.8	E939.5	E950.3	E962.0	E980.3
Hyoscine (hydrobromide)	971.1	E855.4	E941.1	E950.4	E962.0	E980.4
Hyoscyamine	971.1	E855.4	E941.1	E950.4	E962.0	E980.4
Hyoscyamus (albus) (niger)	988.2	E865.4	—	E950.9	E962.1	E980.9
Hypaque	977.8	E858.8	E947.8	E950.4	E962.0	E980.4
Hypertussis	964.6	E858.2	E934.6	E950.4	E962.0	E980.4
Hypnotics NEC	967.9	E852.9	E937.9	E950.2	E962.0	E980.2
Hypochlorites — see Sodium, hypochlorite						
Hypotensive agents NEC	972.6	E858.3	E942.6	E950.4	E962.0	E980.4
Ibufenac	965.69	E850.6	E935.6	E950.0	E962.0	E980.0
ibuprofen	965.61	E850.6	E935.6	E950.0	E962.0	E980.0
ICG	977.8	E858.8	E947.8	E950.4	E962.0	E980.4
Ichthammol	976.4	E858.7	E946.4	E950.4	E962.0	E980.4
Ichthyol	976.4	E858.7	E946.4	E950.4	E962.0	E980.4
Idoxuridine	976.5	E858.7	E946.5	E950.4	E962.0	E980.4
IDU	976.5	E858.7	E946.5	E950.4	E962.0	E980.4
Iletin	962.3	E858.0	E932.3	E950.4	E962.0	E980.4
Ilex	988.2	E865.4	—	E950.9	E962.1	E980.9
Illuminating gas — see Gas, utility						
Ilopan	963.5	E858.1	E933.5	E950.4	E962.0	E980.4
Ilotycin	960.3	E856	E930.3	E950.4	E962.0	E980.4
ophthalmic preparation	976.5	E858.7	E946.5	E950.4	E962.0	E980.4
topical NEC	976.0	E858.7	E946.0	E950.4	E962.0	E980.4
Imipramine	969.05	E854.0	E939.0	E950.3	E962.0	E980.3
Immu–G	964.6	E858.2	E934.6	E950.4	E962.0	E980.4
Immuglobin	964.6	E858.2	E934.6	E950.4	E962.0	E980.4
Immune serum globulin	964.6	E858.2	E934.6	E950.4	E962.0	E980.4
Immunosuppressive agents	963.1	E858.1	E933.1	E950.4	E962.0	E980.4
Immu–tetanus	964.6	E858.2	E934.6	E950.4	E962.0	E980.4
Indandione (derivatives)	964.2	E858.2	E934.2	E950.4	E962.0	E980.4
Inderal	972.0	E858.3	E942.0	E950.4	E962.0	E980.4
Indian						
hemp	969.6	E854.1	E939.6	E950.3	E962.0	E980.3
tobacco	988.2	E865.4	—	E950.9	E962.1	E980.9
Indigo carmine	977.8	E858.8	E947.8	E950.4	E962.0	E980.4
Indocin	965.69	E850.6	E935.6	E950.0	E962.0	E980.0
Indocyanine green	977.8	E858.8	E947.8	E950.4	E962.0	E980.4
Indomethacin	965.69	E850.6	E935.6	E950.0	E962.0	E980.0
Industrial						
alcohol	980.9	E860.9	—	E950.9	E962.1	E980.9
fumes	987.8	E869.8	—	E952.8	E962.2	E982.8
solvents (fumes) (vapors)	982.8	E862.9	—	E950.9	E962.1	E980.9
Influenza vaccine	979.6	E858.8	E949.6	E950.4	E962.0	E982.8
Ingested substances NEC	989.9	E866.9	—	E950.9	E962.1	E980.9
INH (isoniazid)	961.8	E857	E931.8	E950.4	E962.0	E980.4
Inhalation, gas (noxious) — see Gas						
Ink	989.89	E866.8	—	E950.9	E962.1	E980.9
Innovar	967.6	E852.5	E937.6	E950.2	E962.0	E980.2
Inositol niacinate	972.2	E858.3	E942.2	E950.4	E962.0	E980.4
Inproquone	963.1	E858.1	E933.1	E950.4	E962.0	E980.4
Insect (sting), venomous	989.5	E905.5	—	E950.9	E962.1	E980.9
Insecticides (see also Pesticides)	989.4	E863.4	—	E950.6	E962.1	E980.7
chlorinated	989.2	E863.0	—	E950.6	E962.1	E980.7
mixtures	989.4	E863.3	—	E950.6	E962.1	E980.7
organochlorine (compounds)	989.2	E863.0	—	E950.6	E962.1	E980.7
organophosphorus (compounds)	989.3	E863.1	—	E950.6	E962.1	E980.7
Insular tissue extract	962.3	E858.0	E932.3	E950.4	E962.0	E980.4

Substance	Poisoning	Accident	Therapeutic Use	Suicide Attempt	Assault	Undetermined
			External Cause (E-Code)			
Insulin (amorphous) (globin) (isophane) (Lente) (NPH) (protamine) (Semilente) (Ultralente) (zinc)	962.3	E858.0	E932.3	E950.4	E962.0	E980.4
Intranarcon	968.3	E855.1	E938.3	E950.4	E962.0	E980.4
Inulin	977.8	E858.8	E947.8	E950.4	E962.0	E980.4
Invert sugar	974.5	E858.5	E944.5	E950.4	E962.0	E980.4
Inza—*see* Naproxen						
Iodide NEC (*see also* Iodine)	976.0	E858.7	E946.0	E950.4	E962.0	E980.4
mercury (ointment)	976.0	E858.7	E946.0	E950.4	E962.0	E980.4
methylate	976.0	E858.7	E946.0	E950.4	E962.0	E980.4
potassium (expectorant) NEC	975.5	E858.6	E945.5	E950.4	E962.0	E980.4
Iodinated glycerol	975.5	E858.6	E945.5	E950.4	E962.0	E980.4
Iodine (antiseptic, external) (tincture) NEC	976.0	E858.7	E946.0	E950.4	E962.0	E980.4
diagnostic	977.8	E858.8	E947.8	E950.4	E962.0	E980.4
for thyroid conditions (antithyroid)	962.8	E858.0	E932.8	E950.4	E962.0	E980.4
vapor	987.8	E869.8	—	E952.8	E962.2	E982.8
Iodized oil	977.8	E858.8	E947.8	E950.4	E962.0	E980.4
Iodobismitol	961.2	E857	E931.2	E950.4	E962.0	E980.4
Iodochlorhydroxyquin	961.3	E857	E931.3	E950.4	E962.0	E980.4
topical	976.0	E858.7	E946.0	E950.4	E962.0	E980.4
Iodoform	976.0	E858.7	E946.0	E950.4	E962.0	E980.4
Iodopanoic acid	977.8	E858.8	E947.8	E950.4	E962.0	E980.4
Iodophthalein	977.8	E858.8	E947.8	E950.4	E962.0	E980.4
Ion exchange resins	974.5	E858.5	E944.5	E950.4	E962.0	E980.4
Iopanoic acid	977.8	E858.8	E947.8	E950.4	E962.0	E980.4
Iophendylate	977.8	E858.8	E947.8	E950.4	E962.0	E980.4
Iothiouracil	962.8	E858.0	E932.8	E950.4	E962.0	E980.4
Ipecac	973.6	E858.4	E943.6	E950.4	E962.0	E980.4
Ipecacuanha	973.6	E858.4	E943.6	E950.4	E962.0	E980.4
Ipodate	977.8	E858.8	E947.8	E950.4	E962.0	E980.4
Ipral	967.0	E851	E937.0	E950.1	E962.0	E980.1
Ipratropium	975.1	E858.6	E945.1	E950.4	E962.0	E980.4
Iproniazid	969.01	E854.0	E939.0	E950.3	E962.0	E980.3
Iron (compounds) (medicinal) (preparations)	964.0	E858.2	E934.0	E950.4	E962.0	E980.4
dextran	964.0	E858.2	E934.0	E950.4	E962.0	E980.4
nonmedicinal (dust) (fumes) NEC	985.8	E866.4	—	E950.9	E962.1	E980.9
Irritant drug	977.9	E858.9	E947.9	E950.5	E962.0	E980.5
Ismelin	972.6	E858.3	E942.6	E950.4	E962.0	E980.4
Isoamyl nitrite	972.4	E858.3	E942.4	E950.4	E962.0	E980.4
Isobutyl acetate	982.8	E862.4	—	E950.9	E962.1	E980.9
Isocarboxazid	969.01	E854.0	E939.0	E950.3	E962.0	E980.3
Isoephedrine	971.2	E855.5	E941.2	E950.4	E962.0	E980.4
Isoetharine	971.2	E855.5	E941.2	E950.4	E962.0	E980.4
Isoflurophate	971.0	E855.3	E941.0	E950.4	E962.0	E980.4
Isoniazid (INH)	961.8	E857	E931.8	E950.4	E962.0	E980.4
Isopentaquine	961.4	E857	E931.4	E950.4	E962.0	E980.4
Isophane insulin	962.3	E858.0	E932.3	E950.4	E962.0	E980.4
Isopregnenone	962.2	E858.0	E932.2	E950.4	E962.0	E980.4
Isoprenaline	971.2	E855.5	E941.2	E950.4	E962.0	E980.4
Isopropamide	971.1	E855.4	E941.1	E950.4	E962.0	E980.4
Isopropanol	980.2	E860.3	—	E950.9	E962.1	E980.9
topical (germicide)	976.0	E858.7	E946.0	E950.4	E962.0	E980.4
Isopropyl						
acetate	982.8	E862.4	—	E950.9	E962.1	E980.9
alcohol	980.2	E860.3	—	E950.9	E962.1	E980.9
topical (germicide)	976.0	E858.7	E946.0	E950.4	E962.0	E980.4
ether	982.8	E862.4	—	E950.9	E962.1	E980.9
Isoproterenol	971.2	E855.5	E941.2	E950.4	E962.0	E980.4

Substance	Poisoning	Accident	Therapeutic Use	Suicide Attempt	Assault	Undetermined
			External Cause (E-Code)			
Isosorbide dinitrate	972.4	E858.3	E942.4	E950.4	E962.0	E980.4
Isothipendyl	963.0	E858.1	E933.0	E950.4	E962.0	E980.4
Isoxazolyl penicillin	960.0	E856	E930.0	E950.4	E962.0	E980.4
Isoxsuprine hydrochloride	972.5	E858.3	E942.5	E950.4	E962.0	E980.4
I–thyroxine sodium	962.7	E858.0	E932.7	E950.4	E962.0	E980.4
Jaborandi (pilocarpus) (extract)	971.0	E855.3	E941.0	E950.4	E962.0	E980.4
Jalap	973.1	E858.4	E943.1	E950.4	E962.0	E980.4
Jamaica						
dogwood (bark)	965.7	E850.7	E935.7	E950.0	E962.0	E980.0
ginger	989.89	E866.8	—	E950.9	E962.1	E980.9
Jatropha	988.2	E865.4	—	E950.9	E962.1	E980.9
curcas	988.2	E865.3	—	E950.9	E962.1	E980.9
Jectofer	964.0	E858.2	E934.0	E950.4	E962.0	E980.4
Jellyfish (sting)	989.5	E905.6	—	E950.9	E962.1	E980.9
Jequirity (bean)	988.2	E865.3	—	E950.9	E962.1	E980.9
Jimson weed	988.2	E865.4	—	E950.9	E962.1	E980.9
seeds	988.2	E865.3	—	E950.9	E962.1	E980.9
Juniper tar (oil) (ointment)	976.4	E858.7	E946.4	E950.4	E962.0	E980.4
Kallikrein	972.5	E858.3	E942.5	E950.4	E962.0	E980.4
Kanamycin	960.6	E856	E930.6	E950.4	E962.0	E980.4
Kantrex	960.6	E856	E930.6	E950.4	E962.0	E980.4
Kaolin	973.5	E858.4	E943.5	E950.4	E962.0	E980.4
Karaya (gum)	973.3	E858.4	E943.3	E950.4	E962.0	E980.4
Kemithal	968.3	E855.1	E938.3	E950.4	E962.0	E980.4
Kenacort	962.0	E858.0	E932.0	E950.4	E962.0	E980.4
Keratolytics	976.4	E858.7	E946.4	E950.4	E962.0	E980.4
Keratoplastics	976.4	E858.7	E946.4	E950.4	E962.0	E980.4
Kerosene, kerosine (fuel) (solvent) NEC	981	E862.1	—	E950.9	E962.1	E980.9
insecticide	981	E863.4	—	E950.6	E962.1	E980.7
vapor	987.1	E869.8	—	E952.8	E962.2	E982.8
Ketamine	968.3	E855.1	E938.3	E950.4	E962.0	E980.4
Ketobemidone	965.09	E850.2	E935.2	E950.0	E962.0	E980.0
Ketols	982.8	E862.4	—	E950.9	E962.1	E980.9
Ketone oils	982.8	E862.4	—	E950.9	E962.1	E980.9
Ketoprofen	965.61	E850.6	E935.6	E950.0	E962.0	E980.0
Kiln gas or vapor (carbon monoxide)	986	E868.8	—	E952.1	E962.2	E982.1
Konsyl	973.3	E858.4	E943.3	E950.4	E962.0	E980.4
Kosam seed	988.2	E865.3	—	E950.9	E962.1	E980.9
Krait (venom)	989.5	E905.0	—	E950.9	E962.1	E980.9
Kwell (insecticide)	989.2	E863.0	—	E950.6	E962.1	E980.7
anti–infective (topical)	976.0	E858.7	E946.0	E950.4	E962.0	E980.4
Laburnum (flowers) (seeds)	988.2	E865.3	—	E950.9	E962.1	E980.9
leaves	988.2	E865.4	—	E950.9	E962.1	E980.9
Lacquers	989.89	E861.6	—	E950.9	E962.1	E980.9
Lacrimogenic gas	987.5	E869.3	—	E952.8	E962.2	E982.8
Lactic acid	983.1	E864.1	—	E950.7	E962.1	E980.6
Lactobacillus acidophilus	973.5	E858.4	E943.5	E950.4	E962.0	E980.4
Lactoflavin	963.5	E858.1	E933.5	E950.4	E962.0	E980.4
Lactuca (virosa) (extract)	967.8	E852.8	E937.8	E950.2	E962.0	E980.2
Lactucarium	967.8	E852.8	E937.8	E950.2	E962.0	E980.2
Laevulose	974.5	E858.5	E944.5	E950.4	E962.0	E980.4
Lanatoside(C)	972.1	E858.3	E942.1	E950.4	E962.0	E980.4
Lanolin (lotion)	976.3	E858.7	E946.3	E950.4	E962.0	E980.4
Largactil	969.1	E853.0	E939.1	E950.3	E962.0	E980.3
Larkspur	988.2	E865.3	—	E950.9	E962.1	E980.9
Laroxyl	969.05	E854.0	E939.0	E950.3	E962.0	E980.3
Lasix	974.4	E858.5	E944.4	E950.4	E962.0	E980.4
Latex	989.82	E866.8	—	E950.9	E962.1	E980.9
Lathyrus (seed)	988.2	E865.3	—	E950.9	E962.1	E980.9
Laudanum	965.09	E850.2	E935.2	E950.0	E962.0	E980.0
Laudexium	975.2	E858.6	E945.2	E950.4	E962.0	E980.4

Substance	Poisoning	Accident	Therapeutic Use	Suicide Attempt	Assault	Undetermined
			External Cause (E-Code)			
Laurel, black or cherry	988.2	E865.4	—	E950.9	E962.1	E980.9
Laurolinium	976.0	E858.7	E946.0	E950.4	E962.0	E980.4
Lauryl sulfoacetate	976.2	E858.7	E946.2	E950.4	E962.0	E980.4
Laxatives NEC	973.3	E858.4	E943.3	E950.4	E962.0	E980.4
emollient	973.2	E858.4	E943.2	E950.4	E962.0	E980.4
L–dopa	966.4	E855.0	E936.4	E950.4	E962.0	E980.4
L Tryptophan—*see* amino acid						
Lead (dust) (fumes) (vapor) NEC	984.9	E866.0	—	E950.9	E962.1	E980.9
acetate (dust)	984.1	E866.0	—	E950.9	E962.1	E980.9
anti–infectives	961.2	E857	E931.2	E950.4	E962.0	E980.4
antiknock compound (tetraethyl)	984.1	E862.1	—	E950.9	E962.1	E980.9
arsenate, arsenite (dust) (insecticide) (vapor)	985.1	E863.4	—	E950.8	E962.1	E980.8
herbicide	985.1	E863.5	—	E950.8	E962.1	E980.8
carbonate	984.0	E866.0	—	E950.9	E962.1	E980.9
paint	984.0	E861.5	—	E950.9	E962.1	E980.9
chromate	984.0	E866.0	—	E950.9	E962.1	E980.9
paint	984.0	E861.5	—	E950.9	E962.1	E980.9
dioxide	984.0	E866.0	—	E950.9	E962.1	E980.9
inorganic (compound)	984.0	E866.0	—	E950.9	E962.1	E980.9
paint	984.0	E861.5	—	E950.9	E962.1	E980.9
iodine	984.0	E866.0	—	E950.9	E962.1	E980.9
pigment (paint)	984.0	E861.5	—	E950.9	E962.1	E980.9
monoxide (dust)	984.0	E866.0	—	E950.9	E962.1	E980.9
paint	984.0	E861.5	—	E950.9	E962.1	E980.9
organic	984.1	E866.0	—	E950.9	E962.1	E980.9
oxide	984.0	E866.0	—	E950.9	E962.1	E980.9
paint	984.0	E861.5	—	E950.9	E962.1	E980.9
paint	984.0	E861.5	—	E950.9	E962.1	E980.9
salts	984.0	E866.0	—	E950.9	E962.1	E980.9
specified compound NEC	984.8	E866.0	—	E950.9	E962.1	E980.9
tetra–ethyl	984.1	E862.1	—	E950.9	E962.1	E980.9
Lebanese red	969.6	E854.1	E939.6	E950.3	E962.0	E980.3
Lente Iletin (insulin)	962.3	E858.0	E932.3	E950.4	E962.0	E980.4
Leptazol	970.0	E854.3	E940.0	E950.4	E962.0	E980.4
Leritine	965.09	E850.2	E935.2	E950.0	E962.0	E980.0
Letter	962.7	E858.0	E932.7	E950.4	E962.0	E980.4
Lettuce opium	967.8	E852.8	E937.8	E950.2	E962.0	E980.2
Leucovorin (factor)	964.1	E858.2	E934.1	E950.4	E962.0	E980.4
Leukeran	963.1	E858.1	E933.1	E950.4	E962.0	E980.4
Levalbuterol	975.7	E858.6	E945.7	E950.4	E962.0	E980.4
Levallorphan	970.1	E854.3	E940.1	E950.4	E962.0	E980.4
Levanil	967.8	E852.8	E937.8	E950.2	E962.0	E980.2
Levarterenol	971.2	E855.5	E941.2	E950.4	E962.0	E980.4
Levodopa	966.4	E855.0	E936.4	E950.4	E962.0	E980.4
Levo–dromoran	965.09	E850.2	E935.2	E950.0	E962.0	E980.0
Levoid	962.7	E858.0	E932.7	E950.4	E962.0	E980.4
Levo–iso–methadone	965.02	E850.1	E935.1	E950.0	E962.0	E980.0
Levomepromazine	967.8	E852.8	E937.8	E950.2	E962.0	E980.2
Levoprome	967.8	E852.8	E937.8	E950.2	E962.0	E980.2
Levopropoxyphene	975.4	E858.6	E945.4	E950.4	E962.0	E980.4
Levorphan, levophanol	965.09	E850.2	E935.2	E950.0	E962.0	E980.0
Levothyroxine (sodium)	962.7	E858.0	E932.7	E950.4	E962.0	E980.4
Levsin	971.1	E855.4	E941.1	E950.4	E962.0	E980.4
Levulose	974.5	E858.5	E944.5	E950.4	E962.0	E980.4
Lewisite (gas)	985.1	E866.3	—	E950.8	E962.1	E980.8
Librium	969.4	E853.2	E939.4	E950.3	E962.0	E980.3
Lidex	976.0	E858.7	E946.0	E950.4	E962.0	E980.4
Lidocaine (infiltration) (topical)	968.5	E855.2	E938.5	E950.4	E962.0	E980.4
nerve block (peripheral) (plexus)	968.6	E855.2	E938.6	E950.4	E962.0	E980.4

Substance	Poisoning	Accident	Therapeutic Use	Suicide Attempt	Assault	Undetermined
			External Cause (E-Code)			
spinal	968.7	E855.2	E938.7	E950.4	E962.0	E980.4
Lighter fluid	981	E862.1	—	E950.9	E962.1	E980.9
Lignocaine (infiltration) (topical)	968.5	E855.2	E938.5	E950.4	E962.0	E980.4
nerve block (peripheral) (plexus)	968.6	E855.2	E938.6	E950.4	E962.0	E980.4
spinal	968.7	E855.2	E938.7	E950.4	E962.0	E980.4
Ligroin(e) (solvent)	981	E862.0	—	E950.9	E962.1	E980.9
vapor	987.1	E869.8	—	E952.8	E962.2	E982.8
Ligustrum vulgare	988.2	E865.3	—	E950.9	E962.1	E980.9
Lily of the valley	988.2	E865.4	—	E950.9	E962.1	E980.9
Lime (chloride)	983.2	E864.2	—	E950.7	E962.1	E980.6
solution, sulferated	976.4	E858.7	E946.4	E950.4	E962.0	E980.4
Limonene	982.8	E862.4	—	E950.9	E962.1	E980.9
Lincomycin	960.8	E856	E930.8	E950.4	E962.0	E980.4
Lindane (insecticide) (vapor)	989.2	E863.0	—	E950.6	E962.1	E980.7
anti–infective (topical)	976.0	E858.7	E946.0	E950.4	E962.0	E980.4
Liniments NEC	976.9	E858.7	E946.9	E950.4	E962.0	E980.4
Linoleic acid	972.2	E858.3	E942.2	E950.4	E962.0	E980.4
Liothyronine	962.7	E858.0	E932.7	E950.4	E962.0	E980.4
Liotrix	962.7	E858.0	E932.7	E950.4	E962.0	E980.4
Lipancreatin	973.4	E858.4	E943.4	E950.4	E962.0	E980.4
Lipo–Lutin	962.2	E858.0	E932.2	E950.4	E962.0	E980.4
Lipotropic agents	977.1	E858.8	E947.1	E950.4	E962.0	E980.4
Liquefied petroleum gases	987.0	E868.0	—	E951.1	E962.2	E981.1
piped (pure or mixed with air)	987.0	E867	—	E951.0	E962.2	E981.0
Liquid petrolatum	973.2	E858.4	E943.2	E950.4	E962.0	E980.4
substance	989.9	E866.9	—	E950.9	E962.1	E980.9
specified NEC	989.89	E866.8	—	E950.9	E962.1	E980.9
Lirugen	979.4	E858.8	E949.4	E950.4	E962.0	E980.4
Lithane	969.8	E855.8	E939.8	E950.3	E962.0	E980.3
Lithium	985.8	E866.4	—	E950.9	E962.1	E980.9
carbonate	969.8	E855.8	E939.8	E950.3	E962.0	E980.3
Lithonate	969.8	E855.8	E939.8	E950.3	E962.0	E980.3
Liver (extract) (injection) (preparations)	964.1	E858.2	E934.1	E950.4	E962.0	E980.4
Lizard (bite) (venom)	989.5	E905.0	—	E950.9	E962.1	E980.9
LMD	964.8	E858.2	E934.8	E950.4	E962.0	E980.4
Lobelia	988.2	E865.4	—	E950.9	E962.1	E980.9
Lobeline	970.0	E854.3	E940.0	E950.4	E962.0	E980.4
Locorten	976.0	E858.7	E946.0	E950.4	E962.0	E980.4
Lolium temulentum	988.2	E865.3	—	E950.9	E962.1	E980.9
Lomotil	973.5	E858.4	E943.5	E950.4	E962.0	E980.4
Lomustine	963.1	E858.1	E933.1	E950.4	E962.0	E980.4
Lophophora williamsii	969.6	E854.1	E939.6	E950.3	E962.0	E980.3
Lorazepam	969.4	E853.2	E939.4	E950.3	E962.0	E980.3
Lotions NEC	976.9	E858.7	E946.9	E950.4	E962.0	E980.4
Lotronex	973.8	E858.4	E943.8	E950.4	E962.0	E980.4
Lotusate	967.0	E851	E937.0	E950.1	E962.0	E980.1
Lowila	976.2	E858.7	E946.2	E950.4	E962.0	E980.4
Loxapine	969.3	E853.8	E939.3	E950.3	E962.0	E980.3
Lozenges (throat)	976.6	E858.7	E946.6	E950.4	E962.0	E980.4
LSD (25)	969.6	E854.1	E939.6	E950.3	E962.0	E980.3
Lubricating oil NEC	981	E862.2	—	E950.9	E962.1	E980.9
Lucanthone	961.6	E857	E931.6	E950.4	E962.0	E980.4
Luminal	967.0	E851	E937.0	E950.1	E962.0	E980.1
Lung irritant (gas) NEC	987.9	E869.9	—	E952.9	E962.2	E982.9
Lutocylol	962.2	E858.0	E932.2	E950.4	E962.0	E980.4
Lutromone	962.2	E858.0	E932.2	E950.4	E962.0	E980.4
Lututrin	975.0	E858.6	E945.0	E950.4	E962.0	E980.4
Lye (concentrated)	983.2	E864.2	—	E950.7	E962.1	E980.6
Lygranum (skin test)	977.8	E858.8	E947.8	E950.4	E962.0	E980.4
Lymecycline	960.4	E856	E930.4	E950.4	E962.0	E980.4
Lymphogranuloma venereum antigen	977.8	E858.8	E947.8	E950.4	E962.0	E980.4

Substance	Poisoning	Accident	Therapeutic Use	Suicide Attempt	Assault	Undetermined
			External Cause (E-Code)			
Lynestrenol	962.2	E858.0	E932.2	E950.4	E962.0	E980.4
Lyovac Sodium Edecrin	974.4	E858.5	E944.4	E950.4	E962.0	E980.4
Lypressin	962.5	E858.0	E932.5	E950.4	E962.0	E980.4
Lysergic acid (amide) (diethylamide)	969.6	E854.1	E939.6	E950.3	E962.0	E980.3
Lysergide	969.6	E854.1	E939.6	E950.3	E962.0	E980.3
Lysine vasopressin	962.5	E858.0	E932.5	E950.4	E962.0	E980.4
Lysol	983.0	E864.0	—	E950.7	E962.1	E980.6
Lytta (vitatta)	976.8	E858.7	E946.8	E950.4	E962.0	E980.4
Mace	987.5	E869.3	—	E952.8	E962.2	E982.8
Macrolides (antibiotics)	960.3	E856	E930.3	E950.4	E962.0	E980.4
Mafenide	976.0	E858.7	E946.0	E950.4	E962.0	E980.4
Magaldrate	973.0	E858.4	E943.0	E950.4	E962.0	E980.4
Magic mushroom	969.6	E854.1	E939.6	E950.3	E962.0	E980.3
Magnamycin	960.8	E856	E930.8	E950.4	E962.0	E980.4
Magnesia magma	973.0	E858.4	E943.0	E950.4	E962.0	E980.4
Magnesium (compounds) (fumes) NEC	985.8	E866.4	—	E950.9	E962.1	E980.9
antacid	973.0	E858.4	E943.0	E950.4	E962.0	E980.4
carbonate	973.0	E858.4	E943.0	E950.4	E962.0	E980.4
cathartic	973.3	E858.4	E943.3	E950.4	E962.0	E980.4
citrate	973.3	E858.4	E943.3	E950.4	E962.0	E980.4
hydroxide	973.0	E858.4	E943.0	E950.4	E962.0	E980.4
oxide	973.0	E858.4	E943.0	E950.4	E962.0	E980.4
sulfate (oral)	973.3	E858.4	E943.3	E950.4	E962.0	E980.4
intravenous	966.3	E855.0	E936.3	E950.4	E962.0	E980.4
trisilicate	973.0	E858.4	E943.0	E950.4	E962.0	E980.4
Malathion (insecticide)	989.3	E863.1	—	E950.6	E962.1	E980.7
Male fern (oleoresin)	961.6	E857	E931.6	E950.4	E962.0	E980.4
Mandelic acid	961.9	E857	E931.9	E950.4	E962.0	E980.4
Manganese compounds (fumes) NEC	985.2	E866.4	—	E950.9	E962.1	E980.9
Mannitol (diuretic) (medicinal) NEC	974.4	E858.5	E944.4	E950.4	E962.0	E980.4
hexanitrate	972.4	E858.3	E942.4	E950.4	E962.0	E980.4
mustard	963.1	E858.1	E933.1	E950.4	E962.0	E980.4
Mannomustine	963.1	E858.1	E933.1	E950.4	E962.0	E980.4
MAO inhibitors	969.01	E854.0	E939.0	E950.3	E962.0	E980.3
Mapharsen	961.1	E857	E931.1	E950.4	E962.0	E980.4
Marcaine	968.9	E855.2	E938.9	E950.4	E962.0	E980.4
infiltration (subcutaneous)	968.5	E855.2	E938.5	E950.4	E962.0	E980.4
nerve block (peripheral) (plexus)	968.6	E855.2	E938.6	E950.4	E962.0	E980.4
Marezine	963.0	E858.1	E933.0	E950.4	E962.0	E980.4
Marihuana, marijuana (derivatives)	969.6	E854.1	E939.6	E950.3	E962.0	E980.3
Marine animals or plants (sting)	989.5	E905.6	—	E950.9	E962.1	E980.9
Marplan	969.01	E854.0	E939.0	E950.3	E962.0	E980.3
Marsh gas	987.1	E869.8	—	E952.8	E962.2	E982.8
Marsilid	969.01	E854.0	E939.0	E950.3	E962.0	E980.3
Matulane	963.1	E858.1	E933.1	E950.4	E962.0	E980.4
Mazindol	977.0	E858.8	E947.0	E950.4	E962.0	E980.4
MDMA	969.72	E854.2	E939.7	E950.3	E962.0	E980.3
Meadow saffron	988.2	E865.3	—	E950.9	E962.1	E980.9
Measles vaccine	979.4	E858.8	E949.4	E950.4	E962.0	E980.4
Meat, noxious or nonbacterial	988.8	E865.0	—	E950.9	E962.1	E980.9
Mebanazine	969.01	E854.0	E939.0	E950.3	E962.0	E980.3
Mebaral	967.0	E851	E937.0	E950.1	E962.0	E980.1
Mebendazole	961.6	E857	E931.6	E950.4	E962.0	E980.4
Mebeverine	975.1	E858.6	E945.1	E950.4	E962.0	E980.4
Mebhydroline	963.0	E858.1	E933.0	E950.4	E962.0	E980.4
Mebrophenhydramine	963.0	E858.1	E933.0	E950.4	E962.0	E980.4
Mebutamate	969.5	E853.8	E939.5	E950.3	E962.0	E980.3
Mecamylamine (chloride)	972.3	E858.3	E942.3	E950.4	E962.0	E980.4
Mechlorethamine hydrochloride	963.1	E858.1	E933.1	E950.4	E962.0	E980.4
Meclizene (hydrochloride)	963.0	E858.1	E933.0	E950.4	E962.0	E980.4

Substance	Poisoning	Accident	Therapeutic Use	Suicide Attempt	Assault	Undetermined
		External Cause (E-Code)				
Meclofenoxate	970.0	E854.3	E940.0	E950.4	E962.0	E980.4
Meclozine (hydrochloride)	963.0	E858.1	E933.0	E950.4	E962.0	E980.4
Medazepam	969.4	E853.2	E939.4	E950.3	E962.0	E980.3
Medicine, medicinal substance	977.9	E858.9	E947.9	E950.5	E962.0	E980.5
specified NEC	977.8	E858.8	E947.8	E950.4	E962.0	E980.4
Medinal	967.0	E851	E937.0	E950.1	E962.0	E980.1
Medomin	967.0	E851	E937.0	E950.1	E962.0	E980.1
Medroxyprogesterone	962.2	E858.0	E932.2	E950.4	E962.0	E980.4
Medrysone	976.5	E858.7	E946.5	E950.4	E962.0	E980.4
Mefenamic acid	965.7	E850.7	E935.7	E950.0	E962.0	E980.0
Megahallucinogen	969.6	E854.1	E939.6	E950.3	E962.0	E980.3
Megestrol	962.2	E858.0	E932.2	E950.4	E962.0	E980.4
Meglumine	977.8	E858.8	E947.8	E950.4	E962.0	E980.4
Meladinin	976.3	E858.7	E946.3	E950.4	E962.0	E980.4
Melanizing agents	976.3	E858.7	E946.3	E950.4	E962.0	E980.4
Melarsoprol	961.1	E857	E931.1	E950.4	E962.0	E980.4
Melia azedarach	988.2	E865.3	—	E950.9	E962.1	E980.9
Mellaril	969.1	E853.0	E939.1	E950.3	E962.0	E980.3
Meloxine	976.3	E858.7	E946.3	E950.4	E962.0	E980.4
Melphalan	963.1	E858.1	E933.1	E950.4	E962.0	E980.4
Menadiol sodium diphosphate	964.3	E858.2	E934.3	E950.4	E962.0	E980.4
Menadione (sodium bisulfate)	964.3	E858.2	E934.3	E950.4	E962.0	E980.4
Menaphthone	964.3	E858.2	E934.3	E950.4	E962.0	E980.4
Meningococcal vaccine	978.8	E858.8	E948.8	E950.4	E962.0	E980.4
Menningovax–C	978.8	E858.8	E948.8	E950.4	E962.0	E980.4
Menotropins	962.4	E858.0	E932.4	E950.4	E962.0	E980.4
Menthol NEC	976.1	E858.7	E946.1	E950.4	E962.0	E980.4
Mepacrine	961.3	E857	E931.3	E950.4	E962.0	E980.4
Meparfynol	967.8	E852.8	E937.8	E950.2	E962.0	E980.2
Mepazine	969.1	E853.0	E939.1	E950.3	E962.0	E980.3
Mepenzolate	971.1	E855.4	E941.1	E950.4	E962.0	E980.4
Meperidine	965.09	E850.2	E935.2	E950.0	E962.0	E980.0
Mephenamin(e)	966.4	E855.0	E936.4	E950.4	E962.0	E980.4
Mephenesin (carbamate)	968.0	E855.1	E938.0	E950.4	E962.0	E980.4
Mephenoxalone	969.5	E853.8	E939.5	E950.3	E962.0	E980.3
Mephentermine	971.2	E855.5	E941.2	E950.4	E962.0	E980.4
Mephenytoin	966.1	E855.0	E936.1	E950.4	E962.0	E980.4
Mephobarbital	967.0	E851	E937.0	E950.1	E962.0	E980.1
Mepiperphenidol	971.1	E855.4	E941.1	E950.4	E962.0	E980.4
Mepivacaine	968.9	E855.2	E938.9	E950.4	E962.0	E980.4
infiltration (subcutaneous)	968.5	E855.2	E938.5	E950.4	E962.0	E980.4
nerve block (peripheral) (plexus)	968.6	E855.2	E938.6	E950.4	E962.0	E980.4
topical (surface)	968.5	E855.2	E938.5	E950.4	E962.0	E980.4
Meprednisone	962.0	E858.0	E932.0	E950.4	E962.0	E980.4
Meprobam	969.5	E853.8	E939.5	E950.3	E962.0	E980.3
Meprobamate	969.5	E853.8	E939.5	E950.3	E962.0	E980.3
Mepyramine (maleate)	963.0	E858.1	E933.0	E950.4	E962.0	E980.4
Meralluride	974.0	E858.5	E944.0	E950.4	E962.0	E980.4
Merbaphen	974.0	E858.5	E944.0	E950.4	E962.0	E980.4
Merbromin	976.0	E858.7	E946.0	E950.4	E962.0	E980.4
Mercaptomerin	974.0	E858.5	E944.0	E950.4	E962.0	E980.4
Mercaptopurine	963.1	E858.1	E933.1	E950.4	E962.0	E980.4
Mercumatilin	974.0	E858.5	E944.0	E950.4	E962.0	E980.4
Mercuramide	974.0	E858.5	E944.0	E950.4	E962.0	E980.4
Mercuranin	976.0	E858.7	E946.0	E950.4	E962.0	E980.4
Mercurochrome	976.0	E858.7	E946.0	E950.4	E962.0	E980.4
Mercury, mercuric, mercurous (compounds) (cyanide) (fumes) (nonmedicinal) (vapor) NEC	985.0	E866.1	—	E950.9	E962.1	E980.9
ammoniated	976.0	E858.7	E946.0	E950.4	E962.0	E980.4
anti–infective	961.2	E857	E931.2	E950.4	E962.0	E980.4

Substance	Poisoning	Accident	Therapeutic Use	Suicide Attempt	Assault	Undetermined
			External Cause (E-Code)			
topical.	976.0	E858.7	E946.0	E950.4	E962.0	E980.4
chloride (antiseptic) NEC.	976.0	E858.7	E946.0	E950.4	E962.0	E980.4
fungicide.	985.0	E863.6	—	E950.6	E962.1	E980.7
diuretic compounds	974.0	E858.5	E944.0	E950.4	E962.0	E980.4
fungicide	985.0	E863.6	—	E950.6	E962.1	E980.7
organic (fungicide)	985.0	E863.6	—	E950.6	E962.1	E980.7
Merethoxylline.	974.0	E858.5	E944.0	E950.4	E962.0	E980.4
Mersalyl	974.0	E858.5	E944.0	E950.4	E962.0	E980.4
Merthiolate (topical)	976.0	E858.7	E946.0	E950.4	E962.0	E980.4
ophthalmic preparation.	976.5	E858.7	E946.5	E950.4	E962.0	E980.4
Meruvax	979.4	E858.8	E949.4	E950.4	E962.0	E980.4
Mescal buttons.	969.6	E854.1	E939.6	E950.3	E962.0	E980.3
Mescaline (salts)	969.6	E854.1	E939.6	E950.3	E962.0	E980.3
Mesoridazine besylate	969.1	E853.0	E939.1	E950.3	E962.0	E980.3
Mestanolone.	962.1	E858.0	E932.1	E950.4	E962.0	E980.4
Mestranol	962.2	E858.0	E932.2	E950.4	E962.0	E980.4
Metacresylacetate.	976.0	E858.7	E946.0	E950.4	E962.0	E980.4
Metaldehyde (snail killer) NEC	989.4	E863.4	—	E950.6	E962.1	E980.7
Metals (heavy) (nonmedicinal) NEC	985.9	E866.4	—	E950.9	E962.1	E980.9
dust, fumes, or vapor NEC	985.9	E866.4	—	E950.9	E962.1	E980.9
light NEC	985.9	E866.4	—	E950.9	E962.1	E980.9
dust, fumes, or vapor NEC	985.9	E866.4	—	E950.9	E962.1	E980.9
pesticides (dust) (vapor)	985.9	E863.4	—	E950.6	E962.1	E980.7
Metamucil.	973.3	E858.4	E943.3	E950.4	E962.0	E980.4
Metaphen	976.0	E858.7	E946.0	E950.4	E962.0	E980.4
Metaproterenol	975.1	E858.6	E945.1	E950.4	E962.0	E980.4
Metaraminol	972.8	E858.3	E942.8	E950.4	E962.0	E980.4
Metaxalone	968.0	E855.1	E938.0	E950.4	E962.0	E980.4
Metformin.	962.3	E858.0	E932.3	E950.4	E962.0	E980.4
Methacycline	960.4	E856	E930.4	E950.4	E962.0	E980.4
Methadone	965.02	E850.1	E935.1	E950.0	E962.0	E980.0
Methallenestril	962.2	E858.0	E932.2	E950.4	E962.0	E980.4
Methamphetamine	969.72	E854.2	E939.7	E950.3	E962.0	E980.3
Methandienone.	962.1	E858.0	E932.1	E950.4	E962.0	E980.4
Methandriol	962.1	E858.0	E932.1	E950.4	E962.0	E980.4
Methandrostenolone.	962.1	E858.0	E932.1	E950.4	E962.0	E980.4
Methane gas.	987.1	E869.8	—	E952.8	E962.2	E982.8
Methanol	980.1	E860.2	—	E950.9	E962.1	E980.9
vapor	987.8	E869.8	—	E952.8	E962.2	E982.8
Methantheline	971.1	E855.4	E941.1	E950.4	E962.0	E980.4
Methaphenilene	963.0	E858.1	E933.0	E950.4	E962.0	E980.4
Methapyrilene	963.0	E858.1	E933.0	E950.4	E962.0	E980.4
Methaqualone (compounds)	967.4	E852.3	E937.4	E950.2	E962.0	E980.2
Metharbital, metharbitone	967.0	E851	E937.0	E950.1	E962.0	E980.1
Methazolamide.	974.2	E858.5	E944.2	E950.4	E962.0	E980.4
Methdilazine.	963.0	E858.1	E933.0	E950.4	E962.0	E980.4
Methedrine	969.72	E854.2	E939.7	E950.3	E962.0	E980.3
Methenamine (mandelate)	961.9	E857	E931.9	E950.4	E962.0	E980.4
Methenolone.	962.1	E858.0	E932.1	E950.4	E962.0	E980.4
Methergine	975.0	E858.6	E945.0	E950.4	E962.0	E980.4
Methiacil	962.8	E858.0	E932.8	E950.4	E962.0	E980.4
Methicillin (sodium)	960.0	E856	E930.0	E950.4	E962.0	E980.4
Methimazole.	962.8	E858.0	E932.8	E950.4	E962.0	E980.4
Methionine	977.1	E858.8	E947.1	E950.4	E962.0	E980.4
Methisazone	961.7	E857	E931.7	E950.4	E962.0	E980.4
Methitural	967.0	E851	E937.0	E950.1	E962.0	E980.1
Methixene.	971.1	E855.4	E941.1	E950.4	E962.0	E980.4
Methobarbital, methobarbitone	967.0	E851	E937.0	E950.1	E962.0	E980.1
Methocarbamol.	968.0	E855.1	E938.0	E950.4	E962.0	E980.4
Methohexital, methohexitone (sodium) . . .	968.3	E855.1	E938.3	E950.4	E962.0	E980.4

TABLE OF DRUGS AND CHEMICALS

Substance	Poisoning	Accident	Therapeutic Use	Suicide Attempt	Assault	Undetermined
			External Cause (E-Code)			
Methoin	966.1	E855.0	E936.1	E950.4	E962.0	E980.4
Methopholine	965.7	E850.7	E935.7	E950.0	E962.0	E980.0
Methorate	975.4	E858.6	E945.4	E950.4	E962.0	E980.4
Methoserpidine	972.6	E858.3	E942.6	E950.4	E962.0	E980.4
Methotrexate	963.1	E858.1	E933.1	E950.4	E962.0	E980.4
Methotrimeprazine	967.8	E852.8	E937.8	E950.2	E962.0	E980.2
Methoxa–Dome	976.3	E858.7	E946.3	E950.4	E962.0	E980.4
Methoxamine	971.2	E855.5	E941.2	E950.4	E962.0	E980.4
Methoxsalen	976.3	E858.7	E946.3	E950.4	E962.0	E980.4
Methoxybenzyl penicillin	960.0	E856	E930.0	E950.4	E962.0	E980.4
Methoxychlor	989.2	E863.0	—	E950.6	E962.1	E980.7
Methoxyflurane	968.2	E855.1	E938.2	E950.4	E962.0	E980.4
Methoxyphenamine	971.2	E855.5	E941.2	E950.4	E962.0	E980.4
Methoxypromazine	969.1	E853.0	E939.1	E950.3	E962.0	E980.3
Methoxypsoralen	976.3	E858.7	E946.3	E950.4	E962.0	E980.4
Methscopolamine (bromide)	971.1	E855.4	E941.1	E950.4	E962.0	E980.4
Methsuximide	966.2	E855.0	E936.2	E950.4	E962.0	E980.4
Methyclothiazide	974.3	E858.5	E944.3	E950.4	E962.0	E980.4
Methyl						
acetate	982.8	E862.4	—	E950.9	E962.1	E980.9
acetone	982.8	E862.4	—	E950.9	E962.1	E980.9
alcohol	980.1	E860.2	—	E950.9	E962.1	E980.9
amphetamine	969.72	E854.2	E939.7	E950.3	E962.0	E980.3
androstanolone	962.1	E858.0	E932.1	E950.4	E962.0	E980.4
atropine	971.1	E855.4	E941.1	E950.4	E962.0	E980.4
benzene	982.0	E862.4	—	E950.9	E962.1	E980.9
bromide (gas)	987.8	E869.8	—	E952.8	E962.2	E982.8
fumigant	987.8	E863.8	—	E950.6	E962.2	E980.7
butanol	980.8	E860.8	—	E950.9	E962.1	E980.9
carbinol	980.1	E860.2	—	E950.9	E962.1	E980.9
cellosolve	982.8	E862.4	—	E950.9	E962.1	E980.9
cellulose	973.3	E858.4	E943.3	E950.4	E962.0	E980.4
chloride (gas)	987.8	E869.8	—	E952.8	E962.2	E982.8
cyclohexane	982.8	E862.4	—	E950.9	E962.1	E980.9
cyclohexanone	982.8	E862.4	—	E950.9	E962.1	E980.9
dihydromorphinone	965.09	E850.2	E935.2	E950.0	E962.0	E980.0
ergometrine	975.0	E858.6	E945.0	E950.4	E962.0	E980.4
ergonovine	975.0	E858.6	E945.0	E950.4	E962.0	E980.4
ethyl ketone	982.8	E862.4	—	E950.9	E962.1	E980.9
hydrazine	983.9	E864.3	—	E950.7	E962.1	E980.6
isobutyl ketone	982.8	E862.4	—	E950.9	E962.1	E980.9
morphine NEC	965.09	E850.2	E935.2	E950.0	E962.0	E980.0
parafynol	967.8	E852.8	E937.8	E950.2	E962.0	E980.2
parathion	989.3	E863.1	—	E950.6	E962.1	E980.7
pentynol NEC	967.8	E852.8	E937.8	E950.2	E962.0	E980.2
peridol	969.2	E853.1	E939.2	E950.3	E962.0	E980.3
phenidate	969.73	E854.2	E939.7	E950.3	E962.0	E980.3
prednisolone	962.0	E858.0	E932.0	E950.4	E962.0	E980.4
ENT agent	976.6	E858.7	E946.6	E950.4	E962.0	E980.4
ophthalmic preparation	976.5	E858.7	E946.5	E950.4	E962.0	E980.4
topical NEC	976.0	E858.7	E946.0	E950.4	E962.0	E980.4
propylcarbinol	980.8	E860.8	—	E950.9	E962.1	E980.9
rosaniline NEC	976.0	E858.7	E946.0	E950.4	E962.0	E980.4
salicylate NEC	976.3	E858.7	E946.3	E950.4	E962.0	E980.4
sulfate (fumes)	987.8	E869.8	—	E952.8	E962.2	E982.8
liquid	983.9	E864.3	—	E950.7	E962.1	E980.6
sulfonal	967.8	E852.8	E937.8	E950.2	E962.0	E980.2
testosterone	962.1	E858.0	E932.1	E950.4	E962.0	E980.4
thiouracil	962.8	E858.0	E932.8	E950.4	E962.0	E980.4
Methylated spirit	980.0	E860.1	—	E950.9	E962.1	E980.9
Methyldopa	972.6	E858.3	E942.6	E950.4	E962.0	E980.4

Substance	Poisoning	Accident	Therapeutic Use	Suicide Attempt	Assault	Undetermined
			External Cause (E-Code)			
Methylene						
blue	961.9	E857	E931.9	E950.4	E962.0	E980.4
chloride or dichloride (solvent) NEC	982.3	E862.4	—	E950.9	E962.1	E980.9
Methylhexabital	967.0	E851	E937.0	E950.1	E962.0	E980.1
Methylparaben (ophthalmic)	976.5	E858.7	E946.5	E950.4	E962.0	E980.4
Methyprylon	967.5	E852.4	E937.5	E950.2	E962.0	E980.2
Methysergide	971.3	E855.6	E941.3	E950.4	E962.0	E980.4
Metoclopramide	963.0	E858.1	E933.0	E950.4	E962.0	E980.4
Metofoline	965.7	E850.7	E935.7	E950.0	E962.0	E980.0
Metopon	965.09	E850.2	E935.2	E950.0	E962.0	E980.0
Metronidazole	961.5	E857	E931.5	E950.4	E962.0	E980.4
Metycaine.	968.9	E855.2	E938.9	E950.4	E962.0	E980.4
infiltration (subcutaneous)	968.5	E855.2	E938.5	E950.4	E962.0	E980.4
nerve block (peripheral) (plexus).	968.6	E855.2	E938.6	E950.4	E962.0	E980.4
topical (surface)	968.5	E855.2	E938.5	E950.4	E962.0	E980.4
Metyrapone	977.8	E858.8	E947.8	E950.4	E962.0	E980.4
Mevinphos	989.3	E863.1	—	E950.6	E962.1	E980.7
Mezereon (berries)	988.2	E865.3	—	E950.9	E962.1	E980.9
Micatin	976.0	E858.7	E946.0	E950.4	E962.0	E980.4
Miconazole	976.0	E858.7	E946.0	E950.4	E962.0	E980.4
Midol	965.1	E850.3	E935.3	E950.0	E962.0	E980.0
Mifepristone	962.9	E858.0	E932.9	E950.4	E962.0	E980.4
Milk of magnesia.	973.0	E858.4	E943.0	E950.4	E962.0	E980.4
Millipede (tropical) (venomous).	989.5	E905.4	—	E950.9	E962.1	E980.9
Miltown	969.5	E853.8	E939.5	E950.3	E962.0	E980.3
Mineral						
oil (medicinal)	973.2	E858.4	E943.2	E950.4	E962.0	E980.4
nonmedicinal	981	E862.1	—	E950.9	E962.1	E980.9
topical.	976.3	E858.7	E946.3	E950.4	E962.0	E980.4
salts NEC	974.6	E858.5	E944.6	E950.4	E962.0	E980.4
spirits	981	E862.0	—	E950.9	E962.1	E980.9
Minocycline	960.4	E856	E930.4	E950.4	E962.0	E980.4
Mithramycin (antineoplastic)	960.7	E856	E930.7	E950.4	E962.0	E980.4
Mitobronitol	963.1	E858.1	E933.1	E950.4	E962.0	E980.4
Mitomycin (antineoplastic)	960.7	E856	E930.7	E950.4	E962.0	E980.4
Mitotane	963.1	E858.1	E933.1	E950.4	E962.0	E980.4
Moderil	972.6	E858.3	E942.6	E950.4	E962.0	E980.4
Mogadon—see Nitrazepam						
Molindone.	969.3	E853.8	E939.3	E950.3	E962.0	E980.3
Monistat	976.0	E858.7	E946.0	E950.4	E962.0	E980.4
Monkshood	988.2	E865.4	—	E950.9	E962.1	E980.9
Monoamine oxidase inhibitors	969.01	E854.0	E939.0	E950.3	E962.0	E980.3
Monochlorobenzene	982.0	E862.4	—	E950.9	E962.1	E980.9
Monosodium glutamate	989.89	E866.8	—	E950.9	E962.1	E980.9
Monoxide, carbon — see Carbon, monoxide						
Moperone.	969.2	E853.1	E939.2	E950.3	E962.0	E980.3
Morning glory seeds	969.6	E854.1	E939.6	E950.3	E962.0	E980.3
Moroxydine (hydrochloride)	961.7	E857	E931.7	E950.4	E962.0	E980.4
Morphazinamide	961.8	E857	E931.8	E950.4	E962.0	E980.4
Morphinans	965.09	E850.2	E935.2	E950.0	E962.0	E980.0
Morphine NEC.	965.09	E850.2	E935.2	E950.0	E962.0	E980.0
antagonists	970.1	E854.3	E940.1	E950.4	E962.0	E980.4
Morpholinylethylmorphine	965.09	E850.2	E935.2	E950.0	E962.0	E980.0
Morrhuate sodium	972.7	E858.3	E942.7	E950.4	E962.0	E980.4
Moth balls (see also Pesticides).	989.4	E863.4	—	E950.6	E962.1	E980.7
naphthalene	983.0	E863.4	—	E950.7	E962.1	E980.6
Motor exhaust gas — see Carbon, monoxide, exhaust gas						
Mouth wash	976.6	E858.7	E946.6	E950.4	E962.0	E980.4
Mucolytic agent	975.5	E858.6	E945.5	E950.4	E962.0	E980.4

Substance	Poisoning	Accident	Therapeutic Use	Suicide Attempt	Assault	Undetermined
			External Cause (E-Code)			
Mucomyst 975.5	E858.6	E945.5	E950.4	E962.0	E980.4
Mucous membrane agents (external) 976.9	E858.7	E946.9	E950.4	E962.0	E980.4
specified NEC 976.8	E858.7	E946.8	E950.4	E962.0	E980.4
Mumps					
immune globulin (human) 964.6	E858.2	E934.6	E950.4	E962.0	E980.4
skin test antigen 977.8	E858.8	E947.8	E950.4	E962.0	E980.4
vaccine 979.6	E858.8	E949.6	E950.4	E962.0	E980.4
Mumpsvax 979.6	E858.8	E949.6	E950.4	E962.0	E980.4
Muriatic acid — *see* Hydrochloric acid					
Muscarine 971.0	E855.3	E941.0	E950.4	E962.0	E980.4
Muscle affecting agents NEC 975.3	E858.6	E945.3	E950.4	E962.0	E980.4
oxytocic 975.0	E858.6	E945.0	E950.4	E962.0	E980.4
relaxants 975.3	E858.6	E945.3	E950.4	E962.0	E980.4
central nervous system 968.0	E855.1	E938.0	E950.4	E962.0	E980.4
skeletal 975.2	E858.6	E945.2	E950.4	E962.0	E980.4
smooth 975.1	E858.6	E945.1	E950.4	E962.0	E980.4
Mushrooms, noxious 988.1	E865.5	—	E950.9	E962.1	E980.9
Mussel, noxious 988.0	E865.1	—	E950.9	E962.1	E980.9
Mustard (emetic) 973.6	E858.4	E943.6	E950.4	E962.0	E980.4
gas 987.8	E869.8	—	E952.8	E962.2	E982.8
nitrogen 963.1	E858.1	E933.1	E950.4	E962.0	E980.4
Mustine 963.1	E858.1	E933.1	E950.4	E962.0	E980.4
M–vac 979.4	E858.8	E949.4	E950.4	E962.0	E980.4
Mycifradin 960.8	E856	E930.8	E950.4	E962.0	E980.4
topical 976.0	E858.7	E946.0	E950.4	E962.0	E980.4
Mycitracin 960.8	E856	E930.8	E950.4	E962.0	E980.4
ophthalmic preparation 976.5	E858.7	E946.5	E950.4	E962.0	E980.4
Mycostatin 960.1	E856	E930.1	E950.4	E962.0	E980.4
topical 976.0	E858.7	E946.0	E950.4	E962.0	E980.4
Mydriacyl 971.1	E855.4	E941.1	E950.4	E962.0	E980.4
Myelobromal 963.1	E858.1	E933.1	E950.4	E962.0	E980.4
Myleran 963.1	E858.1	E933.1	E950.4	E962.0	E980.4
Myochrysin(e) 965.69	E850.6	E935.6	E950.0	E962.0	E980.0
Myoneural blocking agents 975.2	E858.6	E945.2	E950.4	E962.0	E980.4
Myristica fragrans 988.2	E865.3	—	E950.9	E962.1	E980.9
Myristicin 988.2	E865.3	—	E950.9	E962.1	E980.9
Mysoline 966.3	E855.0	E936.3	E950.4	E962.0	E980.4
Nafcillin (sodium) 960.0	E856	E930.0	E950.4	E962.0	E980.4
Nail polish remover 982.8	E862.4	—	E950.9	E962.1	E980.9
Nalidixic acid 961.9	E857	E931.9	E950.4	E962.0	E980.4
Nalorphine 970.1	E854.3	E940.1	E950.4	E962.0	E980.4
Naloxone 970.1	E854.3	E940.1	E950.4	E962.0	E980.4
Nandrolone (decanoate) (phenproprioate) . . . 962.1	E858.0	E932.1	E950.4	E962.0	E980.4
Naphazoline 971.2	E855.5	E941.2	E950.4	E962.0	E980.4
Naphtha (painter's) (petroleum) 981	E862.0	—	E950.9	E962.1	E980.9
solvent 981	E862.0	—	E950.9	E962.1	E980.9
vapor 987.1	E869.8	—	E952.8	E962.2	E982.8
Naphthalene (chlorinated) 983.0	E864.0	—	E950.7	E962.1	E980.6
insecticide or moth repellent 983.0	E863.4	—	E950.7	E962.1	E980.6
vapor 987.8	E869.8	—	E952.8	E962.2	E982.8
Naphthol 983.0	E864.0	—	E950.7	E962.1	E980.6
Naphthylamine 983.0	E864.0	—	E950.7	E962.1	E980.6
Naprosyn—*see* Naproxen					
Naproxen 965.61	E850.6	E935.6	E950.0	E962.0	E980.0
Narcotic (drug) 967.9	E852.9	E937.9	E950.2	E962.0	E980.2
analgesic NEC 965.8	E850.8	E935.8	E950.0	E962.0	E980.0
antagonist 970.1	E854.3	E940.1	E950.4	E962.0	E980.4
specified NEC 967.8	E852.8	E937.8	E950.2	E962.0	E980.2
Narcotine 975.4	E858.6	E945.4	E950.4	E962.0	E980.4
Nardil 969.01	E854.0	E939.0	E950.3	E962.0	E980.3
Natrium cyanide — *see* Cyanide(s)					

Substance	Poisoning	Accident	Therapeutic Use	Suicide Attempt	Assault	Undetermined
			External Cause (E-Code)			
Natural						
blood (product)	964.7	E858.2	E934.7	E950.4	E962.0	E980.4
gas (piped)	987.1	E867	—	E951.0	E962.2	E981.0
incomplete combustion	986	E867	—	E951.0	E962.2	E981.0
Nealbarbital, nealbarbitone	967.0	E851	E937.0	E950.1	E962.0	E980.1
Nectadon	975.4	E858.6	E945.4	E950.4	E962.0	E980.4
Nematocyst (sting)	989.5	E905.6	—	E950.9	E962.1	E980.9
Nembutal	967.0	E851	E937.0	E950.1	E962.0	E980.1
Neoarsphenamine	961.1	E857	E931.1	E950.4	E962.0	E980.4
Neocinchophen	974.7	E858.5	E944.7	E950.4	E962.0	E980.4
Neomycin	960.8	E856	E930.8	E950.4	E962.0	E980.4
ENT agent	976.6	E858.7	E946.6	E950.4	E962.0	E980.4
ophthalmic preparation	976.5	E858.7	E946.5	E950.4	E962.0	E980.4
topical NEC	976.0	E858.7	E946.0	E950.4	E962.0	E980.4
Neonal	967.0	E851	E937.0	E950.1	E962.0	E980.1
Neoprontosil	961.0	E857	E931.0	E950.4	E962.0	E980.4
Neosalvarsan	961.1	E857	E931.1	E950.4	E962.0	E980.4
Neosilversalvarsan	961.1	E857	E931.1	E950.4	E962.0	E980.4
Neosporin	960.8	E856	E930.8	E950.4	E962.0	E980.4
ENT agent	976.6	E858.7	E946.6	E950.4	E962.0	E980.4
ophthalmic preparation	976.5	E858.7	E946.5	E950.4	E962.0	E980.4
topical NEC	976.0	E858.7	E946.0	E950.4	E962.0	E980.4
Neostigmine	971.0	E855.3	E941.0	E950.4	E962.0	E980.4
Neraval	967.0	E851	E937.0	E950.1	E962.0	E980.1
Neravan	967.0	E851	E937.0	E950.1	E962.0	E980.1
Nerium oleander	988.2	E865.4	—	E950.9	E962.1	E980.9
Nerve gases (war)	987.9	E869.9	—	E952.9	E962.2	E982.9
Nesacaine	968.9	E855.2	E938.9	E950.4	E962.0	E980.4
infiltration (subcutaneous)	968.5	E855.2	E938.5	E950.4	E962.0	E980.4
nerve block (peripheral) (plexus)	968.6	E855.2	E938.6	E950.4	E962.0	E980.4
Neurobarb	967.0	E851	E937.0	E950.1	E962.0	E980.1
Neuroleptics NEC	969.3	E853.8	E939.3	E950.3	E962.0	E980.3
Neuroprotective agent	977.8	E858.8	E947.8	E950.4	E962.0	E980.4
Neutral spirits	980.0	E860.1	—	E950.9	E962.1	E980.9
beverage	980.0	E860.0	—	E950.9	E962.1	E980.9
Niacin, niacinamide	972.2	E858.3	E942.2	E950.4	E962.0	E980.4
Nialamide	969.01	E854.0	E939.0	E950.3	E962.0	E980.3
Nickle (carbonyl) (compounds) (fumes) (tetracarbonyl) (vapor)	985.8	E866.4	—	E950.9	E962.1	E980.9
Niclosamide	961.6	E857	E931.6	E950.4	E962.0	E980.4
Nicomorphine	965.09	E850.2	E935.2	E950.0	E962.0	E980.0
Nicotinamide	972.2	E858.3	E942.2	E950.4	E962.0	E980.4
Nicotine (insecticide) (spray) (sulfate) NEC	989.4	E863.4	—	E950.6	E962.1	E980.7
not insecticide	989.89	E866.8	—	E950.9	E962.1	E980.9
Nicotinic acid (derivatives)	972.2	E858.3	E942.2	E950.4	E962.0	E980.4
Nicotinyl alcohol	972.2	E858.3	E942.2	E950.4	E962.0	E980.4
Nicoumalone	964.2	E858.2	E934.2	E950.4	E962.0	E980.4
Nifenazone	965.5	E850.5	E935.5	E950.0	E962.0	E980.0
Nifuraldezone	961.9	E857	E931.9	E950.4	E962.0	E980.4
Nightshade (deadly)	988.2	E865.4	—	E950.9	E962.1	E980.9
Nikethamide	970.0	E854.3	E940.0	E950.4	E962.0	E980.4
Nilstat	960.1	E856	E930.1	E950.4	E962.0	E980.4
topical	976.0	E858.7	E946.0	E950.4	E962.0	E980.4
Nimodipine	977.8	E858.8	E947.8	E950.4	E962.0	E980.4
Niridazole	961.6	E857	E931.6	E950.4	E962.0	E980.4
Nisentil	965.09	E850.2	E935.2	E950.0	E962.0	E980.0
Nitrates	972.4	E858.3	E942.4	E950.4	E962.0	E980.4
Nitrazepam	969.4	E853.2	E939.4	E950.3	E962.0	E980.3
Nitric						
acid (liquid)	983.1	E864.1	—	E950.7	E962.1	E980.6

Substance	Poisoning	Accident	Therapeutic Use	Suicide Attempt	Assault	Undetermined
			External Cause (E-Code)			
vapor	987.8	E869.8	—	E952.8	E962.2	E982.8
oxide (gas)	987.2	E869.0	—	E952.8	E962.2	E982.8
Nitrite, amyl (medicinal) (vapor)	972.4	E858.3	E942.4	E950.4	E962.0	E980.4
Nitroaniline	983.0	E864.0	—	E950.7	E962.1	E980.6
vapor	987.8	E869.8	—	E952.8	E962.2	E982.8
Nitrobenzene, nitrobenzol	983.0	E864.0	—	E950.7	E962.1	E980.6
vapor	987.8	E869.8	—	E952.8	E962.2	E982.8
Nitrocellulose	976.3	E858.7	E946.3	E950.4	E962.0	E980.4
Nitrofuran derivatives	961.9	E857	E931.9	E950.4	E962.0	E980.4
Nitrofurantoin	961.9	E857	E931.9	E950.4	E962.0	E980.4
Nitrofurazone	976.0	E858.7	E946.0	E950.4	E962.0	E980.4
Nitrogen (dioxide) (gas) (oxide)	987.2	E869.0	—	E952.8	E962.2	E982.8
mustard (antineoplastic)	963.1	E858.1	E933.1	E950.4	E962.0	E980.4
Nitroglycerin, nitroglycerol (medicinal)	972.4	E858.3	E942.4	E950.4	E962.0	E980.4
nonmedicinal	989.89	E866.8	—	E950.9	E962.1	E980.9
fumes	987.8	E869.8	—	E952.8	E962.2	E982.8
Nitrohydrochloric acid	983.1	E864.1	—	E950.7	E962.1	E980.6
Nitromersol	976.0	E858.7	E946.0	E950.4	E962.0	E980.4
Nitronaphthalene	983.0	E864.0	—	E950.7	E962.2	E980.6
Nitrophenol	983.0	E864.0	—	E950.7	E962.2	E980.6
Nitrothiazol	961.6	E857	E931.6	E950.4	E962.0	E980.4
Nitrotoluene, nitrotoluol	983.0	E864.0	—	E950.7	E962.1	E980.6
vapor	987.8	E869.8	—	E952.8	E962.2	E982.8
Nitrous	968.2	E855.1	E938.2	E950.4	E962.0	E980.4
acid (liquid)	983.1	E864.1	—	E950.7	E962.1	E980.6
fumes	987.2	E869.0	—	E952.8	E962.2	E982.8
oxide (anesthetic) NEC	968.2	E855.1	E938.2	E950.4	E962.0	E980.4
Nitrozone	976.0	E858.7	E946.0	E950.4	E962.0	E980.4
Noctec	967.1	E852.0	E937.1	E950.2	E962.0	E980.2
Noludar	967.5	E852.4	E937.5	E950.2	E962.0	E980.2
Noptil	967.0	E851	E937.0	E950.1	E962.0	E980.1
Noradrenalin	971.2	E855.5	E941.2	E950.4	E962.0	E980.4
Noramidopyrine	965.5	E850.5	E935.5	E950.0	E962.0	E980.0
Norepinephrine	971.2	E855.5	E941.2	E950.4	E962.0	E980.4
Norethandrolone	962.1	E858.0	E932.1	E950.4	E962.0	E980.4
Norethindrone	962.2	E858.0	E932.2	E950.4	E962.0	E980.4
Norethisterone	962.2	E858.0	E932.2	E950.4	E962.0	E980.4
Norethynodrel	962.2	E858.0	E932.2	E950.4	E962.0	E980.4
Norlestrin	962.2	E858.0	E932.2	E950.4	E962.0	E980.4
Norlutin	962.2	E858.0	E932.2	E950.4	E962.0	E980.4
Normison—see Benzodiazepines						
Normorphine	965.09	E850.2	E935.2	E950.0	E962.0	E980.0
Nortriptyline	969.05	E854.0	E939.0	E950.3	E962.0	E980.3
Noscapine	975.4	E858.6	E945.4	E950.4	E962.0	E980.4
Nose preparations	976.6	E858.7	E946.6	E950.4	E962.0	E980.4
Novobiocin	960.8	E856	E930.8	E950.4	E962.0	E980.4
Novocain (infiltration) (topical)	968.5	E855.2	E938.5	E950.4	E962.0	E980.4
nerve block (peripheral) (plexus)	968.6	E855.2	E938.6	E950.4	E962.0	E980.4
spinal	968.7	E855.2	E938.7	E950.4	E962.0	E980.4
Noxythiolin	961.9	E857	E931.9	E950.4	E962.0	E980.4
NPH Iletin (insulin)	962.3	E858.0	E932.3	E950.4	E962.0	E980.4
Numorphan	965.09	E850.2	E935.2	E950.0	E962.0	E980.0
Nunol	967.0	E851	E937.0	E950.1	E962.0	E980.1
Nupercaine (spinal anesthetic)	968.7	E855.2	E938.7	E950.4	E962.0	E980.4
topical (surface)	968.5	E855.2	E938.5	E950.4	E962.0	E980.4
Nutmeg oil (liniment)	976.3	E858.7	E946.3	E950.4	E962.0	E980.4
Nux vomica	989.1	E863.7	—	E950.6	E962.1	E980.7
Nydrazid	961.8	E857	E931.8	E950.4	E962.0	E980.4
Nylidrin	971.2	E855.5	E941.2	E950.4	E962.0	E980.4
Nystatin	960.1	E856	E930.1	E950.4	E962.0	E980.4
topical	976.0	E858.7	E946.0	E950.4	E962.0	E980.4

Substance	Poisoning	Accident	Therapeutic Use	Suicide Attempt	Assault	Undetermined
		External Cause (E-Code)				
Nytol	963.0	E858.1	E933.0	E950.4	E962.0	E980.4
Oblivion	967.8	E852.8	E937.8	E950.2	E962.0	E980.2
Octyl nitrite	972.4	E858.3	E942.4	E950.4	E962.0	E980.4
Oestradiol (cypionate) (dipropionate) (valerate)	962.2	E858.0	E932.2	E950.4	E962.0	E980.4
Oestriol	962.2	E858.0	E932.2	E950.4	E962.0	E980.4
Oestrone	962.2	E858.0	E932.2	E950.4	E962.0	E980.4
Oil (of) NEC	989.89	E866.8	—	E950.9	E962.1	E980.9
bitter almond	989.0	E866.8	—	E950.9	E962.1	E980.9
camphor	976.1	E858.7	E946.1	E950.4	E962.0	E980.4
colors	989.89	E861.6	—	E950.9	E962.1	E980.9
fumes	987.8	E869.8	—	E952.8	E962.2	E982.8
lubricating	981	E862.2	—	E950.9	E962.1	E980.9
specified source, other — see substance specified						
vitriol (liquid)	983.1	E864.1	—	E950.7	E962.1	E980.6
fumes	987.8	E869.8	—	E952.8	E962.2	E982.8
wintergreen (bitter) NEC	976.3	E858.7	E946.3	E950.4	E962.0	E980.4
Ointments NEC	976.9	E858.7	E946.9	E950.4	E962.0	E980.4
Oleander	988.2	E865.4	—	E950.9	E962.1	E980.9
Oleandomycin	960.3	E856	E930.3	E950.4	E962.0	E980.4
Oleovitamin A	963.5	E858.1	E933.5	E950.4	E962.0	E980.4
Oleum ricini	973.1	E858.4	E943.1	E950.4	E962.0	E980.4
Olive oil (medicinal) NEC	973.2	E858.4	E943.2	E950.4	E962.0	E980.4
OMPA	989.3	E863.1	—	E950.6	E962.1	E980.7
Oncovin	963.1	E858.1	E933.1	E950.4	E962.0	E980.4
Ophthaine	968.5	E855.2	E938.5	E950.4	E962.0	E980.4
Ophthetic	968.5	E855.2	E938.5	E950.4	E962.0	E980.4
Opiates, opioids, opium NEC	965.00	E850.2	E935.2	E950.0	E962.0	E980.0
antagonists	970.1	E854.3	E940.1	E950.4	E962.0	E980.4
Oracon	962.2	E858.0	E932.2	E950.4	E962.0	E980.4
Oragrafin	977.8	E858.8	E947.8	E950.4	E962.0	E980.4
Oral contraceptives	962.2	E858.0	E932.2	E950.4	E962.0	E980.4
Orciprenaline	975.1	E858.6	E945.1	E950.4	E962.0	E980.4
Organidin	975.5	E858.6	E945.5	E950.4	E962.0	E980.4
Organophosphates	989.3	E863.1	—	E950.6	E962.1	E980.7
Orimune	979.5	E858.8	E949.5	E950.4	E962.0	E980.4
Orinase	962.3	E858.0	E932.3	E950.4	E962.0	E980.4
Orphenadrine	966.4	E855.0	E936.4	E950.4	E962.0	E980.4
Ortal (sodium)	967.0	E851	E937.0	E950.1	E962.0	E980.1
Orthoboric acid	976.0	E858.7	E946.0	E950.4	E962.0	E980.4
ENT agent	976.6	E858.7	E946.6	E950.4	E962.0	E980.4
ophthalmic preparation	976.5	E858.7	E946.5	E950.4	E962.0	E980.4
Orthocaine	968.5	E855.2	E938.5	E950.4	E962.0	E980.4
Ortho–Novum	962.2	E858.0	E932.2	E950.4	E962.0	E980.4
Orthotolidine (reagent)	977.8	E858.8	E947.8	E950.4	E962.0	E980.4
Osmic acid (liquid)	983.1	E864.1	—	E950.7	E962.1	E980.6
fumes	987.8	E869.8	—	E952.8	E962.2	E982.8
Osmotic diuretics	974.4	E858.5	E944.4	E950.4	E962.0	E980.4
Ouabain	972.1	E858.3	E942.1	E950.4	E962.0	E980.4
Ovarian hormones (synthetic substitutes)	962.2	E858.0	E932.2	E950.4	E962.0	E980.4
Ovral	962.2	E858.0	E932.2	E950.4	E962.0	E980.4
Ovulation suppressants	962.2	E858.0	E932.2	E950.4	E962.0	E980.4
Ovulen	962.2	E858.0	E932.2	E950.4	E962.0	E980.4
Oxacillin (sodium)	960.0	E856	E930.0	E950.4	E962.0	E980.4
Oxalic acid	983.1	E864.1	—	E950.7	E962.1	E980.6
Oxanamide	969.5	E853.8	E939.5	E950.3	E962.0	E980.3
Oxandrolone	962.1	E858.0	E932.1	E950.4	E962.0	E980.4
Oxaprozin	965.61	E850.6	E935.6	E950.0	E962.0	E980.0
Oxazepam	969.4	E853.2	E939.4	E950.3	E962.0	E980.3

Substance	Poisoning	Accident	Therapeutic Use	Suicide Attempt	Assault	Undetermined
			External Cause (E-Code)			
Oxazolidine derivatives	966.0	E855.0	E936.0	E950.4	E962.0	E980.4
Ox bile extract	973.4	E858.4	E943.4	E950.4	E962.0	E980.4
Oxedrine	971.2	E855.5	E941.2	E950.4	E962.0	E980.4
Oxeladin	975.4	E858.6	E945.4	E950.4	E962.0	E980.4
Oxethazaine NEC	968.5	E855.2	E938.5	E950.4	E962.0	E980.4
Oxidizing agents NEC	983.9	E864.3	—	E950.7	E962.1	E980.6
Oxolinic acid	961.3	E857	E931.3	E950.4	E962.0	E980.4
Oxophenarsine	961.1	E857	E931.1	E950.4	E962.0	E980.4
Oxsoralen	976.3	E858.7	E946.3	E950.4	E962.0	E980.4
Oxtriphylline	975.7	E858.6	E945.7	E950.4	E962.0	E980.4
Oxybuprocaine	968.5	E855.2	E938.5	E950.4	E962.0	E980.4
Oxybutynin	975.1	E858.6	E945.1	E950.4	E962.0	E980.4
Oxycodone	965.09	E850.2	E935.2	E950.0	E962.0	E980.0
Oxygen	987.8	E869.8	—	E952.8	E962.2	E982.8
Oxylone	976.0	E858.7	E946.0	E950.4	E962.0	E980.4
ophthalmic preparation	976.5	E858.7	E946.5	E950.4	E962.0	E980.4
Oxymesterone	962.1	E858.0	E932.1	E950.4	E962.0	E980.4
Oxymetazoline	971.2	E855.5	E941.2	E950.4	E962.0	E980.4
Oxymetholone	962.1	E858.0	E932.1	E950.4	E962.0	E980.4
Oxymorphone	965.09	E850.2	E935.2	E950.0	E962.0	E980.0
Oxypertine	969.09	E854.0	E939.0	E950.3	E962.0	E980.3
Oxyphenbutazone	965.5	E850.5	E935.5	E950.0	E962.0	E980.0
Oxyphencyclimine	971.1	E855.4	E941.1	E950.4	E962.0	E980.4
Oxyphenisatin	973.1	E858.4	E943.1	E950.4	E962.0	E980.4
Oxyphenonium	971.1	E855.4	E941.1	E950.4	E962.0	E980.4
Oxyquinoline	961.3	E857	E931.3	E950.4	E962.0	E980.4
Oxytetracycline	960.4	E856	E930.4	E950.4	E962.0	E980.4
Oxytocics	975.0	E858.6	E945.0	E950.4	E962.0	E980.4
Oxytocin	975.0	E858.6	E945.0	E950.4	E962.0	E980.4
Ozone	987.8	E869.8	—	E952.8	E962.2	E982.8
PABA	976.3	E858.7	E946.3	E950.4	E962.0	E980.4
Packed red cells	964.7	E858.2	E934.7	E950.4	E962.0	E980.4
Paint NEC	989.89	E861.6	—	E950.9	E962.1	E980.9
cleaner	982.8	E862.9	—	E950.9	E962.1	E980.9
fumes NEC	987.8	E869.8	—	E952.8	E962.1	E982.8
lead (fumes)	984.0	E861.5	—	E950.9	E962.1	E980.9
solvent NEC	982.8	E862.9	—	E950.9	E962.1	E980.9
stripper	982.8	E862.9	—	E950.9	E962.1	E980.9
Palfium	965.09	E850.2	E935.2	E950.0	E962.0	E980.0
Palivizumab	979.9	E858.8	E949.6	E950.4	E962.0	E980.4
Paludrine	961.4	E857	E931.4	E950.4	E962.0	E980.4
PAM	977.2	E855.8	E947.2	E950.4	E962.0	E980.4
Pamaquine (naphthoate)	961.4	E857	E931.4	E950.4	E962.0	E980.4
Pamprin	965.1	E850.3	E935.3	E950.0	E962.0	E980.0
Panadol	965.4	E850.4	E935.4	E950.0	E962.0	E980.0
Pancreatic dornase (mucolytic)	963.4	E858.1	E933.4	E950.4	E962.0	E980.4
Pancreatin	973.4	E858.4	E943.4	E950.4	E962.0	E980.4
Pancrelipase	973.4	E858.4	E943.4	E950.4	E962.0	E980.4
Pangamic acid	963.5	E858.1	E933.5	E950.4	E962.0	E980.4
Panthenol	963.5	E858.1	E933.5	E950.4	E962.0	E980.4
topical	976.8	E858.7	E946.8	E950.4	E962.0	E980.4
Pantopaque	977.8	E858.8	E947.8	E950.4	E962.0	E980.4
Pantopon	965.00	E850.2	E935.2	E950.0	E962.0	E980.0
Pantothenic acid	963.5	E858.1	E933.5	E950.4	E962.0	E980.4
Panwarfin	964.2	E858.2	E934.2	E950.4	E962.0	E980.4
Papain	973.4	E858.4	E943.4	E950.4	E962.0	E980.4
Papaverine	972.5	E858.3	E942.5	E950.4	E962.0	E980.4
Para–aminobenzoic acid	976.3	E858.7	E946.3	E950.4	E962.0	E980.4
Para–aminophenol derivatives	965.4	E850.4	E935.4	E950.0	E962.0	E980.0
Para–aminosalicylic acid (derivatives)	961.8	E857	E931.8	E950.4	E962.0	E980.4
Paracetaldehyde (medicinal)	967.2	E852.1	E937.2	E950.2	E962.0	E980.2

Substance	Poisoning	Accident	Therapeutic Use	Suicide Attempt	Assault	Undetermined
			External Cause (E-Code)			
Paracetamol	965.4	E850.4	E935.4	E950.0	E962.0	E980.0
Paracodin	965.09	E850.2	E935.2	E950.0	E962.0	E980.0
Paradione	966.0	E855.0	E936.0	E950.4	E962.0	E980.4
Paraffin(s) (wax)	981	E862.3	—	E950.9	E962.1	E980.9
liquid (medicinal)	973.2	E858.4	E943.2	E950.4	E962.0	E980.4
nonmedicinal (oil)	981	E962.1	—	E950.9	E962.1	E980.9
Paraldehyde (medicinal)	967.2	E852.1	E937.2	E950.2	E962.0	E980.2
Paramethadione	966.0	E855.0	E936.0	E950.4	E962.0	E980.4
Paramethasone	962.0	E858.0	E932.0	E950.4	E962.0	E980.4
Paraquat	989.4	E863.5	—	E950.6	E962.1	E980.7
Parasympatholytics	971.1	E855.4	E941.1	E950.4	E962.0	E980.4
Parasympathomimetics.	971.0	E855.3	E941.0	E950.4	E962.0	E980.4
Parathion	989.3	E863.1	—	E950.6	E962.1	E980.7
Parathormone	962.6	E858.0	E932.6	E950.4	E962.0	E980.4
Parathyroid (derivatives)	962.6	E858.0	E932.6	E950.4	E962.0	E980.4
Paratyphoid vaccine.	978.1	E858.8	E948.1	E950.4	E962.0	E980.4
Paredrine	971.2	E855.5	E941.2	E950.4	E962.0	E980.4
Paregoric	965.00	E850.2	E935.2	E950.0	E962.0	E980.0
Pargyline	972.3	E858.3	E942.3	E950.4	E962.0	E980.4
Paris green	985.1	E866.3	—	E950.8	E962.1	E980.8
insecticide	985.1	E863.4	—	E950.8	E962.1	E980.8
Parnate	969.01	E854.0	E939.0	E950.3	E962.0	E980.3
Paromomycin	960.8	E856	E930.8	E950.4	E962.0	E980.4
Paroxypropione.	963.1	E858.1	E933.1	E950.4	E962.0	E980.4
Parzone.	965.09	E850.2	E935.2	E950.0	E962.0	E980.0
PAS	961.8	E857	E931.8	E950.4	E962.0	E980.4
PCBs.	981	E862.3	—	E950.9	E962.1	E980.9
PCP (pentachlorophenol).	989.4	E863.6	—	E950.6	E962.1	E980.7
herbicide	989.4	E863.5	—	E950.6	E962.1	E980.7
insecticide	989.4	E863.4	—	E950.6	E962.1	E980.7
phencyclidine.	968.3	E855.1	E938.3	E950.4	E962.0	E980.4
Peach kernel oil (emulsion)	973.2	E858.4	E943.2	E950.4	E962.0	E980.4
Peanut oil (emulsion) NEC.	973.2	E858.4	E943.2	E950.4	E962.0	E980.4
topical	976.3	E858.7	E946.3	E950.4	E962.0	E980.4
Pearly Gates (morning glory seeds)	969.6	E854.1	E939.6	E950.3	E962.0	E980.3
Pecazine	969.1	E853.0	E939.1	E950.3	E962.0	E980.3
Pecilocin	960.1	E856	E930.1	E950.4	E962.0	E980.4
Pectin (with kaolin) NEC	973.5	E858.4	E943.5	E950.4	E962.0	E980.4
Pelletierine tannate	961.6	E857	E931.6	E950.4	E962.0	E980.4
Pemoline	969.79	E854.2	E939.7	E950.3	E962.0	E980.3
Pempidine.	972.3	E858.3	E942.3	E950.4	E962.0	E980.4
Penamecillin.	960.0	E856	E930.0	E950.4	E962.0	E980.4
Penethamate hydriodide	960.0	E856	E930.0	E950.4	E962.0	E980.4
Penicillamine	963.8	E858.1	E933.8	E950.4	E962.0	E980.4
Penicillin (any type)	960.0	E856	E930.0	E950.4	E962.0	E980.4
Penicillinase.	963.4	E858.1	E933.4	E950.4	E962.0	E980.4
Pentachlorophenol (fungicide).	989.4	E863.6	—	E950.6	E962.1	E980.7
herbicide	989.4	E863.5	—	E950.6	E962.1	E980.7
insecticide	989.4	E863.4	—	E950.6	E962.1	E980.7
Pentaerythritol	972.4	E858.3	E942.4	E950.4	E962.0	E980.4
chloral	967.1	E852.0	E937.1	E950.2	E962.0	E980.2
tetranitrate NEC	972.4	E858.3	E942.4	E950.4	E962.0	E980.4
Pentagastrin	977.8	E858.8	E947.8	E950.4	E962.0	E980.4
Pentalin.	982.3	E862.4	—	E950.9	E962.1	E980.9
Pentamethonium (bromide).	972.3	E858.3	E942.3	E950.4	E962.0	E980.4
Pentamidine	961.5	E857	E931.5	E950.4	E962.0	E980.4
Pentanol	980.8	E860.8	—	E950.9	E962.1	E980.9
Pentaquine	961.4	E857	E931.4	E950.4	E962.0	E980.4
Pentazocine	965.8	E850.8	E935.8	E950.0	E962.0	E980.0
Penthienate	971.1	E855.4	E941.1	E950.4	E962.0	E980.4

Substance	Poisoning	Accident	Therapeutic Use	Suicide Attempt	Assault	Undetermined
			External Cause (E-Code)			
Pentobarbital, pentobarbitone (sodium)	967.0	E851	E937.0	E950.1	E962.0	E980.1
Pentolinium (tartrate)	972.3	E858.3	E942.3	E950.4	E962.0	E980.4
Pentothal	968.3	E855.1	E938.3	E950.4	E962.0	E980.4
Pentylenetetrazol	970.0	E854.3	E940.0	E950.4	E962.0	E980.4
Pentylsalicylamide	961.8	E857	E931.8	E950.4	E962.0	E980.4
Pepsin	973.4	E858.4	E943.4	E950.4	E962.0	E980.4
Peptavlon	977.8	E858.8	E947.8	E950.4	E962.0	E980.4
Percaine (spinal)	968.7	E855.2	E938.7	E950.4	E962.0	E980.4
topical (surface)	968.5	E855.2	E938.5	E950.4	E962.0	E980.4
Perchloroethylene (vapor)	982.3	E862.4	—	E950.9	E962.1	E980.9
medicinal	961.6	E857	E931.6	E950.4	E962.0	E980.4
Percodan	965.09	E850.2	E935.2	E950.0	E962.0	E980.0
Percogesic.	965.09	E850.2	E935.2	E950.0	E962.0	E980.0
Percorten	962.0	E858.0	E932.0	E950.4	E962.0	E980.4
Pergonal	962.4	E858.0	E932.4	E950.4	E962.0	E980.4
Perhexiline	972.4	E858.3	E942.4	E950.4	E962.0	E980.4
Periactin	963.0	E858.1	E933.0	E950.4	E962.0	E980.4
Periclor	967.1	E852.0	E937.1	E950.2	E962.0	E980.2
Pericyazine	969.1	E853.0	E939.1	E950.3	E962.0	E980.3
Peritrate	972.4	E858.3	E942.4	E950.4	E962.0	E980.4
Permanganates NEC	983.9	E864.3	—	E950.7	E962.1	E980.6
potassium (topical)	976.0	E858.7	E946.0	E950.4	E962.0	E980.4
Pernocton	967.0	E851	E937.0	E950.1	E962.0	E980.1
Pernoston	967.0	E851	E937.0	E950.1	E962.0	E980.1
Peronin(e).	965.09	E850.2	E935.2	E950.0	E962.0	E980.0
Perphenazine	969.1	E853.0	E939.1	E950.3	E962.0	E980.3
Pertofrane	969.05	E854	E939.0	E950.3	E962.0	E980.3
Pertussis						
immune serum (human)	964.6	E858.2	E934.6	E950.4	E962.0	E980.4
vaccine (with diphtheria toxoid) (with						
tetanus toxoid).	978.6	E858.8	E948.6	E950.4	E962.0	E980.4
Peruvian balsam	976.8	E858.7	E946.8	E950.4	E962.0	E980.4
Pesticides (dust) (fumes) (vapor)	989.4	E863.4	—	E950.6	E962.1	E980.7
arsenic	985.1	E863.4	—	E950.8	E962.1	E980.8
chlorinated.	989.2	E863.0	—	E950.6	E962.1	E980.7
cyanide	989.0	E863.4	—	E950.6	E962.1	E980.7
kerosene.	981	E863.4	—	E950.6	E962.1	E980.7
mixture (of compounds)	989.4	E863.3	—	E950.6	E962.1	E980.7
naphthalene	983.0	E863.4	—	E950.7	E962.1	E980.6
organochlorine (compounds)	989.2	E863.0	—	E950.6	E962.1	E980.7
petroleum (distillate) (products)						
NEC	981	E863.4	—	E950.6	E962.1	E980.7
specified ingredient NEC.	989.4	E863.4	—	E950.6	E962.1	E980.7
strychnine	989.1	E863.4	—	E950.6	E962.1	E980.7
thallium	985.8	E863.7	—	E950.6	E962.1	E980.7
Pethidine (hydrochloride)	965.09	E850.2	E935.2	E950.0	E962.0	E980.0
Petrichloral	967.1	E852.0	E937.1	E950.2	E962.0	E980.2
Petrol.	981	E862.1	—	E950.9	E962.1	E980.9
vapor	987.1	E869.8	—	E952.8	E962.2	E982.8
Petrolatum (jelly) (ointment)	976.3	E858.7	E946.3	E950.4	E962.0	E980.4
hydrophilic.	976.3	E858.7	E946.3	E950.4	E962.0	E980.4
liquid	973.2	E858.4	E943.2	E950.4	E962.0	E980.4
topical.	976.3	E858.7	E946.3	E950.4	E962.0	E980.4
nonmedicinal.	981	E862.1	—	E950.9	E962.1	E980.9
Petroleum (cleaners) (fuels) (products)						
NEC	981	E862.1	—	E950.9	E962.1	E980.9
benzin(e) — see Ligroin						
ether — see Ligroin						
jelly — see Petrolatum						
naphtha — see Ligroin						
pesticide.	981	E863.4	—	E950.6	E962.1	E980.7

Substance	Poisoning	Accident	Therapeutic Use	Suicide Attempt	Assault	Undetermined
			External Cause (E-Code)			
solids	981	E862.3	—	E950.9	E962.1	E980.9
solvents	981	E862.0	—	E950.9	E962.1	E980.9
vapor	987.1	E869.8	—	E952.8	E962.2	E982.8
Peyote	969.6	E854.1	E939.6	E950.3	E962.0	E980.3
Phanodorm, phanodorn	967.0	E851	E937.0	E950.1	E962.0	E980.1
Phanquinone, phanquone	961.5	E857	E931.5	E950.4	E962.0	E980.4
Pharmaceutical excipient or adjunct	977.4	E858.8	E947.4	E950.4	E962.0	E980.4
Phenacemide.	966.3	E855.0	E936.3	E950.4	E962.0	E980.4
Phenacetin	965.4	E850.4	E935.4	E950.0	E962.0	E980.0
Phenadoxone.	965.09	E850.2	E935.2	E950.0	E962.0	E980.0
Phenaglycodol	969.5	E853.8	E939.5	E950.3	E962.0	E980.3
Phenantoin	966.1	E855.0	E936.1	E950.4	E962.0	E980.4
Phenaphthazine reagent	977.8	E858.8	E947.8	E950.4	E962.0	E980.4
Phenazocine.	965.09	E850.2	E935.2	E950.0	E962.0	E980.0
Phenazone.	965.5	E850.5	E935.5	E950.0	E962.0	E980.0
Phenazopyridine	976.1	E858.7	E946.1	E950.4	E962.0	E980.4
Phenbenicillin	960.0	E856	E930.0	E950.4	E962.0	E980.4
Phenbutrazate	977.0	E858.8	E947.0	E950.4	E962.0	E980.4
Phencyclidine	968.3	E855.1	E938.3	E950.4	E962.0	E980.4
Phendimetrazine	977.0	E858.8	E947.0	E950.4	E962.0	E980.4
Phenelzine	969.01	E854.0	E939.0	E950.3	E962.0	E980.3
Phenergan.	967.8	E852.8	E937.8	E950.2	E962.0	E980.2
Phenethicillin (potassium)	960.0	E856	E930.0	E950.4	E962.0	E980.4
Phenetsal	965.1	E850.3	E935.3	E950.0	E962.0	E980.0
Pheneturide	966.3	E855.0	E936.3	E950.4	E962.0	E980.4
Phenformin	962.3	E858.0	E932.3	E950.4	E962.0	E980.4
Phenglutarimide	971.1	E855.4	E941.1	E950.4	E962.0	E980.4
Phenicarbazide	965.8	E850.8	E935.8	E950.0	E962.0	E980.0
Phenindamine (tartrate)	963.0	E858.1	E933.0	E950.4	E962.0	E980.4
Phenindione.	964.2	E858.2	E934.2	E950.4	E962.0	E980.4
Pheniprazine	969.01	E854.0	E939.0	E950.3	E962.0	E980.3
Pheniramine (maleate).	963.0	E858.1	E933.0	E950.4	E962.0	E980.4
Phenmetrazine	977.0	E858.8	E947.0	E950.4	E962.0	E980.4
Phenobal	967.0	E851	E937.0	E950.1	E962.0	E980.1
Phenobarbital	967.0	E851	E937.0	E950.1	E962.0	E980.1
Phenobarbitone.	967.0	E851	E937.0	E950.1	E962.0	E980.1
Phenoctide	976.0	E858.7	E946.0	E950.4	E962.0	E980.4
Phenol (derivatives) NEC	983.0	E864.0	—	E950.7	E962.1	E980.6
disinfectant	983.0	E864.0	—	E950.7	E962.1	E980.6
pesticide.	989.4	E863.4	—	E950.6	E962.1	E980.7
red.	977.8	E858.8	E947.8	E950.4	E962.0	E980.4
Phenolphthalein	973.1	E858.4	E943.1	E950.4	E962.0	E980.4
Phenolsulfonphthalein	977.8	E858.8	E947.8	E950.4	E962.0	E980.4
Phenomorphan	965.09	E850.2	E935.2	E950.0	E962.0	E980.0
Phenonyl	967.0	E851	E937.0	E950.1	E962.0	E980.1
Phenoperidine	965.09	E850.2	E935.2	E950.0	E962.0	E980.0
Phenoquin.	974.7	E858.5	E944.7	E950.4	E962.0	E980.4
Phenothiazines (tranquilizers) NEC . . .	969.1	E853.0	E939.1	E950.3	E962.0	E980.3
insecticide	989.3	E863.4	—	E950.6	E962.1	E980.7
Phenoxybenzamine	971.3	E855.6	E941.3	E950.4	E962.0	E980.4
Phenoxymethyl penicillin	960.0	E856	E930.0	E950.4	E962.0	E980.4
Phenprocoumon	964.2	E858.2	E934.2	E950.4	E962.0	E980.4
Phensuximide	966.2	E855.0	E936.2	E950.4	E962.0	E980.4
Phentermine	977.0	E858.8	E947.0	E950.4	E962.0	E980.4
Phentolamine	971.3	E855.6	E941.3	E950.4	E962.0	E980.4
Phenyl						
butazone.	965.5	E850.5	E935.5	E950.0	E962.0	E980.0
enediamine.	983.0	E864.0	—	E950.7	E962.1	E980.6
hydrazine	983.0	E864.0	—	E950.7	E962.1	E980.6
antineoplastic	963.1	E858.1	E933.1	E950.4	E962.0	E980.4

Substance	Poisoning	Accident	Therapeutic Use	Suicide Attempt	Assault	Undetermined
			External Cause (E-Code)			
mercuric compounds — *see* Mercury						
salicylate	976.3	E858.7	E946.3	E950.4	E962.0	E980.4
Phenylephrin	971.2	E855.5	E941.2	E950.4	E962.0	E980.4
Phenylethybiguanide	962.3	E858.0	E932.3	E950.4	E962.0	E980.4
Phenylpropanolamine	971.2	E855.5	E941.2	E950.4	E962.0	E980.4
Phenylsulfthion	989.3	E863.1	—	E950.6	E962.1	E980.7
Phenyramidol, phenyramidon	965.7	E850.7	E935.7	E950.0	E962.0	E980.0
Phenytoin	966.1	E855.0	E936.1	E950.4	E962.0	E980.4
pHisoHex	976.2	E858.7	E946.2	E950.4	E962.0	E980.4
Pholcodine	965.09	E850.2	E935.2	E950.0	E962.0	E980.0
Phorate	989.3	E863.1	—	E950.6	E962.1	E980.7
Phosdrin	989.3	E863.1	—	E950.6	E962.1	E980.7
Phosgene (gas)	987.8	E869.8	—	E952.8	E962.2	E982.8
Phosphate (tricresyl)	989.89	E866.8	—	E950.9	E962.1	E980.9
organic	989.3	E863.1	—	E950.6	E962.1	E980.7
solvent	982.8	E862.4	—	E950.9	E926.1	E980.9
Phosphine	987.8	E869.8	—	E952.8	E962.2	E982.8
fumigant	987.8	E863.8	—	E950.6	E962.2	E980.7
Phospholine	971.0	E855.3	E941.0	E950.4	E962.0	E980.4
Phosphoric acid	983.1	E864.1	—	E950.7	E962.1	E980.6
Phosphorus (compounds) NEC	983.9	E864.3	—	E950.7	E962.1	E980.6
rodenticide	983.9	E863.7	—	E950.7	E962.1	E980.6
Phthalimidogluarimide	967.8	E852.8	E937.8	E950.2	E962.0	E980.2
Phthalylsulfathiazole	961.0	E857	E931.0	E950.4	E962.0	E980.4
Phylloquinone	964.3	E858.2	E934.3	E950.4	E962.0	E980.4
Physeptone	965.02	E850.1	E935.1	E950.0	E962.0	E980.0
Physostigma venenosum	988.2	E865.4	—	E950.9	E962.1	E980.9
Physostigmine	971.0	E855.3	E941.0	E950.4	E962.0	E980.4
Phytolacca decandra	988.2	E865.4	—	E950.9	E962.1	E980.9
Phytomenadione	964.3	E858.2	E934.3	E950.4	E962.0	E980.4
Phytonadione	964.3	E858.2	E934.3	E950.4	E962.0	E980.4
Picric (acid)	983.0	E864.0	—	E950.7	E962.1	E980.6
Picrotoxin	970.0	E854.3	E940.0	E950.4	E962.0	E980.4
Pilocarpine	971.0	E855.3	E941.0	E950.4	E962.0	E980.4
Pilocarpus (jaborandi) extract	971.0	E855.3	E941.0	E950.4	E962.0	E980.4
Pimaricin	960.1	E856	E930.1	E950.4	E962.0	E980.4
Piminodine	965.09	E850.2	E935.2	E950.0	E962.0	E980.0
Pine oil, pinesol (disinfectant)	983.9	E861.4	—	E950.7	E962.1	E980.6
Pinkroot	961.6	E857	E931.6	E950.4	E962.0	E980.4
Pipadone	965.09	E850.2	E935.2	E950.0	E962.0	E980.0
Pipamazine	963.0	E858.1	E933.0	E950.4	E962.0	E980.4
Pipazethate	975.4	E858.6	E945.4	E950.4	E962.0	E980.4
Pipenzolate	971.1	E855.4	E941.1	E950.4	E962.0	E980.4
Piperacetazine	969.1	E853.0	E939.1	E950.3	E962.0	E980.3
Piperazine NEC	961.6	E857	E931.6	E950.4	E962.0	E980.4
estrone sulfate	962.2	E858.0	E932.2	E950.4	E962.0	E980.4
Piper cubeba	988.2	E865.4	—	E950.9	E962.1	E980.9
Piperidione	975.4	E858.6	E945.4	E950.4	E962.0	E980.4
Piperidolate	971.1	E855.4	E941.1	E950.4	E962.0	E980.4
Piperocaine	968.9	E855.2	E938.9	E950.4	E962.0	E980.4
infiltration (subcutaneous)	968.5	E855.2	E938.5	E950.4	E962.0	E980.4
nerve block (peripheral) (plexus)	968.6	E855.2	E938.6	E950.4	E962.0	E980.4
topical (surface)	968.5	E855.2	E938.5	E950.4	E962.0	E980.4
Pipobroman	963.1	E858.1	E933.1	E950.4	E962.0	E980.4
Pipradrol	970.89	E854.3	E940.8	E950.4	E962.0	E980.4
Piscidia (bark) (erythrina)	965.7	E850.7	E935.7	E950.0	E962.0	E980.0
Pitch	983.0	E864.0	—	E950.7	E962.1	E980.6
Pitkin's solution	968.7	E855.2	E938.7	E950.4	E962.0	E980.4
Pitocin	975.0	E858.6	E945.0	E950.4	E962.0	E980.4
Pitressin (tannate)	962.5	E858.0	E932.5	E950.4	E962.0	E980.4
Pituitary extracts (posterior)	962.5	E858.0	E932.5	E950.4	E962.0	E980.4

Substance	Poisoning	Accident	Therapeutic Use	Suicide Attempt	Assault	Undetermined
			External Cause (E-Code)			
anterior	962.4	E858.0	E932.4	E950.4	E962.0	E980.4
Pituitrin.	962.5	E858.0	E932.5	E950.4	E962.0	E980.4
Placental extract	962.9	E858.0	E932.9	E950.4	E962.0	E980.4
Placidyl.	967.8	E852.8	E937.8	E950.2	E962.0	E980.2
Plague vaccine	978.3	E858.8	E948.3	E950.4	E962.0	E980.4
Plant foods or fertilizers NEC	989.89	E866.5	—	E950.9	E962.1	E980.9
mixed with herbicides	989.4	E863.5	—	E950.6	E962.1	E980.7
Plants, noxious, used as food	988.2	E865.9	—	E950.9	E962.1	E980.9
berries and seeds	988.2	E865.3	—	E950.9	E962.1	E980.9
specified type NEC	988.2	E865.4	—	E950.9	E962.1	E980.9
Plasma (blood).	964.7	E858.2	E934.7	E950.4	E962.0	E980.4
expanders	964.8	E858.2	E934.8	E950.4	E962.0	E980.4
Plasmanate	964.7	E858.2	E934.7	E950.4	E962.0	E980.4
Plegicil	969.1	E853.0	E939.1	E950.3	E962.0	E980.3
Podophyllin	976.4	E858.7	E946.4	E950.4	E962.0	E980.4
Podophyllum resin	976.4	E858.7	E946.4	E950.4	E962.0	E980.4
Poison NEC	989.9	E866.9	—	E950.9	E962.1	E980.9
Poisonous berries	988.2	E865.3	—	E950.9	E962.1	E980.9
Pokeweed (any part)	988.2	E865.4	—	E950.9	E962.1	E980.9
Poldine	971.1	E855.4	E941.1	E950.4	E962.0	E980.4
Poliomyelitis vaccine	979.5	E858.8	E949.5	E950.4	E962.0	E980.4
Poliovirus vaccine	979.5	E858.8	E949.5	E950.4	E962.0	E980.4
Polish (car) (floor) (furniture) (metal)						
(silver)	989.89	E861.2	—	E950.9	E962.1	E980.9
abrasive	989.89	E861.3	—	E950.9	E962.1	E980.9
porcelain	989.89	E861.3	—	E950.9	E962.1	E980.9
Poloxalkol.	973.2	E858.4	E943.2	E950.4	E962.0	E980.4
Polyaminostyrene resins	974.5	E858.5	E944.5	E950.4	E962.0	E980.4
Polychlorinated biphenyl—*see* PCBs						
Polycycline	960.4	E856	E930.4	E950.4	E962.0	E980.4
Polyester resin hardener	982.8	E862.4	—	E950.9	E962.1	E980.9
fumes.	987.8	E869.8	—	E952.8	E962.2	E982.8
Polyestradiol (phosphate)	962.2	E858.0	E932.2	E950.4	E962.0	E980.4
Polyethanolamine alkyl sulfate	976.2	E858.7	E946.2	E950.4	E962.0	E980.4
Polyethylene glycol	976.3	E858.7	E946.3	E950.4	E962.0	E980.4
Polyferose.	964.0	E858.2	E934.0	E950.4	E962.0	E980.4
Polymyxin B	960.8	E856	E930.8	E950.4	E962.0	E980.4
ENT agent.	976.6	E858.7	E946.6	E950.4	E962.0	E980.4
ophthalmic preparation.	976.5	E858.7	E946.5	E950.4	E962.0	E980.4
topical NEC	976.0	E858.7	E946.0	E950.4	E962.0	E980.4
Polynoxylin(e)	976.0	E858.7	E946.0	E950.4	E962.0	E980.4
Polyoxymethyleneurea	976.0	E858.7	E946.0	E950.4	E962.0	E980.4
Polytetrafluoroethylene (inhaled)	987.8	E869.8	—	E952.8	E962.2	E982.8
Polythiazide	974.3	E858.5	E944.3	E950.4	E962.0	E980.4
Polyvinylpyrrolidone	964.8	E858.2	E934.8	E950.4	E962.0	E980.4
Pontocaine (hydrochloride) (infiltration)						
(topical)	968.5	E855.2	E938.5	E950.4	E962.0	E980.4
nerve block (peripheral) (plexus).	968.6	E855.2	E938.6	E950.4	E962.0	E980.4
spinal.	968.7	E855.2	E938.7	E950.4	E962.0	E980.4
Pot.	969.6	E854.1	E939.6	E950.3	E962.0	E980.3
Potash (caustic)	983.2	E864.2	—	E950.7	E962.1	E980.6
Potassic saline injection (lactated)	974.5	E858.5	E944.5	E950.4	E962.0	E980.4
Potassium (salts) NEC.	974.5	E858.5	E944.5	E950.4	E962.0	E980.4
aminosalicylate	961.8	E857	E931.8	E950.4	E962.0	E980.4
arsenite (solution)	985.1	E866.3	—	E950.8	E962.1	E980.8
bichromate	983.9	E864.3	—	E950.7	E962.1	E980.6
bisulfate	983.9	E864.3	—	E950.7	E962.1	E980.6
bromide (medicinal) NEC	967.3	E852.2	E937.3	E950.2	E962.0	E980.2
carbonate	983.2	E864.2	—	E950.7	E962.1	E980.6
chlorate NEC.	983.9	E864.3	—	E950.7	E962.1	E980.6

Substance	Poisoning	Accident	Therapeutic Use	Suicide Attempt	Assault	Undetermined
			External Cause (E-Code)			
cyanide — *see* Cyanide						
hydroxide 983.2	E864.2	—	E950.7	E962.1	E980.6
iodide (expectorant) NEC. 975.5	E858.6	E945.5	E950.4	E962.0	E980.4
nitrate. 989.89	E866.8	—	E950.9	E962.1	E980.9
oxalate 983.9	E864.3	—	E950.7	E962.1	E980.6
perchlorate NEC 977.8	E858.8	E947.8	E950.4	E962.0	E980.4
antithyroid 962.8	E858.0	E932.8	E950.4	E962.0	E980.4
permanganate. 976.0	E858.7	E946.0	E950.4	E962.0	E980.4
nonmedicinal 983.9	E864.3	—	E950.7	E962.1	E980.6
Povidone–iodine (anti–infective) NEC 976.0	E858.7	E946.0	E950.4	E962.0	E980.4
Practolol 972.0	E858.3	E942.0	E950.4	E962.0	E980.4
Pralidoxime (chloride). 977.2	E858.8	E947.2	E950.4	E962.0	E980.4
Pramoxine. 968.5	E855.2	E938.5	E950.4	E962.0	E980.4
Prazosin 972.6	E858.3	E942.6	E950.4	E962.0	E980.4
Prednisolone 962.0	E858.0	E932.0	E950.4	E962.0	E980.4
ENT agent. 976.6	E858.7	E946.6	E950.4	E962.0	E980.4
ophthalmic preparation 976.5	E858.7	E946.5	E950.4	E962.0	E980.4
topical NEC 976.0	E858.7	E946.0	E950.4	E962.0	E980.4
Prednisone 962.0	E858.0	E932.0	E950.4	E962.0	E980.4
Pregnanediol. 962.2	E858.0	E932.2	E950.4	E962.0	E980.4
Pregneninolone. 962.2	E858.0	E932.2	E950.4	E962.0	E980.4
Preludin. 977.0	E858.8	E947.0	E950.4	E962.0	E980.4
Premarin 962.2	E858.0	E932.2	E950.4	E962.0	E980.4
Prenylamine 972.4	E858.3	E942.4	E950.4	E962.0	E980.4
Preparation H 976.8	E858.7	E946.8	E950.4	E962.0	E980.4
Preservatives. 989.89	E866.8	—	E950.9	E962.1	E980.9
Pride of China 988.2	E865.3	—	E950.9	E962.1	E980.9
Prilocaine 968.9	E855.2	E938.9	E950.4	E962.0	E980.4
infiltration (subcutaneous) 968.5	E855.2	E938.5	E950.4	E962.0	E980.4
nerve block (peripheral) (plexus). 968.6	E855.2	E938.6	E950.4	E962.0	E980.4
Primaquine 961.4	E857	E931.4	E950.4	E962.0	E980.4
Primidone 966.3	E855.0	E936.3	E950.4	E962.0	E980.4
Primula (veris) 988.2	E865.4	—	E950.9	E962.1	E980.9
Prinadol. 965.09	E850.2	E935.2	E950.0	E962.0	E980.0
Priscol, Priscoline 971.3	E855.6	E941.3	E950.4	E962.0	E980.4
Privet. 988.2	E865.4	—	E950.9	E962.1	E980.9
Privine 971.2	E855.5	E941.2	E950.4	E962.0	E980.4
Pro–Banthine 971.1	E855.4	E941.1	E950.4	E962.0	E980.4
Probarbital 967.0	E851	E937.0	E950.1	E962.0	E980.1
Probenecid 974.7	E858.5	E944.7	E950.4	E962.0	E980.4
Procainamide (hydrochloride) 972.0	E858.3	E942.0	E950.4	E962.0	E980.4
Procaine (hydrochloride) (infiltration)						
(topical) 968.5	E855.2	E938.5	E950.4	E962.0	E980.4
nerve block (peripheral) (plexus). 968.6	E855.2	E938.6	E950.4	E962.0	E980.4
penicillin G 960.0	E856	E930.0	E950.4	E962.0	E980.4
spinal 968.7	E855.2	E938.7	E950.4	E962.0	E980.4
Procalmidol 969.5	E853.8	E939.5	E950.3	E962.0	E980.3
Procarbazine 963.1	E858.1	E933.1	E950.4	E962.0	E980.4
Prochlorperazine 969.1	E853.0	E939.1	E950.3	E962.0	E980.3
Procyclidine 966.4	E855.0	E936.4	E950.4	E962.0	E980.4
Producer gas. 986	E868.8	—	E952.1	E962.2	E982.1
Profenamine 966.4	E855.0	E936.4	E950.4	E962.0	E980.4
Profenil 975.1	E858.6	E945.1	E950.4	E962.0	E980.4
Progesterones 962.2	E858.0	E932.2	E950.4	E962.0	E980.4
Progestin 962.2	E858.0	E932.2	E950.4	E962.0	E980.4
Progestogens (with estrogens). 962.2	E858.0	E932.2	E950.4	E962.0	E980.4
Progestone 962.2	E858.0	E932.2	E950.4	E962.0	E980.4
Proguanil 961.4	E857	E931.4	E950.4	E962.0	E980.4
Prolactin 962.4	E858.0	E932.4	E950.4	E962.0	E980.4
Proloid 962.7	E858.0	E932.7	E950.4	E962.0	E980.4
Proluton 962.2	E858.0	E932.2	E950.4	E962.0	E980.4

Substance	Poisoning	Accident	Therapeutic Use	Suicide Attempt	Assault	Undetermined
			External Cause (E-Code)			
Promacetin	961.8	E857	E931.8	E950.4	E962.0	E980.4
Promazine	969.1	E853.0	E939.1	E950.3	E962.0	E980.3
Promedol	965.09	E850.2	E935.2	E950.0	E962.0	E980.0
Promethazine	967.8	E852.8	E937.8	E950.2	E962.0	E980.2
Promin	961.8	E857	E931.8	E950.4	E962.0	E980.4
Pronestyl (hydrochloride)	972.0	E858.3	E942.0	E950.4	E962.0	E980.4
Pronetalol, pronethalol	972.0	E858.3	E942.0	E950.4	E962.0	E980.4
Prontosil	961.0	E857	E931.0	E950.4	E962.0	E980.4
Propamidine isethionate	961.5	E857	E931.5	E950.4	E962.0	E980.4
Propanal (medicinal)	967.8	E852.8	E937.8	E950.2	E962.0	E980.2
Propane (gas) (distributed in mobile container)	987.0	E868.0	—	E951.1	E962.2	E981.1
distributed through pipes	987.0	E867	—	E951.0	E962.2	E981.0
incomplete combustion of – *see* Carbon monoxide, Propane						
Propanidid	968.3	E855.1	E938.3	E950.4	E962.0	E980.4
Propanol	980.3	E860.4	—	E950.9	E962.1	E980.9
Propantheline	971.1	E855.4	E941.1	E950.4	E962.0	E980.4
Proparacaine	968.5	E855.2	E938.5	E950.4	E962.0	E980.4
Propatyl nitrate	972.4	E858.3	E942.4	E950.4	E962.0	E980.4
Propicillin	960.0	E856	E930.0	E950.4	E962.0	E980.4
Propiolactone (vapor)	987.8	E869.8	—	E952.8	E962.2	E982.8
Propiomazine	967.8	E852.8	E937.8	E950.2	E962.0	E980.2
Propionaldehyde (medicinal)	967.8	E852.8	E937.8	E950.2	E962.0	E980.2
Propionate compound	976.0	E858.7	E946.0	E950.4	E962.0	E980.4
Propion gel	976.0	E858.7	E946.0	E950.4	E962.0	E980.4
Propitocaine	968.9	E855.2	E938.9	E950.4	E962.0	E980.4
infiltration (subcutaneous)	968.5	E855.2	E938.5	E950.4	E962.0	E980.4
nerve block (peripheral) (plexus)	968.6	E855.2	E938.6	E950.4	E962.0	E980.4
Propoxur	989.3	E863.2	—	E950.6	E962.1	E980.7
Propoxycaine	968.9	E855.2	E938.9	E950.4	E962.0	E980.4
infiltration (subcutaneous)	968.5	E855.2	E938.5	E950.4	E962.0	E980.4
nerve block (peripheral) (plexus)	968.6	E855.2	E938.6	E950.4	E962.0	E980.4
topical (surface)	968.5	E855.2	E938.5	E950.4	E962.0	E980.4
Propoxyphene (hydrochloride)	965.8	E850.8	E935.8	E950.0	E962.0	E980.0
Propranolol	972.0	E858.3	E942.0	E950.4	E962.0	E980.4
Propyl						
alcohol	980.3	E860.4	—	E950.9	E962.1	E980.9
carbinol	980.3	E860.4	—	E950.9	E962.1	E980.9
hexadrine	971.2	E855.5	E941.2	E950.4	E962.0	E980.4
iodone	977.8	E858.8	E947.8	E950.4	E962.0	E980.4
thiouracil	962.8	E858.0	E932.8	E950.4	E962.0	E980.4
Propylene	987.1	E869.8	—	E952.8	E962.2	E982.8
Propylparaben (ophthalmic)	976.5	E858.7	E946.5	E950.4	E962.0	E980.4
Proscillaridin	972.1	E858.3	E942.1	E950.4	E962.0	E980.4
Prostaglandins	975.0	E858.6	E945.0	E950.4	E962.0	E980.4
Prostigmin	971.0	E855.3	E941.0	E950.4	E962.0	E980.4
Protamine (sulfate)	964.5	E858.2	E934.5	E950.4	E962.0	E980.4
zinc insulin	962.3	E858.0	E932.3	E950.4	E962.0	E980.4
Protectants (topical)	976.3	E858.7	E946.3	E950.4	E962.0	E980.4
Protein hydrolysate	974.5	E858.5	E944.5	E950.4	E962.0	E980.4
Prothiaden—*see* Dothiepin hydrochloride						
Prothionamide	961.8	E857	E931.8	E950.4	E962.0	E980.4
Prothipendyl	969.5	E853.8	E939.5	E950.3	E962.0	E980.3
Protokylol	971.2	E855.5	E941.2	E950.4	E962.0	E980.4
Protopam	977.2	E858.8	E947.2	E950.4	E962.0	E980.4
Protoveratrine(s) (A) (B)	972.6	E858.3	E942.6	E950.4	E962.0	E980.4
Protriptyline	969.05	E854.0	E939.0	E950.3	E962.0	E980.3
Provera	962.2	E858.0	E932.2	E950.4	E962.0	E980.4
Provitamin A	963.5	E858.1	E933.5	E950.4	E962.0	E980.4

TABLE OF DRUGS AND CHEMICALS

Substance	Poisoning	Accident	Therapeutic Use	Suicide Attempt	Assault	Undetermined
			External Cause (E-Code)			
Proxymetacaine 968.5	E855.2	E938.5	E950.4	E962.0	E980.4
Proxyphylline 975.1	E858.6	E945.1	E950.4	E962.0	E980.4
Prozac—*see* Fluoxetine hydrochloride					
Prunus					
laurocerasus 988.2	E865.4	—	E950.9	E962.1	E980.9
virginiana 988.2	E865.4	—	E950.9	E962.1	E980.9
Prussic acid 989.0	E866.8	—	E950.9	E962.1	E980.9
vapor 987.7	E869.8	—	E952.8	E962.2	E982.8
Pseudoephedrine 971.2	E855.5	E941.2	E950.4	E962.0	E980.4
Psilocin 969.6	E854.1	E939.6	E950.3	E962.0	E980.3
Psilocybin 969.6	E854.1	E939.6	E950.3	E962.0	E980.3
PSP 977.8	E858.8	E947.8	E950.4	E962.0	E980.4
Psychedelic agents 969.6	E854.1	E939.6	E950.3	E962.0	E980.3
Psychodysleptics 969.6	E854.1	E939.6	E950.3	E962.0	E980.3
Psychostimulants 969.70	E854.2	E939.7	E950.3	E962.0	E980.3
Psychotherapeutic agents 969.9	E855.9	E939.9	E950.3	E962.0	E980.3
antidepressants 969.00	E854.0	E939.0	E950.3	E962.0	E980.3
specified NEC 969.8	E855.8	E939.8	E950.3	E962.0	E980.3
tranquilizers NEC 969.5	E853.9	E939.5	E950.3	E962.0	E980.3
Psychotomimetic agents 969.6	E854.1	E939.6	E950.3	E962.0	E980.3
Psychotropic agents 969.9	E854.8	E939.9	E950.3	E962.0	E980.3
specified NEC 969.8	E854.8	E939.8	E950.3	E962.0	E980.3
Psyllium 973.3	E858.4	E943.3	E950.4	E962.0	E980.4
Pteroylglutamic acid 964.1	E858.2	E934.1	E950.4	E962.0	E980.4
Pteroyltriglutamate 963.1	E858.1	E933.1	E950.4	E962.0	E980.4
PTFE 987.8	E869.8	—	E952.8	E962.2	E982.8
Pulsatilla 988.2	E865.4	—	E950.9	E962.1	E980.9
Purex (bleach) 983.9	E864.3	—	E950.7	E962.1	E980.6
Purine diuretics 974.1	E858.5	E944.1	E950.4	E962.0	E980.4
Purinethol 963.1	E858.1	E933.1	E950.4	E962.0	E980.4
PVP 964.8	E858.2	E934.8	E950.4	E962.0	E980.4
Pyrabital 965.7	E850.7	E935.7	E950.0	E962.0	E980.0
Pyramidon 965.5	E850.5	E935.5	E950.0	E962.0	E980.0
Pyrantel (pamoate) 961.6	E857	E931.6	E950.4	E962.0	E980.4
Pyrathiazine 963.0	E858.1	E933.0	E950.4	E962.0	E980.4
Pyrazinamide 961.8	E857	E931.8	E950.4	E962.0	E980.4
Pyrazinoic acid (amide) 961.8	E857	E931.8	E950.4	E962.0	E980.4
Pyrazole (derivatives) 965.5	E850.5	E935.5	E950.0	E962.0	E980.0
Pyrazolone (analgesics) 965.5	E850.5	E935.5	E950.0	E962.0	E980.0
Pyrethrins, pyrethrum 989.4	E863.4	—	E950.6	E962.1	E980.7
Pyribenzamine 963.0	E858.1	E933.0	E950.4	E962.0	E980.4
Pyridine (liquid) (vapor) 982.0	E862.4	—	E950.9	E962.1	E980.9
aldoxime chloride 977.2	E858.8	E947.2	E950.4	E962.0	E980.4
Pyridium 976.1	E858.7	E946.1	E950.4	E962.0	E980.4
Pyridostigmine 971.0	E855.3	E941.0	E950.4	E962.0	E980.4
Pyridoxine 963.5	E858.1	E933.5	E950.4	E962.0	E980.4
Pyrilamine 963.0	E858.1	E933.0	E950.4	E962.0	E980.4
Pyrimethamine 961.4	E857	E931.4	E950.4	E962.0	E980.4
Pyrogallic acid 983.0	E864.0	—	E950.7	E962.1	E980.6
Pyroxylin 976.3	E858.7	E946.3	E950.4	E962.0	E980.4
Pyrrobutamine 963.0	E858.1	E933.0	E950.4	E962.0	E980.4
Pyrrocaine 968.5	E855.2	E938.5	E950.4	E962.0	E980.4
Pyrvinium (pamoate) 961.6	E857	E931.6	E950.4	E962.0	E980.4
PZI 962.3	E858.0	E932.3	E950.4	E962.0	E980.4
Quaalude 967.4	E852.3	E937.4	E950.2	E962.0	E980.2
Quaternary ammonium derivatives 971.1	E855.4	E941.1	E950.4	E962.0	E980.4
Quicklime 983.2	E864.2	—	E950.7	E962.1	E980.6
Quinacrine 961.3	E857	E931.3	E950.4	E962.0	E980.4
Quinaglute 972.0	E858.3	E942.0	E950.4	E962.0	E980.4
Quinalbarbitone 967.0	E851	E937.0	E950.1	E962.0	E980.1
Quinestradiol 962.2	E858.0	E932.2	E950.4	E962.0	E980.4

1745

Substance	Poisoning	Accident	Therapeutic Use	Suicide Attempt	Assault	Undetermined
			External Cause (E-Code)			
Quinethazone	974.3	E858.5	E944.3	E950.4	E962.0	E980.4
Quinidine (gluconate) (polygalacturonate)						
(salts) (sulfate)	972.0	E858.3	E942.0	E950.4	E962.0	E980.4
Quinine.	961.4	E857	E931.4	E950.4	E962.0	E980.4
Quiniobine	961.3	E857	E931.3	E950.4	E962.0	E980.4
Quinolines	961.3	E857	E931.3	E950.4	E962.0	E980.4
Quotane.	968.5	E855.2	E938.5	E950.4	E962.0	E980.4
Rabies						
immune globulin (human)	964.6	E858.2	E934.6	E950.4	E962.0	E980.4
vaccine	979.1	E858.8	E949.1	E950.4	E962.0	E980.4
Racemoramide	965.09	E850.2	E935.2	E950.0	E962.0	E980.0
Racemorphan	965.09	E850.2	E935.2	E950.0	E962.0	E980.0
Radiator alcohol	980.1	E860.2	—	E950.9	E962.1	E980.9
Radio–opaque (drugs) (materials)	977.8	E858.8	E947.8	E950.4	E962.0	E980.4
Ranunculus	988.2	E865.4	—	E950.9	E962.1	E980.9
Rat poison	989.4	E863.7	—	E950.6	E962.1	E980.7
Rattlesnake (venom)	989.5	E905.0	—	E950.9	E962.1	E980.9
Raudixin	972.6	E858.3	E942.6	E950.4	E962.0	E980.4
Rautensin	972.6	E858.3	E942.6	E950.4	E962.0	E980.4
Rautina	972.6	E858.3	E942.6	E950.4	E962.0	E980.4
Rautotal	972.6	E858.3	E942.6	E950.4	E962.0	E980.4
Rauwiloid	972.6	E858.3	E942.6	E950.4	E962.0	E980.4
Rauwoldin	972.6	E858.3	E942.6	E950.4	E962.0	E980.4
Rauwolfia (alkaloids)	972.6	E858.3	E942.6	E950.4	E962.0	E980.4
Realgar	985.1	E866.3	—	E950.8	E962.1	E980.8
Red cells, packed.	964.7	E858.2	E934.7	E950.4	E962.0	E980.4
Reducing agents, industrial NEC	983.9	E864.3	—	E950.7	E962.1	E980.6
Refrigerant gas (freon)	987.4	E869.2	—	E952.8	E962.2	E982.8
not freon	987.9	E869.9	—	E952.9	E962.2	E982.9
Regroton	974.4	E858.5	E944.4	E950.4	E962.0	E980.4
Rela	968.0	E855.1	E938.0	E950.4	E962.0	E980.4
Relaxants, skeletal muscle (autonomic). . . .	975.2	E858.6	E945.2	E950.4	E962.0	E980.4
central nervous system	968.0	E855.1	E938.0	E950.4	E962.0	E980.4
Renese	974.3	E858.5	E944.3	E950.4	E962.0	E980.4
Renografin	977.8	E858.8	E947.8	E950.4	E962.0	E980.4
Replacement solutions	974.5	E858.5	E944.5	E950.4	E962.0	E980.4
Rescinnamine	972.6	E858.3	E942.6	E950.4	E962.0	E980.4
Reserpine	972.6	E858.3	E942.6	E950.4	E962.0	E980.4
Resorcin, resorcinol	976.4	E857	E946.4	E950.4	E962.0	E980.4
Respaire	975.5	E858.6	E945.5	E950.4	E962.0	E980.4
Respiratory agents NEC	975.8	E858.6	E945.8	E950.4	E962.0	E980.4
Retinoic acid	976.8	E858.7	E946.8	E950.4	E962.0	E980.4
Retinol	963.5	E858.1	E933.5	E950.4	E962.0	E980.4
Rh₀ (D) immune globulin (human)	964.6	E858.2	E934.6	E950.4	E962.0	E980.4
Rhodine.	965.1	E850.3	E935.3	E950.0	E962.0	E980.0
RhoGAM	964.6	E858.2	E934.6	E950.4	E962.0	E980.4
Riboflavin.	963.5	E858.1	E933.5	E950.4	E962.0	E980.4
Ricin.	989.89	E866.8	—	E950.9	E962.1	E980.9
Ricinus communis	988.2	E865.3	—	E950.9	E962.1	E980.9
Rickettsial vaccine NEC.	979.6	E858.8	E949.6	E950.4	E962.0	E980.4
with viral and bacterial vaccine	979.7	E858.8	E949.7	E950.4	E962.0	E980.4
Rifampin	960.6	E856	E930.6	E950.4	E962.0	E980.4
Rimifon.	961.8	E857	E931.8	E950.4	E962.0	E980.4
Ringer's injection (lactated)	974.5	E858.5	E944.5	E950.4	E962.0	E980.4
Ristocetin	960.8	E856	E930.8	E950.4	E962.0	E980.4
Ritalin	969.73	E854.2	E939.7	E950.3	E962.0	E980.3
Roach killers — see Pesticides						
Rocky Mountain spotted fever vaccine	979.6	E858.8	E949.6	E950.4	E962.0	E980.4
Rodenticides.	989.4	E863.7	—	E950.6	E962.1	E980.7
Rohypnol	969.4	E853.2	E939.4	E950.3	E962.0	E980.3

Substance	Poisoning	Accident	Therapeutic Use	Suicide Attempt	Assault	Undetermined
			External Cause (E-Code)			
Rolaids	973.0	E858.4	E943.0	E950.4	E962.0	E980.4
Rolitetracycline	960.4	E856	E930.4	E950.4	E962.0	E980.4
Romilar	975.4	E858.6	E945.4	E950.4	E962.0	E980.4
Rose water ointment	976.3	E858.7	E946.3	E950.4	E962.0	E980.4
Rotenone	989.4	E863.7	—	E950.6	E962.1	E980.7
Rotoxamine	963.0	E858.1	E933.0	E950.4	E962.0	E980.4
Rough–on–rats	989.4	E863.7	—	E950.6	E962.1	E980.7
Rubbing alcohol	980.2	E860.3	—	E950.9	E962.1	E980.9
Rubella virus vaccine	979.4	E858.8	E949.4	E950.4	E962.0	E980.4
Rubelogen	979.4	E858.8	E949.4	E950.4	E962.0	E980.4
Rubeovax	979.4	E858.8	E949.4	E950.4	E962.0	E980.4
Rubidomycin	960.7	E856	E930.7	E950.4	E962.0	E980.4
Rue	988.2	E965.4	—	E950.9	E962.1	E980.9
RU486	962.9	E858.0	E932.9	E950.4	E962.0	E980.4
Ruta	988.2	E865.4	—	E950.9	E962.1	E980.9
Sabadilla (medicinal)	976.0	E858.7	E946.0	E950.4	E962.0	E980.4
pesticide	989.4	E863.4	—	E950.6	E962.1	E980.7
Sabin oral vaccine	979.5	E858.8	E949.5	E950.4	E962.0	E980.4
Saccharated iron oxide	964.0	E858.2	E934.0	E950.4	E962.0	E980.4
Saccharin	974.5	E858.5	E944.5	E950.4	E962.0	E980.4
Safflower oil	972.2	E858.3	E942.2	E950.4	E962.0	E980.4
Salbutamol sulfate	975.7	E858.6	E945.7	E950.4	E962.0	E980.4
Salicylamide	965.1	E850.3	E935.3	E950.0	E962.0	E980.0
Salicylate(s)	965.1	E850.3	E935.3	E950.0	E962.0	E980.0
methyl	976.3	E858.7	E946.3	E950.4	E962.0	E980.4
theobromine calcium	974.1	E858.5	E944.1	E950.4	E962.0	E980.4
Salicylazosulfapyridine	961.0	E857	E931.0	E950.4	E962.0	E980.4
Salicylhydroxamic acid	976.0	E858.7	E946.0	E950.4	E962.0	E980.4
Salicylic acid (keratolytic) NEC	976.4	E858.7	E946.4	E950.4	E962.0	E980.4
congeners	965.1	E850.3	E935.3	E950.0	E962.0	E980.0
salts	965.1	E850.3	E935.3	E950.0	E962.0	E980.0
Saliniazid	961.8	E857	E931.8	E950.4	E962.0	E980.4
Salol	976.3	E858.7	E946.3	E950.4	E962.0	E980.4
Salt (substitute) NEC	974.5	E858.5	E944.5	E950.4	E962.0	E980.4
Saluretics	974.3	E858.5	E944.3	E950.4	E962.0	E980.4
Saluron	974.3	E858.5	E944.3	E950.4	E962.0	E980.4
Salvarsan 606 (neosilver) (silver)	961.1	E857	E931.1	E950.4	E962.0	E980.4
Sambucus canadensis	988.2	E865.4	—	E950.9	E962.1	E980.9
berry	988.2	E865.3	—	E950.9	E962.1	E980.9
Sandril	972.6	E858.3	E942.6	E950.4	E962.0	E980.4
Sanguinaria canadensis	988.2	E865.4	—	E950.9	E962.1	E980.9
Saniflush (cleaner)	983.9	E861.3	—	E950.7	E962.1	E980.6
Santonin	961.6	E857	E931.6	E950.4	E962.0	E980.4
Santyl	976.8	E858.7	E946.8	E950.4	E962.0	E980.4
Sarkomycin	960.7	E856	E930.7	E950.4	E962.0	E980.4
Saroten	969.05	E854.0	E939.0	E950.3	E962.0	E980.3
Saturnine – see Lead						
Savin (oil)	976.4	E858.7	E946.4	E950.4	E962.0	E980.4
Scammony	973.1	E858.4	E943.1	E950.4	E962.0	E980.4
Scarlet red	976.8	E858.7	E946.8	E950.4	E962.0	E980.4
Scheele's green	985.1	E866.3	—	E950.8	E962.1	E980.8
insecticide	985.1	E863.4	—	E950.8	E962.1	E980.8
Schradan	989.3	E863.1	—	E950.6	E962.1	E980.7
Schweinfurt (h) green	985.1	E866.3	—	E950.8	E962.1	E980.8
insecticide	985.1	E863.4	—	E950.8	E962.1	E980.8
Scilla — see Squill						
Sclerosing agents	972.7	E858.3	E942.7	E950.4	E962.0	E980.4
Scopolamine	971.1	E855.4	E941.1	E950.4	E962.0	E980.4
Scouring powder	989.89	E861.3	—	E950.9	E962.1	E980.9
Sea						
anemone (sting)	989.5	E905.6	—	E950.9	E962.1	E980.9

Substance	Poisoning	Accident	Therapeutic Use	Suicide Attempt	Assault	Undetermined
			External Cause (E-Code)			
cucumber (sting)	989.5	E905.6	—	E950.9	E962.1	E980.9
snake (bite) (venom)	989.5	E905.0	—	E950.9	E962.1	E980.9
urchin spine (puncture)	989.5	E905.6	—	E950.9	E962.1	E980.9
Secbutabarbital	967.0	E851	E937.0	E950.1	E962.0	E980.1
Secbutabaritone	967.0	E851	E937.0	E950.1	E962.0	E980.1
Secobarbital	967.0	E851	E937.0	E950.1	E962.0	E980.1
Seconal	967.0	E851	E937.0	E950.1	E962.0	E980.1
Secretin	977.8	E858.8	E947.8	E950.4	E962.0	E980.4
Sedatives, nonbarbiturate	967.9	E852.9	E937.9	E950.2	E962.0	E980.2
specified NEC	967.8	E852.8	E937.8	E950.2	E962.0	E980.2
Sedormid	967.8	E852.8	E937.8	E950.2	E962.0	E980.2
Seed (plant)	988.2	E865.3	—	E950.9	E962.1	E980.9
disinfectant or dressing	989.89	E866.5	—	E950.9	E962.1	E980.9
Selective serotonin and norepinephrine reuptake inhibitors (SSNRI)	969.02	E854.0	E939.0	E950.3	E962.0	E980.3
Selective serotonin reuptake inhibitors (SSRI)	969.03	E854.0	E939.0	E950.3	E962.0	E980.3
Selenium (fumes) NEC	985.8	E866.4	—	E950.9	E962.1	E980.9
disulfide or sulfide	976.4	E858.7	E946.4	E950.4	E962.0	E980.4
Selsun	976.4	E858.7	E946.4	E950.4	E962.0	E980.4
Senna	973.1	E858.4	E943.1	E950.4	E962.0	E980.4
Septisol	976.2	E858.7	E946.2	E950.4	E962.0	E980.4
Serax	969.4	E853.2	E939.4	E950.3	E962.0	E980.3
Serenesil	967.8	E852.8	E937.8	E950.2	E962.0	E980.2
Serenium (hydrochloride)	961.9	E857	E931.9	E950.4	E962.0	E980.4
Serepax—see Oxazepam						
Sernyl	968.3	E855.1	E938.3	E950.4	E962.0	E980.4
Serotonin	977.8	E858.8	E947.8	E950.4	E962.0	E980.4
Serpasil	972.6	E858.3	E942.6	E950.4	E962.0	E980.4
Sewer gas	987.8	E869.8	—	E952.8	E962.2	E982.8
Shampoo	989.6	E861.0	—	E950.9	E962.1	E980.9
Shellfish, nonbacterial or noxious	988.0	E865.1	—	E950.9	E962.1	E980.9
Silicones NEC	989.83	E866.8	E947.8	E950.9	E962.1	E980.9
Silvadene	976.0	E858.7	E946.0	E950.4	E962.0	E980.4
Silver (compound) (medicinal) NEC	976.0	E858.7	E946.0	E950.4	E962.0	E980.4
anti–infectives	976.0	E858.7	E946.0	E950.4	E962.0	E980.4
arsphenamine	961.1	E857	E931.1	E950.4	E962.0	E980.4
nitrate	976.0	E858.7	E946.0	E950.4	E962.0	E980.4
ophthalmic preparation	976.5	E858.7	E946.5	E950.4	E962.0	E980.4
toughened (keratolytic)	976.4	E858.7	E946.4	E950.4	E962.0	E980.4
nonmedicinal (dust)	985.8	E866.4	—	E950.9	E962.1	E980.9
protein (mild) (strong)	976.0	E858.7	E946.0	E950.4	E962.0	E980.4
salvarsan	961.1	E857	E931.1	E950.4	E962.0	E980.4
Simethicone	973.8	E858.4	E943.8	E950.4	E962.0	E980.4
Sinequan	969.05	E854.0	E939.0	E950.3	E962.0	E980.3
Singoserp	972.6	E858.3	E942.6	E950.4	E962.0	E980.4
Sintrom	964.2	E858.2	E934.2	E950.4	E962.0	E980.4
Sitosterols	972.2	E858.3	E942.2	E950.4	E962.0	E980.4
Skeletal muscle relaxants	975.2	E858.6	E945.2	E950.4	E962.0	E980.4
Skin						
agents (external)	976.9	E858.7	E946.9	E950.4	E962.0	E980.4
specified NEC	976.8	E858.7	E946.8	E950.4	E962.0	E980.4
test antigen	977.8	E858.8	E947.8	E950.4	E962.0	E980.4
Sleep–eze	963.0	E858.1	E933.0	E950.4	E962.0	E980.4
Sleeping draught (drug) (pill) (tablet)	967.9	E852.9	E937.9	E950.2	E962.0	E980.2
Smallpox vaccine	979.0	E858.8	E949.0	E950.4	E962.0	E980.4
Smelter fumes NEC	985.9	E866.4	—	E950.9	E962.1	E980.9
Smog	987.3	E869.1	—	E952.8	E962.2	E982.8
Smoke NEC	987.9	E869.9	—	E952.9	E962.2	E982.9
Smooth muscle relaxant	975.1	E858.6	E945.1	E950.4	E962.0	E980.4
Snail killer	989.4	E863.4	—	E950.6	E962.1	E980.7

Substance	Poisoning	Accident	Therapeutic Use	Suicide Attempt	Assault	Undetermined
			External Cause (E-Code)			
Snake (bite) (venom) 989.5	E905.0	—	E950.9	E962.1	E980.9
Snuff 989.89	E866.8	—	E950.9	E962.1	E980.9
Soap (powder) (product) 989.6	E861.1	—	E950.9	E962.1	E980.9
medicinal, soft 976.2	E858.7	E946.2	E950.4	E962.0	E980.4
Soda (caustic) 983.2	E864.2	—	E950.7	E962.1	E980.6
bicarb 963.3	E858.1	E933.3	E950.4	E962.0	E980.4
chlorinated — Sodium, hypochlorite					
Sodium					
acetosulfone 961.8	E857	E931.8	E950.4	E962.0	E980.4
acetrizoate 977.8	E858.8	E947.8	E950.4	E962.0	E980.4
amytal 967.0	E851	E937.0	E950.1	E962.0	E980.1
arsenate — see Arsenic					
bicarbonate 963.3	E858.1	E933.3	E950.4	E962.0	E980.4
bichromate 983.9	E864.3	—	E950.7	E962.1	E980.6
biphosphate 963.2	E858.1	E933.2	E950.4	E962.0	E980.4
bisulfate 983.9	E864.3	—	E950.7	E962.1	E980.6
borate (cleanser) 989.6	E861.3	—	E950.9	E962.1	E980.9
bromide NEC 967.3	E852.2	E937.3	E950.2	E962.0	E980.2
cacodylate (nonmedicinal) NEC 978.8	E858.8	E948.8	E950.4	E962.0	E980.4
anti–infective 961.1	E857	E931.1	E950.4	E962.0	E980.4
herbicide 989.4	E863.5	—	E950.6	E962.1	E980.7
calcium edetate 963.8	E858.1	E933.8	E950.4	E962.0	E980.4
carbonate NEC 983.2	E864.2	—	E950.7	E962.1	E980.6
chlorate NEC 983.9	E864.3	—	E950.7	E962.1	E980.6
herbicide 983.9	E863.5	—	E950.7	E962.1	E980.6
chloride NEC 974.5	E858.5	E944.5	E950.4	E962.0	E980.4
chromate 983.9	E864.3	—	E950.7	E962.1	E980.6
citrate 963.3	E858.1	E933.3	E950.4	E962.0	E980.4
cyanide — see Cyanide(s)					
cyclamate 974.5	E858.5	E944.5	E950.4	E962.0	E980.4
diatrizoate 977.8	E858.8	E947.8	E950.4	E962.0	E980.4
dibunate 975.4	E858.6	E945.4	E950.4	E962.0	E980.4
dioctyl sulfosuccinate 973.2	E858.4	E943.2	E950.4	E962.0	E980.4
edetate 963.8	E858.1	E933.8	E950.4	E962.0	E980.4
ethacrynate 974.4	E858.5	E944.4	E950.4	E962.0	E980.4
fluoracetate (dust) (rodenticide) 989.4	E863.7	—	E950.6	E962.1	E980.7
fluoride — see Fluoride(s)					
free salt 974.5	E858.5	E944.5	E950.4	E962.0	E980.4
glucosulfone 961.8	E857	E931.8	E950.4	E962.0	E980.4
hydroxide 983.2	E864.2	—	E950.7	E962.1	E980.6
hypochlorite (bleach) NEC 983.9	E864.3	—	E950.7	E962.1	E980.6
disinfectant 983.9	E861.4	—	E950.7	E962.1	E980.6
medicinal (anti–infective) (external) . . . 976.0	E858.7	E946.0	E950.4	E962.0	E980.4
vapor 987.8	E869.8	—	E952.8	E962.2	E982.8
hyposulfite 976.0	E858.7	E946.0	E950.4	E962.0	E980.4
indigotindisulfonate 977.8	E858.8	E947.8	E950.4	E962.0	E980.4
iodide 977.8	E858.8	E947.8	E950.4	E962.0	E980.4
iothalamate 977.8	E858.8	E947.8	E950.4	E962.0	E980.4
iron edetate 964.0	E858.2	E934.0	E950.4	E962.0	E980.4
lactate 963.3	E858.1	E933.3	E950.4	E962.0	E980.4
lauryl sulfate 976.2	E858.7	E946.2	E950.4	E962.0	E980.4
L–triiodothyronine 962.7	E858.0	E932.7	E950.4	E962.0	E980.4
metrizoate 977.8	E858.8	E947.8	E950.4	E962.0	E980.4
monofluoracetate (dust) (rodenticide) 989.4	E863.7	—	E950.6	E962.1	E980.7
morrhuate 972.7	E858.3	E942.7	E950.4	E962.0	E980.4
nafcillin 960.0	E856	E930.0	E950.4	E962.0	E980.4
nitrate (oxidizing agent) 983.9	E864.3	—	E950.7	E962.1	E980.6
nitrite (medicinal) 972.4	E858.3	E942.4	E950.4	E962.0	E980.4
nitroferricyanide 972.6	E858.3	E942.6	E950.4	E962.0	E980.4
nitroprusside 972.6	E858.3	E942.6	E950.4	E962.0	E980.4
para–aminohippurate 977.8	E858.8	E947.8	E950.4	E962.0	E980.4

Substance	Poisoning	Accident	Therapeutic Use	Suicide Attempt	Assault	Undetermined
			External Cause (E-Code)			
perborate (non-medicinal) NEC	989.89	E866.8	—	E950.9	E962.1	E980.9
medicinal	976.6	E858.7	E946.6	E950.4	E962.0	E980.4
soap	989.6	E861.1	—	E950.9	E962.1	E980.9
percarbonate — see Sodium, perborate						
phosphate	973.3	E858.4	E943.3	E950.4	E962.0	E980.4
polystyrene sulfonate	974.5	E858.5	E944.5	E950.4	E962.0	E980.4
propionate	976.0	E858.7	E946.0	E950.4	E962.0	E980.4
psylliate	972.7	E858.3	E942.7	E950.4	E962.0	E980.4
removing resins	974.5	E858.5	E944.5	E950.4	E962.0	E980.4
salicylate	965.1	E850.3	E935.3	E950.0	E962.0	E980.0
sulfate	973.3	E858.4	E943.3	E950.4	E962.0	E980.4
sulfoxone	961.8	E857	E931.8	E950.4	E962.0	E980.4
tetradecyl sulfate	972.7	E858.3	E942.7	E950.4	E962.0	E980.4
thiopental	968.3	E855.1	E938.3	E950.4	E962.0	E980.4
thiosalicylate	965.1	E850.3	E935.3	E950.0	E962.0	E980.0
thiosulfate	976.0	E858.7	E946.0	E950.4	E962.0	E980.4
tolbutamide	977.8	E858.8	E947.8	E950.4	E962.0	E980.4
tyropanoate	977.8	E858.8	E947.8	E950.4	E962.0	E980.4
valproate	966.3	E855.0	E936.3	E950.4	E962.0	E980.4
Solanine	977.8	E858.8	E947.8	E950.4	E962.0	E980.4
Solanum dulcamara	988.2	E865.4	—	E950.9	E962.1	E980.9
Solapsone	961.8	E857	E931.8	E950.4	E962.0	E980.4
Solasulfone	961.8	E857	E931.8	E950.4	E962.0	E980.4
Soldering fluid	983.1	E864.1	—	E950.7	E962.1	E980.6
Solid substance	989.9	E866.9	—	E950.9	E962.1	E980.9
specified NEC	989.9	E866.8	—	E950.9	E962.1	E980.9
Solvents, industrial	982.8	E862.9	—	E950.9	E962.1	E980.9
naphtha	981	E862.0	—	E950.9	E962.1	E980.9
petroleum	981	E862.0	—	E950.9	E962.1	E980.9
specified NEC	982.8	E862.4	—	E950.9	E962.1	E980.9
Soma	968.0	E855.1	E938.0	E950.4	E962.0	E980.4
Somatotropin	962.4	E858.0	E932.4	E950.4	E962.0	E980.4
Sominex	963.0	E858.1	E933.0	E950.4	E962.0	E980.4
Somnos	967.1	E852.0	E937.1	E950.2	E962.0	E980.2
Somonal	967.0	E851	E937.0	E950.1	E962.0	E980.1
Soneryl	967.0	E851	E937.0	E950.1	E962.0	E980.1
Soothing syrup	977.9	E858.9	E947.9	E950.5	E962.0	E980.5
Sopor	967.4	E852.3	E937.4	E950.2	E962.0	E980.2
Soporific drug	967.9	E852.9	E937.9	E950.2	E962.0	E980.2
specified type NEC	967.8	E852.8	E937.8	E950.2	E962.0	E980.2
Sorbitol NEC	977.4	E858.8	E947.4	E950.4	E962.0	E980.4
Sotradecol	972.7	E858.3	E942.7	E950.4	E962.0	E980.4
Spacoline	975.1	E858.6	E945.1	E950.4	E962.0	E980.4
Spanish fly	976.8	E858.7	E946.8	E950.4	E962.0	E980.4
Sparine	969.1	E853.0	E939.1	E950.3	E962.0	E980.3
Sparteine	975.0	E858.6	E945.0	E950.4	E962.0	E980.4
Spasmolytics	975.1	E858.6	E945.1	E950.4	E962.0	E980.4
anticholinergics	971.1	E855.4	E941.1	E950.4	E962.0	E980.4
Spectinomycin	960.8	E856	E930.8	E950.4	E962.0	E980.4
Speed	969.72	E854.2	E939.7	E950.3	E962.0	E980.3
Spermicides	976.8	E858.7	E946.8	E950.4	E962.0	E980.4
Spider (bite) (venom)	989.5	E905.1	—	E950.9	E962.1	E980.9
antivenin	979.9	E858.8	E949.9	E950.4	E962.0	E980.4
Spigelia (root)	961.6	E857	E931.6	E950.4	E962.0	E980.4
Spiperone	969.2	E853.1	E939.2	E950.3	E962.0	E980.3
Spiramycin	960.3	E856	E930.3	E950.4	E962.0	E980.4
Spirilene	969.5	E853.8	E939.5	E950.3	E962.0	E980.3
Spirit(s) (neutral) NEC	980.0	E860.1	—	E950.9	E962.1	E980.9
beverage	980.0	E860.0	—	E950.9	E962.1	E980.9
industrial	980.9	E860.9	—	E950.9	E962.1	E980.9

Substance	Poisoning	Accident	Therapeutic Use	Suicide Attempt	Assault	Undetermined
			External Cause (E-Code)			
mineral	981	E862.0	—	E950.9	E962.1	E980.9
of salt — *see* Hydrochloric acid						
surgical	980.9	E860.9	—	E950.9	E962.1	E980.9
Spironolactone	974.4	E858.5	E944.4	E950.4	E962.0	E980.4
Sponge, absorbable (gelatin)	964.5	E858.2	E934.5	E950.4	E962.0	E980.4
Sporostacin	976.0	E858.7	E946.0	E950.4	E962.0	E980.4
Sprays (aerosol)	989.89	E866.8	—	E950.9	E962.1	E980.9
cosmetic	989.89	E866.7	—	E950.9	E962.1	E980.9
medicinal NEC	977.9	E858.9	E947.9	E950.5	E962.0	E980.5
pesticides — *see* Pesticides						
specified content — *see* substance						
specified						
Spurge flax	988.2	E865.4	—	E950.9	E962.1	E980.9
Spurges	988.2	E865.4	—	E950.9	E962.1	E980.9
Squill (expectorant) NEC	975.5	E858.6	E945.5	E950.4	E962.0	E980.4
rat poison	989.4	E863.7	—	E950.6	E962.1	E980.7
Squirting cucumber (cathartic)	973.1	E858.4	E943.1	E950.4	E962.0	E980.4
SSNRI (selective serotonin and						
norepinephrine reuptake inhibitors)	969.02	E854.0	E939.0	E950.3	E962.0	E980.3
SSRI (selective serotonin reuptake inhibitors)	969.03	E854.0	E939.0	E950.3	E962.0	E980.3
Stains	989.89	E866.8	—	E950.9	E962.1	E980.9
Stannous — *see also* Tin						
fluoride	976.7	E858.7	E946.7	E950.4	E962.0	E980.4
Stanolone	962.1	E858.0	E932.1	E950.4	E962.0	E980.4
Stanozolol	962.1	E853.0	E932.1	E950.4	E962.0	E980.4
Staphisagria or stavesacre (pediculicide)	976.0	E858.7	E946.0	E950.4	E962.0	E980.4
Stelazine	969.1	E853.0	E939.1	E950.3	E962.0	E980.3
Stemetil	969.1	E853.0	E939.1	E950.3	E962.0	E980.3
Sterculia (cathartic) (gum)	973.3	E858.4	E943.3	E950.4	E962.0	E980.4
Sternutator gas	987.8	E869.8	—	E952.8	E962.2	E982.8
Steroids NEC	962.0	E858.0	E932.0	E950.4	E962.0	E980.4
ENT agent	976.6	E858.7	E946.6	E950.4	E962.0	E980.4
ophthalmic preparation	976.5	E858.7	E946.5	E950.4	E962.0	E980.4
topical NEC	976.0	E858.7	E946.0	E950.4	E962.0	E980.4
Stibine	985.8	E866.4	—	E950.9	E962.1	E980.9
Stibophen	961.2	E857	E931.2	E950.4	E962.0	E980.4
Stilbamide, stilbamidine	961.5	E857	E931.5	E950.4	E962.0	E980.4
Stilbestrol	962.2	E858.0	E932.2	E950.4	E962.0	E980.4
Stimulants (central nervous system)	970.9	E854.3	E940.9	E950.4	E962.0	E980.4
analeptics	970.0	E854.3	E940.0	E950.4	E962.0	E980.4
opiate antagonist	970.1	E854.3	E940.1	E950.4	E962.0	E980.4
psychotherapeutic NEC	969.09	E854.0	E939.0	E950.3	E962.0	E980.3
specified NEC	970.89	E854.3	E940.8	E950.4	E962.0	E980.4
Storage batteries (acid) (cells)	983.1	E864.1	—	E950.7	E962.1	E980.6
Stovaine	968.9	E855.2	E938.9	E950.4	E962.0	E980.4
infiltration (subcutaneous)	968.5	E855.2	E938.5	E950.4	E962.0	E980.4
nerve block (peripheral) (plexus)	968.6	E855.2	E938.6	E950.5	E962.0	E980.4
spinal	968.7	E855.2	E938.7	E950.4	E962.0	E980.4
topical (surface)	968.5	E855.2	E938.5	E950.4	E962.0	E980.4
Stovarsal	961.1	E857	E931.1	E950.4	E962.0	E980.4
Stove gas — *see* Gas, utility						
Stoxil	976.5	E858.7	E946.5	E950.4	E962.0	E980.4
STP	969.6	E854.1	E939.6	E950.3	E962.0	E980.3
Stramonium (medicinal) NEC	971.1	E855.4	E941.1	E950.4	E962.0	E980.4
natural state	988.2	E865.4	—	E950.9	E962.1	E980.9
Streptodornase	964.4	E858.2	E934.4	E950.4	E962.0	E980.4
Streptoduocin	960.6	E856	E930.6	E950.4	E962.0	E980.4
Streptokinase	964.4	E858.2	E934.4	E950.4	E962.0	E980.4
Streptomycin	960.6	E856	E930.6	E950.4	E962.0	E980.4
Streptozocin	960.7	E856	E930.7	E950.4	E962.0	E980.4
Stripper (paint) (solvent)	982.8	E862.9	—	E950.9	E962.1	E980.9

Substance	Poisoning	Accident	Therapeutic Use	Suicide Attempt	Assault	Undetermined
			External Cause (E-Code)			
Strobane	989.2	E863.0	—	E950.6	E962.1	E980.7
Strophanthin	972.1	E858.3	E942.1	E950.4	E962.0	E980.4
Strophanthus hispidus or kombe.	988.2	E865.4	—	E950.9	E962.1	E980.9
Strychnine (rodenticide) (salts)	989.1	E863.7	—	E950.6	E962.1	E980.7
medicinal NEC	970.89	E854.3	E940.8	E950.4	E962.0	E980.4
Strychnos (ignatii) — see Strychnine						
Styramate	968.0	E855.1	E938.0	E950.4	E962.0	E980.4
Styrene	983.0	E864.0	—	E950.7	E962.1	E980.6
Succinimide (anticonvulsant)	966.2	E855.0	E936.2	E950.4	E962.0	E980.4
mercuric — see Mercury						
Succinylcholine	975.2	E858.6	E945.2	E950.4	E962.0	E980.4
Succinylsulfathiazole	961.0	E857	E931.0	E950.4	E962.0	E980.4
Sucrose	974.5	E858.5	E944.5	E950.4	E962.0	E980.4
Sulfacetamide	961.0	E857	E931.0	E950.4	E962.0	E980.4
ophthalmic preparation	976.5	E858.7	E946.5	E950.4	E962.0	E980.4
Sulfachlorpyridazine.	961.0	E857	E931.0	E950.4	E962.0	E980.4
Sulfacytine	961.0	E857	E931.0	E950.4	E962.0	E980.4
Sulfadiazine	961.0	E857	E931.0	E950.4	E962.0	E980.4
silver (topical)	976.0	E858.7	E946.0	E950.4	E962.0	E980.4
Sulfadimethoxine	961.0	E857	E931.0	E950.4	E962.0	E980.4
Sulfadimidine	961.0	E857	E931.0	E950.4	E962.0	E980.4
Sulfaethidole.	961.0	E857	E931.0	E950.4	E962.0	E980.4
Sulfafurazole.	961.0	E857	E931.0	E950.4	E962.0	E980.4
Sulfaguanidine	961.0	E857	E931.0	E950.4	E962.0	E980.4
Sulfamerazine	961.0	E857	E931.0	E950.4	E962.0	E980.4
Sulfameter.	961.0	E857	E931.0	E950.4	E962.0	E980.4
Sulfamethizole	961.0	E857	E931.0	E950.4	E962.0	E980.4
Sulfamethoxazole	961.0	E857	E931.0	E950.4	E962.0	E980.4
Sulfamethoxydiazine	961.0	E857	E931.0	E950.4	E962.0	E980.4
Sulfamethoxypyridazine	961.0	E857	E931.0	E950.4	E962.0	E980.4
Sulfamethylthiazole	961.0	E857	E931.0	E950.4	E962.0	E980.4
Sulfamylon	976.0	E858.7	E946.0	E950.4	E962.0	E980.4
Sulfan blue (diagnostic dye)	977.8	E858.8	E947.8	E950.4	E962.0	E980.4
Sulfanilamide	961.0	E857	E931.0	E950.4	E962.0	E980.4
Sulfanilylguanidine	961.0	E857	E931.0	E950.4	E962.0	E980.4
Sulfaphenazole	961.0	E857	E931.0	E950.4	E962.0	E980.4
Sulfaphenylthiazole	961.0	E857	E931.0	E950.4	E962.0	E980.4
Sulfaproxyline	961.0	E857	E931.0	E950.4	E962.0	E980.4
Sulfapyridine	961.0	E857	E931.0	E950.4	E962.0	E980.4
Sulfapyrimidine	961.0	E857	E931.0	E950.4	E962.0	E980.4
Sulfarsphenamine	961.1	E857	E931.1	E950.4	E962.0	E980.4
Sulfasalazine.	961.0	E857	E931.0	E950.4	E962.0	E980.4
Sulfasomizole	961.0	E857	E931.0	E950.4	E962.0	E980.4
Sulfasuxidine	961.0	E857	E931.0	E950.4	E962.0	E980.4
Sulfinpyrazone	974.7	E858.5	E944.7	E950.4	E962.0	E980.4
Sulfisoxazole	961.0	E857	E931.0	E950.4	E962.0	E980.4
ophthalmic preparation	976.5	E858.7	E946.5	E950.4	E962.0	E980.4
Sulfomyxin	960.8	E856	E930.8	E950.4	E962.0	E980.4
Sulfonal.	967.8	E852.8	E937.8	E950.2	E962.0	E980.2
Sulfonamides (mixtures)	961.0	E857	E931.0	E950.4	E962.0	E980.4
Sulfones	961.8	E857	E931.8	E950.4	E962.0	E980.4
Sulfonethylmethane	967.8	E852.8	E937.8	E950.2	E962.0	E980.2
Sulfonmethane	967.8	E852.8	E937.8	E950.2	E962.0	E980.2
Sulfonphthal, sulfonphthol	977.8	E858.8	E947.8	E950.4	E962.0	E980.4
Sulfonylurea derivatives, oral	962.3	E858.0	E932.3	E950.4	E962.0	E980.4
Sulfoxone	961.8	E857	E931.8	E950.4	E962.0	E980.4
Sulfur, sulfureted, sulfuric, sulfurous,						
sulfuryl (compounds) NEC	989.89	E866.8	—	E950.9	E962.1	E980.9
acid	983.1	E864.1	—	E950.7	E962.1	E980.6
dioxide	987.3	E869.1	—	E952.8	E962.2	E982.8

Substance	Poisoning	Accident	Therapeutic Use	Suicide Attempt	Assault	Undetermined
			External Cause (E-Code)			
ether — *see* Ether(s)						
hydrogen	987.8	E869.8	—	E952.8	E962.2	E982.8
medicinal (keratolytic) (ointment) NEC	976.4	E858.7	E946.4	E950.4	E962.0	E980.4
pesticide (vapor)	989.4	E863.4	—	E950.6	E962.1	E980.7
vapor NEC.	987.8	E869.8	—	E952.8	E962.2	E982.8
Sulkowitch's reagent	977.8	E858.8	E947.8	E950.4	E962.0	E980.4
Sulph — *see also* Sulf–						
Sulphadione	961.8	E857	E931.8	E950.4	E962.0	E980.4
Sulthiame, sultiame	966.3	E855.0	E936.3	E950.4	E962.0	E980.4
Superinone	975.5	E858.6	E945.5	E950.4	E962.0	E980.4
Suramin.	961.5	E857	E931.5	E950.4	E962.0	E980.4
Surfacaine.	968.5	E855.2	E938.5	E950.4	E962.0	E980.4
Surital	968.3	E855.1	E938.3	E950.4	E962.0	E980.4
Sutilains	976.8	E858.7	E946.8	E950.4	E962.0	E980.4
Suxamethoniam (bromide) (chloride) (iodide)	975.2	E858.6	E945.2	E950.4	E962.0	E980.4
Suxethonium (bromide)	975.2	E858.6	E945.2	E950.4	E962.0	E980.4
Sweet oil (birch)	976.3	E858.7	E946.3	E950.4	E962.0	E980.4
Sym–dichloroethyl ether	982.3	E862.4	—	E950.9	E962.1	E980.9
Sympatholytics.	971.3	E855.6	E941.3	E950.4	E962.0	E980.4
Sympathomimetics	971.2	E855.5	E941.2	E950.4	E962.0	E980.4
Synagis	979.6	E858.8	E949.6	E950.4	E962.0	E980.4
Synalar	976.0	E858.7	E946.0	E950.4	E962.0	E980.4
Synthroid	962.7	E858.0	E932.7	E950.4	E962.0	E980.4
Syntocinon	975.0	E858.6	E945.0	E950.4	E962.0	E950.4
Syrosingopine	972.6	E858.3	E942.6	E950.4	E962.0	E980.4
Systemic agents (primarily)	963.9	E858.1	E933.9	E950.4	E962.0	E980.4
specified NEC	963.8	E858.1	E933.8	E950.4	E962.0	E980.4
Tablets (*see also* specified substance)	977.9	E858.9	E947.9	E950.5	E962.0	E980.5
Tace	962.2	E858.0	E932.2	E950.4	E962.0	E980.4
Tacrine	971.0	E855.3	E941.0	E950.4	E962.0	E980.4
Talbutal.	967.0	E851	E937.0	E950.1	E962.0	E980.1
Talc	976.3	E858.7	E946.3	E950.4	E962.0	E980.4
Talcum	976.3	E858.7	E946.3	E950.4	E962.0	E980.4
Tamsulosin	971.3	E855.6	E941.3	E950.4	E962.0	E980.4
Tandearil, tanderil	965.5	E850.5	E935.5	E950.0	E962.0	E980.0
Tannic acid	983.1	E864.1	—	E950.7	E962.1	E980.6
medicinal (astringent)	976.2	E858.7	E946.2	E950.4	E962.0	E980.4
Tannin — *see* Tannic acid						
Tansy.	988.2	E865.4	—	E950.9	E962.1	E980.9
TAO	960.3	E856	E930.3	E950.4	E962.0	E980.4
Tapazole	962.8	E858.0	E932.8	E950.4	E962.0	E980.4
Tar NEC	983.0	E864.0	—	E950.7	E962.1	E980.6
camphor — *see* Naphthalene						
fumes.	987.8	E869.8	—	E952.8	E962.2	E982.8
Taractan	969.3	E853.8	E939.3	E950.3	E962.0	E980.3
Tarantula (venomous)	989.5	E905.1	—	E950.9	E962.1	E980.9
Tartar emetic (anti–infective)	961.2	E857	E931.2	E950.4	E962.0	E980.4
Tartaric acid.	983.1	E864.1	—	E950.7	E962.1	E980.6
Tartrated antimony (anti–infective).	961.2	E857	E931.2	E950.4	E962.0	E980.4
TCA — *see* Trichloroacetic acid						
TDI	983.0	E864.0	—	E950.7	E962.1	E980.6
vapor	987.8	E869.8	—	E952.8	E962.2	E982.8
Tear gas	987.5	E869.3	—	E952.8	E962.2	E982.8
Teclothiazide.	974.3	E858.5	E944.3	E950.4	E962.0	E980.4
Tegretol.	966.3	E855.0	E936.3	E950.4	E962.0	E980.4
Telepaque.	977.8	E858.8	E947.8	E950.4	E962.0	E980.4
Tellurium	985.8	E866.4	—	E950.9	E962.1	E980.9
fumes.	985.8	E866.4	—	E950.9	E962.1	E980.9
TEM	963.1	E858.1	E933.1	E950.4	E962.0	E980.4
Temazepan—*see* Benzodiazepines						

Substance	Poisoning	Accident	Therapeutic Use	Suicide Attempt	Assault	Undetermined
			External Cause (E-Code)			
TEPA	963.1	E858.1	E933.1	E950.4	E962.0	E980.4
TEPP.	989.3	E863.1	—	E950.6	E962.1	E980.7
Terbutaline	971.2	E855.5	E941.2	E950.4	E962.0	E980.4
Teroxalene	961.6	E857	E931.6	E950.4	E962.0	E980.4
Terpin hydrate	975.5	E858.6	E945.5	E950.4	E962.0	E980.4
Terramycin	960.4	E856	E930.4	E950.4	E962.0	E980.4
Tessalon	975.4	E858.6	E945.4	E950.4	E962.0	E980.4
Testosterone	962.1	E858.0	E932.1	E950.4	E962.0	E980.4
Tetanus (vaccine)	978.4	E858.8	E948.4	E950.4	E962.0	E980.4
antitoxin	979.9	E858.8	E949.9	E950.4	E962.0	E980.4
immune globulin (human)	964.6	E858.2	E934.6	E950.4	E962.0	E980.4
toxoid	978.4	E858.8	E948.4	E950.4	E962.0	E980.4
with diphtheria toxoid	978.9	E858.8	E948.9	E950.4	E962.0	E980.4
with pertussis	978.6	E858.8	E948.6	E950.4	E962.0	E980.4
Tetrabenazine	969.5	E853.8	E939.5	E950.3	E962.0	E980.3
Tetracaine (infiltration) (topical)	968.5	E855.2	E938.5	E950.4	E962.0	E980.4
nerve block (peripheral) (plexus)	968.6	E855.2	E938.6	E950.4	E962.0	E980.4
spinal	968.7	E855.2	E938.7	E950.4	E962.0	E980.4
Tetrachlorethylene—see Tetrachloroethylene						
Tetrachlormethiazide	974.3	E858.5	E944.3	E950.4	E962.0	E980.4
Tetrachloroethane (liquid) (vapor)	982.3	E862.4	—	E950.9	E962.1	E980.9
paint or varnish	982.3	E861.6	—	E950.9	E962.1	E980.9
Tetrachloroethylene (liquid) (vapor)	982.3	E862.4	—	E950.9	E962.1	E980.9
medicinal	961.6	E857	E931.6	E950.4	E962.0	E980.4
Tetrachloromethane — see Carbon, tetrachloride						
Tetracycline	960.4	E856	E930.4	E950.4	E962.0	E980.4
ophthalmic preparation	976.5	E858.7	E946.5	E950.4	E962.0	E980.4
topical NEC	976.0	E858.7	E946.0	E950.4	E962.0	E980.4
Tetraethylammonium chloride	972.3	E858.3	E942.3	E950.4	E962.0	E980.4
Tetraethyl lead (antiknock compound)	984.1	E862.1	—	E950.9	E962.1	E980.9
Tetraethyl pyrophosphate	989.3	E863.1	—	E950.6	E962.1	E980.7
Tetraethylthiuram disulfide	977.3	E858.8	E947.3	E950.4	E962.0	E980.4
Tetrahydroaminoacridine	971.0	E855.3	E941.0	E950.4	E962.0	E980.4
Tetrahydrocannabinol	969.6	E854.1	E939.6	E950.3	E962.0	E980.3
Tetrahydronaphthalene	982.0	E862.4	—	E950.9	E962.1	E980.9
Tetrahydrozoline	971.2	E855.5	E941.2	E950.4	E962.0	E980.4
Tetralin	982.0	E862.4	—	E950.9	E962.1	E980.9
Tetramethylthiuram (disulfide) NEC	989.4	E863.6	—	E950.6	E962.1	E980.7
medicinal	976.2	E858.7	E946.2	E950.4	E962.0	E980.4
Tetronal	967.8	E852.8	E937.8	E950.2	E962.0	E980.2
Tetryl	983.0	E864.0	—	E950.7	E962.1	E980.6
Thalidomide	967.8	E852.8	E937.8	E950.2	E962.0	E980.2
Thallium (compounds) (dust) NEC	985.8	E866.4	—	E950.9	E962.1	E980.9
pesticide (rodenticide)	985.8	E863.7	—	E950.6	E962.1	E980.7
THC	969.6	E854.1	E939.6	E950.3	E962.0	E980.3
Thebacon	965.09	E850.2	E935.2	E950.0	E962.0	E980.0
Thebaine	965.09	E850.2	E935.2	E950.0	E962.0	E980.0
Theobromine (calcium salicylate)	974.1	E858.5	E944.1	E950.4	E962.0	E980.4
Theophylline (diuretic)	974.1	E858.5	E944.1	E950.4	E962.0	E980.4
ethylenediamine	975.7	E858.6	E945.7	E950.4	E962.0	E980.4
Thiabendazole	961.6	E857	E931.6	E950.4	E962.0	E980.4
Thialbarbital, thialbarbitone	968.3	E855.1	E938.3	E950.4	E962.0	E980.4
Thiamine	963.5	E858.1	E933.5	E950.4	E962.0	E980.4
Thiamylal (sodium)	968.3	E855.1	E938.3	E950.4	E962.0	E980.4
Thiazesim	969.09	E854.0	E939.0	E950.3	E962.0	E980.3
Thiazides (diuretics)	974.3	E858.5	E944.3	E950.4	E962.0	E980.4
Thiethylperazine	963.0	E858.1	E933.0	E950.4	E962.0	E980.4
Thimerosal (topical)	976.0	E858.7	E946.0	E950.4	E962.0	E980.4
ophthalmic preparation	976.5	E858.7	E946.5	E950.4	E962.0	E980.4

Substance	Poisoning	Accident	Therapeutic Use	Suicide Attempt	Assault	Undetermined
			External Cause (E-Code)			
Thioacetazone 961.8	E857	E931.8	E950.4	E962.0	E980.4
Thiobarbiturates 968.3	E855.1	E938.3	E950.4	E962.0	E980.4
Thiobismol 961.2	E857	E931.2	E950.4	E962.0	E980.4
Thiocarbamide 962.8	E858.0	E932.8	E950.4	E962.0	E980.4
Thiocarbarsone 961.1	E857	E931.1	E950.4	E962.0	E980.4
Thiocarlide 961.8	E857	E931.8	E950.4	E962.0	E980.4
Thioguanine 963.1	E858.1	E933.1	E950.4	E962.0	E980.4
Thiomercaptomerin 974.0	E858.5	E944.0	E950.4	E962.0	E980.4
Thiomerin 974.0	E858.5	E944.0	E950.4	E962.0	E980.4
Thiopental, thiopentone (sodium) 968.3	E855.1	E938.3	E950.4	E962.0	E980.4
Thiopropazate 969.1	E853.0	E939.1	E950.3	E962.0	E980.3
Thioproperazine 969.1	E853.0	E939.1	E950.3	E962.0	E980.3
Thioridazine 969.1	E853.0	E939.1	E950.3	E962.0	E980.3
Thio–TEPA, thiotepa 963.1	E858.1	E933.1	E950.4	E962.0	E980.4
Thiothixene 969.3	E853.8	E939.3	E950.3	E962.0	E980.3
Thiouracil 962.8	E858.0	E932.8	E950.4	E962.0	E980.4
Thiourea 962.8	E858.0	E932.8	E950.4	E962.0	E980.4
Thiphenamil 971.1	E855.4	E941.1	E950.4	E962.0	E980.4
Thiram NEC. 989.4	E863.6	—	E950.6	E962.1	E980.7
medicinal 976.2	E858.7	E946.2	E950.4	E962.0	E980.4
Thonzylamine 963.0	E858.1	E933.0	E950.4	E962.0	E980.4
Thorazine 969.1	E853.0	E939.1	E950.3	E962.0	E980.3
Thornapple 988.2	E865.4	—	E950.9	E962.1	E980.9
Throat preparation (lozenges) NEC 976.6	E858.7	E946.6	E950.4	E962.0	E980.4
Thrombin 964.5	E858.2	E934.5	E950.4	E962.0	E980.4
Thrombolysin 964.4	E858.2	E934.4	E950.4	E962.0	E980.4
Thymol 983.0	E864.0	—	E950.7	E962.1	E980.6
Thymus extract. 962.9	E858.0	E932.9	E950.4	E962.0	E980.4
Thyroglobulin 962.7	E858.0	E932.7	E950.4	E962.0	E980.4
Thyroid (derivatives) (extract). 962.7	E858.0	E932.7	E950.4	E962.0	E980.4
Thyrolar 962.7	E858.0	E932.7	E950.4	E962.0	E980.4
Thyrothrophin, thyrotropin 977.8	E858.8	E947.8	E950.4	E962.0	E980.4
Thyroxin(e) 962.7	E858.0	E932.7	E950.4	E962.0	E980.4
Tigan. 963.0	E858.1	E933.0	E950.4	E962.0	E980.4
Tigloidine 968.0	E855.1	E938.0	E950.4	E962.0	E980.4
Tin (chloride) (dust) (oxide) NEC 985.8	E866.4	—	E950.9	E962.1	E980.9
anti–infectives 961.2	E857	E931.2	E950.4	E962.0	E980.4
Tinactin. 976.0	E858.7	E946.0	E950.4	E962.0	E980.4
Tincture, iodine — *see* Iodine					
Tindal 969.1	E853.0	E939.1	E950.3	E962.0	E980.3
Titanium (compounds) (vapor) 985.8	E866.4	—	E950.9	E962.1	E980.9
ointment. 976.3	E858.7	E946.3	E950.4	E962.0	E980.4
Titroid 962.7	E858.0	E932.7	E950.4	E962.0	E980.4
TMTD — *see* Tetramethylthiuram disulfide					
TNT 989.89	E866.8	—	E950.9	E962.1	E980.9
fumes. 987.8	E869.8	—	E952.8	E962.2	E982.8
Toadstool 988.1	E865.5	—	E950.9	E962.1	E980.9
Tobacco NEC 989.84	E866.8	—	E950.9	E962.1	E980.9
Indian. 988.2	E865.4	—	E950.9	E962.1	E980.9
smoke, second-hand 987.8	E869.4	—	—	—	—
Tocopherol 963.5	E858.1	E933.5	E950.4	E962.0	E980.4
Tocosamine 975.0	E858.6	E945.0	E950.4	E962.0	E980.4
Tofranil. 969.05	E854.0	E939.0	E950.3	E962.0	E980.3
Toilet deodorizer 989.8	E866.8	—	E950.9	E962.1	E980.9
Tolazamide 962.3	E858.0	E932.3	E950.4	E962.0	E980.4
Tolazoline. 971.3	E855.6	E941.3	E950.4	E962.0	E980.4
Tolbutamide 962.3	E858.0	E932.3	E950.4	E962.0	E980.4
sodium 977.8	E858.8	E947.8	E950.4	E962.0	E980.4
Tolmetin 965.69	E850.6	E935.6	E950.0	E962.0	E980.0
Tolnaftate 976.0	E858.7	E946.0	E950.4	E962.0	E980.4
Tolpropamine 976.1	E858.7	E946.1	E950.4	E962.0	E980.4

Substance	Poisoning	Accident	Therapeutic Use	Suicide Attempt	Assault	Undetermined
		External Cause (E-Code)				
Tolserol	968.0	E855.1	E938.0	E950.4	E962.0	E980.4
Toluene (liquid) (vapor)	982.0	E862.4	—	E950.9	E962.1	E980.9
diisocyanate	983.0	E864.0	—	E950.7	E962.1	E980.6
Toluidine	983.0	E864.0	—	E950.7	E962.1	E980.6
vapor	987.8	E869.8	—	E952.8	E962.2	E982.8
Toluol (liquid) (vapor)	982.0	E862.4	—	E950.9	E962.1	E980.9
Tolylene–2,4–diisocyanate	983.0	E864.0	—	E950.7	E962.1	E980.6
Tonics, cardiac	972.1	E858.3	E942.1	E950.4	E962.0	E980.4
Toxaphene (dust) (spray)	989.2	E863.0	—	E950.6	E962.1	E980.7
Toxoids NEC	978.8	E858.8	E948.8	E950.4	E962.0	E980.4
Tractor fuel NEC	981	E862.1	—	E950.9	E962.1	E980.9
Tragacanth	973.3	E858.4	E943.3	E950.4	E962.0	E980.4
Tramazoline	971.2	E855.5	E941.2	E950.4	E962.0	E980.4
Tranquilizers	969.5	E853.9	E939.5	E950.3	E962.0	E980.3
benzodiazepine–based	969.4	E853.2	E939.4	E950.3	E962.0	E980.3
butyrophenone–based	969.2	E853.1	E939.2	E950.3	E962.0	E980.3
major NEC	969.3	E853.8	E939.3	E950.3	E962.0	E980.3
phenothiazine–based	969.1	E853.0	E939.1	E950.3	E962.0	E980.3
specified NEC	969.5	E853.8	E939.5	E950.3	E962.0	E980.3
Trantoin	961.9	E857	E931.9	E950.4	E962.0	E980.4
Tranxene	969.4	E853.2	E939.4	E950.3	E962.0	E980.3
Tranylcypromine (sulfate)	969.01	E854.0	E939.0	E950.3	E962.0	E980.3
Trasentine	975.1	E858.6	E945.1	E950.4	E962.0	E980.4
Travert	974.5	E858.5	E944.5	E950.4	E962.0	E980.4
Trecator	961.8	E857	E931.8	E950.4	E962.0	E980.4
Tretinoin	976.8	E858.7	E946.8	E950.4	E962.0	E980.4
Triacetin	976.0	E858.7	E946.0	E950.4	E962.0	E980.4
Triacetyloleandomycin	960.3	E856	E930.3	E950.4	E962.0	E980.4
Triamcinolone	962.0	E858.0	E932.0	E950.4	E962.0	E980.4
ENT agent	976.6	E858.7	E946.6	E950.4	E962.0	E980.4
ophthalmic preparation	976.5	E858.7	E946.5	E950.4	E962.0	E980.4
topical NEC	976.0	E858.7	E946.0	E950.4	E962.0	E980.4
Triamterene	974.4	E858.5	E944.4	E950.4	E962.0	E980.4
Triaziquone	963.1	E858.1	E933.1	E950.4	E962.0	E980.4
Tribromacetaldehyde	967.3	E852.2	E937.3	E950.2	E962.0	E980.2
Tribromoethanol	968.2	E855.1	E938.2	E950.4	E962.0	E980.4
Tribromomethane	967.3	E852.2	E937.3	E950.2	E962.0	E980.2
Trichlorethane	982.3	E862.4	—	E950.9	E962.1	E980.9
Trichlormethiazide	974.3	E858.5	E944.3	E950.4	E962.0	E980.4
Trichloroacetic acid	983.1	E864.1	—	E950.7	E962.1	E980.6
medicinal (keratolytic)	976.4	E858.7	E946.4	E950.4	E962.0	E980.4
Trichloroethanol	967.1	E852.0	E937.1	E950.2	E962.0	E980.2
Trichloroethylene (liquid) (vapor)	982.3	E862.4	—	E950.9	E962.1	E980.9
anesthetic (gas)	968.2	E855.1	E938.2	E950.4	E962.0	E980.4
Trichloroethyl phosphate	967.1	E852.0	E937.1	E950.2	E962.0	E980.2
Trichlorofluoromethane NEC	987.4	E869.2	—	E952.8	E962.2	E982.8
Trichlorotriethylamine	963.1	E858.1	E933.1	E950.4	E962.0	E980.4
Trichomonacides NEC	961.5	E857	E931.5	E950.4	E962.0	E980.4
Trichomycin	960.1	E856	E930.1	E950.4	E962.0	E980.4
Triclofos	967.1	E852.0	E937.1	E950.2	E962.0	E980.2
Tricresyl phosphate	989.89	E866.8	—	E950.9	E962.1	E980.9
solvent	982.8	E862.4	—	E950.9	E962.1	E980.9
Tricyclamol	966.4	E855.0	E936.4	E950.4	E962.0	E980.4
Tridesilon	976.0	E858.7	E946.0	E950.4	E962.0	E980.4
Tridihexethyl	971.1	E855.4	E941.1	E950.4	E962.0	E980.4
Tridione	966.0	E855.0	E936.0	E950.4	E962.0	E980.4
Triethanolamine NEC	983.2	E864.2	—	E950.7	E962.1	E980.6
detergent	983.2	E861.0	—	E950.7	E962.1	E980.6
trinitrate	972.4	E858.3	E942.4	E950.4	E962.0	E980.4
Triethanomelamine	963.1	E858.1	E933.1	E950.4	E962.0	E980.4

TABLE OF DRUGS AND CHEMICALS

Substance	Poisoning	Accident	Therapeutic Use	Suicide Attempt	Assault	Undetermined
		External Cause (E-Code)				
Triethylene melamine	963.1	E858.1	E933.1	E950.4	E962.0	E980.4
Triethylenephosphoramide	963.1	E858.1	E933.1	E950.4	E962.0	E980.4
Triethylenethiophosphoramide	963.1	E858.1	E933.1	E950.4	E962.0	E980.4
Trifluoperazine	969.1	E853.0	E939.1	E950.3	E962.0	E980.3
Trifluperidol	969.2	E853.1	E939.2	E950.3	E962.0	E980.3
Triflupromazine	969.1	E853.0	E939.1	E950.3	E962.0	E980.3
Trihexyphenidyl	971.1	E855.4	E941.1	E950.4	E962.0	E980.4
Triiodothyronine	962.7	E858.0	E932.7	E950.4	E962.0	E980.4
Trilene	968.2	E855.1	E938.2	E950.4	E962.0	E980.4
Trimeprazine	963.0	E858.1	E933.0	E950.4	E962.0	E980.4
Trimetazidine	972.4	E858.3	E942.4	E950.4	E962.0	E980.4
Trimethadione	966.0	E855.0	E936.0	E950.4	E962.0	E980.4
Trimethaphan	972.3	E858.3	E942.3	E950.4	E962.0	E980.4
Trimethidinium	972.3	E858.3	E942.3	E950.4	E962.0	E980.4
Trimethobenzamide	963.0	E858.1	E933.0	E950.4	E962.0	E980.4
Trimethylcarbinol	980.8	E860.8	—	E950.9	E962.1	E980.9
Trimethylpsoralen	976.3	E858.7	E946.3	E950.4	E962.0	E980.4
Trimeton	963.0	E858.1	E933.0	E950.4	E962.0	E980.4
Trimipramine	969.05	E854.0	E939.0	E950.3	E962.0	E980.3
Trimustine	963.1	E858.1	E933.1	E950.4	E962.0	E980.4
Trinitrin	972.4	E858.3	E942.4	E950.4	E962.0	E980.4
Trinitrophenol	983.0	E864.0	—	E950.7	E962.1	E980.6
Trinitrotoluene	989.89	E866.8	—	E950.9	E962.1	E980.9
fumes	987.8	E869.8	—	E952.8	E962.2	E982.8
Trional	967.8	E852.8	E937.8	E950.2	E962.0	E980.2
Trioxide of arsenic — *see* Arsenic						
Trioxsalen	976.3	E858.7	E946.3	E950.4	E962.0	E980.4
Tripelennamine	963.0	E858.1	E933.0	E950.4	E962.0	E980.4
Triperidol	969.2	E853.1	E939.2	E950.3	E962.0	E980.3
Triprolidine	963.0	E858.1	E933.0	E950.4	E962.0	E980.4
Trisoralen	976.3	E858.7	E946.3	E950.4	E962.0	E980.4
Troleandomycin	960.3	E856	E930.3	E950.4	E962.0	E980.4
Trolnitrate (phosphate)	972.4	E858.3	E942.4	E950.4	E962.0	E980.4
Trometamol	963.3	E858.1	E933.3	E950.4	E962.0	E980.4
Tromethamine	963.3	E858.1	E933.3	E950.4	E962.0	E980.4
Tronothane	968.5	E855.2	E938.5	E950.4	E962.0	E980.4
Tropicamide	971.1	E855.4	E941.1	E950.4	E962.0	E980.4
Troxidone	966.0	E855.0	E936.0	E950.4	E962.0	E980.4
Tryparsamide	961.1	E857	E931.1	E950.4	E962.0	E980.4
Trypsin	963.4	E858.1	E933.4	E950.4	E962.0	E980.4
Tryptizol	969.05	E854.0	E939.0	E950.3	E962.0	E980.3
Tuaminoheptane	971.2	E855.5	E941.2	E950.4	E962.0	E980.4
Tuberculin (old)	977.8	E858.8	E947.8	E950.4	E962.0	E980.4
Tubocurare	975.2	E858.6	E945.2	E950.4	E962.0	E980.4
Tubocurarine	975.2	E858.6	E945.2	E950.4	E962.0	E980.4
Turkish green	969.6	E854.1	E939.6	E950.3	E962.0	E980.3
Turpentine (spirits of) (liquid) (vapor)	982.8	E862.4	—	E950.9	E962.1	E980.9
Tybamate	969.5	E853.8	E939.5	E950.3	E962.0	E980.3
Tyloxapol	975.5	E858.6	E945.5	E950.4	E962.0	E980.4
Tymazoline	971.2	E855.5	E941.2	E950.4	E962.0	E980.4
Typhoid vaccine	978.1	E858.8	E948.1	E950.4	E962.0	E980.4
Typhus vaccine	979.2	E858.8	E949.2	E950.4	E962.0	E980.4
Tyrothricin	976.0	E858.7	E946.0	E950.4	E962.0	E980.4
ENT agent	976.6	E858.7	E946.6	E950.4	E962.0	E980.4
ophthalmic preparation	976.5	E858.7	E946.5	E950.4	E962.0	E980.4
Undecenoic acid	976.0	E858.7	E946.0	E950.4	E962.0	E980.4
Undecylenic acid	976.0	E858.7	E946.0	E950.4	E962.0	E980.4
Unna's boot	976.3	E858.7	E946.3	E950.4	E962.0	E980.4
Uracil mustard	963.1	E858.1	E933.1	E950.4	E962.0	E980.4
Uramustine	963.1	E858.1	E933.1	E950.4	E962.0	E980.4
Urari	975.2	E858.6	E945.2	E950.4	E962.0	E980.4

Substance	Poisoning	Accident	Therapeutic Use	Suicide Attempt	Assault	Undetermined
			External Cause (E-Code)			
Urea	974.4	E858.5	E944.4	E950.4	E962.0	E980.4
topical	976.8	E858.7	E946.8	E950.4	E962.0	E980.4
Urethan(e) (antineoplastic)	963.1	E858.1	E933.1	E950.4	E962.0	E980.4
Urginea (maritima) (scilla) — *see* Squill						
Uric acid metabolism agents NEC	974.7	E858.5	E944.7	E950.4	E962.0	E980.4
Urokinase	964.4	E858.2	E934.4	E950.4	E962.0	E980.4
Urokon	977.8	E858.8	E947.8	E950.4	E962.0	E980.4
Urotropin	961.9	E857	E931.9	E950.4	E962.0	E980.4
Urtica	988.2	E865.4	—	E950.9	E962.1	E980.9
Utility gas — *see* Gas, utility						
Vaccine NEC	979.9	E858.8	E949.9	E950.4	E962.0	E980.4
bacterial NEC	978.8	E858.8	E948.8	E950.4	E962.0	E980.4
with						
other bacterial component	978.9	E858.8	E948.9	E950.4	E962.0	E980.4
pertussis component	978.6	E858.8	E948.6	E950.4	E962.0	E980.4
viral–rickettsial component	979.7	E858.8	E949.7	E950.4	E962.0	E980.4
mixed NEC	978.9	E858.8	E948.9	E950.4	E962.0	E980.4
BCG	978.0	E858.8	E948.0	E950.4	E962.0	E980.4
cholera	978.2	E858.8	E948.2	E950.4	E962.0	E980.4
diphtheria	978.5	E858.8	E948.5	E950.4	E962.0	E980.4
influenza	979.6	E858.8	E949.6	E950.4	E962.0	E980.4
measles	979.4	E858.8	E949.4	E950.4	E962.0	E980.4
meningococcal	978.8	E858.8	E948.8	E950.4	E962.0	E980.4
mumps	979.6	E858.8	E949.6	E950.4	E962.0	E980.4
paratyphoid	978.1	E858.8	E948.1	E950.4	E962.0	E980.4
pertussis (with diphtheria toxoid) (with tetanus toxoid)	978.6	E858.8	E948.6	E950.4	E962.0	E980.4
plague	978.3	E858.8	E948.3	E950.4	E962.0	E980.4
poliomyelitis	979.5	E858.8	E949.5	E950.4	E962.0	E980.4
poliovirus	979.5	E858.8	E949.5	E950.4	E962.0	E980.4
rabies	979.1	E858.8	E949.1	E950.4	E962.0	E980.4
respiratory syncytial virus	979.6	E858.8	E949.6	E950.4	E962.0	E980.4
rickettsial NEC	979.6	E858.8	E949.6	E950.4	E962.0	E980.4
with						
bacterial component	979.7	E858.8	E949.7	E950.4	E962.0	E980.4
pertussis component	978.6	E858.8	E948.6	E950.4	E962.0	E980.4
viral component	979.7	E858.8	E949.7	E950.4	E962.0	E980.4
Rocky Mountain spotted fever	979.6	E858.8	E949.6	E950.4	E962.0	E980.4
rotavirus	979.6	E858.8	E949.6	E950.4	E962.0	E980.4
rubella virus	979.4	E858.8	E949.4	E950.4	E962.0	E980.4
sabin oral	979.5	E858.8	E949.5	E950.4	E962.0	E980.4
smallpox	979.0	E858.8	E949.0	E950.4	E962.0	E980.4
tetanus	978.4	E858.8	E948.4	E950.4	E962.0	E980.4
typhoid	978.1	E858.8	E948.1	E950.4	E962.0	E980.4
typhus	979.2	E858.8	E949.2	E950.4	E962.0	E980.4
viral NEC	979.6	E858.8	E949.6	E950.4	E962.0	E980.4
with						
bacterial component	979.7	E858.8	E949.7	E950.4	E962.0	E980.4
pertussis component	978.6	E858.8	E948.6	E950.4	E962.0	E980.4
rickettsial component	979.7	E858.8	E949.7	E950.4	E962.0	E980.4
yellow fever	979.3	E858.8	E949.3	E950.4	E962.0	E980.4
Vaccinia immune globulin (human)	964.6	E858.2	E934.6	E950.4	E962.0	E980.4
Vaginal contraceptives	976.8	E858.7	E946.8	E950.4	E962.0	E980.4
Valethamate	971.1	E855.4	E941.1	E950.4	E962.0	E980.4
Valisone	976.0	E858.7	E946.0	E950.4	E962.0	E980.4
Valium	969.4	E853.2	E939.4	E950.3	E962.0	E980.3
Valmid	967.8	E852.8	E937.8	E950.2	E962.0	E980.2
Vanadium	985.8	E866.4	—	E950.9	E962.1	E980.9
Vancomycin	960.8	E856	E930.8	E950.4	E962.0	E980.4
Vapor (*see also* Gas)	987.9	E869.9	—	E952.9	E962.2	E982.9

TABLE OF DRUGS AND CHEMICALS

Substance	Poisoning	Accident	Therapeutic Use	Suicide Attempt	Assault	Undetermined
			External Cause (E-Code)			
kiln (carbon monoxide)	986	E868.8	—	E952.1	E962.2	E982.1
lead — *see* Lead						
specified source NEC (*see also*						
specific substance)	987.8	E869.8	—	E952.8	E962.2	E982.8
Varidase	964.4	E858.2	E934.4	E950.4	E962.0	E980.4
Varnish	989.89	E861.6	—	E950.9	E962.1	E980.9
cleaner	982.8	E862.9	—	E950.9	E962.1	E980.9
Vaseline	976.3	E858.7	E946.3	E950.4	E962.0	E980.4
Vasodilan	972.5	E858.3	E942.5	E950.4	E962.0	E980.4
Vasodilators NEC	972.5	E858.3	E942.5	E950.4	E962.0	E980.0
coronary	972.4	E858.3	E942.4	E950.4	E962.0	E980.4
Vasopressin	962.5	E858.0	E932.5	E950.4	E962.0	E980.4
Vasopressor drugs	962.5	E858.0	E932.5	E950.4	E962.0	E980.4
Venom, venomous (bite) (sting)	989.5	E905.9	—	E950.9	E962.1	E980.9
arthropod NEC	989.5	E905.5	—	E950.9	E962.1	E980.9
bee	989.5	E905.3	—	E950.9	E962.1	E980.9
centipede	989.5	E905.4	—	E950.9	E962.1	E980.9
hornet	989.5	E905.3	—	E950.9	E962.1	E980.9
lizard	989.5	E905.0	—	E950.9	E962.1	E980.9
marine animals or plants	989.5	E905.6	—	E950.9	E962.1	E980.9
millipede (topical)	989.5	E905.4	—	E950.9	E962.1	E980.9
plant NEC	989.5	E905.7	—	E950.9	E962.1	E980.9
marine	989.5	E905.6	—	E950.9	E962.1	E980.9
scorpion	989.5	E905.2	—	E950.9	E962.1	E980.9
snake	989.5	E905.0	—	E950.9	E962.1	E980.9
specified NEC	989.5	E905.8	—	E950.9	E962.1	E980.9
spider	989.5	E905.1	—	E950.9	E962.1	E980.9
wasp	989.5	E905.3	—	E950.9	E962.1	E980.9
Ventolin—*see* Salbutamol sulfate						
Veramon	967.0	E851	E937.0	E950.1	E962.0	E980.1
Veratrum						
album	988.2	E865.4	—	E950.9	E962.1	E980.9
alkaloids	972.6	E858.3	E942.6	E950.4	E962.0	E980.4
viride	988.2	E865.4	—	E950.9	E962.1	E980.9
Verdigris (*see also* Copper)	985.8	E866.4	—	E950.9	E962.1	E980.9
Veronal	967.0	E851	E937.0	E950.1	E962.0	E980.1
Veroxil	961.6	E857	E931.6	E950.4	E962.0	E980.4
Versidyne	965.7	E850.7	E935.7	E950.0	E962.0	E980.0
Viagra	972.5	E858.3	E942.5	E950.4	E962.0	E980.4
Vienna						
green	985.1	E866.3	—	E950.8	E962.1	E980.8
insecticide	985.1	E863.4	—	E950.6	E962.1	E980.7
red	989.89	E866.8	—	E950.9	E962.1	E980.9
pharmaceutical dye	977.4	E858.8	E947.4	E950.4	E962.0	E980.4
Vinbarbital, vinbarbitone	967.0	E851	E937.0	E950.1	E962.0	E980.1
Vinblastine	963.1	E858.1	E933.1	E950.4	E962.0	E980.4
Vincristine	963.1	E858.1	E933.1	E950.4	E962.0	E980.4
Vinesthene, vinethene	968.2	E855.1	E938.2	E950.4	E962.0	E980.4
Vinyl						
bital	967.0	E851	E937.0	E950.1	E962.0	E980.1
ether	968.2	E855.1	E938.2	E950.4	E962.0	E980.4
Vioform	961.3	E857	E931.3	E950.4	E962.0	E980.4
topical	976.0	E858.7	E946.0	E950.4	E962.0	E980.4
Viomycin	960.6	E856	E930.6	E950.4	E962.0	E980.4
Viosterol	963.5	E858.1	E933.5	E950.4	E962.0	E980.4
Viper (venom)	989.5	E905.0	—	E950.9	E962.1	E980.9
Viprynium (embonate)	961.6	E857	E931.6	E950.4	E962.0	E980.4
Virugon	961.7	E857	E931.7	E950.4	E962.0	E980.4
Visine	976.5	E858.7	E946.5	E950.4	E962.0	E980.4
Vitamins NEC	963.5	E858.1	E933.5	E950.4	E962.0	E980.4
B_{12}	964.1	E858.2	E934.1	E950.4	E962.0	E980.4

Substance	Poisoning	Accident	Therapeutic Use	Suicide Attempt	Assault	Undetermined
			External Cause (E-Code)			
hematopoietic	964.1	E858.2	E934.1	E950.4	E962.0	E980.4
K	964.3	E858.2	E934.3	E950.4	E962.0	E980.4
Vleminckx's solution	976.4	E858.7	E946.4	E950.4	E962.0	E980.4
Voltaren—*see* Diclofenac sodium						
Warfarin (potassium) (sodium)	964.2	E858.2	E934.2	E950.4	E962.0	E980.4
rodenticide	989.4	E863.7	—	E950.6	E962.1	E980.7
Wasp (sting)	989.5	E905.3	—	E950.9	E962.1	E980.9
Water						
balance agents NEC	974.5	E858.5	E944.5	E950.4	E962.0	E980.4
gas	987.1	E868.1	—	E951.8	E962.2	E981.8
incomplete combustion of — *see* Carbon, monoxide, fuel, utility						
hemlock	988.2	E865.4	—	E950.9	E962.1	E980.9
moccasin (venom)	989.5	E905.0	—	E950.9	E962.1	E980.9
Wax (paraffin) (petroleum)	981	E862.3	—	E950.9	E962.1	E980.9
automobile	989.89	E861.2	—	E950.9	E962.1	E980.9
floor	981	E862.0	—	E950.9	E962.1	E980.9
Weed killers NEC	989.4	E863.5	—	E950.6	E962.1	E980.7
Welldorm	967.1	E852.0	E937.1	E950.2	E962.0	E980.2
White						
arsenic — *see* Arsenic						
hellebore	988.2	E865.4	—	E950.9	E962.1	E980.9
lotion (keratolytic)	976.4	E858.7	E946.4	E950.4	E962.0	E980.4
spirit	981	E862.0	—	E950.9	E962.1	E980.9
Whitewashes	989.89	E861.6	—	E950.9	E962.1	E980.9
Whole blood	964.7	E858.2	E934.7	E950.4	E962.0	E980.4
Wild						
black cherry	988.2	E865.4	—	E950.9	E962.1	E980.9
poisonous plants NEC	988.2	E865.4	—	E950.9	E962.1	E980.9
Window cleaning fluid	989.89	E861.3	—	E950.9	E962.1	E980.9
Wintergreen (oil)	976.3	E858.7	E946.3	E950.4	E962.0	E980.4
Witch hazel	976.2	E858.7	E946.2	E950.4	E962.0	E980.4
Wood						
alcohol	980.1	E860.2	—	E950.9	E962.1	E980.9
spirit	980.1	E860.2	—	E950.9	E962.1	E980.9
Woorali	975.2	E858.6	E945.2	E950.4	E962.0	E980.4
Wormseed, American	961.6	E857	E931.6	E950.4	E962.0	E980.4
Xanthine diuretics	974.1	E858.5	E944.1	E950.4	E962.0	E980.4
Xanthocillin	960.0	E856	E930.0	E950.4	E962.0	E980.4
Xanthotoxin	976.3	E858.7	E946.3	E950.4	E962.0	E980.4
Xigris	964.2	E858.2	E934.2	E950.4	E962.0	E980.4
Xylene (liquid) (vapor)	982.0	E862.4	—	E950.9	E962.1	E980.9
Xylocaine (infiltration) (topical)	968.5	E855.2	E938.5	E950.4	E962.0	E980.4
nerve block (peripheral) (plexus)	968.6	E855.2	E938.6	E950.4	E962.0	E980.4
spinal	968.7	E855.2	E938.7	E950.4	E962.0	E980.4
Xylol (liquid) (vapor)	982.0	E862.4	—	E950.9	E962.1	E980.9
Xylometazoline	971.2	E855.5	E941.2	E950.4	E962.0	E980.4
Yellow						
fever vaccine	979.3	E858.8	E949.3	E950.4	E962.0	E980.4
jasmine	988.2	E865.4	—	E950.9	E962.1	E980.9
Yew	988.2	E865.4	—	E950.9	E962.1	E980.9
Zactane	965.7	E850.7	E935.7	E950.0	E962.0	E980.0
Zaroxolyn	974.3	E858.5	E944.3	E950.4	E962.0	E980.4
Zephiran (topical)	976.0	E858.7	E946.0	E950.4	E962.0	E980.4
ophthalmic preparation	976.5	E858.7	E946.5	E950.4	E962.0	E980.4
Zerone	980.1	E860.2	—	E950.9	E962.1	E980.9
Zinc (compounds) (fumes) (salts)						
(vapor) NEC	985.8	E866.4	—	E950.9	E962.1	E980.9
anti–infectives	976.0	E858.7	E946.0	E950.4	E962.0	E980.4
antivaricose	972.7	E858.3	E942.7	E950.4	E962.0	E980.4

Substance	Poisoning	Accident	Therapeutic Use	Suicide Attempt	Assault	Undetermined
		External Cause (E-Code)				
bacitracin 976.0		E858.7	E946.0	E950.4	E962.0	E980.4
chloride 976.2		E858.7	E946.2	E950.4	E962.0	E980.4
gelatin 976.3		E858.7	E946.3	E950.4	E962.0	E980.4
oxide 976.3		E858.7	E946.3	E950.4	E962.0	E980.4
peroxide. 976.0		E858.7	E946.0	E950.4	E962.0	E980.4
pesticides 985.8		E863.4	—	E950.6	E962.1	E980.7
phosphide (rodenticide) 985.8		E863.7	—	E950.6	E962.1	E980.7
stearate 976.3		E858.7	E946.3	E950.4	E962.0	E980.4
sulfate (antivaricose). 972.7		E858.3	E942.7	E950.4	E962.0	E980.4
ENT agent 976.6		E858.7	E946.6	E950.4	E962.0	E980.4
ophthalmic solution 976.5		E858.7	E946.5	E950.4	E962.0	E980.4
topical NEC 976.0		E858.7	E946.0	E950.4	E962.0	E980.4
undecylenate 976.0		E858.7	E946.0	E950.4	E962.0	E980.4
Zovant 964.2		E858.2	E934.2	E950.4	E962.0	E980.4
Zoxazolamine 968.0		E855.1	E938.0	E950.4	E962.0	E980.4
Zygadenus (venenosus) 988.2		E865.4	—	E950.9	E962.1	E980.9
Zyprexa. 969.3		E853.8	E939.3	E950.3	E962.0	E980.3

TABLE OF DRUGS AND CHEMICALS

Substance	Poisoning	Accident	Therapeutic Use	Suicide Attempt	Assault	Undetermined
			External Cause (E-Code)			

SECTION 3

ALPHABETIC INDEX TO EXTERNAL CAUSES
OF INJURY AND POISONING (E CODE)

This section contains the index to the codes which classify environmental events, circumstances, and other conditions as the cause of injury and other adverse effects. Where a code from the section Supplementary Classification of External Causes of Injury and Poisoning (E800-E998) is applicable, it is intended that the E code shall be used in addition to a code from the main body of the classification, Chapters 1-17.

The alphabetic index to the E codes is organized by main terms which describe the *accident, circumstance, event,* or specific *agent* which caused the injury or other adverse effect.

> *Note—Transport accidents (E800-E848) include accidents involving:*
> *aircraft and space craft (E840-E845)*
> *watercraft (E830-E838)*
> *motor vehicle (E810-E825)*
> *railway (E800-E807)*
> *other road vehicles (E826-E829)*
>
> *For definitions and examples related to transport accidents—see Volume 1, pages 571-585.*
>
> *The fourth-digit subdivisions for use with categories E800-E848 to identify the injured person are found on pages 1447-1451.*
>
> *For identifying the place in which an accident or poisoning occurred (circumstances classifiable to categories E850-E869 and E880-E928)— see the listing in this section under "Accident, occurring."*

See the Table of Drugs and Chemicals (Section 2 of this volume) for identifying the specific agent involved in drug overdose or a wrong substance given or taken in error, and for intoxication or poisoning by a drug or other chemical substance.

The specific adverse effect, reaction, or localized toxic effect to a correct drug or substance properly administered in therapeutic or prophylactic dosage should be classified according to the nature of the adverse effect (e.g.: allergy, dermatitis, tachycardia) listed in Section 1 of this volume.

A

Abandonment
  causing exposure to weather conditions—*see*
    Exposure
  child, with intent to injure or kill E968.4
  helpless person, infant, newborn E904.0
    with intent to injure or kill E968.4
Abortion, criminal, injury to child E968.8
Abuse, (alleged) (suspected)
  adult
    by
      child E967.4
      ex-partner E967.3
      ex-spouse E967.3
      father E967.0
      grandchild E967.7
      grandparent E967.6
      mother E967.2
      non-related caregiver E967.8
      other relative E967.7
      other specified person(s) E967.1
      partner E967.3
      sibling E967.5
      spouse E967.3
      stepfather E967.0
      stepmother E967.2
      unspecified person E967.9
  child
    by
      boyfriend of parent or guardian E967.0
      child E967.4
      father E967.0
      female partner of parent or guardian
        E967.2
      girlfriend of parent or guardian E967.2
      grandchild E967.7
      grandparent E967.6
      male partner of parent or guardian E967.0
      mother E967.2
      non-related caregiver E967.8
      other relative E967.7
      other specified person(s) E967.1
      sibling E967.5
      stepfather E967.0
      stepmother E967.2
      unspecified person E967.9
Accident (to) E928.9
  aircraft (in transit) (powered) E841
    at landing, take-off E840
    due to, caused by cataclysm—*see* categories
      E908, E909
    late effect of E929.1
    unpowered (*see also* Collision, aircraft,
      unpowered) E842
    while alighting, boarding E843
  amphibious vehicle
    on
      land—*see* Accident, motor vehicle
      water—*see* Accident, watercraft
  animal, ridden NEC E828
  animal-drawn vehicle NEC E827
  balloon (*see also* Collision, aircraft,
    unpowered) E842
  caused by, due to
    abrasive wheel (metalworking) E919.3
    animal NEC E906.9
      being ridden (in sport or transport) E828
    avalanche NEC E909.2
    band saw E919.4
    bench saw E919.4

Accident—*continued*
    bore, earth-drilling or mining (land) (seabed)
      E919.1
    bulldozer E919.7
    cataclysmic
      earth surface movement or eruption E909.9
      storm E908.9
    chain
      hoist E919.2
        agricultural operations E919.0
        mining operations E919.1
      saw E920.1
    circular saw E919.4
    cold (excessive) (*see also* Cold, exposure to)
      E901.9
    combine E919.0
    conflagration—*see* Conflagration
    corrosive liquid, substance NEC E924.1
    cotton gin E919.8
    crane E919.2
      agricultural operations E919.0
      mining operations E919.1
    cutting or piercing instrument (*see also* Cut)
      E920.9
    dairy equipment E919.8
    derrick E919.2
      agricultural operations E919.0
      mining operations E919.1
    drill E920.1
      earth (land) (seabed) E919.1
      hand (powered) E920.1
        not powered E920.4
      metalworking E919.3
      woodworking E919.4
    earth(-)
      drilling machine E919.1
      moving machine E919.7
      scraping machine E919.7
    electric
      current (*see also* Electric shock) E925.9
      motor—*see also* Accident, machine, by
        type of machine
        current (of)—*see* Electric shock
    elevator (building) (grain) E919.2
      agricultural operations E919.0
      mining operations E919.1
    environmental factors NEC E928.9
    excavating machine E919.7
    explosive material (*see also* Explosion)
      E923.9
    farm machine E919.0
    fire, flames—*see also* Fire
      conflagration—*see* Conflagration
    firearm missile—*see* Shooting
    forging (metalworking) machine E919.3
    forklift (truck) E919.2
      agricultural operations E919.0
      mining operations E919.1
    gas turbine E919.5
    harvester E919.0
    hay derrick, mower, or rake E919.0
    heat (excessive) (*see also* Heat) E900.9
    hoist (*see also* Accident, caused by, due to,
      lift) E919.2
      chain—*see* Accident, caused by, due to,
        chain
      shaft E919.1

Accident—*continued*
  hot
    liquid E924.0
      caustic or corrosive E924.1
      object (not producing fire or flames)
        E924.8
    substance E924.9
      caustic or corrosive E924.1
      liquid (metal) NEC E924.0
      specified type NEC E924.8
  human bite E928.3
  ignition—*see* Ignition
  internal combustion engine E919.5
  landslide NEC E909.2
  lathe (metalworking) E919.3
    turnings E920.8
    woodworking E919.4
  lift, lifting (appliances) E919.2
    agricultural operations E919.0
    mining operations E919.1
    shaft E919.1
  lightning NEC E907
  machine, machinery—*see also* Accident,
      machine
    drilling, metal E919.3
    manufacturing, for manufacture of
      beverages E919.8
      clothing E919.8
      foodstuffs E919.8
      paper E919.8
      textiles E919.8
    milling, metal E919.3
    moulding E919.4
    power press, metal E919.3
    printing E919.8
    rolling mill, metal E919.3
    sawing, metal E919.3
    specified type NEC E919.8
    spinning E919.8
    weaving E919.8
  natural factor NEC E928.9
  overhead plane E919.4
  plane E920.4
    overhead E919.4
  powered
    hand tool NEC E920.1
    saw E919.4
      hand E920.1
  printing machine E919.8
  pulley (block) E919.2
    agricultural operations E919.0
    mining operations E919.1
    transmission E919.6
  radial saw E919.4
  radiation—*see* Radiation
  reaper E919.0
  road scraper E919.7
    when in transport under its own
        power—*see* categories E810—E825
  roller coaster E919.8
  sander E919.4
  saw E920.4
    band E919.4
    bench E919.4
    chain E920.1
    circular E919.4
    hand E920.4
      powered E920.1
    powered, except hand E919.4
    radial E919.4
  sawing machine, metal E919.3

Accident—*continued*
  shaft
    hoist E919.1
    lift E919.1
    transmission E919.6
  shears E920.4
    hand E920.4
      powered E920.1
    mechanical E919.3
  shovel E920.4
    steam E919.7
  spinning machine E919.8
  steam—*see also* Burning, steam
    engine E919.5
    shovel E919.7
  thresher E919.0
  thunderbolt NEC E907
  tractor E919.0
    when in transport under its own
        power—*see* categories E810-E825
  transmission belt, cable, chain, gear, pinion,
      pulley, shaft E919.6
  turbine (gas) (water driven) E919.5
  under-cutter E919.1
  weaving machine E919.8
  winch E919.2
    agricultural operations E919.0
    mining operations E919.1
  diving E883.0
    with insufficient air supply E913.2
  glider (hang) (*see also* Collision, aircraft,
      unpowered) E842
  hovercraft
    on
      land—*see* Accident, motor vehicle
      water—*see* Accident, watercraft
  ice yacht (*see also* Accident, vehicle NEC)
      E848
  in
    medical, surgical procedure
      as, or due to misadventure—*see*
          Misadventure
      causing an abnormal reaction or later
          complication without mention of
          misadventure—*see* Reaction, abnormal
  kite carrying a person (*see also* Collision,
      aircraft, unpowered) E842
  land yacht (*see also* Accident, vehicle NEC)
      E848
  late effect of—*see* Late effect
  launching pad E845
  machine, machinery (*see also* Accident,
      caused by, due to, by specific type of
      machine) E919.9
    agricultural including animal-powered
        E919.0
    earth-drilling E919.1
    earth moving or scraping E919.7
    excavating E919.7
    involving transport under own power on
        highway or transport vehicle—*see*
        categories E810-E825, E840-E845
    lifting (appliances) E919.2
    metalworking E919.3
    mining E919.1
    prime movers, except electric motors E919.5
      electric motors—*see* Accident, machine, by
          specific type of machine
    recreational E919.8
    specified type NEC E919.8

Accident—*continued*

   transmission E919.6

   watercraft (deck) (engine room) (galley)
     (laundry) (loading) E836

   woodworking or forming E919.4

  motor vehicle (on public highway) (traffic)
   E819

   due to cataclysm—*see* categories E908,
     E909

   involving

     collision (*see also* Collision, motor
       vehicle) E812

     nontraffic, not on public highway—*see*
       categories E820-E825

     not involving collision—*see* categories
       E816-E819

  nonmotor vehicle NEC E829

  nonroad—*see* Accident, vehicle NEC

  road, except pedal cycle, animal-drawn
   vehicle, or animal being ridden E829

  nonroad vehicle NEC—*see* Accident, vehicle
   NEC

  not elsewhere classifiable involving

   cable car (not on rails) E847

     on rails E829

   coal car in mine E846

   hand truck—*see* Accident, vehicle NEC

   logging car E846

   sled(ge), meaning snow or ice vehicle E848

   tram, mine or quarry E846

   truck

     mine or quarry E846

     self-propelled, industrial E846

     station baggage E846

   tub, mine or quarry E846

   vehicle NEC E848

     snow and ice E848

     used only on industrial premises E846

   wheelbarrow E848

  occurring (at) (in)

   apartment E849.0

   baseball field, diamond E849.4

   construction site, any E849.3

   dock E849.8

     yard E849.3

   dormitory E849.7

   factory (building) (premises) E849.3

   farm E849.1

     buildings E849.1

     house E849.0

   football field E849.4

   forest E849.8

   garage (place of work) E849.3

     private (home) E849.0

   gravel pit E849.2

   gymnasium E849.4

   highway E849.5

   home (private) (residential) E849.0

     institutional E849.7

   hospital E849.7

   hotel E849.6

   house (private) (residential) E849.0

     movie E849.6

     public E849.6

   institution, residential E849.7

   jail E849.7

   mine E849.2

   motel E849.6

   movie house E849.6

   office (building) E849.6

Accident—*continued*

   orphanage E849.7

   park (public) E849.4

     mobile home E849.8

     trailer E849.8

   parking lot or place E849.8

   place

     industrial NEC E849.3

     parking E849.8

     public E849.8

       specified place NEC E849.5

     recreational NEC E849.4

     sport NEC E849.4

   playground (park) (school) E849.4

   prison E849.6

   public building NEC E849.6

   quarry E849.2

   railway

     line NEC E849.8

     yard E849.3

   residence

     home (private) E849.0

   resort (beach) (lake) (mountain) (seashore)
     (vacation) E849.4

   restaurant E849.6

   sand pit E849.2

   school (building) (private) (public) (state)
     E849.6

     reform E849.7

     riding E849.4

   seashore E849.8

     resort E849.4

   shop (place of work) E849.3

     commercial E849.6

   skating rink E849.4

   sports palace E849.4

   stadium E849.4

   store E849.6

   street E849.5

   swimming pool (public) E849.4

     private home or garden E849.0

   tennis court E849.4

   theatre, theater E849.6

   trailer court E849.8

   tunnel E849.8

     under construction E849.2

   warehouse E849.3

   yard

     dock E849.3

     industrial E849.3

     private (home) E849.0

     railway E849.3

  off-road type motor vehicle (not on public
   highway) NEC E821

  on public highway—*see* categories
   E810-E819

  pedal cycle E826

  railway E807

   due to cataclysm—*see* categories E908,
     E909

   involving

     avalanche E909.2

     burning by engine, locomotive, train (*see
       also* Explosion, railway engine) E803

     collision (*see also* Collision, railway) E800

     derailment (*see also* Derailment, railway)
       E802

     explosion (*see also* Explosion, railway
       engine) E803

     fall (*see also* Fall, from, railway rolling
       stock) E804

Accident—*continued*
    fire (*see also* Explosion, railway engine)
        E803
    hitting by, being struck by
        object falling in, on, from, rolling stock,
            train, vehicle E806
        rolling stock, train, vehicle E805
    overturning, railway rolling stock, train,
        vehicle (*see also* Derailment, railway)
        E802
    running off rails, railway (*see also*
        Derailment, railway) E802
    specified circumstances NEC E806
    train or vehicle hit by
        avalanche E909
        falling object (earth, rock, tree) E806
            due to cataclysm—*see* categories E908,
                E909
        landslide E909
  roller skate E885.1
  scooter (nonmotorized) E885.0
  skateboard E885.2
  ski(ing) E885.3
    jump E884.9
    lift or tow (with chair or gondola) E847
  snowboard E885.4
  snow vehicle, motor driven (not on public
    highway) E820
    on public highway—*see* categories
        E810-E819
  spacecraft E845
  specified cause NEC E928.8
  street car E829
  traffic NEC E819
  vehicle NEC (with pedestrian) E848
    battery powered
        airport passenger vehicle E846
        truck (baggage) (mail) E846
    powered commercial or industrial (with other
        vehicle or object within commercial or
        industrial premises) E846
  watercraft E838
    with
        drowning or submersion resulting from
            accident other than to watercraft E832
            accident to watercraft E830
        injury, except drowning or submersion,
            resulting from
            accident other than to watercraft—*see*
                categories E833-E838
            accident to watercraft E831
    due to, caused by cataclysm—*see* categories
        E908, E909
    machinery E836
Acid throwing E961
Acosta syndrome E902.0
Activity (involving) E030
  aerobic and step exercise (class) E009.2
  alpine skiing E003.2
  animal care NEC E019.9
  arts and handcrafts NEC E012.9
  athletics NEC E008.9
    played
        as a team or group NEC E007.9
        individually NEC E006.9
  baking E015.2
  ballet E005.0
  barbells E010.2
  BASE (Building, Antenna, Span, Earth)
    jumping E004.2
  baseball E007.3

Activity—*continued*
  basketball E007.6
  bathing (personal) E013.0
  beach volleyball E007.7
  bike riding E006.4
  boogie boarding E002.7
  bowling E006.3
  boxing E008.0
  brass instrument playing E018.3
  building and construction E016.2
  bungee jumping E004.3
  calisthenics E009.1
  canoeing (in calm and turbulent water) E002.5
  capture the flag E007.8
  cardiorespiratory exercise NEC E009.9
  caregiving (providing) NEC E014.9
    bathing E014.0
    lifting E014.1
  cellular
    communication device E011.1
    telephone E011.1
  challenge course E009.4
  cheerleading E005.4
  circuit training E009.3
  cleaning
    floor E013.4
  climbing NEC E004.9
    mountain E004.0
    rock E004.0
    wall climbing E004.0
  combatives E008.4
  computer
    keyboarding E011.0
    technology NEC E011.9
  confidence course E009.4
  construction (building) E016.2
  cooking and baking E015.2
  cooking and grilling NEC E015.9
  cool down exercises E009.1
  cricket E007.9
  crocheting E012.0
  cross country skiing E003.3
  dancing (all types) E005.0
  digging
    dirt E016.0
  dirt digging E016.0
  dishwashing E015.0
  diving (platform) (springboard) E002.1
    underwater E002.4
  dodge ball E007.8
  downhill skiing E003.2
  drum playing E018.1
  dumbbells E010.2
  electronic
    devices NEC E011.9
        hand held interactive E011.1
    game playing (using) (with)
        interactive device E011.1
        keyboard or other stationary device E011.0
  elliptical machine E009.0
  exercise(s)
    machines ((primarily) for)
        cardiorespiratory conditioning E009.0
        muscle strengthening E010.0
    muscle strengthening (non-machine) NEC
        E010.9
  external motion NEC E017.9
    roller coaster E017.0
  field hockey E007.4
  figure skating (pairs) (singles) E003.0
  flag football E007.1

Activity—*continued*
  snow NEC E003.9
    boarding E003.2
    shoveling E016.0
    sledding E003.2
    tubing E003.2
  soccer E007.5
  softball E007.3
  specified NEC E029.9
  spectator at an event E029.1
  sports NEC E008.9
  sports played as a team or group NEC E007.9
  sports played individually NEC E006.9
  springboard diving E002.1
  squash E008.2
  stationary bike E009.0
  step (stepping) exercise (class) E009.2
  stepper machine E009.0
  stove E015.2
  string instrument playing E018.2
  surfing E002.7
  swimming E002.0
  tackle football E007.0
  tap dancing E005.0
  tennis E008.2
  tobogganing E003.2
  touch football E007.1
  track and field events (non-running) E006.6
    running E001.1
  trampoline E005.3
  treadmill E009.0
  trimming shrubs E016.1
  tubing (in calm and turbulent water) E002.5
    snow E003.2
  ultimate frisbee E008.3
  underwater diving E002.4
  unpacking in moving to a new residence
    E013.5
  use of stove, oven and microwave oven
    E015.2
  vacuuming E013.2
  volleyball (beach) (court) E007.7
  wake boarding E002.6
  walking an animal E019.0
  walking (on level or elevated terrain) E001.0
    an animal E019.0
  wall climbing E004.0
  warm up and cool down exercises E009.1
  water NEC E002.9
    aerobics E002.3
    craft NEC E002.9
    exercise E002.3
    polo E002.2
    skiing E002.6
    sliding E002.8
    survival training and testing E002.9
  weeding (garden and lawn) E016.1
  wind instrument playing E018.3
  windsurfing E002.7
  wrestling E008.1
  yoga E005.1
Activity status E000.9
  child assisting in compensated work of other
    family member E000.8
  civilian
    done for
      financial or other compensation E000.0
      pay or income E000.0
  family member assisting in compensated work
    of other family member E000.8
  for income E000.0

Activity status—*continued*
  hobby or leisure E000.8
  off duty military E000.8
  military E000.1
    off duty E000.8
  recreation E000.8
  specified NEC E000.8
  sport not for income E000.8
  student E000.8
  volunteer E000.2
Aeroneurosis E902.1
Aero-otitis media —*see* Effects of, air pressure
Aerosinusitis —*see* Effects of, air pressure
After-effect, late —*see* Late effect
Air
  blast
    in
      terrorism E979.2
      war operations E993.9
  embolism (traumatic) NEC E928.9
    in
      infusion or transfusion E874.1
      perfusion E874.2
  sickness E903
Alpine sickness E902.0
Altitude sickness —*see* Effects of, air pressure
Anaphylactic shock, anaphylaxis (*see also*
    Table of drugs and chemicals) E947.9
  due to bite or sting (venomous)—*see* Bite,
    venomous
Andes disease E902.0
Apoplexy heat—*see* Heat
Arachnidism E905.1
Arson E968.0
Asphyxia, asphyxiation
  by
    chemical
      in
        terrorism E979.7
        war operations E997.2
    explosion—*see* Explosion
    food (bone) (regurgitated food) (seed) E911
    foreign object, except food E912
    fumes
      in
        terrorism (chemical weapons) E979.7
        war operations E997.2
    gas—*see also* Table of drugs and chemicals
      in
        terrorism E979.7
        war operations E997.2
      legal
        execution E978
        intervention (tear) E972
      tear E972
    mechanical means (*see also* Suffocation)
      E913.9
  from
    conflagration—*see* Conflagration
    fire—*see also* Fire E899
      in
        terrorism E979.3
        war operations E990.9
    ignition—*see* Ignition
Aspiration
  foreign body—*see* Foreign body, aspiration
  mucus, not of newborn (with asphyxia,
    obstruction respiratory passage,
    suffocation) E912
  phlegm (with asphyxia, obstruction respiratory
    passage, suffocation) E912

Aspiration—*continued*
vomitus (with asphyxia, obstruction respiratory passage, suffocation) (*see also* Foreign body, aspiration, food) E911
Assassination (attempt) (*see also* Assault) E968.9
Assault (homicidal) (by) (in) E968.9
  acid E961
    swallowed E962.1
  air gun E968.6
  BB gun E968.6
  bite NEC E968.8
    of human being E968.7
  bomb ((placed in) car or house) E965.8
    antipersonnel E965.5
    letter E965.7
    petrol E965.7
  brawl (hand) (fists) (foot) E960.0
  burning, burns (by fire) E968.0
    acid E961
      swallowed E962.1
    caustic, corrosive substance E961
      swallowed E962.1
    chemical from swallowing caustic, corrosive substance NEC E962.1
    hot liquid E968.3
    scalding E968.3
    vitriol E961
      swallowed E962.1
  caustic, corrosive substance E961
    swallowed E962.1
  cut, any part of body E966
  dagger E966
  drowning E964
  explosive(s) E965.9
    bomb (*see also* Assault, bomb) E965.8
    dynamite E965.8
  fight (hand) (fists) (foot) E960.0
    with weapon E968.9
      blunt or thrown E968.2
      cutting or piercing E966
      firearm—*see* Shooting, homicide
  fire E968.0
  firearm(s)—*see* Shooting, homicide
  garrotting E963
  gunshot (wound)—*see* Shooting, homicide
  hanging E963
  injury NEC E968.9
  knife E966
  late effect of E969
  ligature E963
  poisoning E962.9
    drugs or medicinals E962.0
    gas(es) or vapors, except drugs and medicinals E962.2
    solid or liquid substances, except drugs and medicinals E962.1
  puncture, any part of body E966
  pushing
    before moving object, train, vehicle E968.5
    from high place E968.1
  rape E960.1
  scalding E968.3
  shooting—*see* Shooting, homicide
  sodomy E960.1
  stab, any part of body E966
  strangulation E963
  submersion E964
  suffocation E963
  transport vehicle E968.5
  violence NEC E968.9

Assault—*continued*
  vitriol E961
    swallowed E962.1
  weapon E968.9
    blunt or thrown E968.2
    cutting or piercing E966
    firearm—*see* Shooting, homicide
  wound E968.9
    cutting E966
    gunshot—*see* Shooting, homicide
    knife E966
    piercing E966
    puncture E966
    stab E966
Attack by animal NEC E906.9
Avalanche E909.2
  falling on or hitting
    motor vehicle (in motion) (on public highway) E909.2
    railway train E909.2
Aviators' disease E902.1

B

Barotitis, barodontalgia, barosinusitis, barotrauma (otitic) (sinus)—*see* Effects of, air pressure
Battered
  baby or child (syndrome)—*see* Abuse, child; category E967
  person other than baby or child—*see* Assault
Bayonet wound (*see also* Cut, by bayonet) E920.3
  in
    legal intervention E974
    terrorism E979.8
    war operations E995.2
Bean in nose E912
Bed set on fire NEC E898.0
Beheading (by guillotine)
  homicide E966
  legal execution E978
Bending, injury
  due to
    repetitive movement E927.3
    sudden strenuous movement E927.0
Bends E902.0
Bite
  animal (nonvenomous) NEC E906.5
    venomous NEC E905.9
  arthropod (nonvenomous) NEC E906.4
    venomous—*see* Sting
  black widow spider E905.1
  cat E906.3
  centipede E905.4
  cobra E905.0
  copperhead snake E905.0
  coral snake E905.0
  dog E906.0
  fer de lance E905.0
  gila monster E905.0
  human being
    accidental E928.3
    assault E968.7
  insect (nonvenomous) E906.4
    venomous—*see* Sting
  krait E905.0
  late effect of—*see* Late effect
  lizard E906.2
    venomous E905.0

Bite —*continued*
mamba E905.0
marine animal
nonvenomous E906.3
snake E906.2
venomous E905.6
snake E905.0
millipede E906.4
venomous E905.4
moray eel E906.3
rat E906.1
rattlesnake E905.0
rodent, except rat E906.3
serpent—*see* Bite, snake
shark E906.3
snake (venomous) E905.0
nonvenomous E906.2
sea E905.0
spider E905.1
nonvenomous E906.4
tarantula (venomous) E905.1
venomous NEC E905.9
by specific animal—*see* category E905
viper E905.0
water moccasin E905.0
Blast (air)
from nuclear explosion E996
in
terrorism E979.2
from nuclear explosion E979.5
underwater E979.0
war operations E993.9
from nuclear explosion—*see* War
operations, injury due to, nuclear
weapons
underwater E992.9
underwater E992
Blizzard E908.3
Blow E928.9
by law-enforcing agent, police (on duty) E975
with blunt object (baton) (nightstick) (stave)
(truncheon) E973
Blowing up (*see also* Explosion) E923.9
Brawl (hand) (fists) (foot) E960.0
Breakage (accidental)
cable of cable car not on rails E847
ladder (causing fall) E881.0
part (any) of
animal-drawn vehicle E827
ladder (causing fall) E881.0
motor vehicle
in motion (on public highway) E818
not on public highway E825
nonmotor road vehicle, except animal-drawn
vehicle or pedal cycle E829
off-road type motor vehicle (not on public
highway) NEC E821
on public highway E818
pedal cycle E826
scaffolding (causing fall) E881.1
snow vehicle, motor-driven (not on public
highway) E820
on public highway E818
vehicle NEC—*see* Accident, vehicle
Broken
glass
fall on E888.0
injury by E920.8
power line (causing electric shock) E925.1

Bumping against, into (accidentally)
object (moving) E917.9
caused by crowd E917.1
with subsequent fall E917.6
furniture E917.3
with subsequent fall E917.7
in
running water E917.2
sports E917.0
with subsequent fall E917.5
stationary E917.4
with subsequent fall E917.8
person(s) E917.9
with fall E886.9
in sports E886.0
as, or caused by, a crowd E917.1
with subsequent fall E917.6
in sports E917.0
with fall E886.0
Burning, burns (accidental) (by) (from) (on)
E899
acid (any kind) E924.1
swallowed—*see* Table of drugs and
chemicals
airgun E928.7
bedclothes (*see also* Fire, specified NEC)
E898.0
blowlamp (*see also* Fire, specified NEC)
E898.1
blowtorch (*see also* Fire, specified NEC)
E898.1
boat, ship, watercraft—*see* categories E830,
E831, E837
bonfire (controlled) E897
uncontrolled E892
candle (*see also* Fire, specified NEC) E898.1
caustic liquid, substance E924.1
swallowed—*see* Table of drugs and
chemicals
chemical E924.1
from swallowing caustic, corrosive
substance—*see* Table of drugs and
chemicals
in
terrorism E979.7
war operations E997.2
cigar(s) or cigarette(s) (*see also* Fire, specified
NEC) E898.1
clothes, clothing, nightdress—*see* Ignition,
clothes
with conflagration—*see* Conflagration
conflagration—*see* Conflagration
corrosive liquid, substance E924.1
swallowed—*see* Table of drugs and
chemicals
electric current (*see also* Electric shock)
E925.9
fire, flames (*see also* Fire) E899
firearm E928.7
flare, Verey pistol E922.8
heat
from appliance (electrical) E924.8
in local application or packing during
medical or surgical procedure E873.5
homicide (attempt) (*see also* Assault, burning)
E968.0
hot
liquid E924.0
caustic or corrosive E924.1
object (not producing fire or flames) E924.8
substance E924.9
caustic or corrosive E924.1

Burning, burns—*continued*
   liquid (metal) NEC E924.0
   specified type NEC E924.8
   tap water E924.2
ignition—*see also* Ignition
   clothes, clothing, nightdress—*see also*
      Ignition, clothes
   with conflagration—*see* Conflagration
   highly inflammable material (benzine) (fat)
      (gasoline) (kerosine) (paraffin) (petrol)
      E894
inflicted by other person
   stated as
      homicidal, intentional (*see also* Assault,
         burning) E968.0
      undetermined whether accidental or
         intentional (*see also* Burn, stated as
         undetermined whether accidental or
         intentional) E988.1
internal, from swallowed caustic, corrosive
   liquid, substance—*see* Table of drugs and
   chemicals
in
   from nuclear explosion E996
   petrol bomb E990.0
   terrorism E979.3
      from nuclear explosion E979.5
      petrol bomb E979.3
   war operations (from fire-producing device
      or conventional weapon) E990.9
      from nuclear explosion (see also War
         operations, injury due to, nuclear
         weapons) E996.2
      incendiary bomb E990.0
      petrol bomb E990.0
lamp (*see also* Fire, specified NEC) E898.1
late effect of NEC E929.4
lighter (cigar) (cigarette) (*see also* Fire,
   specified NEC) E898.1
lightning E907
liquid (boiling) (hot) (molten) E924.0
   caustic, corrosive (external) E924.1
      swallowed—*see* Table of drugs and
         chemicals
local application of externally applied
   substance in medical or surgical care
   E873.5
machinery—*see* Accident, machine
matches (*see also* Fire, specified NEC) E898.1
medicament, externally applied E873.5
metal, molten E924.0
object (hot) E924.8
   producing fire or flames—*see* Fire
oven (electric) (gas) E924.8
pipe (smoking) (*see also* Fire, specified NEC)
   E898.1
radiation—*see* Radiation
railway engine, locomotive, train (*see also*
   Explosion, railway engine) E803
self-inflicted (unspecified whether accidental
   or intentional) E988.1
   caustic or corrosive substance NEC E988.7
   stated as intentional, purposeful E958.1
      caustic or corrosive substance NEC E958.7
   stated as undetermined whether accidental or
      intentional E988.1
      caustic or corrosive substance NEC E988.7
steam E924.0
   pipe E924.8

Burning, burns—*continued*
substance (hot) E924.9
   boiling or molten E924.0
   caustic, corrosive (external) E924.1
      swallowed—*see* Table of drugs and
         chemicals
suicidal (attempt) NEC E958.1
   caustic substance E958.7
   late effect of E959
tanning bed E926.2
therapeutic misadventure
   overdose of radiation E873.2
torch, welding (*see also* Fire, specified NEC)
   E898.1
trash fire (*see also* Burning, bonfire) E897
vapor E924.0
vitriol E924.1
x-rays E926.3
   in medical, surgical procedure—*see*
      Misadventure, failure, in dosage,
      radiation
Butted by animal E906.8

C

Cachexia, lead or saturnine E866.0
from pesticide NEC (*see also* Table of drugs
   and chemicals) E863.4
Caisson disease E902.2
Capital punishment (any means) E978
Car sickness E903
Casualty (not due to war) NEC E928.9
terrorism E979.8
war (*see also* War operations) E995.9
Cat
bite E906.3
scratch E906.8
Cataclysmic (any injury)
earth surface movement or eruption E909.9
   specified type NEC E909.8
storm or flood resulting from storm E908.9
   specified type NEC E909.8
Catching fire —*see* Ignition
Caught
between
   objects (moving) (stationary and moving)
      E918
   and machinery—*see* Accident, machine
   by cable car, not on rails E847
in
   machinery (moving parts of)—*see* Accident,
      machine
   object E918
Cave-in (causing asphyxia, suffocation (by
   pressure)) (*see also* Suffocation, due to,
   cave-in) E913.3
Cave-in—*continued*
with injury other than asphyxia or suffocation
   E916
   with asphyxia or suffocation (*see also*
      Suffocation, due to, cave-in) E913.3
struck or crushed by E916
   with asphyxia or suffocation (*see also*
      Suffocation, due to, cave-in) E913.3
Change(s) in air pressure—*see also* Effects of,
   air pressure
sudden, in aircraft (ascent) (descent) (causing
      aeroneurosis or aviators' disease) E902.1
Chilblains E901.0
due to manmade conditions E901.1

Choking (on) (any object except food or
  vomitus) E912
  apple E911
  bone E911
  food, any type (regurgitated) E911
  mucus or phlegm E912
  seed E911
Civil insurrection —*see* War operations
Cloudburst E908.8
Cold, exposure to (accidental) (excessive)
  (extreme) (place) E901.9
  causing chilblains or immersion foot E901.0
  due to
    manmade conditions E901.1
    specified cause NEC E901.8
    weather (conditions) E901.0
  late effect of NEC E929.5
  self-inflicted (undetermined whether accidental
    or intentional) E988.3
    suicidal E958.3
  suicide E958.3
Colic, lead, painters', or saturnine —*see*
  category E866
Collapse
  building E916
    burning (uncontrolled fire) E891.8
      in terrorism E979.3
      private E890.8
  dam E909.3
  due to heat—*see* Heat
  machinery—*see* Accident, machine
  man-made structure E909.3
  postoperative NEC E878.9
  structure, burning NEC E891.8
    burning (uncontrolled fire)
      in terrorism E979.3
Collision (accidental)

Note—In the case of collisions between different
types of vehicles, persons and objects, priority in
classification is in the following order:

Aircraft
Watercraft
Motor vehicle
Railway vehicle
Pedal Cycle
Animal-drawn vehicle
Animal being ridden
Streetcar or other nonmotor road vehicle
Other vehicle
Pedestrian or person using pedestrian
  conveyance
Object (except where falling from or set in
  motion by vehicle etc. listed above)

In the listing below, the combinations are listed
only under the vehicle etc. having priority. For
definitions, *see* E code introduction.

---

  aircraft (with object or vehicle) (fixed)
    (movable) (moving) E841
    with
      person (while landing, taking off) (without
        accident to aircraft) E844
      powered (in transit) (with unpowered
        aircraft) E841
        while landing, taking off E840
      unpowered E842
        while landing, taking off E840

Collision—*continued*
  animal being ridden (in sport or transport)
    E828
    and
      animal (being ridden) (herded)
        (unattended) E828
      nonmotor road vehicle, except pedal cycle
        or animal-drawn vehicle E828
      object (fallen) (fixed) (movable) (moving)
        not falling from or set in motion by
        vehicle of higher priority E828
      pedestrian (conveyance or vehicle) E828
  animal-drawn vehicle E827
    and
      animal (being ridden) (herded)
        (unattended) E827
      nonmotor road vehicle, except pedal cycle
        E827
      object (fallen) (fixed) (movable) (moving)
        not falling from or set in motion by
        vehicle of higher priority E827
      pedestrian (conveyance or vehicle) E827
      streetcar E827
  motor vehicle (on public highway) (traffic
    accident) E812
    after leaving, running off, public highway
      (without antecedent collision) (without
      re-entry) E816
    with antecedent collision on public
      highway—*see* categories E810-E815
    with re-entrance collision with another
      motor vehicle E811
    and
      abutment (bridge) (overpass) E815
      animal (herded) (unattended) E815
        carrying person, property E813
      animal-drawn vehicle E813
      another motor vehicle (abandoned)
        (disabled) (parked) (stalled) (stopped)
        E812
        with, involving re-entrance (on same
          roadway) (across median strip) E811
      any object, person, or vehicle off the
        public highway resulting from a
        noncollision motor vehicle nontraffic
        accident E816
      avalanche, fallen or not moving E815
        falling E909
      boundary fence E815
      culvert E815
      fallen
        stone E815
        tree E815
      falling E909.2
      guard post or guard rail E815
      inter-highway divider E815
      landslide, fallen or not moving E815
        moving E909
      machinery (road) E815
      moving E909.2
      nonmotor road vehicle NEC E813
      object (any object, person, or vehicle off
        the public highway resulting from a
        noncollision motor vehicle nontraffic
        accident) E815
        off, normally not on, public highway
          resulting from a noncollision motor
          vehicle traffic accident E816
      pedal cycle E813
      pedestrian (conveyance) E814
      person (using pedestrian conveyance) E814

Collision—*continued*

post or pole (lamp) (light) (signal)
(telephone) (utility) E815
railway rolling stock, train, vehicle E810
safety island E815
street car E813
traffic signal, sign, or marker (temporary)
E815
tree E815
tricycle E813
wall of cut made for road E815
due to cataclysm—*see* categories E908,
E909
not on public highway, nontraffic accident
E822
and
animal (carrying person, property)
(herded) (unattended) E822
animal-drawn vehicle E822
another motor vehicle (moving), except
off-road motor vehicle E822
stationary E823
avalanche, fallen, not moving E823
moving E909
landslide, fallen, not moving E823
moving E909
nonmotor vehicle (moving) E822
stationary E823
object (fallen) (normally) (fixed)
(movable but not in motion)
(stationary) E823
moving, except when falling from, set
in motion by, aircraft or cataclysm
E822
pedal cycle (moving) E822
stationary E823
pedestrian (conveyance) E822
person (using pedestrian conveyance)
E822
railway rolling stock, train, vehicle
(moving) E822
stationary E823
road vehicle (any) (moving) E822
stationary E823
tricycle (moving) E822
stationary E823
moving E909.2
off-road type motor vehicle (not on public
highway) E821
and
animal (being ridden) (-drawn vehicle)
E821
another off-road motor vehicle, except
snow vehicle E821
other motor vehicle, not on public highway
E821
other object or vehicle NEC, fixed or
movable, not set in motion by aircraft,
motor vehicle on highway, or snow
vehicle, motor-driven E821
pedal cycle E821
pedestrian (conveyance) E821
railway train E821
on public highway—*see* Collision, motor
vehicle
pedal cycle E826
and
animal (carrying person, property) (herded)
(unherded) E826
animal-drawn vehicle E826

Collision—*continued*

another pedal cycle E826
nonmotor road vehicle E826
object (fallen) (fixed) (movable) (moving)
not falling from or set in motion by
aircraft, motor vehicle, or railway train
NEC E826
pedestrian (conveyance) E826
person (using pedestrian conveyance) E826
street car E826
pedestrian(s) (conveyance) E917.9
with fall E886.9
in sports E886.0
and
crowd, human stampede E917.1
with subsequent fall E917.6
furniture E917.3
with subsequent fall E917.7
machinery—*see* Accident, machine
object (fallen) (moving) not falling from or
set in motion by any vehicle
classifiable to E800-E848, E917.9
caused by a crowd E917.1
with subsequent fall E917.6
furniture E917.3
with subsequent fall E917.7
in
running water E917.2
with drowning or submersion—*see*
Submersion
sports E917.0
with subsequent fall E917.5
stationary E917.4
with subsequent fall E917.8
vehicle, nonmotor, nonroad E848
in
running water E917.2
with drowning or submersion—*see*
Submersion
sports E917.0
with fall E886.0
person(s) (using pedestrian conveyance) (*see
also* Collision, pedestrian) E917.9
railway (rolling stock) (train) (vehicle) (with
(subsequent) derailment, explosion, fall or
fire) E800
with antecedent derailment E802
and
animal (carrying person) (herded)
(unattended) E801
another railway train or vehicle E800
buffers E801
fallen tree on railway E801
farm machinery, nonmotor (in transport)
(stationary) E801
gates E801
nonmotor vehicle E801
object (fallen) (fixed) (movable) (moving)
not falling from, set in motion by,
aircraft or motor vehicle NEC E801
pedal cycle E801
pedestrian (conveyance) E805
person (using pedestrian conveyance) E805
platform E801
rock on railway E801
street car E801

Crash—*continued*
 glider E842
 motor vehicle—*see also* Accident, motor
  vehicle
  homicidal E968.5
  suicidal E958.5
  undetermined whether accidental or
   intentional E988.5
Crushed (accidentally) E928.9
 between
  boat(s), ship(s), watercraft (and dock or pier)
   (without accident to watercraft) E838
  after accident to, or collision, watercraft
   E831
  objects (moving) (stationary and moving)
   E918
 by
  avalanche NEC E909.2
  boat, ship, watercraft after accident to,
   collision, watercraft E831
  cave-in E916
   with asphyxiation or suffocation (*see also*
    Suffocation, due to, cave-in) E913.3
  crowd, human stampede E917.1
  falling
   aircraft (*see also* Accident, aircraft) E841
    in
     terrorism E979.1
     war operations E994.8
   earth, material E916
    with asphyxiation or suffocation (*see*
     also Suffocation, due to, cave-in)
     E913.3
   object E916
    on ship, watercraft E838
    while loading, unloading watercraft E838
  firearm E928.7
  landslide NEC E909.2
  lifeboat after abandoning ship E831
  machinery—*see* Accident, machine
  railway rolling stock, train, vehicle (part of)
   E805
  slide trigger mechanism, scope or other part
   of gun E928.7
  street car E829
  vehicle NEC—*see* Accident, vehicle NEC
 in
  machinery—*see* Accident, machine
  object E918
  transport accident—*see* categories
   E800-E848
 late effect of NEC E929.9
Cut, cutting (any part of body) (accidental)
  E920.9
 by
  arrow E920.8
  axe E920.4
  bayonet (*see also* Bayonet wound) E920.3
   in war operations E995.2
  blender E920.2
  broken glass E920.8
   following fall E888.0
  can opener E920.4
   powered E920.2
  chisel E920.4
  circular saw E919.4
  cutting or piercing instrument—*see also*
   category E920
   following fall E888.0
   late effect of E929.8
  dagger E920.3

Cut, cutting—*continued*
  dart E920.8
  drill—*see* Accident, caused by drill
  edge of stiff paper E920.8
  electric
   beater E920.2
   fan E920.2
   knife E920.2
   mixer E920.2
  firearm component E928.7
  fork E920.4
  garden fork E920.4
  hand saw or tool (not powered) E920.4
   powered E920.1
  hedge clipper E920.4
   powered E920.1
  hoe E920.4
  ice pick E920.4
  knife E920.3
   electric E920.2
   in war operations E995.2
  lathe turnings E920.8
  lawn mower E920.4
   powered E920.0
   riding E919.8
  machine—*see* Accident, machine
  meat
   grinder E919.8
   slicer E919.8
  nails E920.8
  needle E920.4
   hypodermic E920.5
  object, edged, pointed, sharp—*see* category
   E920
   following fall E888.0
  paper cutter E920.4
  piercing instrument—*see also* category E920
   late effect of E929.8
  pitchfork E920.4
  powered
   can opener E920.2
   garden cultivator E920.1
    riding E919.8
   hand saw E920.1
   hand tool NEC E920.1
   hedge clipper E920.1
   household appliance or implement E920.2
   lawn mower (hand) E920.0
    riding E919.8
   rivet gun E920.1
   staple gun E920.1
  rake E920.4
  saw
   circular E919.4
   hand E920.4
  scissors E920.4
  screwdriver E920.4
  sewing machine (electric) (powered) E920.2
   not powered E920.4
  shears E920.4
  shovel E920.4
  slide trigger mechanism, scope or other part
   of gun E928.7
  spade E920.4
  splinters E920.8
  sword E920.3
   in war operations E995.2
  tin can lid E920.8
  wood slivers E920.8
 homicide (attempt) E966

Cut, cutting—*continued*
inflicted by other person
stated as
intentional, homicidal E966
undetermined whether accidental or
intentional E986
late effect of NEC E929.8
legal
execution E978
intervention E974
self-inflicted (unspecified whether accidental
or intentional) E986
stated as intentional, purposeful E956
stated as undetermined whether accidental or
intentional E986
suicidal (attempt) E956
terrorism E979.8
war operations E995.2
Cyclone E908.1

D

**Death due to injury occurring one year or
more previous** —*see* Late effect
Decapitation (accidental circumstances) NEC
E928.9
homicidal E966
legal execution (by guillotine) E978
Deprivation —*see also* Privation
homicidal intent E968.4
Derailment (accidental)
railway (rolling stock) (train) (vehicle) (with
subsequent collision) E802
with
collision (antecedent) (*see also* Collision,
railway) E800
Derailment (accidental)—*continued*
explosion (subsequent) (without antecedent
collision) E802
antecedent collision E803
fall (without collision (antecedent)) E802
fire (without collision (antecedent)) E802
street car E829
Descent
parachute (voluntary) (without accident to
aircraft) E844
due to accident to aircraft—*see* categories
E840-E842
Desertion
child, with intent to injure or kill E968.4
helpless person, infant, newborn E904.0
with intent to injure or kill E968.4
Destitution —*see* Privation
Dirty bomb (*see also* War operations, injury
due to, nuclear weapons) E996.9
Disability, late effect or sequela of injury
—*see Late effect*
Disease
Andes E902.0
aviators' E902.1
caisson E902.2
range E902.0
Divers' disease, palsy, paralysis, squeeze
E902.0
Dog bite E906.0
Dragged by
cable car (not on rails) E847
on rails E829
motor vehicle (on highway) E814
not on highway, nontraffic accident E825
street car E829

Drinking poison (accidental) —*see* Table of
drugs and chemicals
Drowning —*see* Submersion
Dust in eye E914\

E

Earth falling (on) (with asphyxia or suffocation
(by pressure)) (*see also* Suffocation, due to,
cave-in) E913.3
as, or due to, a cataclysm (involving any
transport vehicle)—*see* categories E908,
E909
not due to cataclysmic action E913.3
motor vehicle (in motion) (on public
highway) E818
not on public highway E825
nonmotor road vehicle NEC E829
pedal cycle E826
railway rolling stock, train, vehicle E806
street car E829
struck or crushed by E916
with asphyxiation or suffocation E913.3
with injury other than asphyxia,
suffocation E916
Earthquake (any injury) E909.0
Effect(s) (adverse) of
air pressure E902.9
at high altitude E902.9
in aircraft E902.1
residence or prolonged visit (causing
conditions classifiable to E902.0)
E902.0
due to
diving E902.2
specified cause NEC E902.8
in aircraft E902.1
cold, excessive (exposure to) (*see also* Cold,
exposure to) E901.9
heat (excessive) (*see also* Heat) E900.9
hot
place—*see* Heat
weather E900.0
insulation—*see* Heat
late—*see* Late effect of
motion E903
nuclear explosion or weapon
in
terrorism E979.5
war operations (*see also* War operations,
injury due to, nuclear weapons) E996.9
radiation—*see* Radiation
terrorism, secondary E979.9
travel E903
Electric shock, electrocution (accidental) (from
exposed wire, faulty appliance, high voltage
cable, live rail, open socket) (by) (in) E925.9
appliance or wiring
domestic E925.0
factory E925.2
farm (building) E925.8
house E925.0
home E925.0
industrial (conductor) (control apparatus)
(transformer) E925.2
outdoors E925.8
public building E925.8
residential institution E925.8
school E925.8
specified place NEC E925.8

Electric shock, electrocution—*continued*
caused by other person
stated as
intentional, homicidal E968.8
undetermined whether accidental or
intentional E988.4
electric power generating plant, distribution
station E925.1
electroshock gun (taser) (stun gun) E925.8
caused by other person E968.8
legal intervention E975
stated as accidental E925.8
stated as intentional E968.8
due to legal intervention E975
stated as intentional self-harm (suicidal
(attempt)) E958.4
stated as undetermined whether accidental or
intentional E988.4
suicide (attempt) E958.4
homicidal (attempt) E968.8
legal execution E978
lightning E907
machinery E925.9
domestic E925.0
factory E925.2
farm E925.8
home E925.0
misadventure in medical or surgical procedure
in electroshock therapy E873.4
self-inflicted (undetermined whether accidental
or intentional) E988.4
stated as intentional E958.4
stated as undetermined whether accidental or
intentional E988.4
suicidal (attempt) E958.4
transmission line E925.1
Electrocution —*see* Electric shock
Embolism
air (traumatic) NEC—*see* Air, embolism
Encephalitis
lead or saturnine E866.0
from pesticide NEC E863.4
Entanglement
in
bedclothes, causing suffocation E913.0
wheel of pedal cycle E826
Entry of foreign body, material, any —*see*
Foreign body
Execution, legal (any method) E978
Exertion, excessive physical, from prolonged
activity E927.2
Exhaustion
cold—*see* Cold, exposure to
due to excessive exertion E927.2
heat—*see* Heat
Explosion (accidental) (in) (of) (on) E923.9
acetylene E923.2
aerosol can E921.8
aircraft (in transit) (powered) E841
at landing, take-off E840
in
terrorism E979.1
war operations
from
enemy fire or explosive(s) (device
placed on aircraft) E994.0
own onboard explosives E994.1
unpowered E842
air tank (compressed) (in machinery) E921.1
anesthetic gas in operating theatre E923.2

Explosion—*continued*
automobile tire NEC E921.8
causing transport accident—*see* categories
E810-E825
blasting (cap) (materials) E923.1
boiler (machinery), not on transport vehicle
E921.0
steamship—*see* Explosion, watercraft
bomb E923.8
in
terrorism E979.2
war operations E993.8
after cessation of hostilities E998.1
atom, hydrogen or nuclear (*see also* War
operations, injury due to, nuclear
weapons) E996.9
injury by fragments from E991.9
antipersonnel bomb E991.3
butane E923.2
caused by
other person
stated as
intentional, homicidal—*see* Assault,
explosive
undetermined whether accidental or
homicidal E985.5
coal gas E923.2
detonator E923.1
dynamite E923.1
explosive (material) NEC E923.9
gas(es) E923.2
missile E923.8
in
terrorism E979.2
war operations E993.1
injury by fragments from E991.9
antipersonnel bomb E991.3
used in blasting operations E923.1
fire-damp E923.2
fireworks E923.0
gas E923.2
cylinder (in machinery) E921.1
pressure tank (in machinery) E921.1
gasoline (fumes) (tank) not in moving motor
vehicle E923.2
grain store (military) (munitions) E923.8
grenade E923.8
in
terrorism E979.2
war operations E993.8
injury by fragments from E991.4
homicide (attempt)—*see* Assault, explosive
hot water heater, tank (in machinery) E921.0
in mine (of explosive gases) NEC E923.2
late effect of NEC E929.8
machinery—*see also* Accident, machine
pressure vessel—*see* Explosion, pressure
vessel
methane E923.2
missile E923.8
in
terrorism E979.2
war operations E993.1
injury by fragments from E991.4
motor vehicle (part of)
in motion (on public highway) E818
not on public highway E825
munitions (dump) (factory) E923.8
in
terrorism E979.2
war operations E993.9

Explosion—*continued*
of mine E923.8
  in
    terrorism
      at sea or in harbor E979.0
      land E979.2
      marine E979.0
    war operations
      after cessation of hostilities E998.0
      at sea or in harbor E992.2
      land E993.8
        after cessation of hostilities E998.0
        injury by fragments from E991.4
      marine E992.2
own weapons
  in
    terrorism (*see also* Suicide) E979.2
    war operations E993.7
      injury by fragments from E991.9
        antipersonnel bomb E991.3
pressure
  cooker E921.8
  gas tank (in machinery) E921.1
  vessel (in machinery) E921.9
    on transport vehicle—*see* categories
      E800-E848
    specified type NEC E921.8
propane E923.2
railway engine, locomotive, train (boiler) (with
  subsequent collision, derailment, fall) E803
  with
    collision (antecedent) (*see also* Collision,
      railway) E800
    derailment (antecedent) E802
    fire (without antecedent collision or
      derailment) E803
secondary fire resulting from—*see* Fire
self-inflicted (unspecified whether accidental
  or intentional) E985.5
  stated as intentional, purposeful E955.5
shell (artillery) E923.8
  in
    terrorism E979.2
    war operations E993.2
      injury by fragments from E991.4
stated as undetermined whether caused
  accidentally or purposely inflicted E985.5
steam or water lines (in machinery) E921.0
suicide (attempted) E955.5
terrorism—*see* Terrorism, explosion
torpedo E923.8
  in
    terrorism E979.0
    war operations E992.0
transport accident—*see* categories E800-E848
war operations—*see* War operations, explosion
watercraft (boiler) E837
  causing drowning, submersion (after jumping
    from watercraft) E830
Exposure (weather) (conditions) (rain) (wind)
  E904.3
with homicidal intent E968.4

Exposure—*continued*
environmental
  to
    algae bloom E928.6
    blue-green algae bloom E928.6
    brown tide E928.6
    cyanobacteria bloom E928.6
    Florida red tide E928.6
    harmful algae
      and toxins E928.6
      bloom E928.6
    pfiesteria piscicida E928.6
    red tide E928.6
excessive E904.3
  cold (*see also* Cold, exposure to) E901.9
    self-inflicted—*see* Cold, exposure to,
      self-inflicted
  heat (*see also* Heat) E900.9
fire—*see* Fire
helpless person, infant, newborn due to
  abandonment or neglect E904.0
noise E928.1
prolonged in deep-freeze unit or refrigerator
  E901.1
radiation—*see* Radiation
resulting from transport accident—*see*
  categories E800-E848
smoke from, due to
  fire—*see* Fire
tobacco, second-hand E869.4
vibration E928.2
External cause status E000.9
child assisting in compensated work of other
  family member E000.8
civilian
  done for
    financial or other compensation E000.0
    pay or income E000.0
family member assisting in compensated work
  of other family member E000.8
for income E000.0
hobby or leisure E000.8
off duty military E000.8
military E000.1
  off duty E000.8
recreation E000.8
specified NEC E000.8
sport not for income E000.8
student E000.8
volunteer E000.2

F

Fall, falling (accidental) E888.9
building E916
  burning E891.8
  private E890.8
down
  escalator E880.0
  ladder E881.0
    in boat, ship, watercraft E833
  staircase E880.9
  stairs, steps—*see* Fall, from, stairs
earth (with asphyxia or suffocation (by
  pressure)) (*see also* Earth, falling) E913.3
from, off
  aircraft (at landing, take-off) (in-transit)
    (while alighting, boarding) E843
    resulting from accident to aircraft—*see*
      categories E840-E842

Fall, falling—*continued*
  wheelies E885.1
  window E882
  in, on
    aircraft (at landing, take-off) (in-transit)
      E843
      resulting from accident to aircraft—*see*
        categories E840-E842
    boat, ship, watercraft E835
      due to accident to watercraft E831
      one level to another NEC E834
      on ladder, stairs E833
    cutting or piercing instrument or machine
      E888.0
    deck (of boat, ship, watercraft) E835
      due to accident to watercraft E831
    escalator E880.0
    gangplank E835
    glass, broken E888.0
    knife E888.0
    ladder E881.0
      in boat, ship, watercraft E833
        due to accident to watercraft E831
    object
      edged, pointed or sharp E888.0
      other E888.1
    pitchfork E888.0
    railway rolling stock, train, vehicle (while
      alighting, boarding) E804
    with
      collision (*see also* Collision, railway) E800
      derailment (*see also* Derailment, railway)
        E802
      explosion (*see also* Explosion, railway
        engine) E803
    scaffolding E881.1
    scissors E888.0
    staircase, stairs, steps (*see also* Fall, from,
      stairs) E880.9
    street car E829
    water transport (*see also* Fall, in, boat) E835
  into
    cavity E883.9
    dock E883.9
      from boat, ship, watercraft (*see also* Fall,
        from, boat) E832
    hold (of ship) E834
      due to accident to watercraft E831
    hole E883.9
    manhole E883.2
    moving part of machinery—*see* Accident,
      machine
    opening in surface NEC E883.9
    pit E883.9
    quarry E883.9
    shaft E883.9
    storm drain E883.2
    tank E883.9
    water (with drowning or submersion) E910.9
    well E883.1
  late effect of NEC E929.3
  object (*see also* Hit by, object, falling) E916
  other E888.8
  over
    animal E885.9
    cliff E884.1
    embankment E884.9
    small object E885.9
  overboard (*see also* Fall, from, boat) E832
  resulting in striking against object E888.1
    sharp E888.0
  rock E916

Fall, falling—*continued*
  same level NEC E888.9
  aircraft (any kind) E843
    resulting from accident to aircraft—*see*
      categories E840-E842
  boat, ship, watercraft E835
    due to accident to, collision, watercraft E831
  from
    collision, pushing, shoving, by or with
      other person(s) E886.9
      as, or caused by, a crowd E917.6
      in sports E886.0
    in-line skates E885.1
    roller skates E885.1
    scooter (nonmotorized) E885.0
    skateboard E885.2
    skis E885.3
    slipping, stumbling, tripping E885.9
    snowboard E885.4
  snowslide E916
    as avalanche E909.2
  stone E916
  through
    hatch (on ship) E834
      due to accident to watercraft E831
    roof E882
    window E882
  timber E916
  while alighting from, boarding, entering,
    leaving
    aircraft (any kind) E843
    motor bus, motor vehicle—*see* Fall, from,
      motor vehicle, while alighting, boarding
    nonmotor road vehicle NEC E829
    railway train E804
    street car E829
Fallen on by
  animal (horse) (not being ridden) E906.8
  being ridden (in sport or transport) E828
Fell or jumped from high place, so stated
  —*see Jumping, from, high place*
Felo-de-se (*see also* Suicide) E958.9
Fever
  heat—*see* Heat
  thermic—*see* Heat
Fight (hand) (fist) (foot) (*see also* Assault,
  fight) E960.0
Fire (accidental) (caused by great heat from
  appliance (electrical), hot object or hot
  substance) (secondary, resulting from
  explosion) E899
  conflagration—*see* Conflagration
  controlled, normal (in brazier, fireplace,
    furnace, or stove) (charcoal) (coal) (coke)
    (electric) (gas) (wood)
    bonfire E897
    brazier, not in building or structure E897
    in building or structure, except private
      dwelling (barn) (church) (convalescent or
      residential home) (factory) (farm
      outbuilding) (hospital) (hotel) (institution
      (educational) (dormitory) (residential))
      (private garage) (school) (shop) (store)
      (theatre) E896
    in private dwelling (apartment) (boarding
      house) (camping place) (caravan)
      (farmhouse) (home (private)) (house)
      (lodging house) (rooming house)
      (tenement) E895
    not in building or structure E897
    trash E897

Fire —*continued*
  forest (uncontrolled) E892
  grass (uncontrolled) E892
  hay (uncontrolled) E892
  homicide (attempt) E968.0
    late effect of E969
  in, of, on, starting in E892
  aircraft (in transit) (powered) E841
    at landing, take-off E840
    stationary E892
    unpowered (balloon) (glider) E842
  balloon E842
  boat, ship, watercraft—*see* categories E830,
    E831, E837
  building or structure, except private dwelling
    (barn) (church) (convalescent or
    residential home) (factory) (farm
    outbuilding) (hospital) (hotel) (institution
    (educational) (dormitory) (residential))
    (school) (shop) (store) (theatre) (*see also*
    Conflagration, building or structure,
    except private dwelling) E891.9
  forest (uncontrolled) E892
  glider E842
  grass (uncontrolled) E892
  hay (uncontrolled) E892
  lumber (uncontrolled) E892
  machinery—*see* Accident, machine
  mine (uncontrolled) E892
  motor vehicle (in motion) (on public
    highway) E818
    not on public highway E825
    stationary E892
  prairie (uncontrolled) E892
  private dwelling (apartment) (boarding
    house) (camping place) (caravan)
    (farmhouse) (home (private)) (house)
    (lodging house) (private garage) (rooming
    house) (tenement) (*see also*
    Conflagration, private dwelling) E890.9
  railway rolling stock, train, vehicle (*see also*
    Explosion, railway engine) E803
    stationary E892
  room NEC E898.1
  street car (in motion) E829
    stationary E892
  terrorism (by fire-producing device) E979.3
    fittings or furniture (burning building)
      (uncontrolled fire) E979.3
    from nuclear explosion E979.5
  transport vehicle, stationary NEC E892
  tunnel (uncontrolled) E892
  war operations (by fire-producing device or
    conventional weapon) E990.9
    from nuclear explosion (*see also* War
      operations, injury due to, nuclear
      weapons) E996.2
    incendiary bomb E990.0
    petrol bomb E990.0
  late effect of NEC E929.4
  lumber (uncontrolled) E892
  mine (uncontrolled) E892
  prairie (uncontrolled) E892
  self-inflicted (unspecified whether accidental
    or intentional) E988.1
    stated as intentional, purposeful E958.1

Fire —*continued*
  specified NEC E898.1
  with
    conflagration—*see* Conflagration
    ignition (of)
      clothing—*see* Ignition, clothes
      highly inflammable material (benzine)
        (fat) (gasoline) (kerosene) (paraffin)
        (petrol) E894
  started by other person
    stated as
      with intent to injure or kill E968.0
      undetermined whether or not with intent to
        injure or kill E988.1
  suicide (attempted) E958.1
    late effect of E959
  tunnel (uncontrolled) E892
Fireball effects from nuclear explosion
  in
    terrorism E979.5
    war operations (see also War operations,
      injury due to, nuclear weapons) E996.2
Fireworks (explosion) E923.0
Flash burns from explosion (*see also*
  Explosion) E923.9
Flood (any injury) (resulting from storm)
  E908.2
  caused by collapse of dam or manmade
    structure E909.3
Forced landing (aircraft) E840
Foreign body, object or material (entrance into
  (accidental))
  air passage (causing injury) E915
    with asphyxia, obstruction, suffocation E912
    food or vomitus E911
    nose (with asphyxia, obstruction, suffocation)
      E912
      causing injury without asphyxia,
        obstruction, suffocation E915
  alimentary canal (causing injury) (with
    obstruction) E915
    with asphyxia, obstruction respiratory
      passage, suffocation E912
    food E911
    mouth E915
      with asphyxia, obstruction, suffocation
        E912
      food E911
    pharynx E915
      with asphyxia, obstruction, suffocation
        E912
      food E911
  aspiration (with asphyxia, obstruction
    respiratory passage, suffocation) E912
    causing injury without asphyxia, obstruction
      respiratory passage, suffocation E915
    food (regurgitated) (vomited) E911
      causing injury without asphyxia,
        obstruction respiratory passage,
        suffocation E915
    mucus (not of newborn) E912
    phlegm E912
  bladder (causing injury or obstruction) E915
  bronchus, bronchi—*see* Foreign body, air
    passages
  conjunctival sac E914
  digestive system—*see* Foreign body,
    alimentary canal
  ear (causing injury or obstruction) E915
  esophagus (causing injury or obstruction) (*see*
    also Foreign body, alimentary canal) E915

Foreign body—*continued*
eye (any part) E914
eyelid E914
hairball (stomach) (with obstruction) E915
ingestion—*see* Foreign body, alimentary canal
inhalation—*see* Foreign body, aspiration
intestine (causing injury or obstruction) E915
iris E914
lacrimal apparatus E914
larynx—*see* Foreign body, air passage
late effect of NEC E929.8
lung—*see* Foreign body, air passage
mouth—*see* Foreign body, alimentary canal,
mouth
nasal passage—*see* Foreign body, air passage,
nose
nose—*see* Foreign body, air passage, nose
ocular muscle E914
operation wound (left in)—*see* Misadventure,
foreign object
orbit E914
pharynx—*see* Foreign body, alimentary canal,
pharynx
rectum (causing injury or obstruction) E915
stomach (hairball) (causing injury or
obstruction) E915
tear ducts or glands E914
trachea—*see* Foreign body, air passage
urethra (causing injury or obstruction) E915
vagina (causing injury or obstruction) E915
Found dead, injured
from exposure (to)—*see* Exposure
on
public highway E819
railway right of way E807
Fracture (circumstances unknown or
unspecified) E887
due to specified external means—*see* manner
of accident
late effect of NEC E929.3
occurring in water transport NEC E835
Freezing —*see* Cold, exposure to
Frostbite E901.0
due to manmade conditions E901.1
Frozen —*see* Cold, exposure to

G

Garrotting, homicidal (attempted) E963
Gored E906.8
Gunshot wound (*see also* Shooting) E922.9

H

Hailstones, injury by E904.3
Hairball (stomach) (with obstruction) E915
Hanged himself (*see also* Hanging,
self-inflicted) E983.0
Hang gliding E842
Hanging (accidental) E913.8
caused by other person
in accidental circumstances E913.8
stated as
intentional, homicidal E963
undetermined whether accidental or
intentional E983.0
homicide (attempt) E963
in bed or cradle E913.0
legal execution E978

Hanging—*continued*
self-inflicted (unspecified whether accidental
or intentional) E983.0
in accidental circumstances E913.8
stated as intentional, purposeful E953.0
stated as undetermined whether accidental or
intentional E983.0
suicidal (attempt) E953.0
Heat (apoplexy) (collapse) (cramps) (effects of)
(excessive) (exhaustion) (fever) (prostration)
(stroke) E900.9
due to
manmade conditions (listed in E900.1,
except boat, ship, watercraft) E900.1
weather (conditions) E900.0
from
electric heating apparatus causing burning E924.8
nuclear explosion
in
terrorism E979.5
war operations (see also War operations,
injury due to, nuclear weapons)
E996.2
generated in, boiler, engine, evaporator, fire
room of boat, ship, watercraft E838
inappropriate in local application or packing in
medical or surgical procedure E873.5
late effect of NEC E989
Hemorrhage
delayed following medical or surgical
treatment without mention of
misadventure—*see* Reaction, abnormal
during medical or surgical treatment as
misadventure—*see* Misadventure, cut
High
altitude, effects E902.9
level of radioactivity, effects—*see* Radiation
pressure effects—*see also* Effects of, air
pressure
from rapid descent in water (causing caisson
or divers' disease, palsy, or paralysis)
E902.2
temperature, effects—*see* Heat
Hit, hitting (accidental) by
aircraft (propeller) (without accident to
aircraft) E844
unpowered E842
avalanche E909.2
being thrown against object in or part of
motor vehicle (in motion) (on public
highway) E818
not on public highway E825
nonmotor road vehicle NEC E829
street car E829
boat, ship, watercraft
after fall from watercraft E838
damaged, involved in accident E831
while swimming, water skiing E838
bullet (*see also* Shooting) E922.9
from air gun E922.4
in
terrorism E979.4
war operations E991.2
rubber E991.0
flare, Very pistol (*see also* Shooting) E922.8
hailstones E904.3
landslide E909.2
law-enforcing agent (on duty) E975
with blunt object (baton) (night stick) (stave)
(truncheon) E973
machine—*see* Accident, machine

Hit, hitting—*continued*
missile
  firearm (*see also* Shooting) E922.9
  in
    terrorism—*see* Terrorism, missile
    war operations—*see* War operations,
      missile
motor vehicle (on public highway) (traffic
  accident) E814
  not on public highway, nontraffic accident
    E822
nonmotor road vehicle NEC E829
object
  falling E916
  from, in, on
    aircraft E844
      due to accident to aircraft—*see*
        categories E840-E842
      unpowered E842
    boat, ship, watercraft E838
      due to accident to watercraft E831
    building E916
      burning E891.8
        in terrorism E979.3
        private E890.8
    cataclysmic
      earth surface movement or eruption
        E909.9
      storm E908.9
    cave-in E916
      with asphyxiation or suffocation (*see*
        also Suffocation, due to, cave-in)
        E913.3
    earthquake E909.0
    motor vehicle (in motion) (on public
      highway) E818
      not on public highway E825
      stationary E916
    nonmotor road vehicle NEC E829
    pedal cycle E826
    railway rolling stock, train, vehicle E806
    street car E829
    structure, burning NEC E891.8
    vehicle, stationary E916
  moving NEC—*see* Striking against, object
  projected NEC—*see* Striking against, object
  set in motion by
    compressed air or gas, spring, striking,
      throwing—*see* Striking against, object
    explosion—*see* Explosion
  thrown into, on, or towards
    motor vehicle (in motion) (on public
      highway) E818
      not on public highway E825
    nonmotor road vehicle NEC E829
    pedal cycle E826
    street car E829
off-road type motor vehicle (not on public
  highway) E821
  on public highway E814
other person(s) E917.9
  with blunt or thrown object E917.9
    in sports E917.0
      with subsequent fall E917.5
    intentionally, homicidal E968.2
    as, or caused by, a crowd E917.1
      with subsequent fall E917.6
    in sports E917.0
pedal cycle E826

Hit, hitting—*continued*
police (on duty) E975
  with blunt object (baton) (nightstick) (stave)
    (truncheon) E973
railway, rolling stock, train, vehicle (part of)
  E805
shot—*see* Shooting
snow vehicle, motor-driven (not on public
  highway) E820
  on public highway E814
street car E829
vehicle NEC—*see* Accident, vehicle NEC
Homicide, homicidal (attempt) (justifiable) (*see
  also* Assault) E968.9
Hot
liquid, object, substance, accident caused
  by—*see also* Accident, caused by, hot, by
  type of substance
late effect of E929.8
place, effects—*see* Heat
weather, effects E900.0
Humidity, causing problem E904.3
Hunger E904.1
resulting from
  abandonment or neglect E904.0
  transport accident—*see* categories
    E800-E848
Hurricane (any injury) E908.0
Hypobarism, hypobaropathy —*see* Effects of,
  air pressure
Hypothermia —*see* Cold, exposure to

I

Ictus
caloris—*see* Heat
solaris E900.0
Ignition (accidental)
anesthetic gas in operating theatre E923.2
bedclothes
  with
    conflagration—*see* Conflagration
    ignition (of)
      clothing—*see* Ignition, clothes
      highly inflammable material (benzine)
        (fat) (gasoline) (kerosene) (paraffin)
        (petrol) E894
benzine E894
clothes, clothing (from controlled fire) (in
  building) E893.9
  with conflagration—*see* Conflagration
  from
    bonfire E893.2
    highly inflammable material E894
    sources or material as listed in E893.8
    trash fire E893.2
    uncontrolled fire—*see* Conflagration
  in
    private dwelling E893.0
    specified building or structure, except
      private dwelling E893.1
  not in building or structure E893.2
  explosive material—*see* Explosion
fat E894
gasoline E894
kerosene E894
material
  explosive—*see* Explosion
  highly inflammable E894
    with conflagration—*see* Conflagration
    with explosion E923.2

Ignition—*continued*
nightdress—*see* Ignition, clothes
paraffin E894
petrol E894
Immersion —*see* Submersion
Implantation of quills of porcupine E906.8
Inanition (from) E904.9
hunger—*see* Lack of, food
resulting from homicidal intent E968.4
thirst—*see* Lack of, water
Inattention after, at birth E904.0
homicidal, infanticidal intent E968.4
Infanticide (*see also* Assault)
Ingestion
foreign body (causing injury) (with
obstruction)—*see* Foreign body, alimentary
canal
poisonous substance NEC—*see* Table of drugs
and chemicals
Inhalation
excessively cold substance, manmade E901.1
foreign body—*see* Foreign body, aspiration
liquid air, hydrogen, nitrogen E901.1
mucus, not of newborn (with asphyxia,
obstruction respiratory passage,
suffocation) E912
phlegm (with asphyxia, obstruction respiratory
passage, suffocation) E912
poisonous gas—*see* Table of drugs and chemicals
smoke from, due to
fire —*see* Fire
tobacco, second-hand E869.4
vomitus (with asphyxia, obstruction respiratory
passage, suffocation) E911
Injury, injured (accidental(ly)) NEC E928.9
by, caused by, from
air rifle (B-B gun) E922.4
animal (not being ridden) NEC E906.9
being ridden (in sport or transport) E828
assault (*see also* Assault) E968.9
avalanche E909.2
bayonet (*see also* Bayonet wound) E920.3
being thrown against some part of, or object in
motor vehicle (in motion) (on public
highway) E818
not on public highway E825
nonmotor road vehicle NEC E829
off-road motor vehicle NEC E821
railway train E806
snow vehicle, motor-driven E820
street car E829
bending
due to
repetitive movement E927.3
sudden strenuous movement E927.0
bite, human E928.3
broken glass E920.8
bullet—*see* Shooting
cave-in (*see also* Suffocation, due to,
cave-in) E913.3
without asphyxiation or suffocation E916
cloudburst E908.8
component of firearm or air gun E928.7
cutting or piercing instrument (*see also* Cut)
E920.9
cyclone E908.1
earth surface movement or eruption E909.9
earthquake E909.0
electric current (*see also* Electric shock) E925.9
explosion (*see also* Explosion) E923.9
of gun part E928.7
fire—*see* Fire

Injury, injured—*continued*
by —*continued*
flare, Very pistol E922.8
flood E908.2
foreign body—*see* Foreign body
gun recoil E928.7
hailstones E904.3
hurricane E908.0
landslide E909.2
law-enforcing agent, police, in course of
legal intervention—*see* Legal intervention
lightning E907
live rail or live wire—*see* Electric shock
machinery—*see also* Accident, machine
aircraft, without accident to aircraft E844
boat, ship, watercraft (deck) (engine room)
(galley) (laundry) (loading) E836
mechanism of firearm or air gun E928.7
missile
explosive E923.8
firearm—*see* Shooting
in
terrorism—*see* Terrorism, missile
war operations—*see* War operations,
missile
moving part of motor vehicle (in motion)
(on public highway) E818
not on public highway, nontraffic accident
E825
while alighting, boarding, entering,
leaving—*see* Fall, from, motor vehicle,
while alighting, boarding
nail E920.8
needle (sewing) E920.4
hypodermic E920.5
noise E928.1
object
fallen on
motor vehicle (in motion) (on public
highway) E818
not on public highway E825
falling—*see* Hit by, object, falling
paintball gun E922.5
radiation—*see* Radiation
railway rolling stock, train, vehicle (part of)
E805
door or window E806
recoil of firearm E928.7
rotating propeller, aircraft E844
rough landing of off-road type motor vehicle
(after leaving ground or rough terrain)
E821
snow vehicle E820
saber (*see also* Wound, saber) E920.3
shot—*see* Shooting
sound waves E928.1
splinter or sliver, wood E920.8
storm E908.9
straining
due to
repetitive movement E927.3
sudden strenuous movement E927.0
street car (door) E829
suicide (attempt) E958.9
sword E920.3
terrorism—*see* Terrorism
third rail—*see* Electric shock
thunderbolt E907
tidal wave E909.4
caused by storm E908.0

Injury, injured—*continued*
  by —*continued*
   tornado E908.1
   torrential rain E908.2
   twisting
    due to
     repetitive movement E927.3
     sudden strenuous movement E927.0
   vehicle NEC—*see* Accident, vehicle NEC
   vibration E928.2
   volcanic eruption E909.1
   weapon burst, in war operations E993.9
   weightlessness (in spacecraft, real or
    simulated) E928.0
   wood splinter or sliver E920.8
  due to
   civil insurrection—*see* War operations
    occurring after cessation of hostilities
     E998.9
   terrorism—*see* Terrorism
   war operations—*see* War operations
    occurring after cessation of hostilities
     E998.9
   weapon of mass destruction [WMD] E997.3
  homicidal (*see also* Assault) E968.9
  in, on
   civil insurrection—*see* War operations
   fight E960.0
   parachute descent (voluntary) (without
    accident to aircraft) E844
    with accident to aircraft—*see* categories
     E840-E842
   public highway E819
   railway right of way E807
   terrorism—*see* Terrorism
   war operations—*see* War operations
  inflicted (by)
   in course of arrest (attempted), suppression
    of disturbance, maintenance of order, by
    law-enforcing agents—*see* Legal
    intervention
   law-enforcing agent (on duty)—*see* Legal
    intervention
   other person
    stated as
     accidental E928.9
     homicidal, intentional—*see* Assault
     undetermined whether accidental or
      intentional—*see* Injury, stated as
      undetermined
   police (on duty)—*see* Legal intervention
   late effect of E929.9
  purposely (inflicted) by other person(s)—*see*
   Assault
  self-inflicted (unspecified whether accidental
   or intentional) E988.9
   stated as
    accidental E928.9
    intentionally, purposely E958.9
  specified cause NEC E928.8

Injury, injured—*continued*
  stated as
   undetermined whether accidentally or
    purposely inflicted (by) E988.9
   cut (any part of body) E986
   cutting or piercing instrument (classifiable
    to E920) E986
   drowning E984
   explosive(s) (missile) E985.5
   falling from high place E987.9
    manmade structure, except residential E987.1
    natural site E987.2
    residential premises E987.0
   hanging E983.0
   knife E986
   late effect of E989
   puncture (any part of body) E986
   shooting—*see* Shooting, stated as undetermined
    whether accidental or intentional
   specified means NEC E988.8
   stab (any part of body) E986
   strangulation—*see* Suffocation, stated as
    undetermined whether accidental or
    intentional
   submersion E984
   suffocation—*see* Suffocation, stated as
    undetermined whether accidental or
    intentional
  to child due to criminal abortion E968.8
Insufficient nourishment —*see also* Lack of,
  food
  homicidal intent E968.4
Insulation, effects —*see* Heat
Interruption of respiration by
  food lodged in esophagus E911
  foreign body, except food, in esophagus E912
Intervention, legal —*see* Legal intervention
Intoxication, drug or poison —*see* Table of
  drugs and chemicals
Irradiation —*see* Radiation

J

Jammed (accidentally)
  between objects (moving) (stationary and
   moving) E918
  in object E918
Jumped or fell from high place, so stated
  —*see Jumping, from, high place, stated as
  in undetermined circumstances*
Jumping
  before train, vehicle or other moving object
   (unspecified whether accidental or
   intentional) E988.0
   stated as
    intentional, purposeful E958.0
    suicidal (attempt) E958.0
  from
   aircraft
    by parachute (voluntarily) (without
     accident to aircraft) E844
    due to accident to aircraft—*see* categories
     E840-E842
   boat, ship, watercraft (into water)
    after accident to, fire on, watercraft E830
     and subsequently struck by (part of) boat
      E831
    burning, crushed, sinking E830
     and subsequently struck by (part of) boat
      E831

Jumping—*continued*
    voluntarily, without accident (to boat) with
        injury other than drowning or
        submersion E883.0
    building—*see also* Jumping, from, high
        place
    burning (uncontrolled fire) E891.8
        in terrorism E979.3
        private E890.8
    cable car (not on rails) E847
        on rails E829
    high place
        in accidental circumstances or in
            sport—*see* categories E880-E884
        stated as
            with intent to injure self E957.9
                man-made structures NEC E957.1
                natural sites E957.2
                residential premises E957.0
            in undetermined circumstances E987.9
                man-made structures NEC E987.1
                natural sites E987.2
                residential premises E987.0
            suicidal (attempt) E957.9
                man-made structures NEC E957.1
                natural sites E957.1
                residential premises E957.0
    motor vehicle (in motion) (on public
        highway)—*see* Fall, from, motor vehicle
    nonmotor road vehicle NEC E829
    street car E829
    structure—*see also* Jumping, from, high
        place
        burning NEC (uncontrolled fire) E891.8
            in terrorism E979.3
    into water
        with injury other than drowning or
            submersion E883.0
        drowning or submersion—*see* Submersion
    from, off, watercraft—*see* Jumping, from,
        boat
Justifiable homicide —*see* Assault

K

Kicked by
    animal E906.8
    person(s) (accidentally) E917.9
        with intent to injure or kill E960.0
        as, or caused by a crowd E917.1
            with subsequent fall E917.6
        in fight E960.0
        in sports E917.0
            with subsequent fall E917.5
Kicking against
    object (moving) E917.9
        in sports E917.0
            with subsequent fall E917.5
        stationary E917.4
            with subsequent fall E917.8
    person—*see* Striking against, person
Killed, killing (accidentally) NEC (*see also*
    Injury) E928.9
    in
        action—*see* War operations
        brawl, fight (hand) (fists) (foot) E960.0
            by weapon—*see also* Assault
                cutting, piercing E966
                firearm—*see* Shooting, homicide

Killed, killing—*continued*
    self
        stated as
            accident E928.9
            suicide—*see* Suicide
        unspecified whether accidental or suicidal
            E988.9
Knocked down (accidentally) (by) NEC E928.9
    animal (not being ridden) E906.8
        being ridden (in sport or transport) E828
    blast from explosion (*see also* Explosion)
        E923.9
    crowd, human stampede E917.6
    late effect of—*see* Late effect
    person (accidentally) E917.9
        in brawl, fight E960.0
        in sports E917.5
    transport vehicle—*see* vehicle involved under
        Hit by
    while boxing E917.5

L

Laceration NEC E928.9
Lack of
    air (refrigerator or closed place), suffocation
        by E913.2
    care (helpless person) (infant) (newborn)
        E904.0
        homicidal intent E968.4
    food except as result of transport accident
        E904.1
        helpless person, infant, newborn due to
            abandonment or neglect E904.0
    water except as result of transport accident
        E904.2
        helpless person, infant, newborn due to
            abandonment or neglect E904.0
Landslide E909.2
    falling on, hitting
        motor vehicle (any) (in motion) (on or off
            public highway) E909.2
        railway rolling stock, train, vehicle E909.2
Late effect of
    accident NEC (accident classifiable to E928.9)
        E929.9
        specified NEC (accident classifiable to
            E910-E928.8) E929.8
    assault E969
    fall, accidental (accident classifiable to
        E880-E888) E929.3
    fire, accident caused by (accident classifiable
        to E890-E899) E929.4
    homicide, attempt (any means) E969
    injury due to terrorism E999.1
    injury undetermined whether accidentally or
        purposely inflicted (injury classifiable to
        E980-E988) E989
    legal intervention (injury classifiable to
        E970-E976) E977
    medical or surgical procedure, test or therapy
        as, or resulting in, or from
            abnormal or delayed reaction or
                complication—*see* Reaction, abnormal
            misadventure—*see* Misadventure
    motor vehicle accident (accident classifiable to
        E810-E825) E929.0
    natural or environmental factor, accident due
        to (accident classifiable to E900-E909)
        E929.5

Late effect of—*continued*
poisoning, accidental (accident classifiable to
 E850-E858, E860-E869) E929.2
suicide, attempt (any means) E959
transport accident NEC (accident classifiable
 to E800-E807, E826-E838, E840-E848)
 E929.1
war operations, injury due to (injury
 classifiable to E990-E998) E999.0
Launching pad accident E845
Legal
execution, any method E978
intervention (by) (injury from) E976
 baton E973
 bayonet E974
 blow E975
 blunt object (baton) (nightstick) (stave)
  (truncheon) E973
 cutting or piercing instrument E974
 dynamite E971
 execution, any method E973
 explosive(s) (shell) E971
 firearms(s) E970
 gas (asphyxiation) (poisoning) (tear) E972
 grenade E971
 late effect of E977
 machine gun E970
 manhandling E975
 mortar bomb E971
 nightstick E973
 revolver E970
 rifle E970
 specified means NEC E975
 stabbing E974
 stave E973
 truncheon E973
Lifting, injury
due to
 repetitive movement E927.3
 sudden strenuous movement E927.0
Lightning (shock) (stroke) (struck by) E907
Liquid (noncorrosive) in eye E914
corrosive E924.1
Loss of control
motor vehicle (on public highway) (without
 antecedent collision) E816
 with
  antecedent collision on public highway
   —*see* Collision, motor vehicle
  involving any object, person or vehicle
   not on public highway E816
  on public highway—*see* Collision, motor
   vehicle
 not on public highway, nontraffic accident
  E825
  with antecedent collision—*see* Collision,
   motor vehicle, not on public highway
 off-road type motor vehicle (not on public
  highway) E821
  on public highway—*see* Loss of control,
   motor vehicle
 snow vehicle, motor-driven (not on public
  highway) E820
  on public highway—*see* Loss of control,
   motor vehicle
Lost at sea E832
with accident to watercraft E830
in war operations E995.8
Low
pressure, effects—*see* Effects of, air pressure
temperature, effects—*see* Cold, exposure to

**Lying before train, vehicle or other moving
 object** (unspecified whether accidental or
 intentional) E988.0
stated as intentional, purposeful, suicidal
 (attempt) E958.0
Lynching (*see also* Assault) E968.9

M

**Malfunction, atomic power plant in water
 transport** E838
Mangled (accidentally) NEC E928.9
Manhandling (in brawl, fight) E960.0
legal intervention E975
Manslaughter (nonaccidental)—*see* Assault
Marble in nose E912
Mauled by animal E906.8
Medical procedure, complication of
delayed or as an abnormal reaction without
 mention of misadventure—*see* Reaction,
 abnormal
due to or as a result of misadventure—*see*
 Misadventure
Melting of fittings and furniture in burning
in terrorism E979.3
Minamata disease E865.2
Misadventure(s) to patient(s) during surgical or
 medical care E876.9
contaminated blood, fluid, drug or biological
 substance (presence of agents and toxins
 as listed in E875) E875.9
 administered (by) NEC E875.9
  infusion E875.0
  injection E875.1
  specified means NEC E875.2
  transfusion E875.0
  vaccination E875.1
cut, cutting, puncture, perforation or
 hemorrhage (accidental) (inadvertent)
 (inappropriate) (during) E870.9
 aspiration of fluid or tissue (by puncture or
  catheterization, except heart) E870.5
 biopsy E870.8
  needle (aspirating) E870.5
 blood sampling E870.5
 catheterization E870.5
  heart E870.6
 dialysis (kidney) E870.2
 endoscopic examination E870.4
 enema E870.7
 infusion E870.1
 injection E870.3
 lumbar puncture E870.5
 needle biopsy E870.5
 paracentesis, abdominal E870.5
 perfusion E870.2
 specified procedure NEC E870.8
 surgical operation E870.0
 thoracentesis E870.5
 transfusion E870.1
 vaccination E870.3
excessive amount of blood or other fluid
 during transfusion or infusion E873.0
failure
 in dosage E873.9
  electroshock therapy E873.4
  inappropriate temperature (too hot or too
   cold) in local application and packing
   E873.5

Misadventure(s)—*continued*
infusion
excessive amount of fluid E873.0
incorrect dilution of fluid E873.1
insulin-shock therapy E873.4
nonadministration of necessary drug or
medicinal E873.6
overdose—*see also* Overdose
radiation, in therapy E873.2
radiation
inadvertent exposure of patient (receiving
radiation for test or therapy) E873.3
not receiving radiation for test or
therapy—*see* Radiation
overdose E873.2
specified procedure NEC 873.8
transfusion
excessive amount of blood E873.0
mechanical, of instrument or apparatus
(during procedure) E874.9
aspiration of fluid or tissue (by puncture or
catheterization, except of heart) E874.4
biopsy E874.8
needle (aspirating) E874.4
blood sampling E874.4
catheterization E874.4
heart E874.5
dialysis (kidney) E874.2
endoscopic examination E874.3
enema E874.8
infusion E874.1
injection E874.8
lumbar puncture E874.4
needle biopsy E874.4
paracentesis, abdominal E874.4
perfusion E874.2
specified procedure NEC E874.8
surgical operation E874.0
thoracentesis E874.4
transfusion E874.1
vaccination E874.8
sterile precautions (during procedure) E872.9
aspiration of fluid or tissue (by puncture or
catheterization, except heart) E872.5
biopsy E872.8
needle (aspirating) E872.5
blood sampling E872.5
catheterization E872.5
heart E872.6
dialysis (kidney) E872.2
endoscopic examination E872.4
enema E872.8
infusion E872.1
injection E872.3
lumbar puncture E872.5
needle biopsy E872.5
paracentesis, abdominal E872.5
perfusion E872.2
removal of catheter or packing E872.8
specified procedure NEC E872.8
surgical operation E872.0
thoracentesis E872.5
transfusion E872.1
vaccination E872.3
suture or ligature during surgical procedure
E876.2
to introduce or to remove tube or instrument
E876.4
foreign object left in body—*see*
Misadventure, foreign object

Misadventure(s)—*continued*
foreign object left in body (during procedure)
E871.9
aspiration of fluid or tissue (by puncture or
catheterization, except heart) E871.5
biopsy E871.8
needle (aspirating) E871.5
blood sampling E871.5
catheterization E871.5
heart E871.6
dialysis (kidney) E871.2
endoscopic examination E871.4
enema E871.8
infusion E871.1
injection E871.3
lumbar puncture E871.5
needle biopsy E871.5
paracentesis, abdominal E871.5
perfusion E871.2
removal of catheter or packing E871.7
specified procedure NEC E871.8
surgical operation E871.0
thoracentesis E871.5
transfusion E871.1
vaccination E871.3
hemorrhage—*see* Misadventure, cut
inadvertent exposure of patient to radiation
(being received for test or therapy) E873.3
inappropriate
temperature (too hot or too cold) in local
application or packing E873.5
infusion—*see also* Misadventure, by specific
type, infusion
excessive amount of fluid E873.0
incorrect dilution of fluid E873.1
wrong fluid E876.1
mismatched blood in transfusion E876.0
nonadministration of necessary drug or
medicinal E873.6
overdose—*see also* Overdose
radiation, in therapy E873.2
perforation—*see* Misadventure, cut
performance of correct operation (procedure)
on wrong
body part E876.7
side E876.7
site E876.7
performance of operation (procedure)
intended for another patient E876.6
on patient not scheduled for surgery E876.6
on wrong patient E876.6
performance of wrong operation on correct
patient E876.5
puncture—*see* Misadventure, cut
specified type NEC E876.8
failure
suture or ligature during surgical operation
E876.2
to introduce or to remove tube or
instrument E876.4
foreign object left in body E871.9
infusion of wrong fluid E876.1
transfusion of mismatched blood E876.0
wrong
fluid in infusion E876.1
placement of endotracheal tube during
anesthetic procedure E876.3
transfusion—*see also* Misadventure, by
specific type, transfusion
excessive amount of blood E873.0
mismatched blood E876.0

Misadventure(s)—*continued*
wrong
  device implanted into correct surgical site
    E876.5
  procedure (operation) performed on the
    correct patient E876.5
  drug given in error—*see* Table of drugs and
    chemicals
  fluid in infusion E876.1
  placement of endotracheal tube during
    anesthetic procedure E876.3
Motion (effects) E903
  sickness E903
Mountain sickness E902.0
**Mucus aspiration or inhalation, not of
  newborn** (with asphyxia, obstruction
  respiratory passage, suffocation) E912
Mudslide of cataclysmic nature E909.2
Murder (attempt) (*see also* Assault) E968.9

N

Nail, injury by E920.8
Needlestick (sewing needle) E920.4
  hypodermic E920.5
Neglect —*see also* Privation
  criminal E968.4
  homicidal intent E968.4
Noise (causing injury) (pollution) E928.1
Nuclear weapon (see also War operations,
  injury due to, nuclear weapons) E996.9

O

Object
falling
  from, in, on, hitting
    aircraft E844
      due to accident to aircraft—*see*
        categories E840-E842
    machinery—*see also* Accident, machine
      not in operation E916
    motor vehicle (in motion) (on public
      highway) E818
      not on public highway E825
    stationary E916
    nonmotor road vehicle NEC E829
    pedal cycle E826
    person E916
    railway rolling stock, train, vehicle E806
    street car E829
    watercraft E838
      due to accident to watercraft E831
set in motion by
  accidental explosion of pressure vessel—*see*
    category E921
  firearm—*see* category E922
  machine(ry)—*see* Accident, machine
  transport vehicle—*see* categories E800-E848
thrown from, in, on, towards
  aircraft E844
  cable car (not on rails) E847
    on rails E829
  motor vehicle (in motion) (on public
    highway) E818
    not on public highway E825
  nonmotor road vehicle NEC E829
  pedal cycle E826
  street car E829
  vehicle NEC—*see* Accident, vehicle NEC

Obstruction
air passages, larynx, respiratory passages
  by
    external means NEC—*see* Suffocation
    food, any type (regurgitated) (vomited)
      E911
    material or object, except food E912
    mucus E912
    phlegm E912
    vomitus E911
digestive tract, except mouth or pharynx
  by
    food, any type E915
    foreign body (any) E915
esophagus
  food E911
  foreign body, except food E912
  without asphyxia or obstruction of
    respiratory passage E915
mouth or pharynx
  by
    food, any type E911
    material or object, except food E912
respiration—*see* Obstruction, air passages
Oil in eye E914
Overdose
anesthetic (drug)—*see* Table of drugs and
  chemicals
drug—*see* Table of drugs and chemicals
Overexertion E927.9
from
  lifting
    repetitive movement E927.3
    sudden strenuous movement E927.0
  maintaining prolonged positions E927.1
    holding E927.1
    sitting E927.1
    standing E927.1
  prolonged static position E927.1
  pulling
    repetitive movement E927.3
    sudden strenuous movement E927.0
  pushing
    repetitive movement E927.3
    sudden strenuous movement E927.0
  specified NEC E927.8
  sudden strenuous movement E927.0
Overexposure (accidental) (to)
cold (*see also* Cold, exposure to) E901.9
  due to manmade conditions E901.1
heat (*see also* Heat) E900.9
radiation—*see* Radiation
radioactivity—*see* Radiation
sun, except sunburn E900.0
weather—*see* Exposure
wind—*see* Exposure
Overheated (*see also* Heat) E900.9
Overlaid E913.0
Overturning (accidental)
animal-drawn vehicle E827
boat, ship, watercraft
  causing
    drowning, submersion E830
    injury except drowning, submersion E831
  machinery—*see* Accident, machine
  motor vehicle (*see also* Loss of control, motor
    vehicle) E816
    with antecedent collision on public
      highway—*see* Collision, motor vehicle
    not on public highway, nontraffic accident
      E825

Overturning—*continued*
with antecedent collision—*see* Collision,
motor vehicle, not on public highway
nonmotor road vehicle NEC E829
off-road type motor vehicle—*see* Loss of
control, off-road type motor vehicle
pedal cycle E826
railway rolling stock, train, vehicle (*see also*
Derailment, railway) E802
street car E829
vehicle NEC—*see* Accident, vehicle NEC

P

Palsy, divers' E902.2
Parachuting (voluntary) (without accident to
aircraft) E844
due to accident to aircraft—*see* categories
E840-E842
Paralysis
divers' E902.2
lead or saturnine E866.0
from pesticide NEC E863.4
Pecked by bird E906.8
Performance of correct operation (procedure)
on wrong
body part E876.7
side E876.7
site E876.7
Performance of operation (procedure)
intended for another patient E876.6
on patient not scheduled for surgery E876.6
on wrong patient E876.6
Performance of wrong operation on correct
patient E876.5
Phlegm aspiration or inhalation (with
asphyxia, obstruction respiratory passage,
suffocation) E912
Piercing (*see also* Cut) E920.9
by slide trigger mechanism, scope or other
part of gun E928.7
Pinched
between objects (moving) (stationary and
moving) E918
by slide trigger mechanism, scope or other
part of gun E928.7
in object E918
Pinned under
machine(ry)—*see* Accident, machine
Place of occurrence of accident —*see*
Accident (to), occurring (at) (in)
Plumbism E866.0
from insecticide NEC E863.4
Poisoning (accidental) (by)—*see also* Table of
drugs and chemicals
carbon monoxide
generated by
aircraft in transit E844
motor vehicle
in motion (on public highway) E818
not on public highway E825
watercraft (in transit) (not in transit) E838
caused by injection of poisons or toxins into
or through skin by plant thorns, spines, or
other mechanism E905.7
marine or sea plants E905.6
fumes or smoke due to
conflagration—*see* Conflagration
explosion or fire—*see* Fire
ignition—*see* Ignition

Poisoning—*continued*
gas
in legal intervention E972
legal execution, by E978
on watercraft E838
used as anesthetic—*see* Table of drugs and
chemicals
in
terrorism (chemical weapons) E979.7
war operations E997.2
late effect of—*see* Late effect
legal
execution E978
intervention
by gas E972
**Pressure, external, causing asphyxia,
suffocation** (*see also* Suffocation) E913.9
Privation E904.9
food (*see also* Lack of, food) E904.1
helpless person, infant, newborn due to
abandonment or neglect E904.0
late effect of NEC E929.5
resulting from transport accident—*see*
categories E800-E848
water (*see also* Lack of, water) E904.2
**Projected objects, striking against or struck
by** —*see* Striking against, object
Prolonged stay in
high altitude (causing conditions as listed in
E902.0) E902.0
weightless environment E928.0
Prostration
heat—*see* Heat
Pulling, injury
due to
repetitive movement E927.3
sudden strenuous movement E927.0
Puncture, puncturing (*see also* Cut) E920.9
by
plant thorns or spines E920.8
toxic reaction E905.7
marine or sea plants E905.6
sea-urchin spine E905.6
Pushing (injury in) (overexertion) E927.8
by other person(s) (accidental) E917.9
as, or caused by, a crowd, human stampede
E917.1
with subsequent fall E917.6
before moving vehicle or object
stated as
intentional, homicidal E968.5
undetermined whether accidental or
intentional E988.8
from
high place
in accidental circumstances—*see*
categories E880-E884
stated as
intentional, homicidal E968.1
undetermined whether accidental or
intentional E987.9
man-made structure, except
residential E987.1
natural site E987.2
residential E987.0
motor vehicle (*see also* Fall, from, motor
vehicle) E818
stated as
intentional, homicidal E968.5
undetermined whether accidental or
intentional E988.8

Pushing—*continued*
  by other person—*continued*
    in sports E917.0
      with fall E886.0
      with fall E886.9
      in sports E886.0
  due to
    repetitive movement E927.3
    sudden strenuous movement E927.0

R

Radiation (exposure to) E926.9
  abnormal reaction to medical test or therapy
    E879.2
  arc lamps E926.2
  atomic power plant (malfunction) NEC E926.9
    in water transport E838
  electromagnetic, ionizing E926.3
  gamma rays E926.3
  in
    terrorism (from or following nuclear
      explosion) (direct) (secondary) E979.5
      laser E979.8
    war operations (see also War operations,
      injury due to, nuclear weapons) E996.3
      laser(s) E997.0
    water transport E838
  inadvertent exposure of patient (receiving test
    or therapy) E873.3
  infrared (heaters and lamps) E926.1
    excessive heat E900.1
  ionized, ionizing (particles, artificially
    accelerated) E926.8
    electromagnetic E926.3
  isotopes, radioactive—*see* Radiation,
    radioactive isotopes
  laser(s) E926.4
    in
      terrorism E979.8
      war operations E997.0
    misadventure in medical care—*see*
      Misadventure, failure, in dosage,
      radiation
  late effect of NEC E929.8
  excessive heat from—*see* Heat
  light sources (visible) (ultraviolet) E926.2
  misadventure in medical or surgical
    procedure—*see* Misadventure, failure, in
    dosage, radiation
  overdose (in medical or surgical procedure)
    E873.2
  radar E926.0
  radioactive isotopes E926.5
    atomic power plant malfunction E926.5
      in water transport E838
    misadventure in medical or surgical
      treatment—*see* Misadventure, failure, in
      dosage, radiation
  radiobiologicals—*see* Radiation, radioactive
    isotopes
  radiofrequency E926.0
  radiopharmaceuticals—*see* Radiation,
    radioactive isotopes
  radium NEC E926.9
  sun E926.2
    excessive heat from E900.0
  tanning bed E926.2
  welding arc or torch E926.2
    excessive heat from E900.1

Radiation—*continued*
  x-rays (hard) (soft) E926.3
    misadventure in medical or surgical
      treatment—*see* Misadventure, failure, in
      dosage, radiation
Rape E960.1
Reaction —abnormal to or following(medical or
  surgical procedure) E879.9
  amputation (of limbs) E878.5
  anastomosis (arteriovenous) (blood vessel)
    (gastrojejunal) (skin) (tendon) (natural,
    artificial material, tissue) E878.2
    external stoma, creation of E878.3
  aspiration (of fluid) E879.4
    tissue E879.8
  biopsy E879.8
  blood
    sampling E879.7
    transfusion
      procedure E879.8
  bypass—*see* Reaction, abnormal, anastomosis
  catheterization
    cardiac E879.0
    urinary E879.6
  colostomy E878.3
  cystostomy E878.3
  dialysis (kidney) E879.1
  drugs or biologicals—*see* Table of drugs and
    chemicals
  duodenostomy E878.3
  electroshock therapy E879.3
  formation of external stoma E878.3
  gastrostomy E878.3
  graft—*see* Reaction, abnormal, anastomosis
  hypothermia E879.8
  implant, implantation (of)
    artificial
      internal device (cardiac pacemaker)
        (electrodes in brain) (heart valve
        prosthesis) (orthopedic) E878.1
      material or tissue (for anastomosis or
        bypass) E878.2
        with creation of external stoma E878.3
      natural tissues (for anastomosis or bypass)
        E878.2
      as transplantion—*see* Reaction, abnormal,
        transplant
      with creation of external stoma E878.3
  infusion
    procedure E879.8
  injection
    procedure E879.8
  insertion of gastric or duodenal sound E879.5
  insulin-shock therapy E879.3
  lumbar puncture E879.4
  perfusion E879.1
  procedures other than surgical operation (*see*
    also Reaction, abnormal, by specific type
    of procedure) E879.9
    specified procedure NEC E879.8
  radiological procedure or therapy E879.2
  removal of organ (partial) (total) NEC E878.6
    with
      anastomosis, bypass or graft E878.2
      formation of external stoma E878.3
      implant of artificial internal device E878.1
      transplant(ation)
        partial organ E878.4
        whole organ E878.0

Reaction—*continued*
sampling
blood E879.7
fluid NEC E879.4
tissue E879.8
shock therapy E879.3
surgical operation (*see also* Reaction,
abnormal, by specified type of operation)
E878.9
restorative NEC E878.4
with
anastomosis, bypass or graft E878.2
formation of external stoma E878.3
implant(ation)—*see* Reaction, abnormal,
implant
transplant(ation)—*see* Reaction,
abnormal, transplant
specified operation NEC E878.8
thoracentesis E879.4
transfusion
procedure E879.8
transplant, transplantation (heart) (kidney)
(liver) E878.0
partial organ E878.4
ureterostomy E878.3
vaccination E879.8
Reduction in
atmospheric pressure—*see also* Effects of, air
pressure
while surfacing from
deep water diving causing caisson or
divers' disease, palsy or paralysis
E902.2
underground E902.8
Repetitive movements NEC E927.8
Residual (effect)—*see* Late effect
Rock falling on or hitting (accidentally)
motor vehicle (in motion) (on public highway)
E818
not on public highway E825
nonmotor road vehicle NEC E829
pedal cycle E826
person E916
railway rolling stock, train, vehicle E806
Running off, away
animal (being ridden) (in sport or transport)
E828
not being ridden E906.8
animal-drawn vehicle E827
rails, railway (*see also* Derailment) E802
roadway
motor vehicle (without antecedent collision)
E816
nontraffic accident E825
with antecedent collision—*see* Collision,
motor vehicle, not on public highway
with
antecedent collision—*see* Collision motor
vehicle
subsequent collision
involving any object, person or vehicle
not on public highway E816
on public highway E811
nonmotor road vehicle NEC E829
pedal cycle E826
Run over (accidentally) (by)
animal (not being ridden) E906.8
being ridden (in sport or transport) E828
animal-drawn vehicle E827
machinery—*see* Accident, machine

Run over—*continued*
motor vehicle (on public highway)—*see* Hit
by, motor vehicle
nonmotor road vehicle NEC E829
railway train E805
street car E829
vehicle NEC E848

S

Saturnism E866.0
from insecticide NEC E863.4
Scald, scalding (accidental) (by) (from) (in)
E924.0
acid—*see* Scald, caustic
boiling tap water E924.2
caustic or corrosive liquid, substance E924.1
swallowed—*see* Table of drugs and
chemicals
homicide (attempt)—*see* Assault, burning
inflicted by other person
stated as
intentional or homicidal E968.3
undetermined whether accidental or
intentional E988.2
late effect of NEC E929.8
liquid (boiling) (hot) E924.0
local application of externally applied
substance in medical or surgical care
E873.5
molten metal E924.0
self-inflicted (unspecified whether accidental
or intentional) E988.2
stated as intentional, purposeful E958.2
stated as undetermined whether accidental or
intentional E988.2
steam E924.0
tap water (boiling) E924.2
transport accident—*see* categories E800-E848
vapor E924.0
Scratch, cat E906.8
Sea
sickness E903
Self-mutilation —*see* Suicide
Sequelai (of)
in
terrorism E999.1
war operations E999.0
Shock
anaphylactic (*see also* Table of drugs and
chemicals) E947.9
due to
bite (venomous)—*see* Bite, venomous NEC
sting—*see* Sting
electric (*see also* Electric shock) E925.9
from electric appliance or current (*see also*
Electric shock) E925.9
Shooting, shot (accidental(ly)) E922.9
air gun E922.4
BB gun E922.4
hand gun (pistol) (revolver) E922.0
himself (*see also* Shooting, self-inflicted)
E985.4
hand gun (pistol) (revolver) E985.0
military firearm, except hand gun E985.3
hand gun (pistol) (revolver) E985.0
rifle (hunting) E985.2
military E985.3
shotgun (automatic) E985.1
specified firearm NEC E985.4
Verey pistol E985.4

Slipping (on)—*continued*
  ladder of ship E833
    due to accident to watercraft E831
  mud E885.9
  oil E885.9
  snow E885.9
  stairs of ship E833
    due to accident to watercraft E831
  surface
    slippery E885.9
    wet E885.9
Sliver, wood, injury by E920.8
Smothering, smothered (*see also* Suffocation) E913.9
Smouldering building or structure in terrorism E979.3
Sodomy (assault) E960.1
Solid substance in eye (any part) or adnexa E914
Sound waves (causing injury) E928.1
Splinter, injury by E920.8
Stab, stabbing E966
  accidental—*see* Cut
Starvation E904.1
  helpless person, infant, newborn—*see* Lack of food
  homicidal intent E968.4
  late effect of NEC E929.5
  resulting from accident connected with transport—*see* categories E800-E848
Stepped on
  by
    animal (not being ridden) E906.8
      being ridden (in sport or transport) E828
    crowd E917.1
    person E917.9
      in sports E917.0
  in sports E917.0
Stepping on
  object (moving) E917.9
    in sports E917.0
      with subsequent fall E917.5
    stationary E917.4
      with subsequent fall E917.8
  person E917.9
    as, or caused by a crowd E917.1
      with subsequent fall E917.6
    in sports E917.0
Sting E905.9
  ant E905.5
  bee E905.3
  caterpillar E905.5
  coral E905.6
  hornet E905.3
  insect NEC E905.5
  jelly fish E905.6
  marine animal or plant E905.6
  nematocysts E905.6
  scorpion E905.2
  sea anemone E905.6
  sea cucumber E905.6
  wasp E905.3
  yellow jacket E905.3
Storm E908.9
  specified type NEC E908.8
Straining, injury
  due to
    repetitive movement E927.3
    sudden strenuous movement E927.0
Strangling —*see* Suffocation
Strangulation —*see* Suffocation
Strenuous movements (in recreational or other activities) NEC E927.8

Striking against
  bottom (when jumping or diving into water) E883.0
  object (moving) E917.9
    caused by crowd E917.1
      with subsequent fall E917.6
    furniture E917.3
      with subsequent fall E917.7
    in
      running water E917.2
        with drowning or submersion—*see* Submersion
      sports E917.0
        with subsequent fall E917.5
    stationary E917.4
      with subsequent fall E917.8
  person(s) E917.9
    with fall E886.9
      in sports E886.0
    as, or caused by, a crowd E917.1
      with subsequent fall E917.6
    in sports E917.0
      with fall E886.0
Stroke
  heat—*see* Heat
  lightning E907
Struck by —*see also* Hit by
  bullet
    in
      terrorism E979.4
      war operation E991.2
        rubber E991.0
  lightning E907
  missile
    in terrorism—*see* Terrorism, missile
  object
    falling
      from, in, on
        building
          burning (uncontrolled fire)
            in terrorism E979.3
  thunderbolt E907
Stumbling over animal, carpet, curb, rug or (small) object (with fall) E885.9
  without fall—*see* Striking against, object
Submersion (accidental) E910.8
  boat, ship, watercraft (causing drowning, submersion) E830
    causing injury except drowning, submersion E831
  by other person
    in accidental circumstances—*see* category E910
    intentional, homicidal E964
    stated as undetermined whether accidental or intentional E984
  due to
    accident
      machinery—*see* Accident, machine
      to boat, ship, watercraft E830
      transport—*see* categories E800-E848
    avalanche E909.2
    cataclysmic
      earth surface movement or eruption E909.9
      storm E908.9
    cloudburst E908.8
    cyclone E908.1

Submersion—*continued*
  fall
    from
      boat, ship, watercraft (not involved in
          accident) E832
        burning, crushed E830
        involved in accident, collision E830
      gangplank (into water) E832
      overboard NEC E832
    flood E908.2
    hurricane E908.0
    jumping into water E910.8
      from boat, ship, watercraft
        burning, crushed, sinking E830
        involved in accident, collision E830
        not involved in accident, for swim
            E910.2
      in recreational activity (without diving
          equipment) E910.2
      with or using diving equipment E910.1
      to rescue another person E910.3
  homicide (attempt) E964
  in
    bathtub E910.4
    specified activity, not sport, transport or
        recreational E910.3
    sport or recreational activity (without diving
        equipment) E910.2
      with or using diving equipment E910.1
      water skiing E910.0
    swimming pool NEC E910.8
    terrorism E979.8
    war operations E995.4
      intentional E995.3
    water transport E832
      due to accident to boat, ship, watercraft
          E830
  landslide E909.2
  overturning boat, ship, watercraft E909.2
  sinking boat, ship, watercraft E909.2
  submersion boat, ship, watercraft E909.2
  tidal wave E909.4
    caused by storm E908.0
  torrential rain E908.2
  late effect of NEC E929.8
  quenching tank E910.8
  self-inflicted (unspecified whether accidental
      or intentional) E984
    in accidental circumstances—*see* category
        E910
    stated as intentional, purposeful E954
  stated as undetermined whether accidental or
      intentional E984
  suicidal (attempted) E954
  while
    attempting rescue of another person E910.3
    engaged in
      marine salvage E910.3
      underwater construction or repairs E910.3
    fishing, not from boat E910.2
    hunting, not from boat E910.2
    ice skating E910.2
    pearl diving E910.3
    placing fishing nets E910.3
    playing in water E910.2
    scuba diving E910.1
      nonrecreational E910.3
    skin diving E910.1
    snorkel diving E910.2
    spear fishing underwater E910.1
    surfboarding E910.2

Submersion—*continued*
  swimming (swimming pool) E910.2
  wading (in water) E910.2
  water skiing E910.0
Sucked
  into
    jet (aircraft) E844
Suffocation (accidental) (by external means) (by
    pressure) (mechanical) E913.9
  caused by other person
    in accidental circumstances—*see* category
        E913
    stated as
      intentional, homicidal E963
      undetermined whether accidental or
          intentional E983.9
        by, in
          hanging E983.0
          plastic bag E983.1
          specified means NEC E983.3
  due to, by
    avalanche E909.2
    bedclothes E913.0
    bib E913.0
    blanket E913.0
    cave-in E913.3
      caused by cataclysmic earth surface
          movement or eruption E909.9
    conflagration—*see* Conflagration
    explosion—*see* Explosion
    falling earth, other substance E913.3
    fire—*see* Fire
    food, any type (ingestion) (inhalation)
        (regurgitated) (vomited) E911
    foreign body, except food (ingestion)
        (inhalation) E912
    ignition—*see* Ignition
    landslide E909.2
    machine(ry)—*see* Accident, machine
    material, object except food entering by nose
        or mouth, ingested, inhaled E912
    mucus (aspiration) (inhalation), not of
        newborn E912
    phlegm (aspiration) (inhalation) E912
    pillow E913.0
    plastic bag—*see* Suffocation, in, plastic bag
    sheet (plastic) E913.0
    specified means NEC E913.8
    vomitus (aspiration) (inhalation) E911
  homicidal (attempt) E963
  in war operations E995.3
  in
    airtight enclosed place E913.2
    baby carriage E913.0
    bed E913.0
    closed place E913.2
    cot, cradle E913.0
    perambulator E913.0
    plastic bag (in accidental circumstances)
        E913.1
      homicidal, purposely inflicted by other
          person E963
      self-inflicted (unspecified whether
          accidental or intentional) E983.1
        in accidental circumstances E913.1
        intentional, suicidal E953.1
      stated as undetermined whether
          accidentally or purposely inflicted
          E983.1
      suicidal, purposely self-inflicted E953.1
    refrigerator E913.2
  war operations E995.3

Suffocation—*continued*
  self-inflicted—*see also* Suffocation, stated as
    undetermined whether accidental or
    intentional E953.9
    in accidental circumstances—*see* category E913
    stated as intentional, purposeful—*see*
      Suicide, suffocation
  stated as undetermined whether accidental or
    intentional E983.9
    by, in
      hanging E983.0
      plastic bag E983.1
      specified means NEC E983.8
  suicidal—*see* Suicide, suffocation
Suicide, suicidal (attempted) (by) E958.9
  burning, burns E958.1
  caustic substance E958.7
    poisoning E950.7
    swallowed E950.7
  cold, extreme E958.3
  cut (any part of body) E956
  cutting or piercing instrument (classifiable to
    E920) E956
  drowning E954
  electrocution E958.4
  explosive(s) (classifiable to E923) E955.5
  fire E958.1
  firearm (classifiable to E922)—*see* Shooting,
    suicidal
  hanging E953.0
  jumping
    before moving object, train, vehicle E958.0
    from high place—*see* Jumping, from, high
      place, stated as, suicidal
  knife E956
  late effect of E959
  motor vehicle, crashing of E958.5
  poisoning—*see* Table of drugs and chemicals
  puncture (any part of body) E956
  scald E958.2
  shooting—*see* Shooting, suicidal
  specified means NEC E958.8
  stab (any part of body) E956
  strangulation—*see* Suicide, suffocation
  submersion E954
  suffocation E953.9
    by, in
      hanging E953.0
      plastic bag E953.1
      specified means NEC E953.8
  wound NEC E958.9
Sunburn E926.2
Sunstroke E900.0
Supersonic waves (causing injury) E928.1
Surgical procedure, complication of
  delayed or as an abnormal reaction without
    mention of misadventure—*see* Reaction,
    abnormal
  due to or as a result of misadventure—*see*
    Misadventure
Swallowed, swallowing
  foreign body—*see* Foreign body, alimentary
    canal
  poison—*see* Table of drugs and chemicals
  substance
    caustic—*see* Table of drugs and chemicals
    corrosive—*see* Table of drugs and chemicals
    poisonous—*see* Table of drugs and
      chemicals
Swimmers cramp (*see also* category E910)
  E910.2
  not in recreation or sport E910.3

Syndrome, battered
  baby or child—*see* Abuse, child
  wife—*see* Assault

T

Tackle in sport E886.0
Terrorism (injury) (by) (in) E979.8
  air blast E979.2
  aircraft burned, destroyed, exploded, shot
    down E979.1
    used as a weapon E979.1
  anthrax E979.6
  asphyxia from
    chemical (weapons) E979.7
    fire, conflagration (caused by fire-producing
      device) E979.3
    from nuclear explosion E979.5
    gas or fumes E979.7
  bayonet E979.8
  biological agents E979.6
  blast (air) (effects) E979.2
    from nuclear explosion E979.5
    underwater E979.0
Terrorism—*continued*
  bomb (antipersonnel) (mortor) (explosion)
    (fragments) E979.2
  bullet(s) (from carbine, machine gun, pistol,
    rifle, shotgun) E979.4
  burn from
    chemical E979.7
    fire, conflagration (caused by fire-producing
      device) E979.3
    from nuclear explosion E979.5
    gas E979.7
  burning aircraft E979.1
  chemical E979.7
  cholera E979.6
  conflagration E979.3
  crushed by falling aircraft E979.1
  depth charge E979.0
  destruction of aircraft E979.1
  disability, as seqelae one year or more after
    injury E999.1
  drowning E979.8
  effect
    of nuclear weapon (direct) (secondary)
      E979.5
    secondary NEC E979.9
    sequelae E999.1
  explosion (artillery shell) (breech-block)
    (cannon block) E979.2
    aircraft E979.1
    bomb (antipersonnel) (mortar) E979.2
      nuclear (atom) (hydrogen) E979.5
    depth-charge E979.0
    grenade E979.2
    injury by fragments from E979.2
    land-mine E979.2
    marine weapon E979.0
    mine (land) E979.2
      at sea or in harbor E979.0
      marine E979.0
    missile (explosive) NEC E979.2
    munitions (dump) (factory) E979.2
    nuclear (weapon) E979.5
      other direct and secondary effects of
        E979.5
    sea-based artillery shell E979.0
    torpedo E979.0

Terrorism—*continued*
  exposure to ionizing radiation from nuclear
    explosion E979.5
  falling aircraft E979.1
  fire or fire-producing device E979.3
  firearms E979.4
  fireball effects from nuclear explosion E979.5
  fragments from artillery shell, bomb NEC,
    grenade, guided missile, land-mine, rocket,
    shell, shrapnel E979.2
  gas or fumes E979.7
  grenade (explosion) (fragments) E979.2
  guided missile (explosion) (fragments) E979.2
    nuclear E979.5
  heat from nuclear explosion E979.5
  hot substances E979.3
  hydrogen cyanide E979.7
  land-mine (explosion) (fragments) E979.2
  laser(s) E979.8
  late effect of E999.1
  lewisite E979.7
  lung irritant (chemical) (fumes) (gas) E979.7
  marine mine E979.0
  mine E979.2
    at sea E979.0
    in harbor E979.0
    land (explosion) (fragments) E979.2
    marine E979.0
  missile (explosion) (fragments) (guided)
    E979.2
    marine E979.0
    nuclear E979.5
  mortar bomb (explosion) (fragments) E979.2
  mustard gas E979.7
  nerve gas E979.7
  nuclear weapons E979.5
  pellets (shotgun) E979.4
  petrol bomb E979.3
  piercing object E979.8
  phosgene E979.7
  poisoning (chemical) (fumes) (gas) E979.7
  radiation, ionizing from nuclear explosion
    E979.5
  rocket (explosion) (fragments) E979.2
  saber, sabre E979.8
  sarin E979.7
  screening smoke E979.7
  sequelae effect (of) E999.1
  shell (aircraft) (artillery) (cannon) (land-based)
    (explosion) (fragments) E979.2
    sea-based E979.0
  shooting E979.4
    bullet(s) E979.4
    pellet(s) (rifle) (shotgun) E979.4
  shrapnel E979.2
  smallpox E979.7
  stabbing object(s) E979.8
  submersion E979.8
  torpedo E979.0
  underwater blast E979.0
  vesicant (chemical) (fumes) (gas) E979.7
  weapon burst E979.2
Thermic fever E900.9
Thermoplegia E900.9
Thirst —*see also* Lack of water
  resulting from accident connected with
    transport—*see* categories E800-E848

Thrown (accidently)
  against object in or part of vehicle
    by motion of vehicle
      aircraft E844
      boat, ship, watercraft E838
      motor vehicle (on public highway) E818
        not on public highway E825
        off-road type (not on public highway)
          E821
          on public highway E818
        snow vehicle E820
          on public highway E818
      nonmotor road vehicle NEC E829
      railway rolling stock, train, vehicle E806
      street car E829
  from
    animal (being ridden) (in sport or transport)
      E828
    high place, homicide (attempt) E968.1
    machinery—*see* Accident, machine
    vehicle NEC—*see* Accident, vehicle NEC
  off—*see* Thrown, from
  overboard (by motion of boat, ship, watercraft)
    E832
    by accident to boat, ship, watercraft E830
Thunderbolt NEC E907
Tidal wave (any injury) E909.4
  caused by storm E908.0
Took
  overdose of drug—*see* Table of drugs and
    chemicals
  poison—*see* Table of drugs and chemicals
Tornado (any injury) E908.1
Torrential rain (any injury) E908.2
Traffic accident NEC E819
Trampled by animal E906.8
  being ridden (in sport or transport) E828
Trapped (accidentally)
  between
    objects (moving) (stationary and moving)
      E918
  by
    door of
      elevator E918
      motor vehicle (on public highway) (while
        alighting, boarding)—*see* Fall, from,
        motor vehicle, while alighting
      railway train (underground) E806
      street car E829
      subway train E806
  in object E918
Trauma
  cumulative
    from
      repetitive
        impact E927.4
        motion or movements E927.3
    sudden from strenuous movements E927.0
Travel (effects) E903
  sickness E903
Tree
  falling on or hitting E916
    motor vehicle (in motion) (on public
      highway) E818
      not on public highway E825
    nonmotor road vehicle NEC E829
    pedal cycle E826
    person E916
    railway rolling stock, train, vehicle E806
    street car E829
Trench foot E901.0

Tripping over animal, carpet, curb, rug, or
    small object (with fall) E885.9
  without fall—see Striking against, object
Tsunami E909.4
Twisting, injury
  due to
    repetitive movement E927.3
    sudden strenuous movement E927.0

V

Violence, nonaccidental (see also Assault)
    E968.9
Volcanic eruption (any injury) E909.1
Vomitus in air passages (with asphyxia,
    obstruction or suffocation) E911

W

War operations (during hostilities) (injury) (by)
    (in) E995.9
  after cessation of hostilities, injury due to
    E998.9
  air blast E993.9
  aircraft burned, destroyed, exploded, shot
    down E994
  asphyxia from
    chemical E997.2
    fire, conflagration (caused by fire-producing
      device or conventional weapon) E990.9
      from nuclear explosion (see also War
        operations, injury due to, nuclear
        weapons) E996.8
      incendiary bomb E990.0
      petrol bomb E990.0
    fumes E997.2
    gas E997.2
  baton (nightstick) E995.1
  battle wound NEC E995.8
  bayonet E995.2
  biological warfare agents E997.1
  blast (air) (effects) E993.9
    from nuclear explosion—see War operations,
      injury due to, nuclear weapons
    underwater E992.9
  bomb (mortar) (explosion) E993.2
    after cessation of hostilities E998.1
    fragments, injury by E991.4
      antipersonnel E991.3
  bullet(s) (from carbine, machine gun, pistol,
    rifle, shotgun) E991.2
    rubber E991.0
  burn from
    chemical E997.2
    fire, conflagration (caused by fire-producing
      device or conventional weapon) E990.9
      from
        conventional weapon E990.3
        flamethrower E990.1
        incendiary bomb E990.0
        incendiary bullet E990.2
        nuclear explosion E996.2
        petrol bomb E990.0
    gas E997.2
  burning aircraft E994.3
  chemical E997.2
  chlorine E997.2
  conventional warfare, specified form NEC E995.8
  crushing by falling aircraft E994.8

War operations—continued
  depth charge E992.1
  destruction of aircraft E994.9
  detonation of own munitions (ammunition)
    (artillery) (mortars), unintentional E993.6
  disability as sequela one year or more after
    injury E999.0
  discharge of own munitions launch device
    (autocannons) (automatic grenade
    launchers) (missile launchers) (small arms),
    unintentional E993.7
  drowning E995.4
  effect, nuclear weapon (see also War
    operations, injury due to, nuclear weapons)
    E996.9
  explosion (breech block) (cannon shell)
    E993.9
    after cessation of hostilities
      bomb placed in war E998.1
      mine placed in war E998.0
    aircraft E994.1
      due to
        enemy fire or explosives E994.0
        own onboard explosives E994.1
    artillery shell E993.2
    bomb (mortar) E993.2
      aerial E993.0
      atom (see also War operations, injury due
        to, nuclear weapons) E996.9
      hydrogen (see also War operations, injury
        due to, nuclear weapons) E996.9
      injury by fragments from E991.4
        antipersonnel E991.3
      nuclear (see also War operations, injury
        due to, nuclear weapons) E996.9
    depth charge E992.1
    injury by fragments from E991.4
      antipersonnel E991.3
    marine weapon NEC E992.8
    mine
      at sea or in harbor E992.2
      land E993.8
        injury by fragments from E991.4
      marine E992.2
    missle, guided E993.1
    mortar E993.2
    munitions (accidental) (being used in war)
      (dump) (factory) E993.9
      own E993.7
        launch device (autocannons) (automatic
          grenade launchers) (missile launchers)
          (small arms) E993.7
    nuclear (weapon) (see also War operations,
      injury due to, nuclear weapons) E996.9
    own weapons (accidental) E993.7
      injury by fragments from E991.9
        antipersonnel E991.3
    sea-based artillery shell E992.3
    specified NEC E993.8
    torpedo E992.0
  exposure to ionizing radiation from nuclear
    explosion (see also War operations, injury
    due to, nuclear weapons) E996.3
  falling aircraft E994.8
  fire or fire-producing device E990.9
    flamethrower E990.1
    incendiary bomb E990.0
    incendiary bullet E990.2
    indirectly caused from conventional weapon
      E990.3
    petrol bomb E990.0

War operations—*continued*
  piercing object E995.2
  restriction of airway, intentional E995.3
  sea based artillery shell E992.3
  shrapnel E991.9
  stave E995.1
  strangulation E995.3
  strike by blunt object (baton) (nightstick)
    (stave) E995.1
  submersion (accidental) (unintentional)
    E995.4
    intentional E995.3
  suffocation E995.3
    accidental E995.4
  torpedo E992.0
  underwater blast E992.9
  weapon of mass destruction [WMD] E997.3
knife E995.2
lacrimator (gas) (chemical) E997.2
land mine (explosion) E993.8
  after cessation of hostilities E998.0
  fragments, injury by E991.4
laser(s) E997.0
late effect of E999.0
lewisite E997.2
lung irritant (chemical) (fumes) (gas) E997.2
marine mine E992.2
mine
  after cessation of hostilities E998.0
  at sea E992.2
  in harbor E992.2
  land (explosion) E993.8
    fragments, injury by E991.4
  marine E992.2
missile (guided) (explosion) E993.1
  fragments, injury by E991.4
  marine E992.8
  nuclear (*see also* War operations, injury due
    to, nuclear weapons) E996.9
mortar bomb (explosion) E993.2
  fragments, injury by E991.4
mustard gas E997.2
nerve gas E997.2
phosgene E997.2
piercing object E995.2
poisoning (chemical) (fumes) (gas) E997.2
radiation, ionizing from nuclear explosion (*see*
  also War operations, injury due to, nuclear
  weapons) E996.3
rocket (explosion) E993.8
  fragments, injury by E991.4
saber, sabre E995.2
screening smoke E997.8
shell (aircraft) (artillery) (cannon) (land based)
  (explosion) E993.2
  fragments, injury by E991.4
  sea-based E992.3
shooting E991.2
  after cessation of hostilities E998.8
  bullet(s) E991.2
    rubber E991.0
  pellet(s) (rifle) E991.1
shrapnel E991.9
stave E995.2
strike by blunt object (baton) (nightstick)
  (stave) E995.1
submersion E995.4
  intentional E995.3
sword E995.2
torpedo E992.0

War operations—*continued*
  unconventional warfare, except by nuclear
    weapon E997.9
  biological (warfare) E997.1
  gas, fumes, chemicals E997.2
  laser(s) E997.0
  specified type NEC E997.8
underwater blast E992.9
vesicant (chemical) (fumes) (gas) E997.2
weapon burst E993.9
Washed
  away by flood—*see* Flood
  away by tidal wave—*see* Tidal wave
  off road by storm (transport vehicle) E908.9
  overboard E832
Weapon of mass destruction [WMD] E997.3
Weather exposure —*see also* Exposure
  cold E901.0
  hot E900.0
Weightlessness (causing injury) (effects of) (in
  spacecraft, real or simulated) E928.0
Wound (accidental) NEC (*see also* Injury)
  E928.9
  battle (*see also* War operation) E995.9
  bayonet E920.3
    in
      legal intervention E974
      war operations E995.2
  gunshot—*see* Shooting
  incised—*see* Cut
  saber, sabre E920.3
    in war operations E995.2
Wrong
  body part, performance of correct operation
    (procedure) on E876.7
  device implanted into correct surgical site
    E876.5
  patient, performance of operation (procedure)
    on E876.6
  procedure (operation) performed on correct
    patient E876.5
  side, performance of correct operation
    (procedure) on E876.7
  site, performance of correct operation
    (procedure) on E876.7

RAILWAY ACCIDENTS (E800–E807)

The following fourth-digit subdivisions are for use with categories E800-E807 to identify the injured person.

.0 Railway employee

Any person who by virtue of his employment in connection with a railway, whether by the railway company or not, is at increased risk of involvement in a railway accident, such as:

catering staff on train	postal staff on train
driver	railway fireman
guard	shunter
porter	sleeping car attendant

.1 Passenger on railway

Any authorized person traveling on a train, except a railway employee

Excludes: intending passenger waiting at station (.8)
unauthorized rider on railway vehicle (.8)

.2 Pedestrian

See definition (r), Vol. 1, E code introduction

.3 Pedal cyclist

See definition (p), Vol. 1, E code introduction

.8 Other specified person

Intending passenger waiting at station

Unauthorized rider on railway vehicle

.9 Unspecified person

MOTOR VEHICLE TRAFFIC AND NONTRAFFIC ACCIDENTS
(E810–825)

The following fourth–digit subdivisions are for use with categories E810–E819 and E820–E825 to identify the injured person:

.0 Driver of motor vehicle other than motorcycle

See definition (l), Vol. 1, E code introduction

.1 Passenger in motor vehicle other than motorcycle

See definition (l), Vol. 1, E code introduction

.2 Motorcyclist

See definition (l), Vol. 1, E code introduction

.3 Passenger on motorcycle

See definition (l), Vol. 1, E code introduction

.4 Occupant of streetcar

.5 Rider of animal; occupant of animal–drawn vehicle

.6 Pedal cyclist

See definition (p), Vol. 1, E code introduction

.7 Pedestrian

See definition (r), Vol. 1, E code introduction

.8 Other specified person

Occupant of vehicle other than above

Person in railway train involved in accident

Unauthorized rider of motor vehicle

.9 Unspecified person

OTHER ROAD VEHICLE ACCIDENTS (E826–E829)

(animal–drawn vehicle, streetcar, pedal cycle, and other nonmotor road vehicle accidents)

The following fourth–digit subdivisions are for use with categories E826–E829 to identify the injured person:

.0 Pedestrian

　　See definition (r), Vol. 1, E code introduction

.1 Pedal cyclist (does not apply to codes E827, E828, E829)

　　See definition (p), Vol. 1, E code introduction

.2 Rider of animal (does not apply to code E829)

.3 Occupant of animal–drawn vehicle (does not apply to codes E828, E829)

.4 Occupant of streetcar

.8 Other specified person

.9 Unspecified person

WATER TRANSPORT ACCIDENTS (E830–E838)

The following fourth–digit subdivisions are for use with categories E830–E838 to identify the injured person:

.0 Occupant of small boat, unpowered

.1 Occupant of small boat, powered

See definition (t), Vol. 1, E code introduction

Excludes: water skier (.4)

.2 Occupant of other watercraft — crew

Persons:

> engaged in operation of watercraft
>
> providing passenger services [cabin attendants, ship's physician, catering personnel]
>
> working on ship during voyage in other capacity [musician in band, operators of shops and beauty parlors]

.3 Occupant of other watercraft — other than crew

Passenger

Occupant of lifeboat, other than crew, after abandoning ship

.4 Water skier

.5 Swimmer

.6 Dockers, stevedores

Longshoreman employed on the dock in loading and unloading ships

.8 Other specified person

Immigration and custom officials on board ship

Person:
accompanying passenger or member of crew
visiting boat

Pilot (guiding ship into port)

.9 Unspecified person

AIR AND SPACE TRANSPORT ACCIDENTS (E840–E845)

The following fourth–digit subdivisions are for use with categories E840–E845 to identify the injured person:

.0 Occupant of spacecraft

.1 Occupant of military aircraft, any

Crew in military aircraft [air force] [army] [national guard] [navy]

Passenger (civilian) (military) in military aircraft [air force] [army] [national guard] [navy]

Troops in military aircraft [air force] [army] [national guard] [navy]

Excludes: occupants of aircraft operated under jurisdiction of police departments (.5)
parachutist (.7).

.2 Crew of commercial aircraft (powered) in surface to surface transport

.3 Other occupant of commercial aircraft (powered) in surface to surface transport

Flight personnel:
not part of crew
on familiarization flight

Passenger on aircraft (powered) NOS

.4 Occupant of commercial aircraft (powered) in surface to air transport

Occupant [crew] [passenger] of aircraft (powered) engaged in activities, such as:
aerial spraying (crops) (fire retardants)
air drops of emergency supplies
air drops of parachutists, except from military craft
crop dusting
lowering of construction material [bridge or telephone pole]
sky writing

.5 Occupant of other powered aircraft

Occupant [crew] [passenger] of aircraft (powered) engaged in activities, such as:
aerobatic flying
aircraft racing
rescue operation
storm surveillance
traffic surveillance

Occupant of private plane NOS

.6 Occupant of unpowered aircraft, except parachutist

Occupant of aircraft classifiable to E842

.7 Parachutist (military) (other)

Person making voluntary descent

Excludes: person making descent after accident to aircraft (.1–.6)

.8 Ground crew, airline employee

Persons employed at airfields (civil) (military) or launching pads, not occupants of aircraft

.9 Other person

> * Any changes for FY2013 released after publication will be distributed via email and available for download on the PMIC website.

010.0 Primary tuberculous infection
Revise exclusion terms

017.0 Skin and subcutaneous cellular tissue
Revise exclusion terms

041.41 Shiga toxin-producing Escherichia coli [E. coli] (STEC) O157
New code

041.42 Other specified Shiga toxin-producing Escherichia coli [E. coli] (STEC)
New code

041.43 Shiga toxin-producing Escherichia coli [E. coli] (STEC), unspecified
New code

041.49 Other and unspecified Escherichia coli [E. coli]
New code

099.3 Reiter's disease
Add inclusion term

140 Malignant neoplasm of lip
Revise exclusion terms

154.2 Anal canal
Revise exclusion terms

154.3 Anus, unspecified
Revise exclusion terms

160.0 Nasal cavities
Revise exclusion terms

160.1 Auditory tube, middle ear, and mastoid air cells
Revise exclusion terms

173 Other and unspecified malignant neoplasm of skin
Revise code, add exclusion term

173.0 Other and unspecified malignant neoplasm of skin of lip
Revise subcategory

173.00 Unspecified malignant neoplasm of skin of lip
New code

173.01 Basal cell carcinoma of skin of lip
New code

173.02 Squamous cell carcinoma of skin of lip
New code

173.09 Other specified malignant neoplasm of skin of lip
New code

173.1 Other and unspecified malignant neoplasm of eyelid, including canthus
Revise subcategory

173.10 Unspecified malignant neoplasm of eyelid, including canthus
New code

173.11 Basal cell carcinoma of eyelid, including canthus
New code

173.12 Squamous cell carcinoma of eyelid, including canthus
New code

173.19 Other specified malignant neoplasm of eyelid, including canthus
New code

173.2 Other and unspecified malignant neoplasm of skin of ear and external auditory canal
Revise subcategory

173.20 Unspecified malignant neoplasm of skin of ear and external auditory canal
New code

173.21 Basal cell carcinoma of skin of ear and external auditory canal
New code

173.22 Squamous cell carcinoma of skin of ear and external auditory canal
New code

173.29 Other specified malignant neoplasm of skin of ear and external auditory canal
New code

173.3 Other and unspecified malignant neoplasm of skin of other and unspecified parts of face
Revise subcategory

173.30 Unspecified malignant neoplasm of skin of other and unspecified parts of face
New code

173.31 Basal cell carcinoma of skin of other and unspecified parts of face
New code

173.32 Squamous cell carcinoma of skin of other and unspecified parts of face
New code

173.39 Other specified malignant neoplasm of skin of other and unspecified parts of face
New code

173.4 Other and unspecified malignant neoplasm of scalp and skin of neck
Revise subcategory

173.40 Unspecified malignant neoplasm of scalp and skin of neck
New code

173.41 Basal cell carcinoma of scalp and skin of neck
New code

173.42 Squamous cell carcinoma of scalp and skin of neck
New code

173.49 Other specified malignant neoplasm of scalp and skin of neck
New code

173.5 Other and unspecified malignant neoplasm of skin of trunk, except scrotum
Revise subcategory

173.50 Unspecified malignant neoplasm of skin of trunk, except scrotum
New code

173.51 Basal cell carcinoma of skin of trunk, except scrotum
New code

173.52 Squamous cell carcinoma of skin of trunk, except scrotum
New code

173.59 Other specified malignant neoplasm of skin of trunk, except scrotum
New code

173.6 Other and unspecified malignant neoplasm of skin of upper limb, including shoulder
Revise subcategory

173.60 Unspecified malignant neoplasm of skin of upper limb, including shoulder
New code

173.61 Basal cell carcinoma of skin of upper limb, including shoulder
New code

173.62 Squamous cell carcinoma of skin of upper limb, including shoulder
New code

173.69 Other specified malignant neoplasm of skin of upper limb, including shoulder
New code

173.7 Other and unspecified malignant neoplasm of skin of lower limb, including hip
Revise subcategory

173.70 Unspecified malignant neoplasm of skin of lower limb, including hip
New code

173.71 Basal cell carcinoma of skin of lower limb, including hip
New code

173.72 Squamous cell carcinoma of skin of lower limb, including hip
New code

173.79 Other specified malignant neoplasm of skin of lower limb, including hip
New code

173.8 Other and unspecified malignant neoplasm of other specified sites of skin
Revise subcategory

173.80 Unspecified malignant neoplasm of other specified sites of skin
New code

173.81 Basal cell carcinoma of other specified sites of skin
New code

173.82 Squamous cell carcinoma of other specified sites of skin
New code

173.89 Other specified malignant neoplasm of other specified sites of skin
New code

173.9 Other and unspecified malignant neoplasm of skin, site unspecified
Revise subcategory

173.90 Unspecified malignant neoplasm of skin, site unspecified
New code

173.91 Basal cell carcinoma of skin, site unspecified
New code

173.92 Squamous cell carcinoma of skin, site unspecified
New code

173.99 Other specified malignant neoplasm of skin, site unspecified
New code

174 Malignant neoplasm of female breast
Revise exclusion terms

175 Malignant neoplasm of male breast
Revise exclusion terms

190 Malignant neoplasm of eye
Revise exclusion terms

202.5 Letterer-Siwe disease
Add exclusion term

209.71 Secondary neuroendocrine tumor of distant lymph nodes
Delete inclusion term

209.74 Secondary neuroendocrine tumor of peritoneum
Add inclusion term

236.1 Placenta
Add, revise inclusion terms

243 Congenital hypothyroidism
Revise "Use additional" note

249.8 Secondary diabetes mellitus with other specified manifestations
Revise "Use additional" note

250.8 Diabetes mellitus with other specified manifestations
Revise "Use additional" note

276.5 Volume depletion
Revise exclusion term

277.89 Other specified disorders of metabolism
Add exclusion term

282.40 Thalassemia, unspecified
New code

282.41 Sickle-cell thalassemia without crisis
Add inclusion term

282.43 Alpha thalassemia
New code

282.44 Beta thalassemia
New code

282.45 Delta-beta thalassemia
New code

282.46 Thalassemia minor
New code

282.47 Hemoglobin E-beta thalassemia
New code

282.49 Other thalassemia
New code

282.5 Sickle-cell trait
Revise exclusion term

282.7 Other hemoglobinopathies
Add exclusion terms

283.11 Hemolytic-uremic syndrome
Add "Use additional code" notes

284.1 Pancytopenia
Delete exclusion term

284.11 Antineoplastic chemotherapy induced pancytopenia
New code

284.12 Other drug induced pancytopenia
New code

284.19 Other pancytopenia
New code

286.5 Hemorrhagic disorder due to intrinsic circulating anticoagulants, antibodies, or inhibitors
Revise subcategory

286.52 Acquired hemophilia
New code

286.53 Antiphospholipid antibody with hemorrhagic disorder
New code

286.59 Other hemorrhagic disorder due to intrinsic circulating anticoagulants, antibodies, or inhibitors
New code

289.81 Primary hypercoagulable state
Add/revise inclusion terms; add exclusion terms

Ch. 5 MENTAL, BEHAVIORAL AND NEURODEVELOPMENTAL DISORDERS (290-319)
Revise Chapter Title

290.0 Senile dementia, uncomplicated
Revise exclusion term

294.1 Dementia in conditions classified elsewhere
Revise "Code first" note

294.11 Dementia in conditions classified elsewhere with behavioral disturbance
Delete inclusion term, add "Use additional" note

294.2 Dementia, unspecified
New subcategory

294.20 Dementia, unspecified, without behavioral disturbance
New code

294.21 Dementia, unspecified, with behavioral disturbance
New code

294.8 Other persistent mental disorders due to conditions classified elsewhere
Delete inclusion term, revise exclusion term

310.2 Postconcussion syndrome
Revise exclusion term

310.8 Other specified nonpsychotic mental disorders following organic brain damage
Delete inclusion terms

310.81 Pseudobulbar affect
New code

310.89 Other specified nonpsychotic mental disorders following organic brain damage
New code

317 Mild intellectual disabilities
Revise title

318 Other specified intellectual disabilities
Revise title

318.0 Moderate intellectual disabilities
Revise title

318.1 Severe intellectual disabilities
Revise title

318.2 Profound intellectual disabilities
Revise title

319 Unspecified intellectual disabilities
Revise title

323.0 Encephalitis, myelitis, and encephalomyelitis in viral diseases classified elsewhere
Add "Code first" note

323.4 Other encephalitis, myelitis, and encephalomyelitis due to other infections classified elsewhere
Revise title

323.41 Other encephalitis and encephalomyelitis due to other infections classified elsewhere
Revise title

323.42 Other myelitis due to other infections classified elsewhere
Revise title

330 Cerebral degenerations usually manifest in childhood
Revise "Use additional code" note

331.6 Corticobasal degeneration
New code

331.83 Mild cognitive impairment, so stated
Revise exclusion terms

345.8 Other forms of epilepsy and recurrent seizures
Delete inclusion term

345.9 Epilepsy, unspecified
Delete inclusion term

346 Migraine
Revise 5th digit classification

348.82 Brain death
New code

348.89 Other conditions of brain
Add exclusion term

358.1 Myasthenic syndromes in diseases classified elsewhere
Delete inclusion term

358.3 Lambert-Eaton syndrome
New subcategory

358.30 Lambert-Eaton syndrome, unspecified
New code

358.31 Lambert-Eaton syndrome in neoplastic disease
New code

358.39 Lambert-Eaton syndrome in other diseases classified elsewhere
New code

365.01 Open angle with borderline findings, low risk
Revise code title, revise inclusion terms

365.02 Anatomical narrow angle
Add inclusion term

365.05 Open angle with borderline findings, high risk
New code

365.06 Primary angle closure without glaucoma damage
New code

365.10 Open-angle glaucoma, unspecified
Add "Use additional code" note

365.11 Primary open angle glaucoma
Add "Use additional code" note

365.12 Low tension glaucoma
Add "Use additional code" note

365.13 Pigmentary glaucoma
Add "Use additional code" note

365.20 **Primary angle-closure glaucoma, unspecified**
Add "Use additional code" note

365.22 **Acute angle-closure glaucoma**
Add inclusion terms

365.23 **Chronic angle-closure glaucoma**
Add inclusion terms, add "Use additional code" note

365.31 **Glaucomatous stage**
Add "Use additional code" note

365.52 **Pseudoexfoliation glaucoma**
Add "Use additional code" note

365.62 **Glaucoma associated with ocular inflammations**
Add "Use additional code" note

365.63 **Glaucoma associated with vascular disorders**
Add "Use additional code" note

365.65 **Glaucoma associated with ocular trauma**
Add "Use additional code" note

365.7 **Glaucoma stage**
New subcategory

365.70 **Glaucoma stage, unspecified**
New code

365.71 **Mild stage glaucoma**
New code

365.72 **Moderate stage glaucoma**
New code

365.73 **Severe stage glaucoma**
New code

365.74 **Indeterminate stage glaucoma**
New code

379.27 **Vitreomacular adhesion**
New code

414.4 **Coronary atherosclerosis due to calcified coronary lesion**
New code

415.1 **Pulmonary embolism and infarction**
Revise exclusion term

415.13 **Saddle embolus of pulmonary artery**
New code

416.2 **Chronic pulmonary embolism**
Revise exclusion term

417.0 **Arteriovenous fistula of pulmonary vessels**
Revise exclusion term

417.1 **Aneurysm of pulmonary artery**
Revise exclusion terms

424.1 **Aortic valve disorders**
Revise exclusion term

425.1 **Hypertrophic cardiomyopathy**
Revise title, delete inclusion term, add exclusion term

425.11 **Hypertrophic obstructive cardiomyopathy**
New code

425.18 **Other hypertrophic cardiomyopathy**
New code

425.4 **Other primary cardiomyopathies**
Delete inclusion terms

430 **Subarachnoid hemorrhage**
Add exclusion term

440.23 **Atherosclerosis of the extremities with ulceration**
Revise "Use additional code" note

440.24 **Atherosclerosis of the extremities with gangrene**
Revise "Use additional code" note

444.0 **Of abdominal aorta**
Delete inclusion terms

444.01 **Saddle embolus of abdominal aorta**
New code

444.09 **Other arterial embolism and thrombosis of abdominal aorta**
New code

444.89 **Other**
Revise exclusion term

449 **Septic arterial embolism**
Revise "Use additional code" note

459.81 **Venous (peripheral) insufficiency, unspecified**
Revise "Use additional code" note

466.1 **Acute bronchiolitis**
Add exclusion term

487 **Influenza**
Revise exclusion terms

488 **Influenza due to certain identified influenza viruses**
Revise exclusion term

488.1 **Influenza due to identified 2009 H1N1 influenza virus**
Revise title, revise inclusion terms, add exclusion terms

488.11 **Influenza due to identified 2009 H1N1 influenza virus with pneumonia**
Revise title, revise inclusion terms

488.12 **Influenza due to identified 2009 H1N1 influenza virus with other respiratory manifestations**
Revise title, revise inclusion terms

488.19 **Influenza due to identified 2009 H1N1 influenza virus with other manifestations**
Revise title, revise inclusion terms

488.8 **Influenza due to novel influenza A**
New subcategory

488.81 **Influenza due to identified novel influenza A virus with pneumonia**
New code

488.82 **Influenza due to identified novel influenza A virus with other respiratory manifestations**
New code

488.89 **Influenza due to identified novel influenza A virus with other manifestations**
New code

506 **Respiratory conditions due to chemical fumes and vapors**
Add "Use additional code" note

507 **Pneumonitis due to solids and liquids**
Add exclusion term

508 **Respiratory conditions due to other and unspecified external agents**
Add "Use additional code" note

508.2 **Respiratory conditions due to smoke inhalation**
New code

512	**Pneumothorax and air leak** Revise title		**518.3**	**Pulmonary eosinophilia** Add exclusion term
512.2	**Postoperative air leak** New code		**518.5**	**Pulmonary insufficiency following trauma and surgery** Delete inclusion terms
512.8	**Other pneumothorax and air leak** Revise title, delete inclusion terms		**518.51**	**Acute respiratory failure following trauma and surgery** New code
512.81	**Primary spontaneous pneumothorax** New code		**518.52**	**Other pulmonary insufficiency, not elsewhere classified, following trauma and surgery** New code
512.82	**Secondary spontaneous pneumothorax** New code			
512.83	**Chronic pneumothorax** New code		**518.53**	**Acute and chronic respiratory failure following trauma and surgery** New code
512.84	**Other air leak** New code		**518.81**	**Acute respiratory failure** Add exclusion term
512.89	**Other pneumothor** New code		**518.82**	**Other pulmonary insufficiency, not elsewhere classified** Revise exclusion terms
514	**Pulmonary congestion and hypostasis** Revise exclusion term			
516.3	**Idiopathic interstitial pneumonia** Revise title, delete inclusion terms		**518.84**	**Acute and chronic respiratory failure** Add exclusion term
516.30	**Idiopathic interstitial pneumonia, not otherwise specified** New code		**536.3**	**Gastroparesis** Revise "Code first" note
			539	**Complications of bariatric procedures** New category
516.31	**Idiopathic pulmonary fibrosis** New code		**539.0**	**Complications of gastric band procedure** New subcategory
516.32	**Idiopathic non-specific interstitial pneumonitis** New code			
516.33	**Acute interstitial pneumonitis** New code		**539.01**	**Infection due to gastric band procedure** New code
516.34	**Respiratory bronchiolitis interstitial lung disease** New code		**539.09**	**Other complications of gastric band procedure** New code
516.35	**Idiopathic lymphoid interstitial pneumonia** New code		**539.8**	**Complications of other bariatric procedure** New subcategory
			539.81	**Infection due to other bariatric procedure** New code
516.36	**Cryptogenic organizing pneumonia** New code			
516.37	**Desquamative interstitial pneumonia** New code		**539.89**	**Other complications of other bariatric procedure** New code
516.4	**Lymphangioleiomyomatosis** New code		**569.49**	**Other** Revise "Use additional code" note
516.5	**Adult pulmonary Langerhans cell histiocytosis** New code		**572.8**	**Other sequelae of chronic liver disease** Add exclusion term
516.6	**Interstitial lung diseases of childhood** New subcategory		**573.5**	**Hepatopulmonary syndrome** New code
516.61	**Neuroendocrine cell hyperplasia of infancy** New code		**574**	**Cholelithiasis** Add exclusion term
			590	**Infections of kidney** Revise "Use additional code" note
516.62	**Pulmonary interstitial glycogenosis** New code		**595**	**Cystitis** Revise "Use additional code" note
516.63	**Surfactant mutations of the lung** New code			
516.64	**Alveolar capillary dysplasia with vein misalignment** New code		**596.8**	**Other specified disorders of bladder** Delete inclusion terms
			596.81	**Infection of cystostomy** New code
516.69	**Other interstitial lung diseases of childhood** New code		**596.82**	**Mechanical complication of cystostomy** New code
516.8	**Other specified alveolar and parietoalveolar pneumonopathies** Revise inclusion terms, add "Code first" note, add "Use additional" note, add exclusion terms		**596.83**	**Other complication of cystostomy** New code

596.89   **Other specified disorders of bladder**
New code

599.0   **Urinary tract infection, site not specified**
Revise "Use additional code" note

604   **Orchitis and epididymitis**
Revise "Use additional code" note

616.10   **Vaginitis and vulvovaginitis, unspecified**
Revise "Use additional code" note

618.04   **Rectocele**
Revise "Use additional code" note

629.3   **Complication of implanted vaginal mesh and other prosthetic materials**
New subcategory

629.31   **Erosion of implanted vaginal mesh and other prosthetic materials to surrounding organ or tissue**
New code

629.32   **Exposure of implanted vaginal mesh and other prosthetic materials into vagina**
New code

631   **Other abnormal product of conception**
Delete inclusion terms

631.0   **Inappropriate change in quantitative human chorionic gonadotropin (hCG) in early pregnancy**
New code

631.8   **Other abnormal products of conception**
New code

632   **Missed abortion**
Revise exclusion terms

646.7   **Liver and biliary tract disorders in pregnancy**
Revise title

649.8   **Onset (spontaneous) of labor after 37 completed weeks of gestation but before 39 completed weeks gestation, with delivery by (planned) cesarean section**
New subcategory

704.4   **Pilar and trichilemmal cysts**
New subcategory

704.41   **Pilar cyst**
New code

704.42   **Trichilemmal cyst**
New code

706.2   **Sebaceous cyst**
Add exclusion terms

713.6   **Arthropathy associated with hypersensitivity reaction**
Revise "Code first" note

718.6   **Unspecified intrapelvic protrusion of acetabulum**
Revise valid fifth digits

726.13   **Partial tear of rotator cuff**
New code

727.61   **Complete rupture of rotator cuff**
Add exclusion term

747.3   **Anomalies of pulmonary artery**
Delete inclusion terms

747.31   **Pulmonary artery coarctation and atresia**
New code

747.32   **Pulmonary arteriovenous malformation**
New code

747.39   **Other anomalies of pulmonary artery and pulmonary circulation**
New code

747.6   **Other anomalies of peripheral vascular system**
Revise exclusion term

747.89   **Other**
Revise exclusion terms

780.93   **Memory loss**
Revise exclusion term

785.52   **Septic shock**
Revise "Code first" notes

785.59   **Other**
Revise exclusion terms

786.09   **Other**
Revise exclusion terms

793.1   **Lung field**
Delete inclusion terms

793.11   **Solitary pulmonary nodule**
New code

793.19   **Other nonspecific abnormal finding of lung field**
New code

795.5   **Nonspecific reaction to test for tuberculosis**
Revise title, delete inclusion terms

795.51   **Nonspecific reaction to tuberculin skin test without active tuberculosis**
New code

795.52   **Nonspecific reaction to cell mediated immunity measurement of gamma interferon antigen response without active tuberculosis**
New code

799.1   **Respiratory arrest**
Revise exclusion terms

808.43   **Multiple closed pelvic fractures with disruption of pelvic circle**
Revise title, add inclusion term

808.44   **Multiple closed pelvic fractures without disruption of pelvic circle**
New code

808.53   **Multiple open pelvic fractures with disruption of pelvic circle**
Revise title, add inclusion term

808.54   **Multiple open pelvic fractures without disruption of pelvic circle**
New code

958   **Certain early complications of trauma**
Revise exclusion terms

958.4   **Traumatic shock**
Revise exclustion terms

964.7   **Natural blood and blood products**
Revise exclusion terms

968.5   **Surface (topical) and infiltration anesthetics**
Revise titlte, revise inclusion term

995.0   **Other anaphylactic reaction**
Revise title, add inclusion terms, revise exclusion terms

995.1   **Angioneurotic edema**
Add inclusion term, revise exclusion term

995.4	**Shock due to anesthesia** Revise exclusion term	**997.41**	**Retained cholelithiasis following cholecystectomy** New code
995.6	**Anaphylactic reaction due to food** Revise title, revise inclusion terms	**997.49**	**Other digestive system complications** New code
995.60	**Anaphylactic reaction due to unspecified food** Revise title	**997.5**	**Urinary complications** Delete inclusion term, add exclusion terms
995.61	**Anaphylactic reaction due to peanuts** Revise title	**998.0**	**Postoperative shock** Revise inclusion and exclusion terms
995.62	**Anaphylactic reaction due to crustaceans** Revise title	**998.00**	**Postoperative shock, unspecified** New code
995.63	**Anaphylactic reaction due to fruits and vegetables** Revise title	**998.01**	**Postoperative shock, cardiogenic** New code
995.64	**Anaphylactic reaction due to tree nuts and see** Revise title	**998.02**	**Postoperative shock, septic** New code
995.65	**Anaphylactic reaction due to fish** Revise title	**998.09**	**Postoperative shock, other** New code
995.66	**Anaphylactic reaction due to food additives** Revise title	**998.31**	**Disruption of internal operation (surgical) wound** Revise exclusion term
995.67	**Anaphylactic reaction due to milk products** Revise title	**999.31**	**Other and unspecified infection due to central venous catheter** Revise code title and inclusion terms
995.68	**Anaphylactic reaction due to eggs** Revise title	**999.32**	**Bloodstream infection due to central venous catheter** New code
995.69	**Anaphylactic reaction due to other specified food** Revise title	**999.33**	**Local infection due to central venous catheter** New code
995.7	**Other adverse food reactions, not elsewhere classified** Revise exclusion term	**999.34**	**Acute infection following transfusion, infusion, or injection of blood and blood products** New code
996	**Complications peculiar to certain specified procedures** Revise exclusion term	**999.4**	**Anaphylactic reaction due to serum** Revise code title, revise inclusion and exclusion terms
996.39	**Other** Delete inclusion term, revise exclusion term	**999.41**	**Anaphylactic reaction due to administration of blood and blood products** New code
996.62	**Due to vascular device, implant and graft** Revise exclusion terms	**999.42**	**Anaphylactic reaction due to vaccination** New code
996.64	**Due to indwelling urinary catheter** Add exclusion terms	**999.49**	**Anaphylactic reaction due to other serum** New code
996.7	**Other complications of internal (biological) (synthetic) prosthetic device, implant, and graft** Revise exclusion term	**999.51**	**Other serum reaction due to administration of blood and blood products** New code
996.76	**Due to genitourinary device, implant, and graft** Add exclusion term	**999.52**	**Other serum reaction due to vaccination** New code
996.88	**Stem cell** New code	**999.59**	**Other serum reaction** New code
997	**Complications affecting specified body systems, not elsewhere classified** Revise exclusion term	**999.6**	**ABO incompatibility reaction due to transfusion of blood or blood products** Revise exclusion term
997.3	**Respiratory complications** Revise exclusion terms	**999.8**	**Other and unspecified infusion and transfusion reaction** Revise exclusion term
997.32	**Postprocedural aspiration pneumonia** New code	**V12.21**	**Gestational diabetes** New code
997.39	**Other respiratory complications** New code		
997.4	**Digestive system complications** Add exclusion terms		

V12.29 Other endocrine, metabolic, and immunity disorders
New code

V12.5 Diseases of circulatory system
Add exclusion term

V12.51 Venous thrombosis and embolism
Delete inclusion term, add exclusion term

V12.55 Pulmonary embolism
New code

V13.81 Anaphylaxis
New code

V13.89 Other specified diseases
New code

V17.0 Psychiatric condition
Revise exclusion term

V18.4 Intellectual disabilities
Revise code title

V19.11 Glaucoma
New code

V19.19 Other specified eye disorder
New code

V23.42 Pregnancy with history of ectopic pregnancy
New code

V23.87 Pregnancy with inconclusive fetal viability
New code

V40.31 Wandering in diseases classified elsewhere
New code

V40.39 Other specified behavioral problem
New code

V54.82 Aftercare following explantation of joint prosthesis
New code

V55 Attention to artificial openings
Revise exclusion term

V58.68 Long term (current) use of bisphosphonates
New code

V58.69 Long-term (current) use of other medications
Revise inclusion term, add exclusion terms

V79.2 Intellectual disabilities
Revise code title

V84 Genetic susceptibility to disease
Add exclusion term

V84.81 Genetic susceptibility to multiple endocrine neoplasia [MEN]
Add exclusion term

V87.02 Contact with and (suspected) exposure to uranium
New code

V88.2 Acquired absence of joint
New subcategory

V88.21 Acquired absence of hip joint
New code

V88.22 Acquired absence of knee joint
New code

V88.29 Acquired absence of other joint
New code

PROCEDURES: TABULAR LIST
AND
ALPHABETIC INDEX

VOLUME 3

This page intentionally left blank.

1. **OPERATIONS ON THE NERVOUS SYSTEM (01-05)**

00 **Procedures and interventions, Not Elsewhere Classified**

00.0 **Therapeutic ultrasound**

> Excludes: *diagnostic ultrasound (non-invasive) (88.71-88.79)*
> *intracardiac echocardiography [ICE] (heart chamber(s)) (37.28)*
> *intravascular imaging (adjunctive) (00.21-00.29)*

00.01 **Therapeutic ultrasound of vessels of head and neck**
Anti-restenotic ultrasound
Intravscular non-ablative ultrasound

> Excludes: *diagnostic ultrasound of:*
> *eye (95.13)*
> *head and neck (88.71)*
> *that of inner ear (20.79)*
> *ultrasonic:*
> *angioplasty of non-coronary vessel (39.50)*
> *embolectomy (38.01, 38.02)*
> *endarterectomy (38.11, 38.12)*
> *thrombectomy (38.01, 38.02)*

00.02 **Therapeutic ultrasound of heart**
Note: real-time imaging of lumen of blood vessel(s) using sound waves
Anti-restenotic ultrasound
Intravascular non-ablative ultrasound

> Excludes: *diagnostic ultrasound of heart (88.72)*
> *ultrasonic angioplasty of coronary vessels (00.66, 36.09)*
> *ultrasound ablation of heart lesion (37.34)*

00.03 **Therapeutic ultrasound of peripheral vascular vessels**
Anti-restenotic ultrasound
Intravascular non-ablative ultrasound

> Excludes: *diagnostic ultrasound of peripheral vascular system (88.77)*
> *ultrasonic angioplasty of:*
> *non-coronary vessel (39.50)*

00.09 **Other therapeutic ultrasound**

> Excludes: *ultrasonic:*
> *fragmentation of urinary stones (59.95)*
> *percutaneous nephrostomy with fragmentation (55.04)*
> *physical therapy (93.35)*
> *transurethral guided laser induced prostatectomy (TULIP) (60.21)*

00.1 **Pharmaceuticals**

00.10 **Implantation of chemotherapeutic agent**
Brain wafer chemotherapy
Interstitial / intracavitary

> Excludes: *injection of infusion of cancer chemotherapeutic substance (99.25)*

00.11 **Infusion of drotrecogin alfa (activated)**
Infusion of recombinant protein

00.12 **Administration of inhaled nitric oxide**
Nitric oxide therapy

00.13 **Injection or infusion of nesiritide**
Human B-type natriuretic peptide (hBNP)

00.14 **Injection or infusion of oxazolidinone class of antibiotics**
Linezolid injection

00.15 **High-dose infusion interleukin-2 [IL-2]**
Infusion (IV bolus, CIV) interleukin
Injection of aldesleukin

> Excludes: *low-dose infusion interleukin-2 (99.28)*

00.16 **Pressurized treatment of venous bypass graft [conduit] with pharmaceutical substance**
Ex-vivo treatment vessel
Hyperbaric pressurized graft [conduit]

00.17 **Infusion of vasopressor agent**

**VOL 3
PROCEDURES**

| | Valid O.R. procedure | | Non-O.R. procedure | | Nonspecific O.R. procedure | | Noncovered O.R. procedure |

00.18 Infusion of immunosuppressive antibody therapy
  Monoclonal antibody therapy
  Polyclonal antibody therapy
  Includes: during induction phase of solid organ transplantation

00.19 Disruption of blood brain barrier via infusion [BBBD]
  Infusion of substance to disrupt blood brain barrier

  Code also chemotherapy (99.25)

Excludes:	*other perfusion (39.97)*

00.2 Intravascular imaging of blood vessels
  Endovascular ultrasonography
  Intravascular [ultrasound] imaging of blood vessels
  Intravascular ultrasound (IVUS)
  Virtual histology intravascular ultrasound [VH-IVUS]
Note: real-time imaging of lumen of blood vessel(s) using sound waves

  Code also any synchronous diagnostic or therapeutic procedures

Excludes:	*adjunct vascular system procedures, number of vessels (00.40-00.43)*
	diagnostic procedures on blood vessels treated (38.21-38.29)
	diagnostic ultrasound of peripheral vascular system (88.77)
	intravascular imaging of vessel(s) by OCT (38.24-38.25)
	magnetic resonance imaging (MRI) (88.91-88.97)
	therapeutic ultrasound (00.01-00.09)

00.21 Intravascular imaging of extracranial cerebral vessels
  Common carotid vessels and branches
  Intravascular ultrasound (IVUS), extracranial cerebral vessels

Excludes:	*diagnostic ultrasound (non-invasive) of head and neck (88.71)*

00.22 Intravascular imaging of intrathoracic vessels
  Aorta and aortic arch
  Intravascular ultrasound (IVUS), intrathoracic vessels
  Vena cava (superior) (inferior)

Excludes:	*diagnostic ultrasound (non-invasive) of other sites of thorax (88.73)*

00.23 Intravascular imaging of peripheral vessels
  Imaging of:
    vessels of arm(s)
    vessels of leg(s)
  Intravascular ultrasound (IVUS), peripheral vessels

Excludes:	*diagnostic ultrasound (non-invasive) of peripheral vascular system (88.77)*

00.24 Intravascular imaging of coronary vessels
  Intravascular ultrasound (IVUS), coronary vessels

Excludes:	*diagnostic ultrasound, (non-invasive) of heart (88.72)*
	intracardiac echocardiography [ICE] (ultrasound of heart chamber(s)) (37.28)

00.25 Intravascular imaging of renal vessels
  Intravascular ultrasound (IVUS), renal vessels
  Renal artery

Excludes:	*diagnostic ultrasound (non-invasive) of urinary system (88.75)*

00.28 Intravascular imaging, other specified vessel(s)

00.29 Intravascular imaging, unspecified vessel(s)

00.3 Computer assisted surgery [CAS]
  CT-free navigation
  Image guided navigation (IGN)
  Image guided surgery (IGS)
  Imageless navigation
  That without the use of robotic(s) technology

  Code also diagnostic or therapeutic procedure

Excludes:	*robotic assisted procedures (17.41-17.49)*
	stereotactic frame application only (93.59)

00.31 Computer assisted surgery with CT/CTA

00.32 Computer assisted surgery with MR/MRA

00.33 Computer assisted surgery with fluoroscopy

00.34 Imageless computer assisted surgery

00.35 **Computer assisted surgery with multiple datasets**

00.39 **Other computer assisted surgery**
Computer assisted surgery NOS

00.4 **Adjunct vascular system procedures**
Note: These codes can apply to both coronary and peripheral vessels. These codes are to be used in conjunction with other therapeutic procedure codes to provide additional information on the number of vessels upon which a procedure was performed and/or the number of stents inserted. As appropriate, code both the number of vessels operated on (00.40-00.43), and the number of stents inserted (00.45-00.48).

Code also any:
angioplasty (00.61-00.62, 00.66, 39.50)
atherectomy (17.53-17.56)
endarterectomy (38.10-38.18)
insertion of vascular stent(s) (00.55, 00.63-00.65, 36.06-36.07, 39.90)
other removal of coronary artery obstruction (36.09)

00.40 **Procedure on single vessel**
Number of vessels, unspecified

Excludes:	*(aorto)coronary bypass (36.10-36.19)*
	intravascular imaging of blood vessels (00.21-00.29)

00.41 **Procedure on two vessels**

Excludes:	*(aorto)coronary bypass (36.10-36.19)*
	intravascular imaging of blood vessels (00.21-00.29)

00.42 **Procedure on three vessels**

Excludes:	*(aorto)coronary bypass (36.10-36.19)*
	intravascular imaging of blood vessels (00.21-00.29)

00.43 **Procedure on four or more vessels**

Excludes:	*(aorto)coronary bypass (36.10-36.19)*
	intravascular imaging of blood vessels (00.21-00.29)

00.44 **Procedure on vessel bifurcation**
Note: This code is to be used to identify the presence of a vessel bifurcation; it does not describe a specific bifurcation stent. Use this code only once per operative episode, irrespective of the number of bifurcations in vessels.

00.45 **Insertion of one vascular stent**
Number of stents, unspecified

00.46 **Insertion of two vascular stents**

00.47 **Insertion of three vascular stents**

00.48 **Insertion of four or more vascular stents**

00.49 **SuperSaturated oxygen therapy**
Aqueous oxygen (AO) therapy
SSO_2
SuperOxygenation infusion therapy

Code also any:
injection or infusion of thrombolytic agent (99.10)
insertion of coronary artery stent(s) (36.06-36.07)
intracoronary artery thrombolytic infusion (36.04)
number of vascular stents inserted (00.45-00.48)
number of vessels treated (00.40-00.43)
open chest coronary artery angioplasty (36.03)
other removal of coronary obstruction (37.09)
percutaneous transluminal coronary angioplasty [PCTA] (00.66)
procedure on vessel bifurcation (00.44)
transluminal coronary atherectomy (17.55)

Excludes:	*other oxygen enrichment (93.96)*
	other perfusion (39.97)

00.5 **Other cardiovascular procedures**

	Valid O.R. procedure		Non-O.R. procedure		Nonspecific O.R. procedure		Noncovered O.R. procedure

00.50 **Implantation of cardiac resynchronization pacemaker without mention of defibrillation, total system [CRT-P]**

Note: Device testing during procedure—*omit code*

Biventricular pacemaker

BiV pacemaker

Biventricular pacing without internal cardiac defibrillator

Implantation of cardiac resynchronization (biventricular) pulse generator pacing device, formation of pocket, transvenous leads including placement of lead into left ventricular coronary venous system, and intraoperative procedures for evaluation of lead signals

That with CRT-P generator and one or more leads

Excludes:	*implantation of cardiac resynchronization defibrillator, total system [CRT-D] (00.51)*
	insertion or replacement of any type pacemaker device (37.80-37.87)
	replacement of cardiac resynchronization defibrillator pulse generator only [CRT-D] (00.54)
	replacement of cardiac resynchronization pacemaker pulse generator only [CRT-P] (00.53)

00.51 **Implantation of cardiac resynchronization defibrillator, total system [CRT-D]**

Note: Device testing during procedure—*omit code*

BiV defibrillator

Biventricular defibrillator

BiV ICD

BiV pacemaker with defibrillator

BiV pacing with defibrillator

Biventricular pacing with internal cardiac defibrillator

Implantation of a cardiac resynchronization (biventricular) pulse generator with defibrillator [AICD], formation of pocket, transvenous leads, including placement of lead into left ventricular coronary venous system, intraoperative procedures for evaluation of lead signals, and obtaining defibrillator threshold measurements

That with CRT-D generator and one or more leads

Excludes:	*implantation of cardiac resynchronization pacemaker, total system [CRT-P] (00.50)*
	implantation or replacement of automatic cardioverter/defibrillator, total system [AICD] (37.94)
	replacement of cardiac resynchronization defibrillator pulse generator only, [CRT-D] (00.54)

00.52 **Implantation or replacement of transvenous lead [electrode] into left ventricular coronary venous sytem**

Excludes:	*implantation of cardiac resynchronization defibrillator, total system [CRT-D] (00.51)*
	implantation of cardiac resynchronization pacemeker, total system [CRT-P] (00.50)
	initial insertion of transvenous lead [electrode] (37.70-37.72)
	replacement of transvenous atrial and/or ventricular lead(s) [electrodes] (37.76)

00.53 **Implantation or replacement of cardiac resynchronization pacemaker pulse generator only [CRT-P]**

Note: Device testing during procedure—*omit code*

Implantation of CRT-P device with removal of any existing CRT-P or other pacemaker device

Excludes:	*implantation of cardiac resynchronization pacemaker, total system [CRT-P] (00.50)*
	implantation or replacement of cardiac resynchronization defibrillator pulse generator only [CRT-D] (00.54)
	insertion or replacement of any type pacemaker device (37.80-37.87)

00.54 **Implantation or replacement of cardiac resynchronization defibrillator pulse generator device only [CRT-D]**

Note: Device testing during procedure—*omit code*

Implantation of CRT-D device with removal of any existing CRT-D, CRT-P, pacemaker, or defibrillator device

Excludes:	*implantation of automatic cardioverter/defibrillator pulse generator only (37.96)*
	implantation of cardiac resynchronization defibrillator, total system [CRT-D] (00.51)
	implantation or replacement of cardiac resynchronization pacemaker pulse generator only [CRT-P] (00.53)

00.55 **Insertion of drug-eluting stent(s) of other peripheral vessel(s)**

Endograft(s)
Endovascular graft(s)
Stent graft(s)

Code also any:
angioplasty of other non-coronary vessel(s) (39.50)
atherectomy of other non-coronary vessel(s) (17.56)
number of vascular stents inserted (00.45-00.48)
number of vessels treated (00.40-00.43)
procedure on vessel bifurcation (00.44)

Excludes:	*drug-coated peripheral stents, e.g., heparin coated (39.90)*
	insertion of cerebrovascular stent(s) (00.63-00.65)
	insertion of drug-eluting coronary artery stent (36.07)
	insertion of drug-eluting stent(s) of superficial femoral artery (00.60)
	insertion of non-drug-eluting stent(s):
	coronary artery (36.06)
	peripheral vessel (39.90)
	that for other endovascular procedure (39.71-39.79)

▲ **00.56** **Insertion or replacement of implantable pressure sensor with lead for intracardiac or great vessel hemodynamic monitoring**

Note: The sensor is physically connected by a lead to a separately implanted monitor

Code also any associated implantation or replacement of subcutaneous monitor (00.57)

Excludes:	*circulatory monitoring (blood gas, arterial or venous pressure, cardiac output and coronary blood flow) (89.60-89.69)*
	insertion of implantable pressure sensor without lead for intracardiac or great vessel hemodynamic monitoring (38.26)

00.57 **Implantation or replacement of subcutaneous device for intracardiac or great vessel hemodynamic monitoring**

Implantation of monitoring device with formation of subcutaneous pocket and connection to intracardiac pressure sensor via lead

Code also any associated insertion or replacement of implanted pressure sensor with lead (00.56)

00.58 **Insertion of intra-aneurysm sac pressure monitoring device (intraoperative)**

Insertion of pressure sensor during endovascular repair of abdominal or thoracic aortic aneurysm(s)

00.59 **Intravascular pressure measurement of coronary arteries**

Includes: fractional flow reserve (FFR)

Code also any synchronous diagnostic or therapeutic procedures

Excludes:	*intravascular pressure measurement of intrathoracic arteries (00.67)*

00.6 **Procedures on blood vessels**

00.60 **Insertion of drug-eluting stent(s) of superficial femoral artery**

Code also any:
angioplasty of other non-coronary vessel(s) (39.50)
atherectomy of other non-coronary vessel(s) (17.56)
non-drug-eluting peripheral stents (39.90)
number of vascular stents inserted (00.45-00.48)
number of vessels treated (00.40-00.43)
procedure on vessel bifurcation (00.44)

Excludes:	*insertion of drug-eluting stent(s) of other peripheral vessel (00.55)*
	that for other endovascular procedure (39.71-39.79)

	Valid O.R. procedure		Non-O.R. procedure		Nonspecific O.R. procedure		Noncovered O.R. procedure

▲ **00.61 Percutaneous angioplasty of extracranial vessel(s)**
        Carotid
        Vertebral

        Code also any:
          injection or infusion of thrombolytic agent (99.10)
          number of vascular stents inserted (00.45-00.48)
          number of vessels treated (00.40-00.43)
          percutaneous atherectomy of extracranial vessel(s) (17.53)
          percutaneous insertion of carotid artery stent(s) (00.63)
          percutaneous insertion of other extracranial artery stent(s) (00.64)
          procedure on vessel bifurcation (00.44)

        | *Excludes:* | *angioplasty of other non-coronary vessel(s) (39.50)* |
        atherectomy of other non-coronary vessel(s) (17.56)
        removal of cerebrovascular obstruction of vessel(s) by open approach
          (38.01-38.02, 38.11-38.12, 38.31-38.32, 38.41-38.42)

▲ **00.62 Percutaneous angioplasty of intracranial vessel(s)**
        Basilar artery
        Intracranial portion of vertebral artery

        Code also any:
          injection or infusion of thrombolytic agent (99.10)
          number of vascular stents inserted (00.45-00.48)
          number of vessels treated (00.40-00.43)
          percutaneous atherectomy of intracranial vessel(s) (17.54)
          percutaneous insertion of intracranial stent(s) (00.65)
          procedure on vessel bifurcation (00.44)

        | *Excludes:* | *angioplasty of other non-coronary vessel(s) (39.50)* |
        atherectomy of other non-coronary vessel(s) (17.56)
         removal of cerebrovascular obstruction of vessel(s) by open approach
          (38.01-38.02, 38.11-38.12, 38.31-38.32, 38.41-38.42)

00.63 Percutaneous insertion of carotid artery stent(s)
        Includes the use of any embolic protection device, distal protection device, filter
          device, or stent delivery system
        Non-drug-eluting stent

        Code also any:
          number of vascular stents inserted (00.45-00.48)
          number of vessels treated (00.40-00.43)
          percutaneous angioplasty of extracranial vessel(s) (00.61)
          percutaneous atherectomy of extracranial vessel(s) (17.53)
          procedure on vessel bifurcation (00.44)

        | *Excludes:* | *angioplasty of other non-coronary vessel(s) (39.50)* |
        atherectomy of other non-coronary vessel(s) (17.56)
        insertion of coil-retention or embolization stent (39.72)
        insertion of drug-eluting peripheral vessel stent(s) (00.55)

▲ **00.64 Percutaneous insertion of other extracranial artery stent(s)**
        Includes the use of any embolic protection device, distal protection device, filter
          device, or stent delivery system
        Vertebral stent

        Code also any:
          number of vascular stents inserted (00.45-00.48)
          number of vessels treated (00.40-00.43)
          percutaneous angioplasty of extracranial vessel(s) (00.61)
          percutaneous atherectomy of extracranial vessel(s) (17.53)
          procedure on vessel bifurcation (00.44)

        | *Excludes:* | *angioplasty of other non-coronary vessel(s) (39.50)* |
        atherectomy of other non-coronary vessel(s) (17.56)
        insertion of coil-retention or embolization stent (39.72)
        insertion of drug-eluting peripheral vessel stent(s) (00.55)

| ● | Code new to 2012 edition | ▲ | Revision of existing code | ④ ⑤ | Fourth or fifth digit required |

00.65 Percutaneous insertion of intracranial vascular stent(s)
Basilar stent
Includes the use of any embolic protection device, distal protection device, filter device, or stent delivery system

Code also any:
number of vascular stents inserted (00.45-00.48)
number of vessels treated (00.40-00.43)
percutaneous angioplasty of intracranial vessel(s) (00.62)
percutaneous atherectomy of intracranial vessel(s) (17.54)
procedure on vessel bifurcation (00.44)

Excludes:	*angioplasty of other non-coronary vessel(s) (39.50)*
	atherectomy of other non-coronary vessel(s) (17.56)
	insertion of coil-retention or embolization stent (39.72)
	insertion of drug-eluting peripheral vessel stent(s) (00.55)

▲ **00.66 Percutaneous transluminal coronary angioplasty [PTCA]**
Balloon angioplasty of coronary artery
Percutaneous coronary angioplasty NOS
PTCA NOS

Code also any:
injection or infusion of thrombolytic agent (99.10)
insertion of coronary artery stent(s) (36.06-36.07)
intracoronary artery thrombolytic infusion (36.04)
number of vascular stents inserted (00.45-00.48)
number of vessels treated (00.40-00.43)
procedure on vessel bifurcation (00.44)
SuperSaturated oxygen therapy (00.49)
transluminal coronary atherectomy (17.55)

00.67 Intravascular pressure measurement of intrathoracic arteries
Assessment of:
aorta and aortic arch
carotid

Code also any synchronous diagnostic or therapeutic procedures

00.68 Intravascular pressure measurement of peripheral arteries
Assessment of:
other peripheral vessels
vessels of arm(s)
vessels of leg(s)

Code also any synchronous diagnostic or therapeutic procedures

00.69 Intravascular pressure measurement, other specified and unspecified vessels
Iliac vessels
Intra-abdominal vessels
Mesenteric vessels
Renal vessels

Code also any synchronous diagnostic or therapeutic procedures

Excludes:	*intravascular pressure measurement of:*
	coronary arteries (00.59)
	intrathoracic arteries (00.67)
	peripheral arteries (00.68)

00.7 Other hip procedures

00.70 Revision of hip replacement, both acetabular and femoral components
Total hip revision

Code also any:
removal of (cement) (joint) spacer (84.57)
type of bearing surface, if known (00.74-00.77)

Excludes:	*revision of hip replacement, acetabular component only (00.71)*
	revision of hip replacement, femoral component only (00.72)
	revision of hip replacement, Not Otherwise Specified (81.53)
	revision with replacement of acetabular liner and/or femoral head only (00.73)

	Valid O.R. procedure		Non-O.R. procedure		Nonspecific O.R. procedure		Noncovered O.R. procedure

00.71 **Revision of hip replacement, acetabular component**
Partial, acetabular component only
That with:
exchange of acetabular cup and liner
exchange of femoral head

Code also any type of bearing surface, if known (00.74-00.77)

> Excludes: *revision of hip replacement, both acetabular and femoral components*
> *(00.70)*
> *revision of hip replacement, femoral component (00.72)*
> *revision of hip replacement, Not Otherwise Specified (81.53)*
> *revision with replacement of acetabular liner and/or femoral head only*
> *(00.73)*

00.72 **Revision of hip replacement, femoral component**
Partial, femoral component only
That with:
exchange of acetabular liner
exchange of femoral stem and head

Code also any type of bearing surface, if known (00.74-00.77)

> Excludes: *revision of hip replacement, acetabular component (00.71)*
> *revision of hip replacement, both acetabular and femoral components*
> *(00.70)*
> *revision of hip replacement, not otherwise specified (81.53)*
> *revision with replacement of acetabular liner and/or femoral head only*
> *(00.73)*

00.73 **Revision of hip replacement, acetabular liner and/or femoral head only**
Code also any type of bearing surface, if known (00.74-00.77)

00.74 **Hip bearing surface, metal-on-polyethylene**

00.75 **Hip bearing surface, metal-on-metal**

00.76 **Hip bearing surface, ceramic-on-ceramic**

00.77 **Hip bearing surface, ceramic-on-polyethylene**
Hip bearing surface, oxidized zirconium-on-polyethylene

00.8 **Other knee and hip procedures**
Note: Report up to two components using 00.81-00.83 to describe revision of knee replacements.
If all three components are revised, report 00.80.

00.80 **Revision of knee replacement, total (all components)**
Replacement of femoral, tibial, and patellar components (all components)

Code also any removal of (cement) (joint) spacer (84.57)

> Excludes: *revision of only one or two components (tibial, femoral or patellar*
> *component) (00.81-00.84)*

00.81 **Revision of knee replacement, tibial component**
Replacement of tibial baseplate and tibial insert (liner)

> Excludes: *revision of knee replacement, total (all components) (00.80)*

00.82 **Revision of knee replacement, femoral component**
That with replacement of tibial insert (liner)

> Excludes: *revision of knee replacement, total (all components) (00.80)*

00.83 **Revision of knee replacement, patellar component**

> Excludes: *revision of knee replacement, total (all components) (00.80)*

00.84 **Revision of total knee replacement, tibial insert (liner)**
Replacement of tibial insert (liner)

> Excludes: *that with replacement of tibial component (tibial baseplate and liner)*
> *(00.81)*

00.85 **Resurfacing hip, total, acetabulum and femoral head**
Hip resurfacing arthroplasty, total

00.86 **Resurfacing hip, partial, femoral head**
Hip resurfacing arthroplasty, NOS
Hip resurfacing arthroplasty, partial, femoral head

> Excludes: *that with resurfacing of acetabulum (00.85)*

00.87 **Resurfacing hip, partial, acetabulum**
Hip resurfacing arthroplasty, partial, acetabulum

> Excludes: *that with resurfacing of femoral head (00.85)*

● Code new
to 2012 edition ▲ Revision of
existing code ④ ⑤ Fourth or fifth
digit required

00.9 **Other procedures and interventions**

00.91 **Transplant from live related donor**
Code also organ transplant procedure

00.92 **Transplant from live non-related donor**
Code also organ transplant procedure

00.93 **Transplant from cadaver**
Code also organ transplant procedure

00.94 **Intra-operative neurophysiologic monitoring**
Includes: Cranial nerve, peripheral nerve and spinal cord testing performed
intra-operatively

Intra-operative neurophysiologic testing
IOM
Nerve monitoring
Neuromonitoring
That by:
brainstem auditory evoked potentials [BAEP]
electroencephalogram [EEG]
electromyogram [EMG]
motor evoked potentials [MEP]
nerve conduction study
somatosensory evoked potentials [SSEP]
transcranial Doppler

> *Excludes:* *brain temperature monitoring (01.17)*
> *intracranial oxygen monitoring (01.16)*
> *intracranial pressure monitoring (01.10)*
> *plethysmogram (89.58)*

● **00.95** **Injection or infusion of glucaridase**
(Valid FY2013)

01 **Incision and excision of skull, brain, and cerebral meninges**

01.0 **Cranial puncture**

01.01 **Cisternal puncture**
Cisternal tap

> *Excludes:* *pneumocisternogram (87.02)*

01.02 **Ventriculopuncture through previously implanted catheter**
Puncture of ventricular shunt tubing

01.09 **Other cranial puncture**
Aspiration of
subarachnoid space
subdural space
Cranial aspiration NOS
Puncture of anterior fontanel
Subdural tap (through fontanel)

01.1 **Diagnostic procedures on skull, brain, and cerebral meninges**

01.10 **Intracranial pressure monitoring**
Includes: insertion of catheter or probe for monitoring

01.11 **Closed [percutaneous] [needle] biopsy of cerebral meninges**
Burr hole approach

01.12 **Open biopsy of cerebral meninges**

01.13 **Closed [percutaneous] [needle] biopsy of brain**
Burr hole approach
Stereotactic method

01.14 **Open biopsy of brain**

01.15 **Biopsy of skull**

01.16 **Intracranial oxygen monitoring**
Includes: insertion of catheter or probe for monitoring
Partial pressure of brain oxygen (PbtO$_2$)

01.17 **Brain temperature monitoring**
Includes: insertion of catheter or probe for monitoring

| Valid O.R. procedure | Non-O.R. procedure | Nonspecific O.R. procedure | Noncovered O.R. procedure |

01.18 Other diagnostic procedures on brain and cerebral meninges

Excludes: *brain temperature monitoring (01.17)*
cerebral:
  arteriography (88.41)
  thermography (88.81)
contrast radiogram of brain (87.01-87.02)
echoencephalogram (88.71)
electroencephalogram (89.14)
intracranial oxygen monitoring (01.16)
intracranial pressure monitoring (01.10)
microscopic examination of specimen from nervous system and of
  spinal fluid (90.01-90.09)
neurologic examination (89.13)
phlebography of head and neck (88.61)
pneumoencephalogram (87.01)
radioisotope scan:
  cerebral (92.11)
  head NEC (92.12)
tomography of head:
  C.A.T. scan (87.03)
  other (87.04)

01.19 Other diagnostic procedures on skull

Excludes: *transillumination of skull (89.16)*
x-ray of skull (87.17)

01.2 Craniotomy and craniectomy

Excludes: *decompression of skull fracture (02.02)*
exploration of orbit (16.01-16.09)
that as operative approach—omit code

01.20 Cranial implantation or replacement of neurostimulator pulse generator
Code also any associated lead implantation (02.93)

Excludes: *implantation or replacement of subcutaneous neurostimulator pulse*
generator (86.94 -86.98)

01.21 Incision and drainage of cranial sinus

01.22 Removal of intracranial neurostimulator lead(s)
Code also any removal of neurostimulator pulse generator (86.05)

Excludes: *removal with synchronous replacement (02.93)*

01.23 Reopening of craniotomy site

01.24 Other craniotomy
Cranial decompression
Cranial exploration
Cranial trephination
Craniotomy NOS
Craniotomy with removal of epidural abscess
Craniotomy with removal of extradural hematoma
Craniotomy with removal of foreign body of skull

Excludes: *removal of foreign body with incision into brain (01.39)*

01.25 Other craniectomy
Debridement of skull NOS
Sequestrectomy of skull

Excludes: *debridement of compound fracture of skull (02.02)*
strip craniectomy (02.01)

01.26 Insertion of catheter(s) into cranial cavity or tissue
Code also any concomitant procedure (e.g. resection (01.59))

Excludes: *placement of intracerebral catheter(s) via burr hole(s) (01.28)*

01.27 Removal of catheter(s) from cranial cavity or tissue

01.28 Placement of intracerebral catheter(s) via burr hole(s)
Convection enhanced delivery
Stereotactic placement of intracerebral catheter(s)
Code also infusion of medication

Excludes: *insertion of catheter(s) into cranial cavity or tissue(s) (01.26)*

● Code new to 2012 edition   ▲ Revision of existing code   ④ ⑤ Fourth or fifth digit required

01.29 Removal of cranial neurostimulator pulse generator

01.3 Incision of brain and cerebral meninges

01.31 Incision of cerebral meninges
Drainage of:
    intracranial hygroma
    subarachnoid abscess (cerebral)
    subdural empyema

01.32 Lobotomy and tractotomy
Division of:
    brain tissue
    cerebral tracts
Percutaneous (radio frequency) cingulotomy

01.39 Other incision of brain
Amygdalohippocampotomy
Drainage of intracerebral hematoma
Incision of brain NOS

> *Excludes:* *division of cortical adhesions (02.91)*

01.4 Operations on thalamus and globus pallidus

01.41 Operations on thalamus
Chemothalamectomy
Thalamotomy

> *Excludes:* *that by stereotactic radiosurgery (92.30-92.39)*

01.42 Operations on globus pallidus
Pallidoansectomy
Pallidotomy

> *Excludes:* *that by stereotactic radiosurgery (92.30-92.39)*

01.5 Other excision or destruction of brain and meninges

01.51 Excision of lesion or tissue of cerebral meninges
Decortication of (cerebral) meninges
Resection of (cerebral) meninges
Stripping of subdural membrane of (cerebral) meninges

> *Excludes:* *biopsy of cerebral meninges (01.11-01.12)*

01.52 Hemispherectomy

01.53 Lobectomy of brain

01.59 Other excision or destruction of lesion or tissue of brain
Amygdalohippocampectomy
Curettage of brain
Debridement of brain
Marsupialization of brain cyst
Transtemporal (mastoid) excision of brain tumor

> *Excludes:* *biopsy of brain (01.13-01.14)*
> *laser interstitial thermal therapy [LITT] of lesion or tissue of brain under guidance (17.61)*
> *that by stereotactic radiosurgery (92.30-92.39)*

01.6 Excision of lesion of skull
Removal of granulation tissue of cranium

> *Excludes:* *biopsy of skull (01.15)*
> *sequestrectomy (01.25)*

02 Other operations on skull, brain, and cerebral meninges

02.0 Cranioplasty

> *Excludes:* *that with synchronous repair of encephalocele (02.12)*

02.01 Opening of cranial suture
Linear craniectomy
Strip craniectomy

02.02 Elevation of skull fracture fragments
Debridement of compound fracture of skull
Decompression of skull fracture
Reduction of skull fracture

> *Code also any synchronous debridement of brain (01.59)*

> *Excludes:* *debridement of skull NOS (01.25)*
> *removal of granulation tissue of cranium (01.6)*

| Valid O.R. procedure | Non-O.R. procedure | Nonspecific O.R. procedure | Noncovered O.R. procedure |

02.03 Formation of cranial bone flap
Repair of skull with flap

02.04 Bone graft to skull
Pericranial graft (autogenous) (heterogenous)

02.05 Insertion of skull plate
Replacement of skull plate

02.06 Other cranial osteoplasty
Repair of skull NOS
Revision of bone flap of skull

02.07 Removal of skull plate

| Excludes: | removal with synchronous replacement (02.05) |

02.1 Repair of cerebral meninges

| Excludes: | marsupialization of cerebral lesion (01.59) |

02.11 Simple suture of dura mater of brain

02.12 Other repair of cerebral meninges
Closure of fistula of cerebrospinal fluid
Dural graft
Repair of encephalocele including synchronous cranioplasty
Repair of meninges NOS
Subdural patch

02.13 Ligation of meningeal vessel
Ligation of:
longitudinal sinus
middle meningeal artery

02.14 Choroid plexectomy
Cauterization of choroid plexus

● **02.2 Ventriculostomy**

● **02.21 Insertion or replacement of external ventricular drain [EVD]**
External ventricular drainage [EVD] setup
Replacement of external ventricular drain
Ventricular catheter placement for:
drainage of cerebrospinal fluid [CSF]
injection of medication or other substance
sampling of cerebrospinal fluid [CSF]

| Excludes: | extracranial ventricular shunt (02.31-02.35, 02.39) intracranial ventricular shunt (02.22) other cranial puncture (01.09) ventricular shunt replacement (02.41-02.43) |

● **02.22 Intracranial ventricular shunt or anastomosis**
Anastomosis of ventricle to:
cervical subarachnoid space
cistern magna
Insertion of Holter valve into intracranial system
Shunt between two intracranial ventricles
That by endoscopy
Third ventriculostomy
Ventriculocisternostomy

02.3 Extracranial ventricular shunt
Includes: that with insertion of valve

02.31 Ventricular shunt to structure in head and neck
Ventricle to nasopharynx shunt
Ventriculomastoid anastomosis

02.32 Ventricular shunt to circulatory system
Ventriculoatrial anastomosis
Ventriculocaval shunt

02.33 Ventricular shunt to thoracic cavity
Ventriculopleural anastomosis

02.34 Ventricular shunt to abdominal cavity and organs
Ventriculocholecystostomy
Ventriculoperitoneostomy

02.35 Ventricular shunt to urinary system
Ventricle to ureter shunt

● Code new
to 2012 edition

▲ Revision of
existing code

④ ⑤ Fourth or fifth
digit required

▲ **02.39 Ventricular shunt to extracranial site NEC**
Ventricle to bone marrow shunt

02.4 Revision, removal, and irrigation of ventricular shunt

> Excludes: revision of distal catheter of ventricular shunt (54.95)

02.41 Irrigation and exploration of ventricular shunt
Exploration of ventriculoperitoneal shunt at ventricular site
Re-programming of ventriculoperitoneal shunt

02.42 Replacement of ventricular shunt
Reinsertion of Holter valve
Revision of ventriculoperitoneal shunt at ventricular site

02.43 Removal of ventricular shunt

02.9 Other operations on skull, brain, and cerebral meninges

> Excludes: operations on:
> pineal gland (07.17, 07.51-07.59)
> pituitary gland [hypophysis] (07.13-07.15, 07.61-07.79)

02.91 Lysis of cortical adhesions

02.92 Repair of brain

02.93 Implantation or replacement of intracranial neurostimulator lead(s)
Implantation, insertion, placement, or replacement of intracranial:
brain pacemaker [neuropacemaker]
depth electrodes
electroencephalographic receiver
epidural pegs
foramen ovale electrodes
intracranial electrostimulator
subdural grids
subdural strips

Code also any:
insertion of cranial implantation or replacement of neurostimulator pulse generator
(01.20)
insertion of subcutaneous neurostimulator pulse generator (86.94-86.98)

02.94 Insertion or replacement of skull tongs or halo traction device

02.95 Removal of skull tongs or halo traction device

02.96 Insertion of sphenoidal electrodes

02.99 Other

> Excludes: chemical shock therapy (94.24)
> electroshock therapy:
> subconvulsive (94.26)
> other (94.27)

03 Operations on spinal cord and spinal canal structures
Code also any application or administration of an adhesion barrier substance (99.77)

03.0 Exploration and decompression of spinal canal structures

03.01 Removal of foreign body from spinal canal

03.02 Reopening of laminectomy site

03.09 Other exploration and decompression of spinal canal
Decompression:
laminectomy
laminotomy
Expansile laminoplasty
Exploration of spinal nerve root
Foraminotomy

*Code also any synchronous insertion, replacement and revision of posterior spinal
motion preservation device(s), if performed (84.80 - 84.85)*

> Excludes: drainage of spinal fluid by anastomosis (03.71-03.79)
> laminectomy with excision of intervertebral disc (80.51)
> spinal tap (03.31)
> that as operative approach—omit code

03.1 Division of intraspinal nerve root
Rhizotomy

	Valid O.R. procedure		Non-O.R. procedure		Nonspecific O.R. procedure		Noncovered O.R. procedure

03.2 **Chordotomy**

03.21 **Percutaneous chordotomy**
Stereotactic chordotomy

03.29 **Other chordotomy**
Chordotomy NOS
Tractotomy (one-stage) (two-stage) of spinal cord
Transection of spinal cord tracts

03.3 **Diagnostic procedures on spinal cord and spinal canal structures**

03.31 **Spinal tap**
Lumbar puncture for removal of dye

Excludes: *lumbar puncture for injection of dye [myelogram] (87.21)*

03.32 **Biopsy of spinal cord or spinal meninges**

03.39 **Other diagnostic procedures on spinal cord and spinal canal structures**

Excludes: *microscopic examination of specimen from nervous system or of spinal*
fluid (90.01-90.09)
x-ray of spine (87.21-87.29)

03.4 **Excision or destruction of lesion of spinal cord or spinal meninges**
Curettage of spinal cord or spinal meninges
Debridement of spinal cord or spinal meninges
Marsupialization of cyst of spinal cord or spinal meninges
Resection of spinal cord or spinal meninges

Excludes: *biopsy of spinal cord or meninges (03.32)*

03.5 **Plastic operations on spinal cord structures**

03.51 **Repair of spinal meningocele**
Repair of meningocele NOS

03.52 **Repair of spinal myelomeningocele**

03.53 **Repair of vertebral fracture**
Elevation of spinal bone fragments
Reduction of fracture of vertebrae
Removal of bony spicules from spinal canal

Excludes: *percutaneous vertebral augmentation (81.66)*
percutaneous vertebroplasty (81.65)

03.59 **Other repair and plastic operations on spinal cord structures**
Repair of:
diastematomyelia
spina bifida NOS
spinal cord NOS
spinal meninges NOS
vertebral arch defect

03.6 **Lysis of adhesions of spinal cord and nerve roots**

03.7 **Shunt of spinal theca**
Includes: that with valve

03.71 **Spinal subarachnoid-peritoneal shunt**

03.72 **Spinal subarachnoid-ureteral shunt**

03.79 **Other shunt of spinal theca**
Lumbar-subarachnoid shunt NOS
Pleurothecal anastomosis
Salpingothecal anastomosis

03.8 **Injection of destructive agent into spinal canal**

03.9 **Other operations on spinal cord and spinal canal structures**

03.90 **Insertion of catheter into spinal canal for infusion of therapeutic or palliative**
substances
Insertion of catheter into epidural, subarachnoid, or subdural space of spine with
intermittent or continuous infusion of drug (with creation of any reservoir)
Code also any implantation of infusion pump (86.06)

03.91 **Injection of anesthetic into spinal canal for analgesia**

Excludes: *that for operative anesthesia—omit code*

● Code new ▲ Revision of ④ ⑤ Fourth or fifth
to 2012 edition existing code digit required

03.92 Injection of other agent into spinal canal
Intrathecal injection of steroid
Subarachnoid perfusion of refrigerated saline

> *Excludes:* *injection of:*
> *contrast material for myelogram (87.21)*
> *destructive agent into spinal canal (03.8)*

03.93 Implantation or replacement of spinal neurostimulator lead(s)
Code also any insertion of neurostimulator pulse generator (86.94-86.98)

03.94 Removal of spinal neurostimulator lead(s)
Code also any removal of neurostimulator pulse generator (86.05)

03.95 Spinal blood patch

03.96 Percutaneous denervation of facet

03.97 Revision of spinal thecal shunt

03.98 Removal of spinal thecal shunt

03.99 Other

04 Operations on cranial and peripheral nerves

04.0 Incision, division, and excision of cranial and peripheral nerves

> *Excludes:* *opticociliary neurectomy (12.79)*
> *sympathetic ganglionectomy (05.21-05.29)*

04.01 Excision of acoustic neuroma
That by craniotomy

> *Excludes:* *that by stereotactic radiosurgery (92.3)*

04.02 Division of trigeminal nerve
Retrogasserian neurotomy

04.03 Division or crushing of other cranial and peripheral nerves

> *Excludes:* *that of:*
> *glossopharyngeal nerve (29.92)*
> *laryngeal nerve (31.91)*
> *nerves to adrenal glands (07.42)*
> *phrenic nerve for collapse of lung (33.31)*
> *vagus nerve (44.00-44.03)*

04.04 Other incision of cranial and peripheral nerves

04.05 Gasserian ganglionectomy

04.06 Other cranial or peripheral ganglionectomy

> *Excludes:* *sympathetic ganglionectomy (05.21-05.29)*

04.07 Other excision or avulsion of cranial and peripheral nerves
Curettage of peripheral nerve
Debridement of peripheral nerve
Resection of peripheral nerve
Excision of peripheral neuroma [Morton's]

> *Excludes:* *biopsy of cranial or peripheral nerve (04.11-04.12)*

04.1 Diagnostic procedures on peripheral nervous system

04.11 Closed [percutaneous] [needle] biopsy of cranial or peripheral nerve or ganglion

04.12 Open biopsy of cranial or peripheral nerve or ganglion

04.19 Other diagnostic procedures on cranial and peripheral nerves and ganglia

> *Excludes:* *microscopic examination of specimen from nervous system (90.01-90.09)*
> *neurologic examination (89.13)*

04.2 Destruction of cranial and peripheral nerves
Destruction of cranial or peripheral nerves by:
cryoanalgesia
injection of neurolytic agent
radiofrequency
Radiofrequency ablation

04.3 Suture of cranial and peripheral nerves

04.4 Lysis of adhesions and decompression of cranial and peripheral nerves

04.41 Decompression of trigeminal nerve root

	Valid O.R. procedure		Non-O.R. procedure		Nonspecific O.R. procedure		Noncovered O.R. procedure

04.42 Other cranial nerve decompression

04.43 Release of carpal tunnel

04.44 Release of tarsal tunnel

04.49 Other peripheral nerve or ganglion decompression or lysis of adhesions
Peripheral nerve neurolysis NOS

04.5 Cranial or peripheral nerve graft

04.6 Transposition of cranial and peripheral nerves
Nerve transplantation

04.7 Other cranial or peripheral neuroplasty

04.71 Hypoglossal-facial anastomosis

04.72 Accessory-facial anastomosis

04.73 Accessory-hypoglossal anastomosis

04.74 Other anastomosis of cranial or peripheral nerve

04.75 Revision of previous repair of cranial and peripheral nerves

04.76 Repair of old traumatic injury of cranial and peripheral nerves

04.79 Other neuroplasty

04.8 Injection into peripheral nerve
| Excludes: | *destruction of nerve (by injection of neurolytic agent) (04.2)*

04.80 Peripheral nerve injection, not otherwise specified

04.81 Injection of anesthetic into peripheral nerve for analgesia
| Excludes: | *that for operative anesthesia—omit code*

04.89 Injection of other agent, except neurolytic
| Excludes: | *injection of neurolytic agent (04.2)*

04.9 Other operations on cranial and peripheral nerves

04.91 Neurectasis

04.92 Implantation or replacement of peripheral neurostimulator lead(s)
Code also any insertion of neurostimulator pulse generator (86.94-86.98)
| Excludes: | *implantation or replacement of carotid sinus stimulation lead(s)*
(39.82)

04.93 Removal of peripheral neurostimulator lead(s)
Code also any removal of neurostimulator pulse generator (86.05)

04.99 Other

05 Operations on sympathetic nerves or ganglia
| Excludes: | *paracervical uterine denervation (69.3)*

05.0 Division of sympathetic nerve or ganglion
| Excludes: | *that of nerves to adrenal glands (07.42)*

05.1 Diagnostic procedures on sympathetic nerves or ganglia

05.11 Biopsy of sympathetic nerve or ganglion

05.19 Other diagnostic procedures on sympathetic nerves or ganglia

05.2 Sympathectomy

05.21 Sphenopalatine ganglionectomy

05.22 Cervical sympathectomy

05.23 Lumber sympathectomy

05.24 Presacral sympathectomy

05.25 Periarterial sympathectomy

05.29 Other sympathectomy and ganglionectomy
Excision or avulsion of sympathetic nerve NOS
Sympathetic ganglionectomy NOS
| Excludes: | *biopsy of sympathetic nerve or ganglion (05.11)*
opticociliary neurectomy (12.79)
periarterial sympathectomy (05.25)
tympanosympathectomy (20.91)

● Code new
to 2012 edition
▲ Revision of
existing code
④ ⑤ Fourth or fifth
digit required

05.3 **Injection into sympathetic nerve or ganglion**

Excludes: *injection of ciliary sympathetic ganglion (12.79)*

05.31 **Injection of anesthetic into sympathetic nerve for analgesia**

05.32 **Injection of neurolytic agent into sympathetic nerve**

05.39 **Other injection into sympathetic nerve or ganglion**

05.8 **Other operations on sympathetic nerves or ganglion**

05.81 **Repair of sympathetic nerve or ganglion**

05.89 **Other**

05.9 **Other operations on nervous system**

| Valid O.R. procedure | Non-O.R. procedure | Nonspecific O.R. procedure | Noncovered O.R. procedure |

This page intentionally left blank.

● Code new
to 2012 edition

▲ Revision of
existing code

④ ⑤ Fourth or fifth
digit required

2. **OPERATIONS ON THE ENDOCRINE SYSTEM (06-07)**

06 **Operations on thyroid and parathyroid glands**
Includes: incidental resection of hyoid bone

06.0 **Incision of thyroid field**

> Excludes: *division of isthmus (06.91)*

06.01 **Aspiration of thyroid field**
Percutaneous or needle drainage of thyroid field

> Excludes: *aspiration biopsy of thyroid (06.11)*
> *drainage by incision (06.09)*
> *postoperative aspiration of field (06.02)*

06.02 **Reopening of wound of thyroid field**
Reopening of wound of thyroid field for:
control of (postoperative) hemorrhage
examination
exploration
removal of hematoma

06.09 **Other incision of thyroid field**
Drainage of hematoma by incision
Drainage of thyroglossal tract by incision
Exploration by incision:
neck
thyroid (field)
Removal of foreign body by incision
Thyroidotomy NOS by incision

> Excludes: *postoperative exploration (06.02)*
> *removal of hematoma by aspiration (06.01)*

06.1 **Diagnostic procedures on thyroid and parathyroid glands**

06.11 **Closed [percutaneous] [needle] biopsy of thyroid gland**
Aspiration biopsy of thyroid

06.12 **Open biopsy of thyroid gland**

06.13 **Biopsy of parathyroid gland**

06.19 **Other diagnostic procedures on thyroid and parathyroid glands**

> Excludes: *radioisotope scan of:*
> *parathyroid (92.13)*
> *thyroid (92.01)*
> *soft tissue x-ray of thyroid field (87.09)*

06.2 **Unilateral thyroid lobectomy**
Complete removal of one lobe of thyroid (with removal of isthmus or portion of other lobe)
Hemithyroidectomy

> Excludes: *partial substernal thyroidectomy (06.51)*

06.3 **Other partial thyroidectomy**

06.31 **Excision of lesion of thyroid**

> Excludes: *biopsy of thyroid (06.11-06.12)*
> *laser interstitial thermal therapy [LITT] of lesion or tissue of neck*
> *under guidance (17.62)*

06.39 **Other**
Isthmectomy
Partial thyroidectomy NOS

> Excludes: *partial substernal thyroidectomy (06.51)*

06.4 **Complete thyroidectomy**

> Excludes: *complete substernal thyroidectomy (06.52)*
> *that with laryngectomy (30.3-30.4)*

06.5 **Substernal thyroidectomy**

06.50 **Substernal thyroidectomy, not otherwise specified**

06.51 **Partial substernal thyroidectomy**

06.52 **Complete substernal thyroidectomy**

| | Valid O.R. procedure | | Non-O.R. procedure | | Nonspecific O.R. procedure | | Noncovered O.R. procedure |

06.6 **Excision of lingual thyroid**
Excision of thyroid by:
submental route
transoral route

06.7 **Excision of thyroglossal duct or tract**

06.8 **Parathyroidectomy**

06.81 **Complete parathyroidectomy**

06.89 **Other parathyroidectomy**
Parathyroidectomy NOS
Partial parathyroidectomy

Excludes: *biopsy of parathyroid (06.13)*

06.9 **Other operations on thyroid (region) and parathyroid**

06.91 **Division of thyroid isthmus**
Transection of thyroid isthmus

06.92 **Ligation of thyroid vessels**

06.93 **Suture of thyroid gland**

06.94 **Thyroid tissue reimplantation**
Autotransplantation of thyroid tissue

06.95 **Parathyroid tissue reimplantation**
Autotransplantation of parathyroid tissue

06.98 **Other operations on thyroid glands**

06.99 **Other operations on parathyroid glands**

07 **Operations on other endocrine glands**
Includes: operations on:
adrenal glands
pineal gland
pituitary gland
thymus

Excludes: *operations on:*
aortic and carotid bodies (39.81-39.89)
ovaries (65.0-65.99)
pancreas (52.01-52.99)
testes (62.0-62.99)

07.0 **Exploration of adrenal field**

Excludes: *incision of adrenal gland (07.41)*

07.00 **Exploration of adrenal field, not otherwise specified**

07.01 **Unilateral exploration of adrenal field**

07.02 **Bilateral exploration of adrenal field**

07.1 **Diagnostic procedures on adrenal glands, pituitary gland, pineal gland, and thymus**

07.11 **Closed [percutaneous] [needle] biopsy of adrenal gland**

07.12 **Open biopsy of adrenal gland**

07.13 **Biopsy of pituitary gland, transfrontal approach**

07.14 **Biopsy of pituitary gland, transsphenoidal approach**

07.15 **Biopsy of pituitary gland, unspecified approach**

07.16 **Biopsy of thymus**

07.17 **Biopsy of pineal gland**

07.19 **Other diagnostic procedures on adrenal glands, pituitary gland, pineal gland, and thymus**

Excludes: *microscopic examination of specimen from endocrine gland*
(90.11-90.19)
radioisotope scan of pituitary gland (92.11)

07.2 **Partial adrenalectomy**

07.21 **Excision of lesion of adrenal gland**

Excludes: *biopsy of adrenal gland (07.11-07.12)*

07.22 **Unilateral adrenalectomy**
Adrenalectomy NOS

Excludes: *excision of remaining adrenal gland (07.3)*

● Code new
to 2012 edition
▲ Revision of
existing code
④ ⑤ Fourth or fifth
digit required

07.29 Other partial adrenalectomy
Partial adrenalectomy NOS

07.3   Bilateral adrenalectomy
Excision of remaining adrenal gland

> *Excludes:* *bilateral partial adrenalectomy (07.29)*

07.4   Other operations on adrenal glands, nerves, and vessels

07.41 Incision of adrenal gland
Adrenalotomy (with drainage)

07.42 Division of nerves to adrenal glands

07.43 Ligation of adrenal vessels

07.44 Repair of adrenal gland

07.45 Reimplantation of adrenal tissue
Autotransplantation of adrenal tissue

07.49 Other

07.5   Operations on pineal gland

07.51 Exploration of pineal field

> *Excludes:* *that with incision of pineal gland (07.52)*

07.52 Incision of pineal gland

07.53 Partial excision of pineal gland

> *Excludes:* *biopsy of pineal gland (07.17)*

07.54 Total excision of pineal gland
Pinealectomy (complete) (total)

07.59 Other operations on pineal gland

07.6   Hypophysectomy

07.61 Partial excision of pituitary gland, transfrontal approach
Cryohypophysectomy, partial, transfrontal approach
Division of hypophyseal stalk, transfrontal approach
Excision of lesion of pituitary [hypophysis], transfrontal approach
Hypophysectomy, subtotal, transfrontal approach
Infundibulectomy, hypophyseal, transfrontal approach

> *Excludes:* *biopsy of pituitary gland, transfrontal approach (07.13)*

07.62 Partial excision of pituitary gland, transsphenoidal approach

> *Excludes:* *biopsy of pituitary gland, transsphenoidal approach (07.14)*

07.63 Partial excision of pituitary gland, unspecified approach

> *Excludes:* *biopsy of pituitary gland NOS (07.15)*

07.64 Total excision of pituitary gland, transfrontal approach
Ablation of pituitary by implantation (strontium-yttrium) (Y), transfrontal approach
Cryohypophysectomy, complete, transfrontal approach

07.65 Total excision of pituitary gland, transsphenoidal approach

07.68 Total excision of pituitary gland, other specified approach

07.69 Total excision of pituitary gland, unspecified approach
Hypophysectomy NOS
Pituitectomy NOS

07.7   Other operations on hypophysis

07.71 Exploration of pituitary fossa

> *Excludes:* *exploration with incision of pituitary gland (07.72)*

07.72 Incision of pituitary gland
Aspiration of:
  craniobuccal pouch
  craniopharyngioma
  hypophysis
  pituitary gland
  Rathke's pouch

07.79 Other
Insertion of pack into sella turcica

07.8   Thymectomy

| Valid O.R. procedure | Non-O.R. procedure | Nonspecific O.R. procedure | Noncovered O.R. procedure |

07.80 Thymectomy, not otherwise specified

07.81 Other partial excision of thymus
Open partial excision of thymus

Excludes: *biopsy of thymus (07.16)*
thoracoscopic partial excision of thymus (07.83)

07.82 Other total excision of thymus
Open total excision of thymus

Excludes: *thoracoscopic total excision of thymus (07.84)*

07.83 Thoracoscopic partial excision of thymus

Excludes: *other partial excision of thymus (07.81)*

07.84 Thoracoscopic total excision of thymus

Excludes: *other total excision of thymus (07.82)*

07.9 Other operations on thymus

07.91 Exploration of thymus field

Excludes: *exploration with incision of thymus (07.92)*

07.92 Other incision of thymus
Open incision of thymus

Excludes: *thoracoscopic incision of thymus (07.95)*

07.93 Repair of thymus

07.94 Transplantation of thymus

07.95 Thoracoscopic incision of thymus

Excludes: *other incision of thymus (07.92)*

07.98 Other and unspecified thoracoscopic operations on thymus

07.99 Other and unspecified operations on thymus
Transcervical thymectomy

Excludes: *other thoracoscopic operations on thymus (07.98)*

● Code new to 2012 edition   ▲ Revision of existing code   ④ ⑤ Fourth or fifth digit required

3. **OPERATIONS ON THE EYE (08-16)**

08 **Operations on eyelids**
Includes: operations on the eyebrow

08.0 **Incision of eyelid**

08.01 **Incision of lid margin**

08.02 **Severing of blepharorrhaphy**

08.09 **Other incision of eyelid**

08.1 **Diagnostic procedures on eyelid**

08.11 **Biopsy of eyelid**

08.19 **Other diagnostic procedures on eyelid**

08.2 **Excision or destruction of lesion or tissue of eyelid**
Code also any synchronous reconstruction (08.61-08.74)
Excludes: *biopsy of eyelid (08.11)*

08.20 **Removal of lesion of eyelid, not otherwise specified**
Removal of meibomian gland NOS

08.21 **Excision of chalazion**

08.22 **Excision of other minor lesion of eyelid**
Excision of:
verruca
wart

08.23 **Excision of major lesion of eyelid, partial-thickness**
Excision involving one-fourth or more of lid margin, partial-thickness

08.24 **Excision of major lesion of eyelid, full-thickness**
Excision involving one-fourth or more of lid margin, full-thickness
Wedge resection of eyelid

08.25 **Destruction of lesion of eyelid**

08.3 **Repair of blepharoptosis and lid retraction**

08.31 **Repair of blepharoptosis by frontalis muscle technique with suture**

08.32 **Repair of blepharoptosis by frontalis muscle technique with fascial sling**

08.33 **Repair of blepharoptosis by resection or advancement of levator muscle or aponeurosis**

08.34 **Repair of blepharoptosis by other levator muscle techniques**

08.35 **Repair of blepharoptosis by tarsal technique**

08.36 **Repair of blepharoptosis by other techniques**
Correction of eyelid ptosis NOS
Orbicularis oculi muscle sling for correction of blepharoptosis

08.37 **Reduction of overcorrection of ptosis**

08.38 **Correction of lid retraction**

08.4 **Repair of entropion or ectropion**

08.41 **Repair of entropion or ectropion by thermocauterization**

08.42 **Repair of entropion or ectropion by suture technique**

08.43 **Repair of entropion or ectropion with wedge resection**

08.44 **Repair of entropion or ectropion with lid reconstruction**

08.49 **Other repair of entropion or ectropion**

08.5 **Other adjustment of lid position**

08.51 **Canthotomy**
Enlargement of palpebral fissure

08.52 **Blepharorrhaphy**
Canthorrhaphy
Tarsorrhaphy

08.59 **Other**
Canthoplasty NOS
Repair of epicanthal fold

08.6 **Reconstruction of eyelid with flaps or grafts**
Excludes: *that associated with repair of entropion and ectropion (08.44)*

Valid O.R.
procedure

Non-O.R.
procedure

Nonspecific
O.R. procedure

Noncovered
O.R. procedure

08.61 Reconstruction of eyelid with skin flap or graft

08.62 Reconstruction of eyelid with mucous membrane flap or graft

08.63 Reconstruction of eyelid with hair follicle graft

08.64 Reconstruction of eyelid with tarsoconjunctival flap
Transfer of tarsoconjunctival flap from opposing lid

08.69 Other reconstruction of eyelid with flap or graft

08.7 Other reconstruction of eyelid

> Excludes: that associated with repair of entropion and ectropion (08.44)

08.70 Reconstruction of eyelid, not otherwise specified

08.71 Reconstruction of eyelid involving lid margin, partial-thickness

08.72 Other reconstruction of eyelid, partial-thickness

08.73 Reconstruction of eyelid involving lid margin, full-thickness

08.74 Other reconstruction of eyelid, full-thickness

08.8 Other repair of eyelid

08.81 Linear repair of laceration of eyelid or eyebrow

08.82 Repair of laceration involving lid margin, partial-thickness

08.83 Other repair of laceration of eyelid, partial-thickness

08.84 Repair of laceration involving lid margin, full-thickness

08.85 Other repair of laceration of eyelid, full-thickness

08.86 Lower eyelid rhytidectomy

08.87 Upper eyelid rhytidectomy

08.89 Other eyelid repair

08.9 Other operations on eyelids

08.91 Electrosurgical epilation of eyelid

08.92 Cryosurgical epilation of eyelid

08.93 Other epilation of eyelid

08.99 Other

09 Operations on lacrimal system

09.0 Incision of lacrimal gland
Incision of lacrimal cyst (with drainage)

09.1 Diagnostic procedures on lacrimal system

09.11 Biopsy of lacrimal gland

09.12 Biopsy of lacrimal sac

09.19 Other diagnostic procedures on lacrimal system

> Excludes: contrast dacryocystogram (87.05)
> soft tissue x-ray of nasolacrimal duct (87.09)

09.2 Excision of lesion or tissue of lacrimal gland

09.20 Excision of lacrimal gland, not otherwise specified

09.21 Excision of lesion of lacrimal gland

> Excludes: biopsy of lacrimal gland (09.11)

09.22 Other partial dacryoadenectomy

> Excludes: biopsy of lacrimal gland (09.11)

09.23 Total dacryoadenectomy

09.3 Other operations on lacrimal gland

09.4 Manipulation of lacrimal passage
Includes: removal of calculus
             that with dilation

> Excludes: contrast dacryocystogram (87.05)

09.41 Probing of lacrimal punctum

09.42 Probing of lacrimal canaliculi

09.43 Probing of nasolacrimal duct

> Excludes: that with insertion of tube or stent (09.44)

● Code new   ▲ Revision of   ④ ⑤ Fourth or fifth
         to 2012 edition   existing code   digit required

09.44 Intubation of nasolacrimal duct
Insertion of stent into nasolacrimal duct

09.49 Other manipulation of lacrimal passage

09.5 Incision of lacrimal sac and passages

09.51 Incision of lacrimal punctum

09.52 Incision of lacrimal canaliculi

09.53 Incision of lacrimal sac

09.59 Other incision of lacrimal passages
Incision (and drainage) of nasolacrimal duct NOS

09.6 Excision of lacrimal sac and passage

> *Excludes:*   *biopsy of lacrimal sac (09.12)*

09.7 Repair of canaliculus and punctum

> *Excludes:*   *repair of eyelid (08.81-08.89)*

09.71 Correction of everted punctum

09.72 Other repair of punctum

09.73 Repair of canaliculus

09.8 Fistulization of lacrimal tract to nasal cavity

09.81 Dacryocystorhinostomy [DCR]

09.82 Conjunctivocystorhinostomy
Conjunctivodacryocystorhinostomy [CDCR]

> *Excludes:*   *that with insertion of tube or stent (09.83)*

09.83 Conjunctivorhinostomy with insertion of tube or stent

09.9 Other operations on lacrimal system

09.91 Obliteration of lacrimal punctum

09.99 Other

10 Operations on conjunctiva

10.0 Removal of embedded foreign body from conjunctiva by incision

> *Excludes:*   *removal of:*
>   *embedded foreign body without incision (98.22)*
>   *superficial foreign body (98.21)*

10.1 Other incision of conjunctiva

10.2 Diagnostic procedures on conjunctiva

10.21 Biopsy of conjunctiva

10.29 Other diagnostic procedures on conjunctiva

10.3 Excision or destruction of lesion or tissue of conjunctiva

10.31 Excision of lesion or tissue of conjunctiva
Excision of ring of conjunctiva around cornea

> *Excludes:*   *biopsy of conjunctiva (10.21)*

10.32 Destruction of lesion of conjunctiva

> *Excludes:*   *excision of lesion (10.31)*
>   *thermocauterization for entropion (08.41)*

10.33 Other destructive procedures on conjunctiva
Removal of trachoma follicles

10.4 Conjunctivoplasty

10.41 Repair of symblepharon with free graft

10.42 Reconstruction of conjunctival cul-de-sac with free graft

> *Excludes:*   *revision of enucleation socket with graft (16.63)*

10.43 Other reconstruction of conjunctival cul-de-sac

> *Excludes:*   *revision of enucleation socket (16.64)*

10.44 Other free graft to conjunctiva

10.49 Other conjunctivoplasty

> *Excludes:*   *repair of cornea with conjunctival flap (11.53)*

| | Valid O.R. procedure | | Non-O.R. procedure | | Nonspecific O.R. procedure | | Noncovered O.R. procedure |

10.5 **Lysis of adhesions of conjunctiva and eyelid**
Division of symblepharon (with insertion of conformer)

10.6 **Repair of laceration of conjunctiva**
Excludes: *that with repair of sclera (12.81)*

10.9 **Other operations on conjunctiva**

10.91 **Subconjunctival injection**

10.99 **Other**

11 **Operations on cornea**

11.0 **Magnetic removal of embedded foreign body from cornea**
Excludes: *that with incision (11.1)*

11.1 **Incision of cornea**
Incision of cornea for removal of foreign body

11.2 **Diagnostic procedures on cornea**

11.21 **Scraping of cornea for smear or culture**

11.22 **Biopsy of cornea**

11.29 **Other diagnostic procedures on cornea**

11.3 **Excision of pterygium**

11.31 **Transposition of pterygium**

11.32 **Excision of pterygium with corneal graft**

11.39 **Other excision of pterygium**

11.4 **Excision or destruction of tissue or other lesion of cornea**

11.41 **Mechanical removal of corneal epithelium**
That by chemocauterization
Excludes: *that for smear or culture (11.21)*

11.42 **Thermocauterization of corneal lesion**

11.43 **Cryotherapy of corneal lesion**

11.49 **Other removal or destruction of corneal lesion**
Excision of cornea NOS
Excludes: *biopsy of cornea (11.22)*

11.5 **Repair of cornea**

11.51 **Suture of corneal laceration**

11.52 **Repair of postoperative wound dehiscence of cornea**

11.53 **Repair of corneal laceration or wound with conjunctival flop**

11.59 **Other repair of cornea**

11.6 **Corneal transplant**
Excludes: *excision of pterygium with corneal graft (11.32)*

11.60 **Corneal transplant, not otherwise specified**
Keratoplasty NOS
Note: To report donor source —*see* codes 00.91-00.93

11.61 **Lamellar keratoplasty with autograft**

11.62 **Other lamellar keratoplasty**

11.63 **Penetrating keratoplasty with autograft**
Perforating keratoplasty with autograft

11.64 **Other penetrating keratoplasty**
Perforating keratoplasty (with homograft)

11.69 **Other corneal transplant**

11.7 **Other reconstructive and refractive surgery on cornea**

11.71 **Keratomileusis**

11.72 **Keratophakia**

11.73 **Keratoprosthesis**

11.74 **Thermokeratoplasty**

11.75 **Radial keratotomy**

11.76 **Epikeratophakia**

● Code new
to 2012 edition
▲ Revision of
existing code
④ ⑤ Fourth or fifth
digit required

11.79 Other

11.9 Other operations on cornea

11.91 Tattooing of cornea

11.92 Removal of artificial implant from cornea

11.99 Other

12 Operation on iris, ciliary body, sclera, and anterior chamber

> Excludes: operations on cornea (11.0-11.99)

12.0 Removal of intraocular foreign body from anterior segment of eye

12.00 Removal of intraocular foreign body from anterior segment of eye, not otherwise specified

12.01 Removal of intraocular foreign body from anterior segment of eye with use of magnet

12.02 Removal of intraocular foreign body from anterior segment of eye without use of magnet

12.1 Iridotomy and simple iridectomy

> Excludes: iridectomy associated with:
> cataract extraction (13.11-13.69)
> removal of lesion (12.41-12.42)
> scleral fistulization (12.61-12.69)

12.11 Iridotomy with transfixion

12.12 Other iridotomy
Corectomy
Discission of iris
Iridotomy NOS

12.13 Excision of prolapsed iris

12.14 Other iridectomy
iridectomy (basal) (peripheral) (total)

12.2 Diagnostic procedures on iris, ciliary body, sclera, and anterior chamber

12.21 Diagnostic aspiration of anterior chamber of eye

12.22 Biopsy of iris

12.29 Other diagnostic procedures on iris, ciliary body, sclera, and anterior chamber

12.3 Iridoplasty and coreoplasty

12.31 Lysis of goniosynechiae
Lysis of goniosynechiae by injection of air or liquid

12.32 Lysis of other anterior synechiae
Lysis of anterior synechiae:
NOS
by injection of air or liquid

12.33 Lysis of posterior synechiae
Lysis of iris adhesions NOS

12.34 Lysis of corneovitreal adhesions

12.35 Coreoplasty
Needling of pupillary membrane

12.39 Other iridoplasty

12.4 Excision or destruction of lesion of iris and ciliary body

12.40 Removal of lesion of anterior segment of eye, not otherwise specified

12.41 Destruction of lesion of iris, nonexcisional
Destruction of lesion of iris by:
cauterization
cryotherapy
photocoagulation

12.42 Excision of lesion of iris

> Excludes: biopsy of iris (12.22)

12.43 Destruction of lesion of ciliary body, nonexcisional

12.44 Excision of lesion of ciliary body

12.5 Facilitation of intraocular circulation

12.51 Goniopuncture without goniotomy

	Valid O.R. procedure		Non-O.R. procedure		Nonspecific O.R. procedure		Noncovered O.R. procedure

12.52 Goniotomy without goniopuncture

12.53 Goniotomy with goniopuncture

12.54 Trabeculotomy ab externo

12.55 Cyclodialysis

12.59 Other facilitation of intraocular circulation

12.6 Scleral fistulization

  Excludes: *exploratory sclerotomy (12.89)*

12.61 Trephination of sclera with iridectomy

12.62 Thermocauterization of sclera with iridectomy

12.63 Iridencleisis and iridotasis

12.64 Trabeculectomy ab externo

12.65 Other scleral fistulization with iridectomy

12.66 Postoperative revision of scleral fistulization procedure
Revision of filtering bleb

  Excludes: *repair of fistula (12.82)*

● 12.67 Insertion of aqueous drainage device
Anterior chamber drainage device
Aqueous drainage shunt or stent
Eye valve implant
Filtration canal shunt or device

12.69 Other fistulizing procedure

12.7 Other procedures for relief of elevated intraocular pressure

12.71 Cyclodiathermy

12.72 Cyclocryotherapy

12.73 Cyclophotocoagulation

12.74 Diminution of ciliary body, not otherwise specified

12.79 Other glaucoma procedures

12.8 Operations on sclera

  Excludes: *those associated with:*
retinal reattachment (14.41-14.59)
scleral fistulization (12.61-12.69)

12.81 Suture of laceration of sclera
Suture of sclera with synchronous repair of conjunctiva

12.82 Repair of scleral fistula

  Excludes: *postoperative revision of scleral fistulization procedure (12.66)*

12.83 Revision of operative wound of anterior segment, not elsewhere classified

  Excludes: *postoperative revision of scleral fistulization procedure (12.66)*

12.84 Excision or destruction of lesion of sclera

12.85 Repair of scleral staphyloma with graft

12.86 Other repair of scleral staphyloma

12.87 Scleral reinforcement with graft

12.88 Other scleral reinforcement

12.89 Other operations on sclera
Exploratory sclerotomy

12.9 Other operations on iris, ciliary body, and anterior chamber

12.91 Therapeutic evacuation of anterior chamber
Paracentesis of anterior chamber

  Excludes: *diagnostic aspiration (12.21)*

12.92 Injection into anterior chamber
Injection of:
air into anterior chamber
liquid into anterior chamber
medication into anterior chamber

● Code new to 2012 edition   ▲ Revision of existing code   ④ ⑤ Fourth or fifth digit required

12.93 **Removal or destruction of epithelial downgrowth from anterior chamber**
Excludes: *that with iridectomy (12.41-12.42)*

12.97 **Other operations on iris**

12.98 **Other operations on ciliary body**

12.99 **Other operations on anterior chamber**

13 **Operations on lens**

13.0 **Removal of foreign body from lens**
Excludes: *removal of pseudophakos (13.8)*

13.00 **Removal of foreign body from lens, not otherwise specified**

13.01 **Removal of foreign body from lens with use of magnet**

13.02 **Removal of foreign body from lens without use of magnet**

13.1 **Intracapsular extraction of lens**
Code also any synchronous insertion of pseudophakos (13.71)

13.11 **Intracapsular extraction of lens by temporal inferior route**

13.19 **Other intracapsular extraction of lens**
Cataract extraction NOS
Cryoextraction of lens
Erysiphake extraction of cataract
Extraction of lens NOS

13.2 **Extracapsular extraction of lens by linear extraction technique**
Code also any synchronous insertion of pseudophakos (13.71)

13.3 **Extracapsular extraction of lens by simple aspiration (and irrigation) technique**
Irrigation of traumatic cataract
Code also any synchronous insertion of pseudophakos (13.71)

13.4 **Extracapsular extraction of lens by fragmentation and aspiration technique**
Code also any synchronous insertion of pseudophakos (13.71)

13.41 **Phacoemulsification and aspiration of cataract**

13.42 **Mechanical phacofragmentation and aspiration of cataract by posterior route**
Code also any synchronous vitrectomy (14.74)

13.43 **Mechanical phacofragmentation and other aspiration of cataract**

13.5 **Other extracapsular extraction of lens**
Code also any synchronous insertion of pseudophakos (13.71)

13.51 **Extracapsular extraction of lens by temporal inferior route**

13.59 **Other extracapsular extraction of lens**

13.6 **Other cataract extraction**
Code also any synchronous insertion of pseudophakos (13.71)

13.64 **Discission of secondary membrane [after cataract]**

13.65 **Excision of secondary membrane [after cataract]**
Capsulectomy

13.66 **Mechanical fragmentation of secondary membrane [after cataract]**

13.69 **Other cataract extraction**

13.7 **Insertion of prosthetic lens [pseudophakos]**
Excludes: *implantation of intraocular telescope prosthesis (13.91)*

13.70 **Insertion of pseudophakos, not otherwise specified**

13.71 **Insertion of intraocular lens prosthesis at time of cataract extraction, one-stage**
Code also synchronous extraction of cataract (13.11-13.69)

13.72 **Secondary insertion of intraocular lens prosthesis**

13.8 **Removal of implanted lens**
Removal of pseudophakos

13.9 **Other operations on lens**

13.90 **Operation on lens, not elsewhere classified (NEC)**

13.91 **Implantation of intraocular telescope prosthesis**
Includes: removal of lens, any method
Implantable miniature telescope
Excludes: *secondary insertion of ocular implant (16.61)*

| | Valid O.R. procedure | | Non-O.R. procedure | | Nonspecific O.R. procedure | | Noncovered O.R. procedure |

14   Operations on retina, choroid, vitreous, and posterior chamber

   14.0   Removal of foreign body from posterior segment of eye

      Excludes: *removal of surgically implanted material (14.6)*

     14.00 Removal of foreign body from posterior segment of eye, not otherwise specified

     14.01 Removal of foreign body from posterior segment of eye with use of magnet

     14.02 Removal of foreign body from posterior segment of eye without use of magnet

   14.1   Diagnostic procedures on retina, choroid, vitreous, and posterior chamber

     14.11 Diagnostic aspiration of vitreous

     14.19 Other diagnostic procedures on retina, choroid, vitreous, and posterior chamber

   14.2   Destruction of lesion of retina and choroid
      Includes: destruction of chorioretinopathy or isolated chorioretinal lesion

      Excludes: *that for repair of retina (14.31-14.59)*

     14.21 Destruction of chorioretinal lesion by diathermy

     14.22 Destruction of chorioretinal lesion by cryotherapy

     14.23 Destruction of chorioretinal lesion by xenon arc photocoagulation

     14.24 Destruction of chorioretinal lesion by laser photocoagulation

     14.25 Destruction of chorioretinal lesion by photocoagulation of unspecified type

     14.26 Destruction of chorioretinal lesion by radiation therapy

     14.27 Destruction of chorioretinal lesion by implantation of radiation source

     14.29 Other destruction of chorioretinal lesion
        Destruction of lesion of retina and choroid NOS

   14.3   Repair of retinal tear
      Includes: repair of retinal defect

      Excludes: *repair of retinal detachment (14.41-14.59)*

     14.31 Repair of retinal tear by diathermy

     14.32 Repair of retinal tear by cryotherapy

     14.33 Repair of retinal tear by xenon arc photocoagulation

     14.34 Repair of retinal tear by laser photocoagulation

     14.35 Repair of retinal tear by photocoagulation of unspecified type

     14.39 Other repair of retinal tear

   14.4   Repair of retinal detachment with scleral buckling and implant

     14.41 Scleral buckling with implant

     14.49 Other scleral buckling
        Scleral buckling with:
          air tamponade
          resection of sclera
          vitrectomy

   14.5   Other repair of retinal detachment
      Includes: that with drainage

     14.51 Repair of retinal detachment with diathermy

     14.52 Repair of retinal detachment with cryotherapy

     14.53 Repair of retinal detachment with xenon arc photocoagulation

     14.54 Repair of retinal detachment with laser photocoagulation

     14.55 Repair of retinal detachment with photocoagulation of unspecified type

     14.59 Other

   14.6   Removal of surgically implanted material from posterior segment of eye

   14.7   Operations on vitreous

     14.71 Removal of vitreous, anterior approach
        Open sky technique
        Removal of vitreous, anterior approach (with replacement)

     14.72 Other removal of vitreous
        Aspiration of vitreous by posterior sclerotomy

     14.73 Mechanical vitrectomy by anterior approach

     14.74 Other mechanical vitrectomy
        Posterior approach

  ● Code new   ▲ Revision of   ④ ⑤ Fourth or fifth
             to 2012 edition   existing code   digit required

14.75 Injection of vitreous substitute

> *Excludes:* *that associated with removal (14.71-14.72)*

14.79 Other operations on vitreous

14.9 Other operations on retina, choroid, and posterior chamber

15 Operations on extraocular muscles

15.0 Diagnostic procedures on extraocular muscles or tendons

15.01 Biopsy of extraocular muscle or tendon

15.09 Other diagnostic procedures on extraocular muscles and tendons

15.1 Operations on one extraocular muscle involving temporary detachment from globe

15.11 Recession of one extraocular muscle

15.12 Advancement of one extraocular muscle

15.13 Resection of one extraocular muscle

15.19 Other operations on one extraocular muscle involving temporary detachment from globe

> *Excludes:* *transposition of muscle (15.5)*

15.2 Other operations on one extraocular muscle

15.21 Lengthening procedure on one extraocular muscle

15.22 Shortening procedure on one extraocular muscle

15.29 Other

15.3 Operations on two or more extraocular muscles involving temporary detachment from globe, one or both eyes

15.4 Other operations on two or more extraocular muscles, one or both eyes

15.5 Transposition of extraocular muscles

> *Excludes:* *that for correction of ptosis (08.31-08.36)*

15.6 Revision of extraocular muscle surgery

15.7 Repair of injury of extraocular muscle
Freeing of entrapped extraocular muscle
Lysis of adhesions of extraocular muscle
Repair of laceration of extraocular muscle, tendon, or Tenon's capsule

15.9 Other operations on extraocular muscles and tendon

16 Operations on orbit and eyeball

> *Excludes:* *reduction of fracture of orbit (76.78-76.79)*

16.0 Orbitotomy

16.01 Orbitotomy with bone flap
Orbitotomy with lateral approach

16.02 Orbitotomy with insertion of orbital implant

> *Excludes:* *that with bone flap (16.01)*

16.09 Other orbitotomy

16.1 Removal of penetrating foreign body from eye, not otherwise specified

> *Excludes:* *removal of nonpenetrating foreign body (98.21)*

16.2 Diagnostic procedures on orbit and eyeball

16.21 Ophthalmoscopy

16.22 Diagnostic aspiration of orbit

16.23 Biopsy of eyeball and orbit

16.29 Other diagnostic procedures on orbit and eyeball

> *Excludes:* *examination of form and structure of eye (95.11-95.16)*
> *general and subjective eye examination (95.01-95.09)*
> *microscopic examination of specimen from eye (90.21-90.29)*
> *objective functional tests of eye (95.21-95.26)*
> *ocular thermography (88.82)*
> *tonometry (89.11)*
> *X-ray of orbit (87.14, 87.16)*

16.3 Evisceration of eyeball

16.31 Removal of ocular contents with synchronous implant into scleral shell

 Valid O.R. procedure   Non-O.R. procedure   Nonspecific O.R. procedure   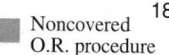 Noncovered O.R. procedure

| | 16.39 | Other evisceration of eyeball |

16.4 **Enucleation of eyeball**

| | 16.41 | Enucleation of eyeball with synchronous implant into Tenon's capsule with attachment of muscles |

Integrated implant of eyeball

| | 16.42 | Enucleation of eyeball with other synchronous implant |

| | 16.49 | Other enucleation of eyeball |

Removal of eyeball NOS

16.5 **Exenteration of orbital contents**

| | 16.51 | Exenteration of orbit with removal of adjacent structures |

Radical orbitomaxillectomy

| | 16.52 | Exenteration of orbit with therapeutic removal of orbital bone |

| | 16.59 | Other exenteration of orbit |

Evisceration of orbit NOS
Exenteration of orbit with temporalis muscle transplant

16.6 **Secondary procedures after removal of eyeball**

Excludes: *that with synchronous:*
enucleation of eyeball (16.41-16.42)
evisceration of eyeball (16.31)

| | 16.61 | Secondary insertion of ocular implant |

| | 16.62 | Revision and reinsertion of ocular implant |

| | 16.63 | Revision of enucleation socket with graft |

| | 16.64 | Other revision of enucleation socket |

| | 16.65 | Secondary graft to exenteration cavity |

| | 16.66 | Other revision of exenteration cavity |

| | 16.69 | Other secondary procedures after removal of eyeball |

16.7 **Removal of ocular or orbital implant**

| | 16.71 | Removal of ocular implant |

| | 16.72 | Removal of orbital implant |

16.8 **Repair of injury of eyeball and orbit**

| | 16.81 | Repair of wound of orbit |

Excludes: *reduction of orbital fracture (76.78-76.79)*
repair of extraocular muscles (15.7)

| | 16.82 | Repair of rupture of eyeball |

Repair of multiple structures of eye

Excludes: *repair of laceration of:*
cornea (11.51-11.59)
sclera (12.81)

| | 16.89 | Other repair of injury of eyeball or orbit |

16.9 **Other operations on orbit and eyeball**

Excludes: *irrigation of eye (96.51)*
prescription and fitting of low vision aids (95.31-95.33)
removal of:
eye prosthesis NEC (97.31)
nonpenetrating foreign body from eye without incision (98.21)

| | 16.91 | Retrobulbar injection of therapeutic agent |

Excludes: *injection of radiographic contrast material (87.14)*
opticociliary injection (12.79)

| | 16.92 | Excision of lesion of orbit |

Excludes: *biopsy of orbit (16.23)*

| | 16.93 | Excision of lesion of eye, unspecified structure |

Excludes: *biopsy of eye NOS (16.23)*

| | 16.98 | Other operations on orbit |

| | 16.99 | Other operations on eyeball |

● Code new to 2012 edition   ▲ Revision of existing code   ④ ⑤ Fourth or fifth digit required

3A   OTHER MISCELLANEOUS DIAGNOSTIC AND THERAPEUTIC PROCEDURES (17)

17   Other miscellaneous procedures

17.1   Laparoscopic unilateral repair of inguinal hernia

| Excludes: | *other and open unilateral repair of hernia (53.00-53.05)* |

> **17.11   Laparoscopic repair of direct inguinal hernia with graft or prosthesis**
> Laparoscopic repair of direct and indirect inguinal hernia with graft or prosthesis

> **17.12   Laparoscopic repair of indirect inguinal hernia with graft or prosthesis**

> **17.13   Laparoscopic repair of inguinal hernia with graft or prosthesis, not otherwise specified**

17.2   Laparoscopic bilateral repair of inguinal hernia

| Excludes: | *other and open bilateral repair of hernia (53.10-53.17)* |

> **17.21   Laparoscopic bilateral repair of direct inguinal hernia with graft or prosthesis**

> **17.22   Laparoscopic bilateral repair of indirect inguinal hernia with graft or prosthesis**

> **17.23   Laparoscopic bilateral repair of inguinal hernia, one direct and one indirect, with graft or prosthesis**

> **17.24   Laparoscopic bilateral repair of inguinal hernia with graft or prosthesis, not otherwise specified**

17.3   Laparoscopic partial excision of large intestine

| Excludes: | *other and open partial excision of large intestine (45.71-45.79)* |

> **17.31   Laparoscopic multiple segmental resection of large intestine**

> **17.32   Laparoscopic cecectomy**

> **17.33   Laparoscopic right hemicolectomy**

> **17.34   Laparoscopic resection of transverse colon**

> **17.35   Laparoscopic left hemicolectomy**

> **17.36   Laparoscopic sigmoidectomy**

> **17.39   Other laparoscopic partial excision of large intestine**

17.4   Robotic assisted procedures
Computer assisted robotic surgery
Computer-enhanced robotic surgery
Robotic procedure with computer assistance
Surgeon-controlled robotic surgery

Code first primary procedure

| Excludes: | *computer assisted surgery (00.31-00.35, 00.39)* |

Note: This category includes use of a computer console with (3-D) imaging, software, camera(s), visualization and instrumentation *combined* with use of robotic arms, device(s), or system(s) at the time of the procedure

> **17.41   Open robotic assisted procedure**
> Robotic assistance in open procedure

> **17.42   Laparoscopic robotic assisted procedure**
> Robotic assistance in laparoscopic procedure

> **17.43   Percutaneous robotic assisted procedure**
> Robotic assistance in percutaneous procedure

> **17.44   Endoscopic robotic assisted procedure**
> Robotic assistance in endoscopic procedure

> **17.45   Thoracoscopic robotic assisted procedure**
> Robotic assistance in thoracoscopic procedure

> **17.49   Other and unspecified robotic assisted procedure**
> Robotic assistance in other and unspecified procedure
>
> | Excludes: | *endoscopic robotic assisted procedure (17.44)* |
> | | *laparoscopic robotic assisted procedure (17.42)* |
> | | *open robotic assisted procedure (17.41)* |
> | | *percutaneous robotic assisted procedure (17.43)* |
> | | *thoracoscopic robotic assisted procedure (17.45)* |

| | Valid O.R. procedure | | Non-O.R. procedure | | Nonspecific O.R. procedure | | Noncovered O.R. procedure |

17.5 **Additional cardiovascular procedures**

17.51 **Implantation of rechargeable cardiac contractility modulation [CCM], total system**

Note: Device testing during procedure – omit code

Implantation of CCM system includes formation of pocket, transvenous leads, including placement of leads, placement of catheter into left ventricle, intraoperative procedures for evaluation of lead signals, obtaining sensing threshold measurements, obtaining defibrillator threshold measurements. Includes implantation of device with removal of existing device

Code also any concomitant:
coronary bypass (36.10 – 36.19)
extracorporeal circulation (39.61)
insertion or replacement of automatic cardioverter/defibrillator, total system [AICD] (37.94)

Excludes:	*implantation of CCM pulse generator only (17.52)*

17.52 **Implantation or replacement of cardiac contractility modulation [CCM] rechargeable pulse generator only**

Note: Device testing during procedure – omit code

Implantation of CCM device with removal of any existing CCM device

Code also any concomitant:
revision of device pocket (37.79)
revision of lead [electrode] (37.75)

● **17.53** **Percutaneous arherectomy of extracranial vessel(s)**
Directional atherectomy
Excimer laser atherectomy
Rotational atherectomy
That by laser
That by transluminal extraction

Code also any:
injection or infusion of thrombolytic agent (99.10)
number of vascular stents inserted (00.45-00.48)
number of vessels treated (00.40-00.43)
percutaneous insertion of carotid artery stent(s) (00.63)
percutaneous insertion of other extracranial artery stent(s) (00.64)
procedure on vessel bifurcation (00.44)

Excludes:	*angioplasty of other non-coronary vessel(s) (39.50)*
	atherectomy of intracranial vessel(s) (17.54)
	atherectomy of other non-coronary vessel(s) (17.56)
	removal of cerebrovascular obstruction of vessel(s) by open approach (38.01-38.02, 38.11-38.12, 38.31-38.32, 38.41-38.42)

● **17.54** **Percutaneous atherectomy of intracranial vessel(s)**
Directional atherectomy
Excimer laser atherectomy
Rotational atherectomy
That by laser
That by transluminal extraction

Code also any:
injection or infusion of thrombolytic agent (99.10)
number of vascular stents inserted (00.45-00.48)
number of vessels treated (00.40-00.43)
percutaneous insertion of intracranial vascular stent(s) (00.65)
procedure on vessel bifurcation (00.44)

Excludes:	*angioplasty of other non-coronary vessel(s) (39.50)*
	atherectomy of extracranial vessel(s) (17.53)
	atherectomy of other non-coronary vessel(s) (17.56)
	removal of cerebrovascular obstruction of vessel(s) by open approach (38.01-38.02, 38.11-38.12, 38.31-38.32, 38.41-38.42)

● Code new to 2012 edition   ▲ Revision of existing code   ④ ⑤ Fourth or fifth digit required

- **17.55 Transluminal coronary atherectomy**
  Directional atherectomy
  Excimer laser atherectomy
  Rotational atherectomy
  That by laser
  That by percutaneous approach
  That by transluminal extraction

  Code also any:
  injection or infusion of thrombolytic agent (99.10)
  insertion of coronary artery stent (36.06-36.07)
  intracoronary artery thrombolytic infusion (36.04)
  number of vascular stents inserted (00.45-00.48)
  number of vessels treated (00.40-00.43)
  procedure on vessel bifurcation (00.44)
  SuperSaturated oxygen therapy (00.49)
  transluminal coronary angioplasty (00.66)

- **17.56 Atherectomy of other non-coronary vessel(s)**
  Percutaneous transluminal atherectomy of:
    lower extremity vessels
    mesenteric artery
    renal artery
    upper extremity vessels
  Includes:
    Directional atherectomy
    Excimer laser atherectomy
    Rotational atherectomy
    That by laser
    That by transluminal extraction

  Code also any:
  injection or infusion of thrombolytic agent (99.10)
  insertion of drug-eluting peripheral vessel stent (00.55)
  insertion of non-drug-eluting peripheral vessel stent(s) or stent graft(s) (39.90)
  number of vascular stents inserted (00.45-00.48)
  number of vessels treated (00.40-00.43)
  procedure on vessel bifurcation (00.44)

Excludes:	*percutaneous angioplasty of extracranial or intracranial vessel(s)*

  percutaneous angioplasty of extracranial or intracranial vessel(s) (00.61-00.62)
  percutaneous angioplasty of other non-coronary vessel(s) (39.50)
  percutaneous atherectomy of extracranial vessel(s) (17.53)
  percutaneous atherectomy of intracranial vessel(s) (17.54)

17.6   Laser interstitial thermal therapy [LITT] under guidance
Focused laser interstitial thermal therapy [f-LITT] under MRI guidance
MRI-guided LITT

17.61 Laser interstitial thermal therapy [LITT] of lesion or tissue of brain under guidance
Focused laser interstitial thermal therapy [f-LITT] under MRI guidance
MRI-guided LITT of lesion or tissue of brain

Excludes:	*laser interstitial thermal therapy [LITT] of lesion or tissue of head under guidance (17.62)*

17.62 Laser interstitial thermal therapy [LITT] of lesion or tissue of head and neck under guidance
Focused laser interstitial thermal therapy [f-LITT] under MRI guidance
MRI-guided LITT of lesion or tissue of head and neck

Excludes:	*laser interstitial thermal therapy [LITT] of lesion or tissue of brain under guidance (17.61)*

17.63 Laser interstitial thermal therapy [LITT] of lesion or tissue of liver under guidance
Focused laser interstitial thermal therapy [f-LITT] under MRI guidance
MRI-guided LITT of lesion or tissue of liver

17.69 **Laser interstitial thermal therapy [LITT] of lesion or tissue of other and unspecified site under guidance**

Focused laser interstitial thermal therapy [f-LITT] under MRI guidance

MRI-guided LITT of lesion or tissue of breast

MRI-guided LITT of lesion or tissue of lung

MRI-guided LITT of lesion or tissue of prostate

Excludes: *laser interstitial thermal therapy [LITT] of lesion or tissue of brain under guidance (17.61)*

laser interstitial thermal therapy [LITT] of lesion or tissue of head and neck under guidance (17.62)

laser interstitial thermal therapy [LITT] of lesion or tissue of liver under guidance (17.63)

17.7 **Other diagnostic and therapeutic procedures**

17.70 **Intravenous infusion of clofarabine**

Excludes: *injection or infusion of cancer chemotherapeutic substance (99.25)*

17.71 **Non-coronary intra-operative fluorescence vascular angiography [IFVA]**

Intraoperative laser arteriogram

SPY arteriogram

SPY arteriography

Excludes: *intra-operative coronary fluorescence vascular angiography (88.59)*

● **17.8** **Other adjunct procedures**

Note: These codes are to be used in conjunction with other therapeutic procedure codes to provide additional information on devices used as part of a procedure.

● **17.81** **Insertion of antimicrobial envelope**

Use of anti-microbial (mesh) (prophylactic antibiotics embedded) envelope with the insertion of cardiovascular implantable electronic devices (CIED)

Code first primary procedure:

Insertion of cardiovascular implantable electronic device(s) [CIED] (00.51, 00.53, 00.54, 37.94, 37.96, 37.98)

● Code new
to 2012 edition
▲ Revision of
existing code
④ ⑤ Fourth or fifth
digit required

4.   OPERATIONS ON THE EAR (18-20)

18   Operations on external ear
Includes: operations on:
external auditory canal
skin and cartilage of:
auricle
meatus

18.0   Incision of external ear

> Excludes: *removal of intraluminal foreign body (98.11)*

18.01   Piercing of ear lobe
Piercing of pinna

18.02   Incision of external auditory canal

18.09   Other incision of external ear

18.1   Diagnostic procedures on external ear

18.11   Otoscopy

18.12   Biopsy of external ear

18.19   Other diagnostic procedures on external ear

> Excludes: *microscopic examination of specimen from ear (90.31-90.39)*

18.2   Excision or destruction of lesion of external ear

18.21   Excision of preauricular sinus
Radical excision of preauricular sinus or cyst

> Excludes: *excision of preauricular remnant [appendage] (18.29)*

18.29   Excision or destruction of other lesion of external ear
Cauterization of external ear
Coagulation of external ear
Cryosurgery of external ear
Curettage of external ear
Electrocoagulation of external ear
Enucleation of external ear
Excision of:
exostosis of external auditory canal
preauricular remnant [appendage]
Partial excision of ear

> Excludes: *biopsy of external ear (18.12)*
> *radical excision of lesion (18.31)*
> *removal of cerumen (96.52)*

18.3   Other excision of external ear

> Excludes: *biopsy of external ear (18.12)*

18.31   Radical excision of lesion of external ear

> Excludes: *radical excision of preauricular sinus (18.21)*

18.39   Other
Amputation of external ear

> Excludes: *excision of lesion (18.21-18.29, 18.31)*

18.4   Suture of laceration of external ear

18.5   Surgical correction of prominent ear
Ear:
pinning
setback

18.6   Reconstruction of external auditory canal
Canaloplasty of external auditory meatus
Construction [reconstruction] of external meatus of ear:
osseous portion
skin-lined portion (with skin graft)

18.7   Other plastic repair of external ear

18.71   Construction of auricle of ear
Prosthetic appliance for absent ear
Reconstruction:
auricle
ear

| Valid O.R. procedure | Non-O.R. procedure | Nonspecific O.R. procedure | Noncovered O.R. procedure |

18.72 Reattachment of amputated ear

18.79 Other plastic repair of external ear
Otoplasty NOS
Postauricular skin graft
Repair of lop ear

18.9 Other operations on external ear

[Excludes:] *irrigation of ear (96.52)*
packing of external auditory canal (96.11)
removal of:
cerumen (96.52)
foreign body (without incision) (98.11)

19 Reconstructive operations on middle ear

19.0 Stapes mobilization
Division, otosclerotic:
material
process
Remobilization of stapes
Stapediolysis
Transcrural stapes mobilization

[Excludes:] *that with synchronous stapedectomy (19.11-19.19)*

19.1 Stapedectomy

[Excludes:] *revision of previous stapedectomy (19.21-19.29)*
stapes mobilization only (19.0)

19.11 Stapedectomy with incus replacement
Stapedectomy with incus:
homograft
prosthesis

19.19 Other stapedectomy

19.2 Revision of stapedectomy

19.21 Revision of stapedectomy with incus replacement

19.29 Other revision of stapedectomy

19.3 Other operations on ossicular chain
Incudectomy NOS
Ossiculectomy NOS
Reconstruction of ossicles, second stage

19.4 Myringoplasty
Epitympanic, type I
Myringoplasty by:
cauterization
graft
Tympanoplasty (type I)

19.5 Other tympanoplasty

19.52 Type II tympanoplasty
Closure of perforation with graft against incus or malleus

19.53 Type III tympanoplasty
Graft placed in contact with mobile and intact stapes

19.54 Type IV tympanoplasty
Mobile footplate left exposed with air pocket between round window and graft

19.55 Type V tympanoplasty
Fenestra in horizontal semicircular canal covered by graft

19.6 Revision of tympanoplasty

19.9 Other repair of middle ear
Closure of mastoid fistula
Mastoid myoplasty
Obliteration of tympanomastoid cavity

20 Other operations on middle and inner ear

20.0 Myringotomy

20.01 Myringotomy with insertion of tube
Myringostomy

20.09 Other myringotomy
Aspiration of middle ear NOS

20.1 Removal of tympanostomy tube

20.2 Incision of mastoid and middle ear

20.21 Incision of mastoid

20.22 Incision of petrous pyramid air cells

20.23 Incision of middle ear
Atticotomy
Division of tympanum
Lysis of adhesions of middle car

> Excludes: *divisions of otosclerotic process (19.0)*
> *stapediolysis (19.0)*
> *that with stapedectomy (19.11-19.19)*

20.3 Diagnostic procedures on middle and inner ear

20.31 Electrocochleography

20.32 Biopsy of middle and inner ear

20.39 Other diagnostic procedures on middle and inner ear

> Excludes: *auditory and vestibular function tests (89.13, 95.41-95.49)*
> *microscopic examination of specimen from ear (90.31-90.39)*

20.4 Mastoidectomy
Code also any:
skin graft (18.79)
tympanoplasty (19.4-19.55)

> Excludes: *that with implantation of cochlear prosthetic device (20.96-20.98)*

20.41 Simple mastoidectomy

20.42 Radical mastoidectomy

20.49 Other mastoidectomy
Atticoantrotomy
Mastoidectomy:
  NOS
  modified radical

20.5 Other excision of middle ear

> Excludes: *that with synchronous mastoidectomy (20.41-20.49)*

20.51 Excision of lesion of middle ear

> Excludes: *biopsy of middle ear (20.32)*

20.59 Other
Apicectomy of petrous pyramid
Tympanectomy

20.6 Fenestration of inner ear

20.61 Fenestration of inner ear (initial)
Fenestration of labyrinth with graft (skin) (vein)
Fenestration of semicircular canals with graft (skin) (vein)
Fenenstration of vestibule with graft (skin) (vein)

> Excludes: *that with tympanoplasty type V (19.55)*

20.62 Revision of fenestration of inner ear

20.7 Incision, excision, and destruction of inner ear

20.71 Endolymphatic shunt

20.72 Injection into inner ear
Destruction by injection (alcohol):
  inner ear
  semicircular canals
  vestibule

20.79 Other incision, excision and destruction of inner ear
Decompression of labyrinth
Drainage of inner ear
Fistulization:
  endolymphatic sac
  labyrinth
Incision of endolymphatic sac
Labyrinthectomy (transtympanic)
Opening of bony labyrinth
Perilymphatic tap

> Excludes: *biopsy of inner ear (20.32)*

	Valid O.R. procedure		Non-O.R. procedure		Nonspecific O.R. procedure		Noncovered O.R. procedure

20.8 **Operations on Eustachian tube**
Catheterization of Eustachian tube
Inflation of Eustachian tube
Injection (Teflon paste) of Eustachian tube
Insufflation (boric acid-salicylic acid) of Eustachian tube
Intubation of Eustachian tube
Politzerization of Eustachian tube

20.9 **Other operations on inner and middle ear**

20.91 **Tympanosympathectomy**

20.92 **Revision of mastoidectomy**

20.93 **Repair of oval and round windows**
Closure of fistula:
oval window
perilymph
round window

20.94 **Injection of tympanum**

20.95 **Implantation of electromagnetic bearing device**
Bone conduction hearing device

Excludes: *cochlear prosthetic device (20.96-20.98)*

20.96 **Implantation or replacement of cochlear prosthetic device, not otherwise specified**
Implantation of receiver (within skull) and insertion of electrode(s) in the cochlea
Includes: mastoidectomy

Excludes: *electromagnetic hearing device (20.95)*

20.97 **Implantation or replacement of cochlear prosthetic device, single channel**
Implantation of receiver (within skull) and insertion of electrode in the cochlea
Includes: mastoidectomy

Excludes: *electromagnetic hearing device (20.95)*

20.98 **Implantation or replacement of cochlear prosthetic device, multiple channel**
Implantation of receiver (within skull) and insertion of electrodes in the cochlea
Includes: mastoidectomy

Excludes: *electromagnetic hearing device (20.95)*

20.99 **Other operations on middle and inner ear**
Attachment of percutaneous abutment (screw) for prosthetic device
Repair or removal of cochlear prosthetic device (receiver) (electrode)

Excludes: *adjustment (external components) of cochlear prosthetic device (95.49)*
fitting of hearing aid (95.48)

● Code new
  to 2012 edition
▲ Revision of
  existing code
④ ⑤ Fourth or fifth
  digit required

5. OPERATIONS ON THE NOSE, MOUTH, AND PHARYNX (21-29)

21 Operation on nose

Includes: operations on:
bone of nose
skin of nose

21.0 Control of epistaxis

21.00 Control of epistaxis, not otherwise specified

21.01 Control of epistaxis by anterior nasal packing

21.02 Control of epistaxis by posterior (and anterior) packing

21.03 Control of epistaxis by cauterization (and packing)

21.04 Control of epistaxis by ligation of ethmoidal arteries

21.05 Control of epistaxis by (transantral) ligation of the maxillary artery

21.06 Control of epistaxis by ligation of the external carotid artery

21.07 Control of epistaxis by excision of nasal mucosa and skin grafting on septum and lateral nasal wall

21.09 Control of epistaxis by other means

21.1 Incision of nose

Chondrotomy
Incision of skin of nose
Nasal septotomy

21.2 Diagnostic procedures on nose

21.21 Rhinoscopy

21.22 Biopsy of nose

21.29 Other diagnostic procedures on nose

Excludes: *microscopic examination of specimen from nose (90.31-90.39)*
nasal:
function study (89.12)
x-ray (87.16)
rhinomanometry (89.12)

21.3 Local excision or destruction of lesion of nose

Excludes: *biopsy of nose (21.22)*
nasal fistulectomy (21.82)

21.30 Excision or destruction of nose, not otherwise specified

21.31 Local excision or destruction of intranasal lesion
Nasal polypectomy

21.32 Local excision or destruction of other lesion of nose

21.4 Resection of nose
Amputation of nose

21.5 Submucous resection of nasal septum

21.6 Turbinectomy

21.61 Turbinectomy by diathermy or cryosurgery

21.62 Fracture of the turbinates

21.69 Other turbinectomy

Excludes: *turbinectomy associated with sinusectomy (22.31-22.39, 22.42, 22.60-22.64)*

21.7 Reduction of nasal fracture

21.71 Closed reduction of nasal fracture

21.72 Open reduction of nasal fracture

21.8 Repair and plastic operations on the nose

21.81 Suture of laceration of nose

21.82 Closure of nasal fistula
Nasolabial fistulectomy
Nasopharyngeal fistulectomy
Oronasal fistulectomy

	Valid O.R. procedure		Non-O.R. procedure		Nonspecific O.R. procedure		Noncovered O.R. procedure

21.83 **Total nasal reconstruction**
Reconstruction of nose with:
  arm flap
  forehead flap

21.84 **Revision rhinoplasty**
Rhinoseptoplasty
Twisted nose rhinoplasty

21.85 **Augmentation rhinoplasty**
Augmentation rhinoplasty with:
  graft
  synthetic implant

21.86 **Limited rhinoplasty**
Plastic repair of nasolabial flaps
Tip rhinoplasty

21.87 **Other rhinoplasty**
Rhinoplasty NOS

21.88 **Other septoplasty**
Crushing of nasal septum
Repair of septal perforation

> | Excludes: | *septoplasty associated with submucous resection of septum (21.5)*

21.89 **Other repair and plastic operations on nose**
Reattachment of amputated nose

21.9 **Other operations on nose**

21.91 **Lysis of adhesions of nose**
Posterior nasal scrub

21.99 **Other**

> | Excludes: | *dilation of frontonasal duct (96.21)*
> *irrigation of nasal passages (96.53)*
> *removal of:*
>   *intraluminal foreign body without incision (98.12)*
>   *nasal packing (97.32)*
> *replacement of nasal packing (97.21)*

22 **Operations on nasal sinuses**

22.0 **Aspiration and lavage of nasal sinus**

22.00 **Aspiration and lavage of nasal sinus, not otherwise specified**

22.01 **Puncture of nasal sinus for aspiration or lavage**

22.02 **Aspiration or lavage of nasal sinus through natural ostium**

22.1 **Diagnostic procedures on nasal sinus**

22.11 **Closed [endoscopic] [needle] biopsy of nasal sinus**

22.12 **Open biopsy of nasal sinus**

22.19 **Other diagnostic procedures on nasal sinuses**
Endoscopy without biopsy

> | Excludes: | *transillumination of sinus (89.35)*
> *x-ray of sinus (87.15-87.16)*

22.2 **Intranasal antrotomy**

> | Excludes: | *antrotomy with external approach (22.31-22.39)*

22.3 **External maxillary antrotomy**

22.31 **Radical maxillary antrotomy**
Removal of lining membrane of maxillary sinus using Caldwell-Luc approach

22.39 **Other external maxillary antrotomy**
Exploration of maxillary antrum with Caldwell-Luc approach

22.4 **Frontal sinusotomy and sinusectomy**

22.41 **Frontal sinusotomy**

22.42 **Frontal sinusectomy**
Excision of lesion of frontal sinus
Obliteration of frontal sinus (with fat)

> | Excludes: | *biopsy of nasal sinus (22.11-22.12)*

22.5   Other nasal sinusotomy

    22.50   Sinusotomy, not otherwise specified

    22.51   Ethmoidotomy

    22.52   Sphenoidotomy

    22.53   Incision of multiple nasal sinuses

22.6   Other nasal sinusectomy
    Includes: that with incidental turbinectomy

    | Excludes: | biopsy of nasal sinus (22.11-22.12)

    22.60   Sinusectomy, not otherwise specified

    22.61   Excision of lesion of maxillary sinus with Caldwell-Luc approach

    22.62   Excision of lesion of maxillary sinus with other approach

    22.63   Ethmoidectomy

    22.64   Sphenoidectomy

22.7   Repair of nasal sinus

    22.71   Closure of nasal sinus fist
        Repair of oro-antral fistula

    22.79   Other repair of nasal sinus
        Reconstruction of frontonasal duct
        Repair of bone of accessory sinus

22.9   Other operations on nasal sinuses
    Exteriorization of maxillary sinus
    Fistulization of sinus

    | Excludes: | dilation of frontonasal duct (96.21)

23   Removal and restoration of teeth

23.0   Forceps extraction of tooth

    23.01   Extraction of deciduous tooth

    23.09   Extraction of other tooth
        Extraction of tooth NOS

23.1   Surgical removal of tooth

    23.11   Removal of residual root

    23.19   Other surgical extraction of tooth
        Odontectomy NOS
        Removal of impacted tooth
        Tooth extraction with elevation of mucoperiosteal flap

23.2   Restoration of tooth by filling

23.3   Restoration of tooth by inlay

23.4   Other dental restoration

    23.41   Application of crown

    23.42   Insertion of fixed bridge

    23.43   Insertion of removable bridge

    23.49   Other

23.5   Implantation of tooth

23.6   Prosthetic dental implant
    Endosseous dental implant

23.7   Apicoectomy and root canal therapy

    23.70   Root canal not otherwise specified

    23.71   Root canal therapy with irrigation

    23.72   Root canal therapy with apicoectomy

    23.73   Apicoectomy

24   Other operations on teeth, gums, and alveoli

24.0   Incision of gum or alveolar bone
    Apical alveolotomy

24.1   Diagnostic procedures on teeth, gums, and alveoli

    24.11   Biopsy of gum

    24.12   Biopsy of alveoli

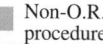 Valid O.R.
procedure

Non-O.R.
procedure

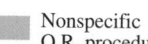 Nonspecific
O.R. procedure

Noncovered
O.R. procedure

24.19 Other diagnostic procedures on teeth, gums, and alveoli

> Excludes: *dental:*
> *examination (89.31)*
> *x-ray:*
> *full-mouth (87.11)*
> *other (87.12)*
> *microscopic examination of dental specimen (90.81-90.89)*

24.2 Gingivoplasty
Gingivoplasty with bone or soft tissue graft

24.3 Other operations on gum

24.31 Excision of lesion or tissue of gum

> Excludes: *biopsy of gum (24.11)*
> *excision of odontogenic lesion (24.4)*

24.32 Suture of laceration of gum

24.39 Other

24.4 Excision of dental lesion of jaw
Excision of odontogenic lesion

24.5 Alveoloplasty
Alveolectomy (interradicular) (intraseptal) (radical) (simple) (with graft or implant)

> Excludes: *biopsy of alveolus (24.12)*
> *en bloc resection of alveolar process and palate (27.32)*

24.6 Exposure of tooth

24.7 Application of orthodontic appliance
Application, insertion, or fitting of:
  arch bars
  orthodontic obturator
  orthodontic wiring
  periodontal splint

> Excludes: *nonorthodontic dental wiring (93.55)*

24.8 Other orthodontic operation
Closure of diastema (alveolar) (dental)
Occlusal adjustment
Removal of arch bars
Repair of dental arch

> Excludes: *removal of nonorthodontic wiring (97.33)*

24.9 Other dental operations

24.91 Extension or deepening of buccolabial or lingual sulcus

24.99 Other

> Excludes: *dental:*
> *debridement (96.54)*
> *examination (89.31)*
> *prophylaxis (96.54)*
> *scaling and polishing (96.54)*
> *wiring (93.55)*
> *fitting of dental appliance [denture] (99.97)*
> *microscopic examination of dental specimen (90.81-90.89)*
> *removal of dental:*
> *packing (97.34)*
> *prosthesis (97.35)*
> *wiring (97.33)*
> *replacement of dental packing (97.22)*

25 Operations on tongue

25.0 Diagnostic procedures on tongue

25.01 Closed [needle] biopsy of tongue

25.02 Open biopsy of tongue
Wedge biopsy

25.09 Other diagnostic procedures on tongue

● Code new to 2012 edition　　▲ Revision of existing code　　④ ⑤ Fourth or fifth digit required

25.1 **Excision or destruction of lesion or tissue of tongue**

> Excludes: *biopsy of tongue (25.01-25.02)*
> *frenumectomy:*
> *labial (27.41)*
> *lingual (25.92)*

25.2 **Partial glossectomy**

25.3 **Complete glossectomy**
Glossectomy NOS

Code also any neck dissection (40.40-40.42)

25.4 **Radical glossectomy**

> *Code also any:*
> neck dissection (40.40-40.42)
> tracheostomy (31.1-31.29)

25.5 **Repair of tongue and glossoplasty**

25.51 **Suture of laceration of tongue**

25.59 **Other repair and plastic operations on tongue**
Fascial sling of tongue
Fusion of tongue (to lip)
Graft of mucosa or skin to tongue

> Excludes: *lysis of adhesions of tongue (25.93)*

25.9 **Other operations on tongue**

25.91 **Lingual frenotomy**

> Excludes: *labial frenotomy (27.91)*

25.92 **Lingual frenectomy**

> Excludes: *labial frenectomy (27.41)*

25.93 **Lysis of adhesions of tongue**

25.94 **Other glossotomy**

25.99 **Other**

26 **Operations on salivary glands and ducts**
Includes: operations on:
lesser salivary gland and duct
parotid gland and duct
sublingual gland and duct
submaxillary gland and duct

Code also any neck dissection (40.40-40.42)

26.0 **Incision of salivary gland or duct**

26.1 **Diagnostic procedures on salivary glands and ducts**

26.11 **Closed [needle] biopsy of salivary gland or duct**

26.12 **Open biopsy of salivary gland or duct**

26.19 **Other diagnostic procedures on salivary glands and ducts**

> Excludes: *x-ray of salivary gland (87.09)*

26.2 **Excision of lesion of salivary gland**

26.21 **Marsupialization of salivary gland cyst**

26.29 **Other excision of salivary gland lesion**

> Excludes: *biopsy of salivary gland (26.11-26.12)*
> *salivary fistulectomy (26.42)*

26.3 **Sialoadenectomy**

26.30 **Sialoadenectomy, not otherwise specified**

26.31 **Partial sialoadenectomy**

26.32 **Complete sialoadenectomy**
En bloc excision of salivary gland lesion
Radical sialoadenectomy

26.4 **Repair of salivary gland or duct**

26.41 **Suture of laceration of salivary gland**

26.42 **Closure of salivary fistula**

| | Valid O.R. procedure | | Non-O.R. procedure | | Nonspecific O.R. procedure | | Noncovered O.R. procedure |

<table>
<tr><td>26.49</td><td colspan="2">Other repair and plastic operations on salivary gland or duct</td></tr>
</table>

26.49 **Other repair and plastic operations on salivary gland or duct**
Fistulization of salivary gland
Plastic repair of salivary gland or duct NOS
Transplantation of salivary duct opening

26.9 **Other operations on salivary gland or duct**

26.91 **Probing of salivary duct**

26.99 **Other**

27 **Other operations on mouth and face**
Includes: operations on:
lips
palate
soft tissue of face and mouth, except tongue and gingiva

Excludes operations on:
gingiva (24.0-24.99)
tongue (25.01-25.99)

27.0 **Drainage of face and floor of mouth**
Drainage of:
facial region (abscess)
fascial compartment of face
Ludwig's angina

Excludes: drainage of thyroglossal tract (06.09)

27.1 **Incision of palate**

27.2 **Diagnostic procedures on oral cavity**

27.21 **Biopsy of bony palate**

27.22 **Biopsy of uvula and soft palate**

27.23 **Biopsy of lip**

27.24 **Biopsy of mouth, unspecified structure**

27.29 **Other diagnostic procedures on oral cavity**

Excludes: soft tissue x-ray (87.09)

27.3 **Excision of lesion or tissue of bony palate**

27.31 **Local excision or destruction of lesion or tissue of bony palate**
Local excision or destruction of palate by:
cautery
chemotherapy
cryotherapy

Excludes: biopsy of bony palate (27.21)

27.32 **Wide excision or destruction of lesion or tissue of bony palate**
En bloc resection of alveolar process and palate

27.4 **Excision of other parts of mouth**

27.41 **Labial frenectomy**

Excludes: division of labial frenum (27.91)

27.42 **Wide excision of lesion of lip**

27.43 **Other excision of lesion or tissue of lip**

27.49 **Other excision of mouth**

Excludes: biopsy of mouth NOS (27.24)
excision of lesion of:
palate (27.31-27.32)
tongue (25.1)
uvula (27.72)
fistulectomy of mouth (27.53)
frenectomy of:
lip (27.41)
tongue (25.92)

27.5 **Plastic repair of lip and mouth**

Excludes: palatoplasty (27.61-27.69)

27.51 **Suture of laceration of lip**

27.52 **Suture of laceration of other part of mouth**

● Code new
to 2012 edition
▲ Revision of
existing code
④ ⑤ Fourth or fifth
digit required

27.53 Closure of fistula of mouth

> *Excludes:* fistulectomy:
> nasolabial (21.82)
> oro-antral (22.71)
> oronasal (21.82)

27.54 Repair of cleft lip

27.55 Full-thickness skin graft to lip and mouth

27.56 Other skin graft to lip and mouth

27.57 Attachment of pedicle or flap graft to lip and mouth

27.59 Other plastic repair of mouth

27.6 Palatoplasty

27.61 Suture of laceration of palate

27.62 Correction of cleft palate
Correction of cleft palate by push-back operation

> *Excludes:* revision of cleft palate repair (27.63)

27.63 Revision of cleft palate repair
Secondary:
attachment of pharyngeal flap
lengthening of palate

27.64 Insertion of palatal implant

27.69 Other plastic repair of palate
Code also any insertion of palatal implant (27.64)

> *Excludes:* fistulectomy of mouth (27.53)

27.7 Operations on uvula

27.71 Incision of uvula

27.72 Excision of uvula

> *Excludes:* biopsy of uvula (27.22)

27.73 Repair of uvula

> *Excludes:* that with synchronous cleft palate repair (27.62)
> uranostaphylorrhaphy (27.62)

27.79 Other operations on uvula

27.9 Other operations on mouth and face

27.91 Labial frenotomy
Division of labial frenum

> *Excludes:* lingual frenotomy (25.91)

27.92 Incision of mouth, unspecified structure

> *Excludes:* incision of:
> gum (24.0)
> palate (27.1)
> salivary gland or duct (26.0)
> tongue (25.94)
> uvula (27.71)

27.99 Other operations on oral cavity
Graft of buccal sulcus

> *Excludes:* removal of:
> intraluminal foreign body (98.01)
> penetrating foreign body from mouth without incision (98.22)

28 Operations on tonsils and adenoids

28.0 Incision and drainage of tonsil and peritonsillar structures
Drainage (oral) (transcervical) of:
parapharyngeal abscess
peritonsillar abscess
retropharyngeal abscess
tonsillar abscess

28.1 Diagnostic procedures on tonsils and adenoids

28.11 Biopsy of tonsils and adenoids

| | Valid O.R. procedure | | Non-O.R. procedure | | Nonspecific O.R. procedure | | Noncovered O.R. procedure |

28.19 Other diagnostic procedures on tonsils and adenoids

Excludes: soft tissue x-ray (87.09)

28.2 Tonsillectomy without adenoidectomy

28.3 Tonsillectomy with adenoidectomy

28.4 Excision of tonsil tag

28.5 Excision of lingual tonsil

28.6 Adenoidectomy without tonsillectomy
Excision of adenoid tag

28.7 Control of hemorrhage after tonsillectomy and adenoidectomy

28.9 Other operations on tonsils and adenoids

28.91 Removal of foreign body from tonsil and adenoid by incision

Excludes: that without incision (98.13)

28.92 Excision of lesion of tonsil and adenoid

Excludes: biopsy of tonsil and adenoid (28.11)

28.99 Other

29 Operation on pharynx
Includes: operations on:
hypopharynx
nasopharynx
oropharynx
pharyngeal pouch
pyriform sinus

29.0 Pharyngotomy
Drainage of pharyngeal bursa

Excludes: incision and drainage of retropharyngeal abscess (28.0)
removal of foreign body (without incision) (98.13)

29.1 Diagnostic procedures on pharynx

29.11 Pharyngoscopy

29.12 Pharyngeal biopsy
Biopsy of supraglottic mass

29.19 Other diagnostic procedures on pharynx

Excludes: x-ray of nasopharynx:
contrast (87.06)
other (87.09)

29.2 Excision of branchial cleft cyst or vestige

Excludes: branchial cleft fistulectomy (29.52)

29.3 Excision or destruction of lesion or tissue of pharynx

29.31 Cricopharyngeal myotomy

Excludes that with pharyngeal diverticulectomy (29.32)

29.32 Pharyngeal diverticulectomy

29.33 Pharyngectomy (partial)

Excludes laryngopharyngectomy (30.3)

29.39 Other excision or destruction of lesion or tissue of pharynx

29.4 Plastic operation on pharynx
Correction of nasopharyngeal atresia

Excludes: pharyngoplasty associated with cleft palate repair (27.62-27.63)

29.5 Other repair of pharynx

29.51 Suture of laceration of pharynx

29.52 Closure of branchial cleft fistula

29.53 Closure of other fistula of pharynx
Pharyngoesophageal fistulectomy

29.54 Lysis of pharyngeal adhesions

29.59 Other

● Code new
to 2012 edition

▲ Revision of
existing code

④ ⑤ Fourth or fifth
digit required

29.9   **Other operations on pharynx**

    29.91   **Dilation of pharynx**
        Dilation of nasopharynx

    29.92   **Division of glossopharyngeal nerve**

    29.99   **Other**

        | Excludes: | *insertion of radium into pharynx and nasopharynx (92.27)*
                   removal of intraluminal foreign body (98.13)

Valid O.R. procedure   Non-O.R. procedure   Nonspecific O.R. procedure   Noncovered O.R. procedure

This page intentionally left blank.

● Code new
  to 2012 edition

▲ Revision of
  existing code

④ ⑤ Fourth or fifth
  digit required

6. OPERATIONS ON THE RESPIRATORY SYSTEM (30-34)

30 Excision of larynx

30.0 Excision or destruction of lesion or tissue of larynx

30.01 Marsupialization of laryngeal cyst

30.09 Other excision or destruction of lesion or tissue of larynx
Stripping of vocal cords

> *Excludes:* *biopsy of larynx (31.43)*
> *laryngeal fistulectomy (31.62)*
> *laryngotracheal fistulectomy (31.62)*

30.1 Hemilaryngectomy

30.2 Other partial laryngectomy

30.21 Epiglottidectomy

30.22 Vocal cordectomy
Excision of vocal cords

30.29 Other partial laryngectomy
Excision of laryngeal cartilage

30.3 Complete laryngectomy
Block dissection of larynx (with thyroidectomy) (with synchronous tracheostomy)
Laryngopharyngectomy

> *Excludes:* *that with radical neck dissection (30.4)*

30.4 Radical laryngectomy
Complete [total] laryngectomy with radical neck dissection (with thyroidectomy) (with synchronous tracheostomy)

31 Other operations on larynx and trachea

31.0 Injection of larynx
Injection of inert material into larynx or vocal cords

31.1 Temporary tracheostomy
Temporary percutaneous dilatational tracheostomy [PDT]
Tracheotomy for assistance in breathing
Code also any synchronous bronchoscopy, if performed (33.21-33.24, 33.27)

31.2 Permanent tracheostomy

31.21 Mediastinal tracheostomy

31.29 Other permanent tracheostomy
Permanent percutaneous dilatational tracheostomy [PDT]
Code also any synchronous bronchoscopy, if performed (33.21-33.24, 33.27)

> *Excludes:* *that with laryngectomy (30.3-30.4)*

31.3 Other incision of larynx or trachea

> *Excludes:* *that for assistance in breathing (31.1-31.29)*

31.4 Diagnostic procedures on larynx and trachea

31.41 Tracheoscopy through artificial stoma

> *Excludes:* *that with biopsy (31.43-31.44)*

31.42 Laryngoscopy and other tracheoscopy

> *Excludes:* *that with biopsy (31.43-31.44)*

31.43 Closed [endoscopic] biopsy of larynx

31.44 Closed [endoscopic] biopsy of trachea

31.45 Open biopsy of larynx or trachea

31.48 Other diagnostic procedures on larynx

> *Excludes:* *contrast laryngogram (87.07)*
> *microscopic examination of specimen from larynx (90.31-90.39)*
> *soft tissue x-ray of larynx NEC (87.09)*

31.49 Other diagnostic procedures on trachea

> *Excludes:* *microscopic examination of specimen from trachea (90.41-90.49)*
> *x-ray of trachea (87.49)*

Valid O.R. procedure   Non-O.R. procedure   Nonspecific O.R. procedure   Noncovered O.R. procedure

31.5 **Local excision or destruction of lesion or tissue of trachea**

> Excludes: *biopsy of trachea (31.44-31.45)*
> *laryngotracheal fistulectomy (31.62)*
> *tracheoesophageal fistulectomy (31.73)*

31.6 **Repair of larynx**

31.61 **Suture of laceration of larynx**

31.62 **Closure of fistula of larynx**
Laryngotracheal fistulectomy
Take-down of laryngostomy

31.63 **Revision of laryngostomy**

31.64 **Repair of laryngeal fracture**

31.69 **Other repair of larynx**
Arytenoidopexy
Graft of larynx
Transposition of vocal cords

> Excludes: *construction of artificial larynx (31.75)*

31.7 **Repair and plastic operations on trachea**

31.71 **Suture of laceration of trachea**

31.72 **Closure of external fistula of trachea**
Closure of tracheotomy

31.73 **Closure of other fistula of trachea**
Tracheoesophageal fistulectomy

> Excludes: *laryngotracheal fistulectomy (31.62)*

31.74 **Revision of tracheostomy**

31.75 **Reconstruction of trachea and construction of artificial larynx**
Tracheoplasty with artificial larynx

31.79 **Other repair and plastic operations on trachea**

31.9 **Other operations on larynx and trachea**

31.91 **Division of laryngeal nerve**

31.92 **Lysis of adhesions of trachea or larynx**

31.93 **Replacement of laryngeal or tracheal stent**

31.94 **Injection of locally-acting therapeutic substance into trachea**

31.95 **Tracheoesophageal fistulization**

31.98 **Other operations on larynx**
Dilation of larynx
Division of congenital web of larynx
Removal of keel or stent of larynx

> Excludes: *removal of intraluminal foreign body from larynx without incision*
> *(98.14)*

31.99 **Other operations on trachea**

> Excludes: *removal of:*
> *intraluminal foreign body from trachea without incision (98.15)*
> *tracheostomy tube (97.37)*
> *replacement of tracheostomy tube (97.23)*
> *tracheostomy toilette (96.35)*

32 **Excision of lung and bronchus**
Includes: rib resection as operative approach
sternotomy as operative approach
sternum-splitting incision as operative approach
thoracotomy as operative approach

Code also any synchronous bronchoplasty (33.48)

32.0 **Local excision or destruction of lesion or tissue of bronchus**

> Excludes: *biopsy of bronchus (33.24-33.25)*
> *bronchial fistulectomy (33.42)*

32.01 **Endoscopic excision or destruction of lesion or tissue of bronchus**

32.09 **Other local excision or destruction of lesion or tissue of bronchus**

> Excludes: *that by endoscopic approach (32.01)*

● Code new
to 2012 edition

▲ Revision of
existing code

④ ⑤ Fourth or fifth
digit required

32.1 **Other excision of bronchus**
Resection (wide sleeve) of bronchus

> Excludes: radical dissection [excision] of bronchus (32.6)

32.2 **Local excision or destruction of lesion or tissue of lung**

32.20 **Thoracoscopic excision of lesion or tissue of lung**
Thoracoscopic wedge resection

32.21 **Plication of emphysematous bleb**

32.22 **Lung volume reduction surgery**

32.23 **Open ablation of lung lesion or tissue**

32.24 **Percutaneous ablation of lung lesion or tissue**

32.25 **Thoracoscopic ablation of lung lesion or tissue**

> Excludes: thoracoscopic excision of lesion or tissue of lung (32.20)

32.26 **Other and unspecified ablatin of lung lesion or tissue**

> Excludes: bronchoscopic bronchial thermoplasty, ablation of smooth airway muscle (32.27)

32.27 **Bronchoscopic bronchial thermoplasty, ablation of smooth airway muscle**

32.28 **Endoscopic excision or destruction of lesion or tissue of lung**

> Excludes: ablation of lung lesion or tissue:
>   open (32.23)
>   other (32.26)
>   percutaneous (32.24)
>   thoracoscopic (32.25)
>   biopsy of lung (33.26-33.27)

32.29 **Other local excision or destruction of lesion or tissue of lung**
Resection of lung:
  NOS
  wedge

> Excludes: ablation of lung lesion or tissue:
>   open (32.23)
>   other (32.26)
>   percutaneous (32.24)
>   thoracoscopic (32.25)
>   biopsy of lung (33.26-33.27)
>   laser interstitial thermal therapy [LITT] of lesion or tissue of lung under guidance (17.69)
>   that by endoscopic approach (32.28)
>   thoracoscopic excision of lesion or tissue of lung (32.20)
>   wide excision of lesion of lung (32.3)

32.3 **Segmental resection of lung**
Partial lobectomy

32.30 **Thoracoscopic segmental resection of lung**

32.39 **Other and unspecified segmental resection of lung**

> Excludes: thoracoscopic segmental resection of lung (32.30)

32.4 **Lobectomy of lung**
Lobectomy with segmental resection of adjacent lobes of lung

> Excludes: that with radical dissection [excision] of thoracic structures (32.6)

32.41 **Thoracoscopic lobectomy of lung**

32.49 **Other lobectomy of lung**

> Excludes: thoracoscopic lobectomy of lung (32.41)

32.5 **Pneumonectomy**
Excision of lung NOS
Pneumonectomy (with mediastinal dissection)

32.50 **Thoracoscopic pneumonectomy**

32.59 **Other and unspecified pneumonectomy**

> Excludes: thoracoscopic pneumonectomy (32.50)

32.6 **Radical dissection of thoracic structures**
Block [en bloc] dissection of bronchus, lobe of lung, brachial plexus, intercostal structure, ribs (transverse process), and sympathetic nerves

	Valid O.R. procedure		Non-O.R. procedure		Nonspecific O.R. procedure		Noncovered O.R. procedure

32.9 **Other excision of lung**

> Excludes: *biopsy of lung and bronchus (33.24-33.27)*
> *pulmonary decortication (34.51)*

33 **Other operations on lung and bronchus**

Includes: rib resection as operative approach
sternotomy as operative approach
sternum-splitting incision as operative approach
thoracotomy as operative approach

33.0 **Incision of bronchus**

33.1 **Incision of lung**

> Excludes: *puncture of lung (33.93)*

33.2 **Diagnostic procedures on lung and bronchus**

33.20 **Thoracoscopic lung biopsy**

> Excludes: *closed endoscopic biopsy of lung (33.27)*
> *closed [percutaneous] [needle] biopsy of lung (33.26)*
> *open biopsy of lung (33.28)*

33.21 **Bronchoscopy through artificial stoma**

> Excludes: *that with biopsy (33.24, 33.27)*

33.22 **Fiber-optic bronchoscopy**

> Excludes: *that with biopsy (33.24. 33.27)*

33.23 **Other bronchoscopy**

> Excludes: *that for:*
> *aspiration (96.05)*
> *biopsy (33.24, 33.27)*

33.24 **Closed [endoscopic] biopsy of bronchus**

Bronchoscopy (fiberoptic) (rigid) with:
brush biopsy of "lung"
brushing or washing for specimen collection
excision (bite) biopsy
Diagnostic bronchoalveolar lavage (BAL)
Mini-bronchoalveolar lavage [mini-BAL]
Transbronchoscopic needle aspiration [TBNA] of bronchus

> Excludes: *closed biopsy of lung, other than brush biopsy of "lung" (33.26, 33.27)*
> *whole lung lavage (33.99)*

33.25 **Open biopsy of bronchus**

> Excludes: *open biopsy of lung (33.28)*

33.26 **Closed [percutaneous] [needle] biopsy of lung**

Fine needle aspiration (FNA) of lung
Transthoracic needle biopsy of lung (TTNB)

> Excludes: *endoscopic biopsy of lung (33.27)*
> *thoracoscopic lung biopsy (33.20)*

33.27 **Closed endoscopic biopsy of lung**

Fiberoptic (flexible) bronchoscopy with fluoroscopic guidance with biopsy
Transbronchial lung biopsy
Transbronchoscopic needle aspiration [TBNA] of lung

> Excludes: *brush biopsy of lung (33.24)*
> *percutaneous biopsy of lung (33.26)*
> *thoracoscopic lung biopsy (33.20)*

33.28 **Open biopsy of lung**

● Code new
to 2012 edition
▲ Revision of
existing code
④ ⑤ Fourth or fifth
digit required

33.29 Other diagnostic procedures on lung and bronchus

> Excludes: bronchoalveolar lavage [BAL] (33.24)
> contrast bronchogram:
>   endotracheal (87.31)
>   other (87.32)
> endoscopic pulmonary airway flow measurement (33.72)
> lung scan (92.15)
> magnetic resonance imaging (88.92)
> microscopic examination of specimen from bronchus or lung
>   (90.41-90.49)
> routine chest x-ray (87.44)
> ultrasonography of lung (88.73)
> vital capacity determination (89.37)
> x-ray of bronchus or lung NOS (87.49)

33.3 Surgical collapse of lung

33.31 Destruction of phrenic nerve for collapse of lung

33.32 Artificial pneumothorax for collapse of lung
Thoracotomy for collapse of lung

33.33 Pneumoperitoneum for collapse of lung

33.34 Thoracoplasty

33.39 Other surgical collapse of lung
Collapse of lung NOS

33.4 Repair and plastic operation on lung and bronchus

33.41 Suture of laceration of bronchus

33.42 Closure of bronchial fistula
Closure of bronchostomy
Fistulectomy:
    bronchocutaneous
    bronchoesophageal
    bronchovisceral

> Excludes: closure of fistula:
>   bronchomediastinal (34.73)
>   bronchopleural (34.73)
>   bronchopleuromediastinal (34.73)

33.43 Closure of laceration of lung

33.48 Other repair and plastic operation on bronchus

33.49 Other repair ad plastic operations on lung

> Excludes: closure of pleural fistula (34.73)

33.5 Lung transplant

Code also cardiopulmonary bypass [extracorporeal circulation] [heart-lung machine] 39.61
Note: To report donor source—see codes 00.91-00.93

> Excludes: Combined heart-lung transplantation (33.6)

33.50 Lung transplantation, not otherwise specified

33.51 Unilateral lung transplantation

33.52 Bilateral lung transplantation
Double-lung transplantation
En bloc transplantation

33.6 Combined heart-lung transplantation

Code also cardiopulmonary bypass [extracorporeal circulation] [heart-lung machine] (39.61)
Note: To report donor source—see codes 00.91-00.93

33.7 Other endoscopic procedures in bronchus or lung

> Excludes: insertion of tracheobronchial stent (96.05)

33.71 Endoscopic insertion or replacement of bronchial valve(s), single lobe
Endobronchial airflow redirection valve
Intrabronchial airflow redirection valve

> Excludes: endoscopic insertion or replacement of bronchial valve(s), multiple lobes (33.73)

	Valid O.R. procedure		Non-O.R. procedure		Nonspecific O.R. procedure		Noncovered O.R. procedure

33.72 Endoscopic pulmonary airway flow measurement
Assessment of pulmonary airway flow

Code also any diagnostic or therapeutic procedure if performed

33.73 Endoscopic insertion or replacement of bronchial valve(s), multiple lobes
Endobronchial airflow redirection valve
Intrabronchial airflow redirection valve

> Excludes: *endoscopic insertion or replacement of bronchial valve(s), single lobe (33.71)*

33.78 Endoscopic removal of bronchial device(s) or substances

33.79 Endoscopic insertion of other bronchial device or substances
Biologic Lung Volume Reduction NOS (BLVR)

33.9 Other operations on lung and bronchus

33.91 Bronchial dilation

33.92 Ligation of bronchus

33.93 Puncture of lung

> Excludes: *needle biopsy (33.26)*

33.98 Other operations on bronchus

> Excludes: *bronchial lavage (96.56)*
> *removal of intraluminal foreign body from bronchus without incision (98.15)*

33.99 Other operations on lung
Whole lung lavage

> Excludes: *other continuous mechanical ventilation (96.70-96.72)*
> *respiratory therapy (93.90-93.99)*

34 Operations on chest wall, pleura, mediastinum, and diaphragm

> Excludes: *operations on breast (85.0-85.99)*

34.0 Incision of chest wall and pleura

> Excludes: *that as operative approach—omit code*

34.01 Incision of chest wall
Extrapleural drainage

> Excludes: *incision of pleura (34.09)*

34.02 Exploratory thoracotomy

34.03 Reopening of recent thoracotomy site

34.04 Insertion of intercostal catheter for drainage
Chest tube
Closed chest drainage
Revision of intercostal catheter (chest tube) (with lysis of adhesions)

> Excludes: *thoracoscopic drainage of pleural cavity (34.06)*

34.05 Creation of pleuroperitoneal shunt

34.06 Thoracoscopic drainage of pleural cavity
Evacuation of empyema

34.09 Other incision of pleura
Creation of pleural window for drainage
Intercostal stab
Open chest drainage

> Excludes: *thoracoscopy (34.21)*
> *thoracotomy for collapse of lung (33.32)*

34.1 Incision of mediastinum

Code also any biopsy, if performed

> Excludes: *mediastinoscopy (34.22)*
> *mediastinotomy associated with pneumonectomy (32.5)*

34.2 Diagnostic procedures on chest wall, pleura, mediastinum, and diaphragm

34.20 Thoracoscopic pleural biopsy

34.21 Transpleural thoracoscopy

34.22 Mediastinoscopy

Code also any biopsy, if performed

● Code new
to 2012 edition ▲ Revision of
existing code ④ ⑤ Fourth or fifth
digit required

34.23 **Biopsy of chest wall**

34.24 **Other pleural biopsy**

> *Excludes:* *thoracoscopic pleural biopsy (34.20)*

34.25 **Closed [percutaneous] [needle] biopsy of mediastinum**

34.26 **Open biopsy of mediastinum**

34.27 **Biopsy of diaphragm**

34.28 **Other diagnostic procedures on chest wall, pleura, and diaphragm**

> *Excludes:* *angiocardiography (88.50-88.58)*
> *aortography (88.42)*
> *arteriography of:*
> *intrathoracic vessels NEC (88.44)*
> *pulmonary arteries (88.43)*
> *microscopic examination of specimen from chest wall. pleura, and*
> *diaphragm (90.41-90.49)*
> *phlebography of:*
> *intrathoracic vessels NEC (88.63)*
> *pulmonary veins (88.62)*
> *radiological examinations of thorax:*
> *C.A.T. scan (87.41)*
> *diaphragmatic x-ray (87.49)*
> *intrathoracic lymphangiogram (87.34)*
> *routine chest x-ray (87.44)*
> *sinogram of chest wall (87.38)*
> *soft tissue x-ray of chest wall NEC (87.39)*
> *tomogram of thorax NEC (87. 42)*
> *ultrasonography of thorax (88.73)*

34.29 **Other diagnostic procedures on mediastinum**

> *Excludes:* *mediastinal:*
> *pneumogram (87.33)*
> *x-ray NEC (87.49)*

34.3 **Excision or destruction of lesion or tissue of mediastinum**

> *Excludes:* *biopsy or mediastinum (34.25-34.26)*
> *mediastinal fistulectomy (34.73)*

34.4 **Excision or destruction of lesion of chest wall**
Excision of lesion of chest wall NOS (with excision of ribs)

> *Excludes:* *biopsy of chest wall (34.23)*
> *costectomy not incidental to thoracic procedure (77. 91)*
> *excision of lesion of:*
> *breast (85.20-85.25)*
> *cartilage (80.89)*
> *skin (86.2-86.3)*
> *fistulectomy (34. 73)*

34.5 **Pleurectomy**

34.51 **Decortication of lung**

> *Excludes:* *thoracoscopic decortication of lung (34.52)*

34.52 **Thoracoscopic decortication of lung**

34.59 **Other excision of pleura**
Excision of pleural lesion

> *Excludes:* *biopsy of pleura (34.24)*
> *pleural fistulectomy (34.73)*

34.6 **Scarification of pleura**
Pleurosclerosis

> *Excludes:* *injection of sclerosing agent (34.92)*

34.7 **Repair of chest wall**

34.71 **Suture of laceration of chest wall**

> *Excludes:* *suture of skin and subcutaneous tissue alone (86.59)*

34.72 **Closure of thoracostomy**

	Valid O.R. procedure		Non-O.R. procedure		Nonspecific O.R. procedure		Noncovered O.R. procedure

34.73 **Closure of other fistula of thorax**
Closure of:
bronchopleural fistula
bronchopleurocutaneous fistula
bronchopleuromediastinal fistula

34.74 **Repair of pectus deformity**
Repair of:
pectus carinatum (with implant)
pectus excavatum (with implant)

34.79 **Other repair of chest wall**
Repair of chest wall NOS

34.8 **Operations on diaphragm**

34.81 **Excision of lesion or tissue of diaphragm**

Excludes: *biopsy of diaphragm (34.27)*

34.82 **Suture of laceration of diaphragm**

34.83 **Closure of fistula of diaphragm**
Thoracicoabdominal fistulectomy
Thoracicogastric fistulectomy
Thoracicointestinal fistulectomy

34.84 **Other repair of diaphragm**

Excludes: *repair of diaphragmatic hernia (53.7-53.82)*

34.85 **Implantation of diaphragmatic pacemaker**

34.89 **Other operations on diaphragm**

34.9 **Other operations on thorax**

34.91 **Thoracentesis**

34.92 **Injection into thoracic cavity**
Chemical pleurodesis
Injection of cytotoxic agent or tetracycline
Instillation into thoracic cavity
Requires additional code for any cancer chemotherapeutic substance (99.25)

Excludes: *that for collapse of lung (33.32)*

34.93 **Repair of pleura**

34.99 **Other**

Excludes: *removal of:*
mediastinal drain (97.42)
sutures (97.43)
thoracotomy tube (97.41)

● Code new
to 2012 edition

▲ Revision of
existing code

④ ⑤ Fourth or fifth
digit required

7.   **OPERATIONS ON THE CARDIOVASCULAR SYSTEM (35-39)**

35   **Operations on valves and septa of heart**
    Includes: sternotomy (median) (transverse) as operative approach
                  thoracotomy as operative approach
    Code also any cardiopulmonary bypass [extracorporeal circulation] [heart-lung machine] (39.61)

▲ **35.0**   **Closed heart valvotomy or transcatheter replacement of heart valve**
    Excludes: *percutaneous (balloon) valvuloplasty (35.96)*

   35.00 **Closed heart valvotomy, unspecified valve**

   35.01 **Closed heart valvotomy, aortic valve**

   35.02 **Closed heart valvotomy, mitral valve**

   35.03 **Closed heart valvotomy, pulmonary valve**

   35.04 **Closed heart valvotomy, tricuspid valve**

   ● **35.05** **Endovascular replacement of aortic valve**
        Note: Includes that with any balloon valvuloplasty; do not code separately
            Implantation of transcatheter aortic valve
            Replacement of aortic valve with tissue graft (autograft) (bioprosthetic)
                (heterograft) (homograft):
              transarterial approach
              transfemoral approach
            TAVI (transcatheter aortic valve implantation)
            TAVR (transcatheter aortic valve replacement)
        Excludes: *open and other replacement of heart valve (35.20-35.28)*

   ● **35.06** **Transapical replacement of aortic valve**
        Note: Includes that with any balloon valvuloplasty; do not code separately
            Implantation of transcatheter aortic valve
            Replacement of aortic valve with tissue graft (autograft) (bioprosthetic)
                (heterograft) (homograft):
              intercostal approach
              transventricular approach
            That via transthoracic exposure, i.e. thoracotomy, sternotomy, or subxiphoid
                approach
        Excludes: *open and other replacement of heart valve (35.20-35.28)*

   ● **35.07** **Endovascular replacement of pulmonary valve**
        Note: Includes that with any balloon valvuloplasty; do not code separately
            Implantation of transcatheter pulmonary valve
            PPVI (percutaneous pulmonary valve implantation)
            Replacement of pulmonary valve:
              transfemoral approach
              transvenous approach
            That within previously created right ventricle-to pulmonary artery conduit
            TPVI (transcatheter pulmonary valve implantation)
        Excludes: *open and other replacement of heart valve (35.20-35.28)*

   ● **35.08** **Transapical replacement of pulmonary valve**
        Note: Includes that with any balloon valvuloplasty; do not code separately
            Implantation of transcatheter pulmonary valve
            Replacement of pulmonary valve:
              intercostal approach
              transventricular approach
            That via transthoracic exposure, i.e. thoracotomy, sternotomy, or subxiphoid
                approach
        Excludes: *open and other replacement of heart valve (35.20-35.28)*

   ● **35.09** **Endovascular replacement of unspecified heart valve**
        Note: Includes that with any balloon valvuloplasty; do not code separately
            Replacement of valve via:
              intercostal approach
              transventricular approach
        Excludes: *open and other replacement of heart valve (35.20-35.28)*

| | Valid O.R. procedure | | Non-O.R. procedure | | Nonspecific O.R. procedure | | Noncovered O.R. procedure |

35.1 **Open heart valvuloplasty without replacement**
Includes: open heart valvotomy

Excludes: *that associated with repair of:*
endocardial cushion defect (35.54, 35.63, 35.73)
percutaneous (balloon) valvuloplasty (35.96)
valvular defect associated with atrial and ventricular septal defects (35.54, 35.63, 35.73)

Code also cardiopulmonary bypass, if performed [extracorporeal circulation] [heart-lung machine] (39.61)

35.10 Open heart valvuloplasty without replacement, unspecified valve

35.11 Open heart valvuloplasty of aortic valve without replacement

35.12 Open heart valvuloplasty of mitral valve without replacement

35.13 Open heart valvuloplasty of pulmonary valve without replacement

35.14 Open heart valvuloplasty of tricuspid valve without replacement

▲ **35.2** **Open and other replacement of heart valve**
Includes: excision of heart valve with replacement

Code also cardiopulmonary bypass [extracorporeal circulation] [heart-lung machine] (39.61)

Excludes: *that associated with repair of:*
endocardial cushion defect (35.54, 35.63, 35.73)
valvular defect associated with atrial and ventricular septal defects (35.54, 35.63, 35.73)
transapical replacement of heart valve (35.06, 35.08)
transcatheter replacement of heart valve (35.05, 35.07)

▲ **35.20** **Open and other replacement of unspecified heart valve**
That with tissue graft or prosthetic implant

Excludes: *endovascular replacement of unspecified heart valve (35.09)*

▲ **35.21** **Open and other replacement of aortic valve with tissue graft**
Includes that by:
autograft
heterograft
homograft

Excludes: *endovascular replacement of aortic valve (35.05)*
transapical replacement of aortic valve (35.06)

▲ **35.22** **Open and other replacement of aortic valve**
Replacement of aortic valve NOS
That with prosthetic (partial) (synthetic) (total)

Excludes: *endovascular replacement of aortic valve (35.05)*
transapical replacement of aortic valve (35.06)

▲ **35.23** **Open and other replacement of mitral valve with tissue graft**
Includes that by:
autograft
heterograft
homograft

▲ **35.24** **Open and other replacement of mitral valve**
Replacement of mitral valve NOS
That with prosthetic (partial) (synthetic) (total)

Excludes: *percutaneous repair with implant or leaflet clip (35.97)*

▲ **35.25** **Open and other replacement of pulmonary valve with tissue graft**
Includes that by:
autograft
heterograft
homograft

Excludes: *endovascular replacement of pulmonary valve (35.07)*
transapical replacement of pulmonary valve (35.08)

▲ **35.26** **Open and other replacement of pulmonary valve**
Replacement of pulmonary valve, NOS
That with prosthetic (partial) (synthetic) (total)

Excludes: *endovascular replacement of pulmonary valve (35.07)*
transapical replacement of pulmonary valve (35.08)

● Code new
to 2012 edition
▲ Revision of
existing code
④ ⑤ Fourth or fifth
digit required

▲ 35.27 **Open and other replacement of tricuspid valve with tissue graft**
Includes that by:
   autograft
   heterograft
   homograft

▲ 35.28 **Open and other replacement of tricuspid valve**
Replacement of tricuspid valve, NOS
That with prosthetic (partial) (synthetic) (total)

35.3   **Operations on structures adjacent to heart valves**
*Code also cardiopulmonary bypass [extracorporeal circulation] [heart-lung machine]
(39.61)*

35.31 **Operations on papillary muscle**
Division of papillary muscle
Reattachment of papillary muscle
Repair of papillary muscle

35.32 **Operations on chordae tendineae**
Division of chordae tendineae
Repair of chordae tendineae

35.33 **Annuloplasty**
Plication of annulus

35.34 **Infundibulectomy**
Right ventricular infundibulectomy

35.35 **Operations on trabeculae carneae cordis**
Division of trabeculae carneae cordis
Excision of trabeculae carneae cordis
Excision of aortic subvalvular ring

35.39 **Operations on other structures adjacent to valves of heart**
Repair of sinus of Valsalva (aneurysm)

35.4   **Production of septal defect in heart**

35.41 **Enlargement of existing atrial septal defect**
Rashkind procedure
Septostomy (atrial) (balloon)

35.42 **Creation of septal defect in heart**
Blalock-Hanlon operation

35.5   **Repair of atrial and ventricular septa with prosthesis**
Includes: repair of septa with synthetic implant of patch
*Code also cardiopulmonary bypass [extracorporeal circulation] [heart-lung machine]
(39.61)*

35.50 **Repair of unspecified septal defect of heart with prosthesis**
| Excludes: | *that associated with repair of:*
endocardial cushion defect (35.54)
septal defect associated with valvular defect (35.54)

35.51 **Repair of atrial septal defect with prosthesis, open technique**
Atrioseptoplasty with prosthesis
Correction of atrial septal defect with prosthesis
Repair:
   foramen ovale (patent) with prosthesis
   ostium secundum defect with prosthesis
| Excludes: | *that associated with repair of:*
*atrial septal defect associated with valvular and ventricular septal
defects (35.54)*
endocardial cushion defect (35.54)

35.52 **Repair of atrial septal defect with prosthesis, closed technique**
Insertion of atrial septal umbrella [King-Mills]

35.53 **Repair of ventricular septal defect with prosthesis, open technique**
Correction of ventricular septal defect with prosthesis
Repair of supracristal defect with prosthesis
| Excludes: | *that associated with repair of:*
endocardial cushion defect (35.54)
*ventricular defect associated with valvular and atrial septal defects
(35.54)*

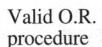 Valid O.R.
procedure

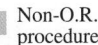 Non-O.R.
procedure

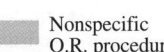 Nonspecific
O.R. procedure

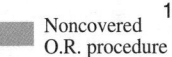 Noncovered
O.R. procedure

35.54 Repair of endocardial cushion defect with prosthesis
Repair:
atrioventricular canal with prosthesis (grafted to septa)
ostium primum defect with prosthesis (grafted to septa)
valvular defect associated with atrial and ventricular septal defects with prosthesis
(grafted to septa)

> Excludes: *repair of isolated:*
> *atrial septal defect (35.51-35.52)*
> *valvular defect (35.20, 35.22, 35.24, 35.26. 35.28)*
> *ventricular septal defect (35.53)*

35.55 Repair of ventricular septal defect with prosthesis, closed technique

35.6 Repair of atrial and ventricular septa with tissue graft
Code also cardiopulmonary bypass [extracorporeal circulation] [heart-lung machine]
(39.61)

35.60 Repair of unspecified septal defect of heart with tissue graft

> Excludes: *that associated with repair of:*
> *endocardial cushion defect (35.63)*
> *septal defect associated with valvular, defect (33.63)*

35.61 Repair of atrial septal defect with tissue graft
Atrioseptoplasty with tissue graft
Correction of atrial septal defect with tissue graft
Repair:
foramen ovale (patent) with tissue graft
ostium secundum defect with tissue graft

> Excludes: *that associated with repair of:*
> *atrial septal defect associated with valvular and ventricular septal*
> *defects (35.63)*
> *endocardial cushion defect (35.63)*

35.62 Repair of ventricular septal defect with tissue graft
Correction of ventricular septal defect with tissue graft
Repair of supracristal defect with tissue graft

> Excludes: *that associated with repair of:*
> *endocardial cushion defect (35.63)*
> *ventricular defect associated with valvular and atrial septal defects*
> *(35.63)*

35.63 Repair of endocardial cushion defect with tissue graft
Repair of:
atrioventricular canal with tissue graft
ostium primum defect with tissue graft
valvular defect associated with atrial and ventricular septal defects, with tissue
graft

> Excludes: *repair of isolated*
> *atrial septal defect (35.61)*
> *valvular defect (35.20-35.21. 35.23, 35.25. 35.27)*
> *ventricular septal defect (35.62)*

35.7 Other and unspecified repair of atrial and ventricular septa
Code also cardiopulmonary bypass [extracorporeal circulation] [heart-lung machine]
(39.61)

35.70 Other and unspecified repair of unspecified septal defect of heart
Repair of septal defect NOS

> Excludes: *that associated with repair of:*
> *endocardial cushion defect (35.73)*
> *septal defect associated with valvular defect (35.73)*

● Code new
   to 2012 edition
▲ Revision of
   existing code
④ ⑤ Fourth or fifth
   digit required

35.71 Other and unspecified repair of atrial septal defect
Repair NOS:
atrial septum
foramen ovale (patent)
ostium secundum defect

> Excludes: *that associated with repair of:*
> *atrial septal defect associated with valvular and ventricular septal*
> *defects (35.73)*
> *endocardial cushion defect (35.73)*

35.72 Other and unspecified repair of ventricular septal defect
Repair NOS:
supracristal defect
ventricular septum

> Excludes: *that associated with repair of:*
> *endocardial cushion defect (35.73)*
> *ventricular septal defect associated with valvular and atrial septal*
> *defects (35.73)*

35.73 Other and unspecified repair of endocardial cushion defect
Repair NOS:
atrioventricular canal
ostium primum defect
valvular defect associated with atrial and ventricular septal defects

> Excludes: *repair of isolated:*
> *atrial septal defect (35.71)*
> *valvular defect (35.20, 35.22, 35.24, 35.26, 35.28)*
> *ventricular septal defect (35.72)*

35.8   Total repair of certain congenital cardiac anomalies
Note: For partial repair of defect [e.g. repair of atrial septal defect in tetralogy of Fallot]— code
to specific procedure

35.81 Total repair of tetralogy of Fallot
One-stage total correction of tetralogy of Fallot with or without:
commissurotomy of pulmonary valve
infundibulectomy
outflow tract prosthesis
patch graft of outflow tract
prosthetic tube for pulmonary artery
repair of ventricular septal defect (with prosthesis)
take-down of previous systemic-pulmonary artery anastomosis

35.82 Total repair of total anomalous pulmonary venous connection
One-stage total correction of total anomalous pulmonary venous connection with or
without:
anastomosis between (horizontal) common pulmonary trunk and posterior wall of
left atrium (side-to-side)
enlargement of foramen ovale
incision [excision] of common wall between posterior left atrium and coronary
sinus and roofing of resultant defect with patch graft (synthetic)
ligation of venous connection (descending anomalous vein) (to left innominate
vein) (to superior vena cava)
repair of atrial septal defect (with prosthesis)

35.83 Total repair of truncus arteriosus
One-stage total correction of truncus arteriosus with or without:
construction (with aortic homograft) (with prosthesis) of a pulmonary artery
placed from right ventricle to arteries supplying the lung
ligation of connections between aorta and pulmonary artery
repair of ventricular septal defect (with prosthesis)

35.84 Total correction of transposition of great vessels, not elsewhere classified
Arterial switch operation [Jatene]
Total correction of transposition of great arteries at the arterial level by switching
the great arteries, including the left or both coronary arteries, implanted in the
wall of the pulmonary artery

> Excludes: *baffle operation [Mustard] [Senning] (35.91)*
> *creation of shunt between right ventricle and pulmonary artery*
> *[Rastelli] (35.92)*

| | Valid O.R. procedure | | Non-O.R. procedure | | Nonspecific O.R. procedure | | Noncovered O.R. procedure |

35.9 Other operations on valves and septa of heart

Code also cardiopulmonary bypass, if performed [extracorporeal circulation] [heart-lung machine] (39.61)

35.91 Interatrial transposition of venous return
Baffle:
  atrial
  interatrial
Mustard's operation
Resection of atrial septum and insertion of patch to direct systemic venous return to tricuspid valve and pulmonary venous return to mitral valve

35.92 Creation of conduit between right ventricle and pulmonary artery
Creation of shunt between right ventricle and (distal) pulmonary artery

Excludes:	*that associated with total repair of truncus arteriosus (35.83)*

35.93 Creation of conduit between left ventricle and aorta
Creation of apicoaortic shunt
Shunt between apex of left ventricle and aorta

35.94 Creation of conduit between atrium and pulmonary artery
Fontan procedure

35.95 Revision of corrective procedure on heart
Replacement of prosthetic heart valve poppet
Resuture or prosthesis of:
  septum
  valve

Excludes:	*complete revision—code to specific procedure*
	replacement of prosthesis or graft of:
	septum (35.50-35.63)
	valve (35.20-35.28)

35.96 Percutaneous balloon valvuloplasty
Balloon dilation of valve

Excludes:	*endovascular replacement of heart valve (35.05, 35.07)*
	mitral valve repair with implant (35.97)
	transapical replacement of heart valve (35.06, 35.08)

35.97 Percutaneous mitral valve repair with implant
Endovascular mitral valve repair
Implantation of mitral valve leaflet clip
Transcatheter mitral valve repair

Code also any transesophageal echocardiography [TEE] (88.72)

Excludes:	*percutaneous balloon valvuloplasty (35.96)*

35.98 Other operations on septa of heart

35.99 Other operations on valves of heart

36 Operations on vessels of heart
Includes: sternotomy (median) (transverse) as operative approach
             thoracotomy as operative approach

Code also any:
  injection or infusion of platelet inhibitor (99.20)
  injection or infusion of thrombolytic agent (99.10)

Code also cardiopulmonary bypass, if performed [extracorporeal circulation] [heart-lung machine] (39.61)

36.0 Removal of coronary artery obstruction and insertion of stent(s)

36.03 Open chest coronary artery angioplasty
Coronary (artery):
  endarterectomy (with patch graft)
  thromboendarterectomy (with patch graft)
Open surgery for direct relief of coronary artery obstruction

Code also any:
  insertion of drug-eluting coronary stent(s) (36.07)
  insertion of non-drug-eluting coronary stent(s) (36.06)
  number of vascular stents inserted (00.45-00.48)
  number of vessels treated (00.40-00.43)
  procedure on vessel bifurcation (00.44)

Excludes:	*that with coronary artery bypass graft (36.10-36.19)*

● Code new
  to 2012 edition
▲ Revision of
  existing code
④ ⑤ Fourth or fifth
  digit required

36.04 Intracoronary artery thrombolytic infusion

That by direct coronary artery injection, infusion, or catheterization
> enzyme infusion
> platelet inhibitor

> | *Excludes:* | *infusion of platelet inhibitor (99.20)* |
> | | *infusion of thrombolytic agent (99.10)* |
> | | *that associated with any procedure in 36.03* |

36.06 Insertion of non-drug-eluting coronary artery stent(s)

Bare stent(s)
Bonded stent(s)
Drug-coated stent(s), i.e. heparin coated
Endograft(s)
Endovascular graft(s)
Stent graft(s)

Code also any:
> number of vascular stents inserted (00.45-00.48)
> number of vessels treated (00.40-00.43)
> open chest coronary artery angioplasty (36.03)
> percutaneous transluminal coronary angioplasty [PTCA] (00.66)
> procedure on vessel bifurcation (00.44)
> transluminal coronary atherectomy (17.55)

> | *Excludes:* | *insertion of drug-eluting coronary artery stent(s) (36.07)* |

36.07 Insertion of drug-eluting coronary artery stent(s)

Endograft(s)
Endovascular graft(s)
Stent graft(s)

Code also any:
> number of vascular stents inserted (00.45-00.48)
> number of vessels treated (00.40-00.43)
> open chest coronary artery angioplasty (36.03)
> percutaneous transluminal coronary angioplasty [PTCA] (00.66)
> procedure on vessel bifurcation (00.44)
> transluminal coronary atherectomy (17.55)

> | *Excludes:* | *drug-coated stent(s), e.g., heparin coated (36.06)* |
> | | *insertion of non-drug-eluting coronary artery stent(s) (36.06)* |

36.09 Other removal of coronary artery obstruction

Coronary angioplasty NOS

Code also any:
> number of vascular stents inserted (00.45-00.48)
> number of vessels treated (00.40-00.43)
> procedure on vessel bifurcation (00.44)

> | *Excludes:* | *that by open angioplasty (36.03)* |
> | | *that by percutaneous transluminal coronary angioplasty [PTCA] (00.66)* |
> | | *transluminal coronary atherectomy (17.55)* |

36.1 Bypass anastomosis for heart revascularization

Note: Do not assign codes from series 00.40-00.43 with codes from series 36.10-36.19

Code also:
> cardiopulmonary bypass [extracorporeal circulation] [heart-lung machine] (39.61)
> pressurized treatment of venous bypass graft [conduit] with pharmaceutical substance, if performed (00.16)

36.10 Aortocoronary bypass for heart revascularization, not otherwise specified

Direct revascularization:
> cardiac with catheter stent, prosthesis, or vein graft
> coronary with catheter stent, prosthesis, or vein graft
> heart muscle with catheter stent, prosthesis, or vein graft
> myocardial with catheter stent, prosthesis, or vein graft

Heart revascularization NOS

36.11 (Aorto)coronary bypass of one coronary artery

36.12 (Aorto)coronary bypass of two coronary arteries

36.13 (Aorto)coronary bypass of three coronary arteries

36.14 (Aorto)coronary bypass of four or more coronary arteries

| Valid O.R. procedure | Non-O.R. procedure | Nonspecific O.R. procedure | Noncovered O.R. procedure |

36.15 Single internal mammary-coronary artery bypass
Anastomosis (single):
mammary artery to coronary artery
thoracic artery to coronary artery

36.16 Double internal mammary-coronary artery bypass
Anastomosis (double):
mammary artery to coronary artery
thoracic artery to coronary artery

36.17 Abdominal-coronary artery bypass
Anastomosis:
gastroepiploic artery to coronary artery

36.19 Other bypass anastomosis for heart revascularization

36.2 Heart revascularization by arterial implant
Implantation of:
aortic branches [ascending aortic branches] into heart muscle
blood vessels into myocardium
internal mammary artery [internal thoracic artery] into:
heart muscle
myocardium
ventricle
ventricular wall
Indirect heart revascularization NOS

36.3 Other heart revascularization

36.31 Open chest transmyocardial revascularization

36.32 Other transmyocardial revascularization

36.33 Endoscopic transmyocardial revascularization
Thorascopic transmyocardial revascularization

36.34 Percutaneous transmyocardial revascularization
Endovascular transmyocardial revascularization

36.39 Other heart revascularization
Abrasion of epicardium
Cardio-omentopexy
Intrapericardial poudrage
Myocardial graft:
mediastinal fat
omentum
pectoral muscles

36.9 Other operations on vessels of heart
Code also cardiopulmonary bypass [extracorporeal circulation] [heart-lung machine]
(39.61)

36.91 Repair of aneurysm of coronary vessel

36.99 Other operations on vessel of heart
Exploration of coronary artery
Incision of coronary artery
Ligation of coronary artery
Repair of arteriovenous fistula

37 Other operations on heart and pericardium
Code also any injection or infusion of platelet inhibitor (99.20)

37.0 Pericardiocentesis

37.1 Cardiotomy and pericardiotomy
Code also cardiopulmonary bypass [extracorporeal circulation] [heart-lung machine]
(39.61)

37.10 Incision of heart, not otherwise specified
Cardiolysis NOS

37.11 Cardiotomy
Incision of:
atrium
endocardium
myocardium
ventricle

37.12 Pericardiotomy
Pericardial window operation
Pericardiolysis
Pericardiotomy

● Code new
to 2012 edition   ▲ Revision of
existing code   ④ ⑤ Fourth or fifth
digit required

37.2   Diagnostic procedures on heart and pericardium

37.20   Noninvasive programmed electrical stimulation [NIPS]

> Excludes: *that as part of intraoperative testing—omit code*
> *catheter based invasive electrophysiologic testing (37.26)*
> *device interrogation only without arrhythmia induction (bedside check) (89.45-89.49)*

37.21   Right heart cardiac catheterization
Cardiac catheterization NOS

> Excludes: *that with catheterization of left heart (37.23)*

37.22   Left heart cardiac catheterization

> Excludes: *that with catheterization of right heart (37.23)*

37.23   Combined right and left heart cardiac catheterization

37.24   Biopsy of pericardium

37.25   Biopsy of heart

37.26   Catheter based invasive electrophysiologic testing
Electrophysiologic studies (EPS)

Code also any concomitant procedure

> Excludes: *that as part of intraoperative testing—omit code*
> *device interrogation only without arrhythmia induction (bedside check) (89.45-89.49)*
> *His bundle recording (37.29)*
> *noninvasive programmed electrical stimulation (NIPS) (37.20)*

37.27   Cardiac mapping

Code also any concomitant procedure

> Excludes: *electrocardiogram (89.52)*
> *His bundle recording (37.29)*

37.28   Intracardiac echocardiography [ICE]
Echocardiography of heart chambers

Code also any synchronous Doppler flow mapping (88.72)

> Excludes: *intravascular imaging of coronary vessels (intravascular ultrasound) (IVUS) (00.24)*

37.29   Other diagnostic procedures on heart and pericardium

> Excludes: *angiocardiography (88.50-88.58)*
> *cardiac function tests (89.41-89.69)*
> *cardiovascular radioisotopic scan and function study (92.05)*
> *coronary arteriography (88.55-88.57)*
> *diagnostic pericardiocentesis (37.0)*
> *diagnostic ultrasound of heart (88.72)*
> *x-ray of heart (87.49)*

37.3   Pericardiectomy and excision of lesion of heart

Code also cardiopulmonary bypass [extracorporeal circulation] [heart-lung machine], if performed (39.61)

37.31   Pericardiectomy
Excision of:
adhesions of pericardium
constricting scar of: epicardium
pericardium

37.32   Excision of aneurysm of heart
Repair of aneurysm of heart

37.33   Excision or destruction of other lesion or tissue of heart, open approach
Ablation or incision of heart tissue (cryoablation) (electrocurrent) (laser) (microwave) (radiofrequency) (resection) (ultrasound), open chest approach
Cox-maze procedure
Maze procedure
That by median sternotomy
That by thoracotomy without use of thoracoscope

> Excludes: *ablation, excision or destruction of lesion or tissue of heart:*
> *endovascular approach (37.34)*
> *thoracoscopic approach (37.37)*
> *excision or destuction of left atrial appendage (LAA) (37.36)*

| | Valid O.R. procedure | | Non-O.R. procedure | | Nonspecific O.R. procedure | | Noncovered O.R. procedure |

37.34 **Excision or destruction of other lesion or tissue of heart, endovascular approach**

Ablation of heart tissue (cryoablation) (electrocurrent) (laser) (microwave) (radiofrequency) (ultrasound), via peripherally inserted catheter

Modified maze procedure, percutaneous approach

> | Excludes: | *ablation, excision or destruction of lesion of tissue of heart:*
> *open approach (37.33)*
> *thoracoscopic approach (37.37)*

37.35 **Partial ventriculectomy**

Ventricular reduction surgery

Ventricular remodeling

Code also any synchronous:
  mitral valve repair (35.02, 35.12)
  mitral valve replacement (35.23-35.24)

▲ **37.36** **Excision, destruction, or exclusion of left atrial appendage (LAA)**

Includes: thoracoscopic approach, minithoracotomy approach, percutaneous approach, endovascular approach, or subxiphoid approach

Clipping of left atrial appendage

Oversewing of left atrial appendage

Stapling of left atrial appendage

That by fastener or suture

Code also any:
  concomitant procedure performed
  fluoroscopy (87.49)
  transesophageal echocardiography (TEE) (88.72)

> | Excludes: | *ablation, excision or destruction of lesion or tissue of heart,*
> *endovascular approach (37.34)*
> *excision or destruction of other lesion or tissue of heart, thoracoscopic*
> *approach (37.37)*
> *insertion of left atrial appendage device (37.90)*

37.37 **Excision or destruction of other lesion or tissue of heart, thoracoscopic approach**

Ablation or incision of heart tissue (cryoablation) (electrocautery) (laser) (microwave) (radiofrequency) (resection) (ultrasound) , via thoracoscope

Modified maze procedure, thoracoscopic approach

That via thoracoscopically-assisted approach (without thoracotomy) (with port access) (with sub-xiphoid incision)

> | Excludes: | *ablation, excision or destruction of lesion or tissue of heart:*
> *open approach (37.33)*
> *endovascular approach (37.34)*
> *thoracoscopic excision or destruction of left atrial appendage [LAA]*
> *(37.36)*

37.4 **Repair of heart and pericardium**

37.41 **Implantation of prosthetic cardiac support device around the heart**

Cardiac support device (CSD)

Epicardial support device

Fabric (textile) (mesh) device

Ventricular support device on surface of heart

Code also any:
  cardiopulmonary bypass [extracorporeal circulation] [heart-lung machine] if
    performed (39.61)
  mitral valve repair (35.02, 35.12)
  mitral valve replacement (35.23-35.24)
  transesophageal echocardiography (88.72)

> | Excludes: | *circulatory assist systems (37.61-37.68)*

37.49 **Other repair of heart and pericardium**

37.5 **Heart replacement procedures**

37.51 **Heart transplantation**

> | Excludes: | *combined heart-lung transplantation (33.6)*

37.52 **Implantation of total internal biventricular heart replacement system**

Artificial heart

> | Excludes: | *implantation of heart assist system [VAD] (37.62, 37.65, 37.66, 37.68)*

Note: This procedure includes substantial removal of part or all of the biological heart. Both ventricles are resected, and the native heart is no longer intact. Ventriculectomy is included in this procedure; do not code separately.

● Code new
to 2012 edition   ▲ Revision of
existing code   ④ ⑤ Fourth or fifth
digit required

37.53 **Replacement or repair of thoracic unit of (total) replacement heart system**

> Excludes: *replacement and repair of heart assist system [VAD] (37.63)*

37.54 **Replacement or repair of other implantable component of (total) replacement heart system**
Implantable battery
Implantable controller
Transcutaneous energy transfer [TET] device

> Excludes: *replacement or repair of heart assist system [VAD] (37.63)*
> *replacement or repair of thoracic unit of (total) replacement heart system (37.53)*

37.55 **Removal of internal biventricular heart replacement system**
Explantation of artificial heart

> *Code also any concomitant procedure, such as:*
> *combined heart-lung transplantation (33.6)*
> *heart transplantation (37.51)*
> *implantation of internal biventricular heart replacement system (37.52)*

> Excludes: *explantation [removal] of external heart assist system (37.64)*
> *explantation [removal] of percutaneous external heart assist device (97.44)*
> *nonoperative removal of heart assist system (97.44)*
> *that with replacement or repair of heart replacement system (37.53, 37.54)*

37.6 **Implantation of heart and circulatory assist system(s)**

> Excludes: *implantation of prosthetic cardiac support system (37.41)*

37.60 **Implantation or insertion of biventricular external heart assist system**
Temporary cardiac support for both left and right ventricles, inserted in the same operative episode
Includes: open chest (sternotomy) procedure for cannulae attachments
Note: Device (outside the body but connected to heart) with external circulation pump.
Ventriculotomy is included; do not code separately

> Excludes: *implantation of internal biventricular heart replacement system (artificial heart) (37.52)*
> *implant of pulsation balloon (37.61)*
> *insertion of percutaneous external heart assist device (37.68)*
> *insertion of temporary non-implantable extracorporeal circulatory assist device (37.62)*

37.61 **Implant of pulsation balloon**

37.62 **Insertion of temporary non-implantable extracorporeal circulatory assist device**
Insertion of:
heart assist system, NOS
heart pump

> Excludes: *implantation of total internal biventricular heart replacement system [artificial heart] (37.52)*
> *implant of external heart assist system (37.65)*
> *insertion of implantable extracorporeal heart assist system (37.66)*
> *insertion of percutaneous external heart assist device (37.68)*
> *removal of heart assist system (37.64)*

Note: Includes explantation of this device; do not code separately

37.63 **Repair of heart assist system**
Replacement of parts of an existing ventricular assist device (VAD)

> Excludes: *replacement or repair of other implantable component of (total) replacement heart system [artificial heart] (37.54)*
> *replacement or repair of thoracic unit of (total) replacement heart system [artificial heart] (37.53)*

37.64 **Removal of external heart assist system(s) or device(s)**
Explantation of external device(s) providing left and right ventricular support
Explantation of single external device and cannulae

> Excludes: *explantation [removal] of percutaneous external heart assist device (97.44)*
> *nonoperative removal of heart assist system (97.44)*
> *temporary non-implantable extracorporeal circulatory assist device (37.62)*
> *that with replacement of implant (37.63)*

	Valid O.R. procedure		Non-O.R. procedure		Nonspecific O.R. procedure		Noncovered O.R. procedure

37.65 Implant of single ventricular (extracorporeal) external heart assist system
        Insertion of one device into one ventricle
Note: Device (outside the body but connected to heart) with external circulation and
        pump.
Note: Insertion or implantation of one external VAD for left or right heart support.
        Includes open chest (sternotomy) procedure for cannulae attachments

> Excludes: *implant of pulsation balloon (37.61)*
>   *implantation of total internal biventricular heart replacement system*
>   *(37.52)*
>   *insertion of implantable heart assist system (37.66)*
>   *insertion or implantation of two external VADs for simultaneous right*
>   *and left heart support (37.60)*
>   *insertion of percutaneous external heart assist device (37.68)*
>   *that without sternotomy (37.62)*

37.66 Insertion of implantable heart assist system
Note: Device directly connected to the heart and implanted in the upper left quadrant of
        peritoneal cavity
Note: This device can be used for either destination therapy (DT) or bridge-to-transplant
        (BTT)

        Axial flow heart assist system
        Diagonal pump heart assist system
        Left ventricular assist device (LVAD)
        Pulsatile heart assist system
        Right ventricular assist device (RVAD)
        Rotary pump heart assist system
        Transportable, implantable heart assist system
        Ventricular assist device (VAD) not otherwise specified

> Excludes: *implant of pulsation balloon (37.61)*
>   *implantation of total internal biventricular heart replacement system*
>   *[artificial heart] (37.52)*
>   *insertion of percutaneous external heart assist device (37.68)*

37.67 Implantation of cardiomyostimulation system
Note: Two-step open procedure consisting of transfer of one end of the latissimus dorsi
        muscle; wrapping it around the heart; rib resection; implantation of epicardial cardiac
        pacing leads into the right ventricle; tunneling and pocket creation for the
        cardiomyostimulator.

37.68 Insertion of percutaneous external heart assist device
        Includes percutaneous [femoral] insertion of cannulae attachments
        Circulatory assist device
        Extrinsic heart assist device
        pVAD
        Percutaneous heart assist device

**37.7   Insertion, revision, replacement and removal of leads; insertion of temporary
        pacemaker system; or revision of cardiac device pocket**
        Code also any insertion and replacement of pacemaker device (37.80-37.87)

> Excludes: *implantation or replacement of transvenous lead [electrode] into left*
>   *ventricular cardiac venous system (00.52)*

37.70 Initial insertion of lead [electrode], not otherwise specified

> Excludes: *insertion of temporary transvenous pacemaker system (37.78)*
>   *replacement of atrial and/or ventricular lead(s) (37.76)*

37.71 Initial insertion of transvenous lead [electrode] into ventricle

> Excludes: *insertion of temporary transvenous pacemaker system (37.78)*
>   *replacement of atrial and/or ventricular lead(s) (37.76)*

37.72 Initial insertion of transvenous leads [electrodes] into atrium and ventricle

> Excludes: *insertion of temporary transvenous pacemaker system (37.78)*
>   *replacement of atrial and/or ventricular lead(s) (37.76)*

37.73 Initial insertion of transvenous lead [electrode] into atrium

> Excludes: *insertion of temporary transvenous pacemaker system (37.78)*
>   *replacement of atrial and/or ventricular lead(s) (37.76)*

● Code new   ▲ Revision of   ④ ⑤ Fourth or fifth
        to 2012 edition   existing code   digit required

37.74 Insertion or replacement of epicardial lead [electrode] into epicardium

Insertion or replacement of epicardial lead by:
sternotomy
thoracotomy

> Excludes: replacement of atrial and/or ventricular lead(s) (37.76)

37.75 Revision of lead [electrode]

Repair of electrode [removal with re-insertion]
Repositioning of lead(s) (AICD) (cardiac device) (CRT-D) (CRT-P) (defibrillator)
(pacemaker) (pacing) (sensing) [electrode]
Revision of lead NOS

> Excludes: repositioning of temporary transvenous pacemaker system—omit code

37.76 Replacement of transvenous atrial and/or ventricular lead(s) [electrode]

Removal or abandonment of existing transvenous or epicardial lead(s) with
transvenous lead(s) replacement

> Excludes: replacement of epicardial lead [electrode] (37.74)

37.77 Removal of lead(s) [electrode] without replacement

Removal:
epicardial lead (transthoracic approach)
transvenous lead(s)

> Excludes: removal of temporary transvenous pacemaker system—omit code
> that with replacement of:
> atrial and/or ventricular lead(s) [electrode] (37.76)
> epicardial lead [electrode] (37.74)

37.78 Insertion of temporary transvenous pacemaker system

> Excludes: intraoperative cardiac pacemaker (39.64)

37.79 Revision or relocation of cardiac device pocket

Debridement and reforming pocket (skin and subcutaneous tissue)
Insertion of loop recorder
Relocation of pocket [creation of new pocket] pacemaker or CRT-P
Removal of cardiac device/pulse generator without replacement
Removal of the implantable hemodynamic pressure sensor (lead) and monitor
device
Removal without replacement of cardiac resynchronization defibrillator device
Repositioning of implantable hemodynamic pressure sensor (lead) and monitor
device
Repositioning of pulse generator
Revision of cardioverter/defibrillator (automatic) pocket
Revision of pocket for intracardiac hemodynamic monitoring
Revision or relocation of CRT-D pocket
Revision or relocation of pacemaker, defibrillator, or other implanted cardiac device
pocket

> Excludes: removal of loop recorder (86.05)

37.8   Insertion, replacement, removal, and revision of pacemaker device

Note: Device testing during procedure—omit code

> Code also any lead insertion, lead replacement, lead removal and/or lead revision
> (37.70-37.77)

> Excludes: implantation of cardiac resynchronication pacemaker [CRT-P] (00.50)
> implantation or replacement of cardiac resynchronization pacemaker pulse
> generator only [CRT-P] (00.53)

**37.80 Insertion of permanent pacemaker, initial or replacement, type of device not
specified**

37.81 Initial insertion of single-chamber device, not specified as rate responsive

> Excludes: replacement of existing pacemaker device (37.85-37.87)

37.82 Initial insertion of a single-chamber device, rate responsive

Rate responsive to physiologic stimuli other than atrial rate

> Excludes: replacement of existing pacemaker device (37.85-37.87)

37.83 Initial insertion of dual-chamber device

Atrial ventricular sequential device

> Excludes: replacement of existing pacemaker device (37.85-37.87)

Valid O.R.   Non-O.R.   Nonspecific   Noncovered
procedure   procedure   O.R. procedure   O.R. procedure

37.85 **Replacement of any type pacemaker device with single-chamber device, not specified as rate responsive**

37.86 **Replacement of any type pacemaker device with single-chamber device, rate responsive**
Rate responsive to physiologic stimuli other than atrial rate

37.87 **Replacement of any type pacemaker device with dual-chamber device**
Atrial ventricular sequential device

37.89 **Revision or removal of pacemaker device**
Removal without replacement of cardiac resynchronization pacemaker device [CRT-P]
Repair of pacemaker device

> Excludes: *removal of temporary transvenous pacemaker system—omit code*
> *replacement of existing pacemaker device (37.85-37.87)*
> *replacement of existing pacemaker device with CRT-P pacemaker device (00.53)*

37.9 **Other operations on heart and pericardium**

37.90 **Insertion of left atrial appendage device**
Left atrial filter
Left atrial occluder
Transseptal catheter technique

37.91 **Open chest cardiac massage**

> Excludes: *closed chest cardiac massage (99.63)*

37.92 **Injection of therapeutic substance into heart**

37.93 **Injection of therapeutic substance into pericardium**

37.94 **Implantation or replacement of automatic cardioverter/defibrillator, total system [AICD]**
Implantation of defibrillator with leads (epicardial patches), formation of pocket (abdominal fascia) (subcutaneous), any transvenous leads, intraoperative procedures for evaluation of lead signals, and obtaining defibrillator threshold measurements
Techniques:
lateral thoracotomy
medial sternotomy
subxiphoid procedure
Note: Device testing during procedure—*omit code*
Code also extracorporeal circulation, if performed (39.61)
Code also any concomitant procedure [e.g., coronary bypass (36.10-36.19) or CCM, total system (17.51)]

> Excludes: *implantation of cardiac resynchronization defibrillator, total system [CRT-D] (00.51)*

37.95 **Implantation of automatic cardioverter/defibrillator lead(s) only**

37.96 **Implantation of automatic cardioverter/defibrillator pulse generator only**
Note: Device testing during procedure—*omit code*

> Excludes: *implantation or replacement of cardiac resynchronization defibrillator, pulse generator device only [CRT-D] (00.54)*

37.97 **Replacement of automatic cardioverter/defibrillator lead(s) only**

> Excludes: *replacement of epicardial lead [electrode] into epicardium (37.74)*
> *replacement of transvenous lead [electrode] into left ventricular coronary venous system (00.52)*

37.98 **Replacement of automatic cardioverter/defibrillator pulse generator only**
Note: Device testing during procedure—*omit code*

> Excludes: *replacement of cardiac resynchronization defibrillator, pulse generator device only [CRT-D] (00.54)*

● Code new to 2012 edition   ▲ Revision of existing code   ④ ⑤ Fourth or fifth digit required

37.99 **Other**

> *Excludes:* cardiac retraining (93.36)
> conversion of cardiac rhythm (99.60-99.69)
> implantation of prosthetic cardiac support device (37.41)
> insertion of left atrial appendage device (37.90)
> maze procedure (Cox-maze), open (37.33)
> maze procedure, endovascular approach (37.34)
> repositioning of pulse generator (37.79)
> revision of lead(s) (37.75)
> revision or relocation of pacemaker, defibrillator or other implanted
>   cardiac device pocket (37.79)

38 **Incision, excision, and occlusion of vessels**

Code also any application or administration of an adhesion barrier substance (99.77)

Code also cardiopulmonary bypass [extracorporeal circulation] [heart-lung machine] (39.61)

Excludes: that of coronary vessels (00.66, 36.03, 36.04, 36.09, 36.10-36.99)

The following fourth-digit subclassification is for use with appropriate categories in sections 38.0, 38.1, 38.3, 38.5, 38.6, 38.8 and 38.9, which are marked with a symbol ④ to identify the site. Valid fourth digits are in [brackets] under each code.

0 unspecified site
1 intracranial vessels
   Cerebral (anterior) (middle)
   Circle of Willis
   Posterior communicating artery
2 other vessels of head and neck
   Carotid artery (common) (external) (internal)
   Jugular vein (external) (internal)
3 upper limb vessels
   Axillary   Radial
   Brachial   Ulnar
4 aorta
5 other thoracic vessels
   Innominate   Subclavian
   Pulmonary (artery) (vein)   Vena cava, superior
6 abdominal arteries
   Celiac   Mesenteric
   Gastric   Renal
   Hepatic   Splenic
   Iliac   Umbilical

> *Excludes:* abdominal aorta (4)

7 abdominal veins
   Iliac   Splenic
   Portal   Vena cava(inferior)
   Renal
8 lower limb arteries
   Femoral (common) (superficial)
   Popliteal
   Tibial
9 lower limb veins
   Femoral   Saphenous
   Popliteal   Tibial

④ **38.0** **Incision of vessel**
[0-9]   Embolectomy
      Thrombectomy

> *Excludes:* endovascular removal of obstruction from head and neck vessel(s) (39.74)
> puncture or catheterization of any:
>   artery (38.91, 38.98)
>   vein (38.92-38.95, 38.99)

Valid O.R.   Non-O.R.   Nonspecific   Noncovered
procedure   procedure   O.R. procedure   O.R. procedure

④ **38.1** **Endarterectomy**
[0-6,8] Endarterectomy with:
  embolectomy
  patch graft
  temporary bypass during procedure
  thrombectomy

  Code also any:
  number of vascular stents inserted (00.45-00.48)
  number of vessels treated (00.40-00.43)
  procedure on vessel bifurcation (00.44)

38.2 **Diagnostic procedures on blood vessels**

  | Excludes: | *adjunct vascular system procedures (00.40-00.43)*

38.21 **Biopsy of blood vessel**

38.22 **Percutaneous angioscopy**

  | Excludes: | *angioscopy of eye (95.12)*

38.23 **Intravascular spectroscopy**
  Includes: spectroscopy of both coronary and peripheral vessels
  Intravascular chemography
  Near infrared (NIR) spectroscopy

  | Excludes: | *intravascular imaging of:*
    coronary vessels (00.24, 38.24)
    peripheral vessels (00.23, 38.25)

38.24 **Intravascular imaging of coronary vessel(s) by optical coherence tomography [OCT]**

38.25 **Intravascular imaging of non-coronary vessel(s) by optical coherence tomography [OCT]**

  | Excludes: | *intravascular imaging of coronary vessel(s) by OCT (38.24)*

● **38.26** **Insertion of implantable pressure sensor without lead for intracardiac or great vessel hemodynamic monitoring**
  Note: The sensor is a standalone device and is not physically connected to a separately implanted monitor.

  Leadless pressure sensor not physically connected to a separately implanted monitor
  Single device combination leadless pressure sensor with integral monitor for
    intracardiac or great vessel (or branch thereof) hemodynamic monitoring
  With or without internal batteries
  Without leads

  | Excludes: | *circulatory monitoring (blood gas, arterial or venous pressure,*
    cardiac output and coronary blood flow) (89.60-89.69)
    hemodynamic monitoring system with sensor and separately implanted
    monitor (00.56 – 00.57)
    insertion or replacement of implantable pressure sensor with lead for
    intracardiac or great vessel hemodynamic monitoring (00.56)

38.29 **Other diagnostic procedures on blood vessels**

  | Excludes: | *blood vessel thermography (88.86)*
    circulatory monitoring (89.61-89.69)
    contrast:
    angiocardiography (88.50-88.58)
    arteriography (88.40-88.49)
    phlebography (88.60-88.67)
    impedance phlebography (88.68)
    peripheral vascular ultrasonography (88.77)
    plethysmogram (89.58)

④ **38.3** **Resection of vessel with anastomosis**
[0-9] Angiectomy with anastomosis
  Excision of:
  aneurysm (arteriovenous) with anastomosis
  blood vessel (lesion) with anastomosis

● Code new   ▲ Revision of   ④ ⑤ Fourth or fifth
    to 2012 edition   existing code   digit required

④ **38.4 Resection of vessel with replacement**
[0-9] Angiectomy with replacement
Excision of
aneurysm (arteriovenous) with replacement
blood vessel (lesion) with replacement
Partial resection with replacement

> Excludes: *endovascular repair of aneurysm (39.71-39.79)*

Requires the use of one of the following fourth-digit subclassifications to identify site:
0 unspecified site
1 intracranial vessels
Cerebral (anterior) (middle)
Circle of Willis
Posterior communicating artery
2 other vessels of head and neck
Carotid artery (common) (external) (internal)
Jugular vein (external) (internal)
3 upper limb vessels
Axillary   Radial
Brachial   Ulnar
4 aorta, abdominal
Code also any thoracic vessel involvement (thoracoabdominal procedure) (38.45)
5 thoracic vessel
Aorta (thoracic)   Subclavian
Innominate   Vena cava (superior)
Pulmonary (artery) (vein)
Code also any abdominal aorta involvement (thoracoabdominal procedure) (38.44)
6 abdominal arteries
Celiac   Mesenteric
Gastric   Renal
Hepatic   Splenic
Iliac   Umbilical

> Excludes: *abdominal aorta (4)*

7 abdominal veins
Iliac   Splenic
Portal   Vena cava (inferior)
Renal
8 lower limb arteries
Femoral (common) (superficial)
Tibial

9 lower limb veins
Femoral   Saphenous
Popliteal   Tibial

④ **38.5 Ligation and stripping of varicose veins**
[0-3,5,7,9]

> Excludes: *ligation of varices:*
> *esophageal (42.91)*
> *gastric (44.91)*

④ **38.6 Other excision of vessels**
[0-9] Excision of blood vessel (lesion) NOS

> Excludes: *excision of vessel for aortocoronary bypass (36.10-36.14)*
> *excision with:*
> *anastomosis (38.30-38.39)*
> *graft replacement (38.40-38.49)*
> *implant (38.40-38.49)*

38.7 Interruption of vena cava
Insertion of implant or sieve in vena cava
Ligation of vena cava (inferior) (superior)
Plication of vena cava

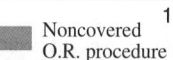

Valid O.R.   Non-O.R.   Nonspecific   Noncovered
procedure   procedure   O.R. procedure   O.R. procedure

[4] **38.8 Other surgical occlusion of vessels**
[0-9]
Clamping of blood vessel
Division of blood vessel
Ligation of blood vessel
Occlusion of blood vessel

[Excludes:] *adrenal vessels (07.43)*
esophageal varices (42.91)
gastric or duodenal vessel for ulcer (44.40-44.49)
gastric varices (44.91)
meningeal vessel (02.13)
percutaneous transcatheter infusion embolization (99.29)
spermatic vein for varicocele (63.1)
surgical occlusion of vena cava (38.7)
that for chemoembolization (99.25)
that for control of (postoperative) hemorrhage:
anus (49.95)
bladder (57.93)
following vascular procedure (39.41)
nose (21.00-21.09)
prostate (60.94)
tonsil (28.7)
thyroid vessel (06.92)

38.9 Puncture of vessel

[Excludes:] *that for circulatory monitoring (89.60-89.69)*

38.91 Arterial catheterization

38.92 Umbilical vein catheterization

38.93 Venous catheterization, not elsewhere classified

[Excludes:] *that for cardiac catheterization (37.21-37.23)*
that for renal dialysis (38.95)
that with guidance (electrocardiogram) (fluoroscopy) (ultrasound) (38.97)

38.94 Venous cutdown

38.95 Venous catheterization for renal dialysis

[Excludes:] *insertion of totally implantable vascular access device [VAD] 86.07*

38.97 Central venous catheter placement with guidance
Includes guidance by:
electrocardiogram
fluoroscopy
ultrasound

38.98 Other puncture of artery

[Excludes:] *that for:*
arteriography (88.40-88.49)
coronary arteriography (88.55-88.57)

38.99 Other puncture of vein
Phlebotomy

[Excludes:] *that for:*
angiography of veins (88.60-88.68)
extracorporeal circulation (39.61, 50.92)
injection or infusion of:
sclerosing solution (39.92)
therapeutic or prophylactic substance (99.11-99.29)
perfusion (39.96-39.97)
phlebography (88.60-88.68)
transfusion (99.01-99.09)

39 Other operations on vessels

[Excludes:] *those on coronary vessels (36.03-36.99)*

39.0 Systemic to pulmonary artery shunt
Descending aorta-pulmonary artery anastomosis (graft)
Left to right anastomosis (graft)
Subclavian-pulmonary anastomosis (graft)

Code also cardiopulmonary bypass [extracorporeal circulation] [heart-lung machine] (39.61)

39.1   Intra-abdominal venous shunt
Anastomosis:
  mesocaval
  portacaval
  portal vein to inferior vena cava
  splenic and renal veins
  transjugular intrahepatic portosystemic shunt (TIPS)

  | Excludes: | *peritoneovenous shunt (54.94)*

39.2   Other shunt or vascular bypass
Code also pressurized treatment of venous bypass graft [conduit] with pharmaceutical substance, if performed (00.16)

39.21   Caval-pulmonary artery anastomosis
Code also cardiopulmonary bypass (39.61)

39.22   Aorta-subclavian-carotid bypass
Bypass (arterial):
  aorta to carotid and brachial
  aorta to subclavian and carotid
  carotid to subclavian

39.23   Other intrathoracic vascular shunt or bypass
Intrathoracic (arterial) bypass graft NOS

  | Excludes: | *coronary artery bypass (36.10-36.19)*

39.24   Aorta-renal bypass

39.25   Aorta-iliac-femoral bypass
Bypass:
  aortofemoral
  aortoiliac
  aortoiliac to popliteal
  aortopopliteal
  iliofemoral [iliac-femoral]

39.26   Other intra-abdominal vascular shunt or bypass
Bypass:
  aortoceliac
  aortic-superior mesenteric
  common hepatic-common iliac-renal
Intra-abdominal arterial bypass graft NOS

  | Excludes: | *peritoneovenous shunt (54.94)*

39.27   Arteriovenostomy for renal dialysis
Anastomosis for renal dialysis
Formation of (peripheral) arteriovenous fistula for renal (kidney] dialysis
Code also any renal dialysis (39.95)

39.28   Extracranial-intracranial (EC-IC) vascular bypass

39.29   Other (peripheral) vascular shunt or bypass
Bypass (graft):
  axillary-brachial
  axillary-femoral [axillofemoral] (superficial)
  brachial
  femoral-femoral
  femoroperoneal
  femoropopliteal (arteries)
  femorotibial (anterior) (posterior)
  popliteal
  vascular NOS

  | Excludes: | *peritoneovenous shunt (54.94)*

39.3   Suture of vessel
Repair of laceration of blood vessel

  | Excludes: | *any other vascular puncture closure device—omit code*
  suture of aneurysm (39.52)
  that for control of hemorrhage (postoperative):
  anus (49.95)
  bladder (57.93)
  following vascular procedure (39.41)
  nose (21.00-21.09)
  prostate (60.94)
  tonsil (28.7)

Valid O.R. procedure   Non-O.R. procedure   Nonspecific O.R. procedure   Noncovered O.R. procedure

39.30 Suture of unspecified blood vessel

39.31 Suture of artery

39.32 Suture of vein

39.4 **Revision of vascular procedure**

39.41 Control of hemorrhage following vascular surgery

> *Excludes:* *that for control of hemorrhage (postoperative):*
> *anus (49.95)*
> *bladder (57.93)*
> *nose (21.00-21.09)*
> *prostate (60.94)*
> *tonsil (28.7)*

39.42 Revision of arteriovenous shunt for renal dialysis
Conversion of renal dialysis:
   end-to-end anastomosis to end-to-side
   end-to-side anastomosis to end-to-end
   vessel-to-vessel cannula to arteriovenous shunt
Removal of old arteriovenous shunt and creation of new shunt

> *Excludes:* *replacement of vessel-to-vessel cannula (39.94)*

39.43 Removal of arteriovenous shunt for renal dialysis

> *Excludes:* *that with replacement [revision] of shunt (39.42)*

39.49 Other revision of vascular procedure
Declotting (graft)
Revision of:
   anastomosis of blood vessel
   vascular procedure (previous)

39.5 **Other repair of vessels**

▲ **39.50** Angioplasty of other non-coronary vessel(s)
Percutaneous transluminal angioplasty (PTA) of non-coronary vessel:
   lower extremity vessels
   mesenteric artery
   renal artery
   upper extremity vessels

> *Code also any:*
> *atherectomy of other non-coronary vessel(s) (17.56)*
> *injection or infusion of thrombolytic agent (99.10)*
> *insertion of drug-eluting peripheral vessel stent (00.55)*
> *insertion of non-drug-eluting peripheral vessel stent(s) or stent graft(s) (39.90)*
> *number of vascular stents inserted (00.45-00.48)*
> *number of vessels treated (00.40-00.43)*
> *procedure on vessel bifurcation (00.44)*

> *Excludes:* *percutaneous angioplasty of extracranial or intracranial vessel(s)*
> *(00.61-00.62)*
> *percutaneous atherectomy of extracranial or intracranial vessel(s)*
> *(17.53-17.54)*

39.51 Clipping of aneurysm

> *Excludes:* *clipping of arteriovenous fistula (39.53)*

39.52 Other repair of aneurysm
Repair of aneurysm by:
   coagulation
   electrocoagulation
   filipuncture
   methyl methacrylate
   suture
   wiring
   wrapping

> *Excludes:* *endovascular repair of aneurysm (39.71-39.79)*
> *re-entry operation (aorta) (39.54)*
> *that with:*
> *graft replacement (38.40-38.49)*
> *resection (38.30-38.49, 38.60-38.69)*

● Code new
to 2012 edition

▲ Revision of
existing code

④ ⑤ Fourth or fifth
digit required

39.53 **Repair of arteriovenous fistula**
Embolization of carotid cavernous fistula
Repair of arteriovenous fistula by:
clipping
coagulation
ligation and division

Excludes:	*repair of:*

arteriovenous shunt for renal dialysis (39.42)
head and neck vessels, endovascular approach (39.72)
that with:
graft replacement (38.40-38.49)
resection (38.30-38.49, 38.60-38.69)

39.54 **Re-entry operation (aorta)**
Fenestration of dissecting aneurysm of thoracic aorta

Code also cardiopulmonary bypass [extracorporeal circulation] [heart-lung machine] (39.61)

39.55 **Reimplantation of aberrant renal vessel**

39.56 **Repair of blood vessel with tissue patch graft**

Excludes:	*that with resection (38.40-38.49)*

39.57 **Repair of blood vessel with synthetic patch graft**

Excludes:	*that with resection (38.40-38.49)*

39.58 **Repair of blood vessel with unspecified type of patch graft**

Excludes:	*that with resection (38.40-38.49)*

39.59 **Other repair of vessel**
Aorticopulmonary window operation
Arterioplasty NOS
Construction of venous valves (peripheral)
Plication of vein (peripheral)
Reimplantation of artery

Code also cardiopulmonary bypass [extracorporeal circulation] [heart-lung machine] (39.61)

Excludes:	*interruption of the vena cava (38.7)*

reimplantation of renal artery (39.55)
that with:
graft (39.56-39.58)
resection (38.30-38.49, 38.60-38.69)

39.6 **Extracorporeal circulation and procedures auxiliary to heart surgery**

39.61 **Extracorporeal circulation auxiliary to open heart surgery**
Artificial heart and lung
Cardiopulmonary bypass
Pump oxygenator

Excludes:	*extracorporeal hepatic assistance (50.92)*

extracorporeal membrane oxygenation [ECMO] (39.65)
hemodialysis (39.95)
percutaneous cardiopulmonary bypass (39.66)

39.62 **Hypothermia (systemic) incidental to open heart surgery**

39.63 **Cardioplegia**
Arrest:
anoxic
circulatory

39.64 **Intraoperative cardiac pacemaker**
Temporary pacemaker used during and immediately following cardiac surgery

39.65 **Extracorporeal membrane oxygenation (ECMO)**

Excludes:	*extracorporeal circulation auxiliary to open heart surgery (39.61)*

percutaneous cardiopulmonary bypass (39.66)

39.66 **Percutaneous cardiopulmonary bypass**
Closed chest

Excludes:	*extracorporeal circulation auxiliary to open heart surgery (39.61)*

extracorporeal hepatic assistance (50.92)
extracorporeal membrane oxygenation [ECMO] (39.65)
hemodialysis (39.95)

	Valid O.R. procedure		Non-O.R. procedure		Nonspecific O.R. procedure		Noncovered O.R. procedure

39.7 **Endovascular procedures on vessel(s)**
 Embolization
 Endoluminal repair
 Implantation
 Occlusion
 Removal
 Repair

> | Excludes: | *angioplasty of other non-coronary vessel(s) (39.50)*
> *atherectomy of other non-coronary vessel(s) (17.56)*
> *insertion of non-drug-eluting peripheral vessel stent(s) (39.90)*
> *other repair of aneurysm (39.52)*
> *percutaneous insertion of carotid artery stent(s) (00.63)*
> *percutaneous insertion of intracranial stent(s) (00.65)*
> *percutaneous insertion of other precerebral artery stent(s) (00.64)*
> *resection of abdominal aorta with replacement (38.44)*
> *resection of lower limb arteries with replacement (38.48)*
> *resection of thoracic aorta with replacement (38.45)*
> *resection of upper limb vessels with replacement (38.43)*
> *temporary therapeutic partial occlusion of vessel (39.77)*

▲ **39.71** **Endovascular implantation of other graft in abdominal aorta**
 Endovascular repair of abdominal aortic aneurysm with graft
 Stent graft(s)

 Code also intra-aneurysm sac pressure monitoring (intraoperative) (00.58)

> | Excludes: | *endovascular implantation of branching or fenestrated graft in aorta (39.78)*

▲ **39.72** **Endovascular (total) embolization or occlusion of head and neck vessels**
 Coil-retention stent
 Embolization stent
 Endograft(s)
 Endovascular grafts(s)
 Liquid tissue adhesive (glue) embolization or occlusion
 Other implant or substance for repair, embolization or occlusion
 That for repair of aneurysm, arteriovenous malformation [AVM] or fistula

> | Excludes: | *embolization of head or neck vessels using bare coils (39.75)*
> *embolization of head or neck vessels using bioactive coils (39.76)*
> *mechanical thrombectomy of pre-cerebral and cerebral vessels (39.74)*

39.73 **Endovascular implantation of graft in thoracic aorta**
 Endograft(s)
 Endovascular graft(s)
 Endovascular repair of defect of thoracic aorta with graft(s) or device(s)
 Stent graft(s) or device(s)
 That for repair of aneurysm, dissection, or injury
 Code also intra-aneurysm sac pressure monitoring (intraoperative) (00.58)

> | Excludes: | *fenestration of dissecting aneurysm of thoracic aorta (39.54)*

39.74 **Endovascular removal of obstruction from head and neck vessel(s)**
 Endovascular embolectomy
 Endovascular thrombectomy of pre-cerebral and cerebral vessels
 Mechanical embolectomy or thrombectomy
 Code also:
  any injection or infusion of thrombolytic agent (99.10)
  number of vessels treated (00.40-00.43)
  procedure on vessel bifurcation (00.44)

> | Excludes: | *endarterectomy of intracranial vessels and other vessels of head and neck (38.11-38.12)*
> *occlusive endovascular embolization of head or neck vessel(s) using bare coils (39.75)*
> *occlusive endovascular embolization of head or neck vessel(s) using bioactive coils (39.76)*
> *open embolectomy or thrombectomy (38.01- 38.02)*

39.75 **Endovascular embolization or occlusion of vessel(s) of head or neck using bare coils**
 Bare metal coils
 Bare platinum coils [BPC]
 That for treatment of aneurysm, arteriovenous malformation [AVM] or fistula

 ● Code new ▲ Revision of ④ ⑤ Fourth or fifth
  to 2012 edition existing code   digit required

39.76 **Endovascular embolization or occlusion of vessel(s) of head or neck using bioactive coils**
Biodegradable inner luminal polymer coils
Coil embolization or occlusion utilizing bioactive coils
Coils containing polyglycolic acid [PGA]
That for treatment of aneurysm, arteriovenous malformation [AVM] or fistula

● **39.77** **Temporary (partial) therapeutic endovascular occlusion of vessel**
Includes that of aorta
That by balloon catheter

Code also any: diagnostic arteriogram (88.40-88.49)

Excludes: *any endovascular head or neck vessel procedure (39.72, 39.74-39.76)*
diagnostic procedures on blood vessels (38.21-38.29)
permanent endovascular procedure (39.79)

● **39.78** **Endovascular implantation of branching or fenestrated graft(s) in aorta**

39.79 **Other endovascular procedures on other vessels**
Endograft(s)
Endovascular graft(s)
Liquid tissue adhesive (glue) embolization or occlusion
Other coil embolization or occlusion
Other implant or substance for repair, embolization or occlusion
Repair of aneurysm

Excludes: *abdominal aortic aneurysm resection [AAA] (38.44)*
endovascular implantation of graft in abdominal aorta (39.71)
endovascular implantation of graft in thoracic aorta (39.73)
endovascular embolization or occlusion of head and neck vessels, bare metal coils (39.75)
endovascular embolization or occlusion of head and neck vessels, bioactive coils (39.76)
insertion of drug-eluting peripheral vessel stent(s) (00.55)
insertion of non-drug-eluting peripheral vessel stent(s) (for other than aneurysm repair) (39.90)
non-endovascular repair of arteriovenous fistula (39.53)
other surgical occlusion of vessels—see category 38.8
percutaneous transcatheter infusion (99.29)
thoracic aortic aneurysm resection (38.45)
transcatheter embolization for gastric or duodenal bleeding (44.44)
uterine artery embolization with coils (68.24)

39.8 **Operations on carotid body, carotid sinus and other vascular bodies**

Excludes: *excision of glomus jugulare (20.51)*

39.81 **Implantation or replacement of carotid sinus stimulation device, total system**
Carotid sinus baroreflex activation device
Implantation of carotid sinus stimulator and lead(s)
Includes: carotid explorations

Excludes: *implantation or replacement of carotid sinus stimulation lead(s) only (39.82)*
implantation or replacement of carotid sinus stimulation pulse generator only (39.83)

39.82 **Implantation or replacement of carotid sinus stimulation lead(s) only**

Excludes: *implantation or replacement of carotid sinus stimulation device, total system (39.81)*

39.83 **Implantation or replacement of carotid sinus stimulation pulse generator only**

Excludes: *implantation or replacement of carotid sinus stimulation device, total system (39.81)*

39.84 **Revision of carotid sinus stimulation lead(s) only**
Repair of electrode [removal with re-insertion]
Repositioning of lead(s) [electrode]

39.85 **Revision of carotid sinus stimulation pulse generator**
Debridement and reforming pocket (skin and subcutaneous tissue)
Relocation of pocket [creation of new pocket]
Repositioning of pulse generator
Revision of carotid sinus stimulation pulse generator pocket

39.86 **Removal of carotid sinus stimulation device, total system**

39.87 **Removal of carotid sinus stimulation lead(s) only**

39.88 **Removal of carotid sinus stimulation pulse generator only**

| | Valid O.R. procedure | | Non-O.R. procedure | | Nonspecific O.R. procedure | | Noncovered O.R. procedure |

39.89 Other operations on carotid body, carotid sinus and other vascular bodies
Chemodectomy
Denervation of:
  aortic body
  carotid body
Glomectomy, carotid

> *Excludes:* excision of glomus jugulare (20.51)

39.9 Other operations on vessels

39.90 Insertion of non-drug-eluting peripheral (non-coronary) vessel stent(s)
Bare stent(s)
Bonded stent(s)
Drug-coated stent(s), i.e., heparing coated
Endograft(s)
Endovascular graft(s)
Endovascular recanalization techniques
Stent graft(s)

Code also any:
  non-coronary angioplasty or atherectomy (39.50)
  number of vascular stents inserted (00.45-00.48)
  number of vessels treated (00.40-00.43)
  procedure on vessel bifurcation (00.44)

> *Excludes:* that for aneurysm repair (39.71-39.79)
>   insertion of drug-eluting peripheral vessel stent(s) (00.55)
>   percutaneous insertion of carotid artery stent(s) (00.63)
>   percutaneous insertion of intracranial stent(s) (00.65)
>   percutaneous insertion of other precerebral artery stent(s) (00.64)

39.91 Freeing of vessel
Dissection and freeing of adherent tissue:
  artery-vein-nerve bundle
  vascular bundle

39.92 Injection of sclerosing agent into vein

> *Excludes:* injection:
>   esophageal varices (42.33)
>   hemorrhoids (49.42)

39.93 Insertion of vessel-to-vessel cannula
Formation of arteriovenous:
  fistula by external cannula
  shunt by external cannula
Code also any renal dialysis (39.95)

39.9 4 Replacement of vessel-to-vessel cannula
Revision of vessel-to-vessel cannula

39.95 Hemodialysis

Artificial kidney	Hemofiltration
Hemodiafiltration	Renal dialysis

> *Excludes:* peritoneal dialysis (54.98)

39.96 Total body perfusion
Code also substance perfused (99.21-99.29)

39.97 Other perfusion
Perfusion NOS
Perfusion, local [regional] of:
  carotid artery
  coronary artery
  head
  lower limb
  neck
  upper limb
Code also substance perfused (99.21-99.29)

> *Excludes:* perfusion of:
>   kidney (55.95)
>   large intestine (46.96)
>   liver (50.93)
>   small intestine (46.95)
>   SuperSaturated oxygen therapy (00.49)

● Code new
  to 2012 edition ▲ Revision of
  existing code ④ ⑤ Fourth or fifth
  digit required

39.98 **Control of hemorrhage, not otherwise specified**
Angiotripsy
Control of postoperative hemorrhage NOS
Venotripsy

> *Excludes:* *control of hemorrhage (postoperative):*
> *anus (49.95)*
> *bladder (57.93)*
> *following vascular procedure (39.41)*
> *nose (21.00-21.09)*
> *prostate (60.94)*
> *tonsil (28.7)*
> *that by:*
> *ligation (38.80-38.89)*
> *suture (39.30-39.32)*

39.99 **Other operations on vessels**

> *Excludes:* *injection or infusion of therapeutic or prophylactic substance*
> *(99.11-99.29)*
> *transfusion of blood and blood components (99.01-99.09)*

Valid O.R.
procedure

Non-O.R.
procedure

Nonspecific
O.R. procedure

Noncovered
O.R. procedure

This page intentionally left blank.

● Code new
to 2012 edition
▲ Revision of
existing code
④ ⑤ Fourth or fifth
digit required

8.   OPERATIONS ON THE HEMIC AND LYMPHATIC SYSTEM (40-41)

40   Operations on lymphatic system

40.0   Incision of lymphatic structures

40.1   Diagnostic procedures on lymphatic structures

40.11   Biopsy of lymphatic structure
Transbronchoscopic needle aspiration [TBNA] of lymph node

40.19   Other diagnostic procedures on lymphatic structures

> Excludes: *lymphangiogram*
> *abdominal (88.04)*
> *cervical (87.08)*
> *intrathoracic (87.34)*
> *lower limb (88.36)*
> *upper limb (88.34)*
> *microscopic examination of specimen (90.71-90.79)*
> *radioisotope scan (92.16)*
> *thermography (88.89)*

40.2   Simple excision of lymphatic structure

> Excludes: *biopsy of lymphatic structure (40.11)*

40.21   Excision of deep cervical lymph node

40.22   Excision of internal mammary lymph node

40.23   Excision of axillary lymph node

40.24   Excision of inguinal lymph mode

40.29   Simple excision of other lymphatic structure
Excision of:
cystic hygroma
lymphangioma
Simple lymphadenectomy

40.3   Regional lymph node excision
Extended regional lymph node excision
Regional lymph node excision with excision of lymphatic drainage area including skin, subcutaneous tissue, and fat

40.4   Radical excision of cervical lymph nodes
Resection of cervical lymph nodes down to muscle and deep fascia

> Excludes: *that associated with radical laryngectomy (30.4)*

40.40   Radical neck dissection, not otherwise specified

40.41   Radical neck dissection, unilateral

40.42   Radical neck dissection, bilateral

40.5   Radical excision of other lymph nodes

> Excludes: *that associated with radical mastectomy (85.45-85.48)*

40.50   Radical excision of lymph nodes, not otherwise specified
Radical (lymph) node dissection NOS

40.51   Radical excision of axillary lymph nodes

40.52   Radical excision of periaortic lymph nodes

40.53   Radical excision of iliac lymph nodes

40.54   Radical groin dissection

40.59   Radical excision of other lymph nodes

> Excludes: *radical neck dissection (40.40-40.42)*

40.6   Operations on thoracic duct

40.61   Cannulation of thoracic duct

40.62   Fistulization of thoracic duct

40.63   Closure of fistula of thoracic duct

40.64   Ligation of thoracic duct

40.69   Other operations on thoracic duct

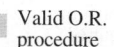 Valid O.R.
procedure

Non-O.R.
procedure

Nonspecific
O.R. procedure

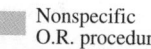 Noncovered
O.R. procedure

40.9   Other operations on lymphatic structures
Anastomosis of peripheral lymphatics
Dilation of peripheral lymphatics
Ligation of peripheral lymphatics
Obliteration of peripheral lymphatics
Reconstruction of peripheral lymphatics
Repair of peripheral lymphatics
Transplantation of peripheral lymphatics
Correction of lymphedema of limb, NOS

> Excludes: reduction of elephantiasis of scrotum (61.3)

41   Operations on bone marrow and spleen

41.0   Bone marrow or hematopoietic stem cell transplant
Note: To report donor source—*see* codes 00.91-00.93

> Excludes: aspiration of bone marrow from donor (41.91)

41.00   Bone marrow transplant, not otherwise specified

41.01   Autologous bone marrow transplant without purging

> Excludes: that with purging (41.09)

41.02   Allogeneic bone marrow transplant with purging
Allograft of bone marrow with in vitro removal (purging) of T-cells

41.03   Allogeneic bone marrow transplant without purging
Allograft of bone marrow NOS

41.04   Autologous hematopoietic stem cell transplant without purging

> Excludes: that with purging (41.07)

41.05   Allogeneic hematopoietic stem cell transplant without purging

> Excludes: that with purging (41.08)

41.06   Cord blood stem cell transplant

41.07   Autologous hematopoietic stem cell transplant with purging
Cell depletion

41.08   Allogeneic hematopoietic stem cell transplant with purging
Cell depletion

41.09   Autologous bone marrow transplant with purging
With extracorporeal purging of malignant cells from marrow
Cell depletion

41.1   Puncture of spleen

> Excludes: aspiration biopsy of spleen (41.32)

41.2   Splenotomy

41.3   Diagnostic procedures on bone marrow and spleen

41.31   Biopsy of bone marrow

41.32   Closed [aspiration] [percutaneous] biopsy of spleen
Needle biopsy of spleen

41.33   Open biopsy of spleen

41.38   Other diagnostic procedures on bone marrow

> Excludes: microscopic examination of specimen from bone marrow (90.61-90.69)
> radioisotope scan (92.05)

41.39   Other diagnostic procedures on spleen

> Excludes: microscopic examination of specimen from spleen (90.61-90.69)
> radioisotope scan (92.05)

41.4   Excision or destruction of lesion or tissue of spleen
Code also any application or administration of an adhesion barrier substance (99.77)

> Excludes: excision of accessory spleen (41.93)

41.41   Marsupialization of splenic cyst

41.42   Excision of lesion or tissue of spleen

> Excludes: biopsy of spleen (41.32-41.33)

41.43   Partial splenectomy

● Code new
  to 2012 edition   ▲ Revision of
                          existing code   ④ ⑤ Fourth or fifth
                                                digit required

41.5 **Total splenectomy**

Code also any application or administration of an adhesion barrier substance (99.77)
Splenectomy NOS

41.9 **Other operations on spleen and bone marrow**

Code also any application or administration of an adhesion barrier substance (99.77)

41.91 **Aspiration of bone marrow from donor for transplant**

Excludes: *biopsy of bone marrow (41.31)*

41.92 **Injection into bone marrow**

Excludes: *bone marrow transplant (41.00-41.03)*

41.93 **Excision of accessory spleen**

41.94 **Transplantation of spleen**

41.95 **Repair and plastic operations on spleen**

41.98 **Other operations on bone marrow**

41.99 **Other operations on spleen**

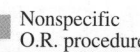

| | Valid O.R. procedure | | Non-O.R. procedure | | Nonspecific O.R. procedure | | Noncovered O.R. procedure |

This page intentionally left blank.

● Code new
   to 2012 edition

▲ Revision of
   existing code

④ ⑤ Fourth or fifth
   digit required

9. OPERATIONS ON THE DIGESTIVE SYSTEM (42-54)

42 Operations on esophagus

42.0 Esophagotomy

42.01 Incision of esophageal web

42.09 Other incision of esophagus
Esophagotomy NOS

> Excludes: esophagomyotomy (42.7)
> esophagostomy (42.10-42.19)

42.1 Esophagostomy

42.10 Esophagostomy, not otherwise specified

42.11 Cervical esophagostomy

42.12 Exteriorization of esophageal pouch

42.19 Other external fistulization of esophagus
Thoracic esophagostomy
Code also any resection (42.40-42.42)

42.2 Diagnostic procedures on esophagus

42.21 Operative esophagoscopy by incision

42.22 Esophagoscopy through artificial stoma

> Excludes: that with biopsy (42.24)

42.23 Other esophagoscopy

> Excludes: that with biopsy (42.24)

42.24 Closed [endoscopic] biopsy of esophagus
Brushing or washing for specimen collection
Esophagoscopy with biopsy
Suction biopsy of the esophagus

> Excludes: esophagogastroduodenoscopy [EGD] with closed biopsy (45.16)

42.25 Open biopsy of esophagus

42.29 Other diagnostic procedures on esophagus

> Excludes: barium swallow (87.61)
> esophageal manometry (89.32)
> microscopic examination of specimen from esophagus (90.81-90.89)

42.3 Local excision or destruction of lesion or tissue of esophagus

42.31 Local excision of esophageal diverticulum

42.32 Local excision of other lesion or tissue of esophagus

> Excludes: biopsy of esophagus (42.24-42.25)
> esophageal fistulectomy (42.84)

42.33 Endoscopic excision or destruction of lesion or tissue of esophagus
Ablation of esophageal neoplasm by endoscopic approach
Control of esophageal bleeding by endoscopic approach
Esophageal polypectomy by endoscopic approach
Esophageal varices by endoscopic approach
Injection of esophageal varices by endoscopic approach

> Excludes: biopsy of esophagus (42.24-42.25)
> fistulectomy (42.84)
> open ligation of esophageal varices (42.91)

42.39 Other destruction of lesion or tissue of esophagus

> Excludes: that by endoscopic approach (42.33)

42.4 Excision of esophagus

> Excludes: esophagogastrectomy NOS (43.99)

42.40 Esophagectomy, not otherwise specified

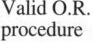 Valid O.R. procedure   Non-O.R. procedure   Nonspecific O.R. procedure   Noncovered O.R. procedure

42.41 Partial esophagectomy

Code also any synchronous:
anastomosis other than end-to-end (42.51-42.69)
esophagostomy (42.10-42.19)
gastrostomy (43.11-43.19)

42.42 Total esophagectomy

Code also any synchronous:
gastrostomy (43.11-43.19)
interposition or anastomosis other than end-to-end (42.51-42.69)

Excludes: *esophagogastrectomy (43.99)*

42.5 Intrathoracic anastomosis of esophagus

Code also any synchronous:
esophagectomy (42.40-42.42)
gastrostomy (43.1)

42.51 Intrathoracic esophagoesophagostomy

42.52 Intrathoracic esophagogastrostomy

42.53 Intrathoracic esophageal anastomosis with interposition of small bowel

42.54 Other intrathoracic esophagoenterostomy
Anastomosis of esophagus to intestinal segment NOS

42.55 Intrathoracic esophageal anastomosis with interposition of colon

42.56 Other intrathoracic esophagocolostomy
Esophagocolostomy NOS

42.58 Intrathoracic esophageal anastomosis with other interposition
Construction of artificial esophagus
Retrosternal formation of reversed gastric tube

42.59 Other intrathoracic anastomosis of esophagus

42.6 Antesternal anastomosis of esophagus

Code also any synchronous:
esophagectomy (42.40-42.42)
gastrostomy (43.1)

42.61 Antesternal esophagoesophagostomy

42.62 Antesternal esophagogastrostomy

42.63 Antesternal esophageal anastomosis with interposition of small bowel

42.64 Other antesternal esophagoenterostomy
Antethoracic:
esophagoenterostomy
esophagoileostomy
esophagojejunostomy

42.65 Antesternal esophageal anastomosis with interposition of colon

42.66 Other antesternal esophagocolostomy
Antethoracic esophagocolostomy

42.68 Other antesternal esophageal anastomosis with interposition

42.69 Other antesternal anastomosis of esophagus

42.7 Esophagomyotomy

42.8 Other repair of esophagus

42.81 Insertion of permanent tube into esophagus

42.82 Suture of laceration of esophagus

42.83 Closure of esophagostomy

42.84 Repair of esophageal fistula, not elsewhere classified

Excludes: *repair of fistula:*
bronchoesophageal (33.42)
esophagopleurocutaneous (34.73)
pharyngoesophageal (29.53)
tracheoesophageal (31.73)

42.85 Repair of esophageal stricture

42.86 Production of subcutaneous tunnel without esophageal anastomosis

● Code new
to 2012 edition
▲ Revision of
existing code
④ ⑤ Fourth or fifth
digit required

42.87 Other graft of esophagus

> *Excludes:* antesternal esophageal anastomosis with interposition of:
>> colon (42.65)
>> small bowel (42.63)
>
> antesternal esophageal anastomosis with other interposition (42.68)
> intrathoracic esophageal anastomosis with interposition of:
>> colon (42.55)
>> small bowel (42.53)
>
> intrathoracic esophageal anastomosis with other interposition (42.58)

42.89 Other repair of esophagus

42.9 Other operations on esophagus

42.91 Ligation of esophageal varices

> *Excludes:* that by endoscopic approach (42.33)

42.92 Dilation of esophagus
Dilation of cardiac sphincter

> *Excludes:* intubation of esophagus (96.03, 96.06-96.08)

42.99 Other

> *Excludes:* insertion of Sengstaken tube (96.06)
> intubation of esophagus (96.03, 96.06-96.08)
> removal of intraluminal foreign body from esophagus without incision
>> (98.02)
>
> tamponade of esophagus (96.06)

43 Incision and excision of stomach
Code also any application or administration of an adhesion barrier substance (99.77)

43.0 Gastrotomy

> *Excludes:* gastrostomy (43.11-43.19)
> that for control of hemorrhage (44.49)

43.1 Gastrostomy

43.11 Percutaneous [endoscopic] gastrostomy [PEG]
Percutaneous transabdominal gastrostomy

43.19 Other gastrostomy

> *Excludes:* percutaneous [endoscopic] gastrostomy [PEG] (43.11)

43.3 Pyloromyotomy

43.4 Local excision or destruction of lesion or tissue of stomach

43.41 Endoscopic excision or destruction of lesion or tissue of stomach
Gastric polypectomy by endoscopic approach
Gastric varices by endoscopic approach

> *Excludes:* biopsy of stomach (44.14-44.15)
> control of hemorrhage (44.43)
> open ligation of gastric varices (44.91)

43.42 Local excision of other lesion or tissue of stomach

> *Excludes:* biopsy of stomach (44.14-44.15)
> gastric fistulectomy (44.62-44.63)
> partial gastrectomy (43.5-43.89)

43.49 Other destruction of lesion or tissue of stomach

> *Excludes:* that by endoscopic approach (43.41)

43.5 Partial gastrectomy with anastomosis to esophagus
Proximal gastrectomy

43.6 Partial gastrectomy with anastomosis to duodenum
Billroth I operation
Distal gastrectomy
Gastropylorectomy

43.7 Partial gastrectomy with anastomosis to jejunum
Billroth II operation

43.8 Other partial gastrectomy

43.81 Partial gastrectomy with jejunal transposition
Henley jejunal transposition operation
Code also any synchronous intestinal resection (45.51)

	Valid O.R. procedure		Non-O.R. procedure		Nonspecific O.R. procedure		Noncovered O.R. procedure

● **43.82 Laparoscopic vertical (sleeve) gastrectomy**

> Excludes: *laparoscopic banding (44.95)*
> *laparoscopic gastric restrictive procedure (44.95)*

▲ **43.89 Open and other partial gastrectomy**
Partial gastrectomy with bypass gastrogastrostomy
Sleeve resection of stomach

> Excludes: *laparoscopic sleeve gastrectomy (43.82)*

43.9 Total gastrectomy

43.91 Total gastrectomy with intestinal interposition

43.99 Other total gastrectomy
Complete gastroduodenectomy
Esophagoduodenostomy with complete gastrectomy
Esophagogastrectomy NOS
Esophagojejunostomy with complete gastrectomy
Radical gastrectomy

44 Other operations on stomach

Code also any application or administration of an adhesion barrier substance (99.77)

44.0 Vagotomy

44.00 Vagotomy, not otherwise specified
Division of vagus nerve NOS

44.01 Truncal vagotomy

44.02 Highly selective vagotomy
Parietal cell vagotomy
Selective proximal vagotomy

44.03 Other selective vagotomy

44.1 Diagnostic procedures on stomach

44.11 Transabdominal gastroscopy
Intraoperative gastroscopy

> Excludes: *that with biopsy (44.14)*

44.12 Gastroscopy through artificial stoma

> Excludes: *that with biopsy (44.14)*

44.13 Other gastroscopy

> Excludes: *that with biopsy (44.14)*

44.14 Closed [endoscopic] biopsy of stomach
Brushing or washing for specimen collection

> Excludes: *esophagogastroduodenoscopy [EGD] with closed biopsy (45.16)*

44.15 Open biopsy of stomach

44.19 Other diagnostic procedures on stomach

> Excludes: *gastric lavage (96.33)*
> *microscopic examination of specimen from stomach (90.81-90.89)*
> *upper GI series (87.62)*

44.2 Pyloroplasty

44.21 Dilation of pylorus by incision

44.22 Endoscopic dilation of pylorus
Dilation with balloon endoscope
Endoscopic dilation of gastrojejunostomy site

44.29 Other pyloroplasty
Pyloroplasty NOS
Revision of pylorus

44.3 Gastroenterostomy without gastrectomy

44.31 High gastric bypass
Printen and Mason gastric bypass

44.32 Percutaneous [endoscopic] gastrojejunostomy
Bypass:
  gastroduodenostomy
  PEGJJ

> Excludes: *percutaneous (endoscopic) feeding jejunostomy (46.32)*

● Code new
to 2012 edition
▲ Revision of
existing code
④ ⑤ Fourth or fifth
digit required

44.38 Laparoscopic gastroenterostomy
Bypass:
gastroduodenostomy
gastroenterostomy
gastrogastrostomy
Laparoscopic gastrojejunostomy without gastrectomy NEC

Excludes: *gastroenterostomy, open approach (44.39)*

44.39 Other gastroenterostomy
Bypass:
gastroduodenostomy
gastroenterostomy
gastrogastrostomy
Gastrojejunostomy without gastrectomy NOS

44.4 Control of hemorrhage and suture of ulcer of stomach or duodenum

44.40 Suture of peptic ulcer, not otherwise specified

44.41 Suture of gastric ulcer site

Excludes: *ligation of gastric varices (44.91)*

44.42 Suture of duodenal ulcer site

44.43 Endoscopic control of gastric or duodenal bleeding

44.44 Transcatheter embolization for gastric or duodenal bleeding

Excludes: *surgical occlusion of abdominal vessels (38.86-38.87)*

44.49 Other control of hemorrhage of stomach or duodenum
That with gastrotomy

44.5 Revision of gastric anastomosis
Closure of:
gastric anastomosis
gastroduodenostomy
gastrojejunostomy
Pantaloon operation

44.6 Other repair of stomach

44.61 Suture of laceration of stomach

Excludes: *that of ulcer site(44.41)*

44.62 Closure of gastrostomy

44.63 Closure of other gastric fistula
Closure of:
gastrocolic fistula
gastrojejunocolic fistula

44.64 Gastropexy

44.65 Esophagogastroplasty
Belsey operation
Esophagus and stomach cardioplasty

44.66 Other procedures for creation of esophagogastric sphincteric competence
Fundoplication
Gastric cardioplasty
Nissen's fundoplication
Restoration of cardio-esophageal angle

Excludes: *that by laparoscopy (44.67)*

44.67 Laparoscopic procedures for creation of esophagogastric sphincteric competence
Fundoplication
Gastric cardioplasty
Nissen's fundoplication
Restoration of cardio-esophageal angle

44.68 Laparoscopic gastroplasty
Banding
Silastic vertical banding
Vertical banded gastroplasty (VBG)

Code also any synchronous laparoscopic gastroenterostomy (44.38)

Excludes: *insertion, laparoscopic adjustable gastric band (restrictive procedure)*
(44.95)
other repair of stomach, open approach (44.61-44.65, 44.69)

Valid O.R.
procedure

Non-O.R.
procedure

Nonspecific
O.R. procedure

Noncovered
O.R. procedure

44.69 Other
Inversion of gastric diverticulum
Repair of stomach NOS

44.9 **Other operations on stomach**

44.91 **Ligation of gastric varices**

> Excludes: that by endoscopic approach (43.41)

44.92 **Intraoperative manipulation of stomach**
Reduction of gastric volvulus

44.93 **Insertion of gastric bubble [balloon]**

44.94 **Removal of gastric bubble [balloon]**

44.95 **Laparoscopic gastric restrictive procedure**
Adjustable gastric band and port insertion

> Excludes: laparoscoipc gastroplasty (44.68)
> other repair of stomach (44.69)

44.96 **Laparoscopic revision of gastric restrictive procedure**
Revision or replacement of:
adjustable gastric band
subcutaneous gastric port device

44.97 **Laparoscopic removal of gastric restrictive device(s)**
Removal of either or both:
adjustable gastric band
subcutaneous port device

> Excludes: nonoperative removal of gastric restrictive device(s) (97.86)
> open removal of gastric restrictive device(s) (44.99)

44.98 **(Laparoscopic) adjustment of size of adjustable gastric restrictive device**
Infusion of saline for device tightening
Withdrawal of saline for device loosening

> Code also any:
> abdominal ultrasound (88.76)
> abdominal wall fluoroscopy (88.09)
> barium swallaw (87.61)

44.99 Other

> Excludes: change of gastrostomy tube (97.02)
> dilation of cardiac sphincter (42.92)
> gastric:
> cooling (96.31)
> freezing (96.32)
> gavage (96.35)
> hypothermia (96.31)
> lavage (96.33)
> insertion of nasogastric tube (96.07)
> irrigation of gastrostomy (96.36)
> irrigation of nasogastric tube (96.34)
> removal of:
> gastrostomy tube (97.51)
> intraluminal foreign body from stomach without incision (98.03)
> replacement of:
> gastrostomy tube (97.02)
> (naso-)gastric tube (97.01)

45 **Incision, excision, and anastomosis of intestine**
Code also any application or administration of an adhesion barrier substance (99.77)

45.0 **Enterotomy**

> Excludes: duodenocholedochotomy (51.41-51.42, 51.51)
> that for destruction of lesion (45.30-45.34)
> that of exteriorized intestine (46.14, 46.24, 46.31)

45.00 **Incision of intestine, not otherwise specified**

45.01 **Incision of duodenum**

45.02 **Other incision of small intestine**

45.03 **Incision of large intestine**

> Excludes: proctotomy (48.0)

● Code new
to 2012 edition   ▲ Revision of
existing code   ④ ⑤ Fourth or fifth
digit required

45.1 **Diagnostic procedures on small intestine**
Code also any laparotomy (54.11-54.19)

45.11 **Transabdominal endoscopy of small intestine**
Intraoperative endoscopy of small intestine

| Excludes: | that with biopsy (45.14) |

45.12 **Endoscopy of small intestine through artificial stoma**

| Excludes: | that with biopsy (45.14) |

45.13 **Other endoscopy of small intestine**
Esophagogastroduodenoscopy [EGD]

| Excludes: | that with biopsy (45.14, 45.16) |

45.14 **Closed [endoscopic] biopsy of small intestine**
Brushing or washing for specimen collection

| Excludes: | esophagogastroduodenoscopy [EGD] with closed biopsy (45.16) |

45.15 **Open biopsy of small intestine**

45.16 **Esophagogastroduodenoscopy [EGD] with closed biopsy**
Biopsy of one or more sites involving esophagus, stomach, and/or duodenum

45.19 **Other diagnostic procedures on small intestine**

Excludes:	microscopic examination of specimen from small intestine (90.91-90.99)
	radioisotope scan (92.04)
	ultrasonography (88.74)
	x-ray (87.61-87.69)

45.2 **Diagnostic procedures on large intestine**
Code also any laparotomy (54.11-54.19)

45.21 **Transabdominal endoscopy of large intestine**
Intraoperative endoscopy of large intestine

| Excludes: | that with biopsy (45.25) |

45.22 **Endoscopy of large intestine through artificial stoma**

| Excludes: | that with biopsy (45.25) |

45.23 **Colonoscopy**
Flexible fiberoptic colonoscopy

Excludes:	endoscopy of large intestine through artificial stoma (45.22)
	flexible sigmoidoscopy (45.24)
	rigid proctosigmoidoscopy (48.23)
	transabdominal endoscopy of large intestine (45.21)

45.24 **Flexible sigmoidoscopy**
Endoscopy of descending colon

| Excludes: | rigid proctosigmoidoscopy (48.23) |

45.25 **Closed [endoscopic] biopsy of large intestine**
Biopsy, closed, of unspecified intestinal site
Brushing or washing for specimen collection
Colonoscopy with biopsy

| Excludes: | proctosigmoidoscopy with biopsy (48.24) |

45.26 **Open biopsy of large intestine**

45.27 **Intestinal biopsy, site unspecified**

45.28 **Other diagnostic procedures on large intestine**

45.29 **Other diagnostic procedures on intestine, site unspecified**

Excludes:	microscopic examination of specimen (90.91-90.99)
	scan and radioisotope function study (92.04)
	ultrasonography (88.74)
	x-ray (87.61-87.69)

45.3 **Local excision or destruction of lesion or tissue of small intestine**

45.30 **Endoscopic excision or destruction of lesion of duodenum**

Excludes:	biopsy of duodenum (45.14-45.15)
	control of hemorrhage (44.43)
	fistulectomy (46.72)

| | Valid O.R. procedure | | Non-O.R. procedure | | Nonspecific O.R. procedure | | Noncovered O.R. procedure |

45.31 Other local excision of lesion of duodenum

[Excludes:] *biopsy of duodenum (45.14-45.15)*
fistulectomy (46.72)
multiple segmental resection (45.61)
that by endoscopic approach (45.30)

45.32 Other destruction of lesion of duodenum

[Excludes:] *that by endoscopic approach (45.30)*

45.33 Local excision of lesion or tissue of small intestine, except duodenum
Excision of redundant mucosa of ileostomy

[Excludes:] *biopsy of small intestine (45.14-45.15)*
fistulectomy (46.74)
multiple segmental resection (45.61)

45.34 Other destruction of lesion of small intestine, except duodenum

45.4 Local excision or destruction of lesion or tissue of large intestine

45.41 Excision of lesion or tissue of large intestine
Excision of redundant mucosa of colostomy

[Excludes:] *biopsy of large intestine (45.25-45.27)*
endoscopic polypectomy of large intestine (45.42)
fistulectomy (46.76)
multiple segmental resection (17.31, 45.71)
that by endoscopic approach (45.42-45.43)

45.42 Endoscopic polypectomy of large intestine

[Excludes:] *that by open approach (45.41)*

45.43 Endoscopic destruction of other lesion or tissue of large intestine
Endoscopic ablation of tumor of large intestine
Endoscopic control of colonic bleeding

[Excludes:] *endoscopic polypectomy of large intestine (45.42)*

45.49 Other destruction of lesion of large intestine

[Excludes:] *that by endoscopic approach (45.43)*

45.5 Isolation of intestinal segment

Code also any synchronous:
anastomosis other than end-to-end (45.90-45.94)
enterostomy (46.10-46.39)

45.50 Isolation of intestinal segment not otherwise specified
Isolation of intestinal pedicle flap
Reversal of intestinal segment

45.51 Isolation of segment of small intestine
Isolation of ileal loop
Resection of small intestine for interposition

45.52 Isolation of segment of large intestine
Resection of colon for interposition

45.6 Other excision of small intestine

Code also any synchronous:
anastomosis other than end-to-end (45.90-45.93, 45.95)
colostomy (46.10-46.13)
enterostomy (46.10-46.39)

[Excludes:] *cecectomy (17.32, 45.72)*
enterocolectomy (17.39, 45.79)
gastroduodenectomy (43.6-43.99)
ileocolectomy (17.33, 45.73)
pancreatoduodenectomy (52.51-52.7)

45.61 Multiple segmental resection of small intestine
Segmental resection for multiple traumatic lesions of small intestine

45.62 Other partial resection of small intestine
Duodenectomy
Jejunectomy
Ileectomy

[Excludes:] *duodenectomy with synchronous pancreatectomy (52.51-52.7)*
resection of cecum and terminal ileum (17.32, 45.72)

45.63 Total removal of small intestine

● Code new to 2012 edition ▲ Revision of existing code ④ ⑤ Fourth or fifth digit required

45.7 **Open and other partial excision of large intestine**

Code also any synchronous:
anastomosis other than end-to-end (45.92-45.94)
enterostomy (46.10-46.39)

| *Excludes:* | *laparoscopic partial excision of large intestine (17.31-17.39)* |

45.71 **Open and other multiple segmental resection of large intestine**
Segmental resection for multiple traumatic lesions of large intestine

45.72 **Open and other cecectomy**
Resection of cecum and terminal ileum

45.73 **Open and other right hemicolectomy**
Ileocolectomy
Right radical colectomy

45.74 **Open and other resection of transverse colon**

45.75 **Open and other left hemicolectomy**

| *Excludes:* | *proctosigmoidectomy (48.41-48.69)* |
| | *second stage Mikulicz operation (46.04)* |

45.76 **Open and other sigmoidectomy**

45.79 **Other and unspecified partial excision of large intestine**
Enterocolectomy NEC

45.8 **Total intra-abdominal colectomy**
Excision of cecum, colon, and sigmoid

| *Excludes:* | *coloproctectomy (48.41-48.69)* |

45.81 **Laparoscopic total intra-abdominal colectomy**

45.82 **Open total intra-abdominal colectomy**

45.83 **Other and unspecified total intra-abdominal colectomy**

45.9 **Intestinal anastomosis**

Code also any synchronous resection (45.31-45.8, 48.41-48.69)

| *Excludes:* | *end-to-end anastomosis – omit code* |

45.90 **Intestinal anastomosis, not otherwise specified**

45.91 **Small-to-small intestinal anastomosis**

45.92 **Anastomosis of small intestine to rectal stump**
Hampton procedure

45.93 **Other small-to-large intestinal anastomosis**

45.94 **Large-to-large intestinal anastomosis**

| *Excludes:* | *rectorectostomy (48.74)* |

45.95 **Anastomosis to anus**
Formation of endorectal ileal pouch (J-pouch) (H-pouch) (S-pouch) with
anastomosis of small intestine to anus

46 **Other operations on intestine**

Code also any application or administration of an adhesion barrier substance (99.77)

46.0 **Exteriorization of intestine**
Includes: loop enterostomy
multiple stage resection of intestine

46.01 **Exteriorization of small intestine**
Loop ileostomy

46.02 **Resection of exteriorized segment of small intestine**

46.03 **Exteriorization of large intestine**
Exteriorization of intestine NOS
First stage Mikulicz exteriorization of intestine
Loop colostomy

46.04 **Resection of exteriorized segment of large intestine**
Resection of exteriorized segment of intestine NOS
Second stage Mikulicz operation

| | Valid O.R. procedure | | Non-O.R. procedure | | Nonspecific O.R. procedure | | Noncovered O.R. procedure |

46.1 **Colostomy**
Code also any synchronous resection (45.49, 45.71-45.79, 45.8)

| Excludes: | loop colostomy (46.03) |

that with abdominoperineal resection of rectum (48.5)
that with synchronous anterior rectal resection (48.62)

46.10 **Colostomy, not otherwise specified**

46.11 **Temporary colostomy**

46.13 **Other permanent colostomy**

46.14 **Delayed opening of colostomy**

46.2 **Ileostomy**
Code also any synchronous resection (45.34, 45.61-45.63)

| Excludes: | loop ileostomy (46.01) |

46.20 **Ileostomy, not otherwise specified**

46.21 **Temporary ileostomy**

46.22 **Continent ileostomy**

46.23 **Other permanent ileostomy**

46.24 **Delayed opening of ileostomy**

46.3 **Other enterostomy**
Code also any synchronous resection (45.61-45.8)

46.31 **Delayed opening of other enterostomy**

46.32 **Percutaneous [endoscopic] jejunostomy [PEJ]**
Endoscopic conversion of gastrostomy to jejunostomy
Percutaneous (endoscopic) feeding enterostomy

| Excludes: | percutaneous [endoscopic] gastrojejunostomy (bypass) (44.32) |

46.39 **Other**
Duodenostomy
Feeding enterostomy

46.4 **Revision of intestinal stoma**

46.40 **Revision of intestinal stoma, not otherwise specified**
Plastic enlargement of intestinal stoma
Reconstruction of stoma of intestine
Release of scar tissue of intestinal stoma

| Excludes: | excision of redundant mucosa (45.41) |

46.41 **Revision of stoma of small intestine**

| Excludes: | excision of redundant mucosa (45.33) |

46.42 **Repair of pericolostomy hernia**

46.43 **Other revision of stoma of large intestine**

| Excludes: | excision of redundant mucosa (45.41) |

46.5 **Closure of intestinal stoma**
Code also any synchronous resection (45.34, 45.49, 45.61-45.8)

46.50 **Closure of intestinal stoma, not otherwise specified**

46.51 **Closure of stoma of small intestine**

46.52 **Closure of stoma of large intestine**
Closure or take-down of:
   cecostomy
   colostomy
   sigmoidostomy

46.6 **Fixation of intestine**

46.60 **Fixation of intestine, not otherwise specified**
Fixation of intestine to abdominal wall

46.61 **Fixation of small intestine to abdominal wall**
Ileopexy

46.62 **Other fixation of small intestine**
Noble plication of small intestine
Plication of jejunum

● Code new
to 2012 edition

▲ Revision of
existing code

④ ⑤ Fourth or fifth
digit required

46.63 **Fixation of large intestine to abdominal wall**
Cecocoloplicopexy
Sigmoidopexy (Moschowitz)

46.64 **Other fixation of large intestine**
Cecofixation
Colofixation

46.7 **Other repair of intestine**

> Excludes: *closure of:*
> *ulcer of duodenum (44.42)*
> *vesicoenteric fistula (57.83)*

46.71 **Suture of laceration of duodenum**

46.72 **Closure of fistula of duodenum**

46.73 **Suture of laceration of small intestine, except duodenum**

46.74 **Closure of fistula of small intestine, except duodenum**

> Excludes: *closure of:*
> *artificial stoma (46.51)*
> *vaginal fistula (70.74)*
> *repair of gastrojejunocolic fistula (44.63)*

46.75 **Suture of laceration of large intestine**

46.76 **Closure of fistula of large intestine**

> Excludes: *closure of:*
> *gastrocolic fistula (44.63)*
> *rectal fistula (48.73)*
> *sigmoidovesical fistula (57.83)*
> *stoma (46.52)*
> *vaginal fistula (70.72-70.73)*
> *vesicocolic fistula (57.83)*
> *vesicosigmoidovaginal fistula (57.83)*

46.79 **Other repair of intestine**
Duodenoplasty

46.8 **Dilation and manipulation of intestine**

46.80 **Intra-abdominal manipulation of intestine, not otherwise specified**
Correction of intestinal malrotation
Reduction of:
intestinal torsion
intestinal volvulus
intussusception

> Excludes: *reduction of intussusception with:*
> *fluoroscopy (96.29)*
> *ionizing radiation enema (96.29)*
> *ultrasonography guidance (96.29)*

46.81 **Intra-abdominal manipulation of small intestine**

46.82 **Intra-abdominal manipulation of large intestine**

46.85 **Dilation of intestine**
Dilation (balloon) of duodenum
Dilation (balloon) of jejunum
Endoscopic dilation (balloon) of large intestine
That through rectum or colostomy

> Excludes: *with insertion of colonic stent (46.86-46.87)*

46.86 **Endoscopic insertion of colonic stent(s)**
Colonoscopy (flexible) (through stoma) with transendoscopic stent placement
Combined with fluoroscopic-guided insertion
Stent endoprosthesis of colon
Through the scope [TTS] technique

> Excludes: *other non-endoscopic insertion of colonic stent (46.87)*

	Valid O.R. procedure		Non-O.R. procedure		Nonspecific O.R. procedure		Noncovered O.R. procedure

46.87 Other insertion of colonic stent(s)
Includes: that by:
  fluoroscopic guidance only
  rectal guiding tube
Non-endoscopic insertion

Code also any synchronous diagnostic procedure(s)

> Excludes: *endoscopic insertion of colonic stent (46.86)*

46.9 Other operations on intestines

46.91 Myotomy of sigmoid colon

46.92 Myotomy of other parts of colon

46.93 Revision of anastomosis of small intestine

46.94 Revision of anastomosis of large intestine

46.95 Local perfusion of small intestine
Code also substance perfused (99.21-99.29)

46.96 Local perfusion of large intestine
Code also substance perfused (99.21-99.29)

46.97 Transplant of intestine
Note: To report donor source—*see* codes 00.91-00.93

46.99 Other
Ileoentectropy

> Excludes: *diagnostic procedures on intestine (45.11-45.29)*
> *dilation of enterostomy stoma (96.24)*
> *intestinal intubation (96.08)*
> *removal of:*
>   *intraluminal foreign body from intestine without incision (98.04)*
>   *intraluminal foreign body from small intestine without incision (98.03)*
>   *tube from large intestine (97.53)*
>   *tube from small intestine (97.52)*
> *replacement of:*
>   *large intestine tube or enterostomy device (97.04)*
>   *small intestine tube or enterostomy device (97.03)*

47 Operations on appendix
Includes: appendiceal stump
Code also any application or administration of an adhesion barrier substance (99.77)

47.0 Appendectomy

> Excludes: *incidental appendectomy, so described (47.11, 47.19)*

47.01 Laparoscopic appendectomy

47.09 Other appendectomy

47.1 Incidental appendectomy

47.11 Laparoscopic incidental appendectomy

47.19 Other incidental appendectomy

47.2 Drainage of appendiceal abscess

> Excludes: *that with appendectomy (47.0)*

47.9 Other operations on appendix

47.91 Appendicostomy

47.92 Closure of appendiceal fistula

47.99 Other
Anastomosis of appendix

> Excludes: *diagnostic procedures on appendix (45.21-45.29)*

48 Operations on rectum, rectosigmoid, and perirectal tissue
Code also any application or administration of an adhesion barrier substance (99.77)

48.0 Proctotomy
Decompression of imperforate anus
Panas' operation [linear proctotomy]

> Excludes: *incision of perirectal tissue (48.81)*

● Code new
to 2012 edition   ▲ Revision of
existing code   ④ ⑤ Fourth or fifth
digit required

48.1   **Proctostomy**

48.2   **Diagnostic procedures on rectum, rectosigmoid, and perirectal tissue**

    48.21   **Transabdominal proctosigmoidoscopy**
Intraoperative proctosigmoidoscopy

> Excludes: *that with biopsy (48.24)*

    48.22   **Proctosigmoidoscopy through artificial stoma**

> Excludes: *that with biopsy (48.24)*

    48.23   **Rigid proctosigmoidoscopy**

> Excludes: *flexible sigmoidoscopy (45.24)*

    48.24   **Closed [endoscopic] biopsy of rectum**
Brushing or washing for specimen collection
Proctosigmoidoscopy with biopsy

    48.25   **Open biopsy of rectum**

    48.26   **Biopsy of perirectal tissue**

    48.29   **Other diagnostic procedures on rectum, rectosigmoid and perirectal tissue**

> Excludes: *digital examination of rectum (89.34)*
> *lower GI series (87.64)*
> *microscopic examination of specimen from rectum (90.91-90.99)*

48.3   **Local excision or destruction of lesion or tissue of rectum**

    48.31   **Radical electrocoagulation of rectal lesion or tissue**

    48.32   **Other electrocoagulation of rectal lesion or tissue**

    48.33   **Destruction of rectal lesion or tissue by laser**

    48.34   **Destruction of rectal lesion or tissue by cryosurgery**

    48.35   **Local excision of rectal lesion or tissue**

> Excludes: *biopsy of rectum (48.24-48.25)*
> *[endoscopic] polypectomy of rectum (48.36)*
> *excision of perirectal tissue (48.82)*
> *hemorrhoidectomy (49.46)*
> *rectal fistulectomy (48.73)*

    48.36   **[Endoscopic] polypectomy of rectum**

48.4   **Pull-through resection of rectum**

Code also any synchronous anastomosis other than end-to-end (45.90, 45.92-45.95)

    48.40   **Pull-through resection of rectum, not otherwise specified**
Pull-through resection NOS

> Excludes: *Abdominoperineal pull-through NOS (48.50)*

    48.41   **Soave submucosal resection of rectum**
Endorectal pull-through operation

    48.42   **Laparoscopic pull-through resection of rectum**

    48.43   **Open pull-through resection of rectum**

    48.49   **Other pull-through resection of rectum**
Abdominoperineal pull-through
Altemeier operation   Swenson proctectomy

> Excludes: *Duhamel abdominoperineal pull-through (48.65)*
> *laparoscopic pull-through resection of rectum (48.42)*
> *open pull-through resection of rectum (48.43)*
> *pull-through resection of rectum, not otherwise specified (48.40)*

48.5   **Abdominoperineal resection of rectum**
Includes: with synchronous colostomy
Combined abdominoendorectal resection
Complete proctectomy

Code also any synchronous anastomosis other than end-to-end (45.90, 45.92-45.95)

> Excludes: *Duhamel abdominoperineal pull-through (48.65)*
> *that as part of pelvic exenteration (68.8)*

    48.50   **Abdominoperineal resection of the rectum, not otherwise specified**

    48.51   **Laparoscopic abdominoperineal resection of the rectum**

    48.52   **Open abdominoperineal resection of the rectum**

	Valid O.R. procedure		Non-O.R. procedure		Nonspecific O.R. procedure		Noncovered O.R. procedure

48.59 Other abdominoperineal resection of the rectum

> Excludes: *abdominoperineal resection of the rectum, NOS (48.50)*
> *laparoscopic abdominoperineal resection of the rectum (48.51)*
> *open abdominoperineal resection of the rectum (48.52)*

48.6 Other resection of rectum

Code also any synchronous anastomosis other than end-to-end (45.90, 45.92-45.95)

48.61 Transsacral rectosigmoidectomy

48.62 Anterior resection of rectum with synchronous colostomy

48.63 Other anterior resection of rectum

> Excludes: *that with synchronous colostomy (48.62)*

48.64 Posterior resection of rectum

48.65 Duhamel resection of rectum
Duhamel abdominoperineal pull-through

48.69 Other
Partial proctectomy
Rectal resection NOS

48.7 Repair of rectum

> Excludes: *repair of:*
> *current obstetric laceration (75.62)*
> *vaginal rectocele (70.50, 70.52, 70.53, 70.55)*

48.71 Suture of laceration of rectum

48.72 Closure of proctostomy

48.73 Closure of other rectal fistula

> Excludes: *fistulectomy:*
> *perirectal (48.93)*
> *rectourethral (58.43)*
> *rectovaginal (70.73)*
> *rectovesical (57.83)*
> *rectovesicovaginal (57.83)*

48.74 Rectorectostomy
Rectal anastomosis NOS
Stapled transanal rectal resection (STARR)

48.75 Abdominal proctopexy
Frickman procedure
Ripstein repair of rectal prolapse

48.76 Other proctopexy
Delorme repair of prolapsed rectum
Proctosigmoidopexy
Puborectalis sling operation

> Excludes: *manual reduction of rectal prolapse (96.26)*

48.79 Other repair of rectum
Repair of old obstetric laceration of rectum

> Excludes: *anastomosis to:*
> *large intestine (45.94)*
> *small intestine (45.92-45.93)*
> *repair of:*
> *current obstetrical laceration (75.62)*
> *vaginal rectocele (70.50, 70.52)*

48.8 Incision or excision of perirectal tissue or lesion
Includes: pelvirectal tissue
rectovaginal septum

48.81 Incision of perirectal tissue
Incision of rectovaginal septum

48.82 Excision of perirectal tissue

> Excludes: *perirectal biopsy (48.26)*
> *perirectofistulectomy (48.93)*
> *rectal fistulectomy (48.73)*

48.9 Other operations on rectum and perirectal tissue

48.91 Incision of rectal stricture

● Code new
to 2012 edition
▲ Revision of
existing code
④ ⑤ Fourth or fifth
digit required

48.92 Anorectal myectomy

48.93 Repair of perirectal fistula

> | Excludes: | that opening into rectum (48.73)

48.99 Other

> | Excludes: | digital examination of rectum (89.34)
> dilation of rectum (96.22)
> insertion of rectal tube (96.09)
> irrigation of rectum (96.38-96.39)
> manual reduction of rectal prolapse (96.26)
> proctoclysis (96.37)
> rectal massage (99.93)
> rectal packing (96.19)
> removal of:
>   impacted feces (96.38)
>   intraluminal foreign body from rectum without incision (98.05)
>   rectal packing (97.59)
> transanal enema (96.39)

49 **Operations on anus**

Code also any application or administration of an adhesion barrier substance (99.77)

49.0 **Incision or excision of perianal tissue**

49.01 Incision of perianal abscess

49.02 Other incision of perianal tissue
Undercutting of perianal tissue

> | Excludes: | anal fistulotomy (49.11)

49.03 Excision of perianal skin tags

49.04 Other excision of perianal tissue

> | Excludes: | anal fistulectomy (49.12)
> biopsy of perianal tissue (49.22)

49.1 **Incision or excision of anal fistula**

> | Excludes: | closure of anal fistula (49.73)

49.11 Anal fistulotomy

49.12 Anal fistulectomy

49.2 **Diagnostic procedures on anus and perianal tissue**

49.21 Anoscopy

49.22 Biopsy of perianal tissue

49.23 Biopsy of anus

49.29 Other diagnostic procedures on anus and perianal tissue

> | Excludes: | microscopic examination of specimen from anus (90.91-90.99)

49.3 **Local excision or destruction of other lesion or tissue of anus**
Anal cryptotomy
Cauterization of lesion of anus

> | Excludes: | biopsy of anus (49.23)
> control of (postoperative) hemorrhage of anus (49.95)
> hemorrhoidectomy (49.46)

49.31 Endoscopic excision or destruction of lesion or tissue of anus

49.39 Other local excision or destruction of lesion or tissue of anus

> | Excludes: | that by endoscopic approach (49.31)

49.4 **Procedures on hemorrhoids**

49.41 Reduction of hemorrhoids

49.42 Injection of hemorrhoids

49.43 Cauterization of hemorrhoids
Clamp and cautery of hemorrhoids

49.44 Destruction of hemorrhoids by cryotherapy

49.45 Ligation of hemorrhoids

49.46 Excision of hemorrhoids
Hemorrhoidectomy NOS

49.47 Evacuation of thrombosed hemorrhoids

| | Valid O.R. procedure | | Non-O.R. procedure | | Nonspecific O.R. procedure | | Noncovered O.R. procedure |

49.49 **Other procedures on hemorrhoids**
Lord procedure

49.5 **Division of anal sphincter**

49.51 **Left lateral anal sphincterotomy**

49.52 **Posterior anal sphincterotomy**

49.59 **Other anal sphincterotomy**
Division of sphincter NOS

49.6 **Excision of anus**

49.7 **Repair of anus**

Excludes: *repair of current obstetric laceration (75.62)*

49.71 **Suture of laceration of anus**

49.72 **Anal cerclage**

49.73 **Closure of anal fistula**

Excludes: *excision of anal fistula (49.12)*

49.74 **Gracilis muscle transplant for anal incontinence**

49.75 **Implantation or revision of artificial anal sphincter**
Removal with subsequent replacement
Replacement during same or subsequent operative episode

49.76 **Removal of artificial anal sphincter**
Explanation or removal without replacement

Excludes: *revision with implantation during same operative episode (49.75)*

49.79 **Other repair of anal sphincter**
Repair of old obstetric laceration of anus

Excludes: *anoplasty with synchronous
hemorrhoidectomy (49.46)
repair of current obstetric laceration (75.62)*

49.9 **Other operations on anus**

Excludes: *dilation of anus (sphincter) (96.23)*

49.91 **Incision of anal septum**

49.92 **Insertion of subcutaneous electrical anal stimulator**

49.93 **Other incision of anus**
Removal of:
foreign body from anus with incision
seton from anus

Excludes: *anal fistulotomy (49.11)
removal of intraluminal foreign body without incision (98.05)*

49.94 **Reduction of anal prolapse**

Excludes: *manual reduction of rectal prolapse (96.26)*

49.95 **Control of (postoperative) hemorrhage of anus**

49.99 **Other**

50 **Operations on liver**
Code also any application or administration of an adhesion barrier substance (99.77)

50.0 **Hepatotomy**
Incision of abscess of liver
Removal of gallstones from liver
Stromeyer-Little operation

50.1 **Diagnostic procedures on liver**

50.11 **Closed (percutaneous) [needle] biopsy of liver**
Diagnostic aspiration of liver

50.12 **Open biopsy of liver**
Wedge biopsy

50.13 **Transjugular liver biopsy**
Transvenous liver biopsy

Excludes: *closed (percutaneous) [needle] biopsy of liver (50.11)
laparoscopic liver biopsy (50.14)*

● Code new
to 2012 edition
▲ Revision of
existing code
④ ⑤ Fourth or fifth
digit required

50.14 Laparoscopic liver biopsy

> *Excludes:* *closed (percutaneous) [needle] biopsy of liver (50.11)*
> *open biopsy of liver (50.12)*
> *transjugular liver biopsy (50.13)*

50.19 Other diagnostic procedures on liver

> *Excludes:* *laparoscopic liver biopsy (50.14)*
> *liver scan and radioisotope function study (92.02)*
> *microscopic examination of specimen from liver (91.01-91.09)*
> *transjugular liver biopsy (50.13)*

50.2 Local excision or destruction of liver tissue or lesion

50.21 Marsupialization of lesion of liver

50.22 Partial hepatectomy
Wedge resection of liver

> *Excludes:* *biopsy of liver, (50.11-50.12)*
> *hepatic lobectomy (50.3)*

50.23 Open ablation of liver lesion or tissue

50.24 Percutaneous ablation of liver lesion or tissue

50.25 Laparoscopic ablation of liver lesion or tissue

50.26 Other and unspecified ablation of liver lesion or tissue

50.29 Other destruction of lesion of liver
Cauterization of hepatic lesion
Enucleation of hepatic lesion
Evacuation of hepatic lesion

> *Excludes:* *ablation of liver lesion or tissue:*
> *laparoscopic (50.25)*
> *open (50.23)*
> *other (50.26)*
> *percutaneous (50.24)*
> *laser interstitial thermal therapy [LITT] of lesion or tissue of liver*
> *under guidance (17.63)*
> *percutaneous aspiration of lesion (50.91)*

50.3 Lobectomy of liver
Total hepatic lobectomy with partial excision of other lobe

50.4 Total hepatectomy

50.5 Liver transplant
Note: To report donor source—*see* codes 00.91-00.93

50.51 Auxiliary liver transplant
Auxiliary hepatic transplantation leaving patient's own liver in situ

50.59 Other transplant of liver

50.6 Repair of liver

50.61 Closure of laceration of liver

50.69 Other repair of liver
Hepatopexy

50.9 Other operations on liver

> *Excludes:* *lysis of adhesions (54.5)*

50.91 Percutaneous aspiration of liver

> *Excludes:* *percutaneous biopsy (50.11)*

50.92 Extracorporeal hepatic assistance
Liver dialysis

50.93 Localized perfusion of liver

50.94 Other injection of therapeutic substance into liver

50.99 Other

51   Operations on gallbladder and biliary tract

Code also any application or administration of an adhesion barrier substance (99.77)

Includes: operations on:
ampulla of Vater
common bile duct
cystic duct
hepatic duct
intrahepatic bile duct
sphincter of Oddi

51.0   Cholecystotomy and cholecystostomy

51.01   Percutaneous aspiration of gallbladder
Percutaneous cholecystotomy for drainage
That by: needle or catheter

Excludes: *needle biopsy (51.12)*

51.02   Trocar cholecystostomy

51.03   Other cholecystostomy

51.04   Other cholecystotomy
Cholelithotomy NOS

51.1   Diagnostic procedures on biliary tract

Excludes: *that for endoscopic procedures classifiable to 51.64, 51.84-51.88, 52.14,
52.21, 52.93-52.94, 52.97-52.98*

51.10   Endoscopic retrograde cholangiopancreatography [ERCP]

Excludes: *endoscopic retrograde:*
cholangiography [ERC] (51.11)
pancreatography [ERP] (52.13)

51.11   Endoscopic retrograde cholangiography [ERC]
Laparoscopic exploration of common bile duct

Excludes: *endoscopic retrograde:*
cholangiopancreatography [ERCP] (51.10)
pancreatography [ERP] (52.13)

51.12   Percutaneous biopsy of gallbladder or bile ducts
Needle biopsy of gallbladder

51.13   Open biopsy of gallbladder or bile ducts

51.14   Other closed [endoscopic] biopsy of biliary duct or sphincter of Oddi
Brushing or washing for specimen collection
Closed biopsy of biliary duct or sphincter of Oddi by procedures classifiable to
51.10-51.11, 52.13

51.15   Pressure measurement of sphincter of Oddi
Pressure measurement of sphincter by procedures classifiable to 51.10-51.11, 52.13

51.19   Other diagnostic procedures on biliary tract

Excludes: *biliary tract x-ray (87.51-87.59)*
microscopic examination of specimen from biliary tract (91.01-91.09)

51.2   Cholecystectomy

51.21   Other partial cholecystectomy
Revision of prior cholecystectomy

Excludes: *that by laparoscope (51.24)*

51.22   Cholecystectomy

Excludes: *laparoscopic cholecystectomy (51.23)*

51.23   Laparoscopic cholecystectomy
That by laser

51.24   Laparoscopic partial cholecystectomy

51.3   Anastomosis of gallbladder or bile duct

Excludes: *resection with end-to-end anastomosis (51.61-51.69)*

51.31   Anastomosis of gallbladder to hepatic ducts

51.32   Anastomosis of gallbladder to intestine

51.33   Anastomosis of gallbladder to pancreas

51.34   Anastomosis of gallbladder to stomach

● Code new
to 2012 edition   ▲ Revision of
existing code   ④ ⑤ Fourth or fifth
digit required

51.35 **Other gallbladder anastomosis**
Gallbladder anastomosis NOS

51.36 **Choledochoenterostomy**

51.37 **Anastomosis of hepatic duct to gastrointestinal tract**
Kasai portoenterostomy

51.39 **Other bile duct anastomosis**
Anastomosis of bile duct NOS
Anastomosis of unspecified bile duct to:
   intestine
   liver
   pancreas
   stomach

51.4 **Incision of bile duct for relief of obstruction**

51.41 **Common duct exploration for removal of calculus**
| Excludes: | percutaneous extraction (51.96) |

51.42 **Common duct exploration for relief of other obstruction**

51.43 **Insertion of choledochohepatic tube for decompression**
Hepatocholedochostomy

51.49 **Incision of other bile ducts for relief of obstruction**

51.5 **Other incision of bile duct**
| Excludes: | that for relief of obstruction (51.41-51.49) |

51.51 **Exploration of common duct**
Incision of common bile duct

51.59 **Incision of other bile duct**

51.6 **Local excision or destruction of lesion or tissue of biliary ducts and sphincter of Oddi**
Code also anastomosis other than end-to-end (51.31, 51.36-51.39)
| Excludes: | biopsy of bile duct (51.12-51.13) |

51.61 **Excision of cystic duct remnant**

51.62 **Excision of ampulla of Vater (with reimplantation of common duct)**

51.63 **Other excision of common duct**
Choledochectomy
| Excludes: | fistulectomy (51.72) |

51.64 **Endoscopic excision or destruction of lesion of biliary ducts or sphincter of Oddi**
Excision or destruction of lesion of biliary duct by procedures classifiable to
   51.10-51.11, 52.13

51.69 **Excision of other bile duct**
Excision of lesion of bile duct NOS
| Excludes: | fistulectomy (51.79) |

51.7 **Repair of bile ducts**

51.71 **Simple suture of common bile duct**

51.72 **Choledochoplasty**
Repair of fistula of common bile duct

51.79 **Repair of other bile ducts**
Closure of artificial opening of bile duct NOS
Suture of bile duct NOS
| Excludes: | operative removal of prosthetic device (51.95) |

51.8 **Other operations on biliary ducts and sphincter of Oddi**

51.81 **Dilation of sphincter of Oddi**
Dilation of ampulla of Vater
| Excludes: | that by endoscopic approach (51.84) |

51.82 **Pancreatic sphincterotomy**
Incision of pancreatic sphincter
Transduodenal ampullary sphincterotomy
| Excludes: | that by endoscopic approach (51.85) |

51.83 **Pancreatic sphincteroplasty**

51.84 **Endoscopic dilation of ampulla and biliary duct**
Dilation of ampulla and biliary duct by procedures classifiable to 51.10-51.11, 52.13

| Valid O.R. procedure | Non-O.R. procedure | Nonspecific O.R. procedure | Noncovered O.R. procedure |

51.85 Endoscopic sphincterotomy and papillotomy
Sphincterotomy and papillotomy by procedures classifiable to 51.10-51.11, 52.13

51.86 Endoscopic insertion of nasobiliary drainage tube
Insertion of nasobiliary tube by procedures classifiable to 51.10-51.11, 52.13

51.87 Endoscopic insertion of stent (tube) into bile duct
Endoprosthesis of bile duct
Insertion of stent into bile duct by procedures classifiable to 51.10-51.11, 52.13

> | Excludes: | nasobiliary drainage tube (51.86)
> | | replacement of stent (tube) (97.05)

51.88 Endoscopic removal of stone(s) from biliary tract
Laparoscopic removal of stone(s) from biliary tract
Removal of biliary tract stone(s) by procedures classifiable to 51.10-51.11, 52.13

> | Excludes: | percutaneous extraction of common duct stones (51.96)

51.89 Other operations on sphincter of Oddi

51.9 Other operations on biliary tract

51.91 Repair of laceration of gallbladder

51.92 Closure of cholecystostomy

51.93 Closure of other biliary fistula
Cholecystogastroenteric fistulectomy

51.94 Revision of anastomosis of biliary tract

51.95 Removal of prosthetic device from bile duct

> | Excludes: | nonoperative removal (97.55)

51.96 Percutaneous extraction of common duct stones

51.98 Other percutaneous procedures on biliary tract
Percutaneous biliary endoscopy via existing T-tube or other tract for:
  dilation of biliary duct stricture
  exploration (postoperative)
  removal of stone(s) except common duct stone
Percutaneous transhepatic biliary drainage

> | Excludes: | percutaneous aspiration of gallbladder (51.01)
> | | percutaneous biopsy and/or collection of specimen by brushing or washing (51.12)
> | | percutaneous removal of common duct stone(s) (51.96)

51.99 Other
Insertion or replacement of biliary tract prosthesis

> | Excludes: | biopsy of gallbladder (51.12-51.13)
> | | irrigation of cholecystostomy and other biliary tube (96.41)
> | | lysis of peritoneal adhesions (54.5)
> | | nonoperative removal of:
> | | cholecystostomy tube (97.54)
> | | tube from biliary tract or liver (97.55)

52 Operations on pancreas
Includes: operations on pancreatic duct
Code also any application or administration of an adhesion barrier substance (99.77)

52.0 Pancreatotomy

52.01 Drainage of pancreatic cyst by catheter

52.09 Other pancreatotomy
Pancreatolithotomy

> | Excludes: | drainage by anastomosis (52.4, 52.96)
> | | incision of pancreatic sphincter (51.82)
> | | marsupialization of cyst (52.3)

52.1 Diagnostic procedures on pancreas

52.11 Closed [aspiration] [needle] [percutaneous] biopsy of pancreas

52.12 Open biopsy of pancreas

52.13 Endoscopic retrograde pancreatography [EPR]

> | Excludes: | endoscopic retrograde:
> | | cholangiography [ERC] (51.11)
> | | cholangiopancreatography [ERCP] (51.10)
> | | that for procedures classifiable to 51.14-51.15, 51.64, 51.84-51.88, 52.14, 52.21, 52.92-52.94, 52.97-52.98

● Code new
to 2012 edition   ▲ Revision of
existing code   ④ ⑤ Fourth or fifth
digit required

52.14 Closed [endoscopic] biopsy of pancreatic duct
Closed biopsy of pancreatic duct by procedures classifiable to 51.10-51.11, 52.13

52.19 Other diagnostic procedure on pancreas

Excludes: *contrast pancreatogram (87.66)*
endoscopic retrograde pancreatography [ERP] (52.13))
microscopic examination of specimen from pancreas (91.01-91.09)

52.2 Local excision or destruction of pancreas and pancreatic duct

Excludes: *biopsy of pancreas (52.11-52.12, 52.14)*
pancreatic fistulectomy (52.95)

52.21 Endoscopic excision or destruction of lesion or tissue of pancreatic duct
Excision or destruction of lesion or tissue of pancreatic duct by procedures
classifiable to 51.10-51.11, 52.13

52.22 Other excision or destruction of lesion or tissue of pancreas or pancreatic duct

52.3 Marsupialization of pancreatic cyst

Excludes: *drainage of cyst by catheter (52.01)*

52.4 Internal drainage of pancreatic cyst
Pancreaticocystoduodenostomy
Pancreaticocystogastrostomy
Pancreaticocystojejunostomy

52.5 Partial pancreatectomy

Excludes: *pancreatic fistulectomy (52.95)*

52.51 Proximal pancreatectomy
Excision of head of pancreas (with part of body)
Proximal pancreatectomy with synchronous duodenectomy

52.52 Distal pancreatectomy
Excision of tail of pancreas (with part of body)

52.53 Radical subtotal pancreatectomy

52.59 Other partial pancreatectomy

52.6 Total pancreatectomy
Pancreatectomy with synchronous duodenectomy

52.7 Radical pancreaticoduodenectomy
One-stage pancreaticoduodenal resection with choledochojejunal anastomosis,
pancreaticojejunal anastomosis, and gastrojejunostomy
Two-stage pancreaticoduodenal resection (first stage) (second stage)
Radical resection of the pancreas
Whipple procedure

Excludes: *radical subtotal pancreatectomy (52.53)*

52.8 Transplant of pancreas
Note: To report donor source—*see* codes 00.91-00.93

52.80 Pancreatic transplant, not otherwise specified

52.81 Reimplantation of pancreatic tissue

52.82 Homotransplant of pancreas

52.83 Heterotransplant of pancreas

52.84 Autotransplantation of cells of Islets of Langerhans
Homotransplantation of islet cells of pancreas

52.85 Allotransplantation of cells of Islets of Langerhans
Heterotransplantation of islet cells of pancreas

52.86 Transplantation of cells of Islets of Langerhans, not otherwise specified

52.9 Other operations on pancreas

52.92 Cannulation of pancreatic duct

Excludes: *that by endoscopic approach (52.93)*

52.93 Endoscopic insertion of stent (tube) into pancreatic duct
Insertion of cannula or stent into pancreatic duct by procedures classifiable to
51.10-51.11, 52.13

Excludes: *endoscopic insertion of nasopancreatic drainage tube (52.97)*
replacement of stent (tube) (97.05)

	Valid O.R. procedure		Non-O.R. procedure		Nonspecific O.R. procedure		Noncovered O.R. procedure

52.94 Endoscopic removal of stone(s) from pancreatic duct
Removal of stone(s) from pancreatic duct by procedures classifiable to 51.10-51.11, 52.13

52.95 Other repair of pancreas
Fistulectomy of pancreas
Simple suture of pancreas

52.96 Anastomosis of pancreas
Anastomosis of pancreas (duct) to:
  intestine
  jejunum
  stomach

Excludes:	*anastomosis to:*
	bile duct (51.39)
	gallbladder (51.33)

52.97 Endoscopic insertion of nasopancreatic drainage tube
Insertion of nasopancreatic drainage tube by procedures classifiable to 51.10-51.11, 52.13

Excludes:	*drainage of pancreatic cyst by catheter (52.01)*
	replacement of stent (tube) (97.05)

52.98 Endoscopic dilation of pancreatic duct
Dilation of Wirsung's duct by procedures classifiable to 51.10-51.11,52.13

52.99 Other
Dilation of pancreatic [Wirsung's] duct by open approach
Repair of pancreatic [Wirsung's] duct by open approach

Excludes:	*irrigation of pancreatic tube (96.42)*
	removal of pancreatic tube (97.56)

53 Repair of hernia

Code also any application or administration of an adhesion barrier substance (99.77)
Includes: hernioplasty
              herniorrhaphy
              herniotomy

Excludes:	*manual reduction of hernia (96.27)*

53.0 Other unilateral repair of inguinal hernia

Excludes:	*laparoscopic unilateral repair of inguinal hernia (17.11-17.13)*

53.00 Unilateral repair of inguinal hernia, not otherwise specified
Inguinal herniorrhaphy NOS

53.01 Other and open repair of direct inguinal hernia
Direct and indirect inguinal hernia

53.02 Other and open repair of indirect inguinal hernia

53.03 Other and open repair of direct inguinal hernia with graft or prosthesis

53.04 Other and open repair of indirect inguinal hernia with graft or prosthesis

53.05 Repair of inguinal hernia with graft or prosthesis, not otherwise specified

53.1 Other bilateral repair of inguinal hernia

Excludes:	*laparoscopic bilateral repair of inguinal hernia (17.21-17.24)*

53.10 Bilateral repair of inguinal hernia, not otherwise specified

53.11 Other and open bilateral repair of direct inguinal hernia

53.12 Other and open bilateral repair of indirect inguinal hernia

53.13 Other and open bilateral repair of inguinal hernia, one direct and one indirect

53.14 Other and open bilateral repair of direct inguinal hernia with graft or prosthesis

53.15 Other and open bilateral repair of indirect inguinal hernia with graft or prosthesis

53.16 Other and open bilateral repair of inguinal hernia, one direct and one indirect, with graft or prosthesis

53.17 Bilateral inguinal hernia repair with graft or prosthesis, not otherwise specified

53.2 Unilateral repair of femoral hernia

53.21 Unilateral repair of femoral hernia with graft or prosthesis

53.29 Other unilateral femoral herniorrhaphy

53.3   **Bilateral repair of femoral hernia**

     53.31   **Bilateral repair of femoral hernia with graft or prosthesis**

     53.39   **Other bilateral femoral herniorrhaphy**

53.4   **Repair of umbilical hernia**

     | Excludes: | *repair of gastroschisis (54.71)*

     53.41   **Other and open repair of umbilical hernia with graft or prosthesis**

     53.42   **Laparoscopic repair of umbilical hernia with graft or prosthesis**

     53.43   **Other laparoscopic umbilical herniorrhaphy**

     53.49   **Other open umbilical herniorrhaphy**

         | Excludes: | *other laparoscopic umbilical herniorrhaphy (53.43)*
                   repair of umbilical hernia with graft or prosthesis (53.41, 53.42)

53.5   **Repair of other hernia of anterior abdominal wall (without graft or prosthesis)**

     53.51   **Incisional hernia repair**

     53.59   **Repair of other hernia of anterior abdominal wall**
           Repair of hernia:
              epigastric
              hypogastric
              spigelian
              ventral
           That by laparoscopic approach

53.6   **Repair of other hernia of anterior abdominal wall with graft or prosthesis**

     53.61   **Other open incisional hernia repair with graft or prosthesis**

         | Excludes: | *laparoscopic incisional hernia repair with graft or prosthesis (53.62)*

     53.62   **Laparoscopic incisional hernia repair with graft or prosthesis**

     53.63   **Other laparoscopic repair of other hernia of anterior abdominal wall with graft or prosthesis**

     53.69   **Other and open repair of other hernia of anterior abdominal wall with graft or prosthesis**

         | Excludes: | *other laparoscopic repair of other hernia of anterior abdominal wall*
                   with graft or prosthesis (53.63)

53.7   **Repair of diaphragmatic hernia, abdominal approach**

     53.71   **Laparoscopic repair of diaphragmatic hernia, abdominal approach**

     53.72   **Other and open repair of diaphragmatic hernia, abdominal approach**

     53.75   **Repair of diaphragmatic hernia, abdominal approach, not otherwise specified**

         | Excludes: | *laparoscopic repair of diaphragmatic hernia (53.71)*
                   other and open repair of diaphragmatic hernia (53.72)

53.8   **Repair of diaphragmatic hernia, thoracic approach**

     53.80   **Repair of diaphragmatic hernia with thoracic approach, not otherwise specified**
           Thoracoabdominal repair of diaphragmatic hernia

     53.81   **Plication of the diaphragm**

     53.82   **Repair of parasternal hernia**

     53.83   **Laparoscopic repair of diaphragmatic hernia, with thoracic approach**

     53.84   **Other and open repair of diaphragmatic hernia, with thoracic approach**

         | Excludes: | *repair of diaphragmatic hernia with thoracic approach NOS (53.80)*

53.9   **Other hernia repair**
       Repair of hernia:
          ischiatic   omental
          ischiorectal   retroperitoneal
          lumbar   sciatic
          obturator

       | Excludes: | *relief of strangulated hernia with exteriorization of intestine (46.01, 46.03)*
                 repair of pericolostomy hernia (46.42)
                 repair of vaginal enterocele (70.92)

| | Valid O.R. procedure | | Non-O.R. procedure | | Nonspecific O.R. procedure | | Noncovered O.R. procedure |

54   Other operations on abdominal region

Code also any application or administration of an adhesion barrier substance (99.77)

Includes: operations on:

epigastric region	mesentery
flank	omentum
groin region	pelvic cavity
hypochondrium	peritoneum
inguinal region	retroperitoneal tissue space
loin region	

Excludes: *hernia repair (53.00-53.9)*
obliteration of cul-de-sac (70.92)
retroperitoneal tissue dissection (59.00-59.09)
skin and subcutaneous tissue of abdominal wall (86.01-86.99)

54.0   Incision of abdominal wall

Drainage of:
abdominal wall
extraperitoneal abscess
retroperitoneal abscess

Excludes: *incision of peritoneum (54.95)*
laparotomy (54.11-54.19)

54.1   Laparotomy

54.11   Exploratory laparotomy

Excludes: *exploration incidental to intra-abdominal surgery—omit code*

54.12   Reopening of recent laparotomy site

Reopening of recent laparotomy site for:
control of hemorrhage
exploration
incision of hematoma

54.19   Other laparotomy

Drainage of intraperitoneal abscess or hematoma

Excludes: *culdocentesis (70.0)*
drainage of appendiceal abscess (47.2)
exploration incidental to intra-abdominal surgery—omit code
Ladd operation (54.95)
percutaneous drainage of abdomen (54.91)
removal of foreign body (54.92)

54.2   Diagnostic procedures of abdominal region

54.21   Laparoscopy

Peritoneoscopy

Excludes: *laparoscopic cholecystectomy (51.23)*
that incidental to destruction of fallopian tubes (66.21-66.29)

54.22   Biopsy or abdominal wall or umbilicus

54.23   Biopsy of peritoneum

Biopsy of:
mesentery
omentum
peritoneal implant

Excludes: *closed biopsy of:*
omentum (54.24)
peritoneum (54.24)

54.24   Closed [percutaneous] [needle] biopsy of intra-abdominal mass

Closed biopsy of:
omentum
peritoneal implant
peritoneum

Excludes: *that of:*
fallopian tube (66.11)
ovary (65.11)
uterine ligaments (68.15)
uterus (68.16)

54.25   Peritoneal lavage

Diagnostic peritoneal lavage

Excludes: *peritoneal dialysis (54.98)*

● Code new
to 2012 edition

▲ Revision of
existing code

④ ⑤ Fourth or fifth
digit required

54.29 **Other diagnostic procedures on abdominal region**

    | Excludes: | *abdominal lymphangiogram (88.04)*
    abdominal x-ray NEC (88.19)
    angiocardiography of venae cavae (88.51)
    C.A.T. scan of abdomen (88.01)
    contrast x-ray of abdominal cavity (88.11-88.15)
    intra-abdominal arteriography NEC (88.47)
    microscopic examination of peritoneal and retroperitoneal specimen
        (91.11-91.19)
    phlebography of:
      intra-abdominal vessels NEC (88.65)
      portal venous system (88.64)
    sinogram of abdominal wall (88.03)
    soft tissue x-ray of abdominal wall NEC (88.09)
    tomography of abdomen NEC(88.02)
    ultrasonography of abdomen and retroperitoneum (88.76)

54.3 **Excision or destruction of lesion or tissue of abdominal wall or umbilicus**
    Debridement of abdominal wall
    Omphalectomy

    | Excludes: | *biopsy of abdominal wall or umbilicus (54.22)*
    size reduction operation (86.83)
    that of skin of abdominal wall (86.22, 86.26, 86.3)

54.4 **Excision or destruction of peritoneal tissue**
    Excision of:
      appendices epiploicae
      falciform ligament
      gastrocolic ligament
      lesion of:
        mesentery
        omentum
        peritoneum
      presacral lesion NOS
      retroperitoneal lesion NOS

    | Excludes: | *biopsy of peritoneum (54.23)*
    endometrectomy of cul-de-sac (70.32)

54.5 **Lysis of peritoneal adhesions**
    Freeing of adhesions of:
      biliary tract
      intestines
      liver
      pelvic peritoneum
      peritoneum
      spleen
      uterus

    | Excludes: | *lysis of adhesions of:*
      bladder (59.11)
      fallopian tube and ovary (65.81, 65.89)
      kidney (59.02)
      ureter (59.01-59.02)

54.51 **Laparoscopic lysis of peritoneal adhesions**

54.59 **Other lysis of peritoneal adhesions**

54.6 **Suture of abdominal wall and peritoneum**

54.61 **Reclosure of postoperative disruption of abdominal wall**

54.62 **Delayed closure of granulating abdomen wound**
    Tertiary subcutaneous wound closure

54.63 **Other suture of abdominal wall**
    Suture of laceration of abdominal wall

    | Excludes: | *closure of operative wound—omit code*

54.64 **Suture of peritoneum**
    Secondary suture of peritoneum

    | Excludes: | *closure of operative wound—omit code*

54.7 **Other repair of abdominal wall and peritoneum**

54.71 **Repair of gastroschisis**

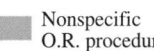

| | Valid O.R. procedure | | Non-O.R. procedure | | Nonspecific O.R. procedure | | Noncovered O.R. procedure |

54.72 **Other repair of abdominal wall**

54.73 **Other repair of peritoneum**
Suture of gastrocolic ligament

54.74 **Other repair of omentum**
Epiplorrhaphy
Graft of omentum
Omentopexy
Reduction of torsion of omentum

> *Excludes:* *cardio-omentopexy (36.39)*

54.75 **Other repair of mesentery**
Mesenteric plication
Mesenteropexy

54.9 **Other operations of abdominal region**

> *Excludes:* *removal of ectopic pregnancy (69.11, 74.3)*

54.91 **Percutaneous abdominal drainage**
Paracentesis

> *Excludes:* *creation of cutaneoperitoneal fistula (54.93)*

54.92 **Removal of foreign body from peritoneal cavity**

54.93 **Creation of cutaneoperitoneal fistula**

54.94 **Creation of peritoneovascular shunt**
Peritoneovenous shunt

54.95 **Incision of peritoneum**
Exploration of ventriculoperitoneal shunt at peritoneal site
Ladd operation
Revision of distal catheter of ventricular shunt
Revision of ventriculoperitoneal shunt at peritoneal site

> *Excludes:* *that incidental to laparotomy (54.11-54.19)*

54.96 **Injection of air into peritoneal cavity**
Pneumoperitoneum

> *Excludes:* *that for:*
> *collapse of lung (33.33)*
> *radiography (88.12-88.13, 88.15)*

54.97 **Injection of locally-acting therapeutic substance into peritoneal cavity**

> *Excludes:* *peritoneal dialysis (54.98)*

54.98 **Peritoneal dialysis**

> *Excludes:* *peritoneal lavage (diagnostic) (54.25)*

54.99 **Other**

> *Excludes:* *removal of:*
> *abdominal wall sutures (97.83)*
> *peritoneal drainage device (97.82)*
> *retroperitoneal drainage device (97.81)*

● Code new
to 2012 edition
▲ Revision of
existing code
④ ⑤ Fourth or fifth
digit required

10. OPERATIONS ON THE URINARY SYSTEM (55-59)

55 Operations on kidney
Code also any application or administration of an adhesion barrier substance (99.77)
Includes: operations on renal pelvis

> **Excludes:** *perirenal tissue (59.00-59.09, 59.21-59.29, 59.91-59.92)*

55.0 Nephrotomy and nephrostomy

> **Excludes:** *drainage by:*
> *anastomosis (55.86)*
> *aspiration (55.92)*
> *incision of kidney pelvis (55.11-55.12)*

55.01 Nephrotomy
Evacuation of renal cyst
Exploration of kidney
Nephrolithotomy

55.02 Nephrostomy

55.03 Percutaneous nephrostomy without fragmentation
Nephrostolithotomy, percutaneous (nephroscopic)
Percutaneous removal of kidney stone(s) by:
  basket extraction
  forceps extraction (nephroscopic)
Pyelostolithotomy, percutaneous (nephroscopic)
With placement of catheter down ureter

> **Excludes:** *percutaneous removal by fragmentation (55.04)*
> *repeat nephroscopic removal during current episode (55.92)*

55.04 Percutaneous nephrostomy with fragmentation
Percutaneous nephrostomy with disruption of kidney stone by ultrasonic energy and
  extraction (suction) through endoscope
With placement of catheter down ureter
With fluoroscopic guidance

> **Excludes:** *repeat fragmentation during current episode (59.95)*

55.1 Pyelotomy and pyelostomy

> **Excludes:** *drainage by anastomosis (55.86)*
> *percutaneous pyelostolithotomy (55.03)*
> *removal of calculus without incision (56.0)*

55.11 Pyelotomy
Exploration of renal pelvis
Pyelolithotomy

55.12 Pyelostomy
Insertion of drainage tube into renal pelvis

55.2 Diagnostic procedures on kidney

55.21 Nephroscopy

55.22 Pyeloscopy

55.23 Closed [percutaneous] [needle] biopsy of kidney
Endoscopic biopsy via existing nephrostomy, nephrotomy, pyelostomy, or
  pyelotomy

55.24 Open biopsy of kidney

55.29 Other diagnostic procedures on kidney

> **Excludes:** *microscopic examination of specimen from kidney (91.21-91.29)*
> *pyelogram:*
>   *intravenous (87.73)*
>   *percutaneous (87.75)*
>   *retrograde (87.74)*
> *radioisotope scan (92.03)*
> *renal arteriography (88.45)*
> *tomography:*
>   *C.A.T. scan (87.71)*
>   *other (87.72)*

55.3 Local excision or destruction of lesion or tissue of kidney

55.31 Marsupialization of kidney lesion

55.32 Open ablation of renal lesion or tissue

55.33 Percutaneous ablation of renal lesion or tissue

	Valid O.R. procedure		Non-O.R. procedure		Nonspecific O.R. procedure		Noncovered O.R. procedure

55.34 Laparoscopic ablation of renal lesion or tissue

55.35 Other and unspecified ablation of renal lesion or tissue

55.39 Other local destruction or excision of renal lesion or tissue
Obliteration of calyceal diverticulum

> | Excludes: | *ablation of renal lesion or tissue:*
> *laparoscopic (55.34)*
> *open (55.32)*
> *other (55.35)*
> *percutaneous (55.33)*
> *biopsy of kidney (55.23-55.24)*
> *partial nephrectomy (55.4)*
> *percutaneous aspiration of kidney (55.92)*
> *wedge resection of kidney (55.4)*

55.4 **Partial nephrectomy**
Calycectomy
Wedge resection of kidney
Code also any synchronous resection of ureter (56.40-56.42)

55.5 **Complete nephrectomy**
Code also any synchronous excision of:
adrenal gland (07.21-07.3)
bladder segment (57.6)
lymph nodes (40.3, 40.52-40.59)

55.51 Nephroureterectomy
Nephroureterectomy with bladder cuff
Total nephrectomy (unilateral)

> | Excludes: | *removal of transplanted kidney (55.53)*

55.52 Nephrectomy of remaining kidney
Removal of solitary kidney

> | Excludes: | *removal of transplanted kidney (55.53)*

55.53 Removal of transplanted or rejected kidney

55.54 Bilateral nephrectomy

> | Excludes: | *complete nephrectomy NOS (55.51)*

55.6 **Transplant of kidney**
Note: To report donor source—*see* codes 00.91-00.93

55.61 Renal autotransplantation

55.69 Other kidney transplantation

55.7 **Nephropexy**
Fixation or suspension of movable [floating] kidney

55.8 **Other repair of kidney**

55.81 Suture of laceration of kidney

55.82 Closure of nephrostomy and pyelostomy

55.83 Closure of other fistula of kidney

55.84 Reduction of torsion of renal pedicle

55.85 Symphysiotomy for horseshoe kidney

55.86 Anastomosis of kidney
Nephropyeloureterostomy
Pyeloureterovesical anastomosis
Ureterocalyceal anastomosis

> | Excludes: | *nephrocystanastomosis NOS (56.73)*

55.87 Correction of ureteropelvic junction

55.89 Other

55.9 **Other operations on kidney**

> | Excludes: | *lysis of perirenal adhesions (59.02)*

55.91 Decapsulation of kidney
Capsulectomy of kidney
Decortication of kidney

● Code new
to 2012 edition ▲ Revision of
existing code ④ ⑤ Fourth or fifth
digit required

55.92 Percutaneous aspiration of kidney (pelvis)
Aspiration of renal cyst
Renipuncture

> Excludes: *percutaneous biopsy of kidney (55.23)*

55.93 Replacement of nephrostomy tube

55.94 Replacement of pyelostomy tube

55.95 Local perfusion of kidney

55.96 Other Injection of therapeutic substance into kidney
Injection into renal cyst

55.97 Implantation or replacement of mechanical kidney

55.98 Removal of mechanical kidney

55.99 Other

> Excludes: *removal of pyelostomy or nephrostomy tube (97.61)*

56   Operations on ureter
Code also any application or administration of an adhesion barrier substance (99.77)

56.0 Transurethral removal of obstruction from ureter and renal pelvis
Removal of:
blood clot from ureter or renal pelvis without incision
calculus from ureter or renal pelvis without incision
foreign body from ureter or renal pelvis without incision

> Excludes: *manipulation without removal of obstruction (59.8)*
> *that by incision (55.11, 56.2)*
> *transurethral insertion of ureteral stent for passage of calculus (59.8)*

56.1 Ureteral meatotomy

56.2 Ureterotomy
Incision of ureter for:
drainage
exploration
removal of calculus

> Excludes: *cutting of ureterovesical orifice (56.1)*
> *removal of calculus without incision (56.0)*
> *transurethral insertion of ureteral stent for passage of calculus (59.8)*
> *urinary diversion (56.51-56.79)*

56.3 Diagnostic procedures on ureter

56.31 Ureteroscopy

56.32 Closed percutaneous biopsy of ureter

> Excludes: *endoscopic biopsy of ureter (56.33)*

56.33 Closed endoscopic biopsy of ureter
Cystourethroscopy with ureteral biopsy
Transurethral biopsy of ureter
Ureteral endoscopy with biopsy through ureterotomy
Ureteroscopy with biopsy

> Excludes: *percutaneous biopsy of ureter (56.32)*

56.34 Open biopsy of ureter

56.35 Endoscopy (cystoscopy) (looposcopy) of ileal conduit

56.39 Other diagnostic procedures on ureter

> Excludes: *microscopic examination of specimen from ureter (91.21-91.29)*

56.4 Ureterectomy
Code also anastomosis other than end-to-end (56.51-56.79)

> Excludes: *fistulectomy (56.84)*
> *nephroureterectomy (55.51-55.54)*

56.40 Ureterectomy, not otherwise specified

56.41 Partial ureterectomy
Excision of lesion of ureter
Shortening of ureter with reimplantation

> Excludes: *biopsy of ureter (56.32-56.34)*

56.42 Total ureterectomy

	Valid O.R. procedure		Non-O.R. procedure		Nonspecific O.R. procedure		Noncovered O.R. procedure

56.5 **Cutaneous uretero-ileostomy**

56.51 **Formation of cutaneous uretero-ileostomy**
Construction of ileal conduit
External ureteral ileostomy
Formation of open ileal bladder
Ileal loop operation
Ileoureterostomy (Bricker's) (ileal bladder)
Transplantation of ureter into ileum with external diversion

> *Excludes:* *closed ileal bladder (57.87)*
> *replacement of ureteral defect by ileal segment (56.89)*

56.52 **Revision of cutaneous uretero-ileostomy**

56.6 **Other external urinary diversion**

56.61 **Formation of other cutaneous ureterostomy**
Anastomosis of ureter to skin
Ureterostomy NOS

56.62 **Revision of other cutaneous ureterostomy**
Revision of ureterostomy stoma

> *Excludes:* *nonoperative removal of ureterostomy tube (97.62)*

56.7 **Other anastomosis or bypass of ureter**

> *Excludes:* *ureteropyelostomy (55.86)*

56.71 **Urinary diversion to intestine**
Anastomosis of ureter to intestine
Internal urinary diversion NOS

> *Code also any synchronous colostomy (46.10-46.13)*

> *Excludes:* *external ureteral ileostomy (56.51)*

56.72 **Revision of ureterointestinal anastomosis**

> *Excludes:* *revision of external ureteral ileostomy (56.52)*

56.73 **Nephrocystanastomosis, not otherwise specified**

56.74 **Ureteroneocystostomy**
Replacement of ureter with bladder flap
Ureterovesical anastomosis

56.75 **Transureteroureterostomy**

> *Excludes:* *ureteroureterostomy associated with partial resection (56.41)*

56.79 **Other**

56.8 **Repair of ureter**

56.81 **Lysis of intraluminal adhesions of ureter**

> *Excludes:* *lysis of periureteral adhesions (59.02-59.03)*
> *ureterolysis (59.02-59.03)*

56.82 **Suture of laceration of ureter**

56.83 **Closure of ureterostomy**

56.84 **Closure of other fistula of ureter**

56.85 **Ureteropexy**

56.86 **Removal of ligature from ureter**

56.89 **Other repair of ureter**
Graft of ureter
Replacement of ureter with ileal segment implanted into bladder
Ureteroplication

56.9 **Other operations on ureter**

56.91 **Dilation of ureteral meatus**

56.92 **Implantation of electronic ureteral stimulator**

56.93 **Replacement of electronic ureteral stimulator**

56.94 **Removal of electronic ureteral stimulator**

> *Excludes:* *that with synchronous replacement (56.93)*

56.95 **Ligation of ureter**

● Code new
to 2012 edition   ▲ Revision of
existing code   ④ ⑤ Fourth or fifth
digit required

56.99 Other

> *Excludes:* *removal of ureterostomy tube and ureteral catheter (97.62)*
> *ureteral catheterization (59.8)*

57 Operations on urinary bladder

Code also any application or administration of an adhesion barrier substance (99.77)

> *Excludes:* *perivesical tissue (59.11-59.29, 59.91-59.92)*
> *ureterovesical orifice (56.0-56.99)*

57.0 Transurethral clearance of bladder

Drainage of bladder without incision
Removal of:
  blood clots from bladder without incision
  calculus from bladder without incision
  foreign body from bladder without incision

> *Excludes:* *that by incision (57.19)*

57.1 Cystotomy and cystostomy

> *Excludes:* *cystotomy and cystostomy as operative approach—omit code*

57.11 Percutaneous aspiration of bladder

57.12 Lysis of intraluminal adhesion with incision into bladder

> *Excludes:* *transurethral lysis of intraluminal adhesions (57.41)*

57.17 Percutaneous cystostomy

Closed cystostomy
Percutaneous suprapubic cystostomy

> *Excludes:* *removal of cystostomy tube (97.63)*
> *replacement of cystostomy tube (59.94)*

57.18 Other suprapubic cystostomy

> *Excludes* *percutaneous cystostomy (57.17)*
> *removal of cystostomy tube (97.63)*
> *replacement of cystostomy tube (59.94)*

57.19 Other cystotomy

Cystolithotomy

> *Excludes:* *percutaneous cystostomy (57.17)*
> *suprapubic cystostomy (57.18)*

57.2 Vesicostomy

> *Excludes:* *percutaneous cystostomy (57.17)*
> *suprapubic cystostomy (57.18)*

57.21 Vesicostomy

Creation of permanent opening from bladder to skin using a bladder flap

57.22 Revision or closure of vesicostomy

> *Excludes:* *closure of cystostomy (57.82)*

57.3 Diagnostic procedures on bladder

57.31 Cystoscopy through artificial stoma

57.32 Other cystoscopy

Transurethral cystoscopy

> *Excludes:* *cystourethroscopy with ureteral biopsy (56.33)*
> *retrograde pyelogram (87.74)*
> *that for control of hemorrhage (postoperative):*
> *bladder (57.93)*
> *prostate (60.94)*

57.33 Closed [transurethral] biopsy of bladder

57.34 Open biopsy of bladder

57.39 Other diagnostic procedures on bladder

> *Excludes:* *cystogram NEC (87.77)*
> *microscopic examination of specimen from bladder (91.31-91.39)*
> *retrograde cystourethrogram (87.76)*
> *therapeutic distention of bladder (96.25)*

57.4 Transurethral excision or destruction of bladder tissue

57.41 Transurethral lysis of intraluminal adhesions

	Valid O.R. procedure		Non-O.R. procedure		Nonspecific O.R. procedure		Noncovered O.R. procedure

57.49 Other transurethral excision or destruction of lesion or tissue of bladder
Endoscopic resection of bladder lesion

| Excludes: | transurethral biopsy of bladder (57.33) |
| | transurethral fistulectomy (57.83-57.84) |

57.5 Other excision or destruction of bladder tissue

| Excludes: | that with transurethral approach (57.41-57.49) |

57.51 Excision of urachus
Excision of urachal sinus of bladder

| Excludes: | excision of urachal cyst of abdominal wall (54.3) |

57.59 Open excision or destruction of other lesion or tissue of bladder
Endometrectomy of bladder
Suprapubic excision of bladder lesion

| Excludes: | biopsy of bladder (57.33-57.34) |
| | fistulectomy of bladder (57.83-57.84) |

57.6 Partial cystectomy
Excision of bladder dome
Trigonectomy
Wedge resection of bladder

57.7 Total cystectomy
Includes: total cystectomy with urethrectomy

57.71 Radical cystectomy
Pelvic exenteration in male
Removal of bladder, prostate, seminal vesicles, and fat
Removal of bladder, urethra, and fat in a female

Code also any:
lymph node dissection (40.3, 40.5)
urinary diversion (56.51-56.79)

| Excludes: | that as part of pelvic exenteration in female (68.8) |

57.79 Other total cystectomy

57.8 Other repair of urinary bladder

Excludes:	repair of:
	current obstetric laceration (75.61)
	cystocele (70.50-70.51)
	that for stress incontinence (59.3-59.79)

57.81 Suture of laceration of bladder

57.82 Closure of cystostomy

57.83 Repair of fistula involving bladder and intestine
Rectovesicovaginal fistulectomy
Vesicosigmoidovaginal fistulectomy

57.84 Repair of other fistula of bladder
Cervicovesical fistulectomy
Urethroperineovesical fistulectomy
Uterovesical fistulectomy
Vaginovesical fistulectomy

| Excludes: | vesicoureterovaginal fistulectomy (56.84) |

57.85 Cystourethroplasty and plastic repair of bladder neck
Plication of sphincter of urinary bladder
V-Y plasty of bladder neck

57.86 Repair of bladder exstrophy

57.87 Reconstruction of urinary bladder
Anastomosis of bladder with isolated segment of ileum
Augmentation of bladder
Replacement of bladder with ileum or sigmoid [closed ileal bladder]
Code also resection of intestine (45.50-45.52)

57.88 Other anastomosis of bladder
Anastomosis of bladder to intestine NOS
Cystocolic anastomosis

| Excludes: | formation of closed ileal bladder (5787) |

● Code new
to 2012 edition

▲ Revision of
existing code

④ ⑤ Fourth or fifth
digit required

57.89 **Other repair of bladder**
Bladder suspension, not elsewhere classified
Cystopexy NOS
Repair of old obstetric laceration of bladder

Excludes: *repair of current obstetric laceration (75.61)*

57.9 **Other operations on bladder**

57.91 **Sphincterotomy of bladder**
Division of bladder neck

57.92 **Dilation of bladder neck**

57.93 **Control of (postoperative) hemorrhage of bladder**

57.94 **Insertion of indwelling urinary catheter**

57.95 **Replacement of indwelling urinary catheter**

57.96 **Implantation of electronic bladder stimulator**

57.97 **Replacement of electronic bladder stimulator**

57.98 **Removal of electronic bladder stimulator**

Excludes: *that with synchronous replacement (57.97)*

57.99 **Other**

Excludes: *irrigation of:*
cystostomy (96.47)
other indwelling urinary catheter (96.48)
lysis of external adhesions (59.11)
removal of:
cystostomy tube (97.63)
other urinary drainage device (97.64)
therapeutic distention of bladder (96.25)

58 **Operations on urethra**
Code also any application or administration of an adhesion barrier substance (99.77)
Includes: operations on:
bulbourethral gland [Cowper's gland]
periurethral tissue

58.0 **Urethrotomy**
Excision of urethral septum
Formation of urethrovaginal fistula
Perineal urethrostomy
Removal of calculus from urethra by incision

Excludes: *drainage of bulbourethral gland or periurethral tissue (58.91)*
internal urethral meatotomy (58.5)
removal of urethral calculus without incision (58.6)

58.1 **Urethral meatotomy**

Excludes: *internal urethral meatotomy (58.5)*

58.2 **Diagnostic procedures on urethra**

58.21 **Perineal urethroscopy**

58.22 **Other urethroscopy**

58.23 **Biopsy of urethra**

58.24 **Biopsy of periurethral tissue**

58.29 **Other diagnostic procedures on urethra and periurethral tissue**

Excludes: *microscopic examination of specimen from urethra (91.31-91.39)*
retrograde cystourethrogram (87.76)
urethral pressure profile (89.25)
urethral sphincter electromyogram (89.23)

58.3 **Excision or destruction of lesion or tissue of urethra**

Excludes: *biopsy of urethra (58.23)*
excision of bulbourethral gland (58.92)
fistulectomy (58.43)
urethrectomy as part of:
complete cystectomy (57.79)
pelvic evisceration (68.8)
radical cystectomy (57.71)

58.31 **Endoscopic excision or destruction of lesion or tissue of urethra**
Fulguration of urethral lesion

	Valid O.R. procedure		Non-O.R. procedure		Nonspecific O.R. procedure		Noncovered O.R. procedure

58.39 Other local excision or destruction of lesion or tissue of urethra
Excision of:
   congenital valve of urethra
   lesion of urethra
   stricture of urethra
Urethrectomy

> *Excludes:* *that by endoscopic approach (58.31)*

58.4 Repair of urethra

> *Excludes:* *repair of current obstetric laceration (75.61)*

58.41 Suture of laceration of urethra

58.42 Closure of urethrostomy

58.43 Closure of other fistula of urethra

> *Excludes:* *repair of urethroperineovesical fistula (57.84)*

58.44 Reanastomosis of urethra
Anastomosis of urethra

58.45 Repair of hypospadias or epispadias

58.46 Other reconstruction of urethra
Urethral construction

58.47 Urethral meatoplasty

58.49 Other repair of urethra
Benenenti rotation of bulbous urethra
Repair of old obstetric laceration of urethra
Urethral plication

> *Excludes:* *repair of:*
>   *current obstetric laceration (75.61)*
>   *urethrocele (70.50-70.51)*

58.5 Release of urethral stricture
Cutting of urethra] sphincter
Internal urethral meatotomy
Urethrolysis

58.6 Dilation of urethra
Dilation of urethrovesical junction
Passage of sounds through urethra
Removal of calculus from urethra without incision

> *Excludes:* *urethral calibration (89.29)*

58.9 Other operations on urethra and periurethral tissue

58.91 Incision of periurethral tissue
Drainage of bulbourethral gland

58.92 Excision of periurethral tissue

> *Excludes:* *biopsy of periurethral tissue (58.24)*
>   *lysis of periurethral adhesions (59.11-59.12)*

58.93 Implantation of artificial urinary sphincter [AUS]
Placement of inflatable:
   bladder sphincter
   urethral sphincter
Removal with replacement of sphincter device [AUS]
With pump and/or reservoir

58.99 Other
Removal of inflatable urinary sphincter without replacement
Repair of inflatable sphincter pump and/or reservoir
Surgical correction of hydraulic pressure of inflatable sphincter device

> *Excludes:* *removal of:*
>   *intraluminal foreign body from urethra without incision (98.19)*
>   *urethral stent (97.65)*

59 Other operations on urinary tract
Code also any application or administration of an adhesion barrier substance (99.77)

59.0 Dissection of retroperitoneal tissue

59.00 Retroperitoneal dissection, not otherwise specified

● Code new
  to 2012 edition
▲ Revision of
  existing code
④ ⑤ Fourth or fifth
    digit required

59.02 Other lysis of perirenal or periureteral adhesions

> Excludes: *that by laparoscope (59.03)*

59.03 Laparoscopic lysis of perirenal or periureteral adhesions

59.09 Other incision of perirenal or periureteral tissue
Exploration of perinephric area
Incision of perirenal abscess

59.1 Incision of perivesical tissue

59.11 Other lysis of perivesical adhesions

59.12 Laparoscopic lysis of perivesical adhesions

59.19 Other incision of perivesical tissue
Exploration of perivesical tissue
Incision of hematoma of space of Retzius
Retropubic exploration

59.2 Diagnostic procedures on perirenal and perivesical tissue

59.21 Biopsy of perirenal or perivesical tissue

59.29 Other diagnostic procedures on perirenal tissue, perivesical tissue, and retroperitoneum

> Excludes: *microscopic examination of specimen from:*
> *perirenal tissue (91.21-91.29)*
> *perivesical tissue (91.31-91.39)*
> *retroperitoneum NEC (91.11-91.19)*
> *retroperitoneal x-ray (88.14-88.16)*

59.3 Plication of urethrovesical junction
Kelly-Kennedy operation on urethra
Kelly-Stoeckel urethral plication

59.4 Suprapubic sling operation
Goebel-Frangenheim-Stoeckel urethrovesical suspension
Millin-Read urethrovesical suspension
Oxford operation for urinary incontinence
Urethrocystopexy by suprapubic suspension

59.5 Retropubic urethral suspension
Burch procedure
Marshall-Marchetti-Krantz operation
Suture of periurethral tissue to symphysis pubis
Urethral suspension NOS

59.6 Paraurethral suspension
Pereyra paraurethral suspension
Periurethral suspension

59.7 Other repair of urinary stress incontinence

59.71 Levator muscle operation for urethrovesical suspension
Cystourethropexy with levator muscle sling
Gracilis muscle transplant for urethrovesical suspension
Pubococcygeal sling

59.72 Injection of implant into urethra and/or bladder neck
Collagen implant
Endoscopic injection of implant
Fat implant
Polytef implant

59.79 Other
Anterior urethropexy
Augmentation urethroplasty
Repair of stress incontinence NOS
Tudor "rabbit ear" urethropexy

59.8 Ureteral catheterization
Drainage of kidney by catheter
Insertion of ureteral stent
Ureterovesical orifice dilation

Code also any synchronous ureterotomy (56.2)

> Excludes: *that for:*
> *retrograde pyelogram (87.74)*
> *transurethral removal of calculus or clot from ureter and renal pelvis (56.0)*

Valid O.R. procedure   Non-O.R. procedure   Nonspecific O.R. procedure   Noncovered O.R. procedure

59.9 Other operations on urinary system

[Excludes:] *nonoperative removal of therapeutic device (97.61-97.69)*

59.91 Excision of perirenal or perivesical tissue

[Excludes:] *biopsy of perirenal or perivesical tissue (59.21)*

59.92 Other operations on perirenal or perivesical tissue

59.93 Replacement of ureterostomy tube

Change of ureterostomy tube
Reinsertion of ureterostomy tube

[Excludes:] *nonoperative removal of ureterostomy tube (97.62)*

59.94 Replacement of cystostomy tube

[Excludes:] *nonoperative removal of cystostomy tube (97.63)*

59.95 Ultrasonic fragmentation of urinary stones

Shattered urinary stones

[Excludes:] *percutaneous nephrostomy with fragmentation (55.04)*
shockwave disintegration (98.51)

59.99 Other

[Excludes:] *instillation of medication into urinary tract (96.49)*
irrigation of urinary tract (96.45-96.48)

● Code new to 2012 edition ▲ Revision of existing code ④ ⑤ Fourth or fifth digit required

11. OPERATIONS ON THE MALE GENITAL ORGANS (60-64)

60 Operations on prostate and seminal vesicles

Code also any application or administration of an adhesion barrier substance (99.77)
Includes: operations on periprostatic tissue

Excludes: *that associated with radical cystectomy (57.71)*

60.0 Incision of prostate
Drainage of prostatic abscess
Prostatolithotomy

Excludes: *drainage of periprostatic tissue only (60.81)*

60.1 Diagnostic procedures on prostate and seminal vesicles

60.11 Closed [percutaneous] [needle] biopsy of prostate
Approach:
transrectal
transurethral
Punch biopsy

60.12 Open biopsy of prostate

60.13 Closed [percutaneous] biopsy of seminal vesicles
Needle biopsy of seminal vesicles

60.14 Open biopsy of seminal vesicles

60.15 Biopsy of periprostatic tissue

60.18 Other diagnostic procedures on prostate and periprostatic tissue

Excludes: *microscopic examination of specimen from prostate (91.31-91.39)*
x-ray of prostate (87.92)

60.19 Other diagnostic procedures on seminal vesicles

Excludes: *microscopic examination of specimen from seminal vesicles*
(91.31-91.39)
x-ray:
contrast seminal vesiculogram (87.91)
other (87.92)

60.2 Transurethral prostatectomy

Excludes: *local excision of lesion of prostate (60.61)*

60.21 Transurethral (ultrasound) guided laser induced prostatectomy (TULIP)
Ablation (contact) (noncontact) by laser

60.29 Other transurethral prostatectomy
Excision of median bar by transurethral approach
Transurethral electrovaporization of prostate (TEVAP)
Transurethral enucleative procedure
Transurethral prostatectomy NOS
Transurethral resection of prostate (TURP)

60.3 Suprapubic prostatectomy
Transvesical prostatectomy

Excludes: *local excision of lesion of prostate (60.61)*
radical prostatectomy (60.5)

60.4 Retropubic prostatectomy

Excludes: *local excision of lesion of prostate (60.61)*
radical prostatectomy (60.5)

60.5 Radical prostatectomy
Prostatovesiculectomy
Radical prostatectomy by any approach

Excludes: *cystoprostatectomy (57.71)*

60.6 Other prostatectomy

60.61 Local excision of lesion of prostate

Excludes: *biopsy of prostate (60.11-60 12)*
laser interstitial thermal therapy [LITT] of lesion or tissue of prostate
under guidance (17.69)

Valid O.R.
procedure

Non-O.R.
procedure

Nonspecific
O.R. procedure

Noncovered
O.R. procedure

60.62 **Perineal prostatectomy**
Cryoablation of prostate
Cryoprostatectomy
Cryosurgery of prostate
Radical cryosurgical ablation of prostate (RCSA)

Excludes: *local excision of lesion of prostate (60.61)*

60.69 **Other**

60.7 **Operations on seminal vesicles**

60.71 **Percutaneous aspiration of seminal vesicle**

Excludes: *needle biopsy of seminal vesicle (60.13)*

60.72 **Incision of seminal vesicle**

60.73 **Excision of seminal vesicle**
Excision of Mullerian duct cyst
Spermatocystectomy

Excludes: *biopsy of seminal vesicle (60.13-60.14)*
prostatovesiculectomy (60.5)

60.79 **Other operations on seminal vesicles**

60.8 **Incision or excision of periprostatic tissue**

60.81 **Incision of periprostatic tissue**
Drainage of periprostatic abscess

60.82 **Excision of periprostatic tissue**
Excision of lesion of periprostatic tissue

Excludes: *biopsy of periprostatic tissue (60.15)*

60.9 **Other operations on prostate**

60.91 **Percutaneous aspiration of prostate**

Excludes: *needle biopsy of prostate (60.11)*

60.92 **Injection into prostate**

60.93 **Repair of prostate**

60.94 **Control of (postoperative) hemorrhage of prostate**
Coagulation of prostatic bed
Cystoscopy for control of prostate hemorrhage

60.95 **Transurethral balloon dilation of the prostatic urethra**

60.96 **Transurethral destruction of prostate tissue by microwave thermotherapy**
Transurethral microwave thermotherapy (TUMT) of prostate

Excludes: *Prostatectomy:*
other (60.61-60.69)
radical (60.5)
retropubic (60.4)
suprapubic (60.3)
transurethral (60.21-60.29)

60.97 **Other transurethral destruction of prostate tissue by other thermotherapy**
Radiofrequency thermotherapy
Transurethral needle ablation (TUNA) of prostate

Excludes: *Prostatectomy:*
other (60.61-60.69)
radical (60.5)
retropubic (60.4)
suprapubic (60.3)
transurethral (60.21-60.29)

60.99 **Other**

Excludes: *prostatic massage (99.94)*

61 **Operations on scrotum and tunica vaginalis**

61.0 **Incision and drainage of scrotum and tunica vaginalis**

Excludes: *percutaneous aspiration of hydrocele (61.91)*

61.1 **Diagnostic procedures on scrotum and tunica vaginalis**

61.11 **Biopsy of scrotum or tunica vaginalis**

61.19 **Other diagnostic procedures on scrotum and tunica vaginalis**

● Code new
to 2012 edition
▲ Revision of
existing code
④ ⑤ Fourth or fifth
digit required

61.2 **Excision of hydrocele (of tunica vaginalis)**
Bottle repair of hydrocele of tunica vaginalis

> Excludes: *percutaneous aspiration of hydrocele (61.91)*

61.3 **Excision or destruction of lesion or tissue of scrotum**
Fulguration of lesion of scrotum
Reduction of elephantiasis of scrotum
Partial scrotectomy of scrotum

> Excludes: *biopsy of scrotum (61.11)*
> *scrotal fistulectomy (61.42)*

61.4 **Repair of scrotum and tunica vaginalis**

61.41 **Suture of laceration of scrotum and tunica vaginalis**

61.42 **Repair of scrotal fistula**

61.49 **Other repair of scrotum and tunica vaginalis**
Reconstruction with rotational or pedicle flaps

61.9 **Other operations on scrotum and tunica vaginalis**

61.91 **Percutaneous aspiration of tunics vaginalis**
Aspiration of hydrocele of tunica vaginalis

61.92 **Excision of lesion of tunica vaginalis other than hydrocele**
Excision of hematocele of tunica vaginalis

61.99 **Other**

> Excludes: *removal of foreign body from scrotum without incision (98.24)*

62 **Operations on testes**

62.0 **Incision of testis**

62.1 **Diagnostic procedures on testes**

62.11 **Closed [percutaneous] [needle] biopsy of testis**

62.12 **Open biopsy or testis**

62.19 **Other diagnostic procedures on testes**

62.2 **Excision or destruction of testicular lesion**
Excision of appendix testis
Excision of cyst of Morgagni in the male

> Excludes: *biopsy of testis (62.11-62.12)*

62.3 **Unilateral orchiectomy**
Orchidectomy (with epididymectomy) NOS

62.4 **Bilateral orchiectomy**
Male castration
Radical bilateral orchiectomy (with epididymectomy)
Code also any synchronous lymph node dissection (40.3, 40.5)

62.41 **Removal of both testes at same operative episode**
Bilateral orchidectomy NOS

62.42 **Removal of remaining testis**
Removal of solitary testis

62.5 **Orchiopexy**
Mobilization and replacement of testis in scrotum
Orchiopexy with detorsion of testis
Torek (-Bevan) operation (orchidopexy) (first stage) (second stage)
Transplantation to and fixation of testis in scrotum

62.6 **Repair of testes**

> Excludes: *reduction of torsion (63.52)*

62.61 **Suture of laceration of testis**

62.69 **Other repair of testis**
Testicular graft

62.7 **Insertion of testicular prosthesis**

62.9 **Other operations on testis**

62.91 **Aspiration of testis**

> Excludes: *percutaneous biopsy of testis (62.11)*

62.92 **Injection of therapeutic substance into testis**

62.99 **Other**

63   Operations on spermatic cord, epididymis, and vas deferens

63.0   Diagnostic procedures on spermatic cord, epididymis and vas deferens

63.01   Biopsy of spermatic cord, epididymis, or vas deferens

63.09   Other diagnostic procedures on spermatic cord, epididymis, and vas deferens

Excludes: *contrast epididymogram (87.93)*
contrast vasogram (87.94)
other x-ray of epididymis and vas deferens (87.95)

63.1   Excision of varicocele and hydrocele of spermatic cord
High ligation of spermatic vein
Hydrocelectomy of canal of Nuck

63.2   Excision of cyst of epididymis
Spermatocelectomy

63.3   Excision of other lesion or tissue of spermatic cord and epididymis
Excision of appendix epididymis

Excludes: *biopsy of spermatic cord or epididymis (63.01)*

63.4   Epididymectomy

Excludes: *that synchronous with orchiectomy (62.3-62.42)*

63.5   Repair of spermatic cord and epididymis

63.51   Suture of laceration of spermatic cord and epididymis

63.52   Reduction of torsion of testis or spermatic cord

Excludes: *that associated with orchiopexy (62.5)*

63.53   Transplantation of spermatic cord

63.59   Other repair of spermatic cord and epididymis

63.6   Vasotomy
Vasostomy

63.7   Vasectomy and ligation of vas deferens

63.70   Male sterilization procedure not otherwise specified

63.71   Ligation of vas deferens
Crushing of vas deferens
Division of vas deferens

63.72   Ligation of spermatic cord

63.73   Vasectomy

63.8   Repair of vas deferens and epididymis

63.81   Suture of laceration of vas deferens and epididymis

63.82   Reconstruction of surgically divided vas deferens

63.83   Epididymovasostomy

63.84   Removal of ligature from vas deferens

63.85   Removal of valve from vas deferens

63.89   Other repair of vas deferens and epididymis

63.9   Other operations on spermatic cord, epididymis and vas deferens

63.91   Aspiration of spermatocele

63.92   Epididymotomy

63.93   Incision of spermatic cord

63.94   Lysis of adhesions of spermatic cord

63.95   Insertion of valve in vas deferens

63.99   Other

64   Operations on penis
Includes: operations on:
corpora cavernosa
glans penis
prepuce

64.0   Circumcision

64.1   Diagnostic procedures on the penis

64.11   Biopsy of penis

64.19   Other diagnostic procedures on penis

● Code new
to 2012 edition   ▲ Revision of
existing code   ④ ⑤ Fourth or fifth
digit required

64.2 **Local excision or destruction of lesion of penis**

  Excludes: *biopsy of penis (64.11)*

64.3 **Amputation of penis**

64.4 **Repair and plastic operation on penis**

  64.41 **Suture of laceration of penis**

  64.42 **Release of chordee**

  64.43 **Construction of penis**

  64.44 **Reconstruction of penis**

  64.45 **Replantation of penis**
    Reattachment of amputated penis

  64.49 **Other repair of penis**

    Excludes: *repair of epispadias and hypospadias (58.45)*

64.5 **Operations for sex transformation, not otherwise classified.**

64.9 **Other operations on male genital organs**

  64.91 **Dorsal or lateral slit of prepuce**

  64.92 **Incision of penis**

  64.93 **Division of penile adhesions**

  64.94 **Fitting of external prosthesis of penis**
    Penile prosthesis NOS

  64.95 **insertion or replacement of non-inflatable penile prosthesis**
    Insertion of semi-rigid rod prosthesis into shaft of penis

    Excludes: *external penile prosthesis (64.94)*
      inflatable penile prosthesis (64.97)
      plastic repair, penis (64.43-64.49)
      that associated with:
        construction (64.43)
        reconstruction (64.44)

  64.96 **Removal of internal prosthesis of penis**
    Removal without replacement of non-inflatable or inflatable penile prosthesis

  64.97 **Insertion or replacement or inflatable penile prosthesis**
    Insertion of cylinders into shaft of penis and placement of pump and reservoir

    Excludes: *external penile prosthesis (64.94)*
      non-inflatable penile prosthesis (64.95)
      plastic repair, penis (64.43-64.49)

  64.98 **Other operations on penis**
    Corpora cavernosa-corpus spongiosum shunt
    Corpora-saphenous shunt
    Irrigation of corpus cavernosum

    Excludes: *removal of foreign body:*
      intraluminal (98.19)
      without incision (98.24)
      stretching of foreskin (99.95)

  64.99 **Other**

    Excludes: *collection of sperm for artificial insemination (99.96)*

Valid O.R. procedure   Non-O.R. procedure   Nonspecific O.R. procedure   Noncovered O.R. procedure

This page intentionally left blank.

● Code new
to 2012 edition

▲ Revision of
existing code

④ ⑤ Fourth or fifth
digit required

12. OPERATIONS ON THE FEMALE GENITAL ORGANS (65-71)

65 Operations on ovary

Code also any application or administration of an adhesion barrier substance (99.77)

65.0 Oophorotomy
Salpingo-oophorotomy

65.01 Laparoscopic oophorotomy

65.09 Other oophorotomy

65.1 Diagnostic procedures on ovaries

65.11 Aspiration biopsy of ovary

65.12 Other biopsy of ovary

65.13 Laparoscopic biopsy of ovary

65.14 Other laparoscopic diagnostic procedures on ovaries

65.19 Other diagnostic procedure on ovaries

> *Excludes:* *microscopic examination of specimen from ovary (91.41-91-49)*

65.2 Local excision or destruction of ovarian lesion or tissue

65.21 Marsupialization of ovarian cyst

> *Excludes:* *that by laparoscope (65.23)*

65.22 Wedge resection of ovary

> *Excludes:* *that by laparoscope (65.24)*

65.23 Laparoscopic marsupialization of ovarian cyst

65.24 Laparoscopic wedge resection of ovary

65.25 Other laparoscopic local excision or destruction of ovary

65.29 Other local excision or destruction of ovary
Bisection of ovary
Cauterization of ovary
Partial excision of ovary

> *Excludes:* *biopsy of ovary (65.11-65.13)*
> *that by laparoscope (65.25)*

65.3 Unilateral oophorectomy

65.31 Laparoscopic unilateral oophorectomy

65.39 Other unilateral oophorectomy

> *Excludes:* *that by laparoscope (65.31)*

65.4 Unilateral salpingo-oophorectomy

65.41 Laparoscopic unilateral salpingo-oophorectomy

65.49 Other unilateral salpingo-oophorectomy

65.5 Bilateral oophorectomy

65.51 Other removal of both ovaries at same operative episode
Female castration

> *Excludes:* *that by laparoscope (65.53)*

65.52 Other removal of remaining ovary
Removal of solitary ovary

> *Excludes:* *that by laparoscope (65.54)*

65.53 Laparoscopic removal of both ovaries at same operative episode

65.54 Laparoscopic removal of remaining ovary

65.6 Bilateral salpingo-oophorectomy

65.61 Other removal of both ovaries and tubes at same operative episode

> *Excludes:* *that by laparoscope (65.63)*

65.62 Other removal of remaining ovary and tube
Removal of solitary ovary and tube

> *Excludes:* *that by laparoscope (65.64)*

65.63 Laparoscopic removal of both ovaries and tubes at same operative episode

65.64 Laparoscopic removal of remaining ovary and tube

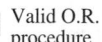 Valid O.R. procedure   Non-O.R. procedure   Nonspecific O.R. procedure   Noncovered O.R. procedure

65.7 **Repair of ovary**

> *Excludes:* *salpingo-oophorostomy (66.72)*

65.71 **Other simple suture of ovary**

> *Excludes:* *that by laparoscope (65.74)*

65.72 **Other reimplantation of ovary**

> *Excludes:* *that by laparoscope (65.75)*

65.73 **Other salpingo-oophoroplasty**

> *Excludes:* *that by laparoscope (65.76)*

65.74 **Laparoscopic simple suture of ovary**

65.75 **Laparoscopic reimplantation of ovary**

65.76 **Laparoscopic salpingo-oophoroplasty**

65.79 **Other repair of ovary**
Oophoropexy

65.8 **Lysis of adhesions of ovary and fallopian tube**

65.81 **Laparoscopic lysis of adhesions of ovary and fallopian tube**

65.89 **Other lysis of adhesions of ovary and fallopian tube**

> *Excludes:* *that by laparoscope (65.81)*

65.9 **Other operations on ovary**

65.91 **Aspiration of ovary**

> *Excludes:* *aspiration biopsy of ovary (65.11)*

65.92 **Transplantation of ovary**

> *Excludes:* *reimplantation of ovary (65.72, 65.75)*

65.93 **Manual rupture of ovarian cyst**

65.94 **Ovarian denervation**

65.95 **Release of torsion of ovary**

65.99 **Other**
Ovarian drilling

66 **Operations on fallopian tubes**
Code also any application or administration of an adhesion barrier substance (99.77)

66.0 **Salpingotomy and salpingostomy**

66.01 **Salpingotomy**

66.02 **Salpingostomy**

66.1 **Diagnostic procedures on fallopian tubes**

66.11 **Biopsy of fallopian tube**

66.19 **Other diagnostic procedures on fallopian tubes**

> *Excludes:* *microscopic examination of specimen from fallopian tubes*
> *(91.41-91.49)*
> *radiography of fallopian tubes (87.82-87.83, 87.85)*
> *Rubin's test (66.8)*

66.2 **Bilateral endoscopic destruction or occlusion of fallopian tubes**
Includes: bilateral endoscopic destruction or occlusion of fallopian tubes by:
culdoscopy
endoscopy
hysteroscopy
laparoscopy
peritoneoscopy
endoscopic destruction of solitary fallopian tube

66.21 **Bilateral endoscopic ligation and crushing of fallopian tubes**

66.22 **Bilateral endoscopic ligation and division of fallopian tubes**

66.29 **Other bilateral endoscopic destruction or occlusion of fallopian tubes**

66.3 **Other bilateral destruction or occlusion of fallopian tubes**
Includes: destruction of solitary fallopian tube

> *Excludes:* *endoscopic destruction or occlusion of fallopian tubes (66.21-66.29)*

66.31 **Other bilateral ligation and crushing of fallopian tubes**

● Code new
to 2012 edition
▲ Revision of
existing code
④ ⑤ Fourth or fifth
digit required

66.32 Other bilateral ligation and division of fallopian tubes
Pomeroy operation

66.39 Other bilateral destruction or occlusion of fallopian tubes
Female sterilization operation NOS

66.4 Total unilateral salpingectomy

66.5 Total bilateral salpingectomy

Excludes: *bilateral partial salpingectomy for sterilization (66.39)*
that with oophorectomy (65.61-65.64)

66.51 Removal of both fallopian tubes at same operative episode

66.52 Removal of remaining fallopian tube
Removal of solitary fallopian tube

66.6 Other salpingectomy
Includes: salpingectomy by:
cauterization
coagulation
electrocoagulation
excision

Excludes: *fistulectomy (66.73)*

66.61 Excision or destruction of lesion of fallopian tube

Excludes: *biopsy of fallopian tube (66.11)*

66.62 Salpingectomy with removal of tubal pregnancy
Code also any synchronous oophorectomy (65.31, 65.39)

66.63 Bilateral partial salpingectomy, not otherwise specified

66.69 Other partial salpingectomy

66.7 Repair of fallopian tube

66.71 Simple suture of fallopian tube

66.72 Salpingo-oophorostomy

66.73 Salpingo-salpingostomy

66.74 Salpingo-uterostomy

66.79 Other repair of fallopian tube
Graft of fallopian tube
Reopening of divided fallopian tube
Salpingoplasty

66.8 Insufflation of fallopian tube
Insufflation of fallopian tube with:
air
dye
gas
saline
Rubin's test

Excludes: *insufflation of therapeutic agent (66.95)*
that for hysterosalpingography (87.82-87.83)

66.9 Other operations on fallopian tubes

66.91 Aspiration of fallopian tube

66.92 Unilateral destruction or occlusion of fallopian tube

Excludes: *that of solitary tube (66.21-66.39)*

66.93 Implantation or replacement of prosthesis of fallopian tube

66.94 Removal of prosthesis of fallopian tube

66.95 Insufflation of therapeutic agent into fallopian tubes

66.96 Dilation of fallopian tube

66.97 Burying of fimbriae in uterine wall

66.99 Other

Excludes: *lysis of adhesions of ovary and tube (65.81, 65.89)*

67 Operations on cervix
Code also any application or administration of an adhesion barrier substance (99.77)

| | Valid O.R. procedure | | Non-O.R. procedure | | Nonspecific O.R. procedure | | Noncovered O.R. procedure |

67.0 Dilation of cervical canal

> *Excludes:* *dilation and curettage (69.01-69.09)*
> *that for induction of labor (73.1)*

67.1 Diagnostic procedures on cervix

67.11 Endocervical biopsy

> *Excludes:* *conization of cervix (67.2)*

67.12 Other cervical biopsy
Punch biopsy of cervix NOS

> *Excludes:* *conization of cervix (67.2)*

67.19 Other diagnostic procedures on cervix

> *Excludes:* *microscopic examination of specimen from cervix (91.41-91.49)*

67.2 Conization of cervix

> *Excludes:* *that by:*
> *cryosurgery (67.33)*
> *electrosurgery (67.32)*

67.3 Other excision or destruction of lesion or tissue of cervix

67.31 Marsupialization of cervical cyst

67.32 Destruction of lesion of cervix by cauterization
Electroconization of cervix
LEEP (loop electrosurgical excision procedure)
LLETZ (large loop excision of the transformation zone)

67.33 Destruction of lesion of cervix by cryosurgery
Cryoconization of cervix

67.39 Other excision or destruction of lesion or tissue of cervix

> *Excludes:* *biopsy of cervix (67.11-67.12)*
> *cervical fistulectomy (67.62)*
> *conization of cervix (67.2)*

67.4 Amputation of cervix
Cervicectomy with synchronous colporrhaphy

67.5 Repair of internal cervical os

67.51 Transabdominal cerclage of cervix

67.59 Other repair of internal cervical os
Cerclage of isthmus uteri
McDonald operation
Shirodkar operation
Transvaginal cerclage

> *Excludes:* *laparoscopically assisted supracervical hysterectomy [LASH] (68.31)*
> *transabdominal cerclage of cervix (67.51)*

67.6 Other repair of cervix

> *Excludes:* *repair of current obstetric laceration (75.51)*

67.61 Suture of laceration of cervix

67.62 Repair of fistula of cervix
Cervicosigmoidal fistulectomy

> *Excludes:* *fistulectomy:*
> *cervicovesical (57.84)*
> *ureterocervical (56.84)*
> *vesicocervicovaginal (57.84)*

67.69 Other repair of cervix
Repair of old obstetric laceration of cervix

68 Other incision and excision of uterus

Code also any application or administration of an adhesion barrier substance (99.77)

68.0 Hysterotomy
Hysterotomy with removal of hydatidiform mole

> *Excludes:* *hysterotomy for termination of pregnancy (74.91)*

68.1 Diagnostic procedures on uterus and supporting structures

● Code new
to 2012 edition
▲ Revision of
existing code
④ ⑤ Fourth or fifth
digit required

68.11 Digital examination of uterus

> *Excludes:* pelvic examination, so described (89.26)
> postpartal manual exploration of uterine cavity (75.7)

68.12 Hysteroscopy

> *Excludes:* that with biopsy (68.16)

68.13 Open biopsy of uterus

> *Excludes:* closed biopsy of uterus (68.16)

68.14 Open biopsy of uterine ligaments

> *Excludes:* closed biopsy of uterine ligaments (68.15)

68.15 Closed biopsy of uterine ligaments
Endoscopic (laparoscopy) biopsy of uterine adnexa, except ovary and fallopian tube

68.16 Closed biopsy of uterus
Endoscopic (laparoscopy) (hysteroscopy) biopsy of uterus

> *Excludes:* open biopsy of uterus (68.13)

68.19 Other diagnostic procedures on uterus and supporting structures

> *Excludes:* diagnostic:
> aspiration curettage (69.59)
> dilation and curettage (69.09)
> microscopic examination of specimen from uterus (91.41-91.49)
> pelvic examination (89.26)
> radioisotope scan of:
> placenta (92.17)
> uterus (92.19)
> ultrasonography of uterus (88.78-88.79)
> x-ray of uterus (87.81-87.89)

68.2 Excision or destruction of lesion or tissue of uterus

68.21 Division of endometrial synechiae
Lysis of intraluminal uterine adhesions

68.22 Incision or excision of congenital septum of uterus

68.23 Endometrial ablation
Dilation and curettage
Hysteroscopic endometrial ablation

● **68.24 Uterine artery embolization [UAE] with coils**

> *Excludes:* that without coils (68.25)

● **68.25 Uterine artery embolization [UAE] without coils**
Includes that by:
gelatin sponge
gelfoam
microspheres
particulate agent NOS
polyvinyl alcohol [PVA]
spherical embolics

> *Excludes:* that with coils (68.24)

68.29 Other excision or destruction of lesion of uterus
Uterine myomectomy

> *Excludes:* biopsy of uterus (68.13)
> uterine fistulectomy (69.42)

68.3 Subtotal abdominal hysterectomy

68.31 Laparoscopic supracervical hysterectomy [LSH]
Classic infrafascial SEMM hysterectomy [CISH]
Laparoscopically assisted supracervical hysterectomy [LASH]

68.39 Other and unspecified subtotal abdominal hysterectomy
Supracervical hysterectomy

> *Excludes:* classic infrafascial SEMM hysterectomy [CISH] (68.31)
> laparoscopic supracervical hysterectomy [LSH] (68.31)

	Valid O.R. procedure		Non-O.R. procedure		Nonspecific O.R. procedure		Noncovered O.R. procedure

68.4 **Total abdominal hysterectomy**
Hysterectomy:
extended

Code also any synchronous removal of tubes and ovaries (65.31-65.64)

| *Excludes:* | *radical abdominal hysterectomy, any approach (68.61-68.69)* |

68.41 **Laparoscopic total abdominal hysterectomy**
Total laparoscopic hysterectomy [TLH]

68.49 **Other and unspecified total abdominal hysterectomy**
Hysterectomy:
Extended

| *Excludes:* | *laparoscopic total abdominal hysterectomy (68.41)* |

68.5 **Vaginal hysterectomy**
Code also any synchronous:
removal of tubes and ovaries (65.31-65.64)
repair of cystocele or rectocele (70.50-70.52)
repair of pelvic floor (70.79)

68.51 **Laparoscopically assisted vaginal hysterectomy (LAVH)**

68.59 **Other and unspecified vaginal hysterectomy**

| *Excludes:* | *laparoscopically assisted vaginal hysterectomy (LAVH) (68.51)* |
| | *radical vaginal hysterectomy (68.7)* |

68.6 **Radical abdominal hysterectomy**
Code also any synchronous:
lymph gland dissection (40.3, 40.5)
removal of tubes and ovaries (65.61-65.64)

| *Excludes:* | *pelvic evisceration (68.8)* |

68.61 **Laparoscopic radical abdominal hysterectomy**
Laparoscopic modified radical hysterectomy
Total laparoscopic radical hysterectomy [TLRH]

68.69 **Other and unspecified radical abdominal hysterectomy**
Modified radical hysterectomy
Wertheim's operation

| *Excludes:* | *laparoscopic total abdominal hysterectomy (68.41)* |
| | *laparoscopic radical abdominal hysterectomy (68.61)* |

68.7 **Radical vaginal hysterectomy**
Code also any synchronous:
lymph gland dissection (40.3, 40.5)
removal of tubes and ovaries (65.61-65.64)

| *Excludes:* | *abdominal hysterectomy, any approach (68.31-68.39, 68.41-68.49,* |
| | *68.61-68.69, 68.9)* |

68.71 **Laparoscopic radical vaginal hysterectomy [LRVH]**

68.79 **Other and unspecified radical vaginal hysterectomy**
Hysterocolpectomy
Schauta operation

68.8 **Pelvic evisceration**
Removal of ovaries, tubes, uterus, vagina, bladder and urethra (with removal of sigmoid
colon and rectum)

Code also any synchronous:
colostomy (46.12-46.13)
lymph gland dissection (40.3, 40.5)
urinary diversion (56.51-56.79)

68.9 **Other and unspecified hysterectomy**
Hysterectomy, NOS

Excludes:	*abdominal hysterectomy, any approach (68.31-68.39, 68.41-68.49,*
	68.61-68.69)
	vaginal hysterectomy, any approach (68.51-68.59, 68.71-68.79)

69 **Other operations on uterus and supporting structures**
Code also any application or administration of an adhesion barrier substance (99.77)

69.0 **Dilation and curettage of uterus**

| *Excludes:* | *aspiration curettage of uterus (69.51-69.59)* |

● Code new ▲ Revision of ④ ⑤ Fourth or fifth
to 2012 edition existing code digit required

69.01 Dilation and curettage for termination of pregnancy

69.02 Dilation and curettage following delivery or abortion

69.09 Other dilation and curettage
Diagnostic D and C

69.1 Excision or destruction of lesion or tissue of uterus and supporting structures

69.19 Other excision or destruction of uterus and supporting structures
Excludes: *biopsy of uterine ligament (68.14)*

69.2 Repair of uterine supporting structures

69.21 Interposition operation
Watkins procedure

69.22 Other uterine suspension
Hysteropexy
Manchester operation
Plication of uterine ligament

69.23 Vaginal repair of chronic inversion of uterus

69.29 Other repair of uterus and supporting structures

69.3 Paracervical uterine denervation

69.4 Uterine repair
Excludes: *repair of current obstetric laceration (75.50-75.52)*

69.41 Suture of laceration of uterus

69.42 Closure of fistula of uterus
Excludes: *uterovesical fistulectomy (57.84)*

69.49 Other repair of uterus
Repair of old obstetric laceration of uterus

69.5 Aspiration curettage of uterus
Excludes: *menstrual extraction (69.6)*

69.51 Aspiration curettage of uterus for termination of pregnancy
Therapeutic abortion NOS

69.52 Aspiration curettage following delivery or abortion

69.59 Other aspiration curettage of uterus

69.6 Menstrual extraction or regulation

69.7 Insertion of intrauterine contraceptive device

69.9 Other operations on uterus, cervix, and supporting structures
Excludes: *obstetric dilation or incision of cervix (73.1, 73.93)*

69.91 Insertion of therapeutic device into uterus
Excludes: *insertion of:*
intrauterine contraceptive device (69.7)
laminaria (69.93)
obstetric insertion of bag, bougie, or pack (73.1)

69.92 Artificial insemination

69.93 Insertion of laminaria

69.94 Manual replacement of inverted uterus
Excludes: *that in immediate postpartal period (75.94)*

69.95 Incision of cervix
Excludes: *that to assist delivery (73.93)*

69.96 Removal of cerclage material from cervix

69.97 Removal of other penetrating foreign body from cervix
Excludes: *removal of intraluminal foreign body from cervix (98.16)*

69.98 Other operations on supporting structures of uterus
Excludes: *biopsy of uterine ligament (68.14)*

Valid O.R. procedure   Non-O.R. procedure   Nonspecific O.R. procedure   Noncovered O.R. procedure

69.99 Other operations on cervix and uterus

> | Excludes: | removal of:
> *foreign body (98.16)*
> *intrauterine contraceptive device (97.71)*
> *obstetric bag, bougie, or pack (97.72)*
> *packing (97.72)*

70   Operations on vagina and cul-de-sac

Code also any application or administration of an adhesion barrier substance (99.77)

70.0   Culdocentesis

70.1   Incision of vagina and cul-de-sac

70.11   Hymenotomy

70.12   Culdotomy

70.13   Lysis of intraluminal adhesion of vagina

70.14   Other vaginotomy
Division of vaginal septum
Drainage of hematoma of vaginal cuff

70.2   Diagnostic procedures on vagina and cul-de-sac

70.21   Vaginoscopy

70.22   Culdoscopy

70.23   Biopsy of cul-de-sac

70.24   Vaginal biopsy

70.29   Other diagnostic procedures on vagina and cul-de-sac

70.3   Local excision or destruction of vagina and cul-de-sac

70.31   Hymenectomy

70.32   Excision or destruction of lesion of cul-de-sac
Endometrectomy of cul-de-sac

> | Excludes: | *biopsy of cul-de-sac (70.23)*

70.33   Excision or destruction of lesion of vagina

> | Excludes: | *biopsy of vagina (70.24)*
> *vaginal fistulectomy (70.72-70.75)*

70.4   Obliteration and total excision of vagina
Vaginectomy

> | Excludes: | *obliteration of vaginal vault (70.8)*

70.5   Repair of cystocele and rectocele

70.50   Repair of cystocele and rectocele

> | Excludes: | *repair of cystocele and rectocele with graft or prosthesis (70.53)*

70.51   Repair of cystocele
Anterior colporrhaphy (with urethrocele repair)

> | Excludes: | *repair of cystocele and rectocele with graft or prosthesis (70.53)*
> *repair of cystocele with graft or prosthesis (70.54)*

70.52   Repair of rectocele
Posterior colporrhaphy

> | Excludes: | *repair of cystocele and rectocele with graft or prosthesis (70.53)*
> *repair of rectocele with graft or prosthesis (70.55)*
> *STARR procedure (48.74)*

70.53   Repair of cystocele and rectocele with graft or prosthesis
Use additional code for biological substance (70.94) or synthetic substance (70.95), if known

70.54   Repair of cystocele with graft or prosthesis
Anterior colporrhaphy (with urethrocele repair)
Use additional code for biological substance (70.94) or synthetic substance (70.95), if known

70.55   Repair of rectocele with graft or prosthesis
Posterior colporrhaphy
Use additional code for biological substance (70.94) or synthetic substance (70.95), if known

70.6 Vaginal construction and reconstruction

70.61 Vaginal construction

70.62 Vaginal reconstruction

70.63 Vaginal construction with graft or prosthesis

Use additional code for biological substance (70.94) or synthetic substance (70.95), if known

Excludes: vaginal construction (70.61)

70.64 Vaginal reconstruction with graft or prosthesis

Use additional code for biological substance (70.94) or synthetic substance (70.95), if known

Excludes: vaginal reconstruction (70.62)

70.7 Other repair of vagina

Excludes: lysis of intraluminal adhesions (70.13)
repair of current obstetric laceration (75.69)
that associated with cervical amputation (67.4)

70.71 Suture of laceration of vagina

70.72 Repair of colovaginal fistula

70.73 Repair of rectovaginal fistula

70.74 Repair of other vaginoenteric fistula

70.75 Repair of other fistula of vagina

Excludes: repair of fistula:
rectovesicovaginal (57.83)
ureterovaginal (56.84)
urethrovaginal (58.43)
uterovaginal (69.42)
vesicocervicovaginal (57.84)
vesicosigmoidovaginal (57.83)
vesicoureterovaginal (56.84)
vesicovaginal (57.84)

70.76 Hymenorrhaphy

70.77 Vaginal suspension and fixation

70.78 Vaginal suspension and fixation with graft or prosthesis

Use additional code for biological substance (70.94) or synthetic substance (70.95), if known

70.79 Other repair of vagina
Colpoperineoplasty
Repair of old obstetric laceration of vagina

70.8 Obliteration of vaginal vault
LeFort operation

70.9 Other operations on vagina and cul-de-sac

70.91 Other operations on vagina

Excludes: insertion of:
diaphragm (96.17)
mold (96.15)
pack (96.14)
pessary (96.18)
suppository (96.49)
removal of:
diaphragm (97.73)
foreign body (98.17)
pack (97.75)
pessary (97.74)
replacement of:
diaphragm (97.24)
pack (97.26)
pessary (97.25)
vaginal dilation (96.16)
vaginal douche (96.44)

	Valid O.R. procedure		Non-O.R. procedure		Nonspecific O.R. procedure		Noncovered O.R. procedure

70.92 Other operations on cul-de-sac
Obliteration of cul-de-sac
Repair of vaginal enterocele

70.93 Other operations on cul-de-sac with graft or prosthesis
Repair of vaginal enterocele with graft or prosthesis

Use additional code for biological substance (70.94) or synthetic substance (70.95), if known

70.94 Insertion of biological graft
Allogenic material or substance
Allograft
Autograft
Autologous material or substance
Heterograft
Xenogenic material or substance

Code first these procedures when done with graft or prosthesis:
Other operations on cul-de-sac (70.93)
Repair of cystocele (70.54)
Repair of cystocele and rectocele (70.53)
Repair of rectocele (70.55)
Vaginal construction (70.63)
Vaginal reconstruction (70.64)
Vaginal suspension and fixation (70.78)

70.95 Insertion of synthetic graft or prosthesis
Artificial tissue

Code first these procedures when done with graft or prosthesis:
Other operations on cul-de-sac (70.93)
Repair of cystocele (70.54)
Repair of cystocele and rectocele (70.53)
Repair of rectocele (70.55)
Vaginal construction (70.63)
Vaginal reconstruction (70.64)
Vaginal suspension and fixation (70.78)

71 Operations on vulva and perineum
Code also any application or administration of an adhesion barrier substance (99.77)

71.0 Incision of vulva and perineum

71.01 Lysis of vulvar adhesions

71.09 Other incision of vulva and perineum
Enlargement of introitus NOS

| Excludes: | removal of foreign body without incision (98.23) |

71.1 Diagnostic procedures on vulva

71.11 Biopsy of vulva

71.19 Other diagnostic procedures on vulva

71.2 Operations on Bartholin's gland

71.21 Percutaneous aspiration of Bartholin's gland (cyst)

71.22 Incision of Bartholin's gland (cyst)

71.23 Marsupialization of Bartholin's gland (cyst)

71.24 Excision or other destruction of Bartholin's gland (cyst)

71.29 Other operations on Bartholin's gland

71.3 Other local excision or destruction of vulva and perineum
Division of Skene's gland

| Excludes: | biopsy of vulva (71.11) |
| | vulvar fistulectomy (71.72) |

71.4 Operations on clitoris
Amputation of clitoris
Clitoridotomy
Female circumcision

71.5 Radical vulvectomy
Code also any synchronous lymph gland dissection (40.3, 40.5)

71.6 Other vulvectomy

71.61 Unilateral vulvectomy

● Code new
  to 2012 edition
▲ Revision of
  existing code
④ ⑤ Fourth or fifth
  digit required

71.62 Bilateral vulvectomy
Vulvectomy NOS

71.7 Repair of vulva and perineum

| Excludes: | repair of current obstetric laceration (75.69) |

71.71 Suture of laceration of vulva or perineum

71.72 Repair of fistula of vulva or perineum

| Excludes: | repair of fistula:
urethroperineal (58.43)
urethroperineovesical (57.84)
vaginoperineal (70.75) |

71.79 Other repair of vulva and perineum
Repair of old obstetric laceration of vulva or perineum

71.8 Other operations on vulva

| Excludes: | removal of:
foreign body without incision (98.23)
packing (97.75)
replacement of packing (97.26) |

71.9 Other operations on female genital organs

Valid O.R.
procedure

Non-O.R.
procedure

Nonspecific
O.R. procedure

Noncovered
O.R. procedure

This page intentionally left blank.

● Code new
to 2012 edition

▲ Revision of
existing code

④ ⑤ Fourth or fifth
digit required

13. OBSTETRICAL PROCEDURES (72-75)

72 Forceps, vacuum, and breech delivery

72.0 Low forceps operation
Outlet forceps operation

72.1 Low forceps operation with episiotomy
Outlet forceps operation with episiotomy

72.2 Mid forceps operation

72.21 Mid forceps operation with episiotomy

72.29 Other mid forceps operation

72.3 High forceps operation

72.31 High forceps operation with episiotomy

72.39 Other high forceps operation

72.4 Forceps rotation of fetal head
DeLee maneuver
Key-in-lock rotation
Kielland rotation
Scanzoni's maneuver
Code also any associated forceps extraction (72.0-72.39)

72.5 Breech extraction

72.51 Partial breech extraction with forceps to aftercoming head

72.52 Other partial breech extraction

72.53 Total breech extraction with forceps to aftercoming head

72.54 Other total breech extraction

72.6 Forceps application to aftercoming head
Piper forceps operation

> Excludes: *partial breech extraction with forceps to aftercoming head (72.51)*
> *total breech extraction with forceps to aftercoming head (72.53)*

72.7 Vacuum extraction
Includes: Malström's extraction

72.71 Vacuum extraction with episiotomy

72.79 Other vacuum extraction

72.8 Other specified instrumental delivery

72.9 Unspecified instrumental delivery

73 Other procedures inducing or assisting delivery

73.0 Artificial rupture of membranes

73.01 Induction of labor by artificial rupture of membranes
Surgical induction NOS

> Excludes: *artificial rupture of membranes after onset of labor (73.09)*

73.09 Other artificial rupture of membranes
Artificial rupture of membranes at time of delivery

73.1 Other surgical induction of labor
Induction by cervical dilation

> Excludes: *injection for abortion (75.0)*
> *insertion of suppository for abortion (96.49)*

73.2 Internal and combined version and extraction

73.21 Internal and combined version without extraction
Version NOS

73.22 Internal and combined version with extraction

73.3 Failed forceps
Application of forceps without delivery
Trial forceps

73.4 Medical induction of labor

> Excludes: *medication to augment active labor—omit code*

73.5 Manually assisted delivery

73.51 Manual rotation of fetal head

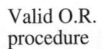 Valid O.R.
procedure

Non-O.R.
procedure

Nonspecific
O.R. procedure

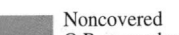 Noncovered
O.R. procedure

73.59 Other manually assisted delivery
Assisted spontaneous delivery
Crede maneuver

73.6 Episiotomy
Episioproctotomy
Episiotomy with subsequent episiorrhaphy

> *Excludes:* *that with:*
> *high forceps (72.31)*
> *low forceps (72.1)*
> *mid forceps (72.21)*
> *outlet forceps (72.1)*
> *vacuum extraction (72.71)*

73.8 Operations on fetus to facilitate delivery
Clavicotomy on fetus
Destruction of fetus
Needling of hydrocephalic head

73.9 Other operations assisting delivery

73.91 External version

73.92 Replacement of prolapsed umbilical cord

73.93 Incision of cervix to assist delivery
Dührssen's incisions

73.94 Pubiotomy to assist delivery
Obstetrical symphysiotomy

73.99 Other

> *Excludes:* *dilation of cervix obstetrical, to induce labor (73.1)*
> *insertion of bag or bougie to induce labor (73.1)*
> *removal of cerclage material (69.96)*

74 Cesarean section and removal of fetus
Code also any synchronous:
hysterectomy (68.3-68.4, 68.6, 68.8)
myomectomy (68.29)
sterilization (66.31-66.39, 66.63)

74.0 Classical cesarean section
Transperitoneal classical cesarean section

74.1 Low cervical cesarean section
Lower uterine segment cesarean section

74.2 Extraperitoneal cesarean section
Supravesical cesarean section

74.3 Removal of extratubal ectopic pregnancy
Removal of:
ectopic abdominal pregnancy
fetus from peritoneal or extraperitoneal cavity following uterine or tubal rupture

> *Excludes:* *that by salpingostomy (66.02)*
> *that by salpingotomy (66.01)*
> *that with synchronous salpingectomy (66.62)*

74.4 Cesarean section of other specified type
Peritoneal exclusion cesarean section
Transperitoneal cesarean section NOS
Vaginal cesarean section

74.9 Cesarian section of unspecified type

74.91 Hysterotomy to terminate pregnancy
Therapeutic abortion by hysterotomy

74.99 Other cesarean section of unspecified type
Cesarean section NOS
Obstetrical abdominouterotomy
Obstetrical hysterotomy

● Code new
to 2012 edition   ▲ Revision of
existing code   ④ ⑤ Fourth or fifth
digit required

75   Other obstetric operations

75.0   Intra-amniotic injection for abortion
Injection of:
    prostaglandin for induction of abortion
    saline for induction of abortion
Termination of pregnancy by intrauterine injection

> Excludes: insertion of prostaglandin suppository for abortion (96.49)

75.1   Diagnostic amniocentesis

75.2   Intrauterine transfusion
Exchange transfusion in utero
Insertion of catheter into abdomen of fetus for transfusion
Code also any hysterotomy approach (68.0)

75.3   Other Intrauterine operations on fetus and amnion
Code also any hysterotomy approach (68.0)

75.31   Amnioscopy
Fetoscopy
Laparoamnioscopy

75.32   Fetal EKG (scalp)

75.33   Fetal blood sampling and biopsy

75.34   Other fetal monitoring
Antepartum fetal nonstress test
Fetal monitoring, not otherwise specified

> Excludes: fetal pulse oximetry (75.38)

75.35   Other diagnostic procedures on fetus and amnion
Intrauterine pressure determination

> Excludes: amniocentesis (75.1)
> diagnostic procedures on gravid uterus
> and placenta (87.81, 88.46, 88.78, 92.17)

75.36   Correction of fetal defect

75.37   Amnioinfusion
Code also injection of antibiotic (99.21)

75.38   Fetal pulse oximetry
Transcervical fetal oxygen saturation monitoring
Transcervical fetal SpO$_2$ monitoring

75.4   Manual removal of retained placenta

> Excludes: aspiration curettage (69.52)
> dilation and curettage (69.02)

75.5   Repair of current obstetric laceration of uterus

75.50   Repair of current obstetric laceration of uterus not otherwise specified

75.51   Repair of current obstetric laceration of cervix

75.52   Repair of current obstetric laceration of corpus uteri

75.6   Repair of other current obstetric laceration
Code also episiotomy, if performed (73.6)

75.61   Repair of current obstetric laceration of bladder and urethra

75.62   Repair of current obstetric laceration of rectum and sphincter ani

75.69   Repair of other current obstetric laceration
Episioperineorrhaphy
Repair of:
    pelvic floor
    perineum
    vagina
    vulva
Secondary repair of episiotomy

75.7   Manual exploration of uterine cavity, postpartum

75.8   Obstetric tamponade of uterus or vagina

> Excludes: antepartum tamponade (73.1)

75.9   Other obstetric operations

| | Valid O.R. procedure | | Non-O.R. procedure | | Nonspecific O.R. procedure | | Noncovered O.R. procedure |

75.91 Evacuation of obstetrical incision hematoma of perineum
Evacuation of hematoma of:
episiotomy
perineorrhaphy

75.92 Evacuation of other hematoma of vulva or vagina

75.93 Surgical correction of inverted uterus
Spintelli operation

> Excludes: *vaginal repair of chronic inversion of uterus (69.23)*

75.94 Manual replacement of inverted uterus

75.99 Other

● Code new
to 2012 edition

▲ Revision of
existing code

④ ⑤ Fourth or fifth
digit required

14. OPERATIONS ON THE MUSCULOSKELETAL SYSTEM (76-84)

76   Operations on facial bones and joints

> *Excludes:*   *accessory sinuses (22.00-22.9)*
> *nasal bones (21.00-21.99)*
> *skull (01.01-02.99)*

76.0   Incision of facial bone without division

76.01   Sequestrectomy of facial bone
Removal of necrotic bone chip from facial bone

76.09   Other incision of facial bone
Reopening of osteotomy site of facial bone

> *Excludes:*   *osteotomy associated with orthognathic surgery (76.61-76.69)*
> *removal of internal fixation device (76.97)*

76.1   Diagnostic procedures on facial bones and joints

76.11   Biopsy of facial bone

76.19   Other diagnostic procedures on facial bones and joints

> *Excludes:*   *contrast arthrogram of temporomandibular joint (87.13)*
> *other x-ray (87.11-87.12 87.14-87.16)*

76.2   Local excision or destruction of lesion of facial bone

> *Excludes:*   *biopsy of facial bone (76.11)*
> *excision of odontogenic lesion (24.4)*

76.3   Partial ostectomy of facial bone

76.31   Partial mandibulectomy
Hemimandibulectomy

> *Excludes:*   *that associated with temporomandibular arthroplasty (76.5)*

76.39   Partial ostectomy of other facial bone
Hemimaxillectomy (with bone graft or prosthesis)

76.4   Excision and reconstruction of facial bones

76.41   Total mandibulectomy with synchronous reconstruction

76.42   Other total mandibulectomy

76.43   Other reconstruction of mandible

> *Excludes:*   *genioplasty (76.67-76.68)*
> *that with synchronous total mandibulectomy (76.41)*

76.44   Total ostectomy of other facial bone with synchronous reconstruction

76.45   Other total ostectomy of other facial bone

76.46   Other reconstruction of other facial bone

> *Excludes:*   *that with synchronous total ostectomy (76.44)*

76.5   Temporomandibular arthroplasty

76.6   Other facial bone repair and orthognathic surgery

Code also any synchronous:
bone graft (76.91)
synthetic implant (76.92)

> *Excludes:*   *reconstruction of facial bones (76.41-76.46)*

76.61   Closed osteoplasty [osteotomy] of mandibular ramus
Gigli saw osteotomy

76.62   Open osteoplasty [osteotomy] of mandibular ramus

76.63   Osteoplasty [osteotomy] of body of mandible

76.64   Other orthognathic surgery on mandible
Mandibular osteoplasty NOS
Segmental or subapical osteotomy

76.65   Segmental osteoplasty [osteotomy] of maxilla
Maxillary osteoplasty NOS

76.66   Total osteoplasty [osteotomy] of maxilla

76.67   Reduction genioplasty
Reduction mentoplasty

| Valid O.R. procedure | Non-O.R. procedure | Nonspecific O.R. procedure | Noncovered O.R. procedure |

76.68 Augmentation genioplasty
Mentoplasty:
NOS
with graft or implant

76.69 Other facial bone repair
Osteoplasty of facial bone NOS

76.7   Reduction of facial fracture
Includes: internal fixation

Code also any synchronous:
bone graft (76.91)
synthetic implant (76.92)

Excludes: *that of nasal bones (21.71-21.72)*

76.70 Reduction of facial fracture, not otherwise specified

76.71 Closed reduction of malar and zygomatic fracture

76.72 Open reduction of malar and zygomatic fracture

76.73 Closed reduction of maxillary fracture

76.74 Open reduction of maxillary fracture

76.75 Closed reduction of mandibular fracture

76.76 Open reduction of mandibular fracture

76.77 Open reduction of alveolar fracture
Reduction of alveolar fracture with stabilization of teeth

76.78 Other closed reduction of facial fracture
Closed reduction of orbital fracture

Excludes: *nasal bone (21.71)*

76.79 Other open reduction of facial fracture
Open reduction of orbit rim or wall

Excludes: *nasal bone (21.72)*

76.9   Other operations on facial bones and joints

76.91 Bone graft to facial bone
Autogenous graft to facial bone
Bone bank graft to facial bone
Heterogenous graft to facial bone

76.92 Insertion of synthetic implant in facial bone
Alloplastic implant to facial bone

76.93 Closed reduction of temporomandibular dislocation

76.94 Open reduction of temporomandibular dislocation

76.95 Other manipulation of temporomandibular joint

76.96 Injection of therapeutic substance into temporomandibular joint

76.97 Removal of internal fixation device from facial bone

Excludes: *removal of:*
dental wiring (97.33)
external mandibular fixation device NEC (97.36)

76.99 Other

● Code new   ▲ Revision of   ④ ⑤ Fourth or fifth
       to 2012 edition   existing code   digit required

77   Incision, excision, and division of other bones

Excludes:	laminectomy for decompression (03.09)
	operations on:
	accessory sinuses (22.00-22.9)
	ear ossicles (19.0-19.55)
	facial bones (76.01-76.99)
	joint structures (80.00-81.99)
	mastoid (19.9-20.99)
	nasal bones (21.00-21.99)
	skull (01.01-02.99)

The following fourth-digit subclassification is for use with appropriate categories in section 77, marked with a symbol to identify the site. Valid fourth-digit categories are in [brackets] under each code.

0   unspecified site
1   scapula, clavicle, and thorax [ribs and sternum]
2   humerus
3   radius and ulna
4   carpals and metacarpals
5   femur
6   patella
7   tibia and fibula
8   tarsals and metatarsals
9   other
      Pelvic bones
      Phalanges (of foot) (of hand)
      Vertebrae

④ **77.0   Sequestrectomy**
[0-9]

④ **77.1   Other incision of bone without division**
[0-9]   Reopening of osteotomy site

Excludes:	aspiration of bone marrow (41.31,41.91)
	removal of internal fixation device (78.60-78.69)

④ **77.2   Wedge osteotomy**
[0-9]

Excludes:	that for hallux valgus (77.51)

④ **77.3   Other division of bone**
[0-9]   Osteoarthrotomy

Excludes:	clavicotomy of fetus (73.8)
	laminotomy or incision of vertebra (03.01-03.09)
	pubiotomy to assist delivery (73.94)
	sternotomy incidental to thoracic operation—omit code

④ **77.4   Biopsy of bone**
[0-9]

77.5   Excision and repair of bunion and other toe deformities

77.51   Bunionectomy with soft tissue correction and osteotomy of the first metatarsal

77.52   Bunionectomy with soft tissue correction and arthrodesis

77.53   Other bunionectomy with soft tissue correction

77.54   Excision or correction of bunionette
      That with osteotomy

77.56   Repair of hammer toe
      Fusion of hammer toe
      Phalangectomy (partial) of hammer toe
      Filleting of hammer toe

77.57   Repair of claw toe
      Fusion of claw toe
      Phalangectomy (partial) of claw toe
      Capsulotomy of claw toe
      Tendon lengthening of claw toe

77.58   Other excision, fusion, and repair of toes
      Cockup toe repair
      Overlapping toe repair
      That with use of prosthetic materials

77.59   Other bunionectomy
      Resection of hallux valgus joint with insertion of prosthesis

	Valid O.R. procedure		Non-O.R. procedure		Nonspecific O.R. procedure		Noncovered O.R. procedure

④ **77.6** **Local excision of lesion or tissue of bone**
[0-9]
> | Excludes: | biopsy of bone (77.40-77.49) |

> debridement of compound fracture (79.60-79.69)

④ **77.7** **Excision of bone for graft**
[0-9]

④ **77.8** **Other partial ostectomy**
[0-9] Condylectomy

> | Excludes: | amputation (84.00-84.19,84.91) |

> arthrectomy (80.90-80.99)
> excision of bone ends associated with:
>   arthrodesis (81.00-81.39, 81.62-81.66)
>   arthroplasty (81.40-81.59, 81.71-81.85)
> excision of cartilage (80.5-80.6, 80.80-80.99)
> excision of head of femur with synchronous replacement (00.70-00.73, 81.51-81.53)
> hemilaminectomy (03.01-03.09)
> laminectomy (03.01-03.09)
> ostectomy for hallux valgus (77.51-77.59)
> partial amputation:
>   finger (84.01)
>   thumb (84.02)
>   toe (84.11)
> resection of ribs incidental to thoracic operation—omit code
> that incidental to other operation—omit code

④ **77.9** **Total ostectomy**
[0-9]
> | Excludes: | amputation of limb (84.00-84.19, 84.91) |

> that incidental to other operation—omit code

78 **Other operations on bones, except facial bones**

> | Excludes: | operations on: |

> accessory sinuses (22.00-22.9)
> facial bones (76.01-76.99)
> joint structures (80.00-81.99)
> nasal bones (21.00-21.99)
> skull (01.01-02.99)

The following fourth-digit subclassification is for use with categories in section 78 to identify the site. Valid fourth-digit categories are in [brackets] under each code.

0 unspecified site
1 scapula, clavicle, and thorax (ribs and sternum]
2 humerus
3 radius and ulna
4 carpals and metacarpals
5 femur
6 patella
7 tibia and fibulas
8 tarsals and metatarsals
9 other
    Pelvic bones
    Phalanges (of foot) (of hand)
    Vertebrae

④ **78.0** **Bone graft**
[0-9] Bone:
    bank graft
    graft (autogenous) (heterogenous)
That with debridement of bone graft site (removal of sclerosed, fibrous, or necrotic bone or tissue)
Transplantation of bone
Code also any excision of bone for graft (77.70-77.79)
> | Excludes: | that for bone lengthening (78.30-78.39) |

④ **78.1** **Application of external fixator device**
[0-9] Fixator with insertion of pins/wires/screws into bone
Code also any type of fixator device, if known (84.71-84.73)
> | Excludes: | other immobilization, pressure, and attention to wound (93.51-93.59) |

● Code new to 2012 edition   ▲ Revision of existing code   ④ ⑤ Fourth or fifth digit required

④ **78.2** **Limb shortening procedures**
[0,2-5,7-9] Epiphyseal stapling
Open epiphysiodesis
Percutaneous epiphysiodesis
Resection/osteotomy

④ **78.3** **Limb lengthening procedures**
[0,2-5,7-9] Bone graft with or without internal fixation devices or osteotomy
Distraction technique with or without corticotomy/osteotomy

Code also any application of an external fixation device (78.10-78.19)

④ **78.4** **Other repair or plastic operations on bone**
[0-9] Other operation on bone NEC
Repair of malunion or nonunion fracture NEC

Excludes:	*application of external fixation device (78.10-78.19)*
	limb lengthening procedures (78.30-78.39)
	limb shortening procedures (78.20-78.29)
	osteotomy (77.3)
	reconstruction of thumb (82.61-82.69)
	repair of pectus deformity (34.74)
	repair with bone graft (78.00-78.09)

④ **78.5** **Internal fixation of bone without fracture reduction**
[0-9] Internal fixation of bone (prophylactic)
Reinsertion of internal fixation device
Revision of displaced or broken fixation device

Excludes:	*arthroplasty and arthrodesis (81.00-81.85)*
	bone graft (78.00-78.09)
	insertion of sternal fixation device with rigid plates (84.94)
	limb shortening procedures (78.20-78.29)
	that for fracture reduction (79.10-79.19, 79.30-79.59)

④ **78.6** **Removal of implanted devices from bone**
[0-9] External fixator device (invasive)
Internal fixation device
Removal of bone growth stimulator (invasive)
Removal of internal limb lengthening device
Removal of pedicle screw(s) used in spinal fusion

Excludes:	*removal of cast, splint, and traction device (Kirschner wire) (Steinmann pin) (97.88)*
	removal of posterior spinal motion preservation (facet replacement, pedicle-based dynamic stabilization, interspinous process) device(s) (80.09)
	removal of skull tongs or halo traction device (02.95)

④ **78.7** **Osteoclasis**
[0-9]

④ **78.8** **Diagnostic procedures on bone, not elsewhere classified**
[0-9]

Excludes:	*biopsy of bone (77.40-77.49)*
	magnetic resonance imaging (88.94)
	microscopic examination of specimen from bone (91.51-91.59)
	radioisotope scan (92.14)
	skeletal x-ray (87.21-87.29, 87.43, 88.21-88.33)
	thermography (88.83)

④ **78.9** **Insertion of bone growth stimulator**
(0-9) Insertion of:
bone stimulator (electrical) to aid bone healing
osteogenic electrodes for bone growth stimulation
totally implanted device (invasive)

Excludes:	*non-invasive (transcutaneous) (surface) stimulator (99.86)*

Valid O.R. procedure	Non-O.R. procedure	Nonspecific O.R. procedure	Noncovered O.R. procedure

79 Reduction of fracture and dislocation

Includes: application of cast or splint
reduction with insertion of traction device (Kirschner wire) (Steinmann pin)

Code also any:
application of external fixator device (78.10-78.19)
type of fixator device, if known (84.71-84.73)

[Excludes:] *external fixation alone for immobilization of fracture (93.51-93.56,93.59)*
internal fixation without reduction of fracture (78.50-78.59)
operations on:
facial bones (76.70-76.79)
nasal bones (21.71-21.72)
orbit (76.78-76.79)
skull (02.02)
vertebrae (03.53)
removal of cast or splint (97.88)
replacement of cast or splint (97.11-97.14)
traction alone for reduction of fracture (93.41-93.46)

The following fourth-digit subclassification is for use with appropriate categories in section 79, marked with a symbol to identify the site. Valid fourth-digit codes are in [brackets] under each code.

0 unspecified site
1 humerus
2 radius and ulna
Arm NOS
3 carpals and metacarpals
Hand NOS
4 phalanges of hand
5 femur
6 tibia and fibula
Leg NOS
7 tarsals and metatarsals
Foot NOS
8 phalanges of foot
9 other specified bone

[4] **79.0 Closed reduction of fracture without internal fixation**
[0-9] [Excludes:] *that for separation of epiphysis (79.40-79.49)*

[4] **79.1 Closed reduction of fracture with internal fixation**
[0-9] [Excludes:] *that for separation of epiphysis (79.40-79.49)*

[4] **79.2 Open reduction of fracture without internal fixation**
[0-9] [Excludes:] *that for separation of epiphysis (79.50-79.59)*

[4] **79.3 Open reduction of fracture with internal fixation**
[0-9] [Excludes:] *that for separation of epiphysis (79.50-79.59)*

[4] **79.4 Closed reduction of separated epiphysis**
[0-2,5,6,9] Reduction with or without internal fixation

[4] **79.5 Open reduction of separated epiphysis**
[0-2,5,6,9] Reduction with or without internal fixation

[4] **79.6 Debridement of open fracture site**
[0-9] Debridement of compound fracture

79.7 Closed reduction of dislocation
Includes: closed reduction (with external traction device)
[Excludes:] *closed reduction of dislocation of temporomandibular joint (76.93)*

79.70 Closed reduction of dislocation of unspecified site

79.71 Closed reduction of dislocation of shoulder

79.72 Closed reduction of dislocation of elbow

79.73 Closed reduction of dislocation of wrist

79.74 Closed reduction of dislocation of hand and finger

79.75 Closed reduction of dislocation of hip

79.76 Closed reduction of dislocation of knee

79.77 Closed reduction of dislocation of ankle

79.78 Closed reduction of dislocation of foot and toe

79.79 Closed reduction of dislocation of other specified sites

79.8 Open reduction of dislocation
Includes: open reduction (with internal and external fixation devices)

Excludes: *open reduction of dislocation of temporomandibular joint (76.94)*

79.80 Open reduction of dislocation of unspecified site

79.81 Open reduction of dislocation of shoulder

79.82 Open reduction of dislocation of elbow

79.83 Open reduction of dislocation of wrist

79.84 Open reduction of dislocation of hand and finger

79.85 Open reduction of dislocation of hip

79.86 Open reduction of dislocation of knee

79.87 Open reduction of dislocation of ankle

79.88 Open reduction of dislocation of foot and toe

79.89 Open reduction or dislocation of other specified sites

④ **79.9 Unspecified operation on bone injury**
[0-9]

80 Incision and excision of joint structures
Includes: operations on:
capsule of joint
cartilage
condyle
ligament
meniscus
synovial membrane

Excludes: *cartilage of:*
ear (18.01-18.9)
nose (21.00-21.99)
temporomandibular joint (76.01-76.99)

The following fifth-digit subclassification is for use with appropriate categories in section 80, that are marked with a symbol to identify the site:

0 unspecified site
1 shoulder
2 elbow
3 wrist
4 hand and finger
5 hip
6 knee
7 ankle
8 foot and toe
9 other specified sites
Spine

④ **80.0 Arthrotomy for removal of prosthesis, without replacement**
Includes: removal of posterior spinal motion preservation (dynamic stabilization, facet replacement, interspinous process) device(s)

Code also any:
insertion of (cement) (joint) (methylmethacrylate) spacer (84.56)
removal of (cement) (joint) (methylmethacrylate) spacer (84.57)

Excludes: *removal of pedicle screws used in spinal fusion (78.69)*

80.00 Arthrotomy for removal of prosthesis without replacement, unspecified site

80.01 Arthrotomy for removal of prosthesis without replacement, shoulder

80.02 Arthrotomy for removal of prosthesis without replacement, elbow

80.03 Arthrotomy for removal of prosthesis without replacement, wrist

80.04 Arthrotomy for removal of prosthesis without replacement, hand and finger

80.05 Arthrotomy for removal of prosthesis without replacement, hip

80.06 Arthrotomy for removal of prosthesis without replacement, knee

80.07 Arthrotomy for removal of prosthesis without replacement, ankle

80.08 Arthrotomy for removal of prosthesis without replacement, foot and toe

80.09 Arthrotomy for removal of prosthesis without replacement, other specified sites

	Valid O.R. procedure		Non-O.R. procedure		Nonspecific O.R. procedure		Noncovered O.R. procedure

④ **80.1** **Other arthrotomy**
Arthrostomy

> Excludes: that for:
> arthrography (88.32)
> arthroscopy (80.20-80.29)
> injection of drug (81.92)
> operative approach—omit code

④ **80.2** **Arthroscopy**

④ **80.3** **Biopsy of joint structure**
Aspiration biopsy

④ **80.4** **Division of joint capsule, ligament, or cartilage**
Goldner clubfoot release
Heyman-Herndon(-Strong) correction of metatarsus varus
Release of:
adherent or constrictive joint capsule
joint
ligament

> Excludes: symphysiotomy to assist delivery (73.94)
> that for:
> carpal tunnel syndrome (04.43)
> tarsal tunnel syndrome (04.44)

80.5 **Excision, destruction and other repair of intervertebral disc**

80.50 **Excision or destruction of intervertebral disc, unspecified**
Unspecified as to excision or destruction

80.51 **Excision of intervertebral disc**
Diskectomy
Levels:
cervical
lumbar (lumbosacral)
thoracic
Removal of herniated nucleus pulposus
That by laminotomy or hemilaminectomy
That with decompression of spinal nerve root at same level
Requires additional code for any concomitant decompression of spinal nerve root at
different level from excision site

> Code also any concurrent spinal fusion (81.00-81.09)
>
> Code also any repair of the anulus fibrosus (80.53-80.54)
>
> Excludes: intervertebral chemonucleolysis (80.52)
> laminectomy for exploration of intraspinal canal (03.09)
> laminotomy for decompression of spinal nerve root only (03.09)
> that for insertion of (non-fusion) spinal disc replacement device
> (84.60-84.69)
> that with corpectomy, (vertebral) (80.99)

80.52 **Intervertebral chemonucleolysis**
Injection of proteolytic enzyme into intervertebral space (chymopapain)
With aspiration of disc fragments
With diskography

> Excludes: injection of anesthetic substance (03.91)
> injection of other substances (03.92)

80.53 **Repair of the anulus fibrosus with graft or prosthesis**
Anular disc repair
Closure (sealing) of the anulus fibrosus defect
Includes:
microsurgical suture repair with fascial autograft
soft tissue re-approximation repair with tension bands
surgical mesh repair

> Code also any"
> application or administration of adhesion barrier substance, if performed (99.77)
> intervertebral discectomy, if performed (80.51)
> locally harvested fascia for graft (83.43)

● Code new
to 2012 edition   ▲ Revision of
existing code   ④ ⑤ Fourth or fifth
digit required

80.54 Other and unspecified repair of the anulus fibrosus
Anular disc repair
Closure (sealing) of the anulus fibrosus defect
Microsurgical suture repair without fascial autograft
Percutaneous repair of the anulus fibrosus

Code also any:
application or administration of adhesion barrier substance, if performed (99.77)
intervertebral discectomy, if performed (80.51)

80.59 Other destruction of intervertebral disc
Destruction NEC
That by laser

80.6 Excision of semilunar cartilage of knee
Excision of meniscus of knee

④ **80.7 Synovectomy**
Complete or partial resection of synovial membrane

| Excludes: | *excision of Baker's cyst (83.39)* |

④ **80.8 Other local excision or destruction of lesion of joint**

④ **80.9 Other excision of joint**

| Excludes: | *cheilectomy of joint (77.80-77.89)* |
| | *excision of bone ends (77.80-77.89)* |

81 Repair and plastic operations on joint structures

81.0 Spinal fusion
Note: Spinal fusion is classified by the anatomic portion (column) fused and the technique
(approach) used to perform the fusion.

For the anterior column, the body (corpus) of adjacent vertebrae are fused (interbody
fusion). The anterior column can be fused using an anterior, lateral, or posterior technique.

For the posterior column, posterior structures of adjacent vertebrae are fused (pedicle,
lamina, facet, transverse process, or "gutter" fusion). A posterior column fusion can be
performed using a posterior, posterolateral, or lateral transverse technique.

Code also any insertion of interbody spinal fusion device (84.51)
Code also any insertion of recombinant bone morphogenetic protein (84.52)
Code also any synchronous excision of (locally) harvested bone for graft (77.70-77.79)
Code also the total number of vertebrae fused (81.62-81.64)
Includes: arthrodesis of spine with:
bone graft
internal fixation

| Excludes: | *correction of pseudarthrosis of spine (81.30-81.39)* |
| | *refusion of spine (81.30-81.39)* |

81.00 Spinal fusion, not otherwise specified

81.01 Atlas-axis spinal fusion
Craniocervical fusion by anterior transoral or posterior technique
C1-C2 fusion by anterior transoral or posterior technique
Occiput-C2 fusion by anterior transoral or posterior technique

81.02 Other cervical fusion of the anterior column, anterior technique
Arthrodesis of C2 level or below:
anterior interbody fusion
anterolateral technique

81.03 Other cervical fusion of the posterior column, posterior technique
Arthrodesis of C2 level or below, posterolateral technique

81.04 Dorsal and dorsolumbar fusion of the anterior column, anterior technique
Arthrodesis of thoracic or thoracolumbar region:
anterior interbody fusion
anterolateral technique
Extracavitary technique

81.05 Dorsal and dorsolumbar fusion of the posterior column, posterior technique
Arthrodesis of thoracic or thoracolumbar region, posterolateral technique

| Valid O.R. procedure | Non-O.R. procedure | Nonspecific O.R. procedure | Bilateral procedure |

81.06 **Lumbar and lumbosacral fusion of the anterior column, anterior technique**
Anterior lumbar interbody fusion (ALIF)
Arthrodesis of lumbar or lumbosacral region:
anterior interbody fusion
anterolateral technique
retroperitoneal
transperitoneal
Direct lateral interbody fusion [DLIF]
Extreme lateral interbody fusion [XLIF]

81.07 **Lumbar and lumbosacral fusion of the posterior column, posterior technique**
Facet fusion
Posterolateral technique
Transverse process technique

81.08 **Lumbar and lumbosacral fusion of the anterior column, posterior technique**
Arthrodesis of lumbar or lumbosacral region, posterior interbody fusion
Axial lumbar interbody fusion [AxiaLIF]
Posterior lumbar interbody fusion (PLIF)
Transforaminal lumbar interbody fusion (TLIF)

81.1 **Arthrodesis and arthroereisis of foot and ankle**
Includes: arthrodesis of foot and ankle with:
bone graft
external fixation device

81.11 **Ankle fusion**
Tibiotalar fusion

81.12 **Triple arthrodesis**
Talus to calcaneus and calcaneus to cuboid and navicular

81.13 **Subtalar fusion**

> Excludes: *arthroereisis (81.18)*

81.14 **Midtarsal fusion**

81.15 **Tarsometatarsal fusion**

81.16 **Metatarsophalangeal fusion**

81.17 **Other fusion of foot**

81.18 **Subtalar joint arthroereisis**

81.2 **Arthrodesis of other joint**
Includes: arthrodesis with:
bone graft
external fixation device
excision of bone ends and compression

81.20 **Arthrodesis of unspecified joint**

81.21 **Arthrodesis of hip**

81.22 **Arthrodesis of knee**

81.23 **Arthrodesis of shoulder**

81.24 **Arthrodesis of elbow**

81.25 **Carporadial fusion**

81.26 **Metacarpocarpal fusion**

81.27 **Metacarpophalangeal fusion**

81.28 **Interphalangeal fusion**

81.29 **Arthrodesis of other specified joints**

● Code new
to 2012 edition

▲ Revision of
existing code

④ ⑤ Fourth or fifth
digit required

81.3   Refusion of spine

Note: Spine fusion is classified by the anatomic portion (column) fused and the technique (approach) used to perform the fusion.

For the anterior column, the body (corpus) of adjacent vertebrae are fused (interbody fusion). The anterior column can be fused using an anterior, lateral, or posterior technique.

For the posterior column, posterior structures of adjacent vertebrae are fused (pedicle, lamina, facet, transverse process, or "gutter" fusion). A posterior column fusion can be performed using a posterior, posterolateral, or lateral transverse technique.

Includes: arthrodesis of spine with:
   bone graft
   internal fixation
   correction of pseudarthrosis of spine

Code also any insertion of interbody spinal fusion device (84.51)

Code also any insertion of recombinant bone morphogenetic protein (84.52)

Code also any synchronous excision of (locally) harvested bone for graft (77.70-77.79)

Code also the total number of vertebrae fused (81.62-81.64)

81.30 Refusion of spine, not otherwise specified

81.31 Refusion of atlas-axis spine
   Craniocervical fusion by anterior, transoral or posterior technique
   C1-C2 fusion by anterior, transoral or posterior technique
   Occiput C2 fusion by anterior, transoral or posterior technique

81.32 Refusion of other cervical spine, anterior column, anterior technique
   Arthrodesis of C2 level or below:
      anterior interbody fusion
      anterolateral technique

81.33 Refusion of other cervical spine, posterior column, posterior technique
   Arthrodesis of C2 level or below, posterolateral technique

81.34 Refusion of dorsal and dorsolumbar spine, anterior column, anterior technique
   Arthrodesis of thoracic or thoracolumbar region, anterior interbody fusion
   Extracavitary technique

81.35 Refusion of dorsal and dorsolumbar spine, posterior column, posterior technique
   Arthrodesis of thoracic and thoracolumbar region, posterolateral technique

81.36 Refusion of lumbar and lumbosacral spine, anterior column, anterior technique
   Anterior lumbar interbody fusion (ALIF)
   Arthrodesis of lumbar or lumbosacral region:
      anterior interbody fusion
      anterolateral technique
      retroperitoneal
      transperitoneal
   Direct lateral interbody fusion [DLIF]
   Extreme lateral interbody fusion [XLIF]

81.37 Refusion of lumbar and lumbosacral spine, posterior column, posterior technique
   Facet fusion
   Posterolateral technique
   Transverse process technique

81.38 Refusion of lumbar and lumbosacral spine, anterior column, posterior technique
   Arthrodesis of lumbar or lumbosacral region, posterior interbody fusion
   Axial lumbar interbody fusion [AxiaLIF]
   Posterior lumbar interbody fusion (PLIF)
   Transforaminal lumbar interbody fusion (TLIF)

81.39 Refusion of spine, not elsewhere classified

81.4   Other repair of joint of lower extremity
   Includes: arthroplasty of lower extremity with:
      external traction or fixation
      graft of bone chips or cartilage
      internal fixation device

81.40 Repair of hip, not elsewhere classified

81.42 Five-in-one repair of knee
   Medial meniscectomy, medial collateral ligament repair, vastus medialis
      advancement, semitendinosus advancement, and pes anserinus transfer

| | Valid O.R. procedure | | Non-O.R. procedure | | Nonspecific O.R. procedure | | Noncovered O.R. procedure |

81.43 **Triad knee repair**
Medial meniscectomy with repair of the anterior cruciate ligament and the medial collateral ligament
O'Donoghue procedure

81.44 **Patellar stabilization**
Roux-Goldthwait operation for recurrent dislocation of patella

81.45 **Other repair of the cruciate ligaments**

81.46 **Other repair of the collateral ligaments**

81.47 **Other repair of knee**

81.49 **Other repair of ankle**

81.5 **Joint replacement of lower extremity**
Note: Removal of prior prosthesis — *omit code*
Includes: arthroplasty of lower extremity with:
external traction or fixation
graft of bone (chips) or cartilage
internal fixation device or prosthesis

81.51 **Total hip replacement**
Replacement of both femoral head and acetabulum by prosthesis
Total reconstruction of hip
Code also any type of bearing surface, if known (00.74-00.77)

81.52 **Partial hip replacement**
Bipolar endoprosthesis
Code also any type of bearing surface, if known (00.74-00.77)

81.53 **Revision of hip replacement, not otherwise specified**
Revision of hip replacement, not specified as to component(s) replaced, (acetabular, femoral or both)
Code also any:
removal of (cement) (joint) spacer (84.57)
type of bearing surface, if known (00.74-00.77)
Excludes: *revision of hip replacement, components specified (00.70-00.73)*

81.54 **Total knee replacement**
Bicompartmental
Partial knee replacement
Tricompartmental
Unicompartmental (hemijoint)

81.55 **Revision of knee replacement, not otherwise specified**
Code also any removal of (cement) spacer (84.57)
Excludes: *arthrodesis of knee (81.22)*
revision of knee replacement, components specified (00.80-00.84)

81.56 **Total ankle replacement**

81.57 **Replacement of joint of foot and toe**

81.59 **Revision of joint replacement of lower extremity, not elsewhere classified**

81.6 **Other procedures on spine**
Note: Number of vertebrae
The vertebral spine consists of 25 vertebrae in the following order and number:
Cervical: C1 (atlas), C2 (axis), C3, C4, C5, C6, C7
Thoracic or Dorsal: T1, T2, T3, T4, T5, T6, T7, T8, T9, T10, T11, T12
Lumbar or Sacral: L1, L2, L3, L4, L5, S1

Coders should report only one code from the series 81.62 or 81.63 or 81.64 to show the total number of vertebrae fused on the patient.
Code also the level and approach of the fusion or refusion (81.00-81.08, 81.30-81.39)

81.62 **Fusion or refusion of 2-3 vertebrae**

81.63 **Fusion or refusion of 4-8 vertebrae**

81.64 **Fusion or refusion of 9 or more vertebrae**

81.65 **Percutaneous vertebroplasty**
Injection of bone void filler (cement) (polymethylmethacrylate) (PMMA) into the diseased or fractured vertebral body
Excludes: *kyphoplasty (81.66)*
percutaneous vertebral augmentation (81.66)

● Code new
to 2012 edition
▲ Revision of
existing code
④ ⑤ Fourth or fifth
digit required

81.66 Percutaneous vertebral augmentation
Insertion of inflatable balloon, bone tamp, or other device displacing (removing) (compacting) bone to create a space (cavity) (void) prior to the injection of bone void filler (cement) (polymethylmethacrylate) (PMMA) or other substance
Arcuplasty
Kyphoplasty
SKyphoplasty
Spineoplasty

| Excludes: | percutaneous vertebroplasty (81.65) |

81.7 Arthroplasty and repair of hand, fingers, and wrist
Includes: arthroplasty of hand and finger with:
external traction or fixation
graft of bone (chips) or cartilage
internal fixation device or prosthesis

| Excludes: | operations on muscle, tendon, and fascia of hand (82.01-82.99) |

81.71 Arthroplasty of metacarpophalangeal and interphalangeal joint with implant

81.72 Arthroplasty of metacarpophalangeal and interphalangeal joint without implant

81.73 Total wrist replacement

81.74 Arthroplasty of carpocarpal or carpometacarpal joint with implant

81.75 Arthroplasty of carpocarpal or carpometacarpal joint without implant

81.79 Other repair of hand, fingers, and wrist

81.8 Arthroplasty and repair of shoulder and elbow
Includes: arthroplasty of upper limb NEC with:
external traction or fixation
graft of bone (chips) or cartilage
internal fixation device or prosthesis

81.80 Other total shoulder replacement

| Excludes: | reverse total shoulder replacement (81.88) |

81.81 Partial shoulder replacement

81.82 Repair of recurrent dislocation of shoulder

81.83 Other repair of shoulder

81.84 Total elbow replacement
Partial elbow replacement

81.85 Other repair of elbow

81.88 Reverse total shoulder replacement
Reverse ball-and-socket of the shoulder

| Excludes: | conversion of prior (failed) total shoulder replacement (arthroplasty) to reverse total shoulder replacement (81.97) |

81.9 Other operations on joint structures

81.91 Arthrocentesis
Joint aspiration

| Excludes: | that for:
arthrography (88.32)
biopsy of joint structure (80.30-80.39)
injection of drug (81.92) |

81.92 Injection of therapeutic substance into joint or ligament

81.93 Suture of capsule or ligament of upper extremity

| Excludes: | that associated with arthroplasty (81.71-81.75, 81.80-81.81, 81.84) |

81.94 Suture of capsule or ligament of ankle and foot

| Excludes: | that associated with arthroplasty (81.56-81.59) |

81.95 Suture of capsule or ligament of other lower extremity

| Excludes: | that associated with arthroplasty (81.51-81.55, 81.59) |

81.96 Other repair of joint

81.97 Revision of joint replacement of upper extremity
Partial   Total
Revision of arthroplasty of shoulder
Includes: removal of cement spacer

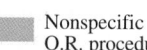

| | Valid O.R. procedure | | Non-O.R. procedure | | Nonspecific O.R. procedure | | Noncovered O.R. procedure |

81.98 Other diagnostic procedures on joint structures

> Excludes: *arthroscopy (80.20-80.29)*
> *biopsy of joint structure (80.30-80.39)*
> *microscopic examination of specimen from joint (91.51-91.59)*
> *thermography (88.83)*
> *x-ray (87.21-87.29, 88.21-88.33)*

81.99 Other

82 Operations on muscle, tendon, and fascia of hand
Includes: operations on:
aponeurosis
synovial membrane (tendon sheath)
tendon sheath

82.0 Incision of muscle, tendon, fascia, and bursa of hand

82.01 Exploration of tendon sheath of hand
Incision of tendon sheath of hand
Removal of rice bodies in tendon sheath of hand

> Excludes: *division of tendon (82.11)*

82.02 Myotomy of hand

> Excludes: *myotomy for division (82.19)*

82.03 Bursotomy of hand

82.04 Incision and drainage of palmar or thenar space

82.09 Other incision of soft tissue of hand

> Excludes: *incision of skin and subcutaneous tissue alone (86.01-86.09)*

82.1 Division of muscle, tendon, and fascia of hand

82.11 Tenotomy of hand
Division of tendon of hand

82.12 Fasciotomy of hand
Division of fascia of hand

82.19 Other division of soft tissue of hand
Division of muscle of hand

82.2 Excision of lesion of muscle, tendon, and fascia of hand

82.21 Excision of lesion of tendon sheath of hand
Ganglionectomy of tendon sheath (wrist)

82.22 Excision of lesion of muscle of hand

82.29 Excision of other lesion of soft tissue of hand

> Excludes: *excision of lesion of skin and subcutaneous tissue (86.21-86.3)*

82.3 Other excision of soft tissue of hand
Code also any skin graft (86.61-86.62, 86.73)

> Excludes: *excision of skin and subcutaneous tissue (86.21-86.3)*

82.31 Bursectomy of hand

82.32 Excision of tendon of hand for graft

82.33 Other tenonectomy of hand
Tenosynovectomy of hand

> Excludes: *excision of lesion of:*
> *tendon (82.29)*
> *sheath (82.21)*

82.34 Excision of muscle or fascia of hand for graft

82.35 Other fasciectomy of hand
Release of Dupuytren's contracture

> Excludes: *excision of lesion of fascia (82.29)*

82.36 Other myectomy of hand

> Excludes: *excision of lesion of muscle (82.22)*

82.39 Other excision of soft tissue of hand

> Excludes: *excision of skin (86.21-86.3)*
> *excision of soft tissue lesion (82.29)*

82.4 Suture of muscle, tendon, and fascia of hand

● Code new
to 2012 edition

▲ Revision of
existing code

④ ⑤ Fourth or fifth
digit required

82.41 Suture of tendon sheath of hand

82.42 Delayed suture of flexor tendon of hand

82.43 Delayed suture of other tendon of hand

82.44 Other suture of flexor tendon of hand

> Excludes: *delayed suture of flexor tendon of hand (82.42)*

82.45 Other suture of other tendon of hand

> Excludes: *delayed suture of other tendon of hand (82.43)*

82.46 Suture of muscle or fascia of hand

82.5 Transplantation of muscle and tendon of hand

82.51 Advancement of tendon of hand

82.52 Recession of tendon of hand

82.53 Reattachment of tendon of hand

82.54 Reattachment of muscle of hand

82.55 Other change in hand muscle or tendon length

82.56 Other hand tendon transfer or transplantation

> Excludes: *pollicization of thumb (82.61)*
> *transfer of finger, except thumb (82.81)*

82.57 Other hand tendon transposition

82.58 Other hand muscle transfer or transplantation

82.59 Other hand muscle transposition

82.6 Reconstruction of thumb
Includes: digital transfer to act as thumb
Code also any amputation for digital transfer (84.01, 84.11)

82.61 Pollicization operation carrying over nerves and blood supply

82.69 Other reconstruction of thumb
"Cocked-hat" procedure [skin flap and bone]
Grafts:
    bone to thumb
    skin (pedicle) to thumb

82.7 Plastic operation on hand with graft or implant

82.71 Tendon pulley reconstruction
Reconstruction for opponensplasty

82.72 Plastic operation on hand with graft of muscle or fascia

82.79 Plastic operation on hand with other graft or implant
Tendon graft to hand

82.8 Other plastic operations on hand

82.81 Transfer of finger, except thumb

> Excludes: *pollicization of thumb (82.61)*

82.82 Repair of cleft hand

82.83 Repair of macrodactyly

82.84 Repair of mallet finger

82.85 Other tenodesis of hand
Tendon fixation of hand NOS

82.86 Other tenoplasty of hand
Myotenoplasty of hand

82.89 Other plastic operations on hand
Plication of fascia
Repair of fascial hernia

> Excludes: *that with graft or implant (82.71-82.79)*

82.9 Other operations on muscle, tendon, and fascia of hand

> Excludes: *diagnostic procedures on soft tissue of hand (83.21-83.29)*

82.91 Lysis of adhesions of hand
Freeing of adhesions of fascia, muscle, and tendon of hand

> Excludes: *decompression of carpal tunnel (04.43)*
> *that by stretching or manipulation only (93.26)*

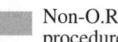 Valid O.R.
procedure

Non-O.R.
procedure

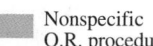 Nonspecific
O.R. procedure

Noncovered
O.R. procedure

82.92 Aspiration of bursa of hand

82.93 Aspiration of other soft tissue of hand
> *Excludes:* *skin and subcutaneous tissue (86.01)*

82.94 Injection of therapeutic substance into bursa of hand

82.95 Injection of therapeutic substance into tendon of hand

82.96 Other injection of locally-acting therapeutic substance into soft tissue of hand
> *Excludes:* *subcutaneous or intramuscular injection (99.11-99.29)*

82.99 Other operations on muscle, tendon, and fascia of hand

83 Operations on muscle, tendon, fascia, and bursa, except hand
Includes: operations on:
    aponeurosis
    synovial membrane of bursa and tendon sheaths
    tendon sheaths

> *Excludes:* *diaphragm (34.81-34.89)*
> *hand (82.01-82.99)*
> *muscles of eye (15.01-15.9).*

83.0 Incision of muscle, tendon, fascia, and bursa

83.01 Exploration of tendon sheath
Incision of tendon sheath
Removal of rice bodies from tendon sheath

83.02 Myotomy
> *Excludes:* *cricopharyngeal myotomy (29.31)*

83.03 Bursotomy
Removal of calcareous deposit of bursa
> *Excludes:* *aspiration of bursa (percutaneous) (83.94)*

83.09 Other incision of soft tissue
Incision of fascia
> *Excludes:* *incision of skin and subcutaneous tissue alone (86.01-86.09)*

83.1 Division of muscle, tendon, and fascia

83.11 Achillotenotomy

83.12 Adductor tenotomy of hip

83.13 Other tenotomy
Aponeurotomy
Division of tendon
Tendon release
Tendon transection
Tenotomy for thoracic outlet decompression

83.14 Fasciotomy
Division of fascia
Division of iliotibial band
Fascia stripping
Release of Volkmann's contracture by fasciotomy

83.19 Other division of soft tissue
Division of muscle
Muscle release
Myotomy for thoracic outlet decompression
Myotomy with division
Scalenotomy
Transection of muscle

83.2 Diagnostic procedures on muscle, tendon, fascia, and bursa, including that of hand

83.21 Open biopsy of soft tissue
> *Excludes:* *biopsy of chest wall (34.23)*
> *closed biopsy of skin and subcutaneous tissue (86.11)*

83.29 Other diagnostic procedures on muscle, tendon, fascia, and bursa, including that of hand
> *Excludes:* *microscopic examination of specimen (91.51-91.59)*
> *soft tissue x-ray (87.09, 87.38-87.39, 88.09, 88.35, 88.37)*
> *thermography of muscle (88.84)*

● Code new to 2012 edition   ▲ Revision of existing code   ④ ⑤ Fourth or fifth digit required

83.3   Excision of lesion of muscle, tendon, fascia, and bursa

> *Excludes:*   biopsy of soft tissue (83.21)

83.31   Excision of lesion of tendon sheath
Excision of ganglion of tendon sheath, except of hand

83.32   Excision of lesion of muscle
Excision of:
heterotopic bone
muscle scar for release of Volkmann's contracture
myositis ossificans

83.39   Excision of lesion of other soft tissue
Excision of Baker's cyst

> *Excludes:*   bursectomy (83.5)
> excision of lesion of skin and subcutaneous tissue (86.3)
> synovectomy (80.70-80.79)

83.4   Other excision of muscle, tendon, and fascia

83.41   Excision of tendon for graft

83.42   Other tenonectomy
Excision of:
aponeurosis
tendon sheath
Tenosynovectomy

83.43   Excision of muscle or fascia for graft

83.44   Other fasciectomy

83.45   Other myectomy
Debridement of muscle NOS
Scalenectomy

83.49   Other excision of soft tissue

83.5   Bursectomy

83.6   Suture of muscle, tendon, and fascia

83.61   Suture of tendon sheath

83.62   Delayed suture of tendon

83.63   Rotator cuff repair

83.64   Other suture of tendon
Achillorrhaphy
Aponeurorrhaphy

> *Excludes:*   delayed suture of tendon (83.62)

83.65   Other suture of muscle or fascia
Repair of diastasis recti

83.7   Reconstruction of muscle and tendon

> *Excludes:*   reconstruction of muscle and tendon associated with arthroplasty

83.71   Advancement of tendon

83.72   Recession of tendon

83.73   Reattachment of tendon

83.74   Reattachment of muscle

83.75   Tendon transfer or transplantation

83.76   Other tendon transposition

83.77   Muscle transfer or transplantation
Release of Volkmann's contracture by muscle transplantation

83.79   Other muscle transposition

83.8   Other plastic operations on muscle, tendon, and fascia

> *Excludes:*   plastic operations on muscle, tendon, and fascia associated with arthroplasty

83.81   Tendon graft

83.82   Graft of muscle or fascia

83.83   Tendon pulley reconstruction

83.84   Release of clubfoot, not elsewhere classified
Evans operation on clubfoot

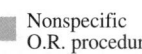 Valid O.R.
procedure

Non-O.R.
procedure

Nonspecific
O.R. procedure

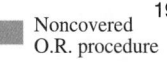 Noncovered
O.R. procedure

83.85 Other change in muscle or tendon length
Hamstring lengthening
Heel cord shortening
Plastic achillotenotomy
Tendon plication

83.86 Quadricepsplasty

83.87 Other plastic operations on muscle
Musculoplasty
Myoplasty

83.88 Other plastic operations on tendon
Myotenoplasty
Tendon fixation
Tenodesis
Tenoplasty

83.89 Other plastic operations on fascia
Fascia lengthening
Fascioplasty
Plication of fascia

83.9 Other operations on muscle, tendon, fascia, and bursa

> Excludes: *nonoperative:*
> *manipulation (93.25-93.29)*
> *stretching (93.27-93.29)*

83.91 Lysis of adhesions of muscle, tendon, fascia,and bursa

> Excludes: *that for tarsal tunnel syndrome (04.44)*

83.92 Insertion or replacement of skeletal muscle stimulator
Implantation, insertion, placement, or replacement of skeletal muscle:
electrodes
stimulator

83.93 Removal of skeletal muscle stimulator

83.94 Aspiration of bursa

83.95 Aspiration of other soft tissue

> Excludes: *that of skin and subcutaneous tissue (86.01)*

83.96 Injection of therapeutic substance into bursa

83.97 Injection of therapeutic substance into tendon

83.98 Injection of locally-acting therapeutic substance into other soft tissue

> Excludes: *subcutaneous or intramuscular injection (99.11-99.29)*

83.99 Other operations on muscle, tendon, fascia and bursa
Suture of bursa

84 Other procedures on musculoskeletal system

84.0 Amputation of upper limb

> Excludes: *revision of amputation stump (84.3)*

84.00 Upper limb amputation, not otherwise specified
Closed flap amputation of upper limb NOS
Kineplastic amputation of upper limb NOS
Open or guillotine amputation of upper limb NOS
Revision of current traumatic amputation of upper limb NOS

84.01 Amputation and disarticulation of finger

> Excludes: *ligation of supernumerary finger (86.26)*

84.02 Amputation and disarticulation of thumb

84.03 Amputation through hand
Amputation through carpals

84.04 Disarticulation of wrist

84.05 Amputation through forearm
Forearm amputation

84.06 Disarticulation of elbow

84.07 Amputation through humerus
Upper arm amputation

84.08 Disarticulation of shoulder

● Code new
to 2012 edition   ▲ Revision of
existing code   ④ ⑤ Fourth or fifth
digit required

84.09 Interthoracoscapular amputation
Forequarter amputation

84.1 Amputation of lower limb

> *Excludes:* revision of amputation stump (84.3)

84.10 Lower limb amputation, not otherwise specified
Closed flap amputation of lower limb NOS
Kineplastic amputation of lower limb NOS
Open or guillotine amputation of lower limb NOS
Revision of current traumatic amputation of lower limb NOS

84.11 Amputation of toe
Amputation through metatarsophalangeal joint
Disarticulation of toe
Metatarsal head amputation
Ray amputation of foot (disarticulation of the metatarsal head of the toe extending
  across the forefoot just proximal to the metatarsophalangeal crease)

> *Excludes:* ligation of supernumerary toe (86.26)

84.12 Amputation through foot
Amputation of forefoot
Amputation through middle of foot
Chopart's amputation
Midtarsal amputation
Transmetatarsal amputation (amputation of the forefoot, including all the toes)

> *Excludes:* ray amputation of foot (84.11)

84.13 Disarticulation of ankle

84.14 Amputation of ankle through malleoli of tibia and fibula

84.15 Other amputation below knee
Amputation of leg through tibia and fibula NOS

84.16 Disarticulation of knee
Batch, Spitler, and McFaddin amputation
Mazet amputation
S.P. Roger's amputation

84.17 Amputation above knee
Amputation of leg through femur
Amputation of thigh
Conversion of below-knee amputation into above-knee amputation
Supracondylar above-knee amputation

84.18 Disarticulation of hip

84.19 Abdominopelvic amputation
Hemipelvectomy
Hindquarter amputation

84.2 Reattachment of extremity

84.21 Thumb reattachment

84.22 Finger reattachment

84.23 Forearm, wrist, or hand reattachment

84.24 Upper arm reattachment
Reattachment of arm NOS

84.25 Toe reattachment

84.26 Foot reattachment

84.27 Lower leg or ankle reattachment
Reattachment of leg NOS

84.28 Thigh reattachment

84.29 Other reattachment

84.3 Revision of amputation stump
Reamputation of stump
Secondary closure of stump
Trimming of stump

> *Excludes:* revision of current traumatic amputation [revision by further amputation of
>   current injury] (84.00-84.19, 84.91)

84.4 Implantation or fitting of prosthetic limb device

84.40 Implantation or fitting of prosthetic limb device not otherwise specified

---

| | Valid O.R. procedure | | Non-O.R. procedure | | Nonspecific O.R. procedure | | Noncovered O.R. procedure |

84.41 Fitting of prosthesis of upper arm and shoulder

84.42 Fitting of prosthesis of lower arm and hand

84.43 Fitting of prosthesis of arm, not otherwise specified

84.44 Implantation of prosthetic device of arm

84.45 Fitting of prosthesis above knee

84.46 Fitting of prosthesis below knee

84.47 Fitting of prosthesis of leg, not otherwise specified

84.48 Implantation of prosthetic device of leg

84.5 Implantation of other musculoskeletal devices and substances

84.51 Insertion of interbody spinal fusion device
Insertion of:
    cages (carbon, ceramic, metal, plastic, or titanium)
    interbody fusion cage
    synthetic cages or spacers
    threaded bone dowels
Code also refusion of spine (81.30-81.39)
Code also spinal fusion (81.00-81.08)

> Excludes: *insertion of (non-fusion) spinal disc replacement device (84.60-84.69)*

84.52 Insertion of recombinant bone morphogenetic protein rhBMP
That via collagen sponge, coral, ceramic and other carriers
Code also primary procedure performed:
    fracture repair (79.00-79.99)
    spinal fusion (81.00-81.08)
    spinal refusion (81.30-81.39)

84.53 Implantation of internal limb lengthening device with kinetic distraction
Code also limb lengthening procedure (78.30-78.39)

84.54 Implantation of other internal limb lengthening device
Implantation of internal limb lengthening device, not otherwise specified (NOS)
Code also limb lengthening procedure (78.30-78.39)

84.55 Insertion of bone void filler
Insertion of:
    acrylic cement (PMMA)
    bone void cement
    calcium based bone void filler
    polymethylmethacrylate (PMMA)

> Excludes: *that with percutaneous vertebral augmentation (81.66)*
> *that with percutaneous vertebroplasty (81.65)*

84.56 Insertion or replacement of (cement) spacer
Insertion or replacement of joint (methylmethacrylate) spacer

84.57 Removal of (cement) spacer
Removal of joint (methylmethacrylate) spacer

84.59 Insertion of other spinal devices

> Excludes: *initial insertion of pedicle screws with spinal fusion-omit code*
> *insertion of facet replacement device(s) (84.84)*
> *insertion of interspinous process device(s) (84.80)*
> *insertion of pedicle-based dynamic stabilization device(s) (84.82)*

84.6 Replacement of spinal disc
Includes: non-fusion arthroplasty of the spine with insertion of artificial disc prosthesis

84.60 Insertion of spinal disc prosthesis, not otherwise specified
Replacement of spinal disc, NOS
Includes: diskectomy (discectomy)

84.61 Insertion of partial spinal disc prosthesis, cervical
Nuclear replacement device, cervical
Partial artificial disc prosthesis (flexible), cervical
Replacement of nuclear disc (nucleus pulposus), cervical
Includes: diskectomy (discectomy)

84.62 Insertion of total spinal disc prosthesis, cervical
Replacement of cervial spinal disc, NOS
Replacement of total spinal disc, cervical
Total artificial disc prosthesis (flexible), cervical
Includes: diskectomy (discectomy)

● Code new
to 2012 edition   ▲ Revision of
existing code   ④ ⑤ Fourth or fifth
digit required

84.63 Insertion of spinal disc prosthesis, thoracic
Artificial disc prosthesis (flexible), thoracic
Replacement of thoracic spinal disc, partial or total
Includes: diskectomy (discectomy)

84.64 Insertion of partial spinal disc prosthesis, lumbosacral
Nuclear replacement device, lumbar
Partial artificial disc prosthesis (flexible), lumbar
Replacement of nuclear disc (nucleus pulposus), lumbar
Includes: diskectomy (discectomy)

84.65 Insertion of total spinal disc prosthesis, lumbosacral
Replacement of lumbar spinal disc, NOS
Replacement of total spinal disc, lumbar
Total artificial disc prosthesis (flexible), lumbar
Includes: diskectomy (discectomy)

84.66 Revision or replacement of artificial spinal disc prosthesis, cervical
Removal of (partial) (total) spinal disc prosthesis with synchronous insertion of new
(partial) (total) spinal disc prosthesis, cervical
Repair of previously inserted spinal disc prosthesis, cervical

84.67 Revision or replacement of artificial spinal disc prosthesis, thoracic
Removal of (partial) (total) spinal disc prosthesis with synchronous insertion of new
(partial) (total) spinal disc prosthesis, thoracic
Repair of previously inserted spinal disc prosthesis, thoracic

84.68 Revision or replacement of artificial spinal disc prosthesis, lumbosacral
Removal of (partial) (total) spinal disc prosthesis with synchronous insertion of new
(partial) (total) spinal disc prosthesis, lumbosacral
Repair of previously inserted spinal disc prosthesis, lumbosacral

84.69 Revision or replacement of artificial spinal disc prosthesis, not otherwise specified
Removal of (partial) (total) spinal disc prosthesis with synchronous insertion of new
(partial) (total) spinal disc prosthesis
Repair of previously inserted spinal disc prosthesis

84.7 Adjunct codes for external fixator devices
Code also any primary procedure performed:
application of external fixator device (78.10, 78.12-78.13, 78.15, 78.17-78.19)
reduction of fracture and dislocation (79.00-79.89)

84.71 Application of external fixator device, monoplanar system

Excludes:	*other hybrid device or system (84.73)*
	ring device or system (84.72)

84.72 Application of external fixator device, ring system
Ilizarov type
Sheffield type

Excludes:	*monoplanar device or system (84.71)*
	other hybrid device or system (84.73)

84.73 Application of hybrid external fixator device
Computer (assisted) (dependent) external fixator device
Hybrid system using both ring and monoplanar devices

Excludes:	*monoplanar device or system, when used alone (84.71)*
	ring device or system, when used alone (84.72)

84.8 Insertion, replacement and revision of posterior spinal motion preservation device(s)
Dynamic spinal stabilization device(s)
Includes: any synchronous facetectomy (partial, total) performed at the same level

Code also any synchronous surgical decompression (foraminotomy, laminectomy, laminotomy), if performed (03.09)

Excludes:	*fusion of spine (81.00 – 81.08, 81.30-81.39)*
	insertion of artificial disc prosthesis (84.60-84.69)
	insertion of interbody spinal fusion device (84.51)

84.80 Insertion or replacement of interspinous process device(s)
Interspinous process decompression device(s)
Interspinous process distraction device(s)

Excludes:	*insertion or replacement of facet replacement device (84.84)*
	insertion or replacement of pedicle-based dynamic stabilization device (84.82)

	Valid O.R. procedure		Non-O.R. procedure		Nonspecific O.R. procedure		Noncovered O.R. procedure

84.81 **Revision of interspinous process device(s)**
Repair of previously inserted interspinous process device(s)

| Excludes: | *revision of facet replacement device(s) (84.85)* |
| | *revision of pedicle-based dynamic stabilization device (84.83)* |

84.82 **Insertion or replacement of pedicle-based dynamic stabilization device(s)**

Excludes:	*initial insertion of pedicle screws with spinal fusion – omit code*
	insertion or replacement of facet replacement device(s) (84.84)
	insertion or replacement of interspinous process device(s) (84.80)
	replacement of pedicle screws used in spinal fusion (78.59)

84.83 **Revision of pedicle-based dynamic stabilization device(s)**
Repair of previously inserted pedicle-based dynamic stabilization device(s)

Excludes:	*removal of pedicle screws used in spinal fusion (78.69)*
	replacement of pedicle screws used in spinal fusion (78.59)
	revision of facet replacement device(s) (84.85)
	revision of interspinous process device(s) (84.81)

84.84 **Insertion or replacement of facet replacement device(s)**
Facet arthroplasty

Excludes:	*initial insertion of pedicle screws with spinal fusion-omit code*
	insertion or replacement of interspinous process device(s) (84.80)
	insertion or replacement of pedicle-based dynamic stabilization device(s) (84.82)
	replacement of pedicle screws used in spinal fusion (78.59)

84.85 **Revision of facet replacement device(s)**
Repair of previously inserted facet replacement device(s)

Excludes:	*removal of pedicle screws used in spinal fusion (78.69)*
	replacement of pedicle screws used in spinal fusion (78.59)
	revision of interspinous process device(s) (84.81)
	revision of pedicle-based dynamic stabilization device(s) (84.83)

84.9 **Other operations on musculoskeletal system**

| Excludes: | *nonoperative manipulation (93.25-93.29)* |

84.91 **Amputation, not otherwise specified**

84.92 **Separation of equal conjoined twins**

84.93 **Separation of unequal conjoined twins**
Separation of conjoined twins NOS

84.94 **Insertion of sternal fixation device with rigid plates**

| Excludes: | *insertion of sternal fixation device for internal fixation of fracture (79.39)* |
| | *internal fixation of bone without fracture reduction (78.59)* |

84.99 **Other**

15. OPERATIONS ON THE INTEGUMENTARY SYSTEM (85-86)

85 Operations on the breast
Includes: operations on the skin and subcutaneous tissue of:
   breast, female or male
   previous mastectomy site, female or male
   revision of previous mastectomy site

85.0 Mastotomy
Incision of breast (skin)
Mammotomy

> Excludes: *aspiration of breast (85.91)*
>   *removal of implant (85.94)*

85.1 Diagnostic procedures on breast

85.11 Closed [percutaneous] [needle] biopsy of breast

85.12 Open biopsy of breast

85.19 Other diagnostic procedures on breast

> Excludes: *mammary ductogram (87.35)*
>   *mammography NEC (87.37)*
>   *manual examination (89.36)*
>   *microscopic examination of specimen (91.61-91.69)*
>   *thermography (88.85)*
>   *ultrasonography (88.73)*
>   *xerography (87.36)*

85.2 Excision or destruction of breast tissue

> Excludes: *mastectomy (85.41-85.48)*
>   *reduction mammoplasty (85.31-85.32)*

85.20 Excision or destruction of breast tissue, not otherwise specified

> Excludes: *laser interstitial thermal therapy [LITT] of lesion or tissue of breast*
>   *under guidance (17.69)*

85.21 Local excision of lesion of breast
Lumpectomy
Removal of area of fibrosis from breast

> Excludes: *biopsy of breast (85.11-8.5.12)*

85.22 Resection of quadrant of breast

85.23 Subtotal mastectomy

> Excludes: *quadrant resection (85.22)*

85.24 Excision of ectopic breast tissue
Excision of accessory nipple

85.25 Excision of nipple

> Excludes: *excision of accessory nipple (85.24)*

85.3 Reduction mammoplasty and subcutaneous mammectomy

85.31 Unilateral reduction mammoplasty
Unilateral:
 amputative mammoplasty
 size reduction mammoplasty

85.32 Bilateral reduction mammoplasty
Amputative mammoplasty
Reduction mammoplasty (for gynecomastia)

85.33 Unilateral subcutaneous mammectomy with synchronous implant

> Excludes: *that without synchronous implant (85.34)*

85.34 Other unilateral subcutaneous mammectomy
Removal of breast tissue with preservation of skin and nipple
Subcutaneous mammectomy NOS

85.35 Bilateral subcutaneous mammectomy with synchronous implant

> Excludes: *that without synchronous implant (85.36)*

85.36 Other bilateral subcutaneous mammectomy

| | Valid O.R. procedure | | Non-O.R. procedure | | Nonspecific O.R. procedure | | Noncovered O.R. procedure |

85.4 **Mastectomy**

85.41 **Unilateral simple mastectomy**
Mastectomy:
NOS
complete

85.42 **Bilateral simple mastectomy**
Bilateral complete mastectomy

85.43 **Unilateral extended simple mastectomy**
Extended simple mastectomy NOS
Modified radical mastectomy
Simple mastectomy with excision of regional lymph nodes

85.44 **Bilateral extended simple mastectomy**

85.45 **Unilateral radical mastectomy**
Excision of breast, pectoral muscles, and regional lymph nodes [axillary, clavicular, supraclavicular]
Radical mastectomy NOS

85.46 **Bilateral radical mastectomy**

85.47 **Unilateral extended radical mastectomy**
Excision of breast, muscles, and lymph nodes [axillary, clavicular, supraclavicular, internal mammary, and mediastinal]
Extended radical mastectomy NOS

85.48 **Bilateral extended radical mastectomy**

85.5 **Augmentation mammoplasty**

Excludes: *that associated with subcutaneous mammectomy (85.33, 85.35)*

85.50 **Augmentation mammoplasty, not otherwise specified**

85.51 **Unilateral injection into breast for augmentation**

Excludes: *injection of fat graft of breast (85.55)*

85.52 **Bilateral injection into breast for augmentation**
Injection into breast for augmentation NOS

Excludes: *injection of fat graft of breast (85.55)*

85.53 **Unilateral breast implant**

85.54 **Bilateral breast implant**
Breast implant NOS

85.55 **Fat graft to breast**
Includes: extraction of fat for autologous graft
Autologous fat transplantation or transfer
Fat graft to breast NOS
Fat graft to breast with or without use of enriched graft
Micro-fat grafting

Excludes: *that with reconstruction of breast (85.70 –85.79)*

85.6 **Mastopexy**

85.7 **Total reconstruction of breast**

85.70 **Total reconstruction of breast, not otherwise specified**
Perforator flap, free

85.71 **Latissimus dorsi myocutaneous flap**

85.72 **Transverse rectus abdominus myocutaneous (TRAM) flap, pedicled**

Excludes: *transverse rectus abdominis myocutaneous (TRAM) flap, free (85.73)*

85.73 **Transverse rectus abdominis myocutaneous (TRAM) flap, free**

Excludes: *transverse rectus abdominis myocutaneous (TRAM) flap, pedicled (85.72)*

85.74 **Deep inferior epigastric artery perforator (DIEP) flap, free**

85.75 **Superficial inferior epigastric artery (SIEA) flap, free**

85.76 **Gluteal artery perforator (GAP) flap, free**

● Code new
to 2012 edition

▲ Revision of
existing code

④ ⑤ Fourth or fifth
digit required

85.79 **Other total reconstruction of breast**

Excludes: *deep inferior epigastric artery perforator (DIEP) flap, free (85.74)*
gluteal artery perforator (GAP) flap, free (85.76)
latissimus dorsi myocutaneous flap (85.71)
perforator flap, free (85.70)
superficial inferior epigastric artery (SIEA) flap, free (85.75)
total reconstruction of breast, NOS (85.70)
transverse rectus abdominus myocutaneous (TRAM) flap, free (85.73)
transverse rectus abdominis myocutaneous (TRAM) flap, pedicled (85.72)

85.8 **Other repair and plastic operations on breast**

Excludes: *that for:*
augmentation (85.50-85.54)
reconstruction (85.70-85.76, 85.79)
reduction (85.31-85.32)

85.81 **Suture of laceration of breast**

85.82 **Split-thickness graft to breast**

85.83 **Full-thickness graft to breast**

85.84 **Pedicle graft to breast**

85.85 **Muscle flap graft to breast**

85.86 **Transposition of nipple**

85.87 **Other repair or reconstruction of nipple**

85.89 **Other mammoplasty**

85.9 **Other operations on the breast**

85.91 **Aspiration of breast**

Excludes: *percutaneous biopsy of breast (85.11)*

85.92 **Injection of therapeutic agent into breast**

Excludes: *that for augmentation of breast (85.51-85.52, 85.55)*

85.93 **Revision of implant of breast**

85.94 **Removal of implant of breast**

85.95 **Insertion of breast tissue expander**

Insertion (soft tissue) of tissue expander (one or more) under muscle or platysma to develop skin flaps for donor use

85.96 **Removal of breast tissue expander(s)**

85.99 **Other**

86 **Operations on skin and subcutaneous tissue**

Includes: operations on:
hair follicles
male perineum
nails
sebaceous glands
subcutaneous fat pads
sudoriferous glands
superficial fossae

Excludes: *those on skin of:*
anus (49.01-49.99)
breast (mastectomy site) (85.0-85.99)
ear (18.01-18.9)
eyebrow (08.01-08.99)
eyelid (08.01-08.99)
female perineum (71.01-71.9)
lips (27.0-27.99)
nose (21.00-21.99)
penis (64.0-64.99)
scrotum (61.0-61.99)
vulva (71.01-71.9)

	Valid O.R. procedure		Non-O.R. procedure		Nonspecific O.R. procedure		Noncovered O.R. procedure

86.0　Incision of skin and subcutaneous tissue

86.01　Aspiration of skin and subcutaneous tissue
Aspiration of:
　abscess of nail, skin, or subcutaneous tissue
　hematoma of nail, skin, or subcutaneous tissue
　seroma of nail, skin, or subcutaneous tissue

86.02　Injection or tattooing of skin lesion or defect
Injection of filling material
Insertion of filling material
Pigmenting of skin

86.03　Incision of pilonidal sinus or cyst
> Excludes: *marsupialization (86.21)*

86.04　Other incision with drainage of skin and subcutaneous tissue
> Excludes: *drainage of:*
> 　*fascial compartments of face and mouth (27.0)*
> 　*palmar or thenar space (82.04)*
> 　*pilonidal sinus or cyst (86.03)*

86.05　Incision with removal of foreign body or device from skin and subcutaneous tissue
Removal of carotid sinus baroreflex activation device
Removal of loop recorder
Removal of neurostimulator pulse generator (single array, dual array)
Removal of tissue expander(s) from skin or soft tissue other than breast tissue
> Excludes: *removal of foreign body without incision (98.20-98.29)*

86.06　Insertion of totally implantable infusion pump
Code also any associated catheterization
> Excludes: *insertion of totally implantable vascular access device (86.07)*

86.07　Insertion of totally implantable vascular access device [VAD]
Totally implanted port
> Excludes: *insertion of totally implantable infusion pump (86.06)*

86.09　Other incision of skin and subcutaneous tissue
Creation of thalamic stimulator pulse generator pocket, new site
Escharotomy
Exploration:
　sinus tract, skin
　superficial fossa
Relocation of subcutaneous device pocket NEC
Reopening subcutaneous pocket for device revision without replacement
Undercutting of hair follicle
> Excludes: *creation of loop recorder pocket, new site and insertion/relocation of*
> 　*device (37.79)*
> 　*creation of pocket for implantable, patient-activated cardiac event*
> 　*recorder and insertion/relocation of device (37.79)*
> 　*removal of catheter from cranial cavity (01.27)*
> 　*that for drainage (86.04)*
> 　*that of cardiac pacemaker pocket, new site (37.79)*
> 　*that of fascial compartments of face and mouth (27.0)*

86.1　Diagnostic procedures on skin and subcutaneous tissue

86.11　Closed biopsy of skin and subcutaneous tissue

86.19　Other diagnostic procedures on skin and subcutaneous tissue
> Excludes: *microscopic examination of specimen from skin and subcutaneous*
> 　*tissue (91.61-91.79)*

86.2　Excision or destruction of lesion or tissue of skin and subcutaneous tissue

86.21　Excision of pilonidal cyst or sinus
Marsupialization of cyst
> Excludes: *incision of pilonidal cyst or sinus (86.03)*

● Code new　　　　▲ Revision of　　　　④ ⑤ Fourth or fifth
　to 2012 edition　　　existing code　　　　　digit required

86.22   Excisional debridement of wound, infection, or burn
Removal by excision of:
  devitalized tissue
  necrosis
  slough

> Excludes: debridement of:
>   abdominal all (wound) (54.3)
>   bone (77.60-77.69)
>   muscle (83.45) of hand (82.36)
>   nail (bed) (fold) (86.27)
>   nonexcisional debridement of wound, infection, or burn (86.28)
>   open fracture site (79.60-79.69)
>   pedicle or flap graft (86.75)

86.23   Removal of nail, nailbed, or nail fold

86.24   Chemosurgery of skin
Chemical peel of skin

86.25   Dermabrasion
That with laser

> Excludes: dermabrasion of wound to remove embedded debris (86.28)

86.26   Ligation of dermal appendage

> Excludes: excision of preauricular appendage (18.29)

86.27   Debridement of nail, nail bed, or nail fold
Removal of:
  necrosis
  slough

> Excludes: removal of nail, nail bed, or nail fold (86.23)

86.28   Nonexcisional debridement of wound, infection, or burn
Debridement NOS
Maggot therapy
Removal of devitalized tissue, necrosis, and slough by such methods as:
  brushing
  irrigation (under pressure)
  scrubbing
  washing
Ultrasonic debridement
Water scalpel (jet)

86.3   Other local excision or destruction of lesion or tissue of skin and subcutaneous tissue
Destruction of skin by:
  cauterization
  cryosurgery
  fulguration
  laser beam
That with Z-plasty

> Excludes: adipectomy (86.83)
>   biopsy of skin (86.11)
>   wide or radical excision of skin (86.4)
>   Z-plasty without excision (86.84)

86.4   Radical excision of skin lesion
Wide excision of skin lesion involving underlying or adjacent structure
Code also any lymph node dissection (40.3-40.5)

86.5   Suture or other closure of skin and subcutaneous tissue

86.51   Replantation of scalp

86.59   Closure of skin and subcutaneous tissue of other sites
Adhesives (surgical) (tissue)
Staples
Sutures

> Excludes: application of adhesive strips (butterfly)—omit code

86.6   Free skin graft
Includes: excision of skin for autogenous graft

> Excludes: construction or reconstruction of:
>   penis (64.43-64.44)
>   trachea (31.75)
>   vagina (70.61-70.64)

	Valid O.R. procedure		Non-O.R. procedure		Nonspecific O.R. procedure		Noncovered O.R. procedure

86.60 **Free skin graft, not otherwise specified**

86.61 **Full-thickness skin graft to hand**

> Excludes: *heterograft (86.65)*
> *homograft (86.66)*

86.62 **Other skin graft to hand**

> Excludes: *heterograft (86.65)*
> *homograft (86.66)*

86.63 **Full-thickness skin graft to other sites**

> Excludes: *heterograft (86.65)*
> *homograft (86.66)*

86.64 **Hair transplant**

> Excludes: *hair follicle transplant to eyebrow or eyelash (08.63)*

86.65 **Heterograft to skin**
Pigskin graft
Porcine graft

> Excludes: *application of dressing only (93.57)*

86.66 **Homograft to skin**
Graft to skin of amnionic membrane from donor
Graft to skin of skin from donor

86.67 **Dermal regenerative graft**
Artificial skin, NOS
Creation of "neodermis"
Decellularized allodermis
Integumentary matrix implants
Prosthetic implant of dermal layer of skin
Regenerate dermal layer of skin

> Excludes: *heterograft to skin (86.65)*
> *homograft to skin (86.66)*

86.69 **Other skin graft to other sites**

> Excludes: *heterograft (86.65)*
> *homograft (86.66)*

86.7 **Pedicle grafts or flaps**

> Excludes: *construction or reconstruction of:*
> *penis (64.43-64.44)*
> *trachea (31.75)*
> *vagina (70.61-70.64)*

86.70 **Pedicle or flap graft, not otherwise specified**

86.71 **Cutting and preparation of pedicle grafts or flaps**
Elevation of pedicle from its bed
Flap design and raising
Partial cutting of pedicle or tube
Pedicle delay

> Excludes: *pollicization or digital transfer (82.61, 82.81)*
> *revision of pedicle (86.75)*

86.72 **Advancement of pedicle graft**

86.73 **Attachment of pedicle or flap graft to hand**

> Excludes: *pollicization or digital transfer (82.61, 82.81)*

86.74 **Attachment of pedicle or flap graft to other sites**
Attachment by: Attachment by:
  advanced flap   rotating flap
  double pedicled flap   sliding flop
  pedicle graft   tube graft

86.75 **Revision of pedicle or flap graft**
Debridement of pedicle or flap graft
Defatting of pedicle or flap graft

86.8 **Other repair and reconstruction of skin and subcutaneous tissue**

86.81 **Repair for facial weakness**

● Code new
to 2012 edition

▲ Revision of
existing code

④ ⑤ Fourth or fifth
digit required

86.82 Facial rhytidectomy
Face lift

> *Excludes:*   *rhytidectomy of eyelid (08.86-08.87)*

86.83 Size reduction plastic operation
Liposuction
Reduction of adipose tissue of:
  abdominal wall (pendulous)
  arms (batwing)
  buttock
  thighs (trochanteric lipomatosis)

> *Excludes:*   *breast (85.31-85.32)*
> *liposuction to harvest fat graft (86.90)*

86.84 Relaxation of scar or web contracture of skin
Z-plasty of skin

> *Excludes:*   *Z-plasty with excision of lesion (86.3)*

86.85 Correction of syndactyly

86.86 Onychoplasty

86.87 Fat graft of skin and subcutaneous tissue
Includes: extraction of fat for autologous graft
Autologous fat transplantation or transfer
Fat graft NOS
Fat graft of skin and subcutaneous tissue with or without use of enriched graft
Micro-fat grafting

> *Excludes:*   *fat graft to breast (85.55)*

86.89 Other repair and reconstruction of skin and subcutaneous tissue

> *Excludes:*   *mentoplasty (76.67-76.68)*

86.9 Other operations on skin and subcutaneous tissue

86.90 Extraction of fat for graft or banking
Harvest of fat for extraction of cells for future use
Liposuction to harvest fat graft

> *Excludes:*   *that with graft at same operative episode (85.55, 86.87)*

86.91 Excision of skin for graft
Excision of skin with closure of donor site

> *Excludes:*   *that with graft at same operative episode (86.60-86.69)*

86.92 Electrolysis and other epilation of skin

> *Excludes:*   *epilation of eyelid (08.91-08.93)*

86.93 Insertion of tissue expander
Insertion (subcutaneous) (soft tissue) of expander (one or more) in scalp (subgaleal space), face, neck, trunk except breast, and upper and lower extremities for development of skin flaps for donor use

> *Excludes:*   *flap graft preparation (86.71)*
> *tissue expander, breast (85.95)*

86.94 Insertion or replacement of single array neurostimulator pulse generator, not specified as rechargeable
Pulse generator (single array, single channel, single port) for intracranial, spinal, and peripheral neurostimulator

Code also any associated lead implantation (02.93, 03.93, 04.92)

> *Excludes:*   *cranial implantation or replacement of neurostimulator pulse generator (01.20)*
> *insertion or replacement of single array rechargeable neurostimulator pulse generator (86.97)*

▲ **86.95 Insertion or replacement of multiple array neurostimulator pulse generator, not specified as rechargeable**
Pulse generator (multiple array, multiple channel, multiple port) for intracranial, spinal, and peripheral neurostimulator

Code also any associated lead implantation (02.93, 03.93, 04.92)

> *Excludes:*   *cranial implantation or replacement of neurostimulator pulse generator (01.20)*
> *insertion or replacement of multiple array rechargeable neurostimulator pulse generator (86.98)*

| | Valid O.R. procedure | | Non-O.R. procedure | | Nonspecific O.R. procedure | | Noncovered O.R. procedure |

86.96 **Insertion or replacement of other neurostimulator pulse generator**

Code also any associated lead implantation (02.93, 03.93, 04.92)

> Excludes: *cranial implantation or replacement of neurostimulator pulse generator (01.20)*
> *insertion of multiple array neurostimulator pulse generator (86.95, 86.98)*
> *insertion of single array neurostimulator pulse generator (86.94, 86.97)*

86.97 **Insertion or replacement of single array rechargeable neurostimulator pulse generator**

Rechargeable pulse generator (single array, single channel, single port) for intracranial, spinal, and peripheral neurostimulator

Code also any associated lead implantation (02.93, 03.93, 04.92)

> Excludes: *cranial implantation or replacement of neurostimulator pulse generator (01.20)*

▲ **86.98** **Insertion or replacement of multiple array (two or more) rechargeable neurostimulator pulse generator**

Rechargeable pulse generator (multiple array, multiple channel, multiple port) for intracranial, spinal, and peripheral neurostimulator

Code also any associated lead implantation (02.93, 03.93, 04.92)

> Excludes: *cranial implantation or replacement of neurostimulator pulse generator (01.20)*

86.99 **Other**

> Excludes: *removal of sutures from:*
> *abdomen (97.83)*
> *head and neck (97.38)*
> *thorax (97.43)*
> *trunk NEC (97.84)*
> *wound catheter:*
> *irrigation (96.58)*
> *replacement (97.15)*

● Code new to 2012 edition   ▲ Revision of existing code   ④ ⑤ Fourth or fifth digit required

16. MISCELLANEOUS DIAGNOSTIC AND THERAPEUTIC PROCEDURES (87-99)

87 Diagnostic Radiology

87.0 Soft tissue x-ray of face, head, and neck

> | Excludes: | *angiography (88.40-88.68)*

87.01 Pneumoencephalogram

87.02 Other contrast radiogram of brain and skull
Pneumocisternogram
Pneumoventriculogram
Posterior fossa myelogram

87.03 Computerized axial tomography of head
C.A.T. scan of head

87.04 Other tomography of head

87.05 Contrast dacryocystogram

87.06 Contrast radiogram of nasopharynx

87.07 Contrast laryngogram

87.08 Cervical lymphangiogram

87.09 Other soft tissue x-ray of face, head, and neck
Noncontrast x-ray of:
adenoid
larynx
nasolacrimal duct
nasopharynx
salivary gland
thyroid region
uvula

> | Excludes: | *x-ray study of eye (95.14)*

87.1 Other x-ray of face, head, and neck

> | Excludes: | *angiography (88.40-88.68)*

87.11 Full-mouth x-ray of teeth

87.12 Other dental x-ray
Orthodontic cephalogram or cephalometrics
Panorex examination of mandible
Root canal x-ray

87.13 Temporomandibular contrast arthrogram

87.14 Contrast radiogram of orbit

87.15 Contrast radiogram of sinus

87.16 Other x-ray of facial bones
X-ray of:
frontal area
mandible
maxilla
nasal sinuses
nose
orbit
supraorbital area
symphysis menti
zygomaticomaxillary complex

87.17 Other x-ray of skull
Lateral projection of skull
Sagittal projection of skull
Tangential projection of skull

87.2 X-ray of spine

87.21 Contrast myelogram

87.22 Other x-ray of cervical spine

87.23 Other x-ray of thoracic spine

87.24 Other x-ray of lumbosacral spine
Sacrococcygeal x-ray

87.29 Other x-ray of spine
Spinal x-ray NOS

Valid O.R. procedure   Non-O.R. procedure   Nonspecific O.R. procedure   Noncovered O.R. procedure

87.3   Soft tissue x-ray of thorax

> | Excludes: | *angiocardiography (88.50-88.58)*
> *angiography (88.40-88.68)*

87.31   Endotracheal bronchogram

87.32   Other contrast bronchogram
Transcricoid bronchogram

87.33   Mediastinal pneumogram

87.34   Intrathoracic lymphangiogram

87.35   Contrast radiogram of mammary ducts

87.36   Xerography of breast

87.37   Other mammography

87.38   Sinogram of chest wall
Fistulogram of chest wall

87.39   Other soft tissue x-ray of chest wall

87.4   Other x-ray of thorax

> | Excludes: | *angiocardiography (88.50-88.58)*
> *angiography (88.40-88.68)*

87.41   Computerized axial tomography of thorax
C.A.T. scan of heart
C.A.T. scan of thorax
Crystal linea scan of x-ray beam of thorax
Electronic substraction of thorax
Photoelectric response of thorax
Tomography with use of computer, x-rays, and camera of thorax

87.42   Other tomography of thorax
Cardiac tomogram

> | Excludes: | *C.A.T. scan of heart (87.41)*

87.43   X-ray of ribs, sternum, and clavicle
Examination for:
cervical rib
fracture

87.44   Routine chest x-ray, so described
X-ray of chest NOS

87.49   Other chest x-ray
X-ray of:
bronchus NOS
diaphragm NOS
heart NOS
lung NOS
mediastinum NOS
trachea NOS

87.5   Biliary tract x-ray

87.51   Percutaneous hepatic cholangiogram

87.52   Intravenous cholangiogram

87.53   Intraoperative cholangiogram

87.54   Other cholangiogram

87.59   Other biliary tract x-ray
Cholecystogram

87.6   Other x-ray of digestive system

87.61   Barium swallow

87.62   Upper GI series

87.63   Small bowel series

87.64   Lower GI series

87.65   Other x-ray of intestine

87.66   Contrast pancreatogram

87.69   Other digestive tract x-ray

87.7   X-ray of urinary system

> | Excludes: | *angiography of renal vessels (88.45, 88.65)*

● Code new
to 2012 edition   ▲ Revision of
existing code   ④ ⑤ Fourth or fifth
digit required

87.71 **Computerized axial tomography of kidney**
C.A.T. scan of kidney

87.72 **Other nephrotomogram**

87.73 **Intravenous pyelogram**
Diuretic infusion pyelogram

87.74 **Retrograde pyelogram**

87.75 **Percutaneous pyelogram**

87.76 **Retrograde cystourethrogram**

87.77 **Other cystogram**

87.78 **Ileal conduitogram**

87.79 **Other x-ray of the urinary system**
KUB x-ray

87.8 **X-ray of female genital organs**

87.81 **X-ray of gravid uterus**
Intrauterine cephalometry by x-ray

87.82 **Gas contrast hysterosalpingogram**

87.83 **Opaque dye contrast hysterosalpingogram**

87.84 **Percutaneous hysterogram**

87.85 **Other x-ray of fallopian tubes and uterus**

87.89 **Other x-ray of female genital organs**

87.9 **X-ray of male genital organs**

87.91 **Contrast seminal vesiculogram**

87.92 **Other x-ray of prostate and seminal vesicles**

87.93 **Contrast epididymogram**

87.94 **Contrast vasogram**

87.95 **Other x-ray of epididymis and vas deferens**

87.99 **Other x-ray of male genital organs**

88 **Other diagnostic radiology and related techniques**

88.0 **Soft tissue x-ray of abdomen**

| Excludes: | angiography (88.40-88.68) |

88.01 **Computerized axial tomography of abdomen**
C.A.T. scan of abdomen

| Excludes: | C.A.T. scan of kidney (87.71) |

88.02 **Other abdomen tomography**

| Excludes: | nephrotomogram (87.72) |

88.03 **Sinogram of abdominal wall**
Fistulogram of abdominal wall

88.04 **Abdominal lymphangiogram**

88.09 **Other soft tissue x-ray of abdominal wall**

88.1 **Other x-ray of abdomen**

88.11 **Pelvic opaque dye contrast radiography**

88.12 **Pelvic gas contrast radiography**
Pelvic pneumoperitoneum

88.13 **Other peritoneal pneumogram**

88.14 **Retroperitoneal fistulogram**

88.15 **Retroperitoneal pneumogram**

88.16 **Other retroperitoneal x-ray**

88.19 **Other x-ray of abdomen**
Flat plate of abdomen

88.2 **Skeletal x-ray of extremities and pelvis**

| Excludes: | contrast radiogram of joint (88.32) |

88.21 **Skeletal x-ray of shoulder and upper arm**

88.22 **Skeletal x-ray of elbow and forearm**

88.23 **Skeletal x-ray of wrist and hand**

Valid O.R. procedure   Non-O.R. procedure   Nonspecific O.R. procedure   Noncovered O.R. procedure

88.24 **Skeletal x-ray of upper limb, not otherwise specified**

88.25 **Pelvimetry**

88.26 **Other skeletal x-ray of pelvis and hip**

88.27 **Skeletal x-ray of thigh, knee, and lower leg**

88.28 **Skeletal x-ray of ankle and foot**

88.29 **Skeletal x-ray of lower limb, not otherwise specified**

88.3 **Other x-ray**

88.31 **Skeletal series**
X-ray of whole skeleton

88.32 **Contrast arthrogram**

Excludes: *that of temporomandibular joint (87.13)*

88.33 **Other skeletal x-ray**

Excludes: *skeletal x-ray of:*
extremities and pelvis (88.21-88.29)
face, head, and neck (87.11-87.17)
spine (87.21-87.29)
thorax (87.43)

88.34 **Lymphangiogram of upper limb**

88.35 **Other soft tissue x-ray of upper limb**

88.36 **Lymphangiogram of lower limb**

88.37 **Other soft tissue x-ray of lower limb**

Excludes: *femoral angiography (88.48, 88.66)*

88.38 **Other computerized axial tomography**
C.A.T. scan NOS

Excludes: *C.A.T. scan of:*
abdomen (88.01)
head (87.03)
heart (87.41)
kidney (87.71)
thorax (87.41)

88.39 **X-ray, other and unspecified**

88.4 **Arteriography using contrast material**
Includes: angiography of arteries
arterial puncture for injection of contrast material
radiography of arteries (by fluoroscopy)
retrograde arteriography

Note: The fourth-digit subclassification identifies the site to be viewed, not the site of injection.

Excludes: *arteriography using:*
radioisotopes or radionuclides (92.01-92.19)
ultrasound (88.71-88.79)
fluorescein angiography of eye (95.12)

88.40 **Arteriography using contrast material, unspecified site**

88.41 **Arteriography of cerebral arteries**
Angiography of:
basilar artery
carotid (internal)
posterior cerebral circulation
vertebral artery

88.42 **Aortography**
Arteriography of aorta and aortic arch

88.43 **Arteriography of pulmonary arteries**

88.44 **Arteriography of other intrathoracic vessels**

Excludes: *angiocardiography (88.50-88.58)*
arteriography of coronary arteries (88.55-88.57)

88.45 **Arteriography of renal arteries**

88.46 **Arteriography of placenta**
Placentogram using contrast material

88.47 **Arteriography of other intra-abdominal arteries**

● Code new
to 2012 edition   ▲ Revision of
existing code   ④ ⑤ Fourth or fifth
digit required

88.48 Arteriography of femoral and other lower extremity arteries

88.49 Arteriography of other specified sites

88.5 Angiocardiography using contrast material
Includes: arterial puncture and insertion of arterial catheter for injection of contrast
material
cineangiocardiography
selective angiocardiography

Code also synchronous cardiac catheterization (37.21-37.23)

Excludes: *angiography of pulmonary vessels (88.43, 88.62)*

88.50 Angiocardiography, not otherwise specified

88.51 Angiocardiography of venae cavae
Interior vena cavography
Phlebography of vena cava (inferior) (superior)

88.52 Angiocardiography of right heart structures
Angiocardiography of:
pulmonary valve
right atrium
right ventricle (outflow tract)

Excludes: *intra-operative fluorescence vascular angiography (88.59)*
that combined with left heart angiocardiography (88.54)

88.53 Angiocardiography of left heart structures
Angiocardiography of:
aortic valve
left atrium
left ventricle (outflow tract)

Excludes: *intra-operative fluorescence vascular angiography (88.59)*
that combined with right heart angiocardiography (88.54)

88.54 Combined right and left heart angiocardiography

Excludes: *intra-operative fluorescence vascular angiography (88.59)*

88.55 Coronary arteriography using a single catheter
Coronary arteriography by Sones technique
Direct selective coronary arteriography using a single catheter

Excludes: *intra-operative fluorescence vascular angiography (88.59)*

88.56 Coronary arteriography using two catheters
Coronary arteriography by:
Judkins technique
Ricketts and Abrams technique
Direct selective coronary arteriography using two catheters

Excludes: *intra-operative fluorescence vascular angiography (88.59)*

88.57 Other and unspecified coronary arteriography
Coronary arteriography NOS

Excludes: *intra-operative fluorescence vascular angiography (88.59)*

88.58 Negative-contrast cardiac roentgenography
Cardiac roentgenography with injection of carbon dioxide

88.59 Intra-operative coronary fluorescence vascular angiography
Intraoperative laser arteriogram (SPY)
SPY arteriogram
SPY arteriography

88.6 Phlebography
Includes: angiography of veins
radiography of veins (by fluoroscopy)
retrograde phlebography
venipuncture for injection of contrast material
venography using contrast material
Note: The fourth-digit subclassification (88.60-88.67) identifies the site to be viewed, not
the site of injection.

Excludes: *angiography using:*
radioisotopes or radionuclides (92.01-92.19)
ultrasound (88.71-88.79)
fluorescein angiography of eye (95.12)

88.60 Phlebography using contrast material, unspecified site

Valid O.R. procedure	Non-O.R. procedure	Nonspecific O.R. procedure	Noncovered O.R. procedure

88.61 Phlebography of veins of head and neck using contrast material

88.62 Phlebography of pulmonary veins using contrast material

88.63 Phlebography of other intrathoracic veins using contrast material

88.64 Phlebography of the portal venous system using contrast material
Splenoportogram (by splenic arteriography)

88.65 Phlebography of other intra-abdominal veins using contrast material

88.66 Phlebography of femoral and other lower extremity veins using contrast material

88.67 Phlebography of other specified sites using contrast material

88.68 Impedance phlebography

88.7 Diagnostic ultrasound
Includes: echography
non-invasive ultrasound
ultrasonic angiography
ultrasonography

Excludes: intravascular imaging (adjunctive) (IVUS) (00.21-00.29)
that for intraoperative monitoring (00.94)
therapeutic ultrasound (00.01-00.09)

88.71 Diagnostic ultrasound of head and neck
Determination of midline shift of brain
Echoencephalography

Excludes: eye (95.13)

88.72 Diagnostic ultrasound of heart
Echocardiography
Transesophageal echocardiography

Excludes: echocardiography of heart chambers (37.28)
intracardiac echocardiography (ICE) (37.28)
intravascular (IVUS) imaging of coronary vessels (00.24)

88.73 Diagnostic ultrasound of other sites of thorax
Aortic arch ultrasonography
Breast ultrasonography
Lung ultrasonography

88.74 Diagnostic ultrasound of digestive system

88.75 Diagnostic ultrasound of urinary system

88.76 Diagnostic ultrasound of abdomen and retroperitoneum

88.77 Diagnostic ultrasound of peripheral vascular system
Deep vein thrombosis ultrasonic scanning

Excludes: adjunct vascular system procedures (00.40-00.43)

88.78 Diagnostic ultrasound of gravid uterus
Intrauterine cephalometry:
echo
ultrasonic
Placental localization by ultrasound

88.79 Other diagnostic ultrasound
Ultrasonography of:
multiple sites
nongravid uterus
total body

88.8 Thermography

88.81 Cerebral thermography

88.82 Ocular thermography

88.83 Bone thermography
Osteoarticular thermography

88.84 Muscle thermography

88.85 Breast thermography

88.86 Blood vessel thermography
Deep vein thermography

88.89 Thermography of other sites
Lymph gland thermography
Thermography NOS

● Code new
to 2012 edition

▲ Revision of
existing code

④ ⑤ Fourth or fifth
digit required

88.9   Other diagnostic imaging

88.90   Diagnostic imaging, not elsewhere classified

88.91   Magnetic resonance imaging of brain and brain stem

> | Excludes: | *intraoperative magnetic resonance imaging (88.96)*
> *laser interstitial thermal therapy [LITT] of lesion or tissue of brain under guidance (17.61)*
> *real-time magnetic resonance imaging (88.96)*

88.92   Magnetic resonance imaging of chest and myocardium
For evaluation of hilar and mediastinal lymphadenopathy

> | Excludes: | *laser interstitial thermal therapy [LITT] of lesion or tissue of breast under guidance (17.69)*
> *laser interstitial thermal therapy [LITT] of lesion or tissue of lung under guidance (17.69)*

88.93   Magnetic resonance imaging of spinal canal
Levels:
  cervical
  lumbar (lumbosacral)
  thoracic
Spinal cord
Spine

88.94   Magnetic resonance imaging of musculoskeletal
Bone marrow blood supply
Extremities (upper) (lower)

88.95   Magnetic resonance imaging of pelvis, prostate, and bladder

> | Excludes: | *laser interstitial thermal therapy [LITT] of lesion or tissue of prostate under guidance (17.69)*

88.96   Other intraoperative magnetic resonance imaging
iMRI
Real-time magnetic resonance imaging

88.97   Magnetic resonance imaging of other and unspecified sites
abdomen   neck
face   eye orbit

> | Excludes: | *laser interstitial thermal therapy [LITT] of lesion or tissue of other and unspecified site under guidance (17.69)*

88.98   Bone mineral density studies
Dual photon absorptiometry
Quantitative computed tomography (CT) studies
Radiographic densitometry
Single photon absorptiometry

89   Interview, evaluation, consultation, and examination

89.0   Diagnostic interview, consultation, and evaluation

> | Excludes: | *psychiatric diagnostic interview (94.11-94.19)*

89.01   Interview and evaluation, described as brief
Abbreviated history and evaluation

89.02   Interview and evaluation, described as limited
Interval history and evaluation

89.03   Interview and evaluation, described as comprehensive
History and evaluation of new problem

89.04   Other interview and evaluation

89.05   Diagnostic interview and evaluation, not otherwise specified

89.06   Consultation, described as limited
Consultation on a single organ system

89.07   Consultation, described as comprehensive

89.08   Other consultation

89.09   Consultation, not otherwise specified

89.1   Anatomic and physiologic measurements and manual examinations—nervous system and sense organs

> | Excludes: | *ear examination (95.41-95.49)*
> *eye examination (95.01-95.26)*
> *the listed procedures when done as part of a general physical examination (89.7)*

| | Valid O.R. procedure | | Non-O.R. procedure | | Nonspecific O.R. procedure | | Noncovered O.R. procedure |

89.10 Intracarotid amobarbital test
Wada test

89.11 Tonometry

89.12 Nasal function study
Rhinomanometry

89.13 Neurologic examination

89.14 Electroencephalogram

> Excludes: that with polysomnogram (89.17)

89.15 Other nonoperative neurologic function tests

89.16 Transillumination of newborn skull

89.17 Polysomnogram
Sleep recording

89.18 Other sleep disorder function tests
Multiple sloop latency test [MSLT]

89.19 Video and radio-telemetered electroencephalographic monitoring
Radiographic EEG monitoring
Video EEG monitoring

> Excludes: intraoperative monitoring (00.94)

89.2 Anatomic and physiologic measurements and manual examinations—genitourinary system

> Excludes: the listed procedures when done as part of a general physical examination (89.7)

89.21 Urinary manometry
Manometry through:
  indwelling urethral catheter
  nephrostomy
  pyelostomy
  ureterostomy

89.22 Cystometrogram

89.23 Urethral sphincter electromyogram

89.24 Uroflowmetry [UFR]

89.25 Urethral pressure profile [UPP]

89.26 Gynecological examination
Pelvic examination

89.29 Other nonoperative genitourinary system measurements
Bioassay of urine
Renal clearance
Urine chemistry

89.3 Other anatomic and physiologic measurements and manual examinations

> Excludes: the listed procedures when done as part of a general physical examination (89.7)

89.31 Dental examination
Oral mucosal survey
Periodontal survey

89.32 Esophageal manometry

89.33 Digital examination of enterostomy stoma
Digital examination of colostomy stoma

89.34 Digital examination of rectum

89.35 Transillumination of nasal sinuses

89.36 Manual examination of breast

89.37 Vital capacity determination

> Excludes: endoscopic pulmonary airway flow measurement (33.72)

89.38 Other nonoperative respiratory measurements
Plethysmography for measurement of respiratory function
Thoracic impedance plethysmography

> Excludes: endoscopic pulmonary airway flow measurement (33.72)

● Code new
  to 2012 edition
▲ Revision of
  existing code
④ ⑤ Fourth or fifth
  digit required

89.39   Other nonoperative measurements and examinations
Basal metabolic rate [BMR]
14 C-Urea breath test
Gastric:
  analysis
  function NEC

> Excludes: *body measurements (93.07)*
>   *cardiac tests (89.41-89.69)*
>   *fundus photography (95.11)*
>   *limb length measurement (93.06)*

89.4   Cardiac stress tests, pacemaker and defibrillator checks

89.41   Cardiovascular stress test using treadmill

89.42   Masters' two-step stress test

89.43   Cardiovascular stress test using bicycle ergometer

89.44   Other cardiovascular stress test
Thallium stress test with or without transesophageal pacing

89.45   Artificial pacemaker rate check
Artificial pacemaker function check NOS
Bedside device check of pacemaker or cardiac resynchronization pacemaker
  [CRT-P]
Interrogation only without arrhythmia induction

> Excludes: *catheter based invasive electrophysiologic testing (37.26)*
>   *noninvasive programmed electrical stimulation [NIPS] (arrhythmia*
>   *induction) (37.20)*

89.46   Artificial pacemaker artifact wave form check

89.47   Artificial pacemaker electrode impedance check

89.48   Artificial pacemaker voltage or amperage threshold check

89.49   Automatic implantable cardioverter/defibrillator (AICD) check
Bedside check of an AICD or cardiac resynchronization defibrillator [CRT-D]
Checking pacing thresholds of device
Interrogation only without arrhythmia induction

> Excludes: *catheter based invasive electrophysiologic testing (37.26)*
>   *noninvasive programmed electrical stimulation [NIPS] (arrhythmia*
>   *induction) (37.20)*

89.5   Other nonoperative cardiac and vascular diagnostic procedures

> Excludes: *fetal EKG (75.32)*

89.50   Ambulatory cardiac monitoring
Analog devices [Holter-type]

89.51   Rhythm electrocardiogram
Rhythm EKG (with one to three leads)

89.52   Electrocardiogram
ECG NOS
EKG (with 12 or more leads)

89.53   Vectorcardiogram (with ECG)

89.54   Electrographic monitoring
Telemetry

> Excludes: *ambulatory cardiac monitoring (89.50)*
>   *electrographic monitoring during surgery—omit code*

89.55   Phonocardiogram with ECG lead

89.56   Carotid pulse tracing with ECG lead

> Excludes: *oculoplethysmography (89.58)*

89.57   Apexcardiogram (with ECG lead)

89.58   Plethysmogram
Penile plethysmography with nerve stimulation

> Excludes: *plethysmography (for):*
>   *measurement of respiratory function (89.38)*
>   *thoracic impedance (89.38)*

89.59   Other nonoperative cardiac and vascular measurements

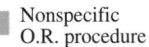 Valid O.R.   Non-O.R.   Nonspecific   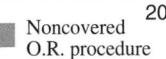 Noncovered
procedure   procedure   O.R. procedure   O.R. procedure

89.6 Circulatory monitoring

[Excludes:] *electrocardiographic monitoring during surgery—omit code*
implantation or replacement of subcutaneous device for intracardiac hemodynamic monitoring (00.57)
insertion or replacement of implantable pressure sensor (lead) for intracardiac hemodynamic monitoring (00.56)

89.60 Continuous intra-arterial blood gas monitoring
Insertion of blood gas monitoring system and continuous monitoring of blood gases through an intra-arterial sensor

89.61 Systemic arterial pressure monitoring

[Excludes:] *intra-aneurysm sac pressure monitoring (intraoperative) (00.58)*
intravascular pressure measurement of intrathoracic arteries (00.67)
intravascular pressure measurement of peripheral arteries (00.68)

89.62 Central venous pressure monitoring

[Excludes:] *intravascular pressure measurement, other specified and unspecified vessels (00.69)*

89.63 Pulmonary artery pressure monitoring

[Excludes:] *pulmonary artery wedge monitoring (89.64)*

89.64 Pulmonary artery wedge monitoring
Pulmonary capillary wedge [PCW] monitoring
Swan-Ganz catheterization

89.65 Measurement of systemic arterial blood gases

[Excludes:] *continuous intra-arterial blood gas monitoring (89.60)*

89.66 Measurement of mixed venous blood gases

89.67 Monitoring of cardiac output by oxygen consumption technique
Fick method

89.68 Monitoring of cardiac output by other technique
Cardiac output monitor by thermodilution indicator

89.69 Monitoring of coronary blood flow
Coronary blood flow monitoring by coincidence counting technique

[Excludes:] *intravascular pressure measurement of coronary arteries (00.59)*

89.7 General physical examination

89.8 Autopsy

90 Microscopic examination—I

The following fourth-digit subclassification is for use with categories in section 90 to identify type of examination:

1 bacterial smear
2 culture
3 culture and sensitivity
4 parasitology
5 toxicology
6 cell block and Papanicolaou smear
9 other microscopic examination

[4] **90.0 Microscopic examination of specimen from nervous system and of spinal fluid**

[4] **90.1 Microscopic examination of specimen from endocrine gland, not elsewhere classified**

[4] **90.2 Microscopic examination of specimen from eye**

[4] **90.3 Microscopic examination of specimen from ear, nose, throat, and larynx**

[4] **90.4 Microscopic examination of specimen from trachea, bronchus, pleura, lung, and other thoracic specimen, and of sputum**

[4] **90.5 Microscopic examination of blood**

[4] **90.6 Microscopic examination of specimen from spleen and of bone marrow**

[4] **90.7 Microscopic examination of specimen from lymph node and of lymph**

[4] **90.8 Microscopic examination of specimen from upper gastrointestinal tract and of vomitus**

[4] **90.9 Microscopic examination of specimen from lower gastrointestinal tract and of stool**

91   Microscopic examination—II

The following fourth-digit subclassification is for use with categories in section 91 to identify type of examination:

    1 bacterial smear
    2 culture
    3 culture and sensitivity
    4 parasitology
    5 toxicology
    6 cell block and Papanicolaou smear
    9 other microscopic examination

④ **91.0   Microscopic examination of specimen from liver, biliary trace and pancreas**

④ **91.1   Microscopic examination of peritoneal and retroperitoneal specimen**

④ **91.2   Microscopic examination of specimen from kidney, ureter, perirenal and periureteral tissue**

④ **91.3   Microscopic examination of specimen from bladder, urethra, prostate, seminal vesicle, perivesical tissue, and of urine and semen**

④ **91.4   Microscopic examination of specimen from female genital tract**
    Amnionic sac
    Fetus

④ **91.5   Microscopic examination of specimen from musculoskeletal system and of joint fluid**
    Microscopic examination of:

bone	ligament
bursa	muscle
cartilage	synovial membrane
fascia	tendon

④ **91.6   Microscopic examination of specimen from skin and other integument**
    Microscopic examination of:
    hair
    nails
    skin

> | Excludes: | *mucous membrane—code to organ site*
> | | *that of operative wound (91.71-91.79)*

④ **91.7   Microscopic examination of specimen from operative wound**

④ **91.8   Microscopic examination of specimen from other site**

④ **91.9   Microscopic examination of specimen from unspecified site**

92   Nuclear Medicine

  92.0   Radioisotope scan and function study

    92.01   Thyroid scan and radioisotope function studies
      Iodine-131 uptake
      Protein-bound iodine
      Radio-iodine uptake

    92.02   Liver scan and radioisotope function study

    92.03   Renal scan and radioisotope function study
      Renal clearance study

    92.04   Gastrointestinal scan and radioisotope function study
      Radio-cobalt B_{12} Schilling test
      Radio-iodinated triolein study

    92.05   Cardiovascular and hematopoietic scan and radioisotope function study
      Bone marrow scan or function study
      Cardiac output scan or function study
      Circulation time scan or function study
      Radionuclide cardiac
        ventriculogram scan or function study
      Spleen scan or function study

    92.09   Other radioisotope function studies

  92.1   Other radioisotope scan

    92.11   Cerebral scan
      Pituitary

    92.12   Scan of other sites of head

> | Excludes: | eye (95.16)

    92.13   Parathyroid scan

    92.14   Bone scan

	Valid O.R. procedure		Non-O.R. procedure		Nonspecific O.R. procedure		Noncovered O.R. procedure

92.15 **Pulmonary scan**

92.16 **Scan of lymphatic system**

92.17 **Placental scan**

92.18 **Total body scan**

92.19 **Scan of other sites**

92.2 **Therapeutic radiology and nuclear medicine**

Excludes: *that for:*
ablation of pituitary gland (07.64-07.69)
destruction of chorioretinal lesion (14.26-14.27)

92.20 **Infusion of liquid brachytherapy radioisotope**
I-125 radioisotope
Intracavitary brachytherapy
Includes: removal of radioisotope

92.21 **Superficial radiation**
Contact radiation [up to 150 KVP]

92.22 **Orthovoltage radiation**
Deep radiation [200-300 KVP]

92.23 **Radioisotopic teleradiotherapy**
Teleradiotherapy using:
cobalt-60
iodine-125
radioactive cesium

92.24 **Teleradiotherapy using photons**
Megavoltage NOS
Supervoltage NOS
Use of:
Betatron
linear accelerator

92.25 **Teleradiotherapy using electrons**
Beta particles

Excludes: *intra-operative electron radiation therapy (92.41)*

92.26 **Teleradiotherapy of other particulate radiation**
Neutrons   Protons NOS

92.27 **Implantation or insertion of radioactive elements**
Intravascular brachytherapy

Code also incision of site

Excludes: *infusion of liquid brachytherapy radioisotope (92.20)*

92.28 **Injection or instillation of radioisotopes**
Injection or infusion of radioimmunoconjugate
Intracavitary injection or instillation
Intravenous injection or instillation
Iodine-131 [I-131] tositumomab
Radioimmunotherapy
Ytrium-90 [Y-90] ibritumomab tiuxetan

Excludes: *infusion of liquid brachytherapy radioisotope (92.20)*

92.29 **Other radiotherapeutic procedure**

92.3 **Stereotactic radiosurgery**

Excludes: *stereotactic biopsy*

Code also stereotactic head frame application (93.59)

92.30 **Stereotactic radiosurgery, not otherwise specified**

92.31 **Single source photon radiosurgery**
High energy x-rays
Linear accelerator (LINAC)

92.32 **Multi-source photon radiosurgery**
Cobalt 60 radiation
Gamma irradiation

92.33 **Particulate radiosurgery**
Particle beam radiation (cyclotron)
Proton accelerator

● Code new
to 2012 edition

▲ Revision of
existing code

④ ⑤ Fourth or fifth
digit required

92.39 Stereotactic radiosurgery, not elsewhere classified

92.4 **Intra-operative radiation procedures**

92.41 **Intra-operative electron radiation therapy**
IOERT
That using a mobile linear accelerator

93 **Physical therapy, respiratory therapy, rehabilitation, and related procedures**

93.0 **Diagnostic physical therapy**

93.01 **Functional evaluation**

93.02 **Orthotic evaluation**

93.03 **Prosthetic evaluation**

93.04 **Manual testing of muscle function**

93.05 **Range of motion testing**

93.06 **Measurement of limb length**

93.07 **Body measurement**
Girth measurement
Measurement of skull circumference

93.08 **Electromyography**

Excludes: *eye EMG (95.25)*
that for intraoperative monitoring (00.94)
that with polysomnogram (89.17)
urethral sphincter EMG (89.23)

93.09 **Other diagnostic physical therapy procedure**

93.1 **Physical therapy exercises**

93.11 **Assisting exercise**

Excludes: *assisted exercise in pool (93.31)*

93.12 **Other active musculoskeletal exercise**

93.13 **Resistive exercise**

93.14 **Training in joint movements**

93.15 **Mobilization of spine**

93.16 **Mobilization of other joints**

Excludes: *manipulation of temporomandibular joint (76.95)*

93.17 **Other passive musculoskeletal exercise**

93.18 **Breathing exercise**

93.19 **Exercise, not elsewhere classified**

93.2 **Other physical therapy musculoskeletal manipulation**

93.21 **Manual and mechanical traction**

Excludes: *skeletal traction (93.43-93.44)*
skin traction (93.45-93.46)
spinal traction (93.41-93.42)

93.22 **Ambulation and gait training**

93.23 **Fitting of orthotic device**

93.24 **Training in use of prosthetic or orthotic device**
Training in crutch walking

93.25 **Forced extension of limb**

93.26 **Manual rupture of joint adhesions**

93.27 **Stretching of muscle or tendon**

93.28 **Stretching of fascia**

93.29 **Other forcible correction of deformity**

93.3 **Other physical therapy therapeutic procedures**

93.31 **Assisted exercise in pool**

93.32 **Whirlpool treatment**

93.33 **Other hydrotherapy**

93.34 **Diathermy**

	Valid O.R. procedure		Non-O.R. procedure		Nonspecific O.R. procedure		Noncovered O.R. procedure

93.35 Other heat therapy
Acupuncture with smouldering moxa
Hot packs
Hyperthermia NEC
Infrared irradiation
Moxibustion
Paraffin bath

Excludes: *hyperthermia for treatment of cancer (99.85)*

93.36 Cardiac retraining

93.37 Prenatal training
Training for natural childbirth

93.38 Combined physical therapy without mention of the components

93.39 Other physical therapy

93.4 Skeletal traction and other traction

93.41 Spinal traction using skull device
Traction using:
caliper tongs
Crutchfield tongs
halo device
Vinke tongs

Excludes: *insertion of tongs or halo traction device (02.94)*

93.42 Other spinal traction
Cotrel's traction

Excludes: *cervical collar (93.52)*

93.43 Intermittent skeletal traction

93.44 Other skeletal traction
Bryant's traction
Dunlop's traction
Lyman Smith traction
Russell's traction

93.45 Thomas' splint traction

93.46 Other skin traction of limbs
Adhesive tape traction
Boot traction
Buck's traction
Gallows traction

93.5 Other immobilization, pressure, and attention to wound

Excludes: *external fixator device (84.71-84.73)*
wound cleansing (96.58-96.59)

93.51 Application of plaster jacket

Excludes: *Minerva jacket (93.52)*

93.52 Application of neck support
Application of:
cervical collar
Minerva jacket
molded neck support

93.53 Application of other cast

93.54 Application of splint
Plaster splint   Tray splint

Excludes: *periodontal splint (24.7)*

93.55 Dental wiring

Excludes: *that for orthodontia (24.7)*

93.56 Application of pressure dressing
Application of:
Gibney bandage
Robert Jones' bandage
Shanz dressing

93.57 Application of other wound dressing
Porcine wound dressing

93.58 **Application of pressure trousers**
Application of:
  anti-shock trousers
  MAST trousers
  vasopneumatic device

93.59 **Other immobilization, pressure and attention to wound**
Elastic stockings
Electronic gaiter
Intermittent pressure device
Oxygenation of wound (hyperbaric)
Stereotactic head frame application
Strapping (non-traction)
Velpeau dressing

93.6 **Osteopathic manipulative treatment**

93.61 **Osteopathic manipulative treatment for general mobilization**
General articulatory treatment

93.62 **Osteopathic manipulative treatment using high-velocity low-amplitude forces**
Thrusting forces

93.63 **Osteopathic manipulative treatment using low-velocity high-amplitude forces**
Springing forces

93.64 **Osteopathic manipulative treatment using isotonic, isometric forces**

93.65 **Osteopathic manipulative treatment using indirect forces**

93.66 **Osteopathic manipulative treatment to move tissue fluids**
Lymphatic pump

93.67 **Other specified osteopathic manipulative treatment**

93.7 **Speech and reading rehabilitation and rehabilitation of the blind**

93.71 **Dyslexia training**

93.72 **Dysphasia training**

93.73 **Esophageal speech training**

93.74 **Speech defect training**

93.75 **Other speech training and therapy**

93.76 **Training in use of lead dog for the blind**

93.77 **Training in braille or Moon**

93.78 **Other rehabilitation for the blind**

93.8 **Other rehabilitation therapy**

93.81 **Recreation therapy**
Diversional therapy
Play therapy
  Excludes: *play psychotherapy (94.36)*

93.82 **Educational therapy**
Education of bed-bound children
Special schooling for the handicapped

93.83 **Occupational therapy**
Daily living activities therapy
  Excludes: *training in activities of daily living for the blind (93.78)*

93.84 **Music therapy**

93.85 **Vocational rehabilitation**
Sheltered employment
Vocational:
  assessment
  retraining
  training

93.89 **Rehabilitation, not elsewhere classified**

93.9 **Respiratory therapy**
  Excludes: *insertion of airway (96.01-96.05)*
        other continuous invasive (through endotracheal tube or tracheostomy)
        mechanical ventilation (96.70-96.72)

Valid O.R. procedure	Non-O.R. procedure	Nonspecific O.R. procedure	Noncovered O.R. procedure

93.90 Non-invasive mechanical ventilation
Bi-level airway pressure
BiPAP without (delivery through) endotracheal tube or tracheostomy
CPAP without (delivery through) endotracheal tube or tracheostomy
Mechanical ventilation NOS
Non-invasive positive pressure (NIPPV)
Non-invasive PPV
NPPV
That delivered by non-invasive interface:
  face mask
  nasal mask
  nasal pillow
  oral mouthpiece
  oronasal mask

> | Excludes: | invasive (through endotracheal tube or tracheostomy) continuous
> mechanical ventilation (96.70-96.72)

Note: Patients admitted on *non-invasive* mechanical ventilation that subsequently require *invasive* mechanical ventilation; code both types of mechanical ventilation

93.91 Intermittent positive pressure breathing [IPPB]

93.93 Nonmechanical methods of resuscitation
Artificial respiration
Manual resuscitation
Mouth-to-mouth resuscitation

93.94 Respiratory medication administered by nebulizer
Mist therapy

93.95 Hyperbaric oxygenation

> | Excludes: | oxygenation of wound (93.59)

93.96 Other oxygen enrichment
Catalytic oxygen therapy
Cytoreductive effect
Oxygenators
Oxygen therapy

> | Excludes: | oxygenation of wound (93.59)
> SuperSaturated oxygen therapy (00.49)

93.97 Decompression chamber

93.98 Other control of atmospheric pressure and composition
Antigen-free air conditioning
Helium therapy

> | Excludes: | inhaled nitric oxide therapy (INO) (00.12)

93.99 Other respiratory procedures
Continuous negative pressure ventilation [CNP]
Postural drainage

94   Procedures related to the psyche

94.0   Psychologic evaluation and testing

94.01 Administration of intelligence test
Administration of:
  Stanford-Binet
  Wechsler Adult Intelligence Scale
  Wechsler Intelligence Scale for Children

94.02 Administration of psychologic test
Administration of:
  Bender Visual - Motor Gestalt Test
  Benton Visual Retention Test
  Minnesota Multiphasic Personality Inventory
  Wechsler Memory Scale

94.03 Character analysis

94.08 Other psychologic evaluation and testing

94.09 Psychologic mental status determination, not otherwise specified

94.1   Psychiatric interviews, consultations, and evaluations

● Code new
to 2012 edition

▲ Revision of
existing code

④ ⑤ Fourth or fifth
digit required

94.11 Psychiatric mental status determination
Clinical psychiatric mental status determination
Evaluation for criminal responsibility
Evaluation for testimentary capacity
Medicolegal mental status determination
Mental status determination NOS

94.12 Routine psychiatric visit, not otherwise specified

94.13 Psychiatric commitment evaluation
Pre-commitment interview

94.19 Other psychiatric interview and evaluation
Follow-up psychiatric interview NOS

94.2 Psychiatric somatotherapy

94.21 Narcoanalysis
Narcosynthesis

94.22 Lithium therapy

94.23 Neuroleptic therapy

94.24 Chemical shock therapy

94.25 Other psychiatric drug therapy

94.26 Subconvulsive electroshock therapy

94.27 Other electroshock therapy
Electroconvulsive therapy (ECT)
EST

94.29 Other psychiatric somatotherapy

94.3 Individual psychotherapy

94.31 Psychoanalysis

94.32 Hypnotherapy
Hypnodrome
Hypnosis

94.33 Behavior therapy
Aversion therapy
Behavior modification
Desensitization therapy
Extinction therapy
Relaxation training
Token economy

94.34 Individual therapy for psychosexual dysfunction
Excludes: that performed in group setting (94.41)

94.35 Crisis intervention

94.36 Play psychotherapy

94.37 Exploratory verbal psychotherapy

94.38 Supportive verbal psychotherapy

94.39 Other individual psychotherapy
Biofeedback

94.4 Psychotherapy and counselling

94.41 Group therapy for psychosexual dysfunction

94.42 Family therapy

94.43 Psychodrama

94.44 Other group therapy

94.45 Drug addiction counselling

94.46 Alcoholism counselling

94.49 Other counselling

94.5 Referral for psychologic rehabilitation

94.51 Referral for psychotherapy

94.52 Referral for psychiatric aftercare
That in:
halfway house
outpatient (clinic) facility

Valid O.R. procedure   Non-O.R. procedure   Nonspecific O.R. procedure   Noncovered O.R. procedure

94.53 Referral for alcoholism rehabilitation

94.54 Referral for drug addiction rehabilitation

94.55 Referral for vocational rehabilitation

94.59 Referral for other psychologic rehabilitation

94.6 Alcohol and drug rehabilitation and detoxification

94.61 Alcohol rehabilitation

94.62 Alcohol detoxification

94.63 Alcohol rehabilitation and detoxification

94.64 Drug rehabilitation

94.65 Drug detoxification

94.66 Drug rehabilitation and detoxification

94.67 Combined alcohol and drug rehabilitation

94.68 Combined alcohol and drug detoxification

94.69 Combined alcohol and drug rehabilitation and detoxification

95 Ophthalmologic and otologic diagnosis and treatment

95.0 General and subjective eye examination

95.01 Limited eye examination
Eye examination with prescription of spectacles

95.02 Comprehensive eye examination
Eye examination covering all aspects of the visual system

95.03 Extended ophthalmologic work-up
Examination (for):
glaucoma
neuro-ophthalmology
retinal disease

95.04 Eye examination under anesthesia
Code also type of examination

95.05 Visual field study

95.06 Color vision study

95.07 Dark adaptation study

95.09 Eye examination, not otherwise specified
Vision check NOS

95.1 Examinations of form and structure of eye

95.11 Fundus photography

95.12 Fluorescein angiography or angioscopy of eye

95.13 Ultrasound study of eye

95.14 X-ray study of eye

95.15 Ocular motility study

95.16 P^{32} and other tracer studies of eye

95.2 Objective functional tests of eye

Excludes: *that with polysomnogram (89.17)*

95.21 Electroretinogram [ERG]

95.22 Electro-oculogram [EOG]

95.23 Visual evoked potential [VEP]

95.24 Electronystagmogram [ENG]

95.25 Electromyogram of eye [EMG]

95.26 Tonography, provocative tests, and other glaucoma testing

95.3 Special vision services

95.31 Fitting and dispensing of spectacles

95.32 Prescription, fitting, and dispensing of contact lens

95.33 Dispensing of other low vision aids

95.34 Ocular prosthetics

95.35 Orthoptic training

95.36 Ophthalmologic counselling and instruction
Counselling in:
  adaptation to visual loss
  use of low vision aids

95.4 Nonoperative procedures related to hearing

95.41 Audiometry
Békésy 5-tone audiometry
Impedance audiometry
Stapedial reflex response
Subjective audiometry
Tympanogram

95.42 Clinical test of hearing
Tuning fork test
Whispered speech test

95.43 Audiological evaluation
Audiological evaluation by:
  Barany noise machine
  blindfold test
  delayed feedback
  masking
  Weber lateralization

95.44 Clinical vestibular function tests
Thermal test of vestibular function

95.45 Rotation tests
Barany chair

95.46 Other auditory and vestibular function tests

95.47 Hearing examination, not otherwise specified

95.48 Fitting of hearing aid

> Excludes: *implantation of electromagnetic hearing device (20.95)*

95.49 Other nonoperative procedures related to hearing
Adjustment (external components) of cochlear prosthetic device

96 Nonoperative intubation and irrigation

96.0 Nonoperative intubation of gastrointestinal and respiratory tracts

96.01 Insertion of nasopharyngeal airway

96.02 Insertion of oropharyngeal airway

96.03 Insertion of esophageal obturator airway

96.04 Insertion of endotracheal tube

96.05 Other intubation of respiratory tract

> Excludes: *endoscopic insertion or replacement of bronchial device or substance (33.71, 33.79)*

96.06 Insertion of Sengstaken tube
Esophageal tamponade

96.07 Insertion of other (naso-)gastric tube
Intubation for decompression

> Excludes: *that for enteral infusion of nutritional substances (96.6)*

96.08 Insertion of (naso-)intestinal tube
Miller-Abbott tube (for decompression)

96.09 Insertion of rectal tube
Replacement of rectal tube

96.1 Other nonoperative insertion

> Excludes: *nasolacrimal intubation (09.44)*

96.11 Packing of external auditory canal

96.14 Vaginal packing

96.15 Insertion of vaginal mold

96.16 Other vaginal dilation

96.17 Insertion of vaginal diaphragm

96.18 Insertion of other vaginal pessary

96.19 Rectal packing

| | Valid O.R. procedure | | Non-O.R. procedure | | Nonspecific O.R. procedure | | Noncovered O.R. procedure |

96.2   Nonoperative dilation and manipulation

96.21   Dilation of frontonasal duct

96.22   Dilation of rectum

96.23   Dilation of anal sphincter

96.24   Dilation and manipulation of enterostomy stoma

96.25   Therapeutic distention of bladder
Intermittent distention of bladder

96.26   Manual reduction of rectal prolapse

96.27   Manual reduction of hernia

96.28   Manual reduction of enterostomy prolapse

96.29   Reduction with intussusception of alimentary tract
With:
Fluoroscopy
Ionizing radiation enema
Ultrasonography guidance
Hydrostatic reduction
Pneumantic reduction

> Excludes: *intra-abdominal manipulation of intestine, not otherwise specified*
> *(46.80)*

96.3   Nonoperative alimentary tract irrigation, cleaning, and local instillation

96.31   Gastric cooling
Gastric hypothermia

96.32   Gastric freezing

96.33   Gastric lavage

96.34   Other irrigation of (naso-)gastric tube

96.35   Gastric gavage

96.36   Irrigation of gastrostomy or enterostomy

96.37   Proctoclysis

96.38   Removal of impacted feces
Removal of impaction:
by flushing
manually

96.39   Other transanal enema
Rectal irrigation

> Excludes: *reduction of intussusception of alimentary tract by ionizing radiation*
> *enema (96.29)*

96.4   Nonoperative irrigation, cleaning, and local instillation of other digestive and genitourinary organs

96.41   Irrigation of cholecystostomy and other biliary tube

96.42   Irrigation of pancreatic tube

96.43   Digestive tract instillation, except gastric gavage

96.44   Vaginal douche

96.45   Irrigation of nephrostomy and pyelostomy

96.46   Irrigation of ureterostomy and ureteral catheter

96.47   Irrigation of cystostomy

96.48   Irrigation of other indwelling urinary catheter

96.49   Other genitourinary instillation
Insertion of prostaglandin suppository

96.5   Other nonoperative irrigation and cleaning

96.51   Irrigation of eye
Irrigation of cornea

> Excludes: *irrigation with removal of foreign body (98.21)*

96.52   Irrigation of ear
Irrigation with removal of cerumen

96.53   Irrigation of nasal passages

96.54   Dental scaling, polishing, and debridement
Dental prophylaxis
Plaque removal

96.55 Tracheostomy toilette

96.56 Other lavage of bronchus and trachea

> *Excludes:* *diagnostic bronchoalveolar lavage (BAL) (33.24)*
> *whole lung lavage (33.99)*

96.57 Irrigation of vascular catheter

96.58 Irrigation of wound catheter

96.59 Other irrigation of wound
Wound cleaning NOS

> *Excludes:* *debridement (86.22, 86.27-86.28)*

96.6 Enteral infusion of concentrated nutritional substances

96.7 Other continuous invasive mechanical ventilation
Includes: BiPAP delivered through endotracheal tube or tracheostomy (invasive interface)
CPAP delivered through endotracheal tube or tracheostomy (invasive interface)
Endotracheal respiratory assistance
Invasive positive pressure ventilation [IPPV]
Mechanical ventilation through invasive interface
That by tracheostomy
Weaning of an intubated (endotracheal tube) patient

> *Excludes:* *continuous negative pressure ventilation [CNP] (iron lung) (cuirass) (93.99)*
> *intermittent positive pressure breathing [IPPB] (93.91)*
> *non-invasive bi-level positive airway pressure (BiPAP) (93.90)*
> *non-invasive continuous positive airway pressure [CPAP] (93.90)*
> *non-invasive positive pressure (NIPPV) (93.90)*
> *that by face mask (93.90-93.99)*
> *that by nasal cannula (93.90-93.99)*
> *that by nasal catheter (93.90-93.99)*

Code also any associated:
endotracheal tube insertion (96.04)
tracheostomy (31.1-31.29)

Note: Endotracheal Intubation
To calculate the number of hours (duration) of continuous mechanical ventilation during a hospitalization, begin the count from the start of the (endotracheal) intubation. The duration ends with (endotracheal) extubation.

If the patient is intubated prior to admission, begin counting the duration from the time of admission. If a patient is transferred (discharged) while intubated, the duration would end at the time of transfer (discharge).

For patients who begin on (endotracheal) intubation and subsequently have a tracheostomy performed for mechanical ventilation, the duration begins with the (endotracheal) intubation and ends when the mechanical ventilation is turned off (after the weaning period).

Tracheostomy
To calculate the number of hours of continuous mechanical ventilation during a hospitalization, begin counting the duration when mechanical ventilation is started. The duration ends when the mechanical ventilator is turned off (after the weaning period).

If a patient has received a tracheostomy prior to admission and is on mechanical ventilation at the time of admission, begin counting the duration from the time of admission. If a patient is transferred (discharged) while still on mechanical ventilation via tracheostomy, the duration would end at the time of the transfer (discharge).

96.70 Continuous invasive mechanical ventilation of unspecified duration
Invasive mechanical ventilation NOS

96.71 Continuous invasive mechanical ventilation for less than 96 consecutive hours

96.72 Continuous invasive mechanical ventilation for 96 consecutive hours or more

97 Replacement and removal of therapeutic appliances

97.0 Nonoperative replacement of gastrointestinal appliance

97.01 Replacement of (naso-)gastric or esophagostomy tube

97.02 Replacement of gastrostomy tube

97.03 Replacement of tube or enterostomy device of small intestine

97.04 Replacement of tube or enterostomy device of large intestine

97.05 Replacement of stent (tube) in biliary or pancreatic duct

97.1 **Nonoperative replacement of musculoskeletal and integumentary system appliance**

97.11 **Replacement of cast on upper limb**

97.12 **Replacement of cast on lower limb**

97.13 **Replacement of other cast**

97.14 **Replacement of other device for musculoskeletal immobilization**
Splinting
Strapping

97.15 **Replacement of wound catheter**

97.16 **Replacement of wound packing or drain**

Excludes: *repacking of:*
dental wound (97.22)
vulvar wound (97.26)

97.2 **Other nonoperative replacement**

97.21 **Replacement of nasal packing**

97.22 **Replacement of dental packing**

97.23 **Replacement of tracheostomy tube**

97.24 **Replacement and refitting of vaginal diaphragm**

97.25 **Replacement of other vaginal pessary**

97.26 **Replacement of vaginal or vulvar packing or drain**

97.29 **Other nonoperative replacements**

97.3 **Nonoperative removal of therapeutic device from head and neck**

97.31 **Removal of eye prosthesis**

Excludes: *removal of ocular implant (16.71)*
removal of orbital implant (16.72)

97.32 **Removal of nasal packing**

97.33 **Removal of dental wiring**

97.34 **Removal of dental packing**

97.35 **Removal of dental prosthesis**

97.36 **Removal of other external mandibular fixation device**

97.37 **Removal of tracheostomy tube**

97.38 **Removal of sutures from head and neck**

97.39 **Removal of other therapeutic device from head and neck**

Excludes: *removal of skull tongs (02.94)*

97.4 **Nonoperative removal of therapeutic device from thorax**

97.41 **Removal of thoracotomy tube or pleural cavity drain**

97.42 **Removal of mediastinal drain**

97.43 **Removal of sutures from thorax**

97.44 **Nonoperative removal of heart assist system**
Explantation [removal] of circulatory assist device
Explantation [removal] of percutaneous external heart assist device
Intra-aortic balloon pump [IABP]
Removal of extrinsic heart assist device
Removal of pVAD
Removal of percutaneous heart assist device

97.49 **Removal of other device from thorax**

Excludes: *endoscopic removal of bronchial device(s) or substances (33.78)*

97.5 **Nonoperative removal of therapeutic device from digestive system**

97.51 **Removal of gastrostomy tube**

97.52 **Removal of tube from small intestine**

97.53 **Removal of tube from large intestine or appendix**

97.54 **Removal of cholecystostomy tube**

97.55 **Removal of T-tube, other bile duct tube, or liver tube**
Removal of bile duct stent

97.56 **Removal of pancreatic tube or drain**

● Code new
to 2012 edition
▲ Revision of
existing code
④ ⑤ Fourth or fifth
digit required

97.59 Removal of other device from digestive system
Removal of rectal packing

97.6 Nonoperative removal of therapeutic device from urinary system

97.61 Removal of pyelostomy and nephrostomy tube

97.62 Removal of ureterostomy tube and ureteral catheter

97.63 Removal of cystostomy tube

97.64 Removal of other urinary drainage device
Removal of indwelling urinary catheter

97.65 Removal of urethral stent

97.69 Removal of other device from urinary system

97.7 Nonoperative removal of therapeutic device from genital system

97.71 Removal of intrauterine contraceptive device

97.72 Removal of intrauterine pack

97.73 Removal of vaginal diaphragm

97.74 Removal of other vaginal pessary

97.75 Removal of vaginal or vulva packing

97.79 Removal of other device from genital tract
Removal of sutures

97.8 Other nonoperative removal of therapeutic device

97.81 Removal of retroperitoneal drainage device

97.82 Removal of peritoneal drainage device

97.83 Removal of abdominal wall sutures

97.84 Removal of sutures from trunk, not elsewhere classified

97.85 Removal of packing from trunk, not elsewhere classified

97.86 Removal of other device from abdomen

97.87 Removal of other device from trunk

97.88 Removal of external immobilization device
Removal of:
  brace
  cast
  splint

97.89 Removal of other therapeutic device

98 Nonoperative removal of foreign body or calculus

98.0 Removal of intraluminal foreign body from digestive system without incision
Excludes: removal of therapeutic device (97.51-97.59)

98.01 Removal of intraluminal foreign body from mouth without incision

98.02 Removal of intraluminal foreign body from esophagus without incision

98.03 Removal of intraluminal foreign body from stomach and small intestine without incision

98.04 Removal of intraluminal foreign body from large intestine without incision

98.05 Removal of intraluminal foreign body from rectum and anus without incision

98.1 Removal of intraluminal foreign body from other sites without incision
Excludes: removal of therapeutic device (97.31-97.49, 97.61-97.89)

98.11 Removal of intraluminal foreign body from ear without incision

98.12 Removal of intraluminal foreign body from nose without incision

98.13 Removal of intraluminal foreign body from pharynx without incision

98.14 Removal of intraluminal foreign body from larynx without incision

98.15 Removal of intraluminal foreign body from trachea and bronchus without incision
Excludes: endoscopic removal of bronchial device(s) or substances (33.78)

98.16 Removal of intraluminal foreign body from uterus without incision
Excludes: removal of intrauterine contraceptive device (97.71)

98.17 Removal of intraluminal foreign body from vagina without incision

98.18 Removal of intraluminal foreign body from artificial stoma without incision

| | Valid O.R. procedure | | Non-O.R. procedure | | Nonspecific O.R. procedure | | Noncovered O.R. procedure |

98.19   Removal of intraluminal foreign body from urethra without incision

98.2   Removal of other foreign body without incision

> Excludes: *removal of intraluminal foreign body (98.01-98.19)*

98.20   Removal of foreign body, not otherwise specified

98.21   Removal of superficial foreign body from eye without incision

98.22   Removal of other foreign body without incision from head and neck
Removal of embedded foreign body from eyelid or conjunctiva without incision

98.23   Removal of foreign body from vulva without incision

98.24   Removal of foreign body from scrotum or penis without incision

98.25   Removal of other foreign body without incision from trunk except scrotum, penis, or vulva

98.26   Removal of foreign body from hand without incision

98.27   Removal of foreign body without incision from upper limb, except hand

98.28   Removal of foreign body from foot without incision

98.29   Removal of foreign body without incision from lower limb, except foot

98.5   Extracorporeal shockwave lithotripsy [ESWL]
Lithotriptor tank procedure
Disintegration of stones by extracorporeal induced shockwaves
That with insertion of stent

98.51   Extracorporeal shockwave lithotripsy [ESWL] of the kidney, ureter and/or bladder

98.52   Extracorporeal shockwave lithotripsy [ESWL] of the gallbladder and/or bile duct

98.59   Extracorporeal shockwave lithotripsy of other sites

99   Other nonoperative procedures

99.0   Transfusion of blood and blood components
Use additional code for that done via catheter or cutdown (38.92-38.94)

99.00   Perioperative autologous transfusion of whole blood or blood components
Intraoperative blood collection
Postoperative blood collection
Salvage

99.01   Exchange transfusion
Transfusion:
   exsanguination
   replacement

99.02   Transfusion of previously collected autologous blood
Blood component

99.03   Other transfusion of whole blood
Transfusion:
   NOS
   blood NOS
   hemodilution

99.04   Transfusion of packed cells

99.05   Transfusion of platelets
Transfusion of thrombocytes

99.06   Transfusion of coagulation factors
Transfusion of antihemophilic factor

99.07   Transfusion of other serum
Transfusion of plasma

> Excludes: *injection [transfusion] of:*
> *antivenin (99.16)*
> *gamma globulin (99.14)*

99.08   Transfusion of blood expander
Transfusion of Dextran

99.09   Transfusion of other substance
Transfusion of:
   blood surrogate
   granulocytes

> Excludes: *transplantation [transfusion] of bone marrow (41.00-41.09)*

● Code new   ▲ Revision of   ④ ⑤ Fourth or fifth
to 2012 edition   existing code   digit required

99.1   Injection or Infusion of therapeutic or prophylactic substance
Includes: injection or infusion given:
hypodermically acting locally or systemically
intramuscularly acting locally or systemically
intravenously acting locally or systemically

99.10   Injection or infusion of thrombolytic agent
Alteplase
Anistreplase
Reteplase
Streptokinase
Tenecteplase
Tissue plasminogen activator (TPA)
Urokinase

Excludes: *aspirin—omit code*
GP IIB/IIIa platelet inhibitors (99.20)
heparin (99.19)
SuperSaturated oxygen therapy (00.49)
warfarin—omit code

99.11   Injection of Rh immune globulin
Injection of:
Anti-D (Rhesus) globulin
RhoGAM

99.12   Immunization for allergy
Desensitization

99.13   Immunization for autoimmune disease

99.14   Injection or infusion of immunoglobulin
Injection of immune sera
Injection or infusion of gamma globulin

99.15   Parenteral infusion of concentrated nutritional substances
Hyperalimentation
Peripheral parenteral nutrition [PPN]
Total parenteral nutrition [TPN]

99.16   Injection of antidote
Injection of:
antivenin
heavy metal antagonist

99.17   Injection of insulin

99.18   Injection or infusion of electrolytes

99.19   Injection of anticoagulant

Excludes: *infusion of drotrecogin alfa (activated) (00.11)*

99.2   Injection or infusion of other therapeutic or prophylactic substance
Includes: injection or infusion given:
hypodermically acting locally or systemically
intramuscularly acting locally or systemically
intravenously acting locally or systemically
Use additional code for:
injection (into):
breast (85.92)
bursa (82.94, 83.96)
intraperitoneal (cavity) (54.97)
intrathecal (03.92)
joint (76.96, 81.92)
kidney (55.96)
liver (50.94)
orbit (16.91)
other sites—see Alphabetic Index
perfusion:
NOS (39.97)
intestine (46.95, 46.96)
kidney (55.95)
liver (50.93)
total body (39.96)

Excludes: *SuperSaturated oxygen therapy (00.49)*

	Valid O.R. procedure		Non-O.R. procedure		Nonspecific O.R. procedure		Noncovered O.R. procedure

99.20 Injection or infusion of platelet inhibitor
Glycoprotein IIB/IIIa inhibitor
GP IIB/IIIa inhibitor
GP IIB-IIIa inhibitor

> Excludes: *infusion of heparin (99.19)*
> *injection or infusion of thrombolytic agent (99.10)*

99.21 Injection of antibiotic

> Excludes: *injection or infusion of oxazolidinone class of antibiotics (00.14)*

99.22 Injection of other anti-infective

> Excludes: *injection or infusion of oxazolidinone class of antibiotics (00.14)*

99.23 Injection of steroid
Injection of cortisone
Subdermal implantation of progesterone

99.24 Injection of other hormone

99.25 Injection or infusion of cancer chemotherapeutic substance
Chemoembolization
Injection or infusion of antineoplastic agent

> *Use additional code for disruption of blood brain barrier, if performed [BBBD]*
> *(00.19)*

> Excludes: *immunotherapy, antineoplastic (00.15, 99.28)*
> *implantation of chemotherapeutic agent (00.10)*
> *injection or infusion of biological response modifier [BRM] as an*
> *antineoplastic agent (99.28)*
> *injection of radioisotopes (92.28)*
> *intravenous infusion of clofarabine (17.70)*

99.26 Injection of tranquilizer

99.27 Iontophoresis

99.28 Injection or infusion of biological response modifier [BRM] as an antineoplastic agent
Low-dose interleukin-2 (IL-2) therapy
Immunotherapy, antineoplastic
Infusion of cintredekin besudotox
Interleukin therapy
Tumor vaccine

> Excludes: *high-dose infusion interleukin-2 [IL-2] (00.15)*

99.29 Injection or infusion of other therapeutic or prophylactic substance

> Excludes: *administration of neuroprotective agent (99.75)*
> *immunization (99.31-99.59)*
> *infusion of blood brain barrier disruption substance (00.19)*
> *injection of sclerosing agent into:*
> *esophageal varices (42.33)*
> *hemorrhoids (49.42)*
> *veins (39.92)*
> *injection or infusion of human B-type natriuretic peptide (hBNP)*
> *(00.13)*
> *injection or infusion of nesiritide (00.13)*
> *injection or infusion of platelet inhibitor (99.20)*
> *injection or infusion of thrombolytic agent (99.10)*
> *uterine artery embolization without coils (68.25)*

99.3 Prophylactic vaccination and inoculation against certain bacterial diseases

99.31 Vaccination against cholera

99.32 Vaccination against typhoid and paratyphoid fever
Administration of TAB vaccine

99.33 Vaccination against tuberculosis
Administration of BCG vaccine

99.34 Vaccination against plague

99.35 Vaccination against tularemia

99.36 Administration of diphtheria toxoid

> Excludes: *administration of:*
> *diphtheria antitoxin (99.58)*
> *diphtheria-tetanus-pertussis combined (99.39)*

99.37 Vaccination against pertussis

> Excludes: *administration of diphtheria-tetanus-pertussis, combined (99.39)*

99.38 Administration of tetanus toxoid

> Excludes: *administration of:*
> *diphtheria-tetanus-pertussis combined (99.39)*
> *tetanus antitoxin (99.56)*

99.39 Administration of diphtheria-tetanus-pertussis, combined

99.4 Prophylactic vaccination and inoculation against certain viral diseases

99.41 Administration of poliomyelitis vaccine

99.42 Vaccination against smallpox

99.43 Vaccination against yellow fever

99.44 Vaccination against rabies

99.45 Vaccination against measles

> Excludes: *administration of measles-mumps-rubella vaccine (99.48)*

99.46 Vaccination against mumps

> Excludes: *administration of measles-mumps-rubella vaccine (99.48)*

99.47 Vaccination against rubella

> Excludes: *administration of measles-mumps-rubella vaccine (99.48)*

99.48 Administration of measles-mumps-rubella vaccine

99.5 Other vaccination and inoculation

99.51 Prophylactic vaccination against the common cold

99.52 Prophylactic vaccination against influenza

99.53 Prophylactic vaccination against arthropod-borne viral encephalitis

99.54 Prophylactic vaccination against other arthropod-borne viral diseases

99.55 Prophylactic administration of vaccine against other disease
Vaccination against:
anthrax
brucellosis
Rocky Mountain spotted fever
Staphylococcus
Streptococcus
typhus

99.56 Administration of tetanus antitoxin

99.57 Administration of botulism antitoxin

99.58 Administration of other antitoxins
Administration of:
diphtheria antitoxin
gas gangrene antitoxin
scarlet fever antitoxin

99.59 Other vaccination and inoculation
Vaccination NOS

> Excludes: *injection of:*
> *gamma globulin (99.14)*
> *Rh immune globulin (99.11)*
> *immunization for:*
> *allergy (99.12)*
> *autoimmune disease (99.13)*

99.6 Conversion of cardiac rhythm

> Excludes: *open chest cardiac:*
> *electric stimulation (37.91)*
> *massage (37.91)*

99.60 Cardiopulmonary resuscitation, not otherwise specified

99.61 Atrial cardioversion

| Valid O.R. procedure | Non-O.R. procedure | Nonspecific O.R. procedure | Noncovered O.R. procedure |

99.62 Other electric countershock of heart
Cardioversion:
  NOS
  external
Conversion to sinus rhythm
Defibrillation
External electrode stimulation

99.63 Closed chest cardiac massage
Cardiac massage NOS
Manual external cardiac massage

99.64 Carotid sinus stimulation

99.69 Other conversion of cardiac rhythm

99.7 Therapeutic apheresis or other injection, administration, or infusion of other therapeutic or prophylactic substance

99.71 Therapeutic plasmapheresis

> *Excludes:* *extracorporeal immunoadsorption [ECI] (99.76)*

99.72 Therapeutic leukopheresis
Therapeutic leukocytapheresis

99.73 Therapeutic erythrocytapheresis
Therapeutic erythropheresis

99.74 Therapeutic plateletpheresis

99.75 Administration of neuroprotective agent

99.76 Extracorporeal immunoadsorption
Removal of antibodies from plasma with protein A columns

99.77 Application or administraion of adhesion barrier substance

99.78 Aquapheresis
Plasma water removal
Ultrafiltration [for water removal]

> *Excludes:* *hemodiafiltration (39.95)*
> *hemodialysis (39.95)*
> *therapeutic plasmapheresis (99.71)*

99.79 Other
Apheresis (harvest) of stem cells
Leech therapy

99.8 Miscellaneous physical procedures

99.81 Hypothermia (central) (local)

> *Excludes:* *gastric cooling (96.31)*
> *gastric freezing (96.32)*
> *that incidental to open heart surgery (39.62)*

99.82 Ultraviolet light therapy
Actinotherapy

99.83 Other phototherapy
Phototherapy of the newborn

> *Excludes:* *extracorporeal photochemotherapy (99.88)*
> *photocoagulation of retinal lesion (14.23-14.25, 14.33-14.35,*
> *14.53-14.55)*

99.84 Isolation
Isolation after contact with infectious disease
Protection of individual from his surroundings
Protection of surroundings from individual

99.85 Hyperthermia for treatment of cancer
Hyperthermia (adjunct therapy) induced by microwave, ultrasound, low energy
  radiofrequency, probes (interstitial), or other means in the treatment of cancer
Code also any concurrent chemotherapy or radiation therapy

99.86 Non-invasive placement of bone growth stimulator
Transcutaneous (surface) placement of pads or patches for stimulation to aid bone
  healing

> *Excludes:* *insertion of invasive or semi-invasive bone growth stimulators (device)*
> *(percutaneous electrodes) (78.90-78.99)*

● Code new   ▲ Revision of   ④ ⑤ Fourth or fifth
     to 2012 edition   existing code   digit required

99.88 **Therapeutic photopheresis**
Extracorporeal photochemotherapy
Extracorporeal photopheresis

Excludes: *other phototherapy (99.83)*
ultraviolet light therapy (99.82)

99.9 **Other miscellaneous procedures**

99.91 **Acupuncture for anesthesia**

99.92 **Other acupuncture**

Excludes: *that with smouldering moxa (93.35)*

99.93 **Rectal massage (for levator spasm)**

99.94 **Prostatic massage**

99.95 **Stretching of foreskin**

99.96 **Collection of sperm for artificial insemination**

99.97 **Fitting of denture**

99.98 **Extraction of milk from lactating breast**

99.99 **Other**
Leech therapy

Valid O.R.
procedure

Non-O.R.
procedure

Nonspecific
O.R. procedure

Noncovered
O.R. procedure

This page intentionally left blank.

● Code new
  to 2012 edition

▲ Revision of
  existing code

④ ⑤ Fourth or fifth
  digit required

A

Abbe operation
construction of vagina 70.61
with graft or prosthesis 70.63
intestinal anastomosis—*see* Anastomosis
intestine
Abciximab, infusion 99.20
Abdominocentesis 54.91
Abdominohysterectomy 68.49
laparoscopic 68.41
Abdominoplasty 86.83
Abdominoscopy 54.21
Abdominouterotomy 68.0
obstetrical 74.99
Abduction, arytenoid 31.69
AbioCor® total replacement heart 37.52
Ablation
biliary ducts (lesion) by ERCP 51.64
endometrial (hysteroscopic) 68.23
inner ear (cryosurgery) (ultrasound) 20.79
by injection 20.72
lesion
esophagus 42.39
endoscopic 42.33
heart
by peripherally inserted catheter 37.34
endovascular approach 37.34
Maze procedure (Cox-maze)
endovascular approach 37.34
open approach 37.33
thoracoscopic approach 37.37
thoracoscopic approach 37.37
liver 50.26
laparoscopic 50.25
open 50.23
percutaneous 50.24
lung 32.26
bronchoscopic thermoplasty 32.27
open 32.23
percutaneous 32.24
thoracoscopic 32.25
renal 55.35
laparoscopic 55.34
open 55.32
percutaneous 55.33
intestine
large 45.49
endoscopic 45.43
large intestine 45.49
endoscopic 45.43
pituitary 07.69
by
Cobalt-60 92.32
implantation (strontium-yttrium) (Y) NEC
07.68
transfrontal approach 07.64
transphenoidal approach 07.65
proton beam (Bragg peak) 92.33
prostate, by
cryoablation 60.62
laser, transurethral 60.21
radical cryosurgical ablation (RCSA) 60.62
radiofrequency thermotherapy 60.97
transurethral needle ablation (TUNA) 60.97
tissue
heart—*see* Ablation, lesion, heart
liver—*see* Ablation, lesion, liver
lung—*see* Ablation, lesion, lung
renal—*see* Ablation, lesion, renal

Abortion, therapeutic 69.51
by
aspiration curettage 69.51
dilation and curettage 69.01
hysterectomy—*see* Hysterectomy
hysterotomy 74.91
insertion
laminaria 69.93
prostaglandin suppository 96.49
intra-amniotic injection (saline) 75.0
Abrasion
corneal epithelium 11.41
for smear or culture 11.21
epicardial surface 36.39
pleural 34.6
skin 86.25
Abscission, cornea 11.49
Absorptiometry
photon (dual) (single) 88.98
Aburel operation (intra-amniotic injection for
abortion) 75.0
Accouchement forcé 73.99
Acetabulectomy 77.85
Acetabuloplasty NEC 81.40
with prosthetic implant 81.52
Achillorrhaphy 83.64
delayed 83.62
Achillotenotomy 83.11
plastic 83.85
Achillotomy 83.11
plastic 83.85
Acid peel, skin 86.24
Acromionectomy 77.81
Acromioplasty 81.83
for recurrent dislocation of shoulder 81.82
partial replacement 81.81
total replacement, NEC 81.80
other 81.80
reverse 81.88
Actinotherapy 99.82
Activities of daily living (ADL)
therapy 93.83
training for the blind 93.78
Acupuncture 99.92
with smouldering moxa 93.35
for anesthesia 99.91
Adams operation
advancement of round ligament 69.22
crushing of nasal septum 21.88
excision of palmar fascia 82.35
Adenectomy —*see also* Excision, by site
prostate NEC 60.69
retropubic 60.4
Adenoidectomy (without tonsillectomy) 28.6
with tonsillectomy 28.3
Adhesiolysis —*see also* Lysis, adhesions
for collapse of lung 33.39
middle ear 20.23
Adipectomy 86.83
Adjustment
cardiac pacemaker program
(reprogramming)—*omit code*
cochlear prosthetic device (external components)
95.49
dental 99.97
gastric restrictive device (laparoscopic) 44.98
occlusal 24.8

Amputation—*continued*
 clitoris 71.4
 Dieffenbach (hip disarticulation) 84.18
 Dupuytren's (shoulder disarticulation) 84.08
 ear, external 18.39
 elbow (disarticulation) 84.06
 finger, except thumb 84.01
  thumb 84.02
 foot (middle) 84.12
 forearm 84.05
 forefoot 84.12
 forequarter 84.09
 Gordon-Taylor (hindquarter) 84.19
 Gritti-Stokes (knee disarticulation) 84.16
 Guyon (ankle) 84.13
 hallux 84.11
 hand 84.03
 Hey's (foot) 84.12
 hindquarter 84.19
 hip (disarticulation) 84.18
 humerus 84.07
 interscapulothoracic 84.09
 interthoracoscapular 84.09
 King-Steelquist (hindquarter) 84.19
 Kirk (thigh) 84.17
 knee (disarticulation) 84.16
 Kutler (revision of current traumatic amputation
   of finger) 84.01
 Larry (shoulder disarticulation) 84.08
 leg NEC 84.10
  above knee (AK) 84.17
  below knee (BK) 84.15
  through
    ankle (disarticulation) 84.13
    femur (AK) 84.17
    foot 84.12
    hip (disarticulation) 84.18
    tibia and fibula (BK) 84.15
 Lisfranc
  foot 84.12
  shoulder (disarticulation) 84.08
 Littlewood (forequarter) 84.09
 lower limb NEC (*see also* Amputation, leg) 84.10
 Mazet (knee disarticulation) 84.16
 metacarpal 84.03
 metatarsal 84.11
  head (bunionectomy) 77.59
 metatarsophalangeal (joint) 84.11
 midtarsal 84.12
 nose 21.4
 penis (circle) (complete) (flap) (partial) (radical)
   64.3
 ray
  finger 84.01
  foot 84.11
  toe (metatarsal head) 84.11
 root (tooth) (apex) 23.73
  with root canal therapy 23.72
 shoulder (disarticulation) 84.08
 Sorondo-Ferré (hindquarter) 84.19
 S.P. Rogers (knee disarticulation) 84.16
 supracondylar, above-knee 84.17
 supramalleolar, foot 84.14
 Syme's (ankle amputation through malleoli of
   tibia and fibula) 84.14
 thigh 84.17
 thumb 84.02
 toe (through metatarsophalangeal joint) 84.11
 transcarpal 84.03
 transmetatarsal 84.12

Amputation—*continued*
 upper limb NEC (*see also* Amputation, arm)
   84.00
 wrist (disarticulation) 84.04
Amygdalohippocampectomy 01.59
Amygdalohippocampotomy 01.39
Amygdalotomy 01.39
Analysis
 cardiac rhythm device (CRT-D) (CRT-P) (AICD)
   (pacemaker)—*see* Interrogation
 character 94.03
 gastric 89.39
 psychologic 94.31
 transactional
  group 94.44
  individual 94.39
Anastomosis
 abdominal artery to coronary artery 36.17
 accessory-facial nerve 04.72
 accessory-hypoglossal nerve 04.73
 anus (with formation of endorectal deal pouch)
   45.95
 aorta (descending)—pulmonary (artery) 39.0
 aorta-renal artery 39.24
 aorta-subclavian artery 39.22
 aortoceliac 39.26
 aorto(ilio)femoral 39.25
 aortomesenteric 39.26
 appendix 47.99
 arteriovenous NEC 39.29
  for renal dialysis 39.27
 artery (suture of distal to proximal end) 39.31
  with
    bypass graft 39.29
      extracranial-intracranial [EC-IC] 39.28
    excision or resection of vessel—*see*
      Arteriectomy, with anastomosis, by site
    revision 39.49
 bile ducts 51.39
 bladder NEC 57.88
  with
    isolated segment of intestine 57.87 *[45.50]*
      colon (sigmoid) 57.87 *[45.52]*
      ileum 57.87 *[45.51]*
    open loop of ileum 57.87 *[45.51]*
    to intestine 57.88
      ileum 57.87 *[45.51]*
 bowel—(*see also* Anastomosis, intestine) 45.90
 bronchotracheal 33.48
 bronchus 33.48
 carotid-subclavian artery 39.22
 caval-mesenteric vein 39.1
 caval-pulmonary artery 39.21
 cervicoesophageal 42.59
 colohypopharyngeal (intrathoracic) 42.55
  antesternal or antethoracic 42.65
 common bile duct 51.39
 common pulmonary trunk and left atrium
   (posterior wall) 35.82
 cystic bile duct 51.39
 cystocolic 57.88
 epididymis to vas deferens 63.83
 esophagocolic (intrathoracic) NEC 42.56
  with interposition 42.55
  antesternal or antethoracic NEC 42.66
    with interposition 42.65
 esophagocologastric (intrathoracic) 42.55
  antesternal or antethoracic 42.65
 esophagoduodenal (intrathoracic) NEC 42.54
  with interposition 42.53

Anastomosis—*continued*
  esophagoenteric (intrathoracic) NEC *see also*
      Anastomosis, esophagus to intestinal
      segment) 42.54
    antesternal or antethoracic NEC (*see also*
        Anastomosis, esophagus, antesternal, to
        intestinal segment) 42.64
  esophagoesophageal (intrathoracic) 42.51
    antesternal or antethoracic 42.61
  esophagogastric (intrathoracic) 42.52
    antesternal or antethoracic 42.62
  esophagus (intrapleural) (intrathoracic)
      (retrosternal) NEC 42.59
    with
      gastrectomy (partial) 43.5
        complete or total 43.99
      interposition (of) NEC 42.58
        colon 42.55
        jejunum 42.53
        small bowel 42.53
    antesternal or antethoracic NEC 42.69
      with
        interposition (of) NEC 42.68
          colon 42.65
          jejunal loop 42.63
          small bowel 42.63
          rubber tube 42.68
      to intestinal segment NEC 42.64
        with interposition 42.68
        colon NEC 42.66
          with interposition 42.65
        small bowel NEC 42.64
          with interposition 42.63
    to intestinal segment (intrathoracic) NEC 42.54
      with interposition 42.58
      antesternal or antethoracic NEC 42.64
        with interposition 42.68
      colon (intrathoracic) NEC 42.56
        with interposition 42.55
        antesternal or antethoracic 42.66
          with interposition 42.65
      small bowel NEC 42.54
        with interposition 42.53
        antesternal or antethoracic 42.64
          with interposition 42.63
  facial-accessory nerve 04.72
  facial-hypoglossal nerve 04.71
  fallopian tube 66.73
    by reanastomosis 66.79
  gallbladder 51.35
    to
      hepatic ducts 51.31
      intestine 51.32
      pancreas 51.33
      stomach 51.34
  gastroepiploic artery (to)
    coronary artery 36.17
  hepatic duct 51.39
  hypoglossal-accessory nerve 04.73
  hypoglossal-facial nerve 04.71
  ileal loop to bladder 57.87 *[45.51]*
  ileoanal 45.95
  ileorectal 45.93
  inferior vena cava and portal vein 39.1
  internal mammary artery (to)
    coronary artery (single vessel) 36.15
      double vessel 36.16
    myocardium 36.2

Anastomosis—*continued*
  intestine 45.90
    large-to-anus 45.95
    large-to-large 45.94
    large-to-rectum 45.94
    large-to-small 45.93
    small-to-anus 45.95
    small-to-large 45.93
    small-to-rectal stump 45.92
    small-to-small 45.91
  intrahepatic 51.79
  intrathoracic vessel NEC 39.23
  kidney (pelvis) 55.86
  lacrimal sac to conjunctiva 09.82
  left-to-right (systemic-pulmonary artery) 39.0
  lymphatic (channel) (peripheral) 40.9
  mesenteric-caval 39.1
  mesocaval 39.1
  nasolacrimal 09.81
  nerve (cranial) (peripheral) NEC 04.74
    accessory-facial 04.72
    accessory-hypoglossal 04.73
    hypoglossal-facial 04.71
  pancreas (duct) (to) 52.96
    bile duct 51.39
    gall bladder 51.33
    intestine 52.96
    jejunum 52.96
    stomach 52.96
  pleurothecal (with valve) 03.79
  portacaval 39.1
  portal vein to inferior vena cava 39.1
  pulmonary-aortic (Pott's) 39.0
  pulmonary artery and superior vena cava 39.21
  pulmonary-innominate artery (Blalock) 39.0
  pulmonary-subclavian artery (Blalock-Taussig)
      39.0
  pulmonary vein and azygos vein 39.23
  pyeloileocutaneous 56.51
  pyeloureterovesical 55.86
  radial artery 36.19
  rectum, rectal NEC 48.74
    stump to small intestine 45.92
  renal (pelvis) 55.86
    vein and splenic vein 39.1
  renoportal 39.1
  salpingothecal (with valve) 03.79
  splenic to renal veins 39.1
  splenorenal (venous) 39.1
    arterial 39.26
  subarachnoid-peritoneal (with valve) 03.71
  subarachnoid-ureteral (with valve) 03.72
  subclavian-aortic 39.22
  superior vena cava to pulmonary artery 39.21
  systemic-pulmonary artery 39.0
  thoracic artery (to)
    coronary artery (single) 36.15
      double 36.16
    myocardium 36.2
  ureter (to) NEC 56.79
    bladder 56.74
    colon 56.71
    ileal pouch (bladder) 56.51
    ileum 56.71
    intestine 56.71
    skin 56.61
  ureterocalyceal 55.86
  ureterocolic 56.71
  ureterovesical 56.74
  urethra (end-to-end) 58.44
  vas deferens 63.82

Angiocardiography—*continued*
 SPY, coronary 88.59
 vena cava (inferior) (superior) 88.51
Angiography (arterial) (*see also* Arteriography)
  88.40
 basilar 88.41
 brachial 88.49
 by C.A.T. —*see* Scan, C.A.T., by site
 by computed tomography —*see* Scan, C.A.T., by
  site
 by magnetic resonance – *see* Imaging, magnetic
  resonance, by site
 by radioisotope—*see* Scan, radioisotope, by site
 by ultrasound—*see* Ultrasonography, by site
 carotid (internal) 88.41
 celiac 88.47
 cerebral (posterior circulation) 88.41
 coronary NEC 88.57
  intra-operative fluorescence vascular 88.59
 eye (fluorescein) 95.12
 femoral 88.48
 heart 88.50
 intra-abdominal NEC 88.47
 intracranial 88.41
 intrathoracic vessels NEC 88.44
 lower extremity NEC 88.48
 neck 88.41
 non-coronary, intra-operative fluorescence 17.71
 placenta 88.46
 pulmonary 88.43
 renal 88.45
 specified artery NEC 88.49
 transfemoral 88.48
 upper extremity NEC 88.49
 veins—*see* Phlebography
 vertebral 88.41
Angioplasty (laser) —*see also* Repair, blood
  vessel

> Note: Also use 00.40, 00.41, 00.42, or 00.43 to
> show the total number of vessels treated. Use
> code 00.44 once to show procedure on a
> bifurcated vessel. In addition, use 00.45, 00.46,
> 00.47, or 00.48 to show the number of vascular
> stents inserted.

 balloon (percutaneous transluminal) NEC 39.50
  coronary artery 00.66
 coronary 36.09
  open chest approach 36.03
  percutaneous transluminal (balloon) 00.66
 percutaneous transluminal (balloon)
  basilar 00.62
  carotid 00.61
  cerebrovascular
   extracranial 00.62
   intracranial 00.61
    carotid 00.61
  coronary (balloon) 00.66
  extracranial 00.61
  femoropopliteal 39.50
  iliac 39.50
  intracranial 00.62
  lower extremity NOS 39.50
  mesenteric 39.50
  peripheral NEC 39.50
  renal 39.50
  subclavian 39.50
  upper extremity NOS 39.50
  vertebral 00.61
   intracranial portion 00.62

Angioplasty (laser)—*continued*
 specified site NEC 39.50
  cerebrovascular
   extracranial 00.62
   intracranial 00.61
  peripheral 39.50
Angiorrhaphy 39.30
 artery 39.31
 vein 39.32
Angioscopy, percutaneous 38.22
 eye (fluorescein) 95.12
Angiotomy 38.00
 abdominal
  artery 38.06
  vein 38.07
 aorta (arch) (ascending) (descending) 38.04
 head and neck NEC 38.02
 intracranial NEC 38.01
 lower limb
  artery 38.08
  vein 38.09
 thoracic NEC 38.05
 upper limb (artery) (vein) 38.03
Angiotripsy 39.98
Ankylosis, production of —*see* Arthrodesis
Annuloplasty (heart) (posteromedial) 35.33
Anoplasty 49.79
 with hemorrhoidectomy 49.46
Anoscopy 49.21
Antibiogram —*see* Examination, microscopic
Antiembolic filter, vena cava 38.7
Antiphobic treatment 94.39
Antrectomy
 mastoid 20.49
 maxillary 22.39
  radical 22.31
 pyloric 43.6
Antrostomy —*see* Antrotomy
Antrotomy (exploratory) (nasal sinus) 22.2
 Caldwell-Luc (maxillary sinus) 22.39
  with removal of membrane lining 22.31
 intranasal 22.2
  with external approach (Caldwell-Luc) 22.39
   radical 22.31
 maxillary (simple) 22.2
  with Caldwell-Luc approach 22.39
   with removal of membrane lining 22.31
  external (Caldwell-Luc approach) 22.39
   with removal of membrane lining 22.31
  radical (with removal of membrane lining) 22.31
Antrum window operation —*see* Antrotomy,
  maxillary
Aorticopulmonary window operation 39.59
Aortogram, aortography (abdominal)
  (retrograde) (selective) (translumbar) 88.42
Aortoplasty (aortic valve) (gusset type) 35.11
Aortotomy 38.04
Apexcardiogram (with ECG lead) 89.57
Apheresis, therapeutic —*see category* 99.7
Apicectomy
 lung 32.39
  thoracoscopic 32.30
 petrous pyramid 20.59
 tooth (root) 23.73
  with root canal therapy 23.72
Apicoectomy 23.73
 with root canal therapy 23.72
Apicolysis (lung) 33.39
Apicostomy, alveolar 24.0
Aponeurectomy 83.42
 hand 82.33

Aponeurorrhaphy (*see also* Suture, tendon) 83.64
  hand (*see also* Suture, tendon, hand) 82.45
Aponeurotomy 83.13
  hand 82.11
Appendectomy (with drainage) 47.09
  incidental 47.19
    laparoscopic 47.11
  laparoscopic 47.01
Appendicocecostomy 47.91
Appendicoenterostomy 47.91
Appendicolysis 54.59
  with appendectomy 47.01, 47.09
  laparoscopic 54.51
Appendicostomy 47.91
  closure 47.92
Appendicotomy 47.2
Application
  adhesion barrier substance 99.77
  anti-shock trousers 93.58
  arch bars (orthodontic) 24.7
    for immobilization (fracture) 93.55
  barrier substance, adhesion 99.77
  Barton's tongs (skull) (with synchronous skeletal traction) 02.94
  bone growth stimulator (surface) (transcutaneous) 99.86
  bone morphogenetic protein (Infuse™) (OP-1™) (recombinant) (rhBMP) 84.52
  Bryant's traction 93.44
    with reduction of fracture or dislocation—*see* Reduction, fracture and Reduction, dislocation
  Buck's traction 93.46
  caliper tongs (skull) (with synchronous skeletal traction) 02.94
  cast (fiberglass) (plaster) (plastic) NEC 93.53
    with reduction of fracture or dislocation—*see* Reduction, fracture and Reduction, dislocation
    spica 93.51
  cervical collar 93.52
    with reduction of fracture or dislocation—*see* Reduction, fracture and Reduction, dislocation
  clamp, cerebral aneurysm (Crutchfield) (Silverstone) 39.51
  croupette, croup tent 93.94
  crown (artificial) 23.41
  Crutchfield tongs (skull) (with synchronous skeletal traction) 02.94
  Dunlop's traction 93.44
    with reduction of fracture or dislocation—*see* Reduction, fracture and Reduction, dislocation
  elastic stockings 93.59
  electronic gaiter 93.59
  external fixator device (bone) 78.10
    carpal, metacarpal 78.14
    clavicle 78.11
    computer assisted (dependent) 84.73
    femur 78.15
    fibula 78.17
    humerus 78.12
    hybrid device or system 84.73
    Ilizarov 84.72
    monoplanar system or device 84.71
    patella 78.16
    pelvic 78.19
    phalanges (foot) (hand) 78.19
    radius 78.13

Application—*continued*
  ring device or system 84.72
  scapula 78.11
  Sheffield type 84.72
  specified site NEC 78.19
  tarsal, metatarsal 78.18
  thorax (ribs) (sternum) 78.11
  tibia 78.17
  ulna 78.13
  vertebrae 78.19
  forceps, with delivery—*see* Delivery, forceps
  graft—*see* Graft
  gravity (G.) suit 93.59
  intermittent pressure device 93.59
  Jewett extension brace 93.59
  Jobst pumping unit (reduction of edema) 93.59
  Lyman Smith traction 93.44
    with reduction of fracture or dislocation—*see* Reduction, fracture and Reduction, dislocation
  MAST (military anti-shock trousers) 93.58
  Minerva jacket 93.52
  minifixator device (bone)—*see category* 78.1
  neck support (molded) 93.52
  obturator (orthodontic) 24.7
  orthodontic appliance (obturator) (wiring) 24.7
  pelvic sling 93.44
    with reduction of fracture or dislocation—*see* Reduction, fracture and Reduction, dislocation
  peridontal splint (orthodontic) 24.7
  plaster jacket 93.51
    Minerva 93.52
  pressure
    dressing (bandage) (Gibney) (Robert Jones') (Shanz) 93.56
    trousers (anti-shock) (MAST) 93.58
  prosthesis for missing ear 18.71
  Russell's traction 93.44
    with reduction of fracture or dislocation—*see* Reduction, fracture and Reduction, dislocation
  splint, for immobilization (plaster) (pneumatic) (tray) 93.54
    with fracture reduction—*see* Reduction, fracture
  stereotactic head frame 93.59
  strapping (non-traction) 93.59
  substance, adhesion barrier 99.77
  Thomas collar 93.52
    with reduction of fracture or dislocation—*see* Reduction, fracture and Reduction, dislocation
  traction
    with reduction of fracture or dislocation—*see* Reduction, fracture and Reduction, dislocation
    adhesive tape (skin) 93.46
    boot 93.46
    Bryant's 93.44
    Buck's 93.46
    Cotrel's 93.42
    Dunlop's 93.44
    gallows 93.46
    Lyman Smith 93.44
    Russell's 93.44
    skeletal NEC 93.44
      intermittent 93.43
    skin, limbs NEC 93.46

Arthrodesis—*continued*
lumbosacral, lumbar NEC 81.08
  anterior column (interbody)
    anterolateral (anterior) technique 81.06
    posterior technique 81.08
  axial lumbar interbody fusion [AxiaLIF] 81.08
  direct lateral interbody fusion [DLIF} 81.06
  extreme lateral interbody fusion [XLIF] 81.06
  facet 81.07
  lateral transverse process technique 81.07
McKeever (metatarsophalangeal) 81.16
metacarpocarpal 81.26
metacarpophalangeal 81.27
metatarsophalangeal 81.16
midtarsal 81.14
pantalar 81.11
PLIF (posterior lumbar interbody fusion) 81.08
sacroiliac 81.08
shoulder 81.23
specified joint NEC 81.29
spinal (*see also* Fusion, spinal) 81.00
subtalar 81.13
tarsometatarsal 81.15
tibiotalar 81.11
TLIF (transforaminal lumbar interbody fusion) 81.08
toe NEC 77.58
  claw toe repair 77.57
  hammer toe repair 77.56
triple 81.12
wrist 81.26
Arthroendoscopy —*see* Arthroscopy
Arthroereisis, subtalar joint 81.18
Arthrogram, arthrography 88.32
temporomandibular 87.13
Arthrolysis 93.26
Arthroplasty (with fixation device) (with prosthesis) (with traction) 81.96
ankle 81.49
carpals 81.75
  with prosthetic implant 81.74
carpocarpal, carpometacarpal 81.75
  with prosthetic implant 81.74
Carroll and Taber (proximal interphalangeal joint) 81.72
cup (partial hip) 81.52
Curtis (interphalangeal joint) 81.72
elbow 81.85
  with prosthetic replacement (partial) (total) 81.84
femoral head NEC 81.40
  with prosthetic implant 81.52
finger(s) 81.72
  with prosthetic implant 81.71
foot (metatarsal) with joint replacement 81.57
Fowler (metacarpophalangeal joint) 81.72
hand (metacarpophalangeal) (interphalangeal) 81.72
  with prosthetic implant 81.71
hip (with bone graft) 81.40
  cup (partial hip) 81.52
  femoral head NEC 81.40
    with prosthetic implant 81.52
      with total replacement 81.51
  partial replacement 81.52
  total replacement 81.51
interphalangeal joint 81.72
  with prosthetic implant 81.71
Kessler (carpometacarpal joint) 81.74

Arthroplasty—*continued*
knee (*see also* Repair, knee) 81.47
  prosthetic replacement (bicompartmental) (hemijoint) (partial) (total) (tricompartmental) (unicompartmental) 81.54
  revision 81.55
metacarpophalangeal joint 81.72
  with prosthetic implant 81.71
shoulder 81.83
  prosthetic replacement (partial) 81.81
    total, NEC 81.80
      other 81.80
      reverse 81.88
  for recurrent dislocation 81.82
temporomandibular 76.5
toe NEC 77.58
  with prosthetic replacement 81.57
  for hallux valgus repair 77.59
wrist 81.75
  with prosthetic implant 81.74
  total replacement 81.73
Arthroscopy 80.20
ankle 80.27
elbow 80.22
finger 80.24
foot 80.28
hand 80.24
hip 80.25
knee 80.26
shoulder 80.21
specified site NEC 80.29
toe 80.28
wrist 80.23
Arthrostomy (*see also* Arthrotomy) 80.10
Arthrotomy 80.10
as operative approach—*omit code*
with
  arthrography—*see* Arthrogram
  arthroscopy—*see* Arthroscopy
  injection of drug 81.92
  removal of prosthesis without replacement —*see* Removal, prosthesis, joint structures
ankle 80.17
elbow 80.12
foot and toe 80.18
hand and finger 80.14
hip 80.15
knee 80.16
shoulder 80.11
specified site NEC 80.19
spine 80.19
wrist 80.13
Artificial
heart 37.52
  AbioCor® 37.52
  CardioWest™ (TAH-t) 37.52
insemination 69.92
kidney 39.95
rupture of membranes 73.09
Arytenoidectomy 30.29
Arytenoidopexy 31.69
Asai operation (larynx) 31.75
Aspiration
abscess—*see* Aspiration, by site
anterior chamber, eye (therapeutic) 12.91
  diagnostic 12.21
aqueous (eye) (humor) (therapeutic) 12.91
  diagnostic 12.21
ascites 54.91
Bartholin's gland (cyst) (percutaneous) 71.21

Aspiration—*continued*
biopsy—*see* Biopsy, by site
bladder (catheter) 57.0
  percutaneous (needle) 57.11
bone marrow (for biopsy) 41.31
  from donor for transplant 41.91
  stem cell 99.79
branchial cleft cyst 29.0
breast 85.91
bronchus 96.05
  with lavage 96.56
bursa (percutaneous) 83.94
  hand 82.92
calculus, bladder 57.0
cataract 13.3
  with
    phacoemulsification 13.41
    phacofragmentation 13.43
    posterior route 13.42
chest 34.91
cisternal 01.01
cranial (puncture) 01.09
craniobuccal pouch 07.72
craniopharyngioma 07.72
cul-de-sac (abscess) 70.0
curettage, uterus 69.59
  after abortion or delivery 69.52
  diagnostic 69.59
  to terminate pregnancy 69.51
cyst—*see* Aspiration, by site
diverticulum, pharynx 29.0
endotracheal 96.04
  with lavage 96.56
extradural 01.09
eye (anterior chamber) (therapeutic) 12.91
  diagnostic 12.21
fallopian tube 66.91
fascia 83.95
  hand 82.93
gallbladder (percutaneous) 51.01
hematoma—*see also* Aspiration, by site
  obstetrical 75.92
    incisional 75.91
hydrocele, tunica vaginalis 61.91
hygroma—*see* Aspiration, by site
hyphema 12.91
hypophysis 07.72
intracranial space (epidural) (extradural)
  (subarachnoid) (subdural) (ventricular) 01.09
  through previously implanted catheter or
    reservoir (Ommaya) (Rickham) 01.02
joint 81.91
  for arthrography—*see* Arthrogram
kidney (cyst) (pelvis) (percutaneous)
  (therapeutic) 55.92
  diagnostic 55.23
liver (percutaneous) 50.91
lung (percutaneous) (puncture) (needle) (trocar)
  33.93
middle ear 20.09
  with intubation 20.01
muscle 83.95
  hand 82.93
nail 86.01
nasal sinus 22.00
  by puncture 22.01
  through natural ostium 22.02
nasotracheal 96.04
  with lavage 96.56
orbit, diagnostic 16.22
ovary 65.91

Aspiration—*continued*
percutaneous—*see* Aspiration, by site
pericardium (wound) 37.0
pituitary gland 07.72
pleural cavity 34.91
prostate (percutaneous) 60.91
Rathke's pouch 07.72
seminal vesicles 60.71
seroma—*see* Aspiration, by site
skin 86.01
soft tissue NEC 83.95
  hand 82.93
spermatocele 63.91
spinal (puncture) 03.31
spleen (cyst) 41.1
stem cell 99.79
subarachnoid space (cerebral) 01.09
subcutaneous tissue 86.01
subdural space (cerebral) 01.09
tendon 83.95
  hand 82.93
testis 62.91
thymus 07.92
  thoracoscopic 07.95
thyroid (field) (gland) 06.01
  postoperative 06.02
trachea 96.04
  with lavage 96.56
  percutaneous 31.99
tunica vaginalis (hydrocele) (percutaneous) 61.91
vitreous (and replacement) 14.72
  diagnostic 14.11
Assessment
fitness to testify 94.11
mental status 94.11
nutritional status 89.39
personality 94.03
temperament 94.02
vocational 93.85
Assistance
cardiac—(*see also* Resuscitation, cardiac
  extracorporeal circulation) 39.61
endotracheal respiratory—*see category* 96.7
hepatic, extracorporeal 50.92
respiratory (endotracheal) (mechanical)—*see*
  Ventilation, mechanical
respiratory (mechanical) NEC —*see category*
  93.9
Astragalectomy 77.98
Asymmetrogammagram —*see* Scan,
  radioisotope
Atherectomy
cerebrovascular
  percutaneous
    extracranial vessel(s) 17.53
    intracranial vessel(s) 17.54
coronary
  percutaneous transluminal 17.55
peripheral (noncoronary) 17.56
Atriocommissuropexy (mitral valve) 35.12
Atrioplasty NEC 37.99
combined with repair of valvular and ventricular
  septal defects—*see* Repair, endocardial
  cushion defect
septum (heart) NEC 35.71
Atrioseptopexy (*see also* Repair, atrial septal
  defect) 35.71
Atrioseptoplasty (*see also* Repair, atrial septal
  defect) 35.71
Atrioseptostomy (balloon) 35.41
Atriotomy 37.11
Atrioventriculostomy (cerebral-heart) 02.32

Attachment
abutment (screw) for prosthetic ear device
  percutaneous 20.99
eye muscle
  orbicularis oculi to eyebrow 08.36
  rectus to frontalis 15.9
pedicle (flap) graft 86.74
  hand 86.73
  lip 27.57
  mouth 27.57
pharyngeal flap (for cleft palate repair) 27.62
  secondary or subsequent 27.63
prosthetic ear device, abutment 20.99
retina—*see* Reattachment, retina
Atticoantrostomy (ear) 20.49
Atticoantrotomy (ear) 20.49
Atticotomy (ear) 20.23
Audiometry (Békésy 5-tone) (impedance)
  (stapedial reflex response) (subjective) 95.41
Augmentation
bladder 57.87
breast—*see* Mammoplasty, augmentation
buttock ("fanny-lift") 86.89
chin 76.68
genioplasty 76.68
Augmentation—*continued*
mammoplasty—*see* Mammoplasty, augmentation
outflow tract (pulmonary valve) (gusset type)
    35.26
  in total repair of tetralogy or Fallot 35.81
  vocal cord(s) 31.0
Auriculectomy 18.39
Autograft —*see* Graft
Autologous —*see* Blood, transfusion
Autopsy 89.8
Autotransfusion (whole blood)—*see* Blood,
  transfusion
Autotransplant, autotransplantation —*see also*
  Reimplantation
adrenal tissue (heterotopic) (orthotopic) 07.45
kidney 55.61
lung—*see* Transplant, transplantation, lung
ovary 65.72
  laparoscopic 65.75
pancreatic tissue 52.81
parathyroid tissue (heterotopic) (orthotopic) 06.95
thyroid tissue (heterotopic) (orthotopic) 06.94
tooth 23.5
Avulsion, nerve (cranial) (peripheral) NEC 04.07
acoustic 04.01
phrenic 33.31
sympathetic 05.29
Azygography 88.63

B

Biopsy—*continued*

   transbronchoscopic needle aspiration (TBNA)
     33.24
     Wang needle (transbronchoscopic) 33.24
     washings 33.24
   bursa 83.21
   cardioesophageal (junction) 44.14
     closed (endoscopic) 44.14
     open 44.15
   cecum 45.25
     brush 45.25
     closed (endoscopic) 45.25
     open 45.26
   cerebral meninges NEC 01.11
     closed 01.11
     open 01.12
     percutaneous (needle) 01.11
   cervix (punch) 67.12
     conization (sharp) 67.2
   chest wall 34.23
   clitoris 71.11
   colon 45.25
     brush 45.25
     closed (endoscopic) 45.25
     open 45.26
   conjunctiva 10.21
   cornea 11.22
   cul-de-sac 70.23
   diaphragm 34.27
   duodenum 45.14
     brush 45.14
     closed (endoscopic) 45.14
     open 45.15
   ear (external) 18.12
     middle or inner 20.32
   endocervix 67.11
   endometrium NEC 68.16
     by
       aspiration curettage 69.59
       dilation and curettage 69.09
     closed (endoscopic) 68.16
     open 68.13
   epididymis 63.01
   esophagus 42.24
     closed (endoscopic) 42.24
     open 42.25
   extraocular muscle or tendon 15.01
   eye 16.23
     muscle (oblique) (rectus) 15.01
   eyelid 08.11
   fallopian tube 66.11
   fascia 83.21
   fetus 75.33
   gallbladder 51.12
     closed (endoscopic) 51.14
     open 51.13
     percutaneous (needle) 51.12
   ganglion (cranial) (peripheral) NEC 04.11
     closed 04.11
     open 04.12
     percutaneous (needle) 04.11
     sympathetic nerve 05.11
   gum 24.11
   heart 37.25
   hypophysis (*see also* Biopsy, pituitary gland)
     07.15
   ileum 45.14
     brush 45.14
     closed (endoscopic) 45.14
     open 45.15

Biopsy—*continued*

   intestine NEC 45.27
     large 45.25
       brush 45.25
       closed (endoscopic) 45.25
       open 45.26
     small 45.14
       brush 45.14
       closed (endoscopic) 45.14
       open 45.15
   intra-abdominal mass 54.24
     closed 54.24
     percutaneous (needle) 54.24
   iris 12.22
   jejunum 45.14
     brush 45.14
     closed (endoscopic) 45.14
     open 45.15
   joint structure (aspiration) 80.30
     ankle 80.37
     elbow 80.32
     foot and toe 80.38
     hand and finger 80.34
     hip 80.35
     knee 80.36
     shoulder 80.31
     specified site NEC 80.39
     spine 80.39
     wrist 80.33
   kidney 55.23
     closed 55.23
     open 55.24
     percutaneous (aspiration) (needle) 55.23
   labia 71.11
   lacrimal
     gland 09.11
     sac 09.12
   larynx 31.43
     brush 31.43
     closed (endoscopic) 31.43
     open 31.45
   lip 27.23
   liver 50.11
     closed 50.11
     laparoscopic 50.14
     open 50.12
     percutaneous (aspiration) (needle) 50.11
     transjugular 50.13
     transvenous 50.13
   lung NEC 33.27
     brush 33.24
     closed (percutaneous) (needle) 33.26
       brush 33.24
       endoscopic 33.27
         brush 33.24
     endoscopic 33.27
       brush 33.24
     open 33.28
     thoracoscopic 33.20
     transbronchial 33.27
     transthoracic 33.26
   lymphatic structure (channel) (node) (vessel)
     40.11
   mediastinum NEC 34.25
     closed 34.25
     open 34.26
     percutaneous (needle) 34.25
   meninges (cerebral) NEC 01.11
     closed 01.11
     open 01.12
     percutaneous (needle) 01.11
     spinal 03.32

C

Closure—*continued*

  atrial septal defect (*see also* Repair, atrial septal
    defect) 35.71
    with umbrella device (King-Mills type) 35.52
    combined with repair of valvular and
      ventricular septal defects—*see* Repair,
      endocardial cushion defect
  bronchostomy 33.42
  cecostomy 46.52
  cholecystostomy 51.92
  cleft hand 82.82
  colostomy 46.52
  cystostomy 57.82
  diastema (alveolar) (dental) 24.8
  disrupted abdominal wall (postoperative) 54.61
  duodenostomy 46.51
  encephalocele 02.12
  endocardial cushion defect (*see also* Repair,
    endocardial cushion defect) 35.73
  enterostomy 46.50
  esophagostomy 42.83
  fenestration
    aorticopulmonary 39.59
    septal, heart (*see also* Repair, heart, septum)
      35.70
  filtering bleb, corneoscleral (postglaucoma) 12.66
  fistula
    abdominothoracic 34.83
    anorectal 48.73
    anovaginal 70.73
    antrobuccal 22.71
    anus 49.73
    aorticopulmonary (fenestration) 39.59
    aortoduodenal 39.59
    appendix 47.92
    biliary tract 51.79
    bladder NEC 57.84
    branchial cleft 29.52
    bronchocutaneous 33.42
    bronchoesophageal 33.42
    bronchomediastinal 34.73
    bronchopleural 34.73
    bronchopleurocutaneous 34.73
    bronchopleuromediastinal 34.73
    bronchovisceral 33.42
    bronchus 33.42
    cecosigmoidal 46.76
    cerebrospinal fluid 02.12
    cervicoaural 18.79
    cervicosigmoidal 67.62
    cervicovesical 57.84
    cervix 67.62
    cholecystocolic 51.93
    cholecystoduodenal 51.93
    cholecystoenteric 51.93
    cholecystogastric 51.93
    cholecystojejunal 51.93
    cisterna chyli 40.63
    colon 46.76
    colovaginal 70.72
    common duct 51.72
    cornea 11.49
      with lamellar graft (homograft) 11.62
        autograft 11.61
    diaphragm 34.83
    duodenum 46.72
    ear, middle 19.9
    ear drum 19.4
    enterocolic 46.74
    enterocutaneous 46.74
    enterouterine 69.42

Closure—*continued*

    enterovaginal 70.74
    enterovesical 57.83
    esophagobronchial 33.42
    esophagocutaneous 42.84
    esophagopleurocutaneous 34.73
    esophagotracheal 31.73
    esophagus NEC 42.84
    fecal 46.79
    gallbladder 51.93
    gastric NEC 44.63
    gastrocolic 44.63
    gastroenterocolic 44.63
    gastroesophageal 42.84
    gastrojejunal 44.63
    gastrojejunocolic 44.63
    heart valve—*see* Repair, heart, valve
    hepatic duct 51.79
    hepatopleural 34.73
    hepatopulmonary 34.73
    ileorectal 46.74
    ileosigmoidal 46.74
    ileovesical 57.83
    ileum 46.74
    in ano 49.73
    intestine 46.79
      large 46.76
      small NEC 46.74
    intestinocolonic 46.74
    intestinoureteral 56.84
    intestinouterine 69.42
    intestinovaginal 70.74
    intestinovesical 57.83
    jejunum 46.74
    kidney 55.83
    lacrimal 09.99
    laryngotracheal 31.62
    larynx 31.62
    lymphatic duct, left (thoracic) 40.63
    mastoid (antrum) 19.9
    mediastinobronchial 34.73
    mediastinocutaneous 34.73
    mouth (external) 27.53
    nasal 21.82
      sinus 22.71
    nasolabial 21.82
    nasopharyngeal 21.82
    oroantral 22.71
    oronasal 21.82
    oval window (ear) 20.93
    pancreaticoduodenal 52.95
    perilymph 20.93
    perineorectal 48.73
    perineosigmoidal 46.76
    perineourethroscrotal 58.43
    perineum 71.72
    perirectal 48.93
    pharyngoesophageal 29.53
    pharynx NEC 29.53
    pleura, pleural NEC 34.93
    pleurocutaneous 34.73
    pleuropericardial 37.49
    pleuroperitoneal 34.83
    pulmonoperitoneal 34.83
    rectolabial 48.73
    rectoureteral 56.84
    rectourethral 58.43
    rectovaginal 70.73
    rectovesical 57.83
    rectovesicovaginal 57.83
    rectovulvar 48.73

Cordotomy
  spinal (bilateral) NEC 03.29
    percutaneous 03.21
  vocal 31.3
Corectomy 12.12
Corelysis 12.35
Coreoplasty 12.35
Corneoconjunctivoplasty 11.53
Corpectomy (vertebral) 80.99
  with diskectomy 80.99
Correction —*see also* Repair
  atresia
    esophageal 42.85
      by magnetic forces 42.99
    external meatus (ear) 18.6
    nasopharynx, nasopharyngeal 29.4
    rectum 48.0
    tricuspid 35.94
  atrial septal defect (*see also* Repair, atrial septal
      defect) 35.71
    combined with repair of valvular and
        ventricular septal defects—*see* Repair,
        endocardial cushion defect
  blepharoptosis (*see also* Repair, blepharoptosis)
      08.36
  bunionette (with osteotomy) 77.54
  chordee 64.42
  claw toe 77.57
  cleft
    lip 27.54
    palate 27.62
  clubfoot NEC 83.84
  coarctation of aorta
    with
      anastomosis 38.34
      graft replacement 38.44
  cornea NEC 11.59
    refractive NEC 11.79
      epikeratophakia 11.76
      keratomileusis 11.71
      keratophakia 11.72
      radial keratotomy 11.75
  esophageal atresia 42.85
    by magnetic forces 42.99
  everted lacrimal punctum 09.71
  eyelid
    ptosis (*see also* Repair, blepharoptosis) 08.36
    retraction 08.38
  fetal defect 75.36
  forcible, of musculoskeletal deformity
      NEC 93.29
  hammer toe 77.56
  hydraulic pressure, open surgery (for) penile
      prosthesis, inflatable 64.99
    urinary sphincter, artificial 58.99
  intestinal malrotation 46.80
    large 46.82
    small 46.81
  inverted uterus—*see* Repair, inverted uterus
  lymphedema (of limb) 40.9
    excision with graft 40.9
    obliteration of lymphatics 40.9
    transplantation of autogenous lymphatics 40.9
  nasopharyngeal atresia 29.4
  overlapping toes 77.58
  palate (cleft) 27.62
  prognathism NEC 76.64
  prominent ear 18.5
  punctum (everted) 09.71
  spinal pseudarthrosis —*see* Refusion, spinal
  syndactyly 86.85

Correction—*continued*
  tetralogy of Fallot
    one-stage 35.81
    partial—*see specific procedure*
    total 35.81
  total anomalous pulmonary venous connection
    one-stage 35.82
    partial—*see specific procedure*
    total 35.82
  transposition, great arteries, total 35.84
  tricuspid atresia 35.94
  truncus arteriosus
    one-stage 35.83
    partial—*see specific procedure*
    total 35.83
  ureteropelvic junction 55.87
  ventricular septal defect (*see also* Repair,
      ventricular septal defect) 35.72
    combined with repair of valvular and atrial
        septal defects—*see* Repair, endocardial
        cushion defect
Costectomy 77.91
  with lung excision—*see* Excision, lung
  associated with thoracic operation—*omit code*
Costochondrectomy 77.91
  associated with thoracic operation—*omit code*
Costosternoplasty (pectus excavatum repair)
    34.74
Costotomy 77.31
Costotransversectomy 77.91
  associated with thoracic operation—*omit code*
Counseling (for) NEC 94.49
  alcoholism 94.46
  drug addiction 94.45
  employers 94.49
  family (medical) (social) 94.49
  marriage 94.49
  ophthalmologic (with instruction) 95.36
  pastoral 94.49
Countershock, cardiac NEC 99.62
Coventry Operation (tibial wedge osteotomy)
    77.27
CPAP (continuous positive airway pressure)
    93.90
  delivered by
    endotracheal tube —*see* category 96.7
    tracheostomy —*see* category 96.7
Craniectomy 01.25
  linear (opening of cranial suture) 02.01
  reopening of site 01.23
  strip (opening of cranial suture) 02.01
Cranioclasis, fetal 73.8
Cranioplasty 02.06
  with synchronous repair of encephalocele 02.12
Craniotomy 01.24
  as operative approach—*omit code*
  fetal 73.8
  for decompression of fracture 02.02
  reopening of site 01.23
Craterization, bone (*see also* Excision, lesion,
    bone) 77.60
Crawford operation (tarso-frontalis sling of
    eyelid) 08.32
Creation —*see also* Formation
  cardiac device (defibrillator) (pacemaker) pocket
    with initial insertion of cardiac device—*omit
      code*
  new site (skin) (subcutaneous) 37.79

Culdoplasty 70.92
  with graft or prosthesis 70.93
Culdoscopy (exploration) (removal of foreign
  body or lesion) 70.22
Culdotomy 70.12
Culp-Deweerd operation (spiral flap
  pyeloplasty) 55.87
Culp-Scardino operation (ureteral flap
  pyeloplasty) 55.87
Culture (and sensitivity)—*see* Examination,
  microscopic
Curettage (with packing) (with secondary
  closure)—*see also* Dilation and curettage
  adenoids 28.6
  anus 49.39
    endoscopic 49.31
  bladder 57.59
    transurethral 57.49
  bone (*see also* Excision, lesion, bone) 77.60
  brain 01.59
  bursa 83.39
    hand 82.29
  cartilage (*see also* Excision, lesion, joint) 80.80
  cerebral meninges 01.51
  chalazion 08.25
  conjunctiva (trachoma follicles) 10.33
  corneal epithelium 11.41
    for smear or culture 11.21
  ear, external 18.29
  eyelid 08.25
  joint (*see also* Excision, lesion, joint) 80.80
  meninges (cerebral) 01.51
    spinal 03.4
  muscle 83.32
    hand 82.22
  nerve (peripheral) 04.07
    sympathetic 05.29
  sclera 12.84
  skin 86.3
  spinal cord (meninges) 03.4
  subgingival 24.31
  tendon 83.39
    hand 82.29
    sheath 83.31
      hand 82.21
  uterus (with dilation) 69.09
    aspiration (diagnostic) NEC 69.59
      after abortion or delivery 69.52
      to terminate pregnancy 69.51
    following delivery or abortion 69.02
Curette evacuation, lens 13.2
Curtis operation (interphalangeal joint
  arthroplasty) 81.72
Cutaneolipectomy 86.83
Cutdown, venous 38.94
Cutting
  nerve (crania]) (peripheral) NEC 04.03
    acoustic 04.01
    auditory 04.01
    root, spinal 03.1
    sympathetic 05.0
    trigeminal 04.02
    vestibular 04.01
  pedicle (flap) graft 86.71
  pylorus (with wedge resection) 43.3
  spinal nerve root 03.1
  ureterovesical orifice 56.1
  urethral sphincter 58.5

CVP (central venous pressure monitoring) 89.62
Cyclectomy (ciliary body) 12.44
  eyelid margin 08.20
Cyclicotomy 12.55
Cycloanemization 12.74
Cyclocryotherapy 12.72
Cyclodialysis (initial) (subsequent) 12.55
Cyclodiathermy (penetrating) (surface) 12.71
Cycloelectrolysis 12.71
Cyclophotocoagulation 12.73
Cyclotomy 12.55
Cystectomy —*see also* Excision, lesion, by site
  gallbladder—*see* Cholecystectomy
  urinary (partial) (subtotal) 57.6
    complete (with urethrectomy) 57.79
    radical 57.71
      with pelvic exenteration (female) 68.8
    total (with urethrectomy) 57.79
Cystocolostomy 57.88
Cystogram, cystography NEC 87.77
Cystolitholapaxy 57.0
Cystolithotomy 57.19
Cystometrogram 89.22
Cystopexy NEC 57.89
Cystoplasty NEC 57.89
Cystoproctostomy 57.88
Cystoprostatectomy, radical 57.71
Cystopyelography 87.74
Cystorrhaphy 57.81
Cystoscopy (transurethral) 57.32
  with biopsy 57.33
  for
    control of hemorrhage
      bladder 57.93
      prostate 60.94
      retrograde pyelography 87.74
  ileal conduit 56.35
  through stoma (artificial) 57.31
Cystostomy
  closed (suprapubic) (percutaneous) 57.17
  open (suprapubic) 57.18
  percutaneous (closed) (suprapubic) 57.17
  suprapubic
    closed 57.17
    open 57.18
Cystotomy (open) (for removal of calculi) 57.19
Cystourethrogram (retrograde) (voiding) 87.76
Cystourethropexy (by) 59.79
  levator muscle sling 59.71
  retropubic suspension 59.5
  suprapubic suspension 59.4
Cystourethroplasty 57.85
Cystourethroscopy 57.32
  with biopsy
    bladder 57.33
    ureter 56.33
Cytology —*see* Examination, microscopic

D

Decompression—*continued*
  pericardium 37.0
  rectum 48.0
  skull fracture 02.02
  spinal cord (canal) 03.09
  tarsal tunnel 04.44
  tendon (sheath) 83.01
    hand 82.01
  thoracic outlet
    by
      myotomy (division of scalenus anticus
        muscle) 83.19
      tenotomy 83.13
  trigeminal (nerve root) 04.41
Decortication
  arterial 05.25
  brain 01.51
  cerebral meninges 01.51
  heart 37.31
  kidney 55.91
  lung (partial) (total) 34.51
    thoracoscopic 34.52
  nasal turbinates—*see* Turbinectomy
  nose 21.89
  ovary 65.29
    laparoscopic 65.25
  periarterial 05.25
  pericardium 37.31
  ventricle, heart (complete) 37.31
Decoy, E2F 00.16
Deepening
  alveolar ridge 24.5
  buccolabial sulcus 24.91
  lingual sulcus 24.91
Defatting, flap or pedicle graft 86.75
Defibrillation, electric (external) (internal) 99.62
  automatic cardioverter/defibrillator —*see*
    category 37.9
de Grandmont operation (tarsectomy) 08.35
Delaying of pedicle graft 86.71
Delivery (with)
  assisted spontaneous 73.59
  breech extraction (assisted) 72.52
    partial 72.52
      with forceps to aftercoming head 72.51
    total 72.54
      with forceps to aftercoming head 72.53
    unassisted (spontaneous delivery)—*omit code*
  cesarean section—*see* Cesarean section
  Credé maneuver 73.59
  De Lee maneuver 72.4
  forceps 72.9
    application to aftercoming head (Piper) 72.6
      with breech extraction
        partial 72.51
        total 72.53
    Barton's 72.4
    failed 73.3
    high 72.39
      with episiotomy 72.31
    low (outlet) 72.0
      with episiotomy 72.1
    mid 72.29
      with episiotomy 72.21
    outlet (low) 72.0
      with episiotomy 72.1
    rotation of fetal head 72.4
    trial 73.3
  instrumental NEC 72.9
    specified NEC 72.8
  key-in-lock rotation 72.4

Delivery—*continued*
  Kielland rotation 72.4
  Malström's extraction 72.79
    with episiotomy 72.71
  manually assisted (spontaneous) 73.59
  spontaneous (unassisted) 73.59
    assisted 73.59
  vacuum extraction 72.79
    with episiotomy 72.71
Delorme operation
  pericardiectomy 37.31
  proctopexy 48.76
  repair of prolapsed rectum 48.76
  thoracoplasty 33.34
Denervation
  aortic body 39.89
  carotid body 39.89
  facet, percutaneous (radio frequency) 03.96
  ovarian 65.94
  paracervical uterine 69.3
  uterosacral 69.3
Denker operation (radical maxillary antrotomy)
  22.31
Dennis-Barco operation —*see* Repair, hernia,
  femoral
Denonvillier operation (limited rhinoplasty)
  21.86
Densitometry, bone (serial)
  (radiographic) 88.98
Depilation, skin 86.92
Derlacki operation (tympanoplasty) 19.4
Dermabond 86.59
Dermabrasion (laser) 86.25
  for wound debridement 86.28
Derotation —*see* Reduction, torsion
Desensitization
  allergy 99.12
  psychologic 94.33
Desmotomy (*see also* Division, ligament) 80.40
Destruction
  breast 85.20
  chorioretinopathy (*see also* Destruction, lesion,
    choroid) 14.29
  ciliary body 12.74
  epithelial downgrowth, anterior chamber 12.93
  fallopian tube 66.39
    with
      crushing (and ligation) 66.31
        by endoscopy laparoscopy) 66.21
      division (and ligation) 66.32
        by endoscopy (culdoscopy) (hysteroscopy)
          (laparoscopy) (peritoneoscopy) 66.22
      ligation 66.39
        with
          crushing 66.31
            by endoscopy (laparoscopy) 66.21
          division 66.32
            by endoscopy (culdoscopy)
              (hysteroscopy) (laparoscopy)
              (peritoneoscopy) 66.22
    unilateral 66.92
  fetus 73.8
  hemorrhoids 49.49
    by
      cryotherapy 49.44
      sclerotherapy 49.42
  inner ear NEC 20.79
    by injection 20.72
  intervertebral disc NOS 80.50
    by injection 80.52
    by other specified method 80.59

Destruction—*continued*
    radiation therapy 14.26
    salivary gland NEC 26.29
      by marsupialization 26.21
    sclera 12.84
    scrotum 61.3
    skin NEC 86.3
    sphincter of Oddi 51.69
      endoscopic 51.64
    spinal cord (meninges) 03.4
    spleen 41.42
      by marsupialization 41.41
    stomach NEC 43.49
      by excision 43.42
        endoscopic 43.41
      endoscopic 43.41
    subcutaneous tissue NEC 86.3
    testis 62.2
    tongue 25.1
    urethra (excisional) 58.39
      endoscopic 58.31
    uterus 68.29
  nerve (cranial) (peripheral) (by cryoanalgesia) (by
    radio frequency) 04.2
    sympathetic, by injection of neurolytic agent
      05.32
    neuroma 04.07
      acoustic
        by craniotomy 04.01
        by radiosurgery 04.07
      cranial 04.07
      Morton's 04.07
      peripheral
      Morton's 04.07
  neuroma
    acoustic 04.01
      by craniotomy 04.01
      by stereotactic radiosurgery 92.30
        cobalt 60 92.32
        linear accelerator (LINAC) 92.31
        multi-source 92.32
        particle beam 92.33
        particulate 92.33
        radiosurgery NEC 92.39
        single source photon 92.31
  prostate (prostatic tissue)
    by
      cryotherapy 60.62
      microwave 60.96
      radiofrequency 60.97
      transurethral microwave thermotherapy
        (TUMT) 60.96
      transurethral needle ablation (TUNA) 60.97
      TULIP (transurethral (ultrasound) guided laser
        induced prostatectomy) 60.21
      TUMT (transurethral microwave
        thermotherapy) 60.96
      TUNA (transurethral needle ablation) 60.97
  semicircular canals, by injection 20.72
  tissue of heart —*see* Excision, lesion, heart
  vestibule, by injection 20.72
Detachment, uterosacral ligaments 69.3
Determination
  mental status (clinical) (medicolegal)
    (psychiatric) NEC 94.11
  psychologic NEC 94.09
  vital capacity (pulmonary) 89.37
Detorsion
  intestine (twisted) (volvulus) 46.80
    large 46.82
      endoscopic (balloon) 46.85
    small 46.81

Detorsion—*continued*
  kidney 55.84
  ovary 65.95
  spermatic cord 63.52
    with orchiopexy 62.5
  testis 63.52
    with orchiopexy 62.5
  volvulus 46.80
    endoscopic (balloon) 46.85
Detoxification therapy 94.25
  alcohol 94.62
    with rehabilitation 94.63
    combined alcohol and drug 94.68
      with rehabilitation 94.69
  drug 94.65
    with rehabilitation 94.66
    combined alcohol and drug 94.68
      with rehabilitation 94.69
Devascularization, stomach 44.99
Device
  CorCap™ 37.41
  external fixator—*see* Fixator, external
Dewebbing
  esophagus 42.01
  syndactyly (fingers) (toes) 86.85
Dextrorotation —*see* Reduction, torsion
Dialysis
  hemodiafiltration, hemofiltration (extracorporeal)
    39.95
  kidney (extracorporeal) 39.95
  liver 50.92
  peritoneal 54.98
  renal (extracorporeal) 39.95
Diaphanoscopy
  nasal sinuses 89.35
  skull (newborn) 89.16
Diaphysectomy —*see* category 77.8
Diathermy 93.34
  choroid—*see* Diathermy, retina
  nasal turbinates 21.61
  retina
    for
      destruction of lesion 14.21
      reattachment 14.51
      repair of tear 14.31
  surgical—*see* Destruction, lesion, by site
  turbinates (nasal) 21.61
Dickson operation (fascial transplant) 83.82
Dickson-Diveley operation (tendon transfer and
  arthrodesis to correct claw toe) 77.57
Dieffenbach operation (hip disarticulation) 84.18
Dilation
  achalasia 42.92
  ampulla of Vater 51.81
    endoscopic 51.84
  anus, anal (sphincter) 96.23
  biliary duct
    endoscopic 51.84
    pancreatic duct 52.99
      endoscopic 52.98
    percutaneous (endoscopy) 51.98
    sphincter
      of Oddi 51.81
        endoscopic 51.84
      pancreatic 51.82
        endoscopic 51.85
  bladder 96.25
    neck 57.92
  bronchus 33.91
  cervix (canal) 67.0
    obstetrical 73.1

Division—*continued*
  muscle 83.19
    hand 82.19
  nasolacrimal duct stricture (with drainage) 09.59
  nerve (cranial) (peripheral) NEC 04.03
    acoustic 04.01
    adrenal gland 07.42
    auditory 04.01
    glossopharyngeal 29.92
    lacrimal branch 05.0
    laryngeal (external) (recurrent) (superior) 31.91
    vestibular 04.01
  phrenic 04.03
    for collapse of lung 33.31
  root, spinal or intraspinal 03.1
  sympathetic 05.0
  tracts
    cerebral 01.32
    spinal cord 03.29
      percutaneous 03.21
    trigeminal 04.02
    vagus (*see also* Vagotomy) 44.00
    vestibular 04.01
  otosclerotic process or material, middle ear 19.0
  papillary muscle (heart) 35.31
  patent ductus arteriosus 38.85
  penile adhesions 64.93
  posterior synechiae 12.33
  pylorus (with wedge resection) 43.3
  rectum (stricture) 48.91
  scalenus anticus muscle 83.19
  Skene's gland 71.3
  soft tissue NEC 83.19
    hand 82.19
  sphincter
    anal (external) (internal) 49.59
      left lateral 49.51
      posterior 49.52
    cardiac 42.7
    of Oddi 51.82
      endoscopic 51.85
    pancreatic 51.82
      endoscopic 51.85
  spinal
    cord tracts 03.29
      percutaneous 03.21
    nerve root 03.1
  symblepharon (with insertion of conformer) 10.5
  synechiae
    endometrial 68.21
    iris (posterior) 12.33
      anterior 12.32
  tarsorrhaphy 08.02
  tendon 83.13
    Achilles 83.11
    adductor (hip) 83.12
    hand 82.11
  trabeculae carneae cordis (heart) 35.35
  tympanum 20.23
  uterosacral ligaments 69.3
  vaginal septum 70.14
  vas deferens 63.71
  vein (with ligation) 38.80
    abdominal 38.87
    head and neck NEC 38.82
    intracranial NEC 38.81
    lower limb 38.89
      varicose 38.59
    thoracic NEC 38.85
    upper limb 38.83

Division—*continued*
  varicose 38.50
    abdominal 38.57
    head and neck NEC 38.52
    intracranial NEC 38.51
    lower limb 38.59
    thoracic NEC 38.55
    upper limb 39.53
  vitreous, cicatricial bands (posterior approach)
    14.74
    anterior approach 14.73
Doleris operation (shortening of round
  ligaments) 69.22
D'Ombrain operation (excision of pterygium
  with corneal graft) 11.32
Domestic tasks therapy 93.83
Dopplergram, Doppler flow mapping —*see
  also* Ultrasonography
  aortic arch 88.73
  head and neck 88.71
  heart 88.72
  intraoperative transcranial 00.94
  thorax NEC 88.73
Dorrance operation (push-back operation for
  cleft palate) 27.62
Dotter operation (transluminal angioplasty)
  39.59
Douche, vagina 96.44
Douglas operation (suture of tongue to lip for
  micrognathia) 25.59
Downstream® System (AO therapy) (aqueous
  oxygen) 00.49
Doyle operation (paracervical uterine
  denervation) 69.3
Drainage
  by
    anastomosis—*see* Anastomosis
    aspiration—*see* Aspiration
    incision—*see* Incision
  abdomen 54.19
    percutaneous 54.91
  abscess—*see also* Drainage, by site and Incision,
    by site
    appendix 47.2
      with appendectomy 47.09
        laparoscopic 47.01
    parapharyngeal (oral) (transcervical) 28.0
    peritonsillar (oral) (transcervical) 28.0
    retropharyngeal (oral) (transcervical) 28.0
    thyroid (field) (gland) 06.09
      percutaneous (needle) 06.01
      postoperative 06.02
    tonsil, tonsillar (oral) (transcervical) 28.0
  antecubital fossa 86.04
  appendix 47.91
    with appendectomy 47.09
      laparoscopic 47.01
    abscess 47.2
      with appendectomy 47.09
        laparoscopic 47.01
  axilla 86.04
  bladder (without incision) 57.0
    by indwelling catheter 57.94
      percutaneous suprapubic (closed) 57.17
      suprapubic NEC 57.18
  buccal space 27.0

Drainage—*continued*
sublingual space 27.0
submental space 27.0
subphrenic space 54.19
   percutaneous 54.91
supraclavicular fossa 86.04
temporal pouches 27.0
tendon (sheath) 83.01
   hand 82.01
thenar space 82.04
thorax (closed) 34.04
   open (by incision) 34.09
   thoracoscopic 34.06
thyroglossal tract (by incision) 06.09
   by aspiration 06.01
thyroid (field) (gland) (by incision) 06.09
   by aspiration 06.01
   postoperative 06.02
tonsil 28.0
tunica vaginalis 61.0
ureter (by catheter) 59.8
   by
      anastomosis NEC (*see also* Anastomosis,
         ureter) 56.79
      incision 56.2
ventricle (cerebral) (incision)
   by
      anastomosis—*see* Shunt, ventricular
      aspiration 01.09
         through previously implanted catheter 01.02
      extracranial ventricular shunt —*see* category
         02.3
vertebral column 03.09
Drawing test 94.08
Dressing
burn 93.57
ulcer 93.56
wound 93.57
Drilling
bone—*see also* Incision, bone 77.10
ovary 65.99
Drotrecogin alfa (activated), infusion 00.11
Ductogram, mammary 87.35
Duhamel operation (abdominoperineal
   pull-through) 48.65
Dührssen's
incisions (cervix, to assist delivery) 73.93
operation (vaginofixation of uterus) 69.22
Dunn operation (triple arthrodesis) 81.12
Duodenectomy 45.62
with
   gastrectomy—*see* Gastrectomy
   pancreatectomy—*see* Pancreatectomy
Duodenocholedochotomy 51.51
Duodenoduodenostomy 45.91
proximal to distal segment 45.62
Duodenoileostomy 45.91
Duodenojejunostomy 45.91
Duodenoplasty 46.79
Duodenorrhaphy 46.71
Duodenoscopy 45.13
through stoma (artificial) 45.12
transabdominal (operative) 45.11
Duodenostomy 46.39
Duodenotomy 45.01
Dupuytren operation
fasciectomy 82.35
fasciotomy 82.12
   with excision 82.35
shoulder disarticulation 84.08
Durabond 86.59

Duraplasty 02.12
Durham (Caldwell) operation (transfer of biceps
   femoris tendon) 83.75
DuToit and Roux operation (staple
   capsulorrhaphy of shoulder) 81.82
DuVries operation (tenoplasty) 83.88
Dwyer operation
fasciotomy 83.14
soft tissue release NEC 83.84
wedge osteotomy, calcaneus 77.28

E

Epididymectomy 63.4
  with orchidectomy (unilateral) 62.3
    bilateral 62.41
Epididymogram 87.93
Epididymoplasty 63.59
Epididymorrhaphy 63.81
Epididymotomy 63.92
Epididymovasostomy 63.83
Epiglottidectomy 30.21
Epikeratophakia 11.76
Epilation
  eyebrow (forceps) 08.93
    cryosurgical 08.92
    electrosurgical 08.91
  eyelid (forceps) NEC 08.93
    cryosurgical 08.92
    electrosurgical 08.91
  skin 86.92
Epiphysiodesis (*see also* Arrest, bone
    growth)—*see* category 78.2
Epiphysiolysis (*see also* Arrest, bone
    growth)—*see* 78.2
Epiploectomy 54.4
Epiplopexy 54.74
Epiplorrhaphy 54.74
Episioperineoplasty 71.79
Episioperineorrhaphy 71.71
  obstetrical 75.69
Episioplasty 71.79
Episioproctotomy 73.6
Episiorrhaphy 71.71
  following episiotomy—*see* Episiotomy
  for obstetrical laceration 75.69
Episiotomy (with subsequent episiorrhaphy) 73.6
  high forceps 72.31
  low forceps 72.1
  mid forceps 72.21
  nonobstetrical 71.09
  outlet forceps 72.1
EPS (electrophysiologic stimulation)
  as part of intraoperative testing —*omit code*
  catheter based invasive electrophysiologic testing
    37.26
  device interrogation only without arrhythmia
    induction (bedside check) 89.45-89.49
  noninvasive programmed electrical stimulation
    (NIPS) 37.20
Eptifibatide, infusion 99.20
Equalization, leg
  lengthening—*see* category 78.3
  shortening—*see* category 78.2
Equilibration (occlusal) 24.8
Equiloudness balance 95.43
ERC (endoscopic) retrograde cholangiography
    51.11
ERCP (endoscopic retrograde
    cholangiopancreatography) 51.10
  cannulation of pancreatic duct 52.93
ERG (electroretinogram) 95.21
ERP (endoscopic retrograde pancreatography)
    52.13
Eruption, tooth, surgical 24.6
Erythrocytapheresis, therapeutic 99.73
Escharectomy 86.22
Escharotomy 86.09
Esophageal voice training (postlaryngectomy)
    93.73
Esophagectomy 42.40
  abdominothoracocervical (combined)
    (synchronous) 42.42

Esophagectomy—*continued*
  partial or subtotal 42.41
  total 42.42
Esophagocologastrostomy (intrathoracic) 42.55
  antesternal or antethoracic 42.65
Esophagocolostomy (intrathoracic) NEC 42.56
  with interposition of Colon 42.55
  antesternal or antethoracic NEC 42.66
    with interposition of colon 42.65
Esophagoduodenostomy (intrathoracic) NEC
    42.54
  with
    complete gastrectomy 43.99
      interposition of small bowel 42.53
Esophagoenterostomy (intrathoracic) NEC (*see
    also* Anastomosis, esophagus, to intestinal
    segment) 42.54
  antesternal or antethoracic (*see also* Anastomosis,
    esophagus, antesternal, to intestinal segment)
    42.64
Esophagoesophagostomy (intrathoracic) 42.51
  antesternal or antethoracic 42.61
Esophagogastrectomy 43.99
Esophagogastroduodenoscopy (EGD) 45.13
  with closed biopsy 45.16
  through stoma (artificial) 45.12
  transabdominal (operative) 45.11
Esophagogastromyotomy 42.7
Esophagogastropexy 44.65
Esophagogastroplasty 44.65
Esophagogastroscopy NEC 44.13
  through stoma (artificial) 44.12
  transabdominal (operative) 44.11
Esophagogastrostomy (intrathoracic) 42.52
  with partial gastrectomy 43.5
  antesternal or antethoracic 42.62
Esophagoileostomy (intrathoracic) NEC 42.54
  with interposition of small bowel 42.53
  antesternal or antethoracic NEC 42.64
    with interposition of small bowel 42.63
Esophagojejunostomy (intrathoracic) NEC 42.54
  with
    complete gastrectomy 43.99
    interposition of small bowel 42.53
  antesternal or antethoracic NEC 42.64
    with interposition of small bowel 42.63
Esophagomyotomy 42.7
Esophagoplasty NEC 42.89
Esophagorrhaphy 42.82
Esophagoscopy NEC 42.23
  with closed biopsy 42.24
  by incision (operative) 42.21
  through stoma (artificial) 42.22
  transabdominal (operative) 42.21
Esophagostomy 42.10
  cervical 42.11
  thoracic 42.19
Esophagotomy NEC 42.09
Estes operation (ovary) 65.72
  laparoscopic 65.75
Estlander operation (thoracoplasty) 33.34
ESWL (extracorporeal shock wave lithotripsy)
    NEC 98.59
  bile duct 98.52
  bladder 98.51
  gallbladder 98.52
  kidney 98.51
  Kock pouch (urinary diversion) 98.51
  renal pelvis 98.51
  specified site NEC 98.59
  ureter 98.51

Ethmoidectomy 22.63
Ethmoidotomy 22.51
Evacuation
  abscess—*see* Drainage, by site
  anterior chamber (eye) (aqueous) (hyphema)
    12.91
Evacuation—*continued*
  cyst—*see also* Excision, lesion, by site
    breast 85.91
    kidney 55.01
    liver 50.29
  hematoma—*see also* Incision, hematoma
    obstetrical 75.92
      incisional 75.91
  hemorrhoids (thrombosed) 49.47
  pelvic blood clot (by incision) 54.19
    by
      culdocentesis 70.0
      culdoscopy 70.22
  retained placenta
    with curettage 69.02
    manual 75.4
  streptothrix from lacrimal duct 09.42
Evaluation (of)
  audiological 95.43
  cardiac rhythm device (CRT-D) (CRT-P) (AICD)
    (pacemaker)—*see* Interrogation
  criminal responsibility, psychiatric 94.11
  functional (physical therapy) 93.01
  hearing NEC 95.49
  orthotic (for brace fitting) 93.02
  prosthetic (for artificial limb fitting) 93.03
  psychiatric NEC 94.19
    commitment 94.13
  psychologic NEC 94.08
  testimentary capacity, psychiatric 94.11
Evans operation (release of clubfoot) 83.84
Evisceration
  eyeball 16.39
    with implant (into scleral shell) 16.31
  ocular contents 16.39
    with implant (into scleral shell) 16.31
  orbit (*see also* Exenteration, orbit) 16.59
  pelvic (anterior) (posterior) (partial) (total)
    (female) 68.8
    male 57.71
Evulsion
  nail (bed) (fold) 86.23
  skin 86.3
  subcutaneous tissue 86.3
Examination (for)
  breast
    manual 89.36
    radiographic NEC 87.37
    thermographic 88.85
    ultrasonic 88.73
  cervical rib (by x-ray) 87.43
  colostomy stoma (digital) 89.33
  dental (oral mucosa) (peridontal) 89.31
    radiographic NEC 87.12
  enterostomy stoma (digital) 89.33
  eye 95.09
    color vision 95.06
    comprehensive 95.02
    dark adaptation 95.07
    limited (with prescription of spectacles) 95.01
    under anesthesia 95.04
  fetus, intrauterine 75.35
  general physical 89.7
  glaucoma 95.03
  gynecological 89.26
  hearing 95.47

Examination—*continued*
  microscopic (specimen) (of) 91.9

Note—Use the following fourth-digit
subclassification with categories 90-91 to
identify type of examination:

1 bacterial smear
2 culture
3 culture and sensitivity
4 parasitology
5 toxicology
6 cell block and Papanicolaou smear
9 other microscopic examination

  adenoid 90.3
  adrenal gland 90.1
  amnion 91.4
  anus 90.9
  appendix 90.9
  bile ducts 91.0
  bladder 91.3
  blood 90.5
  bone 91.5
    marrow 90.6
  brain 90.0
  breast 91.6
  bronchus 90.4
  bursa 91.5
  cartilage 91.5
  cervix 91.4
  chest wall 90.4
  chorion 91.4
  colon 90.9
  cul-de-sac 91.1
  dental 90.8
  diaphragm 90.4
  duodenum 90.8
  ear 90.3
  endocrine gland NEC 90.1
  esophagus 90.8
  eye 90.2
  fallopian tube 91.4
  fascia 91.5
  female genital tract 91.4
  fetus 91.4
  gallbladder 91.0
  hair 91.6
  ileum 90.9
  jejunum 90.9
  joint fluid 91.5
  kidney 91.2
  large intestine 90.9
  larynx 90.3
  ligament 91.5
  liver 91.0
  lung 90.4
  lymph (node) 90.7
  meninges 90.0
  mesentery 91.1
  mouth 90.8
  muscle 91.5
  musculoskeletal system 91.5
  nails 91.6
  nerve 90.0
  nervous system 90.0
  nose 90.3
  omentum 91.1
  operative wound 91.7
  ovary 91.4
  pancreas 91.0

Excision—*continued*

total, except facial—*see* category 77.9

  facial NEC 76.45

    with reconstruction 76.44

    mandible 76.42

      with reconstruction 76.41

brain 01.59

  hemisphere 01.52

  lobe 01.53

branchial cleft cyst or vestige 29.2

breast (*see also* Mastectomy) 85.41

  aberrant tissue 85.24

  accessory 85.24

  ectopic 85.24

  nipple 85.25

    accessory 85.24

  segmental 85.23

  supernumerary 85.24

  wedge 85.21

broad ligament 69.19

bronchogenic cyst 32.09

  endoscopic 32.01

bronchus (wide sleeve) NEC 32.1

buccal mucosa 27.49

bulbourethral gland 58.92

bulbous tuberosities (mandible) (maxilla)

  (fibrous) (osseous) 24.31

bunion (*see also* Bunionectomy) 77.59

bunionette (with osteotomy) 77.54

bursa 83.5

  hand 82.31

canal of Nuck 69.19

cardioma 37.33

carotid body (lesion) (partial) (total) 39.89

cartilage (*see also* Chondrectomy) 80.90

  intervertebral—*see* category 80.5

  knee (semilunar) 80.6

  larynx 30.29

  nasal (submucous) 21.5

caruncle, urethra 58.39

  endoscopic 58.31

cataract (*see also* Extraction, cataract) 13.19

  secondary membrane (after cataract) 13.65

cervical

  rib 77.91

  stump 67.4

cervix (stump) NEC 67.4

  cold (knife) 67.2

  conization 67.2

  cryoconization 67.33

  electroconization 67.32

chalazion (multiple) (single) 08.21

cholesteatoma—*see* Excision, lesion, by site

choroid plexus 02.14

cicatrix (skin) 86.3

cilia base 08.20

ciliary body, prolapsed 12.98

clavicle (head) (partial) 77.81

  total (complete) 77.91

clitoris 71.4

coarctation of aorta (end-to-end anastomosis)

  38.64

  with

    graft replacement (interposition)

      abdominal 38.44

      thoracic 38.45

      thoracoabdominal 38.45 *[38.44]*

Excision—*continued*

common

  duct 51.63

  wall between posterior and coronary sinus (with

    roofing of resultant defect with patch graft)

    35.82

condyle—*see* 77.8

  mandible 76.5

conjunctival ring 10.31

cornea 11.49

  epithelium (with chemocauterization) 11.41

    for smear or culture 11.21

costal cartilage 80.99

cul-de-sac (Douglas') 70.92

  with graft or prosthesis 70.93

cusp, heart valve 35.10

  aortic 35.11

  mitral 35.12

  tricuspid 35.14

cyst—*see also* Excision, lesion, by site

  apical (tooth) 23.73

    with root canal therapy 23.72

  Baker's (popliteal) 83.39

  breast 85.21

  broad ligament 69.19

  bronchogenic 32.09

    endoscopic 32.01

  cervix 67.39

  dental 24.4

  dentigerous 24.4

  epididymis 63.2

  fallopian tube 66.61

  Gartner's duct 70.33

  hand 82.29

  labia 71.3

  lung 32.29

    endoscopic 32.28

    thoracoscopic 32.20

  mesonephric duct 69.19

  Morgagni

    female 66.61

    male 62.2

  mullerian duct 60.73

  nasolabial 27.49

  nasopalatine 27.31

    by wide excision 27.32

  ovary 65.29

    laparoscopic 65.25

  parovarian 69.19

  pericardium 37.31

  periodontal (apical) (lateral) 24.4

  popliteal (Baker's), knee 83.39

  radicular 24.4

  spleen 41.42

  synovial (membrane) 83.39

  thyroglossal (with resection of hyoid bone) 06.7

  urachal (bladder) 57.51

    abdominal wall 54.3

  vagina (Gartner's duct) 70.33

cystic

  duct remnant 51.61

  hygroma 40.29

dentinoma 24.4

diaphragm 34.81

disc, intervertebral NOS 80.50

  herniated (nucleus pulposus) 80.51

  other specified (diskectomy) 80.51

Excision—*continued*
 open and other 45.79
  unspecified 45.83
 small (total) 45.63
  for interposition 45.51
  local 45.33
  partial 45.62
  segmental 45.62
   multiple 45.61
 intraductal papilloma 85.21
 iris prolapse 12.13
 joint (*see also* Arthrectomy) 80.90
 keloid (scar), skin 86.3
 LAA 37.36
 labia—*see* Vulvectomy
 lacrimal
  gland 09.20
   partial 09.22
   total 09.23
  passage 09.6
  sac 09.6
 left atrial appendage 37.36
 lesion (local)
  abdominal wall 54.3
  accessory sinus—*see* Excision, lesion, nasal
   sinus
  adenoids 28.92
  adrenal gland(s) 07.21
  alveolus 24.4
  ampulla of Vater 51.62
  anterior chamber (eye) NEC 12.40
  anus 49.39
   endoscopic 49.31
  apocrine gland 86.3
  artery 38.60
   abdominal 38.66
   aorta (arch) (ascending) (descending thoracic)
    38.64
    with end-to-end anastomosis 38.45
     abdominal 38.44
     thoracic 38.45
     thoracoabdominal 38.45 *[38.44]*
    with interposition graft replacement 38.45
     abdominal 38.44
     thoracic 38.45
     thoracoabdominal 38.45 *[38.44]*
   head and neck NEC 38.62
   intracranial NEC 38.61
   lower limb 38.68
   thoracic NEC 38.65
   upper limb 38.63
  atrium 37.33
  auditory canal or meatus, external 18.29
   radical 18.31
  auricle, ear 18.29
   radical 18.31
  biliary ducts 51.69
   endoscopic 51.64
  bladder (transurethral) 57.49
   open 57.59
   suprapubic 57.59
  blood vessel 38.60
   abdominal
    artery 38.66
    vein 38.67
   aorta (arch) (ascending) (descending) 38.64
   head and neck NEC 38.62
   intracranial NEC 38.61
   lower limb
    artery 38.68
    vein 38.69

Excision—*continued*
   thoracic NEC 38.65
   upper limb (artery) (vein) 38.63
  bone 77.60
   carpal, metacarpal 77.64
   clavicle 77.61
   facial 76.2
   femur 77.65
   fibula 77.67
   humerus 77.62
   jaw 76.2
    dental 24.4
   patella 77.66
   pelvic 77.69
   phalanges (foot) (hand) 77.69
   radius 77.63
   scapula 77.61
   skull 01.6
   specified site NEC 77.69
   tarsal, metatarsal 77.68
   thorax (ribs) (sternum) 77.61
   tibia 77.67
   ulna 77.63
   vertebrae 77.69
  brain (transtemporal approach) NEC 01.59
   by stereotactic radiosurgery 92.30
    cobalt 60 92.32
    linear accelerator (LINAC) 92.31
    multi-source 92.32
    particle beam 92.33
    particulate 92.33
    radiosurgery NEC 92.39
    single source photon 92.31
  breast (segmental) (wedge) 85.21
  broad ligament 69.19
  bronchus NEC 32.09
   endoscopic 32.01
  cerebral (cortex) NEC 01.59
   meninges 01.51
  cervix (myoma) 67.39
  chest wall 34.4
  choroid plexus 02.14
  ciliary body 12.44
  colon 45.41
   endoscopic NEC 45.43
   polypectomy 45.42
  conjunctive 10.31
  cornea 11.49
  cranium 01.6
  cul-de-sac (Douglas) 70.32
  dental (jaw) 24.4
  diaphragm 34.81
  duodenum (local) 45.31
   endoscopic 45.30
  ear, external 18.29
   radical 18.31
  endometrium 68.29
  epicardium 37.31
  epididymis 63.3
  epiglottis 30.09
  esophagus NEC 42.32
   endoscopic 42.33
  eye, eyeball 16.93
   anterior segment NEC 12.40
  eyebrow (skin) 08.20
  eyelid 08.20
   by
    halving procedure 08.24
    wedge resection 08.24

Exploration—*continued*
maxillary antrum or sinus (Caldwell-Luc
    approach) 22.39
mediastinum 34.1
    endoscopic 34.22
middle ear (transtympanic) 20.23
muscle 83.02
    hand 82.02
neck (*see also* Exploration, thyroid) 06.09
nerve (cranial) (peripheral) NEC 04.04
    auditory 04.01
    root (spinal) 03.09
nose 21.1
orbit (*see also* Orbitotomy) 16.09
pancreas 52.09
    endoscopic 52.13
pancreatic duct 52.09
    endoscopic 52.13
pelvis (by laparotomy) 54.11
    by colpotomy 70.12
penis 64.92
perinephric area 59.09
perineum (female) 71.09
    male 86.09
peripheral vessels
    lower limb
        artery 38.08
        vein 38.09
    upper limb (artery) (vein) 38.03
periprostatic tissue 60.81
perirenal tissue 59.09
perivesical tissue 59.19
petrous pyramid air cells 20.22
pilonidal sinus 86.03
pineal (gland) 07.52
    field 07.51
pituitary (gland) 07.72
    fossa 07.71
pleura 34.09
popliteal space 86.09
prostate 60.0
rectum (*see also* Proctoscopy) 48.23
    by incision 48.0
retroperitoneum 54.0
retropubic 59.19
salivary gland 26.0
sclera (by incision) 12.89
scrotum 61.0
shunt
    ventriculoperitoneal at
        peritoneal site 54.95
        ventricular site 02.41
sinus
    ethmoid 22.51
    frontal 22.41
    maxillary (Caldwell-Luc approach) 22.39
    sphenoid 22.52
    tract, skin and subcutaneous tissue 86.09
skin 86.09
soft tissue NEC 83.09
    hand 82.09
spermatic cord 63.93
sphenoidal sinus 22.52
spinal (canal) (nerve rook) 03.09
spleen 41.2
stomach (by incision) 43.0
    endoscopic—*see* Gastroscopy
subcutaneous tissue 86.09
subdiaphragmatic space 54.11
superficial fossa 86.09
tarsal tunnel 04.44

Exploration—*continued*
tendon (sheath) 83.01
    hand 82.01
testes 62.0
thymus (gland) 07.92
    field 07.91
    thoracoscopic 07.95
thyroid (field) (gland) (by incision) 06.09
    postoperative 06.02
trachea (by incision) 31.3
    endoscopic—*see* Tracheoscopy
tunica vaginalis 61.0
tympanum 20.09
    transtympanic route 20.23
ureter (by incision) 56.2
    endoscopic 56.31
urethra (by incision) 58.0
    endoscopic 58.22
uterus (corpus) 68.0
    cervix 69.95
    digital 68.11
    postpartal, manual 75.7
vagina (by incision) 70.14
    endoscopic 70.21
vas deferens 63.6
vein 38.00
    abdominal 38.07
    head and neck NEC 38.02
    intracranial NEC 38.01
    lower limb 38.09
    thoracic NEC 38.05
    upper limb 38.03
vulva (by incision) 71.09
Exposure —*see also* Incision, by site
tooth (for orthodontic treatment) 24.6
Expression, trachoma follicles 10.33
Exsanguination transfusion 99.01
Extension
buccolabial sulcus 24.91
limb, forced 93.25
lingual sulcus 24.91
mandibular ridge 76.43
Exteriorization
esophageal pouch 42.12
intestine 46.03
    large 46.03
    small 46.01
maxillary sinus 22.9
pilonidal cyst or sinus (open excision) (with
    partial closure) 86.21
Extirpation —*see also* Excision, by site
aneurysm—*see* Aneurysmectomy
arteriovenous fistula—*see* Aneurysmectomy
lacrimal sac 09.6
larynx 30.3
    with radical neck dissection (with synchronous
        thyroidectomy) (with synchronous
        tracheostomy) 30.4
nerve, tooth (*see also* Therapy, root canal) 23.70
varicose vein (peripheral) (lower limb) 38.59
    upper limb 38.53
Extracorporeal
circulation (regional), except hepatic 39.61
    hepatic 50.92
    percutaneous 39.66
hemodialysis 39.95
membrane oxygenation (ECMO) 39.65
photopheresis, therapeutic 99.88

Extracorporeal—*continued*
  shock wave lithotripsy (ESWL) NEC 98.59
    bile duct 98.52
    bladder 98.51
    gallbladder 98.52
    kidney 98.51
    renal pelvis 98.51
    specified site NEC 98.59
    ureter 98.51
Extracranial-intracranial bypass [EC-IC]
  39.28
Extraction
  breech (partial) 72.52
    with forceps to aftercoming head 72.51
    total 72.54
      with forceps to aftercoming head 72.53
  cataract 13.19
    after cataract (by)
      capsulectomy 13.65
      capsulotomy 13.64
      discission 13.64
      excision 13.65
      iridocapsulectomy 13.65
      mechanical fragmentation 13.66
      needling 13.64
      phacofragmentation (mechanical) 13.66
    aspiration (simple) (with irrigation) 13.3
    cryoextraction (intracapsular approach) 13.19
      temporal inferior route (in presence of
        fistulization bleb) 13.11
    curette evacuation (extracapsular approach)
      13.2
    emulsification (and aspiration) 13.41
    erysiphake (intracapsular approach) 13.19
      temporal inferior route (in presence of
        fistulization bleb) 13.11
    extracapsular approach (with iridectomy) NEC
      13.59
      by temporal inferior route (in presence of
        fistulization bleb) 13.51
      aspiration (simple) (with irrigation) 13.3
      curette evacuation 13.2
      emulsification (and aspiration) 13.41
      linear extraction 13.2
      mechanical fragmentation with aspiration by
        posterior route 13.42
        specified route NEC 13.43
      phacoemulsification (ultrasonic) (with
        aspiration) 13.41
      phacofragmentation (mechanical)
        with aspiration by
          posterior route 13.42
          specified route NEC 13.43
        ultrasonic (with aspiration) 13.41
      rotoextraction (mechanical) with aspiration
        by
        posterior route 13.42
        specified route NEC 13.43
    intracapsular (combined) (simple) (with
      iridectomy) (with suction) (with
      zonulolysis) 13.19
      by temporal inferior route (in presence of
        fistulization bleb) 13.11
    linear extraction (extracapsular approach) 13.2
    phacoemulsification (and aspiration) 13.41
    phacofragmentation (mechanical)
      with aspiration by
        posterior route 13.42
        specified route NEC 13.43
      ultrasonic 13.41

Extraction—*continued*
  rotoextraction (mechanical)
    with aspiration by
      posterior route 13.42
      specified route NEC 13.43
  secondary membranous (after cataract) (by)
    capsulectomy 13.65
    capsulotomy 13.64
    discission 13.64
    excision 13.65
    iridocapsulectomy 13.65
    mechanical fragmentation 13.66
    needling 13.64
    phacofragmentation (mechanical) 13.66
  common duct stones (percutaneous) (through
    sinus tract) (with basket) 51.96
  fat for grafting or banking 86.90
  foreign body—*see* Removal, foreign body
  kidney stone(s), percutaneous 55.03
    with fragmentation procedure 55.04
  lens (eye) (*see also* Extraction, cataract) 13.19
  Malström's 72.79
    with episiotomy 72.71
  menstrual, menses 69.6
  milk from lactating breast (manual) (pump) 99.98
  tooth (by forceps) (multiple) (single) NEC 23.09
    with mucoperiosteal flap elevation 23.19
    deciduous 23.01
    surgical NEC (*see also* Removal, tooth,
      surgical) 23.19
  vacuum, fetus 72.79
    with episiotomy 72.71
  vitreous (*see also* Removal, vitreous) 14.72

F

Fixation—*continued*
internal
with fracture-reduction—*see* Reduction,
fracture
without fracture-reduction—*see* Fixation, bone,
internal
intestine 46.60
large 46.64
to abdominal wall 46.63
small 46.62
to abdominal wall 46.61
to abdominal wall 46.60
iris (bombé) 12.11
jejunum 46.62
to abdominal wall 46.61
joint—*see* Arthroplasty
kidney 55.7
ligament
cardinal 69.22
palpebrae 08.36
omentum 54.74
parametrial 69.22
plaster jacket 93.51
other cast 93.53
rectum (sling) 48.76
spine, with fusion (*see also* Fusion, spinal) 81.00
spleen 41.95
splint 93.54
tendon 83.88
hand 82.85
testis in scrotum 62.5
tongue 25.59
urethrovaginal (to Cooper's ligament) 70.77
with graft or prosthesis 70.78
uterus (abdominal) (vaginal) (ventrofixation)
69.22
vagina 70.77
with graft or prosthesis 70.78
Fixator, external
computer assisted (dependent) 84.73
hybrid device or system 84.73
Ilizarov type 84.72
monoplanar system 84.71
ring device or system 84.72
Sheffield type 84.72
Flooding (psychologic desensitization) 94.33
Flowmetry, Doppler (ultrasonic)—*see also*
Ultrasonography
aortic arch 88.73
head and neck 88.71
heart 88.72
thorax NEC 88.73
Fluoroscopy —*see* Radiography
Fog therapy (respiratory) 93.94
Folding, eye muscle 15.22
multiple (two or more muscles) 15.4
Foley operation (pyeloplasty) 55.87
Fontan operation (creation of conduit between
right atrium and pulmonary artery) 35.94
Foraminotomy 03.09
Forced extension, limb 93.25
Forceps delivery —*see* Delivery, forceps
Formation
adhesions
pericardium 36.39
pleura 34.6
anus, artificial —*see* Colostomy
duodenostomy 46.39
ileostomy —*see* Ileostomy
jejunostomy 46.39
percutaneous (endoscopic) (PEJ) 46.32

Formation—*continued*
arteriovenous fistula (for kidney dialysis)
(peripheral) (shunt) 39.27
external cannula 39.93
bone flap, cranial 02.03
cardiac device (defibrillator) (pacemaker) pocket
with initial insertion of cardiac device—*omit
code*
new site (skin) (subcutaneous) 37.79
colostomy —*see* Colostomy
conduit
apical-aortic (AAC) 35.93
ileal (urinary) 56.51
left ventricle and aorta 35.93
right atrium and pulmonary artery 35.94
right ventricle and pulmonary (distal) artery
35.92
in repair of
pulmonary artery atresia 35.92
transposition of great vessels 35.92
truncus arteriosus 35.83
endorectal ileal pouch (J-pouch) (H-pouch)
(S-pouch) (with anastomosis to anus) 45.95
fistula
arteriovenous (for kidney dialysis) (peripheral)
shunt) 39.27
external cannula 39.93
bladder to skin NEC 57.18
with bladder flap 57.21
percutaneous 57.17
cutaneoperitoneal 54.93
gastric 43.19
percutaneous (endoscopic)
(transabdominal) 43.11
mucous —*see* Colostomy
rectovaginal 48.99
tracheoesophageal 31.95
tubulovalvular (Beck-Jianu) (Frank's)
(Janeway) (Spivack's) (Ssabanejew-Frank)
43.19
urethrovaginal 58.0
ileal
bladder
closed 57.87 *[45.51]*
open 56.51
conduit 56.51
interatrial fistula 35.42
mucous fistula —*see* Colostomy
pericardial
baffle, interatrial 35.91
window 37.12
pleural window (for drainage) 34.09
pocket
cardiac device (defibrillator) (pacemaker)
with initial insertion of cardiac device—*omit
code*
new site (skin) (subcutaneous) 37.79
loop recorder 37.79
thalamic stimulator pulse generator
with initial insertion of battery package—*omit
code*
new site (skin) (subcutaneous) 86.09
pupil 12.39
by iridectomy 12.14
rectovaginal fistula 48.99
reversed gastric tube (intrathoracic) (retrosternal)
42.58
antesternal or antethoracic 42.68
septal defect, interatrial 35.42
shunt
abdominovenous 54.94
arteriovenous 39.93

Formation—*continued*
  peritoneojugular 54.94
  peritoneo-vascular 54.94
  pleuroperitoneal 34.05
  transjugular intrahepatic portosystemic (TIPS)
    39.1
  subcutaneous tunnel
    esophageal 42.86
      with anastomosis—*see* Anastomosis,
        esophagus, antesternal
    pulse generator lead wire 86.99
      with initial procedure—*omit code*
    thalamic stimulator pulse generator pocket
      with insertion of battery package—*omit code*
    new site (skin) (subcutaneous) 86.09
  syndactyly (finger) (toe) 86.89
  tracheoesophageal 31.95
  tubulovalvular fistula (Beck-Jianu) (Frank's)
    (Janeway) (Spivack's) (Ssabanejew-Frank)
    43.19
  uretero-ileostomy, cutaneous 56.51
  ureterostomy, cutaneous 56.61
    ileal 56.51
  urethrovaginal fistula 58.0
  window
    pericardial 37.12
    pleural (for drainage) 34.09
      thoracoscopic 34.06
Fothergill (Donald) operation (uterine
  suspension) 69.22
Fowler operation
  arthroplasty of metacarpophalangeal joint 81.72
  release (mallet ringer repair) 82.84
  tenodesis (hand) 82.85
  thoracoplasty 33.34
Fox operation (entropion repair with wedge
  resection) 08.43
Fracture, surgical (*see also* Osteoclasis) 78.70
  turbinates (nasal) 21.62
Fragmentation
  lithotriptor—*see* Lithotripsy
  mechanical
    cataract (with aspiration) 13.43
      posterior route 13.42
    secondary membrane 13.66
    secondary membrane (after cataract) 13.66
  ultrasonic
    cataract (with aspiration) 13.41
  stones, urinary (Kock pouch) 59.95
    percutaneous nephrostomy 55.04
Franco operation (suprapubic cystotomy) 57.18
Frank operation 43.19
Frazier (Spiller) operation (subtemporal
  trigeminal rhizotomy) 04.02
Fredet-Ramstedt operation (pyloromyotomy)
  (with wedge resection) 43.3
Freeing
  adhesions—*see* Lysis, adhesions
  anterior synechiae (with injection of air or liquid)
    12.32
  artery-vein-nerve bundle 39.91
  extraocular muscle, entrapped 15.7
  goniosynechiae (with injection of air or liquid)
    12.31
  intestinal segment for interposition 45.50
    large 45.52
    small 45.51
  posterior synechiae 12.33
  synechiae (posterior) 12.33
    anterior (with injection of air or liquid) 12.32
  vascular bundle 39.91
  vessel 39.91

Freezing
  gastric 96.32
  prostate 60.62
Frenckner operation (intrapetrosal drainage)
  20.22
Frenectomy
  labial 27.41
  lingual 25.92
  lip 27.41
  maxillary 27.41
  tongue 25.92
Frenotomy
  labial 27.91
  lingual 25.91
Frenulumectomy —*see* Frenectomy
Frickman operation (abdominal proctopexy)
  48.75
Frommel operation (shortening of uterosacral
  ligaments) 69.22
Fulguration —*see also* Electrocoagulation *and*
  Destruction, lesion, by site
  adenoid fossa 28.7
  anus 49.39
    endoscopic 49.31
  bladder (transurethral) 57.49
    suprapubic 57.59
  choroid 14.21
  duodenum 45.32
    endoscopic 45.30
  esophagus 42.39
    endoscopic 42.33
  large intestine 45.49
    endoscopic 45.43
      polypectomy 45.42
  penis 64.2
  perineum, female 71.3
  prostate, transurethral 60.29
  rectum 48.32
    radical 48.31
  retina 14.21
  scrotum 61.3
  Skene's gland 71.3
  skin 86.3
  small intestine NEC 45.34
    duodenum 45.32
      endoscopic 45.30
  stomach 43.49
    endoscopic 43.41
  subcutaneous tissue 86.3
  tonsillar fossa 28.7
  urethra 58.39
    endoscopic 58.31
  vulva 71.3
Function
  study—*see also* Scan, radioisotope
    gastric 89.39
    muscle 93.08
      ocular 95.25
    nasal 89.12
    pulmonary—*see* categories 89.37-89.38
    renal 92.03
    thyroid 92.01
    urethral sphincter 89.23
Fundectomy, uterine 68.39
Fundoplication (esophageal) (Nissen's) 44.66
  laparoscopic 44.67
Fundusectomy, gastric 43.89

Fusion
  atlas-axis (spine) *—see* Fusion, spinal, atlas-axis
  bone *(see also* Osteoplasty) 78.40
  cervical (spine) (C2 level or below) *—see* Fusion,
    spinal, cervical
  claw toe 77.57
  craniocervical *—see* Fusion, spinal,
    craniocervical
  dorsal, dorsolumbar *—see* Fusion, spinal, dorsal,
    dorsolumbar
  epiphyseal-diaphyseal *(see also* Arrest, bone
    growth) 78.20
  epiphysiodesis *(see also* Arrest, bone growth)
    78.20
  hammer toe 77.56
  joint (with bone graft) *(see also* Arthrodesis)
    81.20
    ankle 81.11
    claw toe 77.57
    foot NEC 81.17
    hammer toe 77.56
    hip 81.21
    interphalangeal, finger 81.28
    ischiofemoral 81.21
    metatarsophalangeal 81.16
    midtarsal 81.14
    overlapping toe(s) 77.58
    pantalar 81.11
    spinal *(see also* Fusion, spinal) 81.00
    subtalar 81.13
    tarsal joints NEC 81.17
    tarsometatarsal 81.15
    tibiotalar 81.11
    toe NEC 77.58
      claw toe 77.57
      hammer toe 77.56
      overlapping toe(s) 77.58
  lip to tongue 25.59
  lumbar, lumbosacral *—see* Fusion, spinal,
    lumbar, lumbosacral
  occiput-C2 (spinal)*—see* Fusion, spinal, occiput
  spinal, NOS (with graft) (with internal fixation)
    (with instrumentation) 81.00
    anterior lumbar interbody fusion (ALIF) 81.06
    atlas-axis (anterior) (transoral) (posterior) 81.01
      for pseudarthrosis 81.31
    axial lumbar interbody fusion [AxiaLIF] 81.08
    cervical (C2 level or below) NEC 81.02
      anterior column (interbody) anterolateral
        (anterior) technique 81.02
        for pseudarthrosis 81.32
      C1-C2 level (anterior) (posterior) 81.01
        for pseudarthrosis 81.31
      for pseudarthrosis 81.32
      posterior column, posterolateral (posterior)
        technique 81.03
        for pseudarthrosis 81.33
    craniocervical (anterior transoral) (posterior)
      81.01
      for pseudarthrosis NEC 81.31
    direct lateral interbody fusion [DLIF] 81.06
    dorsal, dorsolumbar NEC 81.05
      anterior column (interbody) anterolateral
        (anterior) (extracavitary) technique 81.04
        for pseudarthrosis 81.34
      for pseudarthrosis 81.35
      posterior column, posterolateral (posterior)
        technique 81.05
        for pseudarthrosis 81.35
    extreme lateral interbody fusion [XLIF] 81.06
    facet 81.07

Fusion—*continued*
  lumbar, lumbosacral NEC 81.08
    anterior column (interbody)
      anterolateral (anterior) technique 81.06
      for pseudarthrosis 81.36
      posterior technique 81.08
        for pseudarthrosis 81.38
    lateral transverse process technique 81.07
      for pseudarthrosis 81.37
    posterior column, posterior (posterolateral)
      (transverse process) technique 81.07
    number of vertebrae *—see* codes 81.62-81.64
    occiput-C2 (anterior) (transoral) (posterior)
      81.01
    for pseudarthrosis 81.31

> *Note: Also use either 81.62, 81.63 or 81.64 as*
> *an additional code to show the total number of*
> *vertebrae fused*

    posterior lumbar interbody fusion (PLIF) 81.08
    transforaminal lumbar interbody fusion (TLIF)
      81.08
  tongue (to lip) 25.59

G

Graft, grafting—*continued*
tarsal cartilage 08.69
temporalis muscle to orbit 16.63
   with exenteration of orbit 16.59
tendon 83.81
  for joint repair—*see* Arthroplasty
  hand 82.79
testicle 62.69
thumb (for reconstruction) NEC 82.69
tongue (mucosal) (skin) 25.59
trachea 31.79
tubular (tube)—*see* Graft, skin, pedicle
tunnel—*see* Graft, skin, pedicle
tympanum (*see also* Tympanoplasty) 19.4
ureter 56.89
vagina
  biological 70.94
  synthetic 70.95
vein (patch) 39.58
  with
    excision or resection of vessel—*see*
      Phlebectomy, with graft replacement
    synthetic patch (Dacron) (Teflon) 39.57
    tissue patch (vein) (autogenous) (homograft)
      39.56
vermilion border (lip) 27.56
Grattage, conjunctive 10.31
Green operation (scapulopexy) 78.41
Grice operation (subtalar arthrodesis) 81.13
Grip, strength 93.04
Gritti-Stokes operation (knee disarticulation)
  84.16
Gross operation (herniorrhaphy)
laparoscopic 53.43
  with graft or prosthesis 53.42
other and open with graft or prosthesis 53.41
other open 53.49
Group therapy 94.44
Guttering, bone (*see also* Excision, lesion, bone)
  77.60
Guyon operation (amputation of ankle) 84.13

H

Holth operation
iridencleisis 12.63
sclerectomy 12.65
Homan operation (correction of lymphedema)
40.9
Homograft —*see* Graft
Homotransplant, homotransplantation —*see*
Transplant
Hosiery, elastic 93.59
Hutch operation (ureteroneocystostomy) 56.74
Hybinette-Eden operation (glenoid bone block)
78.01
Hydrocelectomy
canal of Nuck (female) 69.19
male 63.1
round ligament 69.19
spermatic cord 63.1
tunica vaginalis 61.2
Hydrotherapy 93.33
assisted exercise in pool 93.31
whirlpool 93.32
Hymenectomy 70.31
Hymenoplasty 70.76
Hymenorrhaphy 70.76
Hymenotomy 70.11
Hyperalimentation 99.15
Hyperbaric oxygenation 93.95
wound 93.59
Hyperextension, joint 93.25
Hyperthermia NEC 93.35
for cancer treatment (interstitial) (local)
(radiofrequency) (regional) (ultrasound)
(whole-body) 99.85
Hypnodrama, psychiatric 94.32
Hypnosis (psychotherapeutic) 94.32
for anesthesia—*omit code*
Hypnotherapy 94.32
Hypophysectomy (complete) (total) 07.69
partial or subtotal 07.63
transfrontal approach 07.61
transsphenoidal approach 07.62
specified approach NEC 07.68
transfrontal approach (complete) (total) 07.64
partial 07.61
transsphenoidal approach (complete) (total) 07.65
partial 07.62
Hypothermia (central) (local) 99.81
gastric (cooling) 96.31
freezing 96.32
systemic (in open heart surgery) 39.62
Hypotympanotomy 20.23
Hysterectomy NOS 68.9
abdominal
laparoscopic (total) (TLH) 68.41
other (total) 68.49
partial or subtotal (supracervical)
(supravaginal) 68.39
radical (modified) (Wertheim's) 68.69
laparoscopic (total) [TLRH] 68.61
laparoscopic
abdominal
radical (total) (TLRH) 68.61
total (TLH) 68.41
supracervical (LASH) (LSH) 68.31
total (TLH) 68.41
vaginal, assisted (LAVH) 68.51
radical (LRVH) 68.71

Hysterectomy—*continued*
radical
abdominal
laparoscopic 68.61
other (modified) (Wertheim's) 68.69
vaginal
laparoscopic (LRVH) 68.71
other 68.79
subterm other 68.79
supracervical 68.39
classic infrafascial SEMM hysterectomy
[CISH] 68.31
laparoscopically assisted [LASH] 68.31
vaginal (complete) (partial) (subtotal) (total)
68.59
laparoscopically assisted (LAVH) 68.51
radical (Schauta) 68.79
laparoscopic [LRVH] 68.71
Hysterocolpectomy (radical) (vaginal) 68.79
abdominal 68.69
laparoscopic 68.61
laparoscopic 68.71
Hysterogram NEC 87.85
percutaneous 87.84
Hysterolysis 54.59
laparoscopic 54.51
Hysteromyomectomy 68.29
Hysteropexy 69.22
Hysteroplasty 69.49
Hysterorrhaphy 69.41
Hysterosalpingography
gas (contrast) 87.82
opaque dye (contrast) 87.83
Hysterosalpingostomy 66.74
Hysteroscopy 68.12
ablation
endometrial 68.23
with biopsy 68.16
Hysterotomy (with removal of foreign body)
(with removal of hydatidiform mole) 68.0
for intrauterine transfusion 75.2
obstetrical 74.99
for termination of pregnancy 74.91
Hysterotrachelectomy 67.4
Hysterotracheloplasty 69.49
Hysterotrachelorrhaphy 69.41
Hysterotrachelotomy 69.95

I

Implant, implantation—*continued*
  Tenon's capsule (with enucleation of eyeball)
    16.42
    with attachment of muscles 16.41
    reinsertion 16.62
  urethra 59.79
  vocal cord(s) 31.0
  infusion pump 86.06
  interbody spinal fusion device 84.51
  intracardiac or great vessel hemodynamic
    monitor, subcutaneous 00.57
  joint (prosthesis) (silastic) (Swanson type) NEC
    81.96
    ankle (total) 81.56
      revision 81.59
    carpocarpal, carpometacarpal 81.74
    elbow (total) 81.84
      revision 81.97
    extremity (bioelectric) (cineplastic)
      (kineplastic) 84.40
      lower 84.48
        revision 81.59
      upper 84.44
        revision 81.97
    femoral (bipolar endoprosthesis) 81.52
      revision NOS 81.53
        acetabular and femoral components (total)
          00.70
        acetabular component only 00.71
        acetabular liner and/or femoral head only
          00.73
        femoral component only 00.72
        femoral head only and/or acetabular liner
          00.73
        total (acetabular and femoral components)
          00.70
    finger 81.71
    hand (metacarpophalangeal) (interphalangeal)
      81.71
      revision 81.97
    hip (partial) 81.52
      revision NOS 81.53
        acetabular and femoral components (total)
          00.70
        acetabular component only 00.71
        acetabular liner and/or femoral head only
          00.73
        femoral component only 00.72
        femoral head only and/or acetabular liner
          00.73
        partial
          acetabular component only 00.71
          acetabular liner and/or femoral head only
            00.73
          femoral component only 00.72
          femoral head only and/or acetabular liner
            00.73
          total (acetabular and femoral components)
            00.70
      total 81.51
        revision (acetabular and femoral
          components) 00.70
    interphalangeal 81.71
      revision 81.97

Implant, implantation—*continued*
  knee (partial) (total) 81.54
    revision NOS 81.55
      femoral component 00.82
      partial
        femoral component 00.82
        patellar component 00.83
        tibial component 00.81
        tibial insert 00.84
      patellar component 00.83
      tibial component 00.81
      tibial insert 00.84
      total (all components) 00.80
  metacarpophalangeal 81.71
    revision 81.97
  shoulder (partial) 81.81
    revision 81.97
    total replacement, NEC 81.80
      other 81.80
      reverse 81.88
  toe 81.57
    for hallux valgus repair 77.59
    revision 81.59
  wrist (partial) 81.74
    revision 81.97
    total replacement 81.73
  kidney, mechanical 55.97
  Lap-Band™ 44.95
  larynx 31.0
  leads (cardiac)—*see* Implant, electrode(s) cardiac
  limb lengthening device, internal (NOS) 84.54
    with kinetic distraction 84.53
  mammary artery
    in ventricle (Vineberg) 36.2
    to coronary artery (single vessel) 36.15
      double vessel 36.16
  M-Brace™ 84.82
  Mulligan hood, fallopian tube 66.93
  nerve (peripheral) 04.79
  neuropacemaker—*see* Implant, neurostimulator,
    by site
  neurostimulator
    brain 02.93
    electrodes
      brain 02.93
      gastric 04.92
      intracranial 02.93
      peripheral nerve 04.92
      sacral nerve 04.92
      spine 03.93
    intracranial 02.93
    peripheral nerve 04.92
    pulse generator (subcutaneous) 86.96
      cranial 01.20
      multiple array 86.95
        rechargeable 86.98
      single array 86.94
        rechargeable 86.97
    spine 03.93
  nose 21.85
  Ommaya reservoir 02.22
  orbit 16.69
    reinsertion 16.62
  outflow tract prosthesis (heart) (gusset type)
    in
      pulmonary valvuloplasty 35.26
      total repair of tetralogy of Fallot 35.81
  ovary into uterine cavity 65.72
    laparoscoic 65.75

Incision—*continued*
  mediastinum 34.1
  perineum (female) 71.09
    male 86.04
  popliteal space 86.04
  scrotum 61.0
  skin 86.04
  space of Retzius 59.19
  subcutaneous tissue 86.04
  vagina (cuff) 70.14
    episiotomy site 75.91
    obstetrical NEC 75.92
  hepatic ducts 51.59
  hordeolum 08.09
  hygroma—*see also* Incision, by site
    cystic 40.0
  hymen 70.11
  hypochondrium 54.0
    intra-abdominal 54.19
  hypophysis 07.72
  iliac fossa 54.0
  infratemporal fossa 27.0
  ingrown nail 86.09
  intestine 45.00
    large 45.03
    small 45.02
  intracerebral 01.39
  intracranial (epidural space) (extradural space)
    01.24
    subarachnoid or subdural space 01.31
  intraperitoneal 54.19
  ischiorectal tissue 49.02
    abscess 49.01
  joint structures (*see also* Arthrotomy) 80.10
  kidney 55.01
    pelvis 55.11
  labia 71.09
  lacrimal
    canaliculus 09.52
    gland 09.0
    passage NEC 09.59
    punctum 09.51
    sac 09.53
  larynx NEC 31.3
  ligamentum flavum (spine)—*omit code*
  liver 50.0
  lung 33.1
  lymphangioma 40.0
  lymphatic structure (channel) (node) (vessel) 40.0
  mastoid 20.21
  mediastinum 34.1
  meibomian gland 08.09
  meninges (cerebral) 01.31
    spinal 03.09
  midpalmar space 82.04
  mouth NEC 27.92
    floor 27.0
  muscle 83.02
    with division 83.19
      hand 82.19
    hand 82.02
      with division 82.19
  myocardium 37.11
  nailbed or nailfold 86.09
  nasolacrimal duct (stricture) 09.59
  neck 86.09
  nerve (cranial) (peripheral) NEC 04.04
    root (spinal) 03.1
  nose 21.1
  omentum 54.19
  orbit (*see also* Orbitotomy) 16.09

Incision—*continued*
  ovary 65.09
    laparoscopic 65.01
  palate 27.1
  palmar space (middle) 82.04
  pancreas 52.09
  pancreatic sphincter 51.82
    endoscopic 51.85
  parapharyngeal (oral) (transcervical) 28.0
  paronychia 86.09
  parotid
    gland or duct 26.0
    space 27.0
  pelvirectal tissue 48.81
  penis 64.92
  perianal (skin) (tissue) 49.02
    abscess 49.01
  perigastric 54.19
  perineum (female) 71.09
    male 86.09
  peripheral vessels
    lower limb
      artery 38.08
      vein 38.09
    upper limb (artery) (vein) 38.03
  periprostatic tissue 60.81
  perirectal tissue 48.81
  perirenal tissue 59.09
  perisplenic 54.19
  peritoneum 54.95
    by laparotomy 54.19
    pelvic (female) 70.12
      male 54.19
  periureteral tissue 59.09
  periurethral tissue 58.91
  perivesical tissue 59.19
  petrous pyramid (air cells) (apex)
    (mastoid) 20.22
  pharynx, pharyngeal (bursa) 29.0
    space, lateral 27.0
  pilonidal sinus (cyst) 86.03
  pineal gland 07.52
  pituitary (gland) 07.72
  pleura 34.09
  popliteal space 86.09
  postzygomatic space 27.0
  pouch of Douglas 70.12
  prostate (perineal approach) (transurethral
    approach) 60.0
  pterygopalatine fossa 27.0
  pulp canal (tooth) 24.0
  Rathke's pouch 07.72
  rectovaginal septum 48.81
  rectum 48.0
    stricture 48.91
  renal pelvis 55.11
  retroperitoneum 54.0
  retropharyngeal (oral) (transcervical) 28.0
  salivary gland or duct 26.0
  sclera 12.89
  scrotum 61.0
  sebaceous cyst 86.04
  seminal vesicle 60.72
  sinus—*see* Sinusotomy
  Skene's duct or gland 71.09
  skin 86.09
    with drainage 86.04
    breast 85.0
    cardiac pacemaker pocket, new site 37.79
    ear 18.09
    nose 21.1

Incision—*continued*
  subcutaneous tunnel for pulse generator lead
    wire 86.99
    with initial procedure—*omit code*
  thalamic stimulator pulse generator pocket, new
    site 86.09
    with initial insertion of battery
      package—*omit code*
  tunnel, subcutaneous for pulse generator lead
    wire 86.99
    with initial procedure —*omit code*
  skull (bone) 01.24
  soft tissue NEC 83.09
    with division 83.19
      hand 82.19
    hand 82.09
      with division 82.19
  space of Retzius 59.19
  spermatic cord 63.93
  sphincter of Oddi 51.82
    endoscopic 51.85
  spinal
    cord 03.09
    nerve root 03.1
  spleen 41.2
  stomach 43.0
  stye 08.09
  subarachnoid space, cerebral 01.31
  subcutaneous tissue 86.09
    with drainage 86.04
    tunnel
      esophageal 42.86
        with anastomosis—*see* Anastomosis,
          esophagus, antesternal
      pulse generator lead wire 86.99
        with initial procedure—*omit code*
  subdiaphragmatic space 54.19
  subdural space, cerebral 01.31
  sublingual space 27.0
  submandibular space 27.0
  submaxillary 86.09
    with drainage 86.04
  submental space 27.0
  subphrenic space 54.19
  supraclavicular fossa 86.09
    with drainage 86.04
  sweat glands, skin 86.04
  temporal pouches 27.0
  tendon (sheath) 83.01
    with division 83.13
      hand 82.11
    hand 82.01
      with division 82.11
  testis 62.0
  thenar space 82.04
  thymus (open) (other) 07.92
    thoracoscopic 07.95
  thyroid (field) (gland) NEC 06.09
    postoperative 06.02
  tongue NEC 25.94
    for tongue tic 25.91
  tonsil 28.0
  trachea NEC 31.3
  tunica vaginalis 61.0
  umbilicus 54.0
  urachal cyst 54.0
  ureter 56.2
  urethra 58.0
  uterus (corpus) 68.0
    cervix 69.95
    for termination of pregnancy 74.91
    septum (congenital) 68.22

Incision—*continued*
  uvula 27.71
  vagina (cull) (septum) (stenosis) 70.14
    for
      incisional hematoma (episiotomy) 75.91
      obstetrical hematoma NEC 75.92
      pelvic abscess 70.12
  vas deferens 63.6
  vein 38.00
    abdominal 38.07
    head and neck NEC 38.02
    intracranial NEC 38.01
    lower limb 38.09
    thoracic NEC 38.05
    upper limb 38.03
  vertebral column 03.09
  vulva 71.09
    obstetrical 75.92
  web, esophageal 42.01
Incudectomy NEC 19.3
  with
    stapedectomy (*see also* Stapedectomy) 19.19
    Tympanoplasty—*see* Tympanoplasty
Incudopexy 19.19
Incudostapediopexy 19.19
  with incus replacement 19.11
Indentation, sclera, for buckling (*see also*
  Buckling, scleral) 14.49
Indicator dilution flow measurement 89.68
Induction
  abortion
    by
      D and C 69.01
      insertion of prostaglandin suppository 96.49
      intra-amniotic injection (prostaglandin)
        (saline) 75.0
  labor
    medical 73.4
    surgical 73.01
      intra- and extra-amniotic injection 73.1
      stripping of membranes 73.1
Inflation
  belt wrap 93.99
  Eustachian tube 20.8
  fallopian tube 66.8
    with injection of therapeutic agent 66.95
Infolding sclera, for buckling (*see also*
  Buckling, scleral) 14.49
Infraction, turbinates (nasal) 21.62
Infundibulectomy
  hypophyseal (*see also* Hypophysectomy, partial)
    07.63
  ventricle (heart) (right) 35.34
    in total repair of tetralogy of Fallot 35.81
Infusion (intra-arterial) (intravenous)
  with
    disruption of blood brain barrier [BBBD] 00.19
  Abciximab 99.20
  antibiotic
    oxazolidinone class 00.14
  antineoplastic agent (chemotherapeutic) 99.25
    biological response modifier [BRM] 99.28
    cintredekin besudotox 99.28
    CLO 17.70
    clofarabine 17.70
    CLOLAR® 17.70
    high-dose interleukin-2 00.15
    low-dose interleukin-2 99.28

Infusion—*continued*
biological response modifier [BRM],
    antineoplastic agent 99.28
  cintredekin besudotox 99.28
  high-dose interleukin-2 00.15
  low-dose interleukin-2 99.28
cancer chemotherapy agent NEC 99.25
cintredekin besudotox 99.28
CLO 17.70
clofarabine 17.70
CLOLAR® 17.70
drotrecogin alfa (activated) 00.11
electrolytes 99.18
enzymes, thrombolytic (streptokinase) (tissue
    plasminogen activator) (TPA) (urokinase)
  direct coronary artery 36.04
  intravenous 99.10
Eptifibatide 99.20
gamma globulin 99.14
glucarpidase 00.95
GP IIB/IIIa inhibitor 99.20
hormone substance NEC 99.24
human B-type natriuretic peptide (hBNP) 00.13
IgG (immunoglobulin) 99.14
immunoglobulin (IgG) (IVIG) (IVIg) 99.14
immunosuppressive antibody therapy 00.18
interleukin-2
  high-dose 00.15
  low-dose 99.28
IVIG (immunoglobulin) (IVIg) 99.14
lymphocyte 99.09
nesiritide 00.13
neuroprotective agent 99.75
nimodipine 99.75
nutritional substance (*see* Nutrition)
platelet inhibitor
  direct coronary artery 36.04
  intravenous 99.20
Proleukin (low-dose) 99.28
  high-dose 00.15
prophylactic substance NEC 99.29
radioimmunoconjugate 92.28
radioimmunotherapy 92.28
radioisotope (liquid brachytherapy) (liquid I-125)
    92.20
recombinant protein 00.11
reteplase 99.10
therapeutic substance NEC 99.29
thrombolytic agent (enzyme) (streptokinase)
    99.10
  with percutaneous transluminal angioplasty

*Note: Also use 00.40, 00.41, 00.42, or 00.43 to
show the total number of vessels treated.*

    coronary 00.66
    non-coronary vessel(s) 39.50
      specified site NEC 39.50
    direct intracoronary artery 36.04
tirofiban (HCl) 99.20
vaccine
  tumor 99.28
vasopressor 00.17
Voraxaze® 00.95
Injection (into) (hypodermically)
    (intramuscularly) (intravenously) (acting
    locally or systemically)
Actinomycin D, for cancer chemotherapy 99.25
adhesion barrier substance 99.77
alcohol
  nerve—*see* Injection, nerve
  spinal 03.8

Injection—*continued*
anterior chamber, eye (air) (liquid) (medication)
    12.92
antibiotic 99.21
  oxazolidinone class 00.14
anticoagulant 99.19
anti-D (Rhesus) globulin 99.11
antidote NEC 99.16
anti-infective NEC 99.22
antineoplastic agent (chemotherapeutic) 99.25
  biological response modifier [BRM] 99.28
  cintredekin besudotox 99.28
  high-dose interleukin-2 00.15
  low-dose interleukin-2 99.28
antivenin 99.16
barrier substance, adhesion 99.77
BCG
  for chemotherapy 99.25
  vaccine 99.33
biological response modifier [BRM],
    antineoplastic agent 99.28
  cintredekin besudotox 99.28
  high-dose interleukin-2 00.15
  low-dose interleukin-2 99.28
bone marrow 41.92
  transplant—*see* Transplant, bone, marrow
breast (therapeutic agent) 85.92
  inert material (silicone) (bilateral) 85.52
  unilateral 85.51
bursa (therapeutic agent) 83.96
  hand 82.94
cancer chemotherapeutic agent 99.25
caudal—*see* Injection, spinal
cintredekin besudotox 99.28
cortisone 99.23
costochondral junction 81.92
dinoprost-tromethine, intra-amniotic 75.0
ear, with alcohol 20.72
electrolytes 99.18
enzymes, thrombolytic (streptokinase) (tissue
    plasminogen activator) (TPA) (urokinase)
  direct coronary artery 36.04
  intravenous 99.10
epidural, spinal—*see* Injection, spinal
esophageal varices or blood vessel
    (endoscopic)(sclerosing agent) 42.33
Eustachian tube (inert material) 20.8
eye (orbit) (retrobulbar) 16.91
  anterior chamber 12.92
  subconjunctival 10.91
fascia 83.98
  hand 82.96
gamma globulin 99.14
ganglion, sympathetic 05.39
  ciliary 12.79
  paravertebral stellate 05.39
gel, adhesion barrier—*see* Injection, adhesion
    barrier substance
globulin
  anti-D (Rhesus) 99.11
  gamma 99.14
  Rh immune 99.11
glucarpidase 00.95
heart 37.92
heavy metal antagonist 99.16
hemorrhoids (sclerosing agent) 49.42
hormone NEC 99.24
human B-type natriuretic peptide (hBNP) 00.13
IgG (immunoglobulin) 99.14
immune sera 99.14
immunoglobulin (IgG) (IVIG) (IVIg) 99.14

Injection—*continued*
inert material—*see* Implant, inert material
inner ear, for destruction 20.72
insulin 99.17
intervertebral space for herniated disc 80.52
intra-amniotic
  for induction of
    abortion 75.0
    labor 73.1
intrathecal—*see* Injection, spinal
IVIG (immunoglobulin) (IVIg) 99.14
joint (therapeutic agent) 81.92
  temporomandibular 76.96
kidney (cyst) (therapeutic substance) NEC 55.96
larynx 31.0
ligament (joint) (therapeutic substance) 81.92
liver 50.94
lung, for surgical collapse 33.32
Methotrexate, for cancer chemotherapy 99.25
nerve (cranial) (peripheral) 04.80
  agent NEC 04.89
    alcohol 04.2
    anesthetic for analgesia 04.81
      for operative anesthesia—*omit code*
    neurolytic 04.2
    phenol 04.2
  laryngeal (external) (recurrent) (superior) 31.91
  optic 16.91
  sympathetic 05.39
    alcohol 05.32
    anesthetic for analgesia 05.31
    neurolytic agent 05.32
    phenol 05.32
nesiritide 00.13
neuroprotective agent 99.75
nimodipine 99.75
orbit 16.91
pericardium 37.93
peritoneal cavity
  air 54.96
  locally-acting therapeutic substance 54.97
platelet inhibitor
  direct coronary artery 36.04
  intravenous 99.20
prophylactic substance NEC 99.29
prostate 60.92
radioimmunoconjugate 92.28
radioimmunotherapy 92.28
radioisotopes (intracavitary) (intravenous) 92.28
renal pelvis (cyst) 55.96
retrobulbar (therapeutic substance) 16.91
  for anesthesia—*omit code*
Rh immune globulin 99.11
RhoGAM 99.11
sclerosing agent NEC 99.29
  esophageal varices 42.33
  hemorrhoids 49.42
  pleura 34.92
    treatment of malignancy (cytotoxic agent)
      34.92 *[99.25]*
      with tetracycline 34.92 *[99.21]*
  varicose vein 39.92
  vein NEC 39.92
semicircular canals, for destruction 20.72
silicone—*see* Implant, inert material
skin (sclerosing agent) (filling material) 86.02
soft tissue 83.98
  hand 82.96

Injection— *continued*
spinal (canal) NEC 03.92
  alcohol 03.8
  anesthetic agent for analgesia 03.91
  for operative anesthesia—*omit code*
  contrast material (for myelogram) 87.21
  destructive agent NEC 03.8
  neurolytic agent NEC 03.8
  phenol 03.8
  proteolytic enzyme (chemopapain)
    (chemodiactin) 80.52
  saline (hypothermic) 03.92
  steroid 03.92
spinal nerve root (intrathecal)—*see* Injection,
  spinal
steroid NEC 99.23
subarachnoid, spinal—*see* Injection, spinal
subconjunctival 10.91
tendon 83.97
  hand 82.95
testis 62.92
therapeutic agent NEC 99.29
thoracic cavity 34.92
thrombolytic agent (enzyme) (streptokinase)
  99.10
  with percutaneous transluminal angioplasty

Note: Also use 00.40, 00.41, 00.42, or 00.43 to
show the total number of vessels treated.

    coronary 00.66
    direct intracoronary artery 36.04
    non-coronary vessel(s) 39.50
    specified site NEC 39.50
  trachea 31.94
  tranquilizer 99.26
  tunica vaginalis (with aspiration) 61.91
  tympanum 20.94
  urethra (inert material)
    for repair of urinary stress incontinence
      collagen implant 59.72
      endoscopic injection of implant 59.72
      fat implant 59.72
      polytef implant 59.72
  vaccine
    tumor 99.28
  varices, esophagus (endoscopic) (sclerosing
    agent) 42.33
  varicose vein (sclerosing agent) 39.92
    esophagus 42.33
  vestibule, for destruction 20.72
  vitreous substitute (silicone) 14.75
    for reattachment of retina 14.59
  vocal cords 31.0
  Voraxaze® 00.95
Inlay, tooth 23.3
Inoculation
  antitoxins—*see* Administration, antitoxins
  toxoids—*see* Administration, toxoids
  vaccine—*see* Administration, vaccine
Insemination, artificial 69.92
Insertion
  airway
    esophageal obturator 96.03
    nasopharynx 96.01
    oropharynx 96.02
  Allen-Brown cannula 39.93
  antimicrobial envelope 17.81
  aqueous drainage device (shunt) (stent) 12.67
  arch bars (orthodontic) 24.7
    for immobilization (fracture) 93.55
  atrial septal umbrella 35.52

Insertion—*continued*
epicardial support device 37.41
Impella® 37.68
pacemaker—*see* Insertion, pacemaker, cardiac
prosthetic cardiac support device 37.41
pump (Kantrowitz) 37.62
valve—*see* Replacement, heart valve
ventricular support device 37.41
hip prosthesis (partial) 81.52
revision NOS 81.53
acetabular and femoral components (total)
00.70
acetabular component only 00.71
acetabular liner and/or femoral head only
00.73
femoral component only 00.72
femoral head only and/or acetabular liner
00.73
partial
acetabular component only 00.71
acetabular liner and/or femoral head only
00.73
femoral component only 00.72
femoral head only and/or acetabular liner
00.73
total (acetabular and femoral components)
00.70
total 81.51
revision
acetabular and femoral components (total)
00.70
total (acetabular and femoral components)
00.70
Holter valve 02.22
Hufnagel valve—*see* Replacement, heart valve
implant—*see* Insertion, prosthesis
infusion pump 86.06
interbody spinal fusion device 84.51
intercostal catheter (with water seal) for drainage
34.04
revision (with lysis of adhesions) 34.04
thoracoscopic 34.06
intra-arterial blood gas monitoring system 89.60
intrauterine
contraceptive device 69.7
radium (intracavitary) 69.91
tamponade (nonobstetric) 69.91
Kantrowitz
heart pump 37.62
pulsation balloon (phase-shift) 37.61
keratoprosthesis 11.73
King-Mills umbrella device (heart) 35.52
Kirschner wire 93.44
with reduction of fracture or dislocation—*see*
Reduction, fracture *and* Reduction,
dislocation
knee prosthesis (partial) (total) 81.54
revision NOS 81.55
femoral component 00.82
partial
femoral component 00.82
patellar component 00.83
tibial component 00.81
tibial insert 00.84
patellar component 00.83
tibial component 00.81
tibial insert 00.84
total (all components) 00.80
laminaria, cervix 69.93
Lap-Band™ 44.95
larynx, valved tube 31.75
leads—*see* Insertion, electrode(s)

Insertion—*continued*
lens, prosthetic (intraocular) 13.70
with cataract extraction, one-stage 13.71
secondary (subsequent to cataract extraction)
13.72
limb lengthening device, internal, NOS 84.54
with kinetic distraction 84.53
loop recorder 37.79
M-Brace™ 84.82
metal staples into epiphyseal plate (*see also*
Stapling, epiphyseal plate) 78.20
minifixator device (bone)—*see* category 78.1
Mobitz-Uddin umbrella, vena cava 38.7
mold, vagina 96.15
Moore (cup) 81.52
myringotomy device (button) (tube) 20.01
with intubation 20.01
nasobiliary drainage tube (endoscopic) 51.86
nasogastric tube
for
decompression, intestinal 96.07
feeding 96.6
naso-intestinal tube 96.08
nasolacrimal tube or stent 09.44
nasopancreatic drainage tube (endoscopic) 52.97
neuropacemaker—*see* Implant, neurostimulator,
by site
neurostimulator—*see* Implant, neurostimulator,
by site
non-coronary vessel
stent(s) (stent graft)

> Note: Also use 00.40, 00.41, 00.42, or 00.43 to
> show the total number of vessels treated. Use
> code 00.44 once to show procedure on a
> bifurcated vessel. In addition, use 00.45, 00.46,
> 00.47, or 00.48 to show the number of vascular
> stents inserted.

basilar 00.64
carotid 00.63
extracranial 00.64
intracranial 00.65
peripheral 39.90
bare, drug-coated 39.90
drug-eluting 00.55
vertebral 00.64
with
angioplasty 39.50
atherectomy 17.56
bypass—*omit code*
non-invasive (transcutaneous) (surface)
stimulator 99.86
obturator (orthodontic) 24.7
ocular implant
with synchronous
enucleation 16.42
with muscle attachment to implant 16.41
evisceration 16.31
following or secondary to
enucleation 16.61
evisceration 16.61
Ommaya reservoir 02.22
orbital implant (stent) (outside muscle cone)
16.69
with orbitotomy 16.02
orthodontic appliance (obturator) (wiring) 24.7
outflow tract prosthesis (gusset type) (heart)
in
pulmonary valvuloplasty 35.26
total repair of tetralogy of Fallot 35.81

Insertion—*continued*
pacemaker
  brain—*see* Implant, neurostimulator, brain
  cardiac (device) (initial) (permanent)
      (replacement) 37.80
    dual-chamber device (initial) 37.83
      replacement 37.87
    during and immediately following cardiac
      surgery 39.64
    resynchronization (biventricular pacemaker)
      (BiV pacemaker) (CRT-P) (device)
      device only (initial) (replacement) 00.53
      total system (device and one or more leads)
          00.50
      transvenous lead into left ventricular
          coronary venous system 00.52
    single-chamber device (initial) 37.81
      rate responsive 37.82
      replacement 37.85
        rate responsive 37.86
    temporary transvenous pacemaker system
        37.78
    during and immediately following cardiac
        surgery 39.64
  carotid 39.89
  gastric 04.92
  heart—*see* Insertion, pacemaker, cardiac
  intracranial—*see* Implant, neurostimulator,
      intracranial
  neural—*see* Implant, neurostimulator, by site
  peripheral nerve—*see* Implant, neurostimulator,
      peripheral nerve
  spine—*see* Implant, neurostimulator, spine
pacing catheter—*see* Insertion, pacemaker,
    cardiac
pack
  auditory canal, external 96.11
  cervix (nonobstetrical) 67.0
    after delivery or abortion 75.8
    to assist delivery or induce labor 73.1
  rectum 96.19
  sella turcica 07.79
  vagina (nonobstetrical) 96.14
    after delivery or abortion 75.8
palatal implant 27.64
penis, prosthetic (non-inflatable) (internal) 64.95
  inflatable (internal) 64.97
peridontal splint (orthodontic) 24.7
peripheral blood vessel—*see* non-coronary
pessary
  cervix 96.18
    to assist delivery or induce labor 73.1
  vagina 96.18
pharyngeal valve, artificial 31.75
port, vascular access 86.07
prostaglandin suppository (for abortion) 96.49

Insertion—*continued*
prosthesis, prosthetic device
  acetabulum (partial) 81.52
  hip 81.52
    revision NOS 81.53
      acetabular and femoral components (total)
          00.70
      acetabular component only 00.71
      acetabular liner and/or femoral head only
          00.73
      femoral component only 00.72
      femoral head only and/or acetabular liner
          00.73
      partial
        acetabular component only 00.71
        acetabular liner and/or femoral head
            only 00.73
        femoral component only 00.72
        femoral head only and/or acetabular
            liner 00.73
      total (acetabular and femoral components)
          00.70
  ankle (total) 81.56
  arm (bioelectric) (cineplastic) (kineplastic)
      84.44
  biliary tract 51.99
  breast (bilateral) 85.54
    unilateral 85.53
  cardiac support device (CSD) (CorCap™)
      37.41
  chin (polyethylene) (silastic) 76.68
  elbow (total) 81.84
    revision 81.97
  extremity (bioelectric) (cineplastic)
      (kineplastic) 84.40
    lower 84.48
    upper 84.44
  fallopian tube 66.93
  femoral head (Austin-Moore) (bipolar) (Eicher)
      (Thompson) 81.52
  hip (partial) 81.52
    revision NOS 81.53
      acetabular and femoral components (total)
          00.70
      acetabular component only 00.71
      acetabular liner and/or femoral head only
          00.73
      femoral component only 00.72
      femoral head only and/or acetabular liner
          00.73
      partial
        acetabular component only 00.71
        acetabular liner and/or femoral head
            only 00.73
        femoral component only 00.72
        femoral head only and/or acetabular
            liner 00.73
      total (acetabular and femoral components)
          00.70
    total 81.51
      revision
        acetabular and femoral components (total)
            00.70
        total (acetabular and femoral components)
            00.70
  joint—*see* Arthroplasty

Insertion—*continued*
  knee (partial) (total) 81.54
    revision NOS 81.55
      femoral component 00.82
      partial
        femoral component 00.82
        patellar component 00.83
        tibial component 00.81
        tibial insert 00.84
      patellar component 00.83
      tibial component 00.81
      tibial insert 00.84
      total (all components) 00.80
  leg (bioelectric) (cineplastic) (kineplastic) 84.48
  lens 13.91
  ocular (secondary) 16.61
    with orbital exenteration 16.42
  outflow tract (gusset type) (heart)
    in
      pulmonary valvuloplasty 35.26
      total repair of tetralogy of Fallot 35.81
  penile (non-inflatable) (internal) 64.95
    inflatable (internal) 64.97
    with
      construction 64.43
      reconstruction 64.44
  Rosen (for urinary incontinence) 59.79
  shoulder
    partial 81.81
    revision 81.97
    total, NEC 81.80
      other 81.80
      reverse 81.88
  spine
    artificial disc, NOS 84.60
      cervical 84.62
        nucleus 84.61
        partial 84.61
        total 84.62
      lumbar, lumbosacral 84.65
        nucleus 84.64
        partial 84.64
        total 84.65
      thoracic (partial) (total) 84.63
    other device 84.59
  testicular (bilateral) (unilateral) 62.7
  toe 81.57
    for hallux valgus repair 77.59
  vagina
    synthetic 70.95
  pseudophakos (*see also* Insertion, lens) 13.70
  pump, infusion 86.06
  radioactive isotope 92.27
  radium 92.27
  radon seeds 92.27
  Reuter bobbin (with intubation) 20.01
  Rickham, reservoir 02.22
  Rosen prosthesis (for urinary incontinence) 59.79
  Scribner shunt 39.93
  Sengstaken-Blakemore tube 96.06
  sensor (lead)
    intra-aneurysm sac pressure monitoring device
      00.58
    intra-arterial, for continuous blood gas
      monitoring 89.60
    intracardiac or great vessel hemodynamic
      monitoring
      with lead 00.56
      without lead 38.26
  shunt—*see* Shunt
  sieve, vena cava 38.7
  skeletal muscle stimulator 83.92

Insertion—*continued*
  skull
    plate 02.05
    stereotactic frame 93.59
    tongs (Barton) (caliper) (Garder Wells) (Vinke)
      (with synchronous skeletal traction) 02.94
  spacer (cement) (joint) (methylmethacrylate)
    84.56
    spine 84.51
  sphenoidal electrodes 02.96
  spine
    bone void filler
      that with percutaneous vertebral
        augmentation 81.66
      that with percutaneous vertebroplasty 81.65
    cage (BAK) 84.51
    facet replacement device(s) 84.84
    interbody spinal fusion device 84.51
    interspinous process decompression device
      84.80
    non-fusion stabilization device —*see* category
      84.8
    pedicle-based dynamic stabilization device(s)
      84.82
    posterior motion preservation device(s) —*see*
      category 84.8
    spacer 84.51
  Spitz-Holter valve 02.2
  Steinmann pin 93.44
    with reduction of fracture or dislocation—*see*
      Reduction, fracture *and* Reduction,
      dislocation
  stent(s) (stent graft)
    aqueous drainage 12.67
    artery (bare) (bonded) (drug-coated)
      (non-drug-eluting)

> *Note: Also use 00.40, 00.41, 00.42, or 00.43 to show the total number of vessels treated. Use code 00.44 once to show procedure on a bifurcated vessel. In addition, use 00.45, 00.46, 00.47, or 00.48 to show the number of vascular stents inserted.*

      basilar 00.64
      carotid 00.63
      cerebrovascular
        cerebral (intracranial) 00.65
        precerebral (extracranial) 00.64
          carotid 00.63
      coronary (bare) (bonded) (drug-coated)
        (non-drug-eluting) 36.06
        drug-eluting 36.07
      extracranial 00.64
        carotid 00.63
      femoral artery, superficial 39.90
        drug-eluting 00.60
        non-drug eluting 39.90
      intracranial 00.65
      non-coronary vessel
        basilar 0.64
        carotid 00.63
        extracranial 00.64
        femoral artery, superficial 39.90
          drug eluting 00.60
          non-drug eluting 39.90
        intracranial 00.65
      peripheral 39.90
        bare, drug-coated 39.90
        drug-eluting 00.55
        femoral artery, superficial, drug eluting
          00.60
      vertebral 00.64

Insertion—*continued*
  bile duct 51.43
    endoscopic 51.87
    percutaneous transhepatic 51.98
  colon
    endoscopic (fluoroscopic guidance) 46.86
    other 46.87
  coronary (artery) (bare) (bonded) (drug-coated)
    (non-drug-eluting) 36.06

*Note: Also use 00.40, 00.41, 00.42, or 00.43 to
show the total number of vessels treated. Use
code 00.44 once to show procedure on a
bifurcated vessel. In addition, use 00.45, 00.46,
00.47, or 00.48 to show the number of vascular
stents inserted.*

    drug-eluting 36.07
  esophagus (endoscopic) (fluoroscopic) 42.81
  mesenteric 39.90
    bare, drug-coated 39.90
    drug-eluting 00.55
  non-coronary vessel

*Note: Also use 00.40, 00.41, 00.42, or 00.43 to
show the total number of vessels treated. Use
code 00.44 once to show procedure on a
bifurcated vessel. In addition, use 00.45, 00.46,
00.47, or 00.48 to show the number of vascular
stents inserted.*

    basilar 00.64
    carotid 00.63
    extracranial 00.64
    intracranial 00.65
    mesenteric 39.90
      bare, drug-coated 39.90
      drug-eluting 00.55
    peripheral 39.90
      bare, drug-coated 39.90
      drug-eluting 00.55
    renal 39.90
      bare, drug-coated 39.90
      drug-eluting 00.55
    vertebral 00.64
    with angioplasty or atherectomy 39.50
  pancreatic duct 52.92
    endoscopic 52.93
  peripheral 39.90

*Note: Also use 00.40, 00.41, 00.42, or 00.43 to
show the total number of vessels treated. Use
code 00.44 once to show procedure on a
bifurcated vessel. In addition, use 00.45, 00.46,
00.47, or 00.48 to show the number of vascular
stents inserted.*

    bare, drug-coated 39.90
    drug-eluting 00.55
  precerebral 00.64

*Note: Also use 00.40, 00.41, 00.42, or 00.43 to
show the total number of vessels treated. Use
code 00.44 once to show procedure on a
bifurcated vessel. In addition, use 00.45, 00.46,
00.47, or 00.48 to show the number of vascular
stents inserted.*

  renal 39.90
    bare, drug-coated 39.90
    drug-eluting 00.55

Insertion—*continued*
  subclavian 39.90

*Note: Also use 00.40, 00.41, 00.42, or 00.43 to
show the total number of vessels treated. Use
code 00.44 once to show procedure on a
bifurcated vessel. In addition, use 00.45, 00.46,
00.47, or 00.48 to show the number of vascular
stents inserted.*

    bare, drug-coated 39.90
    drug-eluting 00.55
  tracheobronchial 96.05
  vertebral 00.64

*Note: Also use 00.40, 00.41, 00.42, or 00.43 to
show the total number of vessels treated. Use
code 00.44 once to show procedure on a
bifurcated vessel. In addition, use 00.45, 00.46,
00.47, or 00.48 to show the number of vascular
stents inserted.*

  sternal fixation device with rigid plates 84.94
  stimoceiver—*see* Implant, neurostimulator, by
    site
  stimulator for bone growth—*see* category 78.9
  subdural
    grids 02.93
    strips 02.93
  suppository
    prostaglandin (for abortion) 96.49
    vagina 96.49
  Swan-Ganz catheter (pulmonary) 89.64
  tampon
    esophagus 96.06
    uterus 69.91
    vagina 96.14
    after delivery or abortion 75.8
  Tandem™ heart 37.68
  telescope (IMT) (miniature) 13.91
  testicular prosthesis (bilateral) (unilateral) 62.7
  tissue expander (skin) NEC 86.93
    breast 85.95
  tissue mandril (peripheral vessel) (Dacron)
    (Spark's type) 39.99
  with
    blood vessel repair 39.56
    vascular bypass or shunt—*see* Bypass,
      vascular
  tongs, skull (with synchronous skeletal traction)
    02.94
  totally implanted device for bone growth
    (invasive)—*see* category 78.9
  tube—*see also* Catheterization *and* Intubation
    bile duct 51.43
      endoscopic 51.87
    chest 34.04
      revision (with lysis of adhesions) 34.04
        thoracoscopic 34.06
      thoracoscopic 34.06
    endotracheal 96.04
    esophagus (nonoperative) (Sengstaken) 96.06
      permanent (silicone) (Souttar) 42.81
    feeding
      esophageal 42.81
      gastric 96.6
      nasogastric 96.6
    gastric
      by gastrostomy—*see* category 43.1
      for
        decompression, intestinal 96.07
        feeding 96.6

Intubation—*continued*
  intestine (for decompression) 96.08
  lacrimal for
    dilation 09.42
    tear drainage, intranasal 09.81
  larynx 96.05
  nasobiliary (drainage) 51.86
  nasogastric
    for
      decompression, intestinal 96.07
      feeding 96.6
  naso-intestinal 96.08
  nasolacrimal (duct) (with irrigation) 09.44
  nasopancreatic drainage (endoscopic) 52.97
  respiratory tract NEC 96.05
  small intestine (Miller-Abbott) 96.08
  stomach (nasogastric) (for intestinal
    decompression) NEC 96.07
    for feeding 96.6
  trachea 96.04
  ventriculocisternal 02.22
Invagination, diverticulum
  gastric 44.69
    laparoscopic 44.68
  pharynx 29.59
  stomach 44.69
    laparoscopic 44.68
Inversion
  appendix 47.99
  diverticulum
    gastric 44.69
      laparoscopic 44.68
    intestine
      large 45.49
        endoscopic 45.43
      small 45.34
    stomach 44.69
      laparoscopic 44.68
  tunica vaginalis 61.49
IOERT (intra-operative electron radiation
  therapy) 92.41
IOM (intra-operative neurophysiologic
  monitoring) 00.94
Ionization, medical 99.27
Iontherapy 99.27
Iontophoresis 99.27
Iridectomy (basal) (buttonhole) (optical)
  (peripheral) (total) 12.14
  with
    capsulectomy 13.65
    cataract extraction—*see* Extraction, cataract
    filtering operation (for glaucoma) NEC 12.65
    scleral
      fistulization 12.65
      thermocauterization 12.62
      trephination 12.61
Iridencleisis 12.63
Iridesis 12.63
Irido-capsulectomy 13.65
Iridocyclectomy 12.44
Iridocystectomy 12.42
Iridodesis 12.63
Iridoplasty NEC 12.39
Iridosclerectomy 12.65
Iridosclerotomy 12.69
Iridotasis 12.63
Iridotomy 12.12
  by photocoagulation 12.12
  with transfixion 12.11
  for iris bombé 12.11
  specified type NEC 12.12

Iron lung 93.99
Irradiation
  gamma, stereotactic 92.32
Irrigation
  anterior chamber (eye) 12.91
  bronchus NEC 96.56
  canaliculus 09.42
  catheter
    ureter 96.46
    urinary, indwelling NEC 96.48
    vascular 96.57
    ventricular 02.41
    wound 96.58
  cholecystostomy 96.41
  cornea 96.51
    with removal of foreign body 98.21
  corpus cavernosum 64.98
  cystostomy 96.47
  ear (removal of cerumen) 96.52
  enterostomy 96.36
  eye 96.51
    with removal of foreign body 98.21
  gastrostomy 96.36
  lacrimal
    canaliculi 09.42
    punctum 09.41
  muscle 83.02
    hand 82.02
  nasal
    passages 96.53
    sinus 22.00
  nasolacrimal duct 09.43
    with insertion of tube or stent 09.44
  nephrostomy 96.45
  peritoneal 54.25
  pyelostomy 96.45
  rectal 96.39
  stomach 96.33
  tendon (sheath) 83.01
    hand 82.01
  trachea NEC 96.56
  traumatic cataract 13.3
  tube
    biliary NEC 96.41
    nasogastric NEC 96.34
    pancreatic 96.42
  ureterostomy 96.46
  ventricular shunt 02.41
  wound (cleaning) NEC 96.59
Irving operation (tubal ligation) 66.32
Irwin operation (*see also* Osteotomy) 77.30
Ischiectomy (partial) 77.89
  total 77.99
Ischiopubiotomy 77.39
Isolation
  after contact with infectious disease 99.84
  ileal loop 45.51
  intestinal segment or pedicle nap
    large 45.52
    small 45.51
Isthmectomy, thyroid (*see also* Thyroidectomy,
  partial) 06.39
IVUS —see Ultrasound, intravascular, by site

J-K

Joulay operation (gastroduodenostomy) 44.39
  laparoscopic 44.38
Janeway operation (permanent gastrostomy)
  43.19
Jatene operation (arterial switch) 35.84
Jejunectomy 45.62
Jejunocecostomy 45.93
Jejunocholecystostomy 51.32
Jejunocolostomy 45.93
Jejunoileostomy 45.91
Jejunojejunostomy 45.91
Jejunopexy 46.61
Jejunorrhaphy 46.73
Jejunostomy (feeding) 46.39
  delayed opening 46.31
  loop 46.01
  percutaneous (endoscopic) (PEJ) 46.32
  revision 46.41
Jejunotomy 45.02
Johanson operation (urethral reconstruction)
  58.46
Jones operation
  claw toe (transfer of extensor hallucis longus
    tendon) 77.57
    modified (with arthrodesis) 77.57
  dacryocystorhinostomy 09.81
  hammer toe (interphalangeal fusion) 77.56
  modified (tendon transfer with arthrodesis) 77.57
  repair of peroneal tendon 83.88
Joplin operation (exostectomy with tendon
  transfer) 77.53

Kader operation (temporary gastrostomy) 43.19
Kasai portoenterostomy 51.37
Kaufman operation (for urinary stress
  incontinence) 59.79
Kazanjiian operation (buccal vestibular sulcus
  extension) 24.91
Kehr operation (hepatopexy) 50.69
Keller operation (bunionectomy) 77.59
Kelly (Kennedy) operation (urethrovesical
  plication) 59.3
Kelly-Stoeckel operation (urethrovesical
  plication) 59.3
Kelotomy 53.9
Keratectomy (complete) (partial) (superficial)
  11.49
  for pterygium 11.39
    with corneal graft 11.32
Keratocentesis (for hyphema) 12.91
Keratomileusis 11.71
Keratophakia 11.72
Keratoplasty (tectonic) (with autograft) (with
  homograft) 11.60
  lamellar (nonpenetrating) (with homograft) 11.62
    with autograft 11.61
  penetrating (full-thickness) (with homograft)
    11.64
    with autograft 11.63
  perforating—*see* Keratoplasty, penetrating
  refractive 11.71
  specified type NEC 11.69
Keratoprosthesis 11.73
Keratotomy (delimiting) (posterior) 11.1
  radial (refractive) 11.75
Kerr operation (low cervical cesarean section)
  74.1
Kessler operation (arthroplasty, carpometacarpal
  joint) 81.74
Kidner operation (excision of accessory
  navicular bone) (with tendon transfer) 77.98
Killian operation (frontal sinusotomy) 22.41
Kineplasty —*see* Cineplasty
King-Steelquist operation (hindquarter
  amputation) 84.19
Kirk operation (amputation through thigh) 84.17
Kock pouch operation
  bowel anastomosis—*omit code*
  continent ileostomy 46.22
  cutaneous uretero-ileostomy 56.51
  ESWL (extracorporeal shockwave lithotripsy)
    98.51
  removal, calculus 57.19
  revision, cutaneous uretero-ileostomy 56.52
  urinary diversion procedure 56.51
Kondoleon operation (correction of
  lymphedema) 40.9
Krause operation (sympathetic denervation)
  05.29
Kroener operation (partial salpingectomy) 66.69
Kroenlein operation (lateral orbitotomy) 16.01
Krönig operation (low cervical cesarean section)
  74.1
Krukenberg operation (reconstruction of
  below-elbow amputation) 82.89
Kuhnt-Szymanowski operation (ectropion
  repair with lid reconstruction) 08.44
Kyphoplasty 81.66

L

LEEP (loop elecrosurgical excision procedure)
   of cervix 67.32
Le Fort operation (colpocleisis) 70.8
LeMesurier operation (cleft lip repair) 27.54
Lengthening
   bone (with bone graft) 78.30
      femur 78.35
      for reconstruction of thumb 82.69
      specified site NEC (*see also* category 78.3) 78.39
      tibia 78.37
      ulna 78.33
   extraocular muscle NEC 15.21
      multiple (two or more muscles) 15.4
   fascia 83.89
      hand 82.89
   hamstring NEC 83.85
   heel cord 83.85
   leg
      femur 78.35
      tibia 78.37
   levator palpebrae muscle 08.38
   muscle 83.85
      extraocular 15.21
         multiple (two or more muscles) 15.4
      hand 82.55
   palate 27.62
      secondary or subsequent 27.63
   tendon 83.85
      for claw toe repair 77.57
      hand 82.55
Leriche operation (periarterial sympathectomy)
   05.25
Leucotomy, leukotomy 01.32
Leukopheresis, therapeutic 99.72
Lid suture operation (blepharoptosis) 08.31
Ligation
   adrenal vessel (artery) (vein) 07.43
   aneurysm 39.52
   appendages, dermal 86.26
   arteriovenous fistula 39.53
      coronary artery 36.99
   artery 38.80
      abdominal 38.86
      adrenal 07.43
      aorta (arch) (ascending) (descending) 38.84
      coronary (anomalous) 36.99
      ethmoidal 21.04
      external carotid 21.06
      for control of epistaxis—*see* Control, epistaxis
      head and neck NEC 38.82
      intracranial NEC 38.81
      lower limb 38.88
      maxillary (transantral) 21.05
      middle meningeal 02.13
      thoracic NEC 38.85
      thyroid 06.92
      upper limb 38.83
   atrium, heart 37.99
   auricle, heart 37.99
   bleeding vessel—*see* Control, hemorrhage
   blood vessel 38.80
      abdominal
         artery 38.86
         vein 38.87
      adrenal 07.43
      aorta (arch) (ascending) (descending) 38.84
      esophagus 42.91
         endoscopic 42.33
      head and neck NEC 38.82
      intracranial NEC 38.81

Ligation—*continued*
   lower limb
      artery 38.88
      vein 38.89
   meningeal (artery) (longitudinal sinus) 02.13
   thoracic NEC 38.85
   thyroid 06.92
   upper limb (artery) (vein) 38.83
   bronchus 33.92
   cisterna chyli 40.64
   coronary
      artery (anomalous) 36.99
      sinus 36.39
   dermal appendage 86.26
   ductus arteriosus, patent 38.85
   esophageal vessel 42.91
      endoscopic 42.33
   ethmoidal artery 21.04
   external carotid artery 21.06
   fallopian tube (bilateral) (remaining)
         (solitary) 66.39
      by endoscopy (culdoscopy) (hysteroscopy)
         (laparoscopy) (peritoneoscopy) 66.29
      with
         crushing 66.31
            by endoscopy (laparoscopy) 66.21
         division 66.32
            by endoscopy (culdoscopy) (laparoscopy)
               (peritoneoscopy) 66.22
         Falope ring 66.39
            by endoscopy (laparoscopy) 66.29
      unilateral 66.92
   fistula, arteriovenous 39.53
      coronary artery 36.99
   gastric
      artery 38.86
      varices 44.91
         endoscopic 43.41
   hemorrhoids 49.45
   longitudinal sinus (superior) 02.13
   lymphatic (channel) (peripheral) 40.9
      thoracic duct 40.64
   maxillary artery 21.05
   meningeal vessel 02.13
   spermatic
      cord 63.72
         varicocele 63.1
      vein (high) 63.1
   splenic vessels 38.86
   subclavian artery 38.85
   superior longitudinal sinus 02.13
   supernumerary digit 86.26
   thoracic duct 40.64
   thyroid vessel (artery) (vein) 06.92
   toes (supernumerary) 86.26
   tooth 93.55
      impacted 24.6
   ulcer (peptic) (base) (bed) (bleeding vessel) 44.40
      duodenal 44.42
      gastric 44.41
   ureter 56.95
   varices
      esophageal 42.91
         endoscopic 42.33
      gastric 44.91
         endoscopic 43.41
      peripheral vein (lower limb) 38.59
         upper limb 38.53
   varicocele 63.1
   vas deferens 63.71

Ligation—*continued*
vein 38.80
  abdominal 38.87
  adrenal 07.43
  head and neck NEC 38.82
  intracranial NEC 38.81
  lower limb 38.89
  spermatic, high 63.1
  thoracic NEC 38.85
  thyroid 06.92
  upper limb 38.83
  varicose 38.50
   abdominal 38.57
   esophagus 42.91
    endoscopic 42.33
   gastric 44.91
    endoscopic 43.41
   head and neck NEC 38.52
   intracranial NEC 38.51
   lower limb 38.59
   stomach 44.91
   thoracic NEC 38.55
   upper limb 38.53
  vena cava, inferior 38.7
  venous connection between anomalous
    vein to
   left innominate vein 35.82
   superior vena cava 35.82
  wart 86.26
Light coagulation —*see* Photocoagulation
Lindholm operation (repair of ruptured tendon)
  83.88
Lingulectomy, lung 32.39
Linton operation (varicose vein) 38.59
Lipectomy (subcutaneous tissue) (abdominal)
  (submental) 86.83
Liposuction 86.83
Lip reading training 95.49
Lip shave 27.43
Lisfranc operation
  foot amputation 84.12
  shoulder disarticulation 84.08
Litholapaxy, bladder 57.0
  by incision 57.19
Lithotomy
  bile passage 51.49
  bladder (urinary) 57.19
  common duct 51.41
   percutaneous 51.96
  gallbladder 51.04
  hepatic duct 51.49
  kidney 55.01
   percutaneous 55.03
  ureter 56.2
Lithotripsy
  bile duct NEC 51.49
   extracorporeal shockwave (ESWL) 98.52
  bladder 57.0
   extracorporeal shockwave (ESWL) 98.51
   with ultrasonic fragmentation 57.0 *[59.95]*
  extracorporeal shockwave (ESWL) NEC 98.59
   bile duct 98.52
   bladder (urinary) 98.51
   gallbladder 98.52
   kidney 98.51
   Kock pouch 98.51
   renal pelvis 98.51
   specified site NEC 98.59
   ureter 98.51
  gallbladder NEC 51.04
   endoscopic 51.88

Lithotripsy—*continued*
  extracorporeal shockwave (ESWL) 98.52
  kidney 56.0
   extracorporeal shock wave (EWSL) 98.51
   percutaneous nephrostomy with fragmentation
    (laser) (ultrasound) 55.04
  renal pelvis 56.0
   extracorporeal shock wave (EWSL) 98.51
   percutaneous nephrostomy with fragmentation
    (laser) (ultrasound) 55.04
  ureter 56.0
   extracorporeal shockwave (ESWL) 98.51
LITT (laser interstitial thermal therapy)
  under guidance
  lesion
   brain 17.61
   breast 17.69
   head and neck 17.62
   liver 17.63
   lung 17.69
   prostate 17.69
   thyroid 17.62
Littlewood operation (forequarter amputation)
  84.09
LLETZ (large loop excision of the
  transformation zone) of cervix 67.32
Lloyd-Davies operation (abdominoperineal
  resection), NOS 48.50
  laparoscopic 48.51
  open 48.52
  other 48.59
Lobectomy
  brain 01.53
   partial 01.59
  liver (with partial excision of adjacent lobes) 50.3
  lung (complete) 32.49
   partial 32.39
    thoracoscopic 32.30
   segmental (with resection of adjacent lobes)
    32.49
    thoracoscopic 32.41
   thoracoscopic 32.41
  thyroid (total) (unilateral) (with removal of
   isthmus) (with removal of portion of
   remaining lobe) 06.2
   partial (*see also* Thyroidectomy, partial) 06.39
   substernal 06.51
   subtotal (*see also* Thyroidectomy, partial) 06.39
Lobotomy, brain 01.32
Localization, placenta 88.78
  by RISA injection 92.17
Longmire operation (bile duct anastomosis)
  51.39
Loop ileal stoma (*see also* Ileostomy) 46.01
Loopogram 87.78
Looposcopy (ileal conduit) 56.35
Lord operation
  dilation of anal canal for hemorrhoids 49.49
  hemorrhoidectomy 49.49
  orchidopexy 62.5
Lower GI series (x-ray) 87.64
Lucas and Murray operation (knee arthrodesis
  with place) 81.22
Lumpectomy
  breast 85.21
  specified site—*see* Excision, lesion, by site
Lymphadenectomy (simple) (*see also* Excision,
  lymph, node) 40.29
Lymphadenotomy 40.0
Lymphangiectomy (radical) (*see also* Excision,
  lymph, node, by site, radical) 40.50

Lymphangiogram
abdominal 88.04
cervical 87.08
intrathoracic 87.34
lower limb 88.36
pelvic 88.04
upper limb 88.34
Lymphangioplasty 40.9
Lymphangiorrhaphy 40.9
Lymphangiotomy 40.0
Lymphaticostomy 40.9
thoracic duct 40.62
Lysis
adhesions

> *Note:*
> *blunt — omit code*
> *digital — omit code*
> *manual — omit code*
> *mechanical — omit code*
> *without instrumentation — omit code*

abdominal 54.59
  laparoscopic 54.51
appendiceal 54.59
  laparoscopic 54.51
artery-vein-nerve bundle 39.91
biliary tract 54.59
  laparoscopic 54.51
bladder (neck) (intraluminal) 57.12
  external 59.11
    laparoscopic 59.12
  transurethral 57.41
blood vessels 39.91
bone—*see* category 78.4
bursa 83.91
  by stretching or manipulation 93.28
  hand 82.91
cartilage of joint 93.26
chest wall 33.99
choanae (nasopharynx) 29.54
conjunctiva 10.5
corneovitreal 12.34
cortical (brain) 02.91
ear, middle 20.23
Eustachian tube 20.8
extraocular muscle 15.7
extrauterine 54.59
  laparoscopic 54.51
eyelid 08.09
  and conjunctiva 10.5
eye muscle 15.7
fallopian tube 65.89
  laparoscopic 65.81
fascia 83.91
  hand 82.91
  by stretching or manipulation 93.26
gallbladder 54.59
  laparoscopic 54.51
ganglion (peripheral) NEC 04.49
  cranial NEC 04.42
hand 82.91
  by stretching or manipulation 93.26
heart 37.10
intestines 54.59
  laparoscopic 54.51
iris (posterior) 12.33
  anterior 12.32
joint (capsule) (structure) (*see also* Division,
  joint capsule) 80.40
kidney 59.02
  laparoscopic 59.03

Lysis—*continued*
labia (vulva) 71.01
larynx 31.92
liver 54.59
  laparoscopic 54.51
lung (for collapse of lung) 33.39
mediastinum 34.99
meninges (spinal) 03.6
  cortical 02.91
middle ear 20.23
muscle 83.91
  by stretching or manipulation 93.27
  extraocular 15.7
  hand 82.91
    by stretching or manipulation 93.26
nasopharynx 29.54
nerve (peripheral) NEC 04.49
  cranial NEC 04.42
  roots, spinal 03.6
  trigeminal 04.41
nose, nasal 21.91
ocular muscle 15.7
ovary 65.89
  laparoscopic 65.81
pelvic 54.59
  laparoscopic 54.51
penile 64.93
pericardium 37.12
perineal (female) 71.01
peripheral vessels 39.91
perirectal 48.81
perirenal 59.02
  laparoscopic 59.03
peritoneum (pelvic) 54.59
  laparoscopic 54.51
periureteral 59.02
  laparoscopic 59.03
perivesical 59.11
  laparoscopic 59.12
pharynx 29.54
pleura (for collapse of lung) 33.39
spermatic cord 63.94
spinal (cord) (meninges) (nerve roots) 03.6
spleen 54.59
  laparoscopic 54.51
tendon 83.91
  by stretching or manipulation 93.27
  hand 82.91
    by stretching or manipulation 93.26
thorax 34.99
tongue 25.93
trachea 31.92
tubo-ovarian 65.89
  laparoscopic 65.81
ureter 59.02
  with freeing or repositioning of ureter 59.02
  intraluminal 56.81
  laparoscopic 59.03
urethra (intraluminal) 58.5
uterus 54.59
  intraluminal 68.21
  laparoscopic 54.51
  peritoneal 54.59
    laparoscopic 54.51
vagina (intraluminal) 70.13
vitreous (posterior approach) 14.74
  anterior approach 14.73
vulva 71.01
goniosynechiae (with injection of air or
  liquid) 12.31
synechiae (posterior) 12.33
  anterior (with injection of air or liquid) 12.32

M

Madlener operation (tubal ligation) 66.31
Magnet extraction
foreign body
anterior chamber, eye 12.01
choroid 14.01
ciliary body 12.01
conjunctiva 98.22
cornea 11.0
eye, eyeball NEC 98.21
anterior segment 12.01
posterior segment 14.01
intraocular (anterior segment) 12.01
iris 12.01
lens 13.01
orbit 98.21
retina 14.01
sclera 12.01
vitreous 14.01
Magnetic resonance imaging (nuclear) *see*
Imaging, magnetic resonance
Magnuson (Stack) operation (arthroplasty for
recurrent shoulder dislocation) 81.82
Mako Tactile Guidance System™ [TSG]—*see*
category 17.4
Malleostapediopexy 19.19
with incus replacement 19.11
Malström's vacuum extraction 72.79
with episiotomy 72.71
Mammaplasty —*see* Mammoplasty
Mammectomy —*see also* Mastectomy
subcutaneous (unilateral) 85.34
with synchronous implant 85.33
bilateral 85.36
with synchronous implant 85.35
Mammilliplasty 85.87
Mammography NEC 87.37
Mammoplasty 85.89
with
full-thickness graft 85.83
muscle flap 85.85
pedicle graft 85.84
split-thickness graft 85.82
amputative (reduction) (bilateral) 85.32
unilateral 85.31
augmentation 85.50
with
breast implant (bilateral) 85.54
unilateral 85.53
injection into breast (bilateral) 85.52
unilateral 85.51
reduction (bilateral) 85.32
unilateral 85.31
revision 85.89
size reduction (gynecomastia) (bilateral) 85.32
unilateral 85.31
Mammotomy 85.0
Manchester (Donald) (Fothergill) operation
(uterine suspension) 69.22
Mandibulectomy (partial) 76.31
total 76.42
with reconstruction 76.41
Maneuver (method)
Bracht 72.52
Credé 73.59
De Lee (key-in-lock) 72.4
Kristeller 72.54

Maneuver—*continued*
Lovset's (extraction of arms
in breech birth) 72.52
Mauriceau (Smellie-Veit) 72.52
Pinard (total breech extraction) 72.54
Prague 72.52
Ritgen 73.59
Scanzoni (rotation) 72.4
Van Hoorn 72.52
Wigand-Martin 72.52
Manipulation
with reduction of fracture or dislocation—*see*
Reduction, fracture *and* Reduction,
dislocation
enterostomy stoma (with dilation) 96.24
intestine (intra-abdominal) 46.80
large 46.82
small 46.81
joint
adhesions 93.26
temporomandibular 76.95
dislocation—*see* Reduction, dislocation
lacrimal passage (tract) NEC 09.49
muscle structures 93.27
musculoskeletal (physical therapy) NEC 93.29
nasal septum, displaced 21.88
osteopathic NEC 93.67
for general mobilization (general articulation)
93.61
high-velocity, low-amplitude forces (thrusting)
93.62
indirect forces 93.65
isotonic, isometric forces 93.64
low-velocity, high-amplitude forces (springing)
93.63
to move tissue fluids 93.66
rectum 96.22
salivary duct 26.91
stomach, intraoperative 44.92
temporomandibular joint NEC 76.95
ureteral calculus by catheter
with removal 56.0
without removal 59.8
uterus NEC 69.98
gravid 75.99
inverted
manual replacement (following delivery)
75.94
surgical—*see* Repair, inverted uterus
Manometry
esophageal 89.32
spinal fluid 89.15
urinary 89.21
Manual arts therapy 93.81
Mapping
cardiac (electrophysiologic) 37.27
doppler (flow) 88.72
electrocardiogram only 89.52
Marckwald operation (cervical os repair) 67.59
Marshall-Marchetti (Krantz) operation
(retropubic urethral suspension) 59.5
Marsupialization —*see also* Destruction, lesion,
by site
cyst
Bartholin's 71.23
brain 01.59
cervical (nabothian) 67.31

Monitoring—*continued*
  intraoperative
    anesthetic effect monitoring and titration
      (IAEMT) 00.94 *[89.14]*
    neurophysiologic (BAEP) (brainstem auditory
      evoked potentials) (EEG)
      (electroencephalogram) (electromyogram)
      (EMG) (MEP) (motor evoked potentials)
      (nerve conduction study) (somatosensory
      evoked potentials) (SSEP) (transcranial
      Doppler) 00.94
    intravascular pressure 00.69
      coronary 00.59
      iliac 00.69
      intra-abdominal 00.69
      intrathoracic 00.67
        aorta 00.67
        aortic arch 00.67
        carotid 00.67
      mesenteric 00.69
      peripheral 00.68
      renal 00.69
    neurophysiologic
      intra-operative 00.94
    partial pressure of brain oxygen (PbtO$_2$) 01.16
    pulmonary artery
      pressure 89.63
      wedge 89.64
    sleep (recording)—*see* categories 89.17-89.18
    systemic arterial pressure 89.61
      intra-aneurysm sac pressure 00.58
    telemetry (cardiac) 89.54
    transesophageal cardiac output (Doppler) 89.68
    ventricular pressure (cardiac) 89.62
Moore operation (arthroplasty) 81.52
Moschowitz
  enterocele repair 70.92
    with graft or prosthesis 70.93
  herniorrhaphy—*see* Repair, hernia, femoral
  sigmoidopexy 46.63
Mountain resort sanitarium 93.98
Mouth-to-mouth resuscitation 93.93
Moxibustion 93.35
MRI —*see* Imaging, magnetic resonance
Muller operation (banding of pulmonary artery)
  38.85
Multiple sleep latency test (MSLT) 89.18
Mumford operation (partial claviculectomy)
  77.81
Musculoplasty (*see also* Repair, muscle) 83.87
  hand (*see also* Repair, muscle, hand) 82.89
Music therapy 93.84
Mustard operation (interatrial transposition of
  venous return) 35.91
Myectomy 83.45
  anorectal 48.92
  eye muscle 15.13
    multiple 15.3
  for graft 83.43
    hand 82.34
  hand 82.36
    for graft 82.34
  levator palpebrae 08.33
  rectal 48.92
Myelogram, myelography (air) (gas) 87.21
  posterior fossa 87.02
Myelotomy
  spine, spinal (cord) (tract) (one-stage) (two-stage)
    03.29
    percutaneous 03.21
Myocardiectomy (infarcted area) 37.33
Myocardiotomy 37.11

Myoclasis 83.99
  hand 82.99
Myomectomy (uterine) 68.29
  broad ligament 69.19
Myoplasty (*see also* Repair, muscle) 83.87
  hand (*see also* Repair, muscle, hand) 82.89
  mastoid 19.9
Myorrhaphy 83.65
  hand 82.46
Myosuture 83.65
  hand 82.46
Myotasis 93.27
Myotenontoplasty (*see also* Repair, tendon)
    83.88
  hand 82.86
Myotenoplasty (*see also* Repair, tendon) 83.88
  hand 82.86
Myotenotomy 83.13
  hand 82.11
Myotomy 83.02
  with division 83.19
    hand 82.19
  colon NEC 46.92
    sigmoid 46.91
  cricopharyngeal 29.31
    that for pharyngeal (pharyngoesophageal)
      diverticulectomy 29.32
  esophagus 42.7
  eye (oblique) (rectus) 15.21
    multiple (two or more muscles) 15.4
  hand 82.02
    with division 82.19
  levator palpebrae 08.38
  sigmoid (colon) 46.91
Myringectomy 20.59
Myringodectomy 20.59
Myringomalleolabyrinthopexy 19.52
Myringoplasty (epitympanic, type I) (by
    cauterization) (by graft) 19.4
  revision 19.6
Myringostapediopexy 19.53
Myringostomy 20.01
Myringotomy (with aspiration) (with drainage)
    20.09
  with insertion of tube or drainage device (button)
    (grommet) 20.01

N

Nailing, intramedullary
  with fracture reduction—*see* Reduction, fracture
    with internal fixation
  internal (without fracture reduction) 78.50
Narcoanalysis 94.21
Narcosynthesis 94.21
Narrowing, palpebral fissure 08.51
Nasopharyngogram 87.09
  contrast 87.06
Necropsy 89.8
Needleoscopy (fetus) 75.31
Needling
  Bartholin's gland (cyst) 71.21
  cataract (secondary) 13.64
  fallopian tube 66.91
  hydrocephalic head 73.8
  lens (capsule) 13.2
  pupillary membrane (iris) 12.35
Nephrectomy (complete) (total) (unilateral)
    55.51
  bilateral 55.54
  partial (wedge) 55.4
  remaining or solitary kidney 55.52
  removal transplanted kidney 55.53
Nephrocolopexy 55.7
Nephrocystanastomosis NEC 56.73
Nephrolithotomy 55.01
Nephrolysis 59.02
  laparoscopic 59.03
Nephropexy 55.7
Nephroplasty 55.89
Nephropyeloplasty 55.87
Nephropyeloureterostomy 55.86
Nephrorrhaphy 55.81
Nephroscopy 55.21
Nephrostolithotomy, percutaneous 55.03
Nephrostomy (with drainage tube) 55.02
  closure 55.82
  percutaneous 55.03
    with fragmentation (ultrasound) 55.04
Nephrotomogram, nephrotomography NEC
    87.72
Nephrotomy 55.01
Nephroureterectomy (with bladder cuff) 55.51
Nephroureterocystectomy 55.51 *[57.79]*
Nerve block (cranial) (peripheral) NEC (*see also*
    Block, by site) 04.81
Neurectasis (cranial) (peripheral) 04.91
Neurectomy (cranial) (infraorbital) (occipital)
    (peripheral) (spinal) NEC 04.07
  gastric (vagus) (*see also* Vagotomy) 44.00
  opticociliary 12.79
  paracervical 05.22
  presacral 05.24
  retrogasserian 04.07
  sympathetic—*see* Sympathectomy
  trigeminal 04.07
  tympanic 20.91
Neurexeresis NEC 04.07
Neuroablation
  radiofrequency 04.2
Neuroanastomosis (cranial) (peripheral) NEC
    04.74
  accessory-facial 04.72
  accessory-hypoglossal 04.73
  hypoglossal-facial 04.71

NeuroFlo™ catheter for partial (temporary)
  abdominal aorta occlusion 39.77
Neurolysis (peripheral nerve) NEC 04.49
  carpal tunnel 04.43
  cranial nerve NEC 04.42
  spinal (cord) (nerve roots) 03.6
  tarsal tunnel 04.44
  trigeminal nerve 04.41
Neuromonitoring
  intra-operative 00.94
Neuroplasty (cranial) (peripheral) NEC 04.79
  of old injury (delayed repair) 04.76
  revision 04.75
Neurorrhaphy (cranial) (peripheral) 04.3
Neurotomy (cranial) (peripheral) (spinal) NEC
    04.04
  acoustic 04.01
  glossopharyngeal 29.92
  lacrimal branch 05.0
  retrogasserian 04.02
  sympathetic 05.0
  vestibular 04.01
Neurotripsy (peripheral) NEC 04.03
  trigeminal 04.02
Nicola operation (tenodesis for recurrent
  dislocation of shoulder) 81.82
Nimodipine, infusion 99.75
NIPS (noninvasive programmed electrical
  stimulation) 37.20
Nissen operation (fundoplication of stomach)
    44.66
  laparoscopic 44.67
Noble operation (plication of small intestine)
    46.62
Norman Miller operation (vaginopexy) 70.77
  with graft or prosthesis 70.78
Norton operation (extraperitoneal cesarean
  section) 74.2
Nuclear magnetic resonance imaging
  —*see* Imaging, magnetic resonance
Nutrition , concentration substances
  enteral infusion (of) 96.6
  parenteral, total 99.15
    peripheral 99.15

O

O

Ober (Yount) operation (gluteal-iliotibial fasciotomy) 83.14
Obliteration
  bone cavity (*see also* Osteoplasty) 78.40
  calyceal diverticulum 55.39
  canaliculi 09.6
  cerebrospinal fistula 02.12
  cul-de-sac 70.92
    with graft or prosthesis 70.93
  frontal sinus (with fat) 22.42
  lacrimal punctum 09.91
  lumbar pseudomeningocele 03.51
  lymphatic structure(s) (peripheral) 40.9
  maxillary sinus 22.31
  meningocele (sacral) 03.51
  pelvic 68.8
  pleural cavity 34.6
  sacral meningocele 03.51
  Skene's gland 71.3
  tympanomastoid cavity 19.9
  vagina, vaginal (partial) (total) 70.4
    vault 70.8
Occlusal molds (dental) 89.31
Occlusion
  artery
    by embolization—*see* Embolization, artery
    by endovascular approach—*see* Embolization, artery
    by ligation—*see* Ligation, artery
  fallopian tube—*see* Ligation, fallopian tube
  patent ductus arteriosus (PDA) 38.85
  vein
    by embolization—*see* Embolization, vein
    by endovascular approach—*see* Embolization, vein
    by ligation—*see* Ligation, vein
  vena cava (surgical) 38.7
Occupational therapy 93.83
OCT (optical coherence tomography) (intravascular imaging)
  coronary vessel(s) 38.24
  non-coronary vessel(s) 38.25
O'Donoghue operation (triad knee repair) 81.43
Odontectomy NEC (*see also* Removal, tooth, surgical) 23.19
Oleothorax 33.39
Olshausen operation (uterine suspension) 69.22
Omentectomy 54.4
Omentofixation 54.74
Omentopexy 54.74
Omentoplasty 54.74
Omentorrhaphy 54.74
Omentotomy 54.19
Omphalectomy 54.3
Onychectomy 86.23
Onychoplasty 86.86
Onychotomy 86.09
  with drainage 86.04
Oophorectomy (unilateral) 65.39
  with salpingectomy 65.49
    laparoscopic 65.41
  bilateral (same operative episode) 65.51
    laparoscopic 65.53
    with salpingectomy 65.61
      laparoscopic 65.63
  laparoscopic 65.31

Oophorectomy—*continued*
  partial 65.29
    laparoscopic 65.25
    wedge 65.22
      that by laparoscope 65.24
  remaining ovary 65.52
    laparoscopic 65.54
    with tube 65.62
      laparoscopic 65.64
Oophorocystectomy 65.29
  laparoscopic 65.25
Oophoropexy 65.79
Oophoroplasty 65.79
Oophororrhaphy 65.71
  laparoscopic 65.74
Oophorostomy 65.09
  laparoscopic 65.01
Oophorotomy 65.09
  laparoscopic 65.01
Opening
  bony labyrinth (ear) 20.79
  cranial suture 02.01
  heart valve
    closed heart technique—*see* Valvulotomy, by site
    open heart technique—*see* Valvuloplasty, by site
  spinal dura 03.09
Operation
  Abbe
    construction of vagina 70.61
      with graft or prosthesis 70.63
    intestinal anastomosis—*see* Anastomosis, intestine
  abdominal (region) NEC 54.99
  abdominoperineal, NOS 48.50
    laparoscopic 48.51
    open 48.52
    other 48.59
  Aburel (intra-amniotic injection for abortion) 75.0
  Adams
    advancement of round ligament 69.22
    crushing of nasal septum 21.88
    excision of palmar fascia 82.35
  adenoids NEC 28.99
  adrenal (gland) (nerve) (vessel) NEC 07.49
  Albee
    bone peg, femoral neck 78.05
    graft for slipping patella 78.06
    sliding inlay graft, tibia 78.07
  Albert (arthrodesis, knee) 81.22
  Aldridge (Studdiford) (urethral sling) 59.5
  Alexander
    prostatectomy
      perineal 60.62
      suprapubic 60.3
    shortening of round ligaments of uterus 69.22
  Alexander-Adams (shortening of round ligaments of uterus) 69.22
  Almoor (extrapetrosal drainage) 20.22
  Altemeier (perineal rectal pull-through) 48.49
  Ammon (dacryocystotomy) 09.53
  Anderson (tibial lengthening) 78.37
  Anel (dilation of lacrimal duct) 09.42
  anterior chamber (eye) NEC 12.99
  anti-incontinence NEC 59.79
  antrum window (nasal sinus) 22.2
    with Caldwell-Luc approach 22.39

Operation—*continued*
Clagett (closure of chest wall following open flap
drainage) 34.72
Clayton (resection of metatarsal heads and bases
of phalanges) 77.88
clitoris NEC 71.4
cocked hat (metacarpal lengthening and transfer
of local flap) 82.69
Cockett (varicose vein)
lower limb 38.59
upper limb 38.53
Cody tack (perforation of footplate) 19.0
Coffey (uterine suspension) (Meigs'
modification) 69.22
Cole (anterior tarsal wedge osteotomy) 77.28
Collis-Nissen (hiatal hernia repair) 53.80
colon NEC 46.99
Colonna
adductor tenotomy (first stage) 83.12
hip arthroplasty (second stage) 81.40
reconstruction of hip (second stage) 81.40
commando (radical glossectomy) 25.4
conjunctive NEC 10.99
destructive NEC 10.33
cornea NEC 11.99
Coventry (tibial wedge osteotomy) 77.27
Cox-maze procedure (ablation or destruction of
heart tissue) —*see* maze procedure
Crawford (tarso-frontalis sling of eyelid) 08.32
cul-de-sac NEC 70.92
Culp-Deweerd (spiral flap pyeloplasty) 55.87
Culp-Scardino (ureteral flap pyeloplasty) 55.87
Curtis (interphalangeal joint arthroplasty) 81.72
cystocele NEC 70.51
Dahlman (excision of esophageal diverticulum)
42.31
Dana (posterior rhizotomy) 03.1
Danforth (fetal) 73.8
Darrach (ulnar resection) 77.83
Davis (intubated ureterotomy) 56.2
de Grandmont (tarsectomy) 08.35
Delorme
pericardiectomy 37.31
proctopexy 48.76
repair of prolapsed rectum 48.76
thoracoplasty 33.34
Denker (radical maxillary antrotomy) 22.31
Dennis-Varco (herniorrhaphy)—*see* Repair,
hernia, femoral
Denonvillier (limited rhinoplasty) 21.86
dental NEC 24.99
orthodontic NEC 24.8
Derlacki (tympanoplasty) 19.4
diaphragm NEC 34.89
Dickson (fascial transplant) 83.82
Dickson-Diveley (tendon transfer and arthrodesis
to correct claw toe) 77.57
Dieffenbach (hip disarticulation) 84.18
digestive tract NEC 46.99
Doleris (shortening of round ligaments) 69.22
D'Ombrain (excision of pterygium with corneal
graft) 11.32
Dorrance (push-back operation for cleft palate)
27.62
Dotter (transluminal angioplasty) 39.59
Douglas (suture of tongue to lip for micrognathia)
25.59
Doyle (paracervical uterine denervation) 69.3
Duhamel (abdominoperineal pull-through) 48.65
Duhrssen (vaginofixation of uterus) 69.22
Dunn (triple arthrodesis) 81.12
duodenum NEC 46.99

Operation—*continued*
Dupuytren
fasciectomy 82.35
fasciotomy 82.12
with excision 82.35
shoulder disarticulation 84.08
Durham (Caldwell) (transfer of biceps femoris
tendon) 83.75
DuToit and Roux (staple capsulorrhaphy of
shoulder) 81.82
DuVries (tenoplasty) 83.88
Dwyer
fasciotomy 83.14
soft tissue release NEC 83.84
wedge osteotomy, calcaneus 77.28
Eagleton (extrapetrosal drainage) 20.22
ear (external) NEC 18.9
middle or inner NEC 20.99
Eden-Hybinette (glenoid bone block) 78.01
Effler (heart) 36.2
Eggers
tendon release (patellar retinacula) 83.13
tendon transfer (biceps femoris tendon)
(hamstring tendon) 83.75
Elliot (scleral trephination with iridectomy) 12.61
Ellis Jones (repair of peroneal tendon) 83.88
Ellison (reinforcement of collateral ligament)
81.44
Elmslie-Cholmeley (tarsal wedge osteotomy)
77.28
Eloesser
thoracoplasty 33.34
thoracostomy 34.09
Emmet (cervix) 67.61
endorectal pull-through 48.41
epididymis NEC 63.99
esophagus NEC 42.99
Estes (ovary) 65.72
laparoscopic 65.75
Estlander (thoracoplasty) 33.34
Evans (release of clubfoot) 83.84
extraocular muscle NEC 15.9
multiple (two or more muscles) 15.4
with temporary detachment from globe 15.3
revision 15.6
single 15.29
with temporary detachment from globe 15.19
eyeball NEC 16.99
eyelid(s) NEC 08.99
face NEC 27.99
facial bone or joint NEC 76.99
fallopian tube NEC 66.99
Farabeuf (ischiopubiotomy) 77.39
Fasanella-Servatt (blepharoptosis repair) 08.35
fascia NEC 83.99
hand 82.99
female (genital organs) NEC 71.9
hysterectomy NEC 68.9
fenestration (aorta) 39.54
Ferguson (hernia repair) 53.00
Fick (perforation of footplate) 19.0
filtering (for glaucoma) 12.79
with iridectomy 12.65
Finney (pyloroplasty) 44.2
fistulizing, sclera NEC 12.69
Foley (pyeloplasty) 55.87
Fontan (creation of conduit between right atrium
and pulmonary artery) 35.94
Fothergill (Donald) (uterine suspension) 69.22

Operation—*continued*
Janeway (permanent gastrostomy) 43.19
Jatene (arterial switch) 35.84
jejunum NEC 46.99
Johanson (urethral reconstruction) 58.46
joint (capsule) (ligament) (structure) NEC 81.99
    facial NEC 76.99
Jones
    claw toe (transfer of extensor hallucis longus
        tendon) 77.57
        modified (with arthrodesis) 77.57
    dacryocystorhinostomy 09.81
    hammer toe (interphalangeal fusion) 77.56
        modified (tendon transfer with arthrodesis)
        77.57
    repair of peroneal tendon 83.88
Joplin (exostectomy with tendon transfer) 77.53
Kader (temporary gastrostomy) 43.19
Kaufman (for urinary stress incontinence) 59.79
Kazanjiian (buccal vestibular sulcus extension)
    24.91
Kehr (hepatopexy) 50.69
Keller (bunionectomy) 77.59
Kelly (Kennedy) (urethrovesical plication) 59.3
Kelly-Stoeckel (urethrovesical plication) 59.3
Kerr (cesarean section) 74.1
Kessler (arthroplasty, carpometacarpal joint)
    81.74
Kidner (excision of accessory navicular bone)
    (with tendon transfer) 77.98
kidney NEC 55.99
Killian (frontal sinusotomy) 22.41
King-Steelquist (hindquarter amputation) 84.19
Kirk (amputation through thigh) 84.17
Kock pouch
    bowel anastomosis—*omit code*
    continent ileostomy 46.22
    cutaneous uretero-ileostomy 56.51
    ESWL (extracorporeal shockwave lithotripsy)
        98.51
    removal, calculus 57.19
    revision, cutaneous uretero-ileostomy 56.52
    urinary diversion procedure 56.51
Kondoleon (correction of lymphedema) 40.9
Krause (sympathetic denervation) 05.29
Kroener (partial salpingectomy) 66.69
Kroenlein (lateral orbitotomy) 16.01
Kronig (low cervical cesarean section) 74.1
Krukenberg (reconstruction of below-elbow
    amputation) 82.89
Kuhnt-Szymanowski (ectropion repair with lid
    reconstruction) 08.44
Labbe (gastrotomy) 43.0
labia NEC 71.8
lacrimal
    gland 09.3
    system NEC 09.99
Ladd (mobilization of intestine) 54.95
Lagrange (iridosclerectomy) 12.65
Lambrinudi (triple arthrodesis) 81.12
Langenbeck (cleft palate repair) 27.62
Lapidus (bunionectomy with metatarsal
    osteotomy) 77.51
Larry (shoulder disarticulation) 84.08
larynx NEC 31.98
Lash
    internal cervical os repair 67.59
    laparoscopic supracervical hysterectomy 68.31
Latzko
    cesarean section, extraperitoneal 74.2
    colpocleisis 70.8

Operation—*continued*
Leadbetter (urethral reconstruction) 58.46
Leadbetter-Politano (ureteroneocystostomy)
    56.74
Le Fort (colpocleisis) 70.8
LeMesurier (cleft lip repair) 27.54
lens NEC 13.90
Leriche (periarterial sympathectomy) 05.25
levator muscle sling
    eyelid ptosis repair 08.33
    urethrovesical suspension 59.71
    urinary stress incontinence 59.71
lid suture (blepharoptosis) 08.31
ligament NEC 81.99
    broad NEC 69.98
    round NEC 69.98
    uterine NEC 69.98
Lindholm (repair of ruptured tendon) 83.88
Linton (varicose vein) 38.59
lip NEC 27.99
Lisfranc
    foot amputation 84.12
    shoulder disarticulation 84.08
Littlewood (forequarter amputation) 84.09
liver NEC 50.99
Lloyd-Davies (abdominoperineal resection), NOS
    48.50
    laparoscopic 48.51
    open 48.52
    other 48.59
Longmire (bile duct anastomosis) 51.39
Lord
    dilation of anal canal for hemorrhoids 49.49
    hemorrhoidectomy 49.49
    orchidopexy 62.5
Lucas and Murray (knee arthrodesis with plate)
    81.22
lung NEC 33.99
lung volume reduction 32.22
    biologic lung volume reduction (BLVR)—*see*
        category 33.7
lymphatic structure(s) NEC 40.9
    duct, left (thoracic) NEC 40.69
Madlener (tubal ligation) 66.31
Magnuson (Stack) (arthroplasty for recurrent
    shoulder dislocation) 81.82
male genital organs NEC 64.99
Manchester (Donald) (Fothergill), (uterine
    suspension) 69.22
mandible NEC 76.99
    orthognathic 76.64
Marckwald (cervical os repair) 67.59
Marshall-Marchetti (Krantz) (retropubic urethral
    suspension) 59.5
Matas (aneurysmorrhaphy) 39.52
Mayo
    bunionectomy 77.59
    herniorrhaphy
        laparoscopic 53.43
            with graft or prosthesis 53.42
        other and open with graft or prosthesis 53.41
        other open 53.49
    vaginal hysterectomy 68.59
        laparoscopically assisted (LAVH) 68.51
Maze procedure (ablation or destruction of heart
    tissue)
    by incision (open) 37.33
    by median sternotomy 37.33
    by peripherally inserted catheter 37.34
    by thoracotomy without thoracoscope 37.33
    endovascular approach 37.34
Mazet (knee disarticulation) 84.16

Operation—*continued*

McBride (bunionectomy with soft tissue correction) 77.53

McBurney—*see* Repair, hernia, inguinal

McCall (enterocele repair) 70.92
  with graft or prosthesis 70.93

McCauley (release of clubfoot) 83.84

McDonald (encirclement suture, cervix) 67.59

McIndoe (vaginal construction) 70.61
  with graft or prosthesis 70.63

McKeever (fusion of first metatarsophalangeal joint for hallux valgus repair) 77.52

McKissock (breast reduction) 85.33

McReynolds (transposition of pterygium) 11.31

McVay
  femoral hernia—*see* Repair, hernia, femoral
  inguinal hernia—*see* Repair, hernia, inguinal

meninges (spinal) NEC 03.99
  cerebral NEC 02.99

mesentery NEC 54.99

Mikulicz (exteriorization of intestine) (first stage) 46.03
  second stage 46.04

Miles (complete proctectomy), NOS 48.50
  laparoscopic 48.51
  open 48.52
  other 48.59

Millard (cheiloplasty) 27.54

Miller
  midtarsal arthrodesis 81.14
  urethrovesical suspension 59.4

Millin-Read (urethrovesical suspension) 59.4

Mitchell (hallux valgus repair) 77.51

Mohs (chemosurgical excision of skin) 86.24

Moore (arthroplasty) 81.52

Moschowitz
  enterocele repair 70.92
    with graft or prosthesis 70.93
  herniorrhaphy—*see* Repair, hernia, femoral
  sigmoidopexy 46.63

mouth NEC 27.99

Muller (banding of pulmonary artery) 38.85

Mumford (partial claviculectomy) 77.81

muscle NEC 83.99
  extraocular—*see* Operation, extraocular
  hand NEC 82.99
  papillary heart NEC 35.31

musculoskeletal system NEC 84.99

Mustard (interatrial transposition of venous return) 35.91

nail (finger) (toe) NEC 86.99

nasal sinus NEC 22.9

nasopharynx NEC 29.99

nerve (cranial) (peripheral) NEC 04.99
  adrenal NEC 07.49
  sympathetic NEC 05.89

nervous system NEC 05.9

Nicola (tenodesis for recurrent dislocation of shoulder) 81.82

nipple NEC 85.99

Nissen (fundoplication of stomach) 44.66
  laparoscopic 44.67

Noble (plication of small intestine) 46.62

node (lymph) NEC 40.9

Norman Miller (vaginopexy) 70.77
  with graft or prosthesis 70.78

Norton (extraperitoneal cesarean operation) 74.2

nose, nasal NEC 21.99
  sinus NEC 22.9

Ober (Yount) (gluteal-iliotibial fasciotomy) 83.14

obstetric NEC 75.99

Operation—*continued*

ocular NEC 16.99
  muscle—*see* Operation, extraocular muscle

O'Donoghue (triad knee repair) 81.43

Olshausen (uterine suspension) 69.22

omentum NEC 54.99

ophthalmologic NEC 16.99

oral cavity NEC 27.99

orbicularis muscle sling 08.36

orbit NEC 16.98

oropharynx NEC 29.99

orthodontic NEC 24.8

orthognathic NEC 76.69

Oscar Miller (midtarsal arthrodesis) 81.14

Osmond-Clark (soft tissue release with peroneus brevis tendon transfer) 83.75

ovary NEC 65.99

Oxford (for urinary incontinence) 59.4

palate NEC 27.99

palpebral ligament sling 08.36

Panas (linear proctotomy) 48.0

Pancoast (division of trigeminal nerve at foramen ovale) 04.02

pancreas NEC 52.99

pantaloon (revision of gastric anastomosis) 44.5

papillary muscle (heart) NEC 35.31

Paquin (ureteroneocystostomy) 56.74

parathyroid gland(s) NEC 06.99

parotid gland or duct NEC 26.99

Partsch (marsupialization of dental cyst) 24.4

Pattee (auditory canal) 18.6

Peet (splanchnic resection) 05.29

Pemberton
  osteotomy of ilium 77.39
  rectum (mobilization and fixation for prolapse repair) 48.76

penis NEC 64.98

Pereyra (paraurethral suspension) 59.6

pericardium NEC 37.99

perineum (female) NEC 71.8
  male NEC 86.99

perirectal tissue NEC 48.99

perirenal tissue NEC 59.92

peritoneum NEC 54.99

periurethral tissue NEC 58.99

perivesical tissue NEC 59.92

pharyngeal flap (cleft palate repair) 27.62
  secondary or subsequent 27.63

pharynx, pharyngeal (pouch) NEC 29.99

pineal gland NEC 07.59

Pinsker (obliteration of nasoseptal telangiectasia) 21.07

Piper (forceps) 72.6

Pirogoff (ankle amputation through malleoli of tibia and fibula) 84.14

pituitary gland NEC 07.79

plastic—*see* Repair, by site

pleural cavity NEC 34.99

Politano-Leadbetter (ureteroneocystostomy) 56.74

pollicization (with nerves and blood supply) 82.61

Polya (gastrectomy) 43.7

Pomeroy (ligation and division of fallopian tubes) 66.32

Poncet
  lengthening of Achilles tendon 83.85
  urethrostomy, perineal 58.0

Porro (cesarean section) 74.99

posterior chamber (eye) NEC 14.9

Operation—*continued*
Potts-Smith (descending aorta-left pulmonary artery anastomosis) 39.0
Printen and Mason (high gastric bypass) 44.31
prostate NEC (*see also* Prostatectomy) 60.69
specified type 60.99
pterygium 11.39
with corneal graft 11.32
Puestow (pancreaticojejunostomy) 52.96
pull-through NEC 48.49
pulmonary NEC 33.99
push-back (cleft palate repair) 27.62
Putti-Platt (capsulorrhaphy of shoulder for recurrent dislocation) 81.82
pyloric exclusion 44.39
laparoscopic 44.38
pyriform sinus NEC 29.99
"rabbit ear" (anterior urethropexy) (Tudor) 59.79
Ramadier (intrapetrosal drainage) 20.22
Ramstedt (pyloromyotomy) (with wedge resection) 43.3
Rankin
exteriorization of intestine 46.03
proctectomy (complete), NOS 48.50
laparoscopic 48.51
open 48.52
other 48.59
Rashkind (balloon septostomy) 35.41
Rastelli (creation of conduit between right ventricle and pulmonary artery) 35.92
in repair of
pulmonary artery atresia 35.92
transposition of great vessels 35.92
truncus arteriosus 35.83
Raz-Pereyra procedure (bladder neck suspension) 59.79
rectal NEC 48.99
rectocele NEC 70.52
re-entry (aorta) 39.54
renal NEC 55.99
respiratory (tract) NEC 33.99
retina NEC 14.9
Ripstein (repair of rectal prolapse) 48.75
Rodney Smith (radical subtotal pancreatectomy) 52.53
Roux-en-Y
bile duct 51.36
cholecystojejunostomy 51.32
esophagus (intrathoracic) 42.54
gastroenterostomy 44.39
laparoscopic 44.38
gastrojejunostomy 44.39
laparoscopic 44.38
pancreaticojejunostomy 52.96
Roux-Goldthwait (repair of patellar dislocation) 81.44
Roux-Herzen-Judine (jejunal loop interposition) 42.63
Ruiz-Mora (proximal phalangectomy for hammer toe) 77.99
Russe (bone graft of scaphoid) 78.04
Saemisch (corneal section) 11.1
salivary gland or duct NEC 26.99
Salter (innominate osteotomy) 77.39
Sauer-Bacon (abdominoperineal resection), NOS 48.50
laparoscopic 48.51
open 48.52
other 48.59
Schanz (femoral osteotomy) 77.35

Operation—*continued*
Schauta (-Amreich) (radical vaginal hysterectomy) 68.79
laparoscopic 68.71
Schede (thoracoplasty) 33.34
Scheie
cautery of sclera 12.62
sclerostomy 12.62
Schlatter (total gastrectomy) 43.99
Schroeder (endocervical excision) 67.39
Schuchardt (nonobstetrical episiotomy) 71.09
Schwartze (simple mastoidectomy) 20.41
sclera NEC 12.89
Scott
intestinal bypass for obesity 45.93
jejunocolostomy (bypass) 45.93
scrotum NEC 61.99
Seddon-Brooks (transfer of pectoralis major tendon) 83.75
Semb (apicolysis of lung) 33.39
seminal vesicle NEC 60.79
Senning (correction of transposition of great vessels) 35.91
Sever (division of soft tissue of arm) 83.19
Sewell (heart) 36.2
sex transformation NEC 64.5
Sharrard (iliopsoas muscle transfer) 83.77
shelf (hip arthroplasty) 81.40
Shirodkar (encirclement suture, cervix) 67.59
sigmoid NEC 46.99
Silver (bunionectomy) 77.59
Sistrunk (excision of thyroglossal cyst) 06.7
Skene's gland NEC 71.8
skin NEC 86.99
skull NEC 02.99
sling
eyelid
fascia lata, palpebral 08.36
frontalis fascial 08.32
levator muscle 08.33
orbicularis muscle 08.36
palpebrae ligament, fascia lata 08.36
tarsus muscle 08.35
fascial (fascia lata)
eye 08.32
for facial weakness (trigeminal nerve paralysis) 86.81
palpebral ligament 08.36
tongue 25.59
tongue (fascial) 25.59
urethra (suprapubic) 59.4
retropubic 59.5
urethrovesical 59.5
Slocum (pes anserinus transfer) 81.47
Sluder (tonsillectomy) 28.2
Smith (open osteotomy of mandible) 76.62
Smith-Peterson (radiocarpal arthrodesis) 81.25
Smithwick (sympathectomy) 05.29
Soave (endorectal pull-through) 48.41
soft tissue NEC 83.99
hand 82.99
Sonneberg (inferior maxillary neurectomy) 04.07
Sorondo-Ferré (hindquarter amputation) 84.19
Soutter (iliac crest fasciotomy) 83.14
Spalding-Richardson (uterine suspension) 69.22
spermatic cord NEC 63.99
sphincter of Oddi NEC 51.89
spinal (canal) (cord) (structures) NEC 03.99
Spinelli (correction of inverted uterus) 75.93
Spivack (permanent gastrostomy) 43.19
spleen NEC 41.99

Oxygenation 93.96
  extracorporeal membrane (ECMO) 39.65
  hyperbaric 93.95
    wound 93.59
  infusion therapy, Super 00.49
Oxygen therapy (catalytic) (pump) 93.96
  hyperbaric 93.95
  SuperSaturated 00.49

P

Pelvimetry 88.25
  gynecological 89.26
Pelviolithotomy 55.11
Pelvioplasty, kidney 55.87
Pelviostomy 55.12
  closure 55.82
Pelviotomy 77.39
  to assist delivery 73.94
Pelvi-ureteroplasty 55.87
Pemberton operation
  osteotomy of ilium 77.39
  rectum (mobilization and fixation for prolapse
    repair) 48.76
Penectomy 64.3
Pereyra operation (paraurethral suspension) 59.6
Perforation
  stapes footplate 19.0
Perfusion NEC 39.97
  carotid artery 39.97
  coronary artery 39.97
  for
    chemotherapy NEC 99.25
    hormone therapy NEC 99.24
  head 39.97
  hyperthermic (lymphatic), localized region
    or site 93.35
  intestine (large) (local) 46.96
    small 46.95
  kidney, local 55.95
  limb (lower) (upper) 39.97
  liver, localized 50.93
  neck 39.97
  subarachnoid (spinal cord) (refrigerated saline)
    03.92
  total body 39.96
Pericardiectomy 37.31
Pericardiocentesis 37.0
Pericardiolysis 37.12
Pericardioplasty 37.49
Pericardiorrhaphy 37.49
Pericardiostomy (tube) 37.12
pericardiotomy 37.12
Peridectomy 10.31
Perilimbal suction 89.11
Perimetry 95.05
Perineoplasty 71.79
Perineorrhaphy 71.71
  obstetrical laceration (current) 75.69
Perineotomy (nonobstetrical) 71.09
  to assist delivery—*see* Episiotomy
Periosteotomy (*see also* Incision, bone) 77.10
  facial bone 76.09
Perirectofistulectomy 48.93
Peritectomy 10.31
Peritomy 10.1
Peritoneocentesis 54.91
Peritoneoscopy 54.21
Peritoneotomy 54.19
Peritoneumectomy 54.4
Phacoemulsification (ultrasonic) (with
  aspiration) 13.41
Phacofragmentation (mechanical) (with
  aspiration) 13.43
  posterior route 13.42
  ultrasonic 13.41
Phalangectomy (partial) 77.89
  claw toe 77.57
  cockup toe 77.58
  hammer toe 77.56
  overlapping toe 77.58
  total 77.99

Phalangization (fifth metacarpal) 82.81
Pharyngeal flop operation (cleft palate repair)
  27.62
  secondary or subsequent 27.63
Pharyngectomy (partial) 29.33
  with laryngectomy 30.3
Pharyngogram 87.09
  contrast 87.06
Pharyngolaryngectomy 30.3
Pharyngoplasty (with silastic implant) 29.4
  for cleft palate 27.62
    secondary or subsequent 27.63
Pharyngorrhaphy 29.51
  for cleft palate 27.62
Pharyngoscopy 29.11
Pharyngotomy 29.0
Phenopeel (skin) 86.24
Phlebectomy 38.60
  with
    anastomosis 38.30
      abdominal 38.37
      head and neck NEC 38.32
      intracranial NEC 38.31
      lower limb 38.39
      thoracic NEC 38.35
      upper limb 38.33
    graft replacement 38.40
      abdominal 38.47
      head and neck NEC 38.42
      intracranial NEC 38.41
      lower limb 38.49
      thoracic NEC 38.45
      upper limb 38.43
  abdominal 38.67
  head and neck NEC 38.62
  intracranial NEC 38.61
  lower limb 38.69
  thoracic NEC 38.65
  upper limb 38.63
  varicose 38.50
    abdominal 38.57
    head and neck NEC 38.52
    intracranial NEC 38.51
    lower limb 38.59
    thoracic NEC 38.55
    upper limb 38.53
Phlebogoniostomy 12.52
Phlebography (contrast) (retrograde) 88.60
  by radioisotope—*see* Scan, radioisotope, by site
  adrenal 88.65
  femoral 88.66
  head 88.61
  hepatic 88.64
  impedance 88.68
  intra-abdominal NEC 88.65
  intrathoracic NEC 88.63
  lower extremity NEC 88.66
  neck 88.61
  portal system 88.64
  pulmonary 88.62
  specified site NEC 88.67
  vena cava (inferior) (superior) 88.51
Phleborrhaphy 39.32
Phlebotomy 38.99
Phonocardiogram, with ECG lead 89.55
Photochemotherapy NEC 99.83
  extracorporeal 99.88
Photocoagulation
  ciliary body 12.73
  eye, eyeball 16.99

Plication—*continued*
  tricuspid valve (with repositioning) 35.14
  ureter 56.89
  urethra 58.49
  urethrovesical junction 59.3
  vein (peripheral) 39.59
  vena cava (inferior) (superior) 38.7
  ventricle (heart)
    aneurysm 37.32
Plicotomy, tympanum 20.23
Plombage, lung 33.39
Pneumocentesis 33.93
Pneumocisternogram 87.02
Pneumoencephalogram 87.01
Pneumogram, pneumography
  extraperitoneal 88.15
  mediastinal 87.33
  orbit 87.14
  pelvic 88.13
  peritoneum NEC 88.13
  presacral 88.15
  retroperitoneum 88.15
Pneumogynecography 87.82
Pneumomediastinography 87.33
Pneumonectomy (extended) (radical) (standard)
  (total) (with mediastinal dissection) 32.59
  partial
    complete excision, one lobe 32.49
    resection (wedge), one lobe 32.39
  thoracoscopic 32.50
Pneumonolysis (for collapse of lung) 33.39
Pneumonotomy (with exploration) 33.1
Pneumoperitoneum (surgically-induced) 54.96
  for collapse of lung 33.33
  pelvic 88.12
Pneumothorax (artificial) (surgical) 33.32
  intrapleural 33.32
Pneumoventriculogram 87.02
Politano-Leadbetter operation
  (ureteroneocystostomy) 56.74
Politzerization, Eustachian tube 20.8
Pollicization (with carry over of nerves and blood
  supply) 82.61
Polya operation (gastrectomy) 43.7
Polypectomy —*see also* Excision, lesion, by site
  esophageal 42.32
    endoscopic 42.33
  gastric (endoscopic) 43.41
  large intestine (colon) 45.42
  nasal 21.31
  rectum (endoscopic) 48.36
Polysomnogram 89.17
Pomeroy operation (ligation and division of
  fallopian tubes) 66.32
Poncet operation
  lengthening of Achilles tendon 83.85
  urethrostomy, perineal 58.0
Porro operation (cesarean section) 74.99
Portoenterostomy (Kasai) 51.37
Positrocephalogram 92.11
Positron emission tomography (PET) —*see*
  Scan, radioisotope
Postmortem examination 89.8
Potts-Smith operation (descending aorta-left
  pulmonary artery anastomosis) 39.0
Poudrage
  intrapericardial 36.39
  pleural 34.6
PPN (peripheral parenteral nutrition) 99.15
PPVI (percutaneous pulmonary valve
  implantation) 35.07

Preparation (cutting), pedicle (flap) graft 86.71
Preputiotomy 64.91
Prescription for glasses 95.31
Pressurized
  graft treatment 00.16
Printen and Mason operation (high gastric
  bypass) 44.31
Probing
  canaliculus, lacrimal (with irrigation) 09.42
  lacrimal
    canaliculi 09.42
    punctum (with irrigation) 09.41
  nasolacrimal duct (with irrigation) 09.43
    with insertion of tube or stent 09.44
  salivary duct (for dilation of duct) (for removal of
    calculus) 26.91
    with incision 26.0
Procedure —*see also* specific procedure
  diagnostic NEC
    abdomen (region) 54.29
    adenoid 28.19
    adrenal gland 07.19
    alveolus 24.19
    amnion 75.35
    anterior chamber, eye 12.29
    anus 49.29
    appendix 45.28
    biliary tract 51.19
    bladder 57.39
    blood vessel (any site) 38.29
    bone 78.80
      carpal, metacarpal 78.84
      clavicle 78.81
      facial 76.19
      femur 78.85
      fibula 78.87
      humerus 78.82
      marrow 41.38
      patella 78.86
      pelvic 78.89
      phalanges (foot) (hand) 78.89
      radius 78.83
      scapula 78.81
      specified site NEC 78.89
      tarsal, metatarsal 78.88
      thorax (ribs) (sternum) 78.81
      tibia 78.87
      ulna 78.83
      vertebrae 78.89
    brain 01.18
    breast 85.19
    bronchus 33.29
    buccal 27.24
    bursa 83.29
    canthus 08.19
    cecum 45.28
    cerebral meninges 01.18
    cervix 67.19
    chest wall 34.28
    choroid 14.19
    ciliary body 12.29
    clitoris 71.19
    colon 45.28
    conjunctiva 10.29
    cornea 11.29
    cul-de-sac 70.29
    dental 24.19
    diaphragm 34.28
    duodenum 45.19

Puncture—*continued*
  spleen 41.1
    for biopsy 41.32
  sternal (for bone marrow biopsy) 41.31
    donor for bone marrow transplant 41.91
  vein NEC 38.99
    for
      phlebography (*see also* Phlebography) 88.60
      transfusion—*see* Transfusion
  ventricular shunt tubing 01.02
Pupillotomy 12.35
Push-back operation (cleft palate repair) 27.62
Putti-Platt operation (capsulorrhaphy of
    shoulder for recurrent dislocation) 81.82
pVAD (percutaneous ventricular assist device)
    37.68
Pyelogram (intravenous) 87.73
  infusion (continuous) (diuretic) 87.73
  percutaneous 87.75
  retrograde 87.74
Pyeloileostomy 56.71
Pyelolithotomy 55.11
Pyeloplasty 55.87
Pyelorrhaphy 55.81
Pyeloscopy 55.22
Pyelostolithotomy, percutaneous 55.03
Pyelostomy 55.12
  closure 55.82
Pyelotomy 55.11
Pyeloureteroplasty 55.87
Pylorectomy 43.6
Pyloroduodenotomy —*see* category 44.2
Pyloromyotomy (Ramstedt) (with wedge
    resection) 43.3
Pyloroplasty (Finney) (Heineke-Mikulicz) 44.29
  dilation, endoscopic 44.22
    by incision 44.21
  not elsewhere classified 44.29
  revision 44.29
Pylorostomy —*see* Gastrostomy

Q-R

Quadrant resection of breast 85.22
Quadricepsplasty (Thompson) 83.86
Quarantine 99.84
Quenuthoracoplasty 77.31
Quotient, respiratory 89.38

Rachicentesis 03.31
Rachitomy 03.09
Radiation therapy —*see also* Therapy, radiation
    teleradiotheraphy—*see* Teleradiotherapy
Radical neck dissection —*see* Dissection, neck
Radicotomy 03.1
Radiculectomy 03.1
Radiculotomy 03.1
Radiography (diagnostic) NEC 88.39
    abdomen, abdominal (flat plate) NEC 88.19
        wall (soft tissue) NEC 88.09
    adenoid 87.09
    ankle (skeletal) 88.28
        soft tissue 88.37
    bone survey 88.31
    bronchus 87.49
    chest (routine) 87.44
        wall NEC 87.39
    clavicle 87.43
    computer assisted surgery (CAS) with
        fluoroscopy 00.33
    contrast (air) (gas) (radio-opaque substance) NEC
        abdominal wall 88.03
        arteries (by fluoroscopy)—*see* Arteriography
        bile ducts NEC 87.54
        bladder NEC 87.77
        brain 87.02
        breast 87.35
        bronchus NEC (transcricoid) 87.32
            endotracheal 87.31
        epididymis 87.93
        esophagus 87.61
        fallopian tubes
            gas 87.82
            opaque dye 87.83
        fistula (sinus tract)—*see also* Radiography,
            contrast, by site
            abdominal wall 88.03
            chest wall 87.38
        gallbladder NEC 87.59
        intervertebral disc(s) 87.21
        joints 88.32
        larynx 87.07
        lymph—*see* Lymphangiogram
        mammary ducts 87.35
        mediastinum 87.33
        nasal sinuses 87.15
        nasolacrimal ducts 87.05
        nasopharynx 87.06
        orbit 87.14
        pancreas 87.66
        pelvis
            gas 88.12
            opaque dye 88.11
        peritoneum NEC 88.13
        retroperitoneum NEC 88.15
        seminal vesicles 87.91
        sinus tract—*see also* Radiography, contrast, by
            site
            abdominal wall 88.03
            chest wall 87.38
            nose 87.15
        skull 87.02
        spinal disc(s) 87.21
        trachea 87.32
        uterus
            gas 87.82
            opaque dye 87.83

Referral (for)
  psychiatric aftercare (halfway house) (outpatient clinic) 94.52
  psychotherapy 94.51
  rehabilitation
    alcoholism 94.53
    drug addiction 94.54
    psychologic NEC 94.59
    vocational 94.55
Reformation
  cardiac pacemaker pocket, new site (skin) (subcutaneous) 37.79
  cardioverter/defibrillator (automatic) pocket, new site (skin) (subcutaneous) 37.79
  chamber of eye 12.99
Refracture
  bone (for faulty union) (*see also* Osteoclasis) 78.70
  nasal bones 21.88
Refusion
  spinal NOS 81.30
    atlas-axis (anterior) (transoral) (posterior) 81.31
    axial lumbar interbody fusion [AxiaLIF] 81.38
    cervical (C2 level or below) NEC 81.32
      anterior column (interbody), anterolateral (anterior) technique 81.32
      C1-C2 level (anterior) (posterior) 81.31
      posterior column, posterolateral (posterior) technique 81.33
    craniocervical (anterior) (transoral) (posterior) 81.31
    direct lateral interbody fusion [DLIF] 81.36
    dorsal, dorsolumbar NEC 81.35
      anterior column (interbody), anterolateral (anterior) (extracavitary) technique 81.34
      posterior column, posterolateral (posterior) technique 81.35
    extreme lateral interbody fusion [XLIF] 81.36
    facet 81.37
    lumbar, lumbosacral NEC 81.38
      anterior column (interbody)
        anterolateral (anterior) technique 81.36
        posterior technique 81.38
      anterior lumbar interbody fusion (ALIF) 81.36
      lateral transverse process technique 81.37
      posterior column, posterior (posterolateral) (transverse process) technique 81.37
      transforaminal lumbar interbody fusion (TLIF) 81.38
    number of vertebrae —*see* codes 81.62-81.64
    occiput — C2 (anterior) (transoral) (posterior) 81.31
    refusion NEC 81.39

> *Note: Also use either 81.62, 81.63 or 81.64 as an additional code to show the total number of vertebrae fused*

Regional blood flow study 92.05
Regulation, menstrual 69.6
Rehabilitation programs NEC 93.89
  alcohol 94.61
    with detoxification 94.63
    combined alcohol and drug 94.67
      with detoxification 94.69
  drug 94.64
    with detoxification 94.66
    combined drug and alcohol 94.67
      with detoxification 94.69
  sheltered employment 93.85
  vocational 93.85

Reimplantation
  adrenal tissue (heterotopic) (orthotopic) 07.45
  artery 39.59
    renal, aberrant 39.55
  bile ducts following excision of ampulla of Vater 51.62
  extremity—*see* Reattachment, extremity
  fallopian tube into uterus 66.74
  kidney 55.61
  lung 33.5
  ovary 65.72
    laparoscopic 65.75
  pancreatic tissue 52.81
  parathyroid tissue (heterotopic) (orthotopic) 06.95
  pulmonary artery for hemitruncus repair 35.83
  renal vessel, aberrant 39.55
  testis in scrotum 62.5
  thyroid tissue (heterotopic) (orthotopic) 06.94
  tooth 23.5
  ureter into bladder 56.74
Reinforcement —*see also* Repair, by site
  sclera NEC 12.88
    with graft 12.87
Reinsertion —*see also* Insertion *or* Revision
  cystostomy tube 59.94
  fixation device (internal) (*see also* Fixation, bone, internal) 78.50
  heart valve (prosthetic) 35.95
  Holter (Spitz) valve 02.42
  implant (expelled) (extruded)
    eyeball (with conjunctival graft) 16.62
    orbital 16.62
  nephrostomy tube 55.93
  pyelostomy tube 55.94
  ureteral stent (transurethral) 59.8
    with ureterotomy 59.8 *[56.2]*
  ureterostomy tube 59.93
  valve
    heart (prosthetic) 35.95
    ventricular (cerebral) 02.42
Relaxation —(*see also* Release)
  training 94.33
Release
  carpal tunnel (for nerve decompression) 04.43
  celiac artery axis 39.91
  central slip, extensor tendon hand (mallet finger repair) 82.84
  chordee 64.42
  clubfoot NEC 83.84
  de Quervain's tenosynovitis 82.01
  Dupuytren's contracture (by palmar fasciectomy) 82.35
    by fasciotomy (subcutaneous) 82.12
      with excision 82.35
  Fowler (mallet finger repair) 82.84
  joint (capsule) (adherent) (constrictive) (*see also* Division, joint capsule) 80.40
  laryngeal 31.92
  ligament (*see also* Division, ligament) 80.40
    median arcuate 39.91
  median arcuate ligament 39.91
  muscle (division) 83.19
    hand 82.19
  nerve (peripheral) NEC 04.49
    cranial NEC 04.42
    trigeminal 04.41
  pressure, intraocular 12.79
  scar tissue
    skin 86.84
    stoma—*see* Revision, stoma
  tarsal tunnel 04.44

Removal—*continued*
  vulva 98.23
    by incision 71.09
  gallstones
    bile duct (by incision) NEC 51.49
      endoscopic 51.88
    common duct (by incision) 51.41
      endoscopic 51.88
      percutaneous 51.96
    duodenum 45.01
    gallbladder 51.04
      endoscopic 51.88
      laparoscopic 51.88
    hepatic ducts 51.49
      endoscopic 51.88
    intestine 45.00
      large 45.03
      small NEC 45.02
    liver 50.0
  Gardner Wells tongs (skull) 02.95
    with synchronous replacement 02.94
  gastric band (adjustable), laparoscopic 44.97
  gastric bubble (balloon) 44.94
  granulation tissue—*see also* Excision, lesion, by
    site
    with repair—*see* Repair, by site
    cranial 01.6
    skull 01.6
  halo traction device (skull) 02.95
    with synchronous replacement 02.94
  heart assist system
    with replacement 37.63
    intra-aortic balloon pump (IABP) 97.44
    nonoperative 97.44
    open removal 37.64
    percutaneous external device 97.44
  heart replacement system
    internal biventricular 37.55
  hematoma—*see* Drainage, by site
  Hoffman minifixator device (bone)—*see* category
    78.6
  hydatidiform mole 68.0
  impacted
    feces (rectum) (by flushing) (manual) 96.38
    tooth 23.19
      from nasal sinus (maxillary) 22.61
  implant
    breast 85.94
    cochlear prosthetic device 20.99
    cornea 11.92
    lens (prosthetic) 13.8
    middle ear NEC 20.99
    ocular 16.71
      posterior segment 14.6
    orbit 16.72
    retina 14.6
    tympanum 20.1
  implantable hemodynamic sensor (lead) and
    monitor device 37.79
  internal biventricular heart replacement system
    37.55
  internal fixation device—*see* Removal, fixation
    device, internal
  intra-aortic balloon pump (IABP) 97.44
  intrauterine contraceptive device (IUD) 97.71
  joint (structure) NOS 80.90
    ankle 80.97
    elbow 80.92
    foot and toe 80.98
    hand and finger 80.94
    hip 80.95

Removal—*continued*
    knee 80.96
    other specified sites 80.99
    shoulder 80.91
    spine 80.99
    toe 80.98
    wrist 80.93
  Kantrowitz heart pump 37.64
    nonoperative 97.44
  keel (tantalum plate), larynx 31.98
  kidney—*see also* Nephrectomy
    mechanical 55.98
    transplanted or rejected 55.53
  laminaria (tent), uterus 97.79
  leads (cardiac)—*see* Removal, electrodes, cardiac
    pacemaker
  lesion—*see* Excision, lesion, by site
  ligamentum flavum (spine)—*omit code*
  ligature
    fallopian tube 66.79
    ureter 56.86
    vas deferens 63.84
  limb lengthening device, internal—*see* category
    78.6
  loop recorder 86.05
  loose body
    bone—*see* Sequestrectomy, bone
    joint 80.10
  mesh (surgical)—*see* Removal, foreign body,
    by site
  lymph node—*see* Excision, lymph, node
  minifixator device (bone)—*see* category 78.6
    external fixation device 97.88
  Mulligan hood, fallopian tube 66.94
    with synchronous replacement 66.93
  muscle stimulator (skeletal) 83.93
    with replacement 83.92
  myringotomy device or tube 20.1
  nail (bed) (fold) 86.23
    internal fixation device—*see* Removal, fixation
      device, internal
  necrosis
    skin 86.28
      excisional 86.22
  neuropacemaker—*see* Removal, neurostimulator,
    by site
  neurostimulator
    brain 01.22
      with synchronous replacement 02.93
    electrodes
      brain 01.22
        with synchronous replacement 02.93
      gastric 04.93
        with synchronous replacement 04.92
      intracranial 01.22
        with synchronous replacement 02.93
      peripheral nerve 04.93
        with synchronous replacement 04.92
      sacral nerve 04.93
        with synchronous replacement 04.92
      spinal 03.94
        with synchronous replacement 03.93
    intracranial 01.22
      with synchronous replacement 02.93
    peripheral nerve 04.93
      with synchronous replacement 04.92

Removal—*continued*

Roger-Anderson minifixator device (bone)—*see* category 78.6

root, residual (tooth) (buried) (retained) 23.11

Rosen prosthesis (urethra) 59.99

Scribner shunt 39.43

scleral buckle or implant 14.6

secondary membranous cataract (with iridectomy) 13.65

secundines (by)
    aspiration curettage 69.52
    D and C 69.02
    manual 75.4

sequestrum—*see* Sequestrectomy

seton, anus 49.93

Shepard's tube (ear) 20.1

Shirodkar suture, cervix 69.96

shunt
    arteriovenous 39.43
        with creation of new shunt 39.42
    lumbar-subarachnoid NEC 03.98
    pleurothecal 03.98
    salpingothecal 03.98
    spinal (thecal) NEC 03.98
    subarachnoid-peritoneal 03.98
    subarachnoid-ureteral 03.98

silastic tubes
    ear 20.1
    fallopian tubes 66.94
        with synchronous replacement 66.93

skin
    necrosis or slough 86.28
        excisional 86.22
    superficial layer (by dermabrasion) 86.25

skull tongs 02.95
    with synchronous replacement 02.94

spacer (cement) (joint) (methylmethacrylate) 84.57

splint 97.88

stent
    bile duct 97.55
    larynx 31.98
    ureteral 97.62
    urethral 97.65

stimoceiver—*see* Removal, neurostimulator

subdural
    grids 01.22
    strips 01.22

supernumerary digit(s) 86.26

suture(s) NEC 97.89
    abdominal wall 97.83
    by incision—*see* Incision, by site
    genital tract 97.79
    head and neck 97.38
    thorax 97.43
    trunk NEC 97.84

symblepharon—*see* Repair, symblepharon

temporary transvenous pacemaker system—*omit code*

testis (unilateral) 62.3
    bilateral 62.41
    remaining or solitary 62.42

Removal—*continued*

thrombus 38.00
    with endarterectomy—*see* Endarterectomy
    abdominal
        artery 38.06
        vein 38.07
    aorta (arch) (ascending) (descending) 38.04
    arteriovenous shunt or cannula 39.49
    bovine graft 39.49
    coronary artery 36.09
    head and neck vessel NEC 38.02
    intracranial vessel NEC 38.01
    lower limb
        artery 38.08
        vein 38.09
    pulmonary (artery) (vein) 38.05
    thoracic vessel NEC 38.05
    upper limb (artery) (vein) 38.0

tissue expander (skin) NEC 86.05
    breast 85.96

toes, supernumerary 86.26

tongs, skull 02.95
    with synchronous replacement 02.94

tonsil tag 28.4

tooth (by forceps) (multiple) (single NEC 23.09
    deciduous 23.01
    surgical NEC 23.19
        impacted 23.19
        residual root 23.11
        root apex 23.73
            with root canal therapy 23.72

trachoma follicles 10.33

T-tube (bile duct) 97.55

tube
    appendix 97.53
    bile duct (T-tube) NEC 97.55
    cholecystostomy 97.54
    cranial cavity 01.27
    cystostomy 97.63
    ear (button) 20.1
    gastrostomy 97.51
    large intestine 97.53
    liver 97.55
    mediastinum 97.42
    nephrostomy 97.61
    pancreas 97.56
    peritoneum 97.82
    pleural cavity 97.41
    pyelostomy 97.61
    retroperitoneum 97.81
    small intestine 97.52
    thoracotomy 97.41
    tracheostomy 97.37
    tympanostomy 20.1
    tympanum 20.1
    ureterostomy 97.62

ureteral splint (stent) 97.62

urethral sphincter, artificial 58.99
    with replacement 58.93

urinary sphincter, artificial 58.99
    with replacement 58.93

utricle 20.79

valve
    vas deferens 63.85
    ventricular (cerebral) 02.43

vascular graft or prosthesis 39.49

ventricular shunt or reservoir 02.43
    with synchronous replacement 02.42

Vinke tongs (skull) 02.95
    with synchronous replacement 02.94

Repair—*continued*

percutaneous repair of intracranial vessel(s) (for stent insertion) 00.62

Note: Also use 00.40, 00.41, 00.42, or 00.43 to show the total number of vessels treated. Use code 00.44 once to show procedure on a bifurcated vessel. In addition, use 00.45, 00.46, 00.47, or 00.48 to show the number of vascular stents inserted.

percutaneous repair of extracranial vessel(s) (for stent insertion) 00.61

Note: Also use 00.40, 00.41, 00.42, or 00.43 to show the total number of vessels treated. Use code 00.44 once to show procedure on a bifurcated vessel. In addition, use 00.45, 00.46, 00.47, or 00.48 to show the number of vascular stents inserted.

non-coronary percutaneous transluminal approach

Note: Also use 00.40, 00.41, 00.42, or 00.43 to show the total number of vessels treated. Use code 00.44 once to show procedure on a bifurcated vessel. In addition, use 00.45, 00.46, 00.47, or 00.48 to show the number of vascular stents inserted.

angioplasty
  basilar 00.62
  carotid 00.61
  femoropopliteal 39.50
  iliac 39.50
  lower extremity NOS 39.50
  mesenteric 39.50
  renal 39.50
  upper extremity NOS 39.50
  vertebral 00.61
    intracranial portion 00.62
  atherectomy 17.56
coronary NEC 36.99
  by angioplasty—*see* Angioplasty, coronary
  by atherectomy
    percutaneous transluminal 17.55
  with
    patch graft 39.58
      with excision or resection of vessel—*see* Arteriectomy, with graft replacement, by site
      synthetic (Dacron) (Teflon) 39.57
      tissue (vein) (autogenous) (homograft) 39.56
    suture 39.31
artificial opening—*see* Repair, stoma
atrial septal defect 35.71
  with
    prosthesis (open heart technique) 35.51
      closed heart technique 35.52
    tissue graft 35.61
  combined with repair of valvular and ventricular septal defects—*see* Repair, endocardial cushion defect
  in total repair of total anomalous pulmonary venous connection 35.82
atrioventricular canal defect (any type) 35.73
  with
    prosthesis 35.54
    tissue graft 35.63
bifid digit (finger) 82.89

Repair—*continued*

bile duct NEC 51.79
  laceration (by suture) NEC 51.79
    common bile duct 51.71
bladder NEC 57.89
  exstrophy 57.86
  for stress incontinence—*see* Repair, stress incontinence
  laceration (by suture) 57.81
    obstetric (current) 75.61
    old 57.89
  neck 57.85
blepharophimosis 08.59
blepharoptosis 08.36
  by
    frontalis muscle technique (with)
      fascial sling 08.32
      suture 08.31
    levator muscle technique 08.34
      with resection or advancement 08.33
    orbicularis oculi muscle sling 08.36
    tarsal technique 08.35
blood vessel NEC 39.59
  with
    patch graft 39.58
      with excision or resection—*see* Angiectomy, with graft replacement
      synthetic (Dacron) (Teflon) 39.57
      tissue (vein) (autogenous) (homograft) 39.56
    resection—*see* Angiectomy
    suture 39.30
  coronary artery NEC 36.99
    by angioplasty—*see* Angioplasty, coronary
    by atherectomy
      percutaneous transluminal 17.55
  peripheral vessel NEC 39.59
    by angioplasty 39.50

Note: Also use 00.40, 00.41, 00.42, or 00.43 to show the total number of vessels treated. Use code 00.44 once to show procedure on a bifurcated vessel. In addition, use 00.45, 00.46, 00.47, or 00.48 to show the number of vascular stents inserted.

by atherectomy 17.56

Note: Also use 00.40, 00.41, 00.42, or 00.43 to show the total number of vessels treated. Use code 00.44 once to show procedure on a bifurcated vessel. In addition, use 00.45, 00.46, 00.47, or 00.48 to show the number of vascular stents inserted.

by endovascular approach 39.79
bone NEC (*see also* Osteoplasty)—*see* category 78.4
  accessory sinus 22.79
  by synostosis technique—*see* Arthrodesis
  cranium NEC 02.06
    with
      flap (bone) 02.03
      graft (bone) 02.04
  for malunion, nonunion, or delayed union of fracture—*see* Repair, fracture, malunion or nonunion
  nasal 21.89
  skull NEC 02.06
    with
      flap (bone) 02.03
      graft (bone) 02.04

Repair—*continued*
  fascia 83.89
    by or with
      arthroplasty—*see* Arthroplasty
      graft (fascial) (muscle) 83.82
        hand 82.72
        tendon 83.81
          hand 82.79
      suture (direct) 83.65
        hand 82.46
    hand 82.89
      by
        graft NEC 82.79
          fascial 82.72
          muscle 82.72
        suture (direct) 82.46
    joint—*see* Arthroplasty
  filtering bleb (corneal) (scleral) (by excision)
      12.82
    by
      corneal graft (*see also* Keratoplasty) 11.60
      scleroplasty 12.82
      suture 11.51
    with conjunctival flap 11.53
  fistula—*see also* Closure, fistula
    anovaginal 70.73
    arteriovenous 39.53
      clipping 39.53
      coagulation 39.53
        endovascular approach 39.79
          head and neck 39.72
      division 39.53
      excision or resection—*see also*
          Aneurysmectomy, by site
        with
          anastomosis—*see* Aneurysmectomy, with
            anastomosis, by site
          graft replacement—*see* Aneurysmectomy,
            with graft replacement, by site
      ligation 39.53
        coronary artery 36.99
      occlusion 39.53
        endovascular approach 39.79
          head and neck 39.72
      suture 39.53
    cervicovesical 57.84
    cervix 67.62
    choledochoduodenal 51.72
    colovaginal 70.72
    enterovaginal 70.74
    enterovesical 57.83
    esophagocutaneous 42.84
    ileovesical 57.83
    intestinovaginal 70.74
    intestinovesical 57.83
    oroantral 22.71
    perirectal 48.93
    pleuropericardial 37.49
    rectovaginal 70.73
    rectovesical 57.83
    rectovesicovaginal 57.83
    scrotum 61.42
    sigmoidovaginal 70.74
    sinus
      nasal 22.71
      of Valsalva 35.39
    splenocolic 41.95
    urethroperineovesical 57.84
    urethrovesical 57.84
    urethrovesicovaginal 57.84
    uterovesical 57.84

Repair—*continued*
    vagina NEC 70.75
    vaginocutaneous 70.75
    vaginoenteric NEC 70.74
    vaginoileal 70.74
    vaginoperineal 70.75
    vaginovesical 57.84
    vesicocervicovaginal 57.84
    vesicocolic 57.83
    vesicocutaneous 57.84
    vesicoenteric 57.83
    vesicointestinal 57.83
    vesicometrorectal 57.83
    vesicoperineal 57.84
    vesicorectal 57.83
    vesicosigmoidal 57.83
    vesicosigmoidovaginal 57.83
    vesicourethral 57.84
    vesicourethrorectal 57.83
    vesicouterine 57.84
    vesicovaginal 57.84
    vulva 71.72
    vulvorectal 48.73
  foramen ovale (patent) 35.71
    with
      prosthesis (open heart technique) 35.51
        closed heart technique 35.52
      tissue graft 35.61
  fracture—*see also* Reduction, fracture
    larynx 31.64
    malunion or nonunion (delayed) NEC—*see*
        category 78.4
      with
        graft—*see* Graft, bone
        insertion (of)
          bone growth stimulator (invasive)—*see*
            category 78.9
          internal fixation device 78.5
        manipulation for realignment—*see*
          Reduction, fracture, by site, closed
      osteotomy
        with
          correction of alignment—*see* category
            77.3
            with internal fixation device—*see*
              categories 77.3 [78.5]
            with intramedullary rod—*see*
              categories 77.3 [78.5]
        replacement arthroplasty—*see* Arthroplasty
        sequestrectomy—*see* category 77.0
        Sofield type procedure—*see* categories 77.3
          [78.5]
        synostosis technique—*see* Arthrodesis
    vertebra 03.53
  funnel chest (with implant) 34.74
  gallbladder 51.91
  gastroschisis 54.71
  great vessels NEC 39.59
    laceration (by suture) 39.30
      artery 39.31
      vein 39.32
  hallux valgus NEC 77.59
    resection of joint with prosthetic implant 77.59
  hammer toe 77.56
  hand 82.89
    with graft or implant 82.79
      fascia 82.72
      muscle 82.72
      tendon 82.79

Repair—*continued*
  muscle NEC 83.87
  by
      graft or implant (fascia) (muscle) 83.82
        hand 82.72
      tendon 83.81
        hand 82.79
      suture (direct) 83.65
        hand 82.46
      transfer or transplantation (muscle) 83.77
        hand 82.58
    hand 82.89
    by
        graft or implant NEC 82.79
          fascia 82.72
        suture (direct) 82.46
        transfer or transplantation (muscle) 82.58
  musculotendinous cuff, shoulder 83.63
  myelomeningocele 03.52
  nasal
    septum (perforation) NEC 21.88
    sinus NEC 22.79
      fistula 22.71
  nasolabial flaps (plastic) 21.86
  nasopharyngeal atresia 29.4
  nerve (cranial) (peripheral) NEC 04.79
    old injury 04.76
    revision 04.75
    sympathetic 05.81
  nipple NEC 85.87
  nose (external) (internal) (plastic) NEC (*see also*
        Rhinoplasty) 21.89
    laceration (by suture) 21.81
  notched lip 27.59
  omentum 54.74
  omphalocele
    laparoscopic 53.43
      with graft or prosthesis 53.42
    other and open with graft or prosthesis 53.41
    other open 53.49
  orbit 16.89
    wound 16.81
  ostium
    primum defect 35.73
      with prosthesis 35.54
      with tissue graft 35.63
    secundum defect 35.71
      with
        prosthesis (open heart technique) 35.51
          closed heart technique 35.52
        tissue graft 35.61
  ovary 65.79
    with tube 65.73
    laparoscopic 65.76
  overlapping toe 77.58
  pacemaker
    cardiac
      device (permanent) 37.89
      electrode(s) (lead) NEC 37.75
      pocket (skin) (subcutaneous) 37.79
  palate NEC 27.69
    cleft 27.62
      secondary or subsequent 27.63
    laceration (by suture) 27.61

Repair—*continued*
  pancreas NEC 52.95
    Wirsung's duct 52.99
  papillary muscle (heart) 35.31
  patent ductus arteriosus 38.85
  pectus deformity (chest) (carinatum) (excavatum)
        34.74
  pelvic floor NEC 70.79
    obstetric laceration (current) 75.69
      old 70.79
  penis NEC 64.49
    for epispadias or hypospadias 58.45
    inflatable prosthesis 64.99
    laceration 64.41
  pericardium 37.49
  perineum (female) 71.79
    laceration (by suture) 71.71
      obstetric (current) 75.69
        old 71.79
    male NEC 86.89
      laceration (by suture) 86.59
  peritoneum NEC 54.73
    by suture 54.64
  pharynx NEC 29.59
    laceration (by suture) 29.51
    plastic 29.4
  pleura NEC 34.93
  postcataract wound dehiscence 11.52
    with conjunctival flap 11.53
  pouch of Douglas 70.52
  primum ostium defect 35.73
    with
      prosthesis 35.54
      tissue graft 35.63
  prostate 60.93
  ptosis, eyelid—*see* Repair, blepharoptosis
  punctum, lacrimal NEC 09.72
    for correction of eversion 09.71
  quadriceps (mechanism) 83.86
  rectocele (posterior colporrhaphy) 70.52
    with graft or prosthesis 70.55
    and cystocele 70.50
      with graft or prosthesis 70.53
  rectum NEC 48.79
    laceration (by suture) 48.71
    prolapse NEC 48.76
      abdominal approach 48.75
      STARR procedure 48.74
  retina, retinal
    detachment 14.59
      by
        cryotherapy 14.52
        diathermy 14.51
        photocoagulation 14.55
          laser 14.54
          xenon arc 14.53
        scleral buckling (*see also* Buckling, scleral)
          14.49
    tear or defect 14.39
      by
        cryotherapy 14.32
        diathermy 14.31
        photocoagulation 14.35
          laser 14.34
          xenon arc 14.33
  retroperitoneal tissue 54.73
  rotator cuff (graft) (suture) 83.63

Repair—*continued*
round ligament 69.29
ruptured tendon NEC 83.88
    hand 82.86
salivary gland or duct NEC 26.49
sclera, scleral 12.89
    fistula 12.82
    staphyloma NEC 12.86
        with graft 12.85
scrotum 61.49
sinus
    nasal NEC 22.79
    of Valsalva (aneurysm) 35.39
skin (plastic) (without graft) 86.89
    laceration (by suture) 86.59
skull NEC 02.06
    with
        flap (bone) 02.03
        graft (bone) 02.04
spermatic cord NEC 63.59
    laceration (by suture) 63.51
sphincter ani 49.79
    laceration (by suture) 49.71
        obstetric (current) 75.62
        old 49.79
spina bifida NEC 03.59
    meningocele 03.51
    myelomeningocele 03.52
spinal (cord) (meninges) (structures) NEC 03.59
    meningocele 03.51
    myelomeningocele 03.52
spleen 41.95
sternal defect 78.41
stoma
    bile duct 51.79
    bladder 57.22
    bronchus 33.42
    common duct 51.72
    esophagus 42.89
    gallbladder 51.99
    hepatic duct 51.79
    intestine 46.40
        large 46.43
        small 46.41
    kidney 55.89
    larynx 31.63
    rectum 48.79
    stomach 44.69
        laparoscopic 44.68
    thorax 34.79
    trachea 31.74
    ureter 56.62
    urethra 58.49
stomach NEC 44.69
    laceration (by suture) 44.61
    laparoscopic 44.68
stress incontinence (urinary) NEC 59.79
    by
        anterior urethropexy 59.79
        Burch 59.5
        cystourethropexy (with levator muscle sling) 59.71
        gracilis muscle transplant 59.71
        injection of implant (collagen) (fat) (polytef) 59.72
        levator muscle sling 59.71
        paraurethral suspension (Pereyra) 59.6
        periurethral suspension 59.6
        plication of urethrovesical junction 59.3
        pubococcygeal sling 59.71
        retropubic urethral suspension 59.5

Repair—*continued*
    suprapubic sling 59.4
    tension free vaginal tape 59.79
    urethrovesical suspension 59.4
subcutaneous tissue (plastic) (without skin graft) 86.89
    laceration (by suture) 86.59
supracristal defect (heart) 35.72
    with
        prosthesis (open heart technique) 35.53
            closed heart technique 35.55
        tissue graft 35.62
symblepharon NEC 10.49
    by division (with insertion of conformer) 10.5
    with free graft 10.41
syndactyly 86.85
synovial membrane, joint—*see* Arthroplasty
telecanthus 08.59
tendon 83.88
    by or with
        arthroplasty—*see* Arthroplasty
        graft or implant (tendon) 83.81
            fascia 83.82
                hand 82.72
            hand 82.79
            muscle 83.82
                hand 82.72
        suture (direct) (immediate) (primary) (*see also* Suture, tendon) 83.64
            hand 82.45
        transfer or transplantation (tendon) 83.75
            hand 82.56
    hand 82.86
        by
            graft or implant (tendon) 82.79
            suture (direct) (immediate) (primary) (*see also* Suture, tendon, hand) 82.45
            transfer or transplantation (tendon) 82.56
    rotator cuff (direct suture) 83.63
    ruptured NEC 83.88
        hand 82.86
    sheath (direct suture) 83.61
        hand 82.41
testis NEC 62.69
tetralogy of Fallot
    partial—*see* specific procedure
    total (one-stage) 35.81
thoracic duct NEC 40.69
thoracostomy 34.72
thymus (gland) 07.93
tongue NEC 25.59
tooth NEC 23.2
    by
        crown (artificial) 23.41
        filling (amalgam) (plastic) (silicate) 23.2
        inlay 23.3
total anomalous pulmonary venous connection
    partial—*see* specific procedure
    total (one-stage) 35.82
trachea NEC 31.79
    laceration (by suture) 31.71
tricuspid atresia 35.94
truncus arteriosus
    partial—*see* specific procedure
    total (one-stage) 35.83
tunica vaginalis 61.49
    laceration (by suture) 61.41
tympanum—*see* Tympanoplasty
ureter NEC 56.89
    laceration (by suture) 56.82

Resection—*continued*

right hemicolon
  laparoscopic 17.33
  open and other 45.73
segmental (large intestine)
  laparoscopic 17.39
  multiple
    laparoscopic 17.31
    open and other 45.71
  open and other 45.79
  small intestine 45.62
    multiple 45.61
sigmoid
  laparoscopic 17.36
  open and other 45.76
small (partial) (segmental) NEC 45.62
  for interposition 45.51
  multiple segmental 45.61
  total 45.63
total
  large intestine
    laparoscopic 45.81
    open 45.82
    other 45.83
    unspecified 45.83
  small intestine 45.63
joint structure NEC (*see also* Arthrectomy) 80.90
kidney (segmental) (wedge) 55.4
larynx—*see also* Laryngectomy
  submucous 30.29
lesion—*see* Excision, lesion, by site
levator palpebrae muscle 08.33
ligament (*see also* Arthrectomy) 80.90
  broad 69.19
  round 69.19
  uterine 69.19
lip (wedge) 27.43
liver (partial) (wedge) 50.22
  lobe (total) 50.3
  total 50.4
lung (wedge) NEC 32.29
  endoscopic 32.28
  segmental (any part) 32.39
    thoracoscopic 32.30
  thoracoscopic 32.20
  volume reduction 32.22
    biologic lung volume reduction (BLVR)
      —*see* category 33.7
meninges (cerebral) 01.51
  spinal 03.4
mesentery 54.4
muscle 83.45
  extraocular 15.13
    with
      advancement or recession of other eye
        muscle 15.3
      suture of original insertion 15.13
    levator palpebrae 08.33
    Müller's for blepharoptosis 08.35
    orbicularis oculi 08.20
    tarsal, for blepharoptosis 08.35
  for graft 83.43
    hand 82.34
  hand 82.36
    for graft 82.34
  ocular—*see* Resection, muscle, extraocular
myocardium 37.33
nasal septum (submucous) 21.5

Resection—*continued*

nerve (cranial) (peripheral) NEC 04.07
  phrenic 04.03
    for collapse of lung 33.31
  sympathetic 05.29
  vagus—*see* Vagotomy
nose (complete) (extended) (partial)
  (radical) 21.4
omentum 54.4
orbitomaxillary, radical 16.51
ovary—(*see also* Oophorectomy
  wedge 65.22
    laparoscopic 65.24
palate (bony) (local) 27.31
  by wide excision 27.32
  soft 27.49
pancreas (total) (with synchronous
  duodenectomy) 52.6
  partial NEC 52.59
    distal (tail) (with part of body) 52.52
    proximal (head) (with part or body) (with
      synchronous duodenectomy) 52.51
    radical subtotal 52.53
  radical (one-stage) (two-stage) 52.7
  subtotal 52.53
pancreaticoduodenal (*see also* Pancreatectomy)
  52.6
pelvic viscera (en masse) (female) 68.8
  male 57.71
penis 64.3
pericardium (partial) (for)
  chronic constrictive pericarditis 37.31
  drainage 37.12
  removal of adhesions 37.31
peritoneum 54.4
pharynx (partial) 29.33
phrenic nerve 04.03
  for collapse of lung 33.31
prostate—*see also* Prostatectomy
  transurethral (punch) 60.29
pterygium 11.39
radial head 77.83
rectosigmoid (*see also* Resection, rectum) 48.69
rectum (partial) NEC 48.69
  with
    pelvic exenteration 68.8
    transsacral sigmoidectomy 48.61
  abdominoendorectal (combined), NOS 48.50
    laparoscopic 48.51
    open 48.52
    other 48.59
  abdominoperineal, NOS 48.50
    laparoscopic 48.51
    open 48.52
    other 48.59
  pull-through NEC 48.49
    laparoscopic 48.42
    not otherwise specified 48.40
    open 48.43
    Duhamel type 48.65
  anterior 48.63
    with colostomy (synchronous) 48.62
  Duhamel 48.65
  endorectal 48.41
    combined abdominal, NOS 48.50
      laparoscopic 48.51
      open 48.52
      other 48.59
  posterior 48.64

Resection—*continued*
  pull-through NEC 48.49
    endorectal 48.41
    laparosopic 48.42
    not otherwise specified 48.40
    open 48.43
  STARR procedure 48.74
  submucosal (Soave) 48.41
    combined abdominal, NOS 48.50
      laparoscopic 48.51
      open 48.52
      other 48.59
  rib (transaxillary) 77.91
    as operative approach—*omit code*
    incidental to thoracic operation—*omit code*
  right ventricle (heart), for infundibular
    stenosis 35.34
  root (tooth) (apex) 23.73
    with root canal therapy 23.72
    residual or retained 23.11
  round ligament 69.19
  sclera 12.65
    with scleral buckling (*see also* Buckling,
      scleral) 14.49
    lamellar (for retinal reattachment) 14.49
      with implant 14.41
  scrotum 61.3
  soft tissue NEC 83.49
    hand 82.39
  sphincter of Oddi 51.89
  spinal cord (meninges) 03.4
  splanchnic 05.29
  splenic flexure (colon) 45.75
  sternum 77.81
  stomach (partial) (sleeve) (subtotal) NEC (*see
    also* Gastrectomy) 43.89
    with anastomosis NEC 43.89
      esophagogastric 43.5
      gastroduodenal 43.6
      gastrogastric 43.89
      gastrojejunal 43.7
    complete or total NEC 43.99
      with intestinal interposition 43.91
    fundus 43.89
    laparoscopic 43.82
    radical NEC 43.99
      with intestinal interposition 43.91
    wedge 43.42
      endoscopic 43.41
  submucous
    larynx 30.29
    nasal septum 21.5
    vocal cords 30.22
  synovial membrane (complete) (partial) (*see also*
    Synovectomy) 80.70
  tarsolevator 08.33
  tendon 83.42
    hand 82.33
  thoracic structures (block) (en bloc) (radical)
    (brachial plexus, bronchus, lobes of lung, ribs,
    and sympathetic nerves) 32.6
  thorax 34.4
  tongue 25.2
    wedge 25.1
  tooth root 23.73
    with root canal therapy 23.72
    apex (abscess) 23.73
      with root canal therapy 23.72
    residual or retained 23.11
  trachea 31.5

Resection—*continued*
  transurethral
    bladder NEC 57.49
    prostate 60.29
  transverse colon
    laparoscopic 17.34
    open and other 45.74
  turbinates—*see* Turbinectomy
  ureter (partial) 56.41
    total 56.42
  uterus—*see* Hysterectomy
  vein—*see* Phlebectomy
  ventricle (heart) 37.35
    infundibula 35.34
  vesical neck 57.59
    transurethral 57.49
  vocal cords (punch) 30.22
Respirator, volume-controlled (Bennett)
  (Byrd)—*see* Ventilation
Restoration
  cardioesophageal angle 44.66
    laparoscopic 44.67
  dental NEC 23.49
    by
      application of crown (artificial) 23.41
      insertion of bridge (fixed) 23.42
        removable 23.43
  extremity—*see* Reattachment, extremity
  eyebrow 08.70
    with graft 08.63
  eye socket 16.64
    with graft 16.63
  tooth NEC 23.2
    by
      crown (artificial) 23.41
      filling (amalgam) (plastic) (silicate) 23.2
      inlay 23.3
Restrictive
  gastric band, laparoscopic 44.95
Resurfacing hip 00.86
  acetabulum 00.87
    with femoral head 00.85
  femoral head 00.86
    with acetabulum 00.85
  partial NOS 00.85
    acetabulum 00.87
    femoral head 00.86
  total (acetabulum and femoral head) 00.85
Resuscitation
  artificial respiration 93.93
  cardiac 99.60
    cardioversion 99.62
      atrial 99.61
    defibrillation 99.62
    external massage 99.63
      open chest 37.91
    intracardiac injection 37.92
  cardiopulmonary 99.60
  endotracheal intubation 96.04
  manual 93.93
  mouth-to-mouth 93.93
  pulmonary 93.93
Resuture
  abdominal wall 54.61
  cardiac septum prosthesis 35.95
  chest wall 34.71
  heart valve prosthesis (poppet) 35.95
  wound (skin and subcutaneous tissue) (without
    graft) NEC 86.59
Retavase, infusion 99.10
Reteplase, infusion 99.10

Revision—*continued*

gastrostomy 44.69
  laparoscopic 44.68
hand replacement (prosthesis) 81.97
heart procedure NEC 35.95
hip replacement NOS 81.53
  acetabular and femoral components (total) 00.70
  acetabular component only 00.71
  acetabular liner and/or femoral head only 00.73
  femoral component only 00.72
  femoral head only and/or acetabular liner 00.73
  partial
    acetabular component only 00.71
    acetabular liner and/or femoral head only 00.73
    femoral component only 00.72
    femoral head only and/or acetabular liner 00.73
  total (acetabular and femoral components) 00.70
Holter (Spitz) valve 02.42
ileal conduit 56.52
ileostomy 46.41
intervertebral disc, artificial (partial) (total) NOS 84.69
  cervical 84.66
  lumbar, lumbosacral 84.68
  thoracic 84.67
jejunoileal bypass 46.93
jejunostomy 46.41
joint replacement 81.59
  acetabular and femoral components (total) 00.70
  acetabular component only 00.71
  acetabular liner and/or femoral head only 00.73
  ankle 81.59
  elbow 81.97
  femoral component only 00.72
  femoral head only and/or acetabular liner 00.73
  foot 81.59
  hand 81.97
  hip 81.53
    acetabular and femoral components (total) 00.70
    acetabular component only 00.71
    acetabular liner and/or femoral head only 00.73
    femoral component only 00.72
    femoral head only and/or acetabular liner 00.73
    partial
      acetabular component only 00.71
      acetabular liner and/or femoral head only 00.73
      femoral component only 00.72
      femoral head only and/or acetabular liner 00.73
    total (acetabular and femoral components) 00.70
  knee replacement NOS 81.55
    femoral component 00.82
    partial
      femoral component 00.82
      patellar component 00.83
      tibial component 00.81
      tibial insert 00.84
    patellar component 00.83
    tibial component 00.81
    tibial insert 00.84
    total (all components) 00.80
  lower extremity NEC 81.59
  toe 81.59
  upper extremity 81.97
  wrist 81.97

Revision—*continued*

knee replacement (prosthesis) NOS 81.55
  femoral component 00.82
  partial
    femoral component 00.82
    patellar component 00.83
    tibial component 00.81
    tibial insert 00.84
  patellar component 00.83
  tibial component 00.81
  tibial insert 00.84
  total (all components) 00.80
laryngostomy 31.63
lateral canthus 08.59
mallet finger 82.84
mastoid antrum 19.9
mastoidectomy 20.92
nephrostomy 55.89
neuroplasty 04.75
ocular implant 16.62
orbital implant 16.62
pocket
  cardiac device (defibrillator) (pacemaker)
    with initial insertion of cardiac device—*omit code*
    new site (cardiac device pocket) (skin) (subcutaneous) 37.79
  carotid sinus stimulation pulse generator 39.85
    with initial insertion of pulse generator—*omit code*
  intracardiac hemodynamic monitoring 37.79
  subcutaneous device pocket NEC
    with initial insertion of generator or device—*omit code*
    new site 86.09
  thalamic stimulator pulse generator
    with initial insertion of battery package—*omit code*
    new site (skin) (subcutaneous) 86.09
previous mastectomy site—*see* categories 85.0-85.99
proctostomy 48.79
prosthesis
  acetabular and femoral components (total) 00.70
  acetabular component only 00.71
  acetabular liner and/or femoral head only 00.73
  ankle 81.59
  breast 85.93
  elbow 81.97
  femoral component only 00.72
  femoral head only and/or acetabular liner 00.73
  foot 81.59
  hand 81.97
  heart valve (poppet) 35.95
  hip 81.53
    acetabular and femoral components (total) 00.70
    acetabular component only 00.71
    acetabular liner and/or femoral head only 00.73
    femoral component only 00.72
    femoral head only and/or acetabular liner 00.73
    partial
      acetabular component only 00.71
      acetabular liner and/or femoral head only 00.73
      femoral component only 00.72
      femoral head only and/or acetabular liner 00.73

Revision—*continued*
    total (acetabular and femoral components)
      00.70
    knee NOS 81.55
      femoral component 00.82
      partial
        femoral component 00.82
        patellar component 00.83
        tibial component 00.81
        tibial insert 00.84
      patellar component 00.83
      tibial component 00.81
      tibial insert 00.84
      total (all components) 00.80
    lower extremity NEC 81.59
    shoulder 81.97
    spine
      facet replacement device 84.85
      interspinous process device(s) 84.81
      pedicle-based dynamic stabilization device(s)
        84.83
    toe 81.59
    upper extremity 81.97
    wrist 81.97
ptosis overcorrection 08.37
pyelostomy 55.12
pyloroplasty 44.29
rhinoplasty 21.84
scar
    skin 86.84
      with excision 86.3
scleral fistulization 12.66
shoulder replacement (prosthesis) 81.97
shunt
    arteriovenous (cannula) (for dialysis) 39.42
    lumbar-subarachnoid NEC 03.97
    peritoneojugular 54.99
    peritoneovascular 54.99
    pleurothecal 03.97
    salpingothecal 03.97
    spinal (thecal) NEC 03.97
    subarachnoid-peritoneal 03.97
    subarachnoid-ureteral 03.97
    ventricular (cerebral) 02.42
    ventriculoperitoneal
      at peritoneal site 54.95
      at ventricular site 02.42
stapedectomy NEC 19.29
    with incus replacement (homograft) (prosthesis)
      19.21
stimulator
    electrode(s)
      carotid sinus 39.84
    pulse generator
      carotid sinus 39.85
stoma
    bile duct 51.79
    bladder (vesicostomy) 57.22
    bronchus 33.42
    common duct 51.72
    esophagus 42.89
    gallbladder 51.99
    hepatic duct 51.79
    intestine 46.40
      large 46.43
      small 46.41
    kidney 55.89
    larynx 31.63
    rectum 48.79
    stomach 44.69
      laparoscopic 44.68

Revision—*continued*
    thorax 34.79
    trachea 31.74
    ureter 56.62
    urethra 58.4
    tack operation 20.79
    toe replacement (prosthesis) 81.59
    tracheostomy 31.74
    tunnel
      pulse generator lead wire 86.99
        with initial procedure—*omit code*
    tympanoplasty 19.6
    uretero-ileostomy, cutaneous 56.52
    ureterostomy (cutaneous) (stoma) NEC 56.62
      ileal 56.52
    urethrostomy 58.49
    urinary conduit 56.52
    vascular procedure (previous) NEC 39.49
    ventricular shunt (cerebral) 02.42
    vesicostomy stoma 57.22
    wrist replacement (prosthesis) 81.97
Rhinectomy 21.4
Rhinocheiloplasty 27.59
    cleft lip 27.54
Rhinomanometry 89.12
Rhinoplasty (external) (internal) NEC 21.87
    augmentation (with graft) (with synthetic
      implant) 21.85
    limited 21.86
    revision 21.84
    tip 21.86
    twisted nose 21.84
Rhinorrhaphy (external) (internal) 21.81
    for epistaxis 21.09
Rhinoscopy 21.21
Rhinoseptoplasty 21.84
Rhinotomy 21.1
Rhizotomy (radio frequency) (spinal) 03.1
    acoustic 04.01
    trigeminal 04.02
Rhytidectomy (facial) 86.82
    eyelid
      lower 08.86
      upper 08.87
Rhytidoplasty (facial) 86.82
Ripstein operation (repair of prolapsed rectum)
    48.75
Robotic assisted surgery
    endoscopic 17.44
    laparosopic 17.42
    open 17.41
    other and unspecified 17.49
    percutaneous 17.43
    thoracoscopic 17.45
Rodney Smith operation (radical subtotal
    pancreatectomy) 52.53
Roentgenography —*see also* Radiography
    cardiac, negative contrast 88.58
Rolling of conjunctiva 10.33
Root
    canal (tooth) (therapy) 23.70
      with
        apicoectomy 23.72
        irrigation 23.71
    resection (tooth) (apex) 23.73
      with root canal therapy 23.72
      residual or retained 23.11
Rotation of fetal head
    forceps (instrumental) (Kielland) (Scanzoni)
      (key-in-lock) 72.4
    manual 73.51

Routine
  chest x-ray 87.44
  psychiatric visit 94.12
Roux-en-Y operation
  bile duct 51.36
  cholecystojejunostomy 51.32
  esophagus (intrathoracic) 42.54
  gastroenterostomy 44.39
    laparoscopic 44.38
  gastrojejunostomy 44.39
    laparoscopic 44.38
  pancreaticojejunostomy 52.96
Roux-Goldthwait operation (repair of recurrent
    patellar dislocation) 81.44
Roux-Herzen-Judine operation (jejunal loop
    interposition) 42.63
Rubin test (insufflation of fallopian tube) 66.8
Ruiz-Mora operation (proximal phalangectomy
    for hammer toe) 77.99
Rupture
  esophageal web 42.01
  joint adhesions, manual 93.26
  membranes, artificial 73.09
    for surgical induction of labor 73.01
  ovarian cyst, manual 65.93
Russe operation (bone graft of scaphoid) 78.04

S

Schede operation (thoracoplasty) 33.34
Scheie operation
  cautery of sclera 12.62
  sclerostomy 12.62
Schlatter operation (total gastrectomy) 43.99
Schroeder operation (endocervical excision)
    67.39
Schuchardt operation (nonobstetrical
    episiotomy) 71.09
Schwartze operation (simple mastoidectomy)
    20.41
Scintiphotography —*see* Scan, radioisotope
Scintiscan —*see* Scan, radioisotope
Sclerectomy (punch) (scissors) 12.65
  for retinal reattachment 14.49
  Holth's 12.65
  trephine 12.61
  with implant 14.41
Scleroplasty 12.89
Sclerostomy (Scheie's) 12.62
Sclerotherapy
  esophageal varices (endoscopic) 42.33
  hemorrhoids 49.42
  pleura 34.92
    treatment of malignancy (cytotoxic agent)
      34.92 *[99.25]*
    with tetracycline 34.92 *[99.21]*
  varicose vein 39.92
  vein NEC 39.92
Sclerotomy (exploratory) 12.89
  anterior 12.89
    with
      iridectomy 12.65
      removal of vitreous 14.71
  posterior 12.89
    with
      iridectomy 12.65
      removal of vitreous 14.72
Scott operation
  intestinal bypass for obesity 45.93
  jejunocolostomy (bypass) 45.93
Scraping
  corneal epithelium 11.41
    for smear or culture 11.21
  trachoma follicles 10.33
Scrotectomy (partial) 61.3
Scrotoplasty 61.49
Scrotorrhaphy 61.41
Scrototomy 61.0
Scrub, posterior nasal (adhesions) 21.91
Sculpturing, heart valve —*see* Valvuloplasty,
    heart
Section —*see also* Division *and* Incision
  cesarean—*see* Cesarean section
  ganglion, sympathetic 05.0
  hypophyseal stalk (*see also* Hypophysectomy,
    partial) 07.63
  ligamentum flavum (spine)—*omit code*
  nerve (cranial) (peripheral) NEC 04.03
    acoustic 04.01
    spinal root (posterior) 03.1
    sympathetic 05.0
    trigeminal tract 04.02
  Saemisch (corneal) 11.1
  spinal ligament 80.49
    arcuate—*omit code*
    flavum—*omit code*
  tooth (impacted) 23.19
Seddon-Brooks operation (transfer of pectoralis
    major tendon) 83.75
Semb operation (apicolysis of lung) 33.39

Senning operation (correction of transposition of
    great vessels) 35.91
Separation
  twins (attached) (conjoined) (Siamese) 84.93
    asymmetrical (unequal) 84.93
    symmetrical (equal) 84.92
Septectomy
  atrial (closed) 35.41
    open 35.42
    transvenous method (balloon) 35.41
  submucous (nasal) 21.5
Septoplasty NEC 21.88
  with submucous resection of septum 21.5
Septorhinoplasty 21.84
Septostomy (atrial) (balloon) 35.41
Septotomy, nasal 21.1
Sequestrectomy
  bone 77.00
    carpals, metacarpals 77.04
    clavicle 77.01
    facial 76.01
    femur 77.05
    fibula 77.07
    humerus 77.02
    nose 21.32
    patella 77.06
    pelvic 77.09
    phalanges (foot) (hand) 77.09
    radius 77.03
    scapula 77.01
    skull 01.25
    specified site NEC 77.09
    tarsals, metatarsals 77.08
    thorax (ribs) (sternum) 77.01
    tibia 77.07
    ulna 77.03
    vertebrae 77.09
  nose 21.32
  skull 01.25
Sesamoidectomy 77.98
Setback, ear 18.5
Sever operation (division of soft tissue of arm)
    83.19
Severing of blepharorrhaphy 08.02
Sewell operation (heart) 36.2
Sharrard operation (iliopsoas muscle transfer)
    83.77
Shaving
  bone (*see also* Excision, lesion, bone) 77.60
  cornea (epithelium) 11.41
    for smear or culture 11.21
  patella 77.66
Shelf operation (hip arthroplasty) 81.40
Shirodkar operation (encirclement suture,
    cervix) 67.59
Shock therapy
  chemical 94.24
  electroconvulsive 94.27
  electrotonic 94.27
  insulin 94.24
  subconvulsive 94.26
Shortening
  bone (fusion) 78.20
    femur 78.25
    specified site NEC (*see* category 78.2)
    tibia 78.27
    ulna 78.23
  endopelvic fascia 69.22
  extraocular muscle NEC 15.22
    multiple (two or more muscles) 15.4
  eyelid margin 08.71
  eye muscle NEC 15.22

Shortening—*continued*
multiple (two or more muscles) (with
lengthening) 15.4
finger (macrodactyly repair) 82.83
heel cord 83.85
levator palpebrae muscle 08.33
ligament—*see also* Arthroplasty
round 69.22
uterosacral 69.22
muscle 83.85
extraocular 15.22
multiple (two or more muscles) 15.4
hand 82.55
sclera (for repair of retinal detachment) 14.59
by scleral buckling (*see also* Buckling, scleral)
14.49
tendon 83.85
hand 82.55
ureter (with reimplantation) 56.41
Shunt —*see also* Anastomosis *and* Bypass,
vascular
abdominovenous 54.94
aorta-coronary sinus 36.39
aorta (descending) pulmonary (artery) 39.0
aortocarotid 39.22
aortoceliac 39.26
aortofemoral 39.25
aortoiliac 39.25
aortoiliofemoral 39.25
aortomesenteric 39.26
aorto-myocardial (graft) 36.2
aortorenal 39.24
aortosubclavian 39.22
apicoaortic 35.93
aqueous drainage 12.67
arteriovenous NEC 39.29
for renal dialysis (by)
anastomosis 39.27
external cannula 39.93
ascending aorta to pulmonary artery (Waterston)
39.0
axillary-femoral 39.29
carotid-carotid 39.22
carotid-subclavian 39.22
caval-mesenteric 39.1
corpora cavernosa-corpus spongiosum 64.98
corpora-saphenous 64.98
descending aorta to pulmonary artery
(Potts-Smith) 39.0
endolymphatic (subarachnoid) 20.71
endolymph-perilymph 20.71
extracranial-intracranial (EC-IC) 39.28
femoroperoneal 39.29
femoropopliteal 39.29
iliofemoral 39.25
ilioiliac 39.25
intestinal
large-to-large 45.94
small-to-large 45.93
small-to-small 45.91
left subclavian to descending aorta
(Blalock-Park) 39.0
left-to-right (systemic-pulmonary artery) 39.0
left ventricle (heart) (apex) and aorta 35.93
lienorenal 39.1
lumbar-subarachnoid (with valve) NEC 03.79
mesocaval 39.1
peritoneal-jugular 54.94
peritoneo-vascular 54.94
peritoneovenous 54.94
pleuroperitoneal 34.05
pleurothecal (with valve) 03.79

Shunt—*continued*
portacaval (double) 39.1
portal-systemic 39.1
portal vein to vena cava 39.1
pulmonary-innominate 39.0
pulmonary vein to atrium 35.82
renoportal 39.1
right atrium and pulmonary artery 35.94
right ventricle and pulmonary artery (distal) 35.92
in repair of
pulmonary artery atresia 35.92
transposition of great vessels 35.92
truncus arteriosus 35.83
salpingothecal (with valve) 03.79
semicircular-subarachnoid 20.71
spinal (thecal) (with valve) NEC 03.79
subarachnoid-peritoneal 03.71
subarachnoid-ureteral 03.72
splenorenal (venous) 39.1
arterial 39.26
subarachnoid-peritoneal (with valve) 03.71
subarachnoid-ureteral (with valve) 03.72
subclavian-pulmonary 39.0
subdural-peritoneal (with valve) 02.34
superior mesenteric-caval 39.1
systemic-pulmonary artery 39.0
transjugular intrahepatic portosystemic (TIPS) 39.1
vena cava to pulmonary artery (Green) 39.21
ventricular (cerebral) (with valve) 02.22
to
abdominal cavity or organ 02.34
bone marrow 02.39
cervical subarachnoid space 02.22
circulatory system 02.32
cisterna magna 02.22
extracranial site NEC 02.39
gallbladder 02.34
head or neck structure 02.31
intracerebral site NEC 02.22
lumbar site 02.39
mastoid 02.31
nasopharynx 02.31
peritoneal 02.34
thoracic cavity 02.33
ureter 02.35
urinary system 02.35
venous system 02.32
ventriculoatrial (with valve) 02.32
ventriculocaval (with valve) 02.32
ventriculocisternal (with valve) 02.22
ventriculolumbar (with valve) 02.39
ventriculomastoid (with valve) 02.31
ventriculonasopharyngeal 02.31
ventriculopleural (with valve) 02.33
Sialoadenectomy (parotid) (sublingual)
(submaxillary) 26.30
complete 26.32
partial 26.31
radical 26.32
Sialoadenolithotomy 26.0
Sialoadenotomy 26.0
Sialodochoplasty NEC 26.49
Sialogram 87.09
Sialolithotomy 26.0
Sieve, vena cava 38.7
Sigmoid bladder 57.87 *[45.52]*
Sigmoidectomy
laparoscopic 17.36
open and other 45.76
Sigmoidomyotomy 46.91
Sigmoidopexy (Moschowitz) 46.63

Sigmoidoproctectomy (*see also* Resection, rectum) 48.69
Sigmoidoproctostomy 45.94
Sigmoidorectostomy 45.94
Sigmoidorrhaphy 46.75
Sigmoidoscopy (rigid) 48.23
  with biopsy 45.25
  flexible 45.24
  through stoma (artificial) 45.22
  transabdominal 45.21
Sigmoidosigmoidostomy 45.94
  proximal to distal segment
    laparoscopic 17.36
    open and other 45.76
Sigmoidostomy (*see also* Colostomy) 46.10
Sigmoidotomy 45.03
Sign language 93.75
Silver operation (bunionectomy) 77.59
Sinogram
  abdominal wall 88.03
  chest wall 87.38
  retroperitoneum 88.14
Sinusectomy (nasal) (complete) (partial) (with turbinectomy) 22.60
  antrum 22.62
    with Caldwell-Luc approach 22.61
  ethmoid 22.63
  frontal 22.42
  maxillary 22.62
    with Caldwell-Luc approach 22.61
  sphenoid 22.64
Sinusotomy (nasal) 22.50
  antrum (intranasal) 22.2
    with external approach (Caldwell-Luc) 22.39
      radical (with removal of membrane lining) 22.31
  ethmoid 22.51
  frontal 22.41
  maxillary (intranasal) 22.2
    external approach (Caldwell-Luc) 22.39
      radical (with removal of membrane lining) 22.31
  multiple 22.53
  perinasal 22.50
  sphenoid 22.52
Sistrunk operation (excision of thyroglossal cyst) 06.7
Size reduction
  abdominal wall (adipose) (pendulous) 86.83
  arms (adipose) (batwing) 86.83
  breast (bilateral) 85.32
    unilateral 85.31
  buttocks (adipose) 86.83
  skin 86.83
  subcutaneous tissue 86.83
  thighs (adipose) 86.83
Skeletal series (x-ray) 88.31
SKyphoplasty 81.66
Sling —*see also* Operation, sling
  fascial (fascia lata)
    for facial weakness (trigeminal nerve paralysis) 86.81
    mouth 86.81
    orbicularis (mouth) 86.81
    tongue 25.59
  levator muscle (urethrocystopexy) 59.71
  pubococcygeal 59.71
  rectum (puborectalis) 48.76
  tongue (fascial) 25.59

Slitting
  canaliculus for
    passage of tube 09.42
    removal of streptothrix 09.42
  lens 13.2
  prepuce (dorsal) (lateral) 64.91
Slocum operation (pes anserinus transfer) 81.47
Sluder operation (tonsillectomy) 28.2
Small bowel series (x-ray) 87.63
Smith operation (open osteotomy of mandible) 76.62
Smith-Peterson operation (radiocarpal arthrodesis) 81.25
Smithwick operation (sympathectomy) 05.29
Snaring, polyp, colon (endoscopic) 45.42
Snip, punctum (with dilation) 09.51
Soave operation (endorectal pull-through) 48.41
Somatotherapy, psychiatric NEC 94.29
Sonneberg operation (inferior maxillary neurectomy) 04.07
Sorondo-Ferré operation (hindquarter amputation) 84.19
Soutter operation (iliac crest fasciotomy) 83.14
Spaulding-Richardson operation (uterine suspension) 69.22
Spectrophotometry NEC 89.39
  blood 89.39
  placenta 89.29
  urine 89.29
Spectroscopy
  intravascular 38.23
  near infrared (NIR) 38.23
Speech therapy NEC 93.75
Spermatocelectomy 63.2
Spermatocystectomy 60.73
Spermatocystotomy 60.72
Sphenoidectomy 22.64
Sphenoidotomy 22.52
Sphincterectomy, anal 49.6
Sphincteroplasty
  anal 49.79
    obstetrical laceration (current) 75.62
      old 49.79
  bladder neck 57.85
  pancreas 51.83
  sphincter of Oddi 51.83
Sphincterorrhaphy, anal 49.71
  obstetrical laceration (current) 75.62
    old 49.79
Sphincterotomy
  anal (external) (internal) 49.59
    left lateral 49.51
    posterior 49.52
  bladder (neck) (transurethral) 57.91
  choledochal 51.82
    endoscopic 51.85
  iris 12.12
  pancreatic 51.82
    endoscopic 51.85
  sphincter of Oddi 51.82
    endoscopic 51.85
  transduodenal ampullary 51.82
    endoscopic 51.85
Spinal anesthesia —*omit code*
Spinelli operation (correction of inverted uterus) 75.93
Spineoplasty 81.66
Spirometry (incentive) (respiratory) 89.37
Spivack operation (permanent gastrostomy) 43.19
Splanchnicectomy 05.29
Splanchnicotomy 05.0

Stripping—*continued*
  subdural membrane (cerebral) 01.51
    spinal 03.4
  varicose veins (lower limb) 38.59
    upper limb 38.53
  vocal cords 30.09
Stromeyer-Little operation (hepatotomy) 50.0
Strong operation (unbridling of celiac artery axis) 39.91
Stryker frame 93.59
Study
  bone mineral density 88.98
  bundle of His 37.29
  color vision 95.06
  conduction, nerve (median) 89.15
  dark adaptation, eye 95.07
  electrophysiologic stimulation and recording, cardiac
    as part of intraoperative testing —*omit code*
    catheter based invasive electrophysiologic testing 37.26
    device interrogation only without arrhythmia induction (bedside check) 89.45-89.49
    noninvasive programmed electrical stimulation (NIPS) 37.20
  function—*see also* Function, study
    radioisotope—*see* Scan, radioisotope
  lacrimal flow (radiographic) 87.05
  ocular motility 95.15
  pulmonary
    airway flow measurement, endoscopic 33.72
    function —*see* categories 89.37-89.38
  radiographic—*see* Radiography
  radio-iodinated triolein 92.04
  renal clearance 92.03
  spirometer 89.37
  tracer—*see also* Scan, radioisotope
    eye (P^{32}) 95.16
  ultrasonic—*see* Ultrasonography
  visual field 95.05
  xenon flow NEC 92.19
    cardiovascular 92.05
    pulmonary 92.15
Sturmdorf operation (conization of cervix) 67.2
Submucous resection
  larynx 30.29
  nasal septum 21.5
Summerskill operation
  (dacryocystorhinostomy by intubation) 09.81
Surgery
  computer assisted (CAS) 00.39
    with robotics —*see* category 17.4
    CAS with CT/CTA 00.31
    CAS with fluoroscopy 00.33
    CAS with MR/MRA 00.32
    CAS with multiple datasets 00.35
      imageless 00.34
      other CAS 00.39
  IGS—*see* Surgery, computer assisted
  image guided—*see* Surgery, computer assisted
  navigation (CT-free, IGN image guided, imageless)—*see* Surgery, computer assisted
  robotic assisted —*see* category 17.4
Surmay operation (jejunostomy) 46.39
Suspension
  balanced, for traction 93.45
  bladder NEC 57.89
  diverticulum, pharynx 29.59
  kidney 55.7
  Olshausen (uterus) 69.22
  ovary 65.79

Suspension—*continued*
  paraurethral (Pereyra) 59.6
  periurethral 59.6
  urethra (retropubic) (sling) 59.5
  urethrovesical
    Goebel-Frangenheim-Stoeckel 59.4
    gracilis muscle transplant 59.71
    levator muscle sling 59.71
    Marshall-Marchetti (Krantz) 59.5
    Millin-Read 59.4
    suprapubic 59.4
  uterus (abdominal or vaginal approach) 69.22
  vagina 70.77
    with graft or prosthesis 70.78
Suture (laceration)
  abdominal wall 54.63
    secondary 54.61
  adenoid fossa 28.7
  adrenal (gland) 07.44
  aneurysm (cerebral) (peripheral) 39.52
  anus 49.71
    obstetric laceration (current) 75.62
      old 49.79
  aorta 39.31
  aponeurosis (*see also* Suture, tendon) 83.64
  arteriovenous fistula 39.53
  artery 39.31
    percutaneous puncture closure—*omit code*
  bile duct 51.79
  bladder 57.81
    obstetric laceration (current) 75.61
  blood vessel NEC 39.30
    artery 39.31
    percutaneous puncture closure—*omit code*
    vein 39.32
  breast (skin) 85.81
  bronchus 33.41
  bursa 83.99
    hand 82.99
  canaliculus 09.73
  cecum 46.75
  cerebral meninges 02.11
  cervix (traumatic laceration) 67.61
    internal os, encirclement 67.59
    obstetric laceration (current) 75.51
      old 67.69
  chest wall 34.71
  cleft palate 27.62
  clitoris 71.4
  colon 46.75
  common duct 51.71
  conjunctiva 10.6
  cornea 11.51
    with conjunctival flap 11.53
  corneoscleral 11.51
    with conjunctival flap 11.53
  diaphragm 34.82
  duodenum 46.71
    ulcer (bleeding) (perforated) 44.42
      endoscopic 44.43
  dura mater (cerebral) 02.11
    spinal 03.59
  ear, external 18.4
  enterocele 70.92
    with graft or prosthesis 70.93
  entropion 08.42
  epididymis (and)
    spermatic cord 63.51
    vas deferens 63.81
  episiotomy—*see* Episiotomy
  esophagus 42.82

Suture—*continued*
  stomach 44.61
    ulcer (bleeding) (perforated) 44.41
      endoscopic 44.43
  subcutaneous tissue (without skin graft) 86.59
    with graft—*see* Graft, skin
  tendon (direct) (immediate) (primary) 83.64
    delayed (secondary) 83.62
      hand NEC 82.43
      flexors 82.42
    hand NEC 82.45
      delayed (secondary) 82.43
      flexors 82.44
    delayed (secondary) 82.42
    ocular 15.7
    rotator cuff 83.63
    sheath 83.61
      hand 82.41
    supraspinatus (rotator cuff repair) 83.63
    to skeletal attachment 83.88
      hand 82.85
  Tenon's capsule 15.7
  testis 62.61
  thymus 07.93
  thyroid gland 06.93
  tongue 25.51
  tonsillar fossa 28.7
  trachea 31.71
  tunics vaginalis 61.41
  ulcer (bleeding) (perforated) (peptic) 44.40
    duodenum 44.42
      endoscopic 44.43
    gastric 44.41
      endoscopic 44.43
    intestine 46.79
    skin 86.59
    stomach 44.41
      endoscopic 44.43
  ureter 56.82
  urethra 58.41
    obstetric laceration (current) 75.61
  uterosacral ligament 69.29
  uterus 69.41
    obstetric laceration (current) 75.50
      old 69.49
  uvula 27.73
  vagina 70.71
    obstetric laceration (current) 75.69
      old 70.79
  vas deferens 63.81
  vein 39.32
  vulva 71.71
    obstetric laceration (current) 75.69
      old 71.79
Suture-ligation —*see also* Ligation
  blood vessel—*see* Ligation, blood vessel
Sweep, anterior iris 12.97
Swenson operation
  bladder reconstruction 57.87
  proctectomy 48.49
Swinney operation (urethral reconstruction)
  58.46
Switch, switching
  coronary arteries 35.84
  great arteries, total 35.84
Syme operation
  ankle amputation through malleoli of tibia and
    fibula 84.14
  urethrotomy, external 58.0

Sympathectomy NEC 05.29
  cervical 05.22
  cervicothoracic 05.22
  lumbar 05.23
  periarterial 05.25
  presacral 05.24
  renal 05.29
  thoracolumbar 05.23
  tympanum 20.91
Sympatheticotripsy 05.0
Symphysiotomy 77.39
  assisting delivery (obstetrical) 73.94
  kidney (horseshoe) 55.85
Symphysis, pleural 34.6
Synchondrotomy (*see also* Division, cartilage)
  80.40
Syndactylization 86.89
Syndesmotomy (*see also* Division, ligament)
  80.40
Synechiotomy
  endometrium 68.21
  iris (posterior) 12.33
    anterior 12.32
Synovectomy (joint) (complete) (partial) 80.70
  ankle 80.77
  elbow 80.72
  foot and toe 80.78
  hand and finger 80.74
  hip 80.75
  knee 80.76
  shoulder 80.71
  specified site NEC 80.79
  spine 80.79
  tendon sheath 83.42
    hand 82.33
  wrist 80.73
Syringing
  lacrimal duct or sac 09.43
  nasolacrimal duct 09.43
    with
      dilation 09.43
      insertion of tube or stent 09.44

T

Therapy—*continued*
educational (bed-bound children) (handicapped)
    93.82
electroconvulsive (ECT) 94.27
electroshock (EST) 94.27
    subconvulsive 94.26
electrotonic (ETT) 94.27
encounter group 94.44
extinction 94.33
family 94.42
fog (inhalation) 93.94
gamma ray 92.23
group NEC 94.44
    for psychosexual dysfunction 94.41
hearing NEC 95.49
heat NEC 93.35
    for cancer treatment 99.85
helium 93.98
hot pack(s) 93.35
hyperbaric oxygen 93.95
    wound 93.59
hyperthermia NEC 93.35
    for cancer treatment 99.85
individual, psychiatric NEC 94.39
    for psychosexual dysfunction 94.34
industrial 93.89
infrared irradiation 93.35
inhalation NEC 93.96
    nitric oxide 00.12
insulin shock 94.24
intermittent positive pressure breathing (IPPB)
    93.91
IPPB (intermittent positive pressure breathing)
    93.91
leech 99.99
lithium 94.22
LITT (laser interstitial thermal therapy) under
    guidance
    lesion
        brain 17.61
        breast 17.69
        head and neck 17.62
        liver 17.63
        lung 17.69
        prostate 17.69
        thyroid 17.62
maggot 86.28
manipulative, osteopathic (*see also* Manipulation,
    osteopathic) 93.67
manual arts 93.81
methadone 94.25
mist (inhalation) 93.94
music 93.84
nebulizer 93.94
neuroleptic 94.23
nitric oxide 00.12
occupational 93.83
oxygen 93.96
    aqueous 00.49
    catalytic 93.96
    hyperbaric 93.95
        wound 93.59
    SuperSaturated 00.49
    wound (hyperbaric) 93.59
paraffin bath 93.35
physical NEC 93.39
    combined (without mention of components)
        93.38
    diagnostic NEC 93.09
play 93.81
    psychotherapeutic 94.36

Therapy—*continued*
positive and expiratory pressure—*see* category 96.7
psychiatric NEC 94.39
    drug NEC 94.25
    lithium 94.22
radiation 92.29
    contact (150 KVP or less) 92.21
    deep (200-300 KVP) 92.22
    electron, intra-operative 92.41
    high voltage (200-300 KVP) 92.22
    low voltage (150 KVP or less) 92.21
    megavoltage 92.24
    orthovoltage 92.22
    particle source NEC 92.26
    photon 92.24
    radioisotope (teleradiotherapy) 92.23
    retinal lesion 14.26
    superficial (150 KVP or less) 92.21
    supervoltage 92.24
radioisotope, radioisotopic NEC 92.29
    implantation or insertion 92.27
    injection or instillation 92.28
    teleradiotherapy 92.23
radium (radon) 92.23
recreational 93.81
rehabilitation NEC 93.89
respiratory NEC 93.99
    bi-level positive airway pressure [BiPAP] 93.90
        delivered by
            endotracheal tube—*see* category 96.7
            tracheostomy—*see* category 96.7
    continuous positive airway pressure [CPAP]
        93.90
        delivered by
            endotracheal tube—*see* category 96.7
            tracheostomy—*see* category 96.7
    endotracheal respiratory assistance—*see*
        category 96.7
    intermittent positive pressure breathing [IPPB]
        93.91
    negative pressure (continuous) [CNP] 93.99
    nitric oxide 00.12
    non-invasive positive pressure (NIPPV) 93.90
    other continuous invasive (unspecified
        duration) 96.70
        for less than 96 consecutive hours 96.71
        for 96 consecutive hours or more 96.72
    positive and expiratory pressure [PEEP]
        invasive—*see* category 96.7
        noninvasive 93.90
root canal 23.70
    with
        apicoectomy 23.72
        irrigation 23.71
shock
    chemical 94.24
    electric 94.27
        subconvulsive 94.26
    insulin 94.24
speech 93.75
    for correction of defect 93.74
SuperOxygenation (SSO$_2$) 00.49
SuperSaturated oxygen 00.49
ultrasound
    heat therapy 93.35
    hyperthermia for cancer treatment 99.85
    physical therapy 93.35
    therapeutic—*see* Ultrasound
    ultraviolet light 99.82
Thermocautery —*see* Cauterization

TRAM (transverse rectus abdominis musculocutaneous) flap of breast
  free 85.73
  pedicled 85.72
Transactional analysis
  group 94.44
  individual 94.39
Transection —*see also* Division
  artery (with ligation) (*see also* Division, artery) 38.80
    renal, aberrant (with reimplantation) 39.55
  bone (*see also* Osteotomy) 77.30
  fallopian tube (bilateral) (remaining) (solitary) 66.39
    by endoscopy 66.22
    unilateral 66.92
  isthmus, thyroid 06.91
  muscle 83.19
    eye 15.13
      multiple (two or more muscles) 15.3
    hand 82.19
  nerve (cranial) (peripheral) NEC 04.03
    acoustic 04.01
    root (spinal) 03.1
    sympathetic 05.0
    tracts in spinal cord 03.29
    trigeminal 04.02
    vagus (transabdominal) (*see also* Vagotomy) 44.00
  pylorus (with wedge resection) 43.3
  renal vessel, aberrant (with reimplantation) 39.55
  spinal
    cord tracts 03.29
    nerve root 03.1
  tendon 83.13
    hand 82.11
  uvula 27.71
  vas deferens 63.71
  vein (with ligation) (*see also* Division, vein) 38.80
    renal, aberrant (with reimplantation) 39.55
    varicose (lower limb) 38.59
Transfer, transference
  bone shaft, fibula into tibia 78.47
  digital (to replace absent thumb) 82.69
  finger (to thumb) (same hand) 82.61
    to
      finger, except thumb 82.81
      opposite hand (with amputation) 82.69 *[84.01]*
    toe (to thumb) (with amputation) 82.69 *[84.11]*
    to finger, except thumb 82.81 *[84.11]*
  fat pad NEC 86.89
  with skin graft—*see* Graft, skin, full-thickness
  finger (to replace absent thumb) (same hand) 82.61
    to
      finger, except thumb 82.81
      opposite hand (with amputation) 82.69 *[84.01]*
  muscle origin 83.77
    hand 82.58
  nerve (cranial) (peripheral) (radial anterior) (ulnar) 04.6
  pedicle graft 86.74
  pes anserinus (tendon) (repair of knee) 81.47
  tarsoconjunctival flap, from opposing lid 08.64
  tendon 83.75
    hand 82.56
    pes anserinus (repair of knee) 81.47
  toe-to-thumb (free) (pedicle) (with amputation) 82.69 *[84.11]*

Transfixion —*see also* Fixation
  iris (bombe) 12.11
Transfusion (of) 99.03
  antihemophilic factor 99.06
  antivenin 99.16
  autologous blood
    collected prior to surgery 99.02
    intraoperative 99.00
    perioperative 99.00
    postoperative 99.00
    previously collected 99.02
    salvage 99.00
  blood (whole) NOS 99.03
    expander 99.08
    surrogate 99.09
  bone marrow 41.00
    allogeneic 41.03
      with purging 41.02
    allograft 41.03
      with purging 41.02
    autograft 41.01
      with purging 41.09
    autologous 41.01
      with purging 41.09
  coagulation factors 99.06
  Dextran 99.08
  exchange 99.01
    intraperitoneal 75.2
    in utero (with hysterotomy) 75.2
  exsanguination 99.01
  gamma globulin 99.14
  granulocytes 99.09
  hemodilution 99.03
  intrauterine 75.2
  packed cells 99.04
  plasma 99.07
  platelets 99.05
  replacement, total 99.01
  serum NEC 99.07
  substitution 99.01
  thrombocytes 99.05
Transillumination
  nasal sinuses 89.35
  skull (newborn) 89.16
Translumbar aortogram 88.42
Transplant, transplantation
  Note: To report donor source:
    cadaver 00.93
    live non-related donor 00.92
    live related donor 00.91
    live unrelated donor 00.92
  artery 39.59
    renal, aberrant 39.55
  autotransplant—*see* Reimplantation
  blood vessel 39.59
    renal, aberrant 39.55
  bone (*see also* Graft, bone) 78.00
    marrow 41.00
      allogeneic 41.03
        with purging 41.02
      allograft 41.03
        with purging 41.02
      autograft 41.01
        with purging 41.09
      autologous 41.01
        with purging 41.09
      stem cell
        allogeneic (hematopoietic) 41.05
          with purging 41.08
        autologous (hematopoietic) 41.04
          with purging 41.07

U

V

W

X

Y

Z

SUMMARY OF ADDITIONS, DELETIONS AND REVISIONS TO VOLUME 3 IN 2012 & 2013

00.4 Adjunct vascular system procedures
Revise code also note; add code also note

00.49 SuperSaturated oxygen therapy
Add code also note

00.55 Insertion of drug-eluting stent(s) of other peripheral vessel(s)
Revise code also note, add code also note

00.56 Insertion or replacement of implantable pressure sensor with lead for intracardiac or great vessel hemodynamic monitoring
Revise code title, add note, revise code also note, add exclusion term

00.57 Implantation or replacement of subcutaneous device for intracardiac or great vessel hemodynamic monitoring
Revise inclusion term, revise code also note

00.60 Insertion of drug-eluting stent(s) of superficial femoral artery
Revise code also note, add code also note

00.61 Percutaneous angioplasty of extracranial vessel(s)
Revise code title, delete inclusion term, add/revise code also note, add/revise exclusion terms

00.62 Percutaneous angioplasty of intracranial vessel(s)
Revise code title, add inclusion terms, add code also note, revise/add exclusion terms

00.63 Percutaneous insertion of carotid artery stent(s)
Revise/add code also notes, revise/add exclusion terms

00.64 Percutaneous insertion of other extracranial artery stent(s)
Revise code title, delete inclusion term, revise/add code also notes, revise/add exclusion terms

00.65 Percutaneous insertion of intracranial vascular stent(s)
Add inclusion term, revise/add code also notes, revise/add exclusion terms

00.66 Percutaneous transluminal coronary angioplasty [PTCA]
Revise code title, delete inclusion term, add code also note

00.77 Hip bearing surface, ceramic-on-polyethylene
Add inclusion term

00.94 Intra-operative neurophysiologic monitoring
Add inclusion terms

00.95 Injection or infusion of glucarpidase
New code fiscal year 2013

02.2 Ventriculostomy
New subcategory, delete inclusion terms

02.21 Insertion or replacement of external ventricular drain [EVD]
New code

02.22 Intracranial ventricular shunt or anastomosis
New code

02.39 Ventricular shunt to extracranial site NEC
Revise code title, delete inclusion term

02.42 Replacement of ventricular shunt
Delete inclusion term

12.67 Insertion of aqueous drainage device
New code

13.65 Excision of secondary membrane [after cataract]
Revise code title, add inclusion term

17.53 Percutaneous atherectomy of extracranial vessel(s)
New code

17.54 Percutaneous atherectomy of intracranial vessel(s)
New code

17.55 Transluminal coronary atherectomy
New code

17.56 Atherectomy of other non-coronary vessel(s)
New code

17.8 Other adjunct procedures
New subcategory

17.81 Insertion of antimicrobial envelope
New code

33.24 Closed [endoscopic] biopsy of bronchus
Add inclusion term, delete exclusion term

35 Operations on valves and septa of heart
Revise code also note

35.0 Closed heart valvotomy or transcatheter replacement of heart valve
Revise subcategory title

35.05 Endovascular replacement of aortic valve
New code

35.06 Transapical replacement of aortic valve
New code

35.07 Endovascular replacement of pulmonary valve
New code

35.08 Transapical replacement of pulmonary valve
New code

35.09 Endovascular replacement of unspecified heart valve
New code

35.2 **Open and other replacement of heart valve**
Revise subcategory title, , add exclusion terms

35.20 **Open and other replacement of unspecified heart valve**
Revise code title, delete/add inclusion terms, add exclusion term

35.21 **Open and other replacement of aortic valve with tissue graft**
Revise code title, delete/add inclusion terms, add exclusion terms

35.22 **Open and other replacement of aortic valve**
Revise code title, delete/add inclusion terms, add exclusion terms

35.23 **Open and other replacement of mitral valve with tissue graft**
Revise code title, delete/add inclusion terms

35.24 **Open and other replacement of mitral valve**
Revise code title, delete/add inclusion terms

35.25 **Open and other replacement of pulmonary valve with tissue graft**
Revise code title, delete/add inclusion terms, add exclusion terms

35.26 **Open and other replacement of pulmonary valve**
Revise code title, delete/add inclusion terms, add exclusion terms

35.27 **Open and other replacement of tricuspid valve with tissue graft**
Revise code title, delete/add inclusion terms

35.28 **Open and other replacement of tricuspid valve**
Revise code title, delete/add inclusion terms

35.96 **Percutaneous balloon valvuloplasty**
Add exclusion terms

36.06 **Insertion of non-drug eluting coronary artery stent(s)**
Revise/add code also notes

36.07 **Insertion of drug-eluting coronary artery stent(s)**
Revise/add code also notes

36.09 **Other removal of coronary artery obstruction**
Revise/add exclusion terms

37.36 **Excision, destruction, or exclusion of left atrial appendage (LAA)**
Revise code title, revise/add/delete inclusion terms, revise/add code also notes, add exclusion term

38.26 **Insertion of implantable pressure sensor without lead for intracardiac or great vessel hemodynamic monitoring**
New code

39.50 **Angioplasty of other non-coronary vessel(s)**
Revise code title, add code also note, revise/add exclusion terms

39.7 **Endovascular procedures on vessel(s)**
Revise/add exclusion terms

39.71 **Endovascular implantation of other graft in abdominal aorta**
Revise code title, add exclusion term

39.72 **Endovascular (total) embolization or occlusion of head and neck vessels**
Revise code title, add inclusion terms

39.77 **Temporary (partial) therapeutic endovascular occlusion of vessel**
New code

39.78 **Endovascular implantation of branching or fenestrated graft(s) in aorta**
New code

39.79 **Other endovascular procedures on other vessels**
Add exclusion term

43.82 **Laparoscopic vertical (sleeve) gastrectomy**
New code

43.89 **Open and other partial gastrectomy**
Revise code title, add exclusion term

68.24 **Uterine artery embolization [UAE] with coils**
New code

68.25 **Uterine artery embolization [UAE] without coils**
New code

68.4 **Total abdominal hysterectomy**
Delete exclusion term

68.49 **Other and unspecified total abdominal hysterectomy**
Add exclusion term

86.28 **Nonexcisional debridement of wound, infection, or burn**
Add inclusion term

86.94 **Insertion or replacement of single array neurostimulator pulse generator, not specified as rechargeable**
Revise inclusion term

86.95 **Insertion or replacement of multiple array neurostimulator pulse generator, not specified as rechargeable**
Revise code title, revise inclusion term, revise exclusion term

86.96 **Insertion or replacement of other neurostimulator pulse generator**
Revise exclusion term

86.97 **Insertion or replacement of single array rechargeable neurostimulator pulse generator**
Revise inclusion term

86.98 **Insertion or replacement of multiple array (two or more) rechargeable neurostimulator pulse generator**
Revise code title, revise inclusion term

88.7   **Diagnostic ultrasound**
Add exclusion term

89.19   **Video and radio-telemetered**
electroencephalographic monitoring
Add exclusion term

93.08   **Electromyography**
Add exclusion term

99.09   **Transfusion of other substance**
Revise exclusion term

99.29   **Injection or infusion of other**
therapeutic or prophylactic substance
Add exclusion term